Fetal and Neonatal
PHYSIOLOGY

Fetal and Neonatal PHYSIOLOGY

VOLUME 1 / THIRD EDITION

Richard A. Polin, M.D.

Professor of Pediatrics
Columbia University College of Physicians and Surgeons
Director, Division of Neonatology
Children's Hospital of New York–Presbyterian
New York, New York

William W. Fox, M.D.

Professor of Pediatrics
University of Pennsylvania School of Medicine
Division of Neonatology
Children's Hospital of Philadelphia
Philadelphia, Pennsylvania

Steven H. Abman, M.D.

Professor of Pediatrics
University of Colorado School of Medicine
Director, Pediatric
Heart Lung Center
The Children's Hospital
Denver, Colorado

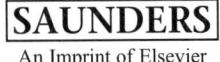

SAUNDERS
An Imprint of Elsevier

SAUNDERS
An Imprint of Elsevier

The Curtis Center
Independence Square West
Philadelphia, Pennsylvania 19106-3399

Volume 1	ISBN	9997628268
Volume 2	ISBN	9997628314
Two-volume set	ISBN	0-7216-9654-6

FETAL AND NEONATAL PHYSIOLOGY

Notice

Medicine is an ever-changing field. Standard safety precautions must be followed, but as new research and clinical experience broaden our knowledge, changes in treatment and drug therapy may become necessary or appropriate. Readers are advised to check the most current product information provided by the manufacturer of each drug to be administered to verify the recommended dose, the method and duration of administration, and contraindications. It is the responsibility of the treating physician, relying on experience and knowledge of the patient, to determine dosages and the best treatment for each individual patient. Neither the Publisher nor the editor assumes any liability for any injury and/or damage to persons or property arising from this publication.

The Publisher

First Edition 1992. Second Edition 1998. Third Edition 2004.

Library of Congress Cataloging-in-Publication Data

Fetal and neonatal physiology/ [edited by] Richard A. Polin, William W. Fox, Steven H. Abman. — 3rd ed.
   p. ; cm.
  Includes bibliographical references and index.
  ISBN 0-7216-9654-6 (set)   ISBN 9997628268 (v. 1)   ISBN 9997628314 (v. 2)
    1. Fetus—Physiology. 2. Infants (Newborn)—Physiology. I. Polin, Richard A. (Richard Alan).
    II. Fox, William W.   III. Abman, Steven H.
   [DNLM: 1. Fetus—physiology. 2. Infant, Newborn—physiology. 3. Maternal-Fetal
   Exchange—physiology. WQ 210.5 F4173 2004]
  RG610.F46 2004
  612.6'47-dc21

            2003042443

Acquisitions Editor: Judith Fletcher
Developmental Editor: Jennifer Shreiner
Project Manager: Jeffrey Gunning

Cover illustration courtesy of Jay S. Greenspan, M.D.

Printed in the United States of America

Last digit is the print number: 9 8 7 6 5 4 3 2 1

This book is dedicated to our wives and children:

Helene, Allison, Mitchell, Jessica, and Gregory Polin
Laurie, Will, Jon, James, and Lauren Fox
Carolyn, Ryan, Lauren, Mark, and Megan Abman

CONTRIBUTORS

Soraya Abbasi, M.D.
Clinical Professor of Pediatrics, University of Pennsylvania
School of Medicine; Neonatologist, Pennsylvania Hospital,
Philadelphia, Pennsylvania
Evaluation of Pulmonary Function in the Neonate

Steven H. Abman, M.D.
Professor of Pediatrics, University of Colorado School of
Medicine; Director, Pediatric Heart Lung Center,
The Children's Hospital, Denver, Colorado

S. Lee Adamson, Ph.D.
Professor of Obstetrics and Gynecology, University of Toronto
Faculty of Medicine; Senior Scientist, Samuel Lunenfeld
Research Institute of Mount Sinai Hospital, Toronto,
Ontario, Canada
Regulation of Umbilical Blood Flow

N. Scott Adzick, M.D.
C. Everett Koop Professor of Pediatric Surgery, University of
Pennsylvania School of Medicine; Surgeon-in-Chief, Children's
Hospital of Philadelphia, Philadelphia, Pennsylvania
Fetal Wound Healing; Pathophysiology of Neural Tube Defects

Kurt H. Albertine, Ph.D.
Professor of Pediatrics, Medicine, and Neurobiology and
Anatomy, and Director, Pediatrics Fellowship Training
Curriculum, University of Utah School of Medicine; Training
Director, Children's Health Research Center, Salt Lake City, Utah
Impaired Lung Growth After Injury in Premature Lung

Benjamin A. Alman, M.D., F.R.C.S.C.
Associate Professor and Canadian Research Chair, University of
Toronto Faculty of Medicine; Surgeon, Hospital for Sick
Children, Toronto, Ontario, Canada
Defective Limb Embryology

Steven M. Altschuler, M.D.
President and Chief Executive Officer, The Children's Hospital
of Philadelphia, Philadelphia, Pennsylvania
Development of the Enteric Nervous System

Page A. W. Anderson, M.D.
Professor of Pediatrics, Department of Pediatrics, Division
of Cardiology, Duke University School of Medicine and
Duke University Medical Center, Durham, North Carolina
**Cardiovascular Function During Development and the Response to
Hypoxia**

Russell V. Anthony, Ph.D.
Hill Professor, Animal Reproduction and Biotechnology
Laboratory, Department of Biomedical Sciences, Colorado State
University, Fort Collins; Perinatal Research Facility, Department
of Pediatrics, University of Colorado Health Sciences Center,
Aurora, Colorado
Angiogenesis

Elisabeth A. Aron, M.D.
Visiting Scientist, Colorado State University, Fort Collins; Senior
Instructor and Women's Reproductive Health Research Scholar,
University of Colorado Health Sciences Center, Denver, Colorado
Angiogenesis

Ahmet R. Aslan, M.D.
Research Scholar in Pediatric Urology, Albany Medical College,
Albany, New York; Attending in Urology, Haydarpasa Numune
Hospital, Istanbul, Turkey
Testicular Development; Testicular Descent

Jeanette M. Asselin, R.R.T., M.S.
Manager, Neonatal Pediatric Research, Children's Hospital and
Research Center at Oakland, Oakland, California
High-Frequency Ventilation

Richard L. Auten, Jr., M.D.
Associate Professor of Pediatrics, Department of Pediatrics,
Duke University School of Medicine, Durham, North Carolina
Mechanisms of Neonatal Lung Injury

Mary Ellen Avery, M.D., Sc.D.(Hon.)
Professor Emeritus, Harvard Medical School; Thomas Morgan
Rotch Distinguished Professor of Pediatrics, Children's Hospital,
Boston, Massachusetts
Historical Perspective [Surfactant]

Ellis D. Avner, M.D.
Gertrude Lee Chandler Tucker Professor and Chairman,
Department of Pediatrics, Case Western Reserve University
School of Medicine; Chief Medical Officer, Rainbow Babies and
Children's Hospital, and Chair for Excellence in Pediatrics,
Rainbow Babies and Children's Corporation, Cleveland, Ohio
Embryogenesis and Anatomic Development of the Kidney

H. Scott Baldwin, M.D.
Katrina Overall McDonald Chair in Pediatrics, Professor of
Pediatrics (Cardiology) and Cell and Development Biology,
Vice Chair of Laboratory Sciences in Pediatrics, Vanderbilt
University Medical Center, Nashville, Tennessee
Molecular Determinants of Embryonic Vascular Development

Philip L. Ballard, M.D., Ph.D.
Professor of Pediatrics, University of Pennsylvania School of
Medicine; Director of Neonatal Research, Children's Hospital of
Philadelphia, Philadelphia, Pennsylvania
Hormonal Therapy for Prevention of Respiratory Distress Syndrome

Eduardo Bancalari, M.D., M.D.
Professor, Departments of Pediatrics and Obstetrics-Gynecology,
University of Miami School of Medicine; Director, Division of
Neonatology, Jackson Memorial Hospital, and Chief, Newborn
Services/Perinatal Intensive Care Unit, Jackson Memorial
Medical Center, Miami, Florida
Pathophysiology of Chronic Lung Disease

David J. P. Barker, M.D., Ph.D., F.R.S
Professor of Clinical Epidemiology, University of Southampton
Faculty of Medicine; Director, Medical Research Council
Environmental Epidemiology Unit, Southampton General
Hospital, Southampton, England
Fetal Origins of Adult Disease

Pierre M. Barker, M.B., Ch.B., M.D., M.R.C.P.
Associate Professor, Department of Pediatrics, University of
North Carolina at Chapel Hill School of Medicine; Medical
Director, Children's Clinics, UNC Children's Hospital, Chapel
Hill, North Carolina
**Regulation of Liquid Secretion and Absorption by the Fetal
and Neonatal Lung**

Frederick C. Battaglia, M.D.
Professor of Pediatrics and Obstetrics-Gynecology, University of
Colorado School of Medicine, Aurora, Colorado
Mechanisms Affecting Fetal Growth

Gary K. Beauchamp, Ph.D.
Adjunct Professor, School of Veterinary Medicine, and School of
Arts and Sciences, University of Pennsylvania; Director and
Member, Monell Chemical Senses Center, Philadelphia,
Pennsylvania
Development of Taste and Smell in the Neonate

Jacqueline Beesley, Ph.D.
Weston Laboratory, Institute of Reproductive and
Developmental Biology, Division of Paediatrics, Obstetrics and
Gynaecology, Imperial College Faculty of Medicine, London,
United Kingdom
Apoptosis and Necrosis

Corinne Benchimol, D.O.
Clinical Assistant Professor, Department of Pediatrics, Division
of Pediatric Nephrology, Mount Sinai School of Medicine of
The City University of New York; Mount Sinai Hospital, New
York, New York
Potassium Homeostasis in the Fetus and Neonate

Laura Bennet, M.D., Ph.D.
Senior Research Fellow, Liggins Institute, University of
Auckland, Auckland, New Zealand
Responses of the Fetus and Neonate to Hypothermia

Robert A. Berg, M.D.
Associate Professor, University of Arizona College of Medicine;
Director, Pediatric Intensive Care Unit, University Medical
Center, Tucson, Arizona
Developmental Pharmacology of Adrenergic Agents

Gerard T. Berry, M.D.
Professor and Vice Dean for Research, Jefferson Medical
College, Thomas Jefferson University, Philadelphia, Pennsylvania
Pathophysiology of Metabolic Disease of the Liver

Carol Lynn Berseth, M.D.
Director, Medical Affairs North America, Mead Johnson
Nutritionals, Evansville, Indiana
Digestion-Absorption Functions in Fetuses, Infants, and Children

Vinod K. Bhutani, M.D.
Professor of Pediatrics, Section of Newborn Pediatrics,
Pennsylvania Hospital; Pediatrician, Pennsylvania Hospital,
and Senior Physician, Children's Hospital of Philadelphia,
Philadelphia, Pennsylvania
Evaluation of Pulmonary Function in the Neonate

Stan R. Blecher, M.D., F.C.C.M.G.
Professor Emeritus, University of Guelph Faculty of Medicine,
Guelph, Ontario, Canada
Genetics of Sex Determination and Differentiation

Arlin B. Blood, B.S.
Research Assistant, Center for Perinatal Biology, Loma Linda
University Medical School, Loma Linda, California
Perinatal Thermal Physiology

David L. Bolender, Ph.D.
Associate Professor, Department of Cell Biology, Neurobiology
and Anatomy, Medical College of Wisconsin, Milwaukee,
Wisconsin
Basic Embryology

**Robert D. H. Boyd, M.B., B.Ch., F.R.C.P., F.F.P.H., F.R.C.P.C.H.,
F.Med.Sci.**
Professor of Pediatrics, University of London Faculty of
Medicine, and Principal, St. George's Hospital Medical School;
Honorary Consultant, St. George's Hospital, London,
England
Mechanisms of Transfer Across the Human Placenta

Robert A. Brace, Ph.D.
Professor Emeritus of Reproductive Medicine, University of
California, San Diego, School of Medicine, La Jolla, California
Fluid Distribution in the Fetus and Neonate

Eileen D. Brewer, M.D.
Professor of Pediatrics and Head, Pediatric Renal Section, Baylor
College of Medicine; Chief Renal Service, Texas Children's
Hospital, Houston, Texas
Urinary Acidification

Patrick D. Brophy, M.D., F.R.C.P.C., F.A.A.P.
Assistant Professor of Pediatrics, University of Michigan Medical
School, Ann Arbor, Michigan
Functional Development of the Kidney *In Utero*

Delma L. Broussard, M.D.
Director, Regulatory Affairs International, Merck Research
Laboratories, Merck & Co., Inc., West Point, Pennsylvania
Development of the Enteric Nervous System

John C. Bucuvalas, M.D.
Professor of Pediatrics, University of Cincinnati College of
Medicine; Medical Director, Liver Transplantation, and
Attending Physician, Cincinnati Children's Hospital Medical
Center, Cincinnati, Ohio
Bile Acid Metabolism During Development

Douglas G. Burrin, Ph.D.
USDA Children's Nutrition Research Center, Baylor College of
Medicine, Houston, Texas
**Trophic Factors and Regulation of Gastrointestinal Tract and Liver
Development**

Bridgette M. P. Byrne, M.D., M.R.C.P.I., M.R.C.O.G.
Senior Lecturer, Royal College of Surgeons in Ireland;
Consultant Obstetrician and Gynaecologist, Coombe Women's
Hospital, Dublin, Ireland
Regulation of Umbilical Blood Flow

Anne Grete Byskov, M.Sc., Ph.D., D.Sc.
Professor of Reproductive Physiology, August Krogh Institute,
University of Copenhagen; Head, Laboratory of Reproductive
Biology, Juliane Marie Centre, Rigshospitalet, Copenhagen,
Denmark
Differentiation of the Ovary

Mitchell S. Cairo, M.D.
Professor of Pediatrics, Medicine, and Pathology, Columbia University College of Physicians and Surgeons; Director, Pediatric Blood and Marrow Transplantation, and Director, Pediatric Cancer Research, Children's Hospital of New York–Presbyterian, New York, New York
Neonatal Neutrophil Normal and Abnormal Physiology

Barbara Cannon, Ph.D.
Professor, The Wenner-Gren Institute, Stockholm University, Stockholm, Sweden
Brown Adipose Tissue: Development and Function

Michael S. Caplan, M.D.
Associate Professor of Pediatrics, Northwestern University Feinberg School of Medicine, Chicago; Chairman, Department of Pediatrics, Evanston Northwestern Healthcare, Evanston, Illinois
Pathophysiology and Prevention of Neonatal Necrotizing Enterocolitis

Neil Caplin, M.B., B.S.
Endocrinology and Diabetes, Princess Margaret Hospital for Children, Perth, Australia
Pathophysiology of Hypoglycemia

Susan E. Carlson, Ph.D.
Professor of Dietetics and Nutrition and Professor of Pediatrics, University of Kansas School of Medicine, Kansas City, Kansas
Long Chain Fatty Acids in the Developing Retina and Brain

David P. Carlton, M.D.
Associate Professor, Department of Pediatrics, University of Wisconsin School of Medicine; Chief, Division of Neonatology, University Hospital, Madison, Wisconsin
Pathophysiology of Edema

William J. Cashore, M.D.
Professor of Pediatrics, Brown University Medical School; Associate Chief of Pediatrics, Women and Infants' Hospital of Rhode Island, Providence, Rhode Island
Bilirubin Metabolism and Toxicity in the Newborn

Tinnakorn Chaiworapongsa, M.D.
Research Fellow, Perinatology Research Branch, National Institute of Child Health and Human Development, National Institutes of Health, Bethesda, Maryland
Fetal and Maternal Responses to Intrauterine Infection

Sylvain Chemtob, M.D., Ph.D., F.R.C.P.C.
Professor of Pediatrics, Pharmacology, and Ophthalmology, University of Montreal, Faculty of Medicine; Neonatologist, Hôpital Ste. Justine, Montreal, Quebec, Canada
Basic Pharmacologic Principles

Robert L. Chevalier, M.D.
Benjamin Armistead Professor and Chair, Department of Pediatrics, University of Virginia School of Medicine, Charlottesville, Virginia
Response to Nephron Loss in Early Development

Sadhana Chheda, M.D., D.T.M.H., M.B.B.S.
Staff Neonatologist, Providence Memorial Hospital, Sierra Medical Center, Las Palmas Medical Center, and Del Sol Medical Center, El Paso, Texas
Immunology of Human Milk and Host Immunity

Robert D. Christensen, M.D.
Professor and Chairman, Department of Pediatrics, University of South Florida College of Medicine; Physician-in-Chief, All Children's Hospital, St. Petersburg, Florida
Developmental Granulocytopoiesis

David H. Chu, M.D., Ph.D.
Teaching Assistant, The Ronald O. Perelman Department of Dermatology, New York University School of Medicine, New York, New York
Structure and Development of the Skin and Cutaneous Appendages

Robert Ryan Clancy, M.D.
Professor of Neurology and Pediatrics, University of Pennsylvania School of Medicine; Director, Pediatric Regional Epilepsy Program, Children's Hospital of Philadelphia, Philadelphia, Pennsylvania
Electroencephalography in the Premature and Full-Term Infant

M. Thomas Clandinin, Ph.D.
Professor of Nutrition, Department of Agricultural Food and Nutritional Science, University of Alberta, Edmonton, Alberta, Canada
Aceretion of Lipid in the Fetus and Newborn

David A. Clark, M.D.
Professor and Chairman, Department of Pediatrics, Albany Medical College; Director, Children's Hospital at Albany Medical Center, Albany, New York
Development of the Gastrointestinal Circulation in the Fetus and Newborn

Jane Cleary-Goldman, M.D.
Maternal-Fetal Medicine Fellow, Columbia Presbyterian Medical Center, Sloane Hospital for Women, New York, New York
Physiologic Effects of Multiple Pregnancy on Mother and Fetus

Ronald I. Clyman, M.D.
Professor of Pediatrics, University of California, San Francisco, School of Medicine; Senior Staff, Cardiovascular Research Institute, San Francisco, California
Mechanisms Regulating Closure of the Ductus Arteriosus

Pinchas Cohen, M.D.
Professor, Department of Pediatrics, David Geffen School of Medicine at UCLA, Los Angeles, California
Growth Factor Regulation of Fetal Growth

Howard E. Corey, M.D.
Director, Children's Kidney Center of New Jersey, Morristown Memorial Hospital, Morristown, New Jersey
Renal Transport of Sodium During Early Development

Robert B. Cotton, M.D.
Professor of Pediatrics, Vanderbilt University School of Medicine, Nashville, Tennessee
Pathophysiology of Hyaline Membrane Disease (Excluding Surfactant)

Beverly J. Cowart, Ph.D.
Adjunct Assistant Professor of Otolaryngology (Research), Jefferson Medical College, Thomas Jefferson University; Member and Director, Monell-Jefferson Taste and Smell Clinic, Monell Chemical Senses Center, Philadelphia, Pennsylvania
Development of Taste and Smell in the Neonate

Richard M. Cowett, M.D.
Professor of Pediatrics, Northeastern Ohio Universities College of Medicine, Rootstown, Ohio
Role of Glucoregulatory Hormones in Hepatic Glucose Metabolism During the Perinatal Period

Timothy M. Crombleholme, M.D.
Associate Professor of Pediatric Surgery, University of
Pennsylvania School of Medicine; Attending Pediatric Surgeon,
Children's Hospital of Philadelphia, and Fetal Surgeon, Center
for Fetal Diagnosis and Therapy at Children's Hospital of
Philadelphia, Philadelphia, Pennsylvania
Pathophysiology of Neural Tube Defects

James E. Crowe, Jr., M.D.
Associate Professor of Pediatrics, Vanderbilt University School
of Medicine, Nashville, Tennessee
B-Cell Development

Leona Cuttler, M.D.
Professor of Pediatrics, Case Western Reserve University School
of Medicine; Division Chief, Pediatric Endocrinology, Rainbow
Babies and Children's Hospital, Cleveland, Ohio
**Luteinizing Hormone and Follicle-Stimulating Hormone Secretion in
the Fetus and Newborn**

Mary E. D'Alton, M.D.
Willard C. Rappeleye Professor of Obstetrics and Gynecology
and Chair, Department of Obstetrics and Gynecology, Columbia
University College of Physicians and Surgeons; Director of
Services, Sloane Hospital for Women, New York Presbyterian
Hospital, New York, New York
Physiologic Effects of Multiple Gestation on Mother and Fetus

Enrico Danzer, M.D.
Fetal Surgery Research Fellow, Center for Fetal Diagnosis and
Treatment/University of Pennsylvania School of
Medicine/Children's Hospital of Philadelphia, Philadelphia,
Pennsylvania
Pathophysiology of Neural Tube Defects

Diva D. De León, M.D.
Assistant Professor of Pediatrics, University of Pennsylvania
School of Medicine; Attending Physician, Children's Hospital of
Philadelphia, Philadelphia, Pennsylvania
Growth Factor Regulation of Fetal Growth

Maria Delivoria-Papadopoulos, M.D.
Professor of Pediatrics, Physiology, and Obstetrics and
Gynecology, Drexel University College of Medicine; Chief,
Division of Neonatal-Perinatal Medicine, St. Christopher's
Hospital for Children, Philadelphia, Pennsylvania
Oxygen Transport and Delivery

George A. Diaz, M.D. Ph.D.
Assistant Professor, Department of Human Genetics and
Pediatrics, Mount Sinai School of Medicine of The City
University of New York, New York, New York
Molecular Genetics: Developmental and Clinical Implications

Chris J. Dickinson, M.D.
Professor of Pediatrics, University of Michigan Medical School,
Ann Arbor, Michigan
Development of Gastric Secretory Function

John P. Dormans, M.D.
Professor of Orthopaedic Surgery, University of Pennsylvania
School of Medicine; Chief, Orthopaedic Surgery, Children's
Hospital of Philadelphia, Philadelphia, Pennsylvania
**The Growth Plate: Embryologic Origin, Structure, and Function;
Common Musculoskeletal Conditions Related to Intrauterine
Compression: Effects of Mechanics on Endochondral
Classification**

David J. Durand, M.D.
Neonatologist, Children's Hospital and Research Center,
Oakland, California
High-Frequency Ventilation

**A. David Edwards, M.A., M.B.B.S., F.R.C.P., F.R.C.P.C.H.,
F.Med.Sci.**
Chairman of Division of Paediatrics, Obstetrics and
Gynaecology, and Professor of Neonatal Medicine, Imperial
College London; Group Head, Medical Research Council
Clinical Sciences Centre, Hammersmith Hospital, London,
United Kingdom
Apoptosis and Necrosis

John F. Ennever, M.D., Ph.D.
Associate Clinical Professor of Pediatrics, Columbia University
College of Physicians and Surgeons; Associate Attending,
Children's Hospital of New York–Presbyterian, New York, New York
Mechanisms of Action of Phototherapy

Robert P. Erickson, M.D.
Professor of Cellular and Molecular Biology and Holsclaw
Family Professor of Human Genetics and Inherited Disease,
Department of Pediatrics, University of Arizona College of
Medicine, Tucson, Arizona
Genetics of Sex Determination and Differentiation

Bulent Erol, M.D.
Attending Surgeon and Fellow, Children's Hospital of
Philadelphia, Philadelphia, Pennsylvania
**The Growth Plate: Embryologic Origin, Structure, and Function;
Common Musculoskeletal Conditions Related to Intrauterine
Compression: Effects of Mechanics on Endochondral
Classification**

Mohamed A. Fahim, Ph.D.
Professor of Physiology, Department of Physiology, Faculty of
Medicine and Health Sciences, Al Ain, United Arab Emirates
Functional Development of Respiratory Muscles

Leonard G. Feld, M.D., Ph.D., M.M.M.
Professor of Pediatrics, UMDNJ–New Jersey Medical School;
Chairman of Pediatrics, Atlantic Health System, Morristown,
New Jersey
Renal Transport of Sodium During Early Development

Miguel Feldman, M.D.
Director, Neonatal Intensive Care Unit, Hillel-Jaffe Medical
Center, Hadera, Israel
Accretion of Lipid in the Fetus and Newborn

Lucas G. Fernandez, M.D.
Postdoctoral Research Assistant, University of Virginia Health
System, Charlottesville, Virginia; Associate Professor, University
of Zulia, Maracaibo, Venezuela
Development of the Renin-Angiotensin System

Douglas G. Field, M.D.
Assistant Professor of Pediatrics, Pennsylvania State University
College of Medicine; Attending, Department of Pediatrics,
Division of Pediatric Gastroenterology and Nutrition, Penn State
Children's Hospital, Milton S. Hershey Medical Center, Hershey,
Pennsylvania
Fetal and Neonatal Intestinal Motility

Delbert A. Fisher, M.D.
Professor Emeritus, Pediatrics and Medicine, David Geffen
School of Medicine at UCLA, Los Angeles, California;
Vice President, Science and Innovation, Quest Diagnostics,
Nichols Institute, San Juan Capistrano, California
Fetal and Neonatal Thyroid Physiology

William W. Fox, M.D.
Professor of Pediatrics, University of Pennsylvania School of
Medicine; Attending, Division of Neonatology, Children's
Hospital of Philadelphia, Philadelphia, Pennsylvania
Assisted Ventilation: Physiologic Implications and Complications

Hans-Georg Frank, Dr. Med.
Associate Professor, Department of Anatomy II, University of
Technology Aachen Medical Faculty, Aachen; CSO, AplaGen
GmbH, Baesweiler, Germany
Placental Development

Philippe S. Friedlich, M.D.
Assistant Professor of Clinical Pediatrics, University of Southern
California Keck School of Medicine; Medical Director,
Neonatal Intensive Care Unit, Children's Hospital Los Angeles,
Los Angeles, California
**Pathophysiology of Shock in the Fetus and Neonate; Regulation of
Acid-Base Balance in the Fetus and Neonate**

Aaron L. Friedman, M.D.
Professor and Chairman, Department of Pediatrics, University of
Wisconsin School of Medicine; Medical Director, University of
Wisconsin Children's Hospital, Madison, Wisconsin
Transport of Amino Acids During Early Development

Joshua R. Friedman, M.D., Ph.D.
Instructor, Department of Pediatrics, University of Pennsylvania
School of Medicine; Fellow, Division of Gastroenterology and
Nutrition, Children's Hospital of Philadelphia, Philadelphia,
Pennsylvania
Pathophysiology of Gastroesophageal Reflux

Marianne Garland, M.B., Ch.B.
Assistant Professor of Pediatrics, Columbia University College
of Physicians and Surgeons; Assistant Attending in Pediatrics,
Children's Hospital of New York–Presbyterian, New York,
New York
Drug Distribution in Fetal Life

Maria-Teresa Gervasi, M.D.
Chief, Operative Unit of Obstetrics, Department of Obstetrics
and Gynecology, Ospedale Regionale Ca' Foncello-Treviso,
Treviso, Italy
Fetal and Maternal Responses to Intrauterine Infection

James B. Gibson, M.D., Ph.D.
Associate Professor, Department of Pediatrics, University of
Arkansas for Medical Sciences; Attending Geneticist, Arkansas
Children's Hospital, Little Rock, Arkansas
Pathophysiology of Metabolic Disease of the Liver

**P. D. Gluckman, M.B., Ch.B., M.Med.Sc., D.Sc., F.R.S.,
F.R.S.N.Z., F.R.A.C.P., F.R.C.P.C.H.**
Director, Liggins Institute for Medical Research, University of
Auckland Faculty of Medicine, Auckland, New Zealand
Growth Hormone and Prolactin

Michael J. Goldberg, M.D.
Professor and Chairman, Department of Orthopaedics, Tufts
University School of Medicine; Orthopaedist in Chief,
Tufts–New England Medical Center, Boston, Massachusetts
Defective Limb Embryology

Armond S. Goldman, M.D.
Emeritus Professor, Department of Pediatrics, Division of
Immunology/Allergy/Rheumatology, University of Texas
Medical Branch, Galveston, Texas
Immunology of Human Milk and Host Immunity

Gary W. Goldstein, M.D.
Professor of Neurology, Pediatrics, and Environmental Health
Sciences, Johns Hopkins University School of Medicine;
President and CEO, Kennedy Krieger Institute, Baltimore,
Maryland
Development of the Blood-Brain Barrier

R. Ariel Gomez, M.D.
Professor of Pediatrics and Biology; Vice President for Research
and Graduate Studies, University of Virginia, Charlottesville,
Virginia
Development of the Renin-Angiotensin System

Bernard Gondos, M.D.
Clinical Professor of Pathology, David Geffen School of
Medicine at UCLA, Los Angeles; Senior Scientist, Sansum
Medical Research Institute, Santa Barbara, California
Testicular Development

Denis M. Grant, Ph.D.
Professor and Chair, Department of Pharmacology, Faculty of
Medicine, and Associate Dean for Research, Faculty of
Pharmacy, University of Toronto; Director, Institute for Drug
Research, Toronto, Ontario, Canada
Pharmacogenetics

Lucy R. Green, Ph.D.
Lecturer, Centre for Fetal Origins of Adult Disease, University of
Southampton; Princess Anne Hospital, Southampton, England
Programming of the Fetal Circulation

Jay S. Greenspan, M.D.
Professor and Vice Chairman, Department of Pediatrics, Jefferson
Medical College, Thomas Jefferson University; Director of
Neonatology, A.I. duPont Hospital for Children, Thomas
Jefferson University Hospital, Philadelphia, Pennsylvania
Assisted Ventilation: Physiologic Implications and Complications

Adda Grimberg, M.D.
Assistant Professor, Department of Pediatrics, University of
Pennsylvania School of Medicine; Attending Physician, Division
of Pediatric Endocrinology, Children's Hospital of Philadelphia,
Philadelphia, Pennsylvania
Hypothalamus: Neuroendometabolic Center

Justin C. Grindley, Ph.D.
Research Instructor, Division of Pediatric Cardiology, Vanderbilt
University School of Medicine, Nashville, Tennessee
Molecular Determinants of Embryonic Vascular Development

Ian Gross, M.D.
Professor of Pediatrics, Yale University School of Medicine;
Director of Perinatal Medicine, Newborn Special Care Unit,
Yale–New Haven Children's Hospital New Haven, Connecticut
Hormonal Therapy for Prevention of Respiratory Distress Syndrome

Jean-Pierre Guignard, M.D.
Professor of Pediatric Nephrology, Lausanne University Faculty
of Medicine; Director, Division of Pediatric Nephrology, Center
Hospitalier Universitaire Vaudois, Lausanne, Switzerland
Postnatal Development of Glomerular Filtration Rate

Alistair J. Gunn, M.B., Ch.B., Ph.D., F.R.A.C.P.
Associate Professor, Liggins Institute, Department of Paediatrics,
University of Auckland, Auckland, New Zealand
Responses of the Fetus and Neonate to Hypothermia

Gabriel G. Haddad, M.D.
Professor of Pediatrics and Neuroscience and University
Chairman, Department of Pediatrics, Albert Einstein College of
Medicine of Yeshiva University; Pediatrician-in-Chief, Children's
Hospital of Montefiore, Bronx, New York
Basic Mechanisms of Oxygen-Sensing and Response to Hypoxia

J. Nathan Hagstrom, M.D.
Assistant Professor of Pediatrics, University of Connecticut
School of Medicine, Farmington; Attending Physician,
Connecticut Children's Medical Center, Hartford, Connecticut
**Developmental Hemostasis; Pathophysiology of Bleeding Disorders
in the Newborn**

Kathrin V. Halpern, B.A.
Research Coordinator, Division of Orthopaedic Surgery,
Children's Hospital of Philadelphia, Philadelphia, Pennsylvania
**Embryologic Origin, Structure, and Function; Common
    Musculoskeletal Conditions Related to Intrauterine Compression:
    Effects of Mechanics on Endochondral Ossification**

K. Michael Hambidge, M.D., Sc.D.
Professor Emeritus, Department of Pediatrics, Section of
Nutrition, University of Colorado School of Medicine;
The Children's Hospital, Denver, Colorado
Zinc in the Fetus and Neonate

Margit Hamosh, Ph.D.
Professor of Pediatrics (Emeritus), Georgetown University
School of Medicine; formerly Chief, Division of Developmental
Biology and Nutrition, Georgetown University Medical Center,
Washington, District of Columbia
Human Milk Composition and Function in the Infant

Mark A. Hanson, M.D., D.Phil., Cert.ED., F.R.C.O.G
British Heart Foundation Professor of Cardiovascular Science,
University of Southampton Faculty of Medicine; Director,
Center for Fetal Origins of Adult Disease, and Director, Fetal
Origins of Adult Disease Research Division, Princess Anne
Hospital, Southampton, England
Programming of the Fetal Circulation

Aviad Haramati, Ph.D.
Professor and Director of Education, Department of Physiology
and Biophysics, Georgetown University School of Medicine,
Washington, District of Columbia
Role of the Kidney in Calcium and Phosphorus Homeostasis

Richard Harding, M.D., D.Sc.
Professor, Department of Physiology, Monash University Faculty
of Medicine, Melbourne, Victoria, Australia
Physiologic Mechanisms of Normal and Altered Lung Growth

Mary Catherine Harris, M.D.
Associate Professor of Pediatrics, University of Pennsylvania
School of Medicine; Attending, Children's Hospital of
Philadelphia, Philadelphia Pennsylvania
Cytokines and Inflammatory Response in the Fetus and Neonate

Musa A. Haxhiu, M.D., Ph.D.
Professor of Pediatrics, Medicine, and Anatomy, Case Western
Reserve University School of Medicine, Cleveland, Ohio;
Professor, Department of Physiology and Biophysics, Howard
University School of Medicine, Washington, District of Columbia
Regulation of Lower Airway Function

William W. Hay, Jr., M.D.
Professor, Department of Pediatrics, University of Colorado
School of Medicine; Director, Neonatal Clinical Research Center,
and Scientific Director, Perinatal Research Center, University of
Colorado Health Sciences Center, Aurora, Colorado
Fetal Requirements and Placental Transfer of Nitrogenous Compounds

Anthony R. Hayward, M.D., Ph.D.
Director, Division of Clinical Research, National Center for
Research Resources, National Institutes of Health, Bethesda,
Maryland
T-Cell Development

William C. Heird, M.D.
Professor of Pediatrics, Children's Nutrition Research Center,
Baylor College of Medicine, Houston, Texas
Protein and Amino Acid Metabolism and Requirements

Emilio Herrera, Ph.D.
Professor of Biochemistry and Molecular Biology, School of
Experimental Sciences and Health, University of San
Pablo–CEU, Madrid, Spain
Maternal-Fetal Transfer of Lipid Metabolites

Harry R. Hill, M.D.
Professor of Pathology, Pediatrics and Internal Medicine,
University of Utah, Salt Lake City, Utah
Host Defense Mechanisms Against Bacteria

A. Craig Hillemeier, M.D.
Professor and Chair, Department of Pediatrics, Pennsylvania
State University College of Medicine; Medical Director, Penn
State Children's Hospital, Milton S. Hershey Medical Center,
Hershey, Pennsylvania
Fetal and Neonatal Intestinal Motility

Kurt Hirschhorn, M.D.
Professor of Pediatrics, Human Genetics, and Medicine, Mount
Sinai School of Medicine of The City University of New York;
Attending Pediatrician, Mount Sinai Hospital, New York,
New York
Molecular Genetics: Developmental and Clinical Implications

Steven B. Hoath, M.D.
Professor of Pediatrics, University of Cincinnati College of
Medicine; Medical Director, Skin Sciences Institute, Children's
Hospital Medical Center, Cincinnati, Ohio
Physiologic Development of the Skin

David A. Horst, M.D.
Assistant Professor, Baylor College of Medicine, Houston,
Texas
Bile Formation and Cholestasis

Tracy E. Hunley, M.D.
Assistant Professor of Pediatrics, Vanderbilt University School of
Medicine; Attending Pediatric Nephrologist, Vanderbilt
Children's Hospital, Nashville, Tennessee
Pathophysiology of Acute Renal Failure in the Neonatal Period

Christian J. Hunter, B.S.
Medical Student/Graduate Student, Loma Linda University
School of Medicine, Loma Linda, California
Perinatal Thermal Physiology

Shahid M. Husain, M.D., F.R.C.P.C.H.
Senior Lecturer, Barts and the London School of Medicine and
Dentistry, Queen Mary College, University of London;
Consultant Neonatologist, Homerton University Hospital,
London, England
**Calcium, Phosphorus, and Magnesium Transport Across
    the Placenta**

Susan M. Hutson, M.D., Ph.D.
Professor of Biochemistry, Wake Forest University School of
Medicine, Winston-Salem, North Carolina
Vitamin K Metabolism in the Fetus and Neonate

Machiko Ikegami, M.D., Ph.D.
Professor of Pediatrics, University of Cincinnati College of
Medicine; Attending, Division of Pulmonary Biology, Cincinnati
Children's Hospital Medical Center, Cincinnati, Ohio
**Pathophysiology of Respiratory Distress Syndrome and Surfactant
    Metabolism**

Terrie E. Inder, M.B., Ch.B., M.D., F.R.A.C.P.
Associate Professor in Pediatrics, University of Melbourne;
Neonatal Neurologist, Royal Women's and Children's Hospitals,
Murdoch Childrens Research Institute, Melbourne, Australia
Pathophysiology of Intraventricular Hemorrhage in the Neonate

Alan H. Jobe, M.D., Ph.D.
Professor of Pediatrics, University of Cincinnati College of
Medicine; Attending, Division of Neonatology Pulmonary
Biology, Cincinnati Children's Hospital, Cincinnati, Ohio
**Antenatal Factors That Influence Postnatal Lung Development and
Injury; Pathophysiology of Respiratory Distress Syndrome and
Surfactant Metabolism; Surfactant Treatment**

Lois H. Johnson, M.D.
Clinical Professor of Pediatrics in the Associated Faculty,
University of Pennsylvania School of Medicine; Associate
Physician, Section of Newborn Pediatrics, Pennsylvania
Hospital, Philadelphia, Pennsylvania
Vitamin E Nutrition in the Fetus and Neonate

Michael V. Johnston, M.D.
Professor of Neurology and Pediatrics, Johns Hopkins
University School of Medicine; Chief Medical Officer, Kennedy
Krieger Institute, Baltimore, Maryland
Development of Neurotransmitters

Richard B. Johnston, Jr., M.D.
Professor of Pediatrics and Associate Dean for Research
Development, University of Colorado School of Medicine,
Denver, Colorado
Host Defense Mechanisms Against Fungi

Deborah P. Jones, M.D.
Associate Professor, Department of Pediatrics, University of
Tennessee Health Sciences Center; Director of Dialysis Services,
Department of Pediatrics, LeBonheur Children's Medical
Center; Attending Physician, St. Jude Children's Research
Hospital, Memphis, Tennessee
Developmental Aspects of Organic Acid Transport

Peter Lloyd Jones, Ph.D.
Assistant Professor of Pediatrics, University of Colorado School
of Medicine, Denver, Colorado
The Extracellular Matrix in Development

Pedro A. Jose, M.D., Ph.D.
Professor of Pediatrics and Physiology and Biophysics,
Georgetown University School of Medicine, Washington,
District of Columbia
Postnatal Maturation of Renal Blood Flow

Satish C. Kalhan, M.B.B.S., F.R.C.P., D.C.H.
Professor, Department of Pediatrics, Case Western Reserve
University School of Medicine; Attending Neonatologist and
Director, Robert Schwartz M. D. Center for Metabolism and
Nutrition, MetroHealth Medical Center, Cleveland, Ohio
**Metabolism of Glucose and Methods of Investigation in the Fetus
and Newborn**

Suhas Kallapur, M.B.B.S., M.D.
Assistant Professor of Pediatrics, University of Cincinnati
College of Medicine; Attending, Cincinnati Children's Hospital,
Cincinnati, Ohio
**Antenatal Factors That Influence Postnatal Lung Development
and Injury**

Stanley Kaplan, Ph.D.
Professor Emeritus, Departments of Cellular Biology,
Neurobiology, and Anatomy, Medical College of Wisconsin,
Milwaukee, Wisconsin
Basic Embryology

Saul J. Karpen, M.D., Ph.D.
Associate Professor of Pediatrics and Molecular and Cellular
Biology, Baylor College of Medicine; Director, Texas Children's
Liver Center, Baylor College of Medicine/Texas Children's
Hospital, Houston, Texas
Bile Formation and Cholestasis

Sudha Kashyap, M.B.B.S., D.C.H.
Professor of Clinical Pediatrics, College of Physicians and
Surgeons, Columbia University; Attending Physician,
Department of Pediatrics, Children's Hospital of New York,
Columbia-Presbyterian Medical Center, New York, New York
Protein and Amino Acid Metabolism and Requirements

Frederick J. Kaskel, M.D., Ph.D.
Professor of Pediatrics and Vice Chairman for Affiliate and
Network Affairs, Albert Einstein College of Medicine of Yeshiva
University; Director of Pediatric Nephrology, Children's Hospital
at Montefiore, Bronx, New York
Role of the Kidney in Calcium and Phosphorus Homeostasis

Lorraine E. Levitt Katz, M.D.
Assistant Professor of Pediatrics, University of Pennsylvania
School of Medicine; Attending, Endocrinology/ Diabetes
Division, Children's Hospital of Philadelphia, Philadelphia,
Pennsylvania
Growth Factor Regulation of Fetal Growth

Peter Kaufmann, M.D.
Professor of Anatomy, University of Technology Aachen
Medical Faculty, Department of Anatomy II, Aachen,
Germany
Placental Development

Susan E. Keeney, M.D.
Associate Professor, Department of Pediatrics, University of
Texas Medical Branch, Galveston, Texas
Immunology of Human Milk and Host Immunity

Laurie Kilpatrick, Ph.D.
Associate Member, Joseph Stokes Jr. Research Institute, Division
of Allergy and Immunology, Children's Hospital of Philadelphia,
Philadelphia, Pennsylvania
Cytokines and Inflammatory Response in the Fetus and Neonate

John P. Kinsella, M.D.
Professor, Department of Pediatrics, University of Colorado
School of Medicine; Attending, Section of Neonatology,
The Children's Hospital; and Director, ECMO Services, and
Director, Pediatric Advisory Group, Flight for Life Emergency
Medical Transport, Denver, Colorado
Physiology of Nitric Oxide in the Developing Lung

Margaret L. Kirby, Ph.D.
Professor of Pediatrics—Neonatology, Duke University School
of Medicine, Durham, North Carolina
Development of the Fetal Heart

Charles S. Kleinman, M.D.
Professor of Pediatrics, Diagnostic Imaging, and Obstetrics and
Gynecology, Yale University School of Medicine; Attending
Pediatrician and Section Chief, Pediatric Cardiology,
Yale–New Haven Hospital, New Haven, Connecticut
**Cardiovascular Function During Development and the Response
to Hypoxia**

Barry A. Kogan, M.D.
Professor of Surgery and Pediatrics, Albany Medical College; Chief,
Division of Urology, Albany Medical Center, Albany, New York
Testicular Development; Testicular Descent

Otakar Koldovský, M.D., Ph.D. (deceased)
Formerly Professor of Pediatrics and Physiology, University of
Arizona College of Medicine, Tucson, Arizona
Digestion-Absorption Functions in Fetuses, Infants, and Children

Valentina Kon, M.D.
Associate Professor of Pediatrics, Vanderbilt University School
of Medicine, Nashville, Tennessee
Pathophysiology of Acute Renal Failure in the Neonatal Period

Ernest A. Kopecky, Ph.D.
Senior Clinical Scientist, Department of Medical Research, Purdue Pharma L.P., Stamford, Connecticut
Maternal Drug Abuse: Effects on Fetus and Neonate

Helen M. Korchak, Ph.D.
Research Professor of Pediatrics and Biochemistry/Biophysics, University of Pennsylvania School of Medicine; Children's Hospital of Philadelphia, Philadelphia, Pennsylvania
Stimulus-Response Coupling in Phagocytic Cells

Gideon Koren, M.D., F.R.C.P.C.
Professor of Pediatrics, Pharmacology, Pharmacy, Medicine, and Medical Genetics, University of Toronto Faculty of Medicine; Director, Motherisk Program, and Senior Scientist, Hospital for Sick Children, Toronto, Ontario, Canada
Maternal Drug Abuse: Effects on Fetus and Neonate

Nancy F. Krebs, M.D.
Associate Professor and Head, Section of Nutrition, Department of Pediatrics, University of Colorado School of Medicine; Medical Director, Department of Nutrition, The Children's Hospital, Denver, Colorado
Zinc in the Fetus and Neonate

Thomas J. Kulik, M.D.
Professor, Department of Pediatrics, University of Michigan Medical School; Medical Director, Pediatric Cardiothoracic Intensive Care Unit, C.S. Mott Children's Hospital, Ann Arbor, Michigan
Physiology of Congenital Heart Disease in the Neonate

Jessica Katz Kutikov, M.D.
Medical student, University of Pennsylvania School of Medicine, Philadelphia, Pennsylvania
Hypothalamus: Neuroendometabolic Center

Timothy R. La Pine, M.D.
Adjunct Assistant Professor of Pathology and Pediatrics, University of Utah School of Medicine, Salt Lake City, Utah
Host Defense Mechanisms Against Bacteria

Miguel Angel Lasunción, Ph.D.
Associate Professor of Biochemistry and Molecular Biology, University of Alcalá Faculty of Medicine, Alcalá de Henares; Head, Biochemical Investigation Service, Hospital Ramón y Cajal, Madrid Spain
Maternal-Fetal Transfer of Lipid Metabolites

John Laterra, M.D., Ph.D.
Professor, Departments of Neurology, Oncology, and Neuroscience, John Hopkins University School of Medicine; Department of Neurology, John Hopkins Hospital; Director of Neuro-Oncology, Kennedy Kriegen Institute, Baltimore, Maryland
Development of the Blood-Brain Barrier

P. C. Lee, Ph.D.
Professor of Pediatrics, Pharmacology and Toxicology, Medical College of Wisconsin; Director, Pediatric Gastrointestinal and Nutrition Laboratory, Medical College of Wisconsin, Milwaukee, Wisconsin
Development of the Exocrine Pancreas

Fred Levine, M.D., Ph.D.
Associate Professor, Department of Pediatrics, University of California, San Diego, School of Medicine; Rebecca and John Moores UCSD Cancer Center, La Jolla, California
Basic Genetic Principles

David B. Lewis, M.D.
Associate Professor of Pediatrics, Stanford University School of Medicine; Attending Physician, Lucile Salter Packard Children's Hospital at Stanford, Palo Alto, California
Host Defense Mechanisms Against Viruses

Chris A. Liacouras, M.D.
Associate Professor, University of Pennsylvania School of Medicine; Attending Physician, Division of Pediatric Gastroenterology, Children's Hospital of Philadelphia, Philadelphia, Pennsylvania
Pathophysiology of Gastroesophageal Reflux

Michael A. Linshaw, M.D.
Associate Professor of Pediatrics, Harvard Medical School; Pediatrician, Massachusetts General Hospital for Children, Boston Massachusetts
Concentration and Dilution of the Urine

George Lister, M.D.
Professor of Pediatrics and Anesthesiology, Department of Pediatrics, Section of Critical Care, Yale University School of Medicine; Director, Pediatric Intensive Care Unit, and Attending Pediatrician and Section Chief, Pediatric Critical Care Medicine, Yale-New Haven Children's Hospital, New Haven, Connecticut
Cardiovascular Function During Development and the Response to Hypoxia

Cynthia A. Loomis, M.D., Ph.D.
Assistant Professor, Department of Dermatology and Cell Biology; Tisch Hospital, Department of Dermatology, NYU School of Medicine, New York, New York
Structure and Development of the Skin and Cutaneous Appendages

John M. Lorenz, M.D.
Professor of Clinical Pediatrics, Columbia University College of Physicians and Surgeons; Attending, Children's Hospital of New York-Presbyterian, New York, New York
Fetal and Neonatal Body Water Compartment Volumes with Reference to Growth and Development

Steven Lobritto, M.D.
Hepatologist, Pediatrics and Adults, New York-Presbyterian Hospital, New York, New York
Organogenesis and Histologic Development of the Liver

Ralph A. Lugo, Pharm.D.
Associate Professor of Pharmacy and Adjunct Associate Professor of Pediatrics, University of Utah College of Pharmacy and School of Medicine, Salt Lake City, Utah
Basic Pharmacokinetic Principles

Akhil Maheshwari, M.D.
Fellow in Neonatal-Perinatal Medicine, University of South Florida College of Medicine, St. Petersburg, Florida
Developmental Granulocytopoiesis

Marilyn J. Manco-Johnson, M.D.
Professor of Pediatrics, University of Colorado School of Medicine; Attending, The Children's Hospital, Denver, Colorado
Pathophysiology of Neonatal Disseminated Intravascular Coagulation and Thrombosis

Carlos B. Mantilla, M.D., Ph.D.
Assistant Professor of Anesthesiology, Mayo Medical School; Senior Associate Consultant, Department of Anesthesiology, Mayo Clinic, Rochester, Minnesota
Functional Development of Respiratory Muscles

M. Michele Mariscalco, M.D.
Assistant Professor of Pediatrics, Baylor College of Medicine, Houston, Texas
Integrins and Cell Adhesion Molecules

László Maródi, M.D., Ph.D., D.Sc.
Professor and Chairman, Department of Pediatrics,
Division of Infectious Disease and Pediatric Immunology,
University of Debrecen Faculty of Medicine, Debrecen,
Hungary
Host Defense Mechanisms Against Fungi

Karel Maršál, M.D., Ph.D.
Professor of Obstetrics and Gynecology, University of Lund
Faculty of Medicine; Attending, Department of Obstetrics and
Gynecology, University Hospital, Lund, Sweden
Fetal and Placental Circulation During Labor

Richard J. Martin, M.B., F.R.A.C.P.
Professor of Pediatrics, Reproductive Biology, Physiology, and
Biophysics, Case Western Reserve University School of
Medicine; Director of Neonatology, Rainbow Babies and
Children's Hospital, Cleveland, Ohio
**Regulation of Lower Airway Function; Pathophysiology of Apnea of
Prematurity**

Dwight E. Matthews, Ph.D.
Professor and Chairman, Department of Chemistry, and
Professor of Medicine, School of Medicine, University of
Vermont, Burlington, Vermont
General Concepts of Protein Metabolism

Marcia McDuffie, M.D.
Associate Professor of Microbiology, University of Virginia
School of Medicine, Charlottesville, Virginia
T-Cell Development

Jane E. McGowan, M.D.
Associate Professor of Pediatrics, Johns Hopkins University
School of Medicine, Baltimore, Maryland
Oxygen Transport and Delivery

James McManaman, Ph.D.
Assistant Professor, Obstetrics and Gynecology, University of
Colorado Health Sciences Center, Denver, Colorado
Physiology of Lactation

Huseyin Mehmet, Ph.D.
Head, Weston Laboratory, Senior Lecturer in Neurobiology,
Imperial College London, London, United Kingdom
Apoptosis and Necrosis

Julie A. Mennella, Ph.D.
Member and Director of Education Outreach, Monell Chemical
Senses Center, Philadelphia, Pennsylvania
Development of Taste and Smell in the Neonate

Andrew Metinko, M.D.
Director, Pediatric Critical Care Services, Swedish Medical
Center, Seattle, Washington
Neonatal Pulmonary Host Defense Mechanisms

Martha J. Miller, M.D., Ph.D.
Associate Professor of Pediatrics, Case Western Reserve
University School of Medicine; Attending, Rainbow Babies and
Children's Hospital, Cleveland, Ohio
Pathophysiology of Apnea of Prematurity

Paul Monagle, M.B.B.S., M.Sc., F.R.A.C.P, F.R.C.P.A., F.C.C.P.
Associate Professor, Department of Paediatrics, University of
Melbourne; Director, Division of Laboratory Services, Head of
Haematology, Royal Children's Hospital, Melbourne, Victoria,
Australia
Developmental Hemostasis

Jacopo P. Mortola, M.D.
Professor of Physiology, McGill University Faculty of Medicine,
Montreal, Quebec, Canada
Mechanics of Breathing

Glen E. Mott, Ph.D.
Professor, Department of Pathology, University of Texas Health
Science Center, San Antonio, Texas
**Lipoprotein Metabolism and Nutritional Programming in the Fetus
and Neonate**

M. Zulficar Mughal, M.B., Ch.B., F.R.C.P., F.R.C.P.C.H., D.C.H.
Department of Child Health, University of Manchester;
Consultant Paediatrician and Honorary Senior Lecturer in Child
Health, Department of Paediatrics, Saint Mary's Hospital for
Women and Children, Manchester, United Kingdom
Calcium, Phosphorus, and Magnesium Transport Across the Placenta

Susan E. Mulroney, Ph.D.
Associate Professor, Department of Physiology, Georgetown
University School of Medicine, Washington, District of Columbia
Role of the Kidney in Calcium and Phosphorus Homeostasis

Upender K. Munshi, M.B.B.S., M.D.
Assistant Professor, Department of Pediatrics, Albany Medical
College, Albany, New York
**Development of the Gastrointestinal Circulation in the Fetus
and Newborn**

Leslie Myatt, Ph.D.
Professor, Department of Obstetrics-Gynecology, Division of
Maternal-Fetal Medicine, University of Cincinnati College of
Medicine, Cincinnati, Ohio
Regulation of Umbilical Blood Flow

Margaret A. Myers, M.D.
Clinical Assistant Professor of Pediatrics, University of
Pennsylvania School of Medicine; Associate Clinical Director,
Newborn Infant Center, Children's Hospital of Philadelphia,
Philadelphia, Pennsylvania
Development of Pain Sensation

Ran Namgung, M.D., Ph.D.
Professor, Department of Pediatrics, Yonsei University College of
Medicine, Seoul, Korea
Neonatal Calcium, Phosphorus, and Magnesium Homeostasis

Michael R. Narkewicz, M.D.
Associate Professor of Pediatrics and Hewit-Andrews Chair in
Pediatric Liver Disease, University of Colorado School of
Medicine; Medical Director, The Pediatric Liver Center,
The Children's Hospital, Denver, Colorado
Neonatal Cholestasis: Pathophysiology, Etiology, and Treatment

Heinz Nau, Ph.D.
Professor, School of Veterinary Medicine, University of
Hannover, Hannover, Germany
**Physicochemical and Structural Properties Regulating Placental Drug
Transfer**

Jan Nedergaard, Ph.D.
Professor, The Wenner-Gren Institute, Stockholm University,
Stockholm, Sweden
Brown Adipose Tissue: Development and Function

Margaret C. Neville, Ph.D.
Professor of Physiology and Biophysics, Professor of Cell and
Developmental Biology, and Professor of Obstetrics and
Gynecology, University of Colorado School of Medicine, Denver,
Colorado
Physiology of Lactation

Heber C. Nielsen, M.D.
Professor of Pediatrics, Tufts University School of Medicine;
Attending, Tufts–New England Medical Center, Boston,
Massachusetts
Homeobox Genes

Lawrence M. Nogee, M.D.
Associate Professor of Pediatrics, Johns Hopkins University
School of Medicine, Baltimore, Maryland
Genetics and Physiology of Surfactant Protein Deficiencies

Shahab Noori, M.D.
Assistant Professor of Pediatrics, University of Southern
California Keck School of Medicine; Neonatologist, USC
Division of Neonatal Medicine, Department of Pediatrics,
Children's Hospital Los Angeles, Women's and Children's
Hospital, and LAC+USC Medical Center, Los Angeles,
California
Pathophysiology of Shock in the Fetus and Neonate

Errol R. Norwitz, M.D., Ph.D., F.A.C.O.G.
Assistant Professor, Harvard Medical School; Attending,
Brigham and Women's Hospital, Boston, Massachusetts
Pathophysiology of Preterm Birth

Victoria F. Norwood, M.D.
Associate Professor of Pediatrics, University of Virginia School
of Medicine; Chief, Pediatric Nephrology, University of Virginia
Health System, Charlottesville, Virginia
Development of the Renin-Angiotensin System

Edward S. Ogata, M.D., M.M.
Professor of Pediatrics and Obstetrics and Gynecology,
Northwestern University Feinberg School of Medicine;
Chief Medical Officer, Children's Memorial Hospital, Chicago,
Illinois
Carbohydrate Metabolism During Pregnancy

Robin K. Ohls, M.D.
Associate Professor of Pediatrics, University of New Mexico
School of Medicine; Director, Neonatal-Perinatal Fellowship
Program, Division of Neonatology, University of New Mexico
Children's Hospital, Albuquerque, New Mexico
Developmental Erythropoiesis

Thomas A. Olson, M.D.
Associate Professor of Pediatric Hematology/Oncology, Emory
University School of Medicine, Atlanta, Georgia
**Developmental Megakaryocytopoiesis in Fetal and Neonatal
   Physiology**

Taher I. Omari, Ph.D.
Affiliate Senior Lecturer, Department of Paediatrics, University
of Adelaide, Adelaide, Australia; Senior Research Officer, Centre
for Paediatric and Adolescent Gastroenterology, Women's and
Children's Hospital, North Adelaide, Australia
Gastrointestinal Motility

James F. Padbury, M.D.
Professor and Vice Chair, Department of Pediatrics, Brown
University Medical School; Chief of Pediatrics, Women and
Infant's Hospital of Rhode Island, Providence, Rhode Island
Developmental Pharmacology of Adrenergic Agents

Mark R. Palmert, M.D., Ph.D.
Assistant Professor of Pediatrics, Case Western Reserve
University School of Medicine; Attending, Division of Pediatric
Endocrinology and Metabolism, Rainbow Babies and Children's
Hospital, University Hospitals of Cleveland, Cleveland, Ohio
**Luteinizing Hormone and Follicle-Stimulating Hormone Secretion in
   the Fetus and Newborn Infant**

Elvira Parravicini, M.D.
Assistant Professor of Pediatrics in Neonatology, Columbia
University College of Physicians and Surgeons;
Attending-Neonatology, Children's Hospital of
New York-Presbyterian, New York, New York
Neonatal Neutrophil Normal and Abnormal Physiology

Gilberto R. Pereira, M.D.
Professor of Pediatrics, University of Pennsylvania School of
Medicine; Neonatologist, Children's Hospital of Philadelphia,
Philadelphia, Pennsylvania
Nutritional Assessment [Intrauterine and Postnatal Growth]

Jeff M. Perlman, M.B., Ch.B.
Professor of Pediatrics, University of Texas Southwestern
Medical Center; Medical Director, Neonatal Intensive Care Unit,
Parkland Hospital, Dallas, Texas
**Cerebral Blood Flow in Premature Infants: Regulation, Measurement,
   and Pathophysiology of Intraventricular Hemorrhage**

Anthony F. Philipps, M.D.
Professor and Chair, Department of Pediatrics, University of
California, Davis, School of Medicine; Attending, UCD Children's
Hospital, Sacramento, California
**Oxygen Consumption and General Carbohydrate Metabolism
   in the Fetus**

Arthur S. Pickoff, M.D.
Professor and Chair, Department of Pediatrics, Wright State
University School of Medicine; Pediatric Cardiologist, Children's
Medical Center, Dayton, Ohio
Developmental Electrophysiology in the Fetus and Neonate

C. S. Pinal, Ph.D.
Biology Santa Cruz Research Fellow, The Liggins Institute,
University of Auckland, Auckland, New Zealand
Growth Factor Regulation of Fetal Growth

David Pleasure, M.D.
Professor of Neurology and Pediatrics, University of
Pennsylvania School of Medicine; Director, Joseph Stokes, Jr.
Research Institute, and Senior VP for Research, Children's
Hospital of Philadelphia, Philadelphia, Pennsylvania
**Trophic Factor and Nutritional and Hormonal Regulation of Brain
   Development**

Jeanette Pleasure, M.D.
Associate Professor of Pediatrics, Drexel University College of
Medicine; Attending Neonatologist, Hahnemann Hospital and
St. Christopher's Hospital for Children, Philadelphia,
Pennsylvania
**Trophic Factor and Nutritional and Hormonal Regulation of Brain
   Development**

Sabine Luise Plonait, M.D., M.R.C.P.(UK), D.C.M.
Private Practice; Instructor, DRU Nursing School; Freelance
Researcher, RUI, Berlin, Germany
**Physicochemical and Structural Properties Regulating Placental Drug
   Transfer**

Richard A. Polin, M.D.
Professor of Pediatrics, Columbia University College of
Physicians and Surgeons; Director, Division of Neonatology,
Children's Hospital of New York-Presbyterian, New York,
New York

Daniel H. Polk, M.D.
Professor of Pediatrics, Northwestern University Feinberg
School of Medicine; Associate Chief, Neonatology, Children's
Memorial Hospital, Chicago, Illinois
Fetal and Neonatal Thyroid Physiology

Scott L. Pomeroy, M.D., Ph.D.
Associate Professor of Neurology, Harvard Medical School;
Senior Associate in Neurology, Children's Hospital, Boston,
Massachusetts
Development of the Nervous System

Fred Possmayer, Ph.D.
Professor, Departments of Obstetrics/Gynaecology and
Biochemistry, University of Western Ontario Faculty of
Medicine; CIHR Group in Fetal and Neonatal Health and
Development, London, Ontario, Canada
Physicochemical Aspects of Pulmonary Surfactant

Martin Post, Ph.D.
Professor of Pediatrics, Physiology, Laboratory Medicine, and
Pathobiology, University of Toronto Faculty of Medicine; Head,
Lung Biology and Integrative Biology Programs, Hospital for
Sick Children, Toronto, Ontario, Canada
**Molecular Mechanisms of Lung Development and Lung Branching
Morphogenesis**

Gordon G. Power, M.D.
Professor of Physiology and Research Professor of Internal
Medicine, Loma Linda University School of Medicine, Loma
Linda, California
Perinatal Thermal Physiology

Jorge A. Prada, M.D.
Assistant Professor, Department of Obstetrics and Gynecology,
Division of Maternal-Fetal Medicine, University of Cincinnati
College of Medicine, Cincinnati, Ohio
Calcium-Regulating Hormones

Guy Putet, M.D.
Professor of Pediatrics, Claude Bernard University Faculty of
Medicine; Head, Department of Neonatology, Hospices Civils de
Lyon, Lyon, France
Lipids as an Energy Source for the Premature and Full-Term Neonate

Theodore J. Pysher, M.D.
Professor (Clinical) of Pathology, University of Utah School of
Medicine; Medical Director of Laboratories, Primary Children's
Medical Center, Salt Lake City, Utah
Impaired Lung Growth After Injury in Premature Lung

Graham E. Quinn, M.D., M.S.C.E.
Professor of Ophthalmology, University of Pennsylvania School
of Medicine; Attending Ophthalmologist, Children's Hospital of
Philadelphia, Philadelphia, Pennsylvania
**Retinal Development and the Pathophysiology of Retinopathy
of Prematurity**

Marlene Rabinovitch, M.D.
Dwight and Vera Dunlevie Professor of Pediatrics and Professor
(by courtesy) of Developmental Biology, Stanford University
School of Medicine; Research Faculty, Cancer Biology Program;
Research Director, Wall Center for Pulmonary Vascular Disease;
Pediatric Cardiologist, Lucile Packard Children's Hospital,
Stanford, California
Developmental Biology of the Pulmonary Vasculature

Scott H. Randell, Ph.D.
Assistant Professor of Medicine and Cell and Molecular
Physiology, University of North Carolina at Chapel Hill School
of Medicine; UNC Cystic Fibrosis/Pulmonary Research and
Treatment Center, Chapel Hill, North Carolina
**Structure of Alveolar Epithelial Cells and the Surface Layer During
Development**

Timothy R. H. Regnault, Ph.D.
Assistant Professor, Department of Pediatrics, Division of
Perinatal Medicine, University of Colorado School of Medicine,
Aurora, Colorado
**Fetal Requirements and Placental Transfer of Nitrogenous
Compounds**

*Michael J. Rieder, M.D., Ph.D., F.R.C.P.C., F.A.A.P., F.R.C.P.
(Glasgow)*
Professor and Chair, Division of Clinical Pharmacology,
Departments of Paediatrics, Physiology, Pharmocology and
Medicine, University of Western Ontario; Section Head,
Paediatric Clinical Pharmacology, Department of Paediatrics,
Children's Hospital of Western Ontario, London, Ontario,
Canada
Drug Excretion During Lactation

Henrique Rigatto, M.D.
Professor of Pediatrics, Physiology, and Reproductive Medicine,
University of Manitoba Faculty of Medicine; Director of
Neonatal Research, Health Sciences Centre, Winnipeg,
Manitoba, Canada
**Control of Breathing in Fetal Life and Onset and Control of Breathing
in the Neonate**

Natalie E. Rintoul, M.D.
Clinical Associate, University of Pennsylvania School of
Medicine; Attending Physician, Division of Neonatology,
Children's Hospital of Philadelphia, Philadelphia,
Pennsylvania
Pathophysiology of Neural Tube Defects

Jean E. Robillard, M.D.
Professor and Dean, University of Iowa Roy J. and Lucille A.
Carver College of Medicine, Iowa City, Iowa
Functional Development of the Kidney *In Utero*

Julian Robinson, M.D.
Assistant Professor of Pediatrics, Columbia University College of
Physicians and Surgeons; Attending, New York–Presbyterian
Hospital, New York, New York
Pathophysiology of Preterm Birth

Roberto Romero, M.D.
Chief, Perinatology Research Branch, National Institute of Child
Health and Human Development, National Institutes of Health,
Bethesda, Maryland
Fetal and Maternal Responses to Intrauterine Infection

Seamus A. Rooney, Ph.D., Sc.D.
Professor of Pediatrics, Yale University School of Medicine,
New Haven, Connecticut
**Regulation of Surfactant-Associated Phospholipid Synthesis
and Secretion**

James C. Rose, Ph.D.
Professor, Department of Obstetrics and Gynecology, Wake
Forest University School of Medicine, Winston-Salem,
North Carolina
**Development of the Corticotropin-Releasing Hormone–Corticotropin/
β-Endorphin System in the Mammalian Fetus**

Charles R. Rosenfeld, M.D.
Professor of Pediatrics and Obstetrics/Gynecology, University of
Texas Southwestern Medical Center; Director of Neonatal
Medicine, Parkland Memorial Hospital; Children's Medical
Center, Dallas, Texas
Regulation of Placental Circulation

Arthur J. Ross III, M.D., M.B.A.
Professor of Surgery and Pediatrics and Associate Dean, Western Clinical Campus, University of Wisconsin Medical School; Director of Medical Education, Gundersen Lutheran Medical Foundation, La Crosse, Wisconsin
Organogenesis of the Gastrointestinal Tract

Colin D. Rudolph, M.D., Ph.D.
Professor, Department of Pediatrics, Medical College of Wisconsin; Chief, Department of Pediatric Gastroenterology, Hepatology and Nutrition, Milwaukee, Wisconsin
Gastrointestinal Motility

Rakesh Sahni, M.B., B.S., M.D.
Associate Professor of Clinical Pediatrics, Columbia University College of Physicians and Surgeons; Associate Attending Pediatrician, Children's Hospital of New York–Presbyterian, New York, New York
Temperature Control in Newborn Infants

Harvey B. Sarnat, M.D., F.R.C.P.C.
Professor of Pediatrics (Neurology) and Pathology (Neuropathology), David Geffen School of Medicine at UCLA; Director, Pediatric Neurology, Cedars-Sinai Medical Center, Los Angeles, California
Ontogenesis of Striated Muscle

Lisa M. Satlin, M.D.
Professor of Pediatrics, Mt. Sinai School of Medicine of The City University of New York; Chief, Division of Pediatric Nephrology, Mount Sinai Medical Center, New York, New York
Potassium Homeostasis in the Fetus and Neonate

Ola Didrik Saugstad, M.D., Ph.D.
Professor of Pediatrics, University of Oslo Faculty of Medicine; Director, Department of Pediatric Research, University of Oslo Hospital, Oslo, Norway
Physiology of Resuscitation

Kurt R. Schibler, M.D.
Associate Professor of Pediatrics, University of Cincinnati College of Medicine; Attending, Children's Hospital Medical Center, Cincinnati, Ohio
Developmental Biology of the Hematopoietic Growth Factors; Mononuclear Phagocyte System

Karl Schulze, M.D.
Associate Professor of Clinical Pediatrics/Special Lecturer in Pediatrics, Columbia University College of Physicians and Surgeons, New York, New York
Temperature Control in Newborn Infants

Jeffrey Schwartz, Ph.D.
Senior Lecturer, School of Molecular and Biomedical Science, University of Adelaide, Adelaide, Australia; Adjunct Assistant Professor, Department of Obstetrics and Gynecology, Wake Forest University School of Medicine, Winston–Salem, North Carolina
Development of the Corticotropin-Releasing Hormone–Corticotropin/β-Endorphin System in the Mammalian Fetus

Gunnar Sedin, M.D., Ph.D.
Professor of Perinatal Medicine, Department of Women's and Children's Health, Perinatal Research Laboratory and Neonatal Intensive Care, Uppsala University; Attending Neonatologist, Uppsala University Children's Hospital, Uppsala, Sweden
Physics and Physiology of Human Neonatal Incubation

Jeffrey L. Segar, M.D.
Associate Professor, Department of Pediatrics, University of Iowa Roy J. and Lucille A. Carver College of Medicine, Iowa City, Iowa
Neural Regulation of Blood Pressure During Fetal and Newborn Life

Istvan Seri, M.D., Ph.D.
Professor of Pediatrics, University of Southern California Keck School of Medicine; Head, USC Division of Neonatal Medicine, Women's and Children's Hospital, USC–LAC Medical Center, and Children's Hospital Los Angeles, Los Angeles, California
Pathophysiology of Shock in the Fetus and Neonate; Regulation of Acid-Base Balance in the Fetus and Neonate

Kenneth Setchell, Ph.D.
Professor of Pediatrics, University of Cincinnati College of Medicine; Professor of Pediatrics, Director, Clinical Mass Spectrometry, Cincinnati Children's Hospital Medical Center, Cincinnati, Ohio
Bile Acid Metabolism During Development

Thomas H. Shaffer, Ph.D.
Professor of Physiology and Pediatrics, Temple University School of Medicine and Professor of Pediatrics, Thomas Jefferson University, Jefferson Medical College, Philadelphia, Pennsylvania; Director, Nemours Research Lung Center, Alfred I. du Pont Hospital for Children, Wilmington, Delaware
Upper Airway Structure: Function, Regulation, and Development; Assisted Ventilation: Physiologic Implications and Complications; Liquid Ventilation

Philip W. Shaul, M.D.
Professor of Pediatrics and Lowe Foundation Professor of Pediatric Critical Care Research, University of Texas Southwestern Medical Center at Dallas, Dallas, Texas
Physiology of Nitric Oxide in the Developing Lung

Jayant P. Shenai, M.D.
Professor of Pediatrics, Vanderbilt University School of Medicine, Nashville, Tennessee
Vitamin A Metabolism in the Fetus and Neonate

Colin P. Sibley, Ph.D.
Professor of Child Health and Physiology, Academic Unit of Child Health, University of Manchester; St. Mary's Hospital, Manchester, England
Mechanisms of Transfer Across the Human Placenta

Gary C. Sieck, Ph.D.
Professor of Physiology and Anesthesiology, Mayo Medical School; Chair, Department of Physiology and Biophysics, Mayo Clinic, Rochester, Minnesota
Functional Development of Respiratory Muscles

Theresa M. Siler-Khodr, Ph.D.
Professor of Obstetrics-Gynecology, University of Texas Health Science Center at San Antonio, San Antonio, Texas
Endocrine and Paracrine Function of the Human Placenta

Faye S. Silverstein, M.D.
Professor of Pediatrics and Neurology, University of Michigan Medical School, Ann Arbor, Michigan
Development of Neurotransmitters

Rebecca A. Simmons, M.D.
Assistant Professor of Pediatrics, University of Pennsylvania School of Medicine; Attending Neonatologist, Children's Hospital of Philadelphia, Philadelphia, Pennsylvania
Cell Glucose Transport and Glucose Handling During Fetal and Neonatal Development

Emidio M. Sivieri, M.S.
Biomedical Engineer, Neonatal Pulmonary Function Laboratory, Newborn Pediatrics, Pennsylvania Hospital/University of Pennsylvania School of Medicine, Philadelphia, Pennsylvania
Evaluation of Pulmonary Function in the Neonate

Harold C. Slavkin, D.D.S.
Dean, University of Southern California School of Dentistry, Los Angeles, California
Regulation of Embryogenesis

Evan Y. Snyder, M.D., Ph.D.
Professor and Director, Program in Stem Cell and Regeneration Biology, The Burnham Institute, La Jolla, California; Attending Neonatologist, Department of Neonatology, University of California, San Diego, La Jolla, California; Attending Neonatologist, Division of Newborn Medicine, Department of Pediatrics, Children's Hospital, Boston, Boston, Massachusetts
Stem Cell Biology

Jeanne M. Snyder, Ph.D.
Professor, Department of Anatomy and Cell Biology, University of Iowa Roy J. and Lucille A. Carver College of Medicine, Iowa City, Iowa
Regulation of Alveolarization

Michael J. Solhaug, M.D.
Professor of Pediatrics and Associate Professor of Physiology, Eastern Virginia Medical School, Norfolk, Virginia
Postnatal Maturation of Renal Blood Flow

Kevin W. Southern, Ph.D., M.B.Ch.B., M.R.C.P.
Senior Lecturer in Pediatric Respiratory Medicine, University of Liverpool Faculty of Medicine; Honorary Consultant in Paediatric Respiratory Medicine, Royal Liverpool Children's Hospital, Liverpool, England
Regulation of Liquid Secretion and Absorption by the Fetal and Neonatal Lung

Adrian Spitzer, M.D.
Professor of Pediatrics, Albert Einstein College of Medicine of Yeshiva University; Attending, Children's Hospital at Montefiore, Montefiore Medical Center, Bronx, New York
Role of the Kidney in Calcium and Phosphorus Homeostasis

Alan R. Spitzer, M.D.
Professor of Pediatrics and Chief, Division of Neonatology, State University of New York at Stony Brook School of Medicine; Director of Neonatology, Stony Brook University Hospital, Stony Brook, New York
Assisted Ventilation: Physiologic Implications and Complications

Charles A. Stanley, M.D.
Professor of Pediatrics, University of Pennsylvania School of Medicine; Chief, Division of Endocrinology/Diabetes, Children's Hospital of Philadelphia, Philadelphia, Pennsylvania
Pathophysiology of Hypoglycemia

F. Bruder Stapleton, M.D.
Ford/Morgan Professor and Chair, University of Washington School of Medicine; Pediatrician-in-Chief, Children's Hospital and Regional Medical Center, Seattle, Washington
Developmental Aspects of Organic Acid Transport

Dennis Styne, M.D.
Professor, Department of Pediatrics, University of California, Davis, School of Medicine; Chief, Pediatric Endocrinology, UCD Medical Center, Sacramento, California
Endocrine Factors Affecting Neonatal Growth

William E. Sweeney, Jr., M.D.
Assistant Professor, Department of Pediatrics, Case Western Reserve University School of Medicine; Director, Renal Development and Center for Childhood PKD Laboratory, Department of Pediatric Nephrology, Rainbow Babies and Children's Hospital, Cleveland, Ohio
Embryogenesis and Anatomic Development of the Kidney

Norman S. Talner, M.D.
Professor of Pediatrics, Department of Pediatrics, Division of Cardiology, Duke University Medical Center, Durham, North Carolina
Cardiovascular Function During Development and the Response to Hypoxia

Paul S. Thornton, M.B., B.Ch., M.R.C.P.I.
Medical Director, Department of Endocrinology and Diabetes, Cook Children's Medical Center, Fort Worth, Texas
Ketone Body Production and Metabolism in the Fetus and Neonate

William Edward Truog, M.D.
Professor of Pediatrics, University of Missouri–Kansas City School of Medicine; Sosland Family Endowed Chair in Neonatal Research and Attending Neonatologist, Children's Mercy Hospital, Kansas City, Missouri
Pulmonary Gas Exchange in the Developing Lung

Reginald C. Tsang, M.B.B.S.
Professor Emeritus of Pediatrics, University of Cincinnati College of Medicine; Children's Hospital Medical Center, Cincinnati, Ohio
Calcium, Phosphorus, and Magnesium Transport Across the Placenta; Neonatal Calcium, Phosphorus, and Magnesium Homeostasis

Alda Tufro, M.D., Ph.D.
Associate Professor of Pediatrics, Department of Pediatrics, Division of Nephrology, Albert Einstein College of Medicine of Yeshiva University, Bronx, New York
Development of the Renin-Angiotensin System

Nicole J. Ullrich, M.D., Ph.D.
Clinical Fellow in Neuro-Oncology, Children's Hospital, Boston, Massachusetts
Development of the Nervous System

Socheata Un, M.A., J.D.
Medical Student, University of Kansas School of Medicine, Kansas City, Kansas
Long Chain Fatty Acids in the Developing Retina and Brain

John E. Van Aerde, M.D., Ph.D.
Clinical Professor of Pediatrics and Director, Division of Neonatology, University of Alberta Faculty of Medicine; Regional Director for Newborn Services, Capital Health, Edmonton, Alberta, Canada
Accretion of Lipid in the Fetus and Newborn

Carmella van de Ven, M.A.
Senior Staff Research Associate, Columbia University, New York, New York
Neonatal Neutrophil Normal and Abnormal Physiology

Johannes B. van Goudoever, M.D., Ph.D.
Attending, Department of Neonatology, Erasmus Medical Center, Sophia Children's Hospital, Rotterdam, The Netherlands
General Concepts of Protein Metabolism

Robert C. Vannucci, M.D.
Professor of Pediatrics (Pediatric Neurology), Pennsylvania State University School of Medicine, Hershey, Pennsylvania
Perinatal Brain Metabolism

Susan J. Vannucci, Ph.D.
Research Director, Pediatric Critical Care Medicine, Morgan Stanley Children's Hospital of New York, New York, New York
Perinatal Brain Metabolism

Minke van Tuyl, M.D.
Research Fellow, Hospital for Sick Children, Toronto, Ontario, Canada
Molecular Mechanisms of Lung Development and Lung Branching Morphogenesis

Joseph J. Volpe, M.D.
Bronson Crothers Professor of Neurology, Harvard Medical School; Neurologist-in-Chief, Children's Hospital, Boston, Massachusetts
Pathophysiology of Intraventricular Hemorrhage in the Neonate

Reidar Wallin, Ph.D.
Professor, Department of Internal Medicine, Wake Forest
University School of Medicine, Winston-Salem, North Carolina
Vitamin K Metabolism in the Fetus and Neonate

David Warburton, D.Sc., M.D., F.R.C.P.
Professor of Pediatrics and Surgery, University of Southern
California Keck School of Medicine; Professor of Craniofacial
Biology, University of Southern California School of Dentistry;
Leader, Developmental Biology Program, Children's Hospital Los
Angeles Research Institute, Los Angeles, California
Regulation of Embryogenesis

Robert M. Ward, M.D.
Professor of Pediatrics, University of Utah School of Medicine;
Director, Pediatric Pharmacology Program, University of Utah
Hospital, Salt Lake City, Utah
Basic Pharmacokinetic Principles

Joern-Hendrik Weitkamp, M.D.
Fellow, Pediatric Infectious Diseases, Vanderbilt University
Medical Center, Nashville, Tennessee
B-Cell Development

Steven L. Werlin, M.D.
Professor of Pediatrics, Medical College of Wisconsin,
Milwaukee, Wisconsin
Development of the Exocrine Pancreas

Lynne A. Werner, Ph.D.
Professor, Department of Speech and Hearing Sciences,
University of Washington School of Medicine, Seattle, Washington
Early Development of the Human Auditory System

Susan E. Wert, Ph.D.
Associate Professor of Pediatrics, University of Cincinnati
College of Medicine; Director, Molecular Morphology Core,
Division of Pulmonary Biology, Cincinnati Children's Hospital
Medical Center, Cincinnati, Ohio
Normal and Abnormal Structural Development of the Lung

Lars Grabow Westergaard, M.D., D.M.Sc.
Associate Professor, Obstetrics and Gynecology, University of
Southern Denmark; Associate Professor, Department of
Obstetrics and Gynecology, Odense University Hospital,
Odense, Denmark
Differentiation of the Ovary

Jeffrey A. Whitsett, M.D.
Professor of Pediatrics, University of Cincinnati College of
Medicine; Director, Neonatology and Pulmonary Biology,
Cincinnati Children's Hospital Medical Center, Cincinnati, Ohio
Composition of Pulmonary Surfactant Lipids and Proteins

Michaelann Wilke, B.Sc.
Doctoral Candidate, Nutrition and Metabolism, University of
Alberta, Edmonton, Alberta, Canada
Accretion of Lipid in the Fetus and Newborn

John V. Williams, M.D.
Assistant Professor, Division of Pediatric Infectious Diseases,
Department of Pediatrics, Vanderbilt University; Assistant
Professor, Division of Pediatric Infectious Diseases, Department
of Pediatrics, Vanderbilt University Medical Center, Nashville,
Tennessee
B-Cell Development

Dermot H. Williamson, D.Phil. (deceased)
Formerly Medical Research Council (UK), External Scientific
Staff, and University Research Lecturer, Metabolic Research
Laboratory, University of Oxford, Radcliffe Infirmary, Oxford,
England
Ketone Body Production and Metabolism in the Fetus and Neonate

Jerry A. Winkelstein, M.D.
Eudowood Professor of Pediatrics and Professor of Medicine
and Pathology, Johns Hopkins University School of Medicine;
Director, Division of Immunology, Department of Pediatrics,
Johns Hopkins Hospital, Baltimore, Maryland
The Complement System of the Fetus and Neonate

Jeremy S. D. Winter, M.D., F.R.C.P.C.
Professor and Head, Section of Endocrinology and Metabolism,
Department of Pediatrics, University of Alberta Faculty of
Medicine, Edmonton, Alberta, Canada
Fetal and Neonatal Adrenocortical Physiology

Douglas A. Woelkers, M.D.
Assistant Professor, Department of Reproductive Medicine,
University of California, San Diego, San Diego, California
**Maternal Cardiovascular Disease and Fetal Growth and
Development**

Marla R. Wolfson, Ph.D.(Physiol.)
Associate Professor of Physiology and Pediatrics and Chair,
Physiology Graduate Studies, Temple University School of
Medicine; Attending, Temple University Children's Hospital,
Philadelphia, Pennsylvania
**Upper Airway Structure: Function, Regulation, and Development;
Liquid Ventilation**

Robert P. Woroniecki, M.D.
Assistant Professor of Pediatrics, Pediatric Nephrology, Albert
Einstein College of Medicine of Yeshiva University; Research
Fellow, Pediatric Nephrology, Children's Hospital at
Monte Fiore, Bronx, New York
Role of the Kidney in Calcium and Phosphorus Homeostasis

Walid K. Yassir, M.D.
Assistant Professor of Orthopaedics, Tufts University School of
Medicine; Pediatric Orthopaedic Surgeon, Tufts–New England
Medical Center, Boston Floating Hospital for Children, Boston,
Massachusetts
Defective Limb Embryology

Stephen Yip, M.D., Ph.D.
Resident, Neurosurgery, Vancouver General Hospital, Vancouver,
British Columbia, Canada
Stem Cell Biology

Mervin C. Yoder, M.D.
Professor of Pediatrics and of Biochemistry and Molecular
Biology, Indiana University School of Medicine; Attending
Hematologist, James Whitcomb Riley Hospital for Children,
Indianapolis, Indiana
**Biology of Stem Cells and Stem Cell Transplantation; Developmental
Biology of the Hematopoietic Growth Factors**

Sharla Young, Ph.D.
Postdoctoral Fellow, National Institute of Child Health and
Human Development, National Institutes of Health, Bethesda,
Maryland
**Development of the Corticotropin-Releasing Hormone–Corticotropin/
β-Endorphin System in the Mammalian Fetus**

Stephen L. Young, M.D.
Professor of Medicine, Duke University School of Medicine,
Durham, North Carolina
**Structure of Alveolar Epithelial Cells and the Surface Layer During
Development**

Dan Zhou, Ph.D.
Instructor, Department of Pediatrics, Albert Einstein College of
Medicine of Yeshiva University, Bronx, New York
Basic Mechanisms of Oxygen-Sensing and Response to Hypoxia

PREFACE TO THE THIRD EDITION

With the publication of the third edition of *Fetal and Neonatal Physiology*, we welcome a new (third) editor, Dr. Steven Abman. Dr. Abman is Professor of Pediatrics at the University of Colorado School of Medicine and Director of the Pediatric Heart Lung Center in the Department of Pediatrics. In addition to his expertise as an editor, he brings considerable experience in basic science investigations in fetal and neonatal pulmonary and cardiovascular physiology.

The challenges posed by preparation of the new edition were immense. Within each major section, the increase in the amount of information—especially at the molecular level—has been staggering. In addition, new topics that were not covered in the second edition needed to be included. Therefore, we faced difficult decisions in determining both the content and the length of the book. As a general rule, we eliminated clinical material that is thoroughly covered in one of the many excellent textbooks of neonatology. However, there are 30 completely new chapters ranging in scope from apoptosis and angiogenesis to stem cells in development. In addition, almost all of the other chapters have been updated and extensively rewritten. As before, advancements in developmental physiology are discussed in the context of changing concepts in normal human physiology.

There are many people to whom we owe special thanks. First of all, we wish to express our gratitude to all the individuals who agreed to write chapters for the third edition. The quality of the chapters is outstanding, and we recognize the time and effort each of them required. We are also indebted to Heidi Kleinbart at the Children's Hospital of New York and to Ellen Ramsay at the Children's Hospital of Philadelphia for their organizational skills and editorial assistance. In addition, we offer our thanks to Jennifer Shreiner at Saunders for her tremendous help with the development and organization of the book. Finally, we want to thank our friend and senior editor Judy Fletcher, who was instrumental in the development of the third edition and served as the "irresistible force" that kept our textbook—the "immovable object"—on target for size and completion date.

Richard A. Polin
William W. Fox
Steven H. Abman

PREFACE TO THE FIRST EDITION

When I was young my teachers were the old.
I gave up fire for form till I was cold.
I suffered like a metal being cast.
I went to school to age to learn the past.

Now I am old my teachers are the young.
What can't be molded must be cracked and sprung.
I strain at lessons fit to start a suture.
I go to school to youth to learn the future.

ROBERT FROST

The first definitive treatise dealing with the care of the newborn infant dates back to the second century A.D. Considering its antiquity, it is startling that Soranus of Ephesus' work persisted as an acceptable way to treat newborn infants until relatively recent times. It is only during the last 100 years that physiologists have directed their attention to the fetus and newborn infant.

The reader of this work will soon appreciate that we have not attempted to reproduce another clinical textbook of neonatal/perinatal medicine. In contrast, we have tried to make our book appropriate for individuals interested in a "readable," in-depth presentation of fetal and neonatal developmental physiology. Clinical topics are presented only when discussion of disease pathophysiology seems appropriate. As can be appreciated from its size (28 sections, 190 chapters), we have tried to make the book both comprehensive and current. Most authors have focused their discussions on the developmental physiology of a single organ system. In addition, we have included several sections (e.g., Genetics and Embryology) that contain information relevant to the development of all body systems. Almost every chapter contains a detailed discussion of the "normal" adult physiology as well as a description of the physiologic differences that exist in the fetus and neonate. Where appropriate, the discussion is directed at biochemical, cellular, or molecular levels. The minor degree of chapter overlap that remains was done purposely so that the reader could obtain viewpoints on the same issue from individuals with different perspectives.

The progress made in fetal and neonatal medicine since the publication of Smith and Nelson's classic textbook, *the Physiology of the Newborn Infant*, has been astounding. At the time of the last edition (1976), infants weighing less than 750 gm rarely survived and most of the survivors demonstrated neurological deficits. Many centers did not even attempt to ventilate infants of that birth weight. Although the lipid composition of surfactant was relatively known at that time, effective artificial surfactant preparations were not available. In 1976, little was understood about the pathophysiology of diseases such as bronchopulmonary dysplasia, intraventricular hemorrhage, and necrotizing enterocolitis. Furthermore, drugs were not routinely available to treat apnea of prematurity or patency of the ductus arteriosus. The last edition of Smith and Nelson's book includes a quote from Dr. Clement Smith that appeared in the third edition: "The very passage of the normal infant through the valley of the shadow (of birth) is a striking example of the physiological resiliency of the newborn infant." Today, clinicians do not have to rely solely upon the inherent resiliency of the newborn infant. We have at our disposal new and better drugs to support the circulation, treat infection, and improve pulmonary function. Even the smallest neonates can be fed intravenously with dextrose and amino acid solutions that are tailored to their physiology and that produce little in the way of metabolic derangements. Technologic advancements in life support (extracorporeal membrane oxygenation and high-frequency ventilation) now allow us to keep infants alive who would previously not have survived. Despite these seeming "breakthroughs," fetal and neonatal medicine ought to be perceived as being in its infancy as a specialty. In the next 10 years, molecular biology techniques should have an enormous impact on the day-to-day practice of our subspecialties. Genetically engineered products are already being used to correct physiologic deficiencies associated with preterm birth, and gene transplantation has recently been used to correct an inborn error of metabolism. We hope this textbook will provide a clear understanding of the physiologic basis for these and future clinical and technologic advancements.

In keeping with the spirit of the poem quoted at the beginning of the preface, we expect this book will be used by both new and established investigators. Young investigators will find the text a comprehensive foundation upon which to formulate new questions. Established investigators will be able to learn not only about future directions of research in their field, but also about alternative approaches taken by other investigators interested in similar problems.

As with the preparation of any large textbook, there are many people who deserve special recognition. First of all, we would like to recognize the help of the section editors, who greatly assisted us in identifying authors considered to be at the "cutting edge" of their respective fields. We would also like to thank each of the chapter authors who expended an enormous amount of time and effort in the preparation of material for their sections. Next we would like to thank Carol Miller for her editorial assistance and help with the typing and re-typing of the manuscripts. We greatly appreciate the many individuals at the W.B. Saunders Company, without whom the project would not have come to fruition. We are especially indebted to Lisette Bralow, who oversaw production of the book from its inception, and Lawrence McGrew, for his advice, assistance, and considerable help in organizing each of the chapters. Lastly, we gratefully acknowledge the contributions of earlier authors (Barcroft, Smith, Dawes, Nelson, and others), for it was their efforts that served as a foundation for the subspecialty of neonatology and that first attracted us (and countless others) to enter the field.

Richard A. Polin
William W. Fox

CONTENTS

VIII

Protein Metabolism 501

IX

Thermoregulation 541

X

Skin 589

XI

Fetal and Neonatal Cardiovascular
Physiology 613

XII

The Lung   783

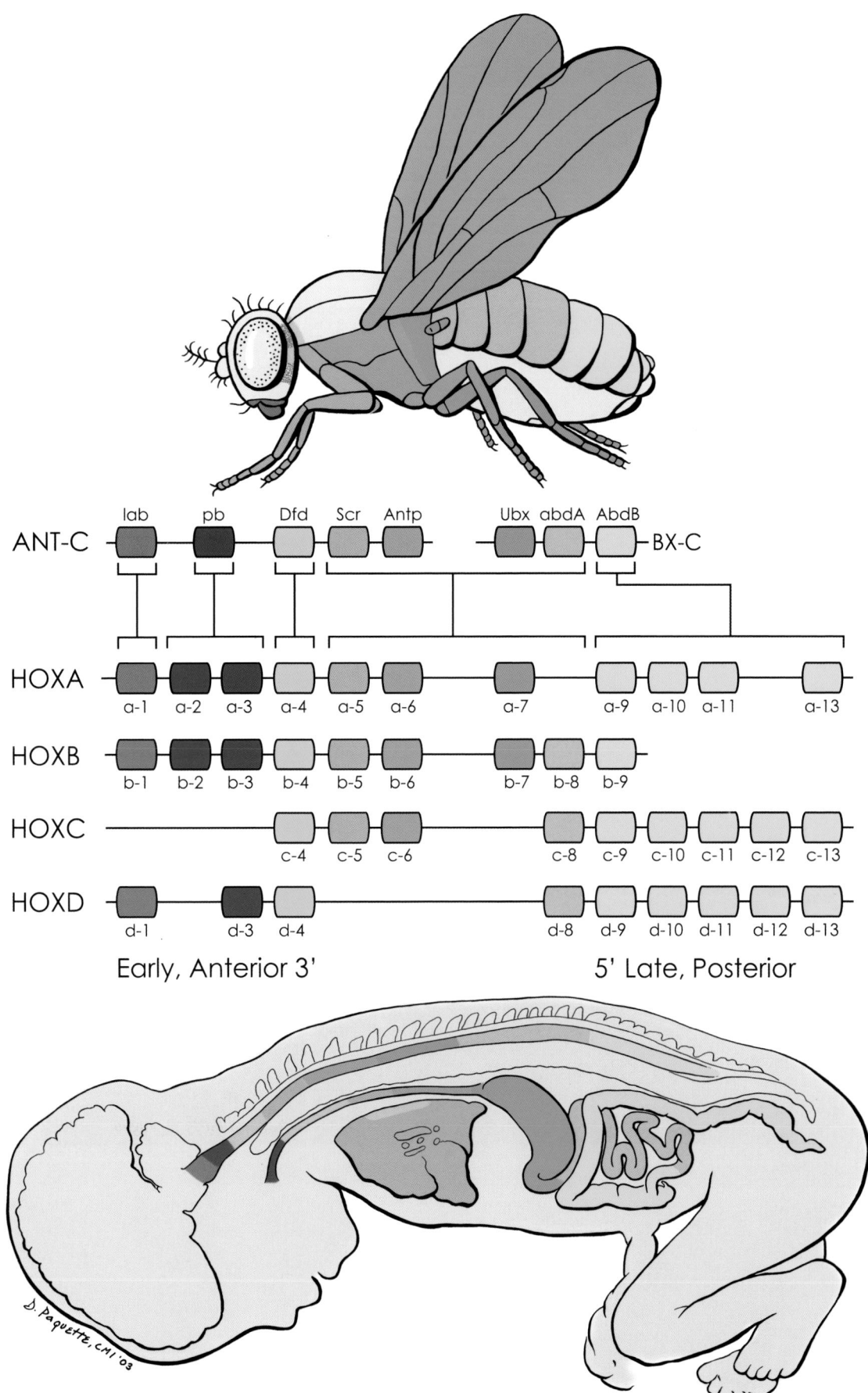

Figure 7–1

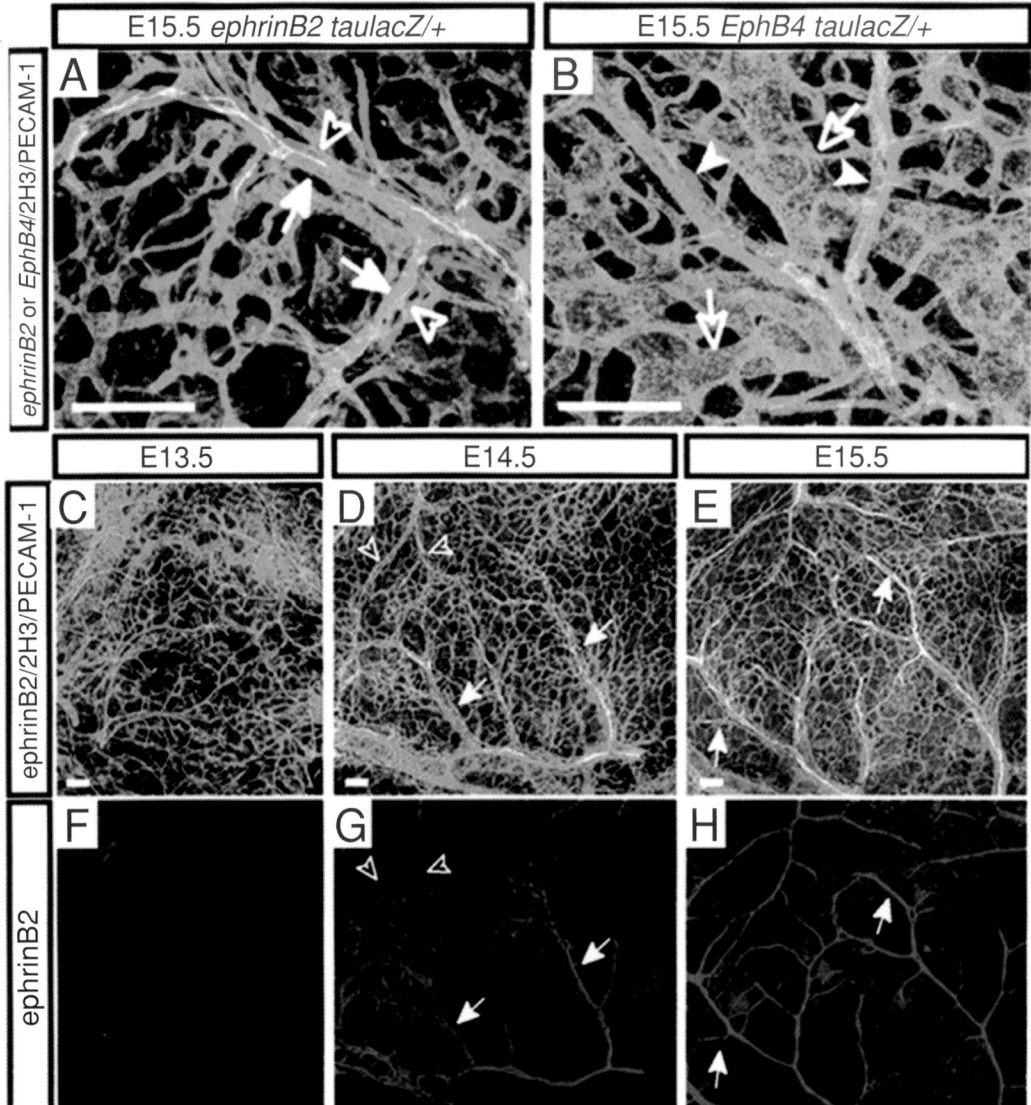

Figure 62–5

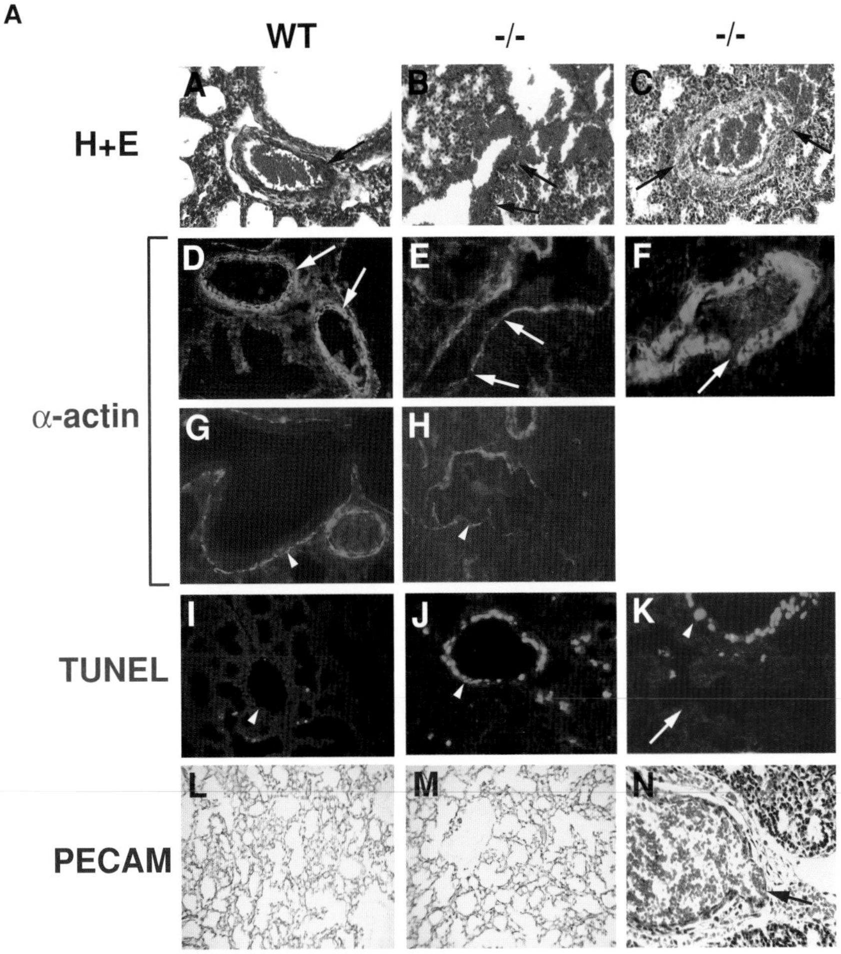

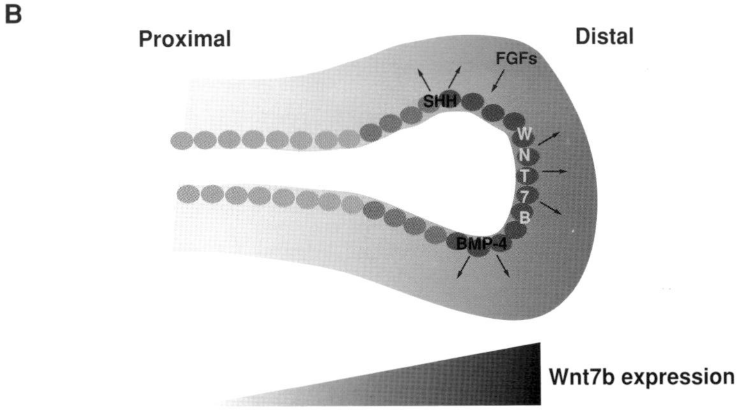

A

	WT	-/-	-/-
H+E	A	B	C
α-actin	D	E	F
	G	H	
TUNEL	I	J	K
PECAM	L	M	N

B

Proximal   Distal

FGFs

SHH

WNT7B

BMP-4

Wnt7b expression

C

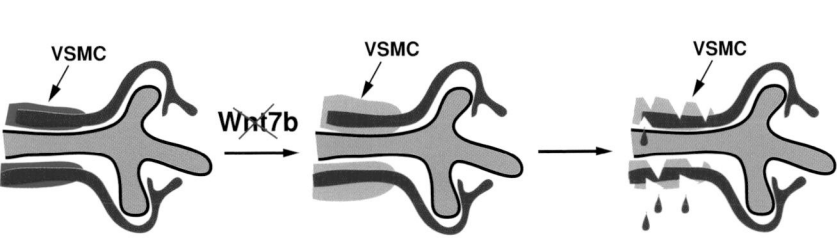

VSMC   VSMC   VSMC

Wnt7b

Figures 65–8A, B and C

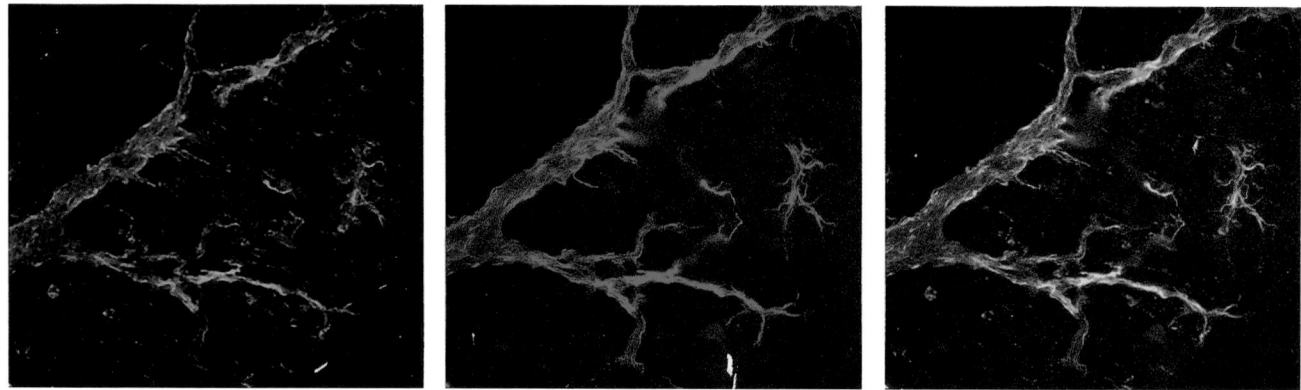

Figure 83–4

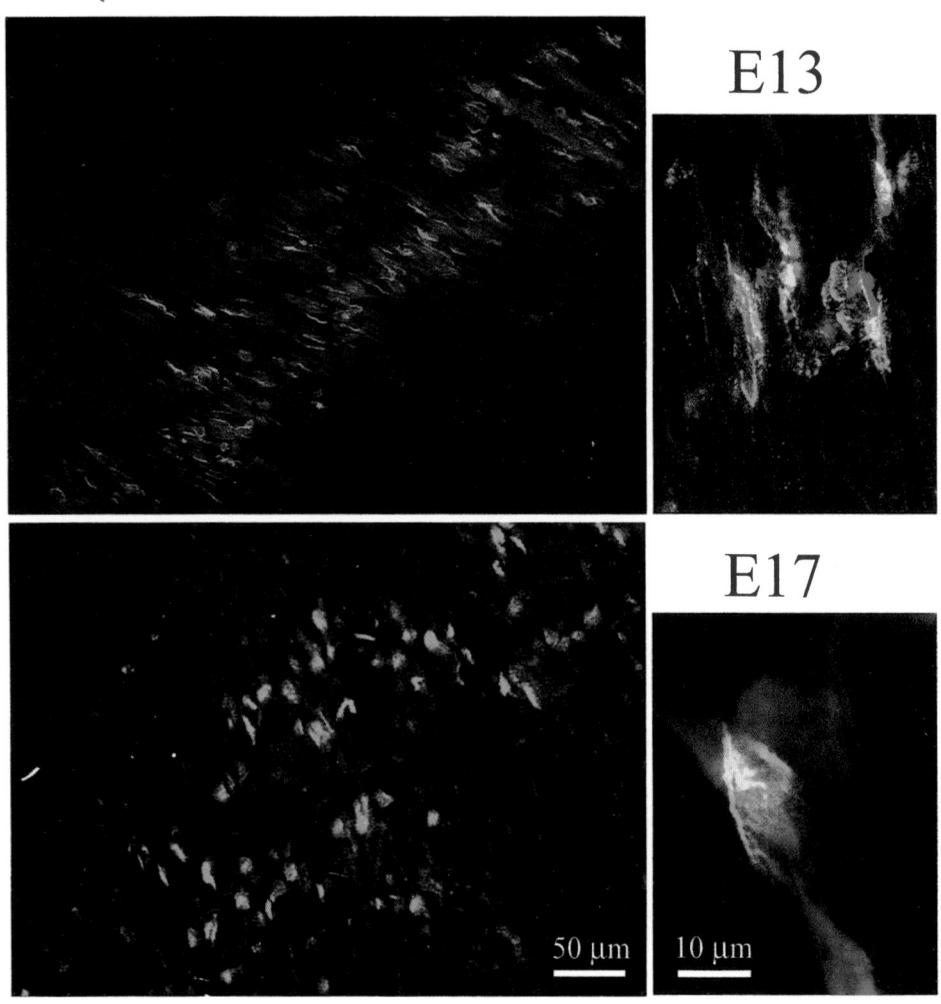

E13

E17

50 μm   10 μm

Figure 83–6

Slow
(Type I)

Fast Fatigable
(Type IIb or IIx)

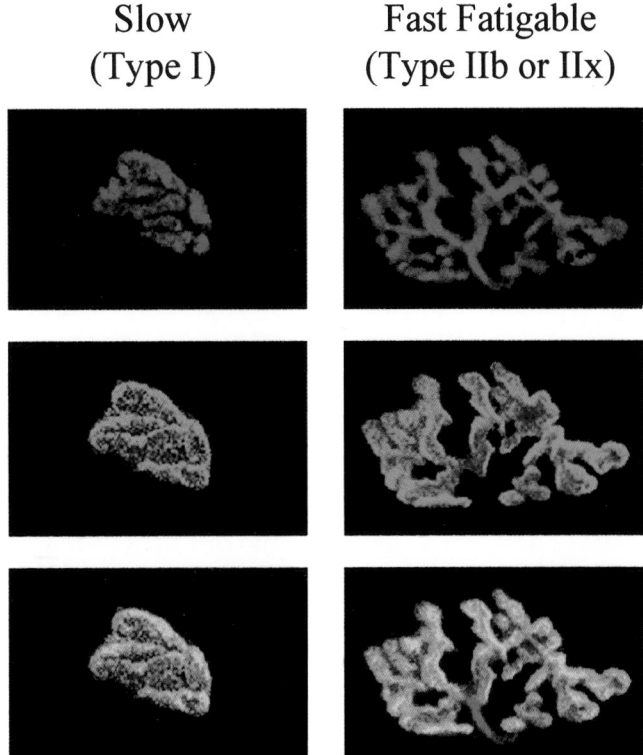

Figure 83–8

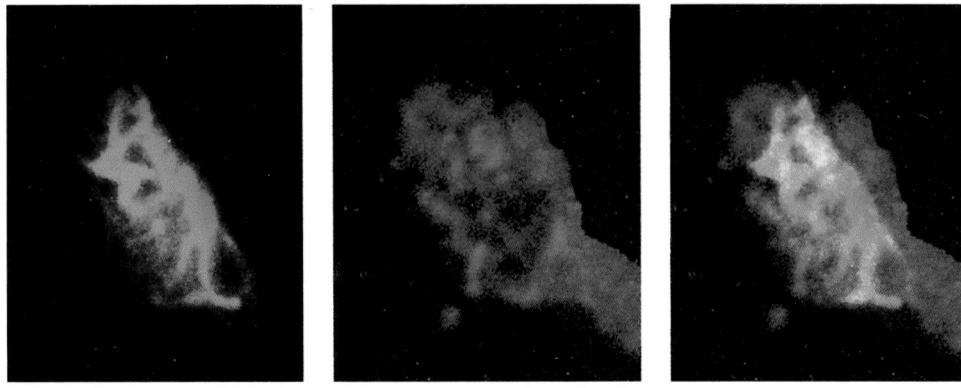

Figure 83–9

Ontogeny

Lung Injury

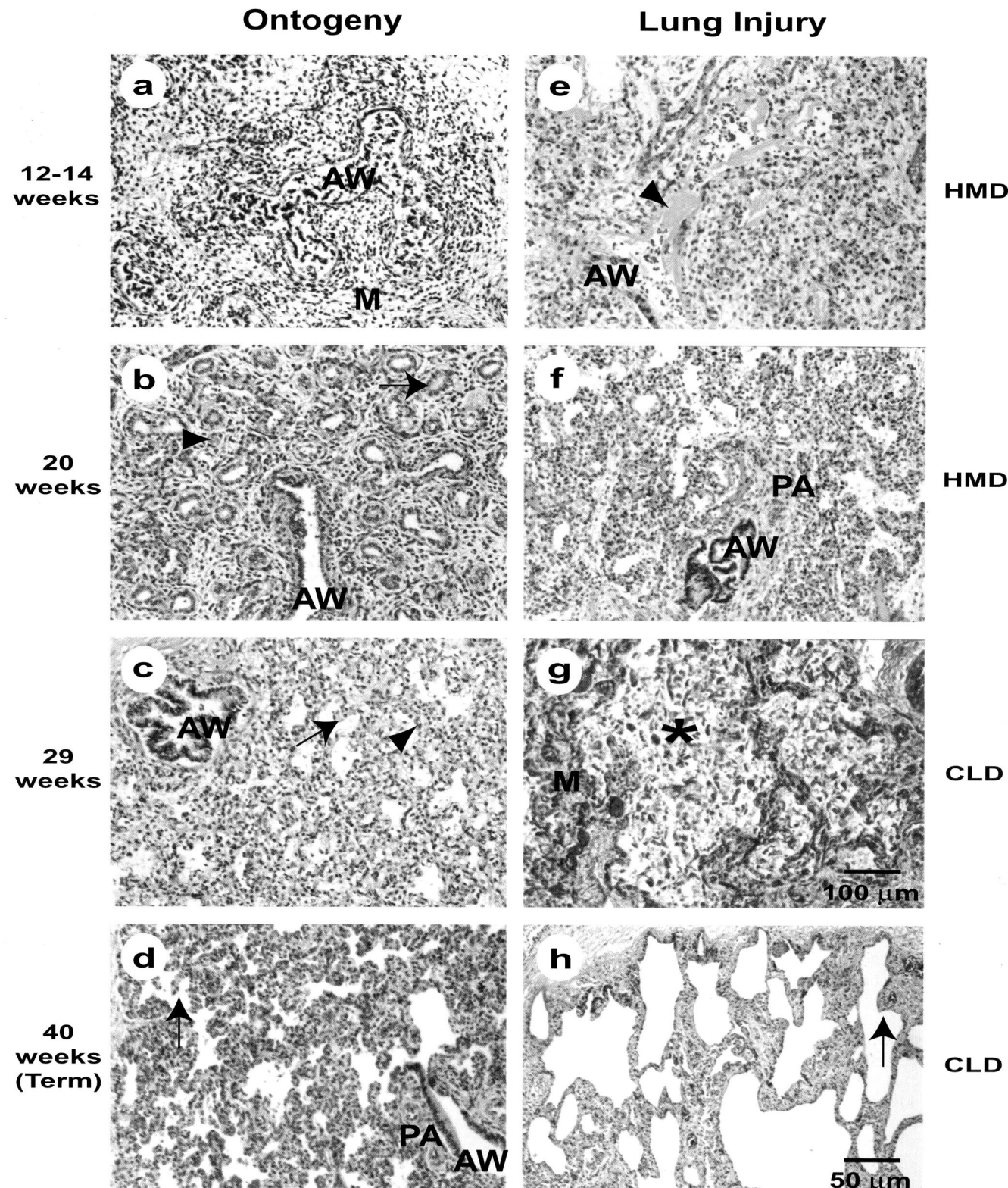

12-14
weeks

20
weeks

29
weeks

40
weeks
(Term)

HMD

HMD

CLD

CLD

100 μm

50 μm

Figure 93–1

Genetics and Embryology

Fred Levine

1

Basic Genetic Principles

PRIMARY STRUCTURE OF NUCLEIC ACID

There are two kinds of nucleic acid—deoxyribonucleic acid (DNA) and ribonucleic acid (RNA)—both of which are composed of recurring monomeric units called *nucleotides*. Each nucleotide has three components (Fig. 1-1A): (1) a phosphate group linked to (2) a five-carbon atom cyclic sugar group, which, in turn, is joined to (3) a purine or pyrimidine base. DNA and RNA are distinguished by their base components and the sugar-phosphate backbones. DNA consists of four deoxyribonucleotides that differ from one another in their base components. The four bases are the purine derivatives adenine (A) and guanine (G) and the pyrimidine derivatives cytosine (C) and thymine (T) (see Fig. 1-1B, C). Similarly, four different ribonucleotides are the major components of RNA; they contain the purine bases adenine and guanine and the pyrimidine bases cytosine and uracil (U). Thus, the major distinction in base composition between RNA and DNA is that RNA contains uracil, whereas DNA contains thymine. The other distinction between RNA and DNA is in their sugar-phosphate backbones: RNA contains ribose, and DNA contains 2-deoxyribose. In both DNA and RNA, the nucleotides are joined together by phosphodiester bonds linking the phosphate group of one nucleotide to a hydroxyl group on the sugar of the adjacent nucleotide. The purine and pyrimidine bases of the nucleotide constitute distinctive side chains and are not present in the backbone structure of nucleic acids.

By analyzing x-ray diffraction patterns of purified DNA and by building models, Watson and Crick deduced that native DNA consists of two antiparallel chains in a structure that can be conceptualized as resembling a spiral staircase, the *double helix* (Fig. 1-2A). The two strands are held together by hydrogen bonds between pairs of bases on the opposing strands, similar to the steps on a spiral staircase (see Fig. 1-2B). The bonding is specific; A always pairs with T, and C always pairs with G. As Watson and Crick noted, a pair of purines would be rather large to fit inside a double helix (which has a thickness of 20 Å), and a pair of pyrimidines would be too far apart to form stable hydrogen bonds with each other. The base pairs AT and GC, however, prove to be not only similar in size, but also similar in shape. Overall, the discovery of the structure of DNA was one of the most important events in biology because it not only provided an explanation for how genetic information is carried, but it also indicated how this information is propagated. As a consequence of the hydrogen bonding between the two DNA strands, also known as *base pairing* or *hybridization,* a DNA molecule can replicate precisely by separation of the two chains followed by synthesis of two new complementary strands. In contrast to the regular structure of DNA, most RNA molecules are single stranded. Base pairing, however, occurs between regions of an RNA strand with complementary sequences, with AU pairs instead of AT, giving RNA molecules a complex secondary structure that is poorly understood in most cases but plays an important role in cellular metabolism (e.g., transfer RNA [tRNA]).

GENOMIC ORGANIZATION

Chromosomes

Each cell in a human being contains an enormous amount of DNA, approximately 3×10^9 base pairs per haploid genome. Obviously, there must be a way for the cell to organize such a large amount of DNA in a compact manner. This is accomplished by organizing the DNA into large macromolecular complexes called *chromosomes*. A major distinguishing feature between prokaryotic organisms such as bacteria and eukaryotic organisms such as humans is the presence of a nucleus, the major function of which is to contain the chromosomes. There are 46 chromosomes in the human nucleus. Of these, the 44 known as autosomes exist in homologous pairs, numbered from 1 to 22 in order of decreasing size, with one member of each pair inherited from one parent. The remaining two chromosomes, known as sex chromosomes because they are involved in sex determination, are designated *X* and *Y*. Normally, females have two X chromosomes, whereas males have one X and one Y. A small segment of the Y chromosome includes the testis-determining factor (TDF) responsible for male development. The lack of this factor results in female development, so it is the presence or absence of the Y chromosome that actually determines a person's sex. The *TDF* gene encodes a sequence-specific DNA binding protein named SRY (sex-determining region Y gene).

Each chromosome consists of one large DNA molecule complexed with large amounts of two types of protein, called *histone* and *nonhistone chromosomal protein*, which serve to condense the DNA into an orderly, compact structure. There are five principal histone types, called *H1, H2a, H2b, H3,* and *H4,* which interact specifically with one another and with DNA to form structures called *nucleosomes*. Each nucleosome consists of a disk-shaped histone core plus a segment of DNA that winds around the core. The core contains two copies of H2a, H2b, H3, and H4, and the DNA wrapped around the histone core is about 140 base pairs in length. H1 binds to the DNA just next to the nucleosomes. The complex of DNA and histones, called *chromatin,* forms coils to produce a fiber with a larger diameter. The

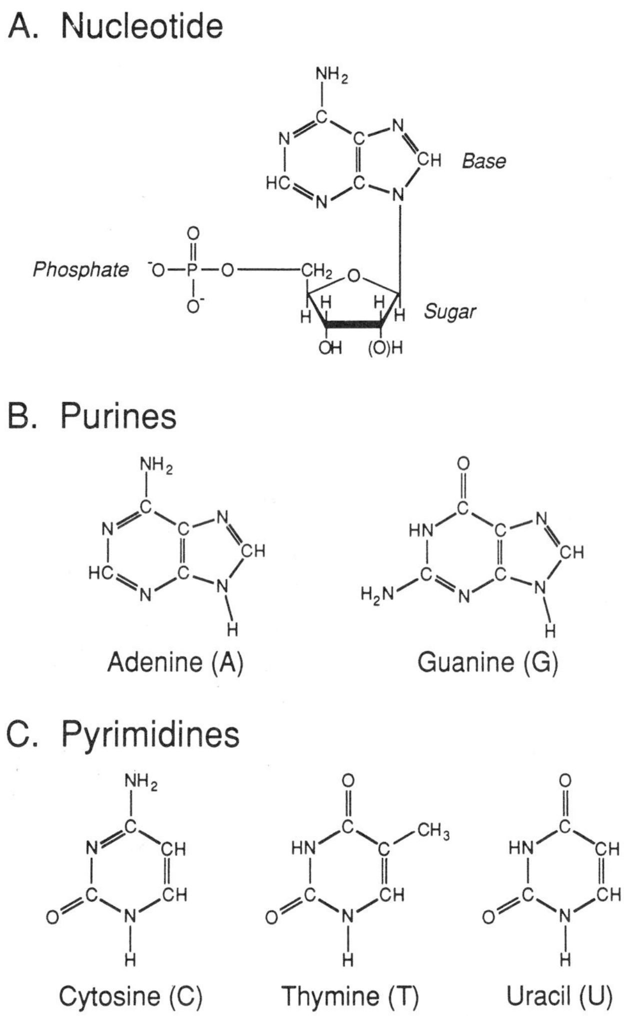

A. Nucleotide

B. Purines

Adenine (A)   Guanine (G)

C. Pyrimidines

Cytosine (C)   Thymine (T)   Uracil (U)

Figure 1–1. Nucleotide structure. A, General structure of nucleotides, consisting of a purine or pyrimidine base (in this case, adenine), a five-carbon atom sugar, and a phosphate group. The oxygen drawn in *parentheses* in the sugar is present in the ribose of RNA but is absent in the deoxyribose of DNA. The plane of the sugar is perpendicular to that of the other subunits. **B,** Structures of the two purines in DNA and RNA. **C,** Structures of the three pyrimidines in nucleic acids. Cytosine is found in both DNA and RNA, thymine is unique to DNA, and uracil is unique to RNA.

nonhistone proteins are much more diverse and complex; 12 to 18 major and many additional minor species have been identified. Nonhistone proteins play important roles, including as chromosomal structural elements and in the control of gene expression, for example, posttranslational modification of histones by acetylation and deacetylation. Histone-depleted metaphase chromosomes have been shown to consist of a non-histone protein scaffold that has the shape characteristic of a metaphase chromosome surrounded by a halo of DNA. In this model of chromosome organization, the nucleoprotein fibers form radially oriented loops that converge to the central scaffolding. Most chromatin fibers undergo a transition between dispersed and condensed configurations during the cell cycle. Before cell division, most chromatin is in the condensed form, with limited but functionally important transcriptional activity. Between cell divisions, the bulk of the chromatin in most cells is dispersed within the nucleus for events such as DNA replication and gene transcription.

Gene Structure

All hereditary information is transmitted from parent to offspring through the inheritance of genes, which are defined as the DNA sequences necessary to produce a functional protein or RNA sequence. It is thought that there are about 50,000 genes on human chromosomes, although this number is the subject of great controversy, even with the completion of the human genome sequence. These genes as well as genes in all eukaryotic cells are divided into regions called *expressed sequences (exons)* and *intervening sequences (introns)*, of which only the exon sequences are present in mature messenger RNA (mRNA) and actually code for proteins (Fig. 1-3, *top*). Although some introns play a role in the control of gene expression, the function of most is unknown, but they can greatly expand the size of genes. For example, the dystrophin gene, involved in Duchenne muscular dystrophy, is about 2300 kilobase (kB) pairs of DNA in length and includes 79 exons accounting for only 14 kB, with the remainder consisting of introns, some more than 100 kB long. In contrast, the α-globin gene, 835 base pairs long, includes two introns that total 261 base pairs.

In addition to the exons and introns of genes, most of the eukaryotic genome consists of long DNA stretches that are not part of genes. In fact, it has been estimated that genes make up only 10% of the human genome, and the actual protein-coding regions account for only 1% of the genome. It is not understood why these long DNA stretches are present. Although some of them may play a role in DNA replication, chromosome pairing, and recombination, most of these stretches apparently serve only to connect genes and complete the integrity of chromosomes. Interspersed throughout the noncoding DNA stretches are many repeated sequences, which are either clustered together or evenly distributed throughout the genome. These sequences can be short and consist only of 5 to 10 nucleotides, or they can be as long as 5000 to 6000 nucleotides. The function of most repeats remains largely a mystery. Some of the longer repeats, such as the so-called Alu or LINE elements, have features similar to viruses and have been shown to be able to move from place to place in the genome. Other repeats are short, consisting of a stretch of two bases, such as CACACA. A feature of short repeats is that they tend to exhibit extreme variability from individual to individual. In essence, the length of repeat units forms a type of fingerprint that can be used to identify any given individual uniquely. This makes them powerful tools for gene mapping studies as well as for forensic applications such as paternity testing and criminal investigations.

HOW GENES FUNCTION

Flow of Genetic Information

Transcription

Because DNA stores genetic information in the nucleus of eukaryotic cells, whereas protein synthesis occurs in the cytoplasm, there must be a mechanism by which the information is carried to the cytoplasm. The first step in gene expression is the production of an RNA molecule from the DNA template. This RNA acts as a molecular messenger, carrying the genetic information out of the nucleus. The synthesis of mRNA is called *transcription* because the genetic information in DNA is transcribed without being changed into a new language. During the process of transcription, the two DNA strands separate, and one functions as a template for the synthesis of single-stranded RNA molecules by the action of enzymes called *RNA polymerases.* The initial RNA transcripts are quite long because they include both intron and exon sequences from the gene (see Fig. 1-3). The intron sequences are cut out by specific enzymes, and the remaining exons are spliced together to form the mature

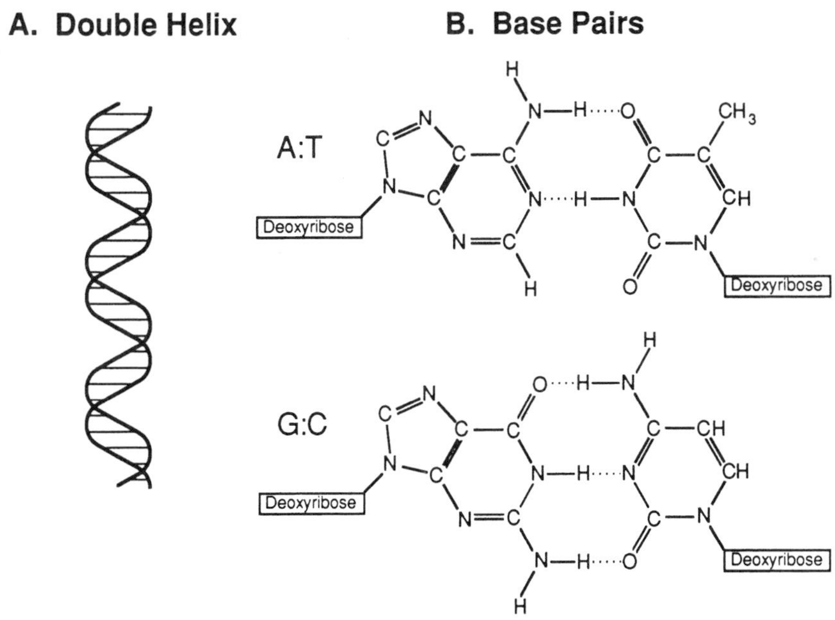

A. Double Helix   ## B. Base Pairs

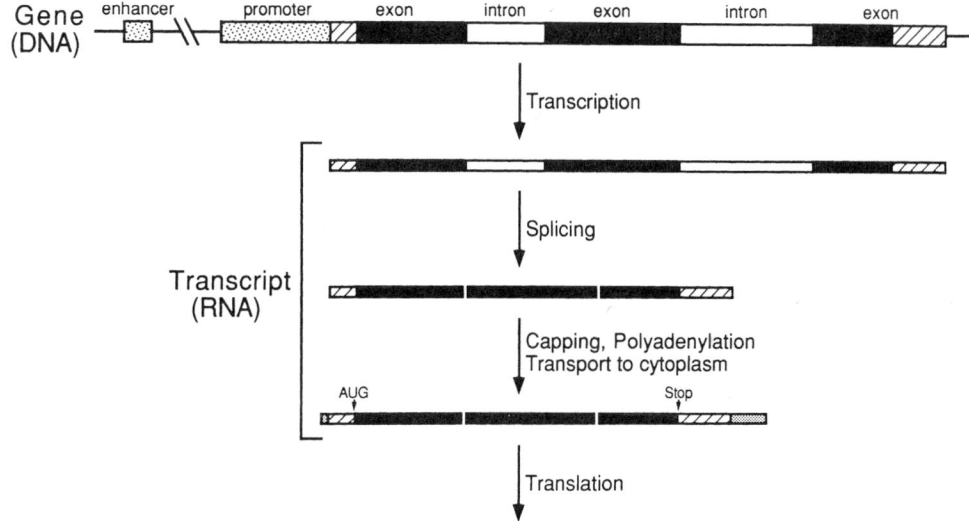

Figure 1–2. DNA structure and base pairing. **A,** Schematic representation of the double helical DNA molecule. **B,** Base pairing of purines and pyrimidines in DNA. Hydrogen bonding between the pairs is indicated by *dotted lines.* The AT and GC base pairs are identical in size and are nearly identical in shape. Also note that the GC base pair has an additional hydrogen bond and therefore is held together more strongly.

Figure 1–3. Gene structure *(top)* and the flow of genetic information from DNA to protein. *Cross-hatched boxes* indicate the regions of exons that do not encode amino acid sequences; *shaded boxes* indicate posttranscriptional modifications.

mRNAs. Before the transcripts leave the nucleus, most are modified in two other ways. A methylated guanine nucleotide, called a *cap*, is added to the beginning in a reverse orientation to the rest of the molecule, and a string of 200 to 250 adenine bases is usually added to the end (see Fig. 1-3). The cap is important for ribosomal binding in the initiation of protein synthesis. The polyadenosine stretch at the end of the mRNA plays a role in the stability of the mRNA and, as discussed later, is quite useful in mRNA purification.

In addition to mRNA, two other major classes of RNA are transcribed from DNA: ribosomal RNA (rRNA) and tRNA. In contrast to mRNA, these classes of RNA do not code for proteins but are required for protein synthesis (see later). Unlike prokaryotic cells, in which a single RNA polymerase makes all types of RNA, eukaryotic cells have three different RNA polymerases that transcribe different classes of RNA: the precursors to 18S and 28S rRNA are made by RNA polymerase I; the precursors to mRNA are made by RNA polymerase II, and 5S rRNA and tRNA are synthesized by RNA polymerase III. RNA polymerase I functions in a specialized region within the nucleus called the *nucleolus.* There has been

great excitement about the discovery of potentially large numbers of small RNA molecules that may play important roles in the control of gene expression by interfering with the expression of mRNA (hence the name "small interfering RNAs" [siRNA]).

Translation and the Genetic Code

The production of protein from an mRNA template is called *translation* because the genetic information that is stored in DNA as a sequence of nucleotides is translated into a sequence of amino acids. The method of storing genetic information is called the *genetic code.* Each member of the code consists of three adjacent bases that constitute a *codon* designating a specific amino acid. Because each of these three sites can be one of four possible nucleotides, there are 4^3 or 64 different codons, all but three of which specify an amino acid. Because there are only 20 amino acids, most amino acids are specified by more than one codon. Thus, the genetic code is referred to as being degenerate. Three codons—UAA, UAG, and UGA—are called nonsense or termination codons because they do not code for amino acids and serve as stop sites for translation.

The process of translating mRNA to produce a protein chain requires two kinds of RNA—rRNA and tRNA—that do not code for polypeptides. The three types of rRNA—28S, 18S, and 5S—associate with more than 50 proteins to form the ribosomes, which are the cytoplasmic sites of translation. The tRNAs are small molecules about 80 nucleotides long whose function is to position the correct amino acid for incorporation into the polypeptide. Before an amino acid can be incorporated into a polypeptide chain, it is first coupled to an appropriate tRNA by an aminoacyl-tRNA synthetase, which is specific for each amino acid-tRNA combination. A three-nucleotide region of each tRNA, designated the *anticodon,* includes a base sequence complementary to the appropriate mRNA codon and therefore hybridizes to it. In this way, each amino acid is brought into proper position and is added sequentially to the growing polypeptide chain by peptidyl transferase, an enzyme that is an integral part of the ribosome. Initiation of transcription almost always occurs at an AUG codon, which codes for methionine (see Fig. 1–3). In many proteins, the initiation methionine is removed posttranslationally. Translation is terminated when a ribosome encounters a nonsense codon (see Fig. 1–3). In the presence of the appropriate factors, the polypeptide chain is released from the last tRNA, and the ribosome disengages from the mRNA to start the cycle of protein synthesis over again.

Regulation of Gene Expression

The ability to control the production of proteins is central to the development and functioning of every organism. Although this control occurs at every stage of protein production, the most important level of control occurs at the level of mRNA production (i.e., transcriptional control). Transcriptional regulation is accomplished via the action of proteins that act on DNA, either by modifying it (e.g., cytosine methylation) or by binding to specific DNA sequences to activate or repress transcription from a gene.

In higher eukaryotes, such as humans, two major types of DNA sequences regulate gene expression promoters and enhancers. Promoters are located immediately adjacent to the start site of transcription, whereas enhancers can be located at large distances from the transcribed regions of the gene (see Fig. 1–3). Several types of regulatory sequences have been identified in promoters that are important in transcriptional initiation by RNA polymerase II, including the *TATA box,* so-called because it consists of a run of T and A base pairs. The TATA box is located about 30 bases before the transcription start site and functions as the binding site for a large, multisubunit complex of transcription factors, which includes RNA polymerase. Other sequence elements that are common to many genes transcribed by RNA polymerase II include the CAAT sequence (*CAT box*) that lies between 50 and 100 bases before the transcription start site and the GGGCGG sequence (*GC box*). Similar to the TATA box, the function of these sequence elements is to serve as binding sites for proteins that are involved in transcriptional control.

Enhancer sequences serve to increase the level of transcription from promoters and have been shown to play pivotal roles in gene regulation, particularly for highly expressed genes such as viral genes and the globins. Many mammalian enhancers are tissue specific in their action. For example, enhancers from the pancreatic amylase, chymotrypsin, and trypsin genes function only in exocrine pancreas, and enhancers from immunoglobulin genes function only in lymphoid cells. In contrast to promoters, which have fixed positions relative to the transcription start site, enhancers have been discovered in various positions, including before the promoter, after the coding region, within introns, and at great distances from the coding sequence, as in the case of the globin enhancer. Another property of enhancers that distinguishes them from promoters is their ability to function in a

position-independent and orientation-independent manner relative to the gene. In addition to enhancer elements that increase the levels of transcription, similar elements, called *silencers,* decrease the level of transcription. Combinations of these elements allow for precise control of the level of gene transcription.

Transcription is regulated by interactions among proteins bound to enhancer and promoter sequences. Such proteins can have either stimulatory or inhibitory functions. For example, the receptors for steroid hormones such as the glucocorticoids, estrogen, and androgens have been isolated and shown to bind to specific sequences near steroid-responsive genes such as vitellogenin and lactalbumin. In addition to the classic transcription factors that bind to specific sequence elements in genes, other proteins play important roles in the control of gene expression. For example, methylases and demethylases regulate the methylation of cytosine residues to affect gene expression. Mutations in MeCP2, a protein that binds to methylated DNA, cause Rett syndrome, an X-linked neurodegenerative disease. Mutations in CREB-binding protein, a transcriptional co-activator that has intrinsic histone acetyltransferase activity, cause Rubinstein-Taybi syndrome, a finding further illustrating the importance of chromatin modifications in regulating gene expression. Overall, it is the complex interplay of positive and negative effects between factors bound to different sites, both near and far from the coding region of the gene, that determines the pattern of gene expression.

Posttranscriptional mechanisms are being increasingly recognized as playing important roles in controlling the level of gene product. Regulation takes place at virtually every level, including alternative splicing, transport of RNA from the nucleus to the cytoplasm, persistence of mRNA in the cytoplasm, translational efficiency, and regulation of the rate of protein degradation. Individual mRNA species differ widely with respect to metabolic stability. The half-lives of some mRNAs span several hours or even days, whereas those of others are extremely short. The rate of turnover of some mRNAs can vary dramatically in response to changes in the cell cycle and in response to treatment with certain hormones. Protein binding and mRNA structural features have also been shown to influence susceptibility to decay. The increasing recognition of the significance of posttranscriptional influences on protein levels has given rise to the field of *proteomics,* in which techniques directed toward measuring protein levels on a global and high-throughput scale are used to define the *proteome* (i.e., the total complement of proteins) within a cell.

Genes and Development

Development, in general terms, is the process by which a single fertilized egg becomes a complete organism. Central to development is the process of *differentiation,* whereby cells acquire different properties to carry out specific functions in separate tissues. To a large extent, differentiation is reflected in the production of tissue-specific proteins that, of course, is the result of specific gene expression. A fundamental question in development is how a group of genetically identical cells comes to express sets of genes in a tissue-specific manner. Much progress in this area has come from the striking similarities between the process of development in organisms such as *Drosophila* and *Caenorhabditis elegans* and in humans. Important principles of development, such as the role of morphogenic gradients, were first described in lower organisms but have proven to be relevant in humans as well. Thus, small molecules such as retinoids and proteins such as transcription factors form concentration gradients that are critical in determining the pattern of body formation.

In addition to knowledge gained from lower organisms, a revolution in understanding of human development and human

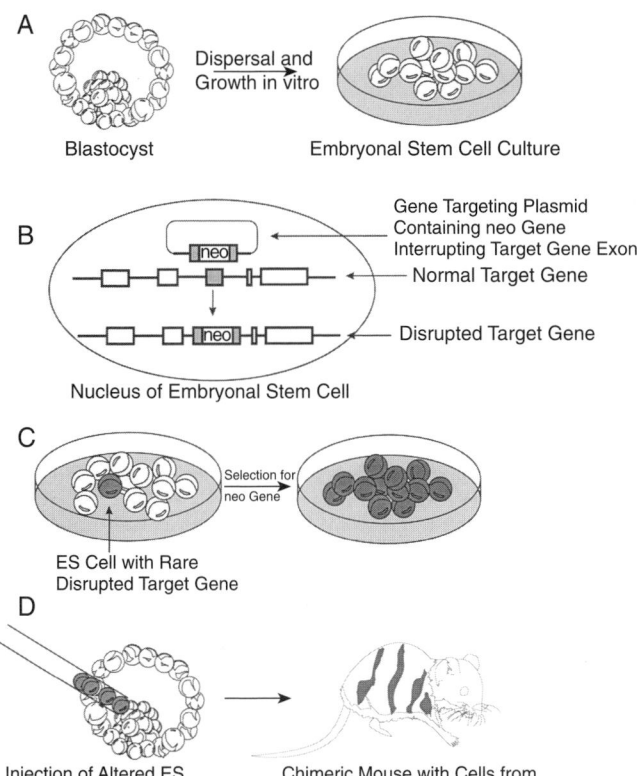

Figure 1–4. Genetic alteration of mice by homologous recombination. ES cell = embryonal stem cell.

genetic disease has come from advances in the ability to manipulate mice genetically. Originally, this was done by introducing genetic material into mice by microinjection of fertilized eggs. The injected eggs give rise to mature animals that integrate the injected genes into their genome resulting in transgenic animals that pass the introduced genetic material through the germline to their offspring. In many cases, the introduced genes are expressed, thus allowing the effect of overexpression or ectopic expression of a gene product to be studied.

More recently, techniques have been developed to inactivate a gene in a mouse. This is done by genetically manipulating embryonic stem (ES) cells derived from the blastocyst (Fig. 1-4). These cells can be grown in culture and thus can be genetically manipulated, while retaining the ability to contribute to both somatic tissues and the germline of mature mice. Using the ability of cells to mediate homologous recombination (Fig. 1-5), genes in ES cells can be "knocked-out," and the genetically manipulated ES cells can then be injected into mouse blastocysts, giving rise to chimeric adult mice. Some of these mice contain the genetically manipulated cells in their germline, thereby giving rise to genetically altered, nonchimeric offspring. A powerful application of this approach in developmental biology is in studying the role of the homeobox family of transcription factors, which plays important roles in development. These genes are systematically being knocked out, to allow investigators to study the role of these genes in development.

Most recently, the ability to express or to knock out genes in a particular tissue has been achieved using tissue-specific promoter elements together with powerful site-specific recombination systems derived from bacterial viruses. This approach allows the study of genetic alterations that could be lethal if present in all the cells of an organism. An example of an application of this technology is the development of a mouse model of cystic fibrosis. In contrast to humans, mice in which the *CFTR* gene has

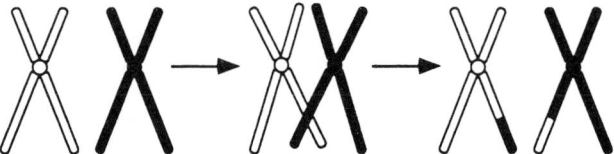

Figure 1–5. Recombination. In this simplified view of recombination, the two members of a homologous pair of chromosomes line up during the first meiotic prophase. Segments of the two chromosomes "cross over," and breakage and rejoining of the DNA strands occur.

been knocked out die shortly after birth, thus making it difficult to study the disease in mice. Efforts are being made to develop mice in which the *CFTR* gene is mutated only in a particular tissue such as the lung.

Finally, the study of vertebrate development is likely to be revolutionized through the development of a new model organism, the zebrafish. Zebrafish have a tremendous advantage over mice in that their embryos can be easily examined during development, thereby making it possible to screen for developmental mutations.

CELL DIVISION AND RECOMBINATION
Cell Cycle and Mitosis

The *cell cycle* is the process by which the cell divides to form two daughter cells. In *mitotic division,* there is a maintenance of the normal complement of 46 chromosomes through a process of DNA replication and subsequent separation of the chromosomes. Additionally, the cytoplasm of the eukaryotic cell cleaves into two approximately equal halves. Mitotic division takes up only a small part of the cell cycle. A complete cell cycle consists of four phases: G_1 (growth or gap 1), S (synthesis), G_2, and M (mitosis). The cycle of each type of cell varies considerably in total duration, from minutes in some cells to weeks or months in others. The G_1 phase begins immediately after a cell division. It is followed by the S phase, during which DNA replication occurs, as described earlier. Immediately after the S phase, the cell has a tetraploid chromosome content, instead of the usual diploid number, so there are 92 chromosomes divided into 46 pairs of sister chromatids. Cells then pass into the premitotic G_2 phase, which ends with the onset of mitosis or actual cell division. The G_1, S, and G_2 phases are called *interphase* because although there is continued cellular growth and synthesis of cellular macromolecules, such as DNA, RNA, and proteins, cell division takes place only during mitosis. DNA and the histone components of the chromatin are synthesized only during the S phase, whereas RNA, the cytoplasmic proteins, and organelles are synthesized continuously during all of interphase. The cell finally divides in the M phase, during which the synthesis of RNA and protein is greatly reduced.

During interphase, chromosomes are not visible by light microscopy because chromatin is dispersed throughout the nucleoplasm. The beginning of mitosis is signaled by the appearance of chromosomes as thin threads inside the nucleus. Mitosis is divided somewhat arbitrarily into four phases: prophase, metaphase, anaphase, and telophase. During *prophase,* the nuclear envelope begins to break up, and each chromosome can be seen to consist of two identical or sister chromatids held together at specific regions called *centromeres.* Another structure that is important for proper segregation of chromosomes is the centriole, an organelle just outside the nuclear membrane. Each cell normally has a pair of centrioles, arranged opposite to one other, but they are duplicated early in the S phase. During mitotic prophase, the two pairs of centrioles separate and migrate to define the poles of the cell. During *metaphase,* the chromosomes move to the equatorial plane of the cell and become attached to the spindle fiber apparatus, which is a structure consisting of microtubules of protein that radiate from the centrioles at either pole and extend from pole to pole. Each chromatid has near its centromere a dense granule called a *kinetochore* to which the spindle fibers attach. Because of the kinetochores and attached spindle fibers, the two sister chromatids are pulled toward opposite poles. During *anaphase,* the centromeres divide, and the two chromatids of each pair, now free of each other, move toward their respective poles by the contraction of spindle fibers. In *telophase,* the chromosomes and spindle fibers disperse and disappear, and new nuclear envelopes are assembled to surround the two sets of daughter chromosomes. Simultaneously, separation and segregation of the cell cytoplasm occur, a process called *cytokinesis,* which results in the formation of a complete membrane around the cell and constitutes the end of the process of forming a new cell.

Progress through the cell is controlled by a complex set of phosphorylation and dephosphorylation steps, mediated by many interacting kinases and phosphatases. Proteins called *cyclins,* so-called because their expression is limited to specific stages of the cell cycle, control the initiation of the kinase-phosphatase cascade. That cascade, in turn, ultimately controls the ability of the cell to progress through the major cell cycle control points (usually called *checkpoints*), at the G_1/S and G_2/M boundaries. Many of the proteins involved in cell cycle control are, not surprisingly, involved in the loss of cell cycle control that is the hallmark of carcinogenesis and so can be classified as oncogenes. In addition to the proteins that are directly involved in cell cycle control, proteins that are important in DNA repair have also been found to be important in carcinogenesis. Most prominently, the *P53* tumor suppressor gene, which seems to be the central monitor of genomic damage, is also the most commonly mutated gene in human cancer, and it has a role in a high percentage of all human cancers.

Meiosis

Meiosis is the process by which germline cells form gametes. In contrast to mitosis, in which a single cell division and an exact duplication of the genetic material in the parent cell occur, meiosis involves two separate cell divisions from a diploid parent cell and a random reassortment and reduction of genetic material so each of the four daughter cells has a haploid DNA content (i.e., 23 chromosomes). In this way, meiosis yields four haploid gametes, the sperm and the egg cells, which support sexual reproduction and a new generation of diploid organisms.

The first meiotic division, similar to mitosis, is separated into four stages: prophase, metaphase, anaphase, and telophase. Before meiosis begins, the chromosomes in the cell are replicated to produce two pairs of sister chromatids, and each pair of sister chromatids remains together throughout the first meiotic division. In metaphase, the spindle fibers attach to chromosomes, and the paired chromosomes align themselves in the equatorial plane of the cell. In anaphase, the paired homologous chromosomes separate and move toward their respective poles. The daughter chromatids, however, remain attached to their centromeres. In telophase, the chromosomes arrive at the poles, and a nuclear membrane forms around each group of chromosomes. The chromatids are still attached by their centromeres. Because the number of chromosomes in each daughter cell is reduced by half, the first mitotic division is called the *reduction division*.

The second meiotic division occurs without DNA replication. The events are similar to those of mitosis; the centromeres divide, and the sister chromatids separate and move toward opposite poles. The result is the production of four haploid cells. Two of these haploid cells carry copies of one set of allelic genes, whereas the other two haploid cells have copies of the homologous allelic set.

Recombination

During prophase of the first meiotic division, homologous pairs of chromosomes are held together by a protein-containing framework called a *synaptonemal complex,* which extends along the entire length of the paired chromosomes. Recombination between chromatids of the homologous chromosomes occurs at this stage and results in the exchange of DNA between the original parental chromosomes (see Fig. 1-5). In males, the X and Y chromosomes are associated only at the tips of their short arms during meiotic prophase. This short associated region is called the *pseudoautosomal region* because recombination between the X and Y chromosomes occurs there (and so it behaves as an autosome in terms of mendelian inheritance). This region probably plays an important role in sex chromosome pairing and segregation as well as in male fertility. Recombination, in conjunction with mutation (see later), is important for generating genetic diversity through the exchange of DNA between different chromosomes, and it plays a critical role in gene mapping studies.

MUTATION AND GENETIC HETEROGENEITY

Mutation is defined broadly as any change in the sequence of DNA. Because most of the human genome does not consist of genes, most mutations are of no apparent functional consequence and thus are termed *silent.* Only mutations that affect the expression or function of a gene or its product are phenotypically apparent. Of these, many are not clinically relevant but instead contribute to normal population heterogeneity. Variations in hair and eye color, for example, originally arose through mutation. Thus, the term *mutation* may be defined differently at the molecular genetic, biologic, and clinical levels. To some extent, mutation should be viewed as a natural, ongoing process that produces population diversity. Along with recombination, it is a central element in the evolutionary process. The mutation rate in humans has been estimated at 1 in 10 million per gene per cell cycle. The mutation rate and the types of mutations that occur, however, can vary dramatically among different loci. The consequence of this rate of mutation is that variations in the human genome are estimated to occur, on average, once per 1000 base pairs. Hence, each genome differs from others at millions of sites. Although mutations occur in both germline and somatic (nongermline) cells, only mutations affecting the germline are inherited. Somatic cell mutations are also of major medical importance, particularly in the development of cancer.

Single-Gene Mutations

Mutations can range from those affecting only a single base pair to major alterations in chromosome structure. Mutations that affect only one nucleotide are called *point mutations* and involve the substitution of one nucleotide for another (Fig. 1-6A). When a point mutation occurs in a part of the gene that codes for a protein and alters the protein by changing the codon of which it is a part, it is called a *missense mutation.* Because the genetic code is degenerate, it is possible to have a point mutation that does not change the amino acid that is encoded. This is another example of a silent mutation. In addition, some missense mutations result in amino acid substitutions that have no effect on protein function but are sometimes detectable by biochemical techniques such as electrophoresis. Insertion or deletion of a nucleotide in the protein-coding portion of a gene is called a *frameshift mutation* because it changes the entire reading frame of the gene at every codon

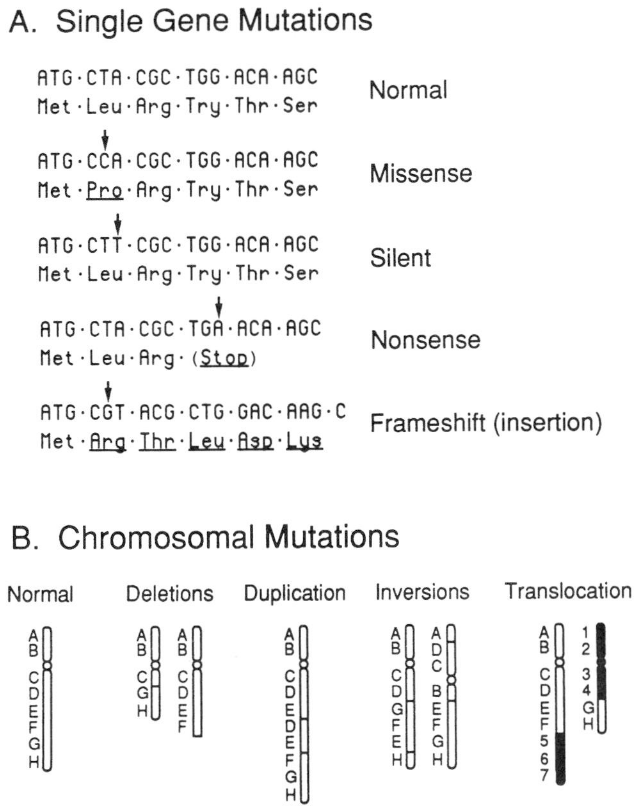

A. Single Gene Mutations

```
ATG·CTA·CGC·TGG·ACA·AGC
Met·Leu·Arg·Try·Thr·Ser      Normal
        ↓
ATG·CCA·CGC·TGG·ACA·AGC
Met·Pro·Arg·Try·Thr·Ser      Missense
     ↓
ATG·CTT·CGC·TGG·ACA·AGC
Met·Leu·Arg·Try·Thr·Ser      Silent
                ↓
ATG·CTA·CGC·TGA·ACA·AGC
Met·Leu·Arg·(Stop)           Nonsense
     ↓
ATG·CGT·ACG·CTG·GAC·AAG·C
Met·Arg·Thr·Leu·Asp·Lys      Frameshift (insertion)
```

B. Chromosomal Mutations

```
Normal    Deletions    Duplication    Inversions    Translocation
```

Figure 1–6. Mutation. A, Single-gene mutations. A prototypical normal gene sequence is shown on the first line, with the corresponding amino acid sequence. Examples of four types of common mutations are shown. The substituted or inserted nucleotides are indicated by *arrows,* and the affected amino acids are *underlined.* **B,** Chromosomal mutations. A prototype normal chromosome is shown, with genes A through H. Examples of gross chromosomal mutations are shown to the *right,* and their effects on gene content and arrangement are indicated. In the translocation example, the two chromosomes are not members of a homologous pair.

distal to the site of the mutation. *Nonsense mutations* are those point mutations that result in the formation of one of the three codons (UAA, UAG, UGA) that do not code for an amino acid and so result in the production of truncated proteins, which usually have little or no activity. Point mutations occurring near the boundaries between introns and exons can cause improper splicing of mRNA precursors, resulting in RNA instability or the production of truncated proteins, or both.

Regulation of gene expression can also be affected by mutations occurring in control elements such as promoters and enhancers. Although this usually results in the production of less protein, such as occurs in some forms of thalassemia, there are also mutations that result in the increased production of a gene product, as in hereditary persistence of fetal hemoglobin.

Another mutational mechanism involves the expansion of triplet repeat sequences. More than 10 disorders have been found to be caused by an increase in the number of copies of CCG or AGC repeats in or near a gene. Examples of diseases caused by triplet repeat expansion are myotonic dystrophy, fragile X syndrome, and Huntington disease. In these disorders, the repeat number tends to increase with succeeding generations, leading to the term *dynamic mutation.* As the repeat number increases, so does the severity of the disease, giving rise to the phenomenon of *anticipation.* First described in myotonic dystrophy, anticipation refers to an increase in disease severity within succeeding generations of an affected family. The mechanism by which triplet repeat expansion disrupts the function of a gene varies, ranging from transcriptional inactivation of the *FMR-1* gene causing fragile X syndrome to an increase in the length of polyglutamine tracts in the gene causing Huntington disease.

Chromosomal Mutations

Mutations involving large alterations in chromosome structure are visible microscopically by karyotypic analysis (see Fig. 1–6*B*). These include deletions, duplications, inversions, and translocations from one chromosome to another. Because chromosomal aberrations usually result in the disruption of multiple genes, they often have profound clinical consequences. *Terminal chromosomal deletions* result from a single chromosomal break with subsequent loss of the piece of chromosome without a centromere. *Duplications* occur when a segment of a chromosome is repeated, either from inappropriate recombination or as a result of meiosis involving chromosomes with inversions or translocations. Most other chromosomal rearrangements, such as interstitial deletions, require multiple breaks and reunion events and so are usually less common. Some common genetic diseases, however, such as Duchenne muscular dystrophy, result primarily from small interstitial deletions, a finding demonstrating that chromosomal regions vary greatly in their propensity to undergo different types of mutational events.

Inversions result from two chromosome breaks followed by reversal of the broken piece of chromosome and subsequent rejoining to form an intact but rearranged chromosome. Although the inversion in and of itself does not have any clinical consequences unless one of the breakpoints affects gene expression, there are significant effects in subsequent generations. When chromosomes with inversions (either pericentric, in which the inverted region includes the centromere, or paracentric, in which the centromere is not involved) go through meiosis and recombination with normal homologues, gametes may be formed that contain duplications and deletions of parts of the involved chromosomes. *Translocations* result from the exchange of genetic material between two nonhomologous chromosomes. Similar to inversions, they do not cause any clinical disease unless the breakpoints occur in a gene. Persons in whom a translocation is present but who have a normal amount of genetic material are called *balanced translocation carriers.* Like inversions, however, translocations can have severe effects in offspring, resulting from the consequent duplication or deficiency syndromes (or both).

GENETIC DISORDERS

Approximately 4500 inherited disorders have been described thus far. More than half of these have been genetically mapped, and the molecular defect is being identified in a rapidly increasing number. Genetic disorders can be classified into three general categories: simple mendelian, chromosomal, and multifactorial. This section discusses these categories of disease as well as factors that contribute to disease heterogeneity.

Mendelian Disorders

Mendelian disorders are caused by mutation of a single gene and so display the simple patterns of inheritance dictated by the mendelian laws. Mendelian disorders can be classified into three categories: autosomal dominant (AD), autosomal recessive (AR), and X-linked. The last category results from mutations on the X chromosome, thus exhibiting a separate inheritance pattern from the other categories, which are the result of mutations on the autosomes. The demonstration that a particular disease or syndrome exhibits simple mendelian inheritance implies that the pathogenesis, no matter how seemingly complex it may be, is an alteration at a single genetic locus. In many cases, a single mutation can lead to numerous, seemingly unrelated defects, a phenomenon known as *pleiotropy*. It has been estimated that about 1% of the population has a monogenic disorder. The simple pattern of inheritance has made it relatively straight-forward to isolate genes for monogenic disorders. Virtually all common monogenic disorders and an increasingly large number of quite rare disorders have had the responsible genes isolated and studied.

Autosomal Dominant Disorders

AD disorders are those in which a patient manifests clinical symptoms when only a single copy of the mutant gene is present (i.e., the patient is heterozygous for the mutation). The following inheritance pattern is characteristic of AD disorders (Fig. 1-7A):

1. Each affected person has an affected parent.
2. Affected persons, on average, have equal numbers of affected and unaffected children.
3. Normal children of affected parents have only unaffected children.
4. Males and females are affected in equal proportions.
5. Each sex is equally likely to transmit the disorder to male and female children.
6. Vertical transmission of the disorder occurs through successive generations.

These general rules of AD inheritance assume that no new mutations occur. This assumption, however, is often not the case, and in some disorders the incidence of new mutations is quite high. For example, up to 50% of the cases of von Recklinghausen neurofibromatosis are estimated to result from new mutations.

Dominant mutations involve types of gene products in which an abnormality in 50% of the protein leads to disease. Although

mutation of genes with many different functions results in AD inheritance, three classes of proteins are frequently involved: (1) proteins that regulate complex metabolic pathways, such as membrane receptors and rate-limiting enzymes in pathways under feedback control; (2) structural proteins; and (3) proteins with alterations that cause a dominant negative function, that is, in which the mutant protein interferes with the function of the protein expressed from the normal allele. Examples of AD disorders include the following: familial hypercholesterolemia, which is caused by mutations in the low-density lipoprotein receptor; osteogenesis imperfecta, caused by mutations in some members of the collagen gene family; and Huntington disease, caused by a triplet repeat expansion in the Huntington gene.

A characteristic of many AD disorders is *incomplete penetrance*. This means that the same gene defect can manifest with widely varying severity. For example, tuberous sclerosis, one of the neurocutaneous disorders, can be clinically silent. Some persons are diagnosed with this disorder only when they have multiple, severely affected children. At that point, careful examination may reveal subtle evidence of tuberous sclerosis, such as a minor abnormality on a computed tomography scan of the head. Similar observations have been made for many different dominant diseases. Incomplete penetrance is a manifestation of the interaction of other gene products with the product of the disease gene. Increasingly, this phenomenon is being recognized as a step in the continuum between simple completely penetrant monogenic disorders and so-called complex disorders in which no single gene is sufficient to cause disease.

The phenomenon of *germline mosaicism* is a complicating factor in incomplete penetrance. Germline mosaicism occurs when a mutation is present in some of the germ cells but not in most other cells. Such a person is completely healthy but is at risk of having multiple affected children. Germline mosaicism is fairly common in Duchenne muscular dystrophy and occurs in other disorders as well. It can sometimes be difficult to distinguish between germline mosaicism and incomplete penetrance, thus making accurate genetic counseling and prenatal diagnosis difficult unless one can assay directly for the presence of a mutated gene.

Autosomal Recessive Disorders

AR disorders are those that are clinically apparent only when the patient is homozygous for the disease (i.e., both copies of the gene are mutant). The following pattern of inheritance is characteristic of AR disorders (see Fig. 1-7B):

1. The parents of affected children may be clinically normal (i.e., carriers).
2. Assuming that the carrier frequency in the population is low, only siblings are affected, and vertical transmission does not occur; the pattern therefore tends to appear horizontal.
3. Males and females are affected in equal proportions.
4. When both parents are heterozygous carriers of the mutation, 25% of their children are affected, 50% are carriers, and 25% are normal.

Every person is a carrier of certain AR mutations. Fortunately, the carrier frequency for most of these mutations is so low that likelihood that carriers will have affected children is low.

Recessive mutations frequently involve enzymes, as opposed to regulatory and structural proteins. This is because 50% of the normal level of enzyme activity is usually sufficient for normal function. Complete enzyme deficiency produces an accumulation of one or more metabolites preceding the enzymatic block, such as the build-up of phenylalanine in phenylketonuria, and a deficiency of metabolites distal to the block. Either, or both, of these abnormalities may be responsible for the disease phenotype. Although many recessive disorders involve enzymes, two of

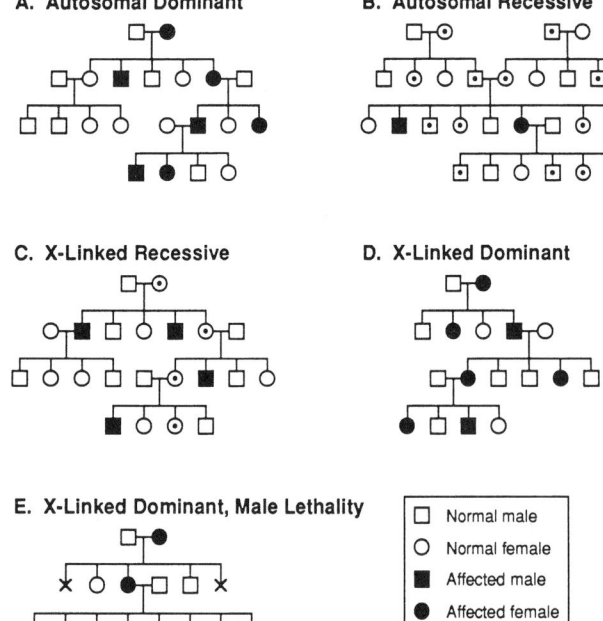

A. Autosomal Dominant

B. Autosomal Recessive

C. X-Linked Recessive

D. X-Linked Dominant

E. X-Linked Dominant, Male Lethality

□ Normal male
○ Normal female
■ Affected male
● Affected female
· Carrier
✕ Abortion

Figure 1–7. A to **E,** Pedigrees for disorders exhibiting the various mendelian modes of inheritance. These are idealized pedigrees, assuming full penetrance and no new mutations.

the most common AR disorders are cystic fibrosis, resulting from a mutation in a chloride channel, and sickle cell anemia, resulting from a mutation in the β-globin gene.

The terms *dominant* and *recessive* refer to phenotypes only and have their greatest application at the clinical level. At the gene level, dominance and recessiveness do not exist. Persons heterozygous for a recessive disorder may be clinically normal, but the reduced level of functional or immunoreactive protein is usually detectable analytically and may lead to other biochemical abnormalities that have no obvious effect on the person's health. In addition, patients homozygous for dominant mutations are usually more severely affected than are heterozygous patients, as is true in familial hypercholesterolemia. In many cases, the homozygous condition results in embryonic lethality and is never seen. Huntington disease stands out as a major exception in that homozygous patients are not clinically different from heterozygous patients.

X-Linked Disorders

The pattern of inheritance of X-linked disorders is distinct because the mutation occurs on the X chromosome, of which females have two copies, whereas males have only one. Thus, the pattern of inheritance of these disorders is distinctive because the clinical risk and disease severity differ between males and females.

The following pattern of inheritance is characteristic of X-linked recessive disorders (see Fig. 1-7C):

1. In contrast to the vertical pattern in AD disorders and the horizontal pattern in AR disorders, the pattern tends to be oblique because patients have unaffected parents but affected cousins and uncles.
2. There is never male-to-male transmission of the disorder because fathers transmit X chromosomes only to daughters.
3. Male children of carrier women have a 50% chance of being affected.
4. All female children of affected men are heterozygous carriers.
5. Unaffected men do not transmit the disease to any children.

Examples of X-linked recessive disorders include hemophilia, color blindness, and the Lesch-Nyhan syndrome (hypoxanthine-guanine phosphoribosyltransferase [HPRT] deficiency).

Although X-linked recessive disorders are generally observed only in male patients, X-linked dominant disorders are approximately twice as prevalent in females as in males and are characterized by transmission of the disorder from affected men to all daughters but to no sons (see Fig. 1-7D). Relatively few of these disorders have been described, but one example is hypophosphatemia (vitamin D-resistant rickets), in which males and females are equally affected even though females carry a normal as well as an abnormal gene. Several X-linked dominant disorders are lethal prenatally in hemizygous males (and presumably in homozygous females). In these disorders, affected mothers transmit the trait to half of their daughters but to no sons (see Fig. 1-7E). There is a high incidence of spontaneous abortions, and the male/female ratio of children is significantly less than 1. Disorders that appear to have this mode of inheritance include focal dermal hypoplasia, incontinentia pigmenti, and orofaciodigital syndrome type I. Aicardi syndrome is a neurodegenerative disorder consisting of agenesis of the corpus callosum with chorioretinal abnormalities that is found only in female patients, a finding suggesting X-linked dominant inheritance. Because of the severity of the phenotype and low reproductive fitness of affected persons, however, it is difficult to define the pattern of inheritance. Presumably, virtually all cases result from new mutations.

An important feature of X-linked disorders is the wide range of clinical expression in heterozygous females. In contrast to the incomplete penetrance of AD disorders, which probably results from interactions among different genes, variability in X-linked disorders is significantly affected by the process of X-inactivation or lyonization (after its discoverer, Mary Lyon). Because females carry two copies of the X chromosome and males carry only one, a mechanism called *dosage compensation* has evolved to equalize the amount of gene product that is produced from genes on the X chromosome. One could envision many ways in which this could be accomplished. For example, X-linked genes in females could be transcribed at one-half the rate of those genes in males, as occurs in insects. The mechanism that operates in humans, however, involves the random inactivation of one of the X chromosomes in every cell of the body. Therefore, there is only one active X chromosome in each cell. This finding has major implications for X-linked diseases. Because the process of inactivation is random, on average half of the cells inactivate the X chromosome carrying the normal gene and half inactivate the abnormal X chromosome. Unfortunately, in some cases, there is a significant deviation from an equal ratio. Female patients in whom a high percentage of the normal X chromosome has been inactivated may demonstrate significant symptoms. This may be one reason for the significant percentage of female carriers of the fragile X syndrome who exhibit varying degrees of mental retardation.

It is also important to distinguish between actual X-linked disorders and sex-influenced disorders. The latter category consists of disorders encoded by autosomal genes that are differentially expressed in the two sexes. Male-pattern baldness, for example, is the result of an AD mutation that requires high testosterone levels to become manifest.

Chromosomal Disorders

Chromosomal disorders fall into two general categories: those involving incorrect chromosome number, called *aneuploidy;* and those that result from large chromosomal mutations, as described earlier. Aneuploidy is the result of nondisjunction during meiosis, in which both members of a homologous pair of chromosomes move to the same daughter cell. As a result of nondisjunction, the fertilized egg receives either one or three copies of the chromosome instead of the usual two. Because they involve numerous genes and upset the normal genomic balance, most disorders affecting chromosome number are lethal prenatally, particularly those involving loss of a chromosome. Those that are not lethal usually result in sterility because they prevent meiosis from proceeding normally. The best known and most common chromosomal disorder is Down syndrome, which generally results from trisomy of chromosome 21 but which can also be caused by a duplication or translocation of a specific region of chromosome 21. Trisomies of chromosomes 13 or 18 also occur but are much less common than Down syndrome. Turner syndrome occurs in women who receive only a single X chromosome, whereas Klinefelter syndrome occurs in men who receive two X chromosomes in addition to the Y chromosome.

Deletions that are too small to be visible using standard cytogenetic techniques (but that still result in the deletion of multiple genes) are called *microdeletion* or *contiguous gene syndromes*. Sometimes, these deletions can be detected using advanced cytogenetic techniques, such as prometaphase banding, in which cells are arrested in mitosis at an earlier stage so that instead of the usual 300 to 400 bands (each containing about 1 megabase of DNA), more than 1000 bands can be visualized. With the availability of cloned genetic markers covering much of the genome, the technique of fluorescent *in situ* hybridization can be used to detect small deletions. In this technique, a cloned DNA probe is labeled with a fluorescent molecule and is then hybridized to a standard chromosome preparation on a microscope slide. The presence of two normal chromosomes can be visualized by the appearance of two fluorescent dots, whereas a heterozygous microdeletion appears as a single dot. Examples of microdeletion syndromes include the DiGeorge syndrome, characterized by T-cell immunodeficiency and cardiac anomalies and caused by a microdeletion of chromosome 22. Prader-Willi syndrome, characterized by mental retardation, infantile hypotonia, and a compulsive eating disorder, is frequently caused by a microdeletion of chromosome 15. A clinically unrelated disorder, Angelman syndrome, characterized by severe mental retardation, seizures, and a movement disorder, can also be caused by a microdeletion in the same region of chromosome 15 as Prader-Willi syndrome. In Prader-Willi syndrome, the deletion is always present on the chromosome inherited from the father, whereas in Angelman syndrome, the deletion is always present on the maternally inherited chromosome. Both Prader-Willi and Angelman syndromes can arise from *uniparental disomy*, which means that both chromosomal homologues are derived from one parent, with no contribution from the other. For example, in about 15% of patients with Prader-Willi syndrome, both copies of chromosome 15 are maternally derived, whereas in Angelman syndrome, both copies can be from the father.

Parent-of-origin effects on the occurrence of a genetic disease are a reflection of the phenomenon of *imprinting*. Imprinting refers to a process in which there is transcriptional inactivation of a region of a chromosome derived from only one parent. The mechanism of this transcriptional inactivation involves methylation of cytosine residues during development. The reason for the existence of imprinting is not known, but it is clear that proper imprinting is necessary for normal development.

Mitochondrial Disorders

Mitochondria, cytoplasmic organelles whose major function is to serve as the sites of oxidative phosphorylation and energy production for the cell, also contain their own genetic material in the form of a small circular piece of DNA. The structure of the mitochondrial genome is similar in this way to bacterial genomes, a finding contributing to the theory that mitochondria originally developed from bacteria that established a symbiotic relationship within eukaryotic cells.

Many different clinical entities are now recognized to be caused by mutations in mitochondrial DNA. Mitochondrial diseases frequently affect organs that are highly dependent on energy production and use, such as the central nervous system, muscle, and also pancreatic β-cells. Examples of mitochondrial diseases include the following: myoclonic epilepsy with ragged red fibers (MERRF) syndrome; mitochondrial encephalomyopathy with lactic acidosis and strokelike (MELAS) syndrome; and Kearns-Sayre syndrome, which has heart block and retinal disease as prominent components. Many of the mutations in the mitochondrial DNA have been defined, with both point mutations and deletions described. The inheritance of mitochondrial DNA is unique because only maternal mitochondria are transmitted to the zygote. Therefore, although both males and females can be equally affected by disorders caused by defects in mitochondrial DNA, the mutation can be passed only through the maternal lineage. This is called *maternal* or *cytoplasmic inheritance* because the mitochondria are located in the cytoplasm.

Multifactorial Disorders

Multifactorial disorders, which are by far the most common form of genetic disease, do not show clear-cut mendelian patterns of inheritance but "tend to run in families." These disorders include common chronic diseases of adults, such as atherosclerosis, hypertension, diabetes, peptic ulcers, and schizophrenia, as well as birth defects, including cleft lip and palate, spina bifida, and congenital heart disease. Multifactorial disorders are

believed to result from the interaction of multiple genes with environmental factors, leading to the observed familial clustering. The polygenic component of these disorders consists of a series of genes interacting in a cumulative manner. A particular combination of genetic and environmental factors pushes persons past a threshold at which they are at risk for the disease. The genes that contribute to a particular polygenic trait such as atherosclerosis can be difficult to define, but advances in gene mapping techniques, combined with increasing understanding of the pathophysiology of these disorders, are leading to rapid advances in understanding of the ways in which genes and the environment interact to cause multifactorial disorders.

Heterogeneity in Genetic Disorders

As discussed earlier, genetic disorders are quite heterogeneous as a result of the complex interactions between multiple genetic loci and environmental factors. This is true for diseases that segregate as simple mendelian traits as well as for multifactorial disorders. There are numerous examples of single-gene disorders in which identical mutations cause widely varying phenotypes. Nongenetic factors can also play roles in mendelian disorders, leading to heterogeneity. Several disorders result from interactions between a mutant gene and an environmental factor. For example, patients with xeroderma pigmentosum are unusually sensitive to sunlight, whereas persons with α_1-antitrypsin deficiency, who have a predisposition to develop emphysema, are more sensitive to the deleterious effects of tobacco smoke. Of particular interest for the clinician, inherited single-gene mutations may produce potentially serious inappropriate responses to certain drugs. These pharmacogenetic disorders exhibit all three mendelian modes of inheritance. The most common is glucose-6-phosphate dehydrogenase deficiency, inherited as an X-linked recessive disorder, which may induce hemolytic anemia in response to various drugs. Without administration of these drugs, such patients otherwise appear to be normal. Genetic differences in drug metabolism are increasingly recognized as important in determining pharmacokinetics. This finding has spurred interest of pharmaceutical companies in the burgeoning field of pharmacogenomics, which is directed at understanding the genetic contribution to pharmacology. Genetic testing for certain alleles of cytochrome P450 that affect drug metabolism are already commercially available.

In addition to the interactions between genetic and nongenetic components in both mendelian and multifactorial disorders, other factors serve to increase the heterogeneity of genetic disorders. As stated earlier, AD disorders are often characterized by varying severity and incomplete penetrance. It is likely that the specific disease locus interacts with the genetic background of the individual patient. Some combinations of genes at other loci may minimize the pathologic consequences of the mutation, whereas other combinations may accentuate them. In addition, disease heterogeneity results from multiple mutant alleles for a single locus. For example, Duchenne muscular dystrophy is caused by mutations in the dystrophin gene that usually lead to complete absence of the protein. The less severe Becker muscular dystrophy results from mutations at the same locus that lead to shortened dystrophin molecules. In addition, mutations that lead to partial deficiency of HPRT activity cause gout, whereas mutations that abolish HPRT activity lead to the severe neurologic manifestations of the Lesch-Nyhan syndrome. These examples of allelic variation and disease are akin to the normal allelic variation that gives rise to the rich diversity of life.

An additional reason for heterogeneity in genetic disease is that mutations in different genes can sometimes have quite similar clinical manifestations. For example, forms of hemophilia are caused by mutations in either the gene for factor VIII (classic hemophilia) or the gene for factor IX (Christmas disease). Both these genes are on the X chromosome, and both conditions are inherited as X-linked recessive disorders. Additional bleeding disorders result from mutations in other genes. Other diseases caused by mutations in multiple gene loci have different modes of inheritance in different families. For example, spastic paraplegia, Charcot-Marie-Tooth syndrome, and retinitis pigmentosa all have AD, AR, and X-linked recessive inheritance forms.

MOLECULAR GENETICS AND MEDICINE

Molecular Genetic Methods

The field of molecular genetics has developed explosively since Watson and Crick's discovery of the structure of DNA in 1953. Two developments in particular made possible recombinant DNA research: the discovery of bacterial restriction enzymes and the invention of blot hybridization methods. Subsequently, the development of DNA and RNA amplification techniques based on the polymerase chain reaction (PCR) revolutionized virtually every area of biology dealing with nucleic acids and had far-reaching effects on society as a whole; for example, forensic DNA testing has had a dramatic effect on criminal investigations.

Restriction Enzymes

Most strains of bacteria possess a class of enzymes known as *endonucleases*, which serve to destroy foreign DNA. Because the function of these endonucleases is to *restrict* viral infection, they are called *restriction enzymes*. These enzymes recognize a specific DNA sequence, most commonly 4 or 6 base pairs long, and they cleave DNA at this site (Fig. 1–8). These enzymes do not cut when the DNA is modified at the recognition site by methylation, and the bacteria protect their own DNA by having methylation enzymes that recognize the same sites, thereby protecting the bacterial genome. Restriction enzymes recognizing many different sequences have been isolated from many species and strains of bacteria. Most of these recognition sites are inverted palindromes, meaning that they have the same sequence on both DNA strands. In addition, most restriction enzymes cut the two strands of DNA in a staggered fashion, leaving two to four bases of single-stranded DNA on both segments of DNA (see Fig. 1–8).

Because of the inverted palindromic nature of most recognition sites, these single-stranded regions are complementary and hybridize to each other whenever pieces of DNA cut with the

same enzyme are mixed together, temporarily joining two segments. If an enzyme called *DNA ligase* is also present, it covalently links the hybridized segments. Thus, the discovery and isolation of restriction enzymes have allowed molecular geneticists to cleave DNA at specific sites and to reconnect the segments in specific arrangements, thus allowing for the creation of *recombinant DNA,* popularly known as genetic engineering.

Blot Hybridization

Various methods, collectively known as *blot hybridization,* have been developed to allow the rapid identification of a segment of nucleic acid containing a particular nucleotide sequence. As first described by Southern in 1975, in blot hybridization, DNA is digested with a restriction enzyme. The now fragmented DNA is separated according to size by electrophoresis through an agarose gel matrix, in which smaller fragments move faster than larger ones. The DNA is then transferred to a filter under conditions that cause the two DNA strands to come apart. The filter is incubated with a radiolabeled RNA or DNA probe including the desired nucleotide sequence. The probe hybridizes to the complementary sequence on the filter, and the labeled DNA band is then visualized by autoradiography (i.e., exposing the filter to x-ray film). This method of identifying DNA sequences is called *Southern blotting*, after its inventor (Fig. 1–9). A similar method

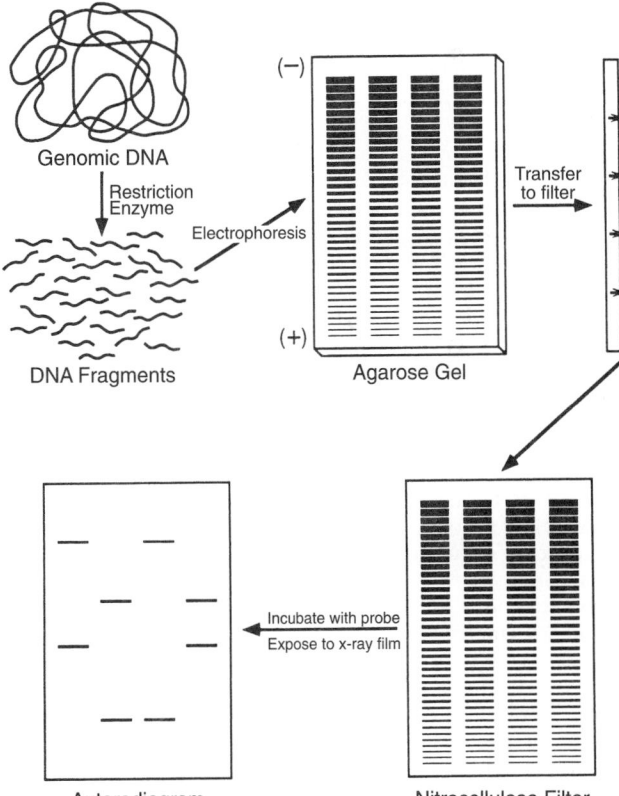

Figure 1–9. Southern blotting. Cellular DNA is cut with a restriction enzyme, to produce small fragments. The cut DNA is separated by size by electrophoresis through an agarose gel. Because DNA is an acid and therefore has a negative charge, it migrates toward the positive electrode, the smaller fragments migrating faster than the larger. The DNA is transferred to a nitrocellulose (or charged nylon) filter, usually by buffer flow (as shown in an edge view), to produce a replica of the gel. The filter is incubated with a radioactive DNA or RNA probe, is washed, and is exposed to x-ray film. The resulting autoradiogram indicates DNA bands that have sequence homology with the probe.

HindIII

```
— A-A-G-C-T-T —              — A          A-G-C-T-T —
— T-T-C-G-A-A —      —→      — T-T-C-G-A          A —
```

SmaI

```
— C-C-C-G-G-G —              — C-C-C      G-G-G —
— G-G-G-C-C-C —      —→      — G-G-G      C-C-C —
```

PstI

```
— C-T-G-C-A-G —              — C-T-G-C-A          G —
— G-A-C-G-T-C —      —→      — G          A-C-G-T-C —
```

Figure 1–8. Restriction enzymes. The recognition sequences for three common restriction enzymes are shown *(left)*. The *vertical arrows* indicate the sites at which each strand is cleaved to produce two ends *(right)*. There are three types of cut ends, differing in which strand, if any, is single stranded.

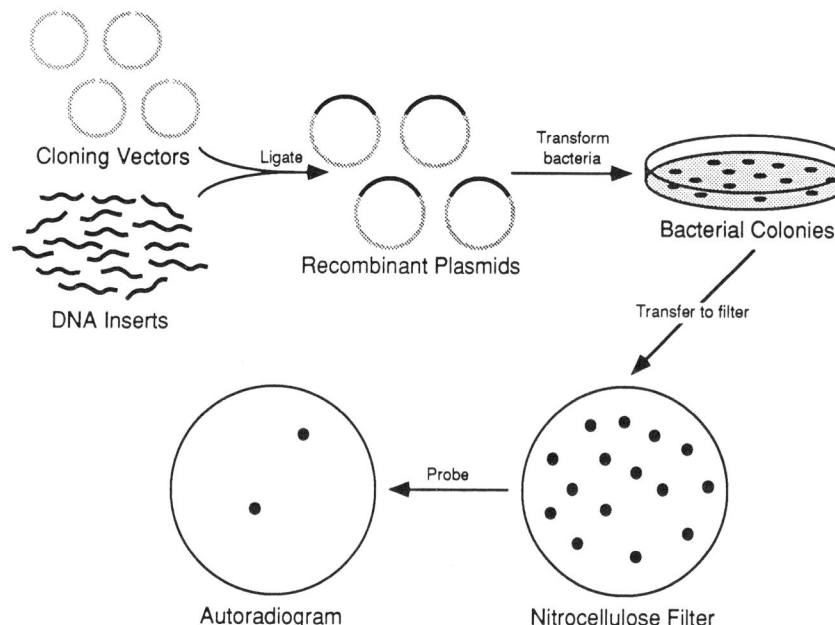

Figure 1–10. Cloning. The desired DNA inserts, either genomic DNA cut with a restriction enzyme or cDNA produced from mRNA, are ligated into cloning vectors that have been cut to accept the inserts. The resulting recombinant plasmids are introduced into bacteria, a process called *genetic transformation,* producing a genetic library. Bacterial colonies grown from the library are transferred to a nitrocellulose filter by simply overlaying the plate. The filter is then probed, either with DNA or RNA, as described for Southern blotting, to look for colonies with homologous sequences, or with labeled antibodies, to look for specific protein production. The resulting autoradiogram indicates the position of colonies containing the desired sequence.

has been developed to identify RNA sequences and is called, in a play on words, *Northern blotting.* (*Western blotting,* in which antibodies directed against specific proteins are used to detect those proteins on blots of cellular extracts, also exists.)

Cloning

The ability to clone genes has greatly facilitated the ability to understand the pathogenesis of inherited disease at the molecular level. In molecular genetics, *cloning* means isolating a particular gene in a form that allows its DNA to be amplified and manipulated. Before the era of genome sequencing (see later), the cloning of a particular gene generally started with what is known as a *DNA library.* There are two classes of such libraries. *Genomic libraries* start with DNA isolated from whole cells. To generate a genomic library, DNA is isolated from cells and is cut with a restriction enzyme, thus generating tens of thousands of unique fragments. Of course, as described earlier, genomic DNA includes not only the DNA contained in genes coding for proteins, but also the introns between the protein-coding exons as well as the vast amount of DNA found between the genes. The fragments of genomic DNA are inserted cloning vectors, which are naturally occurring bacterial viruses or plasmids that have been genetically engineered to accept pieces of foreign DNA. This results in a library containing hundreds of thousands of hybrid DNA molecules, each containing a segment of DNA from the cloning vector as well as a piece of genomic DNA from the starting cell. These hybrid DNA molecules are what are commonly known as *recombinant DNA.* The length of DNA that is usually cloned varies from a few kilobases to a megabase, depending on the vector into which the genomic DNA is inserted. The ability to clone extremely large pieces of DNA greatly facilitated gene mapping and isolation, as well as serving as the starting point for genome sequencing.

Although genomic libraries are fairly easy to construct, they have the disadvantage of containing a large amount of DNA that is not present in genes. Therefore, a method was devised to construct a DNA library that would contain only DNA coding for proteins, which are of the greatest interest. The obvious source of material for such a library is mRNA, which can easily be isolated free of rRNA and tRNA because its polyadenine sequence hybridizes to chemically synthesized polythymidine sequences coupled to solid matrices. It is not possible, however, to construct a library directly from RNA molecules because only DNA can be properly manipulated. A major breakthrough in the ability to construct DNA libraries from mRNA came with the discovery of the enzyme reverse transcriptase, which is essential in the life cycle of a class of viruses called *retroviruses.* These viruses, which have single-stranded RNA genomes, include the human immunodeficiency virus (HIV). The function of reverse transcriptase is to make a DNA copy of the viral genome that can integrate into the cellular DNA and can be replicated. The name *reverse transcriptase* was chosen because it functions counter to the normal DNA-to-RNA direction of transcription. Researchers commonly use reverse transcriptase to make single-stranded DNA molecules complementary to mRNA sequences and therefore called *cDNA.* The single-stranded molecules are converted to normal double-stranded cDNA using DNA polymerase and are then inserted into cloning vectors as described for genomic libraries. The library, either genomic or cDNA, is then inserted into an appropriate strain of *Escherichia coli,* which can then be grown to produce large amounts of the inserted recombinant DNA. Genomic libraries are necessary if one needs to obtain sequences not present in the mRNA, such as promoters, enhancers, or introns.

Once an investigator interested in a particular gene has constructed or otherwise obtained an appropriate library, cloning the gene of interest is a matter of identifying the particular recombinant DNA molecule containing the correct insert. At this stage, cDNA libraries are particularly useful because although genomic libraries contain all the DNA sequences found in an organism, cDNA libraries contain only sequences from genes that are expressed in the starting cells. Thus, an investigator interested in studying growth hormone genes could start with a cDNA library from pituitary tissue. Even knowing the complete human genome sequence, the technology of cDNA libraries remains invaluable for determining the complement of genes that are expressed in a particular cell type. The general approach to cloning gene sequences is summarized in Figure 1-10.

Polymerase Chain Reaction

The development of the *PCR technique,* which allows one to amplify selected pieces of DNA by many orders of magnitude, revolutionized both basic and clinical genetics (Fig. 1-11). Oligonucleotide primers that flank the section of DNA to be amplified are hybridized to a DNA-containing sample. The intervening segment of DNA is then filled in by a heat-stable DNA

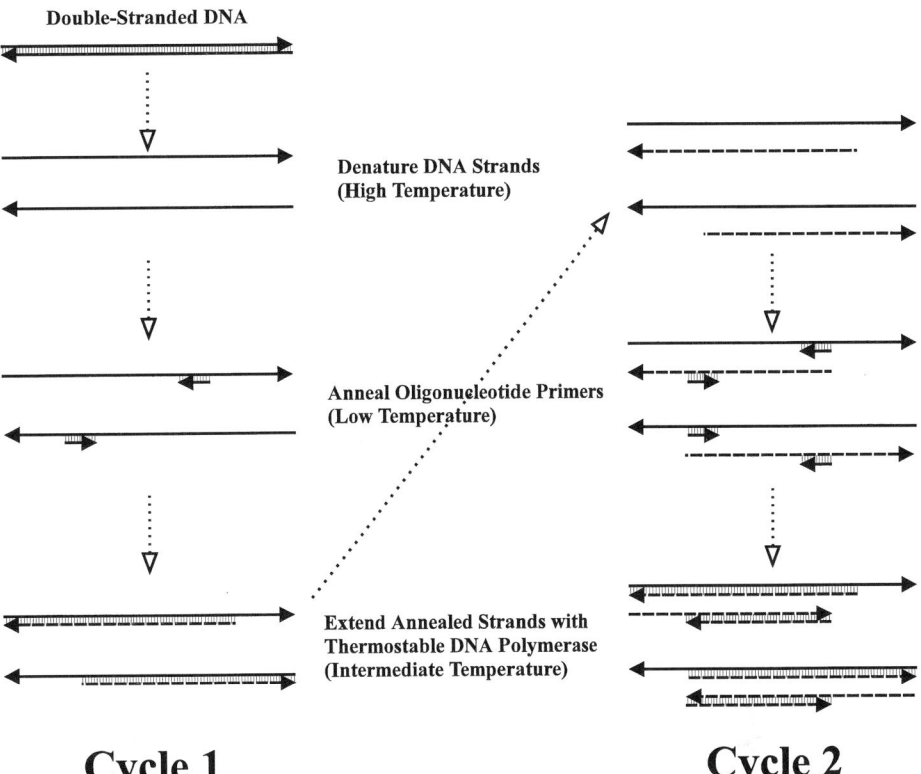

Double-Stranded DNA

Denature DNA Strands
(High Temperature)

Anneal Oligonucleotide Primers
(Low Temperature)

Extend Annealed Strands with
Thermostable DNA Polymerase
(Intermediate Temperature)

Cycle 1   **Cycle 2**

Figure 1–11. Polymerase chain reaction (PCR) amplification of DNA. Double-stranded DNA is subjected to cycles of denaturation, annealing with short, single-stranded, oligonucleotide DNA primers, and extension using a thermostable DNA polymerase. Typically, 20 to 40 cycles of PCR are performed, resulting in exponential amplification of the DNA sequence between the two primers. The high specificity of primer annealing allows a short sequence (typically <1 kB), to be amplified from the 3 million kB present in the human genome. The advantage of a thermostable polymerase is that it can withstand the extreme temperatures (close to boiling) necessary to denature the DNA strands.

polymerase derived from bacteria that are adapted to extremely hot environments. The sample is then heated to separate the strands and is cooled, and the cycle is repeated. In this way, the desired segment of DNA is exponentially amplified, resulting in millionfold increases in the number of copies of a desired segment of DNA after 30 to 40 cycles. This technology has become central to virtually every aspect of genetics and many areas of medicine and biology, including gene mapping, gene cloning, analysis of gene transcription (using reverse-transcribed mRNA as a starting material), prenatal diagnosis (including preimplantation diagnosis from a single cell of an eight-cell embryo), infectious disease detection, and forensic medicine.

Biomedical Applications of Molecular Genetics

Production of Clinically Useful Proteins

Once a gene has been cloned, it is possible to produce virtually unlimited quantities of the encoded protein by introducing the clone (in an appropriate expression vector) into bacterial, yeast, mammalian, or other cell types. Because bacteria do not properly splice eukaryotic mRNA, it is necessary to use cDNA rather than genomic clones to express most genes in bacteria. Another obstacle in producing proteins by recombinant DNA technology is that many eukaryotic proteins undergo posttranslational modification. Most common is proteolytic cleavage at the amino terminus to remove the initiation methionine residue. Other proteolytic cleavages may occur. For example, many proteins that are secreted by cells begin with a region, called a *signal sequence*, that is required for transport into the endoplasmic reticulum. This sequence is removed after the peptide has crossed the membrane. In addition, numerous proteins are synthesized as part of longer precursors, and the active peptides are released by proteolytic cleavage. Additional forms of posttranslational modification include glycosylation, phosphorylation, acylation, and carboxylation. These modifications are frequently required for normal protein function. Rapidly increasing

numbers of recombinant human proteins are in clinical use, including insulin, growth hormone, clotting factors VIII and IX, erythropoietin, hematopoietic colony-stimulating factors, and tissue plasminogen activator, among others. In theory, recombinant proteins should be useful for any replacement therapy involving circulating proteins, the only limitations being the ability to obtain the active protein and the protein's stability.

Genomics and the Genome Project

Perhaps one of the most significant scientific achievements in human history is the complete sequencing of the human genome. The project is still ongoing, and further sequencing and gene identification remain to be done before the sequence will be truly complete, a process that may take many more years. The *genome project* was made possible by the techniques of molecular genetics described earlier as well as the development of automated sequencing machines. Those machines made it possible to achieve the economies of scale necessary to sequence the 3 billion base pairs in the human genome. In addition to the human genome, the genomes of other organisms, including many important human pathogens such as *Mycobacterium tuberculosis,* have been sequenced. Sequencing the genomes of other mammalian and nonmammalian species has led to the realization that most human genes have homologues in other species, including lower organisms such as yeast and worms, thereby justifying the enormous effort that has been devoted to studying those model organisms over the years. The ultimate impact of the genomics revolution has yet to be felt. Much more DNA sequencing and analysis will be required to obtain a complete understanding of how organisms differ from one another at the interspecies and intraspecies level. However, the end result, an understanding of the genetic basis of human variability and predisposition to disease, is certain to produce enormous benefits for human health.

Gene Mapping

Linkage mapping in humans involves examining pedigrees to determine the frequency of co-inheritance of specific traits. As described previously, recombination between chromatids of homologous chromosomes occurs in meiosis, so sections of chromosomes are exchanged with each other. Thus, recombinant chromosomes are produced that contain a segment derived from each of the original homologous chromosomes. The closer together two genes are located on the same chromosome, the less likely it is that recombination will occur between them during meiosis and the more likely it is that particular alleles of these genes will be inherited together. Thus, it is possible to use the recombination frequency between two genes to determine their distance from each other and hence to construct a genetic map. A 1% recombination frequency between two loci is defined as one map unit or 1 centimorgan (cM). Genes located on separate chromosomes are inherited independently and are therefore unlinked. Genes located on the same chromosome but that are so far apart that recombination occurs between them 50% of the time (i.e., 50 cM apart) are also considered unlinked. Although 1 cM corresponds to approximately 1 million base pairs, this physical distance must be considered only a rough estimate because recombination does not occur purely randomly throughout the genome but instead has "hot" and "cold" spots. Regions of decreased recombination give rise to the phenomenon of *linkage disequilibrium,* in which alleles of linked loci are found on the same chromosome more frequently than one would expect with normal levels of recombination occurring over time. Linkage disequilibrium can also arise from selective pressure for the maintenance of linked alleles, as seems to occur for the human leukocyte antigen major histocompatibility complex. The implications of linkage disequilibrium are that two alleles that are not in close physical proximity may nonetheless be co-inherited. A set of alleles inherited as if a single locus is referred to as a *haplotype.*

Until around 1980, linkage mapping relied on the presence of phenotypic traits or markers, such as blood types and polymorphic enzymes (isozymes). Relatively few useful markers were known, meaning that only quite limited regions of the genome could be mapped, thus greatly reducing the usefulness of linkage analysis. The ability to detect and to assay for sequence variations in DNA made feasible the construction of sets of markers that cover the entire genome. When a mutation either occurs within a restriction enzyme's recognition site or changes the distance between two sites, there is a variation between the size of DNA fragments generated by digestion with the enzyme. These *restriction fragment length polymorphisms* (RFLPs) are inherited in simple mendelian fashion and were invaluable in linkage analysis. Later, RFLPs were largely supplanted by the use of simple sequence repeats. Whereas RFLPs are biallelic, there can be numerous alleles for each repeat, each differing only in the number of repeats. Thus, a much higher percentage of the population is heterozygous for a repeat polymorphism as opposed to an RFLP, making mapping efforts much easier. Detection of the repeat length is generally done using PCR with primers flanking the repeat. Because there are many thousands of repeats in the human genome, they have been used to develop detailed linkage maps of the entire human genome. More recently, PCR has been used to assay for single nucleotide polymorphisms, that is, missense mutations that are common in human populations and that may or may not have any phenotypic effect. Because each person differs from another at millions of individual loci, increasingly dense single nucleotide polymorphism maps have been constructed. As the number of polymorphic markers increases, diseases can be mapped with increasing resolution, with the limiting factor becoming the lack of sufficiently large families or sufficient numbers of families to find recombination events between the disease locus and the loci used for mapping.

Linkage maps can be used to locate disease loci by comparing the segregation of the disease phenotype with polymorphic markers in pedigrees. Once an approximate map location is determined for a gene, the genome sequence can be used to search for candidate genes that are known to have sequence elements or biologic functions that suggest that they may be involved in the disease being studied. Moreover, the approximate map locations can be used as the starting point for more detailed studies using a higher density of polymorphic markers from the specific region being studied. Both approaches have been greatly facilitated by the near completion of the human genome sequence, but the dramatic increase in the number of genes that are mapped has particularly benefited the *candidate gene approach.* With this approach, a hypothesis about the function of a gene product from a disease gene is developed from knowledge of the disease phenotype. Once the approximate map location is known, genes with functions that match the hypothesis and map to the proper region are tested for mutations in affected persons.

Linkage analysis and, more recently, direct mutation detection have revolutionized prenatal diagnosis. Fetal cells are obtained from amniotic fluid, and blood or skin samples are obtained from parents and siblings. Analysis of DNA from these samples can then determine in many cases whether the fetus has inherited the disease. This approach was first used for the prenatal diagnosis of sickle cell anemia. It is now used for various inherited disorders and can be applied to any condition for which a linked polymorphic marker or, increasingly commonly, the pathogenic mutation can be identified. Before the advent of molecular genetic techniques, prenatal diagnosis was limited to those few disorders that had diagnostic enzyme assays or that were linked to polymorphic protein markers. Thus, DNA analysis has greatly expanded the number of genetic disorders that can be detected prenatally. The same principles involved in prenatal diagnosis also apply to presymptomatic diagnosis in disorders with late onset and in carrier detection in X-linked and AR disorders.

Gene Therapy

The available therapies for most human genetic diseases are inadequate at best. Treatments such as enzyme replacement for hemophilia and Gaucher disease or dietary restriction as in phenylketonuria have serious limitations, such as high cost or low efficacy. Additionally, protein replacement is applicable to only a few diseases in which delivery into the circulation is efficacious and is problematic when it is necessary to deliver a missing component directly to cells, particularly when tissue specificity is necessary. Therefore, the ultimate treatment for inherited disorders, and the only possible therapy for many, is to use DNA itself as a pharmacologic agent to treat the actual defect, the mutant gene. The development of sophisticated gene transfer methods has made this gene therapy approach a reality.

It is important to distinguish between gene therapy affecting the germline and therapy affecting only somatic tissues. Germline gene therapy would allow genetic modifications to be transmitted to future generations. Even if such modifications were limited to treating specific diseases, there would be serious moral and ethical questions. This situation is further complicated because it would theoretically be possible to alter traits to produce more "desirable" children. Because somatic cell therapy affects only the person treated, the ethical considerations are greatly simplified. All current gene therapy protocols in humans are limited to somatic cell experiments.

Although inherited mutations exist in every cell in the body, most genes are expressed in specific tissues, and, in most cases, gene therapy would need to be directed only toward the proper tissue. Even when a gene is expressed in all tissues, it is possible that only one tissue need be treated to ameliorate the disease phenotype. For example, although the low-density lipoprotein receptor gene is expressed in most cell types, it is likely that only the liver need be treated in familial hypercholesterolemia because the bulk of cholesterol clearance occurs in that organ.

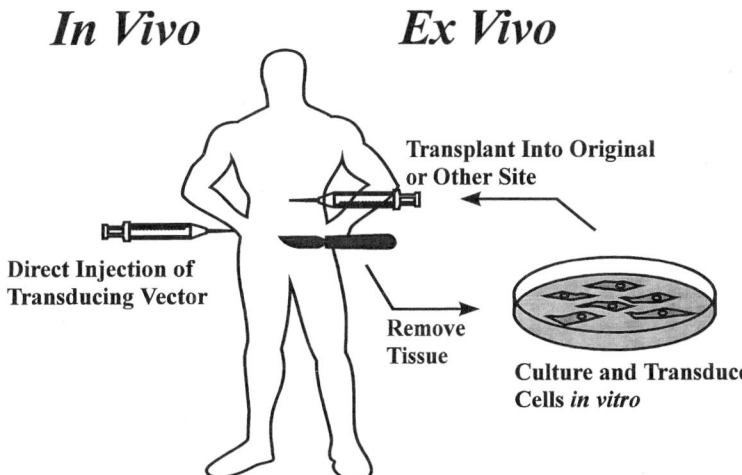

In Vivo   *Ex Vivo*

Direct Injection of Transducing Vector

Transplant Into Original or Other Site

Remove Tissue

Culture and Transduce Cells *in vitro*

Figure 1–12. Models for human gene therapy. *In vivo* gene therapy involves direct introduction of a transducing vector into the patient. *Ex vivo* gene therapy involves removal of tissue and transduction *in vitro*.

For some diseases, such as hemophilia, any cell that can secrete a protein into the circulation is a potential target for gene therapy, even if it is not the normal site of protein production.

In the ideal gene therapy system, the normal gene would be introduced into cells *in vivo* in such a way that it would replace the defective gene through site-specific recombination. This would result in the gene's being in the proper position relative to the various transcriptional regulatory elements. Unfortunately, techniques for site-specific integration are not yet available, and all current methods of gene transfer result in predominantly random integration. This means that gene *replacement* therapy is not yet possible. Instead, gene *augmentation* therapy has been pursued, in which the normal gene supplements the defective gene from a distal site.

The most desirable methods of gene therapy allow for gene transfer directly into the patient (i.e., *in vivo* gene therapy) (Fig. 1-12). For some tissues, such as the central nervous system, this is likely to be the major mode of gene transfer. For organs such as the bone marrow, however, cells can be removed easily, manipulated *in vitro*, and reintroduced into the patient (i.e., *ex vivo* gene therapy) (see Fig. 1-12). The successful treatment of severe combined immune deficiency caused by adenosine deaminase mutations is an example of this approach.

Various biochemical and physical methods have been developed to introduce DNA into mammalian cells, referred to as *transfection* (from *trans*formation and in*fection*). These methods generally suffer from the serious limitation that only a few of the treated cells are permanently genetically modified (1 in 10^3 to 10^7). Direct injection of DNA into some tissues such as muscle results in gene transfer and expression, but this method is inefficient, with only a small number of cells taking up the injected DNA. Regardless of its inefficiency, its simplicity and low cost have made direct injection of DNA a popular approach to vaccine development.

To increase the efficiency of gene transfer, most gene therapy studies have instead used replication-defective genetic transducing vectors derived from viruses. Numerous different viruses have been used, including adenovirus adeno-associated virus, murine retroviruses, and even lentiviruses such as HIV. Viral vectors can infect various cell types from several species at efficiencies often approaching 100%.

Although the initial thrust of research in gene therapy was to correct single-gene defects such as hemophilia and adenosine deaminase deficiency, there has been a shift in the field toward applying gene transfer technology to more common polygenic diseases such as cancer and coronary artery disease. Viral vectors are being used to deliver cytotoxic genes to cancer cells. In some cases, the vectors are designed specifically to target the cancer cells—a so-called magic bullet. Other experiments are using gene transfer techniques to enhance angiogenesis in ischemic cardiac tissue. The appeal of using gene therapy for common polygenic diseases is that these techniques can be applied to many more patients than would be the case if gene therapy were limited to the much rarer monogenic disorders. As with many new technologies, gene therapy went through a phase of unfulfilled promises. However, the increasing number of successful clinical experiments indicates that the field is entering a new phase in which gene therapy will become an important weapon in the physician's armamentarium.

SUGGESTED READINGS

Alberts B, et al: Molecular Biology of the Cell, 4th ed. New York, Garland Publishing, 2002.

Gelehrter TD, et al: Principles of Medical Genetics, 2nd ed. Baltimore, Lippincott Williams & Wilkins, 1998.

Jones KL: Smith's Recognizable Patterns of Human Malformation, 5th ed. Philadelphia, WB Saunders Co, 1997.

Nussbaum RL, et al: Thompson and Thompson Genetics in Medicine, 6th ed. Philadelphia, WB Saunders Co, 2001.

Nyhan WL, et al: Atlas of Metabolic Diseases. Baltimore, Lippincott Williams & Wilkins, 1998.

Rimoin DL, et al: Principles and Practice of Medical Genetics, 3rd ed. New York, Churchill Livingstone, 1997.

Scriver CR, et al (eds): The Metabolic and Molecular Bases of Inherited Disease, 8th ed. New York, McGraw-Hill, 2001.

WEB-BASED RESOURCES

GeneTests·GeneClinics: *http://www.genetests.org/*

McKusick VA: Online Mendelian Inheritance in Man: *http://www.ncbi.nlm.nih.gov/omim/*

George A. Diaz and Kurt Hirshhorn

Molecular Genetics: Developmental and Clinical Implications

The explosive advances in human genetics of the last few decades have been fueled by a powerful set of tools built on a small number of critical scientific developments. Some of these techniques and principles are reviewed briefly in this chapter.

MOLECULAR GENETICS TOOLS

Recombinant DNA Technology

The identification and characterization of enzymes involved in DNA replication, repair, and sequence-specific endonuclease digestion (Table 2–1) have provided tools that allow convenient manipulation of DNA. Restriction endonucleases are a class of enzymes that recognize specific DNA sequences, typically palindromes of six to eight base pairs, and usually cut the DNA backbone at a symmetric point within the recognition sequence on both strands. Digestion of purified genomic DNA with a restriction enzyme yields a collection of fragments with identical end sequences and discrete sizes corresponding to the distance between recognition sites in the DNA sequence. The termini of fragments resulting from a restriction digestion may be single stranded and self-complementary over several bases or completely double stranded, depending on the cleavage site. By using a different enzyme, DNA ligase, digested fragments with compatible complementary or with blunt ends can be spliced together, even if the two pieces were not initially contiguous, generating a recombinant molecule.

Library Construction

The enzymatic tools described earlier allow the direct manipulation of DNA, but additional methods had to be developed to amplify specific fragments efficiently. Small, circular DNA molecules that replicate autonomously in bacterial cells (*plasmids*) have been characterized and developed as vectors to propagate DNA sequences of interest. These reagents make it possible to ligate restriction enzyme-digested DNA fragments into digested plasmids, introduce the recombinant plasmid into bacterial cells, and then select for the presence of a plasmid-encoded antibiotic resistance gene. DNA isolated from the resulting colonies is then analyzed by restriction analysis or sequencing to identify plasmids containing DNA of interest. Cells containing the desired plasmid can then be propagated or stored frozen indefinitely. This process is known as *cloning.*

When complex mixtures of DNA are ligated into a recipient plasmid, the resulting recombinant molecules represent a library of plasmids containing different fragments. Libraries can be generated from digested genomic DNA or from complementary DNA (cDNA) produced by reverse transcription from mRNA. Genomic DNA libraries were critical reagents in the sequencing of the human genome, with improvements made over time in the cloning vectors used (yeast or bacterial artificial chromosomes) and in the stability of the cloned inserts. In contrast to the goal of genomic libraries to represent the full genetic complement of an organism, cDNA libraries are designed to represent the tissue-specific spectrum of genes expressed in the mRNA source tissue. In the creation of such libraries, hybridization methods (see later) are used to normalize the contribution of highly expressed ubiquitous housekeeping genes. Libraries have been generated from a wide range of tissue types and different disease states. Sequence data from clones derived from different libraries, so-called *expressed sequence tags,* have been catalogued in publicly available databases. Identification of transcripts whose expression is restricted to a specific tissue type is a powerful tool for understanding the genetic basis of tissue-specific function. The ability to work with nucleic acids, which are easily manipulated, rather than with the encoded proteins, has allowed a significant acceleration in the understanding of many biologic phenomena.

Polymerase Chain Reaction

The use of thermostable DNA polymerases derived from bacteria that live in extremely high temperature environments represented a revolutionary twist on the use of nucleic acid polymerases. These enzymes retain activity even after heating to temperatures sufficient to denature DNA strands (>96°C.), thus allowing multiple cycles of primer annealing and chain elongation to be carried out in a single reaction. Because each cycle of primer annealing and chain elongation results in double the number of template molecules for the next cycle of primer binding and extension, amplification of the input template DNA occurs exponentially. Polymerase chain reaction (PCR) makes the amplification of large amounts of product from trace amounts of starting material possible and overcomes the technical limitations imposed by the relatively limited number of copies of genomic DNA available in a given human tissue specimen. The extensive range of uses for which PCR is essential, from basic molecular biology research to infectious disease diagnostics and forensic applications, attests to the power of this technique.

Nucleic Acid Hybridization

Alterations in thermal or ionic conditions can disrupt the hydrogen bonding interactions in a DNA double helix and can result in single-stranded DNA. Complementary strands can reanneal with great specificity when reaction conditions are adjusted appropriately, a property that has been exploited to use a cloned DNA as a probe for the presence of related sequences among a mixture of single-stranded DNA or RNA. Target molecules are first separated based on size by gel electrophoresis, transferred to a support matrix, such as a nylon membrane, and are then probed with a DNA fragment labeled with a radioisotope or some other reporter molecule. This procedure is known as a *Southern blot* (Fig. 2–1), after its inventor, Edward Southern. When applied to RNA, the procedure is called a *Northern blot.* Alternatively, a collection of bacterial colonies representing a cDNA library grown on agar plates can be transferred and lysed directly on nylon filters and can allow screening of the entire library for sequences of interest. The thermal energy required to disrupt DNA hydrogen bond interactions is related to the base composition of the nucleic acid duplex, allowing approximate calculations of the melting and annealing temperature of a known sequence. Under appropriate hybridization conditions, even small synthetic oligonucleotides can be used as high-specificity probes to detect single-base mismatches.

Differences between single-stranded and double-stranded nucleic acids in binding to positively charged matrices have been exploited in subtractive hybridization approaches. Single-stranded cDNA from a differentiated or diseased tissue can be hybridized with excess cDNA strands from nondifferentiated precursor or normal tissue. Genes transcribed in both states will be readily available for hybridization with the excess cDNA pool, whereas those induced only in the differentiated or disease condition will remain single stranded. By binding double-stranded molecules on an affinity column, state-specific transcripts can be isolated and enriched in the final library. Modifications of the principles of subtractive hybridization also allow identification of low-abundance transcripts, the expression of which is associated with developmental changes or disease states.

Hybridization-based approaches continue to be employed in various contemporary high-throughput methods, such as those employed in so-called *DNA chips,* in which the hybridization reaction occurs in parallel at an enormous number of individual sites on a small solid support (Fig. 2–2). The ability to perform massive numbers of hybridization reactions in a small volume and to obtain data in a digital format is being used in research settings to assess differences in transcription patterns between normal and diseased tissue or to score for the presence or absence of polymorphisms in genomic DNA. The application of such techniques to the clinical arena offers the promise of therapeutic interventions tailored to an individual's genotype, for example, by aggressive measures for disease prevention (e.g., *BRCA1/BRCA2* testing and in breast and ovarian cancer) or by adjusting medication exposure or dosing based on the presence or absence of polymorphisms affecting the function of metabolic enzymes. This type of approach has also been used to perform molecular characterization of pathologically indistinguishable cancerous cells by the pattern of gene expression exhibited by different specimens on microarray analysis, and this suggests a potentially useful application as a diagnostic and prognostic tool.

HUMAN GENOME PROJECT

The most significant development in molecular genetics of the late 20th century was the commitment to sequence and to identify all the genes in the complete genomes of humans and other important model organisms and pathogens. Use of the basic tools, described earlier, at an industrial level culminated in the development of highly detailed linkage, physical, and sequence maps of the human genome. The following section describes some of the methods that were required to complete the mapping and sequencing of the human genome.

Polymorphic Markers

Although identity at the DNA sequence level between any two humans is greater than 99.9%, many interindividual differences exist. These sequence polymorphisms have been exploited as tools to track the segregation of chromosomal loci through generations in human pedigrees. The first such markers were single-base changes or small insertions or deletions that created or destroyed a restriction enzyme site (restriction fragment length polymorphisms), detectable by Southern blot as bands of altered

---

TABLE 2–1

Commonly Used Molecular Biology Tools.

Restriction Endonucleases	Enzymes that recognize a specific DNA sequence (typically 4–8 base pairs long) then digest the DNA backbone in the target sequence.
Nucleic Acid Polymerases	Single- or multisubunit enzymes that copy a nucleic acid template
DNA polymerase	DNA → DNA
RNA polymerase	DNA → RNA
Reverse transcriptase	RNA → DNA
DNA-Modifying Enzymes	Enzyme functions
Ligase	Religation of DNA fragments
Phosphatase	Removal of 5′ phosphate group
Kinase	Addition of 5′ phosphate group
DNA Plasmid Vectors	Autonomously replicating DNA molecules used to clone and propagate fragments of interest

---

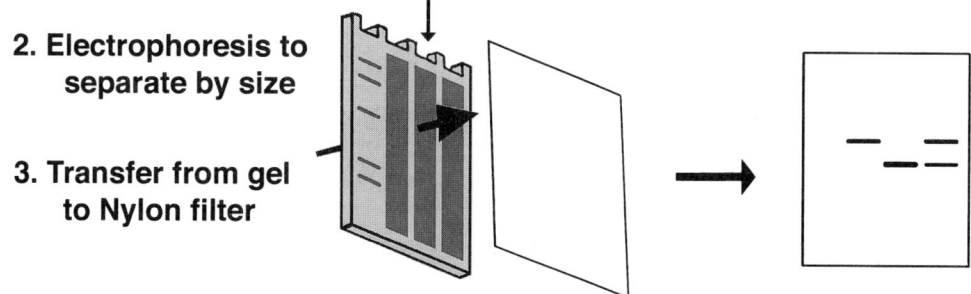

1. Digested DNA loaded in lanes

2. Electrophoresis to separate by size

3. Transfer from gel to Nylon filter

4. Hybridize with labeled probe, autoradiograph

Figure 2–1. Southern blot analysis. Overview of the protocol for hybridization of labeled DNA probes to immobilized DNA affixed to a solid support developed by Dr. Edward Southern. The technique involves separating different-sized DNA fragments produced by restriction enzyme digestion by electrophoresis through a porous gel. After the fragments are separated, the DNA is migrated out of the gel in a perpendicular direction by capillary flow or a second electrophoretic event and onto a positively charged membrane (nitrocellulose or nylon). DNA affixed to this membrane can then be hybridized with a rabiolabeled probe and the filter exposed to x-ray film to detect bands containing DNA sequences with homology to the probe.

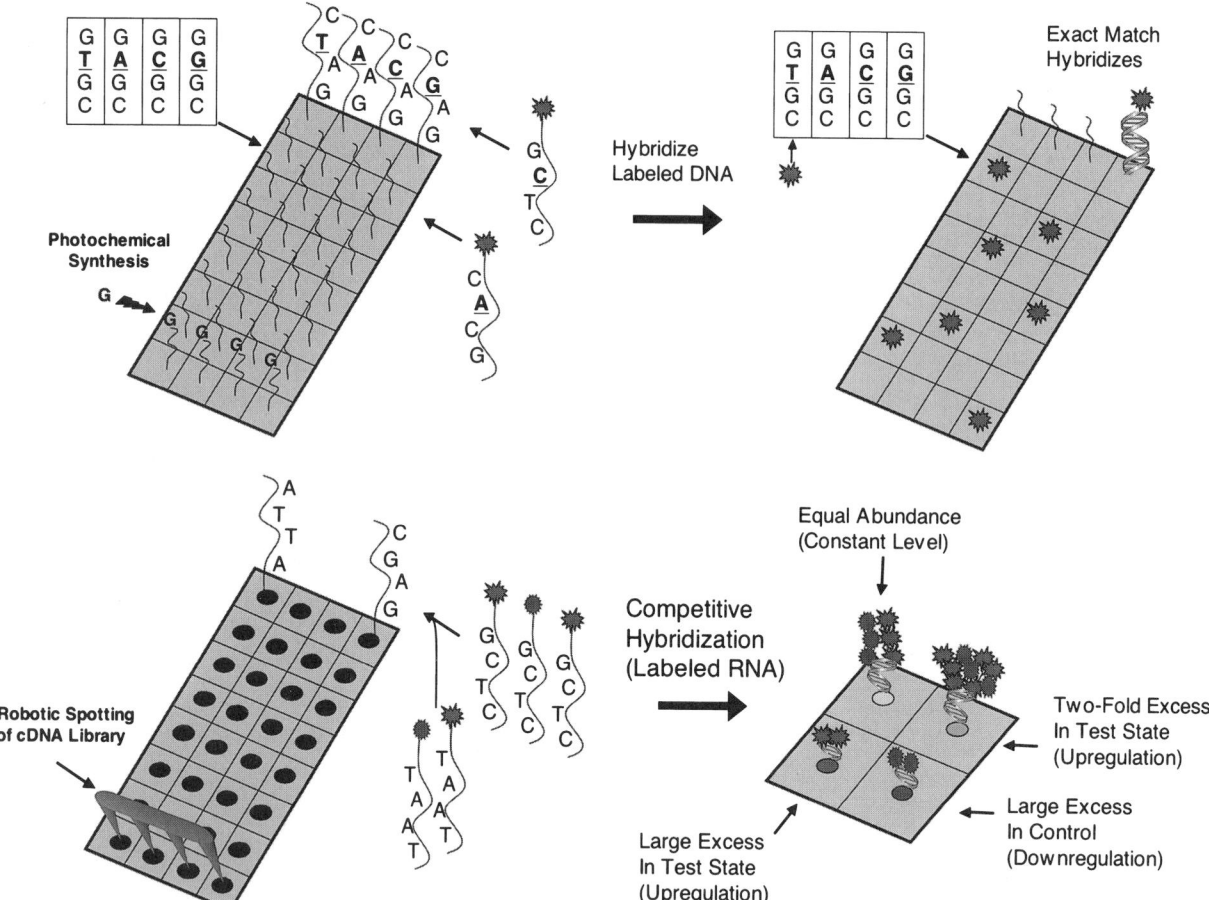

Figure 2–2. Microarrays. The general principles behind two different types of microarrays are illustrated. The *top* cartoon shows the key features of an oligonucleotide array, in which oligomers are synthesized directly on a chip surface by photochemical lithography techniques. By sequential synthesis, a series of overlapping oligomers is produced having all possible single base substitutions introduced at each given position. The DNA sequence to be analyzed (resequenced) is fluorescently labeled and is hybridized to the array, to produce a pattern of hybridization that allows the detection and identification of any point mutations occurring within the portion of a gene represented by the overlapping oligonucleotide array. In the *bottom* cartoon, a cDNA expression array is produced by spotting characterized cDNA clones onto slides. The expression levels of the genes placed on the array are then assayed by a competitive hybridization in which RNA sources from different tissues (i.e., normal versus malignant) or developmental stages are used to generate cDNA labeled fluorescently in two different colors. The ratio of the different fluorescent labels hybridized to the array gives a measure of the relative change in expression level between the different states.

mobility. The discovery of variable number tandem repeat markers provided reagents that were more abundant and more informative (more alleles, corresponding to differences in the number of repeats found in the population). The size of the repeat units typically identified were such that different alleles could differ in size by thousands of base pairs, making Southern blotting a requisite step for genotyping. The marker types used most extensively in the creation of human genetic linkage maps were short tandem repeat markers, in which runs of two to four nucleotides (i.e., CA, AAT, GATA) were repeated approximately 10 to 30 times. Size differences in alleles as small as two base pairs in PCR products ranging in size from approximately 80 to 300 base pairs were resolved easily by electrophoresis of amplification products in polyacrylamide sequencing gels. This process required significantly less labor and sample DNA than Southern blotting and substantially facilitated large-scale genotyping. The most recently developed types of polymorphic markers, single-nucleotide polymorphisms, are single-base changes that occur on average once every 750 base pairs. Single-nucleotide polymorphisms have fewer alleles and are therefore less informative than the repeat markers, but it is anticipated that

their sheer abundance will make them powerful tools in the effort to understand the genetic basis of common complex diseases, such as hypertension and asthma, as well as quantitative traits that affect fetal health, such as birth weight, at the molecular genetic level.

Linkage Analysis

The ability to map genes to specific chromosomal locations was developed in experimental organisms such as *Drosophila melanogaster* in the early 20th century. The construction of genetic maps in model systems required the identification of individuals with traits of interest (e.g., mutations in eye color, wing shape) and subsequent selective mating to generate numbers of progeny suitable for quantitative analysis. This approach was not applicable to humans, so the success of early mapping studies was limited to those diseases in which the genetic locus was tightly linked to the few available polymorphic loci, such as the ABO blood group antigen locus. The discovery of abundant DNA polymorphisms with significant levels of interindividual variation has made linkage mapping feasible in humans.

Linkage analysis is a statistical method in which genotyping data from a pedigree is evaluated for the probability that two loci (markers) are inherited together because they are in physical, and thus genetic, proximity compared with the probability that the data can be explained by the null hypothesis that the markers are not linked and are being inherited independent of each other. The statistic commonly used is the *LOD score,* which represents the logarithm of the probability of linkage divided by the probability of no linkage. An LOD score greater than 3.3 is traditionally taken as the threshold to declare linkage because it represents a 1000:1 probability ratio in favor of linkage, corresponding to a *p* value of approximately .05.

Genetic and Physical Map

An extensive set of polymorphic markers was used to genotype a collection of large multigenerational pedigrees for the construction of a human genetic linkage map. In contrast to the mapping of genes responsible for physical traits in model organisms, the human genetic map established genetic distances among anonymous polymorphic markers. These markers were concurrently mapped to physical locations by various methods such as fluorescence *in situ* hybridization mapping (see later), thus allowing the coordination of genetic loci to physical chromosomal locations. The mapping of markers onto genomic clones (yeast artificial chromosomes [YACs], bacterial artificial chromosomes [BACs]) by hybridization or PCR amplification allowed the identification of clones containing common markers that were therefore overlapping. Collections of overlapping clones were organized by computational analysis into large contiguous assemblages (*contigs*) that allowed the ordering of data generated by sequencing the cloned DNA.

GENETIC BASIS OF HUMAN DISEASE

Identification of Disease-Associated Gene Mutations

The currently available molecular tools allow the efficient mapping and identification of loci underlying single-gene (mendelian) disorders. Families transmitting a disease of interest can be genotyped using polymorphic markers spaced at equal intervals (~10 centiMorgans) across all chromosomes to determine the inheritance of maternal and paternal alleles. The probability that a given marker is close to the disease locus can then be calculated by comparing the inheritance of marker alleles and disease affectation status by linkage analysis. To identify the genetic basis of the trait under study, candidate genes near the disease locus are then analyzed for mutations, with priority given to genes having an expression pattern or known function relevant to the disease manifestations. Before the availability of sequence and map information produced by the Human Genome Project, this latter stage required the construction of a physical map of a YAC or BAC contig spanning the minimal genetic interval containing the locus. These clones were then used to identify new polymorphic markers and to map candidate genes into the region of interest. By eliminating the need to perform these last two laborious and time-intensive steps, the sequence and map information produced by the Human Genome Project dramatically accelerated the rate at which genes underlying mendelian diseases are being identified by this positional cloning approach.

Developmental Genes and Disease

An interesting aspect of the ongoing exploration of the molecular basis of inherited human disease has been the identification of genetic defects in highly conserved developmental pathways leading to malformation syndromes. Work by researchers using

model organisms has elucidated conserved developmental pathways that are critical for normal patterning and organogenesis in both invertebrates and vertebrates. The ability to target genes of interest in mice has provided an opportunity to study the function of conserved gene families in mammals. Although deletion of these genes often results in embryonic lethality or in no phenotype at all, the phenotypes of some knock-outs are informative in defining the role of the targeted gene and reminiscent of human disease states. Discussed in the next three subsections are examples of developmentally important gene families that have been found to result in human malformation syndromes when mutated.

HOX Genes

The Hox family of transcription factors is a set of master control genes that regulate the development of the body plan in invertebrates, such as *Drosophila,* and in vertebrates. Mutations in invertebrate Hox genes can result in striking changes in body segment identity, such as the *Drosophila* Antennapedia phenotype. The duplication of ancestral Hox genes into four distinct clusters in mammals has resulted in redundancy of function, a finding suggesting that mutations in individual genes may be less deleterious. In mammals, Hox genes are important for the appropriate development of axial (central nervous system, axial skeleton, gut, urogenital tract) and peripheral structures (limbs, external genitalia). Mutations in two different genes, *HOXD13* and *HOXA13,* have been discovered in the synpolydactyly and hand-foot-genital syndromes (Fig. 2–3), respectively. Whereas murine models have implicated certain Hox genes in the patterning the hindbrain, no evidence exists at present that mutations of these genes result in human brain malformation syndromes.

PAX Genes

Like the Hox family, Pax genes are also transcriptional regulators defined by a characteristic DNA-binding domain, the paired domain. Emerging data suggest that members of this gene family are involved in different developmental stages of organogenesis in various tissues.[1] The *Pax* genes that have the best-characterized association with human diseases at present are *Pax3* and *Pax6. Pax3* has been shown to be critically important for the appropriate development of neural crest-derived tissues, including the aortic arch and enteric ganglia, in spontaneous murine mutants and in tissue-specific knock-out models. In humans, mutations in *Pax3* cause Waardenburg syndrome, a cause of syndromic deafness associated with white forelock and widely spaced eyes.

The role of *Pax6* in ocular development is the clearest example of the importance of these genes in the regulation of organ development. Strikingly, ablation of *Pax6* function in mice and in *Drosophila* leads to defects in the development of ocular structures in both organisms, a finding demonstrating conservation of function across the evolutionary spectrum. In keeping with this functional conservation, *Pax6* mutations in humans cause various ocular defects ranging from blindness to more subtle structural defects such as cataracts, aniridia, and colobomas.

T-Box Genes

Members of the T-box gene family, characterized by a DNA-binding domain of approximately 200 amino acids, contribute to the development of multiple tissues. In mammals, T-box genes have been shown to contribute to mesoderm determination and to both cardiac and limb morphogenesis. In humans, *Tbx5* is mutated in the Holt-Oram syndrome, in which congenital heart disease is associated with radial-ulnar anomalies. Mutation of the tightly linked gene *Tbx3* results in the ulnar-mammary syndrome, causing limb, apocrine, and genital malformations without cardiac involvement. Although there are no examples of

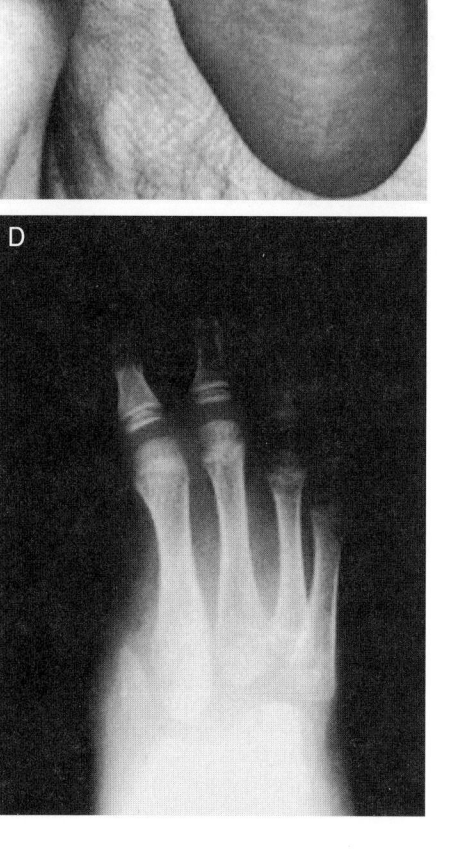

Figure 2–3. Limb malformations in the hand-foot-genital syndrome caused by mutation of *HOXA13*. A and **B,** Digital anomalies (hypoplastic thumb, absent hallux) in a patient heterozygous for a missense mutation in the *HOXA13* homeobox domain. **C** and **D,** Radiographs of the same patient at 5 years of age showing an extremely short first metacarpal, an absent first metacarpal, hypoplasia/aplasia of middle phalanges, delayed ossification of the carpal centers, and abnormal tarsals. (Adapted from Goodman FR, Scambler PJ: Clin Genet 59:1, 2001.)

human T-box gene mutations affecting cardiac, but not limb, development, murine knock-outs of the DiGeorge syndrome critical region gene *Tbx1* recapitulate the cardiac phenotype of that microdeletion syndrome. The gene is therefore an excellent candidate to explain the cardiac manifestations of DiGeorge syndrome, but identification of mutations in patients with a DiGeorge syndrome phenotype lacking the characteristic microdeletion at chromosome 22q11 will be required to establish the role of the gene definitively.

Atypical Inheritance

The mapping of increasing numbers of genetic disease loci has made apparent that numerous diseases can result from mutations at any of several genes, a situation termed *genetic heterogeneity.* Mutation analysis studies of genetically heterogeneous diseases have led to the discovery of interesting exceptions to traditional mendelian inheritance. Aganglionic megacolon (Hirschsprung disease) is a heterogeneous disease that can show autosomal dominant, recessive, or complex inheritance. In

rare cases, inheritance has been found to result from double heterozygosity for single mutant alleles at each of two different genes that can independently cause the phenotype in a mendelian fashion.[2] In some cases of Bardet-Biedl syndrome, a syndrome of mental retardation and obesity, disease expression requires mutation of both alleles of one gene and a single mutant allele at one of two other genes, a situation referred to as *triallelic inheritance.*[3] These situations reflect examples of genetic complexity intermediate between simple monogenic disease inheritance and multigene complex inheritance.

Complex Inheritance

The inheritance of complex traits is thought to involve multiple loci, with environmental factors contributing to phenotypic expression. Trait expression can involve quantitative features such as weight and blood pressure that are distributed in a gaussian fashion in the population or qualitative features that are either present or absent, such as cleft lip and palate. The former are thought to result from interactions among multiple genes with alleles that contribute positively or negatively to the expression of the final phenotype. The favored model for the latter involves the contributions of multiple liability loci, such that the trait is expressed only after a critical liability threshold is passed. Examples of such traits include spina bifida and pyloric stenosis. In this model, traits with marked gender differences in incidence are assumed to reflect sex-specific differences in the liability threshold for disease expression. Occurrence of the condition in the less commonly affected gender implies inheritance of a greater burden of liability alleles, so the recurrence risk for subsequent siblings is higher than if the affected child were of the more commonly affected sex.

Because of the involvement of multiple loci whose relative contribution may differ from pedigree to pedigree, linkage studies have been largely unsuccessful in dissecting the genetic basis of complex traits. However, if a single locus contributes substantially to the heritability of a trait, the locus may be detectable by standard linkage analysis. An encouraging example was the identification of a gene (*NOD2*) contributing to the expression of Crohn's disease.[4,5] Moreover, a collection of families with a subtype of Hirschsprung disease confined to the distal colon and a complex inheritance pattern was studied by linkage and inheritance analysis. The results were consistent with a genetic model in which the interaction of just three loci accounted for the population incidence and recurrence risk of the disease.[6] These examples offer hope that advances in analysis tools and methodologies will allow the genetic dissection of other complex traits in the near future.

DISEASE INHERITANCE AND MOLECULAR PATHOGENESIS

Diseases caused by mutations of single genes may be inherited in either a dominant or a recessive fashion. The observed inheritance pattern depends on the effect of the mutation on the encoded protein. Mutations may inactivate, dysregulate, or enhance protein function. By cataloguing the distribution and types of mutations (e.g., missense, nonsense) causing a given disease phenotype, the effect on protein function can sometimes be deduced.

Null Alleles

Mutations that abolish protein expression or function produce a *null allele*. Potential mechanisms include mutations that interfere with transcription (promoter mutations), prematurely terminate the open reading frame (nonsense, frameshift, splicing mutations), or alter catalytically or structurally critical residues (point mutations, small in-frame insertions or deletions). If cellular function is not compromised by the diminished abundance of wild-type protein, a recessive inheritance pattern is seen. Carriers of a single null allele of a gene encoding an enzyme are usually healthy, but mutation of single alleles encoding structural proteins or transcription factors may cause disease, as discussed later.

Familial cancer syndromes resulting from mutations in tumor suppressor genes are an interesting exception to the rule that mutations in genes for which a single allele is sufficient for normal cellular function will manifest recessive inheritance. Cells carrying a null mutation in a tumor suppressor gene grow normally. Uncontrolled growth occurs when the remaining wild-type allele is mutated by a second, independent event. Because both alleles must be impaired for expression of the phenotype, this is an example of a recessive mechanism at the cellular level. At the level of the organism, the large number of total cells makes the probability of a second mutation event in at least one cell quite high. Thus, despite the recessive mechanism observed at the cellular level, familial cancer syndromes caused by loss of tumor suppressor genes are usually inherited in a dominant fashion.

Haploinsufficiency

For some proteins, such as those expressed as part of highly regulated developmental programs, total abundance may be critical to the execution of their function. When a single copy of an allele is inadequate for normal function or development, carriers of null mutations are symptomatic, a mechanism known as *haploinsufficiency*. Examples include transcription factor mutations, in which decreased transcript abundance results in secondary diminution of downstream effector protein levels, and heteromeric structural protein mutations, such as in collagens, in which the proper stoichiometry of the component subunits is important. Transmission of the null allele is sufficient to cause disease, so dominant inheritance is observed.

Dominant Negative Mutations

Mutations may abolish protein function in a domain-specific manner so that some activities are lost, whereas others are maintained. Potential mechanisms include missense mutations or in-frame deletions that affect a single functional domain or truncations that ablate distal domains. Mutant proteins retaining some aspect of function can be more deleterious for cellular function than complete absence of an allele if the mutant prevents the available wild-type protein from performing its function. This mechanism is exemplified by mutation of a transcription factor so that transactivation is lost, but DNA binding is normal, thus preventing the protein encoded by the wild-type allele from binding to the recognition sequence and activating transcription. Proteins that are components of a multimeric complex, such as the individual collagen chains forming a heterotrimeric collagen fibril, can have dominant negative effects when the incorporation of a mutant subunit impairs the assembly of the functional unit.

Activating Mutations

Mutations can directly (by active site alteration) or indirectly (by disabling a regulatory domain) enhance the activity of a protein. In the case of signal transduction proteins such as kinases, inappropriately regulated enzymatic activity may initiate a signaling cascade that stimulates cell division and sets the stage for cellular transformation. As the abnormal activity of the mutant allele overrides the properly regulated activity of the wild-type allele, dominant inheritance is observed.

TRADITIONAL AND MOLECULAR CYTOGENETICS

Chromosomal abnormalities, numeric or structural, are the leading cause of fetal loss, developmental and congenital abnormalities, and apparent infertility. Although some of these abnormalities result in live births, many are responsible for lack of embryonic implantation, growth, or survival. Of the numeric abnormalities, the only potential survivors are trisomy 21, 13, 18, 22, and, rarely, 9, along with the sex chromosomal abnormalities (XXX, XXY, XYY). The only monosomy capable of survival (although more than 95% abort in the first trimester) is 45,X. Since virtually all these abnormalities are the result of meiotic nondisjunction, we would expect to see trisomies and monosomies of every chromosome. A few trisomies can be found among spontaneous abortions, especially trisomy 16. Calculation of the expected frequency of the discovered and the nonviable trisomies and monosomies predicts that about 75% of fertilized ova are chromosomally abnormal, most of which never implant or are miscarried early in pregnancy, appearing as "late" menstrual periods. In one study,[7] 9 of 10 polar bodies studied by comparative genomic hybridization (discussed later) had either one too many (24) or one too few (22) chromosomes, a proportion not dissimilar from the theoretical prediction. Among the chromosomes involved, some were found that are never seen in viable fetuses, even those studied after spontaneous abortions. Another form of numeric abnormality leading to multiple congenital malformations and fetal demise, stillbirth, or, rarely, neonatal death is triploidy (69 chromosomes). This can result from dispermy in a single ovum or from one sperm with two female germ cells, probably an ovum and a polar body.

Numeric abnormalities can also result from mitotic, postfertilization events, which generally lead to mosaicism. Mosaicism should be distinguished from chimerism resulting from fusion of two separate embryos into one individual embryo. In this latter condition, a live infant will develop, generally normal, but the child can be infertile or a true hermaphrodite if the two initial embryos are of different gender. Mosaicism, conversely, results from either mitotic nondisjunction or anaphase lag. If this occurs in the first cell division after fertilization, an embryo with two cell lines will result: in the case of mitotic nondisjunction, they will both be abnormal (45 and 47 chromosomes each, with monosomy and trisomy for the nondisjoined chromosome), and in the case of anaphase lag, one will have normal cell lines and one will be missing a chromosome. The latter is the cause of many cases of mosaic Turner syndrome, when the involved chromosome is an X or a Y. The source of the nondisjoined chromosome has clinical significance because if is a Y, the resulting mosaic child may have Turner syndrome with testicular rests leading to a risk of gonadal tumors. If mitotic nondisjunction occurs later in embryonic development, it will lead to a child with three cell lines: normal, trisomic and monosomic. This mechanism accounts for patients with mosaic Down syndrome (46 and 47 chromosomes, the latter with trisomy 21), in whom the predicted monosomy 21 cell line dies off because of nonviability of autosomal monosomic cells.

The other major category of chromosomal abnormalities is structural alteration of one or more chromosomes. A single chromosome may be abnormal because of a deletion or a duplication of a piece of chromosomal material ranging from a few genes to whole chromosomal arms. The resulting abnormalities and viability of the fetus will vary depending on the amount and genetic content of the material deleted and duplicated. Breakage and recombination of fragments between two or occasionally more chromosomes result in structural variation. If the exchange is achieved without loss or gain of material, the translocation is balanced and should not result in abnormalities unless a gene is damaged at the breakpoints. However, a normal carrier of such a balanced translocation can produce gametes that have duplications of one of the exchanged fragments, along with deficiency of the other (unbalanced translocation). Because there are virtually infinite possible rearrangements, the phenotype can range from essentially normal or mild anomalies to severe anomalies and death during pregnancy or after birth.

Chromosomal Basis of Nonmendelian Disease

It has become apparent that various mechanisms can lead to nonmendelian behavior of chromosomes and their genes. Some of these mechanisms and their alterations lead to certain developmental defects. Among these are genetic imprinting, uniparental disomy, the formation of neocentromeres, and mitochondrial inheritance.

Imprinting results in the expression of certain genes exclusively from the chromosome derived from one of the two parents in a gender-specific fashion. The allele derived from the parent of the opposite gender is silent (imprinted). This parent-of-origin-specific expression appears to involve differential methylation of the regions controlling imprinted genes during formation of gametes. It is this phenomenon that accounts for the lack of viability of embryos derived from a single parent. Embryos having a chromosomal complement derived only from the male have

poorly functioning placentas, whereas those with entirely female-derived chromosomes do not have a proper embryo and may lead to a hydatid mole. Absence of the active allele by deletion or mutation results in abnormalities of the offspring. The types of abnormalities are determined by which of the imprinted genes is absent. For example, the proximal long arm of chromosome 15 has two adjacent areas, one of which is paternally imprinted and the other maternally imprinted. Deletion of the paternally imprinted genes results in Prader-Willi syndrome, whereas absence of the maternally imprinted genes results in Angelman syndrome, both associated with distinct patterns of developmental defects. Disturbances in an imprinted gene in the short arm of chromosome 11 (most commonly by relaxing imprinting and allowing both alleles to be expressed in an imprinted area) results in an overgrowth syndrome, Beckwith-Wiedemann, which is also associated with tumor formation and other abnormalities. This appears to result from overexpression of a growth factor in this region that is usually imprinted. Chromosomal regions known to contain imprinted genes are shown in Figure 2–4.

One of the mechanisms by which absence of the active allele at an imprinted locus or a double expression of the active allele can occur is *uniparental disomy*. In uniparental disomy, both members of a chromosome, and, in some cases, a part of a pair of chromosomes, are derived from the same parent. If imprinted genes exist in this pair, the phenotypic result will depend on whether the pair derives from the mother or the father and which parent contributes the imprinted gene. As an example, if there is maternal uniparental disomy of chromosome 15, the active allele that is derived from the father will be absent, and the result will be Prader-Willi syndrome, as if the paternal allele were deleted. Similarly, if there is paternal uniparental disomy of chromosome 15, the active maternal allele at the Angelman locus will be absent, and Angelman syndrome will result, just as if the maternal allele had been deleted.

Uniparental disomy comes in two forms. Uniparental heterodisomy occurs if the embryo inherits both members of a pair of chromosomes from one parent, whereas in uniparental isodisomy, two copies of a single chromosome from the pair are transmitted. In addition to the effect on imprinted genes, uniparental isodisomy also results in homozygosity for the entire chromosome or that part which is disomic, including any mutant genes that happen to be on that chromosome. In fact, the first proven case of human uniparental isodisomy was found in a child with cystic fibrosis who had received both members of a single maternal chromosome 7 that happened to contain the cystic fibrosis mutation. The child was also unusually short, because of the presence of an imprinted gene with a strong impact on growth.

None of these observations would be possible without the technical advances allowing detailed examination of the chromosomes. After discovery of methods to produce specific banding patterns in the early 1970s that permitted identification of each chromosome and its major parts, additional breakthroughs led to the ability to identify increasingly smaller parts of chromosomes by fluorescence *in situ* hybridization (Fig. 2–5), identification of each chromosome in a single karyotype by multicolor fluorescence *in situ* hybridization, and, more recently, by comparative genomic hybridization. This last technique involves double hybridization of patient DNA labeled with one fluorochrome and normal DNA labeled with a different fluorochrome to a normal metaphase chromosomes on a slide. Using a computerized camera and microscope, this technique permits the discovery and exact identification of missing and extra material in any sample, even when the sample cannot be grown in culture (e.g., products of conception). The application of comparative genomic hybridization to DNA probes on microarrays has allowed the discovery of the smallest duplications and deletions, even from a single cell. These newer techniques have rapidly led to far more accurate delineation of the causes of developmental and congenital abnormalities.

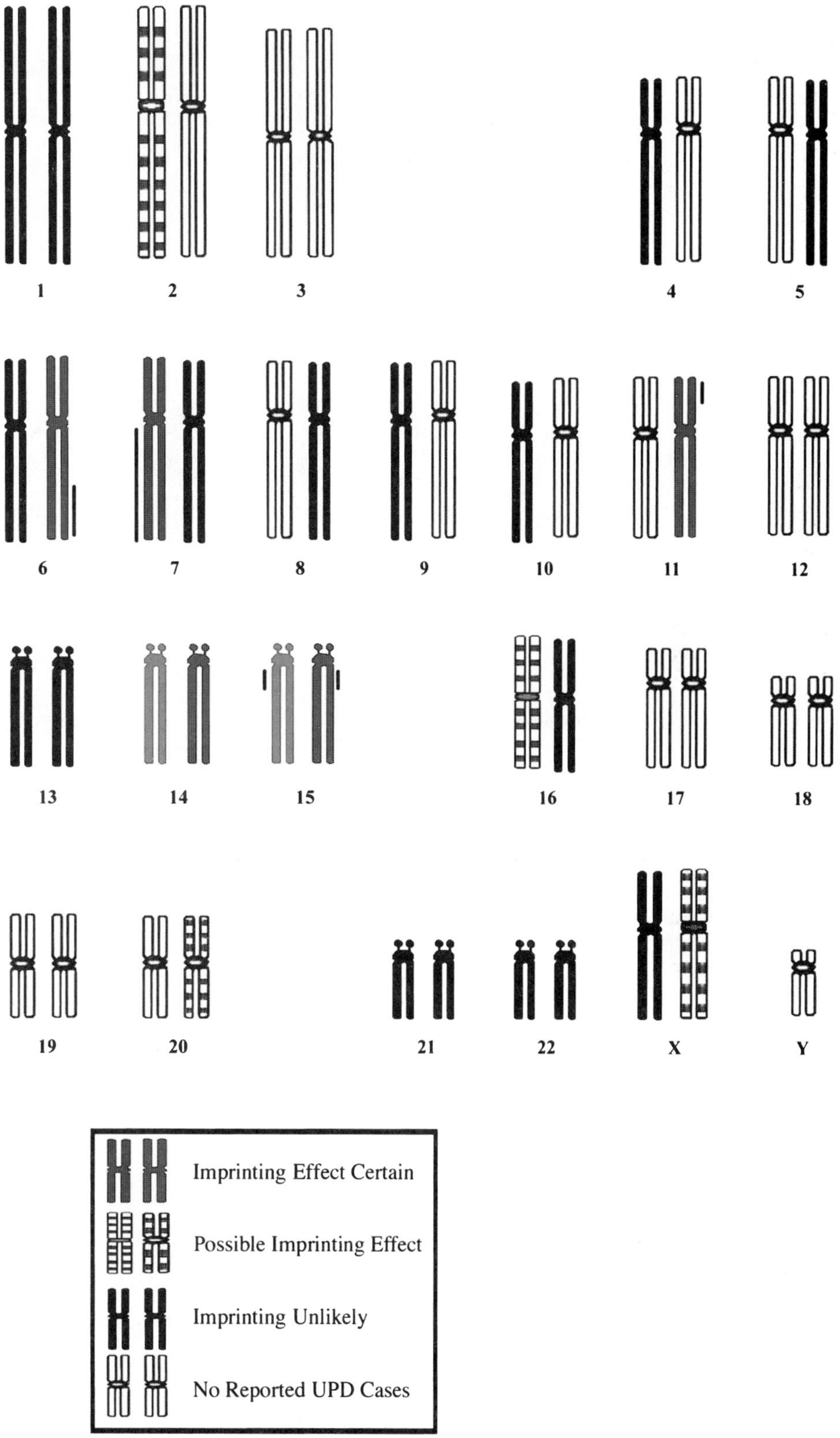

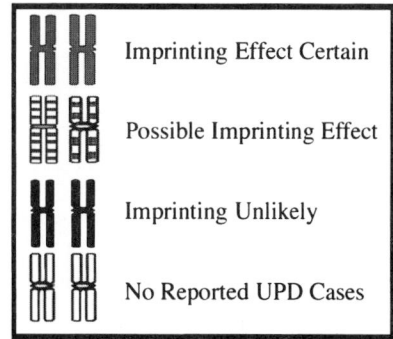

Figure 2–4. Imprinted chromosomal regions. Data are presented from a survey summarizing human chromosomes known to contain imprinted genes and the parent of origin of the imprinted chromosome, if applicable. The figure can be viewed as an interactive Web page document (*http://genes.uchicago.edu/upd*) with links to citations supporting the summary data. UPD = uniparental disomy. (Courtesy of Dr David Ledbetter.)

CONCLUSION AND FUTURE DIRECTIONS

The massive amount of information made available by the Human Genome Project has already shown its power in allowing the mapping of many hundreds of disease genes and the cloning of a high proportion of these. The methods developed by the project, such as high-throughput genotyping, have become widely used and are beginning to be applied to a much broader set of genes associated with susceptibility to common diseases such as cardiovascular disease, diabetes, and obesity. Clearly, numerous conditions applicable to fetal development will fall into this effort, including prematurity, intrauterine growth retardation, and birth weight variability. The search for such genes until now has been primarily by association studies, many of which have not been replicated or replicable. One review[8] showed that of about 200 such associations found in more than

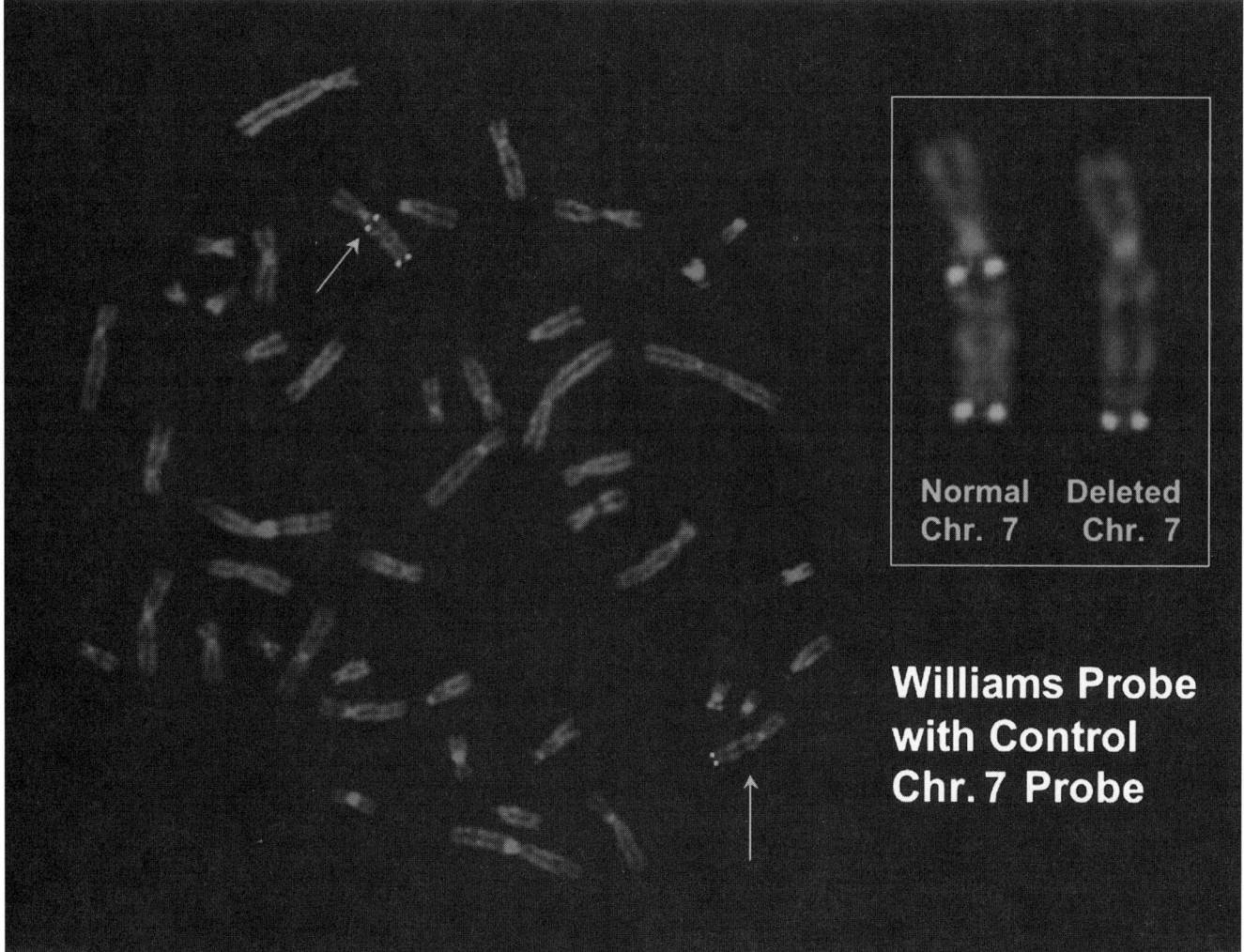

Figure 2–5. Fluorescence *in situ* hybridization. The diagnosis of chromosomal microdeletion syndromes has been revolutionized by molecular cytogenetic techniques allowing metaphase chromosomes to be analyzed for the loss of specific sequences using fluorescently labeled genomic DNA probes. In this example, a control probe specific for a telomeric region of chromosome 7 has hybridized to each replicated chromatid, whereas a second probe specific for a centromeric region that is recurrently deleted in patients with Williams syndrome is absent in one of the chromosome 7 pairs (*arrows*). (Courtesy of Dr Brynn Levy.)

600 references in the literature, only 5 were clearly replicable, and another 20 or so were highly suggestive. Nevertheless, with increasingly powerful methodologies applied to the search for associations between alleles for specific genes and disease susceptibility, it is likely that this number will grow steadily.

Another potentially highly useful outcome of such studies is in the field of pharmacogenomics. Certain genes have already been identified in which polymorphisms lead to large differences in individual responses to therapeutic agents. It is suspected that some of these may even be related to whether a particular drug is teratogenic in a particular fetus. The ability to tailor types and amounts of medications to different patients would be an enormous benefit to therapeutic interventions by reducing the risks of drug reactions or side effects.

Finally, the long hoped-for practical use of gene therapy may grow in the near future. The successful treatment of several children with X-linked severe combined immunodeficiency[9] has given hope for the application of treatment of deleterious mutations by gene replacement. The first success has definitely been helped by the finding that corrected immune cells have a selective advantage over the abnormal cells and therefore replace them to produce a cure of the disease. This success was predictable from prior findings that reversion of deleterious mutations in such

cells led to a reversion to relative normality in an otherwise fatal illness.[10] Prenatal gene therapy has been attempted in immunodeficiency, with some apparent success. Until gene therapy becomes feasible for other diseases, advances in protein product, particularly for lysosomal storage diseases, are expanding and in some cases may also become applicable *in utero*.

REFERENCES

1. Chi N, Epstein JA: Getting your Pax straight: pax proteins in development and disease. Trends Genet *18*:41, 2002.
2. Auricchio A, et al: Double heterozygosity for a RET substitution interfering with splicing and an EDNRB missense mutation in Hirschsprung disease. Am J Hum Genet *64*:1216, 1999.
3. Katsanis N, et al: Triallelic inheritance in Bardet-Biedl syndrome, a Mendelian recessive disorder. Science *293*:2256, 2001.
4. Ogura Y, et al: A frameshift mutation in NOD2 associated with susceptibility to Crohn's disease. Nature *411*:603, 2001.
5. Hugot JP, et al: Association of NOD2 leucine-rich repeat variants with susceptibility to Crohn's disease. Nature *411*:599, 2001.
6. Gabriel SB, et al: Segregation at three loci explains familial and population risk in Hirschsprung disease. Nat Genet *31*:89, 2002.
7. Wells D, et al: First clinical application of comparative genomic hybridization and polar body testing for preimplantation genetic diagnosis of aneuploidy. Fertil Steril *78*:543, 2002.
8. Hirschhorn JN, et al: A comprehensive review of genetic association studies. *Genet Med 4*:45, 2002.

9. Cavazzana-Calvo M, et al: Gene therapy of human severe combined immunodeficiency (SCID)-X1 disease. Science 288:669, 2000.

10. Hirschhorn R, et al: Spontaneous in vivo reversion to normal of an inherited mutation in a patient with adenosine deaminase deficiency. Nat Genet 13:290, 1996.

SUGGESTED READINGS

Alberts B, et al: Molecular Biology of the Cell, 3rd ed. New York, Garland Publishing, 1994.

Brock DJH: Molecular Genetics for the Clinician. New York, Cambridge University Press, 1993.

Emery AEH, Rimoin DL: Principles and Practice of Medical Genetics, 4th ed. New York, Churchill Livingstone, 2002.

Gelehrter TD, et al: Principles of Medical Genetics, 2nd ed. Baltimore, Williams & Wilkins, 1998.

Jones KL: Smith's Recognizable Patterns of Human Malformation, 5th ed. Philadelphia, WB Saunders Co, 1997.

Lewin B: Genes VII. New York, Oxford University Press, 2000.

Miller OJ, Therman E: Human Chromosomes, 4th ed. New York, Springer-Verlag, 2001.

Scriver CR, et al (eds): The Metabolic Basis and Inherited Basis of Inherited Disease, 8th ed. New York, McGraw-Hill, 2001.

Strachan T, Read AP: Human Molecular Genetics, 2nd ed. New York, John Wiley, 1999.

Thompson MW, et al: Genetics in Medicine, 6th ed. Philadelphia, WB Saunders Co, 2001.

Watson JD, et al: Recombinant DNA, 2nd ed. New York, Scientific American Books, 1992.

Weatherall DJ: The New Genetics and Clinical Practice, 3rd ed. Oxford, Oxford University Press, 1991.

WEB-BASED RESOURCES

McKusick VA: Online Mendelian Inheritance in Man: *http://www.ncbi.nlm.nih.gov/Omim/*
A database of human genetic diseases providing clinical overview and survey of relevant literature.

National Center for Biotechnology Information: *http://www.ncbi.nlm.nih.gov/*
A collection of links to literature, genome maps, and genomic analysis tools.

3

David L. Bolender and Stanley Kaplan

Basic Embryology

The human embryo begins as a single large cell, approximately 0.1 mm in diameter, just visible to the unaided eye. During the 266 days of gestation following fertilization, the cell increases in size, weight, and surface area in a rapid and markedly nonlinear fashion. From newly fertilized egg to newborn, length increases by a factor of 5000, surface area by a factor of 61 million, and weight by a factor of nearly 6 billion.[1] During this process the fertilized egg divides and differentiates into more than 200 different morphologically recognizable cell types. Orchestration of the increase in size and specialization in cellular function is a complex process about which much remains unknown. It has been argued, however, that the principles of development are known and that we are missing only details at the molecular level.[2] Although this is an overstatement, it is true that during the last decade or so, our understanding of the molecular control of development has increased substantially. That human embryonic development occurs normally in most pregnancies is a tribute to the design of the control mechanisms that are operating. This chapter includes a brief description of the growth and differentiation of the human embryo along with a limited discussion of certain factors that play a part in control of these activities.

GAMETES AND THEIR MATURATION

The human egg and sperm are two highly specialized cells that share little in common with the other cells of the adult body. They are different in both form and function. Similar to other cells, however, they must achieve a degree of maturity before they can perform their function (i.e., combining to form the zygote). The steps as well as the chronology leading to this maturation are quite different in the male and female, and these differences reflect the diverse pathways of the two sexes, beginning early in human development.[3]

Origin of the Gametes

The human egg and sperm are derived from large, round primordial germ cells that can be identified in the wall of the yolk sac as early as 24 days after fertilization.[4] As the yolk sac begins to be incorporated into the embryo, the germ cells migrate along the dorsal mesentery of the hindgut to the gonadal ridges, which they reach by the end of the fourth or early fifth week (Fig. 3-1). This migration has been observed *in vitro* in pieces of hindgut, mesentery, and gonadal ridges of mouse embryos.[5] It is facilitated in humans by a striking ameboid shape (which persists even after the cells have reached the gonad[6]) and pseudopodia typical of those found in ameboid cells. The pseudopodia disappear later after the migration is complete.[5, 7] In humans, these cells contain glycogen stores that diminish with time and disappear when the cells have reached their destination in the gonad, suggesting that this may be the energy source for their journey.[8]

Organization of the Gonad

The coelomic epithelium covering the medial aspect of the gonadal ridges undergoes proliferation. As these cells multiply, they grow into the underlying mesenchyme in a series of finger-like cords of cells called primitive sex cords. The primordial germ cells associate with these cords. If the embryo is to become a male, these cords continue to be prominent and eventually develop into the seminiferous tubules and rete testis. The early male gonad can also be recognized by the separation of the cords from their parent epithelial covering by a fibrous connective tissue layer, the tunica albuginea that forms just under the epithelium. If the gonad is to become an ovary, the primitive sex cords remain rudimentary. The origin of the follicle cells of the ovary remains unclear, but likely candidates are cells from the coelomic epithelium and the mesonephros. The follicle cells associate with the primordial germ cells to form primordial ovarian follicles.[8]

Development of the Female Gamete (See Chapter 190)

If the gonad develops into an ovary the primordial germ cells become oogonia and continue mitotic division.[9] Mitotic division of these cells has been observed in humans up to the seventh

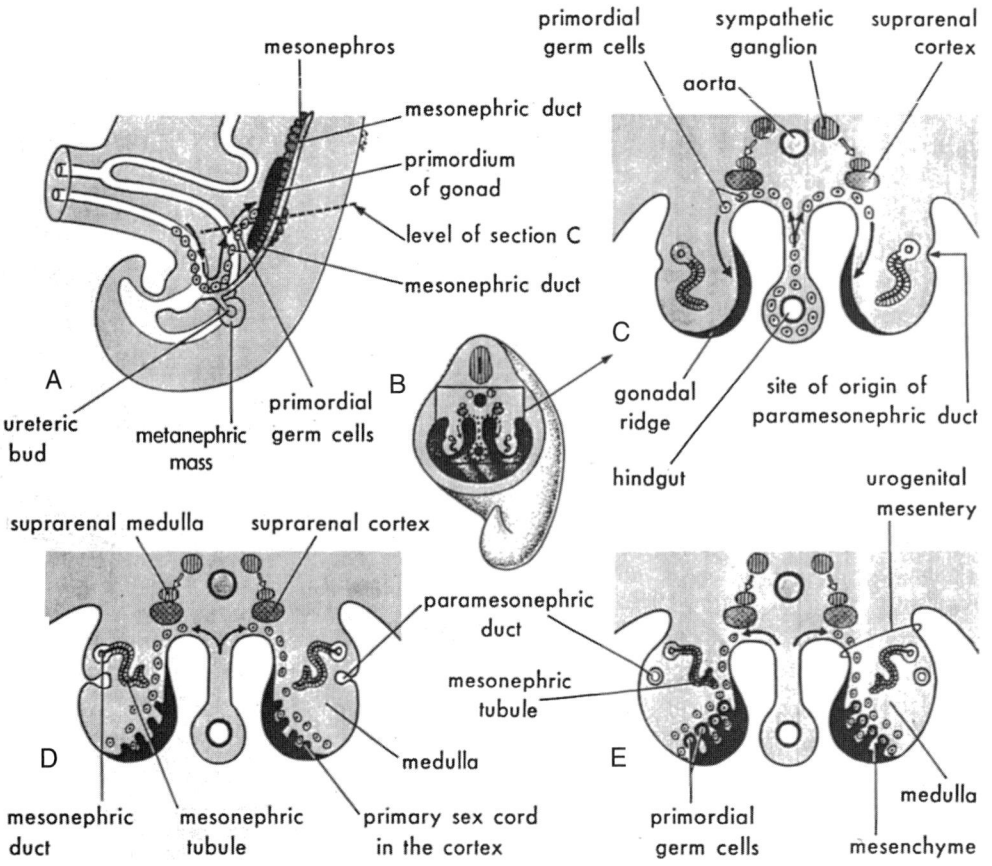

Figure 3–1. A, Sketch of a 5-week embryo, illustrating the migration of primordial germ cells from the yolk sac. **B,** Three-dimensional sketch of the caudal region of a 5-week embryo, showing the location and extent of the gonadal ridges on the medial aspect of the urogenital ridges. **C,** Transverse section showing the primordium of the suprarenal (adrenal) glands, the gonadal ridges, and the migration of primordial germ cells into the developing gonads. **D,** Transverse section through a 6-week embryo, showing the primary sex cords and the developing paramesonephric ducts. **E,** Similar section at a later stage showing the indifferent gonads and the mesonephric and paramesonephric ducts. (From Moore KL, Persaud TVN: The Developing Human: Clinically Oriented Embryology. 5th ed. Philadelphia, WB Saunders Co, 1993: p 281.)

fetal month[10] but ceases sometime shortly before birth. No oogonia form after a normal full-term birth.

In both males and females, the germ cells form a syncytium while dividing.[11,12] These intercellular connections permit communication and facilitate the high degree of synchrony that has been observed during both mitotic and meiotic divisions.[13-15]

By the eighth or ninth week after fertilization, some oogonia enter prophase of meiosis I and become primary oocytes.[9-16] Meiosis begins first deep to the surface of the human ovary and then expands toward the surface. Thus, at an appropriate fetal stage, oogonia are found superficially, oocytes deep to the surface, and small follicles at the inner part of the ovarian cortex.[9] It has been suggested that a diffusible meiosis-activating substance is secreted by rete cells (derived from the mesonephros), which lie in the center of the ovary, and there is good experimental evidence to support this hypothesis.[17-20]

The oocyte goes through the leptotene, zygotene, and pachytene stages of meiosis I, and it then arrests at the diplotene stage. At this point the oocyte becomes surrounded by a single, incomplete layer of flat follicular cells;[9] this unit is called a primordial follicle. The follicle's large central nucleus is known as the germinal vesicle. A crescent-shaped assembly of cellular organelles containing mitochondria, endoplasmic reticulum, the Golgi complex, lysosomes, and annulate lamellae (stacked parallel membrane arrays with pores) remain clustered adjacent to the nucleus.[15,21] Once it has been incorporated into a primordial follicle, the oocyte enters a long period of quiescence, beginning before birth in humans and ending either in atresia or ovulation.

Once sexual maturity is attained, a small number of oocytes begins the process of folliculogenesis or follicle maturation during each menstrual cycle.[22] The oocyte grows and eventually becomes one of the largest cells in the human body.[23] The organelles disperse throughout the cytoplasm and the germinal vesicle (nucleus) enlarges. It increases its complement of nuclear

pores, facilitating transport of molecules between the nucleoplasm and cytoplasm. The follicular cells resume mitosis and increase markedly in size, changing in shape from squamous to cuboidal, and the follicle becomes surrounded by a basement membrane. Those follicles containing an oocyte surrounded by a single layer of cuboidal follicular cells are known as unilaminar primary follicles, to distinguish them from earlier or later stages.[3]

During further growth of the primary follicle, a thick, acellular coat, the zona pellucida, begins to form between the oocyte and the follicular cells. Mitotic activity increases the number of follicle cell layers and the follicle is now called a multilaminar primary follicle. The expanding follicle compresses the surrounding ovarian stoma, which organizes into a compact layer adjacent to the basement membrane of the follicle. This layer of stromal cells is called the theca interna, and its cells have the capacity to produce androgens when stimulated by luteinizing hormone activity (Fig. 3-2). The theca interna is vascularized but the epithelial layers of follicle cells remain avascular.

The zona pellucida is important in the process of fertilization because it contains sperm receptors, takes part in induction of the acrosome reaction, and becomes a block to polyspermy. It may also act after fertilization as a smooth, slippery envelope to contain the sticky ball of cells of the morula staged embryo; these are free to adhere to the uterine endothelium when the zona breaks down, just before implantation.

The zona pellucida (ZP) is made up of three separate filamentous glycoproteins (ZP1 through ZP3), which differ in molecular weight and isoelectric point and which account for virtually all protein in the zona pellucida. ZP1 cross-links these filaments, resulting in a three-dimensional matrix that is permeable to large macromolecules. ZP3 serves as a species-specific sperm receptor and also induces the acrosome reaction in sperm at contact. At or shortly after fertilization, these two characteristics are lost, reducing the likelihood of polyspermy.[24-26] The ZP3 gene has

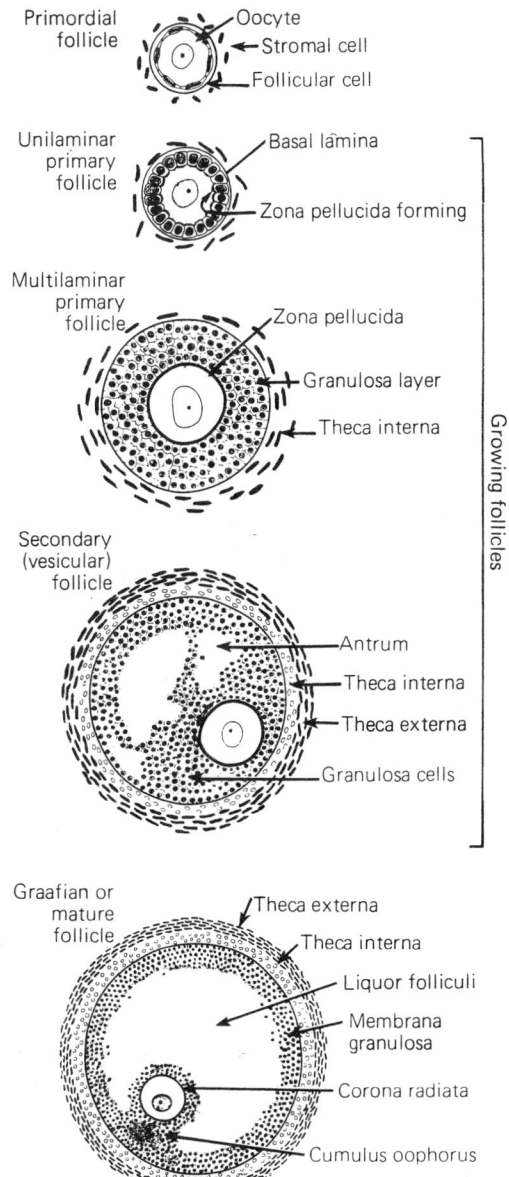

Figure 3–2. Schematic drawing of ovarian follicles, starting with the primordial follicle and ending with mature follicles. (From Junqueira LC, et al: Basic Histology. 7th ed. Norwalk, CT, Appleton & Lange, 1992.)

been cloned; it is expressed only in oocytes and only during the growth phase of oogenesis.[27] The human genes for ZP2 and ZP3 are located on chromosomes 16 and 7, respectively,[28] but the location of ZP1 remains unknown. The interesting story of these ZP proteins has been the subject of a popularized account[29] as well as several reviews.[28,30,31] Radiolabeling studies in mice indicate that all three glycoproteins are synthesized by the oocyte itself, rather than by the follicular cells.[32] Furthermore, immunofluorescence studies show that ZP antigens are present within human oocytes but not in follicular cells.[33] Studies in species other than the mouse, however, suggest that the granulosa cells that surround the oocyte may also play a role in the synthesis of ZP components.[30]

Numerous cytoplasmic projections of the follicular cells penetrate the ZP to contact the cell membrane of the oocyte. In humans, these filopodial extensions of the follicular cell may actually lie deeply buried in the oocyte, in straight invaginations

or pits.[34] These pits are lined by the oocyte cell membrane; however, there is no cytoplasmic continuity between the two cell types. Animal studies have shown that gap junctions exist along the association of these two cell membranes, permitting transfer of small molecules (about 1000 MW) between them.[22]

As the primary follicle enlarges, the follicular cells begin to produce follicular fluid, which collects within the intercellular spaces between follicle cells. These spaces coalesce to form a large fluid-filled cavity called the antrum, which is characteristic of the secondary (vesicular) follicle. The antrum expands, and the oocyte becomes located on one side of the follicle where it is embedded within a mound of follicle cells known as the cumulus oophorus. The layers of follicular cells immediately surrounding the oocyte are termed the *corona radiata*. Because of its increased size, the follicle further compresses the surrounding ovarian stroma. A looser, less organized layer of flattened stromal cells encircles the follicle superficial to the theca interna. This is called the theca externa and its cells have no steroid-secreting activity (see Fig. 3–2). A few days before ovulation, one secondary follicle becomes dominant and inhibits the growth of the remaining secondary follicles. The dominant follicle, now called a graafian follicle, can reach several centimeters in diameter. The oocyte is about 100 μm in diameter at this stage. About a day before ovulation, its nuclear membrane breaks down, the nucleolus disappears, and the first polar body forms, containing one of the two sets of chromosomes. Meiosis I is completed and the oocyte proceeds to meiosis II, but it again arrests when reaching metaphase. In most mammalian species including humans, meiosis II resumes only after the oocyte is penetrated by a sperm.[35,36] Completion of meiosis in the fertilized oocyte results in production of the second polar body.

Follicles of any stage can undergo atresia. Atresia begins in the fetus and continues into menopause until all follicles have disappeared. At birth, approximately 2 million primordial follicles are present within the two ovaries. It has been estimated that half of the 2 million follicles present at birth are atretic at that time.[10] In humans, follicular growth starts before birth and the newborn ovary contains multilaminar primary follicles as well as primordial follicles. Follicular growth and subsequent atresia are continuous during human childhood, and it has been clearly stated that "quiescent ovaries in which follicular growth is absent do not occur in normal children."[37]

Little is known about control of atresia. For example, it is not known whether atresia is initiated by action of the follicular cells, by that of the oocyte, or both.[22] The process of atresia, however, can be manipulated experimentally.[37] About 40,000 follicles are present in the two ovaries of a young adult woman, indicating a reduction to 2% of the pool originally present at birth.[38]

These stages, up to and including the newly fertilized mature ovum, are summarized in Table 3–1. Most or all of the RNA and protein found in a mature oocyte are synthesized during oocyte growth. Those macromolecules present in the oocyte of an atretic follicle are degraded and the degradation products are used for new synthesis.[23]

If one assumes a fertility span of 30 years, about 400 eggs are shed during a woman's lifetime.[35] Thus, about 1 in every 100 of the eggs present in a young adult completes maturation and is ovulated; the rest degenerate. A woman has her full complement of eggs, albeit immature, on the day she is born. This is not the case for sperm development in males.

Early Development of Male Gametes (See Chapter 191)

In male humans, the primordial germ cells migrate into the gonadal ridges as outlined earlier (see Fig. 3–1). Once they have reached the gonad, they divide to form a pool of spermatogonia.[39] Both spermatogonia and their supporting cells (Sertoli cells) can be identified as early as 48 days postfertilization.[40] The germ

TABLE 3-1

Summary of the Developmental Characteristics of the Human Female Germ Cell

Name	Approximate First Recognizable Time (Postfertilization)	Location	Approximate Total Number (Both Ovaries)	Size, Shape, Characteristics	References
Primordial germ cell	During 4th week	Caudal yolk sac, among endoderm cells	500	Large, round 15–20 μm diameter	4, 7
Primordial germ cell	During 5th week	Dorsal mesentery of hindgut and gonadal ridges	500	Ameboid shape, migrating, with pseudopodia; over 20–30 μm in long axis. Alkaline phosphatase positive	4, 7
Oogonium	During 6th week	Sexually indifferent gonad	100,000	Rapid mitosis increases numbers (mitosis signals name change)	4, 9
Oogonium	During 7th week	Gonad recognizable as ovary	100,000	Mitosis continues; almost all primordial germ cells are now in the gonad	7, 38
Oocyte (in primordial follicle)	Weeks 8–9	Ovary	?	Meiosis begins; about 19 μm diameter	16
Quiescent oocyte in primordial follicle	16 weeks	Ovary	?	Arrest of meiosis I at diplotene; 50–70 μm, round-to-ovoid, vitelline body present	34
As above	2 months	Ovary	600,000		10
As above	5 months	Ovary	6,800,000		10
As above	7 months	Ovary		Mitosis of oogonia ceases	10
As above	Birth	Ovary	2,000,000 (50% atretic)		38
As above					10
As above	7 years	Ovary	300,000		10
Primary follicles to mature (graafian)	Puberty on	Ovary	40,000 and declining	From oocyte to mature: comes out of meiotic arrest and enters metaphase of meiosis II, then arrests again	38
Mature ovum	Puberty on	Uterine tube	1 per month	Meiosis is completed and the 2nd polar body is extruded when penetrated by a sperm	38

cells and the supporting cells combine to form seminiferous tubules.

Spermatogonia are located next to the basement membrane of the seminiferous tubule, where they lie quiescent until puberty. Experimental studies with mice have shown that male primordial germ cells are kept in that state by a meiosis-preventing substance, which can also arrest female germ cells in meiosis. Conversely, the female gonad secretes a meiosis-inducing substance, which can induce male germ cells to enter meiosis.[19]

At puberty, the spermatogonia begin differentiation into sperm (spermatogenesis). The process of spermatogenesis occurs in three phases. In the first phase, the spermatogonia divide mitotically. In the second phase, some spermatogonia differentiate into primary spermatocytes and undergo meiosis. In the third phase, spermatids proceed through spermiogenesis to form spermatozoa. In contrast to the female, the cycle of differentiation of gametes in men is essentially continuous throughout life. Studies in which tritiated thymidine was injected into healthy male volunteers indicate that the complete cycle takes approximately 74 days.[41] The various stages of spermatogenesis, however, are not synchronized along the length of the coiled seminiferous tubule in humans, different stages are found at different positions.

FERTILIZATION

Development begins with the fusion of the male and female gametes at fertilization, which takes place in the distal third of the oviduct. Although fertilization is an "internal" process in humans and other mammals, the development of culture systems that support fertilization has made detailed study of the sperm-oocyte interaction possible, as well as providing a basis for *in vitro* fertilization for clinical ends. As a result, the precisely ordered events comprising a "fertilization pathway" have been identified (Fig. 3–3). The mechanisms involved in the fertilization pathway have been the subject of investigation at the molecular level.[29, 31, 42] Most studies on fertilization have been done using mice, but comparative data suggest that the pathway is similar in all mammals, including humans.

The pathway of fertilization begins with binding of the sperm to the surface of the zona pellucida (see Fig. 3–3). On the surface of every sperm, there are thousands of copies of an egg-binding protein, and these are recognized by thousands of copies of sperm receptors on the zona pellucida.[43] Binding is relatively species specific and requires a complete plasma membrane (i.e., an acrosome-intact sperm).[44,45] Once bound to the zona surface, the sperm undergoes a series of dynamic membrane fusions known as the acrosome reaction (see Fig. 3–3).[46] During this phase, the plasma membrane at the apical end of the sperm fuses with the outer membrane of the acrosome, forming a series of membrane-bound vesicles. These are eventually sloughed, which exposes the inner acrosomal membrane and its complement of enzymes.[31, 47]

As a result of enzyme modification of the zona, the sperm is able to tunnel its way through. The first sperm to penetrate the perivitelline space (between the zona pellucida and the oocyte plasma membrane) and fuse with the plasma membrane triggers activation of the egg (see Fig. 3–3). Oocyte activation is a dynamic, multi-step process that includes mechanisms to prevent polyspermy, completion of meiosis by the oocyte,

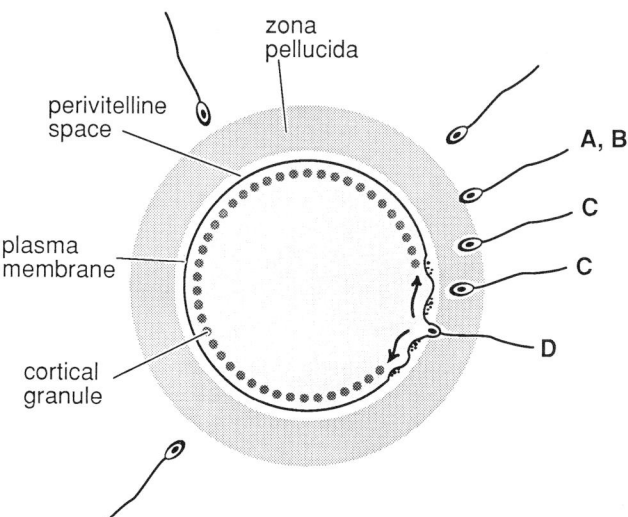

zona
pellucida

perivitelline
space

A, B

C

C

plasma
membrane

cortical
granule

D

Figure 3-3. Pathway of fertilization. A, B, Sperm binding and the acrosome reaction, exposing the zona to acrosomal enzymes. **C,** Penetration of the enzyme-modified zona pellucida by the sperm. **D,** Activation of the egg, including oocyte membrane hyperpolarization and release of enzymes by the cortical granules. (Adapted from Wassarman PM: Sci Am *259*:82, 1988.)

engulfment of the sperm, formation of male and female pronuclei and initiation of the first mitotic division of the embryo. Prevention of fertilization by more than one sperm (polyspermy—a potentially lethal condition) is thought to be a biphasic reaction although the first phase is not well documented in humans. The first phase is rapid and consists of hyperpolarization of the oocyte plasma membrane. The second phase may take several minutes and involves the release of enzymes from the cortical granules that alter the structure of the zona pellucida. As a result, the plasma membrane and zona pellucida become refractory to further penetration by other sperm.

Studies at the molecular level have revealed that a component of the zona pellucida is a key substance in the fertilization pathway. As mentioned earlier, the zona pellucida is an acellular coat that surrounds the oocyte and consists of three glycoproteins (ZP1, ZP2, and ZP3) arranged in an interlacing filamentous network.[43, 48] Interestingly, one of them (ZP3) functions as the sperm receptor, initiates the acrosome reaction, and participates in the zona reaction.[48] Sperm binding is mediated by a subset of the O-linked oligosaccharides associated with ZP3, while a segment of the polypeptide backbone is needed to induce the acrosome reaction.[49, 29]

Several important events necessary for development of the embryo (initially called a zygote after fertilization) are accomplished as a result of fertilization.[38] First, the diploid chromosome number is restored by fusion of the two haploid gametes. Normally, half of the chromosomes come from each parent, and the new complement of chromosomes in the zygote promotes species variation. In addition, the genetic sex of the zygote is determined by the type of sperm that participates in fertilization. Sperm that bear a Y chromosome produce a genetically male zygote (XY) whereas an X-bearing sperm produces a female zygote (XX). Finally, fertilization initiates cleavage, the mitotic division of the zygote. Apposition of the male and female pronuclei forms a metaphase plate, and the first cleavage soon begins. In contrast to some animal species, the human male and female pronuclei never fuse (i.e., form a complete nucleus). Instead, they immediately enter mitotic metaphase.[50]

Parthenogenesis is activation of the unfertilized oocyte, leading thereafter to varying degrees of successful development of the zygote and embryo. In some animal species, this process is well known and may even produce viable offspring. No verified human cases, however, have been reported in the scientific literature.[38]

MORPHOGENESIS

The mechanisms mediating the transformation of a fertilized oocyte into a three-dimensional embryo are complex and still not completely understood. Studies on human embryos have been, for the most part, limited to observations of static images or serial reconstructions on preserved specimens of different stages. Therefore, most knowledge of the mechanisms controlling development has come from animal studies.

During development, cells having different genetic backgrounds are constantly interacting with each other and with a variety of molecules within their extracellular environment. The processes involved in these interactions consist of many well-recognized cell biologic phenomena, including cell division, adhesion, secretion, cytodifferentiation, motility, and cell death. Although the complex interactions that occur during morphogenesis may appear unorganized, they do not occur stochastically, but rather in a precisely ordered sequence of events resulting in recognizable patterns of histogenesis and organogenesis. In the past decade, an abundance of molecular studies have given us a much clearer picture of the complex signaling activity that controls embryonic development.[8]

As a result of fertilization, the zygote undergoes a series of mitotic divisions termed *cleavage.* The cells derived from these repeated mitotic divisions are called *blastomeres.* The first divisions result in a solid mass of blastomeres that are still surrounded by the zona pellucida. Starting at the 8- to 16-cell stage, intercellular spaces between blastomeres coalesce to form a central cavity. The embryo, now termed a *blastocyst,* consists of a regionalized clump of cells termed the *inner cell mass,* which projects into the blastocyst cavity and is surrounded by an outer layer of trophoblast cells (Fig. 3-4A, B). Initially the blastocyst floats freely within the uterine cavity. After shedding the zona pellucida, the blastocyst attaches and implants within the uterine endometrium.[38]

Studies on embryos suggest that the earliest cleavage divisions appear to be driven by maternal messages stored within the oocyte cytoplasm.[51] In mammals (including humans), the embryonic genome is activated by the two- to four-cell stage and begins to synthesize proteins on its own. This is reflected in the steady rise in the synthesis of many intracellular proteins such as actin.[52-54]

During cleavage, several changes fundamental to embryonic development occur at the molecular level. One of the most important processes is the generation of cell diversity. Initially, all blastomeres express a specific transcription factor (oct-4) which reflects the undifferentiated state of these cells. If separated from the others at this stage, each of the blastomeres has the capacity to form a complete embryo. By the 8- and 16-cell stage the embryo is a solid mass of cells called a morula. At this time, the outer cells of the morula are distinguishable from the inner cells because the outer cells no longer express oct-4.[8] The outer cells (now designated the trophoblast) also begin to exhibit epithelial polarity.[55] As a result, the first embryonic tissue (trophoblast epithelium) is formed. Subsequent cytodifferentiation of the trophoblast results in a double-layered membrane, which is a progenitor tissue of the chorion, the fetal portion of the placenta (see Fig. 3-4C). The inner cellular layer is called the *cytotrophoblast,* and the outer layer the *syncytiotrophoblast.* The latter structure, which secretes human chorionic gonadotropin (hCG) and proteolytic enzymes, is critical to implantation.[38]

During the second week of development, the cells of the inner cell mass that face the blastocyst cavity become flattened, forming a second layer of epithelium.[38] The upper layer, located next to the trophoblast, is now designated the epiblast, whereas

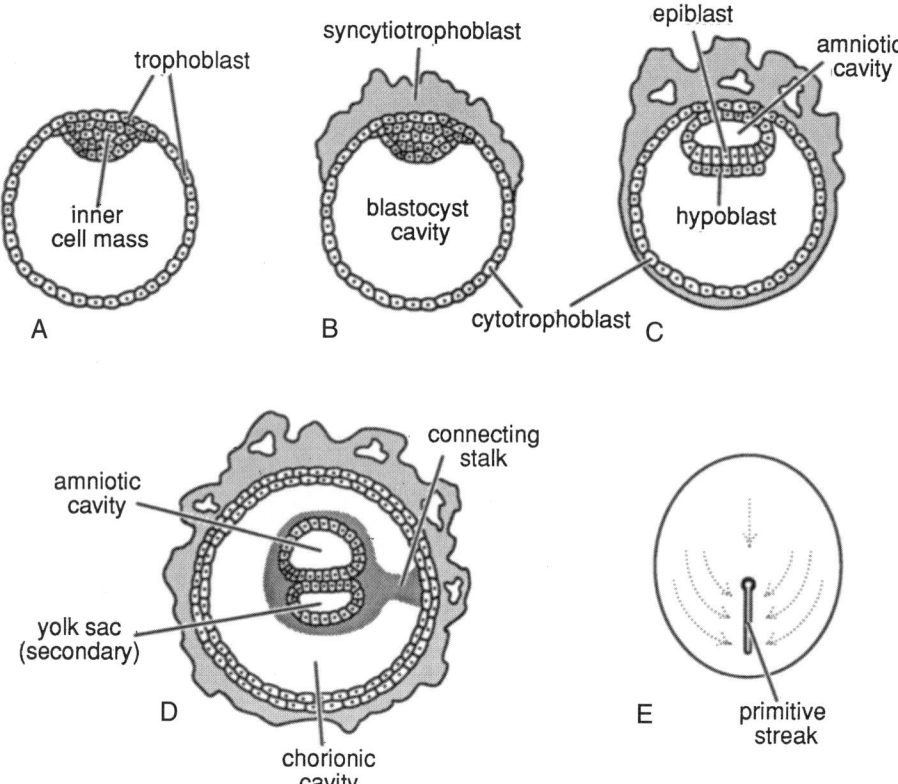

Figure 3–4. A, Blastocyst stage human embryo, exhibiting the inner cell mass as a regionalized mass of cells projecting into the blastocyst cavity. The cavity is surrounded by trophoblast cells. **B,** Slightly older blastocyst than seen in **A.** At this time, the inner cell mass and trophoblast cells are capped by cells of the syncytiotrophoblast, which are buried in the endometrial stroma (not shown). The cellular layer of trophoblast is now called the cytotrophoblast. **C,** An older blastocyst stage human embryo. The cavity is now surrounded by a double-layered membrane, and the inner cell mass has developed into a bilayered embryonic disk capped by a cavity (amniotic cavity). **D,** This somewhat older, completely implanted embryo now exhibits cavities both above and below the embryonic disk, the amniotic cavity, and the yolk sac. No axial features are present in the disk at this time; cephalic and caudal regions cannot be discerned. **E,** Surface view of the embryonic disk, showing the primitive streak. This midline thickening of epiblast cells occurs during the early part of the third week after fertilization and produces a landmark (the primitive streak) that delineates the midline of the embryo and reveals the future cephalic and caudal ends. The thickening of epiblast cells in the midline (primitive streak) is actually an increased population of cells in this region, resulting from both a high mitotic rate in the midline and migration of a subpopulation of epiblast cells to a midline position. The arrows in this diagram indicate migration of the epiblast cells.

the bottom layer of flattened cells is called the primary endoderm or hypoblast (see Fig. 3–4C). Cells of the epiblast become organized into an epithelial disk, the progenitor of all embryonic tissues, as well as the extraembryonic mesoderm, amnion and yolk sac.[53] The cells forming the extraembryonic mesoderm apparently arise from the presumptive caudal end of the epiblast and coat the internal surface of the cytotrophoblast.[56] The extraembryonic mesoderm combined with the trophoblast constitutes the chorion. Even at this early stage of development, it is possible to determine that the surface of the epiblast adjacent to the trophoblast represents the dorsal side of the embryo.[57]

Rearrangement of some of the epiblast cells results in the formation of a small amniotic cavity.[58] It is unclear whether the amnion is derived from epiblast cells adjacent to the newly formed cavity[58] or from the cytotrophoblast.[59] Primary endoderm cells of the hypoblast proliferate and migrate onto the inner surface of the cytotrophoblast, forming the yolk sac or umbilical vesicle.[60] Therefore, by the end of the second week of development, the embryo consists of a circular bilaminar disk located between two fluid-filled cavities (Fig. 3–4C, D). At this time, no axial features are visible within the embryonic disk.

At the outset of the third week of development, dynamic cell movements result in extensive rearrangement of the epiblast cells. In most species, this period (called *gastrulation*) is charac-

terized by morphogenetic movements and the changes resulting from them. A midline thickening of the now elongated epiblast becomes visible, designating the future posterior end of the embryo.[53] This thickening is the primitive streak (see Fig. 3–4E). Cellular activity at the streak results in another fundamental process of morphogenesis, epithelial-mesenchymal transformation. This occurs when some epiblast cells enter the streak while others remain within the epiblast to become the embryonic ectoderm.[61] The transformation from epithelium to mesenchyme consists of a cascade of cellular dynamics, including loss of intercellular connections, cell shape changes, and eventual freedom from the confines of the epiblast. Thus, at the primitive streak, subsets of polarized epithelial cells within the epiblast transform into nonpolarized free cells termed *mesenchyme,* the second embryonic tissue. These events are thought to be mediated by modulation of adhesive molecules located on the cell surface[62] as well as by cytoskeletal rearrangements. In addition, variable expression of homeobox genes as well as of many other signaling molecules also occurs during gastrulation,[8] leading to patterning of axial and nonaxial structures

The primitive streak provides a means by which subsets of epiblast cells can ingress and be distributed to more ventral regions of the embryo as the endoderm and mesoderm.[61] The first cells through the streak probably represent the definitive embryonic endoderm. These are followed by a solid cord of cells, the notochordal process, which extends cranially from the streak. These cells form the notochord, which defines the axis of the embryo and plays a significant role in the induction of the nervous system. Studies suggest that the notochord is an important signaling center for organizing the embryo. It secretes several important morphogenetic signaling molecules such as retinoic acid and sonic hedgehog.[8, 62] Another important signaling center, the prechordal plate, forms just cranial to the notochord. The prechordal plate is an important organizing center for the head of the embryo.[8] Just cranial to the prechordal plate, the endoderm fuses to the to the overlying ectoderm. This region of fused ectoderm and endoderm is the site of the future mouth.[63] The remainder of the cells that pass through the streak become the intraembryonic mesoderm and come to lie between the endoderm and the ectoderm. Thus, the primitive streak provides the embryo with a means to organize epiblast cells, perhaps already partially fate-specified, into three primary germ layers—ectoderm, mesoderm, and endoderm.

As a consequence of cleavage and gastrulation, subpopulations of cells in various states of determination are brought together in new spatial relationships, which permits new tissue interactions. Subsequent histogenesis and organogenesis are driven by these tissue interactions, defined as the action of one dissimilar group of cells on another, resulting in the alteration of cell behavior of one of the component groups in a developmentally significant direction.[64] Tissue interactions often result in induction in which signals from one cell group mediate the change in developmental direction of another cell group that are competent to respond to the inductive signals. These interactions are mediated by a variety of signaling molecules such as growth factors, secreted factors, and transcription factors, secreted by cells and often concentrated in the extracellular matrix.[8]

EMBRYOLOGY OF THE ORGAN SYSTEMS

The following short account of the development of some of the major organs is designed to provide an idea about some of the complex processes that occur as the embryo is built from raw materials. It is an amazing and precisely timed process. That it happens properly in most conceptions is even more remarkable. For a much more complete account, several other excellent and current texts are recommended[8, 38, 63] as well as appropriate chapters in *Fetal and Neonatal Physiology*.

Nervous System (See Chapter 165)

The human nervous system begins to form about 18 days after fertilization,[64] making it the first of the organ systems to initiate development. It begins as a thickening of the ectodermal layer along the craniocaudal axis of the embryo in the area destined to become the cervical region (Fig. 3-5B). This thickening results from an increase in the height of the ectodermal cells as they change shape from cuboidal to tall columnar as well as from intercalatory movements within the local population of cells. The result is an oval or keyhole-shaped area of thickened ectoderm known as the *neural plate*. Two ridges of this neural plate on each side of the midline undergo accelerated growth giving rise to two longitudinal neural folds with a neural groove between. Before this folding, a mesencephalic flexure forms in the cranial portion of the neural plate.[63] This flexure demarcates the future prosencephalon, mesencephalon, and rhombencephalon. These neural folds increase in height, curve toward each other, touch, and fuse to form the rudiment of the neural tube midway along the embryonic axis (see Fig. 3-5B). This fusion then proceeds in both a cranial and caudal direction, as if two zipper fasteners were operating simultaneously but in different directions. The remaining unfused ends of the neural folds

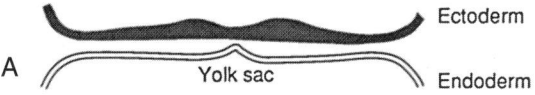

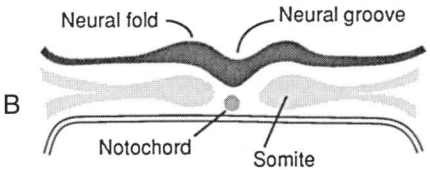

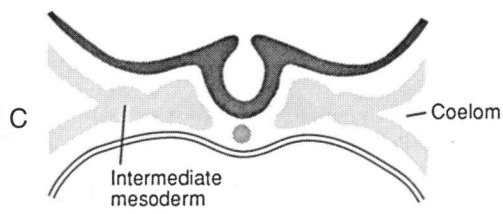

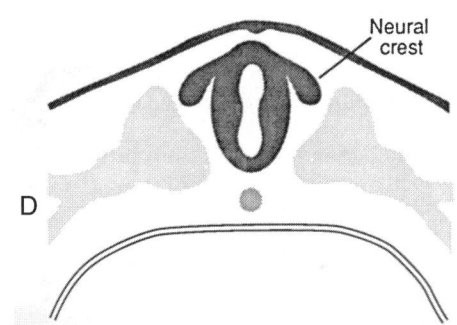

Figure 3-5. Development of the neural tube. Approximate ages: **A,** 15 days; **B,** 18 days; **C,** 20 days; **D,** 23 days. All sections are transverse, approximately midway along the embryonic axis. Note that although the neural tube is completely closed in the section shown in **D,** both the rostral and the caudal neuropores remain open in an embryo of this age. They do not close until near the end of the fourth week.

at each end of the embryo are called the *cranial* and *caudal neuropores* because the neural tube is open at these sites. The cranial neuropore closes on day 25 and the caudal neuropore on day 27 of development.[64] This folding and shaping of the neural tube occur through both intrinsic (cell cycle, cell shape) and extrinsic (proliferation of adjacent tissue) mechanisms.[66, 67] Shortly after fusion of the neural folds in a given region of the embryo, the neural tube separates from the ectoderm and becomes buried in the mesenchyme below the surface.

During this process of neural tube formation, an epithelial-mesenchymal transformation occurs, resulting in formation of a group of cells derived from the crests of the neural folds. These neural crest cells come to lie on the superolateral margins of the tube. The neural tube proper goes on to form the central nervous system, which consists of the brain and spinal cord, whereas the neural crest forms much of the peripheral nervous system, consisting of portions of autonomic, cranial, and spinal ganglia and

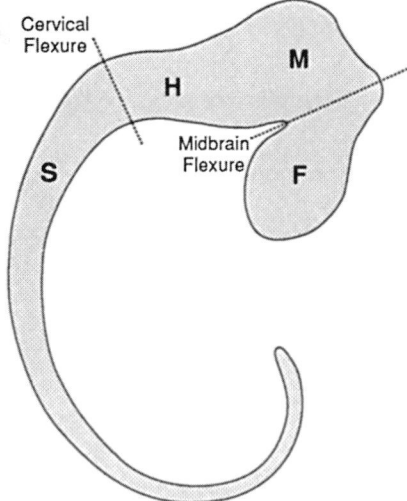

Figure 3–6. Lateral view of the isolated central nervous system of a 28- to 30-day embryo, showing the two flexures and the resulting divisions of the brain and spinal cord at this age. F = forebrain; M = midbrain; H = hindbrain; S = spinal cord.

nerves. The lumen of the neural tube becomes the central canal of the spinal cord and the ventricles of the brain.

Further Development of the Central Nervous System

The spinal cord develops from that part of the neural tube caudal to the cervical flexure, one of two unambiguous bends in an embryo about 30 days old that give the embryonic axis a C-shaped profile in lateral views (Fig. 3-6). The wall of the tube thickens and soon stratifies into a ventricular zone that borders the central canal, an intermediate zone, and a marginal zone. The intermediate zone is actually created by migration of neurons from the ventricular zone. These neurons then send out processes that create the marginal zone, later to become the white matter of the cord.

Proliferation of the cells of these zones is greatly influenced by the somites, mesodermal structures that lie lateral to the neural tube along its craniocaudal axis. Later the roof and floor of the neural tube become thin while the lateral walls thicken. Experiments performed in animals show that this particular organization around the circumference of the neural tube is under the influence of an inductive substance from the somites.[68] Experimental manipulation of the number, size, or position of somites influences the cross-sectional profile of the tube, including the keyhole-shaped profile of the neural canal (Fig. 3-7).

The sulcus limitans is a groove that divides the more dorsal alar plate from the ventral basal plate. The former develops into the dorsal gray horns associated with sensory (afferent) input. The basal plate gives rise to the ventral and lateral gray horns, which function in motor (efferent) output. The floor plate secretes morphogenetic molecules (e.g., retinoic acid, sonic hedgehog), which control the patterning of dorsal sensory and ventral motor elements.[8,69]

The spinal cord extends the entire length of the developing vertebral column during the embryonic period. The spinal cord grows more slowly than the vertebral column, however, so that in the fetal period and beyond, these two structures change position with respect to each other. At 24 weeks, the spinal cord extends caudally to the level of the S1 vertebral body. In the newborn, it extends to L3, and in the adult to L1. This is important clinically with respect to spinal taps and other procedures that require knowledge about where the cord ends.

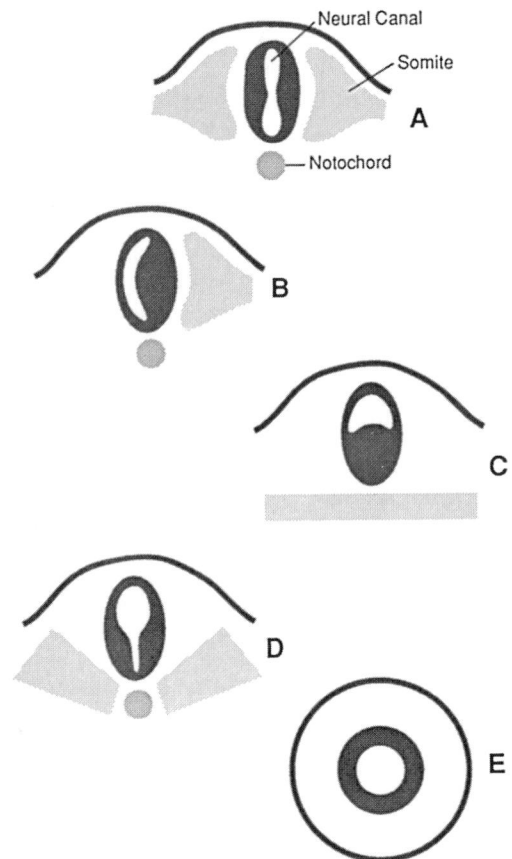

Figure 3–7. Influence of somite mesoderm *(lightly stippled areas)* **on neural tube and neural canal shape. A,** Normal. **B,** One somite removed. **C,** Somite mesoderm transplanted to the ventral surface of the neural tube. **D,** Somite mesoderm transplanted to the ventrolateral surface of the neural tube. **E,** Complete absence of somite mesoderm. Clear areas between structures contain nonsomite mesoderm. (Modified from Saxen L, Toivonen S: Primary Embryonic Induction. London, Logos Press, 1962.)

The brain is divided into forebrain (prosencephalon), midbrain (mesencephalon), and hindbrain (rhombencephalon) when the midbrain flexure appears (see Fig. 3-6). These three divisions of the brain quickly become five by the partitioning of the forebrain into telencephalon and diencephalon and the separation of the hindbrain into metencephalon and myelencephalon. The formation of divisions and their adult derivatives are summarized in Table 3-2. Apparently there are two distinct signaling centers that organize the cranial portion of the neural tube. One organizes the forebrain and the other the hindbrain; each produces its own set of signaling factors. Another important source of signaling molecules for brain regionalization comes from the midbrain/hindbrain signaling center.[8]

The Eye (See Chapter 175)

At about 4 weeks' development, two outpouchings of the forebrain (diencephalon) expand laterally to form the optic vesicles (Fig. 3-8*A*, *B*), progenitors of the eye. Inductive interaction takes place between the optic vesicles and the head ectoderm, which lies closest to the vesicles.[70] The first manifestation of this interaction is the formation of a thickened plate in the head ectoderm, the lens placode (see Fig. 3-8*B*). At about the same time, the lateral surface of the optic vesicles begins to invaginate to form

TABLE 3-2

Brain Vesicles and Their Derivatives

Early Divisions	Later Divisions	Wall Derivatives	Lumen Derivatives
Forebrain (prosencephalon)	Telencephalon	Cerebral hemispheres	Lateral ventricles, rostral part of 3rd ventricle
	Diencephalon	Epithalamus, thalamus, hypothalamus, pineal	Most of 3rd ventricle
Midbrain (metencephalon)	Mesencephalon	Midbrain	Cerebral aqueduct
Hindbrain (rhombencephalon)	Metencephalon	Pons, cerebellum	Superior part of 4th ventricle
	Myelencephalon	Medulla	Inferior part of 4th ventricle

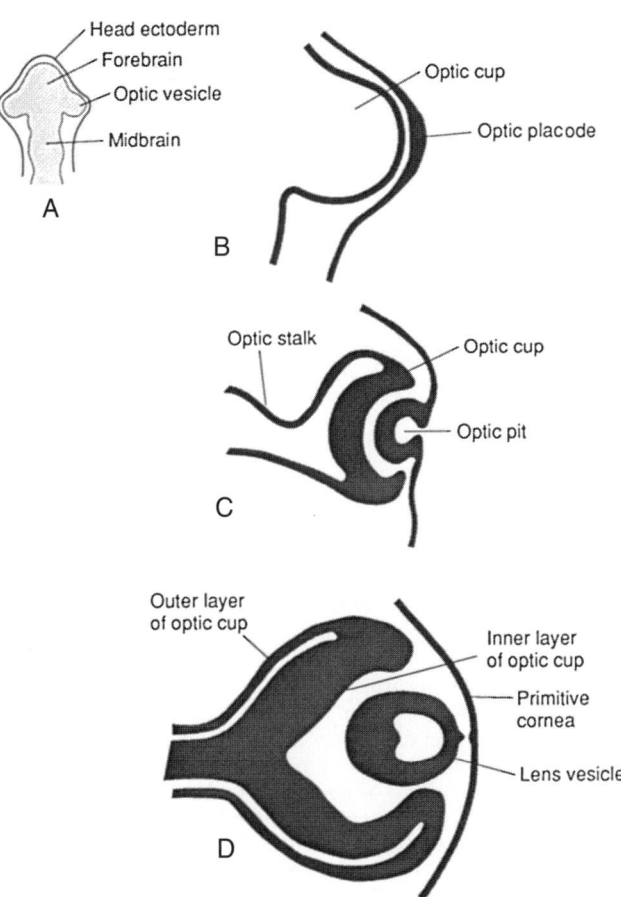

Figure 3–8. Development of the eye. A, Dorsal view showing the head, optic vesicles, and overlying head ectoderm. **B–D,** Magnified view of the right optic vesicle at successively older stages, illustrating the development of the lens placode, pit and vesicle, and the optic cup.

the double-layered optic cup. The lens placode also invaginates creating a lens pit (see Fig. 3-8C). The pit continues to deepen as it follows the profile of the increasingly concave optic cup. Finally the deeply pitted placode pinches off, forming the lens vesicle (Fig. 3-8D). By this time point (around 30 days), the double walls of the optic cup appose each other; fusion of these two layers is completed during the fetal period. The inner layer forms the neural retina, and the outer becomes the pigment epithelium of the retina. The peripheral margin of the optic cup forms the iris

and ciliary apparatus, whereas the optic nerve is formed from the optic stalk. Mesoderm surrounding the optic cup forms the inner vascular choroid and the fibrous outer sclera.

The Ear (See Chapter 176)

Development of the inner ear begins in the fourth week after fertilization as a recognizable thickening of surface ectoderm on either side of the myelencephalon, known as the otic placode (Fig. 3-9A). Similar to the lens vesicle, the placode invaginates (otic pit, see Fig. 3-9B) and pinches off to form the otic vesicle (see Fig. 3-9C). Small diverticula soon bud from each vesicle to form the endolymphatic sac. As growth of the hollow vesicle proceeds, additional regional morphogenesis yields the utricle, semicircular ducts, saccule, and cochlear ducts as well as other sensory receptors and primary sensory neurons (see Fig. 3-9C).

Cardiovascular System (See Chapters 61 and 62)

Heart

Cells destined to form the primitive heart tube are located within two oval areas of mesoderm (Fig. 3-10) on either side of the midline of the embryo.[71,73] Organized as discrete clusters of cells between the ectodermal and endodermal layers, this precardiac mesoderm migrates cranially and fuses in the midline just cranial to the oral membrane. The cell clusters form two more-or-less parallel solid cords of cells on reaching the area just forward of the oral plate (see Fig. 3-10). These soon canalize to form endocardial tubes. The tubes swing together because of lateral body folding and fuse to form the primitive heart tube, which then undergoes additional growth, morphogenesis, and changes in position with time. Initially the primitive chambers of the heart tube are arranged in a linear series with inflow at the caudal end and outflow at the cranial end.

The heart begins beating about 22 days after fertilization, and weak circulatory movement of fluid begins in adjacent vessels about a day later. At this time, the embryo can be compared to an aggregate of cells about $1 \times 1 \times 2$ mm. Tissue culture studies indicate that cells in the center of a mass thicker than about 0.5 mm die of oxygen deprivation because the simple diffusion of oxygen into the core is not sufficient to support cell metabolism. Thus, it appears that the formation of a functional circulatory system is a requisite for the continued life of the embryo. Indeed, the circulatory system is the first organ system to become functional in the human embryo.[75]

There is good evidence from animal experiments that the first contractions of the embryonic heart are initiated by stretching of the heart tube as fluid pressure builds in the developing circulatory system. Isolated hearts do not begin beating on time, unless

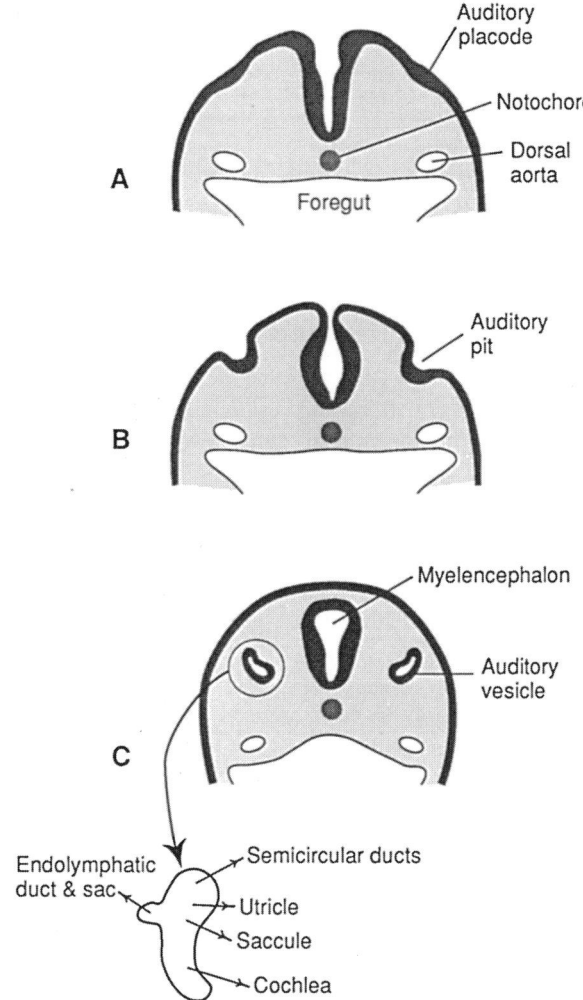

Figure 3–9. Successively older stages (**A–C**) showing development of the inner ear from the auditory placode. Derivative adult structures are shown in the inset in **C.**

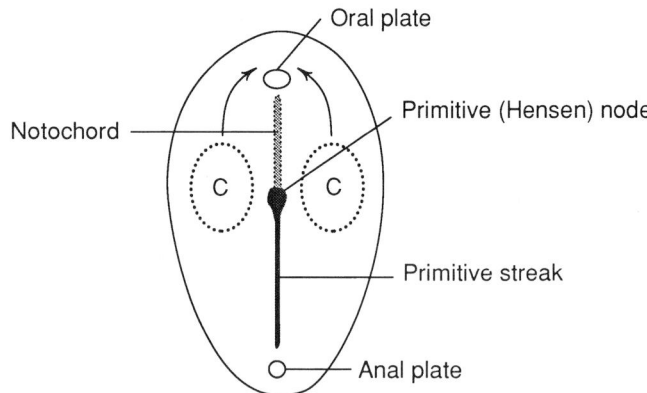

Figure 3–10. Surface view of an embryo at about 16 to 17 days after fertilization. This view is of the ectodermal surface. Structures below the surface are outlined with dotted lines. The anal and oral plates are areas where the ectoderm and endoderm are in tight contact, similar to a "spot weld," with no mesoderm between. Mesoderm is present in other areas. At *C* lie the mesodermal cell clusters that migrate *(arrows)* to an area forward of the oral plate, to form the cardiogenic cords. These two oval areas contain precardiac mesoderm cells.

artificially produced fluid pressure is maintained within the lumen of the heart. Moreover, the heart in intact embryos can be induced to begin beating earlier than normal by the introduction of small amounts of fluid into the lumen, thus increasing intraluminal pressure and causing stretching of the walls of the heart.[76,77]

Almost as soon as the primitive heart tube forms, sulci on its external surface deepen markedly. This begins a process called *cardiac looping,* in which the inflow and outflow regions are brought into approximation. The mechanisms behind the control of looping are poorly understood.

Several concurrent events occur after looping that lead to partitioning of the heart into separate chambers and outflow channels. The sinus venosus, which initially receives all incoming venous blood from the embryo, is remodeled so that all blood enters what will later become the right atrium. Resorption of the sinus venosus forms the smooth area of the definitive right atrium and contributes to atrial septation. Much of the definitive left atrium is formed by resorption of the pulmonary veins.

Separation of the atria begins during week 5 when a sickle-shaped membrane, the septum primum, grows from the roof of the atrium toward the atrioventricular canal. This canal is simultaneously being divided into right and left channels by the fusion of the enlarging superior and inferior endocardial cushions. The opening between right and left sides of the common atrium, now partially divided by the growing septum primum, is called the *foramen* (or *osteum*) *primum.*

Soon the lower edges of the septum primum fuse with the endocardial cushions, and further growth of both the septum and the cushions closes the foramen primum. Before it closes completely, however, several perforations appear in the superior portion of the septum primum. These perforations fuse to form the foramen secundum. Thus, communication between the right and left atrial cavities is maintained during this complex morphogenetic process.

Another septum (the septum secundum) begins to form at about the time the foramen secundum becomes well defined. This septum forms to the right of the septum primum as a crescentic ridge. Further growth produces a thick membrane, but the oval opening in this membrane persists as the foramen ovale. This arrangement of two parallel septa (primum and secundum) with offset holes (secundum and ovale) produces a flap valve between the two atria, ensuring unidirectional flow of blood from right to left.

Fusion of the endocardial cushions (composed of cardiac mesenchyme) forms the septum intermedium. This not only divides the atrioventricular canal into right and left portions but also acts as a central attachment point and reference center for several septation events as already described. The cushion tissue of the septum intermedium contributes to the formation of the membranous portion of the interventricular septum as well as the development of the atrioventricular valves and to the fibrous cardiac skeleton. It is also a fusion point for the cushion tissue derived ridges, which divide the proximal outflow region of the heart.

Even though the heart is enlarging while septation proceeds, the dimensions in this central region around the septum intermedium remain constant. A significant enlargement in this region at this time could lead to congenital heart defects.

Partitioning of the ventricle is primarily accomplished by fusion of trabeculae, which form a muscular interventricular septum. Ventricular septation is completed by formation of the membranous portion of the septum from an outgrowth of endocardial cushion tissue. This occurs simultaneously with division of the proximal outflow area. Initially, there is no direct communication between the right atrium and the right ventricle. Remodeling activities in the inner curvature of the heart create this communication via mechanisms which are still obscure

Division of the outflow tract is complex and still not completely understood. The proximal portion of the outflow tract is

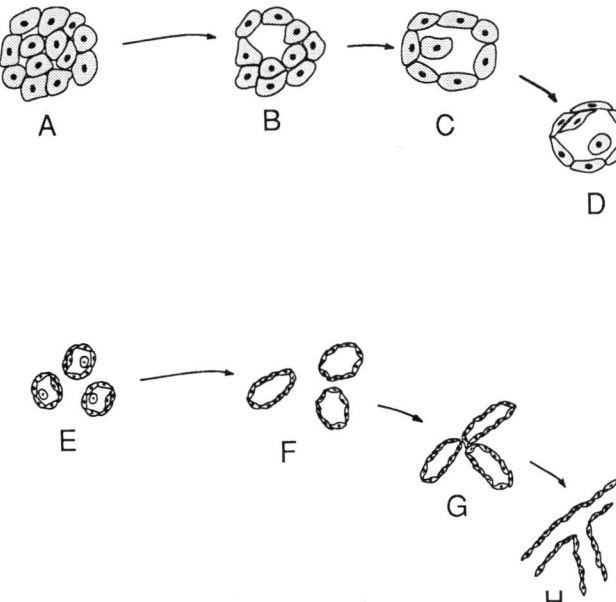

Figure 3–11. Vasculogenesis. A–D, Formation of hollow blood islands from solid clusters of angioblasts. **E–H,** Formation of a portion of a primitive vascular network by fusion of blood islands. Budding (not shown) also contributes to vascular pattern growth.

subdivided into the conus and truncus regions, both of which are divided into left and right halves by ridges of endocardial cushion tissue called the conotruncal or bulbar ridges. Septation of the conus region forms an outflow segment for each ventricle, whereas in the truncus region distinct aortic and pulmonary valves develop. A portion of the conal septum extends down and attaches to the muscular interventricular septum, partially closing the interventricular foramen. Complete closure of the foramen is accomplished by down-growth of cushion tissue from the septum intermedium. In the distal outflow tract (the aortic sac), a wedge of mesenchyme (the aorticopulmonary septum) develops between the fourth and sixth aortic arches. This mesenchyme (thought to be of neural crest origin[78]) grows downward, penetrates, and fuses with the conotruncal ridges.

Vessels

During the third week of development, groups of extraembryonic mesodermal cells in the yolk sac and chorion, known as *angioblasts,* aggregate to form isolated, solid masses called *angioblastic clusters* or *blood islands.* These soon cavitate (Fig. 3–11), and those cells on the periphery of the hollow blood islands differentiate into endothelial cells. Blood cells are formed from those angioblasts remaining in the lumen, as well as by cell division and budding from the primitive endothelial lining. Growth and fusion of the isolated hollow blood islands form tubes, and the tubes fuse to form long interconnected channels. Lateral buds from tubes and channels may also extend the developing vasculature into adjacent areas.

This sequence, based on observations of sectioned embryos, explains how vessels form. It does not explain how the pattern of vessels develops. Little is known concerning how the intricate pattern of anastomosing vessels is established in the early embryo.

The Musculoskeletal System (See Chapter 181)

Muscular System

The three types of muscle tissue (skeletal, smooth, and cardiac) are largely derived from cells of the mesodermal germ layer.

Skeletal muscle forms from paraxial mesoderm, whereas cardiac muscle is a derivative of splanchnic mesoderm. Most smooth muscle is derived from splanchnic mesoderm. However, it seems likely that all mesenchyme, whether derived from mesoderm or from neural crest (as in head mesenchyme), has the potential to form vascular smooth muscle. The dilator and sphincter smooth muscles of the iris as well as the myoepithelial cells that surround sweat glands and mammary glands are thought to be of neural crest origin.

Skeletal Muscle. Mesenchyme cells that are to develop into skeletal muscle elongate and lose their multiple processes. The earliest cell that can be identified as a skeletal muscle precursor is a fusiform cell called a *myoblast* (Fig. 3–12). These cells become postmitotic and fuse into cylindric, multinucleated myotubes. These myotubes start producing actin and myosin myofilaments, which adds to girth. Growth of myotubes may also occur by fusion of additional myoblasts. The skeletal muscles of the head and neck develop from paraxial mesoderm represented by somitomeres in the early embryo. Trunk musculature is derived from the myotome portion of the somites (Fig. 3–13).

Somites themselves are interesting structures—serially repeated paired blocks of condensed (closely packed) paraxial mesoderm cells. About 44 pairs of somites eventually develop in humans, beginning between days 19 and 21.[64] These can be seen in a surface view of the embryo because they produce bulges in the overlying sheet of ectoderm. Each member of a pair of somites lies lateral to the neural tube (see Fig. 3–13). Myoblasts of the myotome portion of each somite divide and spread out deep to the embryonic skin, where they form the musculature. Various morphologic processes including fusion, tangential splitting of layers, reorientation of muscle fibers, and formation of tendon intersections are responsible for the final morphologic form of the named muscles.

The musculature of the limb is also derived from the myotome portion of the somites. These myoblasts migrate into the elongating limb buds and arrange into dorsal and ventral muscle masses, which later become subdivided into the definitive limb muscles.

Cardiac Muscle. This type of muscle develops from splanchnic mesoderm adjacent to the pericardial or transverse portion of the intraembryonic coelom. Myocardial precursor cells undergo mass migration and do not fuse to form myotubes. Rather, the myoblasts differentiate as discrete cells, with closely applied end-to-end junctions, which persist as the adult intercalated disk. They form a layer around the endothelial tube of the heart, which eventually becomes the myocardial or muscular wall of the heart.

Smooth Muscle. Smooth muscle cells form from myoblasts derived primarily from splanchnic mesoderm (see Fig. 3–12).

Skeletal System (See Chapter 178)

Cartilage develops from mesodermally derived mesenchyme except in some areas of the head and neck, where it is of neural crest origin. Chondroblasts aggregate, condense, and begin to produce collagen fibers and ground substance. In the embryo, bone tissue is formed in two distinct ways, depending on the site and type of bone growth. The first consists of *de novo* bone formation, in which mesoderm cells (or, in the case of some skull bones, neural crest cells) first condense (pack) into sheets or membranes. Cells in these sheets then differentiate into osteoblasts, which secrete prebone or osteoid. Osteoid is the extracellular matrix onto which hydroxyapatite crystals (a unique calcium phosphate mineral) form. Once the mineral is present and integrated into the collagen of the matrix, the tissue is considered to be bone. This type of bone formation is called intramembranous ossification because the osteogenesis occurs within these sheets or membranes of condensed mesenchyme. Some of the bones of the cranial vault, face, and jaws form in this way.

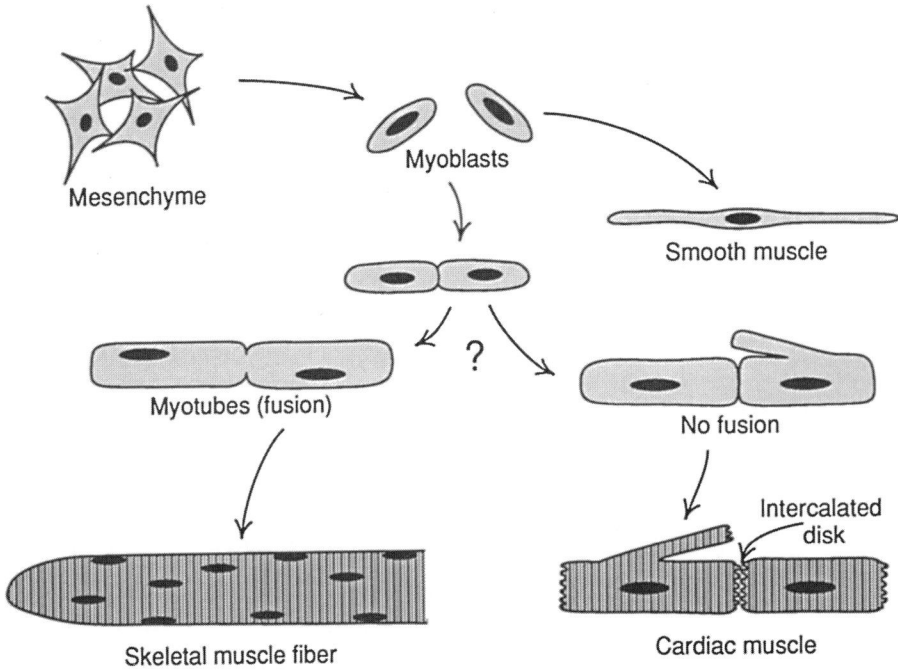

Figure 3–12. Schematic representation of the development of the three types of muscle cells (skeletal, smooth, and cardiac). Some question exists regarding the precursor cells—that is, it currently seems likely that mesenchyme gives rise to a cell type that develops into cardiac and smooth muscle, but that it gives rise to another cell type that develops into skeletal muscle.

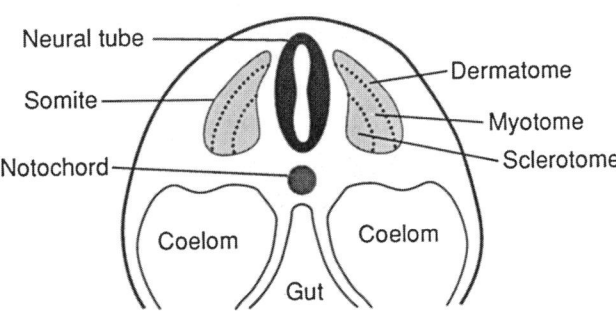

Figure 3–13. Fate map of the somite, showing regions from which cells developing into dermis, muscle, and cartilage and bone are derived.

The second manner in which bone forms in the embryo is called *endochondral ossification.* As implied by the name, bone forms in this case only in sites where preexisting cartilage models are found. The cartilage does not turn into bone. Rather, bone replaces the preexisting cartilage model in a sequence of steps, as follows. Cartilage cells hypertrophy and calcify in an area where bone is to form, that is, they become large and undergo metabolic changes, which lead to infiltration of the surrounding cartilage extracellular matrix with insoluble calcium salts. In this way, the cartilage cells become partitioned from their surroundings by an environment that is presumed to cut off their supply of oxygen and nutrients, and they die. At the same time, local osteoblasts begin to produce osteoid, which then becomes mineralized as described in intramembranous ossification. Once bone has formed in the embryo, it can be remodeled by changes in the balance between addition of more bone by osteoblasts and removal of bone by osteoclasts.

Respiratory System (See Chapter 76)

During the fourth week of development, the embryo forms the shape of a C, and the primitive gastrointestinal tube is already divided into a foregut, midgut, and hindgut (Fig. 3–14). A groove, the respiratory (laryngotracheal) diverticulum, arises as an evagination of the ventral surface of the foregut, close to the region

destined later to become the stomach. As the foregut elongates a wedge of mesoderm, the tracheoesophageal septum, separates the foregut (portion that will become esophagus) from the future lungs. This early association of developing lung and stomach leads to the occasional finding of ectopic lung and cartilage tissue near the esophageal-gastric junction.[79]

The respiratory diverticulum grows caudally and soon splits into two bronchial buds. Each of these buds subdivides to form primitive secondary or lobar bronchi. On the left side, two secondary bronchi supply the developing superior and inferior lobes of the left lung. On the right, the inferior secondary bronchus divides into two, providing a total of three secondary bronchi to supply the three lobes on this side. The third-order branches form the bronchopulmonary segments. Altogether, about 17 generations of branches form. Differentiation of the respiratory passages begins in the fetal stage and proceeds from distal to proximal along the branches of the respiratory diverticulum. Alveolar formation begins towards the end of the fetal period and continues until 2 to 3 years of age.[53]

It should be noted that the endoderm of the foregut gives rise to the epithelial lining of the trachea, bronchi, and lungs, including the alveoli. The surrounding splanchnic mesoderm develops into the cartilage and fibrous connective tissue of the larger airways as well as the blood vessels and supporting tissues of the smaller airways and alveoli.

Digestive System (See Chapters 108 and 109)

The lining of the gastrointestinal tube primarily arises from endoderm, whereas the muscle coats and connective tissue elements are usually derived from splanchnic mesoderm. Toward the end of the third week the embryo folds craniocaudally and laterally, forming a inner gut tube of endoderm that is subdivided into the foregut, midgut (still connected to the degenerating yolk sac), and the hindgut.

Oral Cavity and Anal Regions

Throughout most of the developing gastrointestinal tube, the epithelium and derivative glands arise from the endodermal germ layer, which lines the foregut, midgut, and hindgut (see Fig. 3–14). However, cranial to the foregut and caudal to the hindgut, the relationship of embryonic structure to adult deriva-

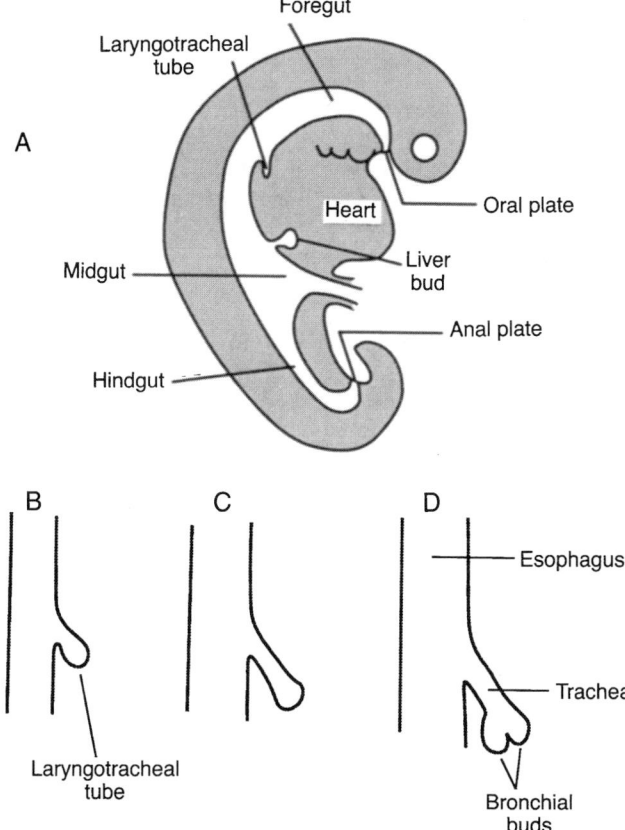

Figure 3–14. Development of the respiratory system. The laryngotracheal (respiratory) tube buds off from the ventral surface of the foregut, as shown in **A.** The tube elongates and splits into two bronchial buds (**B–D**), each of which ultimately gives rise to the epithelial lining of one lung.

tives is less obvious. For example, the oral membrane, which is a fusion of ectoderm and endoderm, is the cranial boundary of the foregut (in the adult this boundary is at the level of the tonsillar fauces). The oral cavity develops cranial to the oral membrane from an ectodermal depression, the stomodeum, bounded by the first pharyngeal arch and the frontal process. Three groups of salivary glands develop in this region. The sublingual and submaxillary glands develop from endoderm, as might be expected, but the parotid is derived from head ectoderm.[38] Similarly, structures below the pectinate line in the adult anal canal are derivatives of the proctodeum, an ectodermal depression in the caudal end of the embryo that is sealed off from the gut tube by the anal plate until the end of the eighth or beginning of the ninth week. Thus, the anal columns (of Morgagni), located above the pectinate line are of endodermal origin, whereas the anocutaneous (white) line and surrounding epithelial structures are from ectoderm.

Liver (See Chapter 118)

The hepatic diverticulum (or liver bud) arises as an outpouching of the lumen of the distal foregut during the fourth week of development (see Fig. 3–14). The liver bud gives rise to the gallbladder and bile ducts as well as to the parenchyma of the liver. The liver bud grows toward the anterior body wall, at first completely buried in the mesenchyme of the septum transversum. Rapid growth causes the liver bud to bulge into the abdominal cavity, freeing it on all but the cephalic surface. There, it remains in contact with the septum transversum as the latter forms part of the diaphragm. After development is complete, this area of contact between the liver and diaphragm is known as the "bare

area of the liver" because it is not covered with capsule or peritoneum.

The liver is connected on its anterior surface to the anterior body wall by the ventral mesentery that becomes the falciform ligament. The hepatocytes are derived from endoderm, as are the bile canaliculi and the epithelial linings of the intrahepatic biliary ducts. The liver sinusoids, larger blood vessels, and connective tissue stroma of the liver are all derived from the mesenchyme of the septum transversum which is of mesodermal origin.

Pancreas (See Chapter 114)

Most of the pancreas develops from the dorsal pancreatic bud, which arises as an outpouch of the dorsal surface of the future duodenum at the caudal end of the foregut. It grows into the mesenchyme of the dorsal mesentery at this site. The ventral pancreatic bud starts as an outgrowth of the future common bile duct, but it fuses with the dorsal pancreatic bud when rotation of the gut brings these two components of the pancreas into contact. Both exocrine and endocrine (islets of Langerhans) elements of the pancreas are derived from endoderm, whereas the blood vessels and connective tissue components arise from splanchnic mesoderm.

Esophagus

The esophagus is a short regional specialization of the embryonic foregut tube that elongates with growth of the body. During the middle of the embryonic period, its lumen is obliterated by proliferation of the endoderm derived lining cells, but cell death (a normal developmental process in many areas of the human embryo) reestablishes the lumen by early fetal life.

Stomach

The stomach begins as a simple fusiform dilation of the foregut. Growth of the dorsal wall of the stomach surpasses that of the ventral wall, leading to the greater curvature and driving a clockwise rotation of the gut that brings the greater curvature (original dorsal surface) to the left and the lesser curvature (original ventral surface) to the right. As a result of differential growth, the cardiac region (cranial) of the stomach moves inferiorly and to the left and the pyloric (caudal) end moves superiorly and to the right. Ultimately, this results in the almost horizontal axis seen in the adult stomach.

Duodenum

The duodenum develops from both the caudal end of the foregut and the cranial end of the midgut. It rapidly elongates into a loop the bend of which is toward the ventral body wall. As the stomach rotates to the right, so does the duodenal loop, bringing it to lie against the dorsal wall of the body cavity. There, it fuses with the dorsal wall and most of it comes to lie in a retroperitoneal position. Similar to the esophagus, the duodenal lumen is transiently obliterated by growth of the endoderm-derived lining cells until the beginning of the fetal period.

Lower Gastrointestinal Tract

Much of the remaining gastrointestinal tube (jejunum, ileum, cecum, ascending colon, and half of the transverse colon) develops from the midgut. The elongating midgut also forms a distinct loop the of which is closest to the anterior body wall. This U-shaped loop herniates (normally) into the extraembryonic coelom of the umbilical cord. While herniated, the loop rotates 90° counterclockwise. Thus, the cranial branch of the U-shaped loop moves to the right. At the same time, growth and elongation create several additional subloops in the cranial portion of the U-shaped loop; these later give rise to the jejunum and ileum.

The herniated small intestine with its subloops returns to the body cavity first. As the large intestine follows, it rotates an additional 180°, bringing the cecum and appendix to their final position in the lower right quadrant of the abdomen.[80] Little is known about how these complex morphogenetic events are controlled. Nevertheless, a thorough knowledge of these events as they occur in a normal embryo can help to explain the numerous anatomic variations and congenital malformations that have been observed. The hindgut contributes to the distal half of the transverse colon, the descending and sigmoid colon, the rectum, and the anal canal down to the white line.

Urinary System (See Chapter 125)

Near the end of the third week after fertilization, the intermediate mesoderm appears as a solid cord of condensed mesenchyme just lateral to the paraxial (somite forming) mesoderm (see Fig. 3-5C). The intermediate mesoderm is bilateral and extends along the length of the body axis as far as the somites do; it gives rise to components of the urinary and genital system.

The intermediate mesoderm is displaced ventrally to a position lateral to the dorsal aorta and notochord when the embryo becomes tubular, owing to growth and formation of the lateral body folds. During this movement, the connection between the somites and intermediate mesoderm is broken. Once this connection is lost, the two bars of intermediate mesoderm are called nephrogenic cords.

The traditional description of kidney development suggests that three successive sets of kidneys form in the embryo—the pronephros, mesonephros, and metanephros. The concept of a pronephros, however, is not relevant to development of humans.[81] Beginning at the level of the eighth or ninth somite,[82] the mesonephric kidney contains primitive tubules associated with glomeruli that empty into a mesonephric (wolffian) duct. The cephalic tubules begin to degenerate even before the more caudal tubules are starting their development. In males, the mesonephric duct becomes associated with the primitive gonad and gives rise to the epididymis, ductus deferens, and ejaculatory ducts; some of the mesonephric tubules persist as the efferent ductules. In females, the mesonephric duct distal to the ureteric bud degenerates. The mesonephros actively produces urine as early as the sixth week of development and continues into the early fetal period.

During the fifth week, the metanephros begins as a small diverticulum near the caudal end of the mesonephric duct—the ureteric bud. The mesoderm at the caudal aspect of the nephrogenic cord condenses around the ureteric bud, forming a metanephric blastema. The ureteric bud plus the metanephric blastema form the metanephric or definitive kidney (see Fig. 3-1A). The nephron from the renal corpuscle to the collecting duct is derived from the metanephric blastema whereas the collecting system and ureter are derived from the ureteric bud. Development of the metanephric kidney depends on mutual inductive signals from the metanephric blastema and the ureteric bud.[68] Signals from the bud result in mesenchymal-epithelial transformation of the metanephric blastema mesenchyme leading to formation of an epithelial vesicle. The vesicle remodels into a tubule, the proximal end of which attaches to the ureteric bud, whereas the distal end becomes associated with vascular precursors of the glomerulus. Signals from the metanephric mesoderm cause the ureteric bud to branch, forming the collecting system. If, for some reason, the ureteric bud does not grow to meet the metanephric blastema, the blastema does not develop nephrons, and renal agenesis results. If the blastema is absent, the ureteric bud does not develop into the collecting system of the kidney.[83]

By the end of the first trimester, the fetal kidneys begin to produce urine.[84] At that time, they have been displaced from their initial pelvic location to the abdomen, and they lie in a retroperitoneal position close to the adrenal glands. The latter develop from coelomic mesoderm (cortex) and neural crest cells (medulla) that have become associated in the abdominal cavity, cephalic to the final position of the kidneys.

The urogenital sinus is an endoderm-lined cavity from which are derived the epithelium of the urinary bladder, all of the female urethra, and most of the male urethra. The muscular coats and connective tissue elements of all these structures are of splanchnic mesoderm origin.

GROWTH AND MATURATION OF THE EMBRYO AND FETUS

Human embryonic development is a continuous process that averages 266 days, or $9\frac{1}{2}$ months, when counted from the day of fertilization. Clinically, the start of gestation is determined by counting from the date of the last menstrual period (LMP). Estimated this way, it averages 280 days or 10 lunar months.[85] Human prenatal development is commonly divided into two periods or phases: the embryonic period and the fetal period (Fig. 3-15). The first 8 weeks after fertilization is the embryonic period. It has been subdivided into 23 developmental stages (Carnegie stages).[53] During the embryonic period, the sinlge-celled zygote is transformed into an embryo. With respect to human embryology, the term embryo means "an unborn human in the first 8 weeks" from fertilization.[53] This period is characterized by several developmental milestones, including cell division of the zygote, formation of a blastocyst, implantation, formation of three primary germ layers, segmentation and axis formation, and initial morphogenesis of organ systems.

It is believed that during the first 2 weeks of development, the embryo is relatively insensitive to the action of agents that cause congenital malformations (teratogens). Retrospective human studies as well as studies in animals suggest that low-to-medium dose of teratogens will not cause abnormal development during the first 2 weeks, but a large dose will kill the embryo. In this 2-week period, defects may develop after treatment with the teratogenic agent, which for some reason remains available to the embryo throughout the period, for example, because of slow metabolism or excretion. The third to eighth week of development is when morphogenesis of most organ systems begins, and for many systems, ends. It is during this portion of the embryonic period that the organs, and therefor the embryo as a whole, are most sensitive to the actions of teratogens. For example, a kidney fails to develop only if, during morphogenesis, the ureteric bud fails to send the proper signals to the metanephric blastema. Moreover, a limb is abnormally foreshortened only if long bones fail to form during that time when the bony elements are due to undergo their primary morphogenesis. Therefore, the third to eighth week of the embryonic period corresponds to the sensitive period in human development with regard to the action of teratogenic agents.

During the fetal period (beyond the end of the eighth week after fertilization or beyond the tenth week of post-LMP pregnancy; see Fig. 3-15), the fetus becomes increasingly resistant to the action of teratogens. This does not mean that no organ system can become malformed during fetal life. An example of such an organ is the brain, which exhibits the longest developmental period of any organ; it continues both physical and functional development throughout the fetal period and beyond, well after birth.[86] This extended period of development also extends its susceptibility; more major congenital defects occur in the brain than any other organ.[87]

Organ systems other than the brain also continue morphogenesis into the fetal period (e.g., palate, ear, external genitalia, lungs). In contrast to the brain, however, most other organ systems essentially complete morphogenesis by the end of the embryonic period.

The fetal period is characterized by rapid growth in weight and size of the conceptus as a whole (Fig. 3-16), which reflects growth in individual organs. All organs expand and undergo histogenesis, or differentiation of the cell populations of which they are composed, but the particular pattern of increase in weight may vary from organ to organ. Hematopoiesis begins in the liver

Figure 3–15. Human development. The upper portion of the figure shows human development divided into periods. The embryonic period extends from fertilization through week 8. The remainder of pregnancy (week 9 through birth) is termed the fetal period. The perinatal period extends from the prenatal week 22 until 4 weeks after birth. The neonatal period is the first 4 weeks after birth. In the bottom portion of the figure, the ages of the embryo/fetus are shown in two time scales. The lower of the two is a clinical scale, with *pregnancy* counted from the date of the last menstrual period. Above it are weeks and months of *development*, counted from fertilization. Note that there is a 2-week difference, with pregnancy lasting 40 weeks. (Modified from Kaplan S: Congenital Defects—An Overview: An Introduction to the Principles of Teratology. Chapel Hill, NC, Health Sciences Consortium, 1981.)

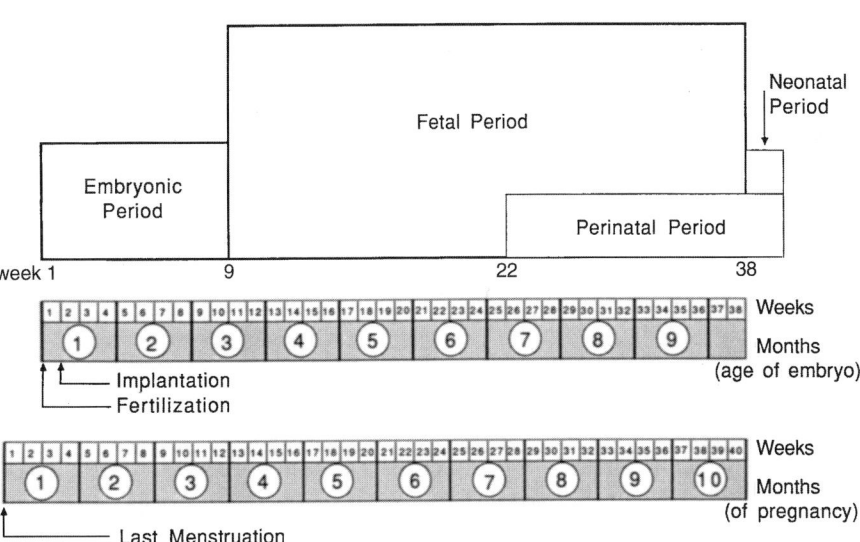

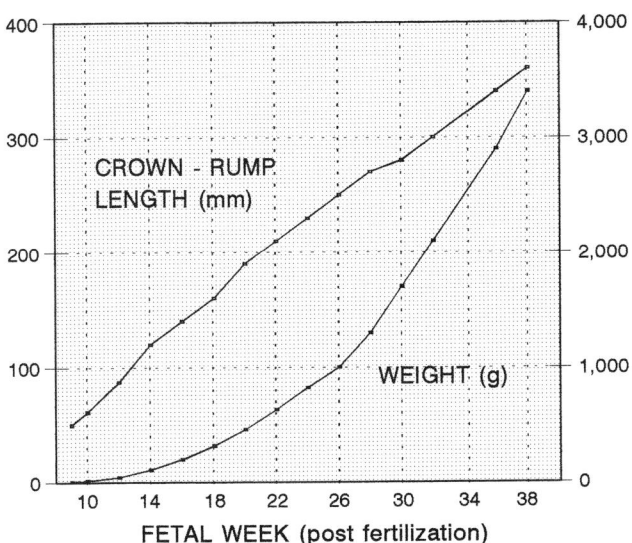

Figure 3–16. Weight and crown-rump length during human development. (Data from Moore KL, Persaud TVN: The Developing Human: Clinically Oriented Embryology, 6th ed. Philadelphia, WB Saunders Co, 1998.)

during the late embryonic period, thus making it a functional organ relatively early in development.[85] Accordingly, it expands rapidly to about 10% of the total body weight by the beginning of fetal life.[38] Thereafter, its growth rate follows that of the whole body so that, as a proportion of body weight, it remains "virtually constant."[88]

The same proportional growth pattern is seen in heart and kidney, but growth of the head is quite different. At the beginning of the fetal period, the head is about one-half the crown-rump length; at 12 weeks, it is about one-third. Thereafter, the rate of growth continues to slow in relation to the rest of the body.

It is important to remember that the establishment of the gross form of an organ does not necessarily correspond to the establishment of function. The human fetal gastrointestinal tube closely resembles that of the newborn infant as early as the middle of the sixth month. By contrast, cell differentiation and the development of complex enzyme systems necessary for the digestive process continue through birth and well beyond.[89]

The early human fetus is about 95% water, and there is a progressive increase in solids throughout fetal growth.[88] Most of the water (ratio of 4:1) is extracellular in early fetal life, but more is found within cells as the fetus matures, so that by birth the ratio is approximately 1:1.[90] Protein is accumulated most rapidly before the fetus weighs 1 kg and slowly declines thereafter. Fat deposition is low until the middle of gestation, when the proportion of fat (especially subcutaneous fat) to total body weight increases exponentially.[91]

REFERENCES

1. Corliss CE: Patten's Human Embryology: Elements of Clinical Development. New York, McGraw-Hill, 1976.
2. Wolpert L: Do we understand development? Science *266*:571, 1994. [See also other relevant articles in this special issue of *Science* devoted to Frontiers of Biology: Development.]
3. Junqueira LC, et al: Basic Histology, 7th ed. Norwalk, CT, Appleton & Lange, 1992.
4. Witschi E: Migration of the germ cells of human embryos from the yolk sac to the primitive gonadal folds. Contrib Embryol Carnegie Inst *32*:67, 1948.
5. Blandau RJ, et al: Observations on the movements of living primordial germ cells in the mouse. Fertil Steril *14*:482, 1963.
6. Gondos B, et al: Ultrastructural observations on germ cells in human fetal ovaries. Am J Obstet Gynecol *110*:644, 1971.
7. Fujimoto T, et al: The origin, migration and fine morphology of human primordial germ cells. Anat Rec *188*:315, 1977.
8. Carlson B. Human Embryology and Developmental Biology, 2nd ed. St Louis, Mosby, 1999.
9. Byskov AG: Sexual differentiation of the mammalian ovary. *In* Motta PM, Hafez ESE (eds): Biology of the Ovary. The Hague, Martinus Nijhoff Publishers, 1980, pp 3–15.
10. Baker TG: A quantitative and cytological study of germ cells in human ovaries. Proc R Soc Lond B *158*:417, 1963.
11. Fawcett DW, et al: The occurrence of intercellular bridges in groups of cells exhibiting synchronous differentiation. J Biophys Biochem Cytol *5*:453, 1959.
12. Zamboni L, Gondos B: Intercellular bridges and synchronization of germ cell differentiation during oogenesis in the rabbit. J Cell Biol *36*:276, 1968.
13. Gondos B, Zamboni L: Ovarian development: the functional importance of germ cell interconnections. Fertil Steril *20*:176, 1969.
14. Peters H: Migration of gonocytes into the mammalian gonad and their differentiation. Philos Trans R Soc Lond (Biol) *259*:91, 1970.
15. Zamboni L: Comparative studies on the ultrastructure of mammalian oocytes. *In* Biggers JD, Scheutz AW (eds): Oogenesis. Baltimore, University Park Press, 1972, pp 5–45.
16. Dvorak M, Tesarik J: Ultrastructure of human ovarian follicles. *In* Motta PM, Hafez ESE (eds): Biology of the Ovary. The Hague, Martinus Nijhoff Publishers, 1980, pp 121–137.

17. Byskov AG: Does the rete ovarii act as a trigger for the onset of meiosis? Nature 252:396, 1974.
18. Byskov AG: The role of the rete ovarii in meiosis and follicle formation in the cat, mink and ferret. J Reprod Fertil 45:201, 1975.
19. Byskov AG, Saxen L: Induction of meiosis in fetal mouse testis in vitro. Devel Biol 52:193, 1976.
20. O WS, Baker TG: Initiation and control of meiosis in hamster gonads in vitro. J Reprod Fertil 48:399, 1976.
21. Kessel RG: Annulate lamellae (porous cytomembranes): With particular emphasis on their possible role in differentiation of the female gamete. In Browder LW (ed): Oogenesis, Vol 1. Developmental Biology: A Comprehensive Synthesis. New York, Plenum Press, 1985, pp 179-233.
22. Schuetz AW: Local control mechanisms during oogenesis and folliculogenesis. In Browder LW (ed): Developmental Biology: A Comprehensive Synthesis. New York, Plenum Press, 1985, pp 3-83.
23. Bachvarova R: Gene expression during oogenesis and oocyte development in mammals. In Browder LW (ed): Developmental Biology: A Comprehensive Synthesis. New York, Plenum Press, 1985, pp 453-524.
24. Van Benedin E: La maturation de l'oeuf, la fecondation et les premieres phases du developpement embryonnaire des mammiferes d'apres des recherches faites le lapin. Bull Acad Belg Cl Su 40:686, 703, 1875.
25. Bliel JD, Wassarman PM: Sperm-egg interactions in the mouse: sequence events and induction of the acrosome reaction by a zona pellucida glycoprotein. Devel Biol 95:317, 1983.
26. Wassarman PM: Fertilization. In Yamada KM (ed): Cell Interactions and Development: Molecular Mechanisms. New York, John Wiley & Sons, 1982, pp 1-27.
27. Dean J, et al: Developmental expression of ZP3, a mouse zona pellucida gene. In Yoshinga K, Mori T (eds): Development of Preimplantation Embryos and Their Environment. New York, Alan R Liss, 1989, pp 21-32.
28. Epifano O, Dean J: Biology and structure of the zona pellucida: a target for immunocontraception. Reprod Fertil Dev 6:319, 1994.
29. Wassarman PM: Fertilization in mammals. Sci Am 259:52, 1988.
30. Dunbar BS, et al: The mammalian zona pellucida: its biochemistry, immunochemistry, molecular biology, and developmental expression. Reprod Fertil Dev 6:331, 1994.
31. Wassarman PM: The biology and chemistry of fertilization. Science 235:553, 1987.
32. Wassarman PM, et al: The mouse egg's extracellular coat: synthesis, structure and function. In Gall JG (ed): Gametogenesis and the Early Embryo. 44th Symp Soc Devel Biol. New York, Alan R Liss, 1986, pp 371-388.
33. Bousquet D, et al: The cellular origin of the zona pellucida antigen in human and hamster. J Exp Zool 215:215, 1981.
34. Baca M, Zamboni L: The fine structure of human follicular oocytes. J Ultrastruct Res 19:354, 1967.
35. Shettles LB: Ovulation: Normal and abnormal. In Grady HG, Smith DE (eds): The Ovary. Baltimore, Williams & Wilkins, 1963, pp 128-142.
36. Austin CR: The Mammalian Egg. Oxford, Blackwell Scientific Publications, 1961.
37. Peters H, McNatty KP: Atresia. In The Ovary: A Correlation of Structure and Function in Mammals. London, Granada Publishing, 1980, pp 98-112.
38. Moore KL, Persaud TVN: The Developing Human: Clinically Oriented Embryology, 6th ed. Philadelphia, WB Saunders Co, 1998.
39. Gwatkin RBL: Fertilization Mechanisms in Man and Mammals. New York, Plenum Press, 1977.
40. van Wagenen G, Simpson ME: Embryology of the Ovary and Testis: Homo sapiens and Macaca mulatta. New Haven, CT, Yale University Press, 1965.
41. Heller CG, Clermont Y: Spermatogenesis in man: an estimate of its duration. Science 140:184, 1963.
42. Wassarman PM: Early events in mammalian fertilization. Ann Rev Cell Biol 3:109, 1987.
43. Wassarman PM, et al: The mouse egg's receptor for sperm: what is it and how does it work? Cold Spring Harbor Symp Quant Biol 50:11, 1985.
44. Anderson E, et al: In vitro fertilization and early embryogenesis: a cytological analysis. J Ultrastruct Res 50:231, 1975.
45. Cherr GN, et al: In vitro studies of golden hamster sperm acrosome reaction: completion on the zona pellucida and induction by homologous soluble zonae pellucidae. Devel Biol 114:119, 1986.
46. Austin CR, Bishop MWH: Fertilization in mammals. Biol Rev 32:296, 1957.
47. Langlais J, Roberts KD: A molecular membrane model of sperm capacitation and the acrosome reaction of mammalian spermatozoa. Gamete Res 12:183, 1985.
48. Bliel JD, Wassarman PM: Structure and function of the zona pellucida: identification and characterization of the proteins of the mouse oocyte's zona pellucida. Devel Biol 76:185, 1980.
49. Florman HM, Wassarman PM: O-linked oligosaccharides of mouse egg ZP3 account for its sperm receptor activity. Cell 41:313, 1985.
50. Szabo SP, O'Day DH: The fusion of sexual nuclei. Biol Rev 58:323, 1983.
51. Flach G, et al: The transition from maternal to embryonic control in the 2-cell mouse embryo. EMBO J 1:681, 1982.
52. Schultz GA: Utilization of genetic information in the preimplantation mouse embryo. In Rossant J, Peterson RA: Experimental Approaches to Mammalian Embryonic Development. New York, Cambridge University Press, 1986, pp 239-265.
53. O'Rahilly R, Muller F: Human Embryology and Teratology, 3rd ed. New York, Wiley-Liss, 2001.
54. O'Rahilly R, Muller F: Developmental stages in human embryos: including a revision of Streeter's "Horizons" and a survey of the Carnegie Collection. Carnegie Institution of Washington Publication 637, 1987.
55. Fleming TP, Johnson MH: From egg to epithelium. Annu Rev Cell Biol 4:313, 1985.
56. Luckett WP: Origin and differentiation of the yolk sac and extraembryonic mesoderm in presomite human and rhesus monkey embryos. Am J Anat 152:59, 1978.
57. O'Rahilly R: The manifestation of the axes of the human embryo. Z Anat Entw 132:50, 1970.
58. Enders AC, et al: Differentiation of the embryonic disc, amnion, and yolk sac in the rhesus monkey. Am J Anat 177:161, 1986.
59. Hertig AT: Human Trophoblast. Springfield, IL, Charles C Thomas, 1968.
60. Luckett WP: Origin and differentiation of the yolk sac and extraembryonic mesoderm in presomite human and rhesus monkey embryos. Am J Anat 152:59, 1978.
61. Bellairs R: The primitive streak. Anat Embryol 174:1, 1986.
62. Edelman GM: Cell adhesion molecules in the regulation of animal form and tissue pattern. Annu Rev Cell Biol 2:81, 1986.
63. Wessels NK: Tissue Interactions and Development. Menlo Park, CA, WA Benjamin Co, 1977, pp 3-5.
64. O'Rahilly R: Developmental stages in human embryos, including a survey of the Carnegie Collection. Part A: embryos of the first three weeks (stages 1 to 9). Carnegie Institution of Washington Publication 631, 1973.
65. Kallen B: Early morphogenesis and pattern formation in the central nervous system. In DeHaan RL, Ursprung H (eds): Organogenesis. New York, Holt Rinehart & Winston, 1965, pp 107-128.
66. Schoenwolf GC: Formation and patterning of the avian neuraxis: one dozen hypotheses. In Neural Tube Defects, Ciba Foundation Symposium 181. Chichester, Wiley, 1994, pp 25-50.
67. Smith JL, Schoenwolf GC: Notochordal induction of cell wedging in the chick neural plate and its role in neural tube formation. J Exp Zool 250:49, 1989.
68. Saxen L, Toivonen S: Primary Embryonic Induction. London, Logos Press, 1962.
69. Yamada T, et al: Control of cell pattern in the developing nervous system: polarizing activity of the floor plate and notochord. Cell 64:635, 1991.
70. Lopashov GV, Stroeva OG: Morphogenesis of the vertebrate eye. In Abercrombie M, Brachet J (eds): Advances in Morphogenesis, Vol 1. New York, Academic Press, 1961, pp 331-377.
71. Ebert JD: An analysis of the synthesis and distribution of the contractile protein, myosin, in the development of the heart. Proc Natl Acad Sci USA 39:333, 1953.
72. Rosenquist GC, DeHaan RL: Migration of precardiac cells in the chick embryo: a radioautographic study. Contrib Embryol 38:111, 1966.
73. Southgate DAT: Fetal measurements. In Falkner F, Tanner JM (eds): Human Growth, Vol 1: Principles and Prenatal Growth. New York, Plenum Press, 1978.
74. Willier BH, Rawles ME: Organ-forming areas of the early chick blastoderm. Proc Soc Exp Biol 32:1293, 1935.
75. Johnson JWC: Cardio-respiratory systems. In Barnes AC: Intrauterine Development. Philadelphia, Lea & Febiger, 1968, pp 176-188.
76. Rajala GM, et al: Evidence that blood pressure controls heart rate in the chick embryo prior to neural control. J Embryol Exp Morph 36:685, 1976.
77. Rajala GM, et al: Response of the quiescent heart tube to mechanical stretch in the intact chick embryo. Devel Biol 61:330, 1977.
78. Kirby ML, et al: Neural crest cells contribute to normal aorticopulmonary septation. Science 220:1059, 1983.
79. Emery J: Embryogenesis. In Emery J (ed): The Anatomy of the Developing Lung. Surrey, England, William Heinemann Medical Books, 1969.
80. Lauge-Hansen N: The Development and Embryonic Anatomy of the Human Gastro-intestinal Tract. Eindhoven, Holland, Centrex Publishing Company, 1960.
81. Torrey TW: The early development of the human nephros. Contrib Embryol Carnegie Inst 35:175, 1954.
82. Davies J: Human Developmental Anatomy. New York, Ronald Press, 1963, p 165.
83. Ebert JD: Interacting Systems in Development. New York, Holt, Rinehart & Winston, 1965, p 181.
84. Walker DG: Functional differentiation of the kidney. In Barnes AC: Intra-uterine Development. Philadelphia, Lea & Febiger, 1968, pp 245-252.
85. Hamilton WJ, Mossman HW: Human Embryology: Prenatal Development of Form and Function, 4th ed. Baltimore, Williams & Wilkins, 1972.
86. Dobbing J: Vulnerable periods in brain growth and somatic growth. In Roberts DF, Thomson AM: The Biology of Human Fetal Growth. Vol 15 of Symposia of the Society for the Study of Human Biology. London, Taylor & Francis, 1976, pp 137-147.
87. Connor JM, Ferguson-Smith MA: Essential Medical Genetics. Oxford, Blackwell Scientific Publications, 1984.
88. Southgate DAT, Hey EN: Chemical and biochemical development of the human fetus. In Roberts DF, Thomson AM: The Biology of Human Fetal Growth. Vol 15 of Symposia of the Society for the Study of Human Biology. London, Taylor & Francis, 1976, pp 195-209.
89. Milla PJ: Intestinal absorption and digestion of nutrients. In Cockburn F (ed): Fetal and Neonatal Growth, Vol 5. In Chamberlain G, Cockburn F (eds): Perinatal Practice. New York, John Wiley & Sons, 1988, pp 93-104.
90. Widdowson EM: Growth and composition of the fetus and newborn. In Assali NS (ed): The Biology of Gestation, Vol 2. New York, Academic Press, 1968, pp 1-49.
91. Widdowson EM, Spray CM: Chemical development in utero. Arch Dis Child 26:205, 1951.

Harold C. Slavkin and David Warburton

4 Regulation of Embryogenesis

The near-completion of the human genome, as well as many animal genomes (e.g., simple worms, fruit flies, lampreys, fish, frogs, mice, and rats), provides a knowledge base that enhances an understanding of regulatory processes required for embryogenesis. The human genome consists of approximately 30,000 different genes; approximately 50% are dedicated to the structure and function of the central nervous system, whereas the other 50% are the structural, functional, and regulatory genes that control all of the stages of human development—from the fertilized ovum through senescence.[1-3] The question of how a single cell, the fertilized egg, develops into a complex multicellular organism, is one of the most fundamental problems in developmental biology. The challenge for human developmental biology is to understand when, where, and how specific genes are expressed during development. It has become increasingly clear that the developmental program resides in the human genome.

Embryogenesis is a highly ordered sequence of processes that requires a precise temporal and spatial control of gene expression. To understand the principles of development, the regulatory genes involved in the control of embryogenesis need to be identified. What are the mechanisms that control the use of genetic information in time-dependent and space-dependent manners? What are the regulatory processes that control embryogenesis? The answers to these questions can provide the knowledge of differential gene activation and serve as the basis for understanding cellular differentiation and specialization. Moreover, enhanced understanding can advance prevention as well as diagnosis, treatment, and therapeutics for human birth defects.

To confound this major problem in human embryogenesis are several often counterintuitive observations. First, all somatic cells contain essentially the same human genome; approximately 9 billion bases or nucleotides (i.e., A, adenosine; T, thymidine; G, guanosine; and C, cytosine) are found in the diploid human somatic cell. Second, the vast majority of the genes found within the human genome individually consist of exons and introns, exons being the sequences of nucleic acids that are encoded within functional gene products and introns being intervening sequences of nucleic acids that are not found within functional transcripts. Third, the sequence of exons within a gene can be rearranged or edited by a process of alternative splicing resulting in different isotypes derived from the original gene (Fig. 4-1). Therefore, one gene can result in multiple and different mRNAs or transcripts. In turn, these multiple transcripts can be translated to produce multiple and different proteins with different biologic functions based on their tertiary or quaternary structures. For example, genes for transcription factors, growth factors, and their cognate receptors can each produce multiple isotypes with different biologic activities. Therefore, the number of transcribed gene products far exceeds the number of genes found within the human genome.[2,3]

The regulation of embryogenesis becomes a problem of when, where, and how specific groups of genes are turned on, turned off, increased, or decreased during development. What regulates the temporal and spatial expression of genes? Regulation becomes a problem of multiple genes, or different isotypes produced from the same gene, functioning in various combinations during development. Sequential developmental processes are regulated by a combinatorial regulatory mechanism.

This chapter provides an integration of several levels of regulation during mammalian embryogenesis with particular emphasis on basic concepts, transcriptional controls, and the elucidation of hormone-mediated and growth factor-mediated signal transduction through their respective cognate receptors. Several clinical abrogations in neonates result from altered regulatory processes required for embryogenesis. This chapter focuses on gene regulation as controlled by transcription factors and signal transduction processes during mammalian embryogenesis.

PRINCIPLES OF REGULATION

During the last decade, significant advances have been made toward understanding the hierarchy of regulatory controls for mammalian embryogenesis.[4-12] In part, the current molecular paradigms for epigenetic regulation of mammalian development stem from three lines of scientific inquiry: (1) critical observations originally made in prokaryotic systems (e.g., *Escherichia coli*); (2) the discovery of homeotic genes, which regulate transcription activities within invertebrate eukaryotic systems (e.g., *Drosophila melanogaster* and *Caenorhabditis elegans*) as well as vertebrate eukaryotic systems (e.g., fish, frogs, alligators, birds, mice, and humans)[9, 13-20]; and (3) the discovery of oncogenes and proto-oncogenes, growth factors, and their cognate receptors associated with vertebrate tumor formation.[8,9,13-24]

Current models describing the cyclic adenosine monophosphate (cAMP) second-messenger pathway and its effects on differential gene expression were originally based on scientific inquiry focusing on prokaryotic systems. In *E. coli*, cAMP regulates the expression of several genes involved in glucose metabolism through binding to a catabolite activator protein (CAP). cAMP binds directly to CAP and induces interactions with specific DNA sequences, thereby activating cAMP-responsive genes. The binding of CAP to specific nucleic acid sequences induces DNA bending, which facilitates transcriptional regulation and RNA polymerase II activity. The cAMP response elements (i.e., specific nucleic acid motifs) function in a distance-independent and orientation-independent fashion and meet the criteria for being enhancers. This line of inquiry resulted in a new understanding of how metabolites (e.g., sugars, vitamins, hormones, growth factors, trace elements) within the microenvironment bind to cell surface receptor molecules and induce specific intracellular metabolic pathways, which regulate differential gene expression.[15-33]

Another line of inquiry resulted in the discovery of homeotic genes (*Hox* genes) in *D. melanogaster* and thereafter in a number of other invertebrates as well as vertebrates. Two types of mutants have been identified during early embryogenesis that affect the spatial organization of the embryo into segments: (1) the segmentation mutants affecting segment number and polarity, and (2) the homeotic mutants, which transform one segment into another or parts of a segment into the corresponding part of another segment.[15] The *Hox* genes are a family of regulatory genes expressed along the anteroposterior axis in most metazoans. These *Hox* genes encode transcription regulators or DNA-binding proteins active in pattern formation during embryogenesis.[34,35] *Hox* genes contain a highly conserved homeodomain or homeobox sequence consisting of 180 base pairs (bp).[15] The experimental strategies of homologous recombinations producing transgenic animals with null mutations for

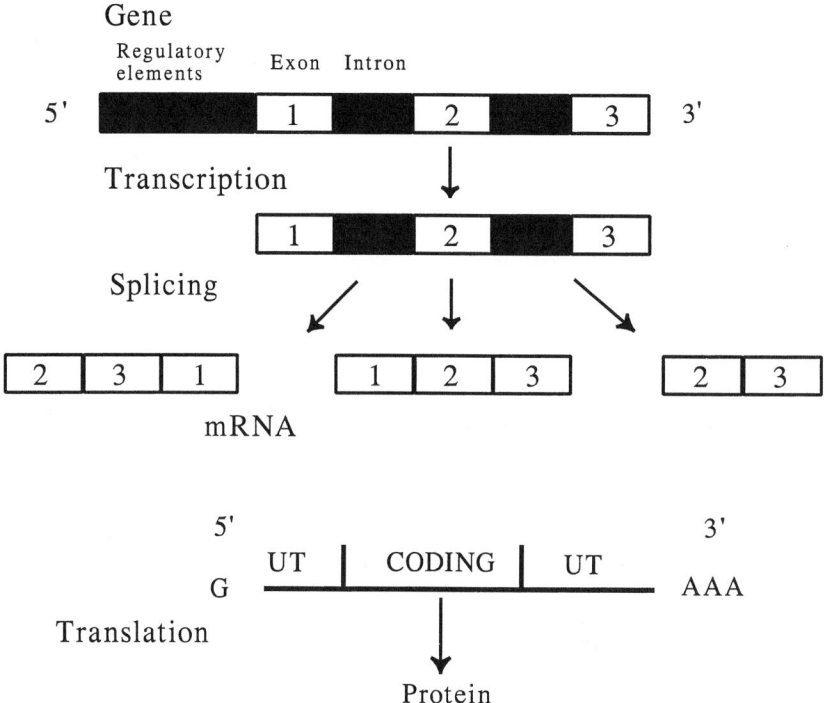

Figure 4–1. Scheme for the transcription and translation of a gene within the human genome resulting in multiple gene products using alternative splicing. The gene consists of a 5′ upstream promoter sequence containing multiple regulatory elements (e.g., retinoic acid, vitamin D, or steroid/thyroxine hormone binding elements), multiple exons (indicated as 1, 2 and 3, which contain the sequence encoding the protein in the mature mRNA), and intervening noncoding nucleic acid sequence within introns. Following transcription, the RNA is processed by splicing out the introns at defined sequence positions and adding a 7′-methyl G residue to the 5′ end and multiple A's (adenosine, a poly-A tail) to the 3′ end of the molecule. This process and that of alternative splicing and rearrangements can produce a number of different mRNAs (transcripts) encoding different proteins as depicted (i.e., transcript$_1$, exons 2-3-1; transcript$_2$, exons 1-2-3; and transcript$_3$, exons 2-3). The designation *UT* is used for noncoding untranslated regions in the mature mRNA, both 5′ and 3′ to the coding sequence. The mature mRNA is subsequently transported to the cytoplasm and translated into the primary structure of a protein. During posttranslational processing, the protein folds and assumes a secondary, tertiary or quaternary structure that facilitates its biologic function(s).

specific *Hox* genes as well as for a number of growth factors and their cognate receptors significantly advanced an understanding of how homeotic DNA-binding proteins regulate time and positional information during embryogenesis.[18] In addition, several *Hox* genes have been found to be highly responsive to vitamins (e.g., retinoic acid) and a number of polypeptide growth factors and hormones during embryonic and fetal stages of mammalian development.[28,36-38] This line of inquiry has provided a rationale for considering master control genes, a master transcription factor that turns on different genes at different times depending on the affinity with which it interacts with protein or nucleic acid targets. These genes control the geometry of mammalian morphogenesis, and a number of levels of biologic regulation that operate during embryogenesis (Fig. 4-2).

The third line of inquiry discovered several oncogenes and proto-oncogenes, growth factors, and their cognate receptors in rapidly growing tumors and subsequently demonstrated that many regulatory molecules are expressed during specific stages of embryogenesis.[21] Oncogenes are genes that are capable of inducing or maintaining cell transformations, and many of these genes induce tumor formation; they were discovered through the study of transforming retroviruses. The progenitors of oncogenes are normal genes called *proto-oncogenes*, which control a number of developmental processes associated with cell growth, cell death (apoptosis), proliferation, and differentiation. Oncogenes encode proteins called *oncoproteins*, which are similar to the normal products of proto-oncogenes except that they have lost key regulatory constraints on their biologic

activity. Oncogenes function as growth factors (e.g., *sis*, *int-2*), trans-membrane growth factor receptors (e.g., *erbB*, *ros*, *kit*), membrane-associated tyrosine kinases (e.g., *src* family), membrane-associated guanine nucleotide binding proteins (e.g., *H-ras*), cytoplasmic serine-threonine kinases (e.g., mos), cytoplasmic hormone receptors (e.g., *erbA*), nuclear DNA-binding proteins (e.g., *c-myc*, *N-myc*, *L-myc*, *c-fos*, *ski*, *ets*), and antitumor suppression proteins (e.g., *bcl-1*, *bcl-2*, *int-1*).

Of equal importance has been the discovery of transforming growth factor β (TGFβ), which has become the prototypic member of a superfamily of growth and differentiation factors identified in a wide variety of organisms ranging from insects to humans.[39,40] Based on their biologic and structural similarities, the members of this superfamily of genes have been subdivided into three groups: (1) the TGFβ (three isotypes, TGFβ$_1$, TGFβ$_2$, and TGFβ$_3$), (2) the activins, and (3) the bone morphogenetic proteins (BMPs).[41-43] These morphoregulatory gene products are multifunctional growth factors with wide-ranging and often opposite effects on numerous cellular processes.[44] TGFβ signals through a heteromeric receptor complex of the Type I and Type II TGFβ receptors. The Type II receptor is a transmembrane serine-threonine kinase. The diversity of the TGFβ cellular responses may reflect an association between the Type I and the Type II receptors, thereby resulting in receptor complexes of differential signaling capacities. This line of inquiry has provided invaluable evidence for signaling by a heteromeric complex resulting in the regulation of disparate cell processes, such as differentiation and proliferation during embryogenesis.[6]

Figure 4–2. Homology between homeotic genes discovered in *Drosophila* and those identified in the mouse and human genomes. Schematic representation of the nomenclature for the four major mammalian *Hox* gene complexes aligned with the homeotic genes originally identified in the *Drosophila melanogaster* genome. The present nomenclature uses four single letters to designate the clusters (A, B, C, and D) followed by the number 1 to 13 representing the individual *Hox* genes in that cluster. Blank spaces indicate that no gene has as yet been identified and characterized. Analysis of the mouse and human *Hox* gene complexes indicates that there are 38 genes organized in four different chromosomal complexes approximately 120 kb in length, and the genes in each cluster are all oriented in the same 5′ to 3′ direction for transcription. Note the colinear relationship between *Hox* gene order along a chromosome and anteroposterior boundaries for *Hox* gene expression along the axis of the embryo. Abbreviations from *D. melanogaster* according to anteroposterior patterns of expression: lab = labial; pb = proboscis; Dfd = dorsal disk; ANT-C = Antennapedia; BX-C = bithorax complex; Ubx = ultrabithorax; abd-A = abdominal-A; abd-B = abdominal-B.

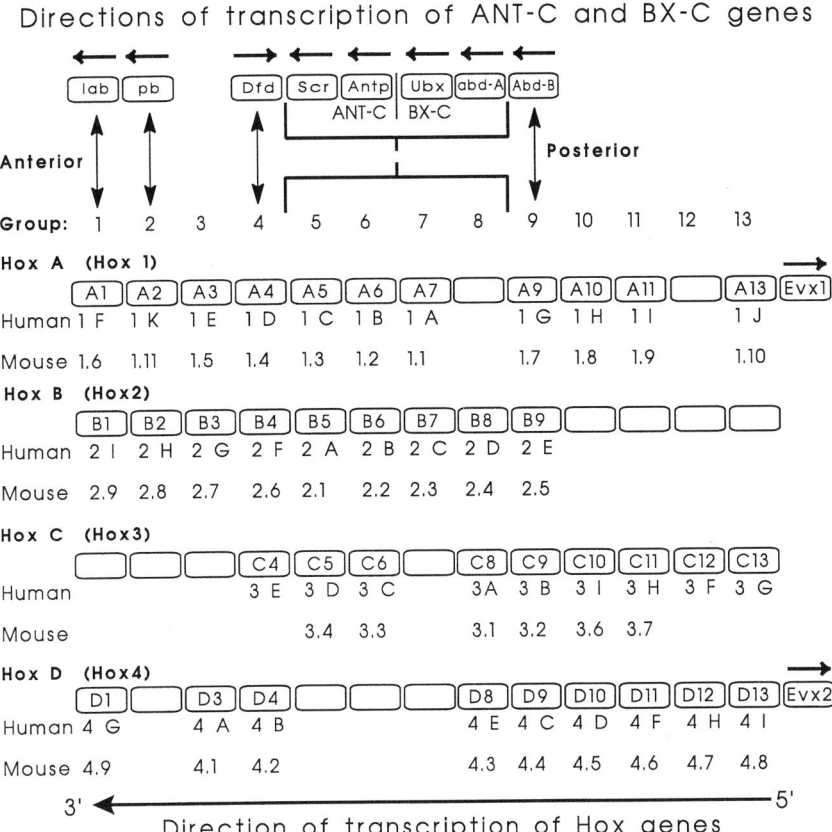

From these three lines of inquiry as well as a number of complementary investigations, several generalities related to the major principles for regulation during embryogenesis have emerged. First, before fertilization, a number of maternally derived morphoregulatory gene products are localized within the ovum (e.g., homeotic gene products, oncogenes, growth factors, cytokines).[11, 12] Second, after fertilization, a number of these gene products or transcripts are translated and become biologically active during the early stages of development. Third, before implantation and during initial stages of gastrulation within the postimplantation embryo, various growth factors and their cognate receptors are expressed and affect numerous transcription factors (e.g., TGF-β, Wnt, fibroblast growth factor, [Fgf]); these regulatory molecules are controlled according to time and position and affect bilateral symmetry, increasing asymmetry during organogenesis, and increasing and disparate rates of cell division within the body form (e.g., cyclin-dependent protein kinases [CDKs]).[31-45] Fourth, in tandem, sequential expression of transcription (e.g., sonic hedgehog [*sonic hh*], distal-less [*Dlx*], homeotic genes ([*Hox*]) and growth factors regulate the anteroposterior axis as well as the dorsal-ventral developmental processes.[36,46-50] In each stage of embryogenesis, a series of biomechanical processes articulate the extracellular microenvironment with the plasma membrane. Transmembrane receptors engage intracellular molecules as well as the cytoskeleton. Similarly, a number of second-messenger pathways facilitate communication between the cytoplasm and the nucleus, and a number of nuclear factors control the cell cycle, cell division, differential gene expression, and cell death.[51-53]

MOLECULAR DETERMINANTS FOR TIMING AND POSITIONAL INFORMATION

A central theme in mammalian embryogenesis is the inductive interactions between two apposed tissues, primary and second- ary embryonic inductions, resulting in the morphologic transformation of one or both of the tissue layers.[13,48,54] These inductive interactions are particularly significant during gastrulation and subsequent postimplantation embryogenesis.[24,55-62] Importantly a number of transcription factors (e.g., homeotic genes, *sonic hh, Dlx,* and proto-oncogenes), growth factors, growth factor receptors, substrate adhesion and cell adhesion molecules, and extracellular matrix molecules have been observed to be transiently expressed during instructive inductive events (Fig. 4–3).[17,34,63-65] The importance of these regulatory molecules has been further elucidated by using experimental strategies designed to analyze overexpression (e.g., dominant-negative effects), underexpression, or null mutations in candidate genes resulting in transgenic animals that do not express the gene products (i.e., knock-out experiments).[18,20,44,66-71] One useful paradigm for understanding the principles of growth factor signaling of transcriptional factors during inductive tissue interactions is that involving TGFβ family gene members or platelet-derived growth factors (e.g., PDGFα) and homeobox genes.[9, 13, 14, 21, 41, 49, 51] For example, a mutation in the PDGFα receptor gene results in the *Patch* mouse mutant that expresses phenotypes, including major craniofacial dysmorphogenesis, dental agenesis, hemifacial microsomia, and prenatal death owing to hemorrhage from the aorta (Fig. 4–4).

Homeobox genes of the *Msx* class have been demonstrated to be transiently expressed during gastrulation, during postimplantation neurulation (e.g., within the neuroectoderm of the rhombomeres of the hindbrain before cranial neural crest emigrations), and in epithelial and mesenchymal tissues associated with inductive processes required for morphogenesis and cytodifferentiation (e.g., tooth, glandular, lung, heart, skeletal, and limb development).[47,63] The *Msx* family of vertebrate *Hox* genes was originally isolated by homology to the *Drosophila msh* (i.e., muscle segment homeobox) gene. Three *Msx* class homeobox genes are identified in mice, and at least two are also identified in the human genome (i.e., *MSX1* and *MSX2*).[72] Homozygous

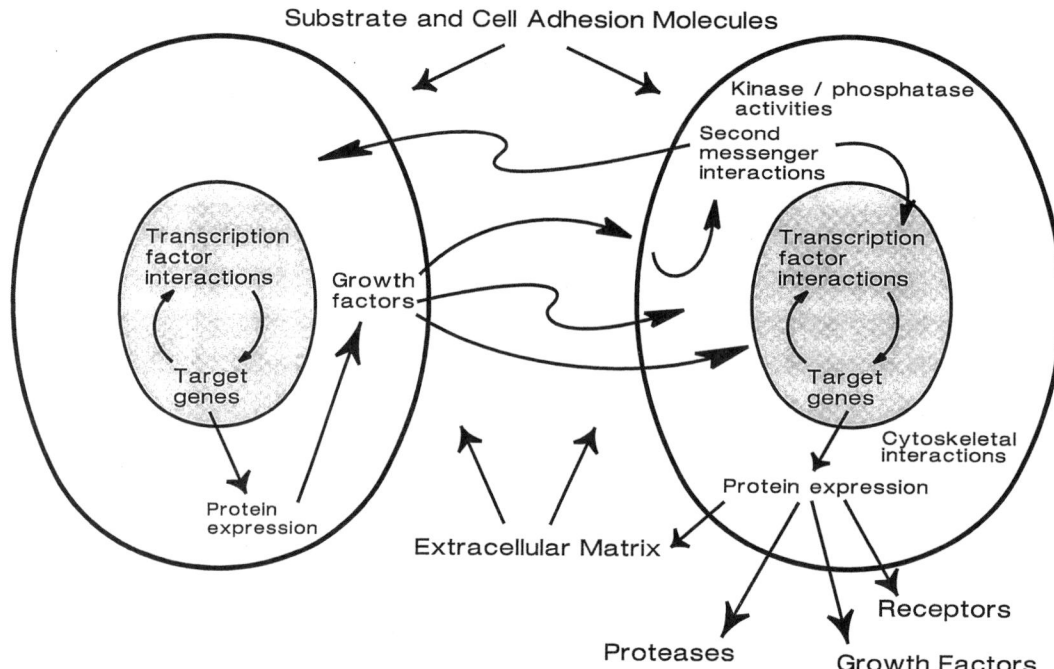

Figure 4-3. A model illustrating molecular regulation at the cellular level during inductive processes. Scheme depicts cell-cell interactions mediated by growth factors or cytokines within the extracellular matrix microenvironment, substrate adhesion molecules and cell adhesion molecules (SAMs, CAMs), growth factor binding to a cognate receptor, signal transduction, and activation of multiple intracellular signaling pathways. A number of cellular responses are shown, including changes in the cell cycle, cytoskeleton, targeted gene expression, protein synthesis, posttranslational processing, and changes in intermediary metabolism.

newborn mice with null mutations of *Msx-1* animals exhibit marked abnormalities in craniofacial development, including a complete cleft of the secondary palate; a failure of tooth and alveolar bone development in the mandible and maxilla; and abnormalities of the skull, malleus, nasal bones, and conchae.[68] Both cleft secondary palate and oligodontia occur in humans in an isolated, nonsyndromic form and also in the Pierre Robin sequence (micrognathia, glossoptosis, and cleft palate).[10,52]

Essentially all phenotypic abnormalities detected in the *Msx-1* null mutation mice represent abnormalities of bone and teeth. *Msx-1* and *Msx-2* are directly implicated in the developmental pathways required for normal differentiation of membrane and alveolar bone of the head and face and in tooth development.[63, 68, 73, 74] Premigratory cranial neural crest transiently express *Msx-2;* subsequently, there is transient expression of *Msx-1, Msx-2, Fgf-8* and *BMP-4* in the odontogenic placode epithelium and in the adjacent mesenchymal tissue associated with tooth and bone formation. One member of the TGFβ gene family *(BMP-4)* appears to be a required epigenetic signal for *Msx-2* gene expression resulting in apoptosis in premigratory crest cells.[47] These selected examples are provided to highlight the combinatorial possibilities suggested for specific inductive interactions in different developmental processes during embryogenesis.

A principle is that many transcription factors (e.g., *Hox* genes, homeobox-containing genes, proto-oncogenes) and growth factors (e.g., Fgfs, TGFβ gene family members, PDGFα) are associated in specific combinations with particular developmental processes; one gene, one protein, one morphogen does not support the current evidence related to the regulation of embryogenesis. Intercellular communication such as during instructive epithelial-mesenchymal interactions is critical to many developmental processes.[34,48,56-62,75] Intercellular communication proceeds in essentially two steps (Figs. 4-5 and 4-6). First, an extracellular molecule (epigenetic signal) binds to a

specific receptor (e.g., insulin, insulinlike growth factor receptor I [IGF-I] or IGF-II) on a target cell, converting the dormant receptor to an active state (Fig. 4-7). Second, the activated receptor stimulates intracellular biochemical pathways leading to one of a number of possible cellular responses: (1) progression through the cell cycle, (2) inhibition of the cell cycle, (3) differential gene expression, (4) changes in the cytoskeletal architecture, (5) changes in protein trafficking, (6) cell-cell adhesion as mediated by substrate adhesion molecules or cell adhesion molecules (SAMs, CAMs), (7) cell migration, and (8) modified intermediary cellular metabolism. One or more growth factors binding to their cognate receptors initiates signal transduction and provides, in part, regulatory features of many distinct signaling pathways during embryogenesis.

CRANIOFACIAL MORPHOGENESIS: A PARADIGM FOR TRANSCRIPTION AND SIGNAL TRANSDUCTION REGULATORY PROCESSES

During gastrulation, positional information for the anteroposterior axis of the mammalian embryo is established within the forming mesoderm. Embryonic mesoderm is formed at the early blastula stage by an inductive interaction between endoderm and ectoderm. This inductive event is facilitated by maternally derived polypeptide growth factors, including members of the *Fgf* and *Tgf*β gene families.[28,34,35,38,49,51,76,77] During subsequent patterning, various transcription factors respond to growth factor signaling along the anteroposterior axis as well as along the dorsoventral axes.[74,78,79]

The discovery of vertebrate *Antennapedia* class homeobox-containing genes has become central toward understanding when, where, and how control genes regulate morphogenesis.[15] Analysis of the mouse and human *Hox* gene complexes indicates that there are 38 genes organized in four different chromosomal

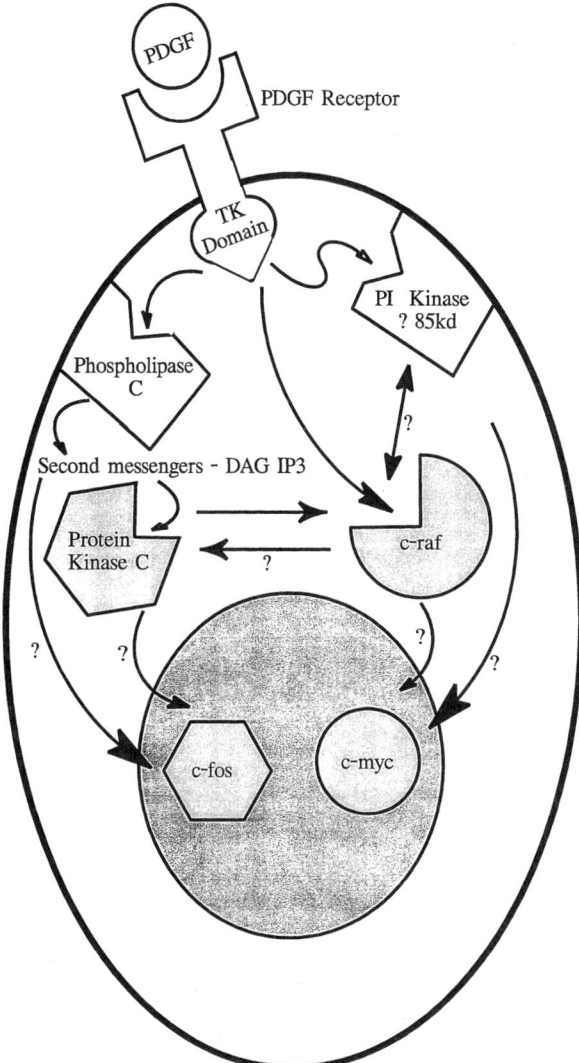

Figure 4–4. Platelet-derived growth factor (PDGF-α)-mediated signal transduction by the transmembrane PDGF-α receptor. A schematic representation of the sequence of events following the binding of PDGF ligand to its cognate PDGF receptor leading to the activation of a number of transcription factors such as homeotic DNA-binding proteins and the proto-oncogenes c-*fos*, c-*myc*, and c-*raf.* This scheme illustrates the articulated molecular processes that transmit an extracellular signal to the nucleus and thereby influence nuclear transcription factor combinations. ? = Indicates pathways currently under investigation. TK = tyrosine kinase; PI = phosphatidylinositol; DAG = diacylglycerol; IP3 = inositol trisphosphate.

complexes approximately 120 kb in length and that the genes in each cluster are all oriented in the same 5′ to 3′ direction of transcription (see Fig. 4–2).[80,81] Figure 4-2 summarizes the organization and homology relationships between the four *Hox* clusters. A key discovery has been the correlation between the physical order of these *Hox* genes along the chromosome and their expression and function along the anteroposterior axis of the mouse and human embryo.[81] Moreover, this property, termed *colinearity,* represents a mechanism for translating genetic information into a combinatorial code for the regulation of regional identity. The colinear relationship between *Hox* gene order along a chromosome and anteroposterior boundaries of *Hox* gene

expression along the axis of the embryo is a fundamental feature for understanding the regulation of embryogenesis.[19,66,80,81] The highly conserved *Hox* genes (e.g., from *Drosophila* to humans) provide patterning codes, codes that represent one component of a specification system in the various regions of the forming embryo.

Embryonic development of the mammalian forebrain, midbrain, and hindbrain is controlled by a number of transcription factors, which pattern the brain into highly ordered structures before synaptic influences are present.[50] These early genes are expressed according to patterns of a transverse domain or a segmentation pattern along the forming neural plate and neural tube.[50] In fact, several homeobox genes (e.g., *Dlx-2, Dlx-14, Gbx-2, Nkx-2, Otx-2, sonic hh*) are expressed according to these segment boundaries[50]; this is a theme that repeats during invertebrate as well as vertebrate development.[13-15,17,18,34,66,69,80,81]

Hindbrain and Branchial Arch Code

Hox genes are involved in patterning structures along an embryonic axis. Along the anteroposterior axis, the neural plate is segmented into forebrain, midbrain, hindbrain, and posterior neural tube.[47,50,52,82] The neural tube of the presumptive hindbrain is organized into a series of repeating segments known as rhombomeres.[47,52] The interface between the hindbrain neural plate and the adjacent dorsal surface ectoderm gives rise to cranial neural crest cells that interact with other cranial tissues, thereby contributing to a series of cranial ganglia and branchial arches.[8] The spatial organization of cranial neural crest emigrations from ectoderm indicates that it is organized on a rhombomeric basis; the crest cells of a specific ganglia and the branchial arch that the ganglia innervates originate from the same rhombomere. Premigratory crest cells within the neuroectoderm are imprinted with a positional value before cell migration.[80,81] The crest cells can transfer this positional information from the rhombomere position within the neuroectoderm to the tissues that surround it, thereby influencing their development.[80,81]

Therefore, early regional specification within hindbrain rhombomere structures vis-à-vis homeoticlike gene expression boundaries provides patterning mechanisms of hindbrain and branchial arch formations. In the embryos of jawed vertebrates (i.e., gnathastomes), the jaw cartilage (Meckel cartilage) develops from the mandibular arch, where *Hox* genes are not expressed. In agnathans (i.e., jawless) such as lampreys and hagfish, *Hox5-6-7* genes are expressed in the mandibular arch. Recent studies suggest that inhibition of these *Hox5-6-7* genes resulted in the transition from jawless to jawed vertebrates.[83]

Transcriptional Factors

"Experiments of nature" as well as experimentally induced mutations have demonstrated that numerous developmental processes are regulated by transcriptional regulatory proteins; in particular, DNA-binding proteins that are expressed in specific cell lineages, at specific times and positions during embryogenesis, participate in the regulation of differential gene expression.[84] Although transcriptional factors have been identified as being restricted to a specific cell lineage (e.g., *MyoD1* and *Myf5* in myogenesis,[85] most are expressed in multiple cell lineages and by often phenotypically unrelated cell types.[47,79,84] This pleiotropic expression suggests that a transcriptional factor (e.g., *Msx-1, Msx-2, c-fos, c-myc, Dlx-2, LEF-1*) can participate in multiple functions through combinatorial association with disparate DNA-binding proteins during remarkably different developmental processes (e.g., neurulation; rhombomere and somite formations; first branchial arch morphogenesis; tooth, heart, lung, and limb development).[50,59,79] Another interpretation of the available information is that the assumed pleiotropic expression may indicate that a specific

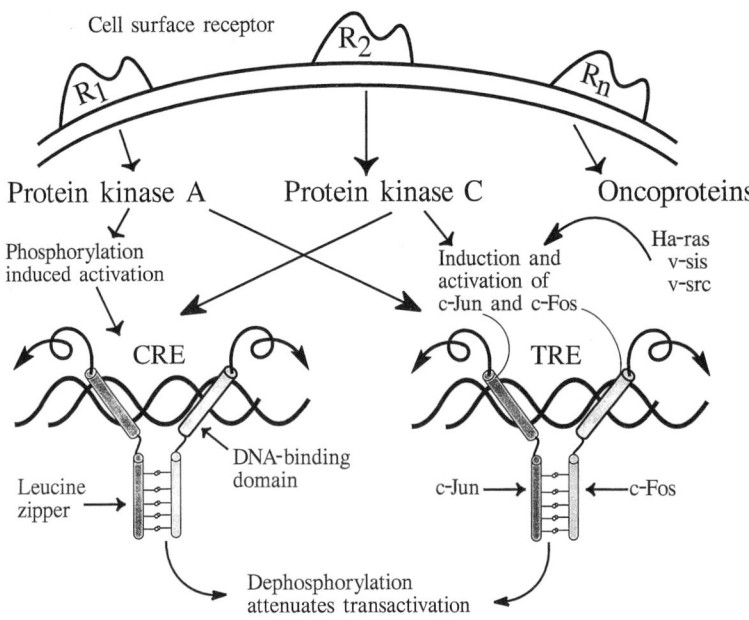

Figure 4–5. Three signal transduction pathways modulate gene transcription: (1) protein kinase A (PKA), (2) protein kinase C (PKC), and (3) oncoproteins. Polypeptide growth factors (e.g., Fgf, TGFβ, PDGF-α, EGF, TGF-α, IGF-I, IGF-II) bind to cell surface transmembrane receptors (R_1, R_2 and R_n), thereby activating the phosphorylation cascade mechanisms. PKC activation increases transcription of AP-1 (i.e., 5′ TGA-GTCA 3′) pathway mediators including proto-oncogene DNA binding proteins *c-jun* and *c-fos*. The *c-jun* activity is also modulated by dephosphorylation of inhibitory sites and phosphorylation of stimulatory sites. Dimerization associated with DNA binding produces transactivation of activator protein 1 (AP-1) responsive genes. Both the PKA and PKC pathways can activate the second-messenger response elements. Cell cycle-regulated kinases (CDKs) and oncoproteins also effect AP-1 activity.
CRE = consensus cAMP response element (5′ TGAC-GTCA 3′); CREB = CRE binding protein; TRE = phorbol ester tumor response element.

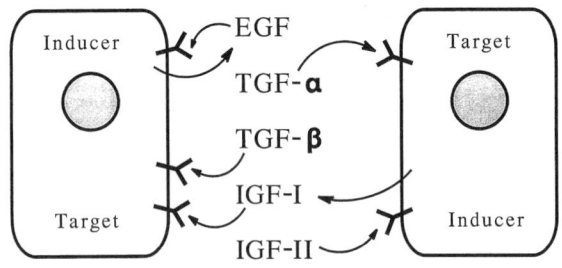

Figure 4–6. Endogenous growth factors mediate autocrine, paracrine, or endocrinelike regulation during embryogenesis.

DNA-binding protein functions within a specific process that is common to many different cell lineages, tissue types, or organ formations during embryogenesis (Fig. 4–8).[79]

Another family of transcription factors that regulates embryogenesis are the nine human paired box genes *(PAX)*. Loss-of-function mutations in *PAX3* result in the craniofacial-deafness-hand Waardenburg syndrome (chromosome 2q35) and loss-of-function mutations in *PAX6* on chromosome 11p13 produce aniridia. Except for *Pax-1* and *Pax-9,* the developing mammalian central nervous system is the primary site of expression for *Pax* genes during mouse embryogenesis. Loss-of-function mutations produce muscle and neural tube defects. *PAX9* loss-of-function mutations result in the congenital absence of molar teeth.[86]

Lymphoid enhancer factor 1 *(LEF-1)* is a sequence-specific DNA-binding protein that is expressed in pre-B and T lymphocytes of adult mice. Curiously, *LEF-1* expression has been identified during mouse embryogenesis in mesencephalon neuroectoderm, cranial neural crest cells, tooth anlagen, whisker follicles, and a number of other developmental sites.[79] *LEF-1* is encoded by a gene located on chromosome 3 in the mouse and chromosome 4 in humans. The sequence-specific recognition of DNA by *LEF-1* protein was found to be controlled by an 85-amino acid region termed the *high mobility group* (HMG) proteins. Transgenic mice carrying a null mutation for *LEF-1* are born with various curious phenotypes, including a lack of the mesencephalic nucleus of the trigeminal ganglion; dental agenesis; and

deficient whiskers, hair, and mammary glands.[79] The animals show no defects in lymphoid cell populations at birth but die within the first 10 days of postnatal life. *LEF-1* appears to be a DNA-binding protein that plays a critical role in a number of inductive epithelial-mesenchymal interactions.

Several regulatory molecules have been identified as intrinsic to the process of myogenesis. Vertebrate somites give rise to virtually all of the muscles of the trunk and limbs, and it is within the somites that the first evidence for determination of the myogenic phenotype is identified in terms of a sequence of myogenic regulatory transcription factors (e.g., *MyoD1, Myf5)*. In contrast to a number of DNA-binding proteins that are transiently expressed in a number of different cell lineages (e.g., *Msx-1, Msx-2, LEF-1, Pax-3, Dlx-2, Ev-2)*, the myogenic DNA-binding proteins are unique to the myogenic cell lineage.[85] Curiously, null mutations of the *MyoD1* gene do not ablate myogenesis, suggesting some degree of developmental redundancy operant during the early determination of the myogenic cell lineage.[85]

Growth Factors and Their Cognate Receptors

Endogenous growth factors and their cognate receptors are expressed throughout embryogenesis: within the fertilized ovum, during early cleavage stages, within the blastocyst, and throughout postimplantation embryonic and subsequent fetal stages of development.[36, 39, 40, 51, 87] These growth factors regulate as autocrine, paracrine (within a few cell diameters' distance), or endocrinelike controls. For example, TGFα is expressed and binds to its cognate receptor within the same cell (i.e., self-regulation, *autocrine).* Fgfs, TGFβ, or PDGFα signals are expressed, secreted, and bind as ligands to their cognate receptors localized on an adjacent cell of the same or of a different phenotype (i.e., *paracrine).* In other instances, growth factors are expressed, secreted, and bind to their cognate receptors at a distance from the source of secretion (i.e., *endocrine)* (Fig. 4–9).

Rieger syndrome is an autosomal dominant disorder of morphogenesis characterized by abnormalities of the anterior segment of the eye, dental hypoplasia, agenesis, as well as a number of other craniofacial malformations.[75] Significant linkage of Rieger syndrome to the region of the epidermal growth factor (EGF) gene on chromosome 4 has been obtained.[88] EGF is a polypeptide that exerts multiple effects on cellular function and maps to chromosome 4q25.[68,89] EGF and its cognate receptor are

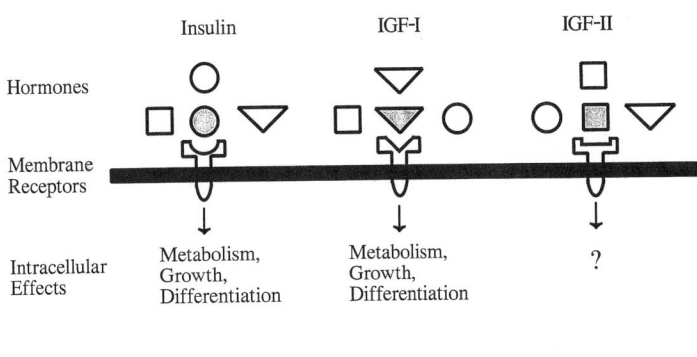

Figure 4–7. Insulin, insulinlike growth factor I (IGF-I), and insulinlike growth factor II (IGF-II) regulate cell proliferation, differentiation, and intermediary metabolism during embryogenesis.

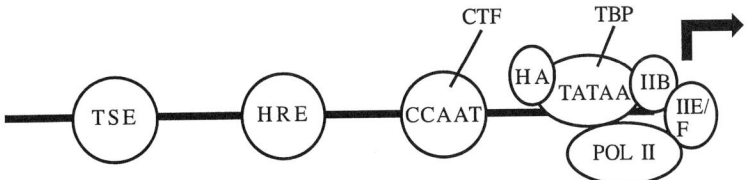

Figure 4–8. Diagram for the canonical transcriptional complex including a number of DNA binding proteins and cofactors. The transcriptional complex is located in the 5′ upstream promoter region of a gene. The 5′ flanking control region of the gene contains consensus sequences for accurate and efficient transcription as well as enhancers, repressors, cell-specific or tissue-specific regulatory elements, and growth factor and hormonal regulatory elements. A number of transcription factors, cofactors, and RNA polymerase II (POL II) are depicted. The *arrow* indicates the direction of transcription downstream toward the 3′ end of the gene. TSE = tissue-specific element (e.g., Pit-1 = pituitary-specific transcription factor); HRE = hormone response element (e.g., thyroid-stimulating hormone-beta); CCAAT = consensus box that controls basal levels of transcription; CTF = a 60-kDa protein that binds to a CCAAT box; TATAA = Goldberg-Hogness consensus sequence 20 to 30 bp upstream from the start of transcription; TBP = TATAA box binding protein; HA, IIB, and IIE/F = transcription factors.

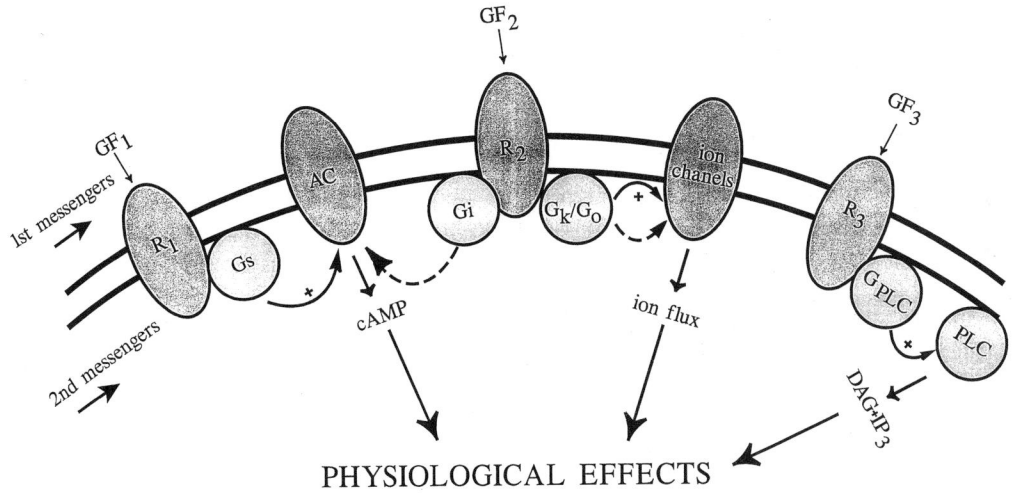

Figure 4–9. Diagram illustrating that different G proteins mediate the regulation of diverse growth factors targeting a single cell type. Three distinct growth factors (GF_1, GF_2, and GF_3) are shown to bind selectively to three distinct transmembrane receptors (R_1, R_2, and R_3). R_1 is coupled to stimulation of adenyl cyclase by Gs. R_2 is coupled to inhibition of adenyl cyclase by G_1 and to regulation of ion channels by G_k and G_O. R_3 is linked by a G protein labeled G_{PLC} to stimulation of phospholipase C (PLC), which produces the dual second messengers diacylglycerol (DAG) and inositol triphosphate (IP3). Each of these pathways can induce cellular responses (e.g., cell proliferation, differentiation) within a single cell type at a specific time and position in development.

expressed in embryonic craniofacial structures, including ophthalmic and dental tissues.[57, 75] Experimental inhibition studies of EGF translation result in dental agenesis, hypodontia, microglossia, and a *fusilli*-form Meckel's cartilage.[57,75]

Retinoids as Regulators of Embryogenesis

Retinoids (RAs) effect cell proliferation, growth, and differentiation through binding to two groups of nuclear receptors, which belong to the steroid/thyroid hormone receptor super-family:

(1) the retinoic acid receptors (RARs) and (2) the retinoid X receptors (RXRs). The RXRs are activated by *9-cis* retinoic acid and form heterodimers with several other nuclear receptors, including the RARs. The RA-activated receptor complexes trans-activate target genes through binding sites known as retinoic acid response elements (RAREs). All-*trans* retinoic acid activated RARs and RXRs are capable of up-regulating or down-regulating the transcription of many target genes, including a number of homeotic genes (e.g., *Msx-1, Msx-2, sonic hh, Dlx-2,* and *Hox* B cluster genes), genes that control apoptosis, growth factors such

as *TGFβ₁* metalloproteinases including collagenase and stromolysin, and a number of SAMs such as laminin and tenascin.

RA is a physiologically active metabolite and a potent teratogen, which, when administered at teratogenic doses, induces a variety of congenital defects, including isotretinoin (Accutane)-induced craniofacial and limb deformities and neural tube defects. During normal embryogenesis, such as during the induction of limb morphogenesis, RA regulates the graded expression of *Hoxb-8* and *sonic hedgehog (hh)* in response to signals from *Fgf-1, Fgf-2,* or *Fgf-4.* Growth factors, *Hox* genes, and RA produce unique combinations that regulate regional specification during embryogenesis.

CLINICAL IMPLICATIONS OF MUTATIONS IN TRANSCRIPTIONAL FACTORS AND FIBROBLAST GROWTH FACTOR RECEPTORS: CRANIOSYNOSTOSIS

Craniosynostosis, the premature fusion of the bones of the skull, is a common birth defect occurring in 1 in 3000 live births.[90] Craniosynostosis is found in more than 100 different craniofacial syndromes. The regulation of calvarial suture formation is complex and involves issues of space-dependent and time-dependent processes during the development of the central nervous system, neurulation, epithelial-mesenchymal cell-cell interactions, chondrogenesis, osteogenesis, extracellular matrix formation, and metalloproteinase-mediated degradation of the extracellular organic matrix.[73] In 1993, the first human homeo-box mutation was identified in the *Msx-2* gene (Pro7His mutation) associated with the autosomal dominant Boston-type craniosynostosis.[72] The human *Msx-2* gene is located on chromosome 5qter. *Msx-2* is expressed in a variety of cell lineages during gastrulation, neurulation, first branchial arch formation, and organogenesis. *Msx-2* is expressed in mesenchymal tissue of presumptive sutures as well as in the underlying cranial neural tissue.[73] The expression of the mouse counterpart of the human mutant gene in the developing skulls of transgenic mice causes both premature fusion of cranial bones (craniosynostosis) and ectopic cranial bone growth.[73]

Several research teams have demonstrated that different mutations in the fibroblast growth factor receptor 2 (Fgfr-2) result in different clinical phenotypes associated with craniosynostosis.[90-94] The *Fgf* gene family comprises nine members in mammals.[30] Through the use of alternative initiation codons for translation (e.g., *Fgf-2* and *Fgf-3),* however, multiple isotypes can be produced. In addition, alternative splicing produces additional isotypes for *Fgfs.*[46] All *Fgf* ligand genes are structurally related; generally, they encode proteins with a mass of 20 to 30 kDa, and these growth factor polypeptides are secreted constitutively.[30] The functions of the *Fgfs* include mitogenesis, cell motility, and differentiation.[49, 55] Studies of the expression patterns, primarily in the mouse, of the *Fgf-1–Fgf-8* genes as well as the four *Fgfr* genes have demonstrated that all these genes are active during embryogenesis.[76, 77] *Fgf* signal transduction pathway plays critical roles in the regulation of growth and patterning in the vertebrate embryo.[91]

Fgfs transduce signals to the cytoplasm through a family of transmembrane receptor tyrosine kinases, the *Fgfrs* four mammalian *Fgfrs* are known.[30, 46, 49, 51] In common with other receptor tyrosine kinase genes (e.g., EGF receptor, IGF-I, IGF-II receptors, PDGFα receptor), the *Fgfrs* are activated by dimerization. Dimerization of receptor tyrosine kinase genes results in their autophosphorylation, which facilitates the recruitment of intracellular signaling proteins that often contain SH2 domains. One response to low-level ligand-induced *Fgfr* binding is a transient activation of cytoplasmic mitogen-activated protein (MAP) kinase.[29] Higher-affinity binding can produce sustained activation of MAP kinase and its translocation to the nucleus of the cell. *Ras* functions upstream of the MAP kinase cascade, and activation of the *Ras* pathway is necessary for the sustained mitogenic response. Several pathways are activated by ligand binding to *Fgfrs,* including phospholipase C-gamma, the regulatory subunit of phosphatidylinositol 3-kinase (Nck), and the activation of Shc. In general, specificity of the response to *Fgf* activation of one of the four *Fgfrs* can be determined by (1) the sum of the SH2 domain proteins and other cytoplasmic signaling molecules that are recruited, (2) the tissue-specific patterns of expression of these same proteins, (3) antagonism by activated protein tyrosine phosphatases within the cell, and (4) by the strength of the signal derived from the ligand-receptor binding.

Mutations in *Fgfr-1, Fgfr-2,* and *Fgfr-3* are associated with craniosynostosis.[51, 55, 90-94] Mutations in different genes (*Fgfr-1* and *Fgfr-2)* can produce the same phenotype (Pfeiffer syndrome).[90, 92-94] *Fgfr-1* is required for embryonic growth, mesodermal patterning during gastrulation, and early postimplantation axial organization during mammalian embryogenesis.[51] In contrast, different mutations in the same gene *(Fgfr-2)* produce different phenotypes (Crouzon syndrome and Apert syndrome).[91] Ironically a mutation such as Cys 342Arg in exon 9 of the *Fgfr-2* gene results in both Crouzon syndrome and Pfeiffer syndrome.[92-94] Mutations of a single amino acid in the transmembrane domains of the *Fgfr-3* gene result in achondroplasia characterized by short-limbed dwarfism and macrocephaly; achondroplasia is the most common cause of chondrodysplasia in humans with a prevalence of 1 in 15,000 live births.[95]

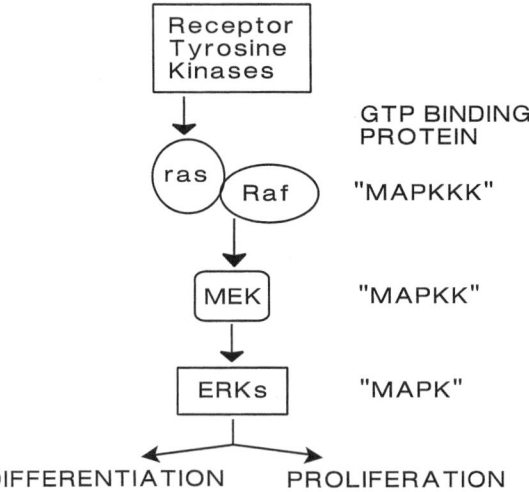

Figure 4–10. The general scheme for the *Ras/Raf*/MEK/ERK pathway; extracellular signal-regulated kinase activation (ERKs) of mitogen-activated protein kinases (MAPKs) as a critical event in signal transduction from transmembrane receptor tyrosine kinases to nuclear factors regulating the cell cycle or targeted gene expression. In this pathway, extracellular signals activate MAPK pathways, which have a three-component protein kinase cascade: (1) a serine/threonine protein kinase (MAPKKK), (2) which phosphorylates and activates a dual-specificity protein kinase (MAPKK), and (3) which in turn phosphorylates and activates another serine/threonine protein kinase (MAPK). *Raf* corresponds to MAPKKK, MEK corresponds to MAPKK, and ERK corresponds to MAPK. These pathways link the cell surface to cytoplasmic and nuclear events and can mediate cell proliferation, apoptosis, differential gene expression, cell shape, osmotic integrity, and responsiveness to other extracellular signals.

MECHANISMS OF SIGNAL TRANSDUCTION

It is the aim of the signal transduction field of study to determine which signaling proteins enable receptor tyrosine kinases to stimulate specific signaling pathways or circuits during embryogenesis. It should also be noted that many of the same genes that determine embryogenesis, when mutated, also play key roles in the induction, progression and suppression of cancer.[96] A number of different intercellular signaling pathways are activated by ligands binding to their cognate receptors (Figs. 4-10 and 4-11). EGF binding to the EGF receptor activates the receptor tyrosine kinase. The activation events include the phospho-

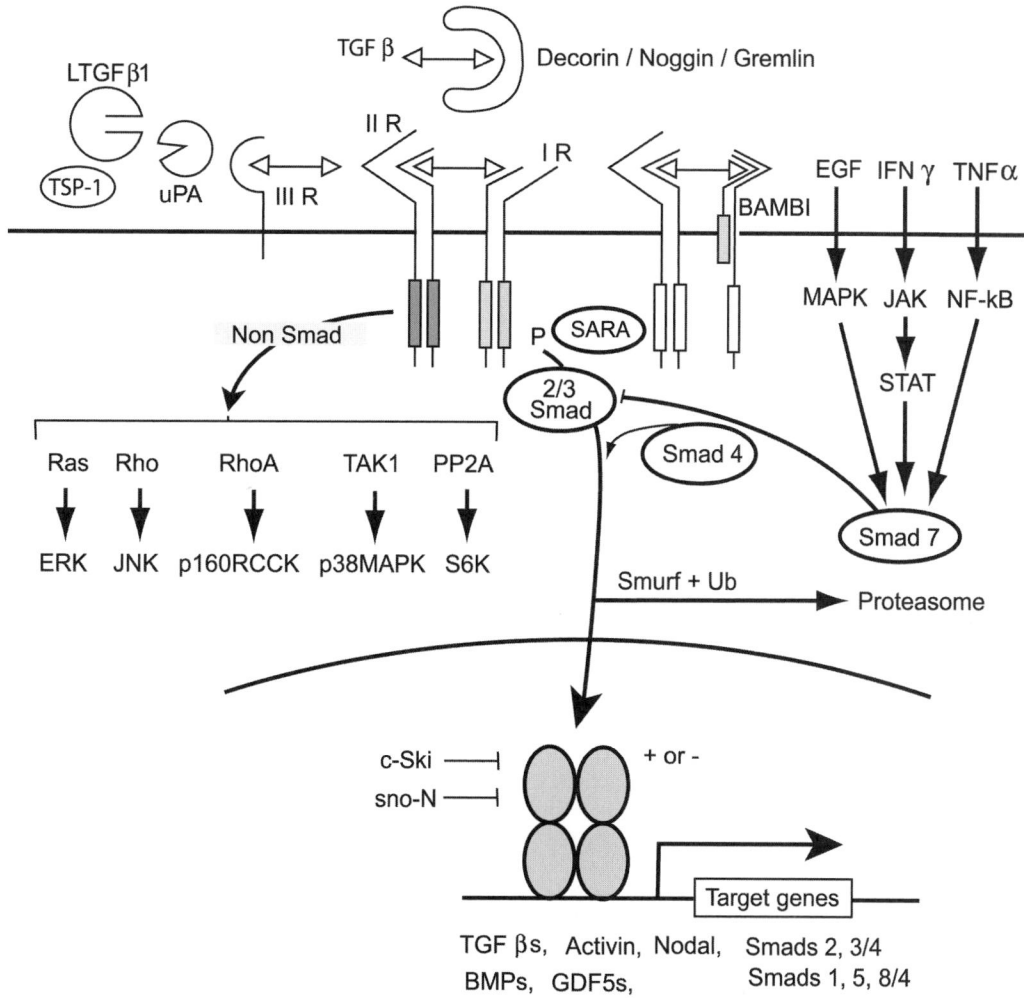

Fig. 4–11. Transforming growth factor β (TGFβ) family peptide signaling in embryonic morphogenesis is finely regulated at many levels, both within and without the cell. As the best studied example, TGFβ$_1$ is secreted as a latent peptide (LTGFβ$_1$), that is cleaved by proteases such as plasmin (uPA) in the presence of thrombospondin-1 (TSP-1) to release an active, dimeric TGFβ$_1$ peptide. Extracellular TGFβ peptide-binding proteins including decorin, noggin, and gremlin, which antagonize TGFβ peptide activity. The Type III TGFβ receptor betaglycan is required for presentation to and increases the affinity of TGFβ$_2$ for the signaling receptor complex. The dimeric ligand binds to and stabilizes a tetrameric cluster of TGFβ Type I and II receptors. In the presence of the dimeric ligand, the constitutively active TGFβ Type II receptor serine/threonine kinase phosphorylates and activates the TGFβ Type I receptor serine/threonine kinase. BAMBI is a naturally occurring dominant negative TGFβ receptor that lacks Smad docking sites, hence blocking the next step in TGFβ signaling. The TGFβ kinase then phosphorylates Smad2/3, which in turn facilitates binding of the common Smad4 to Smad2/3. The Smad 2/3 interaction with TGFβ Type I receptor is stabilized by the FYVE motif in the protein SARA. The complex containing Smad2/3 plus Smad 4 then translocates rapidly into the nucleus. The nuclear Smad complex binds to general transcriptional complexes on specific gene promoters such as PAI-1, collagen I, p21, or cyclin A and respectively activates or represses gene transcription. The stability of the activated Smad complexes is in turn negatively regulated by ubiquitination and proteolytic degradation in the proteosome by the Smurf gene family of ubiquitinases. Smads 6 and 7 are also negative regulators of Smad2/3 binding to and activation by the TGFβ Type I receptor kinase. Smad 7 transcription is rapidly induced by TGFβ, furnishing a rapidly inducible feedback mechanism to control and limit the amplitude of TGFβ signaling. Within the nucleus, c-Ski and Sno-N are transcriptional complex binding factors that negatively regulate Smad complex activity.

EGF, signaling through its cognate tyrosine kinase EGF receptor, which activates the MAPK pathway; interferon γ (IFNγ), which signals via the Janus kinase/STAT transcriptional factor pathway (JAK/STAT); and TNFα, which signals via NFκB, can all also positively regulate Smad 7. However, other possible levels of interaction between these signaling pathways such as Shc 66 are not shown. Non-Smad TGFβ signaling can also act via Ras activation of the ERK pathway. Rho activation of JNK, RhoA activation of p160 RCCK, TAK1 can activate p38 MAPK, whereas PP2A can dephosphorylate and regulate S6 kinase. This figure is freely adapted from the cited reviews.[96,97]

inositide 3-kinase, 70-kDa S6 kinase, mitogen-activated protein kinase (MAPK), phospholipase C-gamma, and the Jak/STAT pathways. Comparative studies using *D. melanogaster, C. elegans,* and a number of different mouse and human cell lines suggest that the extracellular signal-regulated kinase (ERK-regulated) MAPK pathway is common to several signal transduction-induced cellular responses.[22, 27, 29-33, 45, 97]

The principles of signal transduction pathways from receptor tyrosine kinases have been determined. After initial ligand binding (e.g., EGF, IGF-I, IGF-II, FGF, PDGFα), receptor dimerization and autophosphorylation, *Src* homology 2 (SH2) domain-containing proteins are recruited to phosphorylated tyrosine residues on the receptor.[9, 29, 31] These SH2 domain-containing proteins include different constituents in each of the multiple intracellular pathways: (1) the p85 components of the phosphoinositide 3-kinase (PI3-kinase) pathway; (2) the phospholipase C-gamma in the protein kinase C pathway; (3) the *Src* family kinases; and (4) p120-GAP, Shc, and Grb2 in the Ras pathway.[29] The key biochemical reaction is a cascade of phosphorylation or dephosphorylations. Recruitment to phosphorylated tyrosine residues on the EGF receptor, for example, leads to activation of the signaling molecule by a variety of mechanisms. IGF-I and IGF-II signaling regulates preimplantation and postimplantation stages of ernbryogenesis.[25, 32, 98] During mouse lung branching morphogenesis, EGF ligand binding to its cognate receptor mediates both mitogenesis and increased branching morphogenesis.[43, 70, 89, 99] Conversely, the Sprouty gene family has recently been determined to function in flies, mice, and humans as inducible negative regulators of tyrosine kinase receptor activation. Sprouty2 is the closest mammalian orthologue, which functions to modulate FGF pathway negatively signaling in both fly and mouse respiratory organogenesis.[100, 101] This points out the emerging paradigm that positive growth factor signaling must be finely regulated by inducible negative factors such as Sprouty, which inhibits activation of the Ras pathway by the FGF and possibly other tyrosine kinase receptors.

The TGFβ family, which includes various bone morphogenetic proteins (BMPs), signals through a complex of Type I and II serine-threonine kinase receptors (see Fig. 4–11). Ligand is presented to the receptor complex by betaglycan, also known as the type III receptor. Phosphorylation and activation of the type I receptor by the constitutively active type II receptor serine/threonine kinase facilitate direct phosphorylation of specific Smads by the type I receptor serine/threonine kinase. The receptor-Smad interaction is stabilized by the FYVE protein SARA. Smads 1, 5 and 8 mediate BMP and activin signaling, whereas Smads 2 and 3 mediate TGFβ signaling. Smad 4 is the common effector Smad that mediates transcriptional activation or repression by the TGFβ pathway, by interaction with the transcriptional machinery in the 5′ promoter of specific genes. TGFβ and Smads 2, 3, and 4 negatively regulate the cell cycle in epithelial cells by the induction of specific cyclin-dependent kinase inhibitor proteins. Conversely, these pathways also activate matrix genes such as collagen and protease regulatory genes such as PAI-1. Conversely, Smad 7 and Smad 6 are rapidly inducible negative regulators of TGFβ receptor signaling. They function in a similar manner to Sprouty in the FGF pathway as inducible negative modulators in the TGFβ pathway. Smad protein ubiquitination and hence degradation rate are in turn regulated by the Smurf family.[102] TGFβ signaling is also regulated at the extracellular level of ligand binding by extracellular proteoglycans such as decorin and endoglin. Mutations in endoglin are found in families with hereditary ataxia telangiectasia. Recently, cross talk pathways between TGFβ serine/threonine kinase and other peptide growth factor tyrosine kinase receptor pathways have emerged including points of intersection such as Shc, Shp, S6 kinase, and MAP kinase among others.[103] BMPs provide signaling for the induction of osteogenesis involving cell proliferation, cell migration, and cell differentiation.[28, 39, 41, 42, 104] Parallel signal transduction pathways lead to the regulation of DNA synthesis.[27, 29] BMPs are also functionally regulated extracellularly by binding proteins such as gremlin.[105]

In summary, embryogenesis is mediated by finely regulated interactions among many classes of transcription factors, peptide growth factor pathways, and physical forces. Mutations may lead to early lethality if they interfere with cell proliferation, migration, or attachment during implantation or gastrulation. Later, mutations may lead to defects in other key functions such as cilliary beat that lead to defects of lateralization as in cardiac loop defects, situs inversus, malposition of the visceral organs, and lobation defects in the lung. Mutations that affect pulmonary epithelial differentiation and vascularization lead to neonatal respiratory failure and death. Remarkably, in most cases, the genomic embryogenesis program proceeds, leading to the formation of a normal human being. However, in almost every case, minor mistakes lead to birth marks or in other less frequent cases to nonlethal malformations. The recent completion of the human genome project, together with the power of genetics, functional genomics, bioinformatics, and structural biology, now provides a unique opportunity to research, understand, and eventually correct the mutations therapeutically that adversely affect embryogenesis. We rank the developmental biology of the human being as the most exciting scientific endeavor today and for the new century.

ACKNOWLEDGMENTS

The authors wish to acknowledge the invaluable assistance of Eric Bell in the preparation of this manuscript and of Pablo Bringas Jr. for his contributions to the figures.

REFERENCES

1. Collins FS, et al: New goals for the Human Genome Project: 1998–2003. Science *282*:682, 1998.
2. Collins FS, McKusick VA: Implications of the Human Genome Project for medical science. JAMA *285*:540, 2001.
3. Venter JC, et al: The sequence of the human genome. Science *291*:1304, 2001.
4. Altaba ARI, Melton DA: Interaction between peptide growth factors and homeobox genes in the establishment of anteroposterior polarity in frog embryos. Nature (Lond) *341*:33, 1989.
5. Amedee J, et al: Osteogenin (bone morphogenetic protein 3) inhibits proliferation and stimulates differentiation of osteoprogenitors in human bone marrow. Differentiation *58*:157, 1994.
6. Attisano L, et al: TGF-beta receptors and actions. Biochim Biophys Acta *1222*:71, 1994.
7. Baker I, et al: Role of insulin-like growth factors in embryonic and postnatal growth. Cell *75*:73, 1993.
8. Bonner-Fraser M: Environmental influences on neural crest cell migration. J Neurobiol *24*:233, 1993.
9. Burke AC, et al: Hox genes and the evolution of vertebrate axial morphology. Development *121*:333, 1995.
10. Nuckolls GH, et al: Progress towards understanding craniofacial malformations. Cleft Palate Craniofac J *36*:12, 1999.
11. Shum L, et al: Embryogenesis and the classification of craniofacial dysmorphogenesis. *In* Fonseca R (ed): Oral and Maxillofacial Surgery, vol VI. Philadelphia, WB Saunders Co, 2000: p 149.
12. Slavkin HC, et al: Ectodermal dysplasia: a synthesis between evolutionary, development and molecular biology and human clinical genetics. *In* Chuong CM (ed): Molecular Basis of Epithelial Appendage Morphogenesis. New York, Landes Science Publishers, 1999: p 15.
13. De Robertis EM, et al: Determination of axial polarity in the vertebrate embryo: homeodomain proteins and homeogenetic induction. Cell *57*:189, 1989.
14. Fan CM, et al: Patterning of mammalian somites by surface ectoderm and notochord: evidence for sclerotome induction by a hedgehog homolog. Cell *79*:1175, 1994.
15. Gehring WJ: Homeotic genes, the homeobox and the spatial organization of the embryo. The Harvey Lectures, Series 1987. *81*:153, 1987.
16. Gross P, Walther C: *Pax* in development. Cell *69*:719, 1992.
17. Kessel M, Gross P: Murine developmental control genes. Science *249*:374, 1990.
18. Kromlauf R: Hox genes in vertebrate development. Cell *78*:191, 1994.
19. Oliver G, et al: Homeobox genes and connective tissue patterning. Development *121*:693, 1995.

20. Sechrist J, et al: Rhombomere rotation reveals that multiple mechanisms contribute to the segmental pattern of hindbrain neural crest migration. Development *120*:1777, 1994.
21. Druker BI, et al: Oncogenes, growth factors and signal transduction. N Engl J Med *321*:1383, 1989.
22. Flaumenhaft R, Rifkin DB: The extracellular regulation of growth factor action. Mol Biol Cell *3*:1057, 1992.
23. Kiessling AA, Cooper GM: The expression of oncogenesis in mammalian embryogenesis. *In* Rosenblum IY, Heyner S (eds): Growth Factors in Mammalian Development. Boca Raton, FL, CRC Press, 1989, p 167.
24. Nilsen-Hamilton M: Growth factor signaling in early mammalian development. *In* Rosenblum IY, Heyner S (eds): Growth Factors in Mammalian Development. Boca Raton, FL, CRC Press, 1989: p 135.
25. Heyner S, et al: Insulin and insulin-like growth factors in mammalian development. *In* Rosenblum IY, Heyner S (eds): Growth Factors in Mammalian Development. Boca Raton, FL, CRC Press, 1989: p 91.
26. Hill CS, Treisman R: Transcriptional regulation by extracellular signals: mechanisms and specificity. Cell *80*:199, 1995.
27. Hunter T: Signaling: 2000 and beyond. Cell *100*:113, 2000.
28. Lyons KM, et al: The *DVR* gene family in embryonic development. Trends Genet 1991; 7:408.
29. Marshall CJ: Specificity of receptor tyrosine kinase signaling: transient versus sustained extracellular signal-regulated kinase activation. Cell *80*:179, 1995.
30. Mason IJ: The ins and outs of fibroblast growth factors. Cell 78:547, 1994.
31. Morgan DO: Principles of CDK regulation. Nature (Lond) *374*:131, 1995.
32. Okamoto T, Nishimoto I: Analysis of stimulation-G protein sub-unit coupling by using active insulin-like growth factor II receptor peptide. Proc Natl Acad Sci USA *88*:8020, 1991.
33. Pestell RC, Jameson JL: Transcriptional regulation of endocrine genes by second-messenger signaling pathways. *In* Weintraub BD (ed): Molecular Endocrinology: Basic Concepts and Clinical Correlations. New York, Raven Press, 1995: p 59.
34. Melton DA: Pattern formation during animal development. Science *252*:234, 1991.
35. Niehrs C, et al: Mesodermal patterning by a gradient of the vertebrate homeobox gene *goosecoid*. Science *263*:817, 1994.
36. Chen WH, et al: Genesis and prevention of spinal neural tube defects in the curly tail mutant mouse: involvement of retinoic acid and its nuclear receptors RAR-beta and RAR-gamma. Development *121*:681, 1995.
37. Gudas LJ: Retinoids and vertebrate development. J Biol Chem 269:15402, 1994.
38. King MW, Moore MJ: Novel Hox, POU and FKH genes expressed during bFGF-induced mesodermal differentiation in *Xenopus*. Nucleic Acids Res 1994; 22:3990.
39. Chai Y, Slavkin HC: Biology of bone induction and its clinical applications. Oral Maxillofac Surg Clin North Am 7:739, 1995.
40. Chai Y, et al: Specific transforming growth factor-beta subtypes regulate embryonic mouse Meckel's cartilage and tooth development. Dev Biol *162*:85, 1994.
41. Eriebacher A, et al: Toward a molecular understanding of skeletal development. Cell *80*:371, 1995.
42. Jones CM, et al: Involvement of bone morphogenetic protein-4 *(BMP-4)* and *Vgr-1* in morphogenesis and neurogenesis in the mouse. Development *111*:531, 1991.
43. Minoo P, King RJ: Epithelial-mesenchymal interactions in lung development. Annu Rev Physiol *56*:13, 1994.
44. Sanvito F, et al: TGF-beta1 influences the relative development of the exocrine and endocrine pancreas in vitro. Development *120*:3451, 1994.
45. Pawson T: Protein modules and signaling networks. Nature (Lond) *373*:573, 1995.
46. Crossley PH, Martin GR: The mouse Fgf8 gene encodes a family of polypeptides and is expressed in regions that direct outgrowth and patterning in the developing embryo. Development *121*:439, 1995.
47. Graham A, et al: The signaling molecule BMP4 mediates apoptosis in the rhombencephalic neural crest. Nature (Lond) *372*:684, 1994.
48. Gurdon JB: The generation of diversity and pattern in animal development. Cell *68*:185, 1991.
49. Heikinheimo M, et al: Fgf-8 expression in the post-gastrulation mouse suggests roles in the development of the face, limbs and central nervous system. Mech Dev 48:129, 1994.
50. Rubenstein JLR, et al: The embryonic vertebrate forebrain: the prosomeric model. Science *266*:578, 1994.
51. Deng CX, et al: Murine FGFR-1 is required for early postimplantation growth and axial organization. Genes Dev 8:3045, 1994.
52. Gorlin RJ, Slavkin HC: Embryology of the face. *In* Tewfik TL, Der Kaloustian V (eds): Congenital Anomalies of the Ear, Nose, and Throat. London, Oxford University Press, 1997: p 287.
53. Pierce SB, Kimelman D: Regulation of Spemann organizer formation by the intracellular kinase Xgsk-3. Development *121*:755, 1995.
54. Cunha GR, et al: Normal and abnormal development of the male urogenital tract: role of androgens, mesenchymal-epithelial interactions and growth factors. J Androl *13*:465, 1992.
55. Murphy M, et al: FGF-2 regulates proliferation of neural crest cells, with subsequent neuronal differentiation regulated by LIF or related factors. Development *120*:3519, 1994.
56. Sharp R, et al: Transforming growth factor alpha disrupts the normal program of cellular differentiation in the gastric mucosa of transgenic mice. Development *121*:149, 1995.
57. Shum L, et al: EGF abrogation induced *fusilli*-form dysmorphogenesis of Meckel's cartilage during embryonic mouse mandibular morphogenesis in vitro. Development *118*:903, 1993.
58. Slavkin HC: Developmental Craniofacial Biology. Philadelphia, Lea & Febiger, 1979.
59. Slavkin HC: Molecular biology experimental strategies for craniofacial-oral-dental dysmorphology. Connect Tissue Res *31*:1, 1995.
60. Slavkin HC, et al: Early embryonic mouse mandibular morphogenesis and cytodifferentiation in serumless, chemically-defined medium: a model for studies of autocrine and/or paracrine regulatory factors. J Craniofac Genet Dev Biol 9:185, 1989.
61. Slavkin HC, et al: Gene expression, signal transduction and tissue-specific biomineralization during mammalian tooth development. Crit Rev Eukaryotic Gene Expression *2*:315, 1992.
62. Spemann H, Mangold H: Uber Induktionen von Embryonalanlagen durch Implantation artfremder Organisatoren. Arch Entw Mech Org *100*:599, 1924.
63. Jowett AK, et al: Epithelial-mesenchymal interactions are required for Msx-1 and Msx-2 gene expression in the developing murine molar tooth. Development *117*:461, 1991.
64. Lievre CA, et al: Expression of IGF-I and -II mRNA in the brain and craniofacial region of the rat fetus. Development *111*:105, 1991.
65. Mitsiadis TA, et al: Expression of the heparin-binding cytokines, midline (MK) and HB-GAM (pleiotrophin) is associated with epithelial-mesenchymal interactions during fetal development and organogenesis. Development *121*:37, 1995.
66. Holland PWH: Homeobox genes and the vertebrate head. Development *103*:17, 1988.
67. Rijli FM, et al: Insertion of a targeting construct in a *Hoxd-10* allele can influence the control of *Hoxd-9* expression. Dev Dynamics *201*:366, 1994.
68. Satokata I, Maas R: Msx1 deficient mice exhibit cleft palate and abnormalities of craniofacial and tooth development. Nat Genet *6*:348, 1994.
69. Scott MP: Imitations of a creature. Cell *79*:1121, 1994.
70. Seth R, et al: Role of epidermal growth factor expression in early mouse embryo lung branching morphogenesis in culture: antisense oligodeoxynucleotide inhibitory strategy. Dev Biol *158*:555, 1993.
71. Stark K, et al: Epithelial transformation of metanephric mesenchyme in the developing kidney regulated by *Wnt-4*. Nature (Lond) *372*:679, 1994.
72. Jabs EW, et al: A mutation in the homeodomain of the human *MSX-2* gene in a family affected with autosomal dominant craniosynostosis. Cell 75:1, 1993.
73. Liu YH, et al: Premature suture closure and ectopic cranial bone in mice expressing Msx2 transgenes in the developing skull. Proc Natl Acad Sci USA *92*:6137, 1995.
74. Vainio S, et al: Identification of BMP-4 as a signal mediating secondary induction between epithelial and mesenchymal tissues during early tooth development. Cell *75*:45, 1993.
75. Slavkin HC: Rieger syndrome revisited: experimental approaches using pharmacologic and antisense strategies to abrogate EGF and TGF-alpha functions resulting in dysmorphogenesis during embryonic mouse craniofacial morphogenesis. Am J Med Genet 47:689, 1993.
76. Sutherland AE: Expression of syndecan, a putative low affinity fibroblast growth factor receptor, in the early mouse embryo. Development *113*:339, 1991.
77. Yamaguichi TP, et al: fgfr-1 is required for embryonic growth and mesodermal patterning during mouse gastrulation. Genes Dev 8:3032, 1994.
78. Stapleton P, et al: Chromosomal localization of seven *PAX* genes and cloning of a novel member, *PAX-9*. Nat Genet *3*:292, 1993.
79. Van Genderen C, et al: Development of several organs that require inductive epithelial-mesenchymal interactions is impaired in *LEF-I* deficient mice. Genes Dev 8:2691, 1994.
80. Hunt P, Krurnlauf R: *Hox* codes and positional specification in vertebrate embryonic axes. Annu Rev Cell Biol 8:227, 1992.
81. Hunt P, et al: The branchial *Hox* code and its implications for gene regulation, patterning of the nervous system and head evolution. Development 2:63, 1991.
82. Osumi-Yamashita N, et al: The contribution of both forebrain and midbrain crest cells to the mesenchyme in the frontonasal mass of mouse embryos. Dev Biol *164*:409, 1994.
83. Cohn MJ: Lamprey Hox genes and the origin of jaws. Nature *416*:386, 2002.
84. Tijan R, Maniatis T: Transcriptional activation: a complex puzzle with a few easy pieces. Cell *77*:5, 1994.
85. Weintraub H: The *MyoD* family and myogenesis: redundancy, networks and thresholds. Cell *75*:1241, 1993.
86. Stockton DW, et al: Mutation of PAX9 is associated with oligodontia. Nat Genet *24*:18, 2000.
87. Canoun C, et al: Endogenous epidermal growth factor regulates limb development. J Surg Res *54*:638, 1993.
88. Murray JC, et al: Linkage of Rieger syndrome to the region of the epidermal growth factor gene on chromosome 4. Nat Genet *2*:46, 1992.
89. Warburton D, et al: Epigenetic role of epidermal growth factor expression and signalling in embryonic mouse lung morphogenesis. Dev Biol *149*:123, 1992.
90. Cohen MM: Craniosynostosis: phenotypic/molecular correlations. Am J Med Genet *56*:334, 1995.

91. Cohen MM Jr: Fibroblast growth factor receptor mutations. In Cohen MM Jr, MacLean RD (eds): Craniosynostosis. New York, Oxford University Press, 2000: p 77.
92. Jabs EW, et al: Jackson-Weiss and Crouzon syndromes are allelic with mutations in fibroblast growth factor receptor 2. Nat Genet 8:275, 1994.
93. Muenke M, et al: A common mutation in the fibroblast growth factor receptor 1 gene in Pfeiffer syndrome. Nat Genet 8:269, 1994.
94. Reardon W, et al: Mutations in the fibroblast growth factor receptor 2 gene cause Crouzon syndrome. Nat Genet 8:98, 1994.
95. Rousseau F, et al: Mutations in the gene encoding fibroblast growth factor-3 in achondroplasia. Nature (Lond) 371:252, 1994.
96. Derynck R, et al: TGF-beta signaling in tumor suppression and cancer progression. Nat Genet 29:117, 2001.
97. Massague J, Chen YG: Controlling TGFβ signaling. Genes Dev 14:627, 2000.
98. Rappolee DA, et al: Insulin-like growth factor n acts through an endogenous growth pathway regulated by imprinting in early mouse embryos. Genes Dev 6:939, 1992.
99. Warburton D, et al: The molecular basis of lung morphogenesis. Mech Dev 92:55, 2000.
100. Mailluex AA, et al: Evidence that SPROUTY2 functions as an inhibitor of mouse embryonic lung growth and morphogenesis. Mech Dev 102:81, 2001.
101. Tefft JD, et al: Conserves function of mSpry-2, a murine homolog of Drosophila sprouty, which negatively regulates respiratory organogenesis. Curr Biol 9:219, 1999.
102. Zhang Y, et al: Regulation of Smad degradation and activity by Smurf2, an E3 ubiquitin ligase. Proc Natl Acad Sci USA 98:974, 2001.
103. Roberts AB, Derynck R: Meeting report: signaling schemes for TGF-beta. Science's STKE. Available at: www.stke.org/cgi/content/full/OC_sigtrans;2001/113/pe43.
104. Wozney JM, et al: Growth factors influencing bone development. In Waterfield MD (ed): Growth Factors in Cell and Developmental Biology. Cambridge, The Company of Biologists Limited, 1990: p 149.
105. Shi W, Zhao J, Anderson KD, Warburton D: Gremlin negatively modulates BMP-4 induction of mouse lung branching morphogenesis. Am J Physiol 280:L1030, 2001.

Peter Lloyd Jones

5 The Extracellular Matrix in Development

Determining how tissues composed of genetically identical cells acquire and maintain distinct forms and functions within the embryo remains a central goal in developmental biology. One answer to this inquiry lies in the ability of cells within developing tissues to recognize one another, as well as their surrounding tissue microenvironment, which includes the extracellular matrix (ECM). This epigenetic view of development suggests that in addition to its traditional role as a resilient and flexible support for cells within developing and mature tissues, the ECM also behaves as an informational entity that differentially regulates gene expression. One way that cells gain control of gene expression is to surround themselves with specialized, tissue-specific extracellular matrices, which subsequently bind and activate different combinations of cell surface receptors. In this regard, integrin receptors have emerged as major receptors. Adding to this complexity, the ECM and integrins also cross-regulate extra- and intracellular signals emanating from other extrinsic factors, including growth factors, hormones, and biomechanical forces. Additionally, the ECM acts as a reservoir for growth and differentiation factors, and it collaborates with integrins and ECM-degrading proteinases to hide or present these factors to cells within developing tissues. It is also recognized that proteolysis of the ECM generates neoepitopes that confer functions on cells and tissues that are distinct from those specified by their nonproteolyzed counterparts. To illustrate these and other points, it is first essential to appreciate the complex structure of the ECM, and to describe how integrins convey signals from the ECM to the cell interior. Finally, angiogenesis is used as example to show how the ECM controls cell behavior during a fundamental biologic process.

MULTIFUNCTIONAL NATURE OF THE EXTRACELLULAR MATRIX

Normal development requires precise temporal and spatial coordination of cellular proliferation, differentiation, migration, and apoptosis. Deciding which of these programs a cell will ultimately elect is determined, to a large extent, by the ECM. Promotion or suppression of cellular proliferation by the ECM, for example, results in either the stimulation or inhibition of genes involved in the regulation of the cell cycle.[1-3] To counter-

act runaway cellular proliferation, and to sculpt or refine developing tissue structures, cells must also be eliminated from developing tissues. To this end, loss of cell contact with the ECM leads to a specialized form of apoptosis, termed *anoikis*.[4] The ECM also regulates the transcription of genes associated with specialized differentiated functions, including alkaline phosphatase expression in osteoblasts,[5] albumin production in hepatocytes,[6] and intermediate filament protein expression in keratinocytes.[7] These observations are supported by the identification of ECM-responsive transcription factors and *cis*-elements within gene promoter elements.[8, 9] Throughout development, cells need to move from their point of origin to other positions within the embryo, and the ECM represents the template on which migration occurs. Moreover, it is appreciated that stem-cell maintenance, self-renewal, and cell fate determination depend on the ECM.[10, 11] To decipher how the ECM confers so many different functions, it is first essential to appreciate its complex structure.

EXTRACELLULAR MATRIX IS STRUCTURALLY DIVERSE

The ECM is an oligomeric, three-dimensional, network composed of interconnecting proteins that includes four major components: the collagens, structural glycoproteins (e.g., fibronectin, laminin, tenascin-C), proteoglycans (e.g., heparan sulfate proteoglycans, syndecans) and elastic fibers (e.g., elastin, microfibrillar proteins). This is not to suggest that every ECM network contains all these proteins, or that the composition of the ECM remains constant within any particular tissue. Rather, the distribution and organization of the ECM are both dynamic and tissue-specific. For example, mesenchymal cells are surrounded by an interstitial stromal ECM, which includes Type I collagen, Type II collagen, fibronectin, and proteoglycans. The basement membrane represents another specialized ECM that is predominantly composed of laminin, Type IV collagen, heparan sulfate proteoglycan, and entactin. However, not all basement membranes are created equal: they can exist as an amorphous sheetlike structure connected to an underlying collagenous stroma by anchoring fibrils composed of Type VII collagen. Alternatively, basement membrane material may lie between different cell layers, as is the case in the kidney glomerulus where epithelial and endothelial cells are segregated by a basement membrane that functions as a filter.

Cells within certain tissues (e.g., skin, arteries) need to be especially resilient to environmental factors, such as mechanical force. In this respect, extracellular matrices reinforced with elastin fibers represent a suitable ECM.

Within these different extracellular matrices, additional structural and functional diversity is generated through the use of alternative gene promoters, RNA splicing, and by posttranslational modifications, including glycosylation and sulfation of newly synthesized ECM proteins. Furthermore, after individual ECM proteins have been secreted into the extracellular space, they need to be integrated into a functional network. Identifying binding partners for ECM proteins is therefore a prerequisite toward understanding its bulk properties. For example, one structural ECM glycoprotein, tenascin-C, has the potential to interact directly or indirectly with fibronectin, perlecan, neurocan, heparin, phophacan, syndecan, and glypican,[12] albeit in a tissue-specific fashion. Understanding the biology of a single ECM component therefore requires an appreciation of the structure and functions of numerous other affiliated proteins. Given the number of steps involved in coordinating ECM expression, secretion, and assembly, it is easy to appreciate that deciphering how individual ECM proteins contribute to morphogenesis during development represents a formidable task.

GENETIC APPROACHES TO DISSECT EXTRACELLULAR MATRIX FUNCTIONS

Mapping and identifying gene mutations that lead to heritable connective tissue disorders, as well the generation of animal models in which ECM genes have been mutated or ablated, represent two approaches that have been successfully used to ascertain the functions of individual ECM proteins within specific tissues. For the most part, many phenotypes produced by ECM gene mutations reflect their structural nature. For example, mutations in collagen VII, which is normally expressed within anchoring fibrils of the skin, has been linked to the skin-blistering disease epidermolysis bullosa,[13] whereas mutations in Type I collagen genes cause osteogenesis imperfecta and certain forms of Ehlers-Danlos syndrome.[14] Additionally, mutations in elastin and associated microfibrillar proteins lead to Williams-Beuren syndrome and Marfan syndrome,[15] whereas mutations that cause a failure in the synthesis of the proteoglycan, keratan sulfate, result in corneal macular dystrophy.[16]

Apart from mutations in laminin-2 and laminin-5, which have been linked to muscular dystrophies and epidermolysis bullosa, respectively,[17] relatively few heritable disorders involving alterations in ECM glycoproteins have been described. This suggests that structural ECM glycoproteins are essential for embryonic or fetal survival, such that mutations in these genes do not produce a detectable phenotype at birth. Alternatively, structural ECM glycoproteins may be functionally redundant. Indeed, targeted inactivation of genes encoding structural ECM glycoproteins fully supports both these ideas. For example, inactivation of the fibronectin gene in mice results in embryonic death due to mesodermal, neural tube, and vascular developmental defects.[18] In addition, fibronectin has also been shown to be required for normal gastrulation, at least in amphibians.[19] Clearly, the generation of conditional transgenic animals in which ECM genes can be ablated at chosen time points in a tissue-specific manner will help to resolve how fibronectin and other ECM genes function at later stages of development. In the meantime, other approaches have been used to surmount this problem. Injection of peptides or antibodies into normal, postgastrulation embryos have been used to show that preventing cellular interactions with fibronectin inhibits neural crest migration.[20] Similarly, *in utero* suppression of fibronectin expression using a decoy RNA introduced into the ductus arteriosus of lambs at 90-days' gestation prevents cell migration, resulting in the formation of a patent ductus at birth.[21] In contrast to fibronectin, knockout of the tenascin-C gene in mice results in viable and fertile adults,[22] suggesting that other ECM proteins might be able to compensate for tenascin-C deficiency. Consistent with this, experiments using isolated adult hypertensive pulmonary arteries, in which tenascin-C expression has been suppressed, indicate that osteopontin substitutes for tenascin-C in promoting smooth muscle cell proliferation.[23]

Another important lesson that remains to be learned from ECM null mice is whether these animals are truly normal when they interact with the environment. The simple point remains that many of these animals have not been analyzed in sufficient detail to rule out the possibility that they are entirely free from developmental defects. In fact, TN-C knockout mice suffer from several neurologic defects, including hyperactivity, poor sensorimotor coordination, clinging, and freezing behavior, as well as poor performance in passive avoidance tests.[24] Other defects in TN-C knockouts have subsequently been detected, including reduced corneal wound healing and hematopoiesis.[25, 26] Thus, it is apparent that any ECM gene knockout animal with a subtle phenotype must be analyzed under challenging conditions.

Reverse genetics have also been useful in revealing unexpected functions for other ECM genes. For instance, it could be predicted that ablation of the elastin gene would lead to major structural defects in the overall three-dimensional structure of blood vessels. Elastin-null animals, however, die of obstructive arterial disease characterized by proliferation of subendothelial smooth muscle.[27] Thus, elastin exerts an unexpected growth inhibitory role during normal morphogenesis.

EXTRACELLULAR MATRIX RECEPTORS

Integrins

Another way to understand how the ECM controls development and tissue homeostasis is to study its receptors. Cell adhesion or antiadhesion to the ECM is mediated by various cell surface receptors, including cell surface proteoglycans and integrins, which represent the major and most widely studied class of ECM receptors. Integrins are noncovalently linked, heterodimeric, transmembrane proteins composed of one α- and one β-subunit.[28] At the structural level, the α- and β-subunits are unrelated, but within each subunit there is between 40 and 50% homology. For the most part, the large extracellular domains of integrins interact with ECM ligands in the extracellular space, whereas their small intracellular domains associate with the actin cytoskeleton and affiliated proteins, including vinculin, talin, and α-actinin.[29] The $\alpha_6\beta_4$ integrin is an exception to this rule, because it possesses an unusually long cytoplasmic domain that interacts with intermediate filaments within hemidesmosomes, rather than with actin microfilaments. Thus, as their name signifies, integrins integrate the outside of the cell with its inside.

To date, 18 α- and 8 β-subunits have been identified, and these are able to assemble into 24 distinct integrins, which recognize different ECM ligands. For example, certain integrins recognize specific ECM proteins, including fibronectin, vitronectin, and tenascin-C, which contain a small tripeptide sequence, designated RGD (Arg-Gly-Asp). In contrast, $\beta 4$ integrins interacting with α_3-, α_6-, and α_7-subunits recognize laminins; whereas the β_1-integrin subunit interacting with a_1, α_2, α_{10}, and α_{11} represent collagen receptors. This apparent redundancy in ligand binding specificity might at first suggest that integrins would display overlapping functions. Gene knockout experiments in mice, however, have shown that individual integrin subunits possess nonredundant functions.[28, 30] For example, although the $\alpha_3\beta_1$ and $\alpha_7\beta_1$ integrins both recognize laminins, knockout of the α_3 receptor subunit leads to kidney defects and reduced lung branching morphogenesis, whereas $\alpha 7$-null animals develop muscular dystrophy. $\alpha_v\beta_3$ and $\alpha_v\beta_8$ integrins each interact with RGD-containing ECM proteins, yet ablation of the β_3-subunit leads to hemorrhage, due to an inability to aggregate platelets and osteosclerosis, whereas β_8-null mice die during embryogenesis because of placental defects or they exhibit cerebral deficits. Keratinocytes use both $\alpha_3\beta_1$ and $\alpha_6\beta_4$ integrins to adhere to laminin. In contrast to wild-type animals, mice lacking the $\alpha_3\beta_1$ integrin exhibit a poorly organized basement membrane; however, the ability to adhere to the basement membrane is maintained through the $\alpha_6\beta_4$ integrin. These findings suggest that the primary function of the $\alpha_3\beta_1$ laminin receptor is to organize the basement membrane, whereas the $\alpha_6\beta_4$ integrin functions primarily to mediate stable adhesion in hemidesmosomes. Overall, these studies indicate that each member of the integrin family has evolved to subserve specialized and distinct functions throughout development. Determining how integrins transmit signals to the cell interior is clearly fundamental for understanding how this specificity is attained.

Signaling Through Integrins

Integrin clustering and occupancy by ECM ligands result in the formation of multimolecular protein complexes composed of bundles of cytoskeletal protein, as well as numerous intracellular proteins that are recruited to the inner surface of the plasma membrane.[31] These complexes congregate within a specialized signaling center termed a *focal adhesion*. Different types of focal adhesions are known to exist (i.e., fibrillar adhesions and three-dimensional matrix adhesions), depending on whether they are formed within cultured cells or *in vivo*.[32] In this chapter, all these structures are referred to as focal adhesions.

Given that inhibitors of tyrosine kinase activity block the formation of focal adhesions, and given also that integrins lack intrinsic tyrosine kinase activity, the proteins comprising focal adhesions have been analyzed to identify potential tyrosine kinases that could initiate focal adhesion assembly and intracellular signaling pathways.[33] A ubiquitous and major protein found in focal adhesions, which undergoes rapid tyrosine phosphorylation following integrin ligation and clustering, is a 120-kDa nonreceptor tyrosine kinase known as focal adhesion kinase (FAK).[34, 35] Integrin-dependent autophosphorylation of FAK allows it to interact with docking or adaptor proteins, including paxillin, tensin, and Grb2/Son of Sevenless, which in turn are able activate downstream signaling mediators that are known to control fundamental cellular processes.[36]

Many observations strongly suggest that activation of FAK by integrins plays a central role in initiating many of the signals that regulate proliferation. For example, mutation of tyrosine residues critical for FAK activation prevent integrin-mediated proliferation.[37] Additionally, oncogenic transformation of cells, which abolishes the requirement for anchorage-dependent growth, activates FAK.[38] Consistent with this, introduction of constitutively active FAK leads to cell transformation, anchorage-independent growth, and the suppression of apoptosis.[39]

Cross-Talk Between Integrins and Growth Factors

Various soluble growth factors activate FAK, indicating that integrin and growth factor signaling pathways intersect at FAK.[40] Consistent with this, integrin clustering leads to recruitment and activation of growth-factor receptors within focal adhesion complexes. For example, treatment of endothelial cells with beads coated either with RGD tripeptide or with fibronectin leads to coaggregation of $\beta1$ integrins and FAK, as well as with high-affinity receptors for basic fibroblast growth factor (FGF)-2 within newly formed focal adhesions.[41] Parallel studies using similar approaches have extended these findings to show that integrin activation can also lead to recruitment of a more exten-

sive repertoire of growth-factor receptors, including those for epidermal growth factor (EGF) and platelet-derived growth factor (PDGF).[42]

It is not fully understood how integrin ligation leads to the recruitment of receptor tyrosine kinases to the focal adhesion site. However, the fact that high-affinity EGF receptors can directly bind actin, which in turn enhances EGF-dependent autophosphorylation and activation of downstream substrates, indicates a critical role for the F-actin cytoskeleton in coordinating signaling between integrins and growth factors.[43-45] Not surprisingly then, pharmacologic disruption of the actin cytoskeleton not only prevents focal adhesion formation, but this treatment also leads to a failure to activate growth factor receptors.[46, 47] Thus, the actin cytoskeleton and associated proteins may act as a solid-state scaffold that spatially and biochemically coordinates cross-talk between integrins and growth-factor-receptor tyrosine kinases.

In addition to regulating proliferative responses, gene targeting experiments in mice have further revealed the critical role of FAK in mediating other forms of ECM-dependent cell behavior.[48] The phenotype of FAK-deficient mice is embryonic lethality, characterized by delayed embryonic migration, impaired organogenesis, and vascular defects. This phenotype is also reminiscent of fibronectin- or α_5-integrin–deficient mice, supporting the notion that ECM, integrins, and FAK are intimately linked. Unexpectedly, fibroblasts isolated from FAK-null mice are able to assemble focal adhesions and display an enhanced ability to adhere to the ECM substrates in tissue culture. This finding may explain why FAK-deficient cells are unable to migrate *in vivo*.

Finally, although the role of FAK in differentiation of cells and tissues remains unclear, the fact remains that a truncated form of this protein has been detected in the brain, a highly differentiated, largely nonproliferative tissue.[49] Future studies aimed at determining the nature of the signaling molecules that lie downstream from FAK will no doubt reveal how this major integrin-responsive kinase specifies so many functions in different tissues.

EXTRACELLULAR MATRIX AND ANGIOGENESIS

The studies described already fully support the idea that signals generated by the ECM control many, if not all, aspects of cell behavior, at least at some stage during the life-span of a cell. Given this, it is not feasible to describe all the developmental events in which the ECM plays a role within the confines of a single chapter. Instead, I will focus on angiogenesis, an essential process required for normal embryonic growth and development, defined as the growth of new capillaries from preexisting blood vessels. Angiogenesis has also been studied extensively in a variety of pathologic conditions, including neovascularization of solid tumors, and during the growth of new vessels into the retina, as occurs in diabetic retinopathy. Although developmental angiogenesis and pathologic angiogenesis differ somewhat, even a superficial glance at the steps required for generating new capillaries strongly indicates that changes in endothelial cell (EC) adhesion to the ECM are critical in both instances. For example, in response to angiogenic factors, ECs degrade their underlying basement membrane and invade the adjacent perivascular ECM. Catabolism of the ECM also allows serum proteins, including vitronectin, fibronectin, and fibrinogen, to permeate the extracellular space, thereby providing additional ECM components on which ECs migrate. Next, ECs begin to proliferate and to align themselves into vascular networks, a process that requires precise coordination of both cell-cell and cell-ECM adhesion. Finally, to form a patent vessel, ECs become polarized, recruit pericytes, and re-form a basement membrane, which instructs them to exit the cell cycle to become quiescent.

Integrins and Angiogenesis

Although ECs express a variety of integrins, including $\alpha_6\beta_1$, $\alpha_1\beta_1$, $\alpha_2\beta_1$, $\alpha_3\beta_1$, and $\alpha_6\beta_4$, a great deal of attention has been focused on the α_v-subunit–containing receptors. Treatment of ECs with angiogenic factors, including vascular endothelial growth factor (VEGF), stimulates the expression of these integrins.[50] Furthermore, VEGF has been shown to promote EC adhesion to the ECM through $\alpha_v\beta_3$ and $\alpha_v\beta_5$ integrins, demonstrating that VEGF controls integrin activity.[51] In keeping with this, immunoprecipitation experiments have shown that VEGF receptors (i.e., VEGF-R2) associate with $\alpha_v\beta_3$ integrins.[52] At a functional level, blockade of the $\alpha_v\beta_3$ integrins prevents angiogenesis induced by VEGF, whereas inactivating the $\alpha v\beta 5$ integrin inhibits the angiogenic effects of FGF-2.[53] These latter studies not only demonstrate that soluble angiogenic factors and EC integrins communicate with one another, but they also suggest that different soluble angiogenic factors control different aspects of angiogenesis. In support of this, it has been observed that inhibition of protein kinase C[53] disrupts VEGF-induced angiogenesis, yet PKC inhibition has no effect on FGF-2–dependent stimulation of ECs.

A proangiogenic role for the $\alpha_v\beta_3$ integrin is also suggested by a number of other studies. For instance, the $\alpha_v\beta_3$ integrin localizes to newly formed embryonic blood vessels, indicating that it plays a role *in vivo*.[54] This notion is upheld by the finding that blocking the $\alpha v\beta 3$ integrin receptor prevents angiogenesis in various tissue types including the chick chorioallantoic membrane, mouse retina, quail embryo, and rabbit cornea.[54-56] It is fully appreciated that EC survival requires adhesion to the ECM,[57] and the $\alpha_v\beta_3$ integrin receptor has been shown to regulate this process.[58, 59] Interestingly, blocking $\alpha_v\beta_3$ integrins *in vivo* selectively induces apoptosis in newly formed vessels, but this treatment has no effect on pre-existing vessels. In terms of the actual mechanism involved in promoting EC survival, ligation of EC $\alpha_v\beta_3$ integrins suppresses the activity and/or expression of the cell-death mediators, p53 and p21 WAF1/CIP1.[60]

EC motility also depends on the $\alpha_v\beta_3$ integrin receptor. To migrate, ECs must reorganize their cytoskeleton in a manner that allows for the generation of intracellular forces that exert traction on the underlying ECM. It is therefore of interest that activation of the $\alpha_v\beta_3$ integrin receptor is required for sustained activation of the mitogen-activated protein kinases, ERK1 and ERK2,[61] which in turn lead to phosphorylation of myosin light chains, components of the cell motility machinery required for EC motility.[62]

Null mutations of αv integrin subunits have also provided insights about how these receptors function during developmental angiogenesis. Contrary to expectations, vascular development in the αv-null mouse proceeds in a normal manner, and approximately 20% of the animals are born live.[63] After birth, however, these animals succumb to severe intracerebral and intestinal hemorrhages. These studies either reflect redundant and degenerate roles for αv integrins, or they indicate that αv integrins are more essential for vascular integrity, rather than for blood vessel formation.

Matrix Metalloproteinases and Angiogenesis

Movement through the basement membrane and the perivascular tissue microenvironment requires catabolism of the ECM. Certainly, the finding that MMP-2 deficient mice show reduced rates of angiogenesis fully supports this idea.[64] Once again, the $\alpha v\beta 3$ integrin appears to be involved, because interaction of this receptor with MMP-2 leads to MMP-2 activation on the surface of invasive ECs.[65] Furthermore, treatment of angiogenic ECs with a peptide that prevents binding of MMP-2 to $\alpha_v\beta_3$ integrins not only blocks collagenolytic activity, but also inhibits angiogenesis.[66]

Another way that MMPs contribute to angiogenesis is degradation of the pre-existing ECM, revealing neoepitopes that provoke alternative forms of EC behavior. For example, proteolytic cleavage of type IV collagen by MMP-9 results in the exposure of a functionally important proangiogenic $\alpha_v\beta_3$ integrin-binding site that is usually hidden within the native structure of collagen.[67] This mechanism may allow ECs to modify and respond to microenvironmental cues rapidly without the need to wait for *de novo* gene expression.

Experiments involving tissues isolated from MMP-deficient mice have provided additional clues as to how MMPs promote angiogenesis. Ablation of the gene encoding membrane-type matrix metalloproteinase I (MT1-MMP), an enzyme required for MMP-2 activation, leads to an impairment of skeletal development, due to a deficiency in angiogenesis within remodeling cartilage.[68] Similarly, homozygous mice with a null mutation in MMP-9 exhibit an abnormal pattern of skeletal growth plate vascularization and ossification.[69] In each case, tissues explanted from these null mice show delayed release of angiogenic factors, including FGF-2 and VEGF, reinforcing the idea that the MMP-cleavage of the EC ECM promotes the bioavailability of angiogenic growth factors.

Biomechanical Force and Angiogenesis

Cells within developing embryos are constantly exposed to mechanical forces that maintain and modify their biologic behavior. Given their proximity to the bloodstream, ECs are not exempt from this situation. For example, stretching ECs increases β_3 integrin mRNA levels, as well as reorganization of β_1, α_5, and α_2 integrins.[70,71] Studies in vascular smooth muscle cells demonstrate that biomechanical-dependent cellular proliferation relies on β_3 and $\alpha_v\beta_5$ integrins.[72] Whether EC integrins behave in a similar way awaits further investigation, yet the idea that integrins detect biomechanical signals is further supported by the recent finding that FAK is involved in mechanosensing during cell migration.[73] Biomechanical force also modulates the expression and activities of ECM components and proteases that have already been identified as potential positive regulators of angiogenesis, including TN-C and MMP-2.[74] Collectively, these studies indicate that biomechanical signals are not only detected by the ECM and its receptors, but also that intracellular signals generated by these receptors modulate cell adhesion components used to survey and interact with this mechanical microenvironment. Additional studies are clearly needed to determine how local force differentials modulate EC behavior during angiogenesis within the developing embryo.

Extracellular Matrix–Dependent Changes in Cell Shape and Angiogenesis

A frequently overlooked function of the ECM is its ability to maintain or modify cell morphology within developing, remodeling, and differentiated tissues. Moreover, the way in which cell shape imposes itself on signaling pathways generated by the ECM and integrins is not well understood. Nevertheless, a seminal study by Folkman and Moscona in 1978[75] showed that aortic EC proliferation is tightly coupled to EC shape. In essence, the greater the extent of EC spreading, the greater the extent of proliferation. Subsequently, a role for cell shape impacting on integrin-dependent signaling pathways has been demonstrated in angiogenic ECs. The proliferation and subsequent survival of ECs depend on a provisional ECM through the $\alpha_v\beta_3$ integrin, given that blockade of this receptor results in a failure to proliferate due to unscheduled apoptosis.[55] However, occupation and ligation of $\alpha_v\beta_3$ integrins using anti-integrin fail to support EC proliferation and survival if the cells are prevented from acquiring a spread morphology.[76] It could be postulated, then, that EC rounding leads to apoptosis due to decreased integrin ligation, and therefore less signaling through integrins and FAK. However, by culturing ECs on a defined concentration and area of different ECM ligands, it has been shown that cell spreading alone was conducive to proliferation, whereas cellular rounding was associated with apoptosis.[77] Thus, EC shape, specified by the ECM, appears to profoundly modulate signals generated by identical ECM-integrin interactions.

To understand further how ECM/integrin–dependent EC shape changes operate to control angiogenesis, it will be necessary to identify additional proteins that are able to coordinate both intracellular signaling pathways and cell shape. To this end, the discovery that the Rho family of small GTPases triphosphatases (e.g., RhoA, Rac1, Cdc42) are able to relay integrin-derived signals, as well as organize the cytoskeleton,[78,79] suggest that these proteins are well poised to integrate EC shape and function. In fact, recent studies have shown that VEGF-dependent EC motility is critically dependent on Rac1,[80] and that Rac1 integrates signaling through both the actin and microtubule cytoskeletons to promote capillary tube assembly in a tissue culture model of angiogenesis.[81]

CONCLUSION

Clearly, cell-ECM interactions play a fundamental role in development, yet many questions remain. The phenotypic analysis of mice bearing null mutations in ECM genes and receptors has not provided all of the answers. Furthermore, a basic understanding of how different combinations of ECM proteins generate tissue-specific forms of behavior is still lacking. Regardless of the outcomes of such experiments, the development of rapid screening techniques for the detection of ECM gene mutations, as well the development of diagnostic DNA and protein microarrays, will no doubt aid in determining whether the results gleaned from experimental systems are relevant to developmental defects detected in human embryos and fetuses.

ACKNOWLEDGMENT

Peter Lloyd Jones is supported by the American Heart Association (GIA 9950622N) and National Institutes of Health (2 P50 HL57144-06 & 1 R01 HL68798-01).

REFERENCES

1. Boudreau N, et al: Suppression of apoptosis by basement membrane requires three-dimensional tissue organization and withdrawal from the cell cycle. Proc Natl Acad Sci USA 93:3509, 1996.
2. Zhu X, Assoian RK: Integrin-dependent activation of MAP kinase: a link to shape-dependent cell proliferation. Mol Biol Cell 6:273, 1995.
3. Dike LE, Ingber DE: Integrin-dependent induction of early growth response genes in capillary endothelial cells. J Cell Sci 109:2855, 1996.
4. Frisch SM, Screaton RA: Anoikis mechanisms. Curr Opin Cell Biol 13:555, 2001.
5. Mackie EJ, Ramsey S: Modulation of osteoblast behaviour by tenascin. J Cell Sci 109:1597, 1996.
6. Mooney D, et al: Switching from differentiation to growth in hepatocytes: control by extracellular matrix. J Cell Physiol 151:497, 1992.
7. Adams JC, Watt FM: Fibronectin inhibits the terminal differentiation of human keratinocytes. Nature 340:307, 1989.
8. Schmidhauser C, et al: A novel transcriptional enhancer is involved in the pro-lactin- and extracellular matrix-dependent regulation of beta-casein gene expression. Mol Biol Cell 3:699, 1992.
9. Jones PL, et al: Induction of vascular smooth muscle cell tenascin-C gene expression by denatured type I collagen is dependent upon a beta3 integrin-mediated mitogen-activated protein kinase pathway and a 122-base pair promoter element. J Cell Sci 112:435, 1999.
10. Chang C, Werb Z: The many faces of metalloproteases: cell growth, invasion, angiogenesis and metastasis. Trends Cell Biol 11:S37, 2001.
11. Heissig B, et al: Recruitment of stem and progenitor cells from the bone marrow niche requires MMP-9 mediated release of kit-ligand. Cell 109:625, 2002.
12. Jones PL, Jones FS: Tenascin-C in development and disease: gene regulation and cell function. Matrix Biol 19:581, 2000.
13. Bruckner-Tuderman L: Blistering skin diseases: models for studies on epidermal-dermal adhesion. Biochem Cell Biol 74:729, 1996.
14. Prockop DJ, Kivirikko KI: Collagens: molecular biology, diseases, and potentials for therapy. Annu Rev Biochem 64:403, 1995.
15. Milewicz DM, et al: Genetic disorders of the elastic fiber system. Matrix Biol 19:471, 2000.
16. Klintworth GK, Smith CF: Abnormal product of corneal explants from patients with macular corneal dystrophy. Am J Pathol 101:143, 1980.
17. Engvall E: Structure and function of basement membranes. Int J Dev Biol 39:781, 1995.
18. George EL, et al: Defects in mesoderm, neural tube and vascular development in mouse embryos lacking fibronectin. Development 119:1079, 1993.
19. Ramos JW, DeSimone DW: Xenopus embryonic cell adhesion to fibronectin: position-specific activation of RGD/synergy site-dependent migratory behavior at gastrulation. J Cell Biol 134:227, 1996.
20. Boucaut JC, et al: Prevention of gastrulation but not neurulation by antibodies to fibronectin in amphibian embryos. Nature 307:364, 1984.
21. Mason CA, et al: Gene transfer in utero biologically engineers a patent ductus arteriosus in lambs by arresting fibronectin-dependent neointimal formation. Nat Med 5:176, 1999.
22. Saga Y, et al: Mice develop normally without tenascin. Genes Dev 6:1821, 1992.
23. Cowan KN, et al: Elastase and matrix metalloproteinase inhibitors induce regression, and tenascin-C antisense prevents progression, of vascular disease. J Clin Invest 105:21, 2000.
24. Fukamauchi F, et al: Abnormal behavior and neurotransmissions of tenascin gene knockout mouse. Biochem Biophys Res Commun 221:151, 1996.
25. Ohta M, Sakai T, Saga Y, et al: Suppression of hematopoietic activity in tenascin-C-deficient mice. Blood 91:4074, 1998.
26. Talts JF, et al: Tenascin-C modulates tumor stroma and monocyte/macrophage recruitment but not tumor growth or metastasis in a mouse strain with spontaneous mammary cancer. J Cell Sci 112:1855, 1999.
27. Li DY, et al: Elastin is an essential determinant of arterial morphogenesis. Nature 393:276, 1998.
28. Hynes R. Integrins: bidirectional, allosteric signaling machines. Cell 110:673, 2002.
29. Dedhar S, Hannigan GE: Integrin cytoplasmic interactions and bidirectional transmembrane signalling. Curr Opin Cell Biol 8:657, 1996.
30. Sheppard D: In vivo functions of integrins: lessons from null mutations in mice. Matrix Biol 19:203, 2000.
31. Schwartz MA, Ginsberg MH: Networks and crosstalk: integrin signalling spreads. Nat Cell Biol 4:E65, 2002.
32. Cukierman E, et al: Taking cell-matrix adhesions to the third dimension. Science 294:1708, 2001.
33. Burridge K, et al: Tyrosine phosphorylation of paxillin and pp125FAK accompanies cell adhesion to extracellular matrix: a role in cytoskeletal assembly. J Cell Biol 119:893, 1992.
34. Schaller MD, et al: pp125FAK a structurally distinctive protein-tyrosine kinase associated with focal adhesions. Proc Natl Acad Sci USA 89:5192, 1992.
35. Hanks SK, et al: Focal adhesion protein-tyrosine kinase phosphorylated in response to cell attachment to fibronectin. Proc Natl Acad Sci USA 89:8487, 1992.
36. Juliano R: Cooperation between soluble factors and integrin-mediated cell anchorage in the control of cell growth and differentiation. Bioessays 18:911, 1996.
37. Schlaepfer DD, et al: Integrin-mediated signal transduction linked to Ras pathway by GRB2 binding to focal adhesion kinase. Nature 372:786, 1994.
38. Guan JL, Shalloway D. Regulation of focal adhesion-associated protein tyrosine kinase by both cellular adhesion and oncogenic transformation. Nature 1992; 358(6388):690.
39. Frisch SM, et al: Control of adhesion-dependent cell survival by focal adhesion kinase. J Cell Biol 134:793, 1996.
40. Zachary I, et al: Bombesin, vasopressin, and endothelin stimulation of tyrosine phosphorylation in Swiss 3T3 cells. Identification of a novel tyrosine kinase as a major substrate. J Biol Chem 267:19031, 1992.
41. Plopper GE, et al: Convergence of integrin and growth factor receptor signaling pathways within the focal adhesion complex. Mol Biol Cell 6:1349, 1995.
42. Miyamoto S, et al: Integrins can collaborate with growth factors for phosphorylation of receptor tyrosine kinases and MAP kinase activation: roles of integrin aggregation and occupancy of receptors. J Cell Biol 135:1633, 1996.
43. den Hartigh JC, et al: The EGF receptor is an actin-binding protein. J Cell Biol 119:349, 1992.
44. Gronowski AM, Bertics PJ: Modulation of epidermal growth factor receptor interaction with the detergent-insoluble cytoskeleton and its effects on receptor tyrosine kinase activity. Endocrinology 136:2198, 1995.
45. Diakonova M, et al: Epidermal growth factor induces rapid and transient association of phospholipase C-gamma 1 with EGF-receptor and filamentous actin at membrane ruffles of A431 cells. J Cell Sci 108:2499, 1995.
46. Defilippi P, et al: p125FAK tyrosine phosphorylation and focal adhesion assembly: studies with phosphotyrosine phosphatase inhibitors. Exp Cell Res 221:141, 1995.
47. Abedi H, Zachary I: Vascular endothelial growth factor stimulates tyrosine phosphorylation and recruitment to new focal adhesions of focal adhesion kinase and paxillin in endothelial cells. J Biol Chem 272:15442, 1997.
48. Ilic D, et al: Reduced cell motility and enhanced focal adhesion contact formation in cells from FAK-deficient mice. Nature 377:539, 1995.
49. Andre E, Becker-Andre M: Expression of an N-terminally truncated form of human focal adhesion kinase in brain. Biochem Biophys Res Commun 190:140, 1993.

50. Suzuma K, et al: Hypoxia and vascular endothelial growth factor stimulate angiogenic integrin expression in bovine retinal microvascular endothelial cells. Invest Ophthalmol Vis Sci *39*:1028, 1998.
51. Byzova TV, et al: A mechanism for modulation of cellular responses to VEGF: activation of the integrins. Mol Cell *6*:851, 2000.
52. Soldi R, et al: Role of alpha vbeta3 integrin in the activation of vascular endothelial growth factor receptor-2. Embo J *18*:882, 1999.
53. Friedlander M, et al: Definition of two angiogenic pathways by distinct alpha v integrins. Science *270*:1500, 1995.
54. Drake CJ, et al: An antagonist of integrin alpha v beta 3 prevents maturation of blood vessels during embryonic neovascularization. J Cell Sci *108*:2655, 1995.
55. Brooks PC, et al: Requirement of vascular integrin alpha v beta 3 for angiogenesis. Science *264*:569, 1994.
56. Hammes HP, et al: Subcutaneous injection of a cyclic peptide antagonist of vitronectin receptor-type integrins inhibits retinal neovascularization. Nat Med *2*:529, 1996.
57. Meredith JE Jr, et al: The extracellular matrix as a cell survival factor. Mol Biol Cell *4*:953, 1993.
58. Brooks PC, et al: Integrin alpha v beta 3 antagonists promote tumor regression by inducing apoptosis of angiogenic blood vessels. Cell *79*:1157, 1994.
59. Stupack DG, Cheresh DA: Get a ligand, get a life: integrins, signaling and cell survival. J Cell Sci *115*:3729, 2002.
60. Stromblad S, et al: Suppression of p53 activity and p21WAF1/CIP1 expression by vascular cell integrin alpha Vbeta3 during angiogenesis. J Clin Invest *98*:426, 1996.
61. Eliceiri BP, et al: Integrin alpha v beta3 requirement for sustained mitogen-activated protein kinase activity during angiogenesis. J Cell Biol *140*:1255, 1998.
62. Klemke RL, et al: Regulation of cell motility by mitogen-activated protein kinase. J Cell Biol *137*:481, 1997.
63. Bader BL, et al: Extensive vasculogenesis, angiogenesis, and organogenesis precede lethality in mice lacking all alpha v integrins. Cell *95*:507, 1998.
64. Itoh T, et al: Reduced angiogenesis and tumor progression in gelatinase A-deficient mice. Cancer Res *58*:1048, 1998.
65. Brooks PC, et al: Localization of matrix metalloproteinase MMP-2 to the surface of invasive cells by interaction with integrin alpha v beta 3. Cell *85*:683, 1996.
66. Brooks PC, et al: Disruption of angiogenesis by PEX, a noncatalytic metalloproteinase fragment with integrin binding activity. Cell *92*:391, 1998.
67. Hangai M, et al: Matrix metalloproteinase-9-dependent exposure of a cryptic migratory control site in collagen is required before retinal angiogenesis. Am J Pathol *161*:1429, 2002.
68. Zhou Z, et al: Impaired endochondral ossification and angiogenesis in mice deficient in membrane-type matrix metalloproteinase I. Proc Natl Acad Sci USA *97*:4052, 2000.
69. Vu TH, et al: MMP-9/gelatinase B is a key regulator of growth plate angiogenesis and apoptosis of hypertrophic chondrocytes. Cell *93*:411, 1998.
70. Suzuki M, et al: Up-regulation of integrin beta 3 expression by cyclic stretch in human umbilical endothelial cells. Biochem Biophys Res Commun *239*:372, 1997.
71. Yano Y, et al: Cyclic strain induces reorganization of integrin alpha 5 beta 1 and alpha 2 beta 1 in human umbilical vein endothelial cells. J Cell Biochem *64*:505, 1997.
72. Wilson E, et al: Mechanical strain of rat vascular smooth muscle cells is sensed by specific extracellular matrix/integrin interactions. J Clin Invest *96*:2364, 1995.
73. Wang HB, et al: Focal adhesion kinase is involved in mechanosensing during fibroblast migration. Proc Natl Acad Sci USA *98*:11295, 2001.
74. Jones PL, et al: Altered hemodynamics controls matrix metalloproteinase activity and tenascin-C expression in neonatal pig lung. Am J Physiol Lung Cell Mol Physiol *282*:L26, 2002.
75. Folkman J, Moscona A: Role of cell shape in growth control. Nature *273*:345, 1978.
76. Re F, et al: Inhibition of anchorage-dependent cell spreading triggers apoptosis in cultured human endothelial cells. J Cell Biol *127*:537, 1994.
77. Chen CS, et al: Geometric control of cell life and death. Science *276*:1425, 1997.
78. Nobes CD, Hall A: Rho, rac, and cdc42 GTPases regulate the assembly of multimolecular focal complexes associated with actin stress fibers, lamellipodia, and filopodia. Cell *81*:53, 1995.
79. Kheradmand F, et al: Role of Rac1 and oxygen radicals in collagenase-1 expression induced by cell shape change. Science *280*:898, 1998.
80. Soga N, et al: Rho family GTPases regulate VEGF-stimulated endothelial cell motility. Exp Cell Res *269*:73, 2001.
81. Connolly JO, et al: Rac regulates endothelial morphogenesis and capillary assembly. Mol Biol Cell *13*:2474, 2002.

6

Evan Y. Snyder and Stephen Yip

Stem Cell Biology

CONCEPTS AND NOMENCLATURE

Stem cells have entered the consciousness of both the medical community and the lay public because their tremendous regenerative capabilities may offer great therapeutic potentials.[1] However, it is important to realize that these cells are actually the building blocks of organogenesis and hence must actually be viewed in the context of fundamental developmental biology. If certain aspects of this biology fill therapeutic niches, then it should be viewed as "translational developmental biology." Restoration of tissue or the replacement of damaged or defective cells via the recapitulation of developmental processes or a repetition of organogenesis is an extremely powerful concept, if realized. It represents a paradigm shift in medicine and helps give birth to the emerging field of regenerative medicine. Probably during the perinatal periods—when developmental processes are normally at their most intensive—this approach might find its first and most successful expression. A partial glimpse of the potential of stem cell biology is offered by the current success of hematopoietic stem cell transplantations for selected diseases.[2]

A stem cell is the most primitive cell of a given organ or tissue that is able to differentiate into all the more mature and specialized daughter cells of that tissue (multipotency) and to self-renew (i.e., the ability to give rise to some daughter cells with exactly the same potential). *Asymmetric cellular division*—when a stem cell divides into another identical stem cell and a specialized daughter cell—is responsible for this unique developmental dynamic of a stem cell.[3] In addition, stem cells can undergo *symmetric division*, in which one stem cell gives rise to two identical stem cells. The ability to undergo prolonged self-renewal means that a stem cell population can be expanded indefinitely. Teleologically, this is significant for the persistence of stem cell pools into adulthood for maintaining homeostasis throughout life. Taking advantage of this biologic attribute, however, should permit indefinite expansion of stem cells *in vitro* once they have been abstracted from a tissue and placed in culture. *In vivo*, the environment surrounding the stem cell, including the extracellular matrix and the supporting stromal cells, in conjunction with intrinsic stem cell developmental programs, appears to control the various stem cell decision pathways that ultimately lead to the creation of a given organ[4,5]; our attempt to recreate those signals on command and outside their normal window of expression will be the tools of regenerative medicine, or *translational developmental biology* (see Fig. 6-11).

The zygote, when implanted into the uterus, is considered to be a "totipotent" cell because it can give rise to the complete mammalian organism when it combines with another zygote. Each zygote, however, is not self-renewing, hence it is not really a "stem cell" (Fig. 6-1). The coming together of two zygotes yields a fertilized egg, which begins to divide, yielding daughter cells that, if given the appropriate maternal support, will not only

POTENTIAL STEM CELLS WITH NEURAL CAPABILITY

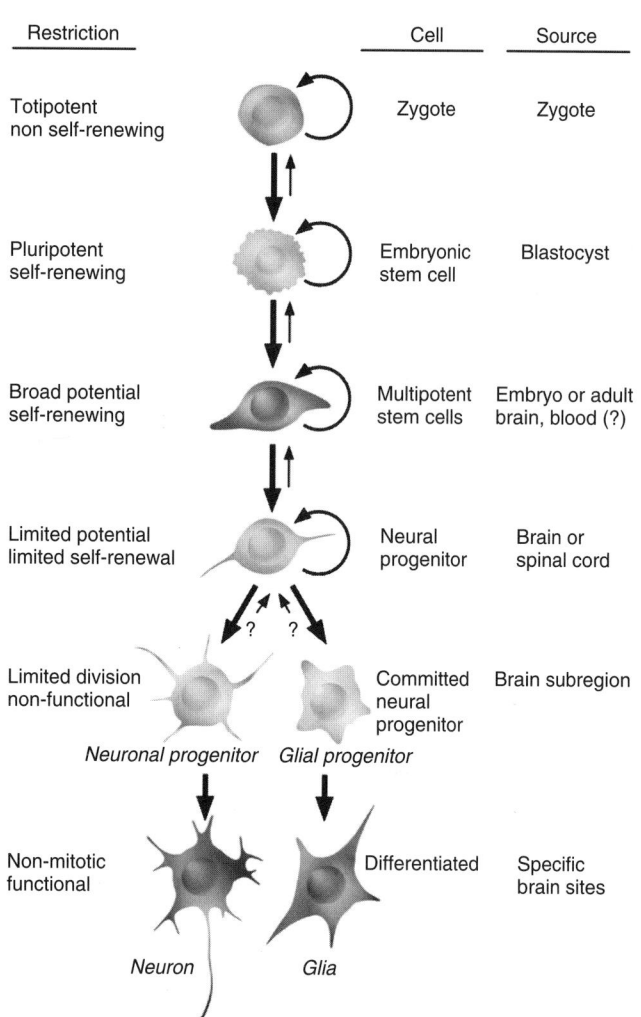

Restriction	Cell	Source
Totipotent non self-renewing	Zygote	Zygote
Pluripotent self-renewing	Embryonic stem cell	Blastocyst
Broad potential self-renewing	Multipotent stem cells	Embryo or adult brain, blood (?)
Limited potential limited self-renewal	Neural progenitor	Brain or spinal cord
Limited division non-functional	*Neuronal progenitor* *Glial progenitor* / Committed neural progenitor	Brain subregion
Non-mitotic functional	*Neuron* *Glia* / Differentiated	Specific brain sites

Figure 6–1. The developmental potential of mammalian stem cells into neurons. The developmental hierarchy of the stem cells is shown; pluripotentiality becomes much more restricted with maturation of the stem cell. (From Gage FH: Science *287*:1433, 2000.)

yield a complete organism but also daughter cells ostensibly with equal potential to yield a complete organism. The fertilized cells go through a 2-cell, then 4-cell, then 8-cell stage, ultimately yielding a morula, and then a blastocyst. The blastocyst becomes asymmetric in its appearance and function. Toward one pole of the blastocyst, a group of stem cells begin to accumulate to form the inner cell mass (ICM), or the future embryo, which is called the "fetal pole." The ICM is composed of embryonic stem cells (ESCs), which within 1 week will begin to generate daughter cells that become partitioned to one of three fundamental germ layers: ectodermal, mesodermal, or endodermal. The ectoderm ultimately gives rise to cells of the neural crest lineage, the central and peripheral nervous system; the mesoderm gives rise to muscle, bone marrow, blood vessels, and the urogenital system, as well as the connective tissues of the body; the endoderm gives rise to the epithelial lining of the gastrointestinal tract, parenchymal pancreas, thyroid, parathyroid, and liver. ESCs are situated at the apex of the stem cell hierarchy, owing to their primacy in the developmental sequence (Fig. 6–2).

Pluripotent stem cells (PSCs) can be isolated from the blastocyst (discussed later) and can give rise to cells of the three primary germ layers in the organism except for the tropho-

blasts. PSCs have been isolated from embryonic tissues—i.e., the ICM. Whether vestiges of such cells can still be isolated from adult tissues remains extremely controversial. Some investigators have claimed that such cells remain in the bone marrow mesenchyme, for example. However, definitive and convincing proof of this, independent of confounding experimental artifacts, remains lacking for now. Multipotent stem cells are stem cells that have "learned their address"; i.e., they have been allocated to residence within a given tissue. These cells are clearly present in the embryonic version of these mature tissues and organs and persist throughout gestation into fetal life and likely into adulthood following birth. They are usually restricted to developmental pathways within their particular organ of residence and certainly to their fundamental germ layer of derivation. They are more developmentally mature or somewhat more restricted in their potential than are either PSCs or totipotent stem cells. For example, a multipotent stem cell of ectodermal origin can give rise to daughter cells that belong to this germ layer only (although that orthodoxy recently has been challenged in a series of controversial and not widely accepted experiments; for practical purposes, however, this tenet most likely holds). Committed progenitor cells, such as the colony-forming unit granulocyte-macrophage (CFU-GM), are even more restricted in their developmental potential. These cells are limited in their ability for self-renewal and are programmed to give rise to a very limited repertoire of specialized cells within a germ layer.

Thus, stem cells may be divided into two main groups: ICM-derived and tissue-derived, or tissue-resident, stem cells. The latter designation can be further modified by specifying the particular tissue and the particular age or developmental stage from which the stem cell was observed or isolated, (e.g., a fetal neural stem cell, an adult neural stem cell, or a newborn hematopoietic stem cell).

These concepts will be discussed in greater detail in the following sections.

Embryo-Derived Stem Cells

Embryonic Development

Differentiation of a 3- to-5-day-old preimplantation embryo, at this stage known as the *blastocyst*, generates the ICM and the trophectoderm.[6] The trophectoderm lacks stem cells but contains trophoblastic precursor cells that later become the fetal part of the placenta. During the preimplantation stage, the outer trophectodermal epithelium pumps fluid to form the bastocoel, a hollow cystic structure that defines the blastocyst.[7] The ICM, located at one end of the blastocoel, consists of approximately 30 pluripotent cells that can give rise to all types of tissue in the fetus (Fig. 6–3). ESCs are derived from the *in vitro* expansion of these cells, which is accomplished by growing the cells on specialized feeder cell layers or in the presence of the cytokine leukemic inhibitory factor (LIF). Immunosurgery is sometimes used to isolate cells from the ICM and to deplete it of contaminating trophoblasts. ESCs can be maintained in an undifferentiated state in the laboratory indefinitely and can be expanded numerically as ESC lines. Once removed from the feeder cell layer or LIF and with the appropriate stimuli, they can be made to differentiate into cells belonging to all three primary germ layers *in vitro*. In addition, teratomas and teratocarcinomas are generated from the implantation of ESCs into immunodeficient animals.[8] Indeed, the ability to form such neoplasms is part of the definition of an ESC. ESCs from primates (both monkey and human) are much harder to grow and to keep in an undifferentiated, proliferative state than are ESCs from mice.

Implantation of the embryo (days 5.5 to 7 in a mouse and days 7 to 12 in humans) is associated with further cellular differentiation and the impending disappearance of the pluripotent state.

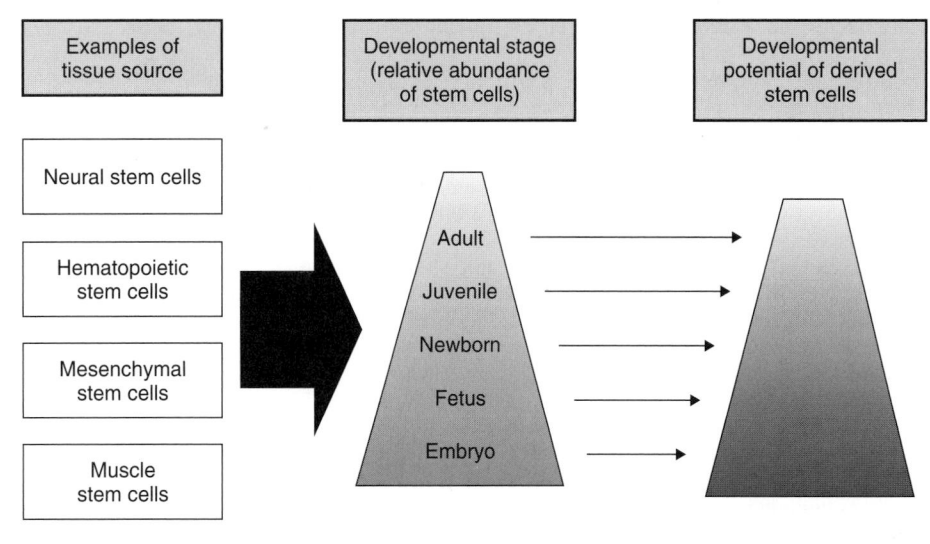

Figure 6–2. Examples of tissue-derived stem cells from different stages of development. Stem cells can be obtained from many different tissues but their abundance and developmental potential follow a strict hierarchy in which embryo-derived stem cells have the highest pluripotentiality.

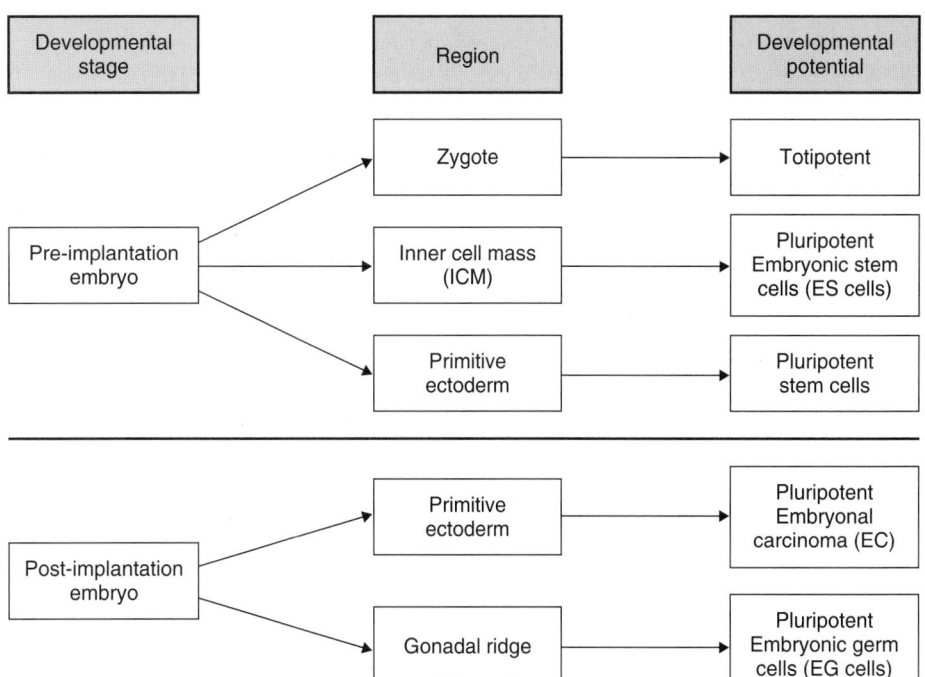

Figure 6–3. Major sources of stem cells from the embryo. Embryo-derived stem cells can be classified as from preimplantation or post-implantation stages. They can be further subcategorized from different regions or origin, which ultimately will affect the developmental potential.

Next comes establishment of the primitive endoderm that contains precursors to cells of the embryonic yolk sac, a nutritive organ for the developing embryo. The field of ESC research was initiated with the study of teratocarcinomas in the 1970s. It was noted that these tumors contain differentiated cells belonging to all three primary germ layers and also to a population of PSCs, which, when transplanted to a receptive host, would form a second tumor. In addition, teratocarcinomas could also proliferate *in vitro* as undifferentiated embryonal carcinoma (EC) cell lines in the presence of a feeder cell layer. These tumors could be generated artificially by transferring cells from the postimplantation epiblasts or ICM into immune sanctuary sites, such as the testis or inside the kidney capsule.[9] As noted earlier, the ability to form a teratoma became part of the operative definition of an ESC.

Embryonic Stem Cells of Mouse Origin

Murine-derived ESCs were originally isolated in 1981 by Evans and Kaufman.[10] Successive groups have refined the isolation and culture techniques. Essentially, ESC lines were generated by the successive replating of undifferentiated ESCs with subsequent numerical expansion. The use of a suitable feeder cell layer was initially indispensable to the maintenance of an undifferentiated state. It was subsequently learned that LIF could be used in place of the feeder cell layer, and this cytokine appears to be important in maintaining the viability of PSCs in the preimplantation embryo.[11,12] LIF also has pleiotrophic actions on the organism, including effects on hematopoiesis, osteogenesis, lipid transport in adipocytes, neurogenesis, and neuronal survival.[13] LIF binds to a heterodimeric transmembrane receptor and shares the *gp130* subunit with the receptor for interleukin-6 (IL-6), oncostatin M, cardiotrophin-1, and ciliary neurotrophic factor (CNTF). Signaling by LIF appears to activate the STAT3 pathway. The feeder cell layer appears to provide a mixture of secreted soluble cytokines, membrane-associated factors, and factors associated with the extracellular matrix (ECM). These factors, in turn, maintain the growth of the ESC lines in an undifferentiated state. Attempts have been made to analyze systemically the biochemical composition of these factors.[14] Ultimately, one would like to replace completely the need for feeder layers (especially for the *in vitro* maintenance of human ESC lines).

Mouse ESC lines have not only been extensively studied and characterized as objects of study in themselves, but also have given rise to a valuable biologic tool, the "transgenic mouse" in which specific genes of interest can be "knocked-out" or "knocked-in" to a mouse at its earliest stages of embryogenesis. A mouse develops with expression of the gene of interest altered—either overexpressed or underexpressed. The advent of transgenic mouse technology has revolutionized studying the molecular basis of both development and disease.

As mentioned previously, ESCs should be able to differentiate into cell types belonging to the three primary germ layers once removed from the feeder layer or from LIF. Furthermore, ESC lines should contain a normal complement of chromosomes and be karyotypically normal and stable, a requirement for meiosis and hence the generation of functional gametes. When introduced into the embryos of recipient animals, ESCs should be able to form all the tissues in the organism, including the germ cells, creating essentially chimeric animals. Further, injection of ESCs into immunodeficient hosts will result in the formation of teratomas or teratocarcinomas. Mouse ESCs have been induced to differentiate into a great variety of cell types, including neurons, glia, adipocytes, islet cells, hepatocytes, and osteoblasts *in vitro*.[15] Kyba and associates were able to engender long- term engraftment of lymphoid-myeloid precursors from genetically modified murine ESCs.[16]

It is thought that, in directing an ESC toward becoming a mature cell type, it passes—even fleetingly—through a stage of being a tissue-derived stem cell. In other words, when one directs an ESC to become a neuron, it first passes through a stage of becoming a neural stem cell, a cell equivalent to that populating the neuroectoderm and lining the neural tube. Various methods have been devised to control the fate of differentiating ESCs. Obviously, one would not want to transplant pluripotential ESCs that could potentially form tumors (e.g., teratomas or teratocarcinomas) or give rise to cell types inappropriate to a given organ (e.g., teeth in the brain). Restricting the potential of these very pluripotent cells has also been a challenge. To take full advantage of ESCs, the mechanisms underlying cellular differentiation and lineage development must be understood. Different groups are already making dramatic progress in this area. Okabe and co-workers reported the preferential expansion of neuroepithelial precursors from murine ESCs using basic fibroblast growth factor (bFGF) in serum-free condition.[17] This cytokine is a well-known mitogenic and trophic factor for developing neuronal precursor cells.[18, 19] The investigators then enforced neuronal and glial differentiation in the enriched neuroepithelial precursor cell population by the withdrawal of bFGF and growth in serum-containing medium. They were able to demonstrate generation of postmitotic functional neurons and glial cells. By taking advantage of the known molecular physiology of a particular cellular lineage, the investigators were able to create the desired cell population. Later, the same group expanded ESCs *in vitro* and directed their differentiation into oligodendroglial and astrocyte precursors which, when transplanted into a myelin-deficient rodent host, were able to induce remyelination of the host neurons,[20] much as neural stem cells were able to do.[21]

Embryonic Stem Cells of Human Origin

Isolation, growth, and characterization of human ESCs was reported in 1998.[22] Characterization of this cell line and other subsequent human ESC lines revealed pluripotentiality, chromosomal euploidy, surface expression of multiple early stem cell antigens such as the stage-specific embryonic antigens (SSEAs), and expression of the early stem cell transcription factor OCT- 4. These characteristics are similar to those of murine ESCs. Human ESCs also displayed significant developmental plasticity and have the ability to undergo indefinite self-renewal in the laboratory in an undifferentiated state.[23] Henderson and colleagues showed a similar antigen expression profile between long-term human ESCs and preimplantation human embryos.[24]

However, some differences exist between human and murine ESCs. Human ESCs grow as flat colonies, whereas mouse ESCs grow in round, amorphous masses. In addition, mouse ESCs are more robust *in vitro* and are able to regenerate all the tissues in a living mouse created by the formation of ESC chimera with host tetraploid embryonic cells.[25] The latter experiment obviously cannot be done in human subjects because of ethical restraints. Human ESCs are very difficult to manipulate and, to date, have not been able to be grown reliably without a mouse feeder layer, making transplantation of cells derived from human ESCs problematic (essentially making them a xenograft). There is significant cross-pollination of knowledge and technical expertise between the fields of ESC research and the rapidly evolving area of assisted reproductive research, especially the subspecialty of *in vitro* fertilization (IVF).[12] The rapid development of preimplantation diagnostics is an example of such a marriage between scientific and technical advances.[26] However, the source of material, namely preimplantation embryos, used to generate human ESC lines remains quite controversial.[27] Society will need to come to a decision regarding the utility of human ESCs.

Recently, Zwaka and Thomson reported the successful homologous recombinations of *hprt1*, the gene encoding hypoxanthine phosphoribosyl transferase-1 (HPRT1), as well as several other developmentally important genes in human ESCs *in vitro*.[28] The power to effect stable *in vitro* targeted genetic changes in human ESCs can be integrated with the techniques of therapeutic cloning and gene therapy as a method of correcting inherited diseases that have been demonstrated in the rodent model.[29, 30] The ability to perpetuate embryonic pluripotent stem cells *in vitro* and to retain the ability to differentiate as directed is an extremely powerful concept with therapeutic potential theoretically, (Fig. 6–4).[31] However, the realization of this goal relies on solving a myriad of scientific and technical problems, one of which is immunoreactivity of allogeneic PSC lines.[32] Another hurdle is the ability to obtain the desired cell population(s) with differentiation. Progress is being made in this area. Schuldiner and co-workers studied eight cytokines and their ability to effect forced differentiation of human ESCs.[33] They found that combinations of growth factors were needed to enforce differentiation and noted the absence of restricted cell type differentiation—i.e., the absence of pure populations of one cell lineage and the spontaneous emergence of cell type heterogeneity. In addition to the technical and supply hurdles, there is ongoing debate on the ethical dilemma posed by the concept of therapeutic cloning: generation of clonal ESC lines for the purpose of scientific research and medical advancement. As demonstrated in Figure 6–5, somatic cell nuclear transfer (SCNT) is a potentially powerful technique that allows for the generation of autologous ESCs from adult somatic cells.[29]

Embryonic Germ Cells (EGCs)

Another source of embryo-derived pluripotent stem cells is the gonadal and germinal ridge from the 7- to 10-day-old embryo. These primordial germ cells (PGCs) can be expanded *in vitro* to generate embryonic germ cell (EGC) lines. Transplantation of mouse PGCs (which persist through midgestation) into susceptible recipients gave rise to teratocarcinomas. Shamblott and associates isolated human PGCs and characterized the subsequently derived EGC line.[34] They harvested and isolated gonadal ridges and mesenteries from weeks 5 to 9 postfertilization embryos, obtained from products of therapeutic termination of pregnancy, using a protocol that was approved by the institution. Extensive characterization of the resultant EGCs demonstrated that they satisfied all the criteria previously set for human ESC lines. Namely, they could be maintained as unspecialized cells *in vitro* in co-cultures with mouse feeder

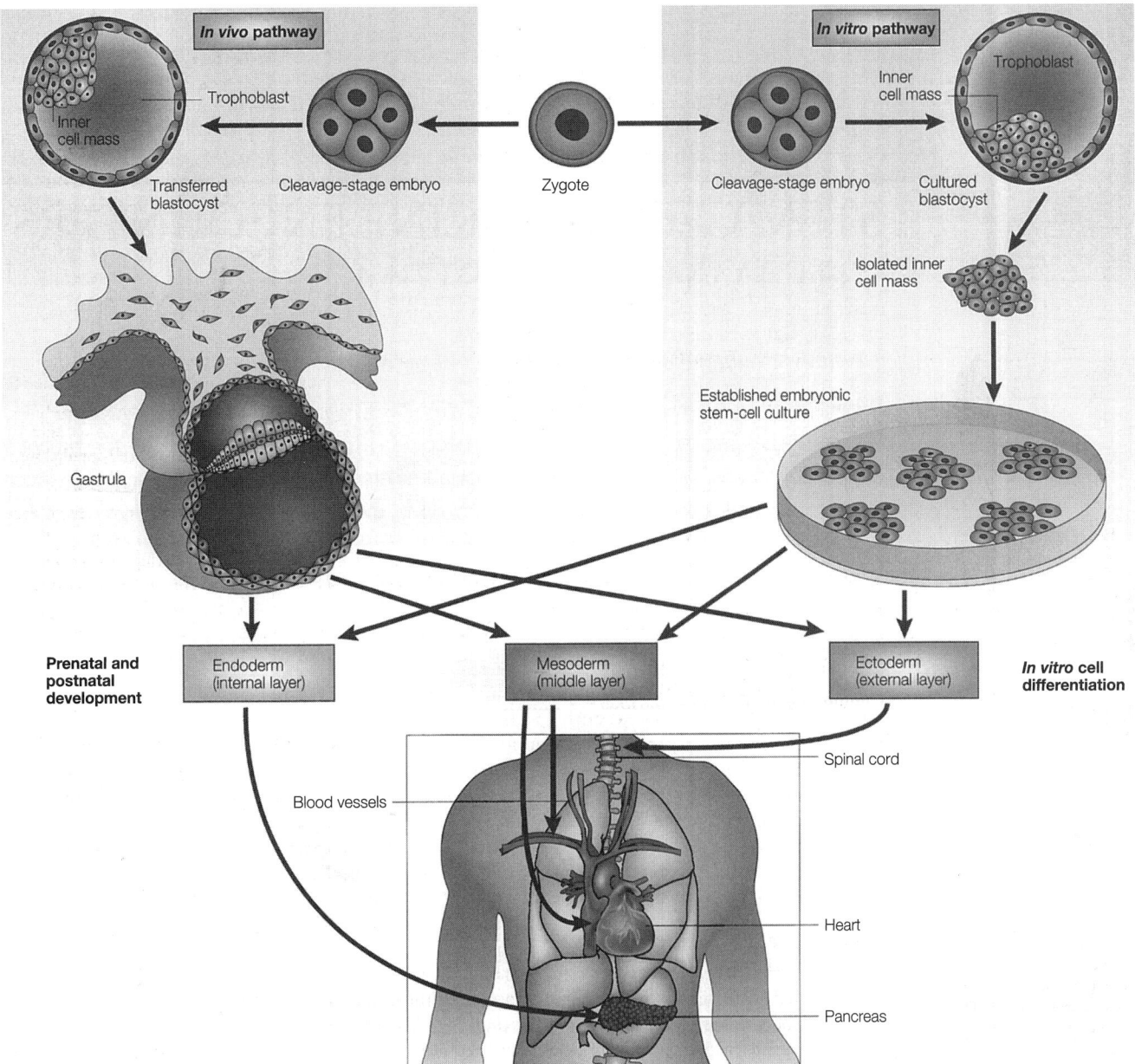

Figure 6–4. Alternative fates for an *in vitro*–fertilized zygote: intrauterine versus *in vitro* development. There are two possible developmental pathways for an embryo generated by *in vitro* fertilization. When an embryo is transferred to the uterus at the cleavage or blastocyst stage, its development can result in the birth of a child. When an embryo is cultured exclusively *in vitro*, it can result in the derivation of stem cells. These two divergent pathways could converge ultimately in the use of stem cells and their derivatives for cell-based transplantation therapies. *In vitro* fertilization was used first as a treatment for infertility, a procedure in which the resulting embryos are transplanted to the uterus at the early cleavage or blastocyst stage. This *in vivo* pathway can result (in approximately one-third of cases) in the implantation of the embryo into the wall of the uterus, where it undergoes gastrulation and subsequent prenatal development. Recent successes in the derivation of human embryonic stem (hES) cells have opened up a second, *in vitro*, pathway for the development of human zygotes. Isolation and culture of the inner cell mass can result (in up to 50% of cases) in the prolonged growth of cells that have the capacity to differentiate into all three cell types of the body—endoderm, mesoderm, and ectoderm. Human ES cells have been shown to be capable of differentiating *in vitro* into insulin-producing cells, heart cells, blood-vessel cells and nerve cells, as have their mouse counterparts. Therefore, hES cells are a promising source of tissue for transplantation for the treatment of, for example, diabetes, lung disease, cardiovascular disease, anemia and other diseases of the blood, and diseases or injuries of the central nervous system. (From Bradley JA, et al: Stem cell medicine encounters the immune system. Nat Rev Immunol *2*:859–871, 2002.)

layers and, when induced to differentiate, were able to generate daughter cells belonging to all three germ layers. The EGCs have normal karyotypes, can be clonally isolated, and demonstrate immunohistochemical profiles similar to those of other embryo-derived stem cells.

The same group subsequently characterized the differentiated progenies of the established EGC lines and demonstrated a wide range of developmental markers associated with neuronal, vascular, hematopoietic, muscle, and endodermal lineages.[35] It is interesting that, as with ESCs, heterogeneous populations of

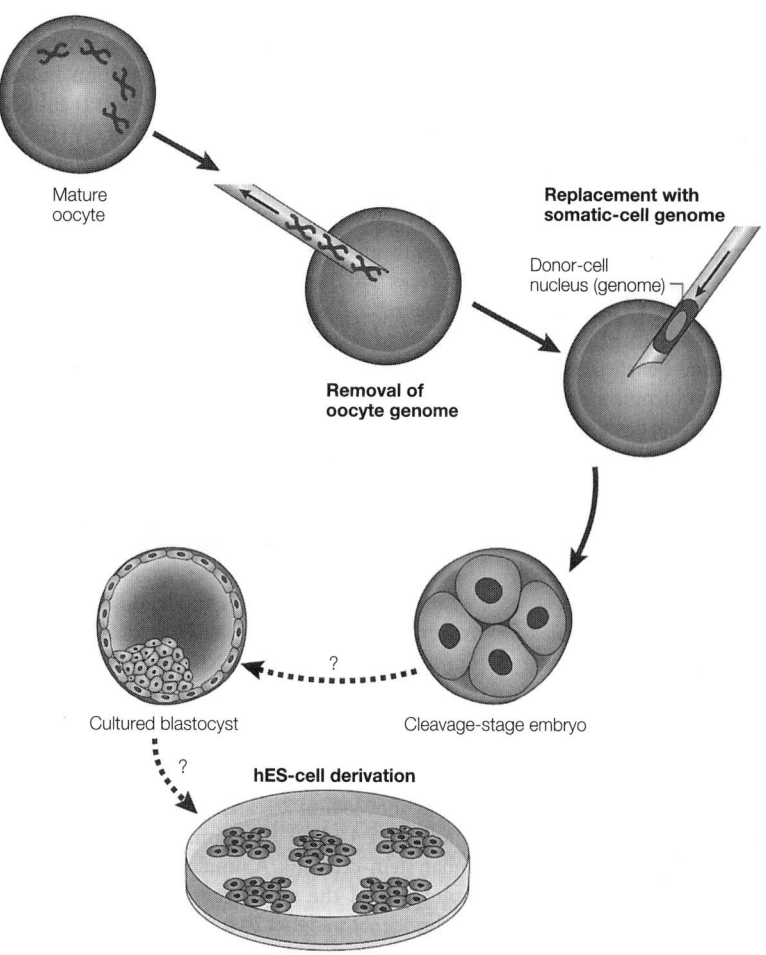

Mature
oocyte

Removal of
oocyte genome

**Replacement with
somatic-cell genome**

Donor-cell
nucleus (genome)

Cultured blastocyst

Cleavage-stage embryo

hES-cell derivation

Figure 6–5. Genomic replacement (somatic-cell nuclear transfer) as a way of matching stem cell-derived tissues with their intended recipient. Replacing the genetic material (genome) of an oocyte with that of a somatic cell generates a near-perfect match between the resulting donor cells and the graft recipient (donor of the somatic-cell genome). For this purpose, the oocyte genome is removed and replaced with the nucleus of a cell from any one of several possible somatic (body) tissues of the graft recipient, using a micropipette. The oocyte cytoplasm enables the donor genome from a somatic cell to support embryonic development by a poorly understood process known as reprogramming. The resulting embryo is cultured to the blastocyst stage, from which embryonic stem cells are derived. It should be noted that, owing to minor histocompatibility antigens encoded by the DNA of egg-derived mitochondria, grafts derived from stem cells grown from such embryos might not be strictly identical to the graft recipient. hES = human embryonic stem cell. (From Bradley JA, et al: Stem cell medicine encounters the immune system. Nat Rev Immunol 2:859–871, 2002.)

multiple lineages persisted or re-emerged. As illustrated in Figure 6-1, ESCs and EGCs are ICM- and gonadal ridge–derived pluripotent cells from the embryo. They are derived from preimplantation and postimplantation embryos, respectively, but both cell populations retain pluripotentiality and many other stem cell characteristics.

Tissue-Derived or Tissue-Resident Stem Cells

Tissue-derived or tissue-resident stem cells retain the ability for self-renewal and to differentiate into specialized cells of the tissue of origin. These cells are found in abundance during early fetal development, and their number is believed to decrease as the organism ages (see Fig. 6-2). The first solid-organ, tissue-derived stem cells to be described, isolated, engrafted, and exploited for therapeutic purposes and for developmental insight was the neural stem cell. Indeed, recognition of the existence of the neural stem cell suggested a greater degree of natural plasticity within the central nervous system than had been classically envisioned. The isolation and expansion of human neural stem cells—including those with the ability to be engrafted, to respond to developmental cues, to replace missing neural cell types, and to transport in foreign genes—was first reported in 1998.[36] These human neural stem cells were obtained from germinal zones (ventricular zone) of a human fetal telencephalon. These tissue-resident stem cells, at least those in the human, are somewhat less robust in their proliferative potential than their embryonic counterparts; in other words, whereas ESCs are "naturally immortalized," such tissue-resident stem cells as neural stem cells typically require tonic exposure to a mitogen or augmentation with cell cycle regulatory genes. The

prolonged expansion and propagation of hematopoietic stem cells still remains a significant obstacle; a reliably effective "cocktail" of mitogens has remained elusive (as of this writing).

Palmer and colleagues demonstrated the presence of neuronal progenitor cells in the adult brain, yet they are much less robust than their neonatal counterparts *in vitro*.[37] The adult cells entered cellular senescence much sooner than the neonatal progenitor cells. The investigators postulated that this was partly related to telomere length, which could be due to a discrepancy in telomerase activity. Recent evidence has pointed to the presence of adult stem cells in a great variety of tissues.[38] Many of these cells retain stem cell characteristics but are less vigorous than embryo- and fetus-derived stem cells from the same tissues. Some examples of adult stem cells are hematopoietic stem cells (HSCs) and crypt cells from the intestinal lining. A single HSC is able to reconstitute the entire hematopoietic system of an animal and a human. Indeed, that capacity is part of the operational definition of a tissue-derived stem cell. Ogawa and co-workers were able to effect durable lymphohematopoietic reconstitution in irradiated recipient mice by the transplantation of a single highly purified HSC.[39] This was supported by earlier lineage studies using retroviral marking of purified HSCs.[40] For obvious reasons, most tissue-resident stem cells cannot be tested for this important and defining characteristic; for example, it is not possible to ablate the nervous system in the way one can ablate the hematopoietic system (as one does experimentally in rodents and clinically prior to bone marrow transplantation). However, substantially large lesions can be created in the nervous system. In such cases, neural stem cells have been found to reconstitute the missing parenchyma with a broad range of missing cell types.[41,42]

As mentioned, the development of these tissue-derived stem cells is lineage-restricted to the resident tissue or germ layer. The exact roles of these tissue-resident stem cells is not yet certain. For example, the existence of neural stem cells has been proved beyond a doubt, yet their purpose is still being elucidated. It is presumed that they are a reservoir of immature cells designed to maintain homeostasis of the organ by buffering the forces that cause cell death (toxins, senescence, infection, trauma) throughout the life of the organism by providing a small supply of replacement cells. If so, it is believed that their role can be exploited for even more extensive repair on demand. Other examples of tissue-derived stem cells—including those that persist into adulthood—are those that seem to reside in the stromal and mesenchymal portion of the bone marrow. These stem cells appear to give rise to diverse specialized mesenchymal cells, such as chondrocytes, adipocytes, and osteocytes.[43] Whether these same stem cells play a homeostatic role for other organs, such as liver and heart and pancreas, is being investigated. Initial evidence,[49] however, has recently been called into question by an experimental artifact—that such mesenchymal cells may actually fuse with cells from other organs, such as the liver, and simply give the illusion of having transdifferentiated.[44,45]

Transdifferentiation

Stem cell plasticity, or transdifferentiation, is a hotly debated topic among stem cell biologists. It is a powerful concept, if proved valid biologically, and can be translated efficiently, safely, and effectively to clinical conditions. Theoretically, a supply of abundant, easily obtainable, autologous immunotolerated stem cells (e.g., from the skin or bone marrow) could be directed toward the lineages of tissues from which stem cells are harder to abstract (e.g., from the adult nervous system).[46] For obvious reasons, this is a very attractive concept because it offers a virtually unlimited supply of stem cells, eliminates the need for fetal tissues, and avoids the politically charged topics of therapeutic cloning.[47] Nevertheless, rigorous laboratory evidence demonstrating adult tissue–resident stem cell plasticity is lacking.

Many papers have pointed to the existence of these tissue-resident adult multipotent stem cells that can differentiate into cells within the same germ layer, and to the existence of adult pluripotent stem cells that can give rise to a variety of cell types representing more than one major germ layer.[48,49] If proved true, one's ability to harvest and expand adult stem cells from one tissue and convert it to cells of the desired lineage would be akin to cellular alchemy.[50] The ability to use one's own pluripotent stem cells obviates the problem of immune-rejection of allergenic tissues derived from established ESC or EGC lines and hence the need for powerful immunosuppressive agents in these patients. In addition, this would avoid the ethical and moral minefield of obtaining pluripotent stem cells from preimplantation embryos and also the issue of therapeutic cloning. Recent published papers, however, showed that previously reported transdifferentiations were due to experimental artifacts, and the presence of target cell lineage markers has no bearing on functional equivalency—in other words, the presence of a mature neuronal marker does not equate the cell behaving like a functional neuron.[51,52]

Alternatively, this phenomenon may, indeed, represent a real but aberrant form of cellular development. For example, cellular de-differentiation or lineage reassignment could account for adult stem cell plasticity.[53] This is similar to (or at least the first step in) metaplasia and neoplastic transformation in tumor development.[54] Much more work will need to be done to prove or disprove this phenomenon.[55] The presence of multiple tissue-specific stem cells (passengers?) actually coursing within the systemic circulation could account for the reported pluripotentiality of "hematopoietic cells."[56]

One potential candidate is the multipotent adult progenitor cell (MAPC) isolated from the bone marrow mesenchyme.[57]

These highly purified cells are reported to differentiate into daughter cells belonging to the mesodermal, neuroectodermal, and endodermal lineages *in vitro*. They may represent persistence of partially committed somatic stem cells in the adult. Derivation of MAPCs requires a very stringent culturing condition involving low-density plating. These cells are also not as robust *in vitro* when compared with ECSs and EGCs, or even with stem cells derived from the particular tissue of interest, e.g., neural stem cells. Nevertheless, more work is needed to study the biology and capabilities of MAPC.[58] In summary, although an attractive concept, rigorous scientific evidence is still lacking for demonstrating tissue-resident stem cell plasticity of a sufficient degree to permit transdifferentiation.

CLINICAL UTILITY OF STEM CELLS

Replacement Cell and Gene Therapies—Neural Stem/Progenitor Cells as a Prototype

Neural stem cells (NSCs), by definition, have the potential to undergo self-renewal via asymmetric division, and to generate intermediate and mature cells of all glial and neuronal lineages throughout the neuraxis and at all stages of life.[59-61] The stem cells also can migrate to various parts of the central nervous system (CNS) to effect population or repopulation of developing and diseased brain, respectively. In fact, the transplanted cells have the uncanny ability to seek out areas of pathology.[62] Various studies have shown that the transplanted stem cells respond to local environment cues and undergo developmental changes accordingly, but with great plasticity.[36,63]

Global CNS pathology is prevalent in most neurologic disorders, including inherited and adult-onset neurodegenerative diseases, diffuse axonal injury secondary to trauma and ischemia, and brain neoplasms. These diseases present difficult challenges for the clinician because of their diffuse nature. The intermingling of diseased cells with normal brain cellular architecture, coupled with extensive brain infiltration, makes current treatment paradigms unsatisfactory. Cell transplantation that takes advantage of some of the unique features of multipotential NSCs has helped give credence to the heretofore theoretical concept of *neurorestoration*.[64] Transplanted neural progenitor cells and stem cells have the capacity to migrate to and integrate into the mammalian CNS in an appropriate fashion.[65-68] This can even occur in the subhuman primate using human cells as graft material.[68]

Taking advantage of these characteristics, unmodified and engineered NSCs have been implanted into several rodent disease models to assess for integration and restoration of abnormal CNS architecture and function. Of note, transplanted NSCs integrate throughout the CNS and yield replacement neural cells in a global manner (for example, myelinating cells in a myelin-deficient mutant, such as the *shiverer* mouse)[21]; indeed, the implanted NSCs shifted their fate to yield a greater proportion of myelinating oligodendrocytes than NSCs would in a wild-type environment. Implanted NSCs could similarly distribute missing gene products throughout the brain; for example, they could effect histologic and phenotypical changes in the MPS VII mouse model defective of lysosomal storage,[69] performing the equivalent of a bone marrow transplant to the brain. There are many other examples of multipotential NSCs repopulating a diseased, traumatically injured, or developmentally deranged CNS.[70-73] In addition to their use for cell replacement, NSCs also can be engineered to deliver therapeutic genes and viral vectors throughout the CNS.[42,74] NSCs have a strong affinity for sites of pathology, ischemic areas, and brain tumors. This ability makes them a potentially valuable adjunct in the treatment of the aggressive disseminating gliomas.[75] They may serve as vehicles that can track down glioma cells and deliver therapeutic gene products directly to these widely dispersed and infiltrating neoplastic cells. Finally, it has been recognized that NSCs—even when they do not differentiate into replacement cells—appear to have—even in their undifferentiated state—an intrinsic ability to rescue or protect degenerating host neurons as a result of complex host–stem cell cross-talk and reciprocal interactions.[42, 73] NSCs therefore have biologic attributes that enable their use in the treatment of various CNS diseases by a variety of mechanisms, all of which are components of fundamental stem cell biology.

Cell Replacement Therapies of Other Tissues

ESCs could be directed to differentiate into the desired cell lineages for cellular replacement. Some of the potential uses for human ESCs in cell replacement therapy in cardiology have been reviewed elsewhere.[76]

SUMMARY

Stem cells have the capability to undergo extensive self-renewal and to differentiate into committed progenitor cells and mature specialized cells of multiple organ systems. Stem cells can be isolated from the mammalian embryo and expanded *in vitro*. These embryonic stem cells are quite robust and have the capability to replenish all tissues of the organism. ESCs then give rise to tissue-derived or tissue-resident stem cells, which also can be used as a source for lineage-specific cell replacement therapy. It remains to be determined how the degree of plasticity of these types of stem cells changes as the organism ages—do vestigeal embryo-like or tissue-resident stem cells persist throughout life in various reservoirs throughout the organism? Can they be isolated and used with equal efficiency, efficacy, and safety at all stages? Are the barriers between cell lineages rigid and inviolate? Many of these questions remain unanswered. For the present, the most useful stem cells have been those derived from the ICM of the blastocyst and from embryonic and fetal tissues. Stem cells, endowed with their special biologic characteristics, also provide an invaluable tool for the study of developmental cell biology. Indeed, any therapeutic use of such cells should be viewed as translational developmental biology.

REFERENCES

1. Smith A: Cell therapy: in search of pluripotency. Curr Biol 8:R802, 1998.
2. Thomas ED: Bone marrow transplantation: a review. Semin Hematol 36:95, 1999.
3. Knoblich JA: Mechanisms of asymmetric cell division during animal development. Curr Opin Cell Biol 9:833, 1997.
4. Kiger AA, et al: Somatic support cells restrict germline stem cell self- renewal and promote differentiation. Nature 407:750, 2000.
5. Spradling A, et al: Stem cells find their niche. Nature 414:98, 2001.
6. Rossant J: Stem cells from the mammalian blastocyst. Stem Cells 19:477, 2001.
7. Rossant J, Cross JC: Placental development: lessons from mouse mutants. Nat Rev Genet 2:538, 2001.
8. Smith A: Embryo-derived stem cells: of mice and men. Annu Rev Cell Dev Biol 17:435, 2001.
9. Pera MF, et al: Isolation and characterization of a multipotent clone of human embryonal carcinoma cells. Differentiation 42:10, 1989.
10. Evans MJ, Kaufman MH: Establishment in culture of pluripotential cells from mouse embryos. Nature 292:154, 1981.
11. Nichols J, et al: Physiological rationale for responsiveness of mouse embryonic stem cells to *gp130* cytokines. Development 128:2333, 2001.
12. Rossant J, Cross JC: Placental development: lessons from mouse mutants. Nat Rev Genet 2:538, 2001.
13. Metcalf D: The unsolved enigmas of leukemia inhibitory factor. Stem Cells 21:5, 2003.
14. Lim JWE, Bodnar A: Proteome analysis of conditioned medium from mouse embryonic fibroblast feeder layers which support the growth of human embryonic stem cells. Proteomics 2:1187, 2002.
15. Wobus AM: Potential of embryonic stem cells. Mol Aspects Med 22:149, 2001.
16. Kyba M, et al: HoxB4 confers definitive lymphoid-myeloid engraftment potential on embryonic stem cell and yolk sac hematopoietic progenitors. Cell 109:29, 2002.
17. Okabe S, et al: Development of neuronal precursor cells and functional post-mitotic neurons from embryonic stem cells in vitro. Mech Dev 59:89, 1996.
18. Vicario-Abejon C, et al: Functions of basic-fibroblast growth factor and neurotrophins in the differentiation of hippocampal neurons. Neuron 15:105, 1995.
19. Kitchens DL, et al: FGF and EGF are mitogens for immortalized neural progenitors. J Neurobiol 25:797, 1994.
20. Brustle O, et al: Embryonic stem cell–derived glial precursors: a source of myelinating transplants. Science 285:754, 1999.
21. Yandava B, et al: "Global" cell replacement is feasible via neural stem cell transplantation: evidence from the dysmyelinated shiverer mouse brain. Proc Natl Acad Sci USA 96:7029, 1999.
22. Thomson JA, et al: Embryonic stem cell lines derived from human blastocyst. Science 282:1145, 1998.
23. Odorico JS, et al: Multilineage differentiation from human embryonic stem cell lines. Stem Cells 19:193, 2001.
24. Henderson JK, et al: Preimpantation human embryos and embryonic stem cells show comparable expression of stage-specific embryonic antigens. Stem Cells 20:329, 2002.
25. Nagy A, et al: Derivation of completely cell culture–derived mice from early-passage embryonic stem cells. Proc Natl Acad Sci USA 90:8424, 1993.
26. Braude P, et al: Preimplantation genetic diagnosis. Nat Rev Genet 3:943, 2002.
27. Robertson JA: Human embryonic stem cell research: ethical and legal issues. Nat Rev Genet 2:74-8, 2001.
28. Zwaka TP, Thomson JA: Homologous recombination in human embryonic stem cells. Nat Biotechnol 21:319, 2003.
29. Rideout WM, 3rd, et al: Correction of a genetic defect by nuclear transplantation and combined cell and gene therapy. Cell 109:17, 2002.
30. Rideout WM, 3rd, et al: Nuclear cloning and epigenetic reprogramming of the genome. Science 293:1093, 2001.
31. Eiges R, Benvenisty N: A molecular view on pluripotent stem cells. FEBS Lett 529: 135, 2002.
32. Bradley JA, et al: Stem cell medicine encounters the immune system. Nat Rev Immunol 2:859, 2002.
33. Schuldiner M, et al: Effects of eight growth factors on the differentiation of cells derived from human embryonic stem cells. Proc Natl Acad Sci USA 97:11307, 2000.
34. Shamblott MJ, et al: Derivation of pluripotent stem cells from cultured human primordial germ cells. Proc Natl Acad Sci USA 95:13726, 1998.
35. Shamblott MJ, et al: Human embryonic germ cell derivatives express a broad range of developmentally distinct markers and proliferate extensively in vitro. Proc Natl Acad Sci USA 98:113, 2001.
36. Flax JD, et al: Engraftable human neural stem cells respond to developmental cues, replace neurons, and express foreign genes Nat Biotechnol 16: 1033, 1998.
37. Palmer TD, et al: Progenitor cells from human brain after death. Nature 411:42, 2001.
38. Presnell SC, et al: Stem cells in adult tissues. Semin Cell Dev Biol 13:369, 2002.
39. Ogawa M, et al: Long- term lymphohematopoietic reconstitution by a single 34-low/negative hematopoietic stem cell. Science 273: 242, 1996.
40. Szilvassy SJ, et al: Retrovirus-mediated gene transfer to purified hemopoietic stem cells with long-term lymphomyelopoietic repopulating ability. Proc Natl Acad Sci U S A 86:8798, 1989.
41. Park KI, et al: Transplantation of neural progenitor and stem cells: developmental insights may suggest new therapies for spinal cord and other CNS dysfunction. Neurotrauma 16:675, 1999.
42. Park KI, et al: Global gene and cell replacement strategies via stem cells. Gene Ther 9:613, 2002.
43. Liechty KW, et al: Human mesenchymal stem cells engraft and demonstrate site-specific differentiation after in utero transplantation in sheep. Nat Med 6:1282, 2000.
44. Wang X, et al: Cell fusion is the principal source of bone marrow–derived hepatocytes. Nature 422:897, 2003.
45. Vassilopoulos G, et al: Transplanted bone marrow regenerates liver by cell fusion. Nature 422:901, 2003.
46. Verfaillie CM: Adult stem cells: assessing the case for pluripotency. Trends Cell Biol 12:502, 2002.
47. Moore MAS: "Turning brain into blood"—clinical applications of stem-cell research in neurobiology and hematology. N Engl J Med 341:605, 1999.
48. Bjornson CRR, et al: Turning brain into blood: a hematopoietic fate adopted by adult stem cells in vivo. Science 283:534, 1999.
49. Orkin SH: Stem cell alchemy. Nat Med 6:1212, 2000.
50. Odelberg SJ: Inducing cellular dedifferentiation: a potential method for enhancing endogenous regeneration in mammals. Semin Cell Dev Biol 19:335, 2002.
51. Tarada N, et al: Bone marrow cells adopt the phenotype of other cells by spontaneous cell fusion. Nature 416:542, 2002.
52. Wagers AJ, et al: Little evidence for developmental plasticity of adult hematopoietic stem cells. Science 297:2256, 2002.
53. Shen CN, et al: Molecular basis of transdifferentiation of pancreas to liver. Nat Cell Biol 2:879, 2000.
54. Morshead CM, et al: Hematopoietic competence is a rare property of neural stem cells that depend on genetic and epigenetic alterations. Nat Med 8:268, 2002.
55. Snyder, EY, Vescovi AL: The possibilities/perplexities of stem cells. Nat Biotechnol 18:827, 2000.
56. Mezey E, et al: Transplanted bone marrow generates new neurons in human brains. Proc Natl Acad Sci U S A 100:1364, 2003.

57. Jiang Y, et al: Pluripotency of mesenchymal stem cells derived from adult marrow. Nature *418*:41, 2002.
58. Grompe M: Adult versus embryonic stem cells: it's still a tie. Mol Ther; *6*:303, 2002.
59. McKay R: Stem cells in the central nervous system. Science *276*:66, 1997.
60. Snyder EY, et al: Multipotent neural precursors can differentiate toward replacement of neurons undergoing targeted apoptotic degeneration in adult mouse neocortex. Proc Natl Acad Sci U S A *94*:11663-8, 1997.
61. Gage FH: Mammalian neural stem cells. Science *287*:1433, 2000.
62. Vescovi AL, Snyder EY: Establishment and properties of neural stem cell clones: plasticity in vitro and in vivo. Brain Pathol *9*:569, 1999.
63. Temple S. Stem cell plasticity—building the brain of our dreams. Nat Rev Neurosci *2*:513, 2001.
64. Pincus DW, et al: Neural stem and progenitor cells: a strategy for gene therapy and brain repair. Neurosurgery *42*:858, 1998.
65. Lacorazza HD, et al: Expression of human β-hexosaminidase α-subunit gene (the gene defect of Tay-Sachs disease) in mouse brains upon engraftment of transduced progenitor cells. Nat Med *4*:424, 1996.
66. Brüstle O, et al: Chimeric brains generated by intraventricular transplantation of fetal human brain cells into embryonic rats. Nat Biotechnol *11*:1040, 1998.
67. Brüstle O, et al: In vitro–generated neural precursors participate in mammalian brain development, Proc Natl Acad Sci U S A *94*:14809, 1997.
68. Ourednik V, et al: Segregation of human neural stem cells in the developing primate forebrain. Science *293*:1820, 2001.
69. Snyder EY, et al: Neural progenitor cell engraftment corrects lysosomal storage throughout the MPS VII mouse brain. Nature *374*:367, 1995.
70. Rosario CM, et al: Differentiation of engrafted multipotent neural progenitors towards replacement of missing granule neurons in meander tail cerebellum may help determine the locus of mutant gene action. Development *124*:4213, 1997.
71. Snyder EY, et al: Potential of neural stem-like cells for gene therapy and repair of the central nervous system. Adv Neurol *72*:121, 1997.
72. Riess P, et al: Transplanted neural stem cells survive, differentiate, and improve neurological motor function after experimental traumatic brain injury. Neurosurgery *51*:1043, 2002.
73. Ourednik J, et al: Neural stem cells display an inherent mechanism for rescuing dysfunctional neurons. Nature Biotechnol *20*:1103, 2002.
74. Lynch WP, et al: Neural stem cells as engraftable packaging lines optimize viral vector-mediated gene delivery to the CNS: evidence from studying retroviral env-related neurodegeneration. J Virol *73*:6841, 1999.
75. Aboody KS, et al: Neural stem cells display extensive tropism for pathology in the adult brain: evidence from intracranial gliomas. Proc Natl Acad Sci U S A *97*:12846, 2000.
76. Gepstein L: Derivation and potential applications of human embryonic stem cells. Circ Res *91*:866, 2002.

7

Heber C. Nielsen

Homeobox Genes

In 1894, Bateson coined the term *homeosis* to describe inherited mutations in *Drosophila melanogaster*, in which significant alteration of morphogenesis was observed.[1] Evidence that these alterations were the result of single gene mutations led to the definition of homeotic genes, i.e., genes that control the formation of the body plan. With the development of gene cloning, these genes were among the first to be defined and sequenced. This showed that homeotic genes are transcription factors, many of which contain within the gene a conserved 180-base pair sequence. This internal 180-base pair sequence codes for a 60 amino acid DNA binding region within the resulting protein. The protein binds to DNA, allowing the transcription factor to regulate the expression of other genes. This specific conserved region is known as the homeobox. Genes containing the homeobox are thus called homeobox genes (reviewed in reference 2). Generally, homeobox genes are expressed in cells of mesodermal origin.

Because of their unique and interesting genomic and genetic characteristics, one group of homeobox genes has received particular attention from developmental biologists. These are the hox genes. In *Drosophila* the eight hox genes are organized in a specific cluster termed *the HOM-C complex*, where they are arranged according to their spatial and temporal expression patterns during larval development (Fig. 7-1). In the HOM-C complex, the hox genes are organized on the *Drosophila* chromosome from 3′ to 5′, corresponding to their anterior (rostral) to posterior (caudal) larval expression pattern (spatial colinearity) and the timing in larval development when expression begins (temporal colinearity)(reviewed in reference 3). Identical to each other within the homeobox region, the hox genes also possess some sequence similarity outside the homeobox region. The degree of similarity is related to the proximity of genes within the cluster.

Hox genes are expressed with a definitive anterior boundary. The level of this boundary is progressively more caudal for each successive gene in the cluster, going in the 5′ direction.[4,5] Within a given area, there may be overlap of more proximal genes with the more distal gene. Hox genes act to define specific body segments of the developing *Drosophila* larvae by the process of posteriorization, in which the most 5′ gene expressed in a given body region actively identifies that region as more posterior than the region just rostral to it. This is termed *posterior dominance*, and explains why, in the presence of overlapping expression, one gene is instructive in determining body segment identity.[6]

Mutations causing ectopic expression of individual hox genes result in altered body segmental identity (homeotic transformation), producing seemingly bizarre deformities in *Drosophila*. Such mutations "posteriorize" an anterior segment through ectopic expression of a posterior gene in an anterior position.[7] Classic examples of posterior homeotic transformation are represented by the Antennapedia and Ultrabithorax mutations. In the Antennapedia mutant, the Antennapedia gene is misexpressed in a more rostral position, causing identification of part of the head structure as mesothorax such that the fly grows a leg instead of an antenna from the head. In the Ultrabithorax mutant, ectopic expression of the Ultrabithorax gene in the second thoracic segment redefines this segment as a duplication of the third thoracic segment, and the fly grows a second pair of halteres instead of the wings, which would normally develop from this body area. It is important to understand that hox genes and the other homeobox genes do not actually code for specific body structures. Antennapedia, for example, does not code for a leg. Rather, these genes act as master control genes, giving specific embryonic cells positional and spatial cues that define their regional identity and fate and regulating the expression of genes that do code for the development of structures specific to the region defined by that homeobox gene.

The discovery that the homeobox is found in many genes throughout the vertebrate kingdom created intense interest in the importance of homeobox genes as master control genes of many aspects of embryonic development. A large number of *Drosophila* homeobox genes have mammalian counterparts that are frequently closely conserved in gene or protein sequence to the *Drosophila* "parent" gene. Generally, the homeobox portion of the gene is either 100% or very close to 100% conserved in the DNA and/or the amino acid sequence. Other mammalian genes

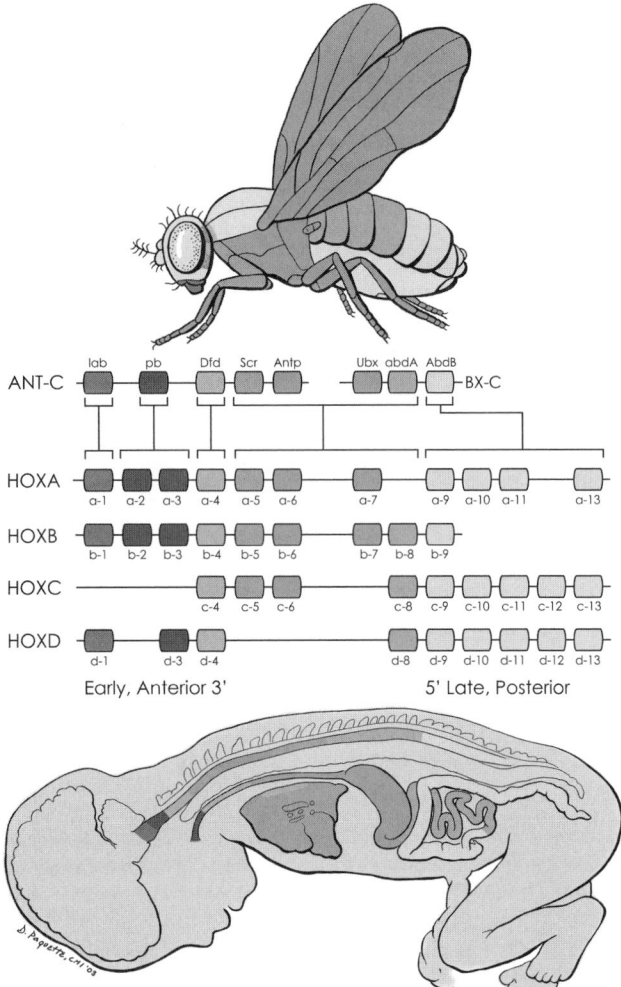

Figure 7–1. Relationship of the *Drosophila* HOM-C homeobox gene cluster and the mammalian Hox complex (see also color plates). Genes are depicted in their 3′ to 5′ organization on the *Drosophila* and each of the mammalian chromosomes. Missing boxes on the mammalian chart reflect that the specific gene is not present within that cluster. Specific colors denote the mammalian genes paralogous to their *Drosophila* counterparts. Colors also illustrate in the adult fly the body regions affected by expression of that specific hox gene during embryonic development. In general, these regions correspond to the most anterior area of expression of that gene in the embryo. Loss of function mutations alter embryonic morphogenesis, resulting in defects of that particular body region. An exception is the pattern of the pb gene, which is *stippled* to indicate that while this is the most anterior region of expression in the embryo, there is no apparent phenotype in this region when the gene is mutated. Colors in the human infant similarly indicate the anterior region where that group of paralogous genes is expressed during embryonic development. For simplicity, only the nervous system, lungs, and intestinal tract are represented. These are not the only systems in which hox genes are important.

Data for the human infant are mostly derived from studies of mouse embryogenesis. Figure drawn after data and charts by Roberts DJ, et al: Development *121*:3163, 1995; Coletta PL, et al: J Anat *184*:15, 1994; McGinnis W, et al: Cell *68*:283, 1992; Mavilio F, et al: Eur J Biochem 212:273, 1993; Mark M, et al: Pediatr Res *42*:421, 1997; Bogue CW, et al: Am J Resp Cell Mol Biol *15*:163, 1996. (© 2003 by Darisse Paquette, CMI, and Heber C. Nielsen, MD.)

containing a strongly conserved homeobox sequence have been discovered that have no counterpart in *Drosophila*. Well over 100 homeobox genes have been identified in humans; it has been estimated that this may represent only half the total number within the human genome.[7] Thus, homeobox genes may account for 0.5% of the approximately 30,000 genes in the human genome.

Homeobox genes are increasingly understood to function as regulators active in the development of embryonic organ morphogenesis and cell fate of all vertebrate species, with activity in the development of nearly all organs. Most studies of mammalian homeobox genes have been done in mice because of the ability to manipulate and study the mouse genome, but available evidence indicates conservation of function across diverse species. Because the number of homeobox and homeobox-like genes is large, this chapter focuses on the role of hox genes in mammalian development, although some related homeobox genes of particular interest are discussed.

In mammals, the *Drosophila* HOM-C gene cluster was duplicated onto four separate chromosomes and is called the HOX-C cluster. Although the genes are located on separate chromosomes, the unique organization and expression patterns, including spatial and temporal colinearity, are completely retained (see Fig. 7–1). Just as in *Drosophila*, the order of 3′ to 5′ chromosomal organization corresponds precisely with the anterior limit of gene expression within the embryo somite stage and ultimate organ structural development. The more 3′ the chromosomal location, the more rostral is the anterior limit of gene expression.[8] The mammalian hox genes retain identity (homology) of the homeobox region at the amino acid level and near or complete identity at the DNA level. Chromosomal order within the mammalian clusters is identical to that of the *Drosophila* complex, allowing the classification of genes within the HOX-C complex as homologues of their *Drosophila* counterpart. Counterpart genes in each of the four complexes, for example hoxa-4, hoxb-4, hoxc-4, and hoxd-4, are termed paralogues. Of great interest is that the HOX-C complex genes also retain characteristics of expression and apparent function of their *Drosophila* homologues. Thus, body segments that are likely to be controlled by mammalian hox genes are similar to the segments controlled by their corresponding *Drosophila* counterpart.[3]

In addition to the HOX-C cluster of homeobox genes in mammals, a number of other homeobox genes are scattered throughout the genome. Some exist in clusters, such as the so-called Para-hox cluster that contains Gsh-1, Pdx-1, and Cdx-2, and possibly other as-yet undiscovered genes. Others can be grouped into families based on sequence similarities outside the homeobox, such as the Nkx family of genes, or based on their similarity to other *Drosophila* homeobox genes, such as the Pax family.

Homeobox genes may exhibit three phases of expression during mammalian development.[9] First is expression in the very early embryo at gastrulation, likely to induce initial patterning. The second phase is during organ morphogenesis, with organ-specific expression that helps establish both organ structure and development of specific cell types. The third phase may begin in late fetal development or later in postnatal life. Expression is generally limited to specific cell types within an organ, such as the insulin-producing beta cell of the pancreatic islets. This expression appears necessary to maintain a differentiated functional phenotype of the particular cell.

Various knockout and transgenic mice models have been created in an attempt to learn the developmental function of many HOX-C and other homeobox genes. Compared with the dramatic homeotic alterations caused by mutations in *Drosophila*, the results in mammals often have been much more modest, especially considering the significant developmental role these genes are felt to play. Knockout models of individual hox genes frequently exhibit changes in vertebral body identity (e.g., transformation of a cervical vertebra into a thoracic vertebra), changes in rib number and/or identity, and shoulder girdle alterations.[4] The reason for such comparatively restricted homeotic changes is unclear but may relate to the fact that the hox genes are reproduced four times in mammals. This may allow paralogues or homologues of the targeted gene to replace some of the missing function, allowing a more normal morphogenesis.[10] This explanation is consistent with the proposed role of the HOX-C genes. In other words, nature has provided multiple back-up possibilities to allow normal development. Indeed, recent strategies in which multiple hox genes have been targeted show more significant homeotic changes in the developing animal.[11, 12] Thus the rule of posterior dominance used in *Drosophila* to determine which hox gene is instructive within a particular segment becomes more complex in mammals. In addition to posterior dominance, likely there are combinatorial and gradient rules that influence gene dominance, a feature called *quantitative colinearity*.[11]

Of interest to those caring for the fetus and newborn infant is the fact that many homeobox genes, and hox genes in particular, are stimulated by retinoic acid.[13, 14] Retinoic acid stimulation of hox gene expression preserves temporal colinearity (the more 5′ hox genes require progressively longer exposure times for stimulation), but spatial colinearity can be violated. Retinoic acid may induce hox gene expression in body regions and cell types, where they are not normally expressed. An *in vitro* example of this phenomenon in lung tissue is described later. With the interest in the potential use of retinoic acid to assist maturation or effect repair from injury in the premature human infant, it is clear that a careful and thorough examination of developmental effects must be made before such treatment is clinically tested. Many of the teratogenic effects of retinoic acid are postulated to be mediated by induced hox expression.

Much of the work on HOX-C genes has focused on development of the nervous system, since this organ system requires spatial identification, patterning, and determination of cell identity and fate that are unique to different somite regions. The anteroposterior expression gradients of each of the four HOX-C gene clusters are relatively easily demonstrated within the developing neural system. However, the development of other embryonic structures also requires spatial identification, patterning, and determination of cell identity (e.g., limb morphogenesis, and the development of the embryonic foregut into different structures, including the lung, stomach, intestinal tract, liver, and pancreas). In these systems, the unique expression features of the HOX-C gene clusters are similarly evident. This review focuses on the role of HOX-C and some other homeobox genes on determination and morphogenesis of the foregut-derived organs. This focus does not mean that more is known about foregut processes, or that development of this system depends more on homeobox genes. Rather, this system is of particular interest to neonatologists, as many neonatal diseases involve foregut-derived organs. An understanding of how their formation is controlled may provide new insights into development of new therapeutic strategies.

HOMEOBOX GENES AND FOREGUT AND HINDGUT DEVELOPMENT

Lung

The embryonic lung develops as an evaginating diverticulum from the embryonic foregut. The diverticulum then becomes bilobate to form the early right and left lungs. Branching morphogenesis, driven by a number of growth factor signals and regulatory molecules, then establishes the respiratory tree. The initial branching of the right and left lung primordia involves fibroblast growth factors. The development of continued branching requires a complex interaction of fibroblast growth factors and morphogenetic proteins, such as sonic hedgehog and BMP4[15] (reviewed in reference 16). The complex pulmonary structure is populated by over 40 different cell types arising from foregut, endoderm, and surrounding mesoderm. This complexity of structure and cell determination and differentiation clearly requires master control genes to establish positional identity and cell fate. Thus, homeobox genes are prime candidates for significant roles in many aspects of lung formation.

Early surveys of individual hox gene expression in mouse embryos using in situ hybridization revealed expression of a few genes in the mesenchyme of developing lung, especially of hoxa-5 and hoxb-5, homologues of the *Drosophila* sex combs reduced (Scr) gene.[17, 18] Scr, among other functions in the *Drosophila* larva, identifies the pharyngeal and upper respiratory region. As a result, several groups interested in lung morphogenesis are focusing on these Scr paralogues and their close neighbors within the HOX-C complex in lung development. Bogue and coworkers surveyed hox genes expressed in developing mouse lung using polymerase chain reaction (PCR) with degenerate primers.[19] They found 15 hox genes, with hoxa-5 and hoxb-5 most prominently expressed. Many of these genes were stimulated by retinoic acid treatment in vivo. Using in situ hybridization, Bogue and coworkers evaluated the temporal and spatial expression of hoxb cluster genes along the foregut just proximal and distal to the developing lung primordium, as well as within the developing lung itself.[20] In agreement with the general proximal-distal patterning and overlapping expression of hox genes, hoxb-3 and hoxb-4 showed anterior expression boundaries in the foregut proximal to, and hoxb-5 just at the position of, the budding lung diverticulum. Within the lung, anterior/posterior expression gradients were also observed, with hoxb-3 and hoxb-4 expressed in mesenchyme underlying tracheal, proximal, and distal airway structures, but hoxb-5 only in mesenchyme of distal airway structures and in the pleura. Curiously, hoxb-2 was also expressed in distal lung mesenchyme, so in this respect spatial colinearity was not completely conserved.

Hoxb-5. Volpe and coworkers have focused on the expression and function of hoxb-5 protein. Earlier studies by Wall and colleagues showed that the fetal organ with highest hoxb-5 protein expression was the spinal cord, followed closely by the lung.[21] Volpe identified the developmental expression of hoxb-5 protein in embryonic mouse lung.[22] Expression increases during branching morphogenesis, becoming maximal at d15 (female lung) and d16 (male lung), declining afterward to become very low at term and only minimally detectable in adult lung. The importance of the observed male-female difference in timing of peak expression is unclear. Structurally, hoxb-5 protein was located diffusely in mesoderm during branching morphogenesis. Then it became localized to mesenchyme underlying conducting airways, especially at apparent developing branch points. It is interesting that at late gestation, hoxb-5 protein was also seen in occasional columnar epithelial cells.

These findings in mouse lung development have been confirmed in human lung development, with maximal expression in the pseudoglandular phase of lung morphogenesis; waning expression and localization to mesenchyme under conducting airways and at branch points in the canalicular stage; further decreasing to occasional mesenchymal cells in the saccular and alveolar stages; and no apparent expression in the adult lung.[23]

The function of hoxb-5 was studied *in vitro* using embryonic mouse lung cultures. Overexpression of hoxb-5 (using retinoic acid stimulation) and knockout of hoxb-5 (using antisense oligonucleotides) each altered the development of branching morphogenesis. Knockout produced reduced proximal branching, and overexpression resulted in elongated proximal airways and reduced ability to form distal branches.[24] Additional studies in mouse lung organotypic cultures showed that growth factors and hormones that prematurely induce the differentiation of distal airway epithelium also significantly reduce expression of hoxb-5 in distal lung mesenchyme.[25, 26]

Results from the overexpression studies suggested a relationship of hoxb-5 to congenital lung malformations. Studies of bronchopulmonary sequestrations and congenital cystic adenomatoid malformations show significantly increased hoxb-5 expression underlying the abnormal airways and persisting in tissue removed at surgery during infancy.[23, 27] It remains to be determined whether this abnormal persistence of high hoxb-5 protein expression is causal to the development of these lung malformations, or whether some other signal initiated the formative process and hoxb-5 expression participated in determining the structural development of the already-initiated malformation.

Hoxa-5. Studies of hoxa-5 in lung development have concentrated on gene expression, although some data on protein expression are available. Like its homologue hoxb-5, hoxa-5 mRNA is diffusely expressed strongly in developing lung mesenchyme during the embryonic to pseudoglandular stages of lung morphogenesis. Some studies described a decrease in late gestation; others reported that both mRNA and protein remain high throughout gestation.[17, 19, 28] *In vitro* blockade of hoxa-5 expression using antisense oligonucleotide technology causes abnormal branching morphogenesis of the embryonic lung, resulting in foreshortened and aberrant branches.[29]

A transgenic knockout of the hoxa-5 gene has produced the most significant *in vivo* pulmonary phenotype of any hox gene knockout. The newborn pups homozygous for the hoxa-5 deletion died an early neonatal death of respiratory failure.[30] The lung is present but structurally abnormal in these animals. Abnormalities seen include upper airway obstruction associated with cricoid cartilage abnormalities and abnormal tracheal rings, altered bronchial epithelium, and decreased production of surfactant proteins, particularly surfactant protein B. It is unclear whether the reason for the lethal respiratory failure is upper airway obstruction, malformed lung airway or saccular formation, abnormal Type II cell surfactant production, or possibly secondary to alterations in rib cage or skeletal muscle that make respirations ineffective.

Studies in cell culture confirm the ability of retinoic acid to strongly stimulate hoxa-5 expression in fetal lung fibroblasts.[28] Of potential concern, this study also found that retinoic acid strongly stimulated hoxa-5 expression in the Type 2 cell-like MLE-12 cell line, in which hoxa-5 expression is not normally apparent. Since lung epithelial cells are not known to express hoxa-5 under normal conditions, this suggests the concern that high doses of retinoic acid may have an undesirable effect on developing pulmonary epithelium by induction of hox genes.

Nkx2.1. This divergent homeobox gene clearly has importance in both lung branching morphogenesis and determination of cell differentiation. Blockade of Nkx2.1 significantly inhibits lung branching morphogenesis, both *in vitro* and *in vivo*, especially of distal branching.[31, 32] In addition, Nkx2.1 is an important transcription factor regulating the differentiation and function of pulmonary epithelium. It specifically activates transcription of the surfactant protein C and surfactant protein B genes in Type 2 cells and the Clara cell secretory protein gene in Clara cells. It appears also to control the determination of these cell types (reviewed in reference 33). An interesting case report described an infant with unexplained respiratory distress, hypothyroidism (Nkx2.1 is also involved in thyroid morphogenesis), and a haplotypic deletion of chromosome 14q13–21, which included the Nkx2.1 gene.[34] The infant's problems may have been due to loss of Nkx2.1, but since the deletion included many more genes such a conclusion remains speculative.

Liver

Much like the lung, the embryonic liver hepatocytes develop from the endoderm of the foregut, invading the surrounding mesenchyme to form the developing liver structure. The process of hepatocyte determination is driven by fibroblast growth factors (FGFs) produced by the closely appositioned embryonic heart.[35] The target genes for these FGFs are not known but may include specific homeobox genes. Homeobox genes are known to be important in the morphogenesis of the liver. In particular, the divergent homeobox gene Hex is necessary for liver formation. Hex is normally expressed in the third pharyngeal pouch and subsequently in developing forebrain, thymus, thyroid, lung, pancreas, and liver, and in adult thyroid, lung, and liver.[36-38] A knockout of the Hex gene results in fetal mortality around embryonic day 12.5.[39] Examination of Hex knockout embryos shows the absence of hepatocytes and the absence of liver formation but the presence of the liver capsule. The lack of commitment of foregut endoderm to hepatocyte endoderm indicates that Hex is necessary for this commitment process and suggests that Hex is a target, either directly or through a pathway, of the cardiac FGFs that initiate liver formation.

Although specific roles of hox genes from the HOX-C cluster remain to be demonstrated, evidence suggests they are involved and important in regulation of hepatocyte maturation and function. For example, overexpression of hoxa-5 in transgenic mice using regulatory elements from hoxb-2, a more proximal gene, caused significant growth repression in the first few postnatal weeks, resulting in a proportionate dwarflike phenotype.[40] This was associated with a profound increase in liver expression of the insulin-like growth factor binding protein-1 (IGFBP-1) and marked decreases in both liver expression of insulin-like growth factor 1 (IGF-1) mRNA and in circulating levels of IGF-1. Additional studies in cultured cells showed that hoxa-5 interacts with other transcription proteins in strongly enhancing IGFBP-1 gene expression. This study represents a good example of how hox genes may act in the developed animal to help maintain cell differentiation in a tissue-specific manner.

Pancreas

A number of homeobox genes are known to be critical in pancreas morphogenesis and cellular differentiation and function. The pancreas develops from ventral and dorsal buds that evaginate from the distal foregut endoderm. Of primary importance in this process is the divergent homeobox gene Pdx-1, a member of the Parahox cluster. During differentiation of the foregut endoderm in the normal embryo, the ventral pancreas bud and the liver bud arise from adjacent nonoverlapping regions of the ventral foregut endoderm.[35] It is the proximity to the embryonic heart that drives the foregut endoderm toward the liver primordium through action of FGFs produced by cardiac mesoderm. If removed from the presence of the heart, this region of the foregut endoderm will default to expression of Pdx-1 and engender pancreatic tissue.[41]

Although it was originally thought that Pdx-1 was necessary only for ventral and dorsal bud growth, recent studies make it clear that Pdx-1 is necessary for bud formation, growth and morphogenesis, and cell differentiation. Using a transgenic approach in which the Pdx-1 gene was placed under the control of a gene promoter that can be turned off by administration of doxycycline, Holland and coworkers interrupted Pdx-1 expression at various stages of pancreatic development, as well as in the adult after normal pancreatic development and function were established.[41] Interruption of Pdx-1 expression at developmental intervals blocked the processes of bud formation, organ growth and morphogenesis, and the identification, differentiation, and function of the islets, including the endocrine and exocrine cell lineages within the islets. Pdx-1 regulates several genes involved in islet cell identity and function, including insulin, glucose transporter 2, glucokinase, islet amyloid polypeptide, and somatostatin expression (reviewed in reference 42). Studies of islet cell regeneration following injury indicate that Pdx-1 regulates the differentiation of a population of stem cells to produce new islet endocrine cells, particularly insulin-producing beta cells.

Pdx-1 gene abnormalities have been described in several human diseases. The extremely rare condition of congenital agenesis of the pancreas was found to be associated with a homozygous mutation in Pdx-1 that produced a truncated, nonfunctional protein product.[43] Family members heterozygous for this mutation manifested an autosomal dominant form of maturity-onset diabetes of the young (MODY type 4). Other studies have documented different mutations in Pdx-1 in families manifesting MODY type 4.[44] In all cases, the mutations alter the ability of Pdx-1 to regulate the maintenance of beta cell identity and function.

Other divergent homeobox genes also exhibit functional regulation of pancreatic islet cell function. Nkx2.2, a member of the Nkx homeobox family, is expressed in three of the types of islet cells, namely alpha, beta, and PP cells, but not in delta cells. Mice in which the Nkx2.2 gene has been knocked out lack beta cells and have marked reductions in the glucagon-producing alpha and PP cells.[45] In addition, there are many islet cells that do not produce any of the four pancreatic endocrine hormones. In other studies, deletion or disruption of the homeobox genes Pax-4 or Pax-6 shows that these genes are vital for islet endocrine cell differentiation, specifically insulin and glucagon-producing cells, respectively.[46,47]

Intestinal Tract

A number of hox and divergent homeobox genes are expressed to influence intestinal development (reviewed in reference 48). Like the central nervous system, the development of stomach, small intestine, and large intestine exhibits a detailed representation of the spatial and temporal colinearity of expression of genes in the HOX-C complex. Several studies have documented groups of hox gene expression in the developing gut.[49,50] Expression is seen early in development of the foregut and hindgut structures and is primarily confined to the mesoderm. In the developing esophagus, stomach, and cloacal region, there is evidence of endodermal cell hox expression.

Functions of hox genes in intestinal development are less clear. Some evidence suggests that they interact with other homeobox genes in providing positional information to direct development of region-specific gut endoderm and structural morphogenesis. The temporal expression of the hox genes also reflects the three waves of expression with peaks in early embryonic mesoderm as the gut tube forms; in midgestation as determination of stomach, duodenum, small intestine, and large intestine is accomplished; and in late gestation/early postnatal period as villous structures develop and are propagated.

Although the specific functions of the hox genes in intestinal development are not understood, several clues have been obtained from gene knockout and transgenic overexpression mouse models. Inactivation of hoxc-4 caused disruption of esophageal muscle development and blockage of the esophageal lumen, similar but not identical to esophageal atresia of the human.[51] Overexpression of hoxa-4 created an extended region of high hoxa-4 expression into the large bowel and resulted in mice with megacolon suggestive of that found in Hirschprung disease.[52] Anterior overexpression of hoxc-8 created the development of multiple hamartomas within the gastric mucosa.[53] The epithelium of these hamartomas resembled that of colonic

mucosa, suggesting that anterior expression of this posterior hox gene caused development of posterior mucosal characteristics.

Studies have suggested that D cluster hox genes are important in the development of intestinal sphincters. A multiple transgenic mouse in which the D cluster of hox genes from hoxd-4 to hoxd-13 was deleted exhibited abnormalities of both pyloric and anal sphincter development.[54] Subsequent studies by Kondo and colleagues[55] showed that deletions of either hoxd-12 or hoxd-13 caused anal sphincter abnormalities and rectal prolapse.

Divergent homeobox genes are also critical for intestinal development. These include the members of the Parahox cluster Cdx-2 and Pdx-1, as well as Nkx2.3. Cdx-2 is a mammalian homologue of the *Drosophila* homeobox gene *caudal*, which acts to posteriorize the rostral *Drosophila* larva. Cdx-2 is expressed in the early embryo in the trophoblast cells; homozygous mutant embryos lacking Cdx-2 fail to implant and so do not survive.[56] After d12 of mouse development, expression of Cdx-2 is confined to gut epithelium where it appears responsible for posterior axial specification of the developing epithelium. Expression begins just anterior to the developing liver bud and extends posterior to the distal colon. In adult animals, expression at high levels is found in the proximal colon, decreasing as one progresses either rostrally into the ileum and jejunum or caudally into the terminal colon.[57] Studies of hox genes in context with Cdx-2 suggest that Cdx proteins may participate in establishing hox expression boundaries in the developing gut.[58,59] As do many homeobox genes in various organs, Cdx-2 induces several extracellular matrix proteins consistent with a proposed role of inducing enterocyte maturation on the intestinal villus.[59]

Despite the fact that homozygous deletion of Cdx-2 causes lethality at implantation, it has been possible to use gene deletion to demonstrate the role of Cdx-2 in gut development in vivo. Transgenic mice that are heterozygous for the Cdx-2 deletion develop multiple polyp-like intestinal lesions, most prominently in the cecum, where Cdx-2 normally becomes most prominently expressed. They extend proximally and distally with decreasing frequency but are found only within the normal expression domain of the Cdx-2 gene.[60] Histologically, these lesions have normal gastric mucosa. As one examines the polyps both proximally and distally from the cecum, the lesions demonstrate an orderly progression of cell type from stratified squamous epithelium typical of the forestomach, through the mucous glands of the cardia, the gastric glands of the corpus, to mucous cells with the appearance of antral cells. Between polyp lesions is an intercalation of villi and Paneth cells, structures that lack Cdx-2 expression. As Beck and associates[60] have pointed out, this is a remarkable presentation of an anterior homeotic shift, the only example of homeosis which to date has been demonstrated for the intestine, and it is also the first report of intercalary regeneration in mammals. Thus, Cdx-2 works within the developing gut similar to the function of its *Drosophila* homologue to create a posterior phenotype that replaces a more proximal default program.

Patients with Hirschprung disease–associated enterocolitis (HDEC) were found to have significantly reduced expression of both Cdx-2 and Cdx-1 in the enterocolitis lesions. In contrast, other intestinal colitis diseases such as necrotizing enterocolitis did not display such a reduction, nor did Hirschprung disease intestine without enterocolitis.[61] Another possible clinical correlate is that of intestinal-type gastric cancer, which is often preceded in humans by metaplasia of gastric-type mucosa in the intestinal tract. The anterior homeosis observed in the heterozygous Cdx-2 knockout mice resemble these types of lesions. Studies in humans suggest that reduced Cdx-2 expression may be an antecedent cause of this type of intestinal cancer.[57]

The important role of the Parahox gene Pdx-1 in pancreatic development has already been discussed. Pdx-1 is expressed in distal foregut, where it not only defines pancreatic endoderm but also affects duodenal development. In Pdx-1 deletion animals, the rostral duodenum does not form villi or Brunner glands and remains lined by a cuboidal epithelium.[62] Abnormalities are very closely restricted to the specific domain of Pdx-1 expression in the distal foregut.

Members of the Nkx group of homeobox genes are expressed in intestinal mesoderm, where they appear to act on the overlying epithelium to direct differentiation. For example, inactivation of Nkx2.3, which is expressed in gut mesoderm, causes abnormalities of adult intestinal epithelium.[63] These abnormalities include delayed villous development, increased growth of crypt cells, and hyperproliferation of epithelium, primarily in the jejunum. These findings support the general hypothesis that one important function of mesodermally expressed homeobox genes in general is to provide positional cues for overlying epithelium that defines their function and structural organization.

In addition, the divergent homeobox genes Cdx-1 and Cdx-4, relatives of Cdx-2 but not members of the Parahox cluster, are expressed in developing gut endoderm and mesoderm, respectively.[64] It is not known whether they are critical for development.

HUMAN DISEASES ASSOCIATED WITH HOMEOBOX GENE ANOMALIES

In the preceding paragraphs several human conditions associated with homeobox gene anomalies have already been mentioned. Table 7–1 summarizes human conditions in which homeobox gene anomalies are known. These represent two categories of findings. In the first category are conditions in which a genome mutation in a homeobox gene has been documented in humans and appears to be responsible for the disease. Many of these are specific syndromes presenting at or shortly after birth. Others are diseases that arise in childhood or adult-

hood, including cancer. Interest in homeobox gene mutations in cancer has been engendered by their role in determining cell fate. The table shows specific cancers in which a mutation of a homeobox gene has been identified. In these diseases, as well as some others in the table, there are likely other causes of the disease separate from homeobox gene abnormalities. The second category includes diseases in which a homeobox gene appears to be normal, but is misexpressed, either overexpressed or underexpressed. In these situations it is not clear whether the abnormal expression is the proximate cause of the disease or whether another insult is the proximate cause, which leads to abnormal expression of homeobox gene(s). In the latter case, abnormal homeobox expression would help establish the phenotype of the disease.

SUMMARY

Several classes of genes are responsible for the development and differentiation of the embryo into the complex adult organ system. A major class of such genes is the group of homeobox genes, which control axial patterning and rostral-caudal definition, as well as influencing the patterning of specific organs and the differentiation and function of specialized cells. As more is understood about the role of homeobox genes, more opportunity will develop for understanding the proximal causes of congenital malformations, as well as diseases in which cell identity is lost. Although it is yet too early to predict treatments of diseases based on homeobox gene functions, there is good reason to hope that understanding the varied and complex function of these genes will provide unique insights that will translate into novel approaches to a variety of human disease conditions.

ACKNOWLEDGMENTS

The assistance and suggestions of Dr. M.V. Volpe, Dr. R. Vosatka, C. Nielsen, and E. Haltiwanger are appreciated. Supported by NIH HD38419 and HL37930.

TABLE 7–1

Homeobox Genes and Human Diseases

Disease	Gene	Reference
Diseases Caused by Homeobox Gene Mutations		
Birth Defects		
Hand-foot-genital syndrome	Hoxa-13	65
Synpolydactyly	Hoxd-13	66
Schizencephaly	Emx-2	67
Aniridia, Peter anomaly, anophthalmia, isolated foveal dysplasia	Pax-6	68, 69
Waardenburg syndrome (Type I, Type III)	Pax-3	48, reviewed in 70
Hypodontia	Msx-1	Reviewed in 71
Craniosynostosis (Boston type)	Msx-2	Reviewed in 72
Rieger syndrome	Rieg	73
Combined pituitary hormone deficiency	Pit-1	Reviewed in 74
Deafness with fixation of the stapes	Pou3F4	75
Congenital absence of pancreas	Pdx-1	43
Other Diseases		
Maturity-onset diabetes of the young Type 4	Pdx-1	43
Acute myelogenous leukemia	Hoxa-9	Reviewed in 76
Pre-B-cell acute lymphocytic leukemia	Pbx-1	Reviewed in 77
T-cell acute lymphocytic leukemia	Hox11	Reviewed in 77
Rhabdomyosarcoma	Pax-3, Pax-7	Reviewed in 78
Diseases Associated with Homeobox Gene Misexpression		
Congenital cystic adenomatoid malformation of the lung	Hoxb-5	23
Bronchopulmonary sequestration	Hoxb-5	23, 27
Hirschprung disease–associated enterocolitis	Cdx-1, Cdx-2	61
Gastric intestinal metaplasia	Cdx-2	57

REFERENCES

1. Bateson W: Materials for the Study of Variation. London, Macmillan, 1894.
2. Gehring WJ: Exploring the homeobox. Gene *135*:215, 1993.
3. Coletta PL, et al: The molecular anatomy of Hox gene expression. J Anat *184*:15, 1994.
4. McGinnis W, Krumlauf R: Homeobox genes and axial patterning. Cell *68*:283, 1992.
5. Lawrence PA, Morata G: Homeobox genes: their function in *Drosophila* segmentation and pattern formation. Cell *78*:181, 1994.
6. Duboule D, Morata G: Colinearity and functional hierarchy among genes of the homeotic complexes. Trends Genet *10*:358, 1994.
7. Mark M, et al: Homeobox genes in embryogenesis and pathogenesis. Pediatr Res *42*:421, 1997.
8. Graham A, et al: The murine and Drosophila homeobox complexes have common features of organization and expression. Cell *57*:367, 1989.
9. Deschamps J, et al: Initiation, establishment and maintenance of *Hox* gene expression patterns in the mouse. Int J Dev Biol *43*:635, 1999.
10. Kostic D, Capecchi MR: Targeted disruptions of the murine Hoxa-4 and Hoxa-6 genes result in homeotic transformations of components of the vertebral column. Mech Dev *46*:231, 1994.
11. Kmita M, et al: Serial deletions and duplications suggest a mechanism for the collinearity of Hoxd genes in limbs. Nature *420*:145, 2002.
12. Condie BG, Capecchi MR: Mice with the targeted disruptions in the paralogous genes hoxa-3 and hoxd-3 reveal synergistic interactions. Nature *370*:304, 2002.
13. Simeone A, et al: Differential regulation by retinoic acid of the homeobox genes of the four HOX loci in human embryonal carcinoma cells. Mech Dev *33*:215, 1991.
14. Mavilio F: Regulation of vertebrate homeobox-containing genes by morphogens. Eur J Biochem *212*:273, 1993.
15. Lebeche D, et al: Fibroblast growth factor interactions in the developing lung. Mech Dev *86*:125, 1999.
16. Warburton D, et al: The molecular basis of lung morphogenesis. Mech Dev *92*:55, 2000.
17. Dony C, Gruss P: Specific expression of the Hox 1.3 homeobox gene in murine embryonic structures originating from or induced by the mesoderm. EMBO J *6*:2965, 1987.
18. Krumlauf, R, et al: Developmental and spatial patterns of expression of the mouse homeobox gene *Hox 2.1*. Development *99*:603, 1987.
19. Bogue CW, et al: Identification of *Hox* genes in newborn lung and effects of gestational age and retinoic acid on their expression. Am J Physiol (Lung Cell Mol Physiol) *266*:L448, 1994.
20. Bogue CW, et al: Expression of *Hoxb* genes in the developing mouse foregut and lung. Am J Respir Cell Mol Biol *15*:163, 1996.
21. Wall NA, et al: Expression and modification of Hox 2.1 protein in mouse embryos. Mech Dev *37*:111, 1992.
22. Volpe MV, et al: Hoxb-5 expression in the developing mouse lung suggests a role in branching morphogenesis and epithelial cell fate. Histochem Cell Biol *108*:405, 1997.
23. Volpe MV, Nielsen HC: Expression of Hoxb-5 during human lung development and in congenital lung malformations. Birth Defects Research: Clinical and Molecular Teratology, In Press, 2003.
24. Volpe MV, et al: Hoxb-5 control of proximal airway formation during branching morphogenesis. Biochim Biophys Acta *1475*:337, 2000.
25. Chinoy MR, et al: Growth factors and dexamethasone regulate Hoxb-5 protein in cultured murine fetal lungs. Am J Physiol (Lung Cell Mol Physiol) *274*:L610, 1998.
26. Archavachotikul K, et al: Thyroid hormone affects embryonic mouse lung branching morphogenesis and cellular differentiation. Am J Physiol (Lung Cell Mol Physiol) *282*:L359, 2001.
27. Volpe MV, et al: Association of bronchopulmonary sequestration with expression of the homeobox protein Hoxb-5. J Pediatr Surg *35*:1817, 2000.
28. Kim C, Nielsen HC: Hoxa-5 in mouse developing lung: cell-specific expression and retinoic acid regulation. Am J Physiol (Lung Cell Mol Physiol) *279*:L863, 2000.
29. Volpe MV, et al: Homeobox genes regulate morphogenesis in the embryonic mouse lung. Pediatr Res *37*:72A, 1995.
30. Aubin J, et al: Early postnatal lethality in *hoxa-5* mutant mice is attributable to respiratory tract defects. Dev Biol *192*:432, 1997.
31. Minoo P, et al: TTF-1 regulates lung epithelial morphogenesis. Dev Biol *172*:694, 1995.
32. Yuan B, et al: Inhibition of distal lung morphogenesis in Nkx2.1(-/-) embryos. Dev Dyn *217*:180, 2000.
33. Warburton D, et al: Commitment and differentiation of lung cell lineages. Biochem Cell Biol *76*:971, 1998.
34. Devriendt K, et al: Deletion of thyroid transcription factor-1 gene in an infant with neonatal thyroid dysfunction and respiratory failure. N Engl J Med *338*:1317, 1998.
35. Deutsch G, et al: A bipotential precursor population for pancreas and liver within the embryonic endoderm. Development (Suppl) *128*:871, 2001.
36. Bogue CW, et al: Hex expression suggests a role in the development and function of organs derived from foregut endoderm. Dev Dyn *219*:84, 2000.
37. Martinez Barbera JP, et al: The homeobox gene Hex is required in definitive endodermal tissues for normal forebrain, liver and thyroid formation. Development (Suppl) *127*:2433, 2000.
38. Ghosh B, et al: Immunocytochemical characterization of murine *Hex*, a homeobox-containing protein. Pediatr Res *48*:634, 2000.
39. Keng VW, et al: Homeobox gene *Hex* is essential for onset of mouse embryonic liver development and differentiation of the monocyte lineage. Biochem Biophys Res Commun *276*:1155, 2000.
40. Foucher I, et al: Hoxa5 overexpression correlates with IGFBP1 upregulation and postnatal dwarfism; evidence for an interaction between Hoxa5 and Forkhead box transcription factors. Development (Suppl) *129*:4065, 2002.
41. Holland AM, et al: Experimental control of pancreatic development and maintenance. Proc Natl Acad Sci USA *99*:12236, 2002.
42. Hui H, Perfetti R: Pancreas duodenum homeobox-1 regulates pancreas development during embryogenesis and islet cell function in adulthood. Eur J Endocrinol *146*:129, 2002.
43. Stoffers DA, et al: Pancreatic agenesis attributable to a single nucleotide deletion in the human *IPF1* gene coding sequence. Nat Genet *15*:106, 1997.
44. McKinnon CM, Docherty K: Pancreatic duodenal homeobox-1, PDX-1, a major regulator of beta cell identity and function. Diabetologia *44*:1203, 2001.
45. Sussel L, et al: Mice lacking the homeodomain transcription factor Nkx2.2 have diabetes due to arrested differentiation of pancreatic beta cells. Development (Suppl) *125*:2213, 1998.
46. Sosa-Pineda B, et al: The Pax4 gene is essential for differentiation of insulin-producing beta cells in the mammalian pancreas. Nature *386*:399, 1997.
47. St-Onge L, et al: Pax6 is required for differentiation of glucagon-producing alpha-cells in mouse pancreas. Nature *387*:406, 1997.
48. Morell R, et al: Three mutations in the paired homeodomain of PAX3 that cause Waardenburg syndrome type 1. Hum Hered *47*:38, 1997.
49. Beck F, et al: Homeobox genes and gut development. BioEssays, *22*:431, 2000.
50. Sekimoto T, et al: Region-specific expression of murine *Hox* genes implies the *Hox* code-mediated patterning of the digestive tract. Genes Cells *3*:51, 1998.
51. Boulet AM Capecchi MR: Targeted disruption of Hoxc-4 causes esophageal defects and vertebral transformations. Dev Biol *177*:232, 1996.
52. Wolgemuth DJ, et al: Transgenic mice overexpressing the mouse homeobox-containing gene *Hox-1.4* exhibit abnormal gut development. Nature *337*:464, 1989.
53. Pollock RA, et al: Altering the boundaries of Hox3.1 expression: evidence for antipodal gene regulation. Cell *71*:911, 1992.
54. Zakany J, Duboule D: Hox genes and the making of sphincters. Nature *401*:761, 1999.
55. Kondo T, et al: Function of posterior HoxD genes in the morphogenesis of the anal sphincter. Development (Suppl) *122*:2651, 1996.
56. Van Den Akker E, et al: Cdx1 and Cdx2 have overlapping functions in antero-posterior patterning and posterior axis elongation. Development (Suppl) *129*:2181, 2002.
57. Silberg DG, et al: Cdx2 ectopic expression induces gastric intestinal metaplasia in transgenic mice. Gastroenterology *122*:689, 2002.
58. Gaunt SJ: Gradients and forward spreading of vertebrate Hox gene expression detected by using a Hox/lacZ transgene. Dev Dyn *221*:26, 2002.
59. Lorentz O, et al: Key role of the *Cdx2* homeobox gene in extracellular matrix-mediated intestinal cell differentiation. J Cell Biol *139*:1553, 1997.
60. Beck F, et al: Reprogramming of intestinal differentiation and intercalary regeneration in Cdx2 mutant mice. Proc Natl Acad Sci USA *96*:7318, 1999.
61. Lui VC, et al: CDX-1 and CDX-2 are expressed in human colonic mucosa and are down-regulated in patients with Hirschsprung's disease-associated enterocolitis. Biochim Biophys Acta *153*:89, 2001.
62. Offield MF, et al: PDX-1 is required for pancreatic outgrowth and differentiation of the rostral duodenum. Development (Suppl) *122*:983, 1996.
63. Pabst O, et al: Targeted disruption of the homeobox transcription factor Nkx2-3 in mice results in postnatal lethality and abnormal development of the small intestine and spleen. Development *126*:2215, 1999.
64. Beck F: Homeobox genes in gut development. Gut *51*:450, 2002.
65. Mortlock DP, Innis JW: Mutation of *HOXD13* in hand-foot-genital syndrome. Nat Genet *15*:179, 1997.
66. Muragaki Y, et al: Altered growth and branching patterns in synpolydactyly caused by mutations in *HOXD13*. Science *272*:548, 1996.
67. Brunelli S, et al: Germline mutations in the homeobox gene *EMX2* in patients with severe schizencephaly. Nat Genet *12*:94, 1996.
68. Glaser T, et al: *PAX6* gene dosage effect in a family with congenital cataracts, anophthalmia and central nervous system defects. Nat Genet *7*:463, 1994.
69. Azuma N, et al: *PAX6* missense mutation in isolated foveal hypoplasia. Nat Genet *13*:141, 1996.
70. Stuart ET, et al: Mammalian *Pax* genes. Annu Rev Genet *27*:219, 1993.
71. Thesleff I, Nieminen P: Tooth morphogenesis and cell differentiation. Curr Opin Cell Biol *8*:844, 1996.
72. Richman JM: Craniofacial genetics makes headway. Curr Biol *5*:345, 1995.
73. Semina EV, et al: Cloning and characterization of a novel *bicoid*-related homeobox transcription factor gene, *RIEG*, involved in Rieger syndrome. Nat Genet *14*:392, 1996.
74. Rhodes SJ, et al: Transcriptional mechanisms in anterior pituitary cell differentiation. Curr Opin Genet Dev *4*:709, 1994.
75. Kok YJM, et al: Association between X-linked mixed deafness and mutations in the POU domain *POU3F4*. Science *267*:685, 1995.
76. Lawrence HJ, et al: The role of *HOX* homeobox genes in normal and leukemic hematopoiesis. Stem Cell *14*:281, 1996.
77. Nakamura T, et al: Cooperative activation of *Hoxa* and *Pbx1*-related genes in murine myeloid leukaemias. Nat Genet *12*:149, 1996.
78. Sorensen PHB, Triche TJ: Gene fusions encoding chimaeric transcription factors in solid tumors. Semin Cancer Biol *7*:3, 1996.

Huseyin Mehmet, Jacqueline Beesley, and A. David Edwards

8
Apoptosis and Necrosis

Apoptosis is a highly regulated form of cell death that is required for both the development and homeostasis of multicellular organisms. Therefore, dysregulation of apoptosis can result in a range of diseases.[1] Originally identified by its characteristic morphologic features—membrane blebbing, cell shrinkage, and chromatin condensation—apoptosis can now also be defined by the biochemical signaling pathways involved.

In contrast to passive cell necrosis, apoptotic cell death is an active process leading to the ordered dismantling of cellular components such as proteins and DNA. Specialized *cysteinyl aspartate*-specific prote*ases* termed *caspases* have been shown to be key components of the apoptotic pathway.[2] Synthesized in the cytoplasm as inactive proenzymes, caspases are activated during apoptosis, cleaving key cellular proteins, including DNA repair enzymes, regulators of the cell cycle, and structural components, resulting in disassembly of the cell. Genetic studies in the nematode *Caenorhabditis elegans* identified a number of genes involved in apoptosis, including ced-3, which has now been shown to be a member of the caspase family. Some caspases (e.g., caspase-8 and caspase-9) act either as upstream initiators in the apoptotic pathway by processing and activating other caspases (such as caspase-3); or these then, in turn, act as downstream executioners cleaving cellular proteins.

There are at least two[3] and possibly three[4] pathways to apoptosis. Initiator caspases are most commonly activated by an extrinsic death receptor pathway or by the intrinsic mitochondrial pathway. In the former, ligand binding to death receptors such as Fas or tumor necrosis factor (TNF) receptor in the cell membrane leads to receptor oligomerization. The activated trimeric death receptors undergo specific conformational changes on the cytoplasmic face of the plasma membrane, allowing the subsequent recruitment of adaptor molecules and, ultimately, an initiator caspase. These sequential protein-protein interactions lead to the formation of a death-inducing signaling complex (DISC) and caspase activation.[5]

In contrast, in the cell-intrinsic pathway of apoptosis, cytochrome c is released from the mitochondrial intermembrane space into the cytosol following membrane depolarization and forms a complex (termed the *apoptosome*) with Apaf-1 (the equivalent of ced-4 in *C. elegans*), adenosine triphosphate (ATP), and procaspase-9, which is then activated. Active caspase-8 (and possibly caspase-10) from the DISC or caspase-9 (from the mitochondrial pathway) can then process and activate downstream caspases such as -3, -6, and -7. Apoptosis thus proceeds by an ordered cascade of protolysis by which initiator caspases cleave and activate the executioner caspases, which in turn act as downstream executioners by processing cellular proteins in order to facilitate disassembly of the cell. In some cases, executioner caspases can inactivate proteins that would disrupt apoptosis. For example, the DNA repair enzyme, poly(adenosine diphosphate [ADP]-ribose) polymerase (PARP), which catalyzes attachment of ADP ribose units from NAD to nuclear proteins, is inactivated by caspase-3–mediated cleavage, resulting in an increase in the ATP available for energy-demanding apoptosis. In other cases, active downstream caspases can trigger enzyme activation. For example, caspase-3 cleaves the inhibitor of the caspase-activated DNase (ICAD), thus destroying its ability to bind and repress the apoptotic endonuclease CAD. The end result of ICAD cleavage is CAD activation, resulting in the initiation of DNA fragmentation, a key feature of apoptosis.[6]

Several regulators of apoptosis have now been identified as normal resident proteins in healthy cells. Bcl-2 was originally identified in follicular lymphoma as an anti-apoptotic protein, supporting the concept that it is the combination of impaired apoptosis and increased proliferation in the same cell that ultimately leads to tumor formation. All members of the Bcl-2 family share at least one conserved region, termed the Bcl-2 homology (BH) domain. Other members of the Bcl-2 family that possess only the BH3 domain have now been shown to be pro-apoptotic (e.g., Egl-1 and Bax). Some BH3-only proteins (e.g., Bid) are thought to act by binding to and preventing the action of anti-apoptotic Bcl-2 family members, whereas others (possibly Bax) may integrate into the outer mitochondrial membrane and increase its permeability to pro-apoptotic messengers such as cytochrome c.[7]

Anti-apoptotic family members also associate with the mitochondrial membrane as well as the endoplasmic reticulum and nuclear membranes. It is speculated that they act by maintaining membrane integrity and possibly preventing cytochrome c release from mitochondria. Inhibitor of apoptosis (IAP) family members act as endogenous caspase inhibitors.[8] They contain between one and three survivin (BIR) motifs that interact with caspases, blocking their catalytic sites. Some IAPs also possess C-terminal ring finger (RING) domains that enable polyubiquitination of proteins and thus their destruction in the proteasome. Recently, a number of other proteins have been identified that are released from mitochondria following membrane depolarization and that activate apoptosis.[9] Among these, Smac/DIABLO and HtrA2/Omi each bind to and inhibit IAPs, thus removing the block on caspase activation. HtrA2/Omi is also thought to activate caspase-independent cell death through its serine protease activity. Other proteins released from the mitochondria can activate apoptosis independently of caspases. These include endonuclease G and apoptosis-inducing factor (AIF), an activator of the nucleases that cause chromatin condensation and high molecular weight DNA fragmentation. The AIF knockout mouse has shown that this protein is rate limiting for apoptosis both *in vitro* and *in vivo*.[10] More recently, a third pathway involving activation of caspase-12, which localizes to the endoplasmic reticulum and is activated following ER stress, including release of intracellular calcium stores, has been described.[11] However, caspase-12 protein is not expressed in human cells, and so it is unclear how relevant it is to human disease unless another caspase functions in its place.

APOPTOSIS IN THE MORPHOLOGIC DEVELOPMENT OF THE EMBRYO AND FETUS

Apoptosis is an essential component of animal development, contributing to the establishment and maintenance of tissue architecture. This involves the elimination of unwanted cells and thus either the sculpting of structures or their complete removal. For example, apoptosis removes cells between developing digits such that if apoptosis is blocked with caspase inhibitors, digit formation is prevented.[12]

In many organs, cells are overproduced and then later eliminated to achieve appropriate numbers. For example, it is estimated that up to half the neurons in the central nervous system (CNS) die during development. It is thought that immature neurons compete for target-derived trophic factors, which are in limited supply, so that only neurons that make correct synaptic connections will survive.

APOPTOSIS IN NEURONAL DAMAGE

There is accumulating evidence that alterations in apoptosis can contribute to the pathogenesis of a number of human diseases, including cancer, viral infections, autoimmune diseases, neurodegenerative disorders, and acquired immunodeficiency syndrome (AIDS). Although trophic factor withdrawal has a prominent role during nervous system development, it is not thought to be the primary pathogenic mechanism in adult neurodegenerative diseases in which toxic insults are more likely to trigger the apoptotic pathway.

MODES OF CELL DEATH IN TISSUE INJURY

Cell death can proceed by different routes, each with characteristic morphologic criteria as an end point. In necrosis, cell death is triggered by an overwhelming external insult damaging cellular organelles such as mitochondria, resulting in the loss of membrane integrity and leaking of cytoplasmic contents into the extracellular matrix. In contrast, cells dying by apoptosis carry out a well-conserved and highly regulated genetic program of cell death. They do not lose membrane integrity, and the organelles remain largely intact. In the final stages, cell fragments are "shrink-wrapped" in the contracting plasma membrane and bud off as apoptotic bodies that are subsequently phagocytozed by healthy neighboring cells. Since the apoptotic response to damage largely circumvents inflammatory responses, this mode of cell death would be particularly beneficial following injury to the brain, which has only a limited capacity for repair and regeneration.

On the other hand, apoptosis as a biochemically and genetically programmed cell death requires time, energy, and, in some cases, new gene transcription and translation. However, as discussed later, the distinction between apoptosis and necrosis is not always clear-cut and, in many instances, these two modes of cell death can be regarded as a continuum of a single cell fate following injury. There is increasing opinion of a continuum of death running from apoptosis to necrosis, but encompassing poorly understood intermediate forms.

Apoptosis and Necrosis Following Hypoxia-Ischemia

Both apoptotic and necrotic cells are found in tissue after hypoxia-ischemia. Necrosis can occur during hypoxia-ischemia or immediately following resuscitation when blood flow is very low, and when an acute deficit in substrate delivery can result in a rapid reduction in cerebral energy production, membrane pump failure, and severe ionic imbalances, with cell swelling and necrotic cell death.[13] These acute early changes may be particularly associated with an increase in excitatory amino acid levels and free radical production, the damaging effects of which can be blocked by specific receptor antagonists and scavengers.[14]

Apoptotic cells are also seen following hypoxic-ischemic injury in both the immature.[15-17] and adult brain.[18, 19] Administration of the anti-apoptotic growth factor insulin-like growth factor-1 (IGF-1) after the primary insult ameliorates delayed injury, while glutamate receptor blockade is only partially protective.[20, 21] Apoptosis has been shown to be involved in human perinatal brain injury. Infants who die after intrauterine injury, either with or without evidence of hypoxia-ischemia, have a significant number of cells in the brain with the morphologic characteristics of apoptosis.[22, 23]

Relation Between Apoptotic and Necrotic Death in Cerebral Injury

It might be convenient to consider immediate cell death following hypoxia-ischemia as necrotic and delayed cell death as apoptotic. However, published data do not entirely support such a simplifying concept. In experimental hypoxia-ischemia, apoptosis and necrosis can occur in adjacent populations of neurons and glial cells in the cingulate sulcus, whereas quantitative analysis of cell death showed that the numbers of both apoptotic and necrotic cells were linearly related to the severity of ATP depletion during hypoxia-ischemia.[24] Human infants who have suffered secondary energy failure have a preponderance of necrotic cells, while those dying *in utero* show a higher proportion of apoptotic cells.[22]

These complexities may arise in part from the fact that some necrotic cells represent the secondary degradation of apoptotic cells. In this context, primary cell necrosis can be regarded as an acute response to severe injury and is the common pattern of change in cerebral infarcts. Secondary cell necrosis can occur in cells triggered to apoptosis but unable to complete the program.[25] Cell necrosis thus should be distinguished from tissue necrosis, in which a large number of cells undergo necrosis together, which may be primary, secondary, or both. Oxygen-glucose deprivation may induce first apoptosis and then secondary necrosis in cerebellar granule cells.[26] Similarly, primary apoptosis precedes secondary necrosis following the injection of excitatory amino acid receptor agonists into the adult rat brain[27] and in rat dorsal root ganglion cell cultures treated with oxidized low-density lipoprotein.[28]

Studies with cultured neurons subjected to oxygen deprivation have confirmed that necrosis and apoptosis can occur in a single cell population.[29] In one study, the administration of Trolox, which interferes with lipid peroxidation, prevented necrosis but allowed neurons to undergo apoptosis.[30] In a separate study, the induction of apoptosis in target cells by cytotoxic T lymphocytes was blocked by inhibitors of transcription or translation; instead, the target cells underwent necrosis.[31] Thus it may be possible to switch the fate of damaged cells between necrosis and apoptosis.

MOLECULAR EVIDENCE OF APOPTOSIS FOLLOWING BRAIN INJURY

A number of molecular signals associated with apoptotic death are induced by impaired oxidative phosphorylation and oxidative injury.

Caspases and Poly(ADP Ribose) Polymerase Cleavage

The nuclear enzyme poly(ADP ribose) polymerase (PARP) provides one of the most apparent links between oxidative stress, impaired energy metabolism, and cell damage. Free radicals such as nitric oxide and peroxynitrite can damage DNA, leading to activation of PARP, which catalyzes attachment of ADP ribose units from NAD to nuclear proteins. However, excessive activation of PARP can deplete NAD^+ and ATP (which is consumed in NAD regeneration), leading to an increase in the $NADH/NAD^+$ ratio and eventually cell death by energy depletion.[32] PARP is induced by hypoxia-ischemia, and genetic disruption of PARP provides profound protection against both glutamate-mediated excitotoxic insults *in vitro* and major decreases in infarct volume after reversible middle cerebral artery occlusion.[33] These results provide compelling evidence for a primary involvement of PARP activation in neuronal damage.

Genetic deletion of PARP or PARP inhibition by 3-aminobenzamide reduced infarct size after transient cerebral ischemia[34] but did not reduce the density of apoptotic cells.[35] The susceptibility of primary neurons toward apoptosis is unaffected in PARP-/- mice, suggesting that PARP activation is not necessary for apoptosis.[36, 37] Thus in cerebral ischemia, PARP may contribute to cell death by NAD^+ depletion and primary energy failure without direct involvement in apoptotic responses.

However, PARP is involved in apoptosis in another way. Specific proteolytic cleavage of PARP by caspase-3 is an important event in at least one pathway to apoptosis,[38] possibly as a mechanism to maintain the ATP needed for successful completion of the apoptotic program. Both caspase activity[39] and PARP cleavage[40] have been shown to increase immediately following ischemic injury *in vivo*, followed several hours later by morphologic features of apoptosis.

Caspase inhibition can reduce neuronal loss following oxygen-glucose deprivation of cortical neurons[41] and following hypoxic ischemic injury (HII) *in vivo*.[42,43] However some results suggest that while caspase inhibition may prevent the cellular manifestations of apoptosis, it does not prevent cell death.[44] The precise roles of PARP cleavage and caspase activity in cell death after hypoxia-ischemia need to be defined further.

Gene Expression and Activation

Apoptotic death is often preceded by the induction and activation of a considerable variety of genes, including immediate early genes,[45-47] zinc finger genes, heat-shock proteins [HSPs], β-amyloid precursor protein,[48,49] and nuclear factor-kappa B (NF-κB).[50]

A number of these genes have been shown to possess either pro- or anti-apoptotic functions.[51] For example, NF-κB[52] and HSPs[53] are thought to be protective against oxidative stress, while c-Jun, which is phosphorylated by stress-activated protein kinases (SAPKs), is strongly implicated in triggering neuronal apoptosis.[45]

In vivo studies of ischemic injury to the heart, kidney, liver, and brain have shown that several SAPKs are activated by injury.[54-58] However, it remains to be determined whether these kinases are pro- or anti-apoptotic. Early activation of p38 SAPK has been shown to protect cells from apoptotic death following TNF treatment,[59] whereas studies of CD40 and B-cell receptor signaling have shown that Jun N-terminal kinase (JNK) and P38 activation do not precede apoptosis triggered by the engagement of these receptors.[60] Conversely, the JNK inhibitor CEP-1347 is able to rescue motoneurons from apoptosis following the withdrawal of neurotrophic factors,[61] whereas the p38 inhibitor SB203580 is able to prevent glutamate-induced apoptosis in cerebellar granule neurons.[62] In the context of oxidative brain injury, the anti-apoptotic protein Bcl-2 is a substrate for JNK but not p38.[63] Although this phosphorylation is specific, the function is not clear, since the protective effects of Bcl-2 appear to be independent of this posttranslational modification.

ACTIVATION OF APOPTOSIS THROUGH DEATH RECEPTORS AFTER TISSUE INJURY

The activation of SAPKs as one of the earliest signals downstream of death receptor activation provides evidence that intercellular signaling may be involved in triggering cell death during tissue injury. Receptors for pro-apoptotic signals, including TNF and interleukin-1β (IL-1β), are expressed acutely in the injured brain and may contribute to the progression of neuronal damage following hypoxia-ischemia.[64-67] A recombinant human IL-1β receptor antagonist markedly protects against focal cerebral ischemia in the rat.[68]

The Fas pathway is apparently involved not only in the death of the immune cells, where it was first described, but also in other tissues such as the brain, and provides an example of the ontologic importance of the apoptotic mechanism in homeostasis and development. Fas is expressed in developing brain tissues, where it may have a role in signaling development. However, it is highly up-regulated after hypoxia-ischemia when it is a functional death receptor. Fas expression is paralleled by expression of several factors of the extrinsic apopotic pathway, including FLICE-like inhibitory protein (FLIP), Fas-associated death domain (FADD), and caspases-8 and -3, and by the translocation of cytochrome c from the mitochondria.[69]

Further observations implicate endogenous inflammatory cytokines in HII. Mice lacking NF-κB are more susceptible to TNF-induced damage.[70] On the other hand, TNF null mice are more susceptible to HII,[71] whereas intracerebroventricular injection of recombinant IL-6 significantly reduces ischemic brain damage, suggesting that the large increases in TNF and IL-6 following cerebral ischemia are endogenous neuroprotective responses.[72]

FACTORS DETERMINING THE CHOICE BETWEEN APOPTOSIS AND NECROSIS

A number of different factors influence whether a cell will undergo apoptosis or necrosis, including development, cell type, severity of injury, and availability of ATP.

Developmental Age, Differentiation, and Cell Type

A general principle of development in multicellular organisms is that excess numbers of cells are made, and then those surplus to requirement are selected to undergo programmed cell death by apoptosis during the maturation of functional organs.[12] In the developing nervous system, more than 50% of neurons are lost during development owing to limiting trophic support from target tissues that they innervate.[73]

The stage of cell development may be a particular determinant of apoptosis versus necrosis. For example, cerebellar Purkinje cells differentiate early in brain development. In the porcine model of HII, these cells are very sensitive indicators of HII but undergo only necrosis, never apoptosis. In contrast, cerebellar granule cells (that continue to divide and migrate after birth) undergo apoptosis on a large scale following HII.[24] Similarly, following excitotoxic injury to the newborn rat striatum, neuronal death occurs by apoptosis, whereas in the adult the same insult produces rapid cytoplasmic disintegration, consistent with necrosis.[74]

The mode of cell death also may depend on the degree of differentiation of the cell. Dividing progenitor cells are particularly sensitive to apoptotic stimuli, because the cell cycle machinery is intimately linked to apoptosis.[75] This is illustrated by the observation that axotomy can lead to apoptotic death in some neurons and proliferation in others.[76]

A number of separate studies have also indicated that specific cell types may be particularly sensitized to either necrosis or apoptosis.[77-79]

Severity of Injury

The same cell type can be triggered to undergo apoptosis following mild injury, but necrosis if the damage is severe.[80] This has been demonstrated in a number of *in vitro* systems (Table 8-1).

It is not clear precisely how the severity of injury dictates apoptosis or necrosis. One possibility is that the degree of damage to cell organelles influences the mode of cell death. Mitochondria are particularly sensitive to hypoxic injury and play a central role in both apoptosis and necrosis. For example, inhibitors of complex I trigger apoptosis at low concentrations and necrosis at high concentrations in neuronal cell lines in culture.[81] Indeed, Kroemer and colleagues have suggested that the severity of mitochondrial damage is the most important deciding factor between these two modes of cell death[82]; in this scenario, a small increase in mitochondrial membrane permeability can result in the controlled release of apoptogenic factors through the outer membrane, while severe mitochondrial damage releases a flood of Ca^{2+} and reactive oxygen species into the cytosol, leading to the disruption of plasma membrane integrity and cell necrosis. The importance of oxidative damage in this process is underlined by the finding that complex I

TABLE 8-1

Examples of Apoptosis or Necrosis Determined by the Severity of Injury

Model	Insult	Reference
PC12 cells (rat pheochromocytoma)	6-Hydroxydopamine	47 (1995)
Neonatal rat cerebrocortical slices	NMDA excitotoxicity	81 (1994)
Embryonic hippocampal rat neurons	Lysophosphatidic acid	136 (1984)
AR4-2J cells (rat pancreatic acinar line)	Menadione	137 (1998)
INS-1 (mouse pancreatic beta cell line)	Streptozotocin	138 (1998)
Rat cortical neurons	Peroxynitrite	139 (1995)
Mastocytoma cell line	Heat	140 (1988)
SK-N-MC (dopaminergic cell line)	Respiratory chain complex; complex I inhibitors	141 (1990)
Molt-4 (human T cell line)	Gamma irradiation	142 (1993)

NMDA = N-methyl-D-aspartate.

TABLE 8-2

Antioxidant Strategies Against Ischemic Injury in the Neonatal Rat

Neuroprotective Strategy	Treatment	Reference
Xanthine oxidase inhibition	Allopurinol	116 (1998); 143 (1990)
Xanthine oxidase inhibition	Oxypurinol	39 (1998)
Reactive oxygen species scavenging	Lazaroids	144 (1991)
Metal chelation	Deferoxamine	99 (1993)
Nitric oxide synthase inhibition	L-NAME	145 (1995); 146 (1998)
Nitric oxide synthase inhibition	Aminoguanidine	110 (1993)
Nitric oxide synthase inhibition	7-Nitroindazole	110 (1993)

inhibitor-dependent apoptosis is decreased by pretreatment with free radical scavengers,[83] although it remains to be determined whether free radical accumulation results directly from the block in the mitochondrial respiratory chain or indirectly from the apoptotic process itself.

Availability of ATP

Apoptosis requires energy,[84] while complete ATP depletion causes necrosis; thus ATP availability is likely to be a significant determinant of apoptotic or necrotic death. If cells sustain a lethal insult, they will be able to execute the apoptotic program if ATP levels are sufficient, whereas in situations of limiting ATP, the same degree of cellular injury can result only in necrosis. Consistent with this possibility, glutamate excitotoxicity has been shown to induce either necrosis or apoptosis, depending on mitochondrial function. During and shortly after exposure to glutamate, neurons that died by necrosis had reduced mitochondrial membrane potential ($\Delta\psi$m) and swollen nuclei. In contrast, neurons that recovered $\Delta\psi$m and ATP levels subsequently underwent apoptosis.[85] Consumption of ATP by cell repair enzymes may thus also influence the mode of cell death. Inhibition of PARP prevents necrosis and triggers apoptosis in cells exposed to hydrogen peroxide.[86,87]

Perhaps the most direct demonstration of the importance of ATP is in cultured mouse proximal tubular cells, where ATP depletion itself caused apoptosis or necrosis depending on the levels: cells subjected to antimycin A to deplete ATP to below 15% of controls died of necrosis, while cells with ATP levels between 25% and 70% of controls all died by apoptosis.[88] Extending these observations, it is also possible to alter the mode of cell death by manipulating cellular ATP levels.[89,90]

Preserving ATP levels can thus reduce the proportion of necrotic cells following HII and increase the relative amount of apoptosis. Choi and colleagues[91] demonstrated that following severe ischemia, primary cell necrosis is reduced by the addition of the N-methyl-D-aspartate antagonist MK-801. Residual neurons underwent a form of cell death with the hallmarks of apoptosis. On the other hand, protection from apoptosis can condemn cells to a necrotic death. Thus, cells treated with agents that reduce $\Delta\psi$m alone underwent apoptosis, whereas those kept in identical conditions in the presence of the caspase inhibitor Z-VADfmk died from necrosis.[92]

Oxidative Stress

The newborn infant, particularly the preterm infant, is thought to be particularly prone to tissue damage from oxidative stress because of reduced total antioxidant capacity, and several studies have looked at the possibility of reducing morbidity by ameliorating the effects of oxidative stress in the neonate.[93]

Oxidative stress is considered to be a major mediator of apoptosis in several cellular systems, including neurons. Stimuli that cause oxidative stress, including culture in high oxygen,[94] exposure to β-amyloid,[95-97] and transient hypoxia-ischemia,[17,18,98,99] all trigger apoptosis. Both H_2O_2 and nitric oxide (NO) species can induce apoptosis when applied exogenously and are produced in toxic concentrations by cells that are undergoing apoptosis by other physiologic stimuli.

Oxidative signals for apoptosis can originate both extracellularly and intracellularly and can also be generated by reduced concentrations of antioxidants. Indeed, a number of cerebroprotective strategies are directed specifically at reducing oxidative stress (Table 8-2). Thus, glutathione depletion in immature embryonic cortical neurons leads to oxidative stress and cell death by apoptosis that can be prevented by antioxidants.[100] The use of cyclosporin A, an inhibitor of pro-oxidant-induced Ca^{2+} release from mitochondria, has demonstrated a role for mitochondrial alterations in apoptotic processes. Cyclosporin A can protect against loss of cell viability induced by pro-oxidants or by NO, can favorably alter mitochondrial function after ischemia,[101] and can protect neuronal cells against apoptosis induced by Fe^{2+}, amyloid β-peptide, or NO generating compounds.[102]

THE ROLE OF MITOCHONDRIA IN APOPTOSIS AND NECROSIS

Although mitochondrial failure and falling ATP levels might be either the trigger or the consequence of death, it has been understood for many years that mitochondrial failure can cause necrosis, while direct inhibition of mitochondrial metabolism can also trigger apoptosis.[81,103] Precise mechanisms are beginning to be elucidated,[82,104] and much current interest is focused upon the mitochondrial membrane permeability transition.

The Mitochondrial Permeability Transition Pore

One of the possible effects of free radical damage on mitochondria was first put forward in a hypothesis by Skulachev[105] and confirmed later by direct experimentation. The hypothesis suggested that the mitochondrial megachannel or permeability transition (PT) pore is involved in preventing reactive oxygen species (ROS) accumulation. High concentrations of ROS in the mitochondria would trigger opening of the pore, allowing release of free radicals into the cytosol. The resulting decrease in mitochondrial ROS subsequently would allow pore closure. Conversely, persistent free radical accumulation in mitochondria would prevent pore closure and eventually lead to the release of the apoptosis-inducing proteins. In this way, cells producing excess amounts of free radicals would be eliminated by apoptosis. In favor of this hypothesis, it is clear that the mitochondrial PT pore is activated by ROS.[106]

The opening of the megachannel also can be triggered independently of ROS, although the result in all cases is a sudden increase in the permeability of the inner mitochondrial membrane to small molecules.[107] Although transient opening of the PT pore may be involved in calcium homeostasis or free radical release, sustained PT causes uncoupling of the respiratory chain enzymes, failure of ATP generation, and the release of specific apoptosis-initiating proteins such as cytochrome c into the cytosol (see later).

Although the exact composition of the PT pore is not known, experiments using specific inhibitors of mitochondrial protein function have identified key components. For example, bongkrekic acid, a ligand of the mitochondrial adenine nucleotide translocator (ANT), abolishes mitochondrial permeability transition and inhibits p53-dependent thymocyte apoptosis induced by DNA damage.[108] Similarly, the protective effects of cyclosporin A implicate cyclophilin D as a key component of the PT pore. Other members include cytosolic hexokinase, porin (the voltage-dependent anion channel), creatine kinase, and at least one member of the Bcl-2 family of proteins.[82]

Bcl-2 Family Members and Mitochondria

Bcl-2 is a mitochondrial membrane protein that blocks the apoptotic death of many cell types.[74] The precise mechanism of Bcl-2 protection is unclear. There is some evidence that Bcl-2 regulates an antioxidant pathway at sites of free radical generation.[109-112] However, new data indicating that Bcl-2 family members prevent the mitochondrial permeability transition[113] suggest that the inhibition of free radical generation may be a secondary effect.

Consistent with this role, cytochrome c release can be initiated by the pro-apoptotic protein Bax[114] and blocked by Bcl-2.[115] Furthermore, Bcl-XL can physically interact with another mitochondrion–derived protein Apaf-1, to inhibit its association (and subsequent activation) of caspase-9.[116, 117] On the other hand, in some cell types, Bcl-2 cannot prevent or delay the decrease of the cellular ATP level subsequent to metabolic inhibition, suggesting that it blocks apoptosis at a point downstream of the collapse of cellular-energy homeostasis.[118]

Figure 8–1. Schematic diagram of mitochondrial proteins involved in apoptosis. Stress signals such as DNA damage, accumulation of calcium ions (Ca2+), and reactive oxygen species (ROS) in the mitochondria trigger the release of apoptogenic proteins, including cytochrome c, apoptosis-inducing factor, endonuclease G, and HtrA2/Omi. Release of at least some of these factors is inhibited by anti-apoptotic Bcl-2 proteins. Once in the cytosol, cytochrome c can form a complex with Apaf-1 and caspase-9. The serine protease HtrA2/Omi can sequester the X-linked inhibitor of apoptosis protein (XIAP), leading to enhanced caspase-9 activity. Both cytochrome c and HtrA2/Omi in the cytosol enhance the activation of caspase-9, which, in turn, proteolytically activates caspase-3. Active caspase-3 then triggers apoptotic execution by activating downstream caspases and endonucleases. Apoptosis-inducing factor (AIF) translocation from mitochondria to nuclei in response to death stimuli triggers cellular changes, such as phosphatidyl serine exposure and chromatin condensation, that are independent of Apaf-1 and caspase-9. Endonuclease G is mitochondrion-specific nuclease that translocates to the nucleus during apoptosis and cleaves chromatin-associated DNA into nucleosomal fragments independently of caspases. AIF = apoptosis-inducing factor; Bid = Bcl-2 family member; CAD = caspase-activated DNAse; FADD = Fas-associated death domain; FLIP = FLICE-like inhibitory protein; ICAD = inhibitor of CAD.

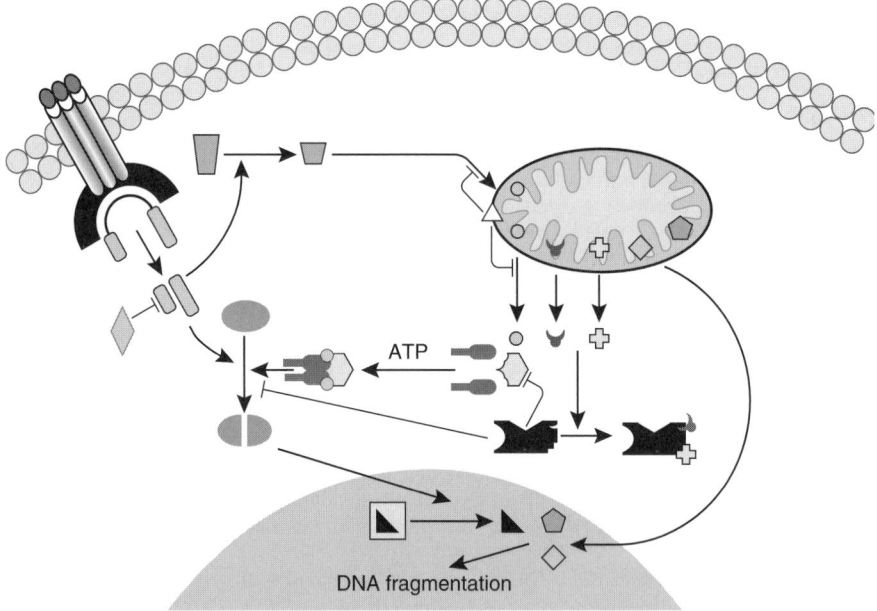

ATP

DNA fragmentation

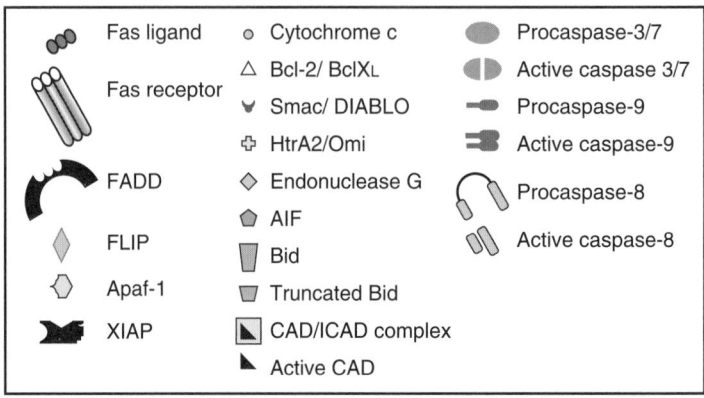

Fas ligand		○ Cytochrome c		Procaspase-3/7	
Fas receptor		△ Bcl-2/ BclXL		Active caspase 3/7	
		⩒ Smac/ DIABLO		Procaspase-9	
FADD		✛ HtrA2/Omi		Active caspase-9	
FLIP		◇ Endonuclease G		Procaspase-8	
Apaf-1		⬠ AIF			
		Bid		Active caspase-8	
XIAP		Truncated Bid			
		CAD/ICAD complex			
		Active CAD			

Although the precise mechanism of Bcl-2 protection is a matter of some debate, it has been shown to protect neurons from apoptosis following cerebral ischemia. Overexpression of the human Bcl-2 protein under the control of neuron-specific promoters reduced neuronal loss following permanent middle cerebral artery occlusion.[119]

Mitochondrial Permeability Transition and Cell Death

In intact cells, an early consequence of mitochondrial permeability transition is a reduction in mitochondrial membrane potential, a process that can be measured using specific fluorogenic dyes.[120] At later time points, a disruption of outer membrane integrity leads to the release of proteins that are involved in apoptotic execution.[121] The finding that supernatants from mitochondria undergoing the permeability transition can cause apoptotic changes in isolated nuclei supports this proposal.[122]

Much of the information regarding the identity of mitochondrial factors involved in apoptosis has been obtained from cell-free systems established to reproduce the apoptotic program *in vitro*.[123] In one such model, apoptosis could be initiated by addition of dATP but cytochrome c was also required. Intact cells undergoing apoptosis showed a translocation of cytochrome c (which normally functions as an electron carrier in the respiratory chain) from mitochondria to the cytosol,[124] which in turn results in the activation of specific caspases,[125] proteases that are specifically involved in apoptotic execution. Among these enzymes, caspase-3 is thought to be pivotal in apoptotic execution, since cells that lack detectable levels of this enzyme fail to undergo cytochrome c–dependent apoptosis.[126] Although caspase inhibitors substantially reduce mitochondrial membrane potential and cell death, they do not prevent the passage of cytochrome c from mitochondria to the cytosol, which must occur upstream of caspase activation.

Along with cytochrome c and dATP, Apaf-1 has been identified as an important protein that participates in the activation of caspase-3.[127] Apaf-1 shares significant homology with *Caenorhabditis elegans* CED-4, a protein that is required for apoptosis in the nematode. A third protein factor, Apaf-3, is also required for caspase-3 activation *in vitro*. Apaf-3 was identified as a member of the caspase family, caspase-9.[128] Genetic studies suggest that caspase-9 is the most upstream member of the apoptotic protease cascade, and the formation of an Apaf-1/caspase-9 complex activates caspase-3 in a cytochrome c– and dATP–dependent manner (Fig. 8–1).

The effects of cytochrome c translocation to the cytosol are paradoxic. Although ATP is required for apoptotic execution, the mitochondrial cytochrome c deficit eventually will result in shutdown of the respiratory chain, and consequently ATP synthesis will cease. Thus, Fas-driven apoptosis in Jurkat cells results in the inactivation of cytochrome c with cessation of oxygen consumption.[129] However, the converse is not always true; we have recently found that apoptosis induced by branched-chain amino acids is preceded by a fall in oxygen consumption without cytochrome c release.[130] Other reports have confirmed that apoptosis can proceed in the absence of cytosolic translocation of cytochrome c.[131,132]

Nevertheless, cytochrome c release is an important link between mitochondria and apoptosis in at least some systems. Consistent with this concept of the mitochondria as a controller of apoptosis, mitochondrial changes precede the activation of cytosolic enzymes involved in apoptotic execution, and inhibitors of the permeability transition pore can prevent apoptosis.[92]

CONCLUSIONS

Both apoptotic and necrotic cell death are important components of neuronal loss. However, the distinction between apoptosis and necrosis is becoming less clear. The mode of cell death is determined by a number of cellular factors, including developmental status, the severity of injury, and mitochondrial function. The complexity of the events involved in oxidative damage to the brain underlines the need for therapeutic approaches that will combat multiple mechanisms of damage and interrupt both apoptotic and necrotic processes.[133-135]

REFERENCES

1. Nijhawan D, et al: Apoptosis in neural development and disease. Annu Rev Neurosci 23:73, 2000.
2. Salvesen GS: Programmed cell death and the caspases. APMIS 107:73, 1999.
3. Hengartner MO: The biochemistry of apoptosis. Nature 407:770, 2000.
4. Mehmet H: Caspases find a new place to hide. Nature 403:29, 2000.
5. Krammer PH: CD95's deadly mission in the immune system. Nature 407:789, 2000.
6. Nagata S, et al: Degradation of chromosomal DNA during apoptosis. Cell Death Differ 10:108, 0003.
7. Korsmeyer SJ, et al: Pro-apoptotic cascade activates BID, which oligomerizes BAK or BAX into pores that result in the release of cytochrome c. Cell Death Differ 2000 7:1166, 2001.
8. Salvesen GS, Duckett CS: IAP proteins: blocking the road to death's door. Nat Rev Mol Cell Biol 6:401, 2002.
9. van Loo G, et al: The role of mitochondrial factors in apoptosis: a Russian roulette with more than one bullet. Cell Death Differ. 9:1031, 2002.
10. Ferri KF, Kroemer G: Organelle-specific initiation of cell death pathways. Nat Cell Biol 3:E255, 2001.
11. Nakagawa T, et al: Caspase-12 mediates endoplasmic-reticulum-specific apoptosis and cytotoxicity by amyloid-beta. Nature 403:98, 2000.
12. Jacobson MD, et al: Programmed cell death in animal development. Cell 88:347, 1997.
13. MacDonald RL, Stoodley M: Pathophysiology of cerebral ischemia. Neurol Med Chir Tokyo 38:1, 1998.
14. Perez-Velazquez JL, et al: In vitro ischemia promotes glutamate-mediated free radical generation and intracellular calcium accumulation in hippocampal pyramidal neurons. J Neurosci 17:9085, 1997.
15. Beilharz EJ, et al: Insulin-like growth factor II is induced during wound repair following hypoxic-ischemic injury in the developing rat brain. Brain Res Mol Brain Res 29:81, 1995.
16. Ferrer I, et al: Evidence of nuclear DNA fragmentation following hypoxia-ischemia in the infant rat brain, and transient forebrain ischemia in the adult gerbil. Brain Pathol 4:115, 1994.
17. Mehmet H, et al: Increased apoptosis in the cingulate sulcus of newborn piglets following transient hypoxia-ischaemia is related to the degree of high energy phosphate depletion during the insult. Neurosci Lett 181:121, 1994.
18. Linnik MD, et al: Evidence supporting a role for programmed cell death in focal cerebral ischemia in rats. Stroke 24:2002, 1993.
19. MacManus JP, et al: Global ischemia can cause DNA fragmentation indicative of apoptosis in rat brain. Neurosci Lett 164:89, 1993.
20. Gluckman PD, et al: A role for IGF-1 in the rescue of CNS neurons following hypoxic-ischemic injury. Biochem Biophys Res Commun 182:593, 1992.
21. Tan WK, et al: Suppression of postischemic epileptiform activity with MK-801 improves neural outcome in fetal sheep. Ann Neurol 32:677, 1992.
22. Edwards AD, et al: Apoptosis in the brains of infants suffering intrauterine cerebral injury. Pediatr Res 42:684, 1997.
23. Scott RJ, Hegyi L: Cell injury in perinatal hypoxic-ischaemic brain injury. Neuropathol Appl Neurobiol 23:307, 1997.
24. Yue X, et al: Apoptosis and necrosis in the newborn piglet brain following transient cerebral hypoxia-ischaemia. Neuropathol Appl Neurobiol 23:16, 1997.
25. Majno G, Joris I: Apoptosis, oncosis, and necrosis. An overview of cell death [see comments]. Am J Pathol 146:3, 1995.
26. Kalda A, et al: Medium transitory oxygen-glucose deprivation induced by both apoptosis and necrosis in cerebellar granule cells. Neurosci Lett 240:21, 1998.
27. Ferrer I, et al: Both apoptosis and necrosis occur following intrastriatal administration of excitotoxins. Acta Neuropathol Berl 90:504, 1995.
28. Papassotiropoulos A, et al: Induction of apoptosis and secondary necrosis in rat dorsal root ganglion cell cultures by oxidized low density lipoprotein. Neurosci Lett 209:33, 1996.
29. Villalba M, et al: Concomitant induction of apoptosis and necrosis in cerebellar granule cells following serum and potassium withdrawal. Neuroreport 8:981, 1997.
30. Copin JC, et al: Trolox and 6,7-dinitroquinoxaline-2,3-dione prevent necrosis but not apoptosis in cultured neurons subjected to oxygen deprivation. Brain Res 784:25, 1998.
31. Zychlinsky A, et al: Cytolytic lymphocytes induce both apoptosis and necrosis in target cells. J Immunol 146:393, 1991.
32. Bolanas JP, et al: Nitric oxide–mediated mitochondrial damage in the brain: mechanisms and implication for neurodegenerative diseases J Neurochem 68:2227, 1997.

33. Eliasson MJ, et al: Poly(ADP-ribose) polymerase gene disruption renders mice resistant to cerebral ischemia. Nat Med 3:1089, 1997.

34. Takahashi K, et al: Neuroprotective effects of inhibiting poly(ADP-ribose) synthetase on focal cerebral ischemia in rats. J Cereb Blood Flow Metab 17:1137, 1997.

35. Endres M, et al: Ischemic brain injury is mediated by the activation of poly (ADP-ribose) polymerase. J Cereb Blood Flow Metab 17:1143, 1997.

36. Leist M, et al: Apoptosis in the absence of poly-(ADP-ribose) polymerase. Biochem Biophys Res Commun 233:518, 1997.

37. Wang ZQ, et al: PARP is important for genomic stability but dispensable in apoptosis. Genes Dev 11:2347, 1997.

38. Lazebnik YA, et al: Cleavage of poly(ADP-ribose) polymerase by a proteinase with properties like ICE. Nature 371:346, 1994.

39. Namura S, et al: Activation and cleavage of caspase-3 in apoptosis induced by experimental cerebral ischemia. J Neurosci 18:3659, 1998.

40. Joashi UC, et al: Poly (ADP ribose) polymerase cleavage precedes neuronal death in the hippocampus and cerebellum following injury to the developing rat forebrain (in press) .

41. Gottron FJ, et al: Caspase inhibition selectively reduces the apoptotic component of oxygen-glucose deprivation-induced cortical neuronal cell death. Mol Cell Neurosci 9:159, 1997.

42. Endres M, et al: Attenuation of delayed neuronal death after mild focal ischemia in mice by inhibition of the caspase family. J Cereb Blood Flow Metab 18:238, 1998.

43. Loddick SA, et al: An ICE inhibitor, z-VAD-DCB, attenuates ischaemic brain damage in the rat. Neuroreport 7:1465, 1996.

44. McCarthy NJ, et al: Inhibition of Ced-3/ICE–related proteases does not prevent cell death induced by oncogenes, DNA damage, or the Bcl-2 homologue Bak. J Cell Biol 136:215, 1997.

45. Dragunow M, Preston K: The role of inducible transcription factors in apoptotic nerve cell death. Brain Res Brain Res Rev 21:1, 1995.

46. Kogure K, Kato H: Altered gene expression in cerebral ischemia. Stroke 24:2121, 1993.

47. Morooka H, et al: Ischemia and reperfusion enhance ATF-2 and c-Jun binding to cAMP response elements and to an AP-1 binding site from the c-jun promoter. J Biol Chem 270:30084, 1995.

48. BadenAmissah K, et al: Induction of beta-amyloid precursor protein (β-APP) expression after neonatal hypoxic ischaemic cerebral injury (HII). J Pathol 182:A49, 1997.

49. Lesort M, et al: NMDA induces apoptosis and necrosis in neuronal cultures. Increased APP immunoreactivity is linked to apoptotic cells. Neurosci Lett 221:213, 1997.

50. Clemens JA, et al: Global cerebral ischemia activates nuclear factor-kappa B prior to evidence of DNA fragmentation. Brain Res Mol Brain Res 48:187, 1997.

51. MacManus JP, Linnik MD: Gene expression induced by cerebral ischemia: an apoptotic perspective. J Cereb Blood Flow Metab 17:815, 1997.

52. Clemens JA, et al: Global ischemia activates nuclear factor-kappa B in forebrain neurons of rats. Stroke 28:1073, discussion 1080, 1997.

53. Polla BS, et al: Mitochondria are selective targets for the protective effects of heat shock against oxidative injury. Proc Natl Acad Sci U S A 93:6458, 1996.

54. Hu Y, et al: Discordant activation of stress-activated protein kinases or c-Jun NH$_2$-terminal protein kinases in tissues of heat-stressed mice. J Biol Chem 272:9113, 1997.

55. Mizukami Y, Yoshida KI: Tissue-specific pattern of stress kinase activation in ischemic/reperfused heart and kidney. J Biol Chem 272:19943, 1997.

56. Walton KM, et al: Activation of p38(MAPK) in microglia after ischemia. J Neurochem 70:1764, 1998.

57. Wang Y, et al: Cardiac hypertrophy induced by mitogen-activated protein kinase 7, a specific activator for c-Jun NH$_2$-terminal kinase in ventricular muscle cells. J Biol Chem 273:5423, 1998.

58. Wang Y, et al: Cardiac muscle cell hypertrophy and apoptosis induced by distinct members of the p38 mitogen-activated protein kinase family. J Biol Chem 273:2161, 1998.

59. Roulston A, et al: Early activation of c-Jun N-terminal kinase and p38 kinase regulates cell survival in response to tumor necrosis factor alpha. J Biol Chem 273:10232, 1998.

60. Sutherland CL, et al: Differential activation of the ERK, JNK and p38 mitogen-activated protein kinases by CD40 and the B-cell antigen receptor. J Immunol 57:3381, 1996.

61. Marks KA, et al: Delayed vasodilation and altered oxygenation after cerebral ischemia in fetal sheep. Pediatr Res 39:48, 1996.

62. Kawasaki H, et al: Activation and involvement of p38 mitogen-activated protein kinase in glutamate-induced apoptosis in rat cerebellar granule cells. J Biol Chem 272:18518, 1997.

63. Maundrell K, et al: Bcl-2 undergoes phosphorylation by c-Jun N-terminal kinase/stress-activated protein kinases in the presence of the constitutively active GTP-binding protein Rac1. J Biol Chem 272:25238, 1997.

64. Botchkina GI, et al: Expression of TNF and TNF receptors (p55 and p75) in the rat brain after focal cerebral ischemia. Mol Med 3:765, 1997.

65. Kato H, et al: Progressive expression of immunomolecules on activated microglia and invading leucocytes following focal cerebral ischemia in the rat. Brain Res 734:203, 1996.

66. Silverstein F, et al: Cytokines and perinatal brain injury. Neurochem Int 30:375, 1997.

67. Szaflarski J, et al: Cerebral hypoxia-ischemia stimulates cytokine gene expression in perinatal rats. Stroke 26:1093, 1995.

68. Loddick SA, Rothwell NJ: Neuroprotective effects of human recombinant interleukin-1 receptor antagonist in focal cerebral ischaemia in the rat. J Cereb Blood Flow Metab 16:932, 1996.

69. Northington FJ, et al: Delayed neurodegeneration in neonatal rat thalamus after hypoxia-ischemia is apoptosis. J Neurosci 21:1931, 2001.

70. Beg AA, Baltimore D: An essential role for NF-kappaB in preventing TNF-alpha-induced cell death [see comments]. Science 274:782, 1996.

71. Bruce AJ, Altered neuronal and microglial responses to excitotoxic and ischemic brain injury in mice lacking TNF receptors. Nat Med 2:788, 1996.

72. Loddick SA, Cerebral interleukin-6 is neuroprotective during permanent focal cerebral ischemia in the rat. J Cereb Blood Flow Metab 18:176, 1998.

73. Oppenheim RW: Cell death during development of the nervous system. Annu Rev Neurosci 14:453, 1991.

74. Portera-Cailliau C, et al: Non-NMDA and NMDA receptor mediated excitotoxic neuronal deaths in adult brain are morphologically distinct: further evidence for an apoptosis-necrosis continuum. J Comp Neurol 378:88, 1997.

75. Ross ME: Cell division and the nervous system: regulating the cycle from neural differentiation to death. Trends Neurosci 19:62, 1996.

76. Herdegen T, et al: The c-Jun transcription factor—bipotential mediator of neuronal death, survival and regeneration. Trends Neurosci 20:227, 1997.

77. Fiers W, et al: TNF-induced intracellular signaling leading to gene induction or to cytotoxicity by necrosis or by apoptosis. J Inflamm 47:67, 1995–96.

78. Kato H, et al: Neuronal apoptosis and necrosis following spinal cord ischemia in the rat. Exp Neurol 148:464, 1997.

79. Sloviter RS, et al: Apoptosis and necrosis induced in different hippocampal neuron populations by repetitive perforant path stimulation in the rat. J Comp Neurol 366:516, 1996.

80. Raffray M, Cohen GM: Apoptosis and necrosis in toxicology: a continuum or distinct modes of cell death? Pharmacol Ther 75:153, 1997.

81. Hartley A, et al: Complex I inhibitors induce dose-dependent apoptosis in PC12 cells: relevance to Parkinson's disease. J Neurochem 63:1987, 1994.

82. Kroemer G, et al: The mitochondrial death/life regulator in apoptosis and necrosis. Annu Rev Physiol 60:619, 1998.

83. Seaton TA, et al: Free radical scavengers protect dopaminergic cell lines from apoptosis induced by complex I inhibitors. Brain Res 777:110, 1997.

84. Kass GE, et al: Chromatin condensation during apoptosis requires ATP. Biochem J 318(Pt 3):749, 1996.

85. Ankarcrona M, et al: Glutamate-induced neuronal death: a succession of necrosis or apoptosis depending on mitochondrial function. Neuron 15:961, 1995.

86. Palomba L, et al: Prevention of necrosis and activation of apoptosis in oxidatively injured human myeloid leukemia U937 cells. FEBS Lett 390:91, 1996.

87. Watson AJ, et al: Poly (adenosine diphosphate ribose) polymerase inhibition prevents necrosis induced by H$_2$O$_2$ but not apoptosis. Gastroenterology 109:472, 1995.

88. Lieberthal W, et al: Graded ATP depletion can cause necrosis or apoptosis of cultured mouse proximal tubular cells. Am J Physiol 274:F315, 1998.

89. Eguchi Y, et al: Intracellular ATP levels determine cell death fate by apoptosis or necrosis. Cancer Res 57:1835, 1997.

90. Leist M, et al: Intracellular adenosine triphosphate (ATP) concentration: a switch in the decision between apoptosis and necrosis. J Exp Med 85:1481, 1997.

91. Gwag BJ, et al: Blockade of glutamate receptors unmasks neuronal apoptosis after oxygen-glucose deprivation in vitro. Neuroscience 68:615, 1995.

92. Hirsch T, et al: Mitochondrial permeability transition in apoptosis and necrosis. Cell Biol Toxicol 14:141, 1998.

93. Saugstad OD: Mechanisms of tissue injury by oxygen radicals: implications for neonatal disease. Acta Paediatr 85:1, 1996.

94. Enokido Y, Hatanaka H: Apoptotic cell death occurs in hippocampal neurons cultured in a high oxygen atmosphere. Neurosci 57:965, 1993.

95. Behl C, et al: Hydrogen peroxide mediates amyloid β protein neurotoxicity. Cell 77:817, 1994.

96. Forloni G, et al: Apoptosis-mediated neurotoxicity induced by chronic application of β-amyloid fragment 25–35. Neuroreport 4:523, 1993.

97. Loo DT, et al: Apoptosis is induced by β-amyloid in cultured central nervous system neurons. Proc Natl Acad Sci U S A 90:7951, 1993.

98. MacManus JP, et al: DNA damage consistent with apoptosis in transient focal ischaemic neocortex. Neuroreport 5:493, 1994.

99. Okamoto M, et al: Internucleosonal DNA cleavage involved in ischemia-induced neuronal death. Biochem Biophys Res Commun 196:1356, 1993.

100. Ratan RR, et al: Oxidative stress induces apoptosis in embryonic cortical neurons. J Neurochem 62:376, 1994.

101. Halestrap AP, et al: Cyclosporin A binding to mitochondrial cyclophilin inhibits the permeability transition pore and protects hearts from ischaemia/reperfusion injury. Mol Cell Biochem 174:167, 1997.

102. Keller JN, et al: Mitochondrial manganese superoxide dismutase prevents neural apoptosis and reduces ischemic brain injury: suppression of peroxynitrite production, lipid peroxidation, and mitochondrial dysfunction J Neurosci 18:687, 1998.

103. Wolvetang EJ, et al: Mitochondrial respiratory chain inhibitors induce apoptosis. FEBS Lett 339:40, 1994.

104. Mignotte B, Vayssiere JL: Mitochondria and apoptosis. Eur J Biochem 252:1, 1998.

105. Skulachev VP: Why are mitochondria involved in apoptosis? Permeability transition pores and apoptosis as selective mechanisms to eliminate superoxide: producing mitochondria and cell. FEBS Lett *397*:7, 1996.

106. Chernyak BV: Redox regulation of the mitochondrial permeability transition pore. Biosci Rep *17*:293, 1997.

107. Kroemer G, et al: Mitochondrial control of apoptosis. Immunol Today *18*:44, 1997.

108. Marchetti P, et al: Mitochondrial permeability transition is a central coordinating event of apoptosis. J Exp Med *184*:1155, 1996.

109. Hennet T, et al: Expression of BCL-2 protein enhances the survival of mouse fibrosarcoid cells in tumor necrosis factor–mediated cytotoxicity. Cancer Res *53*:1456, 1993.

110. Hennet T, et al: Tumour necrosis factor-alpha induces superoxide anion generation in mitochondria of L929 cells. Biochem J *289*(Pt 2):587, 1993.

111. Hockenbery DM, et al: Bcl-2 functions in an antioxidant pathway to prevent apoptosis. Cell *75*:241, 1993.

112. Kane DJ, et al: Bcl-2 inhibition of neural death: decreased generation of reactive oxygen species. Science *262*:1274, 1993.

113. Vander Heiden MG, et al: Bcl-xL regulates the membrane potential and volume homeostasis of mitochondria [see comments]. Cell *91*:627, 1997.

114. Skulachev VP: Cytochrome c in the apoptotic and antioxidant cascades. FEBS Lett *423*:275, 1998.

115. Yang NN, et al: Correction: raloxifene response needs more than an element (letter). Science *275*:1249, 1997.

116. Hu Y, et al: Bcl-XL interacts with Apaf-1 and inhibits Apaf-1-dependent caspase-9 activation. Proc Natl Acad Sci U S A *95*:4386, 1998.

117. Pan G, et al: Caspase-9, Bcl-XL, and Apaf-1 form a ternary complex. J Biol Chem *273*:5841, 1998.

118. Marton A, et al: Apoptotic cell death induced by inhibitors of energy conservation—Bcl-2 inhibits apoptosis downstream of a fall of ATP level. Eur J Biochem *250*:467, 1997.

119. Martinou JC, et al: Overexpression of BCL-2 in transgenic mice protects neurons from naturally occurring cell death and experimental ischemia. Neuron *13*:1017, 1994.

120. Petit PX, et al: Mitochondria and programmed cell death: back to the future. FEBS Lett *396*:7, 1996.

121. Petit PX, et al: Disruption of the outer mitochondrial membrane as a result of large amplitude swelling: the impact of irreversible permeability transition. FEBS Lett *426*:111, 1998.

122. Scarlett JL, Murphy MP: Release of apoptogenic proteins from the mitochondrial intermembrane space during the mitochondrial permeability transition. FEBS Lett *418*:282, 1997.

123. Ellerby HM, et al: Establishment of a cell-free system of neuronal apoptosis: comparison of premitochondrial, mitochondrial, and postmitochondrial phases. J Neurosci *17*:6165, 1997.

124. Liu X, et al: Induction of apoptotic program in cell-free extracts: requirement for dATP and cytochrome c. Cell *86*:147, 1996.

125. Bossy-Wetzel E, et al: Mitochondrial cytochrome c release in apoptosis occurs upstream of DEVD-specific caspase activation and independently of mitochondrial transmembrane depolarization. EMBO J *17*:37, 1998.

126. Li F, et al: Cell-specific induction of apoptosis by microinjection of cytochrome c. Bcl-xL has activity independent of cytochrome c release. J Biol Chem *272*:30299, 1997.

127. Zou H, et al: Apaf-1, a human protein homologous to *C. elegans* CED-4, participates in cytochrome c–dependent activation of caspase-3 (see comments). Cell *90*:405, 1997.

128. Li P, et al: Cytochrome c and dATP-dependent formation of Apaf-1/caspase-9 complex initiates an apoptotic protease cascade. Cell *91*:479, 1997.

129. Adachi S, et al: Bcl-2 and the outer mitochondrial membrane in the inactivation of cytochrome c during Fas-mediated apoptosis. J Biol Chem *272*:21878, 1997.

130. Jouvet P, et al: Maple syrup urine disease metabolites induce apoptosis in neural cells without cytochrome c release or changes in mitochondrial membrane potential. Biochem Soc Trans *26*:S341, 1998.

131. Chauhan D, et al: Cytochrome c–dependent and –independent induction of apoptosis in multiple myeloma cells. J Biol Chem *272*:29995, 1997.

132. Tang DG, et al: Apoptosis in the absence of cytochrome c accumulation in the cytosol. Biochem Biophys Res Commun. *242*:380, 1998.

133. Kato H, et al: Protection of rat spinal cord from ischemia with dextrorphan and cycloheximide: effects on necrosis and apoptosis. J Thorac Cardiovasc Surg *114*:609, 1997.

134. Koh JY, et al: Potentiated necrosis of cultured cortical neurons by neurotrophins [see comments]. Science *268*:573, 1995.

135. Pang Z, Geddes JW: Mechanisms of cell death induced by the mitochondrial toxin 3-nitropropionic acid: acute excitotoxic necrosis and delayed apoptosis. J Neurosci *17*:3064, 1997.

136. Hope PL, et al: Cerebral energy metabolism studied with phosphorus NMR spectroscopy in normal and birth-asphyxiated infants. Lancet *2*:366, 1984.

137. Robertson NJ, et al: Persistent lactate following perinatal hypoxic-ischaemic encephalopathy and its relationship to energy failure studied by magnetic resonance spectroscopy (abstract). Early Hum Dev *5*:73, 1998.

138. Reddy K, et al: Maturational change in the cortical response to hypoperfusion injury in the fetal sheep. Pediatr Res *43*:674, 1998.

139. Bonfoco E, et al: Apoptosis and necrosis: two distinct events induced, respectively, by mild and intense insults with *N*-methyl-D-aspartate or nitric oxide/superoxide in cortical cell cultures. Proc Natl Acad Sci U S A *92*:7162, 1995.

140. Hansen AJ, Nedergaard M: Brain ion homeostasis in cerebral ischemia. Neurochem Pathol *9*:195, 1988.

141. Harmon BV, et al: Cell death induced in a murine mastocytoma by 42–47 degrees C heating in vitro: evidence that the form of death changes from apoptosis to necrosis above a critical heat load. Int J Radiat Biol *58*:845, 1990.

142. Akagi Y, et al: Radiation-induced apoptosis and necrosis in Molt-4 cells: a study of dose-effect relationships and their modification. Int J Radiat Biol *64*:47, 1993.

143. Obrenovitch TP, et al: A rapid redistribution of hydrogen ions is associated with depolarization and repolarization subsequent to cerebral ischaemia/reperfusion. J Neurophysiol *64*:1125, 1990.

144. Bagenholm R, et al: Effects of 21-aminosteroid U74006F on brain damage and edema following perinatal hypoxia-ischemia in the rat. J Cereb Blood Flow Metab *11*:S134, 1991.

145. Ashwal S, et al: *L*-NAME reduces infarct volume in a filament model of transient middle cerebral artery occlusion in the rat pup. Pediatr Res *38*:652, 1995.

146. Ochu EE, et al: Caspases mediate 6-hydroxydopamine–induced apoptosis but not necrosis in PC12 cells. J Neurochem *70*:2637, 1998.

Elisabeth A. Aron and Russell V. Anthony

9

Angiogenesis

Development of any tissue or organ requires the formation of a vascular network within the tissue, such that vascular network formation within any tissue or organ can be viewed as a developmental requisite. Formation of tissue vasculature requires two distinct but related processes: vasculogenesis and angiogenesis. *Vasculogenesis* involves the formation of vessel tubes from the association of endothelial cell precursors or angioblasts, occurs solely in the embryo, and generally involves tissue of endodermal origin, including the heart tube and dorsal aorta, lung, pancreas, and spleen.[1] *Angiogenesis* is defined as the formation of new blood vessels from existing vessels,[2,3] is not limited to embryonic development, and is induced by inflammation, immune reactions, neoplasia, and wound healing.[4,5] Whereas these two pro-

cesses are distinct, they are both critical to embryonic development and the successful outcome of pregnancy, and they rely on many of the same molecular regulators.

At least 20 activators, and a comparable number of inhibitors, are involved in the regulation of vasculogenesis and angiogenesis.[6] During vasculogenesis, these factors induce differentiation of angioblasts to endothelial cells, within embryonic and extraembryonic mesoderm, to form the initial vascular network (Fig. 9-1).[7] The addition of new vessel segments to this vascular mesh, that is, angiogenesis, is required for the formation of a functional vascular system.[8] Formation of new capillaries, by both sprouting and nonsprouting (intussusception) angiogenesis, coupled with the remodeling and pruning of existing vessels,[8]

Vasculogenesis

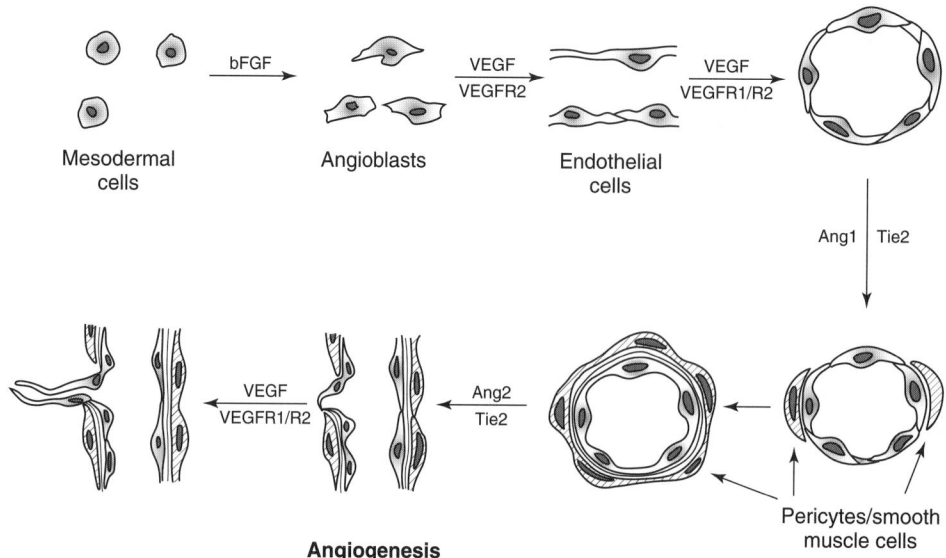

Angiogenesis

Figure 9–1. Schematic of blood vessel formation (vasculogenesis) and remodeling (angiogenesis). Embryonic mesodermal cells are stimulated by basic fibroblast growth factor (bFGF) to form angioblasts, which, under the influence of vascular endothelial growth factor (VEGF), form endothelial cells and vascular tubes. VEGF acts first through the VEGFR-2 receptor and then through VEGFR-1 and VEGFR-2. Angiopoietin (Ang1), acting through Tie2, attracts pericytes around the primitive vessel, thereby stabilizing the vessel. The combined effects of VEGF and angiopoietin 2 (Ang2) provide for disruption of the vessel wall and for new vessel outgrowth or angiogenesis.

provides for the extension and modification of the primitive vascular network (see Fig. 9-1). At the same time, recruitment of perivascular cells (pericytes and smooth muscle cells) and deposition of the basement membrane provide stability and maturation of the developing vascular system (see Fig. 9-1).

Although angiogenesis and the factors regulating it are important in postnatal tissues, this chapter focuses on the fetus and placenta and on the way in which deficits in angiogenesis may cause human disease. Furthermore, we focus on the principal regulators of endothelium growth and morphogenesis.

EMBRYONIC ANGIOGENESIS

Formation of the initial vascular plexus begins quite early, while the embryo is still being nourished by diffusion,[9] but is becoming sufficiently large and complex that simple diffusion is no longer adequate.[10] Early on, angioblastic and hematopoietic cells can be detected within the population of epiblasts that invaginate during the process of gastrulation to form the mesoderm. These cells migrate toward the space between the epiblast and hypoblast.[9] After the angioblasts arrive within the lateral mesoderm of the yolk sac, they differentiate into solid clumps of epithelioid cells called *blood islands*.[9] The condensed extraembryonic angioblasts that form cords and clusters give rise to primitive blood cells and endothelial cells.[10] Centrally located cells give rise to blood cells, whereas those located in the periphery give rise to endothelial cells.[11] Coalescence of endothelial cells from neighboring blood islands provides a *vascular network* consisting of primitive endothelial tubes.[9] Further coalescence of blood islands provides vascular network formation.[10]

Although the cells derived from the yolk sac contribute only to a transient population of blood cells,[9] somite-derived angioblasts migrate throughout the embryo, differentiate into endothelial cells, and aggregate into solid endothelial strands.[12-16] However, only a few of the angioblasts have hemangioblastic potency, and they are localized to the floor of the dorsal aorta. From this location, cells bud off and subsequently

populate various sites of hematopoiesis (liver, spleen, bone marrow).[17] Once the developing vascular network is perfused by cardiac activity, cells from the blood islands are released into circulation and are gradually replaced by definitive blood cells.[9]

Because of the invasive nature of the angioblasts, they can move throughout the embryonic tissues, but they are driven along genetically predetermined paths.[18] The vessels formed along this path of migration are continually remodeled by progressive growth and regression, such that the direction of blood flow can change many times.[19] Accompanying this remodeling is pressure-induced wall stress, generated from blood flow, and this stress also plays a role in developing the vascular system.[20]

PLACENTAL ANGIOGENESIS

Vasculogenesis and angiogenesis within the placenta is likely as important as embryonic angiogenesis for successful pregnancy outcome. Placental development begins early in pregnancy, and continues throughout gestation, as increased blood flow to the placenta is necessary to support the needs of the growing fetus. Beginning at the time of implantation, lacunae develop within the syncytiotrophoblast, coalescing to form the intervillous space which will eventually fill with maternal blood. During this time frame, day 8 to 13 post coitus, the lacunae are separated by trabeculae composed of syncytiotrophoblasts. On about day 13 post coitus, maternal blood cells can be observed in the lacunae, and concomitantly the trabeculae are invaded by proliferating cytotrophoblasts, giving rise to the primary villi. Primary villi are quickly transformed into secondary villi as a result of mesenchyme cell invasion from the primary chorionic plate. Between days 18 and 20 post coitus, the first fetal capillaries are present within the mesenchyme, marking the development of the first tertiary villi.[21]

Early growth of the capillaries forms a primitive capillary network, and by 6 weeks post coitus, the basal lamina begins to form around the capillaries.[22] This primitive network is constantly being modified; the larger villi develop endothelial tubes serving as precursors of arterioles and venules. These tubes become surrounded by cells expressing α and γ smooth muscle actins, vimentin and desmin.[23] Tertiary villi are transformed into immature intermediate villi, and after 15 weeks, the immature intermediate villi are transformed into stem villi. As the loose stroma becomes fibrotic and condensed, the peripheral capillary network condenses while the central capillaries differentiate into arterioles and venules.[24] This villous tree expands from its peripheral ends and gives rise to new villous outgrowth with new capillary networks.[22]

Increasing blood flow and pressure within the primitive vessels aid in stimulating further vessel development.[22] The first half of pregnancy is characterized by branching angiogenesis, whereas from 26 weeks until term, angiogenesis within the placenta is predominantly nonbranching. Mature intermediate villi are produced in conjunction with increasing endothelial proliferation,[22] to form the main unit for nutrient exchange within the placenta. When the length of the intermediate villi vessels begins to exceed the length of the villi, formation of terminal villi occurs. Within the terminal villi, placental vessels lie very close to the intervillous space, such that placental and maternal blood supplies are separated only by a thin layer of syncytiotrophoblast. This arrangement provides a thin diffusion barrier, aiding in the transport of nutrients to the fetus.

ANGIOGENIC GROWTH FACTORS AND RECEPTORS

Angiogenesis is regulated through a complex balance between angiogenic and angiostatic substances, exerting their influence at numerous levels. Promoters of angiogenesis include, but are not limited to, acidic and basic fibroblast growth factors, angiopoietin 1 and 2 (Ang1 and Ang2), placenta growth factor, platelet-derived growth factor, transforming growth factor-β, tumor necrosis factor-α, and vascular endothelial growth factor. Inhibitors of angiogenesis include, but are not limited to, angiostatin, endostatin, interferons, and platelet factor 4. For the purposes of this chapter, we focus on the vascular endothelial growth factor (VEGF) family and their receptors.

Vascular Endothelial Growth Factor Family

VEGF is a 40,000- to 45,000-M_r disulfide-linked homodimeric glycoprotein that acts on endothelial cells as a chemoattractant, mitogen, and morphogen.[25] However, VEGF is not a single protein and is truly a family of gene products, including VEGF-A,[26] VEGF-B,[27] VEGF-C,[28] VEGF-D,[29] and VEGF-E.[30] As a result of differential splicing of the primary VEGF-A gene transcript, five isoforms of human VEGF-A are produced: $VEGF_{121}$, $VEGF_{145}$, $VEGF_{165}$, $VEGF_{189}$, and $VEGF_{206}$. The larger isoforms, $VEGF_{165}$, $VEGF_{189}$, and $VEGF_{206}$, contain heparin binding domains,[31] and although $VEGF_{121}$ and $VEGF_{165}$ are readily diffusible and are the predominant secreted isoforms, $VEGF_{189}$ and $VEGF_{206}$ remain membrane-associated[32] but retain their biologic activity. $VEGF_{145}$ appears to be specific to human endometrium.[33] An additional member of this gene family is placenta growth factor (PlGF), and through alternative splicing, three isoforms are generated: $PlGF_{149}$ (PlGF-1), $PlGF_{170}$ (PlGF-2), and $PlGF_{219}$ (PlGF-3).[34]

Adding to the functional complexity of this family are the ligand-receptor interactions that have been identified. Receptors for this growth factor family include three kinase-domain receptors: fms-like tyrosine kinase 1 (Flt-1 or VEGFR-1),[35] kinase insert domain–containing receptor (KDR, Flk-1, or VEGFR-2)[35] and fms-like tyrosine kinase 4 (Flt-4 or VEGFR-3).[28] The receptor VEGFR-1 binds homodimers of VEGF-A, VEGF-B, PlGF, or VEGF/PlGF heterodimers,[35] whereas VEGFR-2 appears to be specific for homodimers of VEGF. The third receptor, VEGFR-3, acts as the receptor for VEGF-C and VEGF-D, but it does not interact with VEGF-A.[36] Beyond the three classic receptors for the

VEGF family, some tissues produce a soluble form of VEGFR-1, which could act as a functional antagonist.[37] Furthermore, the neuropilins (NP-1 and NP-2), previously described as receptors for semaphorins,[38] exist in human umbilical vein endothelial cells and act as receptors for VEGF-A and PlGF.[39] NP-1 also acts as a receptor for VEGF-B[40] and VEGF-E.[41] The neuropilins could add another layer of regulation to the actions of VEGF and PlGF, because NP-1 and NP-2 act as receptors for $VEGF_{165}$ and $PlGF_2$, but only NP-2 acts as a receptor for $VEGF_{145}$.[39,42] NP-1 not only binds $VEGF_{165}$, but also it complexes with VEGFR-1,[43] a finding that led to the suggestion that VEGFR-1 acts as a negative regulator of angiogenesis by competing for NP-1.

Regulation

Various cytokines and hormones have been shown to stimulate production of VEGF, but the primary regulator of this family of angiogenic growth factors may well be oxygen tension. Low oxygen tension results in the up-regulation of VEGF-A, the down-regulation of PlGF,[44] and the up-regulation of VEGFR-1 and VEGFR-2.[45] Although this regulation has not been entirely characterized for all four of these proteins, hypoxic regulation of VEGF-A expression is mediated at both transcriptional and posttranscriptional levels. In the presence of low oxygen tension, VEGF-A mRNA is stabilized by the interaction of heterogenous nuclear ribonucleoprotein L with the 3'-untranslated region of VEGF-A mRNA,[46] thereby increasing the mRNA half-life. At the transcriptional level, low oxygen tension allows hypoxia-inducible factor-1 (HIF-1), a basic helix-loop-helix transcription factor, to interact with a hypoxia response element (HRE) in hypoxia-induced genes such as VEGF-A, thereby stimulating transcription.[47] HIF-1 is a heterodimeric protein composed of HIF-1α or HIF-2α combined with HIF-1β. The HIF-1β subunit is constitutively expressed, whereas HIF-1α and HIF-2α are regulated by oxygen tension. Under low oxygen tension, HIF-1 is stabilized, allowing it to interact with HREs in the promoters of responsive genes. However, under normal oxygen tensions, conserved proline residues in HIF-1α and HIF-2α are hydroxylated.[48] Prolyl hydroxylation allows targeting of HIF-1α and HIF-2α by the von Hippel–Landau tumor suppressor gene product (pVHL).[49] The HIF-1α and HIF-2α chains are captured by a pVHL-ubiquitin E3 ligase complex, are ubiquitylated, and are destroyed by cellular proteasomes.[50] The importance of this regulatory system is borne out by targeted mutations in mice, in which inactivation of both alleles of *HIF-1A, HIF-2A, HIF-1B,* or *VHL* results in embryonic lethality,[51-55] associated with defects in cardiac function, angiogenesis, vascular remodeling, and placental vascularization. However, additional regulation of HIF-1 activity may also result from increases in HIF-1α or HIF-2α mRNA concentrations, from translocation of HIF-1 to the nucleus, and from recruitment of transactivators.[50]

Angiopoietins and Their Receptor

Ang1 and Ang2, although not part of the VEGF family, act to potentiate the actions of VEGF-A; Ang2 expression is induced by hypoxia and VEGF-A.[56] Ang1 acts synergistically with VEGF-A to stimulate angiogenesis,[57] whereas Ang2 is an antagonist to Ang1, and in the absence of VEGF, Ang2 is thought to destabilize or regress blood vessels.[58] It is believed that Ang1 is important in angiogenesis (rather than vasculogenesis[59]), during the remodeling of the vasculature into a hierarchical network of mature vessels composed of endothelial and adventitial cells, by recruiting and sustaining perivascular cells.[60] Both Ang1 and Ang2 interact with the receptor Tie2, with equal affinity,[58] and whereas Ang1 induces maturation and stabilization of developing neovasculature,[61] Ang2 causes destabilization required for additional sprout formation[58] and branching angiogenesis. Ang1 and Ang2 are true antagonists, competing with equal affinity for Tie2,[58] and it is believed that Ang1 is the natural agonist for Tie2. This concept is supported by the similar phenotypes exhibited by targeted inactivation of either the Ang1[61] or Tie2[62] genes, both resulting in defective vascular development and subsequent embryonic death. In contrast, transgenic mice overexpressing Ang1 appeared generally healthy; however, their skin exhibited greater numbers of large blood vessels.[61] Further studies with mice overexpressing Ang1 indicated that these mice had a greater incidence of leakage-resistant blood vessels.[63] Transgenic mice overexpressing Ang2[58] die during embryogenesis, with similar defects as mice harboring inactivated Ang1 and Tie2 genes,[61,62] a finding further supporting the concept that Ang2 is a natural antagonist to Ang1.

Vascular Endothelial Growth Factor and Angiopoietins in Fetal and Placental Development

The impact of disrupting Ang1, Ang2, or Tie2 (see earlier) infers that these factors, although important, are not involved in the initiating steps of vasculogenesis or angiogenesis. However, disruption of the genes encoding HIF-1α, HIF-2α, HIF-1β, or VHL resulted in phenotypes that infer the necessity of these genes in vasculogenesis, as well as angiogenesis. Because these genes, or their respective gene products, are involved in regulating VEGF-A and its receptors, one could predict similar phenotypes on disruption of the genes encoding VEGF-A, VEGFR-1, or VEGFR-2. Indeed, disruption of a single VEGF-A allele impairs early-stage vascular development, resulting in embryonic lethality around embryonic day 10.[64,65] Included in the processes impaired by VEGF-A deficiency are vasculogenesis, large vessel formation, capillary sprouting, and remodeling of the yolk sac vascular network. The severity of this phenotype[64,65] indicates that VEGF-A acts in a dose-dependent manner to maintain angioblast differentiation and survival. When expression of the primary receptors for VEGF-A was disrupted,[66,67] mice lacking functional VEGFR-2[66] had the more severe phenotype. VEGFR-2–deficient mice exhibited a complete failure of vasculogenesis, endothelial cell differentiation, and hematopoiesis,[66] whereas disruption of VEGR-1[67] resulted in enlarged blood vessels as well as embryonic lethality. Disruption of the PlGF gene[68] resulted in normal development, potentially discrediting a critical role of PlGF in embryonic angiogenesis.

When VEGF-A binds VEGFR-2, rather than VEGFR-1, efficient mitogenic and chemotactic responses occur with endothelial cells. In addition, the lack of a potent mitogenic response from PlGF binding VEGFR-1 suggested that the receptor was ineffective in mediating endothelial cell mitogenesis.[35] PlGF expression has been localized to villous syncytiotrophoblast,[44,69] and although both VEGFR-1 and VEGFR-2 are expressed in placental villous endothelium,[70,71] VEGFR-1 is also expressed in extravillous trophoblast cells.[72] The presence of functional VEGFR-1 receptors on normal human trophoblast suggests that VEGF-A or PlGF binding to trophoblast VEGFR-1 may play a role in the invasion and differentiation of these cells.[44,72] Supporting this hypothesis is the finding that early placental development occurs in a hypoxic environment,[73] a known stimulator of VEGF-A expression.[74]

Demonstration of nonendothelial cell targets for VEGF-A, coupled with the concept that a lack of extravillous trophoblast invasion of the spiral arteries[75-77] results in placental ischemia and the development of preeclampsia or intrauterine growth restriction, led to the investigation of VEGF-A and PlGF expression in these placental disorders. Three distinct types of hypoxia may occur in the fetoplacental unit.[78] These are as follows: (1) preplacental hypoxia, in which the mother, placenta, and fetus are hypoxic, as may occur at high altitude or as a result of maternal anemia or asthma; (2) uteroplacental hypoxia, in which

maternal oxygenation is normal, but impaired uteroplacental circulation results in placental and fetal hypoxia, with preserved end-diastolic flow in the umbilical arteries, as in preeclampsia; and (3) postplacental hypoxia, in which only the fetus is believed to be hypoxic, with reduced, absent, or reversed end-diastolic flow of the umbilical arteries. With preplacental hypoxia and uteroplacental hypoxia, angiogenesis within the placental villi shifts predominantly to branching angiogenesis (Fig. 9-2). Conversely, with postplacental hypoxia, angiogenesis within the placental villi shifts predominantly to nonbranching angiogenesis (see Fig. 9-2). Another way of classifying these pregnancies resulting in fetal growth restriction is early-onset or late-onset intrauterine growth restriction,[24] with late-onset generally encompassing the preplacental and uteroplacental hypoxic groups. In preeclamptic pregnancies, placental VEGF-A is reported to be reduced.[79,80] Reduced placental VEGF-A in preeclamptic pregnancies[79,80] does not coincide with an expectation of placental hypoxia stimulating VEGF-A expression. The reason VEGF-A expression is reduced in these reports[79,80] is not readily apparent, but it may indicate that the near-term placenta may not always be able to respond to hypoxic conditions. Alternatively, because VEGF-A is expressed by both endothelial and trophoblast cells, tissue analysis of the placenta may be affected by the relative abundance of each cell type and by possible discordance in the response by the individual cell types. Supporting the concept that the preeclamptic placenta is hypoxic is the reduction of PlGF in maternal blood observed in preeclamptic pregnancies.[81,82] In cases of postplacental hypoxia associated with early-onset intrauterine growth restriction, the placental villi are believed to be exposed to greater oxygen tension.[78] This concept is supported by the observations that the oxygen content of uterine venous blood is close to arterial values in pregnancies characterized by severe intrauterine growth restriction,[83] and VEGF expression is reduced and PlGF expression is increased.[80,84]

Not only are VEGF-A, VEGFR-1, and VEGFR-2 produced within the placenta by nonendothelial cells, but Ang1 also has been localized in the cyto/syncytiotrophoblast bilayer in first trimester human placenta.[85] Ang2 was found in the cytotrophoblast layer[85] or in the syncytiotrophoblast,[86] and their common receptor, Tie2, was found in the cyto/syncytiotrophoblast bilayer[85] and in endovascular invasive trophoblasts.[86] Whereas Ang1 acts synergistically with VEGF-A[57] to stimulate angiogenesis, Ang 2 is an antagonist to Ang1, and in the absence of VEGF-A, it is thought to destabilize or regress blood vessels.[58] However, this destabilization process,[58] in the presence of VEGF-A, provides for sprouting or branching angiogenesis such that Ang2 should not be considered antiangiogenic. At term gestation, Ang2 mRNA concentrations in placenta from pregnancies characterized by severe intrauterine growth restriction[85] were not different from those in the normal placenta, but the tissue concentration of Ang2 was significantly decreased. Reduction in placental Ang2,[85] coupled with reduced VEGF-A expression and increased PlGF expression,[80,84] fits with the concept of postplacental hypoxia in severe or early-onset intrauterine growth restriction.[78]

SUMMARY

In this chapter, we present an overview of angiogenesis within the fetus and placenta, and in so doing we focus our discussion on a few of the many factors that may affect fetal and placental vascular development. Later chapters deal with angiogenesis within specific organs. Although we limit our discussion to the VEGF family and the angiopoietins, their receptors, and some of the regulatory mechanisms, it should still be obvious that the regulation of vasculogenesis and angiogenesis is extremely complex. Mice harboring functionally disrupted genes encoding these growth factors, receptors, or regulators have provided

Placental Villi   **Umbilical Doppler Waveforms**

Normal
Balanced placental angiogenesis
Placental normoxia

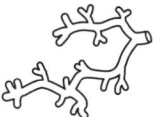

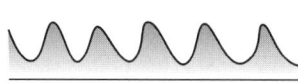

Late-onset IUGR
Predominantly branching angiogenesis
Pre-placental hypoxia
Utero-placental hypoxia

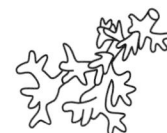

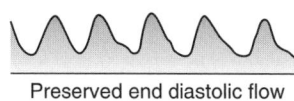

Preserved end diastolic flow

Early-onset IUGR
Predominantly nonbranching
angiogenesis
Post-placental hypoxia

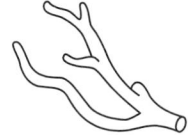

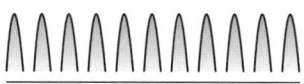

Absent or reversed end
diastolic flow (ARED)

Figure 9–2. Relationship between placental oxygen tension and intrauterine growth restriction (IUGR), placental villi development, and umbilical artery Doppler waveforms. Late-onset IUGR is characterized predominantly by branching angiogenesis within the placenta and preserved end-diastolic flow within the umbilical artery, whereas early-onset IUGR is characterized predominantly by nonbranching angiogenesis within the placenta and absent or reduced end-diastolic flow within the umbilical artery.

invaluable insight into the absolute necessity for some of the vascular growth factors and their receptors in embryonic development and have underlined the importance of vasculogenesis and angiogenesis in embryonic development and survival. Finally, not only are VEGF-A and the angiopoietins important in vascular development of the embryo and placenta, but they are also produced and act on nonendothelial cells within the placenta. Associated with these activities are alterations in vascular growth factor expression in placenta compromised by preeclampsia and intrauterine growth restriction, again highlighting the importance of these factors for successful pregnancy outcome. Although angiogenesis during fetal and placental development is a complex topic and is difficult to examine experimentally, it holds great potential as an area for therapeutic development aimed at improving pregnancy outcome.

REFERENCES

1. Pardanaud L, et al: Relationship between vasculogenesis, angiogenesis and haemopoiesis during avian ontogeny. Development *105*:473, 1989.
2. Fox SB: Tumor angiogenesis and prognosis. Histopathology, *30*:294, 1997.
3. Polverini PJ: Cellular adhesion molecules: newly identified mediators of angiogenesis. Am J Pathol *148*:1023, 1996.
4. Folkman J: How is blood vessel growth regulated in normal and neoplastic tissue? Cancer Res *46*:467, 1986.
5. Folkman J: What is the evidence that tumors are angiogenesis dependent? J Natl Cancer Inst *82*:4, 1990.
6. Conway EM, et al: Molecular mechanisms of blood vessel growth. Cardiovasc Res 49:507, 2001.
7. Risau W, Flamme I: Vasculogenesis. Annu Rev Cell Dev Biol *11*:73, 1995.
8. Risau W: Mechanisms of angiogenesis. Nature 386:671, 1997
9. Flamme I, et al: Molecular mechanisms of vasculogenesis and embryonic angiogenesis. J Cell Physiol *173*:206, 1997.
10. Polverni PJ: The pathophysiology of angiogenesis. Crit Rev Oral Biol Med 6:230, 1995.
11. Gonzalez Crussi F: Vasculogenesis in the chick embryo: an ultrastructural study. Am J Anat *130*:441, 1971.
12. Huang R, et al: The fate of somitocoele cells in avian embryos. Anat Embryol *190*:243, 1994.
13. Wilting J, et al: Angiogenic potential of the avian somite. Dev Dyn *202*:165, 1995.
14. Klessinger S, Christ B: Axial structures control laterality in the distribution pattern of endothelial cells. Anat Embryol 193:319, 1996.
15. Huang R, et al: The fate of the first avian somite. Anat Embryol *195*:435, 1997.
16. Pardanaud L, et al: Vasculogenesis in the early quail blastodisc as studied with a monoclonal antibody recognizing endothelial cells. Development 100:339, 1987.
17. Dieterlen LF, et al: Early haemopoietic stem cells in the avian embryo. J Cell Sci *10*(Suppl):29, 1988.
18. Wagner RC: Endothelial cell embryology and growth. Adv Microcirc 9:47, 1980.
19. Noden DM: Development of craniofacial blood vessels. *In* Feinberg RN, et al (eds): The Development of the Vascular System. Basel, S. Karger, 1991, pp 1–24.
20. Tomanek RJ, et al: Rate of coronary vascularization during embryonic chicken development is influenced by the rate of myocardial growth. Cardiovasc Res *41*:663, 1999.
21. Demir R, et al: Fetal vasculogenesis and angiogenesis in human placental villi. Acta Anat *136*:190, 1989.
22. Ahmed A, Perkins J: Angiogenesis and intrauterine growth restriction. Baillieres Clin Obstet Gynecol *14*:981, 2000.
23. Kohnen G, et al: Placental villous stroma as a model system for myofibroblast differentiation. Histochem Cell Biol *105*:415, 1996.
24. Kingdom J, et al: Development of the placental villous tree and its consequences for fetal growth. Eur J Obstet Gynecol *92*:35, 2000.
25. Neufield G, et al: Vascular endothelial growth factor and its receptors. Prog Growth Factor Res 5:89, 1994.
26. Ferrara N, et al: The vascular endothelial growth factor family of polypeptides. J Cell Biochem *47*:211, 1991.
27. Olofsson B, et al: Vascular endothelial growth factor B, a novel growth factor for endothelial cells. Proc Natl Acad Sci USA 93:2576, 1996.
28. Joukov V, et al: A novel vascular endothelial growth factor, VEGF-C, is a ligand for the Flt4 (VEGFR-3) and KDR (VEGFR-2) receptor tyrosine kinases. EMBO J *15*:290, 1996.
29. Achen MG, et al: Vascular endothelial growth factor D (VEGF-D) is a ligand for the tyrosine kinases VEGF receptor 2 (Flk1) and VEGF receptor 3 (Flt4). Proc Natl Acad Sci USA 95:548, 1998.
30. Ogawa S, et al: A novel type of vascular endothelial growth factor, VEGF-E (NZ-7 VEGF), preferentially utilizes KDR/Flk-1 receptor and carries a potent mitotic activity without heparin-binding domain. J Biol Chem 273:31273, 1998.
31. Firbrother WJ, et al: Solution structure of the heparin-binding domain of vascular endothelial growth factor. Structure 6:637, 1998.
32. Torry DS, Torry RJ: Angiogenesis and the expression of vascular endothelial growth factor in endometrium and placenta. Am J Reprod Immunol *37*:21, 1997.
33. Charnock-Jones DS, et al: Identification and localization of alternatively spliced mRNAs for vascular endothelial growth factor in human uterus and estrogen regulation in endometrial cell lines. Biol Reprod *48*:1120, 1993.

34. Cao Y, et al: Placenta growth factor: identification and characterization of a novel isoform generated by RNA alternative splicing. Biochem Biophys Res Commun 235:493, 1997.

35. Thomas KA: Vascular endothelial growth factor, a potent and selective angiogenic agent. J Biol Chem 271:603, 1996.

36. Veikkola T, Alitalo K: VEGFs, receptors and angiogenesis. Semin Cancer Biol 9:211, 1999.

37. Clark DK, et al: A vascular endothelial growth factor antagonist is produced by the human placenta and released into the maternal circulation. Biol Reprod 59:1540, 1998.

38. He Z, Tessier-Lavigne M: Neuropilin is a receptor for the axonal chemorepellent Semaphorin III. Cell 90:739, 1997.

39. Gluzman-Poltorak Z, et al: Neuropilin-2 and neuropilin-1 are receptors for the 165-amino acid form of vascular endothelial growth factor (VEGF) and of placenta growth factor-2, but only neuropilin-2 functions as a receptor for the 145-amino acid form of VEGF. J Biol Chem 275:18040, 2000.

40. Makinen T, et al: Differential binding of vascular endothelial growth factor B splice and proteolytic isoforms to neuropilin-1. J Biol Chem 274:21217, 1999.

41. Wise LM, et al: Vascular endothelial growth factor (VEGF)–like protein from orf virus NZ2 binds to VEGFR2 and neuropilin-1. Proc Natl Acad Sci USA 96:3071, 1999

42. Migdal M, et al: Neuropilin-1 is a placenta growth factor-2 receptor. J Biol Chem 273:22272, 1998.

43. Fuh G, et al: The interaction of neuropilin-1 with vascular endothelial growth factor and its receptor Flt-1. J Biol Chem 275:26690, 2000.

44. Shore VH, et al: Vascular endothelial growth factor, placenta growth factor and their receptors in isolated human trophoblast. Placenta 18:657, 1997.

45. Tudor RM, et al: Increased gene expression for VEGF and the VEGF receptors KDR/Flk and Flt in lungs exposed to acute or to chronic hypoxia: modulation of gene expression by nitric oxide. J Clin Invest 95:1798, 1995.

46. Shih SC, Claffey KP: Regulation of human vascular endothelial growth factor mRNA stability in hypoxia by heterogenous nuclear ribonucleoprotein L. J Biol Chem 274:1359, 1999.

47. Wang GL, et al: Hypoxia inducible factor 1 is a basic helix-loop-helix PAS heterodimer regulated by cellular O$_2$ tension. Proc Natl Acad Sci USA 92:5510, 1995.

48. Ivan M, et al: HIFα targeted for VHL-mediated destruction by proline hydroxylation: implications for O$_2$ sensing. Science 292:464, 2001.

49. Maxwell PH, et al: The tumor suppressor protein VHL targets hypoxia-inducible factors for oxygen-dependent proteolysis. Nature 399:271, 1999.

50. Maxwell PH, Ratcliffe PJ: Oxygen sensors and angiogenesis. Semin Cell Dev Biol 13:29, 2002.

51. Gnarra JR, et al: Defective placental vasculogenesis causes embryonic lethality in VHL-deficient mice. Proc Natl Acad Sci USA 94:9102, 1997.

52. Iyer NV, et al: Cellular and developmental control of O$_2$ homeostasis by hypoxia-inducible factor 1α. Genes Dev 12:149, 1998.

53. Maltepe E, et al: Abnormal angiogenesis and responses to glucose and oxygen deprivation in mice lacking the protein ARNT. Nature 386:403, 1997.

54. Peng J, et al: The transcription factor EPAS-1/hypoxia-inducible factor 2α plays an important role in vascular remodeling. Proc Natl Acad Sci USA 97:8386, 2000.

55. Tian H, et al: The hypoxia responsive transcription factor EPAS1 is essential for catecholamine homeostasis and protection against heart failure during embryonic development. Genes Dev 12:3320, 1998.

56. Oh H, et al: Hypoxia and vascular endothelial growth factor selectively up-regulate angiopoietin-2 in bovine microvascular endothelial cells. J Biol Chem 274:15732, 1999.

57. Koblizek TI, et al: Angiopoietin-1 induces sprouting angiogenesis in vitro. Curr Biol 8:529, 1998.

58. Maisonpierre PC, et al: Angiopoietin-2, a natural antagonist for Tie-2 that disrupts in vivo angiogenesis. Science 277:50, 1997.

59. Yancopoulos GD, et al: Vasculogenesis, angiogenesis and growth factors: ephrins enter the fray at the border. Cell 93:661, 1998.

60. Ashara T, et al: Tie2 receptor ligands, angiopoietin-1 and angiopoietin-2, modulate VEGF-induced postnatal neovascularization. Circ Res 83:233, 1998.

61. Suri C, et al: Required role of angiopoietin-1, a ligand for the Tie 2 receptor, during embryonic angiogenesis. Cell 87:1171, 1996.

62. Sato TN, et al: Distinct roles of the receptor tyrosine kinases Tie-1 and Tie-2 in blood vessel formation. Nature 376:70, 1995.

63. Thurston G, et al: Leakage-resistant blood vessels in mice transgenically overexpressing angiopoietin-1. Science 286:2511, 1999.

64. Ferrara N, et al: Heterozygous embryonic lethality induced by targeted inactivation of the VEGF gene. Nature 380:439, 1996.

65. Carmeliet P, et al: Abnormal blood vessel development and lethality in embryos lacking a single VEGF allele. Nature 380:435, 1996.

66. Shalaby F, et al: Failure of blood-island formation and vasculogenesis in Flk-1-deficient mice. Nature 376:62, 1995.

67. Fong GH, et al: Role of the Flt-1 receptor tyrosine kinase in regulating the assembly of vascular endothelium. Nature 376:66, 1995.

68. Carmeliet P, Collen D: Role of vascular endothelial growth factor and vascular endothelial growth factor receptors in vascular development. Curr Topics Microbiol Immunol 237:133, 1997.

69. Vuorela P, et al: Expression of vascular endothelial growth factor and placenta growth factor in human placenta. Biol Reprod 56:489, 1997.

70. Charnock-Jones DS, et al: Localization and activation of the receptor for vascular endothelial growth factor on human trophoblast and choriocarcinoma cells. Biol Reprod 51:524, 1994.

71. Vuckovic M, et al: Expression of vascular endothelial growth factor receptor, KDR, in human placenta. J Anat 188:361, 1996.

72. Ahmed AS, et al: Colocalisation of vascular endothelial growth factor and its flt-1 receptor in human placenta. Growth Factors 12:235, 1995.

73. Kingdom JC, Kaufmann P: Oxygen and placental vascular development. Adv Exp Med Biol 474:259, 1999.

74. Schweiki D, et al: Vascular endothelial growth factor induced by hypoxia may mediate hypoxia initiated angiogenesis. Nature 359:843, 1992.

75. Meekins JW, et al: A study of placental bed spiral arteries and trophoblast invasion in normal and severe pre-eclamptic pregnancies. Br J Obstet Gynaecol 101:669, 1994.

76. Redline RW, Patterson P: Pre-eclampsia is associated with an excess of proliferative immature intermediate trophoblast. Hum Pathol 26:594, 1995.

77. Roberson WB, et al: Uteroplacenta vascular pathology. Eur J Obstet Gynecol Reprod Biol 5:47, 1975.

78. Kingdom JC, Kaufmann P: Oxygen and placental villous development: origins of fetal hypoxia. Placenta 18:613, 1997.

79. Cooper JC, et al: VEGF mRNA levels in placentae from pregnancies complicated by pre-eclampsia. Br J Obstet Gynaecol 103:1191, 1996.

80. Lyall F, et al: Placental expression of vascular endothelial growth factor in placentae from pregnancies complicated by pre-eclampsia and intrauterine growth restriction does not support placental hypoxia at delivery. Placenta 18:269, 1997.

81. Torry DS, et al: Preeclampsia is associated with reduced serum levels of placenta growth factor. Am J Obstet Gynecol 179:1539, 1998.

82. Tidwell SC, et al: Low maternal serum levels of placenta growth factor as an antecedent of clinical preeclampsia. Am J Obstet Gynecol 184:1267, 2001.

83. Pardi G, et al: Venous drainage of the human uterus: respiratory gas studies in normal and fetal growth-retarded pregnancies. Am J Obstet Gynecol 166:699, 1992.

84. Khaliq A, et al: Hypoxia down-regulates placenta growth factor, whereas fetal growth restriction up-regulates placenta growth factor expression: molecular evidence for "placental hyperoxia" in intrauterine growth restriction. Lab Invest 79:151, 1999.

85. Dunk C, et al: Angiopoietin-1 and angiopoietin-2 activate trophoblast Tie-2 to promote growth and migration during placental development. Am J Pathol 156:2185, 2000.

86. Goldman-Wohl DS, et al: Tie-2 and angiopoietin-2 expression at the fetal-maternal interface: a receptor ligand model for vascular remodeling. Mol Hum Reprod 6:81, 2000.

Placenta and Intrauterine Environment

Peter Kaufmann and Hans-Georg Frank

10

Placental Development

EARLY DEVELOPMENT

The placenta is defined as the apposition or fusion of fetal membranes with the uterine mucosa for the purpose of maternofetal exchange of nutrients, gases, and waste substances. According to this definition, placental development starts at the time of implantation around day 6 to 7 postconception, as soon as the blastocyst starts invasion of the endometrium. At this stage, the blastocyst consists of an outer vesicular cellular cover, called the *trophoblast*, and of an inner cell mass, called the *embryoblast* (Fig. 10-1A). The placenta and the membranes are mainly derived from the trophoblast, whereas the embryoblast develops into the umbilical cord and the fetus and adds the mesenchyme to the placenta.[1]

Implantation and Lacunar Period

Before adhesion to the uterine mucosa, the blastocystic wall consists of a single layer of trophoblast cells (cytotrophoblast). Those parts of the trophoblast that adhere to the mucosa and later invade it show an increased proliferation, resulting in a trophoblastic wall, which is mostly double layered. At the same time, the outer of the two layers shows disintegration of the lateral intercellular membranes. Thus, it is transformed into a superficial layer of syncytiotrophoblast[2] (see Fig. 10-1A). Continuous proliferation of the inner cellular trophoblastic layer, together with subsequent syncytial fusion of some of the daughter cells with the covering syncytium, is responsible for an enormous increase in volume (prelacunar period) (see Fig. 10-1B). Those parts of the blastocystic wall that are not yet implanted consist only of a single layer of cytotrophoblast.[3]

At day 8 postconception, in the syncytiotrophoblast (at the implantation pole), a system of confluent vacuoles appears.[2] Their appearance marks the beginning of the lacunar period, which lasts from day 8 to day 13 postconception. These lacunae are formed only in the more central parts of the syncytiotrophoblast. The surrounding and separating lamellae and pillars of syncytiotrophoblast are called *trabeculae* (see Fig. 10-1C). This system of trabeculae and lacunae is covered by two uninterrupted syncytial layers: the basal layer, facing the endometrium, is called the *trophoblastic shell*; the superficial layer, facing the blastocystic cavity, is called the *primary chorionic plate*.

Starting at the primary chorionic plate at day 12 postconception, the cytotrophoblast invades the syncytial trabeculae and finally reaches the trophoblastic shell (see Fig. 10-1D). Trophoblastic proliferation inside the trabeculae is responsible for considerable longitudinal growth and for branching of the

latter. The branches that end blindly and protrude into the lacunae are the primary villi (see Fig. 10-1D). The trabeculae, from which they are derived, are called the *anchoring villi* because they connect the villous system with the trophoblastic shell. With the appearance of the first primary villi, the still-expanding lacunar system is called the *intervillous space*.

In parallel to these events, the trophoblast of the trophoblastic shell erodes maternal endometrial vessels as early as day 12 postconception. Maternal blood leaving the eroded vessels enters the lacunar system through holes in the shell and thus establishes a first primitive maternal placental circulation (see Fig. 10-1D).

Meanwhile, the blastocyst is completely embedded in the endometrium and surrounded by endometrial stroma from all sides. The parts of the blastocyst surface that are implanted later, pass through the same developmental steps as the implantation pole. All data given in the following description are valid only for the development at the implantation pole.

Villous Development

At day 14 postconception, mesenchymal cells from the embryonic disk spread along the inner trophoblastic surface of the blastocystic cavity, where they transform into a loose network of branching cells, the extraembryonic mesenchyme.[1,4] From this date onward, the primary chorionic plate consists of three layers: the mesenchyme (the future connective tissue); a middle, discontinuous layer of cytotrophoblast; and a layer of syncytiotrophoblast facing the intervillous space (see Fig. 10-1E). Between days 15 and 20 postconception, cells of the extraembryonic mesenchyme invade the primary villi, transforming the latter into secondary villi. This mesenchyme never reaches the trophoblastic shell so that the segments of the anchoring villi that connect them to the trophoblastic shell remain merely trophoblastic. These trophoblastic segments are called the *cell columns* and consist of a voluminous cytotrophoblastic core and a thin, incomplete syncytial cover (see Fig. 10-1E). Their high share of cytotrophoblast is the main source for longitudinal growth of the anchoring villi. Some of the cytotrophoblast cells achieve an invasive phenotype, migrate across the trophoblastic shell, and invade deeply into the endometrium, forming an admixture with maternal tissue components, the so-called junctional zone.

Within a few hours of the mesenchymal invasion of the villi, some of these mesenchymal cells are transformed into macrophages and others into hemangioblastic cell cords. Around day 20 postconception, the first fetal capillaries are derived from the latter (see Fig. 10-1F).[5] The fetally vascularized villi are

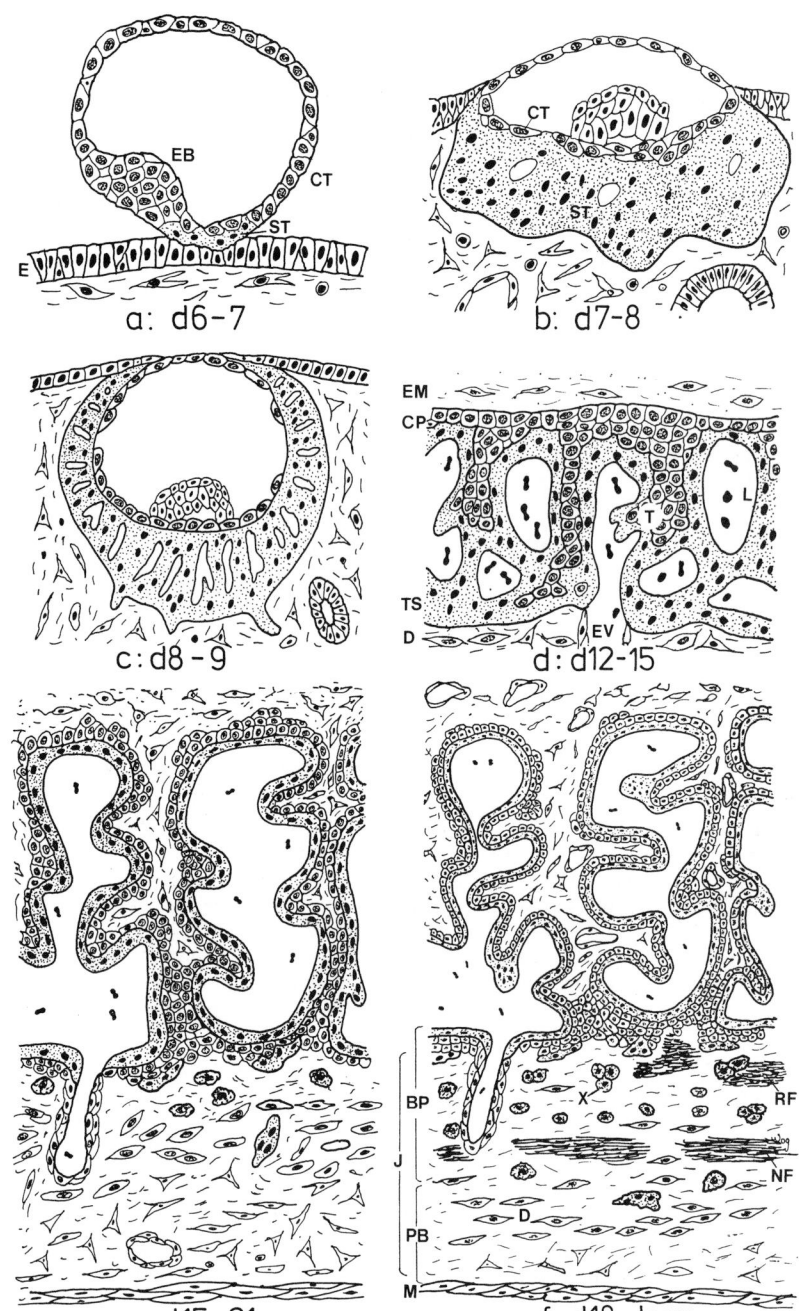

Figure 10–1. A to **F**, Typical stages of placental development. E = endometrial epithelium; D = decidua; EB = embryoblast; CT = cytotrophoblast; ST = syncytiotrophoblast; EM = extraembryonic mesoderm; CP = primary chorionic plate; T = trabeculae and primary villi; L = maternal blood lacunae; TS = trophoblastic shell; EV = endometrial vessel; RF = Rohr fibrinoid; NF = Nitabuch fibrinoid; BP = basal plate; PB = placental bed; J = junctional zone; M = myometrium; X = extravillous trophoblast (X cells). (Modified from Kaufmann P: Entwicklung der Plazenta. *In* Becker V, et al (eds): Die Plazenta des Menschen. Stuttgart, Thieme, 1981, pp 13–50.)

henceforth termed *tertiary villi*. Hematopoietic stem cells are derived from the same hemangiogenetic cell cords, which start blood formation inside the capillaries.

At the same time, the fetally vascularized allantois reaches the chorionic plate.[6] Allantoic vessels extend into the chorionic plate and even into the larger villi. There they fuse with the spreading intravillous capillary bed. A complete fetoplacental circulation is established around the end of the fifth week postconception.[6] In newly formed villous capillaries, hematopoiesis can be observed even later.

Development of the Maternofetal Barrier

As soon as an intraplacental fetal circulation is established in the tertiary villi, fetal blood in the villi and maternal blood in the intervillous space come into close contact with each other

(Fig. 10-2). They are always separated by the placental barrier, which is made up of the following layers (see Fig. 10-3): (1) a continuous layer of syncytiotrophoblast, covering the villi and thus lining the intervillous space; (2) an initially complete (first trimester) but later on discontinuous (second and third trimester) layer of cytotrophoblast; (3) a trophoblastic basal lamina; (4) connective tissue derived from the extraembryonic mesoderm; and (5) fetal endothelium, which is surrounded by an endothelial basal lamina only in the last trimester. Throughout the following months of pregnancy, this barrier undergoes quantitative rather than qualitative changes; the syncytiotrophoblast is reduced in thickness from more than 15 µm to a mean of 4.1 µm (Table 10-1).[6] Due to the expansion of the villous surfaces, the cytotrophoblast is relatively rarified and, at term, can be found in only 20% of the villous surface. The mean villous diameter decreases because the newly formed generations of villi are

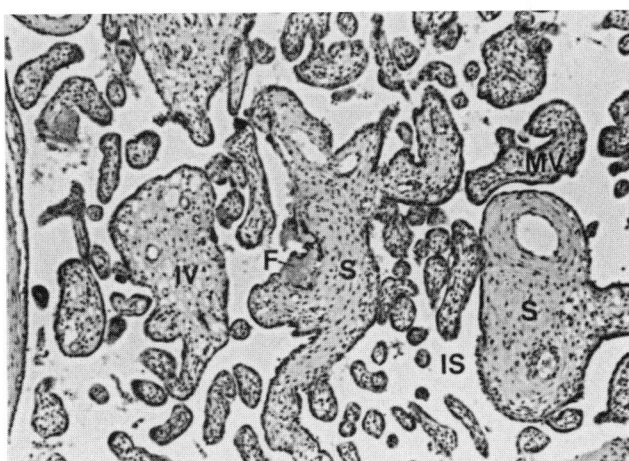

Figure 10–2. Paraffin section of placental villi, twenty-eighth week postmenstruation. The assortment of villi of varying caliber is typical for the last trimester. Larger villi as stem villi (S), immature intermediate villi (IV), and mature intermediate villi (MV) are easily recognizable. The group of smaller villi in between, too small for identification in this figure, is composed of terminal villi, mesenchymal villi, and villous sprouts. IS = intervillous space; F = fibrinoid, attached to the villous surface, resulting from trophoblastic degeneration. × 70.

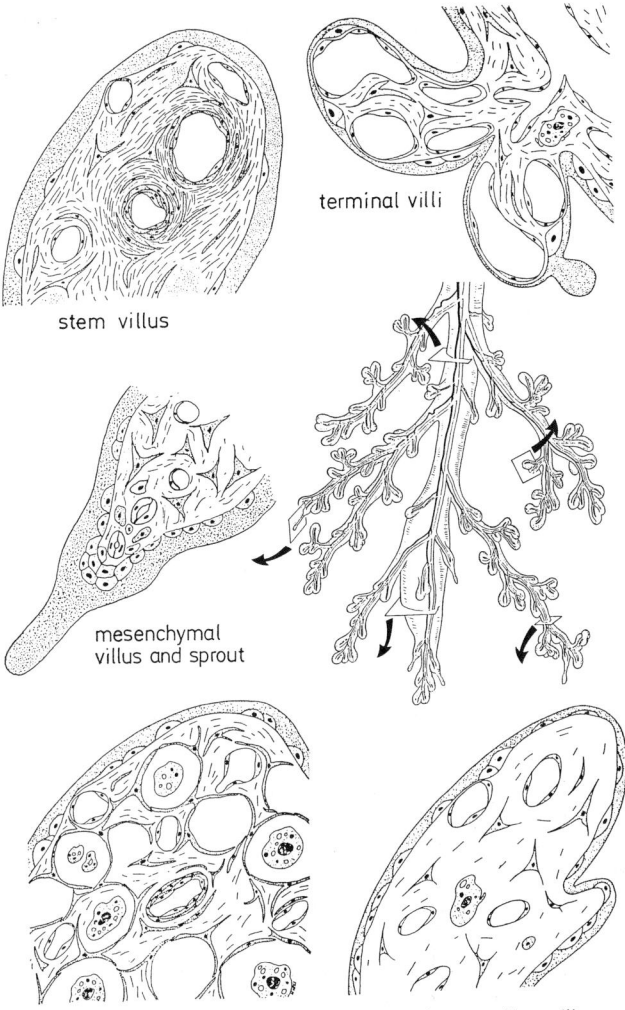

Figure 10–3. A peripheral part of the mature placental villous tree and typical cross-sections of the various villous types. (Modified from Kaufmann P: Contrib Gynecol Obstet *13*:517, 1985. S. Karger AG, Basel.)

generally smaller than the previous generation. Because of this, with advanced maturation, the intravillous position of the fetal capillaries is nearer to the villous surface. All these factors result in a reduction of the mean maternofetal diffusion distance from between 50 and 100 µm in the second month, down to between 4 and 5 µm at term gestation.[6]

PLACENTAL VILLI

The basic morphology of the placental villi can be seen in Figures 10-2 and 10-3. The villous core consists of fixed connective tissue cells, connective tissue fibers, macrophages (Hofbauer cells), some occasional mast cells, and fetal vessels. The stromal core is surrounded by the trophoblastic basal lamina, on which can be found varying numbers of cytotrophoblast (Langhans cells) and an outer, complete layer of syncytiotrophoblast.

Fetal Endothelium

Maternofetal exchange across the placental villi is focused on those villi (terminal villi and mature intermediate villi, see below) which are richly supplied with fetal capillaries. The capillaries are lined by a continuous endothelium without pores or fenestrations[6]; this cell layer acts as a passive filter, limiting macromolecular transfer across the vessel wall to a certain molecular size (below 20,000 daltons).[7,8] In addition, permeability seems to be influenced by molecular charge.[9,10] The cells that surround the walls of the larger vessels (i.e., the pericytes and smooth muscle cells) are active in vasoregulation. Because nerves have never been observed in the placenta, vasoregulation must be accomplished by humoral means or by local mechanisms (or both).[11]

Villous Stroma

The connective tissue cells of the vessel adventitia shade into the components of the surrounding villous stroma without any sharp demarcation line. Depending on villous type and age, mesenchy-

mal cells, fibroblasts or myofibroblasts are the prevailing cell type.[12] They produce connective tissue fibers, which increase the mechanical stability of the villous core. Macrophages (Hofbauer cells) can be observed in varying numbers. In addition to their phagocytotic activity, these are active paracrine cells that produce growth factors that regulate growth and differentiation of all villous components.[6]

Trophoblast

The trophoblastic cover of the villi is the main site for maternofetal transfer and for secretory functions. Most of these take place in the syncytiotrophoblast. The villous cytotrophoblast (Langhans cells) serves as a kind of stem cell, proliferating, differentiating, and afterward fusing with the syncytiotrophoblast.[13] Quantitative assessment of trophoblast proliferation and syncytial fusion have shown that it exceeds the needs for growth of syncytiotrophoblast by more than a factor of 5.[14] Throughout the last month of pregnancy about 3.6 g of cytotrophoblast fuse syncytially per day. However, in this stage of pregnancy, the syncytiotrophoblast grows only by about 0.6 g per day. The daily excess production of 3 g syncytiotrophoblast is shed into the maternal circulation as syncytial knots that mainly contain aged

TABLE 10-1

Summary of Mean Data on Placental Development*

Pregnancy week (postconception)	1, 2	3-6	7-10	11-14	15-18	19-22	23-26	27-30	31-34	35-38
Pregnancy month (postmenstruation)	1	2	3	4	5	6	7	8	9	10
Diameter of the chorionic sac (mm)		8, 11, 17, 25	32, 40, 47, 55	62, 75, /,/						
Placental diameter (mm)				70	95	120	145	170	195	220
Placental weight postpartum (g) without clamping of the cord		6	26	65	115	185	250	315	390	470
Placental thickness postpartum (mm)				12	15	18	20	22	24	25
Placental thickness, including uterine wall, measured by ultrasound *in vivo* (mm)					28	34	38	43	45	45
Length of the umbilical cord (mm)				180	300	350	400	450	490	520
Fetal weight (g) per 1 g of placental weight		0.18	0.65	0.92	2.17	3.03	4.00	4.92	5.90	7.23
Villous volume (g) per placenta		5	18	28	63	102	135	191	234	273
Villous surface (cm²) per placenta		830	3020	5440	14,800	28,100	42,200	72,200	101,000	125,000
Villous surface (cm²) per g villous tissue		166	168	194	235	275	313	377	432	458
Maternofetal diffusion distance (μm)		55.9	40.2	27.7	21.6			20.6	11.7	4.8
Villous trophoblastic thickness (μm)		15.4		9.6	9.9	7.4		6.9	5.2	4.1
Fetal vessel lumina per villous volume (%)		1.0	1.1		6.6		7.4		21.3	28.4

*All data refer to the end of the corresponding week after conception or to the end of the corresponding month of pregnancy.
Data from ref 6.

syncytial nuclei and organelles. The reasons for this enormous turnover of trophoblast are not yet fully understood. Likely they are closely related to the apoptotic events underlying the process of syncytial fusion.[14-19]

For syncytial fusion of cells at least two contemporary signals are needed:

- To provide tissue specificity of fusion, the plasmalemmal exposition of fusogenic proteins is required; in the case of trophoblast the retroviral envelope protein HERV-W, also called syncytin,[20] has been identified as one such fusogenic protein.
- To act as the acute fusion signal, phosphatidylserine flips from the inner to the outer plasmalemmal leaflet.[14, 21] The outward flip of phosphatidylserine is provided by intracytotrophoblastic activation of initiator caspases that inactivate flippases and activate floppases.[15, 22] The initiator caspases are intracellular proteases belonging to the molecular machinery of the early, still reversible stages of the apoptosis cascade. Further progression of the apoptosis cascade in the freshly formed syncytiotrophoblast is blocked by the mitochondrial proteins mcl-1 and bcl-2, both of which inhibit cleavage and thus activation of execution caspases by the active initiator caspases. Both inhibitory proteins are transferred in large quantities from the cytotrophoblast into syncytiotrophoblast by the same fusion event.[14, 23]

All cells entering the apoptosis cascade, irreversibly leave the cell cycle and down-regulate transcription. Both kinds of apoptotic events have been demonstrated for syncytiotrophoblast, the nuclei of which neither incorporate ^{3}H-thymidine[24] nor measurable quantities of ^{3}H-uridine.[14, 25] Consequently, the syncytiotrophoblast depends on a continuous incorporation of cytotrophoblast both for its growth and to ensure a continuous supply of mRNA for all translation processes. Moreover, syncytial incorporation by fusion results in a kind of transplantation of fresh organelles and enzyme systems into the syncytium to replace the aged ones (Fig. 10-4).

Removal of aged syncytiotrophoblast also involves apoptosis.[26] The nuclei incorporated by syncytial fusion into the syncytiotrophoblast become aggregated after an unknown interval (see Fig. 10-4). Parallel to this event the apoptosis cascade is restarted and now passes all execution stages until apoptotic death, including activation of execution caspases, local degradation of the cytoskeleton, formation of membrane-protecting protein scaffolds by activation of transglutaminase II, activation of endonucleases with subsequent DNA-degradation, and nuclear collapse.[14] As the final stage of this cascade, the syncytial knots are formed. They are composed of 10 to 50 aggregated apoptotic nuclei, surrounded by some cytoplasm and an intact plasmalemma. They are pinched off and shed into the maternal circulation (see Fig. 10-4). At term about 3 g of this kind of apoptotic trophoblast enter the maternal blood from where they are removed by phagocytosis in the maternal lung. The mean survival time of a nucleus after syncytial fusion until shedding was calculated to be about 3 to 4 weeks.[14]

As a consequence of the various stages of trophoblast turnover described above, the syncytiotrophoblast is composed of mosaiclike patches with varying ultrastructure, enzyme patterns, and functional specializations[6]:

1. The freshly fused, thick syncytial segments with prevailing rough endoplasmic reticulum specialize in the secretion of proteohormones and placental proteins as well as in maternofetal protein transfer, including catabolism and resynthesis.
2. After degradation of ribosomes, the structurally similar segments, with prevailing smooth endoplasmic reticulum, are involved in the metabolism of steroid hormones.
3. The epithelial plates or vasculosyncytial membranes are thin syncytial lamellas (1-2 μm) resulting from nuclear movement and removal. These are the main sites of diffusional transfer of gases, water, and the carrier transfer of glucose.
4. The syncytial knots are later stages of syncytial apoptosis, directly preceding shedding of the apoptotic material. However, it needs to be pointed out that not all syncytial protrusions containing nuclear aggregates represent such knots. Instead most respective structures noted on histologic sections are tangential sections of the villous surfaces.[27-29] Moreover, few of those, mostly seen in early

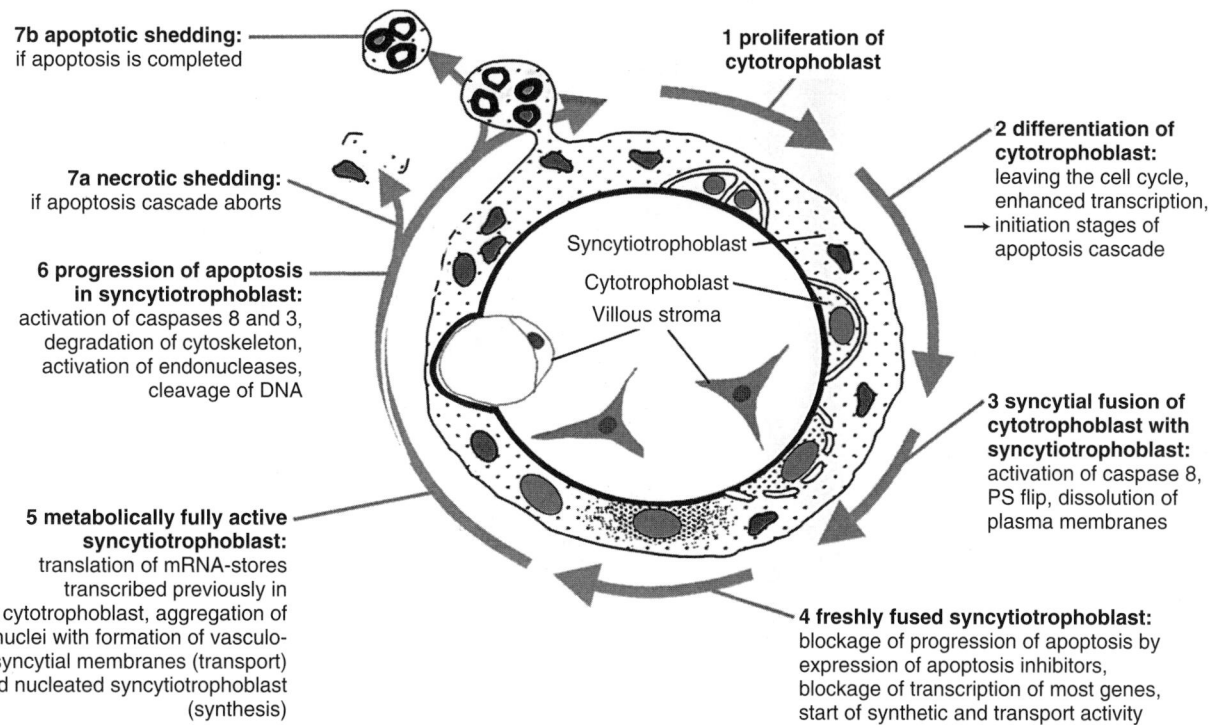

Figure 10–4. Villous trophoblast turnover. The events are arranged in clockwise manner. Proliferation takes place exclusively in the cytotrophoblasts, which act as stem cells. Following differentiation of cytotrophoblasts, syncytial fusion is triggered by molecular mechanisms of early stages of the apoptosis cascade. On syncytial integration of the former cytotrophoblast into the syncytio-trophoblasts, progression of the apoptosis cascade is blocked. As is typical for early apoptotic tissues, transcription is down-regulated to barely measurable levels. Therefore survival of syncytiotrophoblast depends on translation of mRNA that is transferred into the syncytium by continuous syncytial fusion of differentiating cytotrophoblast. After about 3 weeks of aging and restart of apoptosis, the accumulating apoptotic syncytial nuclei are shed into the maternal circulation. When the apoptosis cascade cannot be completed (e.g., in severe hypoxia), shedding is completed by necrosis. The complete cycle takes about 4 weeks.

stages of pregnancy, are true syncytial sprouts that represent trophoblastic proliferation and are thus signs of villous sprouting.[27]

Integrity of the Maternofetal Barrier

It must be pointed out that the syncytiotrophoblast is a continuous, generally uninterrupted syncytial layer that extends over the surfaces of all villous trees. Therefore, it completely lines the intervillous space. Terms such as syncytial cells or syncytiotrophoblasts are therefore inappropriate. Because of its syncytial nature, it is generally believed that every substance passes from the maternal to the fetal circulation under the control of the trophoblast. Despite this view, there is physiologic evidence for the existence of two different routes of transfer across the placental barrier, a transcellular and a paracellular route.[30] The transcellular route involves transfer across the plasma membranes and the cytosol of the syncytiotrophoblast. The paracellular route is thought to be an extracellular, water-filled pathway. Two different structural correlates for the latter have been described:

Integrity and completeness of the syncytiotrophoblastic barrier is not absolute. Gaps in the syncytiotrophoblast caused by degeneration or by mechanical forces are filled by fibrin as a result of blood clotting. About 7% of the villous surfaces in normal term human placentas show corresponding fibrin spots as replacement of the syncytiotrophoblast.[31, 32] Such areas may serve as relevant paratrophoblastic routes for maternofetal macromolecule transfer, thus bypassing the syncytiotrophoblast; *in vitro*, maternally injected horseradish peroxidase (48,000 dalton; 3.0 nm molecular radius) has been shown to pass through the fibrin spots into the fetal villous stroma.[31]

Transtrophoblastic channels provide a paracellular transfer route for smaller molecules.[33-37] Their diameter is approximately 20 nm. The channels pass through the syncytiotrophoblast as winding and branching, membrane-lined tubules from the apical to basal surface. Morphologic evidence for a basoapical membrane flux along these channels suggests that they are likely to be routes for membrane recycling from the basal to the apical syncytiotrophoblastic plasmalemma.[36] Functionally the transtrophoblastic channels are possible sites of transfer for water-soluble, lipid-insoluble molecules with an effective molecular diameter smaller than 1.5 nm.[30,38,39] Moreover, they have been shown to be the sites of fetomaternal fluid shift, which is mediated by hydrostatic and colloid osmotic forces. In the guinea pig and in the isolated human placenta, an elevation of the fetal venous pressure of 5 to 17 mm Hg was sufficient to shift 30 to 50% of the fetal arterial perfusion volumes into the maternal circulation. Under the conditions of fetomaternal fluid shift the channels dilate to several micrometers in diameter.[33, 37] Pressure-dependent dilation and closure of the channels may act as important factors in fetal osmoregulation and water balance. Excessive fetal hydration results in an increase of fetal venous pressure and a decrease of osmotic pressure. Both factors have been experimentally proven to dilate initially narrow channels,[33,37] thus allowing fetomaternal fluid shift and equilibration of the surplus water.

Villous Types

One can typify the human placental villi depending on their position within the villous tree, on the type of fetal vessels, and on their connective tissue structure.[40,41,42,43] Figure 10-3 illustrates a peripheral part of the villous tree, containing all villous types so

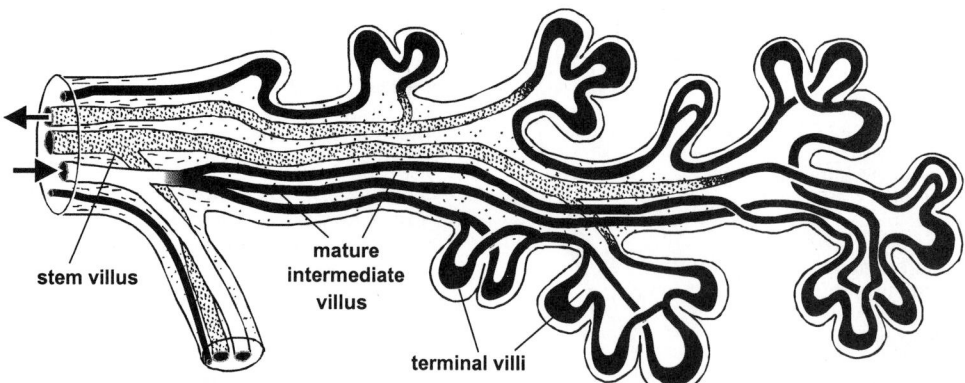

Figure 10–5. Arrangement of fetal vessels in a group of terminal villi (*no shading*) derived from one mature intermediate villus (*shaded*). Note the highly complex loop formation of the terminal fetal capillaries (*black*). Branching is usually followed shortly later by refusioning of the two capillary branches. The branching pattern avoids basal shortcuts in such a way that each erythrocyte has to pass the terminal capillaries of several terminal villi at full length. Local dilatations of the capillaries in the terminal villi, so-called sinusoids, reduce blood flow resistance. Arterioles *unshaded*. Venules *dotted*. (Modified from Benirschke K and Kaufmann P: Pathology of the Human Placenta. New York, Springer, 2000.)

far described. The centrally positioned stem villus is characterized by centrally located arteries and veins or larger arterioles and venules surrounded by a stroma that is rich in connective tissue fibers.[44] Fetal capillaries are poorly developed. Most stromal cells are highly differentiated myofibroblasts that are oriented in parallel to the longitudinal villous axis.[45-47,48] They may be involved in longitudinal contraction of the stem villi (anchoring villi), thus regulating the width of the intervillous space and maternal blood flow impedance.[12] Such a fetal contractile system regulating the intervillous circulation is needed because the uteroplacental arteries are set free from vasomotor influences of the mother by physiologic changes of their walls (see subsequent discussion).[49] About one-third of the total villous volume of the mature placenta consists of this villous type.

The stem villi ramify into bundles of slender, slightly curved villi (see Fig. 10-3), the mature intermediate villi. These villi branch in terminal villi. Most of their vessels are fetal capillaries, between which are some small arterioles and venules.[50, 51] The vessels are embedded in a loose connective tissue, with scant fibers and cells, and occupy more than half of the villous volume. These villi are the main sites of growth and differentiation of terminal villi.[42, 43] Highly active enzyme patterns indicate their metabolic and endocrine activities. About 25% of the villous branches are of this type.

The terminal villi are the final branches of the villous trees. Their bulbous peripheral parts are characterized by numerous dilated capillaries, so-called sinusoids, some with diameters up to 40 μm (Fig. 10-5; see also Fig. 10-3).[50, 51] The extremely high degree of fetal vascularization and the minimal maternofetal diffusion distance (less than 4 μm) make this villous type the most likely place for diffusional exchange. The terminal villous volume amounts to 30 to 40% of the villous tree.

In some of these villous trees, stem villi are continuous with thicker bulbous villi; these are termed *immature intermediate villi* (Fig. 10-6; see also Fig. 10-3).[42, 43] The typical structural features of immature intermediate villi include the presence of arterioles and venules, accompanied by numerous slender capillaries, and a voluminous, reticularly structured connective tissue that is rich in Hofbauer cells and poor in fibers. These villi can be found in the mature placenta only in small restricted groups, which are located in the centers of the villous trees (see Fig. 10-6).[52] In immature placentas, they are the prevailing villous type. The main roles of immature intermediate villi are to act as precursors of stem villi (into which they are transformed continuously) and to provide surface for sprouting of new villous side branches.[42, 43]

The rarest and most inconspicuous villous type in the mature placenta is that of the mesenchymal villi. These villi are transient stages of villous development, derived from villous sprouts (see Fig. 10-3). They differentiate through immature intermediate villi into stem villi or mature intermediate villi. Because new sprouts are formed at the surfaces of mesenchymal and immature intermediate villi, they are normally found grouped in restricted sites. Structurally the mesenchymal villi can be identified by their slender shape, numerous Langhans cells, and poorly developed fetal capillaries. Some of the last-mentioned do not show lumina and are still developing and unperfused.[42, 43]

Fetoplacental Angioarchitecture

Fetal arteries and veins are restricted to the stem villi, whereas arterioles and venules are mainly located in the smaller stem villi and in mature and immature intermediate villi.[44, 50, 51] All the larger fetal vessels are accompanied by a system of long, slender capillaries, the so-called paravascular net.

In the mature intermediate villi, the arterioles and venules turn into long, coiled terminal capillary loops (see Fig. 10-5).[51] At sites of maximum coiling, the capillaries stretch the surface of the mature intermediate villi, producing bulges, the terminal villi. Within the terminal villi, capillaries may dilate considerably, thus resulting in sinusoids (see Figs. 10-3 and 10-5).[50] One capillary loop may supply several terminal villi in series, dilating and narrowing several times for each single terminal villus. The probable function of the sinusoids is to reduce blood flow resistance and, thus, to guarantee an even blood supply to the long terminal capillary loops (mean length, 4000 μm) as well as to the shorter paravascular capillaries (mean length, 1000 μm).

Cotyledons and Villous Trees

The basal surface of the term placenta is characterized by 10 to 40 slightly protruding areas called *maternal cotyledons, lobes,* or *lobules* (Fig. 10-7B).[52] They are scarcely separated from each other by the so-called placental septa (see Fig. 10-6).[52] From the chorionic plate at term, 60 to 70 villous stems (trunci chorii) arise. Each of these trunks branches into a villous tree.[53] Each maternal cotyledon is occupied by at least one villous tree (see Figs. 10-6 and 10-7). As shown in Figure 10-7C, the superficial cotyledonary borderlines are adjacent, to a large extent, to those of a corresponding group of villous trees.[52]

The human placenta belongs to the villous, hemochorial type of placentation: After leaving the spiral arteries, the maternal

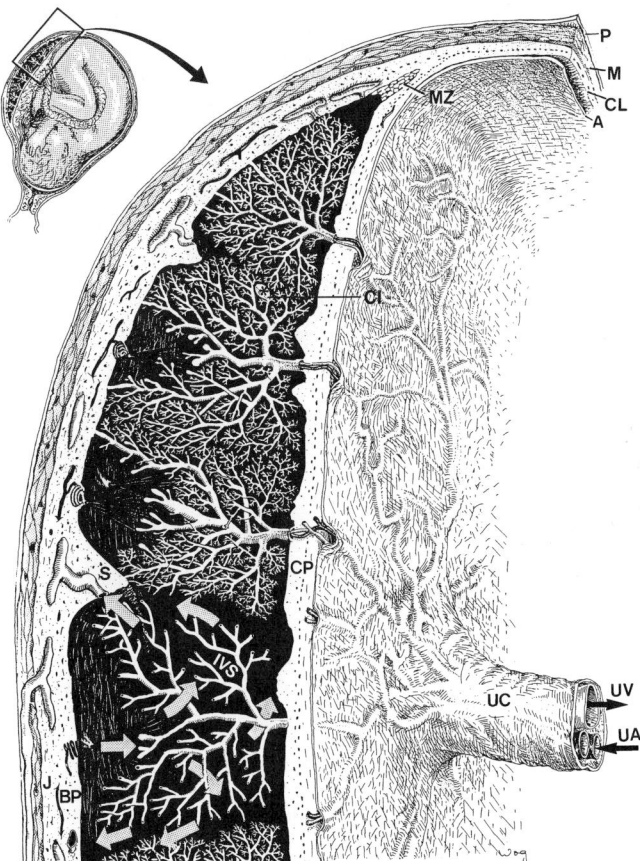

Figure 10–6. Survey diagram of the nearly mature human placenta *in situ*. Loose centers of the villous trees arranged around the maternal arterial inflow area are a frequent feature. These placentome centers usually exhibit immature patterns of villous branching and differentiation. P = perimetrium; M = myometrium; CL = chorion laeve; A = amnion; MZ = marginal zone between placenta and fetal membranes, with obliterated intervillous space and ghost villi; CI = cell island,* connected to the villous tree; S = placental septum; J = junctional zone; BP = basal plate; CP = chorionic plate; IVS =intervillous space; UC = umbilical cord; UV = umbilical vein; UA =umbilical artery.

blood circulates through the diffuse intervillous space, flowing directly around the villous surfaces without any maternal vessel wall (see Fig. 10–6). According to the data of Schuhmann,[54] the arterial inlets are normally situated close to the centers of the villous trees. The venous openings in the basal plate are arranged around the periphery of the villous trees.

One fetomaternal circulatory unit, the placentome, consists of a villous tree and the corresponding part of the intervillous space, which is centrifugally perfused with maternal blood (Fig. 10-6).[54] As depicted in Figure 10-7C, every maternal lobe or cotyledon possesses at least one placentome. Owing to the insufficiency of placental septa, most maternal circulatory units, belonging to the 40 to 60 placentomes, overlap considerably.

The centers of typical placentomes exhibit loosely arranged villi, predominantly of the immature intermediate and mesenchymal types,[52, 55] providing a large intervillous space for maternal arterial inflow. Occasionally the loose villous arrangement results in a central cavity (see Fig. 10-6),[54] which may rapidly collapse after the placenta is delivered because it is a pressure-dependent *in vivo* structure. In the periphery of the placentomes, most villi are mature intermediate and terminal in type. They are separated by narrow intervillous clefts. Here, the mater-

nal blood comes into intimate contact with the villous surface. Near the chorionic plate and at the border of neighboring placentomes, the villous arrangement loosens again, thus providing space for the venous backflow toward the venous openings in the basal plate. The radioangiographic studies of Borell and co-workers[56] in the human placenta and of Ramsey and co-workers[57] in rhesus monkey placenta support this placentome concept. Both studies have revealed a rapid filling of the centers of the maternal circulatory units, called *jet* or *spurt*, and subsequently a slow centrifugal spreading of the blood toward the subchorial, lateral, and basal outflow area of the placentomes. In many places, the placentomes overlap so much that the typical differences between inflow and outflow areas vanish.[52]

As evident from the description of villous types, the immature centers of the placentomes act as growth zones where new formation and differentiation of villi occur. In contrast, the placentomes' periphery represents the metabolically active area and the fetomaternal exchange zone. The placentome centers contain the remainders of completely immature villous trees from earlier stages of pregnancy. In normal pregnancy, they can be observed in at least some placentomes until term. They may disappear completely only in rare cases of preterm hypermaturity of the placenta.[6]

The heterogeneity of the villous trees poses problems for the histopathologic evaluation: neighboring zones of the villous trees differ not only by the presence of different types of villi, but also by different degrees of villous maturation. As a consequence, one histologic section never is representative for all parts of a villous tree or for all villous trees of a placenta.[58] This problem is greater when one uses small tissue samples, for instance, for semithin histology and for electron microscopy. Neither allows a diagnosis of the degree of maturation that is reliable. The same holds true for histologic evaluation of samples obtained by chorionic villus sampling.

With regard to their structural arrangement and effectiveness, the fetomaternal blood flow interrelations are described as a multivillous flow system.[59] This implies that the fetal flow in hairpinlike capillary loops is crossed at varying angles by the intervillous maternal bloodstream. Vessel arrangement and effectiveness, as defined physiologically,[59] ensure that the human placenta does not exhibit a countercurrent flow system as was proposed earlier. The effectiveness of the system is further reduced by the fact that considerable amounts of maternal venous blood are recirculated by the arterial jet before leaving the intervillous space.

Intervillous Space

The usual appearance of the intervillous space of the delivered placenta is that of a system of narrow capillarylike clefts.[3, 60] Boyd and Hamilton[3] questioned these interpretations. According to their experience from *in vivo* radioangiographs, the rapid filling of the intervillous space is not compatible with a cleft system of capillary dimensions. The mean width of the intervillous space (blood volume divided by one-half of the villous surface) ranges from 16.4 to 32 μm (assuming an intervillous blood volume ranging from 23.8-37.9% and a villous surface ranging from 11.0-13.3 m²).[6, 61] One must bear in mind that there is a considerable subchorial lake, and wide spaces also exist in the arterial inflow area (central cavity). Thus, the real intervillous volume in the exchange area is likely to be lower and the intervillous clefts narrower. When one adds the considerable loss of maternal blood during labor,[62] however, these calculations may be nearly true.

TROPHOBLASTIC INVASION

Trophoblast invasion is a peculiarity of all species showing interstitial implantation. It is required for:

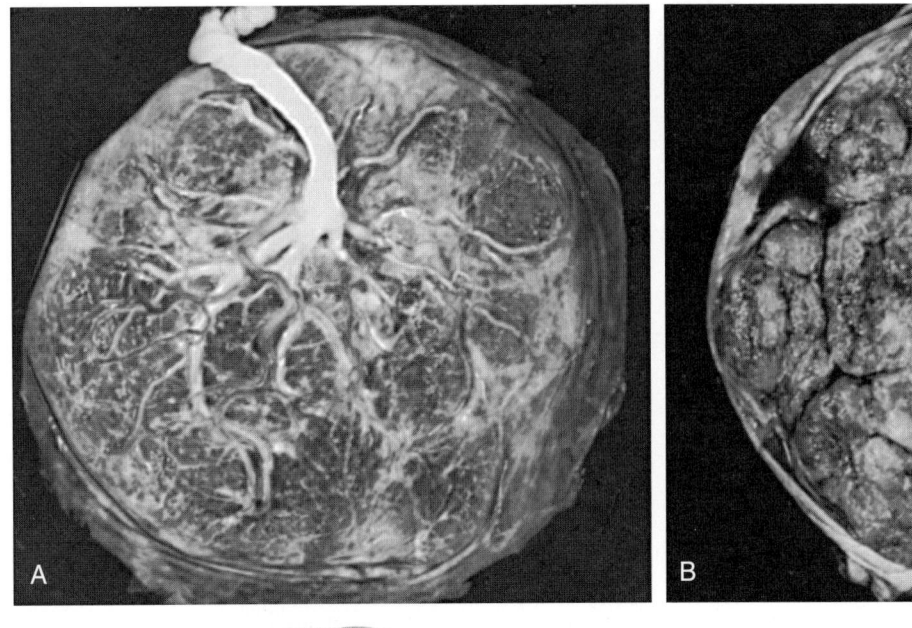

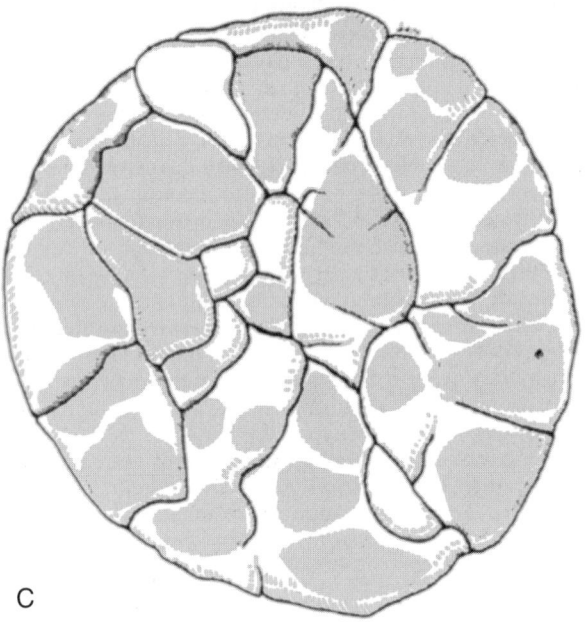

Figure 10–7. Apical (**A**) and basal (**B**) view of a freshly delivered mature human placenta; a corresponding drawing (**C**) combines the basal view with a radiograph of a similar placenta after injection of a radiopaque medium into the fetal vessels. The borderlines of the maternal lobules are marked by lines. The radiographic projections of 29 villous trees are represented by stippled areas. This combination demonstrates a fairly good harmony of villous trees and maternal lobes. (Modified from Kaufmann P: Contrib Gynecol Obstet *13*:517, 1985. S. Karger AG, Basel.)

- Anchorage of the placenta in the uterine wall.
- Adaptation of the uteroplacental circulation to meet the embryonic/fetal requirements.

Interstitial Trophoblast Invasion

Trophoblast invasion starts from the trophoblastic shell which is the base of the lacunar system at day 8 postconception (see Fig. 10-1*C, D*). In the beginning, it is a purely syncytiotrophoblastic layer. From day 13 postconception onward, cytotrophoblast invades the trophoblastic trabeculae and villi. Many of these cells remain in the villi and are the proliferating basis for later development and expansion of the villous trees. Others, the future extravillous trophoblast, reach and focally penetrate the trophoblastic shell (see Fig. 10-1*E*) from where they start invading endometrium and myometrium. The resulting mixture of maternal and fetal tissues stretches from the intervillous space down to the superficial third of the myometrium. It is described as the *junctional zone* (see Fig. 10-1*F*). The superficial part, adhering to the placenta after placental separation, is the *basal plate*. Those

parts that remain in the uterus after delivery are called the *placental bed* and consist mainly of intact and necrotic endometrial tissue, with intermingled trophoblastic cells.

With expansion of the placenta, the trophoblastic shell is disrupted within a few days into multiple clusters of proliferating extravillous trophoblast. Each of these clusters, a *trophoblastic cell column,* is located at the base of an *anchoring villus*, a stem villus that connects the villous trees to the basal plate.[63-65]

Trophoblast invasion is a actual invasive process during which the trophoblast cells penetrate their host tissue using a combination of migratory and proteolytic activities. The latter among others are based on the secretion of various matrix metalloproteinases,[66] serine proteases[67] as well as urokinase and tissue type plasminogen activators.[68] However, unlike tumor invasion, trophoblast invasion stops within few days after delivery of the placenta. This raises the question as to the control of the process. Figure 10-8 summarizes the major differences between tumor and trophoblast invasion, accounting for local and time limitation of trophoblast invasiveness:

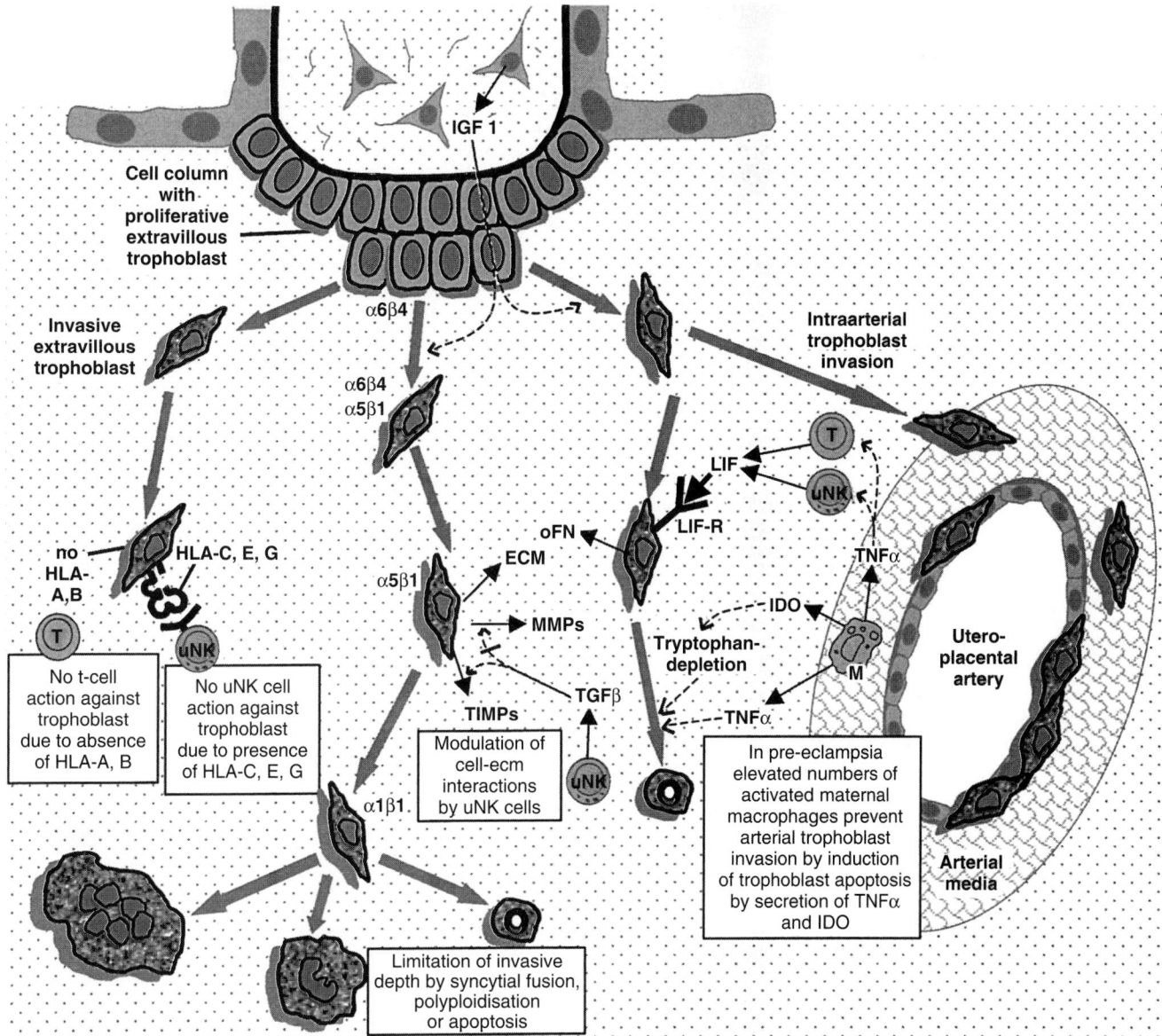

Figure 10–8. Maternofetal interactions between invasive extravillous trophoblast, maternal T cells (T), maternal uterine natural killer cells (uNK) and maternal macrophages (M). *Left invasion route:* Interaction between trophoblastic HLA exposition and maternal lymphocytes. *Central invasion route:* Gradual modification of integrin expression as well as modulation of ECM secretion. *Bottom:* Modes of limitation of invasive depth. *Right invasion route:* Some paracrine interactions between trophoblast and maternal immune cells; intraarterial trophoblast invasion and its inhibition by macrophages. For details, see text.

Although tumor cells *proliferate* and invade at the same time, extravillous trophoblast cells achieve an invasive phenotype only after leaving the cell cycle. They proliferate only for as long as they are resting on the basal lamina of the anchoring villus. This separation of proliferation and invasiveness limits invasive depth to the life-span of each single extravillous trophoblast cell.[69]

Another regulatory factor may be provided by *integrin-matrix interactions*. Shortly after leaving the cell cycle, the majority of trophoblast cells start secreting ample extracellular matrix containing among others laminins, collagen IV, heparan sulfate, vitronectin, cellular and oncofetal fibronectins, and fibrillin.[70-72,73] Interestingly, most invading trophoblast cells in late pregnancy with low invasiveness express only those integrins that are receptors for the respective ECM molecules ($\alpha6\beta4$, $\alpha5\beta1$, $\alpha1\beta1$, and αv integrins).[74] By contrast, in early pregnancy with highly invasive trophoblasts, most cells show mismatch of integrins and surrounding ECM.

It is well known that normal extravillous trophoblast cells *in vitro* show only minimal invasiveness. This has elicited a question about whether cytokines up-regulate and control invasiveness *in vivo*. According to recent *in vitro* data, IGF-I, secreted by placental villous mesenchyme, is a very likely candidate stimulator of trophoblast invasiveness. This paracrine signal would be self-limiting since it diminishes with increasing invasive depth.[76]

Other mechanisms limiting trophoblast invasion probably also include *syncytial fusion* (for review see reference 69). The depth of the invasive zone close to the endometrial/myometrial border is usually marked by a layer of trophoblastic multinucleated giant cells, which are derived from syncytial fusion and show no signs of further invasiveness.

Finally, *apoptosis* of invasive extravillous trophoblast is induced by maternal macrophages by two mechanisms: (a) by secretion of tumor necrosis factor (TNF)α (the trophoblast cells express the respective TNF-receptor I), and (b) by tryptophan depletion (the maternal macrophages secrete tryptophan catabolizing indoleamine 2,3-dioxigenase [IDO]) (see Fig. 10-8).[77]

The interaction between *maternal lymphocytes* and invasive trophoblast is still being discussed (for review see reference 78). The relatively low number of T cells in conjunction with the absence of B cells at the site of implantation make a classic allorecognition reaction of the trophoblast seem unlikely. This view is in agreement with the observation that the invasive trophoblast cells do not express classical polymorphic major histocompatibility complex (MHC) I but rather an unusual combination of human leukocyte antigen (HLA)-C, HLA-E, and HLA-G. The absence of classic semiallogenic MHC-I (HLA-A) molecules prevents attack by T lymphocytes, whereas the presence of the nonpolymorphic HLA-G precludes aggression by the uterine natural killer (NK) cells (large granular lymphocytes) (see Fig. 10-8).

Uterine NK cells are particularly numerous in the decidua basalis at the implantation site where they come into close contact with invading trophoblast cells. Even if they do not interact with trophoblast invasion by direct killing activity, they may control the process by secretion of transforming growth factor β (TGFβ), the receptor of which is expressed by trophoblast cells.[78] TGFβ has been implicated as an immunosuppressive factor in decidua by modulating the response of maternal leukocytes to trophoblast (for review, see reference 78). This cytokine also restricts trophoblast invasion by down-regulation of collagenase secretion and induction of tissue inhibitors of metalloproteinases (TIMPs).[78] The inhibitory effect of TGFβ on trophoblast invasion is mediated by endoglin, a member of the TGFβ receptor complex. Moreover, TGFβ has been reported to enhance the secretion of fibronectins by trophoblast *in vitro* (for review, see reference 6). All these observations suggest that TGFβ is a modulator of trophoblast invasion (see Fig. 10-8).

Arterial Trophoblast Invasion

After erosion of the first endometrial capillaries at day 12 postconception, larger endometrial arteries (spiral arteries) and veins also erode and become connected with the intervillous space. General agreement exists that the number of corresponding maternal vessels that supply the placenta, although originally high, is considerably reduced by obliteration toward term gestation.[3] The final number of spiral arteries present in the term placenta is between 50 and 100.[3,79] According to the same authors, the number of venous openings varies from 50 to 200.

In the second month of pregnancy, pregnancy-induced changes of the uteroplacental vessels start. These primarily affect the uteroplacental arteries and only to a lesser extent affect the respective veins.[80, 81] These changes are obviously induced by invasive extravillous trophoblast approaching the vessel walls. They start with funnel-like dilatation of the arteries (up to a diameter of 2000 μm), followed by dedifferentiation of the media smooth muscle cells, loss of all elastic elements, infiltration of the media with invasive extravillous trophoblast, and replacement of arterial endothelium by so-called intra-arterial trophoblast cells.[49, 79, 82-87] Earlier interpretations that these media changes are degenerative[87] are no longer accepted[83-85]; rather it was shown that the dedifferentiated arterial walls re-differentiate into intact media within few days after delivery including loss of extravillous trophoblast cells.[82]

The trophoblast cells infiltrating the arterial walls and replacing the arterial endothelium, locally form huge intraarterial plugs that were believed to inhibit uteroplacental blood flow. Whether plugging in the first trimester can complete block intervillous blood flow remains subject to further discussion.[6]

Moll and co-workers[49] and Brosens and co-workers[87] have pointed out that because of the degree of physiologic changes in uteroplacental arteries, the latter must be set free from the vaso-motor influences of the mother. This ensures unrestricted maternal blood supply to the placenta, regardless of maternal attempts to regulate the blood flow distribution within her own body; the mother cannot reduce the nutrient supply to the placenta without decreasing the nutrient supply to her own tissues.

Reduced physiologic vessel alterations, including reduced arterial dilatation and reduced intraarterial trophoblast invasion, are regularly observed in pregnancies complicated by preeclampsia, hypertension in pregnancy, and fetal intrauterine growth retardation.[79, 88] There is general agreement that failure of adaptation of the uteroplacental arteries to pregnancy conditions and thus preeclampsia and intrauterine growth restriction (IUGR) are closely related to impaired trophoblast invasion. However, several different hypotheses concerning the nature of this impairment have been proposed. The classic view is that of a general defect of trophoblast invasion,[89, 90] possibly due to impaired integrin expression.[74] The inability of invasive trophoblast cells to express endothelial adhesion receptors, such as VE-cadherin, platelet-endothelial adhesion molecule-1, vascular endothelial adhesion molecule-1, α4-integrins and αvb3-integrin, has been suggested as another possible mechanism.[91, 92] Furthermore, recent data have shown that interstitial trophoblast invasion may be normal. The invasion of vessel walls is inhibited by activated maternal macrophages that secrete TNFα and indoleamine 2,3-dioxygenase (IDO), both inducing apoptosis in those trophoblast cells approaching the arterial walls (see Fig. 10-8).[77,93]

PLACENTAL SEPTA AND CELL ISLANDS

Placental septa and cell islands are oddly shaped conglomerations of fibrinoid, intermingled with groups of trophoblastic and decidual cells. They are not vascularized. If they are connected to the basal plate, they are called *septa*. These septa are columnar or saillike structures rather than real septa.[94] They cannot divide the intervillous space into separate maternally perfused chambers (see Fig. 10-6). They are interpreted as dislocations of basal plate tissue into the intervillous space, caused by lateral movement and folding of the uterine wall and basal plate over each other. Parts of such septa, detached from the basal plate and then attached to neighboring villi, are called *cell islands*. Similar islands, however, without decidual contribution, may be formed from villous tips that have not been opened up by connective tissue and fetal vessels during transition from primary to tertiary villi. In such cases, the cytotrophoblastic core proliferates and, afterward, becomes largely transformed into fibrinoid. These cell islands are growth zones for the attached villous stems comparable to cell columns.[95,96]

CHORIONIC PLATE AND UMBILICAL CORD

At day 14 postconception, the primary chorionic plate consists of three layers: extraembryonic mesenchyme, cytotrophoblast, and syncytiotrophoblast (see Fig. 10-1*E, F*). These layers separate the intervillous space from the blastocystic cavity. Between 8 and 10 weeks' postconception, the amniotic sac has expanded to such a degree that the amniotic mesenchyme comes into close contact with the mesenchymal surface of the chorionic plate and the chorionic laeve (smooth chorion). As soon as amniotic and chorionic plate mesenchyme fuse with each other, the definitive chorionic plate is formed (see Fig. 10-6).[97,98]

As part of the same process, the expanding amniotic sac surrounds the connective stalk and the allantois and joins them to form the umbilical cord. The allantoic vessels—two arteries and one vein—grow in thickness and length and convert into the umbilical vessels. The allantoic epithelium gradually disappears; small vesicular remnants of the allantois, however, may persist until term. The allantoic mesenchyme differentiates into a complex system of myofibroblasts that likely help regulating turgor of the cord and avoid bending of the latter with fatal consequences for the fetus.[99,100] Fusion of the umbilical vessels with the intravillous vessel system establishes a complete fetoplacental circulation at the end of the fifth week postconception. The cord is characterized by a spiral twisting, the number of spiral turns increasing as pregnancy progresses, up to a maximum of 380 turns. In most cases, the twist is leftward, or counterclockwise. The twists have been interpreted as the result of rotary movements of the fetus owing to asymmetric uterine contractions.[6,101]

FETAL MEMBRANES

All developmental steps described thus far are valid only for the implantation pole, which describes that part of the blastocystic circumference that is attached to the endometrium and implanted first. The other parts of the blastocystic circumference, implanted a few days later, undergo a corresponding, although delayed, development that is quickly followed by regressive changes. These parts are called *capsular chorion frondosum.* The first regressive changes can be observed as early as in the fourth week. The newly formed villi degenerate, and the surrounding intervillous space is obliterated. As a consequence of obliteration of the intervillous space, the chorionic plate, villous remnants, and the basal plate fuse, forming a multilayered compact lamella, the smooth chorion (chorion laeve). Formation of the smooth chorion starts opposite to the implantation pole at the so-called anti-implantation pole. From there, it spreads over about 70% of the surface of the chorionic sac until the fourth month of gestation, when this process stops.[3,6] Between the seventh and the 10th weeks of pregnancy, the expanding amniotic sac comes into contact with the smooth chorion. In most places, the mesenchymal layers of both membranes fuse.

With complete implantation, the decidua re-closes over the blastocyst, bulging into the uterine lumen, and is now called the *capsular decidua.* With the increasing diameter of the chorionic sac, the capsular decidua locally touches the parietal decidua of the opposing uterine wall. Between the 15th and the 20th weeks postconception, both decidual layers fuse with each other, thus obstructing the uterine cavity. From this point onward, the smooth chorion has contact over nearly its entire surface with the decidual surface of the uterine wall and may function as a paraplacental exchange organ. Owing to the absence of fetal vascularization in the smooth chorion and the amnion, all paraplacental exchange between fetal membranes and fetus has to pass through the amniotic fluid.

At term, the fetal membranes are structured as follows (see Fig. 10-6)[6,102]: the mean thickness of the membranes, after separation from the uterine wall during labor, is between 200 and 300 μm. The innermost layer, the *amniotic epithelium,* encloses the amniotic fluid. Amniotic epithelium may be involved in the production of the latter and even partially responsible for its resorption. Moreover, it seems to be involved in pH regulation of the amniotic fluid.[103] Together with the *lamina propria,* it measures 30 to 60 μm in thickness.[104]

The next layer consists of *chorionic connective tissue,* which is directly adherent to a *cytotrophoblastic layer* of varying thickness.[104,105] Connective tissue and cytotrophoblast have a combined thickness of 80 to 120 μm. Near the placental margin, the thickness increases because persisting ghost villi, embedded in fibrinoid, split the cytotrophoblast into two layers. At the placental margin, these two layers completely disjoin by interposition of the intervillous space, and they become the chorionic and the basal plates (see Fig. 10-6). Attached to the outer surface of the cytotrophoblast is a *decidual layer* about 50 μm thick. The latter indicates that the separation of membranes does not take place along the maternofetal interface but instead occurs at a somewhat deeper level.

Apart from the amniotic involvement in the production, resorption, and acid-base balance of the amniotic fluid,[103,106] there is no definite and detailed knowledge about exchange and metabolic functions of the smooth chorion.

REFERENCES

1. Enders AC, King BF: Formation and differentiation of extraembryonic mesoderm in the rhesus monkey. Am J Anat *181*:327, 1988.
2. Enders AC: Trophoblast differentiation during the transition from trophoblastic plate to lacunar stage of implantation in the rhesus monkey and human. Am J Anat *186*:85, 1989.
3. Boyd JD and Hamilton WJ, The Human Placenta. Cambridge, UK, Wm. Heffer & Sons, 1970.
4. Luckett WP: Origin and differentiation of the yolk sac and extraembryonic mesoderm in presomite human and rhesus monkey embryos. Am J Anat *152*:59, 1978.
5. Demir R, et al: Fetal vasculogenesis and angiogenesis in human placental villi. Acta Anat Basel *136*:190, 1989.
6. Benirschke K, Kaufmann P: Pathology of the human placenta. Springer, New York, 2000.
7. Sibley CP, et al: Ultrastructural tracer studies on the protein permeability of the guinea-pig placenta. J Anat *137*:787, 1983.
8. Sibley CP, et al: Permeability of the fetal capillary endothelium of the guinea-pig placenta to haem proteins of various molecular sizes. Cell Tissue Res *223*:165, 1982.
9. Firth JA, et al: Permeability pathways in fetal placental capillaries. Trophoblast Res *3*:163, 1988.
10. Sibley CP, et al: Molecular charge as a determinant of macromolecule permeability across the fetal capillary endothelium of the guinea-pig placenta. Cell Tissue Res *229*:365, 1983.
11. Macara LM, et al: Control of the fetoplacental circulation. Fetal Matern Med Rev *5*:167, 1993.
12. Kohnen G, et al: Placental villous stroma as a model system for myofibroblast differentiation. Histochem Cell Biol *105*:415, 1996.
13. Kaufmann P: Untersuchungen über die Langhanszellen in der menschlichen Placenta. Z Zellforsch *128*:283, 1972.
14. Huppertz B, et al: Villous cytotrophoblast regulation of the syncytial apoptotic cascade in the human placenta. Histochem Cell Biol *110*:495, 1998.
15. Huppertz B, et al: Apoptosis: molecular control of placental function—A workshop report. Placenta *22*:S101, 2001.
16. Huppertz B and Hunt JS: Trophoblast apoptosis and placental development—a workshop report. Placenta *21(Suppl A)*:S74, 2000.
17. Huppertz B et al: The apoptosis cascade—morphological and immunohistochemical methods for its visualization. Anat Embryol *200*:1, 1999.
18. Huppertz B, Kaufmann P: The apoptosis cascade in human villous trophoblast. A review. Trophoblast Res *13*:215, 1999.
19. Huppertz B, et al: Apoptosis and syncytial fusion in human placental trophoblast and skeletal muscle. Int Rev Cytol *205*:215, 2001.
20. Mi S, et al: Syncytin is a captive retroviral envelope protein involved in human placental morphogenesis. Nature *403*:785, 2000.
21. Pötgens AJG, et al: Mechanisms of syncytial fusion: A review. Placenta *23, Suppl A*:S107–S113, 2002.
22. Huppertz B, et al: Apoptosis cascade progresses during turnover of human trophoblast: analysis of villous cytotrophoblast and syncytial fragments in vitro. Lab Invest *79*:1687, 1999.
23. Huppertz B, et al: Hypoxia favours necrotic versus apoptotic shedding of placental syncytiotrophoblast into the maternal circulation. Implications for the pathogenesis of pre-eclampsia. Placenta *24*:181, 2003.
24. Richard R: Studies of placental morphogenesis. I. Radioautographic studies of human placenta utilizing tritiated thymidine. Proc Soc Exp Biol Med *106*:829, 1961.
25. Kaufmann P et al: Die funktionelle Bedeutung der Langhanszellen der menschlichen Placenta. Anat Anz *77*:435, 1983.
26. Nelson DM: Apoptotic changes occur in syncytiotrophoblast of human placental villi where fibrin type fibrinoid is deposited at discontinuities in the villous trophoblast. Placenta *17*:387, 1996.
27. Cantle SJ, et al: Interpretation of syncytial sprouts and bridges in the human placenta. Placenta *8*:221, 1987.
28. Kaufmann P, et al: Cross-sectional features and three-dimensional structure of human placental villi. Placenta *8*:235, 1987.
29. Burton GJ: Intervillous connections in the mature human placenta: instances of syncytial fusion or section artifacts? J Anat *145*:13, 1986.
30. Stulc J: Extracellular transport pathways in the haemochorial placenta. Placenta *10*:113, 1989.
31. Edwards D, et al: Paracellular permeability pathways in the human placenta: a quantitative and morphological study of maternal-fetal transfer of horseradish peroxidase. Placenta *14*:63, 1993.
32. Frank HG, et al: Immunohistochemistry of two different types of placental fibrinoid. Acta Anat Basel *150*:55, 1994.
33. Kaufmann P, et al: Fluid shift across the placenta: II. Fetomaternal transfer of horseradish peroxidase in the guinea pig. Placenta *3*:339, 1982.

34. Kaufmann P: Influence of ischemia and artificial perfusion on placental ultrastructure and morphometry. Contrib Gynecol Obstet 13:18, 1985.

35. Kaufmann P, et al: Are there membrane-lined channels through the trophoblast? A study with lanthanum hydroxide. Trophoblast Res 2:557, 1987.

36. Kertschanska S, et al: Is there morphological evidence for the existence of transtrophoblastic channels in human placental villi? Trophoblast Res 8:581, 1994.

37. Kertschanska S, et al: Pressure dependence of so-called transtrophoblastic channels during fetal perfusion of human placental villi. Microsc Res Technique 38:52, 1997.

38. Thornburg KL, Faber JJ: Transfer of hydrophilic molecules by placenta and yolk sac of the guinea pig. Am J Physiol 233:C111, 1977.

39. Thornburg KL, et al: Permeability of placenta to inulin. Am J Obstet Gynecol 158:1165, 1988.

40. Kaufmann P, et al: Classification of human placental villi. I. Histology and scanning electron microscopy. Cell Tissue Res 200:409, 1979.

41. Sen DK, et al: Classification of human placental villi. II. Morphometry. Cell Tissue Res 200:425, 1979.

42. Castellucci M, et al: The development of the human placental villous tree. Anat Embryol 181:117, 1990.

43. Castellucci M, et al: Villous sprouting: fundamental mechanisms of human placental development. Hum Reprod Update 6:485, 2000.

44. Leiser R, et al: The fetal vascularisation of term human placental villi. I. Peripheral stem villi. Anat Embryol 173:71, 1985.

45. Graf R, et al: The perivascular contractile sheath of human placental stem villi: Its isolation and characterization. Placenta 16:57, 1995.

46. Graf R, et al: The extravascular contractile system in the human placenta. Morphological and immunocytochemical investigations. Anat Embryol 190:541, 1994.

47. Graf R, et al: The extravascular contractile system in the human placenta: morphology and co-localization with different autacoid generating systems. Anat Embryol 1993.

48. Kohnen G, et al: The monoclonal antibody GB 42—a useful marker for the differentiation of myofibroblasts. Cell Tissue Res 281:231, 1995.

49. Moll W, et al: Blood flow regulation in the uteroplacental arteries. Trophoblast Res 3:83, 1988.

50. Kaufmann P, et al: Three-dimensional representation of the fetal vessel system in the human placenta. Trophoblast Res 3:113, 1988.

51. Kaufmann P, et al: The fetal vascularisation of term human placental villi. II. Intermediate and terminal villi. Anat Embryol 173:203, 1985.

52. Kaufmann P: Basic morphology of the fetal and maternal circuits in the human placenta. Contrib Gynecol Obstet 13:5, 1985.

53. Demir R, et al: Classification of human placental stem villi: Review of structural and functional aspects. Microsc Res Technique 38:29, 1997.

54. Schuhmann RA: Plazenton: Begriff, Entstehung, funktionelle Anatomie. In Becker V, et al (eds.): Die Plazenta des Menschen. Stuttgart, Thieme Verlag, 1981: pp 199–207.

55. Castellucci M, et al: The stromal architecture of the immature intermediate villus of the human placenta. Functional and clinical implications. Gynecol Obstet Invest 18:95, 1984.

56. Borell U, et al: Eine arteriographische Studie des Plazentarkreislaufs. Geburtshilfe Frauenheilkd 18:1, 1958.

57. Ramsey EM, Corner et al: Serial and cineradioangiographic visualization of maternal circulation in the primate (hemochorial) placenta. Am J Obstet Gynecol 86:213, 1963.

58. Mayhew TM, Burton GJ: Methodological problems in placental morphometry: apologia for the use of stereology based on sound sampling practice. Placenta 9:565, 1988.

59. Faber JJ, Thornburg KL, Placental Physiology. Structure and Function of Fetomaternal Exchange. New York, Raven Press, 1983.

60. Freese UE: The fetal-maternal circulation of the placenta I. Histomorphologic, plastoid injection, and x-ray cinematographic studies on human placentas. Am J Obstet Gynecol 94:354, 1966.

61. Mayhew TM, et al: Microscopical morphology of the human placenta and its effects on oxygen diffusion: a morphometric model. Placenta 7:121, 1986.

62. Bouw GM, et al: Quantitative morphology of the placenta. I. Standardization of sampling. Eur J Obstet Gynecol Reprod Biol 6:325, 1976.

63. Okudaira Y, et al: Electron microscopic study on the trophoblastic cell column of human placenta. J Electron Microsc Tokyo 20:93, 1971.

64. Enders AC: Fine structure of anchoring villi of the human placenta. Am J Anat 122:419, 1968.

65. Enders AC, et al: Structure of anchoring villi and the trophoblastic shell in the human, baboon and macaque placenta. Placenta 22:284, 2001.

66. Huppertz B, et al: Immunohistochemistry of matrix metalloproteinases (MMP), their substrates, and their inhibitors (TIMP) during trophoblast invasion in the human placenta. Cell Tissue Res 291:133, 1998.

67. Castellucci M, et al: Immunohistochemical localization of serine-protease inhibitors in the human placenta. Cell Tissue Res 278:283, 1994.

68. Hu ZY, et al: Expression of tissue type and urokinase type plasminogen activators as well as plasminogen activator inhibitor type-1 and type-2 in human and rhesus monkey placenta. J Anat 194:183, 1999.

69. Kaufmann P, Castellucci M: Extravillous trophoblast in the human placenta. Trophoblast Res 10:21, 1997.

70. Damsky CH, et al: Distribution patterns of extracellular matrix components and adhesion receptors are intricately modulated during first trimester cytotrophoblast differentiation along the invasive pathway, in vivo. J Clin Invest 89:210, 1992.

71. Blankenship TN, King BF: Developmental changes in the cell columns and trophoblastic shell of the macaque placenta: an immunohistochemical study localizing type IV collagen, laminin, fibronectin and cytoceratins. Cell Tissue Res 274:457, 1993.

72. Huppertz B, et al: Extracellular matrix components of the placental extravillous trophoblast: Immunocytochemistry and ultrastructural distribution. Histochem Cell Biol 106:291, 1996.

73. King BF, Blankenship TN: Immunohistochemical localization of fibrillin in developing macaque and term human placentas and fetal membranes. Microsc Res Technique 38:42, 1997.

74. Damsky CH, et al: Integrin switching regulates normal trophoblast invasion. Development 120:3657, 1994.

75. Kemp B, et al: Invasive depth of extravillous trophoblast correlates with cellular phenotype—a comparison on intra-and extrauterine implantation sites. Histochem Cell Biol 117: 401, 2002.

76. Lacey H, et al: Mesenchymally-derived IGF-I provides a paracrine stimulus for trophoblast migration. BioMed Central-Devel Biol 2: 5, 2002 .

77. Reister F, et al: Macrophage-induced apoptosis limits endovascular trophoblast invasion in the uterine wall of preeclamptic women. Lab Invest 81:1143, 2001.

78. Loke YW, King A: Human Implantation-Cell Biology and Immunology. Cambridge, Cambridge University Press, 1995.

79. Brosens IA: The uteroplacental vessels at term—the distribution and extent of physiological changes. Trophoblast Res 3:61, 1988.

80. Blankenship TN, et al: Trophoblastic invasion and the development of uteroplacental arteries in the macaque: immunohistochemical localization of cytoceratins, desmin, type IV collagen, laminin, and fibronectin. Cell Tissue Res 272:227, 1993.

81. Blankenship TN, et al: Trophoblastic invasion and modification of uterine veins during placental development in macaques. Cell Tissue Res 274:135, 1993.

82. Nanaev AK, et al: Pregnancy-induced de-differentiation of media smooth muscle cells in uteroplacental arteries of the guinea pig is reversible after delivery. Placenta 21:306, 2000.

83. Craven CM, et al: Decidual spiral artery remodelling begins before cellular interaction with cytotrophoblasts. Placenta 19:241, 1998.

84. Craven C, Ward K.: α-smooth muscle actin is preserved in arteries showing physiologic change. Placenta. 17:A17, 1996.

85. Nanaev AK, et al: Physiological dilation of uteroplacental arteries in the guinea pig depends on nitric oxide synthase activity extravillous trophoblast. Cell Tissue Res 282:407, 1995.

86. Hees H, et al: Pregnancy-induced structural changes and trophoblastic invasion in the segmental mesometrial arteries of the guinea pig (Cavia porcellus L.). Placenta 8:609, 1987.

87. Brosens IA, et al: The physiological response of the vessels of the placental bed to normal pregnancy. J Pathol Bacteriol 93:569, 1967.

88. Sheppard BL, Bonnar J: The maternal blood supply to the placenta in pregnancy complicated by intrauterine fetal growth retardation. Trophoblast Res 3:69, 1988.

89. Brosens IA: Morphological changes in the utero-placental bed in pregnancy hypertension. Clin Obstet Gynecol 4:573, 1977.

90. Caniggia I, et al: Inhibition of TGF-beta(3) restores the invasive capability of extravillous trophoblasts in preeclamptic pregnancies. J Clin Invest 103:1641, 1999.

91. Zhou Y, et al: Preeclampsia is associated with failure of human cytotrophoblasts to mimic a vascular adhesion phenotype—One cause of defective endovascular invasion in this syndrome? J Clin Invest 99:2152, 1997.

92. Zhou Y, et al: Human cytotrophoblasts adopt a vascular phenotype as they differentiate—A strategy for successful endovascular invasion? J Clin Invest 99:2139, 1997.

93. Reister F, et al: The distribution of macrophages in spiral arteries of the placental bed in pre-eclampsia differs from that in healthy patients. Placenta 20:229, 1999.

94. Becker V, Jipp P: Über die Trophoblastschale der menschlichen Plazenta. Geburtshilfe Frauenheilkd 23:466, 1963.

95. Castellucci M, et al: The human placenta: a model for tenascin expression. Histochemistry 95:449, 1991.

96. Mühlhauser J, et al: Differentiation and proliferation patterns in human trophoblast revealed by c-erbB-2 oncogene product and EGF-R. J Histochem Cytochem 41:165, 1993.

97. Wiese KH: Licht- und elektronenmikroskopische Untersuchungen an der Chorionplatte der reifen menschlichen Plazenta. Arch Gynecol 218:243, 1975.

98. Weser H and Kaufmann P: Lichtmikroskopische und histochemische Untersuchungen an der Chorionplatte der reifen menschlichen Plazenta. Arch Gynecol 225:15, 1978.

99. Takechi K, et al: Ultrastructural and immunohistochemical studies of Wharton's. Placenta 14:235, 1993.

100. Nanaev AK, et al: Stromal differentiation and architecture of the human umbilical cord. Placenta 18:53, 1997.

101. Edmonds HW: The spiral twist of the normal umbilical cord in twins and in singletons. Am J Obstet Gynecol 67:102, 1954.

102. Bourne GL, The human amnion and chorion. London, Lloyd-Luke, 1962.

103. Mühlhauser J, et al: Immunohistochemistry of carbonic anhydrase in human placenta and fetal membranes. Histochemistry *101*:91, 1994.
104. Aplin JD, et al: The extracellular matrix of human amniotic epithelium: ultrastructure, composition and deposition. J Cell Sci *79*:119, 1985.
105. Aplin JD, Campbell S: An immunofluorescence study of extracellular matrix associated with cytotrophoblast of the chorion laeve. Placenta 6:469, 1985.
106. Schmidt W: The amniotic fluid compartment: the fetal habitat. Adv Anat Embryol Cell Biol *127*:1, 1992.

11

Charles R. Rosenfeld

Regulation of the Placental Circulation

THE PLACENTA

Regulation of the Placental Circulation

Pregnancy is associated with several alterations to the maternal cardiovascular system; however, it is the development of the low-resistance, high-flow placental vascular bed that characterizes this physiologic state. Moreover, this vascular bed is unique in that it is composed of maternal and fetal components separated by several cell layers that differ depending on the species under consideration.[1] Although these two vascular beds are intimately associated with each other in all species, present evidence suggests that they function and respond independently of each other.[2-4] It is important to understand the mechanisms that control their vascular tone and the magnitude of placental blood flow because alterations in either maternal or fetal placental blood flow could modify the delivery of oxygen or nutrients or both to the fetus as well as the removal of carbon dioxide and other fetal metabolic wastes.[5] Thus, the integrity of the uteroplacental and umbilicoplacental vascular beds is important to fetal growth and development, minute-to-minute fetal well-being, and possibly to the subsequent occurrence of adult-onset cardiovascular disease.[6,7]

In view of the importance of the placental vascular beds to fetal well-being and survival of the species, research in this area has been intense since the time of Barcroft's research.[8] Because it remains difficult to study humans, our present understanding reflects in large part studies performed in various animal models and, in particular, the pregnant ewe. Thus, conclusions about the relative importance of the mechanisms responsible for the control of blood flow to these vascular beds in the human continue to be temporized. Nonetheless, recent knowledge obtained from these models has been replicated in humans, thereby providing an excellent starting point in understanding this important aspect of pregnancy and enabling clinicians to better understand data obtained in Doppler flow velocity studies in women.[9]

DEVELOPMENT OF THE UTEROPLACENTAL AND UMBILICAL-PLACENTAL VASCULAR BEDS

It is important to describe how these vascular beds change during the course of normal gestation. In women, the uteroplacental vascular bed is composed of cotyledons, lobes, or placentomes similar to those seen in many species.[1] In contrast to the sheep or cow, however, they adhere to each other rather than as separate entities. Nonetheless, they can be seen as individual structures when viewed from the basal or maternal side of the placenta following its delivery. These placentomes receive their maternal arterial blood via the spiral arteries, and it appears that alterations in the tone of these or more proximal uterine arteries may be responsible for modifying the magnitude and distribution of maternal uteroplacental blood flow.[10] As in pregnant sheep, during normal human pregnancy a fixed number of placentomes are ultimately available. Therefore, the increase in uteroplacental blood flow that occurs during pregnancy is due to the development of the placenta (i.e., implantation and growth) and subsequent vasodilation of the spiral arteries so that perfusion of the intravillous space may increase.[11]

When maternal uteroplacental blood flow is examined throughout ovine gestation,[12] a complex scenario is observed.[10,11] Total uterine blood flow (Fig. 11-1) increases about 40-fold during the course of a normal singleton pregnancy, and levels are even higher in multiple gestations. This increase in uteroplacental blood flow is coincident with a doubling of maternal cardiac output and an increase in the relative amount of cardiac output delivered to the uterus, increasing from less than 1% of cardiac output in nonpregnant sheep to 16 to 25% at term.[13] The pattern of this increase in total uterine blood flow (mL/min) occurs in three phases (see Fig. 11-1*B*). The first is associated with relatively low absolute blood flows, which on the basis of uterine/conceptus wet weight is actually high, achieving values of 0.8 mL/min per gram compared with 0.3 mL/min per gram for the nonpregnant uterus (see Fig. 11-1*C*). This increase in uterine blood flow is believed to reflect vasodilation secondary to the increased production of maternal ovarian and possibly fetal hormones (e.g., estrogen and progesterone), which may be required for survival of the conceptus before implantation and the initial phase of implantation and placentation.[14,15] In primates and women, this occurs in the first days or weeks of pregnancy. The second phase is associated with the development of the placentomes and, in the primate, with the development of the intravillous spaces or the maternal placental vascular bed. At this time point, the maternal placental vascular bed becomes as large as it will ever be. If this does not occur in a normal manner, placentation may be restricted, resulting in a small placenta and a fetus with proportionate growth restriction. In the ewe, total uterine blood flow plateaus at this time, averages about 500 mL/min; however, blood flow expressed on a weight basis at the same point in gestation has fallen nearly 50% to 0.3 to 0.4 mL/min per gram, reflecting the ever-increasing weight of the fetus and placenta (see Fig. 11-1*C*). The final phase in the "growth" of uterine blood flow is exponential and associated with a threefold increase in fetal weight that occurs after 110 days in sheep (75% of gestation) and beyond 30 weeks in humans (75%).[12] Because neither the total number of spiral arteries nor placentomes change, this increase in uterine blood flow must be due to vasodilation.[11,12,15] Recent studies suggest that the mechanisms responsible for this final vasodilation involve activation of vascular smooth muscle potassium channels resulting in membrane hyperpolarization;[16] however, the initiating events are unclear. Importantly, the rise in blood flow in mL/min is proportionate to and parallel with the rise in wet weight of the uterus and its metabolically active tissues, which includes the growing fetus,

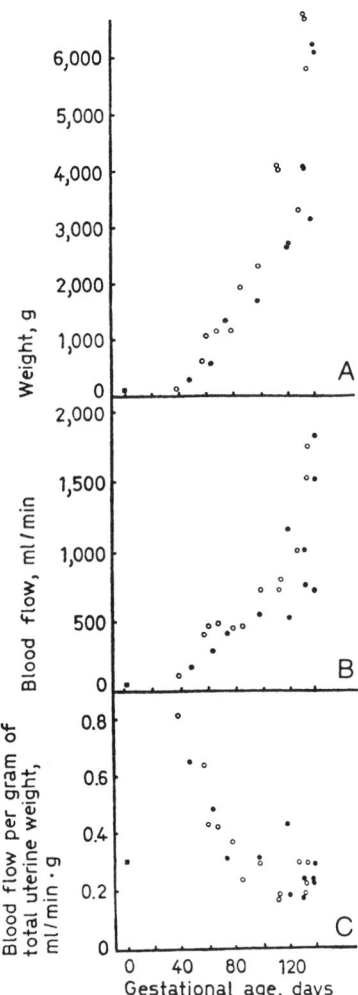

Figure 11–1. Changes in the uterine weight (**A**), blood flow (**B**), and blood flow per gram of total uterine weight (**C**) during ovine pregnancy. Total weight is the sum of all metabolically active tissues. *Square* = nonpregnant; *open circle* = singleton pregnancy; *closed circle* = twin pregnancy. (From Rosenfeld CR, et al: Gynecol Invest 5:252, 1974. S Karger AG, Basel.)

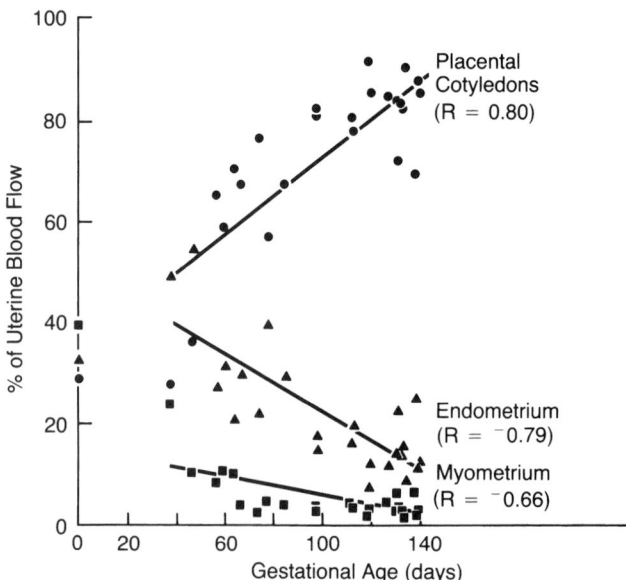

Figure 11–2. The distribution of uterine blood flow during ovine pregnancy (term = 145 days). Blood flow was determined using the microsphere technique. Correlation coefficients are significant at $p < 0.01$. (From Rosenfeld CR: Semin Perinatol 8:42, 1984.)

membranes, and placenta. Thus, blood flow per gram of wet weight remains low (0.2-0.3 mL/min/g) during the remainder of pregnancy. In the fetus with late-onset intrauterine growth restriction (i.e., after 70% of gestation), blood flow per gram of fetoplacental mass is lower and nutrient and oxygen delivery are also decreased. Fetal growth is attenuated until adaptation has occurred and this ratio is reestablished, at which time a new growth curve is established that lies below that of normally growing fetuses.

Although total uterine blood flow increases dramatically during pregnancy, this reflects changes occurring in three separate vascular beds: the placentomes, endometrium, and myometrium. The change in distribution of blood flow to these tissues cannot be determined in women, but it has been studied in sheep and several other species.[11,17] This is an important issue because changes in total uterine blood flow can be measured in women but do not address the issue of primary importance, that is, placental perfusion. As illustrated in Figure 11-2, blood flow to these three tissues is evenly distributed in the nonpregnant uterus, each receiving about one-third. As pregnancy progresses, there is a gradual redistribution of uterine blood flow, and at term the placentomes (cotyledons) receive nearly 90% of total uterine

blood flow. Thus, in the last third of pregnancy, the placentomes account for most of the observed increase in uterine blood flow.

Given that the placentome is the site of nutrient and gas exchange, fetal well-being is determined by changes in placental growth and perfusion. Placental weight is relatively unchanged after the middle third of gestation (Fig. 11-3). This occurs earlier in the human and other primates. The pattern of change in absolute blood flow (see Fig. 11-3*B*) resembles that seen for total uterine blood flow (see Fig. 11-1*B*). This is because placental flow increases disproportionately compared with other uterine tissues (see Fig. 11-2), accounting for more than 80% of uterine blood flow in the last third of gestation. The principal difference between the two patterns is seen when blood flow per gram of metabolically active tissue is examined (see Fig. 11-3*C*). In contrast to the high value for total uterine blood flow early in pregnancy followed by a fall and leveling off, placental blood flow per gram of metabolically active tissue falls in midpregnancy and then increases until term. Thus, placental blood flow rises from 0.5 to 1.0 ml/min per gram to nearly 4 ml/min per gram, a value five times greater than that observed for the total uterus. This rise in placental blood flow must reflect vasodilation because there is no change in either maternal arterial blood pressure (i.e., perfusion pressure) or in the number of maternal placental arteries.[11,18] This rise in maternal placental blood flow also parallels a more general process of functional maturation of the placenta, which involves the simultaneous increase in fetoplacental perfusion[19] and permeability,[20] which are necessary to provide nutrients and oxygen for the rapidly growing fetus. The volume of placental blood flow exceeds that necessary for normal fetal growth,[4,5] and provides a margin of safety that is considered necessary to protect the fetus from episodic decreases in uteroplacental blood flow associated with transient increases in maternal plasma levels of vasoconstrictors (e.g., angiotensin II) or at the time of parturition when increases in myometrial tone may alter placental perfusion.[11]

Although much has been learned about the functional and anatomic aspects of the maternal uteroplacental circulation, few investigators have tried to describe in detail the pattern of change in umbilicoplacental blood flow that occurs over the

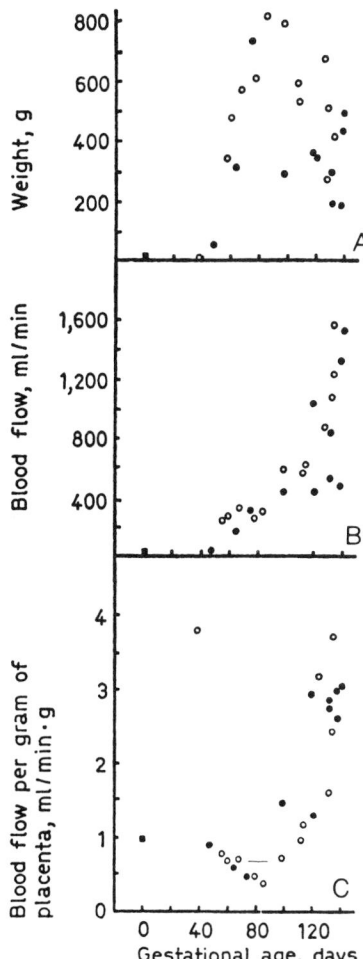

Figure 11–3. Changes in placental weight (**A**), blood flow (**B**), and blood flow per gram of placenta (**C**). Observations on the nonpregnant animals represent the caruncles or future sites of implantation. Placental weight and blood flow in the twin gestations are the sum of the two placentas. Symbols are as noted in Figure 11–1. (From Rosenfeld CR, et al: Gynecol Invest 5:252, 1974. S Karger AG, Basel.)

entire course of pregnancy. This reflects the difficulty in performing such studies even in an animal model. Nonetheless, many similarities exist between species. For example, there is a stem villus originating from the fetal side of the placenta that contains a distal branch of the umbilical artery and vein. As pregnancy progresses, there is development of a villous tree (in the human) or vascular bed originating from the stem villus that subdivides, branches, and grows throughout pregnancy, providing an ever-increasing fetal placental vascular bed with an enormous surface area for nutrient and gas exchange. Although the sheep has no villous tree, there is continued growth of the fetal placental vascular bed similar to that of the human.[1, 18] Thus, in both species, the size of the fetal placental vascular bed and the magnitude of umbilicoplacental blood flow increase, the latter increasing exponentially in the last third of normal pregnancy.[19] In contrast to the rise in uteroplacental blood flow, which reflects vasodilation, the rise in umbilicoplacental blood flow is primarily due to vascular growth and, to a lesser extent, vasodilation. Thus umbilicoplacental blood flow remains approximately 200 mL/min per gram throughout gestation in most species. Conditions that attenuate the growth of the fetal placental vascular bed in the last trimester (e.g., pregnancy-induced

hypertension) or increase fetal placental resistance may result in fetal growth restriction. This, however, has not been well studied.

VASOCONSTRICTORS

Studies of the factors controlling blood flow through the utero-placental and umbilicoplacental vascular beds have centered on the effects of endogenous vasoconstrictors, including angiotensin II, catecholamines, and arginine vasopressin, a hypothalamic-pituitary peptide secreted during episodes of so-called fetal stress. This section reviews how these agents may affect placental perfusion and fetal well-being.

Normotensive pregnant women develop attenuated pressor responses to systemic infusions of angiotensin II early in the midtrimester, and this refractoriness is no longer evident in women who develop hypertension.[21, 22] Pregnant sheep and several other species also develop refractoriness to this vasoconstrictor during pregnancy.[23, 24] In pregnant women and sheep, the uteroplacental vascular bed is more refractory to this agent than the systemic vasculature as a whole.[24-26] Furthermore, as in the peripheral vasculature, this uterine refractoriness is absent in pregnant women who develop hypertension, possibly resulting in placental hypoperfusion.[26] This differential sensitivity is evident when the dose-response curves depicting the relative changes in uterine and systemic vascular resistance are compared (Fig. 11–4). As illustrated, at doses resulting in physiologic blood levels (<1.0 µg/min), systemic infusions of angiotensin II result in greater relative increases in systemic versus uterine vascular resistance. The rise in perfusion pressure also exceeds that of uterine vascular resistance; therefore, uteroplacental blood flow actually increases throughout this dosage range. These observations suggest that the uteroplacental vascular bed is in a sense partially pressure passive and is protected from the vasoconstrictor effects of angiotensin II.[24] This is important because plasma angiotensin II levels are increased in normal pregnancies and may intermittently increase further when pregnant women experience episodes of orthostatic hypotension. Notably, maternal placental blood flow is minimally affected, and the reproductive tissues as a group are more refractory than nonreproductive tissues.[27]

This refractoriness of the uteroplacental circulation to angiotensin II may reflect several mechanisms. In earlier studies, uterine arteries from pregnant ewes demonstrated a threefold rise in the basal synthesis of prostacyclin (a potent vasodilator and angiotensin II antagonist) and a 1.5-fold increase in endothelium-derived prostacyclin synthesis when exposed to angiotensin II *in vivo* or *in vitro* by activating type 1 angiotensin II receptors.[24, 28-30] Uterine arteries from normotensive pregnant women appear to respond similarly, whereas arteries from women with hypertensive disease appear unable to enhance prostacyclin synthesis in the presence of angiotensin II.[31] Because inhibition of cyclooxygenase activity in the uterine vascular bed of pregnant ewes decreased basal prostacyclin synthesis and enhanced constrictor responses to systemic angiotensin II infusions, it was believed this was the predominant mechanism responsible for attenuating uterine vasoconstrictor responses to angiotensin II.[30] Although this differential sensitivity to angiotensin II is not contributed to by preferential down-regulation of angiotensin II receptors in uterine vascular smooth muscle, it was observed that type 2 angiotensin II receptors, which do not mediate vasoconstriction, are the predominant receptor in uterine arteries from women and sheep.[24, 29, 32] Further, local intraarterial infusions of angiotensin II did not increase uterine vascular resistance except at doses that initiated pressor responses before uterine responses, the pattern seen with systemic infusions.[33] It now appears that the attenuated uteroplacental responses to angiotensin II primarily reflect the presence of type 2 receptors, and angiotensin II exerts its effect on uterine blood flow by releasing another agent, for instance, an α-agonist, which is antagonized by local prostacyclin synthesis.[24,33] In addition, the type 2 receptor may antagonize responses to the type 1 receptor.[34] Furthermore, uteroplacental synthesis of endothelial-derived nitric oxide, which is increased in pregnancy and enhanced further by angiotensin II, may provide another route for attenuating responses to angiotensin II.[24, 35] Thus, several local mechanisms appear essential to the maintenance of uteroplacental blood flow while permitting adjustments in the peripheral vascular beds during increases in plasma levels of endogenous angiotensin II in pregnant women. Modification of these agonist-antagonist interactions may occur in hypertensive pregnancies, resulting in uteroplacental hypoperfusion and eventually fetal growth restriction.

The pressor responses to infused catecholamines, epinephrine, and norepinephrine also are attenuated during normal pregnancy,[36] but they are increased in hypertensive pregnant women.[21] In contrast to angiotensin II, however, the uteroplacental vascular responses to α-agonists exceed those seen in the systemic vasculature,[36] that is, increases in uterine vascular resistance exceed simultaneous increases in systemic vascular resistance and perfusion pressure at all dosages of α-agonists (Fig. 11-5). This results in a decline in uterine blood flow at doses of α-agonists that minimally affect maternal blood pressure (Fig. 11-6) and is paralleled by decreases in placental blood flow. Thus, in contrast to angiotensin II, the maternal uteroplacental vascular bed is not protected from endogenous α-agonists, but remains sensitive to them. These differences are physiologically relevant. For example, it would be senseless to put the fetus at risk for placental hypoperfusion and decreased uterine oxygen delivery each time the pregnant woman rises from the supine position to standing and increases her plasma levels of angiotensin II. However, when she is at risk of losing her life (e.g., hemorrhage) and adrenal production and secretion of catecholamines are increased, it is physiologically sound to divert a significant proportion of the excessive volume of uteroplacental blood flow to tissues more relevant to maternal survival. During labor, however, circulating catecholamine levels are elevated and this enhanced responsiveness of the placental arteries to catecholamines might endanger the growth restricted or normally grown fetus whose margin of safety is borderline by decreasing uterine oxygen delivery to dangerous levels, resulting in fetal heart rate decelerations. This problem has been alluded to in Doppler ultrasound studies.[9]

Angiotensin II is a potent vasoconstrictor in the umbilicoplacental circulation.[37,38] It was previously believed that the fetus was more refractory to angiotensin II than the pregnant mother, resulting in the greater circulating levels in the fetus as compared with that of the mother.[38] We now know that the fetal clearance of angiotensin II is 10-fold greater than that in the mother, that 95% of fetal clearance occurs across the placental vascular bed, and that the umbilicoplacental vasculature is more sensitive to the vasoconstricting effects of this peptide than the uteroplacental circulation at similar plasma levels of angiotensin II (Fig. 11-7).[39] This difference between the umbilicoplacental and uteroplacental responses is explained by the predominance of type 1 angiotensin II receptors in the former, and type 2 receptors in the latter in both women and sheep.[29,32,40-42] Further, the umbilical artery smooth muscle demonstrates precocious maturation compared with findings in systemic arteries,[43] which primarily express the type 2 receptor.[40] In contrast, catecholamines minimally alter umbilicoplacental blood flow except at nonphysiologic doses,[44,45] and these decreases in placental perfusion may reflect a fall in fetal cardiac output rather than actual increases in placental vascular resistance. Thus, fetal responses to catecholamines are associated with the maintenance of umbilicoplacental perfusion as well as cerebral and myocardial blood flow. Finally, recent studies suggest that modifications in fetal arterial pressure by angiotensin II are actually due to its effects on umbilicoplacental resistance via type 1 receptors.[46,47]

Arginine vasopressin is a hypothalamic-pituitary hormone with increased secretion during episodes of intrauterine hypoxia and asphyxia.[48] As with adrenal catecholamines, which mediate the primary fetal responses to intrauterine "stress," umbilicoplacental perfusion is not affected substantially by vasopressin.[49] Thus, the maternal and fetal placental vascular beds respond differently to endogenous vasoconstrictors, likely reflecting important mechanisms necessary to ensure adequate fetal oxygen delivery and the survival of the fetus or the mother.

PROSTAGLANDINS

Interest has been considerable in the role of prostanoids in the control and maintenance of uteroplacental and umbilicoplacental blood flows. This interest is derived, in part, from observations in normotensive pregnant women and animals in whom circulating levels of prostanoids, especially vasodilating prostanoids, increase during gestation.[50, 51] In addition, systemic and local infusion of cyclooxygenase inhibitors in pregnant sheep increases both systemic and uterine responses to infused

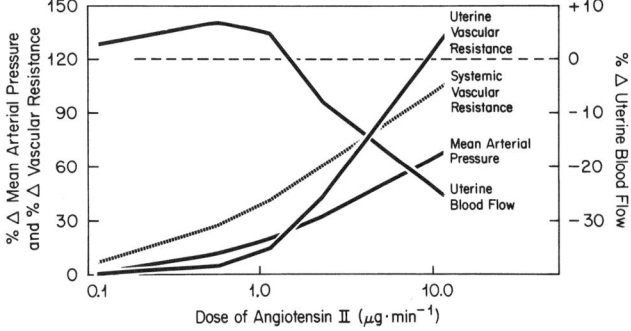

Figure 11–4. The relative changes in uterine blood flow, mean arterial pressure, systemic vascular resistance, and uterine vascular resistance during the systemic infusion of angiotensin II in pregnant sheep. (From Rosenfeld CR: Semin Perinatol *8*:42, 1984.)

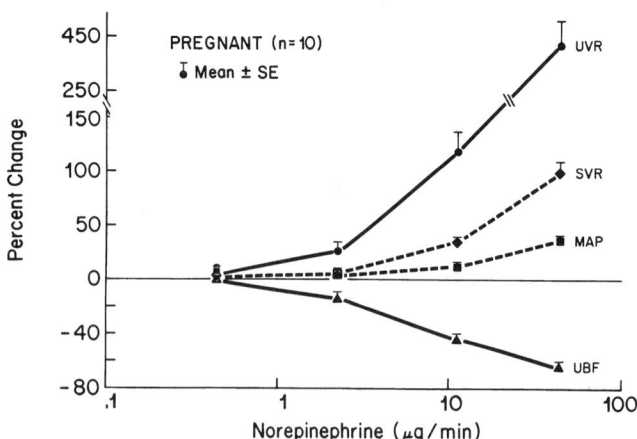

Figure 11–5. The relative changes in uterine blood flow (UBF), mean arterial pressure (MAP), systemic vascular resistance (SVR), and uterine vascular resistance (UVR) during the systemic infusion of norepinephrine in pregnant sheep. (From Magness RR, Rosenfeld CR: Am J Obstet Gynecol *155*:897, 1986.)

angiotensin II.[30] Furthermore, women with pregnancy-induced hypertension exhibit plasma levels of thromboxane (a potent vasoconstricting prostanoid) that exceed those of prostacyclin and that may account for the increased vascular reactivity seen in these women.[50] Because circulating levels of prostacyclin and thromboxane may be of placental origin, it has been suggested that these and other prostanoids may modulate the peripheral and the uterine circulations during pregnancies in normotensive and hypertensive mothers. This hypothesis, however, remains controversial. First, prostanoids may not be circulating hormones, but rather they mediate their effects through paracrine mechanisms. Thus, plasma levels probably provide little physiologic information. Second, increases in vessel perfusion or shear stress increase vascular production of prostacyclin.[52] Therefore, the rise in placental blood flow seen in normal pregnancy may be due to another mechanism, and the increase in prostanoid synthesis is a secondary phenomenon. Third, although cyclooxygenase inhibition enhances systemic and uterine vascular responsiveness in pregnant women and sheep, this does not alter basal uteroplacental blood flow commensurate with the fall in plasma prostaglandin levels.[30,53] Finally, in several studies of low-dose aspirin therapy, pregnancy-induced hypertension was neither ameliorated nor prevented.[54] Thus, the prostanoids may represent a class of stress hormones the primary role of which is to antagonize the vascular responses to increases in circulating placental vasoconstrictors, thereby protecting maternal uterine blood flow.

In the fetal compartment, similar controversy exists. Prostacyclin is a potent placental vasodilator, whereas prostaglandin E_2 (PGE_2) is a vasoconstrictor (in the maternal placental circulation it is a vasodilator). The physiologic role of these two prostanoids, however, is unclear. It was suggested that the differential effects of PGE_2 in the two placental vascular beds may act to autoregulate the two beds so that when umbilicoplacental blood flow falls, maternal placental perfusion increases to maintain fetal oxygen uptake and delivery.[45] More recently, it has been suggested that PGE_2 might potentiate the vasoconstriction seen with angiotensin II, whereas prostacyclin acts to antagonize these effects. These conclusions require further study.

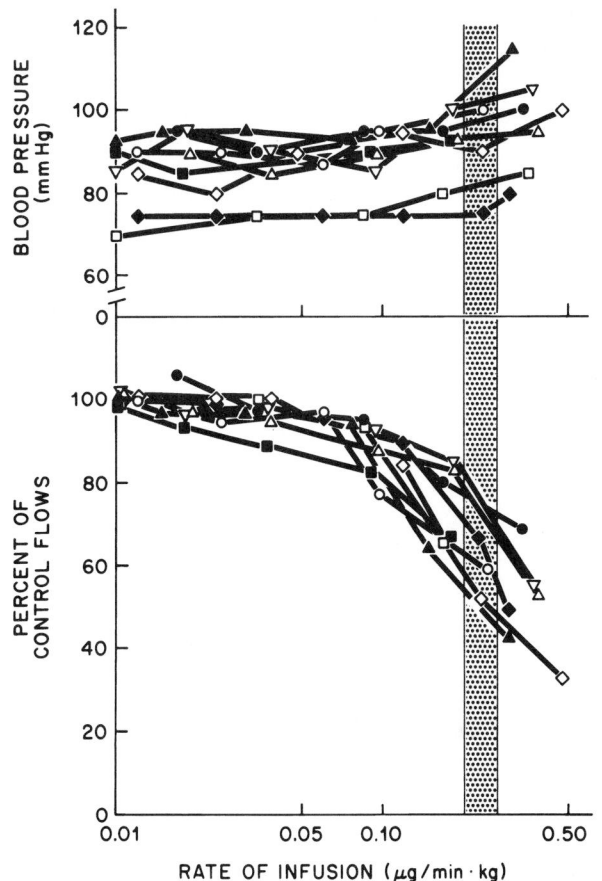

Figure 11–6. Responses of uterine blood flow and mean arterial pressure to increasing doses of norepinephrine. Uterine blood flow is represented as percentage of control flows. Symbols represent responses of separate animals. (From Rosenfeld CR, West J:Am J Obstet Gynecol *127*:376, 1977.)

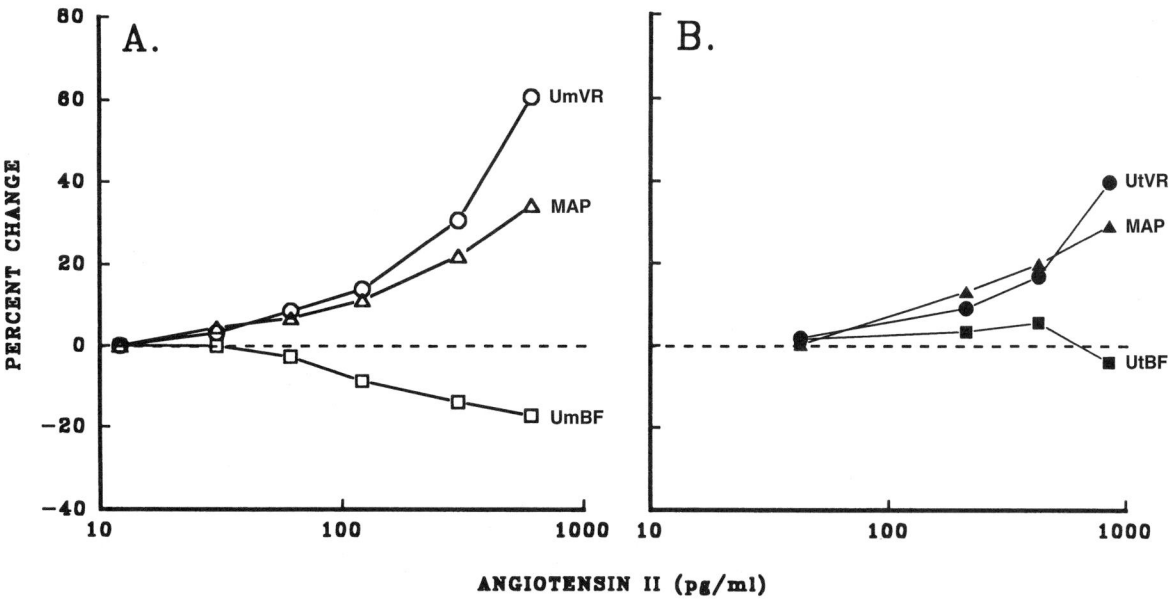

Figure 11–7. Comparison of the relative changes in blood flow, mean arterial pressure, and vascular resistance versus plasma levels of angiotensin II in the umbilicoplacental (**A**) and maternal uteroplacental (**B**) vascular beds during systemic infusions of angiotensin II. (From Rosenfeld CR, et al:Am J Physiol *268*:E237, 1995.)

NITRIC OXIDE

Ten years ago, an endothelium-derived relaxing factor (i.e., not a prostanoid) was identified and shown to promote vascular relaxation by activating smooth muscle guanylate cyclase and the synthesis of cyclic guanosine monophosphate (cGMP). This substance, now known to be nitric oxide, is the product of three isoforms of nitric oxide synthase that are expressed in endothelium and vascular smooth muscle. Evidence exists that nitric oxide synthesis is increased in normotensive pregnancies and may contribute to normal cardiovascular adaptation and increases in urinary or plasma levels of cGMP.[55] Further, maternal administration of a nitric oxide synthase inhibitor results in maternal hypertension and decreased levels of cGMP. Marked increases in uterine venous cGMP and uterine cGMP synthesis have also been observed in pregnant sheep, suggesting that nitric oxide may be essential to the growth in uteroplacental blood flow.[56] Although uterine artery synthesis of nitric oxide is increased in pregnancy, it is unclear what proportion of uterine cGMP synthesis is vascular or placental.[55, 57] Further, the role of nitric oxide in the maintenance or modulation of uteroplacental blood flow is unclear given that nitric oxide synthase inhibition decreases uteroplacental perfusion by no more than 25%.[56, 58]

Although studies of the role of nitric oxide in modulating and maintaining umbilicoplacental blood flow are extensive, it also is unclear to what extent nitric oxide is responsible.[55] Perfused human umbilical arteries and veins release more nitric oxide than prostacyclin.[59] Inhibition of nitric oxide synthase increases umbilicoplacental vascular resistance *in vitro,* and in intact fetal sheep, results in a nearly 50% fall in umbilical blood flow.[60] Increases in nitric oxide generation also attenuate constrictor responses to several agonists. Thus, nitric oxide appears to play an important role in both maintaining and modulating umbilicoplacental blood flow. Because inhibition of nitric oxide synthase does not decrease blood flow completely, nitric oxide may contribute to, but not be totally responsible for, maintaining umbilicoplacental perfusion.

STEROID HORMONES

The placenta is a major site of steroid hormone synthesis, in particular estrogen and progesterone. These hormones have vascular effects and may play an important role in promoting implantation and placentation[15] and modulating placental blood flow and other aspects of maternal cardiovascular adaptation during pregnancy. Unfortunately, few investigators have examined the role of these hormones on umbilicoplacental blood flow. In the ewe, estrogen vasodilates the nonpregnant (increasing blood flow 10- to 15-fold) and pregnant uterus (increasing blood flow by 40–50%).[61] Further, administration of dehydroepiandrosterone (the androgen precursor necessary for placental estrogen synthesis) to the fetus or the ewe increases placental estrogen production and uteroplacental blood flow.[61] No other naturally occurring substance has this effect on uteroplacental perfusion. Because the rise in uterine blood flow occurs in the absence of a change in perfusion pressure,[62] this is a true vasodilatory effect. Progesterone may act to antagonize and modulate these effects of estrogen. Thus, the two steroids may co-regulate the magnitude of maternal uteroplacental blood flow. The effects of estrogen on uterine blood flow are receptor mediated and involve activation and transcriptional regulation of type 1 and type 3 nitric oxide synthases,[63, 64] resulting in increased cGMP synthesis, activation of a cGMP-dependent kinase, and phosphorylation and activation of a potassium channel in uterine artery smooth muscle.[65] This has been observed in nonpregnant and pregnant sheep, and recent data suggest that this potassium channel (BK_{Ca}) also may modulate basal uteroplacental blood flow and the attenuated vasoconstrictor responses seen

in pregnancy.[16] Studies are under way to assess this in uterine arteries from women, which may result in new strategies for treating placental hyoperfusion in the future.

ACKNOWLEDGMENT

This work was supported in part by National Institutes of Health Grant HD-08783.

REFERENCES

1. King BF: The functional anatomy of the placental vasculature. *In* Rosenfeld CR (ed): The Uterine Circulation. Ithaca, Perinatology Press, 1989, pp 17–33.
2. Chez RA, et al: Effects of adrenergic agents on ovine umbilical and uterine blood flows. *In* Longo LD, Reneau DD (eds): Fetal and Newborn Cardiovascular Physiology, vol 2. New York, Garland STPM Press, 1978, pp 1–16.
3. Ehrenkranz RA, et al: Effect of ritodrine infusion on uterine and umbilical blood flow in pregnant sheep. Am J Obstet Gynecol 126:343, 1976.
4. Wilkening RB, et al: Placental transfer as a function of uterine blood flow. Am J Physiol 242:H429, 1982.
5. Wilkening RB: The role of uterine blood flow in fetal oxygen and nutrient delivery. *In* Rosenfeld CR (ed): The Uterine Circulation. Ithaca, Perinatology Press, 1989, pp 191–207.
6. Barker DJP: Fetal programming and public health. *In* O'Brien PMS, et al (eds): Fetal Programming. Influences on Development and Disease in Later Life. London, RCOG Press, 1999, pp 3–11.
7. Couzin J: Quirks of fetal environment felt decades later. Science 296:2167, 2002.
8. Greiss F: Uterine blood flow: an overview since Barcroft. *In* Rosenfeld CR (ed): The Uterine Circulation. Ithaca, Perinatology Press, 1989, pp 3–16.
9. Cohen-Overbeek TE, Campbell S: Doppler ultrasound techniques for the measurement of uterine and umbilical blood flow. *In* Rosenfeld CR (ed): The Uterine Circulation. Ithaca, Perinatology Press, 1989, pp 76–112.
10. Ramsey EM, et al: Serial and cineradioangiographic visualization of maternal circulation in the primate (hemochorial) placenta. Am J Obstet Gynecol 86:213, 1963.
11. Rosenfeld CR: Changes in uterine blood flow during pregnancy. *In* Rosenfeld CR (ed): The Uterine Circulation. Ithaca, Perinatology Press, 1989, pp 135–158.
12. Rosenfeld CR, et al: Circulatory changes in the reproductive tissues of ewes during pregnancy. Gynecol Invest 5:252, 1974.
13. Rosenfeld CR: Distribution of cardiac output in ovine pregnancy. Am J Physiol 232:H231, 1977.
14. Ford SP: Factors controlling uterine blood flow during estrus and early pregnancy. *In* Rosenfeld CR (ed): The Uterine Circulation. Ithaca, Perinatology Press, 1989, pp 113–134.
15. Paria BC, et al: Deciphering the cross-talk of implantation: Advances and challenges. Science 296:2185, 2002.
16. Rosenfeld CR, et al: Ca^{2+}-activated K^+ channels modulate basal and $E_2\beta$-induced rises in uterine blood flow in ovine pregnancy. Am J Physiol Heart Circ Physiol 281:H22, 2001.
17. Rosenfeld CR: Consideration of the uteroplacental circulation in intrauterine growth. Semin Perinatol 8:42, 1984.
18. Teasdale F: Numerical density of nuclei in the sheep placenta. Anat Rec 185:187, 1976.
19. Meschia G, et al: Simultaneous measurements of uterine and umbilical blood flows and oxygen uptakes. J Exp Physiol 52:1, 1967.
20. Kulhanek JF, et al: Changes in DNA content and urea permeability of sheep placenta. Am J Physiol 226:1257, 1974.
21. Chesley LC, et al: Vascular reactivity to angiotensin II and norepinephrine in pregnant and nonpregnant women. Am J Obstet Gynecol 91:837, 1965.
22. Gant NF, et al: A study of angiotensin II pressor response throughout primigravid pregnancy. J Clin Invest 52:2682, 1973.
23. Rosenfeld CR, Gant NF Jr: The chronically instrumented ewe, a model for studying vascular reactivity to angiotensin II in pregnancy. J Clin Invest 67:486, 1981.
24. Rosenfeld CR: Mechanisms regulating angiotensin II responsiveness by the uteroplacental circulation. Am J Physiol Regul Integr Comp Physiol 281:R1025, 2001.
25. Naden RP, Rosenfeld CR: Effect of angiotensin II on uterine and systemic vasculature in pregnant sheep. J Clin Invest 68:468, 1981.
26. Erkkola RU, Pirhonen JP: Uterine and umbilical flow velocity waveforms in normotensive and hypertensive subjects during the angiotensin II sensitivity test. Am J Obstet Gynecol 166:910, 1992.
27. Rosenfeld CR, Naden RP: Responses of uterine and nonuterine tissues to angiotensin II in ovine pregnancy. Am J Physiol 257:H17, 1989.
28. Magness RR, Rosenfeld CR: Calcium modulation of endothelium-derived prostacyclin production in ovine pregnancy. Endocrinology 132:2445, 1993.
29. Cox BE, et al: Tissue specific expression of vascular smooth muscle angiotensin II receptor subtypes during ovine pregnancy. Am J Physiol 271:H212, 1996.
30. Magness RR, et al: Uterine prostaglandin production in ovine pregnancy: effects of angiotensin II and indomethacin. Am J Physiol 263:H188, 1992.
31. Magness RR, et al: *In vitro* prostacyclin production by uterine arteries of normotensive and hypertensive pregnant women. Proceedings of the International Society for the Study of Hypertension in Pregnancy, Montreal, Quebec, Canada, March 22–26, 1988.

32. Cox BE, et al: Angiotensin II receptor characteristics and subtype expression in uterine arteries and myometrium during pregnancy. J Clin Endocrinol Metab 81:49, 1996.
33. Cox BE, et al: Angiotensin II indirectly vasoconstricts the ovine uterine circulation. Am J Physiol 278:R337, 2000.
34. McMullen JR, et al: Interactions between AT₁ and AT₂ receptors in uterine arteries from pregnant ewes. Eur J Pharmacol 378:195, 1999.
35. Magness RR, et al: Endothelial vasodilator production by uterine and systemic arteries. I. Effects of ANG II on PGI₂ and NO in pregnancy. Am J Physiol 270:H1914, 1996.
36. Magness RR, Rosenfeld CR: Systemic and uterine responses to α-adrenergic stimulation in pregnant and nonpregnant ewes. Am J Obstet Gynecol 155:897, 1986.
37. Iwamoto HS, Rudolph AM: Effects of angiotensin II on the blood flow and its distribution in fetal lambs. Circ Res 48:183, 1981.
38. Yoshimura T, et al: Angiotensin II and α-agonist: I. Responses of ovine fetoplacental vasculature. Am J Physiol 259:H464, 1990.
39. Rosenfeld CR, et al: Comparison of ANG II in fetal and pregnant sheep: metabolic clearance and vascular reactivity. Am J Physiol 268:E237, 1995.
40. Cox BE, Rosenfeld CR: Ontogeny of vascular angiotensin II receptor subtype expression in ovine development. Pediatr Res 45:414, 1999.
41. Kalenga MK, et al: Les recepteurs de l'angiotensine II dans le placenta humain sont de type AT₁. Reprod Nutr Dev 31:257, 1991.
42. Knock GA, et al: Angiotensin II (AT₁) vascular binding sites in human placentae from normal-term, preeclamptic and growth retarded pregnancies. JPET 271:1007, 1994.
43. Arens Y, et al: Differential development of umbilical and systemic arteries: II. Contractile proteins. Am J Physiol 274:R1815, 1998.
44. Berman W Jr, et al: Effects of pharmacologic agents on umbilical blood flow in fetal lambs in utero. Biol Neonate 33:225, 1978.
45. Rankin JHG: Interaction between the maternal and fetal placental blood flows. In Rosenfeld CR (ed): The Uterine Circulation. Ithaca, Perinatology Press, 1989, pp 175–190.
46. Kaiser JR, et al: Differential development of umbilical and systemic arteries: I. ANG II receptor subtype expression. Am J Physiol 274:R797, 1998.
47. Adamson SL, et al: Vasomotor responses of the umbilical circulation in fetal sheep. Am J Physiol 256:R1056, 1989.
48. Rosenfeld CR, Porter JC: Arginine vasopressin in the developing fetus. In Albrecht E, Pepe GJ (eds): Research in Perinatal Medicine (IV). Perinatal Endocrinology. Ithaca, Perinatology Press, 1985, pp 91–103.
49. Iwamoto HS, et al: Hemodynamic responses of the sheep fetus to vasopressin infusion. Circ Res 44:430, 1979.
50. Walsh SW, Parisi VM: The role of prostanoids and thromboxane in the regulation of placental blood flow. In Rosenfeld CR (ed): The Uterine Circulation. Ithaca, Perinatology Press, 1989, pp 274–299.
51. Magness RR, et al: Uteroplacental production of eicosanoids in ovine pregnancy. Prostaglandins 39:75, 1990.
52. Frangos JA, et al: Flow effects on prostacyclin production by cultured human endothelial cells. Science 227:1477, 1985.
53. Naden RP, et al: Hemodynamic effects of indomethacin in chronically instrumented pregnant sheep. Am J Obstet Gynecol 151:484, 1985.
54. Italian Study of Aspirin in Pregnancy: Low-dose aspirin in prevention and treatment of intrauterine growth retardation and pregnancy-induced hypertension. Lancet 341:396, 1993.
55. Sladek SM, et al: Nitric oxide and pregnancy. Am J Physiol 272:R441, 1997.
56. Rosenfeld CR, et al: Nitric oxide contributes to estrogen-induced vasodilation of the ovine uterine circulation. J Clin Invest 98:2158, 1996.
57. Conrad KP: Expression of nitric oxide synthase by syncytiotrophobast in human placental villi. FASEB J 7:1268, 1993.
58. Miller SL, et al: Effect of nitric oxide synthase inhibition on the uterine vasculature of the late-pregnant ewe. Am J Obstet Gynecol 180:1138, 1999.
59. Chaudhuri G, et al: NO is more important than PGI₂ in maintaining low vascular tone in feto-placental vessels. Am J Physiol 265:H2036, 1993.
60. Chang J-K, et al: Effect of endothelium-derived relaxing factor inhibition on the umbilical-placental circulation in fetal lambs in utero. Am J Obstet Gynecol 166:727, 1992.
61. Magness RR, Rosenfeld CR: The role of steroid hormones in the control of uterine blood flow. In Rosenfeld CR (ed): The Uterine Circulation. Ithaca, Perinatology Press, 1989, pp 239–273.
62. Magness RR, Rosenfeld CR: Local and systemic estradiol-12β: effects on uterine and systemic vasodilation. Am J Physiol 256:E536, 1989.
63. Salhab W, et al: Regulation of type I and type III nitric oxide synthases by daily and acute estrogen exposure. Am J Physiol Heart Circ Physiol 278:H2134, 2000.
64. Vagnoni KE, et al: Endothelial vasodilator production by uterine and systemic arteries. III. Ovarian and estrogen effects on NO synthase. Am J Physiol Heart Circ Physiol 275:H1845, 1998.
65. Rosenfeld CR: Calcium-activated potassium channels and nitric oxide coregulate estrogen-induced vasodilation. Am J Physiol Heart Circ Physiol 279:H319, 2000.

Julian N. Robinson and Errol R. Norwitz

12 Pathophysiology of Preterm Birth

Labor is the physiologic process by which the products of conception are passed from the uterus to the outside world; it is common to all viviparous species. The classical definition of labor includes an increase in myometrial activity or, more precisely, a switch in the myometrial contractility pattern from irregular so-called contractures (long-lasting, low-frequency activity) to regular contractions (high-intensity, high-frequency activity) leading to effacement or dilatation of the uterine cervix.[1,2] An initial cervical examination of 2-cm dilatation or more and/or 80% or higher effacement in the setting of regular phasic uterine contractions is also accepted as being sufficient for the diagnosis of labor.[3] A bloody discharge (show) is often included in the description of labor, but it is not a prerequisite for the diagnosis. In normal labor, there appears to be a time-dependent relationship between the biochemical connective tissue changes in the cervix that usually precede uterine contractions and cervical dilatation. All these events usually occur before rupture of the membranes.[4]

The mean duration of singleton pregnancy is 40 weeks (280 days) dated from the first day of the last menstrual period. *Term* is defined as two standard deviations from the mean or, more precisely, 37 to 42 completed weeks (266–294 days) of gestation. *Preterm (premature) labor* is defined as labor occurring before 37 completed weeks' gestation.[5]

Preterm birth occurs in 7 to 12% of all deliveries but accounts for over 85% of all perinatal morbidity and mortality.[6,7] Although the ability of physicians to identify women at risk for preterm delivery has improved, overall incidence of preterm birth has not decreased in the last 40 years. Indeed, recent studies have shown that the incidence of preterm delivery in the United States has been increasing steadily from 9.4% in 1981 to 11.8% in 1999.[8] This increase in preterm births and low birth weight infants has been attributed to a combination of factors, including increasing use of early ultrasound dating, preterm induction and preterm cesarean delivery without labor, and an increase in multiple births resulting from assisted reproduction technologies.[8] Preterm birth is now the second leading cause of neonatal mortality in the United States (second only to congenital birth defects),[9] and preterm labor is the cause of most preterm births.[10] Improvements in neonatal intensive care have improved survival rates for babies at the limit of viability, but they have also increased the proportion of survivors with disabilities.[11] A better understanding of the molecular mechanisms responsible for the process of labor, both at term and preterm, will improve our ability to identify and manage women at risk of premature delivery.

ONSET OF LABOR

Historical Perspective

Considerable evidence suggests that, in most viviparous animals, the fetus controls the timing of labor.[2, 12-17] Horse-donkey cross-breeding experiments performed in the 1950s, for example, resulted in a gestational length intermediate between that of horses (340 days) and donkeys (365 days), thereby suggesting a role for the fetal genotype in the initiation of labor.[14, 17] The hypothesis that the fetus is in control of the timing of labor has been elegantly demonstrated in domestic ruminants and involves activation at term of the fetal hypothalamopituitary-adrenal axis leading to a surge in adrenal cortisol production.[13, 17-19] Fetal cortisol then acts to directly up-regulate the activity of placental CYP17 (17α-hydroxylase/17,20-lyase) enzyme, which catalyzes the conversion of pregnenolone to estradiol-17β. The switch in progesterone:estrogen ratio provides the impetus for uterine prostaglandin $F_{2\alpha}$ ($PGF_{2\alpha}$) production and labor. However, human placentas lack glucocorticoid-inducible CYP17, which is critical to this pathway.[14] As such, this mechanism does not apply in humans. The slow progress in our understanding of the biochemical mechanisms involved in the process of labor in humans reflects in large part the difficulty in extrapolating from the endocrine-control mechanisms in various animals to the paracrine-autocrine mechanisms of parturition in humans, processes that, in humans, preclude direct investigation.

Labor at Term

To understand preterm labor, it is important to first understand the factors responsible for the onset of labor at term. The last few decades have seen a marked change in the nature of the hypotheses to explain the onset of labor. Initial investigations centered on changes in the profile of circulating hormone levels in the maternal and fetal circulations (i.e., endocrine events). More recent studies have focused on the dynamic biochemical dialogue that exists between the fetus and the mother (i.e., paracrine-autocrine events) in an attempt to understand in detail the molecular mechanisms that regulate such interactions.

Labor at term may best be regarded physiologically as a release from the inhibitory effects of pregnancy on the myometrium rather than as an active process mediated by uterine stimulants.[20] Strips of quiescent term myometrial tissue placed in an isotonic water bath contract vigorously and spontaneously without added stimuli.[20, 21] *In vivo*, however, it appears that both mechanisms may be important.[22-24] During pregnancy, the uterine musculature is maintained in a state of functional quiescence through the action of various putative inhibitors including, but not limited to, progesterone, prostacyclin (PGI_2), relaxin, parathyroid hormone–related peptide, nitric oxide, calcitonin gene–related peptide, adrenomedullin, and vasoactive intestinal peptide. Regardless of whether the trigger for labor begins within or outside the fetus, the final common pathway for labor ends in the maternal tissues of the uterus and is characterized by increased expression of a series of contraction-associated proteins, including myometrial receptors for prostaglandins and oxytocin, activation of select ion channels, and an increase in connexin-43 (a key component of gap junctions). An increase in gap junctions between adjacent myometrial cells establishes electrical synchrony within the myometrium, thereby allowing for effective coordination of contractions. As in other smooth muscles, myometrial contractions are mediated through the adenosine triphosphatase–dependent binding of myosin to actin. In contrast to vascular smooth muscle, however, myometrial cells have a sparse innervation, which is further reduced during pregnancy.[25] The regulation of the contractile mechanism of the uterus is therefore largely humoral and/or dependent on intrinsic factors within myometrial cells.

It is likely that a so-called parturition cascade exists in the human (Fig. 12-1) which is responsible, at term, for the removal of mechanisms maintaining uterine quiescence and for the recruitment of factors acting to promote uterine activity.[2] In such a model, each element is connected to the next in a sequential fashion, and many of these elements demonstrate positive feed-forward characteristics typical of a cascade mechanism. The sequential recruitment of signals that serve to augment the labor process suggest that it may not be possible to single out any one signaling mechanism as being responsible for the initiation of labor. It may therefore be prudent to describe such mechanisms as being responsible for *promoting*, rather than *initiating*, the process of labor.[26]

A comprehensive analysis of each of the individual paracrine-autocrine pathways implicated in the process of labor has been reviewed in detail elsewhere.[2, 12-18, 23] In brief, human labor at term is a multifactorial physiologic event involving an integrated set of changes within the maternal tissues of the uterus (myometrium, decidua, and uterine cervix) that occur gradually over a period of days to weeks. Such changes include an increase in prostaglandin synthesis and release within the uterus, an increase in myometrial gap junction formation, and up-regulation of myometrial oxytocin receptors. After the myometrium and cervix are prepared, endocrine and/or paracrine-autocrine factors from the fetoplacental unit bring about a switch in the pattern of myometrial activity from irregular contractures to regular contractions. The fetus may coordinate this switch in myometrial activity through its influence on placental steroid hormone production, through mechanical distention of the uterus, and through secretion of neurohypophyseal hormones and other stimulators of prostaglandin synthesis. The final common pathway toward labor appears to be activation of the fetal hypothalamopituitary-adrenal axis, and is probably common to all species. In sheep, this results in an increase in circulating cortisol levels; whereas, in the human, the result is an increase in circulating C-19 steroid (dehydroepiandrosterone) from the intermediate (fetal) zone of the fetal adrenal. This is because the human placenta is an incomplete steroidogenic organ and estrogen synthesis by the human placenta has an obligate need for C-19 steroid precursor[16] (see Fig. 12-1). In the rhesus monkey, infusion of C19 precursor (androstenedione) leads to preterm delivery.[27] This effect is blocked by concurrent infusion of an aromatase inhibitor,[28] demonstrating that conversion to estrogen is important. However, systemic infusion of estrogen fails to induce delivery, suggesting that the action of estrogen is likely paracrine-autocrine based.[27, 29, 30]

PRETERM LABOR

Etiology of Preterm Labor

Preterm labor likely represents a syndrome rather than a diagnosis because its etiologies are varied. Indeed, several investigators have suggested replacing the term *preterm labor* with "preterm birth syndrome." Approximately 20% of preterm deliveries are iatrogenic and are performed for maternal or fetal indications, including intrauterine growth restriction, preeclampsia, placenta previa, and nonreassuring fetal testing.[10] Of the remaining cases of preterm birth, around 30% occur in the setting of preterm premature rupture of the membranes, 20 to 25% result from intra-amniotic infection, and the remaining 25 to 30% are due to spontaneous (unexplained) preterm labor.

Spontaneous preterm labor may reflect a breakdown in the normal mechanisms responsible for maintaining uterine quiescence. For example, the choriodecidua is selectively enriched

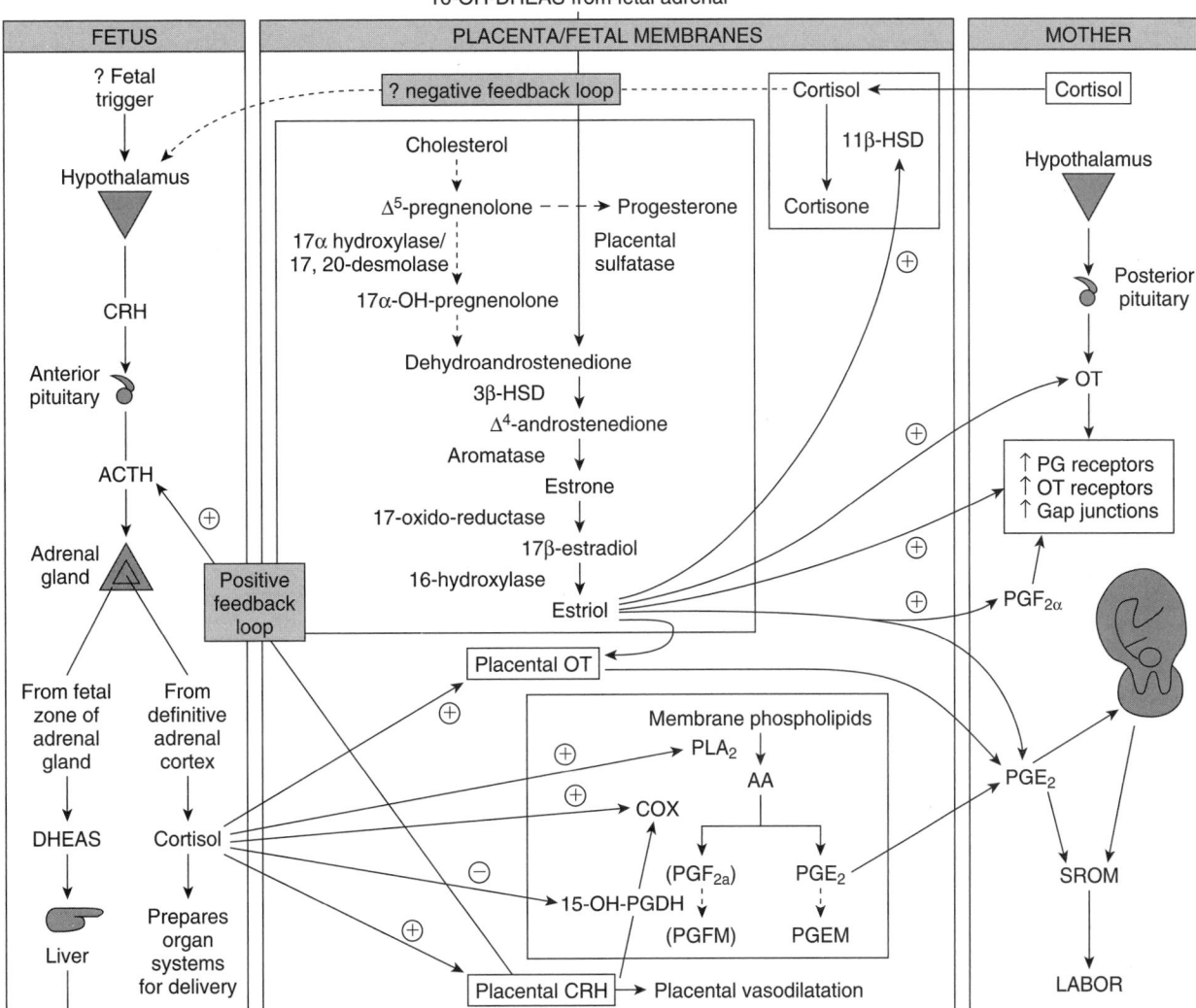

Figure 12–1. Proposed mechanism of labor induction at term. This graphic incorporates the various hormones and paracrine-autocrine factors responsible for promoting uterine contractions at term in an integrated "parturition cascade." (Adapted with permission from Norwitz ER, et al.[23]) AA = arachidonic acid; ACTH = adrenocorticotropic hormone; COX = cyclooxygenase; CRH = corticotropin-releasing hormone; DHEAS = dehydroepiandrosterone sulfate; 3β-HSD = 3β-hydroxy-steroid dehydrogenase; 11β-HSD = 11β-hydroxysteroid dehydrogenase; 15-OH-PGDH = 15-hydroxy-prostaglandin dehydrogenase; OT = oxytocin; PG = prostaglandin; PGE_2 = prostaglandin E_2; PGEM = 13,14-dihydro-15-keto-prostaglandin E_2; $PGF_{2\alpha}$ = prostaglandin $F_{2\alpha}$; PGFM = 13,14-dihydro-15-keto-prostaglandin $F_{2\alpha}$; PLA_2 = phospholipase A_2; SROM = spontaneous rupture of fetal membranes.

with 15-hydroxy-prostaglandin dehydrogenase (15-OH PGDH), the enzyme responsible for degrading the primary prostaglandins. A deficiency in choriodecidual 15-OH PGDH activity may impair the ability of the fetal membranes to metabolize the primary prostaglandins, thereby allowing PGE_2 and lesser amounts of $PGF_{2\alpha}$ to reach the myometrium and initiate contractions. Such a deficiency has been described and may account for up to 15% of instances of idiopathic preterm labor.[12] Alternatively, spontaneous premature labor may represent a short-circuiting or overwhelming of the normal parturition cascade (Fig. 12–2). Indeed, an important feature of the proposed parturition cascade is the ability of the fetoplacental unit to trigger labor prematurely if the intrauterine environment becomes hostile and threatens the well-being of the fetus. For example, up to 25% of preterm labors are thought to result from intraamniotic infection.[10, 31, 32] In many patients with infection,

elevated levels of lipoxygenase and cyclooxygenase pathway products can be demonstrated.[32–34] There are also increased concentrations of cytokines (including interleukin-1β, interleukin-6, and tumor necrosis factor-α) in the amniotic fluid of such women. Cytokines and eicosanoids appear to interact and to accelerate each other's production in a cascadelike fashion, which may act to overwhelm the normal parturition cascade, resulting in preterm labor. Thrombin has been shown to be a powerful uterotonic agent,[35] providing a physiologic mechanism for preterm labor secondary to placental abruption.

Prediction of Preterm Labor

Identification of women at high-risk of preterm delivery is an important goal of modern obstetric management, due to the dramatic consequences of preterm birth and the relatively ineffective treatment options for preterm labor after it occurs. Screening tests for prediction of preterm birth can be divided into four general categories: risk factor scoring, home uterine monitoring, assessment of cervical maturation, and measurements of endocrine-biochemical markers. Numerous risk factors for preterm birth have been identified (Table 12–1), some of which are modifiable (e.g., cigarette smoking, illicit drug use) whereas others are not (e.g., African-American race, maternal age). Several risk factor–based scoring protocols based primarily on historical factors, epidemiologic factors, and daily habits have been developed in an attempt to identify women at risk. However, reliance on risk factor–based screening protocols alone will fail to identify over 50% of pregnancies that end in preterm delivery, and most women who screen positive will ultimately deliver at term.[36, 37] As such, risk factor–based screening protocols have largely fallen out of favor. Similarly, although an increase in uterine activity is a prerequisite for preterm labor, home uterine monitoring of women at high risk of preterm delivery has not been shown to reduce the incidence of preterm birth.[38, 39] However, this approach has been shown to increase visits to the labor and delivery floor, obstetric intervention, and the cost of prepartum care.[38]

Cervical effacement is a prerequisite for preterm birth. Serial digital evaluation of the cervix in women at risk for preterm delivery is useful if the examination remains normal. However, an abnormal cervical finding (shortening alone, or in combination with dilatation) is associated with preterm delivery in only 4% of low-risk women and 12 to 20% of high-risk women.[40] Real-time sonographic evaluation of the cervix, conversely, has demonstrated a strong inverse correlation between cervical length and preterm delivery.[41, 42] If the cervical length is below the 10th percentile for gestational age, the pregnancy is at a sixfold increased

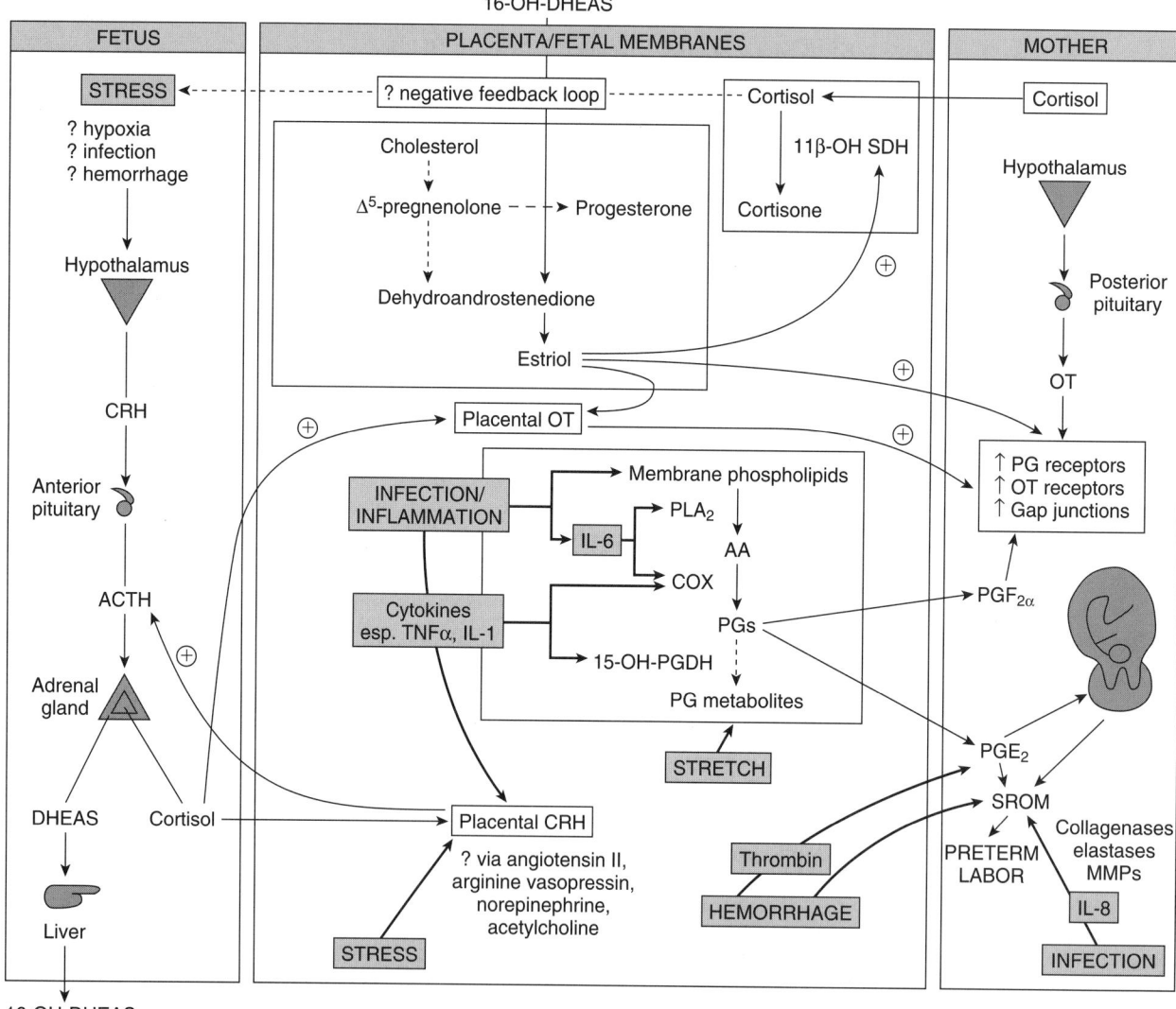

Figure 12–2. Proposed mechanisms of preterm labor. This graphic shows how various factors (including infection, stress, hemorrhage, and uterine stretch) may overwhelm or short-circuit the normal "parturition cascade," leading to preterm labor. (Adapted with permission from Norwitz ER, et al.[23]) AA = arachidonic acid; ACTH = adrenocorticotropic hormone; COX = cyclooxygenase; CRH = corticotropin-releasing hormone; DHEAS = dehydroepiandrosterone sulfate; 3β-HSD = 3β-hydroxy-steroid dehydrogenase; 11β-HSD = 11β-hydroxysteroid dehydrogenase; IL-1 = interleukin-1; IL-6 = interleukin-6; IL-8 = interleukin-8; 15-OH-PGDH = 15-hydroxyprostaglandin dehydrogenase; MMPs = metalloproteinases; OT = oxytocin; PG = prostaglandin; PGE$_2$ = prostaglandin E$_2$; PGEM = 13,14-dihydro-15-keto-prostaglandin E$_2$; PGF$_{2\alpha}$ = prostaglandin F$_{2\alpha}$; PGFM = 13,14-dihydro-15-keto-prostaglandin F$_{2\alpha}$; PLA$_2$ = phospholipase A$_2$; SROM = spontaneous rupture of fetal membranes; TNFα = tumor necrosis factor-α.

risk of delivery before 35 weeks' gestation.[41] A cervical length of 15 mm or less at 23 weeks occurs in fewer than 2% of low-risk women but is predictive of delivery before 28 weeks and 32 weeks in 60% and 90% of cases, respectively.[42] Whether obstetric interventions such as cervical cerclage or prophylactic tocolysis can modify the risk of preterm delivery associated with cervical shortening remains controversial.

Several biochemical markers have been associated with preterm birth, including activin, inhibin, follistatin,[43, 44] fetal fibronectin,[45-47] collagenase,[48] and tissue inhibitors of metallo-proteinases.[49] To date, fetal fibronectin is the only clinically established biochemical screening test for preterm delivery. Elevated levels of fetal fibronectin in cervicovaginal secretions, which may reflect separation of the fetal membranes from the maternal decidua,[45] are associated with premature delivery. However, in a low-risk population, the positive predictive value of a positive fibronectin test at 22 to 24 weeks' gestation for spontaneous preterm delivery before 28 weeks and 37 weeks was only 13% and 36%, respectively.[46] The value of this test may lie in its negative predictive value (99% of patients with a negative fetal fibronectin test do not deliver within 7 days[47]), which may prevent unnecessary hospitalization.

Despite initial disappointments, there has been a recent resurgence of interest in developing endocrine assays to predict preterm labor. Progesterone withdrawal is not a prerequisite for labor in humans and serum progesterone levels or progesterone/estradiol-17β ratios are not predictive of preterm labor. Maternal serum estriol levels, however, accurately reflect activation of the fetal hypothalamopituitary-adrenal axis that occurs before the onset of labor, both at term and preterm.[50] Salivary estriol accurately mirrors the level of biologically active (unconjugated) estriol in the circulation.[51] The detection of elevated levels of estriol in maternal saliva (2.1 ng/mL or more) is predictive of delivery before 37 weeks' gestation in a high-risk population with a sensitivity of 68% to 87%, a specificity of 77%, and a false-positive rate of 23%.[52,53] Several other endocrine predictors of preterm delivery are currently under investigation, including relaxin[54] and corticotropin-releasing hormone.[55, 56]

Prevention of Preterm Labor

Guidelines for the prevention of preterm labor are summarized in Table 12–2. Although numerous risk factors for preterm delivery have been identified (see Table 12–1), it remains unclear whether modification or treatment of these risk factors will affect the overall incidence of preterm birth. It is generally accepted that

TABLE 12–1

Risk Factors for Preterm Delivery

Nonmodifiable Risk Factors	Modifiable Risk Factors
Prior preterm birth	Cigarette smoking
African-American race	Illicit drug use
Age < 18 or > 40 years	Anemia
Poor nutrition	Bacteriuria/urinary tract infection
Low pre-pregnancy weight	Genital infection
Low socioeconomic status	?? Strenuous work
Absent prenatal care	?? High personal stress
Cervical injury or anomaly	
Uterine anomaly or fibroid	
Excessive uterine activity	
Premature cervical dilatation (>2 cm) or effacement (>80%)	
Overdistended uterus (twins, polyhydramnios)	
? Vaginal bleeding	

regular prenatal care is associated with a decrease in the incidence of preterm birth. In 1993, the March of Dimes Multicenter Prematurity Prevention Trial conducted a randomized, controlled trial of 2,395 women at high risk for preterm birth in which women were randomized to either standard of care or enhanced care intervention (which included more frequent prenatal visits, improved patient education regarding signs of preterm labor, and weekly pelvic examinations after 20–24 weeks).[57] There was no significant difference in spontaneous preterm birth rates between the two groups. The authors concluded that "studied interventions are not recommended for similar populations." Bed rest is often recommended for women at high-risk for preterm birth at an estimated cost of over $250 million per year. Even though bed rest has been shown to improve uteroplacental blood flow leading to a slight increase in birth weight, it has not been shown to decrease the incidence of preterm delivery.[58]

The most contentious issue involves screening and treatment of genital infections. Lower genital tract infections (including bacterial vaginosis, *Neisseria gonorrhoeae*, *Chlamydia trachomatis*, Group B *Streptococcus*, *Ureaplasma urealyticum*, and *Trichomonas vaginalis*) have been associated with preterm delivery. Such infections may serve as a marker of upper genital tract infection or may lead to direct migration of organisms to the decidua, fetal membranes, and amniotic fluid. Bacterial vaginosis, for example, complicates 12 to 22% of all pregnancies and is strongly associated with preterm delivery.[59] There is a 40% increased incidence of very low birth weight infants born to women with untreated bacterial vaginosis,[59] and antibiotic treatment has been shown to decrease the rate of preterm labor and premature birth by 33 to 70%.[60,61] It is clear from these studies' results that women with symptomatic bacterial vaginosis should be treated. Whether to screen all asymptomatic women for bacterial vaginosis, however, remains unclear. Indeed, several large prospective randomized controlled trials have suggested that screening and treating asymptomatic women for bacterial vaginosis may be associated with a paradoxical increased risk of preterm birth.[62] As such, this approach has been abandoned.

Obstetric Management of Preterm Labor

The last decade has seen a remarkable transformation in the obstetric management of the parturient with preterm labor. During the 1990s, most authors advocated aggressive short- and long-term tocolysis, maternal bed rest, hydration, and antibiotics, combined with corticosteroid therapy for fetal lung maturation. However, many of these therapies have now been found to be of little benefit and are associated with substantial cost and increased maternal morbidity. For this reason, the current recommendations are far more limited, with short-term tocolysis (<48 hours) to facilitate corticosteroid therapy and possible transfer of the mother to a tertiary care center before delivery.[63]

Guidelines for the management of preterm labor are summarized in Table 12–3. A definitive diagnosis of preterm labor is mandatory before any treatment is initiated. Preterm labor remains a clinical diagnosis and includes regular phasic uterine contractions with progressive cervical effacement and/or

TABLE 12–2

Guidelines for the Prevention of Preterm Delivery

- Prevention and early diagnosis of sexually transmitted diseases and genitourinary infections
- Stop smoking and substance abuse
- Cervical cerclage, if indicated
- Prevention of multifetal pregnancies
- Workforce policies for select women (such as flexible schedules, rest breaks)

dilatation before 37 completed weeks of gestation. Cervical dilatation in the absence of uterine contractions is seen most commonly in the second trimester and is suggestive of cervical incompetence. In this setting, cervical cerclage is the treatment of choice. Similarly, the presence of uterine contractions in the absence of cervical change should be referred to as "premature uterine contractions" or "false labor" but does not meet criteria for the diagnosis of preterm labor. As such, treating such women for preterm labor is likely to be effective, irrespective of the therapeutic regimen selected. The argument that treatment should be initiated before there is evidence of cervical change to prevent the cervix from effacing and dilating is not supported by the literature, and likely represents recollection bias by practitioners who have had great success in treating women with premature uterine contractions.

In many instances, premature labor represents a necessary escape of the fetus from a hostile intrauterine environment and, as such, aggressive intervention to stop labor may be counterproductive. Every effort should be made to exclude contraindications to expectant management and/or tocolysis, including intrauterine infection, unexplained vaginal bleeding, nonreassuring fetal testing results, and intrauterine fetal demise. Indeed, evidence of nonreassuring fetal testing results may prompt emergent cesarean delivery rather than tocolysis. Intraamniotic fluid infection is a clinical diagnosis with evidence of fetal tachycardia, uterine tenderness and contractions, maternal tachycardia, and maternal fever, usually in the setting of an elevated white cell count. Amniocentesis with culture-proven amniotic fluid infection remains the standard criterion for the diagnosis, but it is of limited clinical value because laboratory results usually take a few days to come back. Amniotic fluid Gram stain may be useful but has a sensitivity only of around 50%.[64]

Bed rest and hydration are commonly recommended for the treatment of preterm labor, but without proven efficacy.[58, 65] Although substantial data indicate that broad spectrum antibiotic therapy can prolong latency in the setting of preterm premature rupture of the membranes remote from term, there is no consistent evidence that such an approach can delay delivery in women with preterm labor and intact membranes.[63,66,67]

Pharmacologic therapy remains the cornerstone of modern management. Ethanol (which inhibits oxytocin release from the posterior pituitary) was the first effective tocolytic agent,[68] but adverse maternal side-effects have severely limited its use. Although several alternative agents are now available (Table 12-4), no reliable data suggest that any of these agents are able to delay premature delivery for longer than 48 to 72 hours. Given that no single agent has a clear therapeutic advantage, the side-effect profile of each of the drugs will often determine which to use in a given clinical setting.[2,69-71] Magnesium sulfate (which acts both to suppress nerve transmission to uterine smooth muscle and to lower the concentration of intracellular calcium within myometrial cells, which is necessary for activation of the myosin-actin contractile unit) has a wide margin of safety and, as such, has become the first-line agent for use in preterm labor in North America.[72] β-Adrenergic agonists (which reduce intracellular

calcium levels and decrease the sensitivity of the myosin-actin contractile unit to available calcium through an adenyl cyclase/cyclic adenosine monophosphate–dependent mechanism) are also commonly used. Indeed, ritodrine hydrochloride is the only agent that has received approval from the Food and Drug Administration for the treatment of preterm labor. However, such agents have a higher incidence of major adverse effects compared with magnesium.[73] Nifedipine (a dihydropyridine calcium entry blocker) is as effective as magnesium and β-adrenergic agonists in delaying preterm delivery and is associated with fewer maternal side effects.[74, 75] The major concern limiting the use of calcium channel–blocking agents, however, is the reported adverse effect on uteroplacental blood flow. Prostaglandin synthesis inhibitors such as indomethacin, although capable of delaying premature birth,[76] have been associated with certain serious neonatal complications especially if given shortly before delivery.[77] Promising newer agents include potassium channel openers[78] and oxytocin receptor antagonists,[79] although published reports on the efficacy of the oxytocin receptor antagonist, 1-deamino-2-D-tyr-(OEt)-4-thr-8-orn-vasotocin/oxytocin (Atosiban), in the treatment of preterm labor have been disappointing, showing it to be no more effective than other tocolytics.[80,81]

Maintenance tocolytic therapy longer than 48 hours has not been shown to confer any therapeutic benefit, but it does pose a significant risk of adverse side-effects. In a meta-analysis of 16 randomized trials conducted through the mid-1980's, King and co-workers[82] found only modest prolongation of pregnancy (24-48 hours) and no improvement in neonatal outcome. More recent trials including aggressive adjunctive therapies (including preterm labor education, weekly clinic visits, home uterine contraction assessment, daily phone contact, and 24-hour perinatal nurse access) also failed to demonstrate efficacy of long-term oral or subcutaneous tocolytic therapy.[83,84] As such, maintenance tocolytic therapy is not generally recommended. Oral β-agonist therapy may have a role to play in decreasing uterine irritability and thereby diminishing patient anxiety, physician telephone consultations, and visits to labor and delivery. This effect should not be confused with the use of maintenance β-agonist therapy to "treat" preterm labor. Similarly, the concurrent use of two or more tocolytic agents has not been shown to be more effective than a single agent, and the cumulative risk of side-effects generally precludes this course of management.[85] Sequential therapy, however, may be beneficial.[86] Cyclic therapy (such as treatment with oxytocin receptor antagonists at night and β-agonists during the day) is currently being considered, but there is as yet no evidence that this approach is any more effective than standard tocolytic therapy. In the setting of preterm premature rupture of the fetal membranes, tocolysis has not been shown to be effective and is best avoided.[87]

CONCLUSION

Labor is a complex physiologic process involving fetal, placental, and maternal signals. Considerable evidence suggests that the fetus is in control of the timing of labor and, thus, its birth, but exactly how this is achieved in the human is still unknown. Although the ability of obstetric care providers to identify women at risk for preterm birth has improved, there are as yet no effective strategies available for prevention and treatment in such women.

Obstetric management of pregnancies complicated by preterm labor has evolved slowly over the last two decades, with diminishing emphasis on pharmacological prolongation of gestation and greater emphasis on optimal preparation for delivery should labor continue to progress despite tocolysis. A better understanding of the mechanisms responsible for the process of labor, both at term and preterm, will improve our ability to care for patients at risk for preterm birth.

TABLE 12-3

Guidelines for the Management of Preterm Delivery

- Confirm diagnosis of preterm labor
- Exclude contraindications to expectant management and/or tocolysis
- Administer corticosteroids, if indicated
- Group B Streptococcus chemoprophylaxis, if indicated
- **Pharmacologic tocolysis**
- Consider transfer to tertiary care center

TABLE 12-4

Management of Preterm Labor

Tocolytic Agent	Route of Administration (Dosage)	Efficacy[†]	Major Maternal Side Effects	Major Fetal Side Effects
Magnesium sulfate	IV (4–6 g bolus, then 2–3 g/h infusion)	Effective	Nausea, ileus, headache, weakness	Decreased beat-to-beat variability
	Oral maintenance (100–120 mg q 4 h)	Not effective	Hypotension Pulmonary edema Cardiorespiratory arrest ? Hypocalcemia	Neonatal drowsiness, hypotonia ? Ileus ? Congenital ricketic syndrome (with treatment > 3 weeks)
β-Adrenergic agonists				
Terbutaline sulfate	IV (2 μg/min infusion, maximum 80 μg/min)	Effective	Jitteriness, anxiety, restlessness, nausea,	Fetal tachycardia Hypotension
	SC (0.25 mg q 20 min)	Effective	vomiting, rash	Ileus
	Oral maintenance (2.5–5 mg q 4–6 h)	Not effective	Cardiac dysrhythmias, myocardial	Hyperinsulinemia, hypoglycemia (more
	IV pump (0.05 mL/h)	Not effective	Ischemia, palpitations, chest pain	common with isoxsuprine)
			Hypotension, tachycardia (more common with isoxsuprine)	Hyperbilirubinemia, Hypocalcemia ? Hydrops fetalis
Ritodrine hydrochloride*	IV (50 μg/min infusion, maximum 350 μg/min)	Effective	Pulmonary edema Paralytic ileus	
	IM (5–10 mg q 2–4 h)	Effective	Hypokalemia	
	Oral maintenance (10–20 mg q 3–4 h)	Not effective	Hyperglycemia, acidosis	
Isoxsuprine hydrochloride	IV (0.05–0.5 mg/min)	Effective		
	Oral (10 mg q 8–12 h)	? Effective		
Salbutamol	IV (6–30 μg/min)	Unproven		
	Oral (4 mg q 4–6 h)	Unproven		
Prostaglandin inhibitors				
Indomethacin	Oral (25–50 mg q 4–6 h)	Effective	Gastrointestinal effects (nausea, heartburn),	Transient oliguria, oligohydramnios
	Rectal (100 mg q 12 h)	Effective	headache, rash	Premature closure of the
Naproxen	Oral (375–500 mg q 6 h)	Effective	Interstitial nephritis	neonatal ductus
Fenoprofen	Oral (200–300 mg q 6 h)	Effective	Increased bleeding time	arteriosus and persistent
Aspirin	Oral (375–500 mg q 6–12 h)	Unproven	(most common with	pulmonary hypertension
Meloxicam	(Investigational)	Unproven	aspirin)	? Necrotizing enterocolitis, intraventricular hemorrhage
Calcium channel blockers				
Nifedipine	Oral (20–30 mg q 4–8 h)	Effective	Hypotension, reflex tachycardia (especially with verapamil) Headache, nausea, flushing Potentiates the cardiac depressive effect of	—
Nicardipine	Oral (20–40 mg q 8 h)	Unproven	magnesium sulfate	
Verapamil	Oral (80–120 mg q 8 h)	Unproven	Hepatotoxicity	
Potassium channel openers				
Levcromakalin	(Investigational)	? Effective	?	?
Oxytocin antagonists				
Atosiban	IV (1 μM/min infusion, maximum 32 μM/min)	Effective	Nausea, vomiting, headache, chest pain, arthralgias	? Inhibit lactation
Phosphodiesterase inhibitor				
Aminophylline	Oral (200 mg q 6–8 h)	? Effective	Tachycardia	Fetal tachycardia
	IV (0.5–0.7 mg/kg/h)	? Effective		
Others				
Ethanol	(Historical interest)	Effective	Alcoholic intoxication	? Alcohol toxicity (theoretically)
Nitroglycerine	TD (10–50 mg q day)	Unproven	Hypotension, headache	Fetal tachycardia
	IV (100 μg bolus, 1–10 μg/kg/min infusion)	Unproven		
Diazoxide	IV (1–3 mg/kg infusion)	Unproven	Profound hypotension	Uteroplacental insufficiency

* The only tocolytic agent approved by the Food and Drug Administration.
† Efficacy is defined as proven benefit in delaying delivery by 24–48 hours as compared with placebo or standard control.
IM, intramuscular; IV, intravenous; SC, subcutaneous; TD, transdermal.

REFERENCES

1. Nathanielsz PW, et al: Stimulation of the switch in myometrial activity from contractures to contractions in the pregnant sheep and non-human primate. Equine Vet J 24:838, 1997.
2. Norwitz ER, et al: The control of labor. N Engl J Med 41:660, 1999.
3. Frigoletto FD, et al: A clinical trial of active management of labor. N Engl J Med 333:745, 1995.
4. Duff P, et al: Management of premature rupture of membranes and unfavorable cervix in term pregnancy. Obstet Gynecol 63:697, 1984.
5. American College of Obstetricians and Gynecologists: Assessment of risk factors for preterm birth (ACOG Practice Bulletin Number 31). Washington, D.C.: U.S. Government Printing Office, 2001, pp 709–716.
6. Rush RW, et al: Contribution of preterm delivery to perinatal mortality. BMJ 2:965, 1976.
7. Villar J, et al: Pre-term delivery syndrome: The unmet need. Res Clin Forums 16:9, 1994.
8. Ventura SJ, et al: Births: final data for 1999. Natl Vital Stat Rep 49:1, 2001.
9. Murphy SL: Deaths: final data for 1998. Natl Vital Stat Rep 48:1, 2000.
10. Tucker JM, et al: Etiologies of preterm birth in an indigent population: is prevention a logical expectation? Obstet Gynecol 77:343, 1991.
11. Wood NS, et al: Neurologic and developmental disability after extremely preterm birth. EPICure Study Group. N Engl J Med 343:378, 2000.
12. Challis JRG, Gibb W: Control of parturition. Prenat Neonat Med 1:283, 1996.
13. Flint APF, et al: The mechanism by which fetal cortisol controls the onset of parturition in the sheep. Biochem Soc Trans 3:1189, 1975.
14. Liggins GC: Initiation of labor. Biol Neonate 55:366, 1989.
15. Honnebier MB, Nathanielsz PW: Primate parturition and the role of the maternal circadian system. Eur J Obstet Gynecol Reprod Biol 55:193, 1993.
16. Nathanielsz PW: Comparative studies on the initiation of labor. Eur J Obstet Gynecol Reprod Biol 78:127, 1998.
17. Liggins BJ, et al: The mechanism of initiation of parturition in the ewe. Recent Prog Horm Res 29:111, 1973.
18. Thorburn GD, et al: The trigger for parturition in sheep: Fetal hypothalamus or placenta? J Dev Physiol 15:71, 1991.
19. Matthews SG, Challis JRG: Regulation of the hypothalamo-pituitary-adrenocortical axis in fetal sheep. Trends Endocrinol Metab 4:239, 1996.
20. López Bernal A, et al: Parturition: Activation of stimulatory pathways or loss of uterine quiescence? Adv Exp Med Biol 395:435, 1995.
21. Garrioch DB: The effect of indomethacin on spontaneous activity in the isolated human myometrium and on the response to oxytocin and prostaglandin. Br J Obstet Gynaecol 85:47, 1978.
22. MacDonald PC: Parturition: Biomolecular and Physiologic Process. In Cunningham FG, et al (eds): Williams Obstetrics (19th ed). Norwalk, CT, Appleton & Lange, 1993, pp 298–299.
23. Norwitz ER, et al: The initiation of parturition: A comparative analysis across the species. Current Problems Obstet Gynecol Infertil 22:41, 1999.
24. Blennerhassett MG, Miller SM: Control of myometrial contractility: role and regulation of gap junctions. Oxf Rev Reprod Biol 10:436, 1988.
25. Pauerstein CJ, Zauder HL: Autonomic innervation, sex steroids and uterine contractility. Obstet Gynecol Surv 25(Suppl):617, 1970.
26. Myers DA, Nathanielsz PW: Biologic basis of term and preterm labor. Clin Perinatol 20:9, 1993.
27. Mecenas CA, et al: Production of premature delivery in pregnant rhesus monkeys by androstenedione infusion. Nat Med 2:442, 1996.
28. Nathanielsz PW, et al: Local paracrine effects of estradiol are central to parturition in the rhesus monkey. Nat Med 4:456, 1998.
29. Figueroa JP, et al: Effect of 48 hour intravenous Δ⁴-androstenedione infusion on pregnant rhesus monkeys in the last third of gestation: Changes in maternal plasma estradiol concentrations and myometrial contractility. Am J Obstet Gynecol 161:481, 1989.
30. Nathanielsz PW, et al: Local paracrine effects of estradiol are central to parturition in the rhesus monkey. Nat Med 4:456, 1998.
31. Romero R, et al: The role of systemic and intrauterine infection in pre-term parturition. Ann NY Acad Sci 662:355, 1991.
32. Dudley DJ: Pre-term labor: an intra-uterine inflammatory response syndrome? J Reprod Immunol 36:93, 1997.
33. Romero R, et al: Prostaglandin concentrations in amniotic fluid of women with intra-amniotic infection and preterm labor. Am J Obstet Gynecol 157:1461, 1987.
34. Romero R, et al: Increase in prostaglandin bioavailability precedes the onset of human parturition. Prostaglandins Leukotrienes Essent Fatty Acids 54:187, 1996.
35. Elovitz MA, et al: The mechanisms underlying the stimulatory effects of thrombin on myometrial smooth muscle. Am J Obstet Gynecol 183:674, 2000.
36. Creasy RK, et al: System for predicting spontaneous preterm birth. Am J Obstet Gynecol 55:692, 1980.
37. Mercer BM, et al: The preterm prediction study: A clinical risk assessment system. Am J Obstet Gynecol 174:1885, 1996.
38. Iams JD, et al: A prospective random trial of home uterine activity monitoring in pregnancies at increased risk of preterm labor. Am J Obstet Gynecol 159:595, 1988.
39. Iams JD, et al: Frequency of uterine contractions and the risk of spontaneous preterm delivery. N Engl J Med 346:250, 2002.
40. Mortensen OA, et al: Prediction of preterm birth. Acta Obstet Gynecol Scand 66:507, 1987.
41. Iams JD, et al: The length of the cervix and the risk of spontaneous premature delivery. N Engl J Med 334:567, 1996.
42. Heath VCF, et al: Cervical length at 23 weeks of gestation: prediction of spontaneous preterm delivery. Ultrasound Obstet Gynaecol 12:312, 1998.
43. Petraglia F, et al: Abnormal concentration of maternal serum activin A in gestational diseases. J Clin Endocrinol Metab 80:558, 1995.
44. Petraglia F: Inhibin, activin, and follistatin in the placenta: A new family of regulatory proteins. Placenta 18:3, 1997.
45. Lockwood CJ, et al: Fetal fibronectin in cervical and vaginal secretions as a predictor of preterm delivery. N Engl J Med 325:669, 1991.
46. Goldenberg RL, et al: The preterm prediction study: Fetal fibronectin testing and spontaneous preterm birth. Obstet Gynecol 87:643, 1996.
47. Iams JD, et al: Fetal fibronectin improves the accuracy of diagnosis of preterm labor. Am J Obstet Gynecol 173:141, 1995.
48. Rajabi M, et al: High levels of serum collagenase in preterm labor: A potential biochemical marker. Obstet Gynecol 69:179, 1987.
49. Clark IM, et al: Tissue inhibitor of metallo-proteinases: Serum levels during pregnancy and labor, term and preterm. Obstet Gynecol 83:532, 1994.
50. Goodwin TM: A role for estriol in human labor, term and preterm. Am J Obstet Gynecol 180(Suppl):208, 1999.
51. Voss HF: Saliva as a fluid for measurement of estriol levels. Am J Obstet Gynecol 180(Suppl):226, 1999.
52. McGregor JA, et al: Salivary estriol as risk assessment for preterm labor: a prospective trial. Am J Obstet Gynecol 173:1337, 1995.
53. Heine RP, et al: Accuracy of salivary estriol testing compared to traditional risk factor assessment in predicting preterm birth. Am J Obstet Gynecol 180(Suppl):214, 1999.
54. Petersen LK, et al: Serum relaxin as a potential marker for preterm labour. Br J Obstet Gynaecol 99:292, 1992.
55. Korebrits C, et al: Maternal corticotropin-releasing hormone is increased with impending preterm birth. J Clin Endocrinol Metab 83:1585, 1998.
56. Hobel CJ, et al: Maternal plasma corticotropin-releasing hormone associated with stress at 20 weeks' gestation in pregnancies ending in preterm delivery. Am J Obstet Gynecol 180(Suppl):257, 1999.
57. Multicenter randomized, controlled trial of a preterm birth prevention program. Collaborate Group on Preterm Birth Prevention. Am J Obstet Gynecol 169:352, 1993.
58. Goldenberg RL, et al: Bed rest in pregnancy. Obstet Gynecol 84:131, 1994.
59. Hillier SL, et al: Association between bacterial vaginosis and preterm delivery of a low-birth-weight infant. The Vaginal Infections and Prematurity Study Group. N Engl J Med 333:1737, 1995.
60. Hauth JC, et al: Reduced incidence of preterm delivery with metronidazole and erythromycin in women with bacterial vaginosis. N Engl J Med 333:1732, 1995.
61. McGregor JA, et al: Prevention of premature birth by screening and treatment for common genital tract infections: Results of a prospective controlled evaluation. Am J Obstet Gynecol 173:157, 1995.
62. Goldenberg RL, et al: Intrauterine infection and preterm delivery. N Engl J Med 342:1500, 2000.
63. American College of Obstetricians and Gynecologists. Preterm labor (ACOG Technical Bulletin Number 206). Washington, D.C., U.S. Government Printing Office, 1995, pp 710–719.
64. Romero R, et al: A comparative study of the diagnostic performance of amniotic fluid glucose, white blood cell count, interleukin-6 and Gram stain in the detection of microbial invasion in patients with preterm premature rupture of membranes. Am J Obstet Gynecol 169:839, 1993.
65. Guinn DA, et al: Management options in women with preterm uterine contractions: A randomized clinical trial. Am J Obstet Gynecol 177:814, 1997.
66. Gibbs RS, et al: A review of premature birth and sub-clinical infection. Am J Obstet Gynecol 166:1515, 1992.
67. Romero R, et al: Antibiotic treatment of preterm labor with intact membranes: A multicenter, randomized, double-blind, placebo-controlled trial. Am J Obstet Gynecol 169:764, 1993.
68. Fuchs A-R, Fuchs F: Ethanol for prevention of preterm birth. Semin Perinatol 5:236, 1981.
69. Besinger RE, Niebyl JR: The safety and efficacy of tocolytic agents for the treatment of preterm labor. Obstet Gynecol Surv 45:415, 1990.
70. Higby K, et al: Do tocolytic agents stop preterm labor? A critical and comprehensive review of efficacy and safety. Am J Obstet Gynecol 168:1247, 1993.
71. Hill WC: Risks and complications of tocolysis. Clin Obstet Gynecol 38:725, 1995.
72. Norwitz ER, Robinson JN: The control of labor [Letter]. N Engl J Med 341:2098, 1999.
73. The Canadian Preterm Labor Investigation Group: Treatment of preterm labor with the beta-adrenergic agonist ritodrine. N Engl J Med 327:308, 1992.
74. Glock JL, Morales WJ: Efficacy and safety of nifedipine versus magnesium sulfate in the management of preterm labor: a randomized study. Am J Obstet Gynecol 169:960, 1993.
75. Papatsonis DNM, et al: Nifedipine and ritodrine in the management of preterm labor: a randomized multicenter trial. Obstet Gynecol 90:230, 1997.
76. Zuckerman H, et al: Further study of the inhibition of preterm labor by indomethacin. Part II. Double-blind study. J Perinatol Med 12:25, 1984.
77. Norton ME, et al: Neonatal complications after the administration of indomethacin for preterm labor. N Engl Med J 329:1602, 1993.
78. Morrison JJ, et al: The effects of potassium channel openers on the isolated human pregnant myometrium before and after the onset of labor: Potential for tocolysis. Am J Obstet Gynecol 169:1277, 1993.

79. Anderson LF, et al: Oxytocin receptor blockade: a new principle in the treatment of preterm labor? Am J Perinatol 6:196, 1989.
80. Goodwin TM, et al: Treatment of preterm labor with the oxytocin antagonist atosiban. Am J Perinatol 13:143, 1996.
81. Goodwin TM, Zografyan A: Oxytocin receptor antagonists. Clin Perinatol 25:859, 1998.
82. King JF, et al: Beta-mimetics in preterm labour: An overview of the randomized controlled trials. Br J Obstet Gynaecol 95:211, 1988.
83. Rust OA, et al: The clinical efficacy of oral tocolytic therapy. Am J Obstet Gynecol 175:838, 1996.

84. Guinn DA, et al: Terbutaline pump maintenance therapy for prevention of preterm delivery: A double-blind trial. Am J Obstet Gynecol 179:874, 1998.
85. Ferguson JE, et al: Adjunctive use of magnesium sulfate with ritodrine for preterm labor tocolysis. Am J Obstet Gynecol 148:166, 1984.
86. Valenzuela G, Cline S: Use of magnesium sulfate in premature labor that fails to respond to beta-mimetic drugs. Am J Obstet Gynecol 143:718, 1982.
87. Allen SR: Tocolytic therapy in preterm premature rupture of membranes. Clin Obstet Gynecol 41:842, 1998.

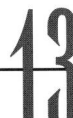

Colin P. Sibley and Robert D. H. Boyd

Mechanisms of Transfer Across the Human Placenta

It has been known since the 18th century that the circulation of the human fetus is kept separate from that of the mother by intervening placental tissue.[1] This chapter reviews transport across the placenta, but there is a less clear and less coherent understanding of placental transfer than there is for more extensively researched transport organs, such as the intestine or the kidney. Also reviewed is the evidence linking altered placental transporter activities with anomalous fetal growth.

Histologically, placentas can be classified broadly into hemochorial types found in the human, rat, rabbit, and guinea pig, in which maternal blood washes directly against fetal chorionic (trophoblastic) tissue, and epitheliochorial types found in the sheep or pig, in which the maternal uterine epithelium is maintained (Fig. 13-1).[2] The dog and some other species are intermediate in structure between these two types (see Fig. 13-1).

Functionally, there are wide differences in the mechanisms and degree of transfer of some solutes, notably γ immunoglobulin G (IgG) (yolk sac in rabbits, placenta in women, and untransported in sheep) and iron (red blood cells in sheep and cats, receptor mediated from plasma transferrin in women). Most other transport systems have been observed in the majority of species studied, but few extensive cross-species sets of data are available. There is an additional major interspecies functional difference in the balance between diffusional and carrier-mediated transplacental transport. Hemochorial placentas (women, rats, guinea pigs) are considerably more permeable to lipid-insoluble molecules for which there are not specific transport systems (and which are presumed to leak across the placenta by diffusion through "pores") than are epitheliochorial placentas (sheep).[3,4] So substantial are the differences that the quantitative balance between specific transport and leak is probably quite different for humans and sheep. The much more restricted leak pathway in sheep (in comparison with humans) suggests that endogenous polypeptides and other lipid-insoluble molecules, in the absence of specific transport systems, cross the sheep placenta much less readily than the human placenta; the same may be predicted for hydrophilic drugs. These differences must be borne in mind when extrapolating conclusions drawn from one species to another.

This chapter reviews examples of the main mechanisms of transplacental transfer. A systematic listing of all transport studies has not been prepared since that of Schultz,[5] although many are considered in the work of Morriss and colleagues[6] and Faber and Thornburg.[4]

This chapter is restricted predominantly to data obtained in the human and to those substances whose net transfer is toward the fetus. In the case of urea, carbon dioxide, and bilirubin, for example, net transfer is in the opposite direction. The methodologic approaches used in humans on which the results discussed hereafter are based are summarized in Table 13-1. Placental nomenclature is sometimes confusing to those from other fields of study. Commonly used anatomic descriptions and terms are therefore defined in Table 13-2.

MECHANISMS OF TRANSFER

The following describes the mechanisms available for transfer across the placenta, summarized diagrammatically in Figures 13-2 and 13-3, together with examples of each process.

Diffusional Transfer

There are several specific transport systems across the placenta that are discussed in subsequent sections, but any molecule for which there is a maternofetal concentration difference also tends to diffuse across the placenta. The net rate (J_{net}) of diffusional transfer of a given solute from maternal to fetal blood within each gram of placenta may be derived from Fick's law:[4]

$$J_{net} = PS\,(\bar{c}_m - \bar{c}_f)\ \mathrm{mol\ sec^{-1}\,g^{-1}} \qquad [1]$$

where P = proportionality constant (placental permeability) (cm² sec⁻¹), S = surface area available for diffusion between the circulations within 1 g placenta (cm² g⁻¹), and $\bar{c}_m$ and $\bar{c}_f$ = mean plasma solute concentrations of the unbound solute in plasma water in maternal and fetal blood flowing past the exchange area. It can be seen from Equation 1 that, in addition to surface area, net diffusional transfer depends on both the permeability constant P and the maternofetal concentration difference. There are two pathways available for diffusion: a hydrophilic route for lipid-insoluble molecules and a lipophilic route. Their relative importance in determining J_{net} is determined by the degree of solubility in lipid of the molecule in question.

J_{net} may be considered as having two components:

$$J_{net} = J_{mf} - J_{fm} \qquad [2]$$

where J_{mf} and J_{fm} = unidirectional transfer rates within 1 g placenta in the maternofetal and fetomaternal directions. This formulation applies to any mechanism of transfer. For molecules crossing by diffusion only:

$$J_{mf} = PS\,(\bar{c}_m)\ \mathrm{mol\ sec^{-1}\,g^{-1}} \qquad [3]$$

$$J_{fm} = PS\,(\bar{c}_f)\ \mathrm{mol\ sec^{-1}\,g^{-1}} \qquad [4]$$

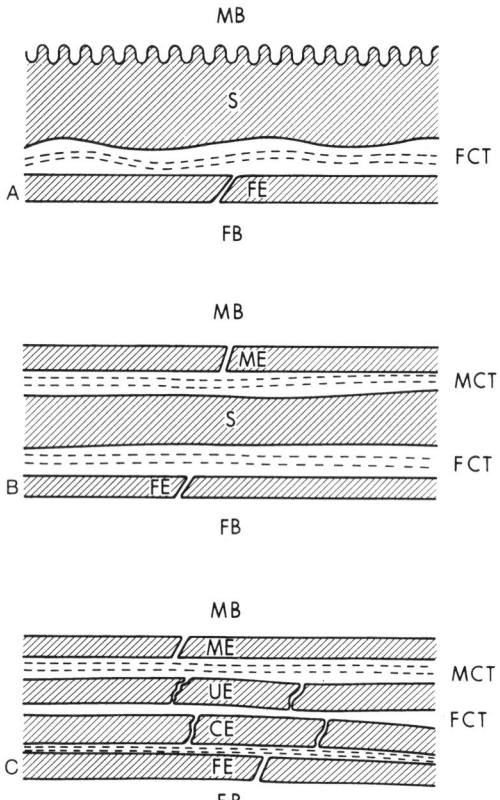

Figure 13–1. Diagrammatic representation of the three main types of placenta classified histologically. **A,** Hemochorial placenta, which has fetal endothelium and syncytiotrophoblast but no maternal endothelium (e.g., human). **B,** Endotheliochorial placenta, which has syncytiotrophoblast and both maternal and fetal endothelium (e.g., dog). **C,** Epitheliochorial placenta, which retains uterine epithelium in close proximity to chorionic epithelium (trophoblast) as well as both maternal and fetal endothelium (e.g., pig). CE = chorionic epithelium; FB = fetal blood; FCT = fetal connective tissue; FE = fetal endothelium; MB = maternal blood; MCT = maternal connective tissue; ME = maternal endothelium; S = syncytiotrophoblast; UE = uterine epithelium. For a fuller account, see Mossman.[154]

Hydrophilic Permeability

In the absence of specific transport mechanisms, lipid-insoluble (hydrophilic) molecules do not permeate the cell membrane of the trophoblast to any extent and are believed to be excluded from the intracellular space of the placenta. Therefore, they are thought to cross the placental barrier by an extracellular porous route of molecular dimensions. Lipid-insoluble molecules cross slowly because the surface area of this pathway is small. Their transfer is limited by P and is said to be membrane limited.[4,7–9]

Mannitol, sucrose, inulin, chromium-labeled ethylenediaminetetraacetic acid, and high-dose vitamin B$_{12}$ have been used together with other hydrophilic inert substances to assess placental permeability. Although these substances are not physiologic permeants, they can be used to evaluate the baseline permeability of the placenta for lipid-insoluble molecules because specific transport systems have not developed (or, as in the case of vitamin B$_{12}$, the transport systems were saturated during studies). Any specific transport mechanisms for other hydrophilic solutes are additive to this baseline.

Table 13-3 lists the permeabilities reported as permeability surface area products (PS) for some such hydrophilic molecules, across the term human placenta *in vivo* and, for comparison, across the term rat placenta. As shown, the permeability of

hydrophilic substances is proportional to their diffusion coefficients in water (although there are differences between the values obtained in two different laboratories).

There is a similar relationship between permeability and diffusion coefficients in water for the hemotrichorial rat placenta (see Table 13-3), which also has a syncytial trophoblast layer, and for the hemochorial guinea pig placenta.[10, 11] Such a relationship is most easily explained by diffusion through paracellular channels or pores sufficiently wide to allow free diffusion unrestricted by molecular size until molecules reach the size of proteins. The permeability of epitheliochorial sheep placenta to similar hydrophilic molecules declines much more rapidly with increasing molecular size.[12] A possible reason for such a permeability difference could be that the channels have a radius some 10 to 20 times smaller in sheep than in humans and other hemochorial placentas.[4] The morphologic nature of the paracellular channels or pores in the syncytiotrophoblast of hemochorial placentas is uncertain, but two possible pathways (not mutually exclusive) have been identified. Kaufmann and colleagues,[13–15] using electron-dense tracers, visualized transtrophoblastic channels lined with tracer after the imposition of a hydrostatic pressure gradient across the perfused guinea pig and human placenta. They hypothesized that, under normal conditions of hydrostatic pressure, the channels are too narrow to be resolved by electron microscopy. They also failed, however, to show channels that are simultaneously open to both the maternal and the fetal sides of the syncytiotrophoblast; this may not be surprising given the small number of channels required to explain the permeability data.[16] A paracellular pathway in the human placenta may also be provided by areas of denudation of the syncytiotrophoblast.[17–20] These are normal features of the human placenta at all stages of gestation, and they are either open or filled with fibrin-containing fibrinoid deposits.[18]

Sodium. The relatively high permeability of hemochorial placentas toward hydrophilic solutes suggests that most sodium transfer across the human placenta occurs by membrane-limited diffusion.[3] If this is true (and assuming electrical forces are unimportant and pores are of only one size), the PS for sodium across human placenta[21] should be the same when it is normalized for its diffusion coefficient as that for extracellular tracers. The available data (see Table 13-3) suggest that this is not the case. There are several possible explanations for such an unexpectedly high sodium permeability.

1. There may be a population of extracellular channels small enough to exclude mannitol (the smallest extracellular tracer so far studied in humans) but large enough to let through some excess sodium (a heterogeneous pore size).[22]

2. Paracellular diffusion of sodium may be accelerated by a transplacental potential difference between the fetal capillary and intervillous space (with the fetal side negative). There is evidence of a potential difference in some species, but other data are contradictory.[9, 22–24] An *in vitro* study, using microelectrodes, measured a transtrophoblast potential difference in mature intermediate villi of human placenta ranging from 2.5 to 10 mV, fetal side negative.[25] This finding is supported by some measurements *in vivo*.[26] Such a fetal side negative potential difference could well explain the apparently anomalous high PS for sodium.

3. Maternofetal sodium transport may be partly transcellular via the various sodium-linked transport systems demonstrable in trophoblast membrane vesicle preparations (described later). This possibility is of interest because it allows potential endocrine control of active sodium transport to the fetus and thus of fetal hydration (see the later discussion of water transfer). In the rat, in which the ratio of PS to diffusion coefficient for sodium is similarly higher than that for extra-

TABLE 13-1

Some Methods of Placental Transfer Study

Method	Variable Measured	Details	Comment	References
Carcass analysis	J_{net}*	Analysis of conceptus content at different gestational ages	Only reliable for nonmetabolized solutes, e.g., Ca; includes all maternofetal routes; poor time resolution	155
Accumulation of exogenous tracer	J_{mf}†	Fetal tracer content estimated after delivery	If fetal plasma concentrations not low, a hybrid of J_{net} and J_{mf} is measured	147, 156–158
Umbilical arteriovenous difference at delivery	J_{mf}† or J_{net}	Cord clamped at cesarean section	Non–steady-state artifact likely	6
Cordocentesis	Maternofetal plasma concentration difference		Midgestation; minimal disturbance; usually only venous sample	57, 142, 159
Cotyledonary perfusion	J_{mf} J_{fm}	Steady-state transfer	Perfusion might alter passive permeability and thus wrongly estimate proportion of specific transport	160
Cotyledonary perfusion	Kinetics of uptake and backflux from maternal and fetal circulation	Single pass, indicator dilution	Can demonstrate transport asymmetry; may not reflect rate-limiting element of transfer	161
Slices; fragments	Kinetics of individual systems	Uptake or efflux studies	May be "housekeeping" rather than transplacental transport systems	62, 65, 162
Membrane vesicles	Kinetics of individual systems	Microvillous (maternal facing); basal (fetal facing)	May be "housekeeping" rather than transplacental transport systems	51, 54, 163
Cultured trophoblast	Uptake		Care needs to be taken that placental cells rather than other lineages are being studied; cells may never terminally differentiate	75, 164
Receptor binding studies	Affinity/number	Many described	May have "housekeeping," endocrine, transport, or other function	9
Microelectrode and patch clamp studies	Transmembrane potential difference and ion channel characteristics		Has implications for ion movements	25, 33, 139, 165–167
Gene knock-out/overexpression	Variety	Mainly mouse	Identify likely mechanisms/regulatory pathways	147

* See Equations 3 and 4 in text.

† The permeability surface area product can be derived from J for diffusional transport when microcirculation plasma water concentrations are known or inferred.[4,9]

TABLE 13-2

Some Anatomic Terms Common in Placental Transport Studies

Term	Meaning
Trophoblast	A fetally derived tissue that comprises a number of different lineages. Within the absorptive part of human placenta, these comprise syncytiotrophoblast, the syncytial layer in immediate contact with maternal blood, and, beneath it, a cytotrophoblast layer from which syncytiotrophoblast is derived. The cytotrophoblast layer is incomplete in later gestation. Other categories of trophoblast outside the exchange area include free cells in the endometrium, trophoblast invading spiral arteries, and trophoblast in nonplacental membranes. There may also be trophoblast free in maternal circulation. The outer surface membrane of syncytiotrophoblast facing maternal blood is microvillous, and vesicular preparations made from this membrane are microvillous membrane (brush-border membrane) vesicles. The fetal surface of syncytial trophoblast is also lined by a cell membrane, which can be isolated and formed into basal membrane vesicles
Umbilical and uterine circulations	The intervillous space (maternal circulation flowing between the placental villi) is supplied by spiral branches of the (maternal) uterine artery. Circulation within the villi is supplied by the (fetal) umbilical artery and vein
Chorion	The outermost layer of the conceptus in early gestation, hence *chorion frondosum*, the chorionic appearance that surrounds all sides of the conceptus in early gestation. As the definitive placenta develops, that part of the frondosum contributing to it becomes more villous; the remainder loses its villi to become *chorion laeve*
Allantois	A fluid-filled compartment adjacent to the umbilical cord, connected to the fetal bladder via a tubular uracus running from the cephalic end of the bladder through the umbilicus. Of considerable size in the sheep, it is rudimentary in the human and disappears in early gestation. However, its tissue contributes to placental formation, hence the description of human placenta as chorioallantoic
Endometrium	The lining of the uterus. In the human, it is shed at menstruation and hence is classified as deciduate. The shed tissue is the decidua
Amnion	A fluid-filled compartment that is bounded internally by the fetal skin and externally by the amniotic membrane closely apposed to overlying chorion, hence, amniochorion. It is rupture of this membrane that allows fetal delivery through the cervix at term. The fetus drinks its contained amniotic fluid and passes lung liquid and urine into it
Fetal membranes	These strictly comprise placenta and amniochorion, the latter being *extraplacental membranes*. Common usage allows fetal membranes to mean amniochorion only
Villus	The fetal component of human placenta arborizes into a large number of small, fingerlike projections or villi; each is bathed by maternal blood flowing through the intervillous space
Cotyledons	The human placenta is partially divided into cotyledons by incomplete septa. In some species, placental elements are quite distinct, as in the sheep, and each element is known as a cotyledon. In human placental perfusion, roughly one cotyledon is perfused. The human placenta as delivered includes some adherent maternal tissue, and the shiny fetal surface from which the umbilical cord projects is known as the chorionic plate, and the maternal tissue surface is known as the basal plate, not to be confused with the converse usage of basal vesicles (see above)
Yolk sac placenta	An important route of immunoglobulin transfer in rodents. The yolk sac is functional only in the first trimester in women, and its contribution, if any, to transfer is uncertain

cellular tracers (see Table 13-3), there is good evidence of active transport, involving sodium/amino acid co-transport and sodium, potassium, adenosine triphosphatase (Na+,K+-ATPase).[27] There is evidence of a similar system in the pig,[28] but as yet no clear evidence that it occurs in the human even though there certainly is sodium/amino acid co-transport and Na+,K+-ATPase activity.[29,30]

Other Ions. Although the paracellular route appears to be large enough in the human to permit some diffusional permeability for all the unbound inorganic ions of plasma, the proportion of their movement that is transcellular is generally unknown. For calcium, *in vitro* data suggest that the paracellular route contributes about 50% of total maternofetal transfer.[31] Furthermore, some data have confirmed the existence in the human placenta of an active transcellular route for transfer of this cation (see Chap. 33). Chloride, phosphate, and sulfate are maintained at higher concentration in fetal than in maternal plasma,[6] and therefore transcellular active transport is likely to be involved in the translocation of these ions; the components of such routes certainly exist.[32-36]

Flow Limitation

Lipid-soluble substances diffuse through the entire trophoblast cell surface. Because of the large surface area involved, P in

Equation 1 is large, and the transport rate depends predominantly on $\bar{c}_m$ and $\bar{c}_f$, which, in turn, depend on the geometric relationships of the maternal and fetal bloodstreams and their flow rates. Therefore, relatively lipophilic molecules, such as respiratory or anesthetic gases, are said to demonstrate *flow limitation* in their permeability pattern.[4,7,8] The hypothetical effect of two different geometric patterns of flow, concurrent and countercurrent, on the profile of c_m and c_f (and thus on $\bar{c}_m$ and $\bar{c}_f$) is illustrated in Figure 13-2.

The human placenta probably belongs to an anatomically intermediate type of exchanger[4] in that, on the fetal side, there are hairpin-like capillary loops, with opposite flow directions in each limb.[13] The maternal circulation in the intervillous space exhibits a *multivillous pool* geometry and lies approximately at 90° to the fetal circulation. This arrangement is intermediate in transfer efficiency.[4]

Oxygen Transfer. It seems probable that oxygen transfer across the human placenta is flow limited as it is in sheep[37] and rabbits.[38] For gases such as oxygen, the terms $\bar{c}_m$ and $\bar{c}_f$ are correctly replaced in the Fick equation by the equivalent partial pressures, and the driving force for net oxygen diffusion is the partial pressure difference for the gas between maternal intervillous space and fetal capillary. Values for partial oxygen pressure (Po_2) in blood taken from large vessels in sheep, monkeys, and humans and from the intervillous space in the humans are

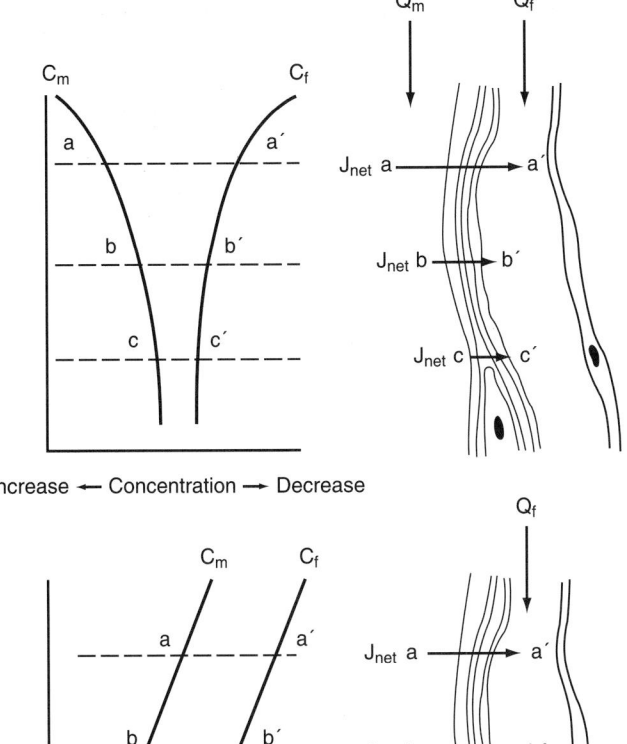

Figure 13–2. Effect of directional relationships of maternal (Q_m) and fetal (Q_f) blood flows on relative concentration differences and net fluxes of a substance crossing the placenta by diffusion under flow-limited conditions. *Top,* Concurrent maternal and fetal flows. *Left,* The maternal (C_m) and fetal (C_f) plasma concentration profiles are shown along the length of the exchange vessel that includes points a, b, and c on the maternal side of the vessel and corresponding points a′, b′, and c′ within the lumen of the fetal vessel. *Right,* The results in net fluxes (J_{net}). The net flux decreases from point a-a′ to point b-b′ to point c-c′ along the length of the exchange vessels. C_m declines along the length of the exchange vessel, and C_f increases along the length of the vessel until the concentration difference that drives net diffusion decreases to almost zero. *Bottom,* Countercurrent maternal and fetal blood flows. *Left,* C_m declines along the length of the exchange vessel, and C_f increases in the exchange vessel along its length. The maternofetal concentration difference is constant along the exchange vessel. *Right,* The net fluxes remain uniform along the length of the capillary. Not illustrated is the membrane-limited situation in which the maternofetal concentration difference and the individual maternal and fetal concentration profiles remain approximately uniform along the length of the capillary; this is true regardless of the directional relationship of maternal and fetal blood flows. (From Morriss FH, et al: *In* Knobil E, Neill J [eds]: Physiology of Reproduction, 2nd ed. New York, Raven Press, 1994, pp 813–861.)

shown in Table 13–4. In the sheep and monkey, it can be seen that the umbilical venous Po_2 is never higher than that in the uterine vein[39] (as would be expected for a concurrent blood flow system).

In an ideal concurrent system, the umbilical venous Po_2 should be identical to the uterine venous Po_2. In the sheep and monkey, however, these two values are not identical (see Table 13–4) because of shunting (some maternal and fetal blood does not pass close to the site of exchange) or uneven perfusion (maternal/fetal blood flow ratios that are different between different segments of the placenta). In addition, the placenta and membranes can consume considerable amounts of oxygen from the uterine circulation. With concurrent flow, the uterine vein Po_2 is the primary determinant of the upper limit of the umbilical venous Po_2; the latter can never be higher than the former.[39]

In the human, the situation is somewhat uncertain. The Po_2 of placental intervillous space samples is slightly higher than that in umbilical samples (see Table 13–4). Because the intervillous space samples are likely to be a mixture of arterial and venous blood (and therefore an overestimate of true venous Po_2), this suggests that the human placenta does not fit the concurrent system model and is most consistent with the proposed multivillous pool arrangement.

It is well known that fetal hemoglobin in most species (including humans but not cats)[4] has a higher affinity for oxygen than maternal hemoglobin (the oxyhemoglobin dissociation curve is shifted to the left). The effect of this shift on placental oxygen transfer and on fetal tissue oxygenation may be complex. In sheep, however, there is direct experimental evidence that the left shift is important because replacement of fetal blood with maternal blood results in a halving of the umbilical venous oxygen saturation and a drop in net transplacental flux of oxygen to the fetus.[40] The observation that fetal acidosis develops in human fetuses transfused with adult blood for Rhesus hemolytic disease is consistent with a similar effect in the human.[41] Because of the left shift in the fetal oxygen-hemoglobin dissociation curve, it is clear that for a given rate of oxygen supply to fetal tissue, the fetal tissue Po_2 is lower than it would be if adult blood at the same Po_2 flowed through it at the same rate.

Transporter Protein–Mediated Transport

The flux of small hydrophilic solutes across the plasma membrane is mediated by transporter proteins. These include carriers, which translocate solute by a saturable mechanism and may use energy either solely from prevailing electrochemical gradients (facilitated diffusion, e.g., glucose) or from the hydrolysis of ATP (active transport, e.g., amino acids, calcium), and channels through which ions diffuse along electrochemical gradients.[42] The transporter protein itself may hydrolyze ATP, or it can co-transport with another solute, a diffusion gradient for which is set up by the hydrolysis of ATP by a separate transporter protein (secondary active transport). Many such transporter proteins in the microvillous (maternal-facing) and basal (fetal-facing) plasma membranes of the human syncytiotrophoblast have been characterized. It is not clear, however, whether most of these transporter proteins are quantitatively important for transplacental transfer or are involved only in solute supply to the trophoblast for its own metabolism. For transplacental transfer to occur by way of this transcellular route, there must clearly be both an entry and an exit step (see Fig. 13–3).

Transplacental active transport can occur via a pump/leak or leak/pump mechanism. In the former process, the active step is located at the microvillous membrane and generates a higher intracellular concentration of the substance than in maternal plasma, followed by a leak across the opposite plasma membrane (probably the case for many amino acids). There may be a leak/pump system in which the substance is pumped out of the

TABLE 13-3

Permeability of the Human and Rat Placenta Near Term

Substance	Diffusion Coefficient in Water at 37°C[a] (cm²sec⁻¹)	Permeability Surface Area Product[g] (μl sec⁻¹ g⁻¹) Human	Rat[a]
Sodium	17.0×10^{-6}	0.56[c]	0.32
Mannitol	9.9×10^{-6}	0.19[d]	0.07
Sucrose	7.5×10^{-6}		0.07
Chromium-labeled ethylenediamine tetraacetic acid	7.0×10^{-6}	0.11[e]	0.05
Cyanocobalamin	4.8×10^{-6f}	0.24[f]	
Inulin	2.6×10^{-6}	0.02[d] 0.15[b]	0.02

[a] Data from ref. 168.
[b] Data from ref. 169.
[c] Data from ref. 170.
[d] Data from ref. 156.
[e] Data from ref. 44.
[f] Data from ref. 158.
[g] See ref. 9 for discussion of the relationship of permeability surface with clearance.

TABLE 13-4

Oxygen Tension of Maternal and Fetal Blood in Sheep, Monkey, and Human

	Sheep* (mm Hg)	Monkey* (mm Hg)	Human† (mm Hg)
Maternal artery	90	108	100
Uterine vein	50	37	55 (Intervillous space sample)
Umbilical artery	22	15	—
Umbilical vein	35	22	51

* Data from ref. 39.
† Data in refs. 159 and 144; umbilical blood obtained by percutaneous blood sampling.

trophoblast at the basal plasma membrane, thus lowering its intracellular concentration so a leak from maternal plasma into the syncytium occurs (perhaps the case for calcium). Two solutes for which it is clear that transporter proteins play an essential role in maternofetal transfer are glucose and amino acids.

Glucose Transfer

Human fetal plasma glucose concentrations are normally lower than those in maternal plasma, and it has been shown that in the isolated perfused human placental cotyledon, net transplacental glucose flux is directly proportional to the maternal arterial concentration.[43] Bain and colleagues[44] (using data on the permeability of the human placenta to extracellular markers) calculated that extracellular diffusion cannot supply sufficient glucose to meet fetal requirements. In fact, it is clear that glucose transfer across the human placenta is saturable, is stereospecific, shows competition, and is independent of energy sources[43,45-48] (i.e., it has all the classic characteristics of a facilitated diffusion system).[49] This finding has been confirmed by the demonstration that the syncytiotrophoblast expresses the GLUT-1–facilitated D-glucose transporter in both the microvillous and the basal plasma membrane.[50,51] GLUT-1 is one of a family of transporter proteins, present in various tissues, which translocate glucose transfer by facilitated diffusion,[52] and other members of the family may also be present in the placenta. Despite the existence of specific receptors for insulin on trophoblast, insulin has no

direct effect on glucose transfer across either the perfused cotyledon[53] or the microvillous membrane vesicles.[54] An insulin effect on metabolism of a glucose analogue by rat placenta has, however, been described.[55] The relationship between glucose transfer and intracellular trophoblast glucose metabolism has not been independently studied in humans; however, it is clear that there must be some pools of glucose within the trophoblast destined for transfer and some for metabolism. The complex behavior of these pools has been demonstrated in sheep.[56]

Amino Acids

Human umbilical venous plasma concentrations of most amino acids are significantly higher than maternal concentrations at mid-gestation[57,58] and at term.[59] Placental tissue concentrations of free amino acids appear to be higher than in either maternal or fetal plasma,[60] presumably because of a high syncytiotrophoblast concentration. A similar situation exists in other species, including guinea pigs and sheep.[61] Uptake of amino acids into human placental slices in vitro is inhibited under anaerobic conditions and in the presence of metabolic inhibitors.[62-64] Anaerobic metabolism, however, can support the uptake of amino acids into slices[65] and can transfer them across the perfused human cotyledon.[66]

It has therefore been assumed that amino acid transport in the maternofetal direction is an active process of the pump/leak type. Energy is required to transport amino acids into the syncytiotrophoblast, followed by a passive leak down the concentration gradient to fetal plasma. There is, however, no intrinsic reason that a passive leak should not also occur from syncytiotrophoblast into maternal plasma. For the observed asymmetric transcellular transport ($J_{mf} > J_{fm}$) to occur, either carriers must be present on the basal plasma membrane of the syncytiotrophoblast that are absent from the microvillous plasma membrane or the kinetic behavior of carriers on opposite faces of the trophoblast must differ. The presence of an asymmetric leak has been demonstrated for dually perfused guinea pig placenta using an indicator dilution technique.[67] In these studies, the uptake of amino acid was similar from both the maternal and the fetal circulations, but backflux (presumed to be efflux from the syncytiotrophoblast) was greater into the fetal circulation.[67]

A similar mechanism may apply to human placenta in that studies with the perfused human placental cotyledon have demonstrated stereospecific transport of the neutral amino acids L-leucine and L-alanine in the maternofetal, but not the fetomaternal, direction.[68] In addition, a faster rate of transport in the maternofetal direction has been demonstrated for aminoisobutyric acid

Figure 13–3. Transfer mechanisms within the placental tissue. A, Simple diffusion of relatively lipophilic substances (e.g., oxygen, anesthetic gases). **B,** Restricted diffusion of hydrophilic substances through hypothesized water-filled transmembrane channels of submicroscopic dimensions (e.g., mannitol). **C,** Facilitated diffusion (e.g., D-glucose). **D,** Active transport (e.g., amino acids). **E,** Receptor-mediated endocytosis (e.g., IgG, fluid-phase endocytosis). **F,** Exit mechanisms into fetal circulation. Not indicated are solvent drag, larger trophoblastic leaks, and the complicating factor of placental metabolism. (From Morriss FH, et al: *In* Knobil E, Neill J [eds]: Physiology of Reproduction, 2nd ed. New York, Raven Press, 1994, pp 813–861.)

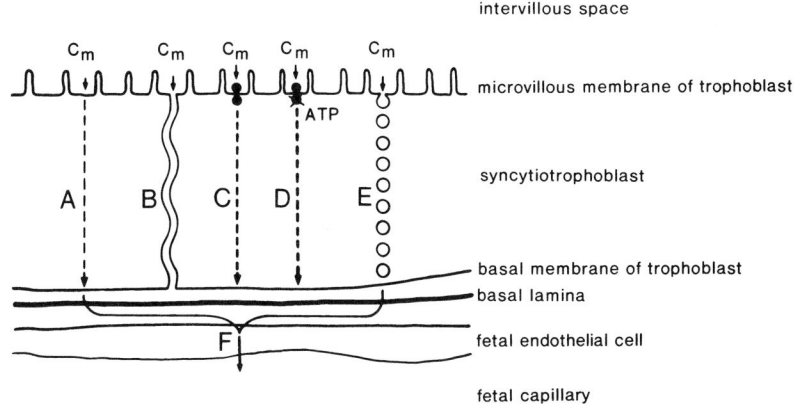

(AIB) (a nonmetabolizable amino acid analogue), L-leucine, and the basic amino acid L-lysine.[69] The fetomaternal transfer rates of AIB, L-leucine, and L-lysine are all nearly half the maternofetal transfer rate. Transport of these amino acids in the fetomaternal direction is thought to occur via the paracellular route because transfer rates are not different from those for the extracellular marker L-glucose. Therefore, paracellular diffusion cannot be ignored when considering net amino acid transfer to the fetus. These experiments have been carried out with equal maternal and fetal perfusate amino acid concentrations, and the importance of paracellular transfer may be even greater *in vivo* because fetal plasma amino acid concentrations are higher than maternal.

Uptake of amino acids by vesicles prepared from either the microvillous membrane or the basal plasma membrane of the syncytiotrophoblast of the human placenta has been extensively investigated.[29] The transporter systems are characterized based on competitive interactions and are analogous to those described for other epithelia.[70]

In both the microvillous and basal membranes, there is the common sodium-dependent System A transporter,[51, 71-74] which can support uptake of neutral amino acids with short polar or linear side chains, such as AIB, methyl-AIB, alanine, serine, proline, glycine, and methionine. Kudo and colleagues[73] also provided evidence of two other sodium-dependent carriers for neutral amino acids in the microvillous plasma membrane: one transporting proline and methionine and another specific for methionine. Neither these authors nor Johnson and Smith,[72] however, could find evidence of a sodium-dependent System ASC–type transporter, distinguished from System A by its relative pH insensitivity, higher stereospecificity, and intolerance of *N*-methylated amino acids (this type prefers large nonpolar branched-chain and aromatic neutral amino acids) similar to those observed using human placental fragments. In fact, the latter observation most probably resulted from the localization of System ASC to basal plasma membranes.[71, 75] There are two sodium-independent neutral amino acid carriers in microvillous plasma membranes, probably of the System 1 type:[72] one has a high affinity for leucine, and the other has a preference for alanine as substrate. System 1 is also present in the basal membrane.[71] Tryptophan, which may have an important role in immune evasion by placenta and fetus,[76] is taken up by microvillous membrane and basal vesicles using System 1;[72,77,78] there is evidence of an additional transporter for this amino acid in the basal membrane.[78]

Taurine has been shown to be taken up by a β-amino acid–specific, sodium/chloride–dependent transporter.[79-81] Cationic amino acids are taken up by syncytiotrophoblast membranes by the sodium-independent transporters System y+, System b0+, and System y+L.[82-84] However, in the term placenta, transport of cationic amino acids across the microvillous plasma membrane is predominantly by Systems y+ and y+L, and that across the basal membrane is predominantly by System y+L.[84]

There is only limited maternofetal transfer of the anionic amino acid glutamate across the perfused cotyledon.[85] Furthermore, there is a negative umbilical artery/umbilical vein concentration difference, suggesting uptake from the fetal circulation into placenta at least under the non–steady-state conditions of delivery.[86] The reasons for the lack of transfer of anionic amino acids are incompletely understood. There is a sodium-dependent, potassium-coupled, anionic amino acid transporter, System X$^-_{AG}$, in both microvillous and basal plasma membranes.[87,88] System X$^-_{AG}$ seems to be efficient because aspartate and glutamate are concentrated 23- and 34-fold by human placental slices, whereas other amino acids tested are concentrated no more than 12-fold.[89]

The sodium-dependent uptake of many amino acids across the microvillous plasma membrane suggests that *in vivo* uptake from the maternal circulation is energized by maintenance of a low sodium concentration within the trophoblast compared with that in the intervillous space. The sodium gradient is maintained by trophoblastic Na+,K+-ATPase activity. In support of this hypothesis is the observation that ouabain (10^{-5} M) inhibits AIB accumulation by the perfused cotyledon.[90] More puzzling, however, is how the accumulation of amino acids such as leucine is energized, when they appear to have only a sodium-independent pathway for uptake.[72] One possibility is that this uptake is energized by exchange transport with amino acids that are concentrated in the syncytiotrophoblast by Na+-dependent co-transport.[91] In fact, even though there is a high concentration of leucine in placental tissue[60] and fetal plasma,[59] ^{14}C-leucine is not concentrated by human placental slices, apparently because of a rapid efflux of leucine from the slices.[89] In contrast, ^{14}C-alanine is concentrated eightfold. It could be that the pump/leak hypothesis is an oversimplification and is not always applicable.

Despite evidence that amino acid handling by the placenta can be modulated by various different effectors,[9,29,61] there is no firm evidence that transfer *in vivo* is substantially reduced or enhanced by any individual hormone or drug. Active transport mechanisms must be operative early because fetal plasma concentrations of amino acids are higher than maternal plasma by 18 to 21 weeks of gestation;[57,58] there is good evidence that System A is present in the microvillous membrane in the first trimester.[92,93]

Amino acid delivery to the fetus is undoubtedly a key regulator of fetal growth[94] and is dependent on metabolic processes as well as transport across the placenta. There is good evidence from both animal models and the human of amino acid metabolism and synthesis in the placenta.[94] Interorgan cycling between liver and placenta of glycine and serine and glutamate and glutamine has also been demonstrated.[94] Placental transfer in relation to fetal growth is considered in more detail later.

Endocytosis and Exocytosis

Endocytosis is an invagination of the cell surface to form an intracellular membrane-bounded vesicle containing extracellular fluid;[95] *exocytosis* may be considered the opposite process, that is, fusion of a plasma membrane-bounded vesicle to the cell surface, followed by release of its contents. Endocytosis is classically divided into two types: *phagocytosis,* the process by which large particles (visible with the light microscope) are ingested; and *pinocytosis,* the process by which small solutes and water are absorbed. Iron transport may use the former process in the sheep,[96] but in the human the latter process is relevant to placental transport. Endocytosis and exocytosis occur in most, if not all, cells. Low-density lipoprotein, the transferrin/iron complex, and IgG all probably gain entry to the human placental syncytiotrophoblast by endocytosis.[97-99] Only IgG seems to be transported intact across the cell and exocytosed. Transfer of iron to the fetus may involve an exocytotic process as well, but not until after some intracellular processing has occurred that results in the return of transferrin to the maternal plasma.[99] The latter is also probably true for the transfer of retinol across the subhuman primate placenta.[100]

Asymmetric transport by endocytosis and exocytosis has three recognized phases, as described in the next sections.

Pinocytosis

This phase of the transport process may be fluid phase (nonselective),[95,101,102] adsorptive with nonspecific solute binding (e.g., that between cationized proteins and anionic sites in the plasma membrane of human and guinea pig placenta),[103,104] or mediated by a specific receptor. In the last, the specific receptors always become associated with specialized regions of the plasma membrane called *coated pits,* which have a coat of the protein clathrin visible on electron microscopy.[105,106] Invaginated coated pits with their associated receptors and receptor-ligand complexes form coated vesicles within the cell. It is also possible, however, that the clathrin coat will remain permanently attached to the plasma membrane and that receptor-bound ligands, after collection in the coated pits, will be transferred to uncoated vesicles.[95]

Transsyncytial Movement of Vesicles

The mechanism by which transsyncytial movement of vesicles occurs remains obscure. In other tissues, many vesicles fuse with lysosomes, and for some macromolecules, such as low-density lipoproteins in fibroblasts, this is the last step of the process.[105] For directed transplacental transport of intact IgG to occur, however, either some vesicles must avoid lysosomal fusion or the transported molecule must be protected from digestion in some other way. Transsyncytial movement of vesicles may occur by diffusion with vesicles moving from the region in which they are in high concentration at the site of endocytosis to the other side. Alternatively, as in secretory cells, microtubules and other components of the cytoskeletal system may direct vesicle shuttling.[107-109] In this regard, there is certainly a well-developed cytoskeletal system in human placental syncytium.[110]

Exocytosis

In the process of exocytosis, vesicles fuse with the plasma membrane at the opposite pole of the syncytium followed by release of the contents by fission. It is unknown how exocytosis occurs in the placenta. Generally, endocytosis cannot occur without exocytosis, in that areas of plasma membrane that are continuously lost from a cell surface must be continuously replaced and vice versa.[95,102] This process becomes even more complex when it is used for asymmetric transport across epithelia in that endocytosis occurring at the apical membrane of the cell is followed by transcytoplasmic movement and exocytosis at the basolateral membrane. The area of apical plasma membrane thus inserted into the basolateral membrane must then be specifically removed and recycled; otherwise, the normal polarity of the epithelial cell will eventually be lost.[102] It is quite obscure how this process takes place in a syncytial transporting epithelium such as human placenta.

Although the consideration of the role of endocytosis and exocytosis in the placental transfer of proteins and other macromolecules has generally focused on the syncytiotrophoblast, the fetal capillary endothelium also provides a considerable barrier to the exchange of such molecules.[111,112] Endocytosis and exocytosis could also be an important mechanism in this layer,[113] but this area requires a considerable amount of further work.

Immunoglobulin G Transfer

The selective transfer of IgG across the placenta confers passive immunity to the fetus. In other species, particularly rabbits, guinea pigs, and rodents, this function is served by the yolk sac placenta, which persists until term, rather than by the chorioallantoic placenta.[101,114] The mechanism of selective IgG transfer across the yolk sac placenta has been studied in depth. The pioneer of these studies, Brambell,[115] suggested that uptake of IgG is by a nonselective process but subsequent binding to receptors selectively prevents its degradation in phagolysosomes, allowing release of the intact molecule on the fetal side. As reviewed by Wild[114] and by Jollie,[101] however, it seems that although there may be some fluid-phase endocytosis of IgG, the most likely mechanism of selective transfer is receptor-mediated endocytosis via specific Fc receptors in coated pits. The IgG is transported through the cytoplasm in microvesicles (possibly coated), which avoid fusion with lysosomes. This model appears to be broadly applicable to selective IgG transfer across the human syncytiotrophoblast.[113] Whether it is also applicable to the fetal capillary endothelium remains a matter for further investigation.

Water Transfer

The human conceptus at term gestation contains 4 l of water (80% by weight of the intrauterine contents[116]); as Barcroft[117] pointed out, the net molar flux of water into the fetus is greater than that of any other substance, including oxygen. From kinetic analysis of plasma and amniotic fluid deuterium oxide concentrations, Hutchinson and colleagues[118] concluded that, at 40 weeks' gestation, the unidirectional flux of water across the human placenta is about 60 ml/minute/placenta in both directions, some 10,000 times the net flux.[119] Unidirectional fluxes from amniotic fluid to fetal plasma and amniotic fluid to maternal plasma (and in the reverse directions) represent only about 5% of the transplacental fluxes.

The main reasons for asymmetric unidirectional fluxes and thus for net water flux across the placenta are likely to be hydrostatic and osmotic pressure differences between fetal and maternal placental microcirculations. For example, acutely increasing the osmotic pressure of either maternal or fetal plasma by injection of hypertonic solutions leads to net flux of water out of the fetus or mother in primates,[120] rabbits,[121] and sheep.[122-124] In less acute experiments in the guinea pig, increasing fetal plasma colloid but not crystalloid osmotic pressure increased water acquisition over 20 hours.[125] Similarly, altering the hydrostatic pressure difference changes flow across both perfused guinea pig[126] and sheep placenta.[127] Despite these observations, the size and direction of osmotic and hydrostatic pressure differences between the microcirculations *in vivo* are unknown.

The factors regulating water acquisition remain somewhat obscure for at least two reasons. First, the reflection coefficients across placenta for the many solutes present in plasma are unknown. This makes calculation of the total effect of osmotic pressure of fetal and maternal plasma from knowledge of their individual solute concentrations[3] or from freezing point depression or colloid osmometry data[128] impossible. The relatively high apparent pore radius in the hemochorial placenta led Faber and Thornburg[3] to suggest that hydrostatic pressure, together with colloid osmotic pressure, rather than small solute osmotic pressures, governs net water flux across these in contrast to epitheliochorial placentas. Second, solute concentrations in plasma of the microcirculation may be different from those in the large vessels from which samples have been collected. Similar problems apply to the measurement of hydrostatic pressure. In women, it is not even clear whether fetal plasma total osmolarity is higher than[129] or equal to[3] maternal plasma osmolarity, whereas hydrostatic pressure in the intervillous space (insofar as it can be estimated) is lower than in the umbilical vein.[116, 130] Both these latter observations, if they reflect the steady state *in vivo,* are, in the absence of other forces, incompatible with the net transplacental acquisition of water by the fetus.

A further area of uncertainty is how far transplacental water flow is transcellular as opposed to paracellular. Both Faber and Hart,[131] using the fetal side perfused rabbit placenta, and Meschia and colleagues,[8] using an *in vivo* sheep preparation, showed that the clearance of ^3H_2O was much greater than would have been predicted based on molecular size alone if water had been restricted to the same paracellular route as, for example, sodium. Illsley and Verkman[132] measured the osmotic water permeability of a microvillous membrane vesicle preparation from which the paracellular route was excluded. Although uptake was found to be low compared with other plasma membranes, these investigators calculated that it was sufficiently high to account for the entire transplacental water flux[119] without the need to invoke a paracellular route for water. Despite the many probable inaccuracies in such a calculation, it does at least appear that a proportion of transplacental water movement in the human placenta is likely to be transcellular. Such transcellular fluxes may be mediated by aquaporins, a family of membrane proteins functioning as water channels and found in the syncytiotrophoblast.[133]

One report suggests that the transfer across the rat placenta of inert hydrophilic tracers is asymmetric, with fetomaternal transfer greater than maternofetal transfer.[134] Such asymmetric transfer is impossible to explain by paracellular diffusion alone, and the authors suggested that it could result from bulk flow of water, creating solvent drag in the fetomaternal direction. On this basis, the authors further suggested that solute-free water is driven transcellularly across the placenta, driven by osmotic gradients set up by active transport of solute. Water and dissolved solute then return from fetus to mother by paracellular filtration across the placenta, the whole system run to ensure that the net flux of water to the fetus is exactly correct. Reports of asymmetric transfer across the perfused human placental cotyledon,[135] together with the hydrostatic gradient as noted previously, suggest that a similar model could apply to the human. Despite this and several other attempts to model fetal water acquisition,[119, 136] the nature and control of water transfer across the placenta are poorly understood at present. It also remains possible that an important fraction of net water transfer between mother and fetus occurs extraplacentally via the amniochorion.

GESTATIONAL CHANGES

Most of the information on mechanisms of transfer across the human placenta has been gleaned from studies on the organ at term. It is important to know whether the same mechanisms apply, quantitatively and qualitatively, throughout gestation. Studies of the microvillous membrane of the syncytiotrophoblast suggest that although the fluidity, the activity of the System A amino acid transporter, the activity of the glucose transporter, and the activity of the Na^+/H^+ exchanger of this membrane are lower in the first trimester than at term,[92,93,137,138,152] its total electrogenic ion transport appears to be higher.[139] Thus, there may be quite selective changes over the course of gestation. The activity of the System A amino acid transporter, the glucose transporter, and the Na^+/H^+ exchanger in the microvillous membrane is similar in second trimester as compared with term placentas,[50,138,152] a finding suggesting that the first trimester is the key time of change. This could be necessary to permit sufficient placental transfer capacity to develop and support normal fetal growth. Regulation of gestational changes is an important area for future investigation.

PLACENTAL TRANSFER AND FETAL GROWTH

Net placental transfer over the course of gestation must (with the addition of any paraplacental transfer—likely to be tiny for most solutes after early gestation) exactly equal the solute and water composition of the baby at term. Placental transfer is thus intimately involved in determining fetal growth. Idiopathic intrauterine growth restriction (IUGR) has therefore been ascribed for many years to placental insufficiency. Because of the importance of oxygen delivery, the tendency of IUGR babies to be hypoxic, and the flow limitation of oxygen transfer (see earlier), placental insufficiency has become almost synonymous in the literature with a reduction in uterine or fetoplacental blood flow. This is also consistent with the association of IUGR with preeclampsia and abnormal uterine Doppler measurements.[140] However, although placental oxygen delivery and blood flow are undoubtedly important in determining fetal growth, more recent data show that this is not the complete picture. IUGR fetuses are hypoaminoacidemic and hyperlacticacidemic, and they also tend to be acidotic.[141-144] Placental transfer of amino acids, lactic acid, and protons is not predominantly flow limited; therefore, the barrier characteristics of the placenta in IUGR also need to be considered. Such a focus has led to the demonstration that the activity and expression of certain transporter proteins in both the microvillous and basal plasma membranes of the syncytiotrophoblast are altered in IUGR. These data, showing that a syncytiotrophoblast transport anomaly is an important facet of the pathophysiology in IUGR resulting from placental insufficiency, are summarized in Table 13–5. Some transporter activities increase, some decrease, and some show no change. This variability shows that the anomaly is complex and does not reflect a general down-regulation of metabolic activity, as could be expected. The reduction in activity of the amino acid transporters is likely to be particularly important in determining fetal growth rate. Human *in vivo* studies with stable isotopes revealed that, in normal pregnancy, the delivery of neutral amino acids is only just sufficient to meet fetal requirements,[94] and, in IUGR, maternofetal ^{13}C-leucine transfer is reduced as compared with normal findings.[145] In normal pregnancy, the activity of the System A amino acid transporter in the microvillous plasma membrane, per milligram of membrane protein, is inversely proportional to fetal size at birth.[146] This finding could reflect a compensatory up-regulation of the transporter in the smaller placentas of small normal babies, a hypothesis that is supported by data from mice in which the placenta-specific insulin-like growth factor II gene has been knocked out.[147] The finding that the same transporter activity is lower than normal in the placentas of IUGR babies[148,149] suggests that they are doubly disadvantaged compared with physiologically normal infants: they have a small placenta and less transporter activity per milligram membrane protein.

Diabetes mellitus during pregnancy can result in fetal overgrowth (macrosomia), and data suggest that syncytiotrophoblast transporter activities are also affected in this condition.[150-153] These observations demonstrate further the need for greater understanding of the regulation of placental transporter activity, in normal pregnancy and in those affected by IUGR and diabetes mellitus, as well as in relation to gestation.

TABLE 13-5

Activity of Transporters in Syncytiotrophoblast Microvillous and Basal Plasma Membranes in Intrauterine Growth Retardation

Transporter	MVM Change	BM Change	References
System A (alanine/glycine)	dec	nc	51, 148, 149, 171–173
Leucine	dec	dec	91
Lysine	nc	dec	91, 174
Sodium-dependent taurine	dec	nc	175
Sodium-independent taurine	nc	dec	175
GLUT1 (glucose)	nc	nc	51
Calcium (ATP-dependent)	Not present	inc	176
Sodium/hydrogen exchanger	dec	Not measured	149, 177

BM = basal plasma membrane; dec = decreased activity; inc = increased activity; MVM = microvillous plasma membrane; nc = no change in activity in comparison with gestation-matched pregnancies with normally grown babies. All data are from studies in which isolated MVM or BM vesicles were used for measurement of transport activity or expression.

REFERENCES

1. Boyd JD, Hamilton WJ: The Human Placenta. Cambridge, W Heffer & Sons, 1970.
2. Wooding FBP, et al: Autoradiographic evidence for migration and fusion of cells in the sheep placenta: resolution of a problem in placental classification. Cell Biol Int Rep 5:821, 1981.
3. Faber JJ, Thornburg KL: The forces that drive inert solutes and water across the epitheliochorial placentae of the sheep and the goat and the haemochorial placentae of the rabbit and the guinea pig. Placenta 2(Suppl):203, 1981.
4. Faber JJ, Thornburg KL: Placental Physiology. New York, Raven Press, 1983.
5. Schultz RL: Placental transport: a review. Obstet Gynecol Surv 25:979, 1970.
6. Morriss FH, et al: Placental transport. In Knobil E, Neill J (eds): Physiology of Reproduction, 2nd ed. New York, Raven Press, 1994, pp 813–861.
7. Faber JJ: Diffusional exchange between foetus and mother as a function of the physical properties of the diffusing materials. In Comline KS, et al (eds): Foetal and Neonatal Physiology. Cambridge, Cambridge University Press, 1973, pp 306–327.
8. Meschia G, et al: Theoretical and experimental study of transplacental diffusion. J Appl Physiol 22:1171, 1967.
9. Sibley CP, Boyd RDH: Control of transfer across the mature placenta. In Clarke JR (ed): Oxford Reviews of Reproductive Biology, Vol 10. Oxford, Oxford University Press, 1988, pp 382–435.
10. Hedley R, Bradbury MWB: Transport of polar non-electrolytes across the intact and perfused guinea-pig placenta. Placenta 1:277, 1980.
11. Thornburg KL, Faber JJ: Transfer of hydrophilic molecules by placenta and yolk sac of the guinea-pig. Am J Physiol 233:C111, 1977.
12. Boyd RDH, et al: Permeability of the sheep placenta to unmetabolized polar nonelectrolytes. J Physiol (Lond) 256:617, 1976.
13. Kaufmann P: Basic morphology of the fetal and maternal circuits in the human placenta. Contrib Gynecol Obstet 13:5, 1985.
14. Kaufmann P, et al: Fluid shift across the placenta. II. fetomaternal transfer of horseradish peroxidase in the guinea-pig. Placenta 3:339, 1982.
15. Kertschanska S, et al: Is there morphological evidence for the existence of transtrophoblastic channels in human placental villi? Troph Res 8:581, 1994.
16. Stulc J: Extracellular transport pathways in the haemochorial placenta. Placenta 10:113, 1989.
17. Edwards D, et al: Paracellular permeability pathways in the human placenta: a quantitative and morphological study of maternal-fetal transfer for horseradish peroxidase. Placenta 14:63, 1993.
18. Nelson DM, et al: Trophoblast interaction with fibrin matrix: epithelialization of perivillous fibrin deposits as a mechanism for villous repair in the human placenta. Am J Pathol 136:855, 1990.
19. Brownbill P, et al: Mechanisms of alphafetoprotein transfer in the perfused human placental cotyledon from uncomplicated pregnancy. J Clin Invest 96:2220, 1995.
20. Brownbill P, et al: Denudations as paracellular routes for alphafetoprotein and creatinine across the human syncytiotrophoblast. Am J Physiol 278:R677, 2000.
21. Stulc J, et al: Estimation of equivalent pore dimensions in the placenta of the rabbit. Life Sci 8:167, 1969.
22. Faber JJ, et al: Electrophysiology of extrafetal membranes. Placenta 8:89, 1988.
23. Stulc J, et al: Electrical potential difference across the mid-term human placenta. Acta Obstet Gynaecol Scand 57:125, 1978.
24. McNaughton TG, Power GG: The maternal-fetal electrical potential difference: new findings and a perspective. Placenta 12:185, 1991.
25. Greenwood SL, et al: Transtrophoblast and microvillous membrane potential difference in mature, intermediate human placental villi. Am J Physiol 265:C460, 1993.

26. Ward S, et al: Electrical potential difference between exocoelomic fluid and maternal blood in early pregnancy. Am J Physiol 43:R1492, 1998.
27. Stulc J, et al: Evidence for active maternal-fetal transport of Na+ across the placenta of the anaesthetised rat. J Physiol (Lond) 470:67, 1993.
28. Sibley CP, et al: Electrical activity and sodium transfer across the in vitro pig placenta. Am J Physiol 250:R474, 1986.
29. Jansson T: Amino acid transporters in the human placenta. Pediatr Res 49:141, 2001.
30. Persson A, et al: Na+/K+-ATPase activity and expression in syncytiotrophoblast plasma membranes in pregnancies complicated by diabetes. Placenta 23:386, 2002.
31. Stulc J, et al: Parallel mechanisms of calcium transfer across the perfused human placental cotyledon. Am J Obstet Gynecol 170:162, 1994.
32. Shennan DB, et al: Chloride transport in human placental microvillous membrane vesicles. Pflugers Arch 406:60, 1986.
33. Brown PD, et al: Chloride channels of high conductance in human placenta. Placenta 4:103, 1993.
34. Brunette MG, Allard S: Phosphate uptake by syncytial brush border membranes of human placenta. Pediatr Res 19:1179, 1985.
35. Cole DEC: Sulfate transport in brush border membrane vesicles prepared from human placental syncytiotrophoblast. Biochem Biophys Res Commun 123:223, 1984.
36. Bustamente JC, et al: A new form of asymmetry in epithelia: kinetics of apical and basal sulphate transport in human placenta. Q J Exp Physiol 73:1013, 1988.
37. Wilkening RB, Meschia G: Fetal oxygen uptake, oxygenation and acid-base balance as a function of uterine blood flow. Am J Physiol 244:H749, 1983.
38. Faber JJ, Hart FM: The rabbit placenta as an organ of diffusional exchange. Circ Res 19:816, 1966.
39. Meschia G: Placental respiratory gas exchange and fetal oxygenation. In Creasy RK, Resnik R (eds): Maternal Fetal Medicine: Principles and Practice. Philadelphia, WB Saunders Co, 1984, pp 274–285.
40. Itskovitz J, et al: Effects of fetal-maternal exchange transfusion on fetal oxygenation and blood flow distribution. Am J Physiol 247:H655, 1984.
41. Soothill PW, et al: The effect of replacing fetal hemoglobin with adult hemoglobin on blood gas and acid-base parameters in human fetuses. Am J Obstet Gynecol 158:66, 1988.
42. Stein WD: Channels, Carriers and Pumps. London, Academic Press, 1990.
43. Haugel S, et al: Glucose uptake, utilization, and transfer by the human placenta as functions of maternal glucose concentration. Pediatr Res 20:269, 1986.
44. Bain MD, et al: Normal placental transfer in the human. Arch Dis Child 63:688, 1988.
45. Carstensen M, et al: Evidence for a specific transport of D-hexoses across the human term placenta in vitro. Arch Gynecol 222:187, 1977.
46. Challier J-C, et al: Placental transport of hexoses: a comparative study with antipyrine and amino acids. Placenta 6:497, 1985.
47. Rice PA, et al: In vitro perfusion studies of the human placenta. IV. Some characterics of the glucose transport system in the human placenta. Gynecol Invest 7:213, 1976.
48. Rice PA, et al: In vitro perfusion studies of the human placenta. Am J Obstet Gynecol 133:649, 1979.
49. Widdas WF: Inability of diffusion to account for placental glucose transfer in the sheep and consideration of the kinetics of a possible carrier transfer. J Physiol (Lond) 118:23, 1952.
50. Jansson T, et al: Glucose transporter expression in placenta throughout gestation and in intrauterine growth retardation. J Clin Endocrinol Metab 77:1554, 1993.
51. Jansson T, et al: Glucose transporter and system A activity in syncytiotrophoblast microvillous and basal plasma membranes in intrauterine growth restriction. Placenta 23:392, 2002.

52. Devaskar SU, Mueckler M: The mammalian glucose transporters. Pediatr Res 31:1, 1992.

53. Challier J-C, et al: Effect of insulin on glucose uptake and metabolism in the human placenta. J Clin Endocrinol Metab 63:803, 1986.

54. Johnson LW, Smith CH: Monosaccharide transport across microvillous membrane of human placenta. Am J Physiol 238:C160, 1980.

55. Leturque A, et al: Glucose utilisation by the placenta of anaesthetised rats: effect of insulin, glucose and ketone bodies. Pediatr Res 22:483, 1987.

56. Hay WW Jr, et al: Maternal-fetal glucose exchange: necessity of a three-pool model. Am J Physiol 246:E528, 1984.

57. McIntosh N: Plasma amino acids of the mid-trimester human fetus. Biol Neonate 45:218, 1984.

58. Soltesz G, et al: The metabolic and endocrine milieu of the human fetus and mother at 18–21 weeks of gestation. I. Plasma amino acid concentrations. Pediatr Res 19:91, 1985.

59. Young M, Prenton MA: Maternal and fetal plasma amino acid concentrations during gestation and in retarded fetal growth. J Obstet Gynaecol Br Commonwlth 76:333, 1969.

60. Pearse WH, Sornson H: Free amino acids of normal and abnormal human placenta. Am J Obstet Gynecol 105:696, 1969.

61. Yudilevich DL, Sweiry JH: Transport of amino acids in the placenta. Biochim Biophys Acta 822:169, 1985.

62. Dancis J, et al: Transport of amino acids by placenta. Am J Obstet Gynecol 101:820, 1968.

63. Litonjua AD, et al: Uptake of alpha-aminoisobutyric acid in placental slices at term. Am J Obstet Gynecol 99:242, 1967.

64. Sybulski S, Tremblay PC: Uptake and incorporation into protein of radioactive glycine by human placentas in vitro. Am J Obstet Gynecol 97:1111, 1967.

65. Longo LD: Anaerobic, glycogen-dependent transport of amino acids by the placenta. Nature 243:531, 1973.

66. Penfold P, et al: Human placental amino acid transfer and metabolism in oxygenated and anoxic conditions. Troph Res 1:27, 1983.

67. Eaton BM, Yudilevich DL: Uptake and asymmetric efflux of amino acids at maternal and fetal sides of the placenta. Am J Physiol 241:C106, 1981.

68. Schneider H, et al: Transfer of amino acids across the in vitro perfused human placenta. Pediatr Res 13:236, 1979.

69. Schneider H, et al: Asymmetrical transfer of α-aminoisobutyric acid (AIB), leucine and lysine across the in vitro perfused human placenta. Placenta 8:141, 1987.

70. Christensen HN: Exploiting amino acid structure to learn about membrane transport. Adv Enzymol 49:41, 1979.

71. Hoeltzli SD, Smith CH: Alanine transport systems in isolated basal plasma membrane of human placenta. Am J Physiol 256:C630, 1989.

72. Johnson LW, Smith CH: Neutral amino acid transport systems of microvillous membrane of human placenta. Am J Physiol 254:C773, 1988.

73. Kudo Y, et al: Characterization of amino acid transport systems in human placental brush-border membrane vesicles. Biochim Biophys Acta 904:309, 1987.

74. Enders RH, et al: Placental amino acid uptake. III. Transport systems for neutral amino acids. Am J Physiol 230:706, 1976.

75. Furesz TC, et al: ASC system activity is altered by development of cell priority in trophoblast from human placenta. Am J Physiol 265:C212, 1993.

76. Kudo Y, Boyd CA: The physiology of immune evasion during pregnancy: the critical role of placental tryptophan metabolism and transport. Pflugers Arch 44:639, 2001.

77. Ganapathy ME, et al: Characterization of tryptophan transport in human placental brush-border membrane vesicles. Biochem J 238:201, 1986.

78. Kudo Y, Boyd CA: Characterisation of L-tryptophan transporters in human placenta: a comparison of brush border and basal membrane vesicles. J Physiol (Lond) 531:405, 2001.

79. Karl PI, Fisher SE: Taurine transport by microvillous membrane vesicles, cultured trophoblasts and isolated perfused human placenta. Am J Physiol 258:C302, 1990.

80. Miyamoto Y, et al: Na$^+$Cl$^-$gradient-driven, high affinity, uphill transport of taurine in human placental brush border membrane vesicles. FEBS Lett 231:263, 1988.

81. Ramamoorthy S, et al: Functional characterisation and chromosomal localisation of cloned taurine transporter from human placenta. Biochem J 300:893, 1994.

82. Furesz TC, et al: Two cationic amino acid transport systems in human placental basal plasma membranes. Am J Physiol 261:C246, 1991.

83. Deves R, et al: Identification of a new transport system (y$^+$L) in human erythrocytes that recognises lycine and leucine with high affinity. J Physiol (Lond) 454:491, 1992.

84. Ayuk P, et al: Development and polarisation of cationic amino acid transporters and regulators in the human placenta. Am J Physiol 278:C1162, 2000.

85. Schneider H, et al: Transfer of glutamic acid across the human placenta perfused in vitro. Br J Obstet Gynaecol 86:299, 1979.

86. Hayashi S, et al: Umbilical vein-artery differences of plasma amino acids in fetal tissues. Biol Neonate 34:11, 1978.

87. Hoeltzli SD, et al: Anionic amino acid transport systems in isolated basal plasma membrane of human placenta. Am J Physiol 259:C47, 1990.

88. Moe AJ, Smith CH: Anionic amino acid uptake by microvillous membrane vesicles from human placenta. Am J Physiol 257:C1005, 1989.

89. Schneider H, Dancis J: Amino acid transport in human placental slices. Am J Obstet Gynecol 120:1092, 1974.

90. Wier PJ, et al: Bidirectional transfer of α-aminoisobutyric acid by the perfused human placental lobule. Troph Res 1:37, 1983.

91. Jansson T, et al: Placental transport of leucine and lycine is reduced in intrauterine growth restriction. Pediatr Res 44:532, 1998.

92. Iioka H, et al: Characterisation of human placental activity of transport of L-alanine using brush border (microvillous) membrane vesicles. Placenta 13:179, 1992.

93. Mahendran D, et al: Na$^+$ transport, H$^+$ concentration gradient dissipation, and system A amino acid transporter activity in purified microvillous plasma membrane isolated from first trimester human placenta: comparison with the term microvillous membrane. Am J Obstet Gynecol 171:1534, 1994.

94. Cetin I: Amino acid interconversions in the fetal-placental unit: the animal model and human studies in vivo. Pediatr Res 49:148, 2001.

95. Besterman JM, Low RB: Endocytosis: a review of mechanisms and plasma membrane dynamics. Biochem J 210:1, 1983.

96. Burton GJ, et al: Ultrastructural studies of the placenta of the ewe: phagocytosis of erythrocytes by the chorionic epithelium at the central depression of the cotyledon. Q J Exp Physiol 61:275, 1976.

97. King BF: Absorption of peroxidase-conjugated immunoglobulin G by human placenta: an in vitro study. Placenta 3:395, 1982.

98. Malassine A, et al: Ultrastructural visualisation of gold low-density lipoprotein endocytosis by human term placental cells (abstract). Placenta 7:485, 1986.

99. van Dijk JP: Regulatory aspects of placental iron transfer: a comparative study. Placenta 9:215, 1988.

100. Vahlquist A, Nilsson S: Vitamin A transfer to the fetus and to the amniotic fluid in rhesus monkey (*Macaca mulatta*). Ann Nutr Metab 28:321, 1984.

101. Jollie WP: Ultrastructural studies of protein transfer across rodent yolk sac. Placenta 7:263, 1986.

102. Steinman RS, et al: Endocytosis and the recycling of plasma membrane. J Cell Biol 96:1, 1983.

103. King BF: The distribution and mobility of anionic sites on the surface of human placental syncytial trophoblast. Anat Rec 199:15, 1981.

104. Sibley CP, et al: Molecular charge as a determinant of macromolecule permeability across the fetal capillary endothelium of the guinea-pig placenta. Cell Tissue Res 229:365, 1983.

105. Goldstein JL, et al: Coated pits, coated vesicles, and receptor-mediated endocytosis. Nature 279:679, 1979.

106. Pearse BMF: Structure of coated pits and vesicles. Ciba Found Symp 92:246, 1982.

107. Aunis D, et al: Tubulin and actin binding proteins in chromaffin cells. Ann NY Acad Sci 493:435, 1987.

108. Knight DE, Baker PF: Exocytosis from the vesicle viewpoint: an overview. Ann NY Acad Sci 493:504, 1987.

109. Sheetz MP, et al: Movement of vesicles on tubules. Ann NY Acad Sci 493:409, 1987.

110. Ockleford CD, et al: Morphogenesis of human placental chorionic villi: cytoskeletal, syncytioskeletal and extracellular matrix proteins. Proc R Soc Lond B Biol Sci 212:305, 1981.

111. Dancis J, et al: Placental transfer of proteins in human gestation. Am J Obstet Gynecol 82:167, 1961.

112. Firth JH, Leach L: Not trophoblast alone: a review of the contribution of the fetal microvasculature to transplacental exchange. Placenta 17:89, 1996.

113. Saji F, et al: Dynamics of immunoglobulins at the feto-maternal interface. Rev Reprod 4:81, 1999.

114. Wild AE: Endocytic mechanisms in protein transfer across the placenta. Placenta 1(Suppl):165, 1981.

115. Brambell FWR: The transmission of immunity from mother to young and the catabolism of immunoglobulins. Lancet 2:1087, 1966.

116. Seeds AE: Water metabolism of the fetus. Am J Obstet Gynecol 92:727, 1965.

117. Barcroft J: Researches on Prenatal Life. Oxford, Blackwell, 1946.

118. Hutchinson DL, et al: The role of the fetus in the water exchange of the amniotic fluid of normal and hydramniotic patients. J Clin Invest 38:971, 1959.

119. Wilbur WJ, et al: Water exchange in the placenta: a mathematical model. Am J Physiol 235:R181, 1978.

120. Bruns PD, et al: Effects of osmotic gradients across the primate placenta upon fetal and placental water contents. Pediatrics 34:407, 1964.

121. Bruns PD, et al: The placental transfer of water from fetus to mother following the intravenous infusion of hypertonic mannitol to the maternal rabbit. Am J Obstet Gynecol 86:160, 1963.

122. Faber JJ, Green TJ: Foetal placental blood flow in the lamb. J Physiol (Lond) 223:375, 1972.

123. Leake RD, et al: Arginine vasopressin and arginine vasotocin inhibit ovine fetal/maternal water transfer. Pediatr Res 17:583, 1983.

124. Woods LL, Brace RA: Fetal blood volume, vascular pressure and heart rate responses to fetal and maternal hyperosmolality. Am J Physiol 251:H716, 1986.

125. Anderson D, Faber J: Water flux due to colloid osmotic pressures across the haemochorial placenta of the guinea-pig. J Physiol (Lond) 332:521, 1982.

126. Schröder H, et al: Fluid shift across the placenta. I. The effect of dextran T40 in the isolated guinea pig placenta. Placenta 3:327, 1982.

127. Power GG, et al: Water transfer across the placenta: hydrostatic and osmotic forces and the control of fetal cardiac output. *In* Longo LD, Reneau DD (eds): Fetal and Newborn Cardiovascular Physiology. New York, Garland Publishing, 1976.

128. Hinkley CM, Blechner JN: Colloidal osmotic pressures of human maternal and fetal blood plasma. Am J Obstet Gynecol 103:71, 1969.

129. Battaglia F, et al: Fetal blood studies. XIII. The effect of the administration of fluids intravenously to mothers upon the concentrations of water and electrolytes in plasma of human fetuses. Pediatrics 25:2, 1960.

130. Reynolds SRM, et al: Multiple simultaneous intervillous space pressures recorded in several regions of the hemochorial placenta in relation to functional anatomy of the fetal cotyledon. Am J Obstet Gynecol 102:1128, 1968.

131. Faber JJ, Hart FM: Transfer of charged and uncharged molecules in the placenta of the rabbit. Am J Physiol 213:890, 1967.

132. Illsley NP, Verkman AS: Serial permeability barriers to water transport in human placental vesicles. J Membr Biol 94:267, 1986.

133. Damiano A, et al: Water channel proteins AQP3 and AQP9 are present in syncytiotrophoblast of human term placenta. Placenta 22:776, 2001.

134. Stulc J, et al: Asymmetrical transfer of inert hydrophilic solutes across the rat placenta. Am J Physiol 265:R670, 1993.

135. Schneider H, et al: Effects of elevated umbilical venous pressure on fluid and solute transport across the isolated perfused human cotyledon. Troph Res 3:189, 1988.

136. Conrad EE, Faber JJ: Water and electrolyte acquisition across the placenta of the sheep. Am J Physiol 233:H475, 1977.

137. Ghosh PK, Mukherje AM: Increasing fluidity of human placental syncytiotrophoblastic brush border membrane with advancement of gestational age: fluorescence polarisation study. Biochim Biophys Acta 1236:317, 1995.

138. Hughes JL, et al: Activity and expression of the Na^+/H^+ exchanger in the microvillous plasma membrane of the syncytiotrophoblast in relation to gestation and small for gestational age birth. Pediatr Res 48: 652, 2000.

139. Birdsey TJ, et al: Microvillous membrane potential (E_m) in isolated placental villi from the first trimester. Placenta 16:A6, 1995.

140. Harrington KF, et al: Doppler velocimetry studies of the uterine artery in the early prediction of pre-eclampsia and intrauterine growth retardation. Eur J Obstet Gynecol Reprod Biol 42(Suppl):S14, 1991.

141. Bernardini I, et al: The fetal concentrating index as a gestational age independent measure of placental dysfunction in intrauterine growth retardation. Am J Obstet Gynecol 164:1481, 1991.

142. Cetin I, et al: Umbilical amino acid concentrations in normal and growth retarded fetuses sampled in utero by cordocentesis. Am J Obstet Gynecol 162:243, 1990.

143. Pardi G, et al: Diagnostic value of blood sampling in fetuses with growth retardation. N Engl J Med 328:692, 1993.

144. Soothill PW, et al: Blood gases and acid base status of the human second trimester fetus. Obstet Gynecol 68:173, 1986.

145. Marconi AM, et al: The steady state maternal-fetal leucine enrichments in normal and fetal growth restricted pregnancies. Pediatr Res 46:114, 1999.

146. Godfrey K, et al: Neutral amino acid uptake by the microvillous plasma membrane of the human placenta is inversely related to fetal size at birth in normal pregnancy. J Clin Endocrinol Metab 83:3320, 1998.

147. Constancia M, et al: Placental-specific IGF2 is a major modulator of placental and fetal growth. Nature 417:945, 2002.

148. Mahendran D, et al: Amino acid (system A) transporter activity in microvillous membrane vesicles from the placentas of appropriate and small for gestational age babies. Pediatr Res 34:661, 1993.

149. Glazier JD, et al: Association between the activity of the system A amino acid transporter in the microvillous plasma membrane of the human placenta and the severity of fetal compromise in intrauterine growth restriction. Pediatr Res 42:514, 1997.

150. Kuruvilla AG, et al: Altered activity of the system A amino acid transporter in microvillous membrane vesicles from placentas of macrosomic babies born to diabetic women. J Clin Invest 94:689, 1994.

151. Gaither K, et al: Diabetes alters the expression and activity of the human placental GLUT1 glucose transporter. J Clin Endocrinol Metab 84:695, 1999.

152. Jansson T: Placental glucose transport and GLUT1 expression in insulin-dependent diabetes. Am J Obstet Gynecol 180:163, 1999.

153. Osmond DT, et al: Placental glucose transport and utilisation is altered at term in insulin treated, gestational-diabetic patients. Diabetologia 44:1133, 2001.

154. Mossman HW: Vertebrate Fetal Membranes. London, Macmillan, 1987.

155. Widdowson EM, Spray CM: Chemical development in utero. Arch Dis Child 26:205, 1951.

156. Bain MD, et al: In vivo permeability of the human placenta to inulin and mannitol. J Physiol (Lond) 399:313, 1988.

157. Flexner LB, Gellhorn A: The comparative physiology of placental transfer. Am J Obstet Gynecol 43:965, 1942.

158. Willis DM, et al: Diffusion permeability of cyanocobalamin in human placenta. Am J Physiol 250:R459, 1986.

159. Nicolaides KH, et al: Ultrasound-guided sampling of umbilical cord and placental blood to assess fetal well being. Lancet 1:1065, 1986.

160. Schneider H, Dancis J (eds): In Vitro Perfusion of Human Placental Tissue. Basel, S. Karger, 1985.

161. Carstensen MH, et al: Lactate carriers in the artificially perfused human term placenta. Placenta 4:165, 1983.

162. Siman CM, et al: The functional regeneration of syncytiotrophoblast in cultured explants of term placenta. Am J Physiol 280:R1116, 2001.

163. Shennan DB, Boyd CAR: Ion transport by the placenta: a review of membrane transport systems. Biochim Biophys Acta 906:437, 1987.

164. Douglas GC, King BF: Receptor mediated endocytosis of ^{125}I-labelled transferrin by human choriocarcinoma (JAR) cells. Placenta 9:252, 1988.

165. Bara M, et al: Membrane potential and input resistance in syncytiotrophoblast of human term placenta in vitro. Placenta 9:139, 1988.

166. Carstensen M, et al: Zellpotentiale in der placenta des Menschen. Arch Gynaecol 215:299, 1973.

167. Birdsey TJ, et al: The effect of hyposmotic challenge on microvillous membrane potential (E_m) in isolated human placental villi. Am J Physiol 276:R1479, 1999.

168. Robinson NR, et al: Permeability of the near-term rat placenta to hydrophilic solutes. Placenta 9:361, 1988.

169. Thornburg KL, et al: Permeability of placenta to inulin. Am J Obstet Gynecol 158:1165, 1988.

170. Flexner LB, et al: The permeability of the human placenta to sodium in normal and abnormal pregnancies and the supply of sodium to the human fetus as determined by radioactive sodium. Am J Obstet Gynecol 55:469, 1948.

171. Dicke JM, Henderson GI: Placental amino acid uptake in normal and complicated pregnancies. Am J Med Sci 295:223, 1988.

172. Dicke JM, Vergas DK: Neutral amino acid uptake by microvillous and basal plasma membrane vesicles from appropriate and small for gestational age human pregnancies. J Matern Fetal Med 3:246, 1994.

173. Harrington B, et al: System A amino acid transporter activity in human placental microvillous membrane vesicles in relation to various anthropometric measurements in appropriate (AGA) and small for gestational age (SGA) babies. Pediatr Res 45:810, 1999.

174. Ayuk PT-Y, et al: L-Arginine transport by the microvillous plasma membrane of the syncytiotrophoblast from human placenta in relation to nitric oxide production: effects of gestation, pre-eclampsia and intrauterine growth restriction. J Clin Endocrinol Metab 87:747, 2002.

175. Norberg S, et al: Intrauterine growth restriction is associated with a reduced activity of placental taurine transporters. Pediatr Res 44:233, 1998.

176. Strid H, et al: ATP-dependent Ca^{2+} transport in pregnancy is complicated by diabetes or intrauterine growth restriction. Placenta 22:A66, 2001.

177. Johansson M., et al: Activity and expression of the Na^+/H^+ exchanger is reduced in syncytiotrophoblast microvillous plasma membranes isolated from preterm intrauterine growth restriction pregnancies. J Clin Endocrinol Metab 87:5686, 2002.

Theresa M. Siler-Khodr

14 Endocrine and Paracrine Function of the Human Placenta

By the early 1900s, the placenta was recognized as an endocrine organ. Reports by Zondek and Aschheim[1] and by Philipp[2] described placental hormone activities similar to both ovarian and hypophyseal hormones, and the significance of placental hormone products for the maintenance of pregnancy was realized. Since that time, the role of placental hormones, which act as endocrine, paracrine, and autocrine regulators of pregnancy, has been defined not only for hypophyseal and gonadal-like hormones but also for multiple hypothalamic-like releasing hormone, cytokines, growth factors, other proteins, peptides, and

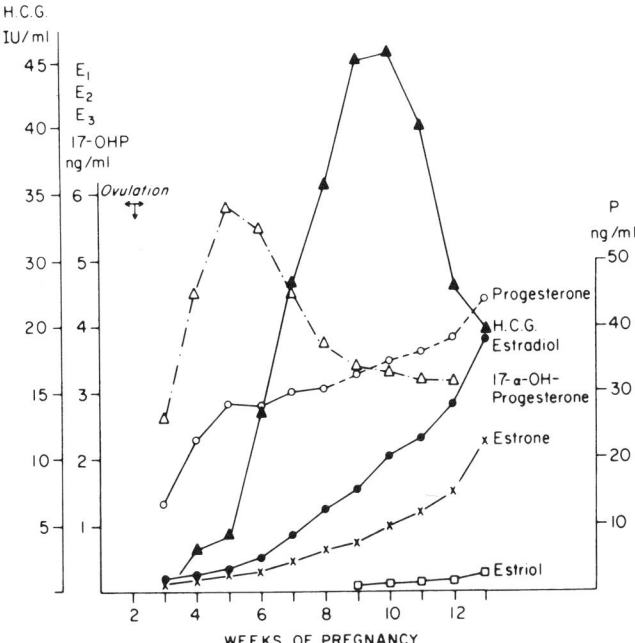

Figure 14–1. Maternal plasma levels of human chorionic gonadotropin (hCG) and steroids during human pregnancy. (From Tulchinsky D, Hobel CJ: Am J Obstet Gynecol *117*:884, 1973.)

eicosanoids. The regulation and function of each of these activities as related to the placenta are discussed in this chapter.

HYPOPHYSEAL-LIKE HORMONES

Possibly the best-known hormone of pregnancy is human chorionic gonadotropin (hCG). Its activity was first reported in the early 1900s.[1, 2] Wislocki and Bennett[3] originally proposed that hCG was synthesized by the cytotrophoblast because its concentrations in pregnancy were parallel to the number and density of cytotrophoblast in the placenta. Since then, it has been demonstrated that after the first few weeks of pregnancy, hCG is primarily synthesized by the syncytiotrophoblastic cells,[4] and a releasing factor, gonadotropin-releasing hormone (GnRH; both mammalian and chicken II isoforms), which is produced largely in the cytophoblast, can regulate its synthesis.[5-7] hCG is a glycoprotein composed of α and β subunits that are translated from separate messenger RNAs.[8] The α subunit is produced in excess of the β subunit, and this ratio increases as gestation progresses. As a result, little free βhCG is secreted, and the hCG in maternal circulation is mostly intact hCG or free αhCG. Intact hCG (i.e., having both α and β subunits) is required for its known biologic activities, which are similar to those of human luteinizing hormone (hLH). In addition, the degree of glycosylation of the hCG molecule decreases as pregnancy advances, and a decreased level of glycosylation in very early pregnancy has been correlated with early pregnancy loss.[9, 10]

hCG can be immunologically distinguished from hLH by using antisera directed against the C-terminal amino acids of its β subunit, which are not present in hLH. Use of β-subunit hCG-specific antisera is the basis for most current pregnancy tests. Increasing hCG secretion can be detected in the maternal circulation by 24 hours after implantation, and it increases with a doubling time averaging 2.11 days. It reaches peak levels of approximately 50 IU/mL at 9 to 10 weeks from the date of the last menstrual period and declines thereafter to 1 IU/mL by midgestation (see Fig. 14–3).[11] In early gestation, the hCG doubling time is an effective way to predict the outcome of a

pregnancy. An abnormally slow doubling time of hCG is considered a poor prognostic sign for pregnancy outcome.[12]

In early pregnancy, hCG has both endocrine and paracrine functions: (1) to stimulate formation of the corpus luteum of pregnancy, which, in turn, produces progesterone; and (2) to stimulate placental steroidogenesis and uterine activities allowing for implantation. As placental function develops, the first role of hCG is to maintain corpus luteal production of progesterone. The ovarian-placental shift occurs at least 2 weeks before attaining peak placental hCG production (35 to 47 days after ovulation) (Fig. 14–1). Another hormonal function ascribed to hCG is that of thyrotropic activity, which may increase thyroid function. Other thyrotropic factors are produced by trophoblastic tissues. In addition, hCG may have an immunosuppressive function. A more complete review of these activities is given by Osathanondh and Tulchinsky.[11]

Multiple factors can influence hCG production, such as GnRH,[13,14] neurotransmitters,[15] cyclic adenosine monophosphate (cAMP),[16] epidermal growth factor,[17] activin,[18] cytokines,[19] hCG itself,[20] and, in some studies, prostaglandins.[21] Each of these is produced by the placenta as well as by other trophoblastic tissue. hCG is known to affect placental steroidogenesis by stimulating both progesterone and estrogen formation. Estrogens can inhibit GnRH stimulation of hCG,[22] thus completing a feedback axis in the paracrine placenta. Other hormones such as inhibin[23] have also been shown to modulate this axis.

Proteins with lactogenic and growth hormone (GH)–like activity were first extracted from human placenta by Higashi in 1961.[24] Shortly thereafter, Josimovich and MacLaren[25] isolated the protein originally named human placental lactogen (hPL). This name was later changed to human chorionic somatomammotropin (hCS) to include in its name its GH-like activity as well as its lactogenic activity. Its amino acid sequence has been determined, and it is known to be a single peptide chain of 192 amino acids having many homologies with human GH and prolactin (PRL). It is synthesized by the syncytiotrophoblasts of the placenta and attains maximal production in late gestation. At that time, it accounts for 10% of the total placental protein synthesis by the placenta. It is the product of two genes, which flank the *hGH-V* gene expressed in the human placenta.[26,27]

Placental concentration of hCS during pregnancy parallels the mass of the placenta throughout gestation. As a result, maternal circulating hCS levels increase throughout gestation and appear to reflect placental function. hCS is secreted into the maternal circulation, where it induces metabolic changes such as mobilization of fatty acids, insulin resistance, decreased utilization of glucose, and increased availability of amino acids through decreased maternal use of protein.[28] In addition, the lactogenic activity of hCS suggests that it may play a synergistic role with PRL and steroids in preparation of the breast for lactation.[29] In the placenta, both hPL and GH-V may regulate insulin-like growth factor I (IGF-I)[30] and may affect fetal growth, most likely by direct action on placental nutrient transport. The absence of hPL and *HGH-V* expression is reported to result in a severely growth-retarded fetus.[28]

Factors that control the release of hCS are poorly defined. Release of hCS is stimulated by high density lipoproteins, apolipoproteins,[27,30] angiotensin,[31] cAMP,[32] and arachidonic acid (AA) and is inhibited by prostaglandin E_2 (PGE_2) and $PGF_{2\alpha}$,[33] catecholamines, phorbol esters, and diacylglycerols.[34] In addition, dopaminergic agents have been shown to inhibit its release.[35] The releasing and inhibiting factors found in the placenta, however, have not yet been shown to affect hCS release.

PRL is also known to increase during pregnancy both in maternal blood and in amniotic fluid.[36] The PRL in maternal blood is thought to be of maternal pituitary origin, whereas that in amniotic fluid is thought to be of decidual origin. The role of these high amniotic fluid PRL levels (up to 3 μg/mL) in pregnancy is not understood. The ability of the decidua to synthesize PRL has been demonstrated. Decidual PRL is stimulated by αhCG.[37]

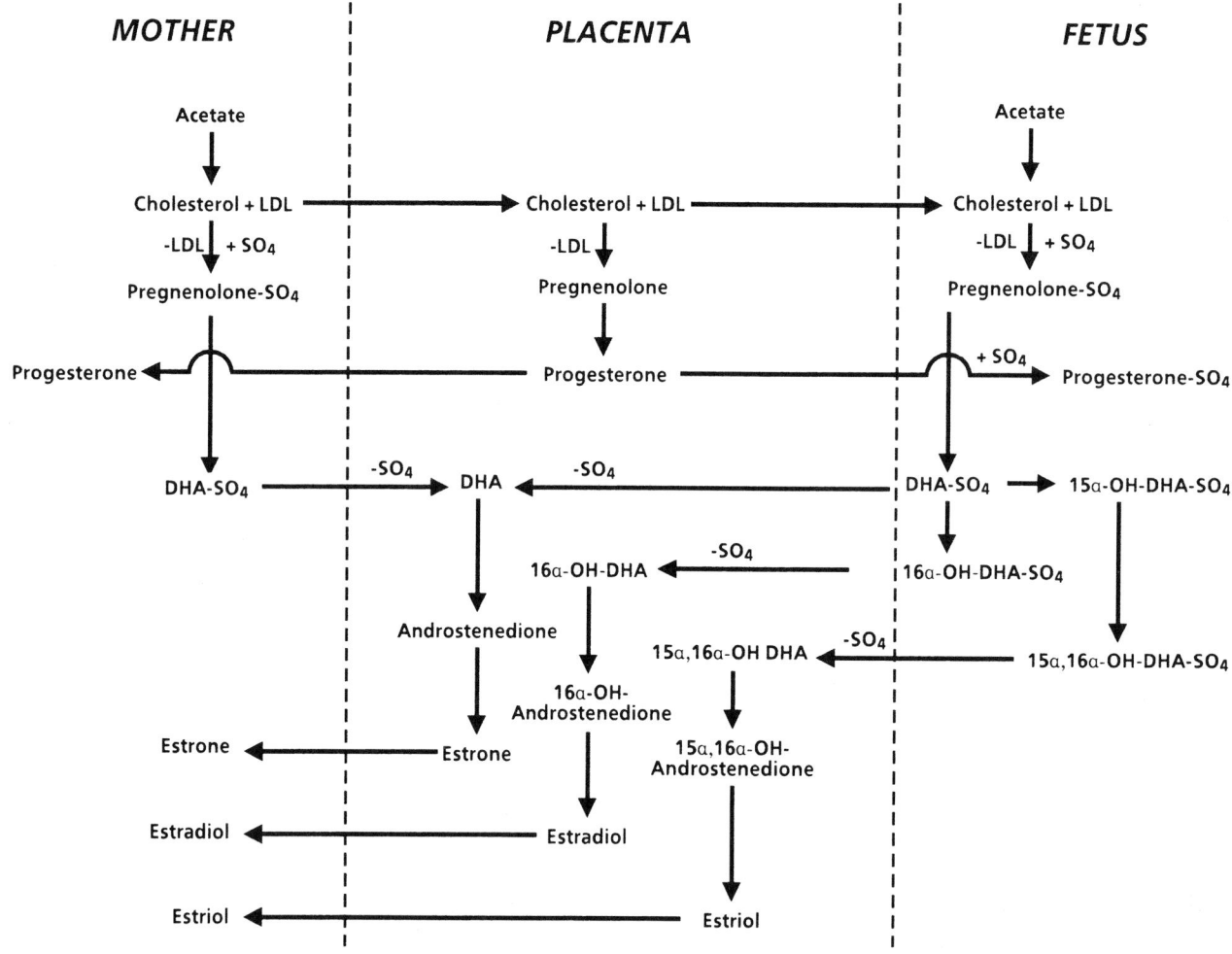

Figure 14–2. Steroidogenic pathways in the human maternal placental-fetal unit. DHA-SO$_4$, dehydroepiandrosterone sulfate.

Other pituitary-like peptides such as corticotropin (ACTH), melanocyte-stimulating hormone, β-endorphins, and β-lipoproteins have been demonstrated in the human placenta by immunologic and biologic assays, although chemical identity of these placental peptides has not been completely defined. This topic is well reviewed by Krieger.[38] Prostaglandins have been found to increase β-lipotropin and β-endorphin levels in amniotic fluid.[39] A chorionic corticotropin-releasing hormone (chorionic CRH) has been described and is discussed in more detail later. CRH has been shown to stimulate the release of chorionic ACTH.[40] The physiologic role of chorionic ACTH has not been defined, but it may affect placental cortisol production or fetal adrenal function or both.

STEROIDOGENESIS AND THE MATERNOFETOPLACENTAL UNIT

Although the placenta has been known to be the source of steroid hormones since the early 1900s, it was not until the late 1950s that it was understood how steroids were synthesized by the placenta. In 1959, Ryan[41] demonstrated that the placenta could convert dehydroepiandrosterone sulfate (DHA-SO$_4$) to estrogens; however, it was not until 5 years later that Diczfalusy[42] proposed and subsequently demonstrated the existence of a fetoplacental unit, in which fetal enzymes and placental enzymes work in concert to produce estrogens. Although the use of maternal cholesterol for placental progesterone synthesis was suggested by Bloch as early as 1945,[43] further studies that

unquestionably confirmed these findings and established that maternal cholesterol was the principal precursor of progesterone production were not completed until 1970.[44] The fetoplacental unit was then expanded to include the mother because maternal cholesterol is needed for placental production of progesterone and for the precursors used for fetal androgen production.[45] Fetal DHA-SO$_4$, in turn, is used as a substrate for placental synthesis of estrogens. Thus, the maternofetoplacental unit functions to produce progesterone and estrogens. These resulting steroids are found largely in the maternal circulation during pregnancy. Comprehensive reviews of the literature defining their synthesis and functions are available.[45]

Figure 14–2 illustrates the tissues and enzymes that participate in the biosynthesis of progesterone and estrogens. Maternal cholesterol, derived from low density lipoprotein, is transported to the placenta and is bound to specific low density lipoprotein receptors on the syncytiotrophoblast, where it is incorporated by endocytosis and is hydrolyzed to free cholesterol in the lysosomes.[8] In the syncytiotrophoblastic cells of the placenta, cholesterol is converted to pregnenolone. This metabolic transformation is catalyzed by mitochondrial enzymes (the 20, 22 desmolase complex). Some of the pregnenolone is sent to the fetus, but much is converted to progesterone by the 3β-hydroxysteroid dehydrogenase–Δ^5-Δ^4-isomerase complex.[10, 11] Approximately 90% of this progesterone goes to the mother and 10% to the fetus. The fetus has the former enzyme activity needed for pregnenolone synthesis but is severely lacking in the latter enzymatic complex, which is needed for progesterone pro-

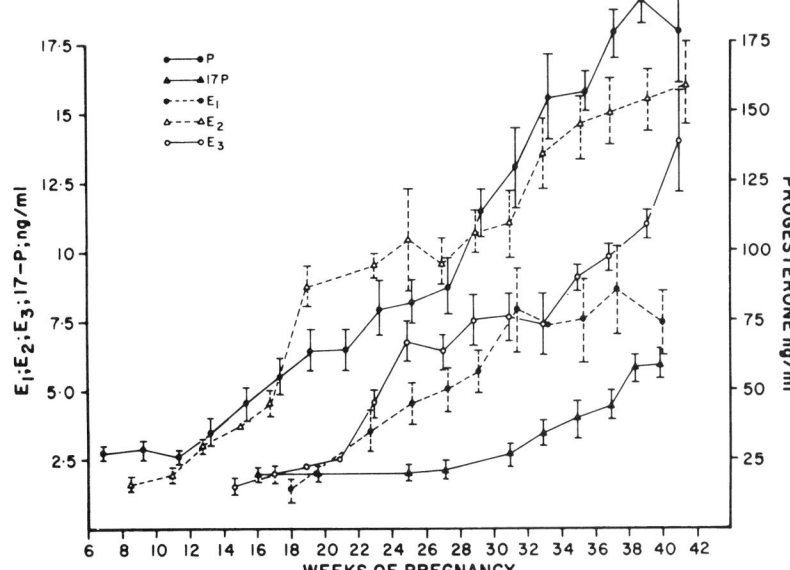

Figure 14–3. Maternal plasma level of progesterone (P) and 17-hydroxyprogesterone (17P) and of estrone (E_1), estradiol (E_2), and estriol (E_3) during human pregnancy. (From Tulchinsky D, et al: Am J Obstet Gynecol *112*:1095, 1972.)

duction. Thus, the progesterone that circulates in the fetus at high levels is of placental origin and may be used as a precursor of Δ^4-3-ketosteroids. Because progesterone is not dependent on fetal enzymes, it is a poor indicator of fetal well-being and is more closely related to placental function.

In the fetus, steroids are rapidly sulfated by an adrenal sulfatase, resulting in steroid sulfates, which make these steroids biologically inactive. This sulfation step may serve as a protective mechanism to ensure that the fetus is not exposed to high levels of active steroids. Pregnenolone-SO_4 is rapidly converted to DHA-SO_4 by fetal adrenal zone enzymes, 17α-hydroxylase and 20,21-desmolase.[46] DHA-SO_4 may be hydroxylated in the fetal liver at the 16α or 15α position or at both positions. These androgens are then transferred to the placenta.

In the placenta, the SO_4 must be cleaved before the 3β-hydroxysteroid dehydrogenase–isomerase complex can convert DHA or the hydroxylated DHAs to androstenedione or hydroxylated androstenediones. These androgens are then aromatized to estrone (E_1), 16α-OH estrone, or 15α-OH estrone and are then converted to estradiol (E_2), estriol (E_3), or estetrol (E_4) by the action of the placental 17β-hydroxylation enzyme.[15-17] Although maternal DHA-SO_4 serves as 40% of the precursor for E_2 synthesis, the latter hormones are predominantly formed from fetal precursors because the maternal liver has limited 15α- or 16α-hydroxylation capabilities.[47] Thus, E_3 and E_4 are good indexes of fetal well-being. Most of the estrogens are then transferred to the mother.

Placental steroidogenic capacity is functional early in pregnancy, but not until 35 to 47 days after ovulation can placental progesterone production solely support the maintenance of pregnancy.[48] Before that time, human pregnancy is dependent on the progesterone produced by the corpus luteum of pregnancy or by exogenous supplementation. Following 35 to 47 days after ovulation, the ovary may be removed, and the pregnancy will continue. This is referred to as the *ovarian-placental shift.*

The concentration of steroid hormones in the maternal circulation increases dramatically throughout gestation (Fig. 14–3).[49] The function of estrogens and progesterone in pregnancy is multiple. Progesterone, as discussed previously, is required for the maintenance of pregnancy because of its suppressant effect on uterine contractions.[48] It also influences breast development while suppressing lactation by inhibiting lactose synthesis.

Progesterone affects glucose homeostasis and water metabolism. In addition, it has been shown to have immunosuppressive activity.[50] Estrogens influence uterine growth, blood flow, and contractility.[22] They also affect metabolism and breast development. Both estrogens and progesterone are thought to modulate the activity of other primary factors involved in the initiation of labor, such as prostaglandins and oxytocin. Before parturition, there is an increase in the estrogen/progesterone ratio within the intrauterine tissues. This may enhance and modulate prostaglandin and oxytocin production and action at the time of parturition.[51] It is now known that placental steroid hormone production is influenced by protein trophic hormones and by other factors such as hypothalamic-like releasing and inhibiting hormones, growth factors, cytokines, and prostaglandins.

Maternal circulating levels of glucocorticoids and mineralocorticoids are increased in pregnancy[52] as a result of increased pituitary ACTH stimulation of the maternal adrenal gland. Although the placenta produces ACTH, its action is primarily localized to the placenta. The placenta has the ability to produce cortisol and to convert it to cortisone, as well as the reverse reaction. The activity of these enzymes differs with the stage of gestation and endocrine milieu.[53] A positive feed-forward axis of cortisol on placental CRH in late gestation (discussed later) increasing CRH may directly affect the fetal adrenal gland and can increase the production of DHEAS (an estrogen precursor). CRH may therefore have an important role in parturition.

HYPOTHALAMIC-LIKE RELEASING AND INHIBITING ACTIVITIES

Although the human placenta has been recognized as an endocrine tissue since the early 1900s, it was not until 1960, (both in protest and in prophecy) that Benirschke and Driscoll[54] stated, "Perhaps even more challenging at this time is the quest for an understanding of the regulatory phenomena which must be responsible for the predictability of levels of various hormones in the secretions of a normal pregnant woman, since it is difficult to conceive that no feedback mechanisms exist for those various rises and declines of hormone titers." In the 1970s, elucidation of such factors began.[5]

Since the mid-1970s, numerous studies have established that trophoblastic tissues contain and produce all the defined hypothalamic releasing and inhibiting activities.[5-7, 14, 55] These data

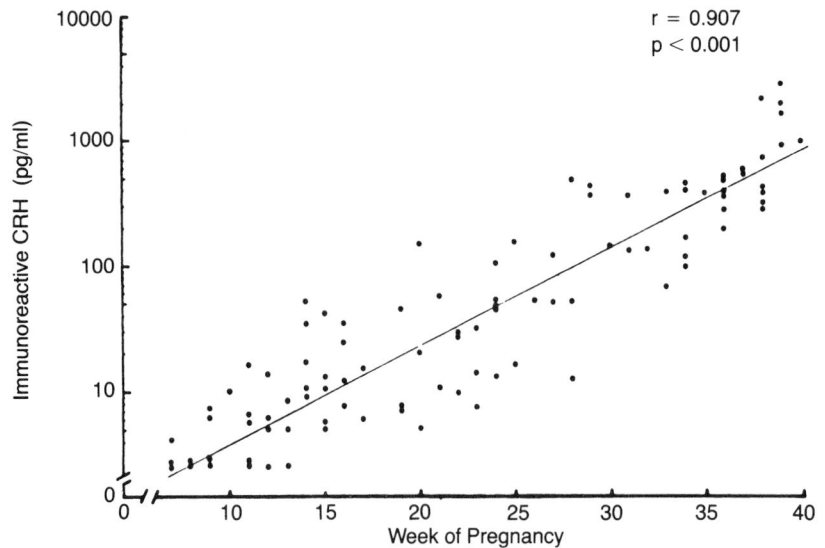

Figure 14–4. Maternal plasma levels of corticotropin-releasing hormone (CRH) during human pregnancy. (From Sasaki A, et al: J Clin Endocrinol Metab *64*:224, 1987.)

have led to the general acceptance of the hypothesis that the classic hormones of the placenta are produced by a controlled paracrine/autocrine system. To a large extent, however, this feedback system remains to be defined.

Human chorionic GnRH, the first described placental hormone with hypothalamic-like activity, has been localized to the cytotrophoblast of the placenta.[5] The human placenta synthesizes peptides having GnRH biologic and immunologic activity.[6] The cDNA that encodes the mammalian GnRH has been defined.[56] This same mRNA contains a 56-amino acid peptide called GnRH-associated peptide, which is thought to have PRL-inhibiting activity (PIF). Thus, the placenta can also make PIF. Further chemical[57] and biologic data[58] suggest that another chorionic GnRH may also exist. My studies with Grayson[7] have demonstrated the expression and action of a chicken II GnRH by the placenta.

GnRH and its analogues bind to specific receptors on the syncytiotrophoblast.[7] GnRH stimulates cAMP[59] and hCG release without affecting hCS release.[13, 14, 60] A role for calcium in the GnRH stimulation of hCG has been indicated.[61] The pattern and degree of hCG release are related to gestational age[13] and to estrogen and progesterone levels[62, 63] and can be modulated by inhibin.[24] A direct action of GnRH on steroid release may also occur.[63] GnRH inhibits certain prostanoid production from the term placenta.[64,65,104-106] In early gestation, GnRH antagonists can inhibit hCG, steroid, and prostaglandin release from placental explants, and because this action can be partially reversed with exogenous GnRH, a specific receptor-mediated action is suggested.[65] The release of GnRH by placenta is affected by cAMP, prostaglandins, epinephrine,[66] and inhibin.[24] Thus, a paracrine axis for chorionic GnRH–hCG-steroids-prostaglandins, inhibin, and PRL has been proposed. In addition, a placental peptidase that can inactivate GnRH has been isolated.[67] This peptidase may play an important role in the metabolism of GnRH and thus may affect the homeostasis of this axis.

Numerous studies in which GnRH analogues or antisera have been administered to pregnant rats, monkeys, or baboons have indicated a possible function of chorionic GnRH in the maintenance of pregnancy.[68] Administration of GnRH analogues in early pregnancy can induce pregnancy failure.[69-71] GnRH-like immunoactivity is increased in the circulation of women with apparently normal pregnancies.[72] Maternal concentrations vary throughout pregnancy and parallel those in the placenta.[14] The serum concentrations of GnRH follow a pattern similar to that of hCG but have an attenuated peak and nadir. Premature labor has

been associated with low levels of circulating GnRH in the first half of gestation. Thus, all these data support the hypothesis that chorionic GnRH plays a significant role in the normal physiology of pregnancy.

Another releasing factor in human placenta and membranes is chorionic thyrotropin-releasing hormone (chorionic TRH). Attempts to define its chemical identity have led to conflicting findings. Shambaugh and colleagues[73] identified chorionic TRH with bioactivity and immunoactivity coincident with TRH. Maternal levels have not been studied; however, exogenous TRH given to the mother passes through the placenta and affects fetal thyroid function.[74] One study reported that low levels of immunoreactive TRH in amniotic fluid correlated with low Apgar scores.[75]

A chorionic somatostatin has also been localized in the cytotrophoblast of the human placenta.[76] Concentrations are highest in first trimester placentas. Amniotic fluid has the capacity to degrade somatostatin rapidly. Somatostatin administered to the mother can cross the placenta;[77] however, the high levels at term in the fetoplacental circulation appear to be of fetal origin.[78] Studies on somatostatin at other times of gestation have not been done. A role for somatostatin in the placental-decidual unit has been reported. Somatostatin is thought to inhibit PRL-releasing factor acutely.[79] PRL-releasing factor is a 24,000-dalton molecule that has been extracted from human placenta and is active in stimulating both long-term and short-term release of decidual PRL. Whether this molecule is transferred to the decidua in an endocrine or a paracrine fashion (or both) is not known. No effect of either somatostatin or PRL-releasing factor on hCS release has been found. A chorionic GH–releasing factor has been identified in both the rat and the porcine placenta, yet its chemical nature or activity remains to be determined.[80, 81]

Chorionic CRH is another hormone with hypothalamic-like activity identified in the placenta.[82,83] It is localized to both the syncytiotrophoblastic and cytotrophoblastic cells of the placenta and is also found in the cytotrophoblasts of the chorion.[84] Its chemical nature appears to be essentially identical to that of hypothalamic CRH, with a placental mRNA that hybridizes with the hypothalamic cDNA. Other studies, however, have also found some larger molecular weight chorionic CRH that await further definition. Human chorionic CRH is transferred to both maternal and fetal circulations.[40, 84, 85] Concentrations in the maternal circulation are greater than those in the fetus and increase throughout pregnancy. There is a rapid increase at term gestation and during labor (Fig. 14-4). In pregnancies complicated by hypertension, the maternal circulating levels of CRH are already elevated by 28 weeks of pregnancy.[86] Chorionic CRH has been shown to be biologically active in stimulating the release of ACTH and β-endorphin.[40, 84, 87] Thus, it is speculated that chorionic CRH may control placental, fetal, or maternal ACTH and endorphin levels. This speculation has not been confirmed. In late-gestation placentas, dexamethasone induces a paradoxical stimulation of mRNA for chorionic CRH.[88]

The increasing CRH released into the maternal circulation has been noted to correlate with the length of gestation and is sometimes referred to as a *placental clock*.[89] Ongoing studies suggest that it may serve as a parameter that can predict preterm delivery.[89, 90] Other studies have demonstrated that CRH can directly stimulate DHEAS production by the fetal adrenal gland.[91] Because DHEAS is the precursor for estrogen, this may be one mechanism by which a favorable endocrine milieu for parturition is effected.

Another hypothalamic hormone thought to play a role in parturition is oxytocin. A review of this topic is presented by Soloff.[92] A placental oxytocinase (cystine aminopeptidase) has been described and may play an important role in the regulation of oxytocin levels. Oxytocin has been shown to increase both prostaglandin[93] and ACTH[87] release from intrauterine tissues.

OTHER CHORIONIC CYTOKINES, GROWTH FACTORS, AND PEPTIDES

Cytokines, such as interferons,[94] tumor necrosis factor-α,[95] and interleukins[96-99] are also produced by the placenta, and their receptors are expressed in the uteroplacental tissues. The cells of the placenta that have been identified to express the many different cytokines include trophoblasts, macrophages, and endothelial cells.[98-102] Expression of these cytokines varies with the stage of gestation, but they are now known to play an important role in implantation and immunosuppression during pregnancy,[103, 104] in regulation of trophoblastic and vascular functions in the placenta during gestation,[105] and in the initiation and process of parturition.[100-102, 106] Cytokines affect these activities through the regulation of other cytokines, growth factors, hormones, and prostanoid production.[107] At the time of implantation, the shift of the ratio of cytokine T-helper type 1 to type 2 cells (Th1/Th2 ratio) toward Th2 is postulated to be of primary importance in suppressing the immune response at the uteroplacental interface.[106] Cytokine production may be a cause of preterm labor (even without intrauterine infection)[101] and may increase prostanoid production.

Another cytokine produced by the placenta is leptin.[110, 111] It is proposed to play a role in the invasive cytotrophoblast at the time of implantation and to participate in regulating fetal growth and placental function.[112, 113] Its increased production in preeclampsia and gestational diabetes has led to the hypothesis that this cytokine may play a role in these diseases of pregnancy.

Another class of hormones described in the placenta and chorionic membranes is that of growth factors. The early blastocyst expresses platelet-derived growth factor A, transforming growth factor-α and β.[114] These factors are thought to be involved in signaling implantation. At this early stage, other growth factors such as epidermal growth factor (EGF), basic fibroblast growth factor, nerve growth factor-β, and granulocyte colony-stimulating factor are not found,[17] but they are expressed by the placenta at later stages of gestation. Receptors for EGF, as well as many other growth factor receptors, have been localized in the placenta and membranes.[116] Most of the EGF receptors in the placenta are localized to the syncytiotrophoblast and correlate with induction of differentiated function of trophoblast rather than proliferation.[117-119] The finding that EGF stimulates hCG secretion supports this hypothesis.[17] EGF also stimulates

prostaglandin synthesis.[119] Another growth factor, hepatocyte growth factor/scatter factor, appears to be essential for placental development.[120, 121]

The production of IGF-I and IGF-II from human placental tissues has also been demonstrated.[122] Within the placenta, IGF-I has been localized predominantly to the syncytiotrophoblast of the fetal villi.[123] IGF-binding proteins (IGFBPs), which are carrier proteins protecting IGF from degradation while blocking its bioactivity, have also been localized in these cells.[122, 123] In addition to placental IGFBP, IGFBP-1 is produced by the decidua in large amounts. Receptors that bind IGFs have been identified in the human placenta; IGF-I receptor is the most dominant.[122-124] Placental GH concentrations correlate with IGF-I throughout pregnancy.[30] IGFs potentiate the action of EGF[125] and stimulate decidual PRL production.[126] The production of progesterone is enhanced, whereas that of estrogen is inhibited.[127] Placental transport of glucose and amino acids is also enhanced by IGFs, and IGFs also regulate both fetal and placental growth.[128-130] In addition, production of placental thromboxane, a potent vasoconstrictor, is specifically inhibited by IGF-I.[131] Thus, the production of placental IGF-I and of its binding proteins is thought to be of major importance for normal intrauterine fetal growth.[129]

Relaxin is also synthesized by the membranes, decidua, and placenta.[132] Receptors for relaxin are present in the syncytiotrophoblast of the placenta.[133] A biologic action for relaxin on the collagenase activity of the chorionic-amnionic membranes has been demonstrated. Relaxin also stimulates prostaglandin release and increases collagenase, the enzyme that degrades collagen. Thus, an important role for relaxin in human parturition has been hypothesized.

Inhibin is also synthesized by the cytotrophoblast of the placenta.[134, 135] Its release by the placenta can be stimulated by 8-Br-cAMP as well as by α-hCG. Inhibin has been shown to inhibit GnRH stimulation of hCG and chorionic GnRH production.[135] Antiserum to inhibin increases hCG release, and this effect can be partially reversed by a GnRH antagonist. Activin potentiates the GnRH-stimulated hCG release.[23] Thus, it appears that activin and inhibin are actively involved in the GnRH-hCG-steroid-prostaglandin axis.

Vasoactive peptides such as vascular endothelial growth factor, endothelin, angiotensin, and arginine vasopressin and their receptors are also expressed by the human placenta. The potent vasoconstrictor peptides, endothelin and endothelin 3, are also produced by the placenta, and both are active and potent vasoconstrictors in the fetoplacental circulation.[136-139] Endothelins also inhibit decidual PRL release.[139] The angiotensin-renin system has been described in the placenta and is thought to be a factor in the regulation of vascular tone in the placental bed through angiotensin II production and action.[140] Other peptide hormones affecting vascular tone, such as atrial natriuretic peptide and its receptors, have been demonstrated in the placenta.[141] Atrial natriuretic peptide is a vasodilatory hormone that is thought to be produced by the cytotrophoblast because secretion decreases as these cells differentiate *in vitro* to syncytiotrophoblast. Atrial natriuretic peptide inhibits the vasoconstrictive action of endothelin and angiotensin, and it induces vasodilatation in the uterus and the placenta.

Neuropeptides, such as enkephalins[142] and dynorphin,[143] have been found in the placenta. There are receptors for opiate-like substances on the syncytial membrane of the placenta. The stimulation of these receptors has been shown to modulate acetylcholine[144] and hCG release.[145, 146] Adrenergic agonists and antagonists affect placental hCG and PRL release,[147] whereas dopaminergic receptor stimulation has been shown to lower hCS[35] and to increase hCG release.[35] A parathyroid-related protein has been extracted from placental tissues[148] and localized to the cytotrophoblastic cells.[149] Parathyroid-related protein has been shown to have potent vasodilatory activity in the fetoplacental circulation.[150]

EICOSANOIDS AND PROSTANOIDS

An important role for eicosanoids, such as thromboxanes, prostacyclins, leukotrienes, and prostanoids, during pregnancy is well recognized. In general, prostanoids and eicosanoids are thought of as products of the decidua and chorionic membranes, which are active in their production. Prostanoids and leukotrienes, however, are also produced in large quantities by the placenta.[151] In the placenta, the chorionic membranes, and decidua, AA must be mobilized (i.e., de-esterified from lipoproteins) before it can be used for production of eicosanoids and prostanoids.[152] Mobilization of AA is induced through two enzymatic pathways. In the first pathway, the hydrolysis of AA from phosphatidylethanolamine is catalyzed by phospholipase A_2. The other pathway releases AA from phosphatidylinositol by the enzymatic activities of phospholipase C, monoacylglycerol lipase, and diacylglycerol lipase. AA is converted to PGG_2 by cyclooxygenase and then by the enzyme, prostaglandin hydroperoxidase, to PGH_2. PGH_2 is the common precursor for PGD_2, PGE_2, and $PGF_{2\alpha}$, which are formed by the enzymatic action of specific endoperoxides (isomerase D and E and F reductase). The levels of PGD_2, $PGF_{2\alpha}$, and PGE_2 can be measured directly. Thromboxanes and prostacyclin are synthesized from PGH_2 by thromboxane and prostacyclin synthetases. Owing to the rapid nonenzymatic conversion of thromboxane A_2 to thromboxane B_2, thromboxane B_2 levels are used as a measure of thromboxane A_2 synthesis. Similarly, prostacyclin is enzymatically metabolized rapidly to 6-keto-$PGF_{1\alpha}$, which can be measured directly.

The level of some prostanoids in term amnion, chorion, decidua, and placenta has been determined.[58, 151] Human term placentas convert AA primarily to thromboxane, PGE_2, and PGD_2. Production of $PGF_{2\alpha}$ is about half that of PGE_2, and that of prostacyclin is one-fifth.[153] Prostaglandins, thromboxanes, and prostacyclin have been implicated as important hormones during pregnancy at the time of implantation, in the regulation of fetal growth, and in the initiation and progress of labor. Their role in implantation has been demonstrated by the inhibitory effect of indomethacin (a cyclooxygenase inhibitor) on implantation Other studies suggest that production of prostaglandins, thromboxane, and, particularly, prostacyclin may enable the trophoblast to invade and colonize the maternal spiral blood vessels of the myometrium.[154] Prostacyclin is known to be a potent vasodilator and inhibitor of platelet aggregation.

After implantation, during the period of fetal growth and development, prostaglandins, thromboxane, and prostacyclin play important roles as vasoregulators of the fetoplacental unit.[155] PGE_2 is known to be a vasodilator of uterine blood flow while constricting the umbilical circulation. $PGF_{2\alpha}$ vasoconstricts both the maternal and the umbilical circulations. In pregnancies associated with hypertension, increased production of thromboxane and reduced prostacyclin production have been demonstrated.[156] Amniotic, chorionic, decidual, and placental tissue levels of PGE_2 and $PGF_{2\alpha}$ are also decreased in pregnancies complicated by hypertension. Similarly, prostacyclin levels in the amnion are diminished in hypertensive pregnancies. Thromboxane production is not increased in pregnancies associated with normotensive intrauterine growth retardation, and in some cases it is reduced.[157]

Another action of prostaglandins in pregnancy is their ability to alter protein synthesis in the placenta and to influence the production of certain other hormones.[158-160] One report found that $PGF_{2\alpha}$ suppresses hCS production. Other studies *in vitro* have shown a direct stimulatory action of AA, but not $PGF_{2\alpha}$ or PGE_2, on hCS. The ability of $PGF_{2\alpha}$ to stimulate hCG release in pregnant women has been reported. In addition, both PGE_2 and prostacyclin have been shown to increase cAMP levels.

An important function of prostaglandins, thromboxanes, and prostacyclin in pregnancy is their role in the initiation and progress of labor. PGE and PGF levels are elevated six- to 12-fold in the amniotic fluid of women in labor.[156, 161] Metabolites of thromboxane and prostacyclins (i.e., thromboxane B_2 and 6-keto-$PGF_{1\alpha}$) are also increased in amniotic fluid (two- to fourfold). It has been shown that infusion of PGE_2 and $PGF_{2\alpha}$ can be used to induce labor. These prostaglandins in larger doses are also effective in inducing midtrimester abortions. Intra-amniotic administration of AA, the precursor of prostanoids, has resulted in the initiation of labor and delivery.[162] Long-term ingestion of aspirin, a cyclooxygenase inhibitor that decreases production of prostanoids from AA, can override this action of AA. Even when aspirin is ingested alone, gestation can be prolonged.[163]

As discussed earlier, factors that are known to stimulate prostanoid production include CRH, cytokines, and growth factors. Both CRH and cytokines are thought to play a primary role in parturition, and increased prostanoid production is believed to be a possible mechanism for this role. Glucocorticoids, progesterone, and estrogens also affect prostaglandin production.[164] Studies have shown that GnRH can affect prostaglandin release from the placenta.[58, 59, 65] Placental prostaglandin release is highest when chorionic GnRH is highest; however, the response of prostaglandins to GnRH varies throughout gestation, as does the basal release of prostaglandins.[88] Basal prostaglandin release can be inhibited by a GnRH antagonist.[65]

The ability of EGF to promote prostaglandin release from amniotic membranes has been mentioned earlier. Another factor known to stimulate prostanoid release is platelet-activating factor (PAF).[165] The mechanism of action of PAF may involve mobilization of calcium. PAF is present in amniotic fluid during active labor but not in women who are not in labor. Thus, a role for PAF in the regulation of prostaglandins at parturition has been hypothesized.[166] A role for PAF at the time of implantation has also been suggested.[167]

ENZYMES THAT REGULATE PLACENTAL ENDOCRINE AND PARACRINE ACTIVITIES

Factors that regulate autocrine, paracrine, and endocrine activities of the placenta are affected not only by factors regulating synthesis and secretion but also by enzymatic activities that affect metabolism. In a few cases for these total activities, the placental autocrine, paracrine, and endocrine activity has been shown to affect the hormonal balance. In the case of GnRH, a highly active postproline peptidase is known to regulate its concentration.[67] The placenta produces large quantities of this enzyme, thus providing a means for compartmentalization and localization of this specific activity. In addition, placental enzymes have been demonstrated to degrade angiotensin II during pregnancy and to regulate conversion of cortisol to cortisone (and vice versa).[53] Furthermore, regulation of the expression of the prostaglandin dehydrogenase has been proposed to participate in the initiation of labor.[168,169]

INTEGRATION OF THE PLACENTA WITH THE INTRAUTERINE TISSUES

The human placenta has multiple physiologic functions, as can be appreciated from the long list of regulatory factors it produces that act on the various cell types. However, the placenta does not act in isolation. Its functions are integrated with those of other intrauterine tissues, such as the maternal uterus, chorion, amnion, decidua, and amniotic fluid and the fetus. These other intrauterine tissues produce or extract some of the same hormones or produce carrier proteins that regulate placental hormone activity. Metabolic signals and precursors as well as hormones are carried by maternal and fetal blood or are transported from cell to cell from the uterus, decidua, chorion, amnion, and amniotic fluid to and from the placenta. Integration of the intrauterine tissues provides for the normal physiology of pregnancy and allows for its maintenance and timely parturition. Aberrations within these intrauterine autocrine, paracrine, and endocrine systems are responsible for many of the disorders that occur during pregnancy. Understanding of this system is rapidly developing and promises to lead to an enhanced ability to regulate this system and thus to maintain pregnancy better and to control the timing of parturition.

REFERENCES

1. Zondek B, Aschheim S: Das Hormon des Hypophysenvorder-lappens. Klin Wochenschr 18:831, 1928.
2. Philipp E: Die innere Schretion der placenta. I. Ihre Beziehungen zum Ovar. Zentralb Gynaekol 44:2754, 1930.
3. Wislocki GB, Bennett HS: The histology and cytology of the human and monkey placenta, with special reference to the trophoblast. Am J Anat 73:335, 1943.
4. Midgley AR, Pierce GB: Immunohistochemical localization of human chorionic gonadotropin. J Exp Med 115:289, 1962.
5. Khodr GS, Siler-Khodr TM: Localization of luteinizing hormone-releasing factor (LRF) in the human placenta. Fertil Steril 29:523, 1978.
6. Khodr GS, Siler-Khodr TM: Placental LRF and its synthesis. Science 207:315, 1980.
7. Siler-Khodr TM, Grayson M: Action of chicken II GnRH on the human placenta. J Clin Endocrinol Metabol 86:804, 2001.
8. Hussa RO: Biosynthesis of human chorionic gonadotropin. Endocr Rev 1:268, 1980.
9. Kovalevskaya G et al: Early pregnancy human chorionic gonadotropin (hCG) isoforms measured by an immunometric assay for choriocarcinomas-like hCG. J Endocrinol 161:99, 1999.
10. O'Connor JF, et al: Differential urinary gonadotropin profiles in early pregnancy and early pregnancy loss. Prenat Diagn 18:1232, 1998.
11. Osathanondh R, Tulchinsky D: Placental polypeptide hormones. In Tulchinsky D, Ryan KJ (eds): Maternal-Fetal Endocrinology. Philadelphia, WB Saunders Co, 1980, pp 17–42.
12. Fritz MA, Guo SM: Doubling time of human chorionic gonadotropin (hCG) in early pregnancy: relationship to hCG concentration and gestational age. Fertil Steril 47:584, 1987.
13. Siler-Khodr TM, et al: GnRH effects on placental hormones during gestation: I. αhCG, hCG and hCS. Biol Reprod 34:245, 1986.
14. Siler-Khodr TM: LHRH and the placenta and fetal membranes. In Rice GE, Brennecke SP (eds): Molecular Aspects of Placental and Fetal Membrane Autocoids. Ann Arbor, CRC Press, 1993, pp 339–360.
15. Shi CZ, et al: Norepinephrine regulates human chorionic gonadotrophin production by first trimester trophoblast tissue in vitro. Placenta 14:683, 1993.
16. Jameson JL, et al: Transcriptional regulation of chorionic gonadotropin α- and β-subunit gene expression by 8-bromoadenosine 3',5'-monophosphate. Endocrinology 119:2560, 1986.
17. Morrish DW, et al: Epidermal growth factor induces differentiation and secretion of human chorionic gonadotropin and placental lactogen in normal human placenta. J Clin Endocrinol Metab 65:1282, 1987.
18. Steele GL, et al: Acute stimulation of human chorionic gonadotropin secretion by recombinant human activin-A in first trimester human trophoblast. Endocrinology 133:297, 1993.
19. Pollack H, et al: Interleukin-2 inhibits the production of human chorionic gonadotropin by trophoblasts in vitro. Placenta 13:A-52, 1992.
20. Licht P, et al: Novel self-regulation of human chorionic gonadotropin biosynthesis in term pregnancy human placenta. Endocrinology 133:3014, 1993.
21. Mukherjee TK, Scerdote A: Studies on hormones controlling hCG production during pregnancy, effect of LRH and PGF₂, preliminary observations. Clin Res 29:297A, 1986.
22. Branchaud CL, et al: Progesterone and estrogen production by placental monolayer cultures: effects of dehydroepiandrosterone and luteinizing hormone-releasing hormone. J Clin Endocrinol Metab 56:761, 1983.
23. Petraglia F, et al: Inhibin and activin modulate the release of gonadotropin-releasing hormone, human chorionic gonadotropin, and progesterone from cultured human placental cells. Proc Natl Acad Sci USA 86:5114, 1989.
24. Higashi K: Studies on the prolactin-like substances in human placenta. 3. Endocrinol Jpn 8:288, 1961.
25. Josimovich JB, MacLaren JA: Presence in the human placenta and term serum of a highly lactogenic substance immunologically related to pituitary growth hormone. Endocrinology 71:209, 1962.
26. Handwerger S, Freemark M: The roles of placental growth hormone and placental lactogen in the regulation of human fetal growth and development. J Pediatr Endocrinol 13:343, 2000.
27. Rygaard K, et al: Absence of human placental lactogen and placental growth hormone (HGH-V) during pregnancy: PCR analysis of the deletion. Hum Genet 102:87, 1998.
28. Grumbach MM, et al: Chorionic growth hormone-prolactin: secretion, disposition, biologic activity in man, and postulated function as the "growth hormone" of the second half of pregnancy. Ann NY Acad Sci 148:501, 1968.
29. Alsat E, et al.: Physiological role of human placental growth hormone. Mol Cell Endocrinol 140:121, 1998.
30. Kanda Y, et al: Apolipoproteins A-I stimulate placental lactogen release by activation of MAP kinase. Mol Cell Endocrinol 143:125, 1998.
31. Petit A, et al: An islet-activating protein-sensitive G-protein is involved in dopamine inhibition of both angiotensin stimulated inositol phosphate production and human placental lactogen release in human trophoblastic cells. J Clin Endocrinol Metab 71:1573, 1990.
32. Harman I, et al: Cyclic adenosine 3',5'-monophosphate stimulates the acute release of placental lactogen from human trophoblast cells. Endocrinology 121:59, 1988.
33. Zeitler P, Handwerger S: Arachidonic acid stimulates phosphoinositide hydrolysis and human placental lactogen release in an enriched fraction of placental cells. Mol Pharmacol 28:549, 1985.
34. Harmon I, et al: Sn 1,2 diacylglycerols and phorbol esters stimulate the synthesis and release of human placental lactogen from placental cells: a role for protein kinase C. Endocrinology 119:1239, 1986.
35. Macaron C, et al: In vitro effect of dopamine and pimozide on human chorionic somatomammotropin (hCS) secretion. J Clin Endocrinol Metab 47:168, 1978.
36. Tyson JE, et al: Studies of prolactin secretion in human pregnancy. Am J Obstet Gynecol 113:14, 1972.
37. Blithe D, et al: Free alpha molecules from pregnancy stimulate secretion of prolactin from human decidual cells: a novel function for free alpha in pregnancy. Endocrinology 129:2257, 1991.
38. Krieger DT: Placenta as a source of 'brain' and 'pituitary' hormones. Biol Reprod 26:55, 1982.
39. Genazzani AR, et al: Prostaglandin-induced mid-pregnancy abortion increases plasma and amniotic fluid levels of β-lipotropin and β-endorphin. Gynecol Obstet Invest 24:23, 1987.
40. Reis FM, et al: Putative role of placental corticotropin-releasing factor in the mechanisms of human parturition. J Soc Gynecol Invest 6:109, 1999.
41. Ryan KJ: Biological aromatization of steroids. J Biol Chem 234:268, 1959.
42. Diczfalusy E: Endocrine functions of the human fetoplacental unit. Fed Proc 23:791, 1964.
43. Bloch K: The biological conversion of cholesterol to pregnanediol. J Biol Chem 157:661, 1945.
44. Hellig H, et al: Steroid production from plasma cholesterol: I. Conversion of plasma cholesterol to placental progesterone in humans. J Clin Endocrinol Metab 30:624, 1970.
45. Ryan KJ: Placental synthesis of steroid hormones. In Tulchinsky D, Ryan KJ (eds): Maternal-Fetal Endocrinology. Philadelphia, WB Saunders Co, 1980, pp 3–16.
46. Bloch E, Hertig AT: Concerning the function of the fetal zone of the human adrenal gland. Endocrinology 58:598, 1956.
47. Madden JD, et al: Study of the kinetics of conversion of maternal plasma dehydroisoandrosterone sulfate to 16α-hydroxydehydroisoandrosterone sulfate, estradiol, and estriol. Am J Obstet Gynecol 132:392, 1978.
48. Csapo AI, et al: Effects of luteectomy and progesterone replacement in early pregnant patients. Am J Obstet Gynecol 115:759, 1973.
49. Tulchinsky D, et al: Plasma estrone, estradiol, estriol, progesterone and 17-hydroxyprogesterone in human pregnancy: I. Normal pregnancy. Am J Obstet Gynecol 112:1095, 1972.
50. Klopper A, Fuchs F: Progestagens. In Fuchs F, Klopper A (eds): Endocrinology of Pregnancy, 3rd ed. Philadelphia, JB Lippincott, 1987, pp 99–122.
51. Romero R, et al: Evidence for a local change in the progesterone/estrogen ratio in human parturition at term. Am J Obstet Gynecol 159:657, 1988.
52. Dorr HG: Longitudinal study of progestins, mineralocorticoids throughout human pregnancy. J Clin Endocrinol Metab 68:863, 1989.
53. Pepe GJ, Albrecht ED: Actions of placental and fetal adrenal steroid hormones in primate pregnancy. Endocrine Rev 16:608, 1995.
54. Benirschke K, Driscoll SG: The hormones of the placenta. In Benirschke K, Driscoll SG (eds): The Pathology of the Human Placenta. New York, Springer-Verlag, 1967, pp 431–456.
55. Siler-Khodr TM: Chorionic peptides. In McNellis D, et al (eds): The Onset of Labor: Cellular and Integrative Mechanisms. New York, Perinatology Press, 1987, pp 213–230.
56. Seeburg PH, Ademan JP: Characterization of cDNA for precursor of human luteinizing hormone-releasing hormone. Nature 311:666, 1986.
57. Gautron JP, et al.: Occurrence of higher molecular forms of LHRH in fractionated extracts from rat hypothalamus cortex and placenta. Mol Cel Endocrinol 24:1, 1981.
58. Siler-Khodr TM, et al: GnRH effects on placental hormones during gestation: III. Prostaglandin E, prostaglandin F and 13, 14-dihydro-15-keto-prostaglandin F. Biol Reprod 35:312, 1986.
59. Haning RV, et al: Effects of prostaglandins, dibutyryl cAMP, LHRH, estrogens, progesterone, and potassium on output of prostaglandin F₂ₐ, 13,14-dihydro-15-keto-prostaglandin F₂ₐ, hCG, estradiol, and progesterone by placental minces. Prostaglandins 24:495, 1982.
60. Siler-Khodr TM, et al: Gestational age related inhibition of placental hCG, αhCG and steroid hormone release in vitro by a GnRH antagonist. Placenta 8:1, 1986.
61. Mathialagan N, Rao AJ: A role for calcium in gonadotropin releasing hormone (GnRH) stimulated secretion of chorionic gonadotropin by first trimester human placental minces in vitro. Placenta 10:61, 1989.

62. Iwashita M, et al: Effect of gonadal steroids on gonadotropin-releasing hormone stimulated human chorionic gonadotropin release from trophoblast cells. Placenta *10*:103, 1989.
63. Siler-Khodr TM, et al: GnRH effects on placental hormones during gestation: II. Progesterone, estrone, estradiol and estriol. Biol Reprod *34*:255, 1986.
64. Kang IS, et al: Dose-related action of GnRH on basal prostanoid production from the human term placenta. Am J Obstet Gynecol *165*:1771, 1991.
65. Siler-Khodr T, et al: Differential inhibition of human placental prostaglandin release in vitro by a GnRH antagonist. Prostaglandins *31*:1003, 1986.
66. Petraglia F, et al: Adenosine 3′,5′-monophosphate, prostaglandins, and epinephrine stimulate the secretion of immunoreactive gonadotropin-releasing hormone from cultured human placental cells. J Clin Endocrinol Metab *65*:1020, 1987.
67. Kang IW, Siler-Khodr TM: Chorionic peptidase inactivates GnRH as a post-proline peptidase. Placenta *13*:81, 1992
68. Sridaran R: Effects of gonadotropin releasing hormone treatment on ovarian steroid production during midpregnancy. Proc Soc Exp Biol Med *182*:120, 1986.
69. Rao AJ, et al: Effect of LHRH agonists and antagonists in male and female bonnet monkeys (*Macaca radiata*). J Steroid Biochem *23*:807, 1985.
70. Das C, Talwar GP: Pregnancy-terminating action of a luteinizing hormone-releasing hormone agonist D-Ser(But)6desGly10ProEA in baboons. Fertil Steril *39*:218, 1983.
71. Kang I-S, et al: Effect of treatment with gonadotropin releasing hormone analogues on pregnancy outcome in the baboon. Fertil Steril *52*:846, 1989.
72. Siler-Khodr TM, et al: Immunoreactive GnRH level in maternal circulation throughout pregnancy. Am J Obstet Gynecol *150*:376, 1984.
73. Shambaugh GD, et al: Thyrotropin-releasing hormone activity in the human placenta. J Clin Endocrinol Metab *48*:483, 1979.
74. Roti E, et al: Human cord blood concentrations of thyrotropin, thyroglobulin, and iodothyronines after maternal administration of thyrotropin-releasing hormone. J Clin Endocrinol Metab *53*:813, 1981.
75. Morley JE, et al: Thyrotropin-releasing hormone and thyroid hormones in amniotic fluid. Obstet Gynecol *134*:581, 1979.
76. Nishihira OM, Yagihashi S: Immunohistochemical demonstration of somato-statin-containing cells in the human placenta. Tohoku J Exp Med *126*:397, 1978.
77. Roti E, et al: Inhibition of foetal growth hormone (GH) and thyrotrophin (TSH) secretion after maternal administration of somatostatin. Endocrinologica *106*:393, 1984.
78. Saito J, et al: Fetal and maternal plasma levels of immunoreactive somatostatin at delivery: evidence for its increase in the umbilical artery and its arterio-venous gradient in the fetoplacental circulation. J Clin Endocrinol Metab *47*:567, 1983.
79. Handwerger S, et al: Purification of decidual prolactin-releasing factor, a placental protein that stimulates prolactin release from human decidual tissue. Biochem Biophys Res Commun *147*:452, 1987.
80. Baird A, et al: Immunoreactive and biologically active growth hormone-releasing factor in the rat placenta. Endocrinology *117*:1598, 1985.
81. Farmer C, Gaudreau P: Presence of a bioactive and immunoreactive growth-hormone-releasing factor-like substance in porcine placenta. Biol Neonate *72*:363, 1997.
82. Shibasaki T, et al: Corticotropin-releasing factor-like activity in human placental extracts. J Clin Endocrinol Metab *55*:384, 1982.
83. Frim FM, et al: Characterization and gestational regulation of corticotropin-releasing hormone messenger RNA in human placenta. J Clin Invest *82*:287, 1988.
84. Riley SC, Challis JRC: Corticotrophin-releasing hormone production by the placenta and fetal membranes. Placenta *12*:105, 1991.
85. Sasaki A, et al: Immunoreactive corticotropin-releasing hormone in human plasma during pregnancy, labor and delivery. J Clin Endocrinol Metab *64*:224, 1987.
86. Dornhorst CD, et al: MA CRF and cortisol in normal and hypertensive pregnancies. Presented at the 69th Annual Meeting of the Endocrine Society, Indianapolis, Abstract 332, 1987.
87. Margioris AN, et al: Corticotropin-releasing hormone and oxytocin stimulate the release of placental proopiomelanocortin peptides. J Clin Endocrinol Metab *66*:922, 1988.
88. Robinson BG, et al: Glucocorticoid stimulates expression of corticotropin-releasing hormone gene in human placenta. Proc Natl Acad Sci USA *85*:5244, 1988.
89. McLean M, Smith R: Corticotrophin-releasing hormone and human parturition. Reproduction *121*:493, 2001.
90. Holzman C, et al.: Second trimester corticotropin-releasing hormone levels in relation to preterm delivery and ethnicity. Obstet Gynecol *97*:657, 2001.
91. Mesiano S, Jaffe RB: Development and functional biology of the primate fetal adrenal cortex. Endocr Rev *18*:378, 1997.
92. Soloff MS: The role of oxytocin in the initiation of labor, and oxytocin-prostaglandin interaction. *In* McNellis D, et al (eds): The Onset of Labor: Cellular and Integrative Mechanisms. Ithaca, Perinatology Press, 1988, pp 87–111.
93. Moore NJ, et al: Oxytocin activates the inositol-phospholipid-protein kinase-C system and stimulates prostaglandin production in human amnion cells. Endocrinology *123*:1771, 1988.
94. Bulmer JN, et al: Immunohistochemical localization of interferons in human placental tissues in normal, ectopic, and molar pregnancy. Am J Reprod Immunol *22*:109, 1990.
95. Starkey PM, et al: The synthesis of tumour necrosis factor by human placental and decidual tissue. Placental Comm Biochem Morphol Cell Aspects *199*:142, 1990.
96. Kojima K, et al: Expression of leukemia inhibitory factor in human endometrium and placenta. Biol Reprod *50*:882, 1994.
97. Chaouat G, et al: A brief review of recent data on some cytokine expressions at the materno-fetal interface which might challenge the classical Th1/Th2 dichotomy. J Reprod Immunol *53*:241, 2002.
98. Sacks GP, et al: Flow cytometric measurement of intracellular Th1 and Th2 cytokine production by human villous and extravillous cytotrophoblast. Placenta *22*:550, 2001.
99. Jokhi PP, et al: Cytokine production and cytokine receptor expression by cells of the human first trimester placental-uterine interface. Cytokine *9*: 126. 1997.
100. Sel'kov SA, Parlov OV, Selyutin AV: Cytokines and placental macrophages in regulation of birth activity. Bull Exp Biol Med *129*:511, 2000.
101. Steinborn A, et al.: Cytokine release from placental endothelial cells, a process associated with preterm labour in the absence of intrauterine infection. Cytokine *11*:66, 1999.
102. Steinborn A, et al.: Identification of placental cytokine-producing cells in term and preterm labor. Obstet Gynecol *91*:329, 1998.
103. Dealtry GB, et al: The Th2 cytokine environment of the placenta. Int Arch Allergy Immunol *123*:107, 2000.
104. Loke YW, King A: Immunological aspects of human implantation. J Reprod Fertil Suppl *55*:83, 2000.
105. Saito S: Cytokine cross-talk between mother and the embryo/placenta. J Reprod Immunol *52*:15, 2001.
106. Keelan JA et al.: Cytokine abundance in placental tissues: evidence of inflammatory activation in gestational membranes with term and preterm parturition. Am J Obstet Gynecol *181*:1530, 1999.
107. Mohan A, et al.: Effect of cytokines and growth factors on the secretion of inhibin A, activin A, and follistatin by term placental villous trophoblast in culture. Eur J Endocrinol *145*:505, 2001.
108. Laham N, et al: Interleukin-8 release from human gestational tissue explants: the effects of lipopolysaccharide and cytokines. Biol Reprod *57*:616, 1997.
109. Lundin-Schiller S, et al: Prostaglandin production by human chorion laeve cells in response to inflammatory mediators. Placenta *12*:353, 1991.
110. Linnerman K, et al.: Physiological and pathological regulation of feto/placento/maternal leptin expression. Biochem Soc Trans *29*:86, 2001.
111. Ashworth CJ, et al.: Placental leptin. Rev Reprod *5*:18, 2000.
112. Henson MC, Castracane VD: Leptin in pregnancy. Biol Reprod *63*:1219, 2000.
113. Gonzalez RR, et al.: Leptin and reproduction. Hum Reprod Update *6*:290, 2000.
114. Rappolee DA, et al: Developmental expression of PDGF, TGF-α, and TGF-β genes in preimplantation mouse embryos. Science *241*:1823, 1988.
115. Maruo T, Mochizuki M: Immunohistochemical localization of epidermal growth factor receptor and myc oncogene product in human placenta: implication for trophoblast proliferation and differentiation. Am J Obstet Gynecol *156*:721, 1987.
116. Chegini N, Rao Ch V: Epidermal growth factor binding to human amnion, chorion, decidua, and placenta from mid- and term pregnancy: quantitative light microscopic autoradiographic studies. J Clin Endocrinol Metab *61*:529, 1985.
117. Maruo T, Mochizuki M: Immunohistochemical localization of epidermal growth factor receptor and myc oncogene product in human placenta: implication for trophoblast proliferation and differentiation. Am J Obstet Gynecol *156*:721, 1987.
118. Hoshina M, et al: Linkage of human chorionic gonadotrophin and placental lactogen biosynthesis to trophoblast differentiation and tumorigenesis. Placenta *6*:163, 1985.
119. Mitchell MD: Epidermal growth factor actions on arachidonic acid metabolism in human amnion cells. Biochim Biophys Acta *928*:240, 1987.
120. Uehara Y, Kitamura N: Hepatocyte growth factor/scatter factor and the placenta. Placenta *17*:97, 1996.
121. Stewart F: Roles of mesenchymal-epithelial interactions and hepatocyte growth factor-scatter factor (HGF-SF in placental development. Rev Reprod *1*:144, 1996.
122. Han K, Carter AM: Spatial and temporal patterns of expression of messenger RNA for insulin-like growth factors and their binding proteins in the placenta of man and laboratory animals. Placenta *21*:289, 2000.
123. Hill DJ, et al: Immunohistochemical localization of insulin-like growth factors (IGFs) and IGF binding proteins -1, -2, -3 in human placenta and fetal membranes. Placenta *14*:1, 1993.
124. Pekonen F, et al: Different insulin-like growth factor binding species in human placenta and decidua. J Clin Endocrinol Metab *67*:1250, 1988.
125. Bhaumick B, et al: Potentiation of epidermal growth factor-induced differentiation of cultured human placental cells by insulin-like growth factor-I. J Clin Endocrinol Metab *74*:1005, 1992.
126. Kubota T, et al:The effects of insulin-like growth factor-I (IGF-I) and IGF-II on prolactin (PRL) release from human decidua and amniotic fluid circulation. Nippon Sanka Fujinka Gakkai Zasshi *43*:1515, 1991.
127. Nestler JE, et al: Modulation of aromatase and P450 cholesterol side-chain cleavage enzyme activities of human placental cytotrophoblasts by insulin and insulin-like growth factor I. Endocrinology *121*:1845, 1987.

128. Kniss DA, et al: Insulinlike growth factors: their regulation of glucose and amino acid transport in placental trophoblasts isolated from first-trimester chorionic villi. J Reprod Med *39*:249, 1994.
129. Zumkeller W: Current topic: the role of growth hormone and insulin-like growth factors for placental growth and development. Placenta *21*:451, 2000.
130. Gluckman PD, Harding JE: The physiology and pathophysiology of intrauterine growth retardation. Hormone Res *48*(Suppl 1):1, 1997.
131. Siler-Khodr TM, et al: Dose-related effect of IGF-1 on placental prostanoid release. Prostaglandins *49*:1, 1995.
132. Sakbun V, et al: Immunocytochemical localization of prolactin and relaxin C-peptide in human decidua and placenta. J Clin Endocrinol Metab *65*:339, 1987.
133. Koay ESC, et al: The human fetal membranes: a target tissue for relaxin. J Clin Endocrinol Metab *62*:513, 1986.
134. Petraglia F: Inhibin, activin and follistatin in the human placenta—a new family of regulatory proteins. Placenta *18*:3, 1997.
135. Petraglia F, et al: Localization, secretion, and action of inhibin in human placenta. Science *237*:187, 1987.
136. Kingdom J et al.: Development of the placental villous tree and its consequences for fetal growth. Eur J Obstet Gynecol Reprod Biol *92*: 35, 2000.
137. Poston L: The control of blood flow to the placenta. Exp Physiol *82*:377, 1997.
138. Myatt L, et al: The comparative effects of big endothelin-1, endothelin-1 and endothelin-3 in the human fetal-placental circulation. Am J Obstet Gynecol *167*:1651, 1992.
139. Chaim H-S, et al: Endothelin inhibits basal and stimulated release of prolactin by human decidual cells. Endocrinology *133*:505, 1993.
140. Nielsen AH, et al: Current topic: the uteroplacental renin-angiotensin system. Placenta *21*:468, 2000.
141. VanWijk MJ, et al: Vascular function in preeclampsia. Cardiovascular Research *47*:38, 2000.
142. Tan L, Yu PH: De novo biosynthesis of enkephalins and their homologues in the human placenta. Biochem Biophys Res Commun *98*:752, 1981.
143. Lemaire S, et al: Purification and identification of multiple forms of dynorphin in human placenta. Neuropeptides *3*:181, 1981.
144. Ahmed MS, Horst MA: Opioid receptors of human placental villi modulate acetylcholine release. Life Sci *39*:535, 1986.
145. Valette A, et al: Placental kappa binding site: interaction with dynorphin and its possible implication in hCG secretion. Life Sci *33*:523, 1983.
146. Belisle S, et al: Functional opioid receptor sites in human placentas. J Clin Endocrinol Metab *66*:283, 1988.
147. Shu-Rong Z, et al: The regulation in vitro of placental release of human chorionic gonadotropin, placental lactogen, and prolactin: effects of an adrenergic beta-receptor agonist and antagonist. Am J Obstet Gynecol *143*:444, 1982.
148. Abbas SK, et al: Measurement of parathyroid hormone-related protein in extracts of fetal parathyroid glands and placental membranes. J Endocrinol *124*:319, 1990.
149. Hellmen P, et al: Parathyroid-like regulation of parathyroid hormone-related protein release and cytoplasmic calcium in cytotrophoblast cells of human placenta. Arch Biochem Biophys *293*:174, 1992.
150. Mandsager NT, et al: Vasodilator effects of parathyroid hormone, parathyroid hormone-related protein, and calcitonin gene-related peptide in the human fetal-placental circulation. J Soc Gynecol Invest *1*:19, 1994.
151. Harper MJK, et al: Prostaglandin production by human term placentas in vitro. Prostaglandins Leukotrienes Med *11*:121, 1983.
152. Bleasdale JE, Johnston JM: Prostaglandins and human parturition: regulation of arachidonic acid mobilization. *In* Scarpell EM, Cosmi EV (eds): Reviews in Perinatal Medicine, Vol 5. New York, Alan R Liss, 1984, pp 151–191.
153. Kang IS, et al: Effect of enzyme inhibitors and exogenous arachidonic acid on placental prostanoids production. Placenta *14*:341, 1993.
154. Lewis P: The role of prostacyclin in preeclampsia. Br J Hosp Med *28*:393, 1982.
155. Ylikorkala O, et al: Maternal prostacyclin, thromboxane, and placental blood flow. Am J Obstet Gynecol *145*:730, 1983.
156. Challis JRG, Patrick JE: The production of prostaglandins and thromboxanes in the feto-placental unit and their effects on the developing fetus. Semin Perinatol *4*:23, 1980.
157. Sorem KA, et al: Placental prostanoids release in severe intrauterine growth retardation. Placenta *16*:503, 1995.
158. Handwerger S, et al: Stimulation of human placental lactogen release by arachidonic acid. Mol Pharmacol *20*:609, 1981.
159. Mukherjee TK, Scerdote A: Studies on hormones controlling hCG production during pregnancy. Effects of LRH and $PGF_{2\alpha}$: preliminary observations. Clin Res *29*:297A, 1986.
160. Kiesel L, et al: The role of prostaglandins, cyclic nucleotides and tricarboxylic acids in the regulation of the human placental 20α-hydroxysteroid dehydrogenase in vitro. Steroids *40*:99, 1982.
161. Casey ML, MacDonald PC: Decidual activation: the role of prostaglandins in labor. *In* McNellis D, et al: (eds): The Onset of Labour: Cellular and Integrative Mechanisms. Ithaca, Perinatology Press, 1988, pp 141–156.
162. MacDonald PC, et al: Initiation of human parturition: I. Mechanism of action of arachidonic acid. Obstet Gynecol *44*:629, 1974.
163. Uzan S, et al: Aspirin during pregnancy. Indications and modalities of prescription after the publication of the later trails. Presse Med *25*:31, 1996.
164. Olson DM et al: Review of steroids on PGs. Estradiol-17β and 2-hydroxyestradiol-17β-induced differential production of prostaglandins by cells dispersed from human intrauterine tissues at parturition. Prostaglandins *25*:639, 1983.
165. Synder F: Platelet-Activating Factor and Related Lipid Mediators. New York, Plenum Publishing, 1987.
166. Angle M, et al: Bioactive metabolites of glycerophospholipid metabolism in relation to parturition. *In* McNellis P, et al (eds): The Onset of Labor: Cellular and Integrative Mechanisms. Ithaca, Perinatology Press, 1988, pp 125–138.
167. Harper MJK, et al: Platelet-activating factor (PAF) and blastocyst-endometrial interactions. *In* Yoshinaga K, Mori T (eds): Development of Preimplantation Embryos and Their Environment. New York, Alan R Liss, 1989.
168. Mizutani S, Tomoda Y: Effects of placental protease on maternal and fetal blood pressure in normal pregnancy and preeclampsia. Am J Hypertension *9*:591, 1996.
169. Challis JR, et al: Prostaglandin dehydrogenase and the initiation of labor. J Perinat Med *27*:26, 1999.

Roberto Romero, Tinnakorn Chaiworapongsa, and Maria-Teresa Gervasi

15 Fetal and Maternal Responses to Intrauterine Infection

Infection has emerged in the last 20 years as an important and frequent mechanism of disease in preterm parturition.[1-8] Indeed, it is the only pathologic process for which a firm causal link with prematurity has been established and a defined molecular pathophysiology is known.[9] Moreover, fetal infection/inflammation has been implicated in the genesis of fetal and neonatal injury,[10,11] leading to cerebral palsy[12] and chronic lung disease.[13] This chapter reviews the evidence showing that infection is causally associated with spontaneous preterm birth, the role of cytokines and other inflammatory mediators in the host response to intrauterine infection, and finally, the fetal and maternal inflammatory response to intrauterine infection.

Systemic maternal infection (i.e., pneumonia, pyelonephritis, malaria, typhoid fever, etc.)[14-24] has been associated with preterm labor and delivery. Yet many of these conditions are rare in developed countries and thus, the attributable risk of systemic maternal infection for prematurity is considered to be low. The recent report of an association between maternal periodontal disease and prematurity may require a re-examination of this view, particularly since some preterm neonates show evidence of a humoral immune response to microorganisms normally present in the oral cavity.[25,26] Recent evidence suggests that some microorganisms isolated in amniotic fluid may have an oral origin.[27]

On the other hand, intrauterine infection/inflammation is frequently associated with preterm labor/delivery. It has been estimated that at least 40% of all preterm births occur to mothers with evidence of intrauterine infection or inflammation, which is largely subclinical in nature.[28-30] Moreover, the lower the gestational age at delivery, the greater the frequency of intrauterine infection[31] and thus the higher the burden of disease attributable to intrauterine infection and inflammation. The first part of the chapter reviews the pathways of intrauterine infection, frequency, microbiology, and rate of fetal infection.

PATHWAYS OF ASCENDING INTRAUTERINE INFECTION

Microorganisms may gain access to the amniotic cavity and fetus through the following pathways: (1) ascending from the vagina and cervix; (2) hematogenous dissemination through the placenta (transplacental infection); (3) retrograde seeding from the peritoneal cavity through the fallopian tubes; and (4) accidental introduction at the time of invasive procedures, such as amniocentesis, percutaneous fetal blood sampling, chorionic villous sampling, or shunting.[32-36] The most common pathway of intrauterine infection is the ascending route.[1,33,34,36] Evidence in support of this includes: (1) histologic chorioamnionitis is more common and severe at the site of membrane rupture than in other locations, such as the placental chorionic plate or umbilical cord[37]; (2) in virtually all cases of congenital pneumonia (stillbirths or neonatal), inflammation of the chorioamniotic membranes is present[32,34,36]; (3) bacteria identified in cases of congenital infections are similar to those found in the lower genital tract[33]; and (4) in twin gestations, histologic chorioamnionitis is more common in the firstborn, and it has not been demonstrated in the second twin only. That the membranes of the first twin are generally opposed to the cervix is taken as evidence in favor of an ascending infection.[33] This observation is consistent with those made during the course of microbiologic studies of the amniotic fluid in twin gestation.[38] When infection is detected, the presenting sac is nearly always involved.[38]

STAGES OF ASCENDING INTRAUTERINE INFECTION

Ascending intrauterine infection is considered to have four stages.[1] Stage I consists of a change in the vaginal/cervical microbial flora or the presence of pathologic organisms (i.e., *Neisseria gonorrhoeae*) in the cervix. Some forms of bacterial vaginosis may be an early manifestation of this initial stage. Once microorganisms gain access to the intrauterine cavity, they reside in the decidua (stage II). A localized inflammatory reaction leads to deciduitis. Microorganisms may then reside in the chorion and amnion. The infection may invade the fetal vessels (choriovasculitis) or proceed through the amnion (amnionitis) into the amniotic cavity, leading to microbial invasion of the amniotic cavity or an intra-amniotic infection (stage III). Rupture of the membranes is not a prerequisite for intra-amniotic infection, as microorganisms are capable of crossing intact membranes.[39] Once in the amniotic cavity, the bacteria may gain access to the fetus by different ports of entry (stage IV). Aspiration of the infected fluid by the fetus may lead to congenital pneumonia. Otitis, conjunctivitis, and omphalitis may occur by direct spreading of microorganisms from infected amniotic fluid. Seeding from any of these sites to the fetal circulation may result in fetal bacteremia and sepsis.

MICROBIOLOGY OF INTRA-AMNIOTIC INFECTION

The most common microbial isolates from the amniotic cavity of women with preterm labor and intact membranes are *Ureaplasma urealyticum*, *Fusobacterium* spp., and *Mycoplasma hominis*.[1,28,40-42] Other microorganisms that have been found in the amniotic fluid include *Streptococcus agalactiae*, *Peptostreptococcus* spp., *Staphylococcus aureus*, *Gardnerella vaginalis*, *Streptococcus viridans*, and *Bacteroides* spp. Occasionally,

Lactobacillus spp., *Escherichia coli*, *Enterococcus faecalis*, *N. gonorrhoeae*, and *Peptococcus* spp. have been encountered. *Haemophilus influenzae*, *Capnocytophaga* spp., *Stomatococcus* spp., and *Clostridium* spp. were rarely identified.[43,44] In 50% of patients with microbial invasion, more than one microorganism is isolated from the amniotic cavity. The inoculum size varies considerably, and in 71% of the cases more than 10^5 colony-forming units per milliliter (cfu/ml) are found.[37]

The role of *Chlamydia trachomatis* as an intrauterine pathogen has not been clearly elucidated. This microorganism is an important cause of cervicitis and has been isolated from amniotic fluid.[45,46] A case report of congenital pneumonia caused by *C. trachomatis* suggests that this microorganism may be involved in the etiology of ascending intra-amniotic infection.[46] The uncertainty about the role of *C. trachomatis* in the etiology of microbial invasion and intrauterine infection seems related to difficulties in isolating the microorganisms from amniotic fluid with standard culture techniques.[47] The use of polymerase chain reaction (PCR) to detect specific sequences for this microorganism should help resolve this problem.[48]

The role of viruses in the etiology of sub-clinical and clinical chorioamnionitis remains unresolved. Yankowitz and colleagues[49] performed PCR for the presence of adenovirus, enterovirus, respiratory syncytial virus, Epstein-Barr virus, parvovirus B-19, cytomegalovirus (CMV), and herpes simplex genomic material in the amniotic fluid of 77 women undergoing midtrimester genetic amniocentesis. Amniotic fluid viral footprints were found in six pregnancies: adenovirus (n = 3), parvovirus (n = 1), CMV (n = 1), and enterovirus (n = 1). Among these six cases were two pregnancy losses: one at 21 weeks (adenovirus) and another at 26 weeks (CMV). Wenstrom and colleagues[50] compared amniotic fluid samples from a group of 62 pregnancy losses following midtrimester amniocentesis with 60 controls from a population of 11,971 women. PCR was performed for the presence of adenovirus, parvovirus, CMV, Epstein-Barr virus, herpes simplex virus, β-actin DNA, enterovirus, and influenza A. No difference in the prevalence of viruses in the amniotic fluid samples was observed [8% of the cases (5/62) vs. 15% of controls (9/60), p = 0.74]. At the time of writing this chapter, no large clinical or epidemiologic study has implicated intrauterine viral infection in the genesis of preterm delivery. However, we have observed acute fetal CMV and herpes viral infection presenting as preterm labor.

FREQUENCY OF INTRA-AMNIOTIC INFECTION IN PRETERM GESTATION

Microbial Invasion of the Amniotic Cavity and Preterm Delivery

Studies examining the clinical circumstances surrounding preterm delivery indicate that one-third of all patients present with preterm labor and intact membranes and one-third with preterm premature rupture of membranes (PROM). The remaining third are the result of indicated delivery because of maternal or fetal indications (i.e., pre-eclampsia, growth restriction, and so on).[51-54] To examine the relationship between microbial invasion of the amniotic cavity and preterm delivery, we shall review the evidence supporting an association between intrauterine infection and spontaneous preterm labor (with or without intact membranes).

Microbial Invasion of the Amniotic Cavity in Patients with Preterm Labor and Intact Membranes

The mean rate of positive amniotic fluid cultures for microorganisms in patients with preterm labor and intact membranes is approximately 12.8% (379/2963), based upon the review of

33 studies.[28,30] Women with positive amniotic fluid cultures generally do not have clinical evidence of infection at presentation. However, they are more likely to develop clinical chorioamnionitis [37.5% (60/160) vs. 9% (27/301)], to be refractory to tocolysis [85.3% (110/129) vs. 16.3% (8/49)], and to rupture their membranes spontaneously [40% (6/15) vs. 3.8% (2/52)], than women with negative amniotic fluid cultures. Several investigators have demonstrated that the rate of neonatal complications is higher in neonates born to women with microbial invasion of the amniotic cavity than in those without infection.[55] Moreover, the earlier the gestational age at preterm birth, the more likely that microbial invasion of the amniotic cavity was present.[31]

Microbial Invasion of the Amniotic Cavity in Patients with Preterm PROM

The rate of positive amniotic fluid cultures for microorganisms is approximately 32.4% (473/1462) in patients with preterm PROM.[28] Clinical chorioamnionitis is present in only 29.7% (49/165) of cases with proven microbial invasion.[9,28] The rate of microbial invasion in preterm PROM reported by these studies is probably an underestimation of the true prevalence of intrauterine infection. Indeed, available evidence indicates that women with PROM and a severely reduced volume of amniotic fluid have a higher incidence of intra-amniotic infection than do those without oligohydramnios.[56,57] Since women with oligohydramnios are less likely to undergo an amniocentesis, the bias in these studies is to underestimate the prevalence of infection. A similar bias is that women with preterm PROM admitted in labor generally do not undergo amniocentesis. These patients have a higher rate of microbial invasion of the amniotic cavity than those admitted without labor [39% (24/61) vs. 25% (41/160), p<0.05].[58] Furthermore, of patients who are not in labor at admission, 75% have a positive amniotic fluid culture at the time of the onset of labor.[58] Therefore, studies restricted to women not in labor provide a lower rate of microbial invasion of the amniotic cavity than those including patients in labor.

Microbial Invasion of the Amniotic Cavity in Patients Presenting with "Acute Cervical Incompetence"

Women presenting with a dilated cervix, intact membranes, and few, if any, contractions before the 24th week are considered to have clinical cervical incompetence. Of these patients, 51.1% have a positive amniotic fluid culture for microorganisms.[59] The outcome of patients with microbial invasion is uniformly poor because they develop subsequent complications (rupture of membranes, clinical chorioamnionitis, or pregnancy loss). Therefore, infection is frequently associated with an acute cervical incompetence.[60] Whether intra-amniotic infection is the cause or consequence of cervical dilatation has not been determined. It is possible that clinical silent cervical dilatation with protrusion of the membranes into the vagina would lead to a secondary intrauterine infection.

Microbial Invasion of the Amniotic Cavity in Patients with Twin Gestations and Preterm Labor

Microbial invasion of the amniotic cavity occurs in 11.9% of twin gestations.[38] This finding is in contrast to the 21.6% of abnormal amniotic fluid cultures observed in singleton gestations with preterm labor and delivery.[37] These data suggest that intra-amniotic infection is a possible cause of preterm labor and delivery in twin gestation, but they do not support the hypothesis that intra-amniotic infection is responsible for the excessive rate of preterm delivery observed in these patients.[61,62]

Chorioamniotic Infection, Histologic Chorioamnionitis, and Preterm Birth

Inflammation of the placenta and chorioamniotic membranes is a nonspecific host-response to a variety of stimuli, including infection. Traditionally, acute inflammation of the chorioamniotic membranes has been considered an indicator of amniotic fluid infection,[32-36,63-65] a view based upon indirect evidence. Several studies have demonstrated an association between acute inflammatory lesions of the placenta and the recovery of microorganisms from the subchorionic plate[66,67] and the chorioamniotic space.[63] Bacteria have been recovered from the subchorionic plate of 72% of placentae with histologic evidence of chorioamnionitis.[40,63,66] Furthermore, there is a strong correlation between positive amniotic fluid cultures for microorganisms and histologic chorioamnionitis.[64,65] Moreover, Cassell and associates have reported an association between positive microbial cultures from material obtained from the chorioamniotic interface and histologic chorioamnionitis.[68,69] The presence of inflammation in the umbilical cord (funisitis) represents evidence of a fetal inflammatory response.[70,71] In contrast, histologic chorioamnionitis reflects a maternal inflammatory response.

Several studies have examined the prevalence of inflammation in placentae from women delivering preterm infants. Collectively, the evidence indicates an association between preterm birth and the occurrence of acute chorioamnionitis, and also that the lower the gestational age at birth, the higher the frequency of histologic chorioamnionitis and funisitis.[40]

Fetal Infection

The most advanced and serious stage of ascending intrauterine infection is fetal infection (stage IV). The overall mortality rate of neonates with congenital neonatal sepsis ranges from 25% to 90%.[72-79] The wide array of results may reflect the effect of gestational age on the likelihood of survival. One study, which focused on infants born before 33 weeks of gestation, found that the mortality rate was 33% for those infected and 17% for noninfected fetuses.[75] Carroll and colleagues have reported that fetal bacteremia is found in 33% of fetuses with positive amniotic fluid culture and in 4% of those with negative amniotic fluid culture.[80] Therefore, subclinical fetal infection is far more common than traditionally recognized.

INTRAUTERINE INFECTION/INFLAMMATION AS A CHRONIC PROCESS

Although intrauterine infection has been traditionally considered an acute complication of pregnancy, accumulating evidence suggests that this may be a chronic condition. The evidence in support of this view is derived from studies of the microbiologic state of the amniotic fluid, as well as the concentration of inflammatory mediators at the time of genetic amniocentesis.

Microbial Invasion of the Amniotic Cavity at the Time of Genetic Amniocentesis

Cassell and associates[68] reported the recovery of genital mycoplasmas from 6.6% (4/61) of amniotic fluid samples collected by amniocentesis between 16 and 21 weeks. Two patients had positive cultures for *Mycoplasma hominis* and two for *Ureaplasma urealyticum*. Patients with *Mycoplasma hominis* delivered at 34 and 40 weeks without neonatal complications, whereas those with *Ureaplasma urealyticum* had premature delivery, neonatal sepsis, and neonatal death at 24 and 29 weeks. Subsequently, Gray and colleagues[81] reported a 0.37% prevalence (9/2461) of positive cultures for *Ureaplasma urealyticum* in amniotic fluid samples obtained during second trimester genetic amniocentesis. Except for one patient who had a therapeutic abortion, all patients (8/8) with positive amniotic fluid cultures had either a fetal loss within 4 weeks of amniocentesis (n = 6) or preterm delivery (n = 2). Furthermore, all had histologic evidence of chorioamnionitis. These observations suggest that microbial invasion could be clinically silent in the midtrimester of pregnancy and that pregnancy loss/preterm delivery could take weeks to occur. A similar finding was reported by Horowitz and associates[82] who detected *Ureaplasma urealyticum* in 2.8% (6/214) of amniotic fluid samples obtained between 16 and 20 weeks of gestation. The rate of adverse pregnancy outcome (fetal loss, preterm delivery, and low birth weight) was significantly higher in patients with a positive amniotic fluid culture than in those with a negative one [3/6 (50%) vs. 15/123 (12%), p = 0.035]. It is interesting that patients with a positive amniotic fluid culture were more likely to have an obstetric history that included more than three previous abortions than those with a negative culture [33% (2/6) vs. 4% (5/123); p = .034].[82]

Chronic Intra-amniotic Inflammation and Preterm Birth

Interleukin (IL)-6 concentrations in amniotic fluid are considered to be a marker of intra-amniotic inflammation frequently associated with microbiologic infection in the amniotic fluid or the chorioamniotic space.[83-86] Romero and colleagues reported the results of a case control study in which IL-6 determinations were conducted in the stored fluid of patients who had a pregnancy loss after a midtrimester amniocentesis and a control group who delivered at term. Patients who had a pregnancy loss had a significantly higher median amniotic fluid IL-6 than those with a normal outcome.[87] Similar findings were reported by Wenstrom and associates.[88] Of note is that maternal plasma concentrations of IL-6 were not associated with adverse pregnancy outcome.

The same approach was subsequently used to test the association between markers of inflammation in midtrimester amniotic fluid of asymptomatic women and preterm delivery. The concentrations of matrix metalloproteinase (MMP)-8,[89] IL-6,[90] tumor necrosis factor alpha (TNFα),[91] and angiogenin[92] in amniotic fluid obtained at the time of midtrimester amniocentesis were significantly higher in patients who subsequently delivered preterm than in those who delivered at term.

Collectively, this evidence suggests that a chronic intra-amniotic inflammatory process is associated with both spontaneous abortion and spontaneous preterm delivery. Whether intra-amniotic inflammation can be detected noninvasively remains to be determined. Recently, Goldenberg and associates[93] demonstrated that the maternal plasma concentration of granulocyte colony–stimulating factor (G-CSF) at 24 and 28 weeks of gestation is associated with early preterm birth. To the extent that G-CSF may reflect an inflammatory process, this finding suggests that a chronic inflammatory process identifiable in the maternal compartment is associated with early preterm birth.

Is the Relationship Between Intrauterine Infection and Spontaneous Premature Birth Causal?

The existence of an association does not mean that infection *causes* preterm delivery. Indeed, it has been argued that microbial invasion of the amniotic cavity is merely the consequence of labor.[94-97] Determining whether or not this relationship is causal is critical, because it has major clinical and therapeutic implications. The evidence supporting a causal role for infection follows the criteria outlined by Sir Branford Hill during his presidential address before the Section of Occupational Medicine of the Royal Society of Medicine in 1965,[98] and includes: (1) biologic plausibility; (2) temporal relationship; (3) consistency and strength of association; (4) dose-response gradient; (5) specificity; and (6) human experimentation.

Animal experimentation indicates that the administration of bacterial products or microorganisms to pregnant animals can lead to premature labor and delivery.[99-108] Three sets of observations suggest that infection precedes the spontaneous onset of preterm labor and delivery: (1) Subclinical microbial invasion of the amniotic cavity or intrauterine inflammation in the midtrimester of pregnancy leads either to spontaneous abortion or premature delivery (see earlier section on intrauterine inflammation/infection as a chronic process), (2) Patients with preterm PROM who on admission had a positive amniotic fluid culture for mycoplasmas (*Ureaplasma urealyticum* or *Mycoplasma hominis*, which are not visible in Gram stain) also had a significantly shorter amniocentesis-to-delivery interval than those with sterile amniotic fluid.[109] This suggests that patients with preterm PROM and microbial invasion of the amniotic cavity are more likely to initiate preterm labor than those with a negative amniotic fluid culture,[109] (3) Colonization of the lower genitourinary tract with microorganisms is a risk factor for preterm delivery. These conditions include asymptomatic bacteriuria, bacterial vaginosis, and infection with *Neisseria gonorrhoeae*.[110-121]

The consistency and strength of association between infection and preterm delivery has been demonstrated by the many studies in which amniotic fluid was cultured for microorganisms in patients with preterm PROM[122] and preterm labor with intact membranes.[37] Moreover, the relative risk is high (> 2) for preterm delivery in patients with preterm labor and intact membranes, and microbial invasion of the amniotic cavity. The hazards ratio is also high for the duration of pregnancy in women with preterm PROM with intrauterine infection.

The likelihood of a causal relationship is increased if a dose-response gradient can be demonstrated. Is there a dose-response gradient between the severity of the infection and the likelihood of preterm delivery? Evidence in support of such a gradient includes: (1) the median concentration of bacterial endotoxin is higher in patients in preterm labor than in patients not in labor;[123] (2) the microbial inoculum is significantly greater in patients with preterm PROM admitted with preterm labor than in those admitted with preterm PROM but not in labor.[58] Specifically, the proportion of patients with an inoculum size of 10^5 cfu/mL or greater was 41.6% in patients with preterm labor and only 15% in patients not in labor (p = .03);[58] (3) the rate of abortion/preterm delivery after the administration of *Escherichia coli* bacterial endotoxin to pregnant mice exhibits a clear dose-response gradient.[124]

One of the criteria for causality that is not met is specificity. Although intrauterine infection appears to be sufficient to induce preterm labor and delivery, it is not specific because many patients have a preterm delivery in the absence of evidence of intrauterine infection/inflammation. However, a high degree of specificity is rare in biologic systems. Although the causal relationship between smoking and lung cancer is widely accepted, it is also nonspecific. Lung cancer occurs in nonsmokers and, of course, smoking can cause diseases other than lung cancer, such as emphysema and chronic bronchitis. Moreover, the formulation of "the necessary and sufficient cause" can inappropriately restrict the conceptualization of causality. In the case of premature labor, we have provided microbiologic, cytologic, biochemical, immunologic, and pathologic data indicating that preterm labor is a syndrome and that infection is only one of its possible causes.[9, 125]

An important criterion for causation is whether eradication of the agent can decrease the frequency of outcome or illness. Many trials of antimicrobial treatment for the prevention of preterm birth have been conducted. There is evidence that treatment of patients with asymptomatic bacteriuria will reduce the rate of prematurity/low birthweight,[119] and that antibiotic treatment of patients with preterm PROM prolongs the latency period and reduces the rate of maternal and neonatal infection.[126-128] However, treatment of patients with preterm labor and intact membranes has not yielded positive results in most trials.[129-132] The reasons for this, complex and reviewed elsewhere,[130, 131] are likely related to the syndromic nature of preterm labor with intact membranes, the chronic nature of the process, and the inclusion in the clinical trials of many patients who do not have intrauterine infection and thus cannot benefit from antimicrobial treatment. This applies to patients presenting with preterm labor, as well as those with bacterial vaginosis.[133,134]

Detection of Microbial Footprints in Amniotic Fluid with Sequence-Based Techniques

Estimates of the frequency and type of microorganisms participating in intrauterine infections (summarized earlier in this chapter) are based upon standard microbiologic techniques (i.e., culture). The estimates are likely to change with the introduction of more sensitive methods for microbial identification. For example, surveys of terrestrial and aquatic ecosystems indicate that more than 99% of existing microorganisms may not be cultivated in the laboratory and that their identification can be performed only with molecular methods.[135] In fact, the identification of infectious agents for the following disorders have, with the aid of molecular diagnosis, only recently been possible: *Helicobacter pylori* for peptic ulcer disease[136,137]; hepatitis C virus for non-A, non-B hepatitis[138]; *Bartonella henselae* for bacillary angiomatosis[139]; *Tropheryma whippelii* for Whipple's disease[140, 141]; Sin Nombre virus for hantavirus pulmonary syndrome[142]; and Kaposi's sarcoma–associated herpes virus for Kaposi's sarcoma.[143] Sequence-based methodologies are likely to demonstrate how insensitive conventional microbiology methods are for the detection of already known and potentially "new" microorganisms in perinatal medicine. Two strategies have been used to detect microorganisms in the amniotic fluid with PCR. The first, also known as broad-range PCR, utilizes primer pairs designed to anneal with highly conserved DNA regions of all bacteria, such as the 16S ribosomal DNA. A positive result indicates the presence of bacteria, but identification of the specific organism requires sequencing of the PCR products. Another approach to molecular diagnosis of infectious diseases is to use specific primers for a particular microorganism. For example, three studies have used primers to the conserved sequence of microorganisms,[43, 144, 145] and three have favored specific primers to recover bacterial DNA from the amniotic fluid.[146-148]

Blanchard and colleagues[146] were the first to report the recovery of *Ureaplasma urealyticum* in amniotic fluid samples using specific primers for the urease structural genes. In their study, 293 amniotic fluid samples collected by amniocentesis at the time of cesarean section were cultured for bacteria, mycoplasmas and chlamydiae and had PCR performed for *Ureaplasma urealyticum*. Among the 10 PCR-positive amniotic fluid samples, only 4 were also culture-positive. Subsequently, Jalava,[144] Hitti[43] and Markenson and their colleagues[145] applied broad-spectrum bacterial 16S rDNA PCR for the detection of bacteria in the amniotic fluid. Jalava and associates[144] studied 20 amniotic fluid samples from patients with PROM and 16 control samples: PCR detected 5 microorganisms [*Ureaplasma urealyticum* (n = 2), *Haemophilus influenzae* (n = 1), *Streptococcus oralis* (n = 1), and *Fusobacterium* spp. (n = 1)]. Only two were positive in a routine bacterial culture; the two patients who developed infectious complications were correctly identified by PCR, and amniotic fluid glucose levels were lower in PCR-positive in comparison to PCR-negative patients. Hitti and associates[43] studied 69 women in preterm labor with intact membranes. PCR was positive in 94% of the culture-positive amniotic fluid samples (15/16) and 36% of the patients with a negative culture,

but in women with elevated IL-6 levels, 5/14 had bacteria detected by PCR. In the study by Markenson[145] 55.5% of the amniotic fluid samples from 54 women in preterm labor with no clinical evidence of infection were PCR-positive, whereas only 9.2% of the cultures recovered a microorganism (p < .05). Of the amniotic fluid samples with elevated IL-6, 66.6% (6/9) were also PCR-positive.

Oyarzun and colleagues[147] described a PCR amplification technique aimed at detecting the 16 microorganisms most commonly cultured from the amniotic fluid of patients in preterm labor (*Ureaplasma urealyticum, Mycoplasma hominis, Gardnerella vaginalis, Escherichia coli, Fusobacterium* spp., *Peptostreptococcus anaerobius, Bacteroides fragilis, Chlamydia trachomatis, Haemophilus influenzae, Neisseria gonorrhoeae* and *Streptococcus* spp.). In 50 patients with preterm labor and intact membranes and 23 patients not in labor, amniotic fluid samples were examined with bacterial culture and PCR. All control samples were both culture-negative and PCR-negative. A higher proportion of samples were positive by PCR when compared with culture [46% (23/50) vs. 12% (6/50)]. The sensitivity of PCR for the prediction of preterm labor before 34 weeks was better than culture [64% (7/11) vs. 18% (4/11), p < .05]. However, there were patients with positive PCR who delivered at term without maternal or neonatal complications.

The clinical implications of the detection of *Ureaplasma urealyticum* by PCR with specific primers in the amniotic fluid of women in preterm PROM have recently been reported.[149] For this study, patients were divided into three groups according to the results of amniotic fluid culture and PCR: culture-negative and PCR-negative (n = 99), culture-negative and PCR-positive (n = 18), and culture-positive regardless of PCR results (n = 37). PCR was more sensitive than culture to detect *Ureaplasma urealyticum* [28% (43/154) vs. 16% (25/154)]. Moreover, patients with a positive PCR assay of amniotic fluid, but a negative culture, had a stronger amniotic fluid inflammatory reaction (amniotic fluid–white blood cell count and amniotic fluid IL-6), a shorter interval to delivery, and a higher rate of histologic chorioamnionitis, funisitis and neonatal morbid events than those with a negative amniotic fluid culture and a negative amniotic fluid PCR assay for *Ureaplasma urealyticum*. This study demonstrated, for the first time, that patients with preterm PROM and a positive PCR assay for *Ureaplasma urealyticum* (but a negative culture) had a worse pregnancy outcome than those with a sterile culture and a negative PCR. Similar results have been observed in the context of preterm labor with intact membranes.[150] Collectively, these studies suggest that PCR is more sensitive than culture for the detection of microorganisms in the amniotic fluid, particularly in patients with evidence of intra-amniotic inflammation. We predict that the application of sequence-based methodology for the identification of microorganisms will lead to increased recognition of the importance of infection in perinatal disease.

MOLECULAR MECHANISMS FOR PRETERM PARTURITION IN THE SETTING OF INTRAUTERINE INFECTION

A considerable body of evidence supports a role for inflammatory mediators in the mechanisms of preterm parturition associated with infection. These factors may also play a part in spontaneous labor at term, though the evidence for this is less compelling. Major attention has focused on the role of proinflammatory cytokines, such as IL-1β, TNF-α, and chemokines, such as IL-8. However, other proinflammatory and anti-inflammatory cytokines may also play a role, for instance, platelet activating factor, prostaglandins, and other inflammatory mediators.[9]

The current understanding of the proposed pathophysiology of preterm parturition in the context of intrauterine infection is summarized here. The interested reader is referred to the references for a comprehensive discussion.[9]

During the course of ascending intrauterine infection, microorganisms may reach the decidua, where they can stimulate a local inflammatory reaction and the production of proinflammatory cytokines and inflammatory mediators (platelet-activating factor, prostaglandins, leukotrienes, reactive oxygen species, nitric oxide, etc.).[1, 9] If this inflammatory process is not sufficient to signal the onset of labor, microorganisms can cross intact membranes into the amniotic cavity, where they can also stimulate the production of inflammatory mediators by resident macrophages and other host cells. Finally, microorganisms that gain access to the fetus may elicit a systemic inflammatory response syndrome, characterized by increased concentrations of IL-6[10, 11] and other cytokines,[151] as well as cellular evidence of neutrophil and monocyte activation.[152]

Prostaglandins and Lipoxygenase Products

Intrauterine prostaglandins (PGs) have been considered to be the key mediators in the biochemical mechanisms regulating the onset of labor. They can induce myometrial contractility[153-156] and changes in the extracellular matrix metabolism associated with cervical ripening,[157-161] and they are thought to participate in decidual/fetal membrane activation.[9]

The evidence traditionally invoked in support of a role for PGs in the initiation of human labor includes (1) administration of PGs can induce early or late termination of pregnancy (abortion or labor)[162-170]; (2) treatment with indomethacin or aspirin can delay spontaneous onset of parturition in animals[171-173]; (3) concentrations of PGs in plasma and amniotic fluid increase during labor[174-180]; and (4) intra-amniotic injection of arachidonic acid can induce abortion.[181] Infection is thought to increase PG production by amnion, chorion, or decidua through the activity of bacterial products, cytokines, growth factors, and other inflammatory mediators. Indeed, amniotic fluid concentrations of PGE2 and PGF2α and their stable metabolites, PGEM and PGFM, are significantly higher in women with preterm labor and microbial invasion of the amniotic cavity than in women with preterm labor alone. Similar observations have been reported in patients with labor and high concentrations of pro-inflammatory mediators in the amniotic cavity (i.e., IL-1β, TNF, IL-6). Moreover, amnion obtained from patients with histologic chorioamnionitis produces higher amounts of PGs than that obtained from patients without documented chorioamnionitis.

Metabolites of arachidonic acid derived through the lipoxygenase pathway, including LTs (leukotrienes) and HETEs (hydroxyeicosatetraenoic [acid]), have also been implicated in the mechanisms of spontaneous preterm and term parturition. Concentrations of 5-HETE, LTB$_4$, and 15-HETE are increased in the amniotic fluid of women with preterm labor and microbial invasion of the amniotic fluid cavity.[182, 183] Similarly, amnion from patients with histologic chorioamnionitis releases more LTB$_4$ *in vitro* than amnion from women who delivered preterm without inflammation.[184] However, the precise role of arachidonate lipoxygenase metabolites in human parturition remains to be determined. 5-HETE and LTC$_4$ can stimulate uterine contractility, and LTB$_4$ is thought to play a role in the recruitment of neutrophils to the site of infection and the regulation of specific arachidonic acid metabolite of the cyclooxygenase (COX) pathway.[185, 186] Additionally, LTB$_4$ has been shown to act as a calcium ionophore (i.e., increases phospholipase activity and enhances the rate of PG biosynthesis in human intrauterine tissues).[187]

Inflammatory Cytokines

Evidence for the participation of IL-1 and TNF-α in preterm parturition includes the following:

1. IL-1β and TNF-α stimulate prostaglandin production by amnion, decidua, and myometrium[188-190]; Prostaglandins have been considered to be central mediators for the onset of labor
2. Human decidua can produce IL-1β and TNF-α in response to bacterial products[189, 191, 192]
3. Amniotic fluid IL-1β and TNF-α bioactivity and concentrations are elevated in women with preterm labor and intra-amniotic infection[193-196] (Fig. 15-1)
4. In women with preterm PROM and intra-amniotic infection, IL-1β and TNF-α concentrations are higher in the presence of labor[187-190]
5. IL-1β and TNF-α can induce preterm parturition when administered systemically to pregnant animals[106, 197]
6. Pretreatment with the natural IL-1 receptor antagonist prior to the administration of IL-1 to pregnant animals prevents preterm parturition[198]
7. Fetal plasma IL-1β is elevated in the context of preterm labor with intrauterine infection[199]
8. Placental tissue obtained from patients in labor, particularly those with chorioamnionitis, produces a larger amount of IL-1β than that obtained from women not in labor[200]

There is, however, considerable redundancy in the cytokine network. Therefore, it is unclear that a particular cytokine is required to signal the onset of labor. Experimental studies in

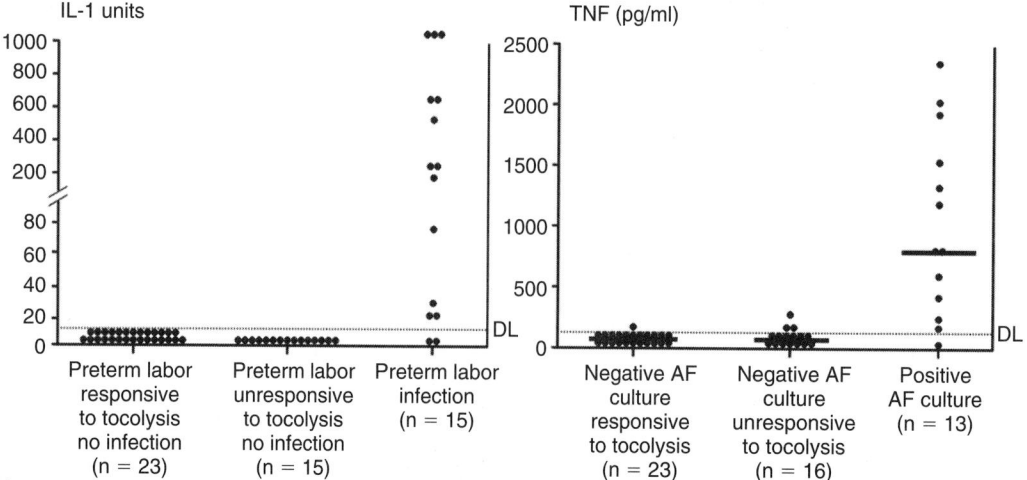

Figure 15-1. Amniotic fluid IL-1β and TNF-α bioactivity and concentrations are elevated in women with preterm labor and intra-amniotic infection.

which anti-TNF and the natural IL-1 receptor antagonist were administered to pregnant animals with intrauterine infection did not prevent preterm delivery.[201] Results of knockout animal experiments suggest that infection-induced preterm labor and delivery occur in animals that lack a particular cytokine.[202]

The precise mechanisms by which IL-1 and TNF participate in the activation of myometrium have been the subject of intensive research, and there is evidence that they involve the participation of cytosolic phospholipase A-2 (PLA-2), cyclooxygenase-2 (COX-2)[203,204] MAP kinases,[205] and NF-kB. A role for thrombin (an enzyme with oxytocin-like properties that is generated during the course of inflammation) has also been postulated by Phillipe's laboratory.[206-210] A novel observation is that labor is associated with increased activity of NF-kB—the transcription factor responsible for many of the actions of IL-1 and TNF in amnion. NF-kB may affect uterine function by blocking factors that promote uterine quiescence (e.g., progesterone).[211]

Matrix-Degrading Enzymes

Preterm PROM accounts for 30% to 40% of all preterm deliveries, and its causal mechanisms are poorly understood. Since the tensile strength and elasticity of the chorioamniotic membranes have been attributed to extracellular matrix proteins, matrix-degrading enzymes have been implicated in preterm PROM. There is now compelling evidence that preterm PROM is associated with increased availability of MMP-1,[211] MMP-8,[213-215] MMP-9,[216-218] and neutrophil elastase,[219] but not MMP-2,[218,220] MMP-3,[221] MMP-7[222] and MMP-13.

Since intrauterine infection is present in 30% of patients with preterm PROM, and proinflammatory cytokines can stimulate the production of MMP-1, MMP-9, and MMP-8, a genetic predisposition to overproduction of MMPs in response to microorganisms has been implicated in the genesis of PROM. Fetal carriage of two functional polymorphisms for MMP-1 and MMP-9 have been associated with preterm PROM.[223,224]

A polymorphism at nt-1607 in the MMP-1 promoter (an insertion of a guanine [G]) creates a core Ets binding site and increases promoter activity.[224] The 2G promoter had greater than two-fold activity compared with the 1G allele in amnion mesenchymal cells and a cloned amnion cell line. Phorbol 12-myristate 13-acetate (PMA) increased mesenchymal cell nuclear protein binding with greater affinity to the 2G allele. Induction of MMP-1 mRNA by PMA is significantly greater in cells with a 1G/2G or 2G/2G genotype compared with cells homozygous for the 1G allele. After treatment with PMA, the 1G/2G and 2G/2G cells produced greater amounts of MMP-1 protein than 1G/1G cells. A significant association was found between the presence of a 2G allele in the fetus and preterm PROM. Thus, the 2G allele has stronger promoter activity in amnion cells, it confers increased responsiveness of amnion cells to stimuli that induce MMP-1, and carriage of this polymorphism augments the risk of preterm PROM.[224]

A second polymorphism implicated in preterm PROM is located within with MMP-9 gene.[223] Functional studies of the 14 CA-repeat allele indicate that this allele is a stronger promoter than the 20 CA-repeat allele in amnion epithelial cells and WISH amnion-derived cells (in monocyte/macrophage cell line, the 14 and 20 CA-repeat alleles have similar activities). A case control study indicated that the 14 CA-repeat allele was more common in neonates delivered to mothers who had preterm PROM than in those delivered at term. Thus, differences in MMP-9 promoter activity are related to the CA-repeat number, and fetal carriage of the 14 CA-repeat allele is associated with preterm PROM.[223]

FETAL INFLAMMATORY RESPONSE SYNDROME

The last stage of ascending intrauterine infection is fetal microbial invasion. There is now clinical and experimental evidence

suggesting that the fetus can be exposed to microorganisms and their products (i.e., bacterial endotoxin)[123,225] that are present in the amniotic cavity, and that the fetus can respond by mounting both a cellular and humoral immunoresponse.[226-228]

The term *fetal inflammatory response syndrome* (FIRS) was coined to define a subclinical condition originally described in fetuses of women presenting with preterm labor and intact membranes, as well as preterm PROM. The operational definition was an elevation of fetal plasma IL-6 concentration above 11 pg/mL.[10] IL-6, a major mediator of the host response to infection and tissue damage, is capable of eliciting biochemical, physiologic, and immunologic changes in the host, including stimulation of the production of C-reactive protein by liver cells, the acute phase plasma protein response, activation of T and natural killer cells, etc. Fetuses with FIRS have a higher rate of neonatal complications[12,13] and are frequently born to mothers with subclinical microbial invasion of the amniotic cavity.[10]

We proposed that fetal microbial invasion results in a systemic fetal inflammatory response that can progress to multiple organ dysfunction, septic shock, and death in the absence of timely delivery. Evidence of multisystemic involvement in cases of a FIRS includes increased concentrations of fetal plasma MMP-9,[229] an enzyme involved in the digestion of type IV collagen. In addition, these fetuses have neutrophilia, a higher number of circulating nucleated red blood cells, and higher plasma concentrations of G-CSF.[151] FIRS is also associated with changes in markers of monocyte and neutrophil activation.[152] Fetuses with elevated concentrations of IL-6 in umbilical cord blood have decreased amniotic fluid volume,[57] and there is evidence that some have cardiac dysfunction.[230,231]

The original work that described FIRS was conducted in samples obtained by cordocentesis.[10,11] However, many of the findings have been confirmed by studying umbilical cord blood at the time of birth, including the elevation of pro-inflammatory cytokines[12,13] and the relationship between these cytokines and the likelihood of clinical and suspected sepsis.[12]

One approach to determine whether fetal inflammation was present before birth is to examine the umbilical cord. Funisitis and chorionic vasculitis inflammation of the umbilical cord or of the fetal vessels on the chorionic plate are the histolopathologic landmarks of FIRS.[70] Neonates with funisitis are at increased risk for neonatal sepsis,[71] as well as long-term handicaps such as bronchopulmonary dysplasia[13] and cerebral palsy.[12] It should also be remembered that normal amniotic fluid does not contain neutrophils, that these cells have been recruited into the amniotic compartment in the course of intrauterine infection, and that their origin is predominantly fetal.[232] Thus, the amniotic fluid white blood cell count is an indirect marker of fetal inflammation.[232]

Among patients with preterm PROM, FIRS is associated with the impending onset of preterm labor, regardless of the inflammatory state of the amniotic fluid[11] (Fig. 15-2). This suggests that the human fetus plays a role in initiating the onset of labor. However, maternal-fetal cooperation must occur for parturition to be completed. Fetal inflammation has been linked to the onset of labor in association with ascending intrauterine infection. However, systemic fetal inflammation may occur in the absence of labor when the inflammatory process does not involve the chorioamniotic membranes and decidua. Such instances may take place in the context of hematogenous viral infections. Three approaches can be used to interrupt the course of FIRS: (1) delivery; (2) antimicrobial treatment of patients in whom FIRS is due to microbial invasion susceptible to treatment; and (3) administration of agents that downregulate the inflammatory response. Delivery in the context of a preterm gestation places the unborn child at risk for the complications of prematurity. Therefore, the risks of prematurity and intrauterine infection need to be balanced. Administration of antimicrobial agents may eradicate microbial invasion of the amniotic cavity in cases of preterm

		n	Procedure-to-delivery interval (median, range, days)
I	AF IL-6 ≤7.9 ng/ml FP IL-6 ≤11 pg/ml	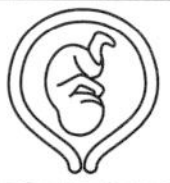 14	5 (0.2-33.6)
II	AF IL-6 >7.9 ng/ml FP IL-6 ≤11 pg/ml	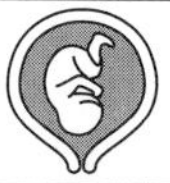 5	7 (1.5-32)
III	AF IL-6 >7.9 ng/ml FP IL-6 >11 pg/ml	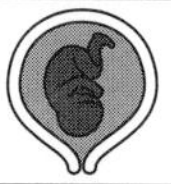 6	1.2 (0.25-2)
IV	AF IL-6 ≤7.9 ng/ml FP IL-6 >11 pg/ml	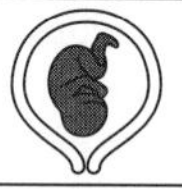 5	0.75 (0.13-1)

Figure 15–2. Among patients with preterm PROM, FIRS is associated with the impending onset of preterm labor, regardless of the inflammatory state of the amniotic fluid.

PROM.[233, 234] Further studies are required to determine whether this strategy is beneficial. The results of the ORACLE I trial suggest that antibiotic administration may not only delay the onset of labor but improve neonatal outcome[126] as well. It is tempting to postulate that this is accomplished by improving/preventing a fetal inflammatory response. Agents that downregulate the inflammatory response, such as anti-inflammatory cytokines [i.e., IL 10[235] and antibody to macrophage migration inhibitory factor (MIF)[236,237]] and antioxidants, may also have a role in preventing labor.[238-240]

Maternal Host Response to Intrauterine Infection

The term clinical chorioamnionitis describes the collection of symptoms and signs associated with the presence of microbial invasion of the amniotic cavity. Yet only 12% of all patients with documented microbial invasion by microbiologic studies will have this clinical syndrome. It has been proposed that normal pregnant women are relatively immunocompromised in order to reduce rejection of the fetal allograft. Recent evidence suggests that normal pregnancy is characterized by activation of the innate limb of the immune response. Indeed, we and others have demonstrated that normal pregnancy is associated with phenotypic and metabolic changes of granulocytes and monocytes, which are traditionally related to a state of activation.[241] It is important to note that we have also found that mothers with preterm labor[242] and preterm PROM[243] have phenotypic and metabolic changes in granulocytes and monocytes that are consistent with activation. Moreover, we have found an inverse relationship between the oxidative burst in monocytes and the time to delivery in preterm labor,[242] suggesting that the maternal immunoresponse may play a role in the onset of parturition. It is possible that the reason why most intrauterine infections are subclinical in nature is that the infection remains largely confined to the amniotic cavity and decidua. Indeed, there is evidence that neutrophils and monocytes of pregnant women change their phenotypic and metabolic characteristics in the context of systemic infections, such as pyelonephritis.[241]

A unique metabolic pattern recently has been identified in the neutrophils of normal pregnant women.[244] Neutrophils have an increase in baseline NADPH oscillations but an inability to modulate the frequency of these oscillations in response to bacterial products. These metabolic changes are coupled with increased production of reactive oxygen species (ROS) but decreased release of intracellular ROS. The cellular basis for this phenomenon appears to be a unique change in the glucose 6-phosphatase dehydrogenase trafficking.[244]

Ascending Intrauterine Infection During Pregnancy: Why?

All women have microorganisms in the lower genital tract (vagina and ectocervix), but the amniotic cavity is sterile. Cervical mucus[245-247] and amniotic fluid[248, 249] are known to have antimicrobial properties. We have proposed that innate immunity conferred by the mucus plug plays a central role in determining susceptibility to infection. Furthermore, we have identified antimicrobial peptides and proteins in the amniotic fluid[250] and cervical secretions[251] of pregnant women, including hematopoietic defensins (human neutrophil defensins 1-3), bacterial permeability-increasing protein, calprotectin[250] and lactoferrin.[252] Studies are in progress to determine the expression of pattern recognition receptors by the epithelium of the lower genital tract. This line of investigation is in the very early stages and requires investment in the study of mucosal immunity in the lower genital tract.

REFERENCES

1. Romero R, Mazor M: Infection and preterm labor. Clin Obstet Gynecol 31:553, 1988.
2. Gibbs RS, et al: A review of premature birth and subclinical infection. Am J Obstet Gynecol 166:1515, 1992.
3. Goldenberg RL, et al: Intrauterine infection and preterm delivery. N Engl J Med 342:1500, 2000.
4. Brocklehurst P: Infection and preterm delivery. BMJ 318:548, 1999.
5. Naeye RL, Ross SM: Amniotic fluid infection syndrome. Clin Obstet Gynaecol 9:593, 1982.
6. Minkoff H: Prematurity: infection as an etiologic factor. Obstet Gynecol 62:137, 1983.
7. Ledger WJ: Infection and premature labor. Am J Perinatol 6:234, 1989.
8. Romero R, et al: Infection in the pathogenesis of preterm labor. Semin Perinatol 12:262, 1988.
9. Romero R: The preterm labor syndrome. Ann N Y Acad Sci 734:414, 1994.
10. Gomez R: The fetal inflammatory response syndrome. Am J Obstet Gynecol 179:194, 1998.
11. Romero R, et al: A fetal systemic inflammatory response is followed by the spontaneous onset of preterm parturition. Am J Obstet Gynecol 179:186, 1998.
12. Yoon BH, et al: Fetal exposure to an intra-amniotic inflammation and the development of cerebral palsy at the age of three years. Am J Obstet Gynecol 182:675, 2000.
13. Yoon BH, et al: A systemic fetal inflammatory response and the development of bronchopulmonary dysplasia. Am J Obstet Gynecol 181:773, 1999.
14. Benedetti TJ, et al: Antepartum pneumonia in pregnancy. Am J Obstet Gynecol 144:413, 1982.
15. Cunningham FG, et al: Acute pyelonephritis of pregnancy: a clinical review. Obstet Gynecol 42:112, 1973.
16. Diddle AW, Stephens RL: Typhoid fever in pregnancy: probable intrauterine transmission of the disease. Am J Obstet Gynecol 37:300, 1938.
17. Fan YD, et al: Acute pyelonephritis in pregnancy. Am J Perinatol 4:324, 1987.
18. Finland M, Dublin TD: Pneumococcic pneumonia complicating pregnancy and the puerperium. JAMA 112:1027, 1939.

19. Gilles HM, et al: Malaria, anaemia and pregnancy. Ann Trop Med Parasitol 63:245, 1969.
20. Heard N, Jordan T: An investigation of malaria during pregnancy in Zimbabwe. Cent Afr J Med 27:62, 1981.
21. Kass E: Maternal urinary tract infection. NY State J Med 1:2822, 1962.
22. Madinger NE, et al: Pneumonia during pregnancy: has modern technology improved maternal and fetal outcome? Am J Obstet Gynecol 161:657, 1989.
23. Oxhorn H: The changing aspects of pneumonia complicating pregnancy. Am J Obstet Gynecol 70:1057, 1955.
24. Wing ES, Troppoli DV: The intrauterine transmission of typhoid. JAMA 95:405, 1930.
25. Madianos PN, et al: Maternal periodontitis and prematurity. Part II: Maternal infection and fetal exposure. Ann Periodonto 6:175, 2001.
26. Offenbacher S, et al: Periodontal infection as a possible risk factor for preterm low birth weight. J Periodontol 67:1103, 1996.
27. Bearfield C, et al: Possible association between amniotic fluid micro-organism infection and microflora in the mouth. Br J Obstet Gynaecol 109:527, 2002.
28. Goncalves LF, et al: Intrauterine infection and prematurity. Ment Retard Dev Disabil Res Rev 8:3, 2002.
29. Romero R, et al: Infection and prematurity and the role of preventive strategies. Semin Neonatol 7:259, 2002.
30. Romero R, et al: The role of infection in preterm labour and delivery. Paediatr Perinat Epidemiol 15(Suppl 2):41, 2001.
31. Watts DH, et al: The association of occult amniotic fluid infection with gestational age and neonatal outcome among women in preterm labor. Obstet Gynecol 79:351, 1992.
32. Benirschke K, Clifford S: Intrauterine bacterial infection of the newborn infant. J Pediatr 54:18, 1959.
33. Benirschke K: Routes and types of infection in the fetus and the newborn. Am J Dis Child 28:714, 1965.
34. Blanc W: Infection amniotique et neonatal. Gynaecologia 136:101, 1953.
35. Driscoll S: Pathology and the developing fetus. Pediatr Clin North Am 12:493, 1965.
36. Blanc W: Pathways of fetal and early neonatal infection: viral placentitis, bacterial and fungal chorioamnionitis. J Pediatr 59:473, 1964.
37. Romero R, et al: Infection and labor. V. Prevalence, microbiology, and clinical significance of intra-amniotic infection in women with preterm labor and intact membranes. Am J Obstet Gynecol 161:817, 1989.
38. Romero R, et al: Infection and labor. VI. Prevalence, microbiology, and clinical significance of intra-amniotic infection in twin gestations with preterm labor. Am J Obstet Gynecol 163:757, 1990.
39. Galask RP, et al: Bacterial attachment to the chorioamniotic membranes. Am J Obstet Gynecol 148:915, 1984.
40. Hillier SL: A case-control study of chorioamnionic infection and histologic chorioamnionitis in prematurity. N Engl J Med 319:972, 1988.
41. Altshuler G, Hyde S: Clinicopathologic considerations of fusobacteria chorioamnionitis. Acta Obstet Gynaecol Scand 67:513, 1988.
42. Leigh J, Garite TJ: Amniocentesis and the management of premature labor. Obstet Gynecol 67:500, 1986.
43. Hitti J, et al: Broad-spectrum bacterial rDNA polymerase chain reaction assay for detecting amniotic fluid infection among women in premature labor. Clin Infect Dis 24:1228, 1997.
44. Alanen A: Polymerase chain reaction in the detection of microbes in amniotic fluid. Ann Med 30:288, 1998.
45. Thomas GB, et al: Isolation of *Chlamydia trachomatis* from amniotic fluid. Obstet Gynecol 76:519, 1990.
46. Thorp JM, Jr, et al: Fetal death from chlamydial infection across intact amniotic membranes. Am J Obstet Gynecol 161:1245, 1989.
47. Pao CC, et al: Intra-amniotic detection of *Chlamydia trachomatis* deoxyribonucleic acid sequences by polymerase chain reaction. Am J Obstet Gynecol 164:1295, 1991.
48. Kay ID, et al: Evaluation of a commercial polymerase chain reaction assay for the detection of *Chlamydia trachomatis*. Diagn Microbiol Infect Dis 28:75, 1997.
49. Yankowitz J, et al: Outcome of low-risk pregnancies with evidence of intra-amniotic viral infection detected by PCR on amniotic fluid obtained at second trimester genetic amniocentesis. J Soc Gynecol Investig 3:132A, 1996.
50. Wenstrom KD, et al: Intrauterine viral infection at the time of second trimester genetic amniocentesis. Obstet Gynecol 92:420, 1998.
51. Kimberlin DF, et al: Indicated versus spontaneous preterm delivery: an evaluation of neonatal morbidity among infants weighing ≤ 1000 grams at birth. Am J Obstet Gynecol 180:683, 1999.
52. Meis PJ, et al: The preterm prediction study: risk factors for indicated preterm births. Maternal-Fetal Medicine Units Network of the National Institute of Child Health and Human Development. Am J Obstet Gynecol 178:562, 1998.
53. Meis PJ, et al: Factors associated with preterm birth in Cardiff, Wales. II. Indicated and spontaneous preterm birth. Am J Obstet Gynecol 173:597, 1995.
54. Arias F, Tomich P: Etiology and outcome of low birth weight and preterm infants. Obstet Gynecol 60:277, 1982.
55. Hillier SL, et al: Microbiologic causes and neonatal outcomes associated with chorioamnion infection. Am J Obstet Gynecol 165:955, 1991.
56. Vintzileos AM, et al: Qualitative amniotic fluid volume versus amniocentesis in predicting infection in preterm premature rupture of the membranes. Obstet Gynecol 67:579, 1986.

57. Yoon BH, et al: Association of oligohydramnios in women with preterm premature rupture of membranes with an inflammatory response in fetal, amniotic, and maternal compartments. Am J Obstet Gynecol 181:784, 1999.
58. Romero R, et al: Intra-amniotic infection and the onset of labor in preterm premature rupture of the membranes. Am J Obstet Gynecol 159:661, 1988.
59. Romero R, et al: Infection and labor. VIII. Microbial invasion of the amniotic cavity in patients with suspected cervical incompetence: prevalence and clinical significance. Am J Obstet Gynecol 167:1086, 1992.
60. Mays JK, et al: Amniocentesis for selection before rescue cerclage. Obstet Gynecol 95:652, 2000.
61. Mazor M, et al: Intra-amniotic infection in patients with preterm labor and twin pregnancies. Acta Obstet Gynaecol Scand 75:624, 1996.
62. Yoon BH, et al: Intra-amniotic infection of twin pregnancies with preterm labor. Am J Obstet Gynecol 176:535, 1997.
63. Chellam VG, Rushton DI: Chorioamnionitis and funiculitis in the placentas of 200 births weighing less than 2.5 kg. Br J Obstet Gynaecol 92:808, 1985.
64. Hillier SL, et al: The relationship of amniotic fluid cytokines and preterm delivery, amniotic fluid infection, histologic chorioamnionitis, and chorioamnion infection. Obstet Gynecol 81:941, 1993.
65. Romero R, et al: The relationship between acute inflammatory lesions of the preterm placenta and amniotic fluid microbiology. Am J Obstet Gynecol 166:1382, 1992.
66. Aquino TI, et al: Subchorionic fibrin cultures for bacteriologic study of the placenta. Am J Clin Pathol 81:482, 1984.
67. Pankuch GA, et al: Placental microbiology and histology and the pathogenesis of chorioamnionitis. Obstet Gynecol 64:802, 1984.
68. Cassell GH, et al: Isolation of *Mycoplasma hominis* and *Ureaplasma urealyticum* from amniotic fluid at 16-20 weeks of gestation: potential effect on outcome of pregnancy. Sex Transm Dis 10:294, 1983.
69. Cassell GH, et al: Chorioamnion colonization: correlation with gestational age in women delivered following spontaneous labor versus indicated delivery. Am J Obstet Gynecol 168:425, 1993.
70. Pacora P, et al: Funisitis and chorionic vasculitis: the histological counterpart of the fetal inflammatory response syndrome. J Matern Fetal Neonatal Med 11:18, 2002.
71. Yoon BH, et al: The relationship among inflammatory lesions of the umbilical cord (funisitis), umbilical cord plasma interleukin 6 concentration, amniotic fluid infection, and neonatal sepsis. Am J Obstet Gynecol 183:1124, 2000.
72. Ohlsson A, Vearncombe M: Congenital and nosocomial sepsis in infants born in a regional perinatal unit: cause, outcome, and white blood cell response. Am J Obstet Gynecol 156:407, 1987.
73. Boyer KM, et al: Selective intrapartum chemoprophylaxis of neonatal group B streptococcal early-onset disease. I. Epidemiologic rationale. J Infect Dis 148:795, 1983.
74. Placzek MM, Whitelaw A: Early and late neonatal septicaemia. Arch Dis Child 58:728, 1983.
75. Thompson PJ, Congenital bacterial sepsis in very preterm infants. J Med Microbiol 36:117, 1992.
76. Philip AG: Diagnosis of neonatal bacteraemia. Arch Dis Child 64:1514, 1989.
77. Philip AG: The changing face of neonatal infection: experience at a regional medical center. Pediatr Infect Dis J 13:1098, 1994.
78. Philip AG: Sepsis + C-reactive protein. Pediatrics 93:693, 1994.
79. Seo K, et al: Preterm birth is associated with increased risk of maternal and neonatal infection. Obstet Gynecol 79:75, 1992.
80. Carroll SG, et al: Lower genital tract swabs in the prediction of intrauterine infection in preterm prelabour rupture of the membranes. Br J Obstet Gynaecol 103:54, 1996.
81. Gray DJ, et al: Adverse outcome in pregnancy following amniotic fluid isolation of *Ureaplasma urealyticum*. Prenat Diagn 12:111, 1992.
82. Horowitz S: Infection of the amniotic cavity with *Ureaplasma urealyticum* in the midtrimester of pregnancy. J Reprod Med 40:375, 1995.
83. Romero R, et al: Interleukin 6 determination in the detection of microbial invasion of the amniotic cavity. Ciba Found Symp 167:205, 1992.
84. Romero R, et al: Amniotic fluid interleukin-6 determinations are of diagnostic and prognostic value in preterm labor. Am J Reprod Immunol 30:167, 1993.
85. Romero R, et al: Amniotic fluid interleukin 6 in preterm labor; association with infection. J Clin Invest 85:1392, 1990.
86. Yoon BH, et al: Amniotic fluid interleukin-6: a sensitive test for antenatal diagnosis of acute inflammatory lesions of preterm placenta and prediction of perinatal morbidity. Am J Obstet Gynecol 172:960, 1995.
87. Romero R, et al: Two thirds of spontaneous abortion/fetal death after genetic amniocentesis are the result of a pre-existing sub-clinical inflammatory process of the amniotic cavity. Am J Obstet Gynecol 172:261, 1995.
88. Wenstrom KD: Elevated second-trimester amniotic fluid interleukin-6 levels predict preterm delivery. Am J Obstet Gynecol 178:546, 1998.
89. Yoon BH, et al: An elevated amniotic fluid matrix metalloproteinase-8 level at the time of mid-trimester genetic amniocentesis is a risk factor for spontaneous preterm delivery. Am J Obstet Gynecol 185:1162, 2001.
90. Wenstrom KD, et al: Elevated amniotic fluid interleukin-6 levels at genetic amniocentesis predict subsequent pregnancy loss. Am J Obstet Gynecol 175:830, 1996.
91. Ghidini A, et al: Elevated mid-trimester amniotic fluid tumor necrosis alpha levels: a predictor of preterm delivery. Am J Obstet Gynecol 174:307, 1996.
92. Spong CY, et al: Angiogenin: a marker for preterm delivery in midtrimester amniotic fluid. Am J Obstet Gynecol 176:415, 1997.

93. Goldenberg RL, et al: The preterm prediction study: granulocyte colony-stimulating factor and spontaneous preterm birth. National Institute of Child Health and Human Development Maternal-Fetal Medicine Units Network. Am J Obstet Gynecol 182:625, 2000.

94. Cox SM, et al: Accumulation of interleukin-1 beta and interleukin-6 in amniotic fluid: a sequela of labour in term and preterm. Hum Reprod Update 3:517, 1997.

95. Cox SM, et al: Interleukin-1 beta, -1 alpha, and -6 and prostaglandins in vaginal/cervical fluids of pregnant women before and during labor. J Clin Endocrinol Metab 77:805, 1993.

96. MacDonald P: Parturition: biomolecular and physiologic processes. In Cunningham FG, et al (eds): Williams Obstetrics. Norwalk, CT, Appleton and Lange, 1993, pp 297–361.

97. MacDonald PC, Casey ML: The accumulation of prostaglandins (PG) in amniotic fluid is an aftereffect of labor and not indicative of a role for PGE2 or PGF2 alpha in the initiation of human parturition. J Clin Endocrinol Metab 76:1332, 1993.

98. Hill AB: The environment and disease: association or causation? Proc R Soc Med 58:295, 1965.

99. Baggia S, et al: Interleukin-1 beta intra-amniotic infusion induces tumor necrosis factor-alpha, prostaglandin production, and preterm contractions in pregnant rhesus monkeys. J Soc Gynecol Investing 3:121, 1996.

100. Brown MB, et al: Genital mycoplasmosis in rats: a model for intrauterine infection. Am J Reprod Immunol 46:232, 2001.

101. Fidel PI, Jr, et al: Bacteria-induced or bacterial product–induced preterm parturition in mice and rabbits is preceded by a significant fall in serum progesterone concentrations. J Matern Fetal Med 7:222, 1998.

102. Gibbs RS, et al: Chronic intrauterine infection and inflammation in the preterm rabbit, despite antibiotic therapy. Am J Obstet Gynecol 186:234, 2002.

103. Gravett MG, et al: Fetal and maternal endocrine responses to experimental intrauterine infection in rhesus monkeys. Am J Obstet Gynecol 174:1725, 1996.

104. Katsuki Y, et al: Ability of intrauterine bacterial lipopolysaccharide to cause in situ uterine contractions in pregnant rabbits. Acta Obstet Gynecol Scand 76:26, 1997.

105. McDuffie RS, Jr, et al: Amniotic fluid tumor necrosis factor-alpha and interleukin-1 in a rabbit model of bacterially induced preterm pregnancy loss. Am J Obstet Gynecol 167:1583, 1992.

106. Romero R, et al: Systemic administration of interleukin-1 induces preterm parturition in mice. Am J Obstet Gynecol 165:969, 1991.

107. Gravett MG, et al: An experimental model for intra-amniotic infection and preterm labor in rhesus monkeys. Am J Obstet Gynecol 171:1660, 1994.

108. Witkin SS, et al: Induction of interleukin-1 receptor antagonist in rhesus monkeys after intra-amniotic infection with group B streptococci or interleukin-1 infusion. Am J Obstet Gynecol 171:1668, 1994.

109. Romero R, et al: The clinical significance of microbial invasion of the amniotic cavity with mycoplasmas in patients with preterm PROM. J Soc Gynecol Investig 70, 1993.

110. Amstey MS, Steadman KT: Asymptomatic gonorrhea and pregnancy. J Am Vener Dis Assoc 3:14, 1976.

111. Carey JC, et al: Antepartum cultures for Ureaplasma urealyticum are not useful in predicting pregnancy outcome. The Vaginal Infections and Prematurity Study Group. Am J Obstet Gynecol 164:728, 1991.

112. Gravett MG, et al: Independent associations of bacterial vaginosis and Chlamydia trachomatis infection with adverse pregnancy outcome. JAMA 256:1899, 1986.

113. Gravett MG, et al: Preterm labor associated with subclinical amniotic fluid infection and with bacterial vaginosis. Obstet Gynecol 67:229, 1986.

114. Handsfield HH, et al: Neonatal gonococcal infection. I. Orogastric contamination with Neisseria gonorrhoeae. JAMA 225:697, 1973.

115. Layton R: Infection of the urinary tract in pregnancy: an investigation of the new routine in antenatal care. Br J Obstet Gynaecol 71:927, 1964.

116. Minkoff H, et al: Risk factors for prematurity and premature rupture of membranes: a prospective study of the vaginal flora in pregnancy. Am J Obstet Gynecol 150:965, 1984.

117. Patrick MJ: Influence of maternal renal infection on the foetus and infant. Arch Dis Child 42:208, 1967.

118. Robertson JG, et al: The management and complications of asymptomatic bacteriuria in pregnancy; report of a study on 8,275 patients. J Obstet Gynaecol Br Commonw 75:59, 1968.

119. Romero R, et al: Meta-analysis of the relationship between asymptomatic bacteriuria and preterm delivery/low birth weight. Obstet Gynecol 73:576, 1989.

120. Sarrel PM, Pruett KA: Symptomatic gonorrhea during pregnancy. Obstet Gynecol 32:670, 1968.

121. Wren BG: Subclinical renal infection and prematurity. Med J Aust 2:596, 1969.

122. Romero R, et al: Microbial invasion of the amniotic cavity in premature rupture of membranes. Clin Obstet Gynecol 34:769, 1991.

123. Romero R, et al: Labor and infection. II. Bacterial endotoxin in amniotic fluid and its relationship to the onset of preterm labor. Am J Obstet Gynecol 158:1044, 1988.

124. Rosenstreich DL, et al: Genetic control of resistance to infection in mice. Crit Rev Immunol 3:263, 1982.

125. Romero R, et al: The preterm labor syndrome: biochemical, cytologic, immunologic, pathologic, microbiologic, and clinical evidence that preterm labor is a heterogeneous disease. Am J Obstet Gynecol 168:288, 1993.

126. Kenyon SL, et al: Broad-spectrum antibiotics for preterm, prelabour rupture of fetal membranes: the ORACLE I randomised trial. ORACLE Collaborative Group. Lancet 357:979, 2001.

127. Mercer BM, et al: Antibiotic therapy for reduction of infant morbidity after preterm premature rupture of the membranes. A randomized controlled trial. National Institute of Child Health and Human Development Maternal-Fetal Medicine Units Network. JAMA 278:989, 1997.

128. Mercer BM, et al: Erythromycin therapy in preterm premature rupture of the membranes: a prospective, randomized trial of 220 patients. Am J Obstet Gynecol 166:794, 1992.

129. Cox SM, et al: Randomized investigation of antimicrobials for the prevention of preterm birth. Am J Obstet Gynecol 174:206, 1996.

130. King J, Flenady V: Antibiotics for preterm labour with intact membranes. Cochrane Database Syst Rev CD000246, 2000.

131. Romero R, et al: Antibiotic treatment of preterm labor with intact membranes: a multicenter, randomized, double-blinded, placebo-controlled trial. Am J Obstet Gynecol 169:764, 1993.

132. Kenyon SL, et al: Broad-spectrum antibiotics for spontaneous preterm labour: the ORACLE II randomised trial. ORACLE Collaborative Group. Lancet 357:989, 2001.

133. Klebanoff MA, et al: Outcome of the Vaginal Infections and Prematurity Study: results of a clinical trial of erythromycin among pregnant women colonized with group B streptococci. Am J Obstet Gynecol 172:1540, 1995.

134. Koumans EH, et al: Indications for therapy and treatment recommendations for bacterial vaginosis in nonpregnant and pregnant women: a synthesis of data. Clin Infect Dis 35:S152, 2002.

135. Relman DA: The search for unrecognized pathogens. Science 284:1308, 1999.

136. Marshall BJ, Warren JR: Unidentified curved bacilli in the stomach of patients with gastritis and peptic ulceration. Lancet 1:1311, 1984.

137. Marshall BJ: The 1995 Albert Lasker Medical Research Award. Helicobacter pylori, the etiologic agent for peptic ulcer. JAMA 274:1064, 1995.

138. Choo QL, et al: Isolation of a cDNA clone derived from a blood-borne non-A, non-B viral hepatitis genome. Science 244:359, 1989.

139. Relman DA, et al: The agent of bacillary angiomatosis. An approach to the identification of uncultured pathogens. N Engl J Med 323:1573, 1990.

140. Relman DA, et al: Identification of the uncultured bacillus of Whipple's disease. N Engl J Med 327:293, 1992.

141. Wilson KH, et al: Phylogeny of the Whipple's-disease-associated bacterium. Lancet 338:474, 1991.

142. Nichol ST, et al: Genetic identification of a hantavirus associated with an outbreak of acute respiratory illness. Science 262:914, 1993.

143. Chang Y, et al: Identification of herpesvirus-like DNA sequences in AIDS-associated Kaposi's sarcoma. Science 266:1865, 1994.

144. Jalava J, et al: Bacterial 16S rDNA polymerase chain reaction in the detection of intra-amniotic infection. Br J Obstet Gynaecol 103:664, 1996.

145. Markenson GR: The use of the polymerase chain reaction to detect bacteria in amniotic fluid in pregnancies complicated by preterm labor. Am J Obstet Gynecol 177:1471, 1997.

146. Blanchard A, et al: Use of the polymerase chain reaction for detection of Mycoplasma fermentans and Mycoplasma genitalium in the urogenital tract and amniotic fluid. Clin Infect Dis 17(Suppl 1):S272, 2003.

147. Oyarzun E, et al: Specific detection of 16 micro-organisms in amniotic fluid by polymerase chain reaction and its correlation with preterm delivery occurrence. Am J Obstet Gynecol 179:1115, 1998.

148. Rizzo G: Ultrasonographic assessment of the uterine cervix and interleukin-8 concentrations in cervical secretions predict intrauterine infection in patients with preterm labor and intact membranes. Ultrasound Obstet Gynecol 12:86, 1998.

149. Yoon BH, et al: Clinical implications of detection of Ureaplasma urealyticum in the amniotic cavity with the polymerase chain reaction. Am J Obstet Gynecol 183:1130, 2000.

150. Shim S, et al: The clinical significance of detecting Ureaplasma urealyticum by PCR in the amniotic fluid of patients with preterm labor and intact membranes. Am J Obstet Gynecol 187:S129, 2003.

151. Berry SM, et al: The role of granulocyte colony stimulating factor in the neutrophilia observed in the fetal inflammatory response syndrome. Am J Obstet Gynecol 178:S202, 1998.

152. Berry SM, et al: Premature parturition is characterized by in utero activation of the fetal immune system. Am J Obstet Gynecol 173:1315, 1995.

153. Bennett PR, et al: The effects of lipoxygenase metabolites of arachidonic acid on human myometrial contractility. Prostaglandins 33:837, 1987.

154. Carraher R, et al: Involvement of lipoxygenase products in myometrial contractions. Prostaglandins 26:23, 1983.

155. Ritchie DM, et al: Smooth muscle contraction as a model to study the mediator role of endogenous lipoxygenase products of arachidonic acid. Life Sci 34:509, 1984.

156. Wiqvist N, et al: L. Prostaglandins and uterine contractility. Acta Obstet Gynaecol Scand Suppl 113:23, 1983.

157. Rajabi M, et al: Hormonal regulation of interstitial collagenase in the uterine cervix of the pregnant guinea pig. Endocrinology 128:863, 1991.

158. Ellwood DA, et al: The in vitro production of prostanoids by the human cervix during pregnancy: preliminary observations. Br J Obstet Gynaecol 87:210, 1980.

159. Calder AA, Greer IA: Pharmacological modulation of cervical compliance in the first and second trimesters of pregnancy. Semin Perinatol 15:162, 1991.

160. Greer I: Cervical ripening. In Drife J, Calder AA (eds): Prostaglandins and the Uterus. London, Springer Verlag, 1992, p 191.

161. Calder AA: Pharmacological management of the unripe cervix in the human. In Naftolin F, Stubblefield P (eds): Dilatation of the Uterine Cervix. New York, Raven Press, 1980, p 317.

162. Karim SM, Filshie GM: Therapeutic abortion using prostaglandin F2alpha. Lancet *1*:157, 1970.

163. Embrey MP: Induction of abortion by prostaglandins E1 and E2. Br Med J *1*:258, 1970.

164. Husslein P: Use of prostaglandins for induction of labor. Semin Perinatol *15*:173, 1991.

165. Macer J, et al: Induction of labor with prostaglandin E2 vaginal suppositories. Obstet Gynecol *63*:664, 1984.

166. MacKenzie IZ: Prostaglandins and midtrimester abortion. *In* Drife J, Calder AA (eds): Prostaglandins and the Uterus. London, Springer-Verlag, 1992, p 119.

167. World Health Organization Task Force: Repeated vaginal administration of 15-methyl PGF2a for termination of pregnancy in the 13th to 20th week of gestation. Contraception *16*:175, 1977.

168. World Health Organization Task Force: Comparison of intra-amniotic prostaglandin F2a and hypertonic saline for second trimester abortion. BMJ *1*:1373, 1976.

169. World Health Organization Task Force: Termination of second trimester pregnancy by intra-muscular injection of 16-phenoxy-w-17,18,19,20-tetranor PGE methyl sulfanilamide. Int J Gynaecol Obstet *20*:383, 1982.

170. Ekman GA, et al: Intravaginal versus intracervical applications of prostaglandin E2 in viscous gel of cervical priming and induction of labor at term in patients with unfavorable cervical state. Am J Obstet Gynecol *47*:657, 1983.

171. Giri SN, et al: Role of eicosanoids in abortion and its prevention by treatment with flunixin meglumine in cows during the first trimester of pregnancy. J Vet Med A*38*:445, 1991.

172. Keirse MJ, Turnbull AC: Prostaglandins in amniotic fluid during pregnancy and labour. J Obstet Gynaecol Br Commonw *80*:970, 1973.

173. Harper MJ, Skarnes RC: Inhibition of abortion and fetal death produced by endotoxin or prostaglandin F2a. Prostaglandins *2*:295, 1972.

174. Sellers SM, et al: The relation between the release of prostaglandins at amniotomy and the subsequent onset of labour. Br J Obstet Gynaecol *88*:1211, 1981.

175. Romero R, et al: Prostaglandin concentrations in amniotic fluid of women with intra-amniotic infection and preterm labor. Am J Obstet Gynecol *157*:1461, 1987.

176. Romero R, et al: Increased amniotic fluid leukotriene C4 concentration in term human parturition. Am J Obstet Gynecol *159*:655, 1988.

177. Romero R, et al: Amniotic fluid concentration of 5-hydroxyeicosatetraenoic acid is increased in human parturition at term. Prostaglandins *35*:81, 1989.

178. Romero R, et al: Amniotic fluid prostaglandin levels and intra-amniotic infections. Lancet *1*:1380, 1986.

179. Romero R, et al: Amniotic fluid prostaglandin E2 in preterm labor. Prostaglandins *34*:141, 1988.

180. Keirse MJ: Endogenous prostaglandins in human parturition. *In* Kerise MA, Gravenhorst J (eds): Human Parturition. Netherlands: The Hague, Martinus Nijhoff Publishers, 1979, p 101.

181. MacDonald PC, et al: Initiation of human parturition. I. Mechanism of action of arachidonic acid. Obstet Gynecol *44*:629, 1974.

182. Romero R, et al: Amniotic fluid 5-hydroxyeicosatetraenoic acid in preterm labor. Prostaglandins *136*:179, 1988.

183. Romero R, et al: Amniotic fluid arachidonate lipoxygenase metabolites in women with preterm labor. Prostaglindins, Leukoc Essent Fatty Acids *36*:60, 1988.

184. Lopez-Bernal A, et al: Prostaglandin, chorioamnionitis and preterm labour. Br J Obstet Gynaecol *94*:1156, 1987.

185. Falco G, et al: Leukotriene C$_4$ stimulates TXA$_2$ formation in isolated sensitized guinea pig lungs. Biochem Pharmacol *30*:2491, 1981.

186. Feuerstein N, et al: Leukotrienes C$_4$ and D$_4$ induce prostaglandin and thromboxane release from rate peritoneal macrophages. Br J Pharmacol *72*:389, 1981.

187. Serhan CD, et al: Leukotriene B4 and phosphatidic acid are calcium ionophores: studies employing arsenazo III in liposomes. J Biol Chem *257*:5746, 1982.

188. Romero R, et al: Interleukin-1: a signal for the initiation of labor in chorioamnionitis. 33rd Annual Meeting for the Society for Gynecologic Investigation. Toronto, Ontario, 1986.

189. Romero R, et al: Human decidua: a source of interleukin-1. Obstet Gynecol *73*:31, 1989.

190. Romero R, et al: Human decidua: a source of cachectin-tumor necrosis factor. Eur J Obstet Gynecol Reprod Biol *41*:123, 1991.

191. Casey ML, et al: Cachectin/tumor necrosis factor-alpha formation in human decidua. Potential role of cytokines in infection-induced preterm labor. J Clin Invest *83*:430, 1989.

192. Gauldie J, et al: Interferon beta 2/B-cell stimulatory factor type 2 shares identity with monocyte-derived hepatocyte-stimulating factor and regulates the major acute phase protein response in liver cells. Proc Natl Acad Sci U S A *84*:7251, 1987.

193. Romero R, et al: Infection and labor. IV. Cachectin-tumor necrosis factor in the amniotic fluid of women with intra-amniotic infection and preterm labor. Am J Obstet Gynecol *161*:336, 1989.

194. Romero R, et al: Infection and labor. III. Interleukin-1: a signal for the onset of parturition. Am J Obstet Gynecol *160*:1117, 1989.

195. Romero R, et al: Tumor necrosis factor in preterm and term labor. Am J Obstet Gynecol *166*:1576, 1992.

196. Romero R, et al: Interleukin-1 alpha and interleukin-1 beta in preterm and term human parturition. Am J Reprod Immunol *27*:117, 1992.

197. Silver RM, et al: Tumor necrosis factor-alpha mediates LPS-induced abortion: evidence from the LPS-resistant murine strain C3H/HeJ. J Soc Gynecol Investig Abstract, 1993.

198. Romero R, Tartakovsky B: The natural interleukin-1 receptor antagonist prevents interleukin-1-induced preterm delivery in mice. Am J Obstet Gynecol *167*:1041, 1992.

199. Gomez R, et al: Two thirds of human fetuses with microbial invasion of the amniotic cavity have a detectable systemic cytokine response before birth. Am J Obstet Gynecol *176*:514, 1997.

200. Taniguchi T, et al: The enhanced production of placental interleukin-1 during labor and intrauterine infection. Am J Obstet Gynecol *165*:131, 1991.

201. Fidel PL Jr, et al: Treatment with the interleukin-1 receptor antagonist and soluble tumor necrosis factor receptor Fc fusion protein does not prevent endotoxin-induced preterm parturition in mice. J Soc Gynecol Investig *4*:22, 1997.

202. Hirsch E, et al: Bacterially induced preterm labor in the mouse does not require maternal interleukin-1 signaling. Am J Obstet Gynecol *186*:523, 2002.

203. Hertelendy F, et al: Interleukin-1 beta-induced prostaglandin E2 production in human myometrial cells: role of a pertussis toxin-sensitive component. Am J Reprod Immunol *45*:142, 2001.

204. Molnar M, et al: Interleukin-1 and tumor necrosis factor stimulate arachidonic acid release and phospholipid metabolism in human myometrial cells. Am J Obstet Gynecol *169*:825, 1993.

205. Molnar M, et al: Oxytocin activates mitogen-activated protein kinase and up-regulates cyclooxygenase-2 and prostaglandin production in human myometrial cells. Am J Obstet Gynecol *181*:42, 1999.

206. Phillippe M, et al: Thrombin-stimulated uterine contractions in the pregnant and nonpregnant rat. J Soc Gynecol Investig *8*:260, 2001.

207. Elovitz MA, et al: The role of thrombin in preterm parturition. Am J Obstet Gynecol *185*:1059, 2001.

208. Elovitz MA, et al: Effects of thrombin on myometrial contractions in vitro and in vivo. Am J Obstet Gynecol *183*:799, 2000.

209. Elovitz MA, et al: The mechanisms underlying the stimulatory effects of thrombin on myometrial smooth muscle. Am J Obstet Gynecol *183*:674, 2000.

210. Chaiworapongsa T, et al: Activation of coagulation system in preterm labor and preterm premature rupture of membranes. J Matern Fetal Neonatal Med *11*:368, 2002.

211. Allport VC, et al: Human labour is associated with nuclear factor-kappaB activity which mediates cyclo-oxygenase-2 expression and is involved with the 'functional progesterone withdrawal'. Mol Hum Reprod 7:581, 2001.

212. Maymon E, et al: Evidence for the participation of interstitial collagenase (matrix metalloproteinase 1) in preterm premature rupture of membranes. Am J Obstet Gynecol *183*:914, 2000.

213. Maymon E, et al: Human neutrophil collagenase (matrix metalloproteinase 8) in parturition, premature rupture of the membranes, and intrauterine infection. Am J Obstet Gynecol *183*:94, 2000.

214. Maymon E, et al: Amniotic fluid matrix metalloproteinase-8 in preterm labor with intact membranes. Am J Obstet Gynecol *185*:1149, 2001.

215. Maymon E, et al: Value of amniotic fluid neutrophil collagenase concentrations in preterm premature rupture of membranes. Am J Obstet Gynecol *185*:1143, 2001.

216. Athayde N, et al: A role for matrix metalloproteinase-9 in spontaneous rupture of the fetal membranes. Am J Obstet Gynecol *179*:1248, 1998.

217. Athayde N, et al: Matrix metalloproteinases-9 in preterm and term human parturition. J Matern Fetal Med *8*:213, 1999.

218. Maymon E, et al: Evidence of in vivo differential bioavailability of the active forms of matrix metalloproteinases 9 and 2 in parturition, spontaneous rupture of membranes, and intra-amniotic infection. Am J Obstet Gynecol *183*:887, 2000.

219. Helmig BR, et al: Neutrophil elastase and secretory leukocyte protease inhibitor in prelabor rupture of membranes, parturition and intra-amniotic infection. J Matern Fetal Neonatal Med *12*:237, 2002.

220. Maymon E, et al: A role for the 72 kDa gelatinase (MMP-2) and its inhibitor (TIMP-2) in human parturition, premature rupture of membranes, and intra-amniotic infection. J Perinat Med *29*:308, 2001.

221. Park KH, et al: Matrix metalloproteinase 3 in parturition, premature rupture of the membranes, and microbial invasion of the amniotic cavity. J Perinat Med *13*:12, 2003.

222. Maymon E, et al: Matrilysin (matrix metalloproteinase 7) in parturition, premature rupture of membranes, and intrauterine infection. Am J Obstet Gynecol *182*:1545, 2000.

223. Ferrand PE, et al: A polymorphism in the matrix metalloproteinase-9 promoter is associated with increased risk of preterm premature rupture of membranes in African Americans. Mol Hum Reprod *8*:494, 2002.

224. Fujimoto T, et al: A single nucleotide polymorphism in the matrix metalloproteinase-1 (MMP-1) promoter influences amnion cell MMP-1 expression and risk for preterm premature rupture of the fetal membranes. J Biol Chem *277*:6296, 2002.

225. Romero R, et al: Infection and labor: the detection of endotoxin in amniotic fluid. Am J Obstet Gynecol *157*:815, 1987.

226. Kramer BW, et al: inflammation, and remodeling in fetal sheep lung after intra-amniotic endotoxin. Am J Physiol Lung Cell Mol Physiol *283*:L452, 2002.

227. Newnham JP, et al: The fetal maturational and inflammatory responses to different routes of endotoxin infusion in sheep. Am J Obstet Gynecol *186*:1062, 2002.

228. Jobe AH, Ikegami M: Antenatal infection/inflammation and postnatal lung maturation and injury. Respir Res *2*:27, 2001.

229. Romero R, et al: The fetal inflammatory response syndrome is characterized by the outpouring of a potent extracellular matrix degrading enzyme into the fetal circulation. Am J Obstet Gynecol 178:S3, 1998.

230. Romero R, et al: A novel form of fetal cardiac dysfunction in preterm premature rupture of membranes. Am J Obstet Gynecol 180:S27, 1999.

231. Yanowitz TD, et al: Hemodynamic disturbances in premature infants born after chorioamnionitis: association with cord blood cytokine concentrations. Pediatr Res 51:310, 2002.

232. Sampson JE, et al: Fetal origin of amniotic fluid polymorphonuclear leukocytes. Am J Obstet Gynecol 176:77, 1997.

233. Mazor M, et al: Successful treatment of preterm labour by eradication of *Ureaplasma urealyticum* with erythromycin. Arch Gynecol Obstet 253:215, 1993.

234. Romero R, et al: Eradication of *Ureaplasma urealyticum* from the amniotic fluid with transplacental antibiotic treatment. Am J Obstet Gynecol 166:618, 1992.

235. Terrone DA, et al: Interleukin-10 administration and bacterial endotoxin-induced preterm birth in a rat model. Obstet Gynecol 98:476, 2001.

236. Calandra T, et al: Protection from septic shock by neutralization of macrophage migration inhibitory factor. Nat Med 6:164, 2000.

237. Chaiworapongsa T, et al: A novel mediator of septic shock, macrophage migration inhibitory factor, is increased in intra-amniotic infection. Am J Obstet Gynecol 187:S73, 2003.

238. Buhimschi IA, et al: Protective effect of *N*-acetylcysteine against fetal death and preterm labor induced by maternal inflammation. Am J Obstet Gynecol 188:203, 2003.

239. Buhimschi IA, et al: Reduction-oxidation (redox) state regulation of matrix metalloproteinase activity in human fetal membranes. Am J Obstet Gynecol 182:458, 2000.

240. Ben Haroush A, et al: Plasma levels of vitamin E in pregnant women prior to the development of preeclampsia and other hypertensive complications. Gynecol Obstet Invest 54:26, 2002.

241. Naccasha N, et al: Phenotypic and metabolic characteristics of monocytes and granulocytes in normal pregnancy and maternal infection. Am J Obstet Gynecol 185:1118, 2001.

242. Gervasi MT, et al: Phenotypic and metabolic characteristics of maternal monocytes and granulocytes in preterm labor with intact membranes. Am J Obstet Gynecol 185:1124, 2001.

243. Gervasi MT, et al: Maternal intravascular inflammation in preterm premature rupture of membranes. J Matern Fetal Neonatal Med 11:171, 2002.

244. Kindzelskii AL, et al: Pregnancy alters glucose-6-phosphate dehydrogenase trafficking, cell metabolism, and oxidant release of maternal neutrophils. J Clin Invest 110:1801, 2002.

245. Eggert-Kruse W, et al: Antimicrobial activity of human cervical mucus. Hum Reprod 15:778, 2000.

246. Hein M, et al: An in vitro study of antibacterial properties of the cervical mucus plug in pregnancy. Am J Obstet Gynecol 185:586, 2001.

247. Hein M: Antimicrobial factors in the cervical mucus plug. Am J Obstet Gynecol 187:137, 2002.

248. Thadepalli H, et al: Amniotic fluid analysis for antimicrobial factors. Int J Gynaecol Obstet 20:1, 1982.

249. Thomas GB, et al: Antimicrobial activity of amniotic fluid against *Chlamydia trachomatis*, *Mycoplasma hominis*, and *Ureaplasma urealyticum*. Am J Obstet Gynecol 158:16, 1988.

250. Espinoza J, et al: Antimicrobial peptides in amniotic fluid: defensins, calprotectin and bacterial/permeability-increasing protein in patients with microbial invasion of the amniotic cavity, intra-amniotic inflammation, preterm labor, and premature rupture of membranes. J Matern Fetal Neonatal Med 13:2, 2003.

251. Svinarich DM, et al: Detection of human defensin 5 in reproductive tissues. Am J Obstet Gynecol 176:470, 1997.

252. Pacora P, et al: Lactoferrin in intrauterine infection, human parturition, and rupture of fetal membranes. Am J Obstet Gynecol 183:904, 2000.

16

Douglas A. Woelkers

Maternal Cardiovascular Disease and Fetal Growth and Development

Within the womb, fetal growth and development depends on inherited genetic potential, environmental factors, and interactions between the two. The importance of the fetal environment is evident in the long-term consequences it imparts on the future health of the adult.[1-3] In crafting the intrauterine environment, both the placenta and the mother play critical roles. The placenta must primarily initiate maternal adaptations to support the growing pregnancy and then successfully distribute substrates and wastes across the uterine interface. For her part, the mother must adequately respond to placental demands for resources by undertaking dramatic cardiovascular adaptations without simultaneously jeopardizing her own health. Disturbances at any of these steps, from implantation to maternal adaptation, may impact the uterine environment and trigger alterations in fetal growth and development.

While essentially all maternal systems undergo some degree of adaptation during pregnancy, the maternal cardiovascular system experiences the most dramatic changes, indicating its critical role in determining the adequacy of the intrauterine environment. By augmenting cardiac output and blood volume, reducing peripheral vascular resistance, and remodeling uterine vasculature, pregnancy triggers a cardiovascular response that increases uterine blood flow more than 10-fold, generating a constant vascular supply designed to withstand moment-to-moment fluctuations in substrate supply and removal.[4-6] In most women, these fetoplacental demands for adaptation are met without compromise to the mother's well-being. But when abnormal placental growth is superimposed on latent or overt maternal cardiovascular disease, these physiologic adaptations may jeopardize maternal health, or fail to occur altogether, compromising fetal growth, development, and survival. In this regard, both fetal growth and maternal cardiovascular function are intimately linked by their dependence on placental function, and disruptions of either process may be related to earlier defects in placental development.

This chapter addresses the associations between maternal cardiovascular disease and aberrant fetal growth and development. Although much has been learned about the regulation of fetal growth, its associations with maternal cardiovascular disease are still largely descriptive. Beyond these clinical associations, this chapter addresses many unique mechanisms by which maternal cardiovascular disease alters the fetal environment and, alternatively, mechanisms by which fetal or placental maldevelopment may trigger maternal vascular disease. One key to understanding the fetomaternal relationship is an appreciation of the essential cardiovascular adaptations to normal pregnancy. This chapter begins, therefore, with an overview of the dramatic changes that pregnancy induces in a women's cardiovascular physiology. Thereafter is a summary of the common vascular diseases of pregnancy, including special mention of preeclampsia, an important condition unique to human pregnancy. The pathophysiology of preeclampsia is considered in some detail to highlight mechanisms by which maternal, fetal, and placental maladaptation may be related to one another. Next, the chapter addresses the associations of disturbed fetal growth with maternal disease and proposes potential mechanisms for this interaction. Finally, mention is given to several long-term consequences that cardiovascular disease in pregnancy may impart to the offspring.

MATERNAL CARDIOVASCULAR ADAPTATIONS TO PREGNANCY

Maternal cardiovascular adaptations in pregnancy serve to augment uterine blood flow by more than 10-fold over the course of pregnancy and are essential for supporting a nutritive intrauterine environment.[6] Most of these vascular adaptations are induced early and progressively by signals from placental hormones, mechanical forces, and physiologic demands placed by other maternal organ systems. The adaptive changes of pregnancy include increases of cardiac output, stroke volume, heart rate, myocardial contractility, plasma volume, blood volume, and total body water and decreases of systemic vascular resistance and blood pressure. A summary of the major cardiovascular changes of pregnancy is presented in Table 16-1.

Cardiac Output

Cardiac output (CO) begins to rise as early as 5 weeks' gestation.[7-9] By 8 weeks, CO is already elevated some 22% above nonpregnant values and increases more slowly thereafter to a maximum increase of 30 to 50% by the third trimester.[7, 8, 10, 11] There is disagreement about when CO peaks in pregnancy, although a review by van Oppen and colleagues of 33 cross-sectional and 19 longitudinal studies suggests a range of between 25 and 30 weeks' gestation.[12] The majority of latent maternal cardiac diseases will become manifest at this same time, potentially impairing uteroplacental blood flow and fetal growth. An exaggerated increase of CO is noted in pregnancies complicated by multiple gestation,[8, 13] anemia,[14, 15] high altitude,[16] hyperthyroidism,[17] and other coincident risk factors for cardiovascular disease. These pregnancies are at increased risk of failed maternal adaptation, fetal growth restriction, and preeclampsia.

Heart Rate and Stroke Volume

Cardiac output is the product of heart rate and stroke volume, both of which increase in pregnancy. The maternal heart rate varies widely in pregnancy but generally rises 10 to 20% above normal values by 32 weeks' gestation.[8,18] The tachycardia of pregnancy (80 to 100 beats per minute) is usually well tolerated but does result in an elevated myocardial oxygen demand and decreased diastolic filling time, two conditions that may be debilitating for women with preexistent cardiac disease. Stroke volume, which increases rapidly to its maximum of 20 to 30% above baseline by 20 weeks' gestation, accounts for much of the early gestational increase in CO.[11, 19, 20]

Contractility and Blood Volume

The hemodynamic factors determining stroke volume include contractility, preload, and afterload. An increase of maternal myocardial contractility in pregnancy is suggested by some studies but is difficult to distinguish from concomitant alterations in preload (i.e., venous return).[20, 21] It is clear, however, that venous return to the heart increases dramatically as total body water, blood volume, and possibly venous tone are augmented within the first few weeks of pregnancy.[11, 22, 23] Water gain is mediated by the nonosmotic release of arginine vasopressin, activation of the renin-angiotensin-aldosterone system, and resetting of the osmolar set point early in pregnancy.[24] It is proposed that rapid vasodilatation in the first weeks of pregnancy induces relative arterial underfilling, which triggers the water- and sodium-sparing response.[25] A woman's total blood volume may increase by 30 to 50% (1.5 to 1.6 L) depending on her response to early placental signals (the so-called hypervolemia of pregnancy).[8, 26, 27] Both plasma and red cell compartments contribute to the increase in total blood volume, although a more rapid and robust increase in plasma volume (40 to 60% by 28 to 32 weeks) compared with red cell volume (25 to 33% at term) results in a physiologic anemia of pregnancy.[28] As with cardiac output, multiple gestations (e.g., twins) induce an earlier and greater blood volume expansion, which may exceed 65% of normal.[29, 30] In the setting of latent or overt pregestational cardiac disease, the hypervolemia of pregnancy may overwhelm right ventricular pump function and lead to heart failure as blood volume approaches its maximum values at 28 weeks. Conversely, failure to achieve this critical augmentation of blood volume and cardiac output early in pregnancy is strongly associated with pregnancy loss and the ultimate development of preeclampsia and fetal growth restriction.[31-38]

TABLE 16-1

Maternal Cardiovascular Adaptation in Normal Pregnancy

Parameter	Modification	Magnitude	Timing
Oxygen consumption (V_{O_2})	↑↑	+20 to 60%	Term
Oxygen delivery (D_{O_2})	↔ to ↑	700 to 1400 ml/min	Term
Blood volume			
Plasma	↑↑↑	+ 45 to 60%	32 weeks
Red blood cells	↑↑	+ 25 to 32%	30 to 32 weeks
Total body water	↑↑	+ 6 to 8 L	Term
Resistance changes			
Systemic (SVR)	↓↓	−20%	16 to 34 weeks
Pulmonary (PVR)	↓↓	−34%	34 weeks
Blood pressure (SVR × CO)			
Systolic	↔ to ↓		
Diastolic	↓	10-15 mm Hg	24 to 32 weeks
Myocardial contractility			
Chronotropism (HR)	↑↑	+20 to 30%	28 to 32 weeks
Inotropism (SV)	↑	+11 to 32%	Term
Cardiac output, CO (HR × SV)	↑↑	+30 to 50%	28 to 32 weeks
Uteroplacental circulation	↑↑↑	> 10-fold	Term
Endometrial	↑↑	10 to 15% of total	
Myometrial	↑	5% of total	
Placental	↑↑↑	80 to 85% of total	

Adapted from Resnik R: *In* Creasy RK, Resnik R (eds): Maternal Fetal Medicine. Philadelphia, WB Saunders Co, 1999, p 91; Ramsey PS, et al: Am J Perinatal *18*:245–266, 2001; and Gei AF, Hankins GD: Obstet Gynecol Clin North Am *28*:465–512, 2001.

Blood Pressure and Systemic Vascular Resistance

Despite substantial increases in blood volume and cardiac output, maternal blood pressure manages to fall gradually to its nadir at 24 to 32 weeks before returning to prepregnancy values at term.[18, 26] This phenomenon is due to an early and sustained fall in the systemic vascular resistance, reaching values 25 to 35% below normal by mid pregnancy.[10, 21, 39] The exact physiology of this response is unknown but probably includes peripheral vasodilation by estrogens, progesterone, atrial natriuretic peptide, prostacyclin (PGI_2), nitric oxide (NO), and the arteriovenous shunt effect of the developing uteroplacental circulation.[21, 22, 25, 40] The peripheral vasodilation is further enhanced by maternal refractoriness to arterial vasoconstrictors, most notably angiotensin II and norepinephrine. A relative loss of this refractoriness to vasopressors in early pregnancy identifies women at risk for the subsequent development of preeclampsia and fetal growth restriction.[41,42]

Regional Blood Flow and the Uteroplacental Circulation

The enhanced cardiac output of pregnancy is not evenly distributed among all organs. Disproportionate increases in blood flow benefit the uterus (and placenta), breasts, kidneys, and skin. The requirement for substantially increased uterine blood flow vis-à-vis nutritional support of the growing fetus and placenta is obvious, and its importance cannot be overstated. Moreover, it has become clear that the uteroplacental circuit is the common factor linking maternal cardiovascular function to fetal growth.

Data from studies in humans suggest that uterine blood flow must increase from a baseline of 40 ml/minute before pregnancy, to greater than 500 ml/minute at term.[4,5,43] By the end of gestation, nearly 90% of flow is directed to the placenta, with approximately 10% reserved for the decidua and 5% for the myometrium.[6] Blood flow through the uterine circulation is critically dependent on maternal cardiac output, because evidence suggests that this circuit is maximally dilated and unable to further increase its flow by autoregulation.[44] This point is well illustrated by the 20% decrease of intervillous blood flow induced by simple changes in maternal posture (e.g., standing or supine recumbency), which can reduce venous return and cardiac output (Fig. 16-1).[45-48] Conditions that decrease maternal cardiac output, and therefore uterine blood flow, are not well tolerated by the fetus and lead to transient or sustained metabolic adjustments. Moreover, the uterine circulation remains sensitive to certain vasoconstrictors during pregnancy (e.g., nicotine), which may impose periodic limitations on placental perfusion and lead to disturbances of fetal growth.[49]

Anatomic Changes of Maternal Uterine Blood Flow in Pregnancy

Anatomically, blood is directed to the uterus primarily through the uterine arteries, which arise from the internal iliac arteries in the pelvis, and secondarily through the ovarian arteries. The uterine arteries arborize in an arcuate pattern (arcuate arteries) to supply the myometrium and then descend in a radial pattern (radial arteries) to the endometrium (decidua) before terminating as the spiral arterioles. The intervillous spaces of the term placenta are supplied by 100 to 200 spiral arterioles and drained by 75 to 175 uterine venules (Fig. 16-2).[50] At the level of the spiral arterioles, pulsatile blood pressure has been largely dissipated (25 mm Hg in spiral arteries, 15 to 20 mm Hg in the intervillous space, and 5 to 10 mm Hg in the uterine veins), allowing slow-moving maternal blood to bathe floating villi in the intervillous spaces.

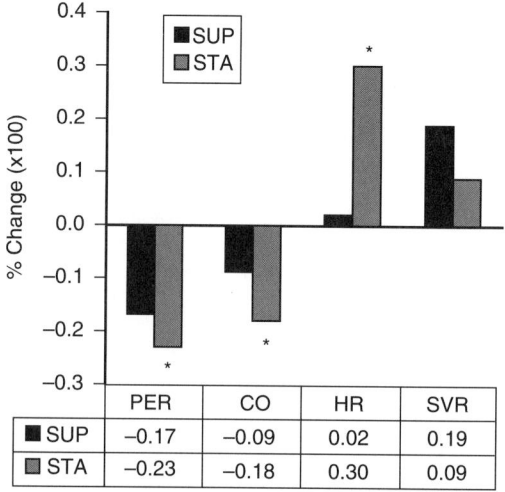

Figure 16–1. Effect of posture on placental and maternal hemodynamics. Percent change of selected hemodynamic parameters with postural change from the left lateral recumbent position to supine recumbency (SUP) or standing (STA). PER = placental perfusion; CO = cardiac output; HR = heart rate; SVR = systemic vascular resistance. *$p < .05$. (Adapted from Clark SL, et al: Am J Obstet Gynecol *164*:883–887, 1991, and Suonio S, et al: Ann Clin Res *8*:22–26, 1976.)

	PER	CO	HR	SVR
■ SUP	−0.17	−0.09	0.02	0.19
■ STA	−0.23	−0.18	0.30	0.09

The spiral arterioles supplying the placenta undergo a critical transformation early in pregnancy to ensure steady and unrestricted blood flow to the intervillous spaces.[51] Direct connections of the arterioles are initially obstructed by endovascular plugs of deep, interstitial cytotrophoblast at 8 weeks' gestation, thus maintaining the hypoxic environment essential for proliferation of the trophoblast.[52,53] Over the ensuing 4 weeks, intervillous blood flow is gradually augmented, concomitant with increasing oxygen tension and aerobic metabolism.[54,55] A second "wave" of arterial transformation is proposed to occur from 14 to 17 weeks' gestation.[56] Through a process of invasion and replacement ("physiologic transformation"), interstitial cytotrophoblasts from the placenta take up residence around and within the vessel walls of the maternal spiral arterioles and induce dramatic anatomic changes (Fig. 16-3). As a result of this endovascular invasion, fetal cells (cytotrophoblast) replace the endothelium and erode the elastic lamina and muscular intima of the maternal arterioles, forming the "uteroplacental arteries."[57] The endovascular trophoblast lining the transformed vessels embed themselves in a fibrinoid extracellular matrix composed of secreted proteins and maternal fibrin, thus creating large, dilated conduits connecting the radial arteries at the inner one third of the myometrium to the intervillous spaces. These low-resistance "uteroplacental arteries" are essentially unresponsive to local vasoconstrictors.[58,59]

Trophoblast differentiation and invasion is regulated by signals at the decidua-placental interface.[60-62] Low oxygen tension in the early placenta enhances the activity of hypoxia inducible factor, which facilitates the expression of transforming growth factor-β3 (TGF-β3), a cytokine that helps maintain the proliferative, "noninvasive phenotype" of the villous cytotrophoblast.[63,64] This phenotype is characterized by the cell surface expression of E-cadherin and integrins αVβ6 and α6β4, which interact with the superficial extracellular matrix proteins of the decidua.[60] The "invasive phenotype" of the extravillous trophoblast is induced in a carefully choreographed manner by local paracrine factors, cell-to-cell contact, extracellular matrix, and oxygen tension.[62,63, 65,66] The access of oxygenated blood to the villous spaces after

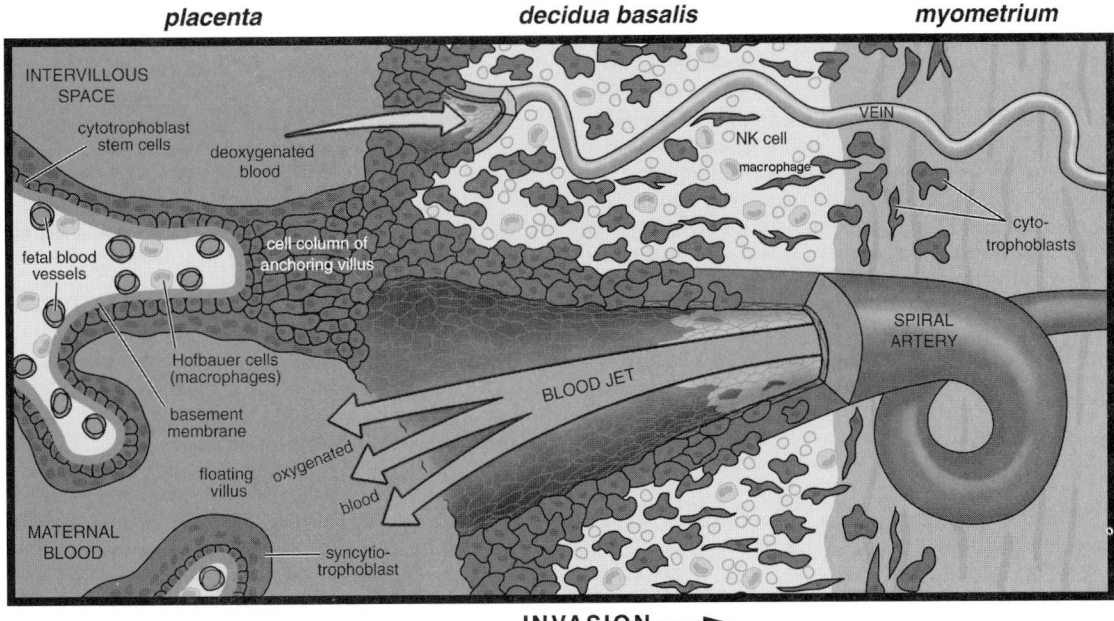

Figure 16–2. Blood supply to the intravillous space. The spiral arteries penetrate the uterine myometrium and decidua basalis beneath the placenta. Invasive trophoblast from columns of anchoring villi migrate toward these vessels and invade their lumina, replacing the normal intima and media. Blood is directed into the intravillous space, where it percolates over the floating villi and is removed by the decidual veins. (Adapted from Zhou Y, et al: Am J Pathol *160*:1405–1423, 2002.)

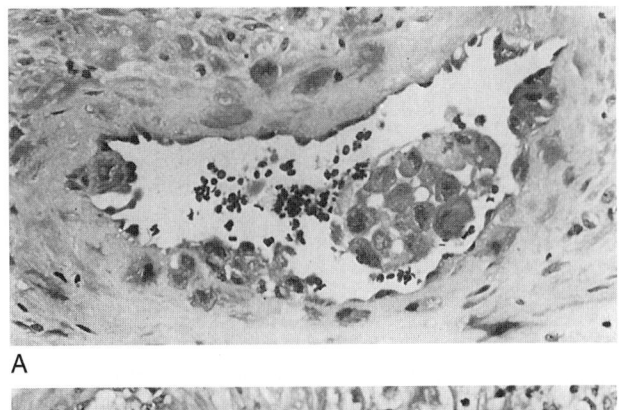

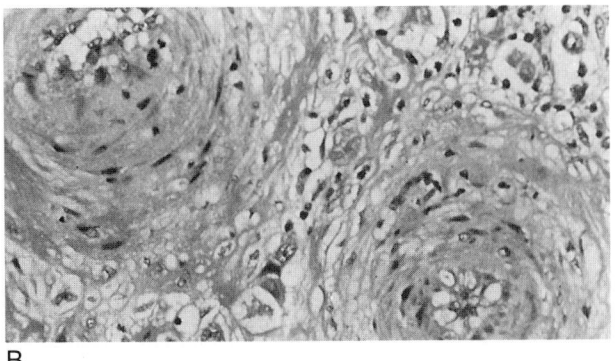

Figure 16–3. Photomicrograph of placental bed spiral arteries. **A,** Normal transformed spiral artery with irregular, dilated shape, attenuated media and intima, and intravascular trophoblasts; **B,** Untransformed basal arteries with medial hyperplasia and restricted lumen. (Adapted from Rushton DI: *In* Perrin EVDK [ed]: Pathology of the Placenta. New York, Churchill Livingstone, 1984, p 57.)

8 weeks' gestation and consequent increase in Pa_{O2} down-regulates activity of hypoxia inducible factor and TGF-β3 expression, thus enabling expression of stage-specific invasive cell surface markers (integrins αVβ3 and α1β1, VE cadherin, PECAM-1) on the trophoblast surface.[52, 67] Simultaneously, the invading trophoblast will begin to express matrix metalloproteinases to facilitate migration through the decidua and into the spiral arterioles.[68,69] On reaching their destination in the lumen of the spiral arteriole, these cells assume an endothelial cell phenotype through the expression of typical surface adhesion molecules such as vascular cell adhesion molecule-1 (VCAM-1) and platelet endothelial cell adhesion molecule-1 (PECAM-1).[60, 70, 71] Disruption of this process leads to shallow implantation and absent or incomplete remodeling of the spiral arterioles. These pathologic findings, which may lead to vascular insufficiency and chronic hypoxia, are described in placental bed biopsies from pregnancies complicated by both preeclampsia and idiopathic intrauterine fetal growth restriction.[50,51,59,72]

Functional and Molecular Changes in Uterine Blood Flow Regulation

Augmented uteroplacental blood flow in pregnancy requires more than just physiologic transformation of the spiral arterioles. Equally important is the functional transformation of the uterine arteries to a low-resistance shunt capable of accepting up to 20% of maternal cardiac output. This is accomplished by two mechanisms: (1) the growth and remodeling of uterine vessels (angiogenesis) throughout pregnancy and (2) the development of uterine vascular refractoriness to vasoconstrictors. With these adaptations, the relative fall in uterine vascular resistance exceeds even the fall in systemic vascular resistance.[73] Data from pregnant animals demonstrate elevations of circulating metabolites of NO and PGI_2 in the uterine circulation, suggesting that an increase in the endogenous production of these endothelium-derived vasodilators may be acting on the uterine vasculature.[74-76] Similar to the maternal systemic circulation, the uterine arteries are resistant to vasoconstrictor actions of angiotensin II and likewise show enhancement of the vasodilator effects of PGI_2 and NO. Consequently, it can be shown that direct uterine artery infusion of inhibitors of PGI_2 or NO synthesis (L-NAME or indomethacin) will decrease ovine uterine blood flow and enhance the local constrictor response to angiotensin II.[77, 78] In humans, as we have noted, systemic circulating PGI_2 metabolites are elevated[79,80] whereas conflicting data suggest the same for NO metabolites (nitrite and nitrate).[40,81,82] Significant arteriovenous gradients of cyclic guanosine monophosphate, the second messenger of nitric oxide, have been documented across the uterine circulation, suggesting an important role for NO in this circuit.[82]

Adaptive Changes That Mimic Cardiovascular Disease

From the preceding discussion it is apparent that virtually all aspects of maternal cardiovascular physiology are altered during the course of a normal pregnancy, some to quite an extreme degree. These changes lead to a number of signs and symptoms that mimic cardiac disease. Dyspnea is experienced by nearly 70% of pregnant women by the third trimester, although it is usually of a mild and nondebilitating nature.[83] Other symptoms include decreased exercise tolerance, occasional orthopnea, fatigue, and syncope. Physical findings that mimic disease include tachycardia, jugular venous distention, and altered heart sounds, such as systolic and diastolic murmurs or ancillary heart sounds. Edema is common to 70% of pregnancies[84] and results from increased venous hydrostatic pressure coupled with decreased colloid oncotic pressure. It is important to recognize that these symptoms arise secondary to normal cardiovascular adaptations in pregnancy and do not necessarily indicate maternal disease.

CARDIOVASCULAR DISEASES IN PREGNANCY

Summary and Definitions

Cardiovascular disease in pregnancy is not rare—despite the fact that reproductive aged women are among the healthiest members of society. This speaks to the physiologic stresses placed on the cardiovascular system by fetal and placental demands for maternal adaptation. Overall, more than 10% of pregnant women in developed countries will manifest some form of pregestational or *de novo* cardiovascular impairment, while an even greater percentage suffer these diseases in underdeveloped regions.[85-88] In total, cardiovascular disorders in pregnancy are associated with nearly 15% of perinatal deaths and more than 15% of preterm deliveries.[87, 89] These disorders are important risk factors for intrauterine growth restriction, stillbirth, and, in some instances, congenital heart disease. Furthermore, there is growing evidence to suggest a link between maternal cardiovascular disease, a suboptimal intrauterine environment, and long-term adverse health outcomes in the offspring.[90-94]

Hypertensive disorders comprise the largest class of cardiovascular disease in pregnancy, affecting 5 to 8% of gestations and having the greatest overall impact on fetal outcomes.[89, 95] The hypertensive disorders of pregnancy include *chronic hypertension* and four unique pregnancy-associated conditions: *preeclampsia*, *superimposed preeclampsia*, *eclampsia*, and *gestational hypertension*.[27] These conditions have in common the element of hypertension—defined most recently as sustained systolic and diastolic blood pressures greater than or equal to

140 over 90 mm Hg, respectively[27]—but differ dramatically in their pathophysiology. Preeclampsia is a syndrome diagnosed clinically as *de novo* hypertension *and* proteinuria after 20 weeks of pregnancy but that pathologically involves activation and dysfunction of the maternal vascular endothelium and leads to diverse manifestations of tissue hypoxia and end organ injury.[96-98] Eclampsia is the occurrence of seizures in the setting of preeclampsia, and superimposed preeclampsia is the occurrence of preeclampsia in the setting of chronic hypertension.[27] A new diagnosis of hypertension in pregnancy without accompanying evidence of preeclampsia is termed *gestational hypertension* and may be found to be transient or may be the first presentation of chronic hypertension (Table 16-2).

Preexistent vascular or congenital cardiac disease affects a much smaller percentage of pregnancies, especially in developed countries. In the United Kingdom the incidence of congenital or acquired heart disease in pregnancy has declined from 3 to 1% and would have fallen farther if it were not for the greater percentage of females with previously lethal congenital cardiac defects now surviving until the reproductive years.[85, 99] Cardiac lesions may adversely affect fetal growth by (1) restricting pregnancy-associated increases in cardiac output or (2) enabling right-to-left shunting of deoxygenated blood (cyanotic heart disease). Examples of restrictive lesions include valvular stenosis, coarctation, or cardiomyopathy. Cyanotic lesions include Eisenmenger syndrome, corrected transpositions, and uncorrected patent ductus arteriosus. Fetal growth restriction accompanies 6% of pregnancies with restrictive congenital lesions but 25% of corrected and 67% of uncorrected cyanotic lesions.[100,101] Because of the multifactorial inheritance pattern of congenital heart disease, infants of women with these lesions also carry an 8 to 14% risk of having a heart defect themselves,[100,102] although the specific lesion is not usually recapitulated in the offspring. Marfan syndrome, however, is a genetic condition which can affect both mother and fetus similarly. Marfan syndrome is an autosomal dominant–inherited defect of the fibrillin-1 gene leading to defective collagen biosynthesis, which may clinically present as aortic valve insufficiency and aortic root dissection in pregnancy.[103] As a genetic model of heart disease, Marfan syndrome illustrates the potential for a maternal cardiac condition to signify a developmental risk in the offspring. Indeed, affected fetuses have been prenatally diagnosed with Marfan syndrome with the typical ultrasound findings of aortic regurgitation and heart failure.[102,104]

Preexistent renovascular disease may also affect fetal growth and development. The rate of small for gestational age infants was nearly 40% in a cohort of pregnancies complicated by moderate or severe renal disease, 20% of whom also developed preeclampsia.[105] Autoimmune conditions such as systemic lupus erythematosus are associated with high rates of fetal growth and developmental aberrations through at least two mechanisms. First, maternal rheumatologic disorders associated with vascular or renal involvement may impair normal cardiovascular adaptation and predispose to inadequate uteroplacental circulation, resulting in fetal loss, growth restriction, and preeclampsia.[106,107] Indeed, rates of fetal growth restriction approach 40% in women with active lupus erythematosus.[108] Placental examination in these cases reveals a high incidence of decidual vasculopathy and villous infarction.[109-111] The exact mechanisms of placental vasculopathy are still unclear but may involve prothrombotic (i.e., thrombophilic) actions of antiphospholipid autoantibodies such as anticardiolipin antibody or the lupus anticoagulant. These autoantibodies are proposed to promote inappropriate intravascular and intravillous thrombosis by disturbing phospholipid/annexin-V association on the surface of endovascular membranes.[112] Second, autoimmune disease in pregnancy has the potential to induce fetal and neonatal rheumatologic disorders through the transplacental passage of self-reactive IgG autoantibodies (e.g., anti-Ro/SSA, anti-La/SSB).[113] The neonatal lupus

TABLE 16-2

Classification of the Hypertensive Disorders of Pregnancy

Classification	Definition and Diagnostic Criteria
Preeclampsia	Hypertension with proteinuria
Hypertension	Blood pressure ≥ 140 mm Hg systolic or 90 mm Hg diastolic after 20 weeks' gestation in a previously normotensive woman
Proteinuria	≥ 300 mg/L in a random specimen or ≥ 300 mg/day in a 24-hr timed collection (*de novo* hypertension with systemic symptoms of preeclampsia in the absence of proteinuria is highly suspicious).
Severe preeclampsia	Includes any of the following: BP > 160/110 mm Hg Proteinuria > 5 g/day or 3+ dipstick Central nervous system symptoms or seizures Liver injury Thrombocytopenia Pulmonary edema Renal failure/oliguria Fetal growth restriction
HELLP syndrome	Variant syndrome of preeclampsia presenting as: *H*emolysis *E*levated *L*iver enzymes *L*ow *P*latelets
Chronic hypertension	Prepregnancy hypertension ≥ 140/90 mm Hg or newly diagnosed hypertension before 20 weeks' gestation that persists more than 6 weeks after pregnancy (new-onset chronic hypertension).
Superimposed preeclampsia	Diagnosis of preeclampsia in setting of chronic hypertension. Suspected when acute worsening of hypertension is accompanied by evidence of accelerating end organ injury (e.g., proteinuria)
Gestational hypertension	Development of hypertension without evidence or symptoms of preeclampsia; resolves shortly after pregnancy.

syndrome is a recognized complication of active maternal disease and may include several transient manifestations, such as lupus dermatitis, anemia, and thrombocytopenia but also permanent congenital heart block secondary to autoimmune-mediated injury of the infant's cardiac conduction fibers.[114,115]

Preeclampsia/Eclampsia

Preeclampsia deserves special attention as a maternal vascular disorder because of its intimate link with fetal growth and development. Preeclampsia is a pregnancy-specific and uniquely human disorder, affecting from 2.6 to 7.3% of gestations and having a predilection for first conceptions, African-American race, multiple gestations, and those pregnancies complicated by medical conditions such as chronic hypertension, diabetes, or collagen vascular disease (where rates may approach 25%).[87,116] The exact etiology of preeclampsia is unknown, although the multitude of documented risk factors and predispositions suggest that it has a multifactorial origin that often involves placental or vascular susceptibility (Table 16-3). More than any other cardiovascular disease of pregnancy, preeclampsia is associated with disruptions of fetal growth and development because of the common involvement of the placenta. Known as the "disease of theories," preeclampsia is perhaps best regarded as a two-stage process in which relative or absolute placental ischemia initiates—by design or accident—a maternal inflammatory response and endothelial dysfunction, whose manifestations include hypertension, proteinuria, and various derangements of end organ performance.[97,117,118] It is not known exactly how placental dysfunction translates into endothelial dysfunction, although many proposed factors have experimental support, including, for example, oxidative stress, cytokine and immune cell activation, prostaglandin imbalance, trophoblast deportation, vascular endothelial growth factor antagonism, and

endocrine disturbances of leptin and insulin.[119-126] In this context, alterations of fetal growth in preeclampsia may arise from (1) primary or acquired placental insufficiency, (2) deficient maternal hemodynamic adaptation and uterine hypoperfusion, (3) pathologic disturbances of fetoplacental growth signaling, and/or (4) shared genetic and environmental constraints. The following summary of the pathophysiology of preeclampsia will serve to illustrate mechanisms by which fetal growth and development are likely impaired.

Placental Origin

A placental origin of preeclampsia is suggested by the many remarkable pathologic and biochemical abnormalities identified,

TABLE 16-3

Risk Factors for Preeclampsia

Nulliparity
History of preeclampsia
History of fetal growth restriction
Preexisting medical conditions
  Chronic hypertension
  Diabetes
  Renal disease
  Thrombophilia
Family history of preeclampsia
Obesity
Multifetal gestation
Molar pregnancy
Dietary deficiencies or excess
Genetic predispositions
  Lipoprotein lipase variant
  Angiotensin receptor polymorphism
  Factor V Leiden mutation

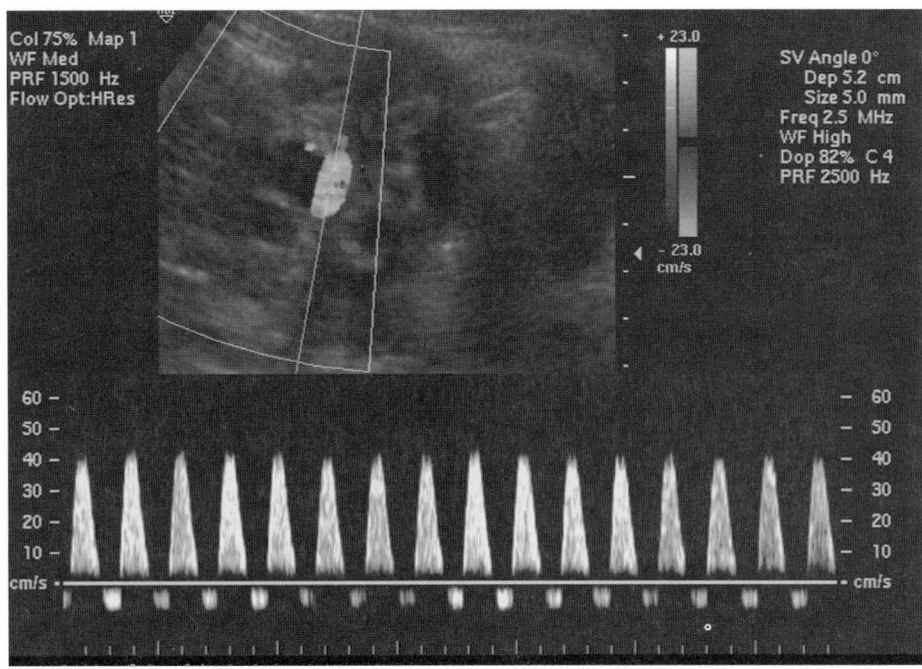

Figure 16–4. Doppler velocimetry of umbilical artery. The Doppler waveform demonstrates reversal of flow in the umbilical artery of this infant with severe preeclampsia at 28 weeks' gestation. (Adapted from Tekay A, Campbell S: *In* Callen PW [ed]: Ultrasound in Obstetrics and Gynecology. Philadelphia, WB Saunders Co, 2000, p 677.)

although these are by no means universal findings. The vascular lesions characteristic of severe or early preterm preeclampsia clearly lead to impairment of uteroplacental blood flow and offer an immediate explanation for the association with fetal growth disturbance.[127] Indeed, many similar lesions are apparent in placentas of growth-restricted infants without preeclampsia.[51, 128] It is important to note, however, that investigation of the placenta is often limited to cases with severe and early-onset disease—the variant of preeclampsia most closely associated with fetal growth restriction. Cases of mild preeclampsia at term are under-represented in many reports and may show no histologic, bio-chemical, or molecular disturbances.

Failed Trophoblast Invasion. Among the pathologic hallmarks of preeclampsia, several placental findings warrant mention. These include decidual atherosis, placental infarction, and failed tro-phoblast invasion and transformation of the spiral arterioles. Examination of placental bed biopsies in preeclampsia reveals shallow decidual penetration of the interstitial trophoblast and absent or severely restricted invasion and transformation of the distal third of the spiral arterioles that feed the placenta.[51, 59] Based on a number of elegant histologic and *in vitro* experi-ments, Zhou and colleagues have proposed that in preeclampsia, cytotrophoblasts fail to switch their cell surface adhesion mole-cules from the proliferating but noninvasive phenotype, to the invasive phenotype, to the endovascular phenotype.[60, 62, 71] Their studies demonstrate that superficial cytotrophoblasts continue to express markers of the early, undifferentiated lineage includ-ing E-cadherin and $\alpha V\beta 6$ and $\alpha 6\beta 4$ integrins and that these cells fail to express markers of the invasive/endovascular phenotype such as $\alpha V\beta 3$, $\alpha 1\beta 1$, VE-cadherin, VCAM-1, and PECAM-1.[71, 129] TGF-$\beta 3$, whose transcription is activated by hypoxia-inducible factor-1α (HIF-1α), is known to suppress expression of the inva-sive phenotype in trophoblast.[63, 130] It has been proposed, although not universally accepted, that impaired oxygen sensing in the nascent placenta maintains activation of HIF-1α and, con-sequently, overexpression of TGF-$\beta 3$, thus preventing the cells from assuming the invasive phenotype.[64, 131, 132] The resulting failure of trophoblast migration and endovascular invasion may allow persistence of the native muscular and intimal layer of the spiral arterioles and impede placental blood flow, a finding that is supported by numerous clinicopathologic studies (Fig. 16–4).[133-135] Indeed, failure of transformation of the spiral

arterioles is also noted in cases of pure intrauterine growth restriction, even without a diagnosis of preeclampsia.[136]

Infarction, Atherosis, Thrombosis. Other pathologic findings of the preeclamptic placenta having relevance for fetal growth include decidual atherosis, villous infarction, and thrombosis (Fig. 16–5).[127] Placental vascular resistance may be markedly increased, even to the point at which uterine artery blood flow is impaired during cardiac diastole.[137, 138] *In vivo* estimates of intervillous blood flow by Doppler ultrasound in severe preeclampsia suggest a reduction approaching 40%.[138, 139] At the subcellular level, preeclamptic placentas may demonstrate ultrastructural abnormalities including increased syncytial knotting, decreased microvillous surface area, and decreased villous arborization—all of which serve to further reduce the effective placental surface area and nutrient exchange.[140, 141] Shedding of syncytiotrophoblast microvillous membranes and cell fragments is increased in preeclampsia and can be meas-ured in the maternal circulation.[123, 142] Villous thrombosis is occasionally noted in the preeclamptic placenta, especially in the setting of growth restriction or early and severe disease.[143] Maternal thrombophilias, such as antiphospholipid antibody

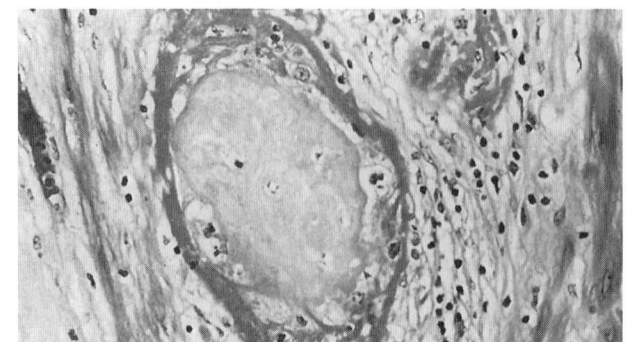

Figure 16–5. Early endothelial atherosis and fibrinoid deposition in a spiral artery from the placental bed. Note the vacuolated foam cells lining the vessel lumen inside a dark band of fibrinoid deposits. (From Rushton DI: *In* Perrin EVDK [ed]: Pathology of the Placenta. New York, Churchill Livingstone, 1984, p 57.)

TABLE 16–4

Placental Factors in Preeclampsia

	Agent	Change	Citation
Growth Factors			
	TGF-β3	Increased	52, 63, 217
	VEGF	Increased or decreased or no change	150, 353, 354
	VEGF receptor		
	FLT-1	Increased	355
	FLT-1	Increased	151
	KDR		
	IFG-I		
	IGF-II	Increased	356
	IGFBPs	Increased	243
	PLGF	Decreased	355
	Angiopoietin-2	Decreased	153
Apoptosis			
	bcl-2	Decreased	357, 358
	Fas	Increased	359
	Fas ligand	Decreased	359
Cytokines			
	TNF-α	Increased	154, 360
	IL-6	Decreased	157
	IL-1β	Increased	154, 155
Oxidative Stress			
	Isoprostanes	Increased	167
	Malondialdehyde	Increased	361
	Lipid peroxides	Increased	362, 363
	Nitrotyrosine	Increased	364, 365
	Xanthine oxidase	Increased	172
	Vitamin E	Decreased	366
	Superoxide dismutase	Decreased	366

syndrome or Factor V Leiden mutation, are associated with increased placental thrombosis and with both preeclampsia and fetal growth restriction.[144, 145] Importantly, certain of the thrombophilias have a genetic origin and may consequently be expressed in the fetus and placenta, thus impacting fetal growth and development in a direct fashion.[146, 147]

The primary cause of placental maldevelopment in preeclampsia is unknown but may include constitutional defects in the trophoblast and/or interactions with a "hostile" maternal decidual environment.[148] Regardless the primary etiology, local imbalances of growth factors, cytokines, prostanoids, and NO will arise in underperfused decidua and placenta, further contributing to vasospasm, shunting, apoptosis, and defective vascularization (Table 16–4).[121, 148] Pathologic activation of these signaling pathways in the placenta is suspected to contribute to the disturbances of fetal growth and development already initiated by deficient uteroplacental blood flow. Angiogenic factors that mediate hypoxic signaling and that are dysregulated in preeclamptic placentas include platelet-derived growth factor (PDGF), vascular endothelial growth factors (VEGFs) and their receptors (FLT-1 and KDR), placental growth factor (PLGF), and angiopoietin-1 and -2 (Ang-1 and Ang-2).[125, 149-153] Altered expression of inflammatory cytokines including tumor necrosis factor-α (TNF-α), interleukin (IL)-1β, and IL-6 has been demonstrated in the placenta of women with preeclampsia by some,[154, 155] but not all, investigators.[156, 157] Vascular reactivity is abnormally regulated in the preeclamptic placenta, and abundant evidence implicates alterations in the production and response of local vasoregulators such as the renin-angiotensin system,[158, 159] endothelin-1,[160-162] NO,[163-166] PGI₂, and thromboxane[167-169] and of peptide hormones such as adrenomedullin and atrial natriuretic peptide.[170, 171] Oxidative stress, which is proposed to arise in the preeclamptic placenta secondarily to

hypoxia and ischemia/reperfusion injury, may have many consequences for placental, maternal, and even fetal well-being.[172] The isoprostane 8-iso-PGF$_{2\alpha}$, a marker of oxidative injury, is elevated in preeclamptic placentas and potentially blocks the invasive capacity of trophoblasts by reducing their metalloproteinase and collagenase expression, thus further exacerbating placental insufficiency.[173] Other markers of oxidation found in the placenta include lipid peroxides, nitrotyrosine, and protein carbonyls. Reactive oxygen species generating enzymes such as NADPH and xanthine oxidase are found at high levels in preeclamptic placentas, accompanied by down-regulation of antioxidant systems.[148] To varying degrees, disturbances of these same vasoregulatory systems may be demonstrated in the cord blood of newborns whose mothers have preeclampsia. For example, soluble IL-8, endothelin, and monocyte and neutrophil activation were elevated, and IL-6 and cell adhesion molecules were decreased in the cord blood of infants born to women with preeclampsia versus controls.[174-176] Although usually thought of as a source of maternal endothelial and inflammatory activation, studies are just now beginning to focus on the potential of placental inflammation to disrupt fetal growth and development.

Maternal Pathophysiology of Preeclampsia

As previously mentioned, the maternal syndrome of preeclampsia is characterized by endothelial dysfunction and intravascular inflammation that is thought to originate in the placenta.[96,97,118,177] Examination of maternal serum at the time of severe or early disease may reveal alterations of numerous factors and homeostatic systems potentially involved in the primary or secondary pathophysiology of this process. The metabolism of NO, PGI₂, thromboxane, endothelin, angiotensin, atrial natriuretic peptide, and other vasoactive substances is disturbed.[178] Lipid hydroperoxides and other reactive oxygen species may be elevated, while antioxidant systems are depleted.[119] Simultaneous activation of the coagulation and fibrinolytic cascades is sometimes evident. Circulating markers of endothelial, platelet, and monocyte activation may be elevated, along with inflammatory cytokines that mediate these responses.[118] The breadth and degree of activation of these systems is generally not seen in other hemodynamic disorders of pregnancy such as chronic or gestational hypertension or congenital or acquired heart disease.

Of particular relevance to fetal growth, however, are maternal metabolic alterations that may precede or accompany preeclampsia. For years it has been known that diabetes is a significant risk factor for preeclampsia. Infants of diabetic mothers display numerous aberrations in growth and development including macrosomia, growth restriction, and congenital anomalies. More recent work confirms that insulin resistance and hyperlipidemia—two components of the heritable metabolic syndrome—also predispose to preeclampsia and tend to worsen during the disease process, and for up to 3 months afterward (Table 16–5).[179, 180] As part of this syndrome, preeclamptic women are found to have elevated levels of triglycerides, free fatty acids, and small dense low-density lipoproteins, all of which are susceptible to oxidative modifications that impair vascular endothelial function.[181, 182] It is not known what effect these metabolic changes would have on the developing fetus, although experimental maternal hyperinsulinemia in late pregnancy is associated with intrauterine growth restriction and altered carbohydrate metabolism in rat pups.[183, 184]

CARDIOVASCULAR DISEASE AND FETAL GROWTH AND DEVELOPMENT

It is now apparent that fetal growth disturbances are associated with maternal cardiovascular diseases in pregnancy. Many clinical studies have estimated the size and prevalence of this effect.[185] Clinical outcome studies categorize birth weight as small for gestational age (SGA—less than the 10th percentile for gestational age), large for gestational age (LGA—greater than 90th percentile for gestational age) or appropriate for gestational age (AGA). In general, cardiovascular disorders of pregnancy are associated with reduced intrauterine growth, although this is not always the case. Depending on the clinical situation, anywhere from 4 to 40% of infants will be SGA.[185] A mixture of growth disturbances that varies with gestational age and associated pregnancy complications has been described for the infants of preeclamptic women.[186,187] Birth weight is but one crude marker of fetal growth and development. Body composition parameters such as body mass index (BMI: weight/height^2) or ponderal index (PI: weight/length^3) are proposed to be more sensitive markers for overgrowth or undergrowth than crude birth weight, although these measurements are not universally reported.[187]

Growth Restriction

Because preeclampsia is a heterogeneous syndrome with multiple potential inciting factors, it is not surprising that the fetal growth effects are also heterogeneous. In a review of the epidemiologic literature, Misra concludes that the best evidence suggests a consistent negative association of preeclampsia with birth weight only when the disease occurs preterm or is of a severe nature.[185, 188] Gestational hypertension without preeclampsia, however, does not appear to be associated with fetal growth restriction.[189] Therefore, when proteinuria is included as a covariate, the association of gestational hypertension with SGA increases two- to fourfold.[185] In a large prospective cohort study at McMaster University Medical Centre, 1948 hypertensive pregnancies were studied.[190] Compared with newborns of women with gestational hypertension only, infants of women with preeclampsia or superimposed preeclampsia were 2.2- and 2.1-fold more likely to be SGA, whereas infants of women with chronic hypertension only were not at risk of SGA. The overall likelihood of SGA in preeclamptic offspring was 25% in this study. The fact that chronic and gestational hypertensive women were delivered of infants without growth restriction suggests that maternal hypertension per se is not the primary determinant of fetal growth in hypertensive pregnancies. Rather, it is likely that the placental defects uniquely associated with preeclampsia determine the fetal outcome and that low birth weight is more closely related to iatrogenic preterm delivery. Illustrating this point, a recent controlled retrospective study reported that 26% of infants born to mothers with preeclampsia were of "low birth weight" (<2500 g), which represented a fourfold increased risk above control pregnancies.[191] The adjusted odds for SGA, on the other hand, were only 2.5, suggesting that much of the excess in low birth weight infants was due to earlier "iatrogenic" delivery. A study by Xiong and associates[192] that controlled for multiple demographic and obstetric factors including race, age, parity, obesity, medical history, anemia, and smoking reported an increased risk of SGA for infants of preeclamptic mothers only when born before 37 weeks of gestation. Those born after 37 weeks did not manifest growth restriction; and as pregnancies passed 40 weeks, the infants from preeclamptic mothers were actually larger than the control infants (Fig. 16-6).

The fetal growth decrements attributed to preeclampsia affect body composition as well as birth weight. A large, population-based study of 672,130 births in Norway demonstrated that infants of preeclamptic mothers were lighter, shorter, and leaner than nonpreeclamptic controls.[187] The fetal growth decrements were accentuated in infants delivered at less than 37 weeks' gestation but persisted even in the term neonates. As would be expected for infants of preeclamptic mothers, the rate of asymmetric SGA was twice that of symmetric SGA, although rates of symmetric SGA were still elevated twofold over controls at both early and late gestational ages, suggesting that a significant proportion of infants began to slip from their growth potential earlier than the second trimester.

On careful evaluation, it is possible to detect abnormal maternal cardiovascular function as soon as fetal growth restriction becomes evident. Vasapollo and colleagues used echocardiography to study 21 otherwise healthy women with newly diagnosed

TABLE 16-5
Correlates of Insulin Resistance Associated with Preeclampsia.

Conditions	Biomarkers
Gestational diabetes	Hyperglycemia
Polycystic ovary syndrome	Hyperinsulinemia
Obesity/excessive weight gain	Hyperlipidemia
	Increased TNF-α
	Elevated PAI-1
	Hyperleptinemia

TNF-α = tumor necrosis factor α; PAI-1 = plasminogen activator inhibitor-1.

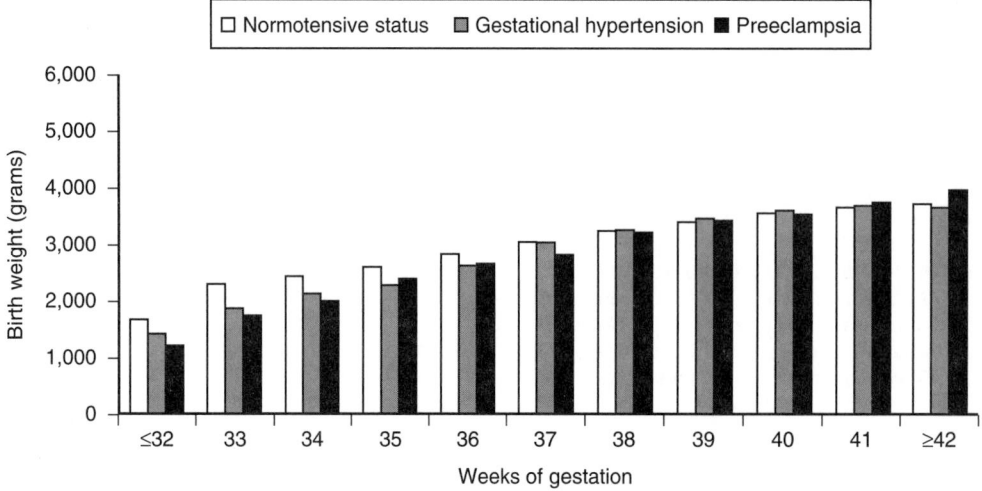

Figure 16–6. Impact of preeclampsia and gestational hypertension on birth weight (n = 87,798), Alberta, Canada, 1991-1996. (From Xiong X, et al: Am J Epidemiol *155*:203-209, 2002.)

growth-restricted fetuses.[193] These women demonstrated higher average blood pressures and peripheral vascular resistance and lower cardiac output, stroke volume, and left ventricular mass as compared with matched controls with AGA fetuses. Similarly, a failure to increase cardiac output in the first weeks of pregnancy was prospectively associated with the development of growth restriction.[36] Very commonly, the failure of maternal cardiovascular adaptation is also associated with abnormal placentation. Of women with Doppler evidence of shallow placentation, 45% also had evidence of suboptimal maternal cardiovascular adaptation and 80% of these patients ultimately developed preeclampsia or fetal growth restriction.[194] These findings lend support to Roberts' two-compartment hypothesis, which predicts the highest rates of preeclampsia in pregnancies with both an underlying maternal vascular impairment and a shallow placentation.[117]

Growth Excess

Contrary to obstetric lore, not all infants of hypertensive pregnancies will suffer from growth restriction. Xiong and colleagues[191] examined a perinatal database from Alberta, Canada, for the years 1991 to 1996 to determine the impact of preeclampsia and gestational hypertension on birth weight. After controlling for multiple factors, they found that, in addition to the expected association with SGA and low birth weight, the offspring of gestational hypertensives and preeclamptics were more likely to be LGA than infants of nonhypertensive mothers. Even though the effect is not large (OR, 1.1 to 1.5), Rasmussen and co-workers were able to demonstrate that the rates of birth weight, length, and ponderal index above the 97.5th percentile are significantly higher in births with preeclampsia than in those without preeclampsia.[187] This finding has been repeated by other investigators[185, 192] and lends support to the idea that near term some infants of preeclamptic and hypertensive women may have enough placental reserve to benefit from increased cardiac output and metabolic manipulations of their mother.

Mechanisms of Growth Impairment

Reduced Placental Perfusion

At first glance, it appears obvious that abnormalities of fetal growth and development in preeclampsia may be immediately related to decreased placental size and perfusion. Direct tracer-technique measurements of blood flow suggest a two- to three-fold decrease in uteroplacental perfusion in hypertensive women compared with normotensive gravidas.[195, 196] These studies, performed at the time of diagnosis, however, do not fully address the variety of growth patterns that may be associated with preeclampsia. More recent studies controlling for gestational age and birth weight, however, suggest that placental mass may be the same, or even greater, in some pregnancies complicated by preeclampsia and growth restriction.[197, 198]

Substrate Deprivation

Very little information exists to describe the transport of substrates across the placenta in preeclampsia. Growth-restricted fetuses without preeclampsia were noted to have lower serum α amino-nitrogenous amino acids such as valine, leucine, isoleucine, lysine, and serine weeks before delivery,[199] and placental homogenates contained significantly more free L-arginine and phenylalanine.[200] Only tyrosine was decreased in free amino acid preparations from preeclamptic placentas.[200] More recently, Powers and associates measured amino acid concentrations in maternal and neonatal blood from pregnancies complicated by preeclampsia.[201] Maternal serum amino acids were elevated in the setting of preeclampsia, as were the fetal blood concentrations. Surprisingly, among the preeclamptic pregnancies, SGA fetuses had significantly higher cord amino acid concentrations than non-SGA fetuses (321 ± 32 μmol/dl vs. 251 ± 17 μmol/dl), suggesting that in contrast to pure intrauterine growth retardation, there may be enhanced placental transport of α-amino acids and/or reduced utilization in preeclampsia, especially among those fetuses with growth restriction.

Cytokines

Transplacental transfer of cytokines has been implicated as a means of altering fetal development in settings of infection and prematurity. Low-dose endotoxin infusion into the pregnant rat has been used as a model for glomerular injury of preeclampsia.[202] The endotoxin induces a generalized Shwartzman reaction in the pregnant rat with fibrin and platelet thrombi in the kidneys that can be reduced with PGI$_2$ infusion.[203] This protocol has also been suggested as a good model for preeclampsia because it results in proteinuria, thrombocytopenia, and hypertension.[204, 205] Infusion of low-dose endotoxin into pregnant rats may lead to fetal death and resorption of fetal anomalies, presumably through reduced uterine blood flow or induction of other humoral factors.[205, 206] The placentas of endotoxin-treated rats display more apoptosis and peroxynitrite, suggesting an overall reduction in effective placental surface area in association with oxidative stress, and this may explain some facets of growth restriction.[207] This finding is also noted in rats infused with the NO synthase inhibitor L-NAME.[207] Endotoxin may or may not cross the placenta from mother to fetus,[208, 209] but a fetal inflammatory response has been documented. Fetal and placental growth restriction demonstrates a dose response to maternal endotoxin administration,[205, 207] but not necessarily at low doses. At subfetotoxic levels, an increase in central nervous system anomalies of the offspring is noted, including periventricular leukomalacia and neuronal necrosis.[210] Expression of proinflammatory cytokines TNF-α and IL-1β are increased within a few hours of maternal lipopolysaccharide administration.[209] More subtle testing of the offspring disclosed no impairment in the maze test but aberrations of male sexual behavior.[211]

Human studies of fetal cytokine concentrations in preeclampsia show conflicting results. TNF-α, IL-6, and IL-1β have been variously reported to be lower[174, 212, 213] or unchanged.[214, 215] In the largest study reported, Odegard and colleagues measured cord IL-6 in 271 cases of preeclampsia and 611 controls and demonstrated a significant decrease, especially in infants with concomitant growth restriction. Although human studies have suggested that inflammatory cytokines are elevated in umbilical cord blood of infants from preeclamptic mothers, there has been no direct association with neurodevelopmental injury.

Growth Factors

Transforming growth factor-β (TGF-β) is a family of cytokines that plays a role in growth and immunology of pregnancy.[216] The three members of the family (TGFβ1–TGFβ3) and their receptors are expressed in the placenta both early in its development and at term.[217, 218] In normal pregnancies, umbilical cord TGF-β levels correlate well with birth weight, presumably owing to its regulation by insulin-like growth factor-I (IGF-I), which also correlates with birth weight.[216] Ostlund and co-workers demonstrated that cord TGF-β1 levels were significantly lower in the cord blood from fetuses with intrauterine growth restriction with or without preeclampsia but not decreased in preeclampsia alone.[216] This suggests that preeclampsia does not *a priori* alter fetal TGB-β1 production, unless other disturbances in growth are also present.

Glucocorticoids

Glucocorticoids may be powerful effectors of fetal growth and development. High fetal concentrations of glucocorticoids are associated with low birth weight and subsequent hypertension

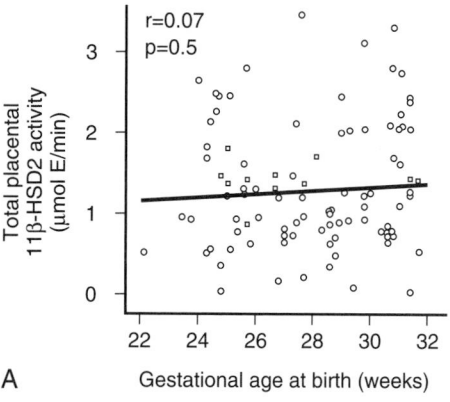
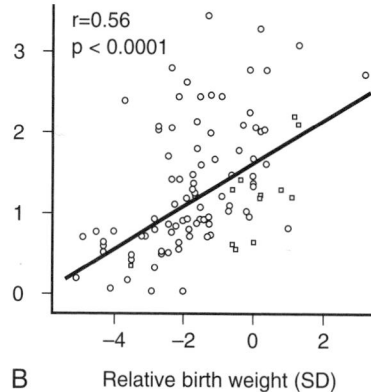

Figure 16–7. Correlation of total placental 11β-HSD2 activity with gestational age (**A**) and relative birth weight (**B**) in preterm, SGA pregnancies. (From Kajantie E, et al: J Clin Endocrinol Metab 88:4979–4983, 2001.)

as adults.[219-221] The fetus has an independent and functioning hypothalamic-pituitary-adrenal axis to regulate its glucocorticoid level, which becomes active at 16 weeks of gestation. The fetal hypothalamic-pituitary-adrenal axis is shielded from excess maternal glucocorticoids and exogenous negative feedback by the placenta, which possesses high levels of the enzyme 11β-hydroxysteroid dehydrogenase (11β-HSD) types 1 and 2.[222, 223] The type 2 isoform efficiently catalyzes the conversion of active corticosterone and cortisol to their inactive metabolite, cortisone, thus preventing high maternal glucocorticoid concentrations from overwhelming the fetal system.[224-226] Maternal cortisol levels are normally several times higher than fetal concentrations and increase near term.[227] Placental 11β-HSD2 activity increases gradually with gestational age in parallel with placental size and maternal cortisol levels, thus protecting the fetus from excess glucocorticoid exposure.[228] Growth-restricted infants demonstrate lower placental 11β-HSD2 activity and mRNA expression and higher circulating cortisol:cortisone ratio, which may result from deficient placental inactivation of maternal compounds.[228-230] Among preterm infants with growth restriction, placental 11β-HSD2 activity does not appear to increase appropriately with gestational age and its inactivity is strongly correlated with low relative birth weight, length, and infant head circumference (Fig. 16–7).[230]

Importantly, there also exists a significant decrease in placental 11β-HSD type 2 activity and an increase in fetal cord cortisol in preeclamptic pregnancies compared with normal controls.[231-233] McCalla and colleagues demonstrated that placental 11β-HSD2 activity was approximately 25% reduced in cases of preeclampsia.[231] Fetal cord cortisol was more than

doubled, and infants of these preeclamptic pregnancies were significantly smaller even when the studies were controlled for gestational age. Kajantie and co-workers also demonstrated reduced total placental 11β-HSD activity and fetal cord cortisone in preterm pregnancies with preeclampsia versus uncomplicated preterm pregnancies.[230] Other investigators have demonstrated a threefold reduction in the level of placental 11β-HSD2 mRNA in hypertensive pregnancies compared with matched controls (Fig. 16–8).[232] The subjects in this study were all near term (37.0 vs. 36.9 weeks) and did not manifest SGA (2462 vs. 2702 g), suggesting that preeclampsia inhibits 11β-HSD expression independently of growth restriction. Why placental 11β-HSD2 function is decreased in preeclampsia is not known, although recent work suggests that hypoxia down-regulates the gene expression and enzyme activity in both early and late placenta, consistent with theories of the pathogenesis of preeclampsia.[233]

Insulin and IGFs

Insulin-like growth factors (IGF-I and IGF-II) are potent regulators of cell division, differentiation, and apoptosis and influence fetal and placental growth.[234-237] Their concentrations in the fetus are strongly correlated with birth weight, and deficiency of either factor in genetically deficient mice is associated with up to a 40% reduction in fetal size.[238] The actions of IGFs are mediated by IGF receptors I and II and are stringently regulated by specific binding proteins (IGFBPs), six of which have been identified.[235,239] IGFBP-3 is the major circulating binding protein, sequestering approximately 80% of IGFs in the plasma. IGFBP-1, on the other hand, has a high affinity for IGF and acts to modulate acute plasma changes or local concentrations of IGF-I by reducing its bioavailability. Consistent with this role, circulating fetal IGFBP-1 concentrations are inversely related to birth weight.[234, 236] IGF-II is important for fetal embryonic development.[240] IGF-II influences pancreatic beta cell proliferation and thus may regulate fetal growth and metabolism by enabling insulin secretion.[241, 242] IGF-I, which predominates in late gestation, is produced mainly in the fetal liver under the influence of insulin and nutritional supply.[241]

IGF signaling is important for decidual development and appears to be critical for proper trophoblast differentiation and invasion in the first trimester and subsequent placental growth in the second and third trimesters.[243-245] Cytotrophoblasts express IGF (especially IGF-II) and high levels of IGF receptors, which promote invasive growth in an autocrine and paracrine fashion.[246] In a coordinated manner, maternal decidua expresses large quantities of IGFBP-1, which potentially acts as a counterregulatory component but which may also induce trophoblast proliferation. Indeed, overexpression of human decidual IGFBP-1 in transgenic mice leads to modest fetal growth restriction and placentomegaly with abnormal, shallow decidual invasion.[247]

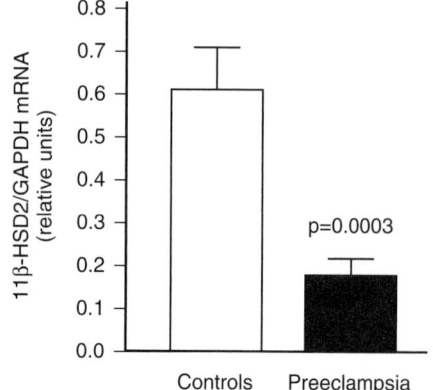

Figure 16–8. Relative expression of placental 11β-HSD2 mRNA in women with preeclampsia (n = 18) or control (n = 20). (From Schoof E, et al: J Clin Endocrinol Metab 86:1313–1317, 2001.)

Normal IGF-IGFBP relationships are disrupted in the maternal, placental, and fetal compartments in preeclampsia and may contribute to fetal growth abnormalities.[243, 245, 248-251] IGFBP-1 immunostaining is reportedly increased in the syncytiotrophoblast and anchoring villi of placentas from women with severe preeclampsia compared with controls.[243] Likewise, maternal plasma IGFBP-1, whose main source is the placenta, is significantly increased in women with severe or early preeclampsia at the time of diagnosis.[243, 252-254] It has been proposed that increased maternal IGFBP-1 production at the decidual interface impairs normal trophoblast invasion and predisposes to the future development of preeclampsia.[243] It is not known why IGFBP-1 expression would be up-regulated in preeclamptic placentas, although hypoxia, which stimulates IGFBP-1 expression in other cell types, has been implicated.[255] Yet at 16 to 24 weeks' gestation, maternal plasma IGFBP-1 concentrations are significantly *decreased* in women destined to develop preeclampsia at term, suggesting that the hypoxic trigger does not develop until later in pregnancy.[251,256,257]

In contrast to IGFBP-1, maternal plasma IGF-I, which normally increases in pregnancy and is derived from hepatic synthesis, is reduced in preeclamptic women.[243, 258, 259] The significance of this decrease for fetal growth is uncertain because while maternal IGF-1 does correlate with fetal size at birth, it appears that fetal and maternal IGF systems function independently of one another.[260] Maternal IGF-II does not change significantly in either normal or preeclamptic placentas.

Most pertinent for fetal growth, of course, are fetal concentrations of the IGFs and their IGFBPs. In a rigorous study of more than 800 infants, Vatten and colleagues demonstrated that cord plasma IGF-I was significantly lower in the setting of severe or early preeclampsia, independent of fetal weight.[261] Conversely, cord IGFBP-1 was elevated in neonates from a pregnancy with severe preeclampsia, replicating many other investigators' findings. After adjustment for birth weight, however, the association of IGFBP-1 with preeclampsia was lost. Thus, it appears that cord IGFBP-1 is regulated primarily by fetal weight and not by processes related to preeclampsia.

Apoptosis

Another potential link between preeclampsia and fetal growth restriction is the process of trophoblast apoptosis, which appears to be up-regulated in both conditions.[262,263] Ishihara and colleagues demonstrated a significant down-regulation of the antiapoptotic protein Bcl-2 in the syncytiotrophoblast of placentas from pregnancies complicated by either SGA or preeclampsia, while other investigators have reported increased evidence of apoptotic activity in pathologic specimens of cytotrophoblast.[262] Fas ligand expression was found to be elevated in trophoblast and in paired maternal/cord blood samples from hypertensive pregnancies.[264, 265] Isolated trophoblast from pregnancies complicated by either intrauterine growth retardation or preeclampsia demonstrates increased susceptibility to induction of apoptosis by hypoxia or TNF-α.[266, 267] It is hypothesized that dysregulated trophoblast apoptosis during the process of endovascular invasion would impair placental perfusion and contribute to both fetal growth restriction and preeclampsia.[266,267] Similarly, inappropriate loss of syncytiotrophoblast from the floating villi nearer to term would reduce the effective villous surface area and restrict transplacental passage of nutrients and oxygen.

Leptin

The disruption of metabolic pathways in preeclampsia may have particular relevance for alterations of fetal growth. Leptin, a 16-kDa hormone secreted by adipocytes, placenta, and select other tissues, is involved in the neuroendocrine regulation of body fat, feeding behavior, energy homeostasis, and reproduction.[268,269] Leptin levels correlate with body mass index in the nonpregnant state, and its production by adipocytes is stimulated by estrogens, progesterone, insulin, and inflammatory cytokines (e.g., TNF-α, IL-1).[268,270,271] Leptin actions include alteration in food intake, sympathetic nervous system activity, fatty acid synthesis, and triglyceride oxidation.[268] In pregnancy, leptin has dual functions in both the maternal and fetal compartment. In the mother, serum leptin levels increase two- to fourfold in normal pregnancy, presumably owing to placental production.[272-274] The increase of maternal leptin in pregnancy is not related to maternal body mass index but rather to placental size.[275, 276] Leptin is actively produced in the syncytiotrophoblast and secreted into the maternal circulation. Leptin and its receptor are also expressed in the early placenta and may play a role in regulating the phenotype of invasive trophoblast.[277,278] The high levels of leptin in pregnancy reflect some degree of leptin resistance at the level of the hypothalamus and serve to augment mobilization of fatty acids in the periphery. Circulating leptin is significantly higher in pregnancies complicated by preeclampsia.[279, 280] The increase predates the clinical diagnosis but rises still farther once the diagnosis is made.[251] The source is likely to be placental, and secretion of leptin by cultured trophoblast is increased by hypoxia and cytokines, which are both present in the preeclamptic placenta.[281-283]

It is widely suspected that leptin plays a role in the regulation of fetal growth.[284, 285] In the fetus, similar to the nonpregnant adult state, leptin reflects adiposity and body composition. Cord leptin levels correlate with placental weight, birth weight, ponderal index, infant length, head circumference, gestational age, and cord insulin levels.[286-292] Cord leptin does not correlate with maternal leptin in normal pregnancies, suggesting a fetoplacental mode of regulation independent from the mother's compartment.[274,288,293] With only 1.6% of placental leptin being secreted into the fetal circulation, it is suspected that fetal adipose tissue is the major source of cord leptin.[294, 295] Cord leptin levels are elevated in LGA infants and decreased in SGA infants[296-298] in proportion to body mass. Alternatively, the lower leptin concentration in SGA infants may be due to placental insufficiency or to lower levels of IGF-I and insulin.[268,274,299]

Severe or early preeclampsia appears to disturb fetal leptin regulation and may be one mechanism of impairing fetal growth.[268] In contrast to uncomplicated pregnancy, a positive correlation between maternal and fetal leptin levels is observed in cases of preeclampsia, suggesting either enhanced placental permeability or basolateral secretion.[279] In the setting of preeclampsia, cord leptin has been reported to be increased, decreased, or unchanged.[279, 282, 300-302] Odegard and colleagues reliably demonstrated that among hypertensive pregnancies, cord leptin was elevated at each gestational age.[302] They suggest that fetal leptinemia may be secondary to uteroplacental hypoxia or a disturbed fetoplacental interface and speculate that a resetting of leptin signaling may result in future insulin resistance and cardiovascular disease in the offspring.

Inherited Thrombophilias

Fetal growth restriction may also be linked to preeclampsia by its association with inherited and acquired thrombophilic conditions.[303, 304] Multiple studies have reported an association between thrombophilic tendencies in women and adverse pregnancy outcomes, including both preeclampsia and intrauterine growth restriction,[145, 303-307] but not all studies agree.[308, 309] It is hypothesized that maternal or fetal predispositions to clotting would lead to thromboses in the placental vasculature, thus restricting oxygen and nutrient exchange resulting in fetal growth impairment. Alternatively, fetal thrombophilia may lead to vascular disruption and potential developmental anomalies.[310] Pathologic inspection of placentas from preeclamptic women with and without known thrombophilic conditions did not, however, disclose a greater frequency of thrombotic or inflammatory lesions,[311] thus leaving in question the means of this association.

Long-Chain Fatty Acid Metabolism

One particularly intriguing genetic association between maternal vascular disease and *in utero* growth restriction concerns a fetal inborn error of metabolism. Long-chain 3-hydroxyacyl-CoA deficiency (LCHAD) is a recessive condition resulting in the interruption of fatty acid β–oxidation and the accumulation of 3-hydroxy fatty acid metabolites.[312,313] Fetal manifestations of the disease include premature delivery, asphyxia, growth restriction, and potentially stillbirth.[314] Mothers of affected infants have an 80% likelihood of developing HELLP syndrome or acute fatty liver of pregnancy (AFLOP), two severe pregnancy complications with similarities to preeclampsia.[313] One possible explanation of this preeclampsia-like response is fetomaternal transmission of accumulated oxidized 3-hydroxy fatty acids and their metabolites. As with preeclampsia, oxidative stress at the placental interface and within the maternal vasculature may lead to both fetal and maternal manifestations.

THERAPEUTICS

In some instances, fetal growth disturbances may be associated with the treatment of cardiovascular disease and not the disease itself. Pregnant women with vascular disease are subject to numerous therapies, including seizure prophylaxis, antihypertensive treatment, immunosuppression, and others.

Magnesium

Magnesium sulfate is administered to nearly all preeclamptic women in the United States as a means of preventing eclamptic seizures in labor and is also commonly used as an inhibitor of preterm labor. Maternal magnesium administration has been associated with decreased rates of cerebral palsy (CP) when used in preterm pregnancies to prevent seizures or labor.[315-319] Other investigators, however, have not found a decrease of CP in preterm infants treated with magnesium whose mothers did not have preeclampsia.[94,320-323] Although preeclampsia and prematurity may be associated with fetal intracranial hemorrhage and subsequent neurodevelopmental delay, magnesium does not reduce objective ultrasound evidence of central nervous system abnormalities,[322,323] although it is associated with lowered cerebral perfusion in preterm infants on the first day of life.[324,325] Most recently, a trial for the prevention of neurologic injury in preterm infants showed that magnesium treatment tended to *increase* the risk of overall morbidity, thus casting doubt on the neuroprotective potential of this treatment.[326]

Antihypertensive Agents

There is substantial accumulated evidence from interventional trials in pregnancy that the β-blocker atenolol increases the risk of intrauterine growth restriction whether used to treat chronic hypertension or to prevent preeclampsia.[327] Other β–blockers, such as labetalol, do not share this effect on fetal growth. Angiotensin-converting enzyme inhibitors are not generally used in pregnancy because of deleterious effects on fetal and neonatal renal function and a potential teratogenic risk.[328] The other commonly used antihypertensives, such as diuretics, calcium channel blockers, and direct vasodilators, have not been associated with disturbances of fetal growth or development.

FUTURE RISKS FOR OFFSPRING OF HYPERTENSIVE PREGNANCIES

Neurodevelopmental Outcomes

Given the "hostile" intrauterine environment supposed by our current models of preeclampsia, one might expect offspring of mothers with preeclampsia or other hypertensive disorders of pregnancy to have increased long-term risks of neurodevelopmental disorders such as neurodevelopmental delay or impaired cognition. There are few well-designed studies to answer this question, and conflicting results have been obtained from retrospective cohort and case-controlled studies. Often, confounders such as gestational age at delivery, the presence or absence of growth restriction, and the peripartum use of medications such as glucocorticoids or magnesium sulfate seizure prophylaxis are not adequately controlled.

Cerebral Palsy

Cerebral palsy is a chronic, nonprogressive disorder of the white matter causing motor function impairment that becomes detectable within months to years after birth.[329,330] The etiology of CP is still elusive but was traditionally thought to stem from asphyxial injury associated with labor and delivery.[329] However, more recent studies suggest that the majority of cases have predelivery antecedents related to early developmental anomalies or infections.[315,329] The association of CP with preeclampsia has been studied in a number of publications. A recent meta-analysis of 10 observational trials from 1966 to 1999 reported that the risk of CP in low birth weight and growth-restricted infants was 50% lower in cases complicated by maternal preeclampsia.[330] This "protective" benefit appeared to persist even after controlling for the use of magnesium sulfate. Preeclampsia seemed to reduce the risk of CP in low birth weight infants even when magnesium was not used.[331-333] It is unclear how preeclampsia, a disorder characterized by "placental hypoxia/ischemia" and inflammatory activation, could protect against CP. One potential explanation is that the early compensatory signals initiated by placental insufficiency (e.g., increased cardiac output[334] or altered uteroplacental blood flow[335]) more than make up for the reduced perfusion later on in pregnancy and prepare the infant for subsequent deprivation.[330] It is illustrative that in term preeclamptic pregnancies, the negative association with CP and preeclampsia is *not* seen, suggesting that longer *in utero* exposure to placental hypoxia may eventually override initial protective effects.[336,337] Recent studies tend to corroborate this possibility by suggesting that birth weights of most infants born of preeclamptic mothers are either appropriate or large compared with gestational age–matched controls.[186,191,192] Alternatively, it is proposed that rather than preeclampsia being protective, the other major cause of preterm delivery and growth restriction (e.g., chorioamnionitis) inflates the risk of CP in study controls.[94,338]

Cognition

Several studies have noted an association between hypertension or preeclampsia in pregnancy and developmental delay.[339] These studies found mild neurodevelopmental abnormalities in SGA infants of hypertensive mothers[340,341] compared with nonhypertensive mothers. Importantly, birth weight and poor fetal growth were more strongly correlated with future deficits than was hypertension per se. Some authors have even suggested that preeclampsia may help prevent cognitive delay because germinal matrix hemorrhage is less common in very low birth weight infants when preeclampsia was present.[342-344] Reduced placental blood flow by itself does not seem to increase the risk of neurodevelopmental or cognition delay, because there was no difference in behavior between preterm preeclamptic children with or without ultrasound evidence of placental blood flow restriction.[345] Thus, other factors associated with early embryonic or fetal development are likely to influence the cognitive outcome.

Hypertension

Several studies suggest a weak association between hypertension in pregnancy and hypertension of the offspring.[346,347]

Seidman and associates demonstrated a 2.3-fold increased risk of systolic hypertension at age 17 in female (but not male) offspring of preeclamptic pregnancies.[346] However, it appears that growth restriction accompanying a hypertensive pregnancy, rather than the hypertension itself, better predicts future cardiovascular risks. In a large epidemiologic survey of the Danish Perinatal Cohort Study, Klebanoff and colleagues reported that pregnant women who were themselves SGA at birth had a 1.8-fold increased risk of developing hypertension in pregnancy compared with women who were AGA at birth.[348] Interestingly, there was no association between hypertension in these women's mothers' pregnancies and in their own pregnancies. Prematurity by itself also predicted an increased risk of hypertension in pregnancy, although this relationship was not statistically significant.

Tenhola and co-workers studied the vascular and metabolic outcomes of a group of children 12 years after their delivery from a normal or preeclamptic pregnancy.[349] They noted that the offspring of the preeclamptic women had significantly elevated systolic and diastolic blood pressure even after adjustment for weight and height. The preeclamptic offspring also had higher circulating epinephrine levels. The blood pressure at 12 years of age was inversely correlated with birth weight in only the preeclampsia group of children. There was no difference in serum lipids, insulin, blood glucose, and adrenocortical hormones or in current weight or height. This suggests that preeclampsia may be related to future hypertension but that birth weight better predicts the future risk of metabolic syndrome.

CONCLUSION

It is apparent that cardiovascular diseases are common in pregnancy and that they constitute a large burden of morbidity for the mother and her fetus. The importance of cardiovascular function in pregnancy relates not only to maternal well-being but also to fetal growth and development. The intimate association between fetal growth and maternal cardiovascular function hinges on the adaptive and maladaptive potential of the placenta, and future investigation of the links between maternal disease and the fetal environment must focus on this interface. As we gain understanding of the compensatory potential of the placenta, we may hope to derive therapies aimed at ameliorating diseases that remain dormant for nearly a lifetime.

REFERENCES

1. Barker DJ, et al: Growth in utero, blood pressure in childhood and adult life, and mortality from cardiovascular disease. BMJ 298:564-567, 1989.
2. Barker DJ, et al: Fetal and placental size and risk of hypertension in adult life. BMJ 301:259-262, 1990.
3. Wilson J: The Barker hypothesis: an analysis. Aust N Z J Obstet Gynaecol 39:1-7, 1999.
4. Assali NS, et al:, Measurement of uterine blood flow and uterine metabolism: IV. Results in normal pregnancy. Am J Obstet Gynecol 66:248-253, 1953.
5. Gant NF, Worley BJ: Measurement of uteroplacental blood flow in the human. In Rosenfeld CR (ed): The Uterine Circulation. Ithaca, NY, Perinatology Press, 1989.
6. Resnik R: Anatomic alterations in the reproductive tract. In Creasy RK, Resnik R (eds): Maternal Fetal Medicine. Philadelphia, WB Saunders Co, 1999, p 91.
7. Capeless EL, Clapp JF: Cardiovascular changes in early phase of pregnancy. Am J Obstet Gynecol 161:1449-1453, 1989.
8. Monga M: Maternal cardiovascular and renal adaptation to pregnancy. In Creasy RK, Resnik R (eds): Maternal Fetal Medicine. Philadelphia, WB Saunders Co, 1999, pp 783-792.
9. Robson SC, et al: Serial study of factors influencing changes in cardiac output during human pregnancy. Am J Physiol 256:H1060-H1065, 1989.
10. Clark SL, et al: Central hemodynamic assessment of normal term pregnancy. Am J Obstet Gynecol 161:1439-1442, 1989.
11. Mabie WC, et al: A longitudinal study of cardiac output in normal human pregnancy. Am J Obstet Gynecol 170:849-856, 1994.
12. van Oppen AC, et al: Cardiac output in normal pregnancy: a critical review. Obstet Gynecol 87:310-38, 1996.
13. Veille JC, et al: Maternal cardiovascular adaptations to twin pregnancy. Am J Obstet Gynecol 153:261-263, 1985.

14. Veille JC, Hanson R: Left ventricular systolic and diastolic function in pregnant patients with sickle cell disease. Am J Obstet Gynecol 170:107-110, 1994.
15. Delpapa EH, et al: Effects of chronic maternal anemia on systemic and uteroplacental oxygenation in near-term pregnant sheep. Am J Obstet Gynecol 166:1007-1012, 1992.
16. Artal R, et al: A comparison of cardiopulmonary adaptations to exercise in pregnancy at sea level and altitude. Am J Obstet Gynecol 172:1170-1178; discussion 1178-1180, 1995.
17. Easterling TR, et al: Maternal hemodynamics in pregnancies complicated by hyperthyroidism. Obstet Gynecol 78:348-352, 1991.
18. Wilson M, et al: Blood pressure, the renin-aldosterone system and sex steroids throughout normal pregnancy. Am J Med 68:97-104, 1980.
19. Thornburg KL, et al: Hemodynamic changes in pregnancy. Semin Perinatol 24:11-14, 2000.
20. Geva T, et al: Effects of physiologic load of pregnancy on left ventricular contractility and remodeling. Am Heart J 133:53-59, 1997.
21. Duvekot JJ, Peeters LL: Maternal cardiovascular hemodynamic adaptation to pregnancy. Obstet Gynecol Surv 49(12 Suppl):S1-14, 1994.
22. Edouard DA, et al: Venous and arterial behavior during normal pregnancy. Am J Physiol 274:H1605-H1612, 1998.
23. Hunter S, Robson SC: Adaptation of the maternal heart in pregnancy. Br Heart J 68:540-543, 1992.
24. Durr JA, Lindheimer M: Control of volume and body tonicity. In Lindheimer M, et al (eds): Chesley's Hypertensive Disorders in Pregnancy Stamford, CT, Appleton & Lange, 1999.
25. Carbillon L, et al: Pregnancy, vascular tone, and maternal hemodynamics: a crucial adaptation. Obstet Gynecol Surv 55:574-581, 2000.
26. Clapp JF, 3rd, et al: Maternal physiologic adaptations to early human pregnancy. Am J Obstet Gynecol 159:1456-1460, 1988.
27. Program N.H.B.P.E: Working group report on high blood pressure in pregnancy. National Heart, Lung, and Blood Institution, 2000.
28. Clark SL, et al: Pregnancy-induced physiologic alterations. In Critical Care Obstetrics. Malden, MA, Blackwell Science, 1997, pp 3-4.
29. Campbell DM: Maternal adaptation in twin pregnancy. Semin Perinatol 10:14-18, 1986.
30. Rovinsky JJ, Jaffin H: Cardiovascular hemodynamics in pregnancy: II. Cardiac output and left ventricular work in multiple pregnancy. Am J Obstet Gynecol 95:781-786, 1996.
31. Silver HM, et al: Comparison of total blood volume in normal, preeclamptic, and nonproteinuric gestational hypertensive pregnancy by simultaneous measurement of red blood cell and plasma volumes. Am J Obstet Gynecol 179:87-93, 1998.
32. Soffronoff EC, et al: Intravascular volume determinations and fetal outcome in hypertensive diseases of pregnancy. Am J Obstet Gynecol 127:4-9, 1977.
33. Redman CW: Maternal plasma volume and disorders of pregnancy. BMJ (Clin Res Ed) 288:955-956, 1984.
34. Hays PM, et al: Plasma volume determination in normal and preeclamptic pregnancies. Am J Obstet Gynecol 151:958-966, 1985.
35. Duvekot JJ, et al: Maternal hemostasis in early pregnancy in relation to fetal growth restriction. Obstet Gynecol 85:361-367, 1995.
36. Duvekot JJ, et al: Severely impaired fetal growth is preceded by maternal hemodynamic maladaptation in very early pregnancy. Acta Obstet Gynecol Scand 74:693-697, 1995.
37. Salas SP, et al: Maternal plasma volume expansion and hormonal changes in women with idiopathic fetal growth retardation. Obstet Gynecol 81:1029-1033, 1993.
38. Rosso P, et al: Maternal hemodynamic adjustments in idiopathic fetal growth retardation. Gynecol Obstet Invest 35:162-165, 1993.
39. Clapp JF, 3rd, Capeless E: Cardiovascular function before, during, and after the first and subsequent pregnancies. Am J Cardiol 80:1469-1473, 1997.
40. Sladek SM, et al: Nitric oxide and pregnancy. Am J Physiol 272:R441-463, 1997.
41. Gant NF, et al: A study of angiotensin II pressor response throughout primigravid pregnancy. J Clin Invest 52:2682-2689, 1973.
42. Gant NF, et al: A clinical test useful for predicting the development of acute hypertension in pregnancy. Am J Obstet Gynecol 120:1-7, 1974.
43. Stock MK, Metcalfe J: Maternal physiology during gestation. In The Physiology of Reproduction. New York, Raven Press, 1994, pp 947-973.
44. Greiss FC, Jr, et al: Uterine pressure-flow relationships during early gestation. Am J Obstet Gynecol 126:799-808, 1976.
45. Ueland K, Hansen JM: Maternal cardiovascular dynamics: II. Posture and uterine contractions. Am J Obstet Gynecol 103:1-7, 1969.
46. Kauppila A, et al: Decreased intervillous and unchanged myometrial blood flow in supine recumbency. Obstet Gynecol 55:203-205, 1980.
47. Easterling TR, et al: The hemodynamic effects of orthostatic stress during pregnancy. Obstet Gynecol 72:550-552, 1980.
48. Clark SL, et al: Position change and central hemodynamic profile during normal third-trimester pregnancy and post partum. Am J Obstet Gynecol 164:883-887, 1991.
49. Resnik R, et al: Catecholamine-mediated reduction in uterine blood flow after nicotine infusion in the pregnant ewe. J Clin Invest 63:1133-1136, 1979.
50. Khong TY, Pearce JM: The Human Placenta: Clinical Perspectives. Lavery JP (ed). Rockville, MD, Aspen, 1987.
51. Brosens JJ, Pijnenborg IA: The myometrial junctional zone spiral arteries in normal and abnormal pregnancies: A review of the literature. Am J Obstet Gynecol 187:1416-1423, 2002.

52. Caniggia I, et al: Oxygen and placental development during the first trimester: implications for the pathophysiology of pre-eclampsia. Placenta *21*(Suppl A):S25–30, 2000.

53. Hustin J, Schaaps JP: Echographic (corrected) and anatomic studies of the maternotrophoblastic border during the first trimester of pregnancy. Am J Obstet Gynecol *157*:162–168, 1987.

54. Rodesch F, et al: Oxygen measurements in endometrial and trophoblastic tissues during early pregnancy. Obstet Gynecol *80*:283–285, 1992.

55. Jauniaux E, et al: Onset of maternal arterial blood flow and placental oxidative stress: a possible factor in human early pregnancy failure. Am J Pathol *157*:2111–2122, 2000.

56. Pijnenborg R, et al: Uteroplacental arterial changes related to interstitial trophoblast migration in early human pregnancy. Placenta *4*:397–413, 1983.

57. Kliman HJ: Uteroplacental blood flow: the story of decidualization, menstruation, and trophoblast invasion. Am J Pathol *157*:1759–1768, 2000.

58. Kam EP, et al: The role of trophoblast in the physiological change in decidual spiral arteries. Hum Reprod *14*:2131–2138, 1999.

59. Brosens IA, et al: The role of the spiral arteries in the pathogenesis of preeclampsia. Obstet Gynecol Annu *1*:177–191, 1972.

60. Zhou Y, et al: Oxygen regulates human cytotrophoblast differentiation and invasion: implications for endovascular invasion in normal pregnancy and in pre-eclampsia. J Reprod Immunol *39*:197–213, 1998.

61. Lyall F: The human placental bed revisited. Placenta *23*:555–562, 2002.

62. Fisher SJ, Damsky CH: Human cytotrophoblast invasion. Semin Cell Biol *4*:183–188, 1993.

63. Caniggia I, et al: Inhibition of TGF-beta 3 restores the invasive capability of extravillous trophoblasts in preeclamptic pregnancies. J Clin Invest *103*:1641–1650, 1999.

64. Caniggia I, Winter JL: Adriana and Luisa Castellucci Award lecture 2001. Hypoxia inducible factor-1: oxygen regulation of trophoblast differentiation in normal and pre-eclamptic pregnancies—a review. Placenta *23*(Suppl A):S47–57, 2002.

65. Damsky CH, Ilic D: Integrin signaling: it's where the action is. Curr Opin Cell Biol *14*:594–602, 2002.

66. Irwin JC, et al: Role of the IGF system in trophoblast invasion and pre-eclampsia. Hum Reprod *14*(Suppl 2):90–96, 1999.

67. Copeman J, et al: Posttranscriptional regulation of human leukocyte antigen G during human extravillous cytotrophoblast differentiation. Biol Reprod *62*:1543–1550, 2000.

68. Graham CH, Lala PK: Mechanism of control of trophoblast invasion in situ. J Cell Physiol *148*:228–234, 1991.

69. Librach CL, et al: 92-kD type IV collagenase mediates invasion of human cytotrophoblasts. J Cell Biol *113*:437–449, 1991.

70. Damsky CH, Fisher SJ: Trophoblast pseudo-vasculogenesis: faking it with endothelial adhesion receptors. Curr Opin Cell Biol *10*:660–666, 1998.

71. Zhou Y, et al: Human cytotrophoblasts adopt a vascular phenotype as they differentiate: a strategy for successful endovascular invasion? J Clin Invest *99*:2139–2151, 1997.

72. Pijnenborg R, et al: Review article: trophoblast invasion and the establishment of haemochorial placentation in man and laboratory animals. Placenta *2*:71–91, 1981.

73. Bird IM, et al: Possible mechanisms underlying pregnancy-induced changes in uterine artery endothelial function. Am J Physiol Regul Integr Comp Physiol *284*:R245–258, 2003.

74. Conrad KP, et al: Identification of increased nitric oxide biosynthesis during pregnancy in rats. FASEB J *7*:566–571, 1993.

75. Magness RR, et al: Endothelial vasodilator production by uterine and systemic arteries: VI. Ovarian and pregnancy effects on eNOS and NO(x). Am J Physiol Heart Circ Physiol *280*:H1692–H1698, 2001.

76. Yang D, et al: Elevation of nitrate levels in pregnant ewes and their fetuses. Am J Obstet Gynecol *174*:573–577, 1996.

77. McLaughlin MK, et al: Effects of indomethacin on sheep uteroplacental circulations and sensitivity to angiotensin II. Am J Obstet Gynecol *132*:430–435, 1978.

78. Rosenfeld CR, et al: Nitric oxide contributes to estrogen-induced vasodilation of the ovine uterine circulation. J Clin Invest *98*:2158–2166, 1996.

79. Fitzgerald DJ, et al: Decreased prostacyclin biosynthesis preceding the clinical manifestation of pregnancy-induced hypertension. Circulation *75*:956–963, 1987.

80. Goodman RP, et al: Prostacyclin production during pregnancy: comparison of production during normal pregnancy and pregnancy complicated by hypertension. Am J Obstet Gynecol *142*:817–822, 1982.

81. Nobunaga T, et al: Plasma nitric oxide levels in pregnant patients with preeclampsia and essential hypertension. Gynecol Obstet Invest *41*:189–193, 1996.

82. Conrad KP, et al: Plasma and 24-h NO(x) and cGMP during normal pregnancy and preeclampsia in women on a reduced NO(x) diet. Am J Physiol *277*:F48–57, 1999.

83. Crapo RO: Normal cardiopulmonary physiology during pregnancy. Clin Obstet Gynecol *39*:3–16, 1996.

84. Davison JM: Edema in pregnancy. Kidney Int Suppl *59*:S90–96, 1997.

85. Ramsey PS, et al: Cardiac disease in pregnancy. Am J Perinatol *18*:245–266, 2001.

86. Gei AF, Hankins GD: Cardiac disease and pregnancy. Obstet Gynecol Clin North Am *28*:465–512, 2001.

87. Saftlas AF, et al: Epidemiology of preeclampsia and eclampsia in the United States, 1979–1986. Am J Obstet Gynecol *163*:460–465, 1990.

88. Ness RB, Roberts JM: Epidemiology of hypertension. *In* Lindheimer M, et al (eds): Chesley's Hypertensive Disorders in Pregnancy. Stamford, CT, Appleton & Lange, 1999, pp 43–66.

89. Roberts JM, et al: Summary of the NHLBI Working Group on Research on Hypertension During Pregnancy. Hypertension *41*:437–445, 2003.

90. Himmelmann A: Blood pressure and left ventricular mass in children and adolescents: the Hypertension in Pregnancy Offspring Study. Blood Press Suppl *3*:1–46, 1994.

91. Innes KE, et al: A woman's own birth weight and gestational age predict her later risk of developing preeclampsia, a precursor of chronic disease. Epidemiology *10*:153–160, 1999.

92. Launer LJ, et al: Relation between birth weight and blood pressure: longitudinal study of infants and children. BMJ *307*:1451–1454, 1993.

93. Palmer L, et al: Antenatal antecedents of moderate and severe cerebral palsy. Paediatr Perinat Epidemiol *9*:171–184, 1995.

94. Wilson-Costello D, et al: Perinatal correlates of cerebral palsy and other neurologic impairment among very low birth weight children. Pediatrics *102*:315–322, 1998.

95. Zhang J, et al: Epidemiology of pregnancy-induced hypertension. Epidemiol Rev *19*:218–232, 1997.

96. Roberts JM, et al: Preeclampsia: an endothelial cell disorder. Am J Obstet Gynecol *161*:1200–1204, 1989.

97. Roberts JM: Preeclampsia: not simply pregnancy-induced hypertension. Hosp Pract (Off Ed) *30*:25–28, 31–36, 1995.

98. Lain KY, Roberts JM: Contemporary concepts of the pathogenesis and management of preeclampsia. JAMA *287*:3183–3186, 2002.

99. Somerville J: Grown-up congenital heart disease—medical demands look back, look forward 2000. Thorac Cardiovasc Surg *49*:21–26, 2001.

100. Whittemore R, et al: Pregnancy and its outcome in women with and without surgical treatment of congenital heart disease. Am J Cardiol *50*:641–651, 1982.

101. Sawhney H, et al: Pregnancy and congenital heart disease—maternal and fetal outcome. Aust N Z J Obstet Gynaecol *38*:266–271, 1998.

102. Rose V, et al: A possible increase in the incidence of congenital heart defects among the offspring of affected parents. J Am Coll Cardiol *6*:376–382, 1985.

103. Simpson LL, et al: Marfan syndrome in pregnancy. Curr Opin Obstet Gynecol *9*:337–341, 1997.

104. Koenigsberg M, et al: Fetal Marfan syndrome: prenatal ultrasound diagnosis with pathological confirmation of skeletal and aortic lesions. Prenat Diagn *1*:241–247, 1981.

105. Jones DC, Hayslett JP: Outcome of pregnancy in women with moderate or severe renal insufficiency. N Engl J Med *335*:226–232, 1996.

106. Persellin RH: The effect of pregnancy on rheumatoid arthritis. Bull Rheum Dis *27*:922–927, 1976.

107. Neely NT, Persellin RH: Activity of rheumatoid arthritis during pregnancy. Tex Med *73*:59–63, 1977.

108. Aggarwal N, et al:, Pregnancy in patients with systemic lupus erythematosus. Aust N Z J Obstet Gynaecol *39*:28–30, 1999.

109. Abramowsky CR, et al:, Decidual vasculopathy of the placenta in lupus erythematosus. N Engl J Med *303*:668–672, 1980.

110. Hanly JG, et al: Lupus pregnancy: a prospective study of placental changes. Arthritis Rheum *31*:358–366, 1988.

111. Out HJ, et al: Histopathological findings in placentae from patients with intrauterine fetal death and anti-phospholipid antibodies. Eur J Obstet Gynecol Reprod Biol *41*:179–86, 1991.

112. Rand JH, et al: Pregnancy loss in the antiphospholipid-antibody syndrome—a possible thrombogenic mechanism. N Engl J Med *337*:154–160, 1997.

113. Lockshin MD, et al: Neonatal lupus erythematosus with heart block: family study of a patient with anti-SS-A and SS-B antibodies. Arthritis Rheum *26*:210–213, 1983.

114. Ramsey-Goldman R, et al: Anti-SS-A antibodies and fetal outcome in maternal systemic lupus erythematosus. Arthritis Rheum *29*:1269–1273, 1986.

115. Buyon JP, et al: Anti-Ro/SSA antibodies and congenital heart block: necessary but not sufficient. Arthritis Rheum *44*:1723–1727, 1981.

116. Levine RJ, et al: Trial of calcium to prevent preeclampsia. N Engl J Med *337*:69–76, 1997.

117. Ness RB, Roberts JM: Heterogeneous causes constituting the single syndrome of preeclampsia: a hypothesis and its implications. Am J Obstet Gynecol *175*:1365–1370, 1996.

118. Sacks GP, et al: Normal pregnancy and preeclampsia both produce inflammatory changes in peripheral blood leukocytes akin to those of sepsis. Am J Obstet Gynecol *179*:80–86, 1998.

119. Hubel CA: Oxidative stress in the pathogenesis of preeclampsia. Proc Soc Exp Biol Med *222*:222–235, 1999.

120. Conrad KP, Benyo DF: Placental cytokines and the pathogenesis of preeclampsia. Am J Reprod Immunol *37*:240–249, 1997.

121. Granger JP, et al: Pathophysiology of hypertension during preeclampsia linking placental ischemia with endothelial dysfunction. Hypertension *38*:718–722, 2001.

122. Liu HS, et al: Thromboxane and prostacyclin in maternal and fetal circulation in pre-eclampsia. Int J Gynaecol Obstet *63*:1–6, 1998.

123. Knight M, et al: Shedding of syncytiotrophoblast microvilli into the maternal circulation in pre-eclamptic pregnancies. Br J Obstet Gynaecol *105*:632–640, 1998.

124. Johansen M, et al: Trophoblast deportation in human pregnancy—its relevance for pre-eclampsia. Placenta 20:531-539, 1999.
125. Maynard SE, et al: Excess placental soluble fms-like tyrosine kinase 1 (sFlt1) may contribute to endothelial dysfunction, hypertension, and proteinuria in preeclampsia. J Clin Invest 111:649-658, 2003.
126. Poston L: Leptin and preeclampsia. Semin Reprod Med 20:131-138, 2002.
127. Benirschke K, Kaufmann P: Maternal diseases complicating pregnancy: diabetes, tumors, preeclampsia, lupus anticoagulant. In Pathology of the Human Placenta. New York, Springer-Verlag, 2000, pp 542-560.
128. Brosens I, et al: Fetal growth retardation and the arteries of the placental bed. Br J Obstet Gynaecol 84:656-663, 1977.
129. Zhou Y, et al: Preeclampsia is associated with failure of human cytotrophoblasts to mimic a vascular adhesion phenotype. One cause of defective endovascular invasion in this syndrome? J Clin Invest 99:2152-2164, 1997.
130. Graham CH, Lala PK: Mechanisms of placental invasion of the uterus and their control. Biochem Cell Biol 70:867-874, 1992.
131. Chakraborty C, et al: Regulation of human trophoblast migration and invasiveness. Can J Physiol Pharmacol 80:116-124, 2002.
132. Lyall F, et al: Transforming growth factor-beta expression in human placenta and placental bed in third trimester normal pregnancy, preeclampsia, and fetal growth restriction. Am J Pathol 159:1827-1838, 2001.
133. Sagol S, et al: The comparison of uterine artery Doppler velocimetry with the histopathology of the placental bed. Aust N Z J Obstet Gynaecol 39:324-329, 1999.
134. Lin S, et al: Uterine artery Doppler velocimetry in relation to trophoblast migration into the myometrium of the placental bed. Obstet Gynecol 85:760-765, 1995.
135. Olofsson P, et al: A high uterine artery pulsatility index reflects a defective development of placental bed spiral arteries in pregnancies complicated by hypertension and fetal growth retardation. Eur J Obstet Gynecol Reprod Biol 49:161-168, 1993.
136. Brosens JJ, et al: The myometrial junctional zone spiral arteries in normal and abnormal pregnancies: a review of the literature. Am J Obstet Gynecol 187:1416-1423, 2002.
137. Karsdorp VH, et al: Placenta morphology and absent or reversed end diastolic flow velocities in the umbilical artery: a clinical and morphometrical study. Placenta 17:393-399, 1996.
138. Harrington K, et al: Doppler fetal circulation in pregnancies complicated by pre-eclampsia or delivery of a small for gestational age baby: 2. Longitudinal analysis. Br J Obstet Gynaecol 106:453-466, 1999.
139. Kaar K, et al: Intervillous blood flow in normal and complicated late pregnancy measured by means of an intravenous 133Xe method. Acta Obstet Gynecol Scand 59:7-10, 1980.
140. Fox H, Agrafojo-Blanco A: Scanning electron microscopy of the human placenta in normal and abnormal pregnancies. Eur J Obstet Gynecol Reprod Biol 4:45-50, 1974.
141. Jones CJ, Fox H: An ultrastructural and ultrahistochemical study of the human placenta in maternal essential hypertension. Placenta 2:193-204, 1981.
142. Redman CW, Sargent IL: Placental debris, oxidative stress and pre-eclampsia. Placenta 21:597-602, 2000.
143. Salafia CM, et al: The very low birthweight infant: maternal complications leading to preterm birth, placental lesions, and intrauterine growth. Am J Perinatol 12:106-110, 1995.
144. Arias F, et al: Thrombophilia: a mechanism of disease in women with adverse pregnancy outcome and thrombotic lesions in the placenta. J Matern Fetal Med 7:277-286, 1998.
145. Kupferminc MJ, et al: Increased frequency of genetic thrombophilia in women with complications of pregnancy. N Engl J Med 340:9-13, 1999.
146. Thorarensen O, et al: Factor V Leiden mutation: an unrecognized cause of hemiplegic cerebral palsy, neonatal stroke, and placental thrombosis. Ann Neurol 42:372-375, 1997.
147. Vern TZ, et al: Frequency of factor V(Leiden) and prothrombin G20210A in placentas and their relationship with placental lesions. Hum Pathol 31:1036-1043, 2000.
148. Myatt L: Role of placenta in preeclampsia. Endocrine 19:103-111, 2002.
149. Gurski MR, et al: Immunochemical localization of platelet-derived growth factor in placenta and its possible role in pre-eclampsia. J Investig Med 47:128-133, 1999.
150. Cooper JC, et al: VEGF mRNA levels in placentae from pregnancies complicated by pre-eclampsia. Br J Obstet Gynaecol 103:1191-1196, 1996.
151. Zhou Y, et al: Vascular endothelial growth factor ligands and receptors that regulate human cytotrophoblast survival are dysregulated in severe preeclampsia and hemolysis, elevated liver enzymes, and low platelets syndrome. Am J Pathol 160:1405-1423, 2002.
152. Taylor RN, et al: Longitudinal serum concentrations of placental growth factor: evidence for abnormal placental angiogenesis in pathologic pregnancies. Am J Obstet Gynecol 188:177-182, 2003.
153. Zhang EG, et al: The regulation and localization of angiopoietin-1, -2, and their receptor Tie2 in normal and pathologic human placentae. Mol Med 7:624-635, 2001.
154. Rinehart BK, et al: Expression of the placental cytokines tumor necrosis factor alpha, interleukin 1beta, and interleukin 10 is increased in preeclampsia. Am J Obstet Gynecol 181:915-920, 1999.
155. Munno I, et al: Spontaneous and induced release of prostaglandins, interleukin (IL)-1beta, IL-6, and tumor necrosis factor-alpha by placental tissue

156. Benyo DF, et al: Expression of inflammatory cytokines in placentas from women with preeclampsia. J Clin Endocrinol Metab 86:2505-2512, 2001.
157. Kauma SW, et al: Preeclampsia is associated with decreased placental interleukin-6 production. J Soc Gynecol Investig 2:614-617, 1995.
158. Glance DG, et al: The effects of the components of the renin-angiotensin system on the isolated perfused human placental cotyledon. Am J Obstet Gynecol 149:450-454, 1984.
159. Ito M, et al: Possible activation of the renin-angiotensin system in the feto-placental unit in preeclampsia. J Clin Endocrinol Metab 87:1871-1878, 2002.
160. Myatt L, et al: Endothelin-1-induced vasoconstriction is not mediated by thromboxane release and action in the human fetal-placental circulation. Am J Obstet Gynecol 165:1717-1722, 1991.
161. Myatt L, et al: The comparative effects of big endothelin-1, endothelin-1, and endothelin-3 in the human fetal-placental circulation. Am J Obstet Gynecol 167:1651-1656, 1992.
162. Myatt L: Control of vascular resistance in the human placenta. Placenta 13:329-341, 1992.
163. Myatt L, et al: Constitutive calcium-dependent isoform of nitric oxide synthase in the human placental villous vascular tree. Placenta 14:373-383, 1993.
164. Morris NH, et al: Nitric oxide synthase activities in placental tissue from normotensive, pre-eclamptic and growth retarded pregnancies. Br J Obstet Gynaecol 102:711-714, 1995.
165. Lyall F, et al: Nitric oxide concentrations are increased in the feto-placental circulation in intrauterine growth restriction. Placenta 17:165-168, 1996.
166. Norris LA, et al: Nitric oxide in the uteroplacental, fetoplacental, and peripheral circulations in preeclampsia. Obstet Gynecol 93:958-963, 1999.
167. Walsh SW, et al: Placental isoprostane is significantly increased in preeclampsia. FASEB J 14:1289-1296, 2000.
168. Walsh SW: Preeclampsia: an imbalance in placental prostacyclin and thromboxane production. Am J Obstet Gynecol 152:335-340, 1985.
169. Walsh SW, et al: Placental prostacyclin production in normal and toxemic pregnancies. Am J Obstet Gynecol 151:110-115, 1985.
170. Jerat S, et al: Effect of adrenomedullin on placental arteries in normal and preeclamptic pregnancies. Hypertension 37:227-231, 2001.
171. Knerr I, et al: Adrenomedullin, calcitonin gene-related peptide and their receptors: evidence for a decreased placental mRNA content in preeclampsia and HELLP syndrome. Eur J Obstet Gynecol Reprod Biol 101:47-53, 2002.
172. Many A, et al: Invasive cytotrophoblasts manifest evidence of oxidative stress in preeclampsia. Am J Pathol 156:321-331, 2001.
173. Staff AC, et al: 8-Iso-prostaglandin f(2alpha) reduces trophoblast invasion and matrix metalloproteinase activity. Hypertension 35:1307-1313, 2000.
174. Odegard RA, et al: Umbilical cord plasma interleukin-6 and fetal growth restriction in preeclampsia: a prospective study in Norway. Obstet Gynecol 98:289-294, 2001.
175. Schiff E, et al: Endothelin-1,2 levels in umbilical vein serum of intra-uterine growth retarded fetuses as detected by cordocentesis. Acta Obstet Gynecol Scand 73:21-24, 1994.
176. Mellembakken JR, et al: Chemokines and leukocyte activation in the fetal circulation during preeclampsia. Hypertension 38:394-398, 2001.
177. Taylor RN, et al: Circulating factors as markers and mediators of endothelial cell dysfunction in preeclampsia. Semin Reprod Endocrinol 16:17-31, 1998.
178. Granger JP, et al: Pathophysiology of pregnancy-induced hypertension. Am J Hypertens 14:178S-185S, 2001.
179. Wolf M, et al: First trimester insulin resistance and subsequent preeclampsia: a prospective study. J Clin Endocrinol Metab 87:1563-1568, 2002.
180. Solomon CG, Seely EW: Brief review: hypertension in pregnancy: a manifestation of the insulin resistance syndrome? Hypertension 37:232-239, 2001.
181. Kaaja R, et al: Serum lipoproteins, insulin, and urinary prostanoid metabolites in normal and hypertensive pregnant women. Obstet Gynecol 85:353-356, 2001.
182. Lorentzen B, et al: Glucose intolerance in women with preeclampsia. Acta Obstet Gynecol Scand 77:22-27, 1998.
183. Gruppuso PA: Chronic maternal hyperinsulinemia and hypoglycemia: a model for experimental intrauterine growth retardation. Biol Neonate 40:113-120, 1981.
184. Ogata ES, et al: Limited maternal fuel availability due to hyperinsulinemia retards fetal growth and development in the rat. Pediatr Res 22:432-437, 1987.
185. Misra DP: The effect of the pregnancy-induced hypertension on fetal growth: a review of the literature. Paediatr Perinat Epidemiol 10:244-263, 1996.
186. Xiong X, et al: Impact of pregnancy-induced hypertension on fetal growth. Am J Obstet Gynecol 180:207-213, 1999.
187. Rasmussen S, Irgens LM: Fetal growth and body proportion in preeclampsia. Obstet Gynecol 101:575-583, 2003.
188. Odegard RA, et al: Preeclampsia and fetal growth. Obstet Gynecol 96:950-955, 2000.
189. Chakravorty AP: Foetal and placental weight changes in normal pregnancy and pre-eclampsia. J Obstet Gynaecol Br Commonw 74:247-253, 1967.
190. Ray JG: MOS HIP: McMaster outcome study of hypertension in pregnancy. Early Hum Dev 64:129-143, 2001.
191. Xiong X, et al: Association of preeclampsia with high birth weight for age. Am J Obstet Gynecol 183:148-155, 2000.

192. Xiong X, et al: Impact of preeclampsia and gestational hypertension on birth weight by gestational age. Am J Epidemiol 155:203-209, 2002.

193. Vasapollo B, et al: Abnormal maternal cardiac function and morphology in pregnancies complicated by intrauterine fetal growth restriction. Ultrasound Obstet Gynecol 20:452-457, 2002.

194. Valensise H, et al: Maternal diastolic function in asymptomatic pregnant women with bilateral notching of the uterine artery waveform at 24 weeks' gestation: a pilot study. Ultrasound Obstet Gynecol 18:450-455, 2001.

195. Browne JCM, Veall NB: The maternal placental blood flow in normotensive and hypertensive women. J Obstet Gynaecol Br Emp 60:141, 1953.

196. Morris NH, et al: Effective uterine bloodflow during exercise in normal and pre-eclamptic pregnancies. Lancet 2:481, 1956.

197. Teasdale F: Histomorphometry of the human placenta in maternal preeclampsia. Am J Obstet Gynecol 152:25-31, 1985.

198. Teasdale F: Histomorphometry of the human placenta in pre-eclampsia associated with severe intrauterine growth retardation. Placenta 8:119-128, 1987.

199. Cetin I, et al: Umbilical amino acid concentrations in normal and growth-retarded fetuses sampled in utero by cordocentesis. Am J Obstet Gynecol 162:253-261, 1990.

200. Morris NH, et al: Free amino acid concentrations in normal and abnormal third trimester placental villi. Eur J Clin Invest 25:796-798, 1995.

201. Powers RW, et al: Increased maternal and fetal amino acid concentrations during preeclampsia and their relationship to fetal growth. In Society for Gynecologic Investigation 50th Annual Meeting. Washington, DC, Elsevier, 2003.

202. Bakker WW, et al: Experimental endotoxemia in pregnancy: in situ glomerular microthrombus formation associated with impaired glomerular adenosine diphosphatase activity. J Lab Clin Med 114:531-537, 1989.

203. Campos A, et al: Prevention of the generalized Shwartzman reaction in pregnant rats by prostacyclin infusion. Lab Invest 48:705-710, 1983.

204. Sakawi Y, et al: Evaluation of low-dose endotoxin administration during pregnancy as a model of preeclampsia. Anesthesiology 93:1446-1455, 2000.

205. Faas MM, et al: A new animal model for human preeclampsia: ultra-low-dose endotoxin infusion in pregnant rats. Am J Obstet Gynecol 171:158-164, 1994.

206. Szocs G, et al: Study of the endotoxin sensitivity of pregnant rats and their fetuses. Acta Chir Hung 31:263-269, 1990.

207. Miller MJ, et al: Fetal growth retardation in rats may result from apoptosis: role of peroxynitrite. Free Radic Biol Med 21:619-629, 1996.

208. Goto M, et al: LPS injected into the pregnant rat late in gestation does not induce fetal endotoxemia. Res Commun Mol Pathol Pharmacol 85:109-112, 1994.

209. Cai Z, et al: Cytokine induction in fetal rat brains and brain injury in neonatal rats after maternal lipopolysaccharide administration. Pediatr Res 47:64-72, 2000.

210. Ornoy A, Altshuler G: Maternal endotoxemia, fetal anomalies, and central nervous system damage: a rat model of a human problem. Am J Obstet Gynecol 124:196-204, 1976.

211. Wijkstra S, et al: Endotoxin treatment of pregnant rats affects sexual behavior of the male offspring. Physiol Behav 49:647-649, 1991.

212. Galazios G, et al: Interleukin-6 levels in umbilical artery serum in normal and abnormal pregnancies. Int J Gynaecol Obstet 78:147-151, 2002.

213. Kupferminc MJ, et al: Tumor necrosis factor-alpha is decreased in the umbilical cord plasma of patients with severe preeclampsia. Am J Perinatol 16:203-208, 1999.

214. Al-Othman S, et al: Differential levels of interleukin 6 in maternal and cord sera and placenta in women with pre-eclampsia. Gynecol Obstet Invest 52:60-65, 2001.

215. Opsjon SL, et al: Interleukin-1, interleukin-6 and tumor necrosis factor at delivery in preeclamptic disorders. Acta Obstet Gynecol Scand 74:19-26, 2001.

216. Ostlund E, et al: Transforming growth factor-beta1 in fetal serum correlates with insulin-like growth factor-I and fetal growth. Obstet Gynecol 100:567-573, 2002.

217. Ando N, et al: Differential gene expression of TGF-beta isoforms and TGF-beta receptors during the first trimester of pregnancy at the human maternal-fetal interface. Am J Reprod Immunol 40:48-56, 1998.

218. Schilling B, Yeh J: Transforming growth factor-beta(1), -beta(2), -beta(3) and their type I and II receptors in human term placenta. Gynecol Obstet Invest 50:19-23, 2000.

219. Bertram CE, Hanson MA: Prenatal programming of postnatal endocrine responses by glucocorticoids. Reproduction 124:459-467, 2002.

220. Stewart PM, et al: Type 2 11-beta-hydroxysteroid dehydrogenase messenger ribonucleic acid and activity in human placenta and fetal membranes: its relationship to birth weight and putative role in fetal adrenal steroidogenesis. J Clin Endocrinol Metab 80:885-890, 1995.

221. Seckl JR: Glucocorticoid programming of the fetus; adult phenotypes and molecular mechanisms. Mol Cell Endocrinol 185:61-71, 2001.

222. Burton PJ, et al: Zonal distribution of 11 beta-hydroxysteroid dehydrogenase types 1 and 2 messenger ribonucleic acid expression in the rat placenta and decidua during late pregnancy. Biol Reprod 55:1023-1028, 1996.

223. Waddell BJ, et al: Tissue-specific messenger ribonucleic acid expression of 11-beta-hydroxysteroid dehydrogenase types 1 and 2 and the glucocorticoid receptor within rat placenta suggests exquisite local control of glucocorticoid action. Endocrinology 139:1517-1523, 1998.

224. Edwards CR, et al: Dysfunction of placental glucocorticoid barrier: link between fetal environment and adult hypertension? Lancet 341:355-357, 1993.

225. Seckl JR, Brown RW: 11-Beta-hydroxysteroid dehydrogenase: on several roads to hypertension. J Hypertens 12:105-112, 1994.

226. Bernal AL, et al: 11 Beta-hydroxysteroid dehydrogenase activity (E.C. 1.1.1.146) in human placenta and decidua. J Steroid Biochem 13:1081-1087, 1980.

227. Lockwood CJ, et al: Corticotropin-releasing hormone and related pituitary-adrenal axis hormones in fetal and maternal blood during the second half of pregnancy. J Perinat Med 24:243-251, 1996.

228. Shams M, et al: 11-Beta-hydroxysteroid dehydrogenase type 2 in human pregnancy and reduced expression in intrauterine growth restriction. Hum Reprod 13:799-804, 1998.

229. McTernan CL, et al: Reduced placental 11-beta-hydroxysteroid dehydrogenase type 2 mRNA levels in human pregnancies complicated by intrauterine growth restriction: an analysis of possible mechanisms. J Clin Endocrinol Metab 86:4979-4983, 2001.

230. Kajantie E, et al: Placental 11-beta-hydroxysteroid dehydrogenase-2 and fetal cortisol/cortisone shuttle in small preterm infants. J Clin Endocrinol Metab 88:493-500, 2003.

231. McCalla CO, et al: Placental 11 beta-hydroxysteroid dehydrogenase activity in normotensive and pre-eclamptic pregnancies. Steroids 63:511-515, 1998.

232. Schoof E, et al: Decreased gene expression of 11-beta-hydroxysteroid dehydrogenase type 2 and 15-hydroxyprostaglandin dehydrogenase in human placenta of patients with preeclampsia. J Clin Endocrinol Metab 86:1313-1317, 1998.

233. Alfaidy N, et al: Oxygen regulation of placental 11 beta-hydroxysteroid dehydrogenase 2: physiological and pathological implications. J Clin Endocrinol Metab 87:4797-4805, 2002.

234. Chard T: Insulin-like growth factors and their binding proteins in normal and abnormal human fetal growth. Growth Regul 4:91-100, 1994.

235. Verhaeghe J, et al: Regulation of insulin-like growth factor-I and insulin-like growth factor binding protein-1 concentrations in preterm fetuses. Am J Obstet Gynecol 188:485-491, 2003.

236. Verhaeghe J, et al: C-peptide, insulin-like growth factors I and II, and insulin-like growth factor binding protein-1 in umbilical cord serum: correlations with birth weight. Am J Obstet Gynecol 169:89-97, 1993.

237. Powell-Braxton L, et al: IGF-I is required for normal embryonic growth in mice. Genes Dev 7:2609-2617, 1993.

238. Baker J, et al: Role of insulin-like growth factors in embryonic and postnatal growth. Cell 75:73-82, 1993.

239. Giudice LC, et al: Insulin-like growth factors and their binding proteins in the term and preterm human fetus and neonate with normal and extremes of intrauterine growth. J Clin Endocrinol Metab 80:1548-1555, 1995.

240. Allan GJ, et al: Insulin-like growth factor axis during embryonic development. Reproduction 122:31-39, 2001.

241. Gluckman PD: Clinical review 68: The endocrine regulation of fetal growth in late gestation: the role of insulin-like growth factors. J Clin Endocrinol Metab 80:1047-1050, 1995.

242. Petrik J, et al: Overexpression of insulin-like growth factor-II in transgenic mice is associated with pancreatic islet cell hyperplasia. Endocrinology 140:2353-2363, 1999.

243. Giudice LC, et al: Insulin-like growth factor binding protein-1 at the maternal-fetal interface and insulin-like growth factor-I, insulin-like growth factor-II, and insulin-like growth factor binding protein-1 in the circulation of women with severe preeclampsia. Am J Obstet Gynecol 176:751-757; discussion 757-758, 1997.

244. Han VK, et al: The expression of insulin-like growth factor (IGF) and IGF-binding protein (IGFBP) genes in the human placenta and membranes: evidence for IGF-IGFBP interactions at the feto-maternal interface. J Clin Endocrinol Metab 81:2680-2693, 1996.

245. Han VK, Carter AM: Spatial and temporal patterns of expression of messenger RNA for insulin-like growth factors and their binding proteins in the placenta of man and laboratory animals. Placenta 21:289-305, 2000.

246. Giudice LC, Irwin JC: Roles of the insulin-like growth factor family in non-pregnant human endometrium and at the decidual:trophoblast interface. Semin Reprod Endocrinol 17:13-21, 1999.

247. Crossey PA, et al: Altered placental development and intrauterine growth restriction in IGF binding protein-1 transgenic mice. J Clin Invest 110:411-418, 2002.

248. Kajantie E, et al: Markers of type I and type III collagen turnover, insulin-like growth factors, and their binding proteins in cord plasma of small premature infants: relationships with fetal growth, gestational age, preeclampsia, and antenatal glucocorticoid treatment. Pediatr Res 49:481-489, 2001.

249. Vatten LJ, et al: Relationship of insulin-like growth factor-I and insulin-like growth factor binding proteins in umbilical cord plasma to preeclampsia and infant birth weight. Obstet Gynecol 99:85-90, 2002.

250. Ostlund E, et al: Insulin-like growth factor I in fetal serum obtained by cordocentesis is correlated with intrauterine growth retardation. Hum Reprod 12:840-844, 1997.

251. Anim-Nyame N, et al: Longitudinal analysis of maternal plasma leptin concentrations during normal pregnancy and pre-eclampsia. Hum Reprod 15:2033-2036, 2000.

252. Iino K, et al: Elevated circulating levels of a decidual protein, placental protein 12, in preeclampsia. Obstet Gynecol 68:58-60, 1986.

253. Howell RJ, et al: Placental proteins 12 and 14 in pre-eclampsia. Acta Obstet Gynecol Scand 68:237-240, 1989.

254. Wang HS, et al: Insulin-like growth factor-binding protein 1 and insulin-like growth factor-binding protein 3 in pre-eclampsia. Br J Obstet Gynaecol 103:654-659, 1996.

255. Krampl E, et al: Maternal serum insulin-like growth factor binding protein-1 in pregnancy at high altitude. Obstet Gynecol 99:594-598, 2002.

256. Hietala R, et al: Serum insulin-like growth factor binding protein-1 at 16 weeks and subsequent preeclampsia. Obstet Gynecol 95:185-189, 2000.

257. de Groot CJ, et al: Biochemical evidence of impaired trophoblastic invasion of decidual stroma in women destined to have preeclampsia. Am J Obstet Gynecol 175:24-29, 1996.

258. Rutanen EM: Insulin-like growth factors in obstetrics. Curr Opin Obstet Gynecol 12:163-168, 2000.

259. Halhali A, et al: Preeclampsia is associated with low circulating levels of insulin-like growth factor I and 1,25-dihydroxyvitamin D in maternal and umbilical cord compartments. J Clin Endocrinol Metab 85:1828-1833, 2000.

260. Boyne MS, et al: The relationship among circulating insulin-like growth factor (IGF)-I, IGF-binding proteins-1 and -2, and birth anthropometry: a prospective study. J Clin Endocrinol Metab 88:1687-1691, 2003.

261. Vatten LJ, et al: Insulin-like growth factor I and leptin in umbilical cord plasma and infant birth size at term. Pediatrics 109:1131-1135, 2002.

262. Levy R, et al: Trophoblast apoptosis from pregnancies complicated by fetal growth restriction is associated with enhanced p53 expression. Am J Obstet Gynecol 186:1056-1061, 2002.

263. Ishihara N, et al: Increased apoptosis in the syncytiotrophoblast in human term placentas complicated by either preeclampsia or intrauterine growth retardation. Am J Obstet Gynecol 186:158-166, 2002.

264. Kuntz TB, et al: Fas and Fas ligand expression in maternal blood and in umbilical cord blood in preeclampsia. Pediatr Res 50:743-749, 2001.

265. Koenig JM, Chegini N: Enhanced expression of Fas-associated proteins in decidual and trophoblastic tissues in pregnancy-induced hypertension. Am J Reprod Immunol 44:347-349, 2000.

266. Crocker IP, et al: The in-vitro characterization of induced apoptosis in placental cytotrophoblasts and syncytiotrophoblasts. Placenta 22:822-830, 2001.

267. Crocker IP, et al: Differences in apoptotic susceptibility of cytotrophoblasts and syncytiotrophoblasts in normal pregnancy to those complicated with preeclampsia and intrauterine growth restriction. Am J Pathol 162:637-643, 2003.

268. Bajoria R, et al: Prospective function of placental leptin at maternal-fetal interface. Placenta 23:103-115, 2002.

269. Sabogal JC, Munoz L: Leptin in obstetrics and gynecology: a review. Obstet Gynecol Surv 56:225-230, 2001.

270. Wabitsch M, et al: Insulin and cortisol promote leptin production in cultured human fat cells. Diabetes 45:1435-1438, 1996.

271. Papaspyrou-Rao S, et al: Dexamethasone increases leptin expression in humans in vivo. J Clin Endocrinol Metab 82:1635-1637, 1997.

272. Schubring C, et al: Longitudinal analysis of maternal serum leptin levels during pregnancy, at birth and up to six weeks after birth: relation to body mass index, skinfolds, sex steroids and umbilical cord blood leptin levels. Horm Res 50:276-283, 1998.

273. Schubring C, et al: Rapid decline of serum leptin levels in healthy neonates after birth. Eur J Pediatr 157:263-264, 1998.

274. Geary M, et al: Leptin concentrations in maternal serum and cord blood: relationship to maternal anthropometry and fetal growth. Br J Obstet Gynaecol 106:1054-1060, 1999.

275. Highman TJ, et al: Longitudinal changes in maternal serum leptin concentrations, body composition, and resting metabolic rate in pregnancy. Am J Obstet Gynecol 178:1010-1015, 1998.

276. Bi S, et al: Identification of a placental enhancer for the human leptin gene. J Biol Chem 272:30583-30588, 1997.

277. Huppertz B, et al: Immunohistochemistry of matrix metalloproteinases (MMP), their substrates, and their inhibitors (TIMP) during trophoblast invasion in the human placenta. Cell Tissue Res 291:133-148, 1991.

278. Castellucci M, et al: Leptin modulates extracellular matrix molecules and metalloproteinases: possible implications for trophoblast invasion. Mol Hum Reprod 6:951-958, 2000.

279. McCarthy JF, Misra DN, Roberts JM: Maternal plasma leptin is increased in preeclampsia and positively correlates with fetal cord concentration. Am J Obstet Gynecol 180:731-736, 1999.

280. Teppa RJ, et al: Free leptin is increased in normal pregnancy and further increased in preeclampsia. Metabolism 49:1043-1048, 2000.

281. Lord GM, et al: Leptin modulates the T-cell immune response and reverses starvation-induced immunosuppression. Nature 394:897-901, 1998.

282. Mise H, et al: Augmented placental production of leptin in preeclampsia: possible involvement of placental hypoxia. J Clin Endocrinol Metab 83:3225-3229, 1998.

283. Sarraf P, et al: Multiple cytokines and acute inflammation raise mouse leptin levels: potential role in inflammatory anorexia. J Exp Med 185:171-175, 1997.

284. Clapp JF 3rd, Kiess W: Cord blood leptin reflects fetal fat mass. J Soc Gynecol Investig 5:300-303, 1998.

285. Manzar S: Leptin concentrations in maternal serum and cord blood: relationship to maternal anthropometry and fetal growth. Br J Obstet Gynecol 107:831, 2000.

286. Matsuda J, et al: Dynamic changes in serum leptin concentrations during the fetal and neonatal periods. Pediatr Res 45:71-75, 1999.

287. Ong KK, et al: Cord blood leptin is associated with size at birth and predicts infancy weight gain in humans. ALSPAC Study Team. Avon Longitudinal Study of Pregnancy and Childhood. J Clin Endocrinol Metab 84:1145-1148, 1999.

288. Schubring C, et al: Levels of leptin in maternal serum, amniotic fluid, and arterial and venous cord blood: relation to neonatal and placental weight. J Clin Endocrinol Metab 82:1480-1483, 1997.

289. Sivan E, et al: Leptin in human pregnancy: the relationship with gestational hormones. Am J Obstet Gynecol 179:1128-1132, 1998.

290. Tamura T, et al: Serum leptin concentrations during pregnancy and their relationship to fetal growth. Obstet Gynecol 91:389-395, 1998.

291. Lin KC, et al: Difference of plasma leptin levels in venous and arterial cord blood: relation to neonatal and placental weight. Kaohsiung J Med Sci 15:679-685, 1999.

292. Ogueh O, et al: The relationship between leptin concentration and bone metabolism in the human fetus. J Clin Endocrinol Metab 85:1997-1999, 2000.

293. Tamas P, et al: Changes of maternal serum leptin levels during pregnancy. Gynecol Obstet Invest 46:169-171, 1998.

294. Linnemann K, et al: Leptin production and release in the dually in vitro perfused human placenta. J Clin Endocrinol Metab 85:4298-4301, 2000.

295. Lepercq J, et al: Prenatal leptin production: evidence that fetal adipose tissue produces leptin. J Clin Endocrinol Metab 86:2409-2413, 2001.

296. Harigaya A, et al: Relationship between concentration of serum leptin and fetal growth. J Clin Endocrinol Metab 82:3281-3284, 1997.

297. Ng PC, et al: Leptin and metabolic hormones in infants of diabetic mothers. Arch Dis Child Fetal Neonatal Ed 83: F193-F197, 2000.

298. Lea RG, et al: Placental leptin in normal, diabetic and fetal growth-retarded pregnancies. Mol Hum Reprod 6:763-769, 2000.

299. Lepercq J, et al: Overexpression of placental leptin in diabetic pregnancy: a critical role for insulin. Diabetes 47:847-850, 1998.

300. Diaz E, et al: Newborn birth weight correlates with placental zinc, umbilical insulin-like growth factor I, and leptin levels in preeclampsia. Arch Med Res 33:40-47, 2002.

301. Gursoy T, et al: Preeclampsia disrupts the normal physiology of leptin. Am J Perinatol 19:303-310, 2002.

302. Odegard RA, et al: Umbilical cord plasma leptin is increased in preeclampsia. Am J Obstet Gynecol 186:427-432, 2002.

303. Grandone E, Margaglione M: Thrombophilia polymorphisms and intrauterine growth restriction. N Engl J Med 347:1530-1531; author reply 1530-1531, 2002.

304. Grandone E, et al: Lower birth-weight in neonates of mothers carrying factor V G1691A and factor II A(20210) mutations. Haematologica 87:177-181, 2002.

305. Kupferminc MJ, et al: Thrombophilia polymorphisms and intrauterine growth restriction. N Engl J Med 347:1530-1531; discussion 1530-1531, 2002.

306. van Pampus MG, et al: High prevalence of hemostatic abnormalities in women with a history of severe preeclampsia. Am J Obstet Gynecol 180:1146-1150, 1999.

307. Alfirevic Z, et al: How strong is the association between maternal thrombophilia and adverse pregnancy outcome? A systematic review. Eur J Obstet Gynecol Reprod Biol 101:6-14, 2002.

308. Livingston JC, et al: Maternal and fetal inherited thrombophilias are not related to the development of severe preeclampsia. Am J Obstet Gynecol 185:153-157, 2001.

309. Infante-Rivard C, et al: Absence of association of thrombophilia polymorphisms with intrauterine growth restriction. N Engl J Med 347:19-25, 2002.

310. Dahms BB, et al: Severe perinatal liver disease associated with fetal thrombotic vasculopathy. Pediatr Dev Pathol 5:80-85, 2002.

311. Sikkema JM, et al: Placental pathology in early onset pre-eclampsia and intrauterine growth restriction in women with and without thrombophilia. Placenta 23:337-342, 2002.

312. Wilcken B, et al: Pregnancy and fetal long-chain 3-hydroxyacyl coenzyme A dehydrogenase deficiency. Lancet 341:407-408, 1993.

313. Ibdah JA, et al: A fetal fatty-acid oxidation disorder as a cause of liver disease in pregnant women. N Engl J Med 340:1723-1731, 1999.

314. Strauss AW, et al: Inherited long-chain 3-hydroxyacyl-CoA dehydrogenase deficiency and a fetal-maternal interaction cause maternal liver disease and other pregnancy complications. Semin Perinatol 23:100-112, 1999.

315. Grether JK, et al: Prenatal and perinatal factors and cerebral palsy in very low birth weight infants. J Pediatr 128:407-414, 1996.

316. Nelson KB, Grether JK: Can magnesium sulfate reduce the risk of cerebral palsy in very low birthweight infants? Pediatrics 95:263-269, 1995.

317. Hirtz DG, Nelson K: Magnesium sulfate and cerebral palsy in premature infants. Curr Opin Pediatr 10:131-137, 1998.

318. Perlman JM: Antenatal glucocorticoid, magnesium exposure, and the prevention of brain injury of prematurity. Semin Pediatr Neurol 5:202-210, 1998.

319. Schendel DE, et al: Prenatal magnesium sulfate exposure and the risk for cerebral palsy or mental retardation among very-low-birth-weight children aged 3 to 5 years. JAMA 276:1805-1810, 1996.

320. Grether JK, et al: Magnesium sulfate for tocolysis and risk of spastic cerebral palsy in premature children born to women without preeclampsia. Am J Obstet Gynecol *183*:717-725, 2000.

321. Paneth N, et al: Magnesium sulfate in labor and risk of neonatal brain lesions and cerebral palsy in low birth weight infants. The Neonatal Brain Hemorrhage Study Analysis Group. Pediatrics *99*:E1, 1997.

322. Leviton A, et al: Maternal receipt of magnesium sulfate does not seem to reduce the risk of neonatal white matter damage. Pediatrics *99*:E2, 1997.

323. Canterino JC, et al: Maternal magnesium sulfate and the development of neonatal periventricular leucomalacia and intraventricular hemorrhage. Obstet Gynecol *93*:396-402, 1999.

324. Rantonen T, et al: Maternal magnesium sulfate treatment is associated with reduced brain-blood flow perfusion in preterm infants. Crit Care Med *29*:1460-1465, 2001.

325. Rantonen T, et al: Antenatal magnesium sulphate exposure is associated with prolonged parathyroid hormone suppression in preterm neonates. Acta Paediatr *90*:278-281, 2001.

326. Mittendorf R, Pryde PG: An overview of the possible relationship between antenatal pharmacologic magnesium and cerebral palsy. J Perinat Med *28*:286-293, 2000.

327. Magee LA, et al: Risks and benefits of beta-receptor blockers for pregnancy hypertension: overview of the randomized trials. Eur J Obstet Gynecol Reprod Biol *88*:15-26, 2000.

328. Magee LA: Drugs in pregnancy. Antihypertensives. Best Pract Res Clin Obstet Gynaecol *15*:827-845, 2001.

329. Palsy AT, et al: Neonatal Encephalopathy and Cerebral Palsy: Defining the Pathogenesis and Pathophysiology. Washington, DC, The American College of Obstetricians and Gynecologists, 2003.

330. Xiong X, et al: Preeclampsia and cerebral palsy in low-birth-weight and preterm infants: implications for the current "ischemic model" of preeclampsia. Hypertens Pregnancy *20*:1-13, 2001.

331. Murphy DJ, et al: Case-control study of antenatal and intrapartum risk factors for cerebral palsy in very preterm singleton babies. Lancet *346*:1449-1454, 1995.

332. Spinillo A, et al: Preeclampsia, preterm delivery and infant cerebral palsy. Eur J Obstet Gynecol Reprod Biol *77*:151-155, 1998.

333. Gray PH, et al: Maternal hypertension and neurodevelopmental outcome in very preterm infants. Arch Dis Child Fetal Neonatal Ed *79*:F88-93, 1998.

334. Easterling TR, et al: Maternal hemodynamics in normal and preeclamptic pregnancies: a longitudinal study. Obstet Gynecol *76*:1061-1069, 1990.

335. Gant NF, et al: Study of the metabolic clearance rate of dehydroisoandrosterone sulfate in pregnancy. Am J Obstet Gynecol *111*:555-563, 1971.

336. Blair E, Stanley F: Intrauterine growth and spastic cerebral palsy: I. Association with birth weight for gestational age. Am J Obstet Gynecol *162*:229-237, 1990.

337. Gaffney G, et al: Case-control study of intrapartum care, cerebral palsy, and perinatal death. BMJ *308*:743-750, 1994.

338. Wilson-Costello D: Risk factors for neurologic impairment among very low-birth-weight infants. Semin Pediatr Neurol *8*:120-126, 2001.

339. Taylor DJ, et al: Do pregnancy complications contribute to neurodevelopmental disability? Lancet *1*:713-716, 1985.

340. Spinillo A, et al: Infant neurodevelopmental outcome in pregnancies complicated by gestational hypertension and intra-uterine growth retardation. J Perinat Med *21*:195-203, 1993.

341. Spinillo A, et al: Two-year infant neurodevelopmental outcome after expectant management and indicated preterm delivery in hypertensive pregnancies. Acta Obstet Gynecol Scand *73*:625-629, 1994.

342. Kuban KC, et al: Maternal toxemia is associated with reduced incidence of germinal matrix hemorrhage in premature babies. J Child Neurol *7*:70-76, 1992.

343. O'Shea TM, et al: Prenatal events and the risk of cerebral palsy in very low birth weight infants. Am J Epidemiol *147*:362-369, 1998.

344. O'Shea TM, et al: Perinatal events and the risk of intraparenchymal echodensity in very-low-birthweight neonates. Paediatr Perinat Epidemiol *12*:408-421, 1998.

345. Kirsten GF, et al: Infants of women with severe early pre-eclampsia: the effect of absent end-diastolic umbilical artery Doppler flow velocities on neurodevelopmental outcome. Acta Paediatr *89*:566-570, 2000.

346. Seidman DS, et al: Pre-eclampsia and offspring's blood pressure, cognitive ability and physical development at 17 years of age. Br J Obstet Gynaecol *98*:1009-1014, 1991.

347. Palti H, Rothschild E: Blood pressure and growth at 6 years of age among offsprings of mothers with hypertension of pregnancy. Early Hum Dev *19*:263-269, 1989.

348. Klebanoff MA, et al: Maternal size at birth and the development of hypertension during pregnancy: a test of the Barker hypothesis. Arch Intern Med *159*:1607-1612, 1999.

349. Tenhola S, et al: Blood pressure, serum lipids, fasting insulin, and adrenal hormones in 12-year-old born with maternal preeclampsia. J Clin Endocrinol Metab *88*:1217-1222, 2003.

350. Suonio S, et al: Effect of the left lateral recumbent position compared with the supine and upright positions on placental blood flow in normal late pregnancy. Ann Clin Res *8*:22-26, 1976.

351. Rushton DI: Placenta as a reflection of maternal disease. *In* Perrin EVDK (Ed): Pathology of the Placenta. New York, Churchill Livingstone, 1984, p 57.

352. Tekay A, Campbell S: Doppler ultrasonography in obstetrics. *In* Callen PW (ed): Ultrasound in Obstetrics and Gynecology. Philadelphia, WB Saunders Co, 2000, p 677.

353. Ranheim T, et al: VEGF mRNA is unaltered in decidual and placental tissues in preeclampsia at delivery. Acta Obstet Gynecol Scand *80*:93-98, 2001.

354. Lyall F, et al: Placental expression of vascular endothelial growth factor in placentae from pregnancies complicated by pre-eclampsia and intrauterine growth restriction does not support placental hypoxia at delivery. Placenta *18*:269-276, 1997.

355. Helske S, et al: Expression of vascular endothelial growth factor receptors 1, 2 and 3 in placentas from normal and complicated pregnancies. Mol Hum Reprod *7*:205-210, 2001.

356. Gratton RJ, et al: The regional expression of insulin-like growth factor II (IGF-II) and insulin-like growth factor binding protein-1 (IGFBP-1) in the placentae of women with pre-eclampsia. Placenta *23*:303-310, 2002.

357. Genbacev O, et al: Hypoxia alters early gestation human cytotrophoblast differentiation/invasion *in vitro* and models the placental defects that occur in preeclampsia. J Clin Invest *97*:540-550, 1996.

358. DiFederico E, et al: Preeclampsia is associated with widespread apoptosis of placental cytotrophoblasts within the uterine wall. Am J Pathol *155*:293-301, 1999.

359. Allaire AD, et al: Placental apoptosis in preeclampsia. Obstet Gynecol *96*:271-276, 2000.

360. Pijnenborg R, et al: Immunolocalization of tumour necrosis factor-alpha (TNF-alpha) in the placental bed of normotensive and hypertensive human pregnancies. Placenta *19*:231-239, 1998.

361. Madazli R, et al: The plasma and placental levels of malondialdehyde, glutathione and superoxide dismutase in pre-eclampsia. J Obstet Gynaecol *22*:477-480, 2002.

362. Gratacos E, et al: Lipid peroxide and vitamin E patterns in pregnant women with different types of hypertension in pregnancy. Am J Obstet Gynecol *178*:1072-1076, 1998.

363. Gratacos E, et al: Serum and placental lipid peroxides in chronic hypertension during pregnancy with and without superimposed preeclampsia. Hypertens Pregnancy *18*:139-146, 1999.

364. Myatt L, et al: Nitrotyrosine residues in placenta. Evidence of peroxynitrite formation and action. Hypertension *28*:488-493, 1996.

365. Lyall F, et al: Increased nitrotyrosine in the diabetic placenta: evidence for oxidative stress. Diabetes Care *21*:1753-1758, 1998.

366. Wang Y, Walsh SW: Antioxidant activities and mRNA expression of superoxide dismutase, catalase, and glutathione peroxidase in normal and preeclamptic placentas. J Soc Gynecol Investig *3*:179-184, 1996.

David J. P. Barker

17 Fetal Origins of Adult Disease

Hitherto the search for the causes of coronary heart disease, and the way to prevent it, has been guided by a "destructive" model. The principal causes to be identified are thought to act in adult life and to accelerate destructive processes—for example, the formation of atheroma, rise in blood pressure, and loss of glucose tolerance. This model, however, has had limited success. Obesity, cigarette smoking, and psychosocial stress have been implicated, and evidence on dietary fat has accumulated to the point at which a public health policy of reduced intake is prudent, if not proved. The effects of modifying adult lifestyle, when formally tested in randomized trials, have, however, been disappointingly small.[1] The model has proved incapable of answering important questions. For example, in Western countries the steep increase in the disease has been associated with rising prosperity, so why do the poorest people in the poorest places have the highest rates.[2]

The recent discovery that people who develop coronary heart disease grew differently compared with other people during fetal life and childhood has led to a new "developmental" model for the disease.[3-5]

THE BIOLOGIC VALUE OF DEVELOPMENTAL PLASTICITY

Like other living creatures in their early life, human beings are "plastic" and able to adapt to their environment. The development of the sweat glands provides a simple example of this. All human beings have similar numbers of sweat glands at birth, but none of them function. In the first 3 years after birth, a proportion of the glands become functional, depending on the temperature to which the child is exposed. The hotter the conditions, the greater the number of sweat glands that are programmed to function. After 3 years the programming is complete and the number of sweat glands is fixed. Thereafter the child who has experienced hot conditions will be better equipped to adapt to similar conditions in later life, because people with more functioning sweat glands cool down faster.

This brief description encapsulates the essence of programming: a critical period when a system is plastic and sensitive to the environment, followed by loss of plasticity and a fixed functional capacity. There are good reasons why it may be advantageous, in evolutionary terms, for the body to remain plastic during development. Why this plasticity is ultimately lost in most tissues and systems is a question to which we have only speculative answers. Some tissues, the trabeculae of bone, for example, do remain plastic throughout life. Bateson and Martin[6] have suggested that plasticity during intrauterine life enables animals, and humans, to receive a "weather forecast" from their mothers that prepares them for the type of world in which they will have to live. If the mother is poorly nourished, she signals to her unborn baby that the environment it is about to enter is likely to be harsh. The baby responds to these signals by adaptations, such as reduced body size and altered metabolism, which help it to survive a shortage of food after birth. In this way programming gives a species the ability to make short-term adaptations, within one generation, in addition to the long-term genetic adaptations that come from natural selection. Since, as Mellanby noted long ago, the ability of a human mother to nourish her baby is partly determined by her own experiences *in utero*, and by her childhood growth,[7] the human fetus receives a "weather forecast" based not only on conditions at the time of the pregnancy, but on conditions a number of decades before. This may be advantageous in places that experience periodic famine.

Until recently we have overlooked a growing body of evidence that systems of the body that are closely related to adult disease, such as the regulation of blood pressure, are also plastic during early development. In animals it is surprisingly easy to produce lifelong changes in the blood pressure and metabolism of a fetus by minor modifications to the diet of the mother before and during pregnancy.

GROWTH AND CORONARY HEART DISEASE

Figure 17-1 shows the growth of 357 men who were either admitted to hospital with coronary heart disease or died from it.[5] They belong to a cohort of 4630 men who were born in Helsinki, and their growth is expressed as Z-scores. The Z-score for the cohort is set at zero, and a boy maintaining a steady posi-

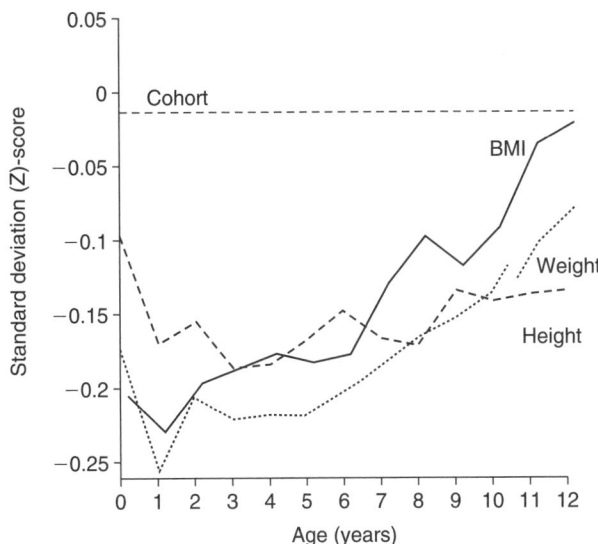

Figure 17-1. This figure shows the growth of 357 men who were either admitted to hospital with coronary heart disease or died from it.[5] They belong to a cohort of 4630 men who were born in Helsinki, and their growth is expressed as SD (Z) scores.

tion as large or small in relation to other boys follows a horizontal path on the figure. Boys who later developed coronary heart disease, however, were small at birth and remained small in infancy but had accelerated gain in weight and body mass index (weight/height[2]) thereafter. In contrast, their heights remained below average. Table 17-1 shows hazard ratios for coronary heart disease according to size at birth. The hazard ratios fall with increasing birth weight and, more strongly, with increasing ponderal index (birth weight/length[3]), a measure of thinness at birth. These trends were found in babies born at term or prematurely and therefore reflect slow intrauterine growth. Table 17-2 shows that the hazard ratios also fell with increasing weight, height, and body mass index at age 1 year. Small size at this age predicts coronary heart disease among men independently of size at birth.

TABLE 17-1

Hazard Ratios for Coronary Heart Disease in Men According to Body Size at Birth

	Hazard Ratios (95% CI)	No. of Cases/No. of Men
Birth Weight (g)		
≤2500	3.63 (2.02-6.51)	24/160
3000	1.83 (1.09-3.07)	45/599
3500	1.99 (1.26-3.15)	144/1775
4000	2.08 (1.31-3.31)	123/1558
>4000	1.00	21/538
P for trend	.006	
Ponderal Index (kg/m³)		
≤25	1.66 (1.11-2.48)	104/1093
27	1.44 (0.97-2.13)	135/1643
29	1.18 (0.78-1.78)	84/1260
>29	1.00	31/578
P for trend	.0006	

CI, confidence interval.

TABLE 17-2

Hazard Ratios for Coronary Heart Disease in Men According to Body Size at 1 Year

	Hazard Ratios (95% CI)	No. of Cases/No. of Men
Weight (kg)		
≤9	1.82 (1.25–2.64)	96/781
10	1.17 (0.80–1.71)	85/1126
11	1.12 (0.77–1.64)	89/1243
12	0.94 (0.62–1.44)	49/852
>12	1.00	38/619
P for trend	<.0001	
Height (cm)		
≤73	1.55 (1.11–2.18)	79/636
75	0.90 (0.63–1.27)	68/962
77	0.94 (0.68–1.31)	87/1210
79	0.83 (0.58–1.18)	64/1011
>79	1.00	59/802
P for trend	.007	
Body Mass Index (kg/m²)		
≤16	1.83 (1.28–2.60)	72/654
17	1.61 (1.15–2.25)	89/936
18	1.29 (0.91–1.81)	83/1136
19	1.12 (0.77–1.62)	59/941
>19	1.00	54/954
P for trend	.0004	

CI, confidence interval.

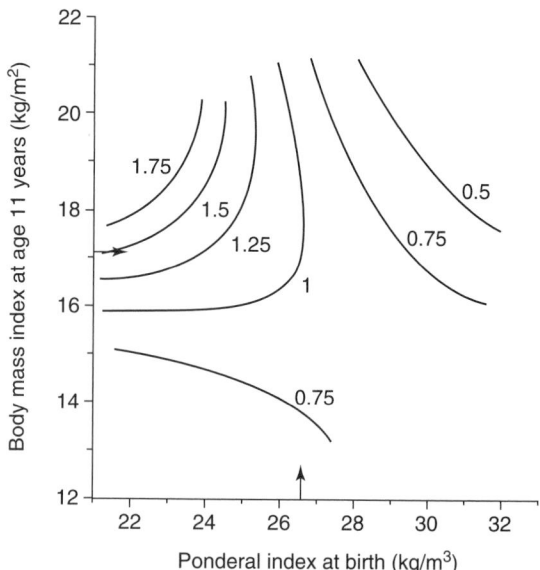

Figure 17-2. Based on the same data used in Figure 17-1, this figure shows the combined effects of ponderal index at birth and body mass index in childhood in the Helsinki cohort.[5] It shows that boys who had a low ponderal index at birth increased their risk of coronary heart disease if they attained even average body mass index in childhood. In contrast, among boys with a high ponderal index no increased risk was associated with a high childhood body mass index. Findings among girls were similar. The risk of coronary heart disease is determined more by the tempo of weight gain than the body size attained.

The association between coronary heart disease and small size at birth has been shown in studies in Europe, North America, and India.[8-12] The association with poor weight gain in infancy was first shown in Hertfordshire[8] and confirmed in Helsinki[5]: the strength of the association was similar in the two studies. The association with rapid childhood weight gain was first shown in a study of an older cohort of men born in Helsinki,[13] and the association with low rates of height growth is consistent with the known association between the disease and short adult stature in men.[14]

Figure 17-2, based on the same data used in Figure 17-1, shows the combined effects of ponderal index at birth and body mass index in childhood in the Helsinki cohort.[5] It shows that boys who had a low ponderal index at birth increased their risk of coronary heart disease if they attained even average body mass index in childhood. In contrast, among boys with a high ponderal index no increased risk was associated with a high childhood body mass index. Findings among girls were similar. The risk of coronary heart disease is determined more by the tempo of weight gain than the body size attained.

GROWTH AND HYPERTENSION AND TYPE 2 DIABETES

There is now a substantial body of evidence showing that people who were small at birth remain biologically different from people who were larger. The differences include an increased susceptibility to hypertension and type 2 diabetes, two disorders closely linked to coronary heart disease.[15,16] Table 17-3 is based on 2997 patients being treated for hypertension and 698 patients being treated for type 2 diabetes in the older and younger Helsinki cohorts combined, totalling 13,517 men and women. These two disorders are associated with the same general pattern of growth as coronary heart disease. Small size at birth is followed by accelerated weight gain. The highest risk for each disease occurs among men and women who had low birth weight but were in the highest body mass index group at 11 years. As with coronary heart disease, the risk of disease is

determined not only by the absolute value of body mass index in childhood but also by the combination of body size at birth and during childhood.[16,17] It is the tempo of growth as well as the attained body size that determines risk.

Associations between low birth weight and hypertension and type 2 diabetes have been found in other studies.[15,18] There is also a substantial literature showing that birth weight is associated with differences in blood pressure and insulin secretion within the normal range.[15,19,20] These differences are found in children and adults but they tend to be small. For example, a 1 kg difference in birth weight is associated with about a 3 mm Hg difference in systolic pressure. The contrast between this small effect and the large effect on hypertension (see Table 17-3) suggests that lesions that accompany poor fetal growth and tend to elevate blood pressure, such as a reduced number of nephrons, have a small influence on blood pressure within the normal range because counterregulatory mechanisms maintain normal blood pressure levels. As the lesions progress, however, these mechanisms are no longer able to maintain homeostasis and blood pressure rises. There may be a cycle of rise in blood pressure resulting in further progression of the lesions and further rise in blood pressure.[21] Possible mechanisms underlying this are described later in the chapter. Studies in South Carolina show that among hypertensive patients the blood pressures of those with low birth weight tend to be more difficult to control by first-line medication with diuretics or beta-blocking agents.[22]

BIOLOGIC MECHANISMS

The associations between altered growth and coronary heart disease suggest that the disease may originate in two phenomena associated with development: "phenotypic plasticity" and "compensatory growth." Phenotypic plasticity is the phenomenon in

TABLE 17-3

Odds Ratios (95% CI) for Hypertension and Type 2 Diabetes According to Birth Weight and Body Mass Index at 11 Years

Birth Weight (g)	Body Mass Index at 11 years (kg/m²)			
	15.7	16.6	17.6	>17.6
Hypertension				
≤3.0	2.0 (1.3–3.2)	1.9 (1.2–3.1)	1.9 (1.2–3.0)	2.3 (1.5–3.8)
3.5	1.7 (1.1–2.6)	1.9 (1.2–2.9)	1.9 (1.2–3.0)	2.2 (1.4–3.4)
4.0	1.7 (1.0–2.6)	1.7 (1.1–2.6)	1.5 (1.0–2.4)	1.9 (1.2–2.9)
>4.0	1.0	1.9 (1.1–3.1)	1.0 (0.6–1.7)	1.7 (1.1–2.8)
Type 2 Diabetes				
≤3.0	1.3 (0.6–2.8)	1.3 (0.6–2.8)	1.5 (0.7–3.4)	2.5 (1.2–5.5)
3.5	1.0 (0.5–2.1)	1.0 (0.5–2.1)	1.5 (0.7–3.2)	1.7 (0.8–3.5)
4.0	1.0 (0.5–2.2)	0.9 (0.4–1.9)	0.9 (0.4–2.0)	1.7 (0.8–3.6)
>4.0	1.0	1.1 (0.4–2.7)	0.7 (0.3–1.7)	1.2 (0.5–2.7)

CI, confidence interval.

which one genotype gives rise to a range of different physiologic or morphologic states in response to different environmental conditions during development.[6, 23] Such gene-environment interactions are ubiquitous in development. Their existence is demonstrated by the numerous experiments showing that minor alterations to the diets of pregnant animals, which may not even change their offspring's body size at birth, can produce lasting changes in their physiology and metabolism—including altered blood pressure and glucose/insulin and lipid metabolism.[24, 25] The evolutionary benefit of phenotypic plasticity is that, in a changing environment, it enables the production of phenotypes that are better matched to their environment than would be possible if one genotype produced the same phenotype in all environments.[23] When undernutrition during development is followed by improved nutrition, many animals stage accelerated or "compensatory" growth in weight or length. This restores the animal's body size but may have long-term costs that include reduced life span.[26]

There are several possible mechanisms by which reduced fetal and infant growth followed by accelerated weight gain in childhood may lead to coronary heart disease. Babies who are thin at birth lack muscle, a deficiency that will persist, as the critical period for muscle growth is around 30 weeks *in utero*, and there is little cell replication after birth.[27] If they develop a high body mass index in childhood, they may have a disproportionately high fat mass. This may be associated with the development of insulin resistance, as children and adults who had low birth weight but are currently heavy are insulin resistant.[19, 28, 29]

Small babies have reduced numbers of nephrons.[21, 30] It has been suggested that this leads to hyperperfusion of each nephron and resulting glomerular sclerosis, further nephron death, and a cycle of increasing blood pressure and nephron death. This may be exacerbated if accelerated growth increases the degree of hyperperfusion. This framework fits with the hypothesis that essential hypertension is a disorder of growth with two separate mechanisms, a growth-promoting process in childhood and a self-perpetuating mechanism in adult life.[31]

People who were small at birth also have a different vascular structure. One aspect of this is that they have reduced elastin in their larger arteries, as a consequence (it is thought) of the hemodynamic changes that accompany growth retardation *in utero*.[32] Elastin is laid down *in utero* and during infancy and thereafter turns over slowly. Reduced elastin leads to less compliant, "stiffer" arteries and to a raised pulse pressure. The gradual loss of elastin and its replacement with collagen, which accompanies aging, tends to amplify the increase in pulse pressure.

Findings in Hertfordshire (UK) suggest that one of the mechanisms linking poor weight gain in infancy with coronary heart disease is altered liver function, reflected in raised serum concentrations of total and low density lipoprotein cholesterol, and raised plasma fibrinogen concentrations.[33, 34] Unlike organs such as the kidney, the liver remains plastic during its development until the age of around 5 years. Its function may be permanently changed by influences that affect its early growth.[35-37] Support for an important role for liver development in the early pathogenesis of coronary heart disease comes from findings in Sheffield, England.[38] Among men and women, a reduced abdominal circumference at birth (a measure that reflects reduced liver size) was a stronger predictor of later elevations of serum cholesterol and plasma fibrinogen than any other measure of body size at birth.

RESPONSES TO ADULT LIVING STANDARDS

Observations on animals show that the environment during development permanently changes not only the body's structure and function but also its responses to environmental influences encountered in later life.[6] Men who had low birth weight are more vulnerable to developing coronary heart disease and type 2 diabetes if they become overweight.[10, 19] Table 17-4 shows the effect of low income in adult life on coronary heart disease among men in Helsinki.[39] As expected, men who had a low taxable income had higher rates of the disease.[2, 40, 41] There is no known explanation for this, and it is a major component of the social inequalities in health in Western countries. The effect of low income, however, is confined to men who had slow fetal growth and were thin at birth, defined by a ponderal index of less than 26 kg/m³. Men who were not thin at birth were resilient to the effects of low income on coronary heart disease, so that there was a statistically significant interaction between the effects of fetal growth and adult income.

One explanation of these findings emphasizes the psychosocial consequences of a low position in the social hierarchy, as indicated by low income and social class, and suggests that perceptions of low social status and lack of success lead to changes in neuroendocrine pathways and hence to disease.[42] The findings in Helsinki seem consistent with this. People who are small at birth are known to have persisting alterations in responses to stress, including raised serum cortisol concentrations.[43] Rapid childhood weight gain could exacerbate these effects.

The effect of a high body mass in childhood is conditioned by size at birth (see Fig. 17-2). In addition, the effect of poor living standards in adult life is conditioned by size at birth (see Table 17-4). The effects of any single influence cannot therefore be quantified as a "small proportion" or "large proportion" of disease. It depends on the path of development that preceded it. The pathogenesis of coronary heart disease or type 2 diabetes

TABLE 17–4

Hazard Ratios (95% CI) for Coronary Heart Disease According to Ponderal Index at Birth and Taxable Income in Adult Life

Household Income 1000 Marks/yr (£)	Ponderal Index ≤26.0 (kg/m³) (n = 1475)	Ponderal Index >26.0 (kg/m³) (n = 2154)
>140 (15,700)	1.00	1.19 (0.65–2.19)
111–140 (15,700)	1.54 (0.83–2.87)	1.42 (0.78–2.57)
96–110 (12,400)	1.07 (0.51–2.22)	1.66 (0.90–3.07)
76–95 (10,700)	2.07 (1.13–3.79)	1.44 (0.79–2.62)
75 (8,400)	2.58 (1.45–4.60)	1.37 (0.75–2.51)
P for trend	<.001	.75

CI, confidence interval.

cannot be understood within a model in which risks associated with adverse influences at different stages of life add to each other.[44] Rather, the consequences of adverse influences depend on events at earlier critical stages of development.[5] This embodies the concept of developmental "switches" triggered by the environment.[6] The effects of any particular birth weight on disease will not only depend on the subsequent path of development but also on the path of growth that led to the birth weight. The same weight can be attained by many different paths of fetal growth, and each is likely to be accompanied by different gene-environment interactions, though this remains to be demonstrated.[45]

The Helsinki studies allow us to estimate the combined effects of birth weight and childhood growth. Men and women who had birth weights above 4 kg, and whose prepubertal body mass index was in the lowest fourth, had around half the risk of coronary heart disease, type 2 diabetes or hypertension, when compared with people who had birth weights below 3 kg but whose body mass index was in the highest fourth.

MOTHERS AND BABIES TODAY

Given the body of evidence showing that coronary heart disease and the related disorders of stroke, hypertension, and type 2 diabetes originate through undernutrition and other adverse influences *in utero*, followed by accelerated weight gain thereafter, protecting the nutrition and health of young women and their babies must be part of any effective strategy for preventing these diseases. The so-call "fetal origins" hypothesis resulted from studies of the geographic association between coronary heart disease and poor living standards in England and Wales and the realization that a poor intrauterine environment played a major role in this association.[46] Areas of the country with high coronary mortality are characterized historically by poor maternal nutrition and health, reflected in high maternal and neonatal mortality.[47]

As yet we do not know the impact of maternal nutrition on fetal development.[48] The relatively disappointing effects of dietary interventions in pregnancy on birth weight in humans have led to the erroneous view that fetal nutrition is little affected by maternal nutrition.[45] It is becoming clear, however, that the concept of maternal nutrition must be extended beyond a mother's diet in pregnancy to include her body composition and metabolism both during pregnancy and at the time of conception. Moreover, birth weight is an inadequate summary measure of fetal experience, and we need a more sophisticated view of optimal fetal development that takes account of the long-term sequelae of fetal responses to undernutrition. If we are to protect babies, we must also protect girls in childhood and adolescence. Body composition is established by childhood growth, and obesity and eating habits are entrained during childhood and adolescence.

CORONARY HEART DISEASE EPIDEMICS

As westernization improves the nutrition of undernourished populations, fetal nutrition improves more slowly than nutrition during childhood or adult life, because the fetus is linked to its mother by a long and precarious supply line that is partly established during the mother's fetal life. It may require more than one generation of improved nutrition before fetal growth responds, whereas child growth responds in one generation. During this phase of development, children who were small at birth undergo accelerated compensatory growth. This is the path of growth that leads to coronary heart disease and, it seems, may generate the epidemics of the disease (see Fig. 17–1). Through phenotypic plasticity and the costs of compensatory growth, people who follow this path are permanently biologically different and at increased risk of coronary heart disease. They are also more vulnerable to the effects of poor living standards (see Table 17–4), obesity, and other adverse influences in adult life.

REFERENCES

1. Ebrahim S, Davey Smith G: Systematic review of randomised controlled trials of multiple risk factor interventions for preventing coronary heart disease. BMJ *314*:1666, 1997.
2. Acheson D: Independent inquiry into inequalities in health. London, HM Stationery Office, 1998.
3. Barker DJP: Fetal origins of coronary heart disease. BMJ *311*:171, 1995.
4. Barker DJP: Mothers, babies, and health in later life, 2nd ed. Edinburgh, Churchill Livingstone, 1998.
5. Eriksson JG, et al: Early growth and coronary heart disease in later life: longitudinal study. BMJ *322*:949, 2001.
6. Bateson P, Martin P: Design for a life: how behaviour develops. London, Jonathan Cape, 1999.
7. Mellanby E: Nutrition and child-bearing. Lancet *2*:1131, 1933.
8. Barker DJP, et al: Weight in infancy and death from ischaemic heart disease. Lancet *2*:577, 1989.
9. Leon D, et al: Reduced fetal growth rate and increased risk of death from ischaemic heart disease: cohort study of 15,000 Swedish men and women born 1915–29. BMJ *317*:241, 1998.
10. Frankel S, Birthweight, body-mass index in middle age, and incident coronary heart disease. Lancet *348*:1478, 1996.
11. Rich-Edwards JW, et al: Birth weight and risk of cardiovascular disease in a cohort of women followed up since 1976. BMJ *315*:396, 1997.
12. Stein CE, et al: Fetal growth and coronary heart disease in South India. Lancet *348*:1269, 1996.
13. Eriksson JG, et al: Catch-up growth in childhood and death from coronary heart disease: longitudinal study. BMJ *318*:427, 1999.
14. Marmot MG, et al: Inequalities in death — specific explanations of a general pattern? Lancet *1*:1003, 1984.
15. Hales CN, et al: Fetal and infant growth and impaired glucose tolerance at age 64. BMJ *303*:1019, 1991.
16. Eriksson JG, et al: Fetal and childhood growth and hypertension in adult life. Hypertension *36*:790, 2000.
17. Forsen T, et al: The fetal and childhood growth of persons who develop type 2 diabetes. Ann Intern Med *133*:176, 2000.
18. Curhan GC, et al: Birth weight and adult hypertension and obesity in women. Circulation *94*:1310, 1996.
19. Lithell HO, et al: Relation of size at birth to non-insulin dependent diabetes and insulin concentrations in men aged 50–60 years. BMJ *312*:406, 1996.

20. Huxley RR, et al: The role of size at birth and postnatal catch-up growth in determining systolic blood pressure: a systematic review of the literature. J Hypertens 18:815, 2000.
21. Brenner BM, Chertow GM: Congenital oligonephropathy and the etiology of adult hypertension and progressive renal injury. Am J Kidney Dis 23:171, 1994.
22. Lackland DT, et al: Associations between birthweight and antihypertensive medication in black and white Americans. Hypertension 39:179, 2002.
23. West-Eberhard MJ: Phenotypic plasticity and the origins of diversity. Ann Rev Ecolo System 20:249, 1989.
24. Kwong WY, et al: Maternal undernutrition during the preimplantation period of rat development causes blastocyst abnormalities and programming of postnatal hypertension. Development 127:4195, 2000.
25. Desai M, Hales CN: Role of fetal and infant growth in programming metabolism in later life. Biol Rev Camb Philos Soc 72:329, 1997.
26. Metcalfe NB, Monaghan P: Compensation for a bad start: grow now, pay later? Trends Ecol Evol 16:254, 2001.
27. Widdowson EM, et al: Cellular development of some human organs before birth. Arch Dis Child 47:652, 1972.
28. Barker DJP, et al: Type 2 (non-insulin-dependent) diabetes mellitus, hypertension and hyperlipidaemia (syndrome X): relation to reduced fetal growth. Diabetologia 36:62, 1993.
29. Bavdekar A, et al: Insulin resistance syndrome in 8-year-old Indian children. Small at birth, big at 8 years, or both? Diabetes 48:2422, 1999.
30. Merlet-benichou C, et al: Retard de croissance intrauterin et deficit en nephrons (Intrauterine growth retardation and inborn nephron deficit). Med Sci 9:777, 1993.
31. Lever AF, Harrap SB: Essential hypertension: a disorder of growth with origins in childhood? J Hypertens 10:101, 1992.
32. Martyn CN, Greenwald SE: Impaired synthesis of elastin in walls of aorta and large conduit arteries during early development as an initiating event in pathogenesis of systemic hypertension. Lancet 350:953, 1997.
33. Fall CHD, et al: Relation of infant feeding to adult serum cholesterol concentration and death from ischaemic heart disease. BMJ 304:801, 1992.
34. Barker DJP, et al: Relation of fetal and infant growth to plasma fibrinogen and factor VII concentrations in adult life. BMJ 304:148, 1992.
35. Gebhardt R: Metabolic zonation of the liver: regulation and implications for liver function. Pharmacol Ther 53:275, 1992.
36. Desai M, et al: Adult glucose and lipid metabolism may be programmed during fetal life. Biochem Soc Trans 23:331, 1995.
37. Kind KL, et al: Restricted fetal growth and the response to dietary cholesterol in the guinea pig. Am J Physiol 277:R1675, 1999.
38. Barker DJP, et al: Growth in utero and serum cholesterol concentrations in adult life. BMJ 307:1524, 1993.
39. Barker DJP, et al: Size at birth and resilience to the effects of poor living conditions in adult life: longitudinal study. BMJ 323:1273, 2001.
40. Marmot M, McDowell ME: Mortality decline and widening social inequalities. Lancet 2:274, 1986.
41. Macintyre K, et al: Relation between socio-economic deprivation and death from a first myocardial infarction in Scotland: population-based analysis. BMJ 322:1152, 2001.
42. Marmot M, Wilkinson RG: Psychosocial and material pathways in the relation between income and health: a response to Lynch et al. BMJ 322:1233, 2001.
43. Phillips DIW, et al: Low birth weight predicts elevated plasma cortisol concentrations in adults from 3 populations. Hypertension 35:1301, 2000.
44. Kuh D, Ben-Shlomo Y: A life-course approach to chronic disease epidemiology. Oxford, Oxford University Press, 1997.
45. Harding JE: The nutritional basis of the fetal origins of adult disease. Int J Epidemiol 30:15, 2001.
46. Barker DJP, Osmond C: Infant mortality, childhood nutrition and ischaemic heart disease in England and Wales. Lancet 1:1077, 1986.
47. Barker DJP, Osmond C: Death rates from stroke in England and Wales predicted from past maternal mortality. BMJ 295:83, 1987.
48. Godfrey KM, Barker DJP: Fetal programming and adult health. Public Health Nutr 4(2B):611, 2001.
49. Mi J, et al: Effects of infant birthweight and maternal body mass index in pregnancy on components of the insulin resistance syndrome in China. Ann Intern Med 132:253, 2000.
50. Campbell DM, et al: Diet in pregnancy and the offspring's blood pressure 40 years later. Br J Obstet Gynaecol 103:273, 1996.
51. Shiell AW, et al: High-meat, low-carbohydrate diet in pregnancy: relation to adult blood pressure in the offspring. Hypertension 38:1282, 2001.
52. Forsen T, et al: Mother's weight in pregnancy and coronary heart disease in a cohort of Finnish men: follow up study. BMJ 315:837, 1997.

Jane Cleary-Goldman and Mary E. D'Alton

18 Physiologic Effects of Multiple Pregnancy on Mother and Fetus

BACKGROUND INFORMATION

Multiple pregnancy, including twins and higher-order multifetal gestations, represents a challenge to obstetricians, perinatologists, and neonatologists. Besides the social, economic, and psychological effects on individual patients and families, multiple pregnancy causes a significant physiologic impact on both the mother and each individual fetus. Multiple births account for a disproportionate share of adverse obstetric and neonatal outcomes. Parturients are at increased risk of preterm labor, preeclampsia, complications of malpresentation, abnormal placentation, and abruption, whereas fetuses are at increased risk of low birth weight, intrauterine growth restriction, intrauterine fetal demise (IUFD), and abnormalities specific to twins, such as the twin-to-twin transfusion syndrome (TTTS).

Maternal and neonatal outcomes may be improved by a better understanding of the physiologic effects of multiple pregnancy on both the mother and the fetus. A multidisciplinary approach to the care of these patients is critical to improve outcomes.[1] In this chapter, we review important physiologic and pathophysiologic aspects of multifetal gestations.

Incidence

In the past, the incidence of twins worldwide was 1 in 80 pregnancies, whereas multiple births were significantly less common.[2] In the United States, however, the incidence of twin and higher-order multiple gestations has increased since the late 1960s because of the use of assisted reproductive techniques (ART), such as superovulation, gamete intrafallopian transfer, and *in vitro* fertilization.[3] In the recent past, some countries have reported a doubling of twin pregnancies.[4] The incidence of multiple pregnancies has been increasing at a greater rate than that of singleton pregnancies. In the United States, between 1973 and 1990, twin births increased by 65% and higher-order births increased by 221%, whereas singleton births increased by only 32%.[3]

Zygosity and Chorionicity

Zygosity refers to the genetic make-up of a pregnancy. Multiple gestations can be monozygotic or dizygotic. Monozygotic twins result from the division of a zygote arising from the fertilization of one ovum by one sperm. These fetuses have an identical phenotype. Dizygotic twins result from the fertilization of separate ova by separate sperm. These fetuses have different genotypes and phenotypes. Approximately two-thirds of twins are dizygotic, whereas one-third are monozygotic.[5]

Chorionicity indicates the membrane composition of the pregnancy—the chorion and amnion. It is determined by the mechanism of fertilization and by the occurrence and timing of embryo division. All dizygotic twins have separate dichorionic diamniotic placentas; that is, each fetus has its own separate placenta and amniotic sac. The reason is that dizygotic twins result from the fertilization of two separate ova by two separate sperm. Monozygous gestations can be dichorionic diamniotic, monochorionic diamniotic, or monochorionic monoamniotic, depending on the timing of embryo division. If the zygote splits during the first 3 days after fertilization (at the morula stage), a dichorionic diamniotic placenta results. Approximately one-third of monozygotic twins have this type of placenta.[5] If the zygote splits between day 3 and day 8 (at the developmental stage), the pregnancy will be monochorionic diamniotic, accounting for approximately two-thirds of monozygous twins.[5] These twins share one placenta but coexist in separate amniotic sacs. Monochorionic monoamniotic twins are formed if the zygote splits after the amnion has formed (the embryonic disc stage) at approximately 9 to 12 days. These twins share the same placenta and amniotic sac, and this phenomenon occurs in approximately 3% of all monozygotic twins.[5] If the yolk sac has already formed and division occurs, the monozygotic pair will be conjoined. Conjoined twins are extremely rare, occurring in 1 in 50,000 births.[6] After the 17th day, a singleton gestation will develop.[7] Higher-order multiples can contain any combination of monozygotic and dizygotic fetuses.[8]

The precise mechanisms causing spontaneous monozygotic and dizygotic twins are not well understood. Dizygotic twins and higher multiples likely derive from multiple ovulations, which result from multiple, simultaneously ongoing, follicle growth.[9] Well-known conditions associated with an increased incidence of dizygotic twins include advanced maternal age, family history, multiparity, and ethnicity.[10-12] Dizygotic twinning may be related to higher baseline levels of gonadotropins in certain women. Ovulation induction and ART are also associated with increased rates of dizygotic twins. Under all these conditions, the ovary is exposed to high levels of gonadotropic hormones resulting in multiple ovulation.[9]

Monozygotic twinning, however, is less understood than dizygotic twinning. Before the use of ART, the frequency of monozygotic twins was constant throughout the world. The incidence was approximately 4 per 1,000 births.[2] Nonetheless, it seems that the incidence of monozygotic twins may be increasing with ART.[13] The mechanism is unknown, but it may be secondary to trauma during the procedure or associated with increased levels of gonadotropins.[14,15]

Determination of Chorionicity

The determination of chorionicity is important in the management of multiple gestations because monochorionic twins are at increased risk of poor outcomes.[16] Prenatally, ultrasound is the best diagnostic method. Chorionicity is most accurately determined in the first trimester (from 6 to 10 weeks) by counting the number of gestational sacs. The presence of two separate gestational sacs, each having one respective heartbeat, suggests a dichorionic diamniotic pregnancy, whereas one gestational sac having two heartbeats suggests a monochorionic pregnancy.[17] The amnion can be visualized via transvaginal ultrasound at approximately 7 to 8 weeks' gestation. Before this time, amnionicity may be difficult to determine. When two separate amniotic sacs, each with a single respective heartbeat, are visualized,

the pregnancy is diamniotic. Conversely, when one amniotic sac with two heartbeats is visualized, the pregnancy is monamniotic.[18] In addition, the number of yolk sacs can be used as an indirect method to indicate the number of amniotic sacs and consequently the amnionicity.[19] At early gestational ages, chorionicity and amnionicity should be confirmed by a repeat ultrasound scan in 2 to 3 weeks because there have been cases of misdiagnosis.[20]

After the first trimester, determination of chorionicity and amnionicity becomes less accurate. As a result, different techniques are needed to determine amnionicity and chorionicity in multiple gestations in the second and third trimesters. These methods include assessing fetal gender, evaluating the placenta, and examining the intertwin membrane.

If the fetuses are of different genders, the pregnancy is almost certainly dichorionic. However, if the gender is unknown or is the same for all fetuses, chorionicity is still unknown. When placentas are clearly separate, the pregnancy is likely dichorionic. If the placentas are adjacent or fused, however, no diagnostic information is gained.

Valuable information may be obtained by assessing the dividing membrane. In dichorionic pregnancies, the membrane contains four layers: two amnions and two chorions. In monochorionic diamniotic pregnancies, the membrane is composed of two layers: two amnions. In dichorionic placentas, a "twin peak" sign has been described in all three trimesters (Fig. 18-1).[21] Placental tissue forms a triangular projection from the chorionic plate into a cleft between the membrane layers. In contrast, a T-shaped junction is present in monochorionic placentas.[22]

Membrane thickness can also be evaluated to help with the diagnosis of chorionicity (Figs. 18-2 and 18-3).[23, 24] Because a dichorionic membrane is composed of four layers, it should appear thicker than a monochorionic membrane. Winn and associates[25] used a 2-mm thickness to indicate a thick, dichorionic membrane. In 32 pregnancies, they found a 95% positive predictive rate for dichorionic pregnancies and an 82% predictive rate for monochorionic pregnancies.[25] Other studies have evaluated both membrane thickness and the number of membrane layers.[26] Examining membranes via ultrasound in the second and third trimesters may be difficult and less accurate. Monochorionic membranes may appear thicker, depending on the ultrasound technique used, and dichorionic membranes can thin out as the pregnancy progresses.[20]

If a dividing membrane is not noted, careful evaluation must be performed to determine amnionicity. The differential diagnosis includes a monochorionic monoamniotic pregnancy versus a

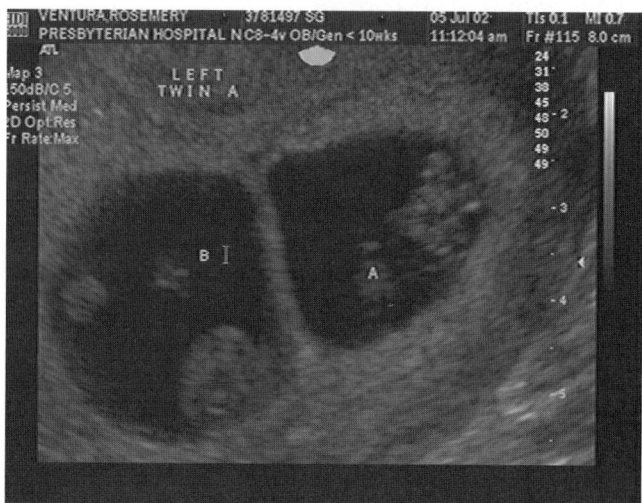

Figure 18–1. Diagnosis of chorionicity: "twin peak" sign.

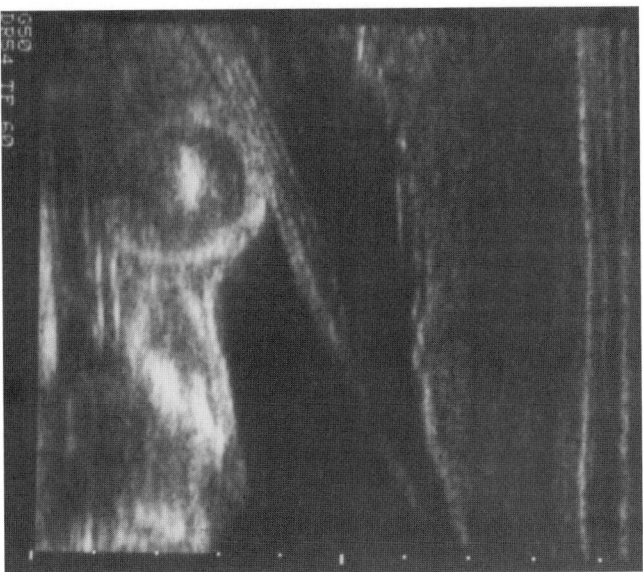

Figure 18–2. Dividing membranes.

monochorionic diamniotic pregnancy, in which one twin has oligohydramnios with an adherent membrane giving the illusion of monoamnionicity. Rare cases have been reported in which monochorionic diamniotic membranes rupture.[27] Nonetheless, in most cases, the pregnancy is a normal monochorionic diamniotic pregnancy, and the intertwin membrane is difficult to visualize.

Although early determination of chorionicity is a primary objective in the management of multifetal pregnancies, extenuating circumstances, such as late diagnosis of a multiple gestation or inconclusive early ultrasound findings, may make this goal unattainable. The optimal management of certain obstetric situations, such as discordant anomalies, requires knowledge of chorionicity. DNA zygosity studies on amniocytes have been used successfully to help with the management of complex cases requiring definitive diagnosis of chorionicity.[28]

MATERNAL PHYSIOLOGY AND MULTIPLE PREGNANCY

The maternal physiologic adaptation to singleton pregnancy is exaggerated in multiple gestations and involves every organ

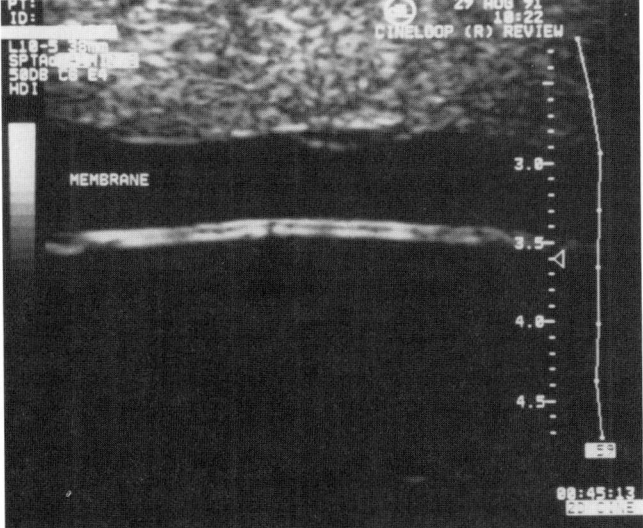

Figure 18–3. Dividing membranes.

system. Although most current teachings on maternal physiology in multiple gestations derive from actual studies on these patients, some concepts have been extrapolated from our knowledge regarding maternal physiology in singleton pregnancies.[29]

Uterine Changes

In both singleton and multiple pregnancies, uterine growth and change begin soon after conception. By 18 weeks, the intrauterine volume of a twin pregnancy is approximately twice that of a singleton pregnancy.[30] This difference in intrauterine volume between singleton and multiple gestations continues until term. As should be appreciated, higher-order multiples have even greater intrauterine volumes.[31]

In singleton pregnancies at term, blood flow to the uterus is approximately 500 to 700 mL/minute. The increased blood flow is directly related to the increasing uterine size and results from a combination of the increased cardiac output of pregnancy and uterine demand. In multiple pregnancies, the increase in uterine blood flow is thought to be even greater.[31] A portion of the increased blood flow may be secondary to the decreased uterine and placental vascular resistance associated with multiple gestations. Doppler studies have indicated that the resistance in the uterine arteries is lower in twins than in singletons.[32]

Uterine activity appears to be increased in multiple pregnancies. After 23 weeks, women with twins report more contractions than do women with singleton pregnancies.[33] Uterine distention is one of many factors that may contribute to the onset of parturition.[34]

Cardiovascular Adaptation

The cardiovascular changes in multiple gestations are similar to those in singletons but are expressed to a greater degree.[35] The maternal heart size in twin pregnancies is the same as in singleton pregnancies; however, the cardiac output is increased to compensate for increased uterine blood flow. As a result, contractility and heart rate are also increased.[35] There is an even greater drop in diastolic blood pressure in the second trimester and a greater rise during the third trimester in patients with twins independent of age, race, or body stature.[36] Blood pressure is dependent on maternal position, and postural changes can lead to hypotension. Because patients with twins have a greater decrease in mean arterial pressure, they seem to have a greater risk of postural hypotension.[31]

Intravascular Volume

Pregnancy is known to be a hypervolemic state, and the increase in plasma volume at term averages approximately 45 to 50% in singletons.[37] Hypervolemia is thought to be a protective mechanism against excessive blood loss.[37] Plasma volume is increased even further in a multiple pregnancy.[38] Depending on the number of fetuses, plasma volume can increase by 50 to 100%.[39] As a result of this increased volume, total concentrations of serum proteins and electrolytes are reduced when compared with singleton pregnancies. However, total intravascular protein mass is unchanged, as are serum sodium, potassium, chloride concentrations, and osmolality.[40]

These physiologic changes are of particular importance when addressing preterm labor and preeclampsia. Because of the slight drop in colloid oncotic pressure associated with β-mimetic medications, women with multiple gestations are at increased risk of volume overload and pulmonary edema when they are given this type of tocolysis.[37, 41] Magnesium sulfate has been associated with fluid overload in women being treated for preterm labor.[42] Other tocolytic agents (especially when used simultaneously) and antenatal steroids have also been associated with an increased risk of pulmonary edema.[43] At our institution, we carefully monitor women with multiple gestations and preterm labor who are receiving tocolytic agents. Fluids are restricted, input and output data are collected rigorously, and frequent physical examinations are performed. If pulmonary edema is diagnosed, aggressive diuresis is initiated.

Although most young healthy women adapt to the cardiac and volume changes associated with multiple pregnancy, women with underlying medical problems and older women may be at increased risk of adverse outcomes such as a myocardial infarction, particularly when they are treated for preterm labor and for preeclampsia.[35] For example, a woman with a multiple gestation and an underlying heart condition may be at increased risk of myocardial infarction resulting from the increased volume status combined with use of β-mimetic tocolytics or magnesium sulfate therapy.[31]

Pulmonary Adaptation

The changes in pulmonary function are similar in both singleton and in multiple gestations. Such changes bring about a state of compensated respiratory alkalosis. The diaphragm level rises approximately 4 cm during a singleton pregnancy, the subcostal angle widens, and the thoracic circumference increases. Consequently, the residual volume decreases, and tidal volume increases. No increase in respiratory rate is noted, although the mother may have a sensation of tachypnea from increased respiratory effort.[44] In multiple gestations, the level of the diaphragm rises higher than in singleton gestations, a change that further reduces residual volume and functional residual capacity while increasing tidal volume.[40] Because of increased tidal volume and oxygen consumption, it is likely that women with multiple gestations have greater pH than women with singleton gestations.[39]

Hematologic Adaptation

Pregnancy is associated with dilutional anemia. Although placental production of chorionic somatomammotropin, progesterone, and prolactin stimulates erythropoiesis, there is only a small increase in red blood cell mass.[37] The increased plasma volume of pregnancy, combined with the smaller increase in red blood cell production, results in maternal dilutional anemia despite adequate iron stores.[45] Anemia (characterized as a hemoglobin concentration lower than 10 g/dL or a hematocrit of less than 30%) occurs 2.4 times more frequently in mothers of twins compared with mothers of singletons.[46] Malone and partners[47] prospectively studied 55 triplet pregnancies at a tertiary care center and found a 27% incidence of anemia in these patients. Multiple gestations have been shown to increase erythropoietin production, perhaps as a physiologic mechanism to improve the anemia associated with pregnancy.[48]

Certain components of the coagulation system are elevated in pregnancy. Factors VII, VIII, IX, and X increase in pregnancy, whereas plasma fibrinolytic activity decreases. These alterations result in a hypercoagulable state until after the postpartum period. The changes are similar in both women with singleton pregnancies and women with multiple gestations.[44] Levels of plasminogen, fibrin split products, antithrombin III, and α_2-macroglobulin are also similar in both types of pregnancies.[49] However, women with twin gestations generally have a greater increase in plasma fibrinogen than do women with singleton pregnancies.[31]

Women with multiple gestations are at increased risk of postpartum hemorrhage, that is, blood loss greater than 500 mL during the first 24 postpartum hours.[50] The risk of such hemorrhage is increased after vaginal and cesarean deliveries. The average blood loss at a twin delivery is approximately 1000 mL.[38] Uterine atony, secondary to overdistention of the uterus, is thought to be the main mechanism contributing to postpartum hemorrhage.[8]

Women with multiple gestations are also at increased risk of placental abruption, which could result in increased blood loss at delivery.[46] However, placenta previa has not been independently associated with multiple gestations.[46]

Endocrine Adaptation

Serum levels of progesterone, estradiol, estriol, human placental lactogen, human chorionic gonadotropin (hCG), α-fetoprotein, cortisol, aldosterone, and free thyroxine are increased in women with multiple gestations compared with levels in singleton pregnancies.[39] To date, it is not known whether carbohydrate metabolism is affected by multiple pregnancy.[46] It seems intuitive that women with multiple gestations would be at increased risk of gestational diabetes because of increased placental lactogen production; however, published studies have been conflicting. Spellacy and associates[46] evaluated 1253 women with twins and did not find an increased risk of gestational diabetes. More recently, Malone and associates[47] found a 7% incidence of gestational diabetes in women pregnant with triplets compared with the 2% incidence in singleton pregnancies. These investigators suggested that the increased risk of gestational diabetes could be secondary to the age of the patients (many were older gravidas; mean age, 32 ± 2.9 years), the weight gain associated with multiple gestations, or the increased serum levels of human placental lactogen.[47]

Renal Adaptation

The normal increase in glomerular filtration rate and size of the renal collecting system is more marked in women with multiple gestations.[39] It is well known that kidney size is increased during pregnancy. Higher levels of progesterone or compression at the pelvic brim, secondary to an overdistended uterus, may lead to increased stasis and an increased incidence of urinary tract infections.[44]

Gastrointestinal Adaptation

The enlarging uterus displaces the stomach and intestines during both singleton and multifetal pregnancies. Increased progesterone levels decrease gastrointestinal tract motility and tone while delaying gastric emptying time. As a result, pregnant women commonly suffer from constipation. The esophageal sphincter has decreased tone resulting in acid reflux. Hemorrhoids are also common secondary to the venous compression and pressure from the enlarged uterus.[44] In addition, nausea and vomiting complicate almost 50% of multiple gestations, likely the result of the higher levels of β-hCG and steroid hormones.[51]

Multiple gestations are a recognized risk factor for the acute fatty liver of pregnancy, a rare condition of unknown origin resulting in elevated liver function tests, nausea, and vomiting.[52] If undiagnosed, this condition is associated with poor outcomes including coma, liver failure, disseminated intravascular coagulopathy, renal failure, metabolic acidosis, and fetal death. Even if it is diagnosed early, maternal mortality is increased (8 to 10%).[53] Treatment includes supportive care and delivery.[39]

The incidence of acute fatty liver is 1 per 13,000 in the general obstetric population.[54] Four series of cases have shown a 16.7% occurrence in twins.[31] Meanwhile, in the series of 55 triplets evaluated by Malone and associates,[47] the disease was present in 7% of patients. It has been postulated that there is an association between this disease and an autosomal recessive order of mitochondrial fatty acid oxidation in the children of affected women.[55-58] A high level of clinical suspicion is needed, when patients with multiple gestations have elevated liver function tests and vague complaints of nausea and vomiting, to diagnose this potentially catastrophic disease.[52]

Nutrition

Weight gain is a physiologic response to pregnancy. The average woman with twins gains between 40 and 45 pounds.[59] Few studies have examined weight gain in triplet and higher-order multiples.[3] The pattern of weight and the amount of weight gain appear to be different in twin than in singleton pregnancies. For example, weight gain occurs faster and earlier in women with multiple gestations.[3] Weight gain and pattern of gain seem to affect pregnancy outcomes.[60] Poor weight gain in early pregnancy (<0.85 lb/week) has been associated with poor intrauterine growth.[3] In contrast, large weight gains have been associated with greater birth weights.[3] Nutritional counseling may improve weight gain in women with twins.[60] Whether better weight gain translates into better perinatal outcomes is yet to be determined.

It is currently recommended that women with multifetal pregnancies increase their daily caloric intake approximately 300 kcal more than that of women with singleton pregnancies.[61] Iron and folic acid supplementation is also recommended.[62] At our institution, patients with multiple gestations receive a nutritional consultation and vitamin supplements, and they are monitored carefully for adequate weight gain.

Gestational Hypertension and Preeclampsia

The risk of pregnancy-induced hypertension or preeclampsia is between 10 and 20% in twin pregnancies and between 25 and 60% in triplet pregnancies, and it may be as high as 90% in quadruplet pregnancies.[39] The cause of these increased rates is unknown, but it may be secondary to high levels of circulating β-hCG.[63] The rates of preeclampsia seem to be the same for both monozygous and dizygous twins.[64] Eclampsia also seems to be increased in multiple pregnancies.[63] In addition, when preeclampsia occurs in higher-order multiple gestations, it seems to occur earlier and is more severe; the clinical presentation is often atypical.[63] Because of the increased risk of preeclampsia, women with multiple gestations require frequent monitoring for early signs and symptoms.[50]

FETAL PHYSIOLOGY AND MULTIPLE PREGNANCIES

Multiple gestations contribute disproportionately to overall perinatal morbidity and mortality. These pregnancies are at risk of both preterm birth and low birth weight. An increased risk of preterm premature rupture of membranes has not been reported for multiple pregnancies.[46,65]

Perinatal outcome is influenced by chorionicity, because dichorionic pregnancies have substantially better outcomes compared with monochorionic ones.[39] The effect of zygosity on outcomes, however, is less clear.[66]

Children of multiple births comprise less than 3% of the U.S. population but are highly represented among the low birth weight (<2500 g) and very low birth weight (<1500 g) populations.[3] Ninety percent of triplets and 50% of twins are of low birth weight compared with 6% of singletons. Preterm birth (less than 37 weeks' gestation) occurs in 88% of triplets and in 48% of twins compared with 11% of singletons. Birth before 32 weeks of gestation occurs in 31% of triplets, 11% of twins, and less than 2% of singletons.[3] More important, the incidence of extreme prematurity in multiple gestations is significant. For triplets, the risk of delivery before 28 weeks may be as high as 14%.[67]

Various interventions have been attempted to decrease the rates of preterm delivery in women with multiple gestations, such as home uterine monitoring, voluntary bed rest, prophylactic tocolytics, and elective cerclage.[1,68-70] Nevertheless, no inter-

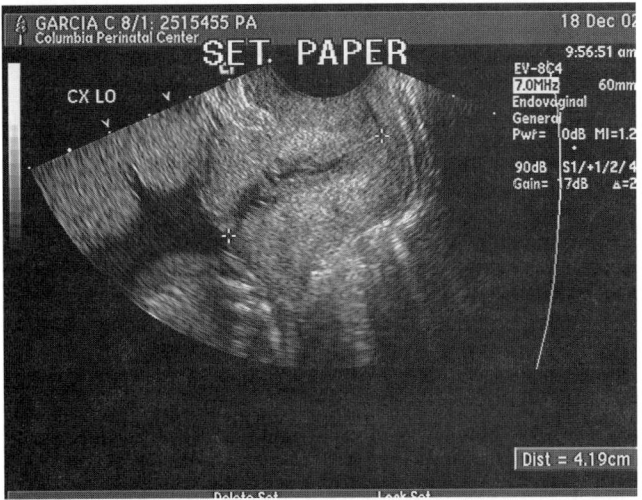

A

B

Figure 18–4. Cervical length. **A,** Normal cervix. **B,** Shortened cervix.

vention has proven successful.[1] Predictors for preterm delivery have been identified. At 24 weeks, a cervical length less than or equal to 25 mm is the best predictor of spontaneous preterm delivery before 32 weeks (Fig. 18-4). Likewise, a positive fetal fibronectin study at 28 weeks is also indicative of spontaneous preterm birth (<32 weeks).[71] If delivery between 24 and 34 weeks is anticipated, maternal steroids are recommended.

Fetal Growth in Multiple Pregnancy

Normal Growth

As suggested earlier, multiple gestations are at increased risk of low birth weight.[72] Part of this increased risk results from preterm labor and delivery, and a portion of this risk is secondary to complications inherent to multiple gestations, such as intrauterine growth restriction, discordant growth, and TTTS. Serial ultrasound is the best method for evaluating fetal growth in a multiple pregnancy, and the biometric parameters used to assess singletons are accurate in multiples.[39] Although individual growth curves for twins and triplets have been described, singleton weight standards are generally used for assessing weight in twins and higher-order multiple births.[39,73]

In twins, each fetus grows at the same rate as singletons up to approximately 32 weeks' gestation. After this gestational age, twins do not gain weight as rapidly as singletons.[74] As a result, multiple gestations are at increased risk of poorer growth than age-matched singletons. After approximately 32 weeks, the combined weight gain in twins is the same as in a singleton at the same gestational age.[75] Nonetheless, head circumferences and body lengths are generally similar. Ultrasound has demonstrated that twin femur length growth patterns are similar to those of singletons throughout gestation, but a reduction in abdominal circumference occurs at about 32 weeks.[76-79] In higher-order pregnancies, this weight difference seems to occur at even earlier gestational ages.[80]

Discordant Growth

Multiple gestations exhibit a significant increase in fetal growth abnormalities directly proportional to the number of fetuses.[81] *Growth discordancy* is the difference in sonographic estimated fetal weight expressed as a percentage in relation to the larger twin.[81] There are various definitions of fetal growth discordancy ranging between 15 and 40%.[81] However, adverse outcomes are generally related to discrepancies of 25% and greater. Discordancy has been associated with a 6.5-fold increased risk of fetal death and a 2.5-fold increased risk of perinatal mortality.[82] The more severe the discordance, the more likely fetal compromise, such as perinatal asphyxia, will occur.[81]

Growth discordancy has different implications depending on chorionicity.[83] Dichorionic diamniotic twins are distinct individuals that exhibit genetically different growth patterns. Therefore, it is not surprising that dichorionic twins have divergent birth weights. Nonetheless, several pathologic conditions result in discordant weight gain in dichorionic pregnancies, including *in utero* crowding, unequal sharing of the placenta, and the combination of a normal fetus with an anomalous fetus. Situations unique to monochorionic twinning, such as TTTS, can also result in growth discordancy.[81]

Two of the most frequent findings in severely discordant twins include small placental weight and umbilical cord abnormalities.[84] For example, velamentous cord insertion—umbilical cord inserting directly into the membranes—occurs 9 to 10 times more frequently in twin gestations than in singletons and 25 to 50 times more frequently in triplets than in singletons[85] (Fig. 18-5). A 13-fold increase in birth weight discordancy has been noted in monoamniotic twins with a velamentous umbilical cord insertion.[83]

In addition to growth discordancy, multiple gestations are at increased risk of intrauterine growth restriction. Uteroplacental insufficiency is thought to be the main cause of growth restriction in multiple gestations. Concordant growth in twins does not rule out intrauterine growth restriction because there are situations in which both twins can have growth restriction.[80] Management of both growth discordancy and intrauterine growth restriction includes intensive antepartum surveillance with delivery at 37 weeks, provided fetal testing is reassuring. Steroids should be administered to the mothers if delivery is anticipated between 24 and 34 weeks, to decrease complications of prematurity.

Multifetal Reduction

The purpose of first trimester multifetal reduction is to improve outcomes by decreasing maternal complications secondary to multiple gestations and by decreasing adverse fetal outcomes associated with preterm delivery[39] (Figs. 18-6 and 18-7). Intracardiac injection with potassium chloride is performed between 10 and 13 weeks of gestation in dichorionic pregnancies.[86] This procedure is contraindicated in monochorionic pregnancies because vascular communications between these fetuses can

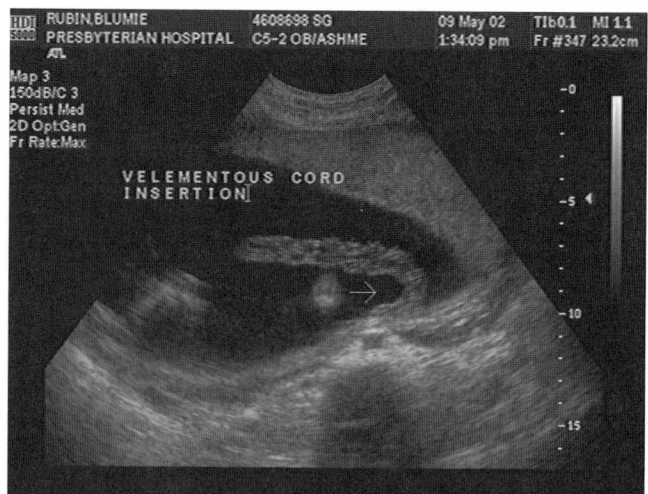

Figure 18–5. Velamentous cord.

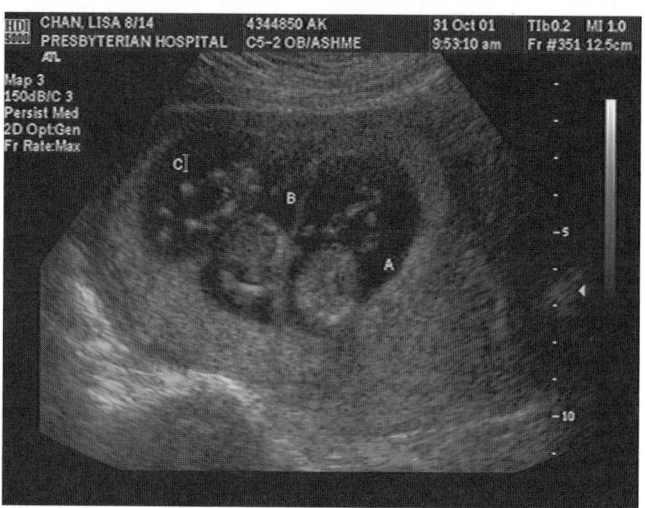

Figure 18–6. Triplets.

result in long-term adverse sequelae for the surviving fetus.[87] Adverse outcomes, such as pregnancy loss, are decreased with provider experience.[88] In addition, the procedure does not appear to be associated with adverse outcomes, such as intrauterine growth restriction.[89]

Stone and colleagues[90] reported on a series of 1000 cases of multifetal reduction. In each case, multifetal reduction was performed transabdominally at 10 to 13 weeks' gestation. This series demonstrated a loss rate of 6.2%. Although the loss rate was highest among patients reducing from six or more fetuses, the rate did not differ for starting numbers of three, four, or five fetuses. Birth weights demonstrated a linear decline with increasing starting and finishing numbers of fetuses. Gestational ages of delivery for finishing numbers of one, two, and three fetuses were similar to those of nonreduced pregnancies.

The same group demonstrated improved outcomes when twin pregnancies were reduced to singleton pregnancies. Stone and colleagues[91] compared 101 twin pregnancies reduced to singleton pregnancies with 365 patients reduced from triplet to twin pregnancies. These investigators found a threefold decrease in the spontaneous loss rate in the group reduced to singleton pregnancies compared with the group reduced to twin pregnancies. Reduction to singleton pregnancy was also associated

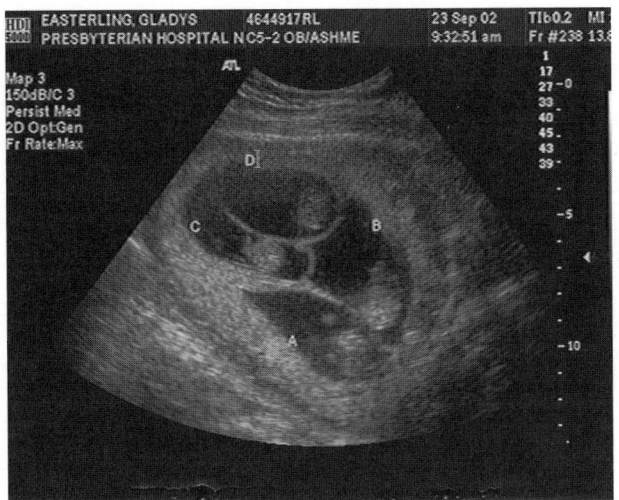

Figure 18–7. Higher-order multiple pregnancy: quadruplets.

with statistically significant increased birth weight and gestational age at delivery. In addition, cesarean section rates were decreased in the patients reduced to singleton pregnancies.

Multifetal reduction is an ethical dilemma.[92] The starting number of fetuses needed to justify the procedure is controversial. There have been conflicting studies regarding whether multifetal reduction from triplets to twins results in improved perinatal outcomes versus expectant management.[93-95] Triplet and higher-order multiple pregnancies have been associated with increased costs derived from antepartum hospital stays, missed work hours, and neonatal intensive care in the postpartum period. As would be expected, multifetal reduction greatly reduces such costs.[96] However, regardless of the cost savings, some women suffer from depression and grief after their decision to reduce their pregnancies.[97]

At our institution, we present women who have three or more fetuses in the first trimester with both options: multifetal reduction and expectant management. We discuss the risks and benefits of these options, so each woman can make her own informed decision.

Fetal Lung Maturity in Multiple Gestation

At this point, there is no consensus on whether pulmonary maturation differs between singleton and multiple pregnancies. In one study of singleton and twin pregnancies, it was found that after 31 weeks of gestation, twins exhibited higher TDx-fetal lung maturity fluorescence polarization assay values compared with singletons. The reason that twin gestations may have accelerated changes in pulmonary maturity index values is unknown. Likewise, it is not known whether this reflects a difference in the risk of respiratory distress syndrome between singleton and multiple pregnancies. If age-specific risks of respiratory distress syndrome are similar for twins and for singletons, new guidelines will be needed to avoid false-positive prediction of adequate lung maturity in twins.[98]

When assessing lung maturity in multiple gestations, there is a debate regarding whether all amniotic sacs or just one sac should be tapped. Investigators believe that, in certain situations, one fetus may attain pulmonary maturity before the others.[80] Two series found lecithin/sphingomyelin ratios to be similar in 34 sets of twins.[99, 100] In another study of 8 sets of twins (6 of 8 twins were delivered vaginally), a significant difference was noted in phospholipid profiles from the tracheal aspirates in the postpartum period.[101] Other studies have shown a significant discrepancy between lecithin/sphingomyelin ratios in the pre-

senting fetus of a multiple pregnancy and the other fetuses irrespective of delivery mode.[102, 103] Because of the conflicting data, at our institution, we generally tap all sacs to determine lung maturity.

Fetal Pathophysiology and Multiple Pregnancy

Pathophysiology Specific to Multifetal Gestations

Certain pathophysiologic situations are unique to multiple pregnancies. These include early pregnancy loss, fetus papyraceus, monochorionic monoamniotic twins, conjoined twins, TTTS, and twin reversed arterial perfusion (TRAP).

Early Pregnancy Loss

The incidence of early pregnancy loss in multiple gestations is higher than initially thought.[44] The routine use of ultrasound has shown that early fetal wastage is common in multiple gestations. In patients with twin gestations scanned in the first trimester, rates of demise ranged from 13 to 78%.[104] This phenomenon has been termed the *vanishing twin*. The explanations for this occurrence include physiologic resorption, versus artifact, and sonographic error.[44] Although this phenomenon may be associated with first trimester bleeding and spotting, it has not been associated with adverse pregnancy outcomes.[80]

Fetus Papyraceus

Fetal papyraceus, also known as fetus compressus, develops when one twin dies at approximately 15 to 20 weeks. The fetus loses all water content and becomes compressed by the continued development of the surviving twin. Such pregnancies rarely enter birth statistics. Thus, along with the vanishing twin phenomenon, fetus papyraceus may result in an underestimation of the incidence of twinning.[7]

Monoamniotic Twins

Monoamniotic twins are a rare form of monozygous twins in which both fetuses occupy the same sac. The diagnosis is made by ultrasound. No amniotic membrane is visualized in a same-sex pregnancy with one placental mass (Fig. 18–8). Unexplained rupture of a dividing membrane has also been observed. However, these pregnancies should be managed like true monoamniotic twins, because they have been found to have similar outcomes.[27] The diagnosis of monoamniotic twins has been confirmed by observing cord entanglement.[105]

Monoamniotic twins are associated with a high rate of perinatal mortality. Past studies indicated a fetal mortality rate ranging from 30 to 68%.[106-108] Monoamniotic pregnancies are associated with preterm delivery, growth restriction, vascular anastomosis, congenital anomalies, cord entanglement, and cord accidents[109] (Figs. 18–9 and 18–10). The management of these pregnancies has been controversial, particularly regarding the optimal timing of delivery and protocol for antenatal surveillance.[108, 110, 111] Delivery is generally performed via cesarean section. Although vaginal delivery is not contraindicated, it should be undertaken with caution.[112] There have been reports of inadvertent severing of the second twin's umbilical cord at delivery of the presenting twin.[113]

Data suggest better outcomes with intensive surveillance. In a study by House and colleagues,[114] 22 patients were managed at one tertiary care center over a 10-year period. Management included close fetal surveillance with daily testing starting at 24 to 26 weeks' gestation. Steroids were routinely used, and elective delivery occurred at 34 to 35 weeks, provided the results of testing were reassuring. No fetal mortality occurred in this group of patients. Nevertheless, monoamniotic twins were more likely to deliver prematurely and had more respiratory problems compared with monochorionic diamniotic and dichorionic diamniotic pregnancies.

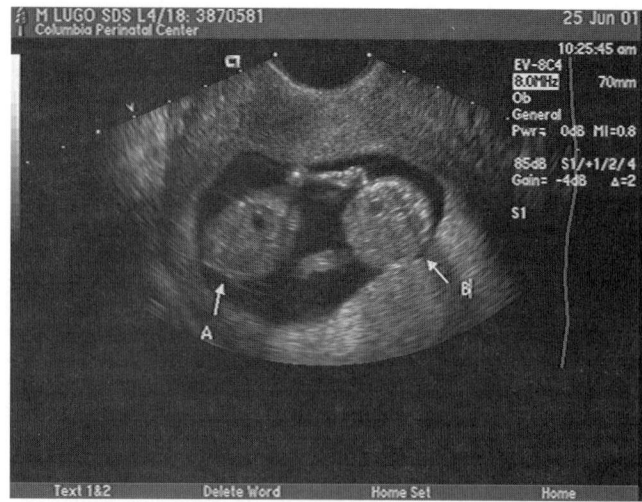

Figure 18–8. Monoamniotic twins: no dividing membrane. (From Weiss JL, Devine PC: Ultrasound Obstet Gynecol 2002;20:516.)

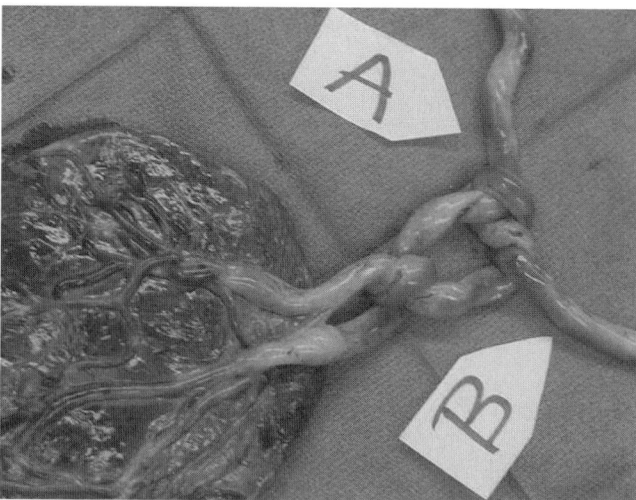

Figure 18–10. A and **B**, Monoamniotic twin placenta with cord entanglement. (From Weiss JL, Devine PC: Ultrasound Obstet Gynecol 2002;20:516.)

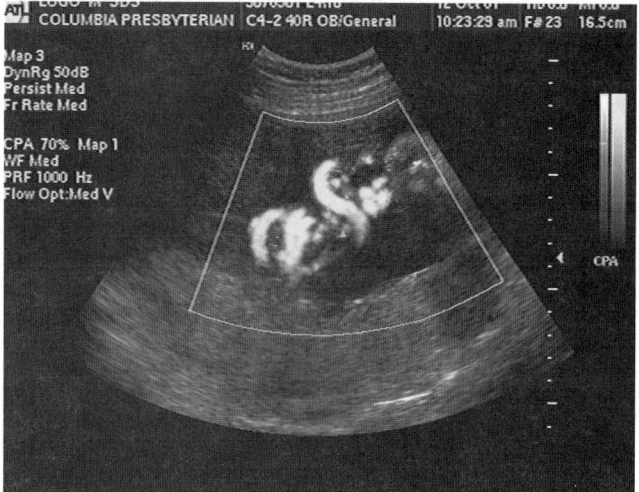

Figure 18–9. Monoamniotic twins: cord entanglement. (From Weiss JL, Devine PC: Ultrasound Obstet Gynecol 2002;20:516.)

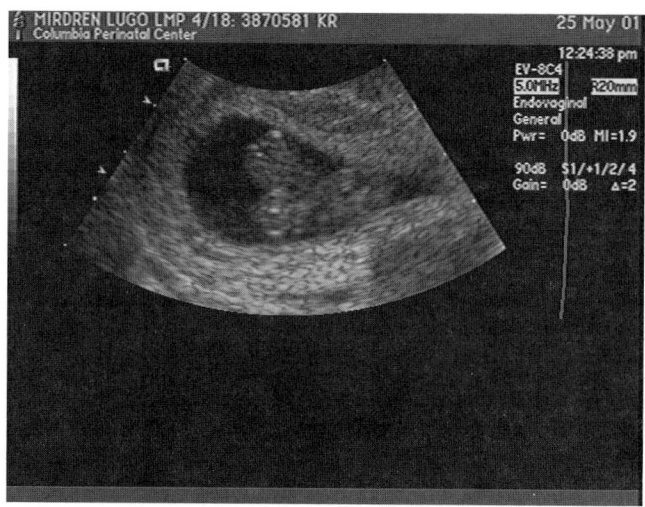

Figure 18–11. First trimester ultrasound scan: conjoined twins versus monoamniotic twins.

Conjoined Twins

Conjoined twins are an extremely rare form of monoamniotic twins, occurring in 1 in 50,000 pregnancies.[6] The diagnosis is made ultrasonographically. If the diagnosis is suspected early in the first trimester, a follow-up scan is needed for confirmation, because there have been incorrect diagnoses made at early gestational ages[115] (Fig. 18-11).

Conjoined twins may be joined at various anatomic locations. Five distinct types have been recognized.[39] The first type is thoracopagus, accounting for 75% of conjoined twins. The fetuses face each other and usually have a common sternum, diaphragm, upper abdominal wall, liver, pericardium, and gastrointestinal tract.[116] The second type is omphalopagus, also known as xiphopagus, which is a rare form of thoracophagus, in which the abdominal wall is connected and there is a common liver. The third type, pygopagus, comprises 20% of conjoined twins. The fetuses face away from one another and share a sacrum, bladder, and rectum.[116] In the fourth type, ischiopagus, the twins share a bony pelvis. This accounts for 5% of conjoined twins.[116] Finally, the fifth type, craniopagus (cephalopagus), is classified by partial or complete fusion of the skull, meninges, and vascular structures and comprises 1 to 2% of these cases.[115]

If conjoined twins are diagnosed early, parents should be counseled about the option for termination of the pregnancy. Depending on the type of conjoined twin and the gestational age, this procedure can be performed by dilatation and curettage, dilatation and evacuation, induction, or hysterotomy.[115] If expectant management is desired, care should be transferred to a referral center. Generally, delivery should be performed via cesarean section as near to term as possible, with a multidisciplinary team.[115] Vaginal delivery is possible in selected cases of extreme prematurity or if survival is improbable. Successful separation of the twins depends on the degree of organ and vascular sharing between the two fetuses.[117]

Twin-to-Twin Transfusion Syndrome

TTTS is a complication of monochorionic pregnancies in which there is an imbalance in the blood flow across a shared placenta of two fetuses. The net effect of this blood flow imbalance is a large hyperperfused recipient twin and a small, hypoperfused, anemic donor twin (Fig. 18-12). If the condition is untreated, the prognosis is poor, with a 60 to 100% mortality rate for both twins.[118-120] When one twin dies *in utero*, the surviving twin is

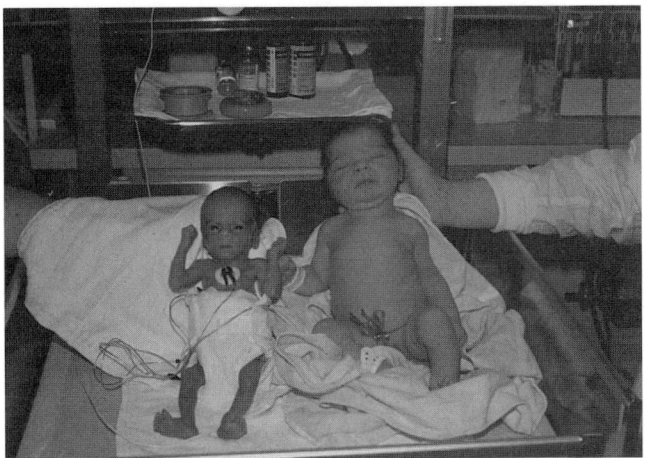

Figure 18–12. Twin-twin transfusion syndrome: donor and recipient twins.

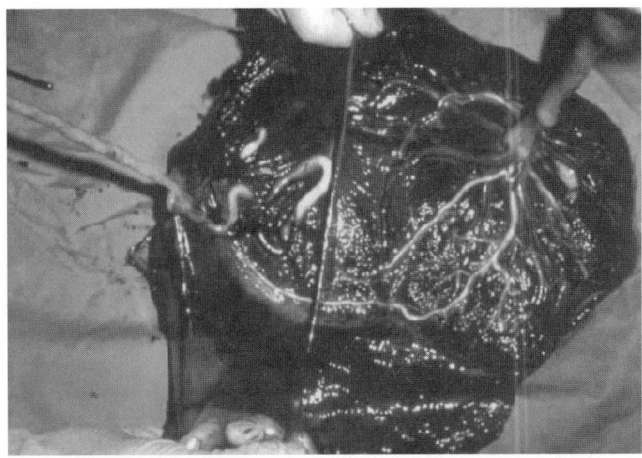

Figure 18–13. Vascular anastomoses in twin-twin transfusion syndrome. (Courtesy of Dr. Alfred Z. Abuhamad, Norfolk, VA.)

at risk of severe neurologic damage. The true incidence of TTTS is unknown, because many of these pregnancies result in early loss.[116]

Although all monochorionic twins share a portion of their vasculature, only 5 to 15% will develop TTTS.[2] TTTS occurs predominantly in monochorionic pregnancies.[116] There are a few rare case reports of TTTS in dichorionic pregnancies.[121, 122] Although the exact origin is not known, Bajoria and colleagues[123] proposed the following mechanism. In monochorionic placentas, there can be three types of vascular communications: arteriovenous communications, arterioarterial communications, and venovenous communications. One cotyledon near the dividing membrane may receive arterial blood supply from one fetus and yet may drain directly by a vein to the other side. The arteriovenous shunt is usually deep in the placenta and is unidirectional. Superficial arterioarterial and venovenous connections are crucial for maintaining the bidirectional flow.[115] According to the theory proposed by Bajoria and associates,[123] TTTS results from the absence of the superficial anastomoses, which maintain balanced blood flow (Fig. 18–13).

Diagnosis of TTTS is made via ultrasound. The four requirements for the diagnosis of TTTS are (1) the presence of a single placenta, (2) same-gender fetuses, (3) weight discordance of greater than 20%, and (4) significant amniotic fluid discordance often with a stuck twin[115] (Fig. 18–14). The recipient twin may exhibit signs of heart failure and hydrops. On echocardiography, the recipient twin may have decreased ventricular function, tricuspid regurgitation, and cardiomegaly.[124] Doppler studies may be abnormal for both twins. A staging system has evolved for the purpose of describing this disease progression. Stage I occurs when the bladder of the donor twin is still visible; Stage II occurs when the bladder of the donor is not visible; Stage III refers to abnormal Doppler studies; Stage IV is hydrops; and Stage V is IUFD.[125]

Weight and hematologic discordances are no longer considered diagnostic of TTTS.[116] Likewise, a stuck twin is not pathognomic for TTTS because it has been observed in cases of structural fetal anomalies, congenital infection, chromosomal abnormalities, and premature rupture of membranes.[116] The differential diagnosis of TTTS includes abnormal cord insertion or uteroplacental insufficiency with poor fetal growth and decreased urine output in one twin and fetal anomalies, such as bladder obstruction and aneuploidy.[115]

Because of the poor outcomes associated with this disorder, expectant management is rarely employed. Medical management has been reported using digoxin.[126] Indomethacin is no longer

recommended after reports appeared of fetal demise after its use.[127, 128]

One management option for TTTS is serial reduction amniocentesis.[129-136] Under ultrasound guidance, an 18-gauge spinal needle is placed into the sac with polyhydramnios. The fluid is removed until the amniotic fluid level returns to normal (provided the patient can tolerate the procedure). This procedure is repeated as often as necessary to maintain a normal amniotic fluid volume. The mechanism by which this procedure restores the amniotic fluid balance is unknown. It is possible that removing fluid from the sac with polyhydramnios results in decreased pressure on the sac with oligohydramnios. This may result in increased perfusion to the stuck twin and an improved amniotic fluid volume for this twin.[115]

Amniotic septostomy is another management option.[137] In this procedure, a 20-gauge spinal needle is inserted through the dividing membrane under ultrasound guidance. The amniotic fluid equilibrates across the two sacs. As in serial amnioreduction, it is uncertain how this technique improves outcomes.[115] It is possible that the donor swallows a large fluid volume, resulting in restoration of circulating blood volume and better perfusion. Studies regarding the effectiveness of this treatment technique have been conflicting. In one report of 12 cases, pregnancy was prolonged by 8 weeks, with an 83% survival rate.[138] In a second study of 3 cases, 100% of the pregnancies were lost in 5 days as a result of preterm premature rupture of membranes.[139]

Serial reduction amniocentesis and amniotic septostomy do not affect the placental anastomoses. As a result, neither of these techniques is thought to prevent the neurologic complications associated with this disease entity.[115] Laser ablation of placental anastomoses is an experimental treatment that may correct TTTS and reduce the neurologic complications associated with these pregnancies.[126, 132, 140-143] In this procedure, a fetoscope is placed in the sac with polyhydramnios under ultrasound guidance, and the anatomy of the placental vessels is studied. An arteriovenous shunt is diagnosed by identifying an artery, supplying a cotyledon without a vein returning on the same side of the dividing membrane. A vein may be seen on the other side of the dividing membrane draining the cotyledon of the other fetus. A 0.4-mm neodymium:yttrium-aluminum-garnet laser fiber is then placed in the fetoscope to ablate these vessels. A reduction amniocentesis is simultaneously performed. A multicenter trial is currently in progress.

Until this trial is completed, antenatal management includes serial ultrasound scans with assessment of cardiac function, amniotic fluid, and weight discordancy. Treatment should be

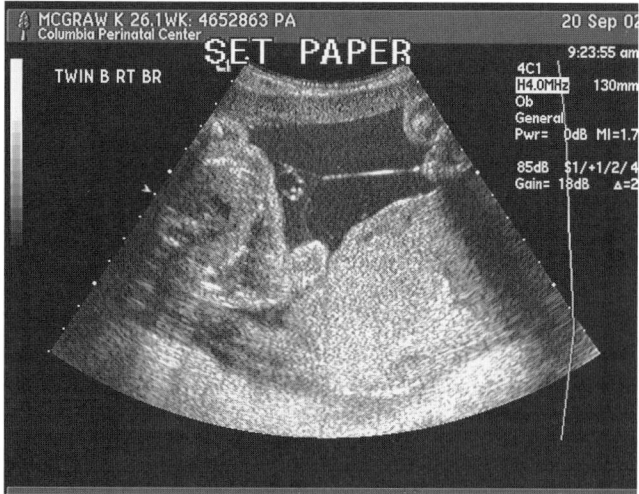

A

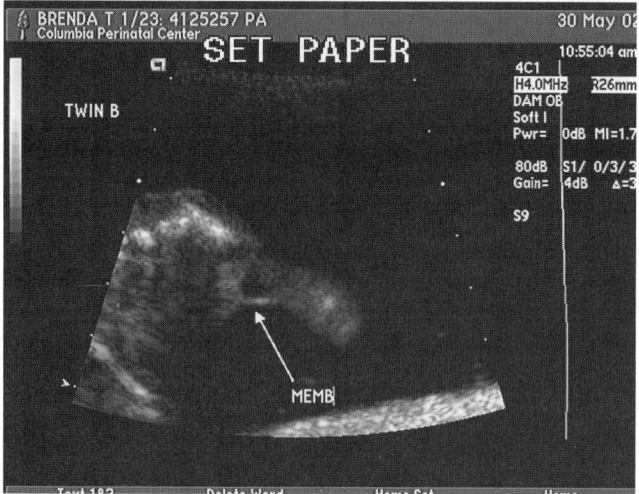

B

Figure 18–14. **A** and **B**, Twin-twin transfusion syndrome: stuck twin.

tailored to each clinical situation; however, reduction amniocentesis may be performed as the first therapeutic intervention. For patients with severe and early-onset TTTS, referral to a center performing laser therapy may be warranted. Antenatal corticosteroids should be administered if delivery is anticipated between 24 and 34 weeks. If either fetus shows compromise between 32 to 34 weeks, immediate delivery should be considered.[115]

Twin Reversed Arterial Perfusion Syndrome

TRAP, also known as acardia, is defined by the absence of a normally functioning heart in one fetus of a multiple pregnancy (Fig. 18-15). The incidence is estimated to be 1% of monozygotic twins.[109] The true incidence is unknown because many cases of TRAP may result in early pregnancy loss.[116] The normal fetus perfuses the acardiac twin by an umbilical artery to umbilical artery anastomosis at the placental surface. There is reversal of blood flow in the umbilical artery of the recipient twin, and deoxygenated blood is brought from the pump twin to the acardiac twin. As a result, there is a normal twin and an amorphous twin. A range of anomalies can be seen in the acardiac twin including anencephaly, absent limbs, intestinal atresia, abdominal wall defects, and absent organs.[144] Because of the increased cardiac work load, the normal twin can develop heart failure.[39]

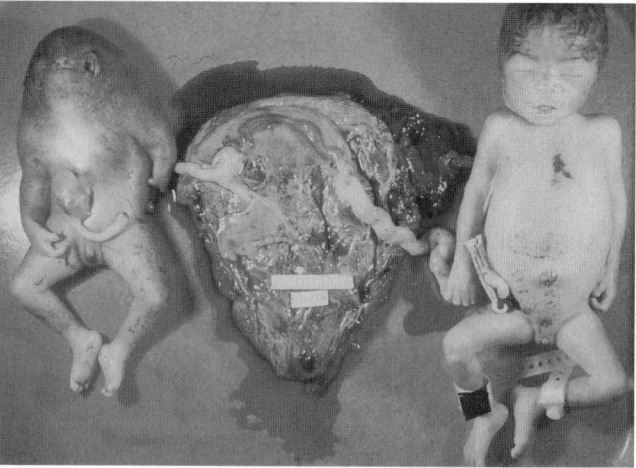

Figure 18–15. Twin reversed arterial perfusion syndrome sequence. (From Bianchi DW, et al: Fetology, Diagnosis, and Management of the Fetal Patient. New York, McGraw-Hill, 2000, p 922.)

Ultrasound is used for diagnosis, and the differential diagnosis of acardia includes IUFD or anencephaly in one twin.[116] The cause is thought to be the development of arterial to arterial vascular anastomoses between the umbilical arteries of twins in early embryogenesis.[116] Seventy-four percent of cases are monochorionic diamniotic gestations, and 24% of cases are monochorionic monoamniotic pregnancies. Cases are rarely dichorionic.[145] The pump twin is generally morphologically normal, but approximately 9% of these twins have trisomy. Thirty-three percent of acardiac twins have an abnormal karyotype, including monosomy, trisomy, deletions, mosaicism, and polyploidy.[145]

The goal of management is to maximize the outcome of the normal twin. Poor prognosis has been associated with polyhydramnios and congestive heart failure in the pump twin. Prognosis for the pump twin depends on the ratio of the weight of the perfused twin to the weight of the pump twin. Standard biometric measurements cannot be used to measure the acardiac twin. As a result, a second-order regression equation has been devised: weight in grams = $(-1.66 \times \text{length}) + (1.21 \times \text{length}^2)$.[146] When the twin weight ratio is greater than 0.70, there is a 30% risk of congestive heart failure for the pump twin.[39]

In the absence of poor prognostic indicators (congestive heart failure, polyhydramnios, and a twin weight ratio of greater than 0.70), expectant management with serial ultrasound is suggested.[109] Steroids are advised if delivery is anticipated between 24 and 34 weeks, and tocolysis is suggested to stop preterm labor.[116] Medical management with indomethacin and digoxin has been reported.[147, 148] More invasive management has included hysterotomy of the acardiac twin followed by interval delivery of the pump twin.[149,150]

Percutaneous interruption of the circulation in the acardiac twin has also been described. Procedures have included insertion of a thrombogenic coil into the recipient twin's umbilical cord, endoscopic ligation of the cord, injection of silk soaked in alcohol into the cord, injection of absolute alcohol into the cord, and radioablation.[151-160] These methods are usually reserved for when the pump twin has already developed cardiac failure before reaching a viable age.[39]

Pathophysiology with Special Considerations in Multiple Pregnancy

Intrauterine Fetal Demise of One Twin

IUFD of one fetus during the first trimester is common and appears to have no adverse impact on the surviving fetus or fetuses. IUFD of one fetus in the second or third trimester is less common, occurring in 2.6% of twin pregnancies and in 4.3% of triplet pregnancies.[161] This phenomenon can result in morbidity for the surviving co-twin as a result of preterm delivery.[109] Eglowstein and D'Alton[162] and D'Alton and Simpson[109] reviewed 20 cases and found the mean gestational age at delivery to be 30.6 weeks for monochorionic pregnancies and 32.9 weeks for dichorionic pregnancies.

Neurologic morbidity may be increased in monochorionic twins after IUFD of one twin.[109] Studies report a 12 to 20% risk of multicystic encephalomalacia in the twin survivor of a monochorionic pregnancy.[109,163] The proposed mechanism is a hypotensive event at the time of death resulting in acute blood loss into the dying twin, rather than thromboembolic arterial occlusion.[164-167] Most neurologic damage occurs after demise of the twin during the late second trimester.[109] Neurologic morbidity has been reported after demise of the twin as early as 18 weeks.[109]

Management of IUFD in one twin depends on the gestational age and the chorionicity of the pregnancy. Unfortunately, in a monochorionic pregnancy, the risk of neurologic handicap may be present from the moment of the twin's demise. As a result, immediate delivery after the demise of one twin may not prevent an adverse outcome in the surviving twin. Furthermore, multicystic encephalomalacia may not be evident on ultrasound or from fetal heart rate tracing.[39] Management recommendations include close fetal surveillance and delivery at 37 weeks (or when lung maturity has been established). Steroids should be given if delivery is expected to occur between 24 and 34 weeks. For maternal or fetal indications, delivery should occur before 37 weeks.[39]

There is a theoretical risk of maternal coagulopathy when an IUFD occurs in one twin and delivery of the surviving twin is delayed.[168] In two series of twin gestations complicated by a single intrauterine demise, none of the patients developed coagulopathy, whereas only two patients demonstrated transient biochemical evidence of coagulopathy.[162,169] Laboratory surveillance of these patients with coagulation profiles is probably unnecessary.[109]

Congenital Anomalies

Congenital anomalies appear to be more common in multiple than in singleton gestations.[170] Discordancy of structural anomalies can occur in both monochorionic and dichorionic pregnancies.[39]

When a multiple gestation is complicated by a fetal anomaly in one fetus, the patient has three options: (1) expectant management and, depending on the gestational age at diagnosis, either (2) termination of the entire pregnancy or (3) selective termination of the anomalous fetus.[171] Counseling must take into account the patient's religious and moral beliefs, as well as the chorionicity of the pregnancy, the severity of the anomaly, and the effect the anomaly will have on the normal co-twin.[172]

If a patient elects expectant management, the patient and the family should be counseled about possible outcomes. Malone and colleagues[171] studied 14 twin pregnancies complicated by an anomalous fetus over a 5-year period at one tertiary care center and compared them to 78 normal twin pregnancies from the same center during a 2-year period. The obstetric management was similar for all patients. Gestational age at delivery and birth weight were significantly lower in the study group. The mean gestational age at delivery for the study group was 33.6 weeks, whereas it was 35.6 weeks for the controls. The risk of delivering at 36 weeks or less was 78.6% for the anomalous twin group compared with 59% for the normal twin group. Likewise, the mean birth weight for the study group was 1864 g, versus 2318 g for the controls. The lower birth weights resulted from the higher incidence of prematurity in the study group. The study infants also appeared to be at increased risk of delivery via cesarean section. There was no difference in perinatal mortality

between the two groups.[171] Thus, it is important to counsel patients that conservative management can result in adverse outcomes for the healthy twin.[172]

Some patients may opt for selective termination of the pregnancy after counseling. In dichorionic pregnancies, ultrasound-guided intracardiac injection of potassium chloride is used. Eddelman and colleagues[173] reported favorable outcomes on 200 cases, including 164 twins, 32 triplets, and 4 quadruplets. The average gestational age at time of the procedure was 19 2/7 weeks, with a range of 12 to 23 6/7 weeks. The reasons for selective reduction included chromosomal abnormalities, structural abnormalities, mendelian disorders, placental insufficiency, and cervical incompetence. The unintended pregnancy loss rate was 4%. The loss rate was almost fivefold higher in triplets than in twins. The average gestational age at delivery was 36 1/7 weeks. Approximately 84% delivered after 32 weeks of gestation.[173] According to this study, selective termination may result in good outcomes for the surviving twin.

In monochorionic twins, selective termination is more challenging. Complete ablation of the umbilical cord of the anomalous fetus is needed to avoid neurologic morbidity to the remaining normal fetus. Techniques used have included fetoscopic cord ligation, fetoscopic laser ablation of umbilical vessels, percutaneous injection of alcohol or occlusive materials into the umbilical cord or into the umbilical vein, and radioablation.[154,155,157-159,174,175]

Chromosomal Anomalies

Most known chromosomal anomalies have been reported in multiple gestations.[39] Both monozygotic and dizygotic twins can be discordant for these anomalies. In dizygotic pregnancies, the maternal age-related risk of chromosomal abnormalities for each twin may be the same as in a singleton pregnancy.[39] It has been suggested that the chance of at least one fetus' being affected by a chromosomal defect is twice as high as in a singleton. At our institution, invasive genetic testing, such as amniocentesis, is offered to all women aged 32 years and older with dichorionic twins. Mothers with trichorionic triplets are offered invasive testing if they are 28 years old and older. Patients with higher-order multiple pregnancies are offered testing at progressively younger ages. In monozygotic twins, the risk of a chromosomal abnormality is the same as for a singleton, and in most cases, both fetuses are affected. These patients are offered genetic testing if they are 35 years old and older. As previously stated, there are cases reported of monozygotic twins discordant for abnormalities of autosomal or sex chromosomes resulting from postzygotic nondisjunction. In the most common situation, one fetus has Turner syndrome, and the other fetus has either a normal male or a normal female phenotype with a mosaic karyotype.[80]

As a result of increased risk of both genetic and structural abnormalities, patients with multiple gestations should be offered both genetic testing and prenatal diagnosis. In the first trimester, ultrasound nuchal translucency can be used to help determine whether a patient is at risk of a genetic or structural abnormality.[39] At our institution, second trimester screening for Down syndrome and for open neural tube defects with maternal serum α-fetoprotein, hCG, and unconjugated estriol is generally not performed, because these tests are not as reliable for multiple gestations.[39] If invasive testing, such as amniocentesis or chorionic villus sampling, is used, all fetuses should be tested, because there can be discordancy for genetic abnormalities despite monozygosity.[39]

SUMMARY

Multifetal pregnancy has a physiologic impact on both the mother and the fetus. Accordingly, a multidisciplinary approach is needed for the management of these patients. The mother is at increased risk of adverse outcomes, such as anemia, postpartum hemorrhage, and preterm delivery. The fetus is at increased risk of low birth weight, growth abnormalities, and several problems particular to multiple gestations, such as discordant anomalies, monoamnionicity, IUFD of one twin, TTTS, and TRAP.

Fetal outcomes are dependent on gestational age at delivery and on chorionicity, because adverse outcomes are more commonly associated with monochorionicity. Ultrasound is imperative for the management of these patients. It is critical for diagnosis of chorionicity and structural abnormalities, as well as for surveillance of fetal growth and well-being. To date, no strategies have proven useful to prevent adverse outcomes in these pregnancies. However, maternal steroids should be administered if preterm delivery is anticipated. Further, complex issues unique to multiple gestations should be referred to a tertiary care center with perinatologists, neonatalogists, and pediatric specialists proficient at caring for these complex patients.

REFERENCES

1. Newman RB, Ellings JM: Antepartum management of the multiple gestation: the case for specialized care. Semin Perinatol 1995;19(5):387-403.
2. Benirschke K, Kim CK: Multiple pregnancy. I. N Engl J Med 1973; 288(24):1276-84.
3. Luke B: The changing pattern of multiple births in the United States: maternal and infant characteristics, 1973 and 1990. Obstet Gynecol 1994;84(1):101-6.
4. Cain JM: Ethical guidelines in the prevention of iatrogenic multiple pregnancy. Int J Gynaecol Obstet 2000;71(3):293-4.
5. Benirschke K: Remarkable placenta. Clin Anat 1998;11(3):194-205.
6. Hanson JW: Letter: Incidence of conjoined twinning. Lancet 1975;2(7947):1257.
7. Benirschke K: The biology of the twinning process: how placentation influences outcome. Semin Perinatol 1995;19(5):342-50.
8. Reece EA, Hobbins JC: Medicine of the Fetus and Mother. Philadelphia, Lippincott-Raven, 1999.
9. Lambalk CB, Schoemaker J: Hypothetical risks of twinning in the natural menstrual cycle. Eur J Obstet Gynecol Reprod Biol 1997;75(1):1-4.
10. White C, Wyshak G: Inheritance in human dizygotic twinning. N Engl J Med 1964;271:1003.
11. Waterhouse JAH: Twinning in twin pedigrees. Br J Soc Med 1950;4:197.
12. Nylander PP: Ethnic differences in twinning rates in Nigeria. J Biosoc Sci 1971;3(2):151-7.
13. Chow JS, et al: Frequency of a monochorionic pair in multiple gestations: relationship to mode of conception. J Ultrasound Med 2001;20(7):757-60.
14. Derom C, et al: Increased monozygotic twinning rate after ovulation induction. Lancet 1987;1(8544):1236-8.
15. Schachter M, et al: Monozygotic twinning after assisted reproductive techniques: a phenomenon independent of micromanipulation. Hum Reprod 2001;16(6):1264-9.
16. D'Alton ME, Mercer BM: Antepartum management of twin gestation: ultrasound. Clin Obstet Gynecol 1990;33(1):42-51.
17. Barss VA, et al: Ultrasonographic determination of chorion type in twin gestation. Obstet Gynecol 1985;66(6):779-83.
18. Warren WB, et al: Dating the early pregnancy by sequential appearance of embryonic structures. Am J Obstet Gynecol 1989;161(3):747-53.
19. Bromley B, Benacerraf B: Using the number of yolk sacs to determine amnionicity in early first trimester monochorionic twins. J Ultrasound Med 1995;14(6):415-9.
20. Callen P: Ultrasonography in Obstetrics and Gynecology. Philadelphia, WB Saunders Co, 2000.
21. Finberg HJ: The "twin peak" sign: reliable evidence of dichorionic twinning. J Ultrasound Med 1992;11(11):571-7.
22. Monteagudo A, et al: Early and simple determination of chorionic and amniotic type in multifetal gestations in the first fourteen weeks by high-frequency transvaginal ultrasonography. Am J Obstet Gynecol 1994; 170(3):824-9.
23. Hertzberg BS, et al: Significance of membrane thickness in the sonographic evaluation of twin gestations. AJR Am J Roentgenol 1987;148(1):151-3.
24. Townsend RR, et al: Membrane thickness in ultrasound prediction of chorionicity of twin gestations. J Ultrasound Med 1988;7(6): 327-32.
25. Winn HN, et al: Ultrasonographic criteria for the prenatal diagnosis of placental chorionicity in twin gestations. Am J Obstet Gynecol 1989;161 (6 Pt 1):1540-2.
26. D'Alton ME, Dudley DK: The ultrasonographic prediction of chorionicity in twin gestation. Am J Obstet Gynecol 1989;160(3):557-61.
27. Gilbert WM: Chorionicity morbidity associated with prenatal disruption of the dividing membrane in twin gestations. Obstet Gynecol 1991;78(4):623-30.
28. Norton ME, et al: Molecular zygosity studies aid in the management of discordant multiple gestations. J Perinatol 1997;17(3):202-7.
29. Yeast JD: Maternal physiologic adaptation to twin gestation. Clin Obstet Gynecol 1990;33(1):10-7.
30. Redford DH: Uterine growth in twin pregnancy by measurement of total intrauterine volume. Acta Genet Med Gemellol 1982;31(3-4):145-8.
31. Gall SA: Multiple Pregnancy and Delivery. St. Louis, CV Mosby, 1996.
32. Rizzo G, et al: Uterine artery Doppler velocity waveforms in twin pregnancies. Obstet Gynecol 1993;82(6):978-83.
33. Newman RB, et al: Uterine activity during pregnancy in ambulatory patients: comparison of singleton and twin gestations. Am J Obstet Gynecol 1986;154(3):530-1.
34. Norwitz ER, Robinson JN, Challis JR: The control of labor. N Engl J Med 1999;341(9):660-6.
35. Veille JC, et al: Maternal cardiovascular adaptations to twin pregnancy. Am J Obstet Gynecol 1985;153:261-3.
36. Campbell DM, Campbell AJ: Arterial blood pressure: the pattern of change in twin pregnancies. Acta Genet Med Gemellol 1985;34(3-4):217-23.
37. Clark SL, et al: Critical Care Obstetrics. Malden, MA, Blackwell Science, 1997.
38. Pritchard JA: Changes in blood volume during pregnancy and delivery. Anesthesiology 1965;26:393.
39. Creasy RK, Resnik R: Maternal-Fetal Medicine. Philadelphia, WB Saunders Co, 1999.
40. MacGillivray I, et al: Maternal metabolic response to twin pregnancy in primigravidae. J Obstet Gynaecol Br Commonw 1971;78(6):530-4.
41. Tatara T, et al: Pulmonary edema after long-term beta-adrenergic therapy and cesarean section. Anesth Analg 1995;81(2):417-8.
42. Yeast JD, et al: The risk of pulmonary edema and colloid osmotic pressure changes during magnesium sulfate infusion. Am J Obstet Gynecol 1993;169(6):1566-71.
43. Ogburn PL, Jr., et al: The use of magnesium sulfate for tocolysis in preterm labor complicated by twin gestation and betamimetic-induced pulmonary edema. Acta Obstet Gynecol Scand 1986;65(7):793-4.
44. Keith LG, et al: Multiple Pregnancy, Epidemiology, Gestation and Perinatal Outcome. New York, Parthenon Publishing Group, 1995.
45. Cavill I: Iron and erythropoiesis in normal subjects and in pregnancy. J Perinat Med 1995;23(1-2):47-50.
46. Spellacy WN, et al: A case-control study of 1253 twin pregnancies from a 1982-1987 perinatal data base. Obstet Gynecol 1990;75(2):168-71.
47. Malone FD, et al: Maternal morbidity associated with triplet pregnancy. Am J Perinatol 1998;15(1):73-7.
48. Goldstein JD, et al: Obstetric conditions and erythropoietin levels. Am J Obstet Gynecol 2000;182(5):1055-7.
49. Condie R, Campbell D: Components of the haemostatic mechanism in twin pregnancy. Br J Obstet Gynaecol 1978;85(1):37-9.
50. Campbell D: A review of maternal complications of multiple pregnancy. Twin Res 2001;4(3):146-9.
51. Seoud MA, et al: Outcome of twin, triplet, and quadruplet in vitro fertilization pregnancies: the Norfolk experience. Fertil Steril 1992;57(4):825-34.
52. Davidson KM, et al: Acute fatty liver of pregnancy in triplet gestation. Obstet Gynecol 1998;91(5 Pt 2):806-8.
53. Usta IM, et al: Acute fatty liver of pregnancy: an experience in the diagnosis and management of fourteen cases. Am J Obstet Gynecol 1994; 171(5):1342-7.
54. Pockros PJ, et al: Idiopathic fatty liver of pregnancy: findings in ten cases. Medicine (Baltimore) 1984;63(1):1-11.
55. Sims HF, et al: The molecular basis of pediatric long chain 3-hydroxyacyl-CoA dehydrogenase deficiency associated with maternal acute fatty liver of pregnancy. Proc Natl Acad Sci USA 1995;92(3):841-5.
56. Treem WR, et al: Acute fatty liver of pregnancy and long-chain 3-hydroxyacyl-coenzyme A dehydrogenase deficiency. Hepatology 1994;19(2):339-45.
57. Treem WR, et al: Acute fatty liver of pregnancy, hemolysis, elevated liver enzymes, and low platelets syndrome, and long 3-hydroxyacyl-coenzyme A dehydrogenase deficiency. Am J Gastroenterol 1996;91(11):2293-300.
58. Isaacs JD, Jr., et al: Maternal acute fatty liver of pregnancy associated with fetal trifunctional protein deficiency: molecular characterization of a novel maternal mutant allele. Pediatr Res 1996;40(3):393-8.
59. Luke B, et al: The ideal twin pregnancy: patterns of weight gain, discordancy, and length of gestation. Am J Obstet Gynecol 1993;169(3):588-97.
60. Luke B, et al: Maternal nutrition in twin gestations: weight gain, cravings and aversions, and sources of nutrition advice. Acta Genet Med Gemellol 1997;46(3):157-66.
61. Monsen ER: The 10th edition of the Recommended Dietary Allowances: what's new in the 1989 RDAs? J Am Diet Assoc 1989;89(12):1748-52.
62. ACOG educational bulletin. Special problems of multiple gestation. Number 253, November 1998 (Replaces Number 131, August 1989). American College of Obstetricians and Gynecologists. Int J Gynaecol Obstet 1999; 64(3):323-33.
63. Hardardottir H, et al: Atypical presentation of preeclampsia in high-order multifetal pregnancies. Obstet Gynecol 1996;87(3):370-4.
64. Maxwell CV, et al: Relationship of twin zygosity and risk of preeclampsia. Am J Obstet Gynecol 2001;185(4):819-21.
65. Kovacs BW, et al: Twin gestations: I. Antenatal care and complications. Obstet Gynecol 1989;74(3 Pt 1):313-7.
66. Dube J, et al: Does chorionicity or zygosity predict adverse perinatal outcomes in twins? Am J Obstet Gynecol 2002;186(3):579-83.
67. Devine PC, et al: Maternal and neonatal outcome of 100 consecutive triplet pregnancies. Am J Perinatol 2001;18(4):225-35.
68. Crowther CA: Hospitalisation and bed rest for multiple pregnancy. Cochrane Database Syst Rev 2001;1.
69. Dyson DC, et al: Monitoring women at risk for preterm labor. N Engl J Med 1998;338(1):15-9.

70. Dor J, et al: Elective cervical suture of twin pregnancies diagnosed ultrasonically in the first trimester following induced ovulation. Gynecol Obstet Invest 1982;13(1):55–60.
71. Goldenberg RL, et al: The preterm prediction study: risk factors in twin gestations. National Institute of Child Health and Human Development Maternal-Fetal Medicine Units Network. Am J Obstet Gynecol 1996;175 (4 Pt 1):1047–53.
72. Blickstein I, et al: Risk for one or two very low birth weight twins: a population study. Obstet Gynecol 2000;96(3):400–2.
73. Min SJ, et al: Birth weight references for twins. Am J Obstet Gynecol 2000;182(5):1250–7.
74. McKeown T, et al: Influences on fetal growth. J Reprod Fertil 1976;47(1):167–81.
75. Daw E, Walker J: Growth differences in twin pregnancy. Br J Clin Pract 1975;29(6):150–2.
76. Shah YG, et al: Biparietal diameter growth in uncomplicated twin gestation. Am J Perinatol 1987;4(3):229–32.
77. Crane JP, et al: Ultrasonic growth patterns in normal and discordant twins. Obstet Gynecol 1980;55(6):678–83.
78. Grumbach K, et al: Twin and singleton growth patterns compared using US. Radiology 1986;158(1):237–41.
79. Socol ML, et al: Diminished biparietal diameter and abdominal circumference growth in twins. Obstet Gynecol 1984;64(2):235–8.
80. Gabbe SV, et al: Obstetrics: Normal and Problem Pregnancies. New York, Churchill Livingstone, 2002.
81. Sherer DM, Divon MY: Fetal growth in multifetal gestation. Clin Obstet Gynecol 1997;40(4):764–70.
82. Erkkola R, et al: Growth discordancy in twin pregnancies: a risk factor not detected by measurements of biparietal diameter. Obstet Gynecol 1985;66(2):203–6.
83. Hanley ML, et al: Placental cord insertion and birth weight discordancy in twin gestations. Obstet Gynecol 2002;99(3):477–82.
84. Victoria A, et al: Perinatal outcome, placental pathology, and severity of discordance in monochorionic and dichorionic twins. Obstet Gynecol 2001;97(2):310–5.
85. Feldman DM, et al: Clinical implications of velamentous cord insertion in triplet gestations. Am J Obstet Gynecol 2002;186(4):809–11.
86. Berkowitz RL, et al: The current status of multifetal pregnancy reduction. Am J Obstet Gynecol 1996;174(4):1265–72.
87. Golbus MS, et al: Selective termination of multiple gestations. Am J Med Genet 1988;31(2):339–48.
88. Evans MI, et al: Improvement in outcomes of multifetal pregnancy reduction with increased experience. Am J Obstet Gynecol 2001;184(2):97–103.
89. Torok O, et al: Multifetal pregnancy reduction is not associated with an increased risk of intrauterine growth restriction, except for very-high-order multiples. Am J Obstet Gynecol 1998;179(1):221–5.
90. Stone J, et al: A single center experience with 1000 consecutive cases of multifetal pregnancy reduction (MPR). Am J Obstet Gynecol 2002;185:S96.
91. Stone J, et al: Does elective reduction to a singleton have a better outcome than reduction to twins? Am J Obstet Gynecol 2002;185:S237.
92. Berkowitz RL: Ethical issues involving multifetal pregnancies. Mt Sinai J Med 1998;65(3):185–90; discussion 215–23.
93. Boulot P, et al: Multifetal reduction of triplets to twins: a prospective comparison of pregnancy outcome. Hum Reprod 2000;15(7):1619–23.
94. Leondires MP, et al: Triplets: outcomes of expectant management versus multifetal reduction for 127 pregnancies. Am J Obstet Gynecol 2000;183(2):454–9.
95. Yaron Y, et al: Multifetal pregnancy reductions of triplets to twins: comparison with nonreduced triplets and twins. Am J Obstet Gynecol 1999;180(5):1268–71.
96. Miller VL, et al: Multifetal pregnancy reduction: perinatal and fiscal outcomes. Am J Obstet Gynecol 2000;182(6):1575–80.
97. Papiernik E, et al: Should multifetal pregnancy reduction be used for prevention of preterm deliveries in triplet or higher order multiple pregnancies? J Perinatol Med 1998;26(5):365–70.
98. McElrath TF, et al: Differences in TDx fetal lung maturity assay values between twin and singleton gestations. Am J Obstet Gynecol 2000;182(5):1110–2.
99. Sims CD, et al: The lecithin/sphingomyelin (L/S) ratio in twin pregnancies. Br J Obstet Gynaecol 1976;83(6):447–51.
100. Spellacy WN, Buhi WC: Amniotic fluid lecithin-sphingomyelin ratio as an index of fetal maturity. Obstet Gynecol 1972;39(6):852–60.
101. Obladen M, Gluck L: RDS and tracheal phospholipid composition in twins: independent of gestational age. J Pediatr 1977;90(5):799–802.
102. Wilkinson AR, et al: Uterine position and fetal lung maturity in triplet and quadruplet pregnancy. Lancet 1982;2(8299):663.
103. Norman RJ, et al: Amniotic fluid phospholipids and glucocorticoids in multiple pregnancy. Br J Obstet Gynaecol 1983;90(1):51–5.
104. Landy HJ, et al: The vanishing twin. Acta Genet Med Gemellol 1982;31(3–4):179–94.
105. Nyberg DA, et al: Entangled umbilical cords: a sign of monoamniotic twins. J Ultrasound Med 1984;3(1):29–32.
106. Salerno LJ: Monoamniotic twinning: a survey of the American literature since 1935 with a report of four new cases. Obstet Gynecol 1959;14:205–13.
107. Quigley JK: Monoamniotic twin pregnancy: a case record with review of the literature. Am J Obstet Gynecol 1935;29: 354–62.
108. Carr SR, et al: Survival rates of monoamniotic twins do not decrease after 30 weeks' gestation. Am J Obstet Gynecol 1990;163(3):719–22.
109. D'Alton ME, Simpson LL: Syndromes in twins. Semin Perinatol 1995;19(5):375–86.
110. Rodis JF, et al: Monoamniotic twins: improved perinatal survival with accurate prenatal diagnosis and antenatal fetal surveillance. Am J Obstet Gynecol 1997;177(5):1046–9.
111. Tessen JA, Zlatnik FJ: Monoamniotic twins: a retrospective controlled study. Obstet Gynecol 1991;77(6):832–4.
112. Kantanka KS, Buchmann EJ: Vaginal delivery of monoamniotic twins with umbilical cord entanglement: a case report. J Reprod Med 2001;46(3):275–7.
113. McLeod FN, McCoy DR: Monoamniotic twins with an unusual cord complication. Case report. Br J Obstet Gynaecol 1981;88(7):774–5.
114. House M, et al: Intensive management of monoamniotic twin pregnancies improves perinatal outcome. Am J Obstet Gynecol 2002;185:S113.
115. Malone FD, D'Alton ME: Anomalies peculiar to multiple gestations. Clin Perinatol 2000;27(4):1033–46.
116. Bianchi DW, et al: Fetology: Diagnosis and Management of the Fetal Patient. New York, McGraw-Hill, 2000.
117. Filler RM: Conjoined twins and their separation. Semin Perinatol 1986;10(1):82–91.
118. Rausen AR, et al: Twin transfusion syndrome. J Pediatr 1965;66:613–628.
119. Gonsoulin W, et al: Outcome of twin-twin transfusion diagnosed before 28 weeks of gestation. Obstet Gynecol 1990;75(2):214–6.
120. Chescheir NC, Seeds JW: Polyhydramnios and oligohydramnios in twin gestations. Obstet Gynecol 1988;71(6 Pt 1):882–4.
121. Robertson EG, Neer KJ: Placental injection studies in twin gestation. Am J Obstet Gynecol 1983;147(2):170–4.
122. Lage JM, et al: Vascular anastomoses in fused, dichorionic twin placentas resulting in twin transfusion syndrome. Placenta 1989;10(1):55–9.
123. Bajoria R, et al: Angioarchitecture of monochorionic placentas in relation to the twin-twin transfusion syndrome. Am J Obstet Gynecol 1995;172(3):856–63.
124. Simpson LL, et al: Cardiac dysfunction in twin-twin transfusion syndrome: a prospective, longitudinal study. Obstet Gynecol 1998;92(4 Pt 1):557–62.
125. Quintero RA, et al: Staging of twin-twin transfusion syndrome. J Perinatol 1999;19(8 Pt 1):550–5.
126. De Lia J, et al: Twin transfusion syndrome: successful in utero treatment with digoxin. Int J Gynaecol Obstet 1985;23(3):197–201.
127. Lange IR, et al: Twin with hydramnios: treating premature labor at source. Am J Obstet Gynecol 1989;160(3):552–7.
128. Jones JM, et al: Indomethacin in severe twin-to-twin transfusion syndrome. Am J Perinatol 1993;10(1):24–6.
129. Dennis LG, Winkler CL: Twin-to-twin transfusion syndrome: aggressive therapeutic amniocentesis. Am J Obstet Gynecol 1997;177(2):342–7; discussion 347–9.
130. Dickinson JE, Evans SF: Obstetric and perinatal outcomes from the Australian and New Zealand twin-twin transfusion syndrome registry. Am J Obstet Gynecol 2000;182(3):706–12.
131. Elliott JP, et al: Aggressive therapeutic amniocentesis for treatment of twin-twin transfusion syndrome. Obstet Gynecol 1991;77(4):537–40.
132. Hecher K, et al: Endoscopic laser surgery versus serial amniocenteses in the treatment of severe twin-twin transfusion syndrome. Am J Obstet Gynecol 1999;180(3 Pt 1):717–24.
133. Mahony BS, et al: The "stuck twin" phenomenon: ultrasonographic findings, pregnancy outcome, and management with serial amniocenteses. Am J Obstet Gynecol 1990;163(5 Pt 1):1513–22.
134. Pinette MG, et al: Treatment of twin-twin transfusion syndrome. Obstet Gynecol 1993;82(5): 841–6.
135. Reisner DP, et al: Stuck twin syndrome: outcome in thirty-seven consecutive cases. Am J Obstet Gynecol 1993;169(4):991–5.
136. Saunders NJ, et al: Therapeutic amniocentesis in twin-twin transfusion syndrome appearing in the second trimester of pregnancy. Am J Obstet Gynecol 1992;166(3):820–4.
137. Johnson JR, et al: Amnioreduction versus septostomy in twin-twin transfusion syndrome. Am J Obstet Gynecol 2001;185(5):1044–7.
138. Saade GR, et al: Amniotic septostomy for the treatment of twin oligohydramnios-polyhydramnios sequence. Fetal Diagn Ther 1998;13(2):86–93.
139. Pistorius LR, Howarth GR: Failure of amniotic septostomy in the management of 3 subsequent cases of severe previable twin-twin transfusion syndrome. Fetal Diagn Ther 1999;14(6):337–40.
140. Ville Y, et al: Endoscopic laser coagulation in the management of severe twin-to-twin transfusion syndrome. Br J Obstet Gynaecol 1998;105(4):446–53.
141. Ville Y, et al: Preliminary experience with endoscopic laser surgery for severe twin-twin transfusion syndrome. N Engl J Med 1995;332(4):224–7.
142. De Lia JE, et al: Fetoscopic laser ablation of placental vessels in severe previable twin-twin transfusion syndrome. Am J Obstet Gynecol 1995;172 (4 Pt 1):1202–8; discussion 1208–11.
143. De Lia JE, et al: Fetoscopic neodymium:YAG laser occlusion of placental vessels in severe twin-twin transfusion syndrome. Obstet Gynecol 1990;75(6):1046–53.
144. Van Allen MI, et al: Twin reversed arterial perfusion (TRAP) sequence: a study of 14 twin pregnancies with acardius. Semin Perinatol 1983;7(4):285–93.
145. Healey MG: Acardia: predictive risk factors for the co-twin's survival. Teratology 1994;50(3): 205–13.

146. Moore TR, et al: Perinatal outcome of forty-nine pregnancies complicated by acardiac twinning. Am J Obstet Gynecol 1990;163(3):907–12.

147. Simpson PC, et al: The intrauterine treatment of fetal cardiac failure in a twin pregnancy with an acardiac, acephalic monster. Am J Obstet Gynecol 1983;147(7):842–4.

148. Ash K, et al: TRAP sequence: successful outcome with indomethacin treatment. Obstet Gynecol 1990;76(5 Pt 2):960–2.

149. Fries MH, et al: Treatment of acardiac-acephalus twin gestations by hysterotomy and selective delivery. Obstet Gynecol 1992;79(4):601–4.

150. Robie GF, et al: Selective delivery of an acardiac, acephalic twin. N Engl J Med 1989;320(8):512–3.

151. Ville Y, et al: Endoscopic laser coagulation of umbilical cord vessels in twin reversed arterial perfusion sequence. Ultrasound Obstet Gynecol 1994;4:396–8.

152. Rodeck C, et al: Thermocoagulation for the early treatment of pregnancy with an acardiac twin. N Engl J Med 1998;339(18):1293–5.

153. Porreco RP, et al: Occlusion of umbilical artery in acardiac, acephalic twin. Lancet 1991;337(8737):326–7.

154. Nicolini U, et al: Complicated monochorionic twin pregnancies: experience with bipolar cord coagulation. Am J Obstet Gynecol 2001;185(3):703–7.

155. Quintero RA, et al: In utero percutaneous umbilical cord ligation in the management of complicated monochorionic multiple gestations. Ultrasound Obstet Gynecol 1996;8(1):16–22.

156. Holzgreve W, et al: A simpler technique for umbilical-cord blockade of an acardiac twin. N Engl J Med 1994;331(1):56–7.

157. Denbow ML, et al: High failure rate of umbilical vessel occlusion by ultrasound-guided injection of absolute alcohol or enbucrilate gel. Prenat Diagn 1999;19(6):527–32.

158. Deprest JA, et al: Bipolar coagulation of the umbilical cord in complicated monochorionic twin pregnancy. Am J Obstet Gynecol 2000;182(2):340–5.

159. Deprest JA, et al: Endoscopic cord ligation in selective feticide. Lancet 1996;348(9031):890–1.

160. Arias F, et al: Treatment of acardiac twinning. Obstet Gynecol 1998;91(5 Pt 2):818–21.

161. Johnson CD, Zhang J: Survival of other fetuses after a fetal death in twin or triplet pregnancies. Obstet Gynecol 2002;99(5):698–703.

162. Eglowstein M, D'Alton ME: Intrauterine demise in multiple gestation: theory in management. J Matern Fetal Med 1993;2:272–5.

163. Pharoah PO, Cooke RW: A hypothesis for the aetiology of spastic cerebral palsy: the vanishing twin. Dev Med Child Neurol 1997;39(5):292–6.

164. Fusi L, Gordon H: Twin pregnancy complicated by single intrauterine death. Problems and outcome with conservative management. Br J Obstet Gynaecol 1990;97(6):511–6.

165. D'Alton ME: Antepartum and intrapartum management of multiple pregnancy. Curr Opin Obstet Gynecol 1991;3(6):792–5.

166. Nicolini U, Poblete A: Single intrauterine death in monochorionic twin pregnancies. Ultrasound Obstet Gynecol 1999;14(5):297–301.

167. Okamura K, et al: Funipuncture for evaluation of hematologic and coagulation indices in the surviving twin following co-twin's death. Obstet Gynecol 1994;83(6):975–8.

168. Romero R, et al: Prolongation of a preterm pregnancy complicated by death of a single twin in utero and disseminated intravascular coagulation: effects of treatment with heparin. N Engl J Med 1984;310(12):772–4.

169. Santema JG, et al: Expectant management of twin pregnancy with single fetal death. Br J Obstet Gynaecol 1995;102(1):26–30.

170. Kohl SG, Casey G: Twin gestation. Mt Sinai J Med 1975;42(6):523–39.

171. Malone FD, et al: Outcome of twin gestations complicated by a single anomalous fetus. Obstet Gynecol 1996;88(1):1–5.

172. Malone FD, D'Alton ME: Management of multiple gestations complicated by a single anomalous fetus. Curr Opin Obstet Gynecol 1997;9(3):213–6.

173. Eddleman K, et al: Selective termination (ST) of anomalous fetuses in multifetal pregnancies: 200 cases at a single center. Am J Obstet Gynecol 2002;185:S79.

174. Bebbington MW, et al: Selective feticide in twin transfusion syndrome using ultrasound-guided insertion of thrombogenic coils. Fetal Diagn Ther 1995;10(1):32–6.

175. Dommergues M, et al: Twin-to-twin transfusion syndrome: selective feticide by embolization of the hydropic fetus. Fetal Diagn Ther 1995;10(1):26–31.

Developmental Pharmacology and Pharmacokinetics

19

Sylvain Chemtob

Basic Pharmacologic Principles

PRINCIPLES OF DRUG ABSORPTION, BIOAVAILABILITY, AND DISTRIBUTION

Drug Absorption

Most drugs administered to the premature newborn are injected by the intravenous route and thus are not affected by factors that govern systemic absorption. Some agents are administered intramuscularly (e.g., vitamin K), are administered by an enteral route (e.g., thiazides, caffeine), or applied topically (e.g., topical antiseptics, anesthetics, nitric oxide, bronchodilators). Regardless of the route of administration, drugs must often cross cell membranes to reach their sites of action. Therefore, the mechanisms governing the passage of drugs across cell membranes and the physicochemical properties of molecules and membranes are important to consider in drug transfer. Among the most important physicochemical properties of the drug molecule are lipid solubility, degree of ionization (pKa), molecular weight, and protein binding.

Although some drugs (<200 daltons) cross the cellular lipid membranes by diffusion,[1] it is now well known that many require transporters.[2] The greater the lipid solubility and the lower degree of ionization, the more easily drugs transfer across the cell membrane. Furthermore, because it is believed that the active molecule is the non–protein-bound portion, drugs that have lower protein binding have greater access to their site of action.

Transport Mechanisms

Other than the physicochemical properties of the drug molecules, numerous physiologic transport processes influence the mechanism by which a drug traverses the cell membrane:[3]

1. *Passive diffusion* is the principal transmembrane process for many small drugs. According to Fick's law of diffusion, drug molecules diffuse from a region of high drug concentration to a region of low drug concentration according to the following equation:

$$dQ/dt = DAK/h\ (C_1 - C_2)$$

where dQ/dt = rate of diffusion, D = diffusion coefficient, K = partition coefficient, A = surface area of membrane, h = membrane thickness, and $C_1 - C_2$ = concentration gradient across the membrane. Because D, A, K, and h are

constants under usual conditions, a combined constant P or permeability coefficient may be defined: P = DAK/h. Therefore, the previous equation can be simplified to the following:

$$dQ/dt = P(C_1 - C_2)$$

This equation does not take into account the ionization state of the drug molecule, the effect of regional blood flow, or the influence of tissue affinity on drug partitioning. The ionization state is affected by the pH on both sides of the membrane, according to the Henderson-Hasselbalch equation:

$$pH = pKa + \log\ (base/acid)$$

Therefore, acidic compounds, such as salicylic acid, diffuse across cell membranes more readily when the environmental pH is low because they are less ionized at low pH. Regional blood flow also influences the rate of diffusion because this alters the delivery and consequently the local concentration of drug. Finally, some drugs demonstrate increased affinity for a particular tissue component, which influences the concentration of drug on either side of the membrane. For example, tetracycline forms a complex with calcium in the bones and teeth.

2. *Active transport* is a carrier-mediated transmembrane process that plays an important role in the renal, intestinal, and biliary secretion and absorption of many drugs and metabolites. Active transport is characterized by a transfer of molecules against a concentration gradient. Thus, energy must be consumed to achieve this process. An example of this transport system is contributed by the adenosine triphosphate (ATP)-dependent secretion of organic acids in the renal tubule that permits secretion of indomethacin.[4] This process, in contrast to diffusion, is saturable and therefore follows Michaelis-Menten kinetics.

3. *Facilitated diffusion* is also a carrier-mediated transport system, in which, in contrast to active transport, molecules move along a concentration gradient. This system does not require energy input but is also saturable and selective. A major class of transporters involved in facilitated diffusion includes the organic cation transporters, the organic anion transporters, and the dipeptide transporters, including

PEPT1, that incorporate in cells numerous drugs[2,5,6]; examples of drugs transported by these transporters include corticosterone, ethacrynic acid, and captopril, respectively.

4. *Pinocytosis* is the process of engulfing large molecules such as immunoglobins.[7]

Membrane Transporters

Transporters are membrane-integrated proteins that facilitate movement of nutrients such as amino acids, dipeptides and tripeptides, sugars, nucleosides, vitamins, and bile acids into cells. In the intestine, it has now become increasingly clear that several of these transporters play a significant role in drug absorption. Cellular import of numerous nutrients and drugs depends on transporters that use voltage and ion gradients generated by primary transporters and exchangers. Sodium (Na^+) and protons are frequently cotransported with the compound of interest. Because the activity of a given transporter is a function of the electrochemical gradient driving force, the efficiency of the transport is influenced by the activity of the Na^+/H^+ antiporter and of the Na^+/HCO_3^- symporter.

Certain membrane transporters play key roles in drug import. These include the H^+/dipeptide symporters, facilitative glucose transporter-related proteins, Na^+/glucose and Na^+/nucleoside cotransporters, amino acid transporters, Na^+/neurotransmitter symporters, and the organic cation and anion transporters.[2,5,6,8] The H^+/dipeptide symporters carry cephalosporins and angiotensin-converting enzyme inhibitors, the organic cation transporters carry antihistaminics and β-blockers, and the organic anion transporters carry aspirin, indomethacin, and methotrexate. These ports of entry along with their structural polymorphisms may pose an additional challenge to pharmacokinetics and drug delivery.

Kinetics of Absorption

Most pharmacokinetic models assume that drug absorption and elimination follow *first-order kinetics* (i.e., the rate of change in the concentration of a drug depends on the amount of drug present at that particular time). This process is described in the following equation:

$$dD_B/dt = FK_aD_{si} - K_{el}D_B$$

where dD_B/dt = rate of change of drug in the body (D_B), F = fraction absorbed (bioavailability term), K_a and K_{el} = absorption and elimination constants, and D_{si} = drug concentration at the site of absorption. This equation assumes a single-compartment pharmacokinetic model. In a single-compartment model, the drug rapidly equilibrates with tissues of the body. Therefore, changes in the concentration of the drug in serum or plasma mirror those in the tissues. Although many drugs follow multiple-compartment kinetics, the K_a may still be calculated from a one-compartment model.[9] The importance of the K_a lies in the design of a multiple dosage regimen. Knowledge of the K_a and K_{el} allows for the prediction of the peak and trough steady-state plasma drug concentrations ($C_{ss\ max}$ and $C_{ss\ min}$) after multiple dosing concentrations (see the later section on clinical pharmacokinetics and Fig. 19–3)[10]:

$$C_{ss\ max} = (FD_{si}/V_d)/(1 - e^{-Kelt}); C_{ss\ min} = C_{ss\ max} \cdot e^{-Kelt}$$

where τ = dosing interval. From these equations, it is evident that peak and trough concentrations depend on the absorption rate, the volume of distribution, the elimination rate constant, and the dosing interval.

Factors Affecting Absorption of Drugs

The systemic absorption of a drug from its site of administration depends on the variables discussed previously, which constitute the physicochemical properties of the agent and of the membrane. Other factors can also influence the efficiency of drug absorption, including the following: the disintegration, dissolution, and solubility of the compound; the blood flow to the site of absorption; the surface area available for absorption; the transit time of the drug through the gastrointestinal tract; the export of drugs by P-glycoproteins in enterocytes; and *in situ* metabolism of the agent, including the first-pass effect. A *first-pass effect* is defined as the rapid uptake and metabolism of an agent into inactive compounds by the liver, immediately after enteric absorption and before the agent reaches the systemic circulation. Drugs that exhibit a first-pass effect include morphine, isoproterenol, propranolol, and hydralazine. Each of the factors affecting absorption, taken separately or in conjunction, may have profound effects on the efficacy and toxicity of a drug.

When evaluating absorption of drugs through the gastrointestinal tract of the newborn, the developmental stages of this organ must be taken into account.[11] Gastric acid secretion is low in premature infants.[12] The increased pH results in a reduced absorption of weak acids and bases. In contrast, lipid-soluble drugs (e.g., methylxanthines) are more easily absorbed in newborns than in older children.[13] Bile salt secretion is also diminished in the newborn infant,[14] and this can secondarily reduce the absorption of fats and lipid-soluble vitamins, such as vitamins D and E;[15,16] conversely, vitamin E is adequately absorbed in premature infants,[17] probably because of a lower intake of iron.[18]

Enzymatic development of the gastrointestinal tract may also alter drug absorption. The elevated activity of β-glucuronidase in the brush border of newborn intestine may deconjugate drug-glucuronide conjugates,[19] thus resulting in enhanced reabsorption of free unconjugated drug into the systemic circulation; this may prolong the pharmacologic activity of certain agents, such as indomethacin.[20] In contrast, the presence of P-glycoproteins, highly distributed in the gastrointestinal tract epithelium apical brush border as well as in the bile canalicular face of hepatocytes, can reduce drug absorption and bioavailability;[21] lower expression of P-glycoproteins in the immature subject may contribute to variable bioavailability.[22] Although modulators of P-glycoproteins, primarily cyclosporin A and verapamil, have been used with marginal efficacy to enhance drug action such as in cancer,[23,24] these drugs exert their own toxicity; selective inhibitors of P-glycoproteins and related multidrug resistance proteins have yet to be developed. Another factor that influences drug absorption and access to the target organ is the presence of metabolizing enzymes in intestinal epithelium; this is especially the case for cytochrome P450 enzymes.[25] Depending on their activity, limited or excess bioavailability may be observed.

In comparison with adults, newborn infants also exhibit qualitative and quantitative differences in the bacterial colonization of their gastrointestinal tracts. The development of the intestinal flora has been clearly shown to affect the absorption of vitamin K.[26] Thus, maturation of the gastrointestinal tract may also explain some of the characteristics of intestinal absorption of drugs in the growing child.

Finally, in addition to the physiologic changes in the gastrointestinal tract that occur during development, drug absorption can also be altered by disease processes. Diseases of genetic (e.g., cystic fibrosis) and microbial or circulatory (e.g., necrotizing enterocolitis) origin may alter the intestinal mucosa and may result in a reduced absorptive surface.

Bioavailability

Drug bioavailability is the fraction of the administered dose that reaches the systemic circulation. For the clinician, the most relevant consideration is the percentage of active drug that reaches the central compartment. Bioavailability does not take into account the rate at which the drug is absorbed. Bioavailability is affected by factors that influence absorption. The absolute availability of a drug may be determined by comparing the respective area under the plasma concentration curves (AUC) after oral (PO) and intravenous (IV) administration.

$$\text{Absolute availability} = [\text{AUC}_{PO}/\text{dose}_{PO}] / [\text{AUC}_{IV}/\text{dose}_{IV}]$$

This measurement may be performed as long as the volume of distribution (V_d) and the elimination rate constant (K_{el}) are independent of the route of administration.

Distribution

The *disposition* of a drug refers to its passage in the body from absorption to excretion. After absorption, a drug is distributed to various body compartments. This distribution determines its efficacy as well as its toxicity. The distribution of drugs is influenced by several factors, including the size of the body water and lipid compartments, regional hemodynamic features, and the degree of binding of drugs to plasma and tissue proteins. The initial phase of distribution reflects regional blood flow. Organs that are well perfused, such as the brain, heart, and kidneys, are the first exposed to the drug. The second phase of distribution involves a large fraction of the body mass, including the muscle and adipose mass. Thus, the various distribution compartments form the apparent volume of distribution (V_d), which is expressed by the following equation:

$$V_d = \text{total drug in the body / concentration of drug in plasma}$$

Assuming instant equilibration of the drug after administration, V_d can be determined by extrapolating the drug concentration to time zero (C_0) and dividing the dose of drug administered by the concentration of drug at time zero (C_0). This equation, however, can be applied only to a single-compartment model. V_d may also be calculated using the following equation, which is independent of the model used:

$$V_d = \text{Dose} / K_{el} [\text{AUC}]_0^\infty$$

Physiologic and Pathologic Factors Affecting Distribution of Drugs

The factors that influence the distribution of drugs in the body are subject to developmental changes. The amount and distribution of total body water undergo marked changes in the perinatal period.[27] Total body water and extracellular fluid volume decrease with increasing gestational age. Consequently, the volume of distribution of many drugs has been observed to increase in preterm neonates.[28] After birth, total body water decreases, and the volume of intracellular fluid increases relative to that of the extracellular fluid. In the term newborn, as reported for the older child,[29] the degree of insensible water loss is linked to the metabolic rate of the infant. In contrast, in the preterm newborn, there is no fixed relationship between metabolic rate and insensible water loss, and in the very low birth weight infant, evaporative heat loss is substantially greater than heat produced by basal metabolic rate.[17,30]

Many disorders of the newborn as well as drugs administered to critically ill newborn infants (e.g., diuretics[31,32]) can affect total body water and, secondarily, the distribution of drugs. For instance, renal and hepatic dysfunctions may have important consequences on both elimination and distribution of xenobiotics. Similarly, diseases that lead to increased total body water (e.g., congestive heart failure, syndrome of inappropriate secretion of antidiuretic hormone) can have profound effects on drug pharmacokinetics and pharmacodynamics. Therefore, any change in either total body water content or the relationship between extracellular and intracellular fluid volume may have significant effects on the distribution of drugs within the body.

The extent and disposition of the lipid mass in the body also contribute to the distribution of drugs. The adipose tissue mass changes markedly during development. Between 28 and 40 weeks of gestation, the amount of adipose tissue (expressed as a percentage of total body mass) increases from 1% to 15%,[33] and by 1 year of age, it represents 25% of body mass.

The nervous system contains a high proportion of lipids. Normally, the maximal increment in weight of the human brain occurs in the few weeks preceding term gestation; however, a substantial part of myelination (and lipid deposition) occurs postnatally.[34] The entry of drugs into the central nervous system is generally restricted. In contrast to capillaries elsewhere in the body, endothelial cells of brain capillaries exhibit a predominance of tight junctions producing nonfenestrated capillaries, which restrict the penetration of hydrophilic substances into the brain. Consequently, ionized molecules, such as quaternary amines (e.g., neostigmine), exhibit limited capacity to diffuse into the central nervous system, whereas lipid-soluble compounds, such as chloramphenicol and pentobarbital, traverse the blood-brain barrier.

The distribution of drugs into brain and other organs is also dependent on specific transporters of nutrients and endogenous compounds, as described earlier. Furthermore, efflux carriers present in brain endothelium and glia, primarily P-glycoproteins, limit drug concentration in brain. This is well described for a number of drugs including human immunodeficiency virus (HIV) protease inhibitors, vinca alkaloids, and anthracyclines.[35] P-glycoproteins are also present in placenta and function as export transporters to limit fetal exposure to potentially toxic agents.

A major determinant of drug distribution is the cardiac output and blood flow to various organs.[36] Marked changes in the neonatal circulation take place during the perinatal period.[37,38] In addition, regional blood flow may also change acutely as a result of congestive heart failure (secondary to patent ductus arteriosus or other congenital heart diseases),[36] as a result of sudden changes in acid-base balance (especially respiratory acidosis), or secondary to the limited ability of the stressed preterm neonate to autoregulate regional blood flow.[39]

The affinity of a drug for plasma proteins is another important variable affecting drug distribution. The degree of binding is inversely related to the volume of distribution, such that increased protein binding tends to maintain the drug within the vascular space. Protein binding affects renal and plasma clearance, the half-life, and the efficacy of the agent at its site of action. Table 19-1 lists the protein binding of some commonly used agents in the neonate.

Several factors modify the binding of drugs to plasma proteins:

1. The amount of plasma binding proteins
2. The number of binding sites
3. The affinity of the drug for the protein
4. Pathophysiologic conditions that alter drug-protein binding, such as blood pH, free fatty acids, bilirubin, other drugs, and disease states (e.g. renal failure, liver failure)

Albumin binds principally acidic drugs, whereas basic agents are bound to lipoproteins, β-globulins, and α_1-acid glycoproteins.[40] Albumin contains a few high-affinity and several low-affinity binding sites.[41] In the preterm newborn, both albumin and α_1-acid glycoprotein concentrations and binding affinities are deficient, resulting in an increased fraction of free drug[42] and increased distribution of free drug outside the vascular compartment.[43] Numerous conditions may further reduce the binding of drugs to proteins. For example, a decrease in pH may enhance the dissociation of weak acids from their albumin binding sites. Thus, the frequent occurrence of acidosis in premature infants may significantly change the binding of drugs to plasma proteins. The elevated plasma free fatty acid content of the newborn may also alter drug binding to plasma proteins;[44,45] this effect, however,

TABLE 19-1

Plasma Protein Binding of Commonly Used Drugs in the Newborn

Drug	Percentage of Drug Protein-Bound
Ampicillin	≈10
Atropine	25
Caffeine	25
Cefotaxime	25–50
Dexamethasone	65
Digoxin	20
Ethacrynic acid	95
Furosemide	95
Gentamicin	45
Hydrochlorothiazide	40
Indomethacin	95
Morphine	30
Phenobarbital	≈20
Phenytoin	≈80
Theophylline	35

Data from refs. 76–79.

TABLE 19-2

Drugs That Cause Significant Displacement of Bilirubin from Albumin *in Vitro*

Sulfonamides
Moxalactam
Fusidic acid
Radiographic contrast media for cholangiography (sodium iodipamide, sodium ipodate, iopanoic acid, meglumine ioglycamate)
Aspirin
Apazone
Tolbutamide
Albumin preservatives (sodium caprylate and *N*-acetyl tryptophan: rapid infusions *in vivo*)
High concentrations of ampicillin (rapid infusions *in vivo*)
Long-chain free fatty acids (FFA) at high molar ratios of FFA to albumin

may be questionable.[46] In a similar fashion, maternal drugs that have crossed the placenta or other agents concomitantly administered to the infant may also compete for the same plasma protein binding sites of drugs given to the newborn.

The potential interference of endogenous compounds, particularly unconjugated bilirubin, on drug-protein binding has been well addressed.[47] A displacement of bilirubin from its albumin binding site may result in free circulating unconjugated bilirubin, which can penetrate into the brain and ultimately cause injury. Bilirubin itself, however, is tightly bound to albumin and may displace drugs from their protein binding sites.[47] In addition, free bilirubin is only sparingly lipophilic. Thus, the drug-induced displacement of bilirubin from albumin binding sites possibly plays a minor role in the development of bilirubin-induced encephalopathy. Nonetheless, a few drugs can alter the binding affinity of albumin for bilirubin (Table 19-2).[47]

The volume of distribution of certain compounds is also affected by their binding to proteins outside the vascular space. For instance, digoxin exhibits a higher degree of binding to myocardial and skeletal proteins in the newborn than in the adult.[48, 49] This results in an increase in the volume of distribution of digoxin.

Numerous factors influence the distribution of drugs in the body. These factors are themselves affected by development and disease conditions of the newborn infant. Major changes in the distribution of fluids and fat and their proportion relative to body mass occur at the end of gestation and during the neonatal period. Perinatal and neonatal alterations in cardiac output and regional blood flow, secondary to physiologic and pathophysiologic changes, also occur. Furthermore, the degree of drug binding to plasma proteins between the newborn and adult varies for several drugs. These variables should be taken into account when deciding on the appropriate drug dosage for a newborn.

PRINCIPLES OF DRUG ELIMINATION

The relatively high lipophilicity of many drugs does not permit their rapid elimination. After filtration through the glomerulus or passage into the bile, these agents are readily absorbed by the renal tubule or gastrointestinal mucosa. Consequently, the elimination of most drugs from the body involves the process of biotransformation followed by excretion. This section reviews the different biotransformation processes that take place in the human body and the mechanisms of renal drug excretion, with particular reference to developmental aspects.

Drug Biotransformation

Drug biotransformation converts drug molecules into more polar derivatives that are less able to diffuse across cell membranes. As a consequence of biotransformation, these converted molecules do not reach their receptors and, in addition, are not reabsorbed by the renal tubule. Thus, biotransformation of drugs not only facilitates their excretion from the body but also may diminish their pharmacologic activity.

The metabolism of drugs does not always produce inactive compounds. Initial biotransformation of certain agents results in the formation of active metabolites. For instance, codeine is demethylated to morphine, acetylsalicylic acid is hydrolyzed to salicylic acid, and theophylline is methylated to caffeine. Furthermore, oxidation of certain aromatic compounds produces highly reactive *electrophiles* (compounds that serve as electron acceptors). This latter reaction may be primary (aromatic hydrocarbons) or it may be an increasingly active secondary reaction resulting from an inhibited or overwhelmed primary metabolic pathway (e.g., due to an excessive dose of the agent, as in acetaminophen overdose). Therefore, biotransformation can produce relatively innocuous metabolites or highly toxic compounds.

The mechanisms affecting the biotransformation of drugs are usually the same as those that metabolize endogenous products (e.g., hormones). Most biotransformation takes place in the liver, but some may occur at other sites, such as the kidneys, intestinal mucosa, and lungs. Biotransformation reactions are classically divided into two phases: phase I, the nonsynthetic reactions; and phase II, the synthetic or conjugation reactions (Table 19-3). Each phase has reactions that can take place in the microsomes or outside the microsomal system. Most phase I reactions (oxidation, reduction, and hydrolysis) are catalyzed by microsomal enzymes; other than glucuronidation, phase II reactions are extramicrosomal.

Phase I Reactions (Nonsynthetic Reactions)

Microsomal. The portion of microsomes that contain the enzymes that metabolize drugs is localized in the smooth endoplasmic reticulum. The oxidative enzymes of this system have attracted particular attention. This group of enzymes has been called mixed-function oxidases or monooxygenases. They consist of three principal components: an electron transporter, nicotinamide adenine dinucleotide phosphate (NADPH)-cytochrome P450 reductase (a flavoprotein), and one of the many cytochrome P450 isozymes (designated by CYP and a

TABLE 19-3

Biotransformation Reactions

Reaction	Examples of Drug Substrates
Phase I (Nonsynthetic Reactions)	
(a) *Oxidation*	
Aromatic ring hydroxylation	Phenytoin, phenobarbital
Aliphatic hydroxylation	Ibuprofen
N-hydroxylation	Acetaminophen
N-, *O*-, *S*-dealkylation	Morphine, codeine
Deamination	Diazepam
Sulfoxidation, *N*-oxidation	Cimetidine
(b) *Reduction*	
Azoreduction	Prontosil
Nitroreduction	Chloramphenicol
Alcohol dehydrogenase	Ethanol
(c) *Hydrolysis*	
Ester hydrolysis	Acetylsalicylic acid
Amide hydrolysis	Indomethacin
Phase I (Enzymes)	
CYP1A1	Caffeine, theophylline
CYP2C	Warfarin, ibuprofen, phenytoin, omeprazole, diazepam
CYP2D6	Codeine, imipramine, propranolol, timolol, tamoxifen
CYP2E1	Acetaminophen, caffeine, tamoxifen
CYP3A	Erythromycin, midazolam, 6β-hydroxycortisol
Phase II (Synthetic Reactions: Conjugations)	
(a) Glucuronide conjugation	Morphine, acetaminophen
(b) Glycine conjugation	Salicylic acid
(c) Sulfate conjugation	Acetaminophen, α-methyldopa
(d) Glutathione conjugation	Ethacrynic acid
(e) Methylation	Dopamine, epinephrine
(f) Acetylation	Sulfonamides, clonazepam

Adapted from ref. 80.

TABLE 19-4

Ontogeny of Human Phase I and Phase II Metabolizing Enzymes

Enzyme	Fetus	Newborn	Infant	Adult
Phase I				
CYP1A1	+	–	–	–
CYP1A2	–	–	+	+
CYP2C	–	+	+	+
CYP2D6	+/–	+	+	+
CYP2E1	+/–	+	+	+
CYP3A7	+	+	–	–
CYP3A4/5	–	+	+	+
Phase II				
UGT1A1	–	+	+	+
UGT1A3	+/–	+/–	+	+
UGT2B7	+/–	+/–	+	+
GSTA	+/–	+/–	+	+
SULT1A1	+/–	+/–	+	+
SULT1A3	+	+	+	+/–

UGT = UDP-glucuronosyltransferase; GST = glutathione *S*-transferase; SULT = sulfotransferase.

There are approximately 1000 known cytochrome P450s; only about 50 are functionally active in humans. Seventeen families and many subfamilies have been sequenced. CYP1, CYP2, and CYP3 families are involved in the majority of all drug metabolism reactions; members of the other families are important in the synthesis and degradation of steroids, fatty acids, vitamins, and other endogenous compounds. Individual CYP isoforms tend to have substrate specificities, but overlap is common. CYP3A4 and CYP3A5 are similar isoforms, which together are involved in metabolism of approximately 50% of drugs. CYP2C and CYP2D6 are also involved in metabolism of many drugs. CYP1A1/2, CYP2A6, CYP2B1, and CYP2E1 are not extensively involved in drug metabolism but, rather, in activation of procarcinogenic agents including aromatic amines and aromatic hydrocarbons.

The cytochrome P450–dependent monooxygenase system develops in fetal life, but in general its activity in the fetus and newborn remains considerably lower than that found in adult liver.[25, 51] The diminished enzyme activity may be clinically important because drugs that are oxygenated slowly by these enzymes (e.g., phenobarbital and phenytoin) can exhibit a prolonged half-life in the young infant;[52] this is especially the case for CYP2A, CYP2B6, CYP2C, and CYP3A4/5 (Table 19–4). However, there are significant differences in the developmental expression of the three important gene families implicated in xenobiotic metabolism; accordingly, drugs converted by CYP2D6 and CYP3A7 such as carbamazepine, dextromethorphan, and tricyclic antidepressants are eliminated in the newborn nearly as rapidly as in the adult.[25] CYP2E1 is induced and metabolized by ethanol in the fetus and has been proposed to be implicated in the development of fetal alcohol syndrome.[53]

Extramicrosomal. A few of the oxidative and reductive reactions are mediated by enzymes in the mitochondria and cytosol of the liver and other tissues. These enzymes include the following: those involved in oxidation of alcohols and aldehydes; alcohol and aldehyde dehydrogenases; and enzymes that partake in the metabolism of catecholamines, tyrosine hydroxylase, and monoamine oxidase. Although the activity of some of these enzymes can be detected early in gestation, their full activity is reached only in early childhood.[25] However, once again, marked ontogenic differences among enzymes are observed. For instance, class I alcohol dehydrogenase, the major ethanol-metabolizing enzyme, tends to be well expressed in fetal liver, whereas class III alcohol dehydrogenase is relatively deficient in the fetus.[25]

number that refers to the gene family and subfamily to which they belong), which are oxidase hemoproteins.[50] The system requires both a reducing agent, NADPH, and molecular oxygen. The end result of the reactions catalyzed by cytochrome P450 is the incorporation of one oxygen atom into the endogenous or exogenous compound being metabolized (hence the name *monooxygenase*) and the formation of water after reduction of the second oxygen atom.

The reactions catalyzed by the microsomal monooxygenases include aromatic ring and aliphatic side chain hydroxylation, *N*-, *O*-, and *S*-dealkylation, deamination, dehalogenation, sulfoxidation, *N*-oxidation, *N*-hydroxylation, nitroreduction, and azoreduction. Epoxides are also formed by monooxygenases, thus converting aromatic moieties of agents to arene and alkene oxides, which are, in turn, detoxified by epoxide hydrolases present in endoplasmic reticulum. These electrophilic compounds react avidly with proteins and nucleic acids and exert potential mutagenic and carcinogenic effects; polychlorinated and polybrominated biphenyls exert their toxicity through their metabolites.[50]

Several drugs, including cimetidine, spironolactone, and propylthiouracil, can inhibit cytochrome P450 enzyme activity. This inhibition reduces the metabolism of potential substrates and secondarily retards their elimination. In contrast, other substrates can act as inducers of the cytochrome P450 system. Prototypes of the most extensively studied inducers of separate cytochrome P450 isozymes are phenobarbital (CYP3A), rifampin (CYP1A, CYP2C), and the polycyclic aromatic hydrocarbon 3-methylcholanthrene (CYP1A).

Phase II Reactions (Synthetic Reactions)

In phase II reactions, molecules that are naturally present in the body are conjugated or combined with the drug or other endogenous compounds. The drug may have first undergone a phase I reaction, or the original drug may be directly conjugated. Conjugation converts drugs into more polar compounds, which are pharmacologically less active and are more readily excreted; an exception applies to acetylation, whereby the metabolite is often less water soluble. Although it was previously thought that conjugation reactions represented true inactivation and detoxification reactions, it is currently known that certain conjugation reactions may lead to the formation of reactive species responsible for hepatotoxicity (N-acetylation of isoniazid). The major conjugation reactions are listed in Table 19-4.

Glucuronidation. The formation of glucuronides is the principal conjugation reaction in the body. Natural substrates of this pathway include bilirubin and thyroxine. Many drugs containing hydroxyl, amino, carboxyl, thiol, and phenolic groups, however, also use the same pathway (e.g., morphine, acetaminophen, phenytoin, sulfonamides, chloramphenicol, salicylic acid, and indomethacin).

The conjugation of a compound with glucuronic acid results in the production of a strongly acidic substance that is more water soluble at physiologic pH than the parent compound. This reduces its transfer across membranes, facilitates its dissociation with its receptor, and enhances its elimination in urine and bile. The fate of the glucuronidated drugs in urine or bile depends on their molecular size. Compounds with relatively low molecular weights are almost completely excreted in urine, whereas those with high molecular weights (>500 molecular weight) are eliminated almost entirely in bile.

Glucuronides are eliminated by the kidneys predominantly by glomerular filtration; however, tubular secretion and tubular reabsorption followed by secretion represent alternative pathways. Biliary excretion of drugs conjugated to glucuronic acid occurs by simple diffusion or by active secretion. Once in the intestine, these drugs may be reabsorbed after being deconjugated (hydrolyzed) by glucuronidase, which exhibits an elevated activity in the fetus and newborn.[19]

Drugs or conditions that inhibit formation of glucuronides are likely to prolong the pharmacologic activity of these agents. Inhibition may occur at the level of the synthesis of glucuronic acid (e.g., by certain steroid hormones) or at the level of the uridine diphosphate glucuronyl transferase activity itself, which consists of 16 different isoforms in humans. In the human fetus and newborn, glucuronide conjugation reactions have reduced activity, and fetal underexpression of the 2B isoform is responsible for the gray baby syndrome associated with chloramphenicol intake. Postnatal development proceeds relatively rapidly, as occurs with the metabolism of bilirubin.[54,55]

Other Synthetic Conjugation Reactions. Other kinds of conjugation reactions that occur in the body are listed in Table 19-4. As is the case with glucuronyl transferase, the activity of the other various transferases is also lower in the fetus and newborn, in contrast to those of the adult.[54,55]

Overall, available data permit the following generalizations regarding drug metabolism in the fetus and newborn:

1. The rates of drug biotransformation and overall elimination are slow.
2. The rate of drug elimination from the body exhibits marked interpatient variability.
3. The maturational changes in drug metabolism and disposition as a function of postnatal age are extremely variable and depend on the substrate (or drug) used.
4. Neonatal drug biotransformation and elimination are vulnerable to pathophysiologic states.
5. Neonates may exhibit activation of alternate biotransformation pathways.

Factors Affecting Biotransformation in the Liver

Several factors may alter the rate, extent, and type of biotransformation reactions in the liver. The issues of enzyme activity that may be modified by development and by endogenous or exogenous compounds have been addressed. Environmental influences also significantly affect drug metabolism; this includes the inducing or inhibitory effects of drugs per se on enzyme activities. For instance, calcium channel blockers, antifungal agents, and macrolide antibiotics are potent inhibitors of CYP3A enzymes, quinidine inhibits CYP2D6, and other compounds such as cimetidine, amiodarone, and fluoxetine reduce activity of many cytochrome P450 enzymes. Conversely, numerous agents, including anticonvulsants and aromatic hydrocarbons, can stimulate induction of certain CYP subfamilies and isoforms.

Metabolic enzyme activity is also affected by genetic factors; this is the rule rather than the exception. However, the interplay between ontogeny and genetics remains largely unknown in drug metabolism. There exist approximately 70 single nucleotide polymorphisms and other genetic variants of the *CYP2D6* gene, many of which yield diminished enzyme activity; this may significantly affect drugs metabolized by CYP2D6 such as β-blockers and certain opiates. In the case of CYP3A enzymes, no significant functional polymorphisms have been yet identified; hence factors regulating gene expression are more important to explain the interindividual variability (>10-fold). Because genetic factors and environmental influences exert greater effects on drug metabolism than they do on renal excretion, drugs that are metabolized are considerably more strongly affected by interpersonal differences than those not requiring biotransformation.

Other factors that affect biotransformation include blood flow to the liver, gender, and disease states. For certain drugs (e.g., morphine, meperidine, propranolol, and verapamil), blood flow may be the limiting factor controlling drug elimination. These drugs (often termed *flow-limited* drugs) are so readily metabolized by the liver that hepatic clearance is essentially equal to liver blood flow. In contrast, the biotransformation of *capacity-limited* drugs (e.g., phenytoin, theophylline, diazepam, and chloramphenicol) is determined by the liver's metabolizing capacity rather than by hepatic blood flow.[56] The effect of gender in newborn infants remains unclear, but it may not be as important as in the adult.

Renal Excretion of Drugs

The renal excretion of drugs and their metabolites occurs through three major processes: glomerular filtration, active tubular secretion, and passive tubular reabsorption. After the entry of a drug into a renal tubule, its elimination is dependent on its lipophilicity and ionization state.

Glomerular Filtration of Drugs

The amount of drug filtered through the glomerulus depends on a molecular size less than that of albumin (molecular weight 69,000) and the degree of protein binding. Hence, nearly all non–protein-bound drugs are filtered. Glomerular filtration rate increases during fetal development, but in the newborn it remains far less than that observed in the adult.[57-60] Furthermore, conditions that lead to decreased glomerular filtration rate, such as asphyxia, severe respiratory insufficiency, renal failure, and patent ductus arteriosus, are associated with reduced drug excretion. Certain agents (e.g., indomethacin, tolazoline) may hamper their own excretion by reducing glomerular filtration rate.[61-63]

Active Tubular Transport of Drugs

Numerous transport systems found in the proximal tubule are involved in the energy-dependent secretion of organic compounds (endogenous or xenobiotic).[64] These carrier systems are relatively nonselective. One such system transports organic anions, including drug conjugates with glucuronic acid, glycine, and sulfates; examples of drugs that use this excretory system include penicillins, furosemide, and chlorothiazide. The other transport system secretes organic cations, such as histamine and choline. Multidrug resistance proteins 1, 3, 5, and 6 are localized at the basolateral membrane, whereas multidrug resistance proteins 2 and 4 are found at the brush-border membrane of tubular epithelium. Generally, these transporters operate as efflux pumps. A counteracting mechanism involves the peptide transporters PEPT1 and especially PEPT2 localized at the proximal tubular epithelium apex, which operate as influx pumps of filtered drugs. All transporters described are energy dependent. In the case of organic cation, organic anion, and peptide transporters, cellular import requires an electrochemical gradient, especially of Na^+, which is largely maintained by the Na^+/K^+ ATPase pump, whereas multidrug resistance proteins are directly ATP dependent.[64] Membrane transporters, mainly located in the distal tubule, actively reabsorb drugs from the tubular lumen back into the systemic circulation. Most such reabsorption occurs by nonionic diffusion.

Tubular secretion of organic anions and cations is also lower in newborns than it is in adults. This developmental characteristic explains the prolonged half-life of certain agents that use this system of elimination, such as furosemide, penicillins, and glucuronidated drugs, in the newborn.

Passive Tubular Reabsorption of Drugs

In both proximal and distal tubules, nonionized forms of weak acids and bases undergo net passive reabsorption. Accordingly, this form of renal reabsorption of drugs is regulated by three factors: the concentration gradient across the tubular membrane, the ionization state of the compound in the tubular fluid (which depends on the drug's pKa and the tubular fluid pH), and the lipid solubility of the drug. Manipulation of these physicochemical properties can be used to enhance renal excretion. For instance, alkalinization of the urine can increase the elimination of salicylic acid by up to sixfold.

Overall, patterns of renal excretion of drugs can be summarized as follows:

1. Renal excretion of lipid-soluble drugs depends largely on urine volume.
2. Elimination of polar drugs depends on glomerular filtration rate.
3. The renal elimination of drugs that ionize readily is principally dependent on the activity of the tubular secretory systems and the urine pH.

Effect of Disease on Drug Elimination

Most pharmacokinetic parameters are determined on healthy or moderately ill persons. In neonatal intensive care units, as in other similar environments, drugs are often administered to very sick patients. Life-threatening illnesses produce remarkable variation in pharmacokinetic behavior. Adjustment in drug dosage in the presence of a changing disease is critical to avoid toxicity.[11, 65] For this reason, an understanding of the pathophysiology of a disease and its pharmacologic consequences becomes of utmost importance for appropriate pharmacologic therapy. This section addresses the issue of diseases as applied to drug disposition in the newborn.

Cardiovascular Disease

Cardiac output is a major determinant of drug elimination. Heart failure produces a decrease in cardiac output that alters the regional distribution of blood flow. Significant decreases in cardiac output or oxygen delivery can result in adverse effects on liver function and consequently can diminish drug clearance.[66]

Congestive heart failure is also associated with a reduction in renal blood flow and glomerular filtration rate. This compromise in renal function contributes to a decrease in drug elimination. In newborns with congestive heart failure, elevated plasma levels of digoxin have been observed, a finding suggesting a decreased clearance of the drug.

Renal Disease

Because the kidneys are a major source of drug elimination, alterations in their function can significantly influence drug pharmacokinetics.[58] The pharmacologic consequences of renal dysfunction depend on the fraction of drug cleared by the kidneys and on the degree of renal failure. Under these circumstances, drugs for which the kidneys represent their primary route of elimination (e.g., aminoglycosides, cephalosporins) accumulate in the body; this is especially true when renal clearance is greater than 90% of total clearance.

As glomerular filtration rate falls, there is a decrease in drugs eliminated principally by this route, such as digoxin, aminoglycosides, and cephalosporins. Reduction in tubular function can significantly affect the elimination of drugs that depend on tubular reabsorption or secretion, such as penicillins and furosemide. In addition, changes in plasma and urine pH alter the excretion of ionized drugs. The development of uremia may be associated with changes in cardiac output, liver function, and blood-brain barrier permeability, all of which can further disturb drug disposition.

The clinical significance of drug accumulation depends on whether the unexcreted products are pharmacologically active or toxic. Nomograms have been developed to allow modification of drug dosage in patients with renal failure. However, most nomograms primarily apply to adults and not to infants and thus must be used with caution.

Liver Disease

Because the liver is a major site of drug disposition, hepatic insufficiency is associated with defects in multiple liver functions, many of which have the potential to alter drug excretion. Hepatic insufficiency can affect drug elimination by (1) reducing plasma protein binding, (2) decreasing liver blood flow, and (3) disturbing intrinsic biotransformation reactions.

A decrease in plasma protein concentration influences the disposition of drugs extensively bound to proteins. Drugs with liver uptake and metabolism can be categorized into two groups: one dependent on liver blood flow (*flow-limited* drugs) and the other dependent on the liver's metabolic capacity (*capacity-limited* drugs). Drugs belonging to the first group exhibit a more uniform change in drug elimination during hepatic failure. In contrast, drugs dependent on the metabolic activity of the liver exhibit heterogeneic changes in biodisposition. This results from inconsistent qualitative and quantitative changes in liver enzyme activity in the presence of liver disease of variable severity.

Because of the marked variability in the severity of liver dysfunction, it is difficult to formulate rules for dosage modification. Marked changes in pharmacokinetics (as noted with renal insufficiency) are generally not observed in liver failure.[67] Nonetheless, dosages of drugs eliminated mainly by hepatic biotransformation should be reduced in infants with severe liver disease.

The consequences of intercurrent disease on the pharmacokinetics and pharmacodynamics of drugs are irrefutably complex. An accurate prediction of drug disposition in the presence of interacting intricate individual variables is virtually impossible. The paucity of information on pharmacokinetics of drugs in infants with cardiac, renal, and hepatic dysfunction and the often changing and transient nature of these disorders render careful clinical observations and appropriate therapeutic monitoring imperative under these circumstances.

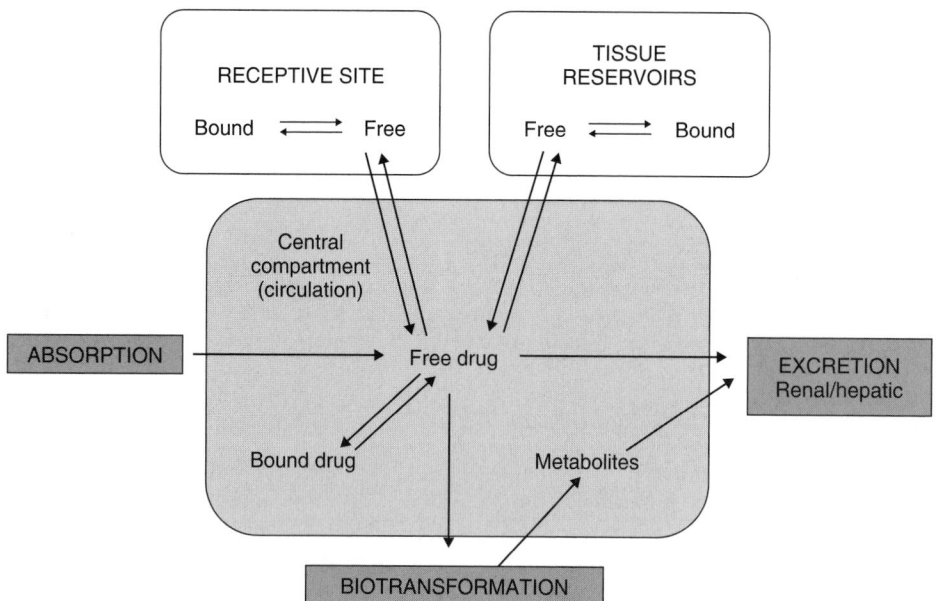

Figure 19–1. Schema of possible drug disposition to various compartments in the body.

CLINICAL PHARMACOKINETICS

The fundamental assumption of *clinical pharmacokinetics* is that a relationship exists between the concentration of a drug at its site of action and its serum or plasma level. The concentration of a drug in the blood enables one to monitor the dose-response relationship and to predict its pharmacokinetics. Thus, drug levels in blood permit appropriate individual dosing adjustments.

Pharmacokinetic principles can be understood only with respect to the various compartments into which a drug is distributed (Fig. 19-1). A *compartment* is not necessarily a defined physiologic or anatomic site but is considered one or many tissues that exhibit similar affinity for a drug.

The factors that determine the movement of a drug into and out of compartments are those that affect distribution. Therefore, the lipophilicity, ionization state, transporters (both influx and efflux carriers), and protein binding of a drug, as well as regional blood flow, regulate the extent and rate of passage of an agent into and out of a compartment.

Single-Compartment Distribution

The simplest model is the *single-compartment model*. In this model, it is assumed that after administration of the drug, immediate equilibration of drug concentration is achieved in all major tissues. First-order kinetics apply to this model, meaning that the rate of changes in the amount of drug in the body is a constant fraction of the amount of drug present at the time. Thus, the higher the dose, the greater is the elimination rate from the compartment. The rate of disappearance of a drug concentration using first-order kinetics can be expressed as follows:

$$dC/dt = -kC$$

where C = concentration of the drug and k = first-order elimination rate constant, expressed in units of time^{-1} (e.g., h^{-1}). Integration of this equation yields the drug concentration at a time, t:

$$\log C = -kt/2.3 + \log C_0 \text{ or } C = C_0\, e^{-kt}$$

where C_0 = concentration at time = 0. Thus, the slope of the log of the concentration-time curve = $-k/2.3$.

Drug Half-Life

From the previous equation ($\log C = -kt/2.3 + \log C_0$), the first-order half-life can be obtained:

$$t_{1/2} = 0.693/k$$

Regardless of the initial concentration of drug, the time required for the concentration to decrease by one-half is a constant determined by k. Thus, the time it takes to achieve a steady-state plasma concentration or the time it takes to eliminate the near totality of the drug is equal to approximately five half-lives (Fig. 19-2). In newborns, because the elimination rate is decreased for many drugs, the half-life is often prolonged compared with that of the adult (Table 19-5).

To minimize the onset time a drug takes to achieve average steady-state plasma concentrations ($C_{ss\ av}$), a loading dose (D_L) can be given. This dose is equal to the following:

$$D_L = C_{ss\ av} \times V_d$$

Maintenance Dose

After steady-state concentration is achieved (after a loading dose), the dose necessary to maintain this concentration (maintenance dose, D_{ss}) can be calculated from the following equation:

$$D_{ss} = (0.693 \times C_{ss\ av} \times V_d \times \tau) / t_{1/2}$$

TABLE 19-5

Comparative Plasma Half-Lives of Miscellaneous Drugs in Newborns and Adults

	Plasma Half-Life (hours)	
	Newborn	*Adult*
Acetaminophen	3.5	2.2
Phenylbutazone	21–34	12–30
Indomethacin	7.5–51.0	6
Meperidine	22	3.5
Phenytoin	21	11–29
Carbamazepine	8–28	21–36
Phenobarbital	82–199	24–140
Caffeine	100	6
Theophylline	30	6
Chloramphenicol	14–24	2.5
Salicylates	4.5–11.5	2.7
Digoxin	52	31–40

Data from refs. 20, 77, 81.

where τ = dosing interval. Thus, D_{ss} is also equal to the rate of drug elimination during the dosing interval.

Optimal Dosing Schedule

Knowledge of the half-life permits the clinician to determine an optimal dosing schedule, having set the maximum and minimum effective steady-state concentrations during a multiple dosing regimen (see Fig. 19-2). By using the same equation to calculate the concentration at a time, t ($\log C = -kt/2.3 + \log C_0$), an optimal dosing interval, τ, can also be determined. By substituting C with $C_{ss\ min}$ and C_0 with $C_{ss\ max}$, the following equation is obtained:

$$\log C_{ss\ min} - \log C_{ss\ max} = -kt/2.3$$

By further substituting k by $0.693/t_{1/2}$, the dosing interval, τ, which is the time it takes for the drug concentration to decrease from $C_{ss\ max}$ to $C_{ss\ min}$, can be determined by the following equation:

$$\tau = \log(C_{ss\ max}/C_{ss\ min}) \times 3.3 \times t_{1/2}$$

Drug Clearance

Drug clearance can be defined as the plasma volume in the vascular compartment that is cleared of drug per unit of time. Total clearance gives an indication of drug elimination from the central compartment without reference to the mechanism of this process. For drugs that are eliminated by first-order kinetics, clearance is constant.

Clearance by the kidneys is called *renal clearance*, and that by all other organs is referred to as *nonrenal clearance*. The latter most often represents clearance by the liver. *Total clearance* is the sum of all body clearances. The same factors that determine renal and hepatic elimination of drugs affect drug clearance.

Clearance (Cl) is mathematically defined as excretion rate/plasma concentration. Over a drug excretion time, clearance can be expressed by the following equation:

$$Cl = D_0 / [AUC]_0^t$$

Rearrangement of this formula according to the equation expressing V_d (see distribution earlier) yields the following:

$$Cl = V_d \times k$$

Multicompartment Distribution

Many drugs distribute in the body according to the kinetics of a *multicompartment model.* Consequently, after intravenous administration of the drug, the plasma concentration does not decline linearly as a first-order rate process but exhibits a non-linear elimination (Fig. 19-3). The first part of the curve with its sharper slope, the α-phase, represents the distribution of drug to highly perfused areas, including the blood. This area consists of the central compartment. With time and depending on the affinity of the drug for certain tissues, the agent distributes to the peripheral compartment or compartments. After equilibration, the tissues are saturated with the drug, and its decline in blood usually occurs by a first-order elimination process, the β-phase (see Fig. 19-3). Usually, the half-life of drugs that distribute according to a two-compartment model is determined during the β-phase.

To apply kinetic analysis of a multicompartment model, one assumes that all rate processes for the passage of drug from one compartment to another exhibit first-order kinetics. Therefore, the plasma level–time curve for a drug that follows a multi-compartment model is described by the summation of several first-order rate processes.

Zero-Order Kinetics

When elimination processes become saturated, disposition of certain drugs occurs through *zero-order kinetics.* In contrast to a first-order process, in which the fraction of drug eliminated is constant, in zero-order kinetics the elimination rate itself is constant. Thus, the drug is eliminated at a constant rate. Consequently, the zero-order half-life is not constant but is proportional to the initial amount or concentration of the drug:

$$t_{1/2} = 0.5C_0/k_0$$

where k_0 = zero-order rate constant. Many drugs exhibit zero-order kinetics with elevated concentrations, and as these decline, first-order kinetics prevails. Examples of drugs that exhibit saturation kinetics include salicylates, phenylbutazone, phenytoin, diazepam, and chloramphenicol.

The determination of drug pharmacokinetics has not been widely accepted as an essential part of newborn intensive care. The amount of reliable pharmacokinetic data for drugs used in the ill neonate has lagged considerably behind knowledge of

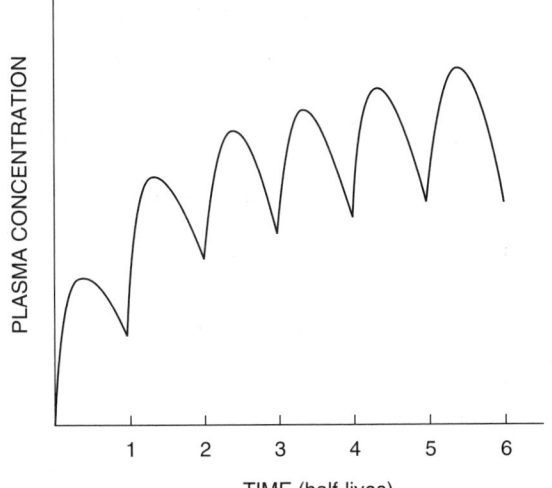

Figure 19–2. Pharmacokinetic relationships of a multiple dosing regimen. From this graph, it can easily be appreciated that the time required to attain steady-state drug concentrations is equal to approximately five half-lives, when first-order rates of absorption, distribution, and elimination are in process.

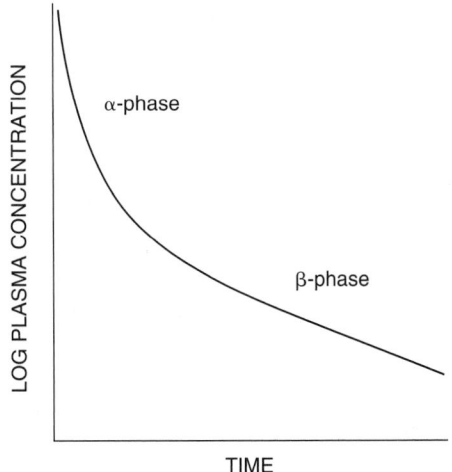

Figure 19–3. Two-compartment model for serum drug disappearance curve. The α-phase represents the distribution phase, and the β-phase represents the elimination phase.

pathophysiology. There is little doubt that this information, as well as monitoring of serum levels, can optimize drug dosage. When one considers the risks of therapeutic failure and toxicity, the rationale for drug monitoring is obvious. In addition, the many complex development-related and disease-related dynamic processes that take place in the sick newborn provide sufficient justification to measure drug blood levels to obtain an indication of its kinetics.

PRINCIPLES OF PHARMACODYNAMICS: DRUG-RECEPTOR INTERACTION

Pharmacodynamics is defined as the biochemical and physiologic effects of drugs. This aspect of pharmacology is the raison d'être of pharmacotherapeutics. The mechanism of action of drugs at the receptive site has received much attention since the 1980s. This section reviews some of the issues regarding drug-receptor interaction; the term *receptive site* refers to the molecular entity with which the agent is presumed to interact.

SITES OF DRUG ACTION

Drugs may act outside the cell, at the cell membrane, or inside the cell. Regardless of cell localization, the drug action may be mediated by receptors or can be independent of receptors. Certain agents do not act on cellular sites but instead act on extracellular products of cells. Most drugs bind to specific receptor sites, whereas the action of others does not seem to be mediated by receptors. For instance, chelating agents, such as dimercaprol, penicillamine, and desferrioxamine, bind circulating metals. The action of these agents can be considered truly extracellular.

Drugs that bind to physiologic receptors and mimic the regulatory effects of the endogenous ligands are termed *agonists*. Compounds that block the effects of endogenous ligands are termed *antagonists*, and these may be partial or inverse; the latter applies to drugs that stabilize the receptor in its inactive conformation. *Localization of drug action* refers both to drug distribution and to the specificity of the drug action. Such specificity implies the existence of receptors. Receptors consist of macromolecules that recognize and bind specific ligands and translate this binding into propagation of an intracellular message, either directly (e.g., nicotinic receptor: ion transport) or indirectly by virtue of a second messenger (e.g., protein kinase C: angiotensin II). This concept of receptor characteristics has led some investigators to suggest the existence of functional domains on the receptor molecule: a ligand-binding domain and an effector domain. Such conceptualization of the receptor is consistent with the mode of action of agonists and antagonists.

Receptor Classification

Receptors have traditionally been classified pharmacologically by their response to specific antagonists. The precise classification of receptors with respect to structure-activity relationship, however, relies on multiple approaches, which include physiologic, biochemical, biophysical, and immunologic techniques. The last-mentioned scheme delineates more precisely the action of drugs and facilitates the development of therapeutic agents having selectivity for specific receptors. This also provides the clinician with an appropriate basis for therapeutics, by ameliorating efficacy and limiting toxicity.

Receptor Regulation

The concentration and affinity of receptors are physiologically regulated by ligand-receptor binding and activation. *Receptor down-regulation* is the process by which the concentration and affinity of receptors are decreased. This regulation of receptor function can be classified on the basis of the time course, short term and long term. Short-term regulation occurs in the order of seconds to minutes, and long-term regulation takes place over hours to days. The mechanisms responsible for short-term regulation appear to involve conformational changes, transient intracellular receptor sequestration (e.g., nicotinic and α-adrenergic receptors), and phosphorylation of receptors. *Protein phosphorylation* is the mechanism by which most receptors are regulated, although myristoylation and palmytoylation are also involved in the regulation of expression of certain receptors. Long-term receptor down-regulation involves initial protein phosphorylation (myristoylation or palmytoylation) followed by internalization and degradation.

The term *receptor up-regulation* refers to the process of increasing receptor number. An example of up-regulation is the phenomenon of denervation supersensitivity of nicotinic receptors. The process of up-regulation is less clearly understood. Alterations in transcription of mRNA, translation, or posttranslational modifications seem to contribute to receptor up-regulation. Thus, changes in receptor number and affinity may well explain certain forms of drug tolerance, tachyphylaxis, and desensitization.

Changes in receptor binding, density, and coupling events can also occur with development. For instance, in the brain of the rat and pig, marked ontogenic changes in cholinergic muscarinic, α-adrenergic, and prostaglandin receptor density have been observed.[68-70] In addition, the pathophysiology of diseases such as testicular feminization, pseudohypoparathyroidism, myasthenia gravis, and certain forms of diabetes seems to involve receptor-associated dysfunctions.[71-73] Similarly, mutations of receptors can increase vulnerability to certain conditions and can accelerate desensitization to receptor agonists as reported for β-adrenoceptor agonists.[74] Thus, developmental and pathologic considerations must be accounted for by the clinicians and investigators when they evaluate a response.

Relationship Between Drug Dose and Response

According to the *receptor occupancy theory,* response is proportional to receptor binding.[75] Thus, maximal response is achieved when all receptors are bound. Although this concept is valid, interpretation of receptor binding is often difficult, particularly when the coupling events encompass a complex sequence of reactions. Such is the case when further receptor occupancy does not produce greater response; this has led to the concept of *spare receptors,* wherein a maximal response is achieved when a relatively small proportion of the receptors is occupied.

The common relationship between drug dose and response can often be displayed by a sigmoidal curve (Fig. 19–4). This is, of course, not the only dose-response relationship, and others can be more complex. Three characteristics can be used to describe dose-response curves: slope, potency, and maximal efficacy. A fourth one, individual variation, influences all the others.

The slope and shape of the curve reflect the mechanism of action of a drug. *Potency* describes the location of the curve along the x-axis and is influenced by the inherent affinity of the drug for its receptor and the latter's ability to couple with the postreceptor mechanisms. *In vivo*, potency is also influenced by disposition of the drug. In the clinical setting, potency per se should not be a determining factor in the selection of an agent. In contrast, *maximal efficacy* must be taken into consideration when choosing drugs. In all cases, *toxicity* of the agent must be taken into account. Under all therapeutic circumstances, the drug chosen should ideally provide the greatest margin of safety. This selectivity has been termed the *therapeutic index,* which is usually defined as the ratio of the median toxic dose to median

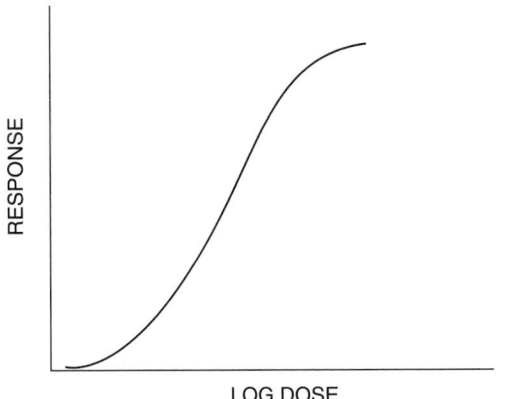

Figure 19–4. The dose-response relationship. The potency is reflected by the position of the curve along the abscissa. The slope and shape of the curve reflect the mechanism of action of the drug. The maximum efficacy is reflected by the uppermost position of the curve along the ordinate.

effective dose (TD_{50}/ED_{50}) and in laboratory studies as the ratio of the median lethal dose to effective dose (LD_{50}/ED_{50}).

CONCLUSION

Marked differences in drug disposition and action exist between newborns and adults. Greater differences exist for the ill preterm neonate. These differences must be taken into consideration when applying therapies to newborns. Appropriate application of basic principles in pharmacology and adequate drug monitoring allow individualization of drug dosage and ameliorate the treatment of neonates by reducing adverse drug effects.[65]

REFERENCES

1. Schanker LS: Passage of drugs across body membranes. Pharmacol Rev *14*:501, 1962.
2. Lee VH, et al: Pharmacogenomics of drug transporters: the next drug delivery challenge. Adv Drug Deliv Rev *50*:S33, 2001.
3. Jollow DJ, Brodie BB: Mechanisms of drug absorption and drug solution. Pharmacology *8*:21, 1972.
4. Quamme GA: Loop diuretics. In Dirks JH, Sutton RAL (eds): Diuretics: Physiology, Pharmacology and Clinical Use. Philadelphia, WB Saunders Co, 1986, p 86.
5. Zhang L, et al: Role of organic cation transporters in drug absorption and elimination. Ann Rev Pharmacol Toxicol *38*:431, 1998.
6. Burckhardt G, Wolff NA: Structure of renal organic anion and cation transporters. Am J Physiol *278*:F853, 2000.
7. Bode F: Analysis of the pinocytic process in rat. Biochim Biophys Acta *433*:294, 1976.
8. Sadee W, et al: Biology of membrane transporter proteins. Pharm Res *12*:1823, 1995.
9. Shargell L, Yu ABC: Applied Biopharmaceutics and Pharmacokinetics. New York, Appleton-Century-Crofts, 1980, p 68.
10. Winter ME: Basic Clinical Pharmacokinetics. San Francisco, Applied Therapeutics, 1980.
11. Bearer CF: The special and unique vulnerability of children to environmental hazards. Neurotoxicology *21*:925, 2000.
12. Euler AR, et al: Basal pentagastrin-stimulated acid secretion in newborn human infants. Pediatr Res *13*:36, 1979.
13. Neese AL, Soyka LF: Development of a radioimmunoassay for theophylline: application to studies in premature infants. Clin Pharmacol Ther *21*:633, 1977.
14. Watkins JB, et al: Bile salt metabolism in the human premature infant: preliminary observations of pool size and synthesis rate following prenatal administration of dexamethasone and phenobarbital. Gastroenterology *69*: 706, 1975.
15. Hillman LS: Absorption and maintenance dosage of 25-hydroxycholecalciferol (25-HCC) in premature infants. Pediatr Res *13*:400, 1979.
16. Melhorn DK, Gross S: Vitamin E-dependent anemia in the premature infant: II. relationships between gestational age and absorption of vitamin E. J Pediatr *79*:581, 1971.
17. Bell EF, et al: Vitamin E absorption in small premature infants. Pediatrics *63*:830, 1979.
18. Graeber JE, et al: The use of intramuscular vitamin E in the premature infant: optimum dose and iron interaction. J Pediatr *90*:282, 1977.
19. Yaffe SJ, Stern L: Clinical implications of perinatal pharmacology. *In* Mirkin BL (ed): Perinatal Pharmacology and Therapeutics. New York, Academic Press, 1976, p 382.
20. Morselli PL, et al: Clinical pharmacokinetics in newborns and infants: age-related differences and therapeutic implications. Clin Pharmacokinet *5*:485, 1980.
21. Matheny CJ, et al: Pharmacokinetic and pharmacodynamic implications of P-glycoprotein modulation. Pharmacotherapy *21*:778, 2001.
22. Tsai CE, et al: P-glycoprotein expression in mouse brain increases with maturation. Biol Neonate *81*:58, 2002.
23. Relling MV: Are the major effects of P-glycoprotein modulators due to altered pharmacokinetics of anticancer drugs? Ther Drug Monit *18*:350, 1996.
24. Lehne G: P-glycoprotein as a drug target in the treatment of multidrug resistant cancer. Current Drug Targets *1*:85, 2000.
25. Hines RN, McCarver DG: The ontogeny of human drug-metabolizing enzymes: phase I oxidative enzymes. J Pharmacol Exp Ther *300*:355, 2002.
26. Gustaffson BE: Effects of vitamin K-active compounds and intestinal microorganisms in vitamin K–deficient germ-free rats. J Nutr *78*:461, 1962.
27. Costarino A, Baumgart S: Modern fluid and electrolyte management of the critically ill premature infant. Pediatr Clin North Am *33*:153, 1986.
28. Yaffe SJ, Aranda J: Pediatric Pharmacology: Therapeutic Principles in Practice. Philadelphia, WB Saunders Co, 1992.
29. Winters RW: Maintenance fluid therapy. *In* Winters RW (ed): The Body Fluids in Pediatrics. Boston, Little, Brown and Co, 1973, p 113.
30. Williams PR, Oh W: Effects of radiant warmer on insensible water loss in newborn infants. Am J Dis Child *128*:511, 1974.
31. Chemtob S, et al: Alternating sequential dosing with furosemide and ethacrynic acid in drug tolerance in the newborn. Am J Dis Child *143*:850, 1989.
32. Chemtob S, et al: Cumulative increase in serum furosemide concentration following repeated doses in the newborn. Am J Perinatol *4*:203, 1987.
33. Widdowson EM: Growth and composition of the fetus and newborn. In Assali NS (ed): Biology of Gestation, Vol 2. New York, Academic Press, 1968, p 1.
34. Davison N, Dobbing J: Myelination as a vulnerable period in brain development. Br Med Bull *22*:40, 1966.
35. Lee G, et al: Drug transporters in the central nervous system: brain barriers and brain parenchyma considerations. Pharmacol Rev 53:569, 2001.
36. Calligaro IL, Burman CA: Pharmacologic considerations in the neonate with congenital heart disease. Clin Perinatol *28*:209, 2001.
37. Iwamoto HS, et al: Effects of birth-related events on blood flow distribution. Pediatr Res *22*:634, 1987.
38. Klopfenstein HS, Rudolph AM: Postnatal changes in the circulation, and the responses to volume loading in sheep. Circ Res *42*:839, 1978.
39. Lou HC, et al: Impaired autoregulation of cerebral blood flow in the distressed newborn infant. J Pediatr *94*:118, 1979.
40. Dayton PG, et al: Influence of binding on drug metabolism and distribution. Ann NY Acad Sci *226*:172, 1973.
41. Vallner JJ: Binding of drugs by albumin and plasma protein. J Pharm Sci *66*:447, 1977.
42. Piafsky KM, Mpamugo L: Dependence of neonatal drug binding on α_1-acid glycoprotein concentration. Clin Pharmacol Ther *29*:272, 1981.
43. Boreus LO: Principles of pediatric pharmacology. *In* Boreus LO (ed): Monographs in Clinical Pharmacology. New York, Churchill Livingstone, 1982.
44. Friedman Z, et al: Cord blood fatty acid composition in infants and in their mothers during the third trimester. J Pediatr *92*:461, 1978.
45. Thiessen H, et al: Displacement of albumin-bound bilirubin by fatty acids. Acta Paediatr Scand *61*:285, 1972.
46. Fredholm BB: Diphenylhydantoin binding to proteins in plasma and its dependence on free fatty acid and bilirubin concentration in dogs and newborn infants. Pediatr Res *9*:26, 1975.
47. Brodersen R, et al: Drug-induced displacement of bilirubin from albumin in the newborn. Dev Pharmacol Ther *6*:217, 1983.
48. Andersson KE, et al: Post-mortem distribution and tissue concentrations of digoxin in infants and adults. Acta Paediatr Scand *64*:497, 1975.
49. Lang D, et al: Postmortem tissue and plasma concentrations of digoxin in newborns and infants. Eur J Pediatr *128*:151, 1978.
50. Guengerich FP, et al: Twenty years of biochemistry of human P450s: purification, expression, mechanism, and relevance to drugs. Drug Metab Dispos *26*:1175, 1998.
51. de Wildt SN, et al: Cytochrome P450 3A: ontogeny and drug disposition. Clin Pharmacokinet *37*:485, 1999.
52. Battino D, et al: Clinical pharmacokinetics of antiepileptic drugs in paediatric patients. Part I: phenobarbital, primidone, valproic acid, ethosuximide and mesuximide. Clin Pharmacokinet *29*:257, 1995.
53. Lieber CS: Cytochrome P-4502E1: its physiological and pathological role. Physiol Rev *77*:517, 1997.
54. McCarver DG, Hines RN: The ontogeny of human drug-metabolizing enzymes: phase II conjugation enzymes and regulatory mechanisms. J Pharmacol Exp Ther *300*:361, 2002.
55. de Wildt SN, et al: Glucuronidation in humans. Pharmacogenetic and developmental aspects. Clin Pharmacokinet *36*:439, 1999.
56. Wilkinson GR, Shand DG: A physiological approach to hepatic drug clearance. Clin Pharmacol Ther *18*:377, 1975.

57. Jose PA, et al: Neonatal renal function and physiology. Curr Opinion Pediatr *6*:172, 1994.
58. Van den Anker JN: Pharmacokinetics and renal function in preterm infants. Acta Paediatr *85*:1393, 1996.
59. Modi N: Development of renal function. Br Med Bull *44*:935, 1988.
60. Robillard JE, et al: Maturational changes in the fetal glomerular filtration rate. Am J Obstet Gynecol *122*:601, 1975.
61. Tóth-Heyn P, et al: The stressed neonatal kidney: from pathophysiology to clinical management of neonatal vasomotor nephropathy. Pediatr Nephrol *14*:227, 2000.
62. Catterton Z, et al: Inulin clearance in the premature infant receiving indomethacin. J Pediatr *96*:737, 1980.
63. Ward RM: Pharmacology of tolazoline. Clin Perinatol *11*:703, 1984.
64. Russel FG, et al: Molecular aspects of renal anionic drug transport. Annu Rev Physiol *64*:563, 2002.
65. Koren G: Therapeutic drug monitoring principles in the neonate. National Academy of Clinical Biochemistry. Clin Chem *43*:222, 1997.
66. Nies AS, et al: Altered hepatic blood flow and drug disposition. Clin Pharmacokinet *1*:135, 1976.
67. Wilkinson GR: Influences of liver disease on pharmacokinetics. In Evans WE, et al (eds): Applied Pharmacokinetics: Principles of Therapeutic Drug Monitoring. San Francisco, Applied Therapeutics, 1980, p 57.
68. Dausse JP, et al: α_1- and α_2-adrenoceptors in rat cerebral cortex: effects of neonatal treatment with 6-hydroxydopamine. Eur J Pharmacol *78*:15, 1982.
69. Li D-Y, et al: Fewer PGE_2 and $PGF_{2\alpha}$ receptors in brain synaptosomes of newborn than of adult pigs. J Pharmacol Exp Ther *267*:1292, 1993.
70. Nordberg A, Winblad B: Cholinergic receptors in human hippocampus-regional distribution and variance with age. Life Sci *29*:1937, 1981.
71. Kolterman OG, et al: Evidence for receptor and postreceptor defects. J Clin Invest *65*:1272, 1980.
72. Levine MA, et al: Deficient guanine nucleotide regulation unit activity in cultured fibroblast membranes from patients with pseudohypoparathyroidism type I: a cause of impaired synthesis of 3',5'-cyclic AMP by intact and broken cells. J Clin Invest *72*:316, 1983.
73. Schilling EE: Primary defect of insulin receptors in skin fibroblasts cultured from an infant with leprechaunism and insulin resistance. Proc Natl Acad Sci USA *76*:5877, 1979.
74. Turki J, et al: Genetic polymorphisms of the beta 2-adrenergic receptor in nocturnal and nonnocturnal asthma. Evidence that Gly16 correlates with the nocturnal phenotype. J Clin Invest *95*:1635, 1995.
75. Ruffolo RR Jr: Important concepts of receptor theory. J Auton Pharmacol *2*:277, 1982.
76. Radde IC: Drug metabolism. *In* MacLeod SM, Radde IC (eds): Textbook of Pediatric Clinical Pharmacology. Littleton, MA, PSG Publishing Co, 1985, p 56.
77. Morselli PL: Clinical pharmacokinetics in neonates. Clin Pharmacokinet *1*:81, 1976.
78. Krasner J, Yaffe SJ: Drug-protein binding in the neonate. *In* Morselli PL, et al (eds): Basic and Therapeutic Aspects of Perinatal Pharmacology. New York, Raven Press, 1975, p 357.
79. Roberts RJ: Drug Therapy in Infants: Pharmacologic Principles and Clinical Experience. Philadelphia, WB Saunders Co, 1984, p 3.
80. Correia MA, Castagnoli N: Pharmacokinetics: II. Drug biotransformation. *In* Katzung BG (ed): Basic and Clinical Pharmacology. Norwalk, Appleton & Lange, 1986.
81. Aranda JV, et al: Drug monitoring in the perinatal patient: uses and abuses. Ther Drug Monit *2*:39, 1980.

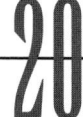 *Ralph A. Lugo and Robert M. Ward*

Basic Pharmacokinetic Principles

Pharmacokinetics describes the absorption, distribution, metabolism, and excretion of drugs. The pharmacokinetic parameters of a drug are used to characterize the drug concentrations reached within the body after a dose and the changes in those concentrations over time.[1] Clinical pharmacokinetics is the discipline that applies pharmacokinetic principles to individualize dosage regimens, optimize the therapeutic effects of a medication, and minimize the chances of an adverse drug reaction. These goals are accomplished by achieving an effective concentration of unbound drug at the site of action. Clinically important sites of action include receptors, membrane transport systems, intracellular enzymes, interstitial tissues where infections may occur, and many others. Correlations have been made between drug concentrations in the circulation and effective and toxic drug concentrations at various sites of action.[2] Depending on the strength of those correlations, ranges of effective, toxic, and ineffective circulating drug concentrations have been defined for many drugs. Pharmacokinetics serves as a guide to effective therapy, but achieving specific concentrations is not the goal of therapy. Effective therapy can be best judged by improvements in function, not just by reaching the desired peak and trough concentrations in the circulation.

Although the mathematical principles used to describe pharmacokinetics have become quite sophisticated with advanced mathematical modeling, statistical-arm theory,[3] and complex noncompartmental analysis,[4] the clinical issues in dosing are simple. Once a drug has been selected, three primary factors must be decided: what route to use for administration, how large a dose to administer, and how often to administer the dose. The size of the dose relates to its distribution within the body, and the frequency of administration relates to clearance or the rate of removal of active drug from the body. The factors needed to determine these parameters of drug therapy are presented mathematically and then are simplified for bedside application.

PHARMACOKINETIC MODELS

Mathematical principles may be used to describe pharmacokinetic processes to predict a drug's behavior in the body. To apply these principles using a compartmental approach requires selection of a compartmental model that best represents a drug's distribution and rate(s) of concentration change in the body.[1] Compartmental models may be classified as one-compartment, two-compartment, or multicompartment models, depending on the number of exponential equations required to describe the concentration changes. Seldom does a drug require more than three exponential equations to characterize its kinetics. These "compartments" theoretically represent a group of similar tissues, fluids, or organs and may be correlated with different anatomic fluids and tissues. In a one-compartment model, all body tissues are included in the model, and an intravenously administered drug is assumed to distribute instantaneously and homogeneously throughout the compartment.[2] In general, drugs that do not distribute widely into extravascular tissues can be described by a one-compartment model, such as aminoglycosides or very large molecules. This approach simplifies the calculations necessary for therapeutic drug monitoring of these agents because only two or three concentrations may be needed to characterize the pharmacokinetics for dosage adjustments adequately.

Many drugs, however, do not fit a one-compartment model because of slow distribution from the blood into other fluids and tissues. Accordingly, a drug reaches the central compartment made up of blood/plasma and highly perfused organs, such as the heart, liver, kidneys, and lungs, and diffuses out to peripheral sites such as adipose tissue, cerebral spinal fluid, and muscles.[2] The disposition of these drugs is best described using a multicompartment approach. Examples of drugs with such behavior include vancomycin, digoxin, and lipophilic drugs (e.g., fentanyl, midazolam, propofol). For the purposes of therapeutic drug monitoring in which only two or three plasma concentrations are obtained around an administered dose, characterization of the multicompartmental pharmacokinetics is not feasible or accurate. Thus, this multicompartment approach is reserved for more detailed pharmacokinetic study, when more frequent plasma sampling can be obtained.

FIRST-ORDER ELIMINATION

The change in drug amount within the body can be described with the following general equation in which A is the amount of drug within the body, k is the rate constant of change for A within the body, and n defines the order (e.g., zero, first, second) of the process.[5]

$$\frac{dA}{dt} = -kA^n \qquad [1]$$

Most drugs are eliminated by first-order exponential rates (k) in which a constant fraction of the drug is eliminated per unit of time. If the kinetics is characterized by first-order elimination, the rate of change of drug in the body (dA/dt) is proportional to the amount in the body. Thus, at high concentrations, a greater amount of drug is eliminated per hour than at low concentrations. This results in an exponential decline in plasma concentration (Fig. 20-1), which can be represented by the following equation:

$$C_t = C_0 \times e^{-kt} \qquad [2]$$

where C_t is the concentration at some time t, C_0 is the initial concentration at time 0, and e^{-kt} represents the exponential decline in plasma concentration associated with first-order elimination. The plasma concentration versus time relationship may be made linear by taking the natural logarithm of each side of Equation 2:

$$Ln\ C_t = Ln\ C_0 - kt \qquad [3]$$

The slope of this straight line is the elimination rate constant k (time^{-1}), which may be calculated by rearranging Equation 3:

$$k = (Ln\ C_1 - Ln\ C_2) / \Delta t \qquad [4]$$

where C_1 is the higher concentration and C_2 is the lower concentration measured some time later. If the logarithm (base 10) of concentration is graphed versus time, the slope will be k/2.303. The half-life of a drug exhibiting first-order elimination is the time

necessary for the concentration in the plasma to decrease by one-half. The relationship between the elimination rate constant and the half-life for a first-order process may be derived mathematically from Equation 3. For a drug whose initial concentration is 100 mg/L, the concentration at one half-life is 50 mg/L.

$$Ln\ 50 = Ln\ 100 - kt$$
$$kt = Ln\ (100/50)$$

which can be rearranged to

$$k = Ln\ 2 / t$$

where t represents one half-life; therefore,

$$k = 0.693 / T_{1/2} \qquad [5]$$

To illustrate the concept that the amount of drug removed per unit time decreases with declining amounts (or concentrations) of drug in the body, the amount of drug in the body at different times can be calculated with Equation 2 by substituting plasma concentration with the amount of drug in the body. For example, if a 100-mg dose of a drug with first-order elimination is administered by rapid intravenous bolus, and it has a 2-hour half-life (k = 0.693/2 h = 0.347 h^{-1}), a constant fraction of drug will be removed each hour = $e^{(0.347)(1)}$ = 29.3% of the amount of drug in the body. The amount of drug in the body each hour can be calculated to show the decreasing amount of drug removed each hour (Table 20-1).

First-Order Multicompartment Kinetics

If drug clearance from the circulation is studied thoroughly, with concentration measurements made multiple times soon after intravenous administration as well as during the terminal elimination phase, two or more exponential rates of clearance are often detected by a change in slope of a semilogarithmic graph of concentration versus time (Fig. 20-2). The number and nature of the compartments for the clearance of a drug do not necessarily correspond to specific body fluids or tissues. When two first-order exponential equations are required to describe the clearance of drug from the circulation, the kinetics is designated first-order and two-compartment or biexponential.[6] Such kinetics is commonly observed for drugs that rapidly distribute from the central compartment (blood and highly perfused organs) to peripheral compartments after intravenous administration. Figure 20-2 illustrates the kinetics for such drugs. The initial rapid decrease in concentration is referred to as the α distribution phase and is primarily the result of drug distribution to tissues; however, elimination is also occurring. Accordingly, the slope of this initial decrease in concentration is determined by

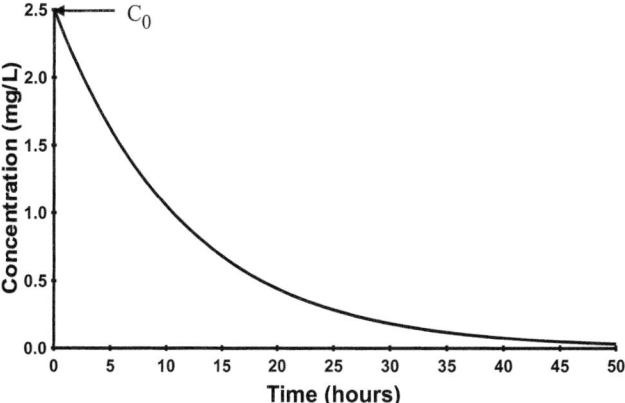

Figure 20-1. Exponential decrease in drug concentration after a rapid intravenous bolus injection graphed on linear-linear axes. The initial concentration (C_0) of 2.5 mg/L declines with a half-life of 8 hours.

TABLE 20-1

Amount of Drug Remaining in the Body Each Hour for a Drug Eliminated by First-Order Kinetics with a Half-Life of 2 Hours (k = 0.347 h^{-1})

Time (h)	Amount of Drug in Body (mg)	Drug Eliminated over Preceding Hour (mg)	Fraction of Drug Eliminated During Preceding Hour
0	100	0	0
1	70.7	29.3	0.293
2	50	20.7	0.293
3	35.4	14.6	0.293
4	25	10.4	0.293
5	17.7	7.3	0.293
6	12.5	5.2	0.293

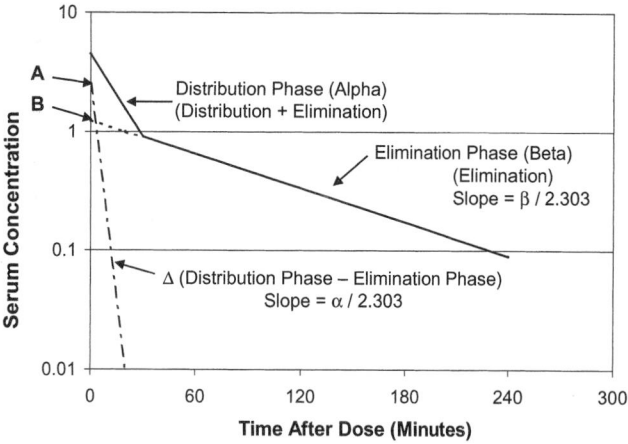

Figure 20–2. Two-compartment or biexponential kinetics graphed as a *solid line* on semilogarithmic axes with the initial rapid decrease in concentration resulting from distribution and elimination during the distribution phase (alpha) followed by the slower decrease in concentration during the elimination phase (beta) with a slope of the elimination rate constant β/2.303. B is the intercept of the elimination phase extrapolated with a *dashed line* to time 0. The concentration difference (Δ) between the distribution and elimination phases is graphed with *dashes alternating with dots* with intercept A and a slope of the distribution rate constant α/2.303.

both drug elimination and drug distribution. After the inflection point in the slope and during the terminal (β) elimination phase of the curve, elimination accounts for most of the change in drug concentration and has a rate constant of β. The α distribution rate constant can be determined by subtracting the concentration during the initial period after drug administration from concentrations extrapolated to time zero from the β elimination phase (see Fig. 20–2). The rate constant α is the slope of the natural logarithm of the concentration difference (Δ) versus time curve shown as the line of alternating dashes and dots in Figure 20–2. A more detailed mathematical discussion can be found elsewhere.[6, 7] The equation that represents a first-order, two-compartment model is as follows:

$$C_t = Ae^{-\alpha t} + Be^{-\beta t} \qquad [6]$$

where C_t is concentration at time t after the dose, A is the concentration at time 0 for the distribution rate represented by the broken line graph, α is the rate constant for the initial distribution phase, B is the concentration at time 0 for the terminal elimination phase, and β is the rate constant for terminal elimination. When concentration is graphed on semilogarithmic axes using logarithm (base 10) of concentration, the slope of the lines for α and β = α/2.303 and β/2.303, respectively.

Although many drugs demonstrate multicompartment kinetics, the intensive blood sampling required to fit data to more than one compartment is usually not clinically feasible, particularly in the newborn patient. Furthermore, the mathematical complexity of two-compartment models makes this kinetic approach clinically impractical. To minimize cost and to simplify pharmacokinetic calculations, only two plasma concentrations (peak and trough) are usually obtained for therapeutic monitoring of commonly used drugs, such as gentamicin and vancomycin. Accordingly, a one-compartment model is assumed, and the elimination rate constant (k) is determined from the slope of these points plotted on a semilogarithmic scale. Because the elimination rate constant should be determined during the terminal elimination phase, it is important that peak concentra-

tions of multicompartment drugs not be drawn prematurely, that is, during the initial distribution phase. If they are drawn too early, the high initial predistribution concentration will result in an overestimation of the slope and terminal elimination rate constant. Clinically, this is not usually problematic with gentamicin because the initial distribution phase commonly occurs during the 30- to 60-minute infusion.[8] Thus, a peak concentration obtained 30 to 60 minutes after the end of infusion usually reflects the terminal phase of elimination. However, with vancomycin, the half-life of the initial distribution phase is approximately 0.5 hours.[9] Thus, a peak vancomycin concentration drawn prematurely may lead to error in estimating the pharmacokinetic parameters.

ZERO-ORDER ELIMINATION

Elimination of some drugs occurs with loss of a constant amount of drug per time, rather than a constant fraction per time as with first-order kinetics. When the rate of change in the amount or concentration of a drug is constant, these rates are described as zero-order rates, and the concentration can be calculated using the following equation:

$$C_t = C_0 - k_0 t \qquad [7]$$

In this equation, C_t equals the concentration at time t, C_0 is the initial concentration, and k_0 (amount/time) is the rate constant for this process. Zero-order elimination may occur when the elimination process of a drug becomes saturated, that is, the eliminating organ has reached the maximum capacity for drug removal. This may be referred to as *saturation kinetics*. Some drugs administered to newborns that are eliminated, at least in part, by zero-order kinetics include caffeine, chloramphenicol, diazepam, furosemide, indomethacin, and phenytoin.[10] Such elimination may occur for other drugs after excess doses or when the organ responsible for drug elimination becomes dysfunctional. When kinetics changes from first-order to zero-order kinetics (dose-dependent kinetics), continuation of the same dosage usually leads to a rapid accumulation of drug, resulting in toxic drug concentrations.[10]

APPARENT VOLUME OF DISTRIBUTION

The *apparent volume of distribution* (Vd) is a mathematical term that relates the total amount of drug in the body to the drug concentration in the circulation. After a rapid intravenous bolus dose and assuming a one-compartment model, the following equation may be used to relate Vd, dose, and the change in circulating concentration.

$$\Delta \text{ Circulating drug concentration (mg/L)} = \frac{\text{Dose (mg/kg)}}{\text{Vd (L/kg)}} \quad [8]$$

Vd may be viewed as the volume of dilution into which the dose is added to produce the observed change in concentration. The larger the volume of distribution, the greater the dilution of a dose, and the smaller the increase in circulating concentration. Volume of distribution does not necessarily correspond to a true physiologic body fluid or tissue volume, hence the designation "apparent." For drugs that are extensively distributed to peripheral tissues, the Vd derived from changes in concentration within the circulation may be very large. For example, the Vd of digoxin in neonates and infants may reach 10 L/kg, an anatomic impossibility.[11] Large volumes of distribution indicate that tissue concentrations of drug may greatly exceed the concentration in the plasma, often because of protein binding in tissues or fat solubility. Drugs that distribute primarily into extracellular fluid (e.g., gentamicin) have small volumes of distribution (0.25 to 0.35 L/kg in adults) that significantly increase in fluid overload states. In addition, because extracellular water makes up a larger percentage of body weight in premature and term infants, their volumes of distribution at birth will be larger for these drugs.

When administering a rapid intravenous bolus dose, Equation 8 serves as the basis for other pharmacokinetic calculations because it is easily rearranged to solve for Vd and dose. If a dose is infused over a longer period, a significant portion of the dose may be cleared from the body during the infusion, in particular for drugs with half-lives that are only three to four times longer than the infusion time. Accordingly, a more complex exponential equation that accounts for concurrent drug administration and drug elimination is required to describe the change in concentration. However, such equations are needed only when the drug is rapidly eliminated and the duration of infusion approaches the drug's half-life. In neonates, who often have relatively slow rates of drug elimination, only a small fraction of drug is eliminated during the time of infusion, and such adjustments often can be omitted. Accordingly, the simpler and more practical equation to estimate pharmacokinetic parameters may be used.

CLEARANCE

Clearance represents the capacity for drug removal by various organs and is defined as the volume of blood from which all drug is removed per unit of time. Both clearance and distribution volume are model-independent parameters, and thus plasma drug concentrations are determined by the rate at which drug is administered, its clearance, and the volume of distribution. Similarly, rate of elimination is determined from clearance and Vd.

$$k = CL/Vd \qquad [9]$$

Drugs can be cleared through numerous pathways, although most drugs are cleared by some combination of renal clearance (CL_R), hepatic clearance (CL_H), and biliary clearance (CL_B) (Fig. 20-3). Thus, the total systemic clearance of a drug is the sum of all the clearances by various mechanisms and can be calculated using the following equation:

$$CL_S = CL_R + CL_H + CL_B + CL_{other} \qquad [10]$$

Because it is seldom possible to calculate each organ's clearance of drug, total systemic clearance (CL_S) is often determined by measuring the area under the plasma concentration-time curve (AUC) after a single dose:

$$CL_S = Dose / AUC \qquad [11]$$

During a continuous infusion, clearance may be determined easily by the relationship between the rate of infusion and the resultant steady-state concentration:

$$CL_S = \text{Rate of drug administration / Steady-state}$$
$$\text{drug concentration}$$
$$[12]$$

FIRST-PASS CLEARANCE

A special situation occurs for some drugs in which dramatic differences in concentrations and effects occur between enteral and parenteral administration as a result of first-pass effect or presystemic drug clearance. During enteral absorption, drug passes through the intestinal wall, enters the portal venous circulation, and passes through the liver before reaching the systemic circulation (see Fig. 20-3). Nearly complete metabolism may occur in the intestinal wall or the liver (especially for drugs

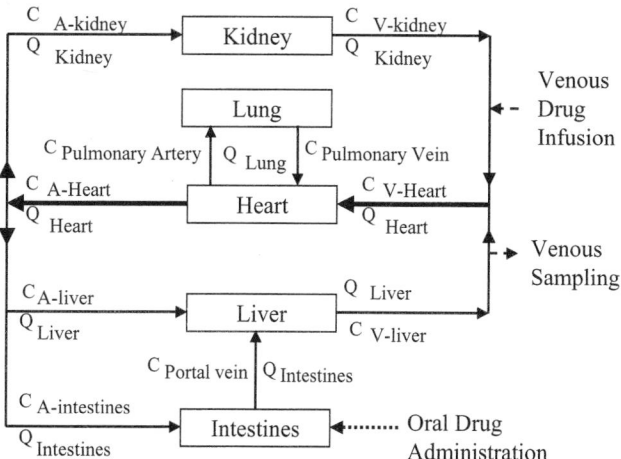

Figure 20–3. Drug clearance by several organs that combine to produce total body clearance in which C_A is arterial concentration, C_V is venous concentration, and Q is organ blood flow. First-pass clearance may occur during drug absorption from the intestines or during circulation of portal venous blood through the liver before reaching systemic circulation.

metabolized by cytochrome P450 3A4), so the amount of parent drug reaching the systemic circulation is only a small fraction of the dose administered.[12,13] The fraction (F) of the oral dose that reaches the systemic circulation is that which remains after hepatic or intestinal metabolism and is expressed as the extraction ratio (ER) in the following equation:

$$F = 1 - ER \qquad [13]$$

The F is determined from the ratio of the area under the plasma concentration curve after oral administration compared with that after intravenous administration. After an intravenous dose of medication, drug enters either the inferior or superior vena caval circulation, returns to the heart, and enters the systemic circulation before perfusing the liver. Drugs that undergo almost complete hepatic or intestinal metabolism before reaching the systemic circulation are described as having a high hepatic or intestinal intrinsic clearance. Some drugs used in the care of newborns that exhibit moderate to significant first-pass, presystemic clearance in adults and infants include midazolam,[14] morphine,[15] and propranolol.[16]

STEADY STATE

Steady-state conditions occur when plasma and tissue concentrations are in equilibrium and the amount of drug removed per unit time is equal to the amount administered per unit time. For drugs administered intermittently, peak and trough concentrations at steady state are unchanged after each dose. For drugs administered by continuous infusion, serum concentrations are constant. Constant serum concentrations, however, do not define steady state because distribution between tissues and the circulation may still be occurring.

The time to reach steady state is dependent only on the elimination rate constant and therefore half-life. If drug is administered repeatedly at a fixed dosing interval, the time to reach greater than 90% of steady state is four or more half-lives (Table 20-2).

During long-term drug treatment, dose adjustments should be made when concentrations are close to steady state and generally not less than three half-lives after a prior dose adjustment, unless organ dysfunction is altering the half-life or volume of distribution.

Percentage of Steady-State Concentration Reached after Drug Administration for One to Five Half-Lives

Number of Half-Lives That Drug is Administered	Percentage of Steady-State Concentration (%)
1	50
2	75
3	87.5
4	93.75
5	96.88

SINGLE-DOSE ADMINISTRATION BY SHORT-DURATION INFUSION

When drugs are infused over a period approaching 25 to 50% of the half-life, significant drug elimination occurs during the infusion process, and thus the standard intravenous bolus equation (e.g., Equation 8) is no longer accurate in calculating the change in concentration or the volume of distribution. A more complex mathematical model must be used to account for drug elimination during drug infusion.

To determine the concentration immediately at the end of the first infusion for a one-compartment model, Equation 14, which is commonly used to calculate concentration during a continuous infusion, may be modified:[17]

$$C_t = (R_0 / CL) \times (1 - e^{-kt}) \qquad [14]$$

where C_t is the concentration at any time (t) during the continuous infusion, R_0 is the rate of infusion, and k is the first-order elimination rate constant. During a continuous infusion, steady state (C_{ss}) is defined by the relationship between infusion rate (R_0) and clearance (Fig. 20-4):

$$C_{ss} = R_0 / CL \qquad [15]$$

In Equation 14, it is intuitive to think of the factor $[(1 - e^{-kt})]$ as the percentage of steady state that is achieved at time t. Thus, the concentration at any time t during the infusion process is the steady-state concentration (C_{ss}) multiplied by the percentage of steady state achieved at time t. As t becomes larger, the factor $[(1 - e^{-kt})]$ in Equation 14 approaches 1, resulting in steady-state Equation 15.

Equation 14 can be adapted easily for a single short-duration infusion. Accordingly, the duration of the infusion is represented by t, and C_t therefore represents the concentration immediately at the end of the infusion. Plasma concentrations anytime thereafter can be calculated by multiplying C_t by the decay factor ($e^{-kt'}$) for a first-order process (see Equation 2). Thus, the concentration measured at any time (t′) after the completion of a single short-duration infusion can be calculated by the following equation:[17]

$$C_{t'} = Ro / CL \times [(1 - e^{-kt_{inf}})] \times e^{-kt'} \qquad [16]$$

where $C_{t'}$ is the concentration measured at some time t′ after the end of infusion. The infusion time is represented by t_{inf} and is often 0.5 hour or 1 hour, and Ro is the rate of infusion defined by [dose/time of infusion]. This single-dose equation is commonly used to calculate the measured peak and trough concentrations after administration of the first dose of an aminoglycoside or vancomycin.

Because $CL = Vd \times k$ (derived from Equation 9), Equation 16 can be rearranged to solve for Vd after a single short-duration infusion.

$$Vd = [Ro / (C_{t'} \times k)] \times (1 - e^{-kt_{inf}}) \times e^{-kt'} \qquad [17]$$

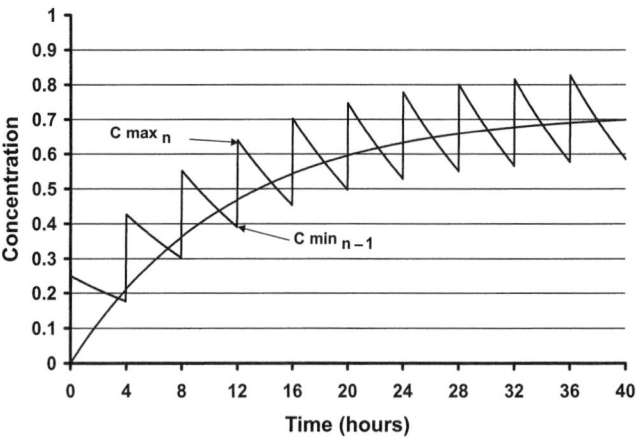

Figure 20–4. Plasma drug concentrations over time during a continuous intravenous infusion and during repeated dosing. For a continuous infusion, the rate of infusion and the clearance of the drug define the steady-state concentration, a plateau reached when the rate of elimination matches the rate of input. For multiple drug dosing using the same daily dose, the average steady-state concentration is the same as the steady-state concentration for a continuous infusion. During multiple drug dosing, the increase in concentration between the trough immediately before the nth dose, $Cmin_{n-1}$, and the peak immediately after the nth dose, $Cmax_n$, is the same increase noted after a single (i.e., first) dose of drug.

This equation represents the calculation of Vd after a single dose of drug. If pharmacokinetic parameters are calculated after multiple doses, the accumulation of drug must be taken into account.

MULTIPLE-DOSE ADMINISTRATION

In most clinical situations, pharmacokinetic parameters are calculated and dosage adjustments are made after multiple doses are administered. When multiple doses are administered at a fixed dosage interval (τ), concentrations will accumulate until steady state is achieved some five half-lives later (see Fig. 20-4). The maximum concentration after the nth dose may be determined by adding the minimum concentration just before the nth dose (n − 1) and the maximum concentration achieved after the first dose is administered (see Fig. 20-4). Mathematically, an *accumulation factor* may be derived that relates the maximum drug concentration after a single dose to drug concentration after n doses administered at a fixed dosage interval (τ). A full mathematical derivation is beyond the scope of this chapter and may be found elsewhere.[18] This accumulation factor (R) may be calculated with the following equation:[17]

$$R = (1 - e^{-nk\tau}) / (1 - e^{-k\tau}) \qquad [18]$$

As $n \to \infty$ (i.e., steady state), the numerator of the accumulation factor approaches 1. Thus, the steady-state accumulation factor is represented by the following equation:

$$\text{Steady-state accumulation factor} = 1 / (1 - e^{-k\tau}) \qquad [19]$$

Thus, to calculate the maximum concentration after the nth dose of drug, the maximum concentration after a single dose ($Cmax_1$) is multiplied by the accumulation factor:

$$Cmax (n) = Cmax_1 \times [(1 - e^{-nk\tau}) / (1 - e^{-k\tau})] \qquad [20]$$

Similarly, to calculate the maximum concentration at steady state, multiply the maximum concentration after the first dose by the steady-state accumulation factor:

$$\text{Cmax (steady state)} = \text{Cmax}_1 \times [1 / (1 - e^{-k\tau})] \quad [21]$$

The accumulation factor can also be used to calculate the minimum concentration after any number (n) of doses or at steady state by multiplying the minimum concentration after a single dose (Cmin_1) by the appropriate accumulation factor.

$$\text{Cmin (n)} = \text{Cmin}_1 \times [(1 - e^{-nk\tau}) / (1 - e^{-k\tau})] \quad [22]$$

$$\text{Cmin (steady state)} = \text{Cmin}_1 \times [1 / (1 - e^{-k\tau})] \quad [23]$$

From Equation 2, $\text{Cmin}_1 = \text{Cmax}_1 \times e^{-kt'}$, where $e^{-kt'}$ accounts for the first-order decline in concentration between the maximum concentration and the minimum concentration during time t′. Therefore, from Equations 22 and 23 the following equations are derived:

$$\text{Cmin (n)} = [\text{Cmax}_1 \times e^{-kt'}] \times [(1 - e^{-nk\tau}) / (1 - e^{-k\tau})] \quad [24]$$

$$\text{Cmin (steady state)} = [\text{Cmax}_1 \times e^{-kt'}] \times [1 / (1 - e^{-k\tau})] \quad [25]$$

Accumulation After Multiple Intravenous Boluses

After a single, rapid intravenous bolus dose, $\text{Cmax}_1 = \text{Dose}/\text{Vd}$ (derived from Equation 8); therefore, the maximum concentration after the nth intravenous bolus dose [Cmax (n)] is determined by substituting Cmax_1 into Equation 20, which is the product of the maximum concentration after a single dose (Dose/Vd) multiplied by the accumulation factor[17]:

$$\text{Cmax (n)} = \text{Dose}/\text{Vd} \times [(1 - e^{-nk\tau}) / (1 - e^{-k\tau})] \quad [26]$$

To calculate the concentration at any time t′ after administration of the nth dose, Equation 26 is multiplied by the exponential term for a first-order process:

$$C_{t'}(n) = \text{Dose}/\text{Vd} \times [(1 - e^{-nk\tau}) / (1 - e^{-k\tau})] \times e^{-kt'} \quad [27]$$

At steady state, the accumulation factor term in the numerator $(1 - e^{-nk\tau})$ is equal to 1, which results in the following equation:

$$C_{t'}(ss) = \text{Dose}/\text{Vd} \times [1 / (1 - e^{-k\tau})] \times e^{-kt'} \quad [28]$$

This equation may be rearranged to solve for dose and Vd as long as k and the concentration are known.

Accumulation After Multiple Administrations of Short-Duration Infusions

For a short-duration infusion, the Cmax_1 after a single dose equals $\text{Ro} / \text{CL} \times [(1 - e^{-kt_{inf}})]$, which adjusts for the amount of drug eliminated during the infusion. Thus, the maximum concentration after the nth dose is the Cmax_1 after a single dose multiplied by the accumulation factor; that is, substitute Cmax_1 into Equation 20:[17]

$$\text{Cmax (n)} = [\text{Ro} / \text{CL}] \times (1 - e^{-kt_{inf}}) \times [(1 - e^{-nk\tau}) / (1 - e^{-k\tau})] \quad [29]$$

To calculate the concentration at any time t′ after completing the infusion of the nth dose, Equation 29 is multiplied by the exponential term for a first-order process:

$$C_{t'}(n) = [\text{Ro} / \text{CL}] \times (1 - e^{-kt_{inf}}) \times [(1 - e^{-nk\tau}) / (1 - e^{-k\tau})] \times e^{-kt'} \quad [30]$$

At steady state, the accumulation factor term in the numerator $(1 - e^{-nk\tau})$ is equal to 1, which results in the following equation:

$$C_{t'}(ss) = [\text{Ro} / \text{CL}] \times (1 - e^{-kt_{inf}}) \times [1 / (1 - e^{-k\tau})] \times e^{-kt'} \quad [31]$$

In the hospital setting, pharmacokinetics is often calculated for aminoglycosides and vancomycin and is usually measured at steady state. Therefore, Equation 31 represents the most important equation for the purposes of therapeutic drug monitoring. Equation 31 may be rearranged to solve for any desired parameter, including Vd and dose. Recall that $\text{CL} = \text{Vd} \times k$ (derived from Equation 9); thus,

$$\text{Vd} = [\text{Ro} / (C_{t'}(ss) \times k)] \times (1 - e^{-kt_{inf}}) \times [1 / (1 - e^{-k\tau})] \times e^{-kt'} \quad [32]$$

Similarly, because $\text{Ro} = \text{dose} / \text{time of infusion} (t_{inf})$, Equation 31 can be rearranged to solve for dose:

$$\text{Dose} = [\text{Vd} \times t_{inf} \times C_{t'}(ss) \times k \times (1 - e^{-k\tau})] / [(1 - e^{-kt_{inf}}) \times e^{-kt'}] \quad [33]$$

where $C_{t'}(ss)$ is a steady-state concentration measured at time t′ after the end of the infusion. In clinical practice, this is often the *measured peak concentration* (e.g., 1 hour after the end of infusion), a random concentration, or a *measured trough concentration*.

EXAMPLES OF MATHEMATICAL PHARMACOKINETIC DOSE ADJUSTMENTS

The foregoing equations may be used to adjust the dose and dosing intervals to attain desired peak and trough concentrations. We recommend a simple four-step approach: (1) calculate k (and half-life), (2) calculate Vd, (3) calculate a dosing interval and dose based on a desired peak and trough, and (4) check the peak and trough of the new dosage regimen.

Example 1

In this example, 100 mg of a drug is administered by rapid intravenous bolus every 8 hours. At steady state, the peak concentration measured 1 hour after the bolus is 10 mg/L, and the trough concentration measured immediately before the next dose is 2 mg/L. Calculate k, Vd, and the new dose to achieve a measured peak of 15 mg/L and a trough of 1 mg/L.

Step 1

Equations 4 and 5 are used to calculate the elimination rate constant and half-life, respectively.

$$k = [\text{Ln}(10) - \text{Ln}(2)] / 7 \text{ h} = 0.2299 \text{ h}^{-1}$$

Because the peak concentration was measured 1 hour after the IV bolus, the Δt is 7 and not 8 hours.

$$T_{1/2} = 0.693 / 0.2299 \text{ h}^{-1} = 3.0 \text{ h}$$

Step 2

Equation 28 may be rearranged to solve for Vd.

$$\text{Vd} = [\text{Dose}/ C_{t'}(ss)] \times [1 / (1 - e^{-k\tau})] \times e^{-kt'}$$

$C_{t'}(ss)$ is the measured peak concentration at steady state (10 mg/L), and $e^{-kt'}$ represents the decline in concentration between the end of the bolus and the measured peak, that is, 1 hour.

$$\text{Vd} = [100 \text{ mg} / (10 \text{ mg/L})] \times [1 / (1 - e^{-(0.2299)(8)})] \times e^{-(0.2299)(1)}$$
$$= 9.45 \text{ L}$$

Step 3

Equation 4 can be rearranged to solve for Δt for a desired peak (15 mg/L) and desired trough (1 mg/L) concentration with a known k. This term is represented as the new dosing interval (τ).

$$\tau = [Ln(15) - Ln(1)] / 0.2299 \text{ h}^{-1} = 11.8 \text{ h}$$

Because this desired peak concentration is measured 1 hour after the dose is administered, the dosing interval must include the additional hour. Thus, the optimal $\tau = 12.8$ hours, which can be rounded to a 12-hour dosing interval.

Equation 28 can be rearranged to solve for the new dose with a known Vd, k, and τ.

$$\text{Dose} = [C_{t'}(ss) \times Vd \times (1 - e^{-k\tau})] / e^{-kt'}$$

$C_{t'}(ss)$ is equal to the new desired measured peak concentration at steady state; that is, 15 mg/L and $e^{-kt'}$ represents the decline in concentration between the end of the bolus and the measured peak, that is, 1 hour. Therefore,

$$\text{Dose} = [15 \text{ mg/L} \times 9.45 \text{ L} \times (1 - e^{-(0.2299)(12)})] / e^{-(0.2299)(1)}$$
$$= 167 \text{ mg every } 12 \text{ h}$$

Step 4

The new steady-state peak and trough can be measured by using Equation 28.

$$C_{t'}(\text{ss peak}) = 167 \text{ mg}/9.45 \text{ L} \times [1/(1 - e^{-(0.2299)(12)})] \times e^{-(0.2299)(1)}$$
$$= 15.0 \text{ mg/L}$$

The trough is determined by changing t' from 1 to 12 hours.

$$C_{t'}(\text{ss trough}) = 167 \text{ mg}/9.45 \text{ L} \times [1/(1 - e^{-(0.2299)(12)})] \times e^{-(0.2299)(12)}$$
$$= 1.2 \text{ mg/L}$$

Example 2

In this example, 100 mg of the same drug is infused over 60 minutes every 8 hours. The peak concentration measured 1 hour after the end of infusion is 10 mg/L, and the trough concentration measured immediately before the next dose is 2 mg/L. Calculate k, Vd, and the new dose to achieve a measured peak of 15 mg/L and a trough of 1 mg/L.

Step 1

Equations 4 and 5 are used to calculate the elimination rate constant and half-life, respectively.

$$k = [Ln(10) - Ln(2)] / 6 \text{ h} = 0.2682 \text{ h}^{-1}$$

$$T_{1/2} = 0.693 / 0.2682 \text{ h}^{-1} = 2.6 \text{ h}$$

Step 2

Equation 32 is used to solve for Vd.

$$Vd = [Ro / (C_{t'}(ss) \times k)] \times (1-e^{-kt_{inf}}) \times [1 / (1-e^{-k\tau})] \times e^{-kt'}$$

$$Vd = \frac{(100 \text{ mg/1 h}) \times [1-e^{-(0.2682)(1)}] \times e^{-(0.2682)(1)}}{[10 \text{ mg/L} \times 0.2682 \text{ h}^{-1}] \times [1-e^{-(0.2682)(8)}]}$$

$$Vd = 7.6 \text{ L}$$

Step 3

Equation 4 can be rearranged to solve for Δt for a desired peak (15 mg/L) and desired trough (1 mg/L) concentration with a known k. This term is represented as the new dosing interval (τ).

$$\tau = [Ln(15) - Ln(1)] / 0.2682 \text{ h}^{-1} = 10.1 \text{ h}$$

Because this desired peak concentration is measured 1 hour after a 1-hour infusion, the dosing interval must include the additional 2 hours. Thus, the optimal $\tau = 12.1$ hours, which can be rounded to a 12-hour dosing interval.

The new dose is calculated using Equation 33:

$$\text{Dose} = [Vd \times t_{inf} \times C_{t'}(ss) \times k \times (1 - e^{-k\tau})] / [(1 - e^{-kt_{inf}}) \times e^{-kt'}]$$

$$\text{Dose} = \frac{[7.6 \text{ L} \times 1 \text{ h} \times 15 \text{ mg/L} \times 0.2682 \text{ h}^{-1} \times (1 - e^{-(0.2682)(12)})]}{[(1-e^{-(0.2682)(1)}) \times e^{-(0.2682)(1)}]}$$

$$\text{Dose} = 164 \text{ mg every } 12 \text{ h}$$

Step 4

The new steady-state peak and trough can be measured by using Equation 31.

$$C_{t'}(ss) = [Ro / CL] \times (1 - e^{-kt_{inf}}) \times [1 / (1 - e^{-k\tau})] \times e^{-kt'}$$

$$C_{t'}(\text{ss peak}) = [(164 \text{ mg/1 h})/(7.6 \text{ L} \times 0.2682 \text{ h}^{-1})] \times$$
$$(1 - e^{-(0.2682)(1)}) \times [1 / (1 - e^{-(0.2682)(12)})] \times e^{-(0.2682)(1)}$$

$$C_{t'}(\text{ss peak}) = 15.0 \text{ mg/L}$$

The trough is determined by changing t' from 1 to 11 hours. This represents the Δt between the end of infusion and the measured trough.

$$C_{t'}(\text{ss trough}) = 1.03 \text{ mg/L}$$

EXAMPLES OF SIMPLIFIED BEDSIDE PHARMACOKINETIC DOSE ADJUSTMENTS

In the clinical setting, in which drugs are administered according to dosing intervals of 4, 6, 8, 12, 18, or 24 hours, approximations of pharmacokinetic values can be used to adjust dosages at the bedside using the simple equation for bolus doses (e.g., Equation 8) and calculators without linear regression or logarithmic functions. This approach only applies, however, to drugs that have half-lives that are severalfold longer than the time required for drug administration. Because drugs administered to neonates often have prolonged half-lives compared with the duration of administration, these bedside techniques are readily applicable, particularly for aminoglycosides and vancomycin. At steady state, volume of distribution can be calculated from the trough preceding a dose and the subsequent peak concentration as outlined earlier without adjusting for drug eliminated during administration. The half-life can be closely approximated by dividing the time between the peak and trough concentration (Δt) by the number of times the concentration decreased in half. When a fraction of a half-life has elapsed, the half-life can be approximated by assuming a linear process, whereas in fact it is really exponential. If the exact fall in concentration is calculated, the concentration decreases during the first half of a half-life by about 59% of the total decrease during that half-life. This introduces a small error, but it is seldom large enough to alter the outcome of the dosage adjustment, because times for drug administration are rounded off to fit fractions of the 24-hour clock.

Example 1

Gentamicin, in a dose of 2.5 mg/kg, is infused over 30 minutes every 12 hours, resulting in a steady-state trough concentration of 1.9 mg/L and a peak of 4.5 mg/L, which was sampled 30 minutes after the end of the infusion. Recall that at steady state, the next trough (11 hours after the peak) will also be 1.9 mg/L.

Calculation of Vd

$$\Delta \text{ Concentration (mg/L)} = \frac{\text{Dose (mg/kg)}}{\text{Vd (L/kg)}}$$

$$C_{peak} - C_{trough} = \frac{2.5 \text{ mg/kg}}{\text{Vd (L/kg)}}$$

$$\text{Vd (L/kg)} = \frac{2.5 \text{ (mg/kg)}}{4.5 - 1.9 \text{ (mg/L)}} = 0.96 \text{ L/kg}$$

Calculation of Half-Life

The half-life can be calculated from the time between the peak concentration of 4.5 mg/L and the next trough concentration of 1.9 mg/L.

$T_{1/2}$ # 1 = Concentration decreases from 4.5 to 2.25 mg/L

$T_{1/2}$ # 2 = Concentration decreases from 2.25 to 1.12 mg/L

In this example, the concentration decreases from 2.25 to 1.9 mg/L, which represents a decline of 0.35 mg/L during the second half-life or 31% of the expected decline of 1.12 mg/L (0.35/1.12 = 31%). Thus, an estimated 1.31 half-lives has elapsed.

$$T_{1/2} = 11 \text{ h} / 1.31 \text{ half-lives} = 8.4 \text{ h}$$

This compares closely with the mathematically purer calculation of half-life using Equation 4:

$$T_{1/2} = 0.693 / [(\text{Ln } 4.5 - \text{Ln } 1.9) / 11 \text{ h}] = 8.8 \text{ h}$$

Dosage Adjustment

If the desired peak concentration is 6 mg/L for effective treatment of infection, the volume of distribution can be used to adjust the next dose after reaching the trough of 1.9 mg/L to reach that concentration.

$$\Delta \text{ Concentration (mg/L)} = \frac{\text{Dose (mg/kg)}}{\text{Vd (L/kg)}}$$

$$C_{peak} - C_{trough} = \frac{\text{Dose (mg/kg)}}{0.96 \text{ (L/kg)}}$$

$$0.96 \text{ L/kg} \times (6 - 1.9) \text{ (mg/L)} = \text{Dose (mg/kg)}$$

$$3.9 \text{ mg/kg} = \text{Dose (mg/kg)}$$

If the half-life and dosing interval remain constant, increasing the peak to 6 mg/L will raise the subsequent trough concentration to a level associated with nephrotoxicity (i.e., >2 mg/L). To maintain a trough of approximately 1.5 mg/L, the dosing interval must be increased to two half-lives or 16.8 hours (one half-life elapses as the concentration decreases from 6 to 3 mg/L and the second as the concentration decreases from 3 to 1.5 mg/L). An additional hour must be added because the dose is infused over 30 minutes and the peak is obtained 30 minutes after the end of infusion. Thus, the dosing interval of 17.8 hours is rounded to 18 hours. This regimen will maintain a trough of 1 to 2 mg/L and will achieve a peak of approximately 6 mg/L.

REFERENCES

1. Gibaldi M, Perrier D: Pharmacokinetics. New York, Marcel Dekker, 1982.
2. Wilkinson GR: Pharmacokinetics: the dynamics of drug absorption, distribution, and elimination. *In* Hardman JG, et al (eds): Goodman & Gilman's The Pharmacological Basis of Therapeutics. New York, McGraw-Hill, 2001, pp 3–29.
3. Krzyzanski W, Jusko WJ: Application of moment analysis to the sigmoid effect model for drug administered intravenously. Pharm Res *14*:949, 1997.
4. Cheng H, Jusko WJ: Noncompartmental determination of the mean residence time and steady-state volume of distribution during multiple dosing. J Pharm Sci *80*:202, 1991.
5. Notari RE: Rate processes in biological systems. *In* Biopharmaceutics and Clinical Pharmacokinetics: An Introduction, 3rd ed. New York, Marcel Dekker, 1980, pp 5–44.
6. Greenblatt DJ, Koch-Weser J: Clinical pharmacokinetics. N Engl J Med *293*:702, 1975.
7. Galinsky RE, Svvensson CK: Basic pharmacokinetics. *In* Gennaro AR, et al (eds): Remington: The Science and Practice of Pharmacy, Vol 1. Easton, MD, Mack Publishing, 1995, pp 724–760.
8. Zaske DE: Aminoglycosides. *In* Evans WE, et al (eds): Applied Pharmacokinetics: Principles of Therapeutic Drug Monitoring. Vancouver, WA, Applied Therapeutics, 1992, pp 1–14.
9. Matzke G: Vancomycin. *In* Evans W, et al (eds): Applied Pharmacokinetics: Principles of Therapeutic Drug Monitoring. Vancouver, WA, Applied Therapeutics, 1992, pp 15–11.
10. Ward RM: Pharmacologic principles and practicalities. *In* Taeusch HW, Ballard RA (eds): Avery's Diseases of the Newborn. Philadelphia, WB Saunders Co, 1998, pp 404–412.
11. Hastreiter AR, et al: Maintenance digoxin dosage and steady-state plasma concentration in infants and children. J Pediatr *107*:140, 1985.
12. Heizmann P, et al: Pharmacokinetics and bioavailability of midazolam in man. Br J Clin Pharmacol *16*(Suppl 1):43S, 1983.
13. Paine MF, et al: First-pass metabolism of midazolam by the human intestine. Clin Pharmacol Ther *60*:14, 1996.
14. de Wildt SN, et al: Pharmacokinetics and metabolism of oral midazolam in preterm infants. Br J Clin Pharmacol *53*:390, 2002.
15. Penson RT, et al: The bioavailability and pharmacokinetics of subcutaneous, nebulized and oral morphine-6-glucuronide. Br J Clin Pharmacol *53*:347, 2002.
16. Borchard U: Pharmacokinetics of beta-adrenoceptor blocking agents: clinical significance of hepatic and/or renal clearance. Clin Physiol Biochem *8*(Suppl 2):28, 1990.
17. DiPiro JT, et al: Concepts in Clinical Pharmacokinetics, 2nd ed. Bethesda, MD, American Society of Health-System Pharmacists, 1996.
18. Bouroujerdi M: Pharmacokinetics: Principles and Applications. New York, McGraw-Hill, 2002, pp 205–231.

Sabine Luise Plonait and Heinz Nau

21

Physicochemical and Structural Properties Regulating Placental Drug Transfer

Evidence has accumulated that essentially all pharmacologic agents, and other exogenous substances as well, are transferred to the embryo and fetus, regardless of whether this transfer is wanted, as in intrauterine nutrition[1] or medical treatment of the fetus,[2–4] or unwanted, with possible teratogenic or toxic fetal effects.[4,5] Because of the increasing numbers of readily available over-the-counter drugs taken as self-medication by women who may be unaware of an early pregnancy or of possible adverse effects to a fetus, demands on public information are growing.[6,7] A better understanding of these aspects can provide support in designing meaningful toxicokinetic and drug disposition studies.[8] It is desirable to identify parameters that determine the extent (total amount) and rate (amount per time) of the placental transfer of a certain specific compound.

METHODOLOGIC APPROACHES

Although investigations of the pharmacokinetics of clinically indicated drugs in the maternal circulation can easily be performed, fetal sampling in earlier gestational stages is restricted to rare procedures (e.g., ultrasound-guided exchange transfusions, termination of pregnancy after maternal ingestion of the drug) and the moment of delivery, when cord blood samples can be obtained. Thus, serial sampling is not usually possible, and the transplacental kinetics must be pieced together from many different subjects studied at various times.

Analysis of amniotic fluid leaking after premature rupture of membranes may allow an indirect approach to the distribution of xenobiotics from the mother to the fetus. As an alternative to fetal blood sampling, Jauniaux and Gulbis[9] introduced coelocentesis to study placental drug transfer in the first trimester when coelomic and amniotic fluid are important compartments and the permeability of the placenta is greater than at term. The presence or absence of compounds or their metabolites in meconium samples gained from the newborns after birth can also be helpful to obtain qualitative data on intrauterine exposure; this method is already used to detect maternal drug abuse in pregnancy.[10,11] These methods, however, do not allow use of kinetic models based on blood or plasma samples. Kinetic models are necessary to allow for extrapolating quantitative drug transfer to the fetus and subsequent risk assessment.

When more than one isolated sample is needed to establish a kinetic model (distribution between maternal and fetal circulation), the use of animal models is helpful. Their relevance with regard to human kinetics may be limited, however, because of difficulties in extrapolating the experimental results to humans.[12] Humans and guinea pigs have a hemomonochorial placenta; the rabbit has a hemodichorial placenta, and the rat has a hemotrichorial placenta.

In the rodent, the yolk sac placenta is of paramount importance during the entire period of organogenesis, as well as later in development; the hemoendothelial (chemotrichorial) placenta starts to function from the late organogenesis stage onward.[13-15] This is quite different in monkeys and humans. In these species, the yolk sac plays a much more limited, and poorly understood, role, and the hemomonochorial placenta starts to function at an early stage.[13-15] It is not completely understood how the species differences of the placental morphology influence the transfer of exogenous compounds to the embryo and fetus. If extrapolations from toxicologic *in vitro* models are planned, then the maternofetal interface must be taken into consideration.[16] The presence of membrane barriers around the developing embryo in the whole embryo culture system could prevent the transfer of the water-soluble all-*trans*-retinoyl-β-D-glucuronide from reaching the conceptus and exerting its teratogenic potential, which, in other models without such lipophilic barrier (e.g., the limb bud organ culture), is equal to the lipid-soluble all-*trans*-retinoic acid.[17] Positron emission tomographic studies on placenta transfer using radiolabeled drugs (e.g., ^{11}C-labeled heroin) may become a useful technique, but it will probably not be suitable for investigations in pregnant women.[18]

Human placenta obtained atraumatically at birth provides a way to investigate the human organ in *in vitro* perfusion studies.[19] Both maternofetal clearance and fetomaternal clearance can be standardized by comparison with antipyrine clearance. Limitations of these models include the following: the

experimental period is limited to a few hours; the only available material is human placenta at term (not in early gestational stages that may be more relevant with regard to toxic effects); and this type of model does not allow the observation of physiologically relevant parameters, such as blood flow (important for rapidly transferred compounds) or plasma protein binding.

PLACENTAL TRANSFER

The rate as well and extent of transfer depend on the physicochemical and structural characteristics of the drugs as well as on physiologic characteristics of the maternal-placental-embryonic-fetal unit.[20-26] The concept of the placenta as lipoid membrane is useful to describe the influence of physicochemical characteristics of the drugs on their placental transfer. Most drugs cross the placental membranes by diffusion, the rate of which is governed mainly by physicochemical factors according to Fick's law:[20-24,26]

$$\text{rate of diffusion} = D \times \Delta c \times \frac{A}{d} \qquad [1]$$

where A = area of exchange, d = membrane thickness, Δc = drug concentration gradient across the membrane (e.g., difference between maternal and fetal plasma drug concentrations), and D = diffusion constant of the drug.

From this equation, it may be predicted that a large area of placental exchange (A) consisting of membranes with limited thickness (d) favors placental transfer of drugs. Although A, d, and Δc can be determined in a model, D is far more difficult to predict because it results from the interactions between the membrane and the molecule. The resistance within the tissue layers interposed between maternal and fetal circulations (compartments) limits the diffusion, which is significant for hydrophilic molecules. In the human placenta, two layers contribute to diffusional resistance: the trophoblast and the endothelium. Hydrophilic molecules either have to partition through these layers (membrane hypothesis) or find their way through water-filled channels that extend through the trophoblast and communicate with the intracellular channels of the endothelial layer (*aqueous pores hypothesis*). Such a process is known to be present, but it is not efficient in the intestinal mucosa.[27] Rapid placental transfer is therefore related to better lipid solubility and low ionization and protein binding of drugs with a molecular weight lower than 500.

The permeability of lipid-soluble substances is much higher. Therefore, their placental flux rates are mainly limited by their availability (resulting in the initial maternofetal concentration gradient = Δc) at the area of exchange, which is determined by uterine and umbilical blood flow.[28] *In vivo*, however, the placenta cannot be described by area and thickness. Indeed, earlier studies noted that as placental thickness and the number of placental layers decreased and the area of exchange increased during gestation, increased placental transfer occurred.[20,22-26] Thornburg and Faber[27] found that in rabbit placenta, the fetal endothelium, which is not markedly altered during pregnancy, is the layer defining the transfer rate of many drugs; A and d were apparently of secondary importance. The diffusion of drugs across the hemotrichorial placenta (mouse, rat) is often faster than across hemomonochorial placenta (monkey, human) despite larger numbers of placental membranes. The sheep epitheliochorial placenta allows only small molecules to pass its "aqueous pores."

This chapter is mostly concerned with a discussion of the influence of such physicochemical parameters of drugs on their placental transfer. The statements made previously are a useful concept but represent an oversimplification of a complex situation. Thus, structural characteristics of drugs must play an important role, although little is known about this important aspect.

PHARMACOKINETIC MODELS OF MATERNOFETAL DRUG EXCHANGE

The rate and extent of drug transfer to the embryo and fetus are determined by numerous variables, listed in Table 21-1.[12] Several general types of pharmacokinetic concentration time curves can therefore be observed in the maternofetal unit (Fig. 21-1).[12,29,30] Furthermore, the rate of transfer may change during the course of treatment.[31] Model A in Figure 21-1 is applicable if a drug crosses the placenta rapidly and distributes rapidly within a single fetal compartment that is in rapid equilibrium with the maternal compartment. Fetal concentrations rapidly rise to reach maternal plasma levels; after this time, the fetal and maternal curves overlap. When maternofetal exchange is rapid, two additional models are possible. After equilibrium between the maternal and fetal compartment has been attained, fetal concentrations may exceed maternal plasma levels (curve C), or they may be less than corresponding maternal plasma levels (see curve E in Fig. 21-1). As discussed later, differential protein binding or a pH gradient in the maternofetal unit may be responsible for the relatively high (curve C) or low (curve E) extent of fetal drug exposure after equilibrium between the maternal and fetal compartment has been attained.

When the rate of placental transfer is slow, model D is often applicable in the maternofetal unit. The rise of drug concentration in the fetus is slow. However, because the transport of drug from the fetus back to the mother is also slow, fetal concentrations exceed maternal plasma levels after the cross-over point of the two curves. Thus, the fetus can be considered as a "deep" or "slow" compartment. A protein binding or pH gradient may affect the fetomaternal concentration gradient after postdistribution equilibrium in model D. In model F, the fetal concentrations never reach the corresponding maternal plasma values because the plasma protein binding or the pH gradient may favor higher maternal than fetal concentrations. Alternatively, efficient metabolism by the fetus or fetal excretion (e.g., into amniotic fluid) may also be responsible for the relatively low fetal drug levels. Model B is seldom observed. In this model, drug transport is slow from mother to fetus but rapid from fetus to mother. This situations implies an active or facilitated transport system that is not typically present with therapeutic agents.

Such considerations of models may appear on first glance to be of theoretical interest only. These models are of extreme importance, however, when results from experimental and clinical studies are interpreted. When kinetic curves are inadequately defined, results may be completely misinterpreted. Owing to ethical and practical limitations, often only one or a few fetomaternal sample pairs are available for analysis in clinical studies. If these samples were taken before cross-over (model C), for example, the wrong conclusion (of relatively low fetal exposure) could be reached. For an adequate description of fetal exposure, both the maternal and the fetal concentration time curves must be defined. Although such complete data on placental transfer are rare, an attempt was made to assign tentatively the kinetics of some drugs to the models defined in Figure 21-1; the results are compiled in Table 21-2.

From this discussion, it also becomes clear why it is so difficult to identify parameters that determine the placental transfer of drugs. The selection of the correct model is the prerequisite for a rational interpretation of the relative importance of parameters, such as physicochemical properties of drugs.[32] Drugs have the greatest chance of crossing the placenta if they (1) are lipid soluble, (2) are weak acids, and (3) have a low molecular weight (<500 Da). Another important factor is protein binding.[8]

LIPID SOLUBILITY OF DRUGS

According to the basic concept of drug diffusion through a lipoid barrier, lipophilic drugs (high lipid/water partition coefficient K; poor water solubility) should be rapidly transferred across the placenta (panels on the *left* in Fig. 21-1); the reverse should be true for hydrophilic drugs (low lipid/water partition coefficient K; high water solubility).[20-24,27,33] Thus, substances such as thiopental, secobarbital, propofol, and antipyrine cross the placenta extremely rapidly.[20,26,34] In the pregnant rat, the parathion metabolite *p*-nitrophenol is rapidly transferred into the fetus, where its elimination half-time is the longest of all tissues examined.[35] Bisphenol A reaches peak levels in maternal blood and fetus 20 minutes after single oral administration to the rat, with the fetal concentration reaching about 60% of the level detected in maternal blood.[36] Cocaine, a weak base characterized by high lipid solubility, low molecular weight (MW = 305), and low plasma protein binding (8 to 10%), quickly equilibrates between the maternal and fetal compartment, as does its metabolite cocaethylene.[37-40] More polar compounds, such as the barbiturates butethal and phenobarbital or the more hydrophilic cocaine metabolite benzoylgonine, cross the placenta more

---

TABLE 21-1

Factors Determining Rate and Extent of Drug Transfer to the Embryo/Fetus

	Characteristics	
Transfer	***Drug***	***Maternal/Placental/ Fetal Unit***
Rate	Lipid solubility	Placental structure and
	Molecular weight	function
	Structural	Placental blood flow
	characteristics	Thickness of placental
	Protein binding*	membranes
	Type of transfer†	
Extent	Degree of ionization	Maternal/fetal pH gradient
	(pKa)	
	Protein binding	
	Type of transfer†	

* If transfer is relatively slow.
† Passive diffusion, facilitated or active transport, pinocytosis.

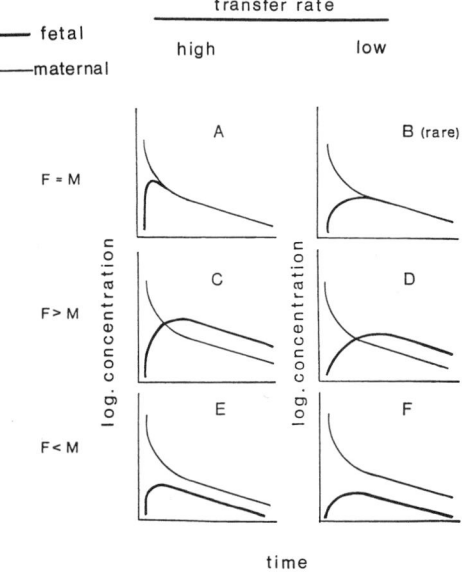

Figure 21-1. Simulation of maternal (M) and fetal (F) plasma concentration time curves from various transplacental pharmacokinetic models. Examples are listed in Table 21-2.

TABLE 21-2

Examples of Drugs with Transplacental Pharmacokinetics According to Models A–F in Figure 21–1*

Model A (or B)	Model C	Model D	Model E	Model F
Some barbiturates	**Some benzodiazepines**	Ascorbate	**Amide-type local anesthetic agents**	Heparin
Thiopental	Diazepam	Colistimethate†		TCDD
Pentobarbital	Lorazepam	Furosemide	Lidocaine	
Secobarbital	Desmethyldiazepam	Meperidine	Bupivacaine	**Quaternary ammonium compounds**
	Oxazepam			
Antipyrine		**Some cephalosporins**	**Some β-adrenoceptor blockers**	Tubocurarine
Promethazine	Valproate	Cephalothin		Succinylcholine
Ritodrine	Salicylate	Cefazolin	Propranolol	Vecuronium
Magnesium (sulfate)	Nalidixic acid	Cephapirin	Sotalol	Pancuronium
Thiamphenicol	Nicotine	Cephalexin	Labetalol	Fazadinium
Digoxin	Urea			Alcuronium
		Some aminoglycosides	Dexamethasone	
	Some penicillins	Gentamicin	Cimetidine	**Elementary ions: Cd, Hg**
	Ampicillin	Kanamycin	Ranitidine	Fenoterol
	Penicillin G		Methadone	Chlorthalidone
	Methicillin			Etozolin (ozolinone)
	Azidocillin		**Some sulfonamides‡**	Dicloxacillin
				Erythromycin
				Nitrofurantoin

* Differentiation between models A and B, C and D, and E and F is often uncertain because of incomplete data on the initial phase of drug distribution across the placenta; model B is rarely applicable.
† Polypeptide antibiotic. MW 1200 Da.
‡ First and second trimester.
TCDD = 2,3,7,8-tetrachlorodibenzo-p-dioxin.
Data from refs. 20–26, 30, 55, 60, 65, 71, 77, 82, 90, 111, 172, 174–176, 178–180, 196.

slowly. The highly lipid-soluble benzodiazepine receptor agonist abecarnil (log P = 4.6) reaches higher concentrations in the rabbit fetus compared with maternal blood levels, whereas its highly polar and subsequently hydrophilic metabolites cannot pass the placental barrier to the same extent.[40] Whereas no particular influence of lipophilia or other chemicostructural properties determining the extent of maternofetal transfer of a group of opioids (fentanyl > alfentanil > sufentanil) was observed, especially in the event of fluctuations in maternal flow, lipophilicity was found to be an important factor when the opioid transfer is compared with that of antipyrine.[41] Another highly lipophilic opiate, buprenorphine (MW = 504.1, high binding to α- and β-globulins but hardly to albumin), shows high sequestration to tissues including the placenta, but only a low transplacental transfer (<10%), in spite of its high lipid solubility. This could explain why neonates born to mothers treated with buprenorphine during pregnancy rarely show signs of withdrawal symptoms.[42]

Comparison of the *in vitro* maternofetal gradients of antibiotics used to treat mother and fetus for perinatal infections (e.g., chorioamnionitis) or conditions associated with an increased risk of infection (e.g., prolonged rupture of membranes) revealed that clavulanate and ticarcillin hardly cross the placenta despite low plasma protein binding (9 and 45%) and molecular weights (236 and 428 kDa). The equally large but more lipophilic molecule ceftizoxime (<30%, MW = 406) reaches higher concentrations in the fetus as compared with the mother.[43,44] Exogenous bases, such as 2′,3′-dideoxyinosine and 2′,3′-dideoxycytidine, and the more lipophilic antiviral drug azidothymidine cross the placental barrier rapidly by simple diffusion.[45-47] The purine derivative 2′,3′-dideoxyinosine, however, crosses the placental barrier more slowly than the pyrimidines.[45,48] Again, there is a marked difference between their partition coefficients, with $P_{azidothymidine} = 0.86$ to 1.26, as opposed to $P_{dideoxyinosine} = 0.07$ to 0.32.[48] *In vitro* and in women before termination of pregnancy, therapeutic maternal levels of azidothymidine resulted in fetal levels within the therapeutic range as well.[49,50] In one study, umbilical cord sample levels even ranged from 113 to 127% of maternal levels, probably reflecting the prolonged elimination half-life in the newborn.[51]

This finding suggests that sufficient preventive treatment of the conceptus would be possible, but also that there is a high potential of adverse fetal effects. Within the human placenta, the drug is metabolized to more polar and yet undefined metabolites, which are not released into the perfusates, probably as a consequence of their reduced lipid solubility.[52] A more polar glucuronidated metabolite could cross the human perfused placenta at about half the rate of azidothymidine.[52] Tuntland and colleagues[53] proposed models that predict the extent of placental transfer of dioxynucleoside drugs. Predicted fetal/maternal steady-state plasma concentration ratios using their *in vitro* partition-coefficient model deviated from observed values only by 3.9 ± 79% (mean, %±SD). *In vivo* and *in vitro* clearance indexes were highly and significantly related to the drug octanol-water partition coefficient (Fig. 21-2A).[53] Another drug in the same group of compounds is acyclovir, which is taken orally by women with recurrent genital herpes simplex infections during late pregnancy to reduce the risk of transmission of herpes simplex to the fetus. As a lipophilic compound with low plasma binding (22 to 33%), it also appears to be quickly transferred by simple diffusion.[54] The highest levels of this compound were measured in the amniotic fluid, probably secondary to unchanged renal excretion of the drug by the fetus, thus providing additional protection against ascending viral infection.[54] Placental transfer of hydrophilic substances is proportional to the coefficient of free diffusion in water, with some evidence of steric restriction of larger molecules (Fig. 21-2B).[27]

The relationship between partition coefficients and placental transfer does not hold for drugs with a high or low partition coefficient (K). If K is high, the substance may be so tightly bound to membranes or other cell constituents (proteins, lipids) that it cannot readily cross into an aqueous phase from the lipid phase. Examples of drugs in this category are cyclosporine and chlorinated aromatics, such as 2,3,7,8,-tetrachlorodibenzo-p-dioxin (TCDD), which are extremely lipophilic but are transferred to the embryo and fetus in minute amounts only.[55,56] These drugs are stored in maternal liver and fat. Therefore, the low fat content of the conceptus may be an additional factor

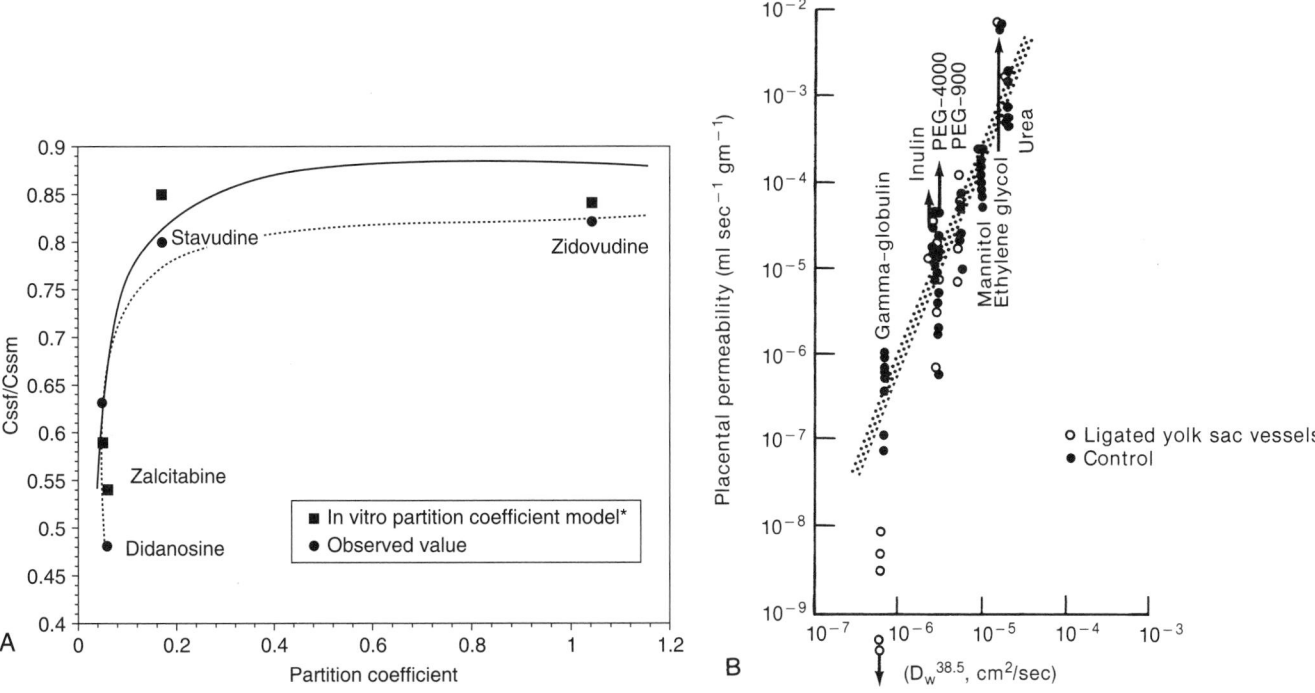

Figure 21–2. A, Comparison of an observed and *in vitro* partition coefficient model predicted fetal/maternal steady-state plasma concentration ratios (Cssf/Cssm). Details regarding the model are to be found in the original publication.[53] The octanol-water partition coefficient is taken as mean from reference 53. **B,** Permeability of guinea pig placenta in fetuses with (*closed circles*) and without (*open circles*) intact vitelline circulations, as functions of coefficients of free diffusion in water at 38.5°C. The linear regression line is a least squares fit of a logarithmically transformed datum, and the *shaded area* is the 95% confidence interval of means. γ-Globulin data are shown but were not used in computation of regression because γ-globulin transfer is not a diffusional process in chorioallantoic placenta. (**A,** Modified from Tuntland T, et al: Am J Obstet Gynecol *180*:198, 1999; **B,** from Thornburg KL, et al: Am J Physiol *2*:C111, 1977.)

limiting the placental transfer of these compounds. This concept is supported by the finding that TCDD is efficiently transferred by mother's milk, which contains a high amount of fat.[57] Phylloquinone (vitamin K_1, supplemented in pregnant women whose infants are at risk of spontaneous hemorrhage) is another compound that, despite its high lipophilicity, is only slowly and in minor quantities transferred through the human placenta (22 to 34 gestational weeks).[58] Data suggest, however, that if one permits an adequate lag period between maternal supplementation and delivery, maternofetal transport of the vitamin can be enhanced.[58]

In the perfused term rat placenta, hydrophilic *p*-aminobenzoic acid crosses to the fetal compartment more readily than lipophilic antipyrine. The mechanism of its transplacental passage is not clear.[59]

IONIZATION OF DRUGS

Most drugs are weakly acidic or basic substances and are thus ionized at physiologic pH. Passive diffusion across lipophilic membranes depends on the degree of ionization. Only the nonionized (lipophilic) portion of the drug is assumed to pass readily through the lipoid barriers, whereas the ionized form carries a charge (and is therefore polar) and cannot pass through the membranes.

This generalization is true for quaternary ammonium compounds, such as neuromuscular blocking agents, which are fully ionized (dimethyltubocurarine, pancuronium, succinylcholine).[60-64] After maternal administration, fetal drug levels increase slowly up to levels that are only about 10% of corresponding maternal plasma concentrations (see model F in Fig. 21-1 and Table 21-2), both during early[60] and late[61] gesta-

tion. The transfer of these compounds is confined to water-filled pores within the lipid membranes, a mechanism much less efficient than the transfer across the lipid portions of the membranes.

This rule does not apply to all highly ionized substances. Weak acids, which constitute an important group of drugs, appear to be rapidly transferred across the placenta. Salicylate[65, 66] and valproate (VPA),[5,67-69] two drugs essentially fully ionized at physiologic pH, are rapidly transported to the conceptus. Fetal salicylate concentrations reach corresponding maternal levels about 1 hour after administration;[66] in mouse and rat, transplacental equilibrium of VPA between embryonic and maternal compartments was reached in less than 0.5 hour.[70-72] Similar observations have been made for the antibiotics ampicillin and methicillin.[4] It seems that the small portions of nonionized drug are responsible for the efficient transport across the membranes; the equilibrium between the ionized and nonionized form is rapidly reestablished for further transfer of the nonionized form.

The importance of ionization is supported by studies using the perfused human placenta. We compared the maternal/fetal clearance ratios of VPA and its glucuronides (β-glucuronidase susceptible = VPA-G and non-β-glucuronidase susceptible = VPA-GR). The glucuronidated acids characterized by partition coefficients of 0.0141 and 0.219 (compared with 1.6 for VPA) were expected to have negative log of dissociation constant (pKa) values between 3 and 4, resulting in higher ionization compared with VPA. As expected, the placental transfer was found to be significantly lower for the glucuronides (13 and 17% compared with 95% for VPA acid). Furthermore, although transport was positively correlated with log (partition coefficient), there was no significant dependence on molecular weight.[73] *In vivo*, similar observations were made concerning lower placental transfer of glucuronidated retinoids in the rabbit.[74] Barbiturates[20] and ascorbate[75] are also efficiently transferred to the fetus.

Similar reasons may explain the efficient transfer of some basic substances, such as the tertiary phenothiazines, meperidine, nicotine,[39,76,77] and lysergic acid diethylamide.[78] As noted earlier, the nonionized portion (in rapid equilibrium with the ionized form) of the drugs may cross to the conceptus. Lead and metallic mercury can be transferred from the blood of occupationally exposed mothers to the fetus.[79,80]

In late gestation, the pH of fetal blood is 0.1 to 0.15 units lower than the pH in maternal blood.[20] This pH gradient between fetal and maternal blood influences the extent of transfer of acidic and basic drugs. As discussed earlier, only the nonionized form of the drugs can readily pass the lipoid membranes. Because basic drugs are ionized at the relatively low (acidic) pH of fetal blood to a higher degree than in maternal blood, this class of drugs accumulates in fetal blood (*ion trapping*) (models C and D in Fig. 21-1). The reverse is true for acidic drugs, which reach lower concentrations in fetal than in maternal blood in late gestation (models E and F in Fig. 21-1). The ratio between the fetal and maternal concentrations ($C_{fetal}/C_{maternal}$) for a particular drug can be calculated with the Henderson-Hasselbalch equation from the pKa of the drug and the fetal and maternal blood pH:

$$\frac{C_{fetal,\ free}}{C_{maternal,\ free}} = \frac{1 + 10^{\ (pKa\ -\ pH,\ fetal)}}{1 + 10^{\ (pKa\ -\ pH,\ maternal)}} \qquad [2]$$

The pH gradient determines the concentration gradient of *free* concentrations, which are unbound to plasma proteins. The *total* concentrations (free and protein-bound) are determined by the protein-binding gradient across the placenta (see later). Basic drugs such as amide-type local anesthetic agents are ionized to a higher degree in fetal blood than in maternal blood. Therefore, the free concentrations of drugs such as lidocaine, bupivacaine, 2-chloroprocaine, ropivacaine, and pethidine accumulate in fetal blood by a considerable factor (about 1.5; Table 21-3).[81,82] An obvious influence of the fetal pH on maternofetal clearance of bupivacaine and ropivacaine was demonstrated *in vitro*.[83] The total concentrations of these drugs are, however, much lower in fetal than in maternal blood because of low fetal protein binding (see later).

Low fetal/maternal total concentration ratios do not imply low or no effects on the fetus. Both the pharmacologic effects and the toxicologic actions of a drug are usually associated with the free, and not the total, drug concentrations. Indeed, fetal side effects of amide-type local anesthetic agents are related to the pH gradient across the placenta and not to the protein-binding gradient.[82] A fall in fetal pH (fetal acidosis as in fetal distress), particularly if accompanied by a rise in maternal pH (maternal alkalosis from hyperventilation), increases the fetomaternal pH gradient and increases fetal drug accumulation and possible fetal side effects. This has been found in experimental and clinical studies for both lidocaine[84-86] and bupivacaine.[87-89] The reverse would be expected with regard to the effects of the fetomaternal pH gradient on the extent of placental transfer of acidic drugs. In agreement with the pH partition hypothesis, the fetal free concentrations of VPA were lower than the corresponding maternal values (fetomaternal free concentration gradient = 0.82 ± 0.34 in one study).[90] Again, the concentration gradient of the total levels was quite different. Owing to decreased maternal plasma protein binding (see later), the total concentrations in fetal plasma exceeded those in maternal plasma by a factor of 1.7.[68,90] The pH partition hypothesis is supported by data in experimental animals that indicate that the transplacental distribution of salicylate is affected by maternal acidosis. Treatment of pregnant rats with ammonium chloride decreases maternal pH and increases the fetomaternal concentration gradient.[91] Maternal acidosis during treatment with VPA can be expected during or after prolonged epileptic seizures. Acetylsalicylic acid is often taken by patients suffering from pyrexia, which under certain conditions can also be associated with acidosis. Low-dose aspirin is used to treat pregnancy-induced hypertension. Acetylsalicylic acid transfers rapidly and reaches a steady state in the perfused placental cotyledon model.[92] Maternal acidosis in the course of the illness may cause a significant fetomaternal gradient.

Little is known of the plasma and embryonic tissue pH during early human gestational periods. The period between week 3 and weeks 6 to 8 after conception may be particularly important for the formation of major malformations, such as those found after intake of thalidomide or retinoids. Studies during similar early periods of organogenesis in mouse, rat, and monkey have yielded surprising and potentially important results. The intracellular pH (pH_i as determined by distribution of the weak acid dimethadione) is surprisingly high during early organogenesis.[70,93,94] Embryonic pH_i considerably exceeded corresponding maternal plasma pH at that period and decreased during later developmental periods to approach values similar to other tissues. In comparison, maternal muscle pH remained low (6.9 and 7.0) during all developmental periods.

An acidic drug, such as VPA, would be expected to be ionized to a higher degree in the relatively basic milieu of the early embryo. Based on the pKa of VPA (4.7), the pH partition hypothesis would predict a concentration of the drug in the embryo twice as high as that in maternal plasma, and this has been found experimentally (Table 21-4).[70,93] The pH_i of the embryo decreases with advancing gestation and, thus, in agreement with the pH partition hypothesis, so does the embryonic-maternal concentration gradient. Salicylate, dimethadione, metabolites of

TABLE 21-3

Extent of Transplacental Distribution of Amide-Type Local Anesthetic Agents

Drug	Total Concentration Ratio F/M	% Protein Binding		Protein-Binding Ratio F/M	Free Concentration F/M*	Total Concentration F/M†
		Maternal	*Fetal*			
Lidocaine	0.4-0.7	63	34	0.54	1.4	0.80
		64	24		1.4	0.66
Bupivacaine	0.18-0.56	91	51	0.56	1.5	0.27
		92	72	0.78	1.5	0.42
Etidocaine	0.09-0.37	92	—	—	1.4	—
Mepivacaine	0.5-0.8	5	36	0.65	1.4	0.71
Prilocaine	1.0-1.3	55	—	—	1.4	—

* Predicted according to formula 2.
† Predicted according to formula 4.
F/M = fetal/maternal.
Data from refs. 82, 84-89 and literature citations therein.

halothane (trichloroacetic acid) and methoxyethanol (methoxyacetic acid), and acidic thalidomide metabolites also accumulate in the early rodent embryo (see Table 21-4).[70] It has been hypothesized that acidic metabolites formed by hydrolysis of thalidomide within the embryo may be trapped there because of their high polarity.[95-97] The pH hypothesis is just as likely to provide an explanation for the embryonic accumulation of these acidic metabolites.

Neutral drugs, such as the anticonvulsants valpromide and ethosuximide (see Table 21-4), should not be affected by transplacental pH gradient. Concentrations of these two drugs in the embryo are essentially the same as corresponding concentrations in maternal plasma.

Certain human teratogens or their metabolites are weakly acidic substances, such as VPA, trimethadione (metabolite dimethadione), phenytoin, thalidomide (glutamic acid derivatives as metabolites), warfarin, isotretinoin, and etretinate (metabolite etretin). Basic drugs are not represented in lists of human teratogens. Perhaps the reason for the predominance of acidic drugs in the list of human teratogens stems is that these substances accumulate in the early embryo, resulting in unexpectedly high "exposure" of the embryo as compared with the maternal organism. Some weak acids may be teratogenic because they can alter the pH_i of the embryonic cell. This concept is attractive as a general mechanism of teratogenesis because the pH controls numerous cellular functions, including proliferation and intercellular communication. Structure-activity studies must answer some of these questions. Certainly, the finding that some related substances without an acid function do not accumulate in the embryo and exhibit low teratogenic potency supports the hypothesis of a special significance of the acid function in teratogenicity.

PROTEIN BINDING OF DRUGS

Protein binding of xenobiotics can occur in maternal blood plasma and other maternal tissues, in placental tissues, and in fetal blood plasma and other fetal tissues. Therefore, not only may drugs from the maternal plasma cross the placenta, but also a portion that initially was bound to placental proteins acting as a temporary sink may diffuse to the conceptus later. In the human placenta, the transfer of some drugs including vinblastine,[98] vincristine,[98] cyclosporine,[99] and digoxin[98, 100] appears to

be regulated by an adenosine triphosphate–dependent membrane protein, P-glycoprotein, apparently protecting the fetus from toxic substances.[98] Rifabutin, being more lipophilic than rifampin, has a greater clearance in the single cotyledon perfusion system; however, because of its trend toward greater disposition in the placental tissue, there may be proportionately less accumulation in the fetal circulation.[101] Placental binding and metabolism are not discussed in this chapter.

Plasma protein binding may affect both the rate and the extent of placental drug transfer (see Table 21-1). The plasma proteins have two functions: for the drugs bound to them they serve as *vehicles* allowing the drug to be transported, but depending on the affinity of compound they may impair transfer. Conversely, they offer binding sites on the other side of the placental barrier, *acceptors* that potentially allow for additional transfer.

Maternal plasma protein binding is a limiting factor for drugs that are transferred through placental membranes relatively slowly. Only the portion of the drugs unbound to proteins ("free drug") is available for placental transfer, and it takes considerable time to reach distribution equilibrium between the maternal and fetal compartments. Here the permeability across the placenta is rate-limiting, and plasma protein binding can be considered as a storage or reservoir of drug.

Many lipophilic drugs, which are highly protein bound, actually permeate the placenta rapidly. Plasma protein binding is rapidly reversible and may even increase the amount transferred by presenting more drug to the placenta. Here, plasma protein binding plays a transport role and serves as a vehicle that is especially important for drugs with poor water solubility that otherwise would not reach the placenta in high amounts. Protein binding depends on the concentration of the protein (P) to which the drug is bound as well as on the binding affinity constant (Ka) and the number of binding sites available (n):

$$B/F = n \times Ka \times P \qquad [3]$$

B/F = bound concentration/free concentration of drug.

The importance of protein binding, however, depends on the degree of binding; a clinically significant effect is expected only when it exceeds about 80%.[102] This may account for the failure to detect differences in transplacental transfer between methimazole (no binding to plasma proteins) and propylthiouracil (67% bound

---

TABLE 21-4

Teratogenicity and Embryo/Maternal Concentration Ratios of Acidic, Neutral, and Basic Substances

Type of Compound	Drug	Species	Period of Gestation	E/M Ratio	Teratogenic
			Placental Transfer		
Acids	Valproic acid	Mouse	Day 9	1.6-2.3	Yes
	Valproic acid	Rat	Day 11	1.5-1.7	Yes
	Salicylic acid	Rat	Day 10	1.3-1.7	Yes
	Thalidomide (acid metabolite)	Rabbit	Day 8 (blastocyst)	1.2	Yes
	Dimethadione	Mouse	Day 9	1.4-1.7	Yes
		Rat	Day 11		Yes
	Halothane (trichloroacetic acid)	Mouse	Day 11	Accumulation of radioactivity	Yes
	Methoxyethanol (methoxyacetic acid)	Rat	Day 12	2	Yes
		Monkey	Day 28	1	Yes
	Hydrochloric acid (acidified sea water)	Sea urchin embryo, *in vitro*	5 h (32 cells)	—	Yes
	2-en-valproic acid	Mouse	Day 9	1.2-1.5	No
Neutral substances	Valpromide	Mouse	Day 9	1	No
	Ethosuximide	Mouse	Day 9	1	No
Basic substances	Nicotine	Mouse	Day 9	3	No
	Doxylamine	Mouse	Day 9	5	No

E/M = embryo/maternal.
Data from refs. 70, 93, 159, and citations therein.

to albumin) *in vitro*.[103] Little information is available on the effects of maternal or fetal hypoproteinemia on placental drug transfer. In a study by Brown and colleagues,[104] fetal (umbilical cord) serum concentrations of the antibiotic cefazolin in human newborns suffering from hydrops fetalis were not different from those obtained from nonhydropic infants. Conversely, no transfer was observed in the presence of little albumin (1 mg/mL) in the perfused human placental cotyledon,[105] and indeed, low digoxin levels have been found in transplacentally treated human fetuses suffering from severe rhesus disease, resulting in hypoproteinemia.[106] *In vitro*, the transplacental transfer of olanzapine (plasma binding *in vitro*: albumin, 90%; α_1-acid glycoprotein, 77%) was largely dependent on the concentration of acceptor proteins on the opposite side of initial drug placement.[107]

There is convincing evidence that the binding affinity or the number of binding sites of fetal proteins is similar to that of maternal proteins (see later).[108-110] Therefore, the extent of placental transfer is determined by the relative concentrations of the binding proteins in maternal and fetal blood.[111] There are two major binding proteins: albumin and α_1-acid glycoprotein. The fetal/maternal concentration ratios of these two proteins differ greatly from each other (Table 21-5). At the end of the first trimester and the beginning of the second, fetal albumin concentrations are about 30% of corresponding maternal levels and increase during gestation to reach maternal levels during the third trimester. At the time of birth, fetal albumin levels even exceed corresponding maternal values (Fig. 21-3).[112-115] Fetal α_1-acid glycoprotein concentrations are low during early gestation (10% of maternal values at the end of first and beginning of

second trimester) and then slowly increase to reach about one-third of corresponding maternal concentrations during late gestation (see Table 21-5).[112,114]

Therefore, the development of a fetomaternal plasma protein-binding gradient (and thus the extent of the placental transfer) for a particular drug depends greatly on the nature of the binding protein. This is exemplified by a comparison of fetal and maternal protein binding of diazepam,[114] VPA,[113] and propranolol (Table 21-6).[114] The first two drugs are bound predominantly to albumin; consequently, protein binding is low in fetal plasma during early to midgestation but increases steadily to reach an extent that exceeds maternal binding at term (Fig. 21-4; see also Fig. 21-3). Propranolol is predominantly bound to α_1-acid glycoprotein; consequently, protein binding is low in fetal plasma during early and midgestation but does not significantly increase during later gestational periods.

Protein binding is defined either as the percentage of drug bound ($C_{bound}/C_{total} \times 100$) or as the unbound (free) fraction ($C_{unbound}/C_{total}$). The fetal/maternal concentration ratio of total drug at postdistributive equilibrium can therefore be predicted as follows:

$$\frac{C_{fetal,\ total}}{C_{maternal,\ total}} = \frac{\text{unbound fraction (mother)}}{\text{unbound fraction (fetus)}} \quad [4]$$

If the drug is an electrolyte, the pH difference between fetal and maternal blood has to be taken into account:

TABLE 21-5

Human Maternal and Fetal Serum Albumin and α_1-Acid Glycoprotein Concentrations During Gestation

Week of Gestation	Albumin Concentration (g/L)			α_1-Acid Glycoprotein Concentration (g/L)		
	Maternal	*Fetal*	*F/M*	*Maternal*	*Fetal*	*F/M*
12–15	28	11	0.28	0.57	0.05	0.09
16–25	34	19	0.66	0.73	0.08	0.11
26–35	28	26	0.97	0.53	0.16	0.24
35–41	29	34	1.20	0.60	0.21	0.37

F/M = fetal/maternal.
Data assembled from refs. 111–115.

TABLE 21-6

Dependence of Plasma Protein Binding of Some Drugs on Gestational Age in Humans

Drug	Binding Protein	% Bound During Week of Gestation					
		16		*23*		*37*	
		M	F	M	F	M	F
Diazepam	Albumin	90	97	96	97	98.5	97
Valproic acid	Albumin	90	50	85	80	80	90
Propranolol	α_1-Acid glycoprotein	63	85	70	85	71	85

F = fetal; M = maternal.
Data from refs. 69, 113, 114.

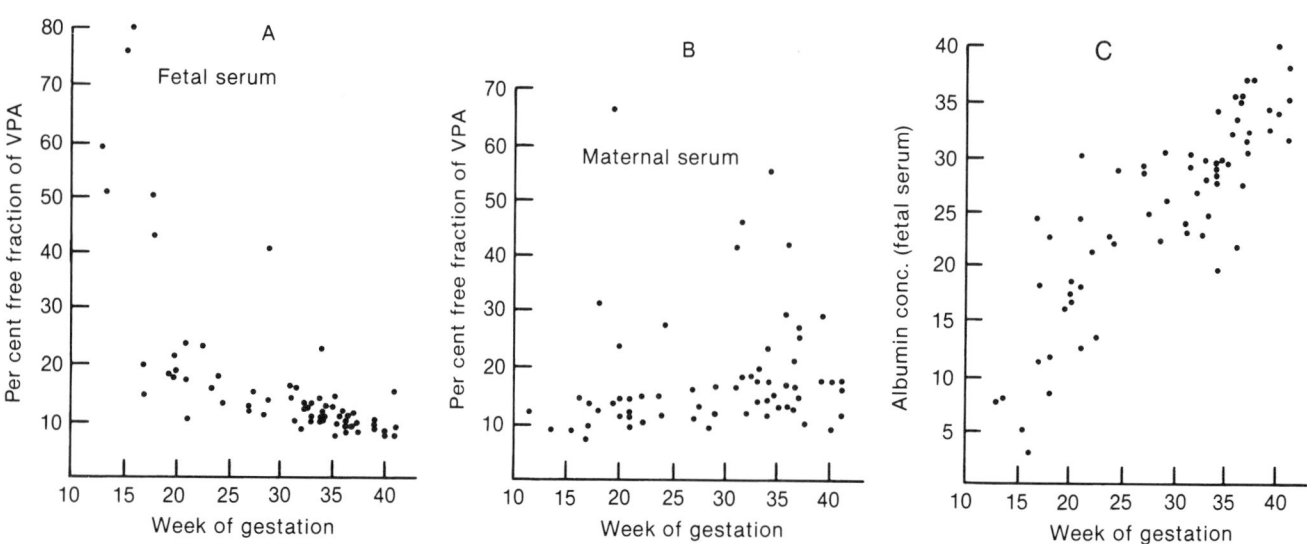

Figure 21–3. A–C, Percentage of free fraction of valproic acid (VPA) in fetal serum (**A**) and maternal serum (**B**) as well as albumin concentrations in fetal serum versus gestational age (**C**). (From Nau H, Krauer B: J Clin Pharmacol *26*:215, 1986.)

A
Early Gestation

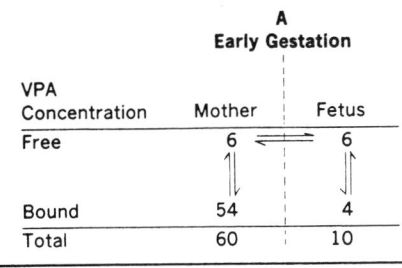

B
Late Gestation

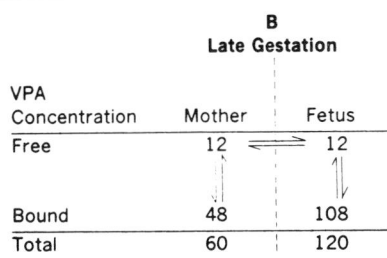

Figure 21–4. A and **B,** Valproic acid (VPA) free and bound concentration gradients in the mother and fetus during early gestation (**A**) and late gestation (**B**). The *dashed line* represents the placental membranes. Concentrations are measured in milligrams per liter. (From Nau H, Krauer B: J Clin Pharmacol *26*:215, 1986.)

$$\frac{C_{\text{fetal, total}}}{C_{\text{maternal, total}}} =$$

$$\frac{1+10^{(\text{pKa fetal})}}{1+10^{(\text{pKa} - \text{pH, maternal})}} \quad \frac{\text{unbound fraction (mother)}}{\text{unbound fraction (fetus)}} \quad [5]$$

Such predicted fetal/maternal concentration ratios are indeed in gross agreement with those found in clinical studies for numerous drugs (Table 21-7; Fig. 21-5; see also Fig. 21-4).[111]

Owing to the low fetal albumin concentrations during early pregnancy, fetal concentrations of drugs such as VPA are much lower in fetal blood than in maternal plasma during this period (see Fig. 21-4).[113] The concentration pattern of albumin and free fatty acids in the maternofetal unit has important implications for the placental transfer of some drugs that are predominantly bound to albumin and the binding of which can be modified by free fatty acids. Free fatty acid concentrations in maternal plasma rise slowly during pregnancy. The free fractions of those drugs, which may be displaced from albumin binding sites, would therefore also be expected to rise during pregnancy. Decreasing maternal albumin concentrations amplify this effect.[115-118] During birth, maternal plasma free fatty acid concentrations rise sharply to levels two to three times higher than normal concentrations: the free fractions of salicylate,[119-121] diazepam,[116-122] VPA,[69] and N-desmethyl diazepam[118] in maternal plasma also rise sharply to values about three times those observed in adult controls or cord plasma.[115-118] This increases the amount of "free" drug available for placental transfer. In the fetus, the fatty acid concentrations remain at low levels, and binding of these drugs is therefore not compromised by endogenous ligands.[123,124] Consequently, the fetus acts as a sink for these drugs, and fetomaternal plasma concentration gradients for VPA (see Figs. 21-4 and 21-5), diazepam, N-desmethyl diazepam, and salicylate[125] are significantly higher than unity. Fetal and neonatal distress may be a result of this unexpectedly high total drug load and its partial displacement after birth. Such adverse effects have been found in the case of neonates of VPA-treated mothers,[126] as well as in the case of neonates and infants of mothers who received relatively high doses of diazepam (*floppy infant syndrome*).[127-130] This situation may be especially serious for the neonate because the

TABLE 21-7

Fetal-Maternal Plasma Protein Binding and Total Concentration Ratios of Selected Drugs During Late Human Gestation

Drug	Primary Binding Protein	% Bound		Fetal-Maternal Total Plasma Concentration Ratio
		M	*F*	
Betamethasone	AGP	60	41	0.33
Bupivacaine	AGP	91	51	0.27
Diazepam	ALB	97	98.5	1.6
Lidocaine	AGP	64	24	0.66
Mepivacaine	AGP	55	36	0.71
N-Desmethyl diazepam	ALB	95	97	1.7
Phenobarbital	ALB	41	36	1.0
Phenytoin	ALB	87	82	1.0
Salicylate	ALB	43	54	1.2
Valproic acid	ALB	73	88	1.7

AGP = α_1-acid glycoprotein; ALB = albumin.
Data from refs. 65, 69, 71, 82, 93, 108-122, 175.

increased free concentrations of these drugs may persist for a prolonged time because of the known deficiency of the neonatal drug elimination mechanisms. This effect could be particularly pronounced in critically ill and preterm neonates.

The pattern of protein binding of warfarin[118] in fetal, maternal, and neonatal plasma mirrors that of VPA, diazepam, and salicylate. It may be that free fatty acids increase the albumin binding of warfarin by allosteric interaction. The free fractions of drugs such as phenytoin, phenobarbital, furosemide, and indomethacin are also increased in neonatal and infant plasma;[118] the reasons for these effects are not clear, and other endogenous displacing agents, such as bilirubin, may play a role. Lethargy has been observed, particularly in those neonates with elevated plasma free fraction values of phenobarbital.[131]

MOLECULAR WEIGHT OF DRUGS

Placental transfer cannot be predicted on the basis of protein binding, lipid solubility (partition coefficient), or ionization (dissociation constant) alone. Although warfarin has a good placental passage, the lipophilic superwarfarin brodifacoum appears not to cross the human placenta, which may result from its large molecular structure with a long polycyclic hydrocarbon side chain.[132] Most authors agree that drugs with molecular weights greater than 500 to 600 Da have an incomplete transfer across the human placenta.[2,4] Therefore, the high molecular weight of erythropoietin is believed to be the reason for its poor placental transfer in the placental perfusion model *ex vivo*.[133] When four oral hypoglycemic agents were compared with regard to their maternofetal transport in the recirculating single cotyledon human placenta model, it was found that glyburide (MW = 494) did not cross the human placenta in significant amounts. Compared with tolbutamide (with a tolbutamide/antipyrine transport ratio of 0.74:1.05), the glyburide/antipyrine transport ratio (0.11:0.21) was much lower (Fig. 21-6). The investigators found a highly significant relationship between the mean drug (tolbutamide, chlorpropamide, glipizide, and glyburide)/antipyrine transport ratios obtained in their experiment and the independent variables (molecular weight, log partition coefficient, and selected dissociation constants [$R^2 = 0.91$, $p < .0001$]). This relationship was described by the following formula:

$$T^d/T^a = -4.90 + 0.5 \log (P^d) + 1.26 \text{ pKa} - 0.0073 \text{ MW}^d \quad [6]$$

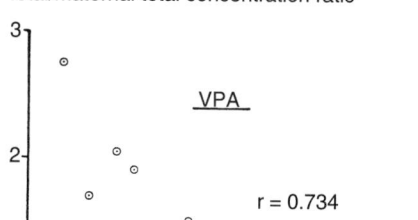
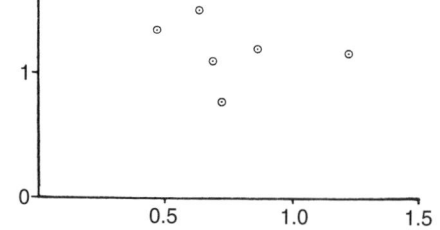

Figure 21–5. Correlation between valproic acid (VPA) total concentration ratio cord serum/maternal serum at birth (ordinate) and VPA free fraction ratio cord serum/maternal serum (abscissa). Accumulation of VPA in the fetus correlates with low free fractions (high protein binding) of this drug in the fetus as compared with the mother. (From Nau H, et al: Valproic acid in the neonatal period. J Pediatr *104*:627, 1984.)

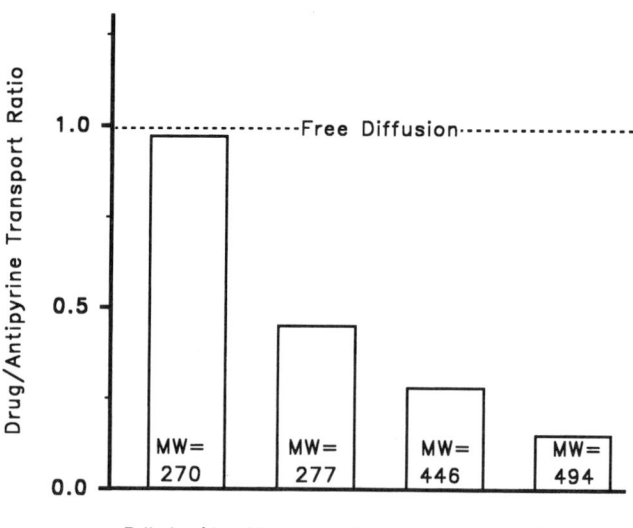

Figure 21–6. Comparative transport of oral hypoglycemic agents in reference to the freely diffusible substance antipyrine (mean values are given). MW = molecular weight. (Modified from Elliott BD, et al: Am J Obstet Gynecol *171*:653, 1994.)

where T^d = placental transport of the drug and T^a = placental transport of antipyrine.

Molecular weight was the most important variable in this regression ($F = 61,75, p < .001$) and determined the cumulative percentage of transport of the drugs tested. Neither the log partition coefficient nor the dissociation constant individually provided significant associations by simple regression with either the drug/antipyrine ratio or the cumulative percentage of transport of these drugs. Furthermore, the high plasma protein binding of glyburide (99%) could account for this finding, as discussed by Koren.[134] Diazepam has similar physicochemical properties, but it crosses the placental barrier rapidly.[135, 136] These results are consistent with the aqueous pore hypothesis noted previously, according to which higher molecular weights and "unsuitable" molecular structures result in steric inhibition. Frequently used drugs, such as the nonsteroidal antiinflammatory drug diclofenac (MW = 318.15) cross the placenta in the first trimester readily.[137]

In vitro heparin does not cross the human term placenta;[138] no biologic activity and very low fractions of radioactivity used for labeling were found in the fetal circulation in the human perfused placental cotyledon model of unfractionated heparin, low molecular weight heparin CY 216, and dermatan sulfate.[139] This finding corresponds with clinical observations in newborns whose mothers had been treated with unfractionated heparin or low molecular weight heparin.[140] The naturally occurring coagulation inhibitor dermatan sulfate (Desmin 370) (MW = 370) cannot pass the ovine placenta at all. Although both molecular weight and charge density of the glycosaminoglycan could account for the placental barrier to heparin, these factors do not explain the failure of the low molecular weight dermatan sulfate, which is characterized not only by a smaller molecular size, but also by a lower charge density.[141]

STEREOSELECTIVITY

Amino acids circulating in the maternal plasma are the primary source of protein synthesis by the fetus and contribute to the fetal energy supply. Amino acids are transferred across the placenta from mother to fetus against a concentration gradient by active, stereospecific placental transport, which functions unidirec-tionally from the maternal to the fetal side.[142-144] The transfer of neutral branched-chain amino acids is faster than that of neutral straight chains or basic amino acids.[145,146] According to the results of *in vitro* studies, taurine, β-alanine, and hypotaurine share a specific putative membrane carrier. Histidine is also quickly transported, reaching a maternofetal gradient of 1:2 (it is known to be 1:3 to 4 *in vivo*). It has been suggested that intracellular partitioning or preferential release (transport asymmetry) at the fetal-facing surface of the syncytiotrophoblast may play a role in the placental transport of amino acids.[144] In the guinea pig, the transfer is stereoselective for L-alanine compared with D-alanine.[147] In the perfused human placenta, S(+)-γ-vinyl-γ-aminobutyric acid was cleared from the maternal circulation more effectively than the R(–)-enantiomer. Even if this did not result in higher levels in the fetal circulation, it suggests either stereoselective sodium-dependent placental uptake on the maternal side of the placenta (as it is known to exist in other tissues) or stereoselective binding to enzymes, such as γ-aminobutyric acid transaminase.[148] The chiral nonsteroidal antiinflammatory drug ketotifen is known to be transferred to the fetus with S/R plasma concentrations averaging 2.3 in premature neonates given rac-ketoprofen as a tocolytic agent. Maternal S/R plasma concentrations are close to 1. Because the R(–)-enantiomer does not undergo substantial metabolic inversion in humans, another mechanism had to account for this finding; it appears that stereoselective protein binding results in a higher "free" S-(+)-ketotifen concentration with a therefore increased transfer across the placenta (compared with R-(–)-ketotifen).[149] Placental transfer of the water-soluble antiepileptic drug vigabatrin (MW = 129), which is unbound to plasma proteins, is low and occurs by simple diffusion. In a human case report, however, it appeared that there may be a slight difference between the kinetics of the entantiomers.[150] The anthelmintic drug albendazole sulfoxide has a chiral center. The formulations used are racemic. After single-dose oral administration in the last trimester in the ewe, area under the curve ratios between the (–)- and (+)- enantiomers of 0.36 (dam) and 0.64 (fetus) were determined, indicating a higher impairment for (+)-albendazole sulfoxide in its placental transfer to the fetus.[151]

The placental transport of retinol and related substances (retinoids) is highly structure specific. Although in the mouse, rat, and rabbit, retinoids with a free carboxyl group in the 13-*cis* configuration are only poorly transferred early in pregnancy,[152-158] a significant increase in transfer has been demonstrated for later gestational periods in the mouse and in the rat.[159] The β-glucuronide conjugates also show very limited placental transfer (mouse, rat, rabbit, monkey).[160] The placental transfer of all-trans-retinoic acid (rat) and all-trans-4-oxoretinoic acid (rabbit) are efficient.[151, 158, 159, 161] It may be that the high affinity of the retinoids with the all-trans configuration for certain plasma and embryonic cellular binding proteins may be the reason for the efficient transport of these compounds. Binding to plasma albumin cannot explain these differential transports because all retinoids with free carboxyl groups bind avidly to albumin and other plasma macromolecules. The increase of glucuronide transfer in later gestational periods may result from the change in the rodent placental structure from a choriovitelline to a chorioallantoic placenta. In the cynomolgus monkey, a relatively efficient transport for 13-cis-retinoic acid has been observed at a time when the chorioallantoic placenta is fully established.[162] This placenta type is functional at earlier developmental stages in the monkey (and presumably in the human) as compared with the rodent species, and this may explain the efficient placental transfer and high teratogenicity of 13-cis-retinoic acid when it is administered during early primate organogenesis. The racemic antiepileptic drug ethosuximide appears to be transferred by nonstereoselective diffusion.[163]

SELECTIVE TRANSFER MECHANISMS: ACTIVE TRANSPORT, FACILITATED DIFFUSION, AND PINOCYTOSIS

There is little evidence that therapeutic agents can be transferred to the embryo or fetus by active transport. Such a transport would function against a concentration gradient and at the expense of metabolic energy; furthermore, it would be saturable at high substrate concentrations, and it would be competitively inhibited by similar compounds that use the same carrier. Active transport, however, is of great importance for the transfer of endogenous compounds and nutrients, such as amino acids, acetylcholine, vitamin B_{12}, vitamin H (biotin), creatine, and ions such as sodium, potassium, calcium, magnesium, and iron.[164] Folate is preferentially transferred to the fetus.[165] A folate receptor in the placenta may play a crucial role in the transfer of folate to the fetus.[166]

Even though many dideoxynucleosides are at least partially actively transported across cell membranes, this appears not to be the case for antiviral drugs, such as acyclovir, azidothymidine, dideoxyinosine, and ganciclovir in the human placenta.[167-170] There is evidence, however, in favor of a carrier-dependent, nucleobase-type uptake in the placenta in addition to diffusional transfer of the drug.[171]

There is some indication that dexamethasone is actively transported across the placenta. In experimental animals (rat, sheep), fetal levels of this steroid are much lower than corresponding maternal values, even after prolonged treatment.[143, 172] This low fetal/maternal concentration ratio has also been observed after fetal administration of this glucocorticoid. Furthermore, sex differences mediated by differential placental transport from the mother have been observed.[173] This concentration gradient is not the result of differential protein binding or metabolism. Placental clearance of dexamethasone from the fetus to the mother is 8.5 times higher than in the reverse direction.[174] The fetomaternal concentration gradient of betamethasone is also low in the human;[175] the reasons for this effect have not been established. Pteridine is also actively transported from the sheep fetus to the mother at a rate that greatly exceeds transport in the reverse direction.[176] [1-β-3H]Calcitriol and its metabolites hardly cross the placenta of the rat.[177] The placenta also plays the role

of a "metabolic barrier" for endogenous, but not synthetic, estrogens.[178-180] Maternal estradiol does not appear in the fetus but is present there as the less potent estrone and its sulfate conjugate. Placental metabolism may therefore protect the fetus from potent estradiol. In contrast, the synthetic estrogen diethylstilbestrol is transferred to the fetus as the potent parent compound.[178-180] The phytoestrogen daidzen is transferred across the placenta of the rat.[181]

The placental transfer of polypeptides is extremely limited. This has been demonstrated for thyroid hormones, growth hormones, corticotropin, chorionic gonadotropin, erythropoietin,[182] oxytocin,[183, 184] interferon,[185] placental lactogen,[29] and protein C.[186] Maternal hormones therefore cannot necessarily influence the development of fetal organ systems when the fetus is deficient in synthesis of its own hormones. Thus, fetal endocrine systems function autonomously, and the placenta protects the fetus from exposure to maternal hormones.[29]

The polypeptide atosiban, a synthetic oxytocin antagonist used as a tocolytic agent in preterm labor, is transferred minimally to the ovine fetus and under steady-state conditions reaches only 10% of maternal levels in the umbilical cord blood.[183, 184] Insulin complexed to antibodies, however, can be transferred to the fetus.[187] This is of clinical significance because extremely high concentrations of animal (bovine or porcine) insulin-antibody complex levels were measured in samples of cord blood from infants with macrosomia whose mothers were treated with animal insulin. This finding indicates that the transferred insulin has biologic activity and may even account for harmful effects such as macrosomia, which is known to be associated with an increased risk of respiratory distress syndrome and hypoglycemia.[188] As the transport of insulin-antibody complexes suggests, proteins are transferred to the fetus to some extent.[189-191] There is considerable selectivity, however, in the placental transport of proteins. Molecular weight does not play a major role. As discussed previously, polypeptides do not enter the fetal circulation to a significant extent, whereas much larger macromolecules, such as γ-globulins (immunoglobulin G [IgG]) and polyvinylpyrrolidone, are transported. Relatively small fragments of IgG (MW = 20,000 to 50,000) are poorly transported, as compared with larger fragments (MW = 50,000 to 82,000) and intact IgG.[192] Therefore, binding of IgG is high, resulting in relatively extensive transport of this protein as compared with other proteins, such as albumin, transferrin, IgE, IgM, IgA, insulin, and growth hormone, all of which pass the placental membranes to a much lower degree.[190] The process by which antibodies are transported across the placenta appears to be highly selective.

Retinol (vitamin A) is transported to the embryo or fetus, at least in part, bound to retinol-binding protein.[192-194] This transport mechanism appears to be especially important during early gestation because the early embryo is not able to synthesize its own binding protein.[192] In addition, lipoproteins as well as retinol-binding protein present in large amounts in the yolk sac may play a role in placental transport of retinol.[193, 194]

Water-soluble vitamins are present in fetal blood in higher concentrations than in maternal blood, and active transport mechanisms have been suggested for some of these substances.[185, 196] The most extensive data are available for vitamin B_{12}, a polar, high molecular weight substance (MW = 1355) that is not expected to transfer by simple diffusion. A receptor-mediated endocytosis process has been identified as a carrier mechanism for this compound.[164]

In the rabbit placenta, maternal iron is concentrated by a facilitated process as an iron-transferrin complex. This is followed by a release of iron into the placental cells and return of the apoprotein to the maternal circulation. Thus, the rabbit placenta may have a carrier protein for iron transport involved in the process of facilitated diffusion.

In the term human placenta, an electroneutral anion-exchange mechanism mediating the transfer of conjugated bile acids across the brush border of the syncytiotrophoblast has been identified.[197] This could explain previous observations demonstrating higher serum bile acid levels in the umbilical artery (versus the umbilical vein) in human newborns at the time of delivery and suggests a transport of bile acids from the fetal to the maternal circulation.[198]

CLINICAL APPLICATIONS

In a group of drugs with similar pharmacodynamic properties, the placental transfer can differ considerably. If no further information is available, the comparison of lipid solubility, protein binding, ionization, and molecular weight may help to select the drug with efficient placental transfer for fetal therapy and the drug with limited placental transfer to prevent effects on the fetus. An example of these considerations has been published in the field of antihypertensive treatment in pregnancy.[199] Oral hypoglycemic agents and biologically active insulin-antibody complexes cross the placental barrier and can induce harmful fetal effects such as macrosomia. Newer oral hypoglycemic agents (characterized by a higher molecular weight) cannot pass the placenta and could therefore be a future alternative to the more invasive insulin therapy in some patients even in pregnancy.[135, 200] This finding indicates that identification of structural properties responsible for pharmacodynamic and pharmacokinetic difference is helpful in estimating which drug will be the least hazardous for the fetus if delivery is imminent and maternal pain relief is unavoidable.

A successful reduction in placental transfer of the cytostatic cisplatin was achieved by coupling the drug to cholylglycinate (Bamet-R2);[201] this finding may suggest the possibility of treating certain maternal tumors during pregnancy with a lower risk to the fetus. Liposome encapsulation of VPA reduced placental transfer in the perfused placenta model by 30%, and microencapsulation of chloramphenicol reduced maternal transfer by 85%.[202]

To treat intrauterine infection, broad-spectrum antibiotics that cross the placenta and concentrate in the fetus are desirable (e.g., the lipophilic ceftizoxime).[203, 204] Some investigations have been performed to identify antibiotics with efficient placental transfer rates in the human perfused placenta.[205-212] If only maternal treatment is desired, antibiotics with relatively low placental transfer, such as macrolids, are favorable.[213] Another example is the treatment of toxoplasmosis. In early pregnancy, spiramycin is preferred because it hardly crosses the placenta and accumulates in the placenta. Later, however, when treatment of the fetus is necessary, pyrimethamine is used, because this drug is efficiently transferred to the fetus.[2]

Other indications for intrauterine drug treatment are intentional or accidental drug poisoning. Once its is known that the ingested compound is transferred to the fetus in potentially harmful quantities, it is essential to ensure that both mother and fetus are sufficiently treated with an available antidote. Acetaminophen and warfarin-like compounds are frequently used for intentional drug poisonings. Whether the antidotes (N-acetylcysteine and vitamin K, respectively) sufficiently cross the placenta is still a matter of discussion.[58,132,214,215]

In the *ex vivo* placenta model, an inhalant (birch pollen major antigen Bet v1; MW = 17 kDa) and a nutrient allergen (cow's milk whey protein BLG; MW = 18.5 kDa) appear to be actively and selectively transferred across the human placenta. We have discussed the possible use of this phenomenon for induction of tolerance to specific allergens in the fetus by controlled intrauterine exposure as a new preventive strategy.[216] Estimations regarding the placental transfer of substances of abuse have been made by Little and VanBeveren using the chemical properties discussed in this chapter.[217]

ACKNOWLEDGMENT

Work in our laboratory was supported by grants from the Deutsche Forschungsgemeinschaft, Bundesministerium für Bildung und Forschung, the Bundesinsitut für Gisundheiteioru Vesauderschutz und Vesraudeschutz and the European Commission.

REFERENCES

1. Luke B: Maternal-fetal nutrition. Clin Obstet Gynecol 37:93, 1994.
2. Chauoi R, Bollmann R: The indirect transplacental therapy of the fetus. Geburtshilfe Frauenheilkd 55:99, 1995.
3. Ward RM: Pharmacological treatment of the fetus. Clin Pharmacokinet 28:343, 1995.
4. Pacifici GM, Nottoli R: Placental transfer of drugs administered to the mother. Clin Pharmacokinet 28:235, 1995.
5. Yerby MS: Pregnancy, teratogenesis, and epilepsy. Neurol Clin 12:749, 1994.
6. Kacew S: Effect of over-the-counter drugs on the unborn child: what is known and how should this influence prescribing? Paediatr Drugs 1:75, 1999.
7. Jacqz-Aigrain E: Placental transfer and fetal risks. Paediat Perinat Drug Ther 3:36,1999.
8. Schwarzt S: Providing toxicokinetic support for reproductive toxicology studies in pharmaceutical development. Arch Toxicol 75:381, 2001.
9. Jauniaux E, Gulbis B: In vivo investigation of placental transfer early in human pregnancy. Eur J Obstet Gynecol Reprod Biol 92:45, 2000.
10. Ostrea EM, et al: The detection of heroin, cocaine, and cannaboid metabolites in meconium of infants of drug-dependent mothers. Ann NY Acad Sci 562:373, 1989.
11. Ostrea EM, et al: A new method for the rapid isolation and detection of drugs in the stools (meconium) of drug dependent infants. Ann NY Acad Sci 562:372, 1989.
12. Nau H: Species differences in pharmacokinetics and drug teratogenesis. Environ Health Perspect 70:113, 1986.
13. Garbis-Berkvens JM, Peters PWJ: Comparative morphology and physiology of embryonic and fetal membranes. In Nau H, Scott WJ Jr (eds): Pharmacokinetics in Teratogenesis, Vol 1. Boca Raton, FL, CRC Press, 1987, pp 13–44.
14. Heap RB: Placenta structure and function. J Reprod Fertil 31(Suppl):1, 1982.
15. Ramsey EM: The Placenta: Human and Animal. New York, Praeger, 1982.
16. DeSesso JM: Anatomical and developmental aspects of the maternal-embryonal/fetal interface. Teratology 61:468, 2000.
17. Ruehl R, et al: Effects of all-*trans*-retinoic acid an all-*trans*-retinoyl glucuronide in two in vitro systems of distinct biological complexity. Arch Toxicol 75:497, 2001.
18. Hartvig M, et al: Positron emission tomographic studies on placenta transfer and in teratology. Teratology 58:20A, 1998.
19. Bourget P, et al: Models for placental transfer studies of drugs. Clin Pharmacokinet 28:161, 1995.
20. Mirkin BL, Singh S: Placental transfer of pharmacologically active molecules. In Mirkin BL (ed): Perinatal Pharmacology and Therapeutics. New York, Academic Press, 1976, pp 1–69.
21. Miller RK, et al: The transport of molecules across placenta membranes. In Poste G, Nicolson GL (eds): The Cell Surface in Animal Embryogenesis and Development. Amsterdam, Elsevier North Holland Biomedical Press, 1976, pp 145–223.
22. Nau H, Liddiard C: Placental transfer of drugs during early human pregnancy. In Neubert D, et al (eds): Role of Pharmacokinetics in Prenatal and Perinatal Toxicology. Stuttgart, Georg Thieme, 1978, pp 465–481.
23. Green TP, et al: Determinants of drug disposition and effect in the fetus. Annu Rev Pharmacol Toxicol 19:285, 1979.
24. Waddel WJ, Marlowe C: Biochemical regulation of the accessibility of teratogens to the developing embryo. In Juchau MR (ed): The Biochemical Basis of Chemical Teratogenesis. New York, Elsevier, 1981, pp 1–62.
25. Dencker L, Danielsson BRG: Transfer of drugs to the embryo and fetus after placentation. In Nau H, Scott WJ (eds): Pharmacokinetics in Teratogenesis, Vol 1. Boca Raton, FL, CRC Press, 1987, pp 55–69.
26. Nau H, Mirkin BL: Fetal and maternal clinical pharmacology. In Avery GS (ed): Drug Treatment: Principles and Practice of Clinical Pharmacology, 3rd ed. Sydney, Adis Press, 1982, pp 117–119.
27. Thornburg KL, Faber JJ: Transfer of hydrophilic molecules by placenta and yolk sac of the guinea pig. Am J Physiol 2:C111, 1977.
28. Bassily M, et al: Determinants of placental drug transfer: studies in the perfused human placenta. J Pharm Sci 84:1054, 1995.
29. Waddell WJ, Marlowe C: Transfer of drugs across the placenta. Pharmacol Ther 14:375, 1981.
30. Krauer B, Drauer F, Hytten FE: Drug disposition and pharmacokinetics in the maternal placental fetal unit. Pharmacol Ther 10:301, 1980.
31. Schoondermark Van-de-Ven E, et al: Pharmacokinetics of spiramycin in the rhesus monkey: transplacental passage and distribution in tissue in the fetus. Antimicrob Agents Chemother 38:1922, 1994.
32. Slikker W Jr, Miller RK: *Placental* metabolism and transfer. In Kimmel CA, Buelke-Sam J (eds): Role in developmental toxicology. Developmental Toxicology, 2nd ed. New York, Raven Press, 1994, p 245.
33. Maickel RP, Snodgrass WR: Physicochemical factors in maternal-fetal distribution of drugs. Toxicol Appl Pharmacol 26:218, 1973.

34. Sanchez-Alcaraz A, et al: Placental transfer and neonatal effects of propofol in caesarean section. J Clin Pharm Ther *23*:19, 1998.
35. Abu-Quare AW, et al: Placental transfer and pharmacokinetics of a single dermal dose of (^{14}C)methyl-parathion in rats. Toxicol Sci *53*:5, 2000.
36. Takahashi O, Oish S: Disposition of orally administered bisphenol A in pregnancy rats and the placental transfer to fetuses. J Toxicol Sci *24*:297, 1999.
37. Schenker S, et al: The transfer of cocaine and its metabolites across the term human placenta. Clin Pharmacol Ther *53*:329, 1993.
38. Simone C et al: Transfer of cocaethylene across the human term placenta. FASEB J *9*:A693, 1995.
39. Pastrakuljic A, et al: Maternal cocaine use and cigarette smoking in pregnancy in relation to amino acid transport and fetal growth. Placenta *20*:499, 1999.
40. Krause W, Mechelke B: Placental transfer of the anxiolytic β-carboline abecarnil in rabbit. Arzneimittelforschung *42*:1079, 1992.
41. Giroux M, et al: Influence of maternal blood flow on the placental transfer of three opioids—fentanyl, alfentanil, sufentanil. Biol Neonate *72*:133, 1997.
42. Nanovskaya T, et al: Transplacental transfer and metabolism of buprenorphine. J Pharmacol Exp Ther *300*:26, 2002.
43. Fortunato SJ, et al: Transfer of ceftizoxime surpasses that of cefoperazone by the isolated human placenta perfused in vitro. Obstet Gynecol *75*:830, 1990.
44. Fortunato SJ, et al: Transfer of Timentin (ticarcillin and clavulanic acid) across the in vitro perfused human placenta: comparison with other agents. Am J Obstet Gynecol *167*:1595, 1992.
45. Liebes L, et al: Transfer of zidovudine (AZT) by human placenta. J Infect Dis *161*:203, 1990.
46. Patterson TA, et al : Transplacental pharmacokinetics and fetal distribution of azidothymidine, its glucuronide, and phosphorylated metabolites in late-term rhesus macaques after maternal infusion. Drug Metab Dispos *25*:453, 1997.
47. Boal JH, et al: Pharmacokinetic and toxicity studies of AZT (zidovudine) following perfusion of human term placenta for 14 hours. Toxicol Appl Pharmacol *143*:13, 1997.
48. Pereira CM, et al: Transplacental pharmacokinetics of dideoxyinosine in pigtailed macaques. Antimicrob Agents Chemother *38*:781, 1994.
49. Bawdon RE, et al: The transfer of anti-human immunodeficiency virus nucleoside compounds by the term human placenta. Am J Obstet Gynecol *167*:1570, 1992.
50. Pons JC, et al: Placental passage of azidothymidine (AZT) during the second trimester of pregnancy: study by direct fetal blood sampling under ultrasound. Eur J Obstet Gynaecol Reprod Biol *40*:229, 1991.
51. Watts DH, et al: Pharmacokinetic disposition of zidovudine during pregnancy. J Infect Dis *163*:226, 1991.
52. Liebes L, et al: Further observations on zidovudine transfer and metabolism by human placenta. AIDS *7*:590, 1993.
53. Tuntland T, et al: In vitro models to predict the in vivo mechanism, rate and extent of placental transfer of dideoxynucleoside drugs against human immunodeficiency virus. Am J Obstet Gynecol *180*:198, 1999.
54. Frenkel LM, et al: Pharmacokinetics of acyclovir in the term human pregnancy and neonate. Am J Obstet Gynecol *164*:569, 1991.
55. Nau H, Bass R: Transfer of 2,3,7,8-tetrachlorodibenzo-p-dioxin (TCDD) to the mouse embryo and fetus. Toxicology *20*:299, 1981.
56. Bourget P, et al: Transplacental passage of cyclosporine after liver transplantation. Transplantation *49*:663, 1990.
57. Nau H, et al: Transfer of 2,3,7,8-tetrachlorodibenzo-*p*-dioxin (TCDD) via placenta and milk, and postnatal toxicity in the mouse. Arch Toxicol *59*:36, 1986.
58. Kazzi NJ, et al: Placental transfer of vitamin K_1 in preterm pregnancy. Obstet Gynecol *75*:334, 1990.
59. Staud F, et al: Pharmacokinetic examination of *p*-aminobenzoic acid passage through the placenta and the small intestine in rats. J Drug Target *5*:57, 1997.
60. Kivalo I, Saarikoski S: Placental transmission and foetal uptake of ^{14}C-dimethyltubocurarine. Br J Anaesth *44*:557, 1972.
61. Kivalo I, Saarikoski S: Placental transfer of ^{14}C-dimethyltubocurarine during caesarean section. Br J Anaesth *48*:239, 1976.
62. Booth PN, et al: Pancuronium and the placental barrier. Anaesthesia *32*:320, 1977.
63. Abouleish E, et al: Pancuronium in caesarean section and its placental transfer. Br J Anaesth *52*:531, 1980.
64. Demetriou M, et al: Placental transfer of ORG NC54 in women undergoing caesarean section. Br J Anaesth *54*:643, 1982.
65. Nöschel H, et al: Plazentapassage von Natriumsalizylat. Zentralbl Gynakol *94*:437, 1972.
66. Tagashira E, et al: Correlation of teratogenicity of aspirin to the stage specific distribution of salicylic acid in rats. Jpn J Pharmacol *31*:563, 1981.
67. Nau H, et al: Valproic acid and its metabolites: placental transfer, neonatal pharmacokinetics, transfer via mother's milk and clinical status in neonates of epileptic mothers. J Pharmacol Exp Ther *219*:768, 1981.
68. Kaneko S, et al: Transplacental passage and half-life of sodium valproate in infants born to epileptic mothers. Br J Clin Pharmacol *15*:503, 1983.
69. Nau H, et al: Valproic acid in the perinatal period: decreased maternal serum protein binding results in fetal accumulation and neonatal displacement of the drug and some metabolites. J Pediatr *104*:627, 1984.
70. Nau H, Scott WJ: Teratogenicity of valproic acid and related substances in the mouse: drug accumulation and pH$_i$ in the embryo during organogenesis and structure-activity considerations. Arch Toxicol *11*:128, 1987.
71. Hendrickx AG, et al: Valproic acid developmental toxicity and pharmacokinetics in the rhesus-monkey: an interspecies comparison. Teratology *38*:329, 1988.
72. Binkerd PE, et al: Evaluation of valproic acid (VPA) developmental toxicity and pharmacokinetics in Sprague-Dawley rats. Fundam Appl Toxicol *11*:485, 1988.
73. Fowler DW, et al: Transplacental transfer and biotransformation studies of valproic acid and its glucuronide(s) in the perfused human placenta. J Pharmacol Exp Ther *24*:318, 1989.
74. Tzimas G, et al: The high sensitivity of the rabbit to the teratogenic effects of 13-*cis*-retinoic acid (isotretinoin) is a consequence of prolonged exposure of the embryo to 13-*cis*-retinoic acid and 13-*cis*-4-oxo-retinoic acid. Arch Toxicol *68*:119, 1994.
75. Worsaschk HJ, et al: Zur diaplazentaren Passage von 1-Askobrinsäure. Zentralbl Gynakol *96*:910, 1974.
76. Greenberg RA, et al: Measuring the exposure of infants to tobacco smoke: nicotine and cotinine in urine and saliva. N Engl J Med *310*:1075, 1984.
77. Luck W, et al: Extent of nicotine and cotinine transfer to the human fetus, placenta and amniotic fluid of smoking mothers. Dev Pharmacol Ther *8*:384, 1985.
78. Back DJ, Singh JKG: LSD: the distribution of [^{3}H]LSD in the reproductive system of the male rat and placental transfer in the female rat. Experientia *15*:501, 1977.
79. Li PJ, et al: Transfer of lead via placenta and breast milk in human. Biomed Environ Sci *13*:85, 2000.
80. Yang J, et al : Maternal-fetal transfer of metallic mercury via the placenta and milk. Ann Clin Lab Sci *27*:135, 1997.
81. Carson RJ, Reynolds F: Elimination of bupivacaine and pethidine from the rabbit feto-placental unit. Br J Anaesth *69*:150, 1992.
82. Nau H: Clinical pharmacokinetics in pregnancy and perinatology. Dev Pharmacol Ther *8*:149, 1985.
83. Johnson RF, et al: A comparison of the placental transfer of ropivacaine versus bupivacaine. Anesth Analg *89*:703, 1999.
84. Biehl D, et al: Placental transfer of lidocaine. Anesthesiology *48*:409, 1978.
85. Brown WU, et al: Acidosis, local anesthetics and the newborn. Obstet Gynecol *48*:27, 1976.
86. Morishima HO, Cavino BTG: Toxicity and distribution of lidocaine in nonasphyxiated and asphyxiated baboon fetuses. Anesthesiology *54*:182, 1981.
87. Datta S, et al: Epidural anesthesia for cesarean section in diabetic parturients: maternal and neonatal acid-base status and bupivacaine concentration. Anesth Analg *60*:574, 1981.
88. Denson DD, et al: Bupivacaine protein binding in the term parturient: effects of lactic acidosis. Clin Pharmacol Ther *35*:702, 1984.
89. Kennedy RL, et al: Effects of changes in maternal-fetal pH on the transplacental equilibrium of bupivacaine. Anesthesiology *51*:50, 1979.
90. Froescher W, et al: Protein binding of valproic acid in maternal and umbilical cord serum. Epilepsia *25*:244, 1984.
91. Varma DR: Modification of transplacental distribution of salicylate in rats by acidosis and alkalosis. Br J Pharmacol *93*:978, 1988.
92. Jacobson RL, et al: Transfer of aspirin across the perfused humasn placental cotyledon. Am J Obstet Gynecol *164*:290, 1991.
93. Nau H, Scott WJ Jr: Weak acids may act as teratogens by accumulating in the basic milieu of the early mammalian embryo. Nature *323*:276, 1986.
94. Nau H, et al: Estimation of intracellular pH (pH$_i$) in primate embryos by transplacental distribution of DMO (5,5′ dimethyloxazolidine-2,4 dione). Teratology *37*:479, 1988.
95. Keberle H, et al: Biochemical effects of drugs in the mammalian conceptus. Ann NY Acad Sci *123*:253, 1965.
96. Nau H, et al: Pharmacokinetic and chiral aspects of thalidomide and EM12 teratogenesis in monkey and rat. *In* Neubert D, et al (eds): Non Human Primates: Developmental Biology and Toxicology. Vienna, Überreuter, 1988, pp 461–476.
97. Schmahl HJ, et al: The enantiomers of the teratogenic thalidomide analogue EM 12. I. Chiral inversion and plasma pharmacokinetics in the marmoset monkey. Arch Toxicol *62*:200, 1988.
98. Ushigome F, et al: Human placental transport of vinblastine, vincristine, digoxin and progesterone: contribution of p-glycoprotein. Eur J Pharmacol *408*:1, 2000.
99. Pavek P, et al: Influence of P-glycoprotein on the transplacental passage of cyclosporin. J Pharm Sci *90*:1583, 2001.
100. Ito S: Transplacental treatment of fetal tachycardia: implication of drug transporting proteins in the placenta. Semin Perinatol *25*:196, 2001.
101. Magee KP, et al: Ex vivo human placental transfer of rifampin and rifabutin. Infect Dis Obstet Gynecol *4*:319, 1996.
102. Wise T, et al: The influence of protein binding upon tissue fluid levels of six beta-lactams. J Infect Dis *142*:77, 1980.
103. Mortimer RH, et al: Methimazole and propylthiouracil equally cross the perfused human term placental lobule. J Clin Endocrinol Metab 1997 *82*:3099, 1997.
104. Brown CEL, et al: Placental transfer of cefazolin and piperacillin in pregnancies remote from term complicated by Rh isoimmunization. Am J Obstet Gynecol *163*:938, 1990.
105. Tsadkin M, et al: Albumin-dependent digoxin transfer in isolated perfused human placenta. Int J Pharmacol Ther *39*:158, 2001.
106. Kanhai HHH, et al: Transplacental passage of digoxin in severe rhesus immunization. J Perinat Med *18*:339, 1990.

107. Schenker S, et al: Olanzapine transfer by human placenta. Clin Exp Pharmacol Physiol 26:691, 1999.
108. Kurz H, et al: Differences in the binding of drugs to plasma proteins from newborn and adult man. I. Eur J Clin Pharmacol 11:463, 1977.
109. Kurz H, et al: Differences in the binding of drugs to plasma proteins from newborn and adult man. II. Eur J Clin Pharmacol 11:469, 1977.
110. Lovecchio JL, et al: Serum protein binding of salicylate during pregnancy and the puerperium. Dev Pharmacol Ther 2:172, 1981.
111. Hill MD, Abramson FP: The significance of plasma protein binding on the fetal/maternal distribution of drugs at steady-state. Clin Pharmacokinet 14:156, 1988.
112. Krauer B, et al: Changes in serum albumin and α₁-acid glyco-protein concentrations during pregnancy: an analysis of fetal-maternal pairs. Br J Obstet Gynaecol 91:875, 1984.
113. Nau H, Krauer B: Serum protein binding of valproic acid in fetus-mother pairs throughout pregnancy: correlation with oxytocin administration and albumin and free fatty acid concentrations. J Clin Pharmacol 26:215, 1986.
114. Krauer B, et al: Serum protein binding of diazepam and propranolol in the feto-maternal unit from early to late pregnancy. Br J Obstet Gynaecol 93:322, 1986.
115. Dean M, et al: Serum protein binding of drugs during and after pregnancy in humans. Clin Pharmacol Ther 28:253, 1980.
116. Kuhnz W, Nau H: Differences in in vitro binding of diazepam and N-desmethyldiazepam to maternal and fetal plasma proteins at birth: relation to free fatty acid concentration and other parameters. Clin Pharmacol Ther 34:220, 1983.
117. Ridd MJ, et al: Differential transplacental binding of diazepam: causes and implications. Eur J Clin Pharmacol 24:595, 1983.
118. Nau H, et al: Serum protein binding of desmethyldiazepam, furosemide, indomethacin, warfarin, and phenobarbital in human fetus, mother, and newborn infants. Pediatr Pharmacol 3:219, 1983.
119. Wegener S, et al: Salicylate protein binding in the serum of the neonate during the first postnatal week: comparison with maternal and fetal binding at birth. IRCS J Med Sci 12:685, 1984.
120. Hamar C, Levy G: Serum protein binding of drugs and bilirubin in newborn infants and their mothers. Clin Pharmacol Ther 28:58, 1980.
121. Hamar C, Levy G: Factors affecting the serum protein binding of salicylic acid in newborn infants and their mothers. Pediatr Pharmacol 1:31, 1980.
122. Nau H, et al: Decreased serum protein binding of diazepam and its major metabolite in the neonate during the first postnatal week related to increased free fatty acid levels. Br J Clin Pharmacol 17:92, 1984.
123. Elphick MC, et al: Concentrations of free fatty acids in maternal and umbilical cord blood during elective caesarean section. Br J Obstet Gynaecol 83:539, 1976.
124. Ogburn PL, et al: Levels of free fatty acids and arachidonic acid in pregnancy and labor. J Lab Clin Med 95:943, 1980.
125. Itami T, Kanoh S: A possible mechanism for the potentiation of the fetal toxicities of salicylates by bacterial pyrogen. In Nau H, Scott WJ Jr (eds): Pharmacokinetics in Teratogenesis, Vol 2. Boca Raton, FL, CRC Press, 1987, pp 27–39.
126. Jäger-Roman E, et al: Fetal growth, major malformations, and minor anomalies in infants born to women receiving valproic acid. J Pediatr 108:997, 1986.
127. Gonzales de Dios J, et al: "Floppy infant" syndrome in twins secondary to the use of benzodiazepines during pregnancy. Rev Neurol 29:121, 1999.
128. Gillberg C: "Floppy infant syndrome" and maternal diazepam. Lancet 1:244, 1977.
129. Rementeria JL, Bhatt K: Withdrawal symptoms in neonates from intrauterine exposure to diazepam. J Pediatr 90:123, 1977.
130. Speight ANP: Floppy infant syndrome and maternal diazepam and/or nitrazepam. Lancet 2:878, 1977.
131. Kuhnz W, et al: Primidone and phenobarbital during lactation period in epileptic women: total and free drug serum levels in the nursed infants and their effects on neonatal behavior. Dev Pharmacol Ther 11:147, 1988.
132. Prybys KM: Life-threatening superwarfarin ingestion in a second trimester pregnancy. J Toxicol Clin Toxicol 34:567, 1997.
133. Reisenberger K, et al: Transfer of erythropoietin across the placenta perfused in vitro. Obstet Gynecol 89:738, 1997.
134. Koren G: Glyburide and fetal safety: transplacental pharmacokinetic considerations. Reprod Toxicol 15:227, 2001.
135. Elliott BD, et al: Comparative placental transport of oral hypoglycemic agents in humans: a model of human placental drug transfer. Am J Obstet Gynecol 171:653, 1994.
136. Jauniaux E et al: In-vivo study of diazepam transfer across the first trimenon human placenta. Hum Reprod 11:889, 1996.
137. Siu SS, et al: A study on placental transfer of diclofenac in the first trimester of human pregnancy. Hum Reprod 15:2423, 2000.
138. Simone C, et al: Transfer of heparin across the human term placenta. Clin Invest Med 18: B18, 1995.
139. Saivin S, et al: Placental transfer of glycosaminoglycans in the human perfused placental cotyledon model. Eur J Obstet Reprod Biol 42:221, 1991.
140. Schneider D, et al: Placental transfer of low-molecular weight heparin. Geburtshilfe Frauenheilkd 55:93, 1995.
141. Dawes J, Lumbers ER: Low molecular weight dermatan sulphate (Desmin 370) does not cross the ovine placenta. Br J Haematol 84:90, 1993.
142. Schneider H, et al: Transfer of amino acids across the in vitro perfused human placenta. Pediatr Res 13:236, 1979.
143. Schneider H, et al: Transfer of glutamic acid across the human placenta perfused in vitro. Br J Obstet Gynaecol 86:299, 1979.
144. Karl PI, Fisher SE: Taurine transport by microvillous membrane vesicles and the perfused cotyledon of the human placenta. Am J Physiol 258:C443, 1990.
145. Dancis J, et al: Transfer of riboflavin by the perfused human. Pediatr Res 19:1143, 1985.
146. Carrol MJ, et al: The relationship between placental protein synthesis and transfer of amino acids. Biochem J 210:99, 1983.
147. Kihlstrom I, Kihlstrom JE: An improved technique for perfusion of the guniea pig placenta in situ giving viable conditions demonstrated by placental transport of amino-acids (L- and D-alanine). Biol Neonate 39:150, 1981.
148. Challier JC, et al: Passage of S(+) and R(−) γ-vinyl-GABA across the human - isolated perfused placenta. Br J Clin Pharmacol 34:139, 1992.
149. Lagrange F, et al: Passage of S-(+)- and R-(−)-ketotifen across the human isolated perfused placenta. Fundam Clin Pharmacol 12:286, 1998.
150. Tran A, et al: Vigabatrin: placental transfer in vivo and excretion into breast milk of the enantiomers. Br J Clin Pharmacol 45:409, 1998.
151. Capece BP, et al: Placental transfer of albendazole sulphoxide enantiomers in sheep. Vet J 163:155, 2002.
152. Nau H: Teratogenicity of isotretinoin revisited: species variation and the role of all-trans-retinoic acid. J Am Acad Dermatol 45:S183, 2001.
153. Soprano DR, et al: Retinol-binding protein synthesis and secretion by the rat visceral yolk sac. J Biol Chem 263:2934, 1988.
154. Creech Kraft J, et al: Low teratogenicity of 13-cis-retinoic acid (isotretinoin) in the mouse corresponds to low embryo concentrations during organogenesis: comparison to the all-trans isomer. Toxicol Appl Pharmacol 87:474, 1987.
155. Kochhar DM, et al: Teratogenicity and disposition of various retinoids in vivo and in vitro. In Nau H, Scott WJ Jr (eds): Pharmacokinetics in Teratogenesis, Vol 2. Boca Raton, FL, CRC Press, 1987, pp 173–186.
156. Reiners J, et al: Transplacental pharmacokinetics of teratogenic doses of etretinate and other aromatic retinoids in mice. Reprod Toxicol 2:19, 1988.
157. Nau H, et al: Teratogenesis of retinoids: aspects of species differences and transplacental pharmacokinetics. In Welsch F (ed): Approaches to Elucidate Mechanisms in Teratogenesis. Washington, DC, Hemisphere, 1986, pp 1–15.
158. Eckhoff C, et al: Teratogenicity and transplacental pharmacokinetics of 13-cis-retinoic acid in rabbits. Toxicol Appl Pharmacol 125:34, 1994.
159. Tzimas G, et al: Developmental stage-associated differences in the transplacental distribution of 13-cis and all-trans-retinoic acid as well as their glucuronides in rats and mice. Toxicol Appl Pharmacol 113:91, 1995.
160. Nau H: Chemical structure–teratogenicity relationship in risk assessment of developmental toxicants. Hum Exp Toxicol 14:683, 1995.
161. Collins MD, et al: Comparative teratology and transplacental pharmacokinetics of all-trans-retinoic acid, 13-cis-retinoic acid, and retinyl palmitate following daily administrations in rats. Toxicol Appl Pharmacol 127:132, 1994.
162. Hummler H, et al: Maternal pharmacokinetics, metabolism, and embryo exposure following a teratogenic dosing regimen with 13-cis-retinoic acid (isotretinoin) in the cynomolgus monkey. Teratology 50:184, 1994.
163. Tomson T, Villeán T: Ethosuximide enantiomers in pregnancy and lactation. Ther Drug Monit 16:621, 1994.
164. Ng WW, Miller RK: Transport of nutrients in the early human placenta: amino acid, creatine, vitamin B₁₂. Trophoblast Res 1:121, 1983.
165. Henderson GI, et al: Folate transport by the human placenta: normal transport and role of short-term exposure to ethanol. Placenta 12:397, 1991.
166. Holm J, et al : Characterization of the folate receptor in human molar placenta. Biosci Rep 16:379, 1996.
167. Bawdon RE, et al: The transfer of anti-human immunodeficiency virus nucleoside compounds by the term placenta. Am J Obstet Gynecol 167:1570, 1992.
168. Liebes L, et al: Further observations on zidovudine transfer and metabolism by human placenta. AIDS 7:590, 1993.
169. Poms JC, et al: Placental passage of azidothymidine (AZT) during the second trimester of pregnancy: study by direct fetal sampling under ultrasound. Eur J Obstet Gynaecol Reprod Biol 40:229, 1999.
170. Gilstrap LC, et al: The transfer of the nucleoside analóg ganciclovir across the perfused human placenta. Am J Obstet Gynecol 170:967, 1994.
171. Henderson GI, et al: Acyclovir transport by the human placenta. J Lab Clin Med 120:885, 1992.
172. Varma DR: Investigation of the maternal to foetal serum concentration gradient of dexamethasone in the rat. Br J Pharmacol 88:815, 1986.
173. Montano MM, et al: Sex differences in plasma corticosterone in mouse fetuses are mediated by differential placental transport from the mother and eliminated by maternal adrenalectomy or stress. J Reprod Fertil 99:283, 1993.
174. Funkhouser JD, et al: Distribution of dexamethasone between mother and fetus after maternal administration. Pediatr Res 12:1053, 1978.
175. Petersen MC, et al: The placental transfer of betamethasone. Eur J Clin Pharmacol 18:245, 1980.
176. McNay JL, Dayton PG: Placental transfer of a substituted pteridine from fetus to mother. Science 167:988, 1970.
177. Nakayama S, et al: Pharmacokinetic study on calcitriol injectable in rats. III. Transfer into the fetus and milk in rats after single intravenous administration. Yakuri Chiro 23:315, 1995.
178. Miller RK, et al: Diethylstilbestrol: placental transfer, metabolism, covalent binding and fetal distribution in the Wistar rat. J Pharmacol Exp Ther 220:358, 1981.

179. Slikker W Jr, et al: Comparison of the transplacental pharmacokinetics of 17β-estradiol and diethylstilbestrol in the subhuman primate. J Pharmacol Exp Ther 221:173, 1978.
180. Slikker W Jr: Disposition of selected naturally occurring and synthetic steroids in the pregnant rhesus monkey. In Nau H, Scott WJ Jr (eds): Pharmacokinetics in Teratogenesis, Vol 1. Boca Raton, FL, CRC Press, 1987, pp 149–176.
181. Degen GH, et al: Transplacental transfer of the phytoestrogen daizein in DA/Han rats. Arch Toxicol 76:23, 2002.
182. Huch R, Huch A: Erythropoietin in obstetrics. Hematol Oncol Clin North Am 8:1021, 1994.
183. Valenzuela GJ, et al: Maternal and fetal cardiovascular effects and placental transfer of the oxytocin antagonist atosiban in late-gestational pregnant sheep. Am J Obstet Gynecol 169:897, 1993.
184. Valenzuela GJ, et al: Newborn oxytocin antagonist (atosibam) levels during maternal infusion. Am J Obstet Gynecol 169:374, 1993.
185. Waysbort A, et al: Experimental study of transplacental passage of alpha interferon by two assay techniques. Antimicrob Agents Chemother 37:1232, 1993.
186. Simone C, et al: Protein C transfer and secretion by the human term placenta perfused in vitro. Clin Invest Med 18:B16, 1995.
187. Bauman WA, Yalow RS: Transplacental passage of insulin complexed to antibody. Proc Natl Acad Sci USA 78:4588, 1981.
188. Menon RK, et al: Transplacental passage of insulin in pregnant women with insulin-dependent diabetes mellitus. N Engl J Med 323:309, 1990.
189. Masters CL, et al: Plasma protein metabolism and transfer to the fetus during pregnancy in the rat. Am J Physiol 216:876, 1969.
190. Gitlin JD, Gitlin D: Protein binding by specific receptors on human placenta, murine placenta, and suckling murine intestine in relation to protein transport across these tissues. J Clin Invest 54:1155, 1974.
191. Balfour AH, Jones EA: The binding of plasma proteins to human placental cell membranes. Clin Sci Mol Med 52:383, 1977.
192. Brambell FWR: The transmission of immunity from mother to young and the catabolism of immunoglobulins. Lancet 2:1087, 1966.
193. Vahlquist A, Nilsson S: Vitamin A transfer to the fetus and to the amniotic fluid in rhesus monkey (Macaca mulatta). Ann Nutr Metab 28:321, 1984.
194. Takahashi YI, et al: Vitamin A and retinol-binding protein metabolism during fetal development in the rat. Am J Physiol 233:E263, 1977.
195. Soprano DR, et al: Retinol-binding protein and transthyretin mRNA levels in visceral yolk sac and liver during fetal development in the rat. Proc Natl Acad Sci USA 83:7330, 1986.
196. Strelling MK: Transfer of folate to the fetus. Dev Med Child Neurol 18:533, 1976.
197. Dumaswala R, et al: An anion exchanger mediates bile acid transport across the placental microvillous membrane. Am J Physiol 264:G1016, 1993.
198. Itoh S, et al: Foetal maternal relationship of bile acid pattern estimated by high-pressure liquid chromatography. Biochem J 204:1411, 1982.
199. Khedun SM, et al: Effects of antihypertensive drugs on the unborn child: what is known, and how should this influence prescribing? Paediatr Drugs 2:419, 2000.
200. Elliott BD, et al: Insignificant transfer of glyburide occurs across the human placenta. Am J Obstet Gynecol 165:807, 1991.
201. Pascual MJ, et al: Enhanced efficiency of the placental barrier to cisplatin through binding to glycolic acid. Anticancer Res 21:2703, 2001.
202. Barzago MM, et al: Placental transfer of valproic acid after liosome encapsulation during in vitro human placenta perfusion. J Pharmacol Exp Ther 277:79, 1996.
203. Fortunato SJ, et al: Placental transfer of cefoperazone and sulfbactam in the isolated in vitro perfused human placenta. Am J Obstet Gynecol 159:1002, 1988.
204. Maberry MC, et al: Antibiotic concentration in maternal blood, cord blood and placental tissue in women with chorioamnionitis. Gynecol Obstet Invest 33:185, 1992.
205. Heikkilä A, Erkkola R: Review of β-lactam antibiotics in pregnancy. Clin Pharmacokinet 27:49, 1994.
206. Heikkilä A, et al: The pharmacokinetics of mecillinam and pivmecillinam in pregnant and non-pregnant women. Br J Clin Pharmacol 33:629, 1992.
207. Heikkilä A, et al: Pharmacokinetics and transplacental passage of imipenem during pregnancy. Antimicrob Agents Chemother 36:2652, 1992.
208. Leeuw JW, et al: Achievement of therapeutic concentrations of cefuroxime in early preterm gestations with premature rupture of the membranes. Obstet Gynecol 81:255, 1993.
209. Fernandez H, et al: Fetal levels of tobramycin following maternal administration. Obstet Gynecol 76:992, 1990.
210. Mattie H: Clinical pharmacokinetics of aztreonam. Clin Pharmacokinet 26:99, 1994.
211. Fernandez H, et al: Fetal levels of tobramycin following maternal administration. Obstet Gynecol 76:992, 1990.
212. Gilstrap LC, et al: Antibiotic concentration in maternal blood, cord blood, and placental membranes in chorioamnionitis. Obstet Gynecol 72:124, 1988.
213. Heikkinen T, et al: The transplacental transfer of the macrolide antibiotics erythromycin, roxithromycin and azithromycin. Br J Obstet Gynaecol 197:770, 2000.
214. Johnson D, et al : N-acetylcysteine does not cross the human term placenta. FASEB J 9:A693, 1995.
215. Horowitz RS, et al: Placental transfer of N-acetylcysteine following human maternal acetaminophen toxicity. J Toxicol Clin Toxicol 35:447, 1997.
216. Szefalusi Z, et al: Direct evidence for placental allergen transfer. Pediatr Res 48:404, 2000.
217. Little BB, VanBeveren: Placental transfer of selected substances of abuse. Semin Perinatol 20:147, 1996.

22

Denis M. Grant

Pharmacogenetics

Pharmacogenetic disorders are a special subclass of genetic disorders (see Chapter 1) that happen to involve proteins functioning in drug metabolism or action.[1] A key distinguishing feature of pharmacogenetic defects is that they are often phenotypically innocuous in the absence of a drug challenge. This means that pharmacogenetic variants are not life-threatening per se, obviating the need for prenatal genetic diagnosis. For the perinatal pharmacologist, however, genetically based variation in drug disposition in the fetus, the mother, and the neonate must be included among many variables, such as developmental changes in fetal and neonatal gene expression, organ maturation, placental transfer and metabolism of drugs, and a host of hormonal and environmental influences that can combine to produce specific patterns of toxicity in mother and child upon exposure to xenobiotics. Therefore, knowledge of potential genetic contributions to drug-induced toxicity in pregnancy and neonatal life can be important in ascertaining drug involvement in observed pathophysiologic states and to prevent their further occurrence in patients.

We have recently witnessed both an explosion of interest in the field of pharmacogenetics and the birth of the related field of "pharmacogenomics," as a result of technologic advances in genetic analysis capability and the availability of the essentially complete consensus human genome sequence. The terms *pharmacogenetics* and *pharmacogenomics* are often used interchangeably, and the distinction between the two is largely related to differences in experimental approach.[2,3] Classic pharmacogenetics—the study of the role of inheritance in producing interindividual differences in drug response—is a "phenotype to genotype" approach that starts with a clinical observation of unexpected drug response, employs a range of biochemical and molecular genetic methods to elucidate its underlying mechanisms, and uses this information in the development of predictive tests that can be applied to the individualization of therapy. Pharmacogenomics, on the other hand, is a "genotype to phenotype" approach that takes advantage of the availability of human genome sequences and modern genomic analysis methods to discover novel disease susceptibility genes and potential drug targets using whole-genome association and linkage methods or more focused candidate gene approaches.

A number of excellent recent reviews have summarized our current state of knowledge of the molecular biology of pharmacogenetic defects and our understanding of their clinical consequences and practical potential and ethical implications.[4-14] Many of the best studied examples are of genetic alterations that affect the biotransformation of drugs,[3, 15] although much research is also focusing on how genetic differences in intended drug targets can directly influence drug efficacy.[6] The following sections provide an overview and examples of some selected pharmacogenetic traits that influence the metabolism[16] of drugs

and hence their *pharmacokinetics* (Table 22–1); briefly discussed are some that alter drug targets[17] and hence directly affect their *pharmacodynamics* (Table 22–2). Polymorphic variation in drug transporters[18] (Table 22–1), although also an important determinant of drug distribution and disposition at sites of action, will not be discussed in detail here.

PHARMACOGENETIC DEFECTS AFFECTING DRUG PHARMACOKINETICS

Variation in the function of drug-metabolizing enzymes among human populations results in variable drug and metabolite con-

---

TABLE 22-1

Some Genetically Polymorphic Enzymes Associated with Variable Drug Pharmacokinetics

Enzyme	Representative Chemical Affected
Cytochromes P450	
CYP1A1	Benzo[a]pyrene
CYP1A2	Caffeine
CYP1B1	17β-Estradiol
CYP2A6	Nicotine
CYP2A13	NNK
CYP2B6	Bupropion
CYP2C8	Paclitaxel
CYP2C9	Warfarin
CYP2C19	Omeprazole
CYP2D6	Codeine
CYP2E1	Halothane
CYP2J2	Arachidonic acid
CYP3A4	Cyclosporine
CYP3A5	Nifedipine
CYP3A7	
CYP4B1	2-Aminofluorene
Flavin-dependent monooxygenase (FMO3)	Trimethylamine
Dihydropyrimidine dehydrogenase (DPD)	5-Fluorouracil
NAD(P)H: quinone oxidoreductase (NQO1)	Benzene
Myeloperoxidase (MPO)	Benzo[a]pyrene
Microsomal epoxide hydrolase (EPHX1)	Benzo[a]pyrene-4,5-oxide
Endothelial nitric oxide synthase (eNOS)	Nitric oxide
Butyrylcholinesterase (BCHE)	Succinylcholine
Paraoxonase (PON1)	Paraoxon
Glutathione *S*-transferases	
GSTM1	Nitrogen mustard
GSTT1	Dichloromethane
GSTM3	
GSTP1	
GSTA3	
Arylamine *N*-acetyltransferases	
NAT1	Sulfamethoxazole
NAT2	Isoniazid
Thiopurine *S*-methyltransferase	
TPMT	6-Mercaptopurine
UDP-glucuronsyltransferases	
UGT1A1	Irinotecan
UGT1A6	
UGT1A7	Benzo[a]pyrene
UGT2B4	
UGT2B7	Oxazepam
UGT2B15	
Histamine *N*-methyltransferase (HNMT)	Histamine
Sulfotransferases	
SULT1A1	Troglitazone
SULT1A2	Hydroxy-2-acetylaminofluorene
SULT1C1	
Catechol *O*-methyltransferase (COMT)	Levodopa
Transporters	
MDR1	
OCT2	
MRP1	

TABLE 22-2

Some Genetically Polymorphic Drug Targets Associated with Variable Pharmacodynamics

Target	Representative Drug
μ-Opioid receptor	Opiates, e.g., morphine-6-glucuronide
β₂-Adrenergic receptor	β-Agonists, e.g., albuterol; antagonists, e.g., metoprolol
5-Lipoxygenase	5-LO inhibitors, e.g., montelukast
Bradykinin B2 receptor	ACE inhibitors, e.g., enalapril
Dopamine receptors	Dopamine antagonists, e.g., clozapine
Serotonin transporter	SSRIs, e.g., fluoxetine, paroxetine
Estrogen receptor-α	Conjugated estrogens

centrations, and thus has effects directly attributable to altered tissue drug levels. Genetic defects in a number of drug-metabolizing enzymes have been well characterized with respect to both their molecular mechanisms and clinical correlates, although evidence is now accumulating that altered drug transporter function also may produce significant phenotypic variation in drug response. In general, the clinical consequences associated with genetically polymorphic drug-metabolizing enzymes may come under four main classifications:

1. Functional drug overdose in persons unable to eliminate an active drug efficiently
2. Lack of therapeutic effect either in persons who metabolize an active drug too quickly or in those unable to convert a pro-drug to its pharmacologically active metabolite
3. Idiosyncratic drug toxicity unrelated to the intended effect of a therapeutic agent (e.g., hypersensitivity reactions, drug-induced lupus, drug-induced birth defects), which may occur more frequently in persons of a particular metabolizer phenotype
4. Apparently spontaneous disorders for which the cause is unknown but presumably is complex and multifactorial, and which may involve drug or chemical exposures

POLYMORPHISMS OF PHASE I DRUG OXIDATION

Considering that the majority of lipid-soluble drugs are metabolized at least to some extent via oxidation, predominantly by members of the liver microsomal monooxygenase (cytochrome P450) enzyme system,[19] it is somewhat surprising that until the mid-1970s, only a few isolated reports of inherited defects of drug oxidation had been published. This may be largely due to the known multiplicity and overlapping substrate specificity of this enzyme superfamily,[20] implying that for many drugs multiple biotransformation pathways exist. Thus, compensatory metabolism by alternate pathways could prevent the clinical manifestations that would be associated with a defect in a particular metabolic reaction. Nonetheless, in the almost three decades since the first discovery of a cytochrome P450 oxidation defect, a large number of polymorphisms of drug oxidation have been characterized in considerable detail.* Selected examples drawn from known polymorphisms in the cytochrome P450 monooxygenase superfamily will be summarized here.

Cytochrome P4502D6 (CYP2D6) Oxidation Polymorphism

This example, reviewed in detail recently,[1] provided the first clear demonstration of polymorphic drug oxidation involving a cytochrome P450 enzyme. It also illustrates the classic experimental phenotype to genotype paradigm of pharmacogenetic investigation, progressing from an initial clinical observation of

variable drug response to an understanding of the biochemical and molecular mechanisms that produce the clinically distinct phenotypes. Such fundamental knowledge can now be applied back to the development and clinical use of predictive tests that may be of value to the clinician in choosing the appropriate type and dose of drug to prescribe to individual patients.

The first clinical observations leading to this discovery were provided during independent studies of the antihypertensive drug debrisoquine[21] and the oxytocic agent sparteine.[22] Wide interpatient variations in the dose of debrisoquine required to achieve a hypotensive response were shown to result from genetic differences in the extent to which the drug is hydroxylated to 4-hydroxydebrisoquine. Using a metabolic ratio of the parent drug to its hydroxylated metabolite excreted in urine following a single oral dose, it was possible to observe a bimodal population frequency histogram that divided subjects into extensive metabolizers (EMs) and poor metabolizers (PMs), with PM phenotype frequencies ranging from 3% to 10% in various white populations.[1] At the same time, studies of variations in the response to sparteine showed that a similar percentage of German subjects were almost entirely unable to metabolize the compound to its dehydro metabolites.[22] Correlation studies subsequently established that defective metabolism of debrisoquine and sparteine is under identical genetic control.[23] Since these initial observations, the polymorphism has been shown to control, either fully or partially, the rate of oxidation of a number of other clinically useful drugs as well[1] (Table 22-3). The fact that the debrisoquine/sparteine polymorphism is not a generalized drug oxidation defect, however, is supported by numerous reports showing unimpaired metabolism of a wide variety of other drugs whose metabolic fate depends in general on cytochrome P450 oxidation.

The clinical consequences of the debrisoquine drug oxidation defect have been thoroughly investigated for a number of the affected drugs in Table 22-3.[1,24] One interesting example is that of codeine, which exerts its analgesic effect predominantly via its conversion to morphine—a reaction mediated by the debrisoquine-oxidizing cytochrome P450. Thus in poor metabolizers of debrisoquine, codeine is ineffective in the relief of pain.[25] It is important to recognize that although the biotransformation of each of the compounds listed in Table 22-3 is measurably affected by the debrisoquine oxidase polymorphism, not all result in the occurrence of altered drug responses. For example, genetically poor metabolizers experience a greater incidence of excessive β-blockade and loss of cardioselectivity because of elevated plasma drug concentrations after administration of the β-adrenergic antagonist metoprolol[26] but not after the closely related propranolol,[27] even though both are linked to the oxidation defect. The reason for this is that propranolol follows several additional metabolic pathways, which, along with renal elimination, can compensate for defective biotransformation by the debrisoquine-oxidizing enzyme. Also, certain drugs such as quinidine and certain neuroleptic agents are potent inhibitors of the polymorphic enzyme without necessarily being significantly metabolized by it. Co-administration of these with any of the drugs in Table 22-3 could then lead to potentially significant drug-drug interactions or even misclassification (phenocopying) of normal individuals as genetically poor metabolizers.

Much progress has been made in determining the biochemical and molecular mechanisms leading to the occurrence of the debrisoquine poor metabolizer phenotype in human populations. The cytochrome P450 isoform that is now known to responsible for the biotransformation of debrisoquine and other affected compounds is designated as CYP2D6. As of this writing, a total of 76 different alleles at the gene locus (*CYP2D6*) encoding the CYP2D6 protein have been detected in human populations, many of which contain sequence alterations that contribute to the occurrence of extensive and poor metabolizer phenotypes.* It is notable that the underlying basis of a clinical

---

* http://www.imm.ki.se/CYPalleles; see also Table 22-1.

* http://www.imm.ki.se/CYPalleles/cyp2d6.htm.

TABLE 22-3

Some Drugs Affected by the Debrisoquine Oxidation (CYP2D6) Polymorphism

Antiarrhythmics	Other Drugs
Encainide	Cinnarizine
Flecainide	Codeine
N-Propylajmaline	Debrisoquine
Propafenone	Dexfenfluramine
Sparteine	Dextromethorphan
Aprindine	Dihydrocodeine
Exiletine	Dolasetron
β-Adrenergic Receptor Blockers	Funarizine
Alprenolol	Guanoxan
Burfuralol	Hydrocodone
Carvedilol	Indoramin
Metoprolol	MDMA (ecstasy)
Propranolol	Meguitozine
Timolol	Methoxyphenamine (MPTP)
Methoxyamphetamine	Nicergoline
Bunitrolol	Orphenadrine
	Perhexiline
Neuroleptics	Phenformin
Haloperidol	Terodiline
Perphenazine	Tolterodine
Risperidone	Tramadol
Sertindole	Tropisetron
Thioridazine	Tamoxifen
Zuclopenthixol	
Antidepressants	
Amitriptyline	
Brofaromine	
Citalopram	
Clomipramine	
Desipramine	
Fluoxetine	
Ifoxetine	
Imipramine	
Maprotiline	
Mianserin	
Nortriptyline	
Paroxetine	
Selegiline	
Tomoxetine	

phenotype that is generally considered by clinicians to be rather homogeneous—the poor metabolizer of debrisoquine—is based on a large and heterogeneous set of molecular defects ranging from single nucleotide substitutions (SNPs), insertions or deletions that change single amino acids and alter enzyme stability or kinetics, to entire gene deletions or duplications that produce either completely absent or elevated function, respectively. As a result, it is now also clear that significant phenotypic differences may exist within as well as between the so-called metabolizer phenotypes. Although such a high degree of allelic multiplicity poses practical problems in devising simple yet reliable molecular tests to predict defective drug oxidation by CYP2D6 and its severity, the rarity of many of the known variants coupled with ongoing improvements to high-throughput genotyping technology advances allows for the development of robust and highly predictive tests for large-scale population studies.[28,29]

Cytochrome P4502C9 (CYP2C9) Oxidation Polymorphism

Polymorphic variants of CYP2C9[30] may be of considerable clinical importance because of the role of this enzyme in metabolizing a number of therapeutically useful drugs, including warfarin, phenytoin, glipizide, and tolbutamide.[31,32] A total of 12 allelic variants are currently known to exist at the *CYP2C9* gene locus.* However, by far the most common of the activity-impaired

enzymes arise from the *CYP2C9*2*[33] and *CYP2C9*3*[34] variants, each possessing one SNP that alters a single amino acid and impairs enzyme function significantly. Because of the narrow therapeutic index of the anticoagulant warfarin, significant hypercoagulation-related toxicity from this drug has been observed in individuals possessing CYP2C9 defective alleles,[35,36] although it is evident that other environmental factors also play significant roles in determining warfarin plasma concentrations and therapeutic efficacy.[37,38] Similar observations have been made with the anticonvulsant phenytoin, a drug with saturation kinetics and significant dose-related cognitive side effects that are amplified in poor CYP2C9 metabolizers.[39] On the other hand, it has recently been shown that the antihypertensive response to the angiotensin II type I receptor antagonist irbesartan is actually improved in individuals possessing one defective CYP2C9 allele when compared with those with only wild-type alleles.[40]

Cytochrome P4502C19 (CYP2C19) Oxidation Polymorphism

A well-studied cytochrome P450 polymorphism affects the function of another member of the CYP2 family, CYP2C19. Originally discovered during studies with the seldom-used anticonvulsant mephenytoin, the defect is now known to affect the function of a small number of commonly prescribed drugs, including the proton pump inhibitors omeprazole, lansoprazole, and pantoprazole and the anxiolytic diazepam.[41] A total of 19 allelic forms of the *CYP2C19* gene have been characterized to date,* with two defective alleles making up the bulk of those associated with poor metabolizer status. The frequency of defective alleles (specifically the *CYP2C19*3* variant) is higher in Asian than in other populations,[42] resulting in an incidence of poor-metabolizer individuals approaching 20% in many Asian groups, compared with approximately 3% in Caucasians. The efficacy of omeprazole in increasing intragastric pH and in successfully treating peptic ulcer has been shown to be significantly higher in individuals possessing defective CYP2C19 alleles,[43] suggesting that dosing regimens for this drug in normal extensive metabolizers in fact may be inadequate. On the other hand, although differences in the clearance of diazepam[44] and the bioactivation of the antimalarial proguanil[45] are altered in poor CYP2C19 metabolizers, the clinical consequences of these findings are modest at best.

POLYMORPHISMS OF PHASE II DRUG-CONJUGATING ENZYMES

Arylamine N-Acetyltransferase 2 (NAT2) Polymorphism

This example (reviewed in ref. 2) lends a special historical perspective to the field of pharmacogenetics, since 2003 marks the 50th anniversary of its discovery. In 1953, high interindividual variation was observed in the urinary excretion of the new tuberculostatic drug isoniazid. This observation was followed by the finding that frequency histograms of plasma isoniazid concentrations after a single oral dose in a normal population were distinctly bimodal, allowing for classification of subjects as "rapid" or "slow" eliminators of the drug. It was soon established that the basis of the observed population variations was related to differences in the rate of arylamine and hydrazine N-acetylation taking place, to a large extent, in the liver.[46] The enzymatic reaction is now known to be catalyzed by a cytosolic arylamine N-acetyltransferase (NAT), which uses the essential cofactor acetyl coenzyme A as acetyl group donor to conjugate primary amine and hydrazine nitrogen atoms, or hydroxylamine oxygen atoms with acetate, producing amides, hydrazides, and acetoxy esters.

The clinical and toxicologic consequences of the acetylation polymorphism have been studied in considerable detail. For instance, slow acetylators are more prone to develop a drug-induced systemic lupus erythematosus–like syndrome during

---

prolonged therapy with procainamide or hydralazine, hematologic toxicity from dapsone, or polyneuropathy after isoniazid treatment. The slow acetylator phenotype also appears to be a predisposing factor in the etiology of sulfonamide-induced idiosyncratic adverse drug reactions (ADRs). In addition, epidemiologic studies suggest that there is an increased risk for bladder cancer in slow acetylators who are exposed to carcinogenic arylamines, which are substrates for NAT, whereas rapid acetylators may be at higher risk for colon cancer. Rapid acetylators also encounter therapeutic failure more often on treatment with once-weekly isoniazid dosage regimens and require higher doses of hydralazine to control hypertension or of dapsone for dermatitis herpetiformis.

Molecular cloning experiments have established that two functional human NAT enzymes exist, NAT1 and NAT2, and that genetically based variation in NAT2 is associated with the isoniazid acetylation polymorphism. Work over the past decade has provided direct evidence for the existence of, at last count, 35 variant alleles at the human NAT2 gene locus that are correlated with the acetylator phenotype.* Each of the quantitatively significant human allelic variants possesses a diagnostic combination of nucleotide substitutions (SNPs) at positions 191, 282, 341, 481, 590, 803, and 857 within the intronless 870-bp NAT2 gene-coding region. At the level of protein function, the single I114T amino acid change produced by a T341C mutation common to the nine NAT2*5 alleles drastically reduces V_{max} values for substrate acetylation without altering enzyme affinity or stability, possibly by preventing the proper folding of the nascent polypeptide into its enzymatically active conformation. On the other hand, the mutations causing R197Q (NAT2*6), G286E (NAT2*7) and R64Q (NAT2*14) amino acid substitutions produce proteins with significantly reduced stabilities.[47] The population frequencies of certain of the NAT2 alleles also show marked interethnic differences.[47] For instance, NAT2*5B (I114T) is the most common allele in white populations but is almost entirely absent in Asians, accounting for most of the known interethnic difference in the frequency of the slow acetylator phenotype between these populations. NAT2*7B (G286E), on the other hand, is more prevalent in Asians than in whites.

NAT1 function is also variable in human populations, and at least some of this variation may be genetically determined. The use of the NAT1-selective substrate p-aminosalicylic acid as a probe drug has allowed for the identification of probands from which variant alleles at the NAT1 gene locus have been isolated and characterized.[48] There are now a total of 26 known NAT1 allelic variants,† although those that are known to alter function significantly are rare in most human populations. Association studies have attempted to correlate variation in the more common NAT1 alleles, particularly NAT1*10, with susceptibility to a variety of cancers, with equivocal results; the functional consequences of these variants for enzyme activity in vivo are also still unclear.

Thiopurine S-Methyltransferase (TPMT) Polymorphism

Clinical relevance has been clearly demonstrated for a polymorphism that occurs in the drug-methylating enzyme thiopurine S-methyltransferase (TPMT).[49-51] This enzyme catalyzes the detoxifying methylation of the cytotoxic agent 6-mercaptopurine, a drug commonly used in cancer chemotherapeutic regimens for the treatment of childhood acute lymphoblastic leukemia. The TPMT-catalyzed reaction competes with a reaction that produces cytotoxic thioguanine nucleotides, which are the pharmacologically active principle in producing leukemic cell death. Thus in individuals with impaired TPMT function, excessive production of thioguanine nucleotides leads to a higher incidence of adverse reactions to the

drug, often requiring cessation of therapy and drastic dose reduction.[52] To date, eight variant TPMT alleles have been identified[53]; three of these, TPMT*2, TPMT*3A, and TPMT*3C, account for 95% of the cases of defective function. Although the frequency of each of the seven known activity-impairing variants is quite low, such that the incidence of individuals possessing two defective copies is only about 1 in 300, functional impairment is observed even in heterozygotes, who make up about 11% of a typical Caucasian population. Because of the relatively small number of relevant mutations known to impair function, simple genetic diagnostic assays can be devised as guides to dosing regimens in initiating chemotherapy. On the other hand, the fact that TPMT expression in blood cells is an accurate reflection of tissue enzyme activity, a direct blood enzyme assay is also practically feasible.[54]

PHARMACOGENETIC DEFECTS AFFECTING DRUG PHARMACODYNAMICS

Table 22-2 provides a number of instances in which genetic variation in specific drug targets may influence drug efficacy. Although a detailed discussion of these examples is beyond the scope of this review, a brief summary of one selected instance is presented here. It is worth noting, however, that because of the multifactorial nature of many drug responses and physiologic processes, the clinical significance of many of the genetic variants in drug targets observed so far has yet to be conclusively established.[55] In addition, since most drug targets, such as receptors, have important endogenous physiologic roles, there is a lower likelihood of observing severely function-impairing mutations arising from single-gene defects for many of these proteins.

β-Adrenergic Receptor Polymorphisms

Variations in the genes encoding β-adrenergic receptors have recently been shown to correlate with a variety of responses to β-agonists, as well as to physiologic and pathologic stimuli.[56-59] For instance, recent experimental observations have suggested that allelic variants possessing an arginine at position 16 of the β_2-adrenergic receptor protein impart increased agonist-mediated vascular desensitization, whereas variants with glutamic acid at position 27 have increased agonist-mediated responsiveness.[60] Asthmatic patients who were homozygous for arginine at position 16 of the β_2-adrenergic receptor were also shown to have greater therapeutic response to albuterol for the relief of their airway constriction.[61] Polymorphisms in the β_1-adrenergic receptor have been shown to affect exercise capacity in patients with congestive heart failure[62] and resting hemodynamics in patients undergoing diagnostic testing for ischemia.[63] Finally, it has been suggested that polymorphic variants of the β_3-adrenergic receptor may be risk factors for obesity.[64]

PHARMACOGENETICS IN CONTEXT: GENE REGULATION AND DEVELOPMENT

Pharmacogenetic defects must be considered as only one part of the complex series of genetic and environmental factors that regulate the level and developmental time course of protein expression. Furthermore, many of these variables have potential relevance for the perinatal pharmacologist. For instance, with regard to drug-metabolizing enzymes, differential activation of transcription of cytochrome P450 and other oxidative metabolism genes at varying stages of prenatal and postnatal development has been shown to produce age-specific isozyme patterns.[65] Different P450 genes have been shown to be activated immediately after birth, in the months following birth, at the onset of puberty, or according to neonatal imprinting by sex

---

* http://www.louisville.edu/medschool/pharmacology/NAT2.html.
† http://www.louisville.edu/medschool/pharmacology/NAT1.html.

hormone exposure, most notably in rodent species; certain isoforms also may be specifically suppressed at puberty. Significant differences exist between the forms of P450 expressed before and after birth.[66-68] It is interesting that one isoform of the CYP3A family (CYP3A7), which previously was considered as fetal specific, has been demonstrated to display both expression in all fetal livers tested and polymorphic expression among adult human livers.[69] On the other hand, recent studies suggest that differences in the content and activity of cytochrome P450 in early life are unlikely to account for the increased clearance of many drugs in children.[70]

In addition, it is known that the expression of certain classes of P450 isozymes is induced (at the level of transcriptional activation) by specific drug or hormonal exposures.[71] For example, polycyclic aromatic hydrocarbons present in cigarette smoke may cause elevation in the liver content of CYP1A isozymes; this response has been shown to be both genetically and developmentally variable.[72] Expression of CYP1A2, which appears to be responsible for the metabolism of caffeine, theophylline, phenacetin, and a variety of aromatic amine procarcinogens, develops slowly (possibly via exposure to environmental inducing agents) over the first several months of extrauterine life,[73] whereas in women its activity is drastically impaired during pregnancy.[68] It has also been suggested that a glucocorticoid-inducible P450 isozyme may be involved in the process of oxygen contracture and subsequent closure of the ductus arteriosus at birth.[74]

The consequences of allelic variation in Phase II enzymes for drug therapy may also be important for the pediatric pharmacologist, especially considering that both genetic and regulatory factors may govern the expression of metabolizing capacity during development.[75] For instance, longitudinal NAT2 acetylator phenotyping studies in developing infants[76] have demonstrated that all neonates are phenotypically slow acetylators, suggesting that the manifestation of the isoniazid acetylation polymorphism develops relatively slowly over the first 1 to 2 years of life. NAT1 activity has been detected in human fetal liver, adrenal glands, lung, kidney, and intestine, although at a lower level than that observed in adult tissues.[77] NAT1 is also present in the placenta[78] and in human preimplantation embryos[79]; given its ability to metabolize a catabolite of folic acid,[80] a role for this enzyme in neural tube development has been suggested.[81] Given the different substrate specificities and tissue-selective patterns of expression of NAT1 and NAT2, exposures to certain arylamine chemicals may be expected to result in different patterns of elimination or toxicity (or both), depending on the levels of expression of these enzymes during fetal and neonatal development. Further work is required to delineate these patterns of expression and their consequences for drug therapy and toxicity.

From the previous examples, it is apparent that when genetic factors, which may differ between mother and child, interact with such developmental and gene regulatory processes, a vast potential exists for variation in metabolizing capacities for drugs and xenobiotics. Thus clinical outcomes (adverse drug reactions, fetal toxicity) depend not only on the chemical agent, but also on the genetic constitution of mother and child and the time point of exposure in relation to the functional integrity of the drug biotransformation systems.[8,82,83]

INTERACTION BETWEEN ONTOGENY AND PHARMACOGENETICS: CLINICAL PEDIATRIC PHARMACOGENETICS

The examples just cited provide some insight into how rapidly the field of pharmacogenetics has grown in the last several years, aided greatly by advances in analytic techniques, cellular assays, and most especially genomic technologies. One of the main challenges has been to provide unified approaches to both genotype and phenotype for the handling of specific drugs and other xenobiotics. Recognition of the specificity of drug metabolic pathways and the ability to determine which pathways are critical for handling a new drug before its widespread use in humans may lead to decreased population variability and risk of untoward side effects. Use of *in vitro* techniques employing human hepatic microsomes (with specific inhibitors of drug-metabolizing enzymes) and recombinantly expressed enzymes can determine whether a new drug is likely to be metabolized polymorphically in the population and what other drugs might interact with the new drug to alter its kinetics. *In vivo* probe compounds (such as dextromethorphan for CYP2D6 and caffeine for NAT2) can help map regulation and development of expression of metabolic pathways safely in large populations. As outlined in the previous section, one of the main challenges in pediatric developmental pharmacology is to integrate the growing body of data on specificity of metabolic pathways with their ontogeny.[65,75]

The interaction of genetics and ontogeny of drug metabolism has been reviewed.[8,82-84] For example, the availability of potentially toxic electrophilic metabolites to mediate toxicity often depends on the interaction of several metabolic pathways, one of which might be genetically polymorphic, whereas others are developmentally regulated. Although the genetic abnormality might be critical to the ultimate toxic outcome, risk may be modulated by developmental expression of other pathways, perhaps explaining why some drug-induced toxicities (such as hepatotoxicity from valproic acid[85]) may be more prevalent in younger patients. Knowledge of specificity of metabolic pathways also can help in the design of clinical pharmacokinetic studies of new drugs. For example, if a new drug is metabolized by CYP1A2, an enzyme that appears to develop over the first postnatal year of life and then undergo down-regulation during puberty (at earlier Tanner stages in girls than in boys[86]), grouping patients 6 to 12 years and 13 to 18 years of age includes children in various Tanner stages in both groups, leading to increased and difficult-to-interpret variability. It may make better sense to group patients by Tanner stage, studying smaller numbers of more homogeneous patients to assess the effects of puberty on handling of the compound. A similar approach can be taken for the newborn infant, determining the pathways of clearance for the drug, understanding the ontogeny of those pathways, and thus more rationally choosing doses for clinical studies.

As with any new field during a period of rapid scientific expansion, it is difficult to predict the ultimate impact of pharmacogenetics on "real-life" pharmacotherapy. The advances of the last several years, however, suggest that the field will have a direct impact on patient care.[4,5,11,12,87,88] The field is clearly expanding beyond just drug metabolism. Molecular approaches will lead to (1) disease susceptibility markers, early preclinical "diagnosis" of disease diathesis for early therapeutic intervention; (2) syndrome diagnostic markers, to determine more specific causes of complex human symptoms and thus improve specificity of therapeutic choices; (3) pharmacogenetic markers for drug metabolism and efficacy variants; and (4) markers to individualize idiosyncratic adverse drug reaction risk, minimizing both individual and population risk of adverse drug effects. Routine availability of molecular diagnostics in the clinical laboratory will usher in a new era for clinical pharmacogenetics.

REFERENCES

1. Kalow W, Grant DM: Pharmacogenetics. *In* Scriver CR, et al (eds): The Metabolic and Molecular Bases of Inherited Disease. New York, McGraw-Hill, 2001, pp 225-255.
2. Grant DM, et al: Pharmacogenetics of the human arylamine *N*-acetyltransferases. Pharmacology 61:204, 2000.
3. Weinshilboum R: Inheritance and drug response. N Engl J Med *348*:529, 2003.

4. Evans WE, Relling MV: Pharmacogenomics: translating functional genomics into rational therapeutics. Science 286:487, 1999.
5. Evans WE, Johnson JA: Pharmacogenomics: the inherited basis for interindividual differences in drug response. Annu Rev Genom Hum Genet 2:9, 2001.
6. Evans WE, McLeod HL: Pharmacogenomics—drug disposition, drug targets, and side effects. N Engl J Med 348:538, 2003.
7. Leeder JS: Pharmacogenetics and pharmacogenomics. Pediatr Clin North Am 48:765, 2001.
8. Leeder JS, Kearns GL: Pharmacogenetics in pediatrics. Implications for practice. Pediatr Clin North Am 44:55, 1997.
9. Linder MW, Valdes R Jr: Genetic mechanisms for variability in drug response and toxicity. J Anal Toxicol 25:405, 2001.
10. Roden DM: Principles in pharmacogenetics. Epilepsia 42(Suppl 5):44, 2001.
11. Roses AD: Pharmacogenetics and the practice of medicine. Nature 405:857, 2000.
12. Roses AD: Pharmacogenetics. Hum Mol Genet 10:2261, 2001.
13. Issa AM: Ethical considerations in clinical pharmacogenomics research. Trends Pharmacol Sci 21:247, 2000.
14. Johnson JA, Evans WE: Molecular diagnostics as a predictive tool: genetics of drug efficacy and toxicity. Trends Mol Med 8:300, 2002.
15. Daly AK: Pharmacogenetics of the major polymorphic metabolizing enzymes. Fundam Clin Pharmacol 17:27, 2003.
16. Bertilsson L: Current status: pharmacogenetics/drug metabolism. In Kalow W, et al (eds): Pharmacogenomics. New York, Marcel Dekker, 2001, pp 33–50.
17. Weber WW: Pharmacogenetics—receptors. In Kalow W, et al (eds): Pharmacogenomics. New York, Marcel Dekker, 2001, pp 51–80.
18. Kim RB, Wilkinson GR: Pharmacogenetics of drug transporters. In Kalow W, et al (eds): Pharmacogenomics. New York, Marcel Dekker, 2001, pp 81–108.
19. Danielson PB: The cytochrome p450 superfamily: biochemistry, evolution and drug metabolism in humans. Curr Drug Metab 3:561, 2002.
20. Parkinson A: Biotransformation of xenobiotics. In Klaasen CD (ed): Casarett & Doull's Toxicology: The Basic Science of Poisons. New York, McGraw-Hill Professional 2001, pp 133–224.
21. Mahgoub A, et al: Polymorphic hydroxylation of debrisoquine in man. Lancet 2:584, 1977.
22. Eichelbaum M, et al: Proceedings: N-oxidation of sparteine in man and its interindividual differences. Naunyn Schmiedebergs Arch Pharmacol 287(Suppl):R94, 1975.
23. Inaba T, et al: Deficient metabolism of debrisoquine and sparteine. Clin Pharmacol Ther 27:547, 1980.
24. Bertilsson L, et al: Molecular genetics of CYP2D6: clinical relevance with focus on psychotropic drugs. Br J Clin Pharmacol 53:111, 2002.
25. Sindrup SH, Brosen K: The pharmacogenetics of codeine hypoalgesia. Pharmacogenetics 5:335, 1995.
26. Wuttke H, et al: Increased frequency of cytochrome P450 2D6 poor metabolizers among patients with metoprolol-associated adverse effects. Clin Pharmacol Ther 72:429, 2002.
27. Sowinski KM, Burlew BS: Impact of CYP2D6 poor metabolizer phenotype on propranolol pharmacokinetics and response. Pharmacotherapy 17:1305, 1997.
28. Gaedigk A, et al: Optimization of cytochrome P4502D6 (CYP2D6) phenotype assignment using a genotyping algorithm based on allele frequency data. Pharmacogenetics 9:669, 1999.
29. McElroy S, et al: CYP2D6 genotyping as an alternative to phenotyping for determination of metabolic status in a clinical trial setting. AAPS PharmSci 2:E33, 2000.
30. Lee CR, et al: Cytochrome P450 2C9 polymorphisms: a comprehensive review of the in-vitro and human data. Pharmacogenetics 12:251, 2002.
31. Kidd RS, et al: Pharmacokinetics of chlorpheniramine, phenytoin, glipizide and nifedipine in an individual homozygous for the CYP2C9*3 allele. Pharmacogenetics 9:71, 1999.
32. Goldstein JA: Clinical relevance of genetic polymorphisms in the human CYP2C subfamily. Br J Clin Pharmacol 52:349, 2001.
33. Rettie AE, et al: Impaired (S)-warfarin metabolism catalysed by the R144C allelic variant of CYP2C9. Pharmacogenetics 4:39, 1994.
34. Sullivan-Klose TH, et al: The role of the CYP2C9-Leu359 allelic variant in the tolbutamide polymorphism. Pharmacogenetics 6:341, 1996.
35. Takahashi H, Echizen H: Pharmacogenetics of warfarin elimination and its clinical implications. Clin Pharmacokinet 40:587, 2001.
36. Bloch A, et al: Major bleeding caused by warfarin in a genetically susceptible patient. Pharmacotherapy 22:97, 2002.
37. Verstuyft C, et al: Genetic and environmental risk factors for oral anticoagulant overdose. Eur J Clin Pharmacol 58:739, 2003.
38. Takahashi H, et al: Population differences in S-warfarin metabolism between CYP2C9 genotype-matched Caucasian and Japanese patients. Clin Pharmacol Ther 73:253, 2003.
39. Kidd RS, et al: Identification of a null allele of CYP2C9 in an African-American exhibiting toxicity to phenytoin. Pharmacogenetics 11:803, 2001.
40. Hallberg P, et al: The CYP2C9 genotype predicts the blood pressure response to irbesartan: results from the Swedish Irbesartan Left Ventricular Hypertrophy Investigation vs Atenolol (SILVHIA) trial. J Hypertens 20:2089, 2002.
41. Desta Z, et al: Clinical significance of the cytochrome P450 2C19 genetic polymorphism. Clin Pharmacokinet 41:913, 2002.
42. De Morais SM, et al: Identification of a new genetic defect responsible for the polymorphism of (S)-mephenytoin metabolism in Japanese. Mol Pharmacol 46:594, 1994.

43. Furuta T, et al: Effect of genetic differences in omeprazole metabolism on cure rates for Helicobacter pylori infection and peptic ulcer. Ann Intern Med 129:1027, 1998.
44. Wan J, et al: The elimination of diazepam in Chinese subjects is dependent on the mephenytoin oxidation phenotype. Br J Clin Pharmacol 42:471, 1996.
45. Kaneko A, et al: Proguanil disposition and toxicity in malaria patients from Vanuatu with high frequencies of CYP2C19 mutations. Pharmacogenetics 9:317, 1999.
46. Evans DAP, White TA: Human acetylation polymorphism. J Lab Clin Med 63:394, 1964.
47. Grant DM, et al: Human acetyltransferase polymorphisms. Mutat Res 376:61, 1997.
48. Hughes NC, et al: Identification and characterization of variant alleles of human acetyltransferase NAT1 with defective function using p-aminosalicylate as an in-vivo and in-vitro probe. Pharmacogenetics 8:55, 1998.
49. McLeod HL, et al: Genetic polymorphism of thiopurine methyltransferase and its clinical relevance for childhood acute lymphoblastic leukemia. Leukemia 14:567, 2000.
50. Krynetski EY, Evans WE: Genetic polymorphism of thiopurine S-methyltransferase: molecular mechanisms and clinical importance. Pharmacology 61:136, 2000.
51. McLeod HL, Siva C: The thiopurine S-methyltransferase gene locus—implications for clinical pharmacogenomics. Pharmacogenomics 3:89, 2002.
52. Relling MV, et al: Mercaptopurine therapy intolerance and heterozygosity at the thiopurine S-methyltransferase gene locus. J Natl Cancer Inst 91:2001, 1999.
53. McLeod HL, Evans WE: Pharmacogenomics: unlocking the human genome for better drug therapy. Annu Rev Pharmacol Toxicol 41:101, 2001.
54. Weinshilboum R: Thiopurine pharmacogenetics: clinical and molecular studies of thiopurine methyltransferase. Drug Metab Dispos 29:601, 2001.
55. Johnson JA: Drug target pharmacogenomics: an overview. Am J Pharmacogen 1:271, 2001.
56. Johnson JA, Terra SG: β-Adrenergic receptor polymorphisms: cardiovascular disease associations and pharmacogenetics. Pharm Res 19:1779, 2002.
57. Wood AJ: Variability in beta-adrenergic receptor response in the vasculature: role of receptor polymorphism. J Allergy Clin Immunol 110:S318, 2002.
58. Taylor DR, Kennedy MA: Beta-adrenergic receptor polymorphisms and drug responses in asthma. Pharmacogenomics 3:173, 2002.
59. Palmer LJ, et al: Pharmacogenetics of asthma. Am J Respir Crit Care Med 165:861, 2002.
60. Dishy V, et al: The effect of common polymorphisms of the beta₂-adrenergic receptor on agonist-mediated vascular desensitization. N Engl J Med 345:1030, 2001.
61. Lima JJ, et al: Impact of genetic polymorphisms of the beta₂-adrenergic receptor on albuterol bronchodilator pharmacodynamics. Clin Pharmacol Ther 65:519, 1999.
62. Wagoner LE, et al: Polymorphisms of the beta₁-adrenergic receptor predict exercise capacity in heart failure. Am Heart J 144:840, 2002.
63. Humma LM, et al: Effects of beta₁-adrenoceptor genetic polymorphisms on resting hemodynamics in patients undergoing diagnostic testing for ischemia. Am J Cardiol 88:1034, 2001.
64. Marti A, et al: TRP64ARG polymorphism of the beta₃-adrenergic receptor gene and obesity risk: effect modification by a sedentary lifestyle. Diabetes Obes Metab 4:428, 2002.
65. Hines RN, McCarver DG: The ontogeny of human drug-metabolizing enzymes: phase I oxidative enzymes. J Pharmacol Exp Ther 300:355, 2002.
66. Hakkola J, et al: Expression of xenobiotic-metabolizing cytochrome P450 forms in human adult and fetal liver. Biochem Pharmacol 48:59, 1994.
67. Kitada M, Kamataki T: Cytochrome P450 in human fetal liver: significance and fetal-specific expression. Drug Metab Rev 26:305, 1994.
68. Oesterheld JR: A review of developmental aspects of cytochrome P450. J Child Adolesc Psychopharmacol 8:161, 1998.
69. Lamba JK: Genetic contribution to variable human CYP3A-mediated metabolism. Adv Drug Deliv Rev 54:1271, 2002.
70. Blanco JG, et al: Human cytochrome P450 maximal activities in pediatric versus adult liver. Drug Metab Dispos 28:379, 2000.
71. Schuetz EG: Induction of cytochromes P450. Curr Drug Metab 2:139, 2001.
72. Lin JH, Lu AY: Interindividual variability in inhibition and induction of cytochrome P450 enzymes. Annu Rev Pharmacol Toxicol 41:535, 2001.
73. Aldridge A, et al: Caffeine metabolism in the newborn. Clin Pharmacol Ther 25:447, 1979.
74. Coceani F, et al: Inhibition of the contraction of the ductus arteriosus to oxygen by 1-aminobenzotriazole, a mechanism-based inactivator of cytochrome P450. Br J Pharmacol 117:1586, 1996.
75. McCarver DG, Hines RN: The ontogeny of human drug-metabolizing enzymes; phase II: conjugation enzymes and regulatory mechanisms. J Pharmacol Exp Ther 300:361, 2002.
76. Pariente-Khayat A, et al: Caffeine acetylator phenotyping during maturation in infants. Pediatr Res 29:492, 1991.
77. Pacifici GM, et al: Acetyltransferase in humans: development and tissue distribution. Pharmacology 32:283, 1986.
78. Derewlany LO, et al: Arylamine N-acetyltransferase activity of the human placenta. J Pharmacol Exp Ther 269:756, 1994.
79. Smelt VA, et al: Expression of arylamine N-acetyltransferase in pre-term placentas and in human pre-implantation embryos. Hum Mol Genet 9:1101, 2000.
80. Ward A, et al: Purification of recombinant human N-acetyltransferase type 1 (NAT1) expressed in E. coli and characterization of its potential role in folate metabolism. Biochem Pharmacol 49:1759, 1995.

81. Sim E, et al: An update on genetic, structural and functional studies of arylamine N-acetyltransferases in eucaryotes and procaryotes. Hum Mol Genet 9:2435, 2000.

82. Kearns GL: Pharmacogenetics and development: are infants and children at increased risk for adverse outcomes? Curr Opin Pediatr 7:220, 1995.

83. Leeder JS, Kearns GL: The challenges of delivering pharmacogenomics into clinical pediatrics. Pharmacogenomics J 2:141, 2002.

84. Spielberg SP: Therapeutics and toxicology: editorial overview. Curr Opin Pediatr 7:193, 1995.

85. Appleton RE, et al: The high incidence of valproate hepatotoxicity in infants may relate to familial metabolic defects. Can J Neurol Sci 17:145, 1990.

86. Lambert GH, et al: The effect of age, gender, and sexual maturation on the caffeine breath test. Dev Pharmacol Ther 9:375, 1986.

87. Anderson GM, Cook EH: Pharmacogenetics. Promise and potential in child and adolescent psychiatry. Child Adolesc Psychiatr Clin North Am 9:23, 2000.

88. Ensom MH, et al: Pharmacogenetics: the therapeutic drug monitoring of the future? Clin Pharmacokinet 40:783, 2001.

23

Marianne Garland

Drug Distribution in Fetal Life

Drug distribution determines the concentration that will be attained at the site of drug action whether in plasma, in extracellular spaces, or in the intracellular environment. Drug targets include cell surface receptors, intracellular receptors, enzymes, transcriptional mechanisms, ion channels, and molecular transport systems. These may be within the circulatory system, in well-perfused tissues, in less well-perfused tissues, or behind specialized endothelial or epithelial barriers. The fetus lies behind one of these circulatory barriers—the placenta. The placenta keeps the maternal and fetal circulations separate but brings them into close apposition for transport of nutritional needs and removal of waste products. This interface is also the major route of drug delivery to, and elimination from, the fetus. The fetus has specialized circulatory arrangements designed for intrauterine life that require additional considerations in the understanding of fetal drug distribution. Furthermore, developmental differences in body composition, drug metabolism, renal clearance, and specialized barriers make drug distribution different from that in the infant, child, and adult.

From a practical point of view, most drug action is predicted based on plasma concentrations of drug. It is not easy, even in experimental models, to measure tissue concentrations, particularly when extracellular versus intracellular concentration merits consideration. Hence, major emphasis is placed on the determinants of fetal plasma concentration. This requires an understanding of physicochemical properties of drugs, placental transfer of drugs, and fetal clearance of drugs. Many of these concepts also pertain to tissue distribution, and a discussion relevant to central nervous system distribution of drugs completes the section. It is paramount to remember that, in discussing developmental issues relevant to fetal disposition of drugs, drug targets also have complex developmental trajectories. Understanding fetal drug distribution may allow prediction of drug concentration at the site of drug action, but prediction of drug action, which is the true goal, requires interaction between the drug and its target.

DETERMINANTS OF FETAL PLASMA CONCENTRATION

Maternal plasma concentration is the main determining factor of fetal plasma concentration. Parallels can be drawn to dose in standard pharmacokinetics, with fetal plasma concentrations considered a function of maternal concentration. Figure 23–1 shows the concentrations of zidovudine measured in paired samples of maternal and fetal baboon plasma under steady-state conditions.[1] Doubling the maternal concentration essentially doubles the fetal concentration. The fetal concentration of zidovudine was always slightly less that that in the mother. This result suggests that other factors influence fetal plasma concentration. Understanding how placental permeability, fetal drug

elimination, drug ionization and protein binding, and volumes of distribution (in non–steady-state situations) affect fetal drug levels is a major goal of this chapter. Once maternal concentration is known, fetal distribution can be divided in three phases: transfer across the placenta, modification of fetal plasma concentration, and tissue distribution. To describe how differences in these various contributors affect fetal drug levels (be it plasma, extracellular, or intracellular), an integrated pharmacokinetic approach is used, with graphic representations throughout.

MATERNAL PLASMA CONCENTRATION

Maternal plasma concentration is the driving force for drug delivery to the fetus. Physiologic changes of pregnancy lead to altered drug absorption, distribution, and clearance in the mother and, hence, different plasma concentrations from those seen in the nonpregnant state.[2-5] Overall, plasma drug concentrations tend to be lower in pregnancy. One sees an increase in the volume of distribution from increased plasma volume and increased fat deposition as well as addition of the fetal compartment. Maternal renal clearance is enhanced because of increased cardiac output and renal blood flow. Hepatic clearance may also be enhanced by increased hepatic blood flow or hormonal stimulation of drug metabolizing enzymes.[6] In some cases, however, pregnancy-related hormones may inhibit drug metabolizing enzymes.[3] For fetal considerations, the numerous physiologic changes of pregnancy that alter maternal drug distribution can be bypassed by measuring maternal plasma concentration of the drug.

DRUG TRANSFER ACROSS THE PLACENTA

The *placenta* is the specialized interface between the mother and fetus across which drug distribution occurs. Most drugs are believed to cross the placenta by passive diffusion, and hence the surface area provided by the placenta and the nature of the interface, together with drug characteristics, determine placental permeability. More recent studies suggest that various transporters have a role in modifying placental transfer of several important drugs, and these transporters are discussed in the section on active transport.

Structural Development of the Placenta

The following is a synopsis of placental development highlighting the aspects relevant to drug transport (see Chap. 10). During implantation, the trophoblastic tissue invades and becomes surrounded by decidua. The placenta develops at the embryonic pole, whereas trophoblast in contact with the rest of the decidua eventually breaks down. Spaces develop within

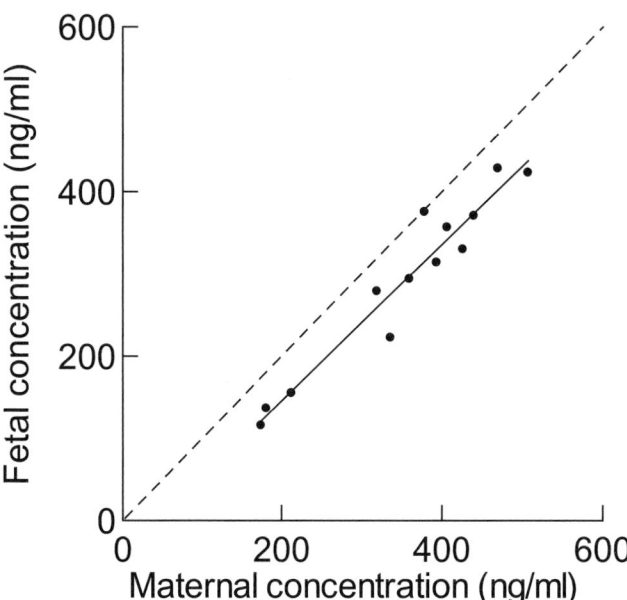

Figure 23–1. Paired fetal and maternal zidovudine concentrations in plasma samples obtained at steady state in the chronically catheterized baboon infused with 150 to 350 µg/minute of zidovudine. (Data from Garland M: Obstet Gynecol Clin North Am *25*:21, 1998.)

the expanding trophoblastic tissue to form the lacunae that lie between the villus structures. The uterine spiral arteries supplying, and the veins draining, the decidua are invaded by trophoblast such that these maternal vessels open directly into the lacunae, and maternal blood bathes the villus structures. Anchoring villi extend the full thickness of the trophoblast layer, whereas most villi resemble treelike structures (Fig. 23-2*A*). As pregnancy advances, placental surface area increases by increasing the number of villi and increasing the number of branches. As with most epithelial transport surfaces, the luminal plasma membrane of the villus trophoblast has microvilli (see Fig. 23-2*C*). Later in gestation, the diffusional capacity of the placenta increases mostly by thinning of the trophoblast layer where it overlies fetal vessels within the villi. The villus structure itself consists of a stromal core to support the fetal blood vessels and is surrounded by a single layer of syncytial trophoblast attached to a basement membrane (see Fig. 23-2*B*). Cytotrophoblasts and some Hofbauer cells (placental tissue macrophages) lie between the two. The syncytial trophoblast is a multinucleated cellular structure formed by the fusion of trophoblastic cells into a syncytium. Underlying cytotrophoblastic cells can add to the syncytiotrophoblast by fusion. Near term, few cytotrophoblasts are present within the villus. The fetal arterioles branch into a capillary bed also surrounded by a basement membrane. The capillaries are nonfenestrated and have variably spaced tight junctions between endothelial cells.[7-9] In the mature placenta, the contact zones between the syncytiotrophoblast and endothelial cells are free of nuclei and are thinner than in other regions (see Fig. 23-2*B*). The layers between maternal and fetal blood over which diffusion occurs are shown in Figure 23-2*C*. The luminal membrane of the syncytiotrophoblast (that in contact with maternal blood) contains clefts in addition to the microvillus surface, and the abluminal membrane also has some infoldings. In view of the continuous nature of the syncytiotrophoblast, there are no intercellular spaces through which transport can occur. In contrast, the endothelium does allow some paracellular transport of low molecular weight hydrophilic substances. Placental

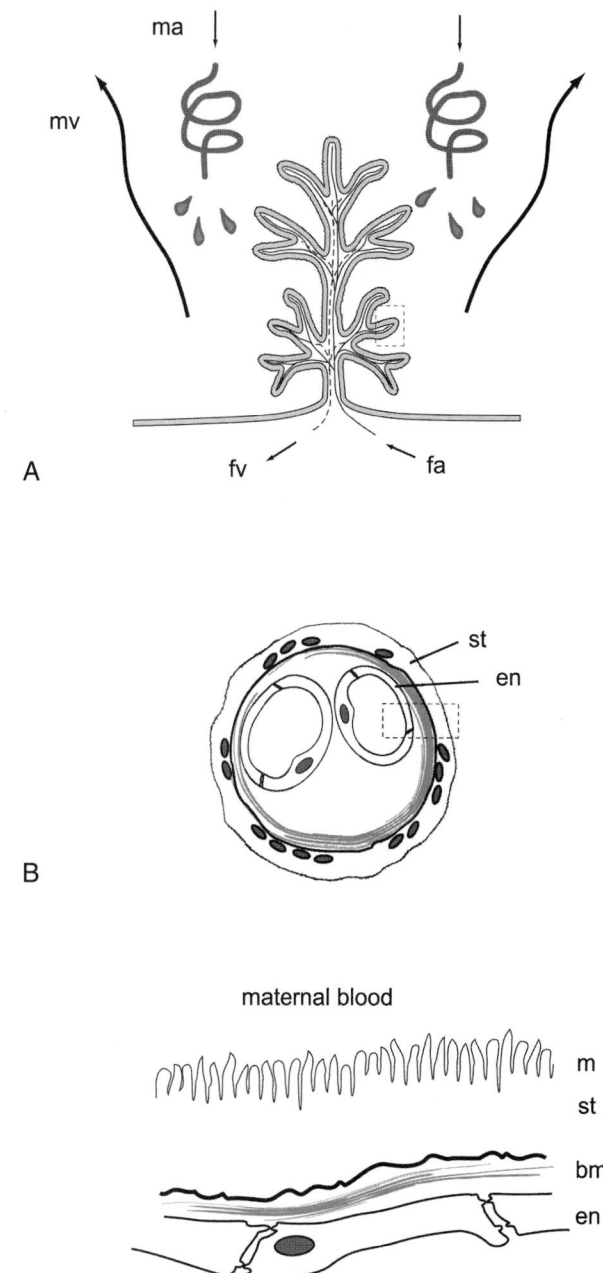

Figure 23–2. Schematic diagrams of mature human placental structure. **A,** The placental villus supports vessels from the fetus and is in direct contact with maternal blood. The *arrows* indicate the direction of blood flow. **B,** The syncytial trophoblast forms a continuous cellular layer over the fetal villi. The areas in close apposition to fetal capillaries are thinner and lack nuclei. **C,** The layers that drugs must cross to transfer from one circulation to the other. The area surrounded by the *dashed line* in **B** is enlarged in **C.** bm = basement membrane; en = endothelium; fa = fetal artery; fv = fetal vein; m = microvilli; ma = maternal artery; mv = maternal vein; st = syncytiotrophoblast.

capillaries are less permeable than most other capillaries present in tissues with continuous capillaries; however, they are still two orders of magnitude more permeable than those present in the brain.[9]

Models of Placental Transfer of Drug

From an anatomic perspective, many placental characteristics are important in the transfer of drug to the fetus. The most striking features are the large exchange surface and the thin syncytial-endothelial barrier between the circulations supporting passive transfer of substances (see Fig. 23–2). Visualizing human placental structure suggests a cross-current exchange interface; however, experimental data at best support a concurrent model (see Chap. 13).

The simplest and perhaps most illustrative way to view the maternofetal dyad with respect to drug distribution is as a two-compartment model (Fig. 23–3).[1, 10–12] This model differs from the standard peripheral compartment model in that the fetal compartment includes an elimination route independent of the placenta. Rate equations for the model describe how the amount of drug in each compartment changes with time and are determined by considering how much drug is entering and leaving each compartment. The amount of drug (D) that leaves in a given time period (mass/time) equals the clearance (Cl, volume/time) multiplied by the mean concentration (c, mass/volume) for that period, as follows (see Fig. 23–3, parameter descriptions):

Rate equation for maternal compartment:

$$\frac{dD_m}{dt} = R_m - Cl_m \cdot c_m - Cl_{mf} \cdot c_m + Cl_{fm} \cdot c_f \qquad [1]$$

Rate equation for fetal compartment:

$$\frac{dD_f}{dt} = Cl_{mf} \cdot c_m - Cl_{fm} \cdot c_f - Cl_f \cdot c_f \qquad [2]$$

Solutions of these rate equations are used to generate concentration-time plots for each compartment, varying fetal and placental clearance parameters to illustrate the effects of placental permeability and nonplacental fetal elimination on fetal drug distribution (Figs. 23–4 and 23–5). Panel A in Figure 23–4 shows the effect of decreasing placental permeability after a single oral bolus of drug and, in Panel A in Figure 23–5, when the drug is administered as a continuous infusion to the mother. In both cases, fetal nonplacental clearance is set at zero, and the only

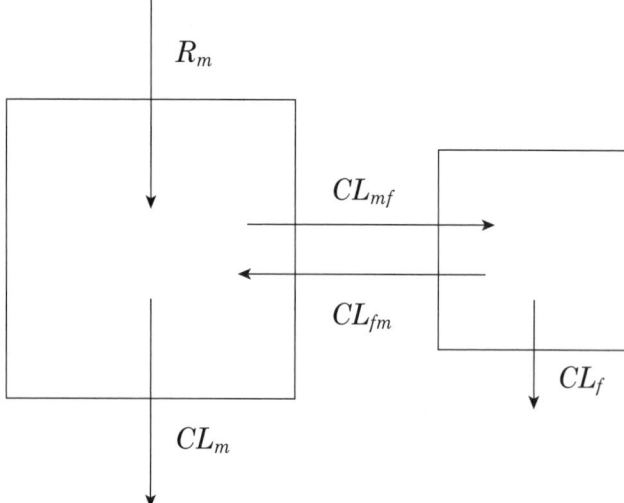

Figure 23–3. The two-compartment model representation of the maternofetal dyad. Drug movement into and out of each compartment is indicated by the *arrows*. Clearance parameters are used to characterize the elimination from or transfer between compartments. Cl = clearance; f = fetal; m = maternal; R = rate of infusion of drug to maternal compartment.

parameter that varies is placental clearance. (Panels B through D are discussed later.) Placental permeability affects peak fetal drug concentrations (when administered by bolus), but total fetal drug exposure, represented by the area under the curve, is the same in each case. Under steady-state conditions (obtained with continuous intravenous infusion), drugs with low placental permeability will achieve fetal levels that are as high as those seen with highly permeable drugs if the infusion continues for long enough.

A much debated question is this: Can active fetal drug concentrations exceed those in the mother with passive placental transfer? During the elimination phase after bolus administration, fetal concentrations are higher than maternal. However, peak fetal concentration will not exceed peak maternal concentration (see Fig. 23–4). Even for rapidly transferred substances, the peak will be blunted. In addition, mean steady-state concentrations will not exceed maternal concentrations, although again, during the elimination phase, fetal concentration exceeds maternal (see Fig. 23–5). Moreover, total drug exposure will not exceed maternal. In panel A in Figures 23–4 and 23–5, in which there is no direct fetal clearance, not only is the area under the curve (measure of total drug exposure) the same in each fetus, but also the area under the curve is the same in the mother as in the fetus. In the absence of direct fetal elimination, mean steady-state concentrations (or areas under the concentration time curves) in the fetus are equal to those in the mother. This is an important concept to grasp because single maternofetal drug determinations after bolus drug administration have caused confusion in the understanding of fetal drug distribution. In contrast, active drug concentrations (after pro-drug administration) and drug metabolite concentrations can be higher in the fetus than in the mother and are explored in more detail later.

Passive Transfer of Drug Across the Placenta

It is believed that most drugs cross the placenta by passive diffusion. *Passive diffusion* is the movement of substances in solution across a *semipermeable membrane*, in this case, the placenta. This process uses the kinetic energy of the molecules rather than any energy provided by cellular mechanisms. As molecules bounce around in solution, a certain percentage will cross to the other side of the membrane. The percentage that crosses is determined by the number of molecules in solution (concentration) and the ease with which molecules cross. Once a molecule has crossed the membrane, the random movements cause a certain percentage to cross back to the other side, again dependent on the concentration and ease of transfer. Because the membrane is essentially the same in both directions, more molecules will cross from the side with the highest concentration, and there will be net transfer to the side of lower concentration. Once equilibrium is reached, the concentrations on the two sides of the membrane will be the same, and there will be no net transfer. Because net transfer is proportional to the concentration gradient across the membrane, it is not a measure of the permeability of the placenta.

Permeability is the ease with which a molecule (or drug) crosses a membrane and is a function of the membrane itself and properties of the molecules. The *placental barrier,* as described earlier, consists of a closely apposed layer of syncytiotrophoblast and fetal endothelial cells. Cell membranes consist of *lipid bilayers* and allow the passage of small, lipid-soluble molecules relatively easily. Tight junctions between endothelial cells in the placenta minimize paracellular transport. Composition of lipid membranes may alter transport characteristics. Known influences on lipid composition include diet, hormones, and pregnancy.[13]

Permeability can be considered per unit of placental tissue or as the placental unit as a whole. Traditional membrane studies express permeability in terms of surface area and thickness of the membrane. In the placenta, the membrane is thin, and permeability is much more dependent on surface area. Because it is extremely difficult to estimate placental surface area, permeability is usually expressed per unit tissue mass or in terms of the whole placenta. For comparisons in different experimental situations, placental perfusion studies often present relative permeabilities comparing test drugs with known substances, usually antipyrine.

Figures 23-4 and 23-5 are examples of passive diffusion systems. The concentration of drug in maternal plasma and the initial lack of drug in fetal plasma provide the gradient across the placenta. In the case of bolus administration, net transfer of drug occurs from mother to fetus, with fetal concentration increasing until the maternal concentration, having begun to fall, equals the fetal concentration. At this point, net transfer is zero. From this point onward, maternal concentration is below fetal concentra-

tion, and net transfer is from the fetus to the mother. In the case of a constant infusion, fetal concentration increases because of net transfer from mother to fetus until steady state is achieved. In panel A, with no elimination from the fetus, an equilibrium is established in which the fetal and maternal concentrations are equal and there is no net transfer in either direction. Drug molecules are still randomly crossing back and forth across the placenta at the same rate as determined by the permeability and drug concentration but at the same rate in both directions. When the drug infusion is stopped, the maternal concentration will fall, setting up a gradient from fetus to mother. Understanding this fundamental process provides the foundation for all distributive properties of drugs.

Rates of transfer from mother to fetus can be determined in experimental models. Measuring the change in concentration over either the uterine circulation or the umbilical circulation at

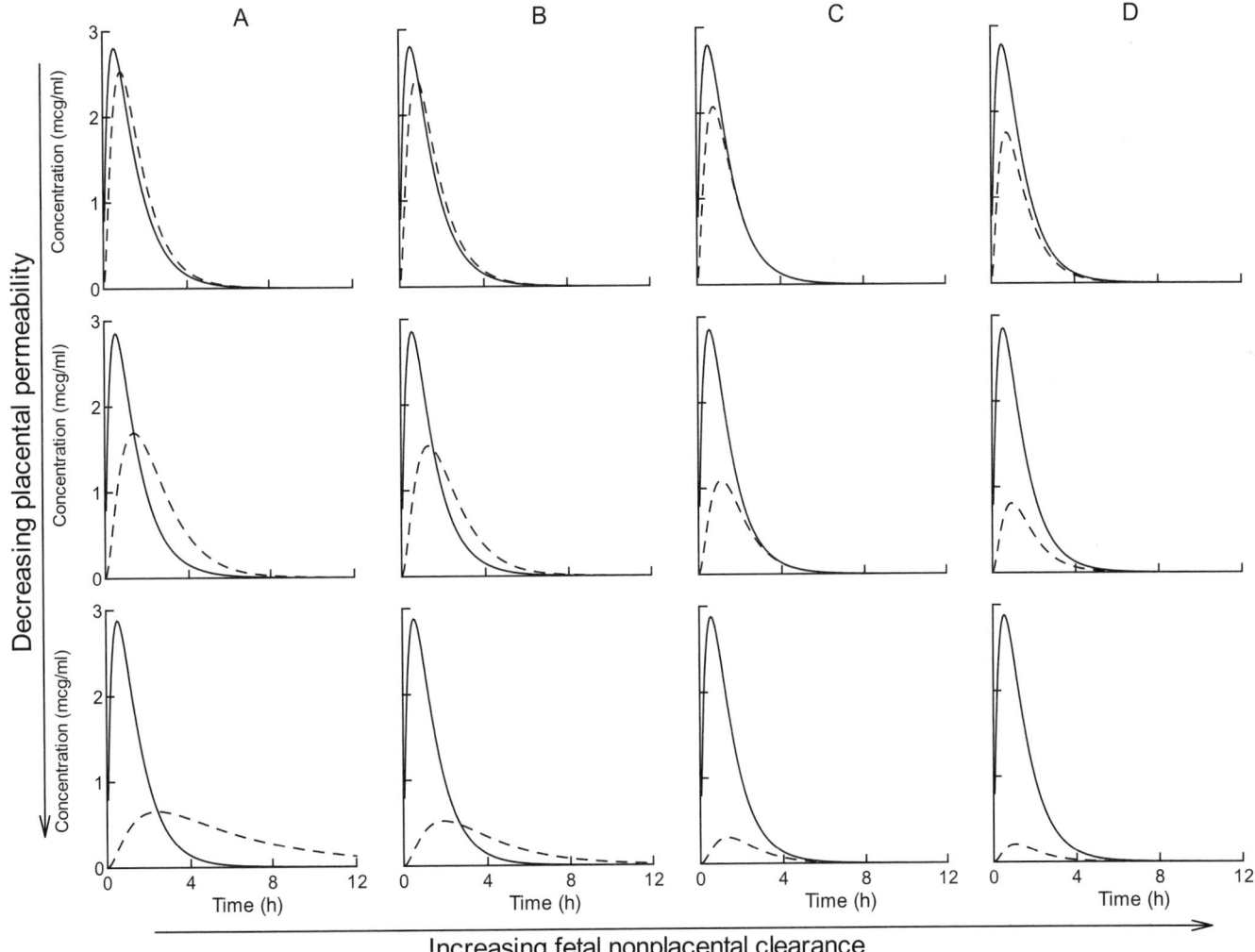

Figure 23–4. Drug concentration time plots for the mother (*solid line*) and fetus (*dashed line*) after an oral bolus of drug. These plots represent the solutions for the rate equations of a two-compartment model after an oral bolus of drug in which placental clearance (a measure of placental permeability) and fetal nonplacental clearance (direct fetal elimination) were varied while all other system parameters remained constant. The general parameters used to make these plots are those obtained experimentally in the pregnant baboon after zidovudine administration.[19,52] The *top row* represents high placental permeability in that placental clearance is 20% of maternal clearance. In the *middle row*, placental clearance is 5% of maternal clearance (that observed experimentally). The *bottom row* represents limited placental permeability in which only 1% of drug administered to the mother will cross the placenta to the fetus. Going across the figure represents increasing levels of direct fetal elimination: in **A**, there is no direct fetal clearance; in **B**, fetal clearance is 1% of maternal clearance (that observed experimentally); in **C**, fetal clearance is 5% of maternal clearance and would approximate when fetal metabolic activity expressed per tissue mass is similar to that in the adult; in **D**, fetal clearance is 10% of maternal clearance and would occur only when fetal enzyme activity is higher than that in the adult.

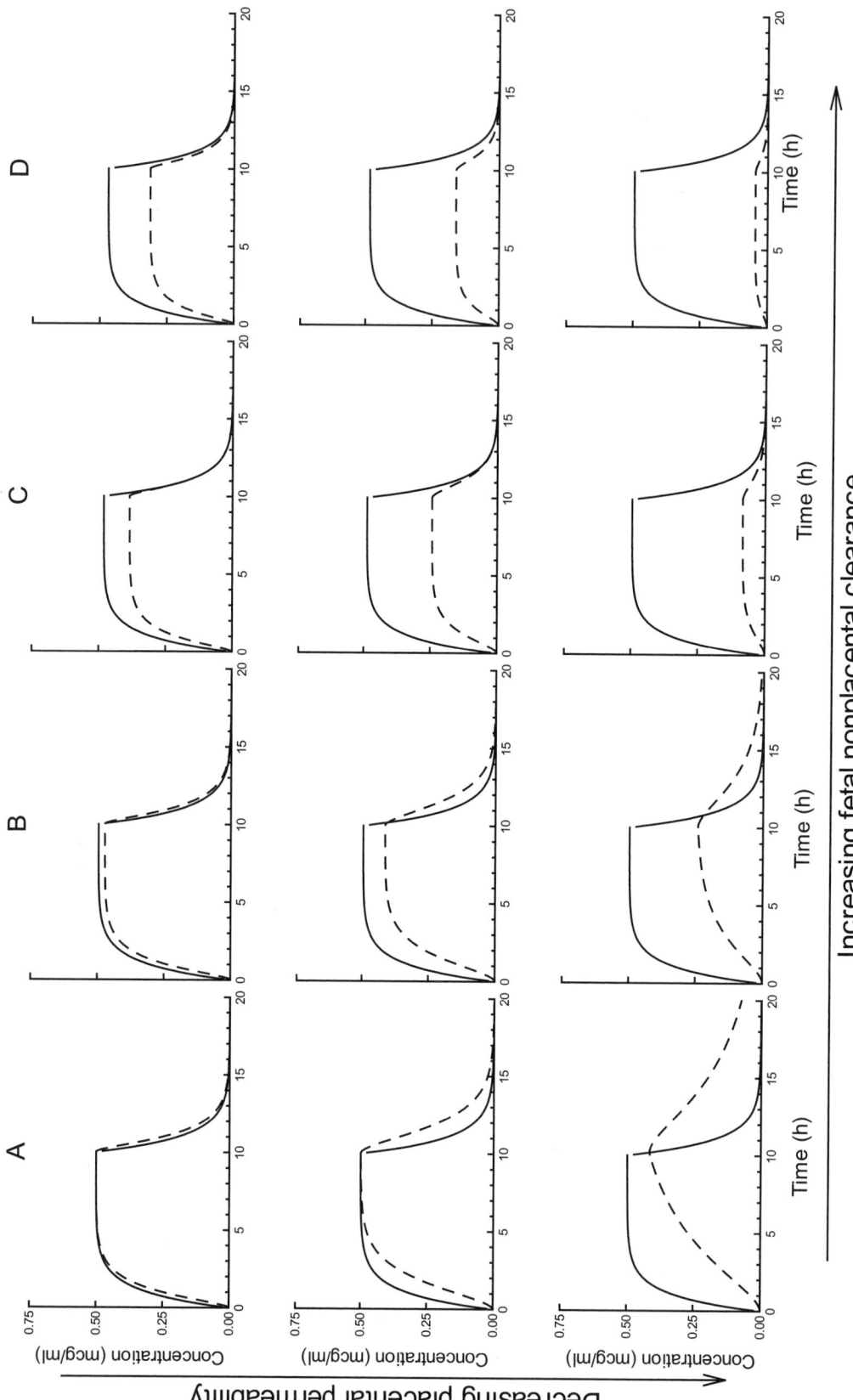

Figure 23–5. Drug concentration time plots for the mother (*solid line*) and fetus (*dashed line*) during and after a constant infusion of drug. These plots represent the solutions for the rate equations of a two-compartment model during and after infusion of drug in which placental clearance (a measure of placental permeability) and fetal nonplacental clearance (direct fetal elimination) were varied while all other system parameters remained constant. Steady-state concentrations provide a good estimate of fetal exposure compared with maternal concentrations. See Figure 23–4 for details on the specific parameter values.

specific flow rates will determine the amount of drug removed from maternal plasma or the amount of drug taken up by fetal plasma. These measurements can be achieved by *in situ* perfusion of whole placentas of small animals by controlling placental and umbilical blood flows or in chronically instrumented sheep models using flow probes on uterine and umbilical circulations.[14] In addition, the human placenta can be perfused *ex vivo*.[15-17] When expressed relative to the transplacental gradient, this provides a measure of placental permeability. This measure has the same units as placental clearance (volume/time). This method can also determine the amount of drug eliminated by the placenta. Another method uses mean steady-state concentrations in the mother and fetus applied to a two-compartment pharmacokinetic model (see Fig. 23-3).[12] This method calculates the placental clearances in both directions across the placenta and is used in sheep and primate models.[18-21] These placental clearances are measures of whole placenta permeability, and if maternal to fetal or fetal to maternal placental clearance exceeds the other, they indicate enhanced transport in one direction. The advantage of this model is that blood flow measurements are not required. It does require drug administration to steady state to both the mother and fetus, with drug determinations from both circulations. Neither of these methods can be used clinically, so extrapolations from animal and *ex vivo* placental perfusion studies are required to predict drug concentrations in the human fetus unless blood samples are obtained during percutaneous umbilical blood sampling. The two-compartment model under steady-state conditions better reflects long-term drug therapy. In addition, parameters derived under steady-state conditions can be used to model single-dose situations. Most of the equations and graphs in this chapter are generated from this model and provide a framework for understanding the effects of physiologic parameters on fetal distribution.

Molecular size and *solubility* are the drug characteristics that determine drug permeability. Lipid-soluble drugs are readily transferred across the placenta up to molecular weights of 600 daltons. Water-soluble drugs up to a molecular weight of 100 daltons also readily cross, whereas larger hydrophilic molecules cross according to their coefficient of diffusion in water.[15] Placental perfusion studies comparing substances of varying sizes and solubilities demonstrate relative permeability rankings that are a combination of the two factors.

Active Drug

When drugs are present in plasma, they may be bound to plasma proteins or, if they are weak acids or bases, may exist in an ionized state. Only drug that is *unbound* and *nonionized* is available for transfer across the placenta and is often referred to as *active* drug. The percentage of drug bound to protein is determined by the number and affinity of binding sites, whereas the percentage of drug ionized is determined by the negative log of the dissociation constant (pKa) of the drug and the pH of the plasma. In both cases, drug will either bind or dissociate, or it will shift between ionized and nonionized forms when the concentration of the active drug changes, as happens when there is an active drug concentration gradient across the placenta. On the maternal side, active drug concentration decreases as it is transferred across the placenta to the fetus, so drug bound to proteins will dissociate, and ionized drug will shift from an ionized to a nonionized form, and newly formed active drug will be available for further transfer. On the fetal side, active drug increases in concentration and will bind to proteins and ionize to achieve the appropriate proportions determined by the conditions. If protein binding attributes and pH were the same in the mother and fetus, total drug concentrations in the mother and the fetus would be the same at equilibrium. Because differences exist in protein binding and fetal pH is slightly less than maternal, both these attributes need to be taken into account.

The two major proteins involved in binding drugs are albumin and α_1-acid glycoprotein, the latter particularly involved in binding basic drugs.[5, 22, 23] During pregnancy, maternal albumin concentration falls, although total albumin is increased.[22, 24, 25] In the fetus, albumin levels increase with gestation and, toward term, exceed those in the mother.[22] α_1-Acid glycoprotein levels tend to be rather variable in both the mother and fetus, but fetal levels are almost always less than maternal levels.[22] *Protein binding* is expressed as the percent protein bound. Equation 3 and Figure 23-6 describe the relationship between protein binding in the mother (M) and fetus (F) and the effect on total drug concentration at steady state (c_{ss}).

$$c_{ssFtotal} = \frac{c_{ssMunbound}/c_{ssMtotal}}{c_{ssFunbound}/c_{ssFtotal}} c_{ssMtotal} \qquad [3]$$

At less than 40 to 60% binding, differences tend to be insignificant, but for drugs with high binding, this can have a major impact. Although bound drug may seem to be of little relevance because it is not active, it serves as a depot of drug that may prolong fetal or newborn exposure, particularly when affinity is high or when drug clearance from the newborn is poor.

The pKa of a drug determines the degree of *ionization* at a specific pH. Usually, there is only 0.1 pH unit difference between mother and fetus and thus minimal difference in ionization. The effect of maternal and fetal pH differences on fetal/maternal concentration ratios of drugs that are weak acids and bases can be calculated from the Henderson-Hasselbalch equation.

The Henderson-Hasselbalch equation is as follows:

$$pH = pK_a + \log\frac{[base]}{[acid]} \qquad [4]$$

For weak acids:

$$c_{ssFtotal} = \frac{1 + 10^{(pH_F - pK_a)}}{1 + 10^{(pH_M - pK_a)}} c_{ssMtotal} \qquad [5]$$

For weak bases:

$$c_{ssFtotal} = \frac{1 + 10^{(pK_a - pH_F)}}{1 + 10^{(pK_a - pH_M)}} c_{ssMtotal} \qquad [6]$$

Weak acids are less ionized and weak bases are more ionized at lower pH. As fetal pH decreases to less than maternal pH, the amount of total drug in the fetus will change (Fig. 23-7); weak acids will be decreased in amount, whereas weak bases will be increased. As long as the pH differential is maintained, the drug effect will not be altered. In the fetus, transition back to a normal pH is likely to be gradual, and placental redistribution will occur without the fetus being exposed to excessive (for basic drugs) or subtherapeutic (for acidic drugs) concentrations of active drug. If at the time of delivery the fetal pH is low, total concentration of basic drugs may be higher than in the mother, and as pH corrects in the newborn and drug quickly returns to an active nonionized state, adverse drug effects may occur. For acidic drugs after delivery, newborn drug concentration may be less that that required for therapeutic benefit after resolution of a fetal acidosis.

Placental Blood Flow

The two sides of the placenta are perfused independently. Maternal placental blood flow is about twice that going through the umbilical circulation (see Chap. 13). Experimental situations show that decreasing blood flow, particularly in the umbilical circulation, will decrease delivery of freely diffusible drugs across the placenta (flow limited) but will have little effect on

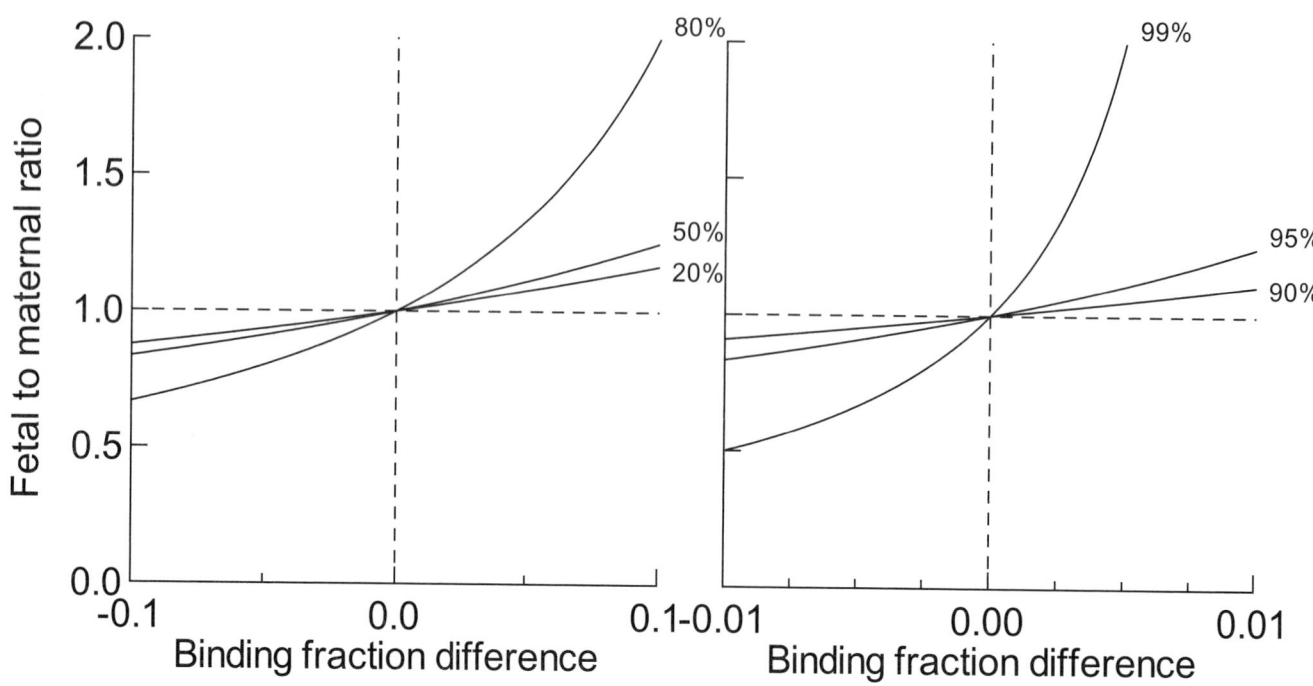

Figure 23–6. Effect of fetal and maternal differences in protein binding on steady-state fetal/maternal total drug concentration ratios. Unbound drug concentrations will be the same in the fetus as in the mother. Drugs that exhibit low protein binding (up to around 50%) exhibit only small differences in the fetal/maternal concentration ratio even with binding differences up to 10%. As binding increases, more marked effects are seen. For drugs that are highly protein bound, even small differences (less than 1%) can have marked effects on the fetal/maternal total drug ratio. These graphs are plotted from Equation 3 for varying levels of maternal protein binding, with fetal protein binding ±10% of maternal for the *left-hand* graph and ±1% of maternal for the *right-hand* graph.

drugs that are permeability limited. Placental circulations are fairly stable at most times in pregnancy but will show gradual increases over gestation. Compromised fetuses and uterine contractions are two situations in which decreased fetal drug transfer has been demonstrated clinically. Changes in blood flow are unlikely to affect steady-state levels achieved unless the increased blood flow enhances nonplacental clearances mechanisms from the mother or fetus.

Active Transport of Drug Across the Placenta

Cell membranes, including those of the syncytiotrophoblast and villous capillary endothelium, contain large numbers of transport proteins that require cellular energy to function. The specificity, orientation (into or out of the cell), and position (whether luminal or basal membrane) are important factors in determining the effect of placental transporters on drug disposition. Few drugs appear to be entirely dependent on active transport for transfer across the placenta to the fetus. Most drugs cross to the fetus by passive diffusion. However, the placental transport proteins may be able to modify the final concentrations achieved. Most work to date has been with P-glycoprotein, one of the multidrug resistance proteins, although organic anion transporters, organic cation transporter, and other multidrug resistance proteins are present in the placenta.[26,27] P-glycoprotein is present in the microvillous membrane of syncytiotrophoblast and transports various drugs (e.g., morphine, digoxin, saquinavir) from the intracellular space to the villous space.[27-29] Drug that passively enters the cell from either the maternal or fetal circulation is

actively transported out to the maternal circulation. This process will enhance placental clearance from the fetus and reduce clearance from mother to fetus. In this situation, fetal steady-state levels will be less than those in the mother. Inhibition of these transporters would decrease fetal placental drug clearance, and fetal steady-state levels would increase toward maternal. For transporters that deliver drugs to the fetus, steady-state levels in the fetus would exceed those in the mother unless direct fetal elimination mechanisms exceeded the active transport activity.

Other Transport Mechanisms

Facilitated diffusion processes are known to occur in the placenta for nutrients and waste products but have not been implicated in drug transfer. Specific macromolecules are taken up across the placenta by *pinocytosis*. An example of this is immunoglobulin G, which can be administered therapeutically.[30] Aquaporins are present in the placenta and may provide bulk flow channels for small hydrophilic drug molecules.[31]

Placental Metabolism

The placenta is a highly metabolic organ, producing and modifying many different hormones. Several members of the cytochrome P450 subclasses are present and can metabolize drugs at the maternofetal interface.[32] Few of the conjugation enzymes are present in the placenta. The placenta acts as a first-pass clearance system and decreases drug concentrations reaching the fetus. However, the fetus may well be exposed to

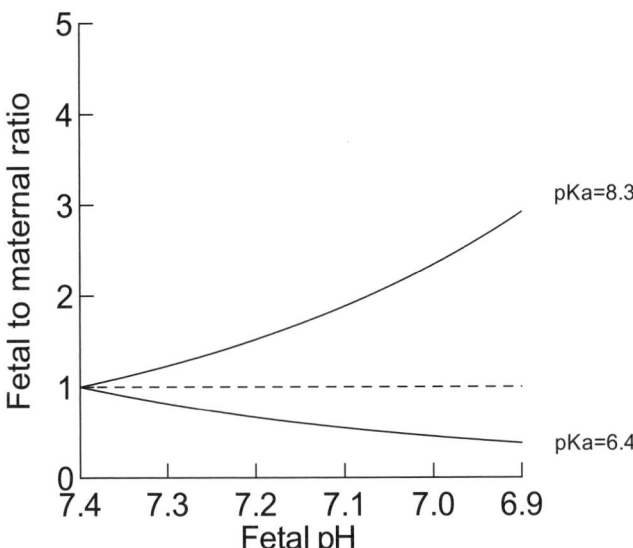

Figure 23-7. The effect of fetal maternal pH differences on steady-state fetal/maternal total drug concentration ratios. Nonionized active drug concentrations will be the same in the fetus as in the mother. Total concentrations of weak acids will be less in the fetus, whereas total concentrations of weak bases will be higher in the fetus. This graph is plotted from Equations 5 and 6, setting maternal pH at 7.4.

metabolites of drugs that are not always harmless.[33] In the two-compartment system, placental metabolism is mostly reflected in fetal nonplacental clearance.

MODIFIERS OF FETAL PLASMA CONCENTRATION

Fetal Circulation

Streaming of oxygenated blood from the umbilical vein, through the ductus venosus and foramen ovale, through the heart leads to more oxygenated blood to the head and upper extremities, so the concept of having different distribution in separate regions is not new (see Chaps. 61 and 63). The high extraction of oxygen from fetal blood maintains this differential across the placenta, and thus the difference in carotid arterial and descending aortic oxygen tensions is able to persist. A similar phenomenon is likely to occur with drugs that cross the placenta, although it has never been clearly documented. This difference will be most pronounced when the umbilical arteriovenous difference is greatest and thus is most likely to occur with bolus administration or for drugs highly metabolized by the fetus.

Another situation in which the fetal circulation affects drug distribution is in the liver.[34] The fetal liver is the first organ that sees fetal blood returning from the placenta. In the healthy fetus, 50 to 70% of blood flow is diverted through the ductus venosus. Pathophysiologic features can lead to redistribution of hepatic blood flow with enhanced hepatic metabolism of drug. Again, the same constraints pertaining to umbilical arteriovenous differences hold.

Fetal Drug Clearance

So far, the discussion has been limited to systems in which the fetal nonplacental clearance is zero. The example of zidovudine levels in the pregnant baboon introduced the idea that fetal steady-state levels can be less than those in the mother. This difference could not be attributed to differences in protein binding or pH or to active transport.[19] In addition, there is clear

evidence that the fetus can metabolize zidovudine to its glucuronide metabolite.[19] Figure 23-3 and Equation 2 include an elimination component directly from the fetus. The effect of direct fetal clearance on fetal drug concentrations is shown in panels B through D in Figures 23-4 and 23-5. Direct fetal clearance lowers fetal drug concentrations, and this is most marked when placental permeability is reduced. This situation differs from the effects of protein binding and ionization in that fetal clearance affects active drug concentrations and hence reduces active drug concentrations in the fetus.

Two-Compartment Model at Steady State

In many of the examples given, the effect of changes in physiologic parameters is best appreciated by comparing steady-state concentrations in the mother and fetus. A relationship between fetal and maternal plasma concentrations can be deduced from the rate equations of the two-compartment model under steady-state conditions. *Steady state* is defined as when the amount of drug in a compartment does not change with time.

Rate equation for the maternal compartment at steady state:

$$\frac{dD_m}{dt} = R_m - Cl_m \cdot c_m - Cl_{mf} \cdot c_m + Cl_{fm} \cdot c_f = 0 \qquad [7]$$

Rate equation for the fetal compartment at steady state:

$$\frac{dD_f}{dt} = Cl_{mf} \cdot c_m - Cl_{fm} \cdot c_f - Cl_f \cdot c_f = 0 \qquad [8]$$

By rearranging the fetal equation, an expression is obtained that relates fetal steady-state plasma concentrations to the maternal concentration:

$$\frac{c_{ssF}}{c_{ssM}} = \frac{Cl_{mf}}{Cl_{fm} + Cl_f} \qquad [9]$$

This expression shows the interdependence of fetal clearance mechanisms and placental permeability in determining fetal drug exposure. For drugs that cross the placenta by passive diffusion, CL_{mf} will be equal to CL_{fm} (clearance being an attribute of the placenta and a measure of placental permeability). When fetal nonplacental clearance and placental clearance are equal, fetal concentration is 50% of maternal concentration (see Fig. 23-5, panel C, *middle row*, and panel B, *bottom row*). Furthermore, the same amount of fetal nonplacental clearance will have a more marked decrease on fetal plasma concentration when placental clearance (or permeability) is low (see Figs. 23-4 and 23-5).

Fetal Elimination Mechanisms

Drug metabolizing enzymes are both present and active in the fetal liver, albeit at reduced levels compared with the adult for most enzymes.[19, 32, 35-38] In addition, as discussed earlier, placental drug metabolizing enzymes also contribute to nonplacental fetal clearance. As seen in the earlier model, even small amounts of fetal clearance can have marked effects on the fetal/maternal drug ratio, depending on placental permeability. It may be expected that drug metabolizing capacity will increase as gestation advances; however, placental permeability also increases with gestation. No experimental data are yet available addressing this issue. Another potential issue is induction of drug metabolizing enzymes. Maternal smoking is known to induce many placental enzymes, but little is known about induction of hepatic enzymes prenatally.[33] Phenobarbital has been used successfully near term to reduce hyperbilirubinemia by induction of glucuronyltransferase UGT1A1.

Also to be considered are the *products of metabolism.* These are often inactive; however, some metabolites are known mutagens, some are pharmacologically active, and others are true drugs in that a *pro-drug* was administered.[39] Rate equations for metabolite formation can be written for the two-compartment model. The solution for these equations is clearly more complex, even at steady state, than those noted earlier, but fetal metabolite concentration can be expressed as a function of maternal concentration.[40] In this case, because metabolite is being formed in the fetus and because placental clearance for metabolites is often less than for the drug, there is a tendency for fetal metabolite concentrations to exceed those in the mother unless other clearance pathways exist.

In adults, the other major route of drug elimination is urinary excretion. The *fetal urinary excretion* system is unique in that fetal urine, a major component of amniotic fluid, is swallowed by the fetus and provides the potential for any drug excreted in fetal urine to be absorbed back into the fetus through the fetal intestinal tract. The extent to which this occurs is not known. Clearly, not all drugs are reabsorbed in their entirety because many can be detected in meconium. Under steady-state conditions, drug excreted into urine that is reabsorbed would not contribute to fetal nonplacental clearance; however, drug that becomes sequestered in meconium would contribute. The influence of fetal nonplacental clearance mechanisms on fetal plasma concentration and hence on subsequent tissue distribution is beginning to be explored quantitatively in animal models.

TISSUE DISTRIBUTION

Volume of distribution is a term used to describe the volume a drug appears to occupy based on the plasma concentration, and it has little bearing on the physical system. Volumes of distribution vary from drug to drug, based on the solubility of the drug in different tissues, reflective of the lipid and water content of the tissues. Individuals also differ in body composition. The fetus has a very high water content, so lipid-soluble drugs would not have a large volume of distribution. Water-soluble drugs would be expected to be higher (per tissue mass) than in adults, particularly if the amniotic fluid compartment cannot be separated. Fat deposition occurs during the last trimester, so during this period there would be a greater capacity for transfer of lipid-soluble drugs. Drug would concentrate into fat tissues until steady state is achieved. Because fetal volume of distribution is small compared with that of the mother, the effect of fetal changes is unlikely to be detectable in plasma concentrations. However, the total amount of drug delivered to the fetus could be substantially higher.

Fetal Blood-Brain Barriers

The brain has evolved a complex set of protections to shield it from external influences and yet still provide passage for the essential nutrients and communication signals. The capillaries that supply the brain are continuous (nonfenestrated), have extremely tight junctions preventing paracellular transport, and are surrounded by astrocytic foot processes. Several transporters that are present in the endothelium transport drugs from the endothelium back to the circulation.[41-43] Pial membranes carry blood vessels across the brain surface. Where the pial membrane comes in contact with the ependyma of the ventricular system, choroidal tissue develops. The capillaries within the choroidal tissue are fenestrated; however, the overlying ependyma is highly specialized with tight junctions, so transfer is essentially all transcellular. Several drug metabolizing enzymes have been identified in choroidal ependymal tissue and are thought to protect the brain from substrates.[44-48] In addition, many transporters are present on both luminal and abluminal sides.[41-43] With respect to drugs, P-glycoprotein is on the abluminal side, removing drugs or

their metabolites from the ependymal cell back to the capillary. Other transporters are present on the luminal and abluminal membranes to transport substances into and out of the ependymal cells. The remainder of the ependyma that is in contact with the ventricular system forms a loose network of cells with minimal barrier function. Thus, once in the cerebrospinal fluid, drugs would have access to target neurons that lie near brain surfaces. Within the brain itself, certain cells have been identified as containing drug metabolizing enzymes, although whether their function is protective or activational is not clear.[47, 49] Transporters are also present on neuronal cells. Although not all the details are known at this time, the distribution of drug metabolizing enzymes and of specific transporters gives some hint of their complexity.[50, 51] Because many drug receptors are present in the brain and because much ongoing research is directed toward neuroprotection, understanding brain distribution of potential agents requires prediction of the concentration at the site of action to optimize effectiveness. Again, plasma concentration is the driving force for drug movement by passive diffusion of drugs down a concentration gradient modulated by metabolism and active transport.

CLINICAL APPLICATIONS

Most drugs taken during pregnancy are for the mother's benefit. However, the use of drugs for fetal benefit is increasing. Various clinical situations are likely to be encountered, with potential ramifications for the patient and the unintentional recipient. Optimally, a drug that achieves therapeutic concentrations in the mother while minimizing fetal concentration will be selected for maternal treatment, whereas a drug that achieves therapeutic concentrations in the fetus while minimizing maternal adverse effects is selected for fetal treatment. Appreciating fetal drug distribution and drug properties will allow selection of appropriate drugs to attain these goals. Drugs are developed for use in nonpregnant adults, and desired characteristics include good oral bioavailability, good tissue distribution, and long half-life, properties that generally lend themselves to placental transfer and hence fetal exposure. Furthermore, what may generally be seen as improvements in drug formulation may alter distributive characteristics unfavorably for the fetus.

REFERENCES

1. Garland M: Pharmacology of drug transfer across the placenta. Obstet Gynecol Clin North Am 25:21, 1998.
2. Cummings AJ: A survey of pharmacokinetic data from pregnant women. Clin Pharmacokinet 8:344, 1983.
3. Luquita MG, et al: Molecular basis of perinatal changes in UDP-glucuronosyl-transferase activity in maternal rat liver. J Pharmacol Exp Ther 298:49, 2001.
4. Mottino AD, et al: Expression of multidrug resistance-associated protein 2 in small intestine from pregnant and postpartum rats. Am J Physiol Gastrointest Liver Physiol 280:G1261, 2001.
5. Pacifici GM, Nottoli R: Placental transfer of drugs administered to the mother. Clin Pharmacokinet 28:235, 1995.
6. Krauer B, et al: Drug disposition and pharmacokinetics in the maternal-placental-fetal unit. Pharmacol Ther 10:301, 1980.
7. Leach L, et al: Molecular organization of tight and adherens junctions in the human placental vascular tree. Placenta 21:547, 2000.
8. Leach L, Firth JA: Fine structure of the paracellular junctions of terminal villous capillaries in the perfused human placenta. Cell Tissue Res 268:447, 1992.
9. Leach L, Firth JA: Advances in understanding permeability in fetal capillaries of the human placenta: a review of organization of the endothelial paracellular clefts and their junctional complexes. Reprod Fertil Dev 7:1451, 1995.
10. Anderson DF, et al: Prediction of fetal drug concentrations. Am J Obstet Gynecol 137:735, 1980.
11. Krauer B, Krauer F: Drug kinetics in pregnancy. Clin Pharmacokinet 2:167, 1977.
12. Szeto HH, et al: The contribution of transplacental clearances and fetal clearance to drug disposition in the ovine maternal-fetal unit. Drug Metab Disp 10:382, 1982.
13. Sen A, et al: Changes in lipid composition and fluidity of human placental basal membrane and modulation of bilayer protein functions with progress of gestation. Mol Cell Biochem 187:183, 1998.

14. Kumar S, et al: Diphenhydramine disposition in the sheep maternal-placental-fetal unit: gestational age, plasma drug protein binding, and umbilical blood flow effects on clearance. Drug Metab Dispos 28:279, 2000.
15. Schneider H, et al: Permeability of the human placenta for hydrophilic substances studied in the isolated dually in vitro perfused lobe. Contrib Obstet Gynecol 13:98, 1985.
16. Liebes L, et al: Transfer of zidovudine (AZT) by human placenta. J Infect Dis 161:203, 1990.
17. Bawdon RE, et al: The ex vivo transfer of the anti-HIV nucleoside compound d4T in the human placenta. Gynecol Obstet Invest 38:1, 1994.
18. Szeto HH, et al: A comparison of morphine and methadone disposition in the maternal-fetal unit. Am J Obstet Gynecol 143:700, 1982.
19. Garland M, et al: Placental transfer and fetal metabolism of zidovudine in the baboon. Pediatr Res 44:47, 1998.
20. Odinecs A, et al: In vivo maternal-fetal pharmacokinetics of stavudine (2′,3′-didehydro-3′-deoxythymidine) in pigtailed macaques (Macaca nemestrina). Antimicrob Agents Chemother 40:196, 1996.
21. Riggs KW, et al: Fetal and maternal placental and nonplacental clearances of metoclopramide in chronically instrumented pregnant sheep. J Pharm Sci 79:1056, 1990.
22. Krauer B, et al: Changes in serum albumin and alpha 1-acid glycoprotein concentrations during pregnancy: an analysis of fetal-maternal pairs. Br J Obstet Gynaecol 91:875, 1984.
23. Perucca E, Crema A: Plasma protein binding of drugs in pregnancy. Clin Pharmacokinet 7:336, 1982.
24. Whittaker PG, Lind T: The intravascular mass of albumin during human pregnancy: a serial study in normal and diabetic women. Br J Obstet Gynaecol 100:587, 1993.
25. Olufemi OS, et al: Albumin metabolism in fasted subjects during late pregnancy. Clin Sci (Lond) 81:161, 1991.
26. St-Pierre MV, et al: Characterization of an organic anion-transporting polypeptide (OATP-B) in human placenta. J Clin Endocrinol Metab 87:1856, 2002.
27. Ganapathy V, et al: Placental transporters relevant to drug distribution across the maternal-fetal interface. J Pharmacol Exp Ther 294:413, 2000.
28. Huisman MT, et al: P-glycoprotein limits oral availability, brain, and fetal penetration of saquinavir even with high doses of ritonavir. Mol Pharmacol 59:806, 2001.
29. Smit JW, et al: Absence or pharmacological blocking of placental P-glycoprotein profoundly increases fetal drug exposure. J Clin Invest 104:1441, 1999.
30. Ellinger I, et al: IgG transport across trophoblast-derived BeWo cells: a model system to study IgG transport in the placenta. Eur J Immunol 29:733, 1999.
31. Damiano A, et al: Water channel proteins AQP3 and AQP9 are present in syncytiotrophoblast of human term placenta. Placenta 22:776, 2001.
32. Hakkola J, et al: Cytochrome P450 3A expression in the human fetal liver: evidence that CYP3A5 is expressed in only a limited number of fetal livers. Biol Neonate 80:193, 2001.
33. Hakkola J, et al: Xenobiotic-metabolizing cytochrome P450 enzymes in the human feto-placental unit: role in intrauterine toxicity. Crit Rev Toxicol 28:35, 1998.
34. Rudolph AM: Hepatic and ductus venosus blood flows during fetal life. Hepatology 3:254, 1983.
35. Pacifici GM, et al: Morphine glucuronidation in human fetal and adult liver. Eur J Clin Pharmacol 22:553, 1982.
36. Ring JA, et al: Fetal hepatic drug elimination. Pharmacol Ther 84:429, 1999.
37. Tonn GR, et al: Hepatic first-pass uptake of diphenhydramine. A comparative study between fetal and adult sheep. Drug Metab Dispos 24:273, 1996.
38. Wang LH, et al: Developmental alterations in hepatic UDP-glucuronosyltransferase: a comparison of the kinetic properties of enzymes from adult sheep and fetal lambs. Biochem Pharmacol 35:3065, 1986.
39. Ritter JK: Roles of glucuronidation and UDP-glucuronosyltransferases in xenobiotic bioactivation reactions. Chem Biol Interact 129:171, 2000.
40. Garland M, et al: Maternal-fetal pharmacokinetics: the two-compartment model revisited. Pediatr Res 39:73A, 1996.
41. Huai-Yun H, et al: Expression of multidrug resistance-associated protein (MRP) in brain microvessel endothelial cells. Biochem Biophys Res Commun 243:816, 1998.
42. Gao B, et al: Localization of the organic anion transporting polypeptide 2 (Oatp2) in capillary endothelium and choroid plexus epithelium of rat brain. J Histochem Cytochem 47:1255, 1999.
43. Zhang Y, et al: Expression of various multidrug resistance-associated protein (MRP) homologues in brain microvessel endothelial cells. Brain Res 876:148, 2000.
44. Ghersi-Egea JF, et al: The activity of 1-naphthol-UDP-glucuronosyltransferase in the brain. Neuropharmacology 26:367, 1987.
45. Ghersi-Egea JF, et al: Subcellular localization of cytochrome P450, and activities of several enzymes responsible for drug metabolism in the human brain. Biochem Pharmacol 45:647, 1993.
46. Ghersi-Egea JF, et al: Localization of drug-metabolizing enzyme activities to blood-brain interfaces and circumventricular organs. J Neurochem 62:1089, 1994.
47. Martinasevic MK, et al: Immunohistochemical localization of UDP-glucuronosyltransferases in rat brain during early development. Drug Metab Dispos 26:1039, 1998.
48. Suleman FG, et al: Uridine diphosphate-glucuronosyltransferase activities in rat brain microsomes. Neurosci Lett 161:219, 1993.
49. King CD, et al: Expression of UDP-glucuronosyltransferases (UGTs) 2B7 and 1A6 in the human brain and identification of 5-hydroxytryptamine as a substrate. Arch Biochem Biophys 365:156, 1999.
50. Strazielle N, Ghersi-Egea JF: Demonstration of a coupled metabolism-efflux process at the choroid plexus as a mechanism of brain protection toward xenobiotics. J Neurosci 19:6275, 1999.
51. Ghersi-Egea JF, Strazielle N: Brain drug delivery, drug metabolism, and multidrug resistance at the choroid plexus. Microsc Res Tech 52:83, 2001.
52. Garland M, et al: Implications of the kinetics of zidovudine in the pregnant baboon following oral administration. J Acquir Immune Defic Syndr Hum Retrovirol 19:433, 1998.

James F. Padbury and Robert A. Berg

24 Developmental Pharmacology of Adrenergic Agents

For hemodynamic responses to adrenergic agents, classic pharmacodynamic theory describes differences among agents in receptor specificity, potency, and pharmacologic profile based on parameters such as the median effective dose (ED_{50}) or half-maximal concentration. These pharmacodynamic parameters, however, are derived exclusively from *in vitro* studies. This chapter describes clinical studies in neonates, infants, and children based on a method of analysis that permits derivation of the *threshold*, or minimum plasma drug concentration, associated with discernible effects. The threshold is derived by graphic analysis of *in vivo* dose-response data. Examples are provided of both animal and human data, which demonstrate agreement of experimental results with predicted responses. This approach permits more direct comparison of studies with different patient populations and studies from different investigators. This chapter also provides evidence of first-order clearance kinetics of dopamine and dobutamine over the ranges of dosages used normally in neonates, infants, and older children.

There are numerous examples in clinical neonatology in which pharmacologic principles developed in adult humans and animals have been used to guide pharmacologic therapy in newborns. However, because newborns are not just small adults, this approach has resulted in many untoward drug-related incidents, including the historic chloramphenicol "gray baby syndrome,"[1-3] errant aminoglycoside drug doses,[4-6] the excessive absorption of topical antiseptics,[7-11] and the benzyl alcohol "gasping syndrome."[12, 13] Inotropic drugs are among several classes of drugs whose initial use in neonates and children was based on data generated in adults. Drug manufacturers have generally avoided costly clinical trials of inotropic agents in neonates and children. Industry has instead relied on the experience of clinicians who care for newborns and who use these drugs based on information generated in adults. Therefore, information on safety and efficacy in newborn and pediatric patients has been the result of practical experience generated in the clinical setting. Adverse effects of drugs that enter the clinical setting in this fashion are reported only after use has become widespread.

To compound this situation further, the plasma concentrations of all the widely used inotropic agents were well below the level of detection of available assays at the time of the initial pharmacologic investigations. This technical problem inhibited assessment of the pharmacokinetics and pharmacodynamics of these inotropic drugs. The development and application of sensitive assays for commonly used inotropic drugs subsequently permitted evaluation of their actions in the clinical setting. We have used this approach to evaluate the pharmacokinetics and pharmacodynamics of inotropic drugs in neonates, older infants, and children. This chapter reviews the results of such studies, which provide a rational basis for the use of inotropic drugs in critically ill newborns and children.

PHARMACOLOGIC PRINCIPLES

Pharmacokinetics

Pharmacokinetics is the study of *in vivo* drug disposition. In most circumstances, plasma drug levels are measured, and their concentrations at different time intervals are analyzed by comparison to classic models. A derived parameter that reflects the rate of drug disposition is then calculated. The most familiar pharmacokinetic parameter to clinicians is the half-life. Figure 24-1 shows a typical concentration versus time graph. Drug is administered as a bolus at time zero. Plasma drug concentration rises rapidly to a short-lived peak concentration. The plasma concentration rapidly decreases as the drug is equilibrating in the plasma compartment. This equilibrium period is referred to as the *distribution phase* or α-*phase*.

A second, more prolonged period of decay in plasma drug concentration is also observed. In this latter period, the rate of decay of plasma drug concentration is dependent on mechanisms for elimination or clearance, such as excretion and metabolism. This is called the *elimination phase* or β-*phase*. For drugs whose mechanisms of elimination have not been saturated, the β or elimination phase of the decay curve is linear when displayed on a semilogarithmic plot. Such drugs are said to have *first-order* or *linear kinetics*. First-order kinetics simply describes nonsaturability within the range of dosages that were studied. Drugs whose elimination kinetics are saturable have nonlinear exponential decay curves.

The plasma half-life, or the time required for drug concentration to decrease by 50%, is determined graphically or by com-

puter analysis of the decay curves. For drugs with extremely rapid rates of disposition, the short half-lives are difficult to determine accurately. Small errors in the timing of samples during the elimination phase create large errors in half-life determination. In addition, drugs with extremely short half-lives, such as inotropic drugs with half-lives of 1 to 2 minutes, are usually administered by continuous infusion. In such circumstances, a more appropriate pharmacokinetic parameter is the *plasma clearance rate*. Clearance is calculated by the following formula:

$$\text{Plasma clearance rate} = \frac{\text{Dose of infusate (g/kg/min)}}{\text{Steady-state concentration} - \text{baseline concentration (g/mL)}}$$

For drugs with first-order kinetics, there is a linear relationship between steady-state plasma drug concentration and dose, and the calculated clearance rate is independent of dose, a finding suggesting nonsaturability of elimination mechanisms over the range of dosage studied. Experimentally, this is determined by measurement of steady-state plasma drug concentration at several different stable infusion rates. Clearance is usually normalized to body weight, whereas half-life is independent of body mass. Although clearance rate is a more appropriate derived parameter for drugs with short half-lives, it is a less familiar concept to clinicians.

We examined elimination kinetics for the inotropic agents dopamine and dobutamine in neonates, older infants, and children in the critical care setting.[14-17] In each study, the drug was infused with a calibrated infusion pump. Samples for measurement of plasma drug concentration were collected at several infusion rates. Data were analyzed by computer-based graphic analysis. Figure 24-2 is a representative plot of plasma dobutamine concentration versus dose in newborns and older children. For each patient, there was a linear relationship between dose and plasma drug concentration, a finding confirming first-order kinetics. The clearance rate of dopamine and dobutamine in neonates and older children is independent of dose, a finding that further supports first-order kinetics over the range of dosages studied.[14-17] The more remarkable observation was the wide range of actual clearance rates. Although mean clearance was 75 to 90 mL/kg/minute, the range was 30 to 170 mL/kg/minute. A similar wide range of dopamine clearance levels has been observed. Figure 24-3 illustrates the mean and range of dopamine and dobutamine clearance rates in multiple studies. Significant interpatient variation was noted for both dopamine and dobutamine plasma clearance rates

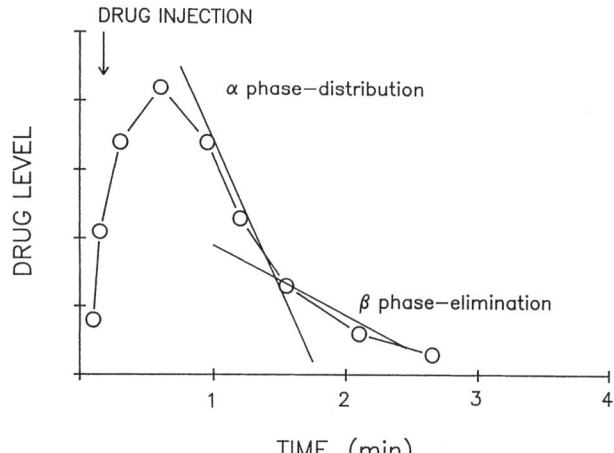

Figure 24-1. Typical concentration versus time result used to generate drug half-life.

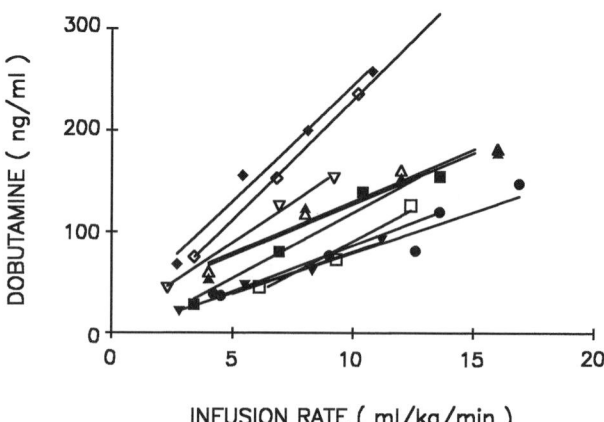

Figure 24-2. Plasma dobutamine level (ng/mL) versus infusion rate. The correlation between dobutamine level and infusion rate was significant (r = 0.97; p < .001). (From Habib DM, et al: Crit Care Med *20*:601,1992.)

in each of the circumstances studied. Initially, it was not clear whether this was the result of specific illnesses in these patients or the result of other factors. Although it is important to generate the pharmacokinetic data under the circumstances of actual drug use in critically ill patients, some feature of their physiologic derangement may have been the source of the high interpatient variation. To address this issue, we examined the clearance rate of dobutamine in a set of healthy normal patient volunteers in an identical fashion to the methods used for sick patients.[17] In each of the individual patients, there was a linear relationship between dose and plasma drug level. The range of clearance rates, 38 to 218 mL/kg/minute, was similar to that seen in critically ill patients. This finding suggests that the high variation in clearance rate among individual patients is not caused by illness itself.

These pharmacokinetic data have significant implications for clinicians using these drugs. The first-order clearance kinetics indicates that plasma drug level is directly and linearly related to dose. In the dosage range studied, clinicians need not be concerned that increasing dose leads to a sudden and exponential increase in plasma level, as seen with drugs with saturable kinetics such as phenytoin or aminoglycosides.

Special Pharmacokinetic Considerations in Neonates: Endotracheal Epinephrine

During cardiopulmonary resuscitation, establishment of an airway and adequate ventilation is generally the first priority. When epinephrine administration is indicated, the endotracheal route is often chosen because of expediency. Animal models and case reports in neonates and children have established that endotracheal epinephrine during cardiopulmonary resuscitation can effectively restore spontaneous circulation.[18-26] In addition, endotracheal epinephrine administration to animals with normal circulatory status, hypovolemia, or asphyxia-induced bradycardia can increase heart rate, mean arterial pressure, and cardiac output.[27-29] The pharmacokinetics of endotracheal epinephrine depends on effective dispersion of the drug over the respiratory mucosa, pulmonary blood flow, and matching of the ventilation (drug dispersal) to perfusion.[21, 26]

During cardiopulmonary resuscitation, gross perturbations of ventilation and perfusion occur. Preexisting conditions, such as pulmonary edema, pneumonia, and airway disease, also affect the pharmacokinetics of endotracheally administered drugs.[30] Furthermore, epinephrine is a local vasoconstrictor and therefore inhibits its own uptake in the local pulmonary vasculature.[27, 31] It should not be surprising that endotracheal

administration results in lower peak plasma concentrations and a prolonged depot effect.[21-33] Administration of typical intravenous emergency epinephrine doses (0.01 mg/kg) via the endotracheal route does not significantly affect arterial epinephrine concentration during cardiopulmonary resuscitation in adults, whereas the same dose intravenously increases arterial epinephrine concentration.[30] Animal models and studies in adult humans demonstrate that 5 to 10 times higher epinephrine doses are generally necessary by the endotracheal route to attain hemodynamic effects comparable to the intravenous route.[19-34] The appropriate endotracheal epinephrine dose for neonates is not known. Higher than intravenous doses are necessary for similar effects, yet prolonged hypertension from depot effects may be particularly dangerous to preterm infants at risk of intracranial hemorrhage. In addition, there are limited data regarding metabolism of catecholamines after cardiopulmonary resuscitation in neonates. Schwab and von Stockhausen[35] demonstrated that premature neonates could effectively inactivate free epinephrine by sulfoconjugation after 0.25 mg/kg was administered endotracheally during cardiopulmonary resuscitation. These investigators did not note any adverse effects, yet they documented 10-fold higher plasma epinephrine concentrations 1 and 2 hours after resuscitation.[32]

Pharmacodynamics

Classic pharmacodynamic theory suggests that the laws of mass action can describe the effects of administered agents such as adrenergic agonists. For a single ligand (e.g., exogenous agonist or endogenous catecholamine) interacting with a single class of receptors, the dose-response relationship is characterized by a sigmoidal dose versus response relationship.[36] The actual data used to derive these curves are usually obtained after cumulative, stepwise increasing doses. Boluses of the drug are most commonly infused. Larger doses are administered after "return of the preparation to steady-state or baseline conditions." Concentrations ranging over 4 to 6 logarithms are needed to construct the sigmoidal dose-response curves. The data are fit either graphically or by computer-based modeling programs to the expected sigmoidal response. Derived parameters such as the concentration necessary for 50% maximal effect or inhibition (ED_{50} or ID_{50}) and potency ratios are then used to define the pharmacologic profile. These parameters are also used to compare individual drugs, to compare subjects in different physiologic or clinical conditions, or to compare subjects at different developmental ages. The assumptions underlying this methodology are as follows: (1) the administered agent achieves a steady-state concentration and effect at the receptor site after the bolus administration; (2) the maximum effect observed experimentally is indeed maximal, accurately measured, and physiologically meaningful; and (3) the maximum effect is relevant to the proposed clinical application of the drug or agent.

These experimental prerequisites preclude their measurement in human subjects *in vivo*. Maximal effects are difficult to achieve, and such doses may lead to dangerous side effects. Clinical administration of drugs rarely varies over a 4 or 5 log concentration range. Pharmacologic literature on the clinical application of newer inotropic agents reveals that the majority of basic information used to define the pharmacologic profile, to determine their potency in comparison with other agents, and to ascertain their potential clinical relevance is derived largely from *in vitro* data.[37-42] It is clear that the generation of data from cumulative responses in isolated tissues is not the method of administration of these agents in clinical use. Nonetheless, a derived parameter is necessary to permit comparison of drug effects from different investigations. There is ample information to suggest that age, diagnosis, and intercurrent clinical problems significantly affect response,[40-43] metabolism,[14-17, 44-45] or side effects[46] of inotropic agents.

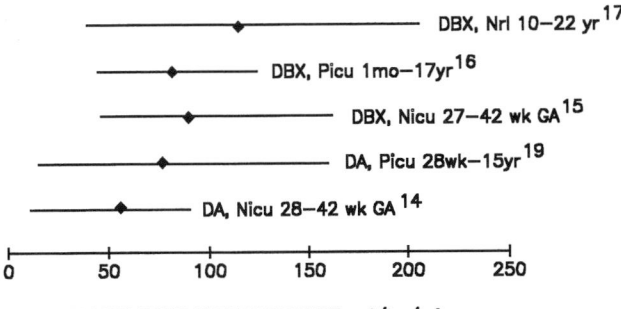

Figure 24–3. Ranges of clearance values in different studies (superscript numbers). Patients were in either neonatal or pediatric intensive care units (Nicu or Picu) at the ages indicated. The references for each published study are shown in superscript. DA = dopamine; DBX = dobutamine; GA = gestational age, Nrl = normal.

Our goal was to develop an alternative approach to study pharmacodynamics of inotropic drugs based on the relationship of the plasma concentration during clinical administration to the hemodynamic effects. Previous investigations comparing responses to infused catecholamines had suggested that there was no change in a particular response until the catecholamine concentration reached or exceeded a "physiologic threshold."[47] Beyond the threshold value, there is a log-linear relationship between the plasma catecholamine concentration and the physiologic response. This concept is illustrated in Figure 24-4. In Figure 24-4, the classic sigmoidal dose-response curve is shown, and the location of the ED_{50} and the threshold on the classic dose-response curve are illustrated. The threshold model at the lower concentrations of the sigmoidal dose-response curve is shown. A zero-order equation $(y = a)$ relates the response to the log of the plasma catecholamine or drug concentration (pg/mL) below the threshold concentration. Above the threshold concentration, there is a linear increase in response to logarithmic increases in plasma catecholamine concentrations $(y = m \log x + b)$. A computerized nonlinear, least-squares regression program was developed to fit experimental data to these assumptions.[48] The *threshold* is defined as the catecholamine concentration at the intersection of these two lines. The program determines the best fit for the baseline value of the response, the threshold drug concentration at the threshold for that response, and the slope and correlation coefficient of the log-linear regression line beyond the threshold value. Goodness of fit to this model can be determined statistically.

To confirm the validity of this approach for *in vivo* studies, we first performed experiments in human infants and children. Preliminary studies confirmed that steady-state plasma concentrations and hemodynamic responses were achieved within 15 minutes. Thresholds for individual hemodynamic responses, including increases in blood pressure, cardiac output, and heart rate, were determined for each patient. There was excellent agreement between the predicted log-linear dose-response relationship and the measured data in newborns as well as older infants and children. Figure 24-5 is a series of representative curves from several children depicting the log-linear relationship of plasma dobutamine concentrations and hemodynamic parameters. Thresholds, similar to clearance rates, varied substantially between patients. Nonetheless, most patients demonstrated the predicted log-linear relationship between plasma inotropic drug concentration and responses. Using the apparent threshold and plasma clearance rate for each patient, one can calculate the minimum infusion rate that would result in plasma drug concentrations equal to or greater than the threshold. The threshold for hemodynamic responses to dopamine occurred at plasma concentrations of dopamine achieved at an infusion rate of approximately 1.0 μg/kg/minute and was fairly uniform among patients. For dobutamine, the plasma threshold was achieved at infusion rates of approximately 2.0 μg/kg/minute.

These results agree with other data demonstrating the effectiveness of dobutamine as an inotropic agent in the newborn[49-51] despite contradictory reports.[43] In most of the patients we studied, dobutamine demonstrated a lower threshold for increases in cardiac output than for changes in blood pressure. This finding suggests that the hemodynamic effects of dobutamine in this age group are the result of a direct inotropic response. Clearer evidence of a direct inotropic effect was the improvement after dobutamine infusions of a load-independent index of myocardial contractility, the relationship of left ventricular end-systolic wall stress to rate-corrected velocity of fiber shortening. Generation of threshold data permits comparisons of different agents or among patients of different gestational ages. For example, comparison of the ratio of the cardiac output threshold to heart rate threshold (inotropic/chronotropic ratio) indicates a ratio of 2.5:1 for dopamine versus 6:1 for dobutamine in neonates.[14, 23] This finding suggests a greater margin of efficacy versus adverse effects for dobutamine in this group of patients. Further analyses of this type may demonstrate a superior pharmacologic profile for dobutamine in comparison with alternative agents.

As noted during the study of the plasma clearance rate of dopamine and dobutamine, there was a wide interpatient variation in the plasma threshold for the cardiovascular effects of both agents. The threshold for increases in systolic blood pressure in neonates in response to dopamine infusion ranged from 3 to 45 ng/mL of dopamine, which would have been achieved at infusion rates from 0.2 to 2.5 μg/kg/minute. For dobutamine, the ranges were similarly quite wide. In infants and children, the threshold for dobutamine-mediated increase in cardiac index was observed at infusion rates from 0.2 to 9 μg/kg/minute. The data are shown graphically in Figure 24-6. The mean and range of thresholds for each study group are shown. The interpatient variation in threshold was nearly 2 logs wide. It was possible that some feature of the physiologic derangement was the source of the high interpatient variation in sensitivity to the pharmacodynamic effects of inotropic drugs. To address this issue, we examined the clearance rate of dobutamine in a set of healthy normal patient volunteers in an identical fashion to the methods used for sick patients.[17] In these normal volunteers, the range of thresholds for improvements in cardiac index was 4 to 20 ng/mL. The mean threshold for the entire group was achieved at dobutamine infusion rates of approximately 2 μg/kg/minute.

The threshold approach provides several important advantages. First, it is based on actual data in clinical subjects. Pharmacologic data suggest that there may be major differences in pharmacokinetics under different clinical situations, such as congestive heart failure, renal disease, or liver dysfunction.[44, 45] Extrapolation of

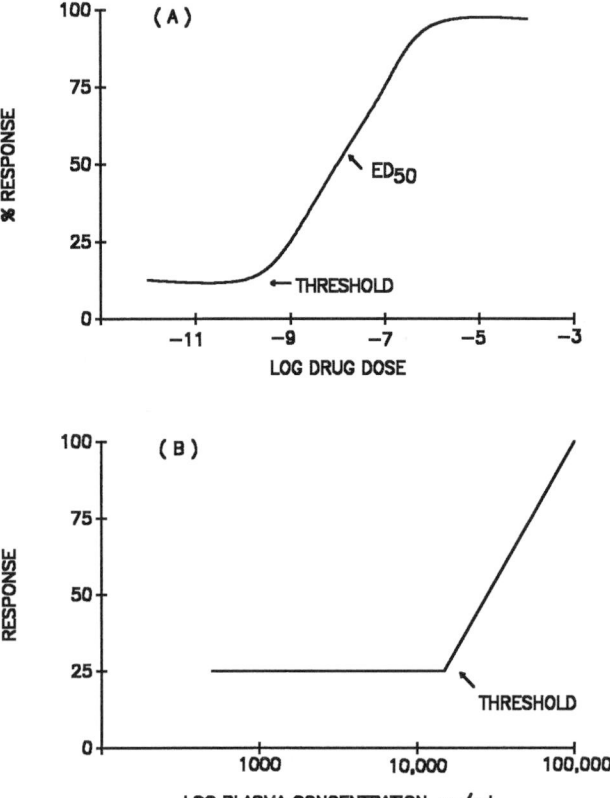

Figure 24-4. A, Dose-response curve showing the approximate location of the median effective dose (ED_{50}) and threshold. **B,** Log transformation of dose-response curve. The location of threshold is indicated as the intersection of the zero-order and log-linear response.

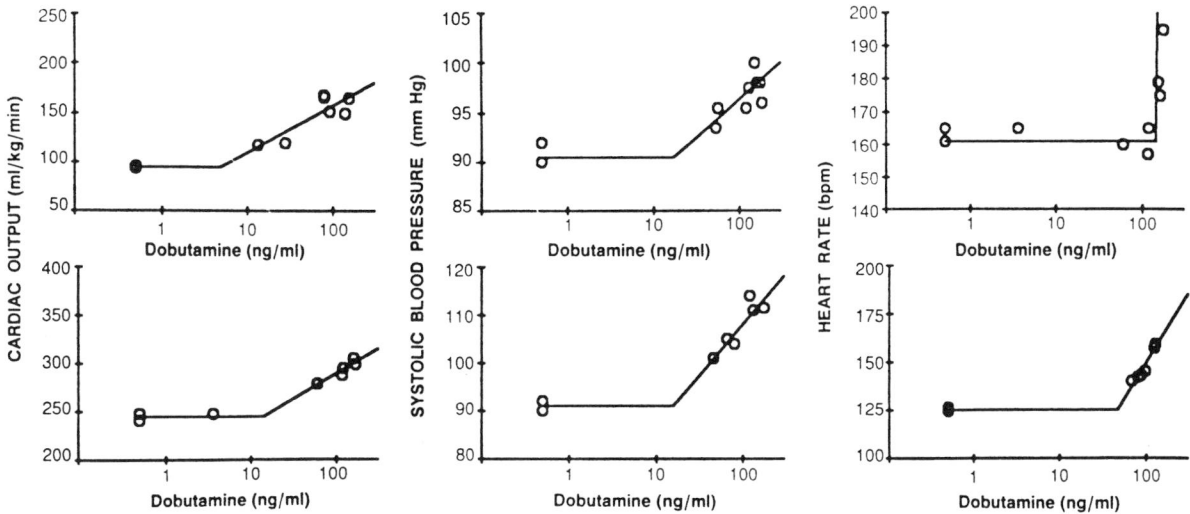

Figure 24–5. Representative dose-response curves. Plasma dobutamine levels are plotted on the logarithmic horizontal axis. Each response is plotted on a vertical linear axis. The *lines* indicate the computer-generated best fit. See Fig. 24–3 for abbreviations. (From Habib DM, et al: Crit Care Med *20*:601, 1992.)

pharmacokinetic or pharmacodynamic data derived in experimental animal preparations may not be applicable to these conditions. Second, the traditional pharmacologic approach uses bolus drug injections for generation of dose-response curves. In this setting, drug doses and presumably plasma level or concentration at the receptor vary over 4 to 6 log units. We and others,[14,15,45,52] however, have shown that plasma concentrations of these agents during clinical use vary only over 1 to 2 log units. For example, plasma dobutamine concentrations in critically ill neonates averaged 23 ng/mL at the recommended starting dose of 2.5 μg/kg/minute and 92 ng/mL at 7.5 μg/kg/minute. Because the ED_{50} is developed from a series of drug doses substantially beyond the range in use clinically, it may represent relations between dose and response quite different from those in the clinical arena. The threshold is based on steady state, *in vivo* conditions and shows the direct relationship between drug dose and effect during actual clinical conditions.

Finally, this experimental approach demonstrates the most rational use of these drugs in the clinical setting. The stepwise increase in dose titrating to desired clinical end-point maximizes

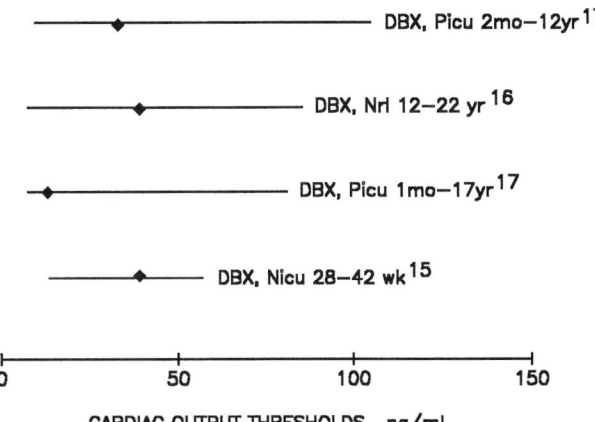

Figure 24–6. Ranges of *threshold* values in different studies. Patients were in either neonatal or pediatric intensive care units (Nicu or Picu) at the ages indicated. The references for each published study are shown in superscript. DBX = dobutamine; Nrl = normal.

the beneficial effects of these agents while minimizing the adverse effects such as tachycardia or other arrhythmias, and it minimizes desensitization. Because there is a log-linear relationship between dose and response, a "doubling dose" response curve, as was used in our dopamine studies (2 to 4 to 8 μg/kg/minute), gives the best results. Likewise, weaning by successive 50% reductions in dose is also more rational than minute decreases with each change.

Special Pharmacodynamic Considerations in Neonates

Developmental changes in myocardial structure and function would be expected to modulate the responses of the newborn to catecholamines. The neonatal myocardium has a greater percentage of noncontractile tissue compared with the myocardium of adults and older children and has incomplete sympathetic innervation.[53] In addition, oxygen consumption and myocardial demands are relatively higher in the neonate. Although neonatal myocardial function is excellent at rest, myocardial reserve is limited. Contractility is near maximal at rest. Preload reserve, contractility reserve, and heart rate reserve are all limited.[53,54] It has been presumed that these issues would limit the neonatal myocardial response to catecholamines, although this is not well documented. Similarly, differences in the degree of peripheral maturation and the mechanisms for vascular constriction and relaxation may affect the newborn's responses to inotropic agents.

When catecholamine infusions are used in neonates, the underlying disease states are often associated with pulmonary hypertension. Studies in infants and adults have demonstrated that higher doses of dopamine can increase pulmonary artery pressure, although these findings are not consistent.[55-57] Pulmonary α-adrenergic receptors lead to pulmonary vasoconstriction, whereas dopaminergic receptors lead to pulmonary vasodilation. In most circumstances, increased cardiac output and aortic blood pressure decrease baroreceptor-mediated sympathetic activity and thereby decrease pulmonary vasoconstriction. In any case, adverse effects on pulmonary vasculature are not well documented in the neonatal population, and their occurrence has not limited the popularity of these agents in critically ill infants with clinical evidence of pulmonary hypertension.

In the neonate, cardiovascular shock is generally the result of intravascular volume depletion and myocardial dysfunction secondary to hypoxic injury. Therefore, intravascular volume repletion is recommended for initial treatment of cardiovascular shock.[55] Myocardial dysfunction or vasoregulatory disturbance,

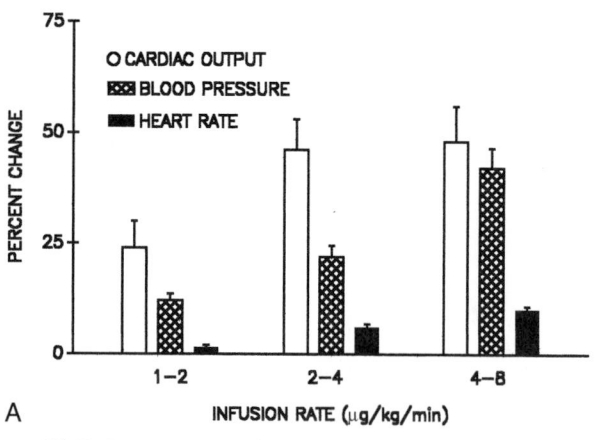
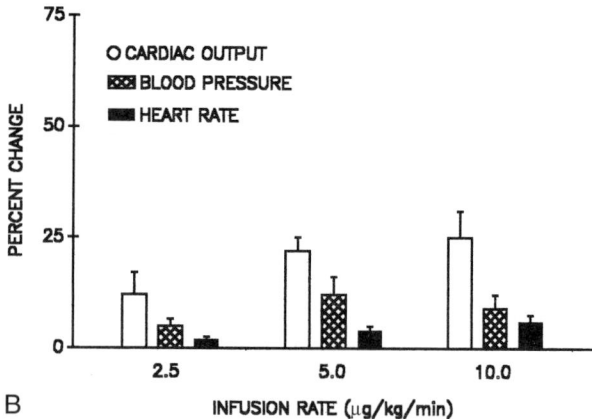

Figure 24–7. Comparison of hemodynamic responses to dopamine and dobutamine in neonates. Results are shown as a percentage of increase in cardiac output *(open bars),* blood pressure *(hatched bars),* or heart rate *(solid bars)* above pretreatment levels. (Data from refs. 14–17.)

however, frequently accompanies shock. In this circumstance, inotropic and vasoactive therapy with catecholamines can improve myocardial function and oxygen delivery.[55-62] We compared the hemodynamic responses of newborns to either dopamine or dobutamine in the studies described earlier to generate the threshold data.[14-17] When expressed as a percentage of improvement in cardiac output, blood pressure, or heart rate above initial level, as shown in Figure 24-7, dopamine has a greater effect on both cardiac output and blood pressure than "equivalent" (equimolar) doses of dobutamine. Dobutamine has a greater proportional effect on cardiac output than on blood pressure, consistent with its "selective inotropic effect" observed in many studies in adults.[63] This finding implies that in clinical disorders such as congestive cardiomyopathy, which frequently accompanies perinatal asphyxia, dobutamine is a preferred inotropic agent. On the contrary, cardiovascular dysfunction secondary to neonatal sepsis may be accompanied by substantial derangements in peripheral vascular function, and thus dopamine, with greater effects on blood pressure and peripheral vascular contractility, is preferred. Other investigators have suggested that dopamine may be more effective than volume expansion or dobutamine for hypotensive preterm infants during the first few days of life.[55, 59-62] In the latter population, hypotension may be more frequently caused by poor peripheral vasoregulation with or without myocardial dysfunction than by volume depletion.[55, 59, 60] The greater chronotropic effect of dopamine can be a clinical limitation to its usefulness. Treatment with both drugs simultaneously is frequent and not necessarily discouraged; however, there is limited direct pharmacodynamic evidence of differences, if any, in dose-response relationships when these drugs are given together.

Neonates in congestive heart failure have high levels of endogenous catecholamines[62] and frequently require exogenous catecholamines for hemodynamic support.[64] Epinephrine infusions in isolated intact newborn piglet hearts resulted in left ventricular systolic and diastolic dysfunction, associated with irreversible ultrastructural abnormalities.[65] The clinical relevance of these worrisome *in vitro* findings is not clear.

CONCLUSION

This chapter has reviewed an approach to pharmacokinetic and pharmacodynamic studies of inotropic agents that we believe provides insights not afforded by more traditional methods. An experimental approach to the generation of a derived parameter,

the threshold, is provided to describe dose-response results for *in vivo* data. This derived parameter permits comparison of responses among different subjects and results of different investigators. This approach avoids some of the flaws inherent in extrapolation of *in vitro* data to the clinical setting and allows new insights into the comparison of drug effects between different agents, in different clinical settings, and at different developmental ages. It also demonstrates the most rational approach to clinical use of these agents. Volume expansion is indicated before administration of inotropic agents. If there is an inadequate response in clinical (perfusion) or physiologic parameters (blood pressure, urine output, acid-base status, or cardiac output or contractility), inotropic support is indicated. The clinician should start at a low dose, near or just above the predicted threshold. The administration rate should be increased by doubling the dose every 15 to 30 minutes until the desired clinical response is observed or until undesired side effects (usually tachycardia) are observed. In a similar fashion, a rational approach to weaning by 50% reductions in dose is based on recognition of the log-linear relationship between dose and response. Therefore, incremental adjustments in dose should be 25 to 50% reductions with continued monitoring of clinical and physiologic responses. These approaches maximize beneficial responses while minimizing both adverse effects and desensitization.

ACKNOWLEDGMENTS

This work is supported by grants from the United States Public Health Service (HD 18014) and the American Heart Association, Los Angeles Affiliate.

REFERENCES

1. Sutherland DM: Fatal cardiovascular collapse of infants receiving large amounts of chloramphenicol. Am J Dis Child *97*:61, 1981.
2. Burns LE, et al: Fatal circulatory collapse in premature infants receiving chloramphenicol. N Engl J Med *26*:1318, 1959.
3. Weiss CF, et al: Chloramphenicol in the newborn infant. N Engl J Med *6*:787, 1960.
4. Finitzo-Hieber T, et al: Prospective controlled evaluation of auditory function in neonates given netilmicin or amikacin. J Pediatr *106*:129, 1985.
5. Odio C, et al: Nephrotoxicity associated with vancomycin-aminoglycoside therapy in four children. J Pediatr *105*:491, 1984.
6. Adelman RD, et al: A controlled study of the nephrotoxicity of mezlocillin and amikacin in the neonate. Am J Dis Child *141*:1175, 1987.
7. Powell H, et al: Hexachlorophene myelinopathy in premature infants. J Pediatr *82*:976, 1973.
8. Shuman RM, et al: Neurotoxicity of hexachlorophene in the human. I. A clinicopathologic study of 248 children. Pediatrics *54*:689, 1974.

9. Shuman RM, et al: Neurotoxicity of hexachlorophene in humans. II. A clinico-pathologic study of 436 premature infants. Arch Neurol *32*:320, 1975.
10. Gowdy JM, Ulsamer AG: Hexachlorophene lesions in newborn infants. Am J Dis Child *130*:247, 1976.
11. Pyati SP, et al: Absorption of iodine in the neonate following topical use of povidone iodine. J Pediatr *91*:825, 1977.
12. Gershank J, et al: The gasping syndrome and benzyl alcohol poisoning. N Engl J Med *307*:1384, 1982.
13. Lovejoy FH: Fatal benzyl alcohol poisoning in neonatal intensive care units. Am J Dis Child *136*:974, 1982.
14. Padbury JF, et al: Pharmacokinetics of dopamine in critically ill newborn infants. J Pediatr *117*:472, 1990.
15. Martinez AM, et al: Dobutamine pharmacokinetics and responses in critically ill neonates. Pediatrics *89*:47, 1992.
16. Habib DM, et al: Dobutamine pharmacokinetics in pediatric intensive care patients. Crit Care Med *20*:601, 1992.
17. Berg RA, et al: Dobutamine pharmacokinetics and pharmacodynamics in normal children and adolescents. J Pharmacol Exp Ther *265*:1232, 1993.
18. Greenberg MI, et al: Use of endotracheally administered epinephrine in a pediatric patient. Am J Dis Child *135*:767, 1981.
19. Lindemann R: Resuscitation of the newborn: endotracheal administration of epinephrine. Acta Paediatr Scand *73*:210, 1984.
20. Polin K, et al: Endotracheal administration of epinephrine and atropine. Pediatr Emerg Care *2*:168, 1986.
21. Ralston SH, et al: Endotracheal versus intravenous epinephrine during electro-mechanical dissociation with CPR in dogs. Ann Emerg Med *14*:1044, 1985.
22. Jasani MS, et al: Effects of different techniques of endotracheal epinephrine administration in pediatric porcine hypoxic-hypercarbic cardiopulmonary arrest. Crit Care Med *22*:1174, 1994.
23. Hornchen U, et al: Influence of the pulmonary circulation on adrenaline pharmacokinetics during cardiopulmonary resuscitation. Eur J Anaesthesiol *9*:85, 1992.
24. Hornchen U, et al: Endobronchial instillation of epinephrine during cardio-pulmonary resuscitation. Crit Care Med *15*:1037, 1987.
25. Redding JS, et al: Effective routes of drug administration during cardiac arrest. Anesth Analg *46*:253, 1967.
26. Hahnel JH, et al: Endobronchial administration of emergency drugs. Resuscitation *7*:261, 1989.
27. Orlowski JP, et al: Endotracheal epinephrine is unreliable. Resuscitation *19*:103, 1990.
28. Roberts JR, et al: Comparison of the pharmacologic effects of epinephrine administered by the intravenous and endotracheal routes. J Am Coll Emerg Phys *7*:260, 1978.
29. Chernow B, et al: Epinephrine absorption after intratracheal administration. Anesth Analg *63*:829, 1984.
30. Quinton DN, et al: Comparison of endotracheal and peripheral intravenous adrenaline cardiac arrest: is the endotracheal route reliable? Lancet *1*:828, 1987.
31. Tang W, et al: Pulmonary ventilation/perfusion defects induced by epinephrine during cardiopulmonary resuscitation. Circulation *84*:2101, 1991.
32. Roberts JR, et al: Blood levels following intravenous and endotracheal epi-nephrine administration. J Am Coll Emerg Phys *8*:53, 1979.
33. Mazkereth R, et al: Epinephrine blood concentrations after peripheral bronchial versus endotracheal administration of epinephrine in dogs. Crit Care Med *20*:1582, 1991.
34. McCrirrick A, Kestin I: Haemodynamic effects of tracheal compared with intra-venous adrenaline. Lancet *340*:868, 1992.
35. Schwab KO, von Stockhausen HB: Plasma catecholamines after endotracheal administration of adrenaline during postnatal resuscitation. Arch Dis Child *70*:F213, 1994.
36. Spector R: The Scientific Basis of Clinical Pharmacology. Boston, Little, Brown and Co, 1986.
37. Colucci WS, et al: New positive inotropic agents in the treatment of congestive heart failure. N Engl J Med *314*:290, 1986.
38. Sorensen EV, Nilesen-Kudsk F: Myocardial pharmacodynamics of dopamine, dobutamine, amrinone and isoprenaline compared in the isolated rabbit heart. Eur J Pharmacol *124*:51, 1986.
39. Driscoll DJ, et al: Inotropic response of the neonatal canine myocardium to dopamine. Pediatr Res *12*:42, 1978.
40. Driscoll DJ, et al: Comparative hemodynamic effects of isoproterenol, dopamine, and dobutamine in the newborn dog. Pediatr Res *13*:1006, 1979.
41. Driscoll DJ, et al: Comparison of the cardiovascular action of isoproterenol, dopamine, and dobutamine in the neonatal and mature dog. Pediatr Cardiol *1*:307, 1980.
42. Park MK, et al: Comparative inotropic response of newborn and adult rabbit papillary muscles to isoproterenol and calcium. Dev Pharmacol Ther *1*:70, 1980.
43. Perkin RM, et al: Dobutamine: a hemodynamic evaluation in children with shock. J Pediatr *100*:977, 1982.
44. Zaritsky A, et al: Steady-state dopamine clearance in critically ill infants and chil-dren. Crit Care Med *16*:217, 1988.
45. Kates RE, Leier CV: Dobutamine pharmacokinetics in severe heart failure. Clin Pharmacol Ther *24*:537, 1978.
46. Guller B, et al: Changes in cardiac rhythm in children treated with dopamine. Crit Care Med *6*:151, 1978.
47. Clutter WE, et al: Epinephrine plasma metabolic clearance rates and physiologic thresholds for metabolic and hemodynamic actions in man. J Clin Invest *66*:94, 1980.
48. Padbury JF, et al: Thresholds for physiological effects of plasma catecholamines in fetal sheep. Am J Physiol *252*:E530, 1987.
49. Stopfkuchen H, et al: Effects of dobutamine on left ventricular performance in newborns as determined by systolic time intervals. Eur J Pediatr *146*:135, 1987.
50. Osborn D, et al: Randomized trial of dobutamine versus dopamine in preterm infants with low systemic blood flow. J Pediatr *140*:183, 2002.
51. Roze JC et al: Response to dobutamine and dopamine in the hypotensive very preterm infant. Arch Dis Child *69*:59, 1993.
52. Jarnberg PO, et al: Dopamine infusion in man: plasma catecholamine levels and pharmacokinetics. Acta Anaesth Scand *25*:328, 1981.
53. Friedman WF, George BL: Treatment of congestive heart failure by altering loading conditions of the heart. J Pediatr *106*:697, 1985.
54. Teitel D, et al: Developmental changes in myocardial contractile reserves in the lamb. Pediatr Res *19*:948, 1985.
55. Seri I: Cardiovascular, renal, and endocrine actions of dopamine in neonates and children. J Pediatr *126*:333, 1995.
56. Lang P, et al: The hemodynamic effects of dopamine in infants after corrective cardiac surgery. J Pediatr *96*:630, 1980.
57. Lucking SE, et al: Shock following generalized hypoxic-ischemic injury in previously healthy infants and children. J Pediatr *108*:359, 1986.
58. Malloy WD, et al: Effects of dopamine on cardiopulmonary function and left ventricular volume in patients with acute respiratory failure. Annu Rev Respir Dis *130*:396, 1984.
59. Seri I, et al: Cardiovascular response to dopamine in hypotensive preterm infants with severe hyaline membrane disease. Eur J Pediatr *142*:3, 1984.
60. Gill AB, Weindling AM: Randomized controlled trial of plasma protein fraction versus dopamine in hypotensive very low birthweight infants. Arch Dis Child *69*:284, 1993.
61. Greenough A, Emery AF: Randomized trial comparing dopamine and dobuta-mine in preterm infants. Eur J Pediatr *152*:925, 1993.
62. Klarr JM, et al: Randomized, blind trial of dopamine versus dobutamine for treatment of hypotension in preterm infants with respiratory distress syndrome. J Pediatr *125*:117, 1994.
63. Majerus TC, et al: Dobutamine: ten years later. Pharmacotherapy *9*:245, 1989.
64. Ross RD, et al: Return of plasma norepinephrine to normal after resolution of congestive heart failure in congenital heart disease. Am J Cardiol *60*:1411, 1987.
65. Caspi J, et al: Heart rate independence of catecholamine-induced myocardial damage in the newborn pig. Pediatr Res *36*:49, 1994.

25

Ernest A. Kopecky and Gideon Koren

Maternal Drug Abuse: Effects on the Fetus and Neonate

GENERAL PRINCIPLES

Women of reproductive age, like many others in society, have been steadily increasing their nonmedical consumption of drugs to the point of abuse for many years. *Substance abuse* is defined as an excessive self-administration of licit and illicit chemicals to alter one's perception of his or her cognitive status.[1] The most commonly abused substances include alcohol, cocaine, marijuana, tobacco, and psychotherapeutic agents. Among the opioids, morphine, heroin, and methadone appear to be the ones most frequently used by women of childbearing age.

Although the effects of substance abuse on the mother may be tolerable and desired, the effects on the fetus and neonate are often serious and manifest in neurobehavioral and physical anomalies. After the thalidomide disaster of the late 1950s and early 1960s, it became evident that the placenta is not a protective barrier against all therapeutic and abused substances. Although several compounds are human teratogens, most agents given to pregnant women do not pose significant reproductive hazards when these agents are used in recommended doses.[2] Moreover, some teratogenic drugs are continued throughout pregnancy because the therapeutic benefit to the woman outweighs the risk to the unborn child.[3]

There have been numerous attempts to describe the nature and extent of maternal drug abuse during pregnancy and its potential impact on the fetus and the neonate. The National Institute on Drug Abuse's National Pregnancy and Health Survey[4] revealed that 5.5% (221,000) of the approximately 4,000,000 women who delivered live babies in the United States in 1992 had used some licit or illicit drug during pregnancy; 18.8% (757,000) of women reported the consumption of alcohol, 1.1% (45,000) reported using cocaine, 0.1% (3600) used heroin, 2.9% (119,000) used marijuana, and 0.1% (3400) used methadone. In addition, 20.4% (820,000) reported that they smoked cigarettes, and 1.5% (61,000) reported the nonmedical use of psychotherapeutic agents at some point during their pregnancy.[4]

Maternal drug abuse during pregnancy is further complicated because the evidence suggests a trend among mothers to decrease the rate of drug consumption from 3 months before pregnancy and throughout the gestational period, rather than to achieve complete discontinuation of drug use.[4] In addition, the tabulated figures provided by the National Pregnancy and Health Survey[4] may actually be underestimates because of the underreporting of live neonates born to substance-abusing women.

Physicians dealing with high-risk pregnancies attributable to maternal drug abuse must recognize that fetal and neonatal complications are confounded by polydrug use in these patients. Studies have indicated a strong association between cigarette smoking and alcohol consumption and use of illicit drugs. For example, of those women who reported both alcohol and cigarette use during pregnancy, 20.4% also used marijuana and 9.5% used cocaine.[4] Therefore, fetal and neonatal dynamic outcomes are a composite of all the substances used by mothers during pregnancy. In addition, maternal drug and polydrug abusers exhibit higher risks for sexually transmitted diseases and poor prenatal care, and they generally lack the appropriate and necessary resources to care for the neonate with complications associated with *in utero* drug exposure.

Significant differences in the total rate of substance use were found among four sociodemographic variables related to pregnant women:[4] marital status, level of education, employment status, and method of hospital payment. The rates of use during pregnancy of marijuana, cocaine, and cigarettes were significantly higher for women who were unmarried, unemployed, had less than 16 years of formal education, or relied on public aid to pay for hospital expenses.[4] Conversely, women using alcohol were employed, had completed college, or had private medical insurance.[4]

It is important for emergency and obstetric medical staff to know that the prevalence of substance abuse differs among ethnic minorities and different age groups so the medical staff can efficiently and correctly decide which management algorithms to implement. Overall, estimated rates of drug use during pregnancy were highest for black women (11.3%) compared with white women (4.5%) and Hispanic women (4.4%).[4] However, the number of white women using drugs during pregnancy was 113,000 compared with 75,000 black and 28,000 Hispanic women.[4] Alcohol and cigarettes were abused by white women more often (22.7 and 24.4%, respectively), and cocaine was most often used by black women (4.5%).[4] Rates of marijuana use were highest (3.5%) in the youngest age group (<25 years), whereas cocaine use was highest (1.6%) among older women (≥25 years).[4]

The purpose of this chapter is to help the reader to understand the magnitude of the problem of substance abuse during pregnancy and the fetal and neonatal effects that may ensue. A general course of treatment is also described for each substance of abuse. In addition, references are provided that explain how drugs of abuse reach the fetus and the neonate eventually to elicit their harmful effects.[5-34]

MATERNAL DRUGS OF ABUSE DURING PREGNANCY

Alcohol

Alcohol is an anxiolytic analgesic with a depressant effect on the central nervous system (CNS). Women who drink heavily (defined as an average of at least 2 drinks per day, or 1 drink per day and occasional binges of 5 or 6 drinks in one sitting, or 45 drinks or more per month)[35] have a higher predilection for polydrug use and exhibit other confounding risk factors—including older age and parity, or, conversely, an increased likelihood of being a younger, single, separated, or divorced woman—that may complicate pregnancy and may jeopardize fetal and neonatal outcome.[36,37]

Fetal alcohol syndrome (FAS) in the children of women who drink heavily before and during pregnancy has been well described. Heavy maternal consumption of alcohol during pregnancy is generally accepted as the factor responsible for FAS.[38] FAS is the most commonly known cause of mental retardation (surpassing Down syndrome) and is characterized by fetal and neonatal growth retardation, severe cognitive impairment because of impaired neural development, microphthalmia, short palpebral fissures, midfacial hypoplasia, abnormal palmar creases, cardiac defects, and joint contractures.[39-42] No single finding is considered pathognomonic, and not all features are present in every neonate who has FAS.

The association of FAS with ethanol dose is not always clearly evident. In many cases, only a few of the typical characteristics of the syndrome manifest themselves. Neonates with partial expression FAS (namely, two or fewer of the syndrome's characteristics) exhibit a condition termed *fetal alcohol effects*. This condition is observed in the infants of women drinking fewer than two drinks per day. However, it remains unexplained why only 10% of fetuses exposed to large amounts of ethanol per day (the ethanol content of six maternal drinks per day) exhibit full-blown FAS. Possible explanations include variations in placental and fetal vasculature, different rates of organogenesis, different rates of ethanol metabolism and elimination by the fetus, and differences in fetal susceptibility to teratogenesis.[43-45] Acetaldehyde has been suggested as a possible causative factor. There is evidence that mothers with alcoholism who give birth to children with FAS have substantially higher levels of acetaldehyde than those mothers who have normal babies.[46] Furthermore, placental perfusion experiments have shown that the human placenta metabolizes alcohol and contributes to the acetaldehyde transferred into the fetal circulation.[47]

FAS occurs in approximately 1 to 2 infants per 1000 live births; 2.5 to 10% of women with alcoholism have a child with FAS.[48,49] It is generally accepted that FAS occurs when drinking reaches six to seven drinks per day (one standard drink is the equivalent of 12 ounces of beer or a 5-ounce glass of wine, or 1.5 ounces of liquor, or approximately 15 g [0.5 oz] of absolute alcohol). It has been shown that having two drinks per day does not increase the risk of FAS; however, having three drinks per day during pregnancy is associated with a lower intelligence quotient when the children of these women are 3 years old.[50]

Pharmacology of Alcohol

The level of blood alcohol (ethanol; C_2H_5OH) depends on the type of beverage (e.g., beer slows absorption) and its ethanol concentration, the gastric contents, and gastrointestinal motility.[51] Eighty to 90% of the absorption of ethanol occurs within 30 to 60 minutes of its consumption. Food may delay absorption for 4 to 6 hours.[51] Absorption occurs primarily in the small intestine, whereas 20 to 30% is rapidly absorbed through the stomach. Ethanol distributes rapidly because it is both water and lipid soluble. Ethanol is a mildly polar molecule that easily crosses cell membranes, the blood-brain barrier, and the placenta, and it is rapidly distributed throughout the fetal circulation. The volume of distribution is estimated to be 0.6 L/kg in adults and 0.7 L/kg in children, and this corresponds to total body water. The volume of distribution is slightly smaller in women because of their lower water and higher fat content than men. Because of the rapid distribution of alcohol, early determination of the blood alcohol concentration provides a reliable estimate of ethanol consumption.

Once ethanol is absorbed into the bloodstream, it is the metabolite acetaldehyde that causes the pharmacodynamic effects in the consumer. Ninety-five per cent of ethanol is con-verted by hepatic oxidized nicotinamide adenine dinucleotide (NAD^+)-alcohol dehydrogenase to the obligate intermediate acetaldehyde, which is more toxic than alcohol. Acetaldehyde is oxidized in the liver by NAD^+-dependent aldehyde dehydrogenase to form acetate. Acetate is also oxidized once in the bloodstream. The kidneys, muscles, lungs, and intestines also contribute to ethanol metabolism. Five to 10% of ethanol is excreted unchanged in the breath, urine, and sweat. The average rate of alcohol metabolism is 10 mL/hour.[52] Alcohol is esterfied with fatty acids to produce fatty acid ethyl esters, which accumulate in neonatal meconium and may be a promising screening test for heavy maternal drinking during pregnancy.

Effects of Alcohol Consumption on the Fetus and Neonate

For a diagnosis of FAS in a neonate or infant, there must be at least one sign in each of the first two categories listed in Table 25-1, and the neonate or infant must have at least two of the three characteristics in category 3.[53] Other features associated with FAS include epicanthal folds, a flat nasal bridge, a thin vermilion border of the upper lip, a hypoplastic maxilla, and a flattened midface. Strabismus, ptosis, poorly formed external ears, congenital heart defects, neural tube defects, renal abnormalities, and unusual palmar creases have also been documented. All infants with FAS have evidence of intrauterine growth retardation (IUGR): birth weight, body length, and head circumference are reduced for gestational age.[54] Infants with FAS may not catch up in growth and may remain small in contrast to small for gestational age opioid-exposed infants.[55] Mild to moderate developmental delays are commonplace, and delays in motor and language development, hyperactivity, hypotonia, hyperacusis, and tremulousness are often described.[1]

Heavy drinkers have an increased risk of spontaneous abortion.[49,56,57] In a study[57] of 1248 women, an estimated minimum harmful dose was 1 oz of absolute alcohol (two drinks) twice per week. The investigators showed a 25% miscarriage rate in women drinking 1 oz of absolute alcohol or more, compared with 14% in those women who drank less. This effect was independent of smoking, gestational age, or a history of spontaneous abortion. In another study[56] of 32,000 women, women consuming one to two drinks per day had a significantly higher risk of second trimester spontaneous abortion than those women who drank less than one drink per day.[56] Women reporting the consumption of more than three drinks per day exhibited an even higher risk.

An increased risk of abruptio placentae has been reported in heavy drinkers.[58,59] There is still considerable controversy about the association of maternal alcohol consumption and the duration of pregnancy with the incidence of stillbirth.[49,60-62] The major problem confounding research efforts to explain poor fetal and neonatal outcomes is the inability to separate high maternal ethanol intake from other confounding variables such as cigarette smoking, polydrug use, and poor prenatal care.

TABLE 25-1

Diagnostic Variables of Fetal Alcohol Syndrome

Category	Variables
1	*Prenatal or postnatal growth retardation*
	Weight, length, or head circumference below 10th percentile after correction for gestational age
2	*Central nervous system involvement*
	Neurologic abnormalities: neonatal irritability and childhood hyperactivity
	Developmental delay
	Cognitive impairment: mild to moderate mental retardation
3	*Characteristic facial dysmorphology*
	Microcephaly: head circumference below third percentile
	Microphthalmia or short palpable fissures
	Poorly developed philtrum and vermilion border, and a flattened or absent maxilla

Many investigators have studied the effects of maternal ethanol use on fetal and neonatal growth, as well as the development of fetuses exposed to ethanol *in utero*. An average of two drinks per day before conception correlated with a marginally lower birth weight (mean of 91 g) (in comparison with the children of lighter drinkers), independent of smoking.[63] A study[1] of 31,600 pregnancies confirmed this observation. In addition, the risk of IUGR is increased with an alcohol consumption of one to two drinks per day.[43-45,64-67] Alcohol interference with the transplacental transfer of amino acids across the placenta may alter embryonic development by inhibiting protein synthesis and prenatal growth. The literature suggests that the level of alcohol consumed by the father may also have an effect on fetal birth weight.[68] A prospective cohort study[69] of 359 neonates that assessed the critical period of alcohol exposure during pregnancy revealed that craniofacial abnormalities are definitively related to first trimester alcohol exposure.

A behavioral study[64] of 124 infants born to women classified according to their alcohol consumption found that tremors, time spent with the neonate's head turned to the left, and low activity levels increased progressively with the level of maternal alcohol intake. Infants of women consuming two to four drinks per day during pregnancy had a lower score for mental and psychomotor development.[66] A 10-year, long-term follow-up study[67] of these children showed severe growth deficiencies and intellectual limitations in those children who developed FAS. In a study[70] of 500 pregnant women who were heavy smokers and drinkers, the children showed a seven-point decrease in intelligence quotient when more than two drinks per day were consumed by the mothers during pregnancy. Postnatal exposure of infants to alcohol may also be harmful. In that regard, infants exposed to alcohol through breast milk scored lower on motor development tasks than unexposed infants at 1 year of age.[71]

Neonatal alcohol withdrawal and neurobehavioral disturbances have been documented in clinically normal neonates born to women who drank throughout pregnancy.[1] Ethanol exposure during the third trimester increased the probability of the newborn's going through postpartum ethanol withdrawal. In a study by Coles and colleagues,[72] abnormalities were observed in motor performance, autonomic regulation, and reflexive behavior during the first postpartum month in neonates exposed to alcohol *in utero*. Hyperactivity, hyperacusis, hypotonia, and tremulousness were commonly described in young infants, in addition to withdrawal symptoms characteristic of narcotic withdrawal in neonates.[64,66]

Clarren and associates[73] described multiple brain malformations attributable to fetal alcohol exposure. The most frequently seen malformations were leptomeningeal and neuroglial heterotopias. These investigators found aberrant neural and glial tissue covering large parts of the surface of the brain, as well as extensive brain disorganization from errors in neuronal and glial migration and rudimentary cerebellum and brain stem disorganization.

Electroencephalographic (EEG) abnormalities encompassing prominent δ bands and atypical slow waves in the posterior head region have been observed in neonates with FAS.[74] The intellectual deficit produced by abnormalities in brain growth is the most important component of FAS. Full expression of FAS generally occurs with long-term consumption of at least 2 g/kg/day of alcohol.

Another investigation[75] studying the effect of maternal alcohol ingestion on the incidence of respiratory distress syndrome suggested that among infants at less than 37 weeks' gestation, the incidence of respiratory distress syndrome decreased with increased maternal alcohol consumption. The researchers proposed that maternal alcohol ingestion enhanced fetal lung maturation. There has been no direct or indirect epidemiologic evidence or basic scientific information supporting or refuting an association between sudden infant death syndrome (SIDS) and maternal alcohol consumption during pregnancy.[76]

Optic nerve hypoplasia is a nonprogressive congenital anomaly associated with a decreased number of axons in the involved nerve.[77,78] The mother's use of alcohol during pregnancy has been associated with the development of optic nerve hypoplasia.[79] Optic nerve hypoplasia has been reported in 48% of children with FAS.[80]

Clinical Management of Heavy Drinkers during Pregnancy

It is well known that self-reports of drinking have a definite tendency to minimize the real incidence of drinking.[81] Given that limitation, accurate determination of the amount of alcohol consumed by the mother during pregnancy is essential because the extent of fetal damage is dose dependent. The age of the mother, other disease conditions, dietary deficiencies, use of other drugs, heavy smoking, and emotional stress are additional teratogenic factors that must be evaluated when the risk to fetal development from maternally consumed alcohol is assessed.

No specific prenatal diagnostic measures exist to identify fetuses with FAS. Serial measurements of α-fetoprotein may suggest the occurrence of FAS because α-fetoprotein is produced by the fetal liver, which, when exposed to alcohol, may be damaged. A decrease in the α-fetoprotein level was seen in most pregnancies of women bearing fetuses with FAS.[82] Currently, the best-established markers for the detection of alcohol abuse in pregnant and non-pregnant women are increased levels of serum γ-glutamyltransferase activity and increased mean blood cell volumes.[83]

Prenatal ultrasonography has been used to visualize and catalog the fetal malformations associated with numerous drugs and chemicals. Prenatal ultrasound examination of fetuses exposed to alcohol may reveal many associated anomalies (Table 25–2).[84,85]

Abstinence should be the desired treatment goal in heavy social drinkers or women who are physically dependent on alcohol. If alcohol consumption totals more than 80 g/day of

---

TABLE 25-2

Fetal Malformations Associated with Maternal Substance Abuse Visualized by Prenatal Ultrasonography

General Anomalies

Microcephaly
Diaphragmatic hernia
Renal defects
Hypospadias
Labial hypoplasia
Fetal growth retardation
Pulmonary atresia

Cardiac Anomalies

Heart malformations
Ventricular septal defect
Atrial septal defect
Double outlet of right ventricle
Dextrocardia
Patent ductus arteriosus
Tetralogy of Fallot

Skeletal Anomalies

Short nose
Hypoplastic philtrum
Hypoplastic maxilla
Micrognathia
Small mandible
Pectus excavatum
Bifid xiphoid
Scoliosis
Poorly formed orbits
Microphthalmia
Cleft lip
Cleft palate
Radioulnar synostosis

absolute ethanol, there should be a gradual reduction in alcohol consumption over 4 days.[48] During detoxification and throughout pregnancy, intense supportive counseling must be provided. A diazepam (Valium)-loading regimen has been used successfully in alcohol withdrawal treatment.[86] β-Blockers can reduce the signs and symptoms of mild to moderate alcohol withdrawal.[87]

Cocaine

Cocaine is the most potent naturally occurring stimulant. Cocaine blocks the reuptake of the biogenic amines serotonin, dopamine, and norepinephrine in the CNS and causes these neurotransmitters to bind with their receptors.[88, 89] Enhanced receptor binding increases neuronal excitability and causes the typical cocaine high. In addition to its effects on the CNS, cocaine acts peripherally to inhibit nerve conduction by blocking the reuptake of norepinephrine at the sympathetic nerve terminals.[90] This action increases norepinephrine levels and causes subsequent vasoconstriction, tachycardia, and hypertension.

Exposure to cocaine decreases blood flow to the fetus by constricting the placental vasculature. In addition, cocaine causes the myometrium to contract, and this potentially increases the risk of premature rupture of the membranes and necessitates the induction of labor.[91, 92] Vasoconstriction of the uterine arteries, causing circulatory insufficiency, has been suggested as the mechanism leading to reduced birth weight, fetal growth retardation, and labor-induced fetal stress.[93]

Initially, cocaine abuse involved concomitant intravenous injections of heroin. Currently, cocaine is insufflated or smoked rather than injected. During the last decade, cocaine use has dramatically increased, especially among young adults. By 1986, it was estimated that 40% of the United States population had tried cocaine.[94] At present, 40% of cocaine addicts use the drug nasally, 30% by free-base smoking, 20% by injection, and the remaining 10% by combining these routes.[95]

Pharmacology of Cocaine

A peak plasma cocaine concentration is attained within 15 to 60 minutes after insufflation.[96] The peak plasma concentration after oral administration of cocaine is reached in 50 to 90 minutes. The bioavailability of cocaine ingested orally is 60%, which is similar to that of cocaine ingested intranasally. Free-base smoking and intravenous cocaine administration have comparable kinetics: both are characterized by rapid and complete absorption of the drug. The elimination half-life of cocaine is between 20 and 90 minutes.[96] After an intranasal dose of 1.5 mg/kg, cocaine can be detected in the urine for 8 hours. Benzoylecgonine, the primary metabolite of cocaine, can be detected in the user's urine for 48 to 72 hours with chromatographic techniques and for 90 to 144 hours with radioimmunoassay.

Cocaine readily diffuses across the blood-brain and placental barriers and also transfers into breast milk. Cocaine rapidly crosses the placenta because of its low molecular weight (MW = 305), high lipid solubility, and low protein binding in human plasma. The rate of transfer of cocaine is approximately 10 times that of benzoylecgonine. Therefore, the majority of the administered dose is available to equilibrate with the fetal circulation.[21] The placenta serves as a reservoir for large amounts of cocaine and consequently offers some protection to the fetus after bolus dosing. Conversely, prolonged fetal exposure may ensue because cocaine and benzoylecgonine leach out of the placenta.[21] Fetal lamb studies[97] also indicate that cocaine and its metabolites in the amniotic fluid may prolong fetal drug exposure. Measurable levels of cocaine and benzoylecgonine have been detected in breast milk as late as 36 hours after consumption of the drug has ceased.

Cocaine is metabolized primarily by esterases and by cytochrome P450 enzymes. Cytochrome P450 accounts for the N-demethylation metabolism (20%) of cocaine into the bioactive metabolite norcocaine, which is more vasoactive than cocaine.[98]

The remainder of the drug is extensively metabolized by plasma and liver cholinesterases that hydrolyze the drug into an active metabolite, ecgonine methyl ester. Cocaine is spontaneously converted to benzoylecgonine in the plasma by nonenzymatic hydrolysis. The metabolites are more polar than cocaine and are readily excreted by the kidney. Less than 10% of cocaine is excreted unchanged in the urine.

The mean cocaine elimination half-life for intranasal administration is 75 minutes, for oral administration 48 minutes, and for intravenous administration 54 minutes. The volume of distribution is 1.2 to 1.9 L/kg. Individual cholinesterase levels explain the variations seen in the half-life of cocaine. The elimination half-life of benzoylecgonine is considerably longer than that of cocaine, but benzoylecgonine is more polar and therefore distributes less rapidly than cocaine.[99]

In adults, more benzoylecgonine than cocaine is found in the blood, brain, and liver.[100] In neonates, the distribution of cocaine in the tissues differs from that in adults. Klein and associates,[99] in their description of the distribution of cocaine and benzoylecgonine in a fetus born to a woman who used cocaine, detected both drugs in the fetal brain, scalp, liver, kidney, heart, placenta, blood, and hair. The neonate's liver contained substantially more cocaine than the other tissues, whereas the brain contained more benzoylecgonine than any other tissues.

Effects of Cocaine Use on the Fetus and Neonate

The potential deleterious effects on the fetus and neonate of mother's cocaine use during pregnancy are numerous. Cocaine use during pregnancy has been associated with an increased risk of spontaneous abortion, abruptio placentae, premature labor, precipitous delivery, stillbirth, and meconium staining.[101-106] After intravenous cocaine use, spontaneous abortion and abruptio placentae are more prevalent.[107] These effects may be associated with increased maternal blood pressure, increased uterine contractility and placental constriction, and decreased uterine blood flow, all of which cause fetal hypoxia.

Decreased birth weight, shorter body length, smaller head circumference, a higher malformation rate, and a greater need for medical support and resuscitation have been documented in newborns exposed to cocaine in utero.[102, 103, 105, 108, 109] These infants also exhibit depressed interactive behavior and poorly organized responses to external stimuli. Marked tremulousness, irritability, and deficiencies in mood control and interactive behavior have also been reported in the literature.[104,107,108,110,111] In a study[110] of 12 infants, 11 infants exhibited poor visual attention and abnormal flash-evoked potentials.

Doberczak and associates[112] studied the relationship between maternal cocaine abuse during pregnancy and neonatal neurologic abnormalities in 39 neonates. These investigators found that 34 neonates displayed CNS irritability, with bursts of sharp waves and spikes that were multifocal in 14 of 17 tracings. EEGs were abnormal in 17 of 38 neonates during the first week of life. Nine of the 17 abnormal EEGs remained abnormal through the second week of life. Between 3 and 12 months later, only 1 of these infants had an abnormal EEG. These findings did not suggest a correlation between fetal cocaine exposure and clinical seizures or neurologic abnormalities.

A rare but serious CNS condition associated with maternal cocaine use near delivery is prenatal cerebral infarction.[113] In the first reported case, a neonate developed right hemiparesis and right-sided focal seizures on the first day of life. The mother had used cocaine excessively 3 days before delivery. The neonate had a computed tomography scan and a lumbar puncture that showed evidence of cerebral infarction.

Neonates exposed in utero to cocaine showed significant differences in organizational response and interactive behavior compared with control neonates when they were assessed with the Brazelton Neurobehavioral Assessment Scale.[103, 114] Oro and Dixon[105] described a prevalence of excessive tremor, hypertonia, hyperreflexia, poor feeding, and sleep disturbances among cocaine-exposed and cocaine-methamphetamine–exposed neonates. It appears that the developing brain is sensitive to cocaine exposure during early development. However, the literature does contain conflicting studies on this issue. Chasnoff and colleagues[114] showed that neonates exposed to cocaine solely in the first trimester exhibited neurobehavioral abnormalities but no growth anomalies. Conversely, the Motherisk group[115] showed that babies exposed to cocaine only during the first trimester had no greater risk of delayed cognitive development than their control groups.

Cocaine-mediated vasoconstriction of the fetal cerebral vasculature decreases cerebral blood flow.[116] Several clinical reports[117-119] described neonatal cerebrovascular accidents after prenatal cocaine exposure in the setting of abruptio placentae or birth asphyxia, each of which is a known risk factor for neonatal cerebrovascular accident. A vascular cause is suggested by the cases of three neonates with porencephaly who were exposed to cocaine *in utero* and that of one neonate with bilateral occipital infarcts after an uncomplicated delivery.[120] Ultrasound examination of the head demonstrated an increased incidence of intracranial hemorrhage and cystic lucencies among cocaine-exposed neonates, at rates (30%) similar to those seen in infants with hypoxic-ischemic encephalopathy.[121] In addition, Doppler examination revealed increased cerebral blood flow in neonates with recent cocaine exposure.[122] Coupled with systemic hypertension, such an increase in cerebral blood flow could elevate intracranial pressure and could indirectly lead to intracranial hemorrhage.

To date, most studies assessing the reproductive neurotoxicity of cocaine have focused on neonatal and infant cognitive function. It is possible, however, that other neurologic damage may occur, causing attention deficit disorders or learning disabilities.[123]

Abnormal sleep patterns in neonates and infants have also been observed after prenatal maternal cocaine use.[105, 124] The risk of SIDS attributable to maternal cocaine use during pregnancy was investigated by several groups. A study[125] of 996 women who used cocaine during pregnancy revealed that of the 175 infants studied, 1 (0.6%) neonate from the cocaine-exposed group died of SIDS, whereas 4 (0.5%) neonates died among the 821 nonexposed control infants. The investigators concluded that cocaine did not increase the risk of SIDS in cocaine-exposed pregnancies.

Conversely, other studies[104, 106] postulated an increased risk of SIDS in neonates who were exposed to cocaine *in utero*. In these studies, 10 (18%) of 56 cocaine-exposed neonates died of SIDS. This figure is substantially different from other reported values and may suggest a sample-size effect or an inclusion or reporting bias. Chasnoff and co-workers[126] conducted a prospective study of cardiorespiratory patterns in 32 cocaine-exposed neonates and in 18 methadone-exposed neonates. Eight of the 32 cocaine-using women also abused heroin and were started on methadone maintenance therapy. Although 12 of 32 cocaine-exposed neonates and 1 of the 18 methadone-exposed neonates had abnormal pneumograms, no deaths were attributable to SIDS. Despite the methodologic weaknesses in the study design, the investigators concluded that prenatal exposure to cocaine appeared to be linked to cardiorespiratory abnormalities. It was not, however, specifically concluded that cocaine exposure was linked directly to SIDS. The same link was previously suggested by Ward and colleagues.[127] The relationship between cocaine use during pregnancy and SIDS is still not clear.[76]

The pathophysiology of SIDS is not completely elucidated. Many studies support the concept of abnormal CNS regulation of breathing as the most plausible mechanism.[128-130] Cocaine-mediated changes in the content of the biogenic amines, which are important respiratory control neurotransmitters, may be responsible for neonatal hypoxia. Alternatively, through the direct effect of cocaine-induced hypertension or, indirectly, through repeated episodes of hypoxia secondary to cocaine-mediated vasoconstriction of the placental vasculature, cocaine may disrupt brain structures essential to respiratory regulation.[131-133]

The effects of maternal cocaine abuse on the neonatal auditory system were studied in 18 newborns.[134] The auditory brain stem responses of neonates exposed to cocaine showed prolonged interpeak and absolute latencies (evoked potentials) compared with those of nonexposed control neonates. These abnormalities suggest a neurologic impairment or dysfunction such as delayed myelination, as well as altered DNA synthesis requiring further audiologic and neurologic follow-up.

The risk of major structural malformations attributable to *in utero* cocaine exposure is still undetermined. Results of a meta-analysis failed to show increased teratogenic risk after controlling for use of other drugs of abuse.[135] Cocaine use during pregnancy has also been associated with the risk that neonates may develop transient myocardial ischemia.[136] Transient ST-segment elevation and a lower ratio of low- to high-frequency power in the spectral analysis for heart rate variability reflected increased vagal activity in cocaine-exposed neonates.[136]

The fetal cardiovascular response to cocaine is postulated to be a combination of direct and indirect effects. There is an indirect effect of placental hypoperfusion, fetal hypoxia, and subsequent catecholamine release.[131] The direct effect of cocaine is at the level of the fetal noradrenergic-nerve terminal.[131]

The principal focus of published research on cocaine use is on the fetal risks associated with heavy maternal cocaine users whose practices and general health also add numerous confounding variables such as polydrug use, concomitant use of cigarettes and alcohol, higher risk of vaginal bleeding, hepatitis B carrier state, and poor prenatal care. Because constituents of smoke such as carbon monoxide and nicotine are known fetotoxicants,[137] Forman and associates[109] examined the outcome of neonates exposed to cocaine alone, and to cocaine and maternal smoking, to ascertain the effects attributable to cocaine, as opposed to those attributable to tobacco. The analysis revealed that most of the detrimental effects on the fetus and neonate were the result of cigarette smoking. These results are in agreement with an earlier meta-analysis.[138]

Very little research has focused on the potential risks of social maternal cocaine use. Most of these social cocaine users seem to discontinue their cocaine use once they are pregnant. A comparison[123] of social cocaine users to drug-free controls produced no evidence that neonates born to social cocaine users have an increased risk of perinatal complications, dysmorphology, or abnormal neurobehavioral development. Analysis of all available studies pertaining to maternal social cocaine consumption suggests that cocaine is not a major human teratogen and that neonates born to social cocaine users are normal in their physical and neurobehavioral development,[123] as evidenced by Bayley scores at 18 months of age.

There is, however, a subgroup of fetuses susceptible to the adverse effects of cocaine, probably because of variability in the maternal metabolism of cocaine,[139] the placental transfer of cocaine,[140] and the placental-vascular response to cocaine, as well as fetal pharmacodynamic variability.[123] Cocaine toxicity tends to reduce the activity of the choline esterase enzyme that metabolizes cocaine. Therefore, women using similar doses of cocaine vary significantly in placental and fetal exposure.

The reliability of the evaluation of the reproductive risks associated with cocaine use during pregnancy is dependent on the verification of fetal drug exposure, or nonexposure in the control groups. Fetal drug exposure is based on the mother's self-reports of gestational cocaine use and a positive result on the neonatal urine test, or a negative result on the neonatal urine test in the control groups. Cocaine has a short elimination half-life. If a woman chooses to deny her cocaine use and the urine tests are negative, her neonate may be erroneously identified as a non-exposed control subject.

To overcome this problem, a cocaine hair test can be used. Cocaine and benzoylecgonine incorporate into a growing hair shaft.[141] As is the case with nutrients, cocaine transfers into the growing hair shaft through the capillaries nourishing it. The cocaine hair test remains positive for the entire life span of the hair shaft of both the mother and the baby, often long after the urine tests are negative.[141]

The detection of cocaine in neonatal hair is an indicator of maternal cocaine use during the last months of pregnancy. The initial fetal hair, lanugo, sheds at 5 to 6 months of gestation. Neonatal hair grows throughout the third trimester of pregnancy and subsequently changes at 4 to 6 months' postnatal age. Therefore, detecting intrauterine drug exposure becomes a problem after this time. Because maternal hair grows at a rate of 1.0 to 1.5 cm per month, the hair test may also be used to determine the time of fetal drug exposure during gestation from an analysis of the maternal hair in sections. The clinician may use the results of this analysis to predict the extent and type of deleterious effects on the fetus attributable to the drug (based on the length of drug exposure *in utero*), to plan a clinical course of treatment for the fetus and neonate.

Neonatal signs such as abnormal sleep-wake cycles, tremulousness, poor feeding, hypotonia, and hyperreflexia have been documented in neonates exposed *in utero* to cocaine.[104, 105, 110] These neonatal signs may reflect the effects of cocaine's slow elimination in the newborn.[113] A study[106] of eight neonates exposed to cocaine *in utero* reported no withdrawal symptoms. Ascertaining the existence of a neonatal cocaine withdrawal syndrome is further complicated by the maternal cocaine abuser's concomitant use of opioids that are known to cause neonatal withdrawal symptoms.

Clinical Management of Pregnant Cocaine Abusers

A clinical management algorithm for the treatment of cocaine abuse is dependent on the extent of the mother's cocaine use and all associated medical and social problems. Irregular use of cocaine does not imply that the dependence on the drug is less severe. Most patients can be managed on an outpatient basis, although some women need hospitalization. Maternal cocaine withdrawal is characterized by periods of depression ranging from hours to days, hypersomnolence, and hyperphagia, followed by a period of high energy and an intense craving for cocaine.[94] Unless the depression is severe, no pharmacologic therapy is recommended. A careful history is always essential because cocaine abusers frequently use other drugs in combination with cocaine, for which treatment may be necessary.

Neonatal symptoms of hyperexcitability can be treated with the administration of benzodiazepines as necessary to effectively control symptoms. Withdrawal symptoms should be managed supportively.

Cigarette Smoking

Epidemiologic data indicate that cigarette smoking in the Western world has been gradually declining, more so in men than in women. The prevalence of smoking during pregnancy decreased from 40 to 25% between 1967 and 1980.[142] This decrease was seen primarily in highly educated populations.

Pharmacology of Nicotine

In addition to the well-described long-term health hazards attributable to smoking, exposure to carbon monoxide from cigarette smoke produces a progressive rise in maternal and fetal carboxyhemoglobin concentrations that parallels a fall in tissue oxygen delivery as the smoking day progresses. Carbon monoxide readily crosses the placenta. Several hours are required for the fetal carboxyhemoglobin concentration to equilibrate with maternal concentrations. Final fetal concentrations eventually become higher than maternal concentrations because fetal hemoglobin has a greater affinity for carbon monoxide and because the elimination half-life from the fetal circulation is longer than that from the maternal circulation.[137] One smoking day may result in a maternal carboxyhemoglobin concentration of 12% and a fetal concentration that is 10 to 15% higher. A 10% carbon monoxide level means that the delivery of oxygen to the fetus may actually be reduced by as much as 20 to 25% because carbon monoxide is also bound to the cytochrome enzymes. In addition, other compounds in tobacco smoke, such as thiocyanate and other cyanides, bind irreversibly to fetal and maternal hemoglobin to reduce oxygen delivery even further.

Intense uterine vasoconstriction[143] and a rapid fall in the uterine blood flow have been attributed to nicotine concentrations similar to those measured in arterial blood after smoke inhalation. These effects are produced by nicotine-mediated catecholamine release from the adrenal glands. Fetal hypoxemia often accompanies this vasoconstrictive effect.

Nicotine is readily absorbed by the oral mucosa, respiratory tract, gastrointestinal tract, and skin. Eighty to 90% of nicotine is metabolized in the liver, and smaller amounts are metabolized in the lung and kidney. The volume of distribution of nicotine is 2.0 L/kg in smokers and 3.0 L/kg in nonsmokers.[144] Nicotine is rapidly transferred from the maternal serum to the breast milk. Nicotine concentrations in breast milk are linearly correlated with those measured in maternal serum.[145] Both nicotine and cotinine (the major metabolite of nicotine) transfer into breast milk.[146-148] The mean elimination half-life of nicotine in breast milk is 92 ± 15 minutes, and in plasma it is 81 ± 9 minutes. Heavy maternal smoking may alter the milk supply and may cause nausea and vomiting in the neonate.[1] Nicotine and its metabolites are excreted primarily by the kidneys. Cotinine has an elimination half-life of 10 to 20 hours.[149]

Effects of Cigarette Smoking on the Fetus and Neonate

Studies[64, 150] have shown an association between maternal smoking throughout pregnancy and increased risks of spontaneous abortion, placenta previa and abruptio placentae, early or late gestational bleeding, and IUGR. Morphologically, placentas in women who smoke are markedly different from those of nonsmoking women. The placenta of a smoker tends to be heavier and has a greater degree of infarction, calcification, and vascular anomalies.

In a review[151] conducted to ascertain whether perinatal fetal mortality was increased among mothers who smoked, 5 of 17 studies found significantly increased risks of stillbirth among infants born to smoking women. The risk of perinatal mortality may not be equally distributed and may vary with maternal age, parity, the ethnic group, and socioeconomic status.[152] A study[153] from Sweden found that smoking was associated with a higher risk of early neonatal mortality.

A reduction in fetal growth has been associated with maternal smoking. In that regard, Scholl and colleagues[154] demonstrated that smokers were 3.1 times more likely than nonsmokers to deliver a small for gestational age neonate. Neonatal weights averaged 272 g less than those in the nonsmoking group. A quantitative dose-and-effect relation between tobacco exposure and decreased gestational age at birth and size of the neonate has been reported.[155] The lower oxygen saturation in infants of heavy smokers may adversely affect fetal growth. Alternatively, a reduction in epidermal growth factor (EGF)–stimulated autophosphorylation may be associated with IUGR.[156] EGF is normally involved in human embryouterine signaling and implantation,[157] *in vitro* stimulation of syncytiotrophoblast formation,[158, 159] and modulation of placental endocrine functions.[158-161] Receptor autophosphorylation is required for EGF to elicit normal placental cell division and differentiation.[156] Conversely, abnormal development of the placenta may interfere with fetal growth.[162] Gabriel and associates[156] and Wang and co-workers[163] showed that EGF receptor autophosphorylation was significantly reduced in the placental membranes of smokers with small for gestational age neonates compared with the placental membranes of smokers who delivered neonates without IUGR and those of nonsmokers. Gabriel and colleagues[156] concluded that IUGR in women who smoked during pregnancy is associated with an alteration in the EGF receptor bioactivity of the placenta and suggested that the regulatory role of EGF in placental growth and differentiation is defective in smokers.

A case-controlled study[164] of childhood cancer described a dose-response relationship between the number of cigarettes smoked per day by the mother during pregnancy and the risk of cancer in her children. A 50% higher incidence of cancer was found in infants exposed prenatally to cigarette smoke than among controls. The risks for the development of Hodgkin disease, acute lymphoblastic leukemia, and Wilms' tumor were also higher. The incidence of neonatal respiratory distress syndrome is reduced by smoking.[165] However, children exposed to smoke during pregnancy tend to manifest a higher incidence of bronchitis and pneumonia during their first year of life.[166-169] A higher incidence of neonatal respiratory tract infections has also been linked to maternal cigarette smoking.[170] Smoking has been shown to decrease the production of breast milk.[171] Said and co-workers[172] reported that maternal smoking during pregnancy may contribute to the incidence of neonatal colic.

Epidemiologic evidence clearly supports a link between maternal smoking and SIDS, but these studies fail to make the critical differentiation between fetal nicotine exposure and passive postpartum nicotine exposure, consequently weakening the association. Naeye and associates[173] stipulated that the strength of this correlation increased with maternal smoking of six or more cigarettes per day. Passive inhalation of smoke also increases the risk of SIDS for infants.[174] In another study,[175] researchers found that maternal smoking during pregnancy doubled the risk of SIDS from 2.3 to 4.6 per 1000 births. None of these studies, however, attempted to differentiate between intrauterine exposure and passive exposure to smoke after birth. Malloy and colleagues[176] studied the relationship between maternal smoking and the age and cause of infant death, rather than using SIDS deaths as the endpoint. This group concluded that maternal smoking was associated with a nearly twofold increase in SIDS. Haglund and Cnattinguis[177] concluded that maternal smoking of up to 9 cigarettes per day doubled the risk of neonatal SIDS, and smoking 10 or more cigarettes per day tripled the risk of SIDS, compared with the risk of nonsmoking controls. Both Malloy and colleagues[176] and Haglund and Cnattinguis[177] acknowledged that a study of passive smoking by either partner after birth was not conducted, and passive smoking may in fact contribute to the incidence of neonatal SIDS.

To study the effects of maternal smoking on the cognitive development of 3-year-old children, a 700 mother-child pair study[178] was conducted. Extensive information on growth and development, including cognitive development test results, was included in the study variables. The investigators concluded that the cognitive performance of infants born to women who continued to smoke throughout their pregnancies was significantly compromised, at least to the third year of life, after correcting for known confounding variables. Relative hypoxemia may have long-term effects on the developing brain.

Clinical Management of Smokers During Pregnancy

The goal of maternal therapy for smoking during pregnancy is to improve fetal outcome by preventing associated prenatal complications. Education and support are required for pregnant smoking women. The use of nicotine replacement therapy in pregnancy has been tried but with low effectiveness.[179] It is possible that this is the result of doubling of the clearance rate of nicotine in late pregnancy, thus rendering levels subtherapeutic.[180-181] Bupropion is an effective agent for smoking cessation. The manufacturer's registry suggests that it is not teratogenic when used in clinical doses.

Marijuana

After alcohol, the second most commonly used recreational drug in the United States is marijuana. Marijuana, or cannabis, is produced from the flowering tops of hemp plants from which at least 61 cannabinoids and more than 300 naturally occurring compounds can be extracted. The isomer 1-Δ^9-tetrahydrocannabinoid (THC) is the most potent psychoactive compound among the cannabinoids. THC and other cannabinoids are C_{21}-substituted monoterpenoid compounds.

The exact mechanism responsible for the pharmacodynamics of marijuana is unknown. Marijuana produces a carbon monoxide level five times higher than that produced by cigarette smoking.[179] The resulting high carboxyhemoglobin concentration may affect fetal oxygenation and hence fetal growth and development.[180]

Pharmacology of Marijuana

The amount of systemically absorbed THC from a single inhaled dose is between 10 and 50% (mean 18%). The bioavailability of an oral dose is substantially lower.[181-187] The peak plasma concentration after oral administration is attained within 45 minutes and remains relatively constant for 4 to 6 hours.[188] The peak plasma concentration after smoking marijuana is attained after 7 to 8 minutes. Thirty to 60 minutes from the initial time the user consumes the drug, tachycardia and euphoria occur.

THC is almost 100% protein bound. The drug is highly lipid soluble. Plasma levels decline rapidly after inhalation, and a slow elimination phase ensues. The volume of distribution is estimated to be 10 L/kg.[106] The elimination half-life in long-term users is 20 hours compared with 25 to 57 hours in nonusers, primarily because of the faster metabolism of the long-term user.[188-191]

THC is almost entirely converted to the active metabolite 11-hydroxy-THC on first pass through the liver. The effect of the active metabolite is identical to that of the parent drug. This metabolite is subsequently biotransformed to inactive metabolites that are excreted by the kidneys. Less than 1% of THC is excreted unchanged in the urine. Metabolites excreted in the bile can be reabsorbed. Fecal excretion is the major route of elimination of unconjugated cannabinoid metabolites.

Both animal and human studies[192-194] have shown that Δ^9-THC crosses the placenta. The maternal blood concentration of the drug is 2.5 to 6 times higher than that of fetal blood. Length of exposure increases the fetal/maternal concentration ratio. In heavy users, there is an eightfold accumulation of Δ^9-THC in breast milk compared with that in maternal plasma.[195, 196] The nursing neonate can therefore consume Δ^9-THC from the mother's breast milk.

Effects of Marijuana Use on the Fetus and Neonate

As with other drugs of abuse, data collected from mothers who use THC must be interpreted cautiously, considering that these users may practice polydrug abuse and that any self-reported statistics may be grossly inaccurate. In fact, polydrug use may account for the poorer prenatal care received by the fetuses of marijuana users.[197]

The effect of THC on pregnancy outcome has received much attention. Documented effects of cannabinoids on pituitary and ovarian function, prolactin secretion, hormonal activity, and uterine contractility have been amassed from animal and human studies.[198] No relationship between marijuana use during pregnancy and the length of gestation, duration of labor, or birth weight is evident.[199] Heightened tremors, abnormal startle responses, and altered visual responsiveness have been observed in neonates born to women who abused THC.

In a study[200] of pregnancy course and outcome in 35 regular marijuana users and 36 age- and parity-matched nonusers, the neonates of marijuana users exhibited a common tendency toward anemia, poor weight gain, and IUGR. However, the results were not statistically significant and may be indicative of confounding variable clustering. A higher proportion of THC users (29 mothers) than nonusers (3 mothers) experienced prolonged, protracted, or arrested labor. These results have been confirmed by other reports.[201-203] Marijuana abusers also exhibited a higher proportion of fetal distress and more often required manual removal of the placenta. The course of labor appeared to be more hazardous in the THC user group than in the nonuser control group.

THC users also were found to have an increased risk of meconium passage by the fetus. This potentially increases the risk of neonatal mortality.[1,204] In contrast, Fried and associates[205] did not find any evidence to support increased meconium staining among neonates born to heavy marijuana users.

The effects of marijuana use during pregnancy on infant birth weight and length of gestation are controversial. In a study by Fried and colleagues,[201] neonates born to women consuming marijuana six or more times per week during pregnancy had a significant reduction of 0.8 week in the length of gestation, after controlling for the effects of nicotine and alcohol, parity, maternal prepregnancy weight, and the gender of the neonate. There was no reduction in the birth weight of these neonates. However, in another study,[202] the investigators reported contradictory results: reduced birth weight and no changes in the length of gestation were associated with marijuana use. The difference between these two study outcomes may be attributed to the women's young age and low socioeconomic status in the latter study. Moreover, it is possible that alcohol may have caused these minor differences because many women abusing THC also consume large amounts of alcohol.[194,205]

Any association between minor physical anomalies and prenatal marijuana exposure is controversial. No difference was observed in the frequency of anomalies in the children of 25 marijuana-using women and the children of 25 matched nonuser controls.[186] Similar observations have been reported in other studies.[206,207]

A link between prenatal marijuana exposure and the associated features of FAS has been demonstrated.[186, 202, 203, 206, 207] Thirty-one (2%) of 1384 neonates born to women who smoked marijuana had typical features of FAS. The incidence of delivering a neonate with FAS is five times higher in cannabinoid users than in nonusers.

The Brazelton Neonatal Behavioral Assessment scale[208] was used to correlate smoking cannabinoids during pregnancy with a decrease in neonates' response to light directed at their eyes. Forty-six per cent of the neonates born to users of cannabinoids did not respond to the light, in contrast with 16% of those born to matched nonusers.[209, 210] Neonates born to methadone-using mothers showed a similarly poor visual response. In the infants with both marijuana and methadone exposure, the neonatal response to auditory stimulation was normal.[211,212] Other characteristic features seen in neonates born to heavy cannabinoid users include marked tremor, mainly around day 9 of postnatal life, and a startle reflex. Cortical electrical responses in the exposed neonates appeared to be slightly slower than those of age-matched controls. Similar neonatal outcomes have been documented in cases of *in utero* exposure to alcohol and nicotine. Other visual abnormalities, including myopia, strabismus, and unusual optic disks, occur at a higher frequency in marijuana-exposed (33%) than in nonexposed (6%) neonates.[213,214]

The findings of neurologic dysfunction could be interpreted as symptoms of neonatal drug withdrawal. In the adult population, however, abstinence after heavy THC use produces mild withdrawal reactions that encompass restlessness, sleeplessness, anorexia, nausea, vomiting, dreaming, and sweating.[1] Neonates exposed *in utero* to THC are not more irritable than neonates born to women in the non–marijuana-smoking control groups.[1]

Clinical Management of Marijuana Smokers During Pregnancy

Marijuana may be consumed concomitantly with multiple drugs and cigarettes, in which case treatment must be initiated to treat the deleterious effects of the more dangerous drugs and chemicals being used during the pregnancy. Education and support for pregnant marijuana smokers are paramount.

Opioids

Opiates are natural compounds derived from the opium poppy; opioids are synthetically derived analgesic compounds that have morphinelike pharmacodynamic activity. In the United States, there are more than 500,000 opiate and opioid addicts, of whom 70,000 are enrolled in methadone maintenance treatment programs.[215] Neonates exposed *in utero* to either heroin or methadone account for 3 to 5% of live births in New York City municipal hospitals.[215]

Heroin or diacetylmorphine is derived from morphine and produces pharmacologic effects identical to those of morphine. Heroin has a greater solubility and crosses into the CNS more rapidly than morphine, thus making heroin the drug of choice among opioid addicts. Methadone is a synthetic opioid that is different from morphine, but it has nearly identical pharmacodynamic effects. Methadone is principally used in clinical medicine to treat heroin addiction[216] and to manage pain.

Low socioeconomic class, a long history of drug abuse, frequent and multiple medical complications, poor diet, heavy smoking, and the concomitant use of alcohol, marijuana, cocaine, barbiturates, or tranquilizers are the characteristic hallmarks of the opioid addict. Adverse effects of heroin and methadone addiction are encountered frequently.

Pharmacology of Opioids

Opioids affect the activity of neurons involved with respiration, pain perception, and affective behavior. Morphine is an opioid analgesic that exerts its primary effect on the CNS and organs containing smooth muscle. The drug functions as an agonist at specific, saturable opioid μ receptors in these regions. Pharmacologic effects include analgesia, decreased gastric motility, suppression of the cough reflex, respiratory depression, CNS depression, nausea and vomiting, euphoria and dysphoria, sedation (fetal), mental clouding, and alterations of the endocrine and autonomic nervous systems.[217]

Morphine is readily absorbed by the gastrointestinal tract and undergoes significant first-pass metabolism in the liver. The oral bioavailability of morphine is less than 5% in most users. Peak blood concentrations after intramuscular or subcutaneous injection are attained within 30 minutes. Tissue concentrations are quite low within 24 hours after the last dose because morphine does not persist in the tissue for extended periods.

The elimination half-life of morphine in adults is between 2 and 3 hours (mean, 1.9 ± 0.5 hours). There are significant variations in the mean duration of action, ranging from 2.5 to 4.2 hours. Morphine is $35 \pm 2\%$ protein bound,[218] and the clearance of the drug is 2.02 L/hour/kg in healthy young adults and 1.66 L/hour/kg in elderly patients.[219] The elimination half-life of morphine in neonates is between 6 and 14 hours.[220-222] The neonatal clearance of morphine is 1.43 L/hour/kg.[222-225] There is no published information on the oral bioavailability of morphine in neonates. However, the neonatal bioavailability of morphine is probably incomplete, as it is in older children.[220]

Ten per cent of an administered dose of morphine is excreted through the bile; the remainder is excreted in the urine as a glucuronide conjugate. Morphine is metabolized primarily by glucuronidation. Glucuronic acid conjugation of the phenolic hydroxyl group via uridine diphosphate–glucuronyltransferase causes the conversion of morphine into morphine-3-glucuronide (M3G), morphine-6-glucuronide (M6G), and normorphine. Although M3G is quantitatively the major metabolite, M6G is up to 40 times more potent than the parent compound and is thought to be the substance responsible for the analgesic properties of morphine. Morphine is O-methylated to produce codeine. Heroin is deacetylated to form morphine and 6-monoacetylmorphine (6-MAM). 6-MAM has been shown to be pharmacologically equipotent to heroin. It is thought that the characteristic pharmacodynamic effects of heroin are mediated by 6-MAM and morphine. Morphine, heroin, and methadone cross the placenta by simple diffusion.

Methadone is well absorbed from the gastrointestinal tract; peak plasma concentrations are attained within 4 hours. There is not a good correlation between plasma levels and analgesia.[226] A plasma level of 211 μg/L has been associated with the best rehabilitation results in patients receiving methadone maintenance therapy.[227] The oral bioavailability of methadone is 92 ± 21%,[218] and the drug is 89% plasma protein bound. Methadone has a volume of distribution of 3.8±0.1 L/kg and a clearance of 0.08±0.03 L/hour/kg. It is metabolized to form pyrrolidines and pyrrolines, which are excreted in the urine and bile; 24 ± 10% of the drug is excreted in the urine unchanged.[218] Methadone has a longer elimination half-life than morphine, 14.3 hours for the α–phase and 54.8 hours for the β–phase,[228] and it causes less sedation and euphoria. Nausea and vomiting are rare.

Effects of Opioid Use on the Fetus and Neonate

A significantly lower birth weight, shorter length, and smaller head circumference have been observed in neonates who have been exposed in utero to heroin or methadone.[229] The effects on infant growth variables are thought to be a direct result of fetal opioid exposure. These infants catch up in weight and length by 1 year of age. The head circumference of the opioid-exposed infant does not exhibit a catch-up to an appropriate size for age until at least 2 years of age.[1]

Early stunting of growth may be methadone's direct effect on the hypothalamic-hypophyseal axis of the neonate.[230] Neonatal recovery is associated with decreased methadone plasma and tissue concentrations.

Growth retardation in infants born to heroin addicts is attributable mainly to a decrease in cell numbers.[181] Neonates born to women addicted to heroin alone and the combination of heroin and methadone had mean birth weights of 2490 and 2535 g, respectively.[231] Neonates in the control group born to women who did not use heroin or methadone had a mean birth weight of 3176 g. In heroin- and methadone-addicted mothers, a higher incidence of small for gestational age neonates (35 and 22%, respectively) has been reported.[232] In contrast, a lower incidence of small for gestational age neonates (16.5%) was reported in 830 neonates born to drug-addicted women.[233] A 20% incidence of Apgar scores less than 7 at 1 minute post partum has been documented for neonates of drug-addicted or heroin- or methadone-addicted women, representing a twofold higher incidence compared with those of controls. A similar trend in Apgar scores has been reported at 5 minutes post partum.[231,234] In addition, a twofold increase in premature deliveries over a 10-year period was observed in 384 neonates born to heroin-addicted mothers.[235] The incidence of premature deliveries was only slightly higher (7%) in methadone-addicted mothers.[184]

Infants born to heroin addicts exhibit a lower incidence of hyaline membrane disease than those born to nonaddicted women.[236] Opioids such as heroin may induce enzymes to accel-

erate the production of pulmonary surfactant in the fetus. In neonates exposed to opioids during pregnancy, there is a shift to the right in the oxyhemoglobin-dissociation curve in umbilical cord samples and increased 2,3-diphosphoglycerate concentrations in the neonatal red blood cells.[237] 2,3-Diphosphoglycerate decreases fetal hemoglobin affinity for oxygen. Therefore, the enhanced ability of red blood cells to deliver more oxygen to the tissues may contribute to the decreased incidence of hyaline membrane disease. Moreover, neonates exhibiting heroin withdrawal symptoms have respiratory alkalosis in the first few days of life. This may be another protective mechanism because acidosis is a predisposing factor for respiratory distress syndrome. In the first 3 days of neonatal life, a less common severe hyperbilirubinemia occurs in neonates of opioid-addicted women.[235,238]

The incidence of SIDS is increased 5- to 10-fold in neonates born to opioid-addicted women.[239,240] However, an association between SIDS and prenatal opioid exposure has not yet been clearly established, primarily because no comparative drug study has been conducted, other than studies of the opioids used by pregnant women. For neonates exposed to opioids in utero, it may be prudent to initiate cardiorespiratory monitoring. Moreover, neonates with apnea may benefit from 1.5 mg/kg of theophylline (Theo-Dur) every 6 hours.[241] In a study[242] of 1760 cases of SIDS, the risk ratio for SIDS was 3.6 for methadone, 2.3 for heroin, 3.2 for methadone and heroin, and 1.1 for cocaine and methadone or heroin consumption (after controlling for the associated high-risk confounding variables). Despite the consensus linking maternal opioid use to SIDS, no proof of causation has been developed. The most plausible hypothesis suggests that morphine and related opioids reduce brain stem responsiveness to carbon dioxide[243] and depress the pontine and medullary centers that control respiratory rhythmicity.[244] Most of these data, however, are derived from adult studies. Studies of the prolonged effects of opioids on infants after intrauterine exposure are scarce. In one such study, Olsen and Lees[245] examined the ventilatory response to carbon dioxide in nine methadone-exposed neonates and four control neonates. The investigators showed a minimal response to carbon dioxide in drug-exposed neonates during the first 4 days of life that persisted for an average of 15 days. No relationship was evident between ventilatory response and the maternal dose of methadone, serum methadone half-life, or the need to treat neonatal abstinence.

A weaker link between maternal opioid use and neonatal SIDS was postulated by Naeye,[246] who suggested that infants dying of SIDS actually were suffering from chronic hypoxia and chronic hypoxemia. The tissue markers noted during autopsies that support this postulate are shown in Table 25-3.[246] However, none of these markers has been specifically studied in opioid-exposed neonates dying of SIDS. In addition, no evidence exists to indicate that chronic postnatal hypoxia occurs in these infants.[76] Prenatal growth retardation and meconium staining are considered hallmarks of fetal hypoxia and have been observed in neonates exposed to heroin.[247] Hence, predisposition of the neonate to SIDS may occur by opioid-induced chronic intrauterine hypoxia,

TABLE 25-3

Tissue Markers of Chronic Hypoxia and Hypoxemia in Infants Dying of Sudden Infant Death Syndrome

Carotid body gliomic tissue changes
Increased tissue in the adrenal medulla
Abnormal gliosis in brain stem centers controlling respiratory drive
Thickened pulmonary arterial walls
Increased weight of the right cardiac ventricle
Retention of periadrenal brown fat
Increased hepatic erythropoiesis

causing damage to the brain centers regulating respiration. This would elicit the brain stem gliosis described by Naeye.[76]

In a study[229] that used the Brazelton Neonatal Behavioral Assessment scale, opioid-exposed neonates exhibited significant impairment of interactive abilities, motor maturity, and organizational response compared with their nonexposed counterparts. These neonates were more irritable and tremulous compared with control neonates who were not exposed to prenatal opioid consumption. Opioid-exposed neonates also demonstrated deficits in general cognitive abilities and in visual, auditory, and tactile perception. Mothers of neonates exposed to methadone have noted sleep disturbances.[248] These disturbances include irritability, excitability, inability to nap, and various other sleep irregularities. A significant reduction in the complications attributable to opioid abuse was demonstrated when addicted, pregnant women were given comprehensive care that included enrollment in a methadone maintenance regimen of 20 mg/day or less.[249]

Rates of malformation in infants of opioid users are typically not different from those of control groups. In addition, no homogenous pattern of malformation has been established. However, in a study of 830 opioid-exposed neonates, 2.4% demonstrated major malformations, compared with 0.5% in a control group.[231] However, the findings of this study should be viewed with caution, because the rates of major malformation are known to range between 1 and 3% in the general population. In another study, Harper and associates[238] found malformations in 5.9% of neonates born to women in a methadone treatment program. These figures may not represent an increased risk, however. Several other studies[232, 250] failed to demonstrate an increased risk of malformation in neonates prenatally exposed to opioids.

There has been no increased frequency or discernible pattern of teratogenic effects in infants born to women abusing heroin.[251, 252] In reports implicating heroin in congenital anomalies, the findings have been questioned, because the patient population was poorly defined for confounding variables such as polydrug use by the pregnant women. Low birth weight and an increased incidence of meconium staining constitute reported perinatal adverse effects associated with maternal heroin use. After prolonged and continuous heroin use by the mother during pregnancy, narcotic withdrawal occurs in many neonates. Strabismus has been observed in 21% of opioid-exposed neonates compared with 2.8 to 5.3% in the general population.[183, 253]

Morphine is believed to be excreted into breast milk in small, clinically insignificant amounts.[254] Despite the widespread licit and illicit use of morphine, there is a paucity of information on exposure to the drug through breast milk. With the advent of highly sensitive radioimmunoassays and specific high-performance liquid chromatography analytical techniques, new data are becoming available to discern morphine kinetics in the nursing neonate. Robieux and colleagues[255] presented a case report of a nursing woman with systemic lupus erythematosus who was receiving morphine therapy to treat severe arthritic back pain. The neonate had a 4 ng/mL morphine plasma concentration; breast milk concentrations ranged from 10 to 100 ng/mL. The dose needed to achieve the observed morphine plasma concentration in the neonate was calculated to range between 0.8 and 12% of the maternal dose. This case demonstrates that neonates have significant exposure to morphine even when the mother consumes morphine at low doses.

Neonatal withdrawal syndrome is evident primarily after maternal heroin and methadone abuse during pregnancy. However, the syndrome can manifest after prenatal codeine, pentazocine, and propoxyphene exposure. The signs and symptoms are similar; however, methadone-exposed neonates experience more frequent and more severe signs than neonates of heroin-addicted women.[232, 256] The amount of methadone consumed by the mother appears to correlate with the severity of the ensuing neonatal withdrawal. Although the onset of symptoms may vary from minutes to 2 weeks post partum, in most neonates, withdrawal manifests within 48 hours. The duration of acute neonatal withdrawal ranges from a few days to several weeks.[185] CNS excitation, altered gastrointestinal tract function, respiratory distress, and autonomic symptoms characterize the neonatal opioid withdrawal syndrome. Irritability is the most common manifestation, followed by tremors and hypertonicity. Seizure activity may appear between 3 and 34 days post partum in 2 to 11% of addicted neonates.[257]

Neonates born to opioid-addicted women occasionally demonstrate seizure activity.[257] It appears that methadone-exposed neonates have a higher incidence of seizure activity compared with neonates exposed to heroin.

Neonates exposed to low doses of morphine *in utero* or through breast milk may not always exhibit the morphine withdrawal syndrome. The reason for this lack of the syndrome may be the extended half-life of morphine during early life, which results in a slow decline in the concentration of morphine in neonatal plasma.[222] Alternatively, the neonate may have developed tolerance to the opioid after long-term exposure *in utero* and throughout the breast-feeding period.[255]

Clinical Management of Opioid-Addicted Women and Neonates

Mild withdrawal from opioids does not usually necessitate treatment. The treatment of neonatal withdrawal syndrome is primarily symptomatic. Symptomatic neonates may require pharmacologic intervention. Pharmacologic preparations used to treat neonatal withdrawal include paregoric (camphorated tincture of opium), morphine (Astramorph), methadone (Dolophine), diazepam (Valium), chlorpromazine (Thorazine), phenobarbital (Barbita), and clonidine (Catapres).[258-260]

The two most popular agents seem to be paregoric and phenobarbital. Paregoric contains 0.4 mg/mL anhydrous morphine and is therefore a more physiologic substance because it substitutes for the drug that is causing the withdrawal symptoms. The recommended dose for full-term neonates is 0.2 to 0.5 mL (0.08 to 0.20 mg anhydrous morphine) administered orally every 3 to 4 hours until the symptoms are well controlled.[261] The initial paregoric dose is dependent on the severity of the withdrawal symptoms. The severity is assessed based on the Finnegan Scoring System.[262] If within 4 hours there is no observed clinical improvement, the paregoric dose is increased by 0.05 mL every 4 hours until it has an effect. When the withdrawal score is sustained for 48 hours, the dose of paregoric should be reduced by 10% each day while a constant dosing interval is maintained. The recommended dose for paregoric in premature infants is 0.05 mL/kg every 4 hours initially, with increments of 0.02 mL/kg every 4 hours until symptoms are controlled. Neonates treated with paregoric exhibited more physiologic sucking patterns, higher caloric intake, better weight gain, and improved control of seizure activity and gastrointestinal disturbances than did neonates who were treated with phenobarbital.[263, 264]

Overall, the opioid paregoric appears to be more effective than diazepam, phenobarbital, or paraldehyde in ameliorating withdrawal. A randomly assigned clinical trial,[265] however, found no significant difference between the clinical efficacy of paregoric and that of phenobarbital. The advantages of using phenobarbital to treat neonatal withdrawal include the drug's ability to mitigate symptoms referable to the CNS and its safety. Phenobarbital is safer than an opioid[266] when sedation is required. The disadvantages include the inability to titrate the dose because of the long elimination half-life, the presence of other chemicals in the formulation, and the lack of standard dosing guidelines for phenobarbital.

The duration of therapy is dependent on the extent of the maternal addiction and the duration of fetal exposure. A treatment regimen spanning 10 to 20 days is required in approximately 50% of opioid-exposed neonates. Twenty-five per cent require treatment for a longer duration, and the remaining 25% require a shorter course of treatment.[267] Paregoric-treated neonates require a significantly longer period of active treatment compared with phenobarbital-treated neonates, probably because of the longer half-life of phenobarbital.

In the clinical management of addicted women during pregnancy, the clinician must be acutely aware that two patients are actually being treated. Therefore, a treatment regimen must be chosen that maximizes the benefits for both mother and fetus. In late pregnancy, abrupt maternal withdrawal may be accompanied by fetal withdrawal, typically characterized by hyperactivity, hypoxia, passage of meconium, and death.[268, 269] Opioid antagonists such as naloxone (Narcan) should be administered to the pregnant woman only if she experiences a life-threatening overdose. Naloxone crosses the placenta to exert its antagonistic effects on the fetus, thus potentially exacerbating the neonate's withdrawal reaction.

Heroin addicts should be encouraged to enroll in a methadone maintenance program.[270] Methadone suppresses withdrawal symptoms and, in high doses, may block the opioid effect. In addition to decreasing illicit drug use, these programs improve fetal and subsequently neonatal outcome. An obstetrician who is skilled in monitoring high-risk pregnancies should be part of the maternal treatment team because of the potential adverse effects on the fetus attributable to maternal detoxification.

Psychotherapeutic Drugs

The psychotherapeutic drugs include amphetamines, sedatives, tranquilizers, and analgesics. Based on the results of the National Pregnancy and Health Survey,[3] it was estimated that 1.5% of women using some illicit substance in the United States during pregnancy used psychotherapeutic drugs. The nonmedical use of these agents was highest in black women (3.1%), followed by women of Hispanic descent (1.8%) and white women of non-Hispanic origin (1.1%).

Benzodiazepines are widely used for therapeutic reasons and are frequently consumed by polydrug users.[271] Abuse of the benzodiazepines in high doses is not as common as it has been, but some women have been maintained on long-term therapeutic doses for many years. Because of the limited availability of these drugs, abuse of barbiturate and nonbarbiturate hypnosedatives is also not as prevalent as was described previously. These drugs include chloral hydrate (Noctec), glutethimide (Doriden), meprobamate (Equanil), and methaqualone. Butalbital (Fiorinal) is the only frequently abused barbiturate.[272] It is available only as a proprietary combination of aspirin and caffeine with or without codeine.

Amphetamines rank about 10th to 11th in the abused-drug groups. Amphetamine levels are found in about 2% of cases amassed from small, random analytical surveys of emergency department toxicology screens.[273] Illicit amphetamine formulations vary dramatically in potency and in impurity.[274]

Pharmacology of Psychotherapeutic Drugs

Benzodiazepines are weakly basic drugs absorbed most effectively at the high pH found in the duodenum. The oral absorption of diazepam and desmethyldiazepam, the active metabolite of clorazepate, is faster than that of the other benzodiazepines. Oral absorption is extremely rapid for triazolam. After intramuscular injection, the bioavailability of several benzodiazepines, including chlordiazepoxide and diazepam, may be unreliable. The barbiturates are weak acids that are very rapidly absorbed into the blood from the stomach and small intestine.[275]

The benzodiazepines and other sedative-hypnotic drugs cross the human placenta, thus exposing the fetus. The rate at which the maternal and fetal blood concentrations equilibrate is slower than the rate at which the maternal blood and CNS equilibrate, partially because of the lower blood flow to the placenta.[275] Benzodiazepines are highly plasma albumin bound; binding ranges from 60% to more than 95%.

The elimination of benzodiazepines occurs through hepatic metabolism. Most benzodiazepines undergo microsomal oxidation reactions such as N-demethylation and aliphatic hydroxylation. The metabolites are conjugated by glucuronosyltransferase to form glucuronides that are excreted in the urine. Many benzodiazepines have pharmacologically active metabolites. There is a wide range (12 to 150 hours) in the elimination half-life of the various benzodiazepines. Only insignificant amounts of barbiturates (except phenobarbital) are excreted unchanged. The major barbiturate metabolic pathway involves oxidation by hepatic enzymes. Few barbiturate metabolites are pharmacologically active. The elimination half-life of the barbiturates ranges from 18 hours (secobarbital and pentobarbital) to 4 to 5 days (phenobarbital).[275]

After an oral dose of 10 to 25 mg, peak plasma levels of amphetamines occur within 1 to 2 hours. Protein binding ranges between 15 and 34%, depending on the specific drug.[276] Amphetamines are rapidly absorbed from the gastrointestinal tract, and absorption is usually complete within 4 to 6 hours.[276] Amphetamines decrease gastric emptying and intestinal motility, thus enabling polydrug users to extend the time for absorption as the drugs pass through the stomach and intestines. The elimination half-life of amphetamines is in the range of 8 to 12 hours after therapeutic dosing, and 18 to 24 hours after abusive consumption. Amphetamines are metabolized by deamination to form phenylacetone that is subsequently oxidized to benzoic acid and excreted as a glucuronide conjugate.[277] β-Hydroxylation produces the active metabolite O-hydroxynorephedrine, which accounts for some of the drug's effects in long-term users.

Effects of Psychotherapeutic Drugs on the Fetus and Neonate

There are reports[278, 279] of increased risk of cleft lip and cleft palate after first trimester exposure to benzodiazepines, although a subsequent case-controlled study[280] did not confirm those observations. Late third trimester use and exposure during labor may be associated with greater risks of the development of floppy infant syndrome or marked neonatal withdrawal symptoms ranging from mild neonatal sedation, hypotonia, and reluctance to suck to apneic episodes, cyanosis, and impaired metabolic responses to cold stress.[281] No specific neonatal abnormalities have been reported in cases of prenatal exposure to the newer benzodiazepines. A fetal benzodiazepine abstinence syndrome[282] was reported in seven cases; however, because of inadequate controls, a causative role remains speculative.[283] There are no published reports of human teratogenicity attributable to benzodiazepine use during pregnancy.[284]

Neonatal benzodiazepine withdrawal symptoms, including seizures, are indistinguishable from narcotic or barbiturate withdrawal symptoms.[285] Neonatal withdrawal symptoms have been reported even when the mother received therapeutic doses of chlordiazepoxide[286, 287] and diazepam.[282, 288] The onset of neonatal symptoms may occur soon or several days after birth. Case reports of neonatal withdrawal from hydroxyzine (Atarax),[289] ethchlorvynol (Placidyl),[290] and glutethimide[291] have been described. Withdrawal from these agents would not be unexpected. However, because of maternal polydrug practices, withdrawal attributable to phenobarbital, diazepam, and heroin, respectively, cannot be excluded. An initial study[292] reported a three- to fourfold greater risk of cleft palate among neonates exposed in utero to diazepam. This observation was supported by other reports in the literature.[293, 294] However, Czeizel[295] and Rosenberg and colleagues[280] could not confirm this association.

Most of the studies from which conclusions were drawn were retrospective case-controlled studies that relied heavily on maternal recall. In a prospective study,[296] a diazepam-mediated cleft palate malformation was not demonstrated in neonates. Furthermore, prenatal exposure to triazolam and alprazolam in more than 600 cases was not associated with adverse neonatal outcome (data on file, Upjohn Pharmaceuticals, Kalamazoo, MI).

Available evidence suggests that barbiturates are not teratogenic.[297] However, the teratogenicity issue is not completely resolved. Butalbital and secobarbital have not been associated with congenital malformations. Information concerning amobarbital is controversial.

Neonates exposed *in utero* to barbiturates may develop the signs and symptoms associated with neonatal abstinence syndrome.[298-300] Desmond and colleagues[298] reported that all 15 neonates prenatally exposed to barbiturates or phenobarbital for sedation, hypertension, or seizure control demonstrated hyperactivity, restlessness, disturbed sleep, and excessive crying, and most of the neonates were also tremulous, hyperreflexic, and hyperphagic. The clinical manifestations of drug withdrawal appeared later (at approximately 1 week post partum) in barbiturate-exposed neonates than in the narcotic-exposed group.[298] This delay is not unexpected because of the long β-elimination half-life of barbiturates. Women receiving secobarbital[299] and butalbital[300] also manifest barbiturate withdrawal. Neonates withdrawing from barbiturates can develop generalized seizures, in addition to exhibiting increased neuromuscular excitability.[301] Maternal abuse of phenobarbital during pregnancy has also been shown to cause a hemorrhagic syndrome in neonates because of hypoprothrombinemia, interference with vitamin K metabolism, and platelet deficiencies.[302] Phenobarbital use during pregnancy increases the incidence of major malformation in neonates born to epileptic women.

Neonates born to women consuming amphetamines during pregnancy have exhibited CNS hyperexcitability.[105] After the hyperexcitable state subsides, some of these neonates manifest marked lethargy and require tube feeding. This state of profound lethargy is thought to be indicative of a true withdrawal syndrome comparable to that observed during cocaine and methamphetamine withdrawal in the adult population.[303] Similar reactions in neonates born to amphetamine-abusing women have been reported by other investigators.[304, 305] Ramer[304] reported a case in which a neonate born to a woman receiving parenteral amphetamine had episodes of diaphoresis, restlessness, and miotic pupils during the first day of life. By day 3, the neonate was listless with decreased muscle tone and had a glassy-eyed stare. Symptoms abated by postpartum day 9. In a prospective study[297] examining 367 neonates exposed to amphetamine during the first trimester, no increased risk of any malformation was found. Conversely, a retrospective study[306] found that congenital heart malformations were more prevalent when infants had been exposed prenatally to amphetamine.

Clinical Management of Maternal Psychotherapeutic Drug Abusers and Exposed Neonates

A tapering regimen with diazepam obviates the drug concentration fluctuations that occur with short-acting benzodiazepines. In a socially stable woman, tapering may be achieved on 5 mg of diazepam per week, with weekly outpatient supportive counseling.[307] Abstinence usually occurs within 6 to 8 weeks. If the outpatient approach fails to result in abstinence, rapid diazepam tapering can be initiated in hospital. In cases of neonatal benzodiazepine withdrawal, 0.1 mg/kg intravenous diazepam every 12 hours is recommended.[285] Adjustments to the dosing interval and dose may be required to control neonatal withdrawal symptoms adequately.

Women consuming more than 400 mg of barbiturates per day are at risk of developing a withdrawal syndrome characterized by tonic-clonic seizures and delirium. These women should be admitted to the hospital for detoxification. Phenobarbital is the drug of choice, administered either on a tapering regimen[308] or by an oral loading technique.[309] Phenobarbital is also the drug used to treat neonates who exhibit signs and symptoms of barbiturate withdrawal.[285] Therapy should be initiated if the neonate manifests seizure activity, moderate to severe hyperreactivity, irritability, poor feeding, or failure to gain weight. An intravenous or intramuscular loading dose of 20 mg/kg, followed by intravenous or oral maintenance therapy at 4 mg/kg/day, should be administered.[285] The maintenance dose may be adjusted as necessary for effective symptom management.[299] It is important to monitor serum phenobarbital concentrations to avoid toxicity. Once withdrawal symptoms have been effectively controlled for a period of 1 week, the dose can be reduced by 25% per week.[285]

CNS hyperexcitability associated with prenatal amphetamine exposure should be treated with benzodiazepines as necessary.[310] Withdrawal symptoms should be managed supportively.

ACKNOWLEDGMENTS

This work was supported, in part, by grants from the Canadian Institutes for Health Research, Health Canada, and the Physicians Service, Inc., Toronto, Canada, and the Research Leadership in Better Pharmacology During Pregnancy and Lactation (Hospital for Sick Children, Toronto). GK is a senior scientist of the Canadian Institutes of Health Research. This chapter was prepared with the assistance of Editorial Services, Hospital for Sick Children, Toronto, Canada.

REFERENCES

1. Levy M, Koren G: Obstetric and neonatal effects of drug abuse. Emerg Med Clin North Am 8:633, 1990.
2. Koren G: Teratogenic drugs and chemicals in humans. *In* Koren G (ed): Maternal-Fetal Toxicology. New York, Marcel Dekker, 1989, p 15.
3. Koren G, Nulman I: Teratogenic drugs and chemicals in humans. *In* Koren G (ed): Maternal-Fetal Toxicology: A Clinician's Guide, 2nd ed. New York, Marcel Dekker, 2nd ed. 1994, pp 33–48.
4. National Institutes of Health: National Pregnancy and Health Survey-Drug Use among Women Delivering Live Births: 1992. Rockville, MD, National Institutes of Health, NIH Publication 96-3819, 1996.
5. Grosser O: Frühentwicklung, Eihautbildung, und Placentation des Menschen und der Säugetiere. *In* Bergmann JF (ed): Deutsche Frauenheilkunde. München, 1927.
6. Simone C, et al: Drug transfer across the placenta: considerations in treatment and research. Fetal Drug Ther 21:463, 1994.
7. Enders AC: A comparative study of the fine structure of the trophoblast in several hemochorial placentas. Am J Anat 116:29, 1965.
8. Szeto HH, et al: Meperidine pharmacokinetics in the maternal-fetal unit. J Pharmacol Exp Ther 206:448, 1978.
9. Derewlany LO, Koren G: The role of the placenta in perinatal pharmacology and toxicology. *In* MacLeod SM, Radde IC (eds): Pediatric Clinical Pharmacology. St. Louis, Mosby–Year Book, 1993, p 405.
10. Scialli AR: The fetoplacental unit. *In* A Clinical Guide to Reproductive and Developmental Toxicology. Boca Raton, CRC Press, 1992, p 45.
11. Kuemmerle HP: Pregnancy and clinical pharmacology: a review. Biol Res Preg 7:139, 1986.
12. Tropper PJ, Petrie RH: Placental exchange. *In* Lavery JP (ed): The Human Placenta: Clinical Perspectives. Rockville, MD, Aspen Publishers, 1987, p 199.
13. Reynolds F: Placental transfer of drugs. *In* Hawkins DF (ed): Drugs and Pregnancy: Human Teratogenesis and Related Problems. Edinburgh, Churchill Livingstone, 1983, p 3.
14. Challier JC, et al: Clearance of compounds of different molecular size in the human placenta in vitro. Biol Neonate 48:143, 1985.
15. Challier JC, et al: Flow-dependent transfer of antipyrine in the human placenta in vitro. Reprod Nutr Dev 23:41, 1983.
16. Miller RK, et al: Human placenta in vitro: characterization during 12 hours of dual perfusion. Contrib Gynecol Obstet 13:77, 1985.
17. Bajoria R, Contractor F: Transfer of heparin across the human perfused placental lobule. J Pharm Pharmacol 44:952, 1992.
18. Benet LZ: Pharmacokinetics. I. Absorption, distribution, and excretion. *In* Katzung BG (ed): Basic and Clinical Pharmacology, 3rd ed. Norwalk, CT, Appleton & Lange, 1987, pp 23–35.
19. Baselt RC, Cravey RH: Disposition of Toxic Drugs and Chemicals in Man, 4th ed. Foster City, CA, Chemical Toxicology Institute, 1995, p 528.
20. Kopecky EA, et al: Naloxone does not alter the transfer of morphine across the human term placenta perfused in vitro (abstract). Clin Invest Med 19:S10, 1996.

21. Simone C, et al: Transfer of cocaine and benzoylecgonine across the perfused human placental cotyledon. Am J Obstet Gynecol 170:1404, 1994.
22. Woods JR, et al: Effect of cocaine on uterine blood flow and fetal oxygenation. JAMA 257:957, 1987.
23. Ward RW: Drug therapy in the fetus. J Clin Pharmacol 33:3177, 1979.
24. Biehl D, et al: Placental transfer of lidocaine: effects of fetal acidosis. Anesthesiology 48:409, 1978.
25. Boreáus LO: Distribution. In Azarnoff DL (ed): Monographs in Clinical Pharmacology: Principles of Pediatric Pharmacology, Vol 6. New York, Churchill Livingstone, 1982, p 46.
26. Cunningham AS, et al: Breast-feeding and health in the 1980s: a global epidemiologic review. J Pediatr 118:659, 1991.
27. WHO Working Group: Determinants of drug excretion in breast milk. In Bennett PN, et al (eds): Drugs and Human Lactation. Amsterdam, Elsevier, 1988, pp 27–48.
28. Taddio A, Ito S: Drug use during lactation. In Koren G (ed): Maternal-Fetal Toxicology: A Clinician's Guide, 2nd ed. New York, Marcel Dekker, 1994, pp 133–219.
29. Ito S, Koren G: A novel index for expressing exposure of the infant to drugs in breast milk. Br J Clin Pharmacol 38:99, 1994.
30. Besunder JB: Principles of drug biodisposition in the neonate. I. A critical evaluation of the pharmacokinetic-pharmacodynamic interface. Clin Pharmacokinet 14:189, 1988.
31. Dutton GJ: Developmental aspects of drug conjugation, with special reference to glucuronidation. Annu Rev Pharmacol Toxicol 18:17, 1978.
32. Atkinson HC, et al: Drugs in human milk: clinical pharmacokinetic considerations. Clin Pharmacokinet 14:217, 1988.
33. Berlin CM: The excretion of drugs and chemicals in human milk. In Yaffe SJ (ed): Pediatric Pharmacology: Therapeutic Principles in Practice. New York, Grune and Stratton, 1980, pp 137–147.
34. Schanker LS: Passage of drugs across body membranes. Pharmacol Rev 14:501, 1962.
35. Pietrantoni M, Knuppel RA: Alcohol use in pregnancy. Chem Depend Preg 18:93, 1991.
36. Mello NK: Some behavioral and biological aspects of alcohol problems in women. In Kalant OJ (ed): Alcohol and Drug Problems in Women. New York, Plenum Press, 1980, pp 263–298.
37. Weiner L, et al: Alcohol consumption by pregnant women. Obstet Gynecol 61:6, 1983.
38. Majewskis F: Die alkoholembryopathie: Fakten und Hypotesen Ergesunn. Med Kinderheilk 43:1, 1979.
39. Clarren SK, Smith DW: The fetal alcohol syndrome. N Engl J Med 298:1063, 1978.
40. Jones KL, et al: Pattern of malformation in offspring of chronic alcoholic mothers. Lancet 1:1267, 1973.
41. Jones KL, Smith DW: Recognition of the fetal alcohol syndrome in early pregnancy. Lancet 2:999, 1973.
42. Berkow R, Fletcher AJ (eds): The Merck Manual of Diagnosis and Therapy, 15th ed. Rahway, NJ, Merck and Co, 1987, pp 1887–1888.
43. Fogel BJ, et al: Discordant abnormalities in monozygotic twins. J Pediatr 66:64, 1965.
44. Lenz W: Malformations caused by drugs in pregnancy. Am J Dis Child 112:99, 1966.
45. Seppala M, et al: Ethanol elimination in a mother and her premature twins. Lancet 1:1188, 1971.
46. Veghelyi PV: Fetal abnormality and maternal ethanol metabolism. Lancet 2:53, 1983.
47. Karl PI, et al: Acetaldehyde production and transfer by the perfused human placental cotyledon. Science 242:273, 1983.
48. Rosett H, Weiner L: Alcohol and the Fetus: A Clinical Perspective. New York, Oxford University Press, 1984.
49. Sokol RJ, et al: Alcohol abuse during pregnancy: an epidemiologic study. Alcohol Clin Exp Res 4:135, 1980.
50. Streissguth PA, et al: IQ at age 4 in relation to maternal alcohol use and smoking during pregnancy. Dev Psychol 25:3, 1989.
51. Ellenhorn MJ, Barceloux DG (eds): Ethanol. In Medical Toxicology: Diagnosis and Treatment of Human Poisoning. New York, Elsevier, 1988, pp 782–798.
52. Chan D, et al: Population baseline of meconium FACE among infants of non-drinking women in Jerusalem and Toronto. Ther Drug Monit 2003, (in press).
53. Rosett HL: A clinical perspective of the fetal alcohol syndrome. Alcohol Clin Exp Res 4:119, 1980.
54. Streissguth AP, et al: Teratogenic effects of alcohol in humans and laboratory animals. Science 209:353, 1980.
55. Chasnoff IJ, et al: Early growth patterns of methadone-addicted infants. Am J Dis Child 143:1049, 1980.
56. Harlap S, Shions PH: Alcohol, smoking, and incidence of spontaneous abortion in the first and second trimester. Lancet 1:173, 1980.
57. Kline J, et al: Drinking during pregnancy and spontaneous abortion. Lancet 1:176, 1980.
58. Goujard J, et al: Maternal smoking, alcohol consumption, and abruptio placenta. Am J Obstet Gynecol 130:738, 1980.
59. Marbury M-C, et al: The association of alcohol consumption with outcome of pregnancy. Am J Public Health 73:1165, 1983.
60. Kaminski M, et al: Moderate alcohol use and pregnancy outcome. Neurobehav Toxicol Teratol 3:173, 1981.
61. Olegard R, et al: Effects on the child of alcohol abuse during pregnancy: retrospective and prospective studies. Acta Paediatr Scand Suppl 275:112, 1979.
62. Silva VA, et al: Alcohol consumption during pregnancy and newborn outcome: a study in Brazil. Neurobehav Toxicol Teratol 3:169, 1981.
63. Little RE: Moderate alcohol use during pregnancy and decreased infant birth weight. Am J Public Health 67:1154, 1977.
64. Landesman-Dwyer S, et al: Naturalistic observation of newborns: effect of maternal alcohol intake. Alcohol Clin Exp Res 2:171, 1978.
65. Mills JL, Graubard BI: Is moderate drinking during pregnancy associated with an increased risk of malformations? Pediatrics 80:309, 1987.
66. Streissguth AP, et al: Effects of maternal alcohol, nicotine, and caffeine use during pregnancy on infant mental and motor development at eight months. Clin Exp Res 4:152, 1980.
67. Streissguth AP, et al: Natural history of the fetal alcohol syndrome: a 10 year follow up of eleven patients. Lancet 2:85, 1985.
68. Little RE, et al: Association of father's drinking and infant's birthweight. N Engl J Med 314:1644, 1986.
69. Emhart CB, et al: Alcohol teratogenicity in the human: a detailed assessment of specificity, critical period, and threshold. Am J Obstet Gynecol 156:33, 1987.
70. Streissguth AP, et al: Neurobehavioral effects of prenatal alcohol. I. Research strategy. Neurotoxicol Teratol 11:461, 1989.
71. Little RE, et al: Maternal alcohol use during breast feeding and infant mental and motor development at one year. N Engl J Med 32:425, 1989.
72. Coles CD, et al: Persistence over the first months of neurobehavioral differences in infants exposed to alcohol prenatally. Infant Behav Dev 10:23, 1987.
73. Clarren SK, et al: Brain malformations related to prenatal exposure to ethanol. J Pediatr 92:64, 1977.
74. Havlicek V, et al: EEG frequency spectral characteristics of sleep states in infants of alcoholic mothers. Neuropediatrie 8:360, 1977.
75. Jaffe S, Chernike V: Maternal alcohol ingestion and the incidence of RDS. Am J Obstet Gynecol 156:1231, 1987.
76. Kandall SR, Gaines J: Maternal substance use and subsequent sudden infant death syndrome (SIDS) in offspring. Neurotoxicol Teratol 13:235, 1991.
77. Hotchkiss ML, Green WR: Optic nerve aplasia and hypoplasia. J Pediatr Ophthalmol Strabismus 16:225, 1979.
78. Mosier MA, et al: Hypoplasia of the optic nerve. Arch Ophthalmol 96:1437, 1978.
79. Spedick MJ, Beauchamp GR: Retinal vascular and optic nerve abnormalities in albinism. J Pediatr Ophthalmol Strabismus 23:58, 1986.
80. Strömland K: Ocular abnormalities in the fetal alcohol syndrome. Acta Ophthalmol Suppl 171:1, 1985.
81. Feldman Y, et al: Determinants of recall and recall bias in studying drug and chemical exposure in pregnancy. Teratology 39:37, 1989.
82. Halmesmaki E, et al: α-Fetoprotein, human placental lactogen, and pregnancy specific β₁-glycoprotein in pregnant women who drink: relation to FAS. Am J Obstet Gynecol 155:598, 1986.
83. Ylikorkala O, et al: γ-Glutamyl transferase and mean cellular volume reveal maternal alcohol abuse and fetal alcohol effects. Am J Obstet Gynecol 157:344, 1987.
84. Koren G, et al: Antenatal sonography of fetal malformations associated with drugs and chemicals: a guide. Am J Obstet Gynecol 156:79, 1987.
85. Koren G, Nulman I: Antenatal visualization of malformations associated with drugs and chemicals. Dev Brain Dysfunc 6:305, 1993.
86. Sellers EM, et al: Diazepam loading: simplified treatment of alcohol withdrawal. Clin Pharmacol Ther 34:822, 1983.
87. Kraus ML: Randomized clinical trial of atenolol in patients with alcohol withdrawal. N Engl J Med 313:905, 1985.
88. Komiskey HL, et al: The isomers of cocaine and tropacocaine: effect on 3H catecholamine uptake by rat brain synaptosomes. Life Sci 21:1117, 1977.
89. Pitts DK, Marwah J: Cocaine modulation of central monoaminergic neurotransmission. Pharmacol Biochem Behav 26:453, 1987.
90. Cooper JR, et al: The Biochemical Basis of Neuropharmacology, 2nd ed. New York, Oxford University Press, 1974.
91. Forman R, et al: Accumulation of cocaine in maternal and fetal hair: the dose response curve. Life Sci 50:1333, 1992.
92. Cunningham FG, et al: William's Obstetrics, 18th ed. Norwalk, CT, Appleton & Lange, 1989.
93. MacGregor SN, et al: Cocaine use during pregnancy: adverse perinatal outcome. Am J Obstet Gynecol 157:686, 1987.
94. Gawin FH, Ellinwood EH: Cocaine and other stimulants: actions, abuse, and treatment. N Engl J Med 318:1173, 1988.
95. Dougherty RJ: Status of cocaine abuse in 1984. J Subst Abuse Treat 1:157, 1984.
96. Hamilton HE, et al: Cocaine and benzoylecgonine excretion in humans. J Forensic Sci 22:697, 1977.
97. Mahone PR, et al: Cocaine and metabolites in amniotic fluid may prolong fetal drug exposure. Am J Obstet Gynecol 171:465, 1994.
98. Hawks RL, et al: Norcocaine: a pharmacologically active metabolite of cocaine found in brain. Life Sci 15:2189, 1974.
99. Klein J, et al: Fetal distribution of cocaine: case analysis. Pediatr Pathol 12:463, 1992.
100. Spiehler VR, Reed D: Brain concentrations of cocaine and benzoylecgonine in fatal cases. J Forensic Sci 30:1003, 1985.

101. Acker D, et al: Abruptio placentae associated with cocaine use. Am J Obstet Gynecol *146*:220, 1983.
102. Bingol N, et al: Teratogenicity of cocaine in humans. J Pediatr *110*:93, 1987.
103. Chasnoff IJ, et al: Cocaine use during pregnancy. N Engl J Med *313*:666, 1985.
104. Chasnoff IJ, et al: Perinatal cerebral infarction and maternal cocaine use. J Pediatr *108*:456, 1986.
105. Oro AS, Dixon SD: Perinatal cocaine and methamphetamine exposure: maternal and fetal correlates. J Pediatr *111*:571, 1987.
106. Ryan L, et al: Cocaine abuse in pregnancy: effect on the fetus and the newborn. Neurotoxicol Teratol *9*:295, 1987.
107. Woods JR, et al: Effects of cocaine on uterine blood flow and fetal oxygenation. JAMA *257*:957, 1987.
108. Maden JD, et al: Maternal cocaine abuse and effect on the newborn. Pediatrics *77*:209, 1986.
109. Forman R, et al: Maternal and neonatal characteristics following exposure to cocaine in Toronto. Reprod Toxicol *7*:619, 1993.
110. Dixon SD, et al: Visual dysfunction in cocaine exposed infants (abstract). Pediatr Res *21*:359A, 1987.
111. Fulroth RF, et al: Description of 72 infants exposed to cocaine prenatally (abstract). Pediatr Res *21*:361A, 1987.
112. Doberczak TM, et al: Neonatal electroencephalographic effect of intrauterine cocaine exposure. J Pediatr *113*:354, 1988.
113. Chasnoff IJ, et al: Cocaine use in pregnancy: perinatal morbidity and mortality. Neurotoxicol Teratol *9*:291, 1987.
114. Chasnoff IJ, et al: Temporal patterns of cocaine use in pregnancy. JAMA *261*:171, 1989.
115. Koren G, Graham K: Cocaine in pregnancy: analysis of fetal risk. Vet Hum Toxicol *34*:263, 1992.
116. Albbuquerque ML, et al: Cocaine-mediated cerebral vasoconstriction in newborn piglets. Pediatr Res *29*:56A, 1991.
117. Chasnoff IJ, et al: Perinatal cerebral infarction and maternal cocaine use. J Pediatr *108*:456, 1986.
118. Manino FL, et al: Strokes in neonates. J Pediatr *102*:605, 1983.
119. Tenorio GM, et al: Intrauterine stroke and maternal polydrug abuse. Clin Pediatr *27*:565, 1988.
120. Dominguez R, et al: Brain and ocular abnormalities in infants with in utero exposure to cocaine and other street drugs. Am J Dis Child *145*:688, 1991.
121. Bejar R, Dixon SD: Echoencephalographic findings in neonates associated with maternal cocaine and methamphetamine use: incidence and clinical correlates. J Pediatr *115*:770, 1989.
122. Ulleland CN: The offspring of chronic alcoholic mothers. Ann NY Acad Sci *197*:167, 1972.
123. Koren G: Cocaine and the human fetus: the concept of teratophilia. Neurotoxicol Teratol *15*:301, 1993.
124. Cregler L, Mark H: Medical complications of cocaine abuse. N Engl J Med *315*:1495, 1986.
125. Bauchner H, et al: Risk of sudden infant death syndrome among infants with in utero exposure to cocaine. J Pediatr *113*:831, 1988.
126. Chasnoff IJ, et al: Prenatal cocaine exposure is associated with respiratory pattern abnormalities. Am J Dis Child *143*:583, 1989.
127. Ward SLD, et al: Abnormal sleeping ventilatory pattern in infants of substance-abusing mothers. Am J Dis Child *140*:1015, 1986.
128. Hunt CE, Brouillette RT: SIDS: 1987 update. J Pediatr *110*:669, 1987.
129. Bergstrom L, et al: Post-mortem analyses of neuro-peptides in brains from sudden infant death victims. Brain Res *323*:279, 1984.
130. Naeye RL: Brainstem and adrenal abnormalities in SIDS. Am J Clin Pathol *66*:526, 1976.
131. Gingras JL, et al: Cocaine and development: mechanisms of fetal toxicity and neonatal consequences of prenatal cocaine exposure. Early Hum Dev *31*:1, 1992.
132. Pritchard JA: Plasma cholinesterase activity in normal pregnancy and in eclamptogenic toxemia. Am J Obstet Gynecol *70*:1083, 1955.
133. Stewart DJ, et al: Hydrolysis of cocaine in human plasma by cholinesterase. Life Sci *20*:1557, 1977.
134. Lucy-Shih BC, Reddix C: Effects of maternal cocaine abuse on the neonatal auditory system. Int J Pediatr Otolaryngol *15*:245, 1988.
135. Addis A, et al: Fetal effects of cocaine, and updated meta-analysis. Reprod Toxicol *15*:341, 2001.
136. Mehta SK, et al: Transient myocardial ischemia in infants prenatally exposed to cocaine. J Pediatr *122*:945, 1993.
137. Longo LD: The biological effects of carbon monoxide on the pregnant woman, fetus, and newborn infant. Am J Obstet Gynecol *129*:69, 1977.
138. Lutiger B, et al: Relationship between gestational cocaine use and pregnancy outcome: a meta-analysis. Teratology *44*:405, 1991.
139. Hoffman RS, et al: Association between life threatening cocaine toxicity and pharmacholinesterase activity. Ann Emerg Med *21*:247, 1992.
140. Simone C, et al: Can the human placenta biotransform cocaine? Clin Invest Med *15*:A19, 1992.
141. Bar-Oz B, et al: Comparison of meconium and neonatal hair analysis for detection of gestation exposure to drugs of abuse. Arch Dis Child *87*:F0, 2002.
142. Kleinman JC, Kopstein A: Smoking during pregnancy 1967–1980. Am J Public Health *77*:823, 1987.
143. Mactutus CF: Developmental neurotoxicity of nicotine, carbon monoxide, and other tobacco smoke constituents. Ann NY Acad Sci *562*:105, 1989.
144. Kyerematen GA, et al: Smoking induced changes in nicotine disposition: application of a new HPLC assay for nicotine and its metabolites. Clin Pharmacol Ther *32*:769, 1982.
145. Luck W, Nau H: Nicotine and cotinine concentrations in serum and milk of nursing smokers. Br J Clin Pharmacol *18*:9, 1984.
146. Ferguson BB, et al: Determination of nicotine concentrations in human milk. Am J Dis Child *130*:837, 1976.
147. Labrecque M, et al: Feeding and urine cotinine values in babies whose mothers smoke. Pediatrics *83*:93, 1989.
148. Schwartz-Bickenbach D, et al: Smoking and passive smoking during pregnancy and early infancy: effects on birth weight, lactation period, and cotinine concentrations in mother's milk and infant's urine. Toxicol Lett *35*:73, 1987.
149. Hall SM, et al: Blood cotinine levels as indicators of smoking treatment outcome. Clin Pharmacol Ther *35*:810, 1984.
150. Murphy JF, Mucahy R: The effect of age, parity and cigarette smoking on baby weight. Am J Obstet Gynecol *111*:22, 1971.
151. McIntosh ID: Smoking and pregnancy. II. Offspring risks. Public Health Rev *12*:29, 1984.
152. Meyer MB, et al: Perinatal events associated with maternal smoking during pregnancy. Am J Epidemiol *103*:464, 1976.
153. Cnattingius S, et al: Cigarette smoking as a risk factor for late fetal and early neonatal death. BMJ *297*:258, 1988.
154. Scholl JO, et al: Smoking and adolescent pregnancy outcome. J Adolesc Health Care *7*:390, 1986.
155. Bardy AH, et al: Objectively measured tobacco exposure during pregnancy: neonatal effects and relation to maternal smoking. Br J Obstet Gynecol *100*:721, 1993.
156. Gabriel R, et al: Alteration of epidermal growth factor receptor in placental membranes of smokers: relationship with intrauterine growth retardation. Am J Obstet Gynecol *170*:1238, 1994.
157. Hofmann GE, et al: Epidermal growth factor and its receptor in human implantation trophoblast: immunohistochemical evidence for autocrine/paracrine function. J Clin Endocrinol Metab *74*:981, 1992.
158. Morrish DW, et al: Epidermal growth factor induces differentiation and secretion of human chorionic gonadotropin and placental lactogen in normal human placenta. J Clin Endocrinol Mebab *65*:1282, 1987.
159. Qu J, et al: Effect of epidermal growth factor on inhibin secretion in human placental cell culture. Endocrinology *131*:2173, 1992.
160. Maruo T, et al: Induction of differentiated trophoblast function by epidermal growth factor: relation of immunohistochemically detected cellular growth factor receptor levels. J Clin Endocrinol Metab *64*:744, 1987.
161. Barnea ER, et al: The dual effect of epidermal growth factor upon human chorionic gonadotropin secretion by the first trimester placenta in vitro. J Clin Endocrinol Metab *71*:923, 1990.
162. Sands J, Dobbing J: Continuing growth and development of the third-trimester human placenta. Placenta *6*:13, 1985.
163. Wang SI, et al: Smoking-related alterations in epidermal growth factor and insulin receptors in human placenta. Mol Pharmacol *34*:265, 1988.
164. Stjernfeldt M, et al: Maternal smoking during pregnancy and risk of childhood cancer. Lancet *1*:1350, 1986.
165. Curett LB, et al: Maternal smoking and respiratory distress syndrome. Am J Obstet Gynecol *147*:446, 1983.
166. Colley JRT, et al: Respiratory symptoms in childhood and parental smoking and phlegm production. BMJ *2*:201, 1974.
167. Harlap S, Davis AM: Infant admissions to hospital and maternal smoking. Lancet *1*:527, 1974.
168. Rantakallio P: Relationship of maternal smoking to morbidity and mortality of the child up to the age of five. Acta Paediatr Scand *67*:621, 1978.
169. Yarnell JWG Sr, Leger AS: Respiratory illness, maternal smoking habit and lung function in children. Br J Dis Chest *73*:230, 1979.
170. Schulte-Hobein B, et al: Cigarette smoking exposure and development of infants throughout the first year of life: Influence of passive smoking and nursing on cotinine levels in breast milk and infant's urine. Acta Paediatr *81*:550, 1992.
171. Vio F, et al: Smoking during pregnancy and lactation and its effects on breast-milk volume. Am J Clin Nutr *54*:1011, 1991.
172. Said G, et al: Infantile colic and parental smoking. BMJ *289*:660, 1984.
173. Naeye RL, et al: Sudden infant death syndrome. Am J Dis Child *130*:1207, 1976.
174. Bergman AB, et al: Relationship of passive cigarette smoking to sudden infant death syndrome. Pediatrics *58*:665, 1976.
175. Lewak N, et al: Sudden infant death syndrome risk factors. Clin Pediatr *18*:404, 1979.
176. Malloy MH, et al: The association of maternal smoking with age and cause of infant death. Am J Epidemiol *128*:46, 1988.
177. Haglund B, Cnattinguis S: Cigarette smoking as a risk factor for sudden infant death syndrome: a population based study. Am J Public Health *80*:29, 1990.
178. Sexton M, et al: Prenatal exposure to tobacco: effects on cognitive functioning at age three. Int J Epidemiol *19*:72, 1990.
179. Wisbarg K, et al: Nicotine patches for pregnant smokers. Obstet Gynecol *96*:967, 2000.
180. Dempsy D, et al: Accelerated metabolism of nicotine and cotinine in pregnant smokers. J Pharmacol Exp Ther *301*:594, 2002.
181. Selby P, et al: Heavily smoking women who cannot quit in pregnancy: evidence of pharmacokinetic predisposition. Ther Drug Monit *23*:189, 2001.

182. Abel EL: Smoking during pregnancy: a review of effects on growth and development of the offspring. Hum Biol *52*:593, 1980.

183. Chiriboga CA: Fetal effects. Neurol Clin *11*:707, 1993.

184. Newman RG, et al: Results of 313 consecutive live births of infants delivered to patients in the New York City Methadone Maintenance Treatment Program. Am J Obstet Gynecol *121*:233, 1974.

185. Neumann LL, Cohen SN: The neonatal narcotic withdrawal syndrome: a therapeutic challenge. Clin Perinatol *2*:99, 1975.

186. O'Connel CM, Fried PA: An investigation of prenatal cannabis exposure and minor physical anomalies in a low risk population. Neurobehav Toxicol Teratol *6*:345, 1984.

187. Ohlson A, et al: Plasma Δ⁹-tetrahydrocannabinol concentrations and clinical effects after oral and intravenous administration and smoking. Clin Pharmacol Ther *28*:409, 1980.

188. Wall ME, et al: Metabolism, disposition, and kinetics of Δ⁹-tetrahydrocannabinol in men and women. Clin Pharmacol Ther *34*:352, 1983.

189. Hunt CA, Jones RT: Tolerance and disposition of tetrahydrocannabinol in man. J Pharmacol Exp Ther *215*:35, 1980.

190. Lemberger L, et al: Marijuana studies on the disposition and metabolism of Δ⁹-tetrahydrocannabinol in man. Science *170*:1320, 1970.

191. Lemberger L, et al: Tetrahydrocannabinol: metabolism and disposition in long term marijuana smokers. Science *178*:72, 1971.

192. Blackard C, Tennes K: Human placental transfer of cannabinoids. N Engl J Med *311*:797, 1984.

193. Harbison R, Mantilla-Plata B: Prenatal toxicity: maternal distribution and placental transfer of tetrahydrocannabinol. J Pharmacol Exp Ther *180*:446, 1972.

194. Idanpaan-Heikkila J, et al: Placental transfer of tritiated 1-Δ⁹-tetrahydrocannabinol. N Engl J Med *281*:330, 1969.

195. Jakusovitch A, et al: Excretion of THC and its metabolites in ewe's milk. Toxicol Appl Pharmacol *28*:38, 1974.

196. Perez Reyes M, Wall ME: Presence of Δ⁹-tetrahydrocannabinol in human milk. N Engl J Med *307*:819, 1982.

197. Fried PA, et al: Changing patterns of soft drug use prior to and during pregnancy. Drug Alcohol Depend *6*:323, 1980.

198. Harclerode J: The effect of marijuana on reproduction and development. *In* National Institute on Drug Abuse Monograph No. 31. Bethesda, MD, National Institute on Drug Abuse, 1980.

199. Fried PA: Marijuana use during pregnancy and perinatal risk factors. Am J Obstet Gynecol *144*:922, 1983.

200. Greenland S, et al: The effects of marijuana use during pregnancy. I. A preliminary epidemiologic study. Am J Obstet Gynecol *143*:408, 1982.

201. Fried PA, et al: Marijuana use during pregnancy and decreased length of gestation. Am J Obstet Gynecol *150*:23, 1984.

202. Hingson R, et al: Effects of maternal drinking and marijuana use on fetal growth and development. Pediatrics *70*:539, 1989.

203. Qazi QH, et al: Is marijuana smoking fetotoxic? (abstract) Pediatr Res *16*:272A, 1982.

204. Greenland S, et al: Effect of marijuana on human pregnancy, labor, and delivery. Neurobehav Toxicol Teratol *4*:447, 1983.

205. Fried PA, et al: Soft drug use prior to and during pregnancy: a comparison of samples over a four year period. Drug Alcohol Depend *13*:161, 1984.

206. Linn S, et al: The association of marijuana use with outcome of pregnancy. Am J Public Health *73*:1161, 1983.

207. Rose HL, et al: Effect of maternal drinking and marijuana use on fetal growth and development. Pediatrics *70*:539, 1982.

208. Brazelton TB: Neonatal Neurobehavioral Assessment Scale. London, Heinemann, 1973.

209. Fried PA: Marijuana use by pregnant women: neurobehavioral effects in neonates. Drug Alcohol Depend *6*:415, 1980.

210. Fried PA: Marijuana use by pregnant women and effects on offspring: an update. Neurobehav Toxicol Teratol *4*:451, 1982.

211. Finnegan LP: The effect of narcotics and alcohol on pregnancy and the newborn. Ann NY Acad Sci *362*:136, 1981.

212. Lodge A: Developmental findings with infants born to mothers on methadone maintenance: a preliminary report. *In* Beschner G, Brothman R (eds): National Institute on Drug Abuse Symposium and Comprehensive Health Care for Addicted Families and their Children. Washington, DC, US Government Printing Office, 1976, pp 79–85.

213. Fried PA: Short and long term effects of prenatal cannabis inhalation upon rat offspring. Psychopharmacology *50*:185, 1976.

214. Fried PA, Charlebois AT: Cannabis administered during pregnancy: First and second generation effects in rats. Physiol Psychol *7*:307, 1979.

215. Zelson C: Infant of the addicted mother. N Engl J Med *288*:1393, 1973.

216. Hutchings DE: A Treatment for Drug Addiction. New York, Chelsea House, 1985.

217. Krogh CME (ed): Canadian Pharmaceutical Association. Compendium of Pharmaceuticals and Specialties, 29th ed. Ottawa, CK Productions, 1994, pp 749–750.

218. Gilman AG, et al (eds): Goodman and Gilman's The Pharmacologic Basis of Therapeutics, 8th ed. Elmsford, NY, Pergamon Press, 1990.

219. Beauclair TR, Stoner CP: Adherence to guidelines for continuous morphine sulfate infusions. Am J Hosp Pharmacol *43*:671, 1986.

220. Koren G, Maurice L: Pediatric use of opioids. Pediatr Clin North Am *36*:1141, 1989.

221. Bray RJ, et al: Plasma morphine levels produced by continuous infusion in children. Anaesthesia *41*:753, 1986.

222. Koren G, et al: Postoperative morphine infusion in newborn infants: assessment of disposition characteristics and safety. J Pediatr *107*:963, 1985.

223. Olkkola KT, et al: Kinetics and dynamics of postoperative intravenous morphine in children. Clin Pharmacol Ther *44*:128, 1988.

224. Dahlstrom B, et al: Morphine kinetics in children. Clin Pharmacol Ther *26*:354, 1979.

225. Lynn AM, et al: Morphine infusion after pediatric cardiac surgery. Crit Care Med *12*:863, 1984.

226. Berkowitz BA: The relationship of pharmacokinetics to pharmacologic activity: morphine, methadone, and naloxone. Clin Pharmacokinet *1*:219, 1976.

227. Holmstrand J, et al: Methadone maintenance: plasma levels and therapeutic outcome. Clin Pharmacol Ther *23*:175, 1978.

228. Verebely K, et al: Methadone in man: pharmacokinetic and excretion studies in acute and chronic treatment. Clin Pharmacol Ther *18*:180, 1976.

229. Chasnoff IJ: Effect of maternal narcotic vs non narcotic addiction on neonatal neurobehavior and infant development. *In* Pinkert TM (ed): Consequences of Maternal Drug Abuse. Washington, DC, National Institute on Drug Abuse, 1985, pp 84–95.

230. Friedler G, Cochin J: Growth retardation in offspring of female rats treated with morphine prior to conception. Science *175*: 654, 1972.

231. Kandall SR, et al: Differential effects of maternal heroin and methadone use on birth weight. Pediatrics *58*:681, 1976.

232. Zelson C, et al: Comparative effects of maternal intake of heroin and methadone. N Engl J Med *289*:1216, 1973.

233. Ostrea EM Jr, Chavez CJ: Perinatal problems (excluding neonatal withdrawal) in maternal drug addiction: a study of 830 cases. J Pediatr *94*:292, 1979.

234. Olofsson M, et al: Investigation of 89 children born by drug dependent mothers. I. Neonatal course. Acta Paediatr Scand *72*:403, 1983.

235. Zelson C, et al: Neonatal narcotic addiction: 10 year observation. Pediatrics *48*:178, 1971.

236. Glass L, et al: Absence of respiratory distress syndrome in premature infants of heroin addicted mothers. Lancet *2*:685, 1971.

237. Glass L, Evans HE: Physiologic effects of intrauterine exposure to narcotics. *In* Rementeria JL (ed): Drug Abuse in Pregnancy and Neonatal Effects. St. Louis, CV Mosby, 1977, pp 108–115.

238. Harper RG, et al: The effect of methadone treatment program upon pregnant heroin addicts and their newborn infants. Pediatrics *54*:300, 1974.

239. Chavez CJ, et al: Sudden infant death syndrome among infants of drug dependent mothers. J Pediatr *95*:407, 1979.

240. Pierson PS, et al: Sudden death in infants born to methadone maintained addicts. JAMA *220*:1733, 1972.

241. Hunt CE, et al: Home pneumograms in normal infants. J Pediatr *106*:551, 1980.

242. Kandall SR, et al: Relationship of maternal substance abuse to subsequent sudden infant death syndrome in offspring. J Pediatr *123*:120, 1993.

243. Martin WR, et al: The respiratory effects of morphine during a cycle of dependence. J Pharmacol Exp Ther *62*:182, 1968.

244. Meuller RA, et al: The neuropharmacology of respiratory control. Pharmacol Rev *34*:225, 1982.

245. Olsen GD, Lees MH: Ventilatory response to carbon dioxide of infants following chronic prenatal methadone exposure. J Pediatr *96*:983, 1980.

246. Naeye RL: Hypoxia and the sudden infant death syndrome. Science *186*:837, 1974.

247. Kandall SR, et al: The narcotic-dependent mother: fetal and neonatal consequences. Early Hum Dev *1/2*:159, 1977.

248. Dinges DF, et al: Fetal exposure to narcotics: neonatal sleep as a measure of nervous system disturbance. Science *209*:619, 1980.

249. Rosner MA, et al: The Lowestein University drug dependence program: the impact of intensive prenatal care on labor and delivery outcomes. Am J Obstet Gynecol *144*:23, 1982.

250. Schardein JL: Chemically Induced Birth Defect. New York, Marcel Dekker, 1985.

251. Stone ML: Narcotic addiction during pregnancy. Am J Obstet Gynecol *109*:716, 1971.

252. Reddy AM, et al: Observations on heroin and methadone withdrawal in the newborn. Pediatrics *48*:353, 1971.

253. Rosen TS, Johnson HL: Children of methadone-maintained mothers: follow up to 18 months of age. J Pediatr *101*:192, 1982.

254. Briggs GG, et al: Drugs in Pregnancy and Lactation, 2nd ed. Baltimore, Williams & Wilkins, 1986, pp 296–298.

255. Robieux I, et al: Morphine excretion in breast milk and resultant exposure of a nursing infant. Clin Toxicol *28*:365, 1990.

256. Rabbar F: Observations on methadone withdrawal in 16 neonates. Clin Pediatr *14*:369, 1975.

257. Herlinger RA, et al: Neonatal seizures associated with narcotic withdrawal. J Pediatr *91*:638, 1977.

258. Carin I, et al: Neonatal methadone withdrawal: effect of two treatment regimens. Am J Dis Child *137*:1166, 1983.

259. Kaltenbach K, Finnegan LP: Neonatal abstinence syndrome: pharmacotherapy and developmental outcome. Neurobehav Toxicol Teratol *8*:353, 1986.

260. Kandall SR, et al: Opiate vs CNS depressant therapy in neonatal drug abstinence syndrome. Am J Dis Child *137*:378, 1983.

261. Committee on Drugs: Neonatal drug withdrawal. Pediatrics *72*:895, 1983.

262. Finnegan LP, et al: A scoring system for evaluation and treatment of the neonatal abstinence syndrome: a new clinical and research tool. *In* Morselli PL, et al (eds): Basic and Therapeutic Aspects of Perinatal Pharmacology. New York, Raven Press, 1975, pp 139–153.

263. Kron RE, et al: Neonatal narcotic abstinence: effects of pharmacotherapeutic agents and maternal drug usage on nutritive sucking behavior. J Pediatr 88:637, 1976.

264. Kandall SR, et al: The comparative effects of opiates versus central nervous system depressant treatment on neonatal drug withdrawal. Am J Dis Child 137:378, 1983.

265. Carin I, et al: Neonatal methadone withdrawal. Am J Dis Child 137:1166, 1983.

266. Kunstadter RH, et al: Narcotic withdrawal symptoms in newborn infants. JAMA 168:1008, 1958.

267. Zelson C: Acute management of neonatal addiction. Addict Dis 2:159, 1975.

268. Rementeria JL, Nunag NN: Narcotic withdrawal in pregnancy: stillbirth incidence with a case report. Am J Obstet Gynecol 116:1152, 1973.

269. Zuspan FP, et al: Fetal stress from methadone withdrawal. Am J Obstet Gynecol 122:43, 1975.

270. Connaughton JF, et al: Perinatal addiction: outcome and management. Am J Obstet Gynecol 129:679, 1977.

271. Schneiderman JF: Nonmedical drug and chemical use in pregnancy. *In* Koren G (ed): Maternal-Fetal Toxicology: A Clinician's Guide, 2nd ed. New York, Marcel Dekker, 1994, pp 301–319.

272. Devenyi P, et al: Abuse of commonly prescribed analgesic preparations. Can Med Assoc J 133:294, 1985.

273. Bailey DN, Manoguerra AS: Survey of drug abuse patterns and toxicology analysis in an emergency room population. J Anal Toxicol 4:199, 1980.

274. Byrne JA, et al: Quantitative analyses of alleged amphetamine formulations obtained from the street market. Proc West Pharmacol Soc 17:210, 1974.

275. Trevor AJ, Way WL: Sedative-hypnotic drugs. *In* Katzung BG (ed): Basic and Clinical Pharmacology, 6th ed. Norwalk, CT, Appleton & Lange, 1995, pp 333–349.

276. Ellenhorn MJ, Barceloux DG: Amphetamines. *In* Medical Toxicology: Diagnosis and Treatment of Human Poisoning. New York, Elsevier, 1988, pp 625–641.

277. Dring LG, et al: The fate of amphetamine in man and other animals. J Pharm Pharmacol 18:402, 1966.

278. Saxen I, Saxen L: Association between maternal intake of diazepam and oral clefts. Lancet 2:298, 1985.

279. Safra MJ, Oakley GP: Association between cleft lip with and without cleft palate and prenatal exposure to diazepam. Lancet 2:478, 1975.

280. Rosenberg L, et al: Lack of relation of oral clefts to diazepam use during pregnancy. N Engl J Med 309:1282, 1983.

281. McElhatton PR: The effects of benzodiazepine use during pregnancy and lactation. Reprod Toxicol 8:461, 1994.

282. Rementeria JL, Bhatt K: Withdrawal symptoms in neonates from intrauterine exposure to diazepam. Pediatr Pharmacol 90:123, 1977.

283. Laegreid L, et al: Abnormalities in children exposed to benzodiazepines in utero. Lancet 1:108, 1987.

284. Weber LWD: Benzodiazepines in pregnancy: academic debate of teratogenic risk? Biol Res Preg 6:151, 1985.

285. Besunder JB, Blumer JL: Neonatal drug withdrawal syndromes. *In* Koren G (ed): Maternal-Fetal Toxicology: A Clinician's Guide, 2nd ed. New York, Marcel Dekker, 1994, pp 321–352.

286. Athinarayanan P, et al: Chlordiazepoxide withdrawal in the neonate. Am J Obstet Gynecol 124:212, 1976.

287. Bitnum S: Possible effect of chlordiazepoxide on the fetus (letter). Can Med Assoc J 100:351, 1969.

288. Mazzi E: Possible neonatal diazepam withdrawal: a case report. Am J Obstet Gynecol 129:586, 1977.

289. Prenner BM: Neonatal withdrawal syndrome associated with hydroxyzine hydrochloride. Am J Dis Child 3:529, 1977.

290. Rumack BH, Walravens PA: Neonatal withdrawal following maternal ingestions of ethchlorvynol (Placidyl). Pediatrics 52: 714, 1973.

291. Reveri M, et al: Neonatal withdrawal symptoms associated with glutethimide (Doriden) addiction in the mother during pregnancy. Clin Pediatr 16:424, 1977.

292. Saxen I: Associations between oral clefts and drugs taken during pregnancy. Int J Epidemiol 4:37, 1975.

293. Safra MJ, Oakley GP Jr: Associations of cleft lip with and without cleft palate and prenatal exposure to diazepam. Lancet 2:478, 1975.

294. Safra MJ, Oakley GP Jr: Valium: an oral cleft teratogen? Cleft Pal J 13:198, 1976.

295. Czeizel A: Letter. Diazepam, phenytoin, and aetiology of cleft lip and/or cleft palate. Lancet 1:810, 1976.

296. Shiono PH, Mills JL: Oral clefts and diazepam use during pregnancy (letter). N Engl J Med 311:919, 1984.

297. Heinonen OP, et al: Birth Defects and Drugs in Pregnancy. Littleton, MA, PSG Publishing, 1977.

298. Desmond MM, et al: Maternal barbiturate utilization and neonatal withdrawal symptomatology. J Pediatr 80:190, 1972.

299. Bleyer WA, Marshall RE: Barbiturate withdrawal syndrome in a passively addicted infant. JAMA 221:185, 1972.

300. Ostrea EM Jr: Neonatal withdrawal from intrauterine exposure to butalbital. Am J Obstet Gynecol 143:597, 1982.

301. Cohen MS: Drug abuse in pregnancy: fetal and neonatal effects. *In* Melmon KL (ed): Drug Therapeutic Concepts for Physicians. New York, Elsevier, 1982, pp 165–179.

302. Onnis A, Grella P (eds): The Biochemical Effects of Drugs in Pregnancy: Drugs Active on the Nervous, Cardiovascular, and Haemopoietic Systems, Vol 1. New York, Ellis Harwood Ltd, 1984, pp 45–64.

303. Weiner N: Norepinephrine, epinephrine, and the sympathomimetic amines. *In* Gilman AG, et al (eds): The Pharmacologic Basis of Therapeutics, 7th ed. New York, MacMillan, 1985, pp 145–180.

304. Ramer CM: The case history of an infant born to an amphetamine-addicted mother. Clin Pediatr 13:596, 1974.

305. Eriksson M, et al: The influence of amphetamine addiction on pregnancy and the newborn infant. Acta Paediatr Scand 67:95, 1978.

306. Nora JJ, et al: Dexamphetamine: a possible environmental trigger in cardiovascular malformations. Lancet 1:1290, 1970.

307. Busto U, et al: Withdrawal reaction after long-term therapeutic use of benzodiazepines. N Engl J Med 315:854, 1986.

308. Smith DE, et al: Phenobarbital technique for treatment of barbiturate dependence. Arch Gen Psychiatry 24:56, 1971.

309. Robinson GM, et al: Barbiturate and hypnosedative withdrawal by a multiple oral phenobarbital loading dose technique. Clin Pharmacol Ther 309:71, 1981.

310. Gay GR: You've come a long way baby! Coke time for the new American lady of the eighties. J Psychoactive Drugs 13:297, 1981.

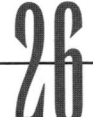

Michael J. Rieder

Drug Excretion During Lactation

BREAST-FEEDING

The optimal feeding of human infants is with breast milk; in addition to psychological benefits, breast-feeding has been shown to decrease the risk of gastrointestinal and respiratory disease in infancy.[1-3] Breast-feeding has been demonstrated to be an effective part of programs to reduce neonatal mortality and there are emerging data that suggest that breast-feeding may influence ultimate neurodevelopmental outcome. Therefore, promotion of breast-feeding has been a major public health initiative in North America and Europe as well as in developing countries.

The incidence of breast-feeding among the mothers of newborn infants in the United States and Canada declined steadily from 1950 to 1970 to reach a nadir at approximately 25%.[4] Since 1970, the incidence of breast-feeding among the mothers of newborn infants has increased steadily until 1984, when more than 60% of mothers breast-fed their newborns. Although a decline in the incidence of breast-feeding in the United States was noted in the early 1980s whereas breast-feeding among newborns continued to increase in Canada, recent data suggests that 75% of women in the United States breast-feed their infants until at least 12 weeks postpartum.[5,6]

Breast-feeding has been recommended as the feeding option of choice for infants in the first 6 to 12 months of life. During this time, it has been estimated that more than 90% of women take medication for the therapy of acute or chronic problems.[7, 8] Many patients are aware of the possibility that medication taken by a lactating mother can pass into breast milk, from which it can be ingested by the nursing infant. Thus, the potential effects of maternal medication transmitted in breast milk on nursing infants are a major concern for families and physicians.[4]

BREAST MILK

Composition

The most abundant component of human breast milk is water, which constitutes approximately 88% of content on average.[9] Milk also contains carbohydrate (5.6 to 6.9%), lipids (3.4 to 4.4%), and protein (1.7 to 2.2%).[10-15] The main carbohydrate present in breast milk is lactose synthesized within the alveolar cell; small amounts of α-glucosides are present as well. The lipids in breast milk are primarily triglycerides, contained in fat globules surrounded by membranes formed from cellular material produced by the alveolar acini (98%). These membranes consist of a complex blend of phospholipids, glycolipids, triglycerides, cholesterol, and proteins, which act to emulsify lipids in the aqueous environment prevalent in breast milk. The protein in human breast milk is a mixture of casein, albumin, lactalbumin, immunoglobulins, and lysozyme with a whey/casein ratio of 60–65:35–40. In addition to protein, human breast milk also contains nonprotein nitrogen in the form of free amino acids and small compounds such as urea.

Breast milk is acidic with reference to plasma; the average pH of human breast milk is 7.08 (range, 6.35 to 7.65). There is a biphasic change in breast milk pH over time. The pH of colostrum is 7.45; it falls to 7.0 in transition milk and then slowly increases to reach an average pH of 7.4 by age 10 months.[4, 16] The pH of breast milk also changes during the course of feeding, with foremilk (expressed during early feeding) having a more acidic pH (as well as a lower fat content) than hindmilk.

The composition of human breast milk is not uniform because the constituents of breast milk change over time and to some extent over the course of feeding. Colostrum, the first milk produced by a lactating mother, is produced in the first 4 or 5 days after birth; transition milk is then produced, followed at 2 or 3 weeks after birth by the production of mature milk.[17]

The protein content of breast milk is subject to changes in both concentration and content. Colostrum has a higher protein content than mature milk, primarily because of increased immunoglobulin content, whereas the albumin content remains relatively constant.[18] The breast milk produced by mothers of preterm infants has approximately twice the protein and less lipid content than that of breast milk produced by mothers of mature infants.[14] The differences between the milk produced by lactating mothers of term and preterm infants are most marked in the immediate perinatal period; changes become less as time from delivery increases.[4] On average, the lipid content of breast milk tends to increase over time.[4]

In addition to changes in composition over time, there is also a diurnal variation in lipid and protein content of breast milk; the fat content and amount of breast milk per feed are highest in the morning and fall to a nadir in the late evening.[19-21] Protein content reaches its nadir in the early afternoon.[20]

Production

Human breast milk is produced in the alveolar acini of mammary tissue located in the breast in response to hormonal stimuli.[22] During the course of gestation, estrogen and progesterone stimulate the maturation of the mammary tissue in the breast.

Estrogen and progesterone, the secretion of which is regulated by follicle-stimulating hormone and luteotrophic hormone, both tend to inhibit milk production. The rapid decrease in estrogen and progesterone secretion immediately before parturition leads to loss of inhibition of milk production.[4] Infants' suckling at the breast stimulates release of prolactin from the pituitary gland; prolactin provides the principal stimulus for milk production and secretion.[23]

Alveolar cells are the component of mammary tissue that produces milk. Clusters of these cells are arranged around a central lumen. Milk flows down the lumen to the ducts, which join in increasing size to meet under the nipple. Milk flow from the acini to the nipple is promoted by oxytocin-mediated contraction of the myoepithelial cells surrounding the acini and ducts.[4]

There is a linear relationship between blood flow and milk production; as blood flow to the alveolar acini increases, so does milk production.[22] Average breast milk production by mothers of 6-month-old infants is approximately 800 mL/day, with production ranging from 600 to 1000 mL/day.[24-26]

PRINCIPLES OF DRUG EXCRETION INTO BREAST MILK

Nursing infants whose mothers consume medications can be exposed to these medications through transfer through breast milk. Drug exposure by this route requires two processes: transfer of the drug into breast milk and then absorption of the drug from breast milk by the infant.[4, 27] In most cases, drug transfer to breast milk requires the presence of the drug in the maternal circulation.[4, 28] The only exception to this rule is when a topical agent is applied directly to the nipple or areola, in which case there may be direct transfer of the drug into breast milk.[29] This is an important but uncommon circumstance.

Transfer of Drug from the Maternal Circulation into Breast Milk

Drugs enter breast milk through the alveolar acini in the mammary gland. A major determinant of the amount of drug transferred to breast milk is the concentration of drug in the maternal circulation. Most drugs taken by lactating women are given orally, although in selected cases drugs may be given by the intravenous, topical, or aerosol routes. The steady-state drug concentration in the maternal circulation is determined by the balance of drug absorption, distribution, metabolism, and excretion (Fig. 26–1).

Drugs can be transferred from the maternal circulation to breast milk by several mechanisms[27]:

1. Transcellular diffusion of small molecules, which are nonionized and have high lipid solubility, such as ethanol, for which plasma and breast milk concentrations are similar.[27,30]
2. Intercellular diffusion of drugs that pass between alveolar cells; this may account for the passage of larger molecules, such as immunoglobulins, into breast milk.[27]
3. Passive diffusion along a concentration gradient.
4. Ionophore diffusion of polar substances by binding to carrier proteins.[27]

In most instances, the passage of drugs from the maternal circulation to breast milk occurs by passive diffusion down a concentration gradient. This concentration gradient is across the capillaries feeding the alveolar acini and into the alveolar cells. To cross from the circulation into the alveolar acini, a drug must be present in the maternal circulation in an unbound, nonionized form. Therefore, the concentration driving diffusion of drugs from the maternal circulation into breast milk is that of the free fraction of drug in the circulation.

It should be recognized that diffusion of drugs into breast milk is a bidirectional process; not only can drugs diffuse into breast

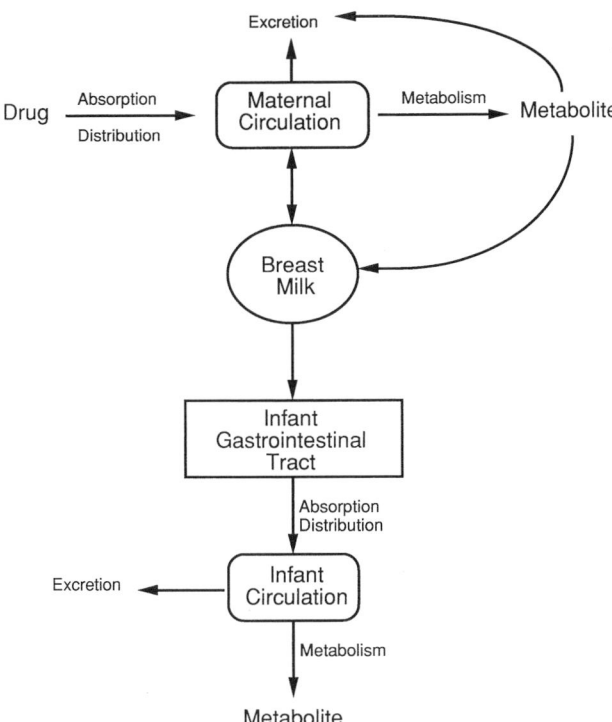

Figure 26–1. Steps involved in transfer of drugs from lactating mothers to nursing infants through breast milk.

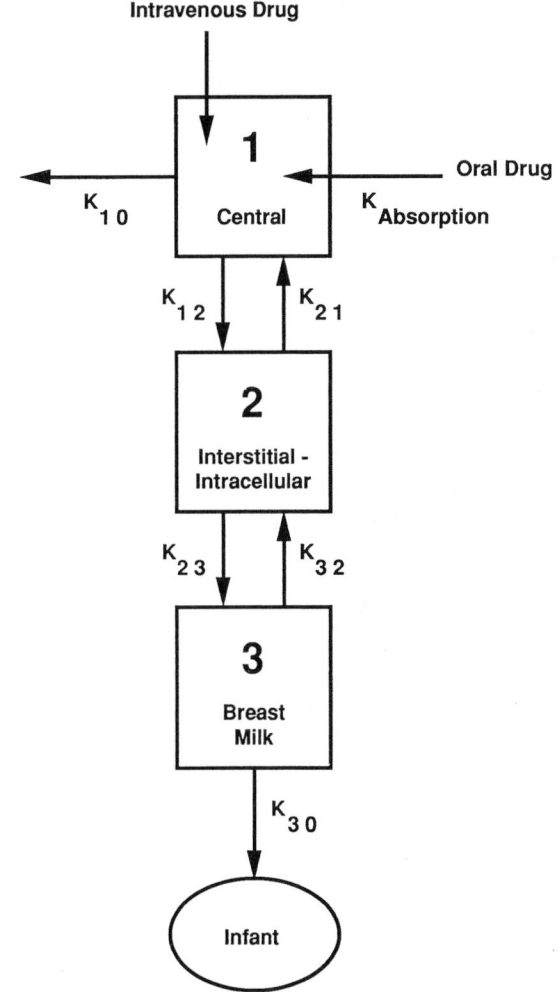

Figure 26–2. Three-compartment model for drug transfer into breast milk. K is rate constant for absorption. (Modified from Wilson JT: Drug Metabol Rev *14*:619, 1983, by courtesy of Marcel Dekker, Inc.)

milk from plasma, but they can also transfer from breast milk back into plasma. In addition, the same principles of drug transfer into and out of breast milk apply equally to drug metabolites.

The free fraction of drug available for transfer into breast milk varies from drug to drug. Some drugs, such as propanolol, are highly protein bound, and thus a relatively smaller amount is available as free drug.[31] In addition, the plasma protein binding of some drugs changes during pregnancy; a decrease in the plasma protein binding of sulfisoxazole, phenytoin, diazepam, and dexamethasone occurs during gestation, with a return to prepregnancy values 1 to 2 months after delivery.[32]

Drug passage across lipid membranes by passive diffusion is a function of molecular size and lipid solubility. Furthermore, for a drug to diffuse from the maternal circulation to the acinar cells, it must be in the nonionized form.

Because most drugs are weakly acidic or basic, drug partitioning between blood and breast milk is at least partially dependent on pH.[4,33-36] The ratio of the drug present in milk (M) versus the amount of the drug present in plasma (P) can be estimated by the following equations[4]:

Drugs that are weak acids:

$$M/P = 1 + 10^{(pHm - pKa)}/1 + 10^{(pHp - pKa)}$$

Drugs that are weak bases:

$$M/P = 1 + 10^{(pKa - pHm)}/1 + 10^{(pKa - pHp)}$$

pHm = the pH of breast milk, pHp = the pH of plasma, and pKa = the pKa of the drug in question.[4] For acidic drugs, the lower pH of breast milk (with reference to plasma) leads to a larger portion of the drug being present in the ionized form in plasma, leading to a lower M/P ratio; this is known as *ion trapping*. For weak bases, the opposite is the case.[4]

The question of whether breast tissue can metabolize drugs present in breast milk is unknown for most compounds.[27] Conjugation has been demonstrated for some animal species, but

human, bovine, and rodent breast tissue does not appear to possess appreciable concentrations of Phase I enzymes such as cytochrome P450.[27] Both ribonuclease and reverse transcriptase have been identified in human milk; the significance of these enzymes is uncertain.[37,38]

A pharmacokinetic model for drug transfer into breast milk has been described for drugs that have low lipid solubility. This model assigns a deep compartment for breast milk, with transfer occurring from a central compartment (maternal circulation) to the deep compartment.[28] A three-compartment model for drug excretion into breast milk has also been described (Fig. 26–2).[22, 28] For most drugs, however, a two-compartment model provides a valid pharmacokinetic model for the study of the transfer of drugs into breast milk.[39,40]

In addition to the mechanisms described above for transfer of drugs from the maternal circulation into breast milk, there is some intriguing preliminary evidence that active transport systems may exist for certain drugs that act to transfer drugs into or out of breast milk.[4]

Transfer of Drug from Breast Milk to the Infant

Given the molecular size and polarity of most drugs in routine clinical use, the processes described previously will predictably lead to a portion of the serum concentration of most drugs passing into breast milk. It must be appreciated, however, that drug absorption from breast milk is not analogous to the enteral administration of drug to an infant for therapeutic purposes. Rather, in the case of drugs in breast milk, drug is present in dilute form in a relatively large volume of liquid, which includes other elements that can interact with the drug and alter the amount of drug available for absorption.

Protein and lipid components of breast milk can interact with drugs present in the aqueous phase. Thus, drugs that undergo protein binding bind to protein in breast milk; for drugs with extensive protein binding, the amount of drug available for absorption can be overestimated.[31] This can be corrected for by calculating M/P ratios for these drugs on the basis of the amount of drug in skim milk.[4,41]

Drugs in breast milk can also interact with the lipid content of milk. The partition of highly lipid-soluble drugs in breast milk can be corrected by calculating the M/P ratio and using a correction factor for the octanol/water partition coefficient of the drug in question.[4,42] Drugs with high lipid solubility, such as phenobarbital, can be trapped in the fat globules in breast milk, with a relative elevation in the amount present in milk versus plasma.[27]

Estimation of the Drug Dose Delivered in Breast Milk

A widely used method to estimate the amount of drug that lactating infants receive through breast milk is to calculate the drug dose in milk using the M/P ratio.[4,28,36,43] To use this method, it is necessary to know the M/P ratio and maternal steady-state plasma or serum drug concentration (C_{ss}) of the drug in question and the volume of milk produced per day. The dose available to the infant can then be calculated using the equation:

Dose (mg/kg/day) = C_{ss} × M/P ratio × milk volume (mL/kg/day)

To use this equation, three pieces of data must be known. The first is the C_{ss}, which can be determined by therapeutic drug monitoring of maternal plasma or serum. The second item is the M/P ratio, which is listed in various reference sources.[4] The final piece of data is an estimate of the milk volume; it has been estimated that, for term infants, the average milk volume is approximately 150 mg/kg/day (in this case, the weight is the weight of the breast-feeding infant[22]).

To illustrate how this equation can be used, one may consider the example of a woman with epilepsy who is taking 300 mg of phenytoin once daily. Therapeutic drug monitoring reveals a steady-state serum concentration of 15 µg/mL. A review of the literature provides two studies that have been used to derive an M/P ratio for phenytoin. In the first study, Rane and colleagues[44] observed an M/P ratio of 0.45 in a group of five infants. Using these values, the amount of drug delivered in breast milk can be calculated:

Dose = 15 µg/mL × 0.45 × 150 mL/kg/day

Dose = 1.01 mg/kg/day

The second study, by Stern and co-workers,[45] was conducted using a sample size of six infants; the M/P ratio derived was 0.13. Using these values, the estimated delivered dose would be

Dose = 15 µg/mL × 0.13 × 150 mL/kg/day

Dose = 0.29 mg/kg/day

Given that the usual therapeutic maintenance dose of phenytoin for children is 5 mg/kg/day, these equations suggest that the dose of phenytoin anticipated in breast milk would be in the range of 6 to 20% of the usual therapeutic dose. In fact, in

the second study, Stern and co-workers[45] were able to detect low serum concentrations of phenytoin (0.12 and 0.18 µg/mL) in two of the six infants studied. Therefore, in considering the implications of these estimates, it is important to note that there was a threefold difference between the M/P ratios in the two studies.

This equation can be useful to estimate the dose available to a nursing infant, but several concerns must be remembered when using any equation involving the M/P ratio.[40] First, for the equation to be accurate, the maternal serum concentration must be at steady state. It is possible that drugs may accumulate in breast milk over time; thus, estimates made before the mother's serum concentration reaches steady state may underestimate the amount of drug present in breast milk.[4] In situations in which the C_{ss} is not available, it may be possible to estimate C_{ss} if the dose rate, bioavailability, and clearance are known.[4]

Another issue affecting the accuracy of this equation is the M/P ratio itself. Although there are many studies describing an M/P ratio for various drugs, some of these studies have derived the M/P ratio from a single, simultaneously obtained determination of plasma (or serum) and milk from small numbers of infants.[4] Therefore, if there are temporal variations in the M/P ratio (as is suggested in the case of phenytoin by the wide variations present), the estimates produced by this equation may not be accurate. The effect of changes in breast milk composition during feeding and of changes in breast composition over time (from colostrum to mature milk) on the M/P ratio has not been evaluated for most drugs.[4,40] A more nearly ideal method of calculating the M/P ratio is to use multiple time points to calculate an area under the curve (AUC) for drug concentrations in milk and plasma and then use the AUCs to calculate the M/P ratio. Additionally, it has been suggested that combining use of the M/P ratio and estimates of drug clearance may be a more relevant evaluation of potential exposure of developing infants to drugs in breast milk.[43]

An additional issue not addressed by the M/P ratio is the effects of drug metabolites, especially for drugs that undergo biotransformation to active metabolites. Given that the same considerations with respect to breast milk transfer apply to drug metabolites, the use of the M/P ratio alone may give a misleading impression of potential biologic effect(s) for compounds that are extensively transformed to active metabolites.

There are many compounds for which no M/P ratios have been described. It is possible to estimate an M/P ratio for these drugs based on the physiochemical nature of the drug, using data such as the acidic strength (pKa) of the drug, the amount of protein binding, and the octanol/water partition coefficient of the drug.[4]

An alternate approach taking advantage of the availability of sensitive analytic technology provides a method for estimation of drug dosage in breast milk by directly measuring the drug in question in breast milk. The drug concentration can then be used to calculate the drug dose presented to the nursing infant. Ideally, multiple determinations should be used to see if there are temporal variations in drug concentration during and between breast feeds. In addition, therapeutic drug monitoring in the infant can be used to follow the plasma or serum drug concentrations.

Clinical Implications of Drug Excretion During Lactation

The most common reason that clinicians estimate drug dose in breast milk is to assess whether it is likely that the drug will exert an adverse effect on a nursing infant. Fortunately the dose in breast milk (in most cases) is much lower than the usual therapeutic dose, and biologic effects (untoward and otherwise) would not be anticipated.

In the usual case, one should be cautious with respect to prescribing drugs for lactating mothers. In cases in which therapy is clearly indicated, however, the demonstrated benefits of maternal therapy almost always outweigh theoretical risks of adverse drug effects in the nursing infant. A useful set of guidelines for a general approach to drug excretion during lactation, based on studies of drug excretion into breast milk, have been proposed by Berlin.[27] In general, it is reasonable to assume the following:

1. The majority of all drugs (and environmental chemicals with molecular weights less than 200 D) cross from maternal plasma to breast milk.
2. The time-concentration profile of drugs in breast milk parallels the time-concentration profile of drugs in plasma, with M/P ratios usually varying from 0.5 to 1.0.
3. The concentration of drugs in breast milk is almost always too low and too unpredictable to treat infants by giving medication to their mothers.
4. The half-life of drugs in plasma and breast milk are similar following a single maternal dose, implying rapid transfer of the drug from plasma to milk.
5. The amount of drug available in breast milk for absorption by the infant is usually less than 1% of the maternal dose. This amount can be minimized by breast-feeding during times when maternal plasma drug concentrations are low, such as just before the next dose.
6. There are few studies that describe drug transfer in the setting of long-term maternal therapy over days or weeks; understanding of how changes in drug transfer may occur over time is limited.
7. In the case of most drugs, even those with potent pharmacologic effects, the risk of adverse drug effects in nursing infants is negligible, especially if attention is given to planning the nursing schedule around the time of minimal drug exposure.

This final point has been reinforced by a prospective study of breast-feeding mothers conducted by the Motherisk Program, a Teratogen Information Service in Toronto. Between 1985 and 1991, 838 mother-infant pairs were assessed for exposure to a number of drugs taken by the mothers; no major adverse events were described among the infants.[4] Minor adverse effects were described in 11% of the infants, but they did not require medical attention.[4]

Although there are many case reports of isolated adverse effects that may be related to drug exposure through breast milk,[46-48] case reports by their nature do not establish causality and in many instances represent rare and possibly nonreproducible events. Furthermore, case reports can sometimes unintentionally give the misleading impression that an adverse effect described in relation to therapy is both causally related and common.[4] Thus, case reports must be interpreted with caution when assessing possible risks associated with therapy of lactating mothers.[46]

Special considerations must be made in the case of long-term therapy, in which the infant may be exposed to the drug in question for a period of weeks or months. In many cases, therapy may have been started before delivery, and in those situations it is likely that the infant will be exposed to smaller concentrations through breast milk than the fetus was exposed to *in utero*. In the case of certain compounds, such as barbiturates, accumulation may occur, and clinicians should monitor such infants for signs of toxicity. For most agents used in long-term therapy, however, taking care and using therapy as indicated to ensure optimal maternal health are of greater importance in maintaining the health of the infant than is a nihilistic policy of drug avoidance regardless of potential effects on maternal health.

DRUGS CONTRAINDICATED FOR NURSING MOTHERS

There are a small number of drugs that are contraindicated during lactation or the use of which contraindicates breast-feeding (Table 26-1).

Antimetabolites

Therapy with antimetabolites, especially for the therapy of neoplastic disease, is contraindicated during lactation. Although the absolute dose present in breast milk is small, the pharmacologic potency of these agents and the potential for serious long-term toxicity is usually believed to preclude lactation when therapy with these agents is required. The two most common agents used for immunosuppressive therapy are azathioprine and methotrexate. Both these drugs (and the methotrexate metabolite 6-mercaptopurine) can be detected in breast milk in low concentrations.[49-51] It has been suggested that it may be safe for mothers on low-dose therapy with methotrexate to breast-feed; however, this remains controversial.[52] When the parents have decided to continue with breast-feeding after being counseled, strong consideration should be given to monitor these infants carefully (with respect to their immunologic and hematologic status) and to determine milk and plasma concentrations of the drug in question.[4]

Anticoagulants

The various warfarin (Coumadin) derivatives appear to be excreted into breast milk in differing amounts. Warfarin has not been detected in breast milk, and the infants of women receiving warfarin therapy have not had problems with coagulation.[53, 54] Similarly, no bleeding was found among the infants of a large cohort of women treated with dicumarol (bishydroxycoumarin) for prevention of thromboembolic complications.[55] This suggests that therapy with warfarin and dicumarol is compatible with breast-feeding.[47, 56] In contrast, the anticoagulant ethyl biscoumacetate has been detected in breast milk, and in one study 5 of 42 nursing infants whose mothers were being treated with ethyl biscoumacetate developed bleeding complications.[57, 58] Phenindione (unavailable in the United States) has been

TABLE 26-1

Drugs Contraindicated for Nursing Mothers

Antimetabolites
  Azathioprine
  Cyclophosphamide
  Doxorubicin
  Methotrexate
Antiocoagulants
  Phenindione
Ergot alkaloids
  Bromocriptine
  Ergotamine
Gold
Iodine-containing compounds
  Amiodarone
  Potassium iodide
  Povidone-iodine (extensive topical use)
Oral contraceptives (relative contraindication)*
Psychoactive drugs
  Lithium
  Phenobarbital
Radiopharmaceuticals†
Recreational chemicals
  Amphetamines
  Cocaine
  Ethanol
  Heroin
  Marijuana
  Phencyclidine (PCP)
  Nicotine (tobacco smoking)

* Relative contraindication; see text.
† See Table 26-2 for specific agents.

detected in the milk of lactating mothers and has been associated with significant bleeding complications in the nursing infant.[56,59,60] Heparin is too large a molecule to be excreted into breast milk.

Ergot Alkaloids

The ergot alkaloid bromocriptine suppresses prolactin and among other indications is used clinically to prevent lactation.[61] Thus, it is not surprising that bromocriptine is contraindicated when planning breast-feeding. Ergotamine is excreted into the breast milk of mothers receiving this agent in doses used to treat migraines, and ergotism, including vomiting, diarrhea, and seizures, has been described among the breast-feeding infants of mothers treated with that drug.[56,62] In addition, ergotamine can suppress lactation.[63] No adverse effects have been described associated with the short-term use of methylergonovine to promote uterine involution.[4]

Gold

Gold can be detected in the breast milk of women treated with that agent.[64-68] It has been estimated that lactating infants can be exposed to as much as 20% of the maternal dose through breast milk.[67] There is controversy, however, with respect to the clinical significance of this exposure. There are reports of gold's being present in breast milk with no apparent adverse effects on the nursing infant. Conversely, there are also reports of infants with a constellation of adverse events, which might be related to exposure to gold in breast milk, although a causal link has not been established.[64,66] Some investigators believe that gold salts are contraindicated during breast-feeding, although the Committee on Drugs of the American Academy of Pediatrics considers these agents compatible with breast-feeding.[56,67] When lactating women are being treated with gold, their infants should be closely observed during follow-up for adverse effects. In addition, gold concentrations should be determined in breast milk and the infant's serum.

Iodine-Containing Compounds

Iodine is excreted into breast milk and can lead to iodine-induced goiter and hypothyroidism in breast-fed infants.[69] This applies both to oral preparations such as potassium iodide and to topical use of povidone-iodine preparations.[56,70,71] Therefore, compounds containing iodine should be avoided during lactation. Amiodarone is an antiarrhythmic agent that contains 75 mg of iodine per each 200-mg dose.[72] Amiodarone is excreted into breast milk, and although there are no reports of adverse effects, the high iodine content of this compound and the long half-life in adults suggest that this agent should be avoided during breast-feeding.[72,73]

Oral Contraceptives

There is a relative contraindication with respect to oral contraceptives, notably for certain groups of mothers. The use of oral contraceptives during the early phases of breast-feeding is associated with shortened duration of lactation, decreased milk production, and decreased nitrogen and protein content in milk (all of which can decrease infant weight gain).[74-78] These changes are less marked with agents containing only progesterone and have not been observed with newer combined oral contraceptives.[78] The effect of oral contraceptives on weight gain may be especially important for the infants of malnourished mothers. Therefore, it has been recommended that oral contraceptives be avoided in nursing mothers who are malnourished.[4,79] For similar reasons, wherever possible, oral contraceptives should be avoided for the first 6 weeks after delivery.[4]

Estrogen and progesterone can both enter breast milk, although with currently available low-dose combination products the estrogen content of breast-fed infants whose mothers are being treated with these products does not appear to be higher than the natural estrogen content of breast milk from women who are not receiving any hormonal agents.[48] There is a single case report of a child who was exposed to a large dose of estrogen who developed mild breast hypertrophy.[48] Use of oral contraceptives is acceptable in women who have successfully established breast-feeding.[56]

Psychoactive Drugs

Lithium can be detected in breast milk in concentrations that can be as high as 40% of the maternal serum concentration.[80-82] This can result in serum concentrations that are approximately equal to those in milk. Fortunately, no adverse effects have been reported. Nonetheless, concerns with respect to possible long-term adverse effects of exposure to lithium have led the Committee on Drugs of the American Academy of Pediatrics to consider lithium contraindicated during lactation.[56] An alternate approach is to perform determinations of the lithium concentration in breast milk and the serum of the nursing infant to determine on an individual basis if lithium therapy can be continued during lactation.

Phenobarbital is excreted into breast milk, with m/p ratios between 0.4 and 0.6.[83,84] Infants exhibit slower elimination of phenobarbital than do adults, and serum phenobarbital concentrations in the infant can actually exceed those of the mother.[84] This has been associated with clinically significant sedation.[85] Therefore, when treating lactating women with phenobarbital, infants should be followed closely for signs of sedation. Additionally the breast milk and serum concentrations of phenobarbital in the infant should be determined at periodic intervals.

Radiopharmaceuticals

Many commonly used radiopharmaceuticals are excreted into breast milk.[56] Therefore, it is generally recommended that breast-feeding be avoided over the time when the radioisotope in question is being excreted into breast milk.[56] The time interval for clearance of the radioisotope varies with the compound used for the investigation in question (Table 26-2). When in doubt, a reference text or a nuclear medicine expert should be consulted. In many cases, it is possible to plan for this eventuality in advance, by banking frozen milk that can be used to feed the infant while the breast milk containing the radioisotope is pumped and discarded until radioactivity has cleared from the milk.[4]

TABLE 26-2

Duration of Excretion of Radioactivity into Milk Following Use of Radiopharmaceuticals

Drug	Duration of Radioactivity in Milk
Copper-64	50 h
Gallium-67	2 w
Indium-111	20 h
Iodine-123	36 h
Iodine-125	12 d
Iodine-131	2-14 d*
Radioactive sodium	96 h
Technetium-99	1-3 d

* Varies depending on type of study.
Modified from Committee on Drugs, American Academy of Pediatrics: The transfer of drugs and other chemicals into human milk. Pediatrics 93: 137, 1994. Used with permission of the American Academy of Pediatrics.

Recreational Chemicals

This group of compounds includes drugs used socially and drugs that are usually used under circumstances of abuse. As a general rule, the active compounds present in these agents can all be excreted into breast milk. Thus, given the potent pharmacology of many of these drugs, the use of these agents should be considered contraindicated during pregnancy and lactation.[4]

Amphetamines can be concentrated in breast milk, with M/P ratios that can range from 2.8 to 7.5.[86] Despite a lack of reports associating neonatal symptoms with amphetamine exposure, the Committee on Drugs of the American Academy of Drugs considers amphetamines to be contraindicated during breast-feeding.[56]

Cocaine enters breast milk readily because of its low molecular weight and high fat solubility. Cocaine and benzoylecgonine, the principal metabolite of cocaine, have been detected in the urine of nursing infants, and some of these infants have had clinical signs compatible with cocaine exposure.[87,88] Symptoms have also been reported in an infant whose mother used cocaine as a topical analgesic on her nipples.[29] Cocaine use should be avoided at all times by lactating mothers.[56]

Ethanol is a small lipid-soluble molecule that freely passes into breast milk at concentrations equivalent to plasma concentrations.[30, 89] In contrast, acetaldehyde, a toxic metabolite of ethanol, apparently does not enter breast milk in appreciable concentrations.[30] The elimination of ethanol from breast milk appears to be similar to that of ethanol in plasma, which follows zero-order kinetics.[30, 89] The consumption of small amounts of ethanol on an infrequent basis does not appear to be associated with untoward effects in nursing infants, given that the amount of ethanol in breast milk is likely to be small.[4] It has been appreciated for some time, however, that ingestion of large amounts of ethanol in a single sitting can result in high concentrations of ethanol in breast milk and cause symptoms, including sedation, in nursing infants.[90] Although controversial, chronic exposure to ethanol in breast milk has been associated with delayed psychomotor development in a single study.[91] Therefore, it would be prudent to recommend that lactating mothers avoid chronic ethanol use while nursing their infants. The Committee on Drugs of the American Academy of Pediatrics considers moderate ethanol use to be compatible with breast-feeding, although caution is recommended.[56] In addition to possible effects on the infant, ethanol in high doses blocks release of oxytocin.[92,93]

Heroin and other opiates can be detected in breast milk. In the case of heroin, sufficient heroin is excreted into breast milk to produce dependence among nursing infants.[94] Heroin and other opiates, especially when used under circumstances of abuse, are contraindicated during lactation.

The active ingredient of marijuana is Δ-9-tetrahydrocannabinol (THC); THC has been found in the breast milk of women who have smoked marijuana.[95] On the basis of finding THC metabolites in the feces of infants in this study, the authors concluded that the infants absorbed THC from breast milk and further metabolized THC.[95] There has been no evidence of adverse clinical consequences following exposure to THC through breast milk.[56] Long-term follow-up studies beyond a year of age, however, have not been performed. The Committee on Drugs of the American Academy of Pediatrics regard marijuana use as being contraindicated when breast-feeding.[56]

Phencyclidine can be detected in the breast milk of women who have used the drug. Furthermore, it can be detected for a considerable time after the last dose.[96, 97] With respect to other hallucinogens, there is little information available regarding transfer into breast milk. Given that these drugs are small molecular weight compounds with considerable potency, however, untoward effect(s) on nursing infants are highly probable. Thus, phencyclidine and other hallucinogens, including lysergic acid diethylamide (LSD), are contraindicated during breast-feeding.

Nicotine and cotinine, the major metabolite of nicotine, have been found in the breast milk of mothers who smoke cigarettes.[98-100] Cotinine has been found in the urine of nursing infants whose mothers smoke, suggesting absorption of nicotine metabolites from breast milk or exposure to second-hand smoke.[4, 101-103] Adverse effects, including increased rates of respiratory illness and possibly an increased rate of colic, have been reported in the infants of mothers who smoke.[103,104] In addition, cigarette smoking may inhibit production of breast milk.[105]

In summary, recreational chemicals pass readily into breast milk and may alter the production, composition, and volume of breast milk; breast-feeding mothers should be advised to restrict their intake of recreational chemicals.[90]

DRUG CLASSES COMMONLY USED BY LACTATING WOMEN

Analgesics

Acetaminophen, aspirin, and nonsteroidal antiinflammatory drugs such as ibuprofen and ketorolac are secreted into breast milk in small concentrations. The use of these agents in usual therapeutic doses has not been associated with adverse effects on nursing infants. There has been a report of salicylism in the nursing infant of a mother treated with aspirin; the pharmacokinetic profile suggests that exposure occurred by routes other than breast milk.[106] Opiates transfer into breast milk; in the case of morphine, transfer to breast milk is limited. Codeine in doses used for the ambulatory patient is compatible with breast-feeding. If therapy is to continue on a long-term basis, however, the clinician should monitor the infant for signs of sedation.

Antiasthma Agents

Asthma is among the most common chronic diseases that women require therapy for during the time that they are breast-feeding their infants. β_2-adrenergic selective agents are the agents of choice for the acute therapy of asthma and are typically given by aerosol. There is minimal absorption of albuterol (salbutamol) (the most commonly used β_2-adrenergic selective agent) when this drug is given by inhalation.[107] Thus, significant excretion of these agents into breast milk is unlikely. The same considerations apply for inhaled adrenocorticosteroids, notably when total dose is less than 1000 μg in a day. Prednisone is excreted into breast milk in small concentrations.[108] Because these concentrations are unlikely to be associated with adverse effects in the nursing infant, use of both prednisone and prednisolone is compatible with breast-feeding.[56] Theophylline is excreted into breast milk in small concentrations, with an estimated infant dose that is less than 1% of maternal dose.[109] There has been a report of irritability in the nursing infant of a mother taking a rapidly absorbed theophylline preparation. This has prompted the suggestion that nursing mothers who require theophylline therapy should be treated with slow-release preparations.[110] Nonetheless, theophylline is considered to be compatible with breast-feeding.[56] Few data are available with respect to the transfer of newer agents such as montelukast into breast milk, but it is reasonable to assume that a small amount is likely to be present.

Antimicrobial and Antiinfective Agents

Essentially all of the antimicrobial and antiinfective drugs transfer into breast milk. The β-lactam antibiotics are compatible with breast-feeding. Tetracycline passes into breast milk in low concentrations, where it can associate with calcium in milk. Absorption of tetracycline from milk appears to be negligible because tetracycline has not been detected in the blood of nursing infants whose mothers were treated with tetracycline.[111, 112] Although use of tetracycline in younger children is normally contraindicated because of the effects on developing teeth and bones, the lack of evidence of absorption has led the Committee on Drugs of the American Academy of Pediatrics to consider tetracycline therapy compatible with breast-feeding.[56] Erythromycin is present in breast milk during maternal therapy but is also compatible with breast-feeding. Azithromycin is excreted into breast milk and may accumulate because of the lipid solubility of the drug and ion trapping.[113]

Caution must be exercised in the use of nalidixic acid, nitrofurantoin, quinine, and sulfonamides for therapy of lactating women who belong to populations at risk for glucose-6-phosphatase deficiency because drug transfer through breast milk may be associated with a risk for hemolysis.[4] Furthermore, it is recommended that sulfonamides be avoided during the first postnatal week because of the theoretical concern that displacement of bilirubin from albumin might lead to kernicterus; this has never been described in a term infant.

The quinolones (norfloxacin, ciprofloxacin, and ofloxacin) appear to be excreted into breast milk in low concentrations.[114] Animal studies demonstrating an arthropathy in a beagle pup model have been cited as a rationale for avoiding use of the quinolones in pregnancy and lactation.[4] The expanding experience with these drugs in pediatrics, however, has not demonstrated adverse effects in humans and suggests that, when clinically indicated, quinolones are compatible with breast-feeding.[115, 116] Chloramphenicol is excreted into breast milk. Caution has been recommended when using chloramphenicol in lactating women because of the possibility of an idiosyncratic reaction or bone marrow toxicity (or both).[4] Therefore, given the severity of potential adverse reactions, chloramphenicol should be used with caution among lactating women. Metronidazole is excreted into breast milk.[117] Although concern has been expressed with respect to the potential mutagenic effects of metronidazole, this has not been demonstrated in humans.[4] In conventional dosages, metronidazole is compatible with breast-feeding. If metronidazole is given in a single large dose (such as the single 2-g dose recommended for therapy of trichomoniasis), however, the breast should be pumped and milk discarded for 12 to 24 hours after the dose, to allow for elimination of metronidazole.[56]

Isoniazid and the isoniazid metabolite acetylisoniazid are excreted into breast milk in large concentrations.[118] Although there are no reports of toxicity among nursing infants of mothers treated with isoniazid, it is recommended that, when treating lactating mothers with isoniazid, the clinician should monitor nursing infants for signs of peripheral neuritis or hepatitis.[119]

Acyclovir has been detected in breast milk in much higher concentrations than would be anticipated given the physiochemical nature of the drug.[120] This suggests that acyclovir may have a unique active or facilitated transport process for entry into breast milk.[120] Based on the poor oral absorption of this agent, it has been estimated that the amount absorbed by nursing infants of mothers treated with acyclovir should be minimal.[120] Therefore, the Committee on Drugs of the American Academy of Pediatrics considers acyclovir therapy to be compatible with breast-feeding.[56]

Recent work has demonstrated that zidovudine appears to transfer into breast milk in concentrations roughly equivalent to those seen in serum.[120] Interestingly, recent research from South Africa has suggested that exclusive breast feeding appears to be associated with a reduction in postnatal transmission of HIV.[121]

Antihypertensives and Diuretics

β-adrenergic blocking agents are excreted into breast milk; the extent of drug transfer is determined by the degree of protein binding. Agents such as atenolol and sotalol, which are relatively less protein bound, pass into breast milk in greater quantities than an agent such as propanolol, which is more highly protein bound.[122-124] Nursing infants of mothers being treated with a β-adrenergic blocking agent should be followed for signs of β-adrenergic blockade, including bradycardia.

Captopril and other angiotensin-converting enzyme inhibitors are excreted into breast milk in low concentrations. The use of these agents and drugs such as hydralazine, methyldopa, and verapamil is considered to be compatible with breast-feeding.[56]

Diuretics such as chlorothiazine and hydrochlorothiazide are excreted into breast milk in low amounts.[33] Although thiazide diuretics can suppress lactation, in the usual therapeutic doses these agents are considered compatible with lactation.[56] Furosemide is also excreted into breast milk and is considered compatible with lactation.[56]

Anticonvulsants and Psychoactive Drugs

Carbamazepine, phenytoin, and valproic acid are excreted into breast milk in small amounts, so that use of these agents is considered compatible with breast-feeding.[56] Ethosuximide is found in breast milk in concentrations roughly equivalent to maternal serum; however, the Committee on Drugs of the American Academy of Pediatrics considers ethosuximide therapy to be compatible with breast-feeding.[56] As described previously, phenobarbital is contraindicated during lactation. Primidone is metabolized to phenobarbital, and the same considerations with respect to phenobarbital therapy apply to primidone.

As described previously, lithium therapy is believed by many authorities to be contraindicated during lactation. Most psychoactive drugs used, including the phenothiazines, benzodiazepines, and antidepressants, are excreted into breast milk. These agents should be used with caution in lactating women.[56]

The selective serotonin reuptake inhibitors, a very widely used class of drugs, are excreted into breast milk in variable and usually small amounts.[125-9] Although isolated case studies of toxicity have been reported, series of mother-infant pairs have demonstrated minimal infant exposure to most of the SSRIs tested, notably paroxetine and venlafaxine.[125-129]

Cardiovascular Drugs

Digoxin is excreted into breast milk in small concentrations and is believed to be compatible with lactation. The same judgment applies to flecainide, mexiletine, and quinidine.[4] Procainamide and its active metabolite N-acetylprocainamide are also excreted into breast milk.[130] Although there are no reports of adverse effects associated with procainamide use by lactating mothers, the effects of long-term exposure are unknown. Therefore, infants of lactating mothers treated with procainamide should be followed closely. Disopyramide is present in milk in relatively high concentrations. Although there have been no adverse effects reported among infants of lactating mothers treated with disopyramide, clinicians should observe these infants closely and consider monitoring breast milk and the infant's blood for drug concentrations.[4] Quinidine is excreted into breast milk and considered to be compatible with breast-feeding.[56, 131] A recent systemic review has suggested that the use of angiotensin-converting enzyme inhibitors and many of the calcium channel blockers would be expected to be safe during breast feeding, but beta-blockers with low protein binding such as atenolol may have the potential for affecting the infants of breast-feeding mothers.[132]

Endocrine and Gastrointestinal Drugs

Thyroid replacement therapy with agents such as levothyroxine is compatible with breast-feeding. The antithyroid agent propylthiouracil is excreted into breast milk in small concentrations; maternal therapy with doses of 50 to 300 mg per day is considered compatible with breast-feeding, although the clinician should monitor the infant's thyroid function on a regular basis.[133]

Tolbutamide and chlorpropamide are excreted into breast milk in low concentrations, which are unlikely to influence the infant's blood glucose concentration.[134] The molecular weight of insulin precludes entry of this agent into breast milk.

Adverse effects have not been described after maternal use of a number of laxatives, including mineral oil, phenolphthalein, and senna derivatives.[4] It has, however, been recommended that lactating mothers who require laxatives should be treated with agents that are poorly absorbed, such as psyllium.[4]

Ranitidine and cimetidine are excreted into breast milk in small amounts, and use of these agents is considered to be compatible with breast-feeding.[56] There is little information on the transfer of omeprazole into breast milk; however, given the potency of this agent, it would be prudent to avoid it if possible. Antacids that contain sodium and aluminum are considered to be compatible with breast-feeding.[135] Metoclopramide and domperidone are both compatible with breast-feeding and have been used to increase milk production.[4]

Over-the-Counter Drugs

Numerous over-the-counter drugs are used for symptomatic relief of common problems, notably self-limited upper respiratory tract infections and environmental allergies. In usual therapeutic doses, these agents are compatible with breast-feeding; however, because these agents have the potential for causing sedation, care should be taken if they are used for a prolonged period.[22, 47, 48] There has been a single case report of an infant who developed irritability and a high-pitched cry while receiving breast milk from a woman taking the antihistamine clemastine.[48] Given that there have been no subsequent reports, this suggests that problems such as this are uncommon with these agents in usual therapeutic doses.[47,48]

Herbal Medicines

Herbal and other traditional medications are frequently used by patients, and recent estimates are that up to one-third of all patients take some type of complementary or alternate medication on a regular basis. Patients often make the assumption that herbal medications are safe because they are natural. However, the active ingredients in herbal medications, like that of most other medications, are likely to be able to enter breast milk. This area is not very well studied. There are two concerns. First, with herbal medication the possibility of adulteration must be borne in mind if infants develop unusual symptoms. Second, it is possible that the active elements of some herbal medications, such as St. John's wort, may be absorbed by breast-feeding infants, and consequently research in this area, given the popularity of these agents, is urgently needed.[136]

REFERENCES

1. Anderson JE, et al: Breast-feeding, birth interval and infant health. Pediatrics 74(Suppl):695, 1984.
2. Cunningham AS, et al: Breast feeding and health in the 1980's: a global epidemiologic review. J Pediatr 118:659, 1991.
3. Kovar MG, et al: Review of the epidemiologic evidence for an association between infant feeding and infant health. Pediatrics 74(Suppl):615, 1984.
4. Ito S: Drug therapy for breast-feeding women. N Engl J Med 343:118, 2000.
5. McNally E, et al: A look at breast-feeding trends in Canada (1963–1982). Can J Public Health 76:101, 1985.
6. Schwartz K, et al: Factors associated with weaning in the first 3 months postpartum. J Fam Pract 51:439, 2002.
7. Matheson I: Drugs taken by mothers in the puerperium. BMJ 290:1588, 1985.
8. Larimore WL, Petrie KA: Drug use during pregnancy and lactation. Prim Care 27:35, 2000.
9. Yong SHY: Monitoring of drugs in breast milk. Ann Clin Lab Sci 15:100, 1985.
10. American Academy of Pediatrics: Composition of human milk: normative data. In Pediatric Nutrition Handbook. Elk Grove, IL, American Academy of Pediatrics, 1985, p 363.
11. Anderson DM, et al: Length of gestation and nutritional composition of milk. Am J Clin Nutr 37:810, 1983.
12. Anderson GH: Human milk feeding. Pediatr Clin North Am 32:325, 1983.
13. Gross SJ, et al: Nutritional composition of milk produced by mothers delivering preterm. J Pediatr 96:641, 1980.
14. Gross SJ, et al: Composition of breastmilk of mothers of preterm infants. Pediatrics 68:490, 1981.
15. Lemons JA, et al: Differences in the composition of preterm and human milk during early lactation. Pediatr Res 16:113, 1982.
16. Morris FH, et al: Relationship of human milk pH during course of lactation to concentrations of citrate and fatty acids. Pediatrics 78:458, 1986.
17. Jennes R: The composition of human milk. Semin Perinatol 3:225, 1979.
18. Lonnerdal B, et al: A longitudinal study of the protein, nitrogen and lactose contents of human milk from Swedish well-nourished mothers. Am J Clin Nutr 29:1127, 1976.
19. Hytten FE: Clinical and chemical studies in human lactation. Br Med J 1954:1, 1954.
20. Lammi-Keefe CJ, et al: Changes in human milk at 0600, 1000, 1400, 1800 and 2200 hr. J Pediatr Gastroenterol Nutr 11:83, 1990.
21. Prentice A, et al: Breast-milk fat concentrations of rural African women: I. Short-term variations within individuals. Br J Nutr 45:483, 1981.
22. Rivera-Calimlim L: The significance of drugs in breast milk. Clin Perinatol 14:51, 1987.
23. Noel GL, et al: Prolactin release during nursing and breast stimulation in postpartum and nonpostpartum subjects. J Clin Endocrinol Metab 38:413, 1974.
24. Beeley L: Drugs and breast feeding. Clin Obstet Gynecol 13:247, 1986.
25. Lucas A, et al: How much energy does the breast fed infant consume and expend? BMJ 295:75, 1987.
26. Neville MC, et al: Studies in human lactation: milk volumes in lactating women during the onset of lactation and full lactation. Am J Clin Nutr 48:1375, 1988.
27. Berlin CM: The excretion of drugs and chemicals in human milk. In Yaffe SJ, Aranda JV (eds): Pediatric Pharmacology, 2nd ed. Philadelphia, WB Saunders Co, 1992, p 205.
28. Wilson JT: Determinants and consequences of drug excretion in breast milk. Drug Metabol Rev 14:619, 1983.
29. Chaney NE, et al: Cocaine convulsions in a breast-feeding baby. J Pediatr 112:134, 1988.
30. Kesaniemi YA: Ethanol and acetaldehyde in the milk and peripheral blood of lactating women after ethanol administration. J Obstet Gynaecol Br Commonw 81:84, 1974.
31. Fleishaker JC, et al: Determination of nicotine concentrations in human milk. Am J Dis Child 130:837, 1976.
32. Dean M, et al: Serum protein binding of drugs during and after pregnancy in humans. Clin Pharmacol Ther 28:253, 1980.
33. Miller ME, et al: Hydrochlorothiazide disposition in a mother and her breast-fed infant. J Pediatr 101:789, 1982.
34. Rasmussen F: Mammary excretion of sulphonamides. Acta Pharmacol (Kbh) 15:139, 1958.
35. Sisodia CS, Stowe CM: The mechanism of drug secretion into bovine milk. Ann NY Acad Sci 111:650, 1964.
36. Wilson JT, et al: Drug excretion in human breast milk: principles, pharmacokinetics and projected consequences. Clin Pharmacokinet 5:1, 1980.
37. Liu DK, et al: Calcium-stimulated ribonuclease. Biochem J 178:241, 1979.
38. McCormick JJ, et al: RNAse inhibition of reverse transcriptase activity in human milk. Nature 251:737, 1974.
39. Benet LZ: General treatment of linear mammillary models with elimination from any compartment as used in pharmacokinetics. J Pharm Sci 61:536, 1972.
40. Wilson JT, et al: Pharmacokinetic pitfalls in the estimation of the breast milk/plasma ratio for drugs. Annu Rev Pharmacol Toxicol 25:667, 1985.
41. Atkinson HC, Begg EJ: Prediction of drug concentrations in human milk from plasma protein binding and acid-base characteristics. Br J Clin 25:495, 1988.
42. Atkison HC, Begg EJ: Prediction of drug distribution into human milk from physiochemical characteristics. Clin Pharmacokinet 18:151, 1990.
43. Ito S, Koren G: A novel index for expressing exposure of the infant to drugs in breast milk. Br J Clin Pharmacol 38:99, 1994.
44. Rane A, et al: Plasma disappearance of transplacentally diphenylhydantoin in the newborn studied by mass fragmentography. Clin Pharmacol Ther 15:39, 1974.
45. Stern B, et al: Phenytoin excretion in human breast milk and plasma levels in nursed infants. Ther Drug Monitor 13:661, 1982.
46. Bennett PN, et al (eds): Drugs and Human Lactation. Amsterdam, Elsevier, 1988.
47. Briggs GG, Yaffe SJ (eds): Drugs in Pregnancy and Lactation, 4th ed. Baltimore, Williams & Wilkins, 1994.
48. Committee on Drugs, American Academy of Pediatrics: Breast-feeding and contraception. Pediatrics 68:138, 1981.
49. Coulam CB, et al: Breast-feeding after renal transplantation. Transplant Proc 13:605, 1982.
50. Grekas DM, et al: Immunosuppressive therapy and breast-feeding after renal transplantation. Nephron 37:68, 1984.
51. Johns DG, et al: Secretion of methotrexate into human milk. Am J Obstet Gynecol 112:978, 1972.
52. Brooks PM, Needs CJ: The use of antirheumatic medication during pregnancy and in the puerperium. Rheum Dis Clin North Am 15:789, 1989.

53. De Swiet M, Lewis PJ: Excretion of anticoagulants in human milk. N Engl J Med 297:1471, 1977.
54. McKenna R, et al: Is warfarin sodium contraindicated in the lactating mother? J Pediatr 103:325, 1983.
55. Brambel CE, Hunter RE: Effect of dicumarol on the nursing infant. Am J Obstet Gynecol 59:1153, 1950.
56. Committee on Drugs, American Academy of Pediatrics: The transfer of drugs and other chemicals into human breast milk. Pediatrics 108:776, 2001.
57. Illingworth RS, Finch E: Ethyl biscoumacetate (Tromexan) in human milk. J Obstet Gynecol Br Commonw 66:487, 1959.
58. Wilson JT (ed): Drugs in Breast Milk. Sydney, ADIS Press, 1981.
59. Eckstein HB, Jack B: Breast-feeding and anticoagulant therapy. Lancet 1:672, 1970.
60. Goguel M, et al: Therapeutique anticoagulante et allaitement: étude du passage de la phenyl-2-dioxo, 1, 3 indane dans le lait maternel. Rev Fr Gynecol Obstet 65:409, 1970.
61. Peters F, et al: Inhibition of lactation by a long-acting bromocriptine. Obstet Gynecol 67:82, 1986.
62. Illingworth RS: Abnormal substances excreted in human milk. Practitioner 171:533, 1953.
63. Varga L, et al: Suppression of puerperal lactation with an ergot alkaloid: a double-blind study. BMJ 2:743, 1972.
64. Bell RAF, Dale IM: Gold secretion in maternal milk. Arthritis Rheum 19:1374, 1976.
65. Bennett PN, et al: Use of a sodium aurothiomalate lactation. Br J Clin Pharmacol 29:777, 1990.
66. Blau SP: Metabolism of gold during lactation. Arthritis Rheum 16:777, 1973.
67. Ostensen M, et al: Excretion of gold into human breast milk. Eur J Clin Pharmacol 31:251, 1986.
68. Rooney TW, et al: Gold pharmacokinetics in breast milk and serum of a lactating woman. J Rheumatol 14:1120, 1987.
69. Braverman LE: Iodine induced thyroid disease. Acta Med Austr 17:29, 1990.
70. Danzinger Y, et al: Transient congenital hypothyroidism after topical iodine in pregnancy and lactation. Arch Dis Child 62:295, 1987.
71. Delange F, et al: Topical iodine, breastfeeding and neonatal hypothyroidism. Arch Dis Child 63:106, 1988.
72. Slotskey GE: Amiodarone: a unique antiarrhythmic agent. Clin Pharmacol 2:230, 1983.
73. McKenna WJ, et al: Amiodarone therapy during pregnancy. Am J Cardiol 51:1231, 1983.
74. Guiloff E, et al: Effect of contraception on lactation. Am J Obstet Gynecol 118:42, 1974.
75. Koetsawang S: The effects of contraceptive methods on the quality and quantity of breast milk. Int J Gynaecol Obstet 25(Suppl):115, 1987.
76. Kora SJ: Effect of oral contraceptives on lactation. Fertil Steril 20:419, 1969.
77. Miller GH, Hughes LR: Lactation and genital involution effects of a new low-dose oral contraceptive on breast-feeding mothers and their infants. Obstet Gynecol 35:44, 1970.
78. World Health Organization Task Force on Oral Contraceptives, Special Programme of Research, Development and Research Training in Human Reproduction: effects of hormonal contraceptives on breast milk composition and infant growth. Stud Fam Plann 19:361, 1988.
79. Laukaran VH: The effects of contraceptive use on the initiation and duration of lactation. Int J Gynaecol Obstet 25(Suppl):129, 1987.
80. Schou M, Amdisen A: Lithium and pregnancy: III. Lithium ingestion by children breast-fed by women on lithium treatment. Br Med J 2:138, 1973.
81. Sykes PA, et al: Lithium carbonate and breast-feeding. BMJ 2:1299, 1976.
82. Tunnessen WW Jr, Hertz CG: Toxic effects of lithium in newborn infants: a commentary. J Pediatr 81:804, 1972.
83. Kaneko S, et al: The levels of anticonvulsants in breast milk. Br J Clin Pharmacol 7:624, 1979.
84. Nau H, et al: Anticonvulsants during pregnancy and lactation: transplacental, maternal and neonatal pharmacokinetics. Clin Pharmacokinet 7:508, 1982.
85. Tyson RM, et al: Drug transmitted through breast milk: II. Barbiturates. J Pediatr 13:86, 1938.
86. Steiner E, et al: Amphetamine secretion in breast milk. Eur J Clin Pharmacol 27:123, 1984.
87. Chasnoff IJ, Lewis DE, Squires L: Cocaine intoxication in a breast-fed infant. Pediatrics 80:836, 1987.
88. Shannon M, et al: Cocaine exposure among children seen at a pediatric hospital. Pediatrics 83:337, 1989.
89. Lawton ME: Alcohol in breast milk. Aust NZ J Obstet Gynaecol 25:71, 1985.
90. Liston J: Breastfeeding and the use of recreational drugs—alcohol, caffeine, nicotine and marijuana. Breastfeed Rev 6: 27, 1998.
91. Little RE, et al: Maternal alcohol use during breast-feeding and infant mental health and motor development at one year. N Engl J Med 321:425, 1989.
92. Carlson HE, et al: Beer-induced prolactin secretion: A clinical and laboratory study of the role of salsolinol. J Clin Endocrinol Metab 60:673, 1985.
93. Cobo E: Effect of different doses of ethanol on the milk-ejecting reflex in lactating women. Am J Obstet Gynecol 115:817, 1973.
94. Lichlenstein PM: Infant drug addiction. NY Med J 102:905, 1915.
95. Perez-Reyes M, Wall ME: Presence of Δ-9-tetrahydrocannabinol in human milk. N Engl J Med 307:819, 1982.
96. Kaufman KR, et al: PCP in amniotic fluid and breast milk: case report. J Clin Psychiatry 44:269, 1983.
97. Nicholas JM, et al: Phencyclidine: its transfer across the placenta as well as into breast milk. Am J Obstet Gynecol 143:143, 1982.
98. Ferguson BB, et al: Determination of nicotine concentrations in human milk. Am J Dis Child 130:837, 1976.
99. Labrecque M, et al: Feeding and urine cotinine values in human milk. Pediatrics 83:93, 1989.
100. Schwartz-Bickenbach D, et al: Smoking and passive smoking during pregnancy and early infancy: effects on birth weight, lactation period and cotinine concentrations in mother's milk and infant's urine. Toxicol Lett 35:73, 1987.
101. Greenberg RA, et al: Measuring the exposure of infants to tobacco smoke: nicotine and cotinine in urine and saliva. N Engl J Med 310:1075, 1984.
102. Luck W, Nau H: Nicotine and cotinine concentrations in serum and urine of infants exposed via passive smoking or milk from smoking mothers. J Pediatr 107:816, 1985.
103. Schulte-Hobein B, et al: Cigarette smoke exposure and development of infants throughout the first year of life: influence of passive smoking and nursing on cotinine levels in breast milk and infants' urine. Acta Paediatr 81:550, 1982.
104. Said G, et al: Infantile colic and parental smoking. BMJ 289:660, 1984.
105. Vio F, et al: Smoking during pregnancy and lactation and its effects on breast-milk volume. Am J Clin Nutr 54:1011, 1991.
106. Clark JH, Wilson WG: A 16-day-old breast-fed infant with metabolic acidosis caused by salicylate. Clin Pediatr 20:53, 1981.
107. Schuh S, et al: Nebulized albuterol in acute childhood asthma—comparison of two doses. Pediatrics 86:509, 1990.
108. Katz FH, Duncan BR: Entry of prednisone into human milk. N Engl J Med 293:1154, 1975.
109. Stec GP, et al: Kinetics of theophylline transfer to breast milk. Clin Pharmacol Ther 28:404, 1980.
110. Berlin CM: Excretion of methylxanthines in human milk. Semin Perinatol 5:389, 1981.
111. Knowles JA: Drugs in milk. Pediatr Curr 21:28, 1972.
112. Posner AC, et al: Further observations on the use of tetracycline hydrochloride in prophylaxis and treatment of obstetric infections. In Wlech H, Marti-Ibanez F (eds): Antibiotic Annual 1954–55. New York, Medical Encyclopedia, 1955, p 594.
113. Kelsey JJ, et al: Presence of azithromycin breast milk concentrations: a case report. Am J Obstet Gynecol 170:1375, 1994.
114. Gardner DK et al: Simultaneous concentrations of ciprofloxacin in breast milk and in serum in mother and breast-fed infant. Clin Pharm 11: 352, 1992.
115. Chysky V, et al: Safety of ciprofloxacin in children: worldwide clinical experience based on compassionate use. Emphasis on joint evaluation. Infection 19:289, 1991.
116. Schaad UB, et al: Clinical, radiologic and magnetic resonance monitoring for skeletal toxicity in pediatric patients with cystic fibrosis receiving a three-month course of ciprofloxacin. Pediatr Infect Dis 10:723, 1991.
117. Heisterberg L, Branebjerg PE: Blood and milk concentrations of metronidazole in mothers and infants. J Perinat Med 11:114, 1983.
118. Berlin CM, Lee C: Isoniazid and acetylisoniazid disposition in human milk, saliva and plasma. Fed Proc 38:429, 1979.
119. Snider DE Jr, Powell KE: Should women taking antituberculosis drugs breast-feed? Arch Intern Med 144:589, 1984.
120. Alcorn J, McNamara PJ: Acyclovir, ganciclovir and zidovudine transfer into rat milk. Animicrob Agents Chemother 46: 1831, 2002.
121. Kuhn L, Peterson I: Options for prevention of HIV transmission from mother to child, with a focus on developing countries. Paediatri Drugs 4: 191, 2002.
122. Boutroy MJ: Fetal and neonatal effects of the beta-adrenoreceptor agents. Dev Pharmacol Ther 10:224, 1987.
123. Riant P, et al: High plasma protein binding as a parameter in the selection of beta blockers for lactating women. Biochem Pharmacol 35:4579, 1986.
124. Schmimmel MS, et al: Toxic effects of atenolol consumed during breast feeding. J Pediatr 114:476, 1989.
125. Misri S, et al: Are SSRIs safe for pregnant and breast-feeding women? Can Fam Physician 46:626, 2000.
126. Epperson N, et al: Maternal sertraline treatment and serotonin transport in breast-feeding mother-infant pairs. Am J Psychiatry 158:1631, 2001
127. Ilett KF, et al: Distribution of venlafaxine and its O-desmethyl metabolite in human milk and their effects in breastfed infants. Br J Clin Pharmacol 53:17, 2002.
128. Hendrick V, et al: Fluoxetine and norfluoxetine concentrations in nursing infants and breast milk. Biol Psychiatry 15: 775, 2001.
129. Misri S, et al: Paroxetine levels in postpartum depressed women, breast milk and infant serum. J Clin Psychiatry 61:828, 2000.
130. Pittard WB III, Glazier H: Procainamide excretion in human milk. J Pediatr 102:631, 1983.
131. Hills LM, Malkasian GD Jr: The use of quinidine sulfate throughout pregnancy. Obstet Gynecol 54:366, 1979.
132. Beardmore KS, et al: Excretion of antihypertensive medication into human breast milk: a systemic review. Hypertens Pregnancy 21:85, 2002.
133. Cooper DS: Antithyroid drugs—to breast-feed or not to breast-feed. N Engl J Med 311:1353, 1984.
134. Moiel RH, Ryan JR: Tolbutamide (Orinase) in human breast milk. Clin Pediatr 6:480, 1967.
135. Lewis JH, Weingold AB, Committee on FDA-Related Matters, American College of Gastroenterology: The use of gastrointestinal drugs during pregnancy and lactation. Am J Gastroenterol 80:912, 1985.
136. Klier CM, et al: St. John's Wort (Hypericum perforatum)—is it safe during breastfeeding? Pharmacopsychiatry 35:29. 2002.

Intrauterine and Postnatal Growth

27

Frederick C. Battaglia

Circulatory and Metabolic Changes Accompanying Fetal Growth Restriction

Fetal growth restriction (FGR) is an important clinical problem in obstetrics and gynecology. As a result, it has stimulated considerable clinical research, which has helped to elucidate aspects of the pathophysiology of FGR and has also led to a better understanding of normal human biology. In this chapter, some of the work directed at describing how the fetus adapts to placental dysfunction is discussed.

Various terms are applied to the problem of FGR. In part, this has a historical foundation. The first attempts to recognize FGR infants came from studies that used gestational age and birth weight information.[1-3] The infants were classified as *small for gestational age* infants if their birth weights fell below the 10th percentile for a given gestational age. Later groups used terms such as *small for dates*, a definition based on standard deviations for the birth weight–gestational age distribution. Many studies brought out the differences in birth weight–gestational age distribution data among different populations. From the beginning however, it was clear that FGR infants were not a homogeneous group, but instead, included some babies who were small but normally grown infants. The term *intrauterine growth retardation* (IUGR) was used initially to identify those who had truly grown more slowly *in utero* because of one or another disease process, usually a disease that affected placental development. Later, because of concerns that retardation is a term parents may associate with mental retardation, the term was modified to *fetal growth restriction*. The term FGR is now used more widely and is interchangeable with IUGR.

The approach to defining FGR infants was changed fundamentally, however, once ultrasound techniques permitted repeated determinations of fetal body size *in utero*. This removed the necessity of using only birth weight data at the completion of a pregnancy. It also permitted estimations of the rate of fetal growth, that is, the change in fetal growth with time in any particular pregnancy. The wide application of ultrasound-derived fetal growth curves made possible the early detection of FGR. Currently, the common practice is to use equations derived from the local population to calculate an estimated fetal weight. Such equations usually rely on measurements of head circumference, abdominal circumference, and femur length. It is not clear, however, that such a calculation of estimated fetal weight is significantly better than relying on the actual measurements made. Alternatively, FGR infants may be defined as those babies with an abdominal circumference 2 standard deviations below the norm for that gestational age.

The diagnosis of FGR can be further sharpened by the use of standards that incorporate maternal and paternal size. Essentially, this approach seeks to identify fetuses who are small because their parents are small versus those with FGR from a pathologic process. Gardosi and colleagues focused on this approach and reviewed the subject extensively.[4] Nomograms for particular countries are available.[5, 6] The most compelling evidence that a fetus is truly growth restricted comes from accumulating functional evidence for those physiologic characteristics that have been shown to be altered in FGR pregnancies.

Sorting out babies who are small but are fulfilling their growth potential (i.e., normally grown) from those with FGR (i.e., growth restricted by disease) is important for several reasons: (1) intensive obstetric surveillance can be applied more effectively to FGR babies, (2) neonatal intensive care can better anticipate problems for FGR babies, and (3) there are long-term implications to development in FGR infants, important not only through childhood but also into adult life. Thus, it behooves us to approach the diagnosis of FGR using all available information.

Studies have begun to sort out normally grown small for gestational age babies from those with FGR by consideration of functional aspects as well as the body size of the fetus and of the parents. These aspects are brought out as we consider some of the vascular and metabolic changes clearly associated with FGR.

PLACENTAL DEVELOPMENT

A great deal of work has been done to delineate the changes in placental development that are associated with FGR pregnancies. The histologic changes in the placenta, including the vascular changes, have been reviewed.[7-9] These changes are consistent with uneven perfusion and diffusion limitations in the small FGR placenta. Surface area is significantly reduced in FGR pregnancies, along with placental mass. The histologic changes led to the hypothesis that these changes may be triggered, in part, by placental hyperoxia in the maternal placental circulation.[8] This hypothesis received support from both animal studies[10] and clinical studies[11] of respiratory gas tensions in the umbilical and uterine circulations of FGR pregnancies. For many years, obstetricians believed that uterine blood flow was reduced in FGR pregnancies. Although this may or may not be true in the earliest stages of pregnancy, it was well established by the study of Pardi and colleagues[11] that uterine blood flow is increased in FGR pregnancies relative to the oxygen (O_2) requirements of the pregnant uterus. This is an important physiologic characteristic of FGR pregnancies and, as stated earlier, is consistent with findings in an ovine model of FGR.[10] The human placenta functions as a venous equilibrator, and this function has implications both for the uterine and the umbilical circulation.[12] Therefore, regardless of the complexity of the fetal circulation and of perfusion patterns within the intervillous space, the human placenta is functioning as an exchange system in which the uterine venous O_2 tension (Po_2) is the major determinant of the umbilical venous Po_2 in the fetal circulation.

FETAL VELOCIMETRY CHANGES

The fetal circulation has been studied extensively in terms of the velocity waveform changes occurring in different fetal vessels.[13] These changes do not occur in all FGR pregnancies. In the classification proposed by Pardi and associates,[14] FGR pregnancies without velocimetry changes represented approximately one-third of all FGR pregnancies. The changes in fetal velocimetry are presumed to reflect two pathophysiologic processes: an increased impedance within the placental vascular bed and a redistribution in fetal cardiac output secondary to fetal hypoxia. Let us consider the evidence for each of these changes.

In normal pregnancies, the umbilical artery pulsatility index starts at a high value in early gestation and decreases until term.[15] However, in FGR pregnancies, the pulsatility index is increased compared with normal values even relatively early in gestation. In the ovine FGR model described previously, the increased pulsatility index is associated with increased blood pressure in the fetal circulation and with reduced umbilical blood flow.[10] This finding provides clear evidence of an increased impedance in the fetal vascular bed. Both an increased pulsatility index and decreased umbilical blood flow[16] have been reported in human FGR pregnancies. Thus, it is not unreasonable to assume increased placental vascular impedance in human FGR pregnancies.

Hypoxia and lacticacidemia occur in a relatively high percentage of FGR pregnancies. Both hypoxia and lacticacidemia were found in approximately two-thirds of the FGR pregnancies in which both umbilical artery velocimetry and fetal heart rate (FHR) were abnormal.[14] Fetal hypoxia has been well studied in animal models. In the ovine fetus, the changes in the distribution of fetal cardiac output that occur with acute fetal hypoxia were well described in 1979.[17] These changes include vasoconstriction to some fetal vascular beds (e.g., skeletal muscle) and vasodilatation to other vascular beds (e.g., cerebral circulation). Other studies have addressed the high perinatal mortality and morbidity associated with these fetal velocimetry changes.[18] However, the same data can provide additional clinical information if one considers the sequence of changes in velocimetry in human FGR fetuses. The physiologic significance of the velocimetry changes in different fetal vessels can only be interpreted properly by viewing them as a sequence of circulatory adjustments by the fetus. The sequence of changes in fetal velocimetry was studied in a group of FGR pregnancies that ultimately required delivery for FHR abnormalities.[19] This study brought out that some vessels show alterations in velocity waveform relatively distant from the time of required delivery of the infant and that others occur much later, within a few days of delivery. Even the "late" changes occurred some days before the FHR became abnormal. In addition, within any single vessel, velocimetry waveforms may show progressive changes, such as in the umbilical artery, progressing from an increased pulsatility index to absent end-diastolic flow to reversed end-diastolic flow. These changes in velocimetry have been described for numerous fetal vessels. It may well be that clinical practice may move toward using fetal velocimetry data for decisions of the optimal delivery time for an FGR infant. This change in practice rests on whether follow-up studies document that leaving an infant *in utero* after "late" velocimetry changes have occurred (but before FHR is abnormal) poses a greater risk for central nervous system injury compared with severe prematurity. At this point, the data are not available to make this decision.

BLOOD FLOW MEASUREMENTS

From a physiologic viewpoint, blood flow is the critical determinant of tissue perfusion, not the velocity of the blood. As techniques have developed to determine the diameter of a vessel accurately, it has become feasible to measure blood flow in the vessel from the diameter and the velocity of blood in the vessel. This approach has been applied in human pregnancies to measure the blood in three important sites:

1. Uterine artery
2. Umbilical vein
3. Ductus venosus

Measurement of blood flow in each of these vessels is very important to an understanding of the disturbed physiology in FGR pregnancies.

Uterine Blood Flow

Measurements of uterine blood flow in human pregnancies were first reported in the 1990s.[20-22] These studies reported estimates of uterine blood flow of approximately 500 mL/minute at term in normal pregnancies. Meschia[12] pointed out that these estimates were likely to be too low, based on the data published for uterine venous O_2 saturation, maternal hemoglobin concentration, and estimates of uterine O_2 consumption. From his calculations, based on these O_2 data, he concluded that uterine blood flow in human pregnancy should be approximately 1 L/minute at term. Konje and colleagues[23] used color power angiography to measure uterine blood flow in uncomplicated human pregnancies. They reported a blood flow at term of 97 ± 193 mL/minute, not significantly different from that estimated by Meschia from the O_2 data. Thus, a blood flow of 1 L/minute appears to be a reliable estimate for normal human pregnancy. Unfortunately, no measurements of uterine blood flow in FGR pregnancies have yet been reported.

Umbilical Blood Flow

Numerous studies have reported the umbilical blood flow at different gestational ages in uncomplicated human pregnancies.[24-29] Umbilical blood flow (mL/minute) increases exponentially during gestation, roughly in a pattern similar to the increase in fetal weight. However, several studies have shown that blood flow does not increase in a fixed proportion to fetal body weight. When umbilical blood flow is expressed per kg fetal weight, it decreases slightly during gestation from approximately 130 mL/minute at 20 weeks' gestation to approximately 100 mL/minute at term. Both the umbilical vein diameter and the mean velocity increase during gestation, although the increase in diameter is the dominant factor leading to the exponential increase in umbilical blood flow during gestation.

For obvious reasons, umbilical blood flow uncorrected for fetal size is low in FGR pregnancies because the fetus is smaller. However, if blood flow is expressed per kilogram of fetal weight or is normalized to fetal body mass by some other biometric index such as fetal head or abdominal circumference, it is still significantly reduced in most FGR pregnancies.[16] This is one of the more important findings in FGR pregnancies, that umbilical blood flow to the placenta is reduced even when it is corrected for fetal body size. Furthermore, the reduction is quite large. For example at 34 weeks' gestation, the umbilical flow (mL/minute) in FGR pregnancies was reduced by approximately 70%. The data presented in Figure 27–1 were taken from the study of Ferrazzi and colleagues.[16] In this figure, blood flow was normalized for estimated fetal weight, which is also reduced in FGR pregnancies. The reduction is even more striking if it is normalized for head circumference because head circumference is spared in FGR pregnancies. The study conducted by Ferrazzi and associ-

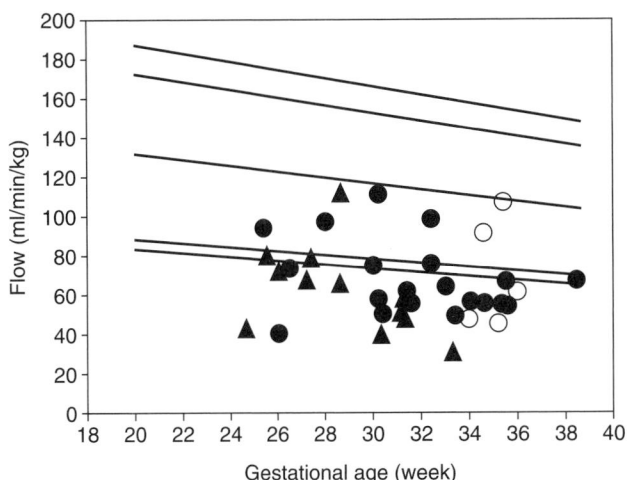

Figure 27-1. Umbilical vein flow per unit head circumference against gestational age in growth-restricted fetuses: group 1, *open circles*; group 2, *closed circles*; group 3, *triangles*. Continuous lines represent the 5th, 10th, 50th, 90th, and 95th percentile from 70 normally grown fetuses. (From Ferrazzi E, et al: Ultrasound Obstet Gynecol *16*:432, 2000.)

ates[16] demonstrated that the decrease in flow is entirely attributable to the decrease in umbilical vein velocity, not in the diameter of the vessel. The reduction in umbilical blood flow can occur quite early in gestation, that is, at the time the diagnosis of FGR is first made by serial ultrasound examinations (24 weeks). As noted in Figure 27-1, some FGR pregnancies have umbilical blood flows within the normal range. It will be important through follow-up studies to determine what differences in outcomes, both long term and short term, are associated with a reduction in umbilical blood flow of this magnitude. These first studies were cross-sectional in design, but a subsequent longitudinal study established that these flow changes were persistent in a pregnancy.[30] A reduced umbilical blood flow makes it more difficult to deliver O_2 and nutrients to the fetal tissues and increases the likelihood of developing fetal hypoxia and acidosis.

Fetal Hepatic and Ductus Venosus Blood Flow

The third fetal vessel for which there are now blood flow data in human pregnancies is the ductus venosus.[31,32] In the human fetus, this is a small, trumpet-shaped vessel connecting the umbilical vein and the inferior vena cava. Its purpose is to shunt some of the highly oxygenated umbilical venous blood away from the fetal liver and directly into the inferior vena cava. Because of its conical shape (its inlet diameter is smaller than its outlet diameter), the velocity waveform changes along the length of the vessel. In a series of studies (some of which were directed at computerized modeling of the velocity waveform as a function of conicity), several groups of investigators measured the blood flow in the ductus venosus.[33-36] This measurement permits determination of the amount of umbilical venous blood shunted through the ductus as well as the amount perfusing the fetal liver. These flows, as well as umbilical flow, have been measured together in normal human pregnancies throughout the latter half of gestation. The percentage of ductal shunt decreases as pregnancy progresses. The change is rather striking, given that ductal flow does not increase as much as umbilical blood flow during gestation. The ductal shunt, expressed as a percentage of umbilical flow, decreases from 40% at 20 weeks to 15% at term. Figure 27-2 abstracts data contained in three studies on blood flows in human pregnancies. The uterine blood flow data are from the study of Konje and colleagues,[23] those for umbilical flow from the study of Barbera and associates,[24] and

those for the ductus are from the study of Bellotti and colleagues.[32] Figure 27-2A presents the flows in milliliters per minute, and Figure 27-2B presents flows per kilogram of fetal body weight. In Figure 27-2B, it is clear that the growth of umbilical flow during gestation most closely approximates the growth of the fetus because flow per kilogram decreases only slightly during gestation in normal pregnancies.

Several studies pointed out that the ductal shunt is increased (for gestational age) in some clinically severe FGR pregnancies. Because fetal hepatic blood flow of well-oxygenated umbilical venous blood is determined by the umbilical blood flow and inversely by the percentage of ductal shunt, an FGR fetus with a reduction in umbilical blood flow and an increased ductal shunt may have an enormous reduction in fetal hepatic blood flow. Bellotti and associates showed that this combined effect does indeed occur in some FGR pregnancies.[37,38] It is not surprising, given these vascular changes, that two different groups have reported FGR newborns with hepatic injury unrelated to infection.[39,40] Obviously, this area needs more study because it may affect the management (particularly nutritional management) of FGR babies in the immediate neonatal period.

METABOLIC CHANGES IN FGR PREGNANCIES

Carbohydrates

Lacticacidemia, hypoxia, and acidosis have already been discussed as frequent complications of FGR pregnancies, particularly in the FGR pregnancies with "late" velocimetry changes such as reversed end-diastolic flow in the umbilical artery. With regard to lacticacidemia and acidosis, it is important to emphasize the unique metabolic characteristics of the fetal liver and placenta with regard to the metabolism and transport of lactate and pyruvate. In animal studies, it has been well established that the fetal liver has a large net output of pyruvate and net uptake of lactate from the fetal circulation. Because the fetal liver is perfused with a high percentage of umbilical venous blood (the best oxygenated blood of the fetus), it is clear that the fetal liver could play an important role in the defense of acid-base balance during fetal hypoxia. Figure 27-3 presents in graphic form some of the changes in acid-base balance and lactate concentration during severe and persistent fetal hypoxia taken from the study of Wilkening and colleagues.[41] The striking finding is that, despite persistent, severe fetal hypoxia for 24 hours, the fetal acidosis is largely corrected, as reflected in fetal arterial pH, although the lactate concentration is still elevated. This correction of metabolic acidosis occurs because of the continued uptake of lactate and release of pyruvate from the fetal liver.[42] This important finding was derived from studies of normal pregnancies, which were then made hypoxic. However, in FGR pregnancies in which the ductus venosus shunt may be increased, this defense mechanism may be further compromised. It is the reduced hepatic perfusion in some FGR pregnancies that makes the FGR fetus particularly vulnerable to fetal hypoxia.

Glucose metabolism is also altered in FGR pregnancies. In ovine FGR pregnancies, glucose uptake into the fetal circulation from the placenta is maintained within the normal range when expressed per kilogram fetal weight or expressed per gram of placental weight.[43] The maintenance of normal glucose uptake despite the small placenta in FGR pregnancies is accomplished by an increase in the transplacental glucose gradient. In human pregnancies, umbilical glucose uptake cannot be measured directly. However, the glucose gradient across the placenta in normal human pregnancies has been well described by numerous investigators.[44-48] Figure 27-4, taken from the study by Marconi and colleagues,[44] presents data obtained at the time of cordocentesis for the maternal "arterialized" and fetal umbilical venous glucose concentration differences throughout gestation

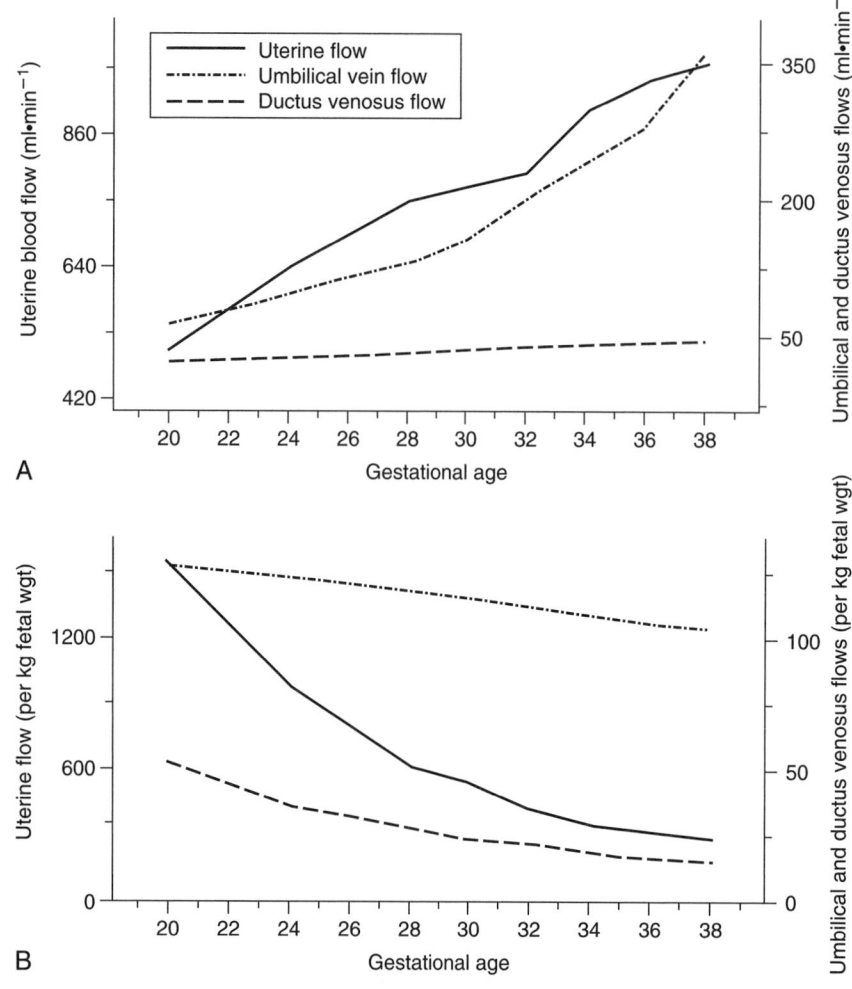

Figure 27–2. The three vessels for which flow measurements are available in human pregnancies are presented with uterine flow as a *solid line,* with umbilical flow as a *dashed-and-dotted line,* and with ductus venosus flow as a *dashed line.* The *upper panel* presents flows in milliliters per minute, and the *lower panel* presents flows in the same three vessels expressed as milliliters per minute per kilogram of fetal weight. In the human, the uterine flow is much greater than the umbilical flow. The umbilical flow in milliliters per minute per kilogram of fetal weight has only a slight decline with gestation, and this finding establishes that the rate of increase in umbilical flow is roughly parallel to the rate of increase in fetal weight.

for normal human pregnancies. It illustrates that the maternal-fetal concentration difference increases with advancing gestation. However, in FGR pregnancies, just as in the ovine model of FGR, the maternal-fetal glucose concentration difference is increased significantly compared with normal pregnancies of the same gestational age. The magnitude of the glucose concentration difference correlates with clinical severity of the FGR pregnancies, defined by umbilical artery velocimetry and FHR data (Fig. 27–5).[44] Thus, the changes in glucose gradients are linked to the fetal velocimetry changes as well.

Scaling of all metabolic data is critically important in studies of FGR pregnancies. Because an FGR baby and the placenta are both smaller than normal, all the uptake data of nutrients and all the blood flow data will be reduced unless the data are normalized for body size. The smaller conceptus mass significantly reduces the metabolic demand on the mother. In human pregnancies, this issue has only been addressed for glucose.[48] Marconi and colleagues[48] examined the relationship among three variables: (1) maternal plasma glucose disposal rate at steady state, a measure of maternal glucose utilization; (2) conceptus mass (fetal plus placental weight); and (3) maternal plasma glucose concentration. Their studies demonstrated that, at comparable maternal glucose concentrations, the smaller the mass of the conceptus, the smaller the maternal glucose utilization rate.

Another aspect of glucose metabolism in FGR pregnancies is the question of whether there is significant gluconeogenesis. Figure 27–6 summarizes the normal fluxes into and out of the fetal liver in the ovine fetus in late gestation (control period) taken from the study of Teng and associates.[49] The fetal liver has a very large

uptake of lactate and gluconeogenic amino acids. Despite this large uptake of potential glucose carbon, there is no significant glucose release from the fetal liver under normal conditions. Instead, carbon leaves the liver primarily as glutamate, serine, and pyruvate. It is only when fetal gluconeogenesis is stimulated by a fetal infusion of glucagon that net glucose release from the liver can be found, and glutamate release is virtually shut off in response. In human FGR pregnancies, stable isotopically labeled glucose has been infused into the maternal circulation to examine whether there was any evidence of dilution of the fetal plasma glucose enrichment in FGR pregnancies.[50] Even though these studies were carried out after an overnight fast, no evidence of dilution of the fetal glucose enrichment could be found. Thus, in this study, an FGR pregnancy did not stimulate detectable fetal gluconeogenesis.

Amino Acid Transport and Metabolism

This aspect of nutrient transport has been the subject of considerable research interest since the mid-1990s. In large part, the research was stimulated by advances in molecular biology that permitted the identification of specific transporter proteins on the two plasma membrane surfaces of the trophoblast. It is not appropriate in this chapter to review the field of placental amino acid transport;[51-53] however, as it applies to human FGR pregnancies, the following characteristics have been reasonably well established.

When microvesicle preparations are prepared from either the basal (fetal) surface or the microvillous (maternal) surface of the trophoblast, FGR placentas have a reduced transport capacity on both surfaces of the placenta.[51] These defects are not present for

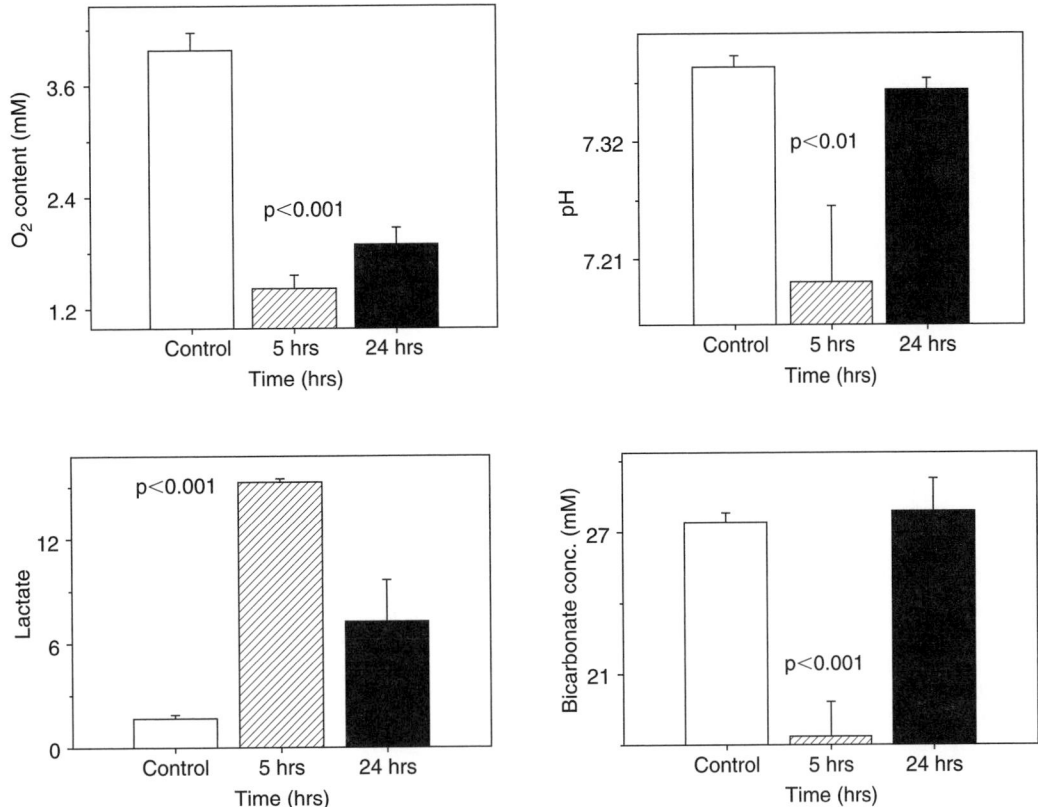

Figure 27–3. Changes in acid-base balance and lactate concentration during acute and prolonged fetal hypoxia. (From Wilkening RB, et al: *Biol Neonate* *63*:129, 1993.)

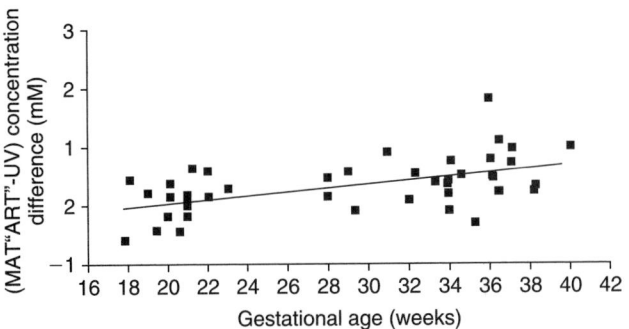

Figure 27–4. Maternal "arterial"-umbilical venous (MAT "ART"-UV) glucose concentration difference versus gestational age in appropriate for gestational age pregnancies. (From Marconi AM, et al: *Obstet Gynecol* *87*:937, 1996.)

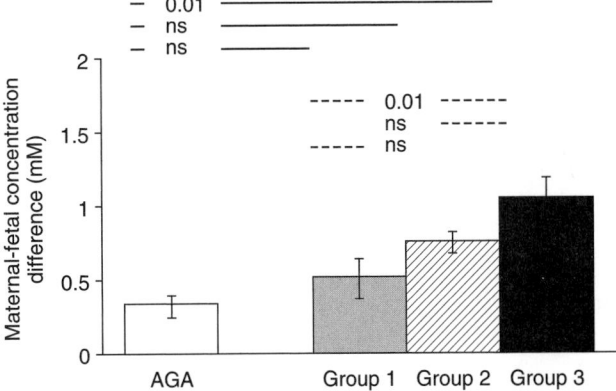

Figure 27–5. Measured mean ± SD values of maternal "arterial" umbilical venous glucose concentration differences in appropriate for gestational age (AGA) fetuses and fetal growth restriction (FGR) cases of groups 1, 2, and 3. The *p* values refer to the significance of the differences for the intercepts of AGA versus FGR groups *(solid lines)* and among groups of FGR *(dashed lines)* for the regression analysis of the maternal-fetal difference versus gestational age, because there were no significant differences (ns) among the slopes of these regressions. (From Marconi AM, et al: *Obstet Gynecol* *87*:937, 1996.)

all transport systems, nor are the problems the same on each surface. Changes of amino acid transport *in vivo* in FGR pregnancies can be a reflection not only of changes in membrane transporter activity but also reflect changes in placental utilization or production of an amino acid as well as changes in perfusion of the placenta.

Figure 27-7 outlines the transplacental fluxes of an essential amino acid, leucine, in diagrammatic form. The data were obtained in normal pregnant sheep in late gestation.[54, 55] The nutritionally important variable, namely, the net uptake of leucine into the fetal circulation, is determined principally by three different fluxes of approximately equal magnitude. These are (1) the transplacental flux from maternal plasma to fetal plasma, (2) the backflux from the fetal plasma into the placenta, and (3) the leucine flux from placental protein breakdown into the fetal plasma. In the ovine model of FGR, it has been shown for two essential amino acids,

leucine and threonine, that the transplacental flux is significantly reduced.[55, 56] This is true even when the flux is expressed per gram of placenta. In those studies, the fetal adaptation to the reduced transplacental flux is a lower fetal plasma amino acid concentration. This, in turn, leads to a lower fetal amino acid oxidation rate and a reduced backflux into the placenta. Both these changes would tend to divert these amino acids to fetal protein synthesis. The reduced transplacental flux in ovine FGR pregnancies results

Net fluxes across the fetal liver
(g-atoms of carbon/mole O2 uptake)

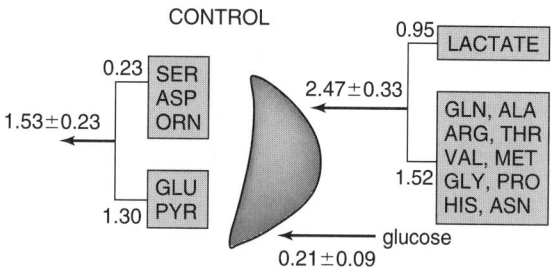

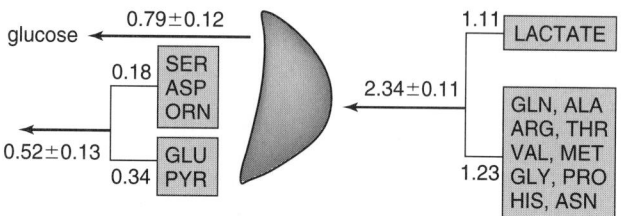

Figure 27–6. Fetal hepatic uptake and output of glucose carbon and glucogenic substrate carbon under normal physiologic conditions (control) and during a glucagon-somatostatin infusion into the fetal circulation. Each number represents a substrate carbon-to-oxygen uptake molar ratio. (From Teng C, et al: Am J Physiol *282*:E542, 2002.)

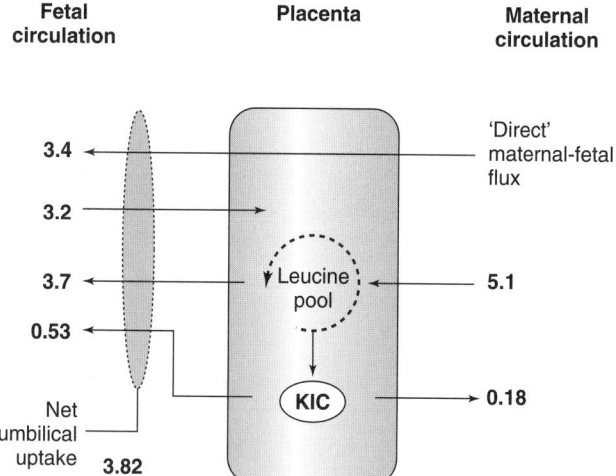

Figure 27–7. The unidirectional fluxes of leucine into and out of the placenta (μmol/min/kg fetal weight) measured *in vivo* under steady-state conditions are presented. The data are abstracted from refs. 54 and 55. The three major fluxes that together determine the umbilical uptake are of approximately equal magnitude. KIC = alpha-ketoisocaproic acid. (From Battaglia FC, Regnault TR: Placenta *22*:145, 2001.)

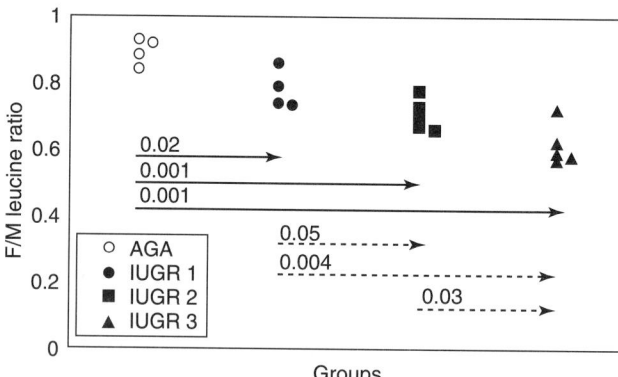

Figure 27–8. Leucine fetal/maternal (F/M) enrichment ratio in appropriate for gestational age (AGA) and intrauterine growth retardation (IUGR) pregnancies at fetal blood sampling. (From Marconi AM, et al: Pediatr Res *46*:114, 1999.)

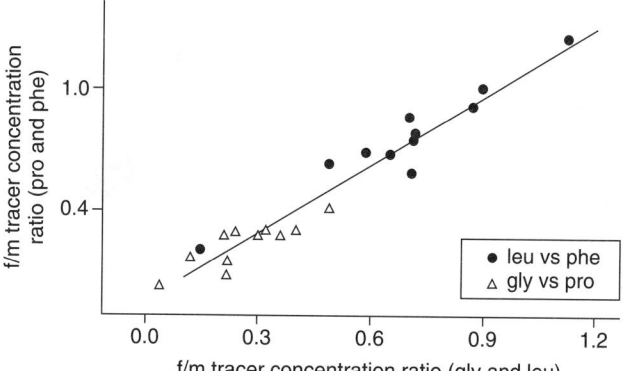

Figure 27–9. The fetal/maternal (F/M) plasma tracer concentration ratios are plotted with the values for glycine and leucine along the abscissa and those for proline and phenylalanine along the ordinate. The regression is highly significant: F/M $y = -0.0511 + 1.1274(F/M) \, x \, R^2 = 0.94, p < .001$. (From Paolini CL, et al: J Clin Endocrinol Metab *86*:5427, 2001.)

in a significantly lower fetal/maternal (F/M) enrichment ratio for both leucine and threonine. The clinical data for the leucine F/M ratio are presented in Figure 27–8 from the study of Marconi and associates.[57] Two aspects of these data are worthy of attention. First, the data clearly demonstrate a significant reduction in the F/M enrichment ratio of leucine in FGR pregnancies, a finding presumably reflecting a significant reduction in the maternofetal transplacental flux. Second, the magnitude of this effect correlated with the classification of clinical severity in FGR pregnancies pro-

posed by Pardi and colleagues,[14] which was based on fetal umbilical arterial velocimetry and FHR data. Just as with glucose data, leucine metabolic data correlated with clinical severity defined by fetal vascular changes.

A previous study, using non–steady-state stable isotope methodology, in normal human pregnancies demonstrated that reasonably good kinetic data could be obtained even in cross-sectional studies,[58] and it emphasized the striking difference in transport rate into the fetal circulation for leucine and glycine. A study by Paolini and colleagues in ovine pregnancy used similar non–steady-state methodology to compare the transport rates of the nine essential amino acids in a normal ovine pregnancy.[59] One of the observations coming from that study was that the three branched-chain amino acids and phenylalanine and methionine appeared to cross at similar rates and much more rapidly than all other essential amino acids. Differences for the pulse fluxes from the maternal to the fetal circulation for these five amino acids were determined by differences in their normal concentrations in maternal plasma (Fig. 27–9). Similar methodology was used in human normal and FGR pregnancies to examine the relative placental transport rates for four amino acids: leucine, phenylalanine, glycine, and proline.[60] Figure 27–9, taken from that study, compares the F/M plasma enrichment ratio of leucine with phenylalanine and that of glycine with proline. It is clear that no significant differences in transport rate were found between leucine and phenylalanine or between glycine and proline. However, leucine and phenylalanine crossed much more quickly than glycine and proline. Furthermore, in FGR pregnancies, the F/M ratios of leucine and phenylalanine were significantly reduced compared with normal pregnancies. Thus, with amino acids, it is now possible to assess placental function in human FGR pregnancies *in vivo*.

In summary, it is clear that FGR pregnancies present problems for the fetus in terms of the transport of O_2 and nutrients. Most of these problems can be attributed directly to the maldevelopment of the placenta, which is not only reduced in size but also has structural abnormalities in its vasculature. These changes in the placenta (complicated by the presence of chronic hypoxia) can lead to fetal circulatory changes in many fetal vascular beds. Circulatory and metabolic studies have made it clear that there is a wide range of clinical severity encompassing the diagnosis of FGR based on fetal size for gestation. The delineation of more homogeneous subsets of FGR pregnancies in terms of their clinical severity can provide the basis for better timing of delivery in severe FGR pregnancies. It can also form the basis of better adjustments in neonatal care for these infants after delivery. Finally, such information can provide the foundation for much more focused follow-up studies in childhood and in adulthood.

REFERENCES

1. Battaglia FC, Lubchenco LO: A practical classification of newborn infants by weight and gestational age. J Pediatr 71:159, 1967.
2. World Health Organization: W.H.O. Manual of International Statistical Classification of Diseases, Injuries and Causes of Death. New York, World Health Organization, 1949 (Adopted 1948.)
3. Battaglia FC, et al: Birth weight, gestational age, and pregnancy outcome, with special reference to high birth weight–low gestational age infant. Pediatrics 37:417, 1966.
4. Gardosi J, et al: Customised antenatal growth charts. Lancet 339:283, 1992.
5. Altman DG, Coles EC: Nomograms for precise determination of birth weight for dates. Br J Obstet Gynaecol 87:81, 1980.
6. Brenner WE, et al: A standard of fetal growth for the United States of America. Am J Obstet Gynecol 126:555, 1976.
7. Kingdom JC, Kaufmann P: Oxygen and placental villous development: origins of fetal hypoxia. Placenta 18:613, 1997.
8. Kingdom JC, et al: Development of the placental villous tree and its consequences for fetal growth. Eur J Obstet Gynecol Reprod Biol 92:35, 2000.
9. Benirschke K, Kaufmann P: Pathology of the Human Placenta. New York, Springer-Verlag, 1995.
10. Regnault TRH, et al: Altered uteroplacental angiogenesis, oxygenation, and hemodynamics in IUGR: setting the stage for fetal damage. Presented at the 8th International Federation of Placenta Associations, Melbourne, Australia, October 2002.
11. Pardi G, et al: Venous drainage of the human uterus: respiratory gas studies in normal and fetal growth-retarded pregnancies. Am J Obstet Gynecol 166:699, 1992.
12. Meschia G: Placental Respiratory Gas Exchange and Fetal Oxygenation. In Creasy R, Resnik R (eds): Maternal-Fetal Medicine. Philadelphia, WB Saunders Co, 1999 pp 260–69.
13. Gudmundsson S, Dubiel M: Doppler velocimetry in the evaluation of fetal hypoxia. J Perinatal Med 29:399, 2001.
14. Pardi G, et al: Diagnostic value of blood sampling in fetuses with growth retardation. N Engl J Med 1993;328:692–96.
15. Wladimiroff JW, et al: Fetal and umbilical flow velocity waveforms between 10–16 weeks' gestation: a preliminary study. Obstet Gynecol 78:812, 1991.
16. Ferrazzi E, et al: Umbilical vein blood flow in growth-restricted fetuses. Ultrasound Obstet Gynecol 16:432, 2000.
17. Peeters LL, et al: Blood flow to fetal organs as a function of arterial oxygen content. Am J Obstet Gynecol 135:637, 1979.
18. Dubiel M, et al: Comparison of power Doppler and velocimetry in predicting outcome of high-risk pregnancy. Eur J Ultrasound 12:197, 2001.
19. Ferrazzi E, et al: Temporal sequence of abnormal Doppler changes in the peripheral and central circulatory systems of the severely growth-restricted fetus. Ultrasound Obstet Gynecol 19:140, 2002.
20. Thaler I, et al: Changes in uterine blood flow during human pregnancy. Am J Obstet Gynecol 162:121, 1990.
21. Dickey RP, Hower JF: Ultrasonographic features of uterine blood flow during the first 16 weeks of pregnancy. Hum Reprod 10:2448, 1995.
22. Bower S, et al: Improved prediction of preeclampsia by two-stage screening of uterine arteries using the early diastolic notch and color Doppler imaging. Obstet Gynecol 82:78, 1993.
23. Konje JC, et al: A longitudinal study of quantitative uterine blood flow with the use of color power angiography in appropriate for gestational age pregnancies. Am J Obstet Gynecol 185:608, 2001.
24. Barbera A, et al: Relationship of umbilical vein blood flow to growth parameters in the human fetus. Am J Obstet Gynecol 181:174, 1999.
25. Sutton MS, et al: Changes in placental blood flow in the normal human fetus with gestational age. Pediatr Res 28:383, 1990.
26. Rasmussen K: Precision and accuracy of Doppler flow measurements: in vitro and in vivo study of the applicability of the method in human fetuses. Scand J Clin Lab Invest 47:311, 1987.
27. Lingman G, Marsal K: Fetal central blood circulation in the third trimester of normal pregnancy: a longitudinal study. II. Aortic blood velocity waveform. Early Hum Dev 13:151, 1986.
28. Chen HY, et al: Antenatal measurement of fetal umbilical venous flow by pulsed Doppler and B-mode ultrasonography. J Ultrasound Med 1986;5:319, 1986.
29. Gill RW, et al: Fetal umbilical venous flow measured in utero by pulsed Doppler and B-mode ultrasound. I. Normal pregnancies. Am J Obstet Gynecol 139:720, 1981.
30. Rigano S, et al: Early and persistent reduction in umbilical vein blood flow in the growth-restricted fetus: a longitudinal study. Am J Obstet Gynecol 185:834, 2001.
31. Kiserud T, et al: Umbilical flow distribution to the liver and the ductus venosus: an in vitro investigation of the fluid dynamic mechanisms in the fetal sheep. Am J Obstet Gynecol 177:86, 1997.
32. Bellotti M, et al: Role of ductus venosus in distribution of umbilical blood flow in human fetuses during second half of pregnancy. Am J Physiol 279:H1256, 2000.
33. Kiserud T, et al: Ultrasonographic velocimetry of the fetal ductus venosus. Lancet 338:1412, 1991.
34. Pennati G, et al: Hemodynamic changes across the human ductus venosus: a comparison between clinical findings and mathematical calculations. Ultrasound Obstet Gynecol 9:383, 1997.
35. Pennati G, et al: Mathematical modelling of the human foetal cardiovascular system based on Doppler ultrasound data. Med Eng Phys 19:327, 1997.
36. Pennati G, et al: Blood flow through the ductus venosus in human fetus: calculation using Doppler velocimetry and computational findings. Ultrasound Med Biol 24:PP, 1998.
37. Pennati G, et al: Umbilical flow distribution to the liver and the ductus venosus in human fetuses during gestation: an anatomy-based mathematical modeling. Med Eng Phys 25:229, 2003.
38. Bellotti M, et al: Dilatation of the ductus venosus in human fetuses: ultrasonographic evidence and mathematical modeling. Am J Physiol 275:H1759, 1998.
39. Baserga M, et al: Prolonged total parenteral nutrition and hepatobiliary dysfunction in extremely low birth weight infants: impact of intrauterine growth retardation. Pediatr Res 49:293A, 2001.
40. el-Hennawy M, et al: Relationship between clinical risk factors and pathological findings of liver injury in neonates receiving total parenteral nutrition (TPN). Pediatr Res 49:3989, 2001.
41. Wilkening RB, et al: Fetal pH improvement after 24 h of severe, nonlethal hypoxia. Biol Neonate 63:129, 1993.
42. Holcomb RG, Wilkening RB: Hepatic metabolism during acute hypoxia in fetal lambs. Pediatr Res 43:49A, 1998.
43. Thureen PJ, et al: Placental glucose transport in heat-induced fetal growth retardation. Am J Physiol 263:R578, 1992.
44. Marconi AM, et al: The impact of gestational age and fetal growth on the maternal-fetal glucose concentration difference. Obstet Gynecol 87:937, 1996.
45. Nicolini U, et al: Maternal-fetal glucose gradient in normal pregnancies and in pregnancies complicated by alloimmunization and fetal growth retardation. Am J Obstet Gynecol 161:924, 1989.
46. Bozzetti P, et al: The relationship of maternal and fetal glucose concentrations in the human from midgestation until term. Metab Clin Exp 37:358, 1988.
47. Economides DL, et al: Relation between maternal-to-fetal blood glucose gradient and uterine and umbilical Doppler blood flow measurements. Br J Obstet Gynaecol 97:543, 1990.
48. Marconi AM, et al: Impact of conceptus mass on glucose disposal rate in pregnant women. Am J Physiol 264:E514, 1993.
49. Teng C, et al: Fetal hepatic and umbilical uptakes of glucogenic substrates during a glucagon-somatostatin infusion. Am J Physiol 282:E542, 2002.
50. Marconi AM, et al: An evaluation of fetal glucogenesis in intrauterine growth-retarded pregnancies. Metab Clin Exp 42:860, 1993.
51. Battaglia FC, Regnault TR: Placental transport and metabolism of amino acids. Placenta 22:145, 2001.
52. Moe AJ: Placental amino acid transport. Am J Physiol 268:C1321, 1995.
53. Jansson T: Amino acid transporters in the human placenta. Pediatr Res 49:141, 2001.
54. Loy GL, et al: Fetoplacental deamination and decarboxylation of leucine. Am J Physiol 259:E492, 1990.
55. Ross JC, et al: Placental transport and fetal utilization of leucine in a model of fetal growth retardation. Am J Physiol 270:E491, 1996.
56. Anderson AH, et al: Placental transport of threonine and its utilization in the normal and growth-restricted fetus. Am J Physiol 272:E892, 1997.
57. Marconi AM, et al: Steady state maternal-fetal leucine enrichments in normal and intrauterine growth-restricted pregnancies. Pediatr Res 46:114, 1999.
58. Cetin I, et al: In vivo placental transport of glycine and leucine in human pregnancies. Pediatr Res 37:571, 1995.
59. Paolini CL, et al: An in vivo study of ovine placental transport of essential amino acids. Am J Physiol 280:E31, 2001.
60. Paolini CL, et al: Placental transport of leucine, phenylalanine, glycine, and proline in intrauterine growth-restricted pregnancies. J Clin Endocrinol Metab 86:5427, 2001.

Dennis M. Styne

Endocrine Factors Affecting Neonatal Growth

PATTERN OF NEONATAL GROWTH

The greatest growth rate occurs during fetal life; in fact, the passage from one fertilized cell to a 3.5-kg neonate encompasses an increase in length of 5000-fold, an increase in surface area by $61 \times 10,^6$ and an increase in weight by $6 \times 10.$[12] The greatest postnatal growth rate occurs just after birth,[1] with slower growth following during midchildhood; growth increases once more in puberty before the final cessation at epiphyseal fusion. The characteristic pattern of postnatal growth in stature and weight has been documented since the Count de Montelbeillard carefully recorded measurements during the growth of his son in 18th century France.[2] Subsequent longitudinal and cross-sectional studies aided our understanding of the growth process until the new-growth charts became available from the Centers for Disease Control and Prevention. These charts demonstrate the 3rd to 97th percentile of length during the first 3 years after birth.* Further analysis of the factors affecting various phases of growth led to the development of the infant-childhood-pubertal (ICP) growth charts,[3] in which the amounts of growth for each of the three phases of growth are considered and their sums plotted together. There are mathematical functions for each component of this model:

Infancy: This slowly decelerating component occurs when the rapid fetal growth phase decreases before birth; it dwindles away by age 3 to 4 years. An infancy-child growth spurt at about 6 to 9 months of age defines the beginning of the childhood phase.[4] The average total gain in height for Swedish boys (the population in whom the plots were originally developed) during this phase is 79.0 cm (44.0% of final height) and for girls, 76.8 cm (46.2%).

Childhood: This phase begins during the first year of life and continues to adult height. It reflects the strengthening endocrine effects of thyroid hormone, growth hormone, and other agents. Average total gain in height for boys is 85.2 cm (47.4%) and for girls is 78.4 cm (47.3%).

Puberty: Average total gain in height for boys is 15.4 cm (8.6%) and for girls is 10.9 cm (6.5%). This phase is dependent upon sex steroids, mainly estrogen.

The accurate measurement of length at birth is as important as the measurement of weight since the determination of growth velocity is not possible without it.[5] Unfortunately, accurate measurement of neonates and infants is honored more in the breech. A study of the measurement of infants, as well as inanimate dolls, led to inaccuracies of up to 25% in length measurements, with weight measurement errors exceeding 10% or more.[6] Even if a measurement is assumed to be accurate, the points plotted on the growth chart are also prone to error due to rounding or to lack of attention to adjustment for gestational age (if the baby is premature).[7,8] Measurement of growth can be performed accurately if two individuals are involved to straighten the infant gently and hold the child against a calipers-like device, such as a neo-infantometer (Graham-Field, Inc. Hauppauge, NY) that expands and contracts to measure the linear distance from a perpendicular plate at the top of the head to a perpendicular plate at the bottom of the feet.[6,9,10]

Knemometry is a technique that measures minute changes in length of the lower leg[11] and is applicable even to seriously ill children in the neonatal intensive care unit.[12] Whereas the yearly growth rate is considered linear and consistent, knemometry demonstrates the waxing and waning pattern of growth in an infant that occurs over days and weeks; the time between peak and nadir growth rate may stretch to 10 to 20 days.[9,13,14] This fluctuating growth in length may be accompanied by changes in the pattern of weight gain; however, since caloric intake does not affect this pattern, it is innate and perhaps genetic in origin.[15] Knemometry was used to demonstrate the effect of dexamethasone or chronic lung disease on growth velocity;[11] glucocorticoid treatment increases weight while decreasing length velocity. Therefore, it is apparent that measuring weight cannot substitute for measuring growth in length.

The length of a full-term neonate is closely correlated with maternal stature, but once free from the constraints of the uterus, the full-term infant often will adjust growth to achieve the growth percentile that will be followed for most of childhood. An increase in percentiles occurs soon after birth as the childhood percentile is reached by 11 to 12 months in children destined to be taller, whereas a downward adjustment will allow the child who will be shorter to reach the new lower percentile by a mean of 13 months of age.[16]

Prematurity, Intrauterine Growth Restriction (IUGR) and Small for Gestational Age (SGA). The definitions of IUGR and SGA are often confused, and even the medical literature is not always clear. The present convention is that IUGR indicates a documented decrease in intrauterine growth noted by ultrasound; an IUGR baby may have a temporary problem that will still allow a normal or near-normal birth weight and length. SGA refers to an infant whose weight (and presumably length) are below a limit, usually the 10th percentile for gestational age. Two descriptors of IUGR are used: symmetrical IUGR denotes normal body proportions (a small head and a small body) and is considered a more severe and long-standing form of IUGR, dating from the second trimester, whereas asymmetrical IUGR denotes small abdominal circumferences (due mostly to a small liver), decreased subcutaneous and abdominal fat, and reduced skeletal muscle mass—probably due to stress effects in the third trimester. The head circumference is in the normal range. A low ponderal index (birth weight/length²) is a marker for asymmetrical growth restriction and also increases the risk for cerebral palsy.[17] Asymmetrical IUGR infants show catch-up growth more frequently than symmetrical IUGR infants, but 10 to 30% of IUGR infants remain short as children and adults. The FDA has approved treating IUGR infants lacking catch-up growth with growth hormone; short-term growth acceleration is demonstrated, but the effect on final height is not yet known.

Standards of height, weight, and weight for height adjusted for gestational age are available for preterm low birth weight infants. These allow determination of appropriate weight gain in the evaluation of failure to thrive, as well as patterns of excessive weight gain in these infants.[18,19] Customized British birth weight percentile charts based upon characteristics of the mother and the physiologic, characteristics of the neonate are available.[20] Although ultrasonographic evidence of fetal growth rate is more specific and accurate for the diagnosis of IUGR, customized

---

* (http://www.cdc.gov/nchs/about/major/nhanes/growthcharts/clinical_charts.htm#Clin%202).

growth charts are considered useful as indications of inadequate fetal growth.[21] Most analyses of mortality are based upon birth weight. However, careful analysis of birth length and mortality in the Swedish population showed the importance of knowing length in preterm infants. Low weight or ponderal index led to a greater risk of early death, but the weight of infants at 4 to 5 days of age did not. A length of more than 1 SD below the mean increased the risk of long-term mortality.[22] Premature infants are expected to have catch-up growth by 2 years; those born after 29 weeks' of gestation exhibit catch-up growth, whereas those born before 29 weeks are more likely to have a decreased rate of length and weight gain, which may be noted in the first week after birth and last up to 2 years.[6,23,24]

Although it had been assumed that SGA babies (in contrast to appropriate for gestational age [AGA] premature babies) did not have catch-up growth in length, there is now evidence from longitudinal, as well as less powerful cross-sectional, studies that the majority (up to 80%) of SGA babies who started with lengths greater than 2 SD below the mean do indeed show catch-up in height for age.[25-27] An acceleration of growth in length is noted in the first 6 months of SGA babies who will catch up.[28] In one study, 44% of infants with neonatal length greater than -1.28 SD (and therefore considered SGA) caught up to less than -1.28 SD by 3 months, 51% caught up by 3 years, and 73% by 6 years.[29] A large (n = 3650) study of SGA infants found that 88% of healthy singleton SGA infants exhibited catch-up growth by 2 years, with most showing the catch-up by age 2 months; those that remained short at 2 years of age had a greater risk of shorter adult stature.[26] In a prospective study of SGA babies, 38% were less than or equal to the 10th percentile of height at 6 months of postnatal age versus 7% of control babies; proportionate SGA infants had greater catch-up than did disproportionate SGA babies, but the differences were in the range of 1 cm increased growth/6 months.[30] In general, children born SGA will achieve an adult height standard deviation score (SDS) equivalent to their SDS in childhood. The risk of having an adult height of less than 2 SD was fivefold higher in children who had a low birth weight and sevenfold higher in those with a low birth length.[26] About one fifth of extremely short children have a history of IUGR.[31,32]

There is controversy in the infantile growth rate of SGA infants of less than 1500 g; some studies show similar growth in length and head circumference in these infants compared with those of the same birth weight but shorter gestation (preterm but weight AGA)[33] while others[34] found the opposite. Of 166 children with birth weight less than 1000 g and SGA, 81% demonstrated catch-up growth in length during childhood, with 78% showing catch-up in length by 3 years of age.[35] Symmetrical SGA infants had less catch up than those with asymmetrical SGA, the opposite of that found in heavier children.[30]

Controversy exists over the long-term effects of SGA on intellectual function. A 26-year follow-up of infants classified as SGA (birth weight < 5th percentile; 1064 SGA compared with 14,189 non-SGA for controls) showed no difference in years of education, employment, marital status, or satisfaction with life.[36] However, the SGA infants were less likely to be in the top 15% of their high school class and more likely to be recommended for special education; the SGA had small but significant defects in academic achievement. The SGA population had shorter adult heights (-.55 SDS). Further, the SGA infants were less likely to hold managerial or professional employment and had less income. Another 20-year longitudinal follow-up of very low birth weight infants (less than 1500 g) demonstrated a lower mean IQ (87 versus 92), lower academic achievement scores, fewer high school graduations and less post secondary school study but, on the positive side, less alcohol and drug abuse than those born at normal weight.[37]

Neonatal growth may be affected by metabolic bone disease in preterm infants. For example, the finding of a peak neonatal alkaline phosphatase level of greater than 1200 IU/L predicted shorter stature up to age 12 years. The effect exceeds that of maternal or paternal height, sex, parental educational achievement, and hypertension during pregnancy, which are other factors known to affect childhood height.[38] Neonatal diet supplementation does not seem to have an effect on bone mineralization,[39] thus treatment of metabolic bone disease in the neonate is of great importance.

Midchildhood Growth Spurt. The striking pubertal growth spurt attracts much attention, but two periods after birth are characterized by brief growth spurts before puberty occurs: the infant-childhood growth spurt between 8 months and 3 years and the midchildhood growth spurt between 6 and 7 years. There is an "adiposity rebound" of accelerating weight gain and rising body mass index (BMI) in midchildhood after a period of relative stability of weight gain. An early adiposity rebound is a risk factor for the development of obesity later in childhood and thereafter (Fig. 28–1).

Hormonal Control of Neonatal Growth

The hormones that mediate postnatal growth do not play the same roles in fetal growth. Growth hormone (GH) is present in very high concentrations in the fetus (Fig. 28–2), in contrast to the limited presence of GH receptors. Although this discrepancy suggests limited activity of GH in the fetus, GH does play a role in fetal growth that is reflected in the poorer growth of GH-deficient infants. Infants with Laron syndrome (GH resistance due to reduced or absent GH receptors) have elevated GH and low serum insulin-like growth factors-1 (IGF-1) levels; they have decreased birth length and weight. Insulin excess, as in the infant of a diabetic mother, causes increased growth. Thyroid hormone deficiency does not directly affect human birth weight, but prolonged gestation is a feature of congenital hypothyroidism, and this factor in itself increases weight. Placental lactogen exerts no apparent effect on birth size in human beings. However, the concentration of placental GH (from the *GHV* gene, see later) is significantly decreased in the serum of a pregnant woman bearing a fetus with IUGR. In the postnatal phase, these hormones have quite important but, in many cases, different roles.

GROWTH HORMONE

The major form of human GH is a single chain of 191 amino acids (about 21,500 daltons), containing two intramolecular disulfide bonds.[40] A 20-kD variant of pituitary growth hormone accounts for 5 to 10% of circulating GH.[41] The genes for a family of GH-related proteins share a common structural organization, with four introns separating five exons. The gene for GH is located on the long arm of chromosome 17 in a cluster of five genes with evolutionary relationships: *GHN* codes for human GH (a single 191-amino acid polypeptide chain with a molecular weight of 22 kD), *GHV* codes for a variant GH produced in the placenta, *CSH1* and *CSH2* code for prolactin, and *CSHP1* codes for a variant prolactin molecule.[42]

GH is released in a pulsatile pattern in which there are rare peaks, measurable by most assays, and nadirs that only the most ultrasensitive assays detect (e.g., values of 0.04 μg/L). These peaks and valleys of GH are under the control of the two hypothalamic regulatory peptides, GH-releasing hormone (GHRH), a stimulatory peptide also released in a pulsatile manner, and somatostatin (or somatotropin release–inhibiting factor, SRIF), an inhibitory factor.[43] GHRH contains 44 amino acids, but alternative forms have 40 and 37 amino acids, although the amino terminus of GHRH must be present for biologic activity. GHRH exerts effects by binding to a G protein–related receptor on the pituitary somatotropes, increasing intracellular cAMP production and subsequently increasing GH synthesis. Somatostatin, however, regulates the timing and amplitude of the pulses of GH

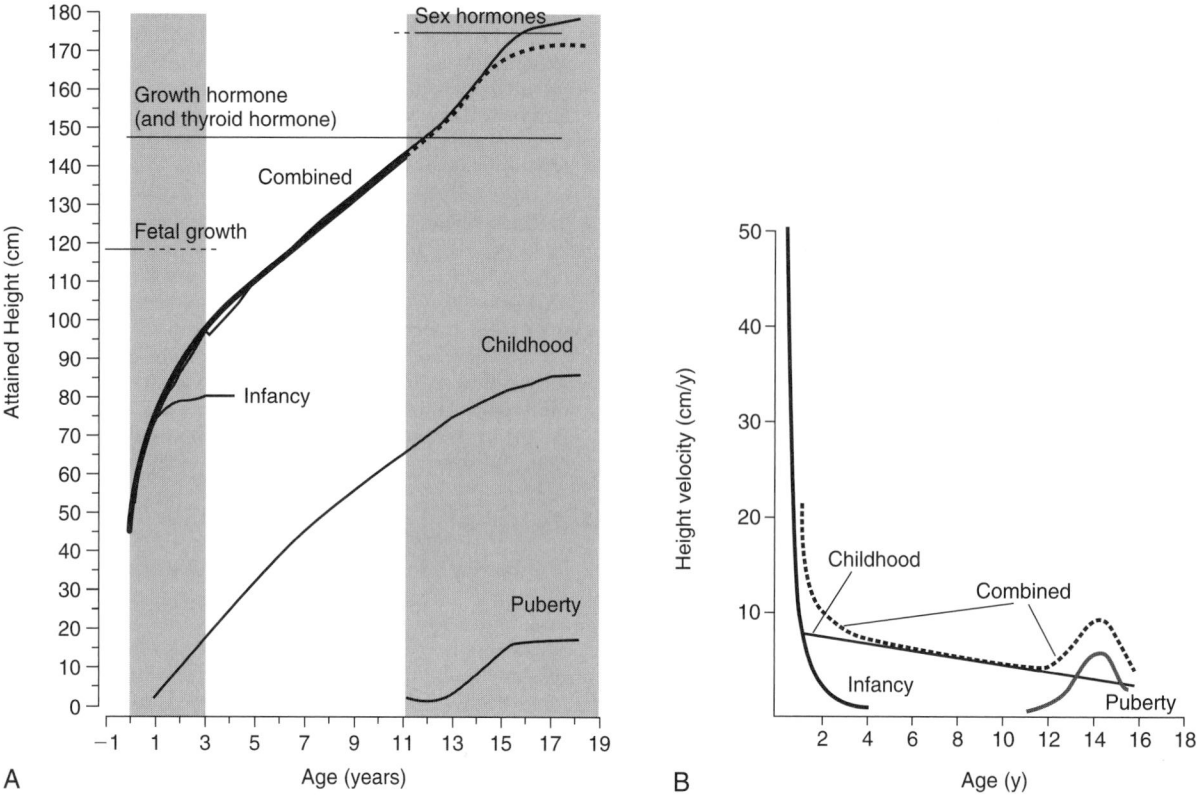

Figure 28–1. The individual components of the infancy, childhood, and puberty growth chart (**A**) and the combined growth curve that results from the sum of them (**B**). (Adapted from Karlberg J: Acta Paediatr Scand [Suppl] *356*:26, 1989; and Larsen PR, et al [eds]: Williams Textbook of Endocrinology, 10th ed. Philadelphia, WB Saunders Co, 2003, p 1129.)

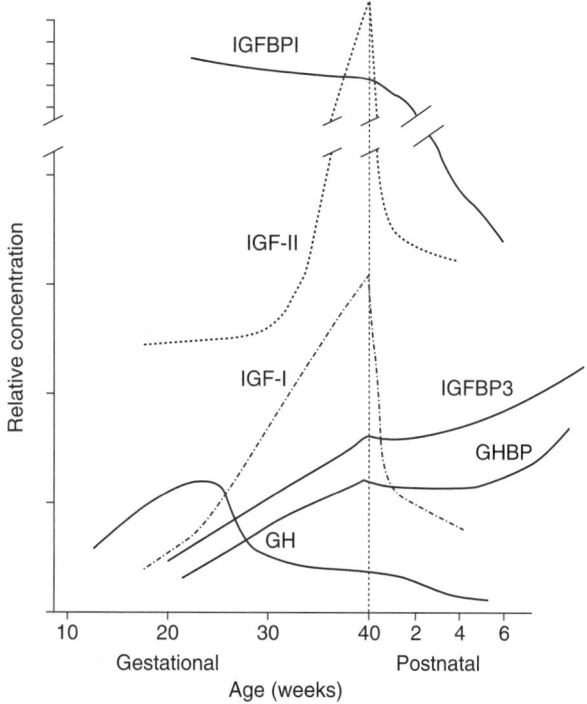

Figure 28–2. Relative concentrations of GH, GHBP, IGFs, and IGFBPs during gestation and perinatally. (Adapted from Wollmann HA: Horm Res *53(Suppl 1)*:50, 2000.)

but has no effect upon synthesis of GH. In contrast to the action of GHRH on the pituitary, when somatostatin binds to its receptor it inhibits adenylate cyclase activity and reduces intracellular calcium levels.[44] Pulses of GH secretion occur when there is a decrease in the release of somatostatin from the hypothalamus and an increase in the release of GHRH; when SRIF is released without GHRH, there is a nadir of the GH pulse.

A plethora of neurotransmitters regulate the release of these hypothalamic factors, including serotonin, histamine, norepinephrine, dopamine, acetylcholine, gamma-aminobutyric acid, thyroid-releasing hormone, vasoactive intestinal peptide, gastrin, neurotensin, substance P, calcitonin, neuropeptide Y, vasopressin, galanin, and corticotropin-releasing hormone.[45] The physiologic state also can increase GH secretion, including stress, sleep (deep sleep during later childhood), hemorrhage, fasting, hypoglycemia, and, at least in older subjects, exercise. GH-stimulatory tests are employed in the evaluation of GH secretory capacity in neonates if indicated. The secretion of GH is also influenced by a variety of hormones, such as estrogen, which in most cases increases basal and stimulated GH secretion (androgens exert their effect through aromatization to estrogens); thyroid hormone, which is essential in allowing GH secretion; and glucocorticoids, which decrease GH secretion when in excess. Small (6 amino acid) peptides, GH-releasing peptides, regulate GH secretion through pituitary and hypothalamic receptors separate from GHRH and SRIF. They have been identified as receptors for ghrelin, a recently discovered gastrointestinal hormone that stimulates GH secretion.[46, 47] IGF peptides exert negative feedback control of GH secretion by interaction with pituitary IGF receptors.

The cell membrane GH receptor has 620 amino acids and a molecular weight of 70 kD. It contains an extracellular, hormone-binding domain; a single membrane-spanning domain; and a cytoplasmic domain. A circulating growth hormone–binding protein (GHBP) that has the same amino acid sequence as the extracellular domain of the GH receptor (approximately 55 kD) is derived from proteolytic cleavage of the extracellular domain of the receptor and is found in the blood.[48] The major GHBP in human plasma binds GH with high specificity and affinity but with relatively low capacity, as about 45% of circulating GH is bound. Levels of GHBP are low in early life, rise through childhood, and plateau during puberty and adulthood. Patients with abnormalities of the GH receptor (e.g., Laron dwarfism) also have the defect reflected in the serum GHBP concentration; those with decreased numbers of GH receptors have decreased serum GHBP concentrations.[49] Nutritional state as well as other factors regulates both GH secretion and GHBP values.

It has long been recognized that cord blood values of GH are higher than those of adults[50] and fall during the 2 weeks to 2 months after birth.[51] Adults exhibit pulsatile GH release, but the sampling of blood for the analysis of pulsatile GH secretion in neonates is problematic. Recently, safe microsampling techniques allowing blood withdrawal every 20 to 30 minutes over 12 hours or longer have been developed.[52] With this technique, a pulsatile pattern of GH release was demonstrated, but infants, unlike adults, have not yet developed entrainment of the GH secretory rhythm with sleep. By 4 days of age, there was a direct correlation of GH and insulin secretion, signifying a relationship between feeding and GH secretion.[53] On the first day after birth, infants from gestational age 33 to 41 weeks demonstrated elevated GH levels (9 to 191 µg/L) released in pulses with 5 to 6 bursts over 6 hours, leading to a pulse periodicity of 73 minutes and a half-life of 18 minutes.[54] This elevation of GH was due to increased secretion rather than decreased clearance. Prolactin was also high, but not released in pulses, and prolactin release was not related to the GH peaks.

In another study, term infants exhibited a higher GH pulse frequency and amplitude soon after birth (8 to 40 hours) compared with 63 to 85 hours, with no difference between boys and girls.[55] Studies of GH secretion at 1 to 13 days after birth revealed higher values of GH in the neonates than in later life, and even higher peaks of GH were found in SGA babies compared with AGA infants.[56,57] Basal, mean, and peak GH values in AGA and SGA babies were 33.9 versus 22.5, 33.9 versus 22.5, and 45 versus 30.7 µg/L, respectively. The pulse frequency was greater in SGA (5.1/12 hours) than AGA (4.0/12 hours) babies, with a pulse periodicity of 180 minutes in AGA and 140 minutes in SGA infants. Premature infants (mean 33 weeks' gestation) sampled at about 40 hours after birth had high basal (24 to 26 µg/L), incremental (20 to 24 µg/L), and peak (45 to 51 µg/L) GH values, with a frequency of 3/12 hours; no difference was seen between boys and girls.[56] Although elevated GH is not related to growth rate in premature infants, persistent elevation of serum GH has been linked to the development of retinopathy of prematurity.[58] Premature infants had higher secretory burst amplitudes, higher production rates, and a higher mass of GH per secretory burst than term infants. The integrated plasma GH concentration exhibited a strong trend toward a higher value in the premature infants.[59] Serum GH is elevated in IUGR infants, and normalizes by 1 month of age. Elevations of growth hormone are related to the pattern of intrauterine growth, but not to postnatal growth.[60]

The bioactivity of GH measured in an Nb2 cell assay changed in a pattern similar to that of the immunoactive GH, with higher values when first measured at 5 days that decreased by 1 and 4 months in term infants.[61] Urinary GH excretion is higher in SGA, AGA, premature, and term infants than in controls.[62]

Although serum GH is high in the neonate, GH receptors are decreased, as reflected in the lower serum GHBP. A rise in GHBP occurs at 6 months of age, which just predates the phase of increasing IGF-binding proteins (IGFBP-1) and IGFBP-3 (after about 10 months), suggesting a greater GH dependence of GH-responsive factors and GH-dependent growth in the infant of this age. It also denotes the end of the infancy phase of growth and the beginning of the childhood phase of growth.[63] Nonetheless, even though infants with congenital GH deficiency are of near-normal length at birth, growth rate rapidly decreases within a few months after birth and may descend to more than 3 to 7 SD below the mean.[64] Treatment with GH increases growth rate, and catch-up growth increases height by 2 years. Children born SGA have a different profile of GH and IGF than normal-weight individuals. At birth and at 3 days of age SGA infants exhibit high basal GH, low peak amplitude, and higher frequency of peaks of GH, while IGF-1, IGFBP-3, and leptin are significantly reduced.[26,57]

Various congenital defects of the pituitary hypothalamic axis lead to deficiency of GH or other pituitary hormones. There is a range of defects from pituitary hypoplasia to other midline defects up to holoprosencephaly; any midline defect of the central nervous system (CNS) should be suspect as an etiology of hypopituitarism. The pituitary gland resides in the sella turcica near the optic chiasm. A decrease in the size of the sella turcica indicates reduced pituitary development. Alternatively, there may be a combined defect in the function of the pituitary gland and visual ability, as found in the syndrome of (septo-)optic dysplasia in which congenital blindness or nystagmus is an indication of potential pituitary defects. This condition is sporadic or rarely due to homozygosity of an inactivating mutation of the *Hesx-1* gene.

The anterior pituitary gland and pituitary stalk are often smaller than normal, and a bright spot representing the posterior pituitary is located in the hypothalamus rather than in its normal location. This finding is referred to as an ectopic posterior pituitary. Congenital hypopituitarism is associated with breech birth, forceps delivery, and intrapartum and maternal bleeding.

Genetic Forms of Hypopituitarism.[65,66] Genetic defects account for more than 5% of isolated GH deficiency or combined pituitary hormone deficiencies.

Isolated Growth Hormone Deficiency (IGHD)

Autosomal recessive complete deletions of the GH1 gene are IGHD type IA. Autosomal recessive IGHD type IB has various sizes and sites of deletions in the GH gene or mutations in the GHRH receptor gene. Autosomal dominant IGHD II is caused by mutations in the GH1 gene. The gene responsible for X-linked IGHD III has not yet been identified. Some subjects have associated immunoglobulin deficiency. In similar terminology, autosomal recessive multiple pituitary hormone deficiency is type I, and the X-linked form is type III.

Mutations may be found in the pituitary transcription factors PROP1 (causing deficiencies of luteinizing hormone [LH] and follicle-stimulating hormone [FSH] as well as GH, prolactin [PRL], and thyroid-stimulating hormone [TSH] and possibly ACTH in a pattern of recessive inheritance) and also POU1F1 (autosomal dominant pattern of GH and PRL deficiency, as well as some degree of TSH deficiency). Children with Laron syndrome lack GH receptor structure or function;[67] affected children will not grow when treated with GH but must receive IGF-1, which is available only in clinical trials. Serum GHBP is decreased in those with GH receptor deficiency, while others have adequate numbers of receptors that are inactive or have lesser activity. One patient with congenital IGF-1 deficiency (not due to GH receptor defects)[68,69] had a birth length 5.4 SD below the mean and was 6.9 SD below the mean for height at age 15 years. Since there was no IGF-1, there was no feedback to GH secretion, and GH values were elevated (similar to findings found in Laron dwarfism).

Insulin-like Growth Factors.[45] The effects of growth hormone are mainly mediated by the IGFs (originally called sulfation factor, subsequently nonsuppressible insulin-like activity [NSILA], and then somatomedin) but GH also has direct effects such as lipolysis, increased amino acid transport into tissues, and increased protein synthesis in liver. Growth hormone produces insulin resistance and is a diabetogenic substance, increasing blood sugar.

The two IGFs, IGF-1 and IGF-2, share 45 of a 73-amino acid sequence and have structures similar to that of the proinsulin molecule. They are 50% homologous with the A and B chains of insulin.[70, 71] Both the IGFs and proinsulin have a connecting peptide or a C chain, although the homology is not complete in terms of the amino acid structure. The IGF-1 C-peptide region is 12 amino acids long and the IGF-2 C-peptide region is 8 amino acids long. Neither shows homology in amino acid sequence with the C-peptide region of proinsulin. Also, the IGFs have a carboxyl terminal extension or D-peptide, unlike proinsulin.

The gene for prepro-IGF-1 is located on the long arm of chromosome 12 and contains at least 5 exons.[72] IGF-1 is produced in most tissues and appears to be exported to neighboring cells to act upon them in a paracrine manner.[73] Thus, serum IGF-1 concentrations may not reflect the most significant actions of this growth factor. The liver is a major site of IGF-1 synthesis, and much of the circulating IGF-1 probably originates in the liver. Serum IGF-1 concentrations vary in liver disease and with the extent of liver destruction. IGF-1 is a progression factor, so that a cell that has been exposed to a competence factor (e.g., platelet-derived growth factor, PDGF) in stage G_0 of the cell cycle and has progressed to G_1 can, with IGF-1 exposure in G_1, undergo division in the S phase of the cell cycle.[74] Aside from the stimulatory effects of IGF-1 on cartilage growth, IGF-1 has stimulatory effects on hematopoiesis, ovarian steroidogenesis, myoblast proliferation and differentiation, and differentiation of the lens.

The IGF-1 cell membrane receptor (the type I receptor) resembles the insulin receptor in its structure of two α and two β chains.[75, 76] Binding of IGF-1 to type I receptors stimulates tyrosine kinase activity and autophosphorylation of tyrosine residues in the receptor. This leads to cell differentiation or division (or both). The type 1 IGF receptor mRNA is present in almost all tissues except liver. IGF-1 receptors are down-regulated by increased IGF-1 concentrations, whereas decreased IGF-1 concentrations lead to an increase in IGF-1 receptors. The structural similarity of the IGFs and insulin explains why IGFs are able to bind to the insulin receptor and why insulin in excess can bind to the type 1 IGF receptor (in physiologic levels, insulin has little binding to the IGF-1 receptor) although the structural differences may explain why insulin cannot bind to the IGFBPs (see later).

IGF molecules may be bound to one of six IGFBPs, some of which are found in the circulation and some of which are found in tissue.[77] IGFBPs generally are considered to be inhibitory to IGF effects, although there is evidence that some IGFBPs can enhance IGF activity in some situations. IGFBP proteases (for IGFBP-2–5), which control the IGFBPs by proteolysis, lead to another level of control. IGFBP-1 is a 25-kD protein, which is suppressed by insulin but not affected by GH. IFGBP-1 inhibits IGF action IGFBP-1 is present in high concentrations in fetal serum and amnionic fluid. Serum values of IFGBP-1 and IGFBP-2 in blood are inversely proportional to birth weight, suggesting that IGFBP-1 suppresses fetal growth. IGF-1 circulates bound to IGFBP-3 and an acid labile subunit in a 150-kD complex. Serum IGFBP-3 concentrations are directly proportional to GH concentrations as well as to IGF-1 concentrations and are also regulated by nutritional status (as is IGF-1). Thus, in malnutrition, IGFBP-3 and IGF-1 levels fall while GH rises. IGFBP-3 rises with advancing age throughout childhood, with highest values achieved during puberty.

IGF-2 is a 67-amino acid acidic peptide coded by a gene on the short arm of chromosome 11, close to the gene for preproinsulin.[72] Information about the function of IGF-2 is limited. The type II IGF receptor preferentially binds IGF-2 and is identical to the mannose 6-phosphate receptor, a single-chain transmembrane protein. Although most of the effects of IGF-2 are mediated by its interaction with the type I receptor, independent actions of IGF-2 via the type II receptor are described. The ratio of IGF-2 to IGF-2R (a soluble form of the type 2 IGF receptor that exhibits inhibitory effects on IGF-2 action) is directly related to birth weight and is even more closely related to placental weight.[78]

IGF-1 in the fetus is regulated by metabolic factors rather than undergoing significant influence by GH, as is the case in postnatal life. One explanation is that there are fewer GH receptors in the fetus than after birth. The GH receptor is first found at about 30 weeks' gestation.[79] In the human fetus, the serum GH level falls during later gestation owing to maturation of CNS negative control, whereas serum IGF-1 and IGFBP-3 rise during gestation, demonstrating their differing pattern and independence from GH stimulation. Serum GH in the last half of gestation falls while IGF-1 increases, as does IGF-2 and IGFBP-3.[60]

Early studies demonstrated that IGF-1 (then measured as NSILA) is directly related to gestational age and birth weight.[80] The serum values of IGF-1 are 50% or less of adult values; IGF-2 values are about 50% of adult values in term neonates. Cord blood IGF-1 values correlate with birth weight in some but not all studies. IGF-1 concentrations are more highly correlated in monozygotic twins than in same-sex dizygotic twins, indicating a genetic effect upon IGF-1 regulation. Premature infants have lower serum IGF-1 and IGFBP-3 and lower GHBP but higher IGFBP-1 and IGFBP-2 than term neonates; there is an inverse correlation with levels of IGFBP-1 and IGFBP-2 and gestational age.[81] In SGA infants, IGF-2 is decreased. The smallest SGA infants evidence increased GH resistance; GH is higher and the GH-dependent growth factors are lower compared with AGA infants.[82] Alternatively, in LGA infants, IGF-1, insulin, and IGFBP-3 are increased while IGFBP-1 is decreased.[83] Preeclampsia further lowers cord blood IGF-1 values after correcting for gestational age and for birth weight.[84] IGFBP-1 and IGF-1 are elevated in SGA infants and decreased in LGA infants. IGF-1 levels are inversely related to birth weight.[85, 86] However, in Spanish infants, IGF-1 and IGFBP-3 had a direct relationship to ponderal index: IGF-1, IGFBP-3, and GHBP rose with gestational age and IGFBP-1 fell.[87]

The relationship between IGF and postnatal growth has been studied. At a mean of 4 days after birth, IGF-1 was higher in AGA than SGA infants, whereas peak, mean, and incremental GH was higher in SGA infants, as was IGFBP-1.[53] Measurements during the first week after birth demonstrated that IGF-1 decreased in term infants for the first 3 days, then rose again at the end of the week, but IGF-1 remained stable in preterm infants. IGFBP-3 and IGF-2 did not change significantly during this first week.[88] In normal term neonates, IGFBP-1 and IGFBP-2 decreased between 1 and 3 months of age; IGF-2 increased by 3 months and GH decreased. GHBP values did not change much during this time period in one study,[89] but a rise over 30 days was demonstrated in others,[61,81] and a rise was seen at 4 and 6 months of age.[61, 89] Values of IGF-1 and IGFBP-3 remain relatively low until a peak is reached during puberty, when values are higher than at any other time in life. Because IGF-1 is so low in the neonate, IGFBP-3 values (which are higher in normal neonates) may serve as a better indication of GH deficiency than serum IGF-1. Cord blood IGF-1 correlates with postnatal growth in SGA and AGA infants during the first month of life.[90] There appears to be a correlation of IGF-2 and IGFBP-3 and catch-up growth over the first year in SGA babies.[91] Some studies show a relationship between catch-up growth and higher IGF-1 and IGFBP-3[60, 91, 92] and others do not.[93] One study has reported a relationship between serum IGF-2 values at 3 months and catch-up growth.[94] IGF-1 and IGFBP-3 are related to length in growing preterm infants receiving enteral nutrition.[95]

Phosphorylated IGFBP-1 is less active and more inhibitory than nonphosphorylated IGFBP-1. The proportion of nonphosphorylated IGFBP-1 to total IGFBP-1 was higher in cord blood than in mothers' serum, and although this form did not vary by gestational age, the concentration was lower in SGA infants. However, phosphorylated isoforms were higher in SGA fetuses. Thus the isoforms vary with fetal growth and may be of importance.[96] Over an 8-week period after birth, the growth of leg length was related to IGF-1 and weight growth related to IGFBP-3 values. The ratio of low phosphorylated IGFBP-1 to high phophorylated IGFBP-1 correlates with weight growth velocity;[97] this ratio also decreases with advancing gestational age. Gene manipulation and infusion of growth factors in animals demonstrate the influence these factors exert on fetal growth.[98, 99] IGF-1 knockout mice (which produce no IGF-1) have reduced late fetal and postnatal growth as well as diaphragmatic muscular hypoplasia (which ultimately causes their death), organ hypoplasia, and delayed ossification of cartilage.[100,101] IGF-2 knockout mice have an earlier fetal growth deficit than IGF-1 knockout mice, although their growth rate is normal later in gestation. This suggests a role for IGF-2 in growth in early gestation and one for IGF-1 in later gestation. Elimination of type 1 receptors (by gene knockout) leads to a more profound growth failure than is found in IGF-1 knockout mice, suggesting that factors other than IGF-1 exert effects upon fetal growth through the type 1 receptor (IGF-2 is one of these factors).

Artificial elevation of maternal IGF-1 can increase growth in mouse and rat fetuses and overcome the restraint imposed by uterine limitations of litter size.[102] Knockout of the maternal gene for the type 2 receptor leads to high birth weight, generalized organomegaly and other anomalies usually leading to rapid postnatal death; the type 2 receptor appears necessary for postnatal life.[103, 104] Transgenic mice over-expressing IGFBP-1 have smaller birth size, lower birth weight, poorer postnatal weight gain (as well as more frequent postnatal death), a proportional decrease in the size of all organs except the brain (which is much smaller in proportion to other organs), fasting hyperglycemia, and impaired glucose tolerance.[105, 106] Early postnatal growth retardation occurs in mice experiencing excess IGFBP-1, suggesting an inhibitory growth role for IGFBP-1 in late gestation and thereafter. Overexpression of IGFBP-3 in mice led to organomegaly of the spleen, liver, and heart, although birth weight was not different from that of wild-type mice.[105,107] Thus excess IGFBP-1 stunts fetal growth, whereas excess IGFBP-3 leads to selective organomegaly. In fetal rhesus monkeys given synthetic IGF-1, spleen, thymus, and kidney weights increased, as well as small intestinal length.[108]

Insulin. While insulin is a major regulatory factor for carbohydrate metabolism, many lines of evidence demonstrate its importance in fetal growth as well. Macrosomia is a well-known effect of fetal hyperinsulinism and may be seen in the infant of the diabetic mother.[109,110] These infants have increased body fat at 1 year[111] and by 10 years of age have a higher prevalence of obesity than nonmacrosomic infants. At the other end of the spectrum are the SGA infants born to diabetic women with vascular disease, extremely tight regulation of glucose levels, or eclampsia or preeclampsia. This demonstrates that limited nutrient delivery compromises the growth of the infant. These SGA infants are at risk for long-term metabolic defects.

Errors in the normal pattern of IGF-2 gene expression from the paternal chromosome and type 2 IGF receptor for IGF-2 from the maternally derived gene may underlie the pathogenesis of Beckwith-Wiedemann syndrome.[112] Affected infants are large with elevated insulin concentrations. In contrast, syndromes of fetal insulin deficiency such as are found in congenital diabetes mellitus, pancreatic dysgenesis, or fetal insulin resistance (e.g. leprechaunism) are characterized by IUGR and decreased muscle and fat mass.[113, 114] The ability of insulin either to signal metabolic processes or to stimulate growth is related to its ability to auto-phosphorylate insulin receptor substrate-1 (IRS-1). Gene knockout of the IRS-1 leads to a growth-retarded fetal mouse that is born viable but has fetal and postnatal growth deficiency and hyperglycemia (knockout of IRS-2 leads to diabetes).[115] Insulin values are lower in SGA than in normals whereas values are elevated in LGA babies.[88]

Two states of decreased insulin effects are known: (1) congenital absence of insulin in pancreatic aplasia, and (2) congenital absence of the insulin receptor as found in Donohue leprechaunism syndrome. Infants lacking insulin receptors have severe postprandial hyperglycemia, as expected from the lack of an insulin effect. Remarkably, they have preprandial hypoglycemia at first but fasting hyperglycemia several months after birth. They also are able to demonstrate some effects of insulin, such as suppression of ketone formation; an inverse relationship between insulin and IGFBP-1 is maintained, suggesting some insulin effects upon the liver.[116] It is possible that the insulin effects are mediated by the extremely elevated insulin concentrations acting through the type 1 IGF receptor. GH levels are also quite low in leprechaunism and survival is limited to a matter of months. Other infants with insulin deficiency due to absence of the islets of Langerhans have severe diabetic ketoacidosis in the untreated state[117] and exhibit poor growth, which may be less related to the lack of insulin effects than to the severe illness the children suffer.

Leptin. Leptin is produced in adipose tissue. In older individuals it is correlated with fat mass, although androgens decrease leptin values so that values are higher in girls than boys.[118] Leptin also correlates with body weight and body fat mass in cord blood.[119-121] SGA infants have lower leptin levels than controls as they have a lower fat mass.[122] This direct relationship to birth weight is independent from IGF-1 control mechanisms.[123] In contrast, 1-year-old children born with IUGR had significantly higher serum leptin levels than normal children, independent of body mass index (BMI).[124] The higher leptin levels in these children suggest a degree of leptin resistance during this period of catch-up growth, or an adipocyte defect.

Thyroid Hormone

Thyroid hormone is a major factor in postnatal growth, although, like GH, it has relatively little effect in the growth in length of the fetus. After birth, an acute release of TSH is followed by a rapid decline during the first 24 hours and a slower decline during the next 5 days. The initial peak of TSH causes a rise in serum T_4 and T_3 (due to increased conversion from T_4) a few hours after birth. Thus thyroid hormone values change by the hour and day in the neonatal period. During the next weeks after birth, serum T_4 and T_3 fall.

The effect of thyroxine in the neonate and infant is best reflected in the growth of patients with untreated and treated congenital hypothyroidism. Endemic goiter due to iodine deficiency is the most common cause of hypothyroidism worldwide but in most of the developed world anatomic or metabolic defects of the thyroid gland prevail, rather than nutritional causes. Congenital hypothyroidism is found in about 1/4000 infants; defects in the development of the thyroid gland (thyroid dysgenesis) account for 90% of affected infants and about one third of those have complete aplasia.[125] The rest of these neonates have an ectopic location of thyroid tissue. The genes TTF-1, TTF-2, and PAX-8 are important transcription factors for thyroid development; mutations of the PAX-8 gene are described in some affected neonates with either hypoplasia or ectopy. Alternatively, blocking antibodies may be transferred from the mother to cause the hypothyroidism. In addition to the anatomic defects, metabolic defects of thyroid function (usually associated with goiter and commonly transmitted in an autosomal recessive fashion) cause congenital hypothyroidism. TSH deficiency may be isolated or may occur in cases with Pit-1 mutations. Infants born with resistance to the actions of thyroid hormone may demonstrate elevated T_4 without euthyroidism and may exhibit growth failure.

Infants with congenital hypothyroidism are of normal length or, as gestation is often prolonged, length might even be increased. Careful study of the growth rate demonstrates a decrease in growth in length in the untreated state during the first few weeks of age, with profound growth failure lasting as long as the infant is not treated. Analysis of infant growth using the ICP chart demonstrated a delay in the onset of the childhood component even if thyroxine therapy is begun early. Thus an effect of thyroxine is exerted in the first months of life upon the onset of the childhood component of growth during the last months of the first year of life.[126] Remarkably, decreased growth is also seen in congenital hypothyroidism compared with normal controls during the first 2 and 4 weeks of thyroid therapy; this demonstrates that the early dependence of neonatal growth upon thyroid hormone lasts for weeks after institution of therapy. There is a greater decrease in growth rate in those infants most deficient in thyroid hormone in the weeks after the onset of therapy.[127]

In addition to a direct effect on epiphyseal cartilage and growth, thyroid hormones have a permissive effect on GH secretion because individuals with hypothyroidism have decreased spontaneous GH secretion and blunted responses to GH provocative tests. A small study of congenital hypothyroid infants demonstrated a decrease in GHBP for the first 6 months of therapy with thyroxine, suggesting a degree of GH resistance in congenital hypothyroidism that continues even after replacement therapy.[128] Serum IGF is so low in normal children that patients with congenital hypothyroidism appear to have no decrease in IGF-1 and IGFBP-3 at the time of diagnosis, if the diagnosis is made within the first month after birth.[129, 130] However, if the diagnosis is not made early, the values of IGF-1 and IGFBP-3 decrease below control levels. With appropriate therapy with thyroxine, the values of IGF-1 and IGFBP-3 rise to age-appropriate levels.[131]

Untreated hypothyroidism starting after the postnatal period can cause profound growth failure and virtual arrest of skeletal maturation, although there is no permanent intellectual impairment. Treatment with thyroid hormone after a long delay results in rapid catch-up growth, which is typically accompanied by marked skeletal maturation; if doses are excessive, there may be overly rapid epiphyseal fusion and compromise of adult height. Epiphyseal dysgenesis is seen when calcification of the epiphyses progresses with thyroxine treatment after an initial delay in development.[132] The normal decrease in the upper to lower segment ratio with age is delayed (and therefore the ratio is elevated), owing to poor limb growth in hypothyroid infants and children.

Congenital hypothyroidism diagnosed at birth and treated appropriately soon thereafter will lead to normal height and weight during infancy. Early-treated congenital hypothyroidism is compatible with normal height at 1 year[133] and 3 to 4 years.[134] If the diagnosis is delayed up to 1 year, there is still a chance the child will achieve a normal height by 10 months after starting therapy;[134-136] even if thyroxine therapy is started as late as 2 years of age, catch-up growth in length appears possible (although an optimal IQ may not occur).[137] However, a study from Canada showed that there is an inverse relationship between bone age at birth and length of time until treatment begins and height at 9 years, demonstrating long-term effects of intrauterine hypothyroidism on growth potential.[138] Adult height is related to genetic potential in early treated congenital hypothyroidism, as there is complete catch-up growth in those treated in the first month of life.[139, 140]

The long-term intellectual development of patients with congenital hypothyroidism treated early is usually normal, although decreased IQ and abnormal coordination or other neurologic manifestations have also been reported. In general, the use of the higher replacement doses of thyroxine (10 to 15 µg/kg/day)[142]

and maintenance of high normal serum T_4 levels (upper one half to one third of the normal range) are usually associated with normal IQ and neurologic functioning[141, 143, 144] in most studies.[126, 141, 143-146]

Neonatal Hyperthyroidism.[147] Neonatal hyperthyroidism is temporary and usually results from the transplacental passage of thyroid-stimulating immunoglobulin from the affected mother to the fetus, causing a temporary disorder. Infants with congenital hyperthyroidism may exhibit IUGR. After birth they have poor weight gain that will tend to limit growth during the temporary hyperthyroid phase.[148, 149] In older children with hyperthyroidism, increased growth may occur if nutrition is adequate, but this tendency is overcome by the hypermetabolic state.

Sex Steroids. Gonadal sex steroids exert an important influence on the pubertal growth spurt, although absence of these factors is not noticeable in prepubertal growth.[150] But even in early life gonadal and adrenal sex steroids in excess can cause a sharp increase in growth rate, as well as the premature appearance and progression of secondary sexual features. Sex steroids exert a direct effect upon long bone growth, but can increase growth hormone secretion through conversion to estrogen. Untreated virilizing congenital adrenal hyperplasia is compatible with survival, sometimes for years, as long as severe hypoglycemia or shock does not develop; in those children remaining clinically stable, growth acceleration may occur early in infancy. When there is also salt loss, the failure to thrive will mask any tendency toward increased growth rate, and the child will grow poorly until treatment is supplied or the child dies from complications of adrenal insufficiency. Familial Leydig and germinal cell maturation also may cause increased growth early in the first year. If unabated, increased sex steroids will cause advancement of skeletal age, premature epiphyseal fusion, and short adult stature. Thus just as growth deceleration requires evaluation, growth acceleration can be just as abnormal and may be a sign of precocious puberty or virilizing congenital adrenal hyperplasia.

Glucocorticoids. Glucocorticoids are necessary for normal metabolic function, but endogenous or exogenous glucocorticoids in excess will quickly decrease or stop growth; this effect occurs more quickly than weight gain. An infant treated with excess glucocorticoids (e.g., incorrect diagnosis of congenital adrenal hyperplasia) will exhibit a remarkable decrease in growth rate.[151] The absence of glucocorticoids has little effect on growth if the individual is clinically well in other respects.

In a preliminary study of normal term infants, cord blood cortisol was inversely related to growth achieved in the first 3 months of life.[152] There is an inverse relationship between serum cortisol and catch-up growth over the first 6 months of postnatal life in IUGR infants.[153]

Socioeconomic and Nutritional Factors. Worldwide, the most common cause of poor growth and short stature is poverty and its effects. Poor nutrition, poor hygiene, and poor health influence growth both before and after birth.

REFERENCES

1. Wollmann HA: Growth hormone and growth factors during perinatal life. Horm Res 53(Suppl 1):50, 2000.
2. Tanner JM: A History of the Study of Human Growth. Cambridge: Cambridge University Press, 1981.
3. Karlberg J: On the construction of the infancy-childhood-puberty growth standard [see comments]. Acta Paediatr Scandinavica Supplement 356:26, 1989.
4. Karlberg J: The infancy-childhood growth spurt. Acta Paediatr Suppl 367:111, 1990.
5. Laron Z: The diagnostic and prognostic importance of neonatal length measurements. Isr Med Assoc J 2:84, 2000.
6. Gibson AT, et al: Neonatal and post-natal growth. Horm Res 53(Suppl 1):42, 2000.
7. Cooney K, et al: Infant growth charts. Arch Dis Child 71:159, 1994.
8. Gairdner D, Pearson J: A growth chart for premature and other infants. Arch Dis Child 46:783, 1971.

9. Wales JK, et al: The measurement of neonates. Horm Res 48:2, 1997.
10. Johnson TS, et al: Reliability of length measurements in full-term neonates. J Obstetri Gynecol Neonat Nurs 27:270, 1998.
11. Gibson AT, et al: Knemometry and the assessment of growth in premature babies. Arch Dis Child 69(5 Spec No):498, 1993.
12. Kaempf DE, et al: Validation of a newly developed mini-knemometer for premature infants. Ann Hum Biol 26:259, 1999.
13. Greco L, et al: Pulsatile weight increases in very low birthweight babies appropriate for gestational age. Arch Dis Child 65(4 Spec No):373, 1990.
14. Kaempf DE, et al: Influence of nutrition on growth in premature infants: assessment by knemometry. Ann Hum Biol 25:127, 1998.
15. Wales JK, Gibson AT: Short-term growth: rhythms, chaos, or noise? Arch Dis Child 71:84, 1994.
16. Smith DW, et al: Shifting linear growth during infancy: illustration of genetic factors in growth from fetal life through infancy. J Pediatr 89:225, 1976.
17. Williams MC, O'Brien WF: Cerebral palsy in infants with asymmetric growth restriction. Am J Perinatol 14:211, 1999.
18. Guo SS, et al: Weight-for-length reference data for preterm, low-birth-weight infants. Arch Pediatr Adolesc Med 150:964, 1996.
19. Guo SS, et al: Growth in weight, recumbent length, and head circumference for preterm low-birthweight infants during the first three years of life using gestation-adjusted ages. Early Hum Dev 47:305, 1997.
20. Gardosi J, et al: Customised antenatal growth charts. Lancet 339:283, 1992.
21. Owen P, et al: Relationship between customised birthweight centiles and neonatal anthropometric features of growth restriction. Br J Obstet Gynecol 109:658, 2002.
22. Cheung YB, et al: Parametric modelling of neonatal mortality in relation to size at birth. Stat Med 20:2455, 2001.
23. Gill A, et al: Postnatal growth in infants born before 30 weeks' gestation. Arch Dis Child 61:549, 1986.
24. Casey PH, et al: Growth patterns of low birth weight preterm infants: a longitudinal analysis of a large, varied sample. J Pediatr 117:298, 1990.
25. Albertsson-Wikland K, Karlberg J: Natural growth in children born small for gestational age with and without catch-up growth. Acta Paediatr Suppl 399:64, 1994.
26. Albertsson-Wikland K, et al: Children born small-for-gestational age: postnatal growth and hormonal status. Horm Res 49:7, 1998.
27. Karlberg J, Albertsson-Wikland K: Growth in full-term small-for-gestational-age infants: from birth to final height. Pediatr Res 38:733, 1995.
28. Fitzhardinge PM, Inwood S: Long-term growth in small-for-date children. Acta Paediatr Suppl 349:27, 1989.
29. Seminara S, et al: Catch-up growth in short-at-birth NICU graduates. Horm Res 53:139, 2000.
30. Nieto A, et al: Different postnatal growth between disproportionate and proportionate fetal growth retardation at term. Zentralb Gynakol 119:633, 1999.
31. Fitzhardinge P: Follow-up studies on small for dates infants. Curr Concepts Nutr 14:147, 1985.
32. Karlberg J, Albertsson-Wikland K: Growth in full-term small-for-gestational-age infants: from birth to final height [published erratum appears in Pediatr Res 39:175, 1996]. Pediatr Res 38:733, 1995.
33. Gutbrod T, et al: Effects of gestation and birth weight on the growth and development of very low birthweight small for gestational age infants: a matched group comparison. Arch Dis Child Fetal Neonatal Ed 82:F208, 2000.
34. Sung IK, et al: Growth and neurodevelopmental outcome of very low birth weight infants with intrauterine growth retardation: comparison with control subjects matched by birth weight and gestational age. J Pediatr 123:618, 1993.
35. Monset-Couchard M, de Bethmann O: Catch-up growth in 166 small-for-gestational age premature infants weighing less than 1,000 g at birth. Biol Neonate 78:161, 2000.
36. Strauss RS, Pollack HA: Epidemic increase in childhood overweight, 1986–1998. JAMA 286:2845, 2001.
37. Hack M, et al: Outcomes in young adulthood for very-low-birth-weight infants. N Engl J Med 346:149, 2002.
38. Fewtrell MS, et al: Neonatal factors predicting childhood height in preterm infants: evidence for a persisting effect of early metabolic bone disease? J Pediatr 137:668, 2000.
39. Fewtrell MS, et al: Bone mineralization and turnover in preterm infants at 8–12 years of age: the effect of early diet. J Bone Miner Res 14:810, 1999.
40. Lewis UJ, et al: Human growth hormone: a complex of proteins. Rec Prog Horm Res 36:477, 1980.
41. Lewis UJ, et al: The 20,000-dalton variant of human growth hormone: location of the amino acid deletions. Biochem Biophys Res Commun 92:511, 1980.
42. Miller WL, Eberhardt NL: Structure and evolution of the growth hormone gene family. Endocr Rev 4:97, 1983.
43. Thorner MO, et al: Neuroendocrine regulation of growth hormone secretion. Neurosci Biobehav Rev 19:465, 1995.
44. Holl RW, et al: Intracellular calcium concentration and growth hormone secretion in individual somatotropes: effects of growth hormone-releasing factor and somatostatin. Endocrinology 122:2927, 1988.
45. Reiter EO, Rosenfeld RG: Normal and aberrant growth. In Wilson JD, et al (eds) Williams Textbook of Endocrinology. Philadelphia, WB Saunders, 1998, 1427–1507.
46. Arvat E, et al: Endocrine activities of ghrelin, a natural growth hormone secretagogue (GHS), in humans: comparison and interactions with hexarelin, a nonnatural peptidyl GHS, and GH-releasing hormone. J Clin Endocrinol Metab 86:1169, 2001.
47. Broglio F, et al: Ghrelin, a natural GH secretagogue produced by the stomach, induces hyperglycemia and reduces insulin secretion in humans. J Clin Endocrinol Metab 86:5083, 2001.
48. Leung DW, et al: Growth hormone receptor and serum binding protein: purification, cloning and expression. Nature 330:537, 1987.
49. Laron Z, Klinger B: Laron syndrome: clinical features, molecular pathology and treatment. Horm Res 42:198, 1994.
50. Hintz RL, et al: Somatomedin and growth hormone in the newborn. Am J Dis Child 131:1249, 1977.
51. Keret R, et al: Correlation between plasma growth hormone and insulin and blood glucose concentrations in premature infants. Horm Res 7:313, 1976.
52. Adcock CJ, et al: The use of an automated microsampling system for the characterization of growth hormone pulsatility in newborn babies. Pediatr Res 42:66, 1997.
53. Ogilvy-Stuart AL, et al: Insulin, insulin-like growth factor I (IGF-I), IGF-binding protein-1, growth hormone, and feeding in the newborn. J Clin Endocrinol Metab 83:3550, 1998.
54. de Zegher F, et al: Properties of growth hormone and prolactin hypersecretion by the human infant on the day of birth. J Clin Endocrinol Metab 76:1177, 1993.
55. Miller JD, et al: Spontaneous growth hormone release in term infants: changes during the first four days of life. J Clin Endocrinol Metab 76:1058, 1993.
56. Miller JD, et al: Spontaneous pulsatile growth hormone release in male and female premature infants. J Clin Endocrinol Metab 75:1508, 1992.
57. Deiber M, et al: Functional hypersomatotropism in small for gestational age (SGA) newborn infants. J Clin Endocrinol Metab 68:232, 1989.
58. Hikino S, et al: Physical growth and retinopathy in preterm infants: involvement of IGF-I and GH. Pediatr Res 50:732, 2001.
59. Wright NM, et al: Elevated growth hormone secretory rate in premature infants: deconvolution analysis of pulsatile growth hormone secretion in the neonate. Pediatr Res 32:286, 1992.
60. Leger J, et al: Growth factors and intrauterine growth retardation. II. Serum growth hormone, insulin-like growth factor (IGF) I, and IGF-binding protein 3 levels in children with intrauterine growth retardation compared with normal control subjects: prospective study from birth to two years of age. Study Group of IUGR. Pediatr Res 40:101, 1996.
61. Bozzola M, et al: Postnatal variations of growth hormone bioactivity and of growth hormone-dependent factors. Arch Pediatr Adolesc Med 150:1068, 1996.
62. Quattrin T, et al: Comparison of urinary growth hormone and IGF-I excretion in small- and appropriate-for-gestational-age infants and healthy children. Pediatr Res 28:209, 1990.
63. Low LC, et al: Onset of significant GH dependence of serum IGF-I and IGF-binding protein 3 concentrations in early life. Pediatr Res 50:737, 2001.
64. Huet F, et al: Long-term results of GH therapy in GH-deficient children treated before 1 year of age. Eur J Endocrinol 140:29, 1999.
65. Parks JS: Hormones of the pituitary and hypothalamus. In Behrman RE, et al (eds): Nelson's Textbook of Pediatrics. Philadelphia, WB Saunders, 2002, pp 1673–1680.
66. Parks JS: Genetic forms of hypopituitarism. In Finberg L (ed): Saunders Manual of Pediatric Practice. Philadelphia, WB Saunders, 2002.
67. Laron Z: The essential role of IGF-1: lessons from the long-term study and treatment of children and adults with Laron syndrome. J Clin Endocrinol Metab 84:4397, 1999.
68. Woods KA, et al: Insulin-like growth factor I gene deletion causing intrauterine growth retardation and severe short stature. Acta Paediatr Suppl 423:39, 1997.
69. Woods KA, et al: Insulin-like growth factor I gene deletion causing intrauterine growth retardation and severe short stature. Acta Paediatr Suppl 423:39, 1997.
70. Rinderknecht E, Humbel RE: The amino acid sequence of human insulin-like growth factor I and its structural homology with proinsulin. J Biol Chem 253:2769, 1978.
71. Rinderknecht E, Humbel RE: Primary structure of human insulin-like growth factor II. FEBS Lett 89:283, 1978.
72. Sussenbach JS: The gene structure of the insulin-like growth factor family. Prog Growth Factor Res 1:33, 1989.
73. Underwood LE, et al: Paracrine functions of somatomedins. Clin Endocrinol Metab 15:59, 1986.
74. Clemmons DR, et al: Sequential addition of platelet factor and plasma to BALB/c 3T3 fibroblast cultures stimulates somatomedin-C binding early in cell cycle. Proc Natl Acad Sci U S A 77:6644, 1980.
75. Massague J, Czech MP: The subunit structures of two distinct receptors for insulin-like growth factors I and II and their relationship to the insulin receptor. J Biol Chem 257:5038, 1982.
76. Ullrich A, et al: Human insulin receptor and its relationship to the tyrosine kinase family of oncogenes. Nature 313:756, 1985.
77. Rosenfeld RG, et al: Insulinlike growth factor-binding proteins. Rec Prog Horm Res 46:99, 1990.
78. Ong K, et al: Size at birth and cord blood levels of insulin, insulin-like growth factor I (IGF-I), IGF-II, IGF-binding protein-1 (IGFBP-1), IGFBP-3, and the soluble IGF-II/mannose-6-phosphate receptor in term human infants. The ALSPAC Study Team. Avon Longitudinal Study of Pregnancy and Childhood. J Clin Endocrinol Metab 85:4266, 2000.

79. Hill DJ, et al: Localization of the growth hormone receptor, identified by immunocytochemistry, in second trimester human fetal tissues and in placenta throughout gestation. J Clin Endocrinol Metab 75:646, 1992.

80. Heinrich UE, et al: NSILA and foetal growth. Acta Endocrinol (Copenh) 90:534, 1979.

81. Radetti G, et al: Growth hormone bioactivity and levels of growth hormone, growth hormone-binding protein, insulinlike growth factor I, and insulinlike growth factor-binding proteins in premature and full-term newborns during the first month of life. Arch Pediatr Adolesc Med 151:170, 1997.

82. Cance-Rouzaud A, et al: Growth hormone, insulin-like growth factor-I and insulin-like growth factor binding protein-3 are regulated differently in small-for-gestational-age and appropriate-for-gestational-age neonates. Biol Neonate 73:347, 1998.

83. Wiznitzer A, et al: Insulin-like growth factors, their binding proteins, and fetal macrosomia in offspring of nondiabetic pregnant women. Am J Perinatol 15:23, 1998.

84. Vatten LJ, et al: Relationship of insulin-like growth factor-I and insulin-like growth factor binding proteins in umbilical cord plasma to preeclampsia and infant birth weight. Obstet Gynecol 99:85, 2002.

85. Hills FA, et al: Circulating levels of IGF-I and IGF-binding protein-1 throughout pregnancy: relation to birthweight and maternal weight. J Endocrinol 148:303, 1996.

86. Wang HS, et al: The concentration of insulin-like growth factor-I and insulin-like growth factor-binding protein-1 in human umbilical cord serum at delivery: relation to fetal weight. J Endocrinol 129:459, 1991.

87. Barrios V, et al: Insulin-like growth factor I, insulin-like growth factor binding proteins, and growth hormone binding protein in Spanish premature and full-term newborns. Horm Res 46:130, 1996.

88. Giudice LC, et al: Insulin-like growth factors and their binding proteins in the term and preterm human fetus and neonate with normal and extremes of intrauterine growth. J Clin Endocrinol Metab 80:1548, 1995.

89. Bernardini S, et al: Plasma levels of insulin-like growth factor binding protein-1, and growth hormone binding protein activity from birth to the third month of life. Acta Endocrinol (Copenh) 127:313, 1992.

90. Orbak Z, et al: Maternal and fetal serum insulin-like growth factor-I (IGF-I), IGF binding protein-3 (IGFBP-3), leptin levels and early postnatal growth in infants born asymmetrically small for gestational age. J Pediatr Endocrinol Metab 14:1119, 2001.

91. Ozkan H, et al: Associations of IGF-I, IGFBP-1 and IGFBP-3 on intrauterine growth and early catch-up growth. Biol Neonate 76:274, 1999.

92. Thieriot-Prevost G, et al: Serum insulin-like growth factor 1 and serum growth-promoting activity during the first postnatal year in infants with intrauterine growth retardation. Pediatr Res 24:380, 1988.

93. Cianfarani S, et al: Intrauterine growth retardation: evidence for the activation of the insulin-like growth factor (IGF)-related growth-promoting machinery and the presence of a cation-independent IGF binding protein-3 proteolytic activity by two months of life. Pediatr Res 44:374, 1998.

94. Garcia H, et al: GH-IGF axis during catch up growth in small for gestational age (SGA) infants. J Pediatr Endocrinol Metab 9:561, 1996.

95. Colonna F, et al: Serum insulin-like growth factor-I (IGF-I) and IGF binding protein-3 (IGFBP-3) in growing preterm infants on enteral nutrition. J Pediatr Endocrinol Metab 9:483, 1996.

96. Iwashita M, et al: Phosphoisoforms of insulin-like growth factor binding protein-1 in appropriate-for-gestational-age and small-for-gestational-age fetuses. Growth Horm IGF Res 8:487, 1998.

97. Kajantie E, et al: IGF-I, IGF binding protein (IGFBP)-3, phosphoisoforms of IGFBP-1, and postnatal growth in very low birth weight infants. J Clin Endocrinol Metab 87:2171, 2002.

98. D'Ercole AJ, et al: Use of transgenic mice for understanding the physiology of insulin-like growth factors. Horm Res 45(Suppl 1):5, 1996.

99. D'Ercole AJ: Insulin-like growth factors and their receptors in growth. Endocrinol Metab Clin North Am 25:573, 1996.

100. Baker J, Role of insulin-like growth factors in embryonic and postnatal growth. Cell 75:73, 1993.

101. Liu JP, et al: Mice carrying null mutations of the genes encoding insulin-like growth factor I (IGF-1) and type 1 IGF receptor (IGF1r). Cell 75:59, 1993.

102. Gluckman PD, et al: Elevating maternal insulin-like growth factor-I in mice and rats alters the pattern of fetal growth by removing maternal constraint. J Endocrinol 134:R1, 1992.

103. Filson AJ, et al: Rescue of the T-associated maternal effect in mice carrying null mutations in Igf-2 and Igf2r, two reciprocally imprinted genes. Development 118:731, 1993.

104. Ludwig T, et al: Mouse mutants lacking the type 2 IGF receptor (IGF2R) are rescued from perinatal lethality in IGF2 and IGF1r null backgrounds. Dev Biol 177:517, 1996.

105. Murphy LJ, et al: Phenotypic manifestations of insulin-like growth factor binding protein-1 (IGFBP-1) and IGFBP-3 overexpression in transgenic mice. Prog Growth Factor Res 6:425, 1995.

106. Rajkumar K, et al: Growth retardation and hyperglycemia in insulin-like growth factor binding protein-1 transgenic mice. Endocrinology 136:4029, 1995.

107. Murphy LJ, et al: Expression of human insulin-like growth factor-binding protein-3 in transgenic mice. J Mol Endocrinol 15:293, 1995.

108. Tarantal AF, Gargosky SE: Characterization of the insulin-like growth factor I. Growth Reg 5:190, 1995.

109. Fowden AL: The role of insulin in prenatal growth. J Dev Physiol 12:173, 1989.

110. Economides DL, et al: Metabolic and endocrine findings in appropriate and small for gestational age fetuses. J Perinat Med 19:97, 1991.

111. Vohr BR, McGarvey ST: Growth patterns of large-for-gestational-age and appropriate-for-gestational-age infants of gestational diabetic mothers and control mothers at age 1 year. Diabetes Care 20:1066, 1997.

112. Fukuzawa R, et al: Nesidioblastosis and mixed hamartoma of the liver in Beckwith-Wiedemann syndrome: case study including analysis of H19 methylation and insulin-like growth factor 2 genotyping and imprinting. Pediatr Dev Pathol 4:381, 2001.

113. Donohue W, Uchida I: Leprechaunism: a euphemism for a rare familial disorder. J Pediatr 45:505, 1954.

114. Bier DM, et al: Glucose kinetics in leprechaunism: accelerated fasting due to insulin resistance. J Clin Endocrinol Metab 51:988, 1980.

115. Tamemoto H, et al: Insulin resistance and growth retardation in mice lacking insulin receptor substrate-1. Nature 372:182, 1994.

116. Ogilvy-Stuart AL, et al: Hypoglycemia and resistance to ketoacidosis in a subject without functional insulin receptors. J Clin Endocrinol Metab 86:3319, 2001.

117. Dodge JA, Laurence KM: Congenital absence of islets of Langerhans. Arch Dis Child 52:411, 1977.

118. Chan JL, et al: Regulation of circulating soluble leptin receptor levels by gender, adiposity, sex steroids, and leptin: observational and interventional studies in humans. Diabetes 51:2105, 2002.

119. Sivan E, et al: Leptin is present in human cord blood. Diabetes 46:917, 1997.

120. Matsuda J, et al: Serum leptin concentration in cord blood: relationship to birth weight and gender. J Clin Endocrinol Metab 82:1642, 1999.

121. Schubring C, et al: Levels of leptin in maternal serum, amniotic fluid, and arterial and venous cord blood: relation to neonatal and placental weight. J Clin Endocrinol Metab 82:1480, 1997.

122. Jaquet D, et al: Ontogeny of leptin in human fetuses and newborns: effect of intrauterine growth retardation on serum leptin concentrations. J Clin Endocrinol Metab 83:1243, 1998.

123. Christou H, et al: Cord blood leptin and insulin-like growth factor levels are independent predictors of fetal growth. J Clin Endocrinol Metab 86:935, 2001.

124. Jaquet D, et al: High serum leptin concentrations during catch-up growth of children born with intrauterine growth retardation. J Clin Endocrinol Metab 84:1949, 1999.

125. LaFranchi S: Congenital hypothyroidism: etiologies, diagnosis, and management. Thyroid 9:735, 1999.

126. Heyerdahl S, et al: Linear growth in early treated children with congenital hypothyroidism. Acta Paediatr 86:479, 1999.

127. Leger J, Czernichow P: Congenital hypothyroidism: decreased growth velocity in the first weeks of life. Biol Neonate 55:218, 1989.

128. Cassio A, et al: Low growth hormone-binding protein in infants with congenital hypothyroidism. J Clin Endocrinol Metab 83:3643, 1998.

129. Mitchell ML, et al: Somatomedin-C/insulin-like growth factor-1 in infants with congenital hypothyroidism during the first week of life. Clin Endocrinol (Oxf) 27:625, 1987.

130. Kandemir N, et al: Age-related differences in serum insulin-like growth factor-I (IGF-I) and IGF-binding protein-3 levels in congenital hypothyroidism. J Pediatr Endocrinol Metab 10:379, 1997.

131. Bona G, et al: IGF-1 and IGFBP in congenital and acquired hypothyroidism after long-term replacement treatment. Minerva Endocrinol 24:51, 1999.

132. Virtanen M, Perheentupa J: Bone age at birth; method and effect of hypothyroidism. Acta Paediatr Scand 78:412, 1989.

133. Casado dF, et al: Evolution of height and bone age in primary congenital hypothyroidism. Clin Pediatr 32:426, 1993.

134. Grant DB: Growth in early treated congenital hypothyroidism. Arch Dis Child 70:464, 1994.

135. Siragusa V, et al: Congenital hypothyroidism: auxological retrospective study during the first six years of age. J Endocrinol Invest 19:224, 1996.

136. Fisher DA: Catch-up growth in hypothyroidism. N Engl J Med 318:632, 1988.

137. Chiesa A, et al: Growth follow-up in 100 children with congenital hypothyroidism before and during treatment. J Pediatr Endocrinol 7:211, 1994.

138. Aronson R, et al: Growth in children with congenital hypothyroidism detected by neonatal screening. J Pediatr 116:33, 1990.

139. Salerno M, et al: Longitudinal growth, sexual maturation and final height in patients with congenital hypothyroidism detected by neonatal screening. Eur J Endocrinol 145:377, 2001.

140. Dickerman Z, De Vries L: Prepubertal and pubertal growth, timing and duration of puberty and attained adult height in patients with congenital hypothyroidism (CH) detected by the neonatal screening programme for CH—a longitudinal study [see comments]. Clin Endocrinol 47:649, 1997.

141. Salerno M, et al: Effect of different starting doses of levothyroxine on growth and intellectual outcome at four years of age in congenital hypothyroidism. Thyroid 12:45, 2002.

142. Hrytsiuk I, et al: Starting dose of levothyroxine for the treatment of congenital hypothyroidism: a systematic review. Arch Pediatr Adolesc Med 156:485, 2002.

143. Dubuis JM, et al: Outcome of severe congenital hypothyroidism: closing the developmental gap with early high dose levothyroxine treatment. J Clin Endocrinol Metab 81:222, 1996.

144. Bongers-Schokking JJ, et al: Influence of timing and dose of thyroid hormone replacement on development in infants with congenital hypothyroidism. J Pediatr *136*:292, 2000.
145. Fisher DA, Foley BL: Early treatment of congenital hypothyroidism. Pediatrics *83*:785, 1989.
146. American Academy of Pediatrics AAP Section on Endocrinology and Committee on Genetics, and American Thyroid Association Committee on Public Health: Newborn screening for congenital hypothyroidism: recommended guidelines. Pediatrics *91*:1203, 1993.
147. Daneman D, Howard NJ: Neonatal thyrotoxicosis: intellectual impairment and craniosynostosis in later years. J Pediatr *97*:257, 1980.
148. Zimmerman D: Fetal and neonatal hyperthyroidism. Thyroid *9*:727, 1999.
149. Krude H, et al: Congenital hyperthyroidism. Exp Clin Endocrinol Diabetes *105* (Suppl 4):6, 1997.
150. Grumbach MM, Styne DM: Puberty, ontogeny, neuroendocrinology, physiology, and disorders. *In* Wilson JD, et al (eds) Williams Textbook of Endocrinology. Philadelphia, WB Saunders 1998, pp 1509-1625.
151. Styne DM: Growth. *In* Greenspan FS, Gardner DG (eds): Basic and Clinical Endocrinology. New York, Lange, 2001, pp 163-200.
152. Cianfarani S, et al: IGF-I and IGF-binding protein-1 are related to cortisol in human cord blood. Eur J Endocrinol *138*:524, 1998.
153. Cianfarani S, et al: Growth, IGF system, and cortisol in children with intrauterine growth retardation: is catch-up growth affected by reprogramming of the hypothalamic-pituitary-adrenal axis? Pediatr Res *51*:94, 2002.

Margit Hamosh

29 Human Milk Composition and Function in the Infant

Human milk, like the milk of many other mammals, is specifically adapted to the needs of the newborn. Transfer of nutrients and bioactive components from mother to infant occurs through the placenta before birth and through colostrum and milk after birth. The substitution of infant formula for human milk deprives the infant not only of nutrients that are more accessible from human milk than from formula, but also of many bioactive and immunoprotective factors directed specifically against pathogens in the infant's environment. In many instances, human milk components compensate for immature function in the newborn and the inability for endogenous production of digestive enzymes, immunoglobulin A (IgA), taurine, nucleotides, and long chain polyunsaturated fatty acids (LC-PUFAs). Many of these components are resistant to pasteurization, a finding indicating that it may be advisable to feed pasteurized human donor milk to infants whose mothers are unable to nurse. The bioactive components are the reason that human milk is superior to even the best infant formulas.

MILK VOLUME

Milk volume seems to be relatively constant regardless of maternal nutritional status. In general, healthy infants have an average daily intake of 750 to 800 mL milk within the first 4 to 5 months after birth.[1,2] There is, however, a much wider range of intake of volumes, from 450 to 1200 mL/day.[1,3] Similar findings were reported from developing countries,[1,3] although maternal nutritional status may be subject to seasonal variation and could be less adequate than in industrialized countries. Increasing the intake of fluid does not seem to affect milk volume; therefore, lactating women should maintain adequate fluid intake, but they should be aware that "fluids consumed in excess of natural thirst have no effect on milk volume."[1]

MILK COMPOSITION

Table 29-1 presents estimates of the concentration of nutrients in mature human milk (i.e., after the colostrum stage of early lactation). The nutrients in milk have three different sources: some are synthesized *de novo* within the lactating mammary gland (e.g., medium chain fatty acids), some are modified within the mammary secretory cells from precursors taken up from the circulation (e.g., long chain fatty acids incorporated into milk triglycerides), and some are transferred into milk directly from plasma (e.g., vitamins and minerals, which are taken up from the circulation, without modification within the mammary gland).

Endocrine changes specific to lactation are known to modulate mammary gland function and milk composition. For example, the marked increase in mammary gland lipoprotein lipase activity and its concomitant sharp decrease in adipose tissue at the onset of lactation[4] (both under the effect of prolactin[5]) result in channeling of dietary fat to the mammary gland for incorporation into milk lipids, rather than deposition in adipose tissue.

Lactose is synthesized within the mammary gland from the precursors galactose and glucose provided from the circulation. Lactose, present at a concentration of 7 g/dL, is the most constant nutrient of human milk and is not affected by maternal nutrition. The protein content of mature human milk is about 0.9 g/dL,[1] and, based on studies in industrialized and developing countries, it seems to be unaffected by maternal diet or body composition.[1] There is, however, limited information that seems to indicate that short-term high-protein diets increase the protein and nonprotein nitrogen content of human milk, whereas limited maternal food supply leads to lower milk protein levels.[1]

Most milk proteins participate in the immune and nonimmune protection of the newborn from infection. These proteins, IgA, IgG, IgM, lactoferrin (LF), and lysozyme, have various functions in the newborn.[6] Whether the level of these protective proteins in milk is affected by maternal diet is not clear at present.[7-10]

Although the amount and composition of carbohydrate and protein remain relatively constant in mature human milk, the composition of fat is highly variable and to a large extent is immediately (within several hours) affected by maternal nutrition. Table 29-2 lists the factors that affect milk fat content and composition. Length of gestation and length of lactation particularly affect the content of lipids that constitute the milk fat globule membrane, phospholipid and cholesterol.[11] The latter are higher in the early stage of lactation (colostrum and transitional milk) because the milk fat globules are much smaller than in mature milk.[12,13] Therefore, the total membrane lipid level is higher in colostrum and transitional milk. LC-PUFAs (C20:4 n-6 and C22:6 n-3, arachidonic acid [AA] and docosahexaenoic acid [DHA]) are essential for growth, brain development, and retinal function.[14] These fatty acids are stored in the fetus only in the last trimester of pregnancy, and preterm infants depend on human milk for the provision of these essential nutrients. Using measurements of mean melting points of plasma phospholipids as an indicator of fatty acid composition, Holman and colleagues[15] reported lower levels of LC-PUFAs in pregnant and lactating women, a finding suggesting preferential transfer of these essential fatty acids from mother to fetus or to the newborn through

TABLE 29-1

Estimates of the Concentrations of Nutrients in Mature Human Milk

Nutrients*		Vitamins	
Major Nutrients	**g/L**	**Fat-soluble**	**mg/L**
Lactose	72.0 ± 2.5	Vitamin A, RE	670 ± 200 (2,230 IU)
Protein	10.5 ± 2.0	Vitamin D	0.55 ± 0.10
Fat	39.0 ± 4.0	Vitamin E	2300 ± 1000
		Vitamin K	2.1 ± 0.1
Minerals			
Macronutrient elements	**mg/L**	**Water-soluble**	**mg/L**
Calcium	280 ± 26	Vitamin B_6	93,000 ± 8000
Chloride	420 ± 60	Vitamin B_{12}	0.97
Magnesium	35 ± 2	Biotin	4 ± 1
Phosphorus	140 ± 22	Vitamin C	40,000 ± 10,000
Potassium	525 ± 35	Folate	85 ± 37
		Niacin	1500 ± 200
Trace elements	**µg/L**		
Chromium	50 ± 5	Pantothenic acid	1800 ± 200
Copper	250 ± 30	Riboflavin	350 ± 25
Fluoride	16 ± 5	Thiamin	210 ± 35
Iodine	110 ± 40		
Iron	300 ± 100		
Manganese	6 ± 2		
Molybdenum	NR		
Selenium	20 ± 5		
Zinc	1200 ± 290		

*Data (means ± SD). NR = not reported; RE = retinol equivalents.
From Hamosh M, et al: Nutrition During Lactation. Washington, DC, National Academy Press, 1991, p 116.

milk, even at the cost of possible depletion of maternal reserves. Studies in lactating and suckling ferrets showed that the adipose tissues of the suckling animals contain about threefold higher concentrations of LC-PUFAs than maternal adipose stores.[16] The latter contain, however, only slightly lower levels of LC-PUFA than the adipose depots of virgin females, a finding suggesting that the suckling ferret's higher LC-PUFA adipose tissue reserves result from increased storage of these fatty acids by the suckling newborn.[16]

It has long been known that milk fat content changes drastically during each feeding,[17, 18] and milk fat composition is markedly affected by maternal diet.[19] Studies have shown that the mechanism for endogenous synthesis of fatty acids seems to be exhausted in women of high parity,[20] that infants who receive low-fat milk tend to nurse more frequently and for longer periods, thereby causing an increase in milk volume,[21] and that

there is a strong positive relationship between weight gain during pregnancy and milk fat content.[22]

As mentioned previously, the vitamin content of human milk depends on the mother's vitamin status, and when maternal intake of specific vitamins is chronically low, these vitamins are also present at lower levels in the milk. With supplementation of vitamins, levels in milk also increase. Water-soluble vitamins in milk are generally more responsive to maternal dietary intake than are fat-soluble vitamins.[1] The relationship between maternal intake and milk concentration varies among vitamins, however. For example, excess vitamin C does not further increase the level in milk (above that associated with adequate intake), whereas milk vitamin B levels continue to rise with higher intakes; milk folate levels remain normal even at the expense of maternal folate stores and do not decrease until the latter are depleted.[1] Based on the concentrations of fat-soluble vitamins in human

TABLE 29-2

Factors That Affect Milk Fat Content and Composition

Variable	Change
Gestation	LC-PUFA higher in preterm* and transitional milk
Lactation	Phospholipid, cholesterol higher in colostrum (preterm > term)
	LC-PUFA decrease during lactation (3 mo–1 y) in term milk, but remains constant in preterm milk for 6 months
Parity	P10 +: lower endogenous synthesis of fatty acids (C_6–C_{16})
Volume	Low–milk fat concentration associated with high volume
Feed	Fat: fore < mid < hind milk
Diet	
High carbohydrate intake	Increase in endogenous synthesis of fatty acids (C_6–C_{16})
Low caloric intake	Increase in palmitic acid (C_{16})
High margarine intake	Increase in *trans*-fatty acids
Pregnancy weight gain	Positively associated with gain in milk fat content
	Weight loss Increase

*Preterm, term refer to milk or colostrum of women who deliver prematurely or at term. LC-PUFA = long chain polyunsaturated fatty acids.
From Hamosh M: Pediatr Clin North Am *42*:839, 1995.

milk and infant needs, it is advised that in the United States all newborns should receive 0.5 to 1.0 mg vitamin K by injection or 1.0 to 2.0 mg orally immediately after birth;[2] infants should receive 5.0 to 7.5 mg vitamin D per day if exposure to sunlight seems inadequate.

The concentration of trace minerals varies as a function of length of lactation (iron, copper, zinc, selenium). Although the concentrations in milk seem to be independent of maternal nutrition for iron[23,24] or fluoride,[25] concentrations of manganese,[26] iodine,[27] and selenium[28] are dependent. Iodine is unique among trace elements in that it is avidly accumulated by the mammary gland. It is recommended that breast-fed infants be supplemented with fluoride if the water supply for their family has a low fluoride content (<0.3 ppm). Because of the high bioavailability of iron in human milk, exclusively breast-fed infants do not need iron supplements during the first 6 months of life. When supplementary foods are introduced (as recommended after 4 to 6 months of exclusive breast-feeding), iron should be supplemented in the diet.

It is important to assess not only the concentration of milk components, but also the amount delivered to the infant. Thus, although some milk components are present at a higher concentration in colostrum than in milk, one has to take into consideration the marked differences in volume: colostrum amounts to about 100 mL/day, whereas average milk volumes are 750 to 850 mL/day.

The recommendation by the American Academy of Pediatrics is that breast-feeding should be of longer duration, 12 months, as compared with the previous recommendation by the Institute of Medicine of the American Academy of Sciences (4 to 6 months).[1] Therefore, the need for proper supplementation after 4 to 6 months of exclusive breast-feeding should be strongly emphasized. This is especially important in view of the resurgence of rickets[29-31] and zinc deficiencies[32] in breast-fed infants. It is known that, in some populations, human milk does not provide sufficient vitamin D during the first 6 months of lactation[33] (e.g., persons with dark skin or limited exposure to sunlight),[34-36] and this deficiency can be overcome by provision of vitamin D supplements. Furthermore, the global increase in atmospheric pollution may put mothers and breast-fed infants everywhere at risk of vitamin D deficiency.[37] The report of hypovitaminosis D—42% in young black women and 4.2% in the same age group of white women[38]—emphasizes the importance of supplementation during pregnancy and lactation.

Zinc supplements are indicated for breast-fed infants during the second half of the first year of life if the complementary foods are low in zinc. Furthermore, some infants may require supplementation even during early lactation because of a low milk zinc content secondary to a defect in zinc transfer from maternal serum to breast milk.[39] Although zinc homeostasis and normal milk levels during the first 2 months of lactation in a population with low zinc intake seem to be achieved by high fractional absorption and intestinal conservation,[40] clinical zinc deficiency during breast-feeding is reported to occur because of a combination of low fetal zinc accumulation and insufficient zinc in breast milk.[41,42]

Although iodine is unique among trace elements in that it is widely accumulated by the mammary gland,[1] the iodine content of human milk varies greatly according to geographic region and maternal intake, from a low of 15 μg/L in areas where iodine deficiency disorders are prevalent to 150 μg/L in areas with sufficient iodine.[43] However, despite the importance of iodine for normal growth and cognitive development, there are only a few studies on its concentration in human milk. In light of the newest recommendations for iodine (minimum 8 μg/100 kcal and maximum 35 μg/100 kcal),[122] further studies worldwide are necessary to estimate accurately the daily intakes of iodine by breast-fed infants throughout lactation.

Growth of Breast-Fed Infants

The growth of breast-fed infants in affluent populations differs from that of formula-fed ones.[44,45] When compared with the 1977 and 2000 National Center for Health Statistics growth charts, breast-fed infants gain weight rapidly during the first 2 to 3 months of life, followed by a downward trend in percentile ranking thereafter.[44,45] The earlier growth charts were obtained by evaluating mainly formula-fed infants, and when breast-fed infants were included, there was no information on exclusivity or duration of breast-feeding. The acceptance of a clear definition of breast-feeding[46] and the availability of newer studies that measured infant growth during breast-feeding of up to 12 to 18 months (exclusively for the first 4 to 6 months, followed by quantified complementary feeding)[44,45] resulted in a reevaluation, led by the World Health Organization, of the specific growth pattern of breast-fed infants, with the aim of creating specific reference growth curves for these infants.[47] The major differences in growth patterns between breast-fed and formula-fed infants can be summarized as follows: for weight, breast-fed infants gain less than formula-fed infants during the first year of life (at 12 months, this difference is 600 to 650 g); for length, linear growth seems to be unaffected by type of feeding, with no difference or only slightly lower gain in the breast-fed group; for head circumference, feeding mode makes no difference. Breast-fed infants are generally leaner than formula-fed ones (after about 4 months of age), a finding consistent with the observed association between duration of breast-feeding and greater decline in weight-for-length Z-scores during the first 12 months of life.[44,45,48] The physiologic reason for lower weight gain is that breast-fed infants self-regulate their energy intake[1,44,45,49,50] at a lower level than do formula-fed infants. This may be related to the lower body temperature and metabolic rate of breast-fed infants.[51] It may also be associated with the different endocrine environment of breast-fed as compared with formula-fed infants[49,51] that could be affected by the marked differences in protein content of human milk and infant formula.[51] The question whether formula feeding (which is regulated by the mother) leads to higher incidence of obesity as compared with breast-feeding (which is infant regulated) is still open, although a difference in adiposity by mode of feeding persists at least until 18 to 24 months of age, with overweight infants amounting to 13% versus 35% in those fed human milk versus formula-fed groups, respectively.[44]

The slower weight gain associated with breast-feeding is, however, not associated with short- or long-term deleterious effects. Indeed, morbidity and mortality from infectious diseases are lower in breast-fed infants, and the cognitive development of breast-fed infants seems to be enhanced by this mode of feeding. Furthermore, there seem to be long-term health benefits of breast-feeding that may become apparent only in childhood and adolescence.[52]

Bioactive Milk Components

This section focuses on milk nutrients that protect the infant against infection.

The relatively immature state at birth of the human infant leads to the production of milk that provides many components that facilitate the postnatal development of specific organs such as the brain, the immune system, and the digestive system. During this critical period when the newborn is exposed to infectious agents, protective factors in the mother's milk are essential to the infant's health. Provision of digestive enzymes facilitates the digestion and absorption of nutrients, and the provision of specific nutrients ensures normal development of the brain and other organs. Thus, what is unique to human milk, and so far has not been duplicated, is the bioactive function of many human milk nutrients.

Many nutrients in human milk have to be considered multifunctional agents. First, they provide an essential bioactive function, and, subsequently, they are digested and used as nutrients.

Protection Against Microorganisms

The antiinfective properties of human milk were recognized millennia ago (see the Indian medical treatise *Susruta*), but only recently has the rationale for this protection from infection (i.e., the immaturity of the immune system in the newborn and the reciprocal relationship between protection by human milk and the postnatal development of the newborn's immune system) been explored extensively. Furthermore, in addition to providing protective agents, human milk components also modulate the development of immune function in the newborn. Indeed, the thymus of breast-fed infants is twice as large as that of formula-fed infants, and a dose-dependent response of thymus size to human milk intake has been reported.[53]

Earlier studies carried out mainly in developing countries that showed protection against diarrhea, infectious diseases, and otitis media were found to be methodologically flawed.[54, 55] However, in the 1990s, carefully designed studies confirmed without any doubt that breast-feeding protects the newborn from diarrhea, respiratory infections, and otitis media not only in developing countries (where inocula may be higher),[56] but also in industrialized countries.[57-59] Furthermore, early observations that, if infection occurs, it is less severe in breast-fed than in formula-fed infants,[1] have been complemented by studies showing that breast-feeding may protect against nosocomial infections.[60]

Ongoing research since the 1980s has started to elucidate the nature of the protective factors in milk as well as the mechanisms by which this protection is provided. These studies have shown that protection from infection is provided by two main mechanisms: classic immune protection provided by IgA, IgG, and IgM in human milk, as well as by many other milk components that act as ligands for bacteria and viruses; and factors that refine the interaction among these agents and that may also enhance the maturation of the infant's own immune potential. The protective agents in milk share several characteristics that enable them to be active in the infant:[61] they act at mucosal sites and are well adapted to resist the environment of the gastrointestinal tract (hydrolytic enzymes, changes in gastric and intestinal pH, presence of bile salts). Furthermore, action on microorganisms is often accomplished synergistically, and protection is achieved without triggering inflammatory reactions. As is the case for many milk components, secretion of many protective factors during lactation is inversely related to the infant's capacity for their release at mucosal sites.

Immunoglobulins

This topic is reviewed in the literature.[62, 63] Briefly, whereas IgG, IgM, and IgD are present in human milk and may protect both the lactating mammary gland and the newborn from infection, polymeric IgA is the main component of human milk (consumption by the infant is 4 g on day 1 and about 1 g/day after day 4 post partum). In addition to the resistance of IgA to proteolysis, the functional advantages of IgA are the presence of four to eight antigen-binding sites, carbohydrate moiety–mediated antiadherence proteins, and inhibition of complement activation. Although the protective effect of IgA is exercised mainly at mucosal surfaces, internalization by cells expressing various IgA receptors suggests additional protective functions.[64]

Nonimmune Protection

Nonimmune protection is provided by many components in human milk that protect in a nonspecific way and thus provide a broad spectrum of antiinfective activity (Tables 29-3 and 29-4). These components are reviewed briefly, because many excellent reviews on this topic appear in the literature.[52,62-70]

Proteins

Lactoferrin (LF), a 79-kDa, 692-amino acid, single chain glycosylated protein, consists of two globular lobes, each containing one iron-binding site (Table 29-5). Although this protein was once considered an iron transporter and its antiinfective function was ascribed to its high affinity for iron (which could deprive microorganisms of needed iron), more recent studies cast doubt on both functions[71,72] and showed that LF-associated protection is provided by several other mechanisms. LF is bactericidal, antiviral, and antiinflammatory, and it modulates cytokine function. The bactericidal activity is provided by an 18-amino acid residue loop formed by a disulfide bond between cysteine residues 20 to 37 of human LF and 19 to 36 of bovine LF. This

---

TABLE 29-3

Multiple Functions of the Major Nutrients of Human Milk in the Infant

Nutrients	Amount	Function
Protein	*mg/dL*	
sIgA	50–100	Immune protection
IgM	2	Immune protection
IgG	1	Immune protection
Lactoferrin	100–300	Antiinfective, growth promoting, iron carrier(?)
Lysozyme	5–25	Antiinfective
α-Lactalbumin	200–300	Induces tumor apoptosis, part of lactose synthase, ion carrier (calcium)
Casein	200–300	Ion carrier, inhibits microbial adhesion to mucosal membranes, growth factor for probiotics
Carbohydrate	*g/L*	
Lactose	6.5–7.3	Energy source
Oligosaccharides	1.0–1.5	Microbial ligands
Glycoconjugates		Microbial and viral ligands
Fat	*g/L*	
Triglyceride	3.0–4.5	Energy source
Long chain polyunsaturated fatty acids		Essential for brain and retinal development and for infant growth
Free fatty acids, monoglycerides*		Antiinfective

* Free fatty acids and monoglycerides produced from triglycerides during fat digestion in the stomach and intestine.

Protective Functions of Minor Nutrients in Human Milk

Immune Protection	Function
IgA, IgG, IgM, IgD	Specific antigen-targeted antiinfective activity
Nonspecific protection	Antibacterial, antiviral and antimicrobial toxin, enhance newborn's immune system maturation
Major nutrients	See Tables 29-1, 29-3, and 29-5
Minor nutrients	
Nucleotides	Enhancement of T-cell maturation, NK cell activity, antibody response to certain vaccines, intestinal maturation and repair after diarrhea, growth factors for probiotics
Vitamins	
A (β-carotene)	Antiinflamatory (scavenging of oxygen radicals)
C (ascorbic acid)	Antiinflamatory (scavenging of oxygen radicals)
E (tocopherol)	Antiinflamatory (scavenging of oxygen radicals)
Enzymes	
Bile salt–dependent lipase	Production of free fatty acids with antiprotozoan and antibacterial activity
Catalase	Antiinflamatory (degrades hydrogen peroxide)
Glutathione peroxidase	Antiinflamatory (prevents lipid peroxidation)
PAF acetylhydrolase	Protects against necrotizing enterocolitis (hydrolysis of PAF)
Hormones	
Prolactin	Enhancement of the development of B and T lymphocytes, affects differentiation of intestinal lymphoid tissue
Cortisol, thyroxine, insulin, and growth factors	Promotion of maturation of the newborn's intestine and development of intestinal host defense mechanism
Cells	
Macrophages, PMNs, and lymphocytes	Microbial phagocytosis, production of lymphokines and cytokines, interaction with and enhancement of other protective agents
Cytokines	Modulation of function and maturation of the immune system

PAF = platelet-activating factor; PMN = polymorphonuclear leukocytes.
Adapted from Hamosh M: Pediatr Clin North Am 45:53, 2001.

domain, called lactoferricin and located in the N-terminus of LF in a region distinct from its iron-binding site, has broad antimicrobial properties.[73] Partial gastric hydrolysis of LF actually enhances antiviral activity against herpes simplex virus (HSV), cytomegalovirus, and human immunodeficiency virus (HIV), and it occurs during the early stage of infection, probably at the stage of virus adsorption or penetration. Immunomodulating activity leads to reduced release of interleukins 1, 2, and 6 and tumor necrosis factor-α from monocytes and of prostaglandin E$_2$ from macrophages. This activity is the result of LF binding to LF receptors on these cells.[74] Other LF activities include activation of natural killer cells, modulation of complement activation, effects on coagulation, and inhibition of adhesion of enterotoxigenic *Escherichia coli*[75] and of adhesion and invasiveness of *Shigella flexneri*. The last is caused by LF-induced disruption of outer membrane virulence proteins required for invasion (IpaB) and for intracellular and extracellular spread (IcsA).[76] Antiinflammatory activity involves scavenging of iron, which inhibits iron-catalyzed formation of hydroxyl radicals from superoxide and hydrogen peroxide,[75] inhibition of lipopolysaccharide-mediated activation of neutrophils,[77] and endotoxin-induced cytokine release.[78] Large fragments of LF are present in the stool[79] and

Protective Function of Human Milk Proteins

Protein	Protective Function
Lactoferrin (500–600 mg/dL in colostrum, 150 mg/dL in mature milk)	Iron chelation: bacteriostatic for siderophilic bacteria and fungi Lactoferricin, 18-amino acid loop has broad-spectrum antimicrobial action Antiviral activity (HIV, CMV, HSV) probably by interfering with virus adsorption or penetration Immunomodulating activity: reduced release of IL-1, IL-2, and IL-6 and TNF-α from monocytes and of prostaglandin E$_2$ from macrophages; activation of NK cells, effect on complement activation and coagulation Antiadhesive for *Escherichia coli* and antiinvasive for *Shigella flexneri* Affects neonatal intestinal growth and recovery from injury, thereby reducing intestinal infections
Lysozyme 5–25 mg/dL increases with prolonged lactation	Bacterial lysis: hydrolysis of β1–4 link between *N*-acetyl-glucosamine and *N*-acetylmuramic acid in bacterial walls Immunomodulating activity: muramyl dipeptide enhances IgA production, macrophage activation Binding to bacterial lipopolysaccharides: reduces endotoxin effect
α-Lactalbumin 200–300 mg/dL	Causes apoptosis in tumor cells after structural change induced by association with oleic acid
k-Casein < 100 mg/dL	Antiadhesive: Inhibits binding of *Helicobacter pylori* to human gastric mucosa and *Streptococcus pneumoniae* and *Haemophilus influenzae* to human respiratory tract epithelial cells
Casein macropeptide	A strong growth-promoting factor for the probiotic *Bifidobacterium bifidum*

CMV = cytomegalovirus; HIV = human immunodeficiency virus; HSV = herpes simplex virus; IL = interleukin; TNF-α = tumor necrosis factor-α.
Adapted from Hamosh M: Pediatr Clin North Am 45:35, 2001.

urine[80] of breast-fed infants, a finding suggesting that protection is provided within the gastrointestinal tract and systemically. Enhancement of neonatal intestinal growth,[81,82] hepatic protein synthesis, intestinal recovery from injury[81,82] (associated with avid LF interaction with nucleic acids),[83] and stimulation of growth of probiotic intestinal bacteria are additional LF-mediated mechanisms to reduce intestinal infections and the development of protein allergy.[84]

Lysozyme, a 14.4-kDa, 130-amino acid containing glycoprotein, hydrolyzes the β1-4 linkage between *N*-acetyl glucosamine and *N*-acetylmuramic acid in bacterial walls. Lysozyme, like LF, is present in other exocrine secretions and lyses gram-positive and a few gram-negative bacteria. Contrary to the other protective proteins in human milk (IgA and LF), concentrations of which decrease during lactation, those of lysozyme increase with prolonged lactation. Concentrations in milk are higher than in serum. In addition, lysozyme concentrations are severalfold higher in human than in bovine milk.[67,85]

k-Casein, a 30- to 40-kDa, 162-amino acid, highly glycosylated human milk protein, has been shown to inhibit adherence of *Helicobacter pylori* to human gastric mucosa and of *Streptococcus pneumoniae* and *Haemophilus influenzae* to human respiratory tract epithelial cells. The C-terminus proteolysis product of k-casein is a strong growth-promoting factor for *Bifidobacterium bifidum*, an acid-producing anaerobe that reduces the growth of intestinal pathogenic microorganisms in breast-fed infants.[67] The genes for the foregoing human milk proteins have been cloned.

α-Lactalbumin and Apoptosis of Malignant Cells

α-Lactalbumin is present in the mammary gland and in human milk and is part of the lactose synthase complex. Studies showed that it may also prevent growth of human adenocarcinoma cells in culture.[86] Detailed structural studies showed that a partial unfolding of the protein and association with oleic acid result in a variant able to induce apoptosis in tumor cells and immature cells, whereas healthy cells are resistant to this effect.[87] Conditions in the newborn's stomach favor formation of this complex and may explain the lower incidence of cancer in breast-fed persons.

Other proteins with potentially protective functions in human milk are fibronectin, protectin, and components of the complement system.[88] The extent to which milk proteins provide protection to the breast-fed newborn has yet to be quantitatively evaluated, although good data are currently available for immunoglobulins and LF. Whether supplementation of infant formula with recombinant human milk proteins will have protective effects remains to be evaluated in the future.

Most proteins in human milk are heavily glycosylated[85] and are therefore resistant to proteolysis after ingestion by the infant,[67,70]

as well as after short-term (4 to 24 hours) storage at elevated ambient temperatures (15° to 38°C).[89]

Glycoconjugates and Oligosaccharides

These milk components act as ligands for microorganisms, viruses, and their toxins and thereby inhibit binding of pathogens to epithelial surfaces (Table 29–6). These components are present in the milk fat globule membrane and in skim milk and amount to 1.5 g/dL. Thus, they are the third most abundant components in human milk. Among the best known components in this group are mucin-1 (400 kDa)[90] and lactadherin (46 kDa);[70] mucin decreases adhesion of S-fimbriated *E. coli* to buccal epithelial cells,[80] and lactadherin inhibits replication of rotavirus *in vitro*[91] and protects infants against symptomatic rotavirus infection.[92] Other glycoconjugates in milk inhibit binding of the HIV envelope glycoprotein gp120 to its host cell receptor CD_4 (chondroitin-rich glycosaminoglycan in the milk fat globule membrane),[93] and they act as receptor analogues for *Vibrio cholerae* and *E. coli* heat-labile toxins, as well as for *V. cholerae* El Tor and enterotoxigenic *E. coli*. Oligosaccharides in human milk prevent the attachment of *H. influenzae* and *S. pneumoniae* to the respiratory epithelium.[67]

There is no significant digestion of milk oligosaccharides during intestinal transit, with resulting excretion of 40 to 50% of intact milk oligosaccharides in the breast-fed infant's stools.[94,95] The presence of these oligosaccharides in urine[95,96] suggests that they provide protection not only in the infant's intestinal tract but also systemically.[95-97] The extent of fucosylation of oligosaccharides that affects the binding and inhibition of bacteria is controlled by fucosyl transferase and fucosidases present in human milk at different levels of activity in the course of lactation.

Milk glycolipids such as the ganglioside Gb_3, the receptor of the β subunit of Shiga toxins, are present in the cream fraction (the milk fat globules) of human milk. Shiga toxin–associated diarrhea and the more serious complications of hemolytic uremic syndrome are caused by *Shigella dysenteriae* and some strains of *E. coli* (0.57:H7 and 011:NM). Protection against this disease may be accomplished by the combined action of Gb_3 and specific IgA antibodies.[98]

Lipids

Milk fat globules, the second most abundant component of human milk, protect the infant from infection by two separate mechanisms. As noted earlier, the membrane glycoconjugates act as specific bacterial and viral ligands, whereas the digestive product of the core triglycerides, free fatty acids, and monoglycerides have a detergent-like lytic action on enveloped viruses, bacteria, and protozoa (Table 29–7).[99,100] Although products of lipolysis are qualitatively similar in formula-fed and breast-fed infants, quantitatively, the breast-fed infant benefits from higher

---

TABLE 29-6

Protective Functions of Oligoconjugates in Human Milk

Structure	Distribution in Milk	Function*
Oligosaccharides	Skim milk	Protect against heat-stable *Escherichia coli* enterotoxin, attachment of *Haemophilus influenzae* and *Streptococcus pneumoniae* to respiratory epithelium, *Vibrio cholerae* hemagglutinin activity
Glycoproteins	MFGM/skim milk	Prevent binding of *V. cholerae* El Tor
Mucin	MFGM	Prevents binding of S-fimbriated *E. coli*
Lactadherin	MFGM/skim milk	Prevents binding of rotavirus
Gangliosides	MFGM	Receptor analogues for heat-labile toxins of *V. cholerae* and *E. coli*
Glycosaminoglycan	MFGM	Inhibits binding of HIV gp 120 to CD4 receptor

MFGM = milk fat globule membrane.
*Most of the listed activities are based on in vitro studies; however, lactadherin prevents rotavirus-caused diarrhea in mice and human infants.
Adapted from Hamosh M: Pediatr Clin North Am 45:53, 2001.

rates of gastric lipolysis[100] and duodenal lipolysis associated with the structure of milk fat globules and the presence of milk bile salt–dependent lipase, respectively.[100] Hydrolysis of milk triglyceride during storage at 4° to 38°C probably contributes to resistance to bacterial and viral growth in milk.[89] Indeed, addition of lipases or free fatty acids and monoglycerides to human milk or formula increases antiviral (respiratory syncytial virus, HSV-1) and anti–gram-positive microbial (*H. influenzae,* group B streptococci) activity.[67, 88, 101] Antiprotozoan activity against *Giardia lamblia* was shown to be directly related to the release of free fatty acids from milk triglycerides by bile salt–dependent lipase and lipoprotein lipase.[67]

The structural determinants associated with the highest level of microbial and protozoan lysis are fatty acid chain length (C12:0), degree of unsaturation (C18:2), and nature of the active group (highest with carboxyl containing lipids, i.e., fatty acids). Lauric acid (C12:0) and linoleic acid (C18:2) amount to 5 and 15% of total fatty acids in human milk and are the most readily released during gastric lipolysis.[67]

Antiinflammatory Components

Antiinflammatory components in human milk that consist of antioxidants (e.g., vitamins A, C, and E and enzymes such as catalase and glutathione peroxidase) are reviewed in detail in the literature.[65, 102] Therefore, they are not discussed here.

Cells in Human Milk

This subject,[62, 63] studied extensively and reviewed in the literature, is not discussed here.

Nucleotides in Human Milk

Nucleotides are considered conditionally essential nutrients because of the insufficient synthesis by the newborn.[103] They differ qualitatively and quantitatively from those in bovine milk and are another agent shown to enhance intestinal repair after injury[104] and to potentiate the immune response to certain vaccines.[105] Certain nucleotides may also promote the growth of *Lactobacillus bifidus,* which is known to suppress the growth of enteropathogens in the newborn's intestine.

Enzymes in Human Milk

Human milk, like the milk of other species, contains many enzymes;[85, 99] however, the specific enzymes and their activity levels vary among species. We discuss briefly only those milk enzymes that may benefit the human infant. Among these enzymes are those involved in protective function (see earlier) such as lysozyme (see Table 29-3), peroxidase, the antiproteases, catalase, glutathione peroxidase, and platelet-activating factor acetyl hydrolase (see Table 29-4). Milk enzymes have been shown to aid in the digestion of carbohydrates and fats during the period of pancreatic exocrine immaturity, which results in low pancreatic lipase levels and the absence of amylase for up to 2 months after full-term delivery.[85, 106, 107] Milk bile salt–dependent lipase and amylase are secreted into human milk and

have been shown to be active in the infant,[85, 106, 108] thus providing the breast-fed premature and full-term infant with better digestive potential (Table 29-8) than that of formula-fed infants.

Probiotics and Prebiotics

These substances have received much attention as potential protective factors. *Probiotics* are viable organisms that have a beneficial effect on intestinal microbial balance. Human milk feeding stimulates the growth of lactobacilli and bifidobacteria, lactic acid–producing microorganisms that generate an intestinal milieu that inhibits the growth of pathogens such as *E. coli* and *Clostridium difficile.*[84] *Prebiotics* are nondigestible food ingredients that enhance the growth or metabolic activity of certain bacteria in the colon. For example, *L. reuteri* produces reuterine, a bacteriocin with broad antimicrobial activity.[84]

Breast-Feeding and Atopic Disease

In contrast to the protective effect of breast-feeding against infectious diseases in infants,[52-63] the relationship between breast-feeding and infant allergy is poorly understood.[109] It seems that allergy-preventing effects, if present, may be limited to infants with a genetically determined increased risk of atopic disease.[109] Deleterious effects of breast-feeding have also been reported; thus, an abnormal ratio between LC-PUFA of the n-6 and n-3 series in mother's milk is associated with the development of allergic disease in infants during the first year of life.[110] Furthermore, although breast-feeding is associated with lower rates of wheezing illnesses in infancy, this effect differs according to maternal asthma status. In children of asthmatic mothers, the development of childhood asthma increases significantly with duration of exclusive breast-feeding.[111] Exclusive breast-feeding and development of cow's milk allergy have also generated controversy. Studies showed that, although early feeding of cow's milk increases the risk of allergy development, exclusive breast-feeding does not seem to reduce the risk.[112]

Late Effects of Breast-Feeding

Among the late-onset diseases that may be affected by the mode of infant feeding are diabetes mellitus, cancer, inflammatory bowel disease, and celiac disease.[52, 113] There is still controversy about the specific role of breast-feeding in the origin of these diseases, which are known to have multifactorial causes, among them environmental factors (e.g., early feeding pattern) and genetic susceptibility.[52, 113-115] The apoptosis-inducing effect of modified α-lactalbumin[87] lends support to the epidemiologic data of lower incidence of certain forms of cancer in infants who were exclusively breast-fed.[113] The controversy about the role of breast-feeding in protection against celiac disease[52] seems to have been resolved by studies showing that the gradual introduction of gluten-containing foods into the diet of infants while they are still being breast-fed reduces the risk of celiac disease in early childhood and probably also subsequently.[116]

TABLE 29-7

Protective Functions of Lipids in Human Milk

Structural determinants of antiinfective activity	Free fatty acids and monoglycerides, most active: lauric acid (C12:0) and linoleic acid (C18:2)
Role of digestion	Milk triglycerides (98% of milk fat) have to be hydrolyzed in the stomach* and intestine† to free fatty acids and monoglycerides
Antiinfective function	Antiprotozoan: *Giardia lamblia*
	Antimicrobial: *Haemophilus influenzae*, group B streptococci, *Staphylococcus epidermidis*
	Antiviral: respiratory syncytial virus, herpes simplex virus 1

*Gastric lipolysis of milk triglycerides is higher in human milk-fed (25%) than formula-fed (14%) infants.
† Human milk bile salt–dependent lipase enhances intestinal fat digestion in breast-fed infants.
Adapted from Hamosh M: Pediatr Clin North Am *45*:53, 2001.

Enzymes with Digestive Function in the Infant

Characteristic	Bile Salt–Dependent Lipase	Amylase
Maternal factors		
Parity (=10)	?	Low activity
Diurnal and within feed activity	Constant	Constant
Secretion		
Prepartum*	Present	?
Postpartum	Constant	Decreases before first month
Preterm versus term delivery†	Equal activity	Equal activity
Milk characteristics		
Distribution	Skim milk	Skim milk
Storage (−20°, −70°C)	Stable years	Stable years
Pasteurization (62°, 30 min)	Inactivated	85% of activity maintained
Storage (15–38°C)	Stable (at least 24 hrs)	Stable (at least 24 h)
Stable at low pH (stomach)	>3.0	>3.0
pH optimum	7.4–8.5	6.5–7.5
Enzyme characteristics	Identical to pancreatic cholesteryl ester lipase	Isoenzyme of salivary amylase
Evidence of activity in infants	Yes	Yes
Present in milk of other species: primates, carnivores, rodents		?

*Prepartum: 2–3 months secretion.
† Infants delivered preterm (26–36 weeks' gestation) and term (37–40 weeks' gestation.)
Adapted from Hamosh M: Pediatr Clin North Am *45*: 53, 2001.

The controversy about whether breast-feeding protects against obesity in later life is, however, still unresolved.[49,117,118] A protective effect of breast-feeding on later obesity, if present, is probably weaker than genetic factors or other environmental factors.[117]

Breast-Feeding, Long Chain Polyunsaturated Fatty Acids, and Cognitive Function

LC-PUFAs are essential for normal growth and development.[119-121] The two families of LC-PUFAs, the n-3 derived from α-linolenic acid and the n-6 originating from linoleic acid, have specific functions. DHA (22:6n3) has an important role in retina and brain development, and AA (20:4n6) is the precursor of prostaglandins, leukotrienes, and other ecosanoids. These highly unsaturated fatty acids affect many aspects of membrane function including membrane order, permeability, and lipid-lipid as well as protein-lipid interactions. Specific interactions of membrane proteins with particular lipids may, in turn, affect receptor function, enzyme activities, signal transduction, and membrane excitability. For the developing infant, DHA is of major importance because it is the major PUFA in cerebral cortex and retinal membranes. The photoreceptor outer segments of the retina contain very high concentrations of DHA, and most molecular species contain at least one DHA moiety. Retinal DHA is important for normal photochemical activity of the visual pigment rhodopsin.

LC-PUFA requirements of the newborn are a major focus of research.[119-122] The reason for this intense interest is based on several observations. Accretion of LC-PUFAs occurs primarily during the last trimester of pregnancy, thereby making the preterm infant particularly vulnerable to LC-PUFA deficiency. Plasma levels of LC-PUFAs decrease markedly after birth in formula-fed preterm infants as compared with nearly constant levels in breast-fed infants of comparable gestational age, and brain levels of DHA are lower in formula-fed than in breast-fed full-term infants.

Studies indicate that the newborn can synthesize LC-PUFAs from essential fatty acid precursors; however, the extent of *de novo* synthesis seems to be insufficient to meet the newborn's demands.[120-122] Postnatally, human milk provides LC-PUFAs to the newborn. Maternal LC-PUFA reserves depend on diet and can be improved by supplementation of DHA and AA during pregnancy and lactation. This, in turn, affects fetal LC-PUFA accretion and postnatal provision through mother's milk. Supplementation of formula-fed preterm or full-term infants with DHA and AA leads to plasma and red blood cell LC-PUFA levels similar to those of breast-fed infants. The higher blood and, presumably, tissue levels of LC-PUFAs after supplementation have only temporary cognitive or visual functional benefits.[120-122]

Studies conducted on larger numbers of formula-fed infants clearly showed that full-term infants do not benefit from supplementation with DHA and AA,[121-123] whereas definite visual and cognitive benefits are found in preterm infants.[124] Indeed, the Life Sciences Research Office's assessment of nutrient requirements for term infant formulas prepared for the United States Food and Drug Administration did not recommend supplementation of formulas for term infants with DHA or AA.[122] DHA and AA are now supplemental to preterm human formulas. Because DHA and AA are present in human milk and not in formulas, it has been inferred that they may be associated with a higher intelligence quotient (IQ) in breast-fed infants. Although this may be true, it seems to be an oversimplification, given the great number of bioactive factors in milk that may affect early cognitive development and the finding that LC-PUFA levels decrease markedly after 2 to 3 months of lactation.[52,120] Furthermore, maternal input may differ between mothers of breast-fed and bottle-fed infants.

The effects of the mode of infant feeding on subsequent cognitive development have been investigated since 1929.[52] Studies since 1977 have shown small benefits in IQ in children and adolescents who were breast-fed.[52] Two studies in large cohorts of young adults (mean age, 18 years[125] and 27 years[126]) showed a dose-response relationship between duration of breast-feeding and higher scores on intelligence tests. Although in many studies the effects of breast-feeding became less apparent when maternal intelligence, level of education, and socioeconomic status were taken into consideration, the consensus points to long-term beneficial effects of breast-feeding for up to 9 months.[127]

REFERENCES

1. Hamosh M, et al: Nutrition During Lactation. Washington, DC, National Academy Press, 1991.
2. Neville MC, et al: Studies in human lactation: milk volumes in lactating women during the onset of lactation and full lactation. Am J Clin Nutr 48:1375, 1988.
3. Prentice A, et al: Crosscultural differences in lactational performance. *In* Hamosh M, Goldman AS (eds): Human Lactation, Vol 2: Maternal and Environmental Factors. New York, Plenum Press, 1986, pp 13–44.
4. Hamosh M, et al: Lipoprotein lipase activity of adipose and mammary tissue and plasma triglyceride in pregnant and lactating rats. Biochim Biophys Acta 210:473, 1970.
5. Zinder O, et al: Effect of prolactin on lipoprotein lipase in mammary gland and adipose tissue of rats. Am J Physiol 226:744, 1974.
6. Hamosh M: Human milk composition and function in the infant. Semin Pediatr Gastroenterol Nutr 3:4, 1992.
7. Cruz JR, et al: Studies in human milk. III. Secretory IgA quantity and antibody levels against *Escherichia coli* in colostrum and milk from underprivileged and privileged mothers. Pediatr Res 16:272, 1982.
8. Reddy V, Srikantia SG: Interaction of nutrition and the immune response. Ind J Med Res 66:48, 1978.
9. Mirahda R, et al: Effect of maternal nutritional status on immunological substances in human colostrum and milk. Am J Clin Nutr 37:632, 1983.
10. Robertson DM, et al: Avidity of IgA antibody to *Escherichia coli* polysaccharide and diphtheria toxin in breast milk from Swedish and Pakistani mothers. Scand J Immunol 28:783, 1988.
11. Bitman J, et al: Comparison of the lipid composition of breast milk from mothers of term and preterm infants. Am J Clin Nutr 38:300, 1983.
12. Ruegg M, Blanc B: The fat globule size distribution in human milk. Biochim Biophys Acta 666:7, 1981.
13. Simonin C, et al: Comparison of the fat content and fat globule size distribution of breast milk from mothers delivering term and preterm. Am J Clin Nutr 40:820, 1984.
14. Hamosh M: Long chain polyunsaturated fatty acids in neonatal nutrition (editorial). J Am Coll Nutr 13:546, 1994.
15. Holman RT, et al: Deficiency of essential fatty acids and membrane fluidity during pregnancy and lactation. Proc Natl Acad Sci USA 88:4835, 1991.
16. Hamosh M, et al: Long chain polyunsaturated fatty acids (LC-PUFA) during early development: Contribution of milk LC-PUFA to accretion rates varies among organs. Adv Exp Med Biol 501:397, 2001.
17. Hytten FE: Clinical and chemical studies in human lactation: variations in major constituents during a feeding. BMJ 1:176, 1954.
18. Macy IG, et al: Human milk studies. VII. Chemical analysis of milk representative of the entire first and last halves of the nursing period. Am J Dis Child 42:569, 1931.
19. Insull W Jr, et al: The fatty acids of human milk: alterations produced by manipulation of caloric balance and exchange of dietary fats. J Clin Invest 38:443, 1959.
20. Prentice A, et al: Breast-milk fatty acids of rural Gambian mothers: effects of diet and maternal parity. J Pediatr Gastroenterol Nutr 8:486, 1989.
21. Tyson J, et al: Adaptation of feeding to a low fat yield in breast milk. Pediatrics 89:215, 1992.
22. Michaelsen KF, et al: The Copenhagen cohort study on infant nutrition and growth: breast milk intake, human milk macronutrient content, and influencing factors. Am J Clin Nutr 59:600, 1994.
23. Dallman PR: Iron deficiency in the weanling: a nutritional problem on the way to resolution. Acta Paediatr Scand Suppl 323:59, 1986.
24. Siimes MA, et al: Exclusive breast-feeding for 9 months: risk of iron deficiency. J Pediatr 104:196, 1984.
25. Ekstrand J, et al: Distribution of fluoride to human breast milk following intake of high doses of fluoride. Caries Res 18:93, 1984.
26. Vuori E, et al: The effects of the dietary intakes of copper, iron, manganese, and zinc on the trace element content of human milk. Am J Clin Nutr 33:227, 1980.
27. Gushurst CA, et al: Breast milk iodide: reassessment in the 1980s. Pediatrics 73:354, 1984.
28. Mannan S, et al: Influence of maternal selenium status on human milk selenium concentration and glutathione peroxidase activity. Am J Clin Nutr 46:95, 1987.
29. Oken E, Lightdale JR: Updates in pediatric nutrition. Curr Opin Pediatr 13:280, 2001.
30. Biser-Rothbaugh A, Hadley-Miller N: Vitamin D deficiency in breast-fed toddlers. J Pediatr Orthop 21:508, 2001.
31. Mughal MZ, et al: Lesson of the week: florid rickets associated with prolonged breast-feeding without vitamin D supplementation. BMJ 318:39, 1999.
32. Krebs NF, Westcott J: Zinc and breast-fed infants: if and when is there a risk of deficiency? Adv Exp Med Biol 503:69, 2002.
33. Green FR: Do breast-fed infants need supplemental vitamins? Pediatr Clin North Am 48:401, 2001.
34. Kreiter SR, et al: Nutritional rickets in African American breast-fed infants. J Pediatr 137:153, 2000.
35. Gessner BD, et al: Nutritional rickets among breast-fed Alaska native children. Alaska Med 29:72, 1997.
36. Msomekela M, et al: A high prevalence in metabolic bone disease in exclusively breast-fed very low birth weight infants in Dar-es-Salaam, Tanzania. Ann Trop Paediatr 19:337, 1999.
37. Agarwal KS, et al: The impact of atmospheric pollution on vitamin D status of infants and toddlers in Delhi, India. Arch Dis Child 87:111, 2002.
38. Nesby-O'Dell S, et al: Hypovitaminosis D prevalence and determinants among African American and White women of reproductive age: Third National Health and Nutrition Examination Survey, 1988–1994. Am J Clin Nutr 76:187, 2002.
39. Stevens J, Lubitz L: Symptomatic zinc deficiency in breastfed term and premature infants. J Paediatr Child Health 34:97, 1998.
40. Sian L, et al: Zinc homeostasis during lactation in a population with a low zinc intake. Am J Clin Nutr 75:99, 2002.
41. Dorea JG: Zinc deficiency in nursing infants. Nutrition 21:84, 2002.
42. Dorea JG: Zinc in human milk. Nutr Res 20:1645, 2000.
43. Semba RD, Delange F: Iodine in human milk: perspectives for infant health. Nutr Rev 59:269, 2001.
44. Dewey KG: Growth characteristics of breastfed compared to formula-fed infants. Biol Neonate 74:94, 1998.
45. Dewey KG: Nutrition, growth and complementary feeding of the breast-fed infant. Pediatr Clin North Am 48:87, 2001.
46. Labbok M, Krasnovec K: Toward consistency in breast feeding definitions. Stud Fam Plan 21:226, 1990.
47. De Onis M, et al: Time for a new growth reference. Pediatrics 100:98, 1998.
48. Dewey KG et al: WHO working group on infant growth: growth of breast-fed infants deviates from current reference data: a pooled analysis of US, Canadian and European data sets. Pediatrics 96:495, 1995.
49. Hamosh M: Does infant nutrition affect adiposity and cholesterol levels in the adult? J Pediatr Gastroenterol Nutr 7:10, 1988.
50. Butte NF: Energy requirements in infants. Eur J Clin Nutr 50(Suppl):24, 1996.
51. Axelsson IE, et al: Protein intake in early infancy: effects of plasma amino acid concentrations, insulin metabolism and growth. Pediatr Res 26:614, 1989.
52. Villalpando S, Hamosh M: Early and late effects on breast-feeding: does breast feeding really matter? Biol Neonate 74:177, 1998.
53. Hasselbalch H, et al: Decreased thymus size in formula-fed infants. Acta Pediatr 85:1029, 1996.
54. Bauchner H, et al: Studies on breast-feeding and infection: how good is the evidence? JAMA 256:887, 1986.
55. Habicht JP, et al: Does breast-feeding really save lives, or are apparent benefits due to biases? Am J Epidemiol 13:279, 1986.
56. Popkin BM, et al: Breast-feeding and diarrheal morbidity. Pediatrics 86:274, 1990.
57. Dewey KG, et al: Differences in morbidity between breast-fed and formula-fed infants. J Pediatr 126:696, 1995.
58. Howie PN, et al: Protective effect of breast-feeding against infection. BMJ 200:11, 1993.
59. Howie PN: Protective effect of breast-feeding against infection in the first and second six months of life. Adv Exp Med Biol 503:141, 2002.
60. El-Mohandes AE, et al: Use of human milk in the intensive care nursery decreases the incidence of nosocomial sepsis. J Perinatol 17:130, 1997.
61. Goldman AS: The immune system of human milk: antimicrobial, anti-inflammatory and immunomodulating properties. Pediatr Infect Dis J 12:226, 1993.
62. Xanthou M, et al: Human milk and intestinal host defenses in newborns: an update. Adv Pediatr 42:171, 1995.
63. Xanthou M: Immune protection of human milk. Biol Neonate 74:121, 1998.
64. Garofalo RP, Goldman AS: Cytokines, chemokines and colony stimulating factors in human milk: the 1997 update. Biol Neonate 74:134, 1998.
65. Garofalo RP, Goldman AS: Expression of functional immunomodulating and anti-inflammatory factors in human milk. Clin Perinatol 26:361, 1999.
66. Hamosh M: Breast-feeding: unraveling the mysteries of mother's milk. In Medscape Women's Health. http//:www.medscape.com, 1996, 23 pages.
67. Hamosh M: Protective functions of proteins and lipids in human milk. Biol Neonate 74:163, 1998.
68. Mestecky J, et al (eds): Immunology of Milk and the Neonate. New York, Plenum Press, 1991, p 483.
69. Newburg DS, Neubauer SH: Carbohydrates in milks: analysis, quantities and significance. *In* Jensen RG (ed): Handbook of Milk Composition. San Diego, Academic Press 1994, pp 273–349.
70. Peterson JA, et al: Glycoproteins of the human milk fat globule in the protection of breast-fed infants against infections. Biol Neonate 74:143, 1998.
71. Davidson LA, et al: Influence of lactoferrin on iron absorption from human milk in infants. Pediatr Res 34:117, 1994.
72. Hanson LH, et al: Does human lactoferrin in the milk of transgenic mice deliver iron to suckling neonates? Adv Exp Med Biol 501:233, 2001.
73. Tomita M, et al: Antimicrobial peptides of lactoferrin. Adv Exp Med Biol 347:209, 1994.
74. Miyazawa K, et al: Lactoferrin lipopolysaccharide interactions: effect of lactoferrin binding to monocyte-macrophage differentiated HL-60 cells. J Immunol 146:723, 1991.
75. Giugliano LG, et al: Free secretory components and lactoferrin of human milk inhibit the adhesion of enterotoxigenic *Escherichia coli*. J Med Microbiol 42:3, 1995.
76. Cleary TG: Human milk feeding provides redundant protection from bacillary dysentery. Pediatr Res 45:742, 1999.
77. Van Berkel PHC, et al: Glycosylated and unglycosylated human lactoferrins can both bind iron and have identical affinities toward human lysozyme and bacterial lipopolysaccharides but differ in their susceptibility towards tryptic proteolysis. Biochem J 312:107, 1995.

78. Hanson LA, et al: Anti-inflammatory capacities of human milk: lactoferrins and secretory IgA inhibit endotoxin-induced cytokine release. *In* Mestecky JC (ed): Advances in Mucosal Immunity. New York, Plenum Press, 1995, p 669.

79. Schanler RJ, et al: Enhanced fecal excretion of selected immune factors in very low birth weight infants. Pediatr Res 20:711, 1986.

80. Schroten H, et al: Inhibition of adhesion of S-fimbriated *Escherichia coli* to buccal epithelial cells by human milk fat globule membrane components: a novel aspect of the protective function of mucin in the non-immunoglobulin fraction. Infect Immun 60:2893, 1992.

81. Nichols BL, et al: Human lactoferrin stimulates thymidine incorporation into DNA of rat crypt cells. Pediatr Res 21:563, 1987.

82. Zhang P, et al: Human lactoferrin in the milk of transgenic mice increases intestinal growth in ten-day-old suckling neonates. Adv Exp Med Biol 501:107, 2001.

83. Hutchens TW, et al: Origin of intact lactoferrin and its DNA binding fragments found in the urine of human milk fed preterm infants. Pediatr Res 29:243, 1991.

84. Pickering LK, Biotherapeutic agents and disease in infants. Adv Exp Med Biol 501:265, 2001.

85. Hamosh M: Enzymes in human milk. *In* Jensen RG (ed): Handbook of Milk Composition. San Diego, Academic Press, 1995, p 388.

86. Sternhagen L, Allen JC: Growth rates of a human colon adenocarcinoma cell line are regulated by the milk protein α-lactalbumin. Adv Exp Med Biol 501:115, 2001.

87. Svensson M, et al: Conversion of α-lactalbumin to a protein inducing apoptosis. Proc Natl Acad Sci USA 97:4211, 2000.

88. Hamosh M: Bioactive factors in human milk. Pediatr Clin North Am 48:69, 2001.

89. Hamosh M, et al: Breastfeeding and the working mother: effect of time and temperature of short-term storage on proteolysis, lipolysis and bacterial growth. Pediatrics 97:492, 1996.

90. Patton S, et al: The epithelial mucin, MUC-1, of milk mammary gland and other tissues. Biochim Biophys Acta 1241:407, 1995.

91. Yolken RH, et al: Human milk mucin inhibits rotavirus replication and prevents experimental gastroenteritis. J Clin Invest 90:1984, 1992.

92. Newburg DS, et al: Human milk lactadherin: nature of its carbohydrate linkage and protection against symptomatic rotavirus infection. Pediatr Res 39:399, 1996.

93. Newburg DS, et al: Human milk glycosaminoglycans inhibit HIV glycoprotein (gp 120) binding to its host cell receptor CD4. J Nutr 124:419, 1995.

94. Coppa GV, et al: Characterization of oligosaccharides in milk and feces of breast-fed infants by high performance anion chromatography. Adv Exp Med Biol 501:307, 2001.

95. Coppa GV, et al: Preliminary study of breast-feeding and bacterial adhesion to uroepithelial cells. Lancet 334:569, 1990.

96. Chaturved P, et al: Survival of human milk oligosaccharides in the intestine of infants. Adv Exp Med Biol 501:315, 2001.

97. Clemens K, Silvia R: Physiology of oligosaccharides in lactating women and breast-fed infants. Adv Exp Med Biol 478:241, 2000.

98. Herrera-Insua I, et al: Human milk lipids bind shigatoxin. Adv Exp Med Biol 501:333, 2001.

99. Hamosh M, et al: Protective function of human milk: The milk fat globule. Semin Perinatol 23:242, 1999.

100. Armand M, et al: Effect of human milk or formula on gastric function and fat digestion in the premature infant. Pediatr Res 40:429, 1996.

101. Isaacs CE: Specific and non-specific protective factors in milk: why don't they prevent viral transmission during breast-feeding? Adv Exp Med Biol 503:173, 2002.

102. Buesdher ES: Anti-inflammatory characteristics of human milk. Adv Exp Med Biol 501:207, 2001.

103. Hamosh M: Conditionally essential nutrients: can long-chain polyunsaturated fatty acids and nucleotides qualify? Adv Exp Med Biol 401:357, 2001.

104. Tanaka M, et al: Exogenous nucleotides alter the proliferation, differentiation and apoptosis of human small intestinal epithelium. J Nutr 126:424, 1996.

105. Pickering LK, et al: Modulation of the immune system by human milk and formula containing nucleotides. Pediatrics 101:242, 1998.

106. Hamosh M: Digestion in the neonate. Clin Perinatol 23:191, 1996.

107. Hamosh M, Hamosh P: Development of secreted digestive enzymes. *In* Sanders IR, Walker WA (eds) Development of the Gastrointestinal Tract. Hamilton, Ontario, Canada, Decker, 2000, pp 201.

108. Hamosh M: Digestion in the premature infant: the effects of human milk. Semin Perinatol 18:485, 1994.

109. Bjorsten B: Is allergy a preventable disease? Adv Exp Med Biol 478:109, 2000.

110. Duchen K, et al: Atopic sensitization during the first year of life in relation to long-chain polyunsaturated fatty acid levels in human milk. Pediatr Res 44:478, 1998.

111. Wright AL, et al: Maternal asthma status alters relation of infant feeding to asthma in childhood. Adv Exp Med Biol 478:131, 2000.

112. Saarinen KM, et al: Breast-feeding and the development of cow's milk protein allergy. Adv Exp Med Biol 478:121, 2000.

113. Davis MK: Breast-feeding and chronic disease in childhood and adolescence. Pediatr Clin North Am 48:125, 2001.

114. Hammond-McKibben D, Dosch H-M: Cow milk, BSA and IDDM: can we settle these controversies? Diabetes Care 20:897, 1997.

115. Dosch H-M, Becker DJ: Infant feeding and autoimmune diabetes. Adv Exp Med Biol 503:133, 2002.

116. Iversson A, et al: Breast-feeding protects against celiac disease. Am J Clin Nutr 75:914, 2002.

117. Butte NF: The role of breast-feeding in obesity. Pediatr Clin North Am 48:189, 2001.

118. Von Kries R, et al: Does breast-feeding protect against childhood obesity? Adv Exp Med Biol 478:29, 2000.

119. Innis SM: Essential fatty acids in growth and development. Prog Lipid Res 30:39, 1991.

120. Hamosh M, Salem N Jr: Long-chain polyunsaturated fatty acids. Biol Neonate 74:106, 1998.

121. Heird WC: The role of polyunsaturated fatty acids in term and preterm infants and breast-feeding mothers. Pediatr Clin North Am 48:173, 2001.

122. Raiten DJ, et al: LSRO report: assessment of nutrient requirements for infant formulas. J Nutr 128(Suppl):115, 1998.

123. Auestad N, et al: Growth and development in term infants fed long-chain polyunsaturated fatty acids: a double-masked, randomized, parallel prospective multivariate study. Pediatrics 108:372, 2001.

124. O'Connor DL, et al: Growth and development in preterm infants fed long-chain polyunsaturated fatty acids: a prospective, randomized controlled trial. Pediatrics 108:259, 2000.

125. Harwood IJ, Fergusson DM. Breast-feeding and later cognitive and academic outcome. Pediatrics 101:1, 1998.

126. Mortensen EL, et al: The association between duration of breast-feeding and adult intelligence. JAMA 287:2365, 2002.

127. Angelsen NK, et al: Breast-feeding and cognitive development at age 1 and 5 years. Arch Dis Child 85:183, 2001.

Margaret C. Neville and James McManaman

30 Physiology of Lactation

Unlike most other organs in the body the breast achieves its mature function, the secretion of milk, only after a developmental program that takes place in the adult, guided by reproductive hormones. For this reason, we first describe this developmental program through puberty and pregnancy to its completion several days after parturition when milk assumes mature composition. The later parts of this program are repeated during each pregnancy because the glandular epithelium responsible for the secretion of milk regresses after weaning is completed to a state resembling that of the condition before pregnancy.

During lactation, a multitude of highly coordinated synthetic and secretory processes combine to produce the complex fluid we call milk, which is capable of fully sustaining the human infant for at least the first 6 months of life. However, without the let-down reflex to eject the milk through the ducts and out the nipple, this fluid is retained in the lumens of the alveoli into which it is secreted. Secretory activation, formerly called lactogenesis II, consists of the functional changes that take place during the first week postpartum and that transform a prepared, but nonsecretory gland, into a fully functioning organ. Most lactation problems arise during this period. Additional information on the hormonal regulation of mammary development and lactation can be found in an excellent on-line chapter by Wysolmerski and Van Houten.[1]

OVERVIEW OF THE DEVELOPMENTAL ANATOMY OF THE BREAST

The breast is composed of a tubuloalveolar parenchyma embedded in a connective and adipose tissue stroma. In the mature breast of the nonpregnant, nonlactating woman 10 to 15 branching ducts form a treelike pattern that extends from the nipple to the edges of a specialized fat pad on the anterior wall of the thorax. Lobules, the origin of the acinar structures that will develop into the milk-secreting organ, extend from the ducts and are referred to by pathologists as *terminal duct lobular units (TDLUs)*. Figure 30–1 depicts the developmental origin of these units starting with embryogenesis, which begins in the 18- to 19-week fetus when a bulb-shaped mammary bud can be discerned extending from the epidermis into the dense subepidermal mesenchyme (see Fig. 30–1A).[2] A nipple forms in the epidermal portion of the structure and ducts invade the fat-pad precursor, branching and canalizing to form the rudimentary system that is present at birth.[2,3] Limited milk secretion occurs in the infant after birth due to changes in maternal hormones. The immature gland remains as nipple with a set of small branching ducts that grow in parallel with the child.

At puberty, estrogen[4] and a pituitary factor that is probably a growth hormone[5] stimulate the further elongation and branching of the mammary ducts. In early puberty, bare ducts course through the fat pad (see Fig. 30–1B). With the onset of menses and ovulatory cycles, the progesterone secreted by the ovary during the luteal phase brings about some lobular development as shown in Figure 30–1C. The lobular clusters are dynamic structures that increase in size and complexity during each luteal phase but tend to regress with the onset of the menses and the loss of hormonal support.[4]

The hormones of pregnancy bring about full alveolar development and differentiation of the epithelium. In addition to increasing levels of progesterone, a lactogenic hormone, either prolactin or human placental lactogen possibly aided by growth hormone, is thought to be essential for the final stages of mammary growth and differentiation.[6] By midpregnancy, the gland has developed extensive lobular clusters (see Fig. 30–1D and E) and indeed, small amounts of secretion product are formed. However, differentiation continues until parturition, with full secretion being inhibited by the high circulating concentrations of progesterone. Secretory activation represents the onset of *copious* milk secretion and takes place during the first 4 days postpartum. A major volume increase that occurs around 40 hours postpartum is often referred as the *coming in* of the milk. The fall in progesterone due to loss of the placenta and maintenance of prolactin secretion from pituitary glands are necessary for milk secretion.

Lactation is the process of milk secretion that will continue as long as milk is removed from the gland on a regular basis. In women prolactin is required to maintain milk secretion and oxytocin is required to produce the let-down that allows the infant to extract milk from the gland. An example of the swollen ducts and alveoli that occur when milk is not removed from the gland is shown in Figure 30–1E. The actual volume of milk secreted is adjusted to the requirements of the infant by local factors. One of these may be the so-called feedback inhibitor of lactation (FIL).[7] Stretching and flattening of the mammary epithelial cells may also be important.

Involution takes place when regular extraction of milk from the gland ceases or in many, but not all, species, when prolactin is withdrawn. Like lactogenesis this stage involves an orderly

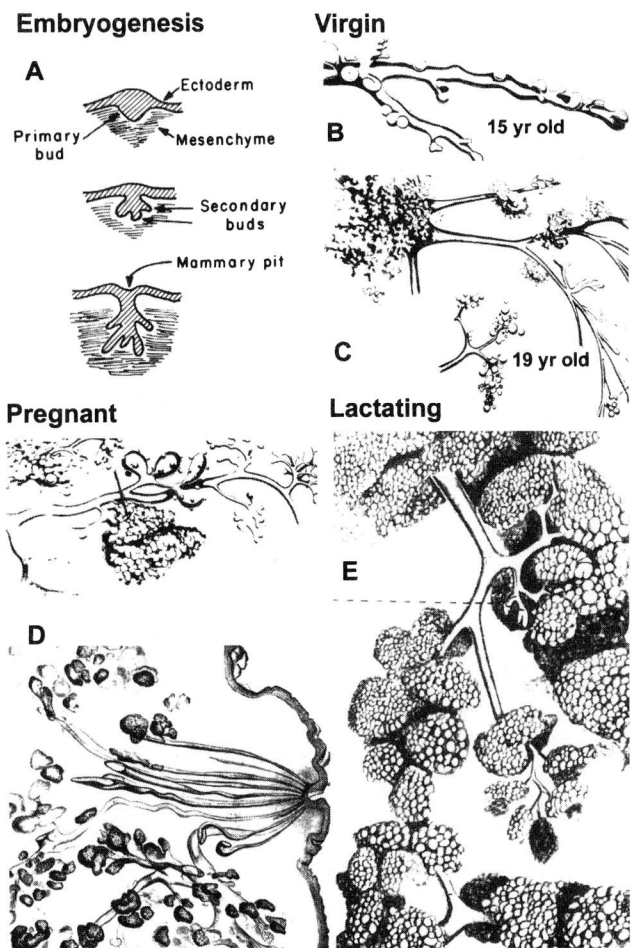

Figure 30–1. Human mammary development. **A,** A thickening of the ectoderm called the placode pushes branches into the underlying stroma to produce the rudimentary mammary gland with the nipple present at birth in both sexes. **B,** At the onset of puberty, ductal structures branch and elongate into the fat pad. **C,** With the onset of the menstrual cycles, progesterone secretion during the luteal phase brings about budding of alveolar complexes called terminal duct lobular units (TDLU) from the sides and ends of the ducts. **D, E,** The TDLUs undergo extensive development during pregnancy. **F,** This picture of the lactating gland was drawn from a section of the breast of a woman who died 2 days after last suckling her infant. Note that each alveolus is engorged with milk. The camera lucida drawings of sections of the human breast are from Dabelow, A: Morphol J 85:361–416 , 1941. (With permission for publication from Springer-Verlag.)

sequence of events that includes cessation of milk secretion, apoptosis of the mammary epithelium,[8] and remodeling of the gland, which return it approximately to a prepregnant state.

CELLULAR MECHANISMS FOR MILK SYNTHESIS AND SECRETION

Milk components are secreted into the alveolar lumina by five distinct pathways as illustrated diagrammatically in Figure 30–2.[9] Four secretory processes are synchronized in the alveolar cell: (1) exocytosis, (2) fat synthesis and secretion, (3) secretion of ions and water, and (4) transcytosis of immunoglobulins and other substances from the interstitial space. These processes are summarized briefly here, followed by an introduction to the role

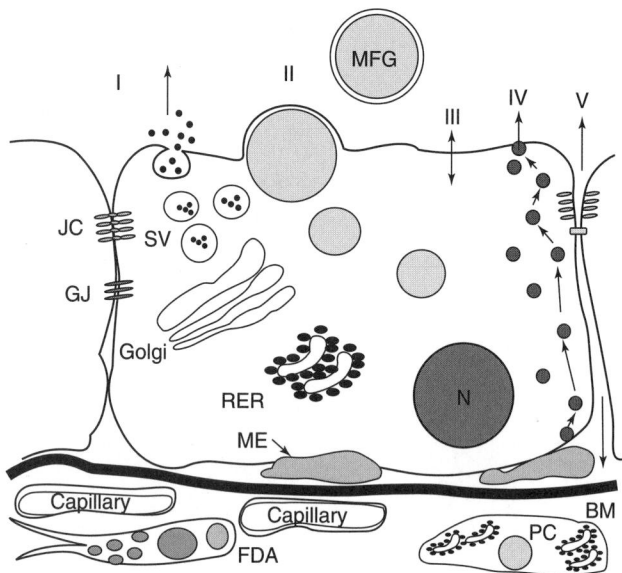

Figure 30–2. Cartoon of a mammary epithelial cell showing pathways for milk secretion. Pathway I. Exocytotic pathway for secretion of milk proteins, lactose, calcium, and other components of the aqueous phase of milk. Pathway II. Milk fat secretion with formation of cytoplasmic lipid droplets that move to the apical membrane to be secreted as a membrane-bound milk fat globule (MFG). Pathway III. Transporters for the direct movement of monovalent ions, water and glucose across the apical membrane of the cell. Pathway IV. Vesicular transcytosis of proteins such as immunoglobulins from the interstitial space. Pathway V. The paracellular pathway for plasma components and leukocytes. Pathway V is open only during pregnancy, involution, and in inflammatory states such as mastitis. Abbreviations: SV = secretory vesicle; RER = rough endoplasmic reticulum; BM = basement membrane; N = nucleus; PC = plasma cell; FDA = fat depleted adipocyte; JC = junctional complex containing the tight and adherens junctions; GJ = gap junction; ME = myoepithelial cell. (Redrawn from Neville MC, Allen JC, Watters C: The mechanisms of milk secretion. *In* Neville MC and Neifert MR: *Lactation: Physiology, Nutrition and Breast-Feeding.* New York, Plenum Press, 1983, p 50. Used by permission)

of a fifth pathway, the paracellular pathway, in determining the composition of the mammary secretion.

Exocytosis

Most components of the aqueous phase of milk are secreted by the exocytotic pathway (see Pathway I, Fig. 30-2). This pathway, like the exocytotic pathway in all cells, ultimately begins in the nucleus with the synthesis of mRNA molecules specific for milk proteins. The mature mRNA serves as a template for protein synthesis. The protein molecules are transported into the endoplasmic reticulum where they are folded and transported through the Golgi system to take part in secretory vesicle formation. Secretory vesicles move to the apical membrane where they discharge their contents into the alveolar lumen by exocytosis. Several specialized reactions in this pathway give milk components their final form. For example, lactose and the oligosaccharides that together comprise almost 8% of the weight of human milk are synthesized here. The formation of casein micelles, which add large quantities of calcium during maturation, also takes place within this pathway.

Lipid Synthesis and Secretion

Triacylglycerols, synthesized in the smooth endoplasmic reticulum of the mammary alveolar cell from precursor fatty acids and glycerol, coalesce into small cytoplasmic lipid droplets that are drawn to the apex of the cell (see Pathway II, Fig. 30-2). These droplets coalesce and gradually become enveloped in apical plasma membrane and bud from the cell as the milk fat globule. The occasional inclusion of a crescent of cytoplasm within the membrane-bound globule[10] enables any substance contained in the cytoplasm to enter milk. The membrane surrounding the milk fat globule has two functions: it is the primary dietary source of phospholipids for the breast-fed infant and it prevents the fat globules from coalescing into large fat droplets that might interfere with milk removal.

Transport of Small Molecules Across the Apical Membrane

Unlike other pathways for milk secretion, the pathways for the direct transport of substances across the apical membrane of the mammary alveolar cell are poorly understood (see Pathway III, Fig. 30-2). Linzell and Peaker[11] devised a clever technique to determine which molecules could use this pathway, infusing isotopes of small molecules up the teat of a goat and calculating how much of the substance left the milk and entered the blood. They found that sodium, potassium, chloride, and certain monosaccharides, as well as water, directly permeated this membrane but calcium, phosphate, and citrate did not. Although the mechanisms are not understood, it is clear that apical membrane transport pathways are limited to a modest number of small molecules that also include glucose and possibly amino acids.

Transcytosis of Interstitial Molecules

Intact proteins in the interstitial space surrounding the basal and lateral surface of the mammary alveolar cell can cross the mammary epithelium in two possible ways: by transcytosis and through the paracellular pathway. Because the paracellular pathway is closed during lactation, plasma proteins must enter milk through transcytosis (see Pathway IV, Fig. 30-2). The best-studied molecule in this regard is immunoglobulin A (IgA).[12] IgA is synthesized by plasma cells that reside in the interstitial spaces of the mammary gland or elsewhere in the body. Dimeric IgA binds to receptors on the basal surface of the mammary alveolar cell, after which the entire IgA-receptor complex is endocytosed and transferred to the apical membrane, where the extracellular portion of the receptor is cleaved and secreted together with the IgA. The many proteins including serum albumin, insulin, prolactin, IGF-1, and possibly other growth factors that find their way into milk from the plasma are also thought to be secreted by a similar, but much less well-studied, mechanism.

The Role of the Paracellular Pathway in Milk Secretion

Pathway V (see Fig. 30-2) involves passage of substances between epithelial cells, rather than through them, and for this reason is designated the *paracellular pathway*. During lactation the passage of even low molecular weight substances between alveolar cells is impeded by a gasketlike structure called the *tight junction* that joins the epithelial cells tightly, one to another.[13] Although immune cells apparently can elicit diapedesia between epithelial cells to reach the milk,[14] the junctions seal tightly behind them and leave no permanent gap. During pregnancy, in the course of mastitis, and after involution, these tight junctions are leaky and allow components of the interstitial space to pass unimpeded into the milk. At the same time, milk components can enter the plasma. This leakiness is useful during these periods, inasmuch as secretion products are allowed to leave the gland, so that inflammatory cells can enter and so that products of the dissolution of the mammary cells during involution can be cleared from the breast. When the junctions are open, mammary secretions have a high concentration of sodium and chloride, a fact that is sometimes useful in diagnosing breast-feeding problems.[15]

REGULATION OF MILK SYNTHESIS, SECRETION, AND EJECTION

Milk is synthesized continuously and secreted into the alveolar lumen where it is stored until it is ejected from the breast by a let-down reflex. This means that two levels of regulation must exist: regulation of the rate of synthesis and secretion and regulation of milk ejection. Although both processes ultimately depend on sucking by the infant or other stimulation of the nipple, the mechanisms involved, both central and local, are very different. Prolactin mediates the central nervous system regulation of milk secretion, but its influence is greatly modified by local factors that depend on milk removal from the breast. Oxytocin, on the other hand, participates in a neuroendocrine reflex that results in stimulation of the myoepithelial cells that surround the alveoli and ducts. When these cells contract, milk is forced out of the alveoli to the nipple. Only then does it become available to the suckling infant. If the letdown reflex is inhibited, milk cannot be removed from the breast and local mechanisms bring about an inhibition of milk secretion. With consistent partial removal of milk, these local factors adjust milk secretion to a new steady state level.[16] If milk removal ceases altogether, involution sets in and the gland loses its competency to secrete milk within days to weeks.

MILK VOLUME PRODUCTION IN LACTATING WOMEN

A meta-analysis of the volume of milk secreted by exclusively breast-feeding women showed that milk volume at 6 months postpartum is remarkably constant at about 800 mL/day in populations throughout the world.[16] Milk volume increases 5 to 15% in women with very low body fat who secrete milk with a lower lipid content, which decreases caloric density of up to 15%. This observation illustrates the important principle that *milk volume secretion in lactating women is regulated by infant demand.* Thus, when the milk has a lower caloric density, increased sucking by the infant is thought to result in increased emptying of the breast, in turn bringing about an increase in milk secretion. Mothers of twins, and occasionally even triplets, are able to produce volumes of milk sufficient for complete nutrition of their multiple infants. Studies of wet nurses, completed in the 1930s, show that at least some women are capable of producing up to 3.5 L of milk per day. Conversely, if infants are supplemented with foods other than breast-milk, milk secretion is proportionally reduced. For example, in countries such as Peru and the Gambia where infants' diets are customarily supplemented with small amounts of food at mealtimes, but given several breast-feeds a day, the daily milk production remains at about 600 mL/day for 12 months or longer.

The mechanisms by which the volume of milk is regulated are still under study. Although prolactin is necessary for milk production, and prolactin levels are consistently above baseline for the duration of lactation,[17] they are not proportional to milk volume secretion. Two local mechanisms have been implicated in the regulation of milk volume production. Wilde and co-workers[7] have produced extensive evidence for the existence in milk of an inhibitor of lactation they call FIL that appears to build up as milk accumulates in the lumen of the mammary gland. This factor can be shown to inhibit milk secretion in both *in vivo* and *in vitro* preparations of fresh mammary glands. Some recent evidence suggests that stretch may have regulatory effects on milk synthesis and secretion but this seemingly reasonable idea currently lacks good experimental support.

OXYTOCIN, MILK EJECTION, AND SUCKLING

Milk removal from the breast is accomplished by the contraction of myoepithelial cells, the processes of which form a basketlike network around the alveoli where milk is stored. When the infant is suckled, afferent impulses from sensory stimulation of nerve terminals in the areolas travel to the central nervous system where they promote release of oxytocin from the posterior pituitary. In the woman, oxytocin release is often associated with such stimuli as the sight or sound, or even the thought, of the infant indicating a significant psychological component in this so-called neuroendocrine reflex. The oxytocin is carried through the bloodstream to the mammary gland where it interacts with specific receptors on myoepithelial cells, initiating their contraction and expelling milk from the alveoli into the ducts and sub-areolar sinuses. The process by which milk is forcibly moved out of the alveoli is called *milk ejection* or *let-down* and is essential to milk removal from the lactating breast.

During correct suckling, the nipple and much of the areola are drawn well into the mouth so that a long teat reaching nearly to the infant's soft palate is formed.[18] The mammary sinuses extend into this teat. Milk is removed not so much by suction as by the stripping motion of the tongue against the hard palate. This motion carries milk through the teat into the baby's mouth. The sinuses refill as the continued action of oxytocin forces milk from the alveoli into the ducts.

It has been known for some time that psychological stress or pain decrease milk output. Recently the basis for this finding was shown by Ueda and colleagues[19] to be inhibition of oxytocin release. In relaxed, undisturbed women suckling their infants, oxytocin release begins with the onset of suckling or even before suckling when the infant cries or becomes restless. When the suckling women were asked to carry out difficult mental calculations or were fed traffic noise through earphones while nursing the infant, the number of oxytocin pulses was significantly reduced. Interestingly, the prolactin response to suckling was not impaired by psychological stress, implicating different neural pathways in the release of the two hormones.

Alcohol and drugs of abuse may have effects on let-down. Building on earlier studies showing that ethanol inhibits milk ejection in a dose-dependent manner, Coiro and colleagues[20] measured plasma oxytocin concentrations in response to breast-stimulation in nonlactating women and found that 50 mL of ethyl alcohol completely abolished the rise in oxytocin levels. Minor effects of chronic maternal ethanol consumption on motor development of breast-fed infants in a well-controlled study in humans[21] were attributed to alcohol transfer to the infant rather than suppression of milk secretion. A potent effect of morphine on oxytocin release has been described in rats,[22] but the effects of opioids and other drugs of abuse on lactation have not been studied in women.

EFFECTS OF LACTATION ON THE MOTHER

Nutritional Effects

In many species such as the high-producing dairy cow and the laboratory mouse, a large portion of the metabolic output is directed to milk synthesis so that careful management of nutrient intake is critical for lactation success. By contrast, in humans the metabolic demands of breast-feeding a single infant require an increase in maternal metabolism about equal to only 20% of the metabolic output of a moderately active woman.[23] For this reason most of the adjustments are small, so that a relatively small increase in food intake or increased weight loss can compensate for the metabolic needs for the secretion of breast milk.

Nonetheless, it is important to remember that, as already stated, the amount of milk produced is almost entirely regulated by infant demand. If a woman is breast-feeding twins, she will produce double the usual volume of about 800 mL per day.[16] Under these circumstances the nutritional demands may be substantial and attention should be paid to nutritional intake, particularly in malnourished women, so that maternal depletion does not result. One maternal effect that seems clear is that lactating women whose menses have not yet returned have a significant loss of calcium from their bones.[24] Both secretion of parathyroid hormone—related peptide (PTHrp) from the mammary epithelium and the lack of estrogen due to postpartum amenorrhea may be involved. That PTHrP plays an active role in mobilizing bone calcium during human lactation is suggested by findings that plasma calcium and alkaline phosphatase are elevated in lactating women and that the calcium regulatory hormone PTH is decreased.[24] After weaning, bone calcium levels return to normal.

Effects of Lactation on Reproduction

The most marked maternal effect of lactation is on fertility. In the early postpartum period, secretions of the ovarian follicle remain suppressed for a period of time the duration of which depends to a substantial extent on the pattern of suckling.[25] In non-breast-feeding women, fertility returns about 6 weeks postpartum as pulsatile secretion of gonadotropin-releasing hormone returns to normal. In breast-feeding women who suckle their infants at regular intervals, follicle-stimulating hormone secretion returns to normal follicular phase levels during the course of lactation, but pulsatile secretion of luteinizing hormone tends to remain in a suppressed state so that the preovulatory surge of luteinizing hormone does not occur.

Postpartum suppression of fertility is thought to play a significant role in birth spacing on a population basis in developing countries where prolonged breast-feeding may be the rule and the use of supplementary feedings delayed. In developed countries, women who wish to ensure against pregnancy during lactation are usually advised to use other contraceptive means, often progesterone-containing compounds that do not interfere with milk secretion.[26]

SECRETORY ACTIVATION

The most critical time in the establishment of lactation is its onset during the transition from pregnancy to lactation, a period we now call *secretory activation* (previously termed *lactogenesis stage II*). Secretory activation takes place after birth in women, in contrast to many animal species where it occurs concomitantly with parturition.[6]

Milk Volume and Composition During the First Week Postpartum

Figure 30-3*A* shows milk volumes in 11 American women who weighed their infants before and after every feed for the first week postpartum. Although there is wide variation among individuals, the trend is revealed by the averaged data in Figure 30-3*B*: volumes of breast secretion of less than 100 mL per day characterize the first 2 days postpartum, after which a rapid increase in milk volume leads to production of an average of 600 mL/day by the fourth day postpartum. A detailed study of milk composition over this period reveals a carefully programmed cascade of events that leads to a mammary secretion product with a composition close to that of mature milk. Although the secretion product in the first few days is usually called *colostrum*, we avoid that term here because it implies a

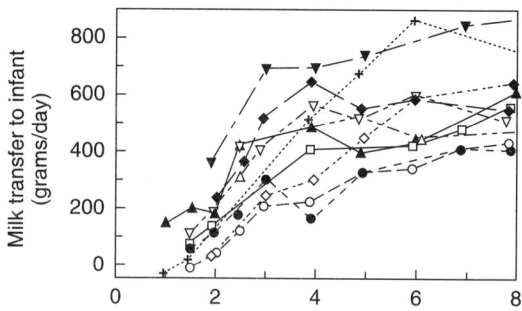

A

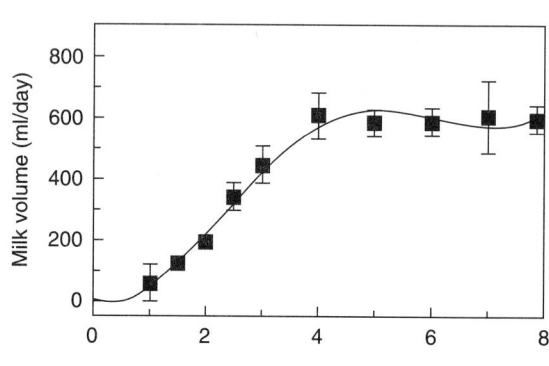

B

Figure 30–3. Milk volumes during the onset of lactation in American women. **A,** Eleven multiparous women weighed their infants before and after every feed for 7 to 8 days postpartum. Milk output was averaged by 0.5-day intervals for the first 3 days and then daily for the remainder of the experiment. All women had successfully breast-fed at least one previous infant. Note the extensive variation in the volumes of milk produced. All these women breast-fed successfully for at least 6 months. **B,** Mean output in the women shown in (**A**). Plotted from data in reference 38. (Graphs from Neville, MC. Lactogenesis in women: A cascade of events revealed by milk composition. *In* Jensen RD (ed): The Composition of Milks. San Diego, Academic Press, 1995, pp 87–98. Used by permission.)

secretion product with a fixed composition. In fact, as we shall see, milk composition changes dramatically during the first 3 to 4 days postpartum.

The first compositional change to occur after delivery is a fall in the sodium and chloride concentrations in the milk and an increase in lactose levels (Fig. 30-4*A*). These modifications commence immediately after delivery and are largely complete by 72 hours postpartum.[6] They precede the rapid increase in milk volume by at least 24 hours and can be explained by closure of the tight junctions that block the paracellular pathway during lactation. With the paracellular pathway closed, lactose, produced by the epithelial cells, can no longer pass into the plasma, and sodium and chloride can no longer pass directly from the interstitial space into the milk space and must be secreted by the cellular route.

The next changes to occur are increases in the concentrations of serum IgA and lactoferrin (see Fig. 30-4*B*).[27] The concentrations of these two important protective proteins remain high for the first 48 hours postpartum, the two together comprising as much as 10% by weight of the milk before they decrease rapidly after day 2 postpartum, as a consequence of both dilution as milk

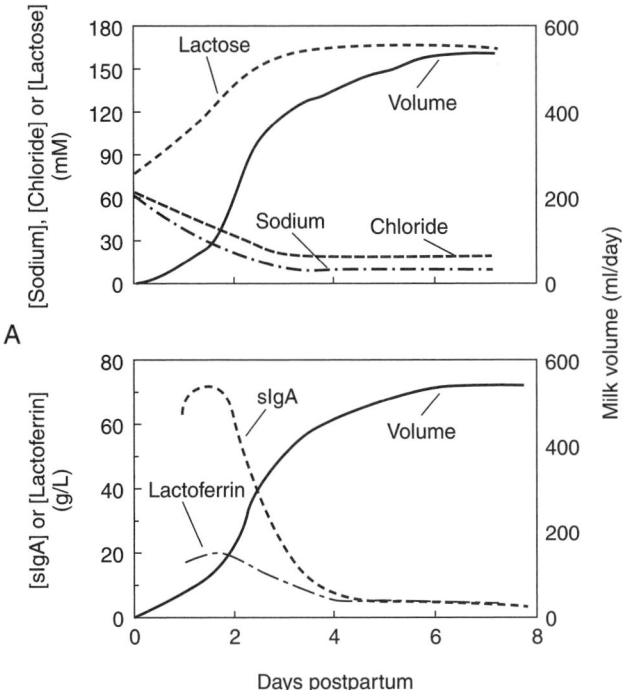

A

B

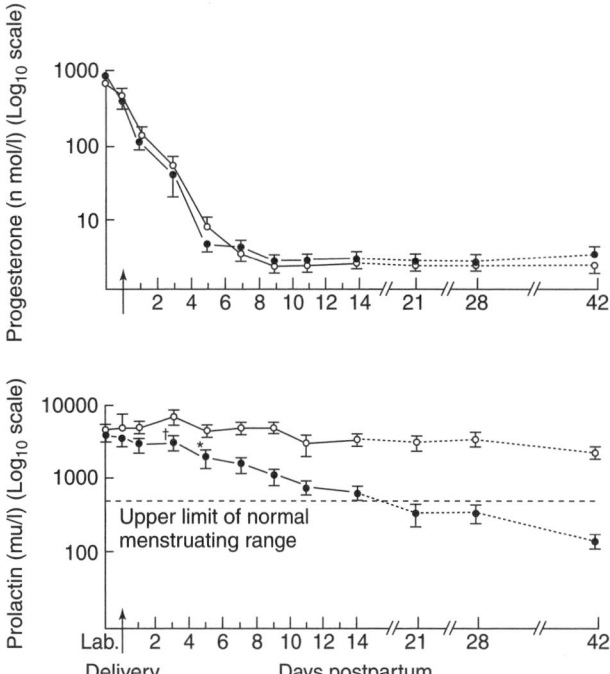

Figure 30–4. Changes in the concentration of certain milk components during the first week postpartum. **A,** Time course of changes in the lactose, chloride and sodium concentrations contrasted with the mean milk volume transfer to the infant. (Data from reference 39.) Changes in these milk components begin immediately postpartum and are complete at least 24 hours before achievement of a steady state in milk volume. As described in the text, the decrease in sodium and chloride and increase in lactose concentration reflect closure of the tight junctions between the mammary epithelial cells. **B,** Changes in the concentration of secretory IgA and lactoferrin during the onset of lactation in women. (Data replotted from reference 27. Figure modified from Neville MC, et al: Pediatr Clin North Am *48*:35, 2001. Used by permission.)

Figure 30–5. Maternal hormone levels after parturition in breast-feeding and non–breast-feeding women. Breast-feeding subjects (n = 10; *open circles*); non-breast-feeding subjects (n = 9; *filled circles*). *P* <0.01. (From Martin RH, et al: Human alpha-lactalbumin and hormonal factors in pregnancy and lactation, Clin Endocrinol *13*:223, 1980. Reprinted with permission.)

volume increases and of an actual decrease in the rate of secretion, particularly in the case of immunoglobulins. By day 8 postpartum, these protective proteins together comprise less than 1% of the total weight of the milk; however, their secretion rate is still substantial, amounting to 2 to 3 g/day for each protein. Concentrations of oligosaccharides in milk are also high in the early secretion product of the mammary gland, amounting to as much as 2% of milk weight on day 4 postpartum. These complex sugars are also considered to have substantial protective effect against a variety of infections.[28]

Finally, 36 to 48 hours postpartum, milk secretion begins in earnest (see Fig. 30-4). This volume increase is perceived by the parturient woman as the coming-in of the milk and reflects a massive increase in the rates of synthesis and secretion of almost all the components of mature milk including but not limited to lactose, protein, lipid, calcium, sodium, magnesium, and potassium.

Hormonal Requirements for Secretory Activation

It has been clear for nearly three decades that the major inhibitor of milk production during pregnancy is progesterone.[6] Once birth occurs, a developed mammary epithelium, the continuing presence of levels of prolactin near 200 ng/mL, and a fall in progesterone are necessary for the onset of copious milk secretion. The levels of these hormones are shown in Figure 30-5.

Evidence is clear for the inhibitory effect of progesterone during pregnancy in women. Thus removal of the placenta, the source of progesterone during pregnancy in this species, has long been known to be necessary for the initiation of milk secretion.[29] Conversely, retained placental fragments with the potential to secrete progesterone have been reported to delay secretory activation.[30] The conundrum that progesterone does not inhibit established lactation was solved when Haslam and Shyamala showed that progesterone receptors are lost in lactating mammary tissues.[31]

In most species high levels of plasma prolactin also appear to be essential for both secretory activation and continued lactation. In women, for example, bromocriptine and other analogues of dopamine, drugs that effectively prevent prolactin secretion, inhibit the onset of lactation when given in appropriate doses.[26] Conversely, an older hypothesis that a prolactin surge is the trigger for secretory activation is probably incorrect. Although a biphasic rise is associated with the stress of parturition in women,[32] it precedes the onset of copious milk secretion by 2 days.

Delays in Secretory Activation

A delay in the onset of milk secretion is a significant problem for the initiation of breast-feeding in a large number of women. For normal women the timing of secretory activation has been determined carefully from milk volume or composition in a few studies of middle-class white women.[6] Most of these data are in reasonable accord but some do suggest that either parity or previous lactation experience may influence the timing of secretory activation. Various pathologic conditions have been reported to delay secretory activation in women including cesarean section, diabetes, obesity,[33] and stress during parturition.[34] The role of cesarean section is controversial, no effect having been found in a large study from the laboratory of Peter Hartmann[35]; a small effect, statistically significant, was found in a more recent study where breast fullness and the appearance of casein in the secretion were measured.[34]

Women with poorly controlled diabetes, studied in both the United States[36] and Australia,[37] often had a delay in secretory activation. In a recent, well-controlled study stress during parturition, accompanied by an increase in cord blood glucose, had the same result and milk production on day 5 postpartum was significantly decreased. The final apparent cause of delayed milk secretion, obesity, has only come to our attention recently. In studies reviewed by Rasmussen and associates,[33] women with a high prepartum body mass index had more difficulty initiating lactation. Is there a common thread in all these conditions? Poorly controlled diabetes is associated with higher blood glucose. Stress and obesity both lead to insulin resistance and higher blood glucose. It is not clear how exposure to increased glucose could alter the onset or course of lactation, but this factor requires serious investigation in the future.

SUMMARY

Milk secretion is a robust process that proceeds according to plan in at least 85% of women postpartum. With assistance in the techniques of breast-feeding, anecdotal evidence suggests that at least 97% of women can successfully breast-feed their infants. The reasons of lack of success in breast-feeding are not well-understood because it is easy to substitute formula when infants fail to thrive on the breast, at least in Western societies. Although this is not the place to discuss possible pathologic mechanisms, it should be noted that breast-feeding failure usually takes place in the first week or so postpartum and a much better understanding of the mechanisms by which milk secretion is initiated during this period may help us to understand why some women have serious problems with lactation. Other areas that require attention are the behavioral correlates of breast-feeding and the transfer of drug and toxins into milk. The latter may have a long-term impact on infant health and should receive additional attention.

ACKNOWLEDGMENT

Preparation of this article was supported in part by grant #HD19547 from the U.S. National Institutes of Health.

REFERENCES

1. Wysolmerski JJ, Van Houten JN: Normal mammary development and disorders of breast development and function. *In* Burrow G (ed.), Endotext.com, *http://www.endotext.org/pregnancy/pregnancy5/pregnancyframe5.htm*, Endotext.org, 2002.
2. Pechoux C, et al: Localization of thrombospondin, CD36 and CD51 during pre-natal development of the human mammary gland. Differentiation, *57*:133, 1994.
3. Russo J, Russo IH: Development of the human mammary gland. *In* Neville MC, Daniel CW (eds.): The Mammary Gland. New York, Plenum, 1987, pp 67–96.
4. Anderson E, et al: Estrogen responsiveness and control of normal human breast proliferation. J Mammary Gland Biol Neoplasia *3*:23, 1998.
5. Kleinberg DL: Early mammary development: growth hormone and IGF-1. J Mammary Gland Biol Neoplasia *2*:49, 1997.
6. Neville MC, et al: Hormonal regulation of mammary differentiation and lacta-tion. J Mammary Gland Biol Neoplasia, 7:49, 2002.
7. Wilde CJ, et al: Autocrine regulation of milk secretion by a protein in milk. Biochem J *305*:51, 1995.
8. Strange R, et al: Apoptotic cell death and tissue remodeling during mouse mammary gland involution. Development *115*:49–58, 1992.
9. Neville MC: Anatomy and Physiology of Lactation. Pediatr Clin North Am *48*:1, 2001.
10. Huston GE, Patton S: Factors related to the formation of cytoplasmic crescents on milk fat globules. J Dairy Sci *73*:2061, 1990.
11. Linzell JL, Peaker M: Mechanism of milk secretion. Physiol Rev *51*:564, 1971.
12. Kraehenbuhl J-P, Hunziker W: Epithelial transcytosis of immunoglobulins. J Mammary Gland Biol Neoplasia *3*:289, 1998.
13. Nguyen D-AD, Neville MC: Tight junction regulation in the mammary gland. J Mammary Gland Biol Neoplasia *3*:233, 1998.
14. Seelig LL Jr., Beer AE: Transepithelial migration of leukocytes in the mammary gland of lactating rats. Biol Reprod *22*:1157, 1981.
15. Morton JA: The clinical usefulness of breast milk sodium in the assessment of lactogenesis. Pediatrics *93*:802, 1994.
16. Neville MC: Volume and caloric density of human milk. In: Jensen RG (ed.): Handbook of Milk Composition. San Diego, Academic Press, 1995, pp 101–113.
17. McNeilly AS, et al: Release of oxytocin and prolactin in response to suckling. BMJ Clin Res *286*:257, 1983.
18. Ardran GM, et al: A cineradiographic study of breast feeding. Br J Radiol *31*:156, 1958.
19. Ueda T, et al: Influence of psychological stress on suckling-induced pulsatile oxytocin release. Obstet Gynecol *84*:259, 1994.
20. Coiro V, et al: Inhibition of oxytocin response to breast stimula-tion in normal women and the role of endogenous opioids. Acta Endocrinol *126*:213, 1992.
21. Little RE, et al: Maternal alcohol use during breast-feeding and infant mental and motor development at one year. New Engl J Med *321*:425, 1989.
22. Rayner VC, et al: Chronic intracerebroventricular morphine and lactation in rats: dependence and tolerance in relation to oxytocin neurones. J Physiol *396*:319, 1995.
23. Prentice AM, Whitehead RG: The energetics of human reproduction. In: Loudon A, Racey T (eds.), Reproductive Energetics in Mammals. Oxford, Oxford University Press, 1987, pp. 275–304.
24. Kalkwarf HJ: Hormonal and dietary regulation of changes in bone density during lactation and after weaning in women. J Mammary Gland Biol Neoplasia *4*:319, 1999.
25. McNeilly AS: Lactational control of reproduction. Reprod Fertil Dev *13*:583, 2001.
26. Neville MC, Walsh CT: Effects of drugs on milk secretion and composition. *In* Bennett PN (ed.): Drugs and Human Lactation. Amsterdam, Elsevier, 1996, pp 15–45.
27. Lewis-Jones DI, et al: Sequential changes in the antimicrobial protein concen-trations in human milk during lactation and its relevance to banked human milk. Pediatr Res *19*:561, 1985.
28. Newburg DS: Oligosaccharides and glycoconjugates of human milk: their role in host defense. J Mammary Gland Biol Neoplasia *1*:271, 1996.
29. Halban J: Die innere Secretion von Ovarium und Placenta und ihre Bedeutung für die Function der Milchdrüse. Arch Gynaekol *75*:353, 1905.
30. Neifert MR, et al: Failure of lactogenesis associated with placental retention. Am J Obstet Gyn *140*:477, 1981.
31. Haslam SZ, Shyamala G: Effect of oestradiol on progesterone receptors in normal mammary glands and its relationship with lactation. Biochem J *182*:127, 1979.
32. Rigg LA, Yen SS: Multiphasic prolactin secretion during parturition in human subjects. Am J Obstet Gynecol *128*:215, 1977.
33. Rasmussen KM, et al: Obesity may impair lactogenesis II. J Nutr *131*:3009, 2001.
34. Chen DC, et al: Stress during labor and delivery and early lactation perform-ance. Am J Clin Nutr *68*:335, 1998.
35. Kulski JK, et al: Normal and Caesarean section delivery and the initiation of lac-tation in women. Aust J Exp Biol Med Sci *59*:405, 1981.
36. Neubauer SH, et al: Delayed lactogenesis in women with insulin-dependent dia-betes mellitus. Am J Clin Nutr *58*:54, 1993.
37. Arthur PG, et al: Milk lactose, citrate and glucose as markers of lactogenesis in normal and diabetic women. J Pediatr Gastroenterol Nutr *9*:488, 1989.
38. Neville MC, et al: Studies in human lactation: milk volumes in lactating women during the onset of lactation and full lactation. Am J Clin Nutr *48*:1375, 1988.
39. Neville MC, et al: Studies in human lactation: milk volume and nutrient com-position during weaning and lactogenesis. Am J Clin Nutr *54*:81, 1991.
40. Martin RH, et al: Human alpha-lactalbumin and hormonal factors in pregnancy and lactation. Clin Endocrinol *13*:223, 1980.

Gilberto R. Pereira

31 Nutritional Assessment

Newborn infants, especially those born prematurely or who are ill, are at great risk for the development of nutritional deficiencies that can adversely affect their postnatal growth. The susceptibility of the neonate to the development of such deficiencies results from the rapid growth velocity of the newborn period, the metabolic immaturity of several organ systems, and the difficulty in meeting the additional nutritional needs imposed by illness, surgical stress, or excessive nutrient losses.

The purpose of this chapter is to outline a practical approach to the nutritional assessment of neonates through the combined evaluation of the following: (1) medical history; (2) physical examination; (3) nutritional intake; (4) body composition; (5) anthropometry; and (6) biochemical markers.

MEDICAL HISTORY

The nutritional evaluation of the newborn infant begins with the analysis of both the maternal medical history during the pregnancy and the neonatal medical history.

The maternal medical history can be obtained by interviewing the mother and by reviewing her medical record. Both are often necessary to retrieve pertinent data, such as (1) maternal weight gain during the pregnancy; (2) maternal nutritional intake before and during the pregnancy; (3) history of chronic illness; (4) family history of chromosomal, metabolic, and endocrinologic disorders; (5) results of amniocentesis and fetal ultrasonographic examinations; (6) use of medications during pregnancy; (7) complications of pregnancy known to cause either retardation or acceleration of fetal growth (Table 31-1); and (8) specific maternal nutrient deficiencies (e.g., iron, folate, and vitamin B_6).

The medical history of the neonate from birth should be reviewed, including the identification of conditions known to increase metabolic demands (respiratory distress, bronchopulmonary dysplasia, congestive heart failure, sepsis, surgery, and cold stress) and nutrient losses (chronic diarrhea, excessive drainage from chest tubes, ostomies and fistulas). In addition, the time during which the infant had been given improper nutritional intake, the mode of alimentation, and the occurrence of feeding intolerance should be noted. Special attention is also paid to the use of medications known to increase metabolic rate (theophylline, corticosteroids) or to interact with nutrient absorption (phenobarbital).

PHYSICAL EXAMINATION

The general physical examination of the newborn infant offers a unique opportunity for the evaluation of nutritional status. By simple inspection, one can assess the lack or presence of physical activity, muscle wasting, and subcutaneous fat. In addition, the examination of the head configuration, skin, hair, and mucous membranes can be instrumental in identifying the deficiency of specific nutrients. By palpation one can assess the presence of craniotabes, raised skin rashes, and bone prominences such as rachitic rosary and healing fractures (Table 31-2). The use of anthropometry for protein-energy assessment is described in a separate section of this chapter.

NUTRITIONAL INTAKE

Optimal nutritional intake by neonates is considered as the diet that supports appropriate growth according to standards without imposing stress on the infants' immature metabolic and excretory functions.[1] Other models for the estimation of nutritional requirements include net uptake of nutrients from the umbilical circulation;[2] nutrient balance studies;[3, 4] infusion of stable isotopes;[5,6] intake of human milk;[7] and the determination of the optimal intake that prevents nutritional deficiencies and allows for favorable growth and developmental outcome.[8] The estimation of dietary intake in neonates is much simpler than that in older children and adults because of the lack of diversity in the neonatal diet, the practice of routinely recording the infant's dietary intake, and the well-documented composition of milk, infant formulas, parenteral nutrition solutions, and nutritional supplements. Accurate estimation of dietary intake in breast-fed infants, however, is more complicated because of the known variability in the composition of human milk among individual mothers and the difficulty of estimating milk intake during feedings. In practice, the composition of human milk is assumed to approximate the average values described for preterm and term human milk, and the volume of breast milk ingested is estimated by weighing the infant immediately before and after feeding, using electronic scales.[9] Computerized programs for assessment of dietary intake are now commonly used by nutrition support services to facilitate the calculation of nutritional intake for patients receiving parenteral and enteral nutrition.

Resting energy expenditure (REE) in premature and in full-term infants can be measured by open circuit indirect calorimetry or by the elimination of stable isotope doubly labeled water ($^2H_2^{18}O$); both methods show comparable results.[10] The estimation of total energy requirement is done by adding the REE to the energy cost of the following: (1) physical activity; (2) thermoregulation; (3) growth; (4) thermic effect of food; and (5) fecal and urinary losses. Energy requirements in full-term neonates receiving enteral feedings vary from 100 to 120 kcal/kg/day.[11] Energy intake as high as 148 kcal/kg/day has been recommended for premature infants to promote weight gain at *in utero* rates.[12] Nevertheless, this level of intake is currently considered excessive because it leads to fat retention at rates significantly greater than those observed in the fetus of similar gestational age.[13] Higher energy requirements than those presented earlier may be present in patients with fever, increased work of breathing,[14] and hypothermia, and in those with ostomy losses or exhibiting catch-up growth. On the contrary, lower energy requirements should be prescribed for patients receiving parenteral nutrition (85 to 100 kcal/kg/day), because energy is neither used for intestinal digestion and absorption of feedings nor lost in the stools, and for infants with limited physical activity due to administration of skeletal muscle relaxants or heavy sedatives. Failure to recognize these changes in energy requirements may have a detrimental effect on the infant's postnatal growth velocity.[15]

The evaluation of nutritional intake in neonates should encompass the period from birth to the time of assessment. The adequacy of nutritional intake can be evaluated by comparing actual intake of a nutrient to a recommended optimal level. Daily

TABLE 31-1

Common Conditions Leading to Acceleration and Retardation of Fetal Growth

Growth Acceleration

Maternal	Diabetes class A and B
	Obesity
	Hyperglycemia resulting from steroid treatment
	Use of lithium during pregnancy
Fetal	Transposition of the aorta
	Beckwith-Wiedemann syndrome
	Soto syndrome (cerebral gigantism)

Growth Retardation

Maternal	Malnutrition
	Pregnancy-induced hypertension
	Chronic hypertension
	Drug addiction (heroin, alcohol)
	Placental insufficiency
	Diabetes class C, D, and E
	Smoking
	High altitude
Fetal	Multiple pregnancy
	Congenital anomaly
	Congenital infection
	Radiation

TABLE 31-2

Clinical Findings in Nutritional Deficiency in Neonates

Clinical Finding	Deficiency
Lethargy	Protein, calorie
Pallor	Iron, copper, folate, vitamin B_{12}
Muscle wasting	Protein, calorie
Edema	Protein, zinc
Craniotabes, frontal bossing	Vitamin D
Hair depigmentation	Protein, zinc
Keratomalacia (eyes)	Vitamin A
Angular stomatitis	Vitamin B_2
Glossitis	Niacin
Goiter	Iodine
Follicular hyperkeratosis	Vitamin A
Dry skin, scaly dermatitis	Essential fatty acids
Acrodermatitis	Zinc
Petechia, ecchymosis	Vitamin C
Rachitic rosary, bone thickening	Vitamin D
Osteopenia	Calcium, phosphorus

TABLE 31-3

Nutritional Needs of the Full-Term and Premature Infant

	Premature		Full-Term
	<1 kg	1–2.5 kg	
	per kg/day		
Protein (g)	4	3.5	2
Na (mEq)	3.5	3	3
Cl (mEq)	3.1	2.5	2.3
K (mEq)	2.5	2.5	2.4
Ca (mg)	210	185	130
P (mg)	140	123	70
Mg (mg)	10	8.5	5
Fe (mg)	2–4	1–2	2
Biotin (µg)	1–1.4	1–2	1–2
Pantothenic acid (mg)	5–9	1–1.4	1–1.4
Choline (mg)	5–9	5–9	5–9
	per day		
Fluoride (mg)	0.1(?)	0.1(?)	0.1(?)
Cu (mg)	0.17	0.1–0.5	0.5–1
Zn (mg)	1.5	1.5–3	3–5
Mn (mg)	0.01–0.02	0.02–0.04	0.5–1
Cr (µg)	2–4	2–6	10–40
I (µg)	5	5–10	10–15
Se (µg)	1.5–2.5	1.5–7.5	10–60
Mo (µg)	2–3	2–7.5	30–80
Vitamin A (IU)	1000	1000	1000
Vitamin D (IU)	400	400	400
Vitamin E (IU)	5–25	5–25	4
Vitamin K (µg)	5	5	5
Vitamin C (mg)	60	60	35
Vitamin B_1 (mg)	0.2	0.2	0.2
Vitamin B_2 (mg)	0.4	5	5
Vitamin B_6 (mg)	0.2	0.2	0.2
Vitamin B_{12} (µg)	0.15	0.15	0.15
Niacin (mg)	5	5	5
Folic acid (µg)	50	50	50

nutritional requirements for premature and full-term infants are given in Table 31-3.

BODY COMPOSITION

At birth, the body composition of the neonate varies both with the length of pregnancy and with the occurrence of intrauterine complications that affect fetal growth. Ziegler and coworkers[16] and Widdowson[17] have been foremost in describing the changes in body composition that fetuses undergo with increasing gestational age. These changes include a progressive decrease in total body water, extracellular water, sodium, and chloride, and a progressive increase in intracellular water, potassium, calcium, and magnesium. In addition, the body stores of protein, fat, glycogen, and mineralized bone also increase with gestational age (Table 31-4). Complications of pregnancy known to either

retard or accelerate fetal growth also can influence the body composition of the neonate. For example, infants who are small for gestational age (SGA) have reduced total body fat, whereas infants who are large for gestational age (LGA) have increased total body fat when compared with infants who are appropriate for gestational age (AGA). Enzi and associates[18] demonstrated that the body fat content approximated 12% in SGA infants, 14% in AGA infants, and 18% in LGA infants. Similarly, Fee and Weil[19] reported a total body fat content of 21% in the LGA infant of a diabetic mother.

Significant changes in body composition are observed with growth during the neonatal period and throughout the first year of life (Fig. 31-1). These changes include (1) a progressive increase in the amount of adipose tissue, which peaks between 4 and 6 months of postnatal life[20] and declines slightly by 12 months of age; and (2) a progressive decrease in total body water, with a relative increase in the amount of intracellular water.[21] The proportion of body weight represented by minerals and protein remains relatively constant from birth to 1 year of age (see Fig. 31-1).

Widdowson and Dickerson[22] described the contributions of various organ systems to the total body mass of premature and full-term infants compared with that of adults (Table 31-5). From their data, it can be seen that certain organ systems such as the heart, bony skeleton, kidneys, and liver maintain the same percentage of total body weight at 24 weeks and 40 weeks of gestational age, as well as during childhood. The skin and the brain make up a larger proportion of neonatal body weight than of adult body weight, whereas skeletal muscle represents a

TABLE 31-4

Water, Protein, Fat, and Mineral Content of the Fetus

Body Weight (g)	Gestational Age (wk)	Water (g)	Fat (g)	Protein (g)	Ca (g)	P (g)	Mg (g)	Na (g)	K (g)	Cl (g)	Fe (mg)	Ca (mg)	Zn (mg)
500	22	433	6	43	2.4	1.5	0.09	1.1	0.8	1.2	30	1.7	8.9
1000	26	850	23	86	5.7	3.4	0.21	2.1	1.7	2.3	64	3.8	17.6
1500	29	1240	60	135	9.8	5.6	0.33	2.9	2.5	3.3	101	6.0	25.9
2000	32	1598	120	188	14.7	8.3	0.45	3.7	3.4	4.2	141	8.1	33.8
2500	35	1925	208	244	19.9	11.0	0.57	4.5	4.2	4.7	183	10.1	41.2
3000	38	2217	330	334	25.1	13.9	0.69	5.5	5.0	5.3	227	12.0	48.1
3500	42	2380	525	446	30.3	17.3	0.80	6.5	5.8	5.7	283	14.3	53.6

Adapted from Widdowson EM: *In* Assali NS (ed): Biology of Gestation. Vol II, The Fetus and Newborn. New York, Academic Press, 1972, pp 1–44.

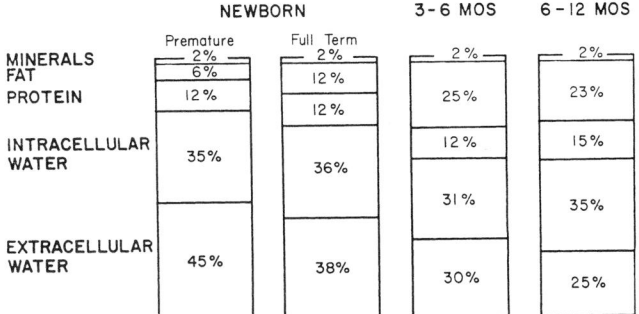

Figure 31–1. Body composition from birth to 12 months of age. (Data from references 19 and 122.)

TABLE 31-5

Contribution of Organs and Major Tissues to Body Weight (%)

Organ or Tissue	Premature (20–24 wk)	Full-Term Newborn	Adult
Skeletal muscle	25.0	25.0	40.0
Skeleton	22.0	18.0	14.0
Heart	0.6	0.5	0.4
Lungs	3.3	1.5	1.4
Liver	4.0	5.0	2.0
Kidneys	0.7	1.0	0.5
Brain	13.0	12.0	2.0

Adapted from Widdowson EM: *In* Assali NS (ed): Biology of Gestation. Volume II. The Fetus and Newborn. New York, Academic Press, 1972, pp 1–44.

relatively lower percentage of neonatal body weight. These studies, performed by chemical analysis of infant cadavers, are still considered the gold standard for measurements of body composition.

Over the past several decades, various methods have been developed for the indirect assessment of body composition in living infants. Although some of these methods have technical limitations, they have the advantages of being noninvasive and applicable for longitudinal measurements in growing infants.

The total body potassium (K40) counter has been used to assess lean body mass, because potassium resides only in the lean body mass (LBM) and not in adipose tissue. This method is based on the supposition that naturally occurring potassium (K39) contains a fixed proportion of the radioactive K40, which can be measured by a counter. Fat mass is determined by subtracting the calculated LBM from total body weight. Limitations to the use of this method include the insufficient sensitivity of the K40 counter for small infants and the variable potassium content of viscera and skeletal muscle in children of different ages. Spady and colleagues[23] used this method to assess the effect of maternal smoking on infant body composition.

Neutral fat does not bind water and, therefore, methods to estimate total body water have been developed to determine the nonfat compartment of the body. The oral administration of doubly labeled water, with a known amount of the stable isotopes deuterium (^{2}H) and oxygen 18 (^{18}O), has been used for the estimation of total body water. This method is based on the dilution of the ^{2}H and ^{18}O isotopes in body fluid such as saliva, urine, or serum, after a period of equilibration.[24] The changes in the water content of the LBM, which occur at various ages and among different individuals, represent a major limitation of this method, which is further explained in the stable isotope section of this chapter.

Total body electrical conductivity (TOBEC) has been used to estimate fat-free mass (FFM) by detecting a change in the electro-

magnetic field. This change is caused by shifts in the amount and volume distribution of electrolytes that are present in the FFM.[25] Fat mass can be estimated by subtracting the FFM from the total body weight. This method is safe, noninvasive, and rapid, but it has some limitations. First, the model used to calibrate this method was the infant miniature pig and not the human neonate. Second, the TOBEC scan is costly, not portable, and not uniformly available. Standard values for FFM and for total body water in infants using TOBEC have been reported by Fiorotto and associates.[25]

A dual-energy x-ray absorptiometry (DEXA) method has been proposed for the determination of lean and fat body masses.[26] This technique employs low-radiation x-ray sources that provide alternating pulses of 70 and 140 kV. After passing through the infant's body, the rays are filtered for analysis. Estimates of body composition derive from the x-ray absorption capacity of different body tissues. This method is safe, rapid, and noninvasive and allows for measurements of bone mineral content, as well as lean and fat body masses.

Magnetic resonance imaging (MRI) is a noninvasive method that allows for fast and reproducible measurements of adipose tissue content in neonates with low intra- and intercoefficients of variability.[27] The MRI measurements of total body fat have been validated against stable isotope dilution methods in term infants with reasonable correlation.[28] A comparison of the various methods of body composition employing different methods is presented in Table 31-6.

ANTHROPOMETRY

Anthropometric assessment provides insight into the quality and quantity of growth in newborn infants. The assessments done at the time of birth reflect the pattern of fetal growth, whereas longitudinal assessments reflect postnatal growth.

The three single measurements most often used for the nutritional assessment of neonates at birth are weight, length, and

TABLE 31-6

Body Composition of Neonates as Assessed by Various Methods

Methods	TBW (%)	ECW (%)	FFM (%)	TBF (%)
Total Body Potassium Counter				
Term Infant[23]	—	—	89.1	10.9
Doubly Labeled Water				
Term Infant[24]	—	—	—	—
TOBEC				
Term Infant[25]	69	—	86.7	13.2
DEXA				
Preterm Infants[134,135]	—	—	—	9–11
Term Infant[26,132,133,134]			82	13.4–18
MRI				
Term Infant[28]	53–69	—	—	17–22

TBW, total body water; ECW, extracellular water; FFM, fat-free mass; TBF, total body fat; TOBEC, total body electrical conductivity; DEXA, dual energy x-ray absorptiometry; MRI, magnetic resonance imaging.

head circumference (HC). When plotted on standard growth charts against gestational age, these measurements indicate whether the infant is AGA, SGA, or LGA. Pathophysiologic conditions that cause aberrant fetal growth increase the risks of perinatal morbidity and mortality.[32] Numerous standard curves for the assessment of birth weight, length, and HC have been published, and major differences among them can be observed.[33-37] These differences appear to be related to the various ethnic, socioeconomic, and environmental characteristics of the reference population. Care must be taken to assess the newborn infant with a growth chart derived from a population with comparable characteristics.

Measurements of weight, length, and HC are also used longitudinally for the assessment of postnatal growth. In the hospitalized neonate, these measurements are performed frequently to determine whether adequate growth is occurring on a particular nutritional regimen. Nevertheless, it should be acknowledged that changes in nutritional intake or in infant needs might take several days to be reflected in anthropometric parameters.

Weight

Weight for age is often considered the gold standard for the assessment of postnatal growth. Hospitalized infants are routinely weighed on a daily basis. However, care must be taken to weigh the infant unclothed and to correct for the weight of attached equipment, such as endotracheal tube, chest tube, intravenous board, gauze, and tape. The assessment of weight gain velocity over time is more useful than one single measurement of weight for age. Premature infants are expected to gain weight at rates comparable to *in utero* standards.[38] Although this appears to be the best approach available, a number of investigators have questioned the validity of this assumption.[39, 40] Dancis and associates published growth curves that take into account the birth weight of the preterm infant and the expected percentage of weight loss during the first 50 days of life.[39] These curves have been modified, demonstrating that advances in medical care and nutritional support have increased the rates of postnatal growth in premature infants.[40] I have studied 50 healthy AGA infants with birth weights less than 2000 g. Despite adequate nutritional intake, 48% of these infants had weight values that fell below the 5th percentile on the growth chart, based on intrauterine standards at some time during their hospital course. In addition, one must be cautious when interpreting weight loss in the first postnatal week, because it is caused predominantly by loss of extracellular water.[41] Weight measurements alone cannot be considered an accurate indicator of lean body mass, nor can they distinguish between gains in lean body mass and fluid gains. The expected rate of fetal weight gain during the last trimester of pregnancy is 10 to 15 g/kg/day.

Length

Length for age is an extremely useful measurement of nutritional status in older children.[42] Neonates, however, are difficult to measure accurately. An accurate length measurement in neonates can be obtained when two trained observers use a rigid surface containing a stationary headboard, a movable footboard, and a built-in centimeter scale. When inter- and intraobserver reliability can be assured, serial measurements of length are excellent for following longitudinal growth. Unlike changes in weight, changes in length are not influenced by fluid status. The expected rate of fetal growth in length during the last trimester of pregnancy is 0.75 cm/week.

Head Circumference

The measurement of HC provides an indirect measurement of brain growth and is, therefore, an important part of the nutritional assessment, both at birth and in longitudinal studies. At birth, the detection of microcephaly indicates retarded brain growth during fetal life, which may result from various causes, such as chromosomal abnormalities, maternal drug addiction, infection, or lack of nutrient availability secondary to placental insufficiency. The lack of brain growth associated with a lower number of cells indicates an insult that occurred during the first trimester of pregnancy. Lack of brain growth caused by small cell size generally indicates a chronic insult throughout pregnancy. Neurologic outcome can be poor in microcephalic infants, particularly if no catch-up head growth is observed during the neonatal period.[43-48]

When measured longitudinally, HC is a useful tool for nutritional assessment, except in the presence of hydrocephalus. Decreases in HC are not unusual during the first few days of life, while head molding and scalp edema are still resolving. For that reason, the HC should be remeasured 3 days postnatally. In the newborn period, the brain is spared during mild to moderate malnutrition. In premature infants, a decrease in nutritional intake that results in slowing of weight and length velocities might not necessarily affect head growth velocity. In addition, in premature infants on a regimen of advancing caloric intake, head growth precedes the onset of growth in weight and length. The maintenance of normal head growth in the neonatal period is important because a rapid period of brain growth, evidenced by DNA synthesis, formation of dendritic synapsis, and myelination, occurs between 28 and 44 weeks postconception.[37-39] Infants

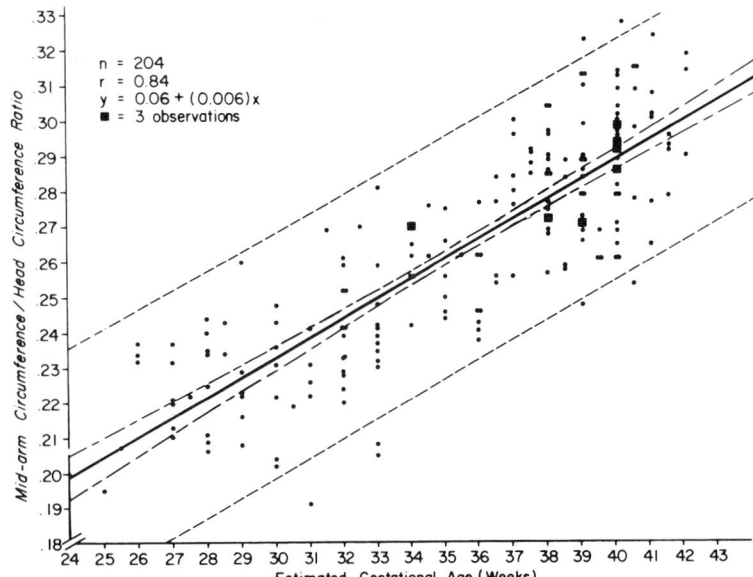

n = 204
r = 0.84
y = 0.06 + (0.006)x
■ = 3 observations

Figure 31-2. Correlation between midarm circumference and gestational age. — represents mean midarm circumference; —- represents 95% confidence limits on predicted mean; ---represents 95% confidence limits for one observation.

who are born with normal head size but who become microcephalic during the postnatal period are at significantly increased risk of poor developmental outcome.[44] The expected rate of fetal head circumference growth during the last trimester of pregnancy is 0.75 cm/week.

Midarm Circumference

The midarm circumference (MAC) reflects the combination of muscle mass and fat stores in the upper arm and rapidly diminishes when protein and fat stores are depleted.[42] Standard values for MAC obtained from neonates born between 24 and 42 weeks of gestation have been reported by Sasanow and colleagues.[49] These data document a predictable linear rise in MAC with increasing birth weight and gestational age (Fig. 31-2). MAC is measured at the midpoint of the upper arm, which is found by measuring the distance between the acromion and the olecranon with the arm held in a horizontal position. In one study, we documented that serial measurements of MAC were more sensitive than those of weight or length for assessing nutritional status in growing premature infants.[50]

Skinfold Thickness

The simplest way to estimate body fat is to measure the thickness of the subcutaneous tissue.[51] Standard measurements of skinfold thickness for premature and term infants have been reported.[52] In addition, serial measurements of skinfold thickness at the triceps or at the scapular site can provide information on the rates of fat accretion in premature and term infants.[53] The correct technique for measurement of skinfold thickness requires firm placement of the calipers without slippage for a minimum of 15 seconds. Several investigators have shown that holding the calipers for 60 seconds while measuring the skinfold thickness of the triceps is useful in eliminating false values resulting from edema.[54,55] Dauncey and colleagues have estimated total body fat percentages from measurements of skinfold thickness from multiple sites.[56] However, the rapidly changing distribution of fat accretion in premature infants makes it difficult to generate a consistent equation for predicting total body fat.[31] Ultrasonography has been used to measure skinfold thickness; however, these measurements appear to be less reproducible than those obtained with skinfold calipers.[57]

Arm Muscle and Arm Fat Areas

Once the measurements of MAC and triceps skinfold thickness at 15 seconds (TSF_{15}) and at 60 seconds (TSF_{60}) are obtained, one can then calculate the arm area (AA), the arm muscle area (AMA), the arm fat area (AFA), and the arm water area (AWA), using the following formulas:[58,59]

$$AA = MAC^2/4\pi$$

$$AMA = (MAC - \pi\,TSF_{15})^2/4\pi$$

$$AFA = AA - (MAC - \pi\,TSF_{60})^2/4\pi$$

$$AWA = AA - AMA - AFA$$

The measurement of TSF_{15} is thought to reflect subcutaneous fat and water; however, the TSF_{60} measurement is thought to reflect fat only, assuming the water has been squeezed out of the subcutaneous tissue.[55] Standard measurements of arm muscle and fat areas for infants at term have been published.[58]

Measurements of arm muscle and fat areas can be useful in the assessment of newborn infants who have experienced either fetal growth retardation or acceleration. For example, these measurements can identify reduced muscle or fat stores in growth-retarded infants who might be classified as AGA by weight criteria. Similarly, the measurements of TSF and AFA are proportionately greater in infants of diabetic mothers.[60, 61] These infants are known to have a greater percentage of their body mass as fat, compared with infants born to nondiabetic mothers.[19]

Ponderal Index and Midarm/Head Circumference Ratio

The ponderal index and the MAC/HC ratio provide information on the proportionality of body growth. As such, they potentially allow the estimation of stunting and wasting that have occurred either *in utero* or postnatally. When measured at birth, both indices have been shown to be more specific than weight for age alone in determining the risk of perinatal morbidity associated with intrauterine growth disorders.[52] When used longitudinally, these indices can assess whether length is spared at the expense of weight, or whether head growth is spared at the expense of somatic growth.

The ponderal index is calculated by using the following formula:[62]

$$weight\ (g) \times 100/length\ (cm^3)$$

The ponderal index has been shown to vary with the gestational age of the infant[63] and is useful for the identification of growth-retarded infants who are at risk for neonatal hypoglycemia.[62] The ponderal index can be greatly misleading if measurements of length are performed inaccurately, because this potential error is cubed during the calculation. The ponderal index has proved not useful for screening macrosomic infants at risk for hypoglycemia;[64] its use for longitudinal assessment of nutritional status in neonates has yet to be studied.

The MAC/HC ratio has proved useful as an index of body proportionality in neonates, because it compares an anthropometric measurement likely to be affected by lack of nutritional intake (MAC) with another measurement that is less likely to be affected by nutritional intake (HC). The rationale for its use is based on the observation that head growth is spared relative to somatic growth in malnourished infants. Standard values for the MAC/HC ratio obtained from infants born between 24 and 42 weeks' gestation have been reported by Sasanow and colleagues.[49] The MAC/HC ratio values increase progressively with the gestational age of the neonate (Fig. 31-3).

When used at birth, the MAC/HC ratio is more sensitive than either the ponderal index or weight for age in identifying neonates at risk of morbidity in association with intrauterine growth retardation or acceleration.[64] We have compared the serial measurements of the MAC/HC ratio and weight and length for age measurements in a large group of premature infants during the first few weeks of life. Although the two indices had comparable sensitivity, the MAC/HC had greater specificity in identifying protein-energy malnutrition in these infants.[65] We have also serially measured the MAC/HC ratio in premature infants to determine the proportionality of body growth throughout the first year of life. Our results indicate that premature infants, despite their small size at birth, maintain proportional growth similar to that of term infants (MAC/HC ratios < 0.3) during the first year, even though they demonstrate no

catch-up weight gain. Thus, it appears that premature infants have a regulatory mechanism that keeps their growth proportional as long as they receive adequate nutritional intake.[65]

Thigh Circumference and Thigh/Head Circumference Ratio

Ultrasonographic measurements of thigh, head, and abdominal circumferences have been used for the estimation of fetal weight during the last trimester of the pregnancy.[66] The chronology of adipose tissue deposition, being last in the lower extremity after occurring in other parts of the body, explains the benefits of the thigh circumference (TC) and the thigh/head ratio (THR) over other fetal parameters. Measurements of the TC are known to be affected by the position of the lower leg at the time that the measurement is being obtained. Ideally, the leg should be maintained at 90° flexion in relation to the thigh. Because of the inability to control leg position *in utero*, Warda and colleagues[67] identified a specific plane in the thigh (transitional plane), at the level of the nutrient foramen of the femur, that allows for ultrasonographic measurements to be performed in an accurate and reproducible manner.

Standard values for TC and THR have been reported for neonates born at gestational ages varying from 27 to 41 weeks and have been plotted against birth weight and gestational age.[68] The same study also reported a good correlation between the THR and the ponderal index. The usefulness of the TC and THR for the evaluation of infants who are either large or small for gestational age needs further study.

BIOCHEMICAL ASSESSMENT

Measurements of various biochemical markers in serum and in whole blood have been used to assess protein, mineral, and vitamin status in newborn infants. Although some of the data on the use of these indices are extrapolated from older children and adults, most of the data presented in this section are derived from studies performed in neonates. A major limitation to the interpretation of the serum concentration of any nutrient as a marker of nutritional status is that the intravascular space generally represents a small portion of the total body pool and, therefore, might not reflect total body stores. This principle can be applied to the majority of minerals, vitamins, and trace elements.

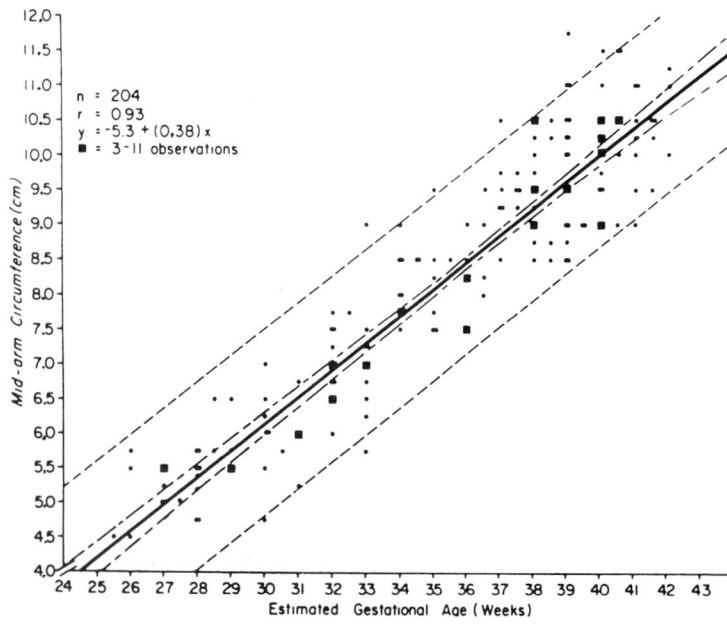

Figure 31-3. Correlation between midarm circumference and head-circumference ratio and gestational age. — represents mean midarm circumference; —- represents 95% confidence limits on predicted mean; --- represents 95% confidence limits for one observation.

The only exceptions are the serum proteins and some electrolytes such as sodium and chloride, which are predominantly concentrated in the extracellular fluid.

Serum Albumin

Serum albumin concentrations have been the mainstay of the biochemical assessment of nutritional status in neonates, children, and adults for several decades.[69] Serum albumin levels are lower in premature infants than in full-term infants because of a more rapid turnover of the albumin pool and a presumed decrease in the rate of synthesis by the immature liver. Albumin levels increase progressively with gestational age, varying from 2.5 to 3.5 g/dL in premature infants to 3.5 to 4.5 g/dL in term infants.[70] The serum half-life of albumin ranges from 14 to 21 days in the full-term neonate and from 5 to 7 days in the premature neonate, which makes it ideal for long-term assessment of nutritional status, but less than optimal for assessing short-term responses to changes in nutritional intake.[71]

Serum Transferrin

The serum concentration of transferrin has been used to assess protein status after nutritional rehabilitation in surgical adult patients and in pediatric cancer patients.[71-73] Transferrin has a serum half-life of 8 to 12 days, which potentially makes it a more responsive marker than albumin to recent changes in protein intake. However, serum transferrin comprises 80% of the total iron-binding capacity, and for that reason the serum level of this protein is elevated during iron deficiency, regardless of the protein status.[74] Serum levels of transferrin range from 90 mg/dL in neonates born at 25 weeks' gestation to 300 mg/dL in those born at term.[75] Like other serum proteins, transferrin concentrations increase with gestational age and body weight. LGA babies have higher concentrations than do AGA babies. Growth-retarded infants also have elevated serum levels of transferrin, most likely on the basis of iron deficiency.[75, 76] In spite of its usefulness for nutritional evaluation in the pediatric population, we were unable to demonstrate a role for serum transferrin in the longitudinal assessment of protein status in premature infants.[76, 77] In our study, changes in serum transferrin concentration, unlike serum transthyretin changes, neither reflected changes in protein intake nor correlated with weight gain velocity.[78-80]

Serum Transthyretin (Prealbumin)

Transthyretin is a minor thyroid-binding globulin and a co-carrier of vitamin A with retinol-binding protein.[81] Its half-life of approximately 2 days makes its serum concentrations responsive to recent changes in protein-energy intake. In contrast, serum transthyretin levels are not particularly useful for long-term nutritional assessment. The serum concentrations of transthyretin at birth range from 5 to 20 mg/dL and are lower in preterm than in term infants.[82, 83] The serum concentrations of this protein in adults are almost twice the values observed in newborn infants.[84] In newborns, increases in the serum concentrations of transthyretin occur rapidly with increases in protein intake, and these increases can predict weight gain velocity more accurately than the actual protein intake per se.[78] Nevertheless, several non-nutritional factors can affect the serum levels of transthyretin, thus limiting its usefulness for nutritional assessment. Transthyretin can act as an acute-phase reactant during neonatal sepsis.[84] In addition, either liver or renal disease can affect the production and degradation of transthyretin, thereby affecting its serum concentrations. Corticosteroids are known to increase the liver synthesis of transthyretin. For this reason, infants who receive dexamethasone for the treatment of bron-

chopulmonary dysplasia and infants whose mothers received betamethasone prenatally have elevated serum concentrations of transthyretin for approximately 2 weeks after these medications are discontinued.[85, 86]

Retinol-Binding Protein

Retinol-binding protein (RBP) is synthesized in the liver and has a serum half-life of approximately 12 hours. RBP is the main carrier of retinol (vitamin A), and its synthesis and release from hepatocytes are modulated by the availability of vitamin A. The serum concentrations of RBP at birth range from 1.2 to 3.5 mg/dL, and the values in premature infants are lower than those in term infants.[83-87] Because premature infants can become relatively vitamin A–deficient after birth, a low serum level of RBP might represent vitamin A deficiency rather than protein deficiency. Like transthyretin, the RBP serum concentrations can be elevated significantly by the administration of corticosteroids.[85, 86] To date, no studies have been undertaken to evaluate the usefulness of RBP in determining protein status in newborn infants.

Plasma Aminogram

The plasma concentration of amino acids is a dynamic function of the following variables: (1) recent protein intake, usually from the previous 24 hours; (2) gastrointestinal assimilation of dietary protein; and (3) uptake of amino acids from the plasma for protein synthesis in the liver. The plasma aminogram pattern has been used for the evaluation of both the quantity and quality of protein ingested by the neonate. The standard pattern of the plasma aminogram has been defined as the one observed postprandially in growing newborn infants fed human milk. It remains to be determined whether this pattern should also be used for nutritional evaluation in sick or malnourished infants. Rassin and colleagues[88, 89] and Gaull and coworkers[90] have studied the plasma aminogram in low birth weight infants fed formula containing either high (3 g/100 kcal) or low (1.5 g/100 kcal) protein content; infant feedings containing two types of protein with a predominance of either whey or casein were also evaluated in these studies. These investigators concluded that low birth weight infants fed formulas containing high protein with a predominance of casein had a higher concentration of plasma amino acids than did infants fed human milk. They also demonstrated that low birth weight infants had a limited capacity to convert methionine to cysteine and taurine, or phenylalanine to tyrosine, thus suggesting that the amino acids cystine, taurine, and tyrosine are essential for the premature infant, but not for the full-term infant. Heird and associates[91] reported a study in which the plasma aminogram was used for the evaluation of a pediatric amino acid solution. The study documented that infants receiving that particular amino acid mixture had plasma amino acid levels within the 95% confidence limits of the plasma concentration observed in breast-fed infants, except for one amino acid, phenylalanine. The study also showed that the ability of low birth weight infants to tolerate parenterally administered amino acids is not as limited as was previously thought.

3-Methylhistidine

This amino acid, a constituent of muscle protein, has unique properties in that it is not available for protein synthesis in the liver, and on its release from the muscle it is excreted unchanged in urine. Therefore, the excretion of this amino acid in the urine has been regarded as a reflection of skeletal muscle catabolism. Although the renal excretion of 3-methylhistidine has been shown to correlate with nitrogen balance in adults,[90, 91] this may not be clinically applicable to the neonate for several reasons: (1) the relative contribution of skeletal to total body mass is smaller in neonates than in adults (25% vs. 40%); (2) the muscle content of 3-methylhistidine in neonates is lower than that in adults (1.7 vs. 4.2 mL/g protein); and (3) the gastrointestinal tract of the neonate might provide a greater portion of 3-methylhistidine than does that of the adult.[92,94-96]

NUTRIENT BALANCE STUDIES

Nutrient balance studies have long been used to estimate nutrient retention in infants.[97,98] One can measure the total body balance of virtually any substance, including nitrogen, minerals, vitamins, and trace elements, by estimating intake and excretion.[97-100] Balance studies are labor intensive because of the need for meticulous methodology. A common goal of balance studies is to define parenteral and enteral nutrient requirements based on accretion and retention of administered compounds. Such studies have been reported for nitrogen,[95] fat,[99] calcium,[99-101] magnesium,[102] zinc, and copper,[103] among others. The techniques employed in these studies are not practical for routine clinical evaluations. Simplified balance studies have been performed with the goal of modifying a patient's nutritional regimen. Most often, these types of studies are used to give an estimate of energy and nitrogen balance, or to document excessive losses of specific nutrients in stools, urine, or other body fluids.

The single greatest limitation to any nutrient balance study is the accuracy with which specimens are collected.[104] This limitation is greater when applying balance techniques to young infants, because the loss of collected specimens, especially urine, is a frequent occurrence. Fomon and Owen[105] have emphasized that a significant overestimation in nitrogen retention can result from a small error either in the measurement of dietary intake or in the volume of urine collected. Another limitation of this method is that, although information can be obtained about net nutrient absorption and retention, no conclusions can be drawn about how the retained nutrient is used.

Balance studies are typically performed by measuring enteral and/or parenteral nutrient intake and subsequent excretion of the whole nutrient or its metabolite in urine, feces, sweat, or exhaled gases. Skin losses, particularly in extremely premature infants, can be large. Urine collections can be performed with relatively simple equipment such as urine bags and diapers, but this approach is fraught with problems because of specimen losses. Bag urine collections from female infants are particularly problematic, especially if the balance study lasts longer than 24 hours.[106,107] The use of metabolic beds ensures accuracy in the quantitation of urine and stool collected during balance studies.[104]

Several factors must be considered when balance studies are being interpreted for clinical or experimental purposes. Assuming adequate collection technique, the next issue is whether the data are representative of the infant's nutritional status. Typically, the shorter the collection period, the greater the chance that the data are not representative. Six-hour urine collections for nitrogen balance have been criticized on this basis. Furthermore, it is important to know the expected length of time that the body will retain a nutrient. If the excretion of a particular nutrient that was administered enterally is to be measured in the stool, one should mark the feedings with a nonabsorbable dye, such as carmine red, to increase the accuracy of the collection period.[104] Balance studies of enterally fed nutrients frequently require 72- to 96-hour collections because of the slow intestinal transit time of the neonate. On the other hand, the balance of exclusively parenterally administered nutrients, particularly in patients who are not stooling, can be done over shorter periods of time and extrapolated to a "daily" nutritional

requirement. This is frequently done when assessing sodium, potassium, and nitrogen balances in critically ill neonates.

Nitrogen balance can be used to determine protein requirements in neonates by determining the difference between nitrogen intake and excretion (urinary and fecal nitrogenous compounds). It is important to measure the total urinary nitrogen, as opposed to the more commonly used, but incomplete, urea urinary nitrogen, when recording urinary nitrogen losses. The estimation of protein requirements from balance studies is predicated on the assumption that the dietary requirement is satisfied once maximal nitrogen retention is attained. Protein requirements in neonates based on nitrogen balance studies range from 1.6 to 4.2 g/kg/day, depending on the type of protein received by the infant, the infant's physiologic status, and the infant's gestational age.[90,108]

Daily energy requirements[104] are not typically assessed by classic balance studies; rather, they are estimated by energy utilization techniques. These include direct and indirect calorimetry. Indirect calorimetry using an open circuit metabolic gas analyzer has been extensively validated in the neonatal literature. These studies can be done in patients who require mechanical ventilation if there is no air leak around the endotracheal tube, or in patients who are in an oxygen tent. Measurements are made of oxygen that is entrained and then removed from the system, with a subsequent calculation of the rate of oxygen consumed by the patient per unit of time. This oxygen consumption rate can then be converted to resting energy expenditure (REE) by using the Weir equation.[107] The REE value approaches, but is not equal to, the basal metabolic rate. Measurements of REE can be used to identify infants with increased energy needs (such as those with bronchopulmonary dysplasia or congestive heart failure) and to then prescribe adequate amounts of energy to meet these infants' basal requirements. It is important to perform the study at various points in a 24-hour period, especially if infants are being enterally fed. This ensures that the thermic effect of feeding and other energy-consuming activities is included in the overall REE value. Infants must be studied in the resting state, because the variance of data generated when they are active renders the values uninterpretable. Typically, less than 5% to 10% variation during the study is the expected norm. Finally, it must be realized that the total energy intake must exceed the REE value by approximately 50 kcal/kg to meet basal energy requirements and to maintain a weight gain of approximately 10 to 15 g/kg/day.

Direct calorimetry can also be performed in neonates. The infant is placed in a chamber and the amount of heat generated is measured. This lost energy is directly related to oxygen consumption. The routine use of this technique in the nursery is precluded by the need for specialized equipment required for the measurement. Longer-term assessment of energy needs can be estimated by using doubly labeled water, a technique that is discussed in the section on stable isotopes.

SPECIAL STUDIES

Stable Isotopes

Stable isotopes are naturally occurring atoms that contain one or more neutrons in their nuclei, which makes them heavier than their parent species (i.e., ^{13}C for ^{12}C [carbon]; ^{15}N for ^{14}N [nitrogen]; and ^{2}H for ^{1}H [hydrogen]). Stable isotopes are suitable for clinical studies because they naturally occur in a predictable ratio to one another, which allows for their quantification in body fluids by measurement of their isotopic ratios using mass spectrometry. The use of stable isotopes in humans is considered safe because they do not decay and, therefore, do not emit ionizing radiation. In general, the stable isotope methodology for

TABLE 31-7

Bone Mineral Content in Premature and Full-Term Infants Measured by Single- and Dual-Photon Absorptiometry

	Site	Bone Mineral Content Full-Term	Bone Mineral Content Premature
Single-Photon Absorptiometry			
Steichen et al, 1976[128]	Distal radius/ulna	103	—
Minton et al, 1979[129]	Distal radius/ulna	91	41 (<32 wk); 58 (>34 wk)
Greer et al, 1983[130]	Distal radius/ulna	94	26 (<24 wk); 71 (37 wk)
Lapillone et al, 1997[131]	Total body scan	65 (41 wk)	20 (32 wk)

	Site	Bone Mineral Content (g)	Bone Density (g/cm)
Dual-Photon Absorptiometry			
Braillon et al, 1992[132]	Lumbar spine (L1 to L5)	1.7 (34 wk) to 2.9 (40 wk)	0.22 (34 wk) to 0.28 (40 wk)
Salle et al, 1992[133]	Lumbar spine (L1 to L5)	1.5 (32 wk) to 2.5 (40 wk)	0.2 (32 wk) to 0.27 (40 wk)
Rigo et al, 1998[134]	Total body scan	10 (1 kg) to 75 (4 kg)	

clinical studies includes the administration of a known amount of an isotope-labeled substrate, followed by the quantification of the isotope present in body fluids, such as blood or urine, to determine the metabolic fate of the labeled substrate.

Several aspects of glucose metabolism in neonates have been studied by using stable isotopes. For instance, continuous administration of a known amount of ^{13}C glucose and the subsequent measurement of the isotopic ratio of ^{13}C glucose in blood, at steady state, allow for the estimation of the rates of endogenous glucose production. Furthermore, the concomitant measurement of the ^{13}C isotopic ratio in expired carbon dioxide (CO_2) allows for the determination of the rates of glucose oxidation. Studies by Bier[110] and Kalhan[111] and their coworkers demonstrated that the rates of glucose production in neonates vary from 4 to 6 mg/kg/min. Studies by Denne and Kalhan[112] estimated that approximately 53% of the glucose produced by the neonate is oxidized. Other studies[113, 114] have shown that the endogenous production of glucose can be suppressed by the exogenous infusion of dextrose at rates exceeding 8 mg/kg/min.

The use of stable isotopes in the form of ^{15}N amino acids provides a method to measure the absolute rates of protein synthesis and degradation. Such studies are based on the assumption that there is a single metabolic pool of nitrogen into which nitrogen enters from either diet or protein catabolism and exits by either protein synthesis or excretion in the form of ammonia or urea. Once the ^{15}N amino acid is administered and a steady state is attained, the flux of nitrogen entering and leaving the pool is equal, thus allowing estimation of the rates of protein synthesis and degradation. ^{15}N-glycine has been safely administered intravenously and intragastrically to newborn infants with a variety of problems.[115] Stable isotope technology has permitted determination of fractional catabolic and synthetic rates for a large number of proteins[116] and can be used to determine which amino acids are essential for the premature neonate.[117]

Doubly labeled water has been used for the determination of rates of CO_2 production and oxygen (O_2) consumption, and values were found to be comparable to those obtained using indirect calorimetry.[118-123] The doubly labeled water technique has been validated for nutritional studies in neonates.[116] This method involves the administration of both ^2H_2O and $H_2^{18}O$ and the subsequent measurement of the enrichment of these isotopes in blood, urine, or saliva. This method is based on the principle that the disappearance of $H_2^{18}O$ from body fluids reflects the elimination of CO_2 and H_2O, whereas the disappearance of ^2H_2O reflects the elimination of H_2O only. The rate of CO_2 production and, therefore, its elimination are represented by the difference between the turnover of H_2O and that of CO_2. A major

concern about the use of doubly labeled water in neonates is that the body composition changes rapidly after birth, and this methodology requires body water volume to remain constant throughout the study period.

Bone Mineralization Measurements

Decreased bone mineralization (osteopenia) has often been reported in sick premature infants.[121-124] Most premature babies with osteopenia are initially asymptomatic and may remain so for several weeks until the occurrence of pathologic fractures or overt rickets. Therefore, the early recognition of osteopenia is of clinical importance for the nutritional assessment of sick premature infants.

Vitamin deficiency has been clearly identified as a potential cause of osteopenia and rickets in premature infants.[125] However, current practices of routinely supplementing vitamin D to parenteral nutrition solutions and to enteral feedings have eliminated vitamin D deficiency as a common etiologic factor. Studies indicate that mineral deficiency is the major cause of osteopenia in premature infants being treated in contemporary neonatal intensive care units. Factors contributing to this mineral deficiency include (1) inability to provide adequate amounts of calcium and phosphorus in parenteral nutrition solutions,[126] and (2) increased renal losses of calcium due to the chronic use of diuretics, such as furosemide.[127]

Assessment of bone mineralization can be performed noninvasively by densitometry with the use of single- or dual-photon absorptiometry techniques.[128-134] Standard values for bone mineral content in premature and full-term infants have been developed by several investigators. Their results are summarized in Table 31-7.

REFERENCES

1. American Academy of Pediatrics Committee on Nutrition: Nutritional needs of low-birth-weight infants. Pediatrics 75:976, 1985.
2. Pohlandt F: Studies on the requirement of amino acids in newborn infants receiving parenteral nutrition. In Visser HKA (ed): Nutrition and Metabolism of the Fetus and Infant. The Hague, Martinus Nijhoff, 1979, pp 341-364.
3. Roy RN, et al: Impaired assimilation of nasojejunal feedings in healthy low birth weight newborn infants. J Pediatr 90:431, 1977.
4. Zlotkin SH, et al: Intravenous nitrogen and energy intakes required to duplicate in utero nitrogen accretion in prematurely born human infants. J Pediatr 99:115, 1981.
5. De Benoist B, et al: The management of whole body protein turnover in the preterm infant with intragastric infusion of L 13 C leucine sampling of the urinary leucine pool. Clin Sci 66:154, 1984.
6. Nissin I, et al: Effect of conceptual age and dietary protein on protein metabolism in premature infants. J Pediatr Gastroenterol Nutr 2:507, 1983.

7. Waterloo JC: Basic concepts of determination of nutritional requirements for normal infants. *In* Tsang RC, et al (eds) Nutrition during Infancy. St. Louis, CV Mosby, 1988, pp 1–19.

8. Lucas A, et al: Early diet in preterm babies and developmental status in infancy. Arch Dis Child *64*:1570, 1989.

9. Meier PP, Lysakowski Y, Engstrom JL, et al: The accuracy of test weighing for preterms. J Pediatr Gastroenterol Nutr *10*:62, 1990.

10. Lafeber HN: Nutritional assessment and measurement of body composition in preterm infants. Clin Perinat *26*:997, 1999.

11. Sinclair JC, et al: Supportive management of the sick neonate. Pediatr Clin North Am *17*:863, 1970.

12. Reichman BL, et al: Partition of energy metabolism and energy cost of growth in the very low birth weight infant. Pediatrics *69*:446, 1982.

13. Reichman BL, et al: Diet, fat accretion, and growth in premature infants. N Engl J Med *305*:1495, 1981.

14. Kurzner SI, et al: Elevated metabolic rates correlate with growth failure in infants with bronchopulmonary dysplasia. Clin Res *35*:235, 1987.

15. Kurzner SI, et al: Growth failure in infants with bronchopulmonary dysplasia: nutrition and elevated resting metabolic expenditure. Pediatrics *81*:379, 1988.

16. Ziegler EE, et al: Nutritional requirements of the premature infant. *In* Susskind RM (ed): Symposium on Pediatric Nutrition. New York, Raven Press, 1980.

17. Widdowson EM: Growth and composition of the fetus and newborn. *In* Assali NS (ed): Biology of Gestation: Volume II, The Fetus and Newborn. New York, Academic Press, 1972, pp 1–44.

18. Enzi G, et al: Intrauterine growth and adipose tissue development. Am J Clin Nutr *34*:1785, 1981.

19. Fee B, Weil WM: Body composition of a diabetic offspring by direct analysis. Am J Dis Child *100*:718, 1960.

20. Fomon SJ: Normal growth, failure to thrive, and obesity. *In* Fomon SJ (ed): Infant Nutrition. Philadelphia, WB Saunders, 1974, pp 34–94.

21. Friis-Hansen B: Body water compartments in children: changes during growth and related changes in body composition. Pediatrics *28*:169, 1961.

22. Widdowson EM, Dickerson JWT: Chemical composition of the body. *In* Cornar CL, Bronner F (eds): Mineral Metabolism. Vol 2, The Elements. New York, Academic Press, 1964, pp 1–247.

23. Spady DW, et al: Effect of maternal smoking on their infants' body composition as determined by total body potassium. Pediatr Res *20*:716, 1986.

24. Schoeller DA, et al: Total body water measurement in humans with ^{18}O and ^2H labeled water. Am J Clin Nutr *33*:2682, 1980.

25. Fiorotto ML, et al: Fat-free mass and total body water of infants estimated from total body electrical conductivity measurements. Pediatr Res *22*:417, 1987.

26. Venkataraman PS, Ahluwalia BW: Total bone mineral content and body composition by x-ray densitometry in newborns. Pediatrics *90*:767, 1992.

27. Harrington TA, et al: Fast and reproducible method for direct quantification of adipose tissue in newborns. Lipids *37*:95, 2000.

28. Olheager E, et al: Description and evaluation of a method on magnetic imaging to estimate adipose tissue volume and total body fat in infants. Pediatr Res *44*:572, 1998.

29. Widdowson EM, Spray CM: Chemical development in utero. Arch Dis Child *26*:205, 1951.

30. Fomon SJ, et al: Body composition of reference children from birth to age 10 years. Am J Clin Nutr *35*:1169, 1982.

31. Ziegler EE, et al: Body composition of the reference fetus. Growth *40*:329, 1976.

32. Lubchenco LO, et al: Neonatal mortality rate: relationship to birth weight and gestational age. J Pediatr *81*:814, 1972.

33. Battaglia FC, Lubchenco LO: A practical classification of newborn infants by weight and gestational age. J Pediatr *71*:159, 1967.

34. Babson SG, et al: Live-born birth weights for gestational age of white middle-class infants. Pediatrics *45*:937, 1970.

35. Brenner WE, et al: A standard of fetal growth for the United States of America. Am J Obstet Gynecol *126*:555, 1976.

36. Bjerkegal T, et al: Percentiles of birth weights of single live births at different gestational periods based on 125,485 births in Norway, 1967 and 1968. Acta Paediatr Scand *62*:449, 1973.

37. Sterky G: Swedish standard curves for intrauterine growth. Pediatrics *46*:7, 1970.

38. Pencharz PB: Nutrition of the low-birth-weight infant. *In* Grand RJ, et al (eds): Pediatric Nutrition Theory and Practice. Boston, Butterworths, 1987, pp 313–326.

39. Dancis J, et al: A grid for recording the weight of premature infants. J Pediatr *33*:570, 1948.

40. Brosius KK, et al: Postnatal growth curve of the infant with extremely low birth weight who was fed enterally. Pediatrics *74*:778, 1984.

41. Shaffer SG, et al: Postnatal changes in total body water and extracellular volume in the preterm infants with respiratory distress syndrome. J Pediatr *109*:1028, 1986.

42. LeLeiko NS, et al: The nutritional assessment of the pediatric patient. *In* Grand RJ, et al (eds): Pediatric Nutritional Theory and Practice. Boston, Butterworths, 1987, pp 396–399.

43. Georgieff MK, et al: Effect of neonatal caloric deprivation on head growth and 1-year developmental status in preterm infants. J Pediatr *107*:5181, 1985.

44. Gross SJ, et al: Head growth and developmental outcome in very low birth weight infants. Pediatrics *71*:70, 1983.

45. Winick M, Rosso P: The effect of severe early malnutrition on cellular growth of human brain. Pediatr Res *3*:181, 1969.

46. Bource JM, et al: Influence of intrauterine malnutrition on brain development: alteration of myelination. Biol Neonate *39*:96, 1974.

47. Takashima S, et al: Retardation of neuronal maturation in premature infants compared with term infants of the same post-conceptional age. Pediatrics *69*:33, 1982.

48. Jackson M: Developmental Neurobiology. New York, Plenum Press, 1978.

49. Sasanow SR, et al: Mid-arm circumference and mid-arm circumference/head ratios: standard curves for anthropometric assessment of neonatal nutritional status. J Pediatr *169*:311, 1986.

50. Moskowitz SR, et al: Mid-arm circumference/head circumference ratio as an anthropometric measure of protein-calorie deprivation in preterm infants. J Am Coll Nutr *2*:284, 1983.

51. Robson JRK, et al: Ethnic differences in skin-fold thickness. Am J Clin Nutr *24*:864, 1971.

52. Vaucher YE, et al: Skinfold thickness in North American infants 24 to 41 weeks of gestation. Hum Biol *56*:713, 1984.

53. Brion LP, et al: Non-invasive assessment of body composition: comparison of low birth weight and normal birth weight infants. Pediatr Res *22*:405A, 1986.

54. Thornton CJ, et al: Dynamic skinfold thickness measurements: a non-invasive estimate of neonatal extracellular water content. Pediatr Res *16*:989, 1982.

55. Brans YW, et al: A non-invasive approach to body composition in the neonate: dynamic skinfold measurements. Pediatr Res *8*:215, 1974.

56. Dauncey MJ, et al: Assessment of total body fat in infancy from skinfold thickness measurements. Arch Dis Child *52*:223, 1977.

57. Borkan GA, et al: Comparison of ultrasound and skinfold measurements in assessment of subcutaneous and total fatness. Am J Phys Anthropol *58*:307, 1982.

58. Sann L, et al: Arm fat and muscle areas in infancy. Arch Dis Child *63*:256, 1988.

59. Gurney JM, Jelliffe D: Arm anthropometry in nutritional assessment: nomogram for rapid calculation of muscle circumference and cross-sectional muscle and fat areas. Am J Clin Nutr *26*:912, 1973.

60. Brans YW, et al: Maternal diabetes and neonatal macrosomia. II. Neonatal anthropometric measurements. Early Hum Dev *8*:297, 1983.

61. Georgieff MK, et al: Mid-arm circumference/head circumference ratios for identification of symptomatic LGA, AGA, and SGA newborn infants. J Pediatr *109*:316, 1986.

62. Lubchenco LO: Intrauterine growth of the normal infant. *In* The High Risk Infant, Volume XIV. Major Problems in Clinical Pediatrics. Philadelphia, WB Saunders, 1976, pp 65–98.

63. Miller-Hassanein K: Diagnosis of impaired fetal growth in newborn infants. Pediatrics *48*:511, 1971.

64. Georgieff MK, et al: A comparison of the mid-arm circumference/head circumference ratio and ponderal index for the evaluation of newborn infants after abnormal intrauterine growth. Acta Pediatr Scand *77*:214, 1988.

65. Georgieff MK, et al: Catch-up growth, muscle and fat accretion, and body proportionality of infants one year after newborn intensive care. J Pediatr *114*:288, 1989.

66. Deter RL, et al: Predicting the birth characteristics of normal fetuses 14 weeks before delivery. J Clin Ultrasound *17*:89, 1989.

67. Warda A, et al: Evaluation of fetal thigh circumference measurements: a comparative ultrasound and anatomical study. J Clin Ultrasound *14*:99, 1986.

68. Merlob P, Sivan Y: Thigh circumference and thigh-to-head ratio in preterm and term infants. J Perinatol *14*:479, 1994.

69. Kelman L, et al: Effect of dietary protein restriction on albumin synthesis, albumin catabolism and the plasma angiogram. Am J Clin Nutr *25*:117, 1972.

70. Thom H, et al: Protein concentrations in the umbilical cord plasma of premature and mature infants. Clin Sci *33*:422, 1967.

71. LeLeiko NS, et al: The nutritional assessment of the pediatric patient. *In* Grand RJ, et al (eds): Pediatric Nutrition Theory and Practice. Boston, Butterworths, 1987, pp 410–411.

72. Richard KA, et al: Serum transferrin: an early indicator of nutritional status in children with advanced cancer. Surg Forum *30*:78, 1979.

73. Howard L, Meguid M: Nutritional assessment in total parenteral nutrition. *In* Labbe RF (ed): Clinics in Laboratory Medicine. Symposium on Laboratory Assessment of Nutritional Status, Vol 1. Philadelphia, WB Saunders, 1981, pp 611–630.

74. Morton AG, Tavill AS: The role of iron in the regulation of hepatic transferrin synthesis. Br J Haematol *36*:383, 1977.

75. Chockalingam UM, et al: The influence of gestational age, size for dates, and prenatal steroids on cord transferrin levels in newborn infants. J Pediatr Gastroenterol Nutr *6*:276, 1987.

76. Chockalingam UM, et al: Cord transferrin and ferritin values in newborn infants at risk for prenatal uteroplacental insufficiency and chronic hypoxia. J Pediatr *111*:283, 1987.

77. Georgieff MK, et al: Serum transferrin levels in the longitudinal assessment of protein-energy status in preterm infants. J Pediatr Gastroenterol Nutr *8*:234, 1989.

78. Georgieff MK, et al: Serum transthyretin levels and protein intake as predictors of weight gain velocity in premature infants. J Pediatr Gastroenterol Nutr *6*:775, 1987.

79. Giacola GP, et al: Rapid turnover transport proteins, plasma albumin and growth in low birth weight infants. J Parenter Enter Nutr *8*:367, 1984.

80. Moskowitz SR, et al: Prealbumin as a biochemical marker of nutritional adequacy in premature infants. J Pediatr *102*:749, 1983.
81. Goodman DS: Retinol-binding protein, prealbumin, and vitamin A transport. Prog Clin Biol Res *5*:313, 1976.
82. Georgieff MK, et al: Cord prealbumin values in newborn infants: effect of prenatal steroids, pulmonary maturity, and size for dates. J Pediatr *108*:972, 1986.
83. Bhatia J, Ziegler EE: Retinol binding protein and prealbumin in cord blood of term and preterm infants. Early Hum Dev *8*:129, 1983.
84. Sann L, et al: Evolution of serum prealbumin, C-reactive protein, and orosomucoid in neonates with bacterial infection. J Pediatr *105*:977, 1984.
85. Georgieff MK, et al: The effect of antenatal betamethasone on cord blood concentrations of retinol-binding protein, transthyretin, transferrin, retinol, and vitamin E. J Pediatr Gastroenterol Nutr 7:713, 1988.
86. Georgieff MK, et al: The effect of postnatal steroid administration of serum vitamin A concentrations in newborn infants with respiratory compromise. J Pediatr *114*:301, 1989.
87. Sasanow SR, et al: The effect of gestational age upon prealbumin and retinol-binding protein in preterm and term infants. J Pediatr Gastroenterol Nutr 5:111, 1986.
88. Rassin DK, et al: Milk protein and quality in low birth weight infants: effects on selected aliphatic amino acids in plasma and urine. Pediatrics *59*:407, 1977.
89. Rassin DK, et al: Milk protein and quantity and quality in low birth weight infants: effects on tyrosine and phenylalanine in plasma and urine. J Pediatr *90*:356, 1977.
90. Gaull GE, et al: Milk protein quantity and quality in low birth weight infants: effects on sulfur amino acids in plasma and urine. J Pediatr *90*:348, 1977.
91. Heird WC, et al: Pediatric parenteral amino acid mixture in low birth weight infants. Pediatrics *81*:41, 1988.
92. Seashore JH, et al: Urinary 3-methylhistidine/creatinine ratio as a clinical tool: correlation between 3-methylhistidine excretion and metabolic and clinical states in healthy and stressed premature infants. Metabolism *30*:959, 1981.
93. Seashore MR, et al: Loss of intellectual function in children with phenylketonuria after relaxation of dietary phenylalanine restriction. Pediatrics *75*:226, 1985.
94. Duffy B, et al: The effect of varying protein quality and energy intake on the nitrogen metabolism of parenterally fed very low birth weight (1600 gm) infants (abstract). Pediatr Res *14*:459, 1980.
95. Millward DJ, et al: Quantitative importance of non-skeletal-muscle sources of *N*-methylhistidine in urine. Biochem J *190*:225, 1980.
96. Young VR, Munro HN: *N*-methylhistidine (3-methylhistidine) and muscle protein turnover: an overview. Fed Proc *37*:2291, 1978.
97. Fomon SJ, et al: Determination of nitrogen balance of infants less than 6 months of age. Pediatrics *22*:94, 1958.
98. Hepner R, Lubchenco LO: A method for continuous urine and stool collection in young infants. Pediatrics *26*:828, 1960.
99. Shenai J: Balance studies in newborn infants. J Pediatr *93*:533, 1978.
100. Schanler RJ, et al: Fortified mother's milk for very low birth weight infants: Results of growth and nutrient balance studies. J Pediatr *107*:437, 1985.
101. Tantibhedhyangkul P, Hashim SA: Medium-chain triglyceride feeding in premature infants: effects on calcium and magnesium absorption. Pediatrics *61*:533, 1978.
102. Wirth FH, et al: Effect of lactose on mineral absorption in preterm infants. J Pediatr *117*:150, 1967.
103. Ehrenkranz RA, et al: Nutrient balance studies in premature infants fed premature formula or fortified preterm human milk. J Pediatr Gastroenterol Nutr *8*:58, 1989.
104. Ernst JA, et al: Metabolic balance studies in premature infants. Clin Perinatol *22*:177, 1995.
105. Fomon SJ, Owen GM: Comment on metabolic balance studies as a method of estimating body composition of infants, with special consideration of nitrogen balance studies. Pediatrics *30*:495, 1962.
106. Wahlig TM, et al: Metabolic response of preterm infants to variable degrees of respiratory illness. J Pediatr *124*:283, 1994.
107. Lopez AM, et al: Estimation of nitrogen balance based on a six-hour urine collection in infants. J Parenter Enter Nutr *10*:517, 1986.
108. Fomon SJ, et al: Requirements for protein and essential amino acids in early infancy; studies with a soy-isolate formula. Acta Paediatr Scand *62*:33, 1973.
109. Weir J: New method for calculating metabolic rate with special reference to protein metabolism. J Physiol *109*:1, 1949.
110. Bier DM, et al: Measurement of "true" glucose production rates in infancy and childhood with 6,6-dideuteroglucose. Diabetes *26*:1016, 1977.
111. Kalhan SC, et al: Measurement of glucose turnover in the human newborn with glucose-1-^{13}C. J Clin Endocrinol Metab *43*:704, 1976.
112. Denne SC, Kalhan SC: Glucose carbon recycling and oxidation in human newborns. Am J Physiol *251*:E71, 1986.
113. Lafeber HN, et al: Glucose production and oxidation in preterm infants during total parenteral nutrition. Pediatr Res *28*:153, 1991.
114. Zarlengo KM, et al: Relationship between glucose utilization rate and glucose concentration in preterm infants. Biol Neonate *49*:181, 1986.
115. Picoe D, Taylor-Roberts T: The measurement of total protein synthesis and catabolism and nitrogen turnover in infants in different nutritional states and receiving different amounts of dietary protein. Clin Sci *36*:283, 1969.
116. Pencharz PB, et al: The effects of human milk and low protein formulae on the rates of total body protein. Clin Sci (Lond) *64*:611, 1983.
117. Jackson AA, et al: Nitrogen balance in preterm infants fed human donor breast milk. The possible essentiality of glycine. Pediatr Res *15*:1454, 1981.
118. Jones PJH, et al: Validation of doubly labeled water for assessing energy expenditure in infants. Pediatr Res *21*:242, 1987.
119. Westerterp KR, et al: Comparison of short-term indirect calorimetry and doubly labeled water method for the assessment of energy expenditure in preterm infants. Biol Neonate *60*:75, 1991.
120. Jensen CL, et al: Determining energy expenditure in preterm infants: comparison of ^{2}H$_2$^{18}O method and indirect calorimetry. Am J Physiol *263*:R685, 1992.
121. Steichen JJ, et al: Osteopenia of prematurity: the cause and possible treatment. J Pediatr *96*:528, 1980.
122. Koo WWK, et al: Skeletal changes in preterm infants. Arch Dis Child *57*:447, 1982.
123. Koo WWK, et al: Osteopenia, rickets and fractures in preterm infants. Am J Dis Child *139*:1045, 1995.
124. James JR, et al: Osteopenia of prematurity. Arch Dis Child *61*:871, 1986.
125. Glaser K, et al: Comparative efficacy of vitamin D preparations in prophylactic treatment of premature infants. Am J Dis Child *77*:1, 1949.
126. MacMahon P, et al: Calcium and phosphorus solubility in neonatal intravenous feeding solutions. Arch Dis Child *65*:352, 1990.
127. Venkataraman PS, et al: Secondary hyperparathyroidism and bone disease in infants receiving long-term furosemide therapy. Am J Dis Child *137*:1157, 1983.
128. Steichen JJ, et al: Bone mineral content in full-term infants measured by direct photon absorptiometry. Am J Roentgenol *126*:1283, 1976.
129. Minton SD, et al: Bone mineral content in term and preterm appropriate for gestational age infants. J Pediatr *95*:1037, 1979.
130. Greer FR, et al: An accurate and reproducible absorptiometry technique for determining bone mineral content in newborn infants. Pediatr Res *17*:259, 1983.
131. Lapillone A, et al: Body composition in appropriate for gestational age infants. Acta Pediatr *86*:196, 1997.
132. Braillon PM, et al: Dual energy x-ray absorptiometry measurement of bone mineral content in newborns: validation of the technique. Pediatr Res *32*:77, 1992.
133. Salle BL, et al: Lumbar mineral content measured by dual energy x-ray absorptiometry in newborns and infants. Acta Paediatr *81*:953, 1992.
134. Rigo J, et al: Reference values for body composition obtained by dual energy xray absorptiometry in preterm and term neonates. J Pediatr Gastrointest Nutr *27*:184, 1998.

SECTION V

Perinatal Iron, Mineral, and Vitamin Metabolism

32

Jorge A. Prada

Calcium-Regulating Hormones

CALCIUM

Calcium (Ca) accounts for 1% to 2% of adult human body weight.[1] Over 99% of total body Ca is found in teeth and bones in hydroxyapatite form, and 1% is in intracellular fluids and soft tissues. Close to 1% of the calcium present in the skeleton serves as a reservoir and is freely transferable with the extracellular fluid. Although this is a small percentage, it is about equal to the total content of calcium in the extracellular fluid and soft tissues.

The extracellular concentration of calcium ions (Ca^{2+}) is approximately 10^{-3} M, whereas the concentration of Ca^{2+} in the cytosol is approximately 10^{-6} M. In the blood, Ca^{2+} exists in three forms: 40% is present as a nondiffusible complex with protein; 5% is a diffusible but undissociated complex with citrate, bicarbonate, and phosphate; and 55% is present as free ionized calcium. The total normal concentration is between 2.25 and 2.75 mM. The nondiffusible complex is bound largely to the carboxyl groups in albumin, and this binding is highly pH-dependent. Acute acidosis decreases binding and increases free ionized calcium, and acute alkalosis increases binding with a decrease in free ionized calcium.

Alteration in extracellular calcium concentration must be sensed to allow rectification by the homeostatic system. The recent cloning of a Ca^{2+}-sensing, G protein–coupled receptor from bovine and human parathyroid, and from rat kidney and brain, has confirmed that Ca^{2+} can function as a conventional first messenger. The calcium-sensing receptor (CaR) is a membrane-bound G protein–coupled receptor present in parathyroid and kidney cells that monitors the level of extracellular calcium and transduces signals involved in serum calcium regulation. Like other family members, it contains 7 hydrophobic helices that anchor it in the plasma membrane. The large (~600 amino acids) extracellular domain is known to be critical to interactions with extracellular calcium. The receptor also has a rather large (~200 amino acids) cytosolic tail (Fig. 32-1) Activation of the calcium sensor has two major signal-transducing effects: (1) activation of phospholipase C, which leads to generation of the second messengers' diacylglycerol and inositol trisphosphate, and (2) inhibition of adenylate cyclase, which suppresses intracellular concentration of cyclic AMP. The sensor can also activate the mitogen-activated protein kinase pathway, suggesting an ability to influence nuclear function. The calcium sensor is expressed in a broad range of cells, including parathyroid cells and C cells in the thyroid gland. Functional studies and investigation of animals with mutations in the calcium sensor gene have confirmed that the calcium sensor directly affects secretion of parathyroid hormone and calcitonin.[2]

The calcium sensor is also expressed in several cell types in the kidney, osteoblasts, a variety of hematopoietic cells in bone marrow, and the gastrointestinal mucosa. It is surprising that it is also present in the squamous epithelial cells of the esophagus. Such a broad distribution of expression supports the concept that calcium, acting as a hormone, has direct effects on the function of many cell types. Understanding the role of the calcium sensor in calcium homeostasis has benefited greatly by the study of mutations in the human gene encoding this receptor.

Inactivating Mutations. A large number of different mutations in the calcium sensor gene have been identified in patients affected by a type of calcium resistance known as familial hypocalciuric hypercalcemia. The different mutations result in a spectrum of calcium sensor dysfunctions, ranging from total inactivation to a moderate decrease in affinity of the receptor for calcium. A prominent clinical consequence of such mutations is an abnormal set point or sensitivity of the parathyroid gland to blood calcium concentration, resulting in hypercalcemia.

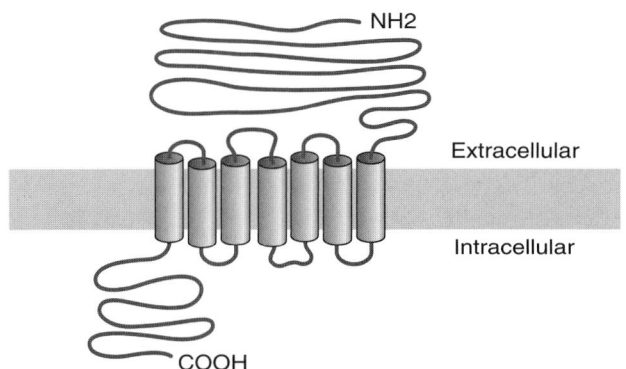

Figure 32–1. Calcium-sensing receptor (CaR). The CaR is a G protein–coupled receptor that contains seven plasma membrane anchoring hydrophobic helices. The large extracellular domain is known to be critical to interactions with extracellular calcium. (Reprinted with permission from Brown EM, Am J Med *106*:238, 1999.)

Abnormalities in renal excretion of calcium are also observed, resulting in hypocalciuria.

Activating Mutations. Certain types of mutations lead to a calcium sensor with an elevated sensitivity to calcium. The clinical consequence of such mutations is familial hypercalciuric hypocalcemia—basically the opposite of what is seen with inactivating mutations in the sensor gene. High blood calcium affects the normal calcium sensor to suppress parathyroid hormone secretion. If the calcium sensor is constitutively more active, then a type of hypoparathyroidism results.

Identification and understanding of the calcium-sensing receptor (CaR) (expressed in the plasma membrane of parathyroid and kidney cells in particular) has been a major advance in understanding mechanisms in control of extracellular calcium homeostasis.[3,4]

Cellular Calcium Metabolism

The control of cellular calcium homeostasis is multifaceted (Fig. 32–2). This section will highlight some of the most important roles of the calcium ion in cellular physiology. Extracellular fluids contain approximately 10^{-3} M of Ca^{2+}, whereas in the cytoplasm, the concentration of ionized calcium is approximately 10^{-6} M, or one thousandth that present in the extracellular fluids. The mitochondria and microsomes contain 90% to 99% of the intracellular calcium. The low calcium concentration in the cytosol is maintained by three pump transport systems: an external system located in the plasma membrane, and two internal systems located in the microsomal membrane and the inner mitochondrial membrane. Each pump acts like a Ca^{2+} outlet from the cytosol and requires energy to operate. Calcium ion is the most important factor linking excitation and contraction in all forms of skeletal and cardiac muscle.[5] Depolarization of the plasma membrane is accompanied by the entry of a small amount of extracellular calcium into the cell. The rise in cytosolic calcium interacts with troponin, a specific calcium-binding protein, leading to a conformational change and the actin-myosin interaction that constitutes muscle contraction. In a number of cells, calcium serves as a second messenger, mediating the effects of membrane signals on the release of secretory products (e.g., neurotransmitters, amylase, insulin, and aldosterone).[5] The calcium messenger system involves two pathways: (1) a calmodulin pathway, and (2) a C-kinase pathway. It is now recognized that the calcium messenger system and the cyclic adenosine monophosphate (cAMP) messenger system are related and integrated in such a way that the net cellular response to a given stimulus is determined by a complex interplay between these two systems.[5]

Many important aspects of our life are regulated by the free cytosolic Ca^{2+} concentration. The regulation of cytosolic Ca^{2+} homeostasis is essential for all cells, particularly vascular smooth

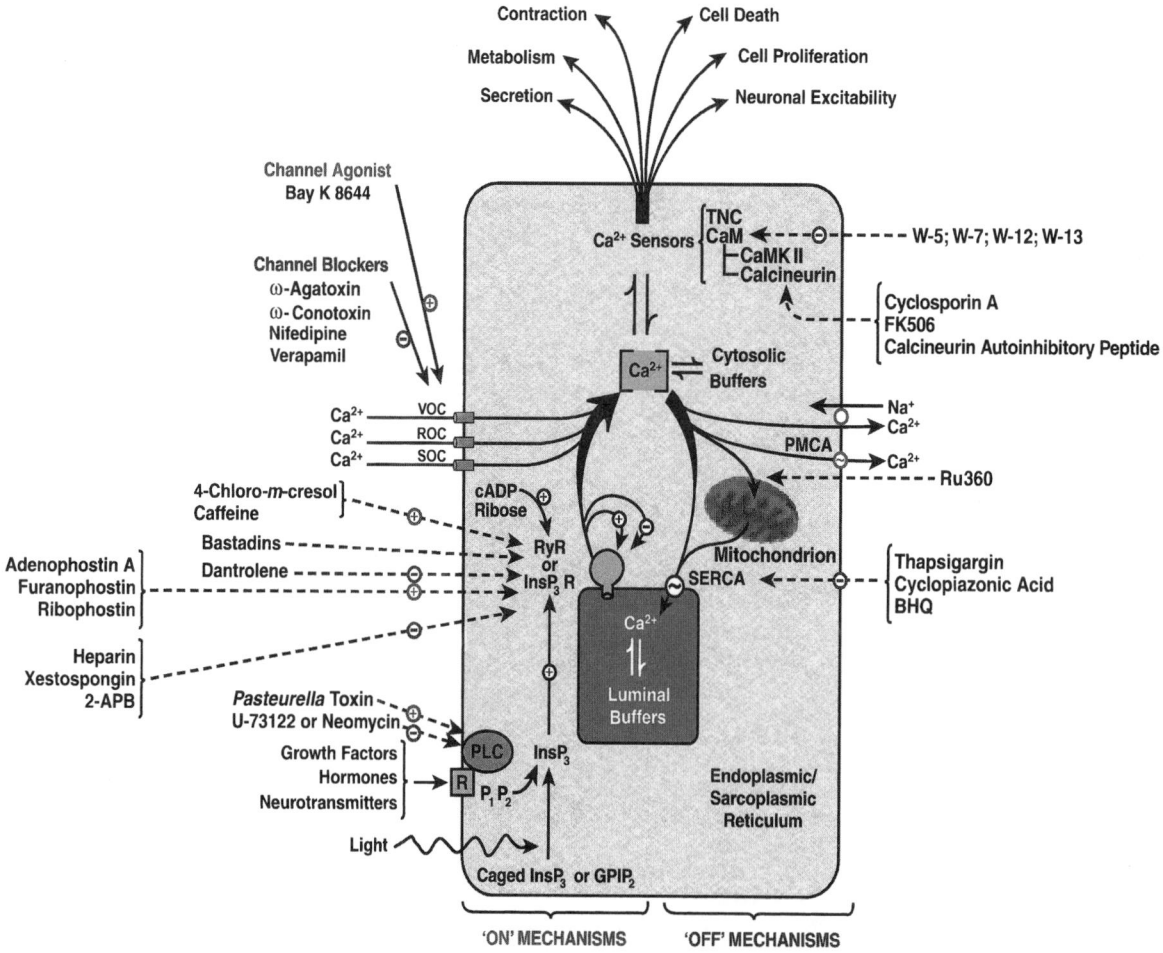

Figure 32–2. ON and OFF mechanisms for modulation of intracellular calcium. Many cellular processes are regulated by the second messenger Ca^{2+} which is derived from two separate sources. The ON mechanisms depend on Ca^{2+} entry through channels in the plasma membrane or Ca^{2+} release through ryanodine receptors (RYRs) or inositol triphosphate receptors (InsP₃Rs). The OFF mechanisms remove Ca^{2+} from the cytoplasm using pumps. (Courtesy of Calbiochem, 2001.)

muscle cells. The extracellular calcium concentration, which itself is the first informative hormone-like messenger in this system, plays an important role. Expression of the calcium-sensing receptor protein, which belongs to the C subfamily of 7 transmembrane-spanning G protein–coupled receptors, in tissues with functions not linked to systemic calcium homeostasis, indicates that extracellular calcium operates as a first messenger to regulate diverse cellular functions.[2, 6] The biology of the low-affinity, G protein–coupled CaR and the effects of its activation in various tissues play a significant role in the regulation of parathyroid hormone secretion and urinary calcium excretion by small changes in extracellular Ca^{2+}. CaR also affects the renal handling of sodium, magnesium, and water.[7-9]

Calcium Ion Balance and Mechanism for Systemic Mineral Homeostasis

The total extracellular amount of calcium in an adult is approximately 900 mg. This amount is in dynamic equilibrium with calcium entering and exiting by way of the intestine, bone, and renal tubules. In zero balance, bone resorption and formation are equivalent, and the net quantity of calcium absorbed by the intestine (approximately 175 mg/day in an adult) is excreted into the urine. Under normal conditions, net calcium absorption provides a surplus of calcium that exceeds systemic requirements. Normal adults lose 1% of their skeleton yearly after 20 years of age; this is the equivalent of a calcium loss of approximately 25 mg/day.

The ionized fraction of calcium is the physiologically important fraction of calcium. It is regulated by fluxes occurring at the levels of bone, kidney, and intestine; these fluxes are controlled by calciotropic hormones, which in turn are controlled by the calcium-sensing receptor protein.[6] The human body is equipped with an efficient protection system against hypocalcemia. Any modification of the extracellular calcium concentration triggers a series of integrated hormonal homeostatic reactions that incorporate parathyroid hormone (PTH), 1,25-dihydroxycholecalciferol (1,25[OH]$_2$D$_3$), and calcitonin.[10]

PARATHYROID HORMONE

Parathyroid hormone (PTH) is a 9500-dalton polypeptide, synthesized and secreted by the chief cells of each of the four parathyroid glands. Its primary role is the maintenance of the normal concentrations of circulating calcium and inorganic phosphate, but many other tissues that are not involved in Ca^{2+} regulation also express PTH receptors.[11] PTH is a single-chain 84-amino-acid polypeptide. The structures of human, bovine, and porcine PTH are shown in Figure 32–3).

The PTH molecule is initially synthesized as a 115-amino acid precursor polypeptide, prepro-parathormone.[12] In the endoplasmic reticulum,[13] the amino terminal 25-amino acid sequence is proteolytically cleaved to form a 90-amino acid polypeptide pro-parathormone, and in the Golgi complex pro-parathormone is successfully cleaved to yield the final hormonal product, the 84-amino acid PTH. The most amino (N)-terminal portion is required for the classic actions of the hormone on mineral ion homeostasis, mediated by type 1 PTH receptor (P1R) activation.[12, 14-17] Proteolysis of the 84-amino acid PTH results in two or more fragments: PTH (37-84) and a large amino terminal fragment PTH (1-36).[18,19] PTH has a half-life of about 4 minutes and is metabolized mainly in the liver by Kupffer cells into a biologically inactive C-terminal fragment and a biologically active N-terminal fragment.[20] PTH is synthesized and secreted continuously at normal plasma calcium concentrations in a pulsatile fashion,[20] with peak plasma levels occurring in the early morning hours.[21, 22]

Human parathyroid glands are functionally active as early as 12 weeks of gestation.[23] PTH does not appear to cross the placenta

in either direction. However, maternal parathyroid dysfunction can adversely affect fetal parathyroid function through variations in calcium concentration. Maternal hyperparathyroidism results in maternal hypercalcemia, which leads to fetal hypercalcemia and suppression of fetal and neonatal parathyroids. Conversely, untreated maternal hypoparathyroidism leads to maternal hypocalcemia, fetal hypocalcemia, and secondary fetal and neonatal hyperparathyroidism. Under normal circumstances, serum PTH levels measured by radioimmunoassay are lower in the fetus than in the mother, due to the relative hypercalcemia that exists during fetal life.[24] After birth, with the abrupt termination of maternal calcium supply, the serum calcium concentration decreases and serum PTH increases correspondingly. Both term and preterm infants show a PTH response to a falling serum calcium concentration.[25] However, infants of diabetic mothers (IDMs) have impaired PTH production during the first days of life.[26] Infants with birth asphyxia may also exhibit a decreased PTH response to hypocalcemia.[27]

Secretion of Parathormone

The extracellular fluid Ca^{2+} concentration sensed by the calcium-sensing receptor is the main determinant of PTH secretion.[28] PTH is secreted in response to small declines in ionized calcium concentration in the extracellular fluid, according to a tight feedback control mechanism. Decreases in ionized calcium of as little as 0.4 mmol/L are transduced via the CaR and expressed in the plasma membrane of the parathyroid gland to stimulate PTH

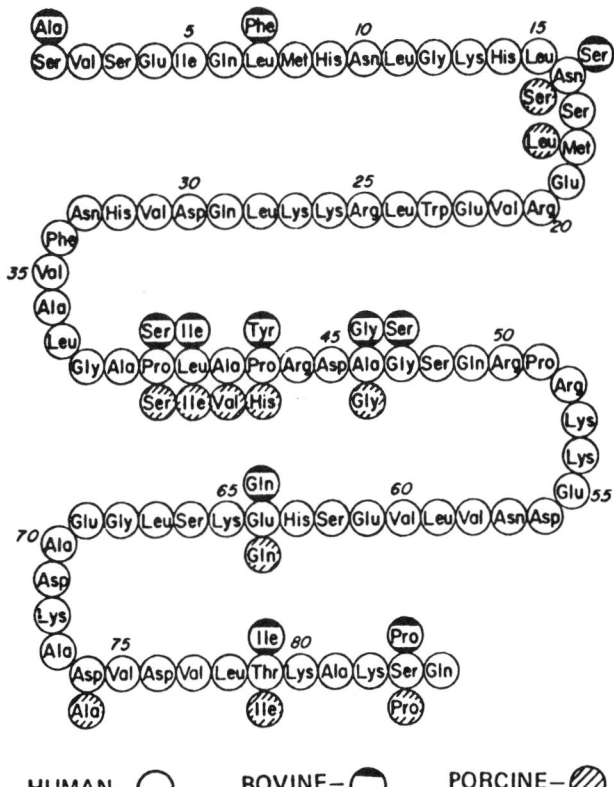

Figure 32–3. The molecular structure of PTH. The human, bovine, and porcine sequences are illustrated. The fully active portion comprises amino acids 1-34. Regions 28-34 and 34-48 are produced by enzymatic cleavage. Positions 48-84 are the biologically inactive C-terminus region. (Reprinted with permission from Keutman HT, et al: Biochemistry *17*:5723, 1978. Copyright 1978, American Chemical Society.)

secretion.[29-31] A recent study demonstrated that extracellular calcium regulates the vitamin D receptor expression by parathyroid cells independently of calcitriol (1,25(OH)$_2$D$_3$) and that by this mechanism hypocalcemia may prevent the feedback of calcitriol on the parathyroids.[32]

Catecholamines,[33] aluminum,[34] histamine,[35,36] and hormones, including active vitamin D metabolites,[37] glucagon,[38] cortisol,[39] and calcitonin[40] also have been shown to influence PTH secretions. Acute decreases in magnesium stimulate PTH secretion[41,42]; however, chronic magnesium deficiency paradoxically decreases PTH secretion, probably by altering the calcium-sensitive magnesium-dependent adenylate cyclase involved in PTH secretion.[43] PTH secretion dramatically increases when Ca^{2+} levels are decreased to approximately 1 mM; however, further lowering of the calcium concentration does not elicit an additional increase in PTH secretion.

Metabolism of Parathyroid Hormone

Intact PTH is cleared rapidly from the circulation by hepatic and renal tissues, with a half-life of less than 4 minutes.[19,44-46] The more efficient hepatic clearance involves three cell types: macrophages, Kupffer cells, and hepatocytes.[47,48] Kupffer cell clearance is high and does not discriminate between active and inactive PTH, whereas uptake by hepatocytes specifically removes active hormone. Renal clearance mechanisms are complex. A small amount of biologically active hormone is removed by the basal-lateral surface of tubule cells. This mechanism may be receptor mediated. However, both intact and C-terminal fragments are removed by glomerular filtration.[49] C-terminal fragments are more abundant than intact PTH and are released into the circulation where they have a half-life several times longer than intact PTH.[50] C-terminal fragments may account for up to 70% to 95% of the circulating immunoreactive PTH.[51] Radioimmunoassays specifically measuring the intact PTH molecule are believed to reflect PTH secretion more accurately.

Parathyroid Hormone Mechanism of Action

Parathyroid hormone regulates calcium homeostasis and phosphate metabolism by a complex interaction affecting both bone turnover and renal excretion of calcium and phosphate. In addition, PTH increases the synthesis of 1,25(OH)$_2$ vitamin D$_3$, which promotes intestinal calcium absorption. PTH administration leads to a release of calcium from the surface of bone.[52] Chronic administration of PTH leads to an increase in the number and activity of osteoclasts[53]; however, intermittent administration results in increased deposition of trabecular bone.[54] PTH increases the serum calcium concentration directly, by increasing bone resorption and by increasing renal calcium reabsorption, and indirectly, by increasing renal synthesis of 1,25(OH)$_2$D$_3$ through activation of 25OHD$_3$-1-hydroxylase in the proximal tubular cell. Administration of PTH also causes a release of phosphate from bone and increased phosphaturia by inhibiting reabsorption of phosphate in the proximal (and in part distal) tubules. Although serum phosphorus may increase from PTH-induced resorption of bone, PTH lowers the serum phosphorus concentration through its phosphaturic action, thus minimizing the possible adverse effect of hyperphosphatemia on calcium homeostasis.[55] The direct result of all these actions is an increase in the concentration of blood calcium and a decrease in the concentration of blood phosphate.

Cellular Actions of Parathormone

Two PTH receptor subtypes, type 1 (PTH1R) and type 2 (PTH2R), have been identified.[56] Type 1 parathyroid hormone receptor binds both parathyroid hormone and amino-terminal

peptides of PTHrP. This molecule is a G protein–coupled receptor with 7 transmembrane segments. The extracellular domain has 6 cysteine residues. Binding of ligand to this receptor activates both adenyl cyclase and phospholipase C systems, generating protein kinase A and protein kinase C signals, respectively. The cyclic AMP/protein kinase A pathway is predominant. As might be expected from the actions of parathyroid hormone, the mRNA encoding the type 1 receptor is most abundant in bone (especially in chondrocytes at growth plates) and kidney. The mRNA is also expressed at lower levels in many other tissues, probably reflecting its use as a receptor for PTHrP. The type 2 parathyroid hormone receptor binds parathyroid hormone but shows very low affinity for PTHrP. This molecule is expressed in only a few tissues, and its structure and physiologic significance are poorly characterized. Like the type 1 receptor, it is coupled to adenyl cyclase, and ligand binding induces a rise in intracellular concentration of cyclic AMP. Their cDNA sequences share 70% similarity are members of a subfamily of G protein–coupled receptors to which the receptors for calcitonin, secretin, and glucagon also belong.[57,58] Expressions of recombinant receptors have established that type 1 and type 2 PTH receptors are each alone capable of stimulating increases in Ca^{2+} and intracellular cyclic AMP.[59-62] Although PTH acts on bone to increase osteoclast number and activity, osteoclasts surprisingly contain no PTH receptors, and PTH has no effect on isolated osteoclasts.[63] PTH receptors are found on bone-forming osteoblasts, which secrete factors that stimulate osteoclast activity. In the kidney, PTH blocks the sodium-dependent phosphate cotransport[64] in proximal and distal tubule cells. However, in the distal tubule cell, PTH also stimulates calcium absorption against an electrochemical gradient.

PTH does not directly act in the cytoplasm of target cells; instead, PTH binds to specific receptors on the surfaces of those cells. This binding stimulates the release of cytoplasmic "second messengers" that mediate the distal effects of PTH. Binding of PTH to its receptors requires the first 34 amino acids of PTH, and the function of the carboxyl portion is unclear. Parathormone-related peptide (PTHrP) produced by certain tumors resembles PTH in its first 13 amino acids.[65] Peptide fragments of this protein bind to PTH receptors in bone and kidney[66]; this explains many activities of the protein and the similarities between hyperparathyroidism and the humoral hypercalcemia of malignancy.

The major mediator of PTH action is cAMP. Exposure of bone or kidney cells to PTH increases intracellular cAMP, and administration of cAMP analogues mimics many of the effects of PTH. Binding of PTH to its receptor on the cell stimulates the release of guanosine diphosphate (GDP) from the G$_s$ protein, and enables the binding of intracellular guanosine triphosphate (GTP) to G$_s$. GTP-G$_s$ then stimulates membrane-bound adenylate cyclase. The cAMP produced by adenylate cyclase binds to the regulatory subunit of cAMP-dependent protein kinase A. This binding causes the regulatory subunit to dissociate from the catalytic subunit. The free catalytic subunit then phosphorylates specific serines and threonines in target proteins.[67] PTH also stimulates phosphatidylinositol turnover in culture cells,[68] causes a rapid rise of free cytosolic calcium,[69] and promotes a shift of protein kinase C to the cell membrane.[70] These effects are different from the actions of cAMP and suggest that multiple second messengers may mediate some actions of PTH. The reader is referred to a recent review of the molecular structure of PTH and its interaction with various receptors, as well as recent technical advances in PTH assays.[71]

PARATHORMONE-RELATED PROTEIN

Parathyroid hormone–related protein (PTHrP) is a family of protein hormones produced by most if not all tissues in the body. PTH and PTHrP bind to the same receptor, but PTHrP also binds to several other receptors. PTHrP was discovered as a protein secreted by certain tumors that caused hypercalcemia in affected patients. It was soon shown that the uncontrolled secretion of PTHrP by many tumor cells induces hypercalcemia by stimulating resorption of calcium from bone and suppressing calcium loss in urine, similar to what is seen with hyperparathyroidism. However, it quickly became apparent that PTHrP had many activities not seen with parathyroid hormone. PTHrP is an important paracrine and autocrine regulator of proliferation, apoptosis, and differentiation of several normal cell types.[72, 73] Many tissues produce PTHrP, which plays a number of physiologic roles, particularly in the mother during pregnancy and in the developing fetus.[73, 74] PTHrP has been isolated from malignant tumors[75, 76] and has been identified as primarily responsible for "humoral" hypercalcemia of malignancy.[77] PTHrP expression in normal and tumor cells may be regulated by glucocorticoids,[78] epidermal growth factor,[79] tumor necrosis factor-α,[80] and vitamin D.[81]

Hormone Structure

PTHrP contains 141 amino acids; 8 of the first 13 are identical to PTH.[82, 83] A single gene that is highly conserved among species encodes PTHrP. It should probably be described as a polyhormone, because a family of peptide hormones is generated by alternative splicing of the primary transcript and through use of alternative post-translational cleavage sites. To make matters even more complex, some cells appear to use alternative translational initiation codons to produce forms of the protein that are targeted either for secretion or nuclear localization.

The diverse activities of PTHrP result not only from processing of the precursor into multiple hormones, but also from use of multiple receptors. It is clear that amino-terminal peptides of PTHrP share a receptor with parathyroid hormone, but they also bind to a type of receptor in some tissues that does not bind parathyroid hormone. In addition to the secreted forms of this hormone, there is considerable evidence that a form of PTHrP is generated in some cells that is not secreted and, via nuclear targeting sequences, is translocated to the nucleus, where it affects nuclear function. The consequences of this "intracrine" mode of action are not yet well characterized but may modulate such important activities as programmed cell death.

PTHrP is secreted from a large and diverse set of cells, during both fetal and postnatal life. Among tissues known to secrete this hormone are several types of epithelium, mesenchyme, vascular smooth muscle, and central nervous system. Although PTHrP is found in serum, a majority of its activity appears to reflect paracrine signaling. PTHrP can interact with PTH receptors in classic PTH target tissues such as bone and kidney.[84, 85] Synthetic peptides that include the N-terminal region PTHrP (1–34) mimic all the classic activities of PTH on bone and kidney, as well as nonclassic activities such as smooth muscle relaxation and vasodilation.[86]

Physiologic Effects of Parathyroid Hormone–Related Protein

One thing to recognize about PTHrP is that its name is inadequate to describe its activities. Like parathyroid hormone, some of the effects of PTHrP result from its effects on transepithelial fluxes of calcium, but many of its actions have nothing to do with calcium homeostasis. Most prominently, PTHrP peptides exert significant control over the proliferation, differentiation, and death of many cell types. They also play a major role in development of several tissues and organs.[87]

Much of our understanding of the biologic effects of PTHrP comes from experiments with genetically altered mice. Mice with targeted deletions in the PTHrP gene (knockout mice), mice that overexpress PTHrP in specific tissues (transgenic mice), and

crosses between knockout and transgenic mice have been critical in delineating many effects of this hormone. Humans with mutations in the PTHrP gene or the parathyroid receptor have also played a role in confirming the activity of PTHrP. Some of the physiologic effects of PTHrP collected from these studies are described here.

Cartilage and Bone Development. Mice with homozygous inactivation of the PTHrP gene die at birth, if not earlier. They manifest severe chondrodysplasia and premature epiphyseal closure, reflecting a developmental defect in proliferation and differentiation of cartilage. These and other types of studies indicate that PTHrP stimulates the proliferation of chondrocytes and suppresses their terminal differentiation. These effects of PTHrP appear due to interaction of the PTH-like peptide with the parathyroid hormone receptor.[74]

Mammary Development and Lactation. The mammary glands of female mice with homozygous inactivation of the PTHrP gene fail to develop, except for the earliest stages. Development of the mammary gland depends upon a complex interaction between epithelial and mesenchymal cells that apparently requires PTHrP. In normal animals, mammary epithelial cells secrete large amounts of PTHrP, which suggests a role of this hormone in adapting maternal metabolism to the calcium demands of lactation. PTHrP concentration in milk is 10,000 times the normal circulating levels and 1000-fold higher than average plasma concentration in hypercalcemic cancer patients.[88] Because PTHrP production can be induced by lactation,[89] it has been suggested that this "milk protein" serves to condition the gastrointestinal absorption of calcium during breast-feeding.[88]

Placental Transfer of Calcium. The "midregion" peptide of PTHrP has been shown to control the normal maternal-to-fetal pumping of calcium across the placenta. In the absence of fetal PTHrP, this gradient is not established. PTHrP and the common PTH/PTHrP receptors have been identified in gestational tissues, including myometrium, fetal membranes, and placenta.[90-97]

Smooth Muscle Functioning. PTHrP is secreted from smooth muscle in many organs, usually in response to stretching. It acts to relax smooth muscle, serving as a vasodilating hormone. Transgenic mice that express PTHrP in vascular smooth muscle manifest hypotension. PTHrP may also have effects on contraction of muscle in the bladder, uterus, and heart. Studies also indicate that endogenous PTHrP is essential for optimal differentiation of keratinocytes.[98, 99] PTHrP and its mRNA have been identified in syncytiotrophoblast and cytotrophoblast cells.[100,101] Potential autocrine, paracrine, and endocrine roles for PTHrP during pregnancy include regulation of cellular growth and differentiation,[102, 103] vasodilation of the uteroplacental vasculature,[91, 104] relaxation of uterine muscle,[105-107] and stimulation of placental calcium transport.[108] Because of its wide distribution, PTHrP may utilize novel (non-PTH) signal transduction systems in autocrine and paracrine fashions in controlling normal physiologic processes.[109]

Other Effects. PTHrP is highly expressed in skin. Transgenic mice that overexpress PTHrP in skin show alopecia, and treatment of mice with a PTHrP antagonist leads to increased numbers of hair follicles and a shaggy appearance. Another interesting defect in PTHrP-knockout mice is that their teeth develop normally but fail to erupt. Finally, both PTHrP and its receptors are widely expressed in the central nervous system and appear to influence neuronal survival by several mechanisms. A recent study has suggested that activation of the calcium-sensing receptor is responsible for increased synthesis and secretion of PTHrP.[110]

VITAMIN D

Vitamin D is synthesized in the skin on exposure to ultraviolet light. The initial step in the production of vitamin D_3, the conversion of 7-DHC to previtamin D_3, requires a UV spectrum that peaks at 295 nm, with conversion dropping to zero at 315 nm.[111] This waveband, known as UVB, is at the short wavelength limit of solar radiation reaching the earth's surface. When the sun is low in the southern sky, the incoming radiation must travel further and is subject to more scattering and absorption than when the sun is directly overhead. Since Rayleigh scattering (scattering of light waves by particles with dimensions much smaller than their wavelengths) and UV absorption at more northern latitudes are strongly wavelength dependent, skin synthesis of previtamin D$_3$ is affected by latitude, season of the year, and weather conditions.

Vitamin D is also absorbed from dietary sources in the duodenum and jejunum, as either vitamin D$_3$ (from animal sources) or vitamin D$_2$ (ergocalciferol, from vegetable sources). The metabolism of vitamin D$_3$ does not differ appreciably from that of vitamin D$_2$. Regardless of its origin, vitamin D is transported to the liver, where it is converted into 25-hydroxyvitamin D, and subsequently to the kidney, where it is transformed to the final, active metabolite 1,25(OH)$_2$ vitamin D. In the liver, 25-hydroxylation is a fairly unregulated process; 25-hydroxyvitamin D is the major circulating vitamin D metabolite and is an indicator of vitamin D status, reflecting both intake and sunshine exposure. In contrast, renal 1-hydroxylation, leading to the active metabolite, appears to be tightly regulated. The main factors increasing the synthesis of 1,25(OH)$_2$D$_3$ are PTH, hypocalcemia, and hypophosphatemia. 1,25(OH)$_2$D$_3$ is a steroid and binds to a receptor in target tissues, leading to synthesis of calcium binding (calbinding-D) proteins.[112]

There are three major sites of action for 1,25(OH)$_2$D$_3$: (1) intestine, where it increases the absorption of calcium and phosphorus; (2) bone, where it mobilizes calcium and phosphorus; and (3) kidneys, where it increases calcium reabsorption. Thus, vitamin D is necessary to maintain normal calcium and phosphorus homeostasis. The most completely studied target tissue for 1,25(OH)$_2$D$_3$ is the intestine, which depends on the hormone for adequate absorption of dietary calcium in adults.[113, 114] In the intestinal mucosa, the steroid receptor complex induces synthesis of a specific calcium-binding protein (molecular weight 28,000). In addition to the endocrine actions of 1,25(OH)$_2$D$_3$ there is interaction of 1,25(OH)$_2$D$_3$ with hematopoietic cells[115] and the immune system.[116] The actions of 1,25(OH)$_2$D$_3$ appear to involve changes in gene expression in target cells.[117-119]

Regulation and Metabolism of Vitamin D

1,25(OH)$_2$D$_3$ is synthesized by the kidney. In the kidney mitochondrion, 25-hydroxyvitamin D$_3$(25[OH]D$_3$), the major circulating form of vitamin D, is hydroxylated to either 1,25(OH)$_2$D$_3$ or 24,25(OH)$_2$D$_3$ by either 1α- or 24-cytochrome P450 hydroxylating enzymes, respectively[120] (Fig. 32–4). The predominant product formed depends on the vitamin D and PTH status of the individual. In the vitamin D–deficient state, 1-hydroxylase activity is high and 24-hydroxylase is low; 1,25(OH)$_2$D$_3$ (the product of 1-hydroxylase) represses 1-hydroxylase and induces 24-hydroxylase activity. Directly or by depleting renal cortical inorganic phosphate concentration, PTH increases 1-hydroxylase activity and decreases 24-hydroxylase activity. cAMP mediates the effect of PTH, but protein kinase C may also be involved in 25(OH)D$_3$ metabolism.

In a vitamin D sufficiency state, 1-hydroxylase activity is low and 24-hydroxylase activity is high. Once synthesized by the kidney, 1,25(OH)$_2$D$_3$ can be converted by enzymatic oxidation into different metabolites. These include 1,24,25(OH)$_3$D$_3$; 1,23,25(OH)$_3$D$_3$; 24 keto-1,23,25(OH)$_3$D$_3$; 1,25(OH)$_2$D$_3$-23–26 lactone; and 1α(OH) 24,25,26-tetranor-23 (COOH) vitamin D$_3$.[121]

Molecular Mechanisms of Action

1α,25(OH)$_2$D$_3$ can generate biologic responses via activation of voltage-dependent Ca^{2+} channels coupled to appropriate signal transduction pathways.[120,122,123] A target cell must have three key components for its genes to be regulated by a steroid hormone: (1) a protein receptor for the hormone that contains a unique binding domain for the steroid *and* a DNA-binding domain for the receptor to locate the genes in the nucleus of the cell it will

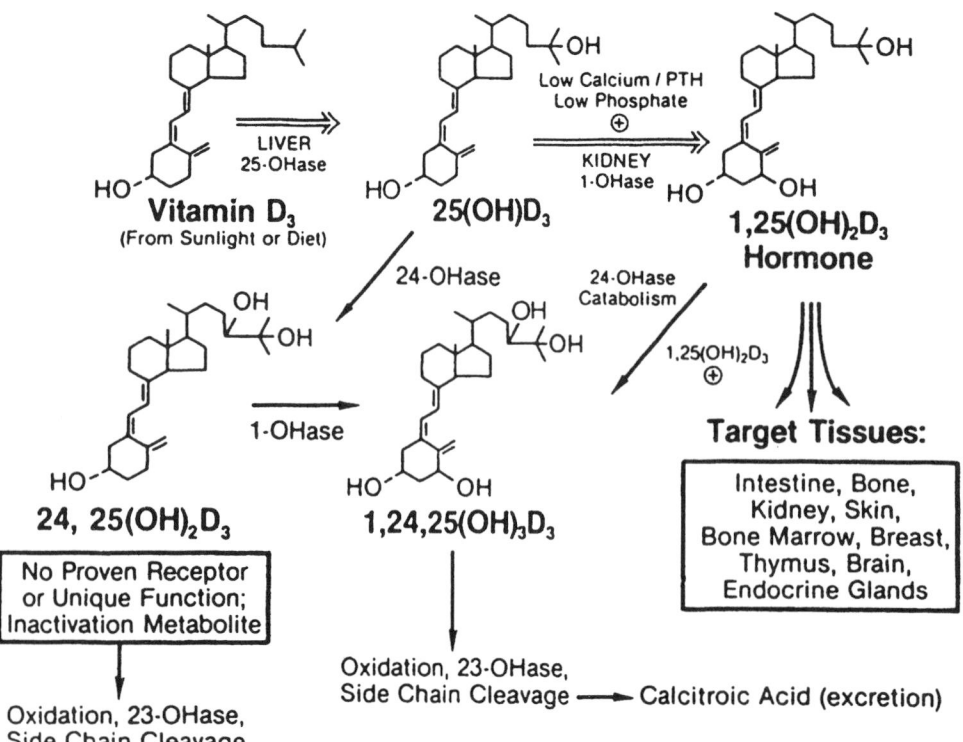

Figure 32–4. Illustration of the metabolic pathways of the vitamin D endocrine system. (From MacDonald PN, et al: Semin Nephrol *14*(2): 101, 1994.)

regulate; (2) responsive elements that consist of specific sequences of DNA nucleotides that promote an interaction between the occupied receptor and the genes to be regulated; and (3) access to the steroid hormone.

The vitamin D receptor is a member of the steroid hormone receptor superfamily.[124] The receptor is primarily a nuclear protein (51,000 daltons) that functions as a transactivating factor.[117] Although this protein is universally termed *vitamin D receptor*, in reality it binds to $1,25(OH)_2D_3$, the metabolite with hormonal activity, with much higher affinity than any other vitamin D metabolite.[125] Vitamin D receptor is a DNA-binding protein, with a typical highly conserved DNA-binding domain located near the *N*-terminus of the molecule and a hormone-binding domain at the carboxyl end.[117, 124] Transcriptional regulation occurs via the variable *N*-terminus domain, which may also be involved in regulating DNA binding. Although the precise mechanisms of protein-DNA interaction are not totally known, it is believed that after binding to $1,25(OH)_2D_3$, the vitamin D receptor undergoes conformational changes that increase its affinity for DNA.[118] The vitamin D receptor is widely distributed in classic and nonclassic target tissues. Tissues in which binding sites have been described include the hematopoietic, lymphatic, and reproductive systems; endocrine glands; the skin, liver, and lungs; and skeletal and smooth muscle.[120] Initial studies for the expression of the cloned vitamin D receptor seem to confirm the hypothesis that a single receptor mediates the protein actions of vitamin D metabolites in the different target cells.[120]

Biologic Actions of Vitamin D

The classic target organs for vitamin D are bone, intestine, and kidney. The actions of $1,25(OH)_2D_3$ on bone cells are essential for bone formation because hypovitaminosis D leads to rickets or osteomalacia. In hematopoietic cells, $1,25(OH)_2D_3$ promotes the differentiation of promonocytes into monocytes and macrophages, and finally into osteoclasts that promote bone resorption, but which are devoid of receptors for $1,25(OH)_2D_3$.[126] However, if administered at high doses, $1,25(OH)_2D_3$ induces bone resorption by a receptor present on osteoblasts. The biologic effects of $1,25(OH)_2D_3$ on bone are indirect and transduced from the osteoblast to the osteoclast.[127] The transduction may occur via the secretion of a soluble factor by the osteoblast. $1,25(OH)_2D_3$ stimulates the synthesis of noncollagenic matrix proteins, such as osteocalcin,[128,129] matrix G1a protein,[130] osteopontin,[131, 132] and fibronectin,[133] and increases alkaline phosphatase activity.[134] It is believed that stimulation of matrix proteins is transcriptional. The regulatory actions of $1,25(OH)_2D_3$ on all these important components of bone matrix imply an important role in bone matrix formation.

$1,25(OH)_2D_3$ stimulates the transcription of the gene encoding for calbindin D,[114, 135] which is a Ca^{2+}-binding protein that mediates Ca^{2+} transport through the intestinal epithelium.[136] $1,25(OH)_2D_3$ also induces nongenomic changes in Ca^{2+} transport in intestinal cells. These include stimulation of Ca^{2+} uptake in the intestinal epithelium,[137] increased net Ca^{2+} transport in duodenal loops,[138] and release of lysosomal enzymes.[139] $1,25(OH)_2D_3$ also stimulates phosphate transport[140] and induction of enterocyte growth and differentiation.[141, 142] The actions of $1,25(OH)_2D_3$ on the kidney have not been studied as well as they have been in other target organs. $1,25(OH)_2D_3$ is involved in calcium and phosphate transport.[120,143] Stimulation of phosphate transport in proximal tubule brush border membranes occurs by altering plasma membrane fluidity.[144] An important action of $1,25(OH)_2D_3$ on the kidney is its feedback inhibition on 1α-hydroxylase activity and the associated stimulation of 24-hydroxylase, the first step in the inactivation pathway of vitamin D metabolites.[145,146]

Knowledge of the spectrum of biologic actions of $1,25(OH)_2D_3$ and broad distribution of vitamin D receptors has

expanded our understanding of the role of the hormone as an important regulator of cell development and proliferation in many tissues, as well as in neoplasia. It is anticipated that there will be further discovery of effects of $1,25(OH)_2D_3$ on tissues other than those regarded as classic targets. The reader is referred to reviews on this subject.[120,147]

Biologic Concentration of Vitamin D and Its Metabolites

The normal adult range for blood $25(OH)D_3$ concentrations for healthy subjects is 10 to 80 ng/mL, and the range for $24,25(OH)_2D_3$ is 1 to 4 ng/mL. The normal circulating concentration of $1,25(OH)_2D_3$ is 15 to 70 pg/mL.[148] $25(OH)D_3$ appears to cross the placenta, whereas little transfer of $1,25(OH)_2D_3$ seems to take place.[149,150] Fetal vitamin D status seems to depend on maternal transfer of $25(OH)D_3$.[151] In term infants, serum $1,25(OH)_2D_3$ concentrations are low at birth but increase to a normal range by 24 hours of life, possibly reflecting the need for increased intestinal absorption of calcium and phosphorus.[149] Studies in the United Kingdom have suggested that maternal vitamin D deficiency might predispose infants to "late" (1 week old) neonatal hypocalcemia. In extremely premature infants, end-organ resistance to $1,25(OH)_2D_3$ may exist and theoretically could predispose to the development of hypocalcemia.[152] The vitamin D concentration is 20 to 60 IU/L in human milk, about 400 IU/L in regular milk (fortified) formulas, and 500 to 1200 IU/L in "preterm" formulas. A daily intake of 200 to 400 IU/day is recommended for both preterm and term infants. Breast-fed term infants with adequate sunshine exposure (30 to 120 minutes per week, with only face and hands exposed) do not appear to require supplemental vitamin D.[153]

CALCITONIN

Calcitonin (CT) is a 32-amino acid peptide with a molecular weight of 3600. It is secreted primarily by the parafollicular or C cells of the thyroid gland (Fig. 32–5). Its main biologic effect is to inhibit osteoclastic bone resorption. Secretion of CT varies with acute changes in serum calcium concentration: it increases when the serum calcium concentration increases and decreases when the serum calcium concentration decreases. The calcitonin receptor has been cloned and shown to be a member of the 7-transmembrane, G protein–coupled receptor family. The U.S. Food and Drug Administration currently approves calcitonin for the treatment of Paget disease, osteoporosis, and the hypercalcemia associated with malignancies. The kidney and the liver metabolize CT.

Physiologic Actions

A diverse set of effects has been attributed to CT, but in many cases, these were seen in response to pharmacologic doses of the hormone. The physiologic effects of calcitonin are opposite to those of PTH; however, CT and PTH share similar target tissues. Calcitonin plays a role in calcium and phosphorus metabolism. Calcitonin can decrease blood calcium concentrations at least in part by effects on two well-studied target organs: bone; calcitonin suppresses resorption of bone by inhibiting the activity of osteoclasts, a cell type that "digests" bone matrix, through production of cAMP, and increments in cytosolic calcium in the osteoclast,[154–156] releasing calcium and phosphorus into blood. Calcitonin inhibits tubular reabsorption of these two ions, leading to increased rates of their loss in urine. In the kidney, CT is involved in transport of ions such as Na^+, K^+, Cl^-, Mg^{2+}, and Ca^{2+}. Calcitonin also enhances calcium excretion in tubule cells.[157] Despite the effects on calcium described earlier, it seems that CT has at best a minor role in regulating blood concentrations of calcium. Evidence to support this statement is that

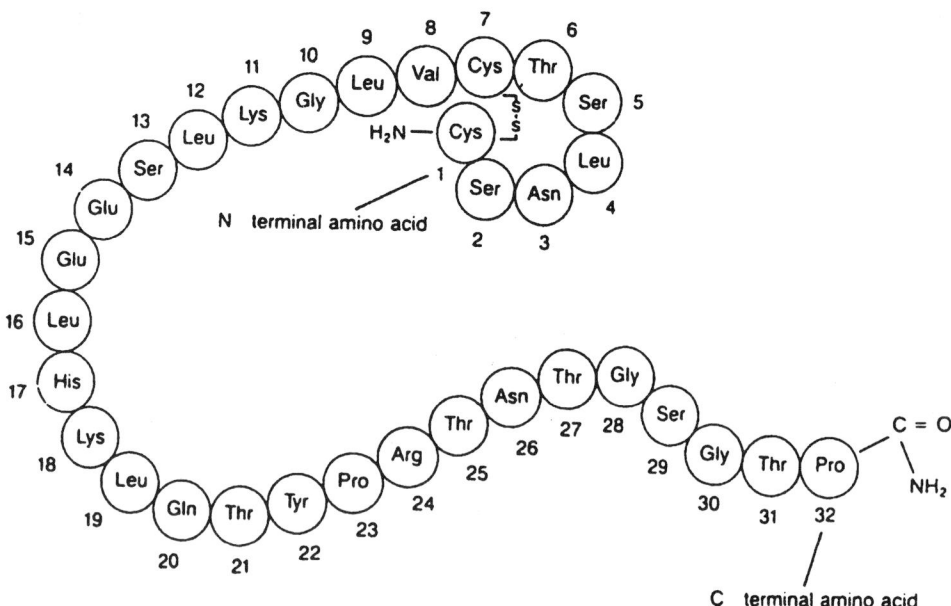

Figure 32–5. The molecular structure of calcitonin. Calcitonin, a hormone produced by the thyroid gland, is a single-chain, 32-amino acid polypeptide with a molecular weight of 3600. (From Miacalcic Calcitonin-Sandoz: A profile of Sandoz's Salmon Calcitonin, Meditext Ltd., London 13, 1989.)

humans with chronically increased (medullary thyroid cancer) or decreased (surgical removal of the thyroid gland) levels of CT in blood do not show alterations from normal in serum calcium.

In the central nervous system, CT may be involved in the modulation of prolactin secretion.[158] Evidence for a physiologic role of CT in the gastrointestinal tract is circumstantial. It is possible that some of the reported actions of CT in the gastrointestinal tract may be secondary to cross-reaction with receptors of structurally related peptides.[159, 160] From recent studies it appears that CT may also play an important role in a variety of processes ranging widely from embryonic or fetal development to sperm function and physiology.[161]

A large number of diseases are associated with abnormally increased or decreased levels of CT, but pathologic effects of abnormal CT secretion per se are not generally recognized. Calcitonin has several therapeutic uses. It is used to treat hypercalcemia resulting from a number of causes and has been a valuable therapy for Paget disease. Calcitonin also appears to be a valuable aid in the management of certain types of osteoporosis. The reader is referred to a recent review on this subject.[161]

Biochemistry

Twelve species of CT have been identified (including human), and common features include a 1-7 amino terminus disulfide bridge that causes the amino terminus to assume the shape of a ring, a C-terminus proline amide residue, and a glycine at residue 28. Five of the nine N-terminus residues are identical among many species.[162] The calcitonin gene encodes two distinct hormones in the initial gene transcript: a 141-amino acid precursor for CT and a 128-amino acid precursor for calcitonin gene-related peptide (Fig. 32-6). Calcitonin is the major processed peptide in C cells, whereas calcitonin gene-related peptide is the processed peptide in neurons.

Biosynthesis and Metabolism

Calcitonin is secreted by mitochondria of thyroid parafollicular C cells. Other tissue sources of CT are the pituitary, neuroendocrine cells, and carcinomatous lesions such as medullary thyroid carcinoma and small cell lung cancer.[163,164] Calcitonin is therefore used as a tumor marker for those cancers. The serum calcium concentration is the most important regulator of CT

secretion.[162] However, the effects of chronic hypercalcemia and chronic hypocalcemia are controversial.[165] C cells respond to hypercalcemia by increasing CT secretion. However, if the hypercalcemia is severe and prolonged, the C cells exhaust their secretory reserve.[162] Women have lower CT concentrations than do men.[166,167] The mechanism responsible for this gender difference is unclear, but the effect of gonadal steroids on CT secretion might play an important role. Newborn infants have high serum concentrations of this hormone, and a significant rise in blood immunoassayable circulating calcitonin (iCT) occurs between ages 6 and 12 years concurrent with a fall in PTH.[168] Calcitonin may condition skeletal remodeling in the growing child by modulating the rate of bone resorption. The metabolism of CT is complex and involves many organ systems. Degradation of the hormone occurs in kidney, liver, bone, and thyroid gland.[169] Inactivation is more important than excretion, and relatively small amounts of CT can be detected in urine. The physiologic significance of calcitonin on calcium homeostasis is not well established.

Calcitonin Gene–Related Peptide

Two calcitonin gene-related peptides (α- and β-CGRP), in addition to CT, form the CT family of regulatory peptides.[170] β-CGRP is the product of a separate gene, but it is structurally similar to α-CGRP, differing only by three amino acids; both peptides have similar biologic properties.[171-173] α-CGRP has been identified in brain, thyroid, heart, smooth muscle, and nerve fibers.[170, 174, 175] Neurons containing CGRP have been identified in the heart, where it is considered an essential regulator of cardiovascular function and vascular tone.[156,174,176] The CT and CGRP molecules are approximately the same size, and both contain a disulfide bridge at the N-terminus. These similarities may account for the ability of these hormones to bind to each other's receptor, and to produce similar *in vivo* biologic responses.[43,159,177]

Because very little CGRP is released into the circulation, CGRP is thought to exert its effects in a paracrine/autocrine fashion.[178] CGRP's potent vasodilatory activity is induced by its binding to two CGRP receptors: CGRP-1, and CGRP-2.[178] CGRP-1 and CGRP-2 receptors have been identified in the human fetoplacental unit[91], however, only CGRP-1 receptors are demonstrable in the human uterine artery.[179] The mechanism of action of CGRP is unclear. It appears that CGRP interacts with receptors on smooth

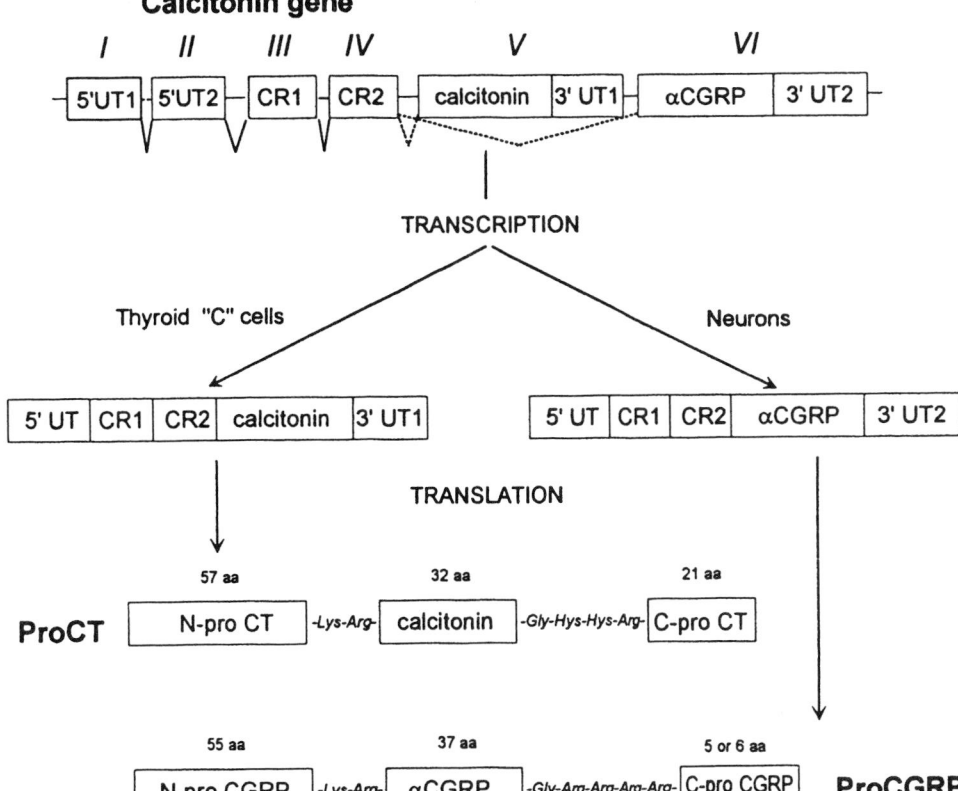

Figure 32–6. The structure of the calcitonin gene. The calcitonin (CT) gene is composed of 6 exons which encode the calcitonin (exon V) and the calcitonin gene–related peptide α (α-CGPR, exon VI). (From Civitelli R, Avioli LV: The biochemistry and function of calciotropic hormones. *In* Crass MF, Avioli LV [eds]: Calcium-Regulating Hormones and Cardiovascular Function. Boca Raton, Florida, CRC Press, 1995.)

muscle cells that are coupled to cAMP production.[180] In rat aorta, CGRP exerts endothelium-dependent relaxant effects by releasing nitric oxide.[178] However, CGRP activity in human placenta is independent of nitric oxide.[91]

REFERENCES

1. Krane SM: Calcium, phosphate, and magnesium. *In* Rasmussen H (ed): International Encyclopedia of Pharmacology and Therapeutics. London, Pergamon Press, 1970, pp 1–19.
2. Brown EM: Physiology and pathophysiology of the extracellular calcium-sensing receptor. Am J Med *106*:238, 1999.
3. Brown EM, MacLeod RJ: Extracellular calcium sensing and extracellular calcium signaling. Physiol Rev *81*:239, 2001.
4. Brauner-Osborne H, et al: Cloning and characterization of a human orphan family C G-protein coupled receptor GPRC5D. Biochim Biophys Acta *1518*:237, 2001.
5. Rasmussen H, et al: Calcium ion as intracellular messenger and cellular toxin. Environ Health Perspect *84*:17, 1990.
6. Lin KI, et al: Elevated extracellular calcium can prevent apoptosis via the calcium-sensing receptor. Biochem Biophys Res Commun *249*:325, 1998.
7. Frazao JM, et al: The calcimimetic agents: perspectives for treatment. Kidney Int Suppl *80*:149, 2002.
8. Coburn JW, et al: Calcium-sensing receptor and calcimimetic agents. Kidney Int Suppl *73*:S52, 1999.
9. Chattopadhyay N: Biochemistry, physiology, and pathophysiology of the extracellular calcium-sensing receptor. Int J Biochem Cell Biol *32*:789, 2000.
10. Fukugawa M, Kurokawa K: Calcium homeostasis and imbalance. Nephron *92*(Suppl 1):1:41, 2002.
11. Short AD, Taylor CW: Parathyroid hormone controls the size of the intracellular Ca(2+) stores available to receptors linked to inositol trisphosphate formation. J Biol Chem *275*:1807, 2000.
12. Habener JF, et al: Parathyroid hormone biosynthesis. Correlation of conversion of biosynthetic precursors with intracellular protein migration as determined by electron microscope autoradiography. J Cell Biol *80*:715, 1979.
13. Milstein C, et al: A possible precursor of immunoglobulin light chains. Nat New Biol *239*:117, 1972.
14. Habener JF, et al: Early events in the cellular formation of proparathyroid hormone. J Cell Biol *85*:292, 1980.
15. Habener JF: Regulation of parathyroid hormone secretion and biosynthesis. Annu Rev Physiol *43*:211, 1981.
16. Shimizu N, et al: Parathyroid hormone (PTH)-(1-14) and -(1-11) analogs conformationally constrained by alpha-aminoisobutyric acid mediate full agonist responses via the juxtamembrane region of the PTH-1 receptor. J Biol Chem *276*:49003, 2001.
17. Divieti P, et al: Human PTH-(7-84) inhibits bone resorption in vitro via actions independent of the type 1 PTH/PTHrP receptor. Endocrinology *143*:171, 2002.
18. MacGregor RR, et al: The degradation of proparathormone and parathormone by parathyroid and liver cathepsin B. J Biol Chem *254*:4428, 1979.
19. Segre GV, et al: Metabolism of parathyroid hormone: physiologic and clinical significance. Am J Med *56*:774, 1974.
20. Harms HM, et al: Pulse amplitude and frequency modulation of parathyroid hormone in primary hyperparathyroidism. J Clin Endocrinol Metab *78*:53, 1994.
21. Jubiz W, et al: Circadian rhythm in serum parathyroid hormone concentration in human subjects: correlation with serum calcium, phosphate, albumin, and growth hormone levels. J Clin Invest *51*:2040, 1972.
22. Calvo MS, et al: Circadian variation in ionized calcium and intact parathyroid hormone: evidence for sex differences in calcium homeostasis. J Clin Endocrinol Metab *72*:69, 1991.
23. Scothorne RJ: Functional capacity of fetal parathyroid glands with reference to their clinical use as homografts. Ann NY Acad Sci *120*:669, 1964.
24. Tsang RC, et al: Possible pathogenetic factors in neonatal hypocalcemia of prematurity. The role of gestation, hyperphosphatemia, hypomagnesemia, urinary calcium loss, and parathormone responsiveness. J Pediatr *82*:423, 1973.
25. Loughead JL, et al: Serum ionized calcium concentrations in normal neonates. Am J Dis Child *142*:516, 1988.
26. Tsang RC, et al: Hypocalcemia in infants of diabetic mothers. Studies in calcium, phosphorus, and magnesium metabolism and parathormone responsiveness. J Pediatr *80*:384, 1972.
27. Tsang RC, et al: Neonatal hypocalcemia in infants with birth asphyxia. J Pediatr *84*:428, 1974.
28. Brown EM: Calcium receptor and regulation of parathyroid hormone secretion. Rev Endocr Metab Disord *1*:307, 2000.
29. Segre G: Secretion, metabolism, and circulating heterogeneity of parathyroid hormone. *In* Favus MJ (ed): Primer on Metabolic Bone Disease and Disorders of Bone Metabolism. New York, Raven Press, 1993, p 55.
30. Breitwieser GE, Gama L: Calcium-sensing receptor activation induces intracellular calcium oscillations. Am J Physiol Cell Physiol *280*:C1412, 2001.
31. Houillier P, et al: [Calcium-sensing receptors: physiology and pathology]. Arch Pediatr *8*:516, 2001.
32. Garfia B, et al: Regulation of parathyroid vitamin D receptor expression by extracellular calcium. J Am Soc Nephrol *13*:2945, 2002.

33. Heath HI: Biogenic amines and the secretion of parathyroid hormone and calcitonin. Endocrinol Rev *1*:319, 1980.

34. Morrissey J, Slatopolsky E: Effect of aluminum on parathyroid hormone secretion. Kidney Int Suppl *18*:S41, 1986.

35. Brown EM: Histamine receptors on dispersed parathyroid cells from pathological human parathyroid tissue. J Clin Endocrinol Metab *51*:1325, 1980.

36. Williams GA, et al: Parathyroid hormone secretion in normal man and in primary hyperparathyroidism: role of histamine H2 receptors. J Clin Endocrinol Metab *52*:122, 1981.

37. Dietel M, et al: Influence of vitamin D3, 1,25-dihydroxyvitamin D3, and 24,25-dihydroxyvitamin D3 on parathyroid hormone secretion, adenosine 3′,5′-monophosphate release, and ultrastructure of parathyroid glands in organ culture. Endocrinology *105*:237, 1979.

38. Windeck R, et al: Effect of gastrointestinal hormones on isolated bovine parathyroid cells. Endocrinology *103*:2020, 1978.

39. Au WY: Cortisol stimulation of parathyroid hormone secretion by rat parathyroid glands in organ culture. Science *193*:1015, 1976.

40. Fischer JA, et al: Calcitonin stimulation of parathyroid hormone secretion in vitro. Horm Metab Res *13*:223, 1971.

41. Habener JF, Potts JT Jr: Relative effectiveness of magnesium and calcium on the secretion and biosynthesis of parathyroid hormone in vitro. Endocrinology *98*:197, 1976.

42. Brown EM, et al: Extracellular calcium potentiates the inhibitory effects of magnesium on parathyroid function in dispersed bovine parathyroid cells. Metabolism *33*:171, 1984.

43. Krahn DD, et al: Effects of calcitonin gene-related peptide on food intake. Peptides *5*:861, 1984.

44. Martin K, et al: Selective uptake of intact parathyroid hormone by the liver: differences between hepatic and renal uptake. J Clin Invest *58*:781, 1976.

45. Hruska KA, et al: Peripheral metabolism of intact parathyroid hormone. Role of liver and kidney and the effect of chronic renal failure. J Clin Invest *67*:885, 1981.

46. D'Amour P, et al: Characteristics of bovine parathyroid hormone extraction by dog liver in vivo. Am J Physiol *241*:E208, 1981.

47. Rouleau MF, et al: Parathyroid hormone binding in vivo to renal, hepatic, and skeletal tissues of the rat using a radioautographic approach. Endocrinology *118*:919, 1986.

48. Segre GV, et al: Metabolism of parathyroid hormone by isolated rat Kupffer cells and hepatocytes. J Clin Invest *67*:449, 1981.

49. Martin KJ, et al: The peripheral metabolism of parathyroid hormone. N Engl J Med *301*:1092, 1979.

50. Segre GV, et al: Edman degradation of radioiodinated parathyroid hormone: application to sequence analysis and hormone metabolism in vivo. Biochemistry *16*:2417, 1977.

51. Goltzman D, et al: Cytochemical bioassay of parathyroid hormone: characteristics of the assay and analysis of circulating hormonal forms. J Clin Invest *65*:1309, 1980.

52. Talmage R: Removal of calcium from bone as influenced by the parathyroids. Endocrinology *62*:717, 1958.

53. Mundy G: Osteoclast ontogeny and function. *In* WAP (ed): Bone and Mineral Research. Amsterdam, Elsevier, 1987, pp 209–210.

54. Slovik DM, et al: Restoration of spinal bone in osteoporotic men by treatment with human parathyroid hormone (1-34) and 1,25-dihydroxyvitamin D. J Bone Miner Res *1*:377, 1986.

55. Agus ZS, et al: Effects of parathyroid hormone on renal tubular reabsorption of calcium, sodium, and phosphate. Am J Physiol *224*:1143, 1973.

56. Mannstadt M, et al: Receptors for PTH and PTHrP: their biological importance and functional properties. Am J Physiol *277*:F665, 1999.

57. Juppner H, et al: AG protein-linked receptor for parathyroid hormone and parathyroid hormone-related peptide. Science *254*:1024, 1991.

58. Schneider H, et al: Cloning and functional expression of a human parathyroid hormone receptor. Eur J Pharmacol *246*:149, 1993.

59. Abou-Samra AB, et al: Expression cloning of a common receptor for parathyroid hormone and parathyroid hormone-related peptide from rat osteoblast-like cells: a single receptor stimulates intracellular accumulation of both cAMP and inositol trisphosphates and increases intracellular free calcium. Proc Natl Acad Sci USA *89*:2732, 1992.

60. Tong Y, et al: Functional expression and signaling properties of cloned human parathyroid hormone receptor in *Xenopus* oocytes. Evidence for a novel signaling pathway. J Biol Chem *271*:8183, 1996.

61. Seuwen K, Boddeke HG: Heparin-insensitive calcium release from intracellular stores triggered by the recombinant human parathyroid hormone receptor. Br J Pharmacol *114*:1613, 1995.

62. Behar V, et al: The human PTH2 receptor: binding and signal transduction properties of the stably expressed recombinant receptor. Endocrinology *137*:2748, 1996.

63. McSheehy PM, Chambers TJ: Osteoblastic cells mediate osteoclastic responsiveness to parathyroid hormone. Endocrinology *118*:824, 1986.

64. Chen L: Sodium gradient-dependent phosphate transport in renal brush border vesicles. J Biol Chem *256*:1556, 1981.

65. Suba L: A parathyroid hormone-related protein implicated in malignant hypercalcemia: cloning and expression. Science *237*:893, 1987.

66. Juppner H, et al: The parathyroid hormone-like peptide associated with humoral hypercalcemia of malignancy and parathyroid hormone bind to the same receptor on the plasma membrane of ROS 17/2.8 cells. J Biol Chem *263*:8557, 1988.

67. Chase LR, Aurbach GD: Parathyroid function and the renal excretion of 3′5′-adenylic acid. Proc Natl Acad Sci U S A *58*:518, 1967.

68. Meltzer V, et al: Parathyroid hormone stimulation of renal phosphoinositide metabolism is a cyclic nucleotide-independent effect. Biochim Biophys Acta *712*:258, 1982.

69. Yamaguchi DT, et al: Parathyroid hormone-activated calcium channels in an osteoblast-like clonal osteosarcoma cell line. cAMP-dependent and cAMP-independent calcium channels. J Biol Chem *262*:7711, 1987.

70. Abou-Samra AB, et al: Parathyroid hormone causes translocation of protein kinase-C from cytosol to membranes in rat osteosarcoma cells. Endocrinology *124*:1107, 1989.

71. Goodman WG, et al: Parathyroid hormone (PTH), PTH-derived peptides, and new PTH assays in renal osteodystrophy. Kidney Int *63*:1, 2003.

72. Massfelder T, et al: Opposing mitogenic and anti-mitogenic actions of parathyroid hormone-related protein in vascular smooth muscle cells: a critical role for nuclear targeting. Proc Natl Acad Sci USA *94*:13630, 1997.

73. Philbrick WM, et al: Defining the roles of parathyroid hormone-related protein in normal physiology. Physiol Rev *76*:127, 1996.

74. Wysolmerski JJ, Stewart AF: The physiology of parathyroid hormone-related protein: an emerging role as a developmental factor. Annu Rev Physiol *60*:431, 1998.

75. Stewart AF, et al: Biochemical evaluation of patients with cancer-associated hypercalcemia: evidence for humoral and nonhumoral groups. N Engl J Med *303*:1377, 1980.

76. Bilezikian JP: Parathyroid hormone-related peptide in sickness and in health. N Engl J Med *322*:1151, 1990.

77. Burtis WJ, et al: Immunochemical characterization of circulating parathyroid hormone-related protein in patients with humoral hypercalcemia of cancer. N Engl J Med *322*:1106, 1990.

78. Lu C, et al: Glucocorticoid regulation of parathyroid hormone-related peptide gene transcription in a human neuroendocrine cell line. Mol Endocrinol *3*:2034, 1989.

79. Heath JK, et al: Epidermal growth factor-stimulated parathyroid hormone-related protein expression involves increased gene transcription and mRNA stability. Biochem J *307*(Pt 1):159, 1995.

80. Rizzoli R, et al: Regulation of parathyroid hormone-related protein production in a human lung squamous cell carcinoma line. J Endocrinol *143*:333, 1994.

81. Merryman JI, et al: Regulation of parathyroid hormone-related protein production by a squamous carcinoma cell line in vitro. Lab Invest *69*:347, 1993.

82. Soifer NE, et al: Parathyroid hormone-related protein. Evidence for secretion of a novel mid-region fragment by three different cell types. J Biol Chem *267*:18236, 1992.

83. Goltzman D: Parathyroid hormone-like peptide: molecular characterization and biological properties. Trends Endocrinol Metab *20*:39, 1989.

84. Fukayama S, et al: Human parathyroid hormone (PTH)–related protein and human PTH: comparative biological activities on human bone cells and bone resorption. Endocrinology *123*:2841, 1988.

85. Torres R, et al: Effects of the (1-34) fragment of synthetic parathyroid hormone-related protein on tartrate-resistant acid phosphatase and alkaline phosphatase and alkaline phosphatase activities, and on osteocalcin synthesis, in cultured fetal rat calvaria. Miner Electrolyte Metab *19*:64, 1993.

86. Kemp BE, et al: Parathyroid hormone-related protein of malignancy: active synthetic fragments. Science *238*:1568, 1987.

87. Strewler GJ: The physiology of parathyroid hormone-related protein. N Engl J Med *342*:177, 2000.

88. Budayr AA, et al: High levels of a parathyroid hormone-like protein in milk. Proc Natl Acad Sci U S A *86*:7183, 1989.

89. Thiede MA, Rodan GA: Expression of a calcium-mobilizing parathyroid hormone-like peptide in lactating mammary tissue. Science *242*:278, 1988.

90. Moseley JM, et al: Immunohistochemical detection of parathyroid hormone-related protein in human fetal epithelia. J Clin Endocrinol Metab *73*:478, 1991.

91. Mandsager NT, et al: Vasodilator effects of parathyroid hormone, parathyroid hormone-related protein, and calcitonin gene-related peptide in the human fetal-placental circulation. J Soc Gynecol Investig *1*:19, 1994.

92. Hellmen P: Parathyroid-like regulation of parathyroid hormone-related protein release and cytoplasmic calcium in cytotrophoblast cells of human placenta. Arch Biochem Biophys *293*:174, 1992.

93. Ferguson JE 2nd, et al: Abundant expression of parathyroid hormone-related protein in human amnion and its association with labor. Proc Natl Acad Sci U S A *89*:8384, 1992.

94. Germain AM, et al: Parathyroid hormone-related protein mRNA in avascular human amnion. J Clin Endocrinol Metab *75*:1173, 1992.

95. Bowden SJ, et al: Parathyroid hormone-related protein in human term placenta and membranes. J Endocrinol *142*:217, 1994.

96. Curtis NE, et al: The expression of parathyroid hormone-related protein mRNA and immunoreactive protein in human amnion and choriodecidua is increased at term compared with preterm gestation. J Endocrinol *154*:103, 1997.

97. Curtis NE, et al: Intrauterine expression of parathyroid hormone-related protein in normal and pre-eclamptic pregnancies. Placenta *19*:595, 1998.

98. Kaiser SM, et al: Antisense-mediated inhibition of parathyroid hormone-related peptide production in a keratinocyte cell line impedes differentiation. Mol Endocrinol *8*:139, 1994.

99. Kremer R, et al: Regulation of parathyroid hormone–like peptide in cultured normal human keratinocytes. Effect of growth factors and 1,25-dihydroxy-vitamin D3 on gene expression and secretion. J Clin Invest 87:884, 1991.
100. Deftos LJ, et al: Neoplastic hormone-producing cells of the placenta produce and secrete parathyroid hormone–related protein. Studies by immunohistology, immunoassay, and polymerase chain reaction. Lab Invest 71:847, 1994.
101. Dunne FP, et al: Parathyroid hormone–related protein (PTHrP) gene expression in fetal and extra-embryonic tissues of early pregnancy. Hum Reprod 9:149, 1994.
102. Alsat E, et al: Increase in epidermal growth factor receptor and its mRNA levels by parathyroid hormone (1-34) and parathyroid hormone–related protein (1-34) during differentiation of human trophoblast cells in culture. J Cell Biochem 53:32, 1993.
103. Lee K, et al: Expression of parathyroid hormone–related peptide and its receptor messenger ribonucleic acids during fetal development of rats. Endocrinology 136:453, 1995.
104. Macgill K, et al: Vascular effects of PTHrP (1-34) and PTH (1-34) in the human fetal-placental circulation. Placenta 18:587, 1997.
105. Thiede MA, et al: Intrauterine occupancy controls expression of the parathyroid hormone–related peptide gene in preterm rat myometrium. Proc Natl Acad Sci U S A 87:6969, 1990.
106. Williams ED, et al: Effect of parathyroid hormone–related protein (PTHrP) on the contractility of the myometrium and localization of PTHrP in the uterus of pregnant rats. J Reprod Fertil 102:209, 1994.
107. Dalle M, et al: Parathyroid hormone–related peptide inhibits oxytocin-induced rat uterine contractions in vitro. Arch Int Physiol Biochim Biophys 100:251, 1992.
108. Kovacs CS, et al: Parathyroid hormone–related peptide (PTHrP) regulates fetal-placental calcium transport through a receptor distinct from the PTH/PTHrP receptor. Proc Natl Acad Sci U S A 93:15233, 1996.
109. Orloff JJ, et al: Parathyroid hormone–related protein as a prohormone: post-translational processing and receptor interactions. Endocr Rev 15:40, 1994.
110. MacLeod RJ, et al: PTHrP stimulated by the calcium-sensing receptor requires MAP kinase activation. Am J Physiol Endocrinol Metab, 284:E435, 2003.
111. MacLaughlin JA, et al: Spectral character of sunlight modulates photosynthesis of previtamin D3 and its photoisomers in human skin. Science 216:1001, 1982.
112. Nemere I, Norman AW: 1,25-Dihydroxyvitamin D3–mediated vesicular transport of calcium in intestine: time-course studies. Endocrinology 122:2962, 1988.
113. Nemere I: Transport of calcium. In Field MF, et al (eds): Handbook of Physiology. Bethesda, MD, American Physiological Society, 1991, pp 337–347.
114. Theofan G, et al: Regulation of calbindin-D28K gene expression by 1,25-dihydroxyvitamin D3 is correlated to receptor occupancy. J Biol Chem 261:16943, 1986.
115. Reichel H, et al: Production of 1 alpha, 25-dihydroxyvitamin D3 by hematopoietic cells. Prog Clin Biol Res 332:81, 1990.
116. Manolagas SC, et al: 1,25-Dihydroxyvitamin D3 and the immune system. Proc Soc Exp Biol Med 191:238, 1989.
117. Pike JW: Vitamin D3 receptors: structure and function in transcription. Annu Rev Nutr 11:189, 1991.
118. Minghetti PP, Norman AW: 1,25(OH)2-vitamin D3 receptors: gene regulation and genetic circuitry. FASEB J 2:3043, 1988.
119. Lowe KE, et al: Vitamin D-mediated gene expression. Crit Rev Eukaryot Gene Expr 2:65, 1992.
120. Walters MR: Newly identified actions of the vitamin D endocrine system. Endocrinol Rev 13:719, 1992.
121. Holic M: Vitamin D metabolism and biological function. In Avioli LK (ed): Metabolic Bone Disease and Clinically Related Disorders. Philadelphia, WB Saunders, 1990, pp 155–156.
122. Caffrey JM, Farach-Carson MC: Vitamin D3 metabolites modulate dihydropyridine-sensitive calcium currents in clonal rat osteosarcoma cells. J Biol Chem 264:20265, 1989.
123. Deboland A: Ca 2+-channel agonist bay K8644 mimics 1,25 (OH)2-vitamin D3 rapid enhancement of Ca2+ transport in chick perfused duodenum. Biochem Biophys Res Commun 166:217, 1990.
124. Evans RM: The steroid and thyroid hormone receptor superfamily. Science 240:889, 1988.
125. Baker AR, et al: Cloning and expression of full-length cDNA encoding human vitamin D receptor. Proc Natl Acad Sci U S A 85:3294, 1988.
126. Suda T, et al: The role of vitamin D in bone and intestinal cell differentiation. Annu Rev Nutr 10:195, 1990.
127. Rodan GA, Martin TJ: Role of osteoblasts in hormonal control of bone resorption—a hypothesis. Calcif Tissue Int 33:349, 1981.
128. Yoon KG, et al: Characterization of the rat osteocalcin gene: stimulation of promoter activity by 1,25-dihydroxyvitamin D3. Biochemistry 27:8521, 1988.
129. Demay MB, et al: Regions of the rat osteocalcin gene which mediate the effect of 1,25-dihydroxyvitamin D3 on gene transcription. J Biol Chem 264:2279, 1989.
130. Fraser JD, et al: 1,25-Dihydroxyvitamin D3 stimulates the synthesis of matrix gamma-carboxyglutamic acid protein by osteosarcoma cells. Mutually exclusive expression of vitamin K-dependent bone proteins by clonal osteoblastic cell lines. J Biol Chem 263:911, 1988.
131. Prince CW, Butler WT: 1,25-Dihydroxyvitamin D3 regulates the biosynthesis of osteopontin, a bone-derived cell attachment protein, in clonal osteoblast-like osteosarcoma cells. Coll Relat Res 7:305, 1987.
132. Noda M, et al: Transcriptional regulation of osteopontin production in rat osteosarcoma cells by type beta transforming growth factor. J Biol Chem 263:13916, 1988.
133. Franceschi RT, et al: 1 Alpha, 25-dihydroxyvitamin D3 specific regulation of growth, morphology, and fibronectin in a human osteosarcoma cell line. J Cell Physiol 123:401, 1985.
134. Majeska RJ, Rodan GA: The effect of 1,25(OH)2D3 on alkaline phosphatase in osteoblastic osteosarcoma cells. J Biol Chem 257:3362, 1982.
135. Dupret JM, et al: Transcriptional and post-transcriptional regulation of vitamin D–dependent calcium-binding protein gene expression in the rat duodenum by 1,25-dihydroxycholecalciferol. J Biol Chem 262:16553, 1987.
136. Christakos S, et al: Vitamin D–dependent calcium-binding proteins: chemistry, distribution, functional considerations, and molecular biology. Endocrinol Rev 10:3, 1989.
137. Nemere I, Szego CM: Early actions of parathyroid hormone and 1,25-dihydroxycholecalciferol on isolated epithelial cells from rat intestine: II. Analyses of additivity, contribution of calcium, and modulatory influence of indomethacin. Endocrinology 109:2180, 1981.
138. Nemere I, et al: Calcium transport in perfused duodena from normal chicks: enhancement within fourteen minutes of exposure to 1,25-dihydroxyvitamin D3. Endocrinology 115:1476, 1984.
139. Nemere I, Szego CM: Early actions of parathyroid hormone and 1,25-dihydroxycholecalciferol on isolated epithelial cells from rat intestine I. Limited lysosomal enzyme release and calcium uptake. Endocrinology 108:1450, 1981.
140. Karsenty G, et al: Early effects of vitamin D metabolites on phosphate fluxes in isolated rat enterocytes. Am J Physiol 248(1 Pt 1):G40, 1985.
141. Birge SJ, Alpers DH: Stimulation of intestinal mucosal proliferation by vitamin D. Gastroenterology 64:977, 1973.
142. Spielvogel AM, et al: Studies on the mechanism of action of calciferol. V. Turnover time of chick intestinal epithelial cells in relation to the intestinal action of vitamin D. Exp Cell Res 74:359, 1972.
143. Reichel H, Norman AW: Systemic effects of vitamin D. Annu Rev Med 40:71, 1989.
144. Kurnick B: Vitamin D metabolites stimulate phosphatidylcholine transfer to renal brush-border membranes. Biochem Biophys Acta 47:858, 1986.
145. Armbrecht HJ, et al: Effect of PTH and 1,25(OH)2D3 on renal 25(OH)D3 metabolism, adenylate cyclase, and protein kinase. Am J Physiol 246(1 Pt 1):E102, 1984.
146. Chandler JS, et al: 1,25-Dihydroxyvitamin D3 induces 25-hydroxyvitamin D3-24-hydroxylase in a cultured monkey kidney cell line (LLC-MK2) apparently deficient in the high affinity receptor for the hormone. J Biol Chem 259:2214, 1984.
147. Rucker RB, Stites T: New perspectives on function of vitamins. Nutrition 10:507, 1994.
148. Seamark DA, et al: The estimation of vitamin D and its metabolites in human plasma. J Steroid Biochem 14:111, 1981.
149. Steichen JJ, et al: Elevated serum 1,25-dihydroxyvitamin D concentrations in rickets of very low-birth-weight infants. J Pediatr 99:293, 1981.
150. Marx SJ, et al: Renal receptors for calcitonin. Binding and degradation of hormone. J Biol Chem 248:4797, 1973.
151. Hollis BW: Evaluation of the total feto-maternal vitamin D relationship at term: evidence for racial differences. J Clin Endocrinol Metab 59:652, 1986.
152. Koo WW, et al: Elevated serum calcium and osteocalcin levels from calcitriol in preterm infants. A prospective randomized study. Am J Dis Child 140:1152, 1986.
153. Specker BL, et al: Sunshine exposure and serum 25-hydroxyvitamin D concentrations in exclusively breast-fed infants. J Pediatr 107:372, 1985.
154. Chambers TJ, et al: The effect of calcium-regulating hormones and prostaglandins on bone resorption by osteoclasts disaggregated from neonatal rabbit bones. Endocrinology 116:234, 1985.
155. Moonga BS, et al: Regulation of cytosolic free calcium in isolated rat osteoclasts by calcitonin. J Endocrinol 132:241, 1992.
156. Deftos LJ: Mechanisms of bone metabolism. In Kem DF (ed): Pathophysiology. Philadelphia, JB Lippincott, 1984, pp 445–462.
157. Marx SJ, et al: Normal intrauterine development of the fetus of a woman receiving extraordinarily high doses of 1,25-dihydroxyvitamin D3. J Clin Endocrinol Metab 51:1138, 1980.
158. Shah GV, et al: Calcitonin inhibits basal and thyrotropin-releasing hormone-induced release of prolactin from anterior pituitary cells: evidence for a selective action exerted proximal to secretagogue-induced increases in cytosolic Ca2+. Endocrinology 127:621, 1990.
159. Goltzman D, Mitchell J: Interaction of calcitonin and calcitonin gene-related peptide at receptor sites in target tissues. Science 227:1343, 1985.
160. Zhu GC, et al: Amylin increases cyclic AMP formation in L6 myocytes through calcitonin gene-related peptide receptors. Biochem Biophys Res Commun 177:771, 1991.
161. Pondel M: Calcitonin and calcitonin receptors: bone and beyond. Int J Exp Pathol 81:405, 2000.
162. Deftos LJ: Calcitonin and medullary thyroid carcinoma. In Wyngaarden J, et al (eds): Cecil Textbook of Medicine. Philadelphia; WB Saunders, 1991, pp. 1420–1421.
163. Deftos LJ: Pituitary cells secrete calcitonin in the reverse hemolytic plaque assay. Biochem Biophys Res Commun 146:1350, 1987.
164. Becker KL, et al: Immunocytochemical localization of calcitonin in Kulchitsky cells of human lung. Arch Pathol Lab Med 104:196, 1980.

165. Austin LA, Heath H 3rd: Calcitonin: physiology and pathophysiology. N Engl J Med *304*:269, 1981.
166. Deftos IJ, et al: Influence of age and sex on plasma calcitonin in human beings. N Engl J Med *302*:1351, 1980.
167. Tiegs RD, et al: Secretion and metabolism of monomeric human calcitonin: effects of age, sex, and thyroid damage. J Bone Miner Res *1*:339, 1986.
168. Tiegs RD, et al: Calcitonin secretion in postmenopausal osteoporosis. N Engl J Med *312*:1097, 1985.
169. Deftos IJ: Calcitonin secretion in humans. *In* Cooper C (ed). Current Research on Calcium Regulating Hormones. Austin, University of Texas Press, 1987, p 79.
170. MacIntyre I: The calcitonin peptide family: relationship and mode of action. Bone Miner *16*:160, 1992.
171. Amara SG, et al: Expression in brain of a messenger RNA encoding a novel neuropeptide homologous to calcitonin gene-related peptide. Science *229*:1094, 1985.
172. Petermann JB, et al: Identification in the human central nervous system, pituitary, and thyroid of a novel calcitonin gene-related peptide, and partial amino acid sequence in the spinal cord. J Biol Chem *262*:542, 1987.
173. Brain SD, et al: Calcitonin gene-related peptide is a potent vasodilator. Nature *313*:54, 1985.
174. Ramana CV, et al: Localization and characterization of calcitonin gene-related peptide mRNA in rat heart. Am J Med Sci *304*:339, 1992.
175. Kawai Y, et al: Topographic localization of calcitonin gene-related peptide in the rat brain: an immunohistochemical analysis. Neuroscience *15*:747, 1985.
176. Bukoski RD, Kremer D: Calcium-regulating hormones in hypertension: vascular actions. Am J Clin Nutr *54*(1 Suppl):220S, 1991.
177. Lenz HJ, et al: Biological actions of human and rat calcitonin and calcitonin gene-related peptide. Regul Pept *12*:81, 1985.
178. Zaidi M, et al: The calcitonin gene peptides: biology and clinical relevance. Crit Rev Clin Lab Sci *28*:109, 1990.
179. Jansen I: Characterization of calcitonin gene-related peptide (CGRP) receptors in guinea pig basilar artery. Neuropeptides *21*:73, 1992.
180. Fiscus RR, et al: hCGRP8-37 antagonizes vasodilations and cAMP responses to rat CGRP in rat caudal artery. Ann N Y Acad Sci *657*:513, 1992.

33

Shahid M. Husain, M. Zulficar Mughal, and Reginald C. Tsang

Calcium, Phosphorus, and Magnesium Transport Across the Placenta

PLACENTAL TRANSPORT OF CALCIUM

During mammalian pregnancy, the placenta transports large amounts of calcium (Ca) to allow rapid fetal skeletal mineralization. In all species that have been studied so far, the rate of maternofetal Ca transfer increases dramatically during the last third of pregnancy. In the human, two-thirds of the 28 g of Ca accumulated in a healthy term fetus is transported during the third trimester.[1] Similarly, in the rat, fetal Ca content increases from 0.45 mg on day 17 of gestation to 12.3 mg at term (22 days).[2]

Active Calcium Transport

In late pregnancy, the concentration of total, ultrafilterable, and ionized Ca in fetal plasma is higher than in maternal plasma (Table 33-1); in the human, this maternofetal gradient is present as early as 20 to 26 weeks' gestation.[3,4] It is likely, therefore, that maternofetal transfer of Ca uses active *transcellular* mechanisms that overcome the concentration gradient across the placenta. However, based on physiologic evidence, there seem to be placental *paracellular* water-filled channels that could be used by any solute, although the morphologic correlate of these channels is difficult to identify. The relative contribution of transcellular and paracellular Ca transport is unclear, but the latter mechanism may be of greater significance in the human.[5] The remainder of this section deals only with active transport of Ca across the placenta.

There is considerable evidence to support the concept of active maternofetal Ca transport in the placenta. Using a method in which the fetal circulation of the *in situ* rat placenta is artificially perfused, Štulc and Štulcová[6] noted that the maternofetal clearance of ^{45}Ca (37.4±0.8 μL/minute) was considerably greater than that of inert, electrically neutral, hydrophilic molecules, such as sucrose (2.6±0.3 μL/minute), which are believed to move across the placenta by passive diffusion. In earlier studies, perfusion of the fetal circulation of the *in situ* guinea pig placenta with plasma from an adult guinea pig[7] and the *in situ* ovine placenta with autologous blood[8] resulted in an increase in the ionized[8] and total[7,8] Ca concentrations of the perfusate effluent compared with the concentration in the inflowing fluid.

TABLE 33-1

Maternal and Fetal Plasma Calcium Concentrations (mmol/L)

	Mother				Fetus			
	Total	*(n)*	*Ultrafilterable/Ionized*	*(n)*	*Total*	*(n)*	*Ultrafilterable/Ionized*	*(n)*
Human	2.13±0.15	(115)	1.12±0.06[i]	(115)	2.65±0.19	(115)	1.41±0.09[i]	(115)
Monkey	2.05±0.008	(7)	1.05±0.006[i]	(5)	2.10±0.008	(7)	1.33±0.005[i]	(5)
Rat	2.23±0.06	(9)	1.10±0.03[i]	(17)	2.75±0.002	(49)	1.42±0.03[i]	(18)
Guinea pig	1.70±0.06	(13)	1.23±0.05[u]	(13)	2.30±0.03	(13)	1.53±0.04[u]	(13)
Sheep	2.12±0.05	(40)	0.99±0.09[i]	(5)	3.30±0.05	(42)	1.59±0.16[i]	(6)
Pig	2.53±0.02	(19)	0.79±0.03[i]	(5)	3.10±0.04	(22)	1.12±0.14	(5)

Values are SEM. u = ultrafilterable; i = ionized.
From Sibley CP, Boyd RDH: Control of transfer across the mature placenta. *In* Clarke JR (ed): Oxford Reviews of Reproductive Biology. Vol 10. By permission of Oxford University Press, 1988.

Further evidence of active maternofetal placental Ca transport has been provided by numerous observations. Shaw and co-workers[9] reported a significant decrease in the unidirectional maternofetal clearance of ^{45}Ca across *in situ* perfused rat placenta after the addition of potassium cyanide (metabolic inhibitor) to perfusion media (Fig. 33–1), or after lowering the temperature of the perfusate (Fig. 33–2), findings confirming the earlier report by Štulc and Štulcová.[6] Using *in vitro* perfusion of

a human placental lobule, Abramovich and colleagues[10] reported an increase in both ionized and total Ca concentrations in the fetal perfusate reservoir during recycling perfusion. Finally, Štulc[5] provided evidence that the transcellular component of unidirectional maternofetal Ca flux ($^{Ca}J_{MF}$) across the isolated human placental cotyledon is saturable and sensitive to cyanide.

Thus, maternofetal transport of Ca across the placenta takes place against a concentration gradient, is temperature dependent,

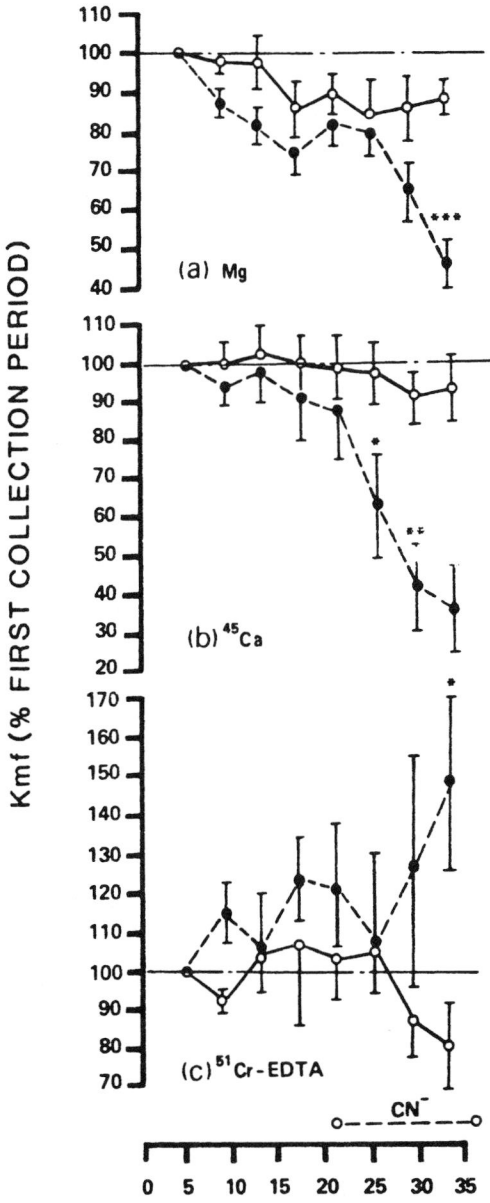

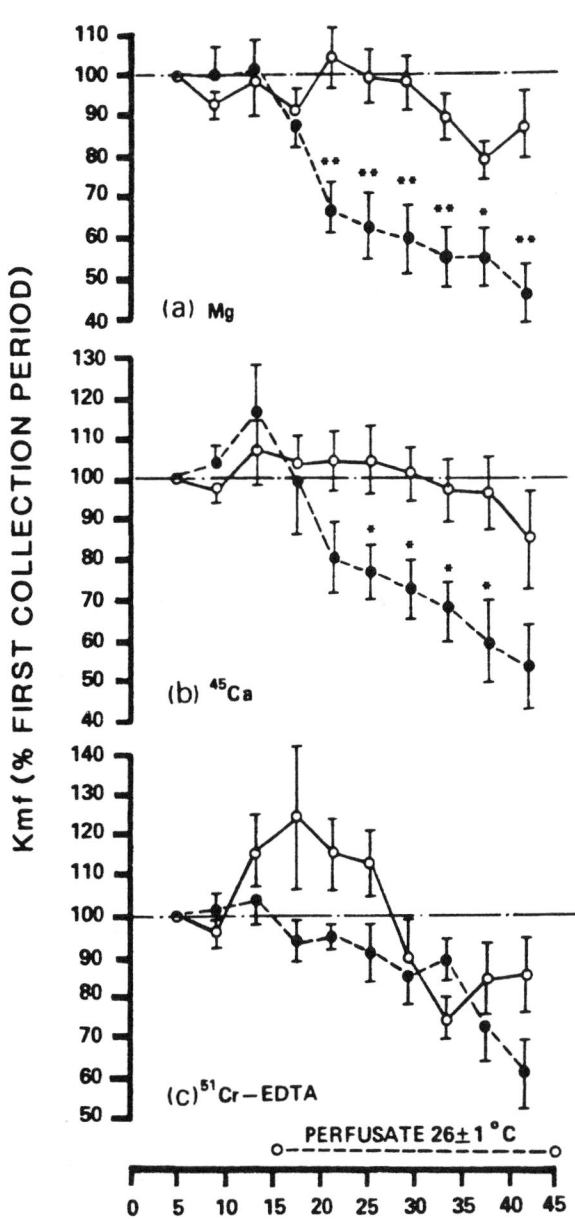

Figure 33–1. Effects of potassium cyanide (CN) (1 mmol/1 final concentration) to perfusate fluid on maternofetal clearance (K_{mf}) of (*a*) magnesium (Mg), (*b*) calcium (^{45}Ca), and (*c*) chromium-51 ethylenediaminetetraacetic acid (^{51}Cr-EDTA) across *in situ*, fetally perfused rat placentas (*n* = 6/group). Mean K_{mf} values ±SEM are normalized to that for the first 4-minute perfusate collection period. Statistical significance between treated (*solid circles*) and control (*open circles*) groups: *p < .05; **p < .01; ***p < .001 (Student's *t*-test, two tails). (From Shaw AJ, et al: Pediatr Res *27*:622, 1990.)

Figure 33–2. Effects of lowering of tempereature of perfusate fluid from 37°C on maternofetal clearance (K_{mf}) of (*a*) magnesium (Mg), (*b*) calcium (^{45}Ca), and (*c*) chromium-51 ethylenediaminetetraacetic acid (^{51}Cr-EDTA) across *in situ*, fetally perfused rat placentas (*n* = 6/group). Mean K_{mf} values ±SEM are normalized to that for the first 4-minute perfusate collection period. Statistical significance between treated (*solid circles*) and control (*open circles*) groups: *p < .05; **p < .01; ***p < .001 (Student's *t*-test, two tails). (From Shaw AJ, et al: Pediatr Res *27*:622, 1990.)

is inhibited by metabolic inhibitors such as cyanide, and is considerably faster than that of molecules that cross the placenta by simple diffusion. All these findings support the conclusion that placental Ca transport involves active transfer processes.

Bidirectional Placental Calcium Transport

Studies employing radioactive isotopes of Ca as tracers have revealed that transport of Ca across the mammalian placenta is bidirectional, with marked species variation in the relative magnitudes of unidirectional maternofetal, unidirectional fetomaternal, and net Ca fluxes. In the sheep near term, placental Ca transport is highly asymmetric, with a calculated $^{Ca}J_{MF}$ of 215 mg/day/kg fetal weight and a $^{Ca}J_{FM}$ of 12 mg/day/kg fetal weight.[11] A similar situation probably prevails in the rat, because the value for net Ca flux estimated from the increase of fetal Ca content between day 20 and day 21 of gestation (100 ± 4 nmol/minute), is close to the $^{Ca}J_{MF}$ (100 ± 7 nmol/minute) estimated in nonanesthetized animals at 21 days.[6] By contrast, in the rhesus monkey, the magnitudes of bidirectional placental Ca fluxes are comparatively similar to one another ($^{Ca}J_{MF}$, 391 mg/kg/day; $^{Ca}J_{FM}$ 326 mg/kg/day).[11] In the human, bidirectional clearances of Ca are also similar (unidirectional maternofetal clearance, 40.9 ± 14.7 μL/g/minute placenta; unidirectional fetomaternal clearance, 39.1 ± 21.8 μL/g/minute).[5] These fluxes and clearances are considerably higher than the rate of daily fetal Ca accumulation or the net flux, which, in the rhesus monkey at term, has been estimated to be 40 mg of Ca per day/kg fetal body weight,[12] and in the human, 200 mg of Ca per day during the last trimester.[1] A similar situation also exists for placental transfer of sodium (Na) across the human placenta.[13]

Mechanisms of Placental Calcium Transport

Although the placental content of total Ca is high,[14] the free cytosolic Ca concentration must be maintained in the submicromolar range, by analogy with other transporting epithelia,[15] if viability is to be preserved. In isolated placental cells, the cytosolic concentration of free Ca is in the nanomolar range.[16] Therefore, the large traffic of Ca ions across the trophoblast poses a threat to normal cellular function, and efficient mechanisms for intracellular Ca buffering and translocation from the maternal-facing cytosol to the fetal-facing cytosol must exist. Whereas bidirectional movements may occur by diffusion through water-filled paracellular channels, asymmetric active transport necessitates a transcellular route. Transcellular placental Ca transport is likely to involve three steps:

1. Influx or entry of Ca^{2+} from maternal plasma across maternal-facing placental membrane.
2. Movement of Ca through trophoblastic cytosol.
3. Efflux or exit of Ca^{2+} from cytosol across the basolateral or fetal-facing placental membrane.

Little is known of the mechanisms involved in Ca influx from maternal plasma into trophoblastic cytosol. The unidirectional influx of Ca is higher on the fetal than the maternal side of the placenta in the guinea pig,[17] and it is equal on both sides of the human placenta.[18] However, the net maternofetal flux is higher than the fetomaternal flux in both placental types. In studies involving uptake of ^{45}Ca from artificial media used to perfuse both the fetal and maternal circulation of guinea pig placenta, van Kreel and van Dijk[19] demonstrated that Ca enters the trophoblast as a charged ion. Thus, placental Ca transport is likely to be similar to that of the intestine, in which entry of Ca ions across the brush-border membrane occurs by passive diffusion down an electrochemical gradient. As in the gut,[15] this process in the placenta is saturable,[5,17] and, therefore, it is likely to involve a specific carrier or a member of the epithelial Ca^{2+} channel family.[20] Evidence of a carrier has been obtained by examining Ca

uptake into human placental microvillous membrane vesicles in which a two-site model was characterized with kinetic estimates of Michaelis constant (Km) of 18 μM and 1.5 mM, and maximum velocity (V_{max}) of 3.2 and 47 nmol/mg/minute, respectively. Using data from isolated placental cells, Bax and colleagues[21] suggested the presence of a Ca-activated Ca channel. The Km of Ca uptake in intestine is approximately 1 mM,[22] much higher than the Km for efflux, which is in micromolar concentrations. Therefore, the rate of Ca influx into the cells is probably the rate-limiting step for transcellular Ca flux. In the intestine, there is evidence that 1,25-dihydroxyvitamin D_3 ($1,25[OH]_2D_3$), the biologically active metabolite of vitamin D, increases the V_{max} of Ca influx, without altering the Km.[23] In other words, $1,25(OH)_2D_3$ probably increases the synthesis of Ca carrier or channel units.

Little is known about passage of Ca through the trophoblastic cytosol. Clearly, in all Ca-transporting epithelial cells, an efficient mechanism for efflux of Ca as well as intracellular compartmentalization or buffering of Ca ions in transit must exist if the cytosolic Ca concentration, which is about 1000 times lower than the extracellular Ca concentration, is to remain unaffected. This may be the role of Ca-binding proteins (CaBPs), a family of proteins involved in the transport and binding of calcium, which may serve as an intracellular Ca buffer or an intracellular shuttle and may thus facilitate transcellular Ca transport.

CaBPs have been identified in numerous species. Placental CaBP in the rat is immunologically identical to the vitamin D–dependent CaBP in the intestine,[24] but it seems to lack the classic dependency of the latter on $1,25(OH)_2D_3$ in intact animals.[25-27] However, the administration of $1,25(OH)_2D_3$ to thyroparathyroidectomized pregnant rats does result in an increase in the concentration of placental CaBP.[28] Thus, the role of maternal vitamin D in control of placental CaBP is not entirely clear.

In the rat, placental concentration of CaBP increases rapidly during the period of increased rate of fetal growth and Ca accumulation in late gestation,[24,29] a finding suggesting a role for this protein in placental Ca transport. This concept is supported by the finding of a temporal relationship between CaBP mRNA expression and $^{Ca}J_{MF}$ of Ca in the placenta of the rat[30] and by the demonstration that uptake of Ca by human placental microsomal membrane vesicles is inhibited by preincubation with antihuman CaBP antibodies.[31] Investigators have shown that CaBP enhances diffusion of Ca through an aqueous compartment,[32] and in the presence of CaBP, the rate of cytosolic Ca diffusion in enterocytes is 60- to 70-fold higher than across cytosol of CaBP-depleted cells.[33] Thus, CaBP may act as an intracellular shuttle to facilitate the diffusion of Ca through trophoblastic cytosol.

Intracellular organelles may serve as cytosolic Ca buffers and reservoirs in the placenta. In the guinea pig placenta, the subcellular distribution of ^{45}Ca is mainly in the nuclear fraction (48%), 28% is bound to cytoplasmic proteins, and approximately 10% is in the mitochondrial fraction.[19] Electron microscopy of human placenta has revealed granular Ca deposits, localized to endoplasmic reticulum and mitochondria, and in vesicles within the trophoblast.[34] Intracellular Ca sequestration is supported by the observation that a human placental microsomal membrane fraction could be reconstituted into vesicles that exhibited a magnesium (Mg^{2+})- and adenosine triphosphate (ATP)–dependent Ca uptake mechanism.[35]

Mechanisms involved in the efflux of Ca from cytosol across the fetal-facing trophoblastic membranes to fetal plasma against a steep concentration gradient are not clearly delineated. In other absorptive epithelia (e.g., the intestine and the kidney), at least two mechanisms are involved in efflux of Ca^{2+} out of the cytosol across the basolateral cell membrane:

1. Ca- and Mg-dependent adenosine triphosphatase (Ca-ATPase).
2. The Ca^{2+}/Na^+ exchanger.

There is growing evidence that, in the placenta, a Ca-ATPase may be responsible for the translocation of Ca from trophoblast cytosol to fetal extracellular fluid across the basal plasma membrane. Hydrolysis of ATP could provide the required energy to overcome the Ca concentration gradient. Ca-ATPase has been identified in placentas of guinea pigs,[36] mice,[37] and humans.[35, 38-40] It is clear that the Ca-ATPases are a heterogeneous group of enzymes,[41] not all of which are involved in Ca transport,[42, 43] and this may explain the reported dissociation between Ca-ATPase transport activity and Ca-ATPase hydrolytic activity.[35, 39] Ca uptake into highly purified human placental basal plasma membrane vesicles has been described.[44,45] This may be mediated by one of the Ca-ATPases. Monoclonal antibodies against the human erythrocyte plasma membrane Ca pump show greater specific staining in the human placental basal membrane and in the fetal-facing membrane of the rat placenta, and they inhibit by 50% transport of Ca into human placental basal plasma membrane vesicles.[46] Expression of Ca-ATPase mRNA and protein[47] in both human[47, 48] and rat[30] placenta shows little change as gestation proceeds; it appears therefore that this protein is not rate limiting in placental Ca transport.

Present evidence indicates that the Ca^{2+}/Na^+ exchange system is unimportant in regulating transplacental Ca movement. van Kreel and van Dijk,[19] who perfused both the maternal and fetal circulations of the term guinea pig placenta with Ca-free media containing ^{22}Na and unlabeled Na, found that the addition of 2 mM Ca to the media after 30 minutes of equilibration did not affect the release of preloaded ^{22}Na from placental cells into the media. The presence of a Ca^{2+}/Na^+ exchanger has been sought in the *in situ* rat placenta by perfusing the fetal circulation and measuring the maternofetal flux of Ca in the presence or absence of Na in the perfusate. In the absence of Na, maternofetal flux of Ca was found to be either unaltered[49] or decreased.[50] However, in the latter study, the effect on $^{Ca}J_{MF}$ was delayed. In addition, $^{Ca}J_{MF}$ was unaffected during perfusion with Na-containing perfusate to which ouabain, a potent $(Na^+ + K^+)$-ATPase inhibitor, had been added; by dissipation of the Na gradient, an effect on Ca flux should have occurred in the presence of a Ca^{2+}/Na^+ exchanger. *In vitro* placental membrane vesicle studies showed a lack of effect of Na or ouabain on Ca uptake.[35, 45] By contrast, in a later study using human placental basal membrane vesicles, the authors suggested the presence of a Ca^{2+}/Na^+ exchanger in this membrane;[51] however, the number of experiments was small, and the orientation of the vesicles (cytoplasmic side inside versus outside) was mixed, features that call into question the significance of this finding in relation to Ca transport across the basal membrane. Using a cDNA probe to cloned human cardiac Ca^{2+}/Na^+ exchanger, Kofuji and co-workers[52] demonstrated that the expression of this gene in human placenta is some 250-fold less than in human heart. The presence of a high-affinity, low-capacity facilitated diffusion transporter in human placental basal membrane vesicles has been reported,[53] but the functional significance of this transporter in relation to maternofetal transfer of Ca is unknown.

Control of Placental Calcium Transport

Factors that may influence the supply of Ca to the fetus include maternal and fetal plasma Ca concentrations, maternal and fetal blood flow, and the capacity and efficiency of placental transport mechanisms. In the rat, the maternofetal clearance of Ca per gram of placental tissue increases 70-fold in the last 6 days of gestation,[30] far more than could be expected by an increase in placental surface area or blood flow; uterine horn blood flow increases fivefold per placenta by day 21 of gestation compared with the virgin state.[54] In the human, over the whole of pregnancy, 170 L of maternal plasma would have to be cleared of its Ca content to account for the total amount of Ca accumulated in a term human fetus.[55] Because the estimated uterine blood flow rate in the human at term gestation is 500 mL/minute,[56] placental Ca transfer appears limited by the area and the efficiency of placental transfer mechanisms, rather than by uteroplacental blood flow.[55] However, Mughal and others[57] observed a marked decrease in the unidirectional maternofetal clearance of ^{45}Ca, but not chromium-51 ethylenediaminetetraacetic acid (^{51}Cr-EDTA, the reference diffusional marker), in growth-retarded rat fetuses induced by uterine artery ligation compared with control fetuses. The authors speculated that placental ischemia from chronic reduction *in utero* placental blood flow could result in depletion of the necessary energy supply for active placental Ca transport. Thus, flow limitation is unlikely to be important for placental Ca transport.

Influence of Maternal Calcium Concentration

Based on indirect evidence from human studies, maternal plasma Ca concentration appears to influence placental Ca transport. Maternal dietary deficiency leading to hypocalcemia can be associated with congenital rickets and neonatal hypocalcemia.[58] Transient congenital hyperparathyroidism has been reported in infants born to mothers with hypocalcemia as a result of poorly treated hypoparathyroidism.[59] It is postulated that, under these conditions, reduced net placental Ca transport leads to fetal hypocalcemia, which, in turn, results in fetal hyperparathyroidism. Conversely, transient neonatal hypoparathyroidism caused by untreated hyperparathyroidism has been reported in infants born to hypercalcemic mothers.[60] Thus, in the pregnant human, placental Ca transport appears to be dependent on the maternal plasma Ca concentration. Similar observations have been made in the guinea pig,[61] pig,[62] and rabbit,[63] but not in the sheep,[64] cow,[65] and rat.[66] In the rat, a doubling of maternal plasma Ca concentration causes only a 30% increase in the $^{Ca}J_{MF}$ across the *in situ* perfused rat placenta. It appears, therefore, that in this species an active placental pump must be working almost at maximal capacity under normal conditions.[6] In contrast, studies using the *in situ* perfused guinea pig placenta have demonstrated that maternal hypercalcemia results in a significant increase in $^{Ca}J_{MF}$,[67] which may result from submaximal saturation of the active Ca pump or from the existence of a quantitatively important and possibly unphysiologic paracellular leak pathway in this preparation.[68]

In sheep, maternal hypocalcemia does not lead to any change in fetal plasma Ca concentrations.[69] In contrast, acute maternal hypocalcemia in the rat[70] and monkey[71] results in a fall in fetal Ca concentrations, but chronic maternal hypocalcemia induced by maternal vitamin D deficiency and thyroparathyroidectomy does not alter the $^{Ca}J_{MF}$ across *in situ* perfused placentas.[72] There is clearly a marked species variation in the fetal response to maternal hypocalcemia or hypercalcemia, which may be physiologic or methodologic.

Hormonal Regulation of Placental Calcium Transport

The placenta has no nerve supply. Therefore, factors that increase placental Ca transport capacity as gestation proceeds must be either genetically preprogrammed or hormones produced by the mother, fetus, or placenta itself. Hormonal signals controlling placental Ca transfer may act on either the maternal or fetal side of the placenta. Possible regulatory hormonal candidates include $1,25(OH)_2D_3$, parathyroid hormone (PTH), calcitonin, and other peptides secreted by the parathyroid glands.

Infants born in summer are reported to have a lower bone mineral content at birth when compared with infants born in winter.[73,74] The reason for this is not entirely clear, but it may be related to seasonal differences in maternal and fetal calciotropic hormones[74,75] and their speculative effect on placental transport of Ca and Mg.

1,25-Dihydroxyvitamin D_3 and 1α-Hydroxycholecalciferol

There are anecdotal clinical reports of maternal vitamin D deficiency causing neonatal rickets,[76] consistent with the thesis that maternal vitamin D may be important for placental Ca transfer. This concept is supported by the presence of cytosolic receptors for $1,25(OH)_2D_3$ in the human and rat.[77] Potential sources of $1,25(OH)_2D_3$ available to the fetus include that transferred from maternal plasma across the placenta,[78] that synthesized by the fetal kidneys,[79] and the placenta itself.[80] Because fetal plasma concentration of $1,25(OH)_2D_3$ falls after fetal nephrectomy in sheep,[81] it appears that in sheep the fetal kidney is a major source of this metabolite of vitamin D.

The data on the role of maternal vitamin D in placental Ca transfer are conflicting. Administration of $1,25(OH)_2D_3$ to pregnant guinea pigs increases fetal Ca content of fetuses and increases maternoplacental, but not maternofetal, transfer of ^{45}Ca.[82] In sheep, maternal treatment with 1α-hydroxycholecalciferol (1α-OHCC) for 12 days leads to a significant increase in fetal Ca content, as well as maternofetal Ca transfer.[83] In the same species, maternal prolactin injections can stimulate placental Ca transfer;[84] this hormone theoretically could exert an effect on the placenta by stimulating production of $1,25(OH)_2D_3$ in the mother. By contrast, in the rat, maternal vitamin D deficiency[72,85] and parathyroidectomy[72] do not affect the maternofetal Ca gradient,[85] the total fetal Ca content,[72,85] or the maternofetal clearance of ^{45}Ca.[72] The concentrations of CaBP[25,26] and its mRNA[27] are significantly reduced in rat maternal intestine, but not placenta, under experimental conditions of maternal vitamin D deficiency. The inconsistent data reported so far may simply reflect interspecies variation.

The effect of fetal $1,25(OH)_2D_3$ on placenta Ca transport is also unclear. Fetal nephrectomy in the rat does not alter the maternofetal total Ca gradient,[86] although injection of a pharmacologic dose of $1,25(OH)_2D_3$ into 19-day rat fetuses increases the fetal Ca concentration on day 21 of gestation, compared with control fetuses.[87] Fetal nephrectomy in sheep leads to a marked decrease in the fetal plasma concentration of $1,25(OH)_2D_3$ associated with reversal of the usual maternofetal Ca gradient that is restored by infusion of $1,25(OH)_2D_3$ into the fetal circulation.[81,88] It is not clear whether these findings represent evidence of control of placental Ca transport by $1,25(OH)_2D_3$ synthesized by fetal kidneys or evidence of short-term dependence of fetal plasma Ca concentrations on mobilization from fetal bone.

In support of a direct permissive effect of fetal $1,25(OH)_2D_3$ on placental Ca transfer is the observation of Robinson and colleagues[89] that $1,25(OH)_2D_3$ stimulates $^{Ca}J_{MF}$ across *in situ* perfused placentas of rat fetuses parathyroidectomized by gross decapitation,[90] but not across placentas of intact fetuses. Because PTH is an important trophic stimulator of $1,25(OH)_2D_3$ synthesis, it is likely that parathyroidectomized rat fetuses have a lower plasma $1,25(OH)_2D_3$ concentration than intact fetuses. Therefore, $1,25(OH)_2D_3$ probably stimulates placental Ca transfer only when fetal plasma concentrations are initially low.

Parathyroid Hormone and Fetal Parathyroid Hormone–Like Peptide

In the rat, fetal parathyroidectomy by decapitation[89,91] or by injection of antibovine PTH serum[92] leads to a fall in fetal plasma total Ca concentration, which is restored by administration of parathyroid extract.[92,93] Similarly, in the sheep, fetal thyroparathyroidectomy with thyroxine replacement results in a rapid fall in fetal Ca^{2+} concentration within 24 hours.[94-96] As previously mentioned, there is a significant fall in maternofetal clearance of ^{45}Ca across the *in situ* perfused placentas of decapitated rat fetuses,[89] and it is increased (but not returned to normal) by sub-

cutaneous administration of bovine PTH(1–84) to the fetuses. This stimulatory effect of PTH(1–84) on maternofetal ^{45}Ca clearance may result from its direct action on the placental Ca pump, or, alternatively, the hormone may increase fetal $1,25(OH)_2D_3$ production. Perfusion of the fetal circulation of intact and decapitated rat fetuses with media containing forskolin (an activator of adenylate cyclase) stimulates maternofetal clearance of ^{45}Ca. However, synthetic rat PTH amide (r[Nle,Tyr])PTH[1–34]) has no effect under these conditions,[98] and because this amide can also increase placental cyclic AMP release,[98] the role of placental adenylate cyclase in Ca transfer is not clear.

Another candidate hormone that may stimulate placental Ca transport is PTH-related protein (PTHrP).[99] The addition of fetal parathyroid gland extract, partially purified PTHrP from a human lung cancer cell line, or recombinant PTHrP, but not bovine PTH(1–84) or rat PTH(1–34),[100] to autologous fetal blood used to perfuse placentas of thyroparathyroidectomized sheep fetuses *in situ* leads to an increase in the rate of Ca accumulation in the fetal blood reservoir.[94,100-102] In sheep, it appears that mid-molecule fragments of PTHrP may be responsible for the stimulation of placental Ca transport.[94,103,104] When human PTHr (hPTHrP) (1–34) or hPTHrP(75–86) is infused into the fetal circulation of the *in situ* rat placenta, these peptides have no effect on Ca transport.[98] However, there is indirect evidence that fetal PTHrP fragments increase maternofetal transport of Ca in murine[105] and human[106] placentas. Surprisingly, net fetal Ca accretion is increased in the absence of fetal PTHrP.[107] Taken together, it appears that, in the absence of fetal PTHrP, maternofetal flux of Ca is decreased, but fetomaternal flux is decreased to a greater extent; the change in the former may be related to PTHrP absence or secondary $1,25(OH)_2D_3$ deficiency in fetal plasma or both.

Calcitonin

In sheep, Barlet[108] demonstrated that chronic maternal calcitonin deficiency (achieved by maternal thyroparathyroidectomy and thyroxine replacement) led to a significant increase in the total fetal Ca content and fetal accumulation of ^{45}Ca on day 140, but not on day 77, of gestation (term gestation, ~150 days). Calcitonin replacement in these ewes led to normalization of both the fetal Ca content and the maternofetal transfer of ^{45}Ca. Thus, in this species, maternal calcitonin deficiency appears to decrease the $^{Ca}J_{MF}$.

PLACENTAL TRANSPORT OF PHOSPHORUS

Provision of an adequate supply of phosphorus (P) to the developing fetus is important because of its role in intermediary metabolism and skeletal mineralization. In mammals during the latter part of gestation, the plasma concentration of P in the fetus is higher than that in the mother (Table 33-2). Thus, placental transfer of P in the maternofetal direction occurs against a con-

TABLE 33-2

Concentrations of Inorganic Phosphorus in Maternal and Fetal Plasma (mmol/L)

Species	Mother	(n)	Fetus	(n)
Human*	1.43±0.5	(115)	1.92±0.4	(115)
Sheep†	1.29±0.16	(6)	1.97±0.4	(6)
Guinea pig‡	1.25±0.1	(6)	1.96±0.13	(6)
Rat§	1.75±0.25	(12)	3.29±0.15	(21)

*Schauberger and Pitkin (1979).[139]
†Mellor and Matheson (1977).[140]
‡Durand, et al (1982).[61]
§Garel, et al (1980).[141]

centration gradient and is likely to involve an active transport process. Most fetal P content is transported to the fetus during the latter stages of pregnancy.[109,110]

Mechanisms of Placental Phosphorus Transport

The flux of P across the placenta is bidirectional, with flux in the maternofetal direction exceeding that in the fetomaternal direction.[49,111] As shown in Figure 33-3, for a 60-g fetus, the calculated net flux of P is 0.7 μmol/minute, a value that is similar to that obtained from retention of P by guinea pig fetuses of comparable weight.[109] Placental uptake of P at both the maternal and fetal faces of guinea pig placenta is reduced by anoxic conditions, by the addition of cyanide, or by the reduction or elimination of Na from the perfusion media.[109] From these results, it appears that the transcellular, bidirectional P transport is highly asymmetric and depends on a Na-dependent active transport mechanism. Maternofetal flux prevails over fetomaternal flux and is reduced by anoxic conditions or addition of cyanide.

In vitro P uptake studies using human placental brush-border membrane vesicles support the presence of a high-affinity (Km, 87 μM; pH, 7; 35°C) Na-dependent transport system[112,113] that is likely to be saturated *in vivo*. At pH 8, the Km increases (500 μM), whereas an increase in the Na concentration of the incubation medium increases P uptake by an increase in V_{max} but not Km. Temperature influences P uptake by changing both Km and V_{max}. The uptake of P by these vesicles is noncompetitively inhibited by glycine, alanine, and proline. Thus, in the human, pH, temperature, Na, and amino acid concentrations appear to modulate the transport of P from maternal plasma into the trophoblastic cytosol.

Hormonal Regulation of Placental Phosphorus Transport

Factors that modulate placental P transport have not been extensively studied. Based on the presence of receptors for

1,25$(OH)_2D_3$[77] and for PTH[114] in the placenta, it has been suggested that these hormones may regulate placental P transport. In the rat, maternal vitamin D deficiency does not affect the maternofetal plasma P concentration gradient or fetal P content at term gestation.[84] In contrast, intravenous administration of 1α-OHCC to pregnant sheep resulted in a significant increase in both maternal and fetal P concentrations.[115] Similarly, Barlet and co-workers[65] observed that feeding of *Solanum glucophyllum* leaves, which contain 1,25$(OH)_2D_3$, to pregnant cows resulted in hyperphosphatemia both in the mother and the fetus. From these studies, it is not clear whether the maternal 1,25$(OH)_2D_3$ or its analogues given to the mother increase fetal serum P concentrations by stimulating net placental P transport or simply by increasing the concentration of P in maternal plasma.

There is some evidence of modulation of placental P transport by vitamin D or its analogues in sheep. Injection of 1α-OHCC to pregnant ewes for 12 days results in increased maternofetal transport of ^{32}P at day 140 of gestation.[83] Lowering of fetal 1,25$(OH)_2D_3$ by fetal nephrectomy leads to increased fetal plasma concentration of P, which can be prevented by daily intravenous injections of 1,25$(OH)_2D_3$ into the fetuses.[88] The authors speculated that unidirectional fetomaternal P transport in this species could be regulated by 1,25$(OH)_2D_3$ produced by fetal kidneys.

The uptake of P by human placental brush-border membrane is inhibited by PTH, with its action possibly mediated by cAMP.[116] Because adenylate cyclase is located in the basal plasma membranes, fetal PTH may reduce placental P transfer in the fetomaternal direction. Thus, 1,25$(OH)_2D_3$, acting on the maternal as well as the fetal side of the placenta, and fetal PTH may regulate placental P transport.

PLACENTAL TRANSPORT OF MAGNESIUM

Toward the end of pregnancy, the plasma concentrations of total and ultrafiltrable Mg[117] in the fetus exceed those of the mother (Table 33-3). Therefore, maternofetal Mg transfer occurs against a concentration gradient and is likely to involve active transport mechanisms. Support for this concept comes from studies by Shaw and others,[9] who observed that the unidirectional maternofetal clearance of Mg across perfused rat placentas *in situ* was considerably higher (26.7 μL/g/minute) than that of ^{51}Cr-EDTA, the reference diffusional marker (3.2 μL/g/minute). They also showed that the maternofetal clearance of Mg was significantly reduced by the addition of cyanide to fetal perfusate (see Fig. 33-1) or by lowering of perfusate temperature (see Fig. 33-2).

In human pregnancy, fetal Mg content increases rapidly after the fifth month of gestation, with net fluxes of about 4.5 mg of Mg per day.[118] Bidirectional Mg flux has been demonstrated in sheep, with maternofetal flux (0.042 mg/kg fetal weight/hour) exceeding fetomaternal flux (0.012 mg/kg/hour).[119]

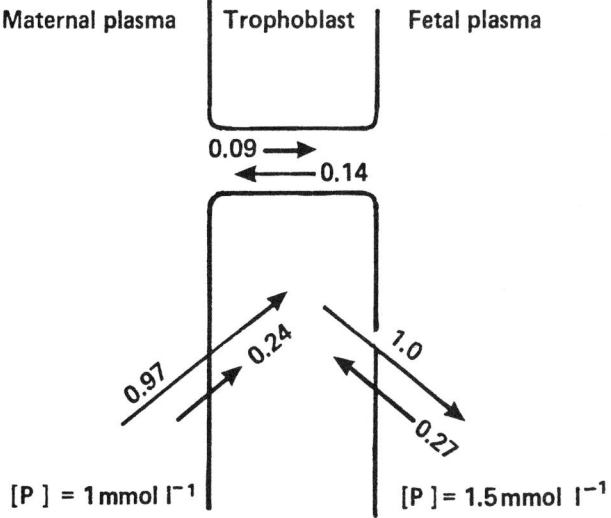

Maternal plasma   Trophoblast   Fetal plasma

0.09 →
← 0.14

0.97   0.24   1.0   0.27

[P] = 1 mmol l^{-1} [P] = 1.5 mmol l^{-1}

Figure 33-3. The components of phosphorus fluxes expressed in micromoles across fetal and maternal faces of a guinea pig placenta (Štulc and colleagues[111] and Štulc and Štulcová[49]). The net phosphorus flux, 0.7 μmol/minute, is similar to the retention of phosphorus by the guinea pig fetus of comparable weight (Fuch and Fuchs[109]). The paracellular fluxes are only a small fraction of the total bidirectional trophoblastic phosphorus fluxes. P = plasma phosphorus concentration. (Adapted from Štulc J, Štulcová: Placenta 5:9, 1984.)

TABLE 33-3

Concentrations of Magnesium in Maternal and Fetal Plasma (mmol/L)

Species	Mother	(n)	Fetus	(n)
Human*	0.66±0.16	(115)	0.71±0.16	(115)
Sheep†	0.71±0.7	(6)	0.99±0.7	(6)
Guinea pig‡	1.11±0.05	(6)	1.20±0.03	(6)
Rat§	0.66±0.02	(15)	0.98±0.03	(23)

*Schauberger and Pitkin (1979).[139]
†Mellor and Matheson (1977).[140]
‡Wood, et al (1978).[142]
§Dancis, et al (1971).[143]

Mechanisms of Placental Magnesium Transport

Little is known of the mechanisms of placental Mg transport. Influx of Mg across the maternal-facing placental membrane may be a passive process depending on the intracellular free Mg concentration and transmembrane potential difference. Membrane proteins mediating this influx have not been identified, but they could be Mg channels or facilitated type carriers. The mechanism by which Mg is translocated across the placental cytoplasm is unknown, but it may be by simple diffusion in either the free or bound state. Mg efflux across the fetal-facing placental membrane is likely to be an energy-dependent process. It is clear that the mechanisms involved in placental Mg transport are separate from those of Ca.[9,120,121]

In the rat, administration of amiloride or furosemide reduces maternofetal Mg flux, consistent with the presence of a Na^+/Mg^{2+} exchanger and Mg^{2+}/HCO_3^- co-transporter.[122] The presence of Na^+/Mg^{2+} is supported by the studies of Shaw and collaborators,[50] who found that the maternofetal clearance of Mg across the *in situ* perfused rat placenta was reduced when the perfusate was either Na free or contained ouabain, both of which would reduce the electrochemical gradient for Na. However, the presence of acetazolamide (a carbonic anhydrase inhibitor) in the perfusate had no effect on the clearance of Mg, and, therefore, the role of an Mg^{2+}/HCO_3^- co-transporter remains speculative.[54]

Control of Placental Magnesium Transport

There is no direct information on the regulation of placental Mg transport. However, insight into placental transfer mechanisms is provided by observing the effect of therapeutic and experimental manipulations of maternal plasma Mg concentrations on fetal plasma and carcass Mg concentrations and the fetomaternal plasma Mg gradient. Treatment of preeclampsia with Mg leads to maternal and fetal hypermagnesemia:[123] either the Mg-transporting pump apparently is not saturated at physiologic plasma Mg concentrations, or there is a high diffusional permeability to Mg in this species. By contrast, in the rat, intraperitoneal administration of Mg leads to a threefold increase in the maternal plasma Mg concentration but only a slight increase in fetal plasma Mg concentration.[124] However, maternal hypomagnesemia in the rat produced by dietary deficiency leads to reduced fetal plasma and carcass Mg concentrations and a loss of the fetomaternal Mg gradient.[117,125] In sheep, neither maternal hypermagnesemia nor maternal hypomagnesemia affects the fetal plasma Mg concentration.[126] Thus, in sheep, placental Mg transport appears to be saturated even when the mother is hypermagnesemic. In addition, any diffusional component of transfer must be small in relation to the carrier-mediated component. The interspecies variation in fetal response to maternal hypomagnesemia and hypermagnesemia may be related to differences in placental structure.

Hormonal Regulation of Placental Magnesium Transport

There is some evidence that in sheep, Mg transport is increased by fetal parathyroid gland extract and mid-molecule fragments of hPTHrP(67–86) and hPTHrP(75–86), whereas the amino-terminal end (hPTHrP[1–34]) has no effect.[94] The same is not true for mid-molecule PTHrP fragments in the rat.[98] These contradictory findings may represent method or species differences.

MINERAL TRANSFER IN DIABETIC PREGNANCIES AND IN INTRAUTERINE GROWTH RETARDATION

Disturbances in fetal growth are commonly encountered in diabetic pregnancy in both animals and humans. In the rat, fetal growth retardation is a consistent finding.[127] This contrasts with the situation in the diabetic pregnant woman, whose children tend to be overgrown at term, although in the first trimester of such pregnancies, the fetus may be growth retarded and may more closely resemble the condition in rats.[128] Many different qualitative and quantitative changes have been reported in placentas of diabetic pregnancies, but there are few data on measurement of placental nutrient flux in such pregnancies.

The bone mineral content in infants of diabetic mothers is reduced by about 10% when compared with infants of nondiabetic mothers.[129] Fetal histomorphometric analysis and ashing studies demonstrated similar findings in the offspring of diabetic rats.[127] From these data, it appears that net fetal accretion of bone minerals and fetal bone mineralization in diabetic pregnancy are reduced. Whereas the increased incidence of hypocalcemia and hypomagnesemia reported in infants of diabetic mothers may result from disturbances in calciotropic hormone responsiveness,[128–132] the reduced fetal bone mineral accretion is likely to be associated with lower net placental transport of bone minerals. We investigated this situation in more detail by measuring the maternofetal flux of Ca and Mg across the *in situ* perfused rat placenta of the streptozocin-induced diabetic rat.[133] Our results indicate that, in the presence of untreated maternal diabetes, the maternofetal flux of both Ca and Mg is reduced by between 20% and 40%, accompanied by lower net fetal accretion of Ca and Mg. These disturbances can be prevented by control of the diabetes with insulin. Fetuses of the untreated diabetic group weighed significantly less than the other groups, but even when an allowance was made for this difference, the Ca content, but not the Mg content, remained significantly lower in the untreated diabetic group of animals. Thus, the net flux of Ca across the diabetic rat placenta is reduced to a greater degree than that expected from growth retardation alone. This is different from the situation in which growth retardation is induced in the rat by reducing uterine blood flow. In that model, net Ca flux is appropriate for fetal size.[57]

The pathophysiology of these disturbances in placental transport of Ca and Mg during diabetic rat pregnancy is not fully understood, and it is likely that a combination of factors leads to altered placental transport and fetal accretion of Ca and Mg. Hypomagnesemia[134] and hypermagnesuria[135] are common in diabetes mellitus, and pregnancy has an additive effect on renal Mg excretion.[136] However, our observations in the untreated diabetic rat pregnancy do not support reduced cation availability as a cause of the reduced maternofetal flux of these cations,[133] although they do support the finding that CaBP is reduced in the placentas of diabetic rats.[137] Our data, confirmed by others,[138] demonstrate that the expression of CaBP mRNA in placentas of diabetic rats is reduced by a factor of 12 to 15.[133]

Infants who are small for gestational age have a lower bone mineral content compared with those whose size is appropriate for gestational age,[74] even after allowing for seasonal variation.[74] The reasons for this are unclear but may be related to differences in calciotropic hormones between infants who are small for gestational age and those who are appropriate for gestational age.[74] Using an experimental model of fetal growth retardation in the rat (uterine artery ligation), we showed that maternofetal transfer of Ca across the placenta is reduced proportional to the reduction in body size.[57] This finding may simply reflect the smaller requirement of Ca in a small fetus, but it may also reflect a depletion of the necessary energy supply for active placental Ca transport secondary to a chronic reduction *in utero* placental blood flow.

REFERENCES

1. Widdowson EM, Spray CM: Chemical development *in utero.* Arch Dis Child 26:205, 1951.
2. Comar CL: Radiocalcium studies in pregnancy. Ann NY Acad Sci 64:281, 1956.
3. Forestier F, et al: Blood chemistry of normal human fetuses at midtrimester of pregnancy. Pediatr Res 21:579, 1987.

4. Moinz CF, et al: Normal reference ranges for biochemical substances relating to renal, hepatic, and bone function in fetal and maternal plasma throughout pregnancy. J Clin Pathol *38*:468, 1985.

5. Štulc J: Parallel mechanisms of Ca^{++} transfer across the perfused human cotyledon. Am J Obstet Gynecol *170*:162, 1994.

6. Štulc J, Štulcová B: Transport of calcium by the placenta of the rat. J Physiol (Lond) *371*:1, 1986.

7. Twardock AR, Austin MK: Calcium transfer in perfused guinea pig placenta. Am J Physiol *219*:540, 1970.

8. Weatherley J, et al: The transfer of calcium during perfusion of the placenta in intact and thyroparathyroidectomized sheep. Placenta *4*:271, 1983.

9. Shaw AJ, et al: Evidence for active maternofetal transfer of magnesium across the *in situ* perfused rat placenta. Pediatr Res *27*:622, 1991.

10. Abramovich DR, et al: Calcium transport across the isolated dually perfused human placental lobule. J Physiol (Lond) *382*:397, 1987.

11. Ramberg CF, et al: Kinetic analysis of calcium transport across the placenta. J Appl Physiol *35*:662, 1973.

12. MacDonald NS, et al: Movement of calcium in both directions across the primate placenta. Proc Soc Exp Biol Med *119*:476, 1965.

13. Flexner LB, et al: The permeability of the human placenta to sodium in normal and abnormal pregnancies and the supply of sodium to the human fetus as determined by radioactive sodium. Am J Obstet Gynecol *55*:469, 1948.

14. Challier JC, et al: The magnesium, calcium, sodium, potassium and chloride contents of the term human placenta. Magnes Res *1*:141, 1988.

15. van Os CH: Transcellular calcium transport in intestinal and renal epithelial cells. Biochem Biophys Acta *906*:195, 1987.

16. Hellman P, et al: Parathyroid-like regulation of parathyroid hormone–related protein release and cytoplasmic calcium in cytotrophoblast cells of human placenta. Arch Biochem Biophys *293*:174, 1992.

17. Sweiry JH, Yudilevich DL: Asymmetric calcium influx and efflux at maternal and fetal sides of the guinea-pig placenta: kinetics and specificity. J Physiol (Lond) *355*:295, 1984.

18. Sweiry JH, et al: Evidence of saturable uptake mechanisms at the maternal and fetal sides of the perfused human placenta by rapid paired-tracer dilution: studies with calcium and choline. J Dev Physiol *8*:435, 1986.

19. van Kreel BK, van Dijk JP: Mechanisms involved in the transfer of calcium across the isolated guinea pig placenta. J Dev Physiol *5*:155, 1983.

20. Hoendrop JGJ, et al: Function and expression of the epithelial Ca^{2+} channel family: comparison of mammalian ECaC1 and 2. J Physiol (Lond) *537*:747, 2001.

21. Bax C, et al: Observations on Ca^{2+} entry into cultured human term trophoblasts via a putative Ca^{2+}-operated Ca^{2+} channel. Placenta *13*:A.4, 1992.

22. Bronner F, et al: Calcium uptake by isolated rat intestinal cells. J Cell Physiol *166*:322, 1983.

23. Laing CT, et al: Characterization of 1,25 dihydroxyvitamin D_3–dependent calcium uptake in isolated chick duodenal cells. J Membr Biol *90*:145, 1986.

24. Bruns MEH, et al: Placental calcium binding protein in rats: apparent identity with vitamin D–dependent calcium binding protein from the rat intestine. J Biol Chem *253*:3186, 1978.

25. Bruns MEH, et al: Regulation of calcium-binding protein in mouse placenta and intestine. Am J Physiol *242*:E47, 1982.

26. Marche P, et al: Intestinal and placental calcium-binding proteins in vitamin D–deprived or supplemented rats. Life Sci *23*:2555, 1978.

27. Glazier JD, et al: Calbindin-D_{9K} gene expression in rat chorioallantoic placenta is not regulated by 1,25-dihydroxyvitamin D_3. Pediatr Res *37*:720, 1995.

28. Garel J-M, et al: Vitamin D_3 metabolite injections to thyroparathyroidectomized pregnant rats: effects on calcium-binding proteins of maternal duodenum and of feto-placental unit. Endocrinology *109*:284, 1981.

29. Delorme AC, et al: Vitamin D–dependent calcium-binding protein: changes during gestation, prenatal and postnatal development in rats. J Dev Physiol *1*:181, 1979.

30. Glazier JD, et al: Gestational changes in Ca^{2+} transport across rat placenta and mRNA for calbindin$_{9K}$ and Ca^{2+}-ATPase. Am J Physiol *263*:R930, 1992.

31. Tuan RS: Calcium-binding protein of the human placenta: characterization, immunohistochemical localization and functional involvement in Ca^{2+} transport. Biochem J *227*:317, 1985.

32. Feher JJ: Facilitated calcium diffusion by intestinal calcium-binding protein. Am J Physiol *244*:C303, 1983.

33. Bronner F, et al: An analysis of intestinal calcium transport across the intestine. Am J Physiol *250*:G561, 1986.

34. Croley TE: The intracellular localization of calcium within the mature human placental barrier. Am J Obstet Gynecol *77*:10, 1973.

35. Whitsett JA, Tsang RC: Calcium uptake and binding by membrane fractions of the human placenta. Pediatr Res *14*:769, 1980.

36. Shami Y, Radde IC: Calcium-stimulated ATPase of guinea-pig placenta. Biochem Biophy Acta *249*:345, 1971.

37. Tuan RS, Bigioni N: Ca^{2+}-activated ATPase of the mouse chorioallantoic placenta: developmental expression, characterization and cytohistochemical localization. Development *110*:505, 1990.

38. Miller RK, Berndt WO: Evidence for Mg^{2+}-dependent (Na^+/K^+)-activated ATPase and Ca^{2+}-ATPase in the human placenta. Proc Soc Exp Biol Med *143*:118, 1973.

39. Treinen KA, Kulkarni AP: High-affinity, calcium-stimulated ATPase in brush border membranes of the human term placenta. Placenta *7*:365, 1986.

40. Tuan RS, Kushner T: Calcium-activated ATPase of the human placenta: identification, characterization, and functional involvement in calcium transport. Placenta *8*:53, 1987.

41. Monteith GR, et al: The plasma membrane calcium pump, its role and regulation: new complexities and possibilities. J Pharmacol Toxicol Methods *40*:183, 1998.

42. Kelley LK, Smith CH: Use of GTP to distinguish calcium transporting ATPase activity from other calcium dependent nucleotide phosphatases in human placental basal plasma membrane. Biochem Biophys Res Commun *148*:126, 1987.

43. Kelley LK, et al: The calcium-transporting ATPase and the calcium- or magnesium-dependent nucleotide phosphatase activities of human placental trophoblast basal plasma membrane are separate enzyme activities. J Biol Chem *265*:5453, 1990.

44. Fisher GH, et al: ATP-dependent calcium transport across basal plasma membranes of human placental trophoblast. Am J Physiol *252*:C38, 1987.

45. Lafond J, et al: Characterization of calcium transport by basal plasma membranes from human placental syncytiotrophoblast. J Cell Physiol *148*:17, 1991.

46. Borke JL, et al: Calcium pump epitopes in placental trophoblast basal plasma membranes. Am J Physiol *257*:C341, 1989.

47. Strid H, Powell TL: ATP-dependent Ca^{2+} transport is up-regulated during third trimester in human syncytiotrophoblast basal membranes. Pediatr Res *48*:58, 2000.

48. Howard A, et al: Plasma membrane calcium pump expression in human placenta and small intestine. Biochem Biophys Res Commun *183*:499, 1992.

49. Štulc J, Štulcová B: Transport of inorganic phosphate by the fetal border of the guinea-pig placenta perfused *in situ*. Placenta *5*:9, 1984.

50. Shaw AJ, et al: Sodium-dependent magnesium transport across *in situ* perfused rat placenta. Am J Physiol *261*:R369, 1991.

51. Kamath SG, Smith CH: Na^+/Ca^{2+} exchange, Ca^{2+} binding, and electrogenic Ca^{2+} transport in plasma membranes of human placental syncytiotrophoblast. Pediatr Res *36*:461, 1994.

52. Kofuji P, et al: Expression of the Na-Ca exchanger in diverse tissues: a study using the cloned human cardiac Na-Ca exchanger. Am J Physiol *263*:C1241, 1990.

53. Kamath SG, et al: ATP independent calcium transport and binding by basal plasma membrane of human placenta. Placenta *15*:147, 1994.

54. Lasuncioán MA, et al: Maternal factors modulating nutrient transfer to fetus. Biol Neonate *51*:86, 1987.

55. Canning JF, Boyd RDH: Mineral and water exchange between mother and fetus. *In* Beard RW, Nathanielsz PW (eds): Fetal Physiology and Medicine. New York, Marcel Dekker, 1984, pp 481–509.

56. Blechner JN, et al: Uterine blood flow in woman at term. Am J Obstet Gynecol *120*:633, 1974.

57. Mughal MZ, et al: Clearance of calcium across *in situ* perfused placentas of intrauterine growth retarded rat fetuses. Pediatr Res *25*:420, 1989.

58. Maxwell JP: Further studies of adult rickets (osteomalacia) and fetal rickets. Proc R Soc Med *28*:265, 1934.

59. Landing BH, Kamoshita S: Congenital hyperparathyroidism secondary to maternal hypoparathyroidism. J Pediatr *77*:842, 1970.

60. Jacobson BB, et al: Neonatal hypocalcemia associated with maternal hyperparathyroidism. Arch Dis Child *53*:308, 1978.

61. Durand D, et al: Plasma calcium homeostasis in the guinea pig during the perinatal period. Biol Neonate *42*:120, 1982.

62. Care AD, et al: Calcium homeostasis in the fetal pig. J Dev Physiol *4*:85, 1982.

63. Graham RW, Porter GP: Fetal maternal plasma calcium relationships in the rabbit. Q J Exp Physiol *56*:160, 1971.

64. Bawden JW, Wolkoff AS: Fetal blood calcium responses to maternal calcium infusion in sheep. Am J Obstet Gynecol *99*:55, 1967.

65. Barlet J-P, et al: Fetal blood calcium response to maternal hypercalcemia induced in the cow by calcium infusion or by *Solanum glucophyllum* ingestion. Horm Metab Res *11*:57, 1979.

66. Chalon S, Garel J-M: Plasma calcium control in the rat fetus, III: Influence of alterations in maternal plasma calcium on fetal plasma calcium levels. Biol Neonate *48*:329, 1985.

67. Derewlany LO, Radda IC: Transplacental ^{45}Ca and ^{32}P flux in the guinea-pig: effect of maternal hypercalcemia and hypocalcemia. Can J Physiol Pharmacol *63*:1577, 1985.

68. Hedley R, Bradbury MWB: Transport of polar nonelectrolytes across the intact and perfused guinea-pig placenta. Placenta *1*:277, 1980.

69. Care AD: Calcium homeostasis in the foetus. J Dev Physiol *2*:85, 1980.

70. Garel J-M, et al: Fetal-maternal calcium relationships in rat and sheep. J Physiol (Paris) *64*:387, 1972.

71. Pitkin RM, et al: Maternal and fetal parathyroid hormone responsiveness in pregnant primates. J Clin Endocrinol Metab *51*:1044, 1980.

72. Mughal MZ, et al: Materno-fetal calcium (Ca) transfer across the *in situ* perfused rat placenta: relation to maternal 1,25-dihydroxyvitamin D (1,25D) administration (abstract). Pediatr Res, 433A, 1987.

73. Namgung R, et al: Low bone mineral content in summer-born compared with winter-born infants. J Pediatr Gastroenterol Nutr *15*:285, 1992.

74. Namgung R, et al: Reduced serum osteocalcin and 1,25-dihydroxyvitamin D concentrations and low bone mineral content in small for gestational age infants: evidence of decreased bone formation rates. J Pediatr *122*:269, 1993.

75. Verity CM, et al: Seasonal changes in perinatal vitamin D metabolism: maternal and cord blood biochemistry in normal pregnancies. Arch Dis Child *56*:943, 1981.

76. Park W, et al: Osteomalacia of the mother—rickets of the newborn. Eur J Pediatr *147*:292, 1987.

77. Pike JW, et al: Biochemical evidence for 1,25-dihydroxyvitamin D receptor macromolecules in parathyroid, pancreatic, pituitary and placental tissues. Life Sci 26:407, 1980.

78. Ron M, et al: Transfer of 25-hydroxyvitamin D_3 and 1,25-dihydroxyvitamin D_3 across the perfused human placenta. Am J Obstet Gynecol 148:370, 1984.

79. Fenton E, Britton HG: 25-Hydroxycholecalciferol 1α-hydroxylase activity in the kidney of the foetal, neonatal and adult guinea pig. Biol Neonate 37:257, 1980.

80. Whitsett JA, et al: Synthesis of 1,25-dihydroxyvitamin D_3 by human placenta in utero. J Clin Endocrinol Metab 53:486, 1981.

81. Ross R, et al: Perinatal 1,25-dihydroxycholecalciferol in the sheep and its role in the maintenance of the transplacental calcium gradient. J Endocrinol 87:17, 1980.

82. Durand D, et al: The influence of 1,25-dihydroxycalciferol on the mineral content of foetal guinea-pigs. Reprod Nutr Dev 23:235, 1983.

83. Durand D, et al: The effect of 1α-hydroxycalciferol on the placental transfer of calcium and phosphate in sheep. Br J Nutr 49:475, 1983.

84. Barlet J-P: Prolactin and calcium metabolism in pregnant ewes. J Endocrinol 107:171, 1985.

85. Brommage R, DeLuca HF: Placental transport of calcium and P is not regulated by vitamin D. Am J Physiol 246:F526, 1984.

86. Chalon S, Garel J-M: Plasma calcium control in the rat fetus, II: Influence of fetal hormones. Biol Neonate 48:313, 1985.

87. Chalon S, Garel J-M: 1,25-Dihydroxyvitamin D_3 injections into rat fetuses: effects on fetal plasma calcium, plasma phosphate and mineral content. Reprod Nutr Dev 23:567, 1983.

88. Moore ES, et al: Role of fetal 1,25-dihydroxyvitamin D production in intrauterine P and calcium metabolism. Pediatr Res 19:566, 1985.

89. Robinson NR, et al: Fetal control of calcium transport across the rat placenta. Pediatr Res 26:109, 1989.

90. Jost A: Experiences de decapitation de l'embryon de lapin. C R Acad Sci Serie B 225:322, 1947.

91. Pic P, et al: Facteurs endocriniens reglant la calcémie et de la phosphorémie du foetus du rat. C R Soc Biol 159:1274, 1965.

92. Garel J-M: Effet de l'injection d'un serum "antiparathormone" chez le foetus de rat. C R Acad Sci Serie D 271:2364, 1970.

93. Garel J-M, et al: Action de la parathormone chez le foetus de rat. Ann Endocrinol 32:253, 1971.

94. Barri M, et al: Fetal magnesium homeostasis in the sheep. Exp Physiol 75:681, 1990.

95. Care AD, Ross R: Fetal calcium homeostasis. J Dev Physiol 6:59, 1984.

96. MacIsaac RJ, et al: Role of the fetal parathyroid glands and parathyroid hormone-related protein in the regulation of placental transport of calcium, magnesium and inorganic phosphate. Reprod Fertil Dev 3:447, 1991.

97. Seamon KB, Daly JW: Forskolin: a unique diterpene activator of cyclic AMP-generating systems. J Cyclic Nucleotide Protein Phosphor Res 7:201, 1981.

98. Shaw AJ, et al: Effects of two synthetic parathyroid hormone-related protein fragments on maternofetal transfer of calcium and magnesium and release of cyclic AMP by the in situ perfused rat placenta. J Endocrinol 129:399, 1991.

99. Clemens TL, et al: Parathyroid hormone-related protein and its receptor: nuclear functions and roles in the renal and cardiovascular systems, the placental trophoblasts and the pancreatic islets. Br J Pharmacol 134:1113, 2001.

100. Rodda CP, et al: Evidence for a novel parathyroid hormone-related protein in fetal lamb parathyroid glands and sheep placenta: Comparisons with a similar protein implicated in humoral hypercalcaemia of malignancy. J Endocrinol 117:261, 1988.

101. Abbas SK, et al: The role of the parathyroid glands in fetal calcium homeostasis in the sheep. J Physiol (Lond) 386:27, 1987.

102. Abbas SK, et al: Stimulation of ovine placental calcium transport by purified natural and recombinant parathyroid hormone-related protein (PTHrP) preparations. Q J Exp Physiol 74:549, 1989.

103. Abbas SK, et al: Measurement of parathyroid hormone-related protein in extracts of fetal parathyroid glands and placental membranes. J Endocrinol 124:319, 1990.

104. Care AD, et al: Stimulation of ovine placental transport of calcium and magnesium by mid-molecule fragments of human parathyroid hormone-related protein. Exp Physiol 75:605, 1990.

105. Kovacs CS, et al: Parathyroid hormone-related peptide (PTHrP) regulates fetal-placental calcium transport through a receptor distinct from the PTH/PTHrP receptor. Proc Natl Acad Sci USA 93:15233, 1996.

106. Farrugia W, et al: Parathyroid hormone (1–34) and parathyroid hormone-related protein (1–34) stimulate calcium release from human syncytiotrophoblast basal membranes via a common receptor. J Endocrinol 166:689, 2000.

107. Tucci J, et al: The role of fetal parathyroid hormone-related protein in transplacental calcium transport. J Mol Endocrinol 17:159, 1996.

108. Barlet J-P: Calcitonin may modulate placental transfer in ewes. J Endocrinol 104:17, 1985.

109. Fuchs F, Fuchs AR: Studies on the placental transfer of phosphate in the guinea pig. Acta Physiol Scand 38:379, 1957.

110. Klem KK: Placental transmission of ^{32}P in late pregnancy and in experimental prolongation of pregnancy in rats. Acta Obstet Gynecol Scand 35:445, 1956.

111. Štulc J, et al: Uptake of inorganic phosphate by the maternal border of the guinea-pig placenta. Pflugers Arch 395:326, 1982.

112. Brunette MG, Allard S: Phosphate uptake by syncytial brush border membranes of human placenta. Pediatr Res 19:1179, 1985.

113. Lajeunesse D, Brunette MG: Sodium gradient-dependent phosphate transport in placental brush border membrane vesicles. Placenta 9:117, 1988.

114. Lafond J, et al: Parathyroid hormone receptor in human placental syncytiotrophoblast brush border and basal plasma membranes. Endocrinology 123:2834, 1988.

115. Barlet J-P, et al: Endocrine regulation of plasma phosphate in sheep fetuses with catheters implanted in utero. In Massry SG, et al (eds): Homeostasis of Phosphate and Other Minerals. New York, Plenum Press, 1978, pp 243–256.

116. Brunette MG, et al: Effect of parathyroid hormone on P transport through the human placental microvilli. Pediatr Res 25:15, 1989.

117. Dancis J, et al: Fetal homeostasis in maternal malnutrition. II. Magnesium deprivation. Pediatr Res 3:131, 1971.

118. Givens MH, Machy IG: The chemical composition of the human fetus. J Biol Chem 102:7, 1933.

119. Care AD, et al: The measurement of transplacental magnesium fluxes in the sheep. Res Vet Sci 27:121, 1979.

120. Cruz ML, et al: Effect of chronic maternal dietary magnesium deficiency on placental calcium transport. J Am Coll Nutr 11:87, 1992.

121. Mimouni F, et al: Placental calcium transport during acute maternal hypermagnesemia in the rat. Am J Obstet Gynecol 168:984, 1993.

122. Günther T, et al: Effects of amiloride and furosemide on ^{28}Mg transport into fetuses and maternal tissues of rats. Magnesium Bull 10:34, 1988.

123. Cruikshank DP, et al: Effects of magnesium sulfate treatment on perinatal calcium metabolism. Am J Obstet Gynecol 134:243, 1979.

124. Garel J-M, Barlet J-P: Calcitonin in mother, fetus and the newborn. Ann Biol Anim Biochim Biophys 18:53, 1978.

125. Vormann J, Günther T: Development of fetal mineral and trace element metabolism in rats with normal as well as magnesium- and zinc-deficient diets. Biol Trace Elem Res 9:37, 1986.

126. Barlet J-P, et al: Foetal plasma magnesium levels during maternal hypo- or hypermagnesaemia in ewes in utero. Br J Nutr 42:559, 1979.

127. Uriu-Hare JY, et al: The effect of maternal diabetes on trace element status and fetal development in the rat. Diabetes 34:1031, 1985.

128. Pedersen JF, Mølsted L: Early growth retardation in diabetic pregnancy. BMJ J 1:18, 1979.

129. Mimouni F, et al: Decreased bone mineral content in infants of diabetic mothers. Am J Perinatol 5:339, 1988.

130. Salle B, et al: Hypocalcemia in infants of diabetic mothers: studies in circulating calciotropic hormone concentrations. Acta Paediatr Scand 71:573, 1982.

131. Tsang RC, et al: Hypocalcemia in infants of diabetic mothers: studies in calcium P and magnesium metabolism and parathormone responsiveness. J Pediatr 80:384, 1972.

132. Tsang RC, et al: Hypomagnesemia in infants of diabetic mothers: perinatal studies. J Pediatr 89:115, 1976.

133. Husain SM, et al: Maternofetal calcium flux and calbindin$_{9k}$ expression in the diabetic rat placenta. Pediatr Res 35:376, 1994.

134. Jackson CE, Meier DW: Routine serum magnesium analysis. Ann Intern Med 69:743, 1968.

135. Garland HO: New experimental data on the relationship between diabetes mellitus and magnesium. Magnes Res 5:193, 1992.

136. Birdsey TJ, et al: The effect of diabetes mellitus on urinary calcium excretion in pregnant rats and their offspring. J Endocrinol 145:11, 1995.

137. Verhaeghe J, et al: 1,25 $(OH)_2D_3$ and Ca-binding protein in fetal rats: relationship to the maternal vitamin D status. Am J Physiol 254:E505, 1988.

138. Hamilton K, et al: Altered calbindin mRNA expression and calcium regulating hormones in rat diabetic pregnancy. J Endocrinol 164:67, 2000.

139. Schauberger CW, Pitkin RM: Maternal-perinatal calcium relationships. Obstet Gynecol 53:74, 1979.

140. Mellor DJ, Matheson IC: Variations in the distribution of calcium, magnesium, and inorganic phosphorus within chronically catheterized sheep conceptuses during the last eight weeks of pregnancy. Q J Exp Physiol 62:55, 1977.

141. garelJ-M, et al: Fetal-maternal calcium relationships in rat and sheep. J Physiol (Paris) 64:387, 1972.

142. Woods LL, et al: Transplacental gradients in the guinea-pig. Am J Physiol 235:H200, 1978.

143. Dancis J, Et al: Fetal homeostasis in maternal malnutrition, II: Magnesium deprivation. Pediatr Res 3:131, 1971.

Ran Namgung and Reginald C. Tsang

34

Neonatal Calcium, Phosphorus, and Magnesium Homeostasis

BODY DISTRIBUTION

Calcium

Calcium (Ca) is the most abundant mineral in the body and the major inorganic constituent of bone. An adult human body contains about 1 to 2 kg Ca.[1] In term newborn infants, the total body Ca is approximately 30 g,[1] most of which (about 80%) accrued during the last trimester of pregnancy at a rate of up to 150 mg/kg of fetal weight/day.[2]

At all ages, 99% of total body Ca is either in bone in the form of hydroxyapatite, integrally associated with collagen fibrils and other components of bone matrix, or in a noncrystalline, amorphous Ca phosphate form (a predominant form in early life).[3] One percent of total body Ca is contained in the extracellular fluid (ECF) and soft tissues. The Ca of the mineral phase (at the surface of the crystals) is in equilibrium with the ECF, but only a minor portion of the skeletal content of Ca (about 1%) is freely exchangeable with the ECF.[4] Although this exchangeable pool represents a small percentage of skeletal content, it is approximately equal to the total content of Ca in the ECF and soft tissues and serves as a reservoir of Ca. In children aged 3 to 16 years, the total exchangeable Ca pool (TEP) size, measured using stable isotope technique, correlates with age independent of variations in body weight. Bone Ca accretion rate (Vo+) and the Vo+/TEP ratio are greater in children than in adults, indicating higher bone flow of Ca associated with relatively higher exchangeable Ca pools in children compared with adults.[5]

The Ca in plasma is in three forms: as free ions (50% of total Ca); bound to plasma protein (40% of total Ca, of which 80% is bound to albumin and the remainder to globulins); and, to a small extent (about 10%), as diffusible complexes (complexed with bicarbonate, phosphate, or citrate).[6] Complexed Ca and free (ionized) Ca are also termed *ultrafiltrable* Ca (or nonprotein-bound Ca), so that about 60% of total Ca in plasma crosses semipermeable membranes. Ca binding to proteins is reduced at acid pH. Alterations in the concentration of serum albumin can exert a major influence on the measured total serum Ca and ionized Ca concentrations. The serum ionized Ca concentration decreases significantly with addition of serum albumin. Thus, a fast infusion of albumin in the human neonate has the potential for acutely lowering the serum ionized Ca concentration.[7] The concentration of free Ca ion (ionized Ca) is the only physiologically active fraction of blood Ca.

Ionized Ca influences many cellular functions and is subjected to tight hormonal control, especially through parathyroid hormone (PTH). Although changes in ionized Ca are frequently reflected in changes in total Ca and there is a general correlation between serum total Ca and serum ionized Ca, total Ca can be a poor predictor of a specific ionized Ca value. Furthermore, ionized Ca values in the neonate are not accurately predicted by the McLean-Hastings nomogram.[8] The ionized Ca can be measured directly with the use of ion-selective electrodes,[9] using capillary blood in newborn infants.[10,11] Several factors, however, may affect ionized Ca determination: higher ionized Ca values are recorded with the ICA-1 Radiometer than with the Orion SS20 electrode; ionized Ca can be decreased proportional to the concentration of heparin used as anticoagulant; ionized Ca concentrations vary inversely with blood pH. The serum sample should

be analyzed immediately or, alternatively, placed in 5% carbon dioxide–containing tubes and frozen, to minimize pH variations.[12]

Ca ions inside the cell mediate a variety of cellular functions. Most of the cellular Ca is in the form of insoluble complexes (99%) at a concentration of about 1×10^{-6} M of cell water. Free Ca (1%) within the cell, which is critical for functional regulation, is present in lower concentrations, approximately 2.5×10^{-7} M.[13] The gradient between plasma and intracellular free Ca is about 10,000:1[14] and is tightly regulated.

The concentration of Ca ions in the ECF is kept constant by processes that constantly feed Ca into and withdraw Ca from the ECF. Calcium enters the plasma via absorption from the intestinal tract and by resorption of ions from bone. In conditions of Ca balance, rates of Ca release from and uptake into bone are equal.[15] In normal adults, the total serum Ca concentration ranges from 2.2 to 2.6 mmol/L (8.8 to 10.4 mg/dL) and is remarkably constant. The ionized Ca concentration, although subject to changes directed by PTH, calcitonin, vitamin D, and blood pH, is also stable within an individual over prolonged periods and ranges from 1.2 to 1.3 mmol/L (4.8 to 5.2 mg/dL).[9]

At birth, an abrupt termination of the maternal-to-fetal Ca supply occurs. To maintain serum Ca homeostasis at this time, it is estimated that an increase of 16 to 20% in Ca flux from bone to extracellular space is required, unless sufficient exogenous intake of Ca is achieved.[16] In term newborn infants, cord blood total Ca concentrations are 2.6 mmol/L (10.2 mg/dL), and ionized Ca concentrations are 1.5 mmol/L (5.8 mg/dL).[17] By 2 hours of age, serum total Ca declines by 5%, and nearly all of this decline is due to a fall in ionized Ca. By 24 to 36 hours, serum Ca reaches its nadir of 2.3 mmol/L (9.0 mg/dL) for total Ca and 1.2 mmol/L (4.9 mg/dL) for ionized Ca, with the change in ionized Ca making up 75% of the change in total Ca (Table 34-1).[17] After a period of stabilization, serum Ca concentration slowly rises, reaching levels by 1 week of age similar to those found in childhood (Table 34-2).[18] In preterm infants, the mean cord serum ionized Ca concentration is 1.45 mmol/L (95% confidence range 1.29 to 1.61 [5.8 (5.74-5.86) mg/dl]), which decreases during the first 24 to 36 hours of life and subsequently rises at about 6 days of age to values that exceed original cord blood concentration.[18,19] The early fall in ionized Ca may be associated with parathyroid glandular unresponsiveness because of prematurity[20] or hypomagnesemia,[21] and severe hypocalcemia may result. Very low birth weight infants are likely to exhibit the lowest nadirs of ionized Ca; however, most are unassociated with tetany or decreased cardiac contractility.[22,23]

Cord serum Ca concentrations differ by season of birth (lower Ca in summer-born versus winter-born newborn infants)[24] and may vary by mode of delivery (lower Ca in elective cesarean section without labor vs. elective cesarean section with labor, spontaneous vaginal delivery, or emergency cesarean section).[25] Cord serum Ca concentrations are unaffected by gender, race, or weight appropriateness for gestation.[26]

Phosphorus

Phosphorus (P) is a major component of bone and of all other tissues and in some form is involved in almost all metabolic processes. The total amount of P in normal adults is about 1 kg.[1]

TABLE 34–1

Serum Concentrations for Total and Ionized Calcium in Term Infants During the First 24 Hours of Life

	Total Ca (mg/dL)		Ionized Ca (mg/dL)	
Age	*Mean*	*95% Confidence Range*	*Mean*	*95% Confidence Range*
Birth (cord blood)	10.2	9.0–11.4	5.82	5.22–6.42
2 h	9.7	8.5–10.9	5.34	4.84–5.84
24 h	9.0	7.8–10.2	4.92	4.40–5.44

Adapted from Loughead JL, et al: Am J Dis Child *142*:516, 1988, copyright 1988, American Medical Association.

In term newborn infants, total body P is approximately 16 g.[1] As with Ca, approximately 80% of the P contained in term newborn infants is accumulated during the last trimester of pregnancy at a rate of approximately 75 mg/kg of fetal weight/day and is closely linked to the accretion of Ca, with a Ca/P ratio of 1.7:1.[1,27]

About 85% of total body P is in bone, primarily as hydroxyapatite but also as more loosely complexed amorphous forms of bone crystal,[3] and thus P plays a key structural role in bone. In contrast to Ca, P is widely distributed in nonosseous tissues both in inorganic form and as a component of various structural macromolecules. About 15% of total body P is present in the ECF, largely in the form of inorganic phosphate ions, and in soft tissues, almost totally in the form of phosphate esters. Intracellular phosphate esters and phosphorylated intermediates are involved in a number of important biochemical processes, including the generation and transfer of cellular energy.

The P in body fluids is divided between an organic fraction composed of phospholipids and phosphoesters and inorganic phosphate (Pi). The latter is composed of two ionic forms, monovalent $H_2PO_4^-$ and divalent HPO_4^{2-}. Divalent HPO_4^{2-} is the major ionic species of P in serum at pH 7.4. Serum inorganic P also exists as three fractions: ionized (about 55%); protein-bound (11%); and complexed to sodium, Ca, and magnesium (Mg) (about 34%).[6] About 90% of the inorganic P in plasma is ultrafiltrable. In contrast to Ca, only a small portion (11%) is protein bound.[6] The intracellular and extracellular concentrations of ionized P (HPO_4^{2-}) are 1×10^{-4} and 2×10^{-4} M.[13] Because so many P species are present, depending on pH and other factors, it is the convention to express concentrations in terms of mass of elemental P (i.e., millimoles per liter or milligrams per deciliter). In contrast to Ca, the serum P concentration varies quite widely, exhibits daily variations of as much as 50%, and is influenced by age, gender, diet, pH, and a variety of hormones. An adequate serum P concentration is important in maintaining a sufficient ion product (with Ca) for normal mineralization.[28]

Serum total P concentrations are higher in children than in adults. Adult concentrations may vary by as much as 100%, with a normal range of 1.24 to 1.86 mmol/L (3.0 to 4.5 mg/dL). At birth, the infant's serum P concentrations are relatively low in comparison to older newborn or childhood values. In normal term appropriate-for-gestational-age infants, cord serum P concentrations do not differ by gender, race, season of birth,[24] weight appropriateness for gestation,[26] or mode of delivery.[25] The relatively low initial values, 2.6 (1.5 to 3.4) mmol/L (6.2 [3.7 to 8.1] mg/dL) begin to rise shortly after birth. The reason for this acute rise is not well understood. The rise may be due to increased gluconeogenesis and endogenous P release or secondary to a low glomerular filtration rate and reduced P excretion. Mean serum P concentrations increase to 3.4 mmol/L (8.1 mg/dL) by 1 week of age and decrease to 1.7 mmol/L (4.1 mg/dL) in childhood (see Table 34–2).[29]

Magnesium

Mg is the fourth most abundant mineral and the most abundant intracellular divalent cation in the body. Adult humans contain about 27 g of Mg.[1] In term newborn infants, the total body Mg is approximately 0.8 g,[1] and about 80% of Mg is accrued during the last trimester of pregnancy at a rate of approximately 3 mg/kg of fetal weight/day.[30]

Mg is distributed in three major compartments in the body: About 65% of the total body Mg is contained in bone in crystalline form, 34% in the intracellular space, and only 1% in the ECF.[31] Mg in bone is not an integral part of the hydroxyapatite lattice structure but appears to be located on the crystal surface. Only a minor fraction of Mg in bone is freely exchangeable with extracellular Mg. In infants aged 4 to 11 months, the calculated apparent Mg exchangeable pool size, measured using the stable isotope[25] Mg, ranges from 5.5 to 7.6 mmol/kg body weight and diminishes with age.[32] Because only 1% of the total body Mg is

TABLE 34–2

Serum Concentrations (mg/dL) for Calcium, Inorganic Phosphorus, and Magnesium in Term Infants Less Than 6 Months of Age*

Age	Type of Feeding	Ca	iCa	Pi	Mg
2 wk	Human milk	10.1 (9.1–11.1)	3.8 (3.6–4.0)	4.2 (3.4–5.0)	
	Human milk + vitamin D	9.9 (9.1–10.7)	3.8 (3.6–4.0)	5.1 (4.5–5.7)	
	Cow's milk-based formula	10.4 (10.0–10.8)	3.7 (3.5–3.9)	4.9 (4.1–5.7)	
16 wk	Human milk	10.4 (10.0–10.8)	3.9 (3.7–4.1)	4.6 (3.8–5.4)	
	Human milk + vitamin D	9.8 (9.2–10.4)	3.9 (3.7–4.1)	5.0 (4.4–5.6)	
	Cow's milk-based formula	10.2 (9.8–10.6)	4.0 (3.8–4.2)	4.7 (4.1–5.3)	
<6 mo	Human milk	9.75 (9.57–9.93)	5.38 (5.32–5.44)	6.44 (6.24–6.64)	2.04 (1.98–2.10)
	Cow's milk-based formula	9.73 (9.61–9.85)	5.27 (5.23–5.31)	6.98 (6.82–7.14)	2.10 (2.04–2.16)

*All data expressed as mean with values in parentheses representing the 95% confidence range.
Adapted from Roberts CC, et al: J Pediatr *99*:192, 1981; and Specker BL, et al: Pediatrics *77*:891, 1986.

located in the extracellular space,[33] its concentration in plasma does not consistently provide a reliable index of either total body or soft tissue Mg content.

The Mg in plasma exists in three forms: as free ion (55%), bound to plasma protein (30%), and complexed to various anions such as phosphate and oxalate (15%).[33] About 70% of the total Mg is ultrafiltrable and freely filtered at the renal glomerulus.[34] The protein-bound fraction interacts with carboxyl groups of albumin and is influenced by pH in a fashion analogous to that of Ca. The ionized fraction of Mg is physiologically important (e.g., to plasma membrane excitability). The extracellular concentration of ionized Mg is tightly controlled by the tubular maximum or threshold for Mg in the nephron.[35]

In contrast to the low concentrations of intracellular Ca, the concentration of free Mg ions (Mg^{2+}) is 5×10^{-4} M in the cytosol, and its concentration is rigidly maintained and stable.[13] This stability is a reflection of the many critical roles that Mg plays in cellular metabolism. Cellular Mg is important as a cofactor for a number of enzymatic reactions and in regulation of neuromuscular excitability.

The serum concentration of Mg is maintained within relatively tight limits and is essentially the same for neonates, infants, children, and adults, with a normal range of 0.62 to 1.16 mmol/L (1.5 to 2.8 mg/dL).[36] In the cord blood of normal term infants, serum Mg concentrations are 0.68 (0.6 to 0.76) mmol/L (1.6 [1.45 to 1.83] mg/dL) and do not vary by gender, race, season of birth,[24] weight appropriateness for gestation,[26] or mode of delivery.[25] Serum ionized Mg concentrations in cord blood appear to be higher in large for gestational age infants and higher in the umbilical vein than in the umbilical artery (the latter values being similar to maternal venous levels).[37] Preterm infants at the eighth month of gestation have cord serum Mg concentrations similar to those of the term infant, with a mean of 0.81 mmol/L (1.95 mg/dL) (range 0.59 to 1.0 mmol/L [1.43 to 2.45 mg/dL]).[38] After birth, both term and preterm infants initially exhibit a decrease in serum Mg concentrations. At 48 hours of life, serum Mg concentrations reach mean concentrations of 0.77 mmol/L (1.87 mg/dL).[38] Subsequently, there is an increase in serum Mg over the first week of life, followed by a decline toward childhood values by the end of the first month (see Table 34–2).[39]

REGULATION OF SERUM CONCENTRATION

Calcium

The homeostasis of Ca in blood is maintained primarily through the interaction of three hormones—parathyroid hormone (PTH), calcitonin (CT), and vitamin D—and their actions on the gastrointestinal tract, kidney, and bone.

Parathyroid Hormone

PTH is a peptide hormone produced in the parathyroid glands. Under normal circumstances, a decrease in the serum ionized Ca concentration stimulates production and secretion of this hormone.[40] PTH, in turn, acts directly on bone, stimulating resorption, thereby releasing Ca and P into the ECF and the circulation.[41] PTH also acts directly on the kidney to increase urinary excretion of P (which removes the P released into the circulation by its bone action) and decreases the urinary excretion of Ca. PTH indirectly enhances the gastrointestinal absorption of Ca,[42] through its effects on synthesis of 1,25-dihydroxyvitamin D (1,25[OH]$_2$D).

The integrated actions of PTH on bone resorption, distal renal tubular Ca reabsorption, and 1,25(OH)$_2$D-mediated intestinal Ca absorption are responsible for the fine regulation of the serum ionized Ca concentration. The precision of this integrated control is such that in a normal individual, serum ionized Ca probably fluctuates by no more than 0.025 mmol/L (0.1 mg/dL)

in either direction from its normal set point value throughout the day. Osteoclastic bone resorption and distal tubular Ca reabsorption are the major control points in serum Ca homeostasis; of these two processes, the effect of PTH on the distal tubule is quantitatively the most important. Together, these effects of PTH on bone and kidney constitute a classic short-loop feedback system on the parathyroid chief cell. Adjustments in the rate of intestinal Ca absorption via the PTH-1,25(OH)$_2$D axis require approximately 24 to 48 hours to become maximal. This axis represents a classic long-loop feedback system. PTH production is closely regulated by the concentration of serum ionized Ca. This feedback system is the critical homeostatic mechanism for maintenance of ECF Ca.[28]

With birth, there is an abrupt interruption of transplacental Ca supply. Regardless of whether the newborn infant is enterally fed or given intravenous fluids, Ca delivery over the first hours to days does not match the Ca delivery rate the fetus has been receiving. This situation sets the stage for a rapid, dramatic decline in serum total and ionized Ca concentrations. In normal term infants, when serum Ca concentrations fall slightly after birth, PTH concentrations increase appropriately (twofold to fivefold increase during the first 48 hours of life) and remain elevated for several days postnatally. The PTH secretion in term newborn infants appears substantial, and blood concentrations negatively correlate with Ca levels.[25] Over the course of the first week of life, the role of PTH appears enhanced, and neonates show an appropriate calcemic response when challenged with PTH. The high circulating concentration of PTH during the first days of life theoretically should result in increased recruitment of osteoclasts and incorporation of a substantial portion of the bone surface into the resorptive process. In a condition of systemic mineral deficit, the integrity of skeletal mineral homeostasis is generally sacrificed to compensate for the deficit (i.e., serum Ca is maintained in the normal range at the expense of bone).

Serum carboxyterminal propeptide of type I procollagen (PICP) and cross-linked carboxyterminal telopeptide of type I collagen (ICTP), liberated during bone type I collagen synthesis and degradation, are new biochemical markers of bone formation and resorption; both PICP and ICTP are significantly correlated with histomorphometric indices of bone formation and resorption.[43,44] Measurements of serum biochemical markers of bone formation and resorption should allow understanding of the changes in bone during the early newborn period. In a study of normal term newborn infants,[45] the serum ICTP concentration, a marker of bone resorption, was reduced at 24 hours of life compared with cord blood values. The early bone formation marker (PICP) was unchanged, but the marker of late bone formation (mineralization), osteocalcin, was reduced. Cord serum ICTP, PICP, and osteocalcin concentrations were high compared with adult normal values, indicating that both osteoclastic and osteoblastic activities were increased during fetal life. These data suggest that there is no substantial increase in bone resorption, with the modest increase of serum PTH at 24 hours of life, and that a major bone effect of PTH might be inhibition of late bone formation (mineralization).[45]

In the cord blood of normal term infants, the mean serum intact PTH concentration is 2.96 (range 0.5 to 18) ng/L or pg/mL. Cord serum intact PTH concentrations do not differ by gender, race, season of birth, or weight appropriateness for gestation[24,26] but may vary by mode of delivery (higher in infants delivered by elective cesarean section without labor versus elective cesarean section with labor, emergency cesarean section, or spontaneous vaginal delivery).[25]

In some preterm infants and infants of diabetic mothers, there is a variable postnatal increase in serum PTH concentrations, even to hyperparathyroid levels, presumably in response to the hypocalcemic stress.[16] In other instances, the PTH response in infants of diabetic mothers appears blunted and may relate to the Mg deficiency state of the diabetic pregnancy. In very low birth weight infants, the serum PTH concentration rises significantly in association with a decline in serum Ca concentration and is suppressed by intravenous Ca infusion, indicating that the parathyroid glands of very low birth weight infants are responsive to changes in serum Ca levels.[22] In infants and young children undergoing cardiac surgery, the PTH response to both hypocalcemia and rising ionized Ca concentrations appears at least as great as that of adults. Thus, in general, the Ca-parathyroid-vitamin D axis functions in infants and young children in a fashion similar to that of adults.[46]

Calcitonin

CT is a hypocalcemic peptide hormone produced by the parafollicular cells of the thyroid,[47] which, in many ways, acts as the physiologic antagonist to PTH. The hypocalcemic activity of CT is accounted for primarily by direct inhibition of osteoclast-mediated bone resorption (decreasing the amount of Ca and P released from bone)[48] and secondarily by increasing renal Ca and P excretion (at high doses).[49] These effects are mediated by receptors on osteoclasts and renal tubular cells and depend on the rate of preexisting bone resorption; the greatest effects of this hormone apparently are seen in circumstances in which bone resorption is increased.[50] The net consequence of the actions of CT is to decrease serum concentrations of Ca and P. The physiologic role of CT in the regulation of Ca homeostasis and the pathophysiologic importance of CT in the human, however, remain unclear.

The secretion of CT is under the direct control of blood Ca: An increase in Ca causes an increase in CT, and a decrease in Ca causes a decrease in CT concentrations.[51] An increase in the production of CT may also be observed with an increase in circulating Mg levels or following ingestion of food (which increases circulating levels of gastrointestinal hormones [gastrin, glucagon, and pancreozymin]). Thus, it has been suggested that this gastrointestinal-thyroid-cell system serves to prevent marked increases in serum Ca during food ingestion.[52] Once secreted, CT disappears from the circulation with a half-life of 2 to 15 minutes.[50]

In the cord blood of normal term infants, cord serum CT concentrations are 44.1 (24.3 to 63.9) ng/L or pg/mL.[24] They do not differ by gender, race, or season of birth[24] but decrease with increasing gestational age. Infants of less than 32 weeks' gestation have nearly three times the cord serum CT concentrations

of term infants.[53] In newborn infants and in fetal animals, cord serum CT concentrations are higher than those of the pregnant mother.[54] In both preterm and term infants, serum CT concentrations further increase after birth, with a peak at 24 to 48 hours of age followed by a decline to childhood values by 1 month of age.[53-55] The physiologic importance of this increase in serum CT is unclear but may relate to its effect on counteracting the bone resorptive action of PTH.

Vitamin D

Vitamin D is either produced in the skin under the influence of ultraviolet light[56] or ingested in the diet and absorbed from the gastrointestinal tract. Before it reaches its final active form, $1,25(OH)_2D$, vitamin D must first undergo two hydroxylation steps—first in the liver and second in the proximal tubule of the kidney.[57] 25-Hydroxylation in the liver is a relatively unregulated process, and serum 25-hydroxyvitamin D (25-OHD) concentrations generally reflect an individual's vitamin D status (reflecting intake and sunlight exposure). The production of $1,25(OH)_2D$ by the renal proximal tubule is enhanced by hypocalcemia, hypophosphatemia, and PTH[58] and appears to be tightly regulated. $1,25(OH)_2D$ is transported through the blood to its target tissues (small intestine and bone), where it regulates Ca homeostasis. $1,25(OH)_2D$ acts on the small intestine to stimulate the active absorption of Ca and P,[59,60] on bone (in conjunction with PTH) to stimulate bone resorption of Ca and P,[61,62] and on kidney to conserve Ca and P. Thus, vitamin D is necessary for maintenance of normal Ca and P homeostasis. The net action of $1,25(OH)_2D$ is to increase the serum concentration of Ca.

In the cord blood of normal term infants, the mean serum $1,25(OH)_2D$ concentration is 76 pmol/L and ranges from 31 to 151 pmol/L (32 [13–63] pg/mL). It varies by season of birth (high in summer-born versus winter-born infants)[24] (Fig. 34–1) and weight in relation to gestation (lower concentrations in small for gestational age infants versus appropriate for gestational age infants[26]) but not by gender or race.[24] These variable concentrations of serum $1,25(OH)_2D$ have been suggested as an adaptive response to low bone mineral content in summer-born newborn infants (in the United States) or may reflect decreased production of $1,25(OH)_2D$ in small for gestational age infants, possibly as a consequence of reduced uteroplacental blood flow. In normal term infants, serum $1,25(OH)_2D$ concentrations are low at birth but increase to adult normal ranges by 24 hours of life, possibly reflecting the need for optimum intestinal Ca and P absorption.[63]

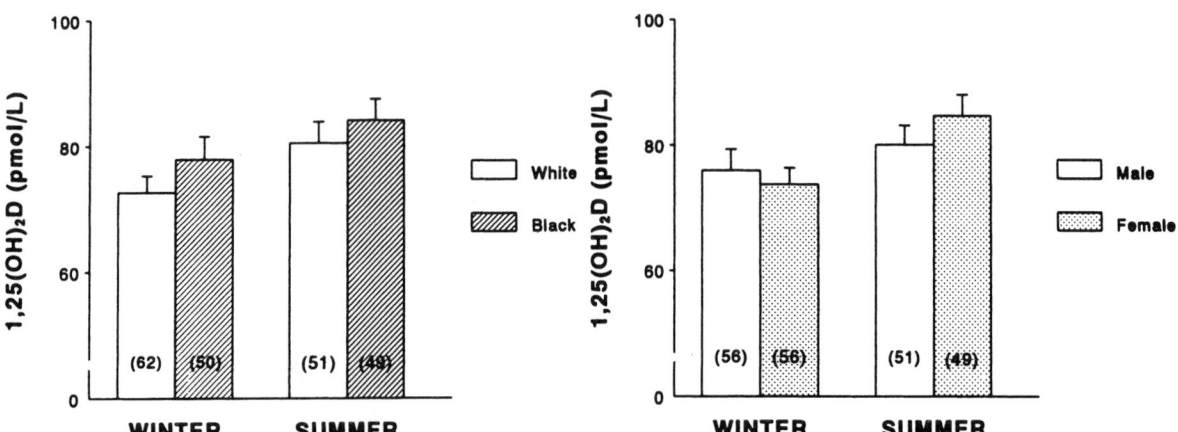

Figure 34–1. Serum $1,25(OH)_2D$ concentrations were higher in summer-born than in winter-born infants ($p = .02$) and did not differ by race or gender. Values are mean ± SE with numbers of newborns in parentheses. (From Namgung R, et al: J Pediatr Gastroenterol Nutr *19*:220, 1994.)

In preterm infants, serum $1,25(OH)_2D$ concentrations at birth are comparable to reference values for healthy children and adults, increase significantly during the first few days of life,[64-66] and are far above reference values between 3 and 12 weeks of life.[66, 67] In preterm infants, serum concentrations of vitamin D–binding protein are lower, serum total $1,25(OH)_2D$ concentrations are higher, and the calculated free $1,25(OH)_2D$ index (total $1,25[OH]_2D/D$ binding protein ratio, which may represent the physiologically active component of $1,25[OH]_2D$) is four to six times higher than in previously studied term infants; the free $1,25(OH)_2D$ index increases significantly with age and does not correlate with serum P or PTH.[68]

Cord serum 25-OHD concentrations are influenced by season of birth and maternal vitamin D status. In Cincinnati, human milk–fed infants in the first year of life have low serum 25-OHD concentrations in winter (33% to 50% of summer values),[69] paralleling measures of actual sunshine exposure.[70] Cord serum 25-OHD concentrations in Cincinnati, however, do not differ by season of birth, possibly because a large percentage of women take prenatal vitamins, which would obscure any sunshine-related effects on vitamin D metabolism.[24] In contrast to Cincinnati, cord serum 25-OHD concentrations of Korean neonates are significantly lower in winter (about one third of summer values), and 97% of winter-born infants have subnormal 25-OHD concentrations (<28 nmol/L; 11 ng/dL), consistent with a low maternal vitamin D nutrition status and reduced seasonal sunlight exposure.[71] The lower vitamin D status in winter may influence fetal bone mineralization during late fetal life; in one study, the total body bone mineral content in winter-born infants was lower (by 6%) than in summer-born infants in Korea.[71]

Phosphorus

The serum concentration of P appears to be primarily regulated through the kidney by means of the tubular reabsorption of Pi; serum P concentrations are maintained at a value close to the tubular P threshold or tubular maximum for P/glomerular filtration rate (TmP/GFR).[28] Because of the normal high efficiency and lack of fine regulation of P absorption in the intestine, only in unusual circumstances is the intestinal absorption of P a limiting factor in P homeostasis.

During P depletion, phosphaturia decreases before the serum P concentration declines. This adaptive response (i.e., increasing tubular transport when luminal concentrations are decreasing) is an intrinsic property of these cells. The following sequence of events is initiated in the face of a hypophosphatemic challenge: (1) stimulation of $1,25(OH)_2D$ synthesis in the kidney, (2) enhanced mobilization of P and Ca from bone, and (3) hypophosphatemia-induced increase in tubular maximum for P (this results in reduced P excretion, the exact mechanism of which is unknown). The increased circulating concentration of $1,25(OH)_2D$ leads to increases in P and Ca absorption in the intestine and provides an additional stimulus to P and Ca mobilization from bone. The increased flow of Ca from bone and intestine inhibits the secretion of PTH. The net result of this series of adjustments is a return of serum P concentration to normal without change in the serum Ca concentration.[28]

The defense against hyperphosphatemia consists largely of a reversal of the events described previously. The principal humoral factor that combats hyperphosphatemia is PTH. An acute rise in the serum P concentration produces a transient fall in the concentration of serum ionized Ca and a stimulation of PTH secretion. This, in turn, reduces TmP/GFR (increasing urinary P excretion) and leads to a readjustment in serum P and Ca concentrations. A prolonged rise in the serum P concentration results in (1) an intrinsic downward adjustment in TmP/GFR that is independent of PTH, and (2) a persistent increase in PTH secretion that ultimately can lead to parathyroid chief cell hyperplasia.[28]

The wide variation in serum P concentrations may be secondary to few direct regulatory mechanisms. PTH, which has the greatest impact on serum P concentrations, primarily responds to changes in ionized Ca concentrations, not P. P is freely filtered at the glomerulus and presents to the renal tubule in high concentrations. The renal tubule reabsorbs P in both the proximal and distal nephron. In states of low PTH concentrations, the renal tubular cells reabsorb up to 95% to 97% of filtered P. In states of high serum PTH concentrations, reabsorption of P in proximal and distal tubules is inhibited, resulting in excretion of high concentrations of urinary P. Although markedly affected by PTH in the usual state, renal tubular cells appear to have a decreased responsiveness to PTH when there is severe P deficiency or overload. Hence, P is reabsorbed in the face of high circulating PTH when there is severe P deficiency, and P is excreted despite low PTH concentrations when serum P is high.[72] Other hormones may also have an effect on the excretion of P by the kidney. Growth hormone, $1,25(OH)_2D$, insulin, and possibly somatomedins (insulin-like growth factors) have all been shown to increase renal tubular reabsorption of P.[72] The extent to which these hormones contribute to the normal regulation of serum P is unclear.

In preterm infants, a P depletion syndrome has been observed in infants fed human milk,[73] in infants with restricted enteral mineral intakes (owing to type of formula), and in infants with chronic illnesses who receive prolonged parenteral nutrition without mineral supplements.[74] In this latter group of patients, biochemical signs of P deficiency are prominent and may be associated with bony, rachitic bone changes; serum $1,25(OH)_2D$ concentrations are increased with evidence of increased bone resorption and turnover (increased serum ICTP and osteocalcin levels in infants with rickets versus controls).[75] These changes appear to be an extreme example of P depletion because of low enteral mineral intakes during the first month of life in very low birth weight infants.

Magnesium

In contrast to Ca and P, systemic Mg homeostasis does not appear to be hormonally regulated. There are no proven hormones that consistently regulate the serum concentration of Mg. Instead, maintenance of the serum Mg concentration seems to result from the combined fluxes of Mg at the levels of intestine, kidney, intracellular fluids, and perhaps the skeleton. With a rise in serum Mg concentration, the fraction of filtered Mg that is excreted increases sharply, whereas a decrease in serum Mg concentration (which occurs when a low-Mg diet is ingested for a few days) leads to the near disappearance of Mg from the urine.[76] The excretion of Mg is directly related to the renal Mg threshold and a tubular maximum-limited process and is primarily responsible for maintaining serum Mg concentration within rather narrow limits.[28]

The body's stores of Mg appear to be important in the maintenance of Ca homeostasis. Mg deficiency may decrease bone Ca release *in vitro*[77] and increase the percentage of bone Ca, compared with that of Mg-replete rats *in vivo*.[78] Congenital rickets may occur in infants whose mothers have received prolonged Mg infusion for tocolysis.[79] Cord serum ICTP concentrations correlated significantly with the duration and cumulative doses of maternal Mg treatment, possibly reflecting increased bone resorption in long-term tocolysis with Mg. This finding is confounded by gestational age, because infants with lower gestational age have higher serum ICTP. By statistical analysis, bone resorption marker was not different when corrected for gestational age.[80] A heteroionic bone exchange of Mg for Ca has been demonstrated *in vitro*.[77] The release of both Ca and Mg from bone is also stimulated by PTH and decreased by CT.[81]

Many of the same hormones that regulate serum Ca concentrations also appear to affect serum Mg, although the relationships are not as well defined as for Ca. Acute changes in serum Mg concentration have similar effects on PTH secretion as acute changes in serum Ca concentrations, but Mg is in general a less potent stimulus than Ca.[82,83] An acute increase in serum Mg concentration leads to a decline in serum PTH.[84] Reduced activity of PTH may increase the tubular clearance of Mg. Conversely, an acute decrease in serum Mg results in an increase in PTH secretion. The increase in PTH secretion results in an increase in serum Mg concentrations, probably via increased bone resorption and, more importantly, decreased losses in the urine. PTH affects tubular reabsorption of Mg, through a mechanism similar to that used for the transport of Ca and P involving cyclic adenosine monophosphate.[76] It has been difficult, however, to identify a direct effect of PTH on tubular Mg transport because concomitant changes in serum or urinary Ca or other factors also can affect tubular Mg transport.[76]

Paradoxically, chronic Mg deficiency results in decreased PTH secretion and a blunting of the action of PTH on target organs,[85-87] partly because of alterations in the Ca-sensitive, Mg-dependent adenylate cyclase system that is involved in the secretion of the hormone.[88] Therefore, Mg deficiency may lead to or exacerbate hypocalcemia by inhibiting the parathyroid response to declining serum Ca concentrations. Although changes in the concentration of Mg can alter the secretion of PTH,[82] further investigations are required to determine the exact physiologic relevance of this relationship with regard to normal Mg homeostasis.

The role of CT in the regulation of serum Mg concentrations appears to be minimal. Elevated serum Mg concentrations increase CT release. In vitro studies have shown that a 100% increase in the Mg concentration of the extracellular bath leads to a discharge of CT from the thyroid parafollicular cells.[89] This compares with a similar calcitonin response with a 20% increase in the Ca concentration. Because CT inhibits bone resorption, the release of Mg from bone is apparently decreased by CT.[90] Calcitonin decreases renal tubular reabsorption of Mg in humans.[91] The physiologic role of CT in the regulation of Mg homeostasis, however, is not well defined, and there are no major difficulties with Mg (or Ca) or skeletal homeostasis in humans with congenital or acquired CT deficiency.[92]

Under physiologic conditions, the role of vitamin D in the regulation of serum Mg concentration is probably of minor importance and appears to have at best an indirect influence on Mg metabolism. There is little effect on intestinal Mg transport at physiologic concentrations of $1,25(OH)_2D$,[93] but increased intestinal Mg absorption occurs at pharmacologic doses of vitamin D.[94-96] Furthermore, no significant correlation exists between Mg absorption and plasma $1,25(OH)_2D$ concentrations[97]; however, Mg is an essential cofactor for the 25-hydroxylation reaction in the hepatic formation of 25-OHD,[98,99] and Mg deficiency is associated with decreased serum $1,25(OH)_2D$ concentrations in adults, presumably because of its role as a cofactor for $25(OH)_2D$-1α-hydroxylase in renal tubular cells.[100]

Other hormones known to have a direct or indirect effect on serum Mg concentrations are estrogens, thyroxine, and aldosterone, which lower serum Mg concentrations, and epinephrine, glucocorticoids, and progesterone, which increase serum Mg concentrations. The overall effect of these hormones in healthy individuals appears to be minimal.[76]

GASTROINTESTINAL TRANSPORT

Calcium

The gastrointestinal tract is generally considered the primary site involved in the long-term regulation of Ca balance. In adults, the average dietary Ca intake is approximately 600 to 800 mg/day, and less than half of dietary Ca is absorbed.[101] In preterm low

birth weight infants, Ca absorption has been reported to range from 50% to 80% at Ca intakes of 80 to 140 mg/kg/day.[102-104] Ca absorption increases during periods of rapid growth in children and decreases with advancing age. The percentage of true Ca absorption in preterm infants, however, does not change with birth weight or gestational age.[105]

Most of the Ca is known to be absorbed in the proximal small intestine, and the efficiency of absorption decreases in the more distal small intestinal segments. Several in vivo studies,[106-108] however, have shown that the bulk of Ca^{2+} absorption can be accomplished in the distal small intestine, in particular the ileum, a segment known to have a limited capacity for active Ca absorption.[109]

Several pathways have been described that may account for cellular mechanism of Ca transport across the intestine. Transepithelial Ca transport in the intestine proceeds by two routes: a transcellular (active) and a paracellular (passive) pathway.[110] The transcellular route is dominant in the proximal intestine, largely the duodenum, whereas paracellular Ca movement takes place throughout the length of the intestine.[109] The transcellular transport is dominant at low levels of Ca at the luminal surface and is down-regulated as total Ca intake rises; paracellular transport is dominant at the highest levels of luminal Ca and is linear over a wide range of Ca concentrations (50 to 200 mmol/L) and unchanged as a result of increasing Ca intake.[109] The passive absorption of Ca does not appear to be a regulated process. There are no recognized hormones that affect net absorption of Ca via this route, and little is known about its modulation. Studies, however, have shown that bile salts and lactose could increase ileal Ca absorption by increasing the permeability of the paracellular pathway.[108,111]

Active transport of Ca in the intestine contrasts markedly with passive absorption. It occurs predominantly in a relatively small portion of the small intestine, the duodenum, and is highly influenced by vitamin D.[106,109] $1,25(OH)_2D$, the active metabolite of vitamin D, is thought to act through a classic steroid hormone mechanism to augment the active absorption of Ca. $1,25(OH)_2D$ is known to interact noncovalently but stereospecifically with an intracellular receptor protein, a DNA-binding protein of 50,000 to 60,000 daltons that binds $1,25(OH)_2D$ with high affinity.[112] This hormone-receptor complex is then associated with DNA in the nucleus of target cells, either to initiate the synthesis of specific RNA encoding proteins that mediate a spectrum of biologic responses or to mediate a selective repression of gene transcription. Thus, $1,25(OH)_2D$ rapidly causes the formation of calbindin-D mRNA either by increasing gene transcription[113] or by a post-transcriptional mechanism.[114] Studies in both humans[115] and animals[116,117] have demonstrated a direct correlation between mucosal concentration of calbindin-D and the rate of intestinal Ca absorption, thus supporting a link between the physiologic action of vitamin D and calbindin-D (Fig. 34-2).

Transcellular movement involves three steps (Fig. 34-3): (1) entry across the brush-border membrane of the enterocyte, (2) intracellular movement, and (3) extrusion across the basolateral membrane. Entry across the brush border of the enterocyte follows an electrochemical gradient, probably via Ca channels.[118] The entry process, although modified by vitamin D, does not appear to be the rate-limiting step because total vitamin D deficiency lowers the rate of entry only by about a third, whereas active Ca transport is wholly inhibited. Ca entry into the cell, as evaluated by uptake measurements that use right-side-out brush-border membrane vesicles, has been described as the sum of a saturable and a nonsaturable step.[119] The saturable step may represent the established and significant binding of Ca to the inner aspect of the brush-border membrane vesicle[120] or a carrier-mediated transport step.[121] Ca extrusion is affected by Ca-ATPase, occurs against an electrochemical gradient, and requires a supply of energy.[122] It is not the rate-limiting step, however,

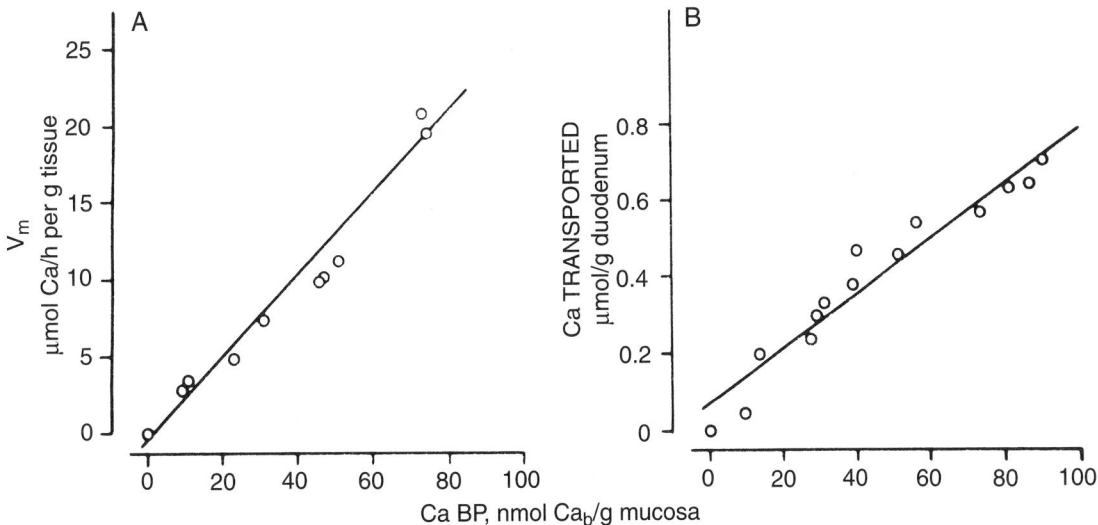

Figure 34–2. The relationship between intestinal calcium transport and calcium-binding protein (CaBP) content. **A**, V_m, calculated from *in situ* duodenal, jejunal, and ileal loop experiments,[109] shown as a function of CaBP content. **B**, Calcium transport, as evaluated from everted duodenal sac experiments,[116] shown as a function of CaBP content. (From Bronner F, et al: Am J Physiol *250*:G561, 1986.)

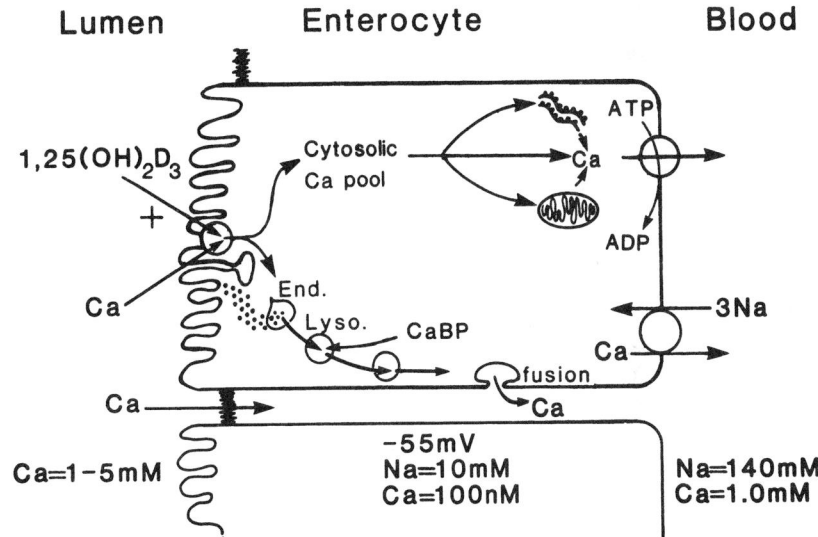

Figure 34–3. The potential pathways, gradients, and mechanisms for calcium transport across intestinal epithelium. End. = endoplasmic reticulum; Lyso. = lysosome. (From Favus MJ, Tembe V: J Nutr *122*:683, 1992. © J Nutr, American Institute of Nutrition.)

because extrusion capacity is more than sufficient to handle the maximum transcellular flux of Ca. It is the flow of Ca inside the cell, from the brush-border pole to the Ca pump at the basolateral side, that is rate limiting.

Basal Ca flow, in the absence of the cytosolic, vitamin D–dependent Ca-binding protein CaBP, is only about 1/70th of the maximum rate in the vitamin D–replete duodenum.[110] CaBP levels vary linearly with the maximum rate. Vitamin D deficiency leads to CaBP deficiency; active transport of Ca is nonexistent when the CaBP concentration is zero.[115] Moreover, interference with Ca binding by CaBP interferes with active Ca transport. Theophylline, when added to the incubation medium of everted duodenal sacs prepared from rats on a low-Ca diet, inhibits transcellular Ca transport in a concentration-dependent manner: Ca binding by CaBP is also depressed by theophylline in a concentration-dependent manner and parallels the inhibition of transcellular Ca transport, supporting a CaBP function as a "Ca ferry" in transcellular transport[123] (Fig. 34–4). Thus, active Ca transport

is totally regulated by vitamin D or processes that modify the action or metabolism of the sterol.

$1,25(OH)_2D_3$ (calcitriol) is the most active hormonal metabolite of vitamin D_3, which stimulates active intestinal Ca (Ca^{2+}) absorption.[124] Apart from calcitriol effects on receptor-mediated genomic protein (calbindin-D_{9k}) induction[115,125] and weak (20% to 40%) enhancement of entry across the brush border,[113,126,127] its presence leads to a doubling or tripling of the basolateral Ca pump activity through an unknown mechanism.[128-130] The effect of calbindin on Ca^{2+} uptake by basolateral membrane vesicles, however, has not been demonstrated in every study.[119,131]

The relative importance of active versus passive intestinal absorption of Ca in the human neonate is uncertain. In rats, it has been observed that during the suckling period, before the time of natural weaning, the absorption of Ca is linearly related to the intraluminal Ca concentration.[132,133] With increasing age, a decrease in the intestinal permeability of Ca is noted, and the relationship between intraluminal Ca concentration and Ca

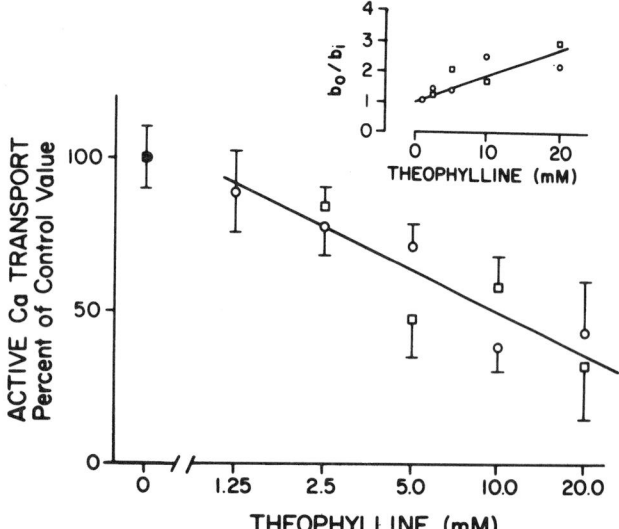

Figure 34–4. Effect of theophylline on transcellular Ca transport as evaluated in everted duodenal sacs. [Ca] in medium: 0.1 mM (○); 0.25 mM (□). Transport ($\mu mol \cdot h^{-1} \cdot g$ tissue^{-1}) in absence of theophylline (●): 0.18 ± 0.02 at 0.1 mM Ca (n = 17), 0.27 ± 0.04 at 0.25 mM Ca (n = 6). *Inset,* $K_i \cdot b_0$ is mean transport without theophylline, and b_i is mean transport inhibited by theophylline. $K_i = 10.8$ mM, based on least-squares relationship. (From Pansu D, et al: Am J Physiol *257* [Gastrointest Liver Physiol 20]: G935, 1989.)

absorption becomes increasingly curvilinear. It is during this time that measurable active intestinal absorption of Ca increases. Just before this increase in active absorption, receptors for $1,25(OH)_2D$ become identifiable,[134] and a marked increase in mucosal vitamin D-dependent Ca-binding protein is observed.[135] Although an increase in active intestinal absorption of Ca is observed around the time of weaning even in vitamin D-deficient rat pups, the marked increase in absorption that is normally observed occurs only in the presence of $1,25(OH)_2D$.[136] Furthermore, the increase in active Ca absorption induced by $1,25(OH)_2D$ is not observed until the appearance of its cytoplasmic receptor.[136]

Neonates of several species are almost insensitive to vitamin D[136,137] and lack detectable concentrations of calcitriol receptor and calbindin in their mucosa.[134,135] The potential importance of calcitriol-independent neonatal Ca absorption is supported by *in vivo* studies of Ca absorption in newborn and weaned piglets suffering from pseudovitamin D-deficiency rickets, type 1 (PVDRI). In this disorder, renal production of calcitriol is absent.[138] Despite the defect, however, affected animals of this strain are normocalcemic and clinically normal at birth and absorb as much Ca from the gut as control animals during the first 4 weeks of life (although the plasma concentrations of calcitriol are already reduced at birth to an unphysiologically low level[139,140]). By the fourth week postpartum, PVDRI piglets develop significant Ca^{2+} malabsorption, hypocalcemia, and typical clinical signs of rickets.[141] In weaned PVDRI piglets, concentrations of Ca^{2+} are significantly lower than those of controls and are associated with significantly lower $1,25(OH)_2D$ concentrations.[140]

A study by Schroder and colleagues[140] demonstrated that the normal absorption of Ca by newborn PVDRI piglets in the early postpartal period occurs via an active mechanism. By measuring unidirectional Ca flux rates using stripped duodenal mucosae (in the absence of an electrochemical gradient), significant net Ca fluxes were found in both newborn (<1 week old) PVDRI and

control piglets, whereas active net Ca absorption was completely absent in weaned (>6 weeks old) PVDRI piglets. Because the impaired Ca^{2+} absorption does not develop during the first 4 weeks postpartum in newborn PVDRI piglets, it is concluded that active Ca^{2+} absorption in neonatal piglets is vitamin D independent. In human neonatal intestine, the possible presence of vitamin D-independent active Ca^{2+} absorption has not been studied.

In newborn PVDRI piglets, active Ca absorption is present despite low $1,25(OH)_2D$ concentrations and decreased numbers of vitamin D receptors, indicating the presence of vitamin D-independent active Ca absorption. In weaned PVDRI piglets, however, active net Ca absorption is absent, with low serum $1,25(OH)_2D$ concentrations but similar vitamin D receptors versus controls.

The timing of similar events in the human is unknown. Because vitamin D-responsive, active Ca absorption occurs in a relatively restricted portion of the small intestine and passive absorption occurs throughout the entire small intestine at similar rates, it should not be surprising that the latter process contributes significantly to the net intestinal absorption of Ca.

In a study of preterm infants 2 to 4 weeks old (mean gestational age of 32 weeks at birth) using metabolic balance techniques, Senterre and Salle[142] demonstrated that human milk-fed and formula-fed infants supplemented with vitamin D exhibited significantly greater absorption of Ca (expressed as a percentage of intake) compared with their unsupplemented counterparts (human milk, supplemented versus unsupplemented—70% versus 49%; formula, supplemented versus unsupplemented—32% versus 20%). Assuming that the absorption of Ca in the unsupplemented groups gives a rough estimate of the passive component, it appears that the passive route accounts for a significant portion of Ca absorption in preterm infants. Likewise, the data from the vitamin D-supplemented groups suggest that vitamin D-responsive, active intestinal absorption of Ca was present at the time of study, and that this component of Ca absorption was present before the normal term date. Alternatively, intestinal maturation with regard to vitamin D responsiveness was accelerated by preterm delivery.

Although these observations do not establish the relative importance of passive and active mechanisms or the timing of intestinal vitamin D responsiveness with regard to Ca absorption, they do indicate that absorption of Ca is not a limiting issue for the preterm infant. With proper attention to dietary manipulation, adequate Ca balance should be attainable.

Generally, fractional Ca absorption can adapt to high Ca intake. Hardwick and colleagues[143] have examined Ca transluminal uptake across intact duodenal epithelium at three different levels of the absorptive processes: net absorption in intact animal, transepithelial transport in everted duodenal sacs, and transapical uptake across intact duodenal epithelium *in vitro*. In the face of a fivefold difference in Ca intake, net Ca absorption remained relatively constant because of a decrease in fractional absorption from 70% with normal Ca intake to 20% under conditions of high Ca intake. This decrease in fractional absorption could be due to a combination of depressed true absorption and increased intestinal secretion of Ca in response to increased dietary Ca. Previous studies, however, have noted that intestinal secretion of Ca is not only negligible compared with intake, but also is not altered by changes in dietary intake.[144] The drop in fractional absorption of Ca is probably due to down-regulation of Ca absorption. This intestinal adaptation to the effect of dietary Ca is well known and is believed to be mediated through changes in $1,25(OH)_2D$ synthesis.[145] High dietary Ca reduces the production of this metabolite and thereby reduces the rate of intestinal Ca absorption.

In contrast to the findings in experimental animals described previously (the apparent adaptation of the Ca absorptive rate to high dietary Ca intake), studies in low birth weight infants have yielded extremely variable results regarding the fractional and total Ca absorbed and retained.[146-152] Early investigations in preterm infants demonstrated a linear relationship between Ca intake and absorption: as Ca intake increases, so does the intestinal absorption of Ca.[153-155] As noted previously, however, more recent balance studies that measure only net absorption (true absorption − endogenous fecal excretion) have shown great variability in Ca retention (80 to 170 mg/kg/day) even when the same preterm formula was used,[146, 147, 150-152] possibly as a result of significant intersubject variability in Ca bioavailability. These variations may represent true differences in the ability of low birth weight infants to absorb Ca, the cause of which may relate to as yet unidentified physiologic or hormonal factors. Based on the findings of Ca absorptive consistency in perimenopausal women,[156] interindividual variability may be an expression of individually different absorptive set points about which each person is operating. There is a consistency in Ca absorption for an individual across differing Ca loads (ranging from 15 to 500 mg): a woman who absorbs Ca poorly with one Ca-containing food is likely to absorb Ca poorly with other foods.

Studies using a dual tracer, stable isotope technique have also shown variable results. Abrams and colleagues[157] have reported that net Ca retention in low birth weight infants fed a high Ca-containing formula is primarily determined by the total dietary Ca absorbed: Net Ca retention correlated closely with true Ca absorption ($r = .98$, $P < .001$). The net Ca retention rate for low birth weight infants weighing 1693 ± 174 g (mean ± standard deviation) at 20 ± 10 days of age was 103 ± 38 mg/kg/day at Ca intakes of 216 ± 13 mg/kg/day, which meets the lower estimates of the *in utero* Ca retention rate (100 to 130 mg/kg/day) during the third trimester.[158] This value was consistent with previous studies of Ca retention obtained using mass balance technique, lower than other reports describing Ca retention rates of 130 to 170 mg/kg/day,[146,147,151,152] and slightly higher than a report of an approximate 80 mg/kg/day retention with this formula.[150] Thus, the use of high Ca-containing formulas could possibly achieve *in utero* rates of Ca retention in low birth weight infants, although some infants retain well below *in utero* rates and may remain at risk for inadequate bone mineralization.[157]

Hillman and colleagues[105] measured the percentage of true absorption and Ca retention rates in low birth weight infants (1400 ± 210 g) fed specially formulated preterm formula with differing Ca contents. The percentage of true Ca absorption from the preterm formula studied was around 50%, the same or slightly higher than that from standard formula (460 mg/L, 47.1%). Increasing the Ca content in formula from the level of 460 mg/L to the levels studied—780 mg/L, 940 mg/L, and 1340 mg/L—resulted in nearly identical levels of true fractional Ca absorption (range: 47.1% to 56.1%) but higher net Ca retention rates with a wide variability. Because multiple factors were different between the formulas studied (e.g., fat composition [content of medium chain triglycerides], whey-predominant protein, Ca/P ratio), however, the effect of increased Ca content alone cannot be assessed in this study.

Significant amounts of endogenous Ca are lost daily through intestinal secretion. Substantial quantities of Ca enter the gastrointestinal tract as constituents of bile and other digestive juices.[159, 160] From studies in rats, it also appears that Ca can be secreted into the gastrointestinal tract via paracellular channels when the serum ionized Ca concentration exceeds the intraluminal Ca concentration.[132, 161] Although the secreted Ca can participate in normal intestinal absorptive mechanisms, it appears that this portion of the intraluminal Ca is reabsorbed at a level of efficiency less than that of dietary Ca.[162]

Simultaneous administration of both intravenous and oral stable isotopic Ca tracers with subsequent monitoring of fecal and urinary tracers has permitted direct calculation of endogenous Ca secretion. In adults, secretion of Ca into the intestinal lumen is small in amount, constant, and independent of absorption.[162] In children (aged 3 to 14 years), endogenous fecal Ca excretion, measured using a stable isotope technique (^{42}Ca), averages 1.4 ± 0.4 mg/kg/day and is lower than urinary Ca excretion,[163] consistent with the values of healthy adults.[4, 162] In preterm infants, endogenous fecal Ca excretion is high and quite variable (4 to 150 mg/day) and may exceed even urinary excretion of Ca.[151, 164, 165] Thus, significant amounts of Ca can be lost via this route, which might explain some of the variability in reported Ca balance studies, because the mass balance technique does not differentiate between unabsorbed and endogenously secreted fecal Ca. In a study of low birth weight infants fed a high Ca-containing formula, endogenous fecal Ca excretion averaged 15 ± 9 mg/kg/day (7.2% ± 4.1% of intake) and was much greater than concurrent urinary Ca excretion.[157] The reasons for these high rates of endogenous fecal Ca excretion in preterm infants are unknown but may be related to gastrointestinal immaturity.[104, 151]

In a study by Hillman and colleagues,[105] endogenous fecal Ca excretion in low birth weight infants fed preterm formula with varying Ca contents ranged from 6.9 to 19.0 mg/kg/day; infants fed human milk excreted 5.1 mg/kg/day. Endogenous fecal excretion is independent of Ca intake (and the true absorption rate), and not related to gestational age or postnatal age at study. A number of carbohydrates (especially lactose) and glucose polymers enhance the intestinal absorption of Ca,[166, 167] probably independent of the actions of vitamin D.[166, 168] *in vitro* studies have established that mucosal lactose directly stimulates ileal[169,170] but not duodenal or jejunal Ca absorption.[171] Lactose, in contrast to other monosaccharides and disaccharides, is not hydrolyzed in the proximal small intestine, and large quantities of this sugar are delivered to the ileum. The observation that lactose feeding can reduce duodenal Ca-binding protein content and Ca absorption[172] may be attributed to increased Ca retention from augmented ileal Ca absorption. Lactose, by itself, does not solubilize precipitated Ca; it does not maintain Ca in a soluble form in the presence of precipitating agents such as phosphate.[111] The lactose effect on Ca absorption may be mediated through its action on the permeability of ileal epithelium, through a paracellular mechanism.[173] The observation that lactose also stimulates intestinal absorption of other divalent cations (e.g., Mg, Ba, Sr, and Ra)[111] further supports the possibility that this sugar may cause a general increase in permeability to divalent ions across the junctional assembly. In rats, osmotic forces that enhance the net intestinal absorption of water also enhance the passive absorption of Ca.[168] It appears from such data that "solvent drag" plays a significant role in the augmentation of Ca absorption and has led to the speculation that this may be the mechanism through which carbohydrates act.

Bile salts stimulate Ca absorption in the chick.[174] The mechanism for bile salt–mediated Ca absorption is not clear, but the stimulatory action is not vitamin D dependent. Bile salts solubilize lipids for absorption through the formation of micelles.[175] The surfaces of micelles bear negative charges, which strongly bind Ca and sodium ions. The process of micellar solubilization may explain the observation that although the physiochemical environment of ileum favors Ca precipitation,[144] the bulk of Ca absorption occurs in this segment *in vivo*.[176] In addition to increasing the amount of Ca available for absorption, bile salts may also influence Ca absorption by acting directly on the intestinal epithelium. In a variety of *in vivo* and *in vitro* perfusion studies[177,178] using isolated, short-circuited rat and rabbit colons, increased permeability of gastrointestinal barriers has been observed with changes in tight-junction complexes. This is reflected by increases in transepithelial conductance[179, 180] and permeation of paracellular pathway markers.[180] In addition to the paracellular action, bile salts can also influence enterocytes directly: bile salts have potent Ca ionophoric effects (thus mimicking the effect of 1,25(OH)$_2$D) across a variety of artificial and plasma membranes, including the jejunal brush border membrane.[181]

As mentioned, the bulk of Ca^{2+} absorption occurs in the distal small intestine, in particular the ileum,[106,107] a segment that is relatively insensitive to 1,25(OH)$_2$D, devoid of Ca^{2+}-binding protein and poorly equipped for active Ca^{2+} absorption.[109] Under *in vivo* postprandial conditions, the simultaneous arrival in ileum of bile salts and Ca^{2+} could foster a highly efficient Ca^{2+} absorptive state. The Ca^{2+} load, solubilized by bile salts,[175] would create a Ca^{2+} concentration gradient in the absorptive direction (i.e., [Ca^{2+}]m > [Ca^{2+}]s). This, in concert with the bile salt–induced increase in the permeability of the intercellular conduit, could promote rapid Ca^{2+} absorption, both economically and in substantial quantities.[108]

Fat malabsorption has the potential to impair intestinal Ca absorption. Preterm infants are not likely to have an intraluminal concentration of bile salts sufficient for the establishment of a micelle phase, which has the potential to reduce the absorption of fat.[182] The unabsorbed free fatty acids would then be available to interact with ionic Ca to form insoluble Ca soaps, which, in turn, would not be available for absorption. Although steatorrhea can be significantly reduced in preterm infants by administering a significant proportion of dietary fat as medium chain triglycerides (which do not require micelle formation for absorption), it is not clear that this practice significantly improves intestinal Ca absorption.[183] Furthermore, despite these general theoretical considerations, the absorption of Ca during this period is high, particularly in comparison with other ages of life.

Fractional intestinal absorption of Ca is enhanced by dietary restriction of Ca or Pi. Under these conditions, rats[184,185] and humans[186] demonstrate increased production of 1,25(OH)$_2$D, with resultant increase in active intestinal absorption of Ca. The effect of short-term moderate dietary P restriction on intestinal net Ca fluxes and external Ca balance was studied in growing rabbits that were fed a P-deficient diet (containing approximately two thirds of the estimated minimum requirement for P) for 10 consecutive days.[187] During P restriction, intestinal Ca absorption rose significantly to reach maximal values within 96 hours; sustained high rates of Ca absorption persisted for the 10 days of P restriction. When the rabbits were consuming the P-replenished control diet, Ca absorption fell to control values during the first 9 days of recovery, implying the persistence of mechanisms for Ca hyperabsorption for at least 1 week following this degree of P restriction. Despite increased intestinal Ca absorption, Ca balance during P restriction was less positive because the increase in urinary Ca excretion was even greater. The increased efficiency of Ca absorption in response to moderate dietary P restriction is consistent with the well-established effect of calcitriol on intestinal Ca transport.[144]

All forms of Ca in the diet may not be equally absorbed. It is generally held that the absorbability of various Ca preparations depends substantially on their solubility in aqueous solution. Heaney and colleagues[188] have shown that Ca absorbability is related to the solubility of Ca salts; however, the association is relatively weak. In the range of concentrations from 0.1 to 10 mmol/L within which most Ca supplement sources fall, there was no detectable effect of solubility on absorption: absorption values varied from 10% for the least soluble preparations (Ca oxalate) to 44% for the most (bisglycinocalcium). When rat diets are constituted with two or more Ca salts of widely differing solubilities, Ca is absorbed from each salt in direct proportion to its solubility. Once dissolved, the quantity of Ca absorbed is largely a function of the intestinal transit time, with the active, transcellular transport process playing a progressively smaller role as the soluble Ca content increases. The solubility of Ca carbonate is low; Ca phosphate is 18 times more soluble than Ca carbonate.

The impaired solubility of Ca carbonate versus Ca phosphate accounts for the diminished Ca absorption observed in rats fed diets high in Ca carbonate.[189] Whether similar events can occur in human neonates has not been studied. If the differing solubilities of Ca salts in infant formulas can truly affect the net Ca absorption in human neonates, this might explain the contradictory data obtained with different formula preparations.

Phosphorus

Compared with Ca, much less is known about the intestinal absorption of Pi. Fewer direct studies have been performed in humans, so that much of the available information has been derived from animal studies. Phosphorus absorption is remarkably efficient, much more than Ca absorption. At low levels of intake (less than 2 mg/kg of body weight per day), 80% to 90% of ingested P in adults is absorbed. Even with levels of intake greater than 10 mg/kg of body weight per day in the form of dairy products, cereals, eggs, and meat, absorption is about 70%.[97] In term and preterm infants, the fractional absorption of P is high, ranging from 86% to 97% regardless of P or Ca intake.[190] Thus, the dietary Pi intake is an important determinant of the amount of P absorbed.

The absorption of Pi occurs throughout the entire small intestine. In early studies using rat isolated intestinal segments, the data suggested that the bulk of Pi absorption occurred in the proximal small intestine,[191,192] whereas little or no active Pi absorption (in both vitamin D–deficient and 1,25(OH)$_2$D-replete rats) took place in the ileum or colon.[193] Only few previous *in vivo* studies[194-196] have evaluated the contributions of different intestinal segments to total intestinal Pi absorption. Because of methodologic problems in these studies (e.g., failure to measure transit and absorption simultaneously in the same animal and disruption of the anatomic and physiologic continuity of intestine) as well as inadequate numbers of data points and lack of information regarding timing of feeding and sample collection,[195,196] it has been difficult to interpret Pi absorption data.

Kayne and associates[197] have developed a new approach to the analysis of *in vivo* segmental Pi absorption using a spontaneously propelled meal in intact rats fed ^{32}P-labeled Pi liquid meal containing a nonabsorbable marker, [^{14}C] polyethylene glycol. The analysis involves a compartmental model describing intersegmental transit and segmental absorption of Pi along the intact intestinal tract over time. The duodenum, which had the highest transit and absorption rates, accounted for a third of total absorption; the terminal ileum, with a lower absorption rate but a longer transit time, also accounted for one third of the total absorption (equal to Pi absorbed in the duodenum); the remaining one third was absorbed by the intervening small intestinal segments. This new technique has provided the opportunity to re-examine many of the important mechanistic and regulatory mechanisms established from experimental models (Fig. 34–5).

The movement of P across the intestinal epithelium can be resolved into two unidirectional fluxes: an absorptive, mucosal-to-serosal flux and a secretory, serosal-to-mucosal flux. Each unidirectional flux, in turn, consists of two components, a transcellular flux and a paracellular flux. The paracellular flux represents a passive, diffusional process and is driven by transepithelial chemical and physical (electrical and hydrostatic) gradients, whereas the transcellular flux represents an active, energy-dependent transport process and is assumed to be unaffected by the transepithelial electrochemical gradients.

The relationship between the intraluminal concentration of Pi and its absorption is curvilinear, supporting the concept that both passive and active processes are involved in the movement of Pi from the intestinal mucosa to serosa.[198] Little is known about the passive absorption of Pi. The active component of Pi absorption involves transcellular transport, with movement

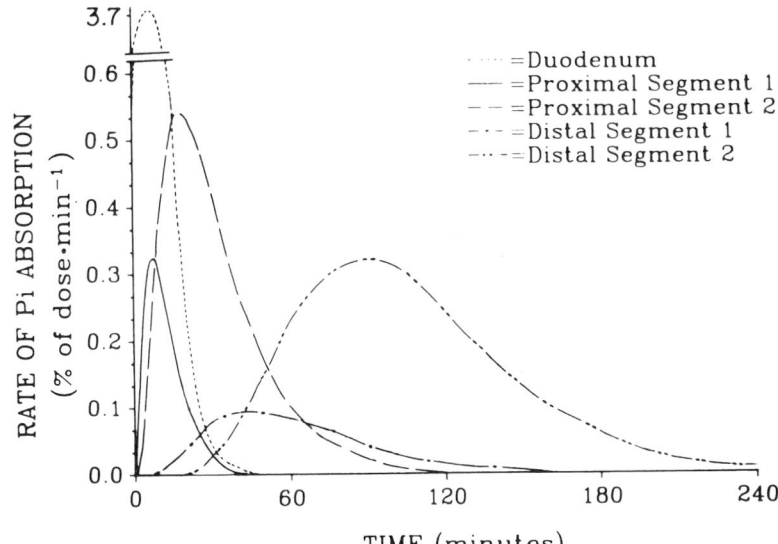

Figure 34–5. Segmental Pi absorption rate profiles. The P_i absorption rates for each segment are shown over time. The rates of Pi absorbed from duodenum through distal segment 2 as a function of time were constructed from the compartmental model: The gastrointestinal tract was divided into duodenum, and four equal-length segments of small intestine (proximal segments 1 and 2 and distal segments 1 and 2). (From Kayne LH, et al: J Clin Invest *91*:915, 1993.)

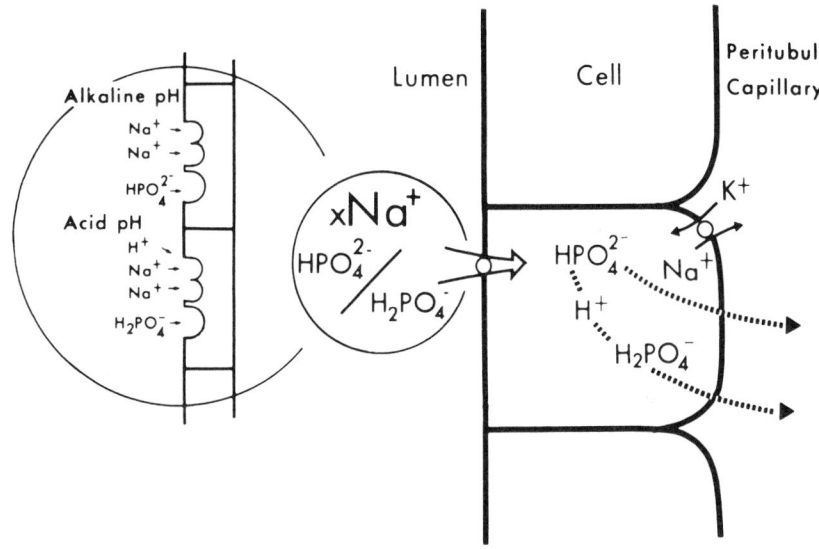

Figure 34–6. Schematic illustration of the sodium-dependent transport of phosphate across the brush-border membrane of the proximal tubule. The *circular inset* provides speculation on the activation of the phosphate carrier by sodium and the interference by hydrogen ions. (From Quamme GA, Shapiro RJ: Can J Physiol *65*:275, 1987.)

across the brush-border membrane appearing to be the rate-limiting step.[198] Lee and colleagues[192] have demonstrated the existence of an active, sodium-dependent transepithelial Pi absorptive mechanism in rat jejunum by measuring net Pi absorptive flux under short-circuited conditions. Sodium stimulates both unidirectional mucosal-to-serosal flux and serosal-to-mucosal flux for Pi (measured in the absence of transepithelial potential differences). Thus, absorption at the brush-border membrane involves the obligate transport of sodium and Pi and occurs in an electroneutral fashion.[199] The absorbed Pi then traverses the cytoplasm via unknown processes; at the basolateral membrane, it moves down its electrochemical gradient by means of simple diffusion[199] or via carrier-mediated facilitated transport (Fig. 34–6).[200]

The regulation of intestinal Pi absorption appears to be centered on the co-transport of sodium and Pi at the brush border. It is at this site that 1,25(OH)$_2$D acts to enhance the intestinal absorption of Pi.[201] The exact mechanism through which 1,25(OH)$_2$D acts is not clear, but it increases the number of trans-

porting sites.[201] Whether this is done through the unmasking of preexisting Na$^+$/Pi co-transporters or through the synthesis of new sites remains to be elucidated. A sodium-dependent 1,25(OH)$_2$D effect on Pi influx across the mucous membrane has been described in rabbit duodenum[202] and brush-border membrane vesicle preparations[203] under short-circuited conditions and under optimized conditions (i.e., [Na] = 90 mM and pH 6.0) for Pi influx. Furthermore, Lee and colleagues[192] have demonstrated that 1,25(OH)$_2$D increases mucosal border Pi entry and that this stimulating action is mediated through the sodium-dependent component of the total measured influx.

Alterations in dietary Pi intake significantly affect intestinal absorption of Pi. With restriction of dietary Pi, fractional intestinal absorption of Pi increases.[184-186, 204] In growing rabbits,[187] moderate short-term dietary P restriction induces both intestinal and renal adaptations to conserve Ca and P: there is net P secretion on the first day of P restriction, but this changes to increased absorption beginning on the second day, indicating intestinal adaptation. With dietary P replenishment, adaptations persist to restore the positive mineral balances that were lost because of dietary P restriction during growth.[187] The mechanisms underlying the increased efficiency (greater fractional absorption) and capacity (hyperabsorption during recovery) of intestinal P absorption in rabbits in response to moderate dietary P restriction are not defined, but it is likely that 1,25(OH)$_2$D plays an important role. It increases the absorptive capacity of this putative Na$^+$/Pi co-transporter,[202, 203] and it may increase the affinity of this transporter for Pi as well.[203] Selective restriction of dietary P decreases plasma [P],[205] minimizes cumulative P balance, and increases plasma 1,25(OH)$_2$D levels in rabbits,[205] humans,[206] and rats.[207] Low P diet-induced increases in 1,25(OH)$_2$D production, however, cannot account for the entire increase in Ca absorption in experimental animals,[208] supporting the contention that the regulation of P absorption is not always predictably a function of 1,25(OH)$_2$D activities.

Vitamin D–deficient or thyroparathyroidectomized rats placed on a Pi-restricted diet demonstrated a 50% increase in intestinal Pi absorption as measured using isolated in situ intestinal loops. The presence of active P absorption in rats severely depleted of vitamin D raises the possibility of non vitamin D–dependent factors in the regulation of active P absorption.[209] Bile salts, lactose, and prolactin are examples of agents that can stimulate P absorption through vitamin D–independent mechanisms.[137] An interesting example of vitamin D–independent regulation of P absorption is the ability of local (perienterocyte) factors to modify or reverse the effect of 1,25(OH)$_2$D. Because there is often marked fluctuation in luminal concentrations of solutes such as P, there might be a need for some local regulation of P absorption to avoid P overloading. In support of a locally mediated vitamin D–independent mechanism, Lee[209] has demonstrated that active jejunal transport of P in vitamin D–deficient rats was not different between rats eating a P-replete diet and rats eating a P-deficient diet.

Hydrogen ion concentration also has been observed to influence the activity of the Na$^+$/Pi co-transport system. Under acidic conditions (media pH ranging from 5.8 to 6.9), rat small intestine brush-border membrane vesicles demonstrate high rates of Pi uptake.[210] In rat jejunum, reduction in extracellular pH from 7.4 to 6.0 is associated with a 150% increase in Pi influx.[192] Because the vesicles are oriented with the intraluminal surface of the brush-border membrane facing the bathing media, these results indicate that intestinal absorption is enhanced when the intraluminal environment is somewhat acidic. In contrast, metabolic acidosis, which should decrease intracellular pH, has been observed to decrease Pi uptake markedly in rats as measured by in situ perfused jejunal loops and jejunal brush-border membrane vesicles.[211] The observed decrease in Pi transport may represent a decrease in the activity of the Na$^+$/Pi co-transport system. Treatment of acidotic rats with 1,25(OH)$_2$D fails to improve the defect in intestinal Pi absorption. In contrast to brush-border membrane vesicle data, however, Lee and colleagues[192] observed a smaller increase (50%) in mucosal Pi influx using intact epithelium when pH was increased from 7.4 to 8.5.

It is unclear how changes in pH specifically alter Pi transport. Alterations in pH change the chemical equilibrium between the monovalent and divalent forms of Pi. It is possible that if one of these forms of Pi is transported in preference to the other, changes in pH could shift the chemical equilibrium to either favor or hinder transport. The effective pH (5.4) at the transporting surface would dictate that all Pi in the immediate ambience would be in the monobasic form. Furthermore, the properties of the Na$^+$/Pi co-transport system may be pH dependent; hence, changes in pH might alter the efficiency of this system to transport Pi. The acidic microenvironment, however, does not explain the observation[192] that Pi influx is also increased when pH is raised from 7.4 to 8.5. One possibility is that alkaline pH may affect P permeation through the tight junc-

tion. This is a reasonable postulate because electrical conductance is increased at this pH. The mechanisms that mediate changes in Pi influx with changes in either extracellular [Na] or pH remain to be elucidated.

In preterm and full-term neonates, numerous studies have demonstrated that Pi is well absorbed from the gastrointestinal tract regardless of the type of feeding given, and it is generally independent of the intake of vitamin D.[211,212] Expressed as a percentage of total Pi intake, intestinal absorption ranges between near 70% to greater than 90%. In general, the percentage of Pi absorbed increases as Pi intake decreases, but the absolute absorption of Pi (measured in mg/kg/day) increases proportionally with increasing intake. In infants fed soy-based formulas, the intestinal absorption of Pi is lower than that of a comparable group of infants fed a similar Pi intake from cow's milk–based formula.[213] Measurements of bone mineral content have also been found to be lower in soy-fed infants compared with cow's milk-based formula-fed infants, consistent with reduced mineral utilization with soy formulas.[214, 215] It is presumed that phytic acid, which is present in soy formulas, complexes with dietary Pi, thereby limiting its bioavailability for absorption. It appears that by increasing the Ca and Pi content of soy formulas, this problem may be overcome.[216]

Magnesium

Intestinal Mg absorption is the normal source through which the body repletes its Mg store or meets the additional demand for Mg imposed by anabolic states such as growth and pregnancy. Minimal information is available with regard to the gastrointestinal handling of Mg. Mg absorption, as with Ca absorption, varies with age. In adults, intestinal absorption of Mg ranges between 34% and 62% of total intake.[97, 217] Term and preterm infants have greater intestinal Mg absorption, in the range of 60% to 86%.[32, 218-221] Mg absorption does not appear to vary with gestational age in low birth weight infants between 29 and 34 weeks' gestation.[220] Mg absorption and retention increase with increasing postnatal age in very low birth weight infants receiving low Ca and P intake or high Mg intake.[221]

Despite considerable research on Mg absorption, there is still uncertainty regarding the site and mechanisms of intestinal Mg transport. Absorption of Mg has been clearly demonstrated to occur in all segments of the intestine. The predominant site of Mg absorption, based on transit time and studies using isolated segments of the intestine, is the distal small intestine, in particular the ileum.[94, 222, 223] Some investigators have reported a higher rate of Mg absorption in duodenum than in ileum.[224, 225] The measurement methods, however, were biased by short incubation time (45 minutes versus 1 to 2 hours), which favors the duodenum in terms of the relative magnitude of Mg transport.[224] Because of its relatively greater length and mass, the distal small intestine is likely to be the principal location in which the bulk of Mg is absorbed. Indeed, the removal of 50% of the distal small intestine results in a 40% drop in Mg absorption in rats.[226]

The colon is also a dominant site for Mg absorption, based on studies in selected segments of the intestine,[227, 228] but not when absorption is measured in the entire undisturbed intestinal tract.[229] Measurements in isolated segments may not adequately reflect Mg absorption in an undisturbed gastrointestinal tract or in the same segment that is in continuity with the rest of the gastrointestinal tract and in contact with a vastly different *in vivo* environment. Both transit time through the gastrointestinal tract and availability of Mg for absorption in various segments may profoundly influence the amount of Mg absorbed along the intestinal tract.

Where and when Mg absorption occurs can be ascertained only in an intestine in which the natural physiologic conditions and regulatory mechanisms are not altered and the transit of the meal is not impeded. Only one study, so far, has attempted to examine Mg absorption under these conditions. In this study, chickens were fed a semipurified diet containing chromic oxide (Cr_2O_3) and 382 ppm of Mg, and absorption of Mg was determined based on the Mg/Cr ratio in each intestinal segment.[230] Greater than 50% of the dietary Mg was absorbed in the duodenum. Jejunal absorption of Mg accounted for 5%, the ileum for 24%, and the colon for 19% of total Mg absorption. These data, however, should be interpreted with caution because there were several potential methodologic problems with this study. First, absorption was measured only at one time point, and Mg absorption in a given segment would likely have varied with time after administration of a meal. Furthermore, it was difficult to interpret the meaning of the Mg/Cr ratio because the intestinal marker used, Cr_2O_3, may not have moved down the intestinal tract at the same rate as Mg. Unfortunately, at this time, there is no effective strategy for accurately determining segmental mineral absorption from a spontaneously propelled meal *in vivo* in an intact intestinal tract.

Kayne and Lee[231] have proposed an indirect solution to this problem using the technique of compartmental modeling to analyze and integrate segmental absorptive events of mineral from a spontaneously propelled liquid meal along the intact intestinal tract, using a labeled mineral in association with nonabsorbable marker. This approach allows the analysis of the mechanism and the regulation of mineral absorption under more authentic *in vivo* conditions. In a compartmental model, the rate constants for intersegmental transit and segmental absorption are estimated. The remarkable correlation between the simulated model and the measured data indicates that the estimated rate constants reflect *in vivo* events. Based on the intestinal transit data of a liquid meal labeled by a nonabsorbable marker, ^{14}C-polyethylene glycol, it is apparent that the proximal small intestine has a short exposure time to the rapidly advancing isotope bolus and is therefore responsible only for the modest Mg absorption observed during the first 2 hours. Thereafter, the food bolus moves more slowly through the ileum and colon, where the bulk of Mg is absorbed at a steady, higher, and more sustained rate. Thus, significant Mg absorption occurs in the distal portions of the intestine (Fig. 34–7).

Available data on the mechanism of Mg absorption are mainly descriptive in nature. There are three mechanisms by which Mg has been shown to cross the intestinal epithelium: passive diffusion, solvent drag, and active transport (saturable Mg absorption) that may[222, 228] or may not[232] require energy. It is not clear, however, which process predominates under normal conditions. These results have been based on tracer techniques,[217, 229, 232] *in vivo* intestinal perfusion preparations,[228, 233, 234] and *in vitro* gut preparations[222, 224] in animals and humans. Conflicting results can be traced to differences in methods between studies using the same technique and to problems inherent to the use of each of these techniques in studying intestinal Mg transport.

Based on studies in both experimental animals and humans, it appears that passive diffusion through the paracellular pathway

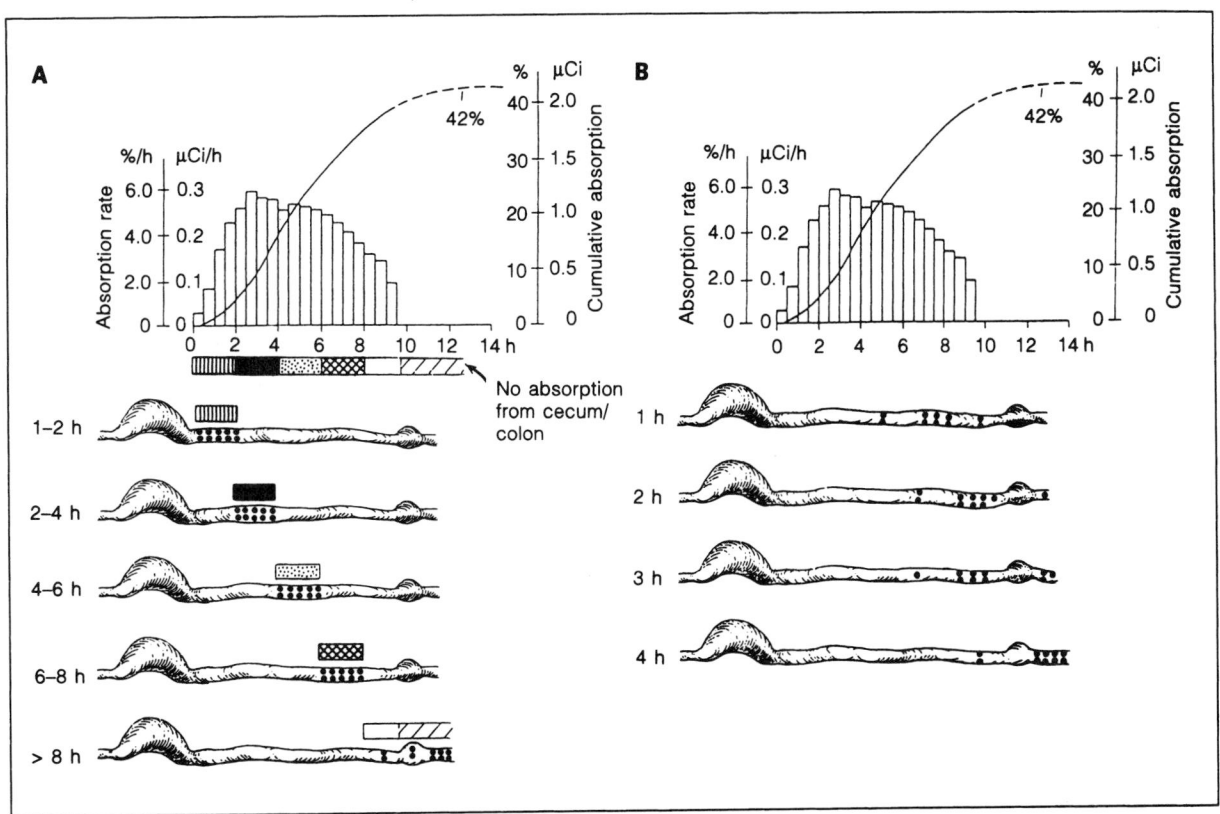

Figure 34–7. **A,** Solid curve in the top graph represents the cumulative absorption of Mg following administration of 5 μCi [28]Mg. Columns represent rates of absorption calculated from the plasma radioactivity. Based on Graham and colleagues'[229] conclusions, the lower diagram schematically depicts the location and distribution of the bolus (*dark dots*) in the intestinal tract over time. Marked boxes represent the sites of absorption at different time intervals: 1–2 hours (*vertical striped box*), 2–4 hours (*black box*), 4–6 hours (*dotted box*), 6–8 hours (*cross-hatched box*), >8 hours (*open/diagonal striped box*). (From Graham L, et al: Metabolism *9*:646, 1960.) **B,** The lower diagram depicts the movement of ^{14}C-polyethylene glycol over time observed in the study by Kayne and associates.[197] (From Kayne LH, et al: J Clin Invest *91*:915, 1993.)

accounts for the majority of Mg absorbed. Passive diffusion is driven by the electrochemical gradient across the epithelium. Absorption by this process is expected to vary with the luminal Mg concentration and not exhibit saturation kinetics. In young, growing rats, luminal Mg uptake in duodenum is a linear, concentration-dependent process, not a saturable Mg absorptive process, and exhibits no age-related changes.[143] This does not mean that Mg absorption is completely unregulated. It is possible that depletion of luminal Mg may loosen the tight junctions, resulting in transepithelial diffusion.[235] Furthermore, a high luminal Mg concentration may reduce transepithelial permeability, the latter accounting for the reduction in fractional Mg absorption observed with a high-Mg diet.[143]

Several investigators have demonstrated that net Mg absorption in adults is linearly related to dietary Mg over a normal range of dietary Mg intake (130 to 490 mg/day).[236-238] This is consistent with a diet-dependent passive process for Mg absorption. Fine and colleagues[239] measured Mg absorption in adults over a wide range of Mg intakes (using a standard meal supplemented with 0 to 80 mEq of Mg acetate). They observed that net Mg absorption rose with each increment in Mg intake but that fractional Mg absorption fell progressively (from 65% at the lowest to 11% at the highest intake) so that the relationship between net Mg absorption and Mg intake was curvilinear. This is consistent with a Mg absorption process that simultaneously uses (1) a mechanism that reaches an absorptive maximum, and (2) a mechanism that endlessly absorbs a defined fraction (7%) of ingested Mg, indicating that Mg absorption is mediated by both a saturable carrier and passive diffusion (Fig. 34–8).

Movement of water across the intestinal epithelium has the ability to transport solutes in the same direction. Solute transport by this process is thus accomplished through solvent drag. Using an *in vivo* perfusion technique in rats, Behar[233] observed a positive correlation between net water absorption and net Mg absorption. Although he proposed that Mg absorption occurs primarily by a solvent drag mechanism, this study did not exclude the presence of other mechanisms of Mg absorption in intestine and, by design, did not evaluate the relation of luminal Mg concentration to Mg uptake. Ross[222] and Brannan and colleagues[234] have demonstrated significant Mg absorption independent of water movement in rats and humans (while keeping net water

movement at zero throughout the study), indicating that other mechanisms are involved.

A saturable component of intestinal Mg absorption has been consistently reported in animal studies.[222, 228] Ross[222] reported curvilinear uptake of Mg in the small intestine of rats when the Mg concentration was varied from 0.1 to 12 mmol/L. Meneely and associates[228] found that Mg absorption was saturable in the colon of adolescent rats but not in the jejunum or ileum. The nature of the saturable component of intestinal Mg absorption is not well understood. It has been speculated that this component is due to down-regulation of active transport of Mg.[222, 240] Active transport has seemed likely because Mg can be absorbed against an electrochemical gradient in the intestine. Studies in rats using the everted gut sac preparation, however, have failed to demonstrate that Mg is actively transported against a concentration gradient in young or adolescent rats.[222-224]

Studies using the Ussing chamber have documented that Mg is actively transported in the descending colon. Karbach and Feldmeier,[241] measuring unidirectional fluxes in the absence of transepithelial electrochemical gradients and under voltage-clamp conditions, have reported active mucosal-to-serosal Mg transport in the ileum and in both the proximal and distal colon of the rat. Because there was no definite evidence supporting either an uphill or an energy-dependent Mg transport process, however, others have proposed that the observed saturation characteristics are mediated by facilitated diffusion.

The presence and characteristics of the proposed carrier-mediated mechanism have not been conclusively demonstrated. Evidence for a saturable process is based on a curvilinear (curved at low intakes and linear at high intakes) relationship between dietary Mg or luminal Mg and Mg uptake in humans. Whether this is due to a carrier-mediated mechanism or due to alterations in absorption through the paracellular route,[231] or to both mechanisms,[239] remains to be determined. Evidence that a Mg transport carrier does exist in the human intestine comes from *in vitro* and *in vivo* studies of human ileum that show saturation of net Mg absorption as Mg concentration in the perfusate is increased.[234, 242] The existence of a recessively inherited disorder of Mg absorption[243, 244] also supports the existence of carrier-mediated Mg absorption in normal subjects.

There is as yet no basal-lateral transport data for Mg in enterocytes or their membrane fractions. Although current data suggest no significant chemical gradient for Mg across the cell membrane, the significant uphill electrical gradient for the exit of a cation such as Mg suggests the participation of an energy-dependent mechanism.[231] The hypothesis that Mg enters the enterocyte by facilitated diffusion mediated by a passive carrier protein and exits the enterocyte by active transport mediated by Mg pump needs to be tested.

Passive diffusion, solvent drag, and active transport all participate in intestinal Mg absorption. Under conditions of usual dietary Mg intake, however, passive diffusion and solvent drag mechanisms of Mg absorption predominate. Thus, absorption of Mg occurs primarily by passive diffusion through the paracellular pathway. Active transport of Mg has been conclusively demonstrated in the colon, although indirect evidence also points to the existence of an active cellular mediated component of Mg transport in the small intestine. This component is probably saturated under conditions of usual dietary Mg intake and, therefore, may be critical only to total Mg absorption in the intestine under conditions of rapid growth or extremely low dietary Mg intake. Further research needs to focus on whether, there is an active component of Mg absorption in the small intestine and determine the role it plays in total Mg absorption.

Absolute intestinal absorption of Mg appears to depend on the Mg content of the diet and on body Mg status.[239] Relatively higher Mg absorption occurs in patients who have previously ingested low-Mg diets or in those individuals with overall nega-

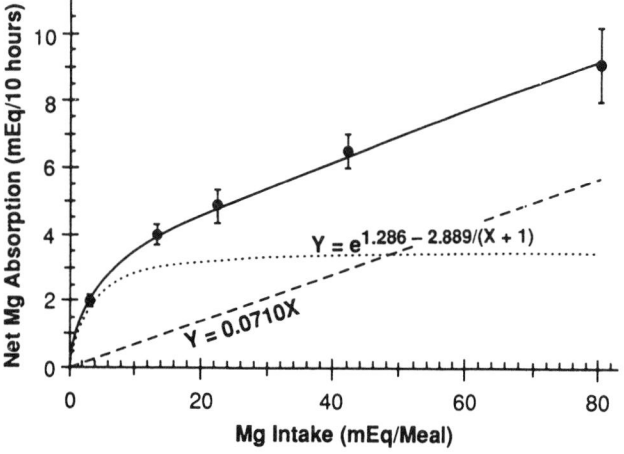

Figure 34–8. Net Mg absorption versus intake as derived by nonlinear regression analysis. The equation for net absorption, $Y = e^{1.286-2.889/(X+1)} + 0.0710X$ represents a hyperbolic function plus a linear function. These separate components and their respective equations are shown. (From Fine KD, et al: J Clin Invest 88:396, 1991.)

tive Mg balance, for instance, in pregnancy, lactation, or excessive renal excretion. The factors controlling intestinal Mg absorption are not well delineated but appear to involve vitamin D metabolites[245] and PTH.[239] A significant amount of Mg absorption, however, is vitamin D independent because it persists under conditions of vitamin D deficiency. Absorption also may be affected by intraluminal complexing agents, such as phytates found in cereal grain.[240]

Repletion of vitamin D in vitamin D–deficient animals and humans is associated with increments in Mg absorption.[94, 95] In vitamin D–replete animals and humans, pharmacologic doses of vitamin D[94-96] appear to increase Mg absorption, whereas spontaneous fluctuations in circulating levels of $1,25(OH)_2D$ have little effect on Mg transport.[93] The importance of vitamin D–stimulated Mg absorption on overall Mg homeostasis remains uncertain,[93-96] particularly in light of the dramatic increases in urinary excretion of Mg that have been associated with vitamin D administration.[245]

For many years, it was assumed that Ca and Mg were handled similarly at different steps in the intestinal absorptive process. Data from Hardwick and colleagues,[143] however, cast doubt on that assumption. In their studies using young, growing (post-weaning) rats, duodenal Ca absorption was mediated both actively and passively (with the former predominating), whereas Mg absorption was predominantly a concentration-dependent mechanism. It appears, therefore, that Ca and Mg are handled differently at various steps of the absorptive process.

In rats, several studies have demonstrated that net absorption of Mg in vivo is depressed by a high Ca intake.[246-248] Karbach and Ewe,[96] however, reported that increasing the Ca concentration in intestinal perfusate from 1.25 to 10 mM/L in vivo had no effect on Mg absorption in the colon of rats. This study does not rule out that Ca at lower concentrations may significantly alter Mg absorption.

In humans, several studies have shown that increasing Ca in the diet significantly depresses Mg absorption.[249, 250] In very low birth weight infants,[221] high dietary Ca intakes that allow retentions equivalent to the in utero accretion rates do limit Mg retention, and a significant Mg deficiency can occur in comparison with intrauterine accretion.[158] Ca and P supplementation reduce Mg absorption and retention; however, with Mg intakes approaching 20 mg/kg/day, appropriate retention is achieved in very low birth weight infants.

The effect of increased Mg intake on Ca absorption and retention is more controversial. In 1987, Karbach and Ewe[96] demonstrated that there was no limitation in Ca absorption when increasing concentrations of Mg (1.25 to 10 mmol/L) were used to perfuse the large intestine of the rat. When Ca and Mg interactions were examined in the descending colon of the rat using the Ussing system, however, Mg exerted a significant negative effect on net Ca absorption. Specifically, increasing the Mg concentration to 1.25 mmol/L decreased the mucosal-to-serosal flux of Ca by 50% and abolished net Ca absorption. The effect was due to a depression of the voltage-dependent component—that is, the paracellular pathway.

Increasing Mg in the diet has been reported to increase fecal Ca significantly in humans.[251-253] Fine and colleagues,[239] however, have demonstrated that an increased Mg intake in adults had no effect on Ca absorption, indicating that Mg does not inhibit active or passive Ca absorption, even when Mg is present in great excess. There is an increase in urine Ca excretion with increased Mg intake and absorption (Fig. 34-9).

Much of the evidence for intestinal interactions between Ca and Mg has come from studies in which transport of one nutrient was studied in the absence of dietary intake of the other nutrient.[246, 254] Moreover, the results of previous studies do not exclude an adaptive effect of Ca on Mg transport in the intestine. The mechanisms by which Ca and Mg interact, however, have

not been well defined. Several possible mechanisms have been proposed. These include competition for a common carrier system, a Ca-induced change in membrane permeability to Mg,[252] and modulation of a specific Mg carrier by Ca.[255] Intestinal membrane permeability is sensitive to alterations in luminal Ca and Mg concentrations[256-258]; depletion of either luminal Mg or Ca increases tight junction permeability and thereby increases diffusion through the paracellular pathway.[235, 259] The physiologic changes in the concentration of Ca or Mg in the lumen might also influence diffusion through the paracellular pathway. Further investigation is required to test this hypothesis and to determine its importance in short-term and long-term regulation of Ca and Mg transport.

Several other factors can affect intestinal Mg absorption. Glucose polymers have been observed to enhance jejunal Mg absorption.[167] The absorption of Mg has been found to be directly related to the net absorption of water, consistent with carbohydrate-enhanced Mg absorption by means of solvent drag. Dietary lactose, a poorly digestible disaccharide, significantly enhances the apparent absorption of Mg in rats.[260, 261] Theoretically, this effect of lactose may involve a decrease in pH in the intestinal lumen, caused by bacterial fermentation,[261] thereby altering the solubility of Mg in the digesta. The observed negative relationship between pH in the ileal lumen and intestinal Mg absorption in the rat supports the notion that the decrease in ileal pH (from 7.5 to 7.2) after lactose feeding is the major mechanism responsible for the improved Mg absorption.[261] In a study investigating the effect of lactose on Mg absorption in term infants,[262] Mg retention was similar between infants fed a formula containing lactose compared with one that was lactose free.

Starch, which is poorly digestible, also influences Mg absorption by a mechanism similar to that of lactose.[263] In rats fed native starch, Mg absorption is increased. Furthermore, the ileal pH is significantly lowered, and Mg concentrations in liquid cecal contents are raised.[263] Whether changing the carbohydrate composition of formula (especially the relatively poorly digestible carbohydrates, e.g., starch) can affect Mg absorption has not been studied in human infants.

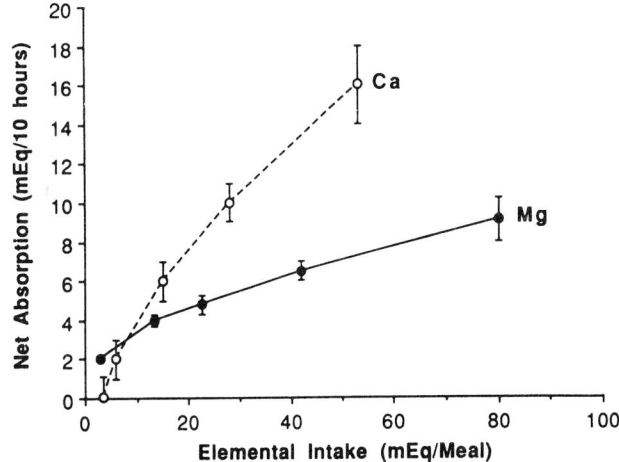

Figure 34-9. Comparison of net Mg absorption with net Ca absorption measured from similar meals supplemented with varying amounts of Ca carbonate or Mg acetate. (Mean ± SE values are shown.) At low levels of intake, more Mg than Ca is absorbed. At intakes greater than 8 mEq, increasingly more Ca than Mg is absorbed. Data based on several studies. (From Fine KD, et al: J Clin Invest 88:396, 1991.)

Mg absorption may be improved with use of easily absorbed fat in the form of medium chain triglyceride.[219] Furthermore, an increase in dietary protein concentration increases apparent Mg absorption in rats[264, 265] and in humans.[266]

Increased P intake may decrease Mg absorption owing to the formation of less soluble P-Mg complexes.[267] In full-term breast-fed infants, however, the addition of P supplements to human milk improved Mg absorption and retention.[268] In very low birth weight infants, increased dietary P resulted in a higher fecal loss of Mg and lower net absorption and retention of Mg.[269]

Finally, it is worth noting that significant amounts of Mg are secreted into the intestinal tract. Bile, pancreatic juice, and gastric juice all contain large amounts of Mg. Almost all the secreted Mg is reabsorbed, so that under normal conditions, secreted Mg accounts for only a small proportion of the total fecal Mg.[33] In rats, a significant portion of Mg in feces is of endogenous origin and is changed by dietary protein intake—high soybean protein causes greater excretion of endogenous Mg.[32, 270, 271] In contrast, endogenous Mg excretion in feces is significantly depressed in rats fed a high-protein diet (threefold higher casein), whereas urinary Mg excretion is increased.[272] It is uncertain why high protein intake depresses the excretion of endogenous Mg in the feces.

Endogenous Mg losses in adult humans[273] range from 6 to 36 mg/day. In term newborn infants, endogenous Mg secretion, measured using radioisotopes, ranged from 6.8 to 16 mg/day, similar to the values noted in adults but much greater if expressed per kilogram of body weight or of percentage total Mg intake.[32]

REFERENCES

1. Widdowson EM, McCance RA: The metabolism of calcium, phosphorus, magnesium and strontium. Pediatr Clin North Am 12:595, 1965.
2. Shaw JCL: Evidence for defective skeletal mineralization in low birth weight infants: the absorption of calcium and fat. Pediatrics 57:16, 1976.
3. Posner AS: Crystal chemistry of bone mineral. Physiol Rev 49:760, 1969.
4. Neer R, et al: Multicompartmental analysis of calcium kinetics in normal adult males. J Clin Invest 46:1364, 1967.
5. Abrams SA, et al: Developmental changes in calcium kinetics in children assessed using stable isotopes. J Bone Miner Res 7:287, 1992.
6. Marshall RW: Plasma fractions. In Nordin BEC (ed): Calcium, Phosphate and Magnesium Metabolism. London, Churchill Livingstone, 1976, pp 162–185.
7. Mimouni A, et al: Effects of albumin on ionized calcium in vitro. Pediatr Emerg Care 7:149, 1991.
8. Brown DM, et al: Serum ionized calcium in newborn infants. Pediatrics 49:841, 1972.
9. Bowers GN, et al: Measurement of ionized calcium in serum with ion-selective electrodes: a mature technology that can meet the daily service needs. Clin Chem 32:1437, 1986.
10. Nelson N, et al: Neonatal reference values for ionized calcium, phosphate, and magnesium: selection of reference population by optimality criteria. Scand J Clin Lab Invest 47:111, 1987.
11. Husain SM, et al: Measurement of ionized calcium concentration in neonates. Arch Dis Child 69:77, 1993.
12. Brauman J, et al: Factors affecting the determination of ionized calcium in blood. Scand J Clin Lab Invest 43(Suppl 165):27, 1983.
13. Rasmussen H, Bordier P: The Physiologic and Cellular Basis of Metabolic Bone Disease. Baltimore, Williams & Wilkins, 1974.
14. Tsien RY, et al: Calcium homeostasis in intact lymphocytes: cytoplasmic free calcium monitored with a new intracellularly trapped fluorescent indicator. J Cell Biol 94:3250, 1982.
15. Holick MF, et al: Calcium, phosphorus, and bone metabolism: calcium regulating hormones. In Isselbacher KJ, et al (eds): Harrison's Principles of Internal Medicine: Section 3. Disorders of Bone and Mineral Metabolism. New York, McGraw-Hill, 1994, pp 2137–2151.
16. Demarini S, Tsang RC: Disorders of calcium and magnesium metabolism. In Fanaroff AF, Martin RJ (eds): Neonatal-Perinatal Medicine: Diseases of the Fetus and Infant, 5th ed. St Louis, Mosby–Year Book, 1992, pp 1181–1195.
17. Loughead JL, et al: Serum ionized calcium concentrations in normal neonates. Am J Dis Child 142:516, 1988.
18. Wandrup J, et al: Age-related reference values for ionized calcium in the first week of life in premature and full-term neonates. Scand J Clin Lab Invest 48:255, 1988.
19. Martinez ME, et al: Ionic calcium levels during pregnancy, at delivery, and in the first hours of life. Scand J Clin Lab Invest 46:27, 1986.
20. Dincsoy MY, et al: The role of postnatal age and magnesium on parathyroid hormone responses during "exchange" blood transfusion in the newborn period. J Pediatr 100:277, 1982.
21. Loughead JL, et al: A role for Mg in neonatal parathyroid gland function? J Am Coll Nutr 10:123, 1991.
22. Venkataraman PS, et al: Postnatal changes in calcium-regulating hormones in very-low-birth-weight infants. Am J Dis Child 139:913, 1985.
23. Venkataraman PS, et al: Effect of hypocalcemia on cardiac function in very-low-birth-weight preterm neonates: studies of blood ionized calcium, echocardiography, and cardiac effect of intravenous calcium therapy. Pediatrics 70:543, 1985.
24. Namgung R, et al: Low bone mineral content and high serum osteocalcin and 1,25-dihydroxyvitamin D in summer- versus winter-born newborn infants: an early fetal effect? J Pediatr Gastroenterol Nutr 19:220, 1994.
25. Bagnoli F, et al: Relationship between mode of delivery and neonatal calcium homeostasis. Eur J Pediatr 149:800, 1990.
26. Namgung R, et al: Reduced serum osteocalcin and 1,25-dihydroxyvitamin D concentrations and low bone mineral content in small for gestational age infants: evidence of decreased bone formation rates. J Pediatr 122:269, 1993.
27. Widdowson EM, Spray CM: Chemical development in utero. Arch Dis Child 26:205, 1951.
28. Broadus AE: Physiological functions of calcium, magnesium, and phosphorus and mineral ion balance. In Favus MJ (ed): Primer on the Metabolic Bone Diseases and Disorders of Mineral Metabolism, 2nd ed. New York, Raven Press, 1993, pp 41–54.
29. David L, Anast CS: Calcium metabolism in newborn infants. J Clin Invest 54:287, 1974.
30. Widdowson EM, et al: Fetal growth and body composition. In Lindblad BS (ed): Perinatal Nutrition. New York, Academic Press, 1988, pp 4–14.
31. Raut SJ, Viswanathan R: Distribution of magnesium in body fluids. Ind J Med Res 60:1272, 1972.
32. Schuette SA, et al: Feasibility of using the stable isotope ^{25}Mg to study Mg metabolism in infants. Pediatr Res 27:36, 1990.
33. Aikawa JK: Magnesium: Its Biological Significance. Boca Raton, FL, CRC Press, 1981, pp 43–56.
34. Silverman SH, Gardner LI: Ultrafiltration studies on serum magnesium. N Engl J Med 250:938, 1954.
35. Rude RK, Singer FR: Magnesium deficiency and excess. Ann Rev Med 32:245, 1981.
36. Tsang RC: Neonatal magnesium disturbances. Am J Dis Child 124:282, 1972.
37. Handwerker SM, et al: Ionized serum magnesium levels in umbilical cord blood of normal pregnant women at delivery: relationship to calcium, demographics, and birth weight. Am J Perinatol 10:392, 1993.
38. Anast CS: Serum magnesium levels in the newborn. Pediatrics 33:969, 1964.
39. Atkinson SA, et al: Macromineral balances in premature infants fed their own mothers' milk or formula. J Pediatr 102:99, 1983.
40. Blum JW, et al: Acute parathyroid hormone response: sensitivity, relationship to hypocalcemia and rapidity. Endocrinology 95:753, 1974.
41. Barnicot NA: The local action of the parathyroid and other tissues on bone in intracerebral grafts. J Anat 82:233, 1948.
42. Kenny AD: Intestinal Calcium Absorption and Its Regulation. Boca Raton, FL, CRC Press, 1981, pp 91–102.
43. Parfitt AM, et al: Procollagen type I carboxy-terminal extension peptide in serum as a marker of collagen biosynthesis in bone: correlation with iliac bone formation rates and comparison with total alkaline phosphatase. J Bone Miner Res 2:427, 1987.
44. Eriksen EF, et al: Serum markers of type I collagen formation and degradation in metabolic bone disease: correlation with bone histomorphometry. J Bone Miner Res 8:127, 1993.
45. Demarini S, et al: Indices of bone formation and resorption in the first 24 hours of life in normal term infants. J Am Coll Nutr 13:526, 1994.
46. Robertie PG, et al: Parathyroid hormone responses to marked hypocalcemia in infants and young children undergoing repair of congenital heart disease. J Am Coll Cardiol 20:672, 1992.
47. Wolfe HJ, et al: Distribution of calcitonin-containing cells in the normal adult human thyroid gland: a correlation of morphology with peptide content. J Clin Endocrinol Metab 38:688, 1974.
48. Holtrop ME, et al: The effects of parathyroid hormone, colchicin, and calcitonin on the ultrastructure and the activity of osteoclasts in organ culture. J Cell Biol 60:346, 1974.
49. Ardailou R: Kidney and calcitonin. Nephron 15:250, 1975.
50. Foster GV, et al: Calcitonin. Clin Endocrinol Metab 1:93, 1972.
51. Parthemore JG, Deftos LJ: Calcitonin secretion in normal human subjects. J Clin Endocrinol Metab 47:184, 1978.
52. Swaminathan R, et al: The relationship between food gastrointestinal hormones and calcitonin secretion. J Endocrinol 59:2217, 1973.
53. Venkataraman PS, et al: Pathogenesis of early neonatal hypocalcemia: studies of serum calcitonin, gastrin and plasma glucagon. J Pediatr 110:599, 1987.
54. Samaan NA, et al: Immunoreactive calcitonin in the mother, neonate, child, and adult. Am J Obstet Gynecol 121:622, 1975.
55. Hillman LS, et al: Serial measurements of serum calcium, magnesium, parathyroid hormone, calcitonin, and 25-hydroxyvitamin D in premature and term infants during the first week of life. Pediatr Res 11:739, 1977.

56. Holick MF: The cutaneous photosynthesis of previtamin D_3: a unique photo-endocrine system. J Invest Dermatol 76:51, 1981.
57. DeLuca HF, Schnoes HK: Metabolism and mechanism of action of vitamin D. Ann Rev Biochem 45:631, 1976.
58. Fraser DR: Regulation of the metabolism of vitamin D. Physiol Rev 60:551, 1980.
59. Holick MF, et al: Identification of 1,25-dihydroxy-cholecalciferol, a form of vitamin D_3 metabolically active in the intestine. Proc Natl Acad Sci USA 68:803, 1971.
60. Harrison HE, Harrison HC: Vitamin D and permeability of intestinal mucosa to calcium. Am J Physiol 208:370, 1965.
61. Raisz LG, et al: 1,25-dihydroxy-cholecalciferol: a potent stimulator of bone resorption in tissue culture. Science 175:768, 1972.
62. Brommage R, Neuman WF: Mechanism of mobilization of bone mineral by 1,25-dihydroxyvitamin D_3. Am J Physiol 237:E113, 1979.
63. Steichen JJ, et al: Vitamin D homeostasis in the perinatal period: 1,25-dihydroxyvitamin D in maternal, cord and neonatal blood. N Engl J Med 302:315, 1980.
64. Salle BL, et al: Vitamin D metabolism in preterm infants: serial serum calcitriol values during the first four days of life. Acta Paediatr Scand 72:203, 1983.
65. Glorieux FH, et al: Vitamin D metabolism in preterm infants: serum calcitriol values during the first five days of life. J Pediatr 99:640, 1981.
66. Markestad T, et al: Plasma concentrations of vitamin D metabolites in premature infants. Pediatr Res 18:269, 1984.
67. Hillman LS, et al: Serum 1,25-dihydroxyvitamin D concentrations in premature infants: preliminary results. Calcif Tissue Int 37:223, 1985.
68. Schilling R, et al: High total and free 1,25-dihydroxyvitamin D concentrations in serum of premature infants. Acta Paediatr Scand 79:36, 1990.
69. Lichtenstein P, et al: Calcium-regulating hormones and minerals from birth to 18 months of age: a cross-sectional study: I. effects of sex, race, age, season, and diets on vitamin D status. Pediatrics 77:883, 1986.
70. Specker BL, et al: Cyclical serum 25-hydroxyvitamin D concentrations paralleling sunshine exposure in exclusively breast-fed infants. J Pediatr 110:744, 1987.
71. Namgung R, et al: Low total body bone mineral content and high bone resorption in Korean winter-born newborn infants: a late fetal effect? (Abstract.) Pediatr Res 37:314A, 1995.
72. Gertner JM: Phosphorus metabolism and its disorders in childhood. Pediatr Ann 16:957, 1987.
73. Lyon AJ, McIntosh N: Calcium and phosphorus balance in extremely low birthweight infants in the first six weeks of life. Arch Dis Child 59:1145, 1984.
74. Namgung R, et al: Radiologic (rickets) and biochemical effects of calcium and phosphorus supplementation of parenteral nutrition in very low birth weight infants. Pediatr Res 33:308A, 1993.
75. Namgung R, et al: High serum osteocalcin and high serum cross-linked carboxyterminal telopeptide of type I collagen in rickets of preterm infants: evidence of increased bone turnover. Pediatr Res 35:317A, 1994.
76. Levine BS, Coburn JW: Magnesium, the mimic/antagonist of calcium. N Engl J Med 310:1253, 1984.
77. MacManus J, Heaton FW: The influence of magnesium on calcium release from bone in vitro. Biochim Biophys Acta 215:360, 1970.
78. Elin RJ, et al: Body fluid electrolyte composition of chronically magnesium-deficient and control rats. Am J Physiol 220:543, 1971.
79. Lamm CI, et al: Congenital rickets associated with magnesium sulfate infusion for tocolysis. J Pediatr 113:1078, 1988.
80. Demarini S, et al: Short-term magnesium sulfate tocolysis effects on fetal indices of bone turnover (abstract). Pediatr Res 41:231A, 1997.
81. Koo WWK, Tsang RC: Bone mineralization in infants. Prog Food Nutr Sci 8:229, 1984.
82. Buckle RM, et al: The influence of plasma magnesium concentration on parathyroid hormone secretion. J Endocrinol 42:529, 1968.
83. Habeber JF, Potts JT Jr: Relative effectiveness of magnesium and calcium on the secretion and biosynthesis of parathyroid hormone in vitro. Endocrinology 98:197, 1976.
84. Cholst IN, et al: The influence of hypermagnesemia on serum calcium and parathyroid hormone levels in human subjects. N Engl J Med 310:1221, 1984.
85. Anast CS, et al: Evidence for parathyroid failure in magnesium deficiency. Science 177:606, 1972.
86. Rude RK, et al: Functional hypoparathyroidism and parathyroid hormone end-organ resistance in human magnesium deficiency. Clin Endocrinol (Oxf) 5:209, 1976.
87. Freitag JJ, et al: Evidence for skeletal resistance to parathyroid hormone in magnesium deficiency. J Clin Invest 64:1238, 1979.
88. Matsuzaki S, Dumont JE: Effect of calcium ion on horse parathyroid gland adenyl cyclase. Biochim Biophys Acta 284:227, 1972.
89. Radde IC, et al: Magnesium and calcitonin: plasma magnesium levels in anemic children and in neonates. Proceedings of XIII International Congress of Pediatrics, Metab Vorlag der Wiener Medizinishen Akademie, Wien, Vol VII, 1971, p 345.
90. Raisz LG, et al: I. Effect of phosphate, calcium and magnesium on bone resorption and hormonal responses in tissue culture. Endocrinology 85:446, 1969.
91. Paillard F, et al: Renal effects of salmon calcitonin in man. J Lab Clin Med 80:200, 1972.
92. Austin LA, Heath H: Calcitonin: physiology and pathophysiology. N Engl J Med 304:269, 1981.
93. Karbach U: Cellular-mediated and diffusive magnesium transport across the descending colon of the rat. Gastroenterology 96:1282, 1989.
94. Krejs GJ, et al: Effect of 1,25-dihydroxyvitamin D_3 on calcium and magnesium absorption in the healthy human jejunum and ileum. Am J Med 75:973, 1983.
95. Hanna S: Influence of large doses of vitamin D on magnesium metabolism in rats. Metabolism 10:734, 1961.
96. Karbach U, Ewe K: Calcium and magnesium transport and influence of 1,25-dihydroxyvitamin D_3. Digestion 37:35, 1987.
97. Wilz DR, et al: Plasma 1,25-dihydroxyvitamin D concentrations and net intestinal calcium, phosphate, and magnesium absorption in humans. Am J Clin Nutr 32:2052, 1979.
98. Horsting M, DeLuca HF: In vitro production of 25-hydroxycholecalciferol. Biochem Biophys Res Commun 36:251, 1969.
99. Bhattacharyya MH, DeLuca HF: Subcellular location of rat liver calciferol-25-hydroxylase. Arch Biochem Biophys 160:58, 1974.
100. Rude RK, et al: Low serum concentrations of 1,25-dihydroxyvitamin D in human magnesium deficiency. J Clin Endocrinol Metab 61:933, 1985.
101. Heaney RP, et al: Calcium absorption as a function of calcium intake. J Lab Clin Med 85:881, 1975.
102. Bronner F, et al: Net calcium absorption in premature infants: results of 103 metabolic balance studies. Am J Clin Nutr 56:1037, 1992.
103. Ehrenkranz RA, et al: Absorption of calcium in premature infants as measured with a stable isotope ^{46}Ca extrinsic tag. Pediatr Res 19:178, 1985.
104. Yergey AL, et al: Recent studies of human calcium metabolism using stable isotope tracers. Can J Physiol Pharmacol 68:973, 1990.
105. Hillman LS, et al: Measurement of true absorption, endogenous fecal excretion, urinary excretion, and retention of calcium in preterm infants by using a dual-tracer, stable-isotope method. J Pediatr 123:444, 1993.
106. Birge SJ, et al: Study of Ca absorption in man: a kinetic analysis and physiologic model. J Clin Invest 48:1705, 1969.
107. Marcus CS, Lengemann FW: Absorption of Ca^{45} and Sr^{85} from solid and liquid food at various levels of alimentary tract of the rat. J Nutr 77:155, 1962.
108. Hu MS, et al: Bile salts and ileal calcium transport in rats: a neglected factor in intestinal calcium absorption. Am J Physiol 264:(2 Pt 1):G319, 1993.
109. Pansu D, et al: Duodenal and ileal calcium absorption in the rat and effects of vitamin D. Am J Physiol 244(Gastrointest Liver Physiol 7):G695, 1983.
110. Bronner F, et al: An analysis of intestinal calcium transport across the rat intestine. Am J Physiol 250:G561, 1986.
111. Wasserman RH: Lactose-stimulated intestinal calcium absorption: a theory. Nature 201:997, 1964.
112. Haussler MR: Vitamin D receptors: nature and function. Annu Rev Nutr 6:527, 1986.
113. Theofan G, et al: Regulation of Calbindin-D_{28k} gene expression by 1,25-dihydroxyvitamin D_3 is correlated to receptor occupancy. J Biol Chem 261:16943, 1986.
114. Dupret JM, et al: Transcriptional and post-transcriptional regulation of vitamin D-dependent calcium-binding protein gene expression in the rat duodenum by 1,25-dihydroxycholecalciferol. J Biol Chem 262:16553, 1987.
115. Staun M: Calbindin-D of human small intestine and kidney. Dan Med Bull 38:271, 1991.
116. Roche C, et al: Localization of vitamin D-dependent active Ca^{2+} transport in rat duodenum and relation to CaBP. Am J Physiol 251(Gastrointest Liver Physiol 14):G314, 1986.
117. Morrissey RL, Wasserman RH: Calcium absorption and calcium binding protein in chicks on differing calcium and phosphate intakes. Am J Physiol 220:1509, 1971.
118. Bronner F: Calcium transport across epithelia. Int Rev Cytol 131:169, 1991.
119. Takito J, et al: Calcium uptake by brush-border and basolateral membrane vesicles in chick duodenum. Am J Physiol 258:G16, 1990.
120. Miller A, et al: Characterization of calcium binding to brush border membranes from rat duodenum. Biochem J 208:773, 1982.
121. Wilson HD, et al: Calcium uptake by brush-border membrane vesicles from the rat intestine. Am J Physiol 257:F446, 1989.
122. Ghijsen WE, et al: ATP-dependent calcium transport and its correlation with Ca^{2+}-ATPase activity in basolateral plasma membranes of rat duodenum. Biochim Biophys Acta 689:327, 1982.
123. Pansu D, et al: Theophylline inhibits transcellular Ca transport in intestine and Ca binding by CaBP. Am J Physiol 257(Gastrointest Liver Physiol 20):G935, 1989.
124. Nemere I, Norman AW: Transcaltachia, vesicular calcium transport, and microtubule-associated calbindin-D_{28k}: emerging views of 1,25-dihydroxyvitamin D_3-mediated intestinal calcium absorption. Miner Electrolyte Metab 16:109, 1990.
125. Gross M, Kumar R: Physiology and biochemistry of vitamin D-dependent calcium binding proteins. Am J Physiol 259(Renal Fluid Electrolyte Physiol 28):F195, 1990.
126. Feher JJ, et al: Role of facilitated diffusion of calcium by calbindin in intestinal calcium absorption. Am J Physiol 262(Cell Physiol 31):C517, 1992.
127. Rasmussen HO, et al: The effect of 1 alpha-hydroxyvitamin D_3 administration on calcium transport in chick intestine brush border membrane vesicles. J Biol Chem 254:2993, 1979.

128. Morgan DW, et al: Specific in vitro activation of Ca, Mg-ATPase by vitamin D-dependent rat renal calcium-binding protein (calbindin D28K). Biochem Biophys Res Commun *138*:547, 1986.

129. Walters JRF: Calbindin-D9K stimulates the calcium pump in rat enterocyte basolateral membranes. Am J Physiol *256*(Gastrointest Liver Physiol 19):G124, 1989.

130. Walters JRF, et al: Stimulation of intestinal basolateral membrane calcium-pump activity by recombinant synthetic calbindin-D9K and specific mutants. Biochem Biophys Res Commun *170*:603, 1990.

131. Ghijsen WEJM: Regulation of duodenal Ca^{2+} pump by calmodulin and vitamin D-dependent Ca^{2+}-binding protein. Am J Physiol *251*(Gastrointest Liver Physiol 14):G223, 1986.

132. Ghishan FK, et al: Maturation of calcium transport in the rat small and large intestine. J Nutr *110*:1622, 1980.

133. Ghishan FK, et al: Kinetics of intestinal calcium transport during maturation in rats. Pediatr Res *18*:235, 1985.

134. Halloran BP, et al: Appearance of the intestinal cytosolic receptor for 1,25-dihydroxyvitamin D_3 during neonatal development in the rat. J Biol Chem *256*:7338, 1981.

135. Bruns MEH, et al: Vitamin D-dependent calcium-binding protein of rat intestine: changes during postnatal development and sensitivity to 1,25-dihydroxycholecalciferol. Endocrinology *105*:934, 1979.

136. Halloran BP, DeLuca HF: Calcium transport in small intestine during early development: role of vitamin D. Am J Physiol *239*:G473, 1980.

137. Lee DBN, et al: Vitamin D-independent regulation of calcium and phosphate absorption. Miner Electrolyte Metab *16*:167, 1990.

138. Winkler I, et al: Absence of renal 25-hydroxycholecalciferol-1-hydroxylase activity in a pig strain with vitamin D-dependent rickets. Calcif Tissue Int *38*:87, 1986.

139. Lachenmaier-Currle U, Harmeyer J: Intestinal absorption of calcium in newborn piglets: role of vitamin D. Biol Neonate *53*:327, 1988.

140. Schroder B, et al: Evidence of vitamin D-independent active calcium absorption in newborn piglets. Calcif Tissue Int *52*:305, 1993.

141. Harmeyer J, Kaune R: Two unique animal models for the study of human metabolic bone diseases. *In* Pliska V, Stranziger G (eds): Farm Animals in Biomedical Research: Advances in Animal Breeding and Genetics, Vol 5. Hamburg, Paul Parey, 1990, pp 111–130.

142. Senterre J, Salle B: Calcium and phosphorus economy of the preterm infant and its interaction with vitamin D and its metabolites. Acta Paediatr Scand *296*(Suppl):85, 1982.

143. Hardwick LL, et al: Comparison of calcium and magnesium absorption: in vivo and in vitro studies. Am J Physiol *259*(Gastrointest Liver Physiol 22):G720, 1990.

144. Allen LH: Calcium bioavailability and absorption: a review. Am J Clin Nutr *35*:783, 1982.

145. Omdahl JL, et al: Regulation of metabolism of 25-hydroxycholecalciferol by kidney tissue in vitro by dietary calcium. Nature New Biol *237*:63, 1972.

146. Shenai JP, et al: Nutritional balance studies in very-low-birth-weight infants: enhanced nutrient retention rates by an experimental formula. Pediatrics *66*:233, 1980.

147. Rowe JC, et al: Achievement of in utero retention of calcium and phosphorus accompanied by high calcium excretion in very low birth weight infants fed a fortified formula. J Pediatr *110*:581, 1987.

148. Schanler RJ, et al: Bioavailability of calcium and phosphorus in human milk fortifiers and formula for very low birth weight infants. J Pediatr *113*:95, 1988.

149. Ehrenkranz RA, et al: Nutritional balance studies in premature infants fed premature formula or fortified preterm human milk. J Pediatr Gastroenterol Nutr *8*:58, 1989.

150. Cooke R, et al: Vitamin D and mineral metabolism in the very low birth weight infant receiving 400 IU of vitamin D. J Pediatr *116*:423, 1990.

151. Wirth FH, et al: Effect of lactose on mineral absorption in preterm infants. J Pediatr *117*:283, 1990.

152. Huston RK, et al: Nutrient and mineral retention and vitamin D absorption in low-birth-weight infants: effect of medium-chain triglycerides. Pediatrics *72*:44, 1983.

153. Barltrop D, et al: Absorption and endogenous faecal excretion of calcium by low birthweight infants on feeds with varying contents of calcium and phosphate. Arch Dis Child *52*:41, 1977.

154. Moya M, Domenech E: Role of calcium-phosphate ratio of milk formulae on calcium balance in low birth weight infants during the first three days of life. Pediatr Res *16*:675, 1982.

155. Day GM, et al: Growth and mineral metabolism in very low birth weight infants: II. effects of calcium supplementation on growth and divalent cations. Pediatr Res *9*:568, 1975.

156. Heaney RP, et al: Calcium absorptive consistency. J Bone Miner Res *5*:1139, 1990.

157. Abrams SA, et al: Dual tracer stable isotopic assessment of calcium absorption and endogenous fecal excretion in low birth weight infants. Pediatr Res *29*:615, 1991.

158. Greer FR, Tsang RC: Calcium, phosphorus, magnesium, and vitamin D requirements for preterm infants. *In* Tsang RC (ed): Vitamin and Mineral Requirements in Preterm Infants. New York, Marcel Dekker, 1985, pp 99–136.

159. Thureborn E: Human hepatic bile: composition changes due to altered enterohepatic circulation. Acta Clin Scand *303*(Suppl):1, 1962.

160. Moore EW, Makhlouf GM: Calcium in normal human gastric juice: a four-component model with speculation on the relation of calcium to pepsin secretion. Gastroenterology *55*:465, 1968.

161. Hansky J: Calcium content of duodenal juice. Am J Dig Dis *12*:725, 1967.

162. Heaney RP, Skillman TG: Secretion and excretion of calcium by the human gastrointestinal tract. J Lab Clin Med *64*:29, 1964.

163. Abrams SA, et al: Stable isotopic measurement of endogenous fecal calcium excretion in children. J Pediatr Gastroenterol Nutr *12*:469, 1991.

164. Moore LJ, et al: Dynamics of calcium metabolism in infancy and childhood: I. methodology and quantification in the infant. Pediatr Res *19*:329, 1985.

165. Senterre J: Calcium and phosphorus retention in preterm infants. *In* Stern L, et al (eds): Intensive Care in the Newborn II. New York, Masson Publishing, 1978, pp 205–215.

166. Lengemann FW, et al: Studies on the enhancement of radiocalcium and radiostrontium absorption by lactose in the rat. J Nutr *68*:443, 1959.

167. Bei L, et al: Glucose polymer increases jejunal calcium, magnesium, and zinc absorption in humans. Am J Clin Nutr *44*:244, 1986.

168. Behar J, Kerstein MD: Intestinal calcium absorption: differences in transport between duodenum and ileum. Am J Physiol *230*:1255, 1976.

169. Favus MJ, Angeid-Backman E: Effects of lactose on calcium absorption and secretion by rat ileum. Am J Physiol *246*:G281, 1984.

170. Armbrecht HJ, Wasserman RH: Enhancement of Ca^{++} uptake by lactose in the rat small intestine. J Nutr *106*:1265, 1976.

171. Chang YO, Hagsted DM: Lactose and calcium transport in gut sacs. J Nutr *82*:297, 1964.

172. Pansu D, et al: Effect of lactose on duodenal calcium-binding protein and calcium absorption. J Nutr *109*:508, 1979.

173. Newberne PM, et al: The influence of food additives and related materials on lower bowel structure and function. Toxicol Pathol *16*:184, 1988.

174. Webing DDA, Holdsworth ES: The effect of bile, bile acids and detergents on calcium absorption in the chick. Biochem J *97*:408, 1965.

175. Olivier AH: The inter-relationship between calcium absorption and bile. Experientia *28*:854, 1970.

176. Marcus CS, Lengemann FW: Absorption of Ca^{45} and Sr^{85} from solid and liquid food at various levels of alimentary tract of the rat. J Nutr *77*:155, 1962.

177. Mekhjian S, et al: Colonic secretion of water and electrolytes induced by bile acids perfusion studies in man. J Clin Invest *50*:1569, 1971.

178. Camilleri M, et al: Pharmacological inhibition of chemodeoxycholate-induced fluid and mucus secretion and mucosal injury in the rabbit colon. Dig Dis Sci *27*:865, 1982.

179. Binder HJ, Rawlins CL: Effect of conjugated dihydroxy bile salts on electrolyte transport in rat colon. J Clin Invest *52*:1460, 1973.

180. Freel RW, et al: Role of tight-junctional pathways in bile salt-induced increases in colonic permeability. Am J Physiol *245*:G816, 1983.

181. Maenz DD, Forsyth GW: Ricinoleate and deoxycholate are calcium ionophores in jejunal brush border vesicles. J Membr Biol *70*:125, 1982.

182. Watkins JB, et al: Bile-salt metabolism in the newborn: measurement of pool size and synthesis by stable isotope technique. N Engl J Med *288*:431, 1973.

183. Huston RK, et al: Nutrient and mineral retention and vitamin D absorption in low-birth-weight infants: effect of medium chain triglycerides. Pediatrics *72*:44, 1983.

184. Edelstein S, et al: Vitamin D metabolism and expression in rats fed on low-calcium and low-phosphorus diets. Biochem J *170*:227, 1978.

185. Tanaka Y, et al: Intestinal calcium transport: stimulation by low phosphorus diets. Science *181*:564, 1973.

186. Portale AA, et al: Oral intake of phosphorus can determine the serum concentration of 1,25-dihydroxyvitamin D by determining its production rate in humans. J Clin Invest *77*:7, 1986.

187. Bourdeau JE, et al: Effects of moderate dietary phosphorus restriction on intestinal absorption and external balances of phosphorus and calcium in growing female rabbits. Miner Electrolyte Metab *16*:378, 1990.

188. Heaney RP, et al: Absorbability of calcium sources: the limited role of solubility. Calcif Tissue Int *46*:300, 1990.

189. Pansu D, et al: Solubility and intestinal transit time limit calcium absorption in rats. J Nutr *123*:1396, 1993.

190. Giles MM, et al: Sequential calcium and phosphorus balance studies in preterm infants. J Pediatr *110*:591, 1987.

191. Lee DBN, et al: Intestinal phosphate absorption: influence of vitamin D and non-vitamin D factors. Am J Physiol *250*:G369, 1986.

192. Lee DBN, et al: Phosphate transport across rat jejunum: influence of sodium, pH, and 1,25-dihydroxyvitamin D. Am J Physiol *251*:G90, 1986.

193. Peterhk M: Intestinal phosphate transport. *In* Martonisi AN (ed): The Enzymes of Biological Membranes, Vol 3. New York, Plenum Press, 1985, pp 287–320.

194. Cramer CF: Progress and rate of absorption of radiophosphorus through the intestinal tract of rats. Can J Biochem Physiol *39*:499, 1961.

195. Hurwitz S, Bar A: Absorption of calcium and phosphorus along the gastrointestinal tract of the laying fowl as influenced by dietary calcium and effective shell formation. J Nutr *86*:433, 1965.

196. Hurwitz S, Bar A: The sites of calcium and phosphate absorption in the chick. Poultry Sci *49*:324, 1970.

197. Kayne LH, et al: Analysis of segmental phosphate absorption in intact rats: a compartmental analysis approach. J Clin Invest *91*:915, 1993.

198. Quamme GA, Shapiro RJ: Membrane controls of epithelial phosphate transport. Can J Physiol Pharmacol *65*:275, 1987.

199. Murer H, Hildman B: Transcellular transport of calcium and inorganic phosphate in the small intestinal epithelium. Am J Physiol *240*:G409, 1981.

200. Kikuchi K, Ghishan FK: Phosphate transport by basolateral plasma membranes of human small intestine. Gastroenterology *93*:106, 1987.

201. Peterlik M, Wasserman RH: Effect of vitamin D on transepithelial phosphate transport in chick intestine. Am J Physiol *234*:E379, 1978.

202. Danish G, et al: Regulation of Na-dependent phosphate influx across the mucosal border of duodenum by 1,25-dihydroxycholecalciferol. Pflugers Arch *388*:227, 1980.

203. Hildmann B, et al: Regulation of Na$^+$-Pi cotransport by 1,25-dihydroxyvitamin D$_3$ in rabbit duodenal brush border membrane. Am J Physiol *242*:G533, 1982.

204. Rizzoli R, et al: Role of 1,25-dihydroxyvitamin D$_3$ on intestinal phosphate absorption in rats with a normal vitamin D supply. J Clin Invest *60*:639, 1977.

205. DePalo D, et al: Renal responses to phosphorus deprivation in young rabbits. Miner Electrolyte Metab *14*:313, 1988.

206. Portale AA, et al: Physiologic regulation of the serum concentration of 1,25-dihydroxyvitamin D by phosphorus in normal man. J Clin Invest *83*:1494, 1989.

207. Gray RW, Napoli JL: Dietary phosphate deprivation increases 1,25-dihydroxyvitamin D$_3$ synthesis in rat kidney in vitro. J Biol Chem *258*:1152, 1983.

208. Baxter LA, DeLuca HF: Stimulation of 25-hydroxyvitamin D$_3$-1 alpha-hydroxylase by phosphate depletion. J Biol Chem *251*:3158, 1976.

209. Lee DBN: Mechanism and regulation of intestinal phosphate transport. Adv Exp Med Biol *208*:207, 1986.

210. Danish G, et al: Effect of pH on phosphate transport into intestinal brush-border membrane vesicles. Am J Physiol *246*:G120, 1984.

211. Senterre J, et al: Effects of vitamin D and phosphorus supplementation on calcium retention in preterm infants fed banked human milk. J Pediatr *103*:305, 1983.

212. Shenai JP, et al: Nutritional balance studies in very-low-birth-weight infants: enhanced nutrient retention rates by an experimental formula. Pediatrics *66*:233, 1980.

213. Shenai JP, et al: Nutritional balance studies in very-low-birth-weight infants: role of soy formula. Pediatrics *67*:631, 1981.

214. Chan GM, et al: Effects of soy formulas on mineral metabolism in term infants. Am J Dis Child *141*:527, 1987.

215. Steichen JJ, Tsang RC: Bone mineralization and growth in term infants fed soy-based or cow milk-based formula. J Pediatr *110*:687, 1987.

216. Chan GM, et al: The effects of soy formula on the growth and mineral metabolism in term infants. Pediatr Res *23*:481A, 1988.

217. Danielson BG, et al: Gastrointestinal magnesium absorption: kinetic studies with ^{28}Mg and a simple method for determination of fractional absorption. Miner Electrolyte Metab *2*:116, 1979.

218. Liu YM, et al: Absorption of calcium and magnesium from fortified human milk by very low birth weight infants. Pediatr Res *25*:496, 1989.

219. Tantibhedhyangkul P, Hashim SA: Medium-chain triglyceride feeding in premature infants: effects on calcium and magnesium absorption. Pediatrics *61*:537, 1978.

220. Okamoto E, et al: Use of medium-chain triglycerides in feeding the low-birth-weight infant. Am J Dis Child *136*:428, 1982.

221. Giles MM, et al: Magnesium metabolism in preterm infants: effects of calcium, magnesium, and phosphorus, and of postnatal and gestational age. J Pediatr *117*:147, 1990.

222. Ross DB: In vitro studies on the transport of magnesium across the intestinal wall of the rat. J Physiol *160*:417, 1962.

223. Hendrix J, et al: Competition between calcium, strontium, and magnesium for absorption in the isolated rat intestine. Clin Chem *9*:734, 1963.

224. Aldor TAM, Moore DW: Magnesium absorption by everted sacs of rat intestine and colon. Gastroenterology *59*:745, 1970.

225. Urban E, Schedl HP: Net movements of magnesium and calcium in the rat small intestine in vivo. Proc Soc Exp Biol Med *132*:1111, 1969.

226. Lopez Aliaga I, et al: Influence of intestinal resection and type of diet on digestive utilization and metabolism of magnesium in rats. Int J Vitam Nutr Res *61*:61, 1990.

227. Chutkow J: Site of magnesium absorption and excretion in the intestinal tract of the rat. J Lab Clin Med *63*:71, 1964.

228. Meneely R, et al: Intestinal maturation: in vivo magnesium transport. Pediatr Res *16*:295, 1982.

229. Graham L, et al: Gastrointestinal absorption and excretion of ^{28}Mg in man. Metabolism *9*:646, 1960.

230. Guenter W, Sell JL: Magnesium absorption and secretion along the gastrointestinal tract of the chicken. J Nutr *103*:875, 1973.

231. Kayne LH, Lee DBN: Intestinal magnesium absorption. Miner Electrolyte Metab *19*:210, 1993.

232. Roth P, Werner E: Intestinal absorption of magnesium in man. Int J Appl Radiat Isot *30*:523, 1979.

233. Behar J: Magnesium absorption by the rat ileum and colon. Am J Physiol *227*:334, 1974.

234. Brannan OB, et al: Magnesium absorption in the human small intestine: results in normal subjects, patients with chronic renal disease, and patients with absorptive hypercalciuria. J Clin Invest *57*:1412, 1976.

235. Cassidy MM, Tidball CS: Cellular mechanism of intestinal permeability: alterations produced by chelation depletion. J Cell Biol *32*:685, 1967.

236. Marshall D, et al: Calcium, phosphorus, and magnesium requirement. Proc Nutr Soc *35*:163, 1976.

237. Heaton F, Pyrah L: Magnesium metabolism in patients with parathyroid disorders. Clin Sci *25*:475, 1963.

238. King R, Stanbury S: Magnesium metabolism in primary hyperparathyroidism. Clin Sci *39*:281, 1970.

239. Fine KD, et al: Intestinal absorption of magnesium from food and supplements. J Clin Invest *88*:396, 1991.

240. Quamme GA: Magnesium metabolism. *In* Maxwell MH, et al (eds): Clinical Disorders of Fluid and Electrolyte Metabolism, 5th ed. New York, McGraw-Hill, 1991.

241. Karbach U, Feldmeier H: New clinical and experimental aspects of intestinal magnesium transport. Magnes Res *4*:9, 1991.

242. Philips JDR, et al: Magnesium absorption in human ileum (abstract). J Am Coll Nutr *8*:459, 1989.

243. Paunier L, et al: Primary hypomagnesemia with secondary hypocalcemia (abstract). J Pediatr *67*:945, 1965.

244. Yamamoto T, et al: Primary hypomagnesemia with secondary hypocalcemia: report of a case and review of the world literature. Magnesium *4*:153, 1985.

245. Hardwick LL, et al: Magnesium absorption: mechanisms and the influence of vitamin D, calcium and phosphate. J Nutr *121*:13, 1991.

246. Behar J: Effect of calcium on magnesium absorption. Am J Physiol *229*:1590, 1975.

247. Ammann P, et al: Calcium absorption in rat large intestine in vivo: availability of dietary calcium. Am J Physiol *251*:G14, 1986.

248. Hardwick LL, et al: Effects of calcium phosphate supplementation on calcium, phosphorus, and magnesium metabolism in the Wistar rat. Nutr Res *7*:787, 1987.

249. Clarkson EM, et al: The effect of a high intake of calcium on magnesium metabolism in normal subjects and patients with chronic renal failure. Clin Sci *32*:11, 1967.

250. Norman DA, et al: Jejunal and ileal adaptation to alteration in dietary calcium: changes in calcium and magnesium absorption and pathogenic role of parathyroid hormone and 1,25-dihydroxyvitamin D. J Clin Invest *67*:1599, 1981.

251. Heaton FW, Parsons FM: The metabolic effect of high magnesium intake. Clin Sci *21*:273, 1961.

252. Leichsenring JM, et al: Magnesium metabolism in college women: observations on the effect of calcium and phosphorus intake levels. J Nutr *45*:477, 1951.

253. Clark I: Importance of dietary Ca:PO$_4$ ratios on skeletal, Ca, Mg, and PO4 metabolism. Am J Physiol *217*:865, 1969.

254. Petith MM, Schedl HP: Divalent cation transport by rat cecum and colon in calcium and magnesium deficiency. Proc Soc Exp Biol Med *155*:225, 1977.

255. Walser M: Magnesium metabolism. Ergeb Physiol *59*:185, 1967.

256. Wright EM, Diamond JM: Effects of pH and polyvalent cations on the selective permeability of gallbladder epithelium to monovalent ions. Biochim Biophys Acta *163*:57, 1968.

257. Fordtran JS, et al: Effect of magnesium on active and passive sodium transport in the human intestine. Gastroenterology *89*:1050, 1985.

258. Smith RH, McAllan AB: Binding of magnesium and calcium in the contents of the small intestine of the calf. Br J Nutr *20*:703, 1966.

259. Tidball CS: Magnesium and calcium as regulators of intestinal permeability. Am J Physiol *206*:243, 1964.

260. Brink EJ, et al: Interaction of calcium and phosphate decreases ileal magnesium solubility and apparent magnesium absorption in rats. J Nutr *122*:530, 1992.

261. Heijnen AMP, et al: Ileal pH and apparent absorption of magnesium in rats fed diets containing either lactose or lactulose. Br J Nutr *70*:747, 1993.

262. Ziegler EE, Fomon SJ: Lactose enhances mineral absorption in infancy. J Pediatr Gastroenterol Nutr *2*:288, 1983.

263. Schulz AGM, et al: Dietary native resistant starch but not retrograded resistant starch raises magnesium and calcium absorption in rats. J Nutr *123*:1724, 1993.

264. Sterck JGH, et al: Inhibitory effect of high protein intake on nephrocalcinogenesis in female rats. Br J Nutr *67*:223, 1992.

265. Van Camp I, et al: Diet-induced nephrocalcinosis and urinary excretion of albumin in female rats. Lab Anim *24*:137, 1990.

266. Lakshmanan FL, et al: Magnesium intakes, balances, and blood levels of adults consuming self-selected diets. Am J Clin Nutr *40*:1380, 1984.

267. Seeling MS: The requirement of magnesium by the normal adult. Am J Clin Nutr *14*:342, 1964.

268. Widdowson EM, et al: Effect of giving phosphate supplements to breast fed babies on absorption and excretion of calcium, strontium, magnesium and phosphorus. Lancet *2*:1250, 1963.

269. Rodder SG, et al: Effects of increased dietary phosphorus on magnesium balance in very low birthweight babies. Magnes Res *5*:273, 1992.

270. Brink EJ, et al: Inhibitory effect of soybean protein vs. casein on apparent absorption of magnesium in rats is due to greater excretion of endogenous magnesium. J Nutr *122*:1910, 1992.

271. Guenther W, Sell JL: Magnesium absorption and secretion along the gastrointestinal tract of the chicken. J Nutr *103*:875, 1973.

272. Verbeek MJF, et al: High protein intake raises apparent but not true magnesium absorption in rats. J Nutr *123*:1880, 1993.

273. Avioli LV, Berman M: ^{28}Mg kinetics in man. J Appl Physiol *21*:1688, 1966.

K. Michael Hambidge and Nancy F. Krebs

35

Zinc in the Fetus and Neonate

In a remarkably short time, our perception of zinc (Zn) has progressed from that of a rather obscure essential trace mineral of doubtful significance for human health to that of a micronutrient of exceptional biologic and public health importance. This is most evident in relation to early development, both prenatal and postnatal. Space provided for an overview of trace minerals, other than iron and Zn, in previous editions will, therefore, be devoted entirely to Zn in this edition, and the reader is referred to other texts for information on other trace minerals.[1, 2] The principal focus of this chapter is the complex biology of Zn that underlies its clinical and public health importance.

BIOCHEMISTRY AND BIOLOGY OF ZINC

The abundance of Zn in the human body (approximately 2 g in the adult)[3] is second only to iron among those trace elements for which a nutritional requirement has been established in humans. In contrast to iron and iodine, however, Zn is located relatively evenly throughout the body, especially as a component of thousands of Zn metalloproteins or Zn-binding proteins, and also of nucleic acids, and it is therefore not so readily detectable. The identification and application of Zn fluorophore sensors are required to assist in the selective and efficient detection of trace Zn^{++}.[4]

With an atomic weight of 65.39, Zn is adjacent to several first-transition elements of biologic importance, yet its biochemical properties are very different from those of other elements of similar atomic weight. One of the properties of the Zn atom that has proved to be of outstanding value in biology is its ability to participate in strong but readily exchangeable ligand binding.[5] Coupled with this feature is the notable flexibility of the coordination geometry of Zn. These two properties are responsible for the unique ability of this metal to interact with a wide range of organic ligands and thus to be incorporated in myriad biologic systems. The principal amino acids supplying ligands that bind with Zn are histidine, glutamic acid, aspartic acid, and cysteine.[6] In catalytic sites, Zn forms complexes with water and with any three nitrogen, oxygen, sulfur donors, especially histidine. Structural Zn sites have four protein ligands, with cysteine the preferred ligand. Zn affects tertiary and quaternary protein structure, and the resulting scaffolding of these Zn coordination spheres is important to the function and reactivity of the metal atom.

Zn can participate in redox reactions in special circumstances,[7] specifically through the biochemistry of Zn, metallothionein (MT) and glutathione. However, the Zn atom per se, in contrast to iron and copper, has no oxidant properties, and it exists virtually entirely in the divalent state. This has simplified the safe transport of Zn, both extracellularly and intracellularly, and its incorporation into biologic systems.

As understanding of its biology evolves, the exceptional importance of this micromineral becomes increasingly impressive. The biologic role of Zn is now recognized in protein structure and function, including enzymes, transcription factors, hormonal receptor sites, and biologic membranes. Zn has numerous central roles in DNA and RNA metabolism,[8] and it is involved in signal transduction, gene expression, and apoptosis.

First to be appreciated were the catalytic properties of Zn, a function of its biochemistry outlined earlier. The number of Zn metalloenzymes with known three-dimensional structures exceeds 200.[9] Although Zn also has a structural role in numerous enzymes, its primary importance is as an active component of the catalytic site. Zn metalloenzymes have been identified in each of the six major enzyme classifications. Several of the key enzymes involved in nucleic acid metabolism, cellular proliferation differentiation, and growth are either Zn metalloenzymes or Zn-dependent enzymes.[10]

A major advance in our understanding of the biology of Zn was the identification of proteins that contain a *Zn finger motif*.[11] Structurally, the Zn finger motif is a recurring pattern of amino acids with conserved residues of cysteine and histidine at the base to which Zn binds in a tetrahedral arrangement. Subsequently, hundreds of Zn finger motifs were identified. More than 1000 genes in the human genome encode members of three protein families with Zn finger domains alone: C2H2 Zn fingers, RING fingers, and LIM domains.[9] The number of genes containing Zn finger domains exceeds 3% of all identified human genes. Although all Zn fingers are quite similar, they vary in their precise conformation. Steroid hormone receptors, for example, have several such domains that are involved in the structure itself, and one each for binding to DNA and RNA polymerase. Among the identified Zn transcription factors are several involved in early intrauterine development.[12]

Many transcription factor proteins have the Zn finger motif, thus giving Zn a broad role in gene expression. This has perhaps been best characterized by the role of this metal in regulating its own metabolism,[13] and that of MT, with which Zn is so closely associated. Gene expression in this context is considered later, in the discussion of Zn metabolism.

Zn is an important regulator of apoptosis.[14] This micronutrient has cytoprotective functions that suppress major pathways leading to apoptosis and also directly influences apoptotic regulators, especially the caspase family of enzymes. In airway epithelial cells, Zn is co-localized with the precursor forms of caspase 3, mitochondria, and microtubules. A decline in intracellular Zn may trigger pathways leading to caspase activation. An early and direct effect of Zn deficiency not only on proliferation and differentiation, but also in inducing apoptosis, has been demonstrated in growth plate chondrocytes of the chick.[15] The development of the human epiphysis is also sensitive to Zn deprivation.[8]

There is evidence of a direct signaling function of Zn on all levels of signal transduction.[16] Zn can modulate cellular signal recognition, second-messenger metabolism, and protein kinase and protein phosphatase activities. In the brain, Zn is sequestered in the presynaptic vesicles of *Zn-containing neurons,* from which Zn is released into the cleft and is then recycled into the presynaptic terminal.[17] Synaptically released Zn functions as a conventional synaptic neurotransmitter or neuromodulator, but also, analogous to calcium, it functions as a transmembrane neural signal. The best-established physiologic role of this vesicular Zn is the tonic modulation of brain excitability. Vesicular-rich regions such as the hippocampus are responsive to dietary Zn deprivation, which causes brain dysfunction, including learning impairment and susceptibility to epileptic seizures. Normal neuronal function is dependent on normal Zn homeostasis in the brain.[18]

The biology of Zn is closely linked with that of MT, a unique small intracellular protein of less than 7 kDa that is strongly conserved across species. Of the 61 to 68 amino acids, more than one-third are cysteine, and it has a unique metal-binding capacity (copper > cadmium > Zn). It consists of two subunits: an α domain that, under typical physiologic circumstances, will bind four Zn atoms, and a more reactive β domain binding three Zn atoms in tetrahedral formation. There are four isoforms, of which 1 and 2 are most abundant and 3 occurs in the brain. MT occurs in all tissues, including those of the conceptus, and is especially abundant in liver and also in pancreas, intestine, and kidney. Zn is the major physiologic inducer of MT. Zn binds directly and reversibly to the Zn finger domains of the metal-response element-binding transcription factor-1 (MTF-1) that functions as a cellular Zn sensor. As a result of this binding, MTF-1 assumes a DNA-binding conformation and translocates to the nucleus, where it binds to metal-response elements of the MT gene and thus initiates transcription.[13] Cytokines, especially interleukin-1, interleukin-6, and tumor necrosis factor-α, and stress hormones (glucocorticoids and catecholamines) are also powerful inducers of MT.[19] This finding suggests a key role for Zn in the inflammatory response, as well as in Zn metabolism and as a metal detoxicant, and several functions for Zn in this context have been hypothesized.[20]

One of these functions is MT's role as an antioxidant. The intracellular redox state is intimately related to MT and intracellular Zn metabolism.[7] Increasing intracellular oxidized glutathione can result in the release of all seven Zn atoms, whereas this is inhibited by reduced glutathione. Oxidants cause greater damage to the liver of MT−/− mice than to that of MT+/+ mice.[21] Despite its central role in Zn metabolism (see later), MT is not essential for survival. Late-gestation MT−/− mice fetuses have decreased hepatic Zn and are prone to obesity in later life.[22] More important, they are disadvantaged when the normal environment is compromised, especially when Zn intake is suboptimal. Factors that increase the induction of maternal hepatic MT during early pregnancy may divert Zn from the conceptus to the maternal liver and may potentially result in a conceptus that is deficient in Zn. This can occur with maternal ingestion of alcohol, which may be an important factor in the origin of the fetal alcohol syndrome.[23] There are close similarities between the teratogenicity of maternal Zn deficiency and alcohol administration to mice in early gestation, and the latter can be diminished by parenteral administration of Zn.[23] Cytokines cause a similar disturbance of maternal Zn metabolism and are also teratogenic in rodents.

PHYSIOLOGY OF ZINC

Intracellular Zinc Metabolism

Zn metabolism is tissue and organ specific. Although this specificity is important to an understanding of Zn metabolism, this review has to be limited to selected aspects of more universal intracellular Zn metabolism. The intracellular concentration of unbound "free" Zn is extremely low. An elaborate homeostatic system of proteins regulates cellular Zn distribution and perhaps controls a hierarchy of Zn-dependent functions.[9] Eukaryotic Zn transporters have a major, but still only partly defined, regulatory role.[24] These transporters are ancient gene families that span all phylogenetic levels. The ZIP family is involved in cellular Zn uptake. One member of this family, Zrt3, is known to transport stored Zn out of a vacuolar intracellular compartment during adaptation to Zn deficiency. The CDF (cation diffusion facilitator) family of transporters mediates efflux of Zn out of cells or facilitates intracellular storage. These transporters are regulated by transcriptional and posttranscriptional mechanisms to maintain Zn homeostasis at a cellular and organ level. ZnT-1 and ZnT-4 are expressed ubiquitously, whereas ZnT-2 is limited to the small intestine, kidney, placenta, and liver. When Zn intake is restricted, intestinal and kidney ZnT-2 is extremely low, and both ZnT-1 and ZnT-2 mRNAs are increased in intestine, kidney, and liver with high Zn intake.[25] Although Zn transporter expression is responsive to variations in dietary Zn, many details of the molecular regulation of Zn metabolism and homeostasis await clarification.

The expression of ZnT-1 and ZnT-2 is comparable to Zn-induced changes in MT mRNA levels, a finding suggesting a similar mode of regulation of these genes. Regulation of MT at the protein level by ligand binding,[26] and at the gene level by multiple inducers, including Zn, provides a means of controlling the intracellular availability of Zn by regulating the quantity of MT and the MT/T ratio. This role of MT is closely linked to both cellular redox and energy status.

Maternal, Placental, Fetal, and Mammary Gland Zinc Metabolism

Maternal Metabolism

There is a physiologic increase in maternal hepatic MT in pregnancy,[23] and it may enhance a maternal store of Zn that is readily available to the conceptus. It is only when Zn is abnormally diverted to the maternal liver, as with alcohol ingestion, that the inappropriately large shift of Zn from the plasma compartment is potentially deleterious to the embryo or fetus. There is also a progressive physiologic decline in maternal plasma Zn as pregnancy progresses,[27] and it is only when this decline is excessive because of maternal Zn deprivation or disturbed metabolism that the embryo or fetus is at risk.

Placental and Fetal Metabolism

Uptake of Zn into placental villous syncytiotrophoblast is the first step in the transfer of this metal from the mother to the fetus, and it is the rate-limiting process.[28] There is evidence that this Zn is derived from the low molecular weight maternal plasma Zn pool, probably by a carrier-mediated process, and also from Zn bound to serum protein, possibly by an endocytic mechanism.[29] A potassium Zn transporter is present in the vesicular membranes.[30] α₂-Macroglobulin binds to human trophoblasts in a specific saturable manner, a finding suggesting the possibility of receptor-mediated uptake of Zn.[31] Affinity for Zn (Km values) by human syncytiotrophoblast microvillous membrane vesicles does not vary with gestational age or with low maternal plasma Zn concentrations. Zn uptake capacity (V_{max}) is higher in preterm than in term placentas and with low maternal plasma Zn.[32] Fetal plasma Zn is higher than maternal concentrations. Short-term changes in fetal Zn status do not influence placental Zn transfer, a finding suggesting that there is no ready mechanism for adjusting to fetal Zn deprivation once (or if) it occurs.[33] As gestation progresses, there are marked increases in fetal hepatic Zn concentration. These concentrations decline as the third trimester progresses. The increase in hepatic Zn concentration early in the third trimester appears to be secondary to hepatic MT induction, rather than its cause.[34]

MT has been localized in fetal amniotic cells, syncytial trophoblasts, and villous interstitial cells.[35] The mammalian embryo is surrounded by cells that actively express MT-1 and MT-2 genes, a finding suggesting that MT has a functional role in the establishment, as well as the maintenance, of normal pregnancy.[36] MT-3 and MT-4 mRNAs are abundant in the maternal deciduum, in contrast to fetal tissues, and these genes are refractory to induction by either Zn or inflammation in the deciduum.[37] MT gene expression may have a physiologic role in placental transport of Zn.[38]

As with the intestine, further research is essential to determine how the roles of these and other factors, such as Zn transporters, are integrated to achieve regulation of placental Zn transport. Only then will it be possible to understand how regulation, and hence the Zn status of the embryo or fetus, may be compromised, especially early in gestation.

Mammary Gland Metabolism

Znt-1 (serosal membrane), ZnT-2, and ZnT-4 (intracellularly) have been identified in the mammary gland. Milk Zn concentration is regulated through co-coordinated regulation of these mammary gland Zn transporters.[39] Vitamin A, which has substantial interactions with Zn,[40] has a role in the maintenance of Zn homeostasis in the mammary gland.[39] The regulatory changes responsible for the notable decline in human milk Zn concentrations as lactation progresses[41, 42] have not been elucidated, but they may be responsive to changes in the hormonal milieu.

Rarely, the mammary gland has a defect in the ZnT-4 gene resulting in impaired secretion of Zn.[43] Breast milk Zn concentrations are less than the normal range at all stages of lactation. Infants breast-fed by these mothers typically develop the classic phenotypic presentation of acrodermatitis enteropathica at about 2 months postnatally. The clinical syndrome responds rapidly and completely to an oral Zn supplement of 2 mg Zn^{++}/kg body weight/day to the infant and then a smaller maintenance dose while breast-feeding continues. This syndrome has been described in term infants but is more likely to occur in those infants born preterm, a finding suggesting an increased vulnerability of the preterm infant to clinically significant Zn deficiency syndromes.[44]

Whole Body Zinc Homeostasis

Postnatally, the small intestine has the major role in maintaining whole body Zn homeostasis.[45, 46] Although Zn transporters have been identified in mammalian intestine, the weight of current evidence based on tracer studies in the human suggests that the quantity of Zn absorbed is not regulated in response to changes in Zn status.[45] Maximal absorption is determined principally by a saturable transport mechanism,[47] and fractional absorption declines accordingly with increasing Zn intake and vice versa. Fractional absorption of Zn from heavily fortified Zn flour products is the same after 7 weeks of consuming these products as it is on day 1, despite a presumptive change in Zn status from the large increase in Zn intake.[48] Passive diffusion also affects total Zn absorption and may be the only mechanism that contributes to increases in absorption once the facilitated diffusion pathway is saturated. The pancreas and small intestine are the major routes of excretion of endogenous Zn. Regulation of the quantity of endogenous Zn excreted has the principal role in maintaining whole body Zn homeostasis in most circumstances.[45, 46, 49] This ability to regulate endogenous Zn losses via the intestine is well developed in early postnatal life in the term infant.[50, 51] The extent of the ability of the intestine of the very low birth weight premature infant to regulate excretion of endogenous Zn remains uncertain. Endogenous Zn losses via the kidneys, although small in comparison with the intestinal losses, are also relatively high in the very low birth weight infant on a body weight basis.

Model-based compartmental analysis of Zn metabolism in the adult[52] has identified several pools of Zn that intermix with Zn in plasma within 3 days. The combined size of these pools (exchangeable Zn pool or EZP) can be estimated from what appears as a single exponential between 3 and 9 days after administration of a Zn tracer and can be estimated from urine enrichment with this Zn-stable isotope tracer.[53] On a body weight basis, the size of the EZP is approximately sevenfold higher in premature infants at 33 weeks post conception (Jalla S, et al: unpublished data) than in adults. This finding may be attributable to more than one possible difference in Zn metabolism

and/or nutrition, but it is explained in part by higher concentrations of MT in the fetal liver earlier in the third trimester.[54]

ZINC DEFICIENCY IN THE CONCEPTUS AND EARLY INFANCY

Embryogenesis

An adequate supply of maternal Zn is critically important for the oocyte and embryo.[12] The teratology in rodents resulting from maternal Zn deficiency is quite exceptional.[55-57] Consequences include high mortality and congenital malformations of nearly all organ systems. Data in the human are very limited and will require prospective trials of Zn supplementation in carefully selected population groups that encompass the perinatal period. There is suggestive evidence that severe maternal Zn deficiency resulting from acrodermatitis enteropathica is causally associated with congenital malformations including neural tube defects.[58] Although one study did not find any evidence of hypozincemia in the first trimester in pregnancies that resulted in neural tube defects,[59] this may not apply in maternal populations in which the dietary supply of available Zn is especially limited.[60] There is also epidemiologic evidence from a presumably well-nourished population of a link between maternal Zn status and neural tube defects.[61] Preliminary data from West Timor, where there is low intake of available Zn and a high incidence of cleft lip or palate, indicate that maternal Zn supplementation commencing by 8 to 10 weeks' gestation is associated with a significant reduction in the incidence of these malformations.[62] The association among maternal alcohol consumption, diversion of maternal Zn from the conceptus, and the fetal alcohol syndrome is discussed earlier. This is also a putative paradigm for any maternal stress or infection that increases cytokine production and consequently increases induction of maternal hepatic MT.

Fetal Development

Maternal Zn restriction during fetal development is associated with intrauterine growth retardation in rodent models.[63] Other effects include decreased nestin, a marker of proliferation of neural stem cell.[64]

In the human, there have been conflicting reports on the effects of maternal Zn supplementation on gestational age at delivery and birth weight.[62, 65-67] It will require multicenter, carefully designed, prospective intervention studies to resolve the question whether maternal Zn deficiency contributes to low birth weight by reducing the duration of gestation or the rate of growth *in utero*. Perhaps unexpectedly, there is more consistent evidence that maternal Zn supplementation starting in the second trimester and discontinued at delivery is associated with decreased infectious disease morbidity during the first 6 months of infancy.[68] This effect, which presumably is mediated through an effect of fetal Zn status on the developing immune system, is itself is an important reason for ensuring optimal maternal Zn intake.

Infancy

The effects of Zn deficiency in infancy require consideration both from a global public health standpoint and from an individual perspective. The latter can usefully be subdivided into acute or severe[69] and mild,[70] but in doing so it is necessary to add that acute or severe Zn deficiency can enter a chronic phase; apparently mild cases with nonspecific clinical features carry the risk of mortality[71] as well as severe morbidity;[72, 73] and there are intermediate clinical presentations, as exemplified by the original descriptions of human Zn deficiency.[74]

The prototype of the acute severe presentation is the autosomal recessively inherited disorder *acrodermatitis enteropathica*,[69] identification of the underlying genetic defect or one of the underlying genetic defects of which is likely to be imminent. The clinical features of this syndrome present between 2 and 6 months of age, although presentation may be delayed with the universal Zn fortification of infant formulas in North America and elsewhere. Before this fortification policy, the onset of the disorder in breast-fed infants was typically later than that in formula-fed infants, and breast milk was found to be of some therapeutic benefit. The single most important diagnostic feature, although not pathognomonic, is the skin rash. This erythematous rash may be widespread but is typically most evident around the body orifices and the extremities. Diarrhea and hair loss, although not inevitable, complete the classical triad of features. Untreated, the infant has anorexia, marked apathy, progressively severe failure to thrive, and recurrent infections resulting in death in later infancy. Similar syndromes have been reported as a result of exclusive breast-feeding by mothers with a genetic defect in their ability to secrete normal quantities of Zn via their mammary gland[42] and secondary to severely restricted Zn intake. The latter was seen quite frequently in parenterally fed patients in the early days of intravenous feeding. Premature infants appeared to be especially vulnerable to a lack of Zn in these infusates.

Many different abnormalities of the immune system have been observed in acrodermatitis enteropathica. Although it has been difficult to separate the effects of Zn deficiency from those of the resulting protein-energy malnutrition, extensive experimental data substantiate the far-reaching effects of Zn deficiency on every aspect of the immune system,[75] defects in which undoubtedly underlie the global public health concerns about Zn deficiency (see later). As one of the systems with the most notable rapid turnover of cells, the immune system is especially vulnerable to the fundamental defects in cellular proliferation, growth, and metabolism that result from an inadequate supply of this mineral.

On a global basis, Zn deficiency is now recognized as a major public health issue. There is solid evidence that as much as 20 to 25% of diarrhea and 40% of pneumonia in developing countries can be prevented by preventing Zn deficiency.[76] The risk of malaria may also be reduced. Acceleration of delayed linear growth and weight gain,[77] and probable improvement in brain development and function,[78] have been documented with correction of Zn deficiency in the same or similar populations of young children and also in North America.[70, 79] Taken together, these features encompass all those, with the exception of human immunodeficient virus, that are of greatest public health concern for young children globally.

Low birth weight infants are at greater risk from Zn deficiency and its sequelae. In India, Zn supplementation from very early postnatal life has resulted in a significant decrease in mortality in infants with intrauterine growth retardation.[71] Improvements in brain function[80] and physical growth velocity and diminution of infectious disease morbidity have also been documented.

EARLY POSTNATAL ZINC REQUIREMENTS OF THE PREMATURE INFANT

For the young, exclusively breast-fed term infant, Zn intake provides an excellent guide to requirements, that is, approximately 2 mg Zn/day.[41] There is an exceptional rate of physiologic decline in breast milk Zn concentration, to give an intake of approximately 1 mg Zn/day for the exclusively breast-fed infant by about 4 months, with subsequent further decline.[41] The jury is still out on the adequacy of this intake after 4 to 6 months,[81] but complementary sources of Zn are clearly required at about this age. For the formula-fed infant, less favorable bioavailability

dictates the apparent need for higher intakes, but these have not been well defined.

Estimation of Zn requirements depends primarily on a factorial approach. Although it is complex in any population, this is especially true in low birth weight infants. One reason is that it remains unclear to what extent it is either necessary or possible for the premature infant to mimic intrauterine accumulation rates[82] at corresponding gestational ages. Using a figure of 17 g/kg body weight/day for postnatal weight gain[83] and 20 µg Zn/g weight gain,[84] the very low birth weight infant needs an average of 340 µg/kg body weight/day. How much needs to be retained to meet this figure depends on the extent to which, and the rate at which, hepatic stores of Zn at birth are or can be used by the neonate and young infant. Although the weight of the premature liver is quite small, Zn concentrations are exceptionally high.[54, 82] Making several assumptions and using complex calculations, the Life Sciences Research Office (LSRO) report included a figure of 130 µg Zn/day (or ~90 µg Zn/kg/day) available from hepatic stores (after 28 weeks' gestation) for postnatal growth.[83] Using these figures, retention of exogenous Zn required for growth is 250 µg Zn/kg/day. With losses of endogenous Zn via feces and urine averaging 215 µg Zn/kg/day in very low birth weight infants fed either breast milk with fortifier or a premature infant formula (Jalla S, et al: unpublished data), the estimated average physiologic Zn requirement (amount of absorbed Zn required) is 465 µg Zn/kg/day. In this study, average fractional absorption from formula and breast milk plus fortifier was 0.25, indicating a dietary requirement approaching 2 mg Zn/kg/day. The quite strong positive correlation between Zn intake and weight gain in this study suggests, but does not prove, that Zn intakes any lower than this can limit growth. Relatively high Zn intakes may need to be maintained for many months if lack of adequate Zn is not to limit growth.[85] The results of Zn supplementation studies in early infancy[71,86] suggest that the early postnatal Zn requirements of the small for gestational age infant are at least as high as those of the premature infant.

At a molecular level, more is known about the regulation of excretion of endogenous Zn in response to high Zn concentrations[25] than is known about the regulation of uptake. The transporter genes that are regulated are ancient, indicating that all eukaryotic cells have developed mechanisms for minimizing the accumulation of Zn in circumstances of environmental excess. This suggests that excess Zn is toxic even though little is known about its deleterious effects. In fact, the margin between optimal and toxic levels of Zn may be quite narrow for individual tissues. Moreover, the maintenance of Zn homeostasis by the gastrointestinal tract, although good, is imperfect.[49] Moreover, excess Zn may not need to reach beyond the enterocyte to be deleterious, at least in terms of metal-metal interactions.[87] Therefore, appropriate caution is required to ensure that the quantity of Zn supplied to the very low birth weight infant is not excessive. The margin between optimal and excessive intake may eventually prove to be quite narrow.[88] However, there is no evidence that the levels of intake from current premature infant formulas and human milk fortifiers are excessive. Rather, the foregoing calculations indicate that these are most reasonable, in light of present knowledge.

CONCLUSIONS

The emergence of the impressive biology of Zn and the public health implications of Zn deficiency in infants and young children[89] are now alerting us to the special attention that we need to confer on this trace element. This is more apparent in the very low birth weight infant than in any other population group. From a practical viewpoint, the most pressing requirement is to delineate the Zn requirements of the infant born very or extremely prematurely, including, as a special subgroup, those with intrauterine growth retardation.

REFERENCES

1. Walker WA, et al: Trace Elements in Human Nutrition. Nutrition in Pediatrics. Hamilton, Canada, BC Decker, 2003.
2. Hambidge KM: Trace minerals. *In* Hay W (ed): Neonatal Nutrition and Metabolism. Chicago, Year Book Medical Publishers, 2003.
3. Hambidge KM, et al: Zinc. *In* Mertz W (ed) Trace Elements in Human and Animal Nutrition, Vol 2. Orlando, FL, Academic Press, 1986, pp 1–137.
4. Kimura E, Aoki S: Chemistry of zinc (II) fluorophore sensors. Biometals *14*:191, 2001.
5. Williams RJP: An introduction to the biochemistry of zinc. *In* Mills CF (ed): Zinc in Human Biology. London, Springer-Verlag, 1989, pp 15–31.
6. Auld DS: Zinc coordination sphere in biochemical zinc sites. Biometals *14*:271, 2001.
7. Maret W: The function of zinc metallothionein in a link between cellular zinc and redox state. J Nutr *130*:1455, 2000.
8. MacDonald RS: The role of zinc in growth and cell proliferation. J Nutr *130*:1500S, 2000.
9. Maret W: Editorial. Biometals *14*:187, 2001.
10. Chesters JK. Biochemical functions of zinc in animals. World Rev Nutr Diet *32*:135, 1978.
11. Miller J, et al: Repetitive Zn-binding domains in the protein transcription factor IIIA from *Xenopus* oocytes. EMBO J *4*:1609, 1985.
12. Falchuk KH, Montorzi M: Zinc physiology and biochemistry in oocytes and embryos. Biometals *14*:385, 2001.
13. Andrews GK: Cellular zinc sensors: MTF-1 regulation of gene expression. Biometals *14*:223, 2001.
14. Truong-Tran AQ, et al: The role of zinc in caspase activation and apoptotic cell death. Biometals *14*:315, 2001.
15. Wang X, et al: Short-term zinc deficiency inhibits chondrocyte proliferation and induces cell apoptosis in the epiphyseal growth plate of young chickens. J Nutr *132*:665, 2002.
16. Beyersmann D, Haase H: Functions of zinc in signaling, proliferation and differentiation of mammalian cells. Biometals *14*:331, 2001.
17. Frederickson CJ, Bush AI: Synaptically released zinc: physiologic functions and pathologic effects. Biometals *14*:335, 2001.
18. Takeda A: Zinc homeostasis and functions of zinc in the brain. Biometals *14*:343, 2001.
19. Coyle P, et al: Metallothionein induction in freshly isolated rat hepatocytes. Biol Trace Elem Res *36*:35, 1993.
20. Coyle P, et al: Metallothionein in a multi-purpose protein. Cell Mol Life Sci *59*:1, 2001.
21. Rofe AM, et al: Paracetamol toxicity in metallothionein-null mice. Toxicology *125*:131, 1998.
22. Beattie JH, et al: Obesity and hyperleptinemia in metallothionein (-I and -II) null mice. Proc Natl Acad Sci USA *95*:358, 1998.
23. Carey LC: Ethanol teratogenicity: the aetiological importance of zinc and metallothionein. Adelaide, Australia, University of Adelaide, Clinical Biochemistry, 2002.
24. Gaither LA, Eide DJ: Eukaryotic zinc transporters and their regulation. Biometals *14*:251, 2001.
25. Liuzzi JP, et al: Differential regulation of zinc transporter 1, 2, and 4 mRNA expression by dietary zinc in rats. J Nutr *131*:46, 2001.
26. Yang Y, et al: Differential fluorescence labeling of cysteinyl clusters uncovers high tissue levels of thionein. Proc Natl Acad Sci USA *98*:5556, 2001.
27. Hambidge KM, et al: Zinc nutritional status during pregnancy: a longitudinal study. Am J Clin Nutr *37*:429, 1983.
28. Mas A, Sarkar B: Binding, uptake and efflux of ^{65}Zn by isolated human trophoblast cells. Biochim Biophys Acta *1092*:35, 1991.
29. Bax CM, Bloxam DL: Two major pathways of zinc (II) acquisition by human placental syncytiotrophoblast. J Cell Physiol *164*:546, 1995.
30. Aslam N, McArdle HJ: Mechanism of zinc uptake by microvilli isolated from human term placenta. J Cell Physiol *151*:533, 1992.
31. Douglas GC, et al: Uptake of ^{125}I-labelled alpha2-macroglobulin and albumin by human placental syncytiotrophoblast in vitro. J Cell Biochem *68*:427, 1998.
32. Vargas Zapata CL, et al: Zinc uptake by human placental microvillous membrane vesicles: effects of gestational age and maternal serum zinc levels. Biol Trace Elem Res *73*:127, 2000.
33. Paterson PG, et al: The effect of zinc levels in fetal circulation on zinc clearance across the in situ perfused guinea pig placenta. Can J Physiol Pharmacol *68*:1401, 1990.
34. Lindsay Y, et al: Zinc levels in the rat fetal liver are not determined by transport across the placental microvillar membrane or the fetal liver plasma membrane. Biol Reprod *51*:358, 1994.
35. Goyer RA, et al: Cellular localization of metallothionein in human term placenta. Placenta *13*:349, 1992.
36. De SK, et al: Cell-specific metallothionein gene expression in mouse decidua and placentae. Development *107*:611, 1989.
37. Liang L, et al: Activation of the complete mouse metallothionein gene locus in the maternal deciduum. Mol Reprod Dev *43*:25, 1996.
38. Huber KL, et al: Maternal zinc deprivation and interleukin-1 influence metallothionein gene expression and zinc metabolism of rats. J Nutr *118*:1570, 1988.
39. Kelleher SL, Lonnerdal B: Zinc transporters in the rat mammary gland respond to marginal zinc and vitamin A intakes during lactation. J Nutr *132*:3280, 2002.
40. Christian P, West KP Jr: Interactions between zinc and vitamin A: an update. Am J Clin Nutr *68*:435S, 1998.
41. Krebs NF, et al: Zinc supplementation during lactation: effects on maternal status and milk zinc concentrations. Am J Clin Nutr *61*:1030, 1995.
42. Krebs NF: Zinc transfer to the breastfed infant. J Mammary Gland Biol Neoplasia *4*:259, 1999.
43. Huang L, Gitschier J: Novel gene involved in zinc transport is deficient in the lethal milk mouse. Nat Genet *17*:292, 1997.
44. Zimmerman AW, et al: Acrodermatitis in breast-fed premature infants: evidence for a defect of mammary zinc secretion. Pediatrics *69*:176, 1982.
45. Krebs NF, Hambidge KM: Zinc metabolism and homeostasis: the application of tracer techniques to human zinc physiology. Biometals *14*:397, 2001.
46. Hambidge KM, Krebs NF: Interrelationships of key variables of human zinc homeostasis: relevance to dietary zinc requirements. Annu Rev Nutr *21*:429, 2001.
47. Steele L, Cousins RJ: Kinetics of zinc absorption by luminally and vascularly perfused rat intestine. Am J Physiol *248*:G46, 1985.
48. Lopez de Romana D, et al: Longitudinal measurements of zinc absorption in Peruvian children receiving different levels of zinc fortification. FASEB J *17*: 2003.
49. Hambidge KM. Underwood Memorial Lecture: Zinc homeostasis: Good but not perfect. J Nutr *133*: 2003.
50. Krebs N, et al: Stable isotope studies of zinc metabolism in infants. *In* Wastney ME, Subramanian KNS (eds): Kinetic Models of Trace Element and Mineral Metabolism during Development. Boca Raton, FL, CRC Press, 1995.
51. Ziegler EE, et al: Effect of low zinc intake on absorption and excretion of zinc by infants studied with 70Zn as extrinsic tag. J Nutr *119*:1647, 1989.
52. Miller LV, et al: Development of a compartmental model of human zinc metabolism: identifiability and multiple studies analyses. Am J Physiol *279*:R1681, 2000.
53. Miller LV, et al: Size of the zinc pools that exchange rapidly with plasma zinc in humans: alternative techniques for measuring and relation to dietary zinc intake. J Nutr *124*:268, 1994.
54. Zlotkin SH, Cherian MG: Hepatic metallothionein as a source of zinc and cysteine during the first year of life. Pediatr Res *24*:326, 1988.
55. Hurley LS: Teratogenic aspects of manganese, zinc, and copper nutrition. Physiol Rev *61*:249, 1981.
56. Keen CL, Hurley LS: Effects of zinc deficiency on prenatal and postnatal development. Neurotoxicology *8*:379, 1987.
57. Record IR, et al: Maternal metabolism and teratogenesis in zinc-deficient rats. Teratology *33*:311, 1986.
58. Hambidge K, et al: Zinc, acrodermatitis enteropathica and congenital malformations. Lancet *1*:577, 1975.
59. Hambidge KM, et al: Neural tube defects and serum zinc. Br J Obstet Gynaecol *100*:746, 1993.
60. Cavdar AO, et al: Zinc status in pregnancy and the occurrence of anencephaly in Turkey. J Trace Elem Electrolytes Health Dis *2*:9, 1988.
61. Velie EM, et al: Maternal supplemental and dietary zinc intake and the occurrence of neural tube defects in California. Am J Epidemiol *150*:605, 1999.
62. Osendarp SJM, et al: The effects of maternal zinc supplementation in developing countries. J Nutr *133*: 2003.
63. Hickory W, et al: Fetal skeletal malformations associated with moderate zinc deficiency during pregnancy. J Nutr *109*:883, 1979.
64. Wang FD, et al: Maternal zinc deficiency impairs brain nestin expression in prenatal and postnatal mice. Cell Res *11*:135, 2001.
65. Hambidge M, et al: Zinc and Human Pregnancy. *In* Roussel AM, Anderson RA, and Favier AE (ed): Trace Elements in Man and Animals 10. New York, Kluwer Academic/Plenum Publishers, 2000.
66. Goldenberg RL, et al: The effect of zinc supplementation on pregnancy outcome. JAMA *274*:463, 1995.
67. Caulfield L, et al: Maternal zinc supplementation does not affect size at birth or pregnancy duration in Peru. J Nutr *129*:1563, 1999.
68. Osendarp SJ, et al: A randomized, placebo-controlled trial of the effect of zinc supplementation during pregnancy on pregnancy outcome in Bangladeshi urban poor. Am J Clin Nutr *71*:114, 2000.
69. Hambidge KM, et al: The role of zinc in the pathogenesis and treatment of acrodermatitis enteropathica. Prog Clin Biol Res *14*:329, 1977.
70. Hambidge K: Mild zinc deficiency in human subjects. *In* Mills C (ed): Zinc in Human Biology. London, Springer-Verlag, 1989.
71. Sazawal S, et al: Effect of zinc and mineral supplementation in small for gestational age infants on growth and mortality. FASEB J *13*:A376, 1999.
72. Bhutta ZA, et al: Prevention of diarrhea and pneumonia by zinc supplementation in children in developing countries: pooled analysis of randomized controlled trials. J Pediatr *135*:689, 1999.
73. Hambidge M, Krebs N: Zinc, diarrhea, and pneumonia (editorial). J Pediatr *135*:661, 1999.
74. Prasad AS, et al: Zinc metabolism in patients with the syndrome of iron deficiency anemia, hepatosplenomegaly, dwarfism and hypogonadism. J Lab Clin *61*:534, 1963.
75. Rink L, Garbriel P: Extracellular and immunological actions of zinc. Biometals *14*:367, 2001.
76. Black RE: Therapeutic and preventive effects of zinc on serious childhood infectious diseases in developing countries. Am J Clin Nutr *68*:476S, 1998.
77. Brown KH, et al: Effect of supplemental zinc on the growth and serum zinc concentrations of prepubertal children: a meta-analysis of randomized controlled trials. Am J Clin Nutr *75*:1062, 2002.

78. Sandstead HH, et al: Effects of repletion with zinc and other micronutrients on neuropsychological performance and growth of Chinese children. Am J Clin Nutr 68(Suppl):470, 1998.
79. Penland J, et al: Zinc, iron, and micronutrients supplementation effects on cognitive and psychomotor function of Mexican-American school children. FASEB J 13:A921, 1999.
80. Black MM: Zinc deficiency and child development. Am J Clin Nutr 68:464S, 1998.
81. Krebs NF, Westcott J: Zinc and breastfed infants: if and when is there a risk of deficiency? In Davis MK, et al (eds): Integrating Population Outcomes, Biological Mechanisms and Research Methods in the Study of Human Milk and Lactation, Vol 503. New York, Kluwer Academic/Plenum Press, 2002, pp 69–76.
82. Widdowson EM, et al: Fetal growth and body composition. In Lindblad BS (ed): Perinatal Nutrition. New York, Academic Press, 1998, pp 3–14.
83. Klein CJ: Minerals: trace elements. J Nutr 132:1472, 2002.
84. Krebs NF, Hambidge KM: Zinc requirements and zinc intakes of breast-fed infants. Am J Clin Nutr 43:288, 1986.
85. Friel J, Andrews WL: Improved growth of very low birthweight infants. Nutr Res 13:611, 1993.
86. Castillo-Duran C, et al: Zinc supplementation and growth of infants born small for gestational age. J Pediatr 127:206, 1995.
87. Food and Nutrition Board Institute of Medicine: Dietary reference intakes for vitamin A, vitamin K, boron, chromium, copper, iodine, iron, manganese, molybdenum, nickel, silicon, vanadium and zinc. In Standing Committee on the Scientific Evaluation of Dietary Reference Intakes. Washington, DC, National Academy Press, 2001, pp 442–501.
88. O'Dell BL, Browning JD: Zinc deprivation and the nervous system. Nutr Neurosci 3:97, 2000.
89. Hambidge M: Human zinc deficiency. J Nutr 130:1344S, 2000.

36

Jayant P. Shenai

Vitamin A Metabolism in the Fetus and Neonate

Vitamin A is a fat-soluble micronutrient recognized since 1912 as a dietary constituent that is essential for growth.[1, 2] The vitamin A compounds (retinoids) are present in three natural forms: retinol, retinaldehyde, and retinoic acid (Fig. 36–1). Retinol (vitamin A alcohol) is a dietary component present in the form of retinyl esters in food sources of animal origin and is also formed *in vivo* from its precursor, β-carotene, which is present in food sources of plant origin. Retinyl esters are derived from esterification of retinol and constitute the principal storage forms of vitamin A; the major retinyl esters found in animal and human tissues include retinyl palmitate and stearate and, to a lesser extent, oleate and linoleate. Retinaldehyde, also called *retinal*, is derived from reversible oxidation of retinol and, in combination with various lipoproteins, forms the visual pigment of the retina.[3] The photoisomerization of retinaldehyde is necessary for vision.[4] Retinoic acid is derived from irreversible oxida-

tion of retinaldehyde in the tissues[5] and is the active metabolite of vitamin A in functions related to growth and differentiation.[6]

VITAMIN A METABOLISM

Transport in Plasma

Vitamin A is transported in plasma as retinol bound to a specific carrier protein, retinol-binding protein, (RBP) (Fig. 36–2). The human RBP molecule consists of a polypeptide chain of about 180 amino acid residues; it has a molecular weight of approximately 21 kD and a single binding site for one molecule of retinol.[7,8] The RBP is synthesized in liver and secreted into plasma as retinol-RBP complex.[9] In plasma, the retinol-RBP complex interacts with another protein, transthyretin, and circulates as an RBP-transthyretin complex.[9] The transthyretin molecule is a

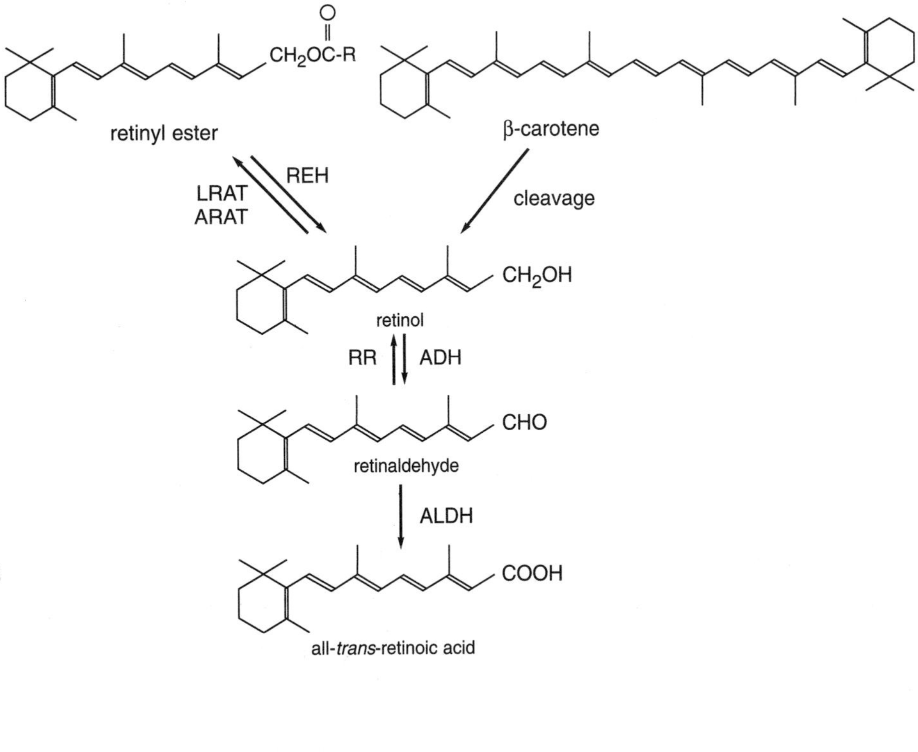

Figure 36–1. Vitamin A compounds.
ADH = alcohol dehydrogenase;
ALDH = aldehyde dehydrogenase;
ARAT = acyl-CoA-retinol acyltransferase;
LRAT = lecithin-retinol acyltransferase;
REH = retinyl ester hydrolase;
RR = retinaldehyde reductase.

stable, symmetrical tetramer composed of four identical subunits and has a molecular weight of approximately 55 kD.[10] Vitamin A is distributed to the target tissues in the form of retinol-RBP complex bound to transthyretin. The cellular uptake of vitamin A depends on a specific plasma membrane receptor that recognizes RBP.[11,12] After delivery of vitamin A to the plasma membrane, RBP is returned to the circulation and is partly reused for vitamin A delivery and partly eliminated by the kidney.[13] The mechanisms involved in the processing of transthyretin are not known.

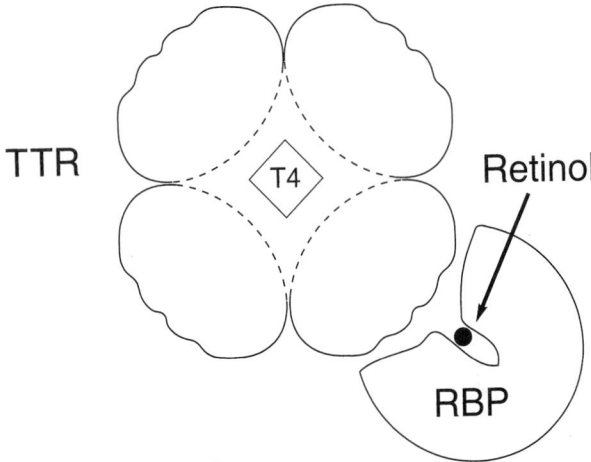

Figure 36–2. Vitamin A (retinol) complexed with its specific carrier proteins in plasma. RBP = retinol-binding protein; TTR = transthyretin; T$_4$ = thyroid hormone.

Metabolism in the Cell

The movement of vitamin A within the tissue cells involves two intracellular vitamin A–binding proteins, cellular retinol-binding protein (CRBP) and cellular retinoic acid–binding protein (CRABP) (Fig. 36–3).[14] The CRBP molecule consists of a polypeptide chain with a molecular weight of approximately 14.6 kD and a single binding site for one molecule of a specific isomer of retinol, all-*trans*-retinol. The CRBP participates in the enzymatic esterification of retinol into retinyl esters for storage in the cell. The CRABP molecule also consists of a polypeptide chain with a molecular weight of approximately 14.6 kD and a single binding site for one molecule of a specific isomer of retinoic acid, all-*trans*-retinoic acid. Given the apparent absence of a plasma delivery system specific for retinoic acid, it seems likely that the retinoic acid within the cell is derived mostly from oxidation of retinol occurring within the cell. The CRABP participates in the interconversion of two specific isomers of retinoic acid, all-*trans*-retinoic acid and 9-*cis*-retinoic acid. Both CRBP and CRABP are suggested as transport proteins for retinoids between the cellular and nuclear membranes.

Processing in the Nucleus

The nuclear uptake of all-*trans*-retinoic acid is mediated exclusively by a family of receptors called *retinoic acid receptors* (RARs) (see Fig. 36–3).[15] Three different isomers of RARs (RAR-α, RAR-β, RAR-γ) exist and are expressed in distinct patterns throughout development. The RARs modulate gene expression by binding as homodimers or heterodimers to specific DNA sequences known as *retinoid acid receptor elements* (RAREs). Contrary to all-*trans*-retinoic acid, the nuclear uptake of 9-*cis*-retinoic acid is mediated partly by RARs but mostly by another

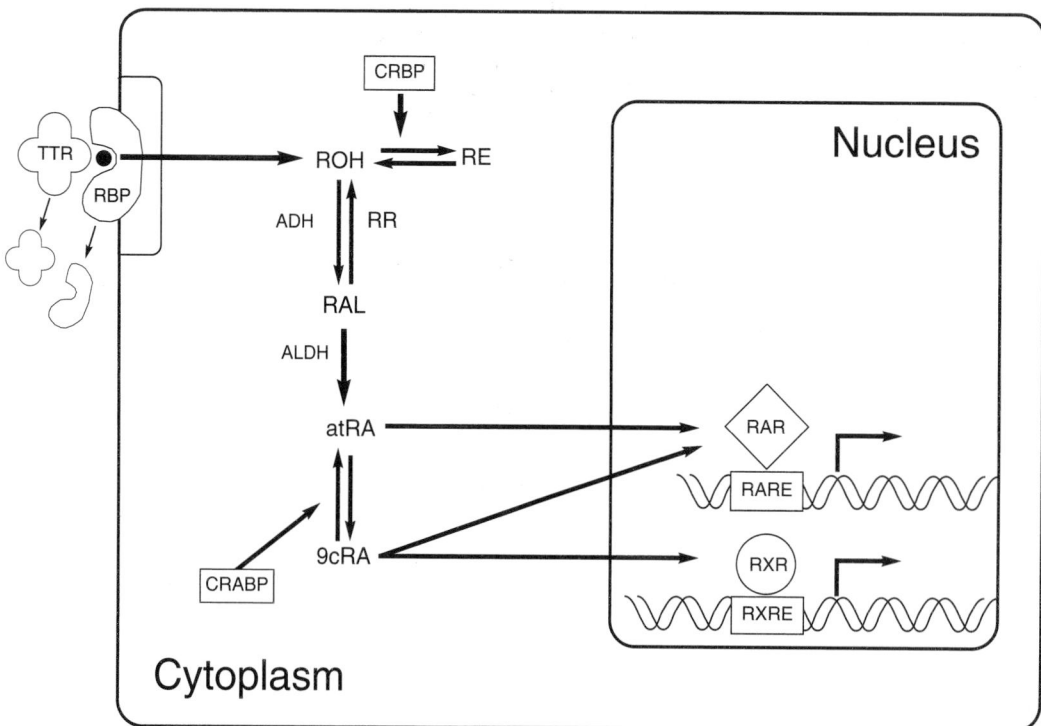

Figure 36–3. Vitamin A metabolism in the cell and nucleus. ADH = alcohol dehydrogenase; ALDH = aldehyde dehydrogenase; atRA = all-*trans*-retinoic acid; CRABP = cellular retinoic acid-binding protein; CRBP = cellular retinol-binding protein; 9cRA = 9-*cis*-retinoic acid; RAL = retinaldehyde; RAR = retinoic acid receptor; RARE = retinoic acid receptor element; RBP = retinol-binding protein; RE = retinyl ester; ROH = retinol; RR = retinaldehyde reductase; RXR = retinoid x receptor; RXRE = retinoid x receptor element; TTR = transthyretin.) (Adapted from Mangelsdorf et al.[15])

family of receptors called *retinoid x receptors* (RXRs).[15] Like RARs, three different isomers of RXRs (RXR-α, RXR-β, RXR-γ) exist, are expressed in distinct patterns throughout development, and modulate gene expression by binding to specific DNA sequences known as *retinoid x receptor elements* (RXREs). The mechanisms by which retinoic acid influences nuclear metabolism, genomic expression, and growth and differentiation of the target tissue remain under investigation.

Vitamin A Excretion

The excretory end products of vitamin A metabolism are derived largely from retinoic acid.[16] Retinoic acid is excreted partly in the ester form of β-glucuronide through the biliary system and is subject to reabsorption in the gut.[17] The enterohepatic circulation of retinoic acid serves to conserve this biologically active form of vitamin A. The rest of the retinoic acid is excreted largely in the urine in the form of oxidation products.[18]

FETAL ACQUISITION OF VITAMIN A

Vitamin A is transferred from the mother to the fetus during pregnancy, particularly in late gestation, in most animal species.[19-25] The transplacental transport of maternal retinol-RBP complex appears to be the predominant source of vitamin A for the fetus in early gestation. In late gestation, RBP synthesized by the fetal liver appears to be involved in extracting vitamin A from the placental circulation. Swallowed amniotic fluid containing vitamin A[26,27] and transfer of maternal lipoproteins containing retinyl esters[23] are other possible sources of vitamin A for the fetus.

The transplacental transfer of vitamin A in humans has been studied by examining paired samples of maternal blood and fetal or cord blood obtained at various gestational ages.[28-32] The ratio of maternal to fetal concentration of plasma vitamin A in healthy human pregnancies is approximately 2:1. In conditions in which the maternal vitamin A status is marginal or deficient, the fetal plasma vitamin A concentration often is maintained within normal limits and may exceed the maternal plasma vitamin A concentration.[28,33,34] Conversely, in studies involving maternal vitamin A supplementation, the cord blood vitamin A concentration in the supplemented cohort remains similar to that in unsupplemented controls.[28,35,36] Thus, the plasma vitamin A concentration in the fetus appears to be maintained within a normal range despite variations in the maternal vitamin A status and intake. The regulatory mechanisms by which this homeostasis is achieved remain unclear, nor is it known whether such mechanisms can compensate successfully for extreme conditions of maternal vitamin A deprivation or excess.

PLASMA VITAMIN A STATUS AT BIRTH

Measurement of plasma concentration of vitamin A is the most commonly used biochemical marker of vitamin A status. In healthy human adults, the plasma vitamin A concentration ranges from 20 to 80 µg/dL.[37] In children, including infants, a plasma vitamin A concentration below 20 µg/dL is indicative of vitamin A deficiency.[38] Most preterm infants, in contrast to those of term gestation, are born with plasma vitamin A concentrations that are in the deficient range.[39,40]

Measurement of plasma concentration of RBP is another biochemical marker of vitamin A status. In healthy human adults, the plasma RBP concentration averages 4.6 mg/dL (± SD 1.0 mg/dL).[41] The plasma RBP concentrations in infants and children are approximately 60% of the adult values,[30] and those below 2.5 mg/dL are indicative of vitamin A deficiency.[42] Most preterm infants, unlike those of term gestation, are born with plasma RBP concentrations that are in the deficient range.[40,43] It is likely that the preterm infants are vitamin A deficient at birth because of deprivation of transplacental vitamin A supply that results from their delivery at an early gestational age.

VITAMIN A STORAGE AT BIRTH

As much as 90% of the total body reserve of vitamin A is stored normally in the liver in most animal species.[44] The liver vitamin A concentration ranges from 100 to 300 µg/g in healthy human adults,[45] and it varies with age in children, being low during infancy relative to later childhood.[46,47] A liver vitamin A concentration below 40 µg/g is indicative of low vitamin A reserve and that below 20 µg/g is considered deficient.[46-48] Most preterm infants, unlike those of term gestation, are born with low liver vitamin A stores.[47,49-52] In the absence of an adequate intake of vitamin A in the postnatal period, therefore, these infants are at an added risk for becoming vitamin A deficient.

Although the liver is the principal storage site for vitamin A, other organs, including the developing lung, are capable of storing vitamin A.[53-55] In the perinatal rat, significant vitamin A storage occurs in the fetal lung during the latter third of prenatal life.[54,55] Depletion of these stores that begins before birth and continues into early postnatal period suggests that the developing lung may depend on these local stores of vitamin A during the period of active growth and differentiation associated with rapid alveolarization of the lung. Prematurely born animals deprived of adequate stores of vitamin A in their lungs may be susceptible to the adverse pulmonary effects of vitamin A deficiency. The fetal lung stores of vitamin A can be augmented by prenatal maternal administration of supplemental vitamin A.[56] Conversely, prenatal interventions, such as maternal glucocorticosteroid treatment, can deplete the fetal lung stores of vitamin A.[57] Whether the developing fetal lung of humans is capable of vitamin A uptake, esterification, and storage remains undetermined. Moreover, the possibility that administration of vitamin A to human mothers with imminent preterm deliveries may augment the lung vitamin A stores of their newborn infants remains unexplored.

VITAMIN A AND ENTERAL NUTRITION

The vitamin A value of a diet is expressed in international units (IU) or retinol equivalents (RE).[37] One IU of vitamin A is equal to 0.3 µg of retinol; one RE of vitamin A is equal to 1.0 µg of retinol.

The vitamin A content of human milk is variable and influenced by several factors, such as age, parity, and socioeconomic status of the mother; postpartum age; and the volume and fat content of the milk.[58] The vitamin A concentration of human milk in colostrum is high (>333 IU/dL), and it decreases gradually in the first few months of lactation.[58-61] The vitamin A concentration of mature human milk ranges from 110 to 257 IU/dL.[58-60,62-64] The milk of mothers giving birth prematurely differs in composition from that of mothers delivering at term gestation. The vitamin A concentration of preterm milk is lower than that of term milk during the first week of lactation, but is higher thereafter.[64-66] At approximately 35 days' postpartum age, the vitamin A concentration of preterm milk ranges from 277 to 333 IU/dL.[65,66] More than 90% of the vitamin A in human milk is in the form of retinyl esters contained in the core of the milk fat globules, whereas less than 10% of the vitamin A is present as free retinol.[63,67-70]

Various infant formulas designed to meet the nutritional needs of a preterm infant are commercially available. The vitamin A content of these formulas varies approximately from 296 to 1,000 IU/dL.[71] Preterm infants receiving full enteral feeds often are given multivitamin supplements. The vitamin A content of a typical multivitamin supplement is 1,500 IU/dL.[71] Like in human milk, most vitamin A in the infant formulas and multivitamin supplements is in the form of retinyl esters. Thus, the efficiency of use of vitamin A in a neonate fed human milk or an infant formula with or without a multivitamin supplement depends largely on the ability of the infant's gastrointestinal tract to process retinyl esters.

VITAMIN A DIGESTION AND ABSORPTION

Dietary retinyl esters are processed by a coordinated series of physical and chemical events in the bowel lumen.[44] These events include dispersion and emulsification of retinyl esters in the stomach, their hydrolysis in the intestinal lumen by pancreatic and other enzymes, and solubilization of retinol (derived from retinyl ester hydrolysis) with bile salts in mixed micelles. These intraluminal events facilitate uptake of vitamin A by the enteral mucosal cells (Fig. 36–4). Retinol within the mucosal cells, also partly derived from β-carotene, is largely reesterified with long-chain fatty acids. The retinyl esters are then incorporated, together with other lipids and apolipoproteins, into chylomicron particles. The chylomicrons are secreted by the enteral mucosal cells into the intestinal lacteals and enter the plasma compartment through the intestinal lymphatics, largely through the thoracic duct. Retinyl esters found in the lymph chylomicron are almost entirely retained in the particle during its processing to a chylomicron remnant. The chylomicron remnants and their retinyl esters are almost completely removed from the circulation by the liver.

The reesterification of retinol in the enteral mucosal cells and its subsequent absorption into the lymph are influenced by a specific carrier protein called *cellular retinol-binding protein type II* (CRBP II) (see Fig. 36–4).[72] The CRBP II molecule consists of a polypeptide chain with a molecular weight of approximately 16 kD. In the adult rat, the CRBP II is present almost exclusively in the absorptive cells of the small intestine.[73] Its concentration in the small intestine appears to be age related; it is lower in immature fetuses relative to findings in mature newborns and adults.[72] A similar gut-specific CRBP II is present in the human small intestine.[74] Its localization in the mature, villus-associated enterocytes of the jejunum suggests that the CRBP II may facilitate vitamin A absorption in the gut. The ontogeny of the CRBP II during fetal and neonatal development in humans has not been studied. It is possible that the lower concentrations

of CRBP II in the small intestine of preterm neonates relative to mature term infants may result in differences in vitamin A absorption by these infants.

VITAMIN A AND PARENTERAL NUTRITION

Preterm infants who experience difficulties with enteral feeding often are sustained exclusively with intravenous nutrition. A protein-dextrose solution and a lipid emulsion are commonly used for intravenous nutrition. Various nutrients, including vitamins, are administered generally through the protein-dextrose solution. The vitamin A concentration of the protein-dextrose solution is estimated at approximately 930 IU/dL.[75] A newborn infant on total parenteral nutrition receiving the protein-dextrose solution at a conventional rate of 120 to 135 mL/kg/day, therefore, is expected to receive a vitamin A intake ranging from 1,116 to 1,256 IU/kg/day. However, vitamin A in protein-dextrose solution is subject to photodegradation, and it binds to intravenous tubing.[76-79] Both photodegradative and adsorptive losses of vitamin A render the intravenous administration of vitamin A inefficient. Until such losses can be reduced substantially or eliminated, either through development of new materials for intravenous tubing or through improved administration of fat-soluble vitamins in the lipid emulsion,[80] alternative methods of vitamin A administration, such as by intramuscular route, may be necessary to optimize the vitamin A status of neonates on long-term parenteral nutrition.

VITAMIN A DEFICIENCY

Vitamin A promotes orderly growth and differentiation of epithelial cells, and its deficiency affects various organ systems, including the lung.[81] The histopathologic changes in the respiratory system generally precede other consequences of vitamin A deficiency involving the genitourinary system, eye, and skin.[81] Vitamin A deficiency results in a progressive sequence of changes in the epithelial lining of pulmonary conducting airways.[81-83] These changes consist of necrotizing tracheobronchitis in early stages and squamous metaplasia in advanced stages of the deficiency. The pathophysiologic consequences of these changes include (1) loss of normal secretions of goblet cells and of other secretory cells; (2) loss of normal water home-

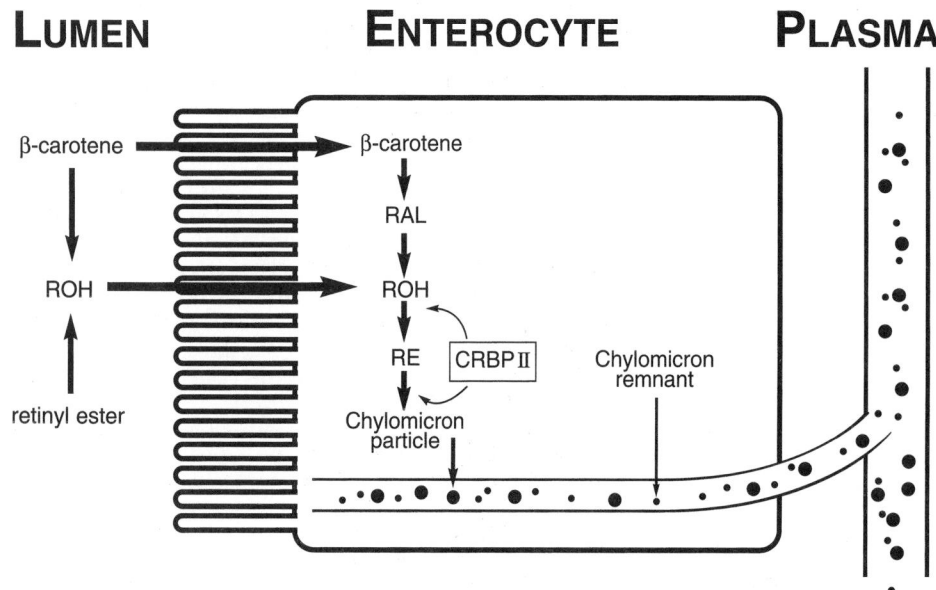

Figure 36–4. Vitamin A absorption in the enterocyte. CRBP II = cellular retinol-binding protein type II.

ostasis across tracheobronchial epithelium; (3) loss of mucociliary transport with resultant predisposition to airway infection; and (4) narrowing of lumina and loss of distensibility of airways with resultant increase in airway resistance and work of breathing. The histopathologic changes of vitamin A deficiency and associated pathophysiologic consequences are reversible with restoration of normal vitamin A status.[84,85]

Preterm infants are susceptible to lung injury from such insults as hyaline membrane disease, barotrauma or volutrauma from mechanical ventilation, oxygen toxicity, and airway infection.[86] These infants are at risk for the development of a form of chronic lung disease called *bronchopulmonary dysplasia* (BPD).[86] The histopathologic changes of BPD, which consist of necrotizing tracheobronchitis in early stages and squamous metaplasia in advanced stages of the disease, are remarkably similar to those seen in vitamin A deficiency.[87] Preterm infants who have BPD, unlike those with no lung disease, often manifest clinical, biochemical, and histopathologic evidence of vitamin A deficiency.[88-91] Vitamin A supplementation from early postnatal life in these infants can improve their vitamin A status and also ameliorate the lung disease, as evidenced by a decreased incidence of BPD and of the associated morbidity.[92,93]

VITAMIN A TOXICITY

Hypervitaminosis A may result from acute intoxication or from chronic ingestion of vitamin A. Administration of a single large dose of vitamin A in excess of 100,000 IU may cause acute intoxication in infants.[37] The clinical manifestations of acute hypervitaminosis A include symptoms and signs of increased intracranial pressure. Prolonged ingestion of vitamin A in excess of 25,000 IU per day may cause chronic intoxication in infants.[37,94,95] The clinical manifestations of chronic hypervitaminosis A include symptoms and signs of increased intracranial pressure, bone and joint pains, and mucocutaneous lesions; hepatomegaly and hepatic injury, hypercalcemia, and hematologic abnormalities are sometimes seen.[96] Radiographic findings of chronic hypervitaminosis A in infants younger than 6 months of age include widened metaphyses, especially of the distal ulna, and radiolucent zones in the radius proximal to the metaphysis.[97] Cortical hyperostosis of multiple long bones and soft tissue changes are seen typically in infants older than 6 months.[97] In hypervitaminosis A, the plasma vitamin A concentration is generally in excess of 100 μg/dL, whereas the plasma RBP concentration usually remains normal.[98]

Hypervitaminosis A is reversible with restriction of vitamin A intake. Infusion of 2-hydroxypropyl-β-cyclodextrin as a means of solubilizing retinoids and enhancing their urinary excretion has been used occasionally as adjunct therapy.[99]

GUIDELINES FOR VITAMIN A NUTRITION

The recommended dietary intake of vitamin A for term newborn infants is 333 IU/kg/day.[100] In preterm infants, a vitamin A intake below 700 IU/kg/day is associated with a marked decline in plasma vitamin A concentrations.[89] Normalization of plasma concentrations of vitamin A and RBP is possible in preterm infants with a vitamin A intake above 1,500 IU/kg/day.[89-92] Lack of clinical and biochemical evidence of toxicity in studies of vitamin A–supplemented infants and maintenance of their plasma vitamin A concentrations below 80 μg/dL suggest that a total vitamin A intake in the range of 1,500 to 2,800 IU/kg/day is safe for preterm infants.[90-92,101]

The potential role of vitamin A in facilitation of healing from lung injury has led to the development of guidelines for optimizing vitamin A nutrition in preterm infants at risk for BPD.[102] According to these guidelines, preterm infants meeting the following criteria are eligible for vitamin A supplementation: birthweight below 1250 g, estimated gestational age at birth earlier

than 31 weeks, appropriate growth for gestational age, need for mechanical ventilation at 24 hours' postnatal age, and no major congenital anomalies. In addition to standard vitamin A intake from parenteral and enteral sources, these infants are given supplemental vitamin A (retinyl palmitate) in two phases. Phase I entails an intramuscular injection of 2,000 IU/kg/dose on postnatal day 1 and on alternate days thereafter until establishment of full enteral feeding. Full enteral feeding is considered established when energy intake by enteral route exceeds 75% of total energy intake. Phase II entails an orogastric administration of 4000 IU/kg/dose on the day of full feeds and daily thereafter until discharge from the neonatal intensive care unit. Each infant is monitored for evidence of vitamin A toxicity by serial measurements of plasma concentrations of vitamin A and RBP, careful physical examination, and periodic blood chemistry profiles, as well as hematologic indexes. Ultrasonographic scanning of the brain to detect intracranial hemorrhage and assessment of intracranial pressure by noninvasive methods such as fontanelle tonometry are also useful.

Dexamethasone, a glucocorticosteroid hormone, is being used increasingly in the postnatal treatment of preterm infants with BPD.[103] Postnatal dexamethasone treatment induces a significant, although short-term, increase in plasma concentrations of both vitamin A and RBP in these infants.[104,105] Thus, in the event dexamethasone treatment is initiated, supplemental vitamin A is withheld throughout the course of the dexamethasone treatment. This precautionary measure is intended to avoid the potential risk of vitamin A toxicity associated with dexamethasone treatment. With the guidelines for vitamin A supplementation already discussed, monitoring of plasma vitamin A indexes, clinical evaluation for potential toxicity, and careful consideration of concomitant therapies, the goal is to optimize vitamin A nutrition in vulnerable preterm infants at risk for lung disease.

REFERENCES

1. Hopkins FG: Feeding experiments illustrating the importance of accessory factors in normal dietaries. J Physiol 44:425, 1912.
2. McCollum EV, Davis M: The influence of certain vegetable fats on growth. J Biol Chem 2:179, 1915.
3. Hubbard R: The molecular weight of rhodopsin and the nature of the rhodopsin-digitonin complex. J Gen Physiol 37:381, 1954.
4. Wald G: Molecular basis of visual excitations. Science 162:230, 1968.
5. Emerick RJ, et al: Formation of retinoic acid from retinol in the rat. Biochem J 102:606, 1967.
6. Blaner WS, Olson JA: Retinol and retinoic acid metabolism. *In* Sporn MB, et al. (eds):The Retinoids: Biology, Chemistry, and Medicine. 2nd edition. New York, Raven Press, 1994, p 229.
7. Kanai M, et al: Retinol-binding protein: the transport protein for vitamin A in human plasma. J Clin Invest 47:2025, 1968.
8. Raz A, et al: Studies on the protein-protein and protein-ligand interactions involved in retinol transport in plasma. J Biol Chem 245:1903, 1970.
9. Soprano DR, Blaner WS: Plasma retinol-binding protein. *In* Sporn MB, et al (eds):The Retinoids: Biology, Chemistry, and Medicine. 2nd edition. New York, Raven Press, 1994, p 257.
10. Kanda Y, et al:The amino acid sequence of human plasma prealbumin. J Biol Chem 249:6796, 1974.
11. Rask L, Peterson PA: In vitro uptake of vitamin A from the retinol-binding plasma protein to mucosal epithelial cells from the monkey's small intestine. J Biol Chem 251:6360, 1976.
12. Bok D, Heller J: Transport of retinol from the blood to the retina: an autoradiographic study of the pigment epithelial cell surface receptor for plasma retinol-binding protein. Exp Eye Res 22:395, 1976.
13. Glover J, et al: Distribution of retinol-binding protein in tissues. Vitamin Horm 32:215, 1974.
14. Chytil F, Ong DE: Cellular retinol- and retinoic acid-binding proteins in vitamin A action. Fed Proc 38:2510, 1979.
15. Mangelsdorf DJ, et al: The retinoid receptors. *In* Sporn MB, et al (eds): The Retinoids: Biology, Chemistry, and Medicine. 2nd edition. New York, Raven Press, 1994, p 319.
16. Sundaresan PR, Sundaresan GM: Studies on the urinary metabolites of retinoic acid in the rat. Internat J Vit Nutr Res 43:61, 1973.
17. Dunagin PE Jr, et al: Retinoyl beta-glucuronic acid: a major metabolite of vitamin A in rat. Science 148:86, 1965.

18. Zile MH, et al: The biological activity of 5,6-epoxyretinoic acid. J Nutr 110:2225, 1980.
19. Moore T: Vitamin A transfer from mother to offspring in mice and rats. Internat J Vit Nutr Res 41:301, 1971.
20. Branstetter RF, et al: Vitamin A transfer from cows to calves. Internat J Vit Nutr Res 43:142, 1973.
21. Mitchell GE Jr, et al: Vitamin A alcohol and vitamin A palmitate transfer from ewes to lambs. Internat J Vit Nutr Res 45:299, 1975.
22. Takahashi YI, et al: Vitamin A and retinol-binding protein metabolism during fetal development in the rat. Am J Physiol 233:E263, 1977.
23. Ismadi SD, Olson JA: Dynamics of the fetal distribution and transfer of vitamin A between rat fetuses and their mother. Internat J Vit Nutr Res 52:112, 1982.
24. Donoghue S, et al: Placental transport of retinol in sheep. J Nutr 112:2197, 1982.
25. Vahlquist A, Nilsson S: Vitamin A transfer to the fetus and to the amniotic fluid in rhesus monkey (Macaca mulatta). Ann Nutr Metab 28:321, 1984.
26. Wallingford JC, et al: Vitamin A and retinol-binding protein in amniotic fluid. Am J Clin Nutr 38:377, 1983.
27. Sklan D, et al: Retinol transport proteins and concentrations in human amniotic fluid, placenta, and fetal and maternal sera. Br J Nutr 54:577, 1985.
28. Lund CJ, Kimble MS: Plasma vitamin A and carotene of the newborn infant with consideration of fetal-maternal relationships. Am J Obstet Gynecol 46:207, 1943.
29. Baker H, et al: Vitamin profile of 174 mothers and newborns at parturition. Am J Clin Nutr 28:59, 1975.
30. Vahlquist A, et al: The concentrations of retinol-binding protein, prealbumin, and transferrin in sera of newly delivered mothers and children of various ages. Scand J Clin Lab Invest 35:569, 1975.
31. Baker H, et al: Vitamin levels in low-birth-weight newborn infants and their mothers. J Obstet Gynecol 129:521, 1977.
32. Jansson L, Nilsson B: Serum retinol and retinol-binding protein in mothers and infants at delivery. Biol Neonate 43:269, 1983.
33. Venketachalam PS, Belavady B, Gopalan C: Studies on vitamin A nutritional status of mothers and infants in poor communities in India. Trop Pediatr 61:262, 1962.
34. Butte NF, Calloway DH: Proteins, vitamin A, carotene, folacin, ferritin and zinc in Navajo maternal and cord blood. Biol Neonate 41:273, 1982.
35. Lewis JM, et al: Supplements of vitamin A and of carotene during pregnancy: their effect on the levels of vitamin A and carotene in the blood of mother and of newborn infant. Am J Dis Child 73:143, 1947.
36. Barnes AC: The placental metabolism of vitamin A. Am J Obstet Gynecol 61:368, 1951.
37. Underwood BA: Vitamin A in human nutrition. In Sporn MB, et al (eds): The Retinoids: Biology, Chemistry, and Medicine. 2nd edition. New York, Raven Press, 1994, p 211.
38. Pitt GAJ: The assessment of vitamin A status. Proc Nutr Soc 40:173, 1981.
39. Brandt RB, et al: Serum vitamin A in premature and term neonates. J Pediatr 92:101, 1978.
40. Shenai JP, et al: Plasma vitamin A and retinol-binding protein in premature and term neonates. J Pediatr 99:302, 1981.
41. Smith FR, Goodman DS: The effects of diseases of liver, thyroid, and kidneys on the transport of vitamin A in human plasma. J Clin Invest 50:2426, 1971.
42. Vahlquist A, et al: Plasma vitamin A transport and visual dark adaptation in diseases of the intestine and liver. Scand J Clin Lab Invest 38:301, 1978.
43. Bhatia J, Ziegler EE: Retinol-binding protein and prealbumin in cord blood of term and preterm infants. Early Hum Dev 8:129, 1983.
44. Goodman DS, Blaner WS: Biosynthesis, absorption, and hepatic metabolism of retinol. In Sporn MB, et al (eds): The Retinoids: Biology, Chemistry, and Medicine. Vol 2. New York, Academic Press, 1984, p 1.
45. Pearson WN: Blood and urinary vitamin levels as potential indices of body stores. Am J Clin Nutr 20:514, 1967.
46. Huque T: A survey of human liver reserves of retinol in London. Br J Nutr 47:165, 1982.
47. Olson JA, et al: Liver concentrations of vitamin A and carotenoids, as a function of age and other parameters, of American children who died of various causes. Am J Clin Nutr 39:903, 1984.
48. Olson JA: Evaluation of vitamin A status in children. World Rev Nutr Diet 31:130, 1978.
49. Iyengar L, Apte SV: Nutrient stores in human foetal livers. Br J Nutr 27:313, 1972.
50. Olson JA: Liver vitamin A reserves of neonates, preschool children and adults dying of various causes in Salvador, Brazil. Arch Latinoam Nutr 26:992, 1979.
51. Montreewasuwat N, Olson JA: Serum and liver concentrations of vitamin A in Thai fetuses as a function of gestational age. Am J Clin Nutr 32:601, 1979.
52. Shenai JP, et al: Liver vitamin A reserves of very low birth weight neonates. Pediatr Res 19:892, 1985.
53. Goodman DS, et al: Tissue distribution and metabolism of newly absorbed vitamin A in the rat. J Lipid Res 6:390, 1965.
54. Zachman RD, et al: Perinatal rat lung retinol (vitamin A) and retinyl palmitate. Pediatr Res 18:1297, 1984.
55. Shenai JP, Chytil F: Vitamin A storage in lungs during perinatal development in the rat. Biol Neonate 57:126, 1990.
56. Shenai JP, Chytil F: Effect of maternal vitamin-A administration on fetal lung vitamin-A stores in the perinatal rat. Biol Neonate 58:318, 1990.
57. Shenai JP, Chytil F: Effect of maternal dexamethasone treatment on fetal lung vitamin A stores in the perinatal rat. Internat J Vit Nutr Res 64:93, 1993.
58. Tarjan R, et al: The effect of different factors on the composition of human milk during lactation. Nutr Diet 7:136, 1965.
59. Lesher M, et al: Human milk studies, XXVI: vitamin A and carotenoid contents of colostrum and mature human milk. Am J Dis Child 70:182, 1945.
60. Hrubetz MC, et al: Studies on carotenoid metabolism, V: the effects of a high vitamin A intake on the composition of human milk. J Nutr 29:245, 1945.
61. Ajans ZA, et al: Influence of vitamin A on human colostrum and early milk. Am J Clin Nutr 17:139, 1965.
62. Chanda R, et al: The composition of human milk with special reference to the relation between phosphorus partition and phosphatase and to the partition of certain vitamins. Br J Nutr 5:228, 1951.
63. Gebre-Medhin M, et al: Breast milk composition in Ethiopian and Swedish mothers: I, vitamin A and β-carotene. Am J Clin Nutr 29:441, 1976.
64. Thomas MR, et al: Vitamin A and vitamin E concentrations of the milk from mothers of preterm infants and milk of mothers of full term infants. Acta Vitaminol Enzymol 3:135, 1981.
65. Chappell JE, et al: Vitamin A and E content of human milk at early stages of lactation. Early Hum Dev 11:157, 1985.
66. Vaisman N, et al: Vitamin A and E content of preterm and term milk. Nutr Res 5:931, 1985.
67. Thompson SY, et al: The application of chromatography to the study of the carotenoids of human and cow's milk. Biochem J 36:17, 1942.
68. Parrish DB, et al: The state of vitamin A in colostrum and in milk. J Biol Chem 167:673, 1947.
69. Fujita A, Kimura K: An improved micromethod for fractional determination of vitamin A alcohol and ester and the changes in both types of vitamin A in blood plasma, milk and liver after loading with both types of the vitamin and β-carotene. J Vitaminol 6:6, 1960.
70. Vahlquist A, Nilsson S: Mechanisms for vitamin A transfer from blood to milk in rhesus monkeys. J Nutr 109:1456, 1979.
71. Denne SC, et al: Nutrition and metabolism in the high-risk neonate: enteral nutrition. In Fanaroff AA, Martin RJ (eds): Neonatal-Perinatal Medicine: Diseases of the Fetus and Infant. Vol 1, 7th ed. St. Louis, Mosby, 2002, p 578.
72. Ong DE: A novel retinol-binding protein from rat: purification and partial characterization. J Biol Chem 259:1476, 1984.
73. Crow JA, Ong DE: Cell-specific immunohistochemical localization of a cellular retinol-binding protein (type two) in the small intestine of rat. Proc Natl Acad Sci USA 82:4707, 1985.
74. Ong DE, Page DL: Cellular retinol-binding protein (type two) is abundant in human small intestine. J Lipid Res 28:739, 1987.
75. Heird WC, Gomez MR: Parenteral nutrition. In Tsang RC, et al (eds): Nutritional Needs of the Preterm Infant: Scientific Basis and Practical Guidelines. Baltimore, Williams and Wilkins, 1993, p 225.
76. Hartline JV, Zachman RD: Vitamin A delivery in total parenteral nutrition solution. Pediatrics 58:448, 1976.
77. Howard L, et al: Vitamin A deficiency from long-term parenteral nutrition. Ann Intern Med 93:576, 1980.
78. Shenai JP, et al: Vitamin A delivery from parenteral alimentation solution. J Pediatr 99:661, 1981.
79. Gillis J, et al: Delivery of vitamins A, D, and E in total parenteral nutrition solutions. J Parenteral Enteral Nutr 7:11, 1983.
80. Greene HL, et al: Persistently low blood retinol levels during and after parenteral feeding of very low birth weight infants: examination of losses into intravenous administration sets and a method of prevention by addition to a lipid emulsion. Pediatrics 79:894, 1987.
81. Wolbach SB, Howe PR: Tissue changes following deprivation of fat-soluble vitamin A. J Exp Med 42:753, 1925.
82. Wong YC, Buck RC: An electron microscopic study of metaplasia of the rat tracheal epithelium in vitamin A deficiency. Lab Invest 24:55, 1971.
83. McDowell EM, et al: Effects of vitamin A-deprivation on hamster tracheal epithelium: a quantitative morphologic study. Virchows Arch Pathol 45:197, 1984.
84. Wolbach SB, Howe PR: Epithelial repair in recovery from vitamin A deficiency. J Exp Med 57:511, 1933.
85. McDowell EM, et al: Restoration of mucociliary tracheal epithelium following deprivation of vitamin A: a quantitative morphologic study. Virchows Arch Pathol 45:221, 1984.
86. Northway WH Jr, et al: Pulmonary disease following respirator therapy of hyaline-membrane disease: bronchopulmonary dysplasia. N Engl J Med 276:357, 1967.
87. Stahlman MT, Gray ME: Lung injury and repair in the neonate. In Brigham KL, Stahlman MT (eds): Respiratory Distress Syndromes: Molecules to Man. Nashville, Vanderbilt University Press, 1990, p 3.
88. Hustead VA, et al: Relationship of vitamin A (retinol) status to lung disease in the preterm infant. J Pediatr 105:610, 1984.
89. Shenai JP, et al: Vitamin A status of neonates with bronchopulmonary dysplasia. Pediatr Res 19:185, 1985.
90. Shenai JP, et al: Plasma retinol-binding protein response to vitamin A administration in infants susceptible to bronchopulmonary dysplasia. J Pediatr 116:607, 1990.
91. Shenai JP, et al: Sequential evaluation of plasma retinol-binding protein response to vitamin A administration in very-low-birth-weight neonates. Biochem Mol Med 54:67, 1995.
92. Shenai JP, et al: Clinical trial of vitamin A supplementation in infants susceptible to bronchopulmonary dysplasia. J Pediatr 111:269, 1987.

93. Tyson JE, et al: Vitamin A supplementation for extremely-low-birth-weight infants. N Engl J Med *340*:1962, 1999.
94. Mahoney CP, et al: Chronic vitamin A intoxication in infants fed chicken liver. Pediatrics *65*:893, 1980.
95. Farris WA, Erdman JW Jr: Protracted hypervitaminosis A following long-term, low-level intake. JAMA *247*:1317, 1982.
96. Goodman DS: Vitamin A and retinoids in health and disease. N Engl J Med *310*:1023, 1984.
97. Persson B, Tunell R, Ekengren K: Chronic vitamin A intoxication during the first half year of life: description of 5 cases. Acta Paediatr Scand *54*:49, 1965.
98. Smith FR, Goodman DS: Vitamin A transport in human vitamin A toxicity. N Engl J Med *294*:805, 1976.
99. Carpenter TO, et al: Severe hypervitaminosis A in siblings: evidence of variable tolerance to retinol intake. J Pediatr *111*:507, 1987.
100. Food and Agriculture Organization/World Health Organization: Requirement of vitamin A, thiamine, riboflavin and niacin: report of a joint FAO/WHO Expert Group. Geneva: FAO/WHO, 1967, p 362.
101. Wang SG, et al: Assessment of vitamin A supplementation in very-low-birth-weight neonates. Pediatr Res *51*:313A, 2002.
102. Shenai JP: Vitamin A supplementation in very low birth weight neonates: rationale and evidence. Pediatrics *104*:1369, 1999.
103. Ng PC:The effectiveness and side effects of dexamethasone in preterm infants with bronchopulmonary dysplasia. Arch Dis Child *68*:330, 1993.
104. Georgieff MK, et al: Effect of postnatal steroid administration on serum vitamin A concentrations in newborn infants with respiratory compromise. J Pediatr *114*:301, 1989.
105. Shenai JP, et al: Vitamin A status and postnatal dexamethasone treatment in bronchopulmonary dysplasia. Pediatrics *106*:547, 2000.

Lois H. Johnson

37 Vitamin E Nutrition in the Fetus and Newborn

Although vitamin E has been shown to be essential to maintenance of pregnancy in female rats, such a role has not been demonstrated in humans. This is perhaps because so severe a deficiency state as can be induced in experimental animals does not occur spontaneously in healthy women of childbearing age. Frank deficiency, however, is not the only concern.[1-3] There is a growing body of evidence documenting the need for protection from oxidant free radical damage throughout life.[2-9] In the case of the fetus, this involves provision of an antioxidant reserve for combating the increased production of reactive oxygen species associated with complications of pregnancy such as placental insufficiency, preeclampsia, and gestational diabetes.[9] Antioxidant reserves are also needed for protection against potential episodes of vascular compromise hypoxemia and ischemia or reperfusion during gestation, delivery, and early postnatal life, which put the fetus at risk for oxidant damage in spite of the low oxygen environment of the fetoplacental unit.[4,10]

This chapter focuses on studies related to the dependence of the human on not only an adequate supply of dietary vitamin E, but also the ability to discriminate among the four naturally occurring tocopherols (α, β, γ, and δ), to maintain at least minimal serum and tissue levels of the α form, by far the most biologically active (Table 37-1). Also discussed are the implications of the physiologic hyperlipidemia of pregnancy for tissue levels of vitamin E in the mother and fetus and the associated requirement for vitamin E in the maternal diet. Finally, this chapter addresses the importance of defining tissue levels of the vitamin in relation to membrane lipid content, composition, and metabolic function, because the need for antioxidant protection varies from tissue to tissue and during different stages of development and environmental conditions.

BRIEF HISTORY OF VITAMIN E

The semipurified diet of Osborne and Mendel (composed of casein, starch, lard, butter fat, salts, and brewer's yeast) was known to contain vitamins A, B, C, and D and to support superior growth and vigor in the laboratory rat. In the pregnant female, however, it was often associated with fetal death and resorption of the conceptus and with testicular degeneration in the young male rat. (The Osborne/Mendel diet was probably not totally deficient in vitamin E because both butter and lard are sources of α-tocopherol.) In 1922, Evans and Bishop demonstrated that the missing dietary factor, termed *factor X*, was present in wheat germ and fresh lettuce. In 1925, they suggested that this "oil of fertility" be given the name *vitamin E*. The classic 1927 monograph of Evans and Burr summarized these early years when vitamin E was recognized solely as a dietary factor necessary for fertility in the rat. The related fertility bioassay quantifies the ability of animal tissues, foods, or preparations of vitamin E to prevent fetal resorption when fed to the pregnant, vitamin E–deficient rat during the first 10 days after impregnation. It remains the standard, but no longer the only, assay for assessing *in vivo* potency of the vitamin.[11,12]

Mechanisms underlying the dependence of mammalian species and nonreproductive as well as reproductive tissues on a dietary supply of vitamin E were poorly understood for many years. In 1928, Evans and Burr described a paralysis in suckling young of mother rats fed a diet low in vitamin E, from which there was occasionally spontaneous recovery. In 1931, Pappenheimer and Goetsch described encephalomalacia in chickens fed the same semipurified diets used by Evans and Burr. In ducklings, this diet caused widespread lesions in the skeletal muscles but no sign of encephalomalacia. These nonreproductive tissue lesions, in all three species, were signs of vitamin E deficiency, but this deficiency was not recognized for another 10 years.

Progress in understanding the role of vitamin E in intermediary metabolism was greatly advanced by the 1936 report of Evans and colleagues on the isolation of an alcohol from wheat germ oil with marked vitamin E biologic activity. They assigned the chemical formula ($C_{29}H_{50}O_2$) to this oil of fertility and proposed the name α-tocopherol from the Greek *tokos*, meaning "childbirth," and *phero*, meaning "to bear or bring forth," with the suffix *ol* to indicate that the substance was an alcohol (Fig. 37-1). In 1937, the same workers isolated β-tocopherol and γ-tocopherol from other vegetable oils and made note of their lesser biologic activity. Almost simultaneously, Olcott and Emerson presented evidence that the tocopherols were effective antioxidants, as suggested by the earlier report of Olcott and Mattill on the association of inhibitols and vitamin E in lettuce oil.

In 1940, Pappenheimer demonstrated that α-tocopherol prevented the myopathy observed in ducklings fed the Evans and Burr diet, and, in the same year, Mackenzie and colleagues presented evidence that the myopathic changes found in vitamin E–deficient rabbits could be prevented by feeding α-tocopherol. They also noted that simultaneous feedings of cod liver oil and other lipids high in unsaturated fatty acids inactivated dietary vitamin E, especially in the presence of pro-oxidant ferric salts.

TABLE 37-1

Nomenclature and Food Sources of Naturally Occurring Vitamin E Compounds: RRR Isomers*

Common Name × Content† μg/mL (US Citizens, 1975)	Chemical Name	Activity Relative to α-Tocopherol (%)	Food Sources	Contribution to Total Vitamin E in US Diets: 1970s (%)
α-Tocopherol Plasma × = 9.6 RBC × = 1.4	5,7,8-Trimethyltocol	100	Nuts, seeds, wheat, rye, rice, vegetable oils, olive, safflower, sunflower Animal fat: butter	20-25
β-Tocopherol Plasma trace RBC n.d.	5,8-Dimethyltocol	25-40	Wheat germ, barley, and oats, lettuce	≤10
γ-Tocopherol Plasma × = 1.6 RBC × = 0.24	7,8-Dimethyltocol	10-20	Many vegetable oils, especially soybean, corn, and coconut	40-50
δ-Tocopherol Plasma trace RBC n.d.	8-Methyltocol	<10	Soybean, coconut, and peanut oil	~20
α-Tocotrienol Plasma trace RBC n.d.	5,7,8-Trimethyltocotrienol	40-50	Oats, barley, rye (whole cereals)	Minimal
β-Tocotrienol Unknown	5,8-Dimethyltocotrienol	~20	Palm oil	Insignificant
γ-Tocotrienol Plasma trace RBC n.d.	7,8-Dimethyltocotrienol	~10	Coconut oil	Minimal
δ-Tocotrienol Plasma trace RBC n.d.	8-Dimethyltocotrienol	<1	Rubber tree oil	None

* Among the naturally occurring tocopherol and tocotrienol RRR isomers, the most important determinants of activity are the number and position of methyl groups in the benzene ring. The fully methylated compound has the greatest biologic activity.
† Data from Chow.[84] By thin-layer chromatography, β-tocotrienol peak could not be separated from α-tocopherol peak. Based on its minimal presence in foods, plasma β-tocotrienol level is judged to be negligible.
n.d. = not detectable.
Data from references 14, 17, and 80 to 84.

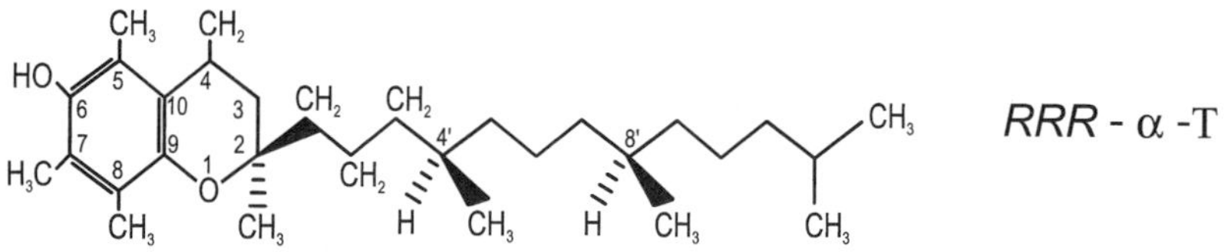

RRR - α -T

Figure 37–1. Structure of RRR α-tocopherol, the most active and abundant form of vitamin E. This schema uses the RS nomenclature for specifying configuration at the three chiral centers at carbon 2, 4′, and 8′. R = clockwise (right-handed) orientation; S = counterclockwise (left-handed) orientation; *solid triangles* = in front of the plane of the paper; *lined triangles* = behind the plane of the paper.

These observations presaged the many studies, still ongoing, addressing the importance and interrelationships of pro-oxidants, oxidant vulnerability, and antioxidant defenses during intermediary metabolism.

ESSENTIALITY OF VITAMIN E AS A CHAIN-BREAKING LIPID ANTIOXIDANT OF CELLULAR MEMBRANES

A large body of work now argues convincingly that the mechanism of action of vitamin E in curing the diverse vitamin E deficiency syndromes depends on its singular effectiveness as a biologic antioxidant, strategically located in every cellular membrane and essential for their structural integrity and function.[13-16] Subtle, radical-mediated perturbations of membrane structure can alter receptor sites, membrane functions, and membrane-bound enzyme activities. Such changes can have serious consequences in some tissues (and some species) and can leave those less vulnerable seemingly unaffected.[16-18] This

would explain much, if not all, of the variability in vitamin E deficiency syndromes among species, organs, developmental periods, dietary intake, and environmental conditions.[13-15]

For example, vitamin E–deficient rabbits typically exhibit muscular dystrophy, but, in contrast to the vitamin E–deficient rat, they have red blood cells (RBCs) that are resistant to peroxidative hemolysis. On standard laboratory chow, the rabbit RBC contains two to three times as much linoleic as arachidonic acid, the more highly unsaturated and readily oxidized of the two. In contrast, rabbit muscle contains up to four times more arachidonate than linoleate. The opposite is true of the rat. Therefore, rabbit muscle is the target tissue in tocopherol deficiency, whereas in the rat it is the RBC. Supplementing the diet of vitamin E–deficient rabbits with arachidonic acid, however, makes the rabbit RBC susceptible to oxidant damage. Specific membrane phospholipid architecture also influences the different patterns of susceptibility displayed by the rabbit and rat RBC.[19] Disruption of function in membranes deficient in vitamin E is also influenced by the physical location of α-tocopherol in the membrane,[16] the degree of local oxidative stress, and the juxtaposition and adequacy of other antioxidant defense systems.[13,15,16,18,19]

NON-ANTIOXIDANT FUNCTIONS OF VITAMIN E

Although some investigators believe that all functions of vitamin E will eventually be explainable on the basis of antioxidant properties, certain actions, especially in invertebrates and lower mammals, appear to be based on other mechanisms. These include the prevention of fetal resorption in the rat and the influence of vitamin E on the growth, phenotype, and reproduction of *Rotifera*, a freshwater metazoan.[15] Of more pertinence to higher primates and humans is the observation that α-tocopherol functions as an ionophore for potassium and rubidium ions in mitochondria but not for sodium and lithium.[15] Further, α-tocopherol and its oxidation product, α-tocopherol quinone, are specific inhibitors of sodium, potassium–adenosine triphosphatase (Na^+,K^+-ATPase) in brain microsomes.[15] Boscoboinik and colleagues[20,21] demonstrated a regulation by the tocopherols of vascular smooth muscle cell proliferation and protein kinase C activity, which is distinct from their activity as antioxidants. Other studies[22,23] observed an effect of vitamin E as an erythropoietic factor in human patients infected with human immunodeficiency virus, especially when they are treated with zidovudine. These observations lend support to the earlier suggestion of Drake and Fitch[24] that humans may have a latent requirement for vitamin E in erythropoiesis. Studies of such possible non-antioxidant functions may lead to a better understanding of the role of vitamin E nutrition during gestation.

FUNCTIONAL REQUIREMENTS FOR VITAMIN E

The earliest marker of vitamin E deficiency in the human, as in the rat, is increased hemolysis of RBCs on exposure to peroxide radicals. This can be seen before, or in the absence of, clinical anemia.[25-27] Membrane susceptibility to oxidant stress is related to the content of readily oxidized unsaturated fatty acids.[28-31] Of greater clinical importance, however, are the slowly developing signs of oxidant damage to the central and peripheral nervous system that are seen when vitamin E nutrition is inadequate for an extended period, especially if such dietary inadequacy begins soon after birth. Susceptibility of the RBC and brain to oxidant damage relates to similarities in the lipid composition of their cellular membranes. Furthermore, in the case of the RBC,[32] it also relates to their oxygen-rich, iron-rich environment and to the lability of their vitamin E content, which is readily exchanged with the vitamin E present in the high density lipoprotein (HDL) and other lipoprotein fractions of the blood.[33,34] It is of considerable clinical importance that the amount of vitamin E in the plasma, the RBC membrane, and other membranes of the body is largely determined by the overall concentration of these lipid-rich components of the blood.[35-38] The rate of equilibration between the plasma vitamin E and that of cellular membranes in different tissues varies greatly, however. For example, the content of α-tocopherol in gray matter from the frontal cortex and thalamus is highest, whereas that in gray matter from the cerebellum and spinal cord is significantly lower.[39] Depletion, when it occurs, is seen first in the cerebellum and spinal cord and last in the cerebral hemispheres and medulla and pons.[39-43] Once depleted, the content of vitamin E in the central nervous system is restored only slowly and in the reverse order. This means that tocopherol therapy for prevention or reversal of nervous system lesions must be continued indefinitely, and signs of improvement cannot be expected until long after correction of the RBC defect.

From a practical standpoint, vitamin E deficiency in humans is usually defined as a plasma ratio of vitamin E to total lipids (in mg/g) of less than 0.8, with RBC hemolysis in the standard hydro-

gen peroxide hemolysis test of greater than 10%. The recommendation for vitamin content of the diet relative to polyunsaturated fatty acid content of dietary lipids is for a vitamin E/polyunsaturated fatty acid ratio of at least 0.7 (in mg/g).[35,36,44,45] Neither of these lipid ratios is entirely satisfactory, owing to the highly variable fatty acid composition and content of dietary lipids and the difficulty in assessing the effect of dietary polyunsaturated fatty acid on membrane antioxidant requirements.[15,16,19,44,45] As discussed later, an assessment of membrane peroxidizability is the best measure of adequacy of vitamin E nutrition for the rapidly growing and differentiating tissues of the fetus and newborn. The RBC has been widely used for this purpose because of its accessibility and because the peroxide hemolysis test (despite its limitations) provides useful information and is simple to do.

HUMAN VITAMIN E DEFICIENCY SYNDROMES

In humans, none of the manifestations of vitamin E deficiency (spinocerebellar degeneration, myopathy, retinopathy, hemolytic anemia) occur in the absence of predisposing conditions such as the following: (1) prematurity coupled with feeding of formulas rich in polyunsaturated fatty acid relative to the tocopherol content,[46-49] especially if the formulas are enriched with iron; (2) chronic pathologic states that interfere with the absorption of fats and fat-soluble vitamins, such as primary biliary atresia, hepatobiliary cholestasis, and fibrocystic disease;[37,38,50-52] and (3) inborn errors of metabolism that interfere with absorption, distribution, and retention of the vitamin, such as the several abetalipoproteinemia syndromes[53-59] and the mutations in the liver α-tocopherol transfer protein, which cause isolated familial vitamin E deficiency (FIVE) and certain of the Friedreich ataxia syndromes.[60-65] Study of the disposition and metabolism of the tocopherols in these disorders has greatly advanced understanding of a complex and highly regulated system that maintains critical levels of RRR (2R, 4′R, 8′α-tocopherol) in plasma and tissues, even under conditions of dietary restriction.

PRESERVATION OF MEMBRANE: α-TOCOPHEROL

This paucity of vitamin E deficiency syndromes in humans is related not only to the widespread availability of tocopherols in diets of the world and the efficient uptake and retention of α-tocopherol in plasma and tissues, but also to the avidity with which membrane content of vitamin E is protected during oxidant stress by other biologic antioxidant systems. Except in the presence of free iron, which is a potent pro-oxidant, the tocopherol peroxy radical formed in the lipid membrane during encounters with oxidant free radicals results in neither propagation of a free radical chain reaction nor formation of the stable oxidized product, tocopherol quinone. This is the case because the tocopherol peroxy radical is returned to its original state by transfer of the radical to vitamin C and the closely linked selenium-dependent glutathione peroxidase, reduced glutathione, glutathione reductase antioxidant network.[6,13,14,39,66-73] Coenzyme Q_{10} is a lipid antioxidant that interacts directly with the aqueous phase, and it also functions to spare vitamin E.[74] Like vitamin C, it is consumed before the membrane content of vitamin E is depleted. For example, in vitamin E–deficient humans and rats, none of these plasma-based systems, the availability of urate or protein SH groups, or up-regulation of glutathione peroxidase or superoxide dismutase activity or coenzyme Q_{10} can substitute for α-tocopherol in its role as antioxidant and structural stabilizer for the complex, lipid-rich cellular membrane.[43,66-69]

These considerations underline the importance of general nutritional support for maintaining the body's antioxidant defenses. This is especially true during periods of rapid growth or illness and in the premature infant, with meager nutrient reserves. With the availability of parenteral amino acids, lipid emulsions, and pediatric multivitamin infusate, which includes generous amounts of vitamin E, the management of sick premature infants from the nutritional standpoint has greatly improved.

INTESTINAL ABSORPTION OF VITAMIN E

Vitamin E is absorbed in the upper intestine, together with digested fats, in particular, the medium chain triglycerides.[75, 76] There is an absolute requirement for micellar solubilization of unesterified vitamin E by intraluminal bile acids before it can be absorbed by the enterocyte.[37, 51] If this requirement is met, α-tocopherol and γ-tocopherol, the major forms of vitamin E in the diet, are equally well absorbed by a process of nonsaturable, non–carrier-mediated passive diffusion.[37, 45] Within the intestinal cell, re-esterified free fatty acids (FFAs), apolipoproteins, phospholipids, cholesterol, α-tocopherol, and γ-tocopherol are incorporated into chylomicrons for secretion via the lymphatics and thoracic duct into the systemic circulation.[77-79] Liver uptake of postabsorptive chylomicrons is discussed later, under plasma transport of vitamin E.

EXCRETION OF VITAMIN E

Although the liver preferentially secretes α-tocopherol in very low density lipoproteins (VLDLs) and γ-tocopherol in bile, both forms are consistently found in the bile after oral intake, with the proportion of γ to α decreasing as increasingly generous amounts of both forms are fed. Between 10 and 75% of an oral dose of vitamin E is excreted in the feces, depending on size of dose and functional health and maturity of the intestinal tract.[77] These phenomena probably explain the relative lack of toxicity of vitamin E compared with that of other fat-soluble vitamins.

SOURCES AND ACTIVITY OF VITAMIN E COMPOUNDS

Vitamin E activity is found in eight naturally occurring compounds in the tocopheryl class, all of which are derivatives of 6-chromanol. Four compounds consist of a tocol structure attached to a saturated phytyl chain, the tocol structure designated αβγδ, depending on the number and position of methyl groups on the benzene ring. Four corresponding tocols with three double bonds in the phytyl side chain are designated tocotrienols (see Table 37-1). The tocopherols have greater biologic activity than the tocotrienols on the basis of standard vitamin E activity assays. Both are widespread in plants such as nuts, seeds, oils, fruits, vegetables, grains, and grasses (mainly in an unesterified form), and they appear to play a developmental role in plant life. For example, the germinating capacity of grain is related to its tocopherol content.[80] Biogenesis of tocopherols in plants is probably through the intermediate of the trienol structure by hydrogenation.[80] Little is known about the importance of tocotrienols for human nutrition, but studies in this regard are in progress and suggest a role for the tocotrienols in suppression of epidermal growth factor and reduction of protein kinase C (α) activation.[81]

The antioxidant activity of the tocopherols and tocotrienols requires the presence of the free alcohol group on the benzene ring.[82-85] Ester forms are totally inactive as antioxidants until hydrolysis has occurred. Because the free alcohol form is highly susceptible to oxidation, commercial preparations are in the form of acetate, succinate, or nicotinate esters (Table 37-2). Ester hydrolysis occurs readily in the intestine but is only slowly accomplished after parenteral injection. In both dogs and humans, measurable levels of the ester (at least 10% of the peak 4- and 8-hour levels) are still present in the bloodstream after intramuscular administration.[86] One stable preparation of free α-tocopherol has been developed but is not commercially available.[86]

TABLE 37-2		
Biologic Activity and Stereochemical Configuration of Vitamin E Compounds		
1 mg	All-racemic-α-tocopheryl acetate 2 RS, 4′ RS, 8′ RS configuration (the synthetic mixture of four mirror image pairs) Formerly (dl)-α-tocopheryl acetate	1.0 IU*
1 mg	RRR-α-tocopheryl acetate 2R, 4′ R, 8′ R configuration (the natural stereoisomer) Formerly (d)-α-tocopheryl	1.36 IU*
1 mg	All Rac-α-tocopherol 2RS, 4′ RS, 8′ RS configuration	1.1 IU†
1 mg	RRR-α-tocopherol 2R, 4′ R, 8′ R configuration	1.49 IU†

* Activity expressed as international units (the USP standard) and based on standard biologic assays as confirmed by several investigators (rat fetal resorption, erythrocyte hemolysis, muscular dystrophy, exudative diathesis, encephalomalacia). Most of the difference in activity of the stereoisomers of α-tocopherol results from differences in the chirality at the 2 carbon position, where the phytyl tail meets the chromanol ring. For example, compared to 2RS, 4′ R, 8′ R-α-tocopherol (2 ambo α-tocopherol) and 2S, 4′ R, 8′ R α-tocopherol (2 epi-α-tocopherol, the International Standard before 1956) have about 60 and 40% activity, respectively, on the basis of the fetal resorption bioassay. Because of their greater stability, currently available commercial preparations of vitamin E are in the ester form, primarily the acetate, but also the succinate and nicotinate.
† Activity calculated on basis of molecular weight compared to the acetate form. The free alcohol forms are available only on an investigative basis.
Data from references 14, 17, 39, 60, 61, 82, and 85.

Each of the four tocopherols and the four tocotrienols can occur in eight stereoisomeric forms related to the chirality (handedness) of carbon atom 2. Only the RRR isomers occur in nature and have been shown by various assays to have significantly greater biologic activity than synthetic preparations of the other isomers. The chemical composition and configuration[39, 87] of free α-tocopherol (MW 430.66) are shown in Figure 37-1. Biologic activity of the free tocopherol alcohols is modified by the number and position of methyl groups on the benzene ring; full methylation, as in the α form, results in the greatest activity (see Table 37-1). Activity also depends on the following: the length of the phytyl side chain (shortening or absence markedly decreases activity); the chirality (stereospecificity) of carbon atom 2, in which the phytyl tail meets the chromanol ring; and, to a lesser extent, the chirality of carbon atoms 4′ and 8′ in the phytyl side chain.

Discrimination in Favor of α-Tocopherol during Intermediary Metabolism

γ-Tocopherol, 7,8-dimethyl tocopherol (MW 416.66), is the major tocopherol found in soy and corn oil. With the increasing substitution of vegetable for animal fats, γ-tocopherol now comprises 40 to 50% of vitamin E content of the average United States diet. Traditional diets of countries such as Brazil[87] contain predominantly the γ form (see Table 37-1). Because γ-tocopherol has only 10% (at most 20%) of the biologic activity of α-tocopherol, however, it makes only a modest contribution (in the range of 10 to 20%) to overall vitamin E nutrition.[83]

The greater biologic activity of RRR-α compared with that of γ-tocopherol (and the non–RRR-α isomers) results from discrimination, during normal intermediary metabolism, in favor of the α form. This discrimination does not occur in the intestine unless esterified forms are fed, in which case there is faster and more complete hydrolysis of the RRR esters.[39] The unesterified α-tocopherol/γ-tocopherol ratio in postabsorptive chylomicrons is similar to that in the diet. Once in the bloodstream, postabsorptive chylomicrons undergo triglyceride hydrolysis by action of endothelial lipoprotein lipase, with the formation of chylomicron remnants, excess surface components, and, to a small extent, FFAs and free γ-tocopherol and α-tocopherol. An interchange occurs between apoprotein E (apo E) of HDL and α-tocopherol and γ-tocopherol in excess surface components and chylomicron remnants. Subsequently, the modified remnants and down-sized chylomicrons (now containing apo E) are taken up by the liver.[60,61]

During liver uptake of chylomicrons and chylomicron remnants, a major discrimination in favor of α-tocopherol over γ-tocopherol occurs, through the action of a liver binding and transfer protein. This protein, first demonstrated in the rat,[88,89] has 10 times the affinity for α-tocopherol versus γ-tocopherol.[61,77,90] It appears to be critical in the uptake and transfer of α-tocopherol to liver organelles for incorporation into nascent VLDL for secretion into the blood. Catabolism of nascent VLDL, enriched in α-tocopherol, results in a sustained increase in the level of α-tocopherol in the plasma and subsequent tocopherol enrichment of low density lipoprotein (LDL) and HDL through interchanges between the various lipoproteins. In contrast, the increase in plasma γ-tocopherol is transitory because of its preferential excretion in the bile after liver uptake. As a result, γ-tocopherol accounts for only about 15% of vitamin E content of the plasma.[60,61,83,84,91]

Patients with the genetic vitamin E deficiency syndrome FIVE have a missense mutation in the gene that codes for this liver uptake and transfer protein.[60-63] Individuals homozygous for this defect have extremely low to undetectable levels of total vitamin E in the plasma, with the level of α-tocopherol consistently less than that required to meet critical tissue needs. As a result, signs of nervous system dysfunction (spinocerebellar degeneration) develop in the absence of any abnormality in fat absorption, lipid metabolism, or dietary deficiency; the age of onset depends on the completeness of the genetic defect. Studies in these patients have shown that the liver transfer protein discriminates not only in favor of α-tocopherol over γ-tocopherol, but also in favor of the natural RRR-α isomer over other synthetically prepared isomeric forms, for example, the 2S epimer (2S,4′R, 8′Rα-tocopherol).[60,61]

Fortunately, in patients with FIVE syndrome, moderately high doses of α-tocopherol (800 to 1200 IU/day), continued over time, can compensate for the defect in tocopherol enrichment of the VLDL.[60,61] This occurs through direct transfer of α-tocopherol in postabsorptive chylomicrons to the HDL and LDL, independent of the liver transfer protein and VLDL.

Discrimination at the Tissue Level

A further discrimination in favor of α-tocopherol occurs at the level of the RBC, brain, and spinal cord, which take up and retain RRR-α-tocopherol in preference to the γ form. As a result, the α/γ ratio in these (but not other) tissues is greater than that in the plasma.[39,91] As in the case of the liver tocopherol transfer protein, the RBC and central nervous system also retain RRR-α-tocopherol in preference to its other isomeric forms. This tissue discrimination relates to the spatial relationship of the tocopherols and their lipoprotein carriers. A moderate chiral selectivity relative to plasma is exhibited by the RBC in favor of the RRR form, presumably because of accentuation of the chiral properties of phospholipids, cholesterol, and proteins by the more structured lipid environment of the RBC, brain, and spinal cord compared with the more relaxed environment of the plasma lipoproteins.[39] As a result, α-tocopherol comprises about 87% of RBC vitamin E compared with 83% in the plasma.[84]

ROLE OF γ-TOCOPHEROL IN HUMAN NUTRITION

The importance of these relationships for the central nervous system has been demonstrated in feeding studies with α-tocopherol and γ-tocopherol and with natural RRR-α-tocopherol and its other stereoisomers. After 3 months on a low–vitamin E diet, rats fed α-tocopherol and γ-tocopherol for only 24 hours demon-

strated 15 times as much α-tocopherol (versus γ-tocopherol) in the brain and 8 times as much α-tocopherol in the adrenal gland.[91] When rats were fed only γ-tocopherol, the brain still contained 3 times as much α-tocopherol as γ-tocopherol, but the adrenal contained 10 times more γ-tocopherol than α-tocopherol.[90] Similarly, Bieri and Evarts,[83] in long-term feeding studies in rats on diets containing up to 4 times as much γ-tocopherol as α-tocopherol, reported that, after 3 months, γ-tocopherol accounted for 60% of vitamin E in adipose tissue, 50% in muscle, and 40% in kidney and spleen. It remained low in the testes (25%), liver (19%), and plasma (27%). Unfortunately, the relative content of α-tocopherol versus γ-tocopherol was not measured in the RBC or the central nervous system, which are the tissues most able to discriminate in favor of the α form.[39,40] One would predict (had they been measured) that the brain and RBC would have shown the least accumulation of γ and the greatest retention of α. This prediction is supported by studies of Ingold and colleagues,[39] in which vitamin E was provided as equal amounts of deuterated RRR and SRR α-tocopherol. All tissues discriminated in favor of the natural isomer. The greatest discrimination, however, occurred in the brain, which accumulated more than five times more deuterated RRR- than SRR-α-tocopherol, with no decrease in rate of RRR accumulation after 5 months on the diet.[39]

γ-Tocopherol and Vitamin E Nutrition in the Fetus and Young Infant

The importance of γ-tocopherol to overall vitamin E nutrition may relate to an ability to spare α-tocopherol for the brain and RBC when dietary intake of the α form is limited. This could have significance for the rapidly growing fetus and newborn, especially under conditions of marginal maternal nutrition. Bieri and Evarts[83] estimated that γ-tocopherol, when present in a diet sufficient in α-tocopherol but at a γ/α ratio of 2 to 3:1, may account for as much as 20% of the total vitamin E activity of the diet. Plasma levels of γ-tocopherol in infants fed a formula (Nutramigen) with three times as much γ-tocopherol as α-tocopherol (total tocopherol content 29.7 μmol/L) were found to have plasma levels in which the γ form contributed 15% of total plasma tocopherol.[92] Cord blood γ-tocopherol levels of infants in Japan, where the intake of soy products is high, have been reported as accounting for 13% of total tocopherols in cord blood.[93]

There is a question, however, about how much γ-tocopherol as opposed to α-tocopherol is advisable in the feedings of infants whose natural food is colostrum and breast milk, both of which are rich in α-tocopherol. At least in young infants, a small study from Japan suggests that the concentration of non-α forms should be limited, even if the amount of α-tocopherol is adequate.[93] This study compared the effect of breast and formula feedings on plasma and RBC concentrations of tocopherol. The formula used contained 2712 μg/dL of total vitamin E, of which large amounts were contributed by β-tocopherol, γ-tocopherol, and δ-tocopherol—2.4%, 45%, and 29% compared with 24% from α-tocopherol. Breast milk collected 5 to 7 days post partum had a total vitamin E content of 749 μg/dL, of which 10% was γ-tocopherol and 90% was α-tocopherol. The actual concentration of α-tocopherol in the two milks was nearly the same, 671 μg/dL for breast and 645 μg/dL for formula milk, but the total vitamin E content was more than three times higher in the latter. Surprisingly, over the first few months after birth, the mean concentration of α-tocopherol in plasma and RBC of breast-fed infants was greater ($p < .05$ for both) than in those fed formula: plasma = 786 μg/dL ± 47 SEM and RBC = 274 μg/dL packed cells ± 22 SEM, and plasma = 596 μg/dL ± 60 SEM and RBC = 154 μg/dL ± 9.4 SEM. (Non-α-tocopherol forms either were not detectable in the RBC or, possibly, were not measured because no values were given for these parameters.) Plasma total vitamin E concentrations were comparable in breast-fed and formula-fed infants at 873 versus

891 µg/dL, with non-α forms accounting for 10% (γ) of total plasma tocopherol in breast-fed and 33% (26% by γ and 7% by δ) in formula-fed infants.[92] These data suggest that, at least in the rapidly growing newborn, there may be a competition among the different vitamers[90, 92] when the amount of α-tocopherol is relatively low compared with other tocopherol forms. This, of course, amounts to yet another argument in favor of breast milk.

PLASMA LIPOPROTEINS

The principal classes of lipoproteins in the blood are the chylomicrons (density gradients <0.95), VLDLs (gradients 0.95 to 1.006), LDLs (gradients 1.006 to 1.063), HDLs (gradients 1.063 to 1.21), and very high density lipoproteins (VHDLs; gradients >1.25). Chylomicrons, on a dry weight basis, are made up of 80 to 95% triglyceride and have a protein content of only 1 to 2%; VLDLs have 40 to 80% triglycerides and 5 to 10% protein; LDLs consist of 10% triglycerides and 25% protein; and HDLs contain 1 to 5% triglycerides and 45 to 50% protein. The primary function of the lipoproteins is transport of lipids, chiefly triglycerides (chylomicrons and VLDLs) and cholesterol (LDLs and HDLs). In addition, the protein component of lipoproteins, the apolipoproteins, has important metabolic functions. The association of apolipoproteins and lipids involves the same sort of noncovalent interactions seen in membrane formation, and the components are quite free to move around, within the lipid aggregates and between different lipoproteins in the circulation. The apolipoproteins fix the general character of the aggregates but do not create exactly reproducible assemblies. Accordingly, the lipoproteins are heterogeneous mixtures that become even more heterogeneous during transit in the bloodstream.[94]

Plasma Transport of Vitamin E

Vitamin E is transported in plasma in association with lipoproteins and chylomicrons. No specific lipoprotein or lipid is solely responsible for this function. Plasma tocopherol concentration largely depends on plasma lipid concentrations, and there is a direct and high correlation between elevated (or depressed) plasma lipid levels and elevated (or depressed) plasma tocopherol levels.[33-38] In patients with primary hyperlipidemia, the lipid primarily responsible for the hyperlipidemia also carries the bulk of the tocopherol. Plasma tocopherol levels may be markedly elevated. To a lesser degree, plasma vitamin E is also elevated in obesity, diabetes mellitus, and hypothyroidism.[51, 93] A study in healthy Japanese schoolchildren found a higher plasma tocopherol level and a significantly lower RBC tocopherol level in obese children than in children of normal weight.[93]

If hyperlipidemia is complicated by impaired intestinal absorption of vitamin E, as in cholestatic liver disease, the elevated plasma lipids may compete so successfully with tissues for the limited supply of vitamin E that signs of RBC and central nervous system vitamin E deficiency appear despite plasma tocopherol levels within or above the normal range. When, however, the plasma vitamin E content is corrected for plasma lipid content, the relative deficiency in the plasma becomes evident. A tocopherol/total lipid ratio of greater than 0.8 (mg/g) has been recommended as an indication of vitamin E sufficiency that takes into account the interdependence of lipid and tocopherol concentrations.[35-38]

Influence of Apolipoproteins on the Distribution of Tocopherol in Plasma

Despite the aforementioned considerations, the distribution of tocopherol between tissue and lipid constituents of the plasma is not entirely passive and nonspecific. The tocopherol content of lipoproteins is influenced by the content of apolipoproteins,

as is clearly shown in the work of Behrens and colleagues (Fig. 37-2).[95]

The apolipoproteins are grouped into five families—A, B, C, D, and E—all of which have important but incompletely understood metabolic functions. Apo B in VLDL, for example, has a primary role in triglyceride transport. Apo C-II and A-I are activators of enzymes involved in lipolysis, lipoprotein lipase, and lecithin cholesterol acyl transferase. Apo E binds to specific liver and endothelial receptors. In adults, the Apo B lipoproteins in LDLs are primarily responsible for cholesterol transport to tissues.[78, 94] Specific LDL receptor sites are present in the plasma membranes of most cells, and cholesterol, together with vitamin E, is delivered to the cells by this mechanism.[96] HDL apolipoproteins are primarily responsible for cholesterol transport to the liver (catabolic).[94]

The different distribution of the apolipoproteins and tocopherol in the HDL and LDL of men and women, as seen in Figure 37-2, has been reported by many investigators. Considering data from men and women together, the correlation of tocopherol with lipoprotein protein is highest for HDL, lowest for LDL, and intermediate for VLDL (HDL, r = .93; VLDL, r = .72; LDL, r = .51). When men and women are considered separately, however, there is a significant correlation of tocopherol with protein (within the LDL class) in men but not in women.[95] Moreover, in a small but probably significant segment of the population, intake of vitamin E seems to influence the proportion of cholesterol carried by HDL relative to LDL.[97, 98] Such a response to increased intake of vitamin E is seen most often in young, nonobese men who have high LDL and low HDL cholesterol levels and in patients with spinal cord injury. In such people, an increased intake of vitamin E has been associated with a redistribution of cholesterol in favor of the HDL to an extent of 10 to 20%.[97, 98] The significance and mechanism of these phenomena are poorly understood, but in rabbits fed a cholesterolemic diet, supplements of vitamin E result in significantly lower concentrations of serum cholesterol, triglycerides, and VLDL than are found in rabbits not supplemented with vitamin E.[99]

Transfer of Tocopherol to Tissues

Several mechanisms have been identified by which α-tocopherol is transferred from human lipoproteins to tissue. A specific high-affinity LDL lipoprotein receptor mechanism has been shown to mediate the delivery of vitamin E from human LDL to fibroblasts.[96] LDL (and tocopherol) can be taken up and degraded by receptor-independent processes. LDL-specific receptor pathways are therefore not the only mechanism for tocopherol delivery to the tissues. For example, human chylomicrons have been shown to transfer tocopherol to human RBCs and fibroblasts during the hydrolysis of triglycerides by lipoprotein lipase. This involves binding of the lipase to the cell membrane.[38, 90, 100] Transfer of tocopherol to tissues by the HDL is less well characterized, but it is known that HDL readily transfers tocopherol to the RBC,[33, 34] and high-affinity receptors have been described for tocopherol in the RBC and adrenals.[18, 90, 101] In adults and newborns, it is probably the HDLs that are the primary means of delivery and exchange of tocopherol with RBCs, which lack LDL receptors.[101]

PATTERN OF PLASMA LIPIDS AND LIPOPROTEINS IN THE NEWBORN

Newborns have low plasma levels of total lipids, apolipoproteins, cholesterol, and tocopherol. Newborn plasma is also characterized by a relatively high content of HDLs, a low content of LDLs, and a very low content of VLDLs, which are poor in triglycerides but rich in cholesterol esters. Newborn HDLs include the subclasses HDL_2 (density gradient 1.063 to 1.092) and HDL_3 of VHDL (gradients >1.125).[102-106] These HDL lipopro-

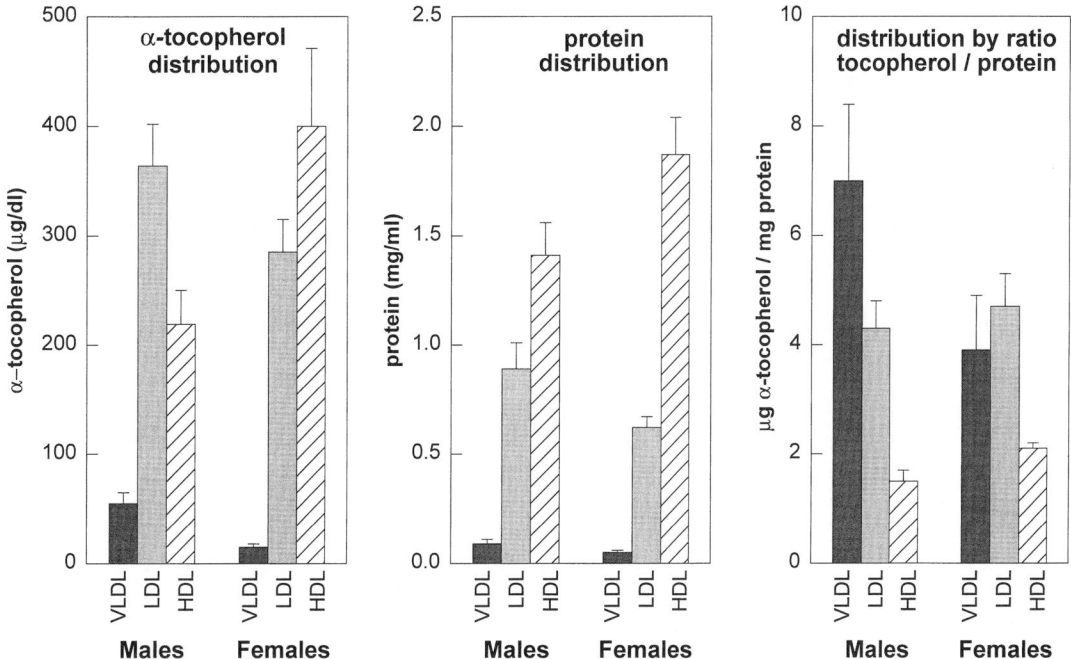

Figure 37–2. α-Tocopherol and protein content of plasma lipoproteins in healthy adults (mean ± SD total tocopherol, μg/dL plasma; males 835 ± 82; females 1035 ± 86.) As has been consistently found by others, more high density lipoprotein (HDL) than low density lipoprotein (LDL) was found in the plasma of women as compared with men in this Canadian study of healthy adults with normal lipid and cholesterol levels. The difference in distribution of tocopherol between the sexes was a reflection of the difference in protein content of the three different lipoprotein classes. Quantitatively very low density lipoproteins (VLDL) account for only a small proportion of total lipoproteins in either sex. They carry the greatest amount of tocopherol, however, relative to protein. This finding may have relevance to the adequacy of vitamin E nutrition during the hyperlipidemia of pregnancy, which is characterized by a disproportionately large increase in triglycerides and VLDL. The study population is from the Ottawa area of Canada. (Data from Behrens WA, et al: Am J Clin Nutr *35*:691, 1981.)

TABLE 37-3

Concentration and Distribution of α-Tocopherol in Red Blood Cells and the Plasma Lipoproteins of Newborns and Pregnant and Nonpregnant Women*

	Nonpregnant Women (μg/dL)	Pregnant (at Term) (μg/dL)	Newborn (Cord) (μg/dL)
Plasma tocopherol	772 ± 144	1417 ± 388	237 ± 62
RBC tocopherol (packed cells)	193 ± 22	201 ± 34	179 ± 33
VLDL tocopherol	60 ± 31 (9%)	332 ± 184 (25%)	14 ± 8 (6%)
LDL tocopherol	271 ± 58 (41%)	558 ± 197 (41%)	68 ± 20 (30%)
HDL tocopherol	331 ± 53 (50%)	454 ± 131 (34%)	143 ± 43 (64%)

* Values are mean ± SD: nonpregnant (n = 8); pregnant (n = 20); newborn (n = 20). In the newborn, 64% of plasma tocopherol is carried by the HDL, which constitutes the major lipoprotein class (>60%) in their plasma. In contrast, only 34% of plasma α-tocopherol in the mother is carried in the HDL, which accounts for a lower proportion of her total plasma lipids. The greatest increase in lipid class during pregnancy occurs in the VLDL, which also shows the greatest increase in tocopherol level. As compared with newborns and their mothers, nonpregnant women have intermediate levels of percentage of (%) distribution for all parameters. Total plasma lipid levels (mg/dL) are much lower in newborns (193 mg/dL ± 52) than in adults (pregnant, 800 ± 131 mg/dL; nonpregnant women, 389 ± 29 mg/dL; adult men, 501 ± 106 mg/dL). The % distribution of VLDL, LDL, and HDL within the total lipids is similar to the % distribution of total vitamin E among the same lipoprotein fractions. In this small sample, there was no significant difference in RBC tocopherol levels between either adult group and the newborn, probably because of the predominance in cord blood of HDL, the primary carrier for α-tocopherol to the RBC. The mean RBC tocopherol level in the newborns, however, was somewhat lower. The study population is from the Osaka area of Japan.
HDL = high density lipoprotein; LDL = low density lipoprotein; RBC = red blood cells; VLDL = very low density lipoprotein;
From Ogihara T, et al: Clin Chem Acta *174*:299, 1988.

teins[107] carry the bulk of plasma tocopherol in the newborn (Table 37–3). After birth, VLDL and LDL concentrations increase dramatically,[108] together with the triglyceride content of VLDL (Fig. 37–3). The proportions of plasma cholesterol, apo A-I, and apo A-II carried by the HDLs in cord blood are high compared with adult values.[105,106] Nevertheless, despite low levels of LDL and cholesterol in the plasma, cholesterol transport to the tissues is high.[103-106]

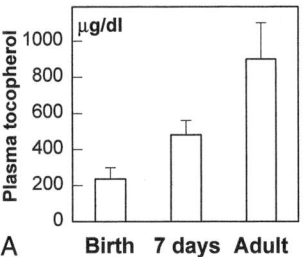

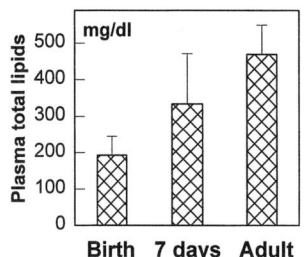

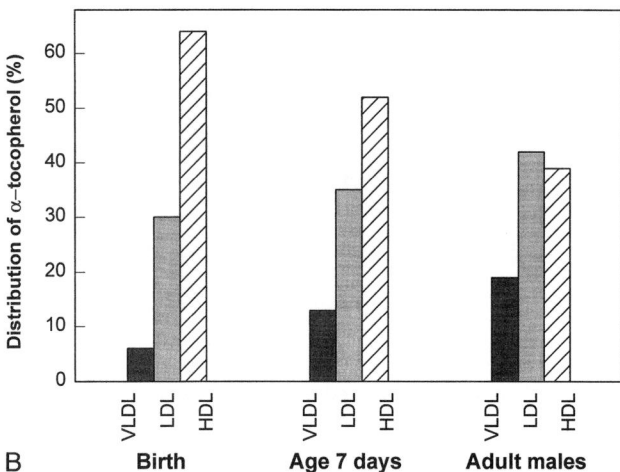

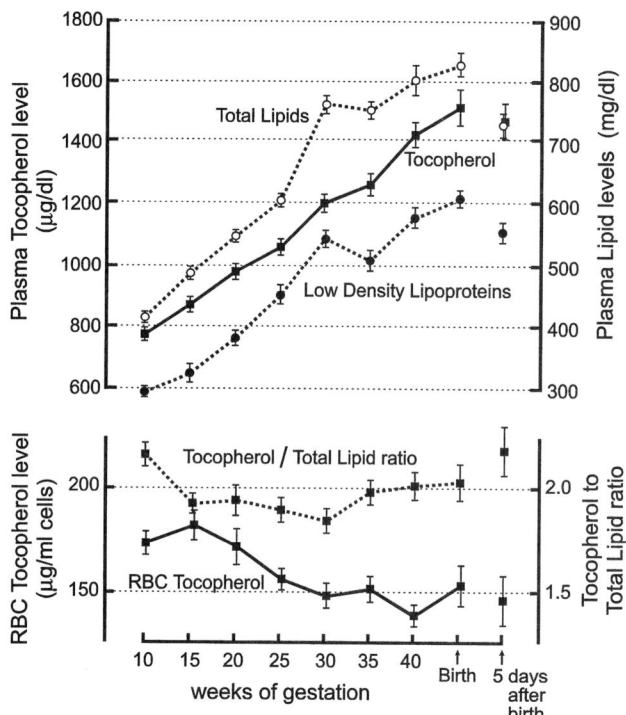

Figure 37–3. A, Age-related changes in plasma α-tocopherol and lipid concentrations. **B,** Age-related changes in distribution of α-tocopherol in plasma lipoproteins. In comparison with adults (n = 20), plasma tocopherol levels in these newborns (n = 11) were even lower than plasma lipid levels. More than 60% of plasma α-tocopherol in the cord blood was carried in the high density lipoprotein (HDL) class. In men, less than 40% of plasma α-tocopherol was carried in the HDL. Newborn very low density lipoproteins (VLDL) and low density lipoprotein (LDL) fractions increased and the HDL fraction decreased over the first 7 days after birth. Lipoprotein fractions were estimated by ultracentrifugation and total lipids by the sum of cholesterol, phospholipid, and triglycerides. The study population is from the Osaka area of Japan. (Data from Ogihara T, et al: Ann NY Acad Sci *570*:487, 1989.)

Figure 37–4. Maternal vitamin E nutrition during pregnancy. This graphic summary shows maternal red blood cell (RBC) α-tocopherol in relation to increasing maternal plasma levels of α-tocopherol, total lipid, and low density lipoproteins during gestation. The greatest relative increase in lipids occurred in the triglyceride class. Despite the rise in plasma E level and the relatively stable α-tocopherol/total lipid ratio, there is a decrease in maternal RBC α-tocopherol as pregnancy progresses. The study population is from the Osaka area of Japan. (Data from Mino M, Nagamatu M: Int J Vit Nutr Res 56:149, 1986.)

Apoprotein E in High Density Lipoprotein of the Fetus and Newborn

The enhanced transport of cholesterol to the tissues by the HDL of cord blood results from the presence of apoprotein E in HDL (not present in the HDL of most children and adults).[109,110] In the neonate, however, and in patients with abetalipoproteinemia (who lack apo-B and LDL and have plasma cholesterol levels <50 mg/dL), the HDL contains a subfraction rich in apo-E and apo E–apo A-II, which migrates with the HDL. This same HDL subfraction, rich in apo-E, is also present in many lower species. Apo-E–containing HDLs bind to apo-B, apo E receptors in fibroblasts, and many other tissues and are responsible for delivering cholesterol to cells and regulating cholesterol metabolism in a manner comparable to the LDLs. These distinctive plasma lipoprotein profiles in the fetus and newborn,[102-110] as well as the rapid changes that occur in the first weeks after birth, are poorly understood. They almost certainly have importance for the transport and delivery of nutrients to the tissues and may

also influence the prenatal and early postnatal transport of vitamin E.

Hyperlipidemia of Pregnancy

Maternal plasma lipids are elevated during pregnancy,[78, 79, 107, 108, 111, 112] and levels of total lipids, triglycerides, cholesterol, and phospholipids are significantly higher than in the neonate (Fig. 37–4). Maternofetal nutrient transfer through the placenta can be accomplished by different mechanisms, including facilitated diffusion, active transport, and simple diffusion. Simple diffusion is the most important mechanism for lipid-derived moieties. Simple diffusion is carried from a high-concentration to a low-concentration region, and the rate of movement is directly proportional to the concentration gradient. The rate of transfer is a direct function of the concentration gradient and decreases with molecular size and hydrosolubility.[78, 79, 111]

The tendency to accumulate fat ceases during late gestation because maternal lipid metabolism changes to a catabolic state. There is also hepatic overproduction of triglycerides and enhanced absorption of dietary lipids, which result in a marked progressive increase in maternal circulating triglycerides. Furthermore, during late gestation (when tissue accretion in the fetus is at a maximum), there is an associated increase in FFAs, glycerol, and triglyceride-rich VLDLs and chylomicrons.[78, 79, 111] The fetus requires not only essential fatty acids from the mother to support growth and brain development, but also nonessential

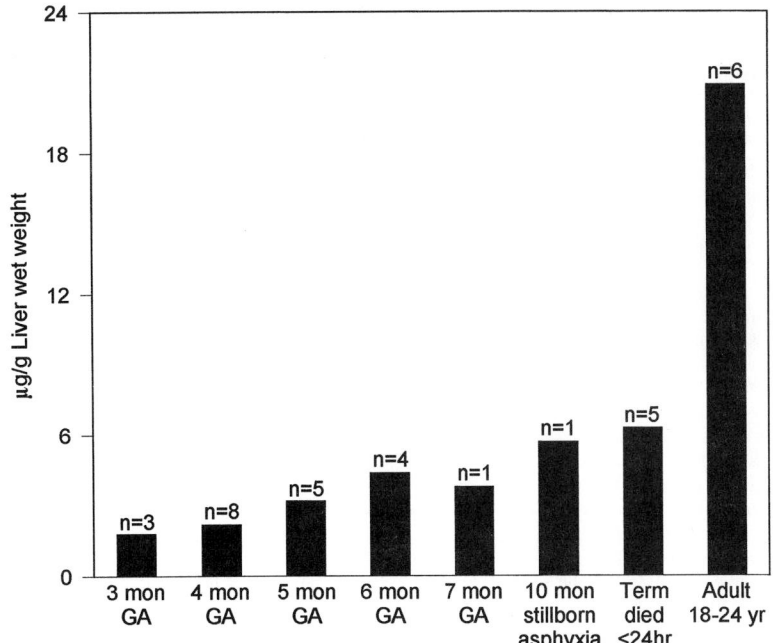

Figure 37–5. Tocopherol concentration in fetal, newborn, and adult human liver. Liver samples were obtained at autopsy after artificial interruption of normal pregnancy, after death from anencephaly or erythroblastosis fetalis on the day of delivery, or after adult accidental death. Liver tocopherol concentrations reported in two studies were in good agreement. GA = gestational age. (Data from Mino M, et al: J Nutr Sci Vitaminol 23:63, 1977; and Dju MY, et al: Etudes Neonatales 1:49, 1952.)

lipids as substrates during early postnatal life. Investigations in guinea pigs, primates, and rats indicate that the amount of fatty acids crossing the placenta exceeds that needed to fulfill lipid storage requirements. Maternal FFAs (esterified fatty acids that have been hydrolyzed at the placental level) and FFAs in unmodified lipoproteins are the potential sources of fatty acids that cross the placenta to the fetus.[78,79,111]

Differences in Fatty Acid Composition of Maternal and Fetal Plasma

Essential and nonessential fatty acids share a common transfer mechanism, regulated by the transplacental nonesterified fatty acid gradient, which consistently favors transport to the fetus. The estimated FFA transfer across the placenta is substantial, although less than for compounds such as glucose and alanine. Placental esterification of FFAs appears to be involved in one type of placental FFA transport. Although maternal circulating triglycerides contribute FFAs directly to the fetal circulation, this probably represents a minor contribution to FFA transport except in conditions of exaggerated maternal hypertriglyceridemia (e.g., in diabetic pregnancies).[111]

The fatty acid mixture entering the fetal circulation from the placenta reflects the maternal FFA concentrations of different fatty acids, with the common exception of arachidonic acid. A higher concentration of arachidonic and docosahexaenoic acid is present in cord blood compared with that in maternal plasma. The opposite is the case for linoleic acid, which is present in higher concentrations in maternal plasma.[79,111,113] The fatty acid composition of adipose tissue triglycerides in the newborn also differs from that of the mother in a manner similar to that of the plasma. Placental arachidonic acid synthesis by an active desaturation and elongation system that synthesizes arachidonic from linoleic acid is believed to be important to the supply of arachidonic acid to the fetus. Tissue enrichment in arachidonic acid plays an important role during fetal life by maintaining normal function of biologic membranes and perhaps by providing a substrate for prostaglandin biosynthesis. Although postnatal brain development is characterized by an increase in linoleic acid content, chain elongation desaturation products do not increase for several weeks, a finding suggesting that placental transfer of

polyenoic fatty acids is of primary importance in fetal accretion of these fatty acids.[79] Such transfer may be compromised under conditions of intrauterine growth restriction.

FETAL ACCUMULATION OF VITAMIN E AND FUNCTIONAL REQUIREMENTS DURING GESTATION

In a series of studies during the 1940s and early 1950s, Mason[114] and Dju and colleagues[115] demonstrated that the concentration of vitamin E, as total tocopherols, in fetal tissues was low and that concentration and body content of vitamin E gradually increased during pregnancy, with a close, direct correlation between content of tocopherol in the body, body weight, and body fat. These early studies were confirmed by Mino and colleagues[116] using more sophisticated biochemical techniques (Fig. 37-5). Despite the long-known increased susceptibility of the newborn RBC to peroxide hemolysis, a state of vitamin E deficiency in newborns has been questioned.[44,117,118] In that regard, the *milligrams total tocopherol/grams total fat* ratios present in the body of the newborn (2.7) and the adult (2.5) are comparable. This calculation does not take into account the greater proportion of unsaturated to saturated fatty acids in the plasma and membranes of newborns compared with that in adults, as described previously and shown in Table 37-4. In addition to being highly unsaturated, the lipid content of membranes in newborns is higher than in adults, in whom lipids reside, to a greater extent, in accumulations of white fat.[31,32,112,113,119]

PATTERNS OF MEMBRANE TOCOPHEROL CONTENT IN THE NEWBORN AND YOUNG INFANT

Because it is easily assessible, a large body of data has been accumulated on the uptake, retention, and functional needs of the RBC. Studies of the tocopherol content of platelets, white blood cells, and buccal mucosal cells have also provided important data, but data are fewer because of greater assay complexity and difficulty in obtaining an adequate sample size. All these studies show a decreased membrane α-tocopherol content in newborns compared with that in 1 year olds, children, and adults (Fig. 37-6).[120-124]

TABLE 37-4

Membrane Fatty Acid Constituents in Cord Maternal and Adult Red Blood Cell Ghosts

	Cord (n = 10)	Maternal (n = 7)	Adults (n = 11)
Total fatty acids (RBC) μmol/2 mg protein	3.74 ± 0.68*	3.17 ± 1.49	2.24 ± 0.41
Distribution of fatty acids			
% Saturated	54.6*	49.5	53.5
% Monounsaturated	10.9*	13.7	4.0
% Polyunsaturated	31.9*	38.4	30.7
% three or more double bonds	27.2*	20.7	20.1
Principal unsaturated fatty acids			
% Linoleic acid (18:2n-6)	4.7 ± 0.8*	12.7 ± 5.0	10.6 ± 0.9
% Dihomo γ linoleic (20:3n-6)	2.4 ± 0.3*	0.8 ± 0.4	0.8 ± 0.3
% Arachidonic (20:4n-6)	16.4 ± 2.1*	11.1 ± 1.5	11.9 ± 1.7
% Docosahexaenoic (22:6n-3)	6.9 ± 1.3*	7.7 ± 1.3	5.9 ± 1.5
Bis-allylic hydrogen atoms†			
× per fatty acid molecule	1.94 ± 0.23*	1.79 ± 0.26	1.53 ± 0.25
× per 2 mg protein	7.25 ± 1.53*	5.60 ± 2.75	3.64 ± 0.79

* $p < .05$ cord as compared to adult values. Maternal values for bis-allylic hydrogen atoms are intermediate between those for newborns and nonpregnant adults. The study population is from the Osaka area of Japan.

† Hydrogen abstraction is the initiating step in the chain reaction of lipid peroxidation. Hydrogen in the bis-allylic position —C=C—C—C=C is highly susceptible to abstraction.

Adapted from Miyake M, et al: Free Radic Res Commun *15*:41, 1991.

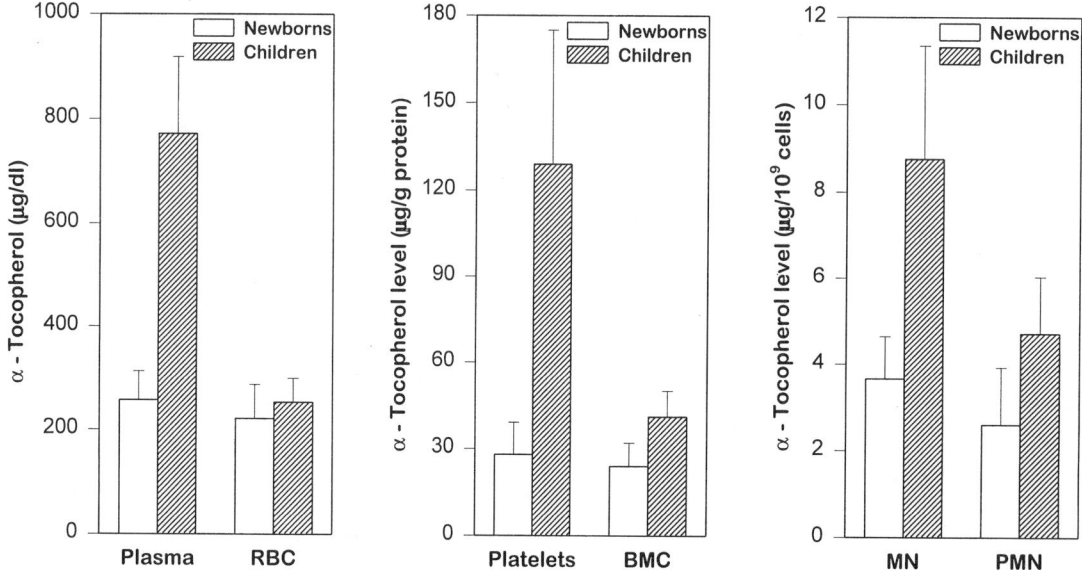

Figure 37–6. Age-related changes in α-tocopherol concentration in plasma, packed red blood cells (RBC), platelets, buccal mucosal cells (BMC), and mononuclear (MN) and polymorphonuclear (PMN) leukocytes in term newborns and children (age 3 to 16 years). The α-tocopherol level in tissues as well as in plasma was significantly lower in newborns than in children except for levels in the RBC, which were comparable. The study population is from the Osaka area of Japan. (Data from Kaempf DE, et al: Int J Vit Nutr Res *64*:185, 1994.)

Figure 37–6 shows the content of vitamin E for several accessible tissues in the newborn, including tissues with and without LDL lipoprotein receptors. All tissues show a low level of α-tocopherol compared with that in older children and adults. Of note is the low concentration of tocopherol in platelets. In human adults and rats, levels of tocopherol in platelets have been shown to reflect changes in the dietary intake of vitamin E more accurately than levels in RBCs, which, in turn, are more sensitive than plasma lipids and lymphocytes.[125] The low levels of vitamin E in platelets of the newborn probably reflect a marginally adequate supply of the vitamin.[120-125] This is suggested by the high concentrations of α-tocopherol in colostrum and breast milk, the first food of the newborn on entry to the oxygen-rich extra-

uterine environment. Breast milk feedings result in a rapid increase in blood and tissue content of vitamin E, with a peak in platelet tocopherol concentration at age 6 months, which is about the time when other foods, less rich in α-tocopherol, are added to the diet.[124]

Healthy breast-fed infants, not uncommonly, have plasma total tocopherol levels of 2.5 to 3.5 mg/dL while they are taking only milk for nourishment. Preliminary studies estimating the delivery of vitamin E to the fetus by measurement of umbilical vein–to–umbilical artery gradients indicate that, over a 24-hour period, a surprisingly large per kilogram transfer occurs to meet the demands of rapid fetal growth. The magnitude of transfer is, of course, greater during the last trimester. This finding is consistent with the much greater difficulty in maintaining plasma vitamin E levels in the sufficient range in small premature infants compared with term infants, who have significantly greater stores of the vitamin.[126-129]

IMPLICATIONS OF MATERNAL HYPERLIPIDEMIA FOR FETAL VITAMIN E NUTRITION

Need for Generous Supplies of Vitamin E in the Maternal Diet

The hyperlipidemia of pregnancy involves an increase in triglycerides in the VLDL and LDL fractions.[79, 111, 112] This increase in plasma lipids is usually associated with an increase in plasma vitamin E level such that the tocopherol/total lipids ratio is maintained above 0.8. Therefore, several laboratories have demonstrated a small decrease in the mean maternal RBC tocopherol content in the last trimester of pregnancy,[112] and in some women (as many as 30% in one study), levels of RBC tocopherol are in the deficient range (Fig. 37-7).[17] This finding suggests that in a significant number of women at term, the plasma lipids have increased their tocopherol content at the expense of the vitamin E content in the mother's RBCs. Data from a Japanese study demonstrating this relationship are shown in Figure 37-4. This finding is relevant to the observation that the concentration of α-tocopherol in maternal RBCs highly correlates with that in her fetus and newborn, after as well as before controlling for differences in lipid levels.[112, 119-121]

Effect of Fatty Acid Composition on Functional Requirements for Vitamin E

The decreased resistance to hydrogen peroxide–induced hemolysis in newborns was first described in the classic studies of Rose and Gyorgy,[25, 26] and of Gordon and colleagues,[27] and it has since been extended and confirmed by other investigators (Tables 37-5 and 37-6 and Figs. 37-8 through 37-12; see also Fig. 37-7).[28, 31, 32, 118-122] The mechanism behind this increased risk of oxidant damage (despite tocopherol RBC concentrations that are at the lower range of normal for adults) was clarified by analysis of the composition of maternal and newborn RBC membranes.[118-122] These studies made it clear that the greater

requirement for antioxidant protection of newborn and maternal RBC membranes results from their increased content of lipid, their greater complement of highly unsaturated fatty acids, and their greater number of active (bisallylic) hydrogen atoms compared with the RBCs of nonpregnant women, older children, and men.[119-121]

These important data and interrelationships are shown in Tables 37-4 through 37-6 and in Figures 37-7 through 37-12, which summarize findings from three different countries on the

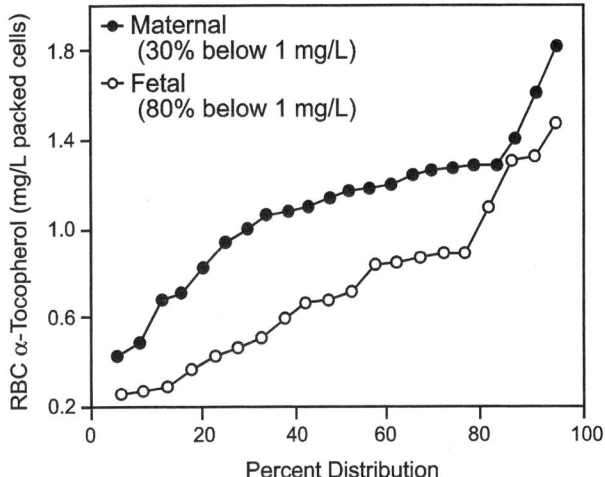

Figure 37–7. Frequency distribution of vitamin E content of centrifugation-packed red blood cells (RBC). Maternal/fetal samples were obtained during percutaneous umbilical blood sample procedures between 20 and 40 weeks' gestation for diagnosis of malformations, intrauterine growth delay, toxoplasmosis, and other viral or parasite infections. The mean RBC α-tocopherol level in these fetuses was 0.74±0.16 mg/L, which is less than the critical level for oxidant protection in the H_2O_2 hemolysis assay. The mean maternal RBC α-tocopherol level was 1.08±0.14 mg/L (i.e., 108 µg/dL). Maternal and fetal levels were significantly correlated (r = .66; p = .002). The study population is from the Montpellier area of France. (Adapted from Cachia O, et al: Am J Obstet Gynecol *173*:42, 1995.)

TABLE 37-5

Effect of Oxidant Stress on Neonatal as Compared with Adult Red Blood Cell Ghosts*

H_2O_2 (mmol/L)	0.0	0.625	0.75	1.0	1.5
α-Tocopherol (µg/mL)					
Neonate	2.27 ± 0.36	2.01 ± 0.33	1.46 ± 0.43[†]	0.60 ± 0.32[†]	0.22 ± 0.30
Adult	2.34 ± 0.34	2.08 ± 0.30	1.95 ± 0.40[†]	0.97 ± 0.31[†]	0.97 ± 0.31
α-Tocopherolquinone (µg/mL)					
Neonate	0.0	0.2 ± 0.09[‡]	0.34 ± 0.10[‡]	0.72 ± 0.14[†]	0.40 ± 0.01
Adult	0.0	0.08 ± 0.07[†]	0.18 ± 0.07[†]	0.45 ± 0.14[†]	0.75 ± 0.20
Malonyldialdehyde (nmol/mL/mL)					
Neonate	0.0	37 ± 9[‡]	37 ± 6[‡]	40 ± 8[‡]	59 ± 7[§]
Adult	0.0	14 ± 4[†]	14 ± 4[†]	14 ± 5[†]	16 ± 7[§]
% hemolysis at 8 h					
Neonate	5% ± 3%	12% ± 4[‡]	16% ± 7[§]	21% ± 10[§]	100% ± 0[§]
Adult	4% ± 1%	4% ± 1[†]	4% ± 2[§]	4% ± 10[§]	6% ± 2[§]

* Washed red blood cells (RBC) (5% hematocrit) in phosphate-buffered saline were incubated with increasing concentrations of hydrogen peroxide. Analyses were carried out after 8 hours for percentage of (%) hemolysis, concentration of α-tocopherol, α-tocopherolquinone, and malonyldialdehyde. Although RBC α-tocopherol levels were comparable in neonates and adults, the susceptibility of neonatal cells to oxidant challenge was much greater. The study population is from Brussels area, Belgium.
[†] p < .05.
[‡] p < .01.
[§] p < .001.
Adapted from Vanderpas J, Vertongen F: Blood *66*:1272, 1985.

TABLE 37–6

α-Tocopherol Levels of Red Blood Cells and Plasma in 26 Paired Mothers and Newborns at Delivery*

	Mothers	Newborns	*p* Value
RBC vitamin E nmol/mL	2.95 ± 0.13	2.77 ± 0.14	.16
Packed cells (26)† nmol/μmol total lipids (25)	0.64 ± 0.04	0.56 ± 0.03	.03
Plasma vitamin E nmol/mL (26)	26.13 ± 1.14	5.46 ± 0.41	.0001
nmol/μmol total lipids (24)	2.57 ± 0.11	1.87 ± 0.12	.0001

* The low plasma α-tocopherol levels in these New Orleans newborns were significantly below those of their respective mothers *after* as well as *before* normalization for their minimal plasma lipid concentrations. Even in these infants, however, the level of tocopherol in the red blood cell (RBC) was not significantly below that of the mother unless the greater lipid content of the newborn RBC membrane was taken into account (i.e., *after* lipid normalization). It is the greater membrane content of lipids, rich in unsaturated fatty acids, in newborn RBC that make them more susceptible to lipid peroxidation than adult RBC at any given concentration of tocopherol per mL of packed cells. Therefore, physiologic characteristics as well as tocopherol concentration determine functional adequacy of vitamin E at the tissue level.
† Number of samples given in parentheses. Values are mean ± SE (5.46 nmol/mL = 2.38 μg/mL = 238 μg/dL).
From Jain SK, et al: J Am Coll Nutr *15*:14, 1996.

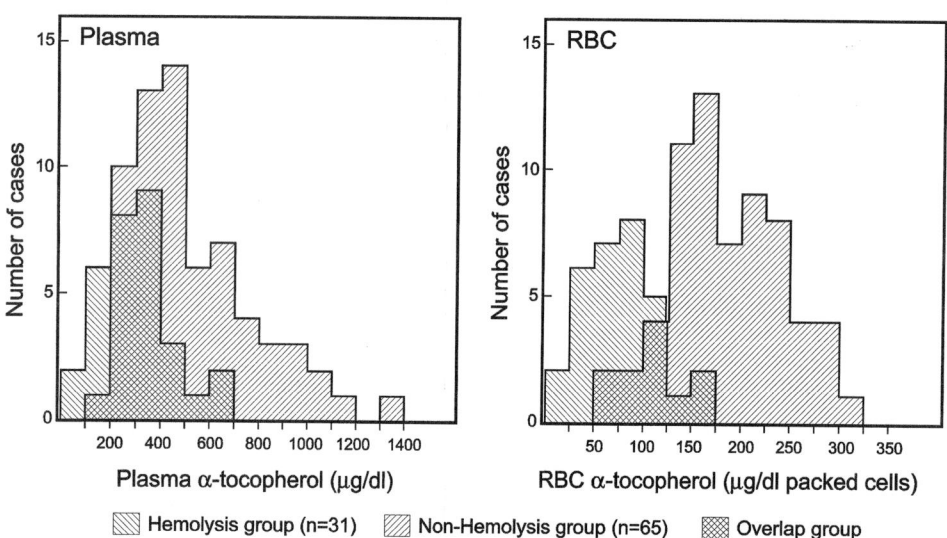

Figure 37–8. Plasma and red blood cell (RBC) α-tocopherol levels as determinants of susceptibility to oxidant stress. Samples from 96 premature and sick infants from birth to age 6 months. Under standard conditions, RBC α-tocopherol level predicts H_2O_2-induced hemolysis better than plasma α-tocopherol level (11.5 versus 25% overlap of RBC versus plasma tocopherol levels associated with presence or absence of hemolysis). The RBC level of α-tocopherol in 90% of infants in the hemolysis group was less than 125 μg/dL. Hemolysis did not occur if the RBC tocopherol level was higher than 175 μg/dL. The study population is from the Osaka area of Japan. (From Mino M, et al: Ann NY Acad Sci *393*:175, 1982.)

increased sensitivity of RBC membranes in the fetus and newborn to peroxide injury. The article by Jain and associates,[121] which is summarized in Table 37-6 and in Figures 37-9 through 37-12, describes data in 26 healthy term newborns and their mothers, from a population with low plasma levels of α-tocopherol. In this study, there were strong correlations between maternal and newborn plasma and RBC tocopherol concentrations (even without controlling for plasma lipids). Plasma α-tocopherol levels, in paired samples, also correlated significantly, but only after lipid normalization. In a much earlier study involving more than 500 infants, a significant correlation of maternal and newborn plasma vitamin E levels was found without consideration of plasma lipid content.[130]

In a study population of women (20 to 40 weeks' gestation) with higher plasma tocopherol levels who required investigation by percutaneous umbilical blood sampling, analysis of the relation between fetal and maternal plasma tocopherol concentrations showed no such correlation.[120] As in the study by Jain and

colleagues,[121] however, there were strong, consistent correlations between concentrations of α-tocopherol in maternal, fetal, and newborn RBCs. Similar data have also been reported by investigators in Japan. This consistent finding (i.e., a correlation between concentrations of tocopherol in maternal and fetal RBC membranes) is important because it means that vitamin E supplements to the mother, continued over time, can increase the content of vitamin E in the RBC membranes of the fetus.[120, 121] Presumably, this would apply to other membranes as well, in particular those of the brain and spinal cord.

In the article by Mino and colleagues,[123] which studied premature and sick term infants for the first 6 months of life, the minimum concentration of RBC α-tocopherol to prevent hemolysis in the peroxide hemolysis test was 100 to 125 μg/dL of packed cells (see Fig. 37-8). Based on these figures, the RBC tocopherol concentrations of 85% of fetuses and 15% of mothers in the study by Cachia and associates[120] mentioned earlier (see Fig. 37-7) were lower than this critical level. As

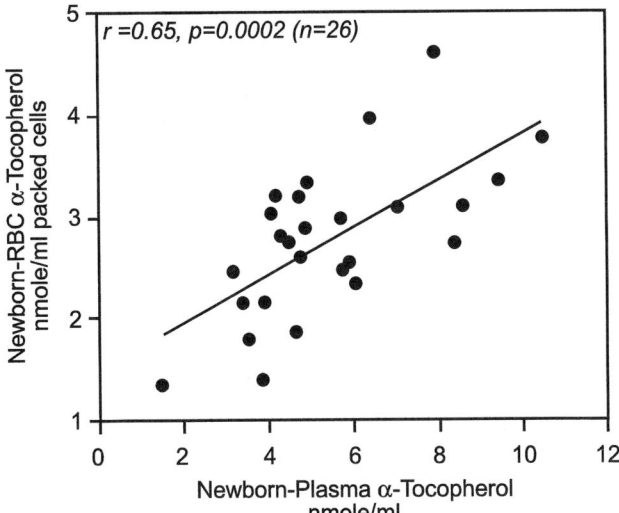

Figure 37–9. Correlation of α-tocopherol concentrations in plasma and red blood cells (RBC) of 26 term newborns. In these newborns, with a mean RBC α-tocopherol level of only 1.18 μg (2.77 nmol) per milliliter of packed cells, there was a good correlation between plasma and RBC α-tocopherol without normalization for plasma and RBC lipid level as shown, as well as with lipid normalization (RBC α-tocopherol as nmol/μmol RBC total lipid in relation to plasma α-tocopherol as nmol/μmol plasma total lipid; r = .63). The study population is from the New Orleans, Louisiana, area. (From Jain SK, et al: J Am Coll Nutr *15*:44, 1996.)

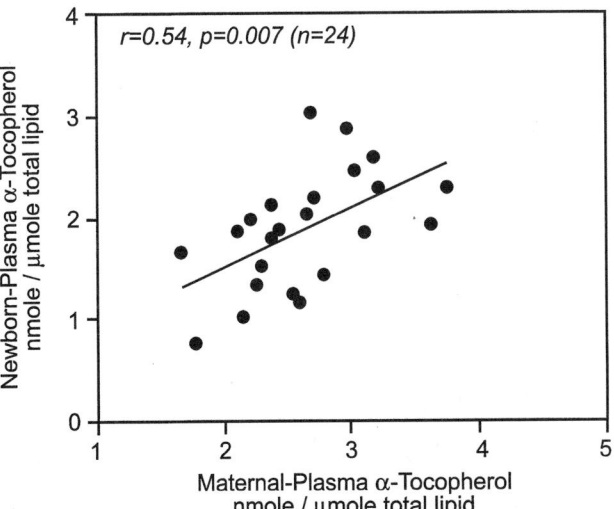

Figure 37–10. Plasma α-tocopherol concentration in 24 mother-infant pairs at term delivery. There was a good correlation between maternal and infant plasma α-tocopherol levels when expressed as nmol tocopherol/μmol total lipid. There was no correlation when levels were expressed as nmol tocopherol/mL plasma (r = .09; data not shown). The study population is from the New Orleans, Louisiana, area. (Adapted from Jain SK, et al: J Am Coll Nutr *15*:44, 1996.)

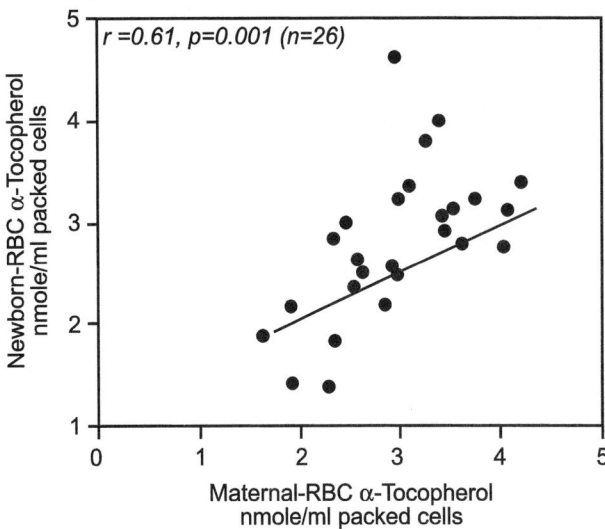

Figure 37–11. Red blood cell (RBC) α-tocopherol concentration in 26 mother-infant pairs at term delivery. As shown in this figure, there was a good correlation between newborn and maternal RBC α-tocopherol levels expressed as nmol/mL packed cells. The correlation was also present when levels were expressed as nmol/μmol total lipid (0.46; *p* = .02). The study population is from the New Orleans, Louisiana, area. (Adapted from Jain SK, et al: J Am Coll Nutr *15*:44, 1996.)

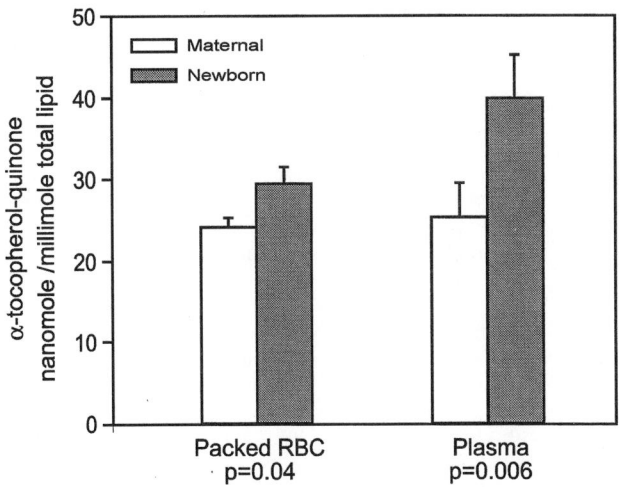

Figure 37–12. α-Tocopherol-quinone levels in 26 mother-infant pairs. Red blood cell (RBC) and plasma levels of α-tocopherol quinone, the oxidation product of α-tocopherol, were measured in mother-infant pairs at birth and were found to be significantly higher in the infant. The mean newborn RBC α-tocopherol level was 2.77±0.14 nM/mL (1.19 μg/mL); in their mothers, it was 2.95±0.13 nM/mL (1.29 μg/mL). Quinone levels in the infant did not correlate with quinone levels in the mother. Blood specimens were protected against oxidant exposure throughout the analytic procedure. The study population is from the New Orleans, Louisiana, area. (Data from Jain SK, et al: J Am Coll Nutr *15*:44, 1996.)

pointed out by the authors, because of the close correlation of the maternal and fetal RBC tocopherol content, it is reasonable to assume that supplementation of the diet of most of these mothers would have benefited the antioxidant defenses of their soon-to-be-born infants.[120]

ESTIMATES OF OXIDANT RISK

In the oxygen-rich, relatively unstable extrauterine environment, antioxidant reserve of the rapidly growing newborn is precarious, even in the absence of perinatal and neonatal complications. For example, in a population of newborns characterized by low plasma and RBC concentrations of vitamin E,[31,32] significant spontaneous peroxidative membrane lipid damage was demonstrated in fresh, untreated RBCs, not exposed to an artificial environmental stress. This peroxidative membrane damage was evidenced by levels of thiobarbituric acid reactivity, lipid fluorescence, and phospholipid:malonyldialdehyde (MDA) adduct formation twice those observed in adult cells under the same conditions. There is also evidence that, at birth, newborn RBCs with their marginal to deficient content of vitamin E exhibit increased coagulability.[31,120] Even in adults, with adequate vitamin E nutrition, decreasing platelet adhesiveness is highly correlated with increasing plasma levels of vitamin E within the physiologic range.[131] These observations may have pertinence to the hypercoagulability of the blood of newborn infants, especially sick newborn.[32,120]

The functional requirement for α-tocopherol in the brain is thought to be at least as great as that of the RBC and probably greater. Membranes of the brain and retina, especially during fetal life and early infancy, have a high lipid content and an even higher complement of highly unsaturated fatty acids, particularly docosahexaenoic acid. The lipids of retinal photoreceptors, for example, are made up of 40 to 50% docosahexaenoic acid.[79,111,132] Even a small decrement in membrane supply of vitamin E places such tissues at risk of oxidant damage. This is true during fetal life, labor and delivery, and the perinatal period because hypoxic or ischemic episodes followed by reoxygenation result in excessive production of oxidant radicals regardless of initial oxygen tensions.[133,134] In the rat, several studies have shown a protective effect of prior supplements of vitamin E on the outcome of episodes of umbilical cord clamping and release *in utero*.[135-144] A similar protective effect against hypoxia has been demonstrated in newborn rats.[135]

CONCLUSION AND FUTURE DIRECTIONS

Thus, there seems to be an absolute membrane requirement for α-tocopherol that varies from tissue to tissue and depends, to a significant extent, on composition of the diet, composition of the cellular membrane, stage of development, and metabolic, constitutional, and environmental stress. In mammals, this requirement cannot be met by any other antioxidant or antioxidant system.[39-43,66-68,74,145] In humans, the most critical requirement is that for the central nervous system, which guards the α-tocopherol content of the cerebral hemispheres, medulla, and pons.[41] Thus, deterioration of mental function[146] and of the retina[51] occurs later than deterioration of spinocerebellar function in patients with childhood cholestasis and abetalipoproteinemia. It will be interesting to observe the effect of vitamin E supplementation on the ability of patients with vitamin E deficiency, especially those with the less severe forms,[60-65] to conceive and carry a pregnancy to term. Such studies may yet identify a role for vitamin E during human gestation.

Finally, with regard to the role of vitamin E in the developing fetus, studies on the effect of metabolic gradients on generation of active oxygen metabolites suggest that these products of cellular oxidation influence gene expression during development.[147-149] Clarification of the importance of regulation of redox state on cellular differentiation and fetal development by antioxidant enzymes, unsaturated lipids, calcium, reduced glutathione, ascorbate, α-tocopherol, and β-carotene is a goal of ongoing investigations.[147-172] So, too, are the definition and pursuit of optimal nutrition during normal gestation and when gestation is complicated by pregnancy-induced hypertension, preeclampsia,[151-158] maternal diabetes,[159-165] smoking,[166-168] intrauterine growth retardation,[169-170] and perhaps premature rupture of membranes.[171] In all these conditions, an increase in reactive oxygen species in the fetoplacental unit and a decrease in fetal morbidity have been found in association with antioxi-

dant treatment. For example, in a controlled clinical trial in a population at high risk of pregnancy-induced hypertension and preeclampsia, dietary supplements of vitamins E and C, initiated at 16 to 22 weeks' gestation, were associated with a significant decrease in the incidence of preeclampsia.[157] However, pregnant women with already established, early-onset preeclampsia did not show benefit from dietary enrichment with these vitamins.[156] With regard to diabetes, numerous studies in experimental diabetic pregnant rats and in rat embryos exposed to diabetic culture media showed a marked decrease in congenital anomalies with addition of vitamins E and C to the maternal diet or to the culture media.[159-165] Such clearly beneficial effects from dietary enrichment, however, have not been found in pregnant women whose insulin-dependent diabetes is managed under current medical protocols.

Enrichment of the maternal diet with vitamin E in the naturally occurring RRR form would be ideal, especially if the fetoplacental unit is already compromised. Similar to the cellular membranes of the brain, RRR-α-tocopherol is transported across the placental membrane more efficiently than the racemic DL or any other form.[172] Nonetheless, placental transport is limited (range of 10%), so prophylactic treatment of high-risk groups must be started very early in pregnancy. As with the degenerative diseases of aging, which are compounded by the cumulative stresses of exposure to an oxygen-rich environment and aggravating diets and lifestyles, the prudent antioxidant enrichment of the mother's diet throughout gestation may enhance the health and vigor of her newborn in infancy and in adult life as well.[173-183]

ACKNOWLEDGMENTS

I would like to thank Emidio Sivieri and Donna Spitz for their help in the preparation of this chapter.

REFERENCES

1. Horwitt MK: Supplementation with vitamin E. Am J Clin Nutr 47:1088, 1988.
2. Cross CE, et al: Oxygen radicals and human disease. Ann Intern Med 107:526, 1987.
3. Lemoyne M, et al: Breath pentane analysis as an index of lipid peroxidation: a functional test of vitamin E status. Am J Clin Nutr 46:267, 1987.
4. McCord JM: Oxygen-derived free radicals in postischemic tissue injury. N Engl J Med 312:159, 1985.
5. Hartmann A, et al: Vitamin E prevents exercise-induced DNA damage. Mutat Res 346:195, 1995.
6. Brown KM, et al: Vitamin E supplementation suppresses indexes of lipid peroxidation and platelet counts in blood of smokers and nonsmokers but plasma lipoprotein concentrations remain unchanged. Am J Clin Nutr 60:383, 1994.
7. DeLorgeril M, et al: The beneficial effect of dietary antioxidant supplementation on platelet aggregation and cyclosporine treatment in heart transplant recipients. Transplantation 58:193, 1994.
8. Nyyssonen K, et al: Increase in oxidation resistance of atherogenic serum lipoproteins following antioxidant supplementation: a randomized double-blind placebo-controlled clinical trial. Eur J Clin Nutr 48:633, 1994.
9. Reaven PD, et al: Effects of vitamin E on susceptibility of low-density lipoprotein and low-density lipoproteins subfractions to oxidation and on protein glycation in NIDDM. Diabetes Care 18:807, 1995.
10. Saugstad OD, et al: Hypoxanthine and oxygen induced lung injury: a possible basic mechanism of tissue damage? Pediatr Res 18:501, 1984.
11. Evans HM: The pioneer history of vitamin E. Vitam Horm 20:379, 1962.
12. Mason KE: The first two decades of vitamin E. Fed Proc 36:1906, 1977.
13. Diplock AT: Possible stabilizing effect of vitamin E on microsomal, membrane-bound, selenide-containing proteins and drug-metabolizing enzyme systems. Am J Clin Nutr 27:995, 1974.
14. Diplock AT, et al: Relationship of tocopherol structure to biological activity, tissue uptake, and prostaglandin biosynthesis. Ann NY Acad Sci 570:75, 1989.
15. McCay PB, King MM: Biochemistry: biochemical function. In Machlin LJ (ed): Vitamin E: A Comprehensive Treatise. New York, Marcel Dekker, 1980, pp 289–312.
16. Lucy JA: Functional and structural aspects of biological membranes: a suggested role for vitamin E in the control of membrane permeability and stability. Ann NY Acad Sci 203:4, 1972.
17. Kasparek S: Chemistry of tocopherols and tocotrienols. In Machlin LJ (ed): Vitamin E: A Comprehensive Treatise. New York, Marcel Dekker, 1980, pp 8–65.

18. Kitabchi AE: Biochemistry: hormonal status in vitamin E deficiency. *In* Machlin LJ (ed): Vitamin E: A Comprehensive Treatise. New York, Marcel Dekker, 1980, pp 348–370.

19. Brin M, et al: Relationship between fatty acid composition of erythrocytes and susceptibility to vitamin E deficiency. Am J Clin Nutr 27:945, 1974.

20. Boscoboinik D, et al: α-tocopherol (vitamin E) regulates vascular smooth muscle cell proliferation and protein kinase C activity. Arch Biochem Biophys 286:264, 1991.

21. Boscoboinik D, et al: Tocopherols and 6-hydroxy-chroman-2-carbonitrile derivatives inhibit vascular smooth muscle cell proliferation by a nonantioxidant mechanism. Arch Biochem Biophys 318:241, 1995.

22. Gogu SR, et al: Protection of zidovudine-vitamin E. Exp Hematol 19:649, 1991.

23. Geissler RG, et al: In vitro improvement of bone-marrow–derived hematopoietic colony formation in HIV-positive patients by alpha-D-tocopherol and erythropoietin. Eur J Haematol 53:201, 1994.

24. Drake JR, Fitch CD: Status of vitamin E as an erythropoietic factor. Am J Clin Nutr 33:2386, 1980.

25. Gyorgy P, et al: Availability of vitamin E in the newborn infant. Proc Soc Exp Biol Med 81:536, 1952.

26. Rose CS, Gyorgy P: Specificity of hemolytic reaction in vitamin E–deficient erythrocytes. Am J Physiol 168:414, 1952.

27. Gordon HH, et al: Studies of tocopherol deficiency in infants and children. Am J Dis Child 90:669, 1955.

28. Vanderpas J, Vertongen F: Erythrocyte vitamin E is oxidized at a lower peroxide concentration in neonates than in adults. Blood 66:1272, 1985.

29. Shahal Y, et al: Oxidative stress in newborn erythrocytes. Pediatr Res 29:119, 1991.

30. Ogihara T, et al: Susceptibility of neonatal lipoproteins to oxidative stress. Pediatr Res 23:39, 1991.

31. Jain SK: Membrane lipid peroxidation in erythrocytes of the newborn. Clin Chim Acta 161:301, 1986.

32. Jain SK: The neonatal erythrocyte and its oxidative susceptibility. Semin Hematol 26:286, 1989.

33. Kayden HJ, Bjornson L: The role of vitamin E in the hematopoietic system. III. The dynamics of vitamin E transport in the human erythrocyte. Ann NY Acad Sci 203:127, 1972.

34. Kayden HJ: The transport and distribution of α-tocopherol in serum lipoproteins and the formed elements of the blood. *In* deDuve C, Hayalshi O (eds): Tocopherol, Oxygen and Biomembranes. Amsterdam, Elsevier/North Holland Biomedical Press, 1978.

35. Horwitt MK, et al: Relationship between tocopherol and serum lipid levels for determination of nutritional adequacy. Ann NY Acad Sci 203:223, 1972.

36. Horwitt MK: Status of human requirements for vitamin E. Am J Clin Nutr 27:1182, 1974.

37. Sokol RJ, et al: Mechanics causing vitamin E deficiency during chronic children cholestasis. Gastroenterology 85:1172, 1983.

38. Sokol RJ, et al: Vitamin E deficiency with normal serum vitamin E concentration in children with chronic cholestasis. N Engl J Med 310:1209, 1984.

39. Ingold KU, et al: Biokinetics of and discrimination between dietary RRR- and SRR-α-tocopherols in the male rat. Lipids 22:163, 1987.

40. Vatassery GT, et al: Concentrations of vitamin E in various neuroanatomical regions and subcellular fractions, and the uptake of vitamin E by specific areas of rat brain. Biochim Biophys Acta 792:118, 1984.

41. Vatassery GT, et al: Vitamin E concentrations in the brains and some selected peripheral tissues of selenium-deficient and vitamin E–deficient mice. J Neurochem 42:554, 1984.

42. Vatassery GT, et al: Effect of high dose of dietary vitamin E on the concentrations of vitamin E in several brain regions, plasma, liver, and adipose tissue of rats. J Neurochem 51:621, 1988.

43. Goss-Sampson MA, et al: Longitudinal studies of the neurobiology of vitamin E and other antioxidant systems, and neurological function in the vitamin E deficient rat. J Neurol Sci 87:25, 1988.

44. Bell EF, Filer LJ: The role of vitamin E in the nutrition of premature infants. Am J Clin Nutr 34:414, 1981.

45. Slagle TA, Gross SJ: Vitamin E. *In* Tsang RC, Nichols BL (eds): Nutrition During Infancy. Philadelphia, Hanley & Belfus, 1988, pp 277–288.

46. Oski FA, Barnes LA: Vitamin E deficiency: a previously unrecognized cause of hemolytic anemia in the premature infant. J Pediatr 70:211, 1967.

47. Melhorn DK, Gross S: Vitamin E–dependent anemia in the premature infant. I. Effects of large doses of medicinal iron. J Pediatr 79:569, 1971.

48. Melhorn DK, Gross S: Vitamin E–dependent anemia in the premature infant. II. Relationship between gestational age and absorption of vitamin E. J Pediatr 79:581, 1971.

49. Williams ML, et al: Role of dietary iron and fat on vitamin E deficiency anemia of infancy. N Engl J Med 292:887, 1975.

50. Sokol RJ, et al: Tocopheryl polyethylene glycol 1000 succinate therapy for vitamin E deficiency during chronic childhood cholestasis: neurologic outcome. J Pediatr 111:830, 1987.

51. Sokol RJ: The coming of age of vitamin E. Hepatology 9:649, 1989.

52. Farrell PM, et al: The occurrence and effects of human vitamin E deficiency: a study in patients with cystic fibrosis. J Clin Invest 60:233, 1977.

53. Guggenheim MA, et al: Progressive neuromuscular disease in children with chronic cholestasis and vitamin E deficiency: diagnosis and treatment with alpha tocopherol. J Pediatr 100:51, 1982.

54. Azizi E, et al: Abetalipoproteinemia treated with parenteral and oral vitamins A and E and with medium chain triglycerides. Acta Paediatr Scand 67:797, 1978.

55. Harding AE, et al: Spinocerebellar degeneration associated with a selective defect of vitamin E absorption. N Engl J Med 313:32, 1985.

56. Kayden HJ: Abetalipoproteinemia. Am Rev Med 23:285, 1972.

57. Malloy MJ, et al: Normotriglyceridemic abetalipoproteinemia: Absence of the B-100 apolipoprotein. J Clin Invest 67:1441, 1981.

58. Kayden HJ, Traber MG: Neuropathies in adults with or without fat malabsorption. Ann NY Acad Sci 570:170, 1989.

59. Sharp D, et al: Cloning and gene defects in microsomal triglyceride transfer protein associated with abetalipoproteinaemia. Nature 365:65, 1993.

60. Traber MG, et al: Impaired ability of patients with familial isolated vitamin E deficiency to incorporate α-tocopherol into lipoproteins secreted to the liver. J Clin Invest 85:397, 1990.

61. Traber MG, et al: Impaired discrimination between stereoisomers of α-tocopherol in patients with familial isolated vitamin E deficiency. J Lipid Res 34:201, 1993.

62. Ouahchi K, et al: Ataxia with isolated vitamin E deficiency is caused by mutations in the α-tocopherol transfer protein. Nat Genet 9:141, 1995.

63. Rosenberg RN: Autosomal dominant cerebellar phenotypes: the genotype has settled the issue. Neurology 45:1, 1995.

64. Ben Hamida C, et al: Localization of Friedreich ataxia phenotype with selective vitamin E deficiency to chromosome 8q by homozygosity mapping. Nat Genet 5:195, 1993.

65. Gotoda T, et al: Adult-onset spinocerebellar dysfunction caused by a mutation in the gene for the α-tocopherol-transfer protein. N Engl J Med 333:1313, 1995.

66. Burton GW, et al: Is vitamin E the only lipid-soluble, chain breaking antioxidant in human blood plasma and erythrocyte membranes? Arch Biochem Biophys 221:281, 1983.

67. Burton GW, et al: Biological antioxidants. Philos Trans R Soc Lond B Biol Sci 311:565, 1985.

68. Burton GW, Ingold KU: Vitamin E as an in vitro and in vivo antioxidant. Ann NY Acad Sci 570:7, 1989.

69. Ingold KU, et al: Vitamin E remains the major lipid-soluble, chain-breaking antioxidant in human plasma even in individuals suffering severe vitamin E deficiency. Arch Biochem Biophys 259:224, 1987.

70. McCay PB, et al: Evidence that alpha-tocopherol functions cyclically to quench free radicals in hepatic microsomes: requirement for glutathione and a heat-labile factor. Ann NY Acad Sci 570:33, 1989.

71. Miki M, et al: Synergistic inhibition of oxidation in RBC ghosts by vitamins C and E. Ann NY Acad Sci 570:474, 1989.

72. Perly B, et al: Estimation of the location of natural alpha-tocopherol in lipid bilayers by 13C-NMR spectroscopy. Biochim Biophys Acta 819:131, 1985.

73. Rotruck J, et al: Selenium: biochemical role as a component of glutathione peroxidase. Science 179:558, 1973.

74. Ingold KU, et al: Autoxidation of lipids and antioxidation by α-tocopherol and ubiquinol in homogeneous solution and in aqueous dispersions of lipids: unrecognized consequences of lipid particle size as exemplified by oxidation of human low density lipoprotein. Proc Natl Acad Sci 90:45, 1993.

75. Gallo-Torres H: Obligatory role of bile acids for the intestinal absorption of vitamin E. Lipids 5:379, 1970.

76. Hollander D, et al: Mechanism and site of small intestinal absorption of α-tocopherol in the rat. Gastroenterology 68:1492, 1975.

77. Traber MG, Kayden HJ: α-tocopherol as compared with γ-tocopherol is preferentially secreted in human lipoproteins. Ann NY Acad Sci 570:95, 1989.

78. Hamosh M: Fat needs for term and preterm infants. *In* Tsang RC, Nichols BL (eds): Nutrition During Infancy. Philadelphia, Hanley & Belfus, 1988, p 133.

79. Herrera E, et al: Placental transport of free fatty acids, glycerol, and ketone bodies. *In* Polin RA, Fox WW (eds): Fetal and Neonatal Physiology, Vol 1. Philadelphia, WB Saunders Co, 1992, pp 291–298.

80. Bauernfeind J: Tocopherols in foods. *In* Machlin LJ (ed): Vitamin E: A Comprehensive Treatise. New York, Marcel Dekker, 1980, pp 100–160.

81. Sylvester PW, et al: Vitamin E inhibition of normal mammary epithelial cell growth is associated with a reduction in protein kinase (alpha) activation. Cell Prolif 34:347, 2001.

82. Desai ID: Assay methods. *In* Machlin LJ (ed): Vitamin E: A Comprehensive Treatise. New York, Marcel Dekker, 1980, pp 68–93.

83. Bieri JG, Evarts RP: Gamma tocopherol: metabolism, biological activity and significance in human vitamin E nutrition. Am J Clin Nutr 27:980, 1974.

84. Chow CK: Distribution of tocopherols in human plasma and red blood cells. Am J Clin Nutr 28:756, 1975.

85. Weiser H, Vecchi M: Stereoisomers of α-tocopheryl acetate. II. Biopotencies of all eight stereoisomers, individually or in mixtures, as determined by rat resorption-gestation tests. Int J Vitam Nutr Res 52:351, 1982.

86. Newmark HL, et al: Biopharmaceutic factors in parenteral administration of vitamin E. J Pharm Sci 64:655, 1975.

87. McGilvery RW, Goldstein G: Citric acid cycle. *In* McGilvery RW, Goldstein G (eds): Biochemistry: A Functional Approach, 2nd ed. Philadelphia, WB Saunders Co, 1979, p 295.

88. Desai ID: Vitamin E status of agricultural migrant workers in Southern Brazil. Am J Clin Nutr 33:2669, 1980.

89. Catignani GL, Bieri JG: Rat liver α-tocopherol binding protein. Biochem Biophys Acta 497:349, 1977.

90. Sato Y, et al: Purification and characterization of the α-tocopherol transfer protein from rat liver. FEBS Lett 288:41, 1991.

91. Behrens WA, Madere R: Transport of αγ-tocopherol in human plasma lipoproteins. Nutr Res 5:167, 1985.

92. Jansson L, et al: The effect of dietary γ-tocopherol on serum tocopherols in formula-fed infants. Acta Paediatr Scand 70:297, 1981.

93. Mino M, et al: Clinical evaluation of red blood cell tocopherol. Ann NY Acad Sci 383:175, 1982.

94. McGilvery RW, Goldstein G: Storage of fats—nature and distribution of fat stores. In McGilvery RW, Goldstein G (eds): Biochemistry: A Functional Approach, 2nd ed. Philadelphia, WB Saunders Co, 1979, pp 511–544.

95. Behrens WA, et al: Distribution of α-tocopherol in human plasma lipoproteins. Am J Clin Nutr 35:691, 1982.

96. Traber MG, Kayden HJ: Vitamin E is delivered to cells via the high affinity receptor for low-density lipoprotein. Am J Clin Nutr 40:747, 1984.

97. Hermann WJ, et al: The effect of tocopherol and high-density lipoprotein cholesterol: a clinical observation. Am J Clin Pathol 72:848, 1979.

98. Barboriak JJ, et al: Plasma high-density lipoprotein cholesterol and vitamin E supplements. Ann NY Acad Sci 383:174, 1982.

99. Viswanathan M, et al: Effect of dietary supplementation of vitamin E on serum lipids and lipoproteins in rabbits fed a cholesterolemic diet. Int J Vitam Nutr Res 49:370, 1979.

100. Cohn W, Kuhn H: Role of the low density lipoprotein receptor for alpha-tocopherol delivery to tissues. Ann NY Acad Sci 570:61, 1989.

101. Kitabchi AE, Wimalasena J: Specific binding sites for D-α-tocopherol on human erythrocytes. Biochem Biophys Acta 684:200, 1982.

102. Carlson SA, Hardell LI: Very-low density lipoproteins in cord blood. Clin Chim Acta 90:295, 1978.

103. Rosseneu M, et al: Quantitative determination of the human plasma apolipoprotein AI by immunonephelometry. Clin Chem 27:856, 1981.

104. Rosseneu M, et al: Isolation and characterization of lipoprotein profiles in newborns by density gradient ultracentrifugation. Pediatr Res 17:788, 1983.

105. VanBiervliet JP, et al: Evolution of lipoprotein patterns in newborns. Acta Paediatr Scand 69:593, 1980.

106. VanBiervliet JP, et al: Plasma apoproteins and lipid patterns in newborns: influence of nutritional factors. Acta Paediatr Scand 70:851, 1981.

107. Ogihara T, et al: Distribution of tocopherol among human plasma lipoproteins. Clin Chem Acta 174:299, 1988.

108. Ogihara T, et al: Tocopherol concentrations of leukocytes in neonates. Ann NY Acad Sci 570:487, 1989.

109. Kirstein P, Carlson K: Determination of the cholesterol content of high-density lipoprotein subfractions HDL2 and HDL3, without contamination of Lp(a) in human plasma. Clin Chem Acta 113:123, 1981.

110. Innerarity TL, et al: Receptor binding activity of high-density lipoproteins containing apoprotein E from abetalipoproteinemic and normal neonate plasma. Metabolism 33:186, 1984.

111. Feldman M, et al: Lipid accretion in the fetus and newborn. In Polin RA, Fox WW (eds): Fetal and Neonatal Physiology, Vol 1. Philadelphia, WB Saunders Co, 1992, pp 299–314.

112. Mino M, Nagamatu M: An evaluation of nutritional status of vitamin E in pregnant women with respect to red blood cell tocopherol level. Int J Vitam Nutr Res 56:149, 1986.

113. Neerhout RC: Erythrocyte lipids in infants with low birth weights. Pediatr Res 5:101, 1971.

114. Mason KE: Distribution of vitamin E in the tissues of the rat. J Nutr 23:71, 1942.

115. Dju MY, et al: Vitamin E (tocopherol) in human fetuses and placentae. Etudes Neo-Natales 1:49, 1952.

116. Mino M, et al: Tocopherol level in human fetal and infant liver. J Nutr Sci Vitaminol 23:63, 1977.

117. Filer LJ Jr: Introductory remarks. Am J Clin Nutr 21:3, 1968.

118. Karp WB, Roberton AF: Vitamin E in neonatology. Adv Pediatr 33:127, 1986.

119. Miyake M, et al: Vitamin E and the peroxidizability of erythrocyte membranes in neonates. Free Radic Res Commun 15:41, 1991.

120. Cachia O, et al: The red blood cell vitamin E concentrations in fetuses are related to but lower than those in mothers during gestation: a possible association with maternal Lp(a) plasma levels. Am J Obstet Gynecol 173:42, 1995.

121. Jain SK, et al: Vitamin E and vitamin E-quinone levels in red blood cells and plasma of newborn infants and their mothers. J Am Coll Nutr 15:44, 1996.

122. Mino M, et al: Red blood cell tocopherol concentrations in a normal population of Japanese children and premature infants in relation to the assessment of vitamin E status. Am J Clin Nutr 41:631, 1985.

123. Mino M, et al: Clinical evaluation of red blood cell tocopherol. Ann NY Acad Sci 383:175, 1982.

124. Kaempf DE, et al: Assessment of vitamin E nutritional status in neonates, infants and children: on the basis of alpha-tocopherol levels in blood components and buccal mucosal cells. Int J Vitam Nutr Res 64:185, 1994.

125. Lehmann J: Comparative sensitivities of tocopherol levels of platelets, red blood cells, and plasma for estimating vitamin E nutritional status in the rat. Am J Clin Nutr 34:2104, 1981.

126. Ianni B, et al: Net placental transport of total carotenoids, retinol and tocopherols in term neonates. Pediatr Res 31:289A, 1992.

127. Ianni BD, et al: Carotenoid, retinol and tocopherol gradients in venous and arterial umbilical cord samples. J Am Coll Nutr 10:557A, 1991.

128. Johnson LH, et al: Umbilical vein to umbilical artery gradient for αγ-tocopherol at term. Pediatr Res 39:312A, 1996.

129. Kelly F, et al: Time course of vitamin E repletion in the premature infants. Br J Nutr 63:631, 1990.

130. Leonard PJ, et al: Levels of vitamin E in the plasma of newborn infants and of the mothers. Am J Clin Nutr 25:480, 1972.

131. Steiner M: Alpha-tocopherol: a potent inhibitor of platelet adhesion. J Nutr Sci Vitaminol (Tokyo) Spec No:191, 1992.

132. Berman ER: Does vitamin E have a protective role in the retina as an antioxidant and free radical scavenger? In BenEzra D, et al (eds): Ocular Circulation and Neovascularization. Lancaster, UK, Martinus Nijhoff & Dr. W. Junk Publishers, 1987, pp 163–167.

133. Bron AM, et al: Modification of vitamin E during ischemia-reperfusion in rat retina. Invest Ophthalmol Vis Sci 36:1084, 1995.

134. Yoshioka T, et al: Lipid peroxidation and vitamin E levels during pregnancy in rats. Biol Neonate 52:223, 1987.

135. Yoshioka T, et al: Protective effect of vitamin E against lipoperoxides in developing rats. Biol Neonate 51:170, 1987.

136. Iwasa H, et al: Protective effect of vitamin E on fetal distress induced by ischemia of the uteroplacental system in pregnant rats. Free Radic Biol Med 8:393, 1990.

137. Tanaka H, et al: The protective effects of vitamin E on microcephaly in rats X-irradiated in utero: DNA, lipid peroxide and confronting cisternae. Brain Res 392:11, 1986.

138. Inan C, et al: The effect of high dose antenatal vitamin E on hypoxia-induced changes in newborn rats. Pediatr Res 38:685, 1995.

139. Pinter E, et al: Fatty acid content of yolk sac and embryo in hyperglycemia-induced embryopathy and effect of arachidonic acid supplementation. Am J Obstet Gynecol 159:1484, 1988.

140. Wentzel P, et al: Diabetes in pregnancy: uterine blood flow and embryonic development in the rat. Pediatr Res 38:598, 1995.

141. Wickens D, et al: Free-radical oxidation (peroxidation) products in plasma in normal and abnormal pregnancy. Ann Clin Biochem 18:158, 1981.

142. Xie Z, Sastry BR: Induction of hippocampal long-term potentiation by α-tocopherol. Brain Res 604:173, 1993.

143. Uotila J, et al: Pregnancy-induced hypertension is associated with changes in maternal and umbilical blood antioxidants. Gynecol Obstet Invest 36:153, 1993.

144. Uotila J, et al: Lipid peroxidation products, selenium-dependent glutathione peroxidase and vitamin E in normal pregnancy. Eur J Obstet Gynaecol Reprod Biol 42:95, 1991.

145. Chan AC, et al: Regeneration of vitamin E in human platelets. J Biol Chem 226:17290, 1991.

146. Arria AM, et al: Vitamin E deficiency and psychomotor performance in adults with primary biliary cirrhosis (abstract). Hepatology 7:1118, 1987.

147. Allen RG, Venkatraj VS: Oxidants and antioxidants in development and differentiation. J Nutr 122:631, 1992.

148. Haendeler J, et al: Vitamin C and E prevent lipopolysaccharide-induced apoptosis in human endothelial cells by modulation of Bcl-2 and Bax. Eur J Pharmacol 317:407, 1996.

149. Takacs P, et al: Increased circulating lipid peroxides in severe preeclampsia activate NF-kappaB and upregulate ICAM-1 in vascular endothelial cells. FASEB J 15:279, 2001.

150. Cheeseman KH, et al: Studies on lipid peroxidation in normal and tumour tissues: the Yoshida rat liver tumour. Biochem J 250:247, 1988.

151. Iioka H: Changes in blood level of lipid peroxide and vitamin E during pregnancy: clinical significance and relation to the pathogenesis of EPH gestosis. Gynecol Obstet Invest 38:173, 1994.

152. Iioka H, et al: Changes in plasma levels of lipid peroxide and vitamin E during pregnancy. Asia Oceania J Obstet Gynaecol 17:357, 1991.

153. Mikhail MS, et al: Preeclampsia and antioxidant nutrients: decreased plasma levels of reduced ascorbic acid, alpha-tocopherol, and beta-carotene in women and preeclampsia. A J Obstet Gynecol 173:673, 1995.

154. Jain SK, Wise R: Relationship between elevated lipid peroxides, vitamin E deficiency and hypertension in preeclampsia. Mol Cell Biochem 151:33, 1995.

155. Hubel CA, et al: Increased ascorbate radical formation and ascorbate depletion in plasma from women with preeclampsia: implications for oxidative stress. Free Radic Biol Med 23:597, 1997.

156. Gulmezoglu AM, et al: Antioxidants in the treatment of severe pre-eclampsia: an explanatory randomised controlled trial. Br J Obstet Gynaecol 104:689, 1997.

157. Chappell LC, et al: Effect of antioxidants on the occurrence of pre-eclampsia in women at increased risk: a randomized trial. Lancet 354:810, 1999.

158. Gratacos E, et al: Serum and placental lipid peroxides in chronic hypertension during pregnancy with and without superimposed preeclampsia. Hypertens Pregnancy 18:139, 1999.

159. Viana M, et al: Teratogenic effects of diabetes mellitus in the rat: prevention by vitamin E. Diabetologia 39:1041, 1996.

160. Sivan E, et al: Dietary vitamin E prophylaxis and diabetic embryopathy: morphologic and biochemical analysis. Am J Obstet Gynecol 175:793, 1996.

161. Siman CM, Eriksson UJ: Vitamin E decreases the occurrence of malformations in the offspring of diabetic rats. Diabetes 46:1054, 1997.

162. Reece EA, Wu YK: Prevention of diabetic embryopathy in offspring of diabetic rats by use of a cocktail of deficient substrates and an antioxidant. Am J Obstet Gynecol 176:790, 1997.

163. Ornoy A, et al: Role of reactive oxygen species (ROS) in the diabetes-induced anomalies in rat embryos in vitro: reduction in antioxidant enzymes and low-

molecular-weight antioxidants (LMWA) may be the causative factor for increased anomalies. Teratology 60:376, 1999.

164. Zaken V, et al: Vitamins C and E improve rat embryonic antioxidant defense mechanism in diabetic culture medium. Teratology 64:33, 2001.

165. Cederberg J, et al: Combined treatment with vitamin E and vitamin C decreases oxidative stress and improves fetal outcome in experimental diabetic pregnancy. Pediatr Res 49:755, 2001.

166. Daube H, et al: DNA adducts in human placenta in relation to tobacco smoke exposure and plasma antioxidant status. J Cancer Res Clin Oncol 123:141, 1997.

167. Laskowska-Klita T, et al: Levels of lipid peroxides and of some antioxidants in placenta and cord blood of newborns whose mothers smoked during pregnancy. Med Wieku Rozwojowego 5:35, 2001.

168. Schwarz KB, et al: Peroxidant effects of maternal smoking and formula in newborn infants. J Pediatr Gastroenterol Nutr 24:68, 1997.

169. Oostenbrug GS, et al: Pregnancy-induced hypertension: maternal and neonatal plasma lipid-soluble antioxidant levels and its relationship with fatty acids unsaturation. Eur J Clin Nutr 52:754, 1998.

170. Cetin I, et al: Intrauterine growth restriction is associated with changes in polyunsaturated fatty acid fetal-maternal relationships. Pediatr Res 52:750, 2002.

171. Woods RJ Jr, et al: Vitamins C and E: missing links in preventing preterm premature rupture of membranes? Am J Obstet Gynecol 185:5, 2001.

172. Schenker S, et al: Antioxidant transport by the human placenta. Clin Nutr 17:159, 1998.

173. Poston L: Intrauterine vascular development: programming effects of nutrition on vascular function in the new born and adult. Nutr Health 15:207, 2001.

174. Delisle H: Foetal programming of nutrition-related chronic diseases. Sante 12:56, 2002.

175. Eriksson JG, et al: Effects of size at birth and childhood growth on the insulin resistance syndrome in elderly individuals. Diabetologia 45:342, 2002.

176. Young LE: Imprinting of genes and the Barker hypothesis. Twin Res 4:307, 2001.

177. Roseboom TJ, et al: Effects of prenatal exposure to the Dutch famine on adult disease in later life: an overview. Twin Res 4:293, 2001.

178. Hales CN, Barker DJ: The thrifty phenotype hypothesis. Br Med Bull 60:5, 2001.

179. Shiell AW, et al: High-meat, low-carbohydrate diet in pregnancy: relation to adult blood pressure in the offspring. Hypertension 38:1282, 2001.

180. Lumbers ER, et al: The selfish brain and the barker hypothesis. Clin Exp Pharmacol Physiol 28:942, 2001.

181. Jackson AA. Nutrients, growth, and the development of programmed metabolic function. Adv Exp Med Biol 478:41, 2000.

182. Tenhola S, et al: Serum lipid concentrations and growth characteristics in 12-year-old children born small for gestational age. Pediatr Res 48:623, 2000.

183. Yajnik C: Interactions of perturbations in intrauterine growth and growth during childhood on the risk of adult-onset disease. Proc Nutr Soc 59:257, 2000.

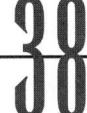

Reidar Wallin and Susan M. Hutson

Vitamin K Metabolism in the Fetus and Neonate

VITAMIN K AND BLOOD COAGULATION

Since the discovery of the pathogenesis of vitamin K deficiency in the 1950s,[1] the importance of prophylactic vitamin K in prevention of hemorrhagic disease in the fetal and neonatal periods has been debated. However, the development of sophisticated high-performance liquid chromatography systems, which can measure low levels of vitamin K and its metabolites in blood and tissues, has provided valuable new information on this subject. These measurements have shown us that placental passage of the vitamin from maternal to fetal blood is restricted.[2-5] Thus, the fetus can acquire a state of vitamin K deficiency.

It is well documented that premature infants and infants at term are all born with reduced levels of many of the essential protein factors of the hemostatic system.[6,7] Among these factors are the vitamin K-dependent clotting factors, prothrombin, Factors VII, IX, and X, protein S, and protein C.[7] Because classic hemorrhagic disease of the newborn has been treated successfully with vitamin K, it has been suggested that neonates begin extrauterine life with a vitamin K deficiency and vitamin K administration is necessary to correct the resulting imbalance of the hemostatic system.[4] Several studies contradict this assumption. Using a procedure for blood sampling *in utero,* Forestier and colleagues[8] found good correlation between procoagulant activity of the vitamin K-dependent clotting factors and the respective antigens in midtrimester fetal blood. Further evidence was the absence of PIVKA (*p*roteins *i*nduced in *v*itamin *K a*bsence) forms of the vitamin K-dependent clotting factors in their samples, a finding arguing against vitamin K deficiency in the fetus.[8] Indeed, in most studies performed on newborns, PIVKA factors have been found in minimal concentrations or are totally absent, even in low birth weight infants.[5,8-12] Thus, classic hemorrhagic disease of the newborn is likely to result from (1) malnutrition by the mother during pregnancy, (2) use of vitamin K antagonists during pregnancy, (3) exhaustion of the liver stores of vitamin K in the newborn, and (4) undefined causes of vitamin K deficiency.

Production of the vitamin K-dependent clotting factors by the liver is related to gestational age.[7,13-15] The blood concentrations of these factors in the neonate are about 30 to 60% of their concentrations in the adult, and these low values gradually increase until they reach normal adult values by 6 weeks of age.[16] Thus, the lower concentrations found in the developing neonate apparently result from immaturity in the system that produces these proteins. Because the hemostatic system requires a fine balance between coagulation on one side and fibrinolysis on the other, abnormal development of the liver system that produces the vitamin K-dependent clotting factors could contribute to hemorrhagic and thrombotic problems in the fetal and neonatal periods. Because vitamin K metabolism and vitamin K function are linked processes in the liver, this review focuses on maturation of the vitamin K-dependent γ-carboxylation system in the fetal and neonatal periods.

FUNCTION AND METABOLISM OF VITAMIN K IN LIVER

The essential steps in vitamin K metabolism and the steps targeted by the anticoagulant drug warfarin were investigated by several laboratories (for review, see ref. 17), including ours,[18-23] in the 1970s and 1980s. The naturally occurring forms of vitamin K are shown in Figure 38-1. Vitamin K_1, or phylloquinone, is found in plants. The plant vitamin is a naphthoquinone with a saturated polyisoprenoid side chain in the 3 position. Vitamin K_2, or the menaquinone family, is found in bacteria and has an unsaturated side chain of variable length in the 3 position. Vitamin K is absorbed in the small intestine and enters the lymphatic system by a process that requires the presence of both bile and pancreatic juice to allow maximum absorption.[17,24] After uptake, the vitamin is distributed ubiquitously among body tissues, but significant quantitative differences have been noted, with the liver being the major organ for uptake. Intracellularly, the vitamin has been found in membranes of mitochondria, the endoplasmic reticulum, and the Golgi apparatus.[25] Although menaquinones have been shown

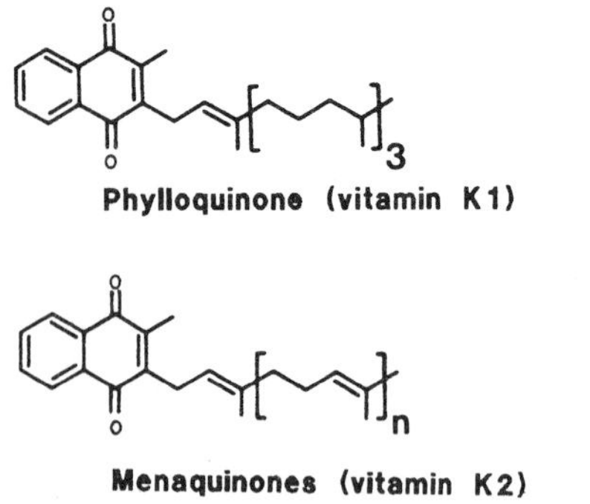

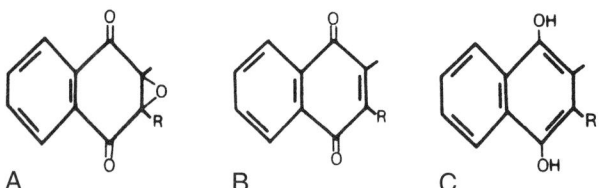

Figure 38–1. Chemical structures of phylloquinone (vitamin K_1) and menaquinones (vitamin K_2). Vitamin K_1 is found in plants. Vitamin K_2 is synthesized with a side chain of variable length by bacteria.

to promote biosynthesis of vitamin K–dependent clotting factors by the liver,[26] the bacterially produced vitamin does not contribute to fetal biosynthesis of vitamin K–dependent clotting factors. There is evidence that the infant is born with essentially no liver stores of menaquinones.[27, 28]

Several theories on the biologic action of vitamin K were proposed before the finding that vitamin K was involved in postribosomal modification of proteins. Stenflo and associates[29] identified the modification as γ-carboxyglutamic acid. Independently, Nelsestuen and co-workers[30] found the modification in a dipeptide (Glu-Ser) from prothrombin. Magnusson and colleagues[31] later showed that the first 10 N-terminal glutamic acid (Glu) residues in prothrombin are γ-carboxylated. The new amino acid formed as a result of vitamin K action was called γ-carboxyglutamic acid and was abbreviated Gla. Its structure is shown in Figure 38–2. The Gla residues bind calcium, and calcium binding by the fully γ-carboxylated clotting factors is essential for optimal activation or activity of these factors in blood.[32]

Vitamin K–dependent γ-carboxylation has been shown to require molecular oxygen, carbon dioxide, and the fully reduced form of vitamin K, vitamin K hydroquinone (Figs. 38–3 and 38–4).[17] Because the normally occurring forms of vitamin K are quinones (see Fig. 38–3), the vitamin must be reduced by liver enzymes before triggering the γ-carboxylation reaction. As illustrated in Figure 38–4, γ-carboxylation of one Glu residue is coupled stoichiometrically to formation of one molecule of the vitamin K metabolite, vitamin K 2,3-epoxide (vitamin K>O). Vitamin K>O is reduced by liver enzymes back to the hydroquinone form, which establishes a redox cycle for vitamin K in liver, known as the vitamin K cycle (see Fig. 38–4).[17, 18] Two pathways for vitamin K reduction are associated with the cycle. Pathway I is physiologically the most important pathway and operates at normal and low liver concentrations of vitamin K.[22] The enzyme involved, vitamin K epoxide reductase, catalyzes reduction of vitamin K>O and vitamin K to the active vitamin KH_2 cofactor (KH_2). The reduced thiol compound dithiothreitol is an excellent

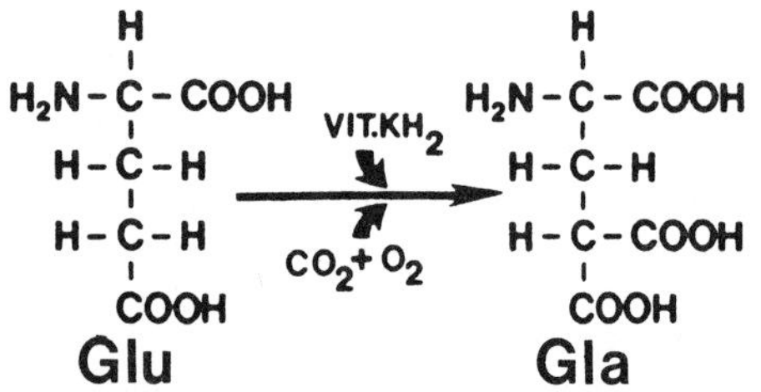

source of electrons for the enzyme-catalyzed (see Fig. 38–4) reaction. However, the thiol compound, which is active *in vivo*, has not yet been identified. It has been documented that vitamin K epoxide reductase is the target for the anticoagulant drug warfarin.[17] Thus, warfarin mediates its anticoagulant effect by preventing production of reduced vitamin KH_2 by pathway I. Inhibition of pathway I by warfarin is essentially irreversible.[33] However, vitamin K is commonly used clinically as an antidote to overcome intoxication with this drug. The antidotal effect of vitamin K is mediated by pathway II,[22] which is operative only at high liver concentrations of vitamin K. Pathway II, which is insensitive to warfarin, has been shown to consist of more than one dehydrogenase that is dependent on the reduced form of nicotinamide adenine nucleotide (NADH) to reduce the quinone form of the vitamin.[19, 20]

Since Bell and Matchiner[34] discovered the warfarin-sensitive vitamin K epoxide reductase of the vitamin K cycle in 1970, much research has focused on this important enzyme. Attempts to purify the enzyme were undertaken by many laboratories (for review, see ref. 33), but all failed because of the extreme difficulty of maintaining enzyme activity during purification. However, the carboxylase, a 92-kDa membrane protein of the endoplasmic reticulum, has been purified[35, 36] and cloned.[37] The successful isolation of the carboxylase has contributed significantly to current understanding of the mechanism by which the carboxylase participates in biosynthesis of vitamin K–dependent clotting factors.

Figure 38–3. Chemical structures of vitamin K metabolites produced by the vitamin K cycle. **A**, Vitamin K 2,3-epoxide (KO). **B**, Vitamin K quinone (K). **C**, Vitamin K hydroquinone (KH_2).

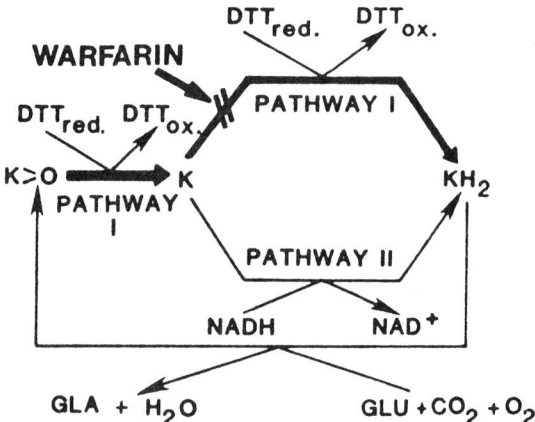

Figure 38–4. Vitamin K metabolism and vitamin K function in liver. Reduction of vitamin K epoxide (K>O) and vitamin K (K) by pathway I is catalyzed by vitamin K epoxide reductase, which requires reduced thiols (dithiothreitol; DTT) for the reaction. Pathway I is inhibited by the anticoagulant drug warfarin. Reduction of vitamin K by pathway II is catalyzed by NAD(P)H-dependent dehydrogenases. This pathway is insensitive to warfarin and mediates the antidotal effect of vitamin K. Reduced vitamin K (KH_2) triggers γ-carboxylation of glutamic acid (GLU) residues and converts them to γ-carboxyglutamic acid (GLA) residues. Formation of GLA is coupled to formation of vitamin K 2,3-epoxide (K>O).

Figure 38–2. Vitamin K-dependent synthesis of γ-carboxyglutamic acid (Gla).

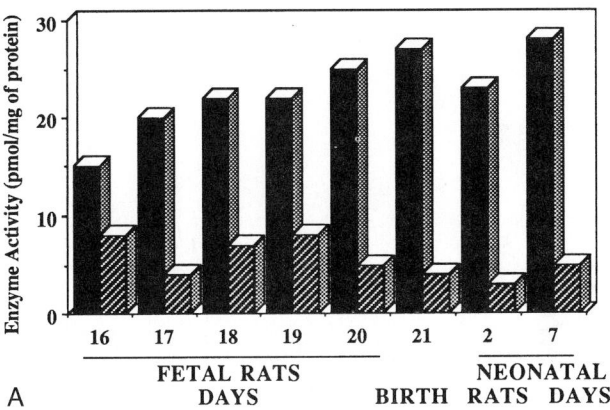

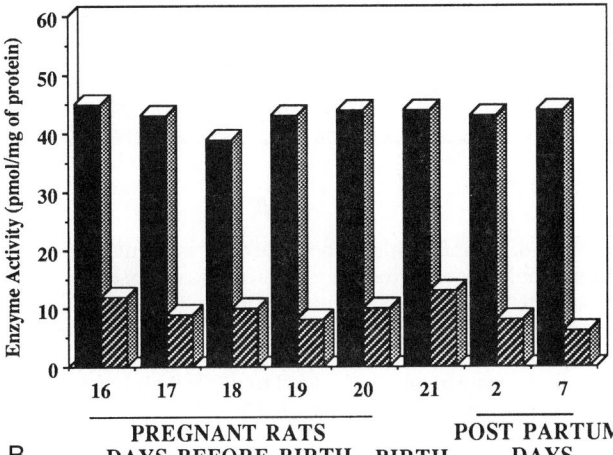

Figure 38–5. Vitamin K epoxide reductase activity in fetal, neonatal (**A**), and maternal (**B**) livers. Before determination of enzyme activity, pregnant rats were injected with saline *(solid bars)* or warfarin *(cross-hatched bars)*. (From Wallin R: Pediatr Res *26*:370, 1989.)

However, because the vitamin K epoxide reductase has not been purified, we have limited knowledge about how vitamin K metabolism is linked to operation of the carboxylase. However, studies in our laboratory have provided evidence that the vitamin K epoxide reductase is a multicomponent enzyme complex in the endoplasmic reticulum and that activity of the complex and its warfarin sensitivity is regulated by the chaperone calumenin.[38]

MATURATION OF THE VITAMIN K–DEPENDENT γ-CARBOXYLATION SYSTEM IN THE FETAL AND NEONATAL PERIODS

The available data on vitamin K metabolism and γ-carboxylation in the fetal and neonatal periods are derived primarily from the rat model. Nevertheless, in one human study,[5] plasma levels of vitamin K_1 and vitamin K_1 2,3-epoxide were measured in 133 term and 26 preterm neonates. The data indicate that the ratio of epoxide to vitamin K increases with gestational age. One possible explanation for this observation could be that maturation of pathway I takes place toward term, and this could lead to underproduction of reduced vitamin KH_2 cofactor and incomplete γ-carboxylation of the vitamin K–dependent clotting factors. Figure 38-5 shows the specific activity profile of the warfarin-sensitive pathway I enzyme, vitamin K epoxide reductase, in 16- to 20-day fetal rats, at birth (day 21), and in 2- and 7-day neonatal rats.[39] As shown, warfarin sensitivity was detected from day 16 in the fetal period, the youngest pups used in these studies. None of

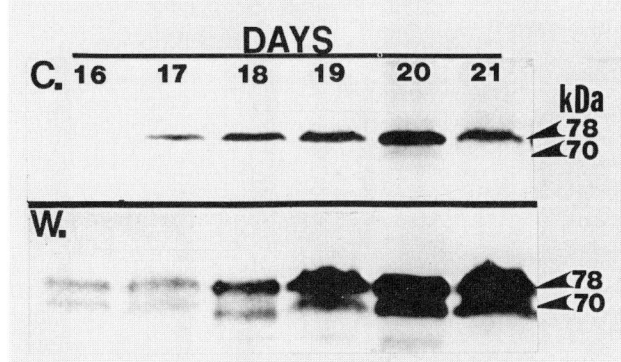

Figure 38–6. Vitamin K–dependent carbon-14 labeling of precursors of prothrombin and factor X in fetal livers. Fetal livers were isolated from day 16 to day 21 pregnant rats injected with saline (**C.**) and warfarin (**W.**). The fluorograms show the prothrombin (78-kDa) and the factor X (70-kDa) precursors. (From Wallin R: Pediatr Res *26*:370, 1989.)

the fetal livers had less than 50% of the specific activity measured in 7-day neonatal rats. These studies indicate that in the rat, significant amounts of vitamin K epoxide reductase are expressed around midterm fetal life (see Fig. 38-5A). Figure 38-5B shows this activity profile in the mothers. The prediction that emerged from the data in Figure 38-5 was that administering warfarin to the mother would affect the developing fetus. This was demonstrated by vitamin K–dependent carbon-14 labeling of prothrombin (78-kDa) and Factor X (70-kDa) precursors in fetal livers. As shown in Figure 38-6, only the pup livers from mothers that had been injected with warfarin demonstrated labeling of the Factor X precursor (70-kDa band, panel *W*), and this provides direct evidence for the effect of warfarin on the vitamin K–dependent carboxylation system.[40] Indeed, the data in Figure 38-6 demonstrate that warfarin passes the placental barrier and anticoagulates the fetus. This finding is consistent with its known effect on human fetal development wherein warfarin intake during pregnancy has been shown to result in an embryopathy characterized by stippled epiphyses, central nervous system abnormalities, optic atrophy, deafness, hypoplasia of the nasal bridge, and distal digital hypoplasia.[41]

Ontogeny of the vitamin K–dependent carboxylase and of its supporting enzymes involved in vitamin K metabolism in the rat is presented in Figure 38-7.[30] There is a dramatic increase (12-fold) in the specific activity of the vitamin K–dependent carboxylase from day 16 in the fetal period to day 7 in the neonatal period. Interestingly, and consistent with our data, Romero and colleagues[42] found, by *in situ* hybridization, that γ-carboxylase mRNA could not be detected before day 16 of fetal life. The activity increases steadily during the fetal period toward birth. At birth, the activity drops, but it increases again to reach adult enzyme activity levels in 7-day neonatal rats. These data are interesting in that human neonates often have a prolonged prothrombin time 2 to 3 days after birth.[14] Jamison and Degen[43] noted a "dip" in rat prothrombin mRNA at birth. Taken together, these data may reflect the dramatic changes in hormonal control that occur around birth,[44] and they may indeed indicate a critical point in development of the coagulation system. Figure 38-7 also shows the carboxylation "capacity" of the vitamin K–dependent carboxylation system during development, when the system is dependent on vitamin K–metabolizing enzymes to provide the reduced vitamin KH_2 cofactor. The cross-hatched bars in Figure 38-7 show carboxylation activity when triggered by pathway I (the warfarin-sensitive pathway), and the diagonal bars show this activity when triggered by the warfarin-insensitive pathway II. The activity of pathway II, which mediates the antidotal effect of vitamin K, could not be

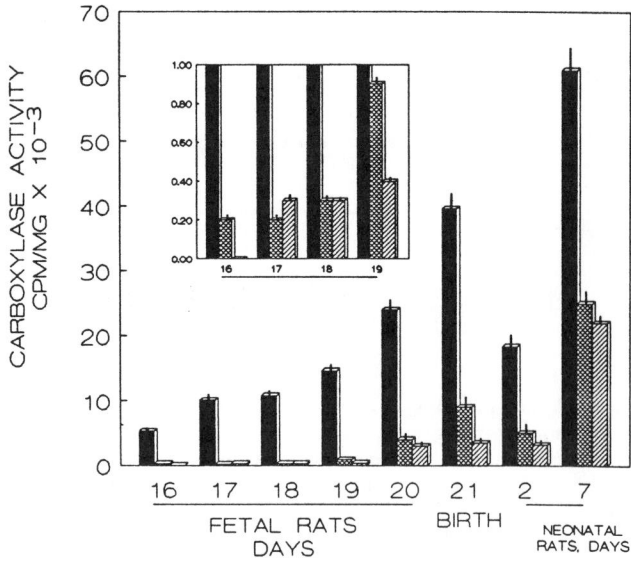

Figure 38–7. Vitamin K–dependent carboxylase activity in fetal and neonatal rat liver. Carboxylase activity was triggered with chemically reduced vitamin K_1H_2 *(solid bars)* or when supported by pathway I *(cross-hatched bars)* and by pathway II *(diagonal bars)*. (From Wallin R: Pediatr Res *26*:370, 1989.)

measured in livers from 16-day rat fetuses. This finding is supported by the observations of Wallin and Martin,[18] who demonstrated that the hepatic enzyme DT-diaphorase (Enzyme Commission number 1.6.99.2), one of the pathway II enzymes, appears late in gestation. These data suggest that vitamin K will not work as efficiently in the fetal liver as in the mature liver by treatment of warfarin intoxication. The vitamin K–dependent carboxylation system has been shown to be similar in rat and human liver.[18]

REGULATION OF DEVELOPMENT OF THE VITAMIN K–DEPENDENT γ-CARBOXYLATION SYSTEM

The stepwise emergence of many enzymes in the developing organism has been shown to be closely related to changes in the hormonal environment, and it is quite reasonable to assume that the vitamin K–dependent carboxylation system is also under the influence of such control. The appearance of enzymes during late fetal life in the rat is believed to be influenced significantly by glucocorticoid secretion and the appearance of the glucocorticoid receptor on day 18 of gestation.[45] The next profound change in the hormonal milieu takes place around birth. Shortly after birth, the insulin/glucagon ratio, which is high in the fetus, drops significantly, and this change induces another cluster of enzymes.[43] Because output of vitamin K–dependent clotting factors from liver to blood is dependent on their γ-carboxylation status in the endoplasmic reticulum,[46] factors that modulate the activities of the carboxylase and the vitamin K–metabolizing enzymes could be used to control development of the hemostatic mechanism. The only information that is available on this issue has been obtained from the rat.[47] As shown in Figure 38–8, fetal rat hepatocytes treated *in vitro* with dexamethasone express significantly higher carboxylase activity than do untreated cells. An effect of insulin on the activity could not be demonstrated. These cell culture data are supported by *in vivo* data from dexamethasone-injected rats, which documented stimulation of γ-carboxylase activity in both liver[39] and lung.[48]

Studies demonstrating dexamethasone stimulation of γ-carboxylase activity in fetal life should be extended to include studies on the effect of the drug on the activities of the vitamin

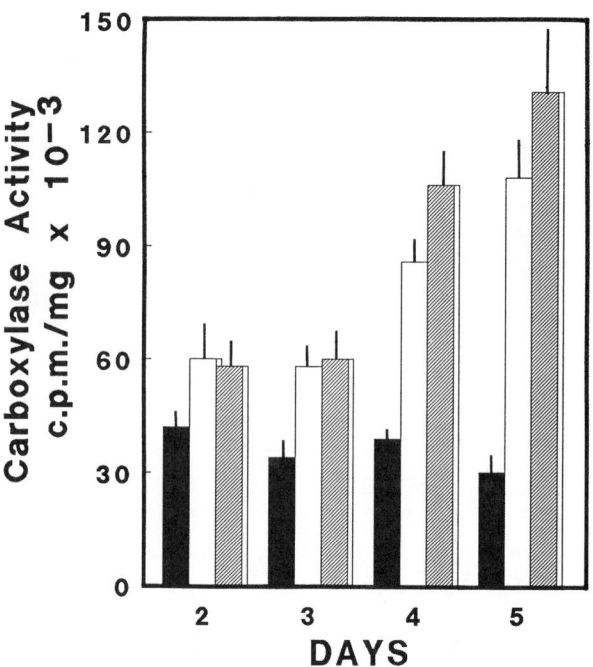

Figure 38–8. Vitamin K–dependent carboxylase activity in cultured fetal hepatocytes treated with dexamethasone. Hepatocytes from day 18 rat fetuses were cultured for 5 days in the absence *(solid bars)* and presence of dexamethasone (0.1 μM, *open bars*; 1 μM, *diagonal shaded bars*). Fresh medium with hormones was added to the cell each day. (From Wallin R, Hutson SM: Pediatr Res *30*:281, 1991.)

K-metabolizing enzymes. The lifesaving effect of dexamethasone on maturation of the lung surfactant system in premature infants (see ref. 49 for review) should stimulate research on the potential use of the drug to control maturation of the vitamin K–dependent γ-carboxylation system in premature neonates with bleeding problems that cannot be corrected by vitamin K administration.

REFERENCES

1. Kisker CT: Pathophysiology of bleeding disorders in the newborn. *In* Polin R, Fox W (eds): Fetal and Neonatal Physiology. Philadelphia, WB Saunders, 1992, pp 1381–1394.
2. Mandelbrot L, et al: Placental transfer of vitamin K_1 and its implications in fetal hemostasis. Thromb Haemost *60*:39, 1988.
3. Yang Y-M, et al: Maternal-fetal transport of vitamin K1 and its effect on coagulation in premature infants. J Pediatr *115*:1009, 1989.
4. Shearer MJ, et al: Plasmal vitamin K_1 in mothers and their newborn babies. Lancet *28*:460, 1982.
5. Bovill EG, et al: Vitamin K_1 metabolism and the production of des-carboxy prothrombin and protein C in the term and preterm neonate. Blood *81*:77, 1993.
6. Buchanan GR: Coagulation disorders in the neonate. Pediatr Clin North Am *33*:102, 1977.
7. Andrew M, et al: Development of the human coagulation system in the full-term infant. Blood *70*:165, 1987.
8. Forestier F, et al: Vitamin K dependent proteins in fetal hemostasis at mid trimester of pregnancy. Thromb Haemost *53*:401, 1985.
9. Corrigan JJ, et al: Factor II levels in cord blood: Correlation of coagulant activity with immunoreactive protein. J Pediatr *97*:979, 1980.
10. van Doorm JM, et al: Vitamin K deficiency in the newborn. Lancet *2*:708, 1977.
11. Maurer HM, et al: Effects of phototherapy on platelet counts in low birth weight infants and on platelet production and life span in rabbits. Pediatrics *57*:506, 1977.
12. Ogata T, et al: Vitamin K effect in low birth weight infants. Pediatrics *81*:423, 1988.
13. Terwiel JP, et al: Coagulation factors in the premature infant born after about 32 weeks of gestation. Biol Neonat *47*:9, 1985.
14. Dube B, et al: Hemostatic parameters in newborn. I. Effect on gestation and rate of intrauterine growth. Thromb Haemost *55*:47, 1986.
15. Kolindewala JK, et al: Hemostatic parameters in newborn. II. Sequential study during the first four weeks of life. Thromb Haemost *55*:51, 1986.
16. Lane PA, Hathaway WE: Vitamin K in infancy. J Pediatr *106*:351, 1985.

17. Suttie JW: Vitamin K. *In* Deluca HF (ed): Handbook of Lipid Research. New York, Plenum Press, 1978, pp 211-277.
18. Wallin R, Martin LF: Vitamin K-dependent carboxylation and vitamin K metabolism in liver: effects of warfarin. J Clin Invest 76:1879, 1985.
19. Wallin R, et al: Vitamin K_1 reduction in human liver: location of the coumarin drug insensitive enzyme. Biochem J 260:879, 1989.
20. Wallin R, Suttie JW: Vitamin K-dependent carboxylation and vitamin K epoxidation; evidence that the warfarin-sensitive microsomal NAD(P)H dehydrogenase reduces vitamin K in these reactions. Biochem J 194:983, 1981.
21. Wallin R: Vitamin K antagonism of coumarin anticoagulation: A dehydrogenase pathway in rat liver is responsible for the antagonistic effect. Biochem J 236:685, 1986.
22. Wallin R, Martin LF: Warfarin poisoning and vitamin K antagonism in rat and human liver: design of a system in vitro that mimics the system in vivo. Biochem J 241:389, 1987.
23. Wallin R, et al: NAD(P)H dehydrogenase and its role in the vitamin K-dependent carboxylation reaction. Biochem J 169:95, 1978.
24. Shearer MJ, et al: Studies on the adsorption and metabolism of phylloquinone (vitamin K_1) in man. Vitam Horm 32:513, 1974.
25. Nyquist SE, et al: Distribution of vitamin K among liver cell fractions. Biochim Biophys Acta 244:645, 1971.
26. Conly JM, et al: The contribution of vitamin K_2 (menaquinones) produced by the intestinal microflora to human nutritional requirements for vitamin K. Am J Gastroenterol 89:915, 1994.
27. Shirahata A, et al: Vitamin K_1 and vitamin K_2 contents in blood, stool and liver tissues of neonates and young infants. *In* Suzuki S, et al (eds): Perinatal Thrombosis and Hemostasis. New York, Springer-Verlag, 1991, pp 213-236.
28. Kayata S, et al: Vitamin K_1 and K_2 in infant human liver. J Pediatr Gastroenterol Nutr 8:304, 1989.
29. Stenflo J, et al: Vitamin K-dependent modifications of glutamic acid residues in prothrombin. Proc Natl Acad Sci USA 71:2730, 1974.
30. Nelsestuen GL, et al: The mode of action of vitamin K: identification of γ-carboxyglutamic acid as a component of prothrombin. J Biol Chem 249:6347, 1974.
31. Magnusson S, et al: Primary structure of the vitamin K-dependent part of prothrombin. FEBS Lett 44:189, 1974.
32. Furie B, Furie BC: The molecular basis of blood coagulation. Cell 53:505, 1988.
33. Suttie JW: The biochemical basis for warfarin therapy. *In* Wessler S, et al (eds): The New Dimensions of Warfarin Prophylaxis. New York, Plenum Press, 1987, pp 3-16.
34. Bell RG, Matchiner JT: Vitamin K activity of phylloquinone oxide metabolite. Arch Biochem Biophys 141:473, 1970.
35. Wu S-M, et al: Identification and purification to near homogeneity of the vitamin K-dependent carboxylase. Proc Natl Acad Sci USA 88:2236, 1991.
36. Berkner KL, et al: Purification and identification of vitamin K-dependent carboxylase. Proc Natl Acad Sci USA 89:6142, 1992.
37. Wu S-M, et al: Cloning and expression of the cDNA for human γ-glutamyl carboxylase. Science 254:1634, 1991.
38. Wallin R, et al: A molecular mechanism for genetic warfarin resistance in the rat. FASEB J 15:2542, 2001.
39. Wallin R: Vitamin K-dependent carboxylation in the developing rat: evidence for a similar mechanism of action of warfarin in fetal and adult livers. Pediatr Res 26:370, 1989.
40. Wallin R, Martin LF: Early processing of prothrombin and factor X by the vitamin K-dependent carboxylase. J Biol Chem 263:9994, 1988.
41. Hall JG, et al: Maternal and fetal sequelae of anticoagulation during pregnancy. Am J Med 68:122, 1980.
42. Romero EE, et al: Cloning of rat vitamin K-dependent γ-glutamyl carboxylase and developmental regulated gene expression in postimplantation embryos. Exp Cell Biol 234:334, 1989.
43. Jamison CS, Degen SJF: Prenatal and postnatal expression of mRNA coding for rat prothrombin. Biochim Biophys Acta 1088:208, 1991.
44. Bohme HJ, et al: Biochemistry of liver development in the perinatal period. Experientia 39:473, 1983.
45. Cake MH, et al: Ontogeny of the glucocorticoid receptor and its relationship to tyrosine aminotransferase induction in cultured foetal hepatocytes. Biochem J 198:301, 1981.
46. Stanton C, Wallin R: Processing and trafficking of clotting factor X in the secretory pathway. Biochem J 284:25, 1992.
47. Wallin R, Hutson SM: Dexamethasone stimulates vitamin K-dependent carboxylase activity in neonatal rats and cultured fetal hepatocytes. Pediatr Res 30:281, 1991.
48. Gallaher KJ, et al: Vitamin K-dependent carboxylase activity in fetal rat lung: developmental effects of dexamethasone and triiodothyronine. Pediatr Res 25:530, 1989.
49. Ballard PL: Antenatal glucocorticoid therapy: hormone concentrations. *In* Gross F, et al (eds): Hormones and Lung Maturation, Vol 28. Heidelberg, Springer, 1986, pp 173-196.

Lipid Metabolism

Emilio Herrera and Miguel Angel Lasunción

39

Maternal-Fetal Transfer of Lipid Metabolites

Changes in maternal lipid metabolism during gestation control the availability of lipid metabolites to the fetus, even though some components do not directly cross the placental barrier. This is the case of maternal plasma lipoproteins, the profile of which during pregnancy differs markedly from that seen in nonpregnant subjects. Although no evidence exists for their transfer to the fetus, placental cells have lipoprotein receptors that allow the uptake and release of their lipid components to the fetus. Other products of maternal lipid metabolism, however, such as free fatty acids (FFA), glycerol, and ketone bodies, are able to cross the placenta and become available to the fetus without prior modification. Although the efficiency of transfer across the placenta differs for each of these metabolites, the major force controlling their actual transfer is the maternal/fetal concentration gradient.

HYPERLIPOPROTEINEMIA IN PREGNANCY AND ITS ROLE AS A SOURCE OF FATTY ACIDS FOR THE FETUS

Maternal hypertriglyceridemia is one of the most striking changes that takes place in lipid metabolism during gestation. The increase in plasma triglycerides during pregnancy is greater than increases in phospholipids and cholesterol,[1, 2] and more triglycerides are found in all the lipoprotein fractions.[3-6] As shown in Figure 39-1, although both triglycerides and cholesterol in very low density lipoproteins (VLDLs), low density lipoproteins (LDLs), and high density lipoproteins (HDLs) are higher in pregnant women in the third trimester of gestation than in the same women during postlactation, the triglyceride/cholesterol ratio remains stable in VLDL despite significant increases in both LDL and HDL. An examination of different HDL subclasses indicates that the rise in triglyceride-enriched HDL_{2b} is mainly responsible for the changes in HDL levels, whereas the small HDL_3 fractions become less abundant.[7]

The mechanisms responsible for these changes in the maternal lipoprotein profile during pregnancy are summarized in Figure 39-2. The increased adipose tissue lipolytic activity during late gestation[8-10] (which is mediated by an insulin-resistant condition[11]) enhances the availability of substrates for triglyceride synthesis in the liver. This action, together with the stimulating effect of estrogen on VLDL production[12] and the decreased extrahepatic lipoprotein lipase (LPL) activity,[7, 13, 14] is in part responsible for the augmented circulating levels of VLDL in the woman in late pregnancy. This change in LPL activity corresponds to its decrease in adipose tissue because, as seen in the rat, this is the body tissue that normally has the highest LPL activity and is the only tissue that shows an intense decrease

during late gestation.[15-19] The decreased adipose tissue LPL activity is also a consequence of the insulin-resistant state present during late pregnancy.[11, 20] Although the abundance of VLDL could justify an enhanced conversion to lipoproteins of higher density, the specific enrichment in triglycerides of the latter seems to be the result of two additional mechanisms (see Fig. 45-2): (1) augmented activity of the cholesteryl ester transfer protein (CETP),[7, 21] which mediates the transfer of triglycerides from triglyceride-rich lipoproteins such as VLDL to the higher density lipoproteins LDL and HDL, and (2) decreased activity of hepatic lipase,[7, 13] which reduces the conversion of triglyceride-rich HDL_{2b} into the lipid-poor HDL_3. The decreased hepatic lipase activity might be a response to an increase in estrogens during late gestation because these hormones are known to inhibit hepatic lipase activity and mRNA expression.[13, 22-24]

The events just summarized are responsible for the sustained hyperlipoproteinemia in the mother during gestation. Because of the impermeability of the placenta to lipoproteins, the precise role that these changes may have on fetal development is as yet unknown; however, the reduction of maternal hyperlipoproteinemia in animals by treatment with hypolipidemic drugs has negative effects on fetal development.[25, 26]

Essential fatty acids (EFAs) derived from maternal diet, which are transported in maternal plasma as triglycerides in triglyceride-rich lipoproteins, must become available to the fetus, despite the lack of a direct placental transfer of maternal lipoproteins. This transfer occurs thanks to the presence of lipoprotein receptors in the placental trophoblast cells that lie at the interface with maternal blood. These cells are therefore positioned to bind maternal lipoproteins and mediate their metabolism and subsequent transfer of the EFAs they deliver to the fetal circulation. VLDL/apo E receptor (VLDLR) as well as LDL receptor (LDLR) and LDLR-related proteins are expressed in human placental tissue.[27-36]

Placental tissue expresses lipoprotein lipase (LPL) activity[37-42] as well as phospholipase A_2[43, 44] and intracellular lipase activities.[45-47] Maternal triglycerides in plasma lipoproteins are therefore hydrolyzed and taken up by the placenta, where their re-esterification and intracellular hydrolysis facilitate the diffusion of released fatty acids (FAs) to the fetus and their subsequent transport to fetal liver. In fact, by using cultured placental trophoblast cells, it has been shown that esterified cellular lipids provide a reservoir of FAs that can be released into the medium.[48]

Once released into fetal plasma, placental transferred FAs bind to a specific oncofetal protein, the α-fetoprotein[49-51] and are rapidly transported to fetal liver. Those FAs taken up by fetal liver

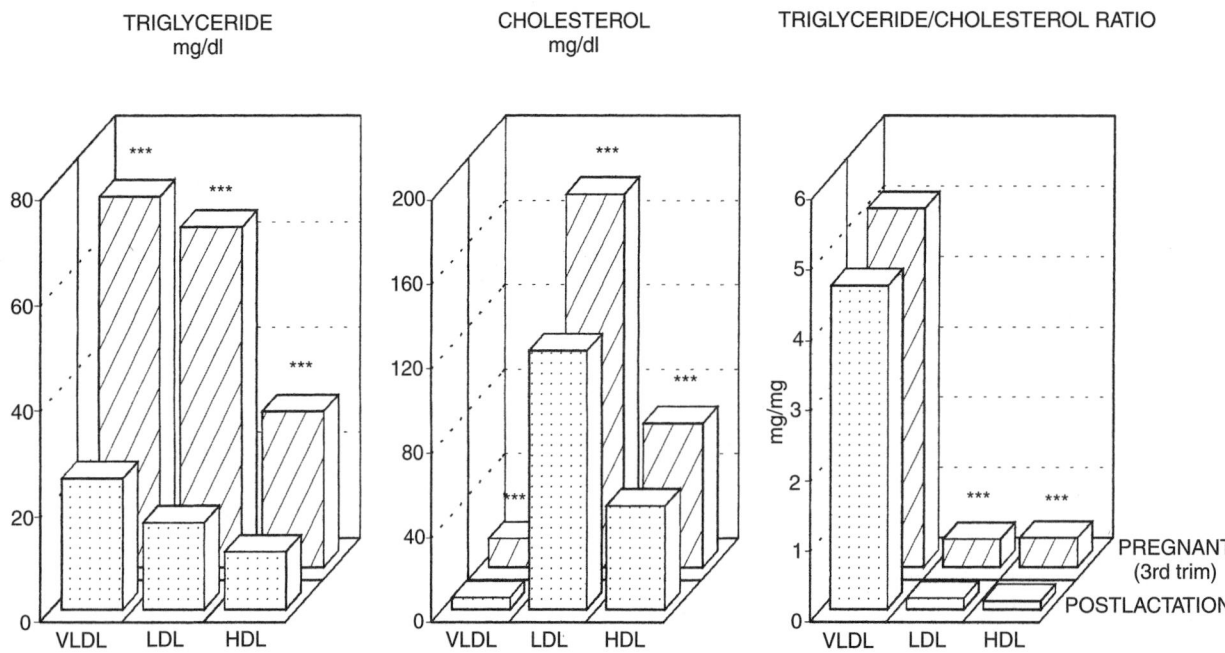

Figure 39–1. Plasma lipoprotein lipids in women in the third trimester of pregnancy and at postlactation. Asterisks indicate significant differences between the two groups.

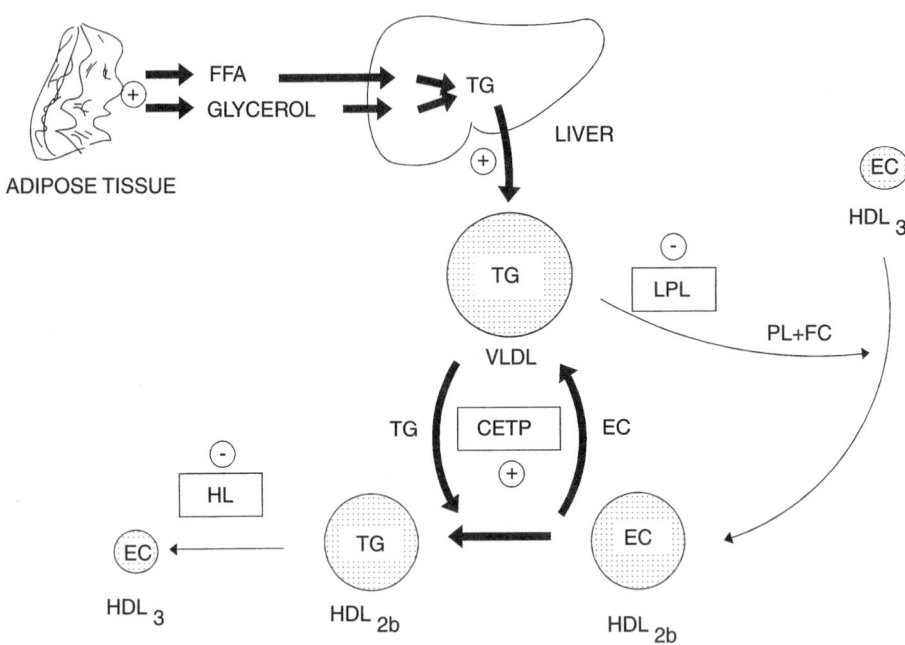

Figure 39–2. Proposed control of major pathways of very low density lipoprotein (VLDL) and high density lipoprotein (HDL) metabolism during late pregnancy. FFA = free fatty acids; LPL = lipoprotein lipase; HL = hepatic lipase; CETP = cholesteryl ester transfer protein; LCAT = lecithin cholesterol acyl transferase; TG = triglycerides; EC = esterified cholesterol; FC = free cholesterol; PL = phospholipids.

are esterified and released back into circulation in the form of triglycerides. This is consistent with the significant linear correlation found for certain long chain polyunsaturated fatty acids (LCPUFAs) between maternal plasma and cord plasma triglycerides during late gestation in humans.[52] A linear correlation has also been found between maternal and fetal plasma triglycerides in the rat.[14,53] This relationship may have important implications in newborn weight, because a direct relationship between maternal triglycerides and newborn weight has been found in humans.[54-56]

MATERNAL LIPID METABOLISM AND PLACENTAL TRANSFER OF FREE FATTY ACIDS, GLYCEROL, AND KETONE BODIES TO THE FETUS

During the first part of gestation, the maternal body accumulates fat[57-59] as the result of combined effects of hyperphagia,[60, 61] enhanced lipogenesis,[62] and unmodified or even increased extrahepatic LPL activity.[7,17,63] The tendency to accumulate fat ceases during late gestation[57,58,64,65] because maternal lipid metabolism changes to a catabolic condition. This is evidenced by increased

MATERNAL LIPID METABOLISM
AT LATE GESTATION

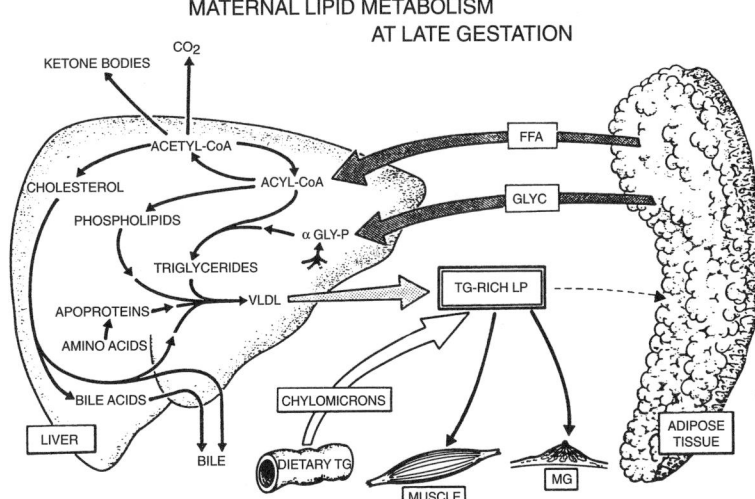

Figure 39–3. Summary of major changes in maternal lipid metabolism at late gestation. FFA = free fatty acids; TG-RICH LP = triglyceride-rich lipoproteins; Glyc = glycerol. (Adapted from Herrera E, et al: Biol Neonate 51:70-77, 1987. S. Karger AG, Basel.)

adipose tissue lipolysis[9, 17, 66] and reduced uptake of circulating triglycerides,[67] secondary to the reduction in adipose tissue LPL activity,[7,13-15,18,19] reviewed earlier in this chapter. These changes, together with hepatic overproduction of triglycerides [68, 69] and the enhanced absorption of dietary lipids,[70] are responsible for the marked progressive increase in maternal circulating triglycerides occurring during late gestation.[3,4,71,72] The major changes in the maternal lipid metabolism are summarized in Figure 39–3, which diagrams the changes in adipose tissue, liver, and intestinal activity that are responsible for the physiologic increase in circulating FFA, glycerol, and triglyceride-rich lipoproteins (VLDL and chylomicrons). Under fed conditions, maternal ketosis is no different from that in nonpregnant subjects, but it increases markedly under fasting conditions.[73,74]

With the exception of glycerol used in gluconeogenesis[75, 76] and the LPL-mediated circulating triglyceride uptake by the mammary gland before labor,[18,70,77,78] no part of the increase in circulating lipid components in the fed mother during late gestation seems to benefit her metabolic needs directly. This increase, however, may benefit the fetus because this gestational period coincides with the rate of maximal fetal accretion, a time when the substrate, metabolic fuel, and essential component requirements of the fetus are greatly enhanced. The lipid component may also constitute a "floating" fuel store for both mother and fetus, easily accessible under conditions of food deprivation, and this may explain the well-known finding of enhanced ketogenesis in the mother under fasting conditions.[73, 79-81] This hypothesis is supported by data demonstrating an increased arrival of FFA in the liver as a result of the greatly enhanced adipose tissue lipolysis[8,9,66] and by studies reporting an increase in liver LPL activity,[16,82,83] which facilitates maternal liver use of circulating triglycerides as ketogenic substrates.

The enhanced availability of ketone bodies to fasted maternal tissues allows them to be used as metabolic fuels and may spare other more limited and essential substrates, such as amino acids and glucose, for transport to the fetus. The fetus also receives maternal ketone bodies through the placenta, and their use plays an important role in the fetal metabolic economy under conditions of maternal food deprivation. Augmented lipolytic activity also increases maternal circulating glycerol levels.[16,75] Glycerol can be used as an efficient gluconeogenic substrate[75,76,84,85] and therefore contributes to the maintenance of glucose production for fetal and maternal tissues. Metabolic adaptations found in the mother during starvation are summarized in Figure 39–4. The transfer of glucose, ketone bodies, and amino acids is empha-

sized in this figure because, quantitatively, they are the major substrates crossing the placenta in this condition.

Understanding FAs, glycerol, and ketone body placental transfer as well as their respective metabolic fates in the fetus provides a clearer insight into the effect on the fetus of these persistently elevated maternal circulating lipid levels. Figure 39–5 compares plasma levels of these metabolites in virgin as well as 24-hour-fasted late pregnant rats and their fetuses. It can be seen that although fetal FFA and glycerol levels are much lower than in their mothers, the concentration of ketone bodies is similar. These maternal/fetal concentration differences probably reflect the efficiency or magnitude of the placental transfer process.

Maternal/fetal nutrient transfer through the placenta may be accomplished by means of different mechanisms, including facilitated diffusion, active transport, and simple diffusion.[86-88] The rate of transfer by simple diffusion seems to be a common mechanism for FAs and related moieties. It is a direct function of the concentration gradient and decreases with the molecular size and hydrosolubility.[89] However, in the case of placental transfer, other factors also participate:[90, 91] uterine and umbilical blood flows, intrinsic placental metabolism, and structural characteristics. As may be expected, some of these factors, such as blood flow, contribute analogously to the transfer of any nutrient, but other factors differ with each nutrient and require specific consideration.

Fatty Acids

The fetus requires not only essential FAs from the mother to support growth[92] and brain development,[93] but also nonessential lipids, which, stored in fetal body fat, become an important substrate during early postnatal life.[94] This is especially true in species such as the guinea pig and human, in which body fat at term represents a substantial percentage of body weight (10% in guinea pigs and 16% in humans),[95] and de novo FA synthesis by fetal tissues cannot fulfill fetal requirements.

Either FFA bound to albumin or esterified FAs transported in lipoproteins are the potential sources of the FAs in the maternal side that cross to the placenta. Early studies in sheep[96] that measured venous-arterial differences across the umbilical circulation of the fetus in utero and across the maternal uterine circulation showed no significant passage of FFA to the fetus and led to the conclusion that FFAs did not appear to constitute a significant part of the metabolic fuel supplied there by the mother.[96] Later

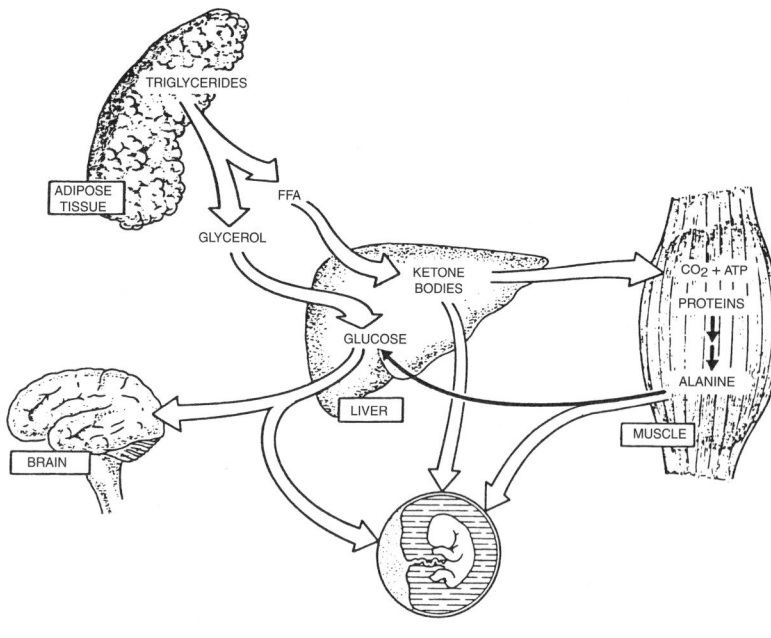

Figure 39–4. Maternal response to starvation. Enhanced adipose tissue lipolysis increases the availability in the liver of glycerol to be used as a preferential substrate for gluconeogenesis and of free fatty acids (FFAs) for ketone body synthesis. By this mechanism, the mother conserves other gluconeogenic substrates, such as alanine, and ensures the adequate availability of fuels and metabolites to the fetus. ATP = adenosine triphosphate (From Herrera E, et al: Biol Neonate *51*: 70–77, 1987. S. Karger AG, Basel.)

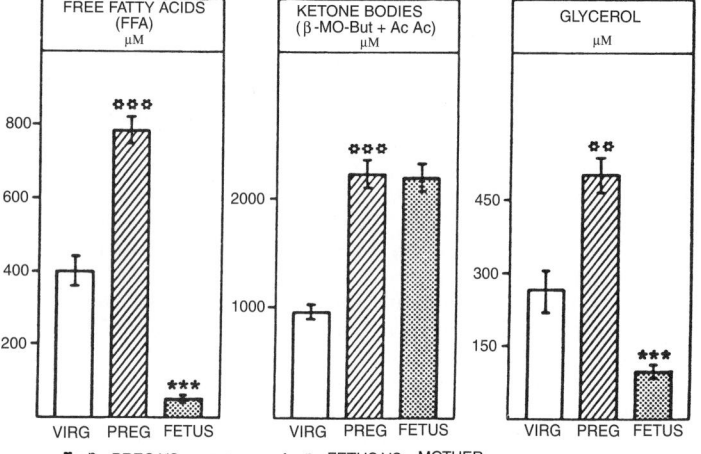

Figure 39–5. Concentration of free fatty acids, ketone bodies, and glycerol in plasma of 48-hour starved virgin rats and 48-hour starved 19-day pregnant rats and thier fetuses. (From Herrera E, et al: Biol Neonate *51*: 70–77, 1987. S. Karger AG, Basel.)

studies demonstrated, however, that the net flux of FAs from mother to fetus across the placenta varies greatly among species. For example, in species with both maternal and fetal layers in the placenta, such as the sheep, pig, and cat, the net transfer of FA to the fetus is generally small.[97-100]

In contrast, in species such as the rabbit,[101] guinea pig,[102,103] primate,[104] and rat[105,106] (in which the placental barrier is formed by only a few layers of fetal origin), the amount of FAs crossing the placenta exceeds even that needed to fulfill lipid storage requirements.[107] In these species, the FA mixture entering fetal circulation from the placenta reflects the maternal FFA concentrations of the different FAs.[97] Furthermore, maternal dietary manipulation with different oil-enriched diets leads to corresponding changes in the FA composition of the fetus.[108,109] These observations, therefore, constitute indirect evidence for the transplacental passage of FAs from mother to fetus.

In humans, although in a smaller proportion than lipoprotein triglycerides, maternal plasma FFAs are an important source of polyunsaturated FAs (PUFA) to the fetus.[110,111] Current evidence suggests that cellular uptake of FFA occurs through a process of facilitated membrane translocation involving a plasma membrane FA-binding protein (FABP$_{pm}$).[112,113] It has been shown that FABP$_{pm}$ is present in human placental membranes[114,115] and is

responsible for the preferential uptake of LCPUFAs by the human placenta.[114,116] The preference for human placental transfer from the maternal to the fetal circulation has been reported as docosahexaenoic⇒ α-linolenic⇒ linoleic⇒ oleic⇒ arachidonic acid.[117] Arachidonic acid was, however, the FA with the highest accumulations in the placenta,[117] and more recently it has been shown that this process of arachidonic uptake by placental syncytiotrophoblast membranes is highly dependent on adenosine triphosphate (ATP) and sodium,[118] implying an active transport mechanism for this FA. A selectivity in the LCPUFA placental transfer may also be exerted at the level of cellular metabolism, given that a certain proportion of arachidonic acid is converted to prostaglandins,[111] a selective incorporation of certain FAs into phospholipids has been found in the ovine placenta,[119] and even selective placental FA oxidation[120,121] and lipid synthesis[122,123] may occur.

The combination of all these processes determines the actual rate of placental FA transfer and its selectivity. Through these mechanisms, the placenta selectively transports arachidonic acid and docosahexaenoic acid from the maternal to the fetal compartment, resulting in a proportional enrichment of these LCPUFAs in circulating lipids in the fetus.[124] This occurs during the third trimester, when the fetal demands for neural and vascular growth are greater.[125-127]

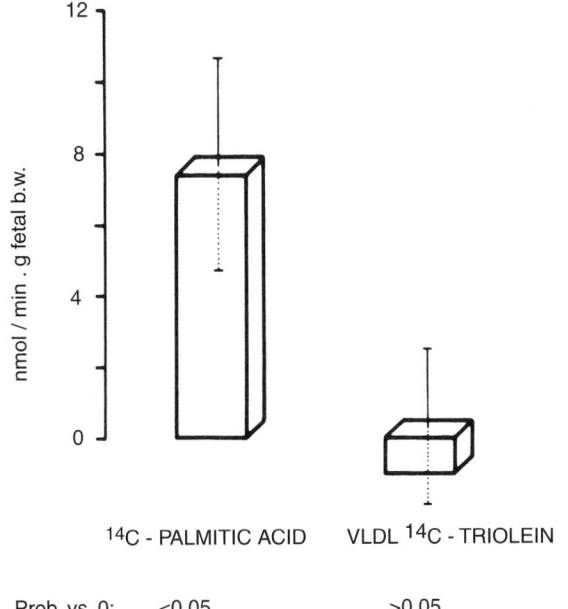

Figure 39–6. Estimation of placental transfer of palmitic acid and VLDL-triolein in the 20-day pregnant rat. Placental transfer to the fetus was determined by measuring the radioactivity appearing in fetuses after infusing ^{14}C-labeled substrates through the left uterine artery and making proper correction of the data for specific activity dilution of the tracer and uterine blood flow, as previously described (see ref. 137).

Although, as commented on earlier, current evidence indicates that FAs are selectively transferred across the placenta, essential and nonessential FAs may also use a common transfer mechanism. Using *in situ* perfused guinea pig or rabbit placentas, several investigations have demonstrated that, within the physiologic range, the net FFA transfer to the fetus correlates with maternal plasma levels of FFA and that this transfer is regulated by the transplacental concentration gradient.[128-130] Furthermore, during maternal fasting, increased amounts of maternal FFA cross the placenta into fetal circulation and are incorporated into fetal stores.[131] These observations suggest that the transfer of several FFA across the placenta is mainly by diffusion. Other factors affecting this transfer process are the uterine and umbilical blood flow rates[128,130] and the fetal plasma albumin concentration.[128,132,133] In this respect, the increase in albumin levels throughout the third trimester in the human fetus[134] may increase its FFA supply.

The authors have studied the placental transfer of palmitic acid in the 20-day pregnant rat by infusing radioactive carbon (^{14}C)-labeled palmitic acid through the left uterine artery for 20 minutes. The amount of label appearing in the placentas and fetuses from the left uterine horn was contrasted with that found in those from the right horn.[135] Although the left uterine horn received the tracer directly, it reached the right horn after dilution in the mother's circulation. Therefore, the amount of substrate transferred to the fetus can be calculated as a function of the values for the concentration of the metabolite studied in maternal plasma, the difference of radioactivity in fetuses between the left and right uterine horns, and the left uterine blood flow.[136-139] As shown in Figure 39-6, the estimated FFA transfer was above 7 nmol/min × g fetal body weight, a value that is lower than the level previously found for other compounds in earlier studies: glucose, 127 nmol/min × g fetal body weight; alanine, 23 nmol/min × g fetal body weight, but higher than that of glycerol, 1 nmol/min × g fetal body weight.[139] When the ^{14}C-labeled lipids that had been retained in the placentas

after (1-^{14}C)-palmitate infusion were measured, it was found that the value was 99 ± 38 nmol/min/g, which is much higher than that found in the fetus. Of those ^{14}C-labeled lipids incorporated into the placenta, 49 ± 3% corresponded to esterified FAs, indicating that a certain proportion of the FFA that reach the placenta is actively esterified. It is not known whether FA esterification participates in the FFA transfer process, but an active placental capacity to form esterified FAs from maternal FFA has also been described in other species[140,141] as well as in humans.[48,142]

As already noted, maternal plasma triglycerides in triglyceride-rich lipoproteins may be considered as an alternative source of FAs for the fetus. We have recently found that the concentration of PUFA in plasma VLDLs in pregnant women during the third trimester of pregnancy is much greater than that in FFA[53] and previous evidence indicates that maternal circulating triglycerides contribute somewhat to plasma fetal FAs of the rat,[143] rabbit,[39] guinea pig,[41,144] and human.[145] The authors applied the *in situ* uterine artery infusion technique[135] described above to test the potential transfer of VLDL-^{14}C-triolein across the placenta and its incorporation into fetal lipids. During the 20-minute study, no significant differences were noted in radioactivity incorporated into fetuses from the left horn as compared to those from the right horn (see Fig. 39-6). Therefore, it was concluded that lipoprotein triglycerides are not a significant direct FA source for placental transfer to the fetus.

Glycerol

As a result of the active lipolytic activity of maternal adipose tissue, plasmatic glycerol levels are consistently elevated during late gestation.[17,75,76] Therefore, the values for plasma glycerol are generally higher in the mother than in the fetus (see Fig. 39-5), but there are some interspecies differences. The maternal/fetal glycerol gradient is greater in those species with an epithelio-chorial placenta (ruminants)[96,146] than in those with a hemochorial placenta.[147-149]

The available experimental data on placental glycerol transfer in any species are scarce. Although the molecular characteristics of glycerol should facilitate easy placental transfer (low weight and uncharged molecule), glycerol transfer is notably lower than for other metabolites with similar molecular characteristics such as glucose or L-alanine.[139,150,151] In contrast with the carrier-mediated process used for these two metabolites, placental glycerol transfer is accomplished by simple diffusion.[146,152] In the sheep fetus, glycerol uptake is low, accounting for no more than 1.5% of the total oxygen consumption of the fetus.[96] In humans, it has not been possible to detect a transfer of glycerol from mother to fetus despite its favorable gradient.[147] When comparing different substrates, and by using the *in situ* infused placental technique in the rat, the authors have found that the transfer of glycerol is much lower than that of glucose and alanine and similar to that of FFA.[139] The authors have also found that the fetal-placental unit converts glycerol into lactate and lipids,[149] and this rapid use may actively contribute to maintaining the high glycerol gradient consistently found between maternal and fetal blood.[81,147-150]

Accelerated turnover of maternal glycerol seems to be influenced by the high liver glycerol kinase activity, which facilitates its rapid phosphorylation and subsequent conversion into glucose.[75,76,84,85] Although this mechanism indirectly benefits the fetus by providing glucose (see Fig. 39-4), it may limit the availability of sufficient glycerol molecules for transfer to the fetus. Figure 39-7 summarizes studies that support this hypothesis. Hepatectomy normally results in increased plasma glycerol levels because of a reduction in glycerol use secondary to absence of the liver, the major receptor organ for this metabolite.[153] In the case of pregnant rats, hepatectomy and nephrectomy produce significant but smaller increases in plasma glycerol levels than in nonpregnant animals. This difference cannot be

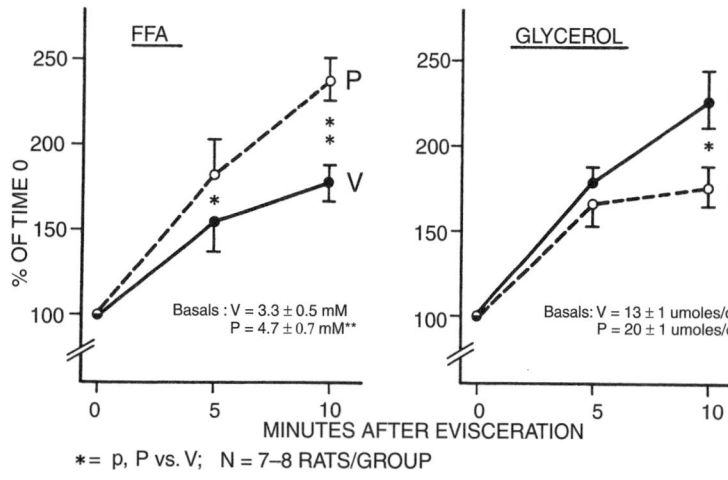

Figure 39–7. Effect of hepatectomy-nephrectomy on plasma free fatty acid and glycerol in virgin (V) and 20-day pregnant rats (P). Experimental details are as indicated in ref. 154.

interpreted as reduced lipolytic activity in the pregnant rat because plasma FFA, the other lipolytic product, increases more than in nonpregnant animals. It might, however, be interpreted as the result of an augmented transfer of glycerol to the fetus because glycerol levels in fetal plasma increase significantly after maternal hepatectomy and nephrectomy.[154]

Therefore, placental glycerol transfer seems to be limited by the effective, rapid use of this substrate for gluconeogenesis by the liver and kidney cortex of the mother. Although the fetal-placental unit actively uses glycerol (which helps to maintain a favorable transfer gradient), its quantitative and physiologic roles in the fetus, except as a preferential substrate for fetal liver glyceride glycerol synthesis,[149] seem to be limited under normal conditions. Under conditions of markedly elevated maternal glycerol levels, however, the placental transfer of glycerol could become an important source of substrates for the fetus.

Ketone Bodies

Although plasma levels of ketone bodies in the fed pregnant mother late in gestation are unchanged under physiologic conditions; with fasting[73, 79, 80, 155-159] or diabetic[3, 160, 161] conditions, they are greatly elevated as a result of increased adipose tissue lipolytic activity and enhanced delivery of FFA to the liver. As noted earlier, when the supply of glucose is limited (e.g., hypoglycemia or reduced insulin levels or sensitivity, or both), ketone bodies are used by some maternal tissues (e.g., skeletal muscle) as alternative substrates. Ketone bodies can also cross the placental barrier and be used as fuels and lipogenic substrates by the fetus.[162-165]

Maternal ketonemia in the poorly controlled pregnant diabetic patient, with or without acidosis, has been associated with an increased stillbirth rate, an increased incidence of congenital malformations, and impaired neurophysiologic development in the infant.[164, 166, 167] These effects are thought to be secondary to placental transfer of maternal ketone bodies to the fetus.[168]

In addition to size and lipid solubility, molecular charge has an important effect on placental membrane permeability. At pH 7.4, most molecules of the two main ketone bodies, β-hydroxybutyrate and acetoacetate, are present in dissociated or ionized form, which retards their diffusion across the placenta. Despite this, in all species studied (human,[157, 158, 169, 170] rat,[79, 80, 171] and sheep[156, 168]), increments in maternal ketone bodies are accompanied by increments in fetal plasma levels, indicating efficient placental transfer; fetal liver ketogenesis is practically negligible.[172]

Placental transfer of ketone bodies occurs either by simple diffusion or by a low specificity carrier-mediated process;[146, 173] the efficiency of which varies among species. Although the

maternofetal gradient for ketone bodies is higher than 10 in sheep,[156, 168] in humans it is about 2,[147] and in rats it is close to 1[79,80,171] (see Fig. 39–5), indicating that the amount of ketone bodies crossing the placenta is much lower in ruminants than in nonruminant species. It has even been proposed that in the fasting condition, the contribution of ketone bodies to the fetal oxidative metabolism accounts for only 2 to 3% of the total oxygen consumption in the case of sheep.[156, 174] In the rat, β-hydroxybutyrate adequately replaces the glucose deficit in the placenta, fetal brain, and liver during fasting hypoglycemia.[165] This suggests a much greater contribution of ketone bodies to the fetal oxidative metabolism in the fasted nonruminant.

Key enzymes for ketone-body utilization—3-hydroxybutyrate dehydrogenase (EC 1.1.1.30), 3-oxoacid-CoA transferase (EC 2.8.3.5), and acetyl-CoA acetyltransferase (EC 2.3.1.9)—have been found in the brain and other tissues in both the human and the rat fetus.[162, 163, 175, 176] Both the human[164] and the rat brain[163] oxidize β-hydroxybutyrate *in vitro* in a form that is dependent on substrate concentration and not on the maternal nutritional state. Other fetal tissue types known to oxidize ketone bodies are kidney, heart, liver, and placenta.[163, 176] Some tissues are even known to use ketone bodies as substrates for FA and cholesterol synthesis, as has been shown in the rat brain, liver, placenta, and lung after *in vivo* administration of ^{14}C-β-hydroxybutyrate to pregnant animals.[177] The activity of ketone-body metabolizing enzymes in fetal tissues (brain, liver, and kidney) can be increased by conditions that result in maternal hyperketonemia, such as starvation during the last days of gestation[178] or high fat feeding.[179] Such a change is especially evident in the fetal brains from starved late pregnant rats[178] and may represent an important fetal adaptation to guarantee brain development under these conditions because fetal brain weight is better preserved than other fetal organ weights.

In conclusion, there is evidence in nonruminant species for efficient placental ketone body transfer and for the fetal use of these materials as substrates for both oxidation and lipogenesis, even in preference to other substrates (glucose, lactate, and amino acids). Because both the placental transfer and the use of ketone bodies are concentration dependent, the quantitative contribution to fetal metabolism is important only under conditions of maternal hyperketonemia (e.g., starvation, high-fat diet, diabetes).

CHOLESTEROL IN THE FETUS

Role of Cholesterol and Related Compounds in Development

Cholesterol plays an important role in fetal development as well as in the general physiology of the organism. First, it is an essential component of cell membranes. By interacting with phospholipids and sphingolipids, cholesterol contributes to the characteristic physicochemical properties of membranes, mainly fluidity and passive permeability.[180] Cholesterol is not homogeneously distributed in the membrane, rather it is concentrated in structures such as rafts and caveolae, where it modulates the function of different integral proteins and receptors. Cholesterol is the precursor of both bile acids and steroid hormones; in the fetus, glucocorticoids are intensely synthesized by the adrenal gland in the last part of development, which represents an important time of cholesterol need. Cholesterol and its oxidized derivatives—oxysterols—are key regulators of different metabolic processes, both by modulating the proteolytic activation of sterol response element binding protein (SREBP) or by acting as ligands of nuclear receptors, such as LXR (liver X receptor).[181,182] Active SREBP and LXR are transcription factors that regulate the expression of multiple genes implicated in intracellular lipid homeostasis and lipoprotein metabolism.[181,183]

Recently, other important actions of cholesterol have become apparent; these actions have special relevance for the fetus because they are related to development, embryogenesis, and differentiation. Cholesterol is required for cell proliferation, not only for membrane formation, but also for the activation of regulatory proteins involved in cell cycle progression, specifically in the transition from the G2 phase to mitosis.[184,185] Cholesterol plays important roles in differentiation and cell-to-cell communication; in fact, it has recently been demonstrated as a key factor in synaptogenesis.[186] Finally, cholesterol is essential in embryonic patterning in both vertebrates and invertebrates.[187] This is attained mainly by activation of hedgehog proteins (i.e., Sonic hedgehog—Shh—in humans), which are involved in cell differentiation.[188]

It is conceivable, thus, that defects affecting cholesterol availability will have deleterious consequences in fetal development. In fact, congenital defects in cholesterol biosynthesis or the reduction of cholesterol synthesis with xenobiotics result in severe malformations and dysfunctions, mainly affecting the craniofacial organs and the central nervous system (CNS), respectively, alterations that are similar to those caused by Shh defficiency.[187,189,190]

It has been observed in pigs that fetal weight is directly correlated to plasma cholesterol concentration in the fetus at late gestation.[191] Similarly, neonatal pigs from lines with genetically low cholesterol levels are smaller at birth and grow more slowly, but the growth rate improved when they were fed with cholesterol.[192,193] An increase in neonatal survival is noted with supplementary dietary fat for the peripartal sow.[194] Thus, cholesterol is essential in body growth and the development of the CNS and fetal requirements must be met either by efficient endogenous cholesterol biosynthesis or transfer from the mother.

Cholesterol Biosynthesis and Congenital Defects

Cholesterol biosynthesis is a multienzymatic pathway that can be separated into three segments according to the type of compounds that are synthesized in each one, that is, mevalonic acid, isoprenoids, and sterols, respectively. In the first, also called the *mevalonate pathway*, three molecules of acetyl-CoA are successively condensed by the action of acetyl-CoA acetyltransferase and cytosolic 3-hydroxy-3-methylglutaryl (HMG)-CoA synthase to form HMG-CoA, which is then reduced with the loss of coenzyme A, rendering mevalonate, a 6-carbon compound[195] (Fig. 39-8). This complex reaction is catalyzed by HMG-CoA reductase, which is present in the endoplasmic reticulum and is the rate-limiting step in cholesterol biosynthesis. In the next series of reactions, mevalonate is converted to squalene (see Fig. 39-8), which is the immediate precursor of sterols. The first sterol formed is lanosterol, which contains 30 carbons (see Fig. 39-8). The transformation of lanosterol into cholesterol occurs in the endoplasmic reticulum and involves at least seven different enzymes (Fig. 39-9).

In humans, six different genetic defects in the cholesterol biosynthesis pathway have been identified. Mevalonic aciduria (MIM 251770) is caused by missense mutations in mevalonate kinase, which impair the formation of both isoprenoids and sterols (see Fig. 39-8). The patients show dysmorphias and failure to thrive. Milder mutations of the enzyme also underlie hyperimmunoglobulinemia D and periodic fever syndrome (MIM 260920). The rest of the disorders are due to defects in the postsqualene segment of the pathway (see Fig. 39-9). Greenberg skeletal dysplasia (MIM 215140), which is associated with short-limb dwarfism, is probably caused by mutations of Δ^{14}-reductase, but confirmation at the molecular level has yet to be observed. CHILD syndrome (MIM 308050) and Conradi-Hünermann-Happle syndrome (CPDX2; MIM 302960) are caused by deficiencies of C4-demethylase and Δ^8-Δ^7-isomerase, respectively; these two disorders are X-linked dominant inherited and carrier males are lethally affected, whereas females present with several skeletal and skin abnormalities. Desmosterolosis (MIM 602398) is an extremely rare and probably autosomal recessive inherited disorder due to the deficiency of Δ^{24}-reductase; the infants affected died shortly after birth and suffered from multiple malformations and dysmorphias. The last of these disorders, and probably the best known and most widely studied, is Smith-Lemli-Opitz syndrome (SLOS; MIM 270400), which is caused by mutations of Δ^7-reductase. The phenotypic expression is highly variable; the most prominent anomalies are microcephalia and facial dysmorphias. All affected patients accumulate 7-dehydrocholesterol in plasma and tissues, but the clinical severity of this syndrome correlates best with its relative level to plasma cholesterol. This suggests that the availability of cholesterol during development is one of the major determinants of the phenotypic expressions in SLOS.

In general, these congenital alterations show the important role of cholesterol and its immediate precursors in morphogenesis and fetal development. The reader is referred to excellent reviews on this subject.[189,190]

Sources of Fetal Cholesterol

The demands for cholesterol in the fetus are relatively high, especially during the last third of gestation when fetal growth is exponential. In principle, the fetus may obtain cholesterol from both endogenous biosynthesis and from the yolk sac and placenta. By following the appearance of radioactivity in the fetus, early experiments demonstrated the placental transfer of maternal cholesterol to the fetus in different species, such as the rat,[196] guinea pig, rabbit,[197] and rhesus monkey.[198] In those studies, the estimated contribution of maternal cholesterol to the fetus varied widely, likely because of methodologic reasons. A more accurate type of study is to compare cholesterol accretion in the fetus with the absolute rate of cholesterol biosynthesis. Measurements of [3H]water incorporation into cholesterol revealed that cholesterol biosynthesis in fetal tissues is highly active; when calculated per mass unit, the rate of cholesterol synthesis in fetal tissues is several times higher than in maternal tissues in different species.[199-203] This is especially the case for the fetal brain, which appears almost completely autonomous in cholesterol accretion, and the liver, the cholesterol biosynthesis of which proceeds at a rate exceeding the need for cholesterol accretion, an excess that is secreted into the plasma for uptake by other developing fetal organs.[202,203] These results are consistent with the near-maximal expression at the level of mRNA of different enzymes involved in cholesterol biosynthesis[204] and the high activity of HMG-CoA reductase—the rate limiting enzyme of cholesterol biosynthesis—in fetal tissues.[205,206]

By comparing the cholesterol synthesis rate with cholesterol accretion in the whole fetus, an estimation of the requirement for exogenous cholesterol can be derived, which would either be directly transferred from maternal plasma or synthesized in the placenta or the yolk sac. In the rat, endogenously synthesized

cont on p 384

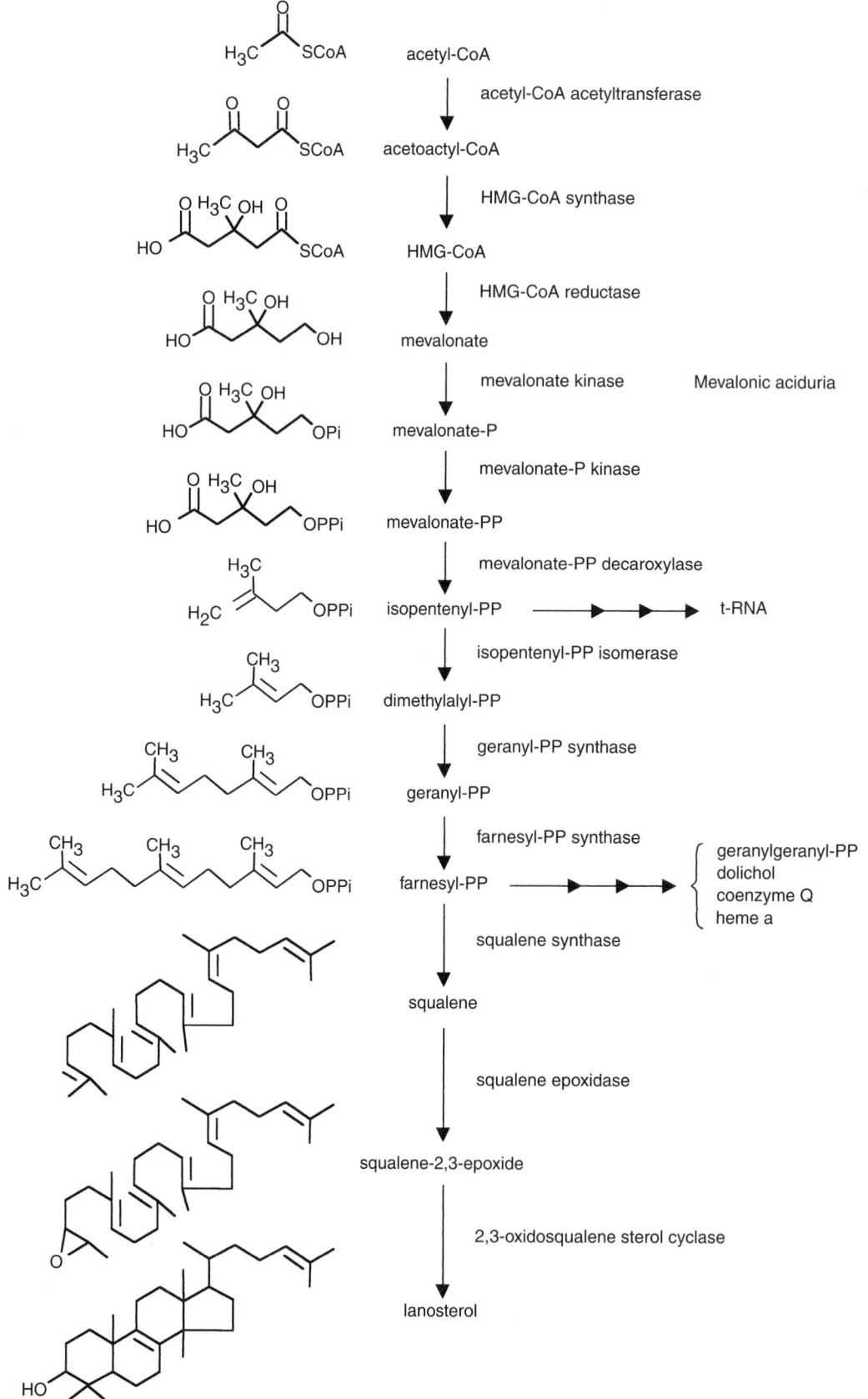

Figure 39–8. Biosynthesis of lanosterol from acetyl-CoA. Aside the route leading to the formation of lanosterol, the first sterol in the cholesterol biosynthesis pathway, the alternative use of isopentenyl-PP for the derivation of certain t-RNA and farnesyl-PP for several isoprenoids is shown. Multiple arrows indicate several reactions. The name of a human inherited disorder is shown in italics beside the affected enzyme.

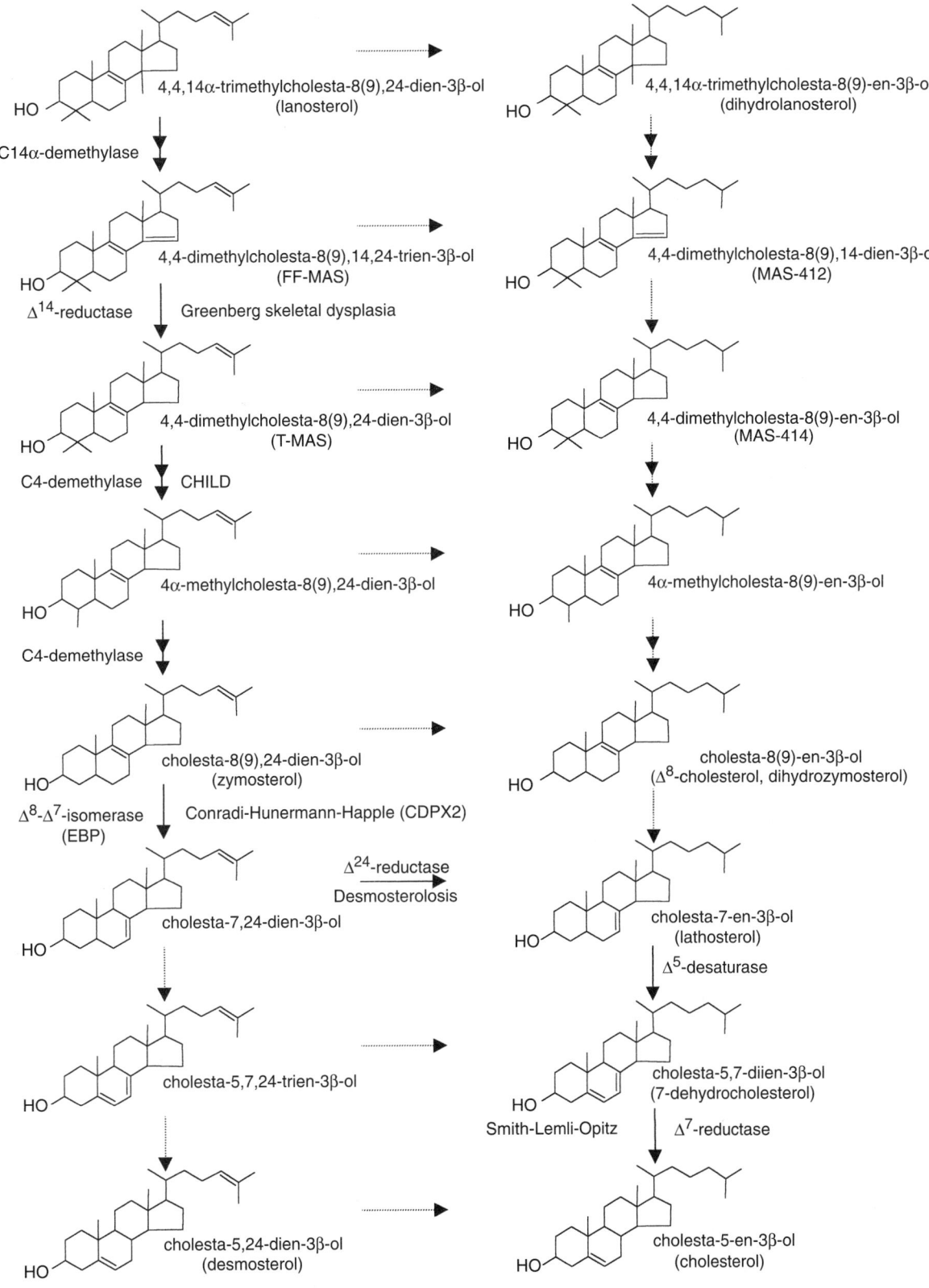

Figure 39–9. Biosynthesis of cholesterol from lanosterol. The main route is indicated by the solid arrows (see text for comments). Double arrows indicate several reactions. The names of the human inherited disorders are shown in italics beside the affected enzymes.

cholesterol appears to account for practically all fetal cholesterol,[202, 203] meaning that the other potential sources are insignificant, at least during the later stages of gestation. In fact, Belknap and Dietschy[200] found that although the rat placenta did take up ^{125}I-cellobiose-labeled lipoprotein from maternal circulation, none of the apolipoprotein or cholesterol was appreciably transferred to the fetus. These studies indicate that the rat fetus receives little or no cholesterol from the mother but, rather, satisfies its need for cholesterol during fetal development through local synthesis. Maneuvers directed to modify cholesterol homeostasis in the mother had no significant effects on cholesterol levels or cholesterol synthesis rates in the fetus. Thus, feeding pregnant rats with cholesterol, which resulted in an increase of plasma cholesterol concentration and reduced cholesterol synthesis in the maternal compartment, did not affect any of these parameters in the fetus.[199,200,207,208] Conversely, treatment of pregnant rats with cholestyramine—a bile acid sequestrant that interferes with intestinal cholesterol absorption and consequently stimulates cholesterol biosynthesis in maternal tissues—did not alter cholesterol accretion in the fetus.[209] All these findings led to the affirmation that in the rat, fetal cholesterol originates mainly from endogenous *de novo* synthesis rather than from placental transfer.

In the early stages of gestation in the rat, however, maternal cholesterol may make a significant contribution to the fetal cholesterol pool. For instance, it is well known that treatment of pregnant rats with AY 9944—an inhibitor of Δ^7-reductase—results in fetal teratogenesis, but the simultaneous oral administration of cholesterol early in gestation completely prevents the characteristic holoprosencephalic brain malformations.[187, 210, 211] In contrast, the anomalies of fetal masculinization caused by AY 9944 when administered late in gestation, are not prevented by the compensatory administration of cholesterol to the mother.[187] These results firmly suggest that maternal cholesterol reaches the fetal compartment at least early in gestation and is of significant physiologic relevance in the rat.

In other species, exogenous cholesterol may constitute an important, quantitative source of cholesterol for the fetus. In the Golden Syrian hamster, Woollett found that endogenous biosynthesis accounted for only 40% of the fetal cholesterol, suggesting that the placenta and/or the yolk sac contributed the remainder.[201] Actually, in hamsters fed increasing amounts of cholesterol, the cholesterol concentration in the fetal tissues was found to be linearly correlated with the maternal plasma cholesterol concentration, while cholesterol synthesis decreased in the reverse way.[212] These studies in hamsters demonstrated that fetal cholesterol homeostasis is affected by maternal plasma cholesterol concentration in a gradient fashion.[212] In the guinea pig, fetal cholesterol homeostasis was found to be relatively insensitive to dietary cholesterol manipulations in the mother throughout gestation.[199] Nevertheless, feeding cholestyramine to the mothers, although producing the expected stimulation of ^{3}H-water incorporation into sterols in maternal liver, also resulted in a 1.4-fold increase in fetal carcass cholesterol synthesis at 60 days' gestation, which demonstrates that fetal cholesterol homeostasis may respond to induction by maternal hypocholesterolemia during the late gestation period.[199]

Data in humans are scarcer and cholesterol biosynthesis in fetal tissues has not been evaluated for obvious reasons. In deliveries at term, Parker and associates[213] measured cholesterol levels in the umbilical venous and the umbilical arterial plasmas and found a highly significant difference between HDL-, LDL-, and total-cholesterol concentrations, venous levels being 7.7 to 12.8% higher than those in arterial plasma. These data were suggestive of the delivery of cholesterol from the placenta to the fetus, which could either be synthesized in the placenta or derived from the maternal plasma. Those same authors, however, estimated that the contribution of such cholesterol to the fetal

plasma cholesterol pool was of minimal quantitative importance in term newborns of women experiencing uncomplicated pregnancies.[213] Several observational studies have addressed this issue by comparing maternal lipoprotein-cholesterol levels with those in mixed umbilical cord blood, reporting either a positive correlation[214, 215] or no correlation between these values.[213, 216-218] The gestational stage, however, could influence these results, because cholesterol plasma concentration has been reported as significantly higher in premature than in full-term newborns.[219, 220] In fact, fetal cholesterol levels show a strong inverse correlation with fetal age, being two-fold higher in 5-month than in 7-month-old fetuses.[221] This has been interpreted as an indication of the greater requirements of cholesterol in the younger, more immature fetuses.[221] Interestingly, in fetuses younger than 6 months, although not in older fetal plasma, cholesterol levels are significantly, directly correlated to the maternal ones.[221] Therefore, available results in humans strongly suggest that maternal cholesterol substantially contributes to fetal cholesterol accretion early in gestation.

Both the placenta and the yolk sac are able to synthesize and remove cholesterol from the maternal circulation. In the pregnant rat it was determined that placenta takes up LDL at rates equal to about one-third of those seen in the maternal liver.[200] In the hamster, LDL clearance rates of the placenta and yolk sac were similar to those in the liver and higher than those in the decidua when studied at mid-gestation (day 10.5).[222] In the same study, it was found that clearance rates for HDL-apoA-I and HDL-cholesteryl ether were similar to those of LDL in the placenta and decidua, whereas rates in the yolk sac were dramatically higher. As gestation progressed to day 14.5, LDL and HDL clearance rates decreased in all three tissues.[222]

Regarding the receptors responsible for the uptake of lipoprotein cholesterol, there are multiple possibilities. Both the placenta[223, 224] and, to a lesser extent, the yolk sac[222] express LDL receptors in their membranes. In correlation with this, several authors documented the use of LDL-cholesterol for progesterone synthesis by trophoblastic cells in vitro.[225, 226] Interestingly, it was found that HDL2-cholesterol stimulated placental progesterone secretion to a greater extent than LDL did, by a mechanism that did not involve the LDL receptor.[226] Further evidence on the role of maternal HDL as an exogenous source of fetal cholesterol comes from studies in apolipoprotein A-I-deficient mice. These animals have markedly reduced HDL-cholesterol levels in plasma, and cholesterol accretion in the fetus was diminished, although cholesterol synthesis in the fetus was not affected.[227] These results were in line with previous observations by Knopp and associates,[228] describing apolipoprotein A-I concentration in maternal plasma as a significant positive predictor of birth length. It appears that HDL could potentially contribute a significant proportion of the cholesterol required for fetal development.

Several lipoprotein receptors, different from the LDL receptor, which can mediate the uptake of HDL cholesterol, have been detected in placental preparations. These include SR-BI/CLA-1—an HDL receptor, megalin/gp330—homologue of the LDL receptor, and cubilin—a protein that binds HDL and acts in conjunction with megalin to mediate HDL endocytosis.[222, 229, 230] These receptors are highly expressed in the yolk sac as well.[222, 231, 232] Taken together, these data confirm the ability of both the placenta and the yolk sac to take up cholesterol from maternal lipoproteins, but the extent to which it is exported to the fetus and the factors that regulate this process remain to be clarified definitively.

SUMMARY

During gestation, both triglyceride and cholesterol increase in all lipoprotein fractions and are associated with an increase in the triglyceride/cholesterol ratio in LDL and HDL. The increase in HDL mainly corresponds to triglyceride-enriched HDL_2. The presence of lipoprotein receptors in the placenta ensures the availability of essential lipoprotein components to the fetus and provides a teleologic reason for maternal hyperlipoproteinemia.

Sustained maternal hyperlipidemia during late pregnancy is of pivotal importance in fetal development. This is especially true during the stage of maximal fetal accretion. Besides using transferred FAs, the fetus also benefits from two other products of maternal lipid metabolism, glycerol and ketone bodies. Although only a small proportion of maternally derived glycerol crosses the placenta, it is quantitatively important as a substrate for maternal gluconeogenesis. Because fetal oxidative metabolism is preferentially sustained by maternal glucose crossing the placenta, the use of glycerol for glucose synthesis actively contributes to the fetal glucose supply.

In nonruminant species, there is an easy transfer of maternal ketone bodies to the fetus, where they can be efficiently used as carbon fuels for oxidative metabolism or as lipogenic substrates. Because all these processes are concentration dependent, they become relevant only under conditions of maternal hyperketonemia. Under healthy physiologic conditions, they constitute an important support for fetal metabolism when the availability of other substrates is more limited (e.g., during periods of maternal starvation). Under conditions of sustained maternal hyperketonemia, such as high-fat feeding, fetal metabolism also adapts to an enhanced consumption of ketone bodies.

Although the contribution of maternal cholesterol to fetal cholesterol appears important during early gestation, it seems to be of minimal quantitative importance during late gestation. This is consistent with the high capacity of all fetal tissues to synthesize cholesterol. In humans, several congenital defects in the cholesterol biosynthesis pathway have been identified, showing the important role of cholesterol in morphogenesis and fetal development.

ACKNOWLEDGMENTS

The present work was carried out in part with grants from the Fondo de Investigación Sanitaria, Instituto de Salud Carlos III (FIS 99/0205 and 99/0286) and Dirección General de Investigación de la Comunidad de Madrid (0023/00), Spain. The editorial help of Linda Hamalainen is greatly appreciated.

REFERENCES

1. Boyd EM: The lipemia of pregnancy. J Clin Invest *13*:347, 1934.
2. Peters JP, et al: The lipids of serum in pregnancy. J Clin Invest *30*:388, 1951.
3. Montelongo A, et al: Longitudinal study of plasma lipoproteins and hormones during pregnancy in normal and diabetic women. Diabetes *41*:1651, 1992.
4. Knopp RH, et al: Lipoprotein metabolism in pregnancy. *In* Herrera E, Knopp RH (eds): Perinatal Biochemistry. Boca Raton, CRC Press, 1992, pp 19–51.
5. Montes A, et al: Physiologic and supraphysiologic increases in lipoprotein lipids and apoproteins in late pregnancy and postpartum: possible markers for the diagnosis of "prelipemia." Arteriosclerosis *4*:407, 1984.
6. Fahraeus L, et al: Plasma lipoproteins including high density lipoprotein subfractions during normal pregnancy. Obstet Gynecol *66*:468, 1985.
7. Alvarez JJ, et al: Longitudinal study on lipoprotein profile, high density lipoprotein subclass, and postheparin lipases during gestation in women. J Lipid Res *37*:299, 1996.
8. Elliott JA: The effect of pregnancy on the control of lipolysis in fat cells isolated from human adipose tissue. Eur J Clin Invest *5*:159, 1975.
9. Knopp RH et al: Carbohydrate metabolism in pregnancy: VIII. metabolism of adipose tissue isolated from fed and fasted pregnant rats during late gestation. J Clin Invest *49*:1438, 1970.
10. Chaves JM, Herrera E: In vitro response of glycerol metabolism to insulin and adrenaline in adipose tissue from fed and fasted rat during pregnancy. Biol Neonate *38*:139, 1980.
11. Ramos P, Herrera E: Reversion of insulin resistance in the rat during late pregnancy by 72-h glucose infusion. Am J Physiol Endocrinol Metab 269:E858, 1995.
12. Weinstein I, et al: Effects of ethynylestradiol on metabolism of (1–14C)-oleate by perfused livers and hepatocytes from female rats. Biochem J *180*:265, 1979.
13. Kinnunen PK, et al: Activities of post-heparin plasma lipoprotein lipase and hepatic lipase during pregnancy and lactation. Eur J Clin Invest *10*:469, 1980.
14. Herrera E, et al: Serum lipid profile in diabetic pregnancy. Adv Diabet *5*(Suppl 1):73, 1992.
15. Otway S, Robinson DS: The significance of changes in tissue clearing-factor lipase activity in relation to the lipaemia of pregnancy. Biochem J *106*:677, 1968.
16. Herrera E, et al: Role of lipoprotein lipase activity on lipoprotein metabolism and the fate of circulating triglycerides in pregnancy. Am J Obstet Gynecol *158*:1575, 1988.
17. Martin-Hidalgo A, et al: Lipoprotein lipase and hormone-sensitive lipase activity and mRNA in rat adipose tissue during pregnancy. Am J Physiol *266*:E930, 1994.
18. Ramos P, Herrera E: Comparative responsiveness to prolonged hyperinsulinemia between adipose tissue and mammary gland lipoprotein lipase activities in pregnant rats. Early Pregnancy Biol Med *2*:29, 1996.
19. Hamosh M, et al: Lipoprotein lipase activity of adipose and mammary tissue and plasma triglyceride in pregnant and lactating rats. Biochim Biophys Acta *210*:473, 1970.
20. Herrera E, et al: Control by insulin of adipose tissue lipoprotein lipase activity during late pregnancy in the rat. *In* Shafrir E (ed): Frontiers in Diabetes Research: Lessons from Animal Diabetes III. London, Smith-Gordon, 1990, pp 551–554.
21. Iglesias A, et al: Changes in cholesteryl ester transfer protein activity during normal gestation and postpartum. Clin Biochem *27*:63, 1994.
22. Applebaum-Bowden D, et al: Lipoprotein, apolipoprotein, and lipolytic enzyme changes following estrogen administration in postmenopausal women. J Lipid Res *30*:1895, 1989.
23. Peinado-Onsurbe J, et al: Effects of sex steroids on hepatic and lipoprotein lipase activity and mRNA in the rat. Horm Res *40*:184, 1993.
24. Brinton EA: Oral estrogen replacement therapy in postmenopausal women selectively raises levels and production rates of lipoprotein A-I and lowers hepatic lipase activity without lowering the fractional catabolic rate. Arterioscler Thromb Vasc Biol *16*:431, 1996.
25. Hrab RV, et al: Prevention of fluvastatin-induced toxicity, mortality, and cardiac myopathy in pregnant rats by mevalonic acid supplementation. Teratology *50*:19, 1994.
26. Soria A, et al: Opposite metabolic response to fenofibrate treatment in pregnant and virgin rats. J Lipid Res. *43*:74, 2002
27. Winkel CA, et al: Uptake and degradation of lipoproteins by human trophoblastic cells in primary culture. Endocrinology *107*:1892, 1980.
28. Albrecht ED, et al: Developmental increase in low density lipoprotein receptor messenger ribonucleic acid levels in placental syncytiotrophoblasts during baboon pregnancy. Endocrinology *136*:5540, 1995
29. Winkel CA, et al: Regulation of cholesterol and progesterone synthesis in human placental cells in culture by serum lipoproteins. Endocrinology *106*:1054, 1980.
30. Alsat E, et al: Low-density lipoprotein binding sites in the microvillous membranes of human placenta at different stages of gestation. Mol Cell Endocrinol *38*:197, 1984.
31. Alsat E, et al: Characterization of specific low-density lipoprotein binding sites in human term placental microvillous membranes. Mol Cell Endocrinol *28*:439, 1982.
32. Winkel CA, et al: Regulation of cholesterol metabolism by human trophoblastic cells in primary culture. Endocrinology *109*:1084, 1981.
33. Henson MC, et al: Developmental increase in placental low density lipoprotein uptake during baboon pregnancy. Endocrinology *130*:1698, 1992.
34. Cummings SW, et al: The binding of high and low density lipoproteins to human placental membrane fractions. J Clin Endocrinol Metab *54*:903, 1982.
35. Furuhashi M, et al: Expression of low density lipoprotein receptor gene in human placenta during pregnancy. Mol Endocrinol *3*:1252, 1989.
36. Malassine A, et al: Ultrastructural visualization of the internalization of low density lipoprotein by human placental cells. Histochemistry *87*:457, 1987.
37. Overbergh L, et al: Expression of mouse alpha-macroglobulins, lipoprotein receptor-related protein, LDL receptor, apolipoprotein E, and lipoprotein lipase in pregnancy. J Lipid Res *36*:1774, 1995.
38. Bonet B, et al: Metabolism of very-low-density lipoprotein triglyceride by human placental cells: the role of lipoprotein lipase. Metabolism *41*:596, 1992.
39. Elphick MC, Hull D: Rabbit placental clearing-factor lipase and transfer to the foetus of fatty acids derived from triglycerides injected into the mother. J Physiol (Lond) *273*:475, 1977.
40. Rotherwell JE, Elphick MC: Lipoprotein lipase activity in human and guinea pig placenta. J Dev Physiol *4*:153, 1982.
41. Thomas CR, Lowy C: The clearance and placental transfer of FFA and triglycerides in the pregnant guinea-pig. J Dev Physiol *4*:163, 1982
42. Clegg RA: Placental lipoprotein lipase activity in the rabbit, rat and sheep. Comp Biochem Physiol *69B*:585, 1981.
43. Farrugia W, et al: Type II phospholipase A2 in human gestational tissues: Subcellular distribution of placental imuno- and catalytic activity. Biochim Biophys Acta *1166*:77, 1993.
44. Rice GE, et al: Contribution of type II phospholipase A_2 to *in vitro* phospholipase A_2 enzymatic activity in human term placenta. J Endocrinol *157*:25, 1998.
45. Biale Y: Lipolytic activity in the placentas of chronically deprived fetuses. Acta Obstet Gynecol Scand *64*:111, 1985.
46. Kaminsky S, et al: Effects of maternal undernutrition and uterine artery ligation on placental lipase activities in the rat. Biol Neonate *60*:201, 1991.

47. Mochizuki M, et al: Lipolytic action of human chorionic somatomammotropin. Endocrinol Jpn 22:123, 1975.
48. Coleman RA, Haynes EB: Synthesis and release of fatty acids by human trophoblast cells in culture. J Lipid Res 28:1335, 1987.
49. Benassayag C, et al: High polyunsaturated fatty acid, thromboxane A₂, and alpha-fetoprotein concentrations at the human feto-maternal interface. J Lipid Res 38:276, 1997.
50. Benassayag C, et al: High affinity of nonesterified polyunsaturated fatty acids for rat alpha-fetoprotein (AFP). Oncodev Biol Med 1:27, 1980.
51. Parmelee DC, et al: The presence of fatty acids in human α-fetoprotein. J Biol Chem 253:2114, 1978.
52. Berghaus TM, et al B: Essential fatty acids and their long-chain polyunsaturated metabolites in maternal and cord plasma triglycerides during late gestation. Biol Neonate 77:96, 2000.
53. Herrera E. Implications of dietary fatty acids during pregnancy on placental, fetal and postnatal development. Placenta (Suppl A, Trophoblast Research) 16:59, 2002.
54. Kitajima M, et al: Maternal serum triglyceride at 24-32 weeks' gestation and newborn weight in nondiabetic women with positive diabetic screens. Obstet Gynecol 97:776, 2001.
55. Knopp RH, et al: Prediction of infant birth weight by GDM screening tests: Importance of plasma triglycerides. Diabetes Care 15:1605, 1992.
56. Skryten A, et al: Studies in diabetic pregnancy. I. Serum lipids. Acta Obstet Gynecol Scand 55:215, 1976.
57. Hytten FE, Leitch I: The Physiology of Human Pregnancy. Oxford, Blackwell Scientific, 1971.
58. Beaton GH, et al: Protein metabolism in the pregnant rat. J Nutr 54:291, 1954.
59. Lopez Luna P, et al: Carcass and tissue fat content in the pregnant rat. Biol Neonate 60:29, 1991.
60. King JC, et al: Energy metabolism during pregnancy: Influence of maternal energy status. Am J Clin Nutr 59 Suppl.: 439S, 1994.
61. Ludeña MC, et al: Effects of alcohol ingestion in the pregnant rat on daily food intake, offspring growth and metabolic parameters. Gen Pharmacol 14:327, 1983.
62. Palacín M, et al: Circulating metabolite utilization by periuterine adipose tissue in situ in the pregnant rat. Metabolism 40:534, 1991.
63. Knopp RH, et al: Lipid metabolism in pregnancy: II. Postheparin lipolytic activity and hypertriglyceridemia in the pregnant rat. Metabolism 24:481, 1975.
64. López-Luna P, et al: Body fat in pregnant rats at mid- and late-gestation. Life Sci 39:1389, 1986.
65. Freinkel N: Metabolic changes in pregnancy. In Wilson JD, Foster DW (eds): Textbook of Endocrinology. Philadelphia, WB Saunders Co, 1985, pp 438–451.
66. Chaves JM, Herrera E: In vitro glycerol metabolism in adipose tissue from fasted pregnant rats. Biochem Biophys Res Commun 85:1299, 1978.
67. Herrera E, et al: Lipid metabolism in pregnancy. Biol Neonate 51:70, 1987.
68. Humphrey JL, et al: Lipid metabolism in pregnancy: VII. Kinetics of chylomicron triglyceride removal in the fed pregnant rat. Am J Physiol 239:E81, 1980.
69. Wasfi I, et al: Hepatic metabolism of [1-¹⁴C]oleate in pregnancy. Biochim Biophys Acta 619:471, 1980.
70. Argiles J, Herrera E: Appearance of circulating and tissue ¹⁴C-lipids after oral ¹⁴C-tripalmitate administration in the late pregnant rat. Metabolism 38:104, 1989.
71. Stemberg L, et al: Serum proteins in parturient mother and newborn: an electrophoretic study. Can Med Assoc J 74:49, 1956.
72. Argilés J, Herrera E: Lipids and lipoproteins in maternal and fetus plasma in the rat. Biol Neonate 39:37, 1981.
73. Herrera E, et al: Carbohydrate metabolism in pregnancy: VI. plasma fuels, insulin, liver composition, gluconeogenesis and nitrogen metabolism during gestation in the fed and fasted rat. J Clin Invest 48:2260, 1969.
74. Rémésy C, Demigné C: Adaptation of hepatic gluconeogenesis and ketogenesis to altered supply of substrates during late pregnancy in the rat. J Dev Physiol 8:195, 1966.
75. Chaves JM, Herrera E: In vivo glycerol metabolism in the pregnant rat. Biol Neonate 37:172, 1980.
76. Zorzano A, et al: Role of the availability of substrates on hepatic and renal gluconeogenesis in the fasted late pregnant rat. Metabolism 35:297, 1986.
77. Ramirez I, et al: Circulating triacylglycerols, lipoproteins, and tissue lipoprotein lipase activities in rat mothers and offspring during the perinatal period: effect of postmaturity. Metabolism 32:333, 1983.
78. Carrascosa JM, et al: Changes in the kinase activity of the insulin receptor account for an increased insulin sensitivity of mammary gland in late pregnancy. Endocrinology 139:520, 1998.
79. Scow RO, et al: Hyperlipemia and ketosis in the pregnant rat. Am J Physiol 206:796, 1964.
80. Scow RO, et al: Ketosis in the rat fetus. Proc Soc Exp Biol Med 98:833, 1958.
81. Girard J, et al: Fetal metabolic response to maternal fasting in the rat. Am J Physiol 232:E456, 1977.
82. Testar X, et al: Increase with starvation in the pregnant rat of the liver lipoprotein lipase. Biochem Soc Trans 13:134, 1985.
83. Vilaró S, et al: Lipoprotein lipase activity in the liver of starved pregnant rats. Biol Neonate 57:37, 1990.
84. Carlson MG, et al: Fuel and energy metabolism in fasting humans. Am J Clin Nutr 60:29, 1994.
85. Vazquez JA, Kazi U: Lipolysis and gluconeogenesis from glycerol during weight reduction with very-low-calorie diets. Metabolism 43:1293, 1994.
86. Palacín M, et al: Transporte de metabolitos a través de la placenta. Rev Esp Pediatr 40:163, 1984.
87. Munro HN, et al: The placenta in nutrition. Rev Nutr 3:97, 1983.
88. Yudilevich DL, Seeiry JH: Transport of amino acids in the placenta. Biochim Biophys Acta 822:169, 1980.
89. Hill EP, Longo LD: Dynamics of maternal-fetal nutrient transfer. Fed Proc 39:239, 1980.
90. Baur R: Morphometric data and questions concerning placental transfer. In Young M, et al (eds): Placental Transfer Methods and Interpretations, Placenta Suppl 2. London, WB Saunders Co, 1981, pp 35–44.
91. Morris FHJ: Placental factors conditioning fetal nutrition and growth. Am J Clin Nutr 34:760, 1981.
92. Burr GO, Burr MM: On the nature and role of the fatty acids essential in nutrition. J Biol Chem 82:345, 1929.
93. Hassam AG, Crawford MA: The differential incorporation of labelled linoleic, T-linolenic, dihomo-T-linolenic and arachidonic acids into the developing brain. J Neurochem 27:967, 1976.
94. Hull D: Total fat metabolism. In Beard RW, Nathaniels G (eds): Fetal Physiology and Medicine. London, WB Saunders Co, 1976, pp 105–120.
95. Widdowson EM: Chemical composition of newly born mammals. Nature (Lond) 166:626, 1950.
96. James E, et al: A-V differences of FFA and glycerol in the ovine umbilical circulation. Proc Soc Exp Biol Med 138:823, 1971.
97. Hull D, Stammers JP: Placental transfer of fatty acids. Biochem Soc Trans 13:821, 1985.
98. Elphick MC, et al: The transfer of fatty acids across the sheep placenta. J Dev Physiol 1:31, 1979.
99. Leat WMF, Harrison FA: Transfer of long chain fatty acids to the fetal and neonatal lamb. J Dev Physiol 2:257, 1980.
100. Hull D, Elphick MC: Transfer of fatty acids across the cat placenta. Biol Neonate 45:15, 1984.
101. Elphick MC, et al: Transfer of fatty acids across the rabbit placenta. J Physiol (Lond) 252:29, 1975.
102. Hershfield MS, Nemeth AM: Placental transport of free palmitic and linoleic acids in the guinea pig. J Lipid Res 9:460, 1968.
103. Bohmer T, Havel RJ: Genesis of fatty liver and hyperlipemia in the fetal guinea pig. J Lipid Res 16:454, 1975.
104. Portman OW, et al: Transfer of free fatty acid across the primate placenta. Am J Physiol 216:143, 1969.
105. Koren Z, Shafrir W: Placental transfer of FFA in the pregnant rat. Proc Soc Exp Biol Med 116:411, 1964.
106. Hummel L, et al: Studies on the lipid metabolism using ¹⁴C-1-palmitate in fetal rats. Biol Neonate 24:298, 1974.
107. Jones CT: Lipid metabolism and mobilization in the guinea pig during pregnancy. Biochem J 156:357, 1976.
108. Stammers JP, et al: Effect of maternal diet during late pregnancy on fetal lipid stores in rabbits. J Dev Physiol 5:395, 1983.
109. Amusquivar E, et al: Low arachidonic acid rather than α-tocopherol is responsible for the delayed postnatal development in offspring of rats fed fish oil instead of olive oil during pregnancy and lactation. J Nutr 130:2855, 2000
110. Coleman RA: The role of the placenta in lipid metabolism and transport. Semin Perinatol 13:180, 1989.
111. Kuhn DC, Crawford M: Placental essential fatty acid transport and prostaglandin synthesis. Prog Lipid Res 25:345, 1986.
112. Abumrad NA, et al: Permeation of long-chain fatty acids into adipocytes. J Biol Chem 259:8945, 1984.
113. Goresky CA, et al: The capillary transport system for free fatty acids in the heart. Circ Res 74:1015, 1994.
114. Campbell FM, et al: Preferential uptake of long chain polyunsaturated fatty acids by isolated human placental membranes. Mol Cell Biochem 155:77, 1996.
115. Campbell FM, et al: Plasma membrane fatty acid binding protein from human placenta: identification and characterization. Biochem Biophys Res Commun 209:1011, 2000.
116. Campbell FM, et al: Uptake of long chain fatty acids by human placental choriocarcinoma (BeWo) cells: role of plasma membrane fatty acid binding protein. J Lipid Res 38:2558–2568, 1997.
117. Haggarty P, et al: Long-chain polyunsaturated fatty acid transport across the perfused human placenta. Placenta 18:635, 1997.
118. Lafond J, et al: Implication of ATP and sodium in arachidonic acid incorporation by placental syncytiotrophoblast brush border and basal plasma membranes in the human. Placenta 21:661, 2000.
119. Shand JH, Noble RC: Incorporation of linoleic and arachidonic acids into ovine placental phospholipids in vitro. Biol Neonate 48:299, 1985.
120. Robertson A, et al: Oxidation of palmitate by human placental tissue slices. Phys Chem Physiol 3:293, 1971.
121. Zimmermann T, et al: Oxidation and synthesis of fatty acids in human and rat placental and fetal tissues. Biol Neonate 36:109, 1979.
122. Robertson A, Sprecher H: Human placental lipid metabolism. III. Synthesis and hydrolysis of phospholipids. Lipids 2:403, 1967.
123. Tulenko TN, Rabinowitz JL: Fatty acid metabolism in human fetal placental vasculature. Am J Physiol 240:E65, 1981.
124. Crawford MA, et al: Essential fatty acids and fetal brain growth. Lancet 1:452, 1976.
125. Innis SM: Essential fatty acids in growth and development. Prog Lipid Res 30:39, 1991.

126. Simopoulos AP: Ω-3 fatty acids in health and disease and in growth and development. Am J Clin Nutr 54:438, 1991.

127. Uauy R, Mena P, Wegher B et al: Long chain polyunsaturated fatty acid formation in neonates: effect of gestational age and intrauterine growth. Pediatr Res 47:127, 2000.

128. Thomas CR, Lowy C: Placental transfer of FFA: factors affecting transfer across the guinea-pig placenta. J Dev Physiol 5:323, 1983.

129. Stephenson TJ, et al: Maternal to fetal transfer of FFA in the "in situ" perfused rabbit placenta. J Dev Physiol 13:117, 1990.

130. Stepien M, et al: Effects of altering umbilical flow and umbilical free fatty acid concentration on transfer of FFA across the rabbit placenta. J Dev Physiol 15:221, 1991.

131. Edson JL, et al: Evidence for increased fatty acid transfer across the placenta during a maternal fast in rabbits. Biol Neonate 27:50, 1975.

132. Stephenson T, et al: Placental transfer of FFA: importance of fetal albumin concentration and acid-base status. Biol Neonate 63:273, 1993.

133. Dancis J, et al: Transfer across perfused human placenta: IV. effect of protein binding on free fatty acids. Pediatr Res 10:5, 1976.

134. Cartlidge PHT, Rutter N: Serum albumin concentrations and oedema in the newborn. Arch Dis Child 61:657, 1986.

135. Lasunción MA, et al: Method for the study of metabolite transfer from rat mother to fetus. Biol Neonate 44:85, 1983.

136. Palacín M, et al: Placental formation of lactate from transferred L-alanine and its impairment by aminooxyacetate in the late-pregnant rat. Biochim Biophys Acta 841:90, 1985.

137. Herrera E, et al: Relationship between maternal and fetal fuels and placental glucose transfer in rats with maternal diabetes of varying severity. Diabetes 34(Suppl 2):42, 1985.

138. Palacín M, et al: Decreased uterine blood flow in the diabetic pregnant rat does not modify the augmented glucose transfer to the fetus. Biol Neonate 48:197, 1985.

139. Lasunción MA, et al: Maternal factors modulating nutrient transfer to fetus. Biol Neonate 51:86, 1987.

140. Elphick MC, Hull D: Incorporation "in vivo" of 1-14C-palmitic acid into placental and fetal liver lipids of the rabbit. Biol Neonate 32:24, 1977.

141. Thomas CR: Placental transfer of non-esterified fatty acids in normal and diabetic pregnancy. Biol Neonate 51:94, 1987.

142. Coleman RA: Placental metabolism and transport of lipid. Fed Proc 45:2519, 1986.

143. Hummel L, et al: Maternal plasma triglycerides as a source of fetal fatty acids. Acta Biol Med Ger 35:1635, 1976.

144. Thomas CR, Lowy C: The interrelationships between circulating maternal esterified and non-esterified fatty acids in pregnant guinea pigs, and their relative contributions to the fetal circulation. J Dev Physiol 9:203, 1987.

145. Elphick MC, et al: The passage of fat emulsion across the human placenta. Br J Obstet Gynaecol 85:610, 1978.

146. Seeds AE, et al: Comparison of human and sheep chorion leave permeability to glucose, beta-hydroxybutyrate and glycerol. Am J Obstet Gynecol 138:604, 1980.

147. Sabata V, et al: The role of FFA, glycerol, ketone bodies and glucose in the energy metabolism of the mother and fetus during delivery. Biol Neonate 13:7, 1968.

148. Gilbert M: Origin and metabolic fate of plasma glycerol in the rat and rabbit fetus. Pediatr Res 11:95, 1977.

149. Palacín M, et al: Lactate production and absence of gluconeogenesis from placental transferred substrates in fetuses from fed and 48-H starved rats. Pediatr Res 22:6, 1987.

150. Battaglia FC, Meschia C: Principal substrates of fetal metabolism. Physiol Rev 58:499, 1978.

151. Herrera E, et al: Carbohydrate-lipid interactions during gestation and their control by insulin. Braz J Med Biol Res 27:2499, 1994.

152. Bissonnette JM: Studies "in vivo" of glucose transfer across the guinea-pig placenta. Placenta 2(Suppl):155, 1981.

153. Mampel T, et al: Changes in circulating glycerol, FFA and glucose levels following liver transplant in the pig. Arch Int Physiol Biochim 89:195, 1981.

154. Mampel T, et al: Hepatectomy-nephrectomy effects in the pregnant rat and fetus. Biochem Biophys Res Commun 131:1219, 1985.

155. Mackay EM, Barnes RH: Fasting ketosis in the pregnant rat as influenced by adrenalectomy. Proc Soc Exp Biol Med 34:683, 1936.

156. Morris FH, et al: Umbilical V-A differences of acetoacetate and beta hydroxybutyrate in fed and starved ewes. Proc Soc Exp Biol Med 145:879, 1974.

157. Kim YJ, Felig P: Maternal and amniotic fluid substrate levels during caloric deprivation in human pregnancy. Metabolism 21:507, 1971.

158. Felig P, Lynch V: Starvation in human pregnancy: hypoglycemia, hypoinsulinemia, and hyperketonemia. Science 170:990, 1970.

159. Williamson DH: Regulation of the utilization of glucose and ketone bodies by brain in the perinatal period. In Camerini-Davalos RA, Cole HS (eds): Early Diabetes in Early Life. New York, Academic Press, 1975, pp 195–202.

160. Persson B, Lunell NO: Metabolic control of diabetic pregnancy: variations in plasma concentrations of glucose, FFA, glycerol, ketone bodies, insulin and human chorionic somato-mammotropin during the last trimester. Am J Obstet Gynecol 122:737, 1975.

161. Butte NF: Carbohydrate and lipid metabolism in pregnancy: normal compared with gestational diabetes mellitus. Am J Clin Nutr 71(Suppl):1256S, 2000.

162. Page MA, Williamson DH: Enzymes of ketone-body utilisation in human brain. Lancet 2:66, 1971.

163. Shambaugh GE, et al: Fetal fuels: III. Ketone utilization by fetal hepatocyte. Am J Physiol 235:E330, 1978.

164. Adam PAJ, et al: Oxidation of glucose and D-hydroxybutyrate by the early human fetal brain. Acta Paediatr Scand 64:17, 1975.

165. Shambaugh GE III, et al: Nutrient metabolism and fetal brain development. In Herrera E, Knopp RH (eds): Perinatal Biochemistry. Boca Raton, CRC Press, 1992, pp 213–231.

166. Drew JH, et al: Congenital malformations, abnormal glucose tolerance, and estriol excretion in pregnancy. Obstet Gynecol 51:129, 1978.

167. Churchill JA, et al: Neuropsychological deficits in children of diabetic mothers. Am J Obstet Gynecol 105:257, 1969.

168. Miodovnik M, et al: Effect of maternal ketoacidemia on the pregnant ewe and the fetus. Am J Obstet Gynecol 144:585, 1982.

169. Paterson P, et al: Maternal and fetal ketone concentrations in plasma and urine. Lancet 1:862, 1967.

170. Smith AL, Scanlon J: Amniotic fluid D(-)-β-hydroxybutyrate and the dysmature newborn infant. Am J Obstet Gynecol 115:569, 1973.

171. Arola L, et al: Effects of 24 hour starvation on plasma composition in 19 and 21 day pregnant rats and their foetuses. Horm Metabol Res 14:364, 1982.

172. Lee LPK, Fritz IB: Hepatic ketogenesis during development. Can J Biochem 49:599, 1971.

173. Alonso de la Torre SR, et al: Carrier-mediated β-hydroxybutyrate transport in brush-border membrane vesicles from rat placenta. Pediatr Res 32:317, 1992.

174. Boyd RD, et al: Growth of glucose and oxygen uptakes by fetuses of fed and starved ewes. Am J Physiol 225:897, 1973.

175. Patel MS, et al: The metabolism of ketone bodies in developing human brain: development of ketone-body utilizing enzymes and ketone bodies as precursors for lipid synthesis. J Neurochem 25:905, 1975.

176. Williamson DH: Ketone body metabolism and the fetus. In Van Assche FA, et al (eds): Fetal Growth Retardation. Edinburgh, Churchill Livingstone, 1981, pp 29–34.

177. Seccombe DW, et al: Fetal utilization of maternally derived ketone bodies for lipogenesis in the rat. Biochim Biophys Acta 438:402, 1977.

178. Thaler MM: Effects of starvation on normal development of beta-hydroxybutyrate dehydrogenase activity in fetal and newborn rat brain. Nature New Biol 236:140, 1972.

179. Dierks-Ventling C: Prenatal induction of ketone-body enzymes in the rat. Biol Neonate 19:426, 1971.

180. Ohvo-Rekilä, H et al.: Cholesterol interactions with phospholipids in membranes. Prog Lipid Res 41:66, 2002.

181. Brown, MS, Goldstein, JL: The SREBP pathway: regulation of cholesterol metabolism by proteolysis of a membrane-bound transcription factor. Cell 89:331, 1997.

182. Schroepfer, GJ: Oxysterols: modulators of cholesterol metabolism and other processes. Physiol Rev 80, 361, 2000.

183. Peet DJ, et al: The LXRs: a new class of oxysterol receptors. Curr Opin Genet Dev 8:571, 1998.

184. Martínez-Botas, J, et al: Cholesterol starvation decreases p34^cdc2 kinase activity and arrests the cell cycle at G2. FASEB J 13:1359, 1999.

185. Suárez, Y et al: Differential effects of ergosterol and cholesterol on Cdk1 activation and SRE-driven transcription: Sterol specificity for cell cycle progression in human cells. Eur J Biochem 269:1761, 2002.

186. Mauch, DH, et al: CNS synaptogenesis promoted by glia-derived cholesterol. Science 294:1354, 2001.

187. Roux, C et al: Role of cholesterol in embryonic development. Am J Clin Nutr 71: 1270s, 2000.

188. Mann, RK, Beachy PA: Cholesterol modification of proteins. Biochim Biophys Acta 1529:188, 2000.

189. Waterham HR, Wanders RJA: Biochemical and genetic aspects of 7-dehydrocholesterol reductase and Smith-Lemli-Opitz syndrome. Biochim Biophys Acta 152:340, 2000.

190. Moebius FF, et al: Genetic defects in postsqualene cholesterol biosynthesis. Trends Endocrinol Metab 11:106, 2000.

191. Wise T, et al: Relationships of light and heavy fetuses to uterine position, placental weight, gestational age, and fetal cholesterol concentrations. J Anim Sci 75:2197, 1997.

192. Schoknecht, PA et al: Dietary cholesterol supplementation improves growth and behavioral response of pigs selected for genetically high and low serum cholesterol. J Nutr 124:305, 1994.

193. Lu, CD et al. Response to dietary fat and cholesterol in young adult boars genetically selected for high or low plasma cholesterol. J Anim Sci 73:2043, 1995.

194. Cieslak, DG, et al: Effect of a high fat supplement in late gestation and lactation on piglet survival and performance. J Anim Sci 57:954, 1983.

195. Schroepfer GJ: Sterol biosynthesis. Annu Rev Biochem 51:555, 1982.

196. Chevallier, F: Transferts et synthèse du cholestérol chez le rat au cours de sa croissance. Biochim Biophys Acta 84:316, 1964.

197. Connor WE, Lin DS: Placental transfer of cholesterol-4-14C into rabbit and guinea pig fetus. J Lipid Res 8:558, 1967.

198. Pitkin RM, et al: Cholesterol metabolism and placental transfer in the pregnant Rhesus monkey. J Clin Invest 51:2584, 1972.

199. Yount NY, McNamara DJ: Dietary regulation of maternal and fetal cholesterol metabolism in the guinea pig. Biochim Biophys Acta 1085:82, 1991.

200. Belknap WM, Dietschy JM Sterol synthesis and low density lipoprotein clearance in vivo in the pregnant rat, placenta, and fetus. Sources for tissue cholesterol during fetal development. J Clin Invest 82:2077, 1988.

201. Woollett LA: Origin of cholesterol in the fetal golden Syrian hamster: contribution of de novo sterol synthesis and maternal-derived lipoprotein cholesterol. J Lipid Res 37:1246, 1996.
202. Jurevics HA, et al: Sources of cholesterol during development of the rat fetus and fetal organs. J Lipid Res 38:723, 1997.
203. Haave NC, Innis SM: Cholesterol synthesis and accretion within various tissues of the fetal and neonatal rat. Metabolism 50:12, 2001.
204. Levin MS, et al: Developmental changes in the expression of genes involved in cholesterol biosynthesis and lipid transport in human and rat fetal and neonatal livers. Biochim Biophys Acta 1003:293, 1989.
205. McNamara DJ, et al: Regulation of hepatic 3-hydroxy-3-methylglutaryl coenzyme A reductase: developmental pattern. J Biol Chem 247:5805, 1972.
206. Ness GC, et al.: Perinatal development of 3-hydroxy-3-methylglutaryl coenzyme A reductase activity in rat lung, liver and brain. Lipids 14:447, 1979.
207. Munilla MA, Herrera E: A cholesterol-rich diet causes a greater hypercholesterolemic response in pregnant than in nonpregnant rats and does not modify fetal lipoprotein profile. J Nutr 127:2239, 1997.
208. Feingold KR, et al.: De novo cholesterogenesis in pregnancy. J Lab Clin Med 101:256, 1983.
209. Haave NC, Innis SM: Hepatic cholesterol and fatty acid synthesis in pregnant and fetal rats: effect of maternal dietary fat and cholestyramine. J Nutr 121:1529, 1991.
210. Gaoua W, et al: Cholesterol deficit but not accumulation of aberrant sterols is the major cause of the teratogenic activity in the Smith-Lemli-Opitz syndrome animal model. J Lipid Res 41:637, 2000.
211. Barbu V, et al. Cholesterol prevents the teratogenic action of AY 9944: importance of the timing of cholesterol supplementation to rats. J Nutr 118:774, 1988.
212. McConihay JA, et al: Effect of maternal hypercholesterolemia on fetal sterol metabolism in the Golden Syrian hamster. J Lipid Res 42:1111, 2001.
213. Parker CR, et al.: Analysis of the potential for transfer of lipoprotein-cholesterol across the human placenta. Early Hum Dev 8:289, 1983.
214. Ortega RM, et al: Influence of maternal serum lipids and maternal diet during the third trimester of pregnancy on umbilical cord blood lipids in two populations of Spanish newborns. Int J Vitam Nutr Res 66:250, 1996.
215. Nakai T, et al.: Plasma lipids and lipoproteins of Japanese adults and umbilical cord blood. Artery 9:132, 1981.
216. Devi CS, et al: Concentration of triglyceride and cholesterol in lipoprotein fractions in maternal and cord blood samples. Clin Chim Acta 123:169, 1982.
217. Ramon y Cajal, J, et al: Plasma lipids and high density lipoprotein cholesterol in maternal and umbilical vessels in twin pregnancies. Artery 15:109, 1988.
218. Neary RH, et al: Fetal and maternal lipoprotein metabolism in human pregnancy. Clin Sci (Colch) 88:311, 1995.
219. Skinner ER, et al: The composition and concentration of umbilical cord plasma lipoproteins; their relationship to the birth weight and other clinical factors of the newborn. Clin Chim Acta 135:219, 1983.
220. Diaz M, et al.: Cord blood lipoprotein-cholesterol: relationship of birth weight and gestational age of newborns. Metabolism 38:435, 1989.
221. Napoli C, et al.: Fatty streak formation occurs in human fetal aortas and is greatly enhanced by maternal hypercholesterolemia: intimal accumulation of low density lipoprotein and its oxidation precede monocyte recruitment into early atherosclerotic lesions. J Clin Invest 100:2680, 1997.
222. Wyne KL, Woollett LA: Transport of maternal LDL and HDL to the fetal membranes and placenta of the Golden Syrian hamster is mediated by receptor-dependent and receptor-independent processes. J Lipid Res 39:518, 1998.
223. Winkel CA, et al: Uptake and degradation of lipoproteins by human trophoblastic cells in primary culture. Endocrinology 107:1892, 1980.
224. Alsat E, et al: Low-density lipoprotein binding sites in the microvillous membranes of human placenta at different stages of gestation. Mol Cell Endocrinol 38:197, 1984.
225. Winkel CA, et al: The role of receptor-mediated low-density lipoprotein uptake and degradation in the regulation of progesterone biosynthesis and cholesterol metabolism by human trophoblasts. Placenta Suppl 3:133, 1981.
226. Lasunción MA, et al: Mechanism of the HDL2 stimulation of progesterone secretion in cultured placental trophoblast. J Lipid Res 32:1073, 1991.
227. McConihay JA, et al: Maternal high density lipoproteins affect fetal mass and extra-embryonic fetal tissue sterol metabolism in the mouse. J Lipid Res 41:424, 2000.
228. Knopp RH, et al: Relationships of infant birth size to maternal lipoproteins, apoproteins, fuels, hormones, clinical chemistries, and body weight at 36 weeks gestation. Diabetes 34:271, 1985.
229. Calvo D, Vega MA: Identification, primary structure, and distribution of CLA-1, a novel member of the CD36/LIMPII gene family. J Biol Chem 268:18929, 1993.
230. Hammad SM, et al: Megalin acts in concert with cubilin to mediate endocytosis of high density lipoproteins. J Biol Chem 275:12003, 2000.
231. Hatzopoulos AK, et al: Temporal and spatial pattern of expression of the HDL receptor SR-BI during murine embryogenesis. J Lipid Res 39:495, 1998.
232. Seetharam B, et al: Identification of rat yolk sac target protein of teratogenic antibodies, gp280, as intrinsic factor-cobalamin receptor. J Clin Invest 99:2317, 1997.

John E. Van Aerde, Michaelann S. Wilke, Miguel Feldman, and M. Thomas Clandinin

40 Accretion of Lipid in the Fetus and Newborn

FETAL FAT METABOLISM

The nutrient and energy requirements of the developing mammalian fetus include the fuels to provide energy for tissue synthesis and the basic nutrients for synthesis of new tissues.[1] From the 26th week of gestation through the 40th week, human fetal weight increases more than fourfold. Part of this increase in weight is water, but the rate of accretion of fat and nonfat components is even greater.[2] Between 26 and 30 weeks' gestation, nonfat and fat calories contribute equally to the energy content of the body;[2] however, beyond that time, fat accumulation considerably exceeds that of the nonfat components.[3] At 36 weeks' gestation, 1.9 g of fat accumulates for each gram of nonfat daily weight gain, and by term gestation, the deposition of fat accounts for more than 90% of the calories accumulated by the fetus.[1] The rate of fat accretion is approximately linear between 36 and 40 weeks' gestation, and by the end of pregnancy, fat accretion ranges from 1.6 to 3.4 g/kg/day.[1] At 28 weeks' gestation, it is slightly less and ranges between 1 and 1.8 g/kg/day.

The main phospholipids of cell membranes contain two of a variety of fatty acids (FAs) and a substituted (amino) alcohol attached to a glycerol phosphate backbone. The nature of the alcohol head group and that of the attached FAs have major effects on the biologic function of that membrane.[4]

The nature and chain length of FAs associated with complex lipids are of particular significance because they determine the structural and functional roles of these lipids in neural membranes.[5] FAs can have no double bonds (saturated), one double bond (monounsaturated), or two or more double bonds (polyunsaturated FAs [PUFAs]). Metabolism of PUFAs results in formation of long chain PUFAs (LCPUFAs; i.e., FAs with more than 18 carbon atoms and multiple double bonds), which are incorporated into complex structural membrane lipids or used for production of biologically active substances (eicosanoids). Biosynthetic pathways producing LCPUFAs consist of a series of desaturation and chain-elongation reactions in which there is no direct cross-over between unsaturated metabolites from one sequence to the other. The type and amount of any given unsaturated FA found in tissue lipids are determined by factors that regulate the synthesis of unsaturated FAs, as well as by control mechanisms dictating the incorporation of a given FA into a lipid.[6]

Eicosanoids are potent compounds that display many different biologic effects.[7] In response to various stimuli, eicosanoids are generated by *de novo* synthesis, are not stored, and are quickly inactivated.[8] The precursor FAs, predominantly arachidonic acid (AA; C20:4n-6), are esterified in the second position of cellular phospholipids and do not exist as free acids to a significant extent. Thus, the generation of free AA from phospholipids is a rate-limiting step for formation of biologically active eicosanoids.[8]

Brain Development

Biochemical Development and Myelination

Brain development is a sequential anatomic process characterized by specific, well-defined stages of growth and maturation.[9] Biochemical development of the brain also appears to be sequential, correlating with anatomic development.[10] The role of lipids during brain development is the subject of a published text.[11] Any defect in the course of brain development can easily result in gross abnormalities of brain function and can cause serious and irreparable damage in the regulation of body activities and expression of behavior.

Lipids are extremely important constituents of the brain. Not only are they essential for the structure and function of the neuronal and glial membranes, but they also constitute the main components of the myelin sheath, which endows the mature axon with its rapid conduction capacity. In myelin, lipids constitute 70 to 75% of dry weight. All the major lipids found in whole brain are also present in myelin, and no lipid components are exclusively present in myelin. However, cerebroside is the most typical lipid found in myelin, and its concentration in brain is proportional to the myelin content.[12] In the adult brain, lipids are the most abundant compounds, constituting about 60% of the total solids or 10 to 20% of the fresh weight of the brain. There is significant regional variation in brain lipid composition; the number of lipids is lower in gray matter and higher in white matter. In cortical gray matter, lipids make up only 7.5% of fresh weight, but in the subcortical white matter, they constitute more than 20%.[13]

The major classes of brain lipids are cholesterol, phospholipids, cerebrosides, sulfatides, and gangliosides. Cerebrosides and sulfatides are found primarily in myelin; the gangliosides are associated with the structure of the external surface of the neuronal membrane, especially in the synaptic region.[14] In myelin, the FAs are predominantly saturated or monounsaturated, whereas in neuronal membranes, particularly synaptosomes, the PUFAs predominate. Each neuron in the cerebral cortex gray matter has more than 10,000 discrete areas of membrane responsible for neurotransmission to other nerve cells through the synaptosomes, which have high concentrations of polyunsaturates, particularly docosahexaenoic acid (DHA; C22:6ω-3). Phosphatidylcholine is quantitatively the most abundant phospholipid in the immature brain, but the major DHA-containing phospholipids in the synaptosomes are phosphatidylserine and phosphatidylethanolamine.[15] In the developing brain, the lipid composition undergoes very significant qualitative and quantitative changes with maturation. During the early stages of development, only those lipids that are part of the general structure of the cell membrane increase. With the onset of myelination, special lipids accumulate in brain tissue and drastically alter its lipid composition, both qualitatively and quantitatively.

In the human brain, myelination begins during the perinatal period, demonstrates a rapid increase during the first year, and continues into the second decade of life. The first structures in the human brain to be myelinated are the motor and sensory roots; the last ones are the reticular formation, nonspecific thalamic projections, and the neocortex.[16, 17] Phylogenetically older structures (e.g., the spinal cord) are myelinated earlier, and the more recently acquired structures follow later.

The total quantity of all classes of lipids increases during brain development. However, not all lipids show the same temporal pattern of increase. For example, phospholipids tend to decrease during brain maturation, whereas others, such as cholesterol, cerebrosides, and sulfatides, are found to increase.[18] This reflects the deposition of myelin in the developing brain and also changes in myelin composition at different ages. The relative proportion of different brain phospholipids and the FA composition of phospholipids in gray and white matter also change with age throughout prenatal life, particularly in the last trimester of pregnancy.

Fatty Acid Deficiency

Prenatal and postnatal essential FA deficiency reduces body and brain weights of the developing progeny even though the mothers are asymptomatic. The extent of these changes in the brain depends on the timing of the deficiency. Compositional changes in myelin parallel or even exceed those observed in whole brain[19] and can be manipulated by dietary FA composition.[20, 21]

The increasing survival of very low birth weight infants has led to study of the development of accretion of essential FAs during the last trimester of fetal development through the early weeks of life. The intrauterine requirements for ω-6 and ω-3 FAs are estimated to be 400 and 50 mg/kg/day, respectively. For the high-risk, low birth weight infant weighing approximately 1300 g, extrauterine tissue synthesis would use about 280 mg/kg/day of ω-6 FAs and about 35 mg/kg/day of ω-3 FAs (based on a projected growth rate, which is similar in composition and amount to the intrauterine rate) (Fig. 40–1).[22]

Clandinin and colleagues[23] determined that during the last trimester of fetal growth, accretion of major tissue FAs occurs earlier and faster in cervical segments than in lumbar regions. There is minimal postnatal accretion of FAs in cervical regions of

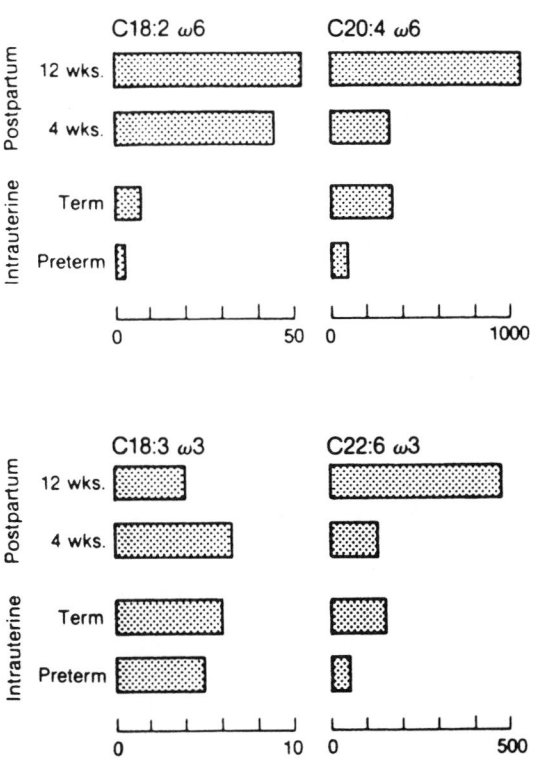

Figure 40–1. Accretion of major essential fatty acids in human brain during intrauterine and early postpartum development.

the spinal cord, with the exception of moderate increases in total ω-9 and saturated FAs, a finding reflecting myelination. Postnatal accretion of FAs in lumbar regions of the spinal cord occurs for approximately 4 weeks, at rates significantly in excess of *in utero* rates.

Changes in Composition of the Brain During Development

Changes in the lipid composition of the brain during development principally reflect accumulation of lipids in myelin sheaths.[24] As a specialized plasma membrane of the myelinating cell, myelin contains large amounts of cholesterol.[25] Cholesterol and sphingolipids (cerebroside, sulfatide, and sphingomyelin) are found mainly in myelin and are the major constituents of total cerebral lipids in the mature brain. On a dry weight basis, approximately 70% of cerebral lipids are contained in myelin. Cerebroside contributes to the stability of the structure of the myelin sheath. In the immature brain, before myelination has occurred, the lipid composition is similar to that in other tissues.[26] At that time, lipid droplets of cholesterol esters are present in glial cell bodies,[27] which rapidly disappear as myelination progresses. Cerebrosides and sulfatides are virtually absent from the brain until myelination begins. At 4 months of gestation, the human fetal brain (which lacks myelin) contains very small amounts of cerebroside and sulfatide, in addition to other glycolipids. The changes in the relative proportions of lipids and the content of individual brain lipids reflect differences in the distribution of lipids in the various cell membranes of the central nervous system. Early in gestation, most cells are devoid of cell processes, and therefore, the lipid content is mainly related to the cell body. Oligodendroglia from the mature brain are characterized by high cerebroside and cholesterol concentrations, but neurons and astrocytes do not change in lipid composition during development.[27]

Ethanolamine phospholipids contain most of the PUFAs esterified in cerebral lipids.[28] Essential FA deficiency in the rat, if imposed during pregnancy, results in significant alterations in the content of LCPUFAs.[29, 30] Conservation of essential FAs in nervous tissue by recycling processes may contribute to stability of the FA composition of cerebral lipids.

LCPUFAs with more than 22 carbon atoms are absent from the human fetal brain but appear in sphingomyelin during the late fetal period where C24:1 predominates.[31] Two classes of sphingomyelin exist: one possesses long chain FAs, with low turnover and localized to myelin; the other is present in nonmyelin membranes. The FA composition of cerebroside also changes with development, as does the FA composition of individual phospholipids (i.e., phosphatidylcholine) from whole brain and from myelin. Phospholipids exhibit an increase in chain length and a greater proportion of unsaturated FAs during maturation. Throughout development, lipid components of the cell membrane undergo continuous turnover, and the lipid components of plasma membranes, including the myelin sheath, are in dynamic equilibrium with intracellular membranes. The enzymes required for lipid biosynthesis exhibit a temporal increase in activity that parallels the rates of accumulation of cerebral lipids.

The ganglioside composition of the brain was reviewed by Ramsey and Nicholas.[24] Gangliosides are important constituents of membranes and are involved in cell differentiation, proliferation, neuritogenesis, growth, inhibition, signaling, and apoptosis.[32-35] The major types of brain gangliosides are fairly consistent between species and include GM_1, GD_3, GD_{1a}, GT_{1a}, GD_{1b}, and GT_{1b}.[36] Gangliosides are present in highest amounts in gray matter and are particularly enriched in synaptic junctions. Rapid changes in the ganglioside composition of the human fetal cortex occur in the latter half of gestation. Vanier and associates[37] revealed that white matter is similar to that of gray matter ganglioside composition of the cerebellum until term, after which GM_1 composition increases to approximately 60% of total

gangliosides. Maximal increase in brain ganglioside content, approximately threefold in the cerebral cortex from the 15th fetal week to the age of 6 months, corresponds to rapid increases in development of neuronal connections at these times. This pattern of increase includes increases in GM_1 and GT_1, with GD_{1a} fractions.[37] Severe maternal protein-calorie deficiency, which lasts throughout gestation and lactation, does not alter prenatal and early postnatal ganglioside accumulation.[38] However, there is a deficit in postnatal ganglioside accumulation after 10 days of age. Stage of development and thus ganglioside amount and composition may relate to membrane ganglioside function. Research by Park and associates[39] showed that, in neonatal rat brain, postnatal ganglioside intake seems to influence ganglioside amount but not composition. Although the ganglioside composition of the diet and enterocyte changed, the plasma and brain composition of the major types of gangliosides measured did not. The functional significance of this preservation of composition is not known.

The fatty acyl-coenzyme A synthetase of cerebral mitochondria is already at maximum activity before birth.[40] There is a correlation between the main FA changes occurring in the brain and those occurring in the liver during early human development. Linoleic acid (LA; C18:2ω-6) and α-linolenic acid (ALA; C18:3ω-3) represent a small proportion of the fatty acyl components of the phosphoglycerides of the fetal brain. In contrast, AA and DHA are readily incorporated into the structural lipids of the developing brain.[41]

Intrauterine Fatty Acid Accretion

Development of the infant brain is accompanied by a rapid rise in cellularity and a declining water content.[42] These changes are associated with an increase in the brain and cerebellar content of LCPUFAs secondary to an increase in the number of plasma membranes.[43] Quantitative analysis of the FA composition of brain lobes indicates rapid accretion of chain elongation and desaturation products during the last trimester of brain growth. Similar analysis of the essential FA composition of cerebrum and cerebellum has indicated how vulnerable the very low birth weight infant is with respect to essential FA deficiency at birth.[43] For example, analysis of the chemical composition of the developing fetus indicates that the total fat content of a 1000-g infant is only 28 g.[44] Levels of LA and ALA are consistently low in brain during the last trimester of development, although a marked accretion of long-chain desaturation products, AA and DHA, occurs at that time (see Fig. 40-1).[43]

During the last trimester of pregnancy, there is a steady increase in the cerebellar content of all FAs, reflecting a general increase in the content of FAs. However, ω-3 FAs represent an exception in that absolute accretion rates, particularly DHA, are greater in the antenatal than in the postnatal period. This finding suggests that the accretion of long-chain ω-3 FAs during the third trimester may be particularly important for the normal rise in brain cellularity.[43]

Examination of intrauterine accretion of ω-6 and ω-3 LCPUFAs has indicated rapid accretion of these components in the fetal brain.[43] In the third trimester, accumulation rates are approximately 43 mg of ω-6 and 22 mg of ω-3 PUFAs per week (Fig 40-2).[22] Thus, during the last trimester, the major FAs to accrue are the chain elongation-desaturation products; only 2.6% of the brain FA content is LA. In term infants during early postnatal brain development, the LA content increases significantly, whereas little increase occurs in brain levels of chain elongation-desaturation products for several weeks postpartum.[45] In humans, the brain undergoes an accelerated growth phase during the last trimester of pregnancy and the first 18 months of postnatal life (Fig. 40-3). During this vulnerable period, essential FAs are required for structural expansion of the brain.

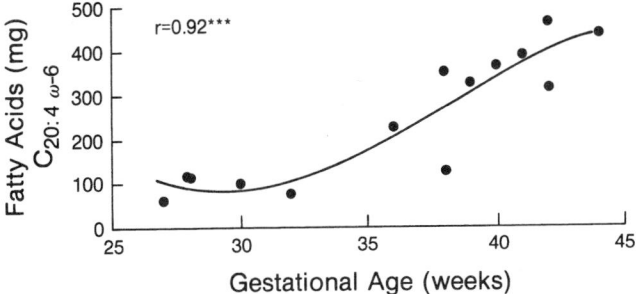

Figure 40–2. Fatty acid content of infant brain expressed as a function of gestational age. Values of r and significance levels are indicated (df = 13). Totals for each fatty acid (mg) are computed where x = gestational age (weeks).

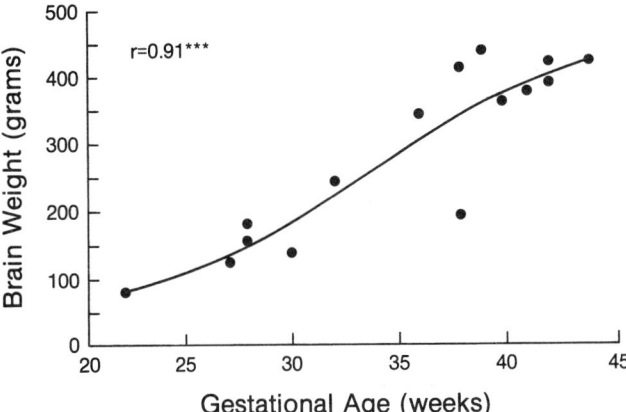

Figure 40–3. Brain weight as a function of gestational age.

PLACENTA

Placental Metabolism and Transport of Lipid

The maternofetal transfer of substances across the placenta involves any of five potential mechanisms (passive diffusion, facilitated diffusion, active transport, ultrafiltration, and pinocytosis); however, FAs, some amino acids, and lipid-soluble vitamins are transferred by a passive diffusion process.[46, 47] Interspecies comparison of fetal fat accretion, with placental permeability for free FAs, demonstrates that the human neonate (who has a high body fat content) has a placenta relatively permeable to free FAs. Most observations suggest that embryonic and fetal lipids in early gestation are derived from maternal FAs that cross the placenta, followed by a gradual shift to *de novo* synthesis from glucose in fetal tissue with advancing gestation.[48]

Free FAs and cholesterol are the only lipid fractions present in maternal blood that are known to cross the placenta.[49] Free FAs are released to the fetus, but the mechanism of release is not known. Maternal free FAs enter the placenta and pass into the fetal circulation;[47] however, the placental permeability for free FAs is low. Although intact complex maternal lipids may not be transported as triacylglycerol, partial glycerides or phospholipids may be synthesized within the placenta and then released into the fetal circulation.[50] Triglycerides and phospholipids are taken up by the placenta but are metabolized to such an extent that neither can be considered a source of free FAs for the fetus.[49] In humans, the levels of free FAs are higher in maternal blood than fetal blood, and their concentrations are highly correlated.[49] Under normal circumstances, the fetal/maternal ratio of free FAs is less than 0.5.[1] "The fetus appears to obtain FAs from a combination of *de novo* synthesis, a passive gradient–dependent

transplacental passage of nonesterified FAs and a selective maternofetal placental transport for certain FAs, such as physiologically important LCPUFAs."[51] Preferential uptake of LCPUFAs by the fetal side of the placenta has been suggested as the main mechanism of incorporation of LCPUFAs in the fetus.[52]

FAs are required by the fetus and the placenta for synthesis of complex lipids.[50] Because fetal tissues can actively synthesize FAs, considerable controversy has existed concerning the relative amounts of FAs synthesized by the fetus and the amounts contributed by the mother.[53] An inverse correlation exists between chain length and transfer rate for FAs. Interpretation of this information is difficult because many factors change coincident with a reduction in chain length, including a decrease in the association constant of the albumin-free FA complex. Observations in animals and estimates of placental transfer of FAs, derived from *in vitro* studies, suggest that approximately 30% of the daily lipid accumulation by the fetus is transported from the maternal circulation;[54] the remainder is synthesized by the fetus. This finding indicates that approximately 1.7 g/day of FAs (including essential FAs) is transferred each day.

Evidence in humans indicates a placental role in preferential accumulation of LCPUFAs in fetal tissues.[55] Selective transfer of monounsaturated and polyunsaturated FAs into fetal circulation seems to occur as a product of a physiologic mechanism, rather than only as a function of free concentration in the maternal perfusate.[56] Selectivity of placental uptake was proposed previously as the result of brush-border and basal membrane concentrations of FA binding proteins in syncytiotrophoblasts,[57] as well as LCPUFA specificity of and competition for FA binding sites.[55] Human placental tissue lacks both the Δ^6 and Δ^5 desaturase activities, and therefore any LCPUFAs in the fetal circulation must come from the maternal plasma.[51, 55, 58] The presence of desaturase and elongase activity in developing fetal liver[58] makes it more difficult to determine the sources of these FAs in the developing fetus. Isotope tracer studies may increase the understanding of these processes *in vivo*.

Examination of intrauterine accretion of ω-6 and ω-3 LCPUFAs has indicated rapid accretion of these components in the fetal brain.[43] In the third trimester, they accumulate at rates of approximately 43 mg of ω-6 and 22 mg of ω-3 PUFAs per week.[22] Thus, during the last trimester, the major FAs to accrue are the chain elongation-desaturation products; only 2.6% of the brain FA content is LA. In term infants during early postnatal brain development, the LA content increases significantly, whereas little increase occurs in brain levels of chain elongation-desaturation products for several weeks postpartum.[45]

The transport of essential FAs derived from the maternal diet appears to be affected by maternal nutrition and varies during the course of gestation. Crawford and associates[59] demonstrated that the proportion of LCPUFA derivatives of parent-essential FAs is greatest in fetal brain, less in fetal liver, and further reduced in cord blood. Maternal blood has an even lower proportion of PUFAs. This biomagnification in the fetal brain indicates that the composition of phospholipids in the fetoplacental unit is the result of alterations designed to achieve a high proportion of LCPUFAs necessary for structural components of the developing brain.[52] Placental prostaglandin synthesis has been assessed in several cellular and subcellular preparations, and it appears that the placenta is capable of producing numerous AA metabolites including prostaglandin D_2, prostaglandin I_2, and several hydroxyacids.[52] Research done with perfused human placentas indicates that the biomagnification of AA may result from fetal synthesis, whereas selective placental transport may be the case for DHA.[56]

Free FAs may cross the placenta in either direction, but the movement of phosphoglycerides and triglycerides is generally restricted or absent. This is especially relevant when one considers that maternally derived LA has been found mostly in the free

FA fraction of fetal circulating lipids, whereas AA is selectively compartmentalized into phosphoglycerides by the placenta and is exported to the fetus mostly in that form. Thus, the selectivity with which the placenta distributes LCPUFAs into a lipid fraction impermeable to the placental barrier may allow those FAs to be preferentially retained in the fetoplacental unit, in relation to shorter chain homologous essential FAs. It is also possible that this mechanism serves to provide the fetus with preformed structural components for inclusion in developing membrane systems.[52] The placenta is able to take up lipids associated with chylomicrons and very low density lipid fractions in maternal plasma through the action of lipoprotein lipase. Triacylglycerol hydrolase may be important for releasing free FAs from intracellular triacylglycerol stores in the placenta.[55] These lipids are subsequently released into the fetal circulation as both esterified and nonesterified FAs.

Although little is known about the processing of FAs accumulated in fetal liver, it has been suggested that they are incorporated into lipoprotein for transport to sites of utilization (i.e., adipose tissue).[60] High rates of lipogenesis have been observed in fetal liver (as compared with lipogenesis after birth), a finding suggesting an important role for the liver in the synthesis of endogenous FAs and indicating that not all of the fetal need for FAs can be met by placental transfer.[61]

Placental Transfer and Cord Polyunsaturated Fatty Acids

Normal growth of infants depends on an adequate supply of essential FAs. The human fetus is unable to synthesize essential FAs, which must be delivered from the maternal circulation via the placenta.[12] Previous reports indicated that maternal plasma lipids are elevated during pregnancy and that levels of total lipids, triglycerides, cholesterol, and phospholipids are also significantly higher than those in the neonate.[62] However, the relationship of maternal nutrition during pregnancy with fetal plasma lipid levels remains controversial.

Friedman and colleagues[63] analyzed the phospholipid, cholesterol ester, triglyceride, and free FA levels in maternal plasma and in cord venous and arterial blood of infants at 28 to 44 weeks' gestation. In that study, there was no difference in the FA composition of phospholipids, cholesterol esters, triglycerides, and free FAs between cord venous and arterial plasma obtained at birth.[63] The concentration of LA in cord plasma phospholipid was less than 40% of the maternal value. Lowest values were noted before 34 weeks' gestation. In contrast, venous and arterial cord plasma contained a higher concentration of AA than maternal plasma in various lipid fractions (phospholipids, cholesterol esters, triglycerides, and free FAs).[62, 63] Similarly, the concentration of DHA was higher in cord plasma at term as compared with levels in maternal plasma.[12] The total levels of FAs of the ALA and LA series in cord plasma phospholipid increased from 25.5% at 24 to 33 weeks to 33.7% at 34 to 37 weeks and 36% at term. In comparison, the maternal plasma level of these FAs was 39.9% at term.[64] Factors that may be responsible for the increased concentrations of AA and DHA in the fetal circulation include preferential transfer of these FAs in later gestation and the presence of enzymatic activity in the fetus, resulting in desaturation and elongation of LA to form AA.

Maternal exposure to *trans*-FAs may be a factor that influences essential FA metabolism in term and preterm infants at birth. Maternal plasma and infant plasma have been found to contain similar percentages of *trans*-FAs.[65] Humans cannot synthesize *trans*-FAs, and therefore these FAs must originate from the maternal diet,[66] and they appear in fetal circulation via placental transport.[55] An inverse relationship has been indicated between *trans*-isomeric FAs and LCPUFAs in cord blood lipids. Research thus far has indicated that total *trans*-FAs in plasma lipid fractions are not related to LA and ALA but are inversely correlated

to ω-3 and ω-6 LCPUFAs and to the product/substrate ratios of long-chain polyunsaturated biosynthesis.[67] *Trans*-FAs may inhibit the transport of LCPUFAs to the placenta by competing for FA binding sites.[55] Existing evidence has not yet shown whether these effects on FA metabolism alter fetal growth or length of gestation.

The FA composition of adipose tissue triglycerides in the newborn infant differs from that of the mother, similar to the observed differences in plasma lipid composition. Body stores of essential FAs are particularly low in low birth weight infants. The concentration of LA in fetal tissue is less than in adults, and the proportion of LA in muscle phospholipids increases with advancing gestational age. Because of the low concentration of LA in fetal adipose tissue, the contribution of LA to the pool of plasma-free FAs during lipolysis is also small.[68] Cord plasma levels of LA are also diminished, a finding reflecting the reduced tissue level of this FA. The low plasma concentrations of LA may have a beneficial effect by increasing the maternofetal gradient for LA and facilitating transfer across the placenta. As noted earlier, the relatively high concentration of AA in fetal tissue could result either from preferential transfer of this FA or from desaturation and elongation of LA in the fetus to produce AA. Tissue enrichment in AA plays an important role during fetal life by maintaining the normal function of biologic membranes and perhaps by providing a substrate for prostaglandin biosynthesis. Postnatal brain development is characterized by an increase in LA content; however, chain elongation-desaturation products do not increase for several weeks postnatally. This finding suggests that placental transfer of LCPUFAs is of primary importance in accretion of these FAs in the fetus.[69]

POSTNATAL LIPID ACCRETION

Fatty Acid Utilization

For most mammalian species, birth represents an abrupt transition from a low-fat to a high-fat diet. The endocrine changes that occur at birth, particularly the surge in the plasma concentration of glucagon, favor mobilization of lipids from peripheral tissues. Blood concentrations of free FAs and glycerol increase, resulting in a higher rate of FA oxidation and increased ketone body production. After birth, milk provides a relatively high-fat diet compared with that consumed by the fetus, and it is clear that lipids play an important role both as metabolic fuels and in fat deposition. Fat is the main energy source of the newborn infant. In addition to providing 40 to 50% of the total calories in human milk or formula, fats are essential to normal development because they provide FAs necessary for brain development; they are an integral part of cell membranes, and they are the sole vehicle for fat-soluble vitamins and hormones in milk.[70]

Using the accretion rate of essential FAs during normal growth of the human fetus and newborn as a reference point, Clandinin and associates[43,71,72] demonstrated a lag in accretion of LCPUFAs in the brain and liver during fetal development and mobilization of PUFA deposits in the liver for a varying period after birth. From these studies, it was concluded that chain-elongation products do not accrue in the neonatal brain for several weeks postnatally. In fact, chain-elongation products are not synthesized at maximal rates for several weeks after birth in the term infant, a finding further supporting the hypothesis that placental transfer of LCPUFAs is of primary importance in their accretion.[72]

Although the composition of FAs contained in brain total lipids and phosphoglycerides demonstrates a characteristic pattern, small alterations in composition of dietary fat intake change the composition of brain membranes during development. When animals are fed ω-3–deficient diets, docosapentaenoic acid (DPA; C22:5ω-6) replaces DHA (C22:ω6ω-3) in neural membranes.[73] The functional effects of this replacement are not yet clear. Even though DPA is a precursor for AA, this substitution does not seem to affect brain AA levels in ω-3–deficient rats.[74] The ω-6/ω-3 balance is also important; hence maternal diets providing a high ratio of LA/ALA (10% corn oil) result in higher levels of DPA and lower levels of DHA in the brains of newborn rats.[75] In similar experiments,[76] weanling rats fed diets supplemented with oil rich either in ω-3 (fish oil) or ω-6 (safflower oil) FAs underwent reciprocal replacement of ω-6 and ω-3 families of FAs in brain ethanolamine phosphoglycerides according to the dietary levels. Jumpsen and associates[77] examined the effects of feeding ALA, AA, and DHA on brain development in neonatal rats. The ω-3/ω-6 ratio at amounts within the recommended limits significantly altered the FA content of the developing rat brain. The amount and rate of AA or DHA accretion into glial and neuronal membranes varied, and ethanolamine phosphoglycerides exhibited the most distinct changes when LCPUFAs were fed.[77] Thus, FA constituents and synthesis of structural lipid in brain membranes that undergo turnover can be altered by changes in the composition of dietary fat intake.[78]

Inclusion of LCPUFAs is currently implemented in infant formulas. The addition of DHA or AA alone is inappropriate because the balanced addition of both ω-6 and ω-3 LCPUFAs (AA and DHA) is required to achieve optimal accretion. The balance between AA and DHA in the diet is a powerful determinant of the level of these FAs in the developing brain. It is becoming increasingly evident that the addition of LA and ALA does not provide optimal ω-3 and ω-6 LCPUFAs, and optimal growth and development require the addition of both AA and DHA. Previous studies had difficulty showing an effect of AA- and DHA-supplemented formulas on growth; however, this difficulty was probably because of a lack of statistical power as a result of insufficient length or size of study or narrow inclusion criteria that eliminated detection of difference. In a double-blind, controlled multicenter study,[79] Clandinin and associates demonstrated that feeding AA and DHA is essential to enhance growth and neurodevelopment in premature infants (<35 weeks' postmenstrual age, <1500 g at birth). Infants fed standard formula supplemented with 34 mg/100 kcal AA and 17 mg/100 kcal DHA from single cell oils (n = 95), had significantly greater mean body weights than the control group (unsupplemented formula, n = 98) at every study time point from 66 weeks' postmenstrual age until the end of study, a similar to or greater length than the control group from 40 to 100 weeks, and by 118 weeks (n = 72) they also had a mean length and weight comparable with those of a reference term group of infants (n = 97). The supplemented group also demonstrated higher mental and psychomotor scores than the control group. It was concluded that formulas supplemented with DHA and AA at median levels found in human milk are safe for very low birth weight premature infants and are essential for optimal growth and development.

Intake

Human Milk

Many physiologic factors influence milk composition, such as stage of lactation, length of gestation, age of the mother, intrafeed regulation of milk release, and the baby's demand for milk.[80] Throughout early lactation, "preterm" milk is 40 to 50% higher in its total fat content than milk from mothers who deliver term infants. As the period of gestation increases and approaches term, differences in the nutrient content between preterm and term breast milk diminish. The stage of lactation may also affect lipid content. Colostrum has 1.19% (w/w) fat, transitional milk has 3% fat, and mature milk has 3.3% fat.[81] Fat provides about 50% of the energy content in human milk.

When compared with cow's milk, the fat content of human milk is characterized by a relatively high proportion of oleic acid,

a higher level of essential FAs, and a relatively lower level of short chain FAs such as butyric, caproic, caprylic, and capric acids.[80] Also notable are the differences in the ganglioside content of human colostrum, later milk, formula, and cow's milk. Human milk and colostrum contain almost twice the total lipid-bound sialic acid levels of cow's milk or formula.[82] The major ganglioside fractions identified in colostrum were GD_3 and GX_1, and later milk also contained a high proportion of GM_3, whereas cow's milk and formula consisted mostly of GD_3.[82] The biologic significance of these differences is not yet fully appreciated.

There is limited quantitative information on the actual amounts of FAs consumed by breast-fed newborn infants. Although better equipment has become available for analysis of FA composition of milk samples, most studies lack basic information, such as lipid content and volume of the milk consumed.[83] Alterations in maternal intake of PUFAs are reflected in milk FA composition, and, secondarily, newborn tissue composition is affected by maternal diet in both animals and humans.[84-87] The LCPUFA status at birth is one of the major determinants of postnatal change in LCPUFA status, with breast milk the most effective diet for maintaining these levels.[88] Consequently, lower LCPUFA status in formula-fed infants compared with breast-fed infants may persist at least until the first year of life.[89]

In well-nourished women (who are in energy balance), the FA composition of breast milk shows a strong relationship with the distribution of fat and carbohydrate calories in the diet. For example, a carbohydrate-rich diet providing 75% of energy requirements may result in an increase in the content of saturated FAs such as lauric acid (C12:0) and myristic acid (C14:0) and a decrease in the LA content.[80] Maternal diet in well-nourished women affects milk lipid constituents, but not the total amount of fat present in milk. Milk from vegetarian mothers exhibits levels of milk fat similar to those in milk from omnivorous women; however, it has a higher proportion of PUFAs derived from increased consumption of vegetable fat, with the primary effect on the milk LA content.[90] In vegetarians, the higher concentration of LA is accompanied by lower concentrations of DHA in the erythrocyte membranes of their breast-fed infants.[90] It is estimated using isotope tracers that about 30% of milk LA is directly transferred from maternal diet, whereas conversion of dietary LA to AA and other longer chain LA homologues (dihomo-γ-linolenic acid; 20:3ω-6) occurs at approximately 1.2% and 11%, respectively.[91] However, the contribution of dietary LA to milk AA may be slightly underestimated because of isotope dilution. Human milk supplies significant amounts of C20 and C22 FAs, which are more effective in supporting tissue AA and DHA accretion than are similar amounts of LA and ALA.[92] A review of articles on human milk FA composition of milk lipids denotes the differences between the DHA content of human milk of Western and non-Western women, with content averaging 0.45% and 0.88% of total FAs respectively, although a wide variation in Western diet was reported.[93] The largest changes in FA composition occur when maternal diet is supplemented with fish oil.[85] For example, high levels of fish consumption by Inuit women increase the breast milk content of ω-3 LCPUFAs.[94] Levels of DHA in human milk have been reported to range from 0.2 to 1.4% of total FAs.[85, 94] Supplementation of maternal diet with DHA also results in markedly increased DHA content in human milk, directly attributable to dietary increase rather than to preferential secretion.[95] Levels of AA remain fairly constant despite wide variation of maternal intake of LA or DHA.[85,94,96]

Because maternal diet affects the FA composition of milk so easily, one may question whether the drastic change in diet over the last few centuries has also modified human milk FA composition. For instance, the dietary ω-6/ω-3 ratio has changed from 1:1 to 10:1 or 20:1, resulting in a higher ratio of ω-6/ω-3 than evolution would have allowed without human interference.[97, 98] Moreover, the proportion of polyunsaturated to saturated FAs present in human milk has been shown to correspond with the ratio of polyunsaturated to saturated FAs in the maternal diet.[84] *Trans*-FA consumption is also noteworthy because *trans*-FA content of milk reflects short-term and long-term maternal diet.[84]

FAs appear in milk not only as a result of maternal dietary intake, but also from factors such as mobilization from maternal fat deposits and endogenous synthesis by the mammary gland.[99] LA and ALA are not synthesized by the mammary gland and are dependent on dietary intake, although to some extent their long chain derivatives may be synthesized in the mammary gland, independent of the length of gestation.[100] Long-term maternal diet is important because mobilization of maternal adipose tissue stores is a major source of milk FAs, including LA, AA, and DHA.[101, 102] Consequently, gestational age and lactational stage influence milk *trans*-FA level, but the rate of maternal postpartum weight loss has the most significant effect.[84]

Interest in human milk and the lipid composition of formulas has primarily focused on "humanized" formulas for premature infants, which have been designed to ensure adequate absorption and metabolism of fat and to promote a satisfactory essential FA status. In this regard, the changes in fat content of milk from mothers of term and preterm infants have been investigated. Chappell and colleagues[103] found that milk from mothers who delivered preterm infants has a higher content of LA and ALA and their LCPUFA derivatives. The prevailing consensus is that early milk produced by women who deliver prematurely is more appropriate for very low birth weight infants than donor milk from the later stages of lactation.[104] LCPUFAs are present in the milk of women who deliver prematurely. Furthermore, the level of these FAs is significantly higher in colostrum and the milk of mothers of premature infants than in the milk of mothers delivering full-term infants.[105] Finally, whereas the supply of DHA and AA remains fairly constant over 26 weeks of lactation in well-nourished, omnivorous mothers who deliver prematurely, the content of these FAs decreases in the milk of mothers who deliver at term. As a result, after 26 weeks of lactation, the relative concentration of AA is 1.5 times higher and that of DHA is twice as high in preterm than in term human milk.[106] Thus, human milk is apparently able to meet the need for LCPUFAs in preterm infants and can efficiently substitute for the diminished supply of FAs to the fetus.

Studies of energy metabolism in low birth weight infants fed mother's own milk indicate that for a net energy intake of 120 kcal/kg/day, approximately 20 kcal/kg/day of fat will be deposited in tissues (i.e., some 2.2 g fat/kg/day). Because human milk contains 1.08 to 2.65% ω-6 FAs and 1.09 to 1.47% ω-3 FAs synthesized from the C18 precursor, it can be estimated that 23.6 to 58.3 mg of ω-6 and 23.9 to 32.3 mg of ω-3 LCPUFAs will be deposited in tissue each day in a low birth weight infant fed adequate amounts of human milk. It is also apparent that human milk contains levels of LCPUFAs sufficient to meet the requirements of neural tissues for these FAs.[45]

Formula for Preterm Infants

Special formulas have been designed to provide adequate intake of calories, fluids, and micronutrients to support the rapid cell division and synthesis of new tissue in the infant.[107, 108] The current trend in infant formula preparation is to use a FA profile that more closely reflects the FA composition of human milk, partly owing to its digestibility by the infant. This is the result of many factors, including the FA composition of human milk fat, the triglyceride positional specificity, and complementary enzymatic activities that originate in the breast milk and in the infant's gastrointestinal tract.[107] For instance, the structure of human milk triglyceride is recognized to be unique with regard to the position of saturated and short chain FAs, the presence of phospholipids containing LCPUFAs, and a triglyceride/phospholipid ratio that undergoes a continuous evolution from birth through weaning at 1 year.[109]

Infant formulas and feeding regimens that differ markedly from the composition of human milk fats are prevalent. In some instances, these formulations have been designed to promote utilization of fats with chain lengths of 8 and 10 carbons for maximal absorption.[110] Quantities of each nutrient in formulas for low birth weight infants have been adjusted to account for the average absorption of that particular nutrient.[111] Fat accretion in the growing formula-fed premature infant is markedly increased in comparison with the fetus of similar weight, rate of weight gain, and postconceptional age. This finding suggests that the weight gain and subsequent body composition of the premature infant differ from those of the comparable placentally nourished fetus.[108]

Interest has focused on the essential FA requirements of preterm infants and the quantities of ALA, AA, and EPA that should be added to formulas in addition to LA. Body stores of essential FAs are diminished in low birth weight infants, and therefore, they theoretically should be at increased risk of developing clinically apparent essential FA deficiency when they are fed a deficient diet.[112] In that regard, Combes and co-workers[113] did not observe gross abnormalities of the skin in premature infants who were fed milk mixtures low in LA; however, they did note histologic features of the skin compatible with LA deficiency and serum dienoic, trienoic, and tetraenoic acid levels that were significantly different from those of infants fed 4% of their calories as linoleate. Similarly, Hansen and associates[114] demonstrated that many babies younger than 6 weeks of age who were fed milk diets deficient in LA (and who remained on that diet for 3 months) developed dry, thick, desquamated skin and retarded growth. Clinical manifestations apparently disappeared after the administration of diets that provided 1% or more of calories as LA.

For term infant formula, the American Academy of Pediatrics recommends a minimum of 3.3 g of fat per 100 kcal (30% of calories) and 300 mg of LA (~2.7% of calories).[115] For preterm infants, the consensus among Europe, the United States, and Canada is 4.4 to 6.0 g of fat per 100 kcal.[116] Several of the most widely used formulas are based on cow's milk protein and also contain lactose. All contain vegetable oils of one type or another, and most contain more LA than human milk. In these vegetable fat blends, palmitic acid is predominantly esterified to the sn-1 and sn-3 positions of the triglycerides, resulting in the release of free palmitic acid after intraluminal hydrolysis by lipases. The absorption of palmitic and stearic acids is low, and their presence in the intestinal lumen results in the formation of soaps with calcium and other divalent cations.[117, 118] To minimize this problem, medium chain triglycerides (MCTs) or coconut oils are sometimes used to replace part of the oils containing a large amount of palmitic and stearic acids. Oleo oils are used to simulate the saturated and monounsaturated FA content of human milk. In this oil, most of the palmitic and stearic acids are esterified in sn-1,3 of the oleo triglycerides. The long-term effects of these types of varied dietary FA regimens used in feeding infants are unknown, but in animal models, physiologic variations in dietary fat intake are known to alter membrane structure and many related membrane functions.

Research has focused on the requirements for LCPUFAs.[4,83,119, 120] Preterm and term infants fed formula without AA and DHA have lower levels of those FAs in plasma and erythrocyte phospholipids than do infants fed human milk.[92, 121] A clear dose response is evident in the levels of AA and DHA found in erythrocyte membrane phospholipids when infant formula is supplemented with increasing levels of AA and DHA.[122] The dietary intake of LA and ALA in infant formulas lacking longer chain homologues of these FAs results in reduced levels of AA and DHA in membrane phospholipids compared with those of infants fed human milk.[121] The currently available formulas with high concentrations of LA or high LA/ALA ratios may be contributing to the low incorporation of DHA, both by providing insufficient substrate (i.e., ALA) and by inhibiting the incorporation of endogenously formed DHA into the membrane. ALA does not seem to act as a competitive inhibitor of the incorporation of AA into membranes,[123] unless the content of ALA is increased to unphysiologic levels.[124, 125] Energy intake may also be an important variable because erythrocyte phosphatidylethanolamine DHA decreases rapidly in preterm infants who receive less than 100 kcal/kg/day, and a similar decrease is seen for AA in erythrocyte phosphatidylethanolamine and phosphatidylcholine.[92] When preterm infants receiving human milk are in energy balance, the levels of erythrocyte DHA remain constant, but they decline in premature infants fed vegetable oil formulas containing ALA but no DHA.[121, 126, 127] This decline is rapid and is associated with electroretinographic changes when the formula contains less than 0.37% kcal ALA; however, both the visual development and the DHA levels in plasma and erythrocytes are comparable to those of breast-fed preterm infants if the formula contains at least 1% kcal ALA.[121, 126, 127] There is evidence from autopsy material that formula-fed infants experience a similar decrease in DHA content in the brain cortex, and this correlates with a similar decrease in the erythrocyte DHA content.[128] Similarly, results in term infants indicate that the lower DHA level in erythrocytes in formula-fed as compared with breast-fed infants correlates with decrease in visual acuity.[129] Similar to preterm infants, a higher intake of ALA (≥1% kcal) should result in similar visual acuity as that seen in breast-fed infants.[130] Supplementing marine oil in formula-fed infants also alters visual acuity, as compared with nonsupplemented formula-fed infants.[131] There is also weak clinical evidence of a higher intelligence test score in breast-fed versus formula-fed infants. In a nonrandomized study, the advantage in intelligence quotient with human milk feeding at 7 to 8 years of age was eight points, which is half one standard deviation of the sample of infants studied.[132] These results, however, could also be explained by group differences in parenting skills and genetic potential.[133] A review by Fleith and Clandinin[134] on dietary PUFA for preterm and term infants provides a thorough review of the clinical evidence regarding factors such as FA status, growth, and visual and cognitive functions.

Whereas the previous section compares several aspects of FA metabolism and functional implications in breast milk versus several types of commercial formula, until recently, there was no commercial formula in North America with essential FAs greater than C20 in chain length. For premature (and term) infants fed synthetic formulations in place of human milk fats, it is important to establish whether they possess the enzymes capable of elongating and desaturating LA and ALA and whether they are capable of producing sufficient amounts of LCPUFAs for optimal synthesis of neural tissues and prostaglandins. This is an especially important question because these infants possess adipose tissue stores adequate for only a few days before essential FA deprivation occurs.[135] Synthesis of AA and DHA therefore depends on adequate desaturase/elongase activity, as well as an adequate supply of dietary LA and ALA and energy. Because specific information on desaturase activity in infants is lacking and because human milk contains a significant amount of AA and DHA, formulas probably need to be supplemented with those FAs as well. There is some evidence that term infants fed formulas without LCPUFAs synthesize sufficient AA and DHA from dietary precursors, although the consensus is that this process may not provide enough DHA to meet accretion demands during rapid brain development.[136–138] Furthermore, in preterm infants, evidence indicates that formula supplemented with AA and DHA is essential for optimal long-term growth and development.[139]

MCTs make up half the fat content of many formulas for preterm infants. These nutrients have been added because it is believed they are better absorbed by the premature gut than long chain triglycerides.[140] Although earlier studies reported improved growth, further studies did not demonstrate an increased gain in weight, head circumference, or linear growth of preterm infants fed a formula containing medium rather than long chain FAs.[141–144] Energy wastage associated with oxidation followed by biosynthesis, compared with direct tissue incorporation of long chain FAs, may explain the absence of improved energy or weight gain in infants fed formulas with MCTs.[145, 146] At higher dietary levels of MCTs, there is some concern that the essential FA balance of the infant may be adversely affected. Lower plasma levels of AA and DHA associated with formula feeding may be exacerbated when MCTs rather than palmitic acid are used as the source of saturated FAs in formula.[147] Although high doses of MCTs do not seem desirable, there is also no overwhelmingly clear evidence that they are harmful. Therefore, there is a need for more extensive studies of the optimal fat blend to use in formulas for low birth weight infants.

In summary, the fat in commercial infant formula is different in many aspects from that in human milk, in that the content of monounsaturated FAs, LA, and ALA varies with the oil blend used, the absence of C20/C22 ω-6/ω-3 FAs, the abundance of MCTs, and the triglyceride FA stereoconfiguration. High levels of LCPUFAs are present in milk lactated by mothers delivering low birth weight infants, whereas current "humanized" formulas are devoid of essential FAs greater than 20 carbons in chain length.[148] Supplementation of infant formulas with very LCPUFAs at levels and ratios similar to those of human milk increases the incorporation of these components into membrane lipids in the developing infant,[149] in a dose-dependent manner.[150] At these physiologic levels, AA and DHA from marine oil sources[151,152] and from single cell oils[150] maintain AA and DHA status in formula-fed infants similar to that of breast-fed infants.

Absorption

Physiologic Phases

Fat absorption improves with gestational age. Most of the dietary fats are triglycerides, and about 2% are phospholipids, free FAs, monoglycerides and diglycerides, cholesterol, and other substances.[153] The absorption of triglycerides is dependent on FA chain length. MCTs can be absorbed directly into the circulation without being hydrolyzed by pancreatic lipase. All other fats, however, are hydrolyzed and are then re-esterified to form triglycerides within the mucosa. Absorption coefficients for unsaturated fats have been demonstrated.[154]

In the newborn infant, pancreatic lipase and bile salt concentrations are diminished, thus impairing emulsification and breakdown of triglyceride.[155] Efficient fat absorption in the newborn depends on lingual and gastric lipases. These have a special role in the hydrolysis of milk fat and can account for hydrolysis of 60% of the ingested fat. Lingual lipase hydrolyzes MCTs and short chain triglycerides,[155] as well as monounsaturated and polyunsaturated, but not saturated, long chain triglycerides.[156–158] Animal studies have shown that short and medium chain FAs can be absorbed directly through the gastric mucosa, a finding suggesting that these products of intragastric lipolysis appear rapidly in the circulation. Free FAs and monoglycerides, the products of intragastric lipolysis, are relatively polar. Therefore, they can locate in the surface layer of the fat globule (dislocate phospholipids and proteins) and make the core triglyceride more accessible to pancreatic lipase and human milk bile salt–stimulated lipase. The latter enzyme hydrolyzes milk fat at pH 7.0 to 8.0, in the presence of bile salts, and thus acts in the intestine to complete the digestive process initiated in the stomach by lingual and gastric lipases.[155]

The breast-fed newborn infant depends on an additional compensatory enzyme, the bile salt–stimulated lipase of human milk.[155] This lipase is present in milk from 26 weeks' gestation, has no positional specificity for triglycerides, and hydrolyzes various triglycerides to free FAs and glycerol in the presence

TABLE 40-1

Compensatory Digestive Lipases Versus Pancreatic Lipase in the Newborn

	Lingual	Gastric	Milk (BSSL)	Pancreatic
Origin	Serous glands	Gastric mucosa	Mammary gland	Acinar cells
TG-site (sn)	sn-3	sn-3	sn-1,2,3	sn-1,3
End products	FFA, DG, (MG)	FFA, DG, (MG)	FFA, glycerol	FFA, MG
pH optimum	2.2–6.0	3.5–6.5	7.0–8.5	6.5–8.0
Bile salts	No	No	Obligatory	Obligatory
Stability	Yes	Yes	Yes	No
(pH 2.5–3.0)				

BSSL = bile salt-stimulated lipase; TG = triglyceride; sn = stereospecific numbering; FFA = free fatty acid; DG = diglyceride; MG = monoglyceride. Modified from Hamosh M, et al: Lipids in human milk and their digestion by the newborn infant. *In* Ghisolfi J, Putet G (eds): Essential Fatty Acids and Infant Nutrition. Paris, J Libbey Eurotext, 1992, pp 119–137.

of bile salts.[159, 160] The major differentiating characteristics of milk lipase and other lipases in gastric aspirates are shown in Table 40-1. It is estimated that milk bile salt–stimulated lipase concentrations are sufficient to hydrolyze 30 to 40% of available triglyceride in 2 hours.[161] Addition of this lipase to formula for preterm infants may be feasible.[162] Given that bile salt–stimulated lipase does not discriminate between FAs and completely hydrolyzes triglycerides, this may aid in efficient release of LCPUFAs, especially in the presence of pancreatic colipase-dependent lipase.[162] The combined action of intragastric lipolysis and intestinal hydrolysis of fat by the bile salt–stimulated lipase of human milk can effectively substitute for low pancreatic lipase activity and low levels of bile salts in the newborn.[155]

It is apparent that a dynamic interrelationship must exist among the products of lipid digestion. The triglyceride emulsion particle, stabilized by the products of intragastric lipolysis and phospholipids, undergoes hydrolysis by pancreatic lipase-colipase and phospholipase A_2. The accumulated lipolytic products are then extruded as unilamellar liposomal vesicles that are in equilibrium with large bile salt mixed micelles. The mechanism of lipid exchange between these phases, particularly for lipids of differing aqueous solubility or chemical composition, is not completely known.[161] Refer to Chapter 115 for more detail regarding digestive and absorptive processes in infants.

Medium and Long Chain Triglycerides

The efficiency of fat absorption in preterm infants is determined not only by maturity of the gastrointestinal tract and pancreas, but also by the dietary fat composition. Preterm infants fed fresh human milk can absorb fat as well as term infants, at an efficiency of 90 to 95% of intake.[163] Only 85 to 92% of the fat in formulas that do not contain MCTs is absorbed by preterm infants.[159] Feeding breast milk has also been shown to promote better fat absorption than that observed in formula-fed infants,[154] not only because of the presence of bile salt–stimulated lipase, but also because of differences in the structure of the milk fat globule and the stereoconfiguration of triglycerides. Feeding of pasteurized or stored human milk eliminates some of these factors.[164] For instance, lipases are completely destroyed by pasteurization, whereas FA levels seem to be unaffected.[165] The stereoconfiguration of triglyceride is important in piglets, in which palmitic acid is absorbed from sow's milk and from formula with rearranged triacylglycerols as an sn-2 monoacylglycerol.[166] Similarly, in full-term infants consuming human milk, palmitic acid is absorbed as sn-2 monopalmityl-glycerol.[167] Positional distribution seems to affect digestion, absorption, and chylomicron triglycerides and has an effect on infant lipoprotein metabolism.[168] However, in preterm infants, randomizing palmitic acid in infant formula triglycerides to improve absorption of fat remains controversial, and there may be no net physiologic benefit conveyed by having

an increased level of palmitic acid in the sn-2 position of the triglyceride. Previous observations indicated that the coefficient for absorption of palmitic and stearic acids is 20 to 30% lower for premature infants fed formula versus infants fed human milk.[154] Some findings suggest that a palmitic acid configuration similar to that of human milk (with C16:0 esterified in the sn-2 position) confers better absorption than when C16:0 is esterified in the sn-1 or sn-3 position.[169] Thus, it is reasonable to expect that if the presence of palmitic acid in the sn-2 position confers improved absorption of palmitic acid, then increasing the content of saturated FA in the sn-2 position of the fed triglyceride could significantly improve absorption of palmitic acid by up to 10%. Significant improvement of net absorption of total FA would probably be difficult to demonstrate because total fat absorption would likely increase only a small amount. In a feeding experiment, the proportion of saturated FAs in the sn-2 position of palm oil was randomized to simulate the positional distribution of FAs in human milk triglyceride closely. FA absorption was assessed in preterm infants fed a commercial formula or a similar formula in which the palmitic acid was randomized into all positions of the triglyceride molecule. Incorporation of approximately one third of the palmitic acid into the sn-2 position of the fed triglyceride improved absorption of fat, but no effect of this triglyceride structure on the net absorption of palmitic acid was observed. Alternatively, other modifications in the triglyceride structure may occur during randomization.[170]

The MCTs are relatively more water soluble and are more completely hydrolyzed by pancreatic lipase. They can also be absorbed directly into mucosal cells. C8:0 and C10:0 are almost 100% absorbed, despite the low lipase and bile salt concentrations. Efficiency of fat absorption increases with the degree of unsaturation, so FAs with more double bonds are absorbed more efficiently (C18:3 > C18:2 > C18:1).[154, 171] Several previous studies[172] demonstrated improved fat absorption but only small differences in weight gain with infant formulas containing MCTs.[173] The effect of MCT diet on energy and macronutrient utilization in very low birth weight infants was studied by Van Aerde,[146] who concluded that the growth of infants fed a formula containing 50% MCTs (at an energy intake of 124 kcal/kg/day) will mirror the intrauterine gain in length, head circumference, and weight. Body composition cannot be simulated because of the higher rate of fat deposition. Further studies could not demonstrate an increased gain in weight, head circumference, or linear growth of preterm infants fed a formula containing medium chain rather than long chain FAs.[141-144] Energy wastage associated with oxidation followed by biosynthesis, compared with direct tissue incorporation of long chain FAs, may explain the absence of improved energy or weight gain in infants fed formulas with MCTs. Premature infants oxidize one-third to two-thirds of the medium chain FAs, a finding indicating that the remaining medium chain FAs are chain elongated.[145, 146] Production of ketones and dicarboxylic acid increases with an increasing amount of MCTs in the preterm infant formula.[174,175] The rapid oxidation of medium chain FAs probably leads to accumulation of acetylcoenzyme A, exceeding the capacity of the tricarboxylic acid cycle. Dicarboxylic acids are the products of ω-oxidation of C8:0 and C10:0.

The absorption coefficient of oleic and LA from vegetable triglycerides is greater than 90%.[176, 154] (For myristic acid, it is only 89%; for palmitic acid, it is 75%; and for stearic acid, it is 62%.) The absorption of oleate and linoleate (unsaturated C18 FAs) is highest in infants fed a formula with a linoleate/oleate ratio similar to the ratio provided by human milk. Therefore, some infant formulas have been designed to provide high linoleate/oleate ratios.[177] There is general agreement in the literature that infant formulas containing cow's milk fat as the sole or principal form of fat are also less well digested by the preterm infant than those containing vegetable oils or MCTs.

Gastric lipolysis,[178] nonnutritive sucking,[179] and a "humanized" lipid formulation for infant feeding can partially compensate for the low birth weight infant's intraluminal immaturity.[154] Human milk triglyceride structure,[180] fat globule integrity,[181] inherent lipase activity,[182] and a substance stimulating expansion of the bile salt pool[183] have been suggested as additional factors responsible for relative efficiency of fat absorption in infants fed human milk. The influence of the composition of free FAs in human milk on fat absorption should also be considered a variable that contributes to efficient absorption of milk fat.[154] Total absorption of FAs and the coefficient of FA absorption are significantly higher in very low birth weight infants fed their mothers' milk than in infants receiving formula.[149]

In the premature infant, the fecal FA pattern generally resembles the FA profile fed; however, an inverse relationship has been found between increasing chain length in saturated FAs and absorption.[154] The marked difference in absorption of C18:0 in preterm mothers' milk and formula-fed infants may indicate that factors in addition to position of FAs on the triglyceride molecule are responsible for the efficient absorption of FAs from preterm mothers' milk.[154] The absorption of specific saturated fats may be low and decreased by the form or perhaps by the method of mineral supplementation.[154] Clandinin and colleagues[149] demonstrated that the overall distribution of individual FAs within an insoluble bound fraction is similar for infants fed breast milk and those fed formula. Insoluble bound C16:0 and C18:0 account for more than 65% of FAs. Calcium supplementation resulted in an unexpected relative increase in fecal C12:0 and C14:0 in formula-fed and breast milk–fed infants and a decrease in C18:0 in the feces of a breast milk–fed group. Providing palmitic acid appropriately esterified in sn-2 of the infant formula triglycerides seemed to improve mineral balance in formula-fed infants.[184]

It is apparent that some FAs (i.e., PUFAs) are readily and efficiently absorbed;[149] however, as much as 25% of dietary LCPUFAs can be lost in the feces of formula and breast-fed preterm infants.[185] In general, longer chain FAs are less well absorbed, possibly because of solubilization and rate limitations of uptake and processing in the enterocyte.[186] Supplementation of formula with AA and DHA has resulted in decreased absorption of these FAs,[187] possibly resulting in variable results in clinical supplementation studies. As previously mentioned, human milk bile salt–stimulated lipase has a role in the utilization of LCPUFAs,[162] and therefore its absence in infant formula may also have an effect. However, it appears that a single cell oil source AA and DHA in formula may be as efficiently absorbed as these FAs are from breast milk.[185] Overall, this finding indicates that the absorption coefficients are not identical for all FAs, and there is a difference between human milk-fed and formula-fed very low birth weight infants.[149]

Metabolism

Oxidation

Our current understanding of the utilization of individual dietary FAs for energy is vague.[149] Because more than 50% of dietary calories of the newborn are derived from fat, metabolic adaptation in the oxidation of long chain FAs and ketone body utilization must occur at the time of birth.[188] It is evident that infants deprived of sufficient fat stores at birth (i.e., premature or growth-restricted infants) lack an important fuel source.[189] In the immediate postnatal period, serum levels of free FAs rise dramatically, indicating active lipolysis of adipose tissue.[190] After 12 to 24 hours, the rate of lipolysis falls rapidly as feeding or intravenous nourishment is initiated. Rates of lipolysis in the first few hours of life appear to be regulated by catecholamine release, resulting in production of cyclic adenosine monophosphate and increased protein kinase C activity. Ultimately, this process leads to activation of adipose tissue lipoprotein lipase.[190, 191] Lipolysis in neonatal adipose tissues may depend more on mobilization of glycogen stores than on catecholamine stimulation. Insulin, growth hormone, thyroxine, sex hormones, and glucagon also have a role in stimulating free FA production in the neonate by increasing lipogenesis.[192] Assuming fecal fat losses of approximately 10 to 15%, one may expect that 40 to 50% of the FA consumed would be potentially available for new tissue synthesis. However, selective β-oxidation of individual dietary acids has been shown in adults.[149] Whether or not this selective β-oxidation of PUFAs also occurs in infants is unknown. Therefore, it is difficult quantitatively to assess or estimate the net oxidation rate for dietary LCPUFAs based on available data.[149]

Relative proportions of major dietary FAs consumed may potentially affect the net contribution of fat oxidation to total energy production. The metabolizable energy of saturated triglycerides has long been known to be less than that observed for unsaturated fats.[193] Studies in animals and humans suggest that the degree of unsaturation of dietary LCPUFAs influences the partitioning of fat between oxidation and storage. Several reports have indicated that LCPUFAs undergo faster oxidation as compared with their saturated counterparts. Thus, as expressed before, human metabolism of dietary fat is not independent of the long chain FA composition of the fat consumed.[194–196] From nutrient balance and energy balance studies, it appears that only a small amount of the absorbed fat is oxidized, and most fat is stored. A faster clearance and a higher rate of oxidation of fats have been observed in hypermetabolic patients than in physiologically normal subjects. In contrast, fat clearance is faster in patients receiving total parenteral nutrition (TPN), but the rate of oxidation is much lower.[197]

In the past, it was generally assumed that medium chain FAs are preferentially oxidized, but more recent studies estimated that preterm infants oxidize only one-third to two-thirds of dietary C8:0.[145] Medium chain FAs, particularly C12:0, are incorporated into adipose tissue of preterm infants, in proportion to the formula content.[198] It is unclear whether this is of benefit to the infant.

Accretion

The lipid content of the brain is fairly constant until 7 months' gestation, when lipid deposition gradually increases, reaching a peak in gray matter at 3 months of postnatal age. In white matter, the process is slower. By 2 years of age, 90% of the adult lipid content has been deposited, and by 10 years of age, 100% has been deposited. White matter accounts for most of the brain lipid, mainly in the form of myelin. Myelin itself contains 50% of the total lipid content and represents 25% of the weight of the mature brain.[199]

Appropriate for gestational age preterm infants (weighing ~1300 g) have a total body FA content of about 30 g, whereas appropriately grown infants born at term have a total body FA content more than 10 times greater (340 g). Quantitative analyses of the FA content of liver and neural tissues have demonstrated a combined FA content of 1.55 g in preterm infants and 4.63 g in term infants. Based on dissection data, the total amount of FAs in white adipose tissue of preterm and term infants can be estimated at approximately 3.45 g and 255.6 g, respectively.[149] During the first 5 weeks of postnatal life, there is an apparent mobilization of total FAs from the liver. Of the essential FAs, only LA and ALA accrue during the initial weeks of life. Significant postnatal accretion of chain elongation-desaturation products does not occur immediately after birth. This finding suggests that, early on, either synthesis in the liver may be limiting or mobilization of LCPUFA homologues of LA and ALA exceeds the capacity of liver to synthesize them from dietary LA and ALA.[149]

Mammalian tissues contain ω-3 FAs primarily in the form of DHA and are mostly concentrated in phospholipids.[200] Although DHA accounts for a small percentage of the FA content of most tissues, very high levels are found in the retina, cerebral cortex, testes, and sperm.[201] Across mammalian species, the levels of DHA in brain and retina phospholipids are remarkably similar despite wide variations in dietary intake. This comparative constancy suggests an important role for DHA in brain and retinal function.[202] DHA occurs almost entirely in the 2-position of phospholipids. The 1-position is characteristically occupied by saturated FAs (stearic and palmitic). The specific role of DHA is not understood, but its chain length and uniquely high degree of unsaturation may help to create a membrane with high fluidity, flexibility, and permeability. However, some studies of model membranes fail to support the long-standing hypothesis that DHA increases membrane fluidity.[203] The role of DHA may be more specific and may involve modulation of the kinetics of carrier-mediated transport systems, the activity of membrane-bound enzymes, or the properties of membrane receptors.[200]

These characteristics of DHA seem to be necessary for the dynamic behavior of rhodopsin (the photosensitive pigment of rod photoreceptors) in the photoreceptive process.[203] Within the retina, DHA is concentrated in specialized membranes, which make up the photoreceptor outer segments. However, it has been shown that visual cell membrane FA composition and thus early retinal development are influenced by small dietary changes in DHA and AA. A diet containing a balanced mixture of both FAs within the physiologic intake range is required to support an ω-3 to ω-6 balance necessary for developing the highest rhodopsin content in the rod outer segments, and this may have important functional implications.[204] Research has begun to delineate a possible role of DHA in promoting optimal G-protein–coupled signaling systems in visual transduction.[205] It has been suggested that early visual experience and input during infancy may be critical to later visual function and may result in lasting consequences.[206] "More generally, delays in the early stages of visual, cognitive, and motor development can have a cascade of effects on later-maturing processes."[206]

In summary, high levels of DHA are found in the photoreceptor outer segment membranes of the retina and in the gray matter of the cerebral cortex. Some evidence, discussed extensively in Chapter 44, suggests a relationship between essential FA intake and the development of visual functions.[207-211] Therefore, it is important to determine whether optimal extrauterine accretion of LCPUFAs requires dietary supply of these FAs (perhaps originating as normal constituents of human milk) or arises sufficiently *in vivo* from chain elongation-desaturation of shorter chain precursors (i.e., LA and ALA). This is discussed in the next section.

APPROPRIATE BALANCE OF DIETARY FATTY ACID INTAKE FOR PRETERM INFANTS

Fat Requirements

"The human neonate and its mammalian counterparts have for millions of years received balanced nutrition during early infancy exclusively through breast-feeding."[212] Unfortunately, by replacing human milk with cow's milk or formula, the nutritional requirements of the infant have become less clear.[213] The caloric requirement of the full-term infant younger than 1 year of age is 100 to 120 kcal/kg/day. For each 100-kcal intake, the term infant requires a minimum of 1.8 g protein, 3.3 to 6 g fat, 300 mg essential FA, and 11 to 17 g carbohydrate.[214] The fat content of preterm infant formulas should be 4.0 to 6.0 g/100 kcal, which would provide 4.8 to 7.2 g/kg/day to infants fed 120 kcal/kg/day.[215] Regardless of the fat content of a particular formula, the fat intake of the infant is generous. A premature infant who receives 180 mL/kg/day of 20 kcal/oz formula will consume 6.2 to 6.8 g/kg/day of fat. In contrast, only 2 g/kg/day of fat must be deposited to simulate the intrauterine fat accretion rate. Some of the excess fat is subjected to oxidation and fecal excretion.[213] Studies of energy requirements indicate that the low birth weight infant requires approximately 80 kcal/kg/day for maintenance. Thus, when the low birth weight infant is fed an energy intake of 120 kcal/kg/day, some 34% of the calories fed will be used for tissue synthesis or growth. Because approximately half of the available calories in human milk are fat, then 36% of fat intake will be used for growth in the preterm infant (assuming 67 kcal/100 mL of milk and 90% fat absorption). In this metabolic situation (if all FAs are used for energy to a similar degree, if fat absorption coefficients are greater than 0.9, and if adipose tissue is synthesized in amounts and composition similar to those of intrauterine growth), the maximum requirements for essential FAs in infants weighing less than 1300 g can be estimated at 1100 mg for ω-6 FAs and 140 mg for ω-3 FAs per day.[216]

In human milk, ω-6 and ω-3 FAs normally represent a consistent percentage by weight of total FAs. Therefore, it has been recommended that these values should be used as a guideline for the composition of infant formulas.[149] Quantitative and qualitative analyses of the composition of human milk lactated by mothers delivering preterm infants indicate that their own milk provides levels of ω-6 and ω-3 essential FAs approximating the predicted requirements at day 16 of life, given intake levels of 120 kcal/kg/day. As the infants' body weight and milk intake increase, the net intake of essential FA will approach and rapidly exceed the predicted requirements.[216] Levels of LCPUFAs in human milk suggest that adequate intakes of mother's own milk also provide quantities of these membrane structural precursors in excess of their reported intrauterine rates of accretion in neural and liver tissues. If the rate of adipose tissue synthesis is projected for the extrauterine growth of a 1300-g low birth weight infant gaining 17 g of body weight per day, it can be estimated that synthesis of adipose tissues would use 185 mg/day of C20ω-6 and C22ω-6 FAs and 30.8 mg/day of C20ω-3 and C22ω-3 FAs. An adequate intake of mother's own milk provides 90 to 130 mg of C20ω-6 and C22ω-6 FAs per day and 55 to 75 mg of C20ω-3 and C22ω-3 FAs per day.[216] It thus seems prudent to feed the preterm infant human milk or formulas with an FA balance similar to that of human milk, containing longer chain homologues of LA and ALA.[217,218] Liu and colleagues,[219] using fish oil as a source of DHA (in a dose of 11 mg/kg/day), maintained red blood cell DHA concentrations in phospholipid in the range observed for human milk-fed infants. The effect of adding marine oil to infant formula has since been investigated in several species and under many different test conditions.[207,220-222] In general, this dietary maneuver causes a reduction of plasma and membrane levels of AA.[222,223] Supplementation of premature infants with long chain homologues of ALA in the absence of long chain homologues of LA not only leads to membrane abnormalities,[224] but also decreases circulating levels of AA and results in a reduction in growth potential during the first year of life.[225,226]

Clandinin and co-workers[149,150] recommended that formulas for premature infants should contain the appropriate balance of ω-6 and ω-3 metabolites of LA and ALA at concentrations that reflect normal human milk levels of these constituents and that will provide a ratio of ω-6 to ω-3 (C20 and C22) FAs of 1 to 1.4:1.[149] A clear dose response is produced in the levels of AA and DHA found in erythrocyte membrane phospholipids when preterm infant formula is supplemented with increasing levels of AA and DHA. It appears that a formula level of 0.32 to 1.1% AA and 0.24 to 0.76% DHA provides sufficient levels of these FAs to achieve a similar membrane phospholipid FA composition to that of infants fed human milk. Approximately 0.6% AA and 0.4% DHA provide sufficient and perhaps optimum levels of these FAs in formula-fed preterm infants.[150]

Composition of Fat

Postnatal growth seems to differ from fetal growth, especially with respect to fat deposition, and net absorption of fat improves with increasing gestational age. In animal models, the brain is sensitive to alteration of dietary lipid intake, even with a nutritionally complete diet. It is therefore reasonable to postulate that dietary lipids fed during the early postnatal period are important determinants of structural and functional components of developing brain tissues.[227]

Although the overall fat content of human and cow's milk appears similar, detailed analyses show marked differences in lipid composition and FA pattern. Cow's milk contains more saturated FAs than does human milk and many fewer essential FAs. Human milk contains somewhat more monounsaturated FAs and LCPUFAs.[213] Current formulations have attempted to simulate the energy and fat content of human milk, resulting in various calorie-dense and fat-dense formulas on the market.[213] To correct dissimilarities in FA composition, bovine milk fat must be augmented or replaced with various vegetable oils to provide mixtures that offer a low saturated FA content and a higher unsaturated FA content, including LA and ALA.

Formulas for premature infants have been further modified by incorporation of MCTs. The result has been that some formulas have FA profiles that are very dissimilar to that of human milk, especially with respect to medium chain FAs (considerably increased) and long chain saturated FAs (decreased). In the newborn infant, synthesis of AA and DHA depends not only on adequate desaturase and sufficient supply of dietary LA and ALA but also on calories to support energy metabolism. Based on the composition of human milk, changes in blood FA levels in preterm infants in energy balance, and studies of other species, one can provide estimates for FA requirements for preterm and term infants. The European Society of Pediatric Gastroenterology and Nutrition (ESPGAN) committee recommended an LA/ALA ratio ranging from 5:1 to 15:1,[228] which is similar to the Canadian recommendation (which ranges from 4:1 to 16:1) when no C20 and C22 FAs are added.[229] This ratio should probably be closer to the lower than to the upper limit, and this can be accomplished by increasing the ALA and decreasing the LA content of commercial formulas.[223] For LA, the recommended intake is 4 to 6% of energy, and for ALA a minimum of 1% of energy for preterm and term infants fed formulas not containing any AA or DHA.[223] Although the addition of 0.25 to 0.5% kcal of long chain ω-3 FAs is sufficient to maintain DHA levels and to keep activities such as retinal function at the same level as observed in breast-fed infants, it also reduces the accretion of AA. Therefore, when ω-3 LCPUFAs are added, ω-6 LCPUFAs should be added

simultaneously.[148,149,223,228,230] Preliminary evidence suggests that the long chain ω-6/ω-3 ratio should be approximately 1.1:1.4.[151,152] The Child Health Foundation Expert Consensus Workshop[231] recommended that infant formulas for term infants should contain at least 0.2% of total FAs as DHA and 0.35% as AA. For preterm infants, because of their lower body stores, formulas should include at least 0.35% DHA and 0.4% AA.

The inclusion of high amounts of medium chain FAs in formulas may not be as important as was previously indicated, because there seems to be no benefit to energy balance and growth, and there is some evidence of abnormal FA metabolism.[141-144,147] Although high doses of MCTs do not seem desirable, there is also no convincing evidence that they are harmful. Consequently, there is a need for more extensive studies of the optimal fat blend to use in formulas for low birth weight infants.

Previous assessments of the essential FA status of the neonate focused on measures of visual function that are different and do not enable analysis of the site of the functional deficit or mechanism involved. Measures of immune function have similar difficulties; however, in neonates, the peripheral immune system is available for analysis. Human milk is known to have many immunologic factors that reduce the incidence of infection and aid in immune development and maturation. One review[232] briefly outlined some of the effects of ω-3 FAs on the immune system. This involves the suppression of inflammatory response through effects on eicosanoids, although it is suggested that ω-3 PUFAs have many noneicosanoid effects on the immune system as well. In rats, dietary saturated FAs have little effect on cytokine production, whereas ω-3 PUFAs are potent inhibitors of the Th1-type (proinflammatory) cytokines.[233,234] Research in humans by Field and colleagues[235,236] indicates that feeding infants with or without AA and DHA alters the composition of functional cells related to maturity of the immune system. By linking changes in the specific cell types with release of subcellular messages (exocytokines) and their receptors, it is possible to develop dynamic measures of cell function that can be used to link known physiologic functions through biochemical mechanisms altered by changes in the essential FA status. The addition of AA and DHA to preterm formula, at levels similar to human milk, can influence the proportion, maturation, and cytokine production of peripheral blood lymphocytes. Improvement of the ability of peripheral mononuclear cells to produce interleukin-10 by supplemented preterm infants as compared with standard formula-fed infants suggests that these dietary modifications may aid induction of tolerance to oral antigens. Further studies will be done to elucidate other aspects of immune development, including antigenic response.[236]

Parenteral Lipid Emulsions and Potential Complicating Factors

TPN is frequently considered when the gastrointestinal tract is not capable of digesting and absorbing nutrients. The basis for calculating nutrient requirements in infants receiving TPN is similar to that for the enterally fed neonate, except malabsorption and the energy cost of the digestion and absorption of food need not be considered. Current research, however, indicates that the enterocyte possesses significant FA desaturation activity.[237] Thus, parenteral feeding of fats may bypass this physiologic control over FA metabolism.

The fat particles in emulsions are similar in size to chylomicrons and, like the latter, are cleared from the circulation by lipoprotein lipase[238] and by hepatic lipase.[239] As compared with the use of 10% lipid emulsions, the use of a 20% lipid emulsion does offer the advantage of more efficient triglyceride clearance with lower cholesterol and phospholipids in low-density lipoproteins.[240,241] This finding suggests that excessive phospholipid liposomes in 10% lipid emulsions, as opposed to the liposome-poor

20% emulsion, impede the removal of triglycerides from plasma. Friedman and colleagues[242] studied sick newborns who were maintained on fat-free intravenous alimentation. These infants developed very rapid biochemical changes in plasma that were compatible with essential FA deficiency during the first week of life and were reversible with oral feedings containing essential FAs. Infusion of lipid emulsions rapidly reversed clinical symptoms of essential FA deficiency and returned plasma phospholipid ω-6 FA levels to normal. However, the erythrocyte and liver phospholipid ω-6 FA content and adipose tissue reserves of ω-6 FAs normalized more slowly. Similar findings have been observed in experimental animals.[243] Innis[244] studied the effect of TPN with LA-rich emulsions on tissue ω-6 and ω-3 FAs in the rat and concluded that intravenous administration of large amounts of LA in parenteral lipid reduces desaturation and elongation of essential FAs but does not competitively inhibit esterification of other FAs into phospholipid. Innis also reported that after 3 days of fat-free parenteral nutrition, not only are DHA and AA both diminished in the red cell membrane phospholipids,[245] but also some biochemical signs of essential FA deficiency develop.[246] Essential FA deficiency is avoided by infusions of 0.5 to 1.0 g/kg/day of intravenous lipid.[247]

Energy metabolism, fat accretion, and oxidation in parenterally fed infants are determined not only by total energy intake,[248] but also by the composition of the nonprotein calories.[249-252] The percentage of nonprotein calories supplied as intravenous fat should probably range between 30 and 50%. Commercial lipid emulsions contain excessive amounts of LA and no long chain derivatives of either LA or ALA in the triglyceride fraction. In adults, the use of MCT and long-chain triglyceride mixtures may alter LCPUFA synthesis, but there is no similar evidence available in neonates.[253] It is also not known whether this alteration in long chain FA metabolism results from a reduction in LA content or from the addition of MCTs to the intravenous lipid emulsion. Research involving structured lipid emulsions in which both medium chain and long chain FAs are esterified to the same glycerol backbone indicates that this could be a safe and well-tolerated approach to TPN.[254]

The physiologic and pharmacologic effects of the LCPUFAs in disease states may result in therapeutic modalities for approach to inflammation, endotoxin effects, liver cholestasis, and pulmonary hypertension.[255-258] There has been some concern regarding the occurrence of hepatic injury with intravenous lipid administration. The current belief is that there is an increase in TPN-associated cholestasis in infants receiving fat emulsions.[259,260] The inclusion of ω-3 PUFAs in intravenous lipid emulsions may be a way to decrease the incidence of TPN-induced cholestasis by improving the bile flow, which is reduced by intravenous soybean oil emulsions.[257] Very significant changes have been found in the FA composition of liver ethanolamine phosphoglycerides and choline phosphoglycerides in infants receiving TPN with a soybean oil emulsion as the lipid source. These alterations have included an increase in LA, a decrease in linoleate elongation-desaturation products, and a decrease in the level of DHA in liver phosphatidylethanolamine and phosphatidylcholine. In the brain, an increase in the LA content of choline phosphoglyceride has been observed; however, it has not been accompanied by any increase in the ω-6 LCPUFAs. Thus, there is a potential for adverse effects of high doses of LA on the tissue levels of LCPUFAs.[261] Conversely, fish oil-enriched emulsions reduced the impairment of bile flow seen in a newborn piglet model of TPN cholestasis.[262] Although feeding the fish oil emulsion resulted in alterations in canalicular and sinusoidal FA composition of membrane phospholipids, the mechanism responsible for the prevention of cholestasis is not known. Changes in eicosanoid metabolites may be partially responsible. More research is required to determine clinical applications of fish oil-enriched emulsions in human neonate TPN.[262]

The necessity of carnitine supplementation for the metabolism of intravenous lipid metabolism remains uncertain, because some studies have demonstrated beneficial effects, which could not be confirmed by others. However, comparisons are difficult to make because the studies used different doses of carnitine.[263] Carnitine is present in human milk,[264,265] and it is essential for FA metabolism, but high doses may have an undesirable effect.[266] There are no convincing data documenting physiologic or metabolic benefit of giving carnitine to infants receiving intravenous lipid. If given, the dose should not exceed the amount a breast-fed infant receives (i.e., 15 μmol/100 kcal).

In summary, the FA composition of commercial lipid emulsions is inappropriate in that it is unphysiologic and results in abnormal FA composition of circulating and tissue membrane lipids. For prevention of essential FA deficiency, 0.5 to 1 g/kg/day of intravenous lipid is required, preferably as a 20% emulsion. To maintain an acceptable energy balance, 0.5 to 1 g/kg/day of intravenous lipid as part of TPN should be introduced by 24 to 48 hours of age. That dose can be progressively increased (by 0.5 to 1 g/kg/day) in incremental daily or alternate-day steps, as tolerated, up to 3 to 4 g/kg/day, while triglyceride clearance is monitored.

REFERENCES

1. Heim T: Energy and lipid requirements of the fetus and the preterm infant. J Pediatr Gastroenterol Nutr 1983;2(Suppl 1):S16.
2. Sparks JW, et al: An estimate of the caloric requirements of the human fetus. Biol Neonate 1980;38(3-4):113.
3. Hahn P, Novak M: Development of brown and white adipose tissue. J Lipid Res 1975;16(2):79.
4. Clandinin MT, et al: Relationship between fatty acid accretion, membrane composition, and biologic functions. J Pediatr 1994;125(5 Pt 2):S25.
5. Sastry PS: Lipids of nervous tissue: composition and metabolism. Prog Lipid Res 1985;24(2):69.
6. Friedman Z: Polyunsaturated fatty acids in the low-birth-weight infant. Semin Perinatol 1979;3(4):341.
7. Granström E: Biochemistry of the eicosanoids: cyclooxygenase and lipoxygenase products of polyunsaturated fatty acids. In Horisberger M, Bracco U (eds): Lipids in Modern Nutrition, Vol 13. New York, Raven Press, 1987, p 59.
8. Seyberth HW, Kuhl PG: The role of eicosanoids in paediatrics. Eur J Pediatr 1988;147(4):341.
9. Gottlieb A, et al: Rodent brain growth stages: an analytical review. Biol Neonate 1977;32(3-4):166.
10. Meisami E, Timiras PS: Normal and abnormal biochemical development of the brain after birth. In Jones CT (ed): The Biochemical Development of the Fetus and Neonate. New York, Elsevier, 1982, p 759.
11. Jumpsen J, Clandinin MT: Brain Development: Relationship to Dietary Lipid and Lipid Metabolism. Champaign, IL, AOCS Press, 1995.
12. Friedman Z: Essential fatty acid consideration at birth in the premature neonate and the specific requirement for preformed prostaglandin precursors in the infant. Prog Lipid Res 1986;25(1-4):355.
13. McIlwain H, Bachelard HS: Cerebral lipids. In McIlwain H, Bachelard HS (eds): Biochemistry and the Central Nervous System. New York, Churchill Livingstone, 1985, p 282.
14. Mandel P: Biochemical correlates of the genetic and environmental determinism of some behaviors. In Brazier MAB (ed): Growth and Development of the Brain: Nutritional, Genetic, and Environmental Factors, Vol 1. New York, Raven Press, 1975, p 203.
15. Ballabriga A: Essential fatty acids and human tissue composition: an overview. Acta Paediatr Suppl 1994;402:63.
16. Davidson AN: Biochemical Correlates of Brain Structure and Function. London, Academic Press, 1977, p 1.
17. Yakovlev PI, Lecours AR: The myelogenetic cycles of regional maturation of the brain. In Minkowski A (ed): Regional Development of the Brain in Early Life. Philadelphia, FA Davis, 1967, p 3.
18. Timiras PS: Developmental Physiology and Aging. New York, Macmillan, 1972, p 129.
19. Menon NK, Dhopeshwarkar GA: Essential fatty acid deficiency and brain development. Prog Lipid Res 1982;21(4):309.
20. Foot M, et al: Influence of dietary fat on the lipid composition of rat brain synaptosomal and microsomal membranes. Biochem J 1982;208(3):631.
21. Hargreaves KM, Clandinin MT: Phosphatidylethanolamine methyltransferase: evidence for influence of diet fat on selectivity of substrate for methylation in rat brain synaptic plasma membranes. Biochim Biophys Acta 1987;918(2):97.
22. Clandinin MT: Fatty acid utilization in perinatal de novo synthesis of tissues. Early Hum Dev 1981;5(4):355.
23. Clandinin MT, et al: Fatty acid accretion in the development of human spinal cord. Early Hum Dev 1981;5(1):1.

24. Ramsey RB, Nicholas JH: Brain lipids. *In* Paoletti R, Kritchevsky D (eds): Advances in Lipid Research. New York, Academic Press, 1972, p 143.

25. Rumsby MG, Crang AJ: The synthesis, assembly and turnover of cell surface component. *In* Poste G, Nicholson GL (eds): Cell Surface Reviews. Amsterdam, Elsevier, 1977, p 247.

26. Carey EM: The biochemistry of fetal brain development and myelination. *In* Jones CT (ed): The Biochemical Development of the Fetus and Neonate. New York, Elsevier, 1982, p 287.

27. Gilles FH: Myelination in the neonatal brain. Hum Pathol 1976;7(3):244.

28. Hansen IB, Clausen J: The fatty acids of the human foetal brain. Scand J Clin Lab Invest 1968;22(3):231.

29. Galli C, et al: Brain lipid modifications induced by essential fatty acid deficiency in growing male and female rats. J Neurochem 1970;17(3):347.

30. Sun GY: Effects of a fatty acid deficiency on lipids of whole brain, microsomes, and myelin in the rat. J Lipid Res 1972;13(1):56.

31. Ställberg-Stenhagen S, Svennerholm L: Fatty acid composition of human brain sphingomyelins: normal variation with age and changes during myelin disorders. J Lipid Res 1965;6:146.

32. Byrne MC, et al: Ganglioside-induced neuritogenesis: verification that gangliosides are the active agents, and comparison of molecular species. J Neurochem 1983;41(5):1214.

33. De Maria R, et al: Requirement for GD3 ganglioside in. Science 1997;277(5332):1652.

34. Ortaldo JR, et al: T cell activation via the disialoganglioside GD3: analysis of signal transduction. J Leukoc Biol 1996;60(4):533.

35. Ledeen RW: Neurobiology of Glycoconjugates. New York, Plenum Press, 1989.

36. Sonnino S, et al: Recognition by two-dimensional thin-layer chromatography and densitometric quantification of alkali-labile gangliosides from the brain of different animals. Anal Biochem 1983;128(1):104.

37. Vanier MT, et al: Developmental profiles of gangliosides in human and rat brain. J Neurochem 1971;18(4):581.

38. Karlsson I: Effects of different dietary levels of essential fatty acids on the fatty acid composition of ethanolamine phosphoglycerides in nyelin and synaptosome plasma membranes. J Neurochem 1975;25(2):101.

39. Park EJ, et al: Diet induced changes in ganglioside content in the intestine, plasma and brain in weanling rats. Unpublished data, 2002.

40. Cantrill RC, Carey EM: Changes in the activities of de novo fatty acid synthesis and palmitoyl-CoA synthetase in relation to myelination in rabbit brain. Biochim Biophys Acta 1975;380(2):165.

41. Crawford MA: Essential fatty acids and the vulnerability of the artery during growth. Postgrad Med J 1978;54:149.

42. Dobbing J, Sands J: Quantitative growth and development of human brain. Arch Dis Child 1973;48(10):757.

43. Clandinin MT, et al: Intrauterine fatty acid accretion rates in human brain: implications for fatty acid requirements. Early Hum Dev 1980;4(2):121.

44. Widdowson EM: Growth and composition of the human fetus and newborn. *In* Assali NS (ed): The Biology of Gestation, Vol 2. New York, Academic Press, 1968, p 1.

45. Clandinin MT, Chappell JE, Heim T: Do low weight infants require nutrition with chain elongation-desaturation products of essential fatty acids? Prog Lipid Res 1981;20:901.

46. Rosso P: Placental function and control of nutrient transfer to the fetus. *In* Grand RJ (ed): Pediatric Nutrition. Boston, Butterworth, 1987, p 239.

47. Dancis J, et al: Transfer across perfused human placenta. II. Free fatty acids. Pediatr Res 1973;7(4):192.

48. Poissonnet CM, et al: Growth and development of adipose tissue. J Pediatr 1988;113(1 Pt 1):1.

49. Bain M: Permeability of the human placenta in vivo. Early Hum Dev 1986;14:147.

50. Coleman RA: Placental metabolism and transport of lipid. Fed Proc 1986;45(10):2519.

51. Berghaus TM, et al: Fatty acid composition of lipid classes in maternal and cord plasma at birth. Eur J Pediatr 1998;157(9):763.

52. Kuhn DC, Crawford M: Placental essential fatty acid transport and prostaglandin synthesis. Prog Lipid Res 1986;25(1–4):345.

53. Hull D, Elphick M: Transfer of fatty acids. *In* Chamberlain GVP, Wilkinson AW (eds): Placental Transfer. Kent, UK, Pitman, 1979, p 159.

54. Rosso P, Lederman SA: Nutrition and fetal growth. *In* Milunsky A (eds): Advances in Perinatal Medicine. New York, Plenum Press, 1981, p 1.

55. Dutta-Roy AK: Transport mechanisms for long-chain polyunsaturated fatty acids in the human placenta. Am J Clin Nutr 2000;71(1 Suppl):315S.

56. Haggarty P, et al: Long-chain polyunsaturated fatty acid transport across the perfused human placenta. Placenta 1997;18(8):635.

57. Lafond J, et al: Linoleic acid transport by human placental syncytiotrophoblast membranes. Eur J Biochem 1994;226(2):707.

58. Chambaz J, et al: Essential fatty acids interconversion in the human fetal liver. Biol Neonate 1985;47(3):136.

59. Crawford MA, et al: Fetal accumulation of long-chain polyunsaturated fatty acids. *In* Bazán NG, et al (eds): Function and Biosynthesis of Lipids: Proceedings of the International Symposium on Function and Biosynthesis of Lipids held at Sierra de la Ventana, Tornquist, Province of Buenos Aires, Argentina, November, 1976. New York, Plenum Press, 1977, p 135.

60. Bohmer T, Havel RJ: Genesis of fatty liver and hyperlipiemia in the fetal guinea pig. J Lipid Res 1975;16(6):454.

61. Smith S, Abraham S: Fatty acid synthesis in developing mouse liver. Arch Biochem Biophys 1970;136(1):112.

62. Olegard R, Svennerholm L: Fatty acid composition of plasma and red cell phosphoglycerides in full term infants and their mothers. Acta Paediatr Scand 1970;59(6):637.

63. Friedman Z, et al: Cord blood fatty acid composition in infants and in their mothers during the third trimester. J Pediatr 1978;92(3):461.

64. Friedman Z: Essential fatty acid requirements for term and preterm infants. *In* Horisberger M, Bracco U (eds): Lipids in Modern Nutrition, Vol 13. Nestlé Nutrition Workshop Series. New York, Raven Press, 1987, p 179.

65. Koletzko B, Muller J: Cis- and trans-isomeric fatty acids in plasma lipids of newborn infants and their mothers. Biol Neonate 1990;57(3–4):172.

66. Decsi T, et al: Inverse association between trans isomeric and long-chain polyunsaturated fatty acids in cord blood lipids of full-term infants. Am J Clin Nutr 2001;74(3):590.

67. Koletzko B: Trans fatty acids may impair biosynthesis of long-chain polyunsaturates and growth in man. Acta Paediatr 1992;81(4):302.

68. Gaull DE: Human milk as food. *In* Friedman E, et al (eds): Advances in Perinatal Medicine. New York, Plenum Medical Book, 1982, p 47.

69. Hamosh M, Hamosh P: Does nutrition in early life have long term metabolic effects? Can animal models be used to predict these effects in the human? *In* Goldman AS, et al (eds): Human Lactation 3: The Effects of Human Milk on the Recipient Infant. New York, Plenum Press, 1987, p 37.

70. Hamosh M: Lipid composition of preterm human milk and its digestion by the infant. *In* Schaub J (ed): Composition and Physiological Properties of Human Milk. Amsterdam, Elsevier, 1985.

71. Clandinin MT, et al: Fatty acid accretion in fetal and neonatal liver: implications for fatty acid requirements. Early Hum Dev 1981;5(1):7.

72. Clandinin MT, et al: Extrauterine fatty acid accretion in infant brain: implications for fatty acid requirements. Early Hum Dev 1980;4(2):131.

73. Salem N, Jr., et al: Mechanisms of action of docosahexaenoic acid in the nervous system. Lipids 2001;36(9):945.

74. Contreras MA, et al: Chronic nutritional deprivation of n-3 alpha-linolenic acid does not affect n-6 arachidonic acid recycling within brain phospholipids of awake rats. J Neurochem 2001;79(5):1090.

75. Ball EG: Some energy relationships in adipose tissue. Ann NY Acad Sci 1965;131(1):225.

76. Galli C, et al: Effects of dietary fatty acids on the fatty acid composition of brain ethanolamine phosphoglyceride: reciprocal replacement of n-6 and n-3 polyunsaturated fatty acids. Biochim Biophys Acta 1971;248:449.

77. Jumpsen J, et al: Small changes of dietary (n-6) and (n-3)/fatty acid content ratio alter phosphatidylethanolamine and phosphatidylcholine fatty acid composition during development of neuronal and glial cells in rats. J Nutr 1997;127(5):724.

78. Hargreaves K, Clandinin MT: Dietary lipids in relation to postnatal development of the brain. Ups J Med Sci (Suppl) 1990;48:79.

79. Clandinin MT, et al: Arachidonic acid and docosahexaenoic acid are essential fatty acids for preterm infants. J Pediatr, 2003, in press.

80. Anderson GH: Human milk feeding. Pediatr Clin North Am 1985;32(2):335.

81. Steichen JJ, et al: Breastfeeding the low birth weight preterm infant. Clin Perinatol 1987;14(1):131.

82. Pan XL, Izumi T: Variation of the ganglioside compositions of human milk, cow's milk and infant formulas. Early Hum Dev 2000;57(1):25.

83. Van Aerde JE, Clandinin MT: Controversy in fatty acid balance. Can J Physiol Pharmacol 1993;71(9):707.

84. Chappell JE, et al: Trans fatty acids in human milk lipids: influence of maternal diet and weight loss. Am J Clin Nutr 1985;42(1):49.

85. Harris WS, et al: Will dietary omega-3 fatty acids change the composition of human milk? Am J Clin Nutr 1984;40(4):780.

86. Jensen RG, et al: Effect of dietary intake of n-6 and n-3 fatty acids on the fatty acid composition of human milk in North America. J Pediatr 1992;120(4 Pt 2):S87.

87. Wainwright PE, et al: The effects of dietary n-3/n-6 ratio on brain development in the mouse: a dose response study with long-chain n-3 fatty acids. Lipids 1992;27(2):98.

88. Guesnet P, et al: Blood lipid concentrations of docosahexaenoic and arachidonic acids at birth determine their relative postnatal changes in term infants fed breast milk or formula. Am J Clin Nutr 1999;70(2):292.

89. Decsi T, et al: Effect of type of early infant feeding on fatty acid composition of plasma lipid classes in full-term infants during the second 6 months of life. J Pediatr Gastroenterol Nutr 2000;30(5):547.

90. Sanders TA, Reddy S: The influence of a vegetarian diet on the fatty acid composition of human milk and the essential fatty acid status of the infant. J Pediatr 1992;120(4 Pt 2):S71.

91. Demmelmair H, et al: Metabolism of U13C-labeled linoleic acid in lactating women. J Lipid Res 1998;39(7):1389.

92. Innis SM: Essential fatty acids in growth and development. Prog Lipid Res 1991;30(1):39.

93. Jensen RG: Lipids in human milk. Lipids 1999;34(12):1243.

94. Innis SM, Kuhnlein HV: Long-chain n-3 fatty acids in breast milk of Inuit women consuming traditional foods. Early Hum Dev 1988;18(2–3):185.

95. Fidler N, et al: Docosahexaenoic acid transfer into human milk after dietary supplementation: a randomized clinical trial. J Lipid Res 2000;41(9):1376.

96. Gibson RA, Kneebone GM: A lack of correlation between linoleate and arachidonate in human breast milk. Lipids 1984;19(6):469.

97. Eaton SB, Konner M: Paleolithic nutrition: a consideration of its nature and current implications. N Engl J Med 1985;312(5):283.
98. Simopoulos AP: Omega-3 fatty acids in health and disease and in growth and development. Am J Clin Nutr 1991;54(3):438.
99. Jensen R: Lipids in human milk: composition and fat-soluble vitamins. *In* Lebenthal E (ed): Textbook of Gastroenterology and Nutrition in Infancy, 2nd ed. New York, Raven Press, 1989, p 157.
100. Hamosh M: Lipids in human milk and their digestion by the newborn infant. *In* Ghisolfi J, Putet G (eds): Essential Fatty Acids and Infant Nutrition. Paris, J Libbey Eurotext, 1992, p 119.
101. Del Prado M, , et al: Contribution of dietary and newly formed arachidonic acid to human milk lipids in women eating a low-fat diet. Am J Clin Nutr 2001;74(2):242.
102. Sauerwald TU, et al: Polyunsaturated fatty acid supply with human milk: physiological aspects and in vivo studies of metabolism. Adv Exp Med Biol 2000;478:261.
103. Chappell JE, et al: Prostanoid content of human milk: relationships to milk fatty acid content. Endocrinol Exp 1983;17(3–4):351.
104. Hopkinson JM, et al: Milk production by mothers of premature infants. Pediatrics 1988;81(6):815.
105. Bitman J, et al: Comparison of the lipid composition of breast milk from mothers of term and preterm infants. Am J Clin Nutr 1983;38(2):300.
106. Luukkainen P, et al: Changes in the fatty acid composition of preterm and term human milk from 1 week to 6 months of lactation. J Pediatr Gastroenterol Nutr 1994;18(3):355.
107. Garza C, et al: Special properties of human milk. Clin Perinatol 1987;14(1):11.
108. Reichman B, et al: Diet, fat accretion, and growth in premature infants. N Engl J Med 1981;305(25):1495.
109. Watkins JB: Lipid digestion and absorption. Pediatrics 1985;75(1 Pt 2):151.
110. Clandinin MT: The effect of dietary fat on milk and tissue lipids. *In* Beare-Rogers J (eds): Dietary Fat Requirements in Health and Development. Champaign, IL, AOCS Press, 1988, p 43.
111. Pencharz PB: Nutrition of the low-birth weight infant. *In* Grand RJ, et al (eds): Pediatric Nutrition: Theory and Practice. Boston, Butterworth, 1987, p 313.
112. Farquharson J, et al: Effect of diet on infant subcutaneous tissue triglyceride fatty acids. Arch Dis Child 1993;69(5):589.
113. Combes M, et al: Essential fatty acids in premature infant feeding. Pediatrics 1962;30:136.
114. Hansen AE, et al: Role of linoleic acid in infant nutrition. Pediatrics 1963;31:171.
115. American Academy of Pediatrics Committee on Nutrition: *In* Kleinman RE (ed): Pediatric Nutrition Handbook, 4th ed. Elk Grove Village, IL, American Academy of Pediatrics, 1998, p 653.
116. Innis S: Fat. *In* Tsang RC (ed): Nutritional Needs of the Preterm Infant: Scientific Basis and Practical Guidelines. Baltimore, Williams & Wilkins, 1993, p 65.
117. Wang Y: Calcium supplementation in premature infants fed breast milk: the effect of timing of calcium supplementation on calcium, phosphorus, magnesium and fat balance and on the absorption coefficients of individual fatty acids. Thesis, University of Alberta, Edmonton, Canada, 1992.
118. Jensen C, et al: Absorption of individual fatty acids from long chain or medium chain triglycerides in very small infants. Am J Clin Nutr 1986;43(5):745.
119. Clandinin MT, et al: Requirements of newborn infants for long chain polyunsaturated fatty acids. Acta Paediatr Scand Suppl 1989;351:63.
120. Clandinin MT: Symposium discussion. J Pediatr 1994;125:S78.
121. Carlson SE, et al: Docosahexaenoic acid status of preterm infants at birth and following feeding with human milk or formula. Am J Clin Nutr 1986;44(6):798.
122. Clandinin MT, et al: Assessment of the efficacious dose of arachidonic and docosahexaenoic acids in preterm infant formulas: fatty acid composition of erythrocyte membrane lipids. Pediatr Res 1997;42(6):819.
123. Gibson RA, et al: Ratios of linoleic acid to alpha-linolenic acid in formulas for term infants. J Pediatr 1994;125(5 Pt 2):S48.
124. Arbuckle LD, et al: Formula 18:2(n-6) and 18:3(n-3) content and ratio influence long-chain polyunsaturated fatty acids in the developing piglet liver and central nervous system. J Nutr 1994;124(2):289.
125. Rioux FM, Innis SM: Arachidonic acid concentrations in plasma and liver phospholipid and cholesterol esters of piglets raised on formulas with different linoleic and linolenic acid contents. Am J Clin Nutr 1992;56(1):106.
126. Innis SM, et al: Plasma and red blood cell fatty acids of low-birth-weight infants fed their mother's expressed breast milk or preterm-infant formula. Am J Clin Nutr 1990;51(6):994.
127. Uauy RD, et al: Effect of dietary omega-3 fatty acids on retinal function of very-low-birth-weight neonates. Pediatr Res 1990;28(5):485.
128. Makrides M, et al: Fatty acid composition of brain, retina, and erythrocytes in breast- and formula-fed infants. Am J Clin Nutr 1994;60(2):189.
129. Makrides M, et al: Erythrocyte docosahexaenoic acid correlates with the visual response of healthy, term infants. Pediatr Res 1993;33(4 Pt 1):425.
130. Innis SM, et al: Development of visual acuity in relation to plasma and erythrocyte omega-6 and omega-3 fatty acids in healthy term gestation infants. Am J Clin Nutr 1994;60(3):347.
131. Carlson SE, et al: Visual-acuity development in healthy preterm infants: effect of marine-oil supplementation. Am J Clin Nutr 1993;58(1):35.
132. Lucas A, et al: Breast milk and subsequent intelligence quotient in children born preterm. Lancet 1992;339(8788):261.
133. Jacobson SW, Jacobson JL: Breastfeeding and intelligence. Lancet 1992;339(8798):926.
134. Fleith M, Clandinin MT: Dietary PUFA for preterm and term infants: a review of clinical studies. Critical Reviews in Food Science and Nutrition (University of Massachusetts), 2002, in press.
135. Widdowson EM, et al: Body fat of British and Dutch infants. Br Med J 1975;1(5959):653.
136. Sauerwald TU, et al: Effect of dietary alpha-linolenic acid intake on incorporation of docosahexaenoic and arachidonic acids into plasma phospholipids of term infants. Lipids 1996;31(Suppl):S131.
137. Salem N, Jr., et al: Arachidonic and docosahexaenoic acids are biosynthesized from their 18-carbon precursors in human infants. Proc Natl Acad Sci USA 1996;93(1):49.
138. Birch EE, et al: A randomized controlled trial of long-chain polyunsaturated fatty acid supplementation of formula in term infants after weaning at 6 wk of age. Am J Clin Nutr 2002;75(3):570.
139. Clandinin MT, et al: Arachidonic acid and docosahexaenoic acid are essential fatty acids for preterm infants. N Engl J Med 2002;139:79.
140. Pencharz PB: Nutrition of the low-birth weight infant. *In* Grand RJ, et al (eds): Pediatric Nutrition: Theory and Practice. Boston, Butterworth, 1987, p 313.
141. Bustamante SA, et al: Growth of premature infants fed formulas with 10%, 30%, or 50% medium-chain triglycerides. Am J Dis Child 1987;141(5):516.
142. Huston RK, et al: Nutrient and mineral retention and vitamin D absorption in low-birth-weight infants: effect of medium-chain triglycerides. Pediatrics 1983;72(1):44.
143. Okamoto E, et al: Use of medium-chain triglycerides in feeding the low-birth-weight infant. Am J Dis Child 1982;136(5):428.
144. Whyte RK, et al: Energy balance in low birth weight infants fed formula of high or low medium-chain triglyceride content. J Pediatr 1986;108(6):964.
145. Sulkers EJ, et al: Quantitation of oxidation of medium-chain triglycerides in preterm infants. Pediatr Res 1989;26(4):294.
146. Van Aerde JE: The effect of medium-chain-triglyceride diet on energy and macronutrient utilisation in very low birth weight infants (abstract). Pediatr Res 1989;91411.
147. Wall KM, et al: Nonessential fatty acids in formula fat blends influence essential fatty acid metabolism and composition in plasma and organ lipid classes in piglets. Lipids 1992;27(12):1024.
148. Clandinin MT, et al: Extrauterine fatty acid accretion in infant brain: implications for fatty acid requirements. Early Hum Dev 1980;4(2):131.
149. Clandinin MT, et al: Requirements of newborn infants for long chain polyunsaturated fatty acids. Acta Paediatr Scand Suppl 1989;351:63.
150. Clandinin MT, et al: Assessment of the efficacious dose of arachidonic and docosahexaenoic acids in preterm infant formulas: fatty acid composition of erythrocyte membrane lipids. Pediatr Res 1997;42(6):819.
151. Clandinin MT, et al: Addition of long-chain polyunsaturated fatty acids to formula for very low birth weight infants. Lipids 1992;27(11):896.
152. Clandinin MT, et al: Feeding preterm infants a formula containing C20 and C22 fatty acids simulates plasma phospholipid fatty acid composition of infants fed human milk. Early Hum Dev 1992;31(1):41.
153. Crawford MA: Essential fatty acids and brain development. *In* Horisberger M, Bracco U (eds): Lipids in Modern Nutrition, Vol 13. New York, Raven Press, 1987, p 67.
154. Chappell JE, et al: Fatty acid balance studies in premature infants fed human milk or formula: effect of calcium supplementation. J Pediatr 1986;108(3):439.
155. Hamosh M, et al: Lipids in milk and the first steps in their digestion. Pediatrics 1985;75(1 Pt 2):146.
156. Hamosh M: Lipids in human milk and their digestion by the newborn infant. *In* Ghisolfi J, Putet G (eds): Essential Fatty Acids and Infant Nutrition. Paris, J Libbey Eurotext, 1992, p 119.
157. Hamosh M, et al: Gastric lipolysis and fat absorption in preterm infants: effect of medium-chain triglyceride or long-chain triglyceride-containing formulas. Pediatrics 1989;83(1):86.
158. Hamosh M, et al: Milk lipids and neonatal fat digestion: relationship between fatty acid composition, endogenous and exogenous digestive enzymes and digestion of milk fat. World Rev Nutr Diet 1994;75:86.
159. Hamosh M: Lipid metabolism in premature infants. Biol Neonate 1987;52(Suppl 1):50.
160. Hernell O: Digestion of human milk fat in early infancy. Acta Paediatr Scand Suppl 1989;351:57.
161. Watkins JB: Lipid digestion and absorption. Pediatrics 1985;75(1 Pt 2):151.
162. Hernell O, Blackberg L: Human milk bile salt-stimulated lipase: functional and molecular aspects. J Pediatr 1994;125(5 Pt 2):S56.
163. Rey J, et al: Fat absorption in low birthweight infants. Acta Paediatr Scand 1982;296(Suppl):81.
164. Lavine M, Clark RM: Changing patterns of free fatty acids in breast milk during storage. J Pediatr Gastroenterol Nutr 1987;6(5):769.
165. Henderson TR, et al: Effect of pasteurization on long chain polyunsaturated fatty acid levels and enzyme activities of human milk. J Pediatr 1998;132(5):876.
166. Innis SM, et al: Palmitic acid is absorbed as sn-2 monopalmitin from milk and formula with rearranged triacylglycerols and results in increased plasma triglyceride sn-2 and cholesteryl ester palmitate in piglets. J Nutr 1995;125(1):73.

167. Innis SM, et al: Evidence that palmitic acid is absorbed as sn-2 monoacylglycerol from human milk by breast-fed infants. Lipids 1994;29(8):541.

168. Nelson CM, Innis SM: Plasma lipoprotein fatty acids are altered by the positional distribution of fatty acids in infant formula triacylglycerols and human milk. Am J Clin Nutr 1999;70(1):62.

169. Verkade HJ, et al: Fat absorption in neonates: comparison of long-chain-fatty-acid and triglyceride compositions of formula, feces, and blood. Am J Clin Nutr 1991;53(3):643.

170. Lien EL: The role of fatty acid composition and positional distribution in fat absorption in infants. J Pediatr 1994;125(5 Pt 2):S62.

171. Friedman HI, Nylund B: Intestinal fat digestion, absorption, and transport: a review. Am J Clin Nutr 1980;33(5):1108.

172. Roy CC, et al: Correction of the malabsorption of the preterm infant with a medium-chain triglyceride formula. J Pediatr 1975;86(3):446.

173. Brooke OG: Energy balance and metabolic rate in preterm infants fed with standard and high-energy formulas. Br J Nutr 1980;44(1):13.

174. Whyte RK, et al: Excretion of dicarboxylic and omega-1 hydroxy fatty acids by low birth weight infants fed with medium-chain triglycerides. Pediatr Res 1986;20(2):122.

175. Wu PY, et al: Medium-chain triglycerides in infant formulas and their relation to plasma ketone body concentrations. Pediatr Res 1986;20(4):338.

176. Jensen C, et al: Absorption of individual fatty acids from long chain or medium chain triglycerides in very small infants. Am J Clin Nutr 1986;43(5):745.

177. Senterre J: Nutrition of Premature Babies. In Stern L (ed): Feeding the Sick Infant, Vol 11. New York, Raven Press, 1987, p 191.

178. Hamosh M: Lingual lipase and fat digestion in the neonatal period. J Pediatr Gastroenterol Nutr 1983;2(Suppl 1):S236.

179. Bernbaum JC, Pereira GR, Watkins JB, et al: Nonnutritive sucking during gavage feeding enhances growth and maturation in premature infants. Pediatrics 1983;71(1):41.

180. Filer LJ, Jr., et al: Triglyceride configuration and fat absorption by the human infant. J Nutr 1969;99(3):293.

181. Dobbing J: Undernutrition and the developing brain: the use of animal models to elucidate the human problem. In Paoletti R, Davidson AN (eds): Chemistry and Brain Development. New York, Plenum Press, 1971, p 399.

182. Hernell O, Blackberg L: Digestion of human milk lipids: physiologic significance of sn-2 monoacylglycerol hydrolysis by bile salt-stimulated lipase. Pediatr Res 1982;16(10):882.

183. Jarvenpaa AL, et al: Feeding the low-birth-weight infant. III. Diet influences bile acid metabolism. Pediatrics 1983;72(5):677.

184. Carnielli VP, et al: Feeding premature newborn infants palmitic acid in amounts and stereoisomeric position similar to that of human milk: effects on fat and mineral balance. Am J Clin Nutr 1995;61(5):1037.

185. Carnielli VP, et al: Intestinal absorption of long-chain polyunsaturated fatty acids in preterm infants fed breast milk or formula. Am J Clin Nutr 1998;67(1):97.

186. Rings EH, et al: Functional development of fat absorption in term and preterm neonates strongly correlates with ability to absorb long-chain fatty acids from intestinal lumen. Pediatr Res 2002;51(1):57.

187. Moya M, et al: Fatty acid absorption in preterms on formulas with and without long-chain polyunsaturated fatty acids and in terms on formulas without these added. Eur J Clin Nutr 2001;55(9):755.

188. Warshaw JB: Cellular energy metabolism during fetal development. IV. Fatty acid activation, acyl transfer and fatty acid oxidation during development of the chick and rat. Dev Biol 1972;28(4):537.

189. Farrell PM, et al: Essential fatty acid deficiency in premature infants. Am J Clin Nutr 1988;48(2):220.

190. Kimura RE, Warshaw JB: Metabolic adaptations of the fetus and newborn. J Pediatr Gastroenterol Nutr 1983;2(Suppl 1):S12.

191. Bahnsen M, et al: Mechanisms of catecholamine effects on ketogenesis. Am J Physiol 1984;247(2 Pt 1):E123.

192. Atkins J, Clandinin MT: Nutritional significance of factors affecting carnitine dependent transport of fatty acids in neonates. Nutr Res 1989;10:117.

193. Jones PJ, et al: Whole body oxidation of dietary fatty acids: implications for energy utilization. Am J Clin Nutr 1985;42(5):769.

194. Clandinin MT, et al: Increasing the dietary polyunsaturated fat content alters whole-body utilization of 16:0 and 10:0. Am J Clin Nutr 1995;61(5):1052.

195. Jones PJ, Schoeller DA: Polyunsaturated:saturated ratio of diet fat influences energy substrate utilization in the human. Metabolism 1988;37(2):145.

196. Jones PJ, et al: Influence of dietary fat polyunsaturated to saturated ratio on energy substrate utilization in obesity. Metabolism 1992;41(4):396.

197. Carpentier YA, Thonnart N: Lipids in clinical nutrition. In Horisberger M, Bracco U (eds): Lipids in Modern Nutrition, Vol 13. New York, Raven Press, 1987, p 147.

198. Sarda P, et al: Storage of medium-chain triglycerides in adipose tissue of orally fed infants. Am J Clin Nutr 1987;45(2):399.

199. Winick M, Morgan BLG: Nutrition and brain development. In Walker WA, Watkins JB (eds): Nutrition in Pediatrics: Basic Science and Clinical Application. Boston, Little, Brown and Co, 1985, p 233.

200. Neuringer M, Connor WE: n-3 fatty acids in the brain and retina: evidence for their essentiality. Nutr Rev 1986;44(9):285.

201. McIlwain H, Bachelard HS: Cerebral lipids. In McIlwain H, Bachelard HS (eds): Biochemistry and the Central Nervous System. New York, Churchill Livingstone, 1985, p 282.

202. Tinoco J: Dietary requirements and functions of alpha-linolenic acid in animals. Prog Lipid Res 1982;21(1):1.

203. Fliesler SJ, Anderson RE: Chemistry and metabolism of lipids in the vertebrate retina. Prog Lipid Res 1983;22(2):79.

204. Suh M, et al: Dietary 20:4n-6 and 22:6n-3 modulates the profile of long- and very-long-chain fatty acids, rhodopsin content, and kinetics in developing photoreceptor cells. Pediatr Res 2000;48(4):524.

205. Litman BJ, et al: The role of docosahexaenoic acid containing phospholipids in modulating G protein-coupled signaling pathways: visual transduction. J Mol Neurosci 2001;16(2-3):237.

206. Neuringer M: Infant vision and retinal function in studies of dietary long-chain polyunsaturated fatty acids: methods, results, and implications. Am J Clin Nutr 2000;71(1 Suppl):256S.

207. Uauy RD, et al: Effect of dietary omega-3 fatty acids on retinal function of very-low-birth-weight neonates. Pediatr Res 1990;28(5):485.

208. Makrides M, et al: Erythrocyte docosahexaenoic acid correlates with the visual response of healthy, term infants. Pediatr Res 1993;33(4 Pt 1):425.

209. Innis SM, et al: Development of visual acuity in relation to plasma and erythrocyte omega-6 and omega-3 fatty acids in healthy term gestation infants. Am J Clin Nutr 1994;60(3):347.

210. Carlson SE, et al: Visual-acuity development in healthy preterm infants: effect of marine-oil supplementation. Am J Clin Nutr 1993;58(1):35.

211. Neuringer M, et al: The role of n-3 fatty acids in visual and cognitive development: current evidence and methods of assessment. J Pediatr 1994;125 (5 Pt 2):S39.

212. Ogra PL, Greene HL: Human milk and breast feeding: an update on the state of the art. Pediatr Res 1982;16(4 Pt 1):266.

213. Heim T: How to meet the lipid requirements of the premature infant. Pediatr Clin North Am 1985;32(2):289.

214. American Academy of Pediatrics. Committee on Nutrition. In Barness LA (ed): Pediatric Nutrition Handbook, 3rd ed. Elk Grove Village, IL, American Academy of Pediatrics, 1993, p 360.

215. Innis S: Fat. In Tsang RC (ed): Nutritional Needs of the Preterm Infant: Scientific Basis and Practical Guidelines. Baltimore, Williams & Wilkins, 1993, p 65.

216. Clandinin MT, Chappell JE, et al: Fatty acid utilization in perinatal de novo synthesis of tissues. Early Hum Dev 1981;5(4):355.

217. Coleman RA: Placental metabolism and transport of lipid. Fed Proc 1986;45(10):2519.

218. Clandinin MT, et al: Fatty acid accretion in fetal and neonatal liver: implications for fatty acid requirements. Early Hum Dev 1981;5(1):7.

219. Liu CC, et al: Increase in plasma phospholipid docosahexaenoic and eicosapentaenoic acids as a reflection of their intake and mode of administration. Pediatr Res 1987;22(3):292.

220. Arbuckle LD, et al: Response of (n-3) and (n-6) fatty acids in piglet brain, liver, and plasma to increasing, but low, fish oil supplementation of formula. J Nutr 1991;121(10):1536.

221. Carlson SE, et al: Effect of fish oil supplementation on the n-3 fatty acid content of red blood cell membranes in preterm infants. Pediatr Res 1987;21(5):507.

222. Carlson SE, et al: Long-term feeding of formulas high in linolenic acid and marine oil to very low birth weight infants: phospholipid fatty acids. Pediatr Res 1991;30(5):404.

223. Van Aerde JE, Clandinin MT: Controversy in fatty acid balance. Can J Physiol Pharmacol 1993;71(9):707.

224. Foote KD, et al: Brain synaptosomal, liver, plasma, and red blood cell lipids in piglets fed exclusively on a vegetable-oil-containing formula with and without fish-oil supplements. Am J Clin Nutr 1990;51(6):1001.

225. Carlson SE, et al: First year growth of preterm infants fed standard compared to marine oil n-3 supplemented formula. Lipids 1992;27(11):901.

226. Carlson SE, et al: Arachidonic acid status correlates with first year growth in preterm infants. Proc Natl Acad Sci USA 1993;90(3):1073.

227. Hargreaves K, Clandinin MT: Dietary lipids in relation to postnatal development of the brain. Ups J Med Sci 1990;48(Suppl):79.

228. Aggett PJ, et al: Comment on the content and composition of lipids in infant formulas: ESPGAN Committee on Nutrition. Acta Paediatr Scand 1991;80(8-9):887.

229. Health and Welfare Canada, Health Protection Branch: Guidelines: Formulas for Low Birthweight Infants. Ottawa, Government of Canada, 1995.

230. Koletzko B, et al: Effects of dietary long-chain polyunsaturated fatty acids on the essential fatty acid status of premature infants. Eur J Pediatr 1989;148(7):669.

231. Koletzko B, et al: Long chain polyunsaturated fatty acids (LC-PUFA) and perinatal development. Acta Paediatr 2001;90(4):460.

232. Calder PC: Dietary fatty acids and the immune system. Lipids 1999;34(Suppl):S137.

233. Wallace FA, et al: Dietary fatty acids influence the production of Th1- but not Th2-type cytokines. J Leukoc Biol 2001;69(3):449.

234. Wallace FA, et al: Dietary fat influences the production of Th1- but not Th2-derived cytokines. Lipids 1999;34(Suppl):S141.

235. Field CJ, et al: Lower proportion of CD45R0+ cells and deficient interleukin-10 production by formula-fed infants, compared with human-fed, is corrected with supplementation of long-chain polyunsaturated fatty acids. J Pediatr Gastroenterol Nutr 2000;31(3):291.

236. Field CJ, et al: Polyunsaturated fatty acids and T-cell function: implications for the neonate. Lipids 2001;36(9):1025.

237. Garg ML, et al: Intestinal microsomes: polyunsaturated fatty acid metabolism and regulation of enterocyte transport properties. Can J Physiol Pharmacol 1990;68(5):636.
238. Garg ML, et al: Dietary cholesterol and/or n-3 fatty acid modulate delta 9-desaturase activity in rat liver microsomes. Biochim Biophys Acta 1988;962(3):330.
239. Grosser J, et al: Function of hepatic triglyceride lipase in lipoprotein metabolism. J Lipid Res 1981;22(3):437.
240. Haumont D, et al: Plasma lipid and plasma lipoprotein concentrations in low birth weight infants given parenteral nutrition with twenty or ten percent lipid emulsion. J Pediatr 1989;115(5 Pt 1):787.
241. Haumont D, et al: Effect of liposomal content of lipid emulsions on plasma lipid concentrations in low birth weight infants receiving parenteral nutrition. J Pediatr 1992;121(5 Pt 1):759.
242. Friedman Z, et al: Rapid onset of essential fatty acid deficiency in the newborn. Pediatrics 1976;58(5):640.
243. Andersen DW, et al: Intravenous lipid emulsions in the treatment of essential fatty acid deficiency: studies in young pigs. Pediatr Res 1984;18(12):1350.
244. Innis SM: Effect of total parenteral nutrition with linoleic acid-rich emulsions on tissue omega 6 and omega 3 fatty acids in the rat. Lipids 1986;21(2):132.
245. Innis SM: Essential fatty acids in growth and development. Prog Lipid Res 1991;30(1):39.
246. Foote KD, et al: Effect of early introduction of formula vs fat-free parenteral nutrition on essential fatty acid status of preterm infants. Am J Clin Nutr 1991;54(1):93.
247. Cooke RJ, et al: Soybean oil emulsion administration during parenteral nutrition in the preterm infant: effect on essential fatty acid, lipid, and glucose metabolism. J Pediatr 1987;111(5):767.
248. Putet G: Energy intake and substrate utilization during total parenteral nutrition in newborn. In Westdorp R, Soeters P (eds): Clinical Nutrition 81. Edinburgh, Blackwell, 1982, p 63.
249. Van Aerde J: Glucose and fat requirements in the intravenously fed neonate. In Stern L, et al (eds): Physiologic Foundations of Perinatal Care. Amsterdam, Elsevier, 1989, p 60.
250. Van Aerde JE, et al: Effect of replacing glucose with lipid on the energy metabolism of newborn infants. Clin Sci (Lond) 1989;76(6):581.
251. Van Aerde J: Intravenous energy support and macronutrient utilization in the neonate. Thesis, Acta Biomedica Lovaniensia 22, 1990, Catholic University of Leuven, Leuven, Belgium.
252. Van Aerde JE, et al: Metabolic consequences of increasing energy intake by adding lipid to parenteral nutrition in full-term infants. Am J Clin Nutr 1994;59(3):659.
253. Dalhan W, et al: Effects of essential fatty acid contents of lipid emulsions on erythrocyte polyunsaturated fatty acid composition on long-term parenteral nutrition. Clin Nutr 1992;11:262.
254. Rubin M, et al: Structured triacylglycerol emulsion, containing both medium- and long-chain fatty acids, in long-term home parenteral nutrition: a double-blind randomized cross-over study. Nutrition 2000;16(2):95.
255. Uauy-Dagach R, Mena P: Nutritional role of omega-3 fatty acids during the perinatal period. Clin Perinatol 1995;22(1):157.
256. Duerksen DR, et al: Total parenteral nutrition impairs bile flow and alters bile composition in newborn piglet. Dig Dis Sci 1996;41(9):1864.
257. Duerksen DR, et al: An omega-3 fatty acid-enriched lipid emulsion normalizes bile flow in newborn piglet model of TPN cholestasis. Gastroenterology 1994;106:A1023.
258. Duerksen DR, et al: Intravenous lipid emulsions with fatty acid compositions similar to milk reduce incidence of neonatal cholestasis induced by total parenteral nutrition. Gastroenterology 1993;104:A1036.
259. Vidyajagar D: Nutritional problems in neonatal intensive care units. In Stern L (ed): Feeding the Sick Infant, Vol 11, 3rd ed. New York, Raven Press, 1987, p 153.
260. Beale EF, et al: Intrahepatic cholestasis associated with parenteral nutrition in premature infants. Pediatrics 1979;64(3):342.
261. Martinez M, Ballabriga A: Effects of parenteral nutrition with high doses of linoleate on the developing human liver and brain. Lipids 1987;22(3):133.
262. Van Aerde JE, et al: Intravenous fish oil emulsion attenuates total parenteral nutrition-induced cholestasis in newborn piglets. Pediatr Res 1999;45(2):202.
263. Lipsky CL, Spear ML: Recent advances in parenteral nutrition. Clin Perinatol 1995;22(1):141.
264. Borum PR: Carnitine. Annu Rev Nutr 1983;3:233.
265. Penn D, et al: Carnitine concentrations in the milk of different species and infant formulas. Biol Neonate 1987;52(2):70.
266. Sulkers EJ, et al: Effects of high carnitine supplementation on substrate utilization in low-birth-weight infants receiving total parenteral nutrition. Am J Clin Nutr 1990;52(5):889.

41

Jan Nedergaard and Barbara Cannon

Brown Adipose Tissue: Development and Function

Mammals such as ourselves are exposed to their greatest temperature-related shock at birth. Coming from a protected and thermoneutral environment, we are suddenly exposed to "cool" surroundings, where to survive we must depend on our own ability to produce sufficient heat to keep warm.

The development of the ability to regulate our body temperature regardless of the temperature of the surroundings (and through this to ensure that our activity as an organism is constant and high) was apparently a necessary step in the evolution of so-called higher animals. A requirement for this development was that newborns be given a physiologic ability to produce the heat essential for survival. To accomplish this, an organ was developed without parallel in cold-blooded animals, an organ endowed with the function of producing heat exactly when required, especially around the time of birth. This organ is brown adipose tissue.

Thus, in evolutionary terms, brown adipose tissue is rather a "new" organ. Even scientifically, brown adipose tissue is a new tissue. Only 40 years ago, the function of the organ as a heat producer in the cold[1] and in newborns[2, 3] was first described. However, during subsequent years, understanding has grown about the events responsible for the heat production in that tissue, and at present researchers are actively elucidating mechanisms underlying the recruitment processes in brown adipose tissue (i.e., those processes that, during perinatal development, are responsible for the growth and differentiation of the tissue).

One of the most important accomplishments in research on brown adipose tissue thermogenesis has been the realization that the ability to produce heat resides in the fact that brown adipose tissue mitochondria are endowed with a unique protein, the original uncoupling protein thermogenin, abbreviated UCP1 in the following text. This protein functions as a regulated protonophore through the mitochondrial membrane. The identification of this protein has in many ways consolidated brown adipose tissue research, and it is understandable that a description of the function and fate of this protein must be a central issue in a review on the perinatal recruitment of brown adipose tissue.

HUMAN INFANTS AND OTHER NEWBORNS

The experiments describing the function of brown adipose tissue in the perinatal animal have generally been performed in rat fetuses and rat pups, and if not specifically stated, the animal referred to here is the rat.

There are, however, significant differences between the perinatal development of brown fat (and many other characteristics) in the newborn of different species. Broadly speaking, three different groups of newborns can be distinguished: altricial newborns, so-called true immature newborns, and precocial newborns.[11]

The *altricial* (literally, nest-dependent) newborns are often whelped as members of litters of more than five pups. They are poorly developed at birth, have no fur, are blind, and move poorly if at all. To keep warm, they huddle together. As discussed later in this chapter, development of brown adipose tissue in these newborns is a slow process that starts just before birth and reaches its maximum some days after birth. The main driving force for this recruitment is probably the (comparatively) low environmental temperature and the attempts by these newborns to activate processes to oppose hypothermia. Rat and mouse pups belong to this group. The morphologic and ultrastructural development of the tissue in these animals has been described in several papers.[16-21]

The *immatures* (not to be confused with prematures) are not able to respond to the environmental temperature at birth and are truly poikilothermic. The recruitment process in brown adipose tissue starts only when their central control systems have developed, after which processes occur that seem similar to those elicited immediately after birth in the altricial newborns. Hamster pups,[22] and possibly the newborns of marsupials,[23, 24] belong to this group. (It is, however, still unclear whether marsupials at any stage of development have brown adipose tissue.)

The *precocial* newborns are normally born singly or in small litters. They are very well developed, their eyes are open, they are furred, and they can walk around shortly after birth. These newborns are born with well-developed brown adipose tissue, which tends to atrophy postnatally. It is unknown how this uterine recruitment of brown adipose tissue is accomplished. Certain small newborns, such as the guinea pig,[25] belong to this group, but more obvious members are the newborns of many larger species, such as lambs,[26, 27] goats,[28] calves,[29] and muskoxen.[30]

The classification of the human infant (or other primate infants[31]) into one or the other of these groups is not self-evident. Although born in a somewhat developed state, the human infant has several traits of immaturity and is probably most akin to the altricial newborns (i.e., human perinatal brown adipose tissue development has similarities to that found in the newborn rat pup).

HOW MANY ADIPOSE TISSUES EXIST?

Experiments concerning the function of most body organs are helped from a practical viewpoint by the fact that most organs are anatomically well-defined entities with a single localization in the body and with structurally homogeneous and stable cells. Unfortunately, such characteristics do not pertain to brown adipose tissue.

Brown adipose tissue is found in many depots within the body; six major depots have been identified in the human infant and constitute 90% of the total brown fat. These include the perirenal depots, interscapular and cervical depots, and periaortic depots. The remaining 10% is found in seven other sites.[32, 33]

The distinction between white and brown fat is not straightforward. When activated, brown adipose tissue can be distinguished from white by its ability to express UCP1. However, as the potential ability to express UCP1 in a given cell (in a given physiologic situation) may not have been invoked at the moment of study, it is likely that each anatomically defined depot contains cells that are genuinely "white," as well as cells that are only disguised as white but that still carry the potential to be brown. Leptin is well expressed in white adipose tissue, but it is not expressed in recruited (i.e., activated) brown adipose tissue.[34] It is, however, expressed in nonactive brown adipose tissue and its expression in both adipose tissues is inhibited by sympathetic stimulation.[35]

Morphologically, even epididymal white adipose tissue can be altered by an intense cold stress to visually resemble brown adipose tissue and to have brown fatlike mitochondria.[36, 37] However, not even under these extreme circumstances has it been possible to detect UCP1 as a protein immunologically or to identify UCP1 mRNA in this tissue.[37] Thus, within this depot, there are apparently only truly white fat cells. Surprisingly, in the parallel female tissue, the parametrial fat pad, there is good evidence for the presence of genuine brown fat cells (i.e., those containing UCP1).[38]

In certain species, even the subcutaneous adipose tissue (which is generally believed to have storage and insulatory properties) can be brown. Thus, based on a functional analysis of the mitochondria in the subcutaneous adipose tissue of newborn seals[39] and in dog pups treated with sympathomimetics,[40] the presence of UCP1 in subcutaneous tissue can be discerned.[41] In these species, the subcutaneous adipose tissue works not only as a blanket, but also as an "electric blanket." Thus, although certain fat depots apparently fully lack any ability to become brown fat, most depots have this potential, and UCP1 may be expressed under certain physiologic or pharmacologic circumstances.

As a general rule, it can be said that there are many more brown adipose tissue depots in the newborn than in the adult, even in comparison with the cold-acclimated adult. It has been stated that in some newborn species all adipose tissue is brown, and these depots are converted to white adipose tissue in the adult. However, the cell biologic meaning of this statement is vague, and no strict lineage relationship between brown and white adipose cells has been clarified. Certainly, the behavior of certain depots that in the adult look white is functionally in the newborn close to that of brown adipose tissue, and these depots retain some potential to again become brown.[42] This tissue does not, however, demonstrate cellular transdifferentiation.

UCP1 AND THERMOGENESIS

Heat production may result from shivering or nonshivering thermogenesis. In the newborn infant and in the adult animal, the first resource used for extra heat production is nonshivering thermogenesis. Only after this capacity is used does shivering begin. In the adult, with little active brown adipose tissue, shivering is the dominant source of extra heat production initially. In the infant, however, the ability to shiver sufficiently and intensively enough to produce substantial amounts of heat does not seem to be fully developed and therefore infants rely on brown adipose tissue for heat production.

There is no doubt that most heat produced during nonshivering thermogenesis results directly from the activity in brown adipose tissue of the unique mitochondrial UCP1 (i.e., thermogenin) and in the absence of this protein, no heat is produced in brown fat cells.[43, 44] Heat production is governed by signals from the hypothalamus. These signals are relayed through the sympathetic nervous system and transmitted to the cell as a norepinephrine stimulus leading to a series of events within the cell (for overview, see Fig. 41-1). Sympathetic innervation to the tissue is dense. One system of fibers, which contains the costored neuropeptide NPY, innervates the numerous blood vessels entering the tissue, and another system innervates the adipocytes.[45] The neuropeptides CGRP and substance P are also found in the tissue, the latter in afferent nerves; however, the localization of CGRP is currently not completely understood, and the functions of these neuropeptides are unknown.[46]

UCP1

Considerable research by several groups has led to the identification of UCP1 as the key enzyme in nonshivering heat production. UCP1, earlier referred to as thermogenin, as the

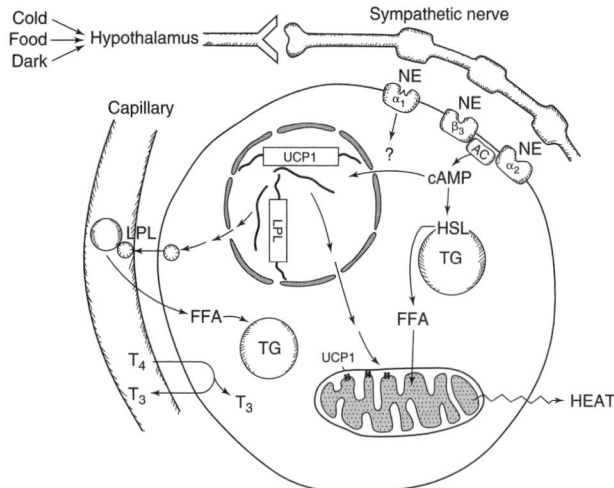

Figure 41–1. Function of the brown fat cell: an overview. When postnatal cold is perceived, the sympathetic nervous system is activated. Norepinephrine (NE) released interacts with adrenergic receptors, leading to release of fatty acids that undergo combustion in the mitochondria. This combustion is possible as a result of the presence of the uncoupling protein 1, UCP1. Further substrate is provided by the action of lipoprotein lipase. Brown adipose tissue may also produce triiodothyronine (T₃) from thyroxine (T₄), leading to local and systemic effects. Dietary factors and darkness also activate centers in the hypothalamus in a manner analogous to that of norepinephrine. AC = adenylyl cyclase; cAMP = cyclic adenosine monophosphate; LPL = lipoprotein lipase; TG = triglycerides; FFA = free fatty acids; HSL = hormone-sensitive lipase.

nucleotide-binding protein (NbP), as the 32-kDa protein of brown fat, or as the guanosine diphosphate (GDP)-binding protein has also been referred to as the proton conductance pathway of brown adipose tissue mitochondria. Much is known

today about this protein (Fig. 41–2A). It has been sequenced both as a protein and from cDNA clones corresponding to the UCP1 mRNA. The amino acid sequence is known from many species of mammals.[47-50] The amino acid sequence of the human protein is 79% homologous to that of the rat protein, thus allowing considerable immunologic cross-reactivity between human UCP1 and rodent UCP1.[51] The human UCP1 gene has also been isolated[52,53] and its organization analyzed.

UCP1 is a member of the superfamily of mitochondrial carrier proteins (see Fig. 41–2B).[54-56] Most closely related to UCP1 are two recently identified but evolutionarily more ancient proteins known as UCP2 and UCP3 because of their high homology with UCP1.[57] The functions of these proteins remain unclear. They are, however, not responsible for any thermoregulatory thermogenesis.[44] Other proteins (e.g., UCP4 and UCP5) are not closely related to UCP1 and therefore functional relationships cannot be expected.

From analysis of the amino acid sequence, it has been proposed that UCP1 may constitute three membrane-spanning "U"s as shown in Figure 41–2A. When functionally inserted into the brown fat mitochondrial inner membrane, UCP1 endows these mitochondria with a series of unique properties, including a high rate of respiration in the absence of adenosine diphosphate (ADP) or uncoupler addition, a high proton conductivity, and a high Cl⁻ conductivity.

THE UCP GENE

The UCP1 gene is found on chromosome 8 in mice[58] and on chromosome 4 in humans.[59] There is only one copy of the gene.[52]

There is an interesting functional and evolutionary connection between the exon/intron pattern of the UCP1 gene and the suggested transmembrane structure of the protein, in that each of the six proposed membrane-spanning segments is represented by one exon.[50,59,60] This pattern is also found in the other UCP genes.

ACUTE REGULATION OF UCP1 ACTIVITY

The function of UCP1 in the mitochondrial membrane is depicted in simplified form in Figure 41–3. UCP1 acts as the equivalent of a

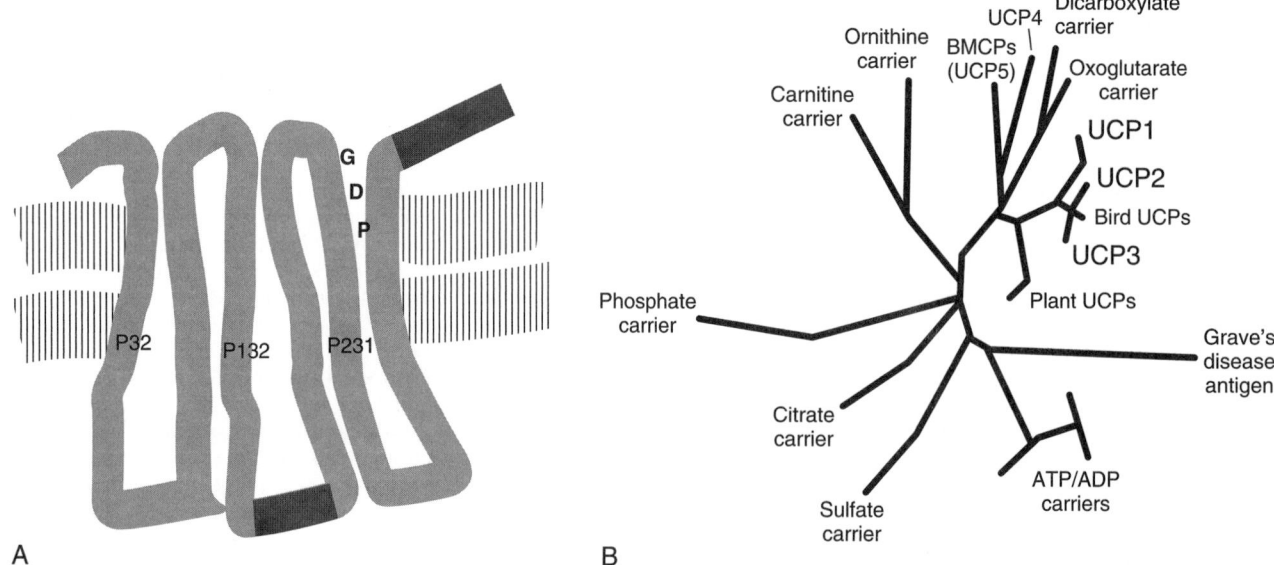

Figure 41–2. A, Suggested structure of the uncoupling protein 1 (UCP1). The tripartite transmembrane structure is common to members of the mitochondrial carrier protein superfamily. P32, P132, and P231 indicate proline residues conserved between all family members, and GDP the general area in which nucleotide binding occurs. **B**, Rootless dendrogram showing similarity between members of the mitochondrial carrier protein superfamily. ATP = adenosine triphosphate; ADP = adenosine diphosphate. (**A**, Adapted and simplified from Nedergaard et al;[8] **B**, from Borecky et al.[204])

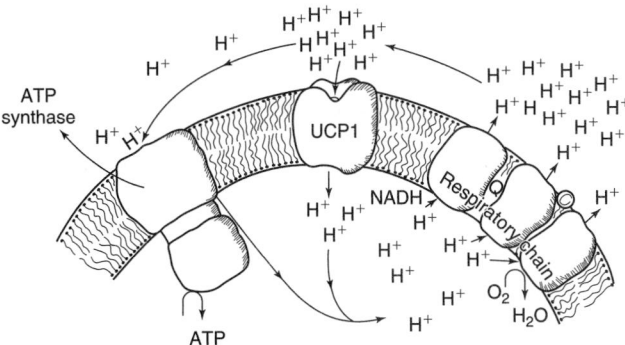

Figure 41–3. Suggested function of the uncoupling protein 1, UCP1, in the brown fat cell. UCP1 functions as a regulated translocator of protons (or proton equivalents) through the mitochondrial membrane, thereby allowing dissipation of the proton gradient built up by the respiratory chain, as a consequence of the oxidation of substrate, e.g., nicotinamide adenine dinucleotide (NADH). Thus, respiration can proceed unlimited by the turnover of adenosine triphosphate (ATP).[205]

proton translocator, allowing dissipation of the proton gradient that has arisen from the functioning of the respiratory chain.

UCP1 cannot be constantly active, because this would lead to a constant high heat production in the tissue, irrespective of the environmental (or ambient) temperature. In experiments with isolated mitochondria, it has been observed that the activity of UCP1 can be inhibited by the addition of purine nucleotides.[61, 62] Traditionally, GDP has been the nucleotide of choice for such experiments, and thus, UCP1 has been known as the GDP-binding protein. (The protein is not related to the G-proteins in signal transduction, nor to the ribosomal GTP-binding proteins, and the term may be considered to be physiologically misleading, because ATP is as good as or better than GDP both for binding and in inhibiting respiration.[63, 64]) Because ATP is present in much higher concentrations in the cytosol of brown fat cells than is GDP,[65] ATP is the physiologically relevant nucleotide that binds to UCP1 and inhibits thermogenesis when thermogenesis is not physiologically required.

The affinity of UCP1 for ATP is so high that the binding site would probably always be saturated with ATP and thermogenesis inhibited if this were the only agent that interacted with UCP1. Thus, it is necessary to postulate the existence of a physiologic activator of UCP1.[62] A long and still ongoing discussion has been conducted concerning the nature of this "positive" modulator. It is outside the scope of this review to analyze the problem in detail, but a few main points can be summarized here.

Although there have been many suggestions, the most simple hypothesis for the nature of this modulator is that it is produced during the release of fatty acids, occurring as an effect of stimulation of the cell. Within this frame, several alternatives have been proposed. The positive modulator could be the free fatty acids themselves.[62, 66, 67] The most telling experiments that indicate a direct effect of free fatty acids are those of Rial and colleagues.[68] Alternatively, the fatty acids have been suggested to have a catalytic function, although in this case a positive modulator may be involved.[69, 70] Another hypothesis along the same line suggested that palmitoyl-CoA could interact directly with UCP1.[71, 72] Each position has advantages and problems. Although conclusive experiments have been published that the modulator is downstream of lipolysis, general agreement on the mechanism has not yet been reached.

POSSIBLE SEMI-ACUTE REGULATION OF UCP1 ACTIVITY

Under certain conditions, there is apparently no direct correlation between the amount of UCP1 (e.g., as measured immunologi-

cally) and the activity of UCP1 (as estimated by GDP binding or proton or Cl⁻ translocation). When the level of activity is found to be lower than expected, the phenomenon has been termed *masking* of UCP1.[73] UCP1 is thus typically masked when it is inactive (as is probably the case *in utero*) but becomes *unmasked* when called into function. Thus, one can speculate that the rapid increase in GDP-binding capacity seen shortly after birth in guinea pigs[25] may be due to this unmasking mechanism.[74]

ADAPTIVE REGULATION OF UCP1 AMOUNT

The total amount of UCP1 in the newborn is expected to be the rate-limiting factor for nonshivering thermogenesis. In newborns and adults, the amount of UCP1 is under precise regulation. Although there is a significant temporal delay between a change in UCP1 mRNA and the ensuing increase in amount of UCP1,[75] the simplest explanation is that the mRNA level determines the protein level.

Receptors Involved

The major stimulus for UCP1 gene expression is from the sympathetic nervous system via the release of norepinephrine. There is no doubt that β-adrenergic receptors are involved in this regulation.[76-78] Further, there are some indications that simultaneous α-stimulation is necessary.[77] Perhaps this α-stimulation is of a permissive nature.

Perinatal UCP1 Expression

Altricial Species

The amount of UCP1 increases around the time of birth (in mice and rats).[21, 79] This is caused by an attendant increase in the amount of UCP1 mRNA (Fig. 41–4A, B).[78, 80, 81] The cause of the postnatal recruitment in brown adipose tissue (and increase in UCP1 mRNA) could be either ontogenic or an effect of the cold stress experienced by the pups at birth.[11] There is no postnatal increase in UCP1 mRNA in the absence of a postnatal cold stress (see Fig. 41–4C); therefore, it may be concluded that in these species, the postnatal brown adipose tissue recruitment is a response to the cold stress experienced by the newborn.[81] This indicates that the increase is mediated by sympathetic activation as in adults.

Immature Newborn Species

In these newborns, the increase in UCP1 occurs rather late.[22, 23] It is conjectured that when the ability to react to environmental cues has developed in these animals, the recruitment of brown adipose tissue takes place in the same way as already described for altricial species.

Precocial Newborn Species

In the precocial newborn, UCP1 is expressed in the fetal state.[25, 29, 82] Because it would be ineffective for the fetus to produce excessive heat, one must also postulate the existence of a uterine inhibitor of thermogenesis, which still allows transmission of the signal for gene expression to occur but inhibits a thermogenic response. If it were not for such an inhibitor, the activation signal might trigger fetal heat production *in utero*. In experiments in which the umbilical cord has been sectioned, some indications for the existence of such an inhibitor have been observed.[83-86]

The central signal that leads to sympathetic stimulation of the tissue *in utero* is unknown. It cannot be a cold stimulus and could hardly be a food stimulus. The only other documented pathway for sympathetic stimulation of brown-fat recruitment is through short day length,[87] probably mediated through the pineal gland and melatonin. It could be argued that the fetus lives its life in darkness, and thus newborns are more sensitive to the

UCP1 mRNA

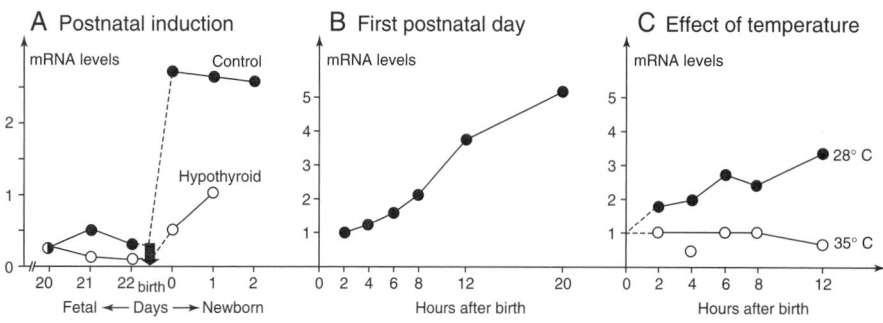

Figure 41–4. Postnatal increase in UCP1 mRNA. **A,** Prenatal to postnatal transition; note the effect of hypothyroidism. **B,** Time resolution of the first postnatal day: pups remaining with their dams. **C,** Effect of temperature on the postnatal increase in UCP1 mRNA. Pups were exposed singly to the indicated environmental temperatures. (**A, B,** and **C** adapted from Obregon et al.[81])

day's elapsed length.[88] Whether such a mechanism could function in precocial species is doubtful, and most available data indicate that it is merely the dam's level of melatonin that is reflected in the fetal blood level. Alternatively, another mechanism of recruitment, independent of sympathetic stimulation, must be postulated.

The Human Newborn

Because the classification of the human newborn as precocial or altricial is not fully clear, it is not evident which animal neonate is the best experimental model to make determinations that may be considered applicable to the human infant. Human brown adipose tissue is present in considerable quantities at term gestation but also demonstrates a postnatal increase.[89] The amount of UCP1 is high in children, and it can even be found in adults.[90-93]

SUBSTRATES FOR THERMOGENESIS

Intracellularly Derived Fatty Acids

During the initial acute phase of thermogenesis, the supply of fatty acids for combustion comes from triglyceride droplets found within the tissue. The release of fatty acids for combustion is caused by a series of events similar to those found in white fat cells, leading to a release of fatty acids in the circulation. Thus, stimulation of β-receptors leads to an increase in intracellular levels of cyclic adenosine monophosphate (cAMP),[94] which in turn leads to activation of the cAMP-dependent protein kinase (see Fig. 41–1). Both these events can be observed during postnatal development: cAMP is elevated in brown adipose tissue,[95,96] and there is an increase in the activity ratio of cAMP-dependent protein kinase, from 0.3 in fetal tissue to 0.7 after birth.[97]

Different Adrenergic Receptors

A β-receptor is the adrenergic receptor type involved in the increase in cAMP in fully differentiated brown adipocytes. In rodents, it is the β3-receptor that is predominantly involved, but the situation in human brown fat is less clearly understood.[98-103] The effects of β-receptor activation on cAMP levels may be counteracted by α2-adrenergic receptors, which are also found in brown adipose tissue of fetuses and newborns.[104-106] Adenosine receptors may also counteract β-stimulation.[107]

Brown fat cells are also endowed with α1-adrenergic receptors.[108] Although some of their intracellular actions are known,[109-111] their significance for thermogenesis is not fully understood. During *in vitro* experiments, only a small fraction of thermogenesis resulting from adrenergic stimulation can be demonstrated to result from stimulation of α1-adrenergic processes. Nonetheless, a large fraction of nonshivering thermogenesis can be inhibited *in vivo* by α1-blockade[112] in the newborn rabbit. This may be secondary to cardiovascular phe-

nomena. In isolated cells, α1-adrenergic stimulation may enhance the effectiveness of cAMP.[113]

Protein Kinase and Hormone-Sensitive Lipase

One substrate for the activated cAMP-dependent protein kinase is the hormone-sensitive lipase found in brown adipose tissue.[114] Activation of this lipase leads to the breakdown of triglycerides already stored in brown fat. The fatty acids released are probably immediately combusted in the mitochondria, whereas glycerol is probably released to the circulation. The decrease in triglyceride droplet size after birth can be seen on electron micrographs.[18]

Whether there is a physiologically significant release of fatty acids from brown adipose tissue into the circulation is still unconfirmed. It was originally suggested that brown fat (unlike white fat) did not release any fatty acids to the circulation,[115] but isolated brown fat cells break down more triglycerides to fatty acids than can be subject to combustion within the cells and release fatty acids *in vitro*.[116] Investigations of the effluent blood from brown adipose tissue have yielded somewhat varying results,[117,118] but it would seem that there is a potential capacity for export.

It is also unknown whether increases in plasma levels of fatty acids observed in cold-stressed animals may be due to an increased release from brown fat and thus reflect the activity of this tissue. Tissue ablation experiments have indicated that this may be the case,[119] especially in newborns in whom a large fraction of the adipose tissue found is in the form of brown adipose tissue.

Fatty Acids from the Circulation

The brown fat cell is endowed with a store of triglycerides that can be used in any situation in which thermogenesis is required. However, this store is found in limited amounts, and in unfed newborn rabbits, the store is sufficient for only 3 days of heat production. After this time, the rabbits die as a result of hypothermia.[120] Similar observations can be made in premature human infants.[121] To ensure a constant supply of substrate for combustion, additional substrate must be supplied by the circulation. Only under conditions of starvation before cold stress has it been reported that the uptake of circulating free fatty acids is significant.[122] The most important source of lipid substrate quantitatively is that found in chylomicrons, which are formed from ingested food. Fatty acids in chylomicron triglycerides are released to the brown fat cells by the enzyme lipoprotein lipase.

Regulation of Lipoprotein Lipase

In contrast to the situation in white adipose tissue, brown adipose tissue lipoprotein lipase activity is increased by adrenergic stimulation.[123,124] (In this respect, the tissue is similar to that of the heart.) This stimulation is mediated by β-adrenergic receptors, resulting in an increase in cAMP and an ensuing increase in the expression of the gene for lipoprotein lipase.[124-127] This is a comparatively slow process, requiring several hours to reach full effect, because the lipase must be synthesized and transported to the capillaries. Thus, the tissue cannot rely on this process to generate an acute thermogenic response.

Insulin can also stimulate lipoprotein lipase activity.[128-130] This insulin stimulation does not seem to be mediated through central effects and the sympathetic nervous system; instead it seems to be a direct effect of insulin on tissue in states of proper nutrition. Insulin stimulation is also mediated through an increased expression of the lipoprotein lipase gene.[126,127]

Perinatal Recruitment of Lipoprotein Lipase

Lipoprotein lipase activity is low in the fetus but it increases postnatally (Fig. 41-5*A*).[131] This postnatal increase can also be seen in premature pups. It is not known whether this increase in lipoprotein lipase activity after birth is an effect of suckling, temperature, or release of an inhibitor transferred through the umbilical cord.

When this "birth-induced" increase in activity is compared with measurements of lipoprotein lipase mRNA, an enigma arises, however (see Fig. 41-5*B*): lipoprotein lipase mRNA is not increased (possibly due to an inhibitory factor in the colostrum).[132] To explain the discrepancy between lipoprotein lipase mRNA level and lipoprotein lipase activity, it has been suggested that there may be a transfer of lipoprotein lipase across gut membranes.[81] This hypothesis requires further investigation. Under conditions of mild cold stress in the absence of the dam, however, lipoprotein lipase mRNA level within brown adipose tissue increases, apparently through processes similar to those described in the adult (see Fig. 41-5*C*).

One effect of this postnatal activation of lipoprotein lipase on the fatty acid composition of tissue triglycerides is that fatty acids become more unsaturated and in this respect reflect the composition of the diet (i.e., the mother's milk).[133-135]

Pathology

No pathologic state that involves activity of lipoprotein lipase in human brown adipose tissue is known, but there is a genetic disease in mice—combined lipase deficiency (cld)—which leads to the synthesis of an inefficient lipoprotein lipase.[136] The absence of lipoprotein lipase activity has the expected effect of reducing the amount of fat droplets in brown adipose tissue.[137]

Glucose

There is uptake of glucose in brown adipose tissue in the newborn rabbit.[122] Based on *in vitro* experiments, it may be envisaged that this uptake of glucose may increase the catabolic capacity of the citric acid cycle through the action of pyruvate carboxylase.[138] Brown adipose tissue shows insulin-sensitive glucose transport through redistribution of the GLUT-4 glucose transporter from intracellular vesicles to the plasma membrane.[139] Glucose uptake in brown adipose tissue is markedly stimulated by cold exposure; this occurs through norepinephrine stimulation rather than through insulin. Although it apparently does not alter GLUT-4 distribution, norepinephrine may increase either GLUT1 or GLUT-4 activity and thus glucose uptake rates.[140,141]

Fatty Acid Synthesis

The significance of lipogenesis in brown adipose tissue has been discussed. The capacity for lipogenesis in brown adipose tissue is high.[142,143] Lipogenesis has also been observed in human infants.[144] However, strong evidence suggests this lipogenesis is not of quantitative or qualitative significance for thermogenesis. Rather, it could be considered a refilling reaction that occurs in tissue after cessation of the thermogenic stimulus. Thus, during the perinatal period, the activity of lipogenesis is low when ther-

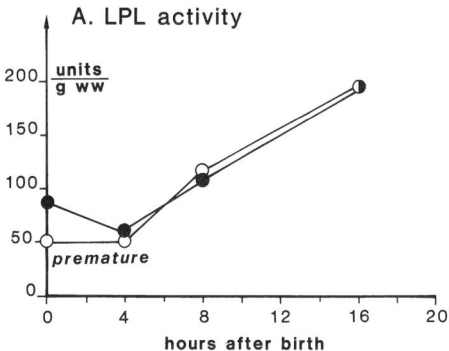

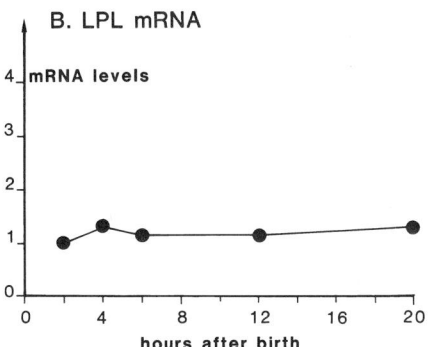

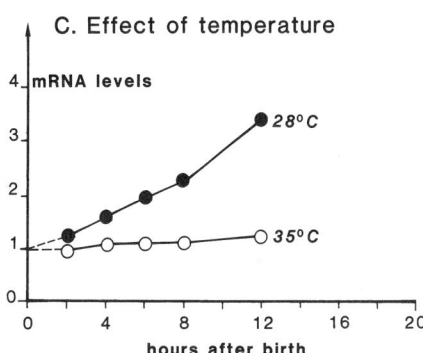

Figure 41–5. Lipoprotein lipase (LPL) activity and gene expression. **A,** Lipoprotein lipase activity in newborns staying with their dams. **B,** Lipoprotein lipase mRNA levels in newborns staying with their dams. **C,** Lipoprotein lipase mRNA levels in single pups exposed to the indicated environmental temperatures. (**A,** Adapted from Cryer et al;[131] **B** and **C** adapted from Obregon et al.[81])

mogenesis is high. This is probably due to the effect of suckling (i.e., a change from a carbohydrate "diet" in the fetal state to a high-lipid diet). There may also be a direct inhibitory effect of increased sympathetic stimulation on lipogenesis.[11] Weaning, which reintroduces a high-carbohydrate diet but also coincides with a reduced demand for thermogenesis, is associated with an increase in lipogenesis.

The so-called lipogenic enzymes (in addition to the fatty acid synthase complex) include pyruvate dehydrogenase, the citrate cleavage enzyme (ATP-citrate lyase), acetyl-CoA carboxylase, glucose-6-phosphate dehydrogenase, 6-phosphogluconate dehydrogenase, and malic enzymes. All these enzymes generally follow the same perinatal pattern. They are high in the fetal state, much reduced during suckling, and return toward high fetal values as suckling ends.[11] For malic enzyme, it has been demonstrated that this is due to a change in the amount of enzyme (not a change in activity of existing enzyme).[145]

The activities of the glycolytic enzymes increase after weaning,[146] indicating that during the time when milk comprises the diet, it is those fatty acids that supply brown adipose tissue and are spent in combustion. Only after weaning to a diet rich in carbohydrates does glycolysis contribute to fatty acid synthesis.

Amino Acid Uptake

The possibility that amino acid uptake occurs has been investigated. It is generally believed that this pathway is of minor importance for the functioning of brown adipose tissue.[147] Amino acid uptake could amount to about one-third of the uptake of glucose. Several amino acids have propionyl-CoA as the end product of oxidation. This 3-carbon fatty acid cannot be degraded through the normal β-oxidation pathway for fatty acid derivatives, and detrimental levels of this fatty acid could accumulate, resulting in a sequestration of all mitochondrial CoA and an ensuing inhibition of thermogenesis. This may be why the mitochondria have a high activity of a propionyl-CoA hydrolase with unusual regulatory properties.[148-150] This hydrolase could also function to recover the CoA otherwise bound up in the propionyl-CoA.

5'-DEIODINASE AND THYROID

In brown adipose tissue, there is a high activity of thyroxine 5'-deiodinase, which produces the active thyroid hormone T_3 (Fig. 41-6).[122] The 5'-deiodinase found in brown adipose tissue has been classified as a type II deiodinase (distinguished from type I by its insensitivity to propylthiouracil *in vitro*[152] and by its being induced by hypothyroidism *in vivo*[153]). The gene has been cloned.[154] It is probably localized to the endoplasmic reticulum. The presence of 5'-deiodinase has been demonstrated in human, lamb, and rodent brown fat.[152,155,156]

Internal Action

It is believed that the activity of the 5'-deiodinase is important both for the normal development of brown adipose tissue and for the rapid increase in brown fat during the perinatal period. The T_3 produced probably binds to T_3 receptors found within the tissue[157,158] (see Fig. 41-6) and in this way influences expression of the UCP1 gene through binding to sequences in the promoter region.[159] Indeed, hypothyroidism leads to a decreased expression of UCP1 in both rats and lambs (see Fig. 41-4A).[80,155] However, in mice in which the nuclear thyroid hormone binding receptors are

ablated, UCP1 expression is high, confirming that the hormone is required primarily to relieve a repression, rather than to cause activation (based on findings reported by Rabelo and colleagues[160] and our unpublished observations).

Systemic Action

The possibility has also been considered that brown adipose tissue 5'-deiodinase is of systemic physiologic significance in that it could release T_3 from brown fat into the circulation.[161] Indeed, such release has been substantiated in the newborn rat.[162]

T_3 could be responsible for the small increase in basal metabolism sometimes found in conditions in which brown fat is stimulated, but no experiments have been performed in which brown fat has been removed to investigate this possibility.

In addition to T_3's metabolic effects, thyroid hormone might also have an important role in promoting differentiation. There are some interesting but as yet unconfirmed observations that removal of brown adipose tissue at a young age affects development of other bodily functions in later life. Thus, in several studies, Jankovic and colleagues have implied such a brown-adipose-tissue effect on the development of the immune response.[163-165]

Regulation of Deiodinase Activity

The activity of 5'-deiodinase is rapidly induced under conditions in which brown adipose tissue is recruited, and this increase in activity is due to an increased synthesis of the enzyme.[166,167]

Adrenergic Regulation

It was originally suggested that the increase in deiodinase activity was mediated through an α_1-adrenergic mechanism.[151] Although an α_1-stimulus is apparently necessary to produce a significant stimulation, it would seem that α- and β-adrenergic stimulation interact synergistically to induce maximal induction of 5'-deiodinase activity. From *in vitro* experiments with isolated cells, it has been suggested that this interaction occurs at the cellular level, and it apparently occurs at a post-cAMP step in the activation pathway.[168,169]

Insulin

Insulin can increase 5'-deiodinase activity when injected into animals[167] and when added to isolated brown fat cells.[170] There are no indications of the physiologic significance of this

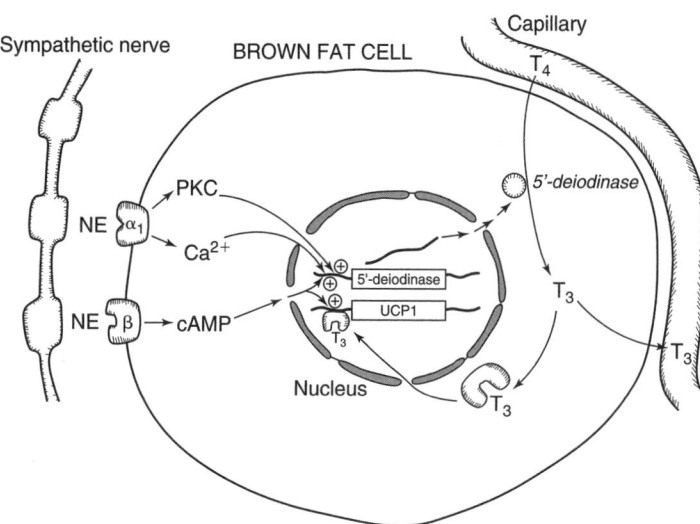

Figure 41-6. The regulation and action of 5'-deiodinase in brown adipose tissue. NE = norepinephrine; cAMP = cyclic adenosine monophosphate; PKC = protein kinase C.

phenomenon, nor of the intracellular pathways involved in the gene activation events.

Perinatal Recruitment of 5′-Deiodinase

The perinatal pattern of development of 5′-deiodinase is unusual. The deiodinase activity rises markedly before birth, after which it spontaneously declines (Fig. 41–7).[171-173] The regulation of this activity and its significance for brown fat recruitment are of interest, but no experimental evidence concerning these questions is available at present.

REGULATION OF RECRUITMENT OF THE TISSUE

The capacity of brown adipose tissue thermogenesis is limited by the amount of UCP1 in the tissue, and this level is governed by the activity of the sympathetic nervous system and norepinephrine. To increase the amount of UCP1 in the tissue, two principal strategies may be employed. In the first, the amount of UCP1 per brown adipocyte is increased. In the second, there is an increase in cell proliferation (i.e., in the number of adipocytes), but each individual adipocyte maintains an unchanged capacity. Although different species appear to use more or less of the first or second modalities, both seem to be employed in all species studied. The situation has not been studied for the human neonate.

The tissue retains a potential proliferative capacity, even in adulthood. Preadipocytes in culture can be stimulated to increase their proliferation by the addition of norepinephrine, and the stimulation is through β_1-receptors and cyclic AMP-coupled mechanisms.[174] This is in contrast to the norepinephrine stimulation of UCP1 gene expression in mature brown adipocytes, which, while also using cAMP as the intracellular messenger, couples to the adenylyl cyclase through β_3-receptors.[175]

Various transcription factors might be expected to be involved in the control of cell proliferation, and many are currently being studied. Notably, an important adipose-related factor, C/EBPα, is transiently decreased as proliferation begins.[176] Other fat-related transcription factors, such as members of the PPAR family, and the coactivator PGC1, appear also to be of importance.[177] A more comprehensive study of the roles of these transcription factors is required to understand the complex control of cell proliferation, both *in utero* and postnatally. It is evident that in the fetal state, growth factors such as insulin-like growth factor-1 (IGF-1),[178,179] are important for cell growth.

CLINICAL IMPLICATIONS

There is good reason to believe that one of the major problems with temperature regulation in small premature infants is that the lipid supply to brown adipose tissue and its recruitment are not sufficiently developed. This deficiency, combined with the larger surface:volume ratio of the small premature infant and the ensuing risk for rapid heat loss, places them at increased risk for hypothermia. Therefore, the main problem resulting from the incomplete development of brown adipose tissue in premature newborns was solved through the introduction of the incubator.[180]

Effects of Environmental Temperature

Convincing evidence exists from animal experiments that the postnatal environmental temperature has a substantial effect on brown adipose tissue development (see Figs. 41–4 and 41–5).[11] Indeed, some anecdotal evidence suggests that children who live in relatively cold environments will acquire or maintain an improved cold tolerance, probably through persistent brown adipose tissue function.

Anesthesia in Infants

During general anesthesia, body temperature regulation is disturbed, and this effect is more marked in young infants. Although there may also be effects on central mechanisms controlling body temperature, it is now apparent that the commonly used inhalation anesthetics halothane and its derivatives are potent inhibitors of brown adipose tissue thermogenesis.[181,182] This is particularly important in young infants in whom the activity of brown adipose tissue is important for body temperature regulation.

Effects of Malnutrition

The effects of prenatal or postnatal malnutrition have been investigated in experimental animals. In general, food restriction reduces the function of brown adipose tissue,[183] although

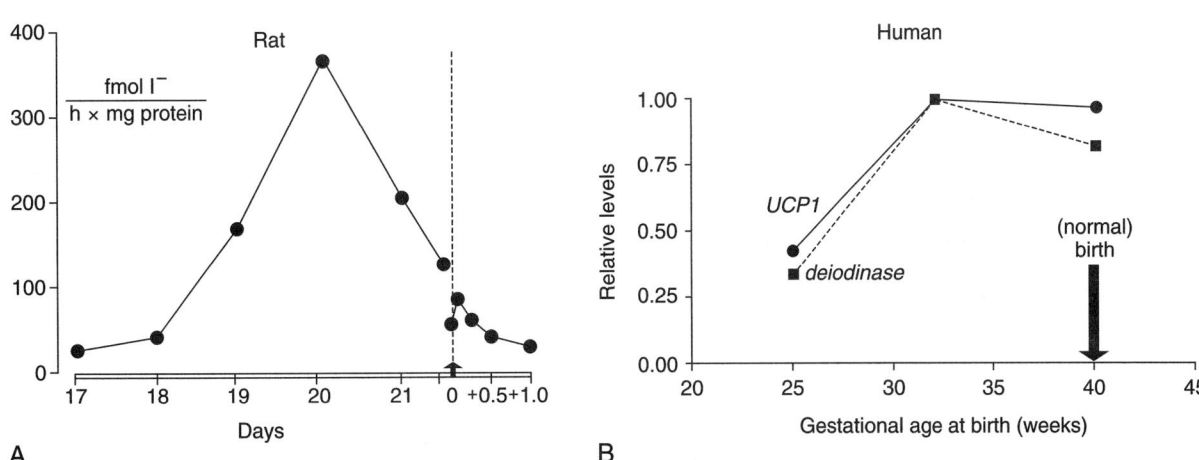

Figure 41–7. Deiodinase activity in the perinatal period. (Data based on rat studies in Giralt et al.[172] Similar data were obtained by Obregon et al.[173] Human data from Houstek et al.[206])

paradoxical observations have been reported.[184] Adverse effects of more specific dietary restrictions (e.g., riboflavin, protein) have also been reported.[185, 186] There are scattered reports in the literature implicating malnutrition as a cause of hypothermia in human newborn infants, presumably because of a lack of substrate available for thermogenesis.[187]

Overfeeding

The presentation of a palatable, so-called cafeteria diet to adult rats results in overfeeding. However, these animals do not gain weight to the extent anticipated by the extent of overfeeding. The brown adipose tissue of such animals is markedly recruited and it has been suggested that the decrease in the animals' whole body efficiency (i.e., lower weight gain than anticipated) could result from increased thermogenesis in brown adipose tissue.[188, 189] Postnatal overfeeding in rats (induced by a reduction in the number of pups per litter) also leads to an activation of brown adipose tissue.[190, 191]

It can be posited that in the human infant overfeeding may cause an activation of brown adipose tissue, leading to an increased thermogenesis that could counteract the effect of the increased food intake.

Genetically Obese Animals

In genetically obese animals (the fa/fa rat and the ob/ob and db/db mice, all of which have problems in the leptin system), the postnatal recruitment process in brown adipose tissue is blunted, before any signs of obesity become evident.[192-194] This inactivity of brown adipose tissue appears to constitute at least one cause of developing obesity. This was apparently confirmed by experiments in which brown adipocytes were molecularly ablated from mice.[53] In these experiments, transgenic animals were produced in which the UCP1-promoter region was coupled to the gene for the diphtheria toxin A chain. This A chain inhibits protein synthesis and thus kills the cells in which it is expressed (e.g., primarily brown adipocytes). The transgenic animals developed obesity and other manifestations associated with obesity, such as insulin resistance. However, mice with an ablation in the UCP1 gene, and thus possessing thermogenically incompetent brown fat, do not become manifestly obese.[195] Thus, these mice would seem competent to regulate food intake to compensate for a decreased ability to combust food substrates.

It is unclear whether some humans may be subject to the same forces as these genetically obese animals. Although it is clear that the potential to develop obesity has a strong genetic component, it is not currently known to what extent brown adipose tissue inactivity contributes to the development of obesity in children.

Diseases Affecting Brown Adipose Tissue

With fever, some heat necessary for an increase in body temperature comes from brown adipose tissue, at least in young experimental animals.[196, 197] It is also clear that brown adipocytes are not only responsive to cytokines released during infections that cause fever but they can also synthesize such cytokines.[198] In a number of relatively rare diseases, such as Duchenne's progressive muscular dystrophy,[199] subcutaneous fat necrosis of the newborn,[200] and sudden infant death syndrome,[201-203] a role for brown adipose tissue has been suggested. However, there is at present no evidence for a causative involvement of brown adipose tissue in any of these syndromes.

REFERENCES

1. Smith RE: Thermogenic activity of the hibernating gland in the cold-acclimated rat. Physiologist 4:113, 1961.
2. Mount LE: Responses to thermal environment in newborn pigs. Fed Proc 22:818, 1963.
3. Dawkins MJR, Hull D: Brown adipose tissue and the response of newborn rabbits to cold. J Physiol 172:216, 1964.
4. Nedergaard J, Lindberg O: The brown fat cell. Int Rev Cytol 74:187, 1982.
5. Nicholls DG, Locke RM: Thermogenic mechanisms in brown fat. Physiol Rev 64:1, 1984.
6. Cannon B, Nedergaard J: The biochemistry of an inefficient tissue: brown adipose tissue. Essays Biochem 20:110, 1985.
7. Himms-Hagen J: Brown adipose tissue metabolism. In Björntorp P, et al (eds): Obesity. New York, JB Lippincott, 1992, pp 15–34.
8. Nedergaard J, et al: UCP1: the only protein able to mediate adaptive non-shivering thermogenesis and metabolic inefficiency. Biochim Biophys Acta 1504:82, 2001.
9. Cannon B, Nedergaard J: Brown adipose tissue: function and physiological significance. Physiol Rev, in press: 2003.
10. Trayhurn P, Nicholls DG (eds): Brown Adipose Tissue. London, Edward Arnold, 1986.
11. Nedergaard J, et al: Brown adipose tissue in the mammalian neonate. In Trayhurn P, Nicholls DG (eds): Brown Adipose Tissue. London, Edward Arnold, 1986, pp 152–213.
12. Cannon B, Nedergaard J: Development of thermogenesis in the fetus. In Thorburn GD, Harding R (eds): Textbook of Fetal Physiology. Oxford, Oxford University Press, 1994, p 388.
13. Skala JP: Mechanisms of hormonal regulation in brown adipose tissue of developing rats. Can J Biochem Cell Biol 62:637, 1984.
14. Benito M: Contribution of brown fat to the neonatal thermogenesis. Biol Neonat 48:245, 1985.
15. Cannon B, et al: Perinatal recruitment of brown adipose tissue. In Kunzel W, Jensen A (eds): The Endocrine Control of the Fetus. Berlin, Springer-Verlag, 1988, pp 306–320.
16. Barnard T: The ultrastructural differentiation of brown adipose tissue in the rat. J Ultrastruct Res 29:311, 1969.
17. Suter ER: The fine structure of brown adipose tissue. II. Perinatal development in the rat. Lab Invest 21:246, 1969.
18. Suter ER: The fine structure of brown adipose tissue. III. The effect of cold exposure and its mediation in newborn rats. Lab Invest 21:259, 1969.
19. Nnodim JO, Lever JD: The pre- and post-natal development and aging of inter-scapular brown adipose tissue in the rat. Anat Embryol 173:215, 1985.
20. Nnodim JO: Stereological assessment of age-related changes in lipid droplet surface area and vascular volume in rat interscapular brown adipose tissue. Anat Rec 220:357, 1988.
21. Houstek J, et al: Uncoupling protein in embryonic brown adipose tissue—existence of nonthermogenic and thermogenic mitochondria. Biochim Biophys Acta 935:19, 1988.
22. Sundin U: Brown fat thermoregulation in developing hamsters (Mesocricetus auratus): a GDP-binding study. Biol Neonat 39:141, 1981.
23. Loudon A, et al: Brown fat, thermogenesis and physiological birth in a marsupial. Comp Biochem Physiol 81A:815, 1985.
24. Hope PJ, et al: Identification of brown fat and mechanisms for energy balance in the marsupial, Sminthopsis crassicaudata. Am J Physiol 273:R161, 1997.
25. Rafael J, Heldt HW: Binding of guanine nucleotides to the outer surface of the inner membrane of guinea pig mitochondria in correlation with the thermogenic activity of the tissue. FEBS Lett 63:304, 1976.
26. Slee J, et al: Comparative methods for inducing and measuring non-shivering thermogenesis in newborn lambs. Anim Prod 45:61, 1987.
27. Slee J, et al: Metabolic rate responses to cold and to exogenous noradrenaline in newborn Scottish blackface lambs genetically selected for high or low resistance to cold. Anim Prod 45:69, 1987.
28. Vatnick I, et al: Regression of brown adipose tissue mitochondrial function and structure in neonatal goats. Am J Physiol 252:E391, 1987.
29. Casteilla L, et al: Characterization of mitochondrial-uncoupling protein in bovine fetus and newborn calf. Am J Physiol 252:E627, 1987.
30. Blix AS, et al: Modes of thermal protection in newborn muskoxen (Ovibos moschatus). Acta Physiol Scand 122:443, 1984.
31. Strieleman PJ, et al: Brown adipose tissue from fetal Rhesus monkey (Macaca mulatta): morphological and biochemical aspects. Comp Biochem Physiol 81B:393, 1985.
32. Merklin RJ: Growth and distribution of human fetal brown fat. Anat Rec 178:637, 1974.
33. Dawkins MJR, Hull D: The production of heat by fat. Sci Am 213:62, 1965.
34. Moinat M, et al: Modulation of obese gene expression in rat brown and white adipose tissue. FEBS Lett 373:131, 1995.
35. Trayhurn P, et al: Acute cold-induced suppression of ob (obese) gene expression in white adipose tissue of mice: mediation by the sympathetic system. Biochem J 311:729, 1995.
36. Loncar D, et al: Epididymal white adipose tissue after cold stress in rats. I. Non-mitochondrial changes. J Ultrastruct Mol Struct Res 101:109, 1988.

37. Loncar D, et al: Epididymal white adipose tissue after cold stress in rats. II. Mitochondrial changes. J Ultrastruct Mol Struct Res *101*:199, 1988.
38. Young P, et al: Brown adipose tissue in the parametrial fat pad of the mouse. FEBS Lett *167*:10, 1984.
39. Grav HJ, Blix AS: Brown adipose tissue: a factor in the survival of harp seal pups. Can J Physiol Pharmacol *54*:409, 1976.
40. Ashwell M, et al: Immunological, histological and biochemical assessment of brown adipose tissue activity in neonatal, control and beta-stimulant-treated adult dogs. Int J Obes *11*:357, 1987.
41. Champigny O, et al: B₃-adrenergic receptor stimulation restores message and expression of brown-fat mitochondrial uncoupling protein in adult dogs. Proc Natl Acad Sci USA *88*:10774, 1991.
42. Kumon A, et al: Effects of catecholamines on the lipolysis of two kinds of fat cells from adult rabbit. J Lipid Res *17*:559, 1976.
43. Matthias A, et al: Thermogenic responses in brown-fat cells are fully UCP1-dependent: UCP2 or UCP3 do not substitute for UCP1 in adrenergically or fatty-acid induced thermogenesis. J Biol Chem *275*:25073, 2000.
44. Golozoubova V, et al: Only UCP1 can mediate adaptive nonshivering thermogenesis in the cold. FASEB J *15*:2048, 2001.
45. Cannon B, et al: 'Neuropeptide tyrosine' (NPY) is co-stored with noradrenaline in vascular but not in parenchymal sympathetic nerves of brown adipose tissue. Exp Cell Res *164*:546, 1986.
46. Norman D, et al: Neuropeptides in interscapular and perirenal brown adipose tissue in the rat: a plurality of innervation. J Neurocytol *17*:305, 1988.
47. Aquila H, et al: The uncoupling protein from brown fat mitochondria is related to the mitochondrial ADP/ATP carrier: analysis of sequence homologies and of folding of the protein in the membrane. EMBO J *4*:2369, 1985.
48. Bouillaud F, et al: Complete cDNA-derived amino acid sequence of rat brown adipose tissue uncoupling protein. J Biol Chem *261*:1487, 1986.
49. Ridley RG, et al: Complete nucleotide and derived amino acid sequence of cDNA encoding the mitochondrial uncoupling protein of rat brown adipose tissue: lack of a mitochondrial targeting presequence. Nucleic Acids Res *14*:4025, 1986.
50. Kozak LP, et al: The mitochondrial uncoupling protein gene: correlation of exon structure to transmembrane domains. J Biol Chem *263*:12274, 1988.
51. Lean MEJ, James WPT: Uncoupling protein in human brown adipose tissue mitochondria: isolation and detection by specific antiserum. FEBS Lett *163*:235, 1983.
52. Bouillaud F, et al: Detection of brown adipose tissue uncoupling protein mRNA in adult patients by a human genomic probe. Clin Sci *75*:21, 1988.
53. Lowell BB, et al: Development of obesity in transgenic mice after genetic ablation of brown adipose tissue. Nature *366*:740, 1993.
54. Aquila H, et al: Solute carriers involved in energy transfer of mitochondria form a homologous protein family. FEBS Lett *212*:1, 1987.
55. Runswick MJ, et al: Sequence of the bovine mitochondrial phosphate carrier protein: structural relationship to ADP/ATP translocase and the brown fat mitochondria uncoupling protein. EMBO J *6*:1367, 1987.
56. Walker JE, Runswick MJ: The mitochondrial transport protein superfamily. J Bioenerg Biomembr *25*:435, 1993.
57. Ricquier D, Bouillaud F: The uncoupling protein homologues: UCP1, UCP2, UCP3, StUCP and AtUCP. Biochem J *345*:161, 2000.
58. Jacobsson A, et al: Mitochondrial uncoupling protein from mouse brown fat: molecular cloning, genetic mapping, and mRNA expression. J Biol Chem *260*:16250, 1985.
59. Cassard AM, et al: Human uncoupling protein gene: structure, comparison with rat gene, and assignment to the long arm of chromosome 4. J Cell Biochem *43*:255, 1990.
60. Bouillaud F, et al: The gene for rat uncoupling protein: complete sequence, structure of primary transcript and evolutionary relationship between exons. Biochem Biophys Res Commun *157*:783, 1988.
61. Rafael J, et al: Mitochondrien aus braunem Fettgewebe: Entkopplung der Atmungskettenphosphorylierung durch langkettige Fettsäuren und rekopplung durch Guanosintriphosphat. Hoppe Seylers Z Physiol Chem *350*:1121, 1969.
62. Cannon B, et al: Purine nucleotides and fatty acids in energy coupling of mitochondria from brown adipose tissue. *In* Azzone GF, et al (ed): Mechanisms in Bioenergetics. New York, Academic Press, 1973, pp 357–364.
63. Nicholls DG, et al: Energy dissipation in non-shivering thermogenesis. *In* Ernster L, et al (eds): Dynamics of Energy-Transducing Membranes. Amsterdam, Elsevier, 1974, pp 529–537.
64. Klingenberg M: Nucleotide binding to uncoupling protein: mechanism of control by protonation. Biochemistry *27*:781, 1988.
65. Prusiner SB, et al: Oxidative metabolism in cells isolated from brown adipose tissue. 2. Catecholamine-regulated respiratory control. Eur J Biochem *7*:51, 1968b.
66. Prusiner SB, et al: Oxidative metabolism in cells isolated from brown adipose tissue. I. Catecholamine and fatty acid stimulation of respiration. Eur J Biochem *6*:15, 1968.
67. Heaton GM, Nicholls DG: Hamster brown-adipose-tissue mitochondria: the role of fatty acids in the control of the proton conductance of the inner membrane. Eur J Biochem *67*:511, 1976.
68. Rial E, et al: Brown adipose tissue mitochondria: the regulation of the 32,000 Mᵥ uncoupling protein by fatty acids and purine nucleotides. Eur J Biochem *173*:197, 1983.
69. Garlid KD: Mitochondrial cation transport: a progress report. J Bioenerg Biomembr *26*:537, 1994.
70. Winkler E, Klingenberg M: Effect of fatty acids on H⁺ transport activity of the reconstituted uncoupling protein. J Biol Chem *269*:2508, 1994.
71. Cannon B, et al: Palmitoyl coenzyme A: a possible physiological regulator of nucleotide binding to brown adipose tissue mitochondria. FEBS Lett *74*:43, 1977.
72. Katiyar SS, Shrago E: Differential interaction of fatty acids and fatty acyl CoA esters with the purified/reconstituted brown adipose tissue uncoupling protein. Biochem Biophys Res Commun *175*:1104, 1991.
73. Desautels M, et al: Increased purine nucleotide binding, altered polypeptide composition, and thermogenesis in brown adipose tissue mitochondria of cold-acclimated rats. Can J Biochem *56*:378, 1978.
74. Nedergaard J, Cannon B: Apparent unmasking of (³H)GDP binding in rat brown-fat mitochondria is due to mitochondrial swelling. Eur J Biochem *164*:681, 1987.
75. Jacobsson A, et al: The uncoupling protein thermogenin during acclimation: indications for pretranslational control. Am J Physiol *267*:R999, 1994.
76. Ricquier D, et al: Rapid increase of mitochondrial uncoupling protein and its mRNA in stimulated brown adipose tissue. FEBS Lett *178*:240, 1984.
77. Jacobsson A, et al: Alpha- and beta-adrenergic control of thermogenin mRNA expression in brown adipose tissue. Biosci Rep *6*:621, 1986.
78. Ricquier D, et al: Expression of uncoupling protein mRNA in thermogenic or weakly thermogenic brown adipose tissue: evidence for a rapid beta-adrenoreceptor-mediated and transcriptionally regulated step during activation of thermogenesis. J Biol Chem *261*:13905, 1986.
79. Sundin U, Cannon B: GDP-binding to the brown fat mitochondria of developing and cold-adapted rats. Comp Biochem Physiol *65B*:463, 1980.
80. Obregon MJ, et al: Euthyroid status is essential for the perinatal increase in thermogenin mRNA in brown adipose tissue of rat pups. Biochem Biophys Res Commun *148*:9, 1987.
81. Obregon M-J, et al: Postnatal recruitment of brown adipose tissue is induced by the cold stress experienced by the pups: an analysis of mRNA levels for thermogenin and lipoprotein lipase. Biochem J *259*:341, 1989.
82. Freeman KB, Patel HV: Biosynthesis of the 32-KDalton uncoupling protein in brown adipose-tissue of developing rabbits. Can J Biochem *62*:479, 1984.
83. Power GG, et al: Oxygen supply and the placenta limit thermogenic responses in fetal sheep. J Appl Physiol *63*:1896, 1987.
84. Gunn TR, et al: Withdrawal of placental prostaglandins permits thermogenic responses in fetal sheep brown adipose tissue. J Appl Physiol *74*:998, 1993.
85. Gunn TR, et al: Reversible umbilical cord occlusion: effects on thermogenesis *in utero*. Pediatr Res *30*:513, 1991.
86. Gunn TR, Gluckman PD: Perinatal thermogenesis. Early Hum Dev *42*:169, 1995.
87. Heldmaier G, et al: Photoperiodic control and effects of melatonin on nonshivering thermogenesis and brown adipose tissue. Science *212*:917, 1981.
88. Vanecek J, Illnerova H: Effect of short and long photoperiods on pineal N-acetyltransferase rhythm and on growth of testes and brown adipose tissue in developing rats. Neuroendocrinology *41*:186, 1985.
89. Karlberg P, et al: The thermogenic response of the newborn infant to noradrenaline. Acta Paediat *51*:284, 1962.
90. Lean MEJ, et al: Brown adipose tissue uncoupling protein content in human infants, children and adults. Clin Sci *71*:291, 1986.
91. Bouillaud F, et al: Detection of brown adipose tissue uncoupling protein mRNA in adult patients by a human genomic probe. Clin Sci *75*:21, 1988.
92. Kortelainen M-L, et al: Immunohistochemical detection of human brown adipose tissue uncoupling protein in an autopsy series. J Histochem Cytochem *41*:759, 1993.
93. Zancanaro C, et al: Immunohistochemical identification of the uncoupling protein in human hibernoma. Biol Cell *80*:75, 1994.
94. Pettersson B, Vallin I: Norepinephrine-induced shift in levels of adenosine 3′:5′-monophosphate and ATP parallel to increased respiratory rate and lipolysis in isolated hamster brown fat cells. Eur J Biochem *62*:383, 1976.
95. Skala J, et al: Changes in interscapular brown adipose tissue of the rat during perinatal and early postnatal development and after cold acclimation. V. Adenyl cyclase, cyclic AMP, protein kinase, phosphorylase, phosphorylase kinase, and glycogen. Int J Biochem *3*:229, 1972.
96. Bertin R, et al: Effect of ambient temperature on perinatal variations of cyclic AMP and cyclic GMP in rat brown adipose tissue. Biochem Syst Ecol *8*:221, 1980.
97. Skala JP, Knight BL: Protein kinases in brown adipose tissue of developing rats. J Biol Chem *252*:1064, 1977.
98. Arch JRS, et al: Atypical beta-adrenoceptor on brown adipocytes as target for anti-obesity drugs. Nature *309*:163, 1984.
99. Mohell N, Nedergaard J: Comparison of the pharmacological profiles of adrenergic drugs at (³H)CGP-12177 binding sites in brown adipose tissue. Comp Biochem Physiol *C94*:229, 1989.
100. Arch J: The brown adipocyte β-adrenoceptor. Proc Nutr Soc *48*:215, 1989.
101. Arch JRS, Kaumann AJ: β₃ and atypical ß-adrenoceptors. Med Res Rev *13*:663, 1993.

102. Lafontan M, Berlan M: Fat cell adrenergic receptors and the control of white and brown fat cell function. J Lipid Res *34*:1057, 1993.
103. Zhao J, et al: Coexisting ß-adrenoceptor subtypes: significance for thermogenic process in brown fat cells. Am J Physiol *267*:C969, 1994.
104. Skala JP, Shaikh IM: Alpha$_2$-adrenergic receptors in brown adipose tissue of infant rats-II. Studies on function and regulation. Int J Biochem *20*:15, 1988.
105. Skala JP, et al: Alpha$_2$-adrenergic receptors in brown adipose tissue of infant rats-I: identification and characteristics of binding sites in isolated plasma membranes. Int J Biochem *20*:7, 1988.
106. Dominguez MJ, et al: Occurrence of alpha$_2$-adrenergic effects on adenylate cyclase activity and (^{3}H)-clonidine specific binding in brown adipose tissue from foetal rats. Biochem Biophys Res Commun *138*:1390, 1986.
107. Woodward JA, Saggerson ED: Effect of adenosine deaminase, N^6-phenylisopropyladenosine and hypothyroidism on the responsiveness of rat brown adipocytes to noradrenaline. Biochem J *238*:395, 1986.
108. Mohell N, et al: Identification of (^{3}H) prazosin binding sites in crude membranes and isolated cells of brown adipose tissue as alpha$_1$-adrenergic receptors. Eur J Pharmacol *92*:15, 1983.
109. Connolly E, et al: Na$^+$ dependent, alpha-adrenergic mobilization of intracellular (mitochondrial) Ca^{2+} in brown adipocytes. Eur J Biochem *141*:187, 1984.
110. Barge RM, et al: Phorbol esters, protein kinase C, and thyroxine 5'-deiodinase in brown adipocytes. Am J Physiol *254*:E323, 1988.
111. Wilcke M, et al: Adrenergic regulation of cytosolic Ca^{2+} in brown fat cells. Biochem Biophys Res Commun *163*:292, 1989.
112. Harris WH, et al: The receptors responsible for heat production in brown adipose tissue in the young rabbit. Can J Physiol Pharmacol *64*:133, 1986.
113. Zhao J, et al: a$_1$-Adrenergic stimulation potentiates the thermogenic action of ß$_3$-adrenoceptor-generated cAMP in brown fat cells. J Biol Chem *272*:32847, 1997.
114. Holm C, et al: Hormone-sensitive lipase in brown adipose tissue: identification and effect of cold exposure. Biosci Rep 7:897, 1987.
115. Hull D, Segall MM: Distinction of brown from white adipose tissue. Nature *212*:469, 1966.
116. Nedergaard J: Catecholamine sensitivity in brown fat cells from cold-adapted hamsters and rats. Am J Physiol *242*:C250, 1982.
117. Hardman MJ, et al: Fat metabolism and heat production in young rabbits. J Physiol *205*:51, 1969.
118. Ma SWY, Foster DO: Uptake of glucose and release of fatty acids and glycerol by rat brown adipose tissue in vivo. Can J Physiol Pharmacol *64*:609, 1986.
119. Heldmaier G, Seidl K: Plasma free fatty acid levels during cold-induced and noradrenaline-induced nonshivering thermogenesis in the Djungarian hamster. J Comp Physiol [B] *155*:679, 1985.
120. Heim T, Kellermayer M: The effect of environmental temperature on brown and white adipose tissue in the starving newborn rabbit. Acta Physiol Acad Sci Hung *31*:339, 1967.
121. Heim T, et al: Thermal conditions and the mobilization of lipids from brown and white adipose tissue in the human neonate. Acta Paediatr Hung *9*:109, 1968.
122. Hardman MJ, Hull D: Fat metabolism in brown adipose tissue in vivo. J Physiol *206*:263, 1970.
123. Radomski MW, Orme T: Response of lipoprotein lipase in various tissues to cold exposure. Am J Physiol *220*:1852, 1971.
124. Carneheim C, et al: Beta-adrenergic stimulation of lipoprotein lipase in rat brown adipose tissue during acclimation to cold. Am J Physiol *246*:E327, 1984.
125. Carneheim C, et al: Cold-induced beta-adrenergic recruitment of lipoprotein lipase in brown adipose tissue is due to increased transcription. Am J Physiol *254*:E155, 1988.
126. Mitchell JR, et al: Regulation of expression of the lipoprotein lipase gene in brown adipose tissue. *In* Rössner S, Björntorp P (eds): Obesity in Europe 88. London, John Libbey, 1989, pp 235–239.
127. Mitchell JR, et al: Lipoprotein lipase is regulated via gene activation in brown adipose tissue. Am J Physiol *263*:E500, 1992.
128. Bartness TJ, et al: Insulin and metabolic efficiency in rats. I. Effects of sucrose feeding and BAT axotomy. Am J Physiol *251*:R1109, 1986.
129. Bartness TJ, et al: Insulin and metabolic efficiency in rats. II. Effects of NE and cold exposure. Am J Physiol *251*:1118, 1986.
130. Carneheim CMH, Alexson SEH: Refeeding-induced increase in lipoprotein lipase activity in brown adipose tissue is mediated by insulin. Am J Physiol *256*:E645, 1989.
131. Cryer A, Jones HM: Developmental changes in the activity of lipoprotein lipase (clearing factor lipase) in rat lung, cardiac muscle, skeletal muscle and brown adipose tissue. Biochem J *174*:447, 1978.
132. Obregon MJ, et al: Postnatal suppression of lipoprotein lipase gene expression in brown adipose tissue. Biochem J *314*:261, 1996.
133. Cogneville AM, et al: Lipid composition of brown adipose tissue as related to nutrition during the neonatal period in hypotrophic rats. J Nutr *105*:982, 1975.
134. Ricquier D, Hemon P: A study of phospholipids and triglycerides in several tissues of the rat during fetal and neonatal development: effect of cretinism. Biol Neonat *28*:225, 1976.
135. Senault C, et al: Cold-induced changes in fatty acid composition of rat brown fat during the perinatal period. Experientia *38*:585, 1982.
136. Olivecrona T, et al: Combined lipase deficiency (cld/cld) in mice. Demonstration that an inactive form of lipoprotein lipase is synthesized. J Biol Chem *260*:2552, 1985.

137. Blanchette-Mackie EJ, et al: Effect of the combined lipase deficiency mutation (cld/cld) on ultrastructure of tissues in mice: diaphragm, heart, brown adipose tissue, lung, and liver. Lab Invest *55*:347, 1986.
138. Cannon B, Nedergaard J: The physiological role of pyruvate carboxylation in hamster brown adipose tissue. Eur J Biochem *94*:419, 1979.
139. Slot JW, et al: Immuno-localization of the insulin regulatable glucose transporter in brown adipose tissue of the rat. J Cell Biol *113*:123, 1991.
140. Omatsu-Kanbe M, Kitasato H: Insulin and noradrenaline independently stimulate the translocation of glucose transporters from intracellular stores to the plasma membrane in mouse brown adipocytes. FEBS Lett *314*:246, 1992.
141. Shimizu Y, et al: Effects of noradrenaline on the cell-surface glucose transporters in cultured brown adipocytes: novel mechanism for selective activation of GLUT1 glucose transporters. Biochem J *330*:397, 1998.
142. McCormack JG, Denton RM: Evidence that fatty acid synthesis in the interscapular brown adipose tissue of cold-adapted rats is increased in vivo by insulin by mechanisms involving parallel activation of pyruvate dehydrogenase and acetyl-coenzyme A carboxylase. Biochem J *166*:627, 1977.
143. Hahn P: Lipid synthesis in various organs of the rat during postnatal development. Biol Neonat *50*:205, 1986.
144. Chakrabarty K, et al: Lipogenic activity and brown fat content of human perirenal adipose tissue. Clin Biochem *21*:249, 1988.
145. Barton CH, Bailey E: Changes in immunoreactive malic enzyme in liver and brown adipose tissue during development of the rat. J Develop Physiol *9*:215, 1987.
146. Simpson MLF, et al: Glycolysis and lipid synthesis in brown adipose tissue during aging in the rat. Biochem Biophys Res Commun *140*:419, 1986.
147. Lopez-Soriano FJ, et al: Amino acid and glucose uptake by rat brown adipose tissue: effect of cold-exposure and acclimation. Biochem J *252*:843, 1988.
148. Alexson SEH, Nedergaard J: A novel type of short- and medium-chain acyl-CoA hydrolases in brown adipose tissue mitochondria. J Biol Chem *263*:13564, 1988.
149. Alexson SEH, et al: NADH-sensitive propionyl-CoA hydrolase in brown-adipose-tissue mitochondria of the rat. Biochim Biophys Acta *1005*:13, 1989.
150. Cannon B, et al: Morphology and biochemical properties of perirenal adipose tissue from lamb (Ovis aries): a comparison with brown adipose tissue. Comp Biochem Physiol *56B*:87, 1977.
151. Silva JE, Larsen PR: Adrenergic activation of triiodothyronine in brown adipose tissue. Nature *305*:712, 1983.
152. Silva JE, et al: Comparison of kidney and brown adipose tissue iodothyronine 5'-deiodinases. Endocrinology *121*:650, 1987.
153. McCann UD, et al: Iodothyronine deiodination reaction types in several rat tissues: effects of age, thyroid status, and glucocorticoid treatment. Endocrinology *114*:1513, 1984.
154. Croteau W, et al: Cloning of the mammalian type II iodothyronine deiodinase. J Clin Invest *2*:405, 1996.
155. Polk DH, et al: Effect of fetal thyroidectomy on newborn thermogenesis in lambs. Pediatr Res *21*:453, 1987.
156. Houstek J, et al: Type II iodothyronine 5'-deiodinase and uncoupling protein in brown adipose tissue of human newborns. J Clin Endocrinol Metab *77*:382, 1993.
157. Bianco AC, Silva JE: Nuclear 3,5,3'- triiodothyronine (T$_3$) in brown adipose tissue: receptor occupancy and sources of T$_3$ as determined by in vivo techniques. Endocrinology *120*:55, 1987.
158. Burgi U, Burgi-Saville ME: Brown fat nuclear triiodothyronine receptors in rats. Am J Physiol *251*:E503, 1986.
159. Bianco AC, Silva JE: Optimal response of key enzymes and uncoupling protein to cold in BAT depends on local T$_3$ generation. Am J Physiol *253*:E255, 1987.
160. Rabelo R, et al: Interactions among receptors, thyroid hormone response elements, and ligands in the regulation of the rat uncoupling protein gene expression by thyroid hormone. Endocrinology *137*:3478, 1996.
161. Silva JE, Larsen PR: Potential of brown adipose tissue type II thyroxine 5'-deiodinase as a local and systemic source of triiodothyronine in rats. J Clin Invest *76*:2296, 1985.
162. Silva JE, Matthews P: Thyroid hormone metabolism and the source of plasma triiodothyronine in 2-week-old rats: effects of thyroid status. Endocrinology *114*:2394, 1984.
163. Jankovic BD, et al: Brown adipose tissue and immunity: effect of neonatal adipectomy on humoral and cellular immune reactions in the rat. Immunology *28*:597, 1975.
164. Jankovic BD, et al: Potentiation of experimental allergic thyroiditis in rats adipectomized at birth. Clin Exp Immunol *29*:173, 1977.
165. Jankovic BD: Brown adipose tissue: its in vivo immunology and involvement in neuroimmunomodulation. *In* Jankovic BD, et al (eds): Neuroimmune Interactions: Proceedings of the Second International Workshop on Neuroimmunomodulation. New York, New York Academy of Science, 1987, pp 3–25.
166. Jones RB, et al: Requirement of gene transcription and protein synthesis for cold- and norepinephrine-induced stimulation of thyroxine deiodinase in rat brown adipose tissue. Biochim Biophys Acta *889*:366, 1986.
167. Silva JE, Larsen PR: Hormonal regulation of iodothyronine 5'- deiodinase in rat brown adipose tissue. Am J Physiol *251*:E639, 1986.
168. Mills I, et al: Effect of thyroid status on catecholamine stimulation of thyroxine 5'-deiodinase in isolated brown adipocytes. Am J Physiol *256*:E74, 1989.

169. Raasmaja A, Larsen PR: Hypothyroidism enhances the alpha$_1$/beta adrenergic synergistic stimulation of the iodothyronine deiodinase in brown adipocytes. Endocrinology 125:2502, 1989.
170. Mills I, et al: Insulin stimulation of iodothyronine 5'-deiodinase in rat brown adipocytes. Biochem Biophys Res Commun 143:81, 1987.
171. Iglesias R, et al: Iodothyronine 5'-deiodinase activity in rat brown adipose tissue during development. Biochim Biophys Acta 923:233, 1987.
172. Giralt M, et al: Evidence for a differential physiological modulation of brown fat iodothyronine 5'-deiodinase activity in the perinatal period. Biochem Biophys Res Commun 156:493, 1988.
173. Obregon MJ, et al: Thyroid hormones and 5'-deiodinase in rat brown adipose tissue during fetal life. Am J Physiol 257:E625, 1989.
174. Bronnikov G, et al: β-Adrenergic, cAMP-mediated stimulation of proliferation of brown fat cells in primary culture: mediation via β$_1$ but not via β$_3$ receptors. J Biol Chem 267:2006, 1992.
175. Rehnmark S, et al: α- and β-adrenergic induction of the expression of the uncoupling protein thermogenin in brown adipocytes differentiated in culture. J Biol Chem 265:16464, 1990.
176. Rehnmark S, et al: Differential adrenergic regulation of C/EBPα and C/EBPβ in brown adipose tissue. FEBS Lett 318:235, 1993.
177. Spiegelman BM, et al: Regulation of adipogenesis and energy balance by PPARgamma and PGC-1. Int J Obes Relat Metab Disord 24 Suppl 4:S8, 2000.
178. Lorenzo M, et al: IGF-I is a mitogen involved in differentiation-related gene expression in fetal rat brown adipocytes. J Cell Biol 123:1567, 1993.
179. Benito M, et al: IGF-I: A mitogen also involved in differentiation processes in mammalian cells. Int J Biochem Cell Biol 28:499, 1996.
180. Editorial: The incubator. Sci Am 1882.
181. Ohlson KBE, et al: Thermogenesis in brown adipocytes is inhibited by volatile anesthetic agents: a factor contributing to hypothermia in infants? Anesthesiology 81:176, 1994.
182. Dicker A, et al: Halothane selectively inhibits nonshivering thermogenesis: possible implications for thermoregulation during anesthesia of infants. Anesthesiology 82:491, 1995.
183. Felipe A, et al: Effects of maternal hypocaloric diet feeding on neonatal rat brown adipose tissue. Biol Neonat 53:105, 1988.
184. Stirling DM, Ashwell M: The effect of diet restriction on the development of prenatal and postnatal brown adipose tissue thermogenesis in the guinea-pig. Proc Nutr Soc 47:75A, 1988.
185. Duerden JM, Bates CJ: Effect of riboflavin deficiency on lipid metabolism of liver and brown adipose tissue of sucking rat pups. Br J Nutr 53:107, 1985.
186. Tyzbir RS, Welsh DL: Brown adipose tissue and liver mitochondrial function in lactating rats fed a protein restricted diet. Nutrition Reports International 33:409, 1986.
187. Brooke OG, et al: The response of malnourished babies to cold. J Physiol 233:75, 1973.
188. Rothwell NJ, Stock MJ: A role for brown adipose tissue in diet-induced thermogenesis. Nature 281:31, 1979.
189. Rothwell NJ, Stock MJ: Brown adipose tissue: does it play a role in the development of obesity? Diabetes Metab Rev 4:595, 1988.
190. Moore BJ, et al: Brown fat mediates increased energy expenditure of cold-exposed overfed neonatal rats. Am J Physiol 251:R518, 1986.
191. Rothwell NJ, Stock MJ: Body weight and brown fat activity in hyperphagic cafeteria-fed female rats and their offspring. Biol Neonat 49:284, 1986.
192. Goodbody AE, Trayhurn P: Studies on the activity of brown adipose tissue in suckling, pre-obese, ob/ob mice. Biochim Biophys Acta 680:119, 1982.
193. Bazin R, et al: Evidence for decreased GDP binding to brown-adipose-tissue mitochondria of obese zucker (fa/fa) rats in the very first days of life. Biochem J 221:241, 1984.
194. Moore BJ, et al: Energy expenditure is reduced in preobese 2-day Zucker fa/fa rats. Am J Physiol 249:R262, 1985.
195. Enerbäck S, et al: Mice lacking mitochondrial uncoupling protein are cold-sensitive but not obese. Nature 387:90, 1997.
196. Blatteis CM: Effect of propranolol on endotoxin-induced pyrogenesis in newborn and adult guinea pigs. J Appl Physiol 40:35, 1976.
197. Harris WH, et al: Evidence for a contribution by brown adipose tissue to the development of fever in the young rabbit. Can J Physiol Pharmacol 63:595, 1985.
198. Cannon B, et al: Brown adipose tissue: more than an effector of thermogenesis? Ann NY Acad Sci 856:171, 1998.
199. Ito M, et al: Brown adipose tissue in Duchenne's progressive muscular dystrophy. Arch Pathol Lab Med 112:550, 1988.
200. Taieb A, et al: Trois cas de cytosteatonecrose neo-natale. Presse Med 15:2197, 1986.
201. Stephenson TJ, Variend S: Visceral brown fat necrosis in postperinatal mortality. J Clin Pathol 40:896, 1987.
202. Stanton AN: Sudden infant death: overheating and cot death. Lancet 2:1199, 1984.
203. Lean MEJ, Jennings G: Brown adipose tissue activity in pyrexial cases of cot death. J Clin Pathol 42:1153, 1989.
204. Borecky J, et al: Mitochondrial uncoupling proteins in mammals and plants. Biosci Rep 21:201, 2001.
205. Nicholls DG: The bioenergetics of brown adipose tissue mitochondria. FEBS Lett 61:103, 1976a.
206. Houstek J, et al: Type II iodothyronine 5'-deiodinase and uncoupling protein in brown adipose tissue of human newborns. J Clin Endocrinol Metab 77:383, 1993.

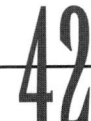

Guy Putet

Lipids as an Energy Source for the Premature and Full-Term Neonate

Fat and carbohydrate are the two major sources of energy for the newborn infant. In human milk and in formula designed for full-term infants, the fat content generally ranges between 3.5 and 4 g/dL and thus provides between 40% and 50% of the total calories. Most of the formulas specially adapted for preterm infants also have a fat content between 3 and 4 g/dL[1] and provide between 35% and 40% of total caloric intake. When only nonprotein energy is considered, fat accounts for more than 50% of energy intake. Even in the very low birth weight infant, fat absorption in the intestine generally exceeds 85% of intake with most modern formulas. In comparison, carbohydrate absorption is always above 95%, even in the smallest infants during the first weeks of life.[2] Therefore, carbohydrate can serve as a readily available nutrient for oxidative metabolism.

It has not been easy to quantify the exact amount of fat oxidized by newborn infants. However, indirect calorimetry measurements performed over several hours have permitted some good estimations of nutrient oxidation.[3,4] In addition, the levels of plasma metabolites also have provided information on the types of fuel oxidized. By critically analyzing both kinds of experimental data, this chapter discusses the importance of fat as a fuel for oxidative metabolism in the term and preterm infant. A comprehensive review of lipid metabolism in the extreme premature infant has been published recently.[5]

FAT OXIDATION IN UTERO AND AT BIRTH

Before birth, glucose is the major energy source for the human fetus. It has been estimated that during fetal life, about 80% of the energy expended is derived from carbohydrate oxidation.[6-9] If one assumes that energy (E) expenditure of the fetus averages 50 kcal/kg/day,[10] the fetus should oxidize about 10 g/kg of carbohydrate each day. The rest of the energy needs are derived in part from amino acid oxidation. Thus, in the human fetus, fat does not seem to be a major source of energy.

At birth, there is an abrupt change in the nutrient supply after the umbilical cord is divided. In term infants, even when oral food is supplied quickly, the amount of energy received during the first hours is low. During the first day of life, the respiratory quotient in human newborn infants drops from approximately 0.9 to below 0.8.[11] At that time, fat provides between 60% and 70% of energy expenditure. The concomitant increase in plasma free fatty acids (FFA) and glycerol also indicates that lipolysis is actively occurring.

FAT OXIDATION RATE IN GROWING INFANTS

After the first week of life, when full feeding has been reached, fat is provided in abundance. There are, however, very minimal data on the respiratory quotient (RQ) in the normally fed and growing full-term infant between 1 week and 1 month of postnatal life. The most careful estimates of RQ place it at around 0.85 or above.[11] Based on those estimates and an oxygen consumption that has been measured at between 7 and 8 mL/kg/min, one can calculate that between 2 and 3 g/kg/day of fat is oxidized. This means that between 40% and 50% of calories oxidized after the first week of life in term infants are derived from fat. (This percentage would range between 30% and 40% for an RQ estimated at 0.9.)

For the growing preterm infant fed either human milk (HM) or a preterm formula (PF), considerably more data on energy balance are available. Table 42-1 summarizes studies from the literature, in which data on metabolizable energy (energy intake minus losses in stools), energy expenditure, nutrient balances, and respiratory quotient have been precisely determined. Very few published reports have provided sufficient data to permit a calculation of the amount of fat oxidized;[12-18] however, several conclusions can be reached concerning the data shown in Table 42-1:

1. Almost all the studies listed in Table 42-1 have observed an RQ greater than 0.9. This value for RQ correlates with values from other investigations[19-21] in which data were not precise enough to be included in this table but in which RQ values were measured in growing infants receiving full oral feedings (lower RQ values have been reported in nongrowing infants[22]).

2. The amount of fat oxidized averages 1.5 g/kg/day (i.e., about 14 kcal/kg/day). This represents approximately 30% of the fat absorbed and 20% (range, 10 to 35%) of the calories oxidized.

3. As shown in Table 42-1, the values for RQ are high but slightly lower with human milk than with preterm formula. A high RQ can result from either a high rate of carbohydrate oxidation (fat being almost nonutilized as a source of energy) or increased storage of carbohydrate as triglyceride.[3,4] With human milk, 35 to 40% of the calories oxidized are derived from fat (1.9 g/kg/day) compared with 10 to 30% with preterm formula (1.1 g/kg/day). It is difficult to assess whether this difference in fat oxidation rate is the consequence of a lower total metabolizable energy intake or of differences in the quality of the human milk. However, if studies that have used only preterm formula are analyzed, it appears that the highest RQ values are consistently observed in infants receiving the highest metabolizable energy intakes. Thus, the lower oxidation rate of fat seen with formula is more likely to be due to the higher caloric intake provided as carbohydrate rather than a difference in the quality of milk. The higher carbohydrate intake in infants receiving formula could also explain the higher urinary C-peptide level observed in artificially fed infants.[23]

Relatively few studies in the literature have made repetitive measurements of energy expenditure in infants. It is, however, interesting to note that Gudinchet and colleagues[24] have demonstrated an increased participation of fat in oxidative metabolism with advancing age in the premature infant fed a constant energy intake of 130 kcal/kg/day (Table 42-2).

Medium Chain Triglycerides (MCTs) as Fuel

MCTs (C8 and C10) were introduced in premature infant nutrition because of the poor absorption of cow's milk fat in these infants. Several studies[25, 26] have demonstrated an improved total fat absorption rate when part of the saturated long chain fatty acids from cow's milk are replaced by MCTs.

In the adult, MCTs appear to be entirely oxidized, but little is known about the metabolism (oxidation and storage) of MCTs in

---

TABLE 42-1

Respiratory Quotients, Energy Balances, and Fat Oxidation Rates in Low Birth Weight Infants Orally Fed Human Milk or Preterm Formulas

Type of Milk (Ref)	Met.E.I.* (kcal/kg/d)	Energy Expenditure (kcal/kg/d)	RQ	Fat Intake g/kg/d	Fat Absorbed g/kg/d	Fat Absorbed % of Met.E.I.	Fat Oxidized g/kg/d	Fat Oxidized % of Absorb.	% of E. Oxidized Derived from: Fat	% of E. Oxidized Derived from: Carbohydrate	At Study Gestational Age (wk)	At Study Postnatal Age (d)
HM (14)	95	49	0.88	5.6	4.6	45	1.6	35	29	67	34.4	31
HM (11)	100	56	0.91	4.7	3.8	35	1.6	42	27	66	33.3	21
HM (15)	87	46	0.91	5.3	3.8	40	1.3	34	26	68	33.2	21
HM (15)	102	51	0.88	5.7	5.2	47	1.9	36	35	61	36	45
PF (12)	110	68	0.96	5.7	4.7	40	0.7	15	10	80	35	21
PF (15)	118	57	0.92	5.3	4.6	36	1.4	30	23	73	33.3	29
PF (15)	123	63	0.92	5.5	5.0	38	1.5	30	22	73	36	46
PF (13)	109	62	0.93	5.4	4.8	41	1.3	27	20	76	35.4	34
PF (16)	130	63	0.96	7.5	6.0	43	0.6	10	9	27	32.3	21
PF (17)	106	60	0.95								>33	≥15†
PF (17)	104	58	0.91								>34	≥19†
PF (17)	137	69	0.97								>34	≥19†

HM = human milk; PF = preterm formula.
* Met. E.I.: metabolizable energy intake.
† From available data.

premature infants. Only small amounts of C8 and C10 are present in human milk,[27, 28] and although there is no evidence that they are harmful, one may be concerned about storage or incorporation of MCTs into structural lipids.

MCT oxidation does occur, and there are data demonstrating increases in the plasma concentrations of β-hydroxybutyrate and acetoacetate when infants receive formula containing these fats.[29, 30] However, when one calculates the total amount of fat oxidized by a preterm infant (in Table 42-1, this amount ranges between 1.3 and 1.5 g/kg/day), it appears that an infant fed 160 mL/kg/day of a formula containing more than 20% of its fat as MCTs has either to oxidize all the MCTs and no other fat, or store some of the medium chain triglycerides if longer chain fatty acids are oxidized simultaneously.

We have assessed MCT oxidation in preterm infants by using indirect calorimetry, nutritional balance techniques, and stable isotope enrichment of expired CO_2 measurement after administration of 13C-trioctanoin.[14] It is important to note that it is difficult to mix MCTs with human milk or formula,[31] and when labeled MCTs are added, care must be taken to achieve a good emulsion that can be appropriately absorbed. Failure to do so may explain the scatter of data in a previous study.[32]

The present study was performed in seven growing premature infants (mean birth weight = 1323 g + 176: gestational age [GA] = 30.6 + 1.4 weeks). At the time of the study, the mean postnatal age of these infants was 34 days + 7 days and the intake of formula (containing 3.4 g/dL of fat, 40% as MCT) was 159 + 4 mL/kg/day. Indirect calorimetry measurements were performed continuously over 24 hours to follow precisely the evolution of the labeled $13CO_2$ in expired air. The mean rate of oxygen consumption was 9.0 + 0.99 mL/kg/min, and the mean RQ was 0.92 + 0.04 during the study period, which is in agreement with data given in Table 42-1.

The results of the energy balance and fat balance are shown in Table 42-3. Isotopic measurement of expired CO_2 indicated that about 54% (range, 46 to 62%) of the labeled octanoic acid was oxidized. Assuming that the oxidation rate of the labeled octanoic acid is representative of the MCT oxidation rate, the investigators calculated that 1.2 g/kg/day of MCT was oxidized (see Table 42-3). This represents more than 80% of the calories derived from fat oxidation, indicating a preferential utilization of C8 and C10 triglycerides. The high rate of utilization of MCTs is likely to be related to their fast absorption; MCTs are the first fats available for oxidation after a meal. MCTs that are not oxidized can either be stored as such in adipose tissue or be elongated to longer chain fatty acids. In our study, the analysis (by isotopic gas chromatography mass spectrometry) of blood, medium chain fatty acids (free and in the form of triglycerides) demonstrated the presence of 13C-octanoic acid in plasma and a low but significant labeling of C12:0. Sarda and associates[33] observed C8:0, C10:0, and C12:0 storage in adipose tissue in association with MCT dietary intake. The biosynthesis of C12 and its storage in the adipose tissue of premature infants were not precisely esti-

TABLE 42-2

Evolution of Energy Expenditure and Respiratory Quotient in Preterm Infants During the First 6 Weeks of Life*

Age (weeks of life)	1	3	6
Weight (g)	1153	1334	1793
RQ	0.97	0.91	0.90
E. expenditure (kcal/kg/d)	40	64	60
% E. derived from:			
Fat oxidation	14%		30%
Carbohydrate oxidation	80%		65%

* From ref. 24. With advancing postnatal age, an increase in energy expenditure and fat oxidation is observed.

TABLE 42-3

Energy and Fat Balances*

	Energy		Fat g/kg/d	
	kcal/kg/d	Total	MCT	Other Fat
Intake	116	5.4	2.2	3.2
Absorbed	109	4.8	2.2	2.6
Oxidized	62	1.3	1.2	0.1
Stored	47	3.5	1.0	2.5

* According to the oxidation rate of the labeled octanoic acid (ref. 14), 54% (i.e., 12 g/kg/d) of the ingested MCTs is oxidized; as indirect calorimetry measurements give a total fat oxidation of 1.3 g/kg/d, the amount of longer chain fatty acids oxidized is assumed to be the difference (i.e., 0.1 g/kg/d).

mated in our study, but both elongation and storage of ingested MCTs may take place when infants are fed MCTs.

A consequence of MCT oxidation is an increased urinary excretion of dicarboxylic acids.[34] The clinical significance of this remains to be determined. There is, however, no evidence that the presence of these oxidation products is harmful. In our study, a significant enrichment of dicarboxylic acids was observed in only four of the seven infants studied, indicating that the MCTs present in the formula were adequately catabolized through β-oxidation. In terms of energy balance, this excretory loss of MCT is negligible.

Fat and Total Parenteral Nutrition (TPN)

Intravenous fat emulsions have been given to newborn infants for several years. There is no doubt that some of the intravenously administered fats are used as a source of energy, as evidenced by changes in the concentrations of free fatty acids and ketone bodies[35, 36] and alterations in the respiratory quotient.[36-38] Even when lipoprotein lipase activity is impaired during the first days of life (especially in low birth weight and small for dates infants), the increase in ketone bodies[35] indicates that fat oxidation occurs during total parenteral nutrition. It is currently recommended that intravenous fat should be administered at a dose of 1 to 3 g/kg/day, given continuously over 20 to 24 hours.[39] However, it is not known how much of the infused lipid is oxidized.

Some studies have indicated that oxidation of intravenous fat may be correlated with total energy intake. As shown in Figure 42-1, as caloric intake is increased, the percentage of oxidized calories derived from fat decreases. We have investi-

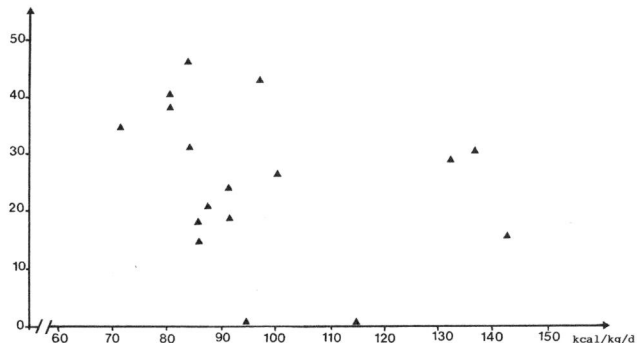

Figure 42–1. Percentage of oxidized calories derived from fat oxidation versus caloric intake during total parenteral nutrition (TPN) with glucose, amino acids, and lipids (data from ref. 40). The increase in energy intake, mostly owing to an increase in fat intake, is obviously not followed by an increase in the oxidation rate of fat. In two infants, fat was almost not oxidized (all infants had triglyceride levels below 100 mg/dL at the time of the study, showing an adequate triglyceride serum clearance).

TABLE 42-4

Difference in Intravenous Fat Oxidation Rates in Neonates (Preterm and Term) on Total Parenteral Nutrition at Two Different Levels of Energy Intake (Calculated from Ref. 40)*

Total Nonprotein Energy Intake (kcal/kg/d)	Fat Intake (g/kg/d)	E. Expenditure (kcal/kg/d)	Fat Oxidation (g/kg/d)	% of E. Expenditure Derived from Fat
102 ± 12 (n = 9)	4.6 ± 1.6	63 ± 12	1.4 ± 0.9	21
73 ± 4 (n = 8)	2.5 ± 0.5	52 ± 3	1.7 ± 0.5	30

* Note that an increase in fat intake (which accounts for almost 70% of the increase of the nonprotein energy intake) is not followed by an increase in fat oxidation rate.

gated this phenomenon in two groups of infants fed glucose, amino acids, and lipids intravenously[40] (Table 42-4); Study Group I received 102 + 12 kcal/kg/day, and Study Group II, 73 + 4 kcal/kg/day as nonprotein energy. All the infants were studied by indirect calorimetry by means of an open-circuit system over several hours. The results of this study indicate that as energy intake in the diet (even as fat) is increased, the portion of energy expenditure derived from fat oxidation and the net amount of fat oxidized are decreased. This information correlates with experimental data in adults demonstrating that an increased oxidation rate of glucose is followed by a decreased oxidation rate of concomitantly infused lipids.[41] When an important part of energy intake is given as glucose, it is likely that glucose oxidation will impair lipid utilization as a fuel during TPN. It is interesting to note that a similar observation has been made in infants receiving oral nutrition (see Table 42-1).

The observation that an increase in fat intake is not followed by a higher rate of fat oxidation when total energy intake is high means that it may not be appropriate to increase the amount of intravenous lipid during total parenteral nutrition (at least when nonprotein energy intake exceeds 80 to 90 kcal/kg/day). When the total nonprotein energy intake is lower, it is possible that more fat will be oxidized and therefore more energy will be provided. Indeed, Rubecz and colleagues[38] have demonstrated a higher rate of fat oxidation when intravenous fat was the only energy provided, and in this experimental design, 85% of the fat infused was oxidized.

REFERENCES

1. Wharton BA: Nutrition and feeding of preterm infants. Oxford, Blackwell, 1987, pp 47–61.
2. Atkinson SA, et al: Human milk feeding in premature infants: protein, fat and carbohydrate balances in the first two weeks of life. J Pediatr 95:617, 1981.
3. Ferrannini E: The theoretical bases of indirect calorimetry: a review. Metabolism 37:287, 1988.
4. Frayn KN: Calculation of substrate oxidation rates in vivo from gaseous exchange. J Appl Physiol 55:628, 1983.
5. Putet G: Lipid metabolism of the micropreemie. Clin Perinatol 27:57, 2000.
6. Battaglia FC, Meschia G: Foetal metabolism and substrate utilization. In Comline RS, et al (eds): Foetal and Neonatal Physiology. Cambridge, Cambridge University Press, 1973, pp 382–397.
7. Battaglia FC, Meschia G: Principal substrates of fetal metabolism. Physiol Rev 58:499, 1978.
8. Girard J, Ferre P: Metabolic and hormonal changes around birth. In Jones CT (ed): Biochemical Development of the Fetus and the Neonate. Amsterdam, Elsevier, 1982, pp 517–551.
9. Girard J, Bougnères P: Adaptations metaboliques à la naissance. In Salle B, Putet G (eds): Alimentation du Nouveau-neá et du Preámatureá. Paris, Doin, 1986, pp 81–102.
10. Sinclair JC: Metabolic rate and temperature control in the newborn. In Goodwin JW, et al (eds): Perinatal Medicine. Toronto, Williams & Wilkins, 1976, pp 558–577.
11. Senterre J, Karlberg P: Respiratory quotient and metabolic rate in normal full-term and small for date newborn infants. Acta Paediatr Scand 59:653, 1970.
12. Chessex P, et al: Quality of growth in premature infants fed their own mother's milk. J Pediatr 102:107, 1983.
13. Freymond D, et al: Energy balance, physical activity and thermogenic effect of feeding in premature infants. Pediatr Res 20:638, 1986.
14. Putet G: Utilisation des triglycéárides à chaine moyenne chez le preámatureá. In Relier JP (ed): Progrès en Neáonatologie. Paris, Karger, 1987, pp 333–344.
15. Putet G, et al: Supplementation of pooled human milk with casein hydrolysate: energy and nitrogen balance and weight gain composition in very low birth weight infants. Pediatr Res 21:458, 1987.
16. Putet G, et al: Nutrient balance, energy utilization and composition of weight gain in very low birth weight infants fed pooled human milk or a preterm formula. J Pediatr 105:79, 1984.
17. Reichman B, et al: Diet, fat accretion and growth in premature infants. N Engl J Med 305:1495, 1981.
18. Schulze K, et al: Energy expenditure, energy balance and composition of weight gain in low birth weight infants fed diets of different protein and energy content. J Pediatr 110:753, 1987.
19. Bell EF, Rios GR: A double walled incubator alters the partition of body heat loss of premature infants. Pediatr Res 17:135, 1983.
20. Marks KH, et al: Day to day energy expenditure variability in low birth weight neonates. Pediatr Res 21:66, 1987.
21. Whyte RK, et al: Energy balance and nitrogen balance in growing low birth weight infants fed human milk or formula. Pediatr Res 17:891, 1983.
22. Mestyan J: Energy metabolism and substrate utilization in the newborn. In Sinclair JC (ed): Temperature Regulation and Energy Metabolism in the Newborn. New York, Grune & Stratton, 1978, pp 39–74.
23. Ginsburg BE, et al: Plasma valine and urinary C-peptide in breast-fed and artificially fed infants up to 6 months of age. Acta Paediatr Scand 73:213, 1984.
24. Gudinchet F, et al: Metabolic cost of growth in very low birth weight infants. Pediatr Res 16:1025, 1982.
25. Huston RK, et al: Nutrient and mineral retention and vitamin D absorption in low birth weight infants: effect of medium chain triglyceride. Pediatrics 72:44, 1983.
26. Roy CC, et al: Correction of the malabsorption of preterm infants with medium chain triglyceride formula. J Pediatr 86:446, 1975.
27. Bitman J, et al: Comparison of the lipid composition of breast milk from mothers of term and preterm infants. Am J Clin Nutr 38:300, 1983.
28. Harzer G, et al: Changing patterns of human milk lipids in the course of lactation and during the day. Am J Clin Nutr 37:612, 1983.
29. Sann L, et al: Effect of oral administration of lipids with 67% medium chain triglycerides on glucose homeostasis in preterm neonates. Metabolism 30:712, 1981.
30. Wu PYK, et al: Medium-chain triglycerides in infant formulas and their relation to plasma and body concentration. Pediatr Res 20:338, 1986.
31. Metha NR, et al: Adherence of medium chain fatty acids to feeding tubes during gavage feeding of human milk fortified with medium-chain triglycerides. J Pediatr 112:474, 1988.
32. Putet G, et al: Medium chain triglycerides as a source of energy in premature infants. In Horisberger M, Bracco U (eds): Lipids in Modern Nutrition. New York, Raven Press, 1987, pp 43–49.
33. Sarda P, et al: Storage of medium chain triglycerides in adipose tissue of orally fed infants. Am J Clin Nutr 45:399, 1987.
34. Whyte RK, et al: Excretion of dicarboxylic acids and ω-1 hydroxy fatty acids by low birth weight infants fed with medium chain triglycerides. Pediatr Res 20:122, 1986.
35. Andrew G, et al: Lipid metabolism in the neonate. III. The ketogenic effect of intralipid infusion in the neonate. J Pediatr 92:995, 1978.
36. Sabel KG, et al: Effects of injected lipid emulsion on oxygen consumption, RQ, triglyceride, free-fatty-acids and β hydroxybutyrate levels in small for gestational age infants. Acta Paediatr Scand 71:63, 1982.
37. Rubecz I, Mestyan J: Energy metabolism and intravenous nutrition of premature infants. II. The response of oxygen consumption respiratory quotient and substrate utilization to infusion of fat emulsion. Biol Neonate 30:66, 1976.
38. Rubecz I, et al: Energy metabolism, substrate utilization and nitrogen balance in parenterally fed post operative neonates and infants. J Pediatr 98:42, 1981.
39. American Academy of Pediatrics, Committee on Nutrition: Use of intravenous fat emulsion in pediatric patients. Pediatrics 68:738, 1981.
40. Putet G, et al: Energy intake and substrate utilization during total parenteral nutrition in newborn. In Wesdrop RIC, Soeters PB (eds): Clinical Nutrition '81. Edinburgh, 1982, pp 63–70.
41. Thiebaud D, et al: Effect of long chain triglyceride infusion on glucose metabolism in man. Metabolism 31:1128, 1982.
42. Sparks JW, et al: An estimate of the caloric requirement of the human fetus. Biol Neonate 38:113, 1980.

Dermot H. Williamson* and Paul S. Thornton

43

Ketone Body Production and Metabolism in the Fetus and Neonate

AVAILABILITY OF KETONE BODIES

Under physiologic conditions, the rate of utilization of ketone bodies is directly proportional to their concentration in the circulation, which in turn represents a balance between production (ketogenesis) by the liver and removal by peripheral tissues. Ketone bodies are excreted in the urine (ketonuria) when the renal threshold is exceeded. The relationship between production and utilization can be disturbed if the utilization of ketone bodies is inhibited by drugs,[1, 2] or if there is a congenital absence of key enzymes required for ketone body utilization (e.g., 3-oxoacid-CoA transferase),[3] or in insulin-deficient states in which there is a metabolic defect in utilization.[4] The concentration of ketone bodies in the blood is extremely sensitive to alterations in the physiologic state. Normoketonemia in humans has been defined as less than 0.2 mmol/L, hyperketonemia as above 0.2 mmol/L, and ketoacidosis (by analogy to the definition of lactic acidosis) as above 7 mmol/L.[5] In adult humans, there are small but characteristic diurnal changes in blood ketone body concentrations.[6] Larger increases in concentration occur in the fasting human and rat, with consumption of a high-fat diet, after exercise, in late pregnancy, and during suckling (Table 43–1). The prevailing blood ketone body concentration in pregnancy will be available to the fetus because the placenta appears to be freely permeable to acetoacetate and 3-hydroxybutyrate.[7,8]

Ketonemia in Pregnancy

The major substrate of the mammalian fetus is considered to be glucose supplied by the mother.[8] However, the concentration of ketone bodies in maternal blood is increased in the last trimester of pregnancy,[5, 7] and high concentrations are attained during delivery, particularly if it is prolonged (ketosis of labor).[7, 8] This increase in blood ketone bodies may, in part, be related to the decrease in food intake around parturition, because women who fast in the second trimester of pregnancy develop hyperketonemia more rapidly than nonpregnant controls.[9, 10] Poorly controlled diabetes during pregnancy (including gestational diabetes) is also likely to lead to wide fluctuations in blood ketone bodies.[11]

Ketonemia in the Neonatal Period

During the suckling period, the neonate is presented with a relatively high-fat and low-carbohydrate diet. Both humans and rats have marked hyperketonemia in the early suckling period, compared with the respective adult fed values (see Table 43–1). In contrast, ketone bodies are not increased to the same extent in the blood of puppies,[12] piglets,[13] and lambs.[14] Nonesterified fatty acids (long and medium chain length) are the major precursors of ketone bodies, and a possible reason for the species differences in neonatal ketonemia may be the fat content of the maternal milk (rat milk contains 14.8 g fat/100 g; sheep milk contains 5.3 g fat/100 g). In addition, the brains of sheep and dogs have a low rate of ketone body utilization, and therefore, the demand for ketone bodies may be less than that in the human or rat.

The hyperketonemia of the neonatal period in the human is a physiologic event, and therefore any change in blood ketone body concentration (decrease or increase) is likely to indicate a pathologic process. Increased ketone bodies may accompany the hypoglycemia associated with certain inborn errors of metabolism, and a decrease may occur in hyperinsulinism. It is therefore advisable to measure blood ketone bodies by a specific enzymatic method[15] in neonates presenting with hypoglycemia or any other abnormality in the concentration of circulating substrates. For example, small for gestational age (SGA) infants have increased blood concentrations of gluconeogenic substrates, in association with decreased blood ketone body concentrations.[16] The latter may be due to defective development of the ketogenic capacity of the liver.

REGULATION OF KETOGENESIS

Our present understanding of the regulation of ketogenesis is mainly based on studies on rats, in particular, during the fed-to-starved transition when there is a large increase (three- to fourfold) in ketogenesis. In addition, a high proportion of the experimental evidence refers to work on perfused livers or isolated hepatocytes from adult rats. Consequently, the regulation of ketogenesis in the adult is briefly reviewed here, and whenever information is available, comparison is made with the neonate or fetus. For further details the reader is referred to more comprehensive reviews.[17-21]

Extrahepatic Regulation

It is convenient to discuss the regulation of ketogenesis in two parts: extrahepatic and intrahepatic. The major precursors of ketone bodies in the postabsorptive state are long chain fatty acids (LCFA), and in all physiologic situations associated with hyperketonemia, including the neonatal period, the plasma concentrations of LCFA are increased (see Table 43–1).[22-25] Extraction of LCFA by the liver is concentration dependent, and a direct relationship between their concentration and the rate of ketogenesis has been shown in rat and man.[26]

Adipose Tissue Lipolysis

In the adult, a key factor in determining the supply of LCFA to the liver is their rate of release (lipolysis) from adipose tissue triacylglycerol stores. Lipolysis is initiated by activation of hormone-sensitive lipase; glucagon, epinephrine, norepinephrine, and thyroxine increase enzyme activity, whereas insulin (and some prostaglandins) have the opposite effect.[27] Isolated human adipocytes from neonates are very sensitive to the lipolytic effects of thyrotropin,[28] which increases in concentration immediately after birth, and therefore may be involved in the regulation of lipolysis in the perinatal period. A decrease in blood glucose (e.g., in starvation, fat feeding) and a concomitant decrease in plasma insulin lead to an increase in lipolysis and efflux of nonesterified fatty acids from adipose tissue. On supplying carbohydrate, the increases in glucose and insulin inhibit lipolysis. The rate of ketogenesis can therefore respond in a reciprocal way to

* Deceased.

Range of Blood Ketone Body Concentrations in Humans and Rats

Situation	Ketone Body Concentration (mmol/L)*	
	Man	*Rat*
Fed normal diet	About 0.1	Up to 0.3
Fed high-fat diet	Up to 3	4-5
Fasted: 12-24 hr	Up to 0.3	1-2
Fasted: 48-72 hr	2-3	2-3
Postexercise	Up to 2	Up to 2
Late pregnancy	Up to 1	Up to 0.3
Late pregnancy: fasted 48 hr	4-6	6-15
Neonate: 0-1 days	0.2-0.5	0.2
Neonate: 5-10 days	0.7-1.0	0.5-1.1
Hypoglycemia	1.5-5	—
Untreated diabetes mellitus	Up to 25	Up to 10

* Concentrations of total ketone bodies (acetoacetate + 3-hydroxybutyrate measured enzymatically) for whole blood.

the availability of glucose in the circulation, and thus an alternative fuel for the brain is provided when needed (Figs. 43-1 and 43-2). During suckling in the rat, the plasma insulin/glucagon ratio is decreased, thus favoring lipolysis.[29-30]

There is evidence that ketone bodies can regulate their own formation by feedback mechanisms on adipose tissue (Fig. 43-3) to decrease lipolysis. Present evidence suggests two mechanisms: direct inhibition of lipolysis by ketone bodies and an indirect effect via stimulation of insulin secretion[31,32] (see Fig. 43-3). Work with the perfused rat pancreas suggests that ketone bodies increase insulin secretion only at concentrations above 1 mM.[33] These feedback mechanisms have not been investigated in neonates.

In the suckling neonate, another important source of precursors for ketogenesis is the medium chain fatty acids (MCFA; 12 or less carbons) of maternal milk.[34] These are in the form of triacylglycerols (one MCFA and two LCFA per triacylglycerol) and are hydrolyzed by the action of lingual lipase. They are rapidly absorbed from the stomach into the portal venous system[35] and are therefore directly available to the liver, unlike LCFA derived from milk lipids, which are transported as triacylglycerols (chylomicrons) via the lymphatic system and initially enter the peripheral circulation (Fig. 43-4).

In the neonatal period, chylomicrons may provide a direct source of LCFA for the liver, because of the presence of lipoprotein lipase (responsible for the hydrolysis of triacylglycerols contained in chylomicrons to LCFA) in neonatal rat liver[36] (see Fig. 43-4). However, the total activity in liver is only a small percentage (3%) of that in the carcass,[34] presumably mainly muscle and adipose tissue.

Intrahepatic Regulation

It is generally considered that liver is the sole tissue capable of synthesis and release of ketone bodies to the circulation. However, ketone bodies can be formed by the intestinal mucosa of neonatal rats; this is due to the presence of an active hydroxymethylglutaryl (HMG)-CoA pathway (Fig. 43-5) during suckling.[37, 38] Research has shown that the expression of the key enzyme, HMG-CoA synthase, in intestinal mucosa is suppressed in weaning suckling rats.[39,40] The rate of intestinal ketogenesis is less than 10% of that in suckling liver, but it does represent an additional strategy for supplying ketone bodies to developing tissues.[34]

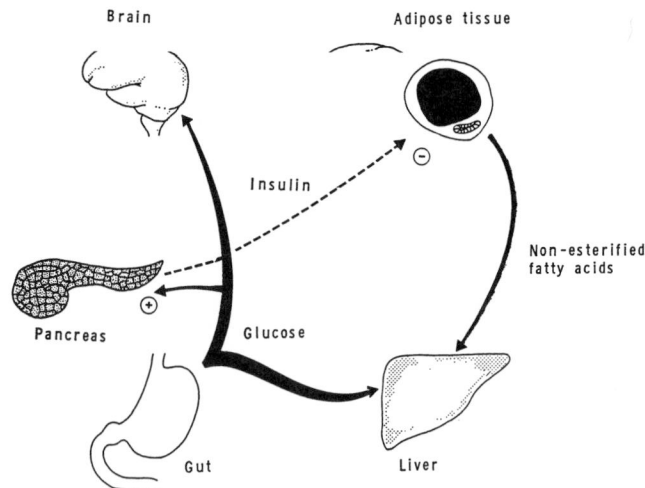

Figure 43-1. Intertissue fluxes in the fed state. Thickness of line denotes rate of flux.

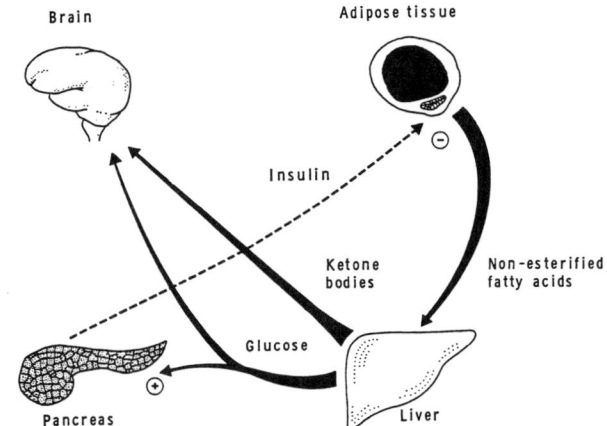

Figure 43-2. Intertissue fluxes in the starved state.

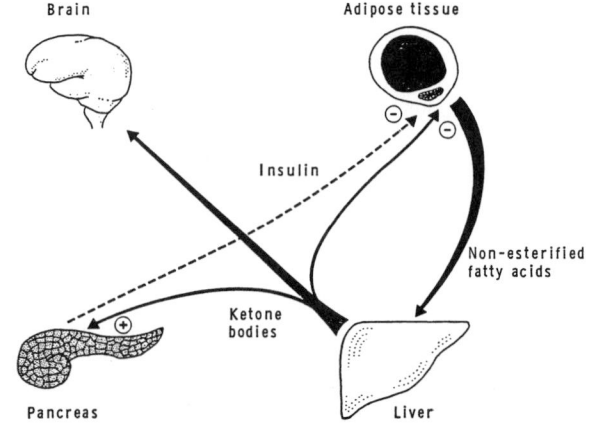

Figure 43-3. Role of ketone bodies as feedback regulators.

Pathway of Fatty Acid Catabolism

LCFA derived from adipose tissue are transported in the plasma bound to albumin, cross the cell membrane as free fatty acids, and then bind again to cytosolic binding proteins.[32] Within the

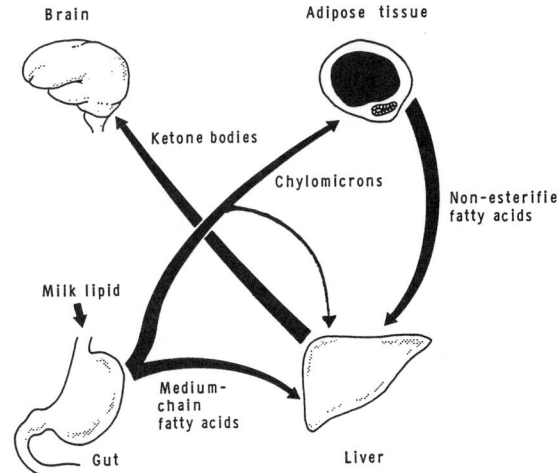

Figure 43–4. Intertissue fluxes in the suckling neonate.

liver, either the LCFA can be re-esterified to form triacylglycerols (for subsequent secretion as very low density lipoprotein) and phospholipids, or they can enter the mitochondria via the carnitine acyltransferase system to undergo β-oxidation. The resultant acetyl-CoA can be converted to ketone bodies (acetoacetate and 3-hydroxybutyrate) via the hydroxymethylglutaryl-CoA (HMG-CoA) pathway, or it can undergo complete oxidation in the tricarboxylic acid cycle (see Fig. 43-5). In contrast, MCFA are not converted to triacylglycerols in mammalian liver and can directly cross the inner mitochondrial membrane, thus bypassing the carnitine acyltransferase system. Within the mitochondrial matrix, the MCFA are converted to the corresponding acyl-CoA derivatives by acyl-CoA synthetases and then undergo β-oxidation (see Fig. 43-5).

Changes in Neonatal Liver

As might be expected because of the relative impermeability of the placenta to LCFA,[41] the concentration of the cytosolic fatty acid binding protein is very low in fetal liver and gradually increases (about 20-fold) to reach adult values; there is no

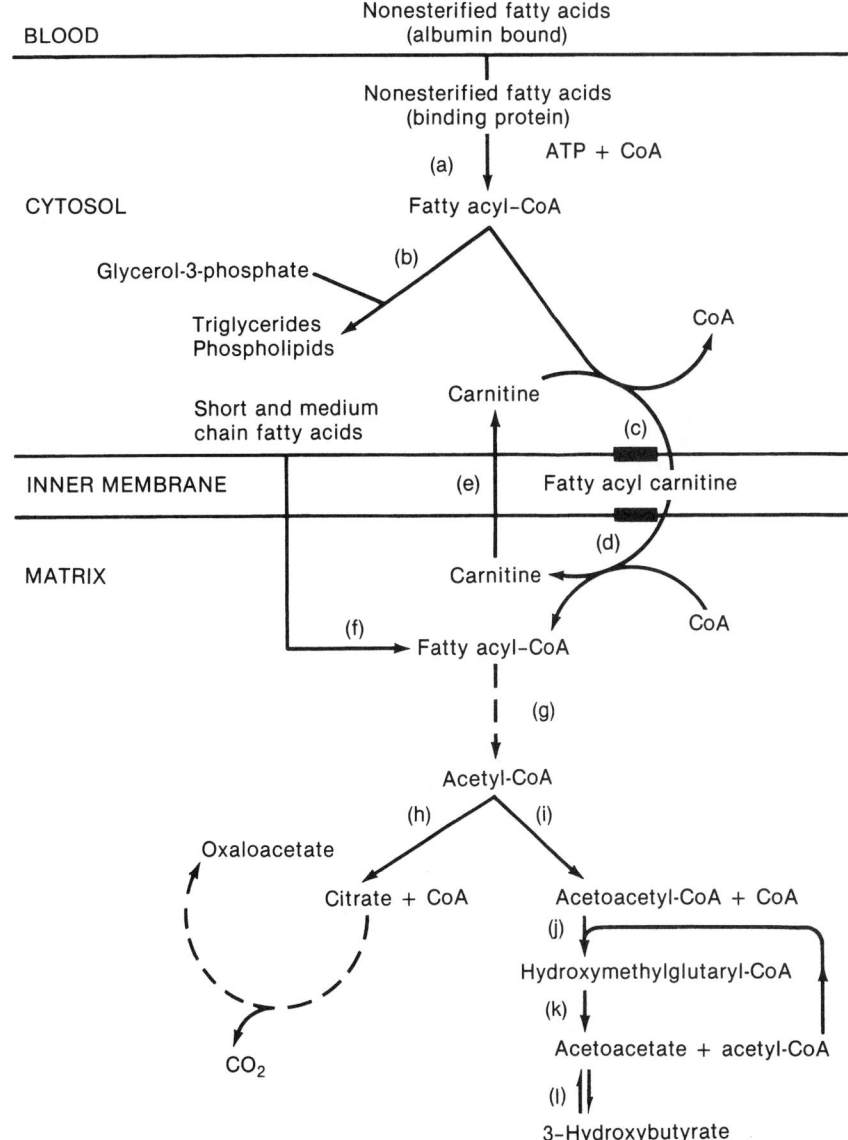

Figure 43–5. Pathway of fatty acid catabolism in liver. Enzymes involved: (*a*) long chain fatty acyl-CoA synthetase; (*b*) glycerol-3-phosphate acyl-transferase; (*c*) carnitine acyltransferase I; (*d*) carnitine acyltransferase II; (*e*) carnitine exchange; (*f*) short and medium chain fatty acyl-CoA synthetase; (*g*) fatty acid oxidation complex; (*h*) citrate synthase; (*i*) acetoacetyl-CoA thiolase; (*j*) hydroxymethylglutaryl-CoA synthase; (*k*) hydroxymethylglutaryl-CoA lyase; (*l*) hydroxybutyrate dehydrogenase.

evidence for a peak concentration of the protein in livers from suckling rats.[42]

Liver of fetal rats has a low capacity for fatty acid catabolism and ketogenesis, and this is rapidly increased after birth. The signals and mechanisms regulating the maturation of ketogenesis in the perinatal period are not completely understood.[43] For a review of this area, see reference[44]. There is evidence that the capacity of the liver for LCFA catabolism is increased in the suckling period. A number of the key enzymes show higher activities,[45-47] particularly carnitine acyltransferase-I [EC 2.3.1.21], which increases at birth and attains values three- to sixfold higher than those of the adult within a few days of parturition; it then declines rapidly on weaning.[47] These increases in enzyme activity[45-47] are paralleled by higher rates of ketogenesis from LCFA in isolated hepatocytes from suckling rats compared with adult rats.[48,49]

The rate of ketogenesis from MCFA is not increased in hepatocytes from suckling rats compared with those from adult animals,[48] which suggests that the increased ketogenesis from LCFA during the neonatal period is connected with either their esterification or entry into the mitochondria via the carnitine acyltransferase transport system.

Role of Malonyl-CoA

In adult liver, carnitine acyltransferase-I is regulated by short-term changes in the concentration of carnitine (a co-substrate) and malonyl-CoA (a potent inhibitor of carnitine acyltransferase-I).[17] Malonyl-CoA is a key intermediate in the conversion of carbohydrate into fat, and the hepatic concentration is directly correlated with the rate of lipogenesis (*de novo* fatty acid synthesis).[50] In liver, the major lipogenic precursor is pyruvate, formed from lactate returning to the liver as a product of glycolysis in peripheral tissues or from hepatic glycogen via glycogenolysis and glycolysis (Fig. 43–6). Therefore, the rate of lipogenesis and the concentration of malonyl-CoA indicate the carbohydrate status of the liver; a high rate of lipogenesis is associated with an elevated malonyl-CoA, inhibition of carnitine acyltransferase-I, and a decreased rate of ketogenesis. Conversely, a decrease in lipogenesis due to lack of substrate or hormonal inactivation of the key enzyme[51] acetyl-CoA carboxylase [EC 6.4.1.2] results in a decrease in malonyl-CoA and a stimulation of ketogenesis owing to increased entry of long chain

acyl-CoA into the mitochondria (see Fig. 43–6). In addition, it appears that the sensitivity of carnitine acyltransferase-I to inhibition by malonyl-CoA is affected by change in the physiologic state[52,53]; it decreases during suckling.[54,55]

In suckling liver, the rate of lipogenesis in isolated hepatocytes[48] and *in vivo*[56] is low, and this is mainly due to the decrease in the activities of key lipogenic enzymes (e.g., acetyl-CoA carboxylase[57] and fatty acid synthetase[58]); this pattern is rapidly reversed on weaning. It is therefore reasonable to assume that hepatic malonyl-CoA is very low during suckling and cannot be altered acutely. This fact, together with the decreased sensitivity of carnitine acyltransferase-I to inhibition by malonyl-CoA,[54,55] suggests that in the suckling neonate, regulation of ketogenesis (once maturation has occurred) depends on both substrate supply and the increased capacity of the mitochondria for fatty acid catabolism, particularly the entry of long chain acyl-CoA. An outstanding question is the nature of the signal or signals which brings about the stimulation of ketogenesis immediately after birth.[43,44,59] One possibility is the acute decrease in the insulin/glucagon ratio.[30,44]

Role of Insulin and Glucagon

The role of hormones in regulating the supply of LCFA to the liver has already been discussed. It might be expected that insulin and glucagon would also act directly on the liver. Glucagon or dibutyryl cAMP (the second messenger) stimulates ketogenesis from LCFA in perfused livers[60,61] and isolated hepatocytes[48] from adult rats. Dibutyryl cAMP or glucagon does not increase ketogenesis from MCFA,[62,63] suggesting that the site of action of glucagon is on the disposition of long chain acyl-CoA between the pathways of esterification and β-oxidation (see Fig. 43–6). A possible mechanism for the effects of glucagon on ketogenesis is the finding that the hormone (or cAMP) inhibits hepatic lipogenesis *in vivo*[64] and *in vitro*[64,65] and, consequently, decreases the concentration of malonyl-CoA.[50] The site of inhibition is acetyl-CoA carboxylase, which is inactivated by glucagon via increased phosphorylation of the protein.[51] However, other sites of action of glucagon cannot be ruled out because cAMP still stimulates ketogenesis and decreases esterification of LCFA in isolated hepatocytes when an inhibitor of lipogenesis is present,[48] and malonyl-CoA is presumably low.

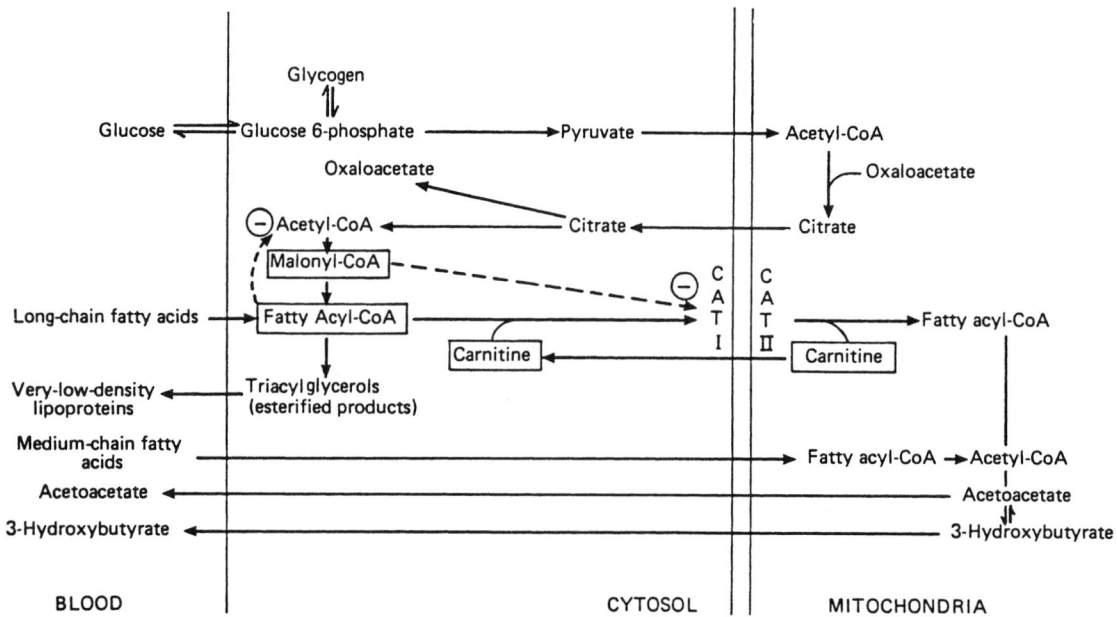

Figure 43–6. Interrelationship between hepatic carbohydrate metabolism, lipogenesis, and ketogenesis. Circled minus signs indicate sites of inhibition by metabolite.

Decreased esterification of LCFA by microsomal fractions isolated from livers of fed rats perfused with dibutyryl cAMP has been reported.[66] Activation of carnitine acyltransferase-I by glucagon (or cAMP) has been described.[67] In hepatocytes from suckling rats, dibutyryl cAMP has no effect on ketogenesis.[48] This may be due to the elevation of cAMP in neonatal hepatocytes[8] and the consequent maximal stimulation of ketogenesis. Alternatively, it can be argued that because of the low rate of lipogenesis in neonatal hepatocytes, glucagon (cAMP) addition does not lead to a further decrease in the already low concentration of malonyl-CoA. Additional evidence that hepatocytes from neonatal rats are maximally stimulated is the finding that starvation of neonatal rats, unlike the situation in adult rats, does not further increase the rate of ketogenesis from LCFA *in vitro*.[49]

By analogy to its potent antilipolytic effect on adipocytes, it might be expected that insulin would exert a direct antiketogenic effect on the liver. However, unlike glucagon, demonstration of direct hepatic effects of insulin has proved comparatively elusive.[63] It is generally considered that in adult liver, insulin stimulates the *de novo* synthesis of fatty acids, in part by activation of acetyl-CoA carboxylase,[51] which in turn increases malonyl-CoA. It is therefore not surprising that in perfused livers of adult rats, insulin decreases the oxidation of LCFA and increases the rate of their esterification.[68] There has been little investigation of the effects of insulin on LCFA catabolism in neonatal liver. Administration of insulin to suckling rat pups decreases blood ketone body concentrations without altering the concentration of plasma LCFA, suggesting a direct antiketogenic effect of the hormone not mediated by a change in LCFA supply to the liver.[69] It is known that livers of suckling rats[31] and human neonates[70] are resistant to the suppressive effects of insulin on glucose production, and this may also extend to its effects on lipid metabolism. It must be emphasized that any putative direct hepatic actions of glucagon or insulin discussed earlier are not likely to affect MCFA metabolism, which appears to have preference over LCFA in suckling liver.[71] This may be important in the formulation of infant feeds.[72]

Thus, a number of changes favor a high rate of ketogenesis in the suckling neonate (Table 43–2); all these are reversed if the neonate is weaned on to a high-carbohydrate diet.

Fatty Acid Catabolism in Fetal Liver

LCFA cannot readily cross the placental barrier,[41] and the capacity of fetal liver to oxidize them and form ketone bodies is very low.[45,73] Ketone body formation by livers of early human fetuses has been demonstrated.[74]

KETONE BODY UTILIZATION

Assuming that ketone bodies are available in the circulation, their rate of utilization is to a large extent regulated by the prevailing concentration.[75] Transport of ketone bodies through the plasma membrane or mitochondrial inner membranes is not considered to limit their utilization in muscle because the tissue concentration is linearly related to the plasma concentration.[76] This may not be true for brain because the ketone body concentrations in rat brain[77] and human cerebrospinal fluid[78] are considerably less than those of blood in hyperketonemic states. Within the cell, the metabolism of ketone bodies depends on the activities of the "initiating" enzymes, which allow their entry into the metabolic pathways of the cell. The acetyl-CoA formed from ketone bodies either is completely oxidized in the tricarboxylic acid cycle to provide energy (ATP) or is used as a precursor of fatty acid or sterol (cholesterol) synthesis. The pathways of ketone body utilization are shown in Figure 43–7. (For a more detailed review of ketone body metabolism in peripheral tissues, refer to reference 32.)

TABLE 43-2

Changes That Favor Ketogenesis in Suckling Rats

Factor	Change *	References
Plasma insulin	Decreased	29, 30, 44
Plasma glucagon	Increased	29, 30, 44
Insulin/glucagon ratio	Decreased	29, 30, 44
Plasma LCFA	Increased	24
Hepatic carnitine acyltransferase–I activity	Increased	47
Sensitivity of carnitine acyltransferase–I to malonyl-CoA inhibition	Decreased	54, 55
Hepatic [carnitine]	Increased	143
Hepatic lipogenesis	Decreased	48, 56
Hepatic [malonyl-CoA]	Decreased†	—

* The comparisons are relative to the adult fed rat, which has a low rate of ketogenesis.
† Malonyl-CoA has not been measured in neonatal rat liver, but it is reasonable to assume that it is low.

Pathways of Ketone Body Utilization

Mitochondrial Pathway

As might be expected in view of its role as an energy-yielding substrate, the major site of ketone body utilization is the mitochondria. The initiating enzyme for acetoacetate metabolism is 3-oxoacid CoA transferase [EC 2.8.3.5], which carries out the following reversible reaction:

$$\text{Acetoacetate} + \text{succinyl-CoA} \rightleftharpoons \text{acetoacetyl-CoA} + \text{succinate}$$

The succinyl-CoA is derived from the tricarboxylic acid cycle and as succinate is returned to the cycle; there is no loss of cycle intermediates. The equilibrium of the reaction is in favor of acetoacetate formation. The K_m value (around 0.2 mM) of 3-oxoacid CoA transferase for acetoacetate and its kinetic properties are similar in different rat tissues.[79] The transferase of rat tissues is inhibited by acetoacetate at concentrations in excess of 5 mM, and this inhibition may depress ketone body utilization in severe hyperketonemic situations.[80]

The acetoacetyl-CoA formed is cleaved by acetoacetyl-CoA thiolase [EC 2.3.1.9] to yield 2 molecules of acetyl-CoA:

$$\text{Acetoacetyl-CoA} + \text{CoA} \rightleftharpoons 2 \text{ acetyl-CoA}$$

The equilibrium of this reaction is strongly in favor of acetyl-CoA formation, and when this reaction is coupled with that of the 3-oxoacid CoA transferase, utilization of acetoacetate is favored. Acetoacetyl-CoA thiolase, unlike the transferase, is present in both the mitochondrial matrix and the cytosol.[81]

D-(-)-3-Hydroxybutyrate is oxidized to acetoacetate by 3-hydroxybutyrate dehydrogenase [EC 1.1.1.30].

$$\text{D-(-)-3-hydroxybutyrate} + \text{NAD}^+ \rightleftharpoons \text{acetoacetate} + \text{NADH} + \text{H}^+$$

The reaction is reversible, but the equilibrium is in favor of acetoacetate reduction. The dehydrogenase is tightly bound to the inner mitochondrial membrane.

Unlike the hepatic hydroxymethylglutaryl-CoA pathway for synthesis of ketone bodies (see Fig. 43–5), the mitochondrial utilization pathway is freely reversible. Assuming that the cell contains sufficient activity of the three enzymes to catalyze near-equilibrium between the three reactions, the utilization of ketone bodies depends on the prevailing concentrations of 3-hydroxybutyrate and acetoacetate and the rate of removal of acetyl-CoA. The latter depends on the activity of the tricarboxylic

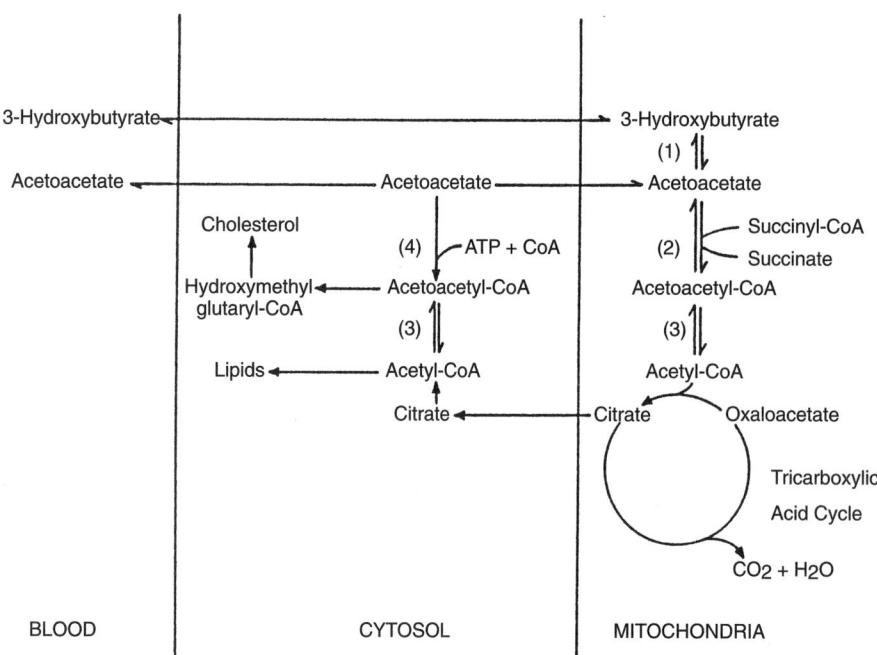

Figure 43–7. Pathways of ketone body utilization in peripheral tissues. (*1*) Hydroxybutyrate dehydrogenase; (*2*) 3-oxoacid–CoA transferase; (*3*) acetoacetyl–CoA thiolase; (*4*) acetoacetyl–CoA synthetase.

acid cycle and on the rate of acetyl-CoA formation from other substrates, mainly oxidation of fatty acids. This explains why it is possible to demonstrate net formation of ketone bodies *in vitro* when kidney slices are incubated with fatty acids.[82] Thus, in certain tissues, the free reversibility of the pathway can be viewed as means of "buffering" the mitochondrial acetyl-CoA pool. Of course, the concentrations of co-substrates (succinyl-CoA, succinate) and cofactors (CoA, NAD+, NADH) may also influence the utilization of ketone bodies.

As already stated, the major role of the mitochondrial pathway is to allow complete oxidation of ketone bodies for energy supply; however, in tissues with active lipogenesis, a portion of the acetyl-CoA is transported to the cytosol in the form of citrate to act as a precursor for lipid synthesis (see Fig. 43-7).

Cytosolic Pathway

The cytosol of all lipogenic tissues (brown and white adipose tissue, developing brain, lactating mammary gland, and liver) contains an enzyme, acetoacetyl-CoA synthetase, that converts acetoacetate into acetoacetyl-CoA:[83-85]

$$\text{Acetoacetate} + \text{ATP} + \text{CoA} \rightarrow \text{acetoacetyl-CoA} + \text{AMP} + \text{pyrophosphate}$$

This reaction is virtually irreversible, and its activity is, at most, 10% of that of the 3-oxoacid CoA transferase. However, the enzyme has a high affinity (K_m 50 μM) for acetoacetate and is therefore probably saturated with substrate even in the fed state.

The presence of 3-hydroxy-3-methylglutaryl-CoA synthase [EC.4.1.3.5] and acetoacetyl-CoA thiolase in the cytosol of the lipogenic tissues allows the acetoacetyl-CoA from acetoacetate to enter the pathway of sterol synthesis (see Fig. 43-7). Evidence for the preferential conversion of acetoacetate to sterols rather than lipids exists in suckling rat brain *in vivo*[86,87] and in adult rat liver *in vitro*.[88] The activity of acetoacetyl-CoA synthetase is very low in suckling rat liver and increases on weaning.[84, 85] Although of comparatively low activity compared with that of the mitochondrial pathway, the cytosolic pathway allows the specific direction of acetoacetate to lipid or sterol synthesis (see Fig. 43-7). The fact that the cytosolic pathway is irreversible means that the flux is unidirectional, and this, together with the delivery of acetoacetyl-CoA and acetyl-CoA at the site of utiliza-

tion, may be the physiologic advantage of this pathway over the mitochondrial pathway.

4.1.3 Utilization of L–(+)-3-Hydroxybutyrate

It is generally accepted that D-(-)-3-hydroxybutyrate, the isomer present in biologic fluids, is the physiologic substrate. However, the L-(+) isomer can also be used by mammalian tissues,[88-91] although its presence in the circulation has not yet been demonstrated. A comprehensive study of the enzymes of L-(+)-3-hydroxybutyrate metabolism in the adult rat has been reported.[92] In suckling rat brain, there is evidence that the L-(+) isomer can be effectively used for synthesis of fatty acids and sterols.[91,92] These findings may be important when DL-3-hydroxybutyrate is administered to humans.

Acetone as a Gluconeogenic Precursor

Acetone is produced by decarboxylation of acetoacetate

$$\text{Acetoacetate} \rightarrow \text{acetone} + CO_2$$

and it can reach high concentrations in blood in states of prolonged hyperketonemia (starvation, diabetic ketoacidosis). The rate of chemical decarboxylation is insufficient to explain the rate of acetone formation, and therefore, tissue acetoacetate decarboxylases have been implicated.[93] A rat kidney enzyme has been studied that has a K_m for acetone around 1 mM and is competitively inhibited by its substrate.[93]

Although early radioactive tracer experiments demonstrated that [2-14C]-acetone can be converted to liver glycogen,[94] only recently has this been investigated in detail,[93,95] and net conversion of acetone to glucose has been measured in rat hepatocytes.[96] The pathways for acetone conversion to glucose are shown in Figure 43-8. Present evidence suggests that at low acetone concentrations (physiologic situations), most of the acetone is converted to glucose, but that at high concentrations (hyperketonemia), the acetone is mainly converted to acetate[95] (see Fig. 43-8). A study in human diabetic ketoacidosis with [2-14C]-acetone indicated that some 10% of the newly gained glucose carbons were derived from acetone.[97] This rate of conversion of fat to carbohydrate (fatty acid oxidation → acetoacetate → acetone → glucose) is not insignificant and deserves investigation in neonatal liver.

Enzyme Activity

Adult Tissues

The relative activities of the enzymes of ketone body utilization in adult rat tissues are given in Table 43–3. The mitochondrial pathway is most active in kidney, heart, brown adipose tissue, and adrenal gland, followed by submaxillary gland, lactating mammary gland, and brain (see Table 43–3). The activities do not change appreciably during short-term fat feeding, starvation, or alloxan-induced diabetes.[22, 98, 99] In contrast, the cytosolic pathway enzyme acetoacetyl-CoA synthetase is more sensitive to alterations of hormonal and nutritional state.[83, 85, 100]

Neonatal Tissues

In contrast to the adult, the enzymes of ketone body utilization show marked changes in activity during development of the rat, and the pattern is tissue-specific. The activities of 3-hydroxybutyrate dehydrogenase and 3-oxoacid transferase increase after birth to reach adult levels by about 5 days' postpartum and then continue to rise until just before weaning, when the values are two- to threefold higher than those of the adult.[22, 24, 47, 101-103] Experiments indicate that the amount of 3-oxoacid-CoA transferase mRNA is threefold higher in suckling rat brain than in fetal or adult brain.[104] Experiments with a modified milk formula low in fat have shown that the physiologic hyperketonemia in the neonatal period is not essential for the normal development of 3-oxoacid-CoA transferase in rat brain.[105]

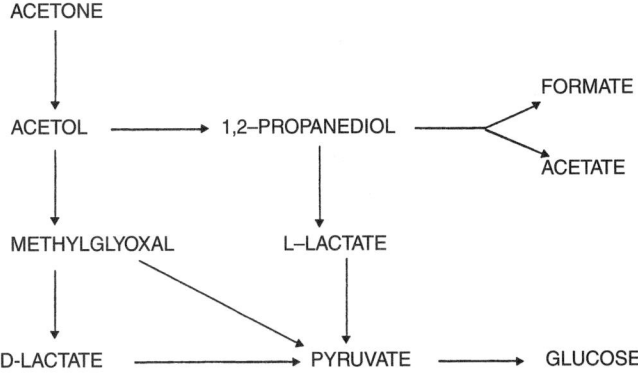

Figure 43–8. Pathways in the conversion of acetone to glucose.

In contrast, in the two adult tissues that have the highest activity of these enzymes, namely kidney and heart (see Table 43–3), the activities remain below the adult values throughout the suckling period. If, in addition, one takes into account the changes in tissue mass during development, it is clear that neonatal brain is the major site for ketone body utilization.

The activities of the cytosolic pathway enzymes (see Fig. 43–7) are also higher in neonatal rat brain,[84, 106] which agrees with their postulated role in lipogenesis (myelinization).

This pattern of increased capacity for utilization of ketone bodies in neonatal rat brain is not shown in other species. In neonatal pigs, the concentration of blood ketone bodies is low,[13, 107] and the brain activity of 3-oxoacid-CoA transferase is barely detectable.[108] In contrast to the rat, the transferase activity in neonatal pig heart and kidney is considerably higher than that in neonatal pig brain.[108] Similarly, the activities of 3-oxoacid-CoA transferase and 3-hydroxybutyrate dehydrogenase remain low throughout the neonatal period in guinea pig brain.[109] There is a lack of data on the activities of the enzymes of ketone body utilization in human neonatal tissues. Where information on postmortem material is available, it suggests that in brain, the activities of the mitochondrial pathway enzymes remain comparatively constant throughout the postnatal period.[110, 111]

Effects of Ketone Bodies on Glucose Metabolism

Glucose Utilization

It is well established that physiologic concentrations of acetoacetate and 3-hydroxybutyrate decrease glucose utilization in a number of adult rat tissues, including heart, soleus muscle, kidney, brain, and lactating mammary gland.[32] These tissues all exhibit high rates of glycolysis and utilization of the pyruvate formed from glucose-6-phosphate. Consequently, if glucose metabolism was not inhibited in situations associated with carbohydrate lack, the animal would rapidly become hypoglycemic. The mechanism for the inhibition of glucose metabolism by ketone bodies was established by the studies of Randle and colleagues[112] and involves inhibition of the enzymes phosphofructokinase [EC 2.7.1.11] and hexokinase [EC 2.7.1.1] and inactivation of pyruvate dehydrogenase [EC 1.2.4.1]. The overall effect is decreased glucose utilization. In addition, a higher proportion of any glucose that still undergoes glycolysis leaves the tissue as lactate and pyruvate and returns to the liver for gluconeogenesis. No systematic investigation of this "sparing" of

TABLE 43-3

Relative Activities of Enzymes of Ketone Body Utilization in Adult Rat Tissues

Tissue	Relative Enzyme Activity*			
	3-Oxoacid-CoA Transferase	Acetoacetyl-CoA Thiolase	3-Hydroxybutyrate Dehydrogenase	Acetoacetyl-CoA Synthetase
Adipose tissue (white)	0.14	0.05	—	1.0
Adipose tissue (brown)	6.9	10.0	—	—
Adrenal gland	2.7	14.8	4.2	—
Brain	1.0	1.0	1.0	1.0
Heart	12.4	4.2	4.2	—
Kidney	12.4	6.9	6.7	—
Liver	0.2	12.9	20.7	6.7[†]
Lung	0.8	0.3	—	—
Mammary gland	2.7	1.2	1.3	10
Muscle (hind limb)	0.4	0.3	1.0	—
Submaxillary gland	3.2	1.1	—	—

* The respective enzyme activities (μmol/min per g fresh wt. at 25°C) of adult rat brain were set at unity (transferase: 2.1; thiolase: 2.1; dehydrogenase: 0.6; synthetase: 0.01). For further details, see refs. 32, 141, 142, 144.
† Higher values reported during dark phase.[48]

glucose by ketone bodies appears to have been made in neonatal tissues. However, in normal children, there is an inverse correlation between glucose flux and the degree of ketonemia.[113] This supports the view that glucose and ketone body interactions operate at the whole body level.

Glucose Production

Ketone bodies can alter hepatic glucose production by their effects on the supply of two important precursors, glycerol and alanine. Ketone bodies decrease flux of glycerol to the liver by their antilipolytic action on adipose tissue and apparently also on muscle triacylglycerol stores.[114] Hypoalaninemia is present in a number of situations associated with hyperketonemia, including starvation, diabetes, and ketotic hypoglycemia of childhood and can be induced by infusion of 3-hydroxybutyrate.[115] The mechanism by which ketone bodies decrease muscle release of alanine is still unknown. There are two possibilities: (1) inhibition of muscle glycolysis decreases pyruvate availability to form alanine by transamination, or (2) a direct inhibition of muscle proteolysis.

Roles of Ketone Bodies in Neonatal Tissues

Only three neonatal tissues of the rat, namely, brain, lung, and brown adipose tissue, have been examined in any detail with regard to ketone body metabolism. The findings are briefly discussed.

Brain

Arteriovenous difference measurements across the brain of adult and suckling rats have shown, for a given arterial concentration of ketone bodies, that the extraction by suckling brain is three- to fourfold higher.[77, 116] This is in agreement with the higher activities of the enzymes of ketone body utilization in suckling brain. A similar increase in ketone body extraction by brain has been demonstrated when human neonates and adults have been compared.[117,118] However, no appreciable increase in the activities of the enzymes of ketone body utilization have been demonstrated in human neonatal brain.[110, 118] Therefore, the increased utilization in the human neonatal brain is likely to be due to another factor. A possibility is increased cerebral permeability to ketone bodies as demonstrated in neonatal rat brain.[119]

The major portion (90%) of the ketone bodies used by suckling brain is likely to be completely oxidized to provide energy[120] and thus spare glucose. However, it is now well established that a portion of the carbon (5 to 10%) is converted to fatty acids and cholesterol.[86,106,111,120,121]

Ketone bodies inhibit glucose utilization in a number of rat tissues, but this is not the case in brain.[122,123] They do, however, decrease glucose oxidation and its conversion to lipid,[122,124] suggesting inhibition of pyruvate dehydrogenase. Support for this hypothesis is the correlation between ketone body extraction by the brain and the proportion of extracted glucose released as lactate and pyruvate in rat[123] and humans.[125]

It must be emphasized that measurements of arteriovenous differences or enzyme activities in whole brain give no information on the regional utilization of ketone bodies within the brain. This question has been addressed in some elegant experiments,[126] and it appears that the telencephalon uses the most ketone bodies and the hind brain the least.[126,127]

Lung

Like neonatal brain, the developing lung has a specific requirement for the synthesis of complex lipids, that is, pulmonary surfactant. *In vivo* synthesis of lipids is more rapid from acetoacetate than from glucose, and the incorporation of ketone bodies appears to occur via direct generation of cytosolic acetyl-CoA.[128] The presence of cytoplasmic aceto-acetyl-CoA synthetase and acetoacetyl-CoA thiolase and their developmental pattern,

which parallels that of acetoacetate incorporation into fatty acids, indicates that the cytoplasmic pathway (see Fig. 43–7) is as important in this tissue in the immediate postnatal period[129] as it is in developing brain.

Fetal Tissues

As already discussed, the fetus is exposed to the concentrations of ketone bodies present in maternal blood. The utilization of ketone bodies as oxidizable substrates has been demonstrated in the fetal human brain[130] and in several tissues of the fetal rat,[131] including liver.[132] However, the interpretation of these findings is not clear because, in some experiments, the tracer used was DL-[3-^{14}C]hydroxybutyrate and the metabolism of the nonphysiologic L-isomer may have made a contribution to $^{14}CO_2$ production. Ketone bodies can also act as lipogenic substrates in the fetus.[133] Injection of D-[3-^{14}C]hydroxybutyrate into the femoral vein of pregnant rats in late gestation results in significant incorporation into the lipids of a number of tissues,[133] the greatest relative incorporation on a per gram basis being into brown adipose tissue.

Ketone Bodies and the Embryo

In contrast to fetal and neonatal tissues, the rates of $^{14}CO_2$ production by mouse conceptuses *in vitro* from DL-[3-^{14}C]hydroxybutyrate are higher than those from the D-isomer, suggesting that utilization of the L-isomer is greater.[134] Of some concern is the finding that DL-3-hydroxybutyrate has a teratogenic effect on rodent embryos in culture,[135-137] and the malformations are similar to those observed in offspring of human diabetics.[138] One potential mechanism appears to be inhibition of the oxidative pentosephosphate pathway of glucose metabolism,[139] which supplies ribose moieties for pyrimidine synthesis. It may be relevant that DL-3-hydroxybutyrate also inhibits the synthesis of pyrimidines in fetal brain slices.[139] Ribose supplementation will maintain the rate of DNA synthesis in embryos exposed to DL-3-hydroxybutyrate,[140] which is consistent with the proposed mechanism of action of the hydroxybutyrate.

It would thus appear that increased maternal blood concentrations of ketone bodies in the first weeks of pregnancy due to malnutrition or insulin deficiency (diabetes mellitus) may lead to malformations in the embryo and subsequent abortion. One can view this as a mechanism for terminating pregnancy in adverse conditions.

REFERENCES

1. Stacpoole PW, et al: Metabolic effects of dichloroacetate in patients with diabetes mellitus and hyperlipoproteinemia. N Engl J Med *298*:526, 1978.
2. Williamson DH, Wilson MB: The effects of cyclopropane derivatives on ketone-body metabolism in vivo. Biochem J *94*:19C, 1965.
3. Tildon JT, Cornblath M: Succinyl-CoA 3-ketoacid CoA transferase deficiency. A cause for ketoacidosis in infancy. J Clin Invest *51*:493, 1972.
4. Sherwin RS, et al: Effect of diabetes mellitus and insulin on the turnover and metabolic response to ketones in man. Diabetes *25*:776, 1976.
5. Williamson DH: The production and utilization of ketone bodies in the neonate. *In* Jones CT (ed): Biochemical Development of the Fetus and Neonate. Amsterdam, Elsevier Biomedical Press 1982, pp 621–650.
6. Wildenhoff KE, et al: Diurnal variation in the concentrations of blood acetoacetate and 3-hydroxybutyrate. Acta Med Scand *195*:25, 1974.
7. Paterson P, et al: Maternal and fetal ketone concentrations in plasma and urine. Lancet *1*:862, 1967.
8. Sabata V, et al: The role of free fatty acids, glycerol, ketone bodies and glucose in the energy metabolism of the mother and fetus during delivery. Biol Neonate *13*:7, 1968.
9. Felig P, Lynch V: Starvation in human pregnancy: hypoglycaemia, hypoinsulinaemia and hyperketonaemia. Science *170*:990, 1970.
10. Kim YJ, Felig P: Maternal and amniotic fluid substrate levels during caloric deprivation in human pregnancy. Metabolism *21*:507, 1972.
11. Persson B, Lunell NO: Metabolic control in diabetic pregnancy. Am J Obstet Gynecol *122*:737, 1975.
12. Spitzer JJ, Weng JT: Removal and utilization of ketone bodies by the brain of newborn puppies. J Neurochem *19*:2169, 1972.

13. Gentz J, et al: Metabolic effects of starvation during the neonatal period in the piglet. Am J Physiol *218*:662, 1976.

14. Varnam GCE, et al: Hepatic ketone body metabolism in developing sheep and pregnant ewes. Br J Nutr *40*:359, 1978.

15. Williamson DH, et al: Enzymic determination of D(-)-β-hydroxybutyric acid and acetoacetic acid in blood. Biochem J *82*:90, 1962.

16. Haymond MW, et al: Increased gluconeogenic substrates in the small for gestational age infant. N Engl J Med *291*:322, 1974.

17. McGarry JD, Foster DW: Regulation of hepatic fatty acid oxidation and ketone body production. Annu Rev Biochem *49*:395, 1980.

18. Sugden MC, Williamson DH: Short-term hormonal control of ketogenesis. *In* Hue L, Van de Werve G (eds): Short-Term Regulation of Liver Metabolism. Amsterdam, Elsevier/North Holland Biomedical Press 1981, pp 291–309.

19. Zammit VA: Regulation of hepatic fatty acid oxidation and ketogenesis. Proc Nutr Soc *42*:289, 1983.

20. Zammit VA: Mechanisms of regulation of the partition of fatty acids between oxidation and esterification in liver. Prog Lipid Res *23*:36, 1984.

21. Zammit VA: Regulation of ketone body metabolism. Diabetes Rev *2*:132, 1994.

22. Dahlquist G, et al: The activity of D-hydroxybutyrate dehydrogenase in fetal, infant and adult rat brain and the influence of starvation. Biol Neonate *20*:40, 1972.

23. Novak M, et al: Release of free fatty acids from adipose tissue obtained from newborn infants. J Lipid Res *6*:91, 1965.

24. Page MA, et al: Activities of enzymes of ketone body utilization in brain and other tissues of suckling rats. Biochem J *121*:49, 1971.

25. Persson B, Gentz J: The pattern of blood lipids, glycerol and ketone bodies during the neonatal period, infancy and childhood. Acta Paediatr Scand *55*:353, 1966.

26. Garber AJ, et al: Hepatic ketogenesis and gluconeogenesis in humans. J Clin Invest *54*:981, 1974.

27. Belfrage P: Hormonal control of lipid degradation. *In* Cryer A, Van RLR (eds): New Perspectives in Adipose Tissue: Structure, Function and Development. London, Butterworths, 1985, pp 121–144.

28. Marcus C, et al: Regulation of lipolysis during the neonatal period: importance of thyrotropin. J Clin Invest *82*:1793, 1988.

29. Beaudry M-A, et al: Gluconeogenesis in the suckling rat. Am J Physiol *233*:E175, 1977.

30. Girard JR, et al: Fuels, hormones and liver metabolism at term and during the early postnatal period in the rat. J Clin Invest *52*:3190, 1973.

31. Issad T, et al: Insulin resistance during suckling period in rats. Am J Physiol *253*:E142, 1987.

32. Robinson AM, Williamson DH: Physiological roles of ketone bodies as substrates and signals in mammalian tissues. Physiol Rev *60*:143, 1980.

33. Ikeda T, et al: Effect of β-hydroxybutyrate and acetoacetate on insulin and glucagon secretion from perfused rat pancreas. Arch Biochem Biophys *257*:140, 1987.

34. Williamson DH, Lund P: Strategies for the supply of lipid substrates during post-natal brain development. Dev Neurosci *15*:156, 1993.

35. Aw TY, Grigor MR: Digestion and absorption of milk triacylglycerols in 14-day-old suckling rats. J Nutr *110*:2133, 1980.

36. Vilaró S, et al: Synthesis of lipoprotein lipase in the liver of newborn rats and localisation of the enzymes by immunofluorescence. Biochem J *249*:549, 1988.

37. Beákeási A, Williamson DH: An explanation for ketogenesis by intestine of the suckling rat: the presence of an active hydroxy-methylglutaryl-coenzyme A pathway. Biol Neonate *58*:110, 1990.

38. Hahn P, Taller M: Ketone formation in the intestinal mucosa of infant rats. Life Sci *41*:1525, 1987.

39. Serra D, et al: Ketogenic mitochondrial 3-hydroxy 3-methylglutaryl-CoA synthase gene expression in intestine and liver of suckling rats. Arch Biochem Biophys *301*:445, 1993.

40. Thumelin S, et al: Developmental changes in mitochondrial 3-hydroxy-3-methylglutaryl-CoA synthase gene expression in rat liver, intestine and kidney. Biochem J *292*:493, 1993.

41. Koren Z, Shafrir E: Placental transfer of free fatty acids in the pregnant rat. Proc Exp Biol Med *116*:411, 1964.

42. Sheridan M, et al: Studies on fatty acid-binding proteins: changes in the concentration of hepatic fatty acid-binding protein during development in the rat. Biochem J *242*:919, 1987.

43. Escriva F, et al: Evidence that the development of hepatic fatty acid oxidation at birth in the rat is concomitant with increased intramitochondrial CoA concentration. Eur J Biochem *156*:603, 1986.

44. Girard J, et al: Adaptations of glucose and fatty acid metabolism during perinatal period and suckling-weaning transition. Physiol Rev *72*:507, 1992.

45. Augenfeld J, Fritz IB: Carnitine palmitoyltransferase activity and fatty acid oxidation by livers from fetal and neonatal rats. Can J Biochem *48*:288, 1970.

46. Foster PC, Bailey E: Changes in the activities of the enzymes of hepatic fatty acid oxidation during development of the rat. Biochem J *154*:49, 1976.

47. Lockwood EA, Bailey E: The course of ketosis and the activity of key enzymes of ketogenesis and ketone body utilization during development of the postnatal rat. Biochem J *124*:249, 1971.

48. Benito M, et al: Regulation of ketogenesis during the suckling-weaning transition in the rat. Studies with isolated hepatocytes. Biochem J *180*:137, 1979.

49. Sly MR, Walker DG: Comparison of lipid metabolism in hepatocytes isolated from fed and starved neonatal and adult rats. Comp Biochem Physiol *61*:501, 1978.

50. McGarry JD, et al: The role of malonyl-CoA in the coordination of fatty acid synthesis and oxidation in isolated hepatocytes. J Biol Chem *253*:8294, 1978.

51. Geelen MJH, et al: Short-term hormonal control of hepatic lipogenesis. Diabetes *29*:1006, 1980.

52. Cook GA, et al: Differential inhibition of ketogenesis by malonyl-CoA in the mitochondria from fed and starved rats. Biochem J *192*:955, 1980.

53. Saggerson ED, Carpenter CA: Effects of fasting, adrenalectomy and streptozotocin-diabetes on sensitivity of hepatic carnitine acyltransferase to malonyl-CoA. FEBS Lett *129*:225, 1981.

54. Peñas M, Benito M: Regulation of carnitine palmitoyltransferase activity in the liver and brown adipose tissue in the newborn rat: effect of starvation and hypothermia. Biochem Biophys Res Commun *135*:589, 1986.

55. Saggerson ED, Carpenter CA: Regulation of hepatic carnitine palmitoyltransferase activity during the foetal-neonatal transition. FEBS Lett *150*:177, 1982.

56. Pillay D, Bailey E: Lipogenesis at the suckling-weaning transition in liver and brown adipose tissue of the rat. Biochem Biophys Acta *713*:663, 1982.

57. Lockwood EA, et al: Factors involved in changes in hepatic lipogenesis during development of the rat. Biochem J *118*:155, 1970.

58. Volpe JJ, Kishimoto Y: Fatty acid synthetase of brain: development, influence of nutritional and hormonal factors and comparison with liver enzyme. J Neurochem *19*:737, 1972.

59. Ferreá P, et al: Development and regulation of ketogenesis in hepatocytes isolated from newborn rats. Biochem J *214*:937, 1983.

60. Cole RA, Margolis S: Stimulation of ketogenesis by dibutyryl cyclic AMP in isolated rat hepatocytes. Endocrinology *94*:1391, 1974.

61. Heimberg M, et al: The effects of glucagon, dibutyryl cyclic adenosine 3,5-monophosphate and concentration of free fatty acid on hepatic lipid metabolism. J Biol Chem *244*:5131, 1969.

62. Raskin P, et al: Independence of cholesterol and fatty acid biosynthesis from cyclic adenosine monophosphate concentration in the perfused rat liver. J Biol Chem *249*:6029, 1974.

63. Witters LA, Trasko CS: Regulation of hepatic free fatty acid metabolism by glucagon and insulin. Am J Physiol *237*:E23, 1979.

64. Cook GA, et al: Effect of glucagon on hepatic malonyl coenzyme A concentration and on lipid synthesis. J Biol Chem *252*:4421, 1977.

65. Allred JB, Roehrig KL: Inhibition of rat liver acetyl coenzyme A carboxylase by N,[6] O[2']-dibutyryl cyclic adenosine 3′,5′-monophosphate *in vitro*. J Biol Chem *248*:4131, 1973.

66. Soler-Argilaga C, et al: Enzymatic aspects of the reduction of microsomal glycerolipid biosynthesis after perfusion of liver with dibutyryl adenosine-3′,5′-monophosphate. Arch Biochem Biophys *190*:367, 1978.

67. Harano Y, et al: Phosphorylation of carnitine palmitoyltransferase and activation by glucagon in isolated hepatocytes. FEBS Lett *188*:267, 1985.

68. Topping DL, Mayes PA: The immediate effects of insulin and fructose on the metabolism of the perfused liver. Biochem J *126*:295, 1972.

69. Yeh Y-Y, Zee P: Insulin, a possible regulator of ketosis in newborn and suckling rats. Pediatr Res *10*:192, 1976.

70. Cowett RM, et al: Persistent glucose production during glucose infusion in the neonate. J Clin Invest *71*:467, 1983.

71. Wells MA: Fatty acid metabolism and ketone formation in the suckling rat. Fed Proc *44*:2365, 1985.

72. Wu PYK, et al: Medium-chain triglycerides in infant formulas and their relation to plasma ketone body concentrations. Pediatr Res *20*:338, 1986.

73. Drahota Z, et al: Acetoacetate formation by liver slices from adult and infant rats. Biochem J *93*:61, 1984.

74. Hahn P, Vavrouskova E: Acetoacetate formation by livers from human fetuses aged 8-17 weeks. Biol Neonate *7*:348, 1964.

75. Balasse EO: Kinetics of ketone body metabolism in fasting humans. Metabolism *28*:41, 1979.

76. Owen OE, et al: Relationship between plasma and muscle concentrations of ketone bodies and free fatty acids in fed, starved and alloxan-diabetic states. Biochem J *134*:499, 1973.

77. Hawkins RA, et al: Ketone-body utilization by adult and suckling rat brain in vivo. Biochem J *122*:13, 1971.

78. Owen OE, et al: Comparative measurements of glucose, beta-hydroxybutyrate, acetoacetate and insulin in blood and cerebrospinal fluid during starvation. Metabolism *23*:7, 1974.

79. Fenselau A, Wallis K: Comparative studies on 3-oxoacid coenzyme A transferase from various rat tissues. Biochem J *142*:619, 1974.

80. Fenselau A, Wallis K: Ketone body usage by mammals: acetoacetate substrate inhibition of CoA transferase from various rat tissues. Life Sci *15*:811, 1974.

81. Middleton P: The oxoacyl-coenzyme A thiolases of animal tissues. Biochem J *132*:717, 1973.

82. Weidemann MJ, Krebs HA: The fuel of respiration of rat kidney cortex. Biochem J *112*:149, 1969.

83. Bergstrom JD, et al: Acetoacetyl-coenzyme A synthetase activity in rat liver cytosol: a regulated enzyme in lipogenesis. Biochem Biophys Res Commun *106*:856, 1984.

84. Buckley BM, Williamson DH: Acetoacetate and brain lipogenesis: developmental pattern of acetoacetyl-CoA synthetase in the soluble fraction of rat brain. Biochem J *132*:653, 1973.

85. Buckley BM, Williamson DH: Acetoacetyl-CoA synthetase: a lipogenic enzyme in rat tissues. FEBS Lett 60:7, 1975.

86. Webber RJ, Edmond J: The *in vivo* utilization of acetoacetate, D-(-)-3-hydroxybutyrate, and glucose for lipid synthesis in brain in the 18-day-old rat: evidence for an acetyl-CoA bypass for sterol synthesis. J Biol Chem 254:3912, 1979.

87. Yeh Y-Y: Partition of ketone bodies into cholesterol and fatty acids *in vivo* in different brain regions of developing rats. Lipids 15:904, 1980.

88. Geelen MJH, et al: Acetoacetate: a major substrate for the synthesis of cholesterol and fatty acids by isolated rat hepatocytes. FEBS Lett 163:269, 1983.

89. Hülsmann WC: Preferential oxidation of fatty acids by rat small intestine. FEBS Lett 17:35, 1971.

90. McCann WP: The oxidation of ketone bodies by mitochondria from liver and peripheral tissues. J Biol Chem 226:15, 1957.

91. Webber RJ, Edmond J: Utilization of L(+)-3-hydroxybutyrate, D(-)-3-hydroxybutyrate, acetoacetate and glucose for respiration and lipid synthesis in the 18 day old rat. J Biol Chem 252:5222, 1977.

92. Reed WD, Ozand PT: Enzymes of L(+)-3-hydroxybutyrate metabolism in the rat. Arch Biochem Biophys 205:94, 1980.

93. Argileás JM: Has acetone a role in the conversion of fat to carbohydrate in mammals? Trends Biochem Sci 11:61, 1986.

94. Sakami W, Lafaye JM: The metabolism of acetone in the intact rat. J Biol Chem 193:199, 1951.

95. Landau BR, Brunengraber H: The role of acetone in the conversion of fat to carbohydrate. Trends Biochem Sci 12:113, 1987.

96. Casazza JP, et al: The metabolism of acetone in the rat. J Biol Chem 259:231, 1984.

97. Reichard GA, et al: Acetone metabolism in humans during diabetic ketoacidosis. Diabetes 35:668, 1986.

98. Dierks-Ventling C, Cone AL: Ketone body enzymes in mammalian tissues: effect of a high fat diet. J Biol Chem 246:5533, 1971.

99. Williamson DH: Activities of enzymes involved in acetoacetate utilization in adult mammalian tissues. Biochem J 121:41, 1971.

100. Robinson AM, Williamson DH: Utilization of D-3-hydroxy [3-14C]butyrate for lipogenesis *in vivo* in lactating rat mammary gland. Biochem J 176:635, 1978.

101. Klee CB, Sokoloff L: Changes in D(-)-β-hydroxybutyric acid dehydrogenase activity during brain maturation in the rat. J Biol Chem 242:3880, 1967.

102. Nehlig A, Pereira de Vasconceles A: Glucose and ketone body utilization by the brain of the neonatal rat. Prog Neurobiol 40:163, 1993.

103. Tildon JT, et al: Coenzyme A transferase activity in rat brain. Biochem Biophys Res Commun 43:225, 1971.

104. Ganapathi MK, et al: Cloning of rat brain succinyl-CoA:3-oxoacid CoA transferase cDNA. Biochem J 248:853, 1987.

105. Haney PM, Patel MS: Regulation of succinyl-CoA:3-oxoacid CoA transferase in developing rat brain: responsiveness associated with prenatal but not postnatal hyperketonaemia. Arch Biochem Biophys 240:426, 1985.

106. Yeh Y-Y, et al: Ketone bodies serve as important precursors of brain lipids in the developing rat. Lipids 12:957, 1977.

107. Pegorier JP, et al: Changes in circulating fuels, pancreatic hormones and liver glycogen concentration in fasting or suckling newborn pig. J Dev Physiol 3:203, 1981.

108. Kahng MW, et al: Substrate oxidation and enzyme activities of ketone body metabolism in the developing pig. Biol Neonate 24:187, 1974.

109. Booth RFG, et al: The development of enzymes of energy metabolism in the brain of a precocial (guinea pig) and non-precocial (rat) species. J Neurochem 34:17, 1980.

110. Page MA, Williamson DH: Enzymes of ketone body utilization in human brain. Lancet 2:66, 1971.

111. Patel MS, et al: The metabolism of ketone bodies in developing human brain: development of ketone-body utilizing enzymes and ketone bodies as precursors for lipid synthesis. J Neurochem 25:905, 1975.

112. Randle PJ, et al: Regulation of glucose uptake by muscle. Biochem J 93:652, 1964.

113. Haymond MW, et al: Effects of ketosis on glucose flux in children and adults. Am J Physiol 245:E373, 1983.

114. Wicklmayr M, et al: Inhibition of muscular triglyceride lipolysis by ketone bodies: a mechanism for energy preservation in starvation. Horm Metab Res 18:476, 1986.

115. Sherwin RS, et al: Effect of ketone infusions on amino acid and nitrogen metabolism in man. J Clin Invest 55:1382, 1975.

116. Dahlquist G, Persson B: The rate of cerebral utilization of glucose, ketone bodies, lactate, pyruvate and amino acids in infant. Pediatr Res 10:910, 1976.

117. Kraus H, et al: Developmental changes of cerebral ketone body metabolism. Hoppe-Seyler's Z Physiol Chem 335:164, 1974.

118. Persson B, et al: Cerebral arteriovenous differences of acetoacetate and D-β-hydroxybutyrate in children. Acta Paediatr Scand 61:273, 1972.

119. Moore TJ, et al: β-Hydroxybutyrate transport in rat brain: developmental and dietary modulations. Am J Physiol 230:619, 1976.

120. Cremer JE, Heath DF: The estimation of rates of utilization of glucose and ketone bodies in the brain of the suckling rat using compartmental analysis of isotopic data. Biochem J 142:527, 1974.

121. Williamson DH: Regulation of the utilization of glucose and ketone bodies by brain in the perinatal period. *In* Camerini-Davalos RA, Cole HS (eds): Early Diabetes in Early Life. New York, Academic Press, 1975, pp 195–202.

122. Itoh T, Quastel JH: Acetoacetate metabolism in infant and adult rat brain in vitro. Biochem J 116:641, 1970.

123. Ruderman NB, et al: Regulation of glucose and ketone body metabolism in brain of anaesthetized rats. Biochem J 138:1, 1974.

124. Patel MS, Owen OE: Development and regulation of lipid synthesis from ketone bodies by rat brain. J Neurochem 28:109, 1977.

125. Dietze G, et al: On the key role of ketogenesis for the regulation of glucose homeostasis during fasting: intrahepatic control, ketone levels and peripheral pyruvate oxidation *In* Söling H-D, Seufert C-D (eds): Biochemical and Clinical Aspects of Ketone Body Metabolism. Stuttgart, Georg Thieme, 1978, pp 213–225.

126. Hawkins RA, et al: Regional ketone body utilization by rat brain in starvation and diabetes. Am J Physiol 250:E169, 1986.

127. Hawkins RA, Biebuyck JF: Ketone bodies are selectively used by individual brain regions. Science 205:325, 1979.

128. Yeh Y-Y: Biosynthesis of lung lipids from acetoacetate and glucose in the developing rat in vivo. Int J Biochem 14:81, 1982.

129. Sheehan PM, Yeh Y-Y: Pathways of acetyl-CoA production for lipogenesis from acetoacetate, β-hydroxybutyrate, pyruvate and glucose in neonatal rat lung. Lipids 19:103, 1984.

130. Adam PA, et al: Oxidation of glucose and D-β-OH butyrate by early human fetal brain. Acta Paediatr Scand 64:17, 1975.

131. Shambaugh GE III, et al: Fetal fuels II: contributions of selected carbon fuels of oxidative metabolism in rat conceptus. Am J Physiol 233:E457, 1977.

132. Shambaugh GE III, et al: Fetal fuels III: ketone utilization by fetal hepatocytes. Am J Physiol 235:E330, 1978.

133. Seccombe DW, et al: Fetal utilization of maternally derived ketone bodies for lipogenesis in the rat. Biochim Biophys Acta 488:402, 1977.

134. Hunter ES III, Sadler TW: Metabolism of D- and DL-β-hydroxybutyrate by mouse embryos *in vitro*. Metabolism 36:558, 1987.

135. Freinkel N, et al: Fuel-mediated teratogenesis during early organogenesis: the effects of increased concentrations of glucose, ketone, or somatomedin inhibitor during embryo culture. Am J Clin Nutr 44:986, 1986.

136. Horton WE Jr, Sadler TW: Effects of maternal diabetes on early embryogenesis: alterations in morphogenesis produced by the ketone body, β-hydroxybutyrate. Diabetes 32:610, 1983.

137. Sheehan EA: Effects of β-hydroxybutyrate on rat embryos grown in culture. Experientia 41:273, 1985.

138. Mills JL, et al: Malformations in infants of diabetic mothers occur before the seventh gestational week; implications for treatment. Diabetes 26:292, 1979.

139. Hunter ES III, et al: A potential mechanism of DL-β-hydroxybutyrate-induced malformations in mouse embryos. Am J Physiol 253:E72, 1987.

140. Bhasin S, Shambaugh GE III: Fetal fuels V: ketone bodies inhibit pyrimidine biosynthesis in fetal rat brain. Am J Physiol 243:E234, 1982.

141. Agius L, Williamson DH: The utilization of ketone bodies by the interscapular brown adipose tissue of the rat. Biochim Biophys Acta 666:127, 1981.

142. Middleton P: The oxoacyl–coenzyme A thiolases of animal tissues. Biochem J 132:717, 1973.

143. Robles-Valdes C, et al: Maternal-fetal carnitine relationships and neonatal ketosis in the rat. J Biol Chem 251:6007, 1976.

144. Zammit VA, et al: The role of 3-oxoacid-CoA transferase in the regulation of ketogenesis in liver. FEBS Lett 105:212, 1979.

Socheata Un and Susan E. Carlson

Long Chain Fatty Acids in the Developing Retina and Brain

The brain and retina contain large quantities of long chain (20 and 22 carbon) n-3 and n-6 polyunsaturated fatty acids (LCPUFAs), particularly docosahexaenoic acid (DHA, 22:6n-3) and arachidonic acid (AA, 20:4n-6).[1,2] During the last intrauterine trimester[3,4] and the first 18 months of postnatal life, DHA and AA accumulate in neural tissue at a high rate supported by selective placental transfer of DHA and AA from mother to fetus,[5,6] transfer from human milk consumption to breast-fed infants,[7,8] and synthesis from the dietary essential fatty acids, α-linolenic acid (18:3n-3), and linoleic acid (18:2n-6),[9-12] respectively. (For a more extensive treatment of these topics, see Chapter 39[13] and Chapter 40.[14])

Diets deficient in α-linolenic acid result in lower brain DHA and a reciprocal increase in docosapentaenoic acid (DPA, 22:5n-6 or n-6 DPA) (Fig. 44–1),[15] abnormal retinal physiology,[16-19] abnormal visual acuity development,[20] and other types of abnormal development.[21-30] As first observed in the late 1970s, it is now well known that infants fed formula without DHA have lower levels of DHA in red blood cell and plasma lipids than breast-fed infants.[7,8] Even though older infant formulas contained the essential fatty acids, these formulas lacked DHA or AA. It was hypothesized that lower DHA in formula-fed infants could decrease DHA accumulation in the brain and retina and could result in less than optimal sensory and cognitive function.

Only randomized studies of DHA supplementation of infants could determine whether functional outcomes such as visual acuity could be improved by adding DHA to infant formula. The first studies focused on preterm infants. Preterm infants were considered more likely than term infants to need dietary DHA, because they are born before maternofetal DHA transfer is complete,[3,4] and many are fed an infant formula rather than human milk. Preliminary reports in 1989 indicated that visual acuity and retinal physiologic development of preterm infants were higher in infants fed experimental formulas with DHA, and these results were subsequently published in full reports.[31-33]

After Makrides and associates[34] reported an association between higher DHA status and visual acuity in term, breast-fed infants, randomized trials were conducted in term infants to determine the potential benefits from the addition of DHA to infant formulas.[35,36] Since the late 1980s, researchers have conducted many randomized trials to compare the growth and development of term infants fed formulas with or without DHA, as discussed later in this chapter. A smaller number of randomized studies have compared growth and development of infants randomized to receive higher DHA through DHA supplementation of their mothers during pregnancy or lactation. Except for the most recent studies, these randomized trials have been reviewed and reported elsewhere.[37,38]

Early studies showed lower growth in preterm infants who were fed DHA and not AA.[39,40] Because AA is important for normal growth,[41] dietary n-3 LCPUFA reduced red blood cell phospholipid AA,[42] and the concentration of AA in circulating lipids was associated with size at birth[43] and first-year growth achievement,[44] many study formulas have included AA and DHA to provide a balance of n-3 and n-6 LCPUFA. Dietary sources of AA were not available for addition to infant formulas when the first randomized studies were conducted. Formulas with both

DHA and AA have resulted in growth of preterm infants similar to that found in infants fed formulas without DHA and AA;[45] however, both DHA and AA were added to term and preterm formulas that became available in the United States in 2002.

Between the first and second editions of this book, formula manufacturers in Europe, Asia, and South America added DHA and AA to some of their products. Since the second edition, DHA and AA were added to infant formulas in the United States after the Food and Drug Administration (FDA) gave generally recognized as safe (GRAS) status to specific single-cell oil sources of DHA and AA (Federal Register). If anything, the addition of DHA and AA to infant formula stimulated an increase in research in this area to address questions regarding the optimal timing for accumulation of DHA, the optimal level of supplementation, and the underlying mechanisms of DHA in the retina and brain.

HISTORICAL PERSPECTIVE

DHA constitutes 30 to 45% of the total fatty acids in some phospholipid classes (specifically ethanolamine and serine phosphoglycerides) in brain gray matter and retina, respectively. In the brain, DHA is especially concentrated in membranes surrounding synapses.[1] In the retina, DHA is concentrated in both synaptic regions and in the disk membranes of photoreceptors.[2] During the last intrauterine trimester, brain DHA increases exponentially and AA decreases linearly, such that the ratio of DHA to AA in the retina doubles between 24 and 40 weeks of gestation and increases further after birth.[46]

Sanders and Naismith[7] were the first to show that formula-fed term infants had lower erythrocyte phospholipid DHA and AA levels compared with breast-fed infants. We made a similar discovery while pursuing another hypothesis.[8] Infants fed an infant formula that contained 5% of total fatty acids as α-linolenic acid had similar amounts of DHA in red blood cell phospholipids compared with infants fed a formula with 1.2% α-linolenic acid. However, the formula-fed groups had lower DHA and AA levels than a comparison group fed milk from their own mothers.

Sinclair and Crawford[47,48] showed, in rats, that DHA and AA were more efficiently incorporated into brain DHA and AA than their essential fatty acid precursors. Rats fed an α-linolenic acid–deficient diet during development had lower DHA accumulation in brain, which was reflected in lower red blood cell phospholipid DHA.[49] Because human milk contains AA, DHA, and other LCPUFAs not found in infant formula at that time, the studies showing higher red blood cell phospholipid DHA levels in infants fed human milk[7,8] suggested that DHA and AA were more effective than their essential fatty acid precursors in increasing membrane DHA and AA.

Clandinin and co-workers[3] had demonstrated that fetal brain DHA and AA accumulated during the third intrauterine trimester. Coupled with studies of α-linolenic acid–deficient rodents and primates, the evidence suggested that preterm infants fed diets without DHA could be at risk of inadequate brain accumulation of DHA, even when their diets contained α-linolenic acid. Formula-fed compared with human milk–fed preterm infants also had lower levels of erythrocyte phospholipid DHA and AA.[50] Preterm infants were surviving with as much as 18 weeks less

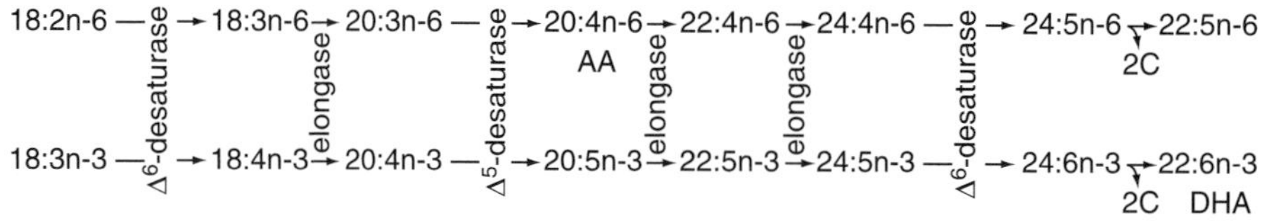

$$18:2n\text{-}6 \xrightarrow{\Delta^6\text{-desaturase}} 18:3n\text{-}6 \xrightarrow{\text{elongase}} 20:3n\text{-}6 \xrightarrow{\Delta^5\text{-desaturase}} \underset{AA}{20:4n\text{-}6} \rightarrow 22:4n\text{-}6 \xrightarrow{\text{elongase}} 24:4n\text{-}6 \xrightarrow{\Delta^6\text{-desaturase}} 24:5n\text{-}6 \underset{2C}{\rightarrow} 22:5n\text{-}6$$

$$18:3n\text{-}3 \xrightarrow{\Delta^6\text{-desaturase}} 18:4n\text{-}3 \xrightarrow{\text{elongase}} 20:4n\text{-}3 \xrightarrow{\Delta^5\text{-desaturase}} 20:5n\text{-}3 \rightarrow 22:5n\text{-}3 \xrightarrow{\text{elongase}} 24:5n\text{-}3 \xrightarrow{\Delta^6\text{-desaturase}} 24:6n\text{-}3 \underset{2C}{\rightarrow} \underset{DHA}{22:6n\text{-}3}$$

Figure 44–1. Elongation and desaturation of the essential fatty acids linoleic acid (18:2ω-6) and linolenic acid (18:3ω-3).

time for intrauterine DHA transfer than term infants. It was hypothesized that formulas containing DHA compared with formulas that contained α-linolenic acid as the only n-3 fatty acid could improve early visual and neural development of infants born at the beginning of the last trimester. The question asked by these studies was whether α-linolenic acid alone could meet developing infants' needs for DHA for brain and retinal function. The human studies, described later in the chapter, compared outcomes in infants fed formulas that contained α-linolenic acid with or without a source of DHA.

FACTORS INFLUENCING ACCUMULATION OF LONG CHAIN POLYUNSATURATED FATTY ACIDS DURING DEVELOPMENT

The timing of brain fatty acid accumulation varies considerably among mammalian species. Researchers have used this variability in studies of essential fatty acid deficiency and function. Humans and pigs accumulate brain DHA both *in utero* and postnatally,[7,8,50-53] whereas guinea pigs receive most maternal LCPUFA during fetal life,[54] and rats receive most maternal LCPUFA postnatally.[48] Differences among species allow researchers to create models for studying the temporal effects of low brain DHA on brain development. For example, newborn rats are a model for human DHA accretion beginning with the third intrauterine trimester, whereas in newborn pigs postnatal DHA accretion resembles that in humans.

Maternal Influences on Accumulation of Arachidonic Acid and Docosahexaenoic Acid in the Fetus and Infant

Arbuckle and Innis[55] found that feeding fish oil DHA to pigs increased DHA levels both in sow milk and in the tissues of piglets. Connor and co-workers,[56] and Harris and associates[57] published the first direct evidence in humans that consumption of fish oil DHA by lactating women increased the amount of postnatal DHA transfer to their infants in milk and increased the DHA status of their infants, that is, increased erythrocyte and plasma phospholipid DHA.

Observational studies showed that maternal DHA status is highly variable during pregnancy and lactation,[58-64] and maternal DHA status is related to DHA status of the infant.[58,59,62,64] Two independent research groups showed that infants fed human milk compared with infant formulas without DHA had more brain DHA at autopsy.[65,66] This evidence suggests that postnatal transfer of DHA can influence infant brain biochemistry and possibly development. Other observational studies associated higher maternal DHA status during pregnancy with higher infant development status.[34,67-71]

Newer experimental studies suggest that maternal DHA status during pregnancy or lactation can enhance infant development.[72,73] Jensen and associates[72] and Helland and associates[73] randomly assigned women to consume DHA from single-cell oil and fish oil during lactation and during pregnancy and lactation, respectively. Jensen and associates[72] reported higher Bayley Psychomotor development at 30 months of age, and Helland and her associates[73] reported a higher intelligence quotient (IQ) at 4 years of age, although neither group could find any develop-

mental advantage of DHA supplementation when these children were infants.[74,75]

Pregnancy itself alters the amount of DHA in circulating blood lipids and red blood cell phospholipids. Otto and colleagues[60] observed that phospholipid DHA in maternal plasma and red blood cells increased in early pregnancy regardless of the initial amount of red blood cell DHA. These data suggest that DHA is mobilized during pregnancy for transfer to the fetus. Regardless, the same group of investigators reported increased maternal n-6 DPA relative to DHA, which they suggested could indicate that pregnant women fall behind with respect to DHA production and transfer to the fetus.[61] Van Houwelingen and colleagues[76] observed similar relative increases in n-6 DPA to DHA in preterm infants, providing further evidence that an increase in n-6 DPA/DHA may be an indicator of inadequate DHA synthesis or accumulation.

In a comparative study of pregnant women from the Netherlands, Hungary, Finland, England, and Ecuador, large differences in the percentage of blood fatty acids as DHA were found among these nationalities.[58] These national differences most likely reflect differences in DHA intake.[58] The number of prior pregnancies has been shown to be inversely related to maternal DHA as well.[52] There do not appear to have been studies of women carrying multiple fetuses, but multiple births would be predicted to reduce maternal DHA transfer to each fetus.

Just as a woman's DHA status during pregnancy affects transfer of DHA to her fetus, a woman's DHA status also influences DHA transfer to her newborn in human milk. DHA content of human milk is quite variable within and among populations. The extremes of milk DHA that have been reported are, as a percentage of total fatty acids, 0.02% in vegans[77] and 2.4% in women from China who consume a diet high in fish.[78] Milk DHA in most populations falls between 0.1 and 0.5% of total fatty acids.[52,53] The variability of DHA in milk of a given woman does not appear to have been studied. Some day-to-day variation would be expected, as with other nutrients; however, it is unlikely that the variability would be sufficient to have much impact on infant status, particularly among women whose DHA consumption is low. In general, women in the United States appear to fall into this category.[79,80]

Like DHA, the reported average amount of AA in human milk encompasses a wide range among cultural groups, from 0.2 to 1.2%. However, the average AA in the milk of most populations falls within the range of 0.4 to 0.6%, and the linoleic acid content ranges from 10 to 17% of total fatty acids.[52,53,81]

Synthesis as a Source of Long Chain Polyunsaturated Fatty Acids

Infants who do not receive dietary DHA must synthesize their DHA from α-linolenic acid (see Fig. 44–1).[55] The question that has been asked by many clinical studies is this: Can infants who consume α-linolenic acid accumulate enough brain DHA for optimal function, or would they benefit from receiving additional dietary DHA? In a later section, the evidence of functional benefits of DHA is discussed. This section provides a brief review of the synthesis of DHA and the relative role that synthesis plays in tissue accumulation regarding preformed DHA.

Voss and colleagues[82] followed stable isotope-labeled fatty acids and demonstrated that the likely pathway for conversion of α-linolenic acid to DHA involves two successive additions of two-carbon units to 20:5n-3 (20:5n-3 to 22:5n-3 to 24:5n-3) followed by a δ^6-desaturation (24:5n-3 to 24:6n-3) and the subsequent removal of a two-carbon segment (24:6n-3 to DHA or 22:6n-3) (see Fig. 44–1). Synthesis of DHA from 22:5n-3 by frog retinal pigment epithelium also generated 24:5n-3 and 24:6n-3.[83] The final step in synthesis of DHA occurs in peroxisomes. Important supporting evidence of the importance of peroxisomes in the supply of DHA comes from Martinez's studies in persons with peroxisomal disorders.[84,85]

DHA can be synthesized from α-linolenic acid by the liver, retina, and brain.[83,86-90] Synthesis in retina has been localized to the retinal pigment epithelium,[83] and synthesis in brain has been localized to astrocytes and cerebral endothelium.[89-91] Retinal photoreceptor cells and neurons do not synthesize DHA.[88-90] Chen and co-workers[92] found that DHA was preferentially incorporated into triglycerides in retinal pigment epithelium. Their observation suggests a role for triglycerides in the DHA enrichment of the retina or recycling of photoreceptor DHA between the retina and the retinal pigment epithelium.[92] Electron microscopic studies of retinal DHA accumulation suggest that DHA is stored in lipid droplets of the pigment epithelium and is transferred to photoreceptors.[93] Moore and coworkers[89] suggested an analogous model for uptake of DHA by neurons. Either preformed DHA or n-3 fatty acid precursors of DHA could be taken up by the cerebral endothelium and incorporated into astrocytes, which could synthesize DHA and transfer it as well as preformed DHA to neurons. Innis and Dyer[91] showed that astrocytes release fatty acids in cholesterol esters.

Early evidence that preterm infants had the capacity to synthesize DHA from α-linolenic acid could be inferred from the results obtained by Uauy and associates.[31] These researchers showed that preterm infants fed formulas containing soybean oil had higher erythrocyte DHA levels than those fed formulas containing corn oil, a fat with much less α-linolenic acid than soybean oil. An early study showed δ^6- and δ^5-desaturase activity in human liver at mid-gestation, a finding suggesting that the fetus could metabolize essential fatty acids to more polyunsaturated forms.[94] Stable isotope studies in human preterm and term infants demonstrated whole body synthesis of DHA,[9-12] as well as a large variability among infants.[11]

Stable isotope studies in humans do not permit quantification of DHA accumulation from new synthesis relative to preformed DHA.[95,96] However, studies with nonhuman primate neonates are helpful for assessing the relative contribution to tissue DHA of newly synthesized versus preformed DHA. Studies with Japanese monkey neonates suggest that the amount of DHA derived from synthesis is relatively minor compared with the amount received from mother's milk.[97] Newborn baboons synthesized DHA from α-linolenic acid;[98] however, preformed DHA was eight times more likely than α-linolenic acid to accumulate in brain. Based on these results, it is unlikely that synthesis of DHA from α-linolenic acid could meet the neonate's need for optimal brain DHA accumulation.[98]

Although pigs,[95] and possibly other species, may have different relative capacities for synthesis of DHA compared with humans, studies with animals are valuable as a means of understanding the relative effects of different tissues and physiologic effects on DHA synthesis. In the rat, the activity of hepatic δ^6- and δ^5-desaturases falls after birth and then peaks after weaning, but brain activities peak around birth and fall steadily through the first several weeks of life.[99] Rat milk, like all mammalian milk, contains DHA. These changes in enzyme activity suggest a classic feedback inhibition of DHA on hepatic enzymes but not on enzymes in the brain. The mouse exhibits a postnatal decline in brain δ^6-desaturase activity similar to that in the rat.[100] After 3 months of age, mouse brain activity of this enzyme is extremely low, but hepatic activity remains fairly high through 9 months of age and then decreases dramatically at later ages.[100] In the fetal pig, δ^5-desaturase activity increases by 7-fold in the brain and by 23-fold in the liver during the last half of gestation.[101,102]

Effects of Dietary Influences on Accumulation of Long Chain Polyunsaturated Fatty Acids

From fatty acid analyses, it is known that diets deficient in α-linolenic acid decrease tissue DHA and increase n-6 DPA. Because of the recognized importance of retinal and neural DHA accumulation, most recent infant formulas in the United States have contained a ratio of linoleic to α-linolenic acid of less than 10 and have provided at least 1.5% of total fatty acids (0.75% energy) as α-linolenic acid. Now that DHA and AA have been added to infant formulas in the United States, it may be time to reassess the high amount of linoleic acid and α-linolenic acid in some formulas. We have reported high levels of 24:2, which appeared to replace 24:1 in red blood cell sphingomyelin, especially in preterm infants.[103] Transfer of essential fatty acids directly to the fetus during gestation appears to be limited, based on low linoleic acid levels in circulating phospholipids of cord blood.[50] Maternal linoleic acid intake was inversely related to infant birth weight in one published study.[104]

An increase in α-linolenic acid intake above some minimal intake does not compensate for the DHA accumulation that occurs in red blood cells, plasma, and the brain with even relatively small intakes of DHA.[42,70,71,105] In the months after birth, infants fed formulas that contain α-linolenic acid but not DHA have progressively lower amounts of circulating DHA.[42] Infants fed formulas with DHA have higher concentrations of red blood cell phospholipid DHA, an indicator of infant DHA status, than infants fed formulas with more than 0.75% energy from α-linolenic acid.[33,42]

Breast-fed human infants have higher brain,[65,66] but not retinal,[66] DHA accumulation compared with infants who were fed formulas without DHA. A functional study by Uauy and co-workers[106] found normal electroretinogram responses in preterm infants at 4 months of corrected age, even though they had been fed a formula low in α-linolenic acid from birth. Thus, although diets deficient in α-linolenic acid lead to reduced retinal DHA in monkeys[18] and piglets,[107] it appears that retinal DHA may be adequate with formulas that contain α-linolenic acid but not DHA. Only infants with impaired DHA synthesis have low retinal DHA.[108]

Many questions remain: Does brain DHA in formula-fed infants eventually catch up to that of milk-fed animals? Is there a critical period for accumulating retinal and brain DHA? What amount of DHA accumulation in retina and brain is optimal for function? Is there a level of DHA intake that could harm the developing infant? Finally, does the answer to these questions depend on gestational age, size at birth, or other maternal or infant factors?

EFFECTS OF ESSENTIAL FATTY ACID DEFICIENCY ON BEHAVIOR

The kinds of behavior in animals subjected to toxic insult or nutrient variation during development can provide useful information about affected behavioral domains, which, in turn, reflect neural function. Behavioral domains include sensory, motivational or arousal, learning, cognitive, and motor. Wainwright[109,110] reviewed the principles governing animal models of behavior and the evidence from these modes that lipids influence behavior. Carlson[111] and Mostofsky[112] reviewed models and methods for studying behavior that have been or could be applied to studies of n-3 fatty acid–deficient animals.

The earliest studies of essential fatty acid deficiency restricted intake of dietary fat, and, therefore, both linoleic and α-linolenic acids were deficient. Diets deficient in both essential fatty acids led to reduced number of brain cells, lower LCPUFAs in brain, and poor growth, probably from AA deficiency.[113] Diets containing linoleic acid but little α-linolenic acid (e.g., made with safflower oil or sunflower oil) reduce DHA accumulation in the retina and brain, with a proportional increase in n-6 DPA compared with diets that contain α-linolenic acid. Animals fed α-linolenic acid (n-3 fatty acid)–deficient diets grow normally and have no evidence of disease; however, they have abnormal retinal responses to light,[16-18] visual acuity,[19,20] and behavior.[21-30]

Behavioral studies of α-linolenic acid–deficient animals differ from studies of DHA adequacy that have been done in human infants. In the animal models, DHA is low because dietary α-linolenic acid is deficient. In the infant studies, α-linolenic acid is not deficient, but synthesis of DHA from α-linolenic acid may not be enough to support optimal brain DHA accumulation and function. Studies of n-3 fatty acid–deficient animals provide clues to the effects of lower brain DHA on behavior regardless of why brain DHA is reduced. Given that infants can synthesize DHA from its essential fatty acid precursor,[9-12] any effects of inadequate conversion would likely be less severe than those found in n-3 fatty acid deficiency, however.

Evidence of the Sensory Effects of n-3 Fatty Acid Deficiency

The physiologic response of the retina evoked by a brief flash of light (electroretinogram [ERG]) has components determined by the photoreceptor outer segments and the synaptic regions of the retina, the a-wave and b-wave, respectively. n-3 Fatty acid–deficient diets have a negative effect on the ERG in rats and monkeys. Wheeler and colleagues[17] reported a higher a-wave amplitude in rats fed linolenic acid compared with linoleic acid. Feeding α-linolenic acid to depleted animals only partially normalized the a-wave amplitude, evidence that the effects of n-3 fatty acid depletion on retinal physiology were not completely reversible.[16] Other investigators have also reported lower a-wave and b-wave amplitudes in n-3 fatty acid–deficient rats[25,114] compared with controls, but there are reports to the contrary in the rat[115] and guinea pig.[116] Among ERG studies, the variability in results may be caused by differences in the duration of light stimulus, interstimulus interval, stimulus intensity, and the degree of n-3 fatty acid deficiency. For example, an effect on amplitude would be suggested in n-3 fatty acid–deficient animals with a recovery latency if the retinas were not allowed to recover fully between stimuli.

In n-3 fatty acid–deficient monkeys, the ERG responses of retinal rods and cones are delayed compared with controls, and the time required for the dark-adapted retina to recover from an initial bright flash of light is doubled.[18,19,117] n-3 Fatty acid–deficient monkeys have also been found to have transiently lower a-wave and b-wave amplitudes compared with controls.[117] When n-3 fatty acid–deficient monkeys were fed fish oil as a source of DHA, the DHA in brain increased to normal levels in both young and adult animals. However, the ERG peak latencies did not return to normal.[117] In fact, even when n-3 fatty acid repletion was started at birth, membrane DHA was reduced, and recovery of the dark-adapted ERG was prolonged, probably because the monkey retina at birth is more developed than the human retina.[19,117]

Visual acuity requires a functioning retina and brain. Monkey infants whose mothers were fed an n-3 fatty acid–deficient diet made with safflower oil during pregnancy had only half as much DHA in phospholipids as those whose mothers were fed a diet with soybean oil. The n-3 fatty acid–deficient animals had lower

visual acuity (determined by forced choice preferential looking) at 4, 8, and 12 weeks of age compared with controls.[20] Bogener and colleagues[118] and Radel and associates[119] studied brain cortical responses evoked by visual and auditory stimuli in a rat model. The brain DHA depletion was similar to that which occurs in human infants fed α-linolenic acid without DHA. In adult rats, visual and auditory brain cortical responses showed increased amplitudes in deficient animals[118,119] in comparison with controls, a finding suggesting decreased ability to inhibit responses to these stimuli. Evidence that the responses were cortical was suggested by the finding that both the ERG and auditory brain responses were normal. Half of the animals in each litter were given a diet with DHA beginning at weaning, and their visual, but not auditory, cortical responses returned to normal as adults.[119] A low pain threshold with n-3 fatty acid deficiency may reflect an effect on sensory function as well.[120,121]

Evidence of the Cognitive Effects of n-3 Fatty Acid Deficiency

Some studies in rodents suggest that n-3 fatty acid–deficient animals may learn more slowly than n-3 fatty acid–sufficient animals. Differences in performance on tasks generally thought to reflect learning could be evidence of effects on ability to learn. However, as Wainwright[109] pointed out, many studies did not control for what are known to be effects of n-3 fatty acid deficiency on visual function, reflex development, and exploratory activity, all of which could influence performance even if the ability to learn were unaffected by n-3 fatty acid deficiency.

Lamptey and Walker[21] noted that the offspring of rats fed safflower oil compared with soybean oil had less ability to discriminate in a black/white Y-maze that used food as reinforcement. Similarly, Yamamoto and colleagues[22-24] demonstrated that n-3–deficient animals had difficulty discriminating between levels of light intensity to obtain food and required longer to extinguish previously reinforced behavior in a new task. Yehuda and associates[121] also reported poorer ability to extinguish a previously learned behavior in n-3–deficient rats.

Reisbick and co-workers[29] reported an inverse relationship between brain DHA accumulation and look duration. The observation could be interpreted as evidence of an effect of higher brain DHA and ability to learn, because shorter-looking human infants have generally superior performance on perceptual-cognitive tasks in infancy and beyond when compared with longer-looking infants. Furthermore, in human infants, short-looking compared with long-looking has been suggested to be an indication of speed of information processing, with greater speed implying higher function.[122] There are alternative explanations for shorter-look duration including increased ability to disengage attention[123] and lower reactivity.[124] However, each of these possible explanations suggests a positive effect of higher brain DHA during development.[125]

Frances and colleagues[126] studied the effects of n-3 deficiency on habituation, a simple form of learning, and found that habituation occurred more slowly in deficient mice. Yoshida and associates[127] observed that deficient mice exhibited inferior learning performance and were unable to rectify incorrect responses through learning sessions with a brightness discrimination task. Ikemoto and co-workers[128] found that altered learning behavior in n-3 fatty acid–deficient mice could be reversed by supplementing with DHA after weaning. Sato and partners[129] reported that altered learning behavior in deficient mice was not associated with substantial changes in the rate of protein synthesis in the brain. Only Greiner and colleagues[130] measured learning through a task that did not require visual function, that is, olfactory function, and found higher performance in rats fed α-linolenic acid compared with an n-3 fatty acid–deficient diet.

Evidence of the Effects of n-3 Fatty Acid Deficiency on Motivation and Arousal

Rats fed n-3 fatty acid–deficient diets were reported to have increased exploratory activity in a novel environment,[131] which Wainwright[109] suggested may reflect greater emotional reactivity. Differences in arousal may also explain the polydipsia and polyuria that have been observed in n-3 fatty acid–deficient monkeys, which have normal renal function, growth and physical health.[132] Reisbick and associates[30] reported evidence of a higher frequency of stereotyped behavior, higher locomotor activity, and higher general behavioral reactivity in n-3 fatty acid–deficient monkeys.

Levant and partners[133] used a model of physiologically relevant reduction in brain DHA content (i.e., modeled after reductions that have been observed in human infants[65,66]) to explore behavioral changes reflective of dopaminergic tone, in particular hyperactivity of the mesolimbic dopamine system.[134] They found higher basal locomotor activity in n-3 fatty acid–deficient adult rats, activity that did not return to normal in deficient rats fed a fish oil source of DHA starting at 21 days of age. An elevated-plus maze was used to assess exploratory behavior in an anxiety-provoking environment. Rats n-3 deficient through adulthood spent significantly more time in the open arms of the maze, a finding suggesting that they experienced less anxiety in a potentially dangerous environment than controls. Wainwright[110] showed that n-3 fatty acid–deficient rats had delayed matching to place in the water maze compared with controls, a task associated with prefrontal dopamine function. Frances and co-workers[135] found a higher increase in morphine-induced locomotor activity in n-3 fatty acid–deficient rats compared with control rats, and the increase also occurred earlier in the deficient animals. Hibbeln and associates[136] reported that DHA and AA supplementation in the diets of infant rhesus monkeys markedly increased heart rate variability. The increase in heart rate variability persisted into adolescence. According to these authors, "low heart rate variability is an indicator of low autonomic arousal and is well established as a longitudinal predictor of disruptive and antisocial behaviors."

Possible Motor Effects of Higher n-3 Long Chain Polyunsaturated Fatty Acid Status

DHA and AA supplementation improved the motor and visual orientation scores of infant rhesus monkeys as well.[136] The scores improved at days 7 and 14, with a ceiling effect noted at day 21.

Possible Mechanisms for Changes in Behavior with Lower Brain Docosahexaenoic Acid Accumulation

Although it is clear from numerous studies that variations in brain DHA influence behavior, the underlying mechanism by which this occurs has not been known. Salem and associates[137] reviewed the evidence for an early theory that a cyclooxygenase or lipoxygenase metabolite of DHA, but not n-6 DPA, played an important role in the function of the central nervous system. These authors concluded that evidence for the theory is currently lacking.

Another hypothesis, for which there is now good evidence, was that phospholipids containing DHA compared with those containing n-6 DPA affected cellular functions. Using a specific example of visual signaling, Salem and associates[137] reported evidence that the signaling pathways depended on the acyl side chains of phospholipids. Cellular studies demonstrated the importance of DHA for the synthesis and accumulation of phosphatidylserine, an aminophospholipid enriched in DHA. Other cellular studies showed that phosphatidylserine accumulation is related to the antiapoptotic effect of DHA (as reviewed by Salem and associates[137]). Finally, biophysical studies of membranes constituted with DHA or DPA n-6 in the sn-2 position by these authors showed that membranes with DHA compared with DPA n-6 have lower-order parameters, a finding reflecting a change in bond geometry and an increase in chain dynamics.[137]

The combined evidence for the effects of variations in DHA accumulation in membrane phospholipids suggests a unifying mechanism that could include effects that have been reported for n-3 fatty acid deficiency on neurotransmitters and their receptors. DHA affected the neural N-methyl-D-aspartate response that relates to calcium influx into postsynaptic neurons.[138] Studies by Chalon and co-workers[134] and by Delion and co-workers[139] pointed to an increase in dopaminergic function in the mesolimbic area of the brain and a decrease in the frontal cortex in adult rats. de la Presa Owens and Innis[140] also observed regional differences in piglet brain monoaminergic neurotransmitters after dietary variations that influenced brain DHA and AA accumulated during development. Presumably, all membrane proteins could be influenced by the DHA/DPA n-6 ratio of the membrane phospholipids, in which case functional effects would probably not be limited to effects on neurotransmitters.

VERY LONG CHAIN POLYUNSATURATED FATTY ACIDS AND THE DEVELOPING HUMAN INFANT

Human infants born at term accumulate DHA during the last intrauterine trimester by maternal transfer of DHA across the placenta.[5,6] The process of maternal transfer continues after birth through human milk feeding, because all samples of human milk contain DHA, albeit in variable amounts.[7,8,51-53,81] Medical advances have made it possible for the fetus to survive even before brain DHA accumulates, and technical advances have permitted feeding alternatives to human milk. The effect of these advances has been that preterm infants fed formulas had to rely on synthesis for any additional postnatal DHA accumulation until the recent addition of DHA and AA to some infant formulas available in the United States.

Breast-fed infants have more DHA and AA in red blood cells than do formula-fed term infants.[7,8,36] Regardless of gestational age at birth or diet (human milk or formula), mean red blood cell phospholipid DHA is higher than levels found in the months after birth. The apparent "physiologic" decline in red blood cell DHA in breast-fed infants raises several questions: Do mothers transfer less DHA to their infants in milk than in utero? Does DHA decrease because of enhanced utilization by other tissues? Is this decline after birth unique to infants in the United States whose mothers have been shown to have milk DHA content among the lowest in the world?[8,50-53,81]

Differences in maternal DHA status reflected by milk DHA content also likely influence an infant's DHA accumulation in utero. The evidence of variable intrauterine DHA accumulation includes (1) the large normal range of values for DHA in cord red blood cell phospholipids of preterm infants,[50] (2) the progressive increase in phospholipid DHA throughout the last intrauterine trimester,[141] (3) the decline in cord red blood cell phospholipid DHA with successive pregnancies,[142] and (4) the variability in brain DHA among preterm infants of the same gestational age.[3]

The addition of DHA to infant formula can prevent declines in red blood cell and plasma phospholipid DHA after birth compared with formulas without DHA. DHA from fish oil,[33,42,143,144] egg phospholipids,[36,145] and single-cell oils[146,147] has been shown to increase DHA in circulating phospholipids, a finding suggesting that these sources could increase DHA supply available for brain. Conversely, infant formulas with α-linolenic acid but no DHA did not prevent the postnatal decline in DHA over several months, and DHA in circulating phospholipids remained low through follow-up to 12 months corrected age.[42, 105]

After birth, AA declines in plasma and red blood cell phospholipids. To some degree, the decline appears to be physiologic. For example, AA is higher in preterm than in term cord blood, and even after 4 to 6 months of breast-feeding, term infants have much lower red blood cell AA than is seen at preterm delivery (8.8% versus 15.7%).[8, 12] AA in the brain and liver also declines during the last intrauterine trimester.[148] However, breast-fed infants have more AA in red blood cell and plasma phospholipids than do infants fed formulas without LCPUFAs, and those fed formulas with n-3 LCPUFAs have still lower phospholipid AA.[149] These declines do not appear to be physiologic.

AA is the source of metabolically important prostaglandins and leukotrienes. Studies correlated AA levels with both intrauterine growth[43, 141] and growth of preterm infants in the first year of life.[44] DHA or total n-3 LCPUFAs added to infant formula reduces AA and alters the balance of n-3 and n-6 LCPUFAs in red blood cell phospholipids.[149] Three randomized trials found some reduction in growth of preterm infants with the addition of fish oil DHA and no AA to infant formula.[39, 40, 150] In one study the effect was limited to a lower weight for length at several ages in the first year.[150] In another study, the growth effects were found only in male infants.[40] No studies in term infants fed DHA have shown lower growth, and no studies in preterm infants that included a source of AA as well as DHA have shown lower growth (for review, see Lapillone and Carlson[45]).

Still, it is possible that long-term feeding of n-3 LCPUFAs without AA could decrease brain AA accumulation and could adversely affect the developing central nervous system. High concentrations of α-linolenate[151] and n-3 LCPUFAs from fish oil[152] decreased brain AA accumulation in rats. Arbuckle and associates[153] reported that piglets fed a diet with 4% of fatty acids as α-linolenic acid, but not one with 1% α-linolenic acid, had lower brain weights and lower levels of AA in membranes of synaptosomes compared with controls. Although experimental evidence for adding AA to the diet of formula-fed infants is lacking, it seems prudent to balance the addition of DHA to infant formulas with AA, as has happened with LCPUFA-supplemented formulas in the United States. The practice can be defended because both these fatty acids are found in all human milk, albeit in variable amounts.

FUNCTIONAL EFFECTS OF DOCOSAHEXAENOIC ACID STATUS: OBSERVATIONAL AND EXPERIMENTAL STUDIES

Retinal and Visual Effects of Feeding Docosahexaenoic Acid to Preterm and Term Infants

Outcomes measured in infant studies of DHA supplementation were modeled after those found to be affected by n-3 fatty acid deficiency in nonhuman primates. Lower retinal and visual development were noted first in n-3 fatty acid–deficient primates,[18-20] and some aspect of visual development has been measured in most infant studies.[37, 38] Retinal physiology is measured by ERG. Visual acuity has been assessed by both a behavioral procedure (Teller Acuity Card) and an electrophysiologic procedure (visual evoked potential [VEP] acuity).[154] Although studies using both procedures have shown higher acuity with higher DHA status in some studies, the electrophysiologic procedure appears to be more sensitive. Two studies that used both procedures found significant effects only with the electrophysiologic procedure.[33, 155]

The first interventions with DHA in infant formula occurred in preterm infants, because these infants were believed to be more likely than term infants to have inadequate brain DHA accumulation. Preliminary reports of higher visual and retinal function, respectively, with DHA supplementation were published in 1989.[156, 157] Full reports of these studies were available at the time of the last edition of this book.[31-33] Most of the trials of DHA supplementation in preterm infants were relatively small (n/group ~20 to 30). However, all the randomized studies in preterm infants that measured visual acuity found higher visual acuity with DHA at some age in the first year of life.[32,33,151,155,158] Unfortunately, one quite large study of DHA and AA supplementation did not include any measure of visual development.[159] Systematic reviews by San Giovanni and associates[160] and by Simmer[161] concluded that supplementing formulas with DHA improves visual development of preterm infants. Both reviews mentioned the absence of long-term evidence of effects of DHA supplementation on visual development of preterm infants. However, as discussed later, positive effects of an intervention at one age may be manifest in other outcomes at later ages.

Compared with preterm infants, the need for supplemental DHA for optimal visual development of term infants has been more difficult to ascertain, because the results of the published studies are mixed.[37, 38] The first suggestion that DHA status played a role in visual development of term infants came from a study by Makrides and colleagues,[34] who showed that higher blood levels of DHA in breast-fed infants were related to higher visual acuity. Observational studies by Jorgensen and co-workers[67] and by Innis and coworkers[68] also showed an association between DHA status of lactating women and visual acuity of their infants. Finally, results of a population-based cohort study suggested that maternal prenatal and postnatal intake of oily fish (a source of both DHA and EPA) was related to higher stereo-acuity in their children at 3.5 years of age.[162]

Only experimental studies that increase DHA transfer to the infant can determine whether infants require DHA for optimal visual function. There have been at least eight published intervention studies with some source of DHA (high eicosapentaenoic acid [EPA] fish oil, low EPA fish oil, egg phospholipid, single-cell oils) with or without AA that measured some aspect of visual development in term formula-fed infants. Six studies were reviewed in one report,[37] and two other studies were also published.[163] One study by Makrides and co-workers[35] found higher VEP acuity, and another one[164] did not. We found higher visual acuity (Teller Acuity Card procedure) at 2 months but not at 4, 6, 9, and 12 months.[36] Jorgensen and colleagues[165] did not find a significant difference between formulas, although the visual acuity in the group fed formula without DHA was significantly less than in the breast-fed group, using the Teller Acuity Card procedure.

Birch and colleagues[147] found higher VEP acuity at 6, 17, and 52 weeks of age, but not at 26 weeks, in infants randomized at birth. More recently, the same group of investigators reported higher sweep VEP acuity at 17, 26, and 52 weeks of age in infants randomly assigned to consume formula with, compared to without, DHA and AA after they were weaned from human milk at 6 weeks of age.[166] Two large multicenter trials conducted in term infants by Ross Laboratories found no effect of DHA supplementation on visual acuity.[163, 167] Most infants were tested with the Teller Acuity Card procedure, but a subgroup was tested with sweep VEP.

Systematic reviews that included all but the most recent Ross Laboratories study reached different conclusions. Simmer[168] concluded that there was little evidence that LCPUFAs conferred any visual development advantage in term infants. San Giovanni and colleagues[169] concluded that significantly higher visual function was associated with LCPUFA intake at 2 and 4 months in both randomized and unrandomized studies. Our group[170] reviewed the evidence more recently and concluded that a middle ground could be supported for DHA supplementation of term infants; that is, some may benefit from supplementation and others may not, depending on the mother's status and possible other factors. However, given that term infants have shown no adverse effects of supplementation and that there is no way to determine in advance who may benefit, it seemed prudent not to delay supplementing formula until further research studies could be done.

Certain international groups have recommended the addition of DHA and AA to infant formula, including the World Health Organization,[171] the International Society for the Study of Fatty Acids and Lipids,[172] and the Child Health Foundation of Germany.[173] The last report came from a consensus conference of the experts who conducted the randomized trials. Even though DHA and AA were added to term formulas in the United States in 2002, the report from the American Society for Nutritional Sciences/Life Sciences Research Office did not recommend a minimum intake of DHA and AA for preterm infants and cited that some of the positive effects noted were small or transient. The report did recommend a maximum concentration of 0.6% AA and 0.35% DHA and cited no adverse effects at these intakes and the possibility that functional changes noted in studies "may be important on a population basis or important for subsequent visual and/or cognitive function."[174]

Although it is true that only about half of the studies showed higher visual acuity in term infants with the addition of DHA to infant formula, a review of the designs and other aspects of these studies led to the conclusion that many studies may lack sufficient statistical power to reject the null hypothesis.[175] Among the factors that likely reduce statistical power in some studies are multiple testers in the multicenter trials and the use of the Teller Acuity Card procedure compared with sweep VEP acuity. Failure to control for variables other than diet that influence visual acuity could lead to an excess of "no effect" studies resulting from increases in the mean group error. Two factors that have not been controlled in any study to date are variability in DHA status at enrollment and certain demographic variables now known to be related to visual function in infants.[176] Of these demographic variables, only gestational age at birth has been controlled and only in two term studies.[36, 147] Both these studies found higher visual acuity in the group supplemented with DHA. The published studies of DHA supplementation include among them differences in ages of assessment and amounts of DHA in the experimental formulas that alone could account for a failure to accept the original hypothesis of higher visual development with DHA supplementation. For excellent reviews that include details of the designs of all but the most recent randomized clinical studies, the reader is referred to Gibson and coworkers[37] and Uauy and coworkers.[38]

Transient effects of DHA supplementation, such as higher visual acuity seen early in infancy but not later, led some investigators to suggest that DHA supplementation of formulas is unnecessary because visual development appears to have "caught up" in several studies. However, catch-up may only be apparent, given that studies have not measured other aspects of visual function that develop later than visual acuity, have used the Teller Acuity Card procedure exclusively, or have studied only a subset of subjects with VEP acuity. Even if effects on visual acuity are actually transient, early differences may set the stage for other differences in development to occur with time. In two studies, preterm infants fed formulas with, compared to without, DHA had shorter duration looks to visual stimuli at 6, 9, and 12 months, even though visual acuity, which had been higher earlier in infancy, was the same.[177, 178] Another study found that higher reported intakes of oily fish during pregnancy were related to higher stereoacuity in childhood.[163] These observations could be used to suggest a possible effect of early differences in visual development on more complex tasks later in infancy.

Reviews by both Wainwright[110] and Colombo[179] include arguments against a static interpretation of development, rather than considering development as "mediated through a series of complex variables across age." Their arguments can be related to developmental systems theory.[180] Both reviewers point out the implications of this theoretical approach for understanding all types of behavioral development in studies that vary LCPUFA status. One of these is the need for investigators to consider other environmental and metabolic factors that may interact with altered LCPUFA status.

Visual Attention: Novelty Preference and Attention Duration in Preterm and Term Infants

Several studies compared novelty preference and attention duration in preterm infants supplemented with DHA. Both novelty preference and shorter look duration in infancy were modestly correlated with higher cognitive function later in childhood.[125] Compared with controls, DHA-supplemented infants had a greater number of discrete looks[181] and a significantly shorter look duration at 6, 9, and 12 months.[177] A second study confirmed these results at 12 months of age, when most infants were tested.[178] These data are analogous to those reported in n-3–sufficient compared with deficient monkeys (i.e., higher membrane DHA correlated with shorter look duration).[29] As in the monkey studies, the results of these studies suggest that DHA supplementation enhances either the speed of visual processing or the ability of the infant to disengage from the stimulus, a possible sign of lower reactivity or impulsivity.

Other support for a relationship between DHA status and visual attention comes from more recent observational studies. Two groups presented evidence of shorter peak look duration at 4 months of age in term infants whose mothers had red blood cell phospholipid DHA higher than compared with lower than the median (2003 Society for Research in Child Development).[70, 71] In our study, the difference in peak look duration disappeared by 6 and 8 months of age,[70] but it reemerged at 12 months of age with a more sophisticated task (Kannass K, personal communication). Given that infants studied were fed little to no DHA after birth, the data suggest that variable DHA accumulation during intrauterine life was the factor that influenced infant development. Experimental studies that manipulate maternal DHA status during pregnancy are needed to test the hypothesis.

Physiologically normal infants have a preference for novel stimuli. In two randomized trials, the Fagan Infantest (Infantest Corporation, Cleveland, OH) was used to measure visual novelty preference at 6, 9, and 12 months of corrected age. A repeated-measures analysis of variance indicated that infants fed control and DHA-supplemented formulas had a similar novelty preference.[177, 178] In contrast, O'Connor[155] found a higher novelty preference but no effect on look duration in one group of infants fed AA and DHA (egg triglyceride and fish oil) compared with the control group at 6 months of age.

Novelty preference and look duration were measured in several studies of term infants,[75, 163, 166] including one that provided additional DHA in the form of fish oil to women during much of pregnancy and the early months after they gave birth.[75] None of these studies found an effect on attention during infancy.

Other Measurements of Infant Development

Willatts and co-workers[182] fed newborn infants formulas with and without DHA for 4 months. At 10 months of age, infants who had received DHA were better able to solve a means-end problem than those fed a formula without DHA. The results may be evidence of increased cognitive ability (ability to learn), but positive effects on other behavioral domains (lower reactivity or impulsivity) cannot be ruled out from the task given. There is evidence of higher reactivity but not lower ability to learn in n-3 fatty acid–deficient monkeys.

Lammi-Keefe and associates[69] reported an association between maternal plasma phospholipid DHA (another indicator of maternal status) and brain maturation in newborn infants based on differences in sleep patterns at birth. With maturation, there is an increase in quiet sleep, a decrease in active sleep, increased wakefulness, and a decrease in the transition from sleep to wake. These authors noted inverse relationships between maternal DHA status and both active sleep and the ratio of active sleep to quiet sleep. They also found that maternal DHA status was associated with more time awake and less time in transition between sleep and wake. Each observation is evidence of more mature function with higher DHA status and adds to the evidence that intrauterine exposure to DHA affects development.

O'Connor[155] found higher vocabulary comprehension at 14 months in preterm infants from English-speaking families who received formulas with, versus without AA and DHA (from either fungal oil and fish oil or egg phospholipids and fish oil). Innis and colleagues[183] studied language comprehension and production of term infants in relation to the range of variation in DHA status within the population. At 9 months, infants were evaluated for their ability to discriminate fine phonetic differences in native and non-native language. At 14 months, language development was assessed with the MacArthur Communicative Inventory. Several indicators of DHA status (plasma phospholipid DHA, red blood cell phosphatidylcholine DHA, and phosphatidylethanolamine DHA) were significantly correlated with the ability to discriminate a non-native language consonant at 9 months and with vocabulary comprehension and production at 14 months of age.

Global Tests of Infant Development

Two tests of global neurodevelopment have been used in studies of DHA supplementation: the Bayley Scales of Infant Development, which was developed in the United States, and the Italian version of the Brunet-Lezine Test, which was developed in France. Both tests are standardized procedures that provide indices of mental and motor age relative to group norms. The most recent version of the Bayley Scales of Infant Development provides several tools for assessing development between 1 and 42 months of age, including the Mental Developmental Index (MDI) and the Psychomotor Developmental Index (PDI).[125]

Because the tests are standardized and are familiar to pediatricians, their use as outcome measures in studies of infant development has been encouraged. However, the tests were designed to identify infants and children who were performing below normal, a major limitation for an outcome used as a measure of an intervention in normal infants. They also include tasks that represent many developmental domains, often two or more within the same task. Because of this, an effect that occurred within a single behavioral domain could be disguised. At older ages (≥ 18 months), there is greater emphasis on language in the Bayley MDI and fine motor development in the Bayley PDI, and performance on the Bayley MDI becomes more closely correlated with later IQ.

Two studies found higher performance on the Bayley MDI at 18 months of age with higher DHA status in observational and intervention studies.[184, 185] The intervention studies were with preterm[184] and term[185] infants. In the only studies specifically powered to detect an effect of LCPUFA supplementation on the Bayley MDI and PDI, no effect of diet was found at 18 months of age in either preterm[159] or term[186] infants.

Three groups reported studies of infants supplemented with DHA by providing additional DHA to their mothers.[72,73,187] In one of these, maternal DHA supplementation began at mid-pregnancy and continued through 3 months after delivery.[73] Most of these infants were also breast-fed. In the other two studies, supplementation occurred during the first 3 or 4 months of lactation.[72, 187] Infants of women supplemented with DHA from fish oil during both pregnancy and lactation showed no developmental advantage in the first year of life,[75] but they scored higher on the Mental Processing Composite of the Kaufman Assessment Battery for Children at 4 years of age.[73] A multiple regression analysis showed that maternal DHA intake during pregnancy was the only variable related to IQ at 4 years of age.[73]

Neither of the groups of infants supplemented through human milk had an advantage for development during the first year of life,[74, 187] but the investigators who studied infants after infancy found a higher Bayley MDI at 30 months of age.[72] The reports by Jensen and colleagues[72] and by Helland and coworkers[73] suggested that even groups of infants previously considered to have the best DHA status (i.e., term, breast-fed) could benefit from additional DHA. The results suggest that optimal levels of DHA for infant development may be higher than previously imagined and higher than currently achievable by diet for most pregnant and lactating women. More studies of the effects of higher maternal DHA intake on infant outcomes are likely. Because there are few data on which to base desirable upper limits for pregnant and lactating women, studies of maternal and infant DHA supplementation should be done as randomized clinical trials that monitor safety as well as efficacy of the intervention.

Many more studies measured Bayley MDI and PDI at 12 months of age. Some groups, including ours, found higher Bayley MDI in some studies and not in others.[181] In general, the studies that have measured the Bayley MDI and PDI at 12 months were not powered to measure this outcome.

Agostoni and co-workers[188] measured psychomotor development of infants randomly assigned to formulas with and without DHA and AA. The Brunet-Lezine test component for psychomotor development was administered at 4, 12, and 24 months. Higher scores were found at 4 months of age with DHA- and AA-supplemented formulas. At 4 months of age, the test evaluates postural, gross motor, and early social performance. Group differences were not found at 12 and 24 months of age.

SUMMARY

Since the last edition of this book, a large study in preterm infants has confirmed smaller randomized studies published earlier that showed higher visual acuity in infants fed formulas with DHA. A number of randomized studies of DHA supplementation have been done in term infants with approximately half showing advantages for visual development. This chapter addresses the possible reasons for the inconsistency of findings in the term studies. The studies in both term and preterm infants have generally concluded after 12 months, with several continuing to 18 months. While long-term effects of DHA supplementation from randomized trials are limited, there are several new reports that suggest early supplementation benefits cognitive and psychomotor function in childhood.

DHA and AA were added to formulas for term and preterm infants in the United States in 2002. The levels of DHA added to study formulas are only slightly higher than DHA provided by milk of U.S. women. While the importance of DHA in infant development is becoming increasingly obvious from human and animal work, the optimal level of DHA intake for pregnant women and infants and the upper level of desirable intake for these groups is not known. Progress in these areas should be expected in the future.

New research since the last edition of this book addresses maternal DHA status during pregnancy and its influence on development of the infant and child. With the exception of one experimental study, these are observational studies that report an association between more mature patterns of sleep, language, peak look duration and global scores on the Bayley MDI with higher maternal DHA status. A positive effect of intervening with DHA during pregnancy and lactation has been found in children as old as 4 years of age, but more studies are needed. To date, most studies of maternal supplementation have been done in countries such as Norway and Denmark, where women have a higher antecedent DHA intake than in the United States.

Experimental studies of infants whose mothers were provided different amounts of DHA during pregnancy are now in progress or planned. In addition to aiding our understanding of the timing and amount of DHA needed for the developing brain, it is hoped that these studies can incorporate novel outcomes that target specific behavioral domains. DHA intake from supplemented foods and formula will be a potential confounder of new studies of intrauterine DHA supplementation. Studies of infant behavior will need to control for postnatal DHA intake.

Animal models continue to be employed to answer questions about the effects of lower brain DHA accumulation on neural development. It seems likely that the results of these studies will aid in targeting new developmental outcomes as well as the effects of DHA on other aspects of physiology. Still other research is being directed toward understanding the mechanisms by which lower DHA accumulation in membranes affects physiologic functions. Readers wishing to have a more extensive treatment of the neural mechanisms of DHA are referred to a recent review by Salem et al.[137]

REFERENCES

1. O'Brien JS, et al: Quantification of fatty acid and fatty aldehyde composition of ethanolamine choline and serine phosphoglycerides in human cerebral gray and white matter. J Lipid Res 5:329, 1964.
2. Anderson RE, et al: Lipids of ocular tissues. X. Lipid composition of subcellular fractions of bovine retina. Vision Res 15:1087, 1975.
3. Clandinin MT, et al: Intrauterine fatty acid accretion rates in human brain: implications for fatty acid requirements. Early Hum Dev 4:121, 1980.
4. Martinez M: Developmental profiles of polyunsaturated fatty acids in the brain of normal infants and patients with peroxisomal diseases: severe deficiency of docosahexaenoic acid in Zellweger's and pseudo-Zellweger's syndromes. World Rev Nutr Diet 66:87, 1991.
5. Ruyle M, et al: Placental transfer of essential fatty acids in humans: venous arterial difference for docosahexaenoic acid in fetal umbilical erythrocytes. Proc Natl Acad Sci USA 78:7902, 1990.
6. Dutta-Roy AK. Transport mechanisms for long-chain polyunsaturated fatty acids in the human placenta. Am J Clin Nutr 71:315S, 2000.
7. Sanders TA, Naismith DJ: A comparison of the influence of breast-feeding and bottle-feeding on the fatty acid composition of the erythrocytes. Br J Nutr 41:619, 1979.
8. Putnam JC, et al: The effect of variations in dietary fatty acids on the fatty acid composition of erythrocyte phosphatidylcholine and phosphatidylethanolamine in human infants. Am J Clin Nutr 36:106, 1982.
9. Demmelmair H, et al: Estimation of arachidonic acid synthesis in full term neonates using natural variation of ^{13}C-abundance. J Pediatr Gastroenterol Nutr 21:31, 1995.
10. Carnielli VP, et al: The very low birth weight premature infant is capable of synthesizing arachidonic acid and docosahexaenoic acid from linoleic and linolenic acids. Pediatr Res 40:169, 1996.
11. Salem N Jr, et al: Arachidonic and docosahexaenoic acids are biosynthesized from their 18-carbon precursors in human infants. Proc Natl Acad Sci USA 93:49, 1996.
12. Sauerwald TU, et al: Intermediates in endogenous synthesis of C22:6ω3 and C20:4ω6 by term and preterm infants. Pediatr Res 41:183, 1997.
13. Herrera E, Lasuncion MA: Maternal-fetal transfer of lipid metabolites. *In* Polin R, et al (eds): Fetal and Neonatal Physiology, 3rd ed. Philadelphia, Elsevier Science, 2003.
14. Van Aerde JE, Accretion of lipid in the fetus and newborn. *In* Polin R, et al (eds): Fetal and Neonatal Physiology, 3rd ed. Philadelphia, Elsevier Science, 2003.
15. Galli C, et al: Effect of dietary fatty acids on the fatty acid composition of brain ethanolamine phosphoglyceride: reciprocal replacement of n-6 and n-3 polyunsaturated fatty acids. Biochim Biophys Acta 248:449, 1971.
16. Benolken RM, et al: Membrane fatty acids associated with the electrical response in visual excitation. Science 182:1253, 1973.
17. Wheeler TG, et al: Visual membranes: specificity of fatty acid precursors for the electrical response to illumination. Science 188:1312, 1975.
18. Neuringer M, et al: Omega-3 fatty acid deficiency in rhesus monkeys: depletion of retinal docosahexaenoic acid and abnormal electroretinograms. Am J Clin Nutr 43:706, 1985.
19. Neuringer M, et al: Electroretinogram abnormalities in young rhesus monkeys deprived of omega-3 fatty acids during gestation and postnatal development or only postnatally. Invest Ophthalmol Vis Sci 29:145, 1988.
20. Neuringer M, et al: Dietary omega-3 fatty acid deficiency and visual loss in infant rhesus monkeys. J Clin Invest 73:272, 1984.
21. Lamptey MS, Walker BL: A possible essential role for dietary linolenic acid in the development of the young rat. J Nutr 106:86, 1976.
22. Yamamoto N, et al: Effect of dietary α-linolenate/linoleate balance on brain lipid compositions and learning ability in rats. J Lipid Res 28:144, 1987.
23. Yamamoto N, et al: Effect of dietary α-linoleate/linoleate balance on lipid compositions and learning ability in rats. J Lipid Res 29:1073, 1988.
24. Yamamoto N, et al: Effects of a high-linoleate and a high-α-linoleate diet on the learning ability of aged rats: evidence against autooxidation-related lipid peroxide therapy of aging. J Gerontol 46:B17, 1991.
25. Bourre JM, et al: The effects of dietary α-linolenic acid on the composition of nerve membranes, enzymatic activity, amplitude of electrophysiological parameters, resistance to poisons and performance of learning tasks in rats. J Nutr 119:1880, 1989.
26. Wainwright PE, et al: Interactive effects of prenatal ethanol and n-3 fatty acid supplementation on brain development in mice. Lipids 24:989, 1989.
27. Wainwright PE, et al: Effects of prenatal ethanol and long chain n-3 fatty acid supplementation on development in mice. I. Body and brain growth, sensori-motor development, and water T-maze reversal learning. Alcohol Clin Exp Res 14:405, 1990.
28. Wainwright PE, et al: The role of n-3 essential fatty acids in brain and behavioral development: a cross-fostering study in the mouse. Lipids 26:203, 1991.
29. Reisbick SW, et al: Visual attention in infant monkeys: effects of dietary fatty acids and age. Dev Psychol 33:387, 1997.
30. Reisbick SW, et al: Home cage behavior of rhesus monkeys with long-term deficiency of omega-3 fatty acids. Physiol Behav 55:231, 1994.
31. Uauy RD, et al: Effect of dietary omega-3 fatty acids on retinal function of very-low-birth-weight neonates. Pediatr Res 38:484, 1990.
32. Carlson SE, et al: Visual acuity development in healthy preterm infants: effect of marine oil supplementation. Am J Clin Nutr 58:35, 1993.
33. Birch EE, et al: Dietary essential fatty acid supply and visual acuity development. Invest Ophthalmol Vis Sci 33:3242, 1992.
34. Makrides M, et al: Erythrocyte docosahexaenoic acid correlated with the visual response of healthy, term infants. Pediatr Res 33:425, 1993.
35. Makrides M, et al: Are long-chain polyunsaturated fatty acids essential nutrients in infancy? Lancet 345:1463, 1995.
36. Carlson SE, et al: Visual acuity and fatty acid status of term infants fed human milk and formulas with and without docosahexaenoate and arachidonate from egg yolk lecithin. Pediatr Res 39:1, 1996.
37. Gibson RA, et al: Randomized trials with polyunsaturated fatty acid interventions in preterm and term infants: functional and clinical outcomes. Lipids 36:873, 2001.
38. Uuay R., et al: Essential fatty acids in visual and brain development. Lipids 36:885, 2001.
39. Carlson SE, et al: First year growth of preterm infants fed standard compared to marine oil n-3 supplemented formula. Lipids 27:901, 1992.
40. Ryan AS, et al: Effect of DHA-containing formula on growth of preterm infants to 59 weeks postmenstrual age. Am J Hum Biol 11:457, 1999.
41. Holman RT: Essential fatty acid deficiency in animals. *In* Rechcigl M Jr (ed): CRC Handbook Series in Nutrition and Food, Nutritional Disorders, Vol 2. Boca Raton, FL, CRC Press, 1978, pp 491–515.
42. Carlson SE, et al: Long-term feeding of formulas high in linolenic acid and marine oil to very low birth weight infants: phospholipid fatty acids. Pediatr Res 30:404, 1991.
43. Koletzko B, Braun M: Arachidonic acid and early human growth: is there a relation? Ann Nutr Metab 35:128, 1991.
44. Carlson SE, et al: Arachidonic acid status correlates with first year growth of preterm infants. Proc Natl Acad Sci USA 90:1073, 1993.
45. Lapillone A and Carlson SE: Polyunsaturated fatty acids and infant growth. Lipids 36:901, 2001.
46. Martinez M: Developmental fatty acid patterns in the human retina. J Neurochem 48(Suppl S):100B, 1987.
47. Sinclair AJ, Crawford MA: Incorporation of radioactive polyunsaturated fatty acids into liver and brain of developing rats. Lipids 10:175, 1975.
48. Sinclair AJ, Crawford MA: The accumulation of arachidonate and docosahexaenoate in the developing rat brain. J Neurochem 19:1753, 1972.
49. Carlson SE, et al: High fat diets varying in ratios of polyunsaturated to saturated fatty acid and linoleic to linolenic acid: a comparison of rat neural and red cell membrane phospholipids. J Nutr 116:718, 1986.
50. Carlson SE, et al: Docosahexaenoic acid status of preterm infants at birth and following feeding with human milk or formula. Am J Clin Nutr 44:798, 1986.
51. Bitman J, et al: Comparison of the lipid composition of breast milk from mothers of term and preterm infants. Am J Clin Nutr 38:300, 1988.
52. Innis SM: Human milk and formula fatty acids. J Pediatr 120:S56, 1992.
53. Koletzko B, et al: The fatty acid composition of human milk in Europe and Africa. J Pediatr 120:S62, 1992.
54. Patel TB, Clark JB: Comparison of the development of the fatty acid content and composition of the brain of a precocial species (guinea pig) and a non-precocial species (rat). J Neurochem 35:149, 1980.
55. Arbuckle LD, Innis SM: Docosahexaenoic acid is transferred through maternal diet to milk and to tissues of natural milk-fed piglets. J Nutr 123:1668, 1993.
56. Connor W, et al: Enhanced Omega-3 Fatty Acid Levels in Newborn Infants by Maternal Omega-3 Fatty Acid Supplementation. Washington, DC, International Society for the Study of Fatty Acids and Lipids, 1995.

57. Harris WS, et al: Will dietary omega-3 fatty acids change the composition of human milk? Am J Clin Nutr 40:780, 1984.

58. Otto SJ, et al: Maternal and neonatal essential fatty acid status in phospholipids: an international comparative study. Eur J Clin Nutr 51: 232, 1997.

59. Al MD, et al: Fat intake of women during normal pregnancy: relationship with maternal and neonatal essential fatty acid status. J Am Coll Nutr 15:49, 1996.

60. Otto SJ, et al: Changes in the maternal essential fatty acid profile during early pregnancy and the relation of the profile to diet. Am J Clin Nutr 73:302, 2001.

61. Al MD, et al: Long-chain polyunsaturated fatty acids, pregnancy, and pregnancy outcome. Am J Clin Nutr 71:285S, 2000.

62. Hornstra G: Essential fatty acids in mothers and their neonates. Am J Clin Nutr 71:1262S, 2000.

63. Zeijdner EE, et al: Essential fatty acid status in plasma phospholipids of mother and neonate after multiple pregnancy. Prostaglandins Leukot Essent Fatty Acids 56:395, 1997.

64. Smuts CM, et al: A randomized trial of docosahexaenoic acid supplementation during the third trimester of pregnancy. J Obstet Gynecol 101:469, 2003.

65. Farquharson J, et al: Infants' cerebral cortex phospholipid fatty-acid composition and diet. Lancet 340:810, 1992.

66. Makrides M, et al: Fatty acid composition of brain, retina, and erythrocytes in breast-fed and formula-fed infants. Am J Clin Nutr 60:189, 1994.

67. Jorgensen MH, et al: Breast-fed (BF) term infants have a better visual acuity than formula fed (FF) infants at the age of 2 and 4 mo. FASEB J 8:A460, 1994.

68. Innis SM, et al: Are human milk long-chain polyunsaturated fatty acids related to visual and neural development in breast-fed term infants? J Pediatr 139:532, 2001.

69. Cheruku SR, et al: Higher maternal plasma docosahexaenoic acid during pregnancy is associated with more mature neonatal sleep-state patterning. Am J Clin Nutr 76:608, 2002.

70. Carlson SE, et al: Maternal DHA levels and the development of infant attention. Soc Res Child Dev Abstr, Tampa, FL, 2003.

71. Willatts P, et al: Maternal DHA status during late pregnancy is related to measures of infant look duration and acuity at age 4 months. Soc Res Child Dev Abstr, Tampa, FL, 2003.

72. Jensen CL, et al: Effects of maternal docosahexaenoic acid (DHA) supplementation on visual function and neurodevelopment of breast-fed infants. Pediatr Res 49:448A, 2001.

73. Helland IB, et al: Maternal supplementation with very long-chain n-3 fatty acids during pregnancy and lactation augments children's IQ at 4 years of age. Pediatrics 111:e39, 2003.

74. Jensen CL, et al: Effects of maternal docosahexaenoic acid (DHA) supplementation on visual function and growth of breast-fed infants. Pediatr Res 43:262A, 1998.

75. Helland IB, et al: Similar effects on infants of n-3 and n-6 fatty acids supplementation to pregnant and lactating women. Pediatrics 108:1, 2001 (http://www.pediatrics.org/cgi/content/full/108/5/e82).

76. Van Houwelingen AC, et al: Essential fatty acid status of fetal plasma phospholipids: similar to postnatal values obtained at comparable gestational ages. Early Hum Dev 46:141, 1996.

77. Sanders TAB, et al: Studies of vegans: the fatty acid composition of plasma phosphoglycerides, erythrocytes, adipose tissue and breast milk and some indications to susceptibility to ischemic heart disease in vegans and omnivores. Am J Clin Nutr 31:805, 1978.

78. Chulei R, et al: Milk composition in women from five different regions of China: the great diversity of milk fatty acids. J Nutr 125:2993, 1995.

79. Henderson RA, et al: Effect of fish oil on the fatty acid composition of human milk and maternal and infant erythrocytes. Lipids 27:863, 1992.

80. Smuts CM, et al: High-docosahexaenoic acid eggs: Feasibility as a means to enhance mother and infant DHA status. Lipids 2003, in press.

81. Jensen RG, et al: Milk lipids A: Human milk lipids. In Jensen RG (ed): Handbook of Milk Composition. San Diego, Academic Press, 1995, pp 495-542.

82. Voss A, et al: The metabolism of 7,10,13,16,19-docosapentaenoic acid to 4,7,19,13,16,19-docosahexaenoic acid in rat liver is independent of a 4-desaturase. J Biol Chem 266:19995, 1991.

83. Wang N, Anderson RE: Synthesis of docosahexaenoic acid by retina and retinal pigment epithelium. Biochemistry 32:13703, 1993.

84. Martinez M: Abnormal profiles of polyunsaturated fatty acids in the brain, liver, kidney and retina of patients with peroxisomal disorders. Brain Res 583:171, 1992.

85. Martinez M: Docosahexaenoic acid therapy in docosahexaenoic acid-deficient patients with disorders of peroxisomal biogenesis. Lipids 31:S145, 1996.

86. Scott BL, Bazan NG: Membrane docosahexaenoate is supplied to the developing brain and retina by the liver. Proc Natl Acad Sci USA 86:2903, 1989.

87. Alvarez RA, et al: Docosapentaenoic acid is converted to docosahexaenoic acid in the retinas of normal and prcd-affected miniature poodle dogs. Invest Ophthalmol Vis Sci 35:402, 1994.

88. Moore SA, et al: Role of the blood-brain barrier in the formation of long chain omega-3 and omega-6 fatty acids from essential fatty acid precursors. J Neurochem 55:391, 1990.

89. Moore SA, et al: Astrocytes, not neurons, produce docosahexaenoic acid (22:5n-3) and arachidonic acid (20:4n-6). J Neurochem 56:518, 1991.

90. Moore SA: Cerebral endothelium and astrocytes cooperate in supplying docosahexaenoic acid to neurons. Adv Exp Med Biol 331:229, 1993.

91. Innis SM, Dyer RA: Brain astrocyte synthesis of docosahexaenoic acid from n-3 fatty acids is limited at the elongation of docosapentaenoic acid. J Lip Res 43:1529, 2002.

92. Chen H, et al: Differential incorporation of docosahexaenoic and arachidonic acids in frog retinal pigment epithelium. J Lipid Res 34:1943, 1993.

93. Gordon WC, Bazan NG: Visualization of [3H] docosahexaenoic acid trafficking through photoreceptors and retinal pigment epithelium by electron microscopic autoradiography. Invest Ophthalmol Vis Sci 34:2402, 1993.

94. Chambaz J, et al: Essential fatty acids in interconversions in the human fetal liver. Biol Neonate 47:136, 1985.

95. Innis SM, et al: Neonatal polyunsaturated fatty acid metabolism. Lipids 34:139, 1999.

96. Emken EA, et al: Stable isotope approaches, applications, and issues related to polyunsaturated fatty acid metabolism studies. Lipids 36:965, 2001.

97. Kanazawa A, et al: Possible essentiality of docosahexaenoic acid in Japanese monkey neonates: occurrence in colostrum and low biosynthetic capacity in neonate brain. Lipids 26:53, 1991.

98. Su HM, et al: Fetal baboons convert 18:3n-3 to 22:6n-3 in vivo. A stable isotope tracer study. J Lip Res 42:581, 2001.

99. Cook HW: In vitro formation of polyunsaturated fatty acids by desaturation in rat brain: some properties of the enzymes in developing brain and comparisons with liver. J Neurochem 30:1327, 1978.

100. Bourre JM, Piciotti M: Delta-6 desaturation of alpha-linolenic acid in brain and liver during development and aging in the mouse. Neurosci Lett 141:65, 1992.

101. Clandinin MT, et al: Delta-5 desaturase activity in liver and brain microsomes during development of the pig. Biochem J 227:1021, 1985.

102. Clandinin MT, et al: Synthesis of chain elongation-desaturation products of linoleic acid by liver and brain microsomes during development of the pig. Biochem J 226:305, 1985.

103. Peeples JM, et al: Effect of LCPUFA and age on red blood cell sphingomyelin 24:1n-9 and 24:2 of preterm infants with reference to term infants. In PUFA in Infant Nutrition: Consensus and Controversies Meeting Abstracts. Barcelona, Spain, AOCS Press, 1996, p 33.

104. Hornstra G: Essential fatty acids in mothers and their neonates. Am J Clin Nutr 71:1262S, 2000.

105. Ponder DL, et al: Docosahexaenoic acid status of term infants fed breast milk or infant formula containing soy oil or corn oil. Pediatr Res. 32:683, 1992.

106. Uauy R, et al: Visual and brain function measurements in studies of n-3 fatty acid requirements of infants. J Pediatr 120:S168, 1992.

107. Arbuckle LD, Innis SM: Docosahexaenoic acid in developing brain and retina of piglets fed high or low alpha-linolenate formula with and without fish oil. Lipids 27:89, 1992.

108. Martinez M: Dietary polyunsaturated fatty acids in relation to neural development in humans. In Galli C, Simopoulos AP (eds): Dietary ω3 and ω6 fatty acids: Biological Effects and Nutritional Essentiality. NATO ASI Series A: Life Sciences, Vol. 171. New York, Plenum Press, 1989, pp 123-133.

109. Wainwright PE: Lipids and behavior: the evidence from animal models. In Dobbing J (ed): Lipids, Learning and the Brain: Fats in Infant Formulas. Report of the 103rd Ross Conference on Pediatric Research. Columbus, OH, Ross Laboratories, 1993, pp 69-88.

110. Wainwright PE: Dietary essential fatty acids and brain function: a developmental perspective on mechanisms. Proc Nutr Soc 61:61, 2002.

111. Carlson SE: Behavioral methods used in the study of long-chain polyunsaturated fatty acid nutrition in primate infants. Am J Clin Nutr 71:268S, 2000.

112. Mostofsky DI: Models and methods for studying behavior in polyunsaturated fatty acid research. Lipids 36:913, 2001.

113. Sun GY, et al: Essential fatty acid deficiency: metabolism of 20:3(n-9) and 22:3(n-9) of major phosphoglycerides in subcellular fractions of developing and mature mouse brain. Lipids 10:365, 1975.

114. Enslen M, et al: Effects of n-3 polyunsaturated fatty acid deficiency during development in the rat: future effects. In Lands WEM (ed): Proceedings of the AOCS Short Course on Polyunsaturated Fatty Acids and Eicosanoids. Biloxi, MS, AOCS Press, 1987, pp 495-497.

115. Leat WMF, et al: Retinal function in rats and guinea pigs reared on diets low in essential fatty acids and supplemented with linoleic and linolenic acids. Ann Metab 30:166, 1986.

116. Cho ES, et al: Electroretinography and retinal phosphatidylcholine fatty acids in omega-3 fatty acid deficient rats. Brighton, UK, XIII International Congress of Nutrition, 1985, p 104.

117. Neuringer M: The relationship of fatty acid composition to function in the retina and visual system. In Dobbing J (ed): Lipids, Learning and the Brain: Fats in Infant Formulas. Report of the 103rd Ross Conference on Pediatric Research. Columbus, OH, Ross Laboratories, 1993, p 134.

118. Bogener J, et al: Effect of a diet deficient in alpha-linolenic acid on adult rat visual evoked potentials. In AOCS PUFA in Maternal and Child Health Meeting Abstracts. Kansas City, MO, AOCS Press, 2000.

119. Radel JD, et al: Effects of developmental DHA deficiency and remediation upon evoked brain activity at maturity in rats. In Program No. 106.5, 2002 Abstracts Viewer/Itinerary Planner. Washington, DC, Society for Neuroscience, 2002 (CD-ROM).

120. Yehuda S, et al: Effects of dietary fat on pain threshold, thermoregulation and motor activity in rats. Pharmacol Biochem Behav 24:1775, 1986.

121. Yehuda S, Carasso RL: Modulation of learning, pain thresholds, and thermoregulation in the rat by preparations of free purified alpha-linolenic and linoleic acids: discrimination of the optimal omega-3-to-omega-6 ratio. Proc Natl Acad Sci USA 90:10345, 1993.

122. Colombo J, et al: Individual differences in infant visual attention: are short lookers fast processors or feature processors? Child Dev 62:1247, 1991.

123. Johnson M, et al: Components of visual orienting in early infancy: Contingency learning, anticipatory looking and disengaging. J Cognitive Neurosci 3:335, 1991.

124. Reisbick S, et al: Effect of n-3 fatty acid deficiency in nonhuman primates. *In* Bindels JG, et al (eds.): Recent Developments in Infant Nutrition. Dordrecht, Netherlands, Kluwer Academic Publishers, 1996, p 157–172.

125. Carlson SE, Neuringer M: Polyunsaturated fatty acid status and neurodevelopment: a summary and critical analysis of the literature. Lipids 34:171, 1999.

126. Frances H, et. al: Effect of dietary alpha-linolenic acid deficiency on habituation. Life Sci 58:1805, 1996.

127. Yoshida S, et al: Synaptic vesicle ultrastructural changes in the rat hippocampus induced by a combination of alpha-linoleate deficiency and a learning task. J Neurochem 68:1261, 1997.

128. Ikemoto A, et al: Reversibility of n-3 fatty acid deficiency-induced alterations of learning behavior in the rat: level of n-6 fatty acids as another critical factor. J Lipid Res 42:1655, 2001.

129. Sato A, et al: Long-term n-3 fatty acid deficiency induces no substantial change in the rate of protein synthesis in rat brain and liver. Biol Pharm Bull 22:775, 1999.

130. Greiner RS, et al: DHA-deficient rats exhibit learning deficits in olfactory-based behavioral tasks. *In* PUFA in Maternal and Child Health Meeting Abstracts. Kansas City, MO, AOCS Press, 2000, p 24.

131. Enslen M, et al: Effect of low intake of n-3 fatty acids during development on brain phospholipid fatty acid composition and exploratory behavior in rats. Lipids 26:203, 1991.

132. Reisbick S, et al: Postnatal deficiency of omega-3 fatty acids in monkeys: fluid intake and urine concentration. Physiol Behav 51:473, 1992.

133. Levant B, et al: Effects of developmental DHA deficiency and remediation on adult behavior in rats. *In* Program No. 106.5 2002. Abstracts Viewer/Itinerary Planner. Washington, DC, Society for Neuroscience, 2002 (CD-ROM).

134. Chalon S, et al. Polyunsaturated fatty acids and cerebral function: focus on monoaminergic neurotransmission. Lipids 36:937, 2001.

135. Frances H, et al: Influences of a dietary alpha-linolenic acid deficiency on learning in the Morris water maze and on the effects of morphine. Eur J Pharmacol 298:217, 1996.

136. Hibbeln JR, et al: DHA and AA supplementation of infant formulas improves motor skills and visual orientation, decrease CSF 5-HIAA in infancy and improve heart rate variability in adolescence. *In* PUFA in Maternal and Child Health Meeting Abstracts. Kansas City, MO, AOCS Press, 2000, p 24.

137. Salem N, et al: Mechanisms of action of docosahexaenoic acid in the nervous system. Lipids 36:945, 2001.

138. Nishikawa M, et al: Facilitatory effect of docosahexaenoic acid on N-methyl-D-aspartate response in pyramidal neurones of rat cerebral cortex. J Physiol 475:1, 1994.

139. Delion S, et al: Chronic dietary α-linolenic acid deficiency alters dopaminergic and serotoninergic neurotransmission in rats. J Nutr 124:2466, 1994.

140. de la Presa Owens S, Innis SM. Diverse, region-specific effects of addition of arachidonic and docosahexaenoic acids to formula with low or adequate linoleic and alpha-linolenic acids on piglet brain monoaminergic neurotransmitters. Pediatr Res 48:125, 2000.

141. Leaf AA, et al: Long chain polyunsaturated fatty acids and fetal growth. Early Hum Dev 30:183, 1992.

142. Spear ML, et al: Milk and blood fatty acid composition during two lactations in the same women. Am J Clin Nutr 56:65, 1992.

143. Carlson SE, et al: Effect of fish oil supplementation on the n-3 fatty acid content of red blood cell membranes in preterm infants. Pediatr Res 21:507, 1987.

144. Liu C-CF, et al: Increase in plasma phospholipid docosahexaenoic and eicosapentaenoic acids as a reflection of their intake and mode of administration. Pediatr Res 22:292, 1987.

145. Koletzko B, et al: Effects of dietary long-chain polyunsaturated fatty acids on the essential fatty acid status of premature infants. Eur J Pediatr 148:669, 1989.

146. Carnielli VP, et al: Long chain polyunsaturated fatty acids (LCP) in low birth weight formula at levels found in human colostrum. Pediatr Res 35:309A, 1994.

147. Birch EE, et al: Visual acuity and the essentiality of docosahexaenoic acid and arachidonic acid in the diet of term infants. Pediatr Res 44:201, 1998.

148. Martinez M, Ballibriga A: Effects of parenteral nutrition with high doses of linoleate on the developing human liver and brain. Lipids 22:133, 1987.

149. Carlson SE: Arachidonic acid status of human infants: influence of gestational age at birth and diets with very long chain n-3 and n-6 fatty acids. J Nutr 126:1092S, 1996.

150. Carlson SE, et al: Effect of long-chain n-3 fatty acid supplementation on visual acuity and growth of preterm infants with and without bronchopulmonary dysplasia. Am J Clin Nutr 63:687, 1996.

151. Mohrhauer H, Holman RT: Alteration of the fatty acid composition of brain lipids by varying levels of dietary essential fatty acids. J Neurochem 10:523, 1963.

152. Witting LA, et al: Dietary alterations of fatty acids of erythrocytes and mitochondria of brain and liver. J Lipid Res 2:412, 1961.

153. Arbuckle LD, et al: Formula 18:2(n-6) and 18:3(n-3) content and ratio influence long-chain polyunsaturated fatty acids in the developing piglet liver and central nervous system. J Nutr 124:289, 1994.

154. Mayer DL, Dobson V. Grating acuity cards: validity, reliability in studies of human visual development. *In* Dobbing J (ed): Developing Brain and Behavior. San Diego, Academic Press, 1997, pp 253–288.

155. O'Connor DL: Growth and development in preterm infants fed long-chain polyunsaturated fatty acids: a prospective, randomized controlled trial. Pediatrics 108:359, 2001.

156. Carlson S, et al: Docosahexaenoate (DHA) and eicosapentaenoate (EPA) supplementation of preterm infants: effects on phospholipid DHA and visual acuity. Fed Proc 3:A1056, 1989.

157. Uauy R, et al: Effect of omega 3 fatty acid (FA) on retinal function of very low birth weight infants. Fed Proc 3:A1247, 1989.

158. Carlson SE, et al: Visual acuity of preterm (PT) infants fed docosahexaenoic acid (DHA) and arachidonic acid (ARA): effect of age at supplementation. Pediatr Res 45:279A, 1999.

159. Fewtrell MS, et al: Double-blind, randomized trial of long-chain polyunsaturated fatty acid supplementation in formula fed to preterm infants. Pediatr 110:73, 2002.

160. SanGiovanni JP, et al: Meta-analysis of dietary essential fatty acids and long-chain polyunsaturated fatty acids as they relate to visual resolution acuity in healthy preterm infants. Pediatr 105:1292, 2000.

161. Simmer K: Long chain polyunsaturated fatty acid supplementation in preterm infants. Cochrane Database Syst Rev 2000.

162. Williams C, et al: Stereoacuity at age 3.5 years in children born full-term is associated with prenatal and postnatal dietary factors: a report from a population-based cohort study. Am J Clin Nutr 73:316:2001.

163. Auestad N, et al: Growth and development in term infants fed long-chain polyunsaturated fatty acids: a double-masked, randomized, parallel, prospective, multivariate study. Pediatrics 108:372, 2001.

164. Makrides M, et al: A critical appraisal of the role of dietary long-chain polyunsaturated fatty acids on neural indices of term infants: a randomized, controlled trial. Pediatrics 105:32, 2000.

165. Jorgensen MH, et al: Effect of formula supplemented with docosahexaenoic acid and γ-linolenic acid on fatty acid status and visual acuity in term infants. J Pediatr Gastroenterol Nutr 26:412, 1998.

166. Birch EE, et al: A randomized controlled trial of long-chain polyunsaturated fatty acid supplementation of formula in term infants after weaning at 6 wk of age. Am J Clin Nutr 75:570, 2002.

167. Auestad N, et al: Visual acuity, erythrocyte fatty acid composition, and growth in term infants fed formulas with long-chain polyunsaturated fatty acids for one year. Pediatr Res 41:1, 1997.

168. Simmer K, Long chain polyunsaturated fatty acid supplementation in infants born at term. Cochrane Database Syst Rev 2000.

169. San Giovanni JP, et al: Dietary essential fatty acids, long-chain polyunsaturated fatty acids, and visual resolution acuity in healthy fullterm infants: a systemic review. Early Hum Dev 57:165, 2000.

170. Forsyth JS, Carlson SE. Long chain polyunsaturated fatty acids in infant nutrition: effects on infant development. Curr Opin Clin Nutr Metab Care 4:1, 2001.

171. World Health Organization: Fats and Oils in Human Nutrition. Report of a Joint Expert Consultation: FAO Food and Nutrition Paper 57. Geneva, World Health Organization, 1994.

172. International Society for the Study of Fatty Acids and Lipids: ISSFAL board statement: recommendations for the essential fatty acid requirement for infant formulas. J Am Coll Nutr 14:213, 1995.

173. Koletzko B, et al: Long chain polyunsaturated fatty acids (LC-PUFA) and perinatal development: report of workshop. Acta Paediatr 90:460, 2001.

174. Nutrient requirements for preterm infant formulas. J Nutr 132:1459S, 2002.

175. Tolley EA, Carlson SE: Considerations of statistical power in infant studies of visual development and docosahexaenoic acid status. Invited editorial. Am J Clin Nutr 71:1, 2000.

176. Makrides M, et al: A randomized trial of different ratios of linoleic to α-linolenic acid in the diet of term infants: effects on visual function and growth. Am J Clin Nutr 71:120, 2000.

177. Werkman SH, Carlson SE: A randomized trial of visual attention of preterm infants fed docosahexaenoic acid until 9 months. Lipids 31:91, 1996.

178. Carlson SE, Werkman SH: A randomized trial of visual attention of preterm infants fed docosahexaenoic acid until 2 months. Lipids 31:85, 1996.11.

179. Colombo J: Recent advances in infant cognition: implications for long-chain polyunsaturated fatty acid supplementation studies. Lipids 36:919, 2001.

180. Gottlieb G: Developmental psychobiological theory. *In* Cairns RB, Elder GH (eds): Developmental Science: Cambridge Studies in Social and Emotional Development. New York, Cambridge University Press, 1998, pp 63–77.

181. Carlson SE: Lipid requirements of very-low-birth-weight infants for optimal growth and development. *In* Dobbing J (ed): Lipids, Learning and the Brain: Fats in Infant Formulas. Report of the 103rd Ross Conference on Pediatric Research. Columbus, OH, Ross Laboratories, 1993, pp 188–214.

182. Willatts P, et al: Effect of long-chain polyunsaturated fatty acids in infant formula on problem solving at 10 months of age. Lancet 352:688, 1998.

183. Innis SM, et al: Early language development and visual acuity are related to docosahexaenoic acid in breast-fed term infants. *In* 93rd AOCS Annual Meeting Abstracts. Montreal, Canada, AOCS Press, 2002, p S73.

184. Clandinin M, et al: Formulas with docosahexaenoic acid (DHA) and arachidonic acid (ARA) promote better growth and development scores in very-low-birth weight infants (VLBW). Pediatr Res 51:187A, 2002.
185. Birch EE, et al: A randomized controlled trial of early dietary supply of long-chain polyunsaturated fatty acids and mental development in term infants. Dev Med Child Neurol 42:174, 2000.
186. Lucas A, et al: Efficacy and safety of long-chain polyunsaturated fatty acid supplementation of infant-formula milk: a randomized trial. Lancet 354:1948:1999.
187. Gibson RA, et al: Effect of increasing breast milk docosahexaenoic acid on plasma and erythrocyte phospholipid fatty acids and neural indices of exclusively breast fed infants. Eur J Clin Nutr 51:578, 1997.
188. Agostoni C, et al: Neurodevelopmental quotient of healthy term infants at 4 months and feeding practice: the role of long-chain polyunsaturated fatty acids. Pediatr Res 38:262, 1995.

Glen E. Mott

45 Lipoprotein Metabolism and Nutritional Programming in the Fetus and Neonate

OVERVIEW

Studies of cholesterol and lipoprotein metabolism in the fetus and infant have dramatically expanded in the past few decades because of their relevance to the etiology and pathogenesis of atherosclerosis. Atherosclerosis, the process leading to coronary heart disease in adult life, is common in young adults and likely has its origins in the arterial fatty streaks found in infants and children. Plasma cholesterol and lipoprotein concentrations, which are associated with the rate of development of these arterial lesions, often track from infancy to adulthood. Furthermore, fetal undernutrition and the type of prenatal and postnatal nutrition can program metabolically an individual to an increased risk of diabetes, the metabolic syndrome, and coronary heart disease in adulthood. Therefore, prenatal and early postnatal nutrition has become the focus of intense investigation in preventive medicine. Because intervention can considerably slow the progression of atherosclerosis in adult life, identifying children at risk and providing follow-up and family counseling are important research goals.

All lipid and lipoprotein cholesterol values are given in milligrams per deciliter. To convert cholesterol values from milligrams per deciliter (mg/dL) to millimoles per liter (mmol/L), multiply by 0.02586. To convert triglyceride concentrations from milligrams per deciliter to millimoles per liter, multiply by 0.01129. Representative conversions are given in Table 45-1.

PRENATAL (FETAL) DEVELOPMENT

Serum Cholesterol, Triglyceride, and Lipoprotein Concentrations

Humans

Early in gestation, serum cholesterol concentrations average 85 ± 31(SD) mg/dL[1] and decrease cyclically to 50 to 75 mg/dL in cord blood of normal term infants,[2-14] which is less than half the normal adult concentration (Fig. 45-1). Serum cholesterol concentrations of preterm infants frequently are elevated and commonly exceed 100 mg/dL,[1, 14-16] possibly because of a second serum cholesterol peak early in the third trimester.[1] Small for gestational age term babies may have slightly higher peak serum cholesterol levels[16] or, if growth retarded and near term, have lower values.[17] Infants with familial hypercholesterolemia have cord blood cholesterol concentrations from 100 to 200 mg/dL.[18] Cord serum triglyceride concentrations average 30 to 50 mg/dL,[5,8,10,11,14,19-27] which are much lower than normal adult values. However, some newborns infants have triglyceride

levels above 200 mg/dL.[19] Most of the variation in plasma lipids at birth is due to genetic factors, gestational age, or disease.

Low density lipoprotein–cholesterol (LDL–C) concentrations also decrease during gestation in the human fetus, from about 65 mg/dL in the first trimester[2] to 25 to 30 mg/dL at term,[2,3,6,25] which is about one fifth the adult level (see Fig. 45-1). Compared with serum cholesterol and LDL-C, high density lipoprotein cholesterol (HDL-C) concentrations in humans are stable during gestation,[2, 3] although a decrease in HDL-C concentration was reported in premature infants.[9] The HDL-C concentration at term gestation is about 25 mg/dL (see Fig. 45-1) compared with adult values of 40 to 50 mg/dL.[2, 7, 9, 25, 27-29] In contrast to the HDL of adults, HDL in cord blood contains higher levels of large HDL$_2$[30-32] and a broader range of particle sizes.[32-34] The very low density lipoprotein (VLDL) of cord blood carries less than one third of the total serum triglyceride concentration,[35,36] and its cholesterol content averages less than 10 mg/dL,[30,31,36] whereas in the adult, VLDL is the principal transport vehicle for triglycerides in fasting plasma. Although some lipoprotein(a) [Lp(a)] protein concentrations at birth may be as high as 20 mg/dL, the average is 4 mg/dL,[8,37-39] compared with average adult values of 15 mg/dL.

The low serum cholesterol and lipoprotein concentrations in the human fetus and neonate compared with those in adults are consistent with the low apolipoprotein B (apo B)[23, 25, 28] and apolipoprotein A-I (apo A-1)[9, 24, 25, 29, 40] concentrations at birth. Although HDL-C concentrations in the human fetus are relatively stable, apo A-I concentrations double between 20 and 40 weeks' gestation and increase the apo A-I/HDL-C ratio.[40] Cord serum apo E, which is principally associated with the lighter density HDL classes,[32, 36] is near or above adult concentrations of

TABLE 45-1

Corresponding Levels of Lipids in Milligrams per Deciliter and Millimoles per Liter

Cholesterol		Triglycerides	
mg/dL	*mmol/L*	*mg/dL*	*mmol/L*
35	0.9	150	1.7
50	1.3	250	2.8
110	2.8	400	4.5
130	3.4	500	5.6
170	4.4	1000	11.3
200	5.2		
240	6.2		

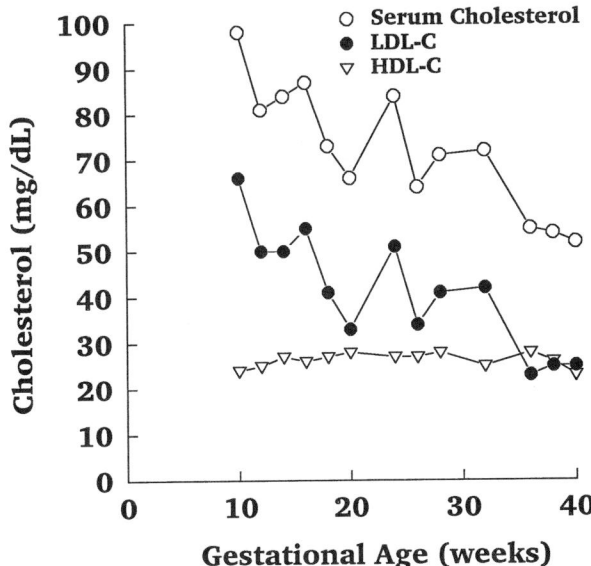

Figure 45–1. Serum cholesterol, low density lipoprotein cholesterol (LDL-C), and high density lipoprotein cholesterol (HDL-C) concentrations of 17 human fetuses by gestational age. (Adapted from Cai H-J, et al: Hepatology *13*:852, 1991.)

TABLE 45-2

Human Apolipoprotein Concentrations in Cord and Adult Serum

Apolipoprotein	Cord (mg/dL)	Adult (mg/dL)	Ratio Cord/Adult
A-I	$73.0 \pm 1.5^*$	134.0 ± 3.4	0.54
A-II	41.0 ± 1.0	68.0 ± 2.5	0.60
B	28.0 ± 0.6	98.0 ± 2.8	0.29
C-I	5.9 ± 0.2	7.0 ± 0.3	0.84
C-II	3.2 ± 0.3	3.7 ± 0.3	0.86
C-III	6.5 ± 0.2	13.0 ± 0.7	0.50
D	3.7 ± 0.1	10.0 ± 0.6	0.37
E	8.3 ± 0.3	10.0 ± 0.6	0.83

* Mean ± standard error.
Adapted from McConathy WJ, Lane DM: Pediatr Res *14*: 757, 1980.

about 10 mg/dL.[8, 23, 24, 28, 36, 41] Apo E polymorphisms affect the metabolism of apo B–containing lipoproteins such that infants with phenotype apo E 2/2 have lower apo B concentrations compared with other apo E phenotypes.[42] At birth, apo C-I and apo C-II levels also approach adult concentrations,[23] but apo C-III and apo A-II are only 40 to 60% of the adult level (Table 45-2).[23,25,43]

Ethnic and racial differences in serum cholesterol, lipoprotein cholesterol, and triglyceride concentrations at birth are small in contrast to later in childhood.[5, 25, 26, 29, 38, 39, 44-48] It is not clear whether the reported ranges of cord serum cholesterol concentrations (50 to 100 mg/dL) among different ethnic groups are related to methodologic variation, maternal diet, or genetic effects. Female infants have slightly higher cord serum cholesterol and lipoprotein concentrations than males[4, 11, 23, 25, 49] but similar triglyceride levels.[5, 11]

Experimental Animals

As in humans, serum cholesterol, LDL-C, and apo B levels are low and decrease during gestation in fetal calves[50, 51] and pigs.[52] HDL-C concentrations are low in fetal calves and do not change with fetal age. In contrast to other large animals, the fetal pig carries less than 1% of the total cholesterol in HDL early in gestation; HDL-C increases gradually until term gestation, when it reaches about 35 to 50% of the adult value.[52,53] As in humans, the serum cholesterol of newborn baboons averages 75 mg/dL,[54, 55] but the ratio of LDL/HDL cholesterol[55] is 0.5 compared with about 1.0 in humans at birth.[2] As observed in newborn humans, apo A-I and B concentrations of neonatal baboons are only about 50% of adult values.[55]

In the rat fetus, serum cholesterol is higher late in gestation compared with that of the adult rat.[56] LDL is the principal carrier of cholesterol in the rat fetus, whereas in the adult rat, HDL is the major lipoprotein class.[15,56] HDL-C concentrations of fetal rats are about 60% and VLDL-C about 10% of adult levels.[57] In contrast to the neonatal rat, the adult rat has high concentrations of apo E-rich HDL, with low levels of LDL.[58] At birth, serum triglyceride levels in the rat are below adult values.[59] Similar to the rat, LDL predominates in the fetal rabbit, and HDL is the major lipoprotein class in the adult.[60] The guinea pig fetus has similar HDL-C and

LDL-C levels, but as an adult, LDL predominates.[15] Newborn rabbits and guinea pigs have higher serum cholesterol levels than their dams unless the dams are fed a high-cholesterol diet.[61-64]

Lipoprotein Metabolism: Humans and Experimental Animals

The development of the LDL-receptor (LDL-R) in humans has a major role in lowering LDL concentrations during gestation.[2] Human fetal liver has a higher LDL-receptor activity by mid-gestation than adult liver[2] (Fig. 45-2), an observation similar to that in the fetal calf compared with the adult cow.[50] In the newborn, LDL-receptor activity is suppressed by the absorption of biliary and dietary cholesterol and by the uptake of bile acids during fat digestion. In the fetus, the absence of these negative regulatory processes probably contributes to the sustained elevation of LDL-receptor activity and low plasma cholesterol and LDL-C levels in humans during the third trimester. The inverse correlation of LDL-receptor activity and serum cholesterol concentration during gestation is consistent with that rationale.[2] The lower level of plasma cholesterol esterification[24] (secondary to reduced lecithin cholesterol acyltransferase activity [LCAT] in the fetus and newborn[9,41,65-67]) also may contribute to differences in lipoprotein composition in the neonate. In the human fetus, hepatic and intestinal genes[68,69] that are essential for cholesterol and apolipoprotein synthesis are transcribed at high levels by 8 to 20 weeks of development.[69] In the human fetus, most cholesterol in tissues probably is derived from endogenous synthesis rather than from the maternal circulation. However, the necessary cholesterol uptake and transport mechanisms are present in the placenta that could transfer cholesterol to the fetus, and there is a high cholesterol content in the yolk sac.[70] The positive association of serum cholesterol in human fetuses with the level of hypercholesterolemia in their mothers through the second trimester also suggests that maternal-fetal transfer of cholesterol occurs in humans at least early in gestation.[71] In pregnant rabbits, dietary-induced hypercholesterolemia increases neonatal serum cholesterol concentrations compared with noncholesterol-fed controls by about 50% in one study[72] and minimally in several others.[73, 74] Considerable maternal-fetal transfer of cholesterol occurs in both the rabbit and guinea pig.[62] In the hamster, tissue cholesterol concentrations of the fetus increase with maternal cholesterol intake but only with very high cholesterol diets.[75]

In fetal rats, LDL metabolism differs considerably from that in the adult. Late in gestation, the rat fetus greatly increases LDL production, leading to higher LDL-C levels and an LDL turnover rate more than 15 times that of the adult.[76] In contrast to humans, lipoprotein binding to hepatic LDL-receptors of the rat fetus is reduced compared with that of the newborn or adult.[77]

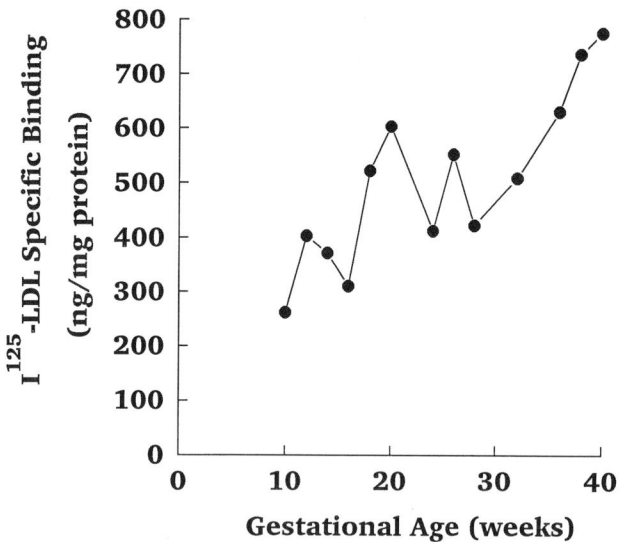

Figure 45–2. Specific binding of I[125]-low density lipoprotein (LDL) by hepatic LDL receptor preparations from 17 human fetuses by gestational age. (Adapted from Cai H-J, et al: *Hepatology 13*:852, 1991.)

In the rat fetus, hepatic cholesterol synthesis[78] and hydroxymethylglutaryl coenzyme A (HMG CoA) reductase activity,[79] the rate-limiting step in cholesterol biosynthesis, markedly increase during the week before parturition but decrease somewhat before birth.[79, 80] The fetal rat increases hepatic and intestinal mRNA concentrations for cholesterol-metabolizing or transport genes a few days before birth or at parturition.[69,81,82]

Summary: Fetal Lipoproteins

In the human fetus, the enzymes for cholesterol and lipoprotein metabolism develop early in gestation. As expression of the LDL receptor increases in gestation, serum cholesterol and LDL-C concentrations decrease to levels much lower than those observed in early postnatal life and adulthood. In the rat, the pathways for cholesterol and lipoprotein production develop rapidly late in gestation and are associated with higher serum cholesterol and LDL-C concentrations in the fetus than in the adult.

POSTNATAL DEVELOPMENT

Serum Cholesterol and Lipoprotein Concentrations

Humans

Serum cholesterol, LDL-C, VLDL-C, and triglyceride concentrations increase rapidly in normal breast-fed infants within a few days after birth.[30, 31, 66, 83, 84] Serum cholesterol concentration increases from an average of 50 to 60 mg/dL on day 1 to greater than 100 mg/dL by 1 week of age, and LDL-C from 25 mg/dL on day 1 to greater than 50 mg/dL by 1 week (Fig. 45–3).[36] Serum cholesterol and LDL-C concentrations are about one-half of the adult level.[28, 36] At 1 month of age, serum cholesterol and LDL-C concentrations[30, 83] are more than double the birth values but decrease after weaning to a typical Western diet.[13,85] In contrast, HDL-C concentrations increase only slightly during the first week of life[28] and thereafter increase to near adult levels (40 to 50 mg/dL) by 1 month of age.[30] Throughout the first month of life, the HDL$_2$/HDL$_3$ cholesterol ratio[31] remains about 1.0 (see Fig. 45–3) but decreases to a ratio of less than 0.5 later in childhood.[86] Apo B and apo A-I levels rise in association with increas-

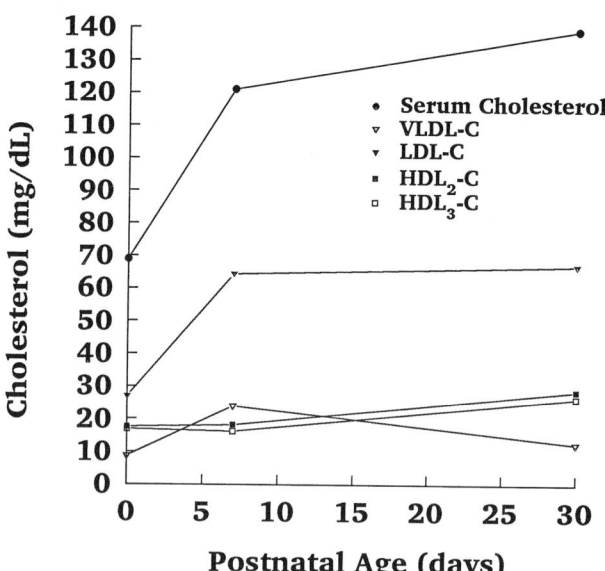

Figure 45–3. Serum cholesterol and lipoprotein cholesterol response of normal human infants that were exclusively breast-fed from birth to 30 days of age. VLDL, very low density lipoprotein; LDL, low density lipoprotein; HDL, high density lipoprotein (subfractions 2 and 3). (Adapted from Rosseneu M, et al: *Pediatr Res 17*:788, 1983.)

ing LDL-C and HDL-C concentrations during the first weeks of life[8] and then stabilize. In contrast, Lp(a) concentrations increase steadily from low levels at birth and reach adult levels by 1 year of age.[37,39] At birth, more than 80% of serum apo E is in the HDL fraction, but by 30 days of age, apo E decreases in HDL to about 60% of the total.[36] The apo E-enriched HDL-C is taken up rapidly by the LDL-receptor, which may facilitate efficient delivery of cholesterol to tissues in the rapidly growing neonate.[87]

Part of the increase in serum cholesterol after birth is attributed to both cholesterol and saturated fat in breast milk, although hemoconcentration during the first 24 hours may account for 10% of the increase.[88] Some of the postnatal increase in serum cholesterol is attributed to other unidentified dietary factors or metabolic maturation, because serum cholesterol and lipoprotein concentrations increase regardless of the diet composition.

Serum cholesterol, LDL-C, HDL-C, and apo B concentrations usually are higher in breast-fed infants compared with those fed typical formulas low in cholesterol and containing fat with a higher polyunsaturated/saturated (P/S) fatty acid ratio than in breast milk.[13, 28, 43, 89, 90-94] Infant formulas of cow's milk or evaporated milk that contain levels of cholesterol and saturated fat similar to those of human milk also increase serum cholesterol concentrations to levels comparable to those of breast-feeding.[4, 44, 95-100] The relative importance of cholesterol versus fat in breast milk in elevating the serum cholesterol concentration is not known because most studies of neonatal dietary cholesterol intake in humans are confounded by differences in fat composition or other factors. Formulas high in saturated fat with 1/2 to 3/4 the level of cholesterol found in breast milk raise the serum cholesterol and apo B levels but have little effect on HDL-C or apo A-I concentrations compared with the same formula low in cholesterol.[30,101,102] Infants fed formula containing cholesterol at twice the level of breast milk have slightly higher LDL-C concentrations but equivalent levels of HDL-C compared with infants fed a similar formula without cholesterol.[103] Generally, more of the lipoprotein response to a preweaning diet is attributed to the type of fat than to the cholesterol content. Serum cholesterol is inversely related to the dietary P/S ratio but is not significantly correlated with cholesterol intake among infants after weaning.[104]

The independent effects of types of fat in diets of the newborn infant have been more thoroughly studied than those of dietary cholesterol. Feeding a formula low in cholesterol with a fatty acid composition similar to that of breast milk increases the serum cholesterol and LDL-C concentrations to about two thirds the level of infants who are breast-fed.[90,105] Feeding low-cholesterol formula containing higher proportions of coconut oil (and therefore more lauric [$C_{12:0}$] and myristic acids [$C_{14:0}$]) increases serum cholesterol,[106] LDL-C, and HDL-C concentrations to nearly the same levels as observed with breast-feeding.[107] Infants fed formulas containing higher concentrations of corn or soy oil (P/S ratio > 3) have about 25 to 35% lower serum cholesterol and LDL-C concentrations[43,108] compared with those fed breast milk. Formulas with more moderate P/S ratios (P/S < 2.0) lower serum cholesterol and LDL-C concentrations by lesser amounts.[90,105,109] The HDL-C level is decreased by a few milligrams per deciliter by high or moderately high P/S formulas.[43,107-109] There is strong evidence that dietary supplementation with long chain polyunsaturated fatty acids is necessary for optimal growth and development, particularly for preterm infants, and possibly should be added to all infant formulas.[110]

Experimental Animals

The serum cholesterol and lipoprotein responses of neonatal nonhuman primates are similar to those described for humans. Breast-fed rhesus monkeys[111] and baboons[54,55] have higher serum cholesterol concentrations than those fed low-cholesterol formulas. In the rhesus monkey, however, breast-feeding principally increases the serum LDL-C fraction, whereas in the baboon, it increases HDL_1-C and HDL_2-C (and therefore HDL-C) levels.[55,112] In the infant rhesus monkey fed a low P/S formula with a cholesterol content similar to that of breast milk, serum cholesterol levels increased to about 100 mg/dL higher than in breast-feeding.[113] In baboons, a high P/S infant formula with a cholesterol content similar to that of breast milk increased the serum cholesterol concentration to the same extent as breast-feeding.[54] Baboons fed formula with a low P/S ratio (similar to that of breast milk) had a higher LDL-C but lower HDL-C level compared with breast-fed baboons.[55] In the suckling pig, serum cholesterol levels increase to about 200 mg/dL by 1 month of age, primarily because HDL levels are more than twofold higher than in the adult.[52,53] Breast-fed piglets have higher serum cholesterol and VLDL+LDL-C concentrations than those fed low-cholesterol[114-116] or high-cholesterol formulas with unsaturated fat.[117] A palm oil–containing, low-cholesterol formula that was similar to sow milk in fatty acid composition raised the serum cholesterol of the piglet only to about 80 mg/dL, nearly half that of piglets fed sow milk; the serum VLDL+LDL-C concentration increased to only 27 mg/dL or about 25% that of piglets fed sow milk.[116] In pigs, neither level of dietary cholesterol nor type of fat accounts for the serum cholesterol or lipoprotein differences between breast-feeding and formula-feeding.[118]

Suckling rabbits have serum cholesterol levels of 300 to 400 mg/dL[61] predominantly as a result of greatly elevated VLDL-C and intermediate density lipoprotein (IDL) concentrations.[119] In the suckling rat, total cholesterol increases from about 60 mg/dL at birth to 100 mg/dL at 10 days[120] and to 170 mg/dL at 3 weeks of age.[121] LDL is the principal carrier of cholesterol in the newborn rat[122] and decreases after 2 to 3 weeks of age.[121-123] In contrast, serum HDL-C concentrations increase from about 20 mg/dL at birth in the neonatal rat to 40 mg/dL by 2 weeks of age.[121,123]

Lipoprotein Metabolism: Humans and Experimental Animals

Breast-feeding increases serum LDL-C concentration and decreases by threefold the cholesterol synthetic rate in human infants[92,93] and by twofold in piglets,[114] compared with those fed low-cholesterol formulas. Consistent with those observations is a lower hepatic HMG-CoA reductase activity in the suckling rat[79,124] compared with the fetus.[79,80] The postpartum increase in serum LDL-C levels is associated with a rapid decrease in the number of LDL receptors during the suckling period in cattle,[50] but a similar decrease in the LDL-receptor–binding capacity is not observed among suckling piglets compared with those fed a high-cholesterol versus a low-cholesterol formula.[118] The rate-limiting step in cholesterol degradation to bile acids (cholesterol 7α-hydroxylase) develops slowly in the fetus, but its activity increases rapidly and the bile acid pool size expands markedly late in gestation and in the early postnatal period (see reviews[125-128]). The role of bile acid metabolism in the lipoprotein responses to early diet are not well understood.

Summary: Postnatal Lipoproteins

In most breast-fed animals, serum cholesterol and lipoprotein concentrations increase rapidly after birth. Although serum cholesterol and lipoprotein concentrations respond to the high cholesterol and saturated fat contents of breast milk, the particular lipoprotein that increases and the timing are species specific. The biochemical and molecular mechanisms responsible for the dramatic neonatal increases in lipoprotein concentrations are only partially understood.

Perinatal Disease and Lipoprotein Concentrations

Familial hypercholesterolemia (FH) is associated with a severalfold increase in LDL-C concentrations in the newborn infant.[18,129] Most neonates with FH can be identified by a cut-off value for LDL-C of 41 mg/dL (95th percentile of control infants). Although no treatment for hypercholesterolemia is generally recommended for infants below the age of 2 years, screening cord blood from infants at risk for FH should be done selectively in anticipation of later follow-up.[130] Aggressive treatment may be indicated for FH-affected children.[131] Maternal diabetes,[132] hypertension,[133] or prenatal treatment with glucocorticoids[134] increases fetal serum cholesterol, LDL-C, HDL-C, or triglyceride levels. Fetal stress and hypoxia may elevate triglyceride and free glycerol concentrations, which imply triglyceride mobilization and lipolysis in these conditions.[20] Premature infants with respiratory distress syndrome (RDS) and birth weight between 1 and 2 kg have lower levels of serum apolipoprotein B and arachidonic acid compared with similar-sized neonates without RDS.[135] A causal relationship among these factors has not been demonstrated. In contrast to adult-onset hypothyroidism, congenital hypothyroidism has only small effects on serum cholesterol or lipoprotein concentrations during the first month of life,[136,137] but nevertheless an inverse association between T3 and LDL-C concentrations was observed.[138]

LONG-TERM CONSEQUENCES OF FETAL AND NEONATAL NUTRITION ON LIPOPROTEIN CONCENTRATIONS

Humans and Experimental Animals

Human fetal undernutrition and low birth weight are associated with type II diabetes and the metabolic syndrome (syndrome X) in adulthood and result in hyperlipidemia.[139,140] The newborn infant with a birth weight less than 6.5 pounds has a ten times greater risk of developing the metabolic syndrome as an adult than do those whose birth weight is greater than 9.5 pounds.[139] Furthermore, low birth weight infants have higher apo B and lower HDL-C concentrations as adults.[139] Maternal malnutrition in early gestation is associated with a higher LDL/HDL cholesterol ratio in adult offspring at midlife.[141] Poor maternal nutrition late in gestation results in a smaller abdominal circumference in the neonate, a condition that may reflect hepatic growth retardation and therefore altered lipoprotein metabolism. For each 1-inch decrease in abdominal circumference at birth, serum cholesterol and LDL-C concentrations of older adults are increased by about 10 mg/dL.[142] Therefore, body proportions at birth may reflect differential timing of gestational malnutrition, resulting in diverse metabolic consequences. Restricted fetal growth without catch-up growth in 8- to 10-year-old children increases LDL-C levels compared with those who grow normally after intrauterine growth retardation.[143] Recent studies in humans report that maternal hypercholesterolemia is positively associated with the serum cholesterol of the fetus through the second trimester,[71] and with the extent of arterial lesions (fatty streaks) in the fetus and also in children who died of multiple causes before age 13.[144] The surprising observation is that the small differences in serum cholesterol levels of children from mothers who were hyper- or normocholesterolemic do not explain the differences in atherosclerosis. The investigators speculated that unidentified "atherogenes" might be programmed by gestational elevation of serum cholesterol concentration.[144]

In guinea pigs, maternal undernutrition lowered the birth weight and also resulted in a higher serum cholesterol and LDL-C in the adult male offspring after a dietary cholesterol challenge.[145] Similarly, pregnant rats that are food restricted produce progeny that have higher levels of serum cholesterol compared with offspring of normally fed mothers.[146] In rats, dietary protein restriction during either gestation or lactation produced offspring with lower serum cholesterol, HDL-C, and triglyceride concentrations compared with controls.[147] In pregnant rabbits, diet-induced maternal hypercholesterolemia does not increase serum cholesterol concentrations in the offspring after birth to 1 year.[73] However, arterial lesion development, which is possibly mediated by oxidative mechanisms, is significantly greater in the offspring of hypercholesterolemic dams compared with normocholesterolemic dams during gestation.[73,74] These findings in humans and experimental animals support the concept that fetal growth retardation, perinatal malnutrition, and hypercholesterolemia during gestation permanently program plasma lipoprotein concentrations or enhance the risks of diseases that cause dyslipoproteinemia. Frequently the lipoprotein changes are associated with an increased risk of cardiovascular disease in adult life.[148,149]

The type of neonatal nutrition also programs or imprints adult lipoprotein concentrations. Elderly men who as infants were breast-fed or fed cow's milk–based formulas compared with those who were weaned before 1 year had higher serum cholesterol, LDL-C, and apo B concentrations.[150] In contrast, women at age 32 years who had been breast-fed had lower plasma cholesterol than those who were bottle-fed.[151] In a study of 6-year-old children, serum cholesterol and LDL-C concentrations increased with the length of breast-feeding up to 6 months of age.[85] Similarly, length of breast-feeding was related to serum cholesterol and the apo B/apo A-1 ratio in adolescents.[152] Short-term prospective studies in children usually have not detected deferred effects of neonatal diet on total serum cholesterol concentrations.[153,154]

Studies of breast-fed versus formula-fed experimental animals also have reported long-term differences in serum cholesterol responses to a high-cholesterol, challenge diet.[155-158] Juvenile and adult baboons that were breast-fed exhibited lower HDL-C levels and higher VLDL + LDL-C/HDL-C ratios compared with those fed formulas as infants.[55,112,159-161] Variation in the type of dietary fat

or the cholesterol content of formulas fed to infant baboons does not affect serum cholesterol or lipoprotein concentrations after weaning.[160,161] Therefore, the long-term effects of breast-feeding versus formula-feeding on serum cholesterol and lipoprotein concentrations are elicited by factors other than the level of cholesterol or the type of fat in the infant diet.

Many of the studies with humans and nonhuman primates were stimulated by results of experiments with rodents in which differences in neonatal diet or premature weaning permanently affected the serum cholesterol response of the adult animal.[155,154] The early studies with experimental animals tested the hypothesis that high cholesterol levels in breast milk affect development of cholesterol homeostasis in adult life (i.e., the cholesterol challenge hypothesis).[155,162,163] Most experiments, however, do not support that supposition.[154] No long-term studies of humans have been performed in which cholesterol intake in the newborn infant was controlled. One recent study of infants fed formulas with or without cholesterol for 6 months does not report a significant difference in serum cholesterol or LDL-C levels before or after a cholesterol challenge at 11 to 12 months. In a parallel study, cholesterol synthesis rates of both formula groups at 4 months of age were about fourfold higher than in a breast-fed group.[164]

Summary: Early Nutritional Programming

These studies provide compelling evidence that nutritional deficiencies during fetal life and the types of newborn feeding program plasma lipoprotein responses and other risk factors affecting the progression of coronary artery disease in the adult. However, the molecular or metabolic basis of these nutritional programming effects on lipoprotein concentrations has not been elucidated.

REFERENCES

1. Johnson HJ Jr, et al: The levels of plasma cholesterol in the human fetus throughout gestation. Pediatr Res 16:682, 1982.
2. Cai H-J, et al: The relationship between hepatic low-density lipoprotein receptor activity and serum cholesterol level in the human fetus. Hepatology 13:852, 1991.
3. Parker CR Jr, et al: Decline in the concentration of low-density lipoprotein-cholesterol in human fetal plasma near term. Metabolism 32:919, 1983.
4. Darmady JM, et al: Prospective study of serum cholesterol levels during first year of life. BMJ 2:685, 1972.
5. Frerichs R, et al: Serum lipids and lipoproteins at birth in a biracial population: the Bogalusa heart study. Pediatr Res 12:858, 1978.
6. Ginsburg B-E, Zetterström R: Serum cholesterol concentrations in newborn infants with gestational ages of 28–42 weeks. Acta Paediatr Scand 69:587, 1980.
7. Van Biervliet JP, et al: Evolution of lipoprotein patterns in newborns. Acta Paediatr Scand 69:593, 1980.
8. Strobl W, et al: Serum apolipoproteins and lipoprotein (a) during the first week of life. Acta Paediatr Scand 72:505, 1983.
9. Amr S, et al: Low levels of apolipoprotein A1 are not contributors to the low lecithin-cholesterol acyl transferase activity in premature newborn infants. Pediatr Res 24:191, 1988.
10. Haumont D, et al: Plasma lipid and plasma lipoprotein concentrations in low birth weight infants given parenteral nutrition with twenty or ten percent lipid emulsion. J Pediatr 115:787, 1989.
11. Hardell LI: Serum lipids and lipoproteins at birth based on a study of 2815 newborn infants. I. Concentrations and distributions of triglycerides and cholesterol. Acta Paediatr Scand Suppl 285:5, 1981.
12. Carlson SE: Plasma cholesterol and lipoprotein levels during fetal development and infancy. In Williams CL, Wynder EL (eds): Hyperlipidemia in Childhood and the Development of Atherosclerosis. Ann NY Acad Sci, New York, The New York Academy of Sciences, 1991, pp 81–89.
13. Kallio MJ, et al: Exclusive breast-feeding and weaning: effect on serum cholesterol and lipoprotein concentrations in infants during the first year of life. Pediatrics 89:663, 1992.
14. Lane DM, McConathy WJ: Factors affecting the lipid and apolipoprotein levels of cord sera. Pediatr Res 17:83, 1983.
15. Innis SM, Hamilton JJ: Effects of developmental changes and early nutrition on cholesterol metabolism in infancy: a review. J Am Coll Nutr 11:63S, 1992.
16. Diaz M, et al: Cord blood lipoprotein-cholesterol: relationship with birth weight and gestational age of newborns. Metabolism 38:435, 1989.

17. Spencer JAD, et al: Third trimester fetal growth and measures of carbohydrate and lipid metabolism in umbilical venous blood at term. Arch Dis Child 76:F21, 1997.
18. Tsang RC, et al: Cholesterol at birth and age 1: comparison of normal hypercholesterolemic neonates. Pediatrics 53:458, 1974.
19. Tsang R, et al: Cord blood hypertriglyceridemia. Am J Dis Child 127:78, 1974.
20. Andersen GE, Friis-Hansen B: Neonatal hypertriglyceridemia: a new index of antepartum-intrapartum fetal stress? Acta Paediatr Scand 65:369, 1976.
21. Christensen NC: Lipids in cord serum and free fatty acids in plasma in healthy newborn term infants. Acta Paediatr Scand 63:711, 1974.
22. Grundt I, et al: Cord blood cholesterol, triglyceride, and lipoprotein pattern from two districts in Norway. Scand J Clin Lab Invest 36:261, 1976.
23. McConathy WJ, Lane DM: Studies on the apolipoproteins and lipoproteins of cord serum. Pediatr Res 14:757, 1980.
24. Dolphin PJ, et al: The lipoproteins of human umbilical cord blood apolipoprotein and lipid levels. Atherosclerosis 51:109, 1984.
25. Averna MR, et al: Lipids, lipoproteins and apolipoproteins AI, AII, B, CII, CIII, and E in newborns. Biol Neonate 60:187, 1991.
26. Valdivielso P, et al: Lipids and lipoproteins in cord blood: analyses of a Hispanic and Arab population. Acta Paediatr 81:439, 1992.
27. Miller NE, et al: Cord blood high density lipoprotein concentration in 1797 births: relationship to family history of coronary disease. J Chron Dis 34:119, 1981.
28. Tenenbaum D, et al: Serum lipoproteins in venous blood serum from birth to the end of the first week: feeding influences. Biol Neonate 53:126, 1988.
29. Taylor GO, et al: Studies of lipoproteins and fatty acids in maternal and cord blood of two racial groups in Trinidad. Lipids 22:173, 1987.
30. Van Biervliet JP, et al: Influence of dietary factors on the plasma lipoprotein composition and content in neonates. Eur J Pediatr 144:489, 1986.
31. Rosseneu M, et al: Isolation and characterization of lipoprotein profiles in newborns by density gradient ultracentrifugation. Pediatr Res 17:788, 1983.
32. Davis PA, et al: Umbilical cord blood lipoproteins: isolation and characterization of high density lipoproteins. Arteriosclerosis 3:357, 1983.
33. Genzel-Boroviczeny O, et al: High-density lipoprotein subclass distribution and human cord blood lipid levels. Pediatr Res 20:487, 1986.
34. Nichols AV, et al: Apolipoprotein-specific populations in high density lipoproteins of human cord blood. Biochim Biophys Acta 1085:306, 1991.
35. Winkler L, et al: Concentration and composition of the lipoprotein classes in human umbilical cord serum. Clin Chim Acta 76:187, 1977.
36. Van Biervliet JP, et al: Apolipoprotein and lipid composition of plasma lipoproteins in neonates during the first month of life. Pediatr Res 20:324, 1986.
37. Van Biervliet JP, et al: Lipoprotein (a) profiles and evolution in newborns. Atherosclerosis 86:173, 1991.
38. Gozlan O, et al: Lipoprotein levels in newborns and adolescents. Clin Biochem 27:305, 1994.
39. Rifai N, et al: Lipoprotein (a) at birth, in blacks and whites. Atherosclerosis 92:123, 1992.
40. Parker CR Jr, et al: Apolipoprotein A-1 in umbilical cord blood of newborn infants: relation to gestational age and high-density lipoprotein cholesterol. Pediatr Res 23:348, 1988.
41. Barkia A, et al: Apolipoprotein A-I-containing lipoproteins in human umbilical cord blood. Biol Neonate 59:352, 1991.
42. Hermann W, et al: The influence of apolipoprotein E polymorphism on plasma concentrations of apolipoprotein B and A-I during the first year of life. Pediatrics 93:296, 1994.
43. Van Biervliet JP, et al: Plasma apoprotein and lipid patterns in newborns: influence of nutritional factors. Acta Paediatr Scand 70:851, 1981.
44. Ballester D, et al: Serum cholesterol in Chilean newborn infants and its evolution during the first months of life. Helv Pediatr Acta 2:227, 1965.
45. Klimov A, et al: Cord blood high density lipoproteins: Leningrad and Cincinnati. Pediatr Res 13:208, 1979.
46. Saha N, Wong HB: Serum HDL cholesterol and apolipoprotein AI, AII, and B levels in Singapore newborns. Biol Neonate 52:93, 1987.
47. Miller GJ: Epidemiological and clinical aspects of high density lipoproteins. In Miller NE, Miller GJ (eds): Metabolic Aspects of Cardiovascular Disease. New York, Elsevier Publishing, 1984, p 48.
48. Glueck CJ, et al: Black-white similarities in cord blood lipids and lipoproteins. Metabolism 26:347, 1977.
49. Carlson LA, Hardell LI: Sex differences in serum lipids and lipoproteins at birth. Eur J Clin Invest 7:133, 1977.
50. Rudling MJ, Peterson CO. LDL receptors in bovine tissues assayed as the heparin-sensitive binding of 125 I-labeled LDL in homogenates: relation between liver LDL receptors and serum cholesterol in the fetus and post term. Biochim Biophys Acta 836:96, 1985.
51. Marcos E, et al: Developmental changes in plasma apolipoproteins B and A-I in fetal bovines. Biol Neonate 59:22, 1991.
52. Johansson MBN, Karlsson BW: Lipoprotein and lipid profiles in the blood serum of the fetal, neonatal, and adult pig. Biol Neonate 42:127, 1982.
53. Johansson MBN: Heterogeneity of serum lipoproteins during the fetal and neonatal development of the pig. Int J Biochem 16:1359, 1984.
54. Mott GE, et al: Diet and sire effects on serum cholesterol and cholesterol absorption in infant baboons (Papio cynocephalus). Circ Res 43:364, 1978.
55. Mott GE, et al: Infant diet affects serum lipoprotein concentrations and cholesterol-esterifying enzymes in baboons. J Nutr 123:155, 1993.
56. Schlag B, Winkler L: Konzentration und Zusammensetzung der Lipoproteinklassen der fetalen Ratte. Acta Biol Med Ger 37:233, 1978.
57. Dargel R, et al: Rat LDL metabolism in the perinatal period. In Parham MJ, Nieman R (eds): Cholesterol-homeostasis. 4th Cologne Atherosclerosis Conference. Basel, Birkhäuser Verlag, 1988, pp 109–115.
58. Oschry Y, Eisenberg S: Rat plasma lipoproteins: re-evaluation of a lipoprotein system in an animal devoid of cholesteryl ester transfer activity. J Lipid Res 23:1099, 1982.
59. Argiles J, Herrera E: Lipids and lipoproteins in maternal and fetus plasma in the rat. Biol Neonate 39:37, 1981.
60. Schlag B, et al: Elektrophoretische Untersuchungen zum pranatalen Status der Serumlipoproteine verschiedener Spezies. Acta Biol Med Ger 41:179, 1982.
61. Friedman M, Byers SO: Effects of diet on serum lipids of fetal, neonatal and pregnant rabbits. Am J Physiol 201:611, 1961.
62. Connor WE, Lin DS: Placental transfer of cholesterol-4-14C into rabbit and guinea pig fetus. J Lipid Res 8:558, 1967.
63. Sisson JA, Plotz EJ: Effect of alloxan diabetes on maternal and fetal serum lipids in the rabbit. Exp Mol Pathol 6:274, 1967.
64. Whatley BJ, et al: Effect of dietary fat and cholesterol on milk composition, milk intake, and cholesterol metabolism in the rabbit. J Nutr 111:432, 1981.
65. Lacko AG, et al: On the rate of cholesterol esterification in cord blood serum. Lipids 7:426, 1972.
66. Lane DM, McConathy WJ: Changes in the serum lipids and apolipoproteins in the first four weeks of life. Pediatr Res 20:332, 1986.
67. Bewer G, et al: Lipide, Lipoproteine, und LCAT im Serum von Säuglingen in den ersten 2 Lebensmonaten unter Berücksichtigung der Ernährungsart—eine Längsschnittuntersuchung. Paediatr Grenzgeb 26:397, 1987.
68. Plonne D, et al: Tracer kinetic studies of the low density lipoprotein metabolism in the fetal rat: an example for estimation of flux rates in the nonsteady state. J Lipid Res 31:747, 1990.
69. Erickson SK, et al: Changes in parameters of lipoprotein metabolism during rat hepatic development. Biochem Biophys Acta 963:525, 1988.
70. Woollett LA: The origins and roles of cholesterol and fatty acids in the fetus. Curr Opin Lipidol 12:305, 2001.
71. Napoli C, et al: Fatty streak formation occurs in human fetal aortas and is greatly enhanced by maternal hypercholesterolemia. J Clin Invest 100:2680, 1997.
72. Montoudis A, et al: Impact of a cholesterol-enriched diet on maternal and fetal plasma lipids and fetal deposition in pregnant rabbits. Life Sci 64:2439, 1999.
73. Napoli C, et al: Maternal hypercholesterolemia enhances atherogenesis in normocholesterolemic rabbits, which is inhibited by antioxidant or lipid-lowering intervention during pregnancy: an experimental model of atherogenic mechanisms in human fetuses. Circ Res 87:946, 2000.
74. Palinski W, et al: Maternal hypercholesterolemia and treatment during pregnancy influence the long-term progression of atherosclerosis in offspring of rabbits. Circ Res 89:991, 2001.
75. McConihay JA, et al: Effect of maternal hypercholesterolemia on fetal sterol metabolism in the Golden Syrian hamster. J Lipid Res 42:1111, 2001.
76. Calandra S, et al: Effect of cholesterol feeding on cholesterol biosynthesis in maternal and foetal rat liver. Eur J Clin Invest 5:27, 1975.
77. McNamara DJ, et al: Regulation of hepatic 3-hydroxy-3-methyl-glutaryl coenzyme A reductase. J Biol Chem 247:5805, 1972.
78. Belknap WM, Dietschy JM: Sterol synthesis and low density lipoprotein clearance in vivo in the pregnant rat, placenta, and fetus. J Clin Invest 82:2077, 1988.
79. Elshourbagy NA, et al: Expression of rat apolipoprotein A-IV and A-I genes: mRNA induction during development and in response to glucocorticoids and insulin. Proc Natl Acad Sci 82:8242, 1985.
80. Levy E, et al: Apolipoprotein synthesis in human fetal intestine: regulation by epidermal growth factor. Biochem Biophys Res Commun 204:1340, 1994.
81. Levin MS, et al: Developmental changes in the expression of genes involved in cholesterol biosynthesis and lipid transport in human and rat fetal and neonatal livers. Biochim Biophys Acta 1003:293, 1989.
82. Demmer LA, et al: Tissue-specific expression and developmental regulation of the rat apolipoprotein B gene. Proc Natl Acad Sci 83:8102, 1986.
83. Rafstedt S: Studies on serum lipids and lipoproteins in infancy and childhood. Acta Paediatr 44(suppl):26, 1955.
84. Kirstein D, et al: Changes in plasma lipoproteins from first day to third week of life in healthy breast-fed infants. Acta Paediatr Scand 74:733, 1985.
85. Štrbák V, et al: Late effects of breast-feeding and early weaning: seven-year prospective study in children. Endocr Regul 25:53, 1991.
86. Moskowitz WB, et al: Lipoprotein and oxygen transport alterations in passive smoking preadolescent children. The MCV Twin Study. Circulation 81:586, 1992.
87. Innerarity TL, et al: Receptor binding activity of high-density lipoproteins containing apoprotein E from abetalipoproteinemic and normal neonate plasma. Metabolism 33:186, 1984.
88. Wegelius R: On the changes in the peripheral blood picture of the newborn infant immediately after birth. Acta Paed 35:1, 1948.
89. Fomon SJ, Bartels DJ: Concentrations of cholesterol in serum of infants in relation to diet. Am J Dis Child 99:27, 1960.

90. Carlson SE, et al: Effect of infant diets with different polyunsaturated to saturated fat ratios on circulating high-density lipoproteins. J Pediatr Gastroenterol Nutr 1:303, 1982.

91. Michaličková J, et al: The effect of natural and artificial nutrition in infants on the metabolism of lipids during oncogenesis. Bratisl lek Listy 87:285, 1987.

92. Cruz MLA, et al: Effects of infant nutrition on cholesterol synthesis rates. Pediatr Res 35:135, 1994.

93. Wong WW, et al: Effect of dietary cholesterol on cholesterol synthesis in breast-fed and formula-fed infants. J Lipid Res 34:1403, 1993.

94. Karlsland Åkeson PM, et al: Plasma lipids and apolipoproteins in breast-fed and formula-fed Swedish infants. Acta Paediatr 88:1, 1999.

95. Lindquist B, Malmcrona R, et al: Dietary fat in relation to serum lipids in the normal infant. J Dis Child 99:39, 1960.

96. Sweeney MJ, et al: Effect of diet during the first six to eight weeks of life on total concentrations of serum protein and on electrophoretic patterns of serum protein and lipoprotein. Pediatrics 26:82, 1962.

97. Paupe J, et al: Influence de l'alimentation sur les variations observees. Arch Fr Pediatr 5:519, 1963.

98. Woodruff CW, et al: Serum lipids in breast-fed infants and in infants fed evaporated milk. Am J Clin Nutr 14:83, 1964.

99. Hodgson PA, et al: Comparison of serum cholesterol in children fed high, moderate, or low cholesterol milk diets during neonatal period. Metabolism 25:739, 1976.

100. Nestel PJ, et al: Changes in cholesterol metabolism in infants in response to dietary cholesterol and fat. Am J Clin Nutr 32:2177, 1979.

101. Van Biervliet JP, et al: Serum cholesterol, cholesteryl ester, and high-density lipoprotein development in newborn infants: response to formulas supplemented with cholesterol and γ-linolenic acid. J Pediatr 120:S101, 1992.

102. Rassin DK, et al: Taurine and cholesterol supplementation in the term infant: responses of growth and metabolism. J Parenter Enter Nutr 14:392, 1990.

103. Wagner V, von Stockhausen HB: The effect of feeding human milk and adapted milk formulae on serum lipid and lipoprotein levels in young infants. Eur J Pediatr 147:292, 1988.

104. Agostoni C, et al: Effects of diet on the lipid and fatty acid status of full-term infants at 4 months. J Am Coll Nutr 13:658, 1994.

105. Andersen GE, et al: Dietary habits and serum lipids during first 4 years of life. Acta Paediatr Scand 68:165, 1979.

106. Sweeney MJ, et al: Dietary fat and concentrations of lipid in the serum during the first six to eight weeks of life. Pediatrics 27:765, 1961.

107. Hayes KC, et al: Modulation of infant formula fat profile alters the low-density lipoprotein/high-density lipoprotein ratio and plasma fatty acid distribution relative to those with breast-feeding. J Pediatr 120:S109, 1992.

108. Wissler RW, et al: Conference on blood lipids in children: optimal levels for early prevention of coronary heart disease. Prev Med 12:888, 1983.

109. Mize CE, Uauy R: Cholesterol in infants' diet. Compr Ther 19:267, 1993.

110. Uauy R, Hoffman DR: Essential fat requirements of preterm infants. Am J Clin Nutr 71(suppl):245S, 2000.

111. Pickering DE, et al: Influence of dietary fatty acids on serum lipids. Am J Dis Child 102:72, 1961.

112. Lewis DS, et al: Deferred effects of preweaning diet on atherosclerosis in adolescent baboons. Arteriosclerosis 8:274, 1988.

113. Greenberg LD, Wheeler P: Influence of fatty-acid composition of infant formulas on the development of arteriosclerosis and on the lipid composition of blood and tissues. Nutr Metab 14:100, 1972.

114. Jones PJH, et al: Comparison of breast-feeding and formula feeding on intestinal and hepatic cholesterol metabolism in neonatal pigs. Am J Clin Nutr 51:979, 1990.

115. Pond WG, Mersmann HJ: Subsequent response to early diet cholesterol and feed restriction in swine. Nutr Res 11:461, 1991.

116. Innis SM, et al: Saturated fatty acid chain length and positional distribution in infant formula: effects on growth and plasma lipids and ketones in piglets. Am J Clin Nutr 57:382, 1993.

117. Rioux FM, Innis SM: Cholesterol and fatty acid metabolism in piglets fed sow milk or infant formula with or without addition of cholesterol. Metabolism 42:1552, 1993.

118. Rioux FM, et al: Cholesterol metabolism in piglets fed formula with or without cholesterol. FASEB J 9:A730, 1995.

119. Roberts DCK, et al: Plasma lipoprotein changes in suckling and weanling rabbits fed semipurified diets. Lipids 14:566, 1979.

120. Fernando-Warnakulasuriya GJP, et al: Studies on fat digestion, absorption, and transport in the suckling rat. I. Fatty acid composition and concentrations of major lipid components. J Lipid Res 22:668, 1981.

121. Mao J, Hamosh M: Postnatal development of plasma-lipid-clearing enzymes (lipoprotein lipase, hepatic lipase, and lecithin: cholesterol acyl transferase) and lipid profiles in suckling rats. Biol Neonate 62:1, 1992.

122. Schlag B, Winkler L: Untersuchungen zur Entwicklung der Serumlipoproteineinverhältnisse vom Fetal-stadium bis zum Erwachsenenalter der Ratte. Acta Biol Med Ger 37:239, 1978.

123. Fernando-Warnakulasuriya GJP, et al: Lipoprotein metabolism in the suckling rat: characterization of plasma and lymphatic lipoproteins. J Lipid Res 24:1626, 1983.

124. Hahn P, Smale F-A: 3-Hydroxy-3-methylglutaryl-CoA reductase activity in liver, brown fat, and small intestine of developing rats. Can J Biochem 60:507, 1982.

125. Subbiah MTR, Hassan AS: Development of bile acid biogenesis and its significance in cholesterol homeostasis. Adv Lipid Res 19:137, 1982.

126. Zimniak P, Lester R: Bile acid metabolism in the perinatal period. In Lebenthal E (ed): Human Gastrointestinal Development. New York, Raven Press, 1989, pp 561–579.

127. Innis SM: The role of diet during development on the regulation of adult cholesterol homeostasis. Can J Physiol Pharmacol 63:557, 1985.

128. Hahn P, Innis SM: Cholesterol oxidation and 7α-hydroxylation during postnatal development of the rat. Biol Neonate 46:48, 1984.

129. Kwiterovich PO, et al: Neonatal diagnosis of familial type II hyperlipoproteinemia. Lancet 1:118, 1973.

130. National Cholesterol Education Program: Report of the expert panel on blood cholesterol levels in children and adolescents. Pediatrics 89:525, 1992.

131. Kronn DF, et al: Management of hypercholesterolemia in childhood and adolescence. Heart Disease 2:348, 2000.

132. Hardell LI: Serum lipids and lipoproteins at birth based on a study of 2815 newborn infants. II. Relations between materno-foetal factors and the concentrations of triglycerides and cholesterol. Acta Pediatr Scand (Suppl) 285:11, 1981.

133. Parker CR Jr, et al: The effect of hypertension in pregnant women on fetal adrenal function and fetal plasma lipoprotein-cholesterol metabolism. Am J Obstet Gynecol 150:263, 1984.

134. Parker CR Jr, et al: The effects of dexamethasone and anencephaly on newborn serum levels of apolipoprotein A-1. J Clin Endocrinol Metab 65:1098, 1987.

135. Lane DM, et al: Cord serum lipid and apolipoprotein levels in preterm infants with the neonatal respiratory distress syndrome. J Matern Fetal Med 11:118, 2002.

136. Moorjani S, et al: Plasma lipid and lipoprotein concentrations are normal in congenital hypothyroidism. Clin Chem 30:159, 1984.

137. Tenenbaum D, et al: Alterations of serum high-density lipoproteins and hepatic lipase activity in congenital hypothyroidism. Biol Neonate 54:241, 1988.

138. Ciomartan T, et al: Serum lipoproteins and apolipoprotein E in infants with congenital hypothyroidism. Pediatr Int 41:249, 1999.

139. Barker DJP, et al: Type 2 (non-insulin–dependent) diabetes mellitus, hypertension, and hyperlipidaemia (syndrome X): relation to reduced fetal growth. Diabetologia 36:62, 1993.

140. Mogren I, et al: Fetal exposure, heredity, and risk indicators for cardiovascular disease in a Swedish welfare cohort. Int J Epidemiol 30:853, 2001.

141. Roseboom TJ, et al: Plasma lipid profiles in adults after prenatal exposure to the Dutch famine. Am J Clin Nutr 72:1101, 2000.

142. Barker DJP, et al: Growth in utero and serum cholesterol concentrations in adult life. BMJ 307:1524, 1993.

143. Cianfarani S, et al: Growth, IGF system, and cortisol in children with intrauterine growth retardation: is catch-up growth affected by reprogramming of the hypothalamic-pituitary-adrenal axis? Pediatr Res 51:94, 2002.

144. Napoli C, et al: Influence of maternal hypercholesterolemia during pregnancy on progression of early atherosclerotic lesions in childhood: fate of early lesions in children (FELIC) study. Lancet 354:1234, 1999.

145. Kind KL, et al: Restricted fetal growth and the response to dietary cholesterol in the guinea pig. Am J Physiol Regul Integr Comp Physiol 277:R1675, 1999.

146. Szitányi P, et al: Influence of intrauterine undernutrition on the development of hypercholesterolemia in an animal model. Physiol Res 49:721, 2000.

147. Lucas A, et al: Nutrition in pregnant or lactating rats programs lipid metabolism in the offspring. Br J Nutr 76:605, 1996.

148. Barker DJP: The intra-uterine origins of disturbed cholesterol homeostasis. Acta Paediatr 88:483, 1999.

149. Osmond C, Barker DJP: Fetal, infant, and childhood growth are predictors of coronary heart disease, diabetes, and hypertension in adult men and women. Environ Health Perspect 108(Supp 3):545, 2000.

150. Fall CHD, et al: Relation of infant feeding to adult serum cholesterol concentration and death from ischaemic heart disease. BMJ 304:801, 1992.

151. Marmot MG, Page CM: Effect of breast-feeding on plasma cholesterol and weight in young adults. J Epidemiol Commun Health 34:164, 1980.

152. Hromadová M, et al: Relationship between the duration of the breast-feeding period and the lipoprotein profile of children at the age of 13 years. Physiol Res 46:21, 1997.

153. Fomon SJ, et al: Indices of fatness and serum cholesterol at age eight years in relation to feeding and growth during early infancy. Pediatr Res 18:1233, 1984.

154. Hamosh M, Hamosh P: Does nutrition in early life have long-term metabolic effects? Can animal models be used to predict these effects in the human? In Goldman AS, et al (eds): Human Lactation. New York, Plenum Press, 1987, pp 37–55.

155. Hahn P, Koldovsky O: Utilization of nutrients during postnatal development. New York, Pergamon Press, 1966, pp 155.

156. Kris-Etherton PM, et al: The influence of early nutrition on the serum cholesterol of the adult rat. J Nutr 109:1244, 1979.

157. Hahn P, Koldovsky R: Late effect of premature weaning of blood cholesterol levels in adult rats. Nutr Reports Intl 13:87, 1976.

158. Reiser R, et al: Studies on a possible function for cholesterol in milk. Nutr Reports Intl 19:835, 1979.

159. Mott GE, et al: Influence of infant and juvenile diets on serum cholesterol, lipoprotein cholesterol, and apolipoprotein concentrations in juvenile baboons. Atherosclerosis *45*:191, 1982.
160. Mott GE, et al: Cholesterol metabolism in adult baboons is influenced by infant diet. J Nutr *120*:243, 1990.
161. Mott GE, et al: Differences in cholesterol metabolism in juvenile baboons are programmed by breast- versus formula-feeding. J Lipid Res *36*:299, 1995.
162. Fomon SJ: A pediatrician looks at early nutrition. Bull NY Acad Med *47*:569, 1971.
163. Reiser R, Sidelman Z: Control of serum cholesterol homeostasis by cholesterol in the milk of the suckling rat. J Nutr *102*:1009, 1972.
164. Bayley TM, et al: Longer-term effects of early dietary cholesterol level on synthesis and circulating cholesterol concentrations in human infants. Metabolism *51*:25, 2002.

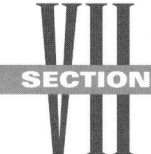

SECTION VII

Carbohydrate Metabolism

46

Satish C. Kalhan

Metabolism of Glucose and Methods of Investigation in the Fetus and Newborn

The metabolism of glucose in the fetus and newborn has been studied extensively, both in animal species and in humans, and several reviews have been published. Our ability to study glucose metabolism has improved significantly owing to the following: (1) the availability of the chronic fetal preparation in sheep, in which fetal blood sampling can be done without causing major changes in the physiologic state of the fetus; (2) the availability of stable, nonradioactive isotopic tracers; and, more recently (3) the application of molecular biology techniques and transgenic animals. In this chapter, the metabolism of glucose in the fetus and newborn is discussed while emphasizing recent developments. Throughout the chapter, emphasis is placed on the available information in humans, supplemented when necessary by animal data.

Since the early 1980s, numerous improvements in the synthesis of stable isotopically labeled tracers and sensitive mass spectrometric methods have allowed investigators to examine glucose metabolism in the human fetus and newborn. Such studies could not be performed in the past because of the lack of availability of these tracers and the risk associated with radioactive tracers. In addition, the development of newer synthetic techniques has increased the number of isotopic tracers, which can be used simultaneously to answer complex questions. By combining these tracer methods along with the measurements of energy consumption, the metabolic fate of substrates and their contribution to overall fuel economy can be quantified.

ISOTOPIC TRACER

Atoms, other than hydrogen, are made of protons (+), electrons (−), and neutrons. Atomic number (Z) represents the number of protons or the number of electrons in an atom; that is, the number of electrons is equal to the number of protons, and the atomic weight is equal to the sum of protons and neutrons. Isotopes are atoms of an element differing from each other only in the number of neutrons. Thus, for a given atomic number (Z), there can be more than one value of atomic weight. The stability of the nucleus of the atom is related to the ratio of neutrons and protons. If there are too many or too few neutrons for the number of protons, the nucleus becomes unstable. To become stable, the nucleus may undergo rearrangement that involves the release of radiation-radioactive nuclei.

The stable, nonradioactive isotopes, by virtue of the lack of radioactivity, have been particularly useful for the study of metabolism in the mother and newborn infant. However, these isotopes also have limitations.

Cost

Initially, because of limited availability, the cost was prohibitive. At the same time, the instruments for their detection, mass spectrometers, were not easily available and were expensive. Now, with relatively easy accessibility and improved sensitivity of the instruments, and with changing attitudes of society toward radioactivity, the use of stable isotopic tracers has become popular, and the cost has continued to decrease.

Natural Abundance

The stable isotopes are naturally occurring nuclides and therefore have a certain background or natural abundance. This is in contrast to the radionuclides whose natural abundance is negligible. Because of this background abundance, and also in part related to the sensitivity of the mass spectrometry, the amount of tracer required for the study of metabolism is more than that used with radioactive tracer.

IDEAL TRACER

Although one could define an ideal tracer in many different ways, the following are some of the most important considerations. Its biologic behavior should be the same as that of the parent compound; that is, it is used in the same manner as the compound traced. This is important for both radioactive and nonradioactive stable tracers. Radioactive-labeled proteins, such as iodine-125 (^{125}I) albumin, are not necessarily metabolized in the same manner as for the native protein. In fact, the labeling may damage or denature the protein.

Stable isotopes, conversely, have their own chemical differences described as isotopic fractionation or isotopic effect. In this process, the isotope behaves differently from the native atom. Two types of isotopic fractionation are important:

1. Temperature: These fractionations are significant in geologic studies in which the changes in the carbon-13 (^{13}C)/^{12}C and oxygen-18 (^{18}O)/^{16}O ratio have been used to study the changes in the earth's temperature.
2. Kinetic/chemical fractionation: These fractionations are the result of isotopic discrimination by various enzyme

systems; that is, the labeled compound is not as rapidly metabolized as the unlabeled compound. Such fractionation will result in the accumulation of the labeled compound in the metabolic pool and will potentially result in errors in measurements. In nature, isotopic fractionation results in differing isotopic composition of nutrients; for example, glucose obtained from sugar cane has different ^{13}C enrichment compared with glucose obtained from beet sugar.[1, 2] The ^{13}C abundance of lipid fractions in several organisms is lower than that of carbohydrates and proteins.[3,4] The basis for these differences has been attributed to isotopic discrimination at certain key enzymatic steps involved in the synthesis of these compounds.[1] DeNiro and Epstein[5] showed that the low ratio of $^{13}C/^{12}C$ of lipids synthesized by *Escherichia coli* grown in minimal media is the result of isotopic fractionation during the oxidation of pyruvate to acetyl coenzyme A (CoA).[5] It is important to recognize these isotopic fractionations when isotopic tracers are used to study metabolism. In general, it is accepted that more heavily labeled tracers such as those labeled with multiple isotopes are likely to be discriminated more than the lightly labeled tracers. In relation to stable isotopes, isotopic fractionation is probably more common with deuterium than with ^{13}C and nitrogen-15 (^{15}N).

The quantity of tracer used should be negligible, so it should have no or minimal pharmacologic effects. This requirement is easily met by the radiolabeled tracers, in which the background radioactivity is essentially zero. In contrast, stable isotope tracers with a significant background natural abundance have to be infused in somewhat larger quantities that are not negligible. The amount of tracer infused is determined by the ability of the analytical instrument to measure the isotopic enrichment above the background in biologic samples. With the newer instruments and better analytical techniques, several of these problems have been resolved, so in most instances, enrichments in the range of 0.5 to 1% above the background can be easily measured. Therefore, the isotopic tracer can be infused at rates approximating 1% of the turnover rate of the tracee. With multiple labeled compounds, in which the background abundance is much lower, even lower rates of tracer infusion can be used and still achieve excellent results.

Isotopic tracers are used *in vivo* to quantify the rate of appearance and disappearance of a substrate, such as glucose and amino acids, or to quantify the utilization and metabolic fate of the substrate, such as oxidation, or the contribution of a substrate to another compound: precursor-product relation.

Quantification of the Rate of Appearance and Disappearance of a Substrate

The usual methods employed involve the administration of the isotopically labeled tracer either as a single bolus (Fig. 46–1) or as a constant-rate infusion (Fig. 46–2). In both instances, the dilution of the tracer in the blood is estimated by measuring the enrichment or specific activity (in case of radioactive tracers) in the blood or plasma. The dilution of the tracer is the function of appearance of the substrate, and the disappearance or utilization of the substrate has no impact on the enrichment because the same proportion of the tracer and tracee will be used. This is a fundamental concept in the tracer studies. The following are the definitions of certain terms used in tracer studies.

Concentration: Amount of substrate per unit of blood or plasma, μmol/ml or mg/ml.

V: Volume of distribution of the substrate or the space in which the substrate is distributed, ml/kg body weight.

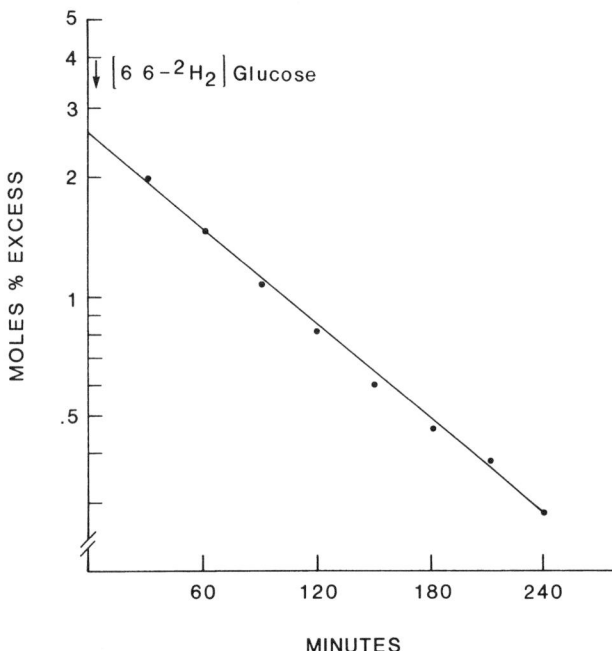

Figure 46–1. Changes in deuterium enrichment of plasma glucose after a single bolus injection of [6,6²H₂]glucose in a physiologically normal man. The rate of glucose appearance is quantified from the rate of decrease (dilution) in the plasma glucose enrichment and the pool size. The latter is quantified from the concentration of glucose, and the volume of distribution is measured by extrapolating the disappearance curve to time zero.

Q: Quantity (moles or grams) of the substrate in the system (body), that is, the size of the substrate pool or pool size, which is equal to the concentration of the substrate times volume of distribution, that is moles (or grams)/mL × mL/kg = moles (or grams)/kg.

Ra: Rate of appearance of the substrate (tracee) in the compartment under study. In most instances, it is the plasma or extracellular fluid compartment, μmoles or mg/minute.

Rd: Rate of disappearance of the substrate from the compartment under study, μmoles or mg/minute. Disappearance is often used as synonymous with utilization. However, utilization is implied in the broad sense of overall utilization and does not necessarily imply a specific pathway.

Steady-state system: The system is said to be in a steady state when the input Ra is equal to output Rd and the concentration remains constant. Conversely, when these parameters are changing, it is called nonsteady state.

Turnover: Rate of turnover of the pool under steady-state conditions, that is, when the concentration is constant: Ra = Rd = turnover, μmol/minute or mg/minute.

Turnover time: Time it takes for the entire pool to turn over, which depends on the size of the pool and the turnover rate: Q (moles)/rate of turnover.

MCR: Metabolic clearance rate, that is, the volume of plasma that is completely cleared of the substrate in a unit time: rate of disappearance Rd (μmol/minute)/Conc. (μmol/ml) = ml/minute. It should be called plasma clearance rate rather than metabolic clearance rate. It does not necessarily mean that the substrate has been *metabolized.*

Two more terms need to be known in relation to tracers:

Specific activity (SA): Radioactivity that is specific to a compound or substrate, expressed in relation to the weight or molecules of the substrate, that is, radioactivity (disinte-

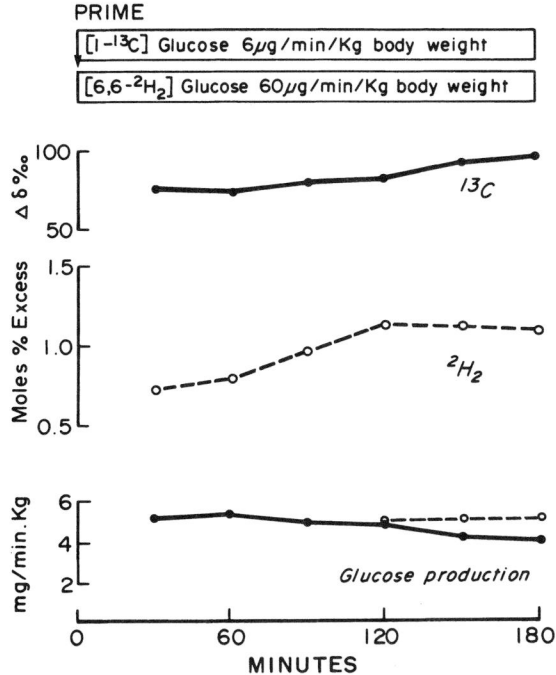

GLUCOSE PRODUCTION RATE IN A NORMAL INFANT WITH SIMULTANEOUS ^{13}C & ^{2}H$_2$ LABELLED GLUCOSE

Figure 46–2. The constant-rate tracer infusion method. As shown, the deuterium-labeled glucose was infused at a constant rate while [1-^{13}C]glucose was administered as a prime-constant-rate infusion. Because of the tracer prime, an early plateau plasma glucose ^{13}C enrichment was achieved. However, a slow continuous increase in enrichment was also seen because of tracer carbon recycling. As shown, the measured rate of glucose production will decrease as the tracer recycling becomes more evident later in the study. (From Kalhan SC, et al: J Clin Endocrinol Metab *50*:456, 1980. Copyright The Endocrine Society.)

grations per minute, or dpm) per mole or gram of substrate = dpm/mole or gram.

Enrichment: Used in relation to stable isotopic tracers to describe the magnitude by which that particular isotope has been increased (enriched) above the background. Enrichment has also been used as synonymous with atom percent excess, that is, how many labeled atoms are present in excess of the background. For practical purposes, enrichment corresponds to specific activity with certain limitations. In relation to stable isotopic tracer, often the tracers are measured as molecules rather than atoms, and therefore, they are described as moles percent excess, that is, the percentage of labeled molecules in excess of the background.

Further, the labeled molecules are designated by the number of labeled atoms added to the parent molecules (m), such as m+1, m+2, and m+3 (or m_0, m_1, m_2, m_3). Therefore, enrichment is described as moles percent excess of these labeled molecules (m+3) enrichment or (m+1) enrichment.

Finally, a tracer is called a *reversible* or *recycling tracer* when, after its disappearance or utilization, it reappears in the plasma. The reappearance results in a second, not easily measurable, source of tracer, and it leads to higher enrichments and underestimation of kinetics. In contrast, when a tracer is lost during its utilization, it is called a *nonrecycling tracer*. In general, when the tracers are labeled with carbon, whether ^{13}C or ^{14}C, the carbon

atoms are likely to be reincorporated (recycle) into newly synthesized substrate; in contrast, when the tracers are labeled with hydrogen ^{2}H, ^{3}H, the hydrogen atoms are lost mostly into water (H$_2$O) during the metabolism of the substrate and are termed *nonrecycling tracers*. Before selecting a tracer to study the kinetics of a tracee, a knowledge of the pathways of metabolism of the tracee can help in the selection of a particular type of label.

During a bolus injection technique, the labeled tracer is administered at zero time, and the rate of change in enrichment or specific activity is measured (see Fig. 46-1). Extrapolation of the decay curve to zero time gives an estimate of the pool size and the volume of distribution of the tracer, and the turnover time is calculated from the rate constant of the disappearance curve.

The constant-infusion technique (see Fig. 46-2), evaluated in detail by Steele and associates,[6] is a commonly used method to quantify tracee kinetics. Steele and colleagues further improved the technique by administering the priming dose of the tracers to achieve early plateau. Thus, it should be called the prime-constant-rate technique. After a priming dose, the tracer is administered at a constant rate throughout the experiment. The size of priming dose depends on the pool size of the tracee and the rate of administration of the tracer. This relation is expressed as follows:

(prime/pool) = (rate of infusion of tracer/rate of appearance of tracee Ra) = enrichment or specific activity

The turnover rate or the rate of appearance and disappearance is calculated from the final asymptote of the enrichment curve and the rate of infusion of the tracer.[6,7]

The methods described earlier assume that the tracer mixes with the tracee in a single compartment instantaneously. Although such an assumption may hold true for a system that is turning over rapidly, it is not necessarily true for slow turnover systems, such as body bicarbonate pool, and it may lead to significant errors. Numerous multiple compartment systems have been used to fit the data most precisely under these circumstances.[8–10] However, at times the physiologic significance of such compartments is not easily understood.

Another problem studied in detail relates to the site of tracer administration and sampling in turnover studies.[11–15] This is particularly true in relation to compounds that are produced by multiple organs and tissues, such as lactate. Thus, a venous sample obtained from a particular vein will not only represent the mixed blood from the body but will also be influenced by the metabolism of the tissues drained by that particular vein. Certain modifications have been proposed, such as retrograde venous sampling, arterial blood, or arterialized venous blood.[12,13] All these have their own limitations and must be recognized during data reduction and interpretation.

Finally, when the concentration of substrate is changing as a result of perturbations, the system is described as being in a *nonsteady state*. Under these conditions, a different set of assumptions and a different data reduction method are employed. The most commonly used method of data reduction is that described by Steele.[16] These equations have been subsequently modified and validated by several investigators.[17,18]

Quantification of Metabolic Fate of the Substrate

An example is oxidation to carbon dioxide (CO$_2$) or the contribution of a substrate to another: precursor-product relationship. This is estimated by the appearance of tracer isotope, usually carbon, in the product. However, the mere appearance of the isotope in the product does not necessarily imply net conversion of the precursor into the product.[19] It may simply represent an exchange of the isotope during biochemical reactions. Second, during the sojourn of the tracer from the precursor to the product, the tracer may be diluted by intermediary compounds. Thus, there would be an underestimation of the contribution of the precursor to the product. The precursor-product relationship is quantified by measuring the turnover of the precursor and product by separate isotopically labeled tracers and by measuring the rate of appearance of the tracer in the product.[9] These concepts of precursor-product relationship are best illustrated using glucose as a model system.

Glucose (precursor) is oxidized to CO_2 (product) by first conversion to pyruvate, which enters the tricarboxylic acid (TCA) cycle via acetyl CoA. During oxidation of pyruvate to CO_2, the three carbons of pyruvate do not appear in CO_2 to the same magnitude. Carbon-1 of pyruvate appears in CO_2 100% during pyruvate's conversion to acetyl CoA by pyruvate dehydrogenase. Carbon-2 and carbon-3 of pyruvate, which form carbon-1 and carbon-2 of acetyl CoA, enter the TCA cycle, and neither of these carbons appears in CO_2 during the first spin of the cycle. It is only in the subsequent turns of the TCA cycle that carbon-2 and carbon-3 appear in CO_2 but not in equal amounts.[20, 21] Wolfe and Jahoor[22] showed, in normal healthy adults by infusing labeled acetate, that only 80% of carbon-1 and 50% of carbon-2 of acetate appeared in CO_2 during isotopic steady state. On the basis of this and other studies, it can be concluded that during glucose/pyruvate oxidation, only 80% of the tracer carbon will appear in CO_2, whereas the remainder is lost via exchange in the TCA cycle. This loss of tracer or the lower appearance of tracer in CO_2 will result in underestimation of oxidation of glucose.

Another example of the loss or exchange of tracer is the synthesis of glucose from pyruvate via gluconeogenesis. During gluconeogenesis, pyruvate is first converted to oxaloacetate, a common intermediate between gluconeogenesis and the TCA cycle. Therefore when carbon labeled precursor is administered for the estimation of gluconeogenesis, some of the tracer will be lost by exchange in the TCA cycle at the oxaloacetate level. Thus, the enrichment or the specific activity of the immediate precursor of glucose, that is, phosphoenol pyruvate, will be less than that of pyruvate, and it will result in a lower estimate of gluconeogenesis.[23] This problem was resolved by Landau and colleagues[24] by using deuterium labeled H_2O, which, in turn, labels the pyruvate pool. Because this method results in constant labeling of pyruvate, and phosphoenol pyruvate without loss of tracer, the appearance of deuterium in glucose can be used to quantify the contribution of gluconeogenesis to total glucose production accurately.

Finally, all these methods of quantification have their own limitations and are near approximations of the actual turnover rates. The assumptions involved in each experimental technique should be recognized when such estimations are done in biologic systems.

MEASUREMENTS OF ENERGY CONSUMPTION

Measurements of energy consumption rate and CO_2 production have become integral components of metabolic studies. Estimation of energy consumption and CO_2 production rate help in the partitioning of the contribution of various substrates to the overall energy utilization. In addition, most studies employing carbon-labeled tracers also estimate the isotopic enrichment of CO_2 either in the blood or in the expired CO_2 to quantify the oxidation rate of the labeled substrate.[25, 26] The major contribution of these estimates has been the ability to accurately quantify as many components of oxidative metabolism as possible and to develop as complete a picture as possible of the fuel metabolism *in vivo*. Two commonly employed methods are briefly discussed here: open-circuit indirect respiratory calorimetry and the doubly labeled H_2O method.

Open-Circuit Indirect Respiratory Calorimetry

In this system, as shown in Figure 46-3, a plastic hood or canopy is placed over the subject's head, and a suction pump is used to draw air through the hood. The air exiting from the hood is mixed by passing through a baffled mixing chamber. The concentration of O_2 and CO_2 is measured in the mixed air by an appropriate device, either an O_2 and CO_2 analyzer or a mass spectrometer, such as the Perkin Elmer medical gas analyzer MGA-1100 (Perkin-Elmer, Pomona, CA). The flow of air through the system is regulated by flow controllers and is measured by a flowmeter. Commercially available servocontrolled flow regulators are appropriate. The rate of O_2 consumption and CO_2 production is measured by multiplying the gradient of these gases across the face with the rate of flow of air and applying Haldane transformations.[27-30] The latter is based on the finding that the volume of air expired is less than the volume of air inspired and that nitrogen is not used or produced by the body. The transformations therefore use the concentration of nitrogen in the inspired and expired air to estimate the inflow of air into the system. The outflow is measured by the flowmeter. The open-circuit method has been validated over many years in large numbers of studies in adults, children, and newborn infants,[31-33] and its limitations have been examined.[34]

Doubly Labeled ($^2H_2^{18}O$) Water Method

This method of measuring energy consumption is based on the estimation of the rate of CO_2 elimination from the body. It has become a popular method because of several distinct advantages:

1. It can be applied to free-living individuals; that is, the subject need not be restrained or confined to bed.
2. CO_2 elimination is measured over a prolonged period, hours to days, and thus it includes a composite measure of energy consumption throughout the entire period.
3. The method is simple and noninvasive. It requires administration of a single dose of labeled H_2O and obtaining a few samples of urine, or saliva, or blood to measure the changes in isotopic enrichment over several days. It can be used in adults, children, and infants with ease, without requiring any major modifications in equipment.

This technique was first described by Lifson and associates[35] to study energy metabolism in small animals and was extensively evaluated in humans, both adults and newborns, by Schoeller and colleagues[36-39] and by other investigators.[40-43] The method is based on the following principles: When H_2O labeled with deuterium (^2H) and ^{18}O is administered to a subject, it equilibrates in all the body H_2O compartments. Then the tracer is eliminated at the same rate as the body H_2O. The deuterium is eliminated from the body as H_2O (^2H_2O). Because oxygen (as well as the

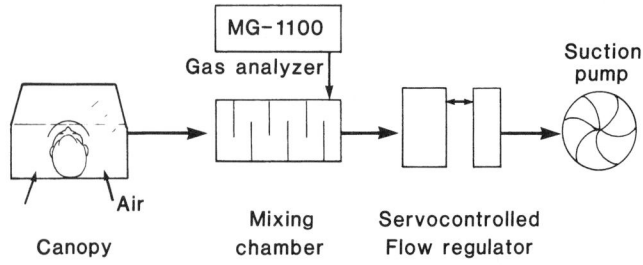

Figure 46-3. Open-circuit indirect respiratory calorimetry. A canopy is placed over the subject's head, and air is drawn through it by a suction pump. Between the canopy and the pump are placed a mixing chamber, a gas analyzer to measure the O_2 and CO_2 concentrations, and a flowmeter and regulator to measure and control the flow rate. For details, see text.

tracer ^{18}O) equilibrates rapidly between H_2O and CO_2 in the presence of carbonic anhydrase, the ^{18}O is eliminated both by CO_2 and H_2O:

$$CO_2 + H_2{}^{18}O \leftrightarrow H_2COO^{18}O \leftrightarrow H_2O + CO^{18}O$$

Thus, the rate of loss of ^{18}O represents the elimination rate of CO_2 plus H_2O, whereas the rate of loss of deuterium from body water represents only the loss of H_2O. Therefore, the difference in the turnover rates of oxygen and hydrogen of H_2O is equal to the CO_2 elimination rate. The mathematical calculations, the limitation of the technique, and related analytical problems were described by Schoeller, and the reader is referred to the excellent review by him.[39]

The partitioning of fuel oxidation is estimated from the stoichiometry of the three oxidative reactions.[27, 28]

$$1 \text{ glucose} + 6\,O_2 = 6\,CO_2 + 6\,H_2O + 673 \text{ kcal}$$

$$\text{respiratory quotient} = \frac{6\,CO_2}{6\,O_2} = 1.0$$

$$1 \text{ palmitate} + 23\,O_2 = 16\,CO_2 + 16\,H_2O + 2398 \text{ kcal}$$

$$\text{respiratory quotient} = \frac{16\,CO_2}{23\,CO_2} = 0.70$$

$$1 \text{ amino acid} + 5.1\,O_2 = 4.1\,CO_2 + 0.7 \text{ urea} + 2.8\,H_2O + 475 \text{ kcal}$$

$$\text{respiratory quotient} = \frac{4.1\,CO_2}{5.1\,O_2} = 0.80$$

Because nitrogen is about 16% protein by weight, the amount of protein oxidized can be estimated from the urinary nitrogen excretion:

$$\text{protein oxidized} = 6.25 \times \text{urinary nitrogen}$$

The contribution of glucose and fat to oxidative metabolism can be estimated from the measured respiratory quotient corrected for protein oxidation.

The limitations in estimation of substrate oxidation by respiratory gas exchange have been discussed by numerous investigators.[21, 27, 28, 44, 45] Respiratory gas exchange measures net utilization or oxidation of the substrates, such as glucose or fat, irrespective of the intermediate steps. For example, if glucose is converted to fatty acids and the fatty acids are oxidized, it will be estimated as glucose oxidation only.[45] Respiratory gas exchange as commonly used and as described earlier does not include other metabolic processes such as gluconeogenesis and lipogenesis.[27, 28] In addition, no net oxidation of fat is assumed to occur at respiratory quotients of less than 1.0.[45] At respiratory quotients greater than 1.0, a calculated negative rate of lipid oxidation is assumed to represent lipid synthesis.[45] Finally, respiratory gas exchange also assumes substrate homogeneity, that is all fatty acids are represented by palmitate with a respiratory quotient of 0.72, and similarly all amino acids and proteins are assumed to have the same respiratory quotient. These limitations should be recognized when data from respiratory calorimetry measurements are interpreted.[20, 21]

GLUCOSE METABOLISM IN THE FETUS

Maternal-Fetal Glucose Relationship

In most species studied, including humans, the fetal plasma glucose concentration has been observed to be significantly lower than that observed in a simultaneously obtained blood sample from the mother.[46, 47] In addition, a significant linear relationship has been observed between the prevailing glucose levels in the mother and that in the fetus.[48, 49] In humans, the fetal blood samples had been obtained mostly at term gestation from fetal scalp blood or at the time of delivery, by cesarean section, from a segment of doubly clamped cord.[48-50] However, because of the effects of labor and delivery on maternal and fetal circulation, these data had been questioned in regard to their representation of fetal metabolism. The technique of percutaneous umbilical blood sampling permits access to fetal circulation without causing any significant perturbations to the physiology of the fetus. Fetal blood samples have been obtained in mid-gestation (18 to 21 weeks) by fetoscopy or late in gestation by ultrasound visualization of the umbilical vessels.[46, 47] Some interesting observations have been made. Bozzetti and colleagues[47] observed a significant correlation between maternal arterialized venous blood glucose and fetal umbilical venous glucose concentrations in 14 fetuses examined between 17 and 21 weeks' gestation, with the fetal glucose concentration lower than that in the mother. Of interest were the findings that in 7 cases, the maternal glucose concentration was less than 4.4 mmol/l (79 mg/dl). These investigators found that, at maternal glucose concentrations lower than 4.4 mmol/l (4.12± 0.11 mmol/l), fetal umbilical venous glucose concentration may exceed the maternal glucose concentration (4.4±0.06 mmol/l) and may be independent of it. Similar suggestions have been made by other investigators when fetal blood samples have been obtained early in gestation.[46] The significance of these findings remains to be defined. However, the higher levels observed were in the umbilical venous sample, whereas the umbilical arterial levels may have been much lower. Later in gestation, and as shown in Figure 46-4, most investigators have observed a close linear relationship between maternal and fetal glucose whether the samples were obtained by percutaneous umbilical blood sampling, by scalp sampling during labor, or from umbilical vessels at the time of elective cesarean section.[48-52] This linear relationship between maternal and fetal glucose concentrations has been observed during euglycemia, during hyperglycemia induced by glucose infusion to the mother, and during hypoglycemia induced by insulin infusion to the mother.

Glucose Transport Across the Placenta

Based on data of *in vivo* studies in animals and isolated perfused placenta, it can be concluded that glucose is transported across

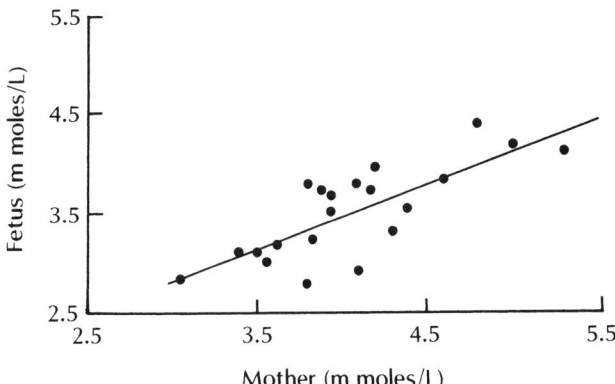

Figure 46-4. Relationship between maternal and fetal glucose concentrations. Simultaneous maternal venous and umbilical venous blood samples (via percutaneous umbilical blood sample) were obtained in the third trimester of pregnancy. (Data from Ashmead GG, et al: Gynecol Obstet Invest 35:18, 1993).

the placenta along a concentration gradient by a facilitated, carrier-mediated diffusion.[53, 54] Furthermore, this process is stereospecific. Although the net transfer is from the mother to fetus, tracer isotope studies have demonstrated a bidirectional diffusion of glucose, that is, from the mother to the fetus and vice versa.[55] Studies of human placenta perfused *in vitro* have shown that the placental glucose uptake from the maternal perfusate and glucose transfer to the fetal perfusate is linearly correlated with maternal glucose concentration up to 20 mmol/L. Beyond this level, glucose is transferred to the fetal perfusate by simple diffusion.[56] Metabolically, the placenta is a very active organ, and glucose transfer to the fetus represents only 40 to 50% of the total glucose uptake by the placenta.[57] The remaining glucose is used by the placental tissue for oxidation, stored as glycogen, or converted to lactate, which is then used by the mother and the fetus.[57-60] As gestation advances, there is an increase in uterine blood flow resulting in an increased delivery of glucose to the fetus.[61] Wilkening and colleagues[62] showed that, in the presence of a constant blood glucose concentration in the pregnant sheep, a reduction of uterine blood flow (from 600 to 300 mL/minute/kg fetus), did not have any effect on fetal glucose uptake or fetal arterial glucose concentration. However, any further decrease in uterine blood flow resulted in decreased fetal glucose uptake and variable fetal arterial glucose concentration. Conversely, a reduction in umbilical blood flow by ligation of one of the umbilical arteries resulted in a decrease in fetal glucose uptake and fetal growth retardation.[63]

Sources of Glucose for the Fetus *in Utero*

Although simultaneous changes in fetal glucose concentration correspond to changes in maternal glucose concentration and are suggestive of fetal dependence on maternal glucose pool, they do not unequivocally indicate that the fetus *in utero* cannot mobilize hepatic glycogen; that is, the fetus does not release glucose from the glycogen stores. To determine whether the fetus *in utero* can regulate glucose metabolism independent of the mother under circumstances in which the maternal metabolism is compromised, two different methods have been applied. The first involves the infusion of glucose labeled with isotopic tracers, to either the mother or the fetus, and examines the isotopic enrichment or specific activity in the maternal and the fetal compartments.[51, 55] In humans, this approach could be applied only in women undergoing elective cesarean section (and therefore minimal maternofetal perturbation) and examining the fetal compartment by obtaining an umbilical arterial and venous blood sample at the time of birth.[51] The second approach, commonly used in animal studies, combines the isotopic tracers with placement of catheters in fetal circulation. Using these techniques, in large as well as small animals, several groups have measured the umbilical blood flow, fetal glucose uptake, fetal glucose utilization, and oxidation.[55,64-69]

Studies in Humans

Only one study has examined the sources of glucose for the human fetus at term gestation.[51] Glucose labeled with ^{13}C was infused at a constant rate to pregnant women undergoing elective cesarean section for clinical indications after an overnight fast. At delivery, simultaneous blood samples were obtained from the maternal vein, cord artery, and cord vein. As shown in Figure 46–5, the ^{13}C enrichment of maternal vein, cord vein, and cord artery was similar in normal and gestationally diabetic women. These data indicate that the fetal glucose pool was in equilibrium with the maternal glucose pool and that maternal glucose was the only source of glucose for the human fetus at term gestation after a brief overnight fast. If the fetus had been producing (releasing) glucose, a lower [^{13}C]glucose enrichment would have been seen in the fetal blood. Whether such a relationship is also

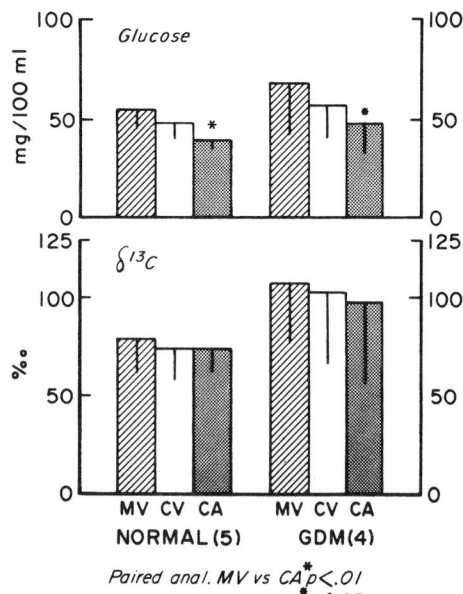

Figure 46–5. Plasma glucose and glucose ^{13}C enrichment (^{13}C) during [1-^{13}C]glucose infusion in maternal venous (MV), cord arterial (CA), and cord venous (CV) blood. Five normal and four gestationally diabetic mothers were infused with [1-^{13}C]glucose tracer for at least 2 hours before elective cesarean section. Simultaneous maternal venous and umbilical blood samples were obtained at delivery. (Reproduced from the Journal of Clinical Investigation, 1979; *63*:388, by copyright permission of the American Society of Clinical Investigation.)

present early in gestation is not known. However, combining isotopic tracer infusion with percutaneous umbilical blood sampling permits an answer to this question at different gestations.

Marconi and colleagues[70] examined whether the fetus could produce glucose in nine patients with pregnancy complicated by intrauterine growth retardation between 29 and 35 weeks' gestation. They administered [U-^{13}C]glucose tracer to the mother and measured the isotopic enrichment in the maternal blood and in fetal blood obtained by cordocentesis. They observed no difference in tracer enrichment in the maternal and fetal compartments, again confirming that even in pregnancies with fetal growth retardation, the maternal glucose is the only source of glucose for the fetus.

Studies in Animals

Examination of the relationship between maternal and fetal glucose pool by measuring maternal and fetal blood glucose concentrations and by infusing isotopic tracer solely in the maternal compartment (as was done in human studies described above) provides only qualitative information regarding maternal and fetal glucose pools. To quantify the magnitude of glucose flux from the mother to the fetus, that is, umbilical glucose uptake and fetal glucose utilization and simultaneous tracer isotopic infusion to the mother and the fetus, measurements of umbilical arterial and venous gradient along with quantification of umbilical blood flow are required. The details of these techniques were described by Krauer and co-workers,[58] Anand and colleagues,[67] and Hay and associates.[68] Because acute perturbations, such as placement of vascular catheters, surgery, or anesthesia, result in major alterations in fetal metabolism, sufficient time must be allowed for the fetus to recover and return to a "normal" basal state. Such studies are not ethically possible in humans.

The sources of fetal glucose have been examined in animal species. The most commonly used animals have been the rat and the sheep. In the pregnant rat examined during the last 3 days of pregnancy (normal rat pregnancy is 21 days) and after a 16-hour fast and with the animal under anesthesia, the fetal glucose specific activity during a constant-rate maternal [14C]glucose tracer infusion was consistently lower than that in the mother, a finding suggesting a fetal source of blood glucose.[64-66] However, such studies should be interpreted with caution because a 16-hour fast in a pregnant rat may be equivalent to a prolonged fast in larger animals.

In contrast to studies in rats, studies in sheep fetuses have shown that, under basal conditions during maternal euglycemia, maternal glucose is the only source of fetal glucose, and fetal glucose production under these circumstances either does not occur or is negligible.[67, 68] The only exception is the study of Hodgson and colleagues,[69] done with the animals in a fed state, which showed that the fetal uptake of glucose from the mother accounted for only approximately 70% of the fetal glucose pool. The reason for this discrepancy is not clear and may be related to feeding in a ruminant mammal. However, it is now accepted that, in most species during basal state, the fetal glucose pool is entirely derived from the maternal glucose pool, and, under these circumstances, the fetus late in gestation does not release endogenous glucose.

Gluconeogenesis *in Utero*

Because in certain animal studies, as stated earlier, the fetus appears to be producing endogenous glucose, and because fetal utilization of placentally produced lactate appears to be a significant component of fetal carbohydrate metabolism, some investigators examined the quantitative contribution of fetal gluconeogenesis. The key gluconeogenesis enzymes, pyruvate carboxylase, phosphoenol pyruvate carboxykinase, and fructose diphosphatase, are present from early fetal life onward in humans.[71, 72] Hepatic cytosolic phosphoenol pyruvate carboxykinase appears for the first time after birth in the rat.[73] In humans, isolated liver tissue (explants) early in gestation can incorporate [14C]alanine and [14C]pyruvate into glucose.[74,75] The recycling of the glucose carbon in isolated human fetal liver preparation, however, is negligible.[76] These observations in humans are similar to those seen in guinea pigs and sheep.[77-81] Gleason and associates[82, 83] and Levitsky and colleagues[84] quantified gluconeogenesis from [14C]lactate in chronically catheterized sheep and baboon fetus. In sheep, although a significant amount of [14C]lactate was taken up by the liver, only a negligible quantity of the tracer was incorporated into glucose, and the lactate/O_2 quotient was 2:1. These studies suggest that lactate in sheep fetal liver is probably used for nonoxidative metabolic processes, such as a source for glycogen.[82,83] In contrast to sheep, the baboon fetus had slightly greater incorporation of tracer lactate into glucose.[84] Finally, Palacin and colleagues[85] demonstrated that even after 48 hours of maternal food deprivation, there was no demonstrable gluconeogenesis from radioactively labeled glycerol or alanine in the rat fetus at 21.5 days of gestation. Thus, in the mammalian species studied, even though the potential for hepatic gluconeogenesis exists, the gluconeogenic capacity is not expressed *in utero* under unperturbed circumstances, and the contribution of gluconeogenesis from lactate, pyruvate, or alanine to glucose is quantitatively negligible. The expression of the regulation of key gluconeogenic enzymes in the fetal and neonatal liver has been reviewed.[86]

Fetal Glucose Utilization

The quantitative aspects of fetal glucose utilization have been studied extensively in large animals, such as sheep, by several investigators.[68,69, 86-89] These data suggest that the fetus of a fed normoglycemic sheep, late in gestation, takes up approximately

5 mg/kg/minute glucose and uses a similar amount, so fetal hepatic glucose production approaches zero.[59, 68, 87] The only exception has been the study by Hodgson and colleagues,[69] which showed a higher utilization rate compared with umbilical uptake, suggesting fetal production of glucose. This difference may be related to the isotopic tracer method employed in which the loss of tracer from the fetal to maternal compartment was not taken into account.[87] In humans, no such estimation of fetal glucose utilization has been possible. The only approximation has been based on the increase in total maternal glucose production, measured in late gestation, and it suggests a fetoplacental glucose utilization rate of 5 to 6 mg/kg/minute.[51] Whether such a magnitude of glucose uptake can account for the oxidative metabolism of the fetus has been examined by calculating glucose/O_2 quotient.[90,91] The glucose/O_2 quotient represents the fraction of the total fetal O_2 consumption required to metabolize aerobically and completely the glucose acquired by the fetus across the placental circulation and is calculated as follows: glucose/O_2 quotient = 6 × [umbilical vein–umbilical artery difference of glucose (mmol)]/[umbilical vein–umbilical artery difference of O_2 (mmol)]. The fetal glucose/O_2 quotient in the fed sheep[91] has been estimated to be approximately 0.5 and in humans approximately 0.8.[90] These data suggest that the maternally acquired glucose could not provide for the entire oxidative metabolism of the fetus and that other substrates, such as lactate and amino acids, may also be used by the fetus *in utero* for its energy needs.

The role of insulin in fetal glucose utilization and fetal glucose production was further evaluated by the following means: (1) infusion of somatostatin, resulting in insulin and glucagon withdrawal from the fetus; (2) infusion of insulin directly to the fetus; and (3) injection of streptozotocin to the fetus, to produce chronic fetal hypoinsulinemia. Acute infusion of somatostatin to the sheep fetus caused a decrease in plasma insulin and glucose concentration without any change in glucagon concentration.[92] Under these circumstances, fetal glucose utilization and umbilical glucose uptake did not change. Exogenous infusion of glucose did not elicit an insulin response; however, glucose utilization increased even though insulin secretion had been suppressed by somatostatin infusion. These data suggest that acute withdrawal of insulin does not affect fetal glucose utilization and that fetal glucose utilization can be increased even in the absence of a significant insulin stimulation.[92] Chronic withdrawal of insulin by streptozotocin injection to the fetus resulted in fetal hypoinsulinism, fetal hyperglycemia, and a decrease in fetal glucose utilization and glucose carbon oxidation.[93-95] There was also an associated decrease in umbilical uptake of glucose, probably as a result of fetal hyperglycemia.[94] Finally, direct infusion of insulin to the fetus increased fetal glucose utilization in both sheep and rat fetus.[96-99] In addition, acute insulin infusion also increased the glucose/O_2 quotient across the hind limb of fetal lamb.[100] These data are important in the context of human infants of diabetic mothers in whom intrauterine hyperinsulinemia results in increased fetal glucose utilization, increased accretion of carbon in insulin sensitive tissue, and increased growth and fetal macrosomia.[101] Such a change in fetal body composition, that is, increased fat deposition and increased hepatic lipogenesis in response to fetal insulin infusion, has been demonstrated in sheep, monkey, and rat.[102-108] The role of other glucose regulatory hormones, such as glucagon, cortisol, and catecholamine, in fetal glucose production, utilization, and umbilical glucose uptake needs to be evaluated.

Utilization of Other Substrates by the Fetus

Because glucose could not account for the total O_2 uptake by the fetus, attention has been focused on the utilization of other substrates such as lactate and amino acids by the fetus. Studies of quantitative aspects of lactic acid metabolism by the fetus are confounded by the rapid changes in the concentration of lactic acid in response to small perturbations in the fetus. Therefore, particularly in humans, in whom previous blood samples had been obtained only at the time of vaginal or elective cesarean delivery, the umbilical arterial concentration of lactate has been observed to be higher than the simultaneously obtained umbilical venous and maternal venous blood concentrations.[109] These data would suggest fetal production and placental clearance of lactate but are subject to criticism because of a lack of steady state and the effect of labor on fetal metabolism. Even in a relatively unperturbed state in which percutaneous umbilical blood samples have been obtained from the fetus *in utero*, the fetal blood lactate concentrations were found to be similar to the simultaneously obtained maternal venous blood concentrations.[46] However, in a more recent study in which fetal blood samples were obtained by cordocentesis late in gestation, no correlation between maternal and fetal blood lactate concentrations was observed (Fig. 46-6).[52]

In contrast to the data in humans, stable chronic preparations in the sheep fetus provide near-optimal conditions to study the maternal-fetal lactate relationship. As shown in Figure 46-7, the umbilical venous and uterine venous concentrations of lactate have been shown to be higher than the simultaneously measured umbilical arterial and uterine arterial lactate concentrations.[59] These data, which have been confirmed by Char and Creasy,[60] indicate uteroplacental production and maternal and fetal utilization of lactate. The metabolic fate of the lactate produced by the uteroplacenta and used by the fetus was not examined in these studies. However, estimation of the lactate/O_2 quotient suggested that complete oxidation of lactate could account for 25% of fetal O_2 consumption.[59] These studies are of interest in that the lactate derived from the placenta could potentially be used by the fetus for both oxidative and nonoxidative purposes such as glycogen synthesis.

In addition to glucose and lactate, amino acids actively transported from the mother to the fetus are an important potential source of energy as well as substrates for glycogen synthesis. Amino acids are actively transported across the human placenta from the mother to the fetus.[110] Lemons and colleagues[111, 112] examined the fetal uptake of amino acids in the unstressed sheep and observed that the fetal uptake of amino acids was far in excess of that found in the carcass. These investigators suggested that a significant amount of amino acids taken up by the fetus was oxidized. Gresham and colleagues[113] estimated that up

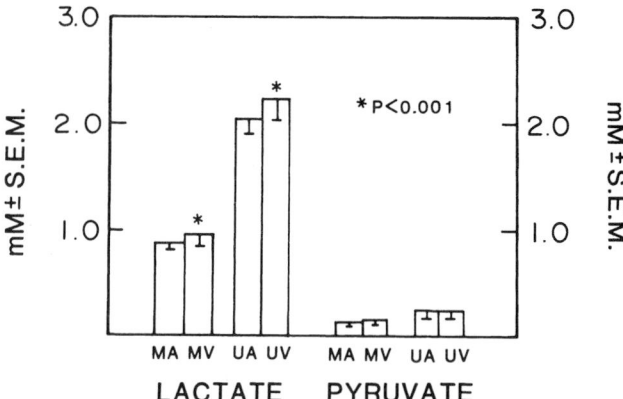

Figure 46–7. Maternal-fetal lactate and pyruvate gradients in the sheep, late in gestation. MA = maternal artery; MV = uterine vein; UA = umbilical artery; UV = umbilical vein. (Reprinted by permission from Nature, vol 254, p 710. Copyright 1975, Macmillan Magazines Ltd.)

to 25% of the total fetal O_2 consumption in the sheep fetus could be accounted for by the oxidation of amino acids. In the human, based on urea concentration gradients across the umbilical circulation, it can be assumed that the human fetus *in utero* catabolizes amino acids and synthesizes urea.[114] Using stable isotopic tracer methods, Gilfillan and colleagues[115] demonstrated synthesis of alanine by the human fetus at term gestation. They estimated that endogenous alanine synthesis could account for approximately 44% of alanine flux in the fetus. Because alanine is a major glucogenic precursor and because alanine nitrogen is a major precursor of urea nitrogen, the major oxidation product of amino acids, these data are consistent with utilization of amino acids by the human fetus for energy metabolism.

Regulation of Umbilical Glucose Uptake and Fetal Glucose Utilization

The fetal uptake of glucose appears to be closely regulated by the maternal plasma glucose concentration. As cited earlier, in human studies, the fetal glucose concentration closely follows maternal glucose concentration. In studies of fetal sheep, when the maternal glucose concentration was decreased by fasting[116] or by acute insulin infusion,[88] the umbilical uptake of glucose also decreased. During acute hypoglycemia produced by insulin infusion, the glucose-specific activity in the maternal and fetal compartment was identical, a finding suggesting no compensatory glucose production by the fetus and hence an associated decrease in fetal glucose utilization.[88] In contrast, in the experiments on fasted sheep, the fetal glucose utilization measured by isotopic tracer did not decline as much as the decrease in umbilical uptake, a finding suggesting a compensatory fetal glucose production.[116] The reason for the difference in these two studies may be that, in the former, hypoglycemia was produced acutely by insulin infusion, whereas in the latter, the hypoglycemia was produced slowly after 5 to 7 days of fasting, which probably permitted the fetus to mount a compensatory response. DiGiacomo and Hay[117] showed that, during chronic maternal hypoglycemia produced by up to 3 weeks of insulin infusion, the sheep fetus increases glucose production and thus maintains glucose utilization. Whether such compensation also occurs in humans is not known. Nevertheless, isolated perfused human liver early in gestation is capable of release and autoregulation of uptake of glucose.[76] In this context, during acute umbilical cord compression in the sheep fetus that resulted in decreased umbilical glucose delivery to the fetus, Rudolph and associates[118] also

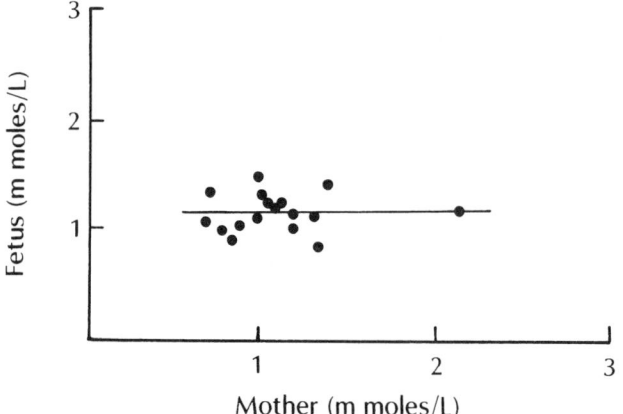

Figure 46–6. Lack of relationship between maternal and fetal blood lactate concentrations. The fetal samples were obtained by percutaneous umbilical blood sampling late in gestation. (Data from Ashmead GG, et al: Gynecol Obstet Invest *35*:18, 1993).

showed an increase in net glucose production by the fetal liver. However, under these circumstances, there was also a decrease in O_2 delivery to the fetus and a decrease in fetal arterial O_2 content, even though umbilical O_2 uptake was maintained. Therefore, the mechanism of compensatory glucose production during these conditions may be different from that seen during sustained hypoglycemia.

Glycogen Metabolism and Sources of Glycogen in the Fetus

The hepatic glycogen content in the human fetus is low early in gestation. As measured by Capkova and Jirasek,[119] the glycogen content of the fetal liver between 51 and 60 days' (average, 8 weeks') gestation was 3.4 mg/g. There was a slow continuous increase in hepatic glycogen, so between 121 and 130 days' gestation, it had reached 24.6 mg/g. In preparation for birth, a rapid steep increase appears to occur at around 36 weeks' gestation. As shown by Shelley and Neligan,[120] in the human fetus at 40 weeks' gestation, the hepatic glycogen content approaches 50 mg/g net weight (Fig. 46–8). Soon after birth, there is a rapid decrease in hepatic glycogen, so by 24 hours of age it has reached a very low concentration. The human data have been obtained from abortions, fresh stillbirths, or infants who died soon after birth. Therefore, the consequences of the events responsible for death should be considered when interpreting these data. It is likely that these estimates are lower than the actual levels in the liver. Similar changes in hepatic glycogen in relation to development have been observed in other animal species.

The fetal liver contains the full complement of enzymes required for the synthesis and breakdown of glycogen.[121] The potential for the synthesis of glucose from three carbon substrates has been demonstrated from early on in gestation in most mammalian species, except the rat. Evidence has been presented in mature animals and in humans suggesting that glucose may not be the immediate precursor of hepatic glycogen and that three carbon substrates—lactate, pyruvate, and alanine—derived from glucose in the periphery are likely to be the precursors for hepatic glycogen.[122-124] Whether a similar "indirect" pathway is also operative in the fetus was examined by Levitsky and associates[125] in chronically catheterized sheep fetus late in gestation. By simultaneously infusing [^{14}C]lactate and [3-^{3}H]glucose in the fetal circulation and measuring ^{14}C- and ^{3}H-specific activity of glycogen, these investigators showed that glycogenesis from glucose, in the ovine fetus, is partly through the "indirect" gluconeogenic route, and lactate may be an important glycogenic precursor. These data are consistent with high lactate turnover rates observed in the sheep fetus.[126, 127]

GLUCOSE METABOLISM IN THE NEWBORN

As discussed in the preceding section, the fetus *in utero* under normal circumstances is entirely dependent on the mother for glucose, and negligible amounts, if any, of fetal glucose production have been observed in most mammalian species studied. At birth, with the discontinuation of the maternal supply of substrates and nutrients as a result of cutting the umbilical cord, the newborn has to mobilize glucose and other substrates to meet energy needs. Therefore, the process of birth involves certain well-orchestrated endocrine and metabolic events that result in adaptive responses for independent existence. Studies in newborn humans and in newborn animals have shown major changes in circulating glucoregulatory hormones, in association with birth and cutting of the umbilical cord. The plasma concentration of epinephrine, norepinephrine, and glucagon has been shown to increase rapidly, whereas the concentration of insulin decreases.[128-132] The net effect of these changes is mobilization of glycogen[133] and fatty acids.[128, 129] After birth in the human newborn, the plasma glucose concentration declines, reaching a nadir by 1 hour of age and then rising spontaneously so plateau levels are reached between 2 and 4 hours.[134-137] The lowest level of glucose observed and the speed with which stable levels are reached are in part dependent on whether the mother received glucose during labor and delivery.[138] With the current obstetric management of the mother and the nutritional practices for the neonate, low blood glucose levels are not seen as often as in the past. In addition, the average glucose levels observed in the nursery are higher than those in the past.[135-137] At present, a full-term healthy neonate in the first 6 hours of life maintains plasma glucose between 40 and 80 mg/dl. The glucose levels increase slightly with the initiation of feeding, so after 24 hours of birth, the normal infant's plasma glucose levels range between 45 and 90 mg/dl. Of course, these data vary with the individual institution's clinical practice regarding nutritional management of the newborn. The data in animal studies are variable depending on the individual species differences. Suffice it that most newborn animals go through a brief period of transient hypoglycemia with spontaneous recovery.

Glucose Kinetics in the Newborn

By using an isotopic tracer dilution method, radioactive tracers in animals, and nonradioactive (stable) tracers in humans, the rates of glucose production and utilization have been quantified in several studies.[139-143] Although these measurements fit within a certain range, these quantitations are influenced by the following factors:

1. The type of tracer used, that is, recycling versus nonrecycling. In general terms, labeled carbon tracers are recycling tracers and result in underestimation of glucose production rate, the only exception being the use of uniformly labeled [^{13}C]glucose and quantitation of only the masses representing the whole molecule of glucose that is uniformly labeled.[142, 144] In contrast to labeled carbon tracers, labeled hydrogen tracers are nonrecycling.[140] However, in some of the later tracers, there may be an excessive loss or exchange of label resulting in an overestimation of the rate of turnover.
2. The clinical condition of the subject. Although it has been described that the subjects were "well," in many of these studies, the infants were receiving intravenous fluids or

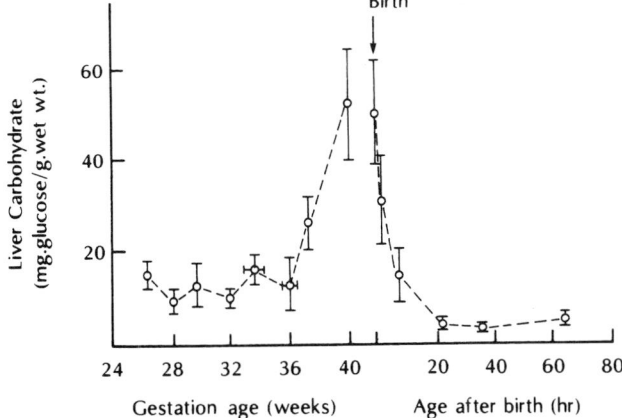

Figure 46–8. Changes in liver glycogen concentration in the human during fetal life and after birth (Adapted from Shelley HJ, Nelligan GA: Br Med Bull *22*:34, 1966.)

were completing a course in antibiotics. In one study, the infants were receiving intravenous glucose, which was discontinued before initiation of isotopic tracers.[140] These infants should not be considered "well" in the strict sense, and their underlying problems may have contributed to the variance in measurements. Similarly, the earlier animal studies were performed either by tying the animals down or administering anesthesia to them.[143] Anesthesia has been documented to have significant effect on glucose metabolism.[145]

3. The blood sampling technique, such as with repeated venipuncture or heel-sticks versus indwelling needles, may influence glucose measurements. It has been well recognized and confirmed[146] that the newborn infant can respond to pain by mounting a "stress"-hormone response, which can result in changes in glucose kinetics.

Glucose Kinetics During Fasting

The rates of glucose production and utilization in the human newborn during fasting, that is, 3 to 4 hours after birth, before feeding, or after 8 to 9 hours after the last feeding, have been estimated to be between 4 and 6 mg/kg/minute.[139-142] These rates are higher than those measured by recycling tracers.[141] The rate of glucose production in the newborn human is somewhat lower than that observed in newborn dog, lamb, or pig,[143,147] and this situation probably is caused by species differences or by experimental conditions.

The rates of glucose production estimated in the newborn are significantly higher than those observed in adult humans and animals and reflect the higher metabolic rate and the higher brain/body weight ratio of the newborn, the brain being the major glucose-using organ. As the newborn grows, the rate of glucose production per unit body weight decreases, so by adolescence, the rates of glucose production approximate the rates in adults, which are one-half to one-third those seen in the newborn.[140]

During steady state, in the presence of a constant blood glucose concentration, the rates of glucose production and utilization are equal. The fate of used glucose and its contribution to oxidative metabolism was quantified in human newborns by Denne and Kalhan.[142] By infusing glucose labeled uniformly with ^{13}C in combination with indirect respiratory calorimetry, these investigators showed that only 53% (range, 40.9 to 68.1) of glucose produced was oxidized to CO_2, and oxidation of plasma glucose contributed up to 38% of the total calorie expenditure. Another interesting finding of this study was the small discrepancy (~20%) between the estimation of total carbohydrate oxidation by respiratory calorimetry and that measured by tracer isotope studies. A similar discrepancy was shown by Sauer and colleagues[148] in their study of glucose-infused newborn infants. This difference has been postulated to result from the inclusion of local glycogen mobilization and oxidation, not included in the tracer isotope estimations.[142] However, this does not explain the observed discrepancy during prolonged fasting conditions.[20]

The study of Denne and Kalhan raises an important question regarding the energy metabolism of the brain in newborn humans during fasting. As demonstrated by studies in adult humans, the brain derives almost all its energy from glucose.[149,150] The calculated amount of glucose necessary to supply the energy for the brain correlates well with the measured oxidation rates of glucose.[151,152] The O_2 consumption rate of the brain in the newborn human has been determined to be 104 μmol/100 g brain tissue/minute.[153] If the average weight of brain in newborn infants is estimated to be 360 g,[154] approximately 3.7 mg/kg/minute of glucose would be required to meet the metabolic needs of the brain. Thus, as shown by Denne and Kalhan, the measured rates of glucose oxidation in the human newborn will

only supply approximately 70% of energy needs of the brain. These data suggest that in the human newborn during fasting, the energy requirements of the brain are supported in part by fuels other than glucose.

Effect of Age

The data presented earlier were obtained in the first 48 hours after birth. Over the next few days, with the introduction of feeding, the normal infant maintains the plasma glucose between 40 and 70 mg/dl during fasting.[155] The endogenous rate of glucose production and utilization, as measured by [1-^{13}C]glucose tracer dilution, also either remains unchanged or decreases slightly (Fig. 46-9). Thus, the glucose production rate in seven infants older than 2 days was 4.1 mg/kg/minute. As shown, in contrast to the physiologically normal infants, in the infant of a diabetic mother, the plasma glucose concentration and endogenous glucose production rate increased and reached those observed in the normal infants. In the infant with intrauterine growth retardation, the endogenous glucose production rate expressed per kilogram of body weight had been noted to be either the same as normal infants or slightly increased, a finding reflecting the higher brain weight/body weight ratio in these infants.

Regulation of Glucose Production in the Newborn

Interest in the regulation of hepatic glucose production in the newborn stems from the observation of marked fluctuation in glucose homeostasis during this period. Both in human and in animal models, hypoglycemia and hyperglycemia have been observed and constitute a significant problem in the clinical management of the infant. The problem is further compounded in the premature newborn and in the presence of intrauterine growth retardation. These responses in the newborn led some investigators to suggest that glucose homeostasis in the newborn is "transitional" as a result of immaturity of the regulatory mechanisms.[147] Evaluation of regulation of glucose homeostasis is rather difficult because of the small size of the newborn infant

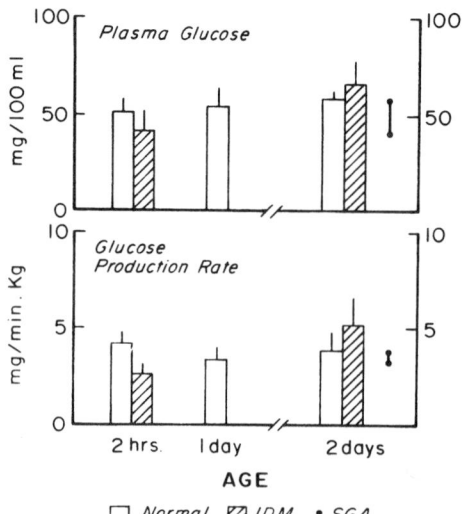

GLUCOSE PRODUCTION RATE IN 28 NEWBORN INFANTS
(mean ± S.D.)

Figure 46–9. Changes in the rate of glucose production and blood glucose concentration in the first 2 days in physiologically normal infants, infants of diabetic mothers (IDM), and small for gestational age infants (SGA).

and animal, the prolonged nature of the experiments, and, finally, the rapid changes in the physiologic state as the newborn adapts to the extrauterine environment.

The role of glucose and the pancreatic hormones insulin and glucagon in the regulation of glucose production has been examined in both adults and newborns. During the basal state in normal adult humans and animals, the hepatic glucose output is regulated by the interaction of insulin and glucagon. An unopposed action of insulin causes a decrease in hepatic glucose output, whereas glucose output increases in the presence of unopposed action of glucagon.[156, 157] When glucose is infused in normal adults, the endogenous glucose production is suppressed as a result of the autoregulatory effect of glucose and the action of insulin on the liver.[158, 159] At low rates of glucose infusion, when the insulin concentrations are similar to those in the basal state, there is 70 to 90% inhibition of endogenous glucose production.[159, 160] However, at higher rates of glucose infusion, with higher levels of circulating insulin, there is complete suppression of endogenous glucose production.[157, 161] Thus, endogenous glucose production in adult animals and humans appears to be regulated by both glucose and insulin. Glucose alone appears to have its effect in suppressing endogenous glucose production on an insulinized liver via its effect on glycogen metabolism.[162-165]

Whether such mechanism of glucose regulation is functional in the newborn infant and animals has been a subject of study for some time. Numerous studies have examined the newborn human's and animal's response to exogenous glucose infusion. Varma and associates[166] observed a continuous increase in plasma glucose concentration during a constant-rate glucose infusion in newborn dogs, while at the same time the rate of endogenous glucose production decreased to a lesser degree than in adult dogs. In this study, the animals were anesthetized with sodium pentobarbital (Nembutal), which may have affected their glucose metabolism; these investigators used [2-³H]glucose tracer, which is lost in excess as compared with other tracers owing to futile cycling; and finally, the newborn dogs had fasted for a very short time, as compared with adults, so they were not in a true fasted state and may have been absorbing glucose from the gut. Sherwood and associates,[167] in a study of rhesus monkey neonates, showed a marked reduction of endogenous glucose output in response to glucose. However, in a group of "sick" newborns, possibly as a result of counterregulatory hormonal responses, marked hyperglycemia developed with no suppression of endogenous glucose output. Finally, in a study of newborn lambs, Cowett and colleagues[147] observed persisting endogenous glucose production until glucose was infused at high rates. However, in this study, the animals had consistently high glucose concentrations, a finding suggesting some influence of counterregulatory hormones, possibly as a result of experiment-related "stress."

In human studies, data have been variable. King and associates[168] observed 80% suppression of endogenous glucose production in term newborn infants. In contrast, Cowett and colleagues[169, 170] observed a variable response—complete suppression in some and incomplete in others. The latter was seen more often in preterm infants. In another study, my colleagues and I[171] examined the role of plasma glucose concentration in the regulation of endogenous glucose production by infusing glucose at 2.6 to 4.6 mg/kg/minute as a continuous infusion to full-term, preterm, and small for gestational age infants. Because of the different rates of exogenous glucose infusion, the measured endogenous glucose production rate was variable. However, the peak glucose concentration was related to the rate of glucose infusion, and a negative correlation between peak glucose concentration and the rate of endogenous glucose production was seen (Fig. 46-10). All infants in this study mounted a significant insulin response, yet the hepatic response in terms of glucose production rate was variable, a finding suggesting that

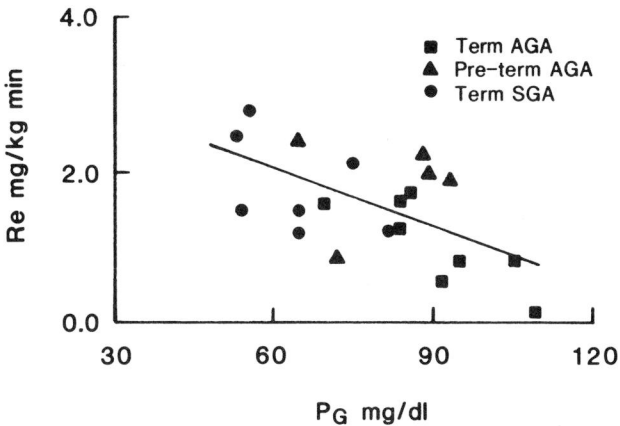

Figure 46–10. Relationship between peak glucose concentration (PG) and endogenous glucose production rate (Re) in newborn infants during intravenous glucose infusion at varying rates. The rate of glucose production was measured by [6,6-²H₂] glucose tracer as a prime–constant-rate infusion. A negative correlation between PG and Re is shown. AGA = appropriate for gestational age; SGA = small for gestational age. $Y = 3.56-0.03x$; $r = 0.59$; $p = .006$. (From Kalhan SC, et al: Pediatr Res 20:49, 1986.)

insulin alone does not appear to be the dominant factor in the regulation of hepatic glucose production. The inverse relationship between plateau glucose concentration and the endogenous glucose production (Re) supports the hypothesis that in the presence of insulin, plasma glucose concentration appears to be the major regulator of hepatic glucose output in the human neonate. Such a regulatory effect of glucose level on hepatic release and uptake of glucose has been demonstrated in the isolated liver from the midterm human fetus.[76] In that study, insulin in physiologic concentration had no detectable effect on hepatic glucose output.

The role of other regulatory hormones, glucagon and catecholamines, in neonatal glucose homeostasis was evaluated in dogs and lambs. As discussed previously, an increase in glucagon concentration and a decrease in insulin are important in the establishment of hepatic glucose production after birth. However, when the role of glucagon was further evaluated in the neonatal dog and lamb by infusing somatostatin (an inhibitor of insulin and glucagon secretion), a variable response was observed.[172-174] This variability was in part the result of "resistance" to somatostatin action on the pancreas, so neonatal pancreas does not show a magnitude of inhibition of insulin and glucagon secretion similar to that seen in adults.[172, 174] Thus, these data remain subject to ambiguity in interpretation. Finally, studies by Cowett[175, 176] suggest that, under normal physiologic conditions, the neonatal liver is more responsive to β-adrenergic stimulation than to α-adrenergic stimulation. The role of hepatic adrenergic receptors in glucose production *in vivo* in the newborn needs further examination.

Gluconeogenesis in the Newborn

Although the capacity for gluconeogenesis is present in the fetal liver with the exception of the rat, and even though the fetus *in utero* as well as the isolated fetal liver preparation can synthesize glucose via gluconeogenesis under certain circumstances, gluconeogenesis, that is, synthesis of new glucose and release in circulation, is a postnatal event in most mammalian species. In the case of rat liver, the key gluconeogenesis enzyme phosphoenol pyruvate carboxykinase appears only after birth, and hence the rat fetus is incapable of gluconeogenesis *in utero*.[86]

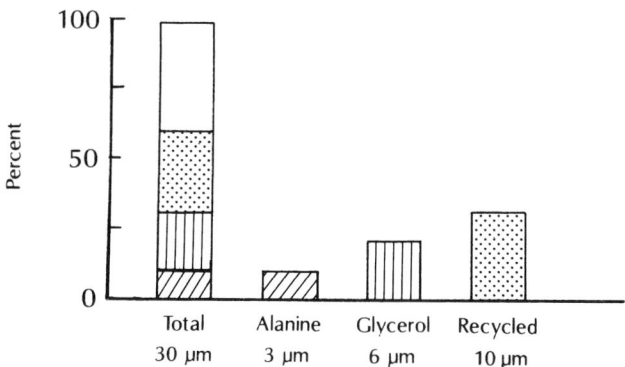

Figure 46–11. Sources of glucose in the human newborn. As measured by tracer isotopes, the major sources of glucose during fasting in the human newborn are glycogen (*unshaded area in the bar*), alanine, glycerol, and recycled glucose carbon.

In the human newborn, a steady plasma glucose concentration maintained by systemic glucose production is evident soon after birth. Although glucose production most likely is initiated at birth, because of technical problems such as infusion of isotopic tracers, the earliest time of measurement has been 2 to 3 hours after birth. The contributors to systemic glucose production are glycogenolysis and various glucogenic substrates—glycerol, lactate, and alanine via gluconeogenesis (Fig. 46–11). Using various isotopic tracer methods, investigators have quantified the kinetics of these gluconeogenic substrates and their contribution to systemic glucose production in healthy newborn infants.

Gluconeogenesis from glycerol has been quantified in healthy full-term infants by simultaneous infusion of carbon-labeled glycerol along with labeled glucose. The appearance of tracer carbon in glucose is used to quantify the contribution of glycerol to glucose.[177-179] Data from two such studies in healthy newborn infants are displayed in Table 46–1. As shown, the rate of appearance of glycerol in healthy full-term infants during the first

48 hours after birth was approximately 9 µmol/kg/minute. Glycerol's contribution to glucose accounted for 10 to 20% of glucose produced. The wide range in estimates of glycerol's contribution to glucose may simply reflect the characteristics of the study population, their time since birth, and relation to the last feeding. Nonetheless, these data show that gluconeogenesis from glycerol is active in the healthy full-term infant immediately after birth, and approximately 10 to 20% of plasma glucose is derived from glycerol. Finally, these data also show that lipolysis in adipose tissue is also active at a high rate in the neonate, because adipose tissue triglyceride depots are the primary source of plasma glycerol.

Because all other gluconeogenic substrates enter the gluconeogenesis pathway via pyruvate, some investigators have examined the contribution of alanine and lactate to glucose production,[86] by using carbon labeled tracers. As discussed previously, all these methods result in an underestimation of the contribution of gluconeogenesis to glucose production because of the loss of tracer carbon via exchange in the TCA cycle. The data on lactate kinetics from one such study[180] are displayed in Table 46–2. The rate of appearance of glucose and lactate were quantified using $[6,6^2H_2]$glucose and $[^{13}C_3]$lactate, respectively. As shown, newborn infants have a relatively high rate of lactate turnover when compared with adults, and approximately 18% of glucose was derived from lactate. However, this estimate of gluconeogenesis from lactate did not correct for the loss of tracer. When corrected for the loss of tracer carbon (correction factor, ~1.5),[181] the lactate's contribution to glucose would be approximately 27%.

Newer techniques have been developed to avoid the errors associated with the loss of tracer carbon in the TCA cycle. These include the deuterium labeling of the body H_2O and mass isotopomer distribution method. These techniques have been applied to quantify gluconeogenesis in full-term and preterm infants.[180, 182, 183] Using the deuterium labeling of body H_2O method, Kalhan and colleagues[180] showed that the contribution of pyruvate to glucose production in healthy full-term infants amounted to 31% or 9.30±1.96 µmol/kg/minute (mean ± SD). These estimates of gluconeogenesis via pyruvate are similar to the

---

TABLE 46–1

Glycerol Metabolism in Healthy Newborn Infants*

	Glycerol Ra (µmol/kg/min)	Glucose Ra (µmol/kg/min)	Fraction, Glucose from Glycerol	Quantity, Glucose from Glycerol (µmol/kg/min)	Reference
n = 6	9.47±2.11	21.09±1.71	0.20±0.06	4.34±1.30	Patel and Kalhan[178]
n = 8	8.7±1.2	25.0±3.5	0.11±0.02	2.75±0.59	Sunehag et al[179]

*Mean ± SD.
Ra = rate of appearance.

TABLE 46–2

Glucose and Lactate Kinetics in Newborn Infants*

	Glucose (mmol/L)	Lactate (mmol/L)	Glucose Ra (µmol/kg/min)	Lactate Ra (µmol/kg/min)	Glucose from Lactate (%)
Normals (n = 10)	2.96±0.51	1.83±0.29	20.66±3.28	38.3±11.90	17.9±5.2
SGA (n = 4)	3.46±0.43	2.22±0.36	17.71±3.34	32.5±5.74	18.0±9.4
IDDM (n = 6)	3.42±1.12	2.14±0.43	25.74±8.92	48.6±10.40	18.4±4.1

*Mean ± SD.
Glucose Ra = rate of appearance of glucose quantified by $[6,6^2H_2]$glucose tracer dilution; IDDM = infants of insulin-dependent diabetic mothers; Lactate Ra = rate of appearance of lactate measured by $[^{13}C_3]$lactate tracer dilution; SGA = small for gestational age infants.

estimate of glucose carbon recycling, approximately 35%,[142] and the measurements of lactate contribution to glucose (see earlier). If the contribution of glycerol (10 to 20%) is also included, then the total gluconeogenesis in a healthy newborn infant will amount to approximately 50% or approximately 15 μmol/kg/minute of the total glucose Ra of 30 μmol/kg/minute. This is significant and implies an important role of gluconeogenesis, even after a brief fast. These data show that gluconeogenesis from pyruvate, and possibly from glycerol, is occurring at all times, although its contribution to glucose varies with feeding and fasting.

These data also suggest that gluconeogenesis is one of the several substrate cycles in the body, like the triglyceride fatty acid cycle and protein turnover, which are active at all times and can be rapidly accelerated at the time of acute demand.[180] The regulation of gluconeogenesis in the human newborn has not been examined, and the reader is referred to a review by Girard for a discussion of regulation in the rat.[73]

Very Low Birth Weight Infant

Low birth weight infants have become the largest clinical population in the neonatal intensive care unit as a result of improved clinical care and enhanced survival.[184] Studies in this population using isotopic tracer methods have shown that low birth weight infants can produce glucose at an appropriate weight-specific rate to meet their metabolic needs, and they respond appropriately to exogenous glucose and amino acid infusions.[185-187] Because several of the studies reported on these infants were performed while the babies were receiving intensive support, the hepatic response to glucose and insulin has been reported to be variable, that is, complete suppression of glucose production in some infants and incomplete in others.[186-191] However, such a response may be related to the stress response in these infants, as documented by persistent increase in circulating catecholamine levels.[192] In relation to glucose production, provision of exogenous lipids (i.e., a source of energy for gluconeogenesis) caused an increase in glucose levels but did not cause an increase in hepatic glucose production.[193, 194] The utilization of glucose by low birth weight infants has been examined both during fasting and in response to intravenous glucose. These data suggest that healthy low birth weight infants can dispose of infused glucose appropriately without developing glycosuria and osmotic diuresis, and glucose disposal is related to both plasma insulin levels and plasma glucose concentrations.[195, 196] Finally, very low birth weight infants less than 28 weeks' gestation show that even this population can regulate endogenous glucose production in response to an infusion of glucose.[196-198]

Quantification of gluconeogenesis in very low birth weight infants has also been done using more newly developed tracer techniques.[180-182] Because the data on low birth weight infants cannot be obtained during fasting, these studies have been performed while the babies were receiving parenteral glucose, glucose plus amino acids with or without lipids. Therefore, these data should be interpreted in view of the specific metabolic and physiologic state. Additionally, low birth weight infants are also receiving other clinical support that may confound the data obtained. These studies on low birth weight infants show that gluconeogenesis is active in these infants, even when they are receiving parenteral nutrients, and it contributes as much as 30 to 70% to endogenous glucose production. Because of the study conditions, that is, parenteral glucose infusion, endogenous glucose production is significantly suppressed. Thus, even under these circumstances with a low rate of appearance of glucose, gluconeogenesis makes a significant contribution to endogenous glucose production.

ACKNOWLEDGMENT

The cited work from my laboratory was supported by grants HD11089 and RR00081 from the National Institutes of Health.

REFERENCES

1. Lefebvre PJ: From plant physiology to human metabolic investigations. Diabetologia 28:255, 1985.
2. Lacroix M, et al: Glucose naturally labeled with carbon-13: use for metabolic studies in man. Science 181:445, 1973.
3. Jacobson BS, et al: The prevalence of carbon-13 in respiratory carbon dioxide as an indicator of the type of endogenous substrate: the change from lipid to carbohydrate during the respiratory rise in potato slices. J Gen Physiol 55:1, 1970.
4. Schoeller DA, et al: ^{13}C abundances of nutrients and the effect of variations in ^{13}C isotopic abundances of test meals formulated for $^{13}CO_2$ breath tests. Am J Clin Nutr 33:2375, 1980.
5. DeNiro MJ, Epstein S: Mechanism of carbon isotope fractionation associated with lipid synthesis. Science 197:261, 1977.
6. Steele R, et al: Measurement of size and turnover rate of body glucose pool by the isotope dilution method. Am J Physiol 187:15, 1956.
7. Katz J, et al: Evaluation of glucose turnover, body mass and recycling with reversible and irreversible tracers. Biochem J 142:161, 1974.
8. DiStefano JJ: Noncompartmental vs. compartmental analysis: some bases for choice. Am J Physiol 243:R1, 1982.
9. Foster DM, et al: A model for carbon kinetics among plasma alanine, lactate and glucose. Am J Physiol 239:E30, 1980.
10. Hall SEH, et al: The turnover and conversion to glucose of alanine in newborn and grown dogs. Fed Proc 36:239, 1977.
11. Katz J, et al: The determination of lactate turnover in vivo with ^{3}H- and ^{14}C-labelled lactate: the significance of sites of tracer administration and sampling. Biochem J 194:513, 1981.
12. McGuire EAH, et al: Effects of arterial versus venous sampling on analysis of glucose kinetics in man. J Appl Physiol 41:565, 1976.
13. Sonnenberg GE, Keller U: Sampling of arterialized heated-hand venous blood as a noninvasive technique for the study of ketone body kinetics in man. Metabolism 31:1, 1982.
14. Abumrad NN, et al: Use of a heated superficial hand vein as an alternative site for the measurement of amino acid concentrations and for the study of glucose and alanine kinetics in man. Metabolism 30:936, 1981.
15. McGuire EAH, et al: Effects of arterial versus venous sampling on analysis of glucose kinetics in man. J Appl Physiol 41:565, 1976.
16. Steele R: Influences of glucose loading and of injected insulin on hepatic glucose output. Ann NY Acad Sci 82:420, 1959.
17. Radziuk J, et al: Experimental validation of measurements of glucose turnover in nonsteady state. Am J Physiol 3:E84, 1978.
18. Cobelli C, et al: Non-steady state: error analysis of Steele's model and developments for glucose kinetics. Am J Physiol 252:E679, 1987.
19. Krebs HA, et al: The fate of isotopic carbon in kidney cortex synthesizing glucose from lactate. Biochem J 101:242, 1966.
20. Glamour TS, et al: Quantification of carbohydrate oxidation by respiratory gas exchange and isotopic tracers. Am J Physiol 268:E799, 1995.
21. Kalhan S: Stable isotopic tracers for studies of glucose metabolism. J Nutr 126:362S, 1996.
22. Wolfe RR, Jahoor F: Recovery of labelled CO_2 during the infusion of C-1 vs. C-2 acetate: implications for tracer studies of substrate oxidation. Am J Clin Nutr 51:248, 1990.
23. Landau BR: Estimating gluconeogenic rates in NIDDM. Adv Exp Med Biol 334:209, 1993.
24. Landau BR, et al: Use of ^2H_2O for estimating rates of gluconeogenesis: application to the fasted state. J Clin Invest 95:172, 1995.
25. Gomez F, et al: Carbohydrate and lipid oxidation in normal human subjects: its influence on glucose tolerance and insulin response to glucose. Metabolism 21:381, 1972.
26. Kalhan SC, et al: Glucose-alanine relationship in normal human pregnancy. Metabolism 37:152, 1988.
27. Frayn KN: Calculation of substrate oxidation rates in vivo from gaseous exchange. J Appl Physiol 55:628, 1983.
28. Ferrannini E: The theoretical bases of indirect calorimetry: a review. Metabolism 37:287, 1988.
29. Wagner JA, et al: Validation of open-circuit method for the determination of oxygen consumption. J Appl Physiol 34:859, 1973.
30. Kappagoda CT, Linden RJ: A critical assessment of an open circuit technique for measuring oxygen consumption. Cardiovasc Res 6:589, 1972.
31. Wilmore JH, Costill DL: Adequacy of the Haldane transformation in the computation of exercise VO2 in man. J Appl Physiol 35:85, 1973.
32. Marks KH, et al: The accuracy and precision of an open-circuit system to measure oxygen consumption and carbon dioxide production in neonates. Pediatr Res 21:58, 1987.
33. Hammarlund K: Measurement of oxygen consumption in preterm infants: assessment of a method using a mass spectrometer. Clin Physiol 4:519, 1984.

34. Kalhan SC, Denne SC: Energy consumption in infants with bronchopulmonary dysplasia. J Pediatr *116*:662, 1990.
35. Lifson N, et al: Measurement of total carbon dioxide production by means of D$_{218}$O. J Appl Physiol 7:704, 1955.
36. Schoeller DA: Energy expenditure from doubly labeled water: some fundamental considerations in humans. Am J Clin Nutr *38*:999, 1983.
37. Schoeller DA, VanSanten E: Measurement of energy expenditure in humans by doubly labeled water method. J Appl Physiol *53*:955, 1982.
38. Schoeller DA, et al: Energy expenditure by doubly labeled water: validation in humans and proposed calculation. Am J Physiol *250*:R823, 1986.
39. Schoeller DA: Measurement of energy expenditure in free-living humans by using doubly labeled water. J Nutr *118*:1278, 1988.
40. Roberts SB, et al: Effect of weaning on accuracy of doubly labeled water method in infants. Am J Physiol *254*:R622, 1988.
41. Roberts SB, et al: Comparison of the doubly labeled water (^{2}H$_2$^{18}O) method with indirect calorimetry and a nutrient-balance study for simultaneous determination of energy expenditure, water intake, and metabolizable energy intake in preterm infants. Am J Clin Nutr *44*:315, 1986.
42. Jones PJH, et al: Evaluation of doubly labeled water for measuring energy expenditure during changing nutrition. Am J Clin Nutr *47*:799, 1988.
43. Jones PJH, et al: Validation of doubly labeled water for assessing energy expenditure in infants. Pediatr Res *21*:242, 1987.
44. Livesey G, Elia M: Estimation of energy expenditure, net carbohydrate utilization, and net fat oxidation and synthesis by indirect calorimetry: evaluation of errors with special reference to the detailed composition of fuels. Am J Clin Nutr *47*:608, 1988.
45. Acheson KJ, et al: Nutritional influences on lipogenesis and thermogenesis after a carbohydrate meal. Am J Physiol *246*:E62, 1984.
46. Aynsley-Green A, et al: The metabolic and endocrine milieu of the human fetus at 18–21 weeks of gestation. Biol Neonate *47*:19, 1985.
47. Bozzetti P, et al: The relationship of maternal and fetal glucose concentrations in the human from midgestation until term. Metabolism *37*:358, 1988.
48. Whaley WH, et al: Correlation between maternal and fetal plasma levels of glucose and free fatty acids. Am J Obstet Gynecol *94*:419, 1966.
49. Tobin JD, et al: Human fetal insulin response after acute maternal glucose administration during labor. Pediatrics *44*:668, 1969.
50. Coltart TM, et al: Blood glucose and insulin relationships in the human mother and fetus before onset of labour. BMJ *4*:17, 1969.
51. Kalhan SC, et al: Glucose production in pregnant women at term gestation: sources of glucose for the human fetus. J Clin Invest *63*:388, 1979.
52. Ashmead GG, et al: Maternal-fetal substrate relationships in the third trimester in human pregnancy. Gynecol Obstet Invest *35*:18, 1993.
53. Young M: Placental transfer of glucose and amino acids. *In* Camerini-Danalos RA, Scole H (eds): Early Diabetes in Early Life. New York, Academic Press, 1975, pp 237–242.
54. Widdas WF: Inability of diffusion to account for placental glucose transfer in the sheep and consideration of the kinetics of a possible carrier transfer. J Physiol (Lond) *118*:23, 1952.
55. Anand RS, et al: Bidirectional placental transfer of glucose and its turnover in fetal and maternal sheep. Pediatr Res *13*:783, 1979.
56. Hauguel S, et al: Glucose uptake, utilization, and transfer by the human placenta as functions of maternal glucose concentration. Pediatr Res *20*:269, 1986.
57. Hauguel S, et al: Metabolism of the human placenta perfused in vitro: glucose transfer and utilization, O$_2$ consumption, lactate and ammonia production. Pediatr Res *17*:729, 1983.
58. Krauer F, et al: The influence of high maternal plasma glucose levels, and maternal blood flow on the placental transfer of glucose in the guinea pig. Diabetologia *9*:453, 1973.
59. Burd LI, et al: Placental production and foetal utilisation of lactate and pyruvate. Nature *254*:710, 1975.
60. Char VC, Creasy RK: Lactate and pyruvate as fetal metabolic substrates. Pediatr Res *10*:231, 1976.
61. Gilbert M, et al: Uterine blood flow and substrate uptake in conscious rabbit during late gestation. Am J Physiol *247*:E574, 1984.
62. Wilkening RB, et al: The relationship of umbilical glucose uptake to uterine blood flow. J Dev Physiol *7*:313, 1985.
63. Oh W, et al: Umbilical blood flow and glucose uptake in lamb fetus following single umbilical artery ligation. Biol Neonate *26*:291, 1975.
64. Goodner CJ, et al: Relation between plasma glucose levels of mother and fetus during maternal hyperglycemia, hypoglycemia, and fasting in the rat. Pediatr Res *3*:121, 1969.
65. Goodner CJ, Thompson DJ: Glucose metabolism in the fetus in utero: the effect of maternal fasting and glucose loading in the rat. Pediatr Res *1*:443, 1967.
66. Bossi E, Greenberg RE: Sources of blood glucose in the rat fetus. Pediatr Res *6*:765, 1972.
67. Anand RJ, et al: Effect of insulin-induced maternal hypoglycemia on glucose turnover in maternal and fetal sheep. Am J Physiol *238*:E524, 1980.
68. Hay WW, et al: Simultaneous measurements of umbilical uptake, fetal utilization rate, and fetal turnover rate of glucose. Am J Physiol *240*:E662, 1981.
69. Hodgson JC, et al: Rates of glucose production and utilization in the foetus in chronically catheterized sheep. Biochem J *186*:739, 1980.
70. Marconi AM, et al: An evaluation of fetal glucogenesis in intrauterine growth-retarded pregnancies. Metabolism *42*:860, 1993.
71. Marsac D, et al: Development of gluconeogenic enzymes in the liver of human newborns. Biol Neonate *28*:317, 1976.
72. Raiha NCR, Lindros KO: Development of some enzymes involved in gluconeogenesis in human liver. Ann Med Exp Biol Fenn *47*:146, 1969.
73. Girard J: Gluconeogenesis in late fetal and early neonatal life. Biol Neonate *50*:237, 1986.
74. Villee CA: The intermediary metabolism of human fetal tissues. Cold Spring Harbor Symp Quant Biol *19*:186, 1954.
75. Schwartz AL, Rall TW: Hormonal regulation of incorporation of alanine-U-^{14}C into glucose in human fetal liver explants. Diabetes *24*:650, 1975.
76. Adam PAJ, et al: Glucose production in midterm human fetus. I. Autoregulation of glucose uptake. Am J Physiol *234*:E560, 1978.
77. Robinson BH: Development of gluconeogenic enzymes in the newborn guinea pig. Biol Neonate *29*:48, 1978.
78. Arinze IJ: On the development of phosphoenolpyruvate carboxykinase and gluconeogenesis in guinea pig liver. Biochem Biophys Res Commun *65*:184, 1975.
79. Jones CT, Ashton IK: The appearance, properties and functions of gluconeogenic enzymes in the liver and kidney of the guinea pig during fetal and early neonatal development. Arch Biochem Biophys *174*:506, 1976.
80. Warnes DM, Seamark RF: Metabolism of glucose, fructose and lactate *in vivo* in chronically cannulated fetuses and suckling lambs. Biochem J *162*:617, 1977.
81. Warnes DM, et al: The appearance of gluconeogenesis at birth in sheep. Biochem J *162*:627, 1977.
82. Gleason CA, et al: Lactate uptake by the fetal sheep liver. J Dev Physiol *7*:177, 1985.
83. Gleason CA, Rudolph AM: Gluconeogenesis by the fetal sheep liver *in vivo*. J Dev Physiol *7*:185, 1985.
84. Levitsky LL, et al: Gluconeogenesis from lactate in the chronically catheterized baboon fetus. Biol Neonate *50*:97, 1986.
85. Palacin M, et al: Lactate production and absence of gluconeogenesis from placental transferred substrates in fetuses from fed and 48-H starved rats. Pediatr Res *22*:6, 1987.
86. Kalhan S, Parimi P: Gluconeogenesis in the fetus and neonate. Semin Perinatol *24*:94, 2000.
87. James EJ, et al: Fetal oxygen consumption, carbon dioxide production, and glucose uptake in a chronic sheep preparation. Pediatrics *50*:361, 1972.
88. Anand RS, et al: Effect of insulin-induced maternal hypoglycemia on glucose turnover in maternal and fetal sheep. Am J Physiol *238*:E524, 1980.
89. Hay WW, et al: Effect of insulin on glucose uptake by the maternal hindlimb and uterus and by the fetus in conscious pregnant sheep. J Endocrinol *100*:119, 1984.
90. Morriss FJ, et al: The glucose/oxygen quotient of the term human fetus. Biol Neonate *25*:44, 1975.
91. Boyd RDH, et al: Growth of glucose and oxygen uptakes by fetuses of fed and starved ewes. Am J Physiol *225*:897, 1973.
92. Bloch CA, et al: Effects of somatostatin and glucose infusion on glucose kinetics in fetal sheep. Am J Physiol *255*:E87, 1988.
93. Hay WW, et al: The effects of streptozotocin on rates of glucose utilization, oxidation, and production in the sheep fetus. Metabolism *38*:30, 1989.
94. Hay WW, Meznarich HK: Use of fetal streptozotocin injection to determine the role of normal levels of fetal insulin in regulating uteroplacental and umbilical glucose exchange. Pediatr Res *24*:312, 1988.
95. Philipps AF, et al: Effects of fetal insulin secretory deficiency on metabolism in fetal lamb. Diabetes *35*:964, 1986.
96. Simmons MA, et al: Insulin effect on fetal glucose utilization. Pediatr Res *12*:90, 1978.
97. Hay WW, et al: Effect of insulin on glucose uptake in near-term fetal lambs. Proc Soc Exp Biol Med *178*:557, 1985.
98. Hay WW, et al: Effects of insulin and glucose concentrations on glucose utilization in fetal sheep. Pediatr Res *23*:381, 1988.
99. Leturque A, et al: Hyperglycemia and hyperinsulinemia increase glucose utilization in fetal rat tissues. Am J Physiol *253*:E616, 1987.
100. Wilkening RB, et al: Effect of insulin on glucose/oxygen and lactate/oxygen quotients across the hindlimb of fetal lambs. Biol Neonate *51*:18, 1987.
101. Kalhan SC, Hertz RH: Diabetes. *In* Gleicher N (ed): Principles of Medical Therapy in Pregnancy. New York, Plenum Medical Books, 1985, pp 239–262.
102. Ogata ES, et al: Insulin injection in the fetal rat: accelerated intrauterine growth and altered fetal and neonatal glucose homeostasis. Metabolism *37*:649, 1988.
103. Milley JR, Papacostas JS: Effect of insulin on metabolism of fetal sheep hindquarters. Diabetes *38*:597, 1989.
104. Susa JB, et al: Somatomedins and insulin in diabetic pregnancies: effects on fetal macrosomia in the human and rhesus monkey. J Clin Endocrinol Metab *58*:1099, 1984.
105. Cha C-J M, et al: Accelerated growth and abnormal glucose tolerance in young female rats exposed to fetal hyperinsulinemia. Pediatr Res *21*:83, 1987.
106. McCormick K, et al: Fetal rat hyperinsulinism and hyperglucagonism: effects on hepatic ketogenesis, lipogenesis, and gluconeogenesis. Endocrinology *116*:1281, 1986.
107. Susa JB, et al: Chronic hyperinsulinemia in the fetal rhesus monkey: effects of physiologic hyperinsulinemia on fetal growth and composition. Diabetes *33*:656, 1984.

108. McCormick KL, et al: Chronic hyperinsulinemia in the fetal rhesus monkey: effects of hepatic enzymes active in lipo- genesis and carbohydrate metabolism. Diabetes 28:1064, 1979.
109. Haberey P, et al: The fate and importance of fetal lactate in the human placenta: a new hypothesis. J Perinat Med 10:127, 1982.
110. Enders RH, et al: Placental amino acids uptake. III. Transport system for neutral amino acids. Am J Physiol 230:706, 1976.
111. Lemons JA, et al: Umbilical uptake of amino acids in the unstressed fetal lamb. J Clin Invest 58:1428, 1976.
112. Lemons JA: Fetal-placental nitrogen metabolism. Semin Perinatol 3:177, 1979.
113. Gresham EL, et al: Production and excretion of urea by the fetal lamb. Pediatrics 50:372, 1972.
114. Gresham EL, et al: Maternal fetal urea concentration difference in man: metabolic significance. J Pediatr 79:809, 1971.
115. Gilfillan CA, et al: Alanine production by the human fetus at term gestation. Biol Neonate 47:141, 1985.
116. Hay WW, et al: Fetal glucose uptake and utilization as functions of maternal glucose concentration. Am J Physiol 246:E237, 1984.
117. DiGiacomo JE, Hay WW: Regulation of placental glucose transfer and consumption by fetal glucose production. Pediatr Res 25:429, 1989.
118. Rudolph CD, et al: Effect of acute umbilical cord compression on hepatic carbohydrate metabolism in the fetal lamb. Pediatr Res 25:228, 1989.
119. Capkova A, Jirasek JE: Glycogen reserves in organs of human foetuses in the first half of pregnancy. Biol Neonate 13:129, 1968.
120. Shelley HJ, Neligan GA: Neonatal hypoglycaemia. Br Med Bull 22:34, 1966.
121. Greengard O: Enzymic differentiation of human liver: comparison with the rat model. Pediatr Res 11:669, 1977.
122. Katz J, McGarry JD: The glucose paradox: is glucose a substrate for liver metabolism? J Clin Invest 74:1901, 1984.
123. Magnusson I, et al: Quantitation of the pathways of hepatic glycogen formation on ingesting a glucose load. J Clin Invest 80:1748, 1987.
124. Newgard CB, et al: Studies on the mechanism by which exogenous glucose is converted into liver glycogen in the rat: a direct or an indirect pathway? J Biol Chem 258:8046, 1983.
125. Levitsky LL, et al: Precursors to glycogen in ovine fetuses. Am J Physiol 255:E743, 1988.
126. Prior RL: Glucose and lactate metabolism in vivo in ovine fetus. Am J Physiol 239:E208, 1980.
127. Sparks JW, et al: Simultaneous measurements of lactate turnover rate and umbilical lactate uptake in the fetal lamb. J Clin Invest 70:179, 1982.
128. Eliot RJ, et al: Plasma catecholamine concentrations in infants at birth and during the first 48 hours of life. J Pediatr 96:311, 1980.
129. Padbury JF, et al: Neonatal adaptation: sympatho-adrenal response to umbilical cord cutting. Pediatr Res 15:1483, 1981.
130. Grajwer LA, et al: Possible mechanisms and significance of the neonatal surge in glucagon secretion: studies in newborn lambs. Pediatr Res 11:833, 1977.
131. Ktorza A, et al: Insulin and glucagon during the perinatal period: secretion and metabolic effects on the liver. Biol Neonate 48:204, 1985.
132. Mayor F, Cuezva JM: Hormonal and metabolic changes in the perinatal period. Biol Neonate 48:185, 1985.
133. Kawai Y, Arinze IJ: Activation of glycogenolysis in neonatal liver. J Biol Chem 156:853, 1981.
134. McCann ML, et al: Effects of fructose on hypoglucosemia in infants of diabetic mothers. N Engl J Med 275:1, 1966.
135. Kalhan SC, Peter-Wohl S: Hypoglycemia: what is it for the neonate? Am J Perinatol 17:11, 2000.
136. Srinivasan G, et al: Plasma glucose values in normal neonates: a new look. J Pediatr 109: 114, 1986.
137. Heck LJ, Erenberg A: Serum glucose levels in term neonates during the first 48 hours of life. J Pediatr 110:119, 1987.
138. Philipson EH, et al: Effects of maternal glucose infusion on fetal acid-base status in human pregnancy. Am J Obstet Gynecol 157:866, 1987.
139. Kalhan SC, et al: Measurement of glucose turnover in the human newborn with glucose-1-¹³C. J Clin Endocrinol Metab 43:704, 1976.
140. Bier DM, et al: Measurement of "true" glucose production rates in infancy and childhood with c, c-dideuteroglucose. Diabetes 26:1016, 1977.
141. Cowett RM, et al: Glucose kinetics in infants of diabetic mothers. Am J Obstet Gynecol 146:781, 1983.
142. Denne SC, Kalhan SC: Glucose carbon recycling and oxidation in human newborns. Am J Physiol 251:E71, 1986.
143. Kornhauser D, et al: Glucose production and utilization in the newborn puppy. Pediatr Res 4:120, 1970.
144. Tserng K-Y, Kalhan SC: Estimation of glucose carbon recycling and glucose turnover with [U-¹³C] glucose. Am J Physiol 245:E476, 1983.
145. Penicaud L, et al: Effect of anesthesia on glucose production and utilization in rats. Am J Physiol 252:E365, 1987.
146. Anand KJS, Hickey PR: Pain and its effects in the human neonate and fetus. N Engl J Med 317:1321, 1987.
147. Cowett RM, et al: Endogenous glucose production during constant glucose infusion in the newborn lamb. Pediatr Res 12:853, 1978.
148. Sauer PJJ, et al: Glucose oxidation rates in newborn infants measured with indirect calorimetry and [U-¹³C] glucose. Clin Sci 70:587, 1986.
149. Owen OE, et al: Brain metabolism during fasting. J Clin Invest 46:1589, 1967.
150. Kalhan C, Kiliç İ: Carbohydrate as nutrient in the infant and child: range of acceptable intake. Eur J Clin Nutr 53:S94, 1999.
151. Paul P, Bortz WM: Turnover and oxidation of plasma glucose in lean and obese humans. Metabolism 18:570, 1969.
152. Wolfe RR, et al: Glucose metabolism in man: responses to intravenous glucose infusion. Metabolism 28:210, 1979.
153. Settergren G, et al: Cerebral blood flow and exchange of oxygen, glucose, ketone bodies, lactate, pyruvate and amino acids in infants. Acta Paediatr Scand 65:343, 1976.
154. Dobbin J, Sands J: Quantitative growth and development of human brain. Arch Dis Child 48:757, 1973.
155. Kalhan SC, Gilfillan CA: Intrauterine nutrition and the newborn. In Jones CT, Nathanielsz PW (eds): The Physiological Development of the Fetus and Newborn. London, Academic Press, 1985, pp 739–746.
156. Sacca L, et al: Influence of continuous physiologic hyperinsulinemia on glucose kinetics and counter regulatory hormones in normal and diabetic humans. J Clin Invest 63:849, 1979.
157. Shulman GI, et al: Glucose disposal during insulinopenia in somatostatin-treated dogs. J Clin Invest 62:487, 1978.
158. Long CL, et al: Carbohydrate metabolism in normal man and effect of glucose infusion. J Appl Physiol 31:102, 1971.
159. Lijenquist JE, et al: Hyperglycemia per se (insulin and glucagon withdrawn) can inhibit hepatic glucose production in man. J Clin Endocrinol Metab 48:171, 1979.
160. Sacca L, et al: Hyperglycemia inhibits glucose production in man independent of changes in glucoregulatory hormones. J Clin Endocrinol Metab 47:1160, 1978.
161. Sacca L, et al: The glucoregulatory response to intravenous glucose infusion in normal man: roles of insulin and glucose. Metabolism 30:457, 1981.
162. Bondy PK, et al: Studies of the role of the liver in human carbohydrate metabolism by the venous catheter techniques. I. Normal subjects under fasting conditions and following the injection of glucose. J Clin Invest 28:238, 1949.
163. Hers HG: The control of glycogen metabolism in the liver. Annu Rev Biochem 45:167, 1976.
164. Stalmans W, et al: The sequential inactivation of phosphorylase and activation of glycogen synthetase in liver after the administration of glucose to mice and rats. Eur J Biochem 41:127, 1974.
165. Bucolo RJ, et al: Dynamics of glucose autoregulation in the isolated, blood-perfused canine liver. Am J Physiol 227:209, 1974.
166. Varma S, et al: Homeostatic responses to glucose loading in newborn and young dogs. Metabolism 22:1367, 1973.
167. Sherwood WG, et al: Glucose homeostasis in preterm rhesus monkey neonates. Pediatr Res 11:874, 1977.
168. King KC, et al: Regulation of glucose production in newborn infants of diabetic mothers. Pediatr Res 16:608, 1982.
169. Cowett RM, et al: Persistent glucose production during glucose infusion in the neonate. J Clin Invest 71:467, 1983.
170. Cowett RM, et al: Glucose kinetics in glucose-infused small for gestational age infants. Pediatr Res 18:74, 1984.
171. Kalhan SC, et al: Role of glucose in the regulation of endogenous glucose production in the human newborn. Pediatr Res 20:49, 1986.
172. Hetenyi G, et al: Plasma glucagon in pups, decreased by fasting, unaffected by somatostatin or hypoglycemia. Am J Physiol 231:1377, 1976.
173. Sperling MA, et al: Effects of somatostatin (SRIF) infusion on glucose homeostasis in newborn lambs: evidence for a significant role of glucagon. Pediatr Res 11:962, 1977.
174. Cowett RM, Tenenbaum D: Hepatic response to insulin in control of glucose kinetics in the neonatal lamb. Metabolism 36:1021, 1987.
175. Cowett RM: Alpha-adrenergic agonists stimulate neonatal glucose production less than beta-adrenergic agonists in the lamb. Metabolism 37:831, 1988.
176. Cowett RM: Decreased response to catecholamines in the newborn: effect on glucose kinetics in the lamb. Metabolism 37:736, 1988.
177. Bougneres PF, et al: Lipid transport in the human newborn: palmitate and glycerol turnover and the contribution of glycerol to neonatal hepatic glucose output. J Clin Invest 70:262, 1982.
178. Patel DG, Kalhan SC: Glycerol metabolism and triglyceride/fatty acid cycling in the human newborn: effect of maternal diabetes and intrauterine growth retardation. Pediatr Res 31:52, 1992.
179. Sunehag A, et al: Glycerol carbon contributes to hepatic glucose production during the first eight hours in healthy term infants. Acta Paediatr 85:1339, 1996.
180. Kalhan SC, et al: Estimation of gluconeogenesis in newborn infants. Am J Physiol 281:E991, 2001.
181. Katz J: Determination of gluconeogenesis in vivo with ¹⁴C-labeled substrates. Am J Physiol 248:R391, 1985.
182. Sunehag AL, et al: Gluconeogenesis in very low birth weight infants receiving total parenteral nutrition. Diabetes. 48:791, 1999.
183. Keshen T, et al: Glucose production and gluconeogenesis are negatively related to body weight in mechanically ventilated, very low birth weight neonates. Pediatr Res 41:132, 1997.
184. Kalhan SC: Metabolism of glucose in very low birth weight infants. In Fanaroff AA, Klaus M (eds): Year Book of Neonatal and Perinatal Medicine. Chicago, Mosby-Year Book, 1994, pp. xix–xxx.
185. Bier DM, et al: In-vivo measurement of glucose and alanine metabolism with stable isotopic tracers. Diabetes 26:1005, 1977.
186. Kalhan SC, et al: Role of glucose in the regulation of endogenous glucose production in the human newborn. Pediatr Res 20:49, 1986.

187. Frazer TE, et al: Direct measurement of gluconeogenesis from [2, 3-$^{13}C_2$] alanine in the human neonate. Am J Physiol 240:E615, 1981.
188. Cowett RM, et al: Ontogeny of glucose homeostasis in low birth weight infants. J Pediatr 112:462, 1988.
189. Van Goudoever JB, et al: Glucose kinetics and glucoregulatory hormone levels in ventilated preterm infants on the first day of life. Pediatr Res 33:583, 1993.
190. Lafeber HN, et al: Glucose production and oxidation in preterm infants during total parenteral nutrition. Pediatr Res 28:153, 1990.
191. Mehandru P, et al: Glucose utilization and kinetics in preterm newborns during parenteral nutrition. Pediatr Res 31:291A, 1992.
192. Mehandru PL, et al: Catecholamine response at birth in preterm newborns. Biol Neonate 64:82, 1993.
193. Vileisis RA, et al: Glycemic response to lipid infusion in the premature infant. J Pediatr 100:108, 1982.
194. Yunis KA, et al: Glucose kinetics following administration of intravenous fat emulsion to low-birth-weight neonates. Am J Physiol 263:E844, 1992.
195. Cowett RM, et al: Glucose disposal of low birth weight infants: steady state hyperglycemia produced by constant intravenous glucose infusion. Pediatrics 63:389, 1979.
196. Hertz DE, et al: Intravenous glucose suppresses glucose production but not proteolysis in extremely premature newborns. J Clin Invest 92:1752, 1993.
197. Sunehag A, et al: Glucose production rate in extremely immature neonates (<28 weeks) studied by use of deuterated glucose. Pediatr Res 33:97, 1993.
198. Sunehag A, et al: Very immature infants (<30 wk) respond to glucose infusion with incomplete suppression of glucose production. Pediatr Res 36:550, 1994.

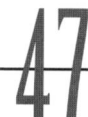

Edward S. Ogata

Carbohydrate Metabolism During Pregnancy

With respect to the effects of pregnancy on maternal metabolism, pregnancy should be considered as two epochs. The first half of gestation is a period of sustained maternal anabolism. During this time, the increased calories ingested by the mother not only sustain fetal growth but also are stored as maternal fat and glucose. Normally expected maternal insulin secretion drives this period of anabolism.[1,2]

The increase in maternal metabolic fuel stores is important for the second half of gestation, a period of logarithmic fetal growth. During this time, the substrate and energy demands of the rapidly growing fetus require not only a greater fraction of maternal fuel intake but also utilization of the maternal energy stores laid down during the first half of pregnancy. Alterations in sensitivity and availability of maternal insulin are central to this process.[3] Because of these changes, pregnancy can unmask a tendency toward diabetes mellitus (gestational diabetes mellitus, pregestational diabetes mellitus).[4,5] The conceptus is responsible for these adaptations. Indeed, these changes parallel the growth of the conceptus.[1] These alterations become increasingly apparent as the conceptus rapidly increases in mass from 20 to 24 weeks of pregnancy onward, and they are promptly reversed after delivery.[1] In the immediate postpartum period, normal glucose tolerance returns, even in those women with gestational diabetes mellitus.

EFFECT OF THE CONCEPTUS ON MATERNAL INSULIN METABOLISM

The fetus and placenta exert multiple metabolic effects. With respect to insulin, maternal insulin does not cross the placenta,[6] although some insulin may be bound there. The placenta clears some maternal insulin by directly degrading it.[7]

Changes in maternal insulin secretion and action are dramatic during the second half of pregnancy.[8] During the first half, basal insulin secretion is normal, and insulin secretion mediates the laying down of metabolic fuels.[9] In the second half of gestation, insulin secretion is greatly exaggerated.[9-11] Intravenous glucose tolerance testing indicates that by the third trimester, physiologically normal pregnant women secrete three times the insulin than they do in the nonpregnant state.[1]

The development of insulin resistance during the second half of pregnancy is responsible for this exaggerated insulin secretion. Responsiveness to insulin is reduced 40 to 60% during the second half of gestation.[9,12] The conceptus causes this insulin resistance in part by the generation of human placental lactogen, progesterone, and estrogen, which become available in ever-increasing amounts as gestation progresses.[13-15] These hormones directly antagonize the effect of maternal insulin. Insulin resistance increases in liver, adipose tissue, and skeletal muscle.[16] Insulin binding appears to be normal during late gestation, a finding indicating that insulin resistance is mediated by events distal to receptor and insulin binding. It is possible that tyrosine kinase inhibition may also contribute to insulin resistance.[17,18]

EFFECT OF THE CONCEPTUS ON MATERNAL FUEL AVAILABILITY

These changes in maternal endocrine controls ensure the availability of metabolic fuels to meet the ever-increasing needs of the fetus during the second half of gestation. This is not trivial, because the energy and substrate needs of the fetus are considerable. Glucose utilization by the human fetus is estimated to be three times that of the adult. Growth of the human fetus during the third trimester requires the net transplacental transfer of 54 mmol of nitrogen per day.[19] The blunted response to insulin ensures that during the postprandial state, glucose and amino acids are made available to the fetus at the mother's expense.

During maternal fasting, the ongoing insulin resistance allows a rapid and profound mobilization of maternal fat stores and stimulates ketogenesis. This also causes a decrease in maternal blood glucose and amino acid concentrations despite increased hepatic gluconeogenesis.[20] The reduction in maternal blood glucose may result in hypoglycemia. This fasting hypoglycemia of pregnancy is a result of a failure of amino acid mobilization to keep up with rates of glucose removal. This "accelerated starvation" of the mother ensures fuel availability to the fetus at the mother's expense during pregnancy.[21,22]

CONSEQUENCES OF MATERNAL FASTING

If maternal fasting is prolonged, maternal ketogenesis as a result of these endocrine changes will be prolonged and exaggerated. The consequences for the fetus are unclear. Ketone bodies readily cross the placenta, and the fetal brain can use ketones as early as 10 to 12 weeks' gestation.[23] Although the capability to use an alternative fuel to glucose may be beneficial for the fetus, limited data suggest that the children of mothers who were ketotic during pregnancy are at risk for cognitive and psychomotor delays during childhood. The mechanisms responsible for this potential association between ketone body oxidation and impaired brain function are unclear.[24]

REFERENCES

1. Freinkel N: The Banting Lecture 1980: of pregnancy and progeny. Diabetes *29*:1023, 1980.
2. Hytten ET, Leitch I: The Physiology of Human Pregnancy. Oxford, Blackwell, 1971, pp 599–636.
3. Freinkel N: The effect of pregnancy on insulin homeostasis. Diabetes *13*:260, 1964.
4. National Diabetes Data Group: Classification and diagnosis of diabetes mellitus and other categories of glucose intolerance. Diabetes *28*:1039, 1979.
5. Metzger BE, et al: Summary and Recommendations of the Fourth International Workshop: Conference on Gestational Diabetes Mellitus. Diabetes Care *21*(Suppl 2):161, 1998.
6. Freinkel N: Effects of the conceptus on maternal metabolism during pregnancy. *In* Leibel BS, Wrenshall GA (eds): On the Nature and Treatment of Diabetes. Amsterdam, Excerpta Medica, 1965, pp 679–688.
7. Katz AI, et al: Peripheral metabolism of insulin, proinsulin, and C-peptide in the pregnant rat. J Clin Invest *56*:1608, 1975.
8. Catalano PM, et al: Longitudinal changes in pancreatic B-cell function and metabolic clearance rate of insulin in pregnant women with normal and abnormal glucose tolerance. Diabetes Care *21*:403, 1998.
9. Catalano PM, et al: Longitudinal changes in insulin release and insulin resistance in nonobese pregnant women. Am J Obstet Gynecol *165*:1667, 1991.
10. Spellacy WN, et al: Plasma insulin in normal "early" pregnancy. Obstet Gynecol *25*:862, 1965.
11. Bleicher SJ, et al: Carbohydrate metabolism in pregnancy. V. The interrelations of glucose, insulin, and free fatty acids in late pregnancy and postpartum. N Engl J Med *271*:866, 1964.
12. Buchanan TA, et al: Insulin sensitivity and B-cell responsiveness to glucose during late pregnancy in lean and moderately obese women with normal glucose tolerance or mild gestational diabetes. Am J Obstet Gynecol *162*:1008, 1990.
13. Grumbach M, et al: Chorionic growth hormone prolactin (CGP) secretion; disposition, biologic activity in man and the postulated function as the "growth hormone" of the second half of pregnancy. Ann NY Acad Sci *140*:501, 1968.
14. Johansson EDB: Plasma levels of progesterone in pregnancy measured by a competitive binding technique. Acta Endocrinol *61*:607, 1969.
15. Kalkhoff RK, et al: Carbohydrate and lipid metabolism during normal pregnancy: relationship to gestational hormone action. Semin Perinatol *2*:291, 1978.
16. Buchanan TA, Catalano PM: The pathogenesis of GDM: implications for diabetes after pregnancy. Diabetes Rev *3*:584, 1995.
17. Tsibris JCM, et al: Insulin receptors in circulating erythrocytes and monocytes from women on oral contraceptives or pregnant women near term. J Clin Endocrinol Metab *51*:711, 1980.
18. Moore P, et al: Insulin binding in human pregnancy: comparisons to the postpartum, luteal and follicular states. J Clin Endocrinol Metab *52*:937, 1981.
19. Puavilai G, et al: Insulin receptors and insulin resistance in human pregnancy: evidence for a post-receptor defect in insulin action. J Clin Endocrinol Metab *54*:247, 1982.
20. Martinez C, et al: Tyrosine kinase activity of liver insulin receptor is inhibited in rats at term gestation. Biochem J *263*:267, 1989.
21. Young M: Placental transfer of glucose and amino acids. *In* Camerini-Davalos RA, Cole HS (eds): Early Diabetes in Early Life. New York, Academic Press, 1975, p 237.
22. Metzger BE, et al: Carbohydrate metabolism in pregnancy. IX. Plasma levels of gluconeogenic fuels during fasting in the rat. J Clin Endocrinol *33*:869, 1971.
23. Williamson DH, et al: Activation of enzymes involved in acetoacetate utilization in adult mammalian tissues. Biochem J *121*:41, 1971.
24. Churchill J, et al: Neuropsychological deficits in children of diabetic mothers. Am J Obstet Gynecol *105*:257, 1969.

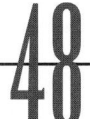

Anthony F. Philipps

Oxygen Consumption and General Carbohydrate Metabolism of the Fetus

This chapter covers those factors related to fetal metabolic processes, with specific reference to fetal energy balance and substrate uptake. Relationships between metabolic rate, whole fetal versus interorgan differences, and differences among fetal oxidative fuels are discussed. Although some direct information regarding human fetal energy metabolism and balance is now available, the subsequent discussion still relies heavily on data from animal experiments as well as theoretical considerations. Because human fetuses of shorter than 30 weeks' gestation are common to most newborn intensive care units, an understanding of those processes involved in determining fetal metabolic demand as well as modifying features may be of use in such settings. The term *metabolism* has been used loosely to denote various biochemical reactions requiring or producing energy. The term is used here in the general sense, that is, to connote chemical processes in the mammalian fetus that alter substrates containing carbon for the goals of either producing more tissue (accretion/growth) or providing the organism with energy necessary for basic life processes (fuel/energy).

FETAL ENERGY REQUIREMENTS

Previously, mammalian fetuses were thought to live in hypoxic environments[1,2] because the normal fetal umbilical venous pO_2 at term had been known to be 25 mm Hg or lower. Several investigators have demonstrated that human and animal umbilical venous blood is hypoxemic relative to adult blood by partial pressure standards. Because of the elevated fetal hemoglobin concentration and a leftward shift of the oxyhemoglobin disso-

ciation curve, however, normal umbilical venous oxygen content, by standards of oxygen content per milliliter of blood, is the rule. In both human cord blood and umbilical venous blood samples from fetuses of a variety of species, fetal oxygen delivery, as measured by fetal blood oxygen content (as opposed to pO_2) is adequate for aerobic metabolic needs.[1,3,4]

It follows that fetal mammals, under steady-state, or unstressed, conditions, ought to achieve adequate oxygen delivery (the product of umbilical venous blood oxygen content and umbilical venous blood flow) and should not exhibit evidence of hypoxia (i.e., low tissue oxygen availability), unless specific organ or total blood flow falls dramatically or if fetal blood oxygen content falls below a critical level. Studies of fetal acid-base or lactate balance indirectly test this hypothesis. The consensus[1,3] is that no current evidence exists to support a hypoxic fetal milieu because (1) umbilical cord blood pH values of unstressed fetal humans, pigs, monkeys, and sheep are all similar to each other and to the normal adult range of 7.35 to 7.45; (2) venoarterial H^+ concentration differences in cord blood of these species are only modest, suggesting relatively small fetomaternal H^+ transfer, inconsistent with hypoxia-induced lactic acid production; (3) positive umbilical venoarterial lactate concentration differences have been observed in sheep[5] and humans,[6-8] indicating net fetal lactate uptake, as opposed to excretion; and (4) experimental production of maternal and therefore relative fetal hyperoxia in the sheep is not associated with an increase in fetal oxygen consumption.

Thus, in the unstressed fetus, energy processes appear to operate for the most part through oxidative pathways. Estimation of fetal oxygen consumption may therefore be used as a direct indicator of the fetal metabolic rate.[3,9] Although rates of substrate uptake and carbon dioxide production provide alternate measurements of fetal metabolic activity, the calculation of each requires a significant number of assumptions. In the case of substrate uptake, the relative partitioning of carbon uptake by the fetus for use as fuel (oxidative needs) or growth (accretion needs) must be considered. In the case of carbon dioxide production measurements, the overall respiratory quotient (RQ) must be estimated (i.e., the relative contributions of carbon from the oxidative metabolism of carbohydrates, amino acids, and fats to carbon dioxide production must be taken into account).[3,10]

FETAL OXYGEN CONSUMPTION

Measurement

Two methods have been used to estimate fetal oxygen consumption (Vo_2) *in vivo*. Because the fetus has little stored oxygen (some is present in muscle and myocardium attached to myoglobin[11]), the vast majority of fetal requirements for oxidative metabolism of substrate is met by transfer of oxygen to the fetus through the placenta and umbilical venous circulation. Little, if any, transfer is thought to occur across the fetal membranes. To measure fetal Vo_2 accurately, several methods have been employed. Among the earliest was Bohr's demonstration that by measuring Vo_2 in the pregnant animal before or after delivery (or in other studies, after either cord occlusion or induced fetal demise), fetal Vo_2 could be calculated as follows:

$$\text{Fetal } Vo_2 = \text{predelivery maternal } Vo_2 \\ - \text{postdelivery maternal } Vo_2 \quad [1]$$

Fetal Vo_2 is usually expressed as either mL O_2/kg or g/minute using fetal weight in the denominator. As shown in Table 48-1, estimates for fetuses of several species, including humans, are available. The major assumption in such studies is that the act of delivery (or cord occlusion) does not measurably alter maternal, uterine, or placental Vo_2. Such assumptions may not be entirely true because of parturition-induced changes in fetal, placental, and maternal rates of metabolism, but the results obtained provide a framework for estimates obtained using other methods.

The second method for measuring fetal Vo_2 relies on Fick's principle, whereby uptake of any substance by an organ (or in this case, the whole fetus) is equal to the product of blood flow to that organ and the arteriovenous concentration difference of the substance in question across the organ. In the case of oxygen consumption for the mammalian fetus, the principle may be restated according to equation 2:

$$\text{Fetal } Vo_2 = \text{Fumb} \times (V - A)_{O_2} \quad [2]$$

where Fumb = umbilical blood flow (mL/minute or mL/kg/minute) and $(V-A)_{O_2}$= the venoarterial difference in O_2 content (mL of O_2/100 mL of blood) across the umbilical circulation.

Newer noninvasive methods for determination of human fetal Vo_2 are being developed, such as magnetic resonance imaging (MRI). This technique makes use of the differences observed in image density between saturated and desaturated hemoglobin and may be particularly useful for assessing specific organ (i.e., liver, brain) oxygen requirements or abnormalities of metabolic function due to maternal or fetal disease states.[12]

Experimental Data

The difficulties involved in obtaining Fick's principle estimates of fetal Vo_2 include the necessity of obtaining samples of umbilical venous and distal aortic blood for oxygen content analysis, which requires use of a relatively large fetus (i.e., sheep, cow, pig) for catheter placement, and the requirement of a reliable estimate of umbilical blood flow. The former problem has been overcome by sampling at these sites either acutely in anesthetized animals or by the implantation of fetal catheters[3,13] for serial measurements under nonstressed conditions. The latter problem has been overcome by the development of several methods for the accurate measurement of umbilical blood flow, which include the use of ultrasonic or electromagnetic flow transducers; radiolabeled microspheres; or steady-state diffusion of substances such as antipyrine, ethanol, or tritiated water across the placenta. The advantages of Fick's method over the original Bohr technique include (1) the ability to perform serial studies in the same animal during late gestation, (2) the ability to measure uptake and excretion of potential fetal metabolites simultaneously with the uptake of oxygen, and (3) the ability to observe changes in metabolic rate before and after experimental manipulation. Other noninvasive methods, such as MRI[12] or the doubly labeled water technique,[14] have been used to estimate long-term oxygen consumption or oxygenation in humans, but significant obstacles in estimating human fetal Vo_2 preclude their use at this time.

As can be seen in Table 48-1, when corrected for fetal weight, fetal Vo_2 as measured in a variety of species at term is remarkably consistent, with a range of 6.5 to 8.5 mL O_2/kg/minute. In a study of fetal Vo_2 in term human fetuses using the Bohr method,[15] the mean value of 6.8 mL/kg/minute obtained fits well within the range observed for other species.

Determining Factors

As stated previously, energy requirements in the fetus may be estimated by considering oxygen consumption as a guide to metabolic processes or by measuring substrate uptake to gauge both fuel and accretion requirements. The factors responsible for control of fetal energy expenditure are not fully understood. Originally formulated for adult mammals by Kleiber[16] was the allometric scaling relationship:

$$\text{Metabolic rate} = (\text{Mass})^{0.75} \quad [3]$$

It has been suggested that as species evolved, there was a general tendency for metabolic rate to increase in proportion to body mass (i.e., to mass$^{1.0}$). However, given that, geometrically speaking, surface area changes are only proportional to the two-thirds power of mass,[17,18] an incongruity existed and the three-quarters-power relationship represents a basic biologic compromise. Interestingly, over the succeeding 70 years since equation 3 was formulated, this basic principle has now been extended and is reasonably predictive of the aerobic metabolic rates not only for a variety of mammals and other vertebrates, but also for single cells and intact mitochondria—and even for the turnover rate for substrates in the respiratory enzyme chain within mitochondria (Fig. 48-1).[19,20]

TABLE 48-1

Fetal Oxygen Consumption in Various Species

Species	Measurement	Vo_2 (mL/kg/min)
Human at term[15]	B	6.8
Human <28 wk[138]	F	5.4
Rhesus monkey 1[139]	F	7.0
Sheep[119]	F	8.0
Cow[140]	F	6.7
Horse[142]	F	7.0
Guinea pig[141]	B	8.8

B = Bohr principle measurement; F = Fick principle measurement.

The general relationship between mass and metabolic rate has been noted and corroborated empirically by a number of observers.[9,17,18] However, West and colleagues[20] have suggested that this scaling relationship is also due to basic limitations in the transport of nutrients and oxygen placed on living cells and related to the geometry of branching networks (i.e., circulation, mitochondrial cristae, and the like). The theory requires that three basic factors be present for the scaling rule to be accurate (1) a space occupying branching network for transport purposes that extends throughout, (2) a "final" size-invariate end branch (such as a capillary) and (3) a requirement for minimization of the energy needed for substrate or oxygen transport purposes.[19,20] The cautions in such a relationship are that the metabolic rate is measured (classically as V_{O_2}) in the resting state as opposed to a "field" metabolic rate (i.e., during normal physical activity and changing milieu), and in nongrowing adults (i.e., does not include subjects that are actively growing, such as the fetus).

Although the basic three-quarters rule would otherwise probably also apply in fetal and early neonatal life, the additional metabolic needs for growth and development clearly increase the demand for energy. As it turns out, mass specific metabolic rate is relatively constant from fertilization through the morula stage[18] and increases dramatically (three- to fourfold) thereafter for the fetus. Metabolic rate (when corrected for body weight) remains higher than the adult by two- to threefold in mammals until after birth, with a slow decline thereafter.[18] In fact, early studies in human infants by various investigators concluded that the relationship between body mass and V_{O_2} falls to "adult" levels [from $(mass)^{1.0}$ to $(mass)^{3/4}$] by about 18 months of age, or at roughly 12 kg.[21] Some of the difference noted relates to growth as previously mentioned, but some is also related to a poorly understood increment in cellular sodium pump activity in the newborn.[22]

At the cellular level, the control of metabolic rate has not been clearly elucidated but involves complex interactions between a number of factors, including (1) the concentration of adenosine 5-triphosphate (ATP), the product of mitochondrial oxidative phosphorylation; (2) the ratio of intracellular adenosine 5-diphosphate (ADP) to ATP; (3) rates of intracellular protein synthesis; and (4) the generation of proton ($[H^+]$) gradients by respiratory enzymes across the mitochondrial and cell membranes.[9,23] For example, it has been estimated that approximately 15% of V_{O_2} of the term fetus might be spent on total active transport processes.

It has been assumed that at the organ or tissue level, metabolic rate is not influenced by oxygen availability, unless the diffusion of oxygen is severely limited. Justification for this view stems from the observation that several mammalian tissues (e.g., liver, kidney) have similar *in vivo* and *in vitro* rates of V_{O_2}, suggesting an intrinsic regulatory mechanism, perhaps related to genetically defined tissue-specific respiratory enzyme activities. In more recent studies, however, certain tissues such as fetal muscle[24] do decrease V_{O_2} in response to change in media pO_2 (Fig. 48-2). This *in vitro* observation is also consistent with *in vivo* studies in fetal sheep[25-27] documenting that carcass V_{O_2} decreases further than fetal whole body V_{O_2} when oxygen delivery to the fetus declines. In fetal brain as well as other organs such as liver and kidney,[24,28,29] similar findings have been observed, contradicting earlier work. In fetal brain,[28] cerebral V_{O_2} is linked to cellular oxygen tension under steady-state conditions. Such studies have important implications for understanding the manner in which the fetus might be protected against sudden changes in oxygen delivery.

INTEGRATION OF FETAL METABOLIC RATE

In terms of integrated metabolic rate of the whole fetus, only studies in animals are available concerning those factors controlling V_{O_2}. Under a wide variety of circumstances, changes in O_2 delivery to the fetus are met by fetal changes in O_2 extraction to meet metabolic demands.[30] In fetal sheep, O_2 extraction may be measured as the ratio between O_2 uptake (as in equation 2) and O_2 delivery (the product of umbilical blood flow and umbilical venous content). In the steady state, this ratio is usually roughly 0.4 in fetal sheep, meaning that only 40% of the oxygen delivered to the fetus through the placental circulation is actually extracted. The ratio during experimental hypoxemia may rise to some extent (to 0.5-0.6). A study in healthy human fetuses during delivery documented an extraction ratio of 0.62.[31]

Of interest is the relative constancy of fetal V_{O_2} across species lines when corrected for fetal weight. In species with fetal weights that differ by as much as a factor of 300, weight-specific fetal V_{O_2} estimates (mL/kg/minute) differ by only 15% with a mean value of 7.4 mL/kg/minute (see Table 48-1).[3] Corroboration of these observations is apparent when resting fetal heart rates of a number of species are compared. Fetal and neonatal heart rates (and therefore cardiac output) have been

Figure 48-1. Basal metabolic rate (W) as a function of mass using a logarithmic scale. The solid line is representative of the Mass[3/4] relationship. The two dashed lines are extrapolations based upon cellular respiration data relative to the corresponding whole animal. *In vivo* data for mitochondria and mitochondrial respiratory enzyme complexes are shown as isolated dots. ((From West GB, et al: Proc Natl Acad Sci USA *99*[Suppl 1]:2473, 2002)

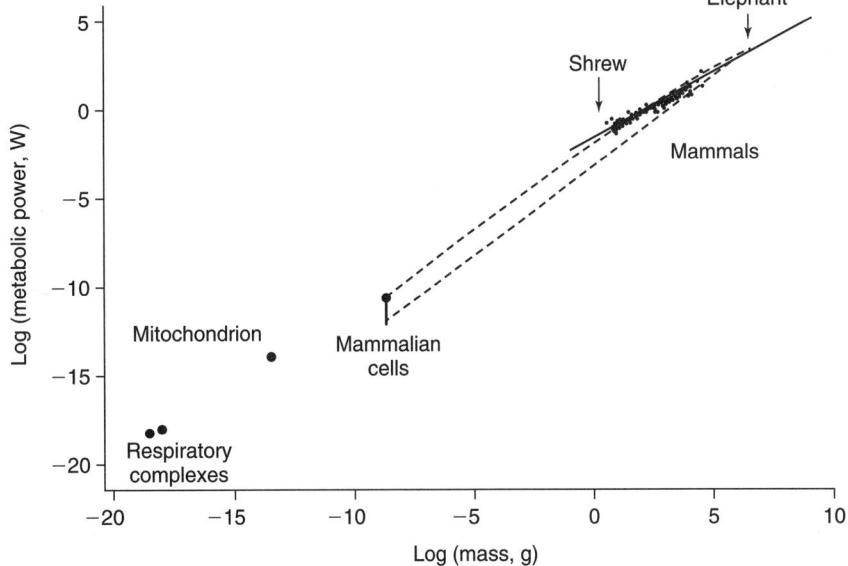

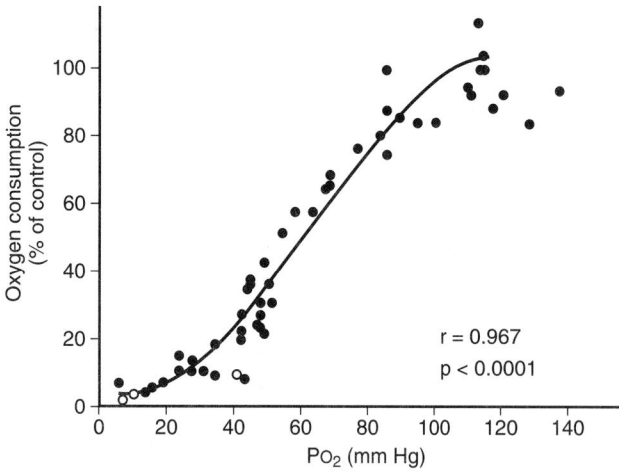

Figure 48–2. Relationship between oxygen tension in media and oxygen consumption in fetal guinea pig skeletal muscle cells. (From Braems G, Jensen A: J Dev Physiol *16*:209, 1991.)

TABLE 48-2

Factors Influencing Fetal Oxygen Consumption

Specific organ metabolism*
Activity
Fetal breathing
Fetal limb movement
Fetal cardiac activity
Fetal sleep state
Fetal growth
Substrate uptake
Maternal exercise
Fetomaternal temperature gradient
Fetal hormonal status
   Thyroid hormones
   Catecholamines
   Insulin

* Including ion pump activity and other processes necessary for cellular homeostasis.

used as reliable indicators of the metabolic rate.[32] Meier and co-workers[33] have observed that fetal heart rate differs little across species lines, in contrast to the adult, in whom heart rate is universally related to body weight. The reasons for such constancy of metabolic rate between various species are unclear but may relate to the already mentioned allometric scaling principles[20] as well as the rapid rate of growth in late gestation. In addition, it has been hypothesized that the fetus is relatively free from the "adult" oxidative demands of temperature homeostasis and, to a lesser extent, gravity and muscular activity, all of which are somewhat dependent on body mass and surface area.

Of those factors influencing fetal V_{O_2}, several are particularly prominent (Table 48-2). The term *specific organ metabolism* refers to those various cellular processes common to most tissues. Under basal conditions, a certain minimal level of V_{O_2} is necessary to maintain cellular homeostasis. Virtually all mitochondrial and plasma membrane ion pumps, vital for maintenance of intracellular and intraorganelle homeostatic reactions, require energy in the form of ATP for their activity and are thus heavily dependent on cellular respiratory activity. Such pumps consist of F-type H^+ pumps (mitochondria), V-type H^+ pumps (lysosomes, storage granules), or P-type Na^+,K^+ or H^+ pumps (plasma membranes).[34] Interestingly, this mitochondrial proton "leakiness" is also allometrically related to body mass among different species.[18] In the adult, overall pump activity has been estimated at approximately 20% of the basal metabolic rate.[35,36] Although it has thus far been difficult to estimate the contribution of such processes to the overall demand on the fetus for oxygen, it is likely that for many tissues, pump activity is important in determining tissue V_{O_2}. For example, in one estimate,[37] ouabain (through inhibition of Na^+,K^+-ATPase pump activity) caused a decline in fetal sheep liver and placental V_{O_2}, which accounted for 20% and for 34% of whole organ V_{O_2}, respectively. Similarly, in the newborn rat, approximately 50% of liver metabolism was due to activity of the sodium pump, with a significant decline in infancy.[22]

Other metabolic processes, such as protein synthesis, clearly add to the cost associated with oxygen demand, but the contributors as well as their specific demands on fetal V_{O_2} are as yet undetermined. Such processes that are common to all cells must make up a significant fraction of what is currently estimated when whole-organ or cellular V_{O_2} is measured.

It is clear that fetal work (i.e., muscle oxidative requirements to perform such activities as fetal breathing movements, limb movements, fetal swallowing, and myocardial contraction during systole) also accounts for a significant fraction of the total fetal V_{O_2}. For example, striated muscle activity (excluding cardiac work), as assessed in the *in vivo* fetal sheep, has been estimated to account for as much as 15% of the total fetal V_{O_2}. Muscle V_{O_2}, *in vitro*, has been measured in the fetus and is approximately 20 μmol/100 g/minute. In the term fetal lamb (in which muscle is approximately 25% of fetal wet weight), this would equate to 10 to 15% of total V_{O_2}, agreeing with the previous estimate. If specific cardiac V_{O_2}, as measured in the lamb, is added, slightly greater than 20% of the fetal requirement for oxygen is necessary for normal striated muscle activity. Unfortunately, further information of tissue-specific oxygen needs in the fetus is limited to several accessible organs in the sheep fetus alone.[4] From estimates in Table 48-3, however, it can be seen that a further 40% of the fetal V_{O_2} is attributable to fetal brain, liver, kidney, and intestine. Finally, the energy cost of growth (i.e., the energy necessary to synthesize new tissue as opposed to the energy stored in new tissue) has been estimated to be approximately 10% of the caloric value of new tissue, which is equivalent to about 6% of the fetal V_{O_2}. Thus, in the sheep fetus, approximately 80% of the fetal V_{O_2} can be accounted for in the resting state. It is assumed that measurement of V_{O_2} in other tissues (e.g., bone marrow, lung, adrenal gland, cartilage) will provide for the remaining 20% of whole fetus oxygen needs.

Several factors may influence the fetal metabolic rate (see Table 48-2). Interestingly, other than active fetal cooling, manipulations such as mild hypoxemia (see later discussion), maternal exercise,[38] or severe maternal starvation[39] do not appear to depress overall fetal metabolic activity. Although not well studied, any maternally administered drug that crosses the placenta and has a depressive effect on fetal activity should be expected to decrease fetal V_{O_2} as well. For example, skeletal muscle paralysis in the fetal lamb causes a 10 to 15% decrease in fetal V_{O_2}.[40] Significant depression of fetal breathing or body movements has been noted with maternal ethanol ingestion, antidepressants, cigarette smoking, hypoxemia, or steroid administration.[41-43]

The fetal metabolic rate can be stimulated by such factors as change in fetal sleep state,[44] excessive fetal muscular activity, and possibly external stimuli, such as sound.[45] Studies regarding changes in fetal behavior are now possible using fetal ultrasound to gauge fetal movement and breathing. Using these techniques, it has been shown that fetal breathing is more prominent after maternal food intake[41] or glucose infusion[41,46] and appears to be stimulated by maternal drug abuse (e.g., cocaine, methadone).[42]

Hormonal milieu of the fetus probably plays a significant role in determination of metabolic rate at rest and when changes occur in the fetal environment. The endocrine milieu influences cellular respiration and metabolic rate. In the adult, changes in

TABLE 48-3

Tissue-Specific Oxygen Needs in the Fetus

Tissue	Vo_2 μmol/100 g/min	Vo_2 μmol/kg/min (ml/kg/min)	% Total Vo_2
Whole fetus	—	360 (8.0)	100.0
Brain[124]	190	30 (0.7)	8.8
Heart[113, 114]	400	25 (0.6)	7.5
Liver[7,29,37]	100–180	58 (1.3)	16.3
Intestine[25]	100	40 (0.9)	11.3
Kidney[3]	100	8 (0.2)	2.5
Adrenal	68	2	0.05
Muscle[*3,111]	20	50 (1.1)	14.0
Growth[3]	—	20 (0.45)	5.6
Activity[*40]	—	54 (1.2)*	15.0
Total	—	285 (6.45)	81

* Data for muscle *(in vitro)* and activity *(in vivo)* must reflect both sedentary and active states of striated muscle respiration.

both sympathetic and parasympathetic nervous activity during meals may be partially responsible for the well-known postprandial increase in metabolic rate. Stimulation of cellular Vo_2 by insulin, thyroid hormones, and adrenal catecholamines has been documented, and, in the case of insulin, direct stimulation of mitochondrial respiratory chain activity has also been observed.[47]

In the steady state, fetal insulin deficiency has not been shown to cause a change in resting umbilical Vo_2.[48] However, fetal thyroid ablation has been shown to cause a 20 to 30% reduction in fetal metabolic rate,[49] without causing any changes in uteroplacental Vo_2. Exogenous thyroxine can be shown to reverse these metabolic changes.

The clinical significance of these changes is unclear, but increases in fetal Vo_2 of 20 to 30% from baseline in fetal lambs have been documented with exogenous infusion of each of the previously mentioned hormones. This may have important implications for such disease states as fetal thyrotoxicosis or maternal diabetes.

FETAL ENERGY SUBSTRATES

As noted in the previous sections, fetal Vo_2 in most species, including humans, has been measured to be approximately 7 to 8 mL/kg/minute, or roughly 11.5 L of oxygen per kg body weight per day. Assuming a "fetal diet" (see later) relatively low in fat intake for most species and a conversion factor of approximately 4.8 to 4.9 kcal energy liberated per liter oxygen consumed, the energy requirement (caloric value of substrate used for oxidation) by the fetus would be equivalent to approximately 55 kcal/kg/day. Because fetal energy requirements dictate a significant source of carbon uptake, it has been of interest to determine the relative uptakes of potential substrates across the fetal circulation. This has been accomplished both by classic Fick's principle physiologic methods in ruminant species and by isotope infusion studies (e.g., radioactive carbon [14C]-labeled glucose, lactate). Although the latter method has been more completely defined in fetal sheep, transfer studies are also available in small mammals such as the guinea pig, rabbit, and rat,[50-52] as well as in human fetuses to a limited extent.[53]

METHODS AND TERMINOLOGY

Uptake

Uptake of a substrate such as glucose may be calculated using the equation derived for fetal Vo_2:

$$U_{substrate} = F_{umb} \times (v - a)_{substrate} \qquad [4]$$

where $U_{substrate}$ = the umbilical uptake of a particular substrate in moles or mg/kg/minute and $(v-a)_{substrate}$ = the umbilical vein-distal aortic concentration difference of substrate in mol/ml or mg/ml. Note that U does not necessarily measure fetal uptake because, theoretically, endogenous production of a particular substrate (e.g., glucose or lactate) from other substrates must be taken into account. U, therefore, measures net umbilical uptake and provides only a minimum estimate of fetal uptake. Another limitation of this method for estimating fetal substrate utilization is the sensitivity of the method used to assay substrate concentration (usually colorimetric or spectrophotometric) relative to the percent extracted from the circulation. For example, in the fetal sheep, the umbilical venous concentration of glucose is approximately 30 mg/dL (1.7 mmol/L), and the extraction coefficient ([uptake/delivery] × 100) ranges from 10 to 15%.[54] The coefficient of variation of the glucose assay is approximately 3%, and, thus, it is possible to measure umbilical glucose uptake with accuracy. By contrast, the umbilical venous concentration for the amino acid serine is 700 μmol/L with a coefficient of variation of the assay of 1%.[55] In this case, however, the extraction coefficient of serine is only 0.6% of the delivery rate. It is therefore obvious that for substances with small extraction coefficients, accuracy in measuring umbilical uptake using Fick's principle may be difficult, if not impossible.

Oxygen Quotient

Previously, it had been difficult to determine directly whether specific fetal substrates were taken up by the umbilical circulation and oxidized completely. The concept of substrate/oxygen quotient was adapted for the fetus,[3] predominantly using the sheep to address this question. To estimate the maximum fraction of fetal oxygen consumption accounted for by the oxidation of any given substrate, the following equation is applied:

$$\text{Substrate/O}_2 \text{ quotient} = \frac{F_{umb} \times (v - a)_{substrate}}{F_{umb} \times (v - a)_{O_2}} \times n \qquad [5]$$

where n = the number of moles of oxygen required for the complete oxidation of substrate:

Substrate	n
Glucose	6.0
Lactate	3.0
Glycerol	3.5
Palmitic acid	23.0
β-Hydroxybutyrate	4.5
Acetoacetate	4.0

Using equation 5, the blood flow terms in numerator and denominator cancel out, leaving the ratio of the venoarterial concentration differences of substrate versus oxygen. Thus, as adapted for fetal metabolic studies under steady-state conditions, this method of estimating substrate requirements for energy has the advantage of not requiring measurement of umbilical blood flow or fetal mass. The demonstration of a substrate/oxygen quotient near or equal to 1.0 suggests that if the particular substrate measured were completely oxidized, it could provide 100% of the carbon necessary for the measured fetal V_{O_2}. A substrate/oxygen quotient significantly less than 1.0 would indicate the requirement for other carbon sources to be used to sustain metabolic rate even if the measured substrate were completely oxidized. It then follows that substrate/oxygen quotients greater than 1.0 indicate use of a significant portion of measured substrate for purposes other than energy production (i.e., for synthesis or transformation into other substrates). In fetal sheep, substrate/oxygen quotients measured under steady-state conditions[3] include glucose, 0.5; total amino acids, 0.25; and lactate, 0.25 with negligible fatty acid uptake. In other species including the human, estimates vary from 0.5 to 0.8 (Table 48-4) for glucose/oxygen quotients.

Although useful conceptually and in situations in which steady-state umbilical blood flow is difficult or impossible to determine, substrate/oxygen quotients that have been measured have had limited usefulness. Major limitations to the interpretation of this method include (1) the inability to trace metabolic pathways of degradation or transformation and (2) the necessity for conditions of steady state to be fulfilled to determine V-A differences accurately. Other more sensitive methods would be of use to overcome these problems.

Substrate Use

The application of radioactive and nonradioactive isotope ("tracer") methodology[56,57] has provided interesting new insights into fetal metabolic processes and added substantially to the body of knowledge obtained from interpreting substrate/oxygen quotients and substrate umbilical uptakes using Fick's method. Fetal infusion of substrates such as glucose or lactate,[58] labeled with such tracers as[13]C or[14]C, can be performed and the fluxes of both radioactive and nonradioactive substrates then measured across the umbilical circulation. In addition, the transformation into other substrates or carbon dioxide can be quantified. Using this method, calculation of fetal glucose utilization (i.e., glucose used for oxidation and storage from exogenous and endogenous sources) can be accomplished. More complete summaries of the methodology and pitfalls inherent in these methods may be found in several reviews.[3,59,60] As discussed later in this chapter, under nonstressed conditions in ruminants, uptake studies are either in agreement with (glucose) or underestimate (lactate, amino acids) actual fetal uptake and use. More recently, limited data have become available[61] in humans using stable isotopes, particularly related to fetal gluconeogenesis (see later discussion). Additional techniques are being perfected for the study of fetal organ metabolism, particularly the brain. For example, positron emission tomography (PET) has been used in fetal sheep to explore cerebral glucose uptake through estimation of intracellular glucose phosphorylation.[62] Additionally, a study by Kok and co-workers[63] has demonstrated that cerebral metabolic information may be obtained noninvasively in human fetuses using proton magnetic resonance spectroscopy.

Respiratory Quotient

In the nongrowing adult mammal, the ratio between generated carbon dioxide and consumed oxygen, the RQ, can provide some indirect information regarding the relative oxidation rates of carbohydrates, fats, and proteins. For example, the RQs of adult subjects oxidizing either carbohydrates or fat are 1.0 or 0.7, respectively, with those on a mixed diet having an RQ of 0.85. In the resting state, the RQ of the fetal lamb is approximately 0.94, suggesting little fetal oxidation of fat. Because of the rapid rate of fetal growth, however, the inequity between carbon uptake and excretion across the umbilical circulation invalidates this method as providing a sensitive measure of differential substrate utilization by the fetus.

Substrate Uptake: Carbohydrate

In most species studied, a significant relationship is present between maternal and fetal levels of glucose, which is the carbohydrate present in highest concentration in fetal blood (Fig. 48-3).[64-66] Other carbohydrates, such as fructose (ruminants) or galactose, are present in fetal blood but appear to play relatively minor roles in oxidative metabolism during fetal life. Maternofetal transfer of glucose has been best studied (although not exclusively so) in ruminant species, in which determinants of transfer include (1) the maternal glucose concentration, (2) the maternofetal glucose gradient, (3) the fetal endocrine milieu (specifically fetal insulin and glucagon secretion), and (4) the degree of placental metabolism of glucose. In several species, including humans, these general determinants of glucose transfer also appear to be applicable. In humans, since the advent of periumbilical blood sampling (PUBS), several investigators have examined maternofetal substrate relationships.[3,7,57,64,65] Bozzetti and colleagues[65] have documented that in both midgestation and late-gestation human pregnancy, a high degree of correlation between maternal and fetal blood glucose concentrations exists under relatively steady-state conditions. Marconi and co-workers[64] have also demonstrated in humans that the maternofetal glucose gradient increases with advancing gestational age in normal pregnancies (Fig. 48-4) and that this difference is more pronounced in growth restricted fetuses. Using ^{13}C-labeled glucose injected

TABLE 48-4

Umbilical Glucose Uptake and Glucose/Oxygen Quotient

Species	Umbilical Glucose Uptake (mg/kg/min)	Umbilical Glucose/O_2
Sheep[35,65]	3.7	
	6.4	0.45
Cow[130]	5.2	0.57
Horse[130]	6.8	0.69
Human[57,58,70]	5.0	0.80

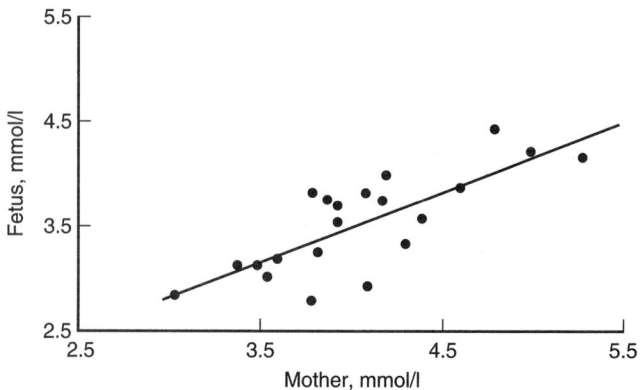

Figure 48–3. Relationship between human maternal and fetal glucose concentrations obtained at the time of cordocentesis ($Y = 0.68 + 0.76x$; p, .001). (From Ashmead G, et al: Gynecol Obstet Invest *35*:18, 1993.)

before cesarean section or PUBS, fetal glucose use has been estimated in pregnant humans.[66] Although the measured glucose disposal rate of the human conceptus included placenta as well as fetus, glucose disposal rate related directly to the maternal plasma glucose concentration and increased with increasing conceptus mass. Furthermore, estimates of fetal glucose disposal were in agreement with studies in neonatal humans as well as fetuses of several other species.

Understanding of mechanisms of placental glucose transport has been expanded with the discovery of at least seven specific bidirectional glucose transporter proteins, now labeled GLUT1 to 5 and sodium-dependent glucose transporters 1-2 (SGLT1-2).[67,68] Specifically the GLUT1 isoform, known also as the *brain erythrocyte glucose transporter*, is expressed on both the maternal and the fetal facing sides[69,70] of human placentas. Although the density of transporters on the maternal side (microvillous membranes) remains constant after the first trimester, the concentration of transporters on the fetal facing (basal) side increases at least twofold after the first trimester.[71] Furthermore, measured rates of placental glucose uptake *in vitro* match the density of placental GLUT1 transcripts. In addition, GLUT1 expression is inhibited by glucose but is not regulated by insulin.[69] In sheep, this carrier can be saturated at maternal glucose concentrations of 10 to 12 mM.[72] In both humans and sheep, it has been estimated that glucose transport capacity is considerably higher than necessary given the normal range for maternal serum glucose concentrations. This suggests that changes in fetal and maternal glucose concentrations or metabolism are key factors in determining fetal glucose transport. Within certain tissues, GLUT expression is important for determining the overall contribution of glucose as a major substrate for the fetus. In addition, various factors including insulin and glucose concentrations may modify synthesis of these transporter proteins. For example, expression of GLUT1 and GLUT4 in fetal skeletal muscle is increased by exogenous infusions of glucose or insulin,[73] and in the fetal rat with defective cardiac myocyte insulin receptors, GLUT1 expression is reduced by 50%.[74] However, the relative roles of these tissue-specific GLUTs in regulation of glucose uptake and use are not yet well understood.

The placenta metabolizes glucose derived from both mother and fetus.[70,75] The rate of placental glucose consumption is not static and appears to be related to maternal, and therefore, fetal, glucose concentration as studied in the fetal sheep.[76,77] Placental contributions to total uterine glucose uptake have been summarized,[78] and approximately 50% of uterine glucose uptake can be accounted for by placental metabolic processes in the sheep.

In addition to concentration gradient, a number of studies have documented that the fetus is capable of exerting some hormonal control over glucose uptake, at least in the last trimester. Philipps and co-workers[54] have shown that fine control of glucose uptake under steady-state conditions is also mediated by changes in the endogenous fetal insulin secretory rate. In addition, surgical or chemical ablation of fetal insulin release induces relative hyperglycemia and a decline in umbilical glucose uptake and fetal glucose use.[54, 79, 80] Other potential glucose regulatory hormones, such as glucagon, cortisol, and thyroid hormones, have been studied to a lesser extent in the fetus. In the absence of maternal or fetal disease, their concentrations in fetal blood do not seem to be related to fetal glucose uptake. Fetal thyroid function, however, may be important in providing glucose homeostasis during times of stress, such as during maternal fasting or malnutrition.[49]

Glucose Uptake and Use

Because of estimates of the fetal RQ approaching 1.0 as well as the relatively high concentrations of glucose in fetal blood, it was previously surmised that a significant fetal uptake of glucose occurred. To test this hypothesis, various investigators measured glucose uptake in the fetus using classic Fick's principle techniques (net umbilical uptake) as well as radiolabeled glucose transfer (fetal uptake and use). In one comparison of the two methods, Hay and colleagues[76] reported essentially identical results—measured net umbilical uptake of glucose was similar to the rate of fetal glucose use in the sheep, and both were related to the maternal glucose concentration. These results in the sheep fetus imply negligible endogenous fetal glucose production in the resting nonstressed state (see later discussion).

Of the studies listed in Table 48-4, the net umbilical glucose uptake near term is approximately 4 to 7 mg (22-39 μmol)/kg/minute. This is equal to roughly 6 to 10 g glucose/kg/day and is equivalent to 32 kcal/kg/day in potential energy production. It is, however, significantly less than the energy estimated to be required by the measured fetal Vo_2 (i.e., approximately 55 kcal/kg/day). In fact, in estimates of umbilical glucose-oxygen quotients obtained in several ruminant species, the complete oxidation of glucose accounted for only roughly 50% of the fetal Vo_2 (i.e., umbilical $G/O_2 = 0.5$; see equation 5). It should again be pointed out that these estimates represent the maximum percent of the fetal Vo_2 accounted for by complete oxidation of

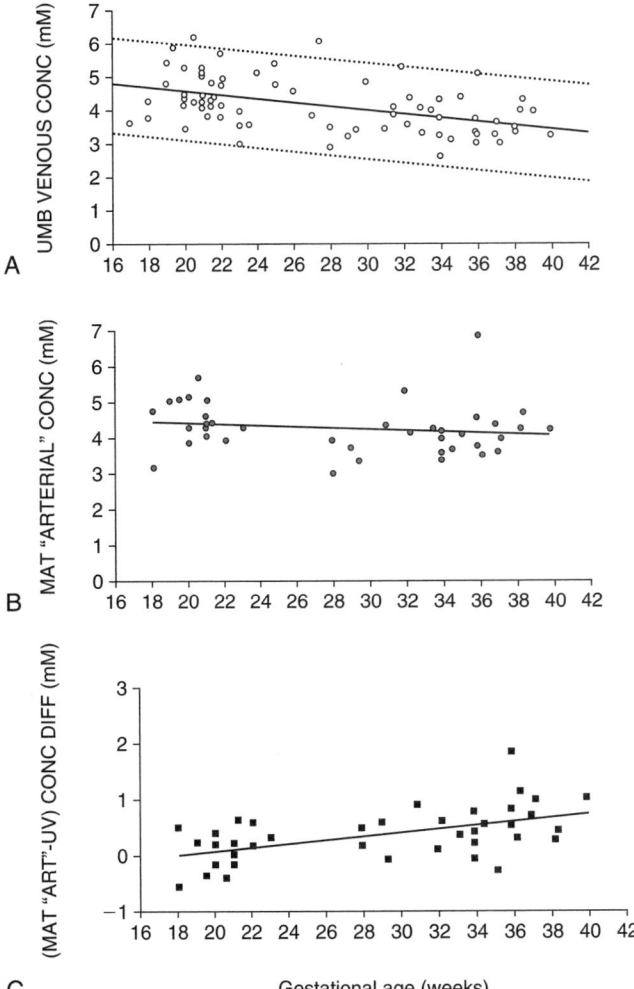

Figure 48-4. Human maternal versus fetal blood glucose concentration changes during gestation. **A**, umbilical venous glucose versus gestational age in normal fetuses, (UV = 5.66 - 0.56 GA), **B**, maternal arterial glucose versus gestational age, **C**, maternal-fetal glucose difference versus gestational age (Marconi, AM, et al: Obstet Gynecol 87:937, 1996.)

glucose and must overestimate the actual fraction if any significant glucose storage (such as conversion to glycogen, fatty acids, or triglycerides) occurs. Only a few similar studies in humans are available for comparison[66,81] (see Table 48-4) but are remarkably similar to data obtained in animals. Thus, although glucose represents a quantitatively significant source of fetal energy (fuel), it probably does not supply enough carbon to support the total oxidative demands of fetal life. As pointed out in one review, estimates of specific organ glucose consumption are incomplete[10] but have been best documented in the sheep fetus. Studies suggest that at least 80% of measured fetal glucose uptake can be accounted for by brain and striated (skeletal plus cardiac) muscle. Although the fetal liver consumes and oxidizes glucose, net consumption as measured in the sheep is nil.[82] Use of other methods may provide more information. For example, Thorngren-Jerneck and co-workers[62] using PET scans, have determined that the global cerebral glucose metabolic rate (rate of intracellular cellular glucose phosphorylation) in near-term fetal lambs was 37.8 μmol/min/100 g. Calculation of the cerebral glucose/O_2 quotient from Table 48-3 and equation 5 yields a value of 1.1, similar to previous estimates measured more directly.

Unfortunately, similar measurements of glucose uptake and oxidation are not available in other species. Less direct work in species such as the rat, pig, or guinea pig,[52,83,84] however, is in agreement with these estimates. In the human, demonstration of glucose uptake and use by fetal brain, liver, and placenta has also been documented. Indirect estimates of glucose production (*not* use) in normal term newborns[85] using stable isotopes have suggested values of 3 to 5 mg/kg/minute. Although cord blood venoarterial differences of glucose in several human studies[65,81] are positive direct measurements of uptake or oxidation are currently limited. As noted previously, however, measurement of glucose disposal rate in human fetuses appears in the range of 5 mg (28 μmol)/kg/minute.[66]

GLUCOSE STORAGE

Glycogen

In the fetus as in the adult, the major storage form of glucose is glycogen, a glucose polymer stored intracellularly as a precipitate, with an average molecular weight of 500,000 daltons or greater. In fetal life, glycogen is stored in significant concentration in liver, skeletal and cardiac muscle, kidney, intestine, brain, and placenta. From the work of Shelley,[86] it is apparent that glycogen storage in most fetal species reaches a maximum concentration at term gestation in organs such as liver and skeletal muscle. In most other storage sites (i.e., lung, myocardium, kidney, and placenta), however, peak values are attained somewhat earlier (50–70% gestation), with a gradual decline near term to adult levels. The factors responsible for glycogen synthesis and induction of enzymes necessary for glycogen synthesis are complex and have been reviewed elsewhere[10] (Fig. 48-5). Of importance are the following generalizations:

1. Activity of the enzyme necessary for glycogen synthesis (glycogen synthase) correlates well with the relative presence or absence of glycogen in fetal tissues.
2. Fetal liver glycogen synthesis appears to be regulated by both endogenous fetal insulin production and intactness of the fetal pituitary-hypothalamic-adrenal axis. Studies show lack of hepatic glycogen accumulation in decapitated fetal rats or rabbits with little effect on glycogen synthesis in other organs.[87,88] Fetal thyroid function may also be an important contributor to hepatic glycogen storage.[49]

3. Significant fetal glycogen turnover with active degradation probably occurs in the last trimester but with relative net accumulation in tissues such as liver.
4. Certain organs, such as placenta, accumulate glycogen in response to maternal stimuli such as human placental lactogen or insulin with little response to changes in fetal hormonal levels.[89]

Maternal nutritional sufficiency plays a major role in late fetal glycogen deposition, but some discrepancies in the literature currently exist, probably as a result of species differences as well as differences in experimental design. In general, when studied in the rat or sheep,[90,91] significant maternal malnutrition causes a decrease in maternal hepatic glycogen stores but inconsistent changes in fetal hepatic glycogen. Fetal hepatic levels of glycogen synthase (rat) and of active and total phosphorylase (sheep) are also unaffected despite significant and prolonged maternal hypoglycemia.

Synthesis of glycogen classically derives from glucose. It has been demonstrated, however, that a significant portion of glycogen in the postabsorptive adult actually is synthesized from precursors of gluconeogenesis such as lactate and pyruvate. This also appears to be the case in the sheep fetus.[92] Another potential pathway for glycogen production involves transformation of glycolytic intermediates through serine (see Fig. 48-5). The production of glycogen from serine has been documented in fetal hepatocytes.[93] This pathway allows for bypass of the gluconeogenic step oxaloacetate to phosphoenolpyruvate (which is rate limiting because of the developmental lag in fetal gluconeogenic enzyme synthesis (see later discussion). It has been estimated that the alternative serine pathway could account for up to 25% of the glycogen produced.[93] In addition, serine and glycine are cycled between fetal liver and placenta,[53,55] providing another convenient source of precursor for fetal glycogen deposition.

Glycogen breakdown (glycogenolysis) with resultant availability of glucose for use as fuel substrate is an important factor contributing to glucose homeostasis during the perinatal period and has significant survival value to the fetus in times of stress. The regulation of the activity of the enzyme involved in glycogenolysis (glycogen phosphorylase) is reciprocal to that of synthase. Thus, when one is stimulated (as when phosphorylase expression is stimulated by catecholamines or glucagon), the other (synthase) is inhibited. In fetal tissues such as liver and kidney, glycogen breakdown can be induced by such hormones as catecholamines or glucagon or by stimuli such as cold stress or hypoxia. In these tissues, the presence of glucose-6-phosphatase allows for glucose dephosphorylation and net exit from intracellular stores. Thus, free glucose can be released into the peripheral circulation for use at sites (e.g., brain) distant from the original storage tissue. In other organs (e.g., lung, placenta, and myocardium), phosphorylase, but not glucose-6-phosphatase, is present, and stored glycogen is available only for intracellular consumption within the storage site. For some tissues (e.g., myocardium and placenta), which have large obligate glucose requirements, this offers a distinct degree of protection against the sudden onset of hypoglycemia. For whatever reason, central nervous system glycogen storage in fetal life is minimal. Of interest is the demonstration of a correlation between the fall in lung glycogen and stimulation of surfactant production, leading to speculation that fetal pulmonary glycogen may be a significant substrate for surfactant synthesis.[94] Local hormonal control of this latter process has been suggested.[95]

In the late-gestation fetus, it is possible to demonstrate glycogenolysis in response to pharmacologic doses of such secretogogues as glucagon.[96] In malnourished sheep, however, as in

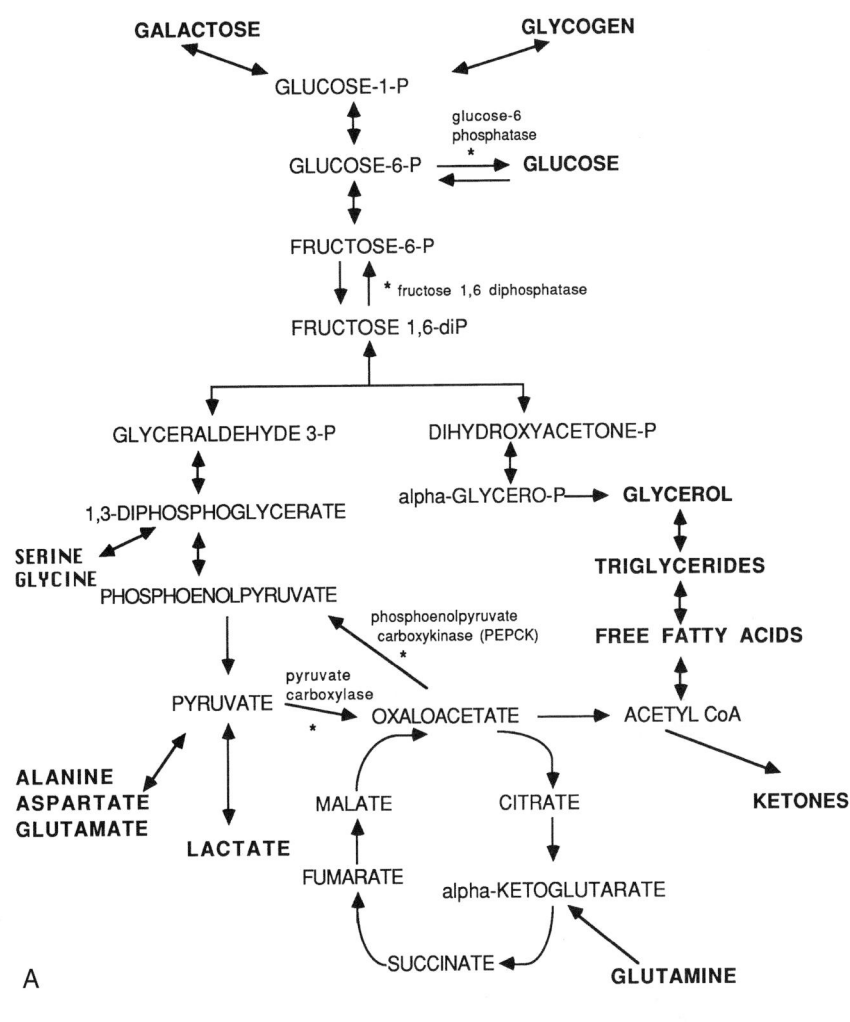

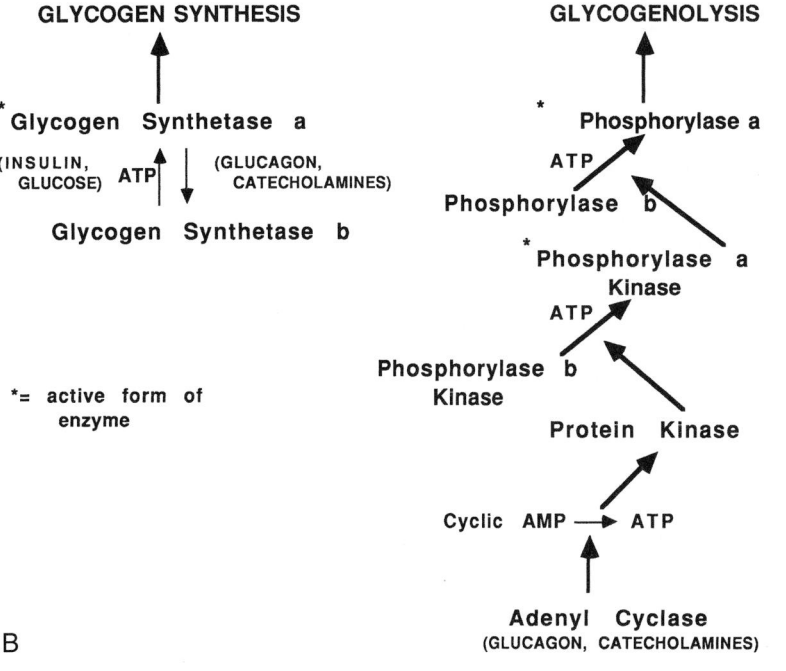

Figure 48–5. A, Metabolic pathways involving fetal metabolic substrates. Key gluconeogenic enzymes (*) include (1) glucose-6-phosphatase, (2) fructose-1, 6-diphosphatase, (3) phosphoenolpyruvate carboxykinase, and (4) pyruvate carboxylase. **B,** Metabolic pathways involved in glycogen synthesis and degradation. (Redrawn after Pagliara AS, et al: J Pediatr 82:365, 1973; Milner RDG: *In* Beard RW, Nathanielsz PW [eds]: Fetal Physiology and Medicine. New York, Marcel Dekker, 1984. Reprinted by courtesy of Marcel Dekker, Inc.)

humans with intrauterine growth retardation, there is inconsistent evidence as to whether significant glucose production may occur from stored glycogen.[61,92]

Other Carbohydrates

In some species, including ruminants and pigs,[97] fetal blood fructose may reach concentrations three- to fourfold above that of glucose.[76] In these species, placental synthesis of fructose from glucose is the major mechanism for production. Negligible fetal fructose uptake from the umbilical circulation, however, suggests that fructose does not play a significant role in fetal metabolism. Fructose concentrations in fetal sheep plasma do rise during fetal hyperglycemia and fall during maternal starvation (with resultant maternal and fetal hypoglycemia), suggesting that fructose in these species may function as a storage form of glucose. Finally, galactose uptake in fetal life has not been well studied, but preliminary data suggest that in tissues such as liver, galactose incorporation into glycogen may be of significantly greater importance than that of glucose.[98] Endogenous production of galactose in the human newborn has been documented.[99]

GLUCONEOGENESIS

Another major pathway for the endogenous production of glucose is through synthesis from nonglucose precursors, such as certain amino acids, lactate, or pyruvate (see Fig. 48–5) (i.e., gluconeogenesis). Although the regulation of gluconeogenesis has been extensively studied in adult humans, significant capacity for gluconeogenesis in the human fetus has not been documented. For glucose to be synthesized from substrates such as glutamate or lactate, key enzymes located largely in liver and kidney must be present. Activities of phosphoenolpyruvate carboxykinase (PEPCK), pyruvate carboxylase (PC), fructose–1, 6-diphosphatase, and glucose-6-phosphatase have been measured in fetal liver from several species, including humans.[100,101] Although glucose-6-phosphatase activity is present from the 12th week of gestation in the human, PEPCK activity is considerably less than in postnatal life and appears to be rate limiting in terms of glucose production. Activities of the other two gluconeogenic enzymes appear to be intermediate. In animal studies of gluconeogenic enzyme capacity, such as in the rat, similar patterns of activity are present. When the rate of gluconeogenesis has been measured through either *in vivo* or *in vitro* studies, variable results have been obtained. For example, even though the liver extracts significant lactate from the umbilical circulation,[82] gluconeogenesis in fetal sheep or rat liver *in vitro* is nil unless stimulated by glucagon in the incubation medium. Small but significant rates of gluconeogenesis have been documented using either fetal rat kidney or liver from pig, guinea pig, and monkey. Even in these species, however, there appears to be a developmental increase in gluconeogenic activity only after approximately 90% of gestation. *In vivo* radiolabeled tracer studies in sheep and rats before term fail to detect significant gluconeogenesis in the resting state,[92,102] although glucagon has been shown to stimulate gluconeogenesis in the near term fetal sheep.[103]

The reasons for these inconsistencies have been elucidated by Fowden and co-workers[92] who have shown in the fetal sheep that the capacity for gluconeogenesis is limited until the last few days of gestation, when it rises to account for roughly 50% of the glucose use rate and parallels the rate of rise in fetal blood concentrations of cortisol and catecholamines. In those studies, maternal fasting induced endogenous glucose production only in late gestation fetuses, but 5 to 6 days earlier than would normally have been observed in nonfasted animals. It has been suggested that in the resting state before term, hepatic interconversion and catabolism of glucogenic substrates occur at the expense of potential glucose production. As noted already, thyroid hormone, cortisol, and catecholamines are all likely to mediate gene regulation and stimulation of synthesis of enzymes involved in hepatic gluconeogenesis, but the role of endogenous glucagon remains unclear.

It is probable (but as yet unproved) that significant endogenous glucose production occurs in the stressed human fetus, such as during maternal hypoglycemia or starvation or in some states of intrauterine growth retardation. In human growth-retarded fetuses exposed to a maternal overnight fast, Marconi and colleagues[61] were unable to detect endogenous fetal glucose production when a maternal infusion of ^{13}C glucose was used. Whether the near-term human fetus has the capacity for significant glucose production under certain conditions, such as during maternal fasting or hypoglycemia, is as yet unknown.

MATERNAL DISORDERS: FETAL EFFECTS

In certain relatively common clinical situations affecting the maternal milieu, fetal metabolic changes may occur. These include fetal hypoxemia induced by maternal hemorrhage or by maternal hypoxemia, fetal hyperglycemia as a consequence of maternal diabetes, and fetal hypoglycemia caused by maternal malnutrition or insulin therapy. Most of the information presented here was derived from studies performed in animals under steady-state conditions. Such studies, in addition to clinical observations, have allowed for better insight into the adaptive mechanisms by which the fetus may respond to potentially damaging insults.

Fetal Hypoxemia

A decline in fetal blood oxygen content may occur through different pathologic events. The predominant factors responsible for oxygen transport across the placenta include uterine and umbilical blood flow, the maternofetal oxygen tension difference, and the hemoglobin concentration in fetal blood.[3] Thus, clinically relevant abnormalities that could affect fetal oxygenation include abnormal uterine or placental blood flow as may occur in hypertensive diseases of pregnancy, abruptio placentae, cord occlusion, or following nicotine or cocaine use; defective maternal oxygenation because of maternal pulmonary or cardiac disease or seizures secondary to eclampsia; and fetal disorders such as sepsis, hemorrhage, anemia, or heart block and certain other arrhythmias.

Acute hypoxemia is known to produce various circulatory adaptations in the fetus that can work to enhance fetal survival (Table 48–5).[25, 30, 104-106] These effects include the development of bradycardia, hypertension, redistribution of blood flow (toward the central nervous system, myocardium,

---

TABLE 48-5

Fetal Response to Hypoxemia or Ischemia

Redistribution of blood flow
To: Brain
         Myocardium
         Adrenal
From: Gastrointestinal tract
         Skin
         Muscle
Increased umbilical O_2 extraction
Decreased fetal movement
Selective decrease in VO_2 (muscle)
Bradycardia
Selective shift toward increased anaerobic glycolysis

and adrenals and away from intestine and muscle), depression of fetal breathing and skeletal muscle activity, and increase in fetal oxygen extraction from umbilical blood. Some of these processes are mediated by endothelial nitric oxide[107] and may be even noted in fetuses at 0.6 of gestation.[108] In addition, Gardner and co-workers[106] have shown that a rapid (10-15%) rise in hemoglobin concentration occurs during controlled cord occlusion, which cannot be explained on the basis of newly generated red blood cells or splenic sequestration. Such an increase could work to ameliorate the concomitant reduction in transplacental oxygen transport.

Less is known about the impact of fetal hypoxemia on fetal metabolic processes. Theoretically, depression of oxygen delivery to respiring tissues increases the ADP:ATP ratio. This acts to stimulate glycolysis (the Pasteur effect), with the effect of subsequently increasing ATP production anaerobically.[109] Thus, hypoxia would be expected to produce relatively high rates of glucose uptake and lactic acid production in most fetal tissues. If hypoxia is severe, both hypoglycemia and metabolic acidosis with ultimate tissue necrosis result. Several factors, however, appear to lessen the impact of hypoxemia on fetal metabolic processes. When oxygen transport is limited experimentally in the sheep fetus, by partial occlusion of uterine blood flow[110] or by mild maternal hypoxia, redistribution of blood flow occurs, but little change in fetal V_{O_2} is noted. In sheep fetuses exposed to severe hypoxemia, whether by occlusion of uterine blood flow or by maternal hypoxia, fetal oxygen consumption declines by 25 to 40%.[25, 26, 111] Because, as mentioned earlier, the metabolic rate of fetal muscle is related to the ambient oxygen tension, it is not surprising that carcass V_{O_2} declines more than that of the whole fetus. Although not yet determined, it is likely that the decline in overall fetal oxygen consumption is due to depressed metabolism in other nonessential organs as well (e.g., fetal intestine, liver, and kidney), and that decreased metabolic work of skeletal muscle (decreased activity) and myocardium (bradycardia)[25, 106] also may play a role. Interestingly, carcass lactate production may be balanced by lactate uptake in relatively nonhypoxic organs and the placenta[111] to avoid a massive accumulation of blood lactate.

In contrast, fetal cerebrum and myocardium appear relatively protected from generalized fetal hypoxemia because of the increase in blood flow to these organs, probably induced by catecholamine secretion as outlined earlier. In studies of hypoxemia in fetal guinea pigs[28] and sheep,[112] relatively small changes in cerebral V_{O_2} occur (at the expense of other organs). An increased rate of anaerobic glycolysis can also be demonstrated, allowing for the ongoing production of high-energy phosphates such as ATP. The fetal heart also has a greater capacity for anaerobic glycolysis than that of the adult.[83, 113] It has also been suggested that elevated levels of adenosine 5-monophosphate (AMP) (the precursor for adenosine) are important regulators of blood flow in brain and heart (i.e., that increased levels of AMP and ADP result in increased local concentrations of adenosine, a potent vasodilator). Several investigators have documented a greater dependence of fetal myocardium (compared with adult myocardium) on energy supplied through glycolysis.[10, 114] Inhibitors of glycolysis affect fetal myocardial function to a much greater degree, but inhibitors of oxidative phosphorylation depress both equally. Furthermore, fetal myocardium, in contrast to fetal muscle, has the capacity to synthesize myoglobin in response to hypoxemia,[11] thus developing a source of storage oxygen for myocardial mitochondrial respiration.

Finally, in states of chronic maternal hypoxemia, such as may occur in a variety of clinical situations, fetal growth retardation is not uncommon.[115] Depression of potent fetal growth factors such as insulin-like growth factor I during hypoxic states may have an important protective effect by conserving fetal substrate for energy as opposed to accretion needs.[116]

Another factor that protects against the effects of hypoxia is an increased fetal availability of glucose, particularly during late gestation. Hypoxia, with secretion of catecholamines, cortisol, and vasopressin, is a major stimulus for glycogenolysis in the adult and probably in fetal life as well.[105, 117] Cardiac glycogen content correlates with fetal ability to withstand anoxia.[1] In fetal lambs and monkeys at term, hypoxia causes a fall in hepatic glycogen content and concomitant rise in blood glucose concentration.[1, 86] In fetal lambs exposed to severe hypoxemia, the net fetal glucose uptake doubles within 30 minutes, as hepatic glucose output rises to equal umbilical glucose uptake and suggests active fetal glycogenolysis. Thus, the simultaneous development of increased cerebral blood flow (to preserve fetal cerebral oxygen delivery), decreased overall fetal oxygen consumption, and rapid fetal glycogen degradation with resultant hyperglycemia ensures adequate substrate and oxygen delivery to vital tissues such as brain and myocardium and provides at least some measure of fetal tolerance to an interruption of placental oxygen transport.

Maternal Hyperglycemia

Diabetes in pregnancy produces several specific fetal and neonatal abnormalities. The development of fetal hyperglycemia as a result of excessive maternofetal glucose transfer has been well documented in a number of species, including the human,[118] and appears to be the major but not sole factor in the development of such neonatal complications as macrosomia, hyperinsulinemia, and postnatal hypoglycemia. Evidence in sheep[119] and monkeys[120] suggests that fetal hyperglycemia or hyperinsulinemia may accelerate fetal metabolism. In the fetal sheep, changes in the circulating concentrations of glucose and insulin appear to have independent stimulatory effects on fetal V_{O_2} and glucose oxidation.[121] In other work, fetal glucose infusion caused increases in fetal glucose and lactate uptake and placental lactate production as well as 30% increase in fetal V_{O_2}, all suggestive of a significant increase in fetal metabolic rate.[119] Severe maternal or fetal hyperglycemia in sheep induces a more pronounced fetal metabolic change, including fetal acidosis and ultimate death. These are all consistent with the effects of hypoxia, as shown in Table 48-6. Some human fetuses of diabetic mothers have been thought to exhibit signs of *in utero* oxygen deprivation, but conclusive proof is not yet available. Glucose infusion in human pregnancy, however, does result in cord blood metabolic changes that mirror those in sheep studied over the long-term.[122] It is presumed that the increase in fetal fuel needs for sustaining the increased V_{O_2} are met by increased uptake of glucose, placentally derived lactate,

---

TABLE 48-6

Fetal Hyperglycemia

Mild-Moderate

Arterial hypoxemia
Hyperinsulinemia
Increased fetal V_{O_2}
Respiratory acidosis
Increased glucose-lactate uptake

Severe

Arterial hypoxemia
Hypoinsulinemia
Increased erythropoietin
Increased fetal V_{O_2}
Metabolic acidosis
Decreased placental perfusion
Fetal demise

Data from Philipps AF, et al: Diabetes *34*(Suppl 2):32, 1985; Crandell SS, et al: Am J Physiol *249*:E454, 1985.

and perhaps amino acids and ketones. Interestingly, although human fetuses of diabetic mothers who exhibit excessive growth *in utero* remain at risk for late fetal demise, macrosomic fetuses of nondiabetic women are not at risk.[123]

The factors responsible for the increase in fetal metabolic rate are unclear. Fetal hyperglycemia is known to increase the rate of fetal breathing movements in sheep and humans,[46] which might serve to increase muscular work and thus increase the V_{O_2}. In addition, specific organ responses to accelerated substrate influx or hyperinsulinemia, particularly in liver and brain, may play important roles. For example, fetal glucose infusion in the sheep may accelerate cerebral V_{O_2} by as much as 70%, with a concomitant increase in cerebral blood flow and glucose entry as well as changes in fetal electrocortical activity.[124] Catecholamine secretion[125] is likely to be responsible for at least some of these changes. The demonstration in prematurely delivered neonates of stimulation of V_{O_2} by intravenously administered nutrients[126] suggests that metabolic rate may be altered by increased delivery of substrate other than glucose.

Maternal Hypoglycemia

Because the major factor responsible for placental glucose transport to the fetus is the maternofetal glucose concentration gradient,[70] it follows that induction of maternal hypoglycemia should depress fetal glucose uptake. In the sheep, maternal hypoglycemia induced by fasting is clearly associated with a decrease in fetal plasma glucose concentration and in depression of both umbilical glucose uptake and fetal glucose use.[57] Because fetal V_{O_2} does not change during hypoglycemia induced by maternal fasting[127] or maternal insulin infusion,[128] other fuel sources, particularly amino acids and endogenously produced glucose and lactate, may be used instead. For example, myocardial lactate uptake in the fetus can account for most oxygen consumption in this organ,[113, 114] even in steady state. Fetal muscle and brain also have the capacity to use ketones.[129] In addition, endogenous glucose production has been demonstrated in fetal sheep,[92, 121] probably secondary to hepatic glycogenolysis. With a more chronic hypoglycemic stress, gluconeogenesis can also be stimulated. For hypoglycemia of short duration, intracellular stores of glycogen, particularly in myocardium, liver, and kidney, clearly offer an available source of glucose for cellular metabolic processes. More prolonged chronic hypoglycemia caused by malnutrition, however, depletes cellular stores of glycogen in a variety of organs, particularly in brain, liver, and heart.[90, 91] This may be the reason for failure to observe any glucogenesis in growth-retarded human fetuses whose mothers were exposed to an overnight fast.[60] Finally, expression of glucose transporter proteins[67, 130, 131] such as GLUT1 in placenta and GLUT4 in muscle may also up-regulate in response to changes in circulating glucose (and insulin) concentration and act to increase the cellular uptake of glucose during relative glucose deprivation.

During induction of maternal hypoglycemia, evidence also suggests that other fetal counterregulatory mechanisms can blunt the fall in fetal blood glucose. Fetal catecholamines rise rapidly in the fetal rat in response to insulin-induced maternal hypoglycemia[132] and may be elevated in some newborn humans with hypoglycemia.[133] These effects act to stimulate both fetal glycogenolysis and gluconeogenesis. During maternal starvation, depressed insulin secretion and elevated glucagon concentrations are noted in the sheep. Hypoglycemia in the fetal monkey, however, was not associated with changes in glucagon concentration.[134] The role that other potential glucose regulatory hormones, such as growth hormone or cortisol, play in defense against fetal hypoglycemia is not known.

The impact of fetal hypoglycemia on fetal metabolism, particularly fetal cerebral metabolism, has not been studied in great depth. As the principal cerebral substrate, glucose is of major importance in maintaining neuronal integrity. Postnatal hypoglycemic brain damage and resultant neuronal and white matter necrosis have been well documented. Theoretically, similar damage should result from fetal hypoglycemia as well. In sheep, however, modest hypoglycemia of 2- to 4-hours' duration produces no changes in fetal cerebral metabolic rate or in cerebral glucose uptake.[135] Richardson and co-workers[136] have proposed an enhancement of cerebral glucose transport in the fetus during hypoglycemia that may have protective value. In addition, fetal brain lactate, fatty acid, and ketone body oxidation are theoretically possible. These substrates could also serve as cerebral metabolic fuels during hypoglycemia induced by maternal malnutrition.[10] Such changes have been documented in studies of cerebral metabolism during hypoglycemia in newborn dogs.[137]

SUMMARY

This chapter includes reviews of basic concepts of studying metabolic function in the fetus, with examples and a summary of both organ and whole fetus information derived from *in vitro* and *in vivo* animal studies. Some discussion of the theoretical allometric relationship between metabolic rate and body mass is also noted. When available, information from human fetal studies has also been presented. In addition, the chapter discusses fetal carbohydrate metabolism, including glycogen deposition and breakdown, gluconeogenesis and potential interconversions of amino acids. Information is taken from studies using both direct and indirect means. Finally, several clinically relevant disorders and the fetal responses are presented, such as fetal hypoxia, maternal hyperglycemia, and maternal hypoglycemia. In conclusion, it is apparent that the fetal mammal in late gestation is able to partition growth and energy needs under most circumstances and through a variety of interconnected means to maintain some degree of homeostasis when the maternal milieu is altered adversely.

REFERENCES

1. Dawes GS: Foetal and Neonatal Physiology. Chicago, Year Book Medical Publishers, 1968.
2. Meschia G: Evolution of thinking in fetal respiratory physiology. Am J Obstet Gynecol *132*:806, 1978.
3. Battaglia FC, Meschia G: An Introduction to Fetal Physiology. New York, Academic Press, 1986.
4. Rudolph AM: Oxygenation in the fetus and neonate—a perspective. Semin Perinatol *8*:158, 1984.
5. Burd LI, et al: Placental production and foetal utilization of lactate and pyruvate. Nature *254*:210, 1975.
6. Bozzetti P, et al: Respiratory gases, acid base balance and lactate concentrations of the midterm human fetus. Biol Neonate *51*:188, 1987.
7. Economides DL, et al: Metabolic and endocrine findings in appropriate and small for gestational age fetuses. J Perinat Med *19*:97, 1991.
8. Pardi G, et al: Diagnostic value of blood sampling in fetuses with growth retardation. N Engl J Med *328*:692, 1993.
9. Adolph EF: Uptakes and uses of oxygen, from gametes to maturity: an overview. Respir Physiol *53*:135,1983.
10. Jones CT, Rolph TP: Metabolism during fetal life: a functional assessment of metabolic development. Physiol Rev *65*:357, 1985.
11. Guiang SF III, et al: The relationship between fetal arterial oxygen saturation and heart and skeletal muscle myoglobin concentrations in the ovine fetus. J Dev Physiol *19*:99, 1993.
12. Semple, SIK et al .The measurement of fetal liver T′$_2$ in utero before and after maternal oxygen breathing: progress towards a non-invasive measurement of fetal oxygenation and placental function. Magn Res Imag *19*:921,2001.
13. Rudolph AM, Heymann MA: Methods for studying the circulation of the fetus in utero. *In* Nathanielsz PW (ed):Animal Models in Fetal Medicine (I). Ithaca, NY, Perinatology Press, 1985, pp 1–58.
14. Jones PJH, et al:Validation of doubly labeled water for assessing energy expenditure in infants. Pediatr Res *21*:242, 1987.
15. Bonds DR, et al: Estimation of human fetal-placental unit metabolic rate by application of the Bohr principle. J Dev Physiol *8*:49, 1986.
16. Kleiber G: The Fire of Life:An Introduction to Animal Energetics. Huntington, NY, RE Krieger, 1975.
17. Heusner AA: Size and power in mammals. J Exp Biol *160*:25, 1991.

18. Hulbert AJ, Else PL: Mechanisms underlying the cost of living in animals. Annu Rev Physiol 62:207, 2000.

19. West GB, et al: A general model for the origin of allometric scaling laws in biology. Science: 276: 122, 1997.

20. West GB, et al: Allometric scaling of metabolic rate from molecules and mitochondria to cells and mammals. Proc Nat Acad Sci. 99:2473, 2002.

21. Hill JR, Rahimtulla KA: Heat balance and the metabolic rate of new-born babies in relation to environmental temperature; and the effect of age and of weight on basal metabolic rate. J Physiol. 180:239, 1965

22. Else PL: Oxygen consumption and sodium pump thermogenesis in a developing mammal. Am J Physiol Regul Integr Comp Physiol 261:R1575, 1991.

23. Senior AE: ATP synthesis by oxidative phosphorylation. Physiol Rev 68:177, 1988.

24. Braems G, Jensen A: Hypoxia reduces oxygen consumption of fetal skeletal muscle cells in monolayer culture. J Dev Physiol 16:209, 1991.

25. Edelstone DI: Fetal compensatory responses to reduced oxygen delivery. Semin Perinatol 8:184, 1984.

26. Jensen A, et al: Effects of reducing uterine blood flow on fetal blood flow distribution and oxygen delivery. J Dev Physiol 15:309, 1991.

27. Newman JP, et al: Hemodynamic and metabolic responses to moderate asphyxia in brain and skeletal muscle of late gestation fetal sheep. J Appl Physiol 88:82, 2000.

28. Berger R, et al: Cerebral energy metabolism in fetal guinea pigs during moderate maternal hypoxemia at 0.75 of gestation. J Dev Physiol 19:193, 1993.

29. Bristow J, et al: A preparation for studying liver blood flow, oxygen consumption, and metabolism in the fetal lamb in utero. J Dev Physiol 3:255, 1981.

30. Carter AM: Factors affecting gas transfer across the placenta and the oxygen supply to the fetus. J Dev Physiol 12:305, 1989.

31. Lackman F, et al: Fetal umbilical cord oxygen values and birth to placental weight ratio in relation to size at birth. Am J Obstet Gynecol 185:674, 2001.

32. Chessex P, et al: Relation between heart rate and energy expenditure in the newborn. Pediatr Res 15:1077, 1981.

33. Meier PR, et al: Fetal heart rate in relation to body mass. Proc Soc Exp Biol Med 172:107, 1983.

34. Lauger P: Electrogenic Ion Pumps. Sunderland, Sinauer Associates, 1991.

35. Elia M: Energy expenditure in the whole body. In Kinney JM, Tucker HN (eds): Energy Metabolism: Tissue Determinants and Cellular Corollaries. New York, Raven Press, 1992, pp 19–31.

36. Kelly JM, McBride BW: The sodium pump and other mechanisms of thermogenesis in selected tissues. J Nutr Soc 49:185, 1990.

37. Vatnick I, Bell AW: Ontogeny of fetal hepatic and placental growth and metabolism in sheep. Am J Physiol 263:R619, 1992.

38. Lotgering FK, et al: Maternal and fetal responses to exercise during pregnancy. Physiol Rev 65:1, 1985.

39. Chandler KD, et al: Effects of undernutrition and exercise during late pregnancy on uterine, fetal, and uteroplacental metabolism in the ewe. Br J Nutr 53:625, 1985.

40. Rurak DW, Gruber NC: The effect of neuromuscular blockade on oxygen consumption and blood gases in the fetal lamb. Am J Obstet Gynecol 145:258, 1983.

41. Mulder EJH, et al: Patterns of breathing movements in the near-term human fetus: relationship to behavioural states. Early Hum Dev 36:127, 1994.

42. Suguihara C, Bancalari E: Substance abuse during pregnancy: effects on respiratory function in the infant. Semin Perinatol 15:302, 1991.

43. Morrison JL, et al: Fetal behavioural state changes following maternal fluoxetine infusion in sheep. Brain Res Dev Brain Res 26:47, 2001.

44. Czikk MJ, et al: Sagittal sinus blood flow in the ovine fetus as a continuous measure of cerebral blood flow: relationship to behavioural state activity. Dev Brain Res 131:103, 2001.

45. Gagnon R: Stimulation of human fetuses with sound and vibration. Semin Perinatol 13:393, 1989.

46. Eller DP, et al: The effect of maternal intravenous glucose administration on fetal activity. Am J Obstet Gynecol 167:1071, 1992.

47. Ida T, et al: Effect of insulin on mitochondrial oxidative phosphorylation and energy charge of the perfused guinea pig liver. J Lab Clin Med 87:925, 1976.

48. Philipps AF, et al: Effects of fetal insulin secretory deficiency on metabolism in fetal lamb. Diabetes 35:964, 1986.

49. Fowden AJ, et al:. Regulation of gluconeogenesis by thyroid hormones in fetal sheep during late gestation. J Endocr 170:461, 2001.

50. Gilbert M: Origin and metabolic fate of plasma glycerol in the rat and rabbit fetus. Pediatr Res 11:95, 1977.

51. Gilbert M, et al: Glucose turnover rate during pregnancy in the conscious guinea pig. Pediatr Res 16:310, 1982.

52. Lasuncion MA, et al: Method for the study of metabolite transfer from rat mother to fetus. Biol Neonate 44:85, 1983.

53. Cetin I: Amino acid interconversions in the fetal-placental unit; the animal model and human studies in vivo. Pediatr Res 49:148, 2001.

54. Philipps AF, et al: Relationship between resting glucose consumption and insulin secretion in the ovine fetus. Biol Neonate 48:85, 1985.

55. Cetin I, et al: Fetal serine fluxes across fetal liver, hindlimb, and placenta in late gestation. Am J Physiol 263:E786, 1992.

56. Anand RS, et al: Effect of insulin-induced maternal hypoglycemia on glucose turnover in maternal and fetal sheep. Am J Physiol 238:E524, 1980.

57. Hay WW Jr, Sparks JW: Placental, fetal, and neonatal carbohydrate metabolism. Clin Obstet Gynecol 28:473, 1985.

58. Hay WW Jr: Glucose and lactate oxidation rates in the fetal lamb. Proc Soc Exp Biol Med 173:553, 1983.

59. Rosenblatt J, Wolfe RR: Calculation of substrate flux using stable isotopes. Am J Physiol 254:E526, 1988.

60. Mao CS, et al: Underestimation of gluconeogenesis by the [U-(13)C(6)] glucose method: effect of lack of isotope equilibrium. Am J Physiol Endocrinol Metab 282:E376, 2002.

61. Marconi AM, et al: An evaluation of fetal glucogenesis in intrauterine growth-retarded pregnancies. Metab Clin Exp 42:860, 1993.

62. Thorngren-Jerneck K, et al: Reduced postnatal cerebral glucose metabolism measured by PET after asphyxia in near term fetal lambs. J Neurosci Res 66:844, 2001.

63. Kok RD, et al: Metabolic information from the human fetal brain obtained with proton magnetic resonance spectroscopy. Am J Obstet Gynecol 185:1011, 2001.

64. Marconi AM, et al: The impact of gestational age and fetal growth on the maternal-fetal glucose concentration difference. Obstet Gynecol 87:937, 1996.

65. Bozzetti P, et al: The relationship of maternal and fetal glucose concentrations in the human from midgestation until term. Metabolism 37:358, 1988.

66. Marconi AM, et al: Impact of conceptus mass on glucose disposal rate in pregnant women. Am J Physiol 264:E514, 1993.

67. Devaskar SU, Mueckler MM: The mammalian glucose transporters. Pediatr Res 31:1, 1992.

68. Brown GK: Glucose transporters: structure, function and consequences of deficiency. J Inherit Metab Dis 23:237, 2000.

69. Haugel-de Mouzon S, et al: Developmental expression of Glut1 glucose transporter and c-fos genes in human placental cells. Placenta 15:35, 1994.

70. Hay WW Jr: Current topic: metabolic interrelationships of placenta and fetus. Placenta 16:19, 1995.

71. Jansson T, et al: Glucose transporter protein expression in human placenta throughout gestation and in intrauterine growth retardation. J Clin Endocrinol Metab 77:1554, 1993.

72. Crandell SS, et al: Effects of ovine maternal hyperglycemia on fetal regional blood flows and metabolism. Am J Physiol 249:E454, 1985.

73. Anderson MS, et al: Effects of selective hyperglycemia and hyperinsulinemia on glucose transporters in fetal ovine skeletal muscle. Am J Physiol Regulatory Integrative Comp Physiol 281:R1256, 2001.

74. Belke DD, et al: Insulin signaling coordinately regulates cardiac size, metabolism, and contractile protein isoform expression. J Clin Invest 109:629, 2002.

75. Philipps AF, et al: The effects of chronic fetal hyperglycemia on substrate uptake by the ovine fetus and conceptus. Pediatr Res 19:659, 1985.

76. Hay WW Jr, et al: Fetal glucose uptake and utilization as functions of maternal glucose concentration. Am J Physiol 246:E237, 1984.

77. Hay WW Jr: Placental transport of nutrients to the fetus. Horm Res 42:215, 1994.

78. Meschia G, et al: Utilization of substrates by the ovine placenta in vivo. Fed Proc 39:245, 1980.

79. Fowden AL, Comline RS: The effects of pancreatectomy on the sheep fetus in utero. Am J Exp Physiol 69:319, 1984.

80. Hay WW Jr, Meznarich HK: Use of fetal streptozotocin to determine the role of normal levels of fetal insulin in regulating uteroplacental and umbilical glucose exchange. Pediatr Res 24:312, 1988.

81. Morriss FH, et al: The glucose oxygen quotient of the term human fetus. Biol Neonate 25:44, 1975.

82. Apatu RSK, Barnes RJ: Blood flow to and the metabolism of glucose and lactate by the liver in vivo in fetal, newborn and adult sheep. J Physiol 436:431, 1991.

83. Lueder FL, et al: Chronic maternal hypoxia retards fetal growth and increases glucose utilization of select tissues in the rat. Metabolism 44:532, 1995.

84. Berger R, et al: Extension of the 2-deoxyglucose method to the fetus in utero: theory and normal values for the cerebral glucose consumption in fetal guinea pigs. J Neurochem 63:271, 1994.

85. Bier DM, et al: Measurement of "true" glucose production rates in infancy and childhood with 6,6 dideuteroglucose. Diabetes 26:1016, 1977.

86. Shelley HJ: Glycogen reserves and their changes at birth and in anoxia. Br Med Bull 17:137, 1961.

87. Bhavnani BR, et al: Regulation of rabbit fetal glycogen: effect of in utero fetal decapitation on the metabolism of glycogen in fetal heart, lung and liver. Biochem Cell Biol 64:405, 1986.

88. Jacquot R, Kretchmer N: Effect of fetal decapitation on enzymes of glycogen metabolism. J Biol Chem 239:1301, 1964.

89. Barash V, et al: Mechanism of placental glycogen deposition in diabetes in the rat. Diabetologia 24:63, 1983.

90. Hsu SD, et al: Maternal malnutrition does not affect fetal hepatic glycogen synthase ontogeny. Dig Dis Sci 38:1500, 1991.

91. Kaneta M, et al: Ovine fetal and maternal glycogen during fasting. Biol Neonate 60:215, 1991.

92. Fowden AL, et al: Developmental regulation of gluconeogenesis in the sheep fetus during late gestation. J Physiol 508:937, 1998.

93. Bismut H, Plas C: Role of serine biosynthesis and its utilization in the alternative pathway from glucose to glycogen during the response to insulin in cultured foetal-rat hepatocytes. Biochem J 276:577, 1991.

94. Maniscalco WM, et al: Development of glycogen and phospho lipid metabolism in fetal and newborn rat lung. Biochim Biophys Acta 530:33, 1978.
95. Bourbon JR, et al: Effect of platelet-activating factor on glycogen metabolism in fetal rat lung. Exp Lung Res 17:789, 1991.
96. Philipps AF, et al: Influence of exogenous glucagon on fetal glucose metabolism and ketone production. Pediatr Res 17:51, 1983.
97. Pere MC: Effects of meal intake on materno-foetal exchanges of energetic substrates in the pig. Reprod Nutr Dev 41:285, 2001.
98. Sparks JW, et al: Regulation of the rat liver glycogen synthesis and activities of glycogen cycle enzymes by glucose and galactose. Metabolism 25:47, 1976.
99. Wilson I, et al: Galactose production by fasting neonates. Pediatr Res 37:323A, 1995.
100. Raiha NCR, Lindros KO: Development of some enzymes involved in gluconeogenesis in human liver. Ann Med Exp Fenn 47:146, 1969.
101. Warnes DM, Seamark RF: The appearance of gluconeogenesis at birth in sheep. Biochem J 162:627, 1977.
102. Townsend SF, et al: Perinatal onset of hepatic gluconeogenesis in the lamb. J Dev Physiol 12:329, 1989.
103. Teng C, et al: Fetal hepatic and umbilical uptakes of glucogenic substrates during a glucagon-somatostatin infusion. Am J Physiol Endocrinol Metab 282:E542, 2002.
104. Peeters LL, et al: Blood flow to fetal organs as a function of arterial oxygen content. Am J Obstet Gynecol 35:637, 1979.
105. Towell ME, et al: The effect of mild hypoxemia maintained for twenty-four hours on maternal and fetal glucose, lactate, cortisol and arginine vasopressin in pregnant sheep. Am J Obstet Gynecol 157:1550, 1987.
106. Gardner DS, et al: A novel method for controlled and reversible long term compression of the umbilical cord in fetal sheep. J Physiol 535:217, 2001.
107. Harris AP, et al: Fetal cerebral and peripheral circulatory responses to hypoxia after nitric oxide synthase inhibition. Am J Physiol Regulatory Integrative Comp Physiol 281:R381, 2001.
108. Kiserud T, et al: Circulatory responses to maternal hyperoxaemia and hypoxaemia assessed non-invasively in fetal sheep at 0.3–0.5 gestation in acute experiments. Br J Obstet Gynecol 108:359, 2001.
109. Lehninger AL: Principles of Biochemistry. New York, Worth, 1982.
110. Bocking AD, et al: Oxygen consumption is maintained in fetal sheep during prolonged hypoxaemia. J Dev Physiol 17:169, 1992.
111. Boyle DW, et al: Metabolic adaptation of fetal hindlimb to severe, nonlethal hypoxia. Am J Physiol 263:R1130, 1992.
112. Assano H, et al: Cerebral metabolism during sustained hypoxemia in preterm fetal sheep. Am J Obstet Gynecol 170:939, 1994.
113. Lopaschuk GD, et al: Developmental changes in energy substrate use by the heart. Cardiovasc Res 26:1172, 1992.
114. Fisher DJ: Oxygenation and metabolism in the developing heart. Semin Perinatol 9:217, 1984.
115. Lowy C: Regulation of intrauterine growth: the role of maternal health. Horm Res 42:203, 1994.
116. Iwamoto HS, et al: Effects of acute hypoxemia on insulin-like growth factors and their binding proteins in fetal sheep. Am J Physiol 263:E1151, 1992.
117. Cohen WR, et al: Plasma catecholamines in the hypoxaemic fetal rhesus monkey. J Dev Physiol 9:507, 1987.
118. Light IJ, et al: Maternal intravenous glucose administration as a cause of hypoglycemia in the infant of the diabetic mother. Am J Obstet Gynecol 13:345, 1972.
119. Philipps AF, et al: Effects of chronic fetal hyperglycemia upon oxygen consumption in the ovine uterus and conceptus. J Clin Invest 74:279, 1984.
120. Susa JB, Schwartz R: Effects of hyperinsulinemia in the primate fetus. Diabetes 34(Suppl 2):36, 1985.
121. Hay WW Jr, et al: Effects of glucose and insulin on fetal glucose oxidation and oxygen consumption. Am J Physiol 256:E704, 1989.
122. Philipson EH, et al: Effects of maternal glucose infusion on fetal acid-base status in human pregnancy. Am J Obstet Gynecol 157:866, 1987.
123. Seeds JW, Peng TC: Does augmented growth impose an increased risk of fetal death? Am J Obstet Gynecol 183:316, 2000.
124. Rosenkrantz TS, et al: Cerebral metabolism and electrocortical activity in the chronically hyperglycemic fetal lamb. Am J Physiol 265:R1262, 1993.
125. Stonestreet BS, et al: Circulatory and metabolic effects of hypoxia in the hyperinsulinemic ovine fetus. Pediatr Res 38:67, 1995.
126. Weinstein MR, et al: Intravenous energy and amino acids in the preterm infant: effects of metabolic rate and potential mechanisms of action. J Pediatr 111:119, 1987.
127. Liechty EA, et al: Effect of hyperinsulinemia on ovine fetal leucine kinetics during prolonged maternal fasting. Am J Physiol 263:E696, 1992.
128. Milley JR: Exogenous substrate uptake by fetal lambs during reduced glucose delivery. Am J Physiol 264:E250, 1993.
129. Harding JE, et al: Effects of β-hydroxybutyrate infusion on hind limb metabolism in fetal sheep. Am J Obstet Gynecol 166:671, 1992.
130. Guillet-Deniau I, et al: Expression and cellular localization of glucose transporters (GLUT1, GLUT3, GLUT4) during differentiation of myogenic cells isolated from rat foetuses. J Cell Sci 107:487, 1994.
131. Takata K, et al: Localization of erythrocyte/HepG2-type glucose transporter (GLUT1) in human placental villi. Cell Tissue Res 267:407, 1992.
132. Phillippe M, Kitzmiller JL: The fetal and maternal catecholamine response to insulin-induced hypoglycemia in the rat. Am J Obstet Gynecol 139:407, 1981.
133. Cornblath M, Schwartz R: Disorders of Carbohydrate Metabolism in Infancy. Boston, Blackwell Scientific, 1991.
134. Chez RA, et al: Glucagon metabolism in nonhuman primate pregnancy. Am J Obstet Gynecol 120:690, 1974.
135. Bissonnette JM, et al: Effect of acute hypoglycemia on cerebral metabolic rate in fetal sheep. J Dev Physiol 7:421, 1985.
136. Richardson BS, et al: Cerebral metabolism in hypoglycemic and hyperglycemic fetal lambs. Am J Physiol 245:R730, 1983.
137. Hernandez MJ, et al: Cerebral blood flow and metabolism during hypoglycemia in newborn dogs. J Neurochem 35:622, 1980.
138. Assali NS, et al: Measurement of uterine blood flow and uterine metabolism. Am J Obstet Gynecol 79:86, 1960.
139. Behrman RE, et al: Distribution of the circulation in the normal and asphyxiated fetal primate. Am J Obstet Gynecol 108:956, 1970.
140. Comline RS, Silver M: Some aspects of foetal and utero-placental metabolism in cows with indwelling umbilical and uterine vascular catheters. J Physiol 260:571, 1976.
141. Moll W, et al: Gas exchange of the pregnant uterus of anesthetized and unanesthetized guinea pigs. Respir Physiol 8:303, 1970.
142. Silver M, Comline RS: Transfer of gases and metabolites in the equine placenta: a comparison with other species. J Reprod Fertil 23(Suppl):589, 1975.

Richard M. Cowett

49

Role of Glucoregulatory Hormones in Hepatic Glucose Metabolism During the Perinatal Period

Relative to metabolism in general and to carbohydrate (glucose) metabolism in particular, the neonate is considered to be in transition (a transitional state) between the complete dependence of the fetus and the complete independence of the adult.[1-3] The neonate must become independent after birth, by balancing between glucose deficiency and excess to maintain euglycemia. The dependence of the conceptus on the mother for continuous substrate delivery *in utero* contrasts with the variable and intermittent exogenous oral intake that is the hallmark of the neonatal period and beyond. Development of carbohydrate homeostasis results from a balance between the specific morbidities to which the neonate is subject and the multiplicity of factors involved in developing regulatory control. The maintenance of euglycemia especially in the sick or low birth weight neonate is difficult. This difficulty reinforces the concept that the neonate is vulnerable to disequilibrium. Because Chapters 46 to 48 discuss carbohydrate metabolism in the fetus, this chapter concentrates on the control of glucose homeostasis in the neonatal period by regulatory hormones.

INSULIN AND GLUCAGON INFLUENCES ON GLUCOSE HOMEOSTASIS

Numerous investigations have focused on the measurement of insulin and glucagon singly and in combination with each other relative to development of glucose homeostasis in the perinatal-neonatal period. Ktorza and associates[4] evaluated insulin and glucagon secretion during the perinatal period. They noted that insulin and glucagon are detected in most species early in gestation. The insulin/glucagon molar ratio is high in the fetus at term, but then it decreases dramatically after birth and remains low during the first hours after birth. This change favors glycogenolysis and gluconeogenesis after birth.

King and colleagues[5] studied postnatal development of insulin secretion in the premature neonate (26 to 30 weeks' gestation) for 110 days after birth and in the full-term neonate for up to 47 days after birth. Insulin was measured before and 30 minutes after the beginning of a glucose infusion given parenterally or enterally. The premature neonate evidenced a small response to glucose on day 1 that gradually increased over the course of the study. The full-term neonate was more responsive. The investigators concluded that the premature neonate may take up to 18 weeks to respond fully to an increase in plasma glucose concentration.

Ghiglione and associates[6] measured immunoreactive glucagon (IRG) levels in dogs between 12 hours and 60 days of age relative to four peaks (IRG >20,000, IRG 9000, IRG 3500, and IRG 2000) obtained by gel filtration. Changes with age were confined to IRG 9000 and IRG 3500. IRG 9000 was nine times higher in 12- to 36-hour-old dogs compared with adults (108± 24 pg/ml versus 12±3 pg/ml) and decreased to two times higher (27±5 pg/ml) at 31 to 60 hours. IRG 3500 was higher in the adult only during the first 36 hours after birth (36±5 pg/ml versus 15±3 pg/ml). Insulin infusion (0.2 U/kg intravenously) produced hypoglycemia, but no change was noted in any IRG component in the neonate. In response to an arginine infusion (0.5 g/kg over 15 minutes) there was an increase in plasma concentrations of IRG 9000 and 3500 in the neonate; however, only IRG 3500 increased in adults. There appeared to be an impaired secretory response to hypoglycemia in the neonate, a conclusion we return to later in this chapter.

Grasso and colleagues[7] infused either glucose (1 g/kg) or saline in 37 term and 35 preterm neonates and measured plasma glucagon, serum insulin, and blood glucose concentrations on the first day of life before feedings were initiated or during the first week after birth. Glucose infusion diminished plasma glucagon secretion by 61±6% in the term neonate and 38±4% in the preterm neonate. Serum insulin response to glucose infusion was variable, data that attest to the heterogeneity that exists in the neonatal period.

Mehta and associates[8] reported four neonates with severe hypoglycemia in whom the glucose production rate and the plasma concentrations of insulin and glucagon were measured. The hepatic glucose production rate was less than 20% of normal, and plasma insulin concentration was never greater than 12 μU/ml. Two of the four neonates had low plasma glucagon concentration as well (i.e., <60 pg/mL); however, a bolus infusion of glucagon restored the glucose production rate toward normal. In one neonate, use of diazoxide further depressed an already low plasma insulin concentration from 4.2 to 1.6 μU/ml. The investigators speculated that the insulin/glucagon ratio may be more important than the absolute concentration of insulin in controlling glucose metabolism.

OTHER COUNTERREGULATORY HORMONE INFLUENCES ON GLUCOSE HOMEOSTASIS

Glucocorticoids and insulin mediate the rate of glycogen accumulation in fetal life. In the presuckling period, muscle glycogenolysis supplies lactate moieties that are subsequently oxidized by neonatal tissue and act as alternative substrate until glucose and ketones are available. The subsequent increase in plasma catecholamines and the decrease in the insulin/glucagon ratio result in liver glycogenolysis and gluconeogenesis to maintain euglycemia postnatally. During suckling, oxidation of free fatty acids, ketone body utilization, and gluconeogenesis supply energy for anabolism. Subsequently, the increase in the insulin/glucagon ratio (which occurs during feeding) promotes lipogenesis.

Padbury and colleagues[9] evaluated the catecholamine surge at birth in the preterm and term lamb using an exteriorized fetal lamb preparation in which the former was treated with surfactant before the first breath. There were similar baseline concentrations of catecholamines and a marked rise in circulating epinephrine and norepinephrine in both groups after cord cutting. However, the preterm lamb evidenced a delayed but exaggerated elevation of both catecholamine concentrations compared with the term group. Changes in heart rate were less profound and more gradual. Likewise, a blunted elevation in blood glucose concentration was noted. These data suggest that the catecholamine surge at birth is an important adaptive physiologic response.

Hägnevik and associates[10] evaluated the immediate postnatal adaptation and sympathoadrenal activation in neonates delivered vaginally compared with those delivered by elective cesarean section. As expected, the vaginally delivered neonates evidenced higher catecholamine concentrations at birth compared with neonates delivered by cesarean section using either epidural or general anesthesia. Likewise, glucose concentration in the umbilical artery was higher in the former group compared with infants delivered by cesarean section. The investigators speculated that, given the marked differences in catecholamine concentrations, the differences in metabolic adaptation were unexpectedly small. This finding implied an attenuated metabolic response to sympathoadrenal stimulation in the neonate.

Finally, Gripois and colleagues[11] evaluated the interrelationships between thyroid secretion and adrenal medullary secretion in the neonatal rat. The adrenal medulla of normal, hypothyroid, and hyperthyroid rats were stimulated by insulin-induced hypoglycemia. In the euthyroid animal, insulin-induced epinephrine secretion increased during the first 10 days of postnatal life. Hypothyroidism retarded the development of that response, and hyperthyroidism accelerated the response. During adrenal medullary depletion after insulin-induced hypoglycemia, recovery was slower for the hyperthyroid animal than for the hypothyroid or euthyroid animal.

KINETIC ANALYSES OF HORMONAL CONTROL OF GLUCOSE HOMEOSTASIS

Kinetic analyses have been employed to evaluate hormonal control of neonatal glucose metabolism. Originally, an indirect technique of stepwise incremental glucose infusion was used to infer the rate of basal glucose output or glucose turnover in the neonate compared with the adult.[12] This inference was dependent on the assumption that the neonate was as sensitive as the adult to minimal changes in glucose concentration. Subsequently, studies in the puppy by Varma and associates[13] indicated that fine control is not developed during the neonatal period. Kornhauser and colleagues[14] first used the Steele steady-state infusion technique to show that basal glucose production in the newborn puppy was two to three times the adult rate when expressed per unit of body weight. The data of Varma and colleagues substantiated this observation.

Cowett and associates[15] hypothesized that the insensitivity of the hepatocyte to insulin appeared to have a dominant effect in controlling the turnover (i.e., production) rate of glucose. In the initial series of experiments, it was expected that the newborn lamb, unlike the adult sheep, would exhibit a developmentally blunted hepatic response with a persistent output of glucose in response to a glucose infusion. After a 7-hour fast, basal plasma glucose, insulin, and glucagon concentrations were determined in term (newborn) lambs and in adult sheep, after which the newborn lambs received 0, 5, 6, 11.7, or 21.7 mg glucose/kg/ minute over a period of 6 hours. Older sheep received either saline or 5.7 mg glucose/kg/minute. Glucose turnover was determined by the prime constant infusion technique of Steele using D-[6-³H]glucose. Both newborn and adult animals maintained a constant plasma glucose concentration and glucose-specific activity during the turnover period. Glucose production rates persisted in the term newborn lambs until an infusion rate of 21.7 mg/kg/minute was reached. In contrast, the adult lambs reduced the glucose production rate with a glucose infusion rate of 5.7 mg/kg/minute. At the point when the glucose production rate was significantly reduced, the plasma insulin concentration in the newborn lamb was fivefold greater than in the adult (270 µU/mL versus 56 µU/mL). Blunted hepatic responsiveness to insulin appeared to be a major factor explaining the inefficiency in glucose homeostasis in the neonatal lamb.

In these studies, hyperglycemia and hyperinsulinemia were produced simultaneously. Therefore, the effect of peripheral hyperinsulinemia could not be differentiated from that of hyperglycemia. Subsequently, varying concentrations of glucose and insulin were infused in six groups of newborn lambs for sufficient time to produce steady-state equilibrium conditions of euglycemia and hyperinsulinemia.[16] Glucose production rates and gluconeogenesis from lactate were measured. The latter was accomplished by determining the ratio of U-[¹⁴C]lactate/D-[6-³H]glucose (noted by "r" in (Fig. 49–1).

Increasing the rate of glucose infusion without administering insulin (Groups II and III) produced a stepwise increase in plasma glucose and insulin concentrations when compared with controls (Group I). Elevation of the plasma insulin concentration

induced by hyperglycemia was associated with a significant reduction in the glucose production rate, but it was seen only when marked hyperglycemia and hyperinsulinemia were achieved (Group III). With insulin administration, a significant and stepwise increase in plasma insulin concentration was observed, depending on the dose of insulin administered. By simultaneous glucose infusion, a state of euglycemia or hyperglycemia was produced with concomitant hyperinsulinemia. With a slight increase in plasma insulin (61 µU/mL; Group IV), a significant reduction in gluconeogenesis was noted, together with a slight but insignificant reduction in the rate of glucose production. When hyperinsulinemia was moderate to marked (236 and 481 µU/ml; Groups V and VI), there was a significant reduction of gluconeogenesis and the rate of glucose production. Insulin is known to inhibit glycogenolysis and gluconeogenesis (while enhancing glycogenesis), and it suppresses glucose production in the adult.[17-19] The data suggested that a moderate elevation of plasma insulin concentration effectively reduced gluconeogenesis (Groups II and IV) but did not influence the endogenous glucose production. The latter was reduced only when a much higher insulin concentration was achieved (Groups II, V, VI). The authors concluded that insulin, rather than glucose, controls the rate of glucose production in newborn lambs.[16]

In neither of the studies cited was the pancreatic β-cell secretory activity evaluated. It was subsequently hypothesized that the pancreatic β-cell response to glucose concentration was comparable in the term neonate and the older adult (i.e., secretory activity by the neonatal β-cell is normal). To confirm this hypothesis, a steady-state insulin secretion study was performed using [¹³¹I]insulin as the tracer.[20] Plasma glucose and insulin concentrations and insulin-specific activity were determined. Endogenous posthepatic insulin secretion and the metabolic clearance rate were derived in the spontaneously delivered term lamb, the betamethasone-treated preterm lamb, and the 4- to 5-month-old adult sheep. After a 7-hour fast, animals received 0.45% saline or glucose (5.7 mg/kg/min) for 6 hours, followed by the tracer insulin infusion for 11 minutes. The posthepatic insulin secretion rate was not different among any of the three groups—term, premature, or adult—under the influence of 0.45% saline infusion. Correspondingly similar posthepatic

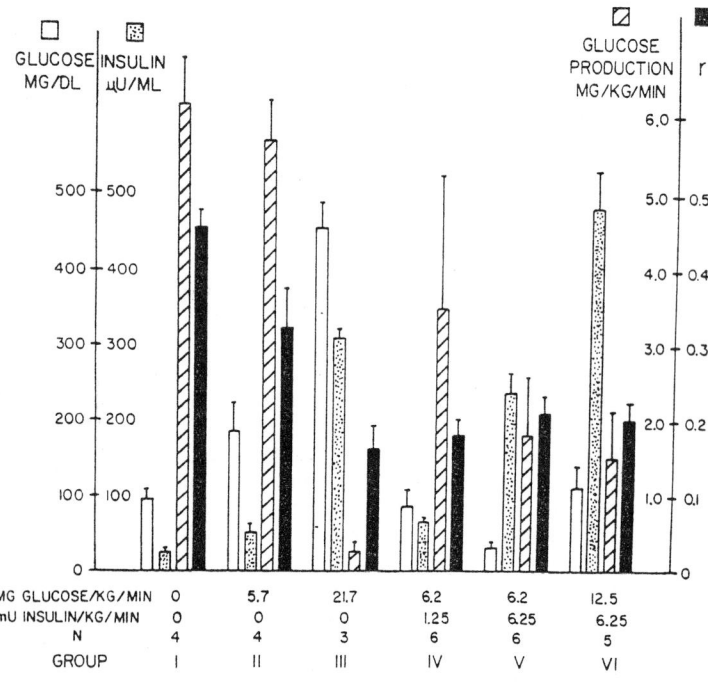

MG GLUCOSE/KG/MIN	0	5.7	21.7	6.2	6.2	12.5
mU INSULIN/KG/MIN	0	0	0	1.25	6.25	6.25
N	4	4	3	6	6	5
GROUP	I	II	III	IV	V	VI

Figure 49–1. Plasma glucose and plasma insulin concentrations, glucose production rates, and ratio of U-[¹⁴C]lactate/D-[6-³H]glucose for all groups. (From Susa JB, et al: Pediatr Res 13:594, 1979.)

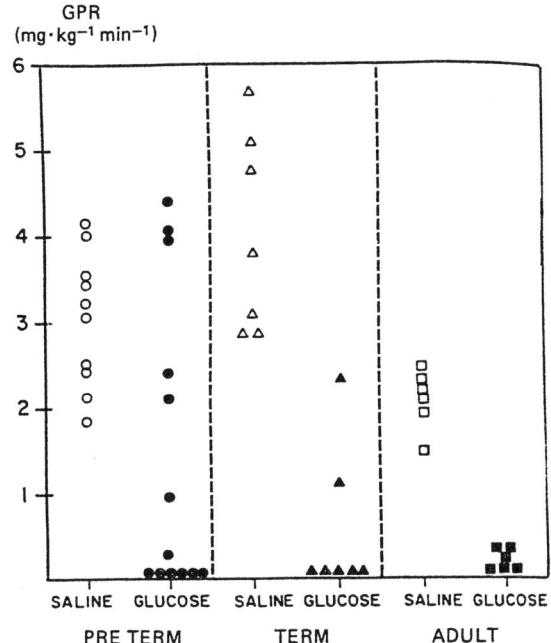

Figure 49–2. Glucose production rate (GPR) for each neonate and adult during saline or glucose infusion. (From Cowett RM, et al: J Clin Invest 71:467, 1983.)

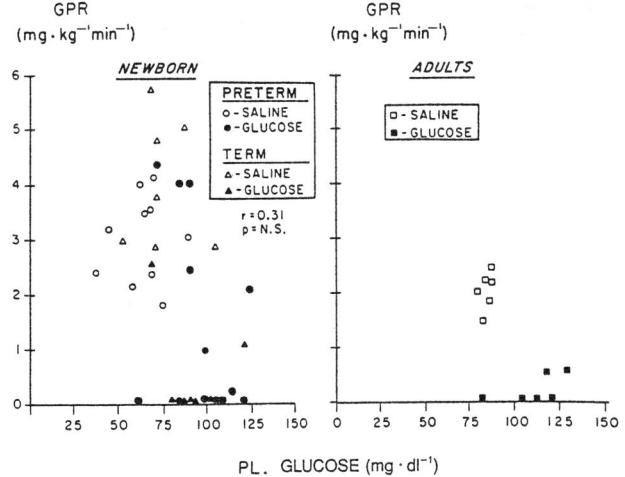

Figure 49–3. Correlation between the plasma glucose concentration during the turnover period and glucose production rate (GPR) in neonates and adults. (From Cowett RM, et al: J Clin Invest 71:467, 1983.)

insulin secretion rates were noted when the three groups were infused with 5.7 mg/kg/minute of glucose. The metabolic clearance rate was not different among the groups. The investigators concluded that the posthepatic insulin secretion rate and the metabolic clearance rate were similar in the term gestation lamb, the prematurely delivered lamb, and the 4- to 5-month-old adult sheep. It had been previously suggested that precise control of the rate of glucose production is characteristic of the mature (adult) animal, whereas the neonate evidences a decreased ability to suppress the rate of glucose production when glucose is infused. The investigators concluded that this immaturity may be explained by hepatic unresponsiveness to insulin in the neonate and is probably not related to secretory capacity of the pancreatic β-cell.

The neonatal lamb is metabolically comparable to the human, and it is frequently used to evaluate perinatal glucose homeostasis. However, kinetic studies in the human neonate are more

physiologically relevant. After the development of stable isotope methodology, it became possible to study the human neonate. Figure 49-2 depicts the glucose production rate for preterm and term neonates and adults who were studied using stable isotopes. Five of 13 preterm and 2 of 7 term neonates had persistent glucose production rates (>1 mg/kg/minute) during glucose infusion. In contrast, the glucose production rate in adults was not measurable. There was no correlation between plasma glucose concentration and the glucose production rate in the neonate or the adult (Fig. 49-3). Both the neonate and the adult demonstrated a correlation between the plasma insulin concentration and the glucose production rate. However, there was considerable variability in the neonate (Fig. 49-4). These data suggest that there are significant developmental differences in neonatal glucose homeostasis and that insulin is important in neonatal hormonal control of glucose production.[21]

The studies described earlier raise the question of when the neonate develops maturation (i.e., adultlike control) of glucose homeostasis. As noted previously, suppression of the endogenous glucose production rate (Ra) is the adult response to glucose infusion. Persistent endogenous glucose production (i.e., ≥1 mg/kg/minute or <80% decrease in Ra) in response to glucose

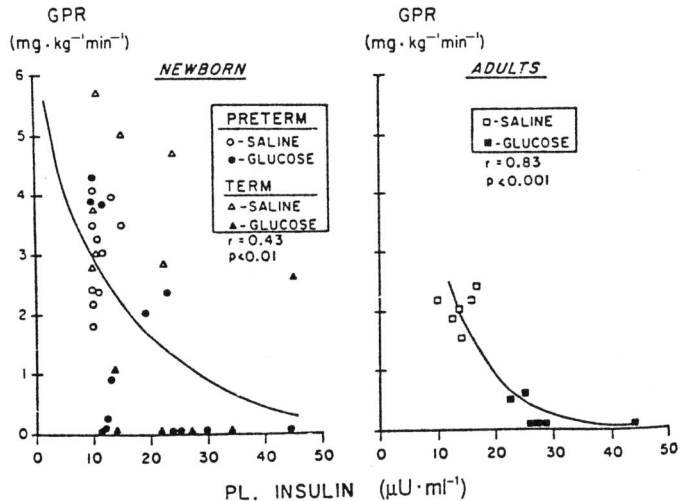

Figure 49–4. Correlation between the peripheral plasma insulin concentration during the turnover period and glucose production rate (GPR) in neonates and adults. (From Cowett RM, et al: J Clin Invest 71:467, 1983.)

infusion is evidence of a transitional homeostatic state in the neonate during the first days after birth. To determine when an adultlike response developed, Ra was measured in 11 prematurely born neonates (33±0.3 weeks) at 2 to 5 weeks after birth. In these paired studies, 4 µg/kg/minute D-[U-13C]glucose tracer was infused by prime constant infusion to determine Ra, during saline or glucose infusion, the latter at a rate of 5.3± 0.2 mg/kg/minute. In comparison with the saline infusion turnover period, the plasma glucose concentration increased significantly during the glucose infusion turnover period, from 88±3 to 101±4 mg/dl. Plasma insulin concentration remained unchanged (12±5 µU/ml versus 8±3 µU/ml). Ra was heterogeneous during glucose infusion, and persistent Ra was present in 6 of 11 neonates (Fig. 49–5). Of the 5 infants who showed decreased Ra during glucose infusion, 3 received glucose at a rate exceeding basal Ra. Of the remaining 6 infants who evidenced persistent Ra during glucose infusion, 3 received glucose at a rate equal to or in excess of basal Ra. These data suggest that glucose homeostasis in low birth weight infants is transitional throughout the neonatal period.[22]

A decreased response to epinephrine in the neonate (a decreased rate of production and decreased plasma glucose concentration) has been reported.[23, 24] This lack of response to epinephrine has been correlated with the lack of response to insulin discussed earlier. It is possible, as noted by Hetenyi and colleagues,[25] that the decreased neonatal response to insulin and other hormones (e.g., glucagon or epinephrine) may protect the neonate from rapid fluctuations in substrate supply and may ensure ready availability of glucose for the developing brain. Diminished responsiveness to both insulin and counterregulatory hormones should assist in maintaining glucose homeostasis in the neonate. More recent studies examined the hypothesis that the imprecise control of glucose production by insulin is mirrored by a corresponding lack of response to the various counterregulatory hormones. Thirty spontaneously delivered term lambs were studied after administration of radiolabeled isotope by the primed constant infusion technique to measure glucose kinetics. Infusion of 2.0 mU/kg/minute insulin produced hyperinsulinemic hypoglycemia. Endogenous insulin, glucagon, and growth hormone release were blocked by administration of somatostatin. The addition of metyrapone blocked cortisol release. The controls received only the isotope. The results suggested that insulin exerted a greater effect on glucose uptake than on glucose production. Glucagon, growth hormone, and cortisol did not affect the Ra during hyperinsulinemic hypoglycemia. The imprecise effect of these counterregulatory hormones on neonatal glucose production mirrors the previously documented imprecise control by insulin.[26]

INSULIN RESISTANCE AND SENSITIVITY IN THE NEONATE

Lack of the precise control of glucose homeostasis in the human neonate has been postulated as secondary to either a decreased sensitivity or resistance to insulin.[21, 27] Although methods for assessing insulin resistance have varied considerably, most studies only evaluated the insulin effect on plasma glucose concentration in the hyperglycemic, stressed neonate.[28–34] Fewer studies have evaluated the effects of insulin on glucose production in the healthy term or preterm neonate.[21,28,35]

Hulman and Kliegman[36] and Kliegman and colleagues[37] are credited with the initial use of the euglycemic hyperinsulinemic clamp in the neonatal period in a beagle puppy model.[38] Graded insulin infusions ranging from 3.75 to 100 mU/kg/minute were used to generate a dose-response curve. The adult group had complete suppression of glucose production, whereas an 80% reduction was achieved in the newborn puppy group. They attributed a lack of complete suppression of glucose production

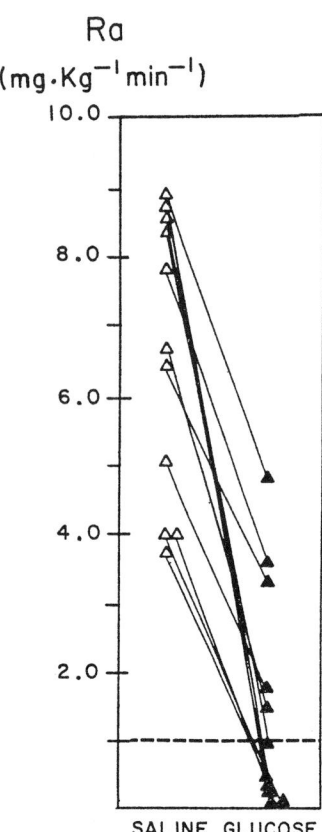

Figure 49–5. Endogenous glucose production rate (Ra) during saline and glucose infusion. (From Cowett RM, et al: J Pediatr *112*:462, 1988.)

in the neonate to hepatic resistance to insulin and persistent gluconeogenesis.

Kahn[39] defined insulin resistance and provided a distinction between insulin insensitivity and insulin unresponsiveness. In the former, there is a shift to the right of insulin dose response curve such that a higher concentration of insulin is necessary to produce a half-maximal effect, with a maximal effect achieved eventually. This is usually the result of decreased affinity or a decreased concentration of insulin receptors. During insulin unresponsiveness, all responses to insulin are reduced (including the maximal response), but the dose-response relationship that exists is normal (i.e., the insulin concentration required to produce a half-maximal response) is normal. This is usually the result of a postreceptor defect. A combination of both forms of insulin resistance may exist simultaneously so a higher insulin concentration would be required to produce a half-maximal effect, and the maximal effect would be reduced compared with that of a normal response.

Farrag and colleagues[40] performed the euglycemic hyperinsulinemic clamp in the human preterm neonate to evaluate insulin sensitivity in the neonatal period. As noted in Figure 49–6, hepatic glucose production was reduced in the preterm neonate at a relatively low insulin concentration. This effect did not significantly change, despite the use of higher insulin infusion rates that resulted in as much as 10-fold higher plasma insulin concentrations. The percentage of reduction of endogenous glucose production ranged from 41 to 58% of basal rates, and persistent glucose production (i.e., ≥1 mg/kg/minute) during steady-state insulin infusion was noted throughout the study. If one considers complete suppression of glucose production to be the maximal effect of insulin on the liver, the data demonstrate that this maximal effect could not be reached in the

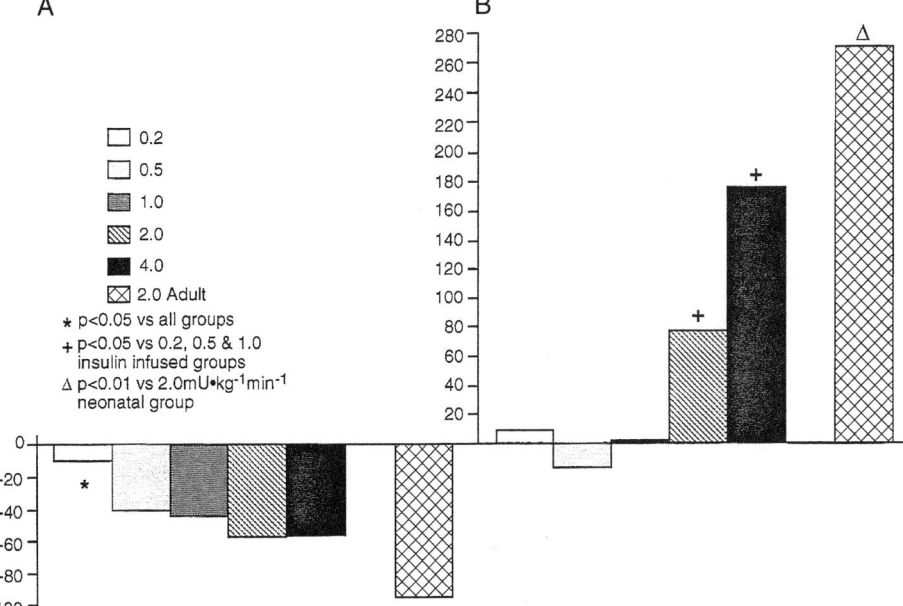

Figure 49–6. The percentage of decrease in endogenous glucose production and the percentage of increase in glucose utilization subdivided by the various insulin infusion rates that were administered to the neonate as well as the 2 mU/kg/minute insulin rate that was administered to the adult. (From Farrag HM, et al: Am J Physiol 272:E86, 1997.)

human preterm neonate. This pattern of response to insulin is most consistent with a postreceptor defect.[41] This mechanism may include factors at the membrane level (aside from receptor concentration and affinity) such as (1) the state of aggregation of the receptor, (2) its ability to interact with other membrane proteins required for signal generation, or (3) a variety of intracellular factors including all the events that occur at steps distal to the membrane. This includes the stimulatory or inhibitory effect of insulin on glucose transporters or key enzymes in the glycolytic, glycogenolytic, or gluconeogenic pathways. Decreased receptor concentration or affinity is an unlikely explanation because, at least in the human adult, there are plenty of "spare" insulin receptors available after the number of receptor sites required to achieve a maximal response is occupied.[36, 42] Second, there is an increase in both receptor concentration and affinity in the human neonate compared with that in the adult.[43] Finally, a reduction in receptor concentration to less than that required for a maximal response will result not only in decreased responsiveness, but also in decreased sensitivity, which was not apparent in the present investigation.[39]

In the studies by Farrag noted earlier, a significant increase in peripheral glucose utilization from basal rates occurred at insulin infusion rates of 2 and 4 mU/kg/minute.[40] It was not possible to determine whether a maximal effect on glucose utilization was achieved, because a plateau was not reached. The data denote a significant increase in glucose utilization at a higher insulin concentration than that required to reduce the rate of glucose production significantly (Fig. 49–7). Even though that plateau was not ultimately reached at these insulin infusion rates, the neonatal glucose utilization response to insulin, even at a lower plasma insulin concentration, far exceeded that reported in the literature as the maximal response in the adult.[42]

The indirect effect of insulin on endogenous glucose production has been evaluated.[44] Inhibition of lipolysis (in adipose tissue) and reduction of free fatty acid concentrations were shown to act as signals to the liver to suppress endogenous glucose production. This particular issue is of current interest, but the limited amount of adipose tissue in the preterm neonate may potentially interfere with the indirect effect of insulin on endogenous glucose production.

As noted previously, Goldman and Hirata[31] suggested that an attenuated response to insulin in the very low birth weight neonate is the reason for the occurrence of hyperglycemia. They attributed this response to insulin resistance rather than lack of the β-cell response. In contrast, abrupt and sustained improvement in glucose tolerance has been reported in response to short-term and long-term insulin infusions.[28-34] Higher insulin infusion rates and plasma insulin concentrations were reported in these studies than in the present study, and no evaluation of glucose production or glucose utilization was documented.

An approximate 50% reduction in glucose production has been reported in response to an exogenous glucose infusion rate of ~4 to 6 mg/kg/minute (i.e., similar to the basal glucose production rate in the neonate) that resulted in a plasma insulin concentration of approximately 19 mU/ml.[22, 35] The literature is unclear whether this reduction in glucose production is primarily a response to a higher plasma insulin concentration or plasma glucose concentration.[21, 35] Kalhan and associates[35] suggested that the decline in the glucose production is secondary to a higher plasma glucose concentration.

The data of Farrag and colleagues[40] are in accord with those reported by Hertz and associates,[45] relative to a strong positive correlation between plasma insulin concentration and glucose utilization. Hertz and associates noted a complete suppression of glucose production in stable, extremely premature infants when a high glucose infusion rate (i.e., 9.5 mg/kg/minute) was used. The glucose load resulted in a significant increase in both plasma glucose and insulin concentrations. At a similar plasma insulin concentration, a 41% reduction in glucose production was noted, so the combined effect of glucose and insulin seems necessary for complete suppression of glucose production. In contrast, a more recent investigation from that laboratory suggested that infusion of glucose at a rate of 5.5 mg/kg/minute resulted in a 90% suppression of glucose production during intravenous infusion administered with or without lipid.[46] Suppression was achieved at a glucose concentration of approximately 90 mg/dL and an extremely low insulin concentration of approximately 6 μU/mL. The mechanisms that explain the dichotomy that exists in the two data sets are unclear.

It is difficult to compare neonatal with adult data, especially when basal glucose production rates, glucose utilization rates, and plasma insulin concentrations are different. Similar to the adult, there is a strong positive linear correlation between plasma insulin concentration and the glucose utilization rate.

A

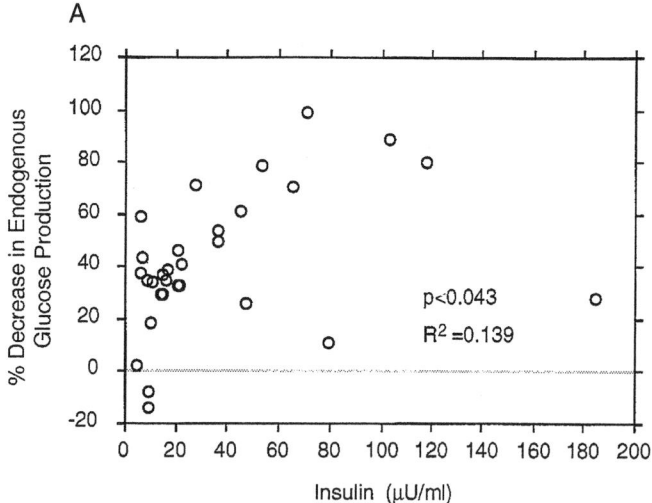

B

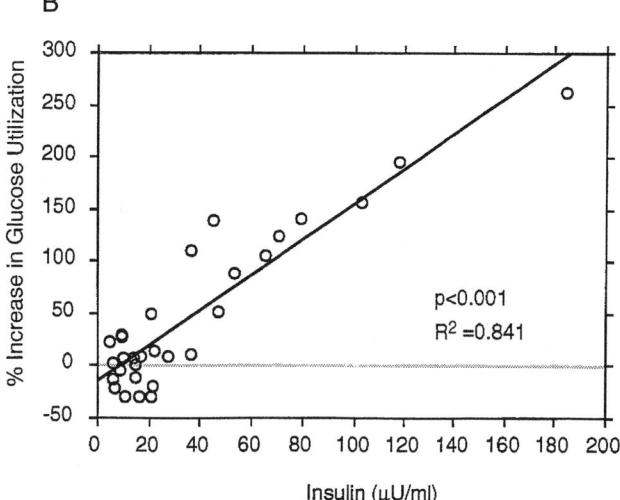

Figure 49–7. A, Regression correlating the percentage of decrease in endogenous glucose production relative to plasma insulin concentration in the neonate. **B,** Regression correlating the percentage of increase in glucose utilization relative to plasma insulin concentration in the neonate. (From Farrag HM, et al: Am J Physiol *272*:E86, 1997.)

The insulin effect on the glucose production rate begins at a lower insulin concentration than that required for the glucose utilization rate. If one calculates insulin sensitivity at euglycemia (that is not confounded by non—insulin-mediated glucose utilization[47]), it is apparent that the neonate has a greater peripheral sensitivity to insulin compared with the adult. This may result from a higher receptor concentration and affinity, provided the postreceptor cascade is intact peripherally. Conversely, unlike in the adult, complete suppression of glucose production could not be achieved in the human neonate by Farrag and colleagues.

Gelardi and associates[48] used a lamb/sheep model and performed the euglycemic hyperinsulinemic clamp studies at two specific ages: 3- to 6-day-old lambs and 31- to 35-day-old sheep. Initially, the younger animals needed a greater rate of glucose infusion (15.87±3.47 mg/kg/minute, $p < .05$) to maintain euglycemia compared with the older animal group (4.30±1.11 mg/kg/minute, receiving the same amount of insulin (100 mU/kg/minute). In fact, endogenous glucose production persisted in both groups; however, the percentage of decrease compared with aged-matched controls receiving no insulin was greater in the younger group compared with the older group (53%, $p < .001$,

versus 34%, $p < .01$). The younger animals evidenced greater glucose utilization compared with the older animals (215% versus 90%, respectively; $p < .01$) (Fig. 49–8). Similar to data in the human neonate, endogenous glucose production was not completely suppressed in the lamb despite very high plasma insulin concentrations. The younger animal group appeared to be more responsive to insulin, resulting in a significantly greater percentage of decrease in endogenous glucose production than in the older animals. The older animals also required significantly lower glucose infusion rates to maintain euglycemia during insulin infusion compared with the 3- to 6-day-old lambs. These data are consistent with data from human preterm neonates who exhibited persistent glucose production and greater peripheral sensitivity to insulin.

The appropriate distribution of whole body glucose is, at least in part, regulated by the tissue-specific expression and regulation of several glucose transporter isoforms with distinct kinetic properties. GLUT2 is the major glucose transporter isoform expressed in hepatocytes, β-cells, and the kidney. The distinguishing feature of this isoform is that it is a low-affinity, high-turnover transport system. GLUT2 forms part of a glucose-sensing apparatus that responds to subtle changes in blood glucose uptake with alterations in the rate of glucose uptake into the cell. GLUT4 glucose transporter is expressed in adipocytes and muscle cells. These are the "insulin-sensitive" cell types, so called because they respond to insulin with a rapid and reversible increase in glucose transport. Glucose transport in insulin-sensitive tissues has received attention because of the importance of this process in the maintenance of whole body glucose homeostasis.[49]

In the study by Gelardi and associates, there appeared to be a developmental increase in GLUT2 in the older animal groups versus the neonatal groups ($p < .05$). This increase may signal the onset of an insulin-resistant state in the ruminant.[50] After an initial decrease, GLUT2 expression increased with time. The reduction in the expression of GLUT2 with euglycemic hyperinsulinemia is in agreement with clamp studies in the diabetic rat. However, acute euglycemic hyperinsulinemia caused no change in the expression of GLUT4. This finding is consistent with previous studies showing that acute hyperinsulinemia does not regulate GLUT4 expression.[51] We speculated that changes in GLUT4 expression are not directly responsible for the changes in insulin sensitivity (Fig. 49–9). Increased GLUT2 expression with age, as well as decreased expression with hyperinsulinemia, is consistent with the development of an insulin-resistant state in the adult.

SUBSTRATE AVAILABILITY IN THE NEONATE

Several investigations have focused on the differential effects of substrate availability versus physiologic hormonal control in the human.[52-54] In the adult, Jahoor and associates[52] suggested that reduction in glucose turnover after an 86-hour fast was not secondary to a lack of gluconeogenic substrates. Conversely, dependence of gluconeogenesis on an adequate supply of precursors was demonstrated. When dichloroacetate was used to reduce lactate and alanine concentrations, a decrease in the rate of glucose production was observed. Bennish and associates[53] suggested that defective gluconeogenesis was the origin of the hypoglycemia in older children with diarrhea. Haymond and colleagues[54] studied differences in circulating gluconeogenic substrates in men, women, and children subjected to short-term fasting and suggested that differences in glucose requirements among the three groups could be responsible for the differences noted in plasma substrate responses to fasting. The men and women evidenced nearly identical plasma lactate and pyruvate concentrations, whereas the initial venous lactate and pyruvate concentrations were highest in children and increased during the 6 hours of fasting. The investigators speculated that lactate

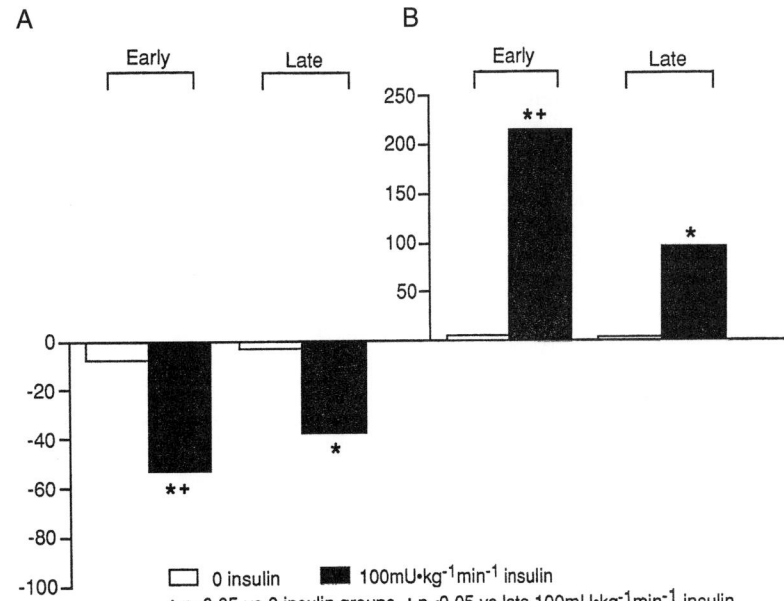

Figure 49–8. The percentage of decrease in endogenous glucose production (**A**) and the percentage of increase in glucose utilization (**B**) during the clamp period in the early and late groups. (From Gelardi NL: Am J Physiol *277*:E1142, 1999.)

production may be accelerated in the pediatric patient, assuming normal hepatic substrate uptake. Neonates were not studied in that investigation. Cowett and Wolfe evaluated the potential for gluconeogenesis from lactate and found it to be accelerated in the preterm neonate compared with the adult.[55] They speculated that substrate acquisition may not be the primary problem in the neonate.

One of the issues of substrate availability related to glucose homeostasis involves the effect of glucose (with or without other substrates) on glucose production. In one series of investigations, the Ra was negligible under conditions in which glucose was infused as part of the hyperalimentation mixture before administration of an intravenous fat emulsion.[56] However, there is still a clear dichotomy in data evaluating the ability of the neonate to diminish endogenous glucose production, which occurs regularly in the adult.[27] In studies in the term neonate,[21,22] the infant of the diabetic mother,[57] and the premature neonate,[21] persistent endogenous glucose production greater than 1.0 mg/kg/minute

was reported in response to administration of exogenous glucose infusion alone. Similar results were observed in the newborn canine model using the euglycemic hyperinsulinemic clamp technique.[36] Other investigators, using different techniques such as the glucose clamp[58] or glucose and amino acid infusion,[59] reported no persistent endogenous glucose production in the neonate. In the latter instance, both an amino acid mixture and a relatively moderate rate of glucose was infused (~8 mg/kg/minute). As pointed out by Lafeber and colleagues,[59] suppression may be incomplete under conditions in which insufficient glucose is administered or it is the sole constituent of the infusate. The data reported in another study supports this latter conclusion. No endogenous glucose production was noted when 6.8 mg/kg/minute was administered during the basal state with amino acids or after administration of glucose, amino acids, and the intravenous fat emulsion combined.[56] Certainly, further work is necessary to determine whether the quantity of glucose administered or the addition of amino acids or lipid emulsion is the

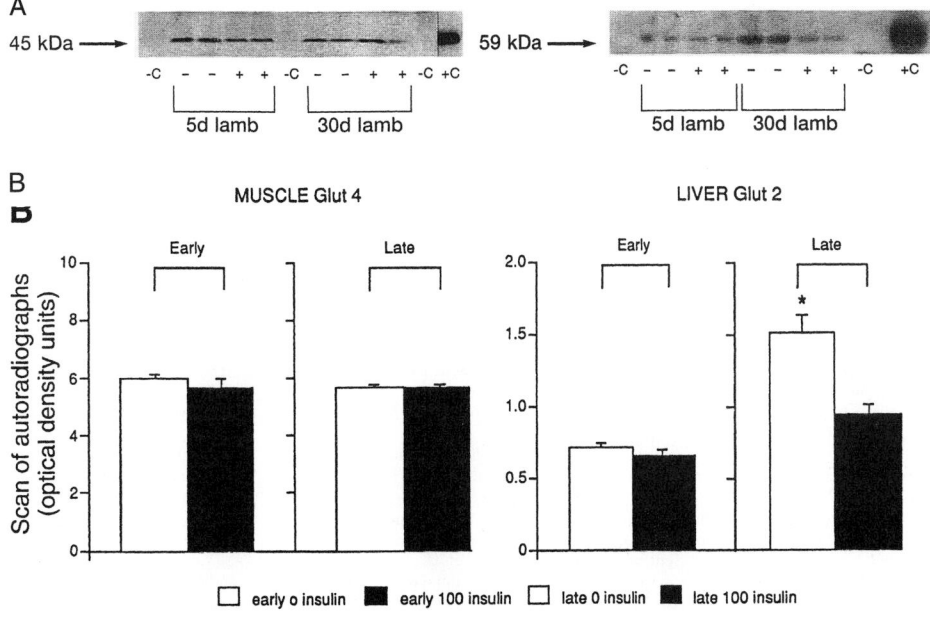

Figure 49–9. A, Representative Western blots for muscle (*left*) and liver (*right*) of 5- and 30-day-old 0 (-) and 100 (+) insulin-infused groups, showing also positive (+C) rat membrane and negative (-C) protein controls. **B,** Results of scans of autoradiograms from Western blots for muscle (*left*) and liver (*right*) for early and late groups. (From Gelardi NL: Am J Physiol *277*:E1142, 1999.)

primary cause of the observed decline in endogenous glucose production in the neonate. Furthermore, the relative role of each of these substrates as a secretagogue for insulin is unknown. Such studies should assist in differentiating hormonal control of neonatal glucose metabolism from availability of substrate as a limiting factor in homeostatic maturation.

In another study, Cowett and associates investigated whether glucose alone tightly controls neonatal glucose homeostasis.[60] Fifteen spontaneously delivered term lambs were studied after receiving radiolabeled glucose as the isotope to measure glucose production. After a baseline period, five lambs received 8.5 mg/kg/minute glucose in combination with the following to isolate the contribution of glucose: somatostatin to block insulin, glucagon, and growth hormone release; metyrapone to block cortisol release; phentolamine to block α-adrenergic release; and propranolol to block β-adrenergic release. Under conditions of glucose infusion at a rate 49% greater than the basal rate, the endogenous glucose production persisted; there was only an evanescent decrease compared with that of the control group that was not statistically different over time. As a substrate, glucose did not tightly control neonatal glucose homeostasis.[60]

In conclusion, it is apparent that hormonal control by glucoregulatory hormones (including insulin and the various counterregulatory hormones) and possibly glucose play a significant role in the developing regulation of glucose homeostasis in the neonatal period. Further research will be required to determine the relative contribution of the multiplicity of factors important in the development of carbohydrate(glucose) homeostasis in the neonatal period.

REFERENCES

1. Cowett RM, Farrag HM: Neonatal glucose metabolism. *In* Cowett RM (ed): Principles of Perinatal Neonatal Metabolism, 2nd ed. New York, Springer-Verlag, 1998, p 683.
2. Farrag HM, Cowett RM: Glucose homeostasis in the micropremie. Clin Perinatol 27:1, 2000.
3. Mayor F, Cuezva JM: Hormonal and metabolic changes in the perinatal period. Biol Neonate 48:185, 1985.
4. Ktorza A, et al: Insulin and glucagon during the perinatal period secretion and metabolic effects on the liver. Biol Neonate 48:204, 1985.
5. King RA, et al: Long term postnatal development of insulin secretion in early premature neonates. Early Hum Dev 13:285, 1986.
6. Ghiglione M, et al: Plasma glucagon immunoreactive components in early life in dogs. Horm Metab Res 17:387, 1985.
7. Grasso S, et al: Inhibiton of glucagon secretion in the human newborn by glucose infusion. Diabetes 32:498, 1983.
8. Mehta A, et al: Effect of diazoxide or glucagon on hepatic glucose production rate during extreme neonatal hypoglycemia. Arch Dis Child 62:924, 1987.
9. Padbury JF, et al: Neonatal adaptation greater sympathoadrenal response in preterm than full term fetal sheep at birth. Am J Physiol 248:E443, 1985.
10. Hägnevik K, et al: Catecholamine surge and metabolic adaptation in the newborn after vaginal delivery and cesarean section. Acta Paediatr Scand 73:602, 1984.
11. Gripois D, et al: Adrenal medullary responses to insulin induced hypoglycemia in the young rat: influence of thyroid hormones. J Auton Nerv Syst 15:165, 1986.
12. Adam PAJ, et al: Model for the investigation of intractable hypoglycemia: insulinglucose interrelationship during steady state infusions. Pediatrics 41:9l, 1968.
13. Varma S, et al: Homeostasis response to glucose loading in newborn and young dogs. Metabolism 22:l367, 1973.
14. Kornhauser D, et al: Glucose production and utilization in the newborn puppy. Pediatr Res 4:120, 1974.
15. Cowett RM, et al: Endogenous glucose production during constant glucose infusion in the newborn lamb. Pediatr Res 12:853, 1978.
16. Susa JB, et al: Suppression of gluconeogenesis and endogenous glucose production by exogenous insulin administration in the newborn lamb. Pediatr Res 13:594, 1979.
17. Clark MG, et al: Gluconeogenesis in isolated intact lamb liver cells. Biochem J 156:671, 1976.
18. Curnow RT, et al: Control of hepatic glycogen metabolism in the rhesus monkey: effect of glucose, insulin, and glucagon administration. Am J Physiol 228:E8O, 1975.
19. Owen OE, et al: Gluconeogenesis in normal, cirrhotic and diabetic humans. *In* Hanson RW, Mehlman MA (eds): Gluconeogenesis: Its Regulation in Mammalian Species. New York, Wiley Interscience, 1965, p 533.
20. Cowett RM, et al: Endogenous post-hepatic secretion and metabolic clearance rates in the neonatal lamb. Pediatr Res 14:1391, 1980.
21. Cowett RM, et al: Persistent glucose production during glucose infusion in the human neonate. J Clin Invest 71:467, 1983.
22. Cowett RM, et al: Ontogeny of glucose homeostasis in low birth weight infants. J Pediatr 112:462, 1988.
23. Cowett RM: Decreased response to catecholamines in the newborn: effect on glucose kinetics in the lamb. Metabolism 37:736, 1988.
24. Cowett RM: Alpha adrenergic agonists stimulate neonatal glucose production less than beta adrenergic agonist in the lamb. Metabolism 37:83, 1988.
25. Hetenyi C, et al: Plasma glucagon in pups, decreased by fasting, unaffected by somatostatin or hyperglycemia. Am J Physiol 231:1377, 1976.
26. Cowett RM, et al: Insulin counterregulatory hormones are ineffective in neonatal hyperinsulinemic hypoglycemia. Metabolism 48:568, 1999.
27. Wolfe R, et al: Glucose metabolism in man: responses to intravenous glucose infusion. Metab Clin Exp 28:210, 1979.
28. Pollak A, et al: Glucose disposal in low birth weight infants during steady state hyperglycemia: effects of exogenous insulin administration. Pediatrics 61:546, 1978.
29. Ostertag SG, et al: Insulin pump therapy in the very low birth weight infant. Pediatrics 78:625, 1986.
30. Vaucher YE, et al: Continuous insulin infusion in hyperglycemic very low birth weight infants. J Pediatr Gastroenterol Nutr 2:211, 1982.
31. Goldman SL, Hirata T: Attenuated responses to insulin in very low birth weight infants. Pediatr Res 14:50, 1980.
32. Heron P, Boucher D: Insulin infusion in infants of birthweight less than 1250 g and with glucose tolerance. Aust Paediatr J 24:362, 1988.
33. Binder ND, et al: Insulin infusion with parenteral nutrition in extremely low birth weight infants with hyperglycemia. J Pediatr 114:273, 1989.
34. Collins JW, et al: A controlled trial of insulin infusion an parenteral nutrition in extremely low birth weight infants with glucose intolerance. J Pediatr 118:921, 1991.
35. Kalhan SC, et al: Role of glucose in the regulation of endogenous glucose production in the human newborn. Pediatr Res 20:49, 1986.
36. Hulman SE, Kliegman RM: Assessment of insulin resistance in newborn beagles with the euglycemic hyperinsulinemic clamp. Pediatr Res 25:219, 1989.
37. Kliegman R, et al: Effects of euglycemic hyperinsulinemia on neonatal canine hepatic and muscle metabolism. Pediatr Res 25:124, 1989.
38. DeFronzo RA, et al: Glucose clamp technique: a method for quantifying insulin secretion and resistance. Am J Physiol 237:E214, 1979.
39. Kahn CR: Insulin resistance, insulin insensitivity and insulin unresponsiveness: a necessary distinction. Metab Clin Exp 27:1893, 1978.
40. Farrag HM, et al: Persistent glucose production and greater peripheral sensitivity to insulin in the neonate vs. the adult. Am J Physiol 272:E86, 1997.
41. Kono T, Barham FW: The relationship between the insulin-binding capacity of fat cells and the cellular response to insulin: studies with intact and trypsintreated fat cells. J Biol Chem 246:6210, 1971.
42. Rizza RA, et al: Dose response characteristics for effects of insulin on production and utilization of glucose in man. Am J Physiol 240:E630, 1981.
43. Thorsson AV, Hintz RL: Insulin receptors in the newborn: increase in receptor affinity and number. N Engl J Med 297:908, 1977.
44. Rebrin K, et al: Free fatty acid as a link in the regulation of hepatic glucose output by peripheral insulin. Diabetes 44:1038, 1995.
45. Hertz DE, et al: Intravenous glucose suppresses glucose production but not proteolysis in extremely premature newborns. J Clin Invest 92:1752, 1993.
46. Denne SC, et al: Effect of intravenous glucose and lipid on proteolysis and glucose production in normal newborns. Am J Physiol 269:E361, 1995.
47. Bergman RN, et al: Assessment of insulin sensitivity in vivo: a critical review. Diabetes Metab Rev 5:411, 1989.
48. Gelardi NL, et al: Insulin resistance and glucose transporter expression during the euglycemic hyperinsulinemic clamp in the lamb. Am J Physiol 277:E1142, 1999.
49. Ramlal T, et al: Muscle subcellular localization and recruitment by insulin of glucose transporters and Na + K+ ATPase subunits in transgenic mice overexpressing the Glut-4 glucose transporter. Diabetes 45:1516, 1996.
50. Hocquette J, et al: Facilitative glucose transporters in ruminants. Proc Nutr Soc 55:221, 1996.
51. Postic C, et al: The effects of hyperinsulinemia and hyperglycemia on Glut-4 and hexokinase II mRNA and protein in rat skeletal muscle and adipose tissue. Diabetes 42:922, 1993.
52. Jahoor F, et al: The relationship between gluconeogenic substrate supply and glucose production in humans. Am J Physiol 258:E288, 1990.
53. Bennish ML, et al: Hypoglycemia during diarrhea in childhood: prevalence pathophysiology and outcome. N Engl J Med 322:1357, 1990.
54. Haymond MW, et al: Differences in circulating gluconeogenic substances during short term fasting in men, women and children. Metabolism 31:33, 1982.
55. Cowett RM, Wolfe RR: The potential for lactate gluconeogenesis is accelerated in the preterm neonate compared to the adult. J Dev Physiol 16:341, 1991.
56. Yunis KA, et al: Glucose kinetics following administration of an intravenous fat emulsion to low birth weight neonates. Am J Physiol 263:E844, 1992.
57. Cowett RM, et al: Glucose kinetics in infants of diabetic mothers. Am J Obstet Gynecol 146:781, 1983.
58. Zarlengo KM, et al: Relationship between glucose utilization rate and glucose concentration in preterm infants. Biol Neonate 49:181, 1986.
59. Lafeber HN, et al: Glucose production and oxidation in preterm infants during total parenteral nutrition. Pediatr Res 28:153, 1990.
60. Cowett RM, et al: The contribution of glucose to neonatal glucose homeostasis in the lamb. Metabolism 47:1239, 1998.

Rebecca A. Simmons

50

Cell Glucose Transport and Glucose Handling During Fetal and Neonatal Development

Glucose is a vital substrate for the growing and developing fetus. It is required by most cells for oxidative and nonoxidative adenosine triphosphate (ATP) production and serves as a precursor for other carbon-containing compounds. It is the primary fuel used for several specialized cells and is the major fuel used by the brain. Its storage in the liver as glycogen provides a means by which glucose homeostasis can be maintained, particularly during the neonatal period. Glycogen stores also represent the primary source of energy for muscle tissue during exercise in postnatal life. Because of the diverse metabolic roles played by glucose, defects in its uptake or metabolism can alter cellular functions and can lead to significant morbidity and mortality. This chapter focuses on the molecular biology and regulation of glucose transporters in the fetus and newborn.

The plasma membranes of most mammalian cells, except those of the proximal kidney and small intestine, have a passively mediated transport system for glucose. Facilitative entry of glucose into the cell is controlled by glucose transporters (GLUTs), structurally related proteins that are encoded by a gene family[1-7] and are expressed in a tissue-specific manner. A different family of proteins, sodium (Na+)-coupled transporters (SLGTs), actively transport glucose across the apical membranes of polarized intestinal and renal epithelial cells.[8-13] The driving force for active glucose absorption is the electrochemical Na+ gradient across the membrane.

Most cells contain at least one glucose transporter isoform, and many contain more than one. In most cell types, glucose transporters mediate a net uptake of glucose. Under some circumstances, glucose is transported out of the cell. For example, the Na+-coupled transporter actively transports glucose into epithelial cells of the small intestine, and a facilitative transporter mediates the efflux of glucose from the cell into the interstitium. In hepatocytes, facilitative glucose transporters are responsible for the uptake of glucose from the portal circulation and for the release of glucose generated by glycogenolysis or gluconeogenesis. Thus, glucose transporters ensure efficient tissue uptake and distribution of glucose.

SODIUM-DEPENDENT GLUCOSE TRANSPORTERS

It has long been known that dietary sugars are actively absorbed from the small intestine; however, only recently has the molecular mechanism been elucidated. Active absorption of glucose across epithelial cells of the small intestine and the kidney proximal tubule is accomplished by Na+-glucose co-transporters located in the brush-border membranes. Transport of each glucose molecule is coupled to the co-transport of two Na+ ions (SGLT1) or of one Na+ ion (SGLT2). This transport system uses the energy from an extracellular to intracellular Na+ ion electrochemical gradient, generated by Na+, potassium–ATPases, to drive the accumulation of glucose into the cell. To date, three Na+-glucose co-transporter isoforms have been isolated. These transporters belong to a major class of membrane proteins called co-transporters (or symporters). These exist in bacteria, plants, and animal membranes, and they actively transport sugars, amino acids, carboxylic acids, and some ions (chloride, phosphate, sulfate, iodide) into cells.

SGLT1 is a hydrophobic integral membrane protein with approximately 12 membrane-spanning domains. The gene encoding the human intestinal SGLT has been localized to the q11.2–q ter region of chromosome 22.[14] It is abundantly expressed in the brush border of the small intestine and at lower levels in kidney, lung, and liver.

Clinical interest in the intestinal brush-border Na+-glucose co-transporter has focused on diarrhea and malabsorption. Glucose-galactose malabsorption is a rare autosomal recessive disorder characterized by onset of severe, watery diarrhea in the newborn period. Unless glucose and galactose are eliminated from the diet, death rapidly ensues. Wright and colleagues demonstrated that a single missense mutation in the gene encoding the intestinal Na+-glucose co-transporter is sufficient to cause life-threatening diarrhea.[15]

SGLT2 complementary DNA (cDNA) was originally isolated by Hediger and colleagues from a human cDNA library.[8] The SGLT amino acid sequences are approximately 60% identical to those of SGLT1, and the proteins have the same predicted secondary structure. The expression of this co-transporter is restricted to the renal cortex and is located in epithelial cells of proximal tubule S1 segments. It is generally thought that the bulk of the filtered glucose is reabsorbed in the proximal convoluted tubule by a low-affinity, high-capacity SGLT2 and that the remainder is reabsorbed by the high-affinity co-transporter SGLT1.

Familial renal glycosuria is an autosomal dominant disorder (an autosomal recessive mode of inheritance has not been excluded in all cases) affecting 0.2 to 0.6% of the general population and is characterized by the excretion of large amounts of glucose into the urine in the presence of normal blood glucose concentrations. The molecular basis of benign renal glycosuria has not been determined. It is possible that mutations in the low-affinity Na+-glucose co-transporter, SGLT2, may be responsible for the defect in renal absorption of filtered glucose.

Na+-glucose co-transporters appear to be active prenatally, and, as a consequence, the intestine is ready to absorb the first ingested glucose.[16] The cloned cDNAs and specific antibodies for the different Na+-glucose co-transporters will be valuable tools for identifying the specific cells in the intestine and kidney that express these proteins and for studying the regulation of their expression during development and in altered metabolic states such as diabetes mellitus or pregnancy.

FACILITATED GLUCOSE TRANSPORTERS

The energy-independent process of transporting glucose across the cell membrane occurs by facilitative diffusion. Transport of glucose is saturable, stereoselective, and bidirectional. The kinetics of glucose transport inward and outward is not necessarily identical,[17] and, in fact, in the erythrocyte, the rate of exchange flux for glucose is faster than net flux. The primary function of the facilitative glucose transporters is to mediate the exchange of glucose between blood and the cytoplasm of the cell. This may involve a net uptake or output of glucose from the cell, depending on the type of cell in question, its metabolic state, and the metabolic state of the organisms. In most cells, cytoplasmic glucose is rapidly phosphorylated by hexokinase or glucokinase, levels of glucose-6-phosphatase are low, and therefore there is little intracellular free glucose. These cells are only involved in net uptake and metabolism of blood glucose. The hepatocyte is also a net producer of glucose in the postabsorptive state. Glycogenolysis and gluconeogenesis increase intracellular free glucose to levels greater than its concentration in the blood and result in net efflux of glucose from the cell. In the postprandial state, glucose is transported into the hepatocyte to replenish glycogen stores.

The facilitative glucose transporters comprise a family of structurally related proteins. Six facilitated glucose transporter isoforms have been identified and are designated GLUT (the gene symbol for facilitative glucose transporter). The human genes encoding these proteins are named *GLUT1* to *GLUT5*.[2, 3, 18-22] Several novel glucose transporters, GLUT8, GLUT9, and GLUT10,

have been identified, and additional glucose transporters may exist.[23-27] Isoforms are expressed in a tissue-specific manner, reflecting the unique glucose requirements of various tissues.

These proteins vary in size from 492 to 524 amino acids. They exhibit 39 to 68% sequence identity and 50 to 76% sequence similarity in pairwise comparisons.[1,3,19,20,28-33] A topology map of the GLUTs has been proposed based on analysis of the primary amino acid sequence of GLUT1.[20] Each isoform consists of 12 membrane-spanning domains, an intracytoplasmic hydrophilic loop, and an exofacial loop bearing a single *N*-glycosylation site. Both the amino and carboxy terminals are exposed intracellularly (Fig. 50–1). Comparisons among the different isoforms have revealed that the sequences of the transmembrane segments and the short cytoplasmic loops connecting these transmembrane regions are highly conserved. Most likely, these regions are

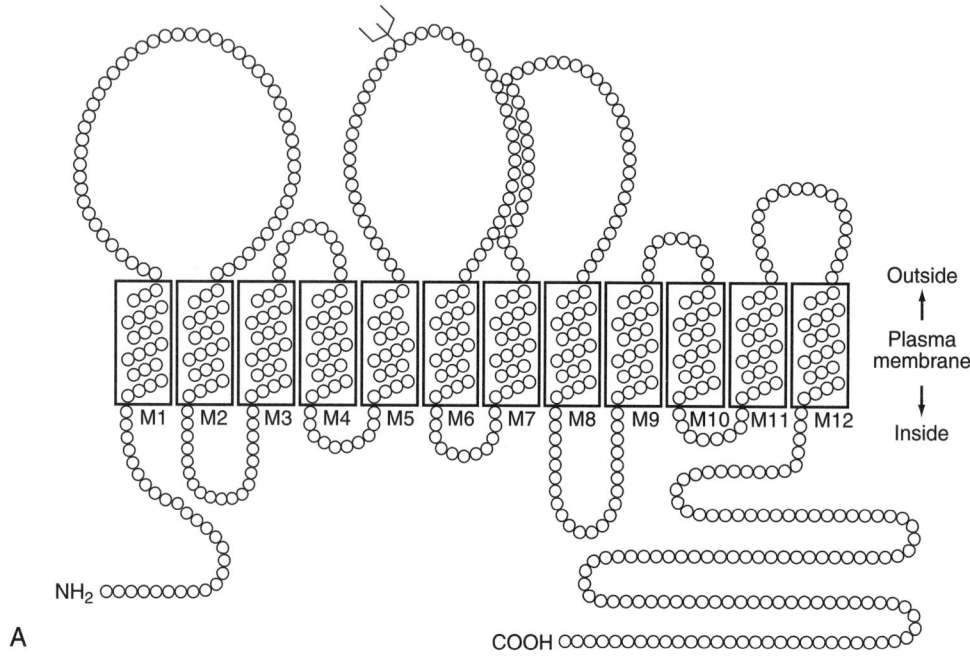

A

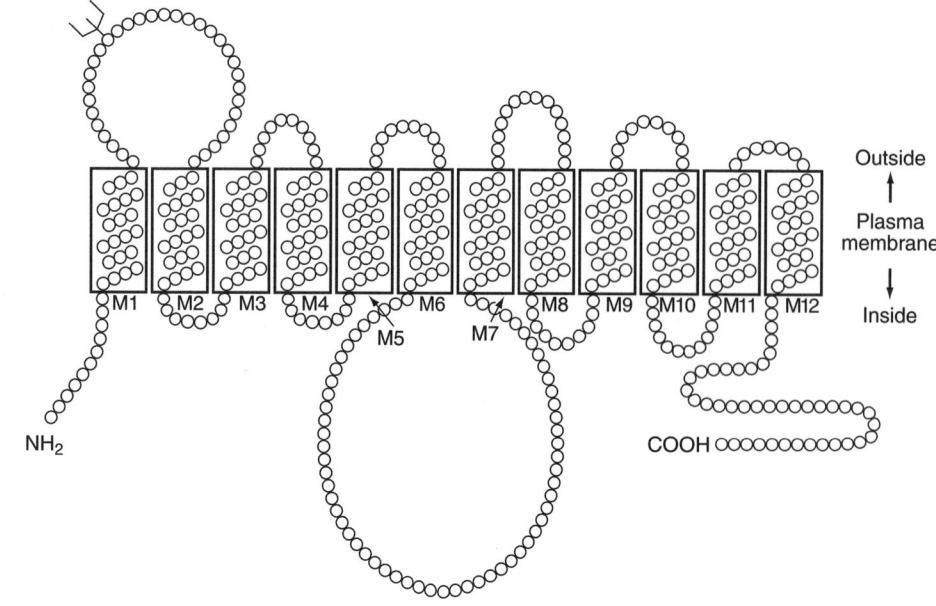

B

Figure 50–1. Models for the orientation of the human sodium/glucose co-transporter SGLT1 (**A**) and members of the facilitative glucose-transporter family (GLUT1 to GLUT5) in the plasma membrane (**B**). The 12 potential membrane-spanning α-helices are shown as *boxes* and are numbered M1 to M12.

responsible for the transport of glucose. The NH_2 and COOH-terminals are unique for each of the different isoforms and may contribute to isoform-specific properties, such as kinetics, hormone sensitivity, and subcellular localization.[1,3,18-20,22,29-32]

STRUCTURE AND PROPERTIES OF FACILITATIVE GLUCOSE TRANSPORTERS

GLUT1

GLUT1 was the first glucose transporter to be cloned. Antibodies were raised against the purified erythrocyte glucose transporter to screen antigen-expression cDNA libraries from RNA from the human hepatoblastoma cell line (HepG2). The amino acid sequence of GLUT1 is highly conserved. There is 98% identity between the sequences of human and rat GLUT1 and 97% identity between the sequences of human and mouse, rabbit, or pig. This high degree of sequence conservation implies that all domains of this 492-residue protein are functionally important.

GLUT1 is the most ubiquitously distributed of the transporter isoforms. It is found in virtually all tissues of the fetus and in many tissues and cell types of the adult.[34-41] GLUT1 has a very high affinity for glucose. These properties make it likely that GLUT1 is responsible for constitutive glucose uptake. In many organs, GLUT1 is concentrated in endothelial cells of blood-tissue barriers. Thus, one of the specialized roles of GLUT1 is to shuttle glucose between blood and organs that have limited access to small solutes via passive diffusion.

GLUT1 is the predominant isoform of the fetus. This transporter is also expressed in fetal tissues that fail to express it significantly in the adult. Most fetal cells exhibit rapid growth and differentiation necessitating an increased supply of energy-producing substrates. This may be the reason for the prevalence of GLUT1 in fetal tissues. After birth, GLUT1 decreases, and other isoforms such as GLUT2 in the liver and GLUT4 in the muscle increase.[34,37,40,41] The signals responsible for the decline in GLUT1 expression during the neonatal period are not known. It is hypothesized that the switch from a carbohydrate to a fat source of fuel may induce this change in some organs.[40]

Most of the studies concerning the regulation of GLUT1 have been carried out in cultured cells and cell lines from humans and rodents. GLUT1 expression is induced by growth factors. Growth factors and hormones such as insulin, insulin-like growth factor I (IGF-I), growth hormone, glucose, estrogen, transforming growth factor-β, thyroid hormone, cyclic adenosine monophosphate, fibroblast growth factor, and oncogenes increase GLUT1 expression in many different cell types.[42-51] Few studies have examined the regulation of GLUT1 *in vivo*, and data regarding GLUT1 regulation in the human fetus are scarce. These reports are discussed later.

GLUT2

GLUT2 is the major transporter isoform expressed in adult liver, pancreatic β-cells, and epithelial cells of the intestinal mucosa and kidney.[29-31] Levels of this isoform are quite low in the fetus. GLUT2 has 55% amino acid identity with sequences of GLUT1, and it has a similar structure and orientation in the plasma membrane. In contrast to GLUT1, whose sequence is highly conserved, there is only 81% identity between the sequences of human and rat GLUT2. The most characteristic feature of this isoform is its low affinity for glucose. GLUT2 and glucokinase form a glucose-sensing apparatus in hepatocytes and β-cells that responds to subtle changes in blood glucose concentrations by altering the rate of glucose transport into the cell. The transport capacity of GLUT2 is in excess of the glucokinase trapping reaction, thus making phosphorylation of glucose the rate-limiting step for glucose uptake in hepatocytes and β-cells. In the intes-

tine and kidney, the high-capacity, low-affinity system is necessary to transport glucose under conditions of large transepithelial substrate fluxes that occur after meals.

Expression of GLUT2 appears to be developmentally regulated. ß-cell content of GLUT2 protein in the fetus is approximately half that of the adult rat.[52] Despite the reduction in GLUT2 content, the blunted insulin secretory response seen in fetal islet cells is not the result of a limitation of glucose transport. At least a 10-fold decrease in transport activity would be required to reduce metabolism of glucose sufficient to perturb glucose-induced insulin secretion.[53,54] Other factors appear to be responsible for the blunted insulin secretory response observed in the fetus.

Studies done in fetal rats have demonstrated that GLUT2 levels are markedly diminished in fetal hepatocytes compared with the adult.[55-58] Shortly after birth, GLUT2 protein content dramatically rises and increases again, coinciding with the newborn pup's weaning from high-fat maternal milk.[51,52] Although an altered hormonal or substrate milieu is often implicated etiologically in the metabolic maturation associated with birth, the mechanism of this change is still unknown.

GLUT3

GLUT3 was first isolated from human fetal skeletal muscle.[59] Human GLUT3 has 64 and 52% identity with human GLUT1 and GLUT2, respectively, with an 83% amino acid sequence identity between the sequences of human and mouse GLUT3. Thus, as with GLUT2, the sequence of GLUT3 is not as highly conserved among species as that of GLUT1. GLUT3 messenger RNA (mRNA) is present at variable levels in all human tissues and is most abundant in brain, kidney, and placenta. The ubiquitous distribution of GLUT3 in human tissues suggests that it, together with GLUT1, may be responsible for basal glucose transport. In other animals such as rats, monkeys, and mice, the pattern of expression of GLUT3 is much different from that observed in humans.[3] In these animals, GLUT3 is abundant only in brain. The expression of GLUT3 in brain indicates that two facilitative glucose transporters are involved in the uptake of glucose. GLUT1 is primarily responsible for transport of glucose across the blood-brain barrier, and GLUT3 controls the uptake of glucose into the neuron.

There is relatively little information available about the regulation of GLUT3. Studies done in fetal rat brain suggest that glucose concentrations do not regulate expression of this transporter isoform.[60] This finding is in contrast to GLUT1, in which high levels of glucose down-regulate GLUT1 protein and mRNA abundance.[44] In contrast to glucose, chronic hypoxia increases GLUT3 mRNA expression in embryonic (day 14) rodent brain.[61]

GLUT4

GLUT4 is primarily expressed in adult tissues that exhibit insulin-stimulated glucose transport, such as adipose tissue and skeletal and cardiac muscle.[44] Low levels are also expressed in fetal rat brain.[61] Compared with the adult, little GLUT4 is expressed in fetal muscle[42] and brown fat,[62] and levels do not increase until well after birth.[38,40,62] The sequence of human GLUT4 is highly conserved, and there is 95 and 96% identity between the sequences of human and rat or mouse GLUT4.[63]

Insulin causes a rapid and reversible increase in glucose uptake in adipocytes and skeletal muscle. This increase results primarily from translocation of a latent pool of glucose transporters from intracellular vesicles[64] to the plasma membrane. Glucose transport in the insulin-sensitive tissues has received considerable attention because of the importance of this process in the maintenance of whole body glucose disposal. The transport step is rate limiting for glucose uptake into fat and muscle under most conditions.[65,66]

GLUT5

GLUT5 is the most divergent member of the glucose transporter family.[22] Human GLUT5 shares 42%, 40%, 39%, and 42% identity with human GLUT1, GLUT2, GLUT3, and GLUT4, respectively.[67] GLUT5 is expressed at high levels in the apical membrane of intestinal enterocytes and mature spermatocytes in adults. Fructose is transported across intestinal epithelial cells by passive transport. There is also a high rate of fructose utilization by testes. In view of these findings, it seems likely that GLUT5 is the major mammalian fructose transporter.

GLUT5 is also found in smaller quantities in adult human kidney, brain, muscle, and adipose tissue.[68, 69] The physiologic significance of GLUT5 in these tissues is unknown.

Novel Glucose Transporters

The facilitative glucose transporters GLUT1 to GLUT4 have considerable sequence similarity and different tissue distributions. Other similar sequences have also been cloned. GLUT6, a pseudogene, is not thought to encode a functional glucose transport protein.[22] GLUT7, originally cloned from a rat liver library, had been proposed to encode an endoplasmic reticulum protein that would facilitate the glucose produced by glucose-6-phosphatase produced in the endoplasmic reticulum lumen to reach the cytosol.[70] However, more recent studies from the same laboratory were unable to demonstrate that neither rat nor human liver RNA normally contains mRNA equivalent to the clone termed GLUT7.[71]

Although the diverse tissue distribution and the specific functions of GLUT1 to GLUT5 appear to indicate that these genes are sufficient to control glucose uptake in all mammalian tissues, it is likely that additional sugar transport facilitators exist. By searching the expressed sequence tag (EST) databases and taking advantage of the conserved sugar transporter signatures, several novel GLUT-like genes have been identified.

GLUT8 exhibits significant sequence similarity with the GLUT1 (29.4%).[23] In human tissues, it is predominantly found in testis, and lower amounts are detected in most other tissues including skeletal muscle, heart, small intestine, and brain.[23] GLUT8 is expressed in testis only from adult, not from prepubertal, rats, and expression is markedly inhibited by estrogen treatment.[23] Thus, GLUT8 may be involved in the provision of glucose required for DNA synthesis in male germ cells. GLUT8 has also been found to be the glucose transporter responsible for insulin-stimulated glucose uptake in the blastocyst.[24]

GLUT9 (44.8% amino acid identity with GLUT8) is detected in human spleen, peripheral leukocytes, and brain.[25, 26] GLUT10 (35% sequence identity with human GLUT1 to GLUT8) is the latest member of the glucose transporter to be cloned and is expressed in human heart, lung, brain, liver, skeletal muscle, kidney, and placenta.[27] It is also detected in fetal brain and liver.[27]

LOCALIZATION AND REGULATION OF FACILITATIVE GLUCOSE TRANSPORTERS

Embryo

Reverse transcriptase polymerase chain reaction, immunofluorescence, and immunoelectron microscopy techniques have confirmed that GLUT1 is expressed in all stages of embryonic development of the mouse, rat, rabbit, cow, and human, including the oocyte and the blastocyst. It is readily detectable in trophectoderm and inner cell mass cells of the mouse blastocyst, and it is associated with intracellular membranes as well as plasma membranes of all cell types.[72-75] During organogenesis in the rat embryo, GLUT1 is localized to the neural tube, as well as the heart tube, gut, and optic vesicle.[76]

GLUT2 also appears to be an important mediator of glucose uptake in the early embryo. GLUT2 is expressed as early as the eight-cell blastocyst stage. It is located on trophoectoderm membranes facing the blastocyst cavity.[72, 74] Expression of GLUT3 appears by day 4 of gestation (in rat), and it is found on the apical membranes of trophoectoderm cells and seems to be responsible for the uptake of maternal glucose.[76, 77] GLUT8 is primarily expressed within vesicles in the cells lining the blastocoele.[24] Insulin and IGF-1 stimulate translocation of GLUT8 to the plasma membrane of these cells via binding to the IGF-1 receptor.[24] Studies suggest that GLUT8 expression and translocation in response to insulin are critical for blastocyst survival.[78] However, the physiologic role that insulin-regulated glucose transporters play *in vivo* in the human blastocyst remains to be determined.

One of the characteristics displayed by preimplantation embryos is the metabolic shift from a dependence on the tricarboxylic acid cycle during the precompactation stages to a metabolism based on glycolysis after compaction.[79] This change in substrate utilization is coincident with the rapid proliferation that occurs during this developmental stage. Similar changes in substrate preference occur in numerous other cells as the undergo proliferation. Therefore, high-affinity glucose transporters such as GLUT1 and GLUT3 are required for glucose uptake.

Pregnant women with diabetes are at increased risk for both first trimester spontaneous abortions and major fetal malformations. Data suggest that hyperglycemia-induced apoptosis in the embryo may contribute to early pregnancy loss.[80, 81] Preimplantation studies have shown that maternal hyperglycemia down-regulates GLUT1, GLUT2, and GLUT3 at the blastocyst stage of development,[82] which is associated with increased apoptosis.[80] Only 40% of the cells showed evidence of apoptosis, which has been shown to result in neural tube defects, limb abnormalities, and abdominal wall malformations, similar to malformations seen among infants of diabetic women.[83]

Placenta

In the human placenta, placental villi are in direct contact with maternal blood. The surface of the placental villi is covered with a single syncytiotrophoblast layer, formed by the fusion of the underlying cytotrophoblast elements. Fetal capillaries lie directly beneath the syncytiotrophoblast. Transfer of glucose from maternal to fetal blood occurs via the placental villi and is most likely mediated by GLUT1. GLUT1 is abundantly expressed in the plasma membranes of both the basal and apical sides of the syncytiotrophoblast. GLUT1 may facilitate the entry of glucose into the cytoplasm of the syncytiotrophoblast from maternal blood, whereas GLUT1 at the basal plasma membrane may aid in the exit of glucose from the cytoplasm of the syncytiotrophoblast to the pericapillary space of the fetus. GLUT1 on the endothelial cell of the capillary then transfers glucose into the fetal circulation.[84-87] Protein and mRNA levels of GLUT1 increase in the placenta as the fetus matures, thus underscoring the importance of this transporter in fetal development.[85]

GLUT3 is distributed throughout placental villous tissue and decreases during gestation.[85, 87-89] Although GLUT3 mRNA is abundantly expressed in villous tissue, GLUT3 protein is primarily localized to the vascular endothelium. GLUT3 may play a role in transporting glucose from mother to fetus after transsyncytial transport.

There are limited data regarding the regulation of glucose transporter expression in human placenta. A few studies have been carried out in placentas from pregnancies complicated by intrauterine growth retardation and diabetes. Growth-retarded fetuses are often hypoglycemic, and impaired placental glucose transport has been implicated as a pathophysiologic mechanism.

Growth-retarded fetuses have a reduced umbilical venoarterial concentration difference in glucose and lower fetal weight-specific umbilical volume flow.[90, 91] However, placentas from preterm and term infants with intrauterine growth retardation have not shown a difference in levels of GLUT1 protein.[92]

Gestational diabetes is associated with placenta overgrowth and an increase in transplacental glucose transfer to the fetus. Levels of GLUT1 protein are increased in the basal membranes and lead to an increase in glucose transport activity of syncytial basal membranes.[93, 94] Microvillous expression and activity are unaffected by hyperglycemia.[95, 96] Likewise, levels of GLUT3 and GLUT4 are not altered in placentas of women with diabetes during pregnancy.[95, 96] Thus, it appears from these studies that increased glucose transport to the fetus of the diabetic mother is facilitated by increased levels of GLUT1. Illsley proposed that this process leads to fetal hyperglycemia, which, in turn, stimulates the production of IGF-1 leading to excess fetoplacental growth.[97]

Brain

Brain glucose utilization accounts for approximately 80% of whole body glucose disposal in humans.[98] Furthermore, there is heterogeneity in glucose utilization among different regions of the brain. Circulating glucose crosses the blood-brain barrier and enters brain parenchyma cells via facilitative glucose transporters. Most studies of GLUT expression in the nervous system of the developing animal have been performed in the rat. Before the formation of the blood-brain barrier, GLUT1 is abundant in the germinal neuroepithelium, which gives rise to both neurons and neuroglia.[99] Just before birth, GLUT1 is abundant in the brain vasculature, meninges, ependyma, and choroid plexus. After birth, GLUT1 is also found in glial cells.[99] GLUT1 is developmentally regulated in rat and rabbit brain.[34-36] Its expression is highest in adult brain, followed by fetal and neonatal brain, respectively.

Few localization studies have been done in the human fetus. One report has demonstrated that the localization of GLUT1 in the mid-gestation to late-gestation human fetus is similar to the rat, that is, it is primarily located in the microvascular endothelial cells that constitute the blood-brain barrier.[69] However, a more recent study suggested a much wider distribution of GLUT1 in the developing brain.[100] From 10 to 21 weeks of gestation, GLUT1 is expressed in all regions of the fetal brain and is primarily present in the endothelial cells of the brain capillaries, in the epithelial cells of the choroid plexus, and in neurons.[100] GLUT 2 is not expressed until mid-gestation (21 weeks), and at that time it is highly expressed in the granular layer of the cerebellum.[100] No study to date has been able to detect GLUT3 or GLUT4 in human fetal brain.

After birth, GLUT3 is found in the cerebellum in neurofilament-positive cellular transverse fibers, cell bodies of Purkinje cells, and other neuronal elements in close proximity to the Purkinje layer.[69] This region-specific pattern of GLUT3 expression may reflect the differing glucose needs of anatomically distinct regions of the brain. Localization of GLUT3 is similar to the distribution of glucose utilization, which during early infancy is mainly infratentorial, and later in development occurs in supratentorial structures as well.[101, 102]

Regulation of glucose transport in the fetal brain is uniquely different from that in the adult. Before birth, low levels of glucose (*in vivo* or *in vitro*) fail to up-regulate glucose transport in whole fetal rat brain[60] or isolated glial cells. However, after birth, hypoglycemia induces a marked increase in GLUT1 expression[103] in whole rat brain isolated glial cells. Furthermore, glucose transport in the fetal brain does not respond to insulin or IGF-I,[42] two hormones that increase GLUT1 expression in glial cells of older animals.[104-105] The mechanisms underlying these differences in regulation of glucose transport that occur with maturation are unknown. In contrast to glucose, hypoxia during gestation does induce a marked increase in GLUT3 levels in fetal rat brain.[61]

Lung

Glucose is an important metabolic substrate for the lung and provides carbon moieties for energy production and synthesis of surfactant. In adult lung, transport of glucose across the apical membrane of the Type II pneumocyte occurs by Na^+-coupled transport,[106-108] and it occurs across the basolateral membrane by facilitative glucose transport. To date, GLUT1 is the only isoform found to be expressed in Type II pneumocytes of fetal rats and humans.[109] It is hypothesized that SGLT1 is also expressed in Type II pneumocytes; however, no study has thus far been able to localize this transporter in fetal lung.

GLUT1 is abundantly expressed in the fetal lung when compared with that of the juvenile and adult rat.[41] Glucose utilization and levels of GLUT1 mRNA and protein dramatically decline as the animal matures.[41,110] By day 14 of life, GLUT1 is undetectable in rat pups. The factors responsible for this significant decrease in the synthesis of GLUT1 are unknown.

Insulin and IGF-I are important modulators of glucose transport in Type II pneumocytes of fetal rats. Physiologic levels of insulin and IGF-I stimulate glucose transport,[42] whereas higher levels of insulin inhibit glucose uptake.[111] Several animal studies suggest that hyperinsulinemia, through its inhibitory effects on glucose transport, contributes to the decrease in surfactant synthesis observed in infants of diabetic mothers. In a model that somewhat mimics human gestational diabetes, diabetes is induced in pregnant rats by streptozotocin. Fetal rats are hyperglycemic, hyperinsulinemic, and large for gestational age. Type II pneumocytes from these animals exhibit markedly diminished glucose uptake and GLUT1 expression.[112] It is possible that the decrease in glucose uptake diminishes the supply of glucose available for surfactant synthesis. This could be one factor that increases the risk of respiratory distress syndrome in infants of diabetic mothers.

Male fetuses exhibit delayed lung maturation and surfactant production in comparison with female fetuses. This delay may be related to sex hormone effects: estrogen enhances and androgens delay lung development. The uptake of glucose, an important precursor for surfactant synthesis, appears to be differently affected by estrogen and androgens. *In vitro* studies performed in fetal rat have shown that estradiol and dehydrotestosterone differentially regulate glucose uptake in fetal rat lung tissue. This regulation of substrate supply (glucose) by estradiol and dehydrotestosterone may be another mechanism for the sexual dimorphism observed in lung development and surfactant synthesis.[113]

Liver

Transport of glucose across the hepatocyte does not appear to be rate limiting for glucose metabolism. However, glucose transport is developmentally regulated in the human and rat, and glucose transport contributes to the changes in glucose metabolic capacity from fetal to extrauterine life. The major glucose transporter in the adult hepatocyte is GLUT2. GLUT1 is expressed only in perivenous hepatocytes.

In contrast, in the fetus, GLUT1 and GLUT2 are abundantly expressed in hepatocytes.[55,56,58] During the fetal to neonatal transition, there is a shift from abundant GLUT1 in the hepatocyte to an adult pattern of little GLUT1 expression.[34,57] Many metabolic and hormonal factors dramatically change during the perinatal period. The factors responsible for the switch in GLUT1 expression remain to be delineated.

Muscle

Most of the studies regarding glucose transport in muscle have been carried out in adults. As described earlier, GLUT4 is the predominant isoform expressed in adult muscle. In response to insulin, this transporter isoform significantly increases the transport of glucose into the myocyte. In contrast to the marked insulin responsiveness observed in the adult, fetal muscle only modestly responds to insulin. Insulin and IGF-I increase GLUT1 expression 1.5-fold in normal fetal rat muscle explants,[42] compared with the 20-fold increase observed in adult muscle.[114, 115] Insulin does not stimulate GLUT1 expression in isolated myoblasts from fetal rats,[40] a finding suggesting that stimulation of glucose transport by insulin requires tissue-specific additional factors.

GLUT1 is localized to the myoblast, and levels are quite high in the fetal and newborn rat pup. GLUT1 decreases significantly during weaning.[40, 116] It appears that the switch from GLUT1 to GLUT4 expression during this period is secondary to dietary factors. If rats are weaned to a diet rich in fat, the normal increase in GLUT4 is prevented.[40, 116, 117] The molecular mechanisms responsible for this observation are unknown.

Kidney

The kidney, small intestine, and liver can all release glucose during periods of decreased glucose availability. Although the liver is the principal supplier of glucose during short fasts, the kidney also produces glucose during prolonged starvation. The Na$^+$-glucose co-transporter, SGLT1, transports glucose into the brush-border cell of the proximal tubule of the kidney. GLUT2, localized on the basolateral membrane of epithelial cells lining renal tubules, is involved in the net release of glucose into the blood during absorption of renal glucose.

No data are available concerning the regulation of glucose transport in the fetal kidney, and only a few reports have described the ontogeny of renal glucose transport. SGLT1 is expressed in lower quantities in fetal compared with adult kidney. GLUT2 is also present in the fetal kidney, and its expression increases with maturation.

SUMMARY

Glucose transporters have acquired distinct physiologic and biochemical properties that allow them to serve specific functions in the tissues in which they are expressed. An understanding of the mechanisms underlying tissue-specific expression of these transporters will facilitate an understanding of *in vivo* glucose utilization and clearance processes that occur normally and in disease states. Although studies in adults provide insight into the regulation of glucose transport, similar studies are required in the fetus and newborn to understand fully the role of the glucose transporter in fetal and neonatal development.

REFERENCES

1. James DE, et al: Molecular cloning and characterization of an insulin-regulatable glucose transporter. Nature 333:83-87, 1989.
2. Fukumoto H, et al: Sequence, tissue distribution, and chromosomal localization of mRNA encoding a human glucose transporter-like protein. Proc Natl Acad Sci USA 85:5434-5438, 1988.
3. Kayano T, et al: Evidence for a family of human glucose transporter-like proteins: sequence and gene localization of a protein expressed in fetal skeletal muscle and other tissues. J Biol Chem 263:15245-15248, 1988.
4. Wheeler TJ, Hinkle PC: The glucose transporter of mammalian cells. Annu Rev Physiol 47:503-517, 1985.
5. Lodish HF: Anion-exchange and glucose transport proteins: structure, function, and distribution. Harvey Lect 82:19-46, 1988.
6. Gould GW, Bell GI: Facilitative glucose transporters: an expanding family. Trends Biochem Sci 15:18-22, 1990.
7. Pilch PF: Glucose transporters: what's in a name? Endocrinology 126:3-5, 1990.
8. Hediger MA, et al: Expression, cloning and cDNA sequencing of the Na$^+$/glucose cotransporter. Nature 330:379-381, 1987.
9. Meddings JB, et al: Glucose transport and microvillus membrane physical properties along the crypt-villus axis of the rabbit. J Clin Invest 85:1099-1107, 1990.
10. Ikeda TS, et al: Characterization of a Na$^+$/glucose cotransporter cloned from rabbit small intestine. J Membr Biol 110:87-95, 1989.
11. Malo C, Berteloot A: Proximo-distal gradient of Na$^+$-dependent D-glucose transport activity in the brush border membrane vesicles from the human fetal small intestine. FEBS Lett 220:201-205, 1987.
12. Turner DJ, Kempner ES: Radiation inactivation studies of the renal brush-border membrane phlorizin-binding protein. J Biol Chem 257:10794-10797, 1982.
13. Takahashi M, et al: Radiation inactivation studies on the rabbit kidney sodium-dependent glucose transporter. J Biol Chem 260:10551-10556, 1985.
14. Hediger MA, et al: Assignment of the human intestinal Na$^+$/glucose gene (SGLT 1) to the q 11.2-q ter region of chromosome 22. Genomics 4:297-300, 1989.
15. Wright EM, et al: Molecular genetics of intestinal glucose transport. J Clin Invest 88:1435-1440, 1991.
16. Buddington RK, Diamond JM: Ontogenetic development of intestinal nutrient transporters. Annu Rev Physiol 51:601-619, 1989.
17. Carruthers A: Facilitative diffusion of glucose. Physiol Rev 70:1135-1176, 1990.
18. Birnbaum MJ: Identification of a novel gene encoding an insulin-responsive glucose transporter protein. Cell 57:305-315, 1989.
19. Birnbaum MJ, et al: Cloning and characterization of cDNA encoding the rat brain glucose-transporter protein. Proc Natl Acad Sci USA 83:5784-5788, 1986.
20. Mueckler M, et al: Sequence and structure of a human glucose transporter. Science 229:941-945, 1985.
21. Bell GI, et al: Structure and function of mammalian facilitative sugar transporters. J Biol Chem 268:19161-19164, 1993.
22. Kayano T, et al: Human facilitative glucose transporters: isolation, functional characterization, and gene localization of cDNAs encoding an isoform (Glut 5) expressed in small intestine, kidney, muscle, and adipose tissue and an unusual glucose transporter pseudo-gene-like sequence (Glut 6). J Biol Chem 265:13276-13282, 1990.
23. Doege H, et al: GLUT8, a novel member of the sugar transport facilitator family with glucose transport activity. J Biol Chem 275:16275-16280, 2000.
24. Carayannopoulos MO, et al: GLUT 8 is a glucose transporter responsible for insulin-stimulated glucose uptake in the blastocyst. Proc Natl Acad Sci USA 97:7313-7318, 2000.
25. Phay JE, et al: Cloning and expression analysis of a novel member of the facilitative glucose transporter family, SLC2A9 (GLUT 9). Genomics 66:217-220. 2000.
26. Doege H, et al: Activity and genomic organization of human glucose transporter 9 (GLUT9), a novel member of the family of sugar-transport facilitators predominantly expressed in brain and leucocytes. Biochem J 350:771-776, 2000.
27. Dawson PA, et al: Sequence and functional analysis of GLUT10: a glucose transporter in the type 2 diabetes-linked region of chromosome 20q12-13.1. Mol Genet Metab 74:186-199, 2001.
28. Shows TB, et al: Polymorphic human glucose transporter gene (Glut) is on chromosome 1p31.3-p35. Diabetes 36:546-549, 1987.
29. Fukumoto H, et al: Identification of a human liver-type glucose transporter: cDNA sequence, expression and localization of the gene to chromosome 3. Proc Natl Acad Sci USA 85:5434-5438, 1988.
30. Thomas B, et al: Cloning and functional expression in bacteria of a novel glucose transporter present in liver, intestine, kidney, and beta pancreatic islet cells. Cell 55:281-290, 1988.
31. Permutt MA, et al: Cloning and functional expression of a human pancreatic islet glucose transporter cDNA. Proc Natl Acad Sci USA 86:8688-8692, 1989.
32. Fukumoto H, et al: Cloning and characterization of the major insulin-responsive glucose transporter expressed in human skeletal muscle and other insulin-responsive tissues. J Biol Chem 264:7776-7779, 1989.
33. Bell GI, et al: Polymorphic human insulin-responsive glucose transporter gene on chromosome 17p13. Diabetes 38:1072-1075, 1989.
34. Werner H, et al: Developmental regulation of rat brain/Hep G2 glucose transporter gene expression. Mol Endocrinol 3:273-279, 1989.
35. Sadiq F, et al: The ontogeny of the rabbit brain glucose transporter. Endocrinology 126:2417-2424, 1990.
36. Sivitz W, et al: Regulation of the glucose transporter in developing rat brain. Endocrinology 124:1875-1880, 1989.
37. Devaskar S, et al: Developmental regulation of the distribution of rat brain insulin-insensitive (Glut 1) glucose transporter. Endocrinology 129:1530-1540, 1991.
38. Santalucia T, et al: Developmental regulation of Glut 1 (erythroid/Hep2) and Glut 4 glucose transporter expression in rat heart, skeletal muscle, and brown adipose tissue. Endocrinology 130:837-846, 1992.
39. Studelska DR, et al: Developmental expression of insulin-regulatable glucose transporter Glut 4. Am J Physiol 263:E102-E106, 1992.
40. Leturque A, et al: Nutritional regulation of glucose transporter and adipose tissue of weaned rats. Am J Physiol 260:E588-E593, 1991.
41. Simmons RA, et al: Glut 1 gene expression in growth-retarded juvenile rats. Pediatr Res 35:382A, 1994.
42. Simmons RA, et al: The effect of insulin and IGF-I upon glucose transport in normal and small for gestational age fetal rats. Endocrinology 133:1361-1368, 1993.

43. Cartee GD, Bohn EE: Growth hormone reduces glucose transport but not Glut-1 or Glut-4 in adult and old rats. Am J Physiol 268:E902-E909, 1995.

44. Simmons RA, et al: Glucose regulated Glut 1 function and expression in fetal rat lung and muscle in vitro. Endocrinology 132:2312-2318, 1993.

45. Hart CD, et al: Modulation of glucose transport in fetal rat lung by estrogen and dihydrotestosterone. Pediatr Res 37:335A, 1995.

46. Kitagawa T, et al: Transforming growth factor-B$_1$ stimulates glucose uptake and the expression of glucose transporter mRNA in quiescent Swiss mouse 3T3 cells. J Biol Chem 266:18066-18071, 1991.

47. Weinstein SP, et al: Thyroid hormone increases basal and insulin-stimulated glucose transport in skeletal muscle. Diabetes 43:1185-1189, 1994.

48. Cornelius P, et al: Regulation of glucose transport as well as glucose transporter and immediate early gene expression in 3T3-L1 preadipocytes by 8-bromo-cAMP. J Cell Physiol 146:298-308, 1991.

49. Leuthner SR, et al: Regulation of Glut 1 gene expression by cAMP in fetal rat brain. Pediatr Res 35:382A, 1994.

50. Hiraki Y, et al: Growth factors rapidly induce expression of the glucose transporter gene. J Biol Chem 263:13655-13662, 1988.

51. Flier JS, et al: Elevated levels of glucose transporter and transporter messenger RNA are induced by ras and src oncogenes. Science 235:1492-1495, 1987.

52. Hughes SJ: The role of reduced glucose transporter content and glucose metabolism in the immature secretory responses of fetal rat pancreatic islets. Diabetologia 37:134-140, 1994.

53. Meglasson MD, Matschinsky FM: Pancreatic islet glucose metabolism and regulation of insulin secretion. Diabetes Metab Rev 2:163-214, 1986.

54. Lenzen S: Glucokinase: signal recognition enzyme for glucose-induced insulin secretion. In Nutrient Regulation of Insulin Secretion. London, Portland Press, 1992, pp 101-125.

55. Lane RH, et al: Localization and quantification of glucose transporters in liver of growth retarded fetal and neonatal rats. Am J Physiol 276:E135-E142, 1998.

56. Lane RH, et al: Measurement of GLUT mRNA in liver of fetal and neonatal rats using a novel method of quantitative polymerase chain reaction. Biochem Mol Med 59:192-9, 1996.

57. Postic C, et al: Development and regulation of glucose transporter and hexokinase expression in rat. Am J Physiol 266:E548-E559, 1994.

58. Levitsky LL, et al: Glut 1 and Glut 2 mRNA, protein, and glucose transporter activity in cultured fetal and adult hepatocytes. Am J Physiol 267:E88-E94, 1994.

59. Yano H, et al: Tissue distribution and species difference of the brain type glucose transporter (Glut 3). Biochem Biophys Res Commun 174:470-477, 1991.

60. Simmons RA, et al: Glucose regulates Glut 1 function and gene expression in fetal rat brain. Pediatr Res 35:71A, 1993.

61. Royer C, et al: Effects of gestational hypoxia on mRNA levels of GLUT3 and GLUT4 transporters, hypoxia inducible factor-1 and thyroid hormone receptors in developing rat brain. Brain Res 856:119-128, 2000.

62. Valverde AM, et al: Insulin and insulin-like growth factor up-regulate GLUT4 gene expression in fetal brown adipocytes, in a phosphoinositide 3-kinase-dependent manner. Biochem J 337:397-405, 1999.

63. James DE, et al: Insulin-regulatable tissue express a unique insulin sensitive glucose transport protein. Nature 333:183-185, 1988.

64. Slot JW, et al: Immunolocalization of the insulin regulatable glucose transporter in brown adipose tissue of the rat. J Cell Biol 113:123-135, 1991.

65. Koranyi LI, et al: Levels of skeletal muscle glucose transporter protein correlate with insulin-stimulated whole body glucose disposal in man. Diabetologia 34:763-765, 1991.

66. Eriksson J, et al: Insulin resistance in type 2 (non–insulin-dependent) diabetic patients and their relatives is not associated with a defect in the expression of the insulin-responsive glucose transporter (GLUT-4) gene in human skeletal muscle. Diabetologia 35:143-147, 1992.

67. Bell GI, et al: Molecular biology of mammalian glucose transporters. Diabetes Care 13:198-208, 1990.

68. Bell GI, et al: Structure and function of mammalian facilitative sugar transporters. J Biol Chem 268:19161-19164, 1993.

69. Mantych GJ, et al: Cellular localization and characterization of Glut 3 glucose transporter isoform in human brain. Endocrinology 131:1270-1278, 1992.

70. Burchell A: Hepatic microsomal glucose transport. Biochem Soc Trans 22:658-663, 1994.

71. Burchell A: A re-evaluation of GLUT7. Biochem J 331:973, 1998.

72. Aghayan M, et al: Developmental expression and cellular localization of glucose transporter molecules during mouse preimplantation development. Development 115:305-312, 1992.

73. Schultz GA, et al: Insulin, insulin-like growth factors and glucose transporters. Reprod Fertil Dev 4:361-371, 1992.

74. Hogan A, et al: Glucose transporter gene expression in early mouse embryos. Development 113:363-372, 1991.

75. Robinson DH, et al: Hexose transport in preimplantation rabbit blastocysts. J Reprod Fertil 89:1-11, 1990.

76. Matsumoto K, et al: Abundant expression of Glut 1 and Glut 3 in rat embryo during the early organogenesis period. Biochem Biophys Res Commun 209:95-102, 1995.

77. Pantaleon M, et al: Glucose transporter GLUT3: ontogeny, targeting, and role in the mouse blastocyst. Proc Natl Acad Sci USA 94:3795-3800, 1997.

78. Pinto AB, et al: Glucose transporter 8 expression and translocation are critical for murine blastocyst survival. Biol Reprod 66:1729–1733, 2002.

79. Gardner DK, Leese HJ: Noninvasive measurement of nutrient uptake by single cultured pre-implantation mouse embryos. Hum Reprod 1:25-27, 1986.

80. Moley KH, et al: Hyperglycemia induces apoptosis in pre-implantation embryos through cell death effector pathways. Nat Med 4:1421-1424, 1998.

81. Phelan SA, et al: Neural tube defects in embryos of diabetic mice: role of the Pax-3 gene and apoptosis. Diabetes 46:1189-1197, 1997.

82. Moley KH, et al: Maternal hyperglycemia alters glucose transport and utilization in mouse preimplantation embryos. Am J Physiol 275:E38-E47, 1998.

83. Polifka JE, et al: Exposure to ethylene oxide during the early zygotic period induces skeletal anomalies in mouse fetuses. Teratology 53:1-9, 1996.

84. Takata K, et al: Localization of erythrocyte/HepG2-type glucose transporter (Glut 1) in human placental villi. Cell Tissue Res 267:407-412, 1992.

85. Arnott G, et al: Immunolocalization of Glut 1 and Glut 3 glucose transporters in human placenta. Biochem Soc Trans 22:272-273, 1994.

86. Reid NA, Boyd R: Further evidence for the presence of 2 facilitative glucose isoforms in the brush border membrane of the syncytiotrophoblast of the human full term placenta. Biochem Soc Trans 22:267, 1994.

87. Sakata M, et al: Increase in human placental glucose transporter-1 during pregnancy. Eur J Endocrinol 132:206-212, 1995.

88. Wolf HJ, Desoye G: Immunohistochemical localization of glucose transporters and insulin receptors in human fetal membranes at term. Histochemistry 100:379-385, 1993.

89. Jansson T, et al: Cellular localization of glucose transporter mRNA in human placenta. Reprod Fertl Dev 7:1425-1430, 1995.

90. Economides DL, Nicolaides KH: Blood glucose and oxygen tension levels in small-for-gestational age fetuses. Am J Obstet Gynecol 160:385-389, 1989.

91. Laurin J, et al: Fetal blood flow in pregnancies complicated by intrauterine growth retardation. Obstet Gynecol 69:895-902, 1987.

92. Jansson TS, et al: Glucose transporter protein expression in human placenta throughout gestation and in intrauterine growth retardation. J Clin Endocrinol Metab 77:1554-1562, 1993.

93. Gaither K, et al: Diabetes alters the expression and activity of the human placental GLUT1 glucose transporter. J Clin Endocr Metab 84:695-701, 1999.

94. Jansson T, et al: Placental glucose transport and GLUT1 expression in insulin-dependent diabetes. Am J Obstet Gynecol 180:163-168, 1999.

95. Kainulainen H, et al: Placental glucose transporters in fetal intrauterine growth retardation and macrosomia. Gynecol Obstet Invest 44:89-92, 1997.

96. Xing AY, et al: Unexpected expression of glucose transporter 4 in villous cells of human placenta. J Clin Endocrinol Metab 83:4097-4101, 1998.

97. Illsley NP: Glucose transporters in the human placenta. Placenta 21:14-22, 2000.

98. Schienberg P: Observations on cerebral carbohydrate metabolism in man. Ann Intern Med 62:367-371, 1963.

99. Bondy CA, et al: Ontogeny and cellular distribution of brain glucose transporter gene expression. Mol Cell Neurosci 3:305-314, 1992.

100. Nualart F, et al: Expression of the hexose transporters GLUT1 and GLUT2 during the early development of the human brain. Brain Res 824:97-104, 1999.

101. Chugani HT, et al: Positron emission tomography study of human brain functional development. Ann Neurol 22:487-497, 1987.

102. Chugani HT, Phelps ME: Maturational changes in cerebral function in infants determined by 18 FD6 positron emission tomography. Science 23:840-843, 1986.

103. Walker PS, et al: Glucose dependent regulation of glucose transport activity, protein, mRNA in primary cultures of rat brain glial cells. J Biol Chem 263:15594-15601, 1988.

104. Clarke DW, et al: Insulin binds to specific receptors and stimulates 2-deoxy-glucose uptake in cultured glial cells from rat brain. J Biol Chem 259:11672-11675, 1984.

105. Werner H, et al: Regulation of rat brain/HepG2 glucose transporter gene expression by insulin and insulin-like growth factor-I in primary cultures of neuronal and glial cells. Endocrinology 125:314-326, 1989.

106. Oelberg DG, et al: Sodium-coupled transport of glucose by plasma membranes of type II pneumocytes. Biochim Biophys Acta 1194:92-98, 1994.

107. Basset G, et al: Apical sodium-sugar transport in pulmonary epithelium in situ. Biochim Biophys Acta 942:11-18, 1988.

108. Clerici C, et al: Sodium-dependent phosphate and alanine transports but sodium-independent hexose transport in type II alveolar epithelial cells in primary culture. Biochim Biophys Acta 1063:27-35, 1991.

109. Simmons RA, et al: Intrauterine growth retardation: fetal glucose transport is diminished in lung but spared in brain. Pediatr Res 31:59-63, 1992.

110. Simmons RA, Charlton VE: Substrate utilization by the fetal sheep lung during the last trimester. Pediatr Res 23:660-611, 1988.

111. Engle MJ, et al: The effects of insulin and hyperglycemia on surfactant phospholipid synthesis in organotypic cultures of type II pneumocytes. Biochim Biophys Acta 753:6-13, 1983.

112. Simmons RA, et al: The effect of maternal diabetes on glut 1 function and expression in fetal lung. Pediatr Res 31:182A, 1992.

113. Hart CD, et al: Modulation of glucose transport in fetal rat lung: a sexual dimorphism. Am J Respir Cell Mol Biol 19:63-70, 1998.

114. Kahn BB, Cushman SW: Mechanisms for markedly hyperresponsive insulin-stimulated glucose transport activity in adipose cells from insulin-treated streptozotocin rats. J Biol Chem 262:5118-5124, 1987.

115. Charron MJ, Kahn BB: Divergent molecular mechanisms for insulin-resistant transport in muscle and adipose cells in vivo. J Biol Chem 240:3237-3244, 1990.

116. Issad T, et al: Insulin resistance during suckling period in rats. Am J Physiol 253:E142-E148, 1987.

117. Wallace S, et al: Development of insulin sensitivity in rat skeletal muscle. FEBS Lett 301:69-72, 1992.

Charles A. Stanley and Neil Caplin

51

Pathophysiology of Hypoglycemia

Hypoglycemia is more common in the newborn than at any other age, particularly in the first 12 to 24 hours of extrauterine life. After the first 24 hours of life, true neonatal hypoglycemia is uncommon; once detected, it must be investigated and treated appropriately. The importance of detecting and treating neonatal hypoglycemia is twofold: first, hypoglycemia deprives the brain of its primary source of metabolic fuel and can lead to seizures and brain damage; and second, hypoglycemia is a presenting feature of numerous endocrine disorders and inborn errors of metabolism that require specific diagnosis and treatment.

The finding of hypoglycemia in a neonate mandates urgent investigation to define the cause, together with rapid restoration of physiologically optimal blood glucose levels. Neonatal hypoglycemia invariably reflects a failure of fasting adaptation; therefore, this chapter focuses on the metabolic and hormonal systems involved in fasting homeostasis and abnormalities of the fasting systems that result in hypoglycemia in the newborn period.

CHARACTERISTICS OF HYPOGLYCEMIA

Despite the frequency with which low blood glucose is encountered, there is considerable controversy regarding the definition of hypoglycemia in the newborn. Based on the finding that low blood glucose levels are common in the first 12 to 24 hours of life, it has been argued that low blood glucose in the neonate represents a physiologic phenomenon[1-4] and that the newborn has unique physiologic adaptation to low blood glucose levels.[5, 6] There is, however, no evidence for this hypothesis. Although transient hypoglycemia occurring in the first 12 to 24 hours can occur in otherwise normal neonates[7] (particularly if there is a delay in feeding), it is essential to ensure that it does not persist. Hypoglycemia not responding to feeding or hypoglycemia occurring after the first 24 hours of life, needs to be investigated to avoid overlooking endocrine disorders or inborn errors of metabolism and exposing the infant to the risk of cerebral damage.

Plasma glucose is determined by a balance between glucose supply and glucose utilization. In the newborn, a large proportion of glucose utilization is accounted for by cerebral metabolism.[8] Glucose transport into the brain occurs by a carrier-mediated facilitated diffusion process dependent on circulating arterial glucose concentration;[9-11] therefore, a fall in the arterial glucose concentration places the infant at risk for neuroglycopenia. By depriving the brain of an important metabolic fuel, hypoglycemia can result in acute symptomatic cerebral dysfunction with manifestations that include lethargy, poor feeding, and seizures (Table 51-1). These findings occur particularly in circumstances in which alternative metabolic fuels such as lactate and ketone bodies are not available. If the hypoglycemia is prolonged, permanent damage to the brain can occur. There is no universally accepted level or duration of hypoglycemia associated with the risk of cerebral damage.[12]

PHYSIOLOGY OF FASTING GLUCOSE HOMEOSTASIS

Studies using radioisotope tracer techniques in fetal sheep[13] and in humans[14] have demonstrated that the fetal glucose supply is derived from the mother with no endogenous glucose production in the fetus. At the time of birth, there is an abrupt change from a high-carbohydrate and low-fat diet to a high-fat and low-carbohydrate diet.[15] At the time of birth, the neonate must make the transition from an environment of continuous glucose supply via the placenta to interrupted periods of feeding and fasting.

The healthy neonate who is able to absorb feedings uses glucose for metabolic processes and stores part of the surplus glucose in the form of glycogen in the liver and muscle and converts the remainder to fat, which is stored in adipose tissue. Hypoglycemia in the newborn occurs in the fasted state. Fasting hypoglycemia can result from developmental delays in establishing fasting metabolic systems, or it may be caused by endocrine disorders or inborn errors of intermediary metabolism. The five systems active during fasting are as follows:

1. Glycogenolysis
2. Gluconeogenesis
3. Adipose tissue lipolysis
4. Fatty acid oxidation and ketogenesis
5. Hormonal regulation of these systems

Glycogenolysis

Breakdown of glycogen stored in the liver occurs as soon as intestinal digestion of carbohydrate is exhausted, 2 to 3 hours postprandially. Glycogenolysis results in the production of glucose-6-phosphate, which can be released as free glucose by the action of glucose-6-phosphatase. Muscle glycogen cannot be released into the circulation because muscle cells lack glucose-6-phosphatase. Conditions that promote glycogenolysis are suppressed insulin levels and elevated glucagon and epinephrine levels. Liver glycogen accumulates *in utero* and is readily available to maintain plasma glucose in the immediate postnatal period. The stored glycogen is, however, depleted in 12 hours in a healthy term neonate, and more rapidly in a preterm or stressed neonate,[16] if there is no other source of glucose. Congenital defects in the enzymes of glycogenolysis are referred to as glycogen storage diseases (GSDs), and the one most likely to be associated with hypoglycemia is GSD Type 3.

Gluconeogenesis

During periods of fasting, the neonate is dependent on active gluconeogenesis to maintain plasma glucose levels. *Gluconeogenesis* is the production of glucose from precursors such as lactate, amino acids, and glycerol, and it requires four enzymes to bypass

TABLE 51-1
Signs of Hypoglycemia in Neonates

Cyanotic episodes
Apnea
Respiratory distress
Refusal to feed
Myoclonic jerks
Wilting spells
Seizures
Somnolence
Subnormal temperature
Sweating

the unidirectional steps in glycolysis. These enzymes are glucose-6-phosphatase, fructose-1,6-bisphosphatase, phosphoenolpyruvate carboxykinase (PEPCK), and pyruvate carboxylase. Most gluconeogenesis occurs in the liver, with a minor contribution from the kidney. Gluconeogenesis requires the provision of gluconeogenic substrates from peripheral tissues. The principal substrates for gluconeogenesis are lactate, alanine, and glutamine; during prolonged fasting in which there is marked lipolysis, glycerol becomes a major substrate.

The normal newborn is not able to carry out gluconeogenesis in the first few hours after birth.[17] Gluconeogenesis increases rapidly after birth in parallel with the appearance of PEPCK, the rate-limiting enzyme of this pathway. The rise in plasma glucagon and the fall in plasma insulin, which occur immediately after birth, are the main determinants of liver PEPCK induction. Liver PEPCK reaches its adult value approximately 24 hours after birth.

Adipose Tissue Lipolysis

The release of free fatty acids from adipose tissue occurs in physiologic conditions similar to those favoring gluconeogenesis (low plasma insulin and elevated plasma epinephrine and growth hormone). Free fatty acid concentrations rise rapidly soon after birth. Although free fatty acids cannot be converted to glucose, they can be oxidized in heart and skeletal muscle. They are oxidized by the liver to produce ketones, acetoacetate, and β-hydroxybutyrate (see later). By supplying an alternative source of fuel, fatty acid oxidation has a glucose-sparing effect.

Hepatic Ketogenesis

The liver produces ketones, β-hydroxybutyrate, and acetoacetate as its major end products of fatty acid oxidation. The ketones are exported and metabolized by the brain, which cannot use fatty acids as a source of fuel. Both appropriate for gestational age and small for gestational age (SGA) newborn infants fail to show the increase in plasma ketone bodies during hypoglycemia that is observed in older children. The delay in development of hepatic ketogenesis is probably the result of delayed expression of two enzymes that catalyze the first and last steps in hepatic ketogenesis: carnitine palmitoyl-transferase-1 and β-hydroxy-β-methylglutaryl–coenzyme A synthase. Delayed expression of these enzymes has been demonstrated in animal models. Fatty acids provided by the first feeding appear to play a critical role in activating transcription of key fatty acid oxidation and ketogenesis enzymes.[18-21]

Hormonal Regulation

A fall in blood glucose is the stimulus for a series of hormonal changes that act to restore blood glucose toward normal and to increase the supply of precursors for gluconeogenesis and alternative fuels.[22-24] The most important mechanism is the suppression of insulin secretion by hypoglycemia. The counterregulatory enzymes become important if blood glucose levels continue to fall; glucagon release is stimulated, followed by the release of epinephrine, cortisol,[25] and growth hormone.[26] The combination of these hormone actions suppresses hepatic glycogenolysis, activates gluconeogenesis, promotes adipose tissue lipolysis, and stimulates ketogenesis. The effects on carbohydrate metabolism serve to increase plasma glucose levels, and the effects on lipolysis and ketogenesis provide an alternative source of fuel for tissue metabolism. The overlapping effects of the counterregulatory hormones means that the loss of one can be partly compensated by other hormones that have a similar counterinsulin action.

At the time of birth, major changes occur in the concentrations of the hormones that regulate plasma glucose concentrations. There is an abrupt increase in glucagon concentration within minutes to hours of birth.[8, 27] This is accompanied by an increase in catecholamine concentrations and a fall in plasma insulin concentration. Together, these hormonal changes promote hepatic glycogenolysis and gluconeogenesis and mobilization of free fatty acids from adipose tissue. The hormonal regulation of fasting systems is summarized in Table 51-2.

TRANSIENT HYPOGLYCEMIA IN NEONATES

Delayed Development of Fasting Systems in Appropriate for Gestational Age Term and Preterm Neonates

Physiologically normal, appropriate for gestational age infants are highly susceptible to developing hypoglycemia on the first day of life if the first feeding is delayed (Table 51-3). For example, if the first feeding is not given until 6 to 8 hours after birth, 30% of term, appropriate for gestational age neonates cannot maintain plasma glucose levels higher than 50 mg/dl, and 10 to 15% may develop glucose values lower than 30 mg/dl. The risk declines quickly after 12 to 24 hours, and by the second day of life in normal newborn infants, the frequency of blood glucose levels lower than 50 mg/dL drops to less than 0.5%.[7, 28] This susceptibility to hypoglycemia is associated with developmental lags in the capacity for both hepatic ketogenesis and gluconeogenesis in the newborn, as described earlier, and it is aggravated in infants who have limited stores of glycogen.[29] Studies performed in the guinea pig and rat have shown delays in expression of the gluconeogenic enzyme, PEPCK, as well as hepatic ketogenic enzymes, carnitine palmitoyl-transferase-1 and β-hydroxy-β-methylglutaryl-coenzyme A synthase, for up to 12 hours after birth.[18,19,30,31]

Premature infants have an increased risk for hypoglycemia. Animal models of SGA infants have demonstrated a reduction in hepatic glycogen stores in addition to the delayed induction of PEPCK noted earlier in normal birth weight animals.[32, 33] Reduced fat stores, impaired fatty acid oxidation, and reduced gluconeogenesis have also been demonstrated in small for gestational age infants on day 1.[34,35]

Hyperinsulinism in Birth Asphyxia and in Small for Gestational Age Infants

Small for gestational age newborns and infants born in circumstances of perinatal stress have an increased incidence of hypoglycemia. In addition to the reduced glycogen stores in SGA

TABLE 51-2

Hormonal Regulation of Fasting Metabolic Systems

	Hepatic Glycogenolysis	Hepatic Gluconeogenesis	Adipose Tissue Lipolysis	Hepatic Ketogenesis
Insulin	Inhibits	Inhibits	Inhibits	Inhibits
Glucagon	Stimulates	—	—	Stimulates
Cortisol	—	Stimulates	—	—
Growth hormone	—	—	Stimulates	—
Epinephrine	Stimulates	Stimulates	Stimulates	Stimulates

TABLE 51-3

Classification of Hypoglycemia in the Newborn

A. Neonatal transient hypoglycemia
  1. Developmental lags in gluconeogenesis and ketogenesis
  2. Transient hyperinsulinism
    Infant of diabetic mother
  3. Perinatal stress-induced hyperinsulinism
    Small for gestational age
    Discordant twin
    Birth asphyxia
    Infant of toxemic mother
B. Neonatal persistent hypoglycemia
  1. Hyperinsulinism
    Potassium-ATP channel hyperinsulinism (recessive, dominant, focal)
    Glucokinase hyperinsulinism (dominant)
    Glutamate dehydrogenase hyperinsulinism (dominant)
    Beckwith-Wiedemann syndrome
  2. Counterregulatory hormone deficiency
    Panhypopituitarism
    Isolated growth hormone deficiency
    Cortisol deficiency
  3. Glycogenolysis disorders
    Debrancher deficiency (GSD 3)
  4. Gluconeogenesis disorders
    Glucose-6-phosphatase deficiency (GSD 1a)
    Glucose-6-phosphatase translocase deficiency (GSD 1b)
    Fructose-1,6-diphosphatase deficiency
    Pyruvate carboxylase deficiency
  5. Fatty acid oxidation disorders

GSD = glycogen storage disease.

infants, there is an increased incidence of hyperinsulinism in these infants that may persist for weeks to months.[36-39] Infants born with erythroblastosis fetalis may also exhibit hyperinsulinism. The origin of hyperinsulinism in SGA infants, those with birth asphyxia, and those with erythroblastosis fetalis is yet to be elucidated.

Infants born to diabetic mothers have an increased incidence of hypoglycemia that results from hyperinsulinism.[40] The fetus increases insulin secretion in response to increased maternal glucose, and, thus, the degree of hyperinsulinemia correlates with maternal diabetic control during pregnancy.[40] It tends to be short lived, and it usually resolves over the first few days of life. Deficiencies of the counterregulatory hormones, epinephrine and glucagon, have also been demonstrated in infants born to diabetic mothers, particularly women with poor control of the disease during pregnancy.[41,42]

CONGENITAL HYPOGLYCEMIC DISORDERS PRESENTING IN THE NEONATE

Congenital Hyperinsulinism

The term *hyperinsulinism* is applied when hypoglycemia results from inadequate suppression of the plasma insulin. Hyperinsulinism in infancy is usually a congenital defect in the regulated release of insulin from pancreatic β-cells associated with inappropriate secretion of insulin. Both sporadic and familial genetic forms of the disease are recognized, with an incidence ranging from 1 in 50,000 births in Western Europe to 1 in 2500 births in societies with high rates of consanguinity.

Congenital hyperinsulinism is a clinically and genetically heterogeneous entity. The clinical heterogeneity ranges from extremely severe, life-threatening disease to very mild clinical symptoms, which may even be difficult to identify. Furthermore, clinical responsiveness to medical and surgical management is extremely variable.[43] Early diagnosis and therapy are essential to prevent brain damage.[44]

The diagnosis of hyperinsulinism cannot rely solely on the measurement of plasma insulin levels at the time of hypoglycemia. This is because the standard assays for insulin are not sufficiently sensitive in the low range to reliably distinguish a normal from an inadequately suppressed insulin level. Insulin secretion is normally suppressed when plasma glucose levels fall to less than 65 mg/dl to values that are undetectable by conventional insulin assays. Thus, an insulin level in the "normal" range when the blood glucose is 50 mg/dl or less is consistent with hyperinsulinism.

Therefore, in addition to plasma insulin measurements at the time of hypoglycemia, other markers of excessive insulin action should be sought, including demonstration of inappropriately low plasma ketones and free fatty acids and an inappropriately large glycemic response to glucagon.[45,46] At a plasma glucose level less than 50 mg/dl, evidence of hyperinsulinism includes the following: plasma insulin level greater than 2 μU/ml, plasma β-hydroxybutyrate less than 2 mmol/l, plasma free fatty acids less than 1.5 mmol/l, and glycemic response to intravenous glucagon 1 mg greater than 30 mg/dl within 15 to 20 minutes.[47] These values reflect insulin suppression of adipose tissue lipolysis and ketone body production and preservation of glycogen stores despite falling plasma glucose levels.

The genetic basis of hyperinsulinism continues to be elucidated; mutations in four different genes have been identified. Most cases are caused by mutations in either of the two subunits of the β-cell adenosine triphosphate (ATP)–sensitive potassium channel (K_{ATP}),[48] whereas others are caused by mutations in the β-cell enzymes glucokinase and glutamate dehydrogenase (GDH). However, for as many as 50% of the cases, no genetic origin has yet been determined.[49]

Insulin Secretion

The regulation of insulin secretion is under the control of at least four mechanisms: (1) substrate mediated mechanisms via glucose and amino acids, (2) neural control by the autonomic nervous system, (3) paracrine control by glucagon and somatostatin secreted within the pancreatic islets, and (4) β-cell autoregulation. Of these mechanisms, abnormalities in the substrate-mediated pathways are known to be associated with genetic forms of hyperinsulinism (Fig. 51-1).

The mechanism of insulin release that is most completely characterized is substrate-mediated insulin release via the K_{ATP} channel and the voltage-gated calcium channel. In the resting state, the membrane potential of the β-cell is dependent on potassium efflux via the K_{ATP} channel. The K_{ATP} channel is regulated by the intracellular ratio of ATP to adenosine diphosphate (ATP/ADP ratio); the channel is closed when this ratio increases. When the cell membrane becomes depolarized (resulting in opening of voltage-gated calcium channels) and an influx of calcium occurs, insulin release is stimulated. The intracellular ATP/ADP ratio is increased by oxidation of substrates in the β-cell. Glucose enters the β-cell and is metabolized via the glycolysis pathway to generate ATP.[50] In the β-cell, glucose phosphorylation carried out by glucokinase is the rate-controlling step in glycolysis.[51] In this manner, glucokinase functions as the pancreatic cell "glucosensor" that governs the dose-response relationship between glucose and insulin release.[52,53]

An increase in the ATP/ADP ratio can also be generated by an increase in the oxidation of glutamate, a reaction catalyzed by the enzyme GDH. GDH activity is controlled allosterically by guanosine triphosphate (GTP) inhibition and is stimulated by ADP or leucine.[54,55] Activating mutations in the GDH gene cause the hyperinsulinism and hyperammonemia syndrome.

Potassium Channel Hyperinsulinism

Recessive Hyperinsulinism. Previously referred to as nesidioblastosis, infants with this form of hyperinsulinism typically present large for gestational age with severe hypoglycemia soon

β-Cell

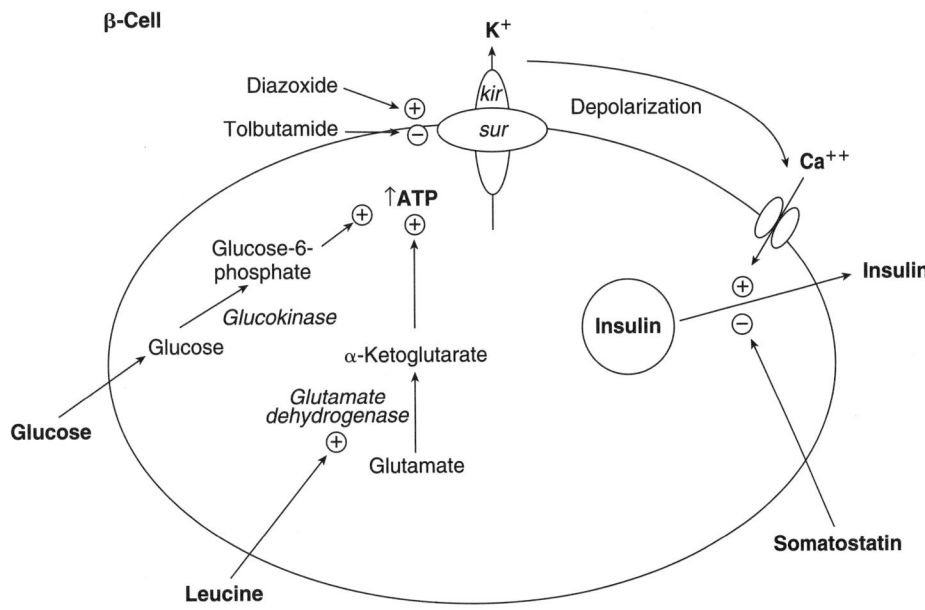

The gene for MCAD is located on chromosome one (1p31)

Figure 51–1. Pancreatic β-cell insulin secretion. Glucose stimulates insulin secretion via its oxidation, which increases levels of intracellular adenosine triphosphate (ATP), which inhibits the potassium efflux through the potassium (K_{ATP}) channel (sur, Kir complex). Closure of the K_{ATP} channel depolarizes the plasma membrane, which activates the voltage-gated calcium channel to increase intracellular calcium and to trigger exocytosis of insulin granules. Leucine is an allosteric activator of glutamate dehydrogenase (GDH); increased activity of GDH increases glutamate oxidation, which also increases intracellular ATP. Diazoxide inhibits insulin release by preventing closure of the K_{ATP} channel. Tolbutamide stimulates insulin secretion by closing the K_{ATP} channel. Somatostatin decreases insulin release by downstream mechanisms.

after delivery. The genetic defect impairs either the SUR1 or Kir6.2 components of the K_{ATP} channel, with most mutations discovered to date affecting the *SUR1* gene.[49, 56, 57] The genes for SUR1 and Kir6.2 are located on chromosome 11p, immediately adjacent to one another, and they have been cloned.[58] Because the mechanism of hyperinsulinism in these cases is an abnormal K_{ATP} channel, therapeutic interventions that act via the SUR such as administration of diazoxide are often ineffective in this condition. Thus, many affected infants require near-total pancreatectomy.

Focal Hyperinsulinism. In the recessive form of hyperinsulinism described earlier, histologic abnormalities of islet nuclear hyperplasia are uniform throughout the pancreas. In the focal form of hyperinsulinism, the area of abnormality is localized to a small, 3- to 5-mm diameter region described as focal adenomatous hyperplasia. The clinical presentation is indistinguishable from the recessive form of hyperinsulinism described earlier. The focal lesions arise as a result of a localized clonal loss of the maternal 11p15 region and expression of a paternally inherited *SUR1* or *Kir6.2* mutation.[59, 60] The loss of the maternal alleles in the 11p15 region is confined to the area of focal adenomatous hyperplasia.[60, 61] The 11p15 region contains several maternally imprinted tumor suppresser genes. It is postulated that the loss of heterozygosity in the region accounts for the focus of hyperplasia.[62, 63] Approximately half of infants with hyperinsulinism requiring surgery may have focal lesions and thus are potentially curable.

Dominant Hyperinsulinism. One family with dominantly inherited congenital hyperinsulinism has been described,[64] associated with a novel *SUR1* mutation. In this report, the patients had a less severe presentation than is typical for other forms of K_{ATP} hyperinsulinism.

Glutamate Dehydrogenase Hyperinsulinism

The hyperinsulinism and hyperammonemia syndrome has been reported as a cause of moderately severe hyperinsulinism with diffuse involvement of the pancreas.[65] As described earlier, GDH is a mitochondrial matrix enzyme that functions in the β-cell in the pathway of leucine-stimulated insulin secretion. The mutations associated with hyperinsulinism impair allosteric inhibition of GDH by GTP and result in a decreased inhibitory effect of GTP on GDH and uninhibited insulin release.[66-68] Clinical manifestations included normal birth weight, late onset of hypoglycemia, diazoxide responsiveness, and protein-sensitive hypoglycemia.[67,69]

Counterregulatory Hormone Deficiencies

Neonatal hypoglycemia occurring secondary to counterregulatory deficiency usually results from pituitary deficiency with various combinations of cortisol and growth hormone deficiency. The clinical presentation of neonates with hypopituitarism can be identical to that seen in hyperinsulinism, requiring a high glucose infusion rate to maintain euglycemia, inappropriate hypoketonemia, and a positive glycemic response to intravenous glucagon at the time of hypoglycemia.

Defects in Gluconeogenesis

GSD 1a (glucose-6-phosphatase deficiency) and GSD 1b (glucose-6-phosphate translocase deficiency) result in a complete inability of the liver to release glucose into the circulation because the formation of glucose from glucose-6-phosphate is a common step in both glycogenolysis and gluconeogenesis. Infants present with hypoglycemia, hepatomegaly, and lactic acidosis.

Deficiency of the enzyme fructose-1,6-diphosphatase results in a blockage of gluconeogenesis from all precursors below the level of fructose-1,6-diphosphate. Infants present with hypoglycemia, lactic acidosis, and hepatomegaly.[70] The disease is inherited as an autosomal recessive condition[71] that can present in neonates and can be fatal. Several cases with possible PEPCK deficiency have been reported;[72, 73] however, this deficiency remains to be confirmed.

Glycogen Storage Diseases

GSDs comprise a group of disorders characterized by abnormal glycogen synthesis or degradation. Hypoglycemia is a feature of several of these disorders, but not all. The two most likely to present in the neonatal period with hypoglycemia are GSD 1 (glucose-6-phosphatase deficiency) and GSD 3 (debrancher deficiency). GSD 1 has been classified as a disorder of gluconeogenesis (see earlier) because the enzyme catalyzes the final common step in glycogenolysis and gluconeogenesis.

Debrancher enzyme deficiency results in an inability to degrade stored glycogen. The disorder is autosomal recessive, with more than 30 mutations reported. The manifestations of the disease include hepatomegaly, hypoglycemia, skeletal myopathy, and cardiomyopathy. Although the disorder usually presents later in infancy, there are reports of neonatal presentation with hypoglycemia.

Fatty Acid Oxidation Defects

Fatty acid oxidation defects is the term applied to errors in the pathway of fatty acid uptake and activation and mitochondrial oxidation. Errors in this pathway disturb oxidative phosphorylation and ATP generation and result in loss of ketogenesis and inhibition of gluconeogenesis.[74] These disorders are provoked by fasting or substrate deprivation and result in hypoglycemia associated with a deficiency in the generation of ketone bodies. The manifestations are usually systemic, involving liver, heart, and skeletal muscle. In severe cases, there may be a Reye-like syndrome resulting in coma and death. Less severe defects can produce a combination of hypotonia or weakness, cardiac hypertrophy, hepatomegaly, nausea, and vomiting with fasting.[75] The diagnosis of suspected disorders of fatty acid oxidation can often be made by determination of the plasma acyl-carnitine profile by mass spectrometry.

Medium chain acyl coenzyme A dehydrogenase (MCAD) deficiency is the most common fatty acid oxidation defect, with a frequency of 1 in 8000.[76, 77] This disorder is now a component of newborn screening protocols in some states. The gene for MCAD is located on chromosome 1 (1p31). A point mutation causing a change from lysine to glutamate at position 304 in the mature MCAD protein has been found in 90% of patients with MCAD who were identified retrospectively,[78] although the frequency of this mutation may be lower in patients identified by neonatal screening.[79, 80] The disorder is readily treated by avoidance of prolonged fasting.

SUMMARY

Hypoglycemia occurring in the neonate reflects an abnormality in fasting adaptation. The endocrine and metabolic systems required during fasting and their normal developmental sequence are emphasized in this chapter. Neonatal hypoglycemia occurring secondary to maturational delay in two of these fasting systems, gluconeogenesis and ketogenesis, is likely to occur if feeding is delayed after birth. Beyond 12 to 24 hours, neonatal hypoglycemia requires specific diagnosis, to institute appropriate treatment and to avoid adverse outcomes. Persistent neonatal hypoglycemia is most commonly the result of transient hyperinsulinism in infants with birth asphyxia, in SGA infants,

and in infants of diabetic mothers. Genetic causes of persistent neonatal hypoglycemia such as congenital hyperinsulinism, hypopituitarism, and gluconeogenesis disorders also need to be considered. Inborn errors of metabolism rarely present with hypoglycemia in the newborn period; of those that do, fatty acid oxidation defects are the most common.

REFERENCES

1. Pildes R, et al: The incidence of neonatal hypoglycemia: a completed survey. J Pediatr 70:76, 1967.
2. Pildes RS, et al: Studies of carbohydrate metabolism in the newborn infant. IX. Blood glucose levels and hypoglycemia in twins. Pediatrics 40:69, 1967.
3. Cornblath M, et al: Hypoglycemia in the newborn. Pediatr Clin North Am 13:905, 1966.
4. Heck LJ, Erenberg A: Serum glucose levels in term neonates during the first 48 hours of life. J Pediatr 110:119, 1987.
5. Cornblath M: Unique metabolic adaptation in the fetus and newborn. N Engl J Med 285:631, 1971.
6. Cornblath M, et al: Metabolic adaptation in the neonate. Isr J Med Sci 8:453, 1972.
7. Lubchenco LO, Bard H: Incidence of hypoglycemia in newborn infants classified by birth weight and gestational age. Pediatrics 47:831, 1971.
8. Menon RK, Sperling MA: Carbohydrate metabolism. Semin Perinatol 12:157, 1988.
9. Settergren G, et al: Cerebral blood flow and exchange of oxygen, glucose, ketone bodies, lactate, pyruvate and amino acids in infants. Acta Paediatr Scand 65:343, 1976.
10. Devaskar SU: The mammalian brain glucose transport system. Adv Exp Med Biol 293:405, 1991.
11. Devaskar SU, Mueckler MM: The mammalian glucose transporters. Pediatr Res 31:1, 1992.
12. Cornblath M, et al: Controversies regarding definition of neonatal hypoglycemia: suggested operational thresholds. Pediatrics 105:1141, 2000.
13. Bloch CA, Sperling MA: Sources and disposition of fetal glucose: studies in the fetal lamb. Am J Perinatol 5:344, 1988.
14. Kalhan SC, et al: Measurement of glucose turnover in the human newborn with glucose-1-13C. J Clin Endocrinol Metab 43:704, 1976.
15. Girard J: Gluconeogenesis in late fetal and early neonatal life. Biol Neonate 50:237, 1986.
16. Girard J, et al: Adaptations of glucose and fatty acid metabolism during perinatal period and suckling-weaning transition. Physiol Rev 72:507, 1992.
17. Kalhan SC, et al: Estimation of glucose turnover and 13C recycling in the human newborn by simultaneous [1-13C]glucose and [6,6-1H2]glucose tracers. J Clin Endocrinol Metab 50:456, 1980.
18. Asins G, et al: Developmental changes in the phospho(enol)pyruvate carboxykinase gene expression in small intestine and liver of suckling rats. Arch Biochem Biophys 329:82, 1996.
19. Pegorier JP, et al: Role of long-chain fatty acids in the postnatal induction of genes coding for liver mitochondrial beta-oxidative enzymes. Biochem Soc Trans 26:113, 1998.
20. Prip-Buus C, et al: Hormonal and nutritional control of liver fatty acid oxidation and ketogenesis during development. Biochem Soc Trans 23:500, 1995.
21. Chatelain F, et al: Cyclic AMP and fatty acids increase carnitine palmitoyltransferase I gene transcription in cultured fetal rat hepatocytes. Eur J Biochem 235:789, 1996.
22. Cryer PE, Gerich JE: Glucose counterregulation, hypoglycemia, and intensive insulin therapy in diabetes mellitus. N Engl J Med 313:232, 1985.
23. Gerich JE, Campbell PJ: Overview of counterregulation and its abnormalities in diabetes mellitus and other conditions. Diabetes Metab Rev 4:93, 1988.
24. Gerich JE: Lilly lecture 1988: glucose counterregulation and its impact on diabetes mellitus. Diabetes 37:1608, 1988.
25. De Feo P, et al: Contribution of cortisol to glucose counterregulation in humans. Am J Physiol 257:E35, 1989.
26. De Feo P, et al: Demonstration of a role for growth hormone in glucose counterregulation. Am J Physiol 256:E835, 1989.
27. Sperling MA, et al: Spontaneous and amino acid-stimulated glucagon secretion in the immediate postnatal period: relation to glucose and insulin. J Clin Invest 53:1159, 1974.
28. Stanley CA, et al: Metabolic fuel and hormone responses to fasting in newborn infants. Pediatrics 64:613, 1979.
29. Fernandez E, et al: Postnatal hypoglycaemia and gluconeogenesis in the newborn rat: delayed onset of gluconeogenesis in prematurely delivered newborns. Biochem J 214:525, 1983.
30. Thumelin S, et al: Developmental changes in mitochondrial 3-hydroxy-3-methylglutaryl-CoA synthase gene expression in rat liver, intestine and kidney. Biochem J 292:493, 1993.
31. Stanley CA, et al: Development of hepatic fatty acid oxidation and ketogenesis in the newborn guinea pig. Pediatr Res 17:224, 1983.
32. Bussey ME, et al: Hypoglycemia in the newborn growth-retarded rat: delayed phosphoenolpyruvate carboxykinase induction despite increased glucagon availability. Pediatr Res 19:363, 1985.

33. Kliegman RM: Alterations of fasting glucose and fat metabolism in intrauterine growth-retarded newborn dogs. Am J Physiol 256:E380, 1989.
34. Sabel KG, et al: Interrelation between fatty acid oxidation and control of gluconeogenic substrates in small-for-gestational-age (SGA) infants with hypoglycemia and with normoglycemia. Acta Paediatr Scand 71:53, 1982.
35. Williams PR, et al: Effects of oral alanine feeding on blood glucose, plasma glucagon and insulin concentrations in small-for-gestational-age infants. N Engl J Med 292:612, 1975.
36. Bhowmick SK, Lewandowski C: Prolonged hyperinsulinism and hypoglycemia in an asphyxiated, small for gestation infant: case management and literature review. Clin Pediatr 28:575, 1989.
37. Collins JE, Leonard JV: Hyperinsulinism in asphyxiated and small-for-dates infants with hypoglycaemia. Lancet 2:311, 1984.
38. Collins JE, et al: Hyperinsulinaemic hypoglycaemia in small for dates babies. Arch Dis Child 65:1118, 1990.
39. Clark W, O'Donovan D: Transient hyperinsulinism in an asphyxiated newborn infant with hypoglycemia. Am J Perinatol 18:175, 2001.
40. Kuhl C, et al: Metabolic events in infants of diabetic mothers during first 24 hours after birth. I. Changes in plasma glucose, insulin and glucagon. Acta Paediatr Scand 71:19, 1982.
41. Artal R, et al: Circulating catecholamines and glucagon in infants of strictly controlled diabetic mothers. Biol Neonate 53:121, 1988.
42. Broberger U, et al: Sympatho-adrenal activity and metabolic adjustment during the first 12 hours after birth in infants of diabetic mothers. Acta Paediatr Scand 73:620, 1984.
43. Stanley CA: Hyperinsulinism in infants and children. Pediatr Clin North Am 44:363, 1997.
44. Meissner T, et al: Persistent hyperinsulinaemic hypoglycaemia of infancy: therapy, clinical outcome and mutational analysis. Eur J Pediatr 156:754, 1997.
45. Stanley CA, Baker L: Hyperinsulinism in infancy: diagnosis by demonstration of abnormal response to fasting hypoglycemia. Pediatrics 57:702, 1976.
46. Stanley CA, Baker L: Hyperinsulinism in infants and children: diagnosis and therapy. Adv Pediatr 23:315, 1976.
47. Finegold DN, et al: Glycemic response to glucagon during fasting hypoglycemia: an aid in the diagnosis of hyperinsulinism. J Pediatr 96:257, 1980.
48. Kane C, et al: Loss of functional KATP channels in pancreatic beta-cells causes persistent hyperinsulinemic hypoglycemia of infancy. Nat Med 2:1344, 1996.
49. Glaser B, et al: Genetics of neonatal hyperinsulinism. Arch Dis Child 82:F79, 2000.
50. Matschinsky FM, et al: Pancreatic beta-cell glucokinase: closing the gap between theoretical concepts and experimental realities. Diabetes 47:307, 1998.
51. Sweet IR, Matschinsky FM: Mathematical model of beta-cell glucose metabolism and insulin release. I. Glucokinase as glucosensor hypothesis. Am J Physiol 268:E775, 1995.
52. Davis EA, et al: Mutants of glucokinase cause hypoglycaemia- and hyperglycaemia syndromes and their analysis illuminates fundamental quantitative concepts of glucose homeostasis. Diabetologia 42:1175, 1999.
53. Matschinsky FM: Glucokinase as glucose sensor and metabolic signal generator in pancreatic beta-cells and hepatocytes. Diabetes 39:647, 1990.
54. Hsu BY, et al: Protein-sensitive and fasting hypoglycemia in children with the hyperinsulinism/hyperammonemia syndrome. J Pediatr 138:383, 2001.
55. Gylfe E: Comparison of the effects of leucines, non-metabolizable leucine analogues and other insulin secretagogues on the activity of glutamate dehydrogenase. Acta Diabetol Lat 13:20, 1976.
56. Thomas PM, et al: The molecular basis for familial persistent hyperinsulinemic hypoglycemia of infancy. Proc Assoc Am Physicians 108:14, 1996.
57. Thomas P, et al: Mutation of the pancreatic islet inward rectifier Kir6.2 also leads to familial persistent hyperinsulinemic hypoglycemia of infancy. Hum Mol Genet 5:1809, 1996.
58. Shepherd RM, et al: Hyperinsulinism of infancy: towards an understanding of unregulated insulin release. European Network for Research into Hyperinsulinism in Infancy. Arch Dis Child 82:F87, 2000.
59. Verkarre V, et al: Paternal mutation of the sulfonylurea receptor (SUR1) gene and maternal loss of 11p15 imprinted genes lead to persistent hyperinsulinism in focal adenomatous hyperplasia. J Clin Invest 102:1286, 1998.
60. Fournet JC, et al: Unbalanced expression of 11p15 imprinted genes in focal forms of congenital hyperinsulinism: association with a reduction to homozygosity of a mutation in ABCC8 or KCNJ11. Am J Pathol 158:2177, 2001.
61. de Lonlay P, et al: Somatic deletion of the imprinted 11p15 region in sporadic persistent hyperinsulinemic hypoglycemia of infancy is specific of focal adenomatous hyperplasia and endorses partial pancreatectomy. J Clin Invest 100:802, 1997.
62. Fournet JC, et al: Loss of imprinted genes and paternal SUR1 mutations lead to focal form of congenital hyperinsulinism. Horm Res 53(Suppl 1):2, 2000.
63. Kassem SA, et al: p57 (KIP2) expression in normal islet cells and in hyperinsulinism of infancy. Diabetes 50:2763, 2001.
64. Huopio H, et al: Dominantly inherited hyperinsulinism caused by a mutation in the sulfonylurea receptor type 1. J Clin Invest 106:897, 2000.
65. Weinzimer SA, et al: A syndrome of congenital hyperinsulinism and hyperammonemia. J Pediatr 130:661, 1997.
66. Stanley CA, et al: Hyperinsulinism and hyperammonemia in infants with regulatory mutations of the glutamate dehydrogenase gene. N Engl J Med 338:1352, 1998.
67. Stanley CA, et al: Molecular basis and characterization of the hyperinsulinism/hyperammonemia syndrome: predominance of mutations in exons 11 and 12 of the glutamate dehydrogenase gene. HI/HA Contributing Investigators. Diabetes 49:667, 2000.
68. MacMullen C, et al: Hyperinsulinism/hyperammonemia syndrome in children with regulatory mutations in the inhibitory guanosine triphosphate–binding domain of glutamate dehydrogenase. J Clin Endocrinol Metab 86:1782, 2001.
69. Kelly A, et al: Acute insulin responses to leucine in children with the hyperinsulinism/hyperammonemia syndrome. J Clin Endocrinol Metab 86:3724, 2001.
70. Baker L, Winegrad AI: Fasting hypoglycaemia and metabolic acidosis associated with deficiency of hepatic fructose-1,6-diphosphatase activity. Lancet 2:13, 1970.
71. Kikawa Y, et al: Identification of genetic mutations in Japanese patients with fructose-1,6-bisphosphatase deficiency. Am J Hum Genet 61:852, 1997.
72. Vidnes J, Sovik O: Gluconeogenesis in infancy and childhood. III. Deficiency of the extramitochondrial form of hepatic phosphoenolpyruvate carboxykinase in a case of persistent neonatal hypoglycaemia. Acta Paediatr Scand 65:307, 1976.
73. Vidnes J, Sovik O: Gluconeogenesis in infancy and childhood. II. Studies on the glucose production from alanine in three cases of persistent neonatal hypoglycaemia. Acta Paediatr Scand 65:297, 1976.
74. Ozand PT: Hypoglycemia in association with various organic and amino acid disorders. Semin Perinatol 24:172, 2000.
75. Hale DE, Bennett MJ: Fatty acid oxidation disorders: a new class of metabolic diseases. J Pediatr 121:1, 1992.
76. Chace DH, et al: Rapid diagnosis of MCAD deficiency: quantitatively analysis of octanoylcarnitine and other acylcarnitines in newborn blood spots by tandem mass spectrometry. Clin Chem 43:2106, 1997.
77. Seymour CA, et al: Newborn screening for inborn errors of metabolism: a systematic review. Health Technol Assess (Winchester) 1:i, 1997.
78. Wang SS, et al: Medium chain acyl-CoA dehydrogenase deficiency human genome epidemiology review. Genet Med 1:332, 1999.
79. Ziadeh R, et al: Medium chain acyl-CoA dehydrogenase deficiency in Pennsylvania: neonatal screening shows high incidence and unexpected mutation frequencies. Pediatr Res 37:675, 1995.
80. Carpenter K, et al: Evaluation of newborn screening for medium chain acyl-CoA dehydrogenase deficiency in 275,000 babies. Arch Dis Child 85:F105, 2001.

Protein Metabolism

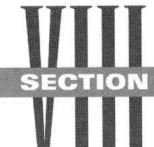

Dwight E. Matthews and Johannes B. van Goudoever

General Concepts of Protein Metabolism

The purpose of this chapter is to describe the methods used to follow dynamic changes in protein metabolism in the newborn. When protein metabolism is discussed, the fundamental point to remember is that amino acids differ from carbohydrate and fat *only* by the inclusion of nitrogen (N). Alanine without its N is pyruvate, which is half a glucose molecule. It is the N atom in amino acids that sets protein apart from carbohydrate and fat, and it is the N aspect of amino acid and protein metabolism that we wish to study. This seemingly obvious point is fundamental.

NITROGEN BALANCE

The oldest (and most widely used) method to follow changes in body N is the *N balance* method. This routine method has been the standard means of defining minimum levels of dietary protein and essential amino acid intake in humans of all ages.[1-3] However, N balance defines only the difference between N going in and N coming out of the body. This is measured by carefully recording all food consumed and collecting all material excreted: urine, feces, sputum, and so on. The N from aliquots of each food, urine, and fecal collection is tediously converted to ammonia by boiling the specimens in concentrated acid. The ammonia is determined, and N intake and excretion are calculated. This simple N balance technique is fraught with technical difficulties: N losses are routinely *underestimated* because of incomplete collections of urine and feces and insensible losses through skin, sweat, and so on, whereas N intake is routinely *overestimated* because of food not consumed, and so on.[4,5]

Alternatively, the anthropometric measure of growth may be used to determine efficacy of the level and quality of protein in the diet of infants. Measurement of growth is an indication of well-being but gives no information specific to protein metabolism. Although measures of N balance and growth have often been used to study infant nutrition,[2,6] both methods require days or weeks to measure effects. Neither method provides any information concerning the turnover of N *within* the body. For example, consider an infant receiving adequate protein, but insufficient energy intake for growth. Assume the infant has a restricted intake, is not growing, and has an N balance of zero. When the infant receives more calories, starts growing, and shows a positive N balance, how did the child's body respond to produce this effect? N balance and growth measurements do not tell us. Figure 52-1 shows four possible responses to the situation. Case 0 is the starting zero N balance. Positive N balance could have been obtained by increasing protein synthesis (case A in Fig. 52-1), decreasing protein breakdown (case C in Fig. 52-1), increasing both but having protein synthesis increase more (case

B in Fig. 52-1), or the opposite (case D in Fig. 52-1). The effect is a positive N balance in all four situations, but the energy implications are considerably different. Because protein synthesis costs energy, cases A and B are more expensive, whereas cases C and D require less energy than the starting case 0. When answers such as these are sought, we have to look directly into the system at rates of protein breakdown, synthesis, and amino acid turnover. For this, we need to be able to look within the system using a labeled tracer.

MODELS FOR WHOLE BODY AMINO ACID AND PROTEIN METABOLISM

The simplest approach to the study of amino acid and protein kinetics is to assume a single, free pool of amino acid N with *two inflows*—amino acid from dietary protein and amino acid released from protein breakdown—and *two outflows*—amino acid oxidation to end products (carbon dioxide [CO_2], urea, and ammonia) and amino acid uptake for protein synthesis (Fig. 52-2). This model can be considered either for whole body protein turnover, in which the pool is the total free amino acid pool (see Fig. 52-2), or for the kinetics of a single amino acid, in which the pools are for a particular amino acid (illustrated for a ^{13}C tracer in Fig. 52-3). The difference between the two approaches is related to how the system is viewed: looking at protein turnover versus looking at the kinetics of a specific amino acid from which inferences to whole body protein turnover are drawn.

All protein in the body (e.g., structural, enzymes) is constantly being made and broken down. Most of the protein in the body turns over slowly (e.g., muscle protein) and can be considered a large amorphous inflow of amino acid via protein breakdown and a large amorphous uptake of amino acid from the fast-turnover free amino acid-N pool. This defines the traditional single-pool model of protein metabolism. The single pool is the free amino acid pool. Because of the size and slow turnover of the protein pool, it is considered to be a *sink* via uptake of amino acids for protein synthesis and is a *source* for amino acid entry via protein breakdown. Whatever tracer enters this protein pool during the time course of the study is not likely to exit. Therefore, even though a "box" or "circle" is drawn in the figures for the models for whole body protein turnover, mathematically it is not considered a pool at all.

Lumping all body protein into a single entity is a gross oversimplification. There are many different tissues, each with a wide range of proteins and each with different turnover rates. However, following the individual rates of hundreds of proteins is an impossible task. Because most of the important stores of N

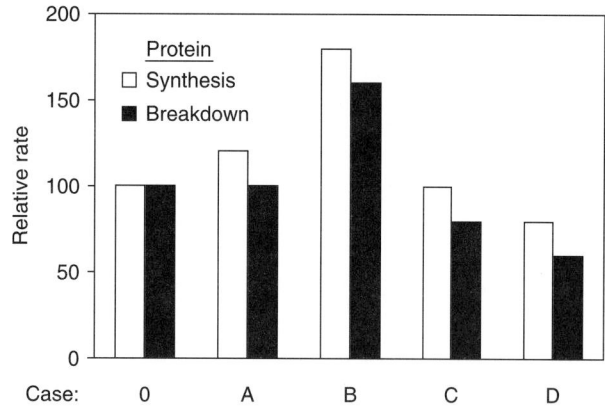

Figure 52–1. Four different hypothetical responses to a change from a zero balance *(case 0)* to a positive nitrogen (N) balance *(cases A to D)*. A positive N balance can be obtained *(A)* by increasing protein synthesis, *(B)* by increasing synthesis more than breakdown, *(C)* by decreasing breakdown, or *(D)* by decreasing breakdown more than synthesis. The N balance method does not distinguish among any of the four possibilities.

in the body turn over at similarly slow rates, it is possible to simplify the system into a conceptual model.

METHODS FOR MEASURING PROTEIN METABOLISM IN HUMANS

Table 52-1 lists the methods used to measure protein and N metabolism in humans. As already discussed, measurements of growth and N balance do not provide information on how protein balance is regulated. Changes in amino acid metabolism for a specific tissue can be inferred by measuring the difference between the amino acids delivered to the tissue (arterial blood levels) and the amino acids released from the tissue (venous blood levels). In adults, this technique has been applied to studies of forearm, leg, liver, kidney, and brain metabolism.[7-9] In animals, this model has been important in dissecting fetal and placental metabolism.[10] However, measuring an arteriovenous difference is similar to the N balance technique—it provides information about the balance across the tissue bed but tells nothing about the mechanism within the tissue affecting the balance. Most exciting is the combination of tracer infusion with the measurement of amino acid balance across the tissue bed. This technique allows for a complete solution of the various pathways operating in the tissue for each amino acid tracer used and can measure tissue-specific rates of protein synthesis and balance.[11-13] However, the use of arterial and venous catheters primarily restricts the applicability of this method to animal models.[10, 14-20] Only a few investigations have addressed human fetal amino acid metabolism by infusing amino acid tracers into

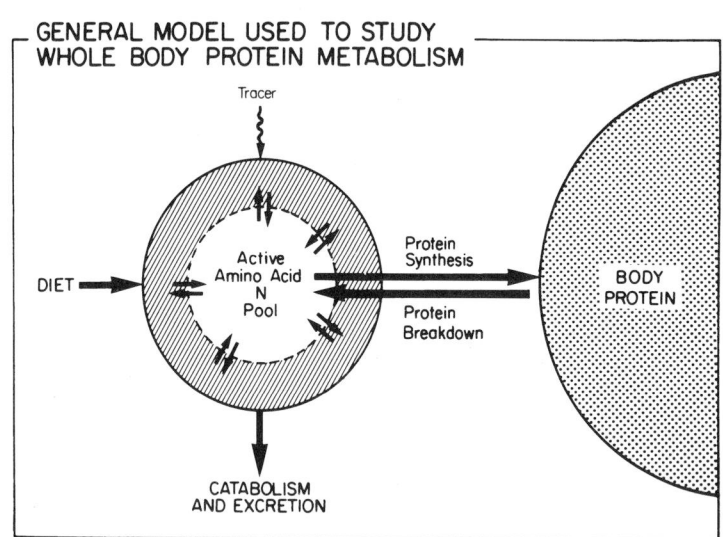

Figure 52–2. Single-pool amino acid model for whole body protein metabolism. The model is applied without requiring definition of individual pools. All free amino acid nitrogen (N) is lumped together. The *shaded outer circle* indicates interchange of free amino acids with various intracellular free amino acid pools and with incorporation into and release from faster-turnover proteins. Slower-turnover protein, such as muscle protein, appears as an exit from the system for free amino acid via protein synthesis and a source of free amino acid entry via protein breakdown. Amino acids also leave the system by oxidation to the end products (carbon dioxide, urea, and ammonia) and can enter via absorption of dietary protein or amino acids. (From Matthews DE: *In* Duncan WP, Susan AB [eds]: Synthesis and Applications of Isotopically Labeled Compounds. Amsterdam, Elsevier Scientific, 1983, pp 279-284.)

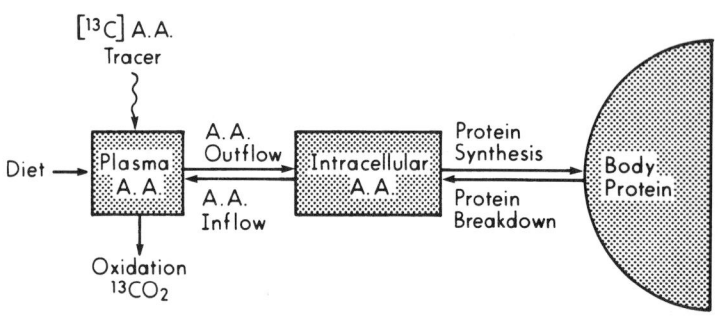

Figure 52–3. Simplified model for following the kinetics of an individual essential amino acid (A.A.) using a ^{13}C label. The ^{13}C-labeled amino acid is infused intravenously. The tracer equilibrates with the free amino acid in plasma and in intracellular compartments. Amino acid is taken up from and released into the intracellular compartment via protein synthesis and breakdown. Amino acid oxidized intracellularly to form carbon dioxide (CO_2) is released into plasma as bicarbonate, and then into exhaled breath as CO_2. (From Bier DM, et al: *In* Garrow JS, Halliday D [eds]: Substrate and Energy Metabolism in Man. London, John Libbey, 1985, pp 27-36.)

TABLE 52-1

Methods for Measuring Protein and Nitrogen Metabolism in Humans

Growth
Nitrogen balance
End-product method
Turnover of individual components
Essential amino acids (index of protein breakdown)
Nonessential amino acids (*de novo* synthesis and gluconeogenesis)
Urea (protein oxidation)
Arteriovenous measurement of amino acids across a tissue bed
Protein synthesis of a specific protein by following tracer incorporation
Protein degradation of a specific protein by following disappearance of
    tracer from the protein

the mother before delivery and obtaining cord blood at delivery to determine fetal metabolism.[21] The closest way to obtain specific tissue amino acid metabolism in human neonates is the simultaneous use of enteral and intravenous tracers. First-pass amino acid metabolism of the small intestine and liver is measured by comparison of the tracer enrichments of both tracers in plasma. The plasma enrichment of the enteral administered tracer will be lower compared with the plasma enrichment of the intravenously infused tracer by the amount of material sequestered by the gut and liver on the first pass during enteral absorption of the tracer. The ratio between the enrichment of the intravenous administered tracer and the enteral administered tracer is used to calculate the first-pass uptake.[22]

End-Product Approach to Measurement of Protein Metabolism

Because glycine is the only amino acid without an optically active α-carbon center, [15N]glycine is the most easily labeled amino acid to synthesize and was the earliest tracer used for measuring protein turnover in the body. Using this tracer, Sprinson and Rittenberg[23] performed pioneering studies of protein metabolism based on a compartmental analysis of a single pool. As indicated in Figure 52-2, the free amino acid-N pool is far too complex to be forced into a single kinetic pool when the metabolism of multiple amino acids is considered. The problem is not in conceptualizing a single amino acid pool, but in applying mathematical equations specific to a single pool. Therefore, almost no progress was made in studying protein metabolism in humans after the initial description by Sprinson and Rittenberg until 1969, when Picou and Taylor-Roberts[24] proposed a significant and simple alternative. Conceptually, the same single-pool approach was used, but no specific single-pool kinetic restriction was applied; that is, the system was viewed in a stochastic fashion.[25] This approach is depicted graphically in Figure 52-4. The [15N]glycine tracer is given, and the [15N]glycine mixes (scatters) among the free amino acids. The 15N in the free amino acid pool is diluted with unlabeled amino acid entering from protein breakdown and from dietary intake. Using the rate of 15N infusion and after measuring the dilution of 15N in the free amino acid pool, the rate of unlabeled N appearance is readily calculated:

$$Q = 100 \bullet i / E$$

where Q is the free amino acid-N pool turnover rate (typically expressed as mg N/kg/day), i is the rate of [15N]glycine infusion (mg 15N/kg/day), and E is the 15N enrichment (dilution of 15N by unlabeled N, expressed as *atom* or *mole percentage of excess*). The 100 factor converts mole percentage to mole fraction. The

dilution of the [15N]glycine tracer (i.e., enrichment in the free amino acid-N pool) is sampled indirectly via either the urea or ammonia end products, which are produced from the free amino acids. According to the standard precursor-product relationship,[25] a product (i.e., urinary urea or ammonia) formed from a single precursor will have an enrichment equal to the precursor (i.e., the free amino acid-N pool).

The rate of whole body protein breakdown (B) is determined from the turnover (Q) by subtracting the known rate of dietary N intake (I):

$$B = Q–I$$

In these calculations, the standard value of 6.25 g protein = 1 g N is used to interconvert protein and N. Attention to the units (grams of *protein* versus grams of *N*) is important, because both units are often used concurrently in the literature.

Like most of the kinetic methods, the end-product method assumes steady-state conditions with respect to the free pool (i.e., the free N pool is neither expanding nor contracting). Obviously, the free pool does both, but over the period of most measurements, increases cancel decreases so the steady-state assumption is reasonable. When *inflows* equal *outflows*:

$$Q = I + B = C + S$$

where the outflows are amino acid-N oxidation (C) to end products urea and ammonia and amino acid-N uptake for protein synthesis (S). Amino acid-N oxidation is simply the sum of the ammonia and urea production rates, which are determined by urine collection. Therefore, the rate of whole body synthesis is

$$S = Q–C$$

Occasionally in the literature,[26] a term called *net protein balance* or *net protein gain* will appear, which is the difference between the measured synthesis and breakdown rates (S–B). Rearranging the balance equation for Q shows that

$$S–B = I–C$$

and I–C is simply the difference between intake and excretion, that is, *N balance*. Therefore, the S–B term is a misnomer in that it is based solely on the N balance measurement and not on the administration of the 15N tracer.

There is no question that the end-product method of Picou and Taylor-Roberts[24] has been the cornerstone method for protein metabolic research in pediatrics. The overwhelming advantage of this method is that it can be completely noninvasive, although the end-product method is not without its problems.

As described by Picou and Taylor-Roberts,[24] the [15N]glycine tracer is given orally at short intervals (e.g., every 3 hours) until a plateau for 15N is reached in urinary urea. The time required to reach this plateau is about 60 hours, regardless of whether adults,[27] children, or infants[28-30] are studied. The delay in attaining a plateau results from the time required for the 15N tracer to equilibrate within the free glycine, serine, and urea pools.[27,31] An additional problem is plateau definition. Often, the urinary urea 15N time course does not show by either visual inspection or curve-fitting regression the anticipated single exponential rise to plateau.

Although [15N]glycine tracer is the cheapest amino acid to purchase, any 15N-labeled amino acid can be used in the end-product method, but widely divergent results have been obtained when different 15N-labeled amino acid tracers have been used for the end-product method.[32-34] Table 52-2 shows the values of protein turnover measured for a single adult subject receiving different 15N-labeled amino acid and protein preparations on different days

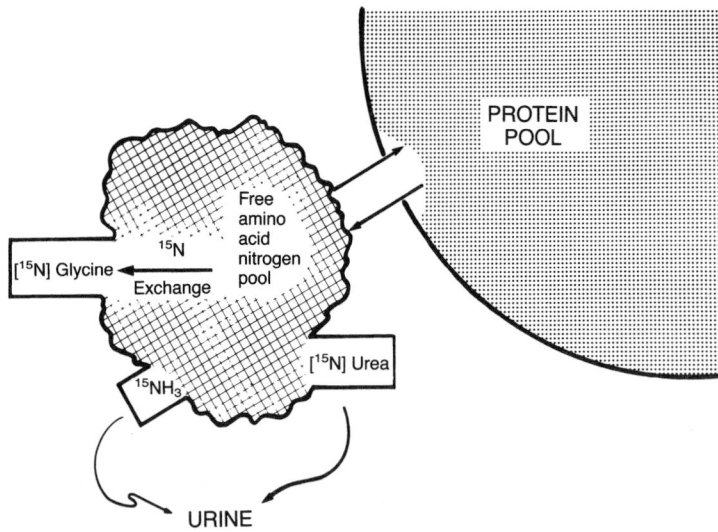

Figure 52–4. Model for distribution of [^{15}N]glycine tracer to free amino acids in the body. Amino acids are taken up via protein synthesis and are released via protein breakdown. Any ^{15}N tracer taken up for protein synthesis is assumed to be removed from the system, that is, not to reenter the free amino acid-N pool during the ^{15}N administration period. Therefore, fast-turnover proteins (e.g., many enzymes) appear as part of the free amino acid-N pool. Amino acids are oxidized to ammonia (NH_3) and urea and are excreted in the urine. The ammonia and urea are formed in different organs in the body and usually have different ^{15}N enrichments. (Reprinted by permission of the FASEB Journal *41*:2679, 1982.)

and highlights the differences in the metabolism of the different amino acid tracers and distribution of the ^{15}N in the free amino acid pool. Glycine, for example, rapidly transfers its ^{15}N to serine, glutamate, and glutamine.[27] That distribution is not changed with changing dietary protein intake.[31] Although it may be fortuitous that [^{15}N]glycine is the best label for use with the end-product method,[35] a change in end product ^{15}N enrichment may be attributable either to a real change in protein turnover *or* to an artifactual change in the distribution of ^{15}N resulting from changes in glycine metabolism, *which can be independent of* changes in protein metabolism. Another clue to difficulties with the end-product method is that the urinary ammonia ^{15}N enrichment is usually different from the urinary urea ^{15}N enrichment[30, 35, 36] because the amino acid-^{15}N precursor for ammonia synthesis is of renal origin, whereas the amino acid-^{15}N precursor for urea synthesis is of hepatic origin. Which enrichment should be used? Urea ^{15}N is probably best, but there is no direct evidence either way.

In two studies,[30, 37] an interesting observation was reported: ^{15}N could not be measured in urinary urea of some preterm infants receiving [^{15}N]glycine, but ^{15}N was observed in urinary ammonia. These results suggest that, in the diet of the preterm infant, glycine may be inadequate to meet the infant's growth requirements.[37] This event could occur only if glycine synthesis were limiting, that is, if glycine were conditionally indispensable.[1,38] Alternatively, the amount of [^{15}N]glycine given could have been too low to produce detectable levels of ^{15}N greater than the

natural abundance in urea. However, other groups[39, 40] have had no difficulty measuring ^{15}N enrichment in urinary urea (when [^{15}N]glycine was administered to infants) or synthesis of glycine,[41] a finding suggesting that glycine can be considered an essential amino acid for preterm and possibly small for gestational age infants.

As with all methods, there are limitations. The best approach with the end-product method is to design the experiment so changes in ^{15}N tracer distribution within the pool or changes in ammonia metabolism are minimized. The utility of the method is readily apparent from its application.[42] For example, Nissim and co-workers used the end-product method to study protein turnover as a function of conceptual age (Fig. 52–5).[43] Energy is required for turnover (i.e., synthesis and breakdown) of protein in the body, and energy is required for accretion of new protein in the growing infant. Therefore, growth is intimately tied to both energy and N intakes, and both must be considered.[6, 26]

TURNOVER OF INDIVIDUAL COMPONENTS OF NITROGEN METABOLISM

Discussion up to now has considered the turnover of whole body protein metabolism itself. Alternatively, the kinetics of individual components can be considered (e.g., Fig. 52–3). As outlined in Table 52–1, the interesting components are (1) the essential (or indispensable) amino acids, (2) the nonessential (or dispensable) amino acids, and (3) end products such as urea. Essential amino acid kinetics can be extrapolated to rates of protein metabolism. An essential amino acid enters the free pool from dietary intake (I_{aa}) and protein breakdown (B_{aa}); it disappears from the free pool by oxidation (C_{aa}) and uptake for protein synthesis (S_{aa}). These are the same components (I, B, C, and S) discussed previously, but cast in terms of the turnover, or flux, of a specific individual amino acid:

$$Q_{aa} = I_{aa} + B_{aa} = C_{aa} + S_{aa}$$

The turnover rate (or flux, Q_{aa}) of a metabolite is measured by the tracer dilution measured directly in the free pool. Typically, a tracer of an essential amino acid is infused until isotopic steady state (constant dilution) is reached in the blood free amino acid pool. By knowing the tracer enrichment and infusion rate and by measuring the tracer dilution in blood from samples taken at plateau, the rate of unlabeled metabolite appearance (Q_{aa}) is determined:

$$Q_{aa} = i_{aa} \cdot [E_i/E_p - 1]$$

TABLE 52-2

Rates of Protein Turnover Determined on Different Occasions for the Same Individual Using the End-Product Method but Different ^{15}N-Labeled Tracers*

	Protein Turnover (g/kg/d)	
^{15}N Tracer	*From Urea*	*From Ammonia*
Glutamine	2.6	3.1
Alanine	2.8	2.6
Wheat protein	3.5	5.8
Glutamate	3.5	8.0
Glycine	4.5	4.8
Leucine	9.6	4.7
Lysine	11.8	21.7
Aspartate	17.8	7.5

* The whole body protein turnover rate was calculated using urinary urea and urinary ammonia ^{15}N enrichments.
Data from Fern EB, et al: Clin Sci *61*:217, 1981.

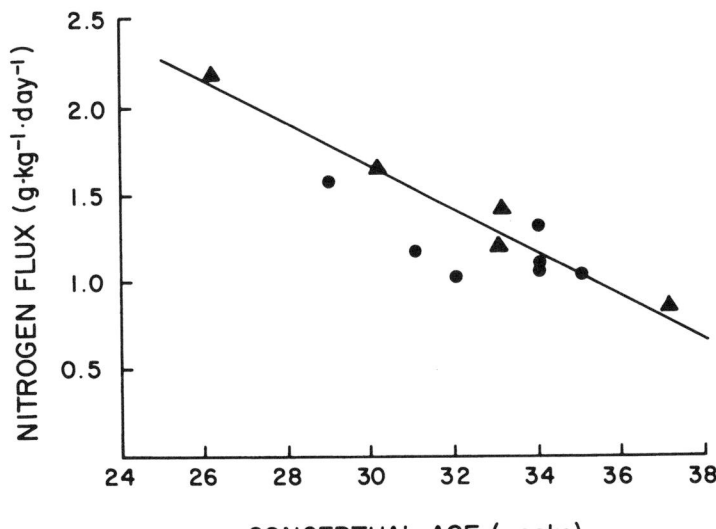

Figure 52–5. Whole body nitrogen flux versus conceptual age measured using a single dose of [^{15}N]glycine given intravenously to eight infants. (From Nissim I, et al: J Pediatr Gastroenterol Nutr *2*:507, 1983.)

where i_{aa} is the infusion rate of tracer with enrichment E_i (mole percentage of excess), and E_p is the blood amino acid enrichment.[44-46]

For a ^{13}C-labeled tracer, the amino acid oxidation rate can be measured from the rate of $^{13}CO_2$ excretion.[44, 45] This approach assumes that the label is *quantitatively* released with the oxidation of the amino acid. For example, the ^{13}C of an L-[1-^{13}C]leucine tracer is removed at the first irreversible step of leucine catabolism (Fig. 52–6),[46] and leucine oxidation is determined directly from $^{13}CO_2$ excretion. Even phenylalanine, whose pathway to oxidation is not direct, has been used to define phenylalanine-tyrosine oxidation.[47-49]

Determining an amino acid flux does not require a ^{13}C label as such. Any label (e.g., ^{15}N, ^{2}H, or ^{18}O) can be used, but the caveat is that the label must follow the metabolic pathway expected. For example, a deuterium label in the tail of leucine or any ^{13}C label will trace leucine metabolism through the critical, irreversible second step of catabolism (see Fig. 52–6), but a [^{15}N]leucine tracer is removed with transamination.[50] Because more than 70% of the leucine transaminated to α-ketoisocaproate (KIC) is immediately reaminated to leucine,[50] the ^{15}N label measures a leucine N turnover rate that is considerably faster than the leucine C flux. Therefore, the [^{15}N]leucine tracer cannot be used to follow leucine C metabolism. For all metabolites to be studied, the biochemistry of the tracer must be carefully considered when choosing an isotopic label.

The rates of amino acid release from protein breakdown (B_{aa}) and uptake for protein synthesis (S_{aa}) are calculated by subtracting dietary intake and oxidation from the flux, respectively, just as is done with the end-product method. The primary distinction is that the measurements are for a specific amino acid, not whole body protein. Flux components are determined typically in units of micromoles per kilogram per hour and are then extrapolated to whole body protein kinetics by dividing the amino acid rates by the assumed concentration of the amino acid in body protein (μmol amino acid/g of protein).

The principal advantages of following individual metabolite kinetics are that (1) the results are specific and improve confidence in the measurement and (2) the turnover time of the free pool is usually fast. By using a priming dose to reduce the time required to come to isotopic steady state, the tracer infusion study can be completed in less than 4 hours.

The principal disadvantages are that (1) the method is invasive, (2) the true intracellular precursor pool is usually not sampled, and (3) dietary intake often enters by a route different from that of the tracer. The amount of blood drawn is not an issue; blood loss can be kept to approximately 2 mL total. However, catheters are necessary for sampling of blood amino acids or for tracer administration. Catheters may already be in place in the seriously ill infant, but invasive procedures are not warranted for studying healthy infants. Yet it is in the healthy infant that the tracer techniques offer the greatest tool for defining normal metabolism and nutritional requirements. The bioavailability of dietary urea N has been determined in infants noninvasively by adding [^{15}N]urea tracer to infants' feeding solution and collecting and measuring the tracer in the urine.[51-53] The purpose of these studies was to determine what fraction of the urea N was retained in the body, rather than passing into the urine. Retention of urea N would reflect gut microorganism hydrolysis of the urea and incorporation of the resulting ammonia (presumably by the liver) into other N-containing compounds, such as amino acids. Because a significant portion of

Protein Metabolism

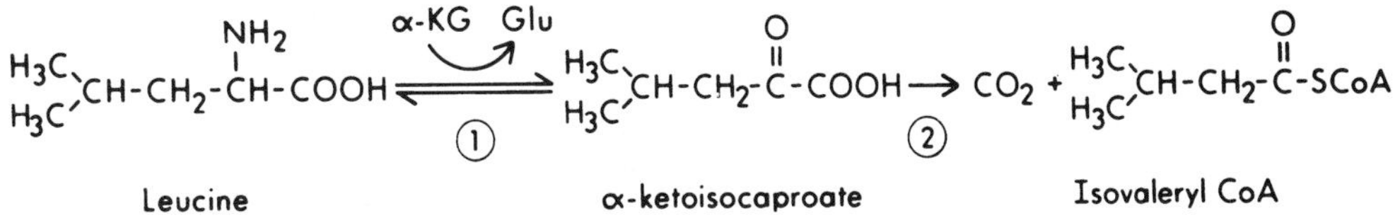

Figure 52–6. Leucine metabolism. *1*, Leucine is first transaminated to α-ketoisocaproate. This reaction is rapid and reversible. *2*, The ketoacid is then decarboxylated, releasing a carbon dioxide and an organic acid, which is further oxidized. The other two branched-chain amino acids, valine and isoleucine, are also metabolized by the same enzymes in these first two metabolic steps.

human milk N is urea N, urea N represents a potentially important N source. These studies demonstrated, however, that the majority of the urea ^{15}N consumed could be recovered in the urine, a finding indicating that little urea N was bioavailable for the infants.

To measure amino acid kinetics, the amino acid tracer is infused into the blood and is sampled from the blood, but the metabolic action takes place within cells. Amino acids do not freely pass through cells as does urea; amino acids are transported.[54, 55] For the neutral amino acids (leucine, isoleucine, valine, phenylalanine, and tyrosine), transport into and out of cells is rapid, and only a small concentration gradient between plasma and intracellular milieus exists.[45] Nonetheless, the intracellular enrichment of leucine, as measured by plasma KIC, which is formed from intracellular leucine and is then released into plasma (Fig. 52–7), is about 20% lower than plasma leucine enrichment.[56] Using the plasma leucine enrichment to calculate leucine turnover underestimates whole body flux by about 20%.

The plasma KIC enrichment can be used during the leucine tracer infusion to resolve the question of intracellular leucine enrichment for calculating leucine kinetics. For amino acids such as glutamate and glutamine, which have extremely large intracellular/extracellular gradients, very little intracellular glutamate or glutamine exchanges with plasma, and the sampled plasma amino acid enrichment reflects primarily interorgan transport of amino acid rather than whole body flux.[57] Therefore, the partitioning of amino acid between intracellular and extracellular milieus must be considered carefully for every individual amino acid studied.

Adults are commonly studied in the postabsorptive state after an overnight fast. The purpose has usually been to study the effect of mediators, such as hormones or specific interventions, on protein metabolism. A few reports of amino acid metabolism using tracers in infants have appeared.[39, 58-72] In terms of nutrition, many of the questions to be addressed in infants are related to oral or enteral feeding. However, the fed state complicates calculating kinetics more than by just adding a dietary intake term to the flux equation. Any dietary amino acid oxidized or taken up for protein synthesis by either gut or liver during absorption of food will not have mixed with the systemic circulation in which the tracer is administered. Therefore, the flux and amino acid released from protein breakdown will be underestimated by an amount equal to that amino acid sequestered on the first pass through the splanchnic bed. It is possible under some circumstances to have a *negative* protein breakdown after dietary amino acid inflow has been subtracted from the flux. This problem is negated if the tracer is administered with food.[73] However, oral feeding will not provide a constant flow of tracer into the system unless tube feeding is used.[73]

Addition of the tracer to the enteral feeding solution solves the problem of following the amino acids from the feeding solution. However, an enteral tracer does not necessarily help when the goal is to compare the effects of parenteral versus enteral feeding regimens. For those kinds of studies, the tracer is administered intravenously with the parenteral nutrition and enterally with the enteral formula. Administering the amino acid tracer by the different feeding routes allows one to compare only apples (enteral feeding with an enteral tracer) with oranges (intravenous feeding with an intravenous tracer).[39] A more elaborate design is required for comparing enteral and parental feeding regimens. For example, if two tracers of the same amino acid are available that give identical measures of metabolism (e.g., [1-^{13}C]leucine and [5,5,5-[2]H$_3$]leucine), they can be administered simultaneously by both enteral and intravenous routes.[22, 45] This approach gives direct measurement of tracers by both routes simultaneously during both parenteral and enteral feeding regimens.[14,66,74]

An alternative to invasive blood sampling is sampling amino acids from urine.[73] Small amounts of amino acids are continually filtered through kidney and normally appear in the urine.

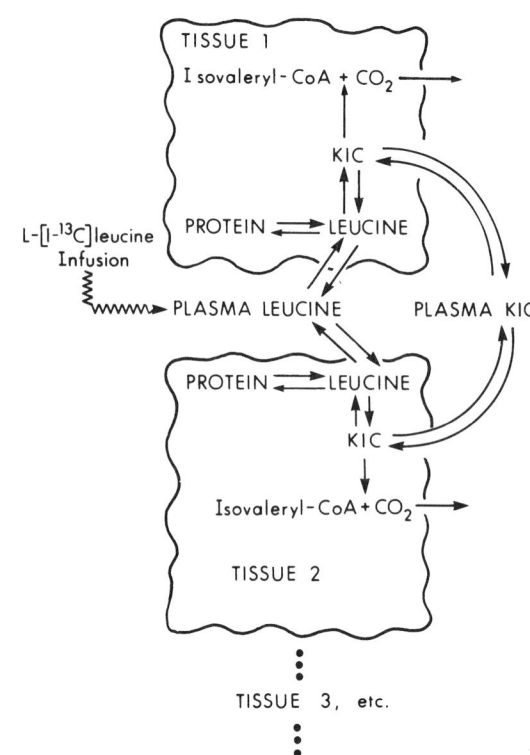

Figure 52–7. Multitissue model of whole body leucine metabolism. Leucine is transported into and out of cells of various tissues in the body (e.g., muscle, kidney, liver, and adipose tissue). α-Ketoisocaproate (KIC), formed within cells from leucine via transamination, is released into plasma. During an infusion of [1-^{13}C]leucine, the plasma KIC ^{13}C enrichment is the weighted average of the intracellular leucine ^{13}C enrichment of those tissues releasing KIC. CoA = coenzyme A; CO_2 = carbon dioxide. (From Matthews DE, et al: Metabolism *31*:1105, 1982.

Because urinary amino acids are derived from blood, they should be a reasonable substitute for measuring blood amino acid tracer enrichments under isotopic steady-state conditions. DeBenoist and colleagues[73] demonstrated in 1984 that urinary leucine enrichments in infants were nearly identical to plasma leucine enrichments during infusion of [1-^{13}C]leucine, a finding indicating that the urinary leucine came directly from plasma and was not contaminated significantly with unlabeled renal-derived leucine. Since then, several applications using this technique have appeared in the literature.[39,69,73,75,76]

REQUIREMENTS OF SPECIFIC AMINO ACIDS

Current dietary recommendations for essential amino acids are based on N balance studies and short-term growth studies. The indicator amino acid oxidation method has been developed to measure specific amino acid requirements.[77-79] It has been validated extensively in animal models of infancy.[80-82] This technique is based on partitioning the essential amino acid outflow under steady-state conditions between oxidation and protein synthesis ($Q_{aa} = C_{aa} + S_{aa}$, as defined earlier). When a single essential amino acid is limited in the diet, the amount of protein that can be synthesized is limited. The limiting amino acid also restricts the use of all other dietary amino acids for protein synthesis; the body has no choice but to oxidize the excess amounts of these amino acids (Fig. 52–8). If we increase the dietary amount of the limiting amino acid, protein synthesis will increase and so will the utilization of the other dietary amino acids; this, in turn, reduces their

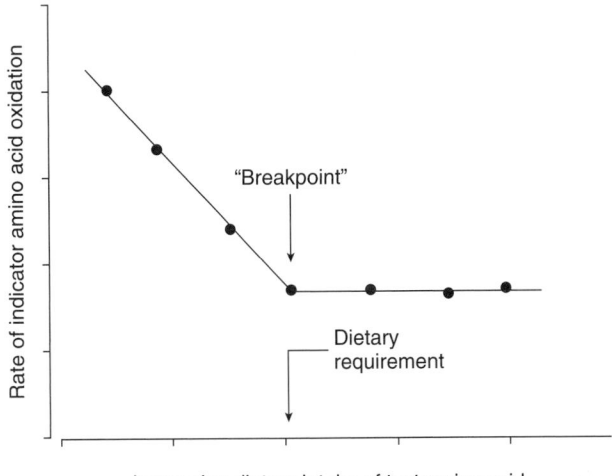

Figure 52–8. The rate of oxidation of an indicator amino acid in response to varying dietary intakes of a test amino acid. The inflection or breakpoint in the rate of indicator oxidation represents the physiologic requirement of the test amino acid for that individual. (From Brunton JA, et al: Curr Opin Clin Nutr Metab Care *1*:449, 1998.)

oxidation. Once the requirement for the limiting amino acid is reached, further increases in its dietary intake will cause no further increase in protein synthesis or decrease in the oxidation of the other essential amino acids.

The indicator amino acid oxidation method works on this principle.[79] Subjects are given a series of diets containing varying amounts of the amino acid for which the requirement is to be determined. The amounts vary below and above requirement. All other amino acids are furnished at constant amounts *above* requirement. At the end of each diet period, a dose of another essential amino acid with a ^{13}C or ^{14}C label (the indicator amino acid) is given, and its oxidation is measured. The oxidation of the labeled indicator amino acid will decrease as the amount of test amino acid increases, until requirements are met, and then the oxidation will plateau. Plotting the oxidation of the labeled indicator amino acid against test amino acid intake should show a breakpoint at the requirement level for the test amino acid.[79]

A slightly different approach is the use of the oxidation rate of the investigated amino acid or its direct metabolite. Such an approach has been used to determine the requirement of tyrosine in parenterally fed infants.[83]

FREE EXTRINSICALLY OR INTRINSICALLY LABELED AMINO ACIDS

Almost all tracer studies have been performed using labeled amino acids as *free* amino acids, rather than amino acid tracers *incorporated into* proteins. When amino acids and proteins are given enterally, there are differences in the time course of hydrolysis and absorption of the amino acids and small peptides.[84] Although it takes time to hydrolyze enterally delivered proteins to peptides, peptides are absorbed more rapidly than free amino acids.[85] The net effect is that free amino acids still appear in systemic blood more quickly than amino acids arising from intact proteins, but different proteins are hydrolyzed at different rates. Thus, an enterally delivered labeled free amino acid will have different absorption kinetics than the corresponding protein-bound amino acids it is meant to trace. Metges and colleagues[86] measured the prandial metabolic fate of ^{13}C-labeled dietary leucine when it was ingested as an intrinsically labeled component of mixed meals either incorporated into casein protein or

as a free amino acid (extrinsically labeled) in a mixture of crystalline free amino acids defined to simulate the casein amino acid pattern. As a control, leucine kinetics was also measured when free labeled leucine was given together with the intact casein. Leucine oxidation was higher for the free ^{13}C]leucine tracer combined with a free amino acid mixture compared with an intrinsically ^{13}C]leucine-labeled casein. This result, together with the finding of a higher uptake of leucine for protein synthesis with the intrinsically labeled casein, suggests that protein-bound leucine was better used for whole body protein synthesis than as a free amino acid. Such studies have not yet been performed in neonates, but they may prove important in defining infant formulas in terms of amino acid and protein composition.

SYNTHESIS OF SPECIFIC PROTEINS

Some proteins are readily sampled. Lipoproteins, albumin, and other plasma proteins are obtained from blood; muscle proteins can be obtained by biopsy. If a protein or group of proteins can be sampled, the synthesis rate can be determined directly from the rate of tracer incorporation into the protein. For proteins that turn over slowly (e.g., muscle protein or albumin), incorporation of tracer is linear with time during the first several hours of tracer infusion.[29,87-89] If the tracer infusion were to be continued for several half-lives of turnover, the tracer concentration would rise exponentially in the protein and match that of its precursor, the intracellular amino acid enrichment.[90,91] For slower-turnover proteins, it is more convenient to measure the synthesis rate from the initial rate of tracer incorporation into the protein.

To convert the initial rate of tracer incorporation in protein into a protein synthesis rate requires knowledge of the intracellular amino acid precursor enrichment for synthesis. For muscle protein synthesis, L-[1-^{13}C]leucine is often used as the tracer[92] because plasma KIC ^{13}C enrichment approximates the intracellular muscle leucine enrichment. Various other schemes have been used to estimate intracellular liver amino acid tracer enrichment.[93-95]

For proteins, such as very low density lipoprotein apoprotein B, that turn over within the period of tracer infusion (typically 4 to 8 hours), tracer incorporation into the protein rises exponentially to a plateau. If the tracer enrichment in the protein does not reach plateau during the time course of the tracer infusion, curve fitting can usually predict the plateau. If the enrichment plateau can be defined, then the precursor enrichment (the enrichment of the intracellular free amino acid from which the protein was made) can be measured directly.[93]

Garlick and colleagues proposed an alternative method to measure protein synthesis of slow-turnover proteins.[96] Their method is to administer a "flooding dose" of tracer amino acid, thus producing a large momentary concentration gradient between extracellular and intracellular spaces. The gradient pushes the amino acid rapidly into cells and floods them with the tracer. This scheme is meant to force the intracellular tracer enrichment (which cannot be readily measured) to equalize with the extracellular enrichment (which can be measured), thereby removing the uncertainty of what is the precursor enrichment for protein synthesis.[97-101] An obvious drawback is that the administered dose is a *pharmacologic* dose of material that may alter metabolism and induce secretion of various hormones (e.g., insulin) and factors that are known to regulate protein metabolism. All this said, the flooding dose is a convenient method for determining protein synthesis of slow-turnover proteins, which can be sampled readily in a short time.

DEGRADATION OF SPECIFIC PROTEINS

Measurement of protein degradation is much more difficult. It usually requires prelabeling a protein and following the disappearance of the labeled protein with time. The first problem is prelabeling the protein. Prelabeling can be done for plasma proteins using radioactive iodine. When the protein degrades, the radioactive iodine disappears from the system. If the protein is labeled by synthesizing it with one or more labeled amino acids, a second problem occurs—recycling of amino acid tracer. As the protein degrades, the newly released amino acids can again be taken up for new protein synthesis; that is, some of the amino acids are *reused* or recycled back into protein. This greatly complicates interpretation of the labeled protein data.

A few amino acids cannot be reused for protein synthesis. Hydroxyproline, methyllysine, and 3-methylhistidine are examples. No transfer RNA exists for these amino acids. Proline is hydroxylated and histidine and lysine are methylated after the protein has been synthesized. This posttranslational process occurs in very specific proteins (e.g., collagen for hydroxyproline and actin and myosin for 3-methylhistidine). When the proteins degrade, these modified amino acids are not reused. Hydroxyproline has been used to follow collagen kinetics,[102] whereas 3-methylhistidine has been used extensively to follow myofibrillar protein breakdown.[103, 104] Because most of the myofibrillar protein is in muscle, muscle should be the principal source of urinary 3-methylhistidine. However, 3-methylhistidine is also in gut actin. Although the gut actin pool is very small relative to muscle protein, gut turns its protein over rapidly and therefore can be a significant contributor to urinary 3-methylhistidine output. Use of urinary 3-methylhistidine to reflect muscle protein breakdown requires cautious interpretation because of the gut 3-methylhistidine source.[105]

ACKNOWLEDGMENTS

This work was supported by grants from the National Institutes of Health (DK38429 and RR00109).

REFERENCES

1. Harper AE: Origin of recommended dietary allowances: an historic overview. Am J Clin Nutr 41:140, 1985.
2. Ziegler EE, Fomon SJ: Methods in infant nutrition research: balance and growth studies. Acta Paediatr Scand 299:90, 1982.
3. Food and Nutrition Board, National Research Council (U.S.): Recommended Dietary Allowances, 10th ed. Washington, DC, National Academy Press, 1989, pp 52-77.
4. Kopple JD: Uses and limitations of the balance technique. JPEN J Parenter Enteral Nutr 11:798, 1987.
5. Tomé D, Bos C: Dietary protein and nitrogen utilization. J Nutr 130:1868S, 2000.
6. Micheli JL, Schutz Y: Protein metabolism and postnatal growth in very low birthweight infants. Biol Neonate 52:25, 1987.
7. Gelfand RA, et al: Removal of infused amino acids by splanchnic and leg tissues in humans. Am J Physiol 250:E407, 1986.
8. Aoki TT, et al: Amino acid levels across normal forearm muscle and splanchnic bed after a protein meal. Am J Clin Nutr 29:340, 1976.
9. Tessari P, Garibotto G: Interorgan amino acid exchange. Curr Opin Clin Nutr Metab Care 3:51, 2000.
10. Lemons JA, et al: Umbilical uptake of amino acids in the unstressed fetal lamb. J Clin Invest 58:1428, 1976.
11. Barrett EJ, et al: An isotopic method for measurement of muscle protein synthesis and degradation in vivo. Biochem J 245:223, 1987.
12. Cheng KN, et al: Direct determination of leucine metabolism and protein breakdown in humans using L-[1-13C,15N]leucine and the forearm model. Eur J Clin Invest 15:349, 1985.
13. Ling PR, et al: Effect of fetal growth on maternal protein metabolism in postabsorptive rat. Am J Physiol Endocrinol Metab 252:E380, 1987.
14. Van Goudoever JB, et al: Adaptive regulation of intestinal lysine metabolism. Proc Natl Acad Sci USA 97:11620, 2000.
15. Stoll B, et al: Substrate oxidation by the portal drained viscera of fed piglets. Am J Physiol 277:E168, 1999.
16. Stoll B, et al: Dietary and systemic phenylalanine utilization for mucosal and hepatic constitutive protein synthesis in pigs. Am J Physiol 276:G49, 1999.
17. Anderson AH, et al: Placental transport of threonine and its utilization in the normal and growth-restricted fetus. Am J Physiol 272:E892, 1997.
18. Cetin I, et al: Fetal serine fluxes across fetal liver, hindlimb, and placenta in late gestation. Am J Physiol 263:E786, 1992.
19. Cetin I, et al: Glycine turnover and oxidation and hepatic serine synthesis from glycine in fetal lambs. Am J Physiol 260:E371, 1991.
20. Loy GL, et al: Measurement of leucine and α-ketoisocaproic acid fluxes in the fetal/placental unit. J Chromatogr 562:169, 1991.
21. Chien PFW, et al: Protein turnover in the human fetus studied at term using stable isotope tracer amino acids. Am J Physiol 265:E31, 1993.
22. Matthews DE, et al: Splanchnic bed utilization of leucine and phenylalanine in humans. Am J Physiol 264:E109, 1993.
23. Sprinson DB, Rittenberg D: The rate of interaction of the amino acids of the diet with the tissue proteins. J Biol Chem 180:715, 1949.
24. Picou D, Taylor-Roberts T: The measurement of total protein synthesis and catabolism and nitrogen turnover in infants in different nutritional states and receiving different amounts of dietary protein. Clin Sci 36:283, 1969.
25. Bier DM: Intrinsically difficult measurements: the kinetics of body proteins and amino acids in man. Diabetes Metab Rev 5:111, 1989.
26. Yudkoff M, Nissim I: Methods for determining the protein requirements of infants. Clin Perinatol 13:123, 1986.
27. Matthews DE, et al: Glycine nitrogen metabolism in man. Metabolism 30:886, 1981.
28. Duffy B, et al: The effect of varying protein quality and energy intake on the nitrogen metabolism of parenterally fed very low birthweight (<1600 g) infants. Pediatr Res 15:1040, 1981.
29. Yudkoff M, et al: Albumin synthesis in premature infants: determination of turnover with [15N]glycine. Pediatr Res 21:49, 1987.
30. Catzeflis C, et al: Whole body protein synthesis and energy expenditure in very low birth weight infants. Pediatr Res 19:679, 1985.
31. Bier DM, Matthews DE: Stable isotope tracer methods for in vivo investigations. Fed Proc 41:2679, 1982.
32. Taruvinga M, et al: Comparison of 15N-labelled glycine, aspartate, valine and leucine for measurement of whole-body protein turnover. Clin Sci 57:281, 1979.
33. Fern EB, et al: Apparent compartmentation of body nitrogen in one human subject: its consequences in measuring the rate of whole body protein synthesis with 15N. Clin Sci 68:271, 1985.
34. Wutzke KD, et al: Whole-body protein parameters in premature infants: a comparison of different 15N tracer substances and different methods. Pediatr Res 31:95, 1992.
35. Fern EB, et al: The excretion of isotope in urea and ammonia for estimating protein turnover in man with [15N]glycine. Clin Sci 61:217, 1981.
36. Pencharz P, et al: A comparison of the estimates of whole-body protein turnover in parenterally fed neonates obtained using three different end products. Can J Physiol Pharmacol 67:624, 1989.
37. Jackson AA, et al: Nitrogen metabolism in preterm infants fed human donor breast milk: the possible essentiality of glycine. Pediatr Res 15:1454, 1981.
38. Jackson AA: The glycine story. Eur J Clin Nutr 45:595, 1991.
39. Wykes LJ, et al: Glycine, leucine, and phenylalanine flux in low-birth-weight infants during parenteral and enteral feeding. Am J Clin Nutr 55:971, 1992.
40. Cauderay M, et al: Energy-nitrogen balances and protein turnover in small and appropriate for gestational age low birthweight infants. Eur J Clin Nutr 42:125, 1988.
41. Miller RG, et al: A new stable isotope tracer technique to assess human neonatal amino acid synthesis. J Pediatr Surg 30:1325, 1995.
42. Matthews DE, Bier DM: Stable isotope methods for nutritional investigation. Annu Rev Nutr 3:309, 1983.
43. Nissim I, et al: Effects of conceptual age and dietary intake on protein metabolism in premature infants. J Pediatr Gastroenterol Nutr 2:507, 1983.
44. Wolfe RR: Radioactive and Stable Isotope Tracers in Biomedicine: Principles and Practice of Kinetic Analysis. New York, Wiley–Liss, 1992, pp 1–471.
45. Matthews DE: Stable isotope methodologies in studying human amino acid and protein metabolism. Ital J Gastroenterol 25:72, 1993.
46. Matthews DE, et al: Measurement of leucine metabolism in man from a primed, continuous infusion of L-[1-13C]leucine. Am J Physiol 238:E473, 1980.
47. Wilson DC, et al: Threonine requirement of young men determined by indicator amino acid oxidation with use of L-[1-13C]phenylalanine. Am J Clin Nutr 71:757, 2000.
48. Marchini JS, et al: Phenylalanine conversion to tyrosine: comparative determination with L-[ring-2H5]phenylalanine and L-[1-13C]phenylalanine as tracers in man. Metabolism 42:1316, 1993.
49. Zello GA, et al: Phenylalanine flux, oxidation, and conversion to tyrosine in humans studied with L-[1-13C]phenylalanine. Am J Physiol 259:E835, 1990.
50. Matthews DE, et al: Regulation of leucine metabolism in man: a stable isotope study. Science 214:1129, 1981.
51. Fomon SJ, et al: Bioavailability of dietary urea nitrogen in the infant. J Pediatr 111:221, 1987.
52. Fomon SJ, et al: Bioavailability of dietary urea nitrogen in the breast-fed infant. J Pediatr 113:515, 1988.
53. Donovan SM, et al: Bioavailability of urea nitrogen for the low birthweight infant. Acta Paediatr Scand 78:899, 1990.
54. Christensen HN: Role of amino acid transport and countertransport in nutrition and metabolism. Physiol Rev 70:43, 1990.
55. Souba WW, Pacitti AJ: How amino acids get into cells: mechanisms, models, menus, and mediators. JPEN J Parenter Enteral Nutr 16:569, 1992.
56. Matthews DE, et al: Relationship of plasma leucine and α-ketoisocaproate during a L-[1-13C]leucine infusion in man: a method for measuring human intracellular leucine tracer enrichment. Metabolism 31:1105, 1982.

57. Darmaun D, et al: Glutamine and glutamate kinetics in humans. Am J Physiol *251*:E117, 1986.
58. Liet JM, et al: Leucine metabolism in preterm infants receiving parenteral nutrition with medium-chain compared with long-chain triacylglycerol emulsions. Am J Clin Nutr *69*:539, 1999.
59. Poindexter BB, et al: Amino acids suppress proteolysis independent of insulin throughout the neonatal period. Am J Physiol *272*:E592, 1997.
60. Battista MA, et al: Effect of parenteral amino acids on leucine and urea kinetics in preterm infants. J Pediatr *128*:130, 1996.
61. Denne SC, et al: Proteolysis and phenylalanine hydroxylation in response to parenteral nutrition in extremely premature and normal newborns. J Clin Invest *97*:746, 1996.
62. Toledo-Eppinga L, et al: Relative kinetics of phenylalanine and leucine in low birth weight infants during nutrient administration. Pediatr Res *40*:41, 1996.
63. Kilani RA, et al: Phenylalanine hydroxylase activity in preterm infants: is tyrosine a conditionally essential amino acid? Am J Clin Nutr *61*:1218, 1995.
64. Van Goudoever JB, et al: Whole-body protein turnover in preterm appropriate for gestational age and small for gestational age infants: comparison of [15N]glycine and [1-13C]leucine administered simultaneously. Pediatr Res *37*:381, 1995.
65. Rivera A Jr, et al: Effect of intravenous amino acids on protein metabolism of preterm infants during the first three days of life. Pediatr Res *33*:106, 1993.
66. Beaufrère B, et al: Leucine kinetics in fed low-birth-weight infants: importance of splanchnic tissues. Am J Physiol *263*:E214, 1992.
67. Denne SC, et al: Leucine kinetics after a brief fast and in response to feeding in premature infants. Am J Clin Nutr *56*:899, 1992.
68. Denne SC, et al: Leucine kinetics during feeding in normal newborns. Pediatr Res *30*:23, 1991.
69. Kandil H, et al: Nitrogen balance and protein turnover during the growth failure in newly born low-birth-weight infants. Am J Clin Nutr *53*:1411, 1991.
70. Mitton SG, et al: Protein turnover rates in sick, premature neonates during the first few days of life. Pediatr Res *30*:418, 1991.
71. Beaufrère B, et al: Whole body protein turnover measured with 13C-leucine and energy expenditure in preterm infants. Pediatr Res *28*:147, 1990.
72. Pencharz P, et al: Total-body protein turnover in parenterally fed neonates: effects of energy source studied by using [15N]glycine and [1-13C]leucine. Am J Clin Nutr *50*:1395, 1989.
73. DeBenoist B, et al: The measurement of whole body protein turnover in the preterm infant with intragastric infusion of L-[1-13C]leucine and sampling of the urinary leucine pool. Clin Sci *66*:155, 1984.
74. Darmaun D, et al: Glutamine metabolism in very low birth weight infants. Pediatr Res *41*:391, 1997.
75. Zello GA, et al: Plasma and urine enrichments following infusion of L-[1-13C]phenylalanine and L-[ring-2H5]phenylalanine in humans: Evidence for an isotope effect in renal tubular reabsorption. Metabolism *43*:487, 1994.
76. Darling PB, et al: Isotopic enrichment of amino acids in urine following oral infusions of L-[1-13C]phenylalanine and L-[1-13C]lysine in humans: confounding effect of D-[13C]amino acids. Metabolism *48*:732, 1999.
77. Zello GA, et al: Dietary lysine requirement of young adult males determined by oxidation of L-[1-13C]phenylalanine. Am J Physiol *264*:E677, 1993.
78. Zello GA, et al: Recent advances in methods of assessing dietary amino acid requirements for adult humans. J Nutr *125*:2907, 1995.
79. Brunton JA, et al: Determination of amino acid requirements by indicator amino acid oxidation: applications in health and disease. Curr Opin Clin Nutr Metab Care *1*:449, 1998.
80. Kim KI, et al: Determination of amino acid requirements of young pigs using an indicator amino acid. Br J Nutr *50*:369, 1983.
81. Kim KI, et al: Oxidation of an indicator amino acid by young pigs receiving diets with varying levels of lysine or threonine, and an assessment of amino acid requirements. Br J Nutr *50*:391, 1983.
82. Ball RO, Bayley HS: Tryptophan requirement of the 2.5-kg piglet determined by the oxidation of an indicator amino acid. J Nutr *114*:1741, 1984.
83. Roberts SA, et al: The effect of graded intake of glycyl-L-tyrosine on phenylalanine and tyrosine metabolism in parenterally fed neonates with an estimation of tyrosine requirement. Pediatr Res *49*:111, 2001.
84. Boirie Y, et al: Slow and fast dietary proteins differently modulate postprandial protein accretion. Proc Natl Acad Sci USA *94*:14930, 1997.
85. Matthews DM: Protein Absorption: Development and Present State of the Subject. New York, Wiley–Liss, 1991, pp 1–414.
86. Metges CC, et al: Kinetics of L-[1-13C]leucine when ingested with free amino acids, unlabeled or intrinsically labeled casein. Am J Physiol *278*:E1000, 2000.
87. Davis TA, et al: Roles of insulin and amino acids in the regulation of protein synthesis in the neonate. J Nutr *128*:347S, 1998.
88. Wagenmakers AJ: Tracers to investigate protein and amino acid metabolism in human subjects. Proc Nutr Soc *58*:987, 1999.
89. Welle S: Human Protein Metabolism. New York, Springer-Verlag, 1999, pp 1–88.
90. Demant T, et al: Sensitive methods to study human apolipoprotein B metabolism using stable isotope-labeled amino acids. Am J Physiol *270*:E1022, 1996.
91. Cryer DR, et al: Direct measurement of apoprotein B synthesis in human very low density lipoprotein using stable isotopes and mass spectrometry. J Lipid Res *27*:508, 1986.
92. Nair KS, et al: Leucine incorporation into mixed skeletal muscle protein in humans. Am J Physiol *254*:E208, 1988.
93. Cayol M, et al: Precursor pool for hepatic protein synthesis in humans: effects of tracer route infusion and dietary proteins. Am J Physiol *270*:E980, 1996.
94. Baumann PQ, et al: Precursor pools of protein synthesis: a stable isotope study in a swine model. Am J Physiol *267*:E203, 1994.
95. Ljungqvist OH, et al: Functional heterogeneity of leucine pools in human skeletal muscle. Am J Physiol *273*:E564, 1997.
96. Garlick PJ, et al: Measurement of the rate of protein synthesis in muscle of postabsorptive young men by injection of a "flooding dose" of [1-13C]leucine. Clin Sci *77*:329, 1989.
97. Davis TA, et al: Aminoacyl-tRNA and tissue free amino acid pools are equilibrated after a flooding dose of phenylalanine. Am J Physiol *277*:E103, 1999.
98. Garlick PJ, et al: Measurement of tissue protein synthesis rates in vivo: a critical analysis of contrasting methods. Am J Physiol *266*:E287, 1994.
99. Garlick PJ, McNurlan MA: Measurement of protein synthesis in human tissues by the flooding method. Curr Opin Clin Nutr Metab Care *1*:455, 1998.
100. Reeds PJ, Davis TA: Of flux and flooding: the advantages and problems of different isotopic methods for quantifying protein turnover in vivo. I. Methods based on the dilution of a tracer. Curr Opin Clin Nutr Metab Care *2*:23, 1999.
101. Rennie MJ: An introduction to the use of tracers in nutrition and metabolism. Proc Nutr Soc *58*:935, 1999.
102. Molnar JA, et al: Synthesis and degradation rates of collagens in vivo in whole skin of rats, studied with 18O2 labelling. Biochem J *240*:431, 1986.
103. Young VR, Munro HN: Nτ-Methylhistidine (3-methylhistidine) and muscle protein turnover: an overview. Fed Proc *37*:2291, 1978.
104. Long CL, et al: Validity of 3-methylhistidine excretion as an indicator of skeletal muscle protein breakdown in humans. Metabolism *37*:844, 1988.
105. Rennie MJ, Millward DJ: 3-Methylhistidine excretion and the urinary 3-methylhistidine/creatinine ratio are poor indicators of skeletal muscle protein breakdown. Clin Sci *65*:217, 1983.

William W. Hay, Jr., and Timothy R. H. Regnault

53

Fetal Requirements and Placental Transfer of Nitrogenous Compounds

INTRAUTERINE GROWTH AND PROTEIN (NITROGEN) ACCRETION

Requirements for fetal protein accretion depend directly on the rate of fetal growth. Human fetal growth has been determined indirectly by inference from anthropometric measurements of infants born at different gestational ages. The better studies have excluded obviously abnormal infants and have involved defined, relatively homogeneous populations. Even with such precautions, however, preterm delivery does not guarantee that an infant has grown normally. Furthermore, anthropometric measurements have their own inherent range of accuracy (or inaccuracy), and cross-sectional, static size for gestational age groupings of neonates may not accurately reflect the dynamics of fetal growth.

In addition, population means of fetal growth rate do not necessarily reflect growth of a given fetus or the changes in body composition with growth that occur with advancing gestational age.[1]

In spite of such concerns about the reliability of data, composite pictures of human fetal growth that have been estimated from neonatal anthropometric measurements at birth have been presented by several investigators. Most mean percentiles among the many different growth curves differ by approximately 5% and can be accounted for largely by factors such as suboptimal pregnancy dating, adverse maternal or fetal medical and obstetric complications of pregnancy, diet, race, ethnicity, socioeconomic status, and altitude differences.[2] Such neonatal-derived fetal weight curves appear as sigmoidal functions of weight versus gestational age. In some studies that accounted for many of the factors that can affect fetal growth and fetal size, fetal weight gain appears to be a linear function of gestational age clear through term (~12 to 13 g/day for pregnancies in white, middle-class women), with only slight increases for male versus female gender, and for maternal obesity.[3] In contrast, weight change (the rate of weight gain/kg body weight/day) is only relatively linear at about 1.5%/day from about 24 to 37 weeks, but it tapers off to a plateau between 37 and 42 weeks, and there may be a decrease after 43 to 44 weeks.

Chemical composition studies of allegedly normal human infants have been accomplished in relatively few cases. Sparks reviewed data from 15 studies accounting for 207 infants.[1] Based on the data from these studies, nonfat dry weight and nitrogen content (both reasonably good predictors of protein content) show a linear relationship with fetal weight (Fig. 53-1) and an exponential relationship with gestational age (Fig. 53-2).[1] However, at each gestational age, various fetal weights are observed. Thus, nonfat dry weight and nitrogen content for a given fetus can also be compared with the "average" fetus. When these comparisons are made, larger fetuses grow faster than smaller fetuses at the same gestational age, and protein accretion follows accordingly.

Tables 53-1 and 53-2 present nitrogen, protein, and selected amino acid composition and accretion rates, respectively, in reportedly normal human fetuses.[4] According to data from sheep and guinea pigs, however, about 80% of the nitrogen content of the fetus in these species is found in protein; the rest is probably found in urea, ammonia, and free amino acids. The data for human fetal protein content and accretion in these tables thus may be high, because they are based solely on nitrogen content.

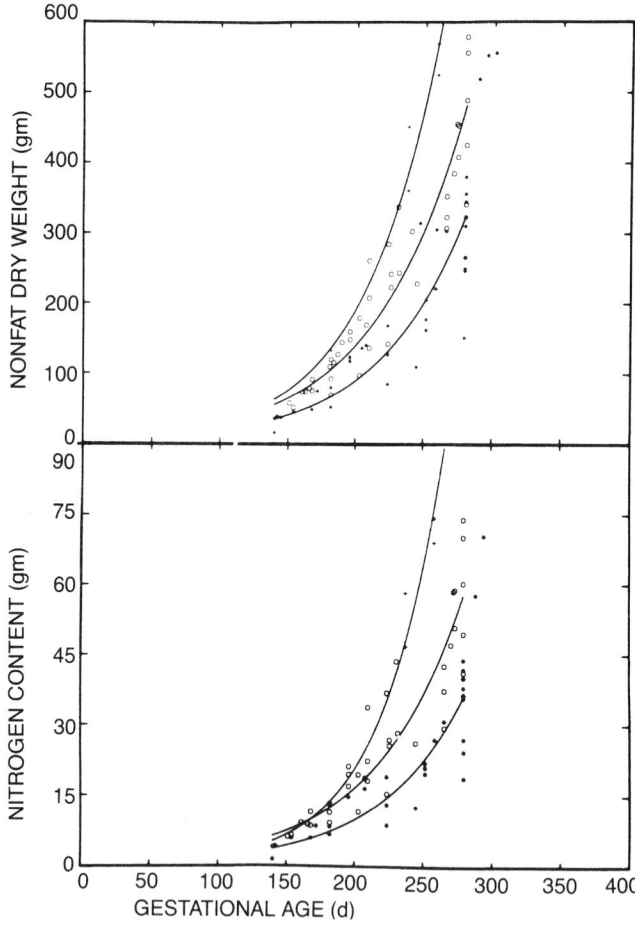

Figure 53-2. *Top,* Relationship of nonfat dry weight (NFDW) to gestational age in 97 human fetuses (see Fig. 53-1 for explanation of symbols). Increase in NFDW:large for gestational age (LGA)-NFDW (g) = 4.78 • $e^{(0.0184 \cdot GA)}$, r = 0.9869; appropriate for gestational age (AGA)-NFDW (g) = 6.38 • $e^{(0.01548 \cdot GA)}$, r = 0.9511; small for gestational age (SGA)-NFDW (g) = 3.60 • $e^{(0.0161 \cdot GA)}$, r = 0.9380. *Bottom,* Relationship of nitrogen (N) content to gestational age in the same infants. Increase in total body N; LGA-N (g) = 0.227 • $e^{(0.0225 \cdot GA)}$, r = 0.9870; AGA-N (g) = 0.703 • $e^{(0.0157 \cdot GA)}$, r = 0.9385; SGA-N (g) = 0.377 • $e^{(0.0163 \cdot GA)}$, r = 0.9351. (Adapted from Sparks JW. Seminars in Perinatology 1984;8[2]:74-93.)

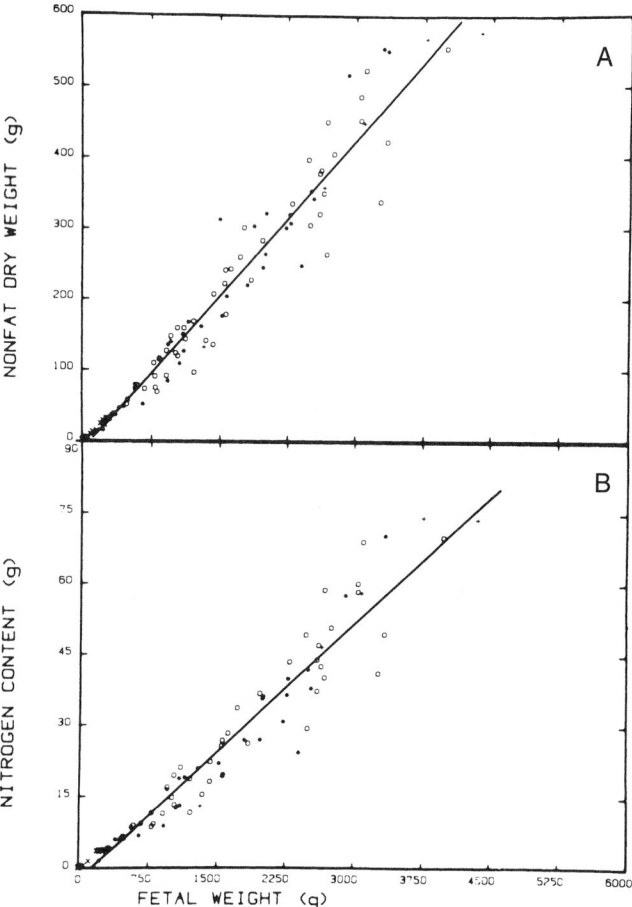

Figure 53-1. A, Relationship of nonfat dry weight (NFDW) to fetal weight in 169 human fetuses. * = small for gestational age infants; + = large for gestational age infants; *open circles* = appropriate for gestational age infants; NFDW (g) = 0.0589 Wt. **B,** Relationship of nitrogen (N) content to fetal weight in the same infants. N (g) = 0.00665 Wt. (Adapted from Sparks JW. Seminars in Perinatology 1984;8[2]:74-93.)

TABLE 53-1

Body Composition of the Human Fetus

Fetal Age (wk)	12	16	20	24	28	32	36	40
Weight (kg)	0.02	0.1	0.3	0.75	1.35	2.0	2.7	3.4
Total Nitrogen (N) and Protein in Fetal Body								
Total N (g)	0.18	1.0	3.6	10.4	19.6	30.2	44.3	64.3
Protein (g) (N × 6.25)	1.1	6.3	22.5	65	1.23	189	227	402
Content of Individual Amino Acids in Fetal Body (g)								
ILE	0.04	0.22	0.77	2.3	4.2	6.5	9.6	13.7
LEU	0.08	0.46	1.7	4.8	9.0	13.9	20.3	29.6
LYS	0.08	0.44	1.6	4.6	8.6	13.3	19.5	28.3
MET	0.02	0.12	0.42	1.2	2.3	3.5	5.2	7.8
PHE	0.05	0.25	0.91	2.6	4.9	7.6	11.1	16.3
TYR	0.04	0.18	0.65	1.9	3.5	5.4	8.0	11.5
THR	0.05	0.25	0.91	2.6	4.9	7.6	11.1	16.3
VAL	0.05	0.28	1.0	3.0	5.6	8.7	12.8	18.6
ARG	0.08	0.47	1.7	4.9	9.2	14.1	20.7	30.3
HIS	0.03	0.16	0.59	1.7	3.2	4.9	7.2	10.4
ALA	0.08	0.44	1.6	4.6	8.6	13.3	19.5	28.5
ASP	0.10	0.56	2.0	5.8	10.9	16.8	24.7	35.7
GLU	0.14	0.80	2.9	8.3	15.7	24.2	35.5	51.4
GLY	0.14	0.73	2.6	7.6	14.3	22.0	32.3	46.6
PRO	0.09	0.51	1.8	5.3	10.1	15.5	22.7	33.2
SER	0.05	0.27	0.97	2.8	5.3	8.2	12.0	17.3

Adapted from Widdowson EM: *In* AEBI H, Whitehead R (eds): Maternal Nutrition During Pregnancy and Lactation. Berne: Hans Huber Press, 1980, pp. 39-48.

Additional nitrogen requirements for urea excretion (and for other possible nitrogen excretion products) are not known for human fetuses. An analysis of complete nitrogen balance of this sort has been accomplished only in fetal sheep and is discussed later in this chapter. Several items of comparative chemical and physical growth in six species are summarized in Table 53-3.[5] The variation among certain parameters is considerable. Growth rate variation is 20-fold and weight-specific content of fat at term varies 16-fold, but nonfat dry weight and protein weight specific contents (as a percentage of total weight) at term are constant. Limited chemical analyses at different gestational ages indicate that in other animals, as in the human, fetal protein content is linearly related to fetal weight. Thus, protein accretion in the fetal rat occurs about 23 times as fast as it does in humans. These species-related differences are remarkable. The rat must possess a placental amino acid transport system with enormous capacity to

TABLE 53-2

Increments per Day of Nutrients in the Fetal Body at Selected Intervals During Gestation

Fetal Age Range (wk)	12–16	16–20	20–24	24–28	28–32	32–36	36–40
Weight Range (kg)	0.02–0.1	0.1–0.3	0.3–0.75	0.75–1.35	1.35–2.0	2.0–2.7	2.7–3.4
Increments of Nitrogen (N) and Protein in Fetal Body/24 (h)							
Total N	29	93	243	326	386	504	714
Protein (g) (N × 6.25)	0.18	0.58	1.52	2.04	2.41	3.15	4.46
Increments of Individual Acids in Fetal Body (mg/d)							
ILE	6	26	53	71	82	109	148
LEU	13	43	111	151	174	231	330
LYS	13	41	107	145	167	222	313
MET	4	11	28	39	44	59	92
PHE	7	23	61	83	95	127	184
TYR	5	17	44	59	68	91	127
THR	7	23	61	83	95	127	184
ARG	14	43	114	154	177	236	340
HIS	5	15	39	53	61	81	112
ALA	13	41	107	145	167	222	319
ASP	17	52	136	183	211	281	392
GLU	23	74	195	263	303	403	568
GLY	21	68	177	240	276	367	513
PRO	15	48	125	168	194	258	300
SER	5	25	66	89	102	136	191

Adapted from Widdowson EM: *In* Aebi H, Whitehead R (eds): Maternal Nutrition During Pregnancy and Lactation. Berne: Hans Huber Press, 1980, pp. 39-48.

TABLE 53-3

Growth Characteristics and Chemical Composition at Term of Selected Mammals and a Representative Human Fetus

	Human	Monkey	Sheep	Guinea Pig	Rabbit	Rat
Gestation (d)	280	163	147	67	30	21.5
Number of fetuses	1	1	1	3-5	4-6	10-12
Growth rate (g/kg/d)	15	44	60	70	300	350
Fetal weight (g)	3500	500	4000	100	60	5
Dry weight (g/%)	1050/30	125/25	760/19	25/25	9/15	0.2/4
Nonfat dry weight (g/%)	490/14	—	640/16	14/14	—	—
Protein (g/%)	490/12	—	480/12	12/12	7.2/12	0.6/12

Adapted from McCance RA, Widdowson EM: *In* Falkner F, Tanner JM (eds): Human Growth, vol 1, 2nd ed. New York: Plenum Press, 1985, p. 139.

support this high protein accretion rate, as well as mechanisms to process and support the high fetal protein synthetic rate.

PLACENTAL AMINO ACID SUPPLY: ACTIVE PLACENTAL TRANSPORT OF AMINO ACIDS

Placental amino acid exchange involves the active, energy-dependent transport of amino acids through transport systems across the placental membranes. The transport of amino acids is altered qualitatively and quantitatively by transport system location and activity, placental metabolism of amino acids, and fetal backflux of amino acids, as well as by changes in the overall size of the placenta, the architecture of the placental tissues, and developmental and pathologic changes in placental transport capacity. In addition, various aspects of placental exchange can be affected by interaction with the fetus, thus demonstrating a unity of function of the conceptus.

For most (but not all) of the amino acids, transport from mother to fetus occurs against a concentration gradient and involves energy-dependent transport mechanisms.[6-10] An increased fetal/maternal ratio of plasma amino acid concentrations has been documented for humans,[11] primates,[12] rats,[13] guinea pigs,[6, 14] sheep,[15, 16] and cows.[17] Although the fetal/maternal concentration ratio is greater than 1.0 for most amino acids measured, there are quantitative differences among species. For example, the fetal/maternal ratio in humans for the basic amino acids lysine and histidine is greater than 1.0, whereas in the sheep the ratio is less than 1.0. Even for amino acids with a fetal/maternal concentration ratio of less than 1.0, overall transport may be energy dependent because the concentration of a specific amino acid (e.g., citrulline) within the trophoblast tissue is greater than in the maternal plasma.[15, 16, 18] This is especially true for the very high intracellular trophoblast concentrations of taurine, glutamate, and aspartate, as well as for moderately increased intracellular concentrations of alanine, glycine, serine, glutamine, and threonine in the trophoblast.[11] For most amino acids, placental transport is sufficiently rapid that in spite of high concentrations of the amino acids in the trophoblast and the requirement for energy to promote amino acid uptake and transport, maternal concentrations of at least some amino acids can affect transport. This has been shown for certain amino acids (e.g., leucine[6, 19] and lysine[8]) in human and guinea pig placentas.

Because placental amino acid transport is energy dependent, it is not surprising that inhibition of both glycolysis and aerobic metabolism can suppress placental amino acid transport and amino acid incorporation into placental proteins. There is less evidence for reduced *in vivo* placental amino acid uptake, transport, or metabolism under conditions of energy substrate or oxygen deficiency or by selected inhibition of glycolysis or aerobic metabolism. However, Milley[20] measured a marked reduction (to 23% of normal) of total amino nitrogen uptake by fetal sheep during 3 to 4 hours of relatively marked hypoxia induced by lowering the maternal inspired oxygen concentration by approximately 50%. This study did not address placental amino acid metabolism or consider individual amino acids, although a subsequent similar study showed reduced fetal tyrosine uptake during maternal and fetal hypoxia.[21]

PLACENTAL AMINO ACID TRANSPORT SYSTEMS

The syncytial epithelium of the human placenta, the syncytiotrophoblast, is a polarized multinucleate epithelium. The maternal-facing, apical surface of this epithelium has a microvillous plasma membrane, whereas the fetal, basal surface is a smooth membrane. The transport of amino acids across the trophoblast involves three steps: (1) uptake from the maternal circulation across the microvillous membrane; (2) transport through the trophoblast cytoplasm; and (3) transport out of the trophoblast, across the basal membrane into the umbilical circulation. Transport systems are required at the two steps that involve transport across plasma membranes, that is, the maternal and fetal surfaces. At least 12 transporter systems for amino acid uptake by placental tissues have been identified (Table 53-4).[9,10,22-24] These are divided generally into sodium (Na+)-dependent and Na+-independent systems, the former designated by upper case letters and the latter by lower case letters. Specific amino acids transported by each system, conditions favoring or inhibiting or affected by each system, and location (maternal or fetal trophoblast membrane) for each system are presented in Table 53-4.

There is considerable overlap among the systems for different amino acids. Competition for a transporter system exists among the amino acids transported by that transporter system, and at least for the L system transporters, finite transport capacity has been demonstrated.[25] Thus, quantitative changes in the balance of amino acids transported by the placenta could be produced by significant alterations in plasma amino acid concentrations. For example, in one study of pregnant rats,[26] leucine was infused into the mother and resulted in a direct correlation between maternal and fetal leucine concentrations but an inverse correlation between the maternal leucine concentration and fetal concentrations of valine, isoleucine, tyrosine, and phenylalanine. All these amino acids share the L transport system. However, other amino acids transported by the L system (alanine, threonine, serine, and glycine) were not affected. Alanine, glutamine, threonine, and serine, four gluconeogenic amino acids found in high concentrations in placental tissues, are also transported by the A, ASC, and N systems.[27, 28] This could represent a uniquely devel-

TABLE 53-4

Placental Amino Acid Transport Systems, Substrates, Conditions, and Location

System	Substrates	Conditions	Membrane
Sodium-Dependent			
A	Neutral amino acids: alanine glycine, serine, proline, threonine, glutamine, MeAIB	Na^+ dependent, slowed by extracellular H^+ Excludes anionic and cationic amino acids, BCH, and leucine	M, F
ASC	Alanine, serine, cysteine, anionic (acidic) amino acids	Na^+ dependent, slowed by extracellular H^+ Excludes MeAIB, cationic amino acids, and proline	F
N	Glutamine, histidine, asparagine	Na^+ dependent Excludes cysteine, MeAIB, transstimulated	M
X^-_{AG}	Anionic (acidic) amino acids, glutamate, aspartate	Na^+ dependent Uptake from fetal blood; noncompetitive with other amino acids Excludes nonanionic amino acids	M, F
β	Taurine	Na^+, Cl^- dependent Highest trophoblast intracellular concentration of all amino acids Excludes α-amino acids	M
B°	Neutral amino acids	Excludes cationic and anionic amino acids	M, F
Gly	Glycine	Na^+ dependent	M
Sodium-Independent			
L(I)	Branched chain amino acids: (leucine, isoleucine, valine), tryptophan, BCH, phenylalanine, tyrosine, alanine, serine, threonine, glutamine	Na^+ independent, enhanced by extracellular H^+ Excludes anionic amino acids, proline, MeAIB	M, F
y^+	Lysine, arginine	Major cationic amino acid transporter excludes anionic amino acids inhibited by neutral amino acids (fetal side >maternal side)	M, (F?)
$b^{\circ,+}$	Lysine, arginine	Excludes anionic amino acids	(F?)
y^+L	Lysine, arginine	Excludes anionic amino acids	(M?),F
Asc	Small neutral amino acids	Excludes cationic and anionic amino acids	ND

BCH = 2-aminobicyclo-(2,2,1)-heptane-2-carboxylic acid; F = fetal; M = maternal; MeAIB = α-(methylamino)isobutyric acid; ND = not determined.
Data from refs. 9, 10, and 22 to 24.

oped protective capacity by which the placenta interacts with the fetus (particularly the fetal liver) to ensure adequate fetal supply of these important amino acids when the supply of glucose to the fetus is severely restricted and diversion of fetal amino acids to fetal gluconeogenesis becomes essential for fetal viability.

A summary of the factors that influence placental amino acid transport and the variety of established mechanisms that have some degree of control over placental amino acid transport are presented in Table 53–5. For systems A, ASC, N, X_{AG}^-, B°, and β, co-transport occurs with inwardly directed Na^+ transport that is energized by Na^+, potassium (K^+)-adenosine triphosphatase (Na^+,K^+-ATPase), producing an outside-inside Na^+ electrochemical gradient. Ganapathy and colleagues[29] observed H^+-amino acid co-transport that is dependent on an H^+ (out)-Na^+ plus amino acid in gradient, and is energized by Na^+,K^+-ATPase; this mechanism

TABLE 53-5

Factors Affecting Placental Amino Acid Transfer

1. Transporter proteins in the trophoblast membranes: ontogeny, location (maternal-facing microvillus, or fetal-facing basal, or both), regulation by local or circulating factors
2. Ion channel activity, ion gradients: Na^+,K^+-ATPase; Na^+, H^+, Cl^- gradients: (e.g., inward Na^+ gradient with system A co-transport)
3. Transport capacity, measured by V_{max} (maximum transport rate, affected by number of active transporters, the number of transporters per unit membrane area, and total membrane surface area)
4. Transporter-substrate binding affinity, measured by K_m (plasma amino acid concentration at half V_{max})
5. Placental disease (e.g., fetal growth restriction and preeclampsia)
6. Intracellular concentrations of amino acids, maternal amino acid concentrations, fetal amino acid concentrations, maternofetal amino acid concentration gradients leading to competition for transporters among amino acids
7. Turnover of transporters (rates of synthesis, degradation, or both)
8. Metabolism of amino acids by the trophoblast (e.g., oxidation of glutamate, conversion to other amino acids or substrates such as serine to glycine and leucine to KIC, protein synthesis, deamination-producing NH_3)
9. Uterine/umbilical blood flows: absolute rates (substrate delivery), the ratio of their flows (substrate delivery versus uptake and transport capacity), and the role of vasoactive substances (local or circulating) that alter uterine and/or umbilical blood flow (e.g., reduction in flow with epinephrine, enhancement of flow with nitric oxide)
10. Circulating hormone concentrations, placental receptors, and second messengers (e.g., hormone stimulation of cAMP-responsive increase in calcium channel and intracellular calcium release, activating amino acid metabolism and transporter activity)
11. Diffusional leaks (1) into or out of cells or (2) via paracellular pathways
12. Inhibitory effects of drugs (e.g., alcohol, nicotine, cocaine)

appears to apply to system L. The remaining transporters are Na+ independent and exclude anionic (acidic) amino acids. These transport mechanisms are active at the maternal microvillus membrane but also may be responsible for transport on the basal membrane. Studies of dually (maternal and fetal side) perfused placentas with paired tracers of amino acids indicate bidirectional transport for many amino acids, but with different transport kinetics, so transplacental transfer is greater in the maternofetal direction for all the amino acids taken up by the placenta.[6] This net flux is largely accounted for by a faster placenta-to-fetus efflux compared with a placenta-to-mother efflux, rather than resulting from different rates of uptake between the maternal and fetal surfaces. It is too simplistic to assume that active transport to high intracellular trophoblast concentrations with purely passive diffusion into the fetus represents the actual trophoblast-to-fetus transport mechanism.

PLACENTAL AMINO ACID TRANSPORTER PROTEINS

Historically, placental amino acid transport was described in terms of systems (see Table 53-4). More recently, the ability to clone, sequence, and study the expression of individual transporter proteins has led to an explosion of data concerning the molecular basis of amino acid transporter systems and their function.[9,22,23,30] Transport systems operate in one of two ways: in a monomeric manner or in a heterodimeric manner.[30-32] Monomeric systems transport amino acids via single membrane proteins, similar to amino acid uptake mechanisms associated with permeases in microorganisms.[33,34] Heterodimeric systems, conversely, involve the grouping together of two proteins to facilitate amino acid transport.[23,30,35] Currently known monomeric transport systems in placental tissues include y+[36] and most likely the X_{AG}^- system, whereas heterodimeric transport systems include system L, system y+L,[37] and the Asc system.[38,39] Those systems that operate in a heterodimeric manner are generally made up of a common heavy chain, a type II membrane glycoprotein, such as 4F2hc (comparable to the CD98 surface antigen, CD98hc),[40,41] NBAT (equivalent to rBAT or D2,[31,42-45]), or as yet undefined heavy chains,[46] which associate with one of a variety of light chain transport proteins to yield a range of differing amino acid transport systems.[32,35,37,39]

The 4F2hc is expressed in placental tissues over gestation, whereas the heavy chain protein, NBAT, has not been found in term human tissues.[41,47,48] During human and rat pregnancy, whole tissue studies have demonstrated the expression of 4F2hc protein to be predominantly located in the microvillous membrane, and protein content increases as gestation advances.[41,47,49] When the heavy chain is coexpressed with a light chain, functional transport occurs after the formation of disulfide bridges between the two chains.[32,50] Both heavy chain and light chain expression and interaction are required for transporter function.[32,48,51] A summary of the traditional transport systems and of their heavy and light chain associations reported in placental tissues and membranes is presented in Table 53-6.

Neutral Amino Acid Transporter Light Chain Proteins

The subcellular location of the light chain proteins and the way in which they interact with the heavy chain 4F2 protein are poorly defined. It is currently believed that an intracellular pool of light chains is available for incorporation within the membrane bound to heavy chains.[23,35,36] Several specific light chains and their amino acid transport system have been identified. System A activity has been demonstrated in microvillous and basal membranes.[52-54] Currently, three subtypes of amino acid system A have been cloned, amino acid transporter (AT) A-1, ATA-2, and ATA-3. The ATA-1 (or GlnT[55,56]) system is expressed predominantly in the placenta and heart and is responsible for the transport of small short chain neutral amino acids, such as alanine, serine, methionine, asparagine, and glutamine.[55] The functional characteristics of ATA-2 are similar to those of ATA1, although it is found in a wider range of tissues including the placenta.[55,57] ATA-3 appears to have a unique tissue distribution predominantly in hepatic and skeletal muscle tissues.[58]

Classic ASC transport of neutral amino acids alanine, serine, and cystine is reported in the microvillous membrane and in the basal membrane.[52,53,59,60] The cDNA ASCT-1 sequences this classic Na+-dependent ASC transport system and has been localized to human placental tissue, but at low expression levels.[61] Another member of this family of Na+-dependent neutral amino acid transport systems, the B° system, is responsible for neutral

TABLE 53-6

Placental Transport Systems and Associated Light Side Chains

Transporter System	Amino Acid Transporter Type	System Interaction	Heavy Chain Protein	Light Chain Protein*	References
A	Neutral			ATA-1	55
	Sodium dependent			ATA-2	57
ASC	Neutral			ASCT-1	61
	Sodium dependent				
B°	Neutral			ATB°	64, 65
	Sodium dependent			(ASCT-2)	
β	Neutral			TAUT	72
	Sodium dependent				
N	Neutral			SN1	
	Sodium dependent				
Asc	Neutral	Heteromeric	4F2hc	Asc-1	38
	Sodium independent		Unknown	Asc-2	46
L	Neutral	Heterodimeric	4F2hc	LAT-1	49, 75
	Sodium independent			LAT-2	39, 76, 77
y+L	Cationic	Heterodimeric	4F2hc	y+LAT-1	84
	Sodium independent			y+LAT-2	
y+	Cationic	Monomeric		CAT-1, CAT-2B, and CAT-4	41, 85, 117
	Sodium independent				
X_{AG}^-	Anionic			EAAT-1, EAAT-2, and EAAT-3	88, 89, 91

* Refer to text for light chain protein expanded abbreviations.

amino acid transport, including the branched chain amino acids.[62-64] The cDNA ATB° (ASCT-2) represents this system in human placental choriocarcinoma cell lines.[64, 65] System N, similar to systems A and ASC, transports neutral amino acids; it differs in its preference for amino acids containing nitrogen-bearing side chains and transports only glutamine, asparagine, and histidine.[66] System N activity has been localized in the human placenta,[67] and the gene *SN1* has been identified as associated with this activity.[23] The β–transporter, which transports taurine, has been found in placental microvillous and basal membrane vesicles.[68-70] Basal membrane activity is only about 6% of that in the microvillous membrane.[71] At present, the cDNA associated with this activity, TAUT, has been reported in placental cell lines.[71,72] The Na⁺-independent ASC system is responsible for the transport of small neutral amino acids and is composed of ASC-1 and ASC-2 components.[38, 46] Although ASC-1 forms a heterodimeric complex with 4F2hc,[38] ASC-2 appears to interact with a currently unknown heavy chain.[46] Light chain proteins also associate with 4F2hc to form the functional L transport system,[48, 51] catalyzing the uptake of neutral amino acids in an Na⁺-independent manner. System L activity has been demonstrated on both microvillous and basal membranes.[53, 73, 74] Two light chain proteins have been reported, L amino acid transporter-1 (LAT-1) and system L amino acid transporter-2 (LAT-2), and both have been identified in placental samples.[36,39,49,51,75-79]

Immunologic and functional studies suggest that at term gestation, the light chain LAT-1 is located predominantly in the microvillous membrane and the syncytiotrophoblast layer of the villi.[49, 79] Furthermore, the L transport system phenotype associated with the microvillous membrane occurs when the LAT-1 catalytic subunit is coexpressed with the 4F2hc, not LAT-2.[80] Human LAT-2 mRNA also has been found in the human choriocarcinoma BeWo cell line and placental villous tissues.[39,76,77,80] Studies on placental basal membrane studies concerning the inhibition of specific amino acid or synthetic amino acid uptake have determined that the basal membrane L transport system phenotype is that which is associated with the coexpression of LAT-2 and 4F2hc, and not LAT-1, as observed to occur in the microvillous membrane.[51,80,81]

Cationic Transport System Light Chain Proteins

System y⁺L activity is localized to both the basal and microvillous membranes.[7,41,82,83] Placental y⁺L system activity is determined by which light chain (system y⁺L amino acid transporter-1 [y⁺LAT-1] or system y⁺L amino acid transporter-2 [y⁺LAT-2]) forms a heterodimer with the 4F2hc.[35, 37, 84] The y⁺LAT-1 mRNA is detected in human placental poly(A)⁺ RNA and when coexpressed with 4F2hc in oocytes, it displays characteristics similar to those of the y⁺L system.[84] It is unclear whether system y⁺LAT light chain proteins display a distribution pattern similar to that of LAT proteins.

The y⁺ transport system currently has three cDNAs that are documented to code for proteins related to this high-capacity cationic, Na⁺-independent amino acid transport system, namely, the cationic amino acid transporters (CAT)-1, CAT-2B, and CAT-4,[41,85] and activity is predominantly localized to the microvillous membrane.[7, 41] The system y⁺ activity is dependent only on the expression of these monomeric proteins (or CAT gene products),[86] unlike systems L and y⁺L, which require expression of both a common heavy chain and a related light chain.[36]

Anionic Transport System Light Chain Proteins

Five cDNAs encoding for proteins capable of mediating high-affinity Na⁺-coupled transport of anionic amino acids have been reported,[87] and three of these have been cloned from rat and human placenta and are present on both the microvillous and basal membranes of the placenta.[87, 88] These proteins, excitatory

amino acid transport (EAAT)-1 (GLAST1), EAAT-2 (GLT1), and EAAT-3 (EAAC1), mediate placental Na⁺-dependent D-aspartate–inhibitable anionic amino acid transport or system X$_{AG}$⁻ activity.[89] EAAT-1 and EAAT-3 have been detected in human placental tissue,[90, 91] whereas these two and EAAT-2 have been detected in HRP.1 cells, a human cell line, and rat placenta.[88,92] The regulation of these proteins appears to be under the control of growth hormone and insulin-like growth factor (IGF) family members,[92] and up-regulation of the system has been demonstrated through nutrient-deprivation studies.[88] These later studies demonstrated that EAAT-1 and EAAT-3 play a key role in the basal anionic amino acid transfer, whereas EAAT-2 may be involved in conditions of amino acid depletion.[88]

With a greater number of studies now using molecular biology to determine the specific transporter proteins in the plasma membranes, it is likely that the identification of individual transporter proteins in the trophoblast will be expanded considerably as sequence data for specific transporters permit rapid identification of other members of the same family of transporters. Thus, the information provided in Table 53–6 should be regarded as an interim report in a rapidly changing field. Moreover, the importance of the heavy/light chain protein interactions in placental amino acid transport and metabolism is highlighted by studies showing that alterations in 4F2hc or y⁺LAT-1 expression may be responsible for lysinuric protein intolerance,[84, 93] cystinuria,[94] alterations in maternoplacental essential amino acid supply,[50, 79] and maternal immune response failures during implantation.[95-97]

DEVELOPMENTAL AND ADAPTIVE CHANGES OF PLACENTAL AMINO ACID TRANSPORT

Development and Growth of Placental Transport Capacity

As pregnancy advances, the increasing nutrient demands of the developing conceptus must be met through an appropriate increase in placental nutrient transport. This enhanced performance is facilitated through alterations in placental perfusion and changes in membrane exchange area together with changes in amino acid transporter concentrations in the plasma membrane. Because amino acids require active transport, they fit into the category of substances transported by the placenta according to diffusion-limited clearance. As such, placental transport rates of amino acids probably are not affected much by moderate fluctuations in uterine or placental blood flow. More severe reductions in flow may affect their transport (but this has not been observed or measured). If it does occur, it may be mediated through flow-reduction effects on placental energetics and ion gradients, rather than by a direct reduction of delivery. Furthermore, changes in flow may alter transport of certain amino acids more than others, potentially leading to changes in the relative proportions of amino acids delivered to the fetus.[98] If changes in blood flow to the placenta are more severe, alterations in amino acid uptake and transport by the placenta may reflect insufficient delivery of energy and oxygen to the Na⁺ and H⁺ ion pumps in the placental membranes, or they may reflect energy-dependent metabolism in the trophoblast cells. Such deficiencies may be as important as, or more important than, amino acid delivery as the means by which amino acid uptake and transport are altered by deficient placental blood flow.

In conjunction with the dramatic increases in uteroplacental blood flow during pregnancy (sixfold in sheep[99]), the developing surface area of the trophoblast is an important factor regulating total placental nutrient transport. Between the 16th week of pregnancy and term, human fetal weight increases approximately 20-fold, whereas the peripheral villous surface area increases only ninefold.[100-102] More important, the multiplication factor of nine actually decreases in late gestation.[102] However, there are only a few careful ontogenetic studies of how total surface area, including microvillous surface, changes over gestation.[101-103] Although some more recent surface area studies have been more detailed,[102-104] they have not yet been conducted in conjunction with *in vivo* amino acid flux studies. The demonstrated increases in total surface area of the placenta alone, however, cannot account for the fetal growth rate occurring over this period. These data suggest that fetal growth is not supported by changes in villous surface area alone; rather, the total transport capacity of the trophoblast is likely to be determined by changes in surface area, aspects of placental permeability, and the concentration of specific amino acid carrier proteins on the cell membrane surface.

In addition to changes in the placental exchange surface area, amino acid transport is also affected by the differing expression and transport parameters of transport systems through gestation.[41,54,105-107] For example, in the term placenta, L-arginine transport in microvillous membrane preparations is mediated through both y+ and y+L systems, whereas in the basal membrane, transport may be restricted to the y+L system. In addition, the kinetic properties of transport systems may also change as gestation advances. The first-trimester microvillous membrane has increased transport activity compared with term placenta vesicles,[106] and 4F2hc protein levels differ between early pregnancy and term placenta.[41] Furthermore, early in gestation, the log Michaelis constant (K_{m1}) of the microvillous high-affinity system y+L is significantly less than in term preparations.[41] Such studies highlight the complex interactions between developing microvillous and basal membranes, within the trophoblast and between the two circulations, to facilitate an increase in nutrient delivery to the growing fetus as gestation advances.

Changes in Amino Acid Transport in Intrauterine Growth Restriction

Both *in vitro* and *in vivo* studies indicate that reduced amino acid concentrations lead to enhanced amino acid transport (increased maximum velocity, reduced K_m).[28,108,109] Furthermore, this adaptive increase in transport can be blocked by selective inhibition of protein synthesis, a finding indicating that the synthesis of new transporter proteins is potentially responsible for this altered amino acid transport pattern. *In vivo* studies have been conducted in pregnant rats made hypoaminoacidemic by glucagon infusion. In these studies, fetal weight was not compromised until the mother became hypoglycemic while fasting.[110] These results indicated that there is placental compensation for the hypoaminoacidemia to maintain fetal amino acid supply and concentrations. In contrast, there was no apparent placental compensation for hypoglycemia (which reduced the fetal energy [glucose] supply) that was unaccompanied by hypoaminoacidemia. These results take on added importance relative to the observations by Cetin and associates,[111] who showed that plasma concentrations of α-amino nitrogen were lower in growth-restricted infants and their mothers. Furthermore, these investigators showed that amino acid concentrations were lower in intrauterine growth-restricted (IUGR) pregnancies, even if the fetuses had normal fetal heart rate and velocimetry monitoring, a finding suggesting that the decrease in amino acid concentrations preceded other clinical pathologic changes in these pregnancies and in the fetuses.[112] Data collected from IUGR babies at delivery show reduced total amino acid concentrations,[113,114] a finding suggesting alterations in amino acid transporter systems.

Placentas from growth-restricted infants display reduced transport of many amino acids, particularly the essential amino acids, with a reduced transport of total α-amino nitrogen. Such clinical observations are supported by *in vitro* observations in which microvillous membrane vesicles from appropriate for gestational age and small for gestational age babies demonstrated markedly lower activity (by 63%) of the A-system transporters in the small for gestational age infants.[115] Studies in rats, in which IUGR is induced through maternal protein deprivation, demonstrate a down-regulation of placental amino acid transport, through reductions in system A, X_{AG}^-, and y+ transport.[116,117] In addition, inhibition of system A transport in rat pregnancies has also shown a decrease in fetal weight.[118] Some investigators have reported that, in cases of human IUGR, system A membrane activity per milligram of microvillous membrane is reduced, a finding suggesting a positive association between fetal growth and system A activity.[105,119,120] The reverse process, a reduction of amino acid transport that occurs *in vitro* with increased amino acid concentrations, may be caused by *trans*-inhibition, that is, substrate binding on the *trans* or opposite side from uptake, limiting carrier mobility.[28] These *in vitro* changes have been observed only for the A system.

The placental changes in IUGR pregnancies are not confined to system A. In IUGR placentas, the Na+-dependent and Na+-independent transport of taurine from maternal to fetal circulation also is reduced, thereby decreasing the fetal taurine concentration.[71] Furthermore, uptake of leucine in both microvillous and basal membranes of the IUGR placenta is reduced, a finding suggesting alterations in the placental L transport system.[83] In these studies, basal membrane uptake was also reduced, suggesting that the changes in the basal membrane could be an important adaptive response by the trophoblast, limiting the backflux from the fetal circulation to the placenta. *In vivo* studies of ovine IUGR placental transport have indeed shown a reduced backflux of leucine and, additionally, threonine from the fetal circulation to the placenta.[121,122] In addition, under steady state in studies of stable isotopic tracer leucine infusion into the mother, the fetal/maternal enrichment ratio of leucine in normal human pregnancies is approximately 0.8, a much higher ratio than that compared with a ratio of 0.4 in sheep.[121,123] However, in both species, this ratio is significantly lower in IUGR pregnancies, a finding suggesting similarly reduced placental transport and metabolism characteristics. Clinical studies have shown that the fetal/maternal leucine enrichment ratio is significantly lower in human IUGR pregnancies compared with normal pregnancies.[123] Furthermore, the magnitude of its reduction correlates with a clinical classification of IUGR severity based on a completely different set of clinical data, namely, fetal arterial velocimetry and fetal heart rate data.[112] In other studies of IUGR placentas, reductions in total villous surface are reported,[103,104] a finding indicating that morphometric changes contribute to the overall reduction in placental amino acid transport capacity. Thus, it appears that both reductions in surface area for exchange and reductions in specific transporter number and activity contribute to the decrease in amino acid transport in IUGR pregnancies.

Other Modifiers of Placental Amino Acid Transport

The placenta contains many hormone receptors (e.g., for insulin, gonadotropin, growth factors, somatomedins, β-adrenergic agents, cholinergics, opiates), but there is little convincing evidence that placental amino acid transport is regulated by these hormones. Acetylcholine, however, perhaps by mediating changes in membrane potential, has been suggested as a potential regulator.[124] Additionally, Greenberg[125] presented preliminary *in vivo* evidence in rats that insulin may enhance placental amino acid uptake, concentration, and transport to the fetus. More recently, Karl and associates[126] found that aminoisobutyric acid (AIB) uptake by *in vitro* cultured trophoblast cells was enhanced by insulin as well as by dexamethasone, glucagon, and 8-bromo-cyclic adenosine monophosphate. These investigators hypothesized that because trophoblasts are known to produce IGF-I,[127] insulin may initially enhance methyl-AIB (MeAIB) uptake via IGF-I receptors. Insulin receptor concentrations are reduced in placentas from small for gestational age infants, and MeAIB uptake is decreased in trophoblast cells in culture,[126-130] although these same studies did not determine whether vectoral transport from maternal to fetal sides of the trophoblast also was reduced. Furthermore, there are no *in vivo* data yet to support these *in vitro* observations.

Ethanol has been shown both *in vitro* and *in vivo* to inhibit placental amino acid transport (primarily in the L system), but at concentrations much greater than those found in chronically alcoholic pregnant women.[131] Whether acute toxic ethanol ingestion impairs amino acid transport remains to be determined. Smoking increases nicotine concentrations in placenta, amniotic fluid, and fetal serum to concentrations higher than those found in maternal serum. Uptake of several amino acids by isolated human placental villi is reduced by nicotine and several components of tobacco smoke. Nicotine also inhibits system A amino acid transport in the placenta (*in vitro* results using MeAIB). One could expect double jeopardy to the fetus from ethanol and nicotine, a common drug combination in pregnant women who produce growth-restricted infants.[132]

Other drugs and toxins of many types may inhibit amino acid transport; mechanisms and clinical changes are still not well defined for most. For example, cocaine use in pregnant women has been associated with fetal growth restriction, and cocaine is known to inhibit placental uptake of amino acids and to bind to a high-affinity binding protein in human placenta.[119, 133-136] Studies with membrane vesicles suggest a potential direct effect of cocaine on Na^+-dependent amino acid transport systems,[119,136] although not the Na^+-independent systems, a finding suggesting possible compensatory mechanisms.[136] Systems L and N have also been demonstrated to be suboptimal when exposed to cocaine,[134,137] although it is recognized that these *in vitro* experiments may oversimplify the *in vivo* actions of cocaine on placental amino acid transport.[136] Complicating the interpretation of these studies are the observations that, *in vivo*, cocaine can reduce uterine and perhaps umbilical blood flow, can produce maternal and fetal hypertension via generalized vasoconstriction, and can impair oxygen transport to the fetus, perhaps through the vascular effects, leading to fetal hypoxemia.[138,139] In addition, there are no known relationships between placental histopathologic abnormalities (e.g., hypertrophy, hypoplasia, inflammation, edema, vascular malformations, or calcium deposition) and reduced amino acid transport.

Amino acid deficiencies or excesses themselves may not be as important as amino acid imbalances. Excess concentrations of some amino acids may interfere with transport and utilization of others,[140] particularly those in low concentration or those with uptake rates by the fetus that are very close to normal accretion rates. However, many of the data for such inferences come from cord blood samples, which are notorious for inaccurate reflection of steady-state, and they must be interpreted with caution. Similar concerns can be raised about interpretations of the relationship of fetal growth abnormalities with changes in fetal or maternal plasma amino acid patterns when such data are obtained from cord blood or maternal blood at the time of delivery. In contrast, experimental data in animals and from prenatal blood samples have demonstrated an association between fetal growth disorders and amino acid imbalances.[141-144]

UTERINE UPTAKE AND PLACENTAL CONSUMPTION OF AMINO ACIDS

Net uptakes of amino acids by the uterus have been difficult to measure because of small arteriovenous concentration differences and relative inaccuracies in the determination of uterine blood flow. In the pregnant sheep, Holzman and colleagues[145] demonstrated positive uterine arteriovenous concentration

differences for all amino acids tested except glutamate and where the ratio of umbilical/uterine arteriovenous differences (1.9:1) was about equal to the uterine/umbilical blood flow ratio. This evidence indicates that most of the uterine amino acid uptake is transported to the fetus, and placental requirements for amino acids are small relative to those of the fetus. There is now increasing evidence, however, to demonstrate that the placenta is also active in amino acid utilization and modification. Examples include leucine, threonine, glycine, alanine, and glutamate,[121, 122, 146-148] and these are discussed in more detail later in this chapter under placental fetal amino acid cycling. In addition, earlier in gestation, the placental/fetal weight ratio is severalfold higher than at term, and placental growth (by surface area increase relative to weight or by actual increase in mass, depending on species and gestational age) may still be significant relative to that of the fetus. However, quantitative aspects of placental amino acid requirements have yet to be worked out at any gestational age. Based on placental nitrogen content at term in the human placenta, Lemons[27] estimated that placental growth over gestation would require about 10.6 g of nitrogen (or 66 g of protein). *In situ* data using perfused guinea pig placenta showed that 12 to 16% of the radiolabeled amino acids were incorporated into placental proteins. This process was inhibited (81 to 96%) by cycloheximide, a finding suggesting that there was, in fact, an active process of placental synthesis of proteins.[149]

The placenta near term contains many different enzymes that are capable of metabolizing amino acids through pathways such as gluconeogenesis, glycogen synthesis, protein synthesis, amino acid oxidation, and ammoniagenesis.[27] Amino acid flux through these pathways has been demonstrated *in vitro*. So far, amino acid oxidation by human placental mitochondria has been demonstrated for alanine, aspartate, glutamate, and glycine.[150] Ammoniagenesis occurs *in vivo* (at least in sheep,[151, 152] rabbit,[153] and guinea pig[154] placentas). Other pathways may operate only under select conditions. Protein requirements include at least a small amount for oxidation and an undetermined amount for synthesis of secreted protein products (e.g., hormones such as human chorionic gonadotropin, luteinizing hormone, and placental lactogen).

UMBILICAL (FETAL) AMINO ACID UPTAKE

The net uptake of amino acids by the umbilical circulation represents the dietary supply of amino acids for fetal growth and protein metabolism. Although peptide uptake has been observed, this additional amount of protein probably provides little nutritional value because total amino nitrogen uptake (at least in the fetal lamb), is not different from the total amino nitrogen uptake in the form of amino acids. Protein molecules as small as albumin and as large as γ-globulin pass from maternal to fetal plasma with increasing efficiency as gestational age progresses.[155,156]

The uptake of amino acids by the umbilical circulation has been studied in only one experimental animal (fetal sheep) because of analytical problems related to the quantification of amino acids. The coefficients of extraction for several amino acids (umbilical venous–umbilical artery concentration/umbilical artery concentration) across the umbilical circulation are close to zero. Therefore, a high degree of accuracy is needed to measure the venous-arterial concentration differences to estimate net uptakes of these amino acids by the Fick principle.[145,157,158] The product of umbilical blood flow times the umbilical venous–arterial blood concentration difference for each amino acid yields the *net* uptake of each amino acid by the fetus. The first measurements of net umbilical amino acid uptake in a healthy, stable, chronically catheterized fetus were made in fetal sheep by Lemons and coworkers.[15] Figure 53-3 shows the net uptake for each amino acid in fetal sheep studied during the last 20% of gestation (net uptake equals the total height of each bar). Together, the net amino acid

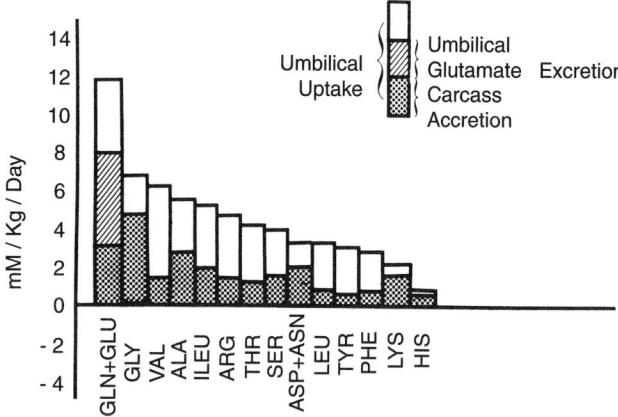

Figure 53–3. Umbilical uptake of individual amino acids by late gestation fetal sheep, partitioned into amino acid utilization for carcass accretion (*lower, dotted portion of bar*) and that presumably used for oxidation (*upper, open portion of bar*). There was a net excretion to the placenta from the fetus for glutamate in this study. ALA = alanine; ARG = arginine; ASN = asparagine; ASP = aspartate; GLN = glutamine; GLU = glutamate; GLY = glycine; HIS = histidine; ILEU = isoleucine; LEU = leucine; LYS = lysine; PHE = phenylalanine; SER = serine; THR = threonine; TYR = tyrosine; VAL = valine. (Adapted from Lemons JA, et al. Journal of Clinical Investigation 1976;58[6]:1428–1434.)

uptakes were estimated to provide 5.3 g/kg/day fetal weight of carbon and 1.6 g/kg/day of nitrogen. The net carbon uptake provided 60 to 70% of fetal carbon requirements (net accretion in carcass protein, glycogen, and fat, and utilization for oxidation yielding carbon dioxide excretion). The nitrogen uptake in this study was about 160% of the nitrogen requirement (net nitrogen accretion plus urea nitrogen excretion). Thus, either there were other excretory forms of nitrogen or the accuracy of estimating nitrogen excretion, accretion, or uptake in this study was limited.

Improved analytical methods for quantifying uterine and umbilical blood flow, and particularly blood amino acid concentrations, have been developed, the latter permitting separation of amino acids that were previously included in the concentration of others. In a study in fetal sheep at term, Marconi and associates[16] demonstrated a total fetal umbilical nitrogen uptake of 0.91 g nitrogen/kg/day (±2 SD, range of 0.56 to 1.27 g nitrogen/kg/day). This value is not very different from the calculated requirement (1 g nitrogen/kg/day) based on nitrogen accretion data and estimated fetal urea production rates in near-term fetal sheep.[16] Figure 53-3 also shows (in the *dotted portion of the bars*) the net accretion of each amino acid in the fetal carcass. The net uptake of most of the basic amino acids exceeds their net accretion by considerable amounts. In contrast, the net uptakes of the two basic amino acids, lysine and histidine, and the neutral amino acid glycine, barely exceed net accretion. Similarly, the combined accretion of asparagine and its product aspartate and the combined accretion of glutamine and its product glutamate are very close to the net uptakes of asparagine and glutamine, respectively. For these amino acid pairs, there is no net uptake of the acidic forms, glutamate and aspartate. This is true not only in the sheep,[158,159] but also in the primate and in humans.[160] These forms are derived in the fetus from deamination. These observations demonstrate that for these amino acids fetal requirements must be met by production within fetal tissues. Limitation of supply of these five amino acids (lysine, histidine, glycine, glutamine, and asparagine) likely would lead to reduced protein accretion and growth.

Placentofetal Amino Acid Cycling

The placenta and fetus interact in various ways to ensure amino acid supply to vital developmental, metabolic, and signaling processes that are unique to fetal growth and development (Fig. 53–4).[161] For example, in addition to net transport of amino acids to the fetus, the placenta may contribute to fetal amino acid and nitrogen balance by contributing to selective interorgan cycling.[8] This is an important concept in fetal physiology; various investigators have focused on placentofetal cycles for several substrates and blood flow patterns. Placentofetal cycling for amino acids were developed conceptually and experimentally by Battaglia and Meschia.[156,162] For example, the placenta actively produces ammonia, which is delivered into both the uterine and umbilical circulation.[152,163] This process appears to be a normal part of mammalian metabolism, occurring in all species studied to date.[156,163] In the fetal sheep, placental production of ammonia occurs over a large part of gestation. Studies by Bell and co-workers demonstrated that the absolute rate of uteroplacental ammonia production (~25 µmol/minute) at 73 to 97 days' gestation is as high as that estimated from data collected in sheep near term.[163,164] These data are consistent with *in vitro* studies demonstrating negligible urea cycle activity in sheep placental tissue over the entire length of gestation.[163,165] This relatively high placental ammonia production rate in mid-gestation probably also accounts for the higher concentration of ammonia (about twofold) in fetal blood at mid-gestation. At that stage of development, fetal weight and the capacity of the fetus to clear ammonia are markedly reduced relative to term,[163,164] in spite of an *in vitro* hepatic capacity for urea synthesis at mid-gestation that is equal to that near term.[166] A fraction of the net umbilical ammonia uptake is extracted by fetal tissues in sheep, perhaps contributing to hepatic urea formation and to other specific metabolic pathways. However, the ammonia taken up by the fetal sheep liver near term (~6.5 µmol/minute) is about 1.5 to 1.8 times that taken up by the umbilical circulation, a finding demonstrating considerable fetal endogenous ammonia production, consistent with observations of net ammonia efflux across the fetal hind limb.[16]

Measurements of umbilical and fetal hepatic concentrations of amino acids in fetal sheep have demonstrated reciprocal relationships among three sets of amino acids.[16] Glutamine and glycine are taken up (in net) by the fetus from the placenta and by the liver from the umbilical vein, whereas their metabolic products glutamate and serine, respectively, are produced (in net) by the fetal liver and are taken up in net by the placenta (although net fetoplacental transfer of serine in the fetal sheep is more characteristic of mid-gestation than near-term gestation). Similar but less marked relationships have been found for net hepatic uptake of asparagine and release of aspartate with a reciprocal change across the umbilical circulation. Thus, for these three amino acids, it is clear that fetal requirements must be met by net production within fetal tissues during all or at least a major portion of gestation.

For serine, preliminary tracer studies in near-term fetal sheep indicate that about 30% of fetal hepatic serine production is derived from glycine, and approximately 30% of the glycine uptake by the fetal liver is directed at serine production.[167] However, only about 5% of fetal plasma serine is derived from plasma glycine, a finding indicating that most of fetal serine is derived from fetal production in peripheral tissues. The bulk of fetal plasma serine oxidation occurs in extrahepatic tissues.[168] These data confirm the interorgan cycling of glycine and serine between the placenta and at least one fetal organ, the liver. Fetal serine production and uptake by the placenta from the umbilical circulation are much larger at 50% of gestation than at term; however, the source of such a relatively higher serine production rate early in gestation (greater synthesis or decreased incorporation into protein) is not known.

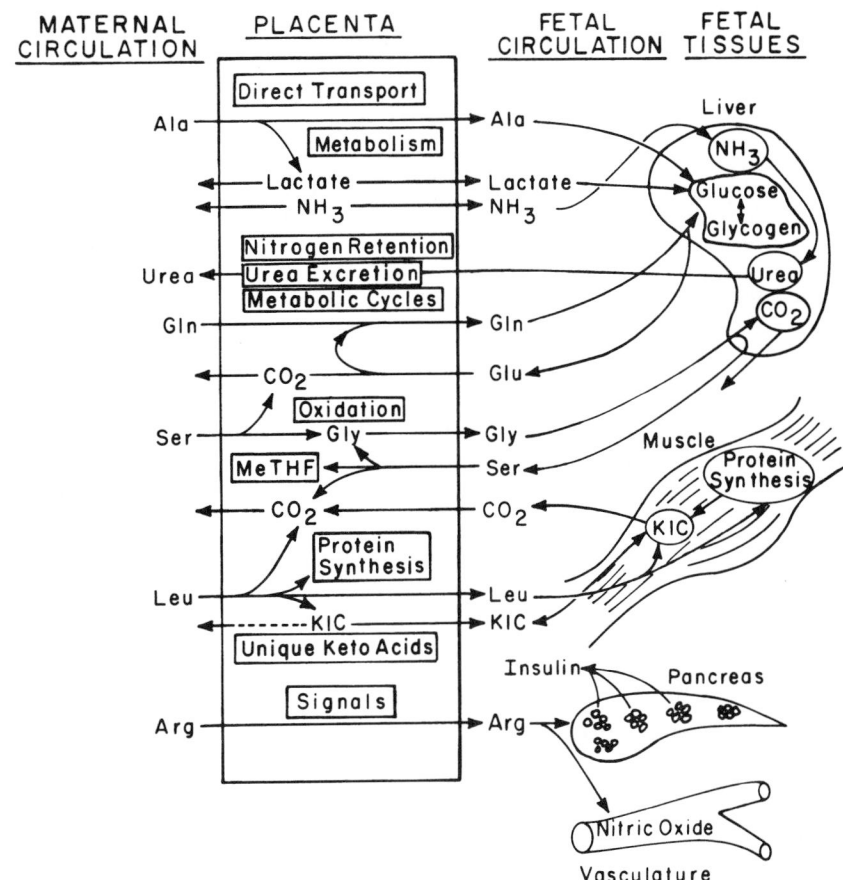

Figure 53–4. Schematic representation of various placentofetal metabolic interactions with respect to amino acid uptake by the placenta, metabolism in the trophoblast cells, direct transfer to the fetus, signaling of fetal vascular and metabolic processes, and utilization in fetal tissues. Ala = alanine; Arg = arginine; Gln = glutamine; Glu = glutamate; Gly = glycine; KIC = α-ketoisocaproic acid; Leu = leucine; MeTHF = methyltetrahydrofolate; NH_3 = ammonia; Ser = serine. (Adapted from Hay WW Jr. Placenta 1995;16[1]:19–30).

Glycine entry into the fetal pool is principally derived from umbilical uptake (about 30%) and from protein breakdown (about 56%). Glycine production in the placenta uses serine derived from both maternal and fetal circulations.[169] An additional source of glycine (about 14%) is derived from fetal glycine synthesis. The production of this nonessential amino acid in late fetal life[170] confirms the importance of the fetal glycine synthetic pathway found in liver and other organs. In their sheep study, Marconi and associates also showed that the hepatic amino acid–oxygen quotient is significantly higher than the umbilical amino acid–oxygen quotient (0.63±0.87 versus 0.13±0.03), a finding that indicates a high rate of amino acid utilization by the fetal liver.[16] The oxidation rate for glycine is high in the fetus, and it occurs almost exclusively in the fetal liver. Fetal hepatic glycine oxidation and serine production from glycine are linked by the enzyme systems, glycine oxidase and serine hydroxymethyl transferase.[171] A byproduct of placental glycine production via serine hydroxymethyl transferase is methylene tetrahydrofolate, which can be involved in various methylation reactions within the placenta.[146, 169]

Moores and colleagues[146, 169] also proposed that the actual release of glutamate and serine from the fetal liver could be a direct reflection of the uncoupling of gluconeogenesis from amino acid oxidation. Ordinarily, glutamine produces glycogen as well as glutamate in the fetal liver.[171] Virtually 100% of fetal glutamate production is accounted for by fetal hepatic production from glutamine.[172] Placental oxidation of glutamate serves as its principal pathway of disposal. At birth, this pattern shifts, so with the loss of the placenta and the development of net hepatic production of glucose, glutamine carbon can be shunted directly to gluconeogenesis. Placental glutamate oxidation also provides nicotinamide adenine dinucleotide phosphate (NADPH), which is required for placental lipid metabolism and steroidogenesis,

particularly that of progesterone.[105] The term human trophoblast lacks an active pentose phosphate pathway, which is another pathway for NADPH production.[105]

The ovine placenta takes up glutamine from maternal plasma. Most is transported directly to the fetus, and some is deaminated to glutamate in the trophoblast.[173,174] The ovine placenta also contains glutamine synthetase, and a small fraction of glutamate that is taken up by the placenta from the fetal circulation is returned to the fetus as glutamine. There is no proof, however, of a direct placentofetal cycle for glutamine and glutamate. Moores[173] demonstrated that the amount of glutamine produced from glutamate in the placenta accounts for less than 10% of the total glutamate uptake by the placenta and represents less than 10% of placental glutamate output. It is the oxidation of glutamate in the placenta that appears to be the predominant pathway of glutamate disposal in the fetoplacental system (70 to 80% of that taken up from the umbilical circulation is oxidized).[173] The ovine placenta receives two major influxes of glutamate: the placental uptake of fetal plasma glutamate, at about 4.8 µmol/kg/minute, and the placental production of glutamate from deamination of branched-chain amino acids, at 3.2 µmol/kg/minute.[173,175] In the sheep, there is practically no uptake of glutamate by the placenta from the maternal circulation, and thus no contribution of maternal plasma glutamate to placentofetal glutamate metabolism. Conditions may be different in the human placenta, which has glutamate transporters on both maternal and fetal surfaces.[176,177]

Another example of placentofetal amino acid cycling involves the relatively high concentrations and activities of branched-chain amino acid aminotransferases found in the placenta (sheep, human).[178,179] The transamination of a branched-chain amino acid provides the placenta with nitrogen, which, in addition to other placental metabolic functions, is used to sustain a high rate of glutamate production rather than the direct placental utilization of branched-chain amino acids as energy substrates.[83,180] Studies in sheep suggest that net placental uptake and transamination to the corresponding α-ketoacid can occur for leucine,[181] with 10 to 15% of leucine carbon transferred to the fetus as ketoisocaproic acid. The existence of these pathways implies a level of regulation in fetoplacental metabolism that is far more complex and sophisticated than was originally thought. It is also clear that the placental free amino acid pool, whether derived from protein breakdown in the placenta or from the maternal circulation, cannot be treated as a single homogeneous pool.[162]

Alanine also is consumed by the ovine placenta.[147,182] Placental metabolism of alanine may contribute significantly to placental lactate production,[183] and also to placental carbon oxidation, and it accounts for 20% of alanine oxidation by the entire conceptus. The placental oxidation of alanine is much higher than the decarboxylation rate of leucine in the placenta.[184] Furthermore, alanine entering the placenta is metabolized and exchanged for placental alanine. In fact, most of the alanine delivered to the fetus is of placental origin.[147] As the fetus matures, fetal hepatic urea cycle enzyme activity and production rates increase, approaching 0.4 g nitrogen excretion/kg/day.[152] In addition, the sheep fetus,[185] like the preterm human infant,[186] responds to an increased intake of ammonia and nitrogen with increased urea production. These observations suggest that the fetus does respond effectively to a varied rate of amino acid supply (uptake or degradation) by appropriate forms of nitrogen excretion (e.g., serine and glutamate uptake by the placenta with placental ammonia and hepatic urea production). The higher ammonia production/urea excretion rate ratio that occurs earlier in gestation may be an advantage to the smaller fetus, providing nitrogen for reincorporation into amino acids and amines essential for rapid fetal growth.[187] The lower urea cycle activity in earlier gestation may also favor conversion of ornithine to polyamines that are essential in development.[188] All five enzymes of the urea cycle are present in the human fetus by 10 to 12 weeks' postconceptional age; however, the levels of arginase are lower than those of the other urea cycle enzymes and may be rate limiting for fetal urea production.[189] Arginase may provide a mechanism in the placenta for urea production from arginine in spite of undetectable levels in the human placenta of ornithine carbamyltransferase.[190] Quantitative aspects of ammonia and urea production in the human fetus are as yet unknown. This knowledge will become important as efforts persist to increase nitrogen intake as a therapy for fetal growth retardation and to help determine the developmental capacity of the preterm infant to use protein and excrete nitrogen effectively in response to allegedly growth-promoting, high-protein diets.

FETAL AMINO ACID OXIDATION

Uptake of neutral amino acids in excess of carcass accretion requirements also implies that this portion of amino acid uptake is used for oxidation. Evidence of the fetal oxidation of amino acids comes from two observations: (1) the high fetal urea production rate and (2) the direct measurement of labeled carbon dioxide production and excretion during fetal infusions of carbon-labeled amino acids.[159]

Although the umbilical arterial-venous concentration difference for urea is too small to measure accurately, the fetal/maternal arterial plasma urea concentration difference is large enough to measure with reasonable accuracy (~4.2 mg/dl in sheep[185] and ~2.5 mg/dl in humans).[191] Thus, the fetal urea production rate can be quantified as the product of placental urea clearance ($Cl_{p)urea}$) times the fetal arterial–maternal arterial plasma urea concentration difference.[151,156] Placental urea clearance has been estimated by the infusion of ^{14}C-labeled urea into the fetus. ^{14}C-urea diffuses rapidly across the placenta from the umbilical circulation to the much larger maternal plasma–extracellular fluid

urea pool and the irreversible maternal urinary urea pool, thus creating a reasonably large and accurately measurable umbilical arterial-venous ^{14}C-urea concentration difference. Calculations have produced estimates of fetal urea production rate ranging from about 0.4 mg/minute/kg in humans[156] and rhesus monkeys[151] to 0.7 mg/minute/kg in sheep.[185] The urea production rate in sheep could account for approximately 0.36 g/kg/day of nitrogen excretion (or ~25% of fetal nitrogen uptake in amino acids) and about 0.2 g/kg/day of carbon (~2% of total fetal carbon uptake or ~6% of fetal carbon uptake in amino acids). Such fetal urea production rates are large, exceeding neonatal and adult body weight–specific rates, indicating relatively rapid protein turnover and oxidation in the fetus.

Direct measurement of fetal amino acid oxidation has been made using carbon-labeled isotopic tracers of selected amino acids, thereby quantifying net excretion of labeled carbon dioxide from the fetus via the umbilical circulation relative to the plasma labeled amino acid–specific activity.[159] An important refinement of this methodology is to use the plasma amino acid reciprocal pool-specific activity; for example, for leucine, the plasma ketoisocaproic acid pool should be used, because it equilibrates with the intracellular specific activity that represents the dilution of intracellular leucine by cellular protein degradation and the final pathway to oxidation.[192] For an amino acid labeled on one carbon, for example, [1-^{14}C]leucine, net excretion of [14]CO_2 can be compared with net fetal [^{14}C]leucine uptake (infusion rate minus diffusional loss to the placenta).[159] This ratio represents the fraction of tracer leucine that is oxidized, and when multiplied by the fetal leucine disappearance rate, it yields the fetal leucine oxidation rate. Dividing the net [14]CO_2 excretion rate by the fetal amino acid reciprocal pool plasma-specific activity (disintegrations per minute per millimole of reciprocal pool amino acid carbon) permits the calculation of the amount of carbon dioxide produced from fetal oxidation of the specific amino acid:

1. Fetal amino acid oxidation fraction = net [14]CO_2 excretion/net ^{14}C-amino acid uptake.
2. Fetal amino acid oxidation rate = amino acid oxidation fraction × amino acid irreversible disposal rate into fetal tissues.
3. Carbon dioxide produced from fetal amino acid oxidation = net [14]CO_2 excretion/amino acid reciprocal pool-specific activity.

Central to this methodology has been the documentation that, at least in the fetal lamb, virtually 100% of fetal carbon dioxide production (e.g., that produced by fetal infusion of NaH[14]CO_3) is excreted via the umbilical circulation.[158] One limitation of this methodology is its overestimation of fetal oxidation of a specific substrate to the extent that carbon-labeled nonoxidative products derived from placental and maternal metabolism of the substrate reenter the fetus and are oxidized.[193] For example, the carbon dioxide production rate from tracer leucine may include carbon dioxide derived from the decarboxylation of ketoisocaproic acid molecules reentering fetal plasma after the placental deamination of fetal leucine.[181] Although estimates of this additional labeled carbon dioxide suggest that it is a fraction of an amino acid's direct oxidation, experimental verification has not been accomplished.

Several ^{14}C-labeled amino acids have been infused into fetuses *in vivo*, documenting [14]CO_2 production (leucine, lysine, alanine, tyrosine, glycine, serine, threonine, glutamate).[121,122,146,169] Oxidation rates have been calculated for leucine (~25% of utilization), lysine (~10% of utilization), and glycine (~13% of utilization), demonstrating that the oxidation/disposal ratio is directly related to the excess of umbilical uptake (which is greater than accretion) and to the plasma concentration of the amino acid.[15,16] Leucine oxidation occurs largely in muscle, whereas glycine oxidation occurs in liver as well. The net umbilical uptake of alanine in the sheep fetus is approximately 5 µmol/kg/minute, which is less than the amount of plasma alanine that is decarboxylated by the fetus (9 µmol/kg/minute), thus emphasizing the need for a relatively high rate of fetal alanine production.[182]

AMINO ACID METABOLISM IN MID-GESTATION

Studies of the fetal lamb in mid-gestation emphasized several important developmental characteristics of fetal amino acid metabolism. First, at mid-gestation, the fetal uptake of amino acid and ammonia nitrogen via the umbilical circulation is comparable to fetal nitrogen requirements estimated from nitrogen accretion and urea excretion data.[164] Second, the contribution of amino acid carbon to energy needs and carbon accretion is comparable to that of glucose.[194] Similar observations have been made near term. However, in relation to fetal dry weight (a comparison made necessary by the large decrease in fetal water content over gestation), the umbilical uptake of amino acid nitrogen at mid-gestation is approximately fourfold greater than it is near term. This much higher dry weight–specific nitrogen uptake at mid-gestation agrees with measurements of protein synthetic rate and oxygen consumption. Third, leucine oxidation at mid-gestation is at least as great as it is at term, a finding indicating that amino acids provide carbon for fetal oxidative metabolism over a large part of gestation.[194,194]

FETAL PROTEIN SYNTHESIS AND TURNOVER

In the growing fetus, net protein synthesis exceeds net protein degradation, although both processes continue simultaneously. The protein synthetic rate has been determined using isotopic tracers of various amino acids. Quite variable rates have been determined, even within a species, largely because of technical differences. The major difference has been the inclusion (incorrectly) or exclusion (correctly) of tracer diffusional loss to the placenta as part of tracer entry.[159] Furthermore, this fractional diffusional loss varies in magnitude among amino acids. Thus, the rate of incorporation of tracer amino acid into proteins is the difference between infusion rate and the combined loss of tracer to catabolic pathways (oxidation) and diffusional loss to the placenta.[129] As discussed earlier, the $^{14}CO_2$ excretion rate varies among amino acids because of unique metabolic pathways, as well as gestational age, nutritional state, and nonprotein caloric supply. The placental tracer loss can also vary by gestational age among amino acids.[184] This tracer methodology also is limited *in vivo* by several factors. First, it calculates a whole body protein synthetic rate, which does not address the markedly different rates of growth and protein synthesis that occur among organs. Moreover, the protein synthetic rate is calculated using the plasma-specific activity (unless a reciprocal pool product is available, such as ketoisocaproic acid for leucine), which may be greater than the intracellular-specific activity because of intracellular reutilization of amino acids released by protein degradation.[195] Thus, the protein synthetic rate is frequently underestimated.

The fractional protein synthetic rate (K_S, or the fraction of body proteins that are synthesized/unit time) can also be calculated and compared with fractional growth rate (K_G). K_S is calculated by infusing an amino acid tracer until a steady-state specific activity (SA) in proteins and in the plasma is reached.[129,156]

$$K_S = SA_{proteins}/(SA_{plasma} \times \text{time of infusion})$$

This calculation can be made more precise by calculating the rate at which steady-state specific activity is obtained and by accounting for the recycling of tracer from degradation of newly synthesized (thus, tracer-containing) proteins. In the fetal lamb, K_S and K_G have been compared using two tracers, ^{14}C-leucine and ^{14}C-lysine, at different gestational ages.[194,196] Figure 53-5 is a

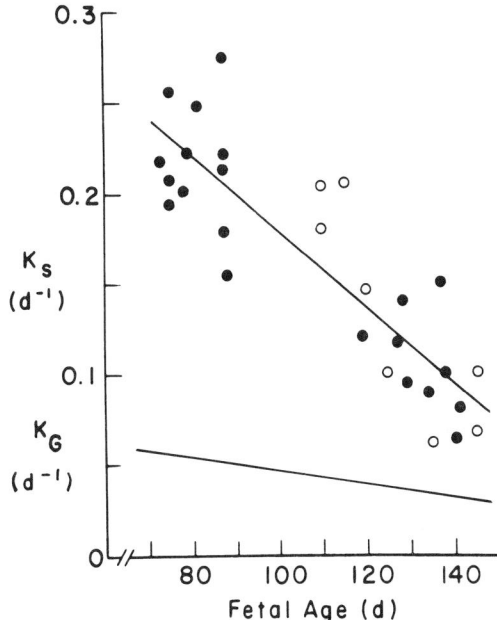

Figure 53–5. Fractional rate of protein synthesis (K_s) over gestation in fetal sheep studied with leucine (*closed circles*) and lysine (*open circles*) radioactive tracers compared with fractional rate of growth (K_G) in the lower portion of the figure (*line*). (Data from refs. 194, 196, and 212.)

composite of data from these studies, demonstrating that both K_S and K_G decrease with gestational age, but the decline in K_S is greater. The higher protein synthetic rate in the mid-gestation fetus is proportional to the higher metabolic rate and the greater glucose uptake and utilization rates at that stage of gestation. Thus, protein synthesis per millimole of oxygen consumed is quite constant from mid-gestation until term.[194] The same appears to be true for the relationship between protein synthesis and glucose consumption.[1] Because other studies in pregnant sheep have shown increasing placental nutrient transport capacity with advancing gestational age, these data suggest that the reduced rate of fetal growth toward term is an intrinsic quality of fetal development and is not the result of placental limitation of nutrient supply. The mechanisms underlying the reduction in protein synthetic rate over gestation remain to be determined. At least a partial explanation can be offered according to the changing proportion of body mass contributed by the major organs (Table 53-7). Based on the relatively increased mass of skeletal muscle (which has a relatively lower fractional synthetic rate in late gestation), for example, it is logical that the whole body fractional synthetic rate should decrease.[160] It is clear, however, that

TABLE 53-7	

Fractional Synthetic Rates Among Organs in Early Postnatal Life

Organ	Percentage of Synthesis/Day (K_s)
Liver	57.0±12.0
Kidney	50.0±10.0
Brain	17.0±3.0
Heart	18.5±4.0
Skeletal muscle	15.2±2.8

Adapted from Waterlow JL, et al: Protein turnover in Mammalian Tissues and in the Whole Body. Amsterdam: Elsevier/North-Holland Biomedical Press, 1978.

a direct relationship with anabolic endocrine-paracrine factors such as insulin, pituitary and placental growth hormone, placental lactogen, IGFs (somatomedins), epidermal growth factors, and so forth, cannot be proposed, because most studies suggest an increasing concentration or secretion of these substances over gestation.[197]

NORMAL FETAL SKELETAL MUSCLE METABOLISM OF AMINO ACIDS

Amino acid metabolism in skeletal muscle has been studied *in vivo* in fetal sheep by measuring blood flow to the hind limb and by sampling for amino acid concentration differences between femoral arterial and venous blood. Under normal physiologic conditions, the fetal hind limb in the sheep has a net uptake of both essential and nonessential amino acids from the circulation to the hind limb,[198] a finding reflecting the relatively high rate of protein synthesis and nitrogen accretion of the fetus. In addition, in the fetal sheep there is a net uptake of serine and glutamate by the hind limb; these are not supplied by placental transfer to the fetal circulation and thus represent a requirement for net hepatic synthesis of these amino acids for disposal in the fetal tissues. Fetal hind limb tissues in the sheep do not release alanine or glutamine under normal conditions, in spite of their large net hepatic uptake rates.

The role of insulin and glucose in fetal hind limb skeletal muscle metabolism of amino acids was studied in the fetal sheep by several groups.[198-203] Under hyperinsulinemic conditions in which glucose and amino acids were also infused to maintain their concentrations relatively in the normal range, there was an increased net uptake of most amino acids by the hind limb, reflecting reduced rates of proteolysis more than increased rates of protein synthesis. Protein synthesis was more strongly regulated by the plasma concentration of amino acids than by insulin alone. Glucose uptake also plays a role, a finding indicating that a positive energy balance, as well as the provision of amino acids, allows insulin to promote nitrogen accretion most effectively.[15, 199, 200] Studies indicate that insulin can enhance the mitogen-activated protein kinase (mitogen-activated pathway) in fetal skeletal muscle,[204] and both insulin and IGF-I regulate protein synthesis through well-recognized intermediates in their signal transduction pathways, including mammalian target of rapamycin and the eukaryotic initiation factors.[205]

FETAL PROTEIN METABOLISM IN RESPONSE TO FASTING

Because protein synthetic and growth rates are quite high in fetal life, it is appropriate that a number of investigators have studied changes in fetal protein and amino acid metabolism in response to maternal conditions that restrict amino acid or energy supply to the fetus. As described earlier, for example, Domenech and co-workers[110] observed sustained fetal amino acid concentrations and fetal growth during selective maternal hypoaminoacidemia in pregnant rats; fetal growth was reduced only when maternal fasting reduced the fetal glucose (energy) supply. Similarly, Lemons and Schreiner[206] observed normal to increased fetal amino acid concentrations during maternal fasting in pregnant sheep. Fetal uptake of amino acids did not change with fasting, a finding indicating either a reduced fetal protein synthetic rate or an enhanced rate of proteolysis that was directly related to fetal glucose energy supply. Liechty and associates[208] and Lemons and Liechty[207] also demonstrated enhanced hind limb release of alanine and glutamine (major potential sources of gluconeogenesis) in fasted sheep. Evidence of fetal gluconeogenesis during prolonged maternal fasting-induced hypoglycemia and reduced glucose supply was demonstrated.[209]

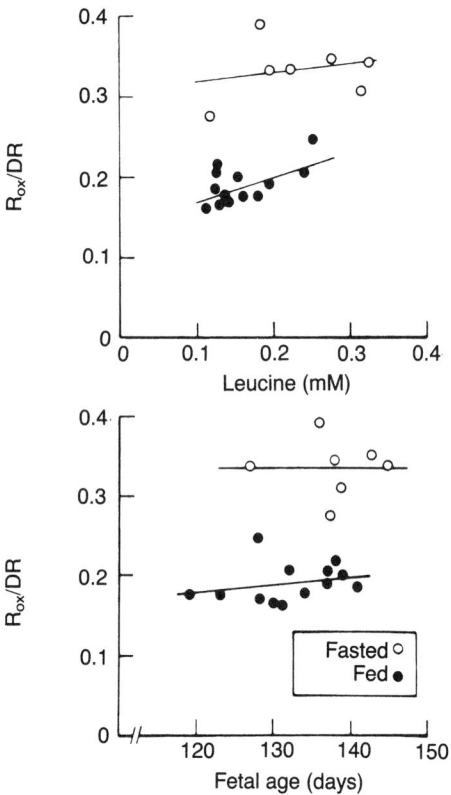

Figure 53–6. Oxidation/disposal rate ratio (R_{ox}/DR) for leucine in fetal sheep near term, studied during fed and fasted conditions compared with (*top*) fetal arterial plasma leucine concentration and (*bottom*) fetal age. (Adapted from van Veen LC, et al. Metabolism: Clinical & Experimental 1987;36[1]:48–53.)

The balance among energy supply, amino acid supply, protein synthesis, and protein catabolism was further investigated in two separate models. In fasted pregnant sheep, van Veen and colleagues[159] demonstrated no change in leucine disposal rate, but a doubling of the leucine oxidation/disposal rate ratio after a week of maternal fasting (Fig. 53–6). In acutely fasted pregnant rats, Johnson and co-workers[210] showed enhanced fetal proteolysis but normal rates of protein synthesis. These animals had relatively normal concentrations of amino acids but markedly reduced glucose concentrations.[210] In a subsequent study, these same investigators showed that prolonged maternal malnutrition with both energy (e.g., glucose) and protein restriction resulted in decreased protein synthesis and proteolysis, but in this case, protein synthesis was reduced to a greater extent.[211] Together, these data support the concept that fetal protein synthesis is both amino acid and energy dependent, whereas fetal protein catabolism may be more specifically regulated by nonprotein energy substrate supply. Furthermore, certain amino acids released by proteolysis can be oxidized to maintain fetal energy balance at the expense of growth, whereas others can be directed toward gluconeogenesis to maintain glucose energy requirements.

AMINO ACID, PROTEIN, NITROGEN, AND CARBON BALANCE

Amino acid balance has been determined for several amino acids, including leucine, glutamine (and glutamate), alanine, glycine, and serine, but thus far in only one species, the fetal sheep. Details of these studies for these amino acids are discussed previously and are presented schematically in Figure 53–4. More complete results for leucine from fetal sheep studied near term and at 50 to 60% of gestation have been determined (Fig. 53–7).[212] Protein turnover/wet weight is higher in the early-gestation fetus, accounted for primarily by relatively increased rates of umbilical leucine uptake (exogenous entry) and protein synthesis. This results in a 50% higher rate of net protein accretion. Table 53–8 summarizes the contributions of amino acids to fetal carbon, calories, and nitrogen balance, compared with other known substrates in late-gestation fetal sheep.[156, 212, 213] Differences among species can be expected based primarily on the capacity of the placenta to transfer fat to the fetus and on the contribution of fat to fetal body composition. Even in those species that take up fat from the placenta and deposit fat in fetal tissues, fatty acid oxidation is presumed low. This presumption has not been tested adequately and may provide a partial explanation for the difference between carbon and caloric requirements and carbon and caloric uptakes.

CONCLUDING REMARKS

There are important lessons for amino acid nutrition of the preterm infant to be learned from evaluation of fetal amino acid uptake and metabolism. As emphasized in this chapter, amino acid supply to the fetus by the placenta is quantitatively large and qualitatively unique. Individual amino acids are actively transported into the fetal circulation at relatively high rates to meet the rapid

TABLE 53-8

Metabolic Balance for the Late Gestation Fetal Sheep

Carbon-Caloric Balance		Carbon (g/kg/d)	Calories (kcal/kg/d)
Requirement			
Accumulation in carcass		3.2	32
Excretion as carbon dioxide		4.4	0
Excretion as urea		0.2	2
Excretion as glutamate		0.3	2
Heat (oxygen consumption)		0.0	50
	TOTAL	8.1	86
Uptake			
Amino acids		3.9	45
Glucose		2.4	17
Lactate		1.4	14
Fructose		1.0	7
Acetate		0.2	3
	TOTAL	8.9	86
Nitrogen Balance Requirement			
Urea nitrogen excretion		0.4	
Nitrogen accretion		0.6	
	TOTAL	1.0	
Uptake (in Amino Acids)		1.0	
	TOTAL	1.0	

Data from refs. 156, 212, 213.

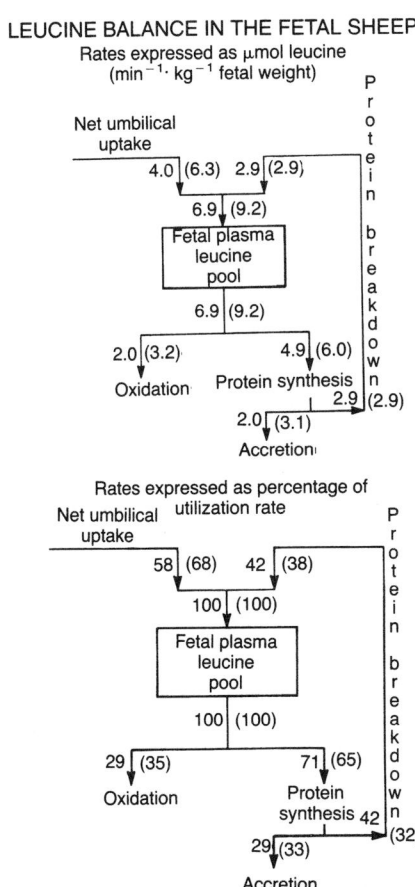

LEUCINE BALANCE IN THE FETAL SHEEP

Figure 53–7. Leucine balance in the fetal sheep. Values in *parentheses* are those measured or calculated at mid-gestation. (Adapted from Battaglia FC, Meschia G. *In* Battaglia FC, Meschia G [eds]. An Introduction to Fetal Physiology. Orlando, FL: Academic Press, 1986, p. 112.)

growth and energy needs of the fetus. The active transport also produces amino acid concentrations in the fetal circulation that are generally higher than those in the maternal circulation. These concentrations also are higher than most preterm infants have in their plasma after birth. By way of comparison, the early third trimester fetal sheep uses about 6 g/kg/day of amino acids. When scaled to the fractional growth rate of lean body mass characteristic of the normally growing human fetus at the same stage of development,[214] this rate of amino acid utilization is about 3.6 to 4.8 g/kg/day. This rate is similar to the required amino acid intake (4.0 g/kg/day) estimated for very preterm infants by the factorial method, but it is noticeably greater than the rate of amino acid or protein intake that these infants are usually fed.[215] Only when amino acid intake rates and plasma concentrations are achieved in preterm infants that meet the fetal values do nitrogen and protein balance as well as oxidation rates of the preterm infant match those of the normally growing fetus.[216] The relative concentrations of amino acids achieved in the fetal circulation also are unique. These concentrations occur as a combined result of (1) unique transport characteristics for each amino acid and for groups of amino acids in the placenta, (2) unique rates of placental metabolism of amino acids, (3) unique amino acid derivatives produced by placental amino acid metabolism, and (4) unique placentofetal hepatic amino acid metabolic cycles. Such information from animal models needs to be expanded by human studies to help determine the optimal supply of each of the amino acids and the unique concentrations that should be achieved in the circulation of the preterm infant to optimize preterm neonatal amino acid metabolism and nitrogen and protein anabolism.

REFERENCES

1. Sparks JW. Human Intrauterine Growth and Nutrient Accretion. Seminars in Perinatology 1984;8(2):74–93.
2. Metcoff J. Fetal Growth and Maternal Nutrition. *In* Falkner F, Tanner JM (eds). Human Growth. 2nd ed. New York: Plenum Press, 1985, pp. 333–388.

3. Nahum GG, et al. Fetal Weight Gain at Term: Linear With Minimal Dependence on Maternal Obesity. American Journal of Obstetrics & Gynecology 1995;172(5):1387–1394.

4. Widdowson EM. Chemical Composition and Nutritional Needs of the Fetus at Different Stages of Gestation. In Aebi H, Whitehead R (eds). Maternal Nutrition During Pregnancy and Lactation. Berne: Hans Huber Press, 1980, pp. 39–48.

5. McCrance RA, Widdowson EM. Glimpses of Comparative Growth and Development. In Falkner F, Tanner JM (eds). Human Growth. 2nd ed. New York: Plenum Press, 1985, pp. 133–151.

6. Eaton BM, Yudilevich DL. Uptake and Asymmetric Efflux of Amino Acids at Maternal and Fetal Sides of Placenta. American Journal of Physiology 1981;241(3):C106–C112.

7. Eleno N, et al. Membrane Potential Dependence of the Kinetics of Cationic Amino Acid Transport Systems in Human Placenta. Journal of Physiology 1994;479(2):291–300.

8. Hill PM, Young M. Net Placental Transfer of Free Amino Acids Against Varying Concentrations. Journal of Physiology 1973;235(2):409–422.

9. Jansson T. Amino Acid Transporters in the Human Placenta. Pediatric Research 2001;49(2):141–147.

10. Moe AJ. Placental Amino Acid Transport. American Journal of Physiology 1995;268(6):C1321–C1331.

11. Phillipps AF. Tissue Concentrations of Free Amino Acids in Term Human Placentas. American Journal of Obstetrics & Gynecology 1978;131:881.

12. Kerr GR. The Free Amino Acids of Serum During Development of Macaca mulatta. II. During Pregnancy and Fetal Life. Pediatric Research 1968;2(6):493–500.

13. Palou A, et al. Plasma Amino Acid Concentrations in Pregnant Rats and in 21-Day Foetuses. Biochemical Journal 1977;166(1):49–55.

14. Reynolds MI, Young M. The Transfer of Free Alpha-Amino Nitrogen Across the Placental Membrane in the Guinea Pig. Journal of Physiology 1971;214:583.

15. Lemons JA, et al. Umbilical Uptake of Amino Acids in the Unstressed Fetal Lamb. Journal of Clinical Investigation 1976;58(6):1428–1434.

16. Marconi AM, et al. A Comparison of Amino Acid Arteriovenous Differences Across the Liver and Placenta of the Fetal Lamb. American Journal of Physiology 1989;257(6):E909–E915.

17. Ferrell CL, Ford SP. Blood Flow Steroid Secretion and Nutrient Uptake of the Gravid Bovine Uterus. Journal of Animal Science 1980;50(6):1113–1121.

18. Morriss FH. Uterine Uptake of Amino Acids Throughout Gestation in the Unstressed Ewe. American Journal of Obstetrics & Gynecology 1979;135:601.

19. Young M. Pathology of the Deprived Fetus and Its Supply Line. Amsterdam: Associated Scientific Publishers, 1974, p.122.

20. Milley JR. Protein Synthesis During Hypoxia in Fetal Lambs. American Journal of Physiology 1987;252(4):E519–E524.

21. Milley JR. Effects of Insulin on Ovine Fetal Leucine Kinetics and Protein Metabolism. Journal of Clinical Investigation 1994;93(4):1616–1624.

22. Battaglia FC, Regnault TR. Placental Transport and Metabolism of Amino Acids. Placenta 2001;22(2–3):145–161.

23. Kudo Y, Boyd CA. Human Placental Amino Acid Transport Genes: Expression and Function. Reproduction 2002;124:593–600.

24. Yudilevich DL, Sweiry JH. Transport of Amino Acids in the Placenta. Biochimica et Biophysica Acta 1985;822(2):169–201.

25. Miller RK, Berndt WO. Characterization of Neutral Amino Acid Accumulation by Human Term Placental Slices. American Journal of Physiology 1974;227(6):1236–1242.

26. Shambaugh GE III. Maternal Amino Acids. Direct and Indirect Arbiters of Transplacental Exchange. Clinical Research 1979;27:660A.

27. Lemons JA. Fetal-Placental Nitrogen Metabolism. Seminars in Perinatology 1979;3(2):177–190.

28. Smith CI. Placental Amino Acid Uptake: Tissue Preparation, Kinetics, and Preincubation Effect. American Journal of Physiology 1973;224:558.

29. Balkovetz DF, et al. Na+-H+ Exchanger of Human Placental Brush-Border Membrane: Identification and Characterization. American Journal of Physiology 1986;251(6):C852–C860.

30. Palacin M, et al. Molecular Biology of Mammalian Plasma Membrane Amino Acid Transporters. Physiological Reviews 1998;78(4):969–1054.

31. Palacin M. A New Family of Proteins (rBAT and 4F2hc) Involved in Cationic and Zwitterionic Amino Acid Transport: a Tale of Two Proteins in Search of a Transport Function. Journal of Experimental Biology 1994;196:123–137.

32. Estevez R, et al. The Amino Acid Transport System Y+L/4F2hc Is a Heteromultimeric Complex. FASEB Journal 1998;12(13):1319–1329.

33. Horak J. Amino Acid Transport in Eucaryotic Microorganisms. Biochimica et Biophysica Acta 1986;864(3–4):223–256.

34. Sophianopoulou V, Diallinas G. Amino Acid Transporters of Lower Eukaryotes: Regulation, Structure and Topogenesis. FEMS Microbiology Reviews 1995;16(1):53–75.

35. Mastroberardino L, et al. Amino-Acid Transport by Heterodimers of 4F2hc/CD98 and Members of a Permease Family. Nature 1998;395(6699):288–291.

36. Kudo Y, Boyd CA. Heterodimeric Amino Acid Transporters: Expression of Heavy But Not Light Chains of CD98 Correlates With Induction of Amino Acid Transport Systems in Human Placental Trophoblast. Journal of Physiology 2000;523(1):13–18.

37. Pfeiffer R, et al. Amino Acid Transport of Y+L-Type by Heterodimers of 4F2hc/CD98 and Members of the Glycoprotein-Associated Amino Acid Transporter Family. EMBO Journal 1999;18(1):49–57.

38. Fukasawa Y, et al. Identification and Characterization of a Na(+)-Independent Neutral Amino Acid Transporter That Associates With the 4F2 Heavy Chain and Exhibits Substrate Selectivity for Small Neutral D- and L-Amino Acids. Journal of Biological Chemistry 2000;275(13):9690–9698.

39. Pineda M, et al. Identification of a Membrane Protein, LAT-2, That Co-Expresses With 4F2 Heavy Chain, an L-Type Amino Acid Transport Activity With Broad Specificity for Small and Large Zwitterionic Amino Acids. Journal of Biological Chemistry 1999;274(28):19738–19744.

40. Bertran J, et al. Stimulation of System Y(+)-Like Amino Acid Transport by the Heavy Chain of Human 4F2 Surface Antigen in Xenopus laevis Oocytes. Proceedings of the National Academy of Sciences of the United States of America 1992;89(12):5606–5610.

41. Ayuk PT, et al. Development and Polarization of Cationic Amino Acid Transporters and Regulators in the Human Placenta. American Journal of Physiology 2000;278(6):C1162–C1171.

42. Bertran J, et al. Expression Cloning of a Human Renal CDNA That Induces High Affinity Transport of L-Cystine Shared With Dibasic Amino Acids in Xenopus Oocytes. Journal of Biological Chemistry 1993;268(20):14842–14849.

43. Markovich D, et al. Two mRNA Transcripts (rBAT-1 and rBAT-2) Are Involved in System B°.(+)-Related Amino Acid Transport. Journal of Biological Chemistry 1993;268(2):1362–1367.

44. Segawa H, et al. Cloning, Functional Expression and Dietary Regulation of the Mouse Neutral and Basic Amino Acid Transporter (NBAT). Biochemical Journal 1997;328(2):657–664.

45. Yao SY, et al. Cloning and Functional Expression of a CDNA From Rat Jejunal Epithelium Encoding a Protein (4F2hc) With System Y+L Amino Acid Transport Activity. Biochemical Journal 1998;330(2):745–752.

46. Chairoungdua A, et al. Identification and Characterization of a Novel Member of the Heterodimeric Amino Acid Transporter Family Presumed to Be Associated With an Unknown Heavy Chain. Journal of Biological Chemistry 2001;276(52):49390–49399.

47. Novak DA, et al. Demonstration of System Y+L Activity on the Basal Plasma Membrane Surface of Rat Placenta and Developmentally Regulated Expression of 4F2HC MRNA. Placenta 1997;18(8):643–648.

48. Fei YJ, et al. The Amino Acid Transport System Y+L Induced in Xenopus Laevis Oocytes by Human Choriocarcinoma Cell (JAR) MRNA Is Functionally Related to the Heavy Chain of the 4F2 Cell Surface Antigen. Biochemistry 1995;34(27):8744–8751.

49. Okamoto Y, et al. Expression and Regulation of 4F2hc and hLAT1 in Human Trophoblasts. American Journal of Physiology 2002;282(1):C196–C204.

50. Wang Y, Tate SS. Oligomeric Structure of a Renal Cystine Transporter: Implications in Cystinuria. FEBS Letters 1995;368(2):389–392.

51. Prasad PD, et al. Human LAT1, a Subunit of System L Amino Acid Transporter: Molecular Cloning and Transport Function. Biochemical & Biophysical Research Communications 1999;255(2):283–288.

52. Hoeltzli SD, Smith CH. Alanine Transport Systems in Isolated Basal Plasma Membrane of Human Placenta. American Journal of Physiology 1989;256(3):C630–C637.

53. Johnson LW, Smith CH. Neutral Amino Acid Transport Systems of Microvillous Membrane of Human Placenta. American Journal of Physiology 1988;254(6):C773–C780.

54. Novak DA, et al. Ontogeny of Amino Acid Transport System A in Rat Placenta. Placenta 1996;17(8):643–651.

55. Wang H, et al. Cloning and Functional Expression of ATA1, a Subtype of Amino Acid Transporter A, From Human Placenta. Biochemical & Biophysical Research Communications 2000;273(3):1175–1179.

56. Varoqui H, et al. Cloning and Functional Identification of a Neuronal Glutamine Transporter. Journal of Biological Chemistry 2000;275(6):4049–40454.

57. Hatanaka T, et al. Primary Structure, Functional Characteristics and Tissue Expression Pattern of Human ATA2, a Subtype of Amino Acid Transport System A. Biochimica et Biophysica Acta 2000;1467(1):1–6.

58. Sugawara M, et al. Cloning of an Amino Acid Transporter With Functional Characteristics and Tissue Expression Pattern Identical to That of System A. Journal of Biological Chemistry 2000;275(22):16473–16477.

59. Karl PI, et al. Na(+)-Dependent Amino Acid Uptake by Human Placental Microvillous Membrane Vesicles: Importance of Storage Conditions and Preservation of Cytoskeletal Elements. Placenta 1991;12(3):239–250.

60. Kudo Y, et al. Characterization of Amino Acid Transport Systems in Human Placental Brush-Border Membrane Vesicles. Biochimica et Biophysica Acta 1987;904(2):309–318.

61. Shafqat S, et al. Cloning and Expression of a Novel Na(+)-Dependent Neutral Amino Acid Transporter Structurally Related to Mammalian Na+/Glutamate Cotransporters. Journal of Biological Chemistry 1993;268(21):15351–15355.

62. Carbo N, et al. Neutral Amino Acid Transport in Placental Plasma Membrane Vesicles in the Late Pregnant Rat. Evidence for a B⁰-Like Transport System. European Journal of Obstetrics, Gynecology, & Reproductive Biology 1997;71(1):85–90.

63. Torres-Zamorano V, et al. Tyrosine Phosphorylation and Epidermal Growth Factor-Dependent Regulation of the Sodium-Coupled Amino Acid Transporter

B⁰ in the Human Placental Choriocarcinoma Cell Line JAR. Biochimica et Biophysica Acta 1997;1356(3):258–270.

64. Kekuda R, et al. Cloning of the Sodium-Dependent, Broad-Scope, Neutral Amino Acid Transporter B⁰ From a Human Placental Choriocarcinoma Cell Line. Journal of Biological Chemistry 1996;271(31):18657–18661.

65. Kudo Y, Boyd CA. Changes in Expression and Function of Syncytin and Its Receptor, Amino Acid Transport System B⁰ (ASCT2), in Human Placental Choriocarcinoma BeWo Cells During Syncytialization. Placenta 2002;23:536–541.

66. Kilberg MS, et al. Characteristics of an Amino Acid Transport System in Rat Liver for Glutamine, Asparagine, Histidine, and Closely Related Analogs. Journal of Biological Chemistry 1980;255(9):4011–4019.

67. Karl PI, et al. Characteristics of Histidine Uptake by Human Placental Microvillous Membrane Vesicles. Pediatric Research 1989;25(1):19–26.

68. Kulanthaivel P, et al. Tyrosine Residues Are Essential for the Activity of the Human Placental Taurine Transporter. Biochimica et Biophysica Acta 1989;985(2):139–146.

69. Kulanthaivel P, et al. Transport of Taurine and Its Regulation by Protein Kinase C in the JAR Human Placental Choriocarcinoma Cell Line. Biochemical Journal 1991;277(1):53–58.

70. Karl PI, Fisher SE. Taurine Transport by Microvillous Membrane Vesicles and the Perfused Cotyledon of the Human Placenta. American Journal of Physiology 1990;258(3):C443–C451.

71. Norberg S, et al. Intrauterine Growth Restriction Is Associated With a Reduced Activity of Placental Taurine Transporters. Pediatric Research 1998;44(2):233–238.

72. Ramamoorthy S, et al. Functional Characterization and Chromosomal Localization of a Cloned Taurine Transporter From Human Placenta. Biochemical Journal 1994;300(3):893–900.

73. Brandsch M, et al. Calmodulin-Dependent Modulation of pH Sensitivity of the Amino Acid Transport System L in Human Placental Choriocarcinoma Cells. Biochimica et Biophysica Acta 1994;1192(2):177–184.

74. Ganapathy ME, et al. Characterization of Tryptophan Transport in Human Placental Brush-Border Membrane Vesicles. Biochemical Journal 1986;238(1):201–208.

75. Kanai Y, et al. Expression Cloning and Characterization of a Transporter for Large Neutral Amino Acids Activated by the Heavy Chain of 4F2 Antigen (CD98). Journal of Biological Chemistry 1998;273(37):23629–23632.

76. Rossier G, et al. LAT2, a New Basolateral 4F2hc/CD98–Associated Amino Acid Transporter of Kidney and Intestine. Journal of Biological Chemistry 1999;274(49):34948–34954.

77. Segawa H, et al. Identification and Functional Characterization of a Na+-Independent Neutral Amino Acid Transporter With Broad Substrate Selectivity. Journal of Biological Chemistry 1999;274(28):19745–19751.

78. Rajan DP, et al. Cloning and Functional Characterization of a Na+-Independent, Broad-Specific Neutral Amino Acid Transporter From Mammalian Intestine. Biochimica et Biophysica Acta 2000;1463:6–14.

79. Ritchie JW, Taylor PM. Role of the System L Permease LAT1 in Amino Acid and Iodothyronine Transport in Placenta. Biochemical Journal 2001;356(3):719–725.

80. Kudo Y, Boyd CA. Characterisation of L-Tryptophan Transporters in Human Placenta: a Comparison of Brush Border and Basal Membrane Vesicles. Journal of Physiology 2001;531(2):405–416.

81. Deves R, Boyd CA. Surface Antigen CD98(4F2): Not a Single Membrane Protein, but a Family of Proteins With Multiple Functions. Journal of Membrane Biology 2000;173(3):165–177.

82. Furesz TC, et al. Lysine Uptake by Human Placental Microvillous Membrane: Comparison of System Y+ With Basal Membrane. American Journal of Physiology 1995;268(3):C755–C761.

83. Jansson T, et al. Placental Transport of Leucine and Lysine Is Reduced in Intrauterine Growth Restriction. Pediatric Research 1998;44(4):532–537.

84. Torrents D, et al. Identification and Characterization of a Membrane Protein (y+L Amino Acid Transporter-1) That Associates With 4F2hc to Encode the Amino Acid Transport Activity Y+L. A Candidate Gene for Lysinuric Protein Intolerance. Journal of Biological Chemistry 1998;273(49):32437–32445.

85. Kamath SG, et al. Identification of Three Cationic Amino Acid Transporters in Placental Trophoblast: Cloning, Expression, and Characterization of hCAT-1. Journal of Membrane Biology 1999;171(1):55–62.

86. Closs EI, et al. Human Cationic Amino Acid Transporters HCAT-1, HCAT-2A, and HCAT-2B: Three Related Carriers With Distinct Transport Properties. Biochemistry 1997;36(21):6462–6468.

87. Danbolt NC. Glutamate Uptake. Progress in Neurobiology 2001;65(1):1–105.

88. Novak D, et al. Regulation of Glutamate Transport and Transport Proteins in a Placental Cell Line. American Journal of Physiology 2001;281(3):C1014–C1022.

89. Matthews JC, et al. Activity and Protein Localization of Multiple Glutamate Transporters in Gestation Day 14 Vs. Day 20 Rat Placenta. American Journal of Physiology 1998;274(3):C603–C614.

90. Fairman WA, et al. An Excitatory Amino-Acid Transporter With Properties of a Ligand-Gated Chloride Channel. Nature 1995;375(6532):599–603.

91. Nakayama T, et al. Expression of Three Glutamate Transporter Subtype mRNAs in Human Brain Regions and Peripheral Tissues. Molecular Brain Research 1996;36(1):189–192.

92. Matthews JC, et al. Placental Anionic and Cationic Amino Acid Transporter Expression in Growth Hormone Overexpressing and Null IGF-II or Null IGF-I Receptor Mice. Placenta 1999;20(8):639–650.

93. Borsani G, et al. SLC7A7, Encoding a Putative Permease-Related Protein, Is Mutated in Patients With Lysinuric Protein Intolerance. Nature Genetics 1999;21(3):297–301.

94. Rosenberg LE, et al. Cystinuria: Biochemical Evidence for Three Genetically Distinct Diseases. Journal of Clinical Investigation 1966;45(3):365–371.

95. Munn DH, et al. Inhibition of T Cell Proliferation by Macrophage Tryptophan Catabolism. Journal of Experimental Medicine 1999;189(9):1363–1372.

96. Kudo Y, et al. Tryptophan Degradation by Human Placental Indoleamine 2,3-Dioxygenase Regulates Lymphocyte Proliferation. Journal of Physiology 2001;535(1):207–215.

97. Kudo Y, Boyd CA. The Role of L-Tryptophan Transport in L-Tryptophan Degradation by Indoleamine 2,3-Dioxygenase in Human Placental Explants. Journal of Physiology 2001;531(2):417–423.

98. Young M. Placental Factors and Fetal Nutrition. American Journal of Clinical Nutrition 1981;34(Suppl 4):738–743.

99. Battaglia FC, Meschia G. Uteroplacental Blood Flow. *In* Battaglia FC, Meschia G (eds). An Introduction to Fetal Physiology. Orlando, FL: Academic Press, 1986, pp. 212–229.

100. Baur R. Morphometry of the Placental Exchange Area. Advances in Anatomy, Embryology & Cell Biology 1977;53(1):3–65.

101. Teasdale F. Gestational Changes in the Functional Structure of the Human Placenta in Relation to Fetal Growth: A Morphometric Study. American Journal of Obstetrics & Gynecology 1980;137(5):560–568.

102. Teasdale F, Jean-Jacques G. Morphometric Evaluation of the Microvillous Surface Enlargement Factor in the Human Placenta From Mid-Gestation to Term. Placenta 1985;6(5):375–381.

103. Woods DL, et al. Placental Size of Small-for-Gestational-Age Infants at Term. Early Human Development 1982;7(1):11–15.

104. Woods DL, Rip MR. Placental Villous Surface Area of Light-for-Dates Infants at Term. Early Human Development 1987;15(2):113–117.

105. Mahendran D, et al. Amino Acid (System A) Transporter Activity in Microvillous Membrane Vesicles From the Placentas of Appropriate and Small for Gestational Age Babies. Pediatric Research 1993;34(5):661–665.

106. Mahendran D, et al. Na+ Transport, H+ Concentration Gradient Dissipation, and System A Amino Acid Transporter Activity in Purified Microvillous Plasma Membrane Isolated From First-Trimester Human Placenta: Comparison With the Term Microvillous Membrane. American Journal of Obstetrics & Gynecology 1994;171(6):1534–1540.

107. Malandro MS, et al. Ontogeny of Cationic Amino Acid Transport Systems in Rat Placenta. American Journal of Physiology 1994;267(3):C804–C811.

108. Smith CH, Depper R. Placental Amino Acid Uptake. II. Tissue Preincubation, Fluid Distribution, and Mechanisms of Regulation. Pediatric Research 1974;8(7):697–703.

109. Smith CH, et al. Nutrient Transport Pathways Across the Epithelium of the Placenta. Annual Review of Nutrition 1992;12:183–206.

110. Domenech M, et al. Preserved Fetal Plasma Amino Acid Concentrations in the Presence of Maternal Hypoaminoacidemia. Pediatric Research 1986;20(11):1071–1076.

111. Cetin I, et al. Umbilical Amino Acid Concentrations in Appropriate and Small for Gestational Age Infants: a Biochemical Difference Present in Utero. American Journal of Obstetrics & Gynecology 1988;158(1):120–126.

112. Pardi G, et al. C. Diagnostic Value of Blood Sampling in Fetuses With Growth Retardation. New England Journal of Medicine 1993;328(10):692–696.

113. Cetin I, et al. Umbilical Amino Acid Concentrations in Normal and Growth-Retarded Fetuses Sampled in Utero by Cordocentesis. American Journal of Obstetrics & Gynecology 1990;162(1):253–261.

114. Cetin I, et al. Fetal Amino Acids in Normal Pregnancies and in Pregnancies Complicated by Intrauterine Growth Retardation. Early Human Development 1992;29(1–3):183–186.

115. Makarewicz W. Mitochondrial Glutamine and Glutamate Metabolism. Placenta 1991;12:416.

116. Rosso P. Maternal-Fetal Exchange During Protein Malnutrition in the Rat. Placental Transfer of Glucose and a Nonmetabolizable Glucose Analog. Journal of Nutrition 1977;107(11):20006–20010.

117. Malandro MS, et al. Effect of Low-Protein Diet-Induced Intrauterine Growth Retardation on Rat Placental Amino Acid Transport. American Journal of Physiology 1996;271(1):C295–C303.

118. Cramer S, et al. Physiological Importance of System A-Mediated Amino Acid Transport to Rat Fetal Development. American Journal of Physiology 2002;282(1):C153–C160.

119. Dicke JM, Henderson GI. Placental Amino Acid Uptake in Normal and Complicated Pregnancies. American Journal of the Medical Sciences 1988;295(3):223–227.

120. Glazier JD, et al. Association Between the Activity of the System A Amino Acid Transporter in the Microvillous Plasma Membrane of the Human Placenta and Severity of Fetal Compromise in Intrauterine Growth Restriction. Pediatric Research 1997;42(4):514–519.

121. Ross JC, et al. Transport and Fetal Utilization of Leucine in a Model of Fetal Growth Retardation. American Journal of Physiology 1996;270(3):E491–E503.

122. Anderson AH, et al. Placental Transport of Threonine and Its Utilization in the Normal and Growth-Restricted Fetus. American Journal of Physiology 1997;272(5):E892–E900.

123. Marconi AM, et al. Steady State Maternal-Fetal Leucine Enrichments in Normal and Intrauterine Growth-Restricted Pregnancies. Pediatric Research 1999;46(1):114–119.

124. Rowell PP, Sastry BV. Human Placental Cholinergic System: Depression of the Uptake of Alpha-Aminoisobutyric Acid in Isolated Human Placental Villi by Choline Acetyltransferase Inhibitors. Journal of Pharmacology & Experimental Therapeutics 1981;216(2):232–238.

125. Greenberg RE. Fetal Insulin Increases Placental Amino Acid Transport. Clinical Research 1989;37:178a.

126. Karl PI, et al. Amino Acid Transport by the Cultured Human Placental Trophoblast: Effect of Insulin on AIB Transport. American Journal of Physiology 1992;262(4):C834–C839.

127. Wang CY, et al. Insulin-Like Growth Factor-I Messenger Ribonucleic Acid in the Developing Human Placenta and in Term Placenta of Diabetics. Molecular Endocrinology 1988;2(3):217–229.

128. Dicke JM, et al. Cocaine Inhibits Alanine Uptake by Human Placental Microvillous Membrane Vesicles. American Journal of Obstetrics & Gynecology 1993;169(3):515–521.

129. Hay WW Jr, Sparks JW. Tracer methods for studying fetal metabolism in vivo. In Nathanielsz P (ed). Animal Models in Fetal Medicine, 6th ed. Ithaca, NY: Perinatology Press, 1987, pp. 134–178.

130. Potau N, et al. Insulin Receptors in Human Placenta in Relation to Fetal Weight and Gestational Age. Pediatric Research 1981;15(5):798–802.

131. Henderson GI, et al. Inhibition of Placental Valine Uptake After Acute and Chronic Maternal Ethanol Consumption. Journal of Pharmacology & Experimental Therapeutics 1981;216(3):465–472.

132. Rowell PP, Sastry BV. The Influence of Cholinergic Blockade on the Uptake of Alpha-Aminoisobutyric Acid by Isolated Human Placental Villi. Toxicology & Applied Pharmacology 1978;45(1):79–93.

133. Ahmed MS, et al. Characterization of a Cocaine Binding Protein in Human Placenta. Life Sciences 1990;46(8):553–561.

134. Barnwell SL, Sastry BVR. Depression of Amino Acid Uptake in Human Placental Villous by Cocaine, Morphine and Nicotine. Trophoblast Research 1983;1:101–105.

135. Slutsker L. Risks Associated With Cocaine Use During Pregnancy. Obstetrics & Gynecology 1992;79(5):778–789.

136. Pastrakuljic A, et al. Maternal Cocaine Use and Cigarette Smoking in Pregnancy in Relation to Amino Acid Transport and Fetal Growth. Placenta 1999;20(7):499–512.

137. Novak DA, et al. Effect of Chronic Cocaine Administration on Amino Acid Uptake in Rat Placental Membrane Vesicles. Life Sciences 1995;56(21):1779–1787.

138. Moore TR, et al. Hemodynamic Effects of Intravenous Cocaine on the Pregnant Ewe and Fetus. American Journal of Obstetrics & Gynecology 1986;154(4):883–888.

139. Woods JR Jr, et al. Effect of Cocaine on Uterine Blood Flow and Fetal Oxygenation. JAMA 1987;257(7):957–961.

140. Harper AE, et al. Effects of Ingestion of Disproportionate Amounts of Amino Acids. Physiological Reviews 1970;50(3):428–558.

141. Metcoff J. Maternal Nutrition and Fetal Development. Early Human Development 1980;4(2):99–120.

142. Metcoff J, et al. Fetal Growth Retardation Induced by Dietary Imbalance of Threonine and Dispensable Amino Acids, With Adequate Energy and Protein-Equivalent Intakes, in Pregnant Rats. Journal of Nutrition 1981;111(8):1411–1424.

143. Metcoff J, , et al. Maternal Nutrition and Fetal Outcome. American Journal of Clinical Nutrition 1981;34(Suppl 4):708–721.

144. Moghissi KS, et al. Relationship of Maternal Amino Acids and Proteins to Fetal Growth and Mental Development. American Journal of Obstetrics & Gynecology 1975;123(4):398–410.

145. Holzman IR, et al. C. Uterine Uptake of Amino Acids and Placental Glutamine-Glutamate Balance in the Pregnant Ewe. Journal of Developmental Physiology 1979;1:137–149.

146. Moores RR Jr, et al. Glutamate Metabolism in Fetus and Placenta of Late-Gestation Sheep. American Journal of Physiology 1994;267(1):R89–R96.

147. Timmerman M, et al. Relationship of Fetal Alanine Uptake and Placental Alanine Metabolism to Maternal Plasma Alanine Concentration. American Journal of Physiology 1998;275(6):E942–E950.

148. Geddie G, et al. Comparison of Leucine, Serine and Glycine Transport Across the Ovine Placenta. Placenta 1996;17(8):619–627.

149. Carroll MJ, Young M. The Relationship Between Placental Protein Synthesis and Transfer of Amino Acids. Biochemical Journal 1983;210(1):99–105.

150. Robertson AF. Human Placental Amino Acid Oxidation. Biology of the Neonate 1972;30:142.

151. Battaglia FC, et al. Clearance of Inert Molecules, Na, and Cl Ions Across the Primate Placenta. American Journal of Obstetrics & Gynecology 1968;102(8):1135–1143.

152. Holzman IR, et al. Ammonia Production by the Pregnant Uterus. Proceedings of the Society for Experimental Biology and Medicine 1977;156(1):27–30.

153. Johnson RL. Uterine Metabolism of the Pregnant Rabbit Under Chronic Steady State Conditions. American Journal of Obstetrics & Gynecology 1985;154:1146.

154. Block SM, et al. C. Metabolic Quotients of the Gravid Uterus of the Chronically Catheterized Guinea Pig. Pediatric Research 1985;19(8):840–845.

155. Dancis J, et al. Placental Transfer of Proteins in Human Gestation. American Journal of Obstetrics & Gynecology 1961;82:167–171.

156. Battaglia FC, Meschia G. Fetal Nutrition. Annual Review of Nutrition 1988;8:43–61.

157. Milley JR. Effect of Insulin on the Distribution of Cardiac Output in the Fetal Lamb. Pediatric Research 1987;22(2):168–72.

158. van Veen LC, et al. Fetal CO_2 Kinetics. Journal of Developmental Physiology 1984;6(4):359–365.

159. van Veen LC, et al. Leucine Disposal and Oxidation Rates in the Fetal Lamb. Metabolism: Clinical & Experimental 1987;36(1):48–53.

160. Waterlow JL. Protein Turnover in Mammalian Tissues and in the Whole Body. Amsterdam: Elsevier/North-Holland Biomedical Press, 1978.

161. Hay WW Jr. Metabolic Interrelationships of Placenta and Fetus. Placenta 1995;16(1):19–30.

162. Battaglia FC, Meschia G. Principal Substrates of Fetal Metabolism. Physiological Reviews 1978;58(2):499–527.

163. Holzman IR, et al. Glucose Metabolism, Lactate, and Ammonia Production by the Human Placenta in Vitro. Pediatric Research 1979;13(2):117–120.

164. Bell AW, et al. Uptake of Amino Acids and Ammonia at Mid-Gestation by the Fetal Lamb. Quarterly Journal of Experimental Physiology 1989;74(5):635–643.

165. Edwards EM, et al. Enzyme Activities in the Sheep Placenta During the Last Three Months of Pregnancy. Biochimica et Biophysica Acta 1977;497(1):133–143.

166. Rattenbury JM, et al. Urea Synthesis in the Liver and Kidney of Developing Sheep. Biochimica et Biophysica Acta 1980;630(2):210–219.

167. Cetin I, et al. Fetal Serine Fluxes Across Fetal Liver, Hindlimb, and Placenta in Late Gestation. American Journal of Physiology 1992;263(4):E786–E793.

168. Cetin I, et al. Glycine Turnover and Oxidation and Hepatic Serine Synthesis From Glycine in Fetal Lambs. American Journal of Physiology 1991;260(3):E371–E378.

169. Moores RR Jr, et al. Metabolism and Transport of Maternal Serine by the Ovine Placenta: Glycine Production and Absence of Serine Transport into the Fetus. Pediatric Research 1993;33(6):590–594.

170. Bender DA. Amino Acid Metabolism. London: Wiley, 1975.

171. Levitsky LL, et al. Glutamine Carbon Disposal and Net Glutamine Uptake in Fetuses of Fed and Fasted Ewes. American Journal of Physiology 1993;265(5):E722–E727.

172. Vaughn PR, et al. Glutamine-Glutamate Exchange Between Placenta and Fetal Liver. American Journal of Physiology 1995;268(4):E705–E711.

173. Markewicz M, et al. The Ontogeny of Serine Hydroxymethyltransferase Isoenzymes in Fetal Sheep Liver, Kidney and Placenta. Mol Genet Metab 1999;68:473–480.

174. Pell JM, et al. Glutamate and Glutamine Metabolism in the Ovine Placenta. Journal of Agricultural Science 1983;101:275–281.

175. Smeaton TC, et al. The Placenta Releases Branched-Chain Keto Acids into the Umbilical and Uterine Circulations in the Pregnant Sheep. Journal of Developmental Physiology 1989;12(2):95–99.

176. Montgomery D, Young M. The Uptake of Naturally Occurring Amino Acids by the Plasma Membrane of the Human Placenta. Placenta 1982;3(1):13–20.

177. Hoeltzli SD, et al. Anionic Amino Acid Transport Systems in Isolated Basal Plasma Membrane of Human Placenta. American Journal of Physiology 1990;259(1):C47–C55.

178. Jaroszewicz L, et al. The Activity of Aminotransferases in Human Placenta in Early Pregnancy. Biochemical Medicine 1971;5:436–439.

179. Goodwin GW, et al. Activities of Branched-Chain Amino Acid Aminotransferase and Branched-Chain 2-Oxo Acid Dehydrogenase Complex in Tissues of Maternal and Fetal Sheep. Biochemical Journal 1987;242(1):305–308.

180. Jozwik M, et al. Contribution of Branched-Chain Amino Acids to Uteroplacental Ammonia Production in Sheep. Biology of Reproduction 1999;61(3):792–796.

181. Loy GL, et al. Fetoplacental Deamination and Decarboxylation of Leucine. American Journal of Physiology 1990;259(4):E492–E497.

182. Guyton TS, et al. Alanine Umbilical Uptake, Disposal Rate, and Decarboxylation Rate in the Fetal Lamb. American Journal of Physiology 1993;265(3):E497–E503.

183. Palacin M, et al. Placental Formation of Lactate From Transferred L-Alanine and Its Impairment by Aminooxyacetate in the Late-Pregnant Rat. Biochimica et Biophysica Acta 1985;841(1):90–96.

184. Loy GL, et al. Versatile Stable Isotope Technique for the Measurement of Amino Acids and Keto Acids: Comparison With Radioactive Isotope and Its Use in Measuring in Vivo Disposal Rates. Analytical Biochemistry 1990;185(1):1–9.

185. Gresham EL, et al. Production and Excretion of Urea by the Fetal Lamb. Pediatrics 1972;50(3):372–379.

186. Raiha NC, et al. Milk Protein Quantity and Quality in Low-Birthweight Infants: I. Metabolic Responses and Effects on Growth. Pediatrics 1976;57(5):659–684.

187. Jones CT, Rolph TP. Metabolism During Fetal Life: A Functional Assessment of Metabolic Development. Physiological Reviews 1985;65(2):357–430.

188. Karsai T, Elodi P. Urea Cycle Enzymes in Human Liver: Ontogenesis and Interaction With the Synthesis of Pyrimidines and Polyamines. Molecular & Cellular Biochemistry 1982;43(2):105–110.

189. Colombo JP, Richterich R. Urea Cycle Enzymes in the Developing Human Fetus. Enzymologia Biologica et Clinica 1968;9(1):68–73.
190. Hagerman DD. Enzymology of the placenta. *In* Kopper A, Diczfalusy E (eds). Foetus and Placenta. Oxford: Blackwell, 1969, pp. 413–469.
191. Gresham EL, et al. Maternal-Fetal Urea Concentration Difference in Man: Metabolic Significance. Journal of Pediatrics 1971;79(5):809–811.
192. Schwenk WF, et al. Use of Reciprocal Pool Specific Activities to Model Leucine Metabolism in Humans. American Journal of Physiology 1985;249(6):E646–E650.
193. Hay WW Jr, et al. Effects of Glucose and Insulin on Fetal Glucose Oxidation and Oxygen Consumption. American Journal of Physiology 1989;256(6):E704–E713.
194. Kennaugh JM, et al. Ontogenetic Changes in the Rates of Protein Synthesis and Leucine Oxidation During Fetal Life. Pediatric Research 1987;22(6):688–692.
195. Nissen S, Haymond MW. Effects of Fasting on Flux and Interconversion of Leucine and Alpha-Ketoisocaproate in Vivo. American Journal of Physiology 1981;241(1):E72–E75.
196. Meier PR, et al. Rates of Protein Synthesis and Turnover in Fetal Life. American Journal of Physiology 1981;240(3):E320–E324.
197. Milner RD, Hill DJ. Interaction Between Endocrine and Paracrine Peptides in Prenatal Growth Control. European Journal of Pediatrics 1987;146(2):113–122.
198. Wilkening RB, et al. Amino Acid Uptake by the Fetal Ovine Hindlimb Under Normal and Euglycemic Hyperinsulinemic States. American Journal of Physiology 1994;266(1):E72–E78.
199. Liechty EA, et al. Increased Fetal Glucose Concentration Decreases Ovine Fetal Leucine Oxidation Independent of Insulin. American Journal of Physiology 1993;265(4):E617–E623.
200. Liechty EA, Lemons JA. Changes in Ovine Fetal Hindlimb Amino Acid Metabolism During Maternal Fasting. American Journal of Physiology 1984;246(5):E430–E435.
201. Milley JR. Uptake of Exogenous Substrates During Hypoxia in Fetal Lambs. American Journal of Physiology 1988;254(5):E572–E578.
202. Milley JR. Effects of insuline on fetal leucine kinetics and protein metabolism. Journal of Clinical Investigations 1994;93:1616–1624.
203. Tsalikien E, Hamilton W. Differential Effect of Hyperinsulinemia on Fetal and Neonatal Amino Acid Kinetics. Pediatric Research 1991;29:54a.
204. Stephens E, et al. Fetal Hyperinsulinemia Increases Farnesylation of P21 Ras in Fetal Tissues. American Journal of Physiology 2001;281:E217–E223.
205. Shen W, et al. IGF-I and Insulin Regulate EIF4F Formation by Different Mechanisms in Muscle and Liver in the Ovine Fetus. American Journal of Physiology 2002;283:E593–E603.
206. Lemons JA, Schreiner RL. Amino Acid Metabolism in the Ovine Fetus. American Journal of Physiology 1983;244(5):E459–E466.
207. Lemons JA, Liechty EA. Nitrogen Flux Across Ovine Maternal and Fetal Hindquarters During Fasting. Journal of Developmental Physiology 1987;9(2):151–158.
208. Liechty EA, et al. Effects of Glucose Infusion on Leucine Transamination and Oxidation in the Ovine Fetus. Pediatric Research 1991;30(5):423–429.
209. Hay WW Jr, et al. Fetal Glucose Uptake and Utilization As Functions of Maternal Glucose Concentration. American Journal of Physiology 1984;246(3):E237–E242.
210. Johnson JD, et al. Protein Turnover in Tissues of the Rat Fetus Following Maternal Starvation. Pediatric Research 1986;20(12):1252–1257.
211. Johnson JD, Dunham T. Protein Turnover in Tissues of the Fetal Rat After Prolonged Maternal Malnutrition. Pediatric Research 1988;23(5):534–538.
212. Battaglia FC, Meschia G. Fetal and placental metabolism. Part II. Amino acids and lipids. *In* Battaglia FC, Meschia G (eds). An Introduction to Fetal Physiology. Orlando, FL: Academic Press, 1986, pp. 100–135.
213. Meier PR, et al. The Rate of Amino Acid Nitrogen and Total Nitrogen Accumulation in the Fetal Lamb. Proceedings of the Society for Experimental Biology & Medicine 1981;167:463–468.
214. Widdowson EM. Changes in body proportions and composition during growth. *In* Davis JA, Dobbing J (eds). Scientific Foundations of Pediatrics. Philadelphia: WB Saunders Co, 1974, pp. 153–163.
215. Ziegler EE. Protein in Premature Feeding. Nutrition 1994;10(1):69–71.
216. Thureen PJ, et al. Effect of Low Versus High Intravenous Amino Acid Intake on Very Low Birth Weight Infants in the Early Neonatal Period. Pediatric Research 2002;53:24–32.

William C. Heird and Sudha Kashyap

54 Protein and Amino Acid Metabolism and Requirements

Proteins are the major structural and functional components of all cells of the body. Enzymes, membrane carriers, blood transport molecules, intracellular matrix, and even hair and fingernails are proteins, as are many hormones. Proteins also constitute a major portion of all membranes, and the constituent amino acids of protein act as precursors of many coenzymes, hormones, nucleic acids, and other essential molecules. An adequate supply of dietary protein is therefore necessary to ensure cellular integrity and function.

In this chapter, some general aspects of the chemistry and metabolism of proteins and amino acids are reviewed. This is followed by discussions of the protein and, then, amino acid needs of preterm, low birth weight (LBW) infants. Finally, the physiologic, pathologic, and environmental factors that affect protein and amino acid needs are discussed, and an attempt is made to reach conclusions concerning the preterm LBW infant's needs for protein and amino acids. Nitrogen, the characteristic element of protein, makes up about 16% of its weight. Thus, nitrogen metabolism is often considered to be synonymous with protein metabolism. Carbon, oxygen, and hydrogen are also abundant elements of proteins, and some contain smaller amounts of sulfur and/or phosphorus.

PROTEIN AND AMINO ACID CHEMISTRY AND METABOLISM

Proteins are among the most complex molecular compounds of the body and of the diet. They consist of chains of amino acid subunits joined together by peptide bonds between the carboxyl group of one amino acid and the amino group of the adjacent amino acid. The chains range from two (dipeptide) to thousands of amino acids, with molecular weights ranging from hundreds to hundreds of thousands of daltons.

Proteins are not simply long straight chains of amino acids. Rather, the chains fold into specific three-dimensional structures, depending on the function of the specific protein and its intended interaction with other molecules. Many proteins have several separate peptide chains held together by ionic or covalent links. From a nutritional perspective, the most important aspect of a protein is its amino acid composition. However, its structure may influence its nutritional availability. Some proteins are insoluble and hence are resistant to digestion, and others are resistant to the hydrolytic enzymes of the intestine.

The amino components of mammalian proteins are α-amino acids. They have a carboxyl group, an amino acid nitrogen group, and a side chain attached to a central α-carbon. The structure of the side chains determines the functional differences among amino acids. The side chains also have different charges at physiologic pH, and they may be either hydrophobic or hydrophilic. The side chains therefore are important determinants of how the protein structure is stabilized and hence how the protein functions. Attractions between positive and negative charges, for example, pull different parts of the molecule together, with hydrophobic groups tending to cluster in the center of globular proteins and hydrophilic groups tending to remain at the periphery. The formation of disulfide bonds between the thiol groups of cysteine is another important factor in stabilization of the folded structure of a polypeptide and is crucial for formation of interpolypeptide bonds. Some proteins contain complex oligosaccharide side chains attached to the hydroxyl and amide groups of amino acids. Ion binding proteins (e.g., calcium binding proteins, iron binding proteins) contain large amounts of histidine and the dicarboxylic acids.

Some amino acids are classified as "indispensable" or "essential," and others are classified as "dispensable" or "nonessential." The carbon skeletons of the former cannot be synthesized by humans from simpler molecules and hence must be provided in the diet, whereas the latter can be synthesized from other amino acids or from other precursors. Some amino acids also are classified as "conditionally indispensable" or "conditionally essential." These can be synthesized from other amino acids, but their synthesis is limited under some conditions.[1-3] These may be particularly important for the preterm LBW infant in whom developmental delays in several enzymes involved in amino acid synthesis have been demonstrated.[4-8] Dietary amino acids classified as essential, nonessential, and conditionally essential are shown in Table 54-1.

Protein Digestion and Absorption

Ingested proteins are denatured by gastric acid and are cleaved into smaller peptides by the enzyme pepsin, which is activated by the feeding-induced increase in gastric acidity. In the small intestine, the peptide bonds of the proteins and peptides are hydrolyzed by various bond-specific proteolytic enzymes of pancreatic origin. This process results in a mixture of free amino acids and small peptides that are transported into the enterocytes by substrate-specific carrier systems. The free amino acids are secreted into the portal blood and pass into the liver, where some are removed and used. The remaining amino acids reach the systemic circulation and are transported to specific sites throughout the body.

The efficiency of digestion of most common dietary proteins (e.g., casein, mixed whey, wheat, and legume proteins) measured as removal of labeled amino acids from the small intestinal

TABLE 54-1

Dispensable, Indispensable, and Conditionally Indispensable Dietary Amino Acids

Indispensable	Dispensable	Conditionally Indispensable
Histidine	Alanine	Arginine
Isoleucine	Aspartic acid	Cysteine
Leucine	Asparagine	Glycine
Lysine	Glutamic acid	Proline
Methionine	Glutamine	Tyrosine
Phenylalanine	Serine	
Threonine		
Tryptophan		
Valine		

lumen is thought to be at least 90%. Nonetheless, nutritionally significant quantities of indispensable amino acids appear to be metabolized by the splanchnic tissues, including the enterocytes.[9] Thus, all amino acids removed from the intestine do not appear to reach the peripheral circulation, and the amounts that do not vary from amino acid to amino acid, with intestinal threonine metabolism being particularly high. Absorbed amino acids that reach the systemic circulation are transported into tissues throughout the body, where they are either metabolized to other amino acids, glycogenic or lipogenic precursors, or are used for protein synthesis.

Protein Synthesis

Amino acids destined for protein synthesis bind with transfer RNA (tRNA). Information concerning the amino acid sequence of each protein to be synthesized is contained in the sequence of nucleotides in messenger RNA (mRNA) molecules that are synthesized in the nucleus from regions of the DNA. The mRNA molecules then interact with different cytoplasmic tRNA molecules to synthesize protein by linking the individual amino acids. The specific proteins expressed in any cell and the rates at which they are synthesized are determined by the relative abundances of the different mRNAs (i.e., the rates of transcription) and the stability of the messages. Changes in the rate of translation alter the number of tRNA molecules or the efficiency of the tRNA and hence alter the rate of synthesis of total cellular protein without altering the composition of the mixture of proteins produced.

Protein synthesis is a continuing process that occurs in most cells of the body. In the absence of either growth or protein loss, it is balanced by an equal amount of protein degradation.

Protein Degradation

The mechanism by which intracellular protein is hydrolyzed to free amino acids is more complex than that of protein synthesis and has not been as well characterized. Although various enzymes that can hydrolyze peptide bonds are present in cells, the bulk of hydrolysis is thought to be shared by two multienzyme systems: the lysosomal and proteasomal systems. The lysosome, a membrane-enclosed intracellular vesicle, contains various proteolytic enzymes called *cathepsins*. This system appears to be relatively unselective, hydrolyzing all engulfed proteins. It is thought to operate when entire areas of the cell or complete organelles need to be degraded (e.g., to provide a rapid supply of free amino acids as substrates for gluconeogenesis).[10] The system is also highly regulated by hormones and amino acids.[10]

The second system, the adenosine triphosphate–dependent ubiquitin-proteasome system, is present in the cytoplasm. The first step is to combine molecules of the very basic 76-amino acid peptide ubiquitin with lysine residues of the target protein. This process, which selectively targets proteins for degradation by a second component, the proteasome, involves several enzymes. The proteasome is a very large complex of proteins with numerous different proteolytic activities. The system is very selective and hence can account for the wide range of degradation rates (e.g., half-lives ranging from minutes to days) among proteins. It is thought to be responsible for degrading abnormal or damaged proteins as well as regulatory proteins, which typically are synthesized and degraded very rapidly.[11, 12]

Protein Turnover

The continuous degradation and resynthesis of all proteins are known as *protein turnover*. It has been estimated that the human adult synthesizes and degrades approximately 250 g of protein daily[13] despite a mean daily protein intake of only 60 to

100 g. The rate of protein turnover on a body weight basis is considerably greater in infants, particularly preterm LBW infants, and is lower in the elderly.[13] The liver and intestine, despite their small contribution to the protein content of the body, are thought to account for approximately 50% of whole body protein turnover.[9, 14] In contrast, skeletal muscle, which comprises about 50% of body protein mass, accounts for only about 25% of total body protein turnover.[13]

Total body protein turnover has been studied in adults as well as both term and preterm infants by using stable isotope tracers. This method assumes a simple two-pool model of protein metabolism in which amino acids are either free or protein bound. Amino acids enter the free pool from the diet (I) from protein breakdown (B) or from endogenous synthesis (e.g., dispensable amino acids). They leave the pool to be incorporated into newly synthesized protein (S) or to be catabolized (E). Because I and E can be measured, S and B can be calculated from the flux of a single amino acid, which also can be measured: $Q = I + B = S + E$. Isotopic tracers of both essential ([1-^{13}C] leucine and [^{13}C] or [^{2}H$_5$] phenylalanine) and nonessential amino acids ([^{15}N] glycine) have been used to label the amino acid pool, which is usually assumed to be represented by plasma. However, use of a single amino acid tracer to calculate body protein kinetics may not adequately represent whole body protein metabolism.[15, 16]

PROTEIN REQUIREMENTS

Methods for studying the protein requirements of any population (including preterm infants) include nitrogen balance, stable isotope tracer kinetics, and the factorial method. All these methods have advantages as well as inherent shortcomings and limitations.

Net gain or loss of protein, that is, the difference between nitrogen intake and nitrogen output, can be determined by the nitrogen balance technique. Although nitrogen intake can be determined precisely, accurate determination of all nitrogen losses, particularly losses from the skin and breath,[17, 18] is difficult. In infants, nitrogen output is usually measured as the sum of nitrogen lost in the urine and stool. Losses from the skin and breath are quantitatively small and either are not taken into account or are estimated.

The stable isotope tracer method allows assessment of the dynamic aspects of protein metabolism and also estimation of protein accretion as the difference between rates of synthesis and breakdown. Protein accretion calculated in this way usually is very close to retention calculated by a carefully conducted, conventional nitrogen balance.

The factorial method requires determining obligatory nitrogen losses (i.e., those that occur on a diet that meets energy needs but lacks protein) and adding to this protein needs for growth, including a correction for incomplete utilization of dietary protein. This latter factor is usually assumed to be approximately 70% (as has been suggested by several sets of data).[19-21]

Alternatively, because human milk is considered the ideal food for infants less than 6 months of age, many equate the protein requirement of infants to that contained in the average intake of human milk by normally growing infants. This is the method used by the Food and Nutrition Board of the Institute of Medicine in establishing a recommended adequate intake of protein for infants less than 6 months of age.

Numerous studies provide considerable insight into the growth and nutrient accretion rates incident to certain protein intakes as well as the effects of various protein intakes on other indices of protein adequacy or excess. Thus, it is possible to define the protein intake required to achieve various goals. In this regard, it is quite clear that the protein intake of preterm infants fed a reasonable volume (i.e., 180 mL/kg/day) of either term (~2 g/kg/day) or preterm human milk (~2.5 g/kg/day) is

insufficient to support the intrauterine rate of nitrogen accretion as recommended by the American Academy of Pediatrics Committee on Nutrition,[22] the Canadian Pediatric Society,[23] and the European Society for Pediatric Gastroenterology, Hepatology, and Nutrition.[24] These intakes also are insufficient to maintain plasma concentrations of albumin and transthyretin at more than 3.25 g/dL and 10 mg/dL, respectively.[25]

Increasing nitrogen retention has been reported with increasing protein intake.[26, 27] It appears that a protein intake of approximately 2.8 g/kg/day is close to the minimal intake needed to ensure rates of weight gain and nitrogen retention at least equal to intrauterine rates and also to maintain acceptable plasma albumin and transthyretin concentrations.[28, 29] Moreover, the blood urea nitrogen concentration and the plasma concentration of most amino acids in infants receiving this intake are only minimally different from concentrations observed in infants fed preterm human milk.[25]

A protein intake of 3.5 to 4 g/kg/day results in rates of both weight gain and nitrogen accretion well in excess of intrauterine rates and also maintains acceptable plasma albumin and transthyretin concentrations.[28, 29] Although blood urea nitrogen and plasma amino acid concentrations of infants fed these intakes are higher than those of infants fed lower intakes, blood urea nitrogen concentrations greater than 10 mg/dL are uncommon, and the plasma concentration of only a few amino acids exceeds the concentration of cord plasma[30] or plasma obtained at fetoscopy.[31]

Today, most LBW infants in the United States are fed either preterm human milk fortified with protein and other nutrients, one of several formulas designed specifically for LBW infants, or a combination of human milk and one of the preterm formulas. When volumes sufficient to provide an energy intake of 120 kcal/kg/day are fed, the LBW infant formulas currently available in the United States provide protein intakes ranging from roughly 3.25 to 3.6 g/kg/day (Table 54-2). Infants fed these formulas gain weight and retain nitrogen at rates equal to or slightly in excess of intrauterine rates,[32-34] without appreciable "metabolic stress." However, data indicate that most conventionally managed infants who weigh less than 1500 g at birth, although of appropriate size for gestational age at birth, weigh less than the 10th percentile of intrauterine standards at hospital discharge.[35] This finding suggests that most of these infants fail to compensate for the lack of growth or actual weight loss during the first 2 to 4 weeks of their life.

The Life Sciences Research Office Expert Panel on Assessment of Nutrient Requirements for Preterm Infant Formulas[36] recommended minimum and maximum protein contents of 2.5 and 3.6 g/100 kcal, respectively. At an energy intake of 120 kcal/kg/day, these recommendations equate to protein intakes of 3 to 4.3 g/kg/day.

SPECIFIC AMINO ACID REQUIREMENTS

The intake of each indispensable amino acid required to maintain nitrogen equilibrium in adults[37, 38] and, to a lesser extent, normal growth and nitrogen retention in term infants[39] has been defined as the amounts necessary to restore growth and nitrogen balance to that observed before elimination of each amino acid from an otherwise adequate diet. Requirements of normal adults also have been defined more recently by Young and Borgonha,[40] based on oxidation of an indicator amino acid in response to various intakes of each amino acid. However, no such studies have been conducted in LBW infants. Rather, the specific amino acid requirements of LBW infants have been estimated by various methods.

Snyderman defined the amino acid requirements of the LBW infant as the amount of each provided by an intake of protein that results in a normal plasma amino acid pattern.[41] Based on

TABLE 54-2

Composition of Available Preterm Infant Formulas

Component	Similac Special Care Advance	Enfamil Premature Lipil
Protein (g/120 kcal)*	3.25	3.6
Fat (g/120 kcal)†	6.5	6.1
Carbohydrate (g/120 kcal)‡	12.7	13.2
Other (amt/120 kcal)		
Calcium (mg)	216	198
Phosphorus (mg)	120	100
Magnesium (mg)	14.4	10.8
Iron (mg)	2.2	2.2
Zinc (mg)	1.8	1.8
Manganese (μg)	14.4	7.6
Copper (μg)	300	144
Iodine (μg)	7.2	30
Sodium (mg)	51.6	69.6
Potassium (mg)	155	118
Chloride (mg)	97	108
Vitamin A (IU)	1500	1500
Vitamin D (IU)	180	288
Vitamin E (IU)	4.8	7.6
Vitamin K (μg)	14.4	9.6
Thiamin B_1 (μg)	300	240
Riboflavin B_2 (μg)	744	360
Vitamin B_6 (μg)	300	180
Vitamin B_{12} (μg)	0.66	0.3
Niacin (μg)	6000	4800
Folic acid (μg)	44.4	48
Pantothenic acid (μg)	2280	1440
Vitamin C (mg)	44.4	24

* Protein content of the formulas is composed of bovine milk and whey proteins with a 60:40 ratio of whey proteins/caseins.
† Similac Special Care Advance contains medium chain triglycerides and a mixture of soy and coconut oils, and Enfamil Premature Lipil contains medium chain triglycerides and a mixture of soy and high oleic vegetable oil; both formulas have less than 0.5% of *C. cohnii* oil and *M. alpina* oil as source of docosahexaenoic acid (DHA) and arachidonic acid (ARA). The DHA and ARA content (mg/120 kcal) of Similac Special Care Advance is 16.3 and 26.1 and of Enfamil Premature Lipil is 20.4 and 40.8, respectively.
‡ Carbohydrate content of the formulas is lactose and corn syrup solids.

observations of "normal" plasma concentrations of most amino acids in LBW infants fed 2 g/kg/day of bovine milk protein, the intake of each amino acid provided by this intake was proposed by Snyderman as the minimum requirement for that amino acid. However, infants receiving this intake have a low plasma concentration of lysine and a somewhat elevated plasma concentration of glycine, findings that are often associated with deficient protein intakes.[42] Thus, considering these plasma amino acid data and the more recent evidence that a protein intake of approximately 2.8 g/kg/day is required to ensure intrauterine rates of nitrogen retention and weight gain as well as "normal" plasma protein concentrations (see earlier),[28] the amount of each amino acid provided by a protein intake of 2.8 g/kg/day seems more reasonable.

This essentially is the approach proposed by Fomon and Filer[43] to define the range of requirements of each amino acid for term infants, that is, the range of intake of each amino acid provided by the amount of commonly used proteins sufficient to support normal growth. For the preterm infant, the range of specific amino acid requirements (per kilogram per day) may reasonably be assumed to encompass the amounts of each amino acid present in 2.8 g of human milk, bovine milk, or modified bovine milk protein. The validity of this approach relies heavily on the assumption that a protein intake of 2.8 g/kg/day is adequate, and this has been demonstrated only for modified bovine milk.[28]

TABLE 54-3

Recommendations for Minimum and Maximum Amino Acid Requirements for Low Birth Weight Infants

Amino Acid Requirement*	Minimum (mg/kg/d)	Maximum (mg/kg/d)
Isoleucine	171	245
Leucine	303	434
Lysine	207	297
Methionine	48	69
Cyst(e)ine	66	95
Phenylalanine	120	172
Tyrosine	141	202
Threonine	141	202
Tryptophan	54	77
Valine	168	241
Histidine	72	103
Arginine	108	155
Alanine	114	163
Aspartate and asparagine	270	387
Glutamate and glutamine	552	791
Glycine	72	103
Proline	258	370
Serine	153	219

* Amino acid content of 3.0 g and 4.3 g of human milk proteins, the minimum and maximum protein contents (g/120 kcal) recommended for preterm infant formulas. Human milk amino acid composition is derived from refs. 45 to 48.

The Life Sciences Research Office Expert Panel on Assessment of the Nutrient Requirements of Term Infant Formulas[44] defined the minimum and maximum contents of each amino acid for these formulas as the amount of each present in the amounts of human milk protein corresponding to the recommended minimum and maximum protein contents, that is, 1.7 and 3.4 g/100 kcal, respectively. The Expert Panel on Assessment of the Nutrient Requirements of Preterm Infant Formulas adapted the same approach, defining the minimum and maximum amino acid contents for preterm infant formulas (mg/100 kcal) as the amounts of each present in 2.5 and 3.6 g/100 kcal of human milk proteins, the minimum and maximum protein contents (g/100 kcal) recommended for preterm infant formulas. Because the panel envisioned the energy intake of the "average" preterm infant to be 120 kcal/kg/day, these recommendations for the amino acid contents of preterm formulas can be translated to a range of requirements (mg/kg/day) as shown in Table 54-3.[45-48]

Widdowson and associates[49] suggested that the amino acid requirements of LBW infants could be estimated as the amount of each that accumulates during normal intrauterine development. These investigators also provided data concerning the accretion of almost all amino acids during intrauterine development, thus making this approach feasible. As illustrated in Table 54-4, the rates of amino acid accretion during different stages of intrauterine development vary somewhat. However, this variation results from variation in rates of protein accretion at different stages of development, rather than from variation in the pattern of amino acid deposited. Thus, the amount of each amino acid deposited during any interval can be calculated by assuming a constant rate of growth over the interval of interest. The amount of each amino acid that accumulates as the fetus grows at a constant rate (~15 g/kg/day) from 900 to 2400 g and the estimated intake of each necessary to ensure deposition rates equal to those of the fetus, assuming retention of 70% of total protein intake, can be calculated. However, the latter estimate does not include an allowance for "maintenance" requirements or obligatory losses (i.e., the amounts necessary to maintain nitrogen equilibrium in the absence of nitrogen intake). According to a recent study, maintenance protein needs of preterm infants are 0.55 to

TABLE 54-4

Accretion of Amino Acids by the Human Fetus

Age (d) Weight (kg)	160–180 0.5–0.9	180–220 0.9–1.4	200–220 1.4–1.9	220–240 1.9–2.4	240–260 2.4–2.9	260–280 2.9–3.4
			Amino Acid Accretion (mg/kg/d)			
Isoleucine	84	62	52	47	45	44
Leucine	181	133	112	102	97	96
Lysine	174	128	107	98	27	92
Methionine	49	35	29	27	25	25
Cyst(e)ine	—	—	—	—	—	—
Phenylalanine	101	74	62	56	53	53
Tyrosine	70	52	44	40	38	37
Threonine	101	74	62	57	54	53
Tryptophan	—	—	—	—	—	—
Valine	116	84	70	64	61	60
Histidine	64	46	39	36	34	33
Arginine	186	137	114	105	99	98
Alanine	176	129	107	99	93	92
Aspartate	220	161	135	123	117	116
Glutamate	317	231	194	178	168	166
Glycine	289	210	176	161	152	151
Proline	206	150	126	115	108	108
Serine	107	78	66	60	57	56
Total nitrogen	393	283	242	221	208	206

Data from Widdowson EM, et al: *In* Visser HKA (ed): Fifth Nutricia Symposium: Nutrition and Metabolism of the Fetus and Infant. The Hague, Martinus Nijhoff, 1979, pp 169–177.

0.75 g/kg/day.[27] Assuming that the amino acid pattern of the maintenance protein needs is the same as that accumulating during development, the intake of each amino acid required to ensure intrauterine rates of growth and nitrogen retention can be calculated. These rates are shown in Table 54-5.

A major assumption inherent in this approach is that the various amino acids contribute proportionally to maintenance needs for protein and the roughly 30% of total nitrogen intake lost in the stool and urine. Another is that the increments of amino acids in the body during development reflect the sole need for amino acids. Both are unlikely to be completely valid. For example, as discussed in more detail later, the content of aromatic amino acids (phenylalanine, tyrosine, tryptophan) in most acute phase proteins is roughly double the content of these amino acids in endogenous protein stores. Hence the stressed infant may require greater intakes of these amino acids to

TABLE 54-5

Amino Acid Requirements (mg/kg/day) of the Low Birth Weight Infant as Predicted from Fetal Rates of Amino Acid Accretion and Obligatory Losses

Amino Acid Requirement*	Accretion Rate (0.9–2.4 kg†)	Obligatory Losses	Estimated Requirement
Isoleucine	52	19	101
Leucine	113	41	220
Lysine	108	40	211
Methionine	30	11	59
Cyst(e)ine	—	—	—
Phenylalanine	62	23	121
Tyrosine	44	13	81
Threonine	62	23	121
Tryptophan	—	—	
Valine	71	26	139
Histidine	39	14	76
Arginine	115	42	224
Alanine	109	40	213
Aspartate	136	50	266
Glutamate	196	72	383
Glycine	178	65	347
Proline	127	46	247
Serine	66	23	127
Total nitrogen	242	86	469‡

* Accretion rate plus obligatory losses/0.7, based on assumption that 70% of intake is retained (see text).
† Data concerning fetal accretion rate of cyst(e)ine and tryptophan as well as asparagine and glutamine are not available.
‡ Equivalent to a protein intake of 2.99 g/kg/day (i.e., 469 mg × 6.38).

support an adequate acute phase protein response to stress without increasing breakdown of endogenous protein stores.

Because of metabolic immaturity, LBW infants require some amino acids (e.g., cysteine and tyrosine) that are not considered indispensable for the older infant and adult. The basis for the LBW infant's and, perhaps, the young term infant's requirement for cyst(e)ine is thought to be low hepatic activity of cystathionase,[4-6] a key enzyme in conversion of methionine to cysteine. In addition, removal of cyst(e)ine from an otherwise complete synthetic diet has been shown to result in decreased rates of weight gain and nitrogen retention as well as a low plasma cyst(e)ine concentration, all of which return to control levels when the cyst(e)ine intake of the control diet (85 mg/kg/day) is restored.[41] In this study, lower cyst(e)ine intakes (44 and 66 mg/kg/day) were not effective; hence it appears that the cyst(e)ine requirement of LBW infants is near 85 mg/kg/day.

The intake of tyrosine necessary to maintain control rates of weight gain and nitrogen retention as well as normal plasma tyrosine concentrations was shown in a similar fashion to be 50 mg/kg/day,[41] slightly less than the estimate based on the intrauterine accretion rate. The reason for the infant's requirement for tyrosine is not as clear as that for the cyst(e)ine requirement. Hepatic activity of phenylalanine hydroxylase, the key enzyme in conversion of phenylalanine to tyrosine, is substantial throughout the last two trimesters of gestation.[50] Moreover, studies using stable isotopes show that even very immature infants can convert phenylalanine to tyrosine.[51,52]

The probable requirement for each amino acid, estimated both as the amount provided by an intake of 2.8 g/kg/day of human milk, bovine milk, or modified bovine milk protein and as the amount theoretically necessary to ensure deposition of each at the intrauterine rate, is shown in Table 54–6. It is obvious that estimates of requirements derived by the various approaches are quite different. In general, the requirements for indispensable amino acids as estimated from the intake of 2.8 g/kg/day of human milk, bovine milk, or modified bovine milk protein are greater than those estimated from fetal accretion rates, whereas the requirements for many dispensable amino acids (arginine, alanine, and, particularly, glycine) are lower. This finding raises

the intriguing possibility that the dispensable amino acid content of proteins commonly used for feeding LBW infants may be limiting, particularly if the infant is unable to synthesize adequate amounts of one or more indispensable amino acid(s). Jackson and co-workers[53] reported that some preterm infants fed banked human milk do not form [15N]urea from administered [15N]glycine, a finding suggesting that the availability of glycine is limited, although perhaps not sufficiently to interfere with growth. Moreover, Miller and colleagues[54] showed that LBW infants have a limited capacity for synthesizing proline from glucose.

Studies in animals and in human adults suggest that glutamine becomes conditionally essential during catabolic illness.[55] The addition of glutamine to enteral feedings of very LBW infants results in no difference in growth, mean hospital stay, or prealbumin concentrations. However, feeding tolerance appears to be better, and the risk for infection is lower.[56]

Obviously, further research concerning the LBW infant's requirement for individual amino acids is needed. Moreover, the requirements are likely to depend on the goal for which the requirements are calculated. For example, if the goal is to produce rates of nitrogen retention and weight gain in excess of the intrauterine rate, the additional requirement for each amino acid over that required to support intrauterine rates of nitrogen retention and weight gain will be greater in proportion to the increase in protein intake necessary to achieve the goal.

AMINO ACID REQUIREMENTS FOR PARENTERAL NUTRITION

Because at least 10% of the nitrogen content of most enterally ingested intakes is lost in stool, whereas fecal loss of parenteral nitrogen intake is minimal, it follows that the minimal parenteral nitrogen intake required to support the intrauterine rate of nitrogen retention should be less than the minimal enteral intake. However, this does not appear to be the case. Zlotkin and co-workers[57] found that the minimal parenteral amino acid intake required to achieve the intrauterine rate of nitrogen retention was 3 g/kg/day, approximately 10% more than the required

TABLE 54–6

Comparison of Amino Acid Requirements (mg/kg/day) of Low Birth Weight Infants as Estimated from Intakes of Various Proteins (2.8 g/kg/day) and from Fetal Accretion Rates of Individual Amino Acids

	Estimates Based on Intakes*			Estimates Based on Accretion† and Obligatory Losses
	Human Milk	Bovine Milk	Modified Bovine Milk	
Isoleucine	160	134	151	101
Leucine	266	274	280	220
Lysine	196	213	235	211
Methionine	59	73	64	59
Cyst(e)ine	53	22	48	—
Phenylalanine	123	120	106	121
Tyrosine	132	123	101	81
Threonine	132	120	162	121
Tryptophan	48	25	48	—
Valine	171	165	157	139
Histidine	67	70	56	76
Arginine	118	98	84	224
Alanine	104	92	118	213
Aspartate	258	218	258	266
Glutamate	504	571	546	383
Glycine	73	53	53	347
Proline	221	277	227	247
Serine	140	154	154	127

* Amino acid content of various proteins provided by Ross Laboratories.
† Data concerning fetal accretion rate of cyst(e)ine and tryptophan as well as asparagine and glutamine are not available.

Amino Acid Patterns (mg/g) of Proteins Commonly Used to Feed Low Birth Weight Infants and of the Developing Fetus

Amino Acid	Human Milk	Bovine Milk	Modified Bovine Milk	Fetal Tissue
Isoleucine	57	48	54	35
Leucine	95	98	100	75
Lysine	70	76	84	72
Methionine	21	26	23	20
Cyst(e)ine	19	8	17	—
Phenylalanine	44	43	38	41
Tyrosine	47	44	36	29
Threonine	47	43	58	41
Tryptophan	17	9	17	—
Valine	61	59	56	47
Histidine	24	25	20	26
Arginine	42	35	30	77
Alanine	37	33	42	72
Aspartate	92	78	92	90
Glutamate	180	204	195	130
Glycine	26	19	19	118
Proline	79	99	81	84
Serine	50	55	55	41

minimal enteral intake (2.8 g/kg/day).[28] The reason appears to be greater urinary nitrogen losses with parenteral versus enteral nutrition. Although 70% or more of most enteral intake is retained despite fecal losses of at least 10%,[19-21] no more than 60 to 65% of most parenteral nitrogen intakes is retained (see later) despite minimal fecal losses. This finding suggests that the quality of available parenteral amino acid mixtures is lower than that of human milk and the proteins commonly used in infant formulas.

In contrast to the relative lack of differences in the overall amino acid pattern of the proteins commonly used in enteral feeding of LBW infants (Table 54-7), the overall quality of available parenteral amino acid mixtures varies considerably, as shown in Table 54-8. In large part, the plasma amino acid pattern of infants receiving parenteral nutrition infusates reflects the pattern of the amino acid mixture used to formulate the infusate.[58,59] Most of the older mixtures, now referred to as general purpose mixtures, result in low plasma concentrations of several indispensable amino acids (e.g., the branched-chain amino acids, tyrosine, and cyst(e)ine) and high concentrations of others (e.g., phenylalanine, methionine), as well as elevated concentrations of some dispensable amino acids (e.g., glycine).[58] Based on conventional theory, these mixtures provide insufficient amounts of the amino acids that are present in low concentrations in plasma and excessive amounts of those that are present in elevated concentrations.

The indispensable amino acid pattern of most early parenteral amino acid mixtures mimicked the pattern of a high-quality dietary protein (e.g., egg yolk protein), and little attention was given to the dispensable amino acid pattern. In fact, glycine composed the bulk of the dispensable amino acid content of many mixtures (see Table 54-8). Currently, numerous parenteral amino acid mixtures designed for use in pediatric patients are available. The amino acid pattern of one of these (Neopham, Kabi-Vitrum, Sweden) is similar to that of human milk protein. The amino acid pattern of another mixture (TrophAmine, Kendall-McGaw Laboratories, Irvine, CA) is that predicted by a mathematical model to result in plasma concentrations of all amino acids similar to those of normally growing, 30-day-old, breast-fed, term infants. The pattern of yet another pediatric parenteral amino acid mixture (Aminosyn-PF, Abbott Laboratories, N. Chicago, IL) is a modification of the pattern of the older, general purpose mixture Aminosyn (Abbott Laboratories).

These pediatric parenteral amino acid mixtures, like human milk protein and the combinations of bovine milk proteins used in most LBW infant formulas (see earlier discussion), provide more indispensable and less dispensable amino acids than the protein deposited by the developing fetus (Table 54-9). Whether a parenteral amino acid mixture with a pattern identical or similar to that of the protein deposited by the fetus may be used more efficiently is not known. The amino acid pattern of TrophAmine is that predicted mathematically to result in "normal" plasma concentrations of all amino acids. Hence, by this criterion, the infant appears to be able to convert the indispensable amino acids, except cyst(e)ine and tyrosine, to the needed dispensable amino acids.

All pediatric parenteral amino acid mixtures contain sufficient taurine to provide at least the amount that would be ingested by

Amino Acid Content (mg/2.5 g) of Commercially Available Amino Acid Mixtures

Amino Acid	Aminosyn (Abbott)	Aminosyn PF (Abbott)	Travasol(B) (Baxter)	FREAmine III (McGaw)	Trophamine (McGaw)	Neopham (Kabi-VITRAM)
Isoleucine	180	191	120	174	204	122
Leucine	235	297	155	227	350	274
Lysine	180	170	145	183	204	207
Methionine	100	45	145	132	83	51
Phenylalanine	110	107	155	141	121	106
Threonine	130	129	105	100	104	141
Tryptophan	40	45	45	38	50	55
Valine	200	161	115	165	196	141
Histidine	75	79	109	74	121	82
Cystine	0	0	0	0	<8	0
Tyrosine	22	16	10	0	58*	20
Taurine	0	18	0	0	6	13
Alanine	320	175	518	176	133	247
Aspartate	0	132	0	0	79	161
Glutamate	0	206	0	0	125	278
Glycine	320	96	518	350	92	82
Proline	215	204	104	280	171	219
Serine	105	124	0	147	96	148
Arginine	245	308	258	238	304	161
Total	2,477	2,503	2,502	2,425	2,505	2,508

* As 17 mg tyrosine and 50 mg *N*-acetyl-L-tyrosine.

TABLE 54-9

Amino Acid Pattern (mg/g) of Pediatric Parenteral Amino Acid Mixtures and the Developing Fetus

Amino Acid	Aminosyn PF	Trophamine	Neopham	Fetal Protein
Isoleucine	76	82	49	35
Leucine	119	140	110	75
Lysine	68	82	83	72
Methionine	18	33	20	20
Cyst(e)ine	0	3	0	—
Phenylalanine	43	48	42	41
Tyrosine	6	23	8	29
Threonine	52	42	56	41
Tryptophan	18	20	22	—
Valine	64	78	56	47
Histidine	32	48	33	26
Arginine	123	122	64	77
Alanine	70	53	99	72
Aspartate	53	32	64	90
Glutamate	82	50	111	130
Glycine	38	37	33	118
Proline	82	68	88	84
Serine	50	38	60	41

a breast-fed infant. However, because tyrosine and cystine are insoluble and cysteine is unstable in aqueous solution, none of the mixtures contains more than trace amounts of these two amino acids, although TrophAmine contains N-acetyl-L-tyrosine, a soluble tyrosine derivative that may at least partially meet the apparent tyrosine needs.[60, 61] Because both tyrosine and cyst(e)ine are thought to be indispensable for the infant and also may be indispensable for all subjects receiving parenteral nutrients exclusively, their absence in parenteral amino acid mixtures may be cause for concern.

Cyst(e)ine, in addition to being a component of protein, also is a component of glutathione, a tripeptide that is an important biologic antioxidant. The plasma concentration of this antioxidant is low in LBW infants,[62] and although cyst(e)ine supplementation does not appear to increase plasma glutathione concentration,[63] it does increase whole blood glutathione concentration.[64] Because oxidant stress has been implicated in certain neonatal disorders, clarification of the role of cyst(e)ine in maintaining plasma and tissue levels of glutathione is important. The lack of adequate tyrosine in parenteral amino acid mixtures may also be important. As already discussed, because of the high content of tyrosine in most acute phase proteins, inadequate tyrosine intake may necessitate endogenous protein breakdown to supply adequate tyrosine for ongoing synthesis of these important proteins.

Few studies have examined directly either the relative efficacy of the available pediatric parenteral amino acid mixtures or the efficacy of any of these mixtures versus that of the general purpose parenteral amino acid mixtures. One exception is the study of Helms and co-workers,[65] showing that LBW infants who received a regimen containing TrophAmine gained weight more rapidly and retained a greater percentage of administered nitrogen than did similar infants who received an isocaloric, isonitrogenous regimen containing a general purpose parenteral amino acid mixture (i.e., 78% versus 66%). The nutritional benefits of TrophAmine were attributed to a greater intake of tyrosine and cyst(e)ine (as cysteine hydrochloride, added when the infusate was prepared). However, other explanations, including the more normal plasma amino acid pattern of the group that received the TrophAmine regimen, are equally feasible. This latter explanation was proposed by Duffy and co-workers[66] to explain the better utilization of a crystalline amino acid mixture versus a protein hydrolysate.

FACTORS AFFECTING PROTEIN UTILIZATION

Many factors can potentially affect protein and amino acid metabolism and, hence protein and amino acid requirements. These include clinical status, quality of protein intake, concomitant energy intake (quantity and quality), concomitant intake of other nutrients, and some hormones. Each of these factors is discussed in the sections that follow.

Clinical Status

Clinical status affects protein metabolism and requirements for protein, as well as requirements for all other nutrients. Although data from infants are limited, it is likely, as has been established for adults, that any type of stress increases protein requirements. In adults, trauma and sepsis result in increased protein degradation (proteolysis) and irreversible catabolism of free amino acids, as reflected by higher rates of urinary nitrogen excretion and higher rates of oxidation of essential amino acids.[67,68] The degree of trauma severity also is directly associated with nitrogen excretion.[69, 70] The increased nitrogen excretion incident to stress appears to be mediated largely by catecholamines and glucocorticoids. Concentrations of both are elevated in stressed subjects, and increased urinary nitrogen excretion has been reported after infusion of these hormones in healthy volunteers.[71] However, although the infusion of glucocorticoids alone results in increased protein degradation,[72] infusion of catecholamines alone does not have a significant effect on proteolysis.[73]

One mechanism by which stress increases urinary nitrogen losses may be related, in part, to synthesis of acute phase proteins. Waterlow[74] estimated that the mixed acute phase protein response of an infected adult is approximately 1.2 g/kg/day. Although similar data for neonates are not available, it is likely that the response of term as well as preterm infants is similar qualitatively, if not quantitatively. Because maintenance of an appropriate acute phase protein response obviously is important for survival, the amino acids needed to support this response, if not provided exogenously, must be derived from breakdown of endogenous protein stores. Reeds and colleagues[75] estimated that roughly 2 g of endogenous protein must be mobilized to support an acute phase protein response of 1 g. Primarily, this is because the aromatic amino acid content of endogenous protein stores is only about half that of most acute phase proteins. Because the other amino acids released from endogenous protein stores cannot be used for endogenous protein synthesis, they are catabolized, thereby increasing urinary nitrogen excretion. The specific cellular and molecular mechanisms involved have not been completely elucidated.

The extensive studies of Knutrud[76] in the 1960s demonstrated that infants subjected to operative stress respond qualitatively in the same manner as adults but to a lesser degree. Although the subjects of these studies were primarily term infants (<1 year of age), there is little reason to believe that the LBW infant does not behave similarly. More recent studies[77] indicated that rates of whole body amino nitrogen flux, synthesis, and breakdown in postsurgical LBW infants are approximately 25% higher than expected. In addition, Boehm and colleagues,[78] comparing the metabolic responses of LBW infants (birth weight <1500 g) who experienced bacterial sepsis during the first week of life with those of healthy control infants and infants with respiratory distress syndrome, found that the urinary nitrogen excretion of infants with septicemia was double that of the other groups. In addition, decreasing nitrogen balance with increasing degree of illness has been reported in infants, with the lowest balances observed in infants with sepsis.[79]

Although many clinicians maintain that it is impossible, regardless of nitrogen intake, to achieve positive nitrogen balance during periods of stress, it is clear that this is not the case. Positive nitrogen balance is achievable in stressed patients, even in adults with severe burns; however, the nitrogen intakes required to achieve positive balance are considerable. The LBW infant with sepsis, for example, would require a nitrogen intake of at least 400 mg/kg/day (equivalent to a protein or amino acid intake of approximately 2.5 g/kg/day) to achieve nitrogen equilibrium and an even greater intake to promote nitrogen accretion. Whether provision of smaller amounts of specific amino acids (e.g., aromatic amino acids as discussed earlier) would be beneficial remains to be determined.

LBW infants who receive no exogenous nitrogen intake during the first week of life excrete, on average, 150 to 200 mg/kg/day of nitrogen,[26, 80-83] equivalent to a daily protein loss of 0.94 to 1.25 g or about 1% of endogenous protein stores. However, these data must be interpreted cautiously because it is likely that the study populations included some nonstressed as well as some moderately (but not severely) stressed infants. Thus, the daily nitrogen losses of some infants may be considerably greater and those of others considerably smaller. However, in the studies cited, a parenteral amino acid intake of 1.5 to 2.5 g/kg/day effectively reversed negative nitrogen balance and, in fact, resulted in achievement of positive balance, although not of the magnitude achieved in older, growing, enterally fed infants. Because conditions associated with greater endogenous excretion of nitrogen are usually short-lived (e.g., infection), such intakes over the short term may be adequate.

Based on the usual interpretation of nitrogen balance, these intakes should preserve lean body mass and should support at least modest rates of protein accretion. Further, because the catecholamines and glucocorticoids released in response to stress also interfere with utilization of energy substrates, particularly carbohydrate, it is unlikely that stressed infants can tolerate the energy intake required for normal growth. If the period of stress is not long, the effects of less than optimal anabolism for a short time usually can be corrected once the infant has recovered from the precipitating clinical insult. Conversely, if the infant can tolerate a nonprotein energy intake of 85 to 90 kcal/kg/day, a greater amino acid intake very likely will result in the intrauterine rate of nitrogen retention.[57]

Although it is clear that the rate of weight gain of infants with chronic conditions such as congenital heart disease and chronic pulmonary disease is less than optimal, it is not clear that the nutrient requirements of these infants are much greater than those of healthy infants. A thorough evaluation of the cause of the less than optimal rate of weight gain often reveals that the infant's intake is less than that of the normally growing infant with no underlying disease. Thus, although the protein requirement of infants with these conditions, as well as their requirements for other nutrients, may be somewhat greater than the requirements of the healthy infant, it is unlikely that they are considerably greater. However, the data on which this statement is based are scarce.

Quality of Protein Intake

An important factor in defining the protein requirement of any population is the overall quality of the protein intake. In large part, this is a function of the amino acid pattern of the protein. For example, the initial use of soy protein formulas resulted in lower rates of weight gain and nitrogen retention than did the use of formulas with a similar content of bovine milk protein.[84] The reason for this was related to the lower methionine content of soy versus bovine milk protein. Hence, the intake of soy protein required to produce a specific rate of nitrogen retention was considerably greater than the required intake of bovine milk protein. Modern soy protein preparations are supplemented with methionine, and their intake results in rates of weight gain and nitrogen retention equivalent to those resulting from a similar intake of bovine milk protein.

LBW infants fed similar intakes of human milk protein, unmodified bovine milk protein, and modified bovine milk protein (whey-predominant) experience similar rates of both weight gain and nitrogen retention. Thus, the overall quality of these three proteins appears to be similar. This finding, of course, is not surprising. Although the amino acid patterns of the three proteins differ somewhat (see Table 54-7), all contain a greater percentage of indispensable amino acids than does the protein synthesized by the fetus during development; further, all contain more of each indispensable amino acid as a percentage of total indispensable amino acid content than does newly synthesized fetal protein. An intake of only approximately 2 g/kg/day of any of the three proteins provides the requirements of all indispensable amino acids, as estimated from fetal accretion rates of individual amino acids (see Table 54-5). This intake does not provide sufficient amounts of some dispensable amino acids (e.g., glycine, alanine, and arginine) to ensure intrauterine accretion rates. This finding raises the intriguing possibility that these proteins may be limiting with respect to dispensable amino acids, particularly if energy intake is sufficient to favor maximal protein deposition. Indeed, as discussed, Jackson and co-workers,[53] studying [15N]glycine turnover in infants fed human milk, found that glycine intake was inadequate (see previous discussion).

Despite the apparent lack of difference in the overall quality of modified and unmodified bovine milk proteins, most currently available LBW infant formulas contain modified bovine milk protein. This probably is because the plasma aminogram of infants fed modified versus unmodified bovine milk protein is somewhat more desirable. For example, because plasma tyrosine concentrations during infancy appear to be related inversely with neurodevelopmental outcome,[85] the lower plasma tyrosine concentration of infants fed modified versus unmodified bovine milk protein[86] may be desirable. In addition, because cyst(e)ine is thought to be an indispensable amino acid for the LBW infant and, perhaps, the term infant, the greater cyst(e)ine content of modified bovine milk protein and the associated higher plasma cyst(e)ine concentrations of infants fed this protein[86] may be another advantage of this protein. Additional data suggest that metabolic acidosis may be less common in infants fed modified versus unmodified bovine milk protein.[87] Modified bovine milk protein, conversely, results in higher plasma threonine concentrations than either human milk or unmodified bovine milk protein.[86]

The quality of protein intake needed in all situations may not be the same. For example, if more aromatic amino acids are needed to support the acute phase protein response to stress (see earlier discussion), a protein with an amino acid pattern resembling the endogenous protein stores of the developing fetus is not likely to be the best quality to provide during periods of stress. However, until the possibility that increasing the intake of aromatic amino acids during stress reduces endogenous nitrogen losses is tested directly, recommendations cannot be made.

Concomitant Energy Intake

The effect of concomitant energy intake on protein, or nitrogen, utilization has been studied extensively in animals and to some extent in human adults,[88,89] but few data from human infants are available. The usual belief is that any nitrogen intake is used better if it is accompanied by a higher versus a lower concomitant energy intake. For any specific nitrogen intake, however, there is a concomitant energy intake beyond which further increases will not improve nitrogen retention. Although the few reported studies of the effect of energy intake on nitrogen utilization of LBW infants fall short of defining the quantitative aspects of this interaction, all suggest that the same principle outlined earlier applies.

Zlotkin and associates,[57] studying LBW infants receiving parenterally delivered nutrients, found that utilization of amino acid intakes of both 3 and 4 g/kg/day was greater when concomitant energy intake was 80 versus 50 kcal/kg/day. Duffy and co-workers[66] and Pineault and associates[90] also observed beneficial effects of intakes of 80 to 90 versus 60 to 70 kcal/kg/day on utilization of parenterally delivered amino acid intakes of 2.5 to 2.9 g/kg/day.

Kashyap and co-workers[29] found no statistically significant difference in nitrogen retention of LBW infants fed an enteral protein intake of 3.5 to 3.6 g/kg/day with a concomitant energy intake of either 120 or 150 kcal/kg/day. However, the blood urea nitrogen concentration and the plasma concentration of several amino acids were somewhat lower in the group that received the higher energy intake, a finding suggesting that the higher energy intake was at least minimally beneficial in enhancing nitrogen utilization. In subsequent studies, these investigators found that nitrogen retention of infants who received enteral protein intakes of either 3.8 to 3.9 g/kg/day or 4.2 to 4.3 g/kg/day with a concomitant energy intake of 140 to 150 kcal/kg/day was significantly higher than that of infants who received the same protein intakes with a concomitant energy intake of 120 kcal/kg/day.[28,91]

These data from LBW infants, summarized in Table 54-10, are insufficient to permit definitive conclusions concerning the precise energy intake required to ensure maximal utilization of a specific protein or amino acid intake. Nonetheless, it appears that a concomitant energy intake of 80 kcal/kg/day is sufficient to ensure near-maximal utilization of a parenterally administered amino acid intake of 2.7 g/kg/day and that a concomitant energy intake of 60 kcal/kg/day is sufficient to ensure reasonable utilization. Similarly, it appears that a concomitant energy intake of 120 kcal/kg/day is sufficient to ensure at least near-maximal utilization of an enterally administered protein intake of 3.6 g/kg/day.

Extrapolating from these data, it seems safe to conclude that utilization of the amino acid content of a parenterally administered regimen will be quite efficient, although perhaps not maximally efficient, if the energy/amino acid ratio of the regimen is at least 20 to 25 kcal/g and, similarly, that utilization of the protein content of an enterally administered regimen will be quite efficient if the energy/protein ratio of the regimen is at least 30 kcal/g. These energy/protein ratios, however, may not be optimal for maximal utilization of protein and amino acid intakes outside the range for which they were calculated. In addition, the ratio may be different if the distribution of energy intake

TABLE 54-10

Nitrogen Retention and Weight Gain of Low Birth Weight Infants Receiving Various Protein (Amino Acid) and Energy Intakes

Protein (Amino Acid) Intake (g/kg/d)	Energy Intake (kcal/kg/d)	Nitrogen Retention (mg/kg/d)	Weight Gain (g/kg/d)
Zlotkin et al.[57]			
3	50	256±20	2.0±4.0
3	80	320±8	16.2±2.4
4	55	274±11	1.5±3.2
4	80	432±21	15.6±1.9
Duffy et al.[66]			
2.6	70	214	—
2.9	96	284	—
Pineault et al.[90]*			
2.7	60	220	11.5±3.2
2.7	80	248	14.6±2.0
Kashyap et al.[28,29]			
3.6	120	422±22	18.3±2.8
3.5	150	425±12	22.0±3.1
3.8	120	420±31	19.1±3.2
3.9	142	473±20	21.5±2.2

* Data from high-fat (3 g/kg/d) groups at each energy intake are combined; there were no effects of quality of energy intake on either nitrogen retention or weight gain.

between carbohydrate and fat is different from the distribution of these nutrients in the regimens for which the ratios were calculated. In this regard, there is considerable evidence that carbohydrate is more effective than fat in promoting nitrogen retention.[89,92,93] There is no apparent benefit of an energy intake much in excess of that necessary to ensure utilization of the concomitant protein intake. Such intakes result simply in excessive fat deposition relative to protein deposition.[21,28,94–97]

Concomitant Intake of Other Nutrients

In theory, an inadequate intake of any nutrient required for production of new tissue also limits the extent to which protein can be deposited as new tissue. The best example of this phenomenon is the study of Rudman and co-workers[98] in adults receiving only parenterally administered nutrients. In this study, withdrawal of sodium, potassium, or phosphorus from an otherwise complete parenteral nutrition regimen resulted in retention of less nitrogen and a lower rate of weight gain. There is no reason to believe that this result is not applicable to all subjects. If so, an inadequate intake of any nutrient required for production of new tissue is likely to interfere with the LBW infant's utilization of protein and amino acid intake.

Kashyap and colleagues[29] suggested this possibility to explain apparent differences between the results of their studies and those of Räihä and associates.[87] The latter investigators found no difference in rates of weight gain of LBW infants fed protein intakes of 2.25 versus 4.5 g/kg/day (with an energy intake of 120 kcal/kg/day), whereas Kashyap and colleagues[29] found a marked difference in rates of weight gain as well as nitrogen retention between infants fed protein intakes of 2.25 g/kg/day versus 3.6 g/kg/day, both with an energy intake of 120 kcal/kg/day. The only apparent difference between the two studies concerned sodium and phosphorus intakes, which were considerably lower in infants studied by Räihä and co-workers. Based on the intrauterine relationships between sodium and phosphorus accretion and the accretion of nitrogen,[99] the sodium and phosphorus intakes of the infants studied by Räihä and co-workers, even if 100% absorbed, were insufficient to permit utilization of the higher protein intake. In contrast, the sodium and phosphorus intakes of the infants studied by Kashyap and associates were generous, and retention of sodium and phosphorus relative to the retention of nitrogen was roughly the same as the intrauterine relationships.

Unfortunately, few data concerning this potentially important relationship are available. Nonetheless, it seems reasonable to conclude that inadequate intake of any nutrient required for synthesis of new tissue is likely to inhibit utilization of nitrogen for production of lean body mass. If so, excessive losses of nutrients required for synthesis of new tissue (e.g., electrolyte losses with chronic diuretic usage) also are likely to inhibit utilization of protein and amino acids for production of new tissue.

Hormones

Insulin and insulin-like growth factor I (IGF-I) are important regulators of fetal and postnatal growth.[100] Secretion of insulin is dependent on the plasma concentration of glucose as well as that of certain amino acids, namely arginine and leucine. In adults, reduction in proteolysis has been reported with plasma insulin concentrations within the physiologic as well as the pharmacologic range.[101, 102] In newborn infants, pharmacologic concentrations of insulin (79±13 μU/mL) result in reduction of proteolysis, but concentrations within the physiologic range do not.[103] Further, the anabolic effect of insulin on protein synthesis has not been demonstrated consistently in infants, possibly because the effect of insulin on protein synthesis may be underestimated if its effect on protein degradation significantly reduces amino acid availability.

IGF-I also has been shown to enhance protein anabolism.[104] Although IGF-I infusion under conditions of adequate substrate supply enhances protein synthesis, it does not affect proteolysis,[105] whereas insulin infusion appears to decrease proteolysis without affecting protein synthesis. When amino acid concentrations are maintained, infusions of both insulin and IGF-I increase protein accretion of the ovine fetus, but the greatest increase are observed with combined infusion.[106]

Growth hormone (GH) increases lean body mass and promotes growth of GH-deficient individuals.[107, 108] It also stimulates muscle and whole body protein synthesis in healthy adults.[109] At least some of these effects of GH are thought to be mediated through increased IGF; however, the exact mechanism for GH-stimulated protein synthesis remains unclear. Although GH has been shown to prevent glucocorticoid-induced protein wasting in adults,[110] administration of recombinant human GH did not prevent the catabolic side effects of dexamethasone in extremely low birth weight infants with bronchopulmonary dysplasia.[111]

CONCLUSIONS

Given the sparsity of available data, and because many of the data available are confusing and are often in conflict with other data, it is difficult to make concrete statements concerning the LBW infant's requirement for protein and amino acids. However, the available data appear to support the following conclusions:

1. The "average" LBW infant who receives no nitrogen intake loses approximately 1% of endogenous protein stores daily.
2. A parenteral amino acid intake of approximately 3 g/kg/day or an enteral protein intake of about 2.8 g/kg/day is required to achieve the intrauterine rate of nitrogen accretion.
3. Enteral protein intakes of 3.5 to 3.6 g/kg/day to 4.2 to 4.3 g/kg/day are well tolerated by LBW infants and result in rates of weight gain and nitrogen accretion exceeding the intrauterine rates.
4. An enteral protein intake in excess of 3.5 to 3.6 g/kg/day is not used maximally unless it is accompanied by an energy intake greater than 120 kcal/kg/day.

5. There are no major differences in the overall quality of the proteins used in modern preterm infant formulas. In addition, the biologic quality of these proteins differs minimally, if at all, from that of human milk protein.
6. The overall quality of most available parenteral amino acid mixtures appears to be less than optimal.

If these conclusions are warranted, it seems reasonable to conclude further that the LBW infant who can tolerate enteral feedings immediately after birth requires a protein intake of at least 2.8 g/kg/day to ensure continued accretion of nitrogen at the intrauterine rate. If the infant cannot be fed enterally, the parenteral amino acid intake required to achieve the same goal is about 3 g/kg/day (this requirement may be somewhat less if a parenteral amino acid mixture designed specifically for infants is used; however, further data are required to confirm the superiority of the pediatric mixtures).

For various reasons, some LBW infants receive little or no protein or amino acids for the first few days of life. Because these infants lose at least 1% of their endogenous protein stores daily (or >1 g/kg/day), their subsequent protein and amino acid needs are greater than required simply to support the intrauterine rate of protein accretion. Otherwise, this early loss will not be replaced until well after discharge. In other words, if the infant receives no protein or amino acid intake for the first several days of life, the minimal requirement is no longer simply the amount required to ensure the intrauterine rate of nitrogen accretion, rather, it is this amount *plus* that required to replace the earlier endogenous losses.

Viewed in this way, the protein (amino acid) requirement of individual infants is quite variable, depending on the extent of endogenous losses before feeding. For example, the infant who receives no amino acid or protein intake for the first week of life sustains endogenous protein losses during this time of at least 7 to 8 g/kg. Assuming that only 70% of intake is retained, these losses increase the infant's subsequent enteral protein requirement by at least 10 g/kg. If this loss is replaced over a period of 40 days, the daily increment in protein requirement is about 0.25 g/kg. If it is replaced over a period of 20 days, the daily increment, of course, is 0.5 g/kg. Thus, once the "average" LBW infant is able to tolerate full enteral feeding, it is likely that the protein requirement will be at least 3 g/kg/day. The protein content of currently available LBW infant formulas is sufficient to provide the minimal protein needs (assuming, of course, that a sufficient volume to provide 120 kcal/kg/day is ingested). A greater protein intake is likely to be tolerated by most LBW infants. Moreover, a greater protein intake also will result in a greater rate of weight gain. Such an intake, therefore, may be particularly desirable for the infant who has sustained extensive endogenous protein losses.

REFERENCES

1. Chipponi JX, et al: Deficiencies of essential and conditionally essential nutrients. Am J Clin Nutr 35(Suppl 5):1112, 1982.
2. Harper AE: Dispensable and indispensable amino acid interrelationships. *In* Blackburn GL, et al (eds): Amino Acids: Metabolism and Medical Applications. Boston: John Wright-PSG, 1983, pp 105–121.
3. Laidlaw SA, Kopple JD: Newer concepts of the indispensable amino acids. Am J Clin Nutr 46:593, 1987.
4. Gaull GE, et al: Development of mammalian sulphur metabolism: absence of cystathionase in human fetal tissues. Pediatr Res 6:538, 1972.
5. Sturman JA, et al: Absence of cystathionase in human fetal liver: is cysteine essential? Science 169:74, 1970.
6. Zlotkin SH, Anderson GH: The development of cystathionase activity during the first year of life. Pediatr Res 16:65, 1982.
7. Greengard O: Enzymic differentiation of human liver: comparison with the rat model. Pediatr Res 11:669, 1977.
8. Raiha NC, Suihkonen J: Development of urea-synthesizing enzymes in human liver. Acta Paediatr Scand 57:121, 1968.
9. Reeds PJ, Davis TA: Of flux and flooding: the advantages and problems of different isotopic methods for quantifying protein turnover in vivo. I. Methods based on the dilution of a tracer. Curr Opin Clin Nutr Metab Care 2:23, 1999.

10. Inubushi T, et al: Hormonal and dietary regulation of lysosomal cysteine proteinases in liver under gluconeogenesis conditions. Biol Chem 377:539, 1996.
11. Ciehanover A, et al: Degradation of nuclear oncoproteins by the ubiquitin system in vitro. Proc Natl Acad Sci USA 88:139, 1991.
12. Goldberg AL, Rock KL: Proteolysis, proteasomes and antigen presentation. Nature 357:375, 1992.
13. Waterlow JC: Protein turnover with special reference to man. Q J Exp Physiol 69:409, 1984.
14. Yu YM, et al: Quantitative role of splanchnic region in leucine metabolism: L-[1-13C,15N] leucine and substrate balance studies. Am J Physiol 259:E36, 1990.
15. Wykes LJ, et al: Glycine, leucine, and phenylalanine flux in low-birth-weight infants during parenteral and enteral feeding. Am J Clin Nutr 55:971, 1992.
16. van Toledo-Eppinga L, et al: Relative kinetics of phenylalanine and leucine in low birth weight infants during nutrient administration. Pediatr Res 40:41, 1996.
17. Calloway DH, et al: Sweat and miscellaneous nitrogen losses in human balance studies. J Nutr 101:775, 1971.
18. Cissik JH, et al: Production of gaseous nitrogen in human steady-state conditions. J Appl Physiol 32:155, 1972.
19. Catzeflis C, et al: Whole body protein synthesis and energy expenditure in very low birth weight infants. Pediatr Res 19:679, 1985.
20. Heird WC, et al: Nutrient utilization and growth in LBW infants. In Goldman A, et al (eds): Human Lactation 3: The Effects of Human Milk on the Recipient Infant. New York, Plenum Press, 1987, pp 9–21.
21. Reichman B, et al: Dietary composition and macronutrient storage in preterm infants. Pediatrics 72:322, 1983.
22. American Academy of Pediatrics Committee on Nutrition: Nutritional needs of preterm infants. In Kleinman RE (ed): Pediatric Nutrition Handbook. Elk Grove Village, IL, American Academy of Pediatrics, 1998, pp 55–87.
23. Canadian Pediatric Society Nutrition Committee: Nutrition needs and feeding of premature infants. Can Med Assoc J 152:1765, 1995.
24. European Society for Gastroenterology, Hepatology, and Nutrition, Committee on Nutrition of the Preterm Infant: Nutrition and feeding of preterm infants. Acta Paediatr Scand Suppl 336:1, 1987.
25. Kashyap S, et al: Growth, nutrient retention and metabolic response of low-birth-weight infants fed supplemented and unsupplemented preterm human milk. Am J Clin Nutr 52:254, 1990.
26. Kashyap S, Heird WC: Protein requirements of low birthweight, very low birthweight, and small for gestational age infants. In Räihä NCR (ed): Protein Metabolism During Infancy: Nestlé Nutrition Workshop Series, Vol 33. New York, Raven Press, 1994, p 133.
27. Zello GA, et al: Minimum protein intake for the preterm neonate determined by protein and amino acid kinetics. Pediatr Res 53:338, 2003.
28. Kashyap S, et al: Growth, nutrient retention and metabolic response in low birth weight infants fed varying intakes of protein and energy. J Pediatr 113:713, 1988.
29. Kashyap S, et al: Effects of varying protein and energy intakes on growth and metabolic response in low birth weight infants. J Pediatr 108:955, 1986.
30. Pittard WB, et al: Cord blood amino acid concentrations from neonates of 23–41 weeks gestational age. JPEN J Parenter Enteral Nutr 12:167, 1988.
31. McIntosh N, et al: Plasma amino acids of the midtrimester human fetus. Biol Neonate 45:218, 1984.
32. Schanler RJ: Nitrogen and mineral balance in preterm infants fed human milks or formula. J Pediatr Gastroenterol Nutr 4:214, 1985.
33. Shenai JP, et al: Nutritional balance studies in very low birth weight infants: enhanced nutrient retention rates by an experimental formula. Pediatrics 66:233, 1980.
34. Tyson JE, et al: Growth, metabolic response and development in very low birth weight infants fed banked human milk or enriched formula. I. Neonatal findings. J Pediatr 103:95, 1983.
35. Ehrenkranz RA, et al: Longitudinal Growth of Hospitalized Very Low Birth Weight Infants. Pediatrics 104:280–289, 1999.
36. Life Sciences Research Office (LSRO) Expert Panel on Assessment of Nutrient Requirements for Preterm Infant Formulas. J Nutr 132(Suppl):1423S, 2002.
37. Rose WC: The amino acid requirements of adult man. Nutr Abstr Rev 27:631, 1957.
38. Young VR, et al: Amino acid kinetics in relation to protein and amino acid requirements: the primary importance of amino acid oxidation. In Garrow JS, Holliday D (eds): Substrate and Energy Metabolism in Man. London, John Libbey, 1985, pp 119–134.
39. Holt LE Jr, Snyderman SE: The amino acid requirements of children. In Nyhan WL (ed): Amino Acid Metabolism and Genetic Variation. New York, McGraw-Hill, 1967, pp 381–390.
40. Young VR, Borgonha S: Nitrogen and amino acid requirements: the Massachusetts Institute of Technology amino acid requirement pattern. J Nutr 130:1841S, 2000.
41. Snyderman SE: The protein and amino acid requirements of the premature infant. In Jonxis JHP, et al (eds): Metabolic Processes in the Foetus and Newborn Infant. Leiden, Holland, Stenfert Kroese, 1971, pp 128–141.
42. Snyderman SE: Amino acid requirements. In Winters RW, Hasselmeyer EG (eds): Intravenous Nutrition in the High Risk Infant. New York, John Wiley & Sons, 1975, pp 205–214.
43. Fomon SJ, Filer LJ Jr: Amino acid requirements for normal growth. In Nyhan WL (ed): Amino Acid Metabolism and Genetic Variation. New York, McGraw-Hill, 1967, pp 391–401.
44. Life Sciences Research Office: Safety of Amino Acids Used as Dietary Supplements: FDA Contract No. 223-88-2124. Washington, DC, Food and Drug Administration (FDA) Center for Food Safety and Applied Nutrition, 1992.
45. Heine WE, et al: The importance of α-lactalbumin in infant nutrition. J Nutr 121:277, 1991.
46. Darragh AJ, Moughan PH: The amino acid composition of human milk corrected for amino acid digestibility. Br J Nutr 80:25, 1998.
47. Davis TA, et al: Amino acid composition of human milk is not unique. J Nutr 124:1126, 1994.
48. Villalpando S, et al: Qualitative analysis of human milk produced by women consuming a maize-predominant diet typical of rural Mexico. Ann Nutr Metab 42:23, 1998.
49. Widdowson EM, et al: Body composition of the fetus and infant. In Visser HKA (ed): Fifth Nutricia Symposium: Nutrition and Metabolism of the Fetus and Infant. The Hague, Martinus Nijhoff, 1979, pp 169–177.
50. Räihä NCR: Biochemical basis for nutritional management of preterm infants. Pediatrics 53:147, 1974.
51. Denne SC, et al: Proteolysis and phenylalanine hydroxylation in response to parenteral nutrition in extremely premature and normal newborns. J Clin Invest 97:746, 1996.
52. Kilani RA, et al: Phenylalanine hydroxylase activity in preterm infants: is tyrosine a conditionally essential amino acid? Am J Clin Nutr 61:1218, 1995.
53. Jackson AA, et al: Nitrogen metabolism in preterm infants fed human donor breast milk: the possible essentiality of glycine. Pediatr Res 15:1454, 1981.
54. Miller RG, et al: Decreased cysteine and proline synthesis in parenterally fed, premature infants. J Pediatr Surg 30:953, 1995.
55. Ziegler TR, et al: Glutamine: from basic science to clinical applications. Nutrition 12(Suppl):S68, 1996.
56. Neu J, et al: Enteral glutamine supplementation for very low birth weight infants decreases morbidity. J Pediatr 131:691, 1997.
57. Zlotkin SH, et al: Intravenous nitrogen and energy intakes required to duplicate in utero nitrogen accretion in prematurely born human infants. J Pediatr 99:115, 1981.
58. Winters RW, et al: Plasma amino acids in infants receiving parenteral nutrition. In Greene HL, et al (eds): Clinical Nutrition Update: Amino Acids. Chicago, American Medical Association, 1977, pp 147–157.
59. Stegink LD, Baker GL: Infusion of protein hydrolysates in the newborn infant: plasma amino acid concentrations. J Pediatr 78:595, 1971.
60. Heird WC, et al: Evaluation of an amino acid mixture designed to maintain normal plasma amino acid patterns in infants and children requiring parenteral nutrition. Pediatrics 80:401, 1987.
61. Heird WC, et al: Pediatric parenteral amino acid mixture in low birth weight infants. Pediatrics 81:41, 1988.
62. Smith CV, et al: Oxidant stress responses in premature infants during exposure to hyperoxia. Pediatr Res 34:360, 1993.
63. Kashyap S, et al: Cysteine supplementation of very low birth weight infants receiving parenteral nutrition. Pediatr Res 31:290A, 1992.
64. Mendoza MR, et al: Cysteine supplementation increases whole blood glutathione concentration in parenterally fed preterm infants. Pediatr Res 33:307A, 1993.
65. Helms RA, et al: Comparison of a pediatric versus standard amino acid formulation in preterm neonates requiring parenteral nutrition. J Pediatr 110:446, 1987.
66. Duffy B, et al: The effect of varying protein quality and energy intake on the nitrogen metabolism of parenterally fed very low birth weight (less than 1600 g) infants. Pediatr Res 15:1040, 1981.
67. Shaw JH, Wolfe RR: An integrated analysis of glucose, fat, and protein metabolism in severely traumatized patients: studies in the basal state and the response to total parenteral nutrition. Ann Surg 209:63, 1989.
68. Biolo G, et al: Metabolic response to injury and sepsis: changes in protein metabolism. Nutrition 13(Suppl):52S, 1997.
69. Moore FD: Metabolic Care of the Surgical Patient. Philadelphia, WB Saunders Co, 1959, pp 409–456.
70. Long CL, et al: Urinary excretion of 3-methylhistidine: an assessment of muscle protein catabolism in adult normal subjects and during malnutrition, sepsis, and skeletal trauma. Metabolism 30:765, 1981.
71. Smeets HJ, et al: Differential effects of counterregulatory stress hormones on serum albumin concentrations and protein catabolism in healthy volunteers. Nutrition 11:423, 1995.
72. Lofberg E, et al: Effects of high doses of glucocorticoids on free amino acids, ribosomes and protein turnover in human muscle. Eur J Clin Invest 32:345, 2002.
73. Ensinger H, et al: Metabolic effects of norepinephrine and dobutamine in healthy volunteers. Shock 18:495, 2002.
74. Waterlow JC: Protein-energy malnutrition: challenges and controversies. Proc Nutr Soc India 37:59, 1991.
75. Reeds PJ, et al: Do the differences between the amino acid compositions of acute-phase and muscle proteins have a bearing on nitrogen loss in traumatic states? J Nutr 124:906, 1994.
76. Knutrud O: The Water and Electrolyte Metabolism in the Newborn Child After Major Surgery. Oslo, Universitets Forlaget, 1965.

77. Duffy B, Pencharz P: The effects of surgery on the nitrogen metabolism of parenterally fed human neonates. Pediatr Res *20*:32, 1986.
78. Boehm G, et al: Effects of bacterial sepsis on protein metabolism in infants during the first week. Biomed Biochim Acta *45*:813, 1986.
79. Mrozek JD, et al: Effect of sepsis syndrome on neonatal protein and energy metabolism. J Perinatol *20*:96, 2000.
80. Anderson TL, et al: A controlled trial of glucose vs. glucose and amino acids in premature infants. J Pediatr *94*:947, 1979.
81. Rivera A Jr, et al: Effect of intravenous amino acids on protein metabolism of preterm infants during the first three days of life. Pediatr Res *22*:106, 1993.
82. van Lingen RA, et al: Effects of early amino acid administration during total parenteral nutrition on protein metabolism in pre-term infants. Clin Sci (Colch) *82*:199, 1992.
83. Saini J, et al: Early parenteral feeding of amino acids. Arch Dis Child *64*:1362, 1989.
84. Fomon SJ, et al: Methionine fortification of a soy protein formula fed to infants. Am J Clin Nutr *32*:2460, 1979.
85. Menkes JH, et al: Relationship of elevated blood tyrosine to the ultimate intellectual performance of premature infants. Pediatrics *49*:218, 1972.
86. Kashyap S, et al: Protein quality in feeding low birth weight infants: a comparison of whey-predominant versus casein-predominant formulas. Pediatrics *79*:748, 1987.
87. Räihä NCR, et al: Milk protein quality in low-birth-weight infants. I. Metabolic response and effects on growth. Pediatrics *57*:659, 1976.
88. Calloway DH, Spector H: Nitrogen balance as related to caloric and protein intake in active young men. Am J Clin Nutr *2*:405, 1954.
89. Munro HN: General aspects of the regulation of protein metabolism by diet and by hormones. III. Influence of dietary carbohydrate and fat on protein metabolism. *In* Munro HN (ed): Mammalian Protein Metabolism. New York, Academic Press, 1964, pp 412–447.
90. Pineault M, et al: Total parenteral nutrition in the newborn: impact of the quality of infused energy on nitrogen metabolism. Am J Clin Nutr *47*:298, 1988.
91. Kashyap S, et al: Evaluation of a mathematical model for predicting the relationship between protein and energy intakes of low-birth-weight infants and the rate and composition of weight gain. Pediatr Res *35*:704, 1994.
92. Long JM, et al: Effect of carbohydrate and fat intake on nitrogen excretion during total intravenous feeding. Ann Surg *185*:417, 1977.
93. Kashyap S, et al: Effects of quality of energy on growth and metabolic response in enterally fed low birth weight infants. Pediatr Res *50*:390, 2001.
94. Millward DJ, et al: The effect of dietary energy and protein on growth as studied in animal models. *In* Fomon SJ, Heird WC (eds): Energy and Protein Needs During Infancy. New York, Academic Press, 1986, pp 127–156.
95. Reichman B, et al: Diet, fat accretion and growth in premature infants. N Engl J Med *305*:1495, 1981.
96. Schulze KF, et al: Energy expenditure, energy balance and composition of weight gain in low birth weight infants fed diets of different protein and energy content. J Pediatr *110*:753, 1987.
97. Whyte RK, et al: Energy balance and nitrogen balance in growing low birth weight infants fed human milk or formula. Pediatr Res *17*:891, 1983.
98. Rudman D, et al: Elemental balances during intravenous hyperalimentation of underweight adult subjects. J Clin Invest *55*:94, 1975.
99. Widdowson EM: Changes in body proportion and composition during growth. *In* Davis J, Dobbing J (eds): Scientific Foundations of Pediatrics. Philadelphia, WB Saunders Co, 1974, pp 153–163.
100. Hill DJ, Milner RDG: Insulin as a growth factor. Pediatr Res *19*:879, 1985.
101. Fukagawa NK, et al: Insulin-mediated reduction of whole body protein breakdown: dose-response effects on leucine metabolism in postabsorptive men. J Clin Invest *76*:2306, 1985.
102. Tessari P, et al: Dose-response curves of effects of insulin on leucine kinetics in humans. Am J Physiol *251*:E334, 1986.
103. Pointdexter BB, et al: Exogenous insulin reduces proteolysis and protein synthesis in extremely low birth weight infants. J Pediatr *132*:948, 1998.
104. Le Roith D, et al: What is the role of circulating IGF-I? Trends Endocrinol Metab *12*:48, 2001.
105. Russell-Jones DL, et al: Use of a leucine clamp to demonstrate that IGF-I actively stimulates protein synthesis in normal humans. Am J Physiol *267*:E591, 1994.
106. Shen W, et al: Protein anabolic effects of insulin and IGF-I in the ovine fetus. Am J Physiol, 2002.
107. Jorgensen JO, et al: Beneficial effects of growth hormone treatment in GH-deficient adults. Lancet *1*:1221, 1989.
108. Salomon F, et al: The effects of treatment with recombinant human growth hormone on body composition and metabolism in adults with growth hormone deficiency. N Engl J Med *321*:1797, 1989.
109. Fryburg DA, et al: Growth hormone acutely stimulates forearm muscle protein synthesis in normal humans. Am J Physiol *260*:E499, 1991.
110. Horber EF, Haymond MW: Human growth hormone prevents the protein catabolic side effects of prednisone in humans. J Clin Invest *86*:265, 1990.
111. Tonini G, et al: Growth hormone does not prevent catabolic side effects of dexamethasone in extremely low birth weight preterm infants with bronchopulmonary dysplasia: a pilot study. J Pediatr Endocrinol Metab *10*:291, 1997.

55

Gordon G. Power, Arlin B. Blood, and Christian J. Hunter

Perinatal Thermal Physiology

OVERVIEW

Fetal tissues are metabolically active compared with similar tissues in adults; they produce relatively large quantities of heat as a by-product. Heat produced within the fetus accumulates until temperature gradients are established that cause the heat to move to the maternal organism. This transfer is remarkably efficient, and in most mammals that have been studied, including the human, a temperature difference of only about 0.5°C is necessary to create a steady state in which the heat produced by the fetus is matched by its rate of dissipation into the mother. Moreover, as maternal temperature varies throughout the day, fetal temperature follows closely, remaining about 0.5°C higher. This tight linkage of maternal and fetal temperatures has been called a *heat clamp*, which, in effect, largely prevents the fetus from independently regulating its body temperature before birth.

After birth, the surrounding temperature falls, and fluids evaporate from the newborn's skin. Cold exposure evokes thermogenic responses that increase basal heat production severalfold. These responses include shivering in skeletal muscle and nonshivering thermogenesis in brown adipose tissue.[1,2] The chain of events that evokes these responses is complex, and includes fundamental metabolic and endocrine alterations with both stimulatory and inhibitory components.

BASAL FETAL HEAT PRODUCTION

The usual method of estimating fetal heat production is based on oxygen (O_2) consumption. Generally, it is assumed that about 5 calories of heat are produced for each milliliter of O_2 used. This assumption has held up well for most metabolic fuels, varying only slightly with growth rate and other factors. Thus a 3-kg fetus, lamb or human, consuming 8 ml O_2/minute per kg is thought to produce 120 cal/minute, or about 9 watts.

In more recent years, it has become possible to measure fetal heat production directly using differential calorimetry.[3] By this method, the rise in fetal temperature that occurs following the introduction of a small quantity of heat is compared with the maternofetal temperature difference that results naturally from basal fetal heat production. An electrically heated, glass-encased nichrome (an alloy of nickel and chromium) wire placed in the inferior vena cava is used to generate heat, expressed as an equation:

$$H_{fetus} = H_{heater} \cdot \Delta T_{fetus} / \Delta T_{heater}$$

Because H_{heater} can be precisely measured from voltage and current readings, and because temperatures can be precisely measured to a few hundredths of a degree Celsius using thermistors, fetal basal heat production is readily calculated. Using this method in fetal sheep, heat production has been found to average 3.3 ± 0.3 watts/kg of fetal tissue.[3] This is equivalent to 47 calories/minute per kg and is about twice the quantity of heat produced by the adult on a per unit weight basis.

Similar experiments have not been attempted in the human fetus, but measurements have been made in newborns a few hours after birth using direct calorimetry. In specially constructed chambers, mean total heat loss was 2.35 watts/kg of body weight when the ambient temperature was 32°C, a temperature at which there was thermal balance.[4]

Alterations in Fetal Heat Production

The rate of oxygen consumption and therefore of heat production is altered in response to changes in oxygen supply to the fetus. Decreases in fetal arterial PO_2, for example, result in decreased fetal oxygen consumption.[5-9] Conversely, increases in fetal arterial PO_2 induce increased oxygen consumption.[9] These findings are in sharp contrast to findings in the adult human[10] and sheep[11] wherein oxygen use is well maintained across the physiologic range of oxygen supply. This direct linkage between oxygen use and oxygen availability strongly suggests that the fetus has mechanisms that allow it to vary metabolic rate to match oxygen availability, a response termed *adaptive hypometabolism* (Fig. 55-1). Among many lower animal species (e.g., turtle and carp particularly, but also more generally in other animals) adaptive hypometabolism is the most prominent defense against hypoxia and anoxia.[12] However, the mechanisms by which adaptive hypometabolism occurs in the mammalian fetus remain uncertain. The fetal liver may be speculated to play a major role because it decreases its oxygen use in response to hypoxia,[13] and because it is a large organ active in protein synthesis, an oxygen-costly process that may be temporarily suspended. Further work is clearly needed to explore the chemical mediators of hypometabolism in the fetus, its biochemical and molecular mechanism(s), and biologic importance, especially during labor.

PLACENTAL AND UTERINE WALL HEAT PRODUCTION

A different method has been devised to measure heat production in tissues of the placenta and uterine wall. This technique posits

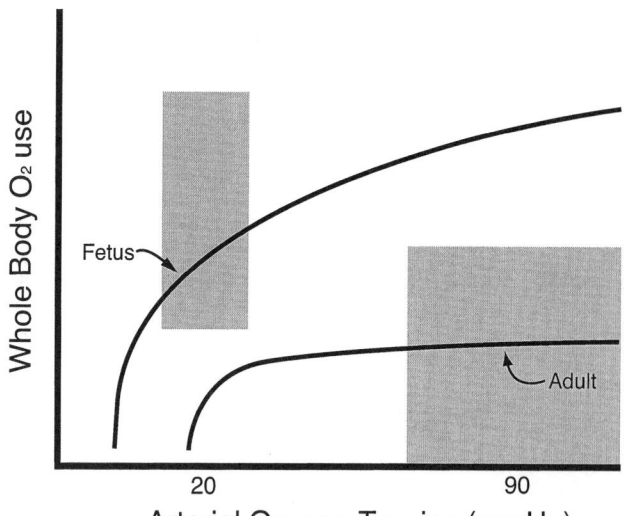

Figure 55–1. A stylized illustration of the relationship between oxygen availability and consumption in the mammalian fetus and adult. Note the stability of adult oxygen consumption over a wide range of arterial PO_2 values above and below the physiologic range in contrast to the fetal values, which vary with arterial PO_2 even within the physiologic range. Shaded areas indicate physiologic range of arterial PO_2 for fetus and adult.

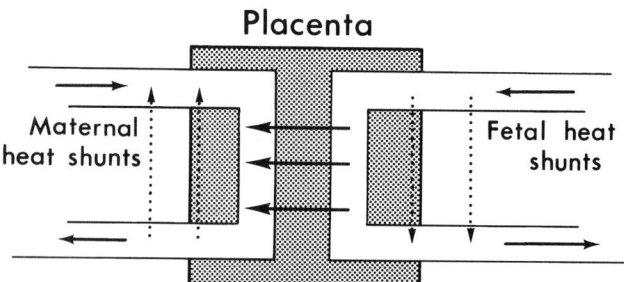

Figure 55–2. Because heat is highly diffusible, shunts may develop between vessels supplying and returning from the placenta. Such shunts diminish the efficiency of the placenta as a heat exchanger.

that the heat output measured from the uterus after fetal death is derived solely from the placenta and uterine wall. Heat output is calculated as the product of uterine blood flow, temperature gain across the uterine vascular bed, and the specific heat of blood. Again using the sheep as the experimental model, it has been demonstrated that the uterus and placenta produce about 2.1 watts/kg of tissue.[14] Thus, the placenta and uterus, as well as the fetus, are responsible for appreciable heat production. This production has been calculated to contribute 10 to 20% of the maternofetal temperature difference.[15] Corresponding measurements have not yet been carried out in the human but may become possible through the advent of noninvasive methods to measure uterine blood flow and metabolism.

PATHWAYS OF HEAT ELIMINATION

The heat produced within the uterus must pass to the maternal body to be eliminated. Heat exits through the umbilical circulation or through the fetal skin, amniotic fluid, and uterine wall. Generally, the umbilical circulation is thought to be the major route of exit because blood flow to the placenta is sizable. Furthermore, the placenta has a large surface area and thin membrane barrier, which should permit rapid temperature equilibration. This theory has been borne out by the demonstration that the temperature of the fetal baboon increases quickly following partial occlusion of the umbilical cord,[16] and it has been further confirmed in fetal sheep, in which the temperature again rose quickly following complete[17] or partial[18] occlusion of the umbilical cord. Likewise, the maternofetal temperature difference widens during uterine contractions in the human.[19] These findings all support the placenta as the major heat excretory pathway.

Placental Heat Transfer

The first direct measurements of placental heat transfer were carried out by Schröder and Hatano[20] using the isolated, artificially perfused guinea pig placenta. These investigators generated arterial temperature differences and measured the transfer of heat under both steady-state and transient conditions. Surprisingly, they found that venous outflow did not reach temperature equilibrium. In comparison with the diffusion of water across the placenta, the exchange of heat appeared less than optimal. One possible explanation is that an exchange of heat occurs between fetal vessels leading to and returning from the placenta. This concept is illustrated in Figure 55–2. This type of arteriovenous transfer of heat would act as a heat shunt, which would function to retain heat within the fetal body and decrease the effectiveness of the placenta as a heat exchanger. As yet, experiments have not been carried out to measure heat flux between umbilical artery and vein in the cord or between smaller vessels within the placenta itself. Such a mechanism should be considered seriously, however, because it could explain, at least in part, the failure of many highly diffusible substances, such as carbon dioxide (CO_2), O_2, and water, as well as heat, to reach equilibrium during placental passage of maternal and fetal blood.

Conductance Through Skin and Uterine Wall

Experiments have been carried out in sheep to measure heat conductance through the fetal skin and uterine wall. Using this method, chilled saline is injected into the amniotic fluid. The time course of temperature changes occurring in the amniotic fluid and maternal and fetal body cores is determined as heat returns to the fluid.[14] By dividing heat flux by the mean temperature gradient, it is possible to calculate a value for conductance, and by comparing results with the fetus alive and dead, the contribution of fetal skin is separated from that of the uterine wall. Skin conductance was found to average 10 watts/degree Celsius, and uterine wall conductance was found to average 3 to 6 watts/degree Celsius.

Direct measurements of heat flux across the human skin are limited. Rudelstorfer and co-workers[21] inserted heat flux–sensing transducers between the presenting fetal part and the vaginal wall during the midstage of labor. They found heat flux varied from 3 watts/m² with breech presentation to 11 watts/m² with head presentation. Moreover, they observed that heat flux across the fetal skin increased when placental exchange was compromised, suggesting a possible compensatory mechanism whereby vasodilation in the skin would enable it to take on a greater role in heat elimination.

Figure 55-3 provides a summary of current thermal information in the fetal sheep. Composite results are tabulated from many sources, and question marks are included to indicate those areas in which information is incomplete.

Changes of Maternal Temperature

The effects of the maternal temperature on the fetus have been tested in sheep by submitting the pregnant ewe to cold and heat stress, exercise, and maternal fever. The temperature of the fetus

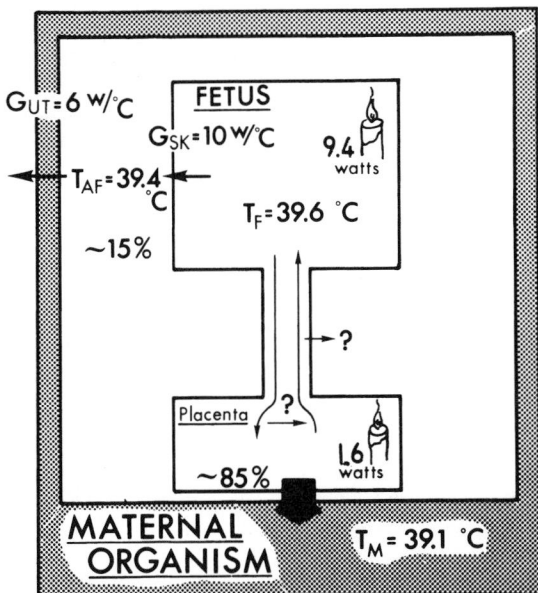

Figure 55–3. Summary of experimental data for heat production (candle symbol), conduction (G), and temperatures in the fetal sheep. About 85% of total heat passes through the placenta, with the remaining 15% passing through the fetal skin, amniotic fluid, and uterine wall. Temperatures average 2°C lower in the human.

does not change as much as that of the ewe when the ewe is either transiently cooled by exposure to cold or warmed by heat exposure[22] or short-term exercise.[22, 23] This thermal buffering may be due to changes in umbilical flow and uterine flow that would eliminate additional heat with warming and would retain additional heat with cooling. Another possibility is adjustments in fetal metabolic rate that would buffer maternal changes. This mechanism, however, appears relatively weak (only a few tenths of a degree Celsius) because the fetus remains thermally tightly linked to the mother by the high efficiency of placental heat transfer.

When heat stress is prolonged, there are detrimental consequences for the fetus. Exposure of the pregnant ewe during the latter part of gestation results in reduced placental blood flow and decreased fetal and placental weight.[24] In addition, maternal fever induced by infusion of lipopolysaccharides causes disproportionate increases of fetal temperature, which increases maternofetal temperature difference to about twice normal.[25] The rise in fetal temperature may be explained by a decrease in umbilical and/or uterine blood flows, increases in fetal metabolic rate, and/or the direct effect of lipopolysaccharides on brown adipose tissue. Thus, long-term maternal hyperthermia and persisting fever during pregnancy may constitute more serious risks for the fetus than brief hyperthermia induced by exercise.

MECHANISMS OF HEAT PRODUCTION

Thermogenic responses fall naturally into several broad categories: shivering of skeletal muscle, nonshivering thermogenesis in brown fat, and futile cycling of ions in specialized heat-producing tissues. Each has a distinctive mechanism of action. During shivering, for example, small random muscle contractions hydrolyze adenosine triphosphate (ATP), stimulate respiration, and dissipate the free energy as heat, without doing useful mechanical work.[26] During nonshivering thermogenesis, oxidative energy is not conserved as ATP but rather is released as heat. During futile ion cycling, respiration remains coupled, but significant amounts of heat are dissipated from specialized tissue

by cycling of Ca^{2+} in the sarcoplasmic reticulum with associated use of ATP.[27] It has been speculated that similar mechanisms may be associated with malignant hyperthermia in humans, but whether aberrant Ca^{2+} cycling contributes to cold-induced thermogenesis in newborn mammals remains unknown. Other nonshivering thermogenic mechanisms include protein synthesis-degradation cycling of proteins and K^+-ATPase cycling, but again their importance in the neonatal period is unknown.[28]

The heat provided by each mechanism varies widely depending on species. In the newborn lamb, shivering accounts for about 60% of the increased heat production during exposure to cold, whereas nonshivering thermogenesis accounts for about 40%.[29] In the human newborn, the relative importance of the different mechanisms is not well established, but it is thought to vary with gestational age and severity of temperature stress. This would be in accord with observations in newborn lambs that nonshivering thermogenesis provides the first line of defense against cold exposure, with shivering commencing only after body temperature falls significantly.[29] Nonshivering thermogenesis is clearly not absolutely essential for survival in all species, demonstrated by the fact that this mechanism is lacking in the newborn pig.

Carbohydrate metabolism is also stimulated by cold exposure. Evidence for augmented carbohydrate metabolism includes a fall in hepatic glycogen stores and increased glucose turnover. During summit metabolism, the maximal O_2 use and heat production that can be evoked upon cold exposure, glucose, glycogen, and lipid energy stores are adequate for 8 to 12 hours in the newborn lamb.

Activation and Regulation of Nonshivering Thermogenesis

Before proceeding further, it seems appropriate to briefly summarize our current understanding of thermal changes at birth. During exposure to cold, increased sympathetic activity causes the release of norepinephrine from nerve endings that terminate on the surface of the brown adipocytes. The catecholamine then acts through adrenergic receptors, largely of type β_3-receptors but also through α_1-receptors, to induce acute effects on brown adipose tissue.[2] Activation of these receptors results in increased hormone-sensitive lipase activity by a cAMP-mediated pathway.[30] Increasing lipase activity then enables rapid hydrolysis of triglycerides and phospholipids with the formation of glycerol and fatty acids. These are both oxidized locally in adipose tissue and they also spill into the circulation to be transported to the periphery, where they are used as metabolic fuel. As fatty acid levels increase within the brown adipocyte, a unique uncoupling protein, UCP1, located in the inner mitochondrial membrane is activated[28] (Fig. 55–4). Oxidation continues with the release of large amounts of heat, but there is now no longer the generation of ATP nor the dampening of metabolic rate that rising levels of ATP would entail. The sequence is unusual in that increasing levels of fatty acids promote their own further release, providing a rare example of a feed-forward loop in biology.

When the stimulation of brown fat is continued for prolonged periods, the expression of UCP1 is increased and heat production continues at a greater than normal rate. Thyroid hormones play an increasing permissive role and help facilitate responses to catecholamines.[31–35] The thyroid hormones also directly modulate the activity of UCP1 through an α_1-dependent mechanism and independently stimulate UCP gene transcription.[31]

In recent years, several protein analogues of UCP1 have been discovered that are widely expressed. They include UCP2, UCP3, UCP4, and UCP5/brain mitochondrial carrier protein-1.[36,37] Some appear to have protective action against oxygen metabolism-derived free radicals,[38] but their presence also raises the possibility that a proton leak and the metabolic rate are regulated not only in brown fat but in other tissue types as well. There is

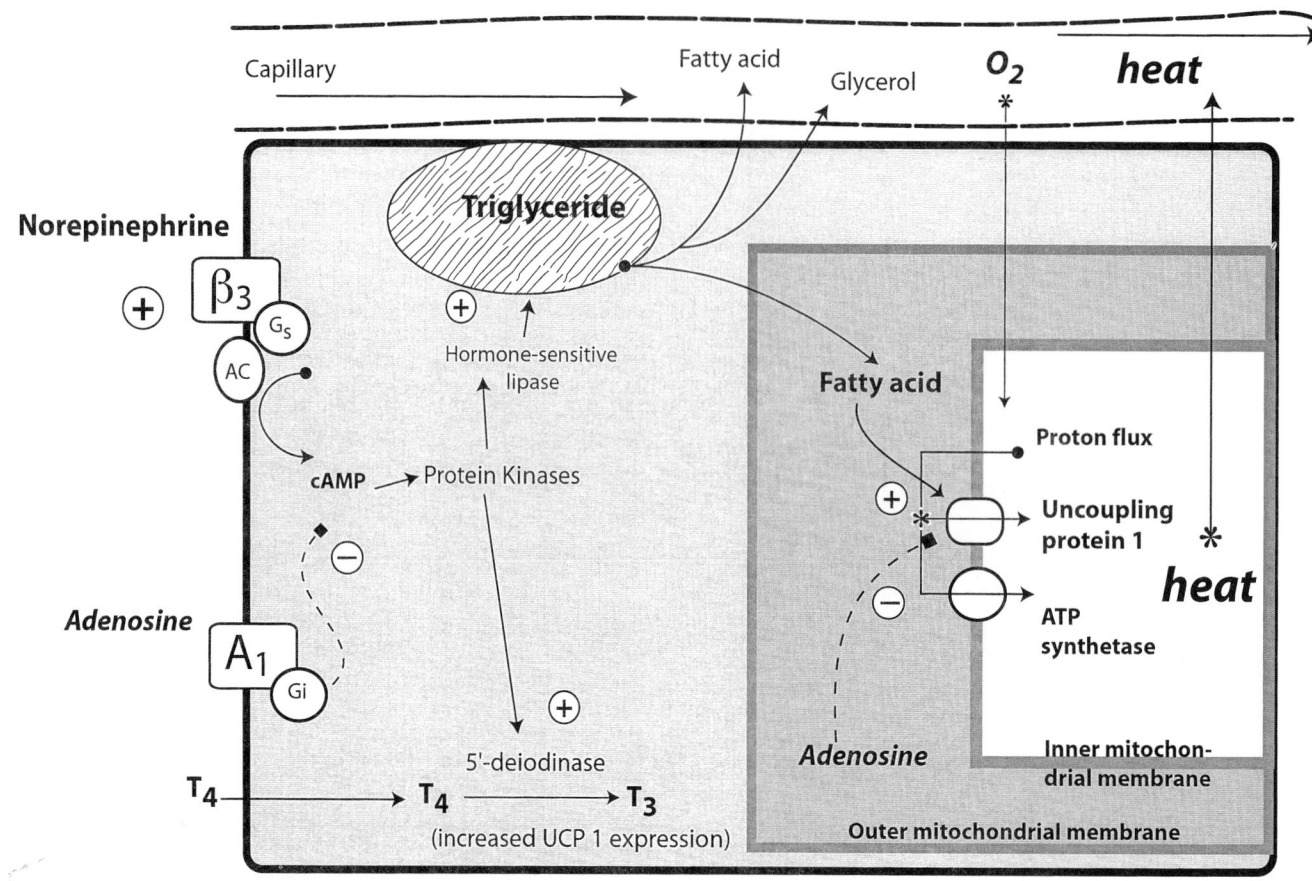

Brown adipose tissue

Figure 55–4. Some metabolic and hormonal controls of brown fat. Control occurs by regulating blood flow; altering the activity of lipase, 5′-deiodinase, and the 32K uncoupling protein 1; and affecting the permeability of the inner mitochondrial membrane to protons. Norepinephrine stimulates thermogenesis through both α_1-receptors and β_3-receptors, but its effects are attenuated *in utero*. Thyroxine T_4 is converted to T_3 within the adipose and increases the expression and activity of the uncoupling protein 1. The means by which brown fat activity is suppressed by adenosine *in utero* remain unknown.

evidence to the contrary during the perinatal period,[28, 36] but further work is needed before the possibility that UCP homologues influence metabolic rate generally can be confirmed or excluded.

Leptin is a hormone produced in brown as well as white fat. Evidence that it may be important in nonshivering thermogenesis is found in adult rats, wherein administration of leptin increases brown fat mass, UCP1 expression, and sympathetic outflow to brown fat. In the newborn rat, maintenance of plasma leptin levels is necessary for increasing oxygen use as a defense against the cold.[39] Furthermore, in the newborn lamb, the administration of leptin helps maintain body temperature.[40] These results indicate that the thermogenic effects of brown fat may not be limited to temperature homeostasis, but may also be important in the regulation of body size and composition. The role of leptin in the fetus and the carryover of early leptin influences into adult life requires further investigation. These pathways are summarized in Figure 55-4.

Whether thermogenic responses help the newborn adapt to extrauterine life immediately after birth, apart from a basic defense against the cold, remains an open question. They may be beneficial because thermogenesis induces dramatic changes in the thyroid, adrenal, and growth hormone axes. An example is the suppression of growth hormone caused by rising fatty acid concentrations that accompany lipolysis and thermogenesis.

INDICATORS OF THERMOGENIC RESPONSE

After birth, the temperature of the mammalian newborn typically falls, and the newborn responds by increasing O_2 consumption and thus heat production. These responses, which begin within a matter of minutes, can persist for many hours.[29, 41] They are particularly strong in the lamb, calf, and rabbit,[42] species in which heat production increases three- to fivefold, and are less powerful in the human, in whom heat production approximately doubles. As noted earlier, when at their maximum level, these responses are termed *summit metabolism*.

Glycerol and fatty acids are the two metabolic products of lipolysis, and hence plasma concentrations of these markers are useful indicators of nonshivering thermogenesis. In the case of glycerol, only negligible quantities of glycerol kinase are present in brown adipose tissue.[2] Therefore, glycerol released within the adipocyte spills into the circulation and is metabolized elsewhere, principally in the liver. Once released into the circulation, glycerol is cleared slowly from the blood and does not pass freely across the ovine placenta.[43] For these reasons, circulating con-

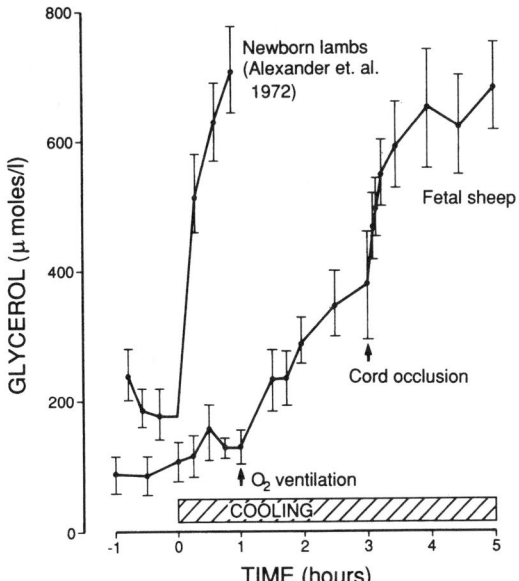

Figure 55–5. Plasma glycerol, an indicator of nonshivering thermogenesis, rises rapidly and markedly in newborn lambs exposed to cold. It rises only negligibly, however, in cooled fetal sheep and only moderately after supplemental oxygen is given. Only after cord occlusion do responses approach newborn levels. This result suggests an intrauterine inhibitor of fetal thermogenesis, possibly of placental origin.

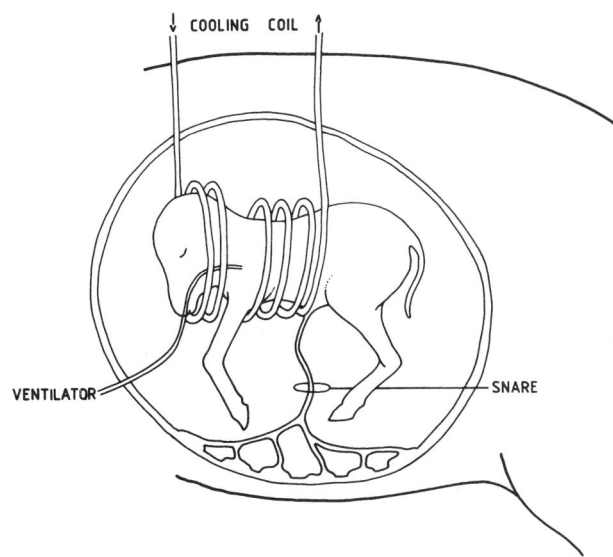

Figure 55–6. Method to study thermogenesis in fetal sheep. Responses to cooling ventilation, oxygenation, cord occlusion, and the infusion of hormones can be tested separately. (From Power GG, et al: J Appl Physiol *63*:1896, 1987.)

centrations of glycerol have proved to be a useful index of lipolysis and hence serve as an index of nonshivering thermogenesis in the fetus and newborn.

Fatty acids differ from glycerol in several important respects. Most are oxidized or reesterified locally within the fat itself. Some, however, enter the circulation, and are transported to the heart, brain, diaphragm, and skeletal muscle, where they provide metabolic fuel and serve as the predominant substrate for shivering. This dispersal of lipid energy reserves permits a more generalized and prolonged thermogenic response than would otherwise be possible and links shivering in skeletal muscle with nonshivering thermogenesis in brown fat. As is the case with glycerol, plasma concentrations of fatty acids are closely related to nonshivering thermogenic activity in the newborn period.[44]

Regulation of Fetal Thermogenesis

Fetal thermogenesis is normally inactive despite the ability of fetal brown fat to respond when studied *in vitro*[45] and despite the fact that even the prematurely delivered lamb can achieve thermoregulation.[41] Several studies indicate that both shivering[46] and nonshivering[47, 48] thermogenic responses are minimal *in utero*. This is clearly shown in Figure 55-5, in which cold-induced responses in plasma glycerol in newborn lambs are compared with those in fetal sheep. Despite intense cooling by artificial means (cold water was circulated through a plastic coil surrounding the fetus *in utero*),[49] as shown in Figure 55-6 and despite reductions in fetal core temperature of more than 2°C, the fetal response can be seen to be relatively weak. Responses in plasma free fatty acids and other indicators of thermogenesis (Table 55-1) are also attenuated and are not stimulated by ventilation of the fetus with either nitrogen or oxygen nor by exogenous triiodothyronine (Fig. 55-7). In other laboratories, only minimal temperature and metabolic responses have been observed after fetal infusions of norepinephrine.[50,51]

This failure to respond despite intense stimulation and supplemental oxygenation raises the possibility that nonshivering thermogenesis is suppressed *in utero*. It can be seen from Figures 55-5 and 55-7 that maximal responses are not observed until the umbilical cord is clamped. In fact, in the presence of cooling and oxygen ventilation *in utero*, activation of brown fat can be turned off and on repeatedly by occlusion of the umbilical cord with a reversible occluder.[52] Likewise, newborn lambs exposed to cold are unable to initiate lipolysis if patency of the umbilical cord is maintained.[53] These studies suggest the presence of one or more circulating inhibitors of thermogenesis (produced by the placenta) that suppress lipolysis in brown fat. Some evidence suggests that adenosine and certain prostaglandins are circulating inhibitors of fetal thermogenesis. Both adenosine[54] and PGE$_2$[55] are produced by the placenta and have short plasma half-lives. The short effective biologic half-life of these compounds would be consistent with the onset of thermogenic responses within minutes after placental separation at birth. Pharmacologic blockade of these compounds *in utero* during oxygenation and cooling stimulates brown fat activation without umbilical cord occlusion.[55,56] Conversely, administration of either of these compounds or their analogues following cord occlusion inhibits the activity of brown fat.[55,57] These findings provide strong evidence of thermogenic inhibitors that circulate before birth. Current knowledge about potential stimuli and suppressors of nonshivering thermogenesis at the time of birth is summarized in Table 55-2.

Caesarean Section and Thermogenesis of the Newborn

The route of delivery influences the strength of thermoregulatory responses immediately following birth. Full-term infants delivered by cesarean section have lower body temperatures that average about 0.3°C less than those delivered vaginally.[58] Brown fat activation and uncoupling protein levels are depressed in newborn lambs delivered by cesarean section compared to those delivered vaginally.[59] Sympathetic activity, plasma levels of catecholamines,[59,60] and plasma levels of thyroid hormones[61] are reduced in infants and lambs delivered by caesarean section. The ability of the newborn lamb to regulate its temperature is improved by intravenous administration of

TABLE 55-1

Indicators of Thermogenic Activity in the Mammalian Fetus and Newborn

Sign	Usefulness and Comment
Plasma free fatty acid concentration	Fatty acids are products of lipolysis; many reesterified without being oxidized; rapid turnover and quick response
Plasma glycerol concentration	Glycerol is also a product of lipolysis; slow turnover and damped response
Body temperature	Nonspecific; thermal inertia causes delays; insensitive
Difference between brown adipose tissue and body core temperature	Highly specific; difficulty arises in verifying location of brown adipose tissue temperature sensor
Oxygen consumption	Relatively nonspecific because measurement includes basal oxygen use as well as shivering and nonshivering components
Direct calorimetry	Research laboratory procedure requiring specialized equipment[4]

norepinephrine, triiodothyronine, or thyrotropin-releasing hormone at the time of caesarean section delivery.[62] The potential benefit of similar treatments in the human newborn appear not to have been tested in a controlled study.

Hypoxia and Thermogenesis of the Newborn

Thermogenic responses are costly in terms of oxygen and substrate use. In the newborn pig, dog, rat, and sheep, exposure to cold can increase oxygen use by 100% or more. This increase in metabolic rate is attenuated if hypoxia accompanies exposure to cold.[63] This inhibition of thermogenic activity by hypoxia appears to be an adaptive response in that it saves oxygen that would otherwise be used to generate heat.[64] Normally the activation of thermogenic activity results when temperature in the hypothalamus drops below the normal thermogenic setpoint. Hypoxia may act by reducing the normal set point and thereby reducing sympathetic outflow in response to cold. Hypoxia also acts locally by suppressing lipolysis in brown fat studied *in vitro*.

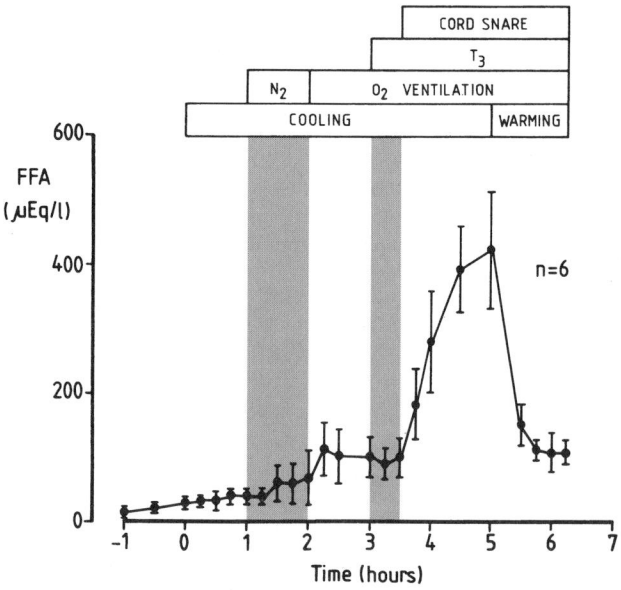

Figure 55–7. Plasma free fatty acids, an index of nonshivering thermogenesis, do not rise appreciably in response to cooling and N_2 ventilation in fetal sheep. Supplemental oxygen and infusion of large quantities of triiodothyronine induce only modest responses. Only after cord occlusion do responses approach a significant fraction of newborn levels. These results suggest that a metabolic inhibitor of placental origin circulates before birth (From Power GG, et al: J Dev Physiol *11*:171, 1989).

By keeping body temperatures lower, the organism not only prevents the use of oxygen for heat production, but also depresses the rate of enzymatic processes due to the effect of temperature on biochemical reactions (Fig. 55-8).

SUMMARY AND CONCLUSIONS

Although the fetus develops in a warm and thermostable environment, its basal heat production is about twice adult levels. Blood flow to the placenta is increased because of the need to maintain adequate respiratory gas exchange, and the placenta functions as a major heat excretory organ. Fetal temperature averages about 0.5°C higher than that of the maternal organism.

A colder environment after birth is sensed by receptors in the skin, spinal cord, and hypothalamus,[65] and the sensory input is then integrated in the hypothalamus. Sympathetic nervous system activity increases and norepinephrine is released from nerve endings in brown adipose tissue. Lipase activity increases[30, 66] and triglycerides are hydrolyzed. Fatty acids are released, which act in a yet incompletely understood manner on a 32-kilodalton uncoupling protein to increase proton conductance across the inner mitochondrial membrane. This process is augmented by triiodothyronine released by intracellular conversion from thyroxine. Most fatty acids are oxidized in the adipocyte with generation of large amounts of heat; some are transported and used as substrate in shivering skeletal muscle, heart, brain, and diaphragm.

Nonshivering thermogenesis does not occur *in utero* because of a lack of O_2 or because of an inability to respond to circulating catecholamines and thyroid hormones. Instead, there is a metabolic inhibition *in utero* caused by placental factors that actively inhibit thermogenesis. Therefore, the placenta provides

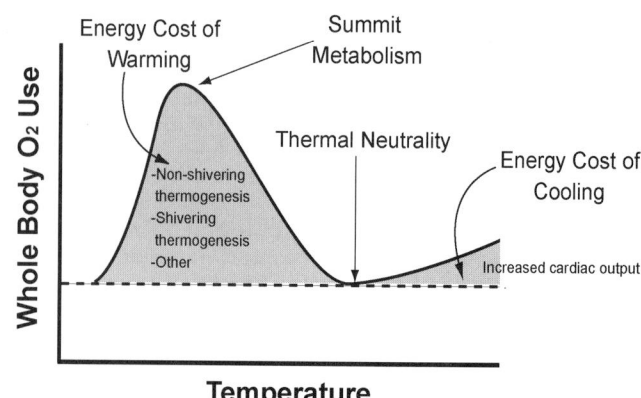

Figure 55-8. A stylized illustration of the relationship between ambient temperature and whole body O_2 use of the newborn.

TABLE 55-2

Sources and Effects of Major Mediators of Nonshivering Thermogenesis in the Mammalian Newborn

Compound	Concentration Changes During Gestation and Parturition	Major Fetal/Newborn Source	Effect on Brown Adipose Tissue
Norepinephrine	Increases after placental separation and in response to cooling	Sympathetic nerve endings within BAT	Stimulates activation of BAT through the β_3 and α_1 receptors
Triiodothyronine	Rises gradually during gestation, then rises sharply at birth	Conversion of thyroxine within BAT by 5′-monodeiodinase	Stimulates production and increases activity of UCP1 within BAT
UCP1	Rises gradually during gestation, peaking at birth, declines thereafter	BAT	Mediates the uncoupling of oxidative phosphorylation in BAT
Prostacyclin	Low during gestation, then increases with onset of ventilation	Lungs	Stimulates lipolysis
Leptin	Rises during gestation, peaking at birth	BAT and white adipose tissue	Stimulates thermogenic activity
Adenosine	High during gestation then falls sharply at birth	Placenta and other organs	Inhibits BAT activation
Prostaglandin E_2	High during gestation, then falls sharply at birth	Placenta and other organs	Inhibits BAT activation

BAT = brown adipose tissue, brown fat.

both the major means of heat transfer for the fetus *in utero* as well as means to limit useless attempts by the fetus to regulate its temperature *in utero*. With this arrangement, clamping of the umbilical cord at birth results in the simultaneous removal of the maternal-fetal heat clamp and activation of thermogenesis by the newborn organism.

ACKNOWLEDGMENT

Support from US Public Health Service Grant HD #65494 is gratefully acknowledged.

REFERENCES

1. Merklin RJ: Growth and distribution of human fetal brown fat. Anat Rec 178:637, 1974.
2. Nedergaard J, Cannon B: Brown adipose tissue: development and function. *In* Polin RA, Fox WW, (eds): Fetal and Neonatal Physiology. 2nd Ed.. Philadelphia, WB Saunders Co, 1998.
3. Power GG, et al: Measurement of fetal heat production using differential calorimetry. J Appl Physiol 57:917, 1984.
4. Ryser G, Jequier E: Study by direct calorimetry of thermal balance on the first day of life. Eur J Clin Invest 2:176, 1972.
5. Dawes GS, Mott JC: The increase in oxygen consumption of the lamb after birth. J Physiol 146:295, 1959.
6. Battaglia FC, et al: The effect of maternal oxygen inhalation upon fetal oxygenation. J Clin Invest 47:548, 1968.
7. Wilkening RB, Meschia G: Fetal oxygen uptake, oxygenation, and acid-base balance as a function of uterine blood flow. Am J Physiol 244:H749, 1983.
8. Itskovitz J, et al: The effect of reducing umbilical blood flow on fetal oxygenation. Am J Obstet Gynecol 145:813, 1983.
9. Asakura H, et al: Interdependence of arterial PO_2 and O_2 consumption in the fetal sheep. J Dev Physiol 13:205, 1990.
10. Dempsey JA, Forster HV: Mediation of ventilatory adaptation. Physiol Rev 62:262, 1962.
11. Parer JT, et al: A quantitative comparison of oxygen transport in sheep and human subjects. Resp Phys 2:196, 1967.
12. Hochachka PW, Lutz PL: Mechanism, origin, and evolution of anoxia tolerance in animals. Comp Biochem Physiol 130:435–459, 2001.
13. Bristow J, et al: Hepatic oxygen and glucose metabolism in the fetal lamb. Response to hypoxia. J Clin Invest 71:1047, 1983.
14. Gilbert RD, Power GG: Fetal and uteroplacental heat production in sheep. J Appl Physiol 61:2018, 1986.
15. Schröder H, et al: Computer model of fetal-maternal heat exchange in sheep. J Appl Physiol 65:460, 1988.
16. Morishima HO, et al: Temperature gradient between fetus and mother as an index for assessing intrauterine fetal condition. Am J Obstet Gynecol 129:443, 1977.
17. Power GG, et al: Temperature responses following ventilation of the fetal sheep in utero. J Dev Physiol 8:477, 1986.
18. Schroder, HJ, Power GG: Increase of fetal arterial blood temperature by reduction of umbilical blood flow in chronically instrumented fetal sheep. Pflug Arch 427:190, 1994.

19. Peltonen R, et al: The difference between fetal and maternal temperatures during delivery (abstract). Uppsala, Sweden, Fifth European Congress of Perinatal Medicine, June, 1976, p 188.
20. Schröder H, Hatano H: Heat transfer across the isolated guinea pig placenta. Pflugers Arch 411(Suppl 1):R205, 1988.
21. Rudelstorfer R, et al: Heatflux from the fetus during delivery. J Perinatol Med 9:311, 1981.
22. Laburn HP, et al: Effects on fetal and maternal body temperatures of exposure of pregnant ewes to heat, cold, and exercise. J Appl Physiol 92:802, 2002.
23. Laburn HP, et al: Effects on fetal and maternal body temperatures of exposure of pregnant ewes to heat, cold, and exercise. J Appl Physiol 92:802, 2002.
24. Bell AW, et al: Some aspects of placental function in chronically heat-stressed ewes. J. Dev Physiol 9:17, 1987.
25. Laburn HP, et al: Fetal and maternal body temperatures measured by radiotelemetry in near-term sheep during thermal stress. J Appl Physiol 72:894, 1992.
26. Hemingway A: Shivering. Physiol Rev 43:397, 1963.
27. Block BA: Billfish brain and eye heater: a new look at nonshivering heat production. News Physiol Sci 2:208, 1987.
28. Lowell BB, Spiegelman BM. Towards a molecular understanding of adaptive thermogenesis. Nature. 404:652, 2000.
29. Alexander G, Williams D: Shivering and non-shivering thermogenesis during summit metabolism in young lambs. J Physiol (Lond) 198:251, 1968.
30. Carneheim C, et al: Cold-induced β-adrenergic recruitment of lipoprotein lipase in brown fat is due to increased transcription. Am J Physiol 254:E155, 1988.
31. Silva JE: The multiple contributions of thyroid hormone to heat production. J Clin Invest 108:35, 2001.
32. Bray GA, Goodman HM: Studies on the early effects of thyroid hormones. Endocrinology 76:323, 1965.
33. Klein AH, et al: Thyroid hormones augment catecholamine-stimulated brown adipose tissue thermogenesis in the ovine fetus. Endocrinology 114:1065, 1984.
34. Swanson HE: Interrelations between thyroxin and adrenalin in the regulation of oxygen consumption in the albino rat. Endocrinology 59:217, 1956.
35. Fisher DA, Kline AH: The ontogenesis of thyroid function and its relationship to neonatal metabolism. *In* Tulchinsky D, Ryan KJ (eds): Maternal-Fetal Endocrinology. Philadelphia, WB Saunders Co, 1980, pp 281–293.
36. Boss O, et al: The uncoupling proteins, a review. Eur J Endocrinol 139:1, 1998.
37. Golozoubova V, et al: Only UCP1 can mediate adaptive nonshivering thermogenesis in the cold. FASEB J. 15:2048, 2001.
38. Echtay KS, et al: Superoxide activates mitochondrial uncoupling proteins. Nature 415:96, 2002.
39. Blumberg MS, Deaver K, Kirby RF. Leptin disinhibits nonshivering thermogenesis in infants after maternal separation. Am J Physiol 276:R606, 1999.
40. Mostyn A, et al: The role of leptin in the transition from fetus to neonate. Proc Nutr Soc 60:187, 2001.
41. Alexander G, et al: Thermogenesis in prematurely delivered lambs. *In* Comline KS, et al (eds): Foetal and Neonatal Physiology. Sir Joseph Barcroft Centenary Symposium. Cambridge, Cambridge University Press, 1973, pp 410–417.
42. Dawkins MJR, Hull D: Brown adipose tissue and the response of new-born rabbits to cold. J Physiol 172:216, 1964.
43. Power G, et al: Unpublished data.
44. Alexander G, et al: The effect of cold exposure on the plasma levels of glucose, lactate, free fatty acids and glycerol and on the blood gas and acid-base status in young lambs. Biol Neonate 20:9, 1972.
45. Klein AH, et al: Development of brown adipose tissue thermogenesis in the ovine fetus and newborn. Endocrinology 112:1662, 1983.

46. Gluckman PD, et al: The effect of cooling on breathing and shivering in unanaesthetized fetal lambs in utero. J Physiol *343*:495, 1983.
47. Gunn TR, et al: Metabolic and hormonal responses to cooling the fetal sheep in utero. J Dev Physiol *8*:55, 1986.
48. Power GG, et al: Oxygen supply and the placenta limit thermogenic response in fetal sheep. J Appl Physiol *63*:1896, 1987.
49. Gluckman PD, et al: Manipulation of the temperature of the fetal lamb in utero. *In* Nathanielsz PW (ed): Animal Models in Fetal Physiology III. Ithaca, NY, Perinatology Press, 1984, pp 37–56.
50. Hodgkin DD, et al: In vivo brown fat response to hypothermia and norepinephrine in the ovine fetus. J Dev Physiol *10*:383, 1988.
51. Schröder H, et al: Fetal sheep temperatures in utero during cooling and application of triiodothyronine, norepinephrine, propranolol and suxamethonium. Pflugers Arch *410*:76, 1987.
52. Gunn TR, et al: Reversible umbilical cord occlusion: Effects on thermogenesis *in utero*. Pediatr Res *30*:513, 1991.
53. Sack J, et al: Umbilical cord cutting triggers hypertriiodothyroninemia and nonshivering thermogenesis in the newborn lamb. Pediatr Res *10*:169, 1976.
54. Sawa R, et al: Changes in plasma adenosine during simulated birth of fetal sheep. J Appl Physiol *70*:1524, 1991.
55. Gunn TR, et al: Withdrawal of placental prostaglandins permits thermogenic responses in fetal sheep brown adipose tissue. J Appl Physiol *74*:998, 1993.
56. Ball KT et al: Suppressive action of endogenous adenosine on ovine fetal nonshivering thermogenesis. J. Appl Physiol *81*:2393, 1996.
57. Ball KT, et al: A potential role for adenosine in the inhibition of nonshivering thermogenesis in the fetal sheep. Ped. Res. *37*:303, 1995.
58. Christensson K, et al: Lower body temperatures in infants delivered by ceasarean section than in vaginally delivered infants. Acta Paediatr *82*:126, 1993.
59. Clarke L, et al: Influence of route of delivery and ambient temperature on thermoregulation in newborn lambs. Am J Physiol *272*:R1931, 1997.
60. Irstedt L, et al: Fetal and maternal plasma catecholamine levels at elective cesarean section under general or epidural anesthesia versus vaginal delivery. Am J Obstet Gynecol *142*:1004, 1982.
61. Symonds ME, et al: Effect of delivery temperature on endocrine stimulation of thermoregulation in lambs born by cesarean section. J Appl Physiol *88*:47, 2000.
62. Heasman L, et al: Influence of thyrotrophin-releasing hormone on thermoregulatory adaptation after birth in near-term lambs delivered by caesarean section. Exp Physiol *84*:979, 1999.
63. Frappell PB, Leon-Velarde F, Aguero L, Mortola JP. Response to cooling temperature in infants born at an altitude of 4,330 meters. Am J Respir Crit Care Med. *158*:1751, 1998.
64. Mortola JP. How newborn mammals cope with hypoxia. Resp Phys *116*:95, 1999.
65. Gunn TR, Gluckman PD: Development of temperature regulation in the fetal lamb. J Dev Physiol *5*:167, 1983.
66. Skala JP, et al: The "second messenger" system in brown adipose tissue of developing rats. Its molecular composition and mechanism of function. Experientia (Suppl) *32*:69, 1978.

Rakesh Sahni and Karl Schulze

56 Temperature Control in Newborn Infants

This chapter is an updated revision of Dr. Kurt Brück's comprehensive treatise on neonatal thermal regulation presented in earlier editions; it is not an original synthesis of the current authors. Brück remains the senior contributor despite his death in 1995. We have immense admiration for his many contributions to our understanding of the physiology of the human neonate. His classic study of temperature regulation[1] provided fundamental knowledge, which has been validated and refined in subsequent years. Using continuous measurements of heat production and cutaneous blood flow, before, during, and after discrete and timed environmental cold stress, Brück defined the fundamental features of the neonatal response to chilling and its dependence on gestational and postnatal ages. These important observations concerning the basic responses of infants to cold—increased heat production and decreased heat loss, as well as the timing of these events and their development pattern—remain central to our understanding of how best to care for human neonates.

CURRENT MODELS AND TERMINOLOGY

It is useful to model the temperature control system of newborn infants using the basic biocybernetic concept of a passive (i.e., controlled) system, the temperature of which depends on metabolic heat production and heat transfer to the environment. The controller consists of sensor, integrator, and effector components (Fig. 56-1). Current understanding provides that information about heat storage and heat gradients within the body is monitored continuously by various central and peripheral thermal sensors. These multiple inputs are transmitted to an integrating neural control network, located in the hypothalamus and limbic systems, which, in turn, is linked by means of efferent neuronal pathways to effector mechanisms that are capable of controlling heat storage. The earlier concept that the controlled variable is a single temperature at a single site within the body has been refined to take into account evidence that temperatures at multiple sites provide important input to the controller.[2-5]

For clarity, the following discussion is structured according to this controller model, reviewing information about the sensors, integrator, and effectors as separate components followed by a consideration of how the integrated control system functions in response to environmental thermal transients, how the system changes during development, and how it operates under special circumstances, such as fever and hypoxia.

PRINCIPLES OF PHYSIOLOGIC TEMPERATURE REGULATION

The maintenance of a stable body temperature that is much warmer than the environmental temperature is a property of the two higher classes of the animal kingdom, birds and mammals. These classes form the group of *homeothermic* beings, all others being designated as *poikilothermic*. A prerequisite of *homeothermy* is a basal rate of metabolism several times higher than that in poikilothermic animals. The former are thus referred to as *tachymetabolic* and the latter as *bradymetabolic* organisms. Furthermore, homeothermy requires a balance among heat production, skin blood flow, sweating, and respiration in such a way that changes in heat loss, or gain, from the environment are precisely compensated.

METABOLISM AND HEAT PRODUCTION

Metabolic processes that provide energy for maintenance of homeostasis and physical exercise are closely linked with heat production. The overall efficiency of energy transformation in homeotherms is only on the order of 10 to 25%, meaning that most of the energy transformed during metabolic activities is liberated as heat and must either be eliminated or stored depending on the needs of the organism. For organisms that are tachymetabolic (including the human neonate), the resting metabolic rate alone is sufficient to increase body temperature by several degrees Celsius above the ambient temperature. The

Control Signals

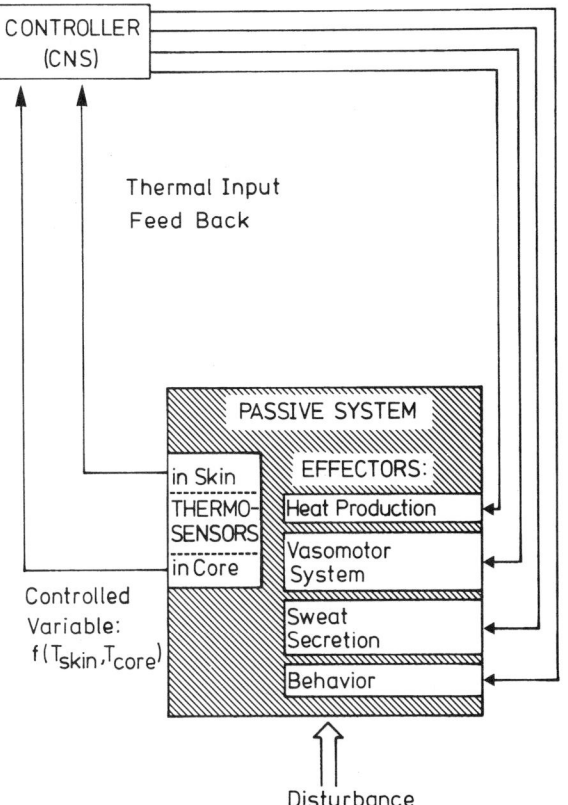

Figure 56–1. Diagram representing the biocybernetic concept of temperature regulation in humans. Temperature is sensed at various sites of the body, and the temperature signals are fed into the central controller *(multiple-input system).*

resting metabolic rate is of great importance for the state of the controlled system (see Fig. 56–1).

Standard Metabolic Rate

The resting metabolic rate depends on several factors, including physical activity, environmental temperature, feeding (thermic effect of food, diet-induced thermogenesis—formerly called *specific dynamic action*), time of day (diurnal rhythmicity), age, and growth rate. By convention, the conditions used for the measurement of resting metabolic rate have been standardized: (1) subjects must be awake and have fasted for at least 12 hours; (2) they must be fully relaxed; and (3) thermoneutral conditions should be maintained.

Metabolic rate measured under these standard conditions is termed the *basal metabolic rate* (BMR). Neonates are unlikely to fulfill the first and second standard conditions at the same time; thus, special conditions for measurement must be defined. The following conditions have been suggested[6]:

1. The infant should remain on a normal feeding schedule (this suggestion is not unreasonable because the maximum increase in energy metabolism in infants is only 4 to 10% after an ordinary feeding).
2. The measurements must be made over a period of 5 to 10 minutes during which the infant is fully relaxed (in contrast with the BMR standard conditions, the infant does not have to be awake). The metabolic rate determination may even be made during postprandial sleep.[7]
3. The measurements must be made under thermoneutral conditions.

The minimum metabolic rate measured in this way is called the standard metabolic rate (SMR) or minimum observed metabolic rate (MOMR).[8] The designation BMR should be used only for determinations performed under standard conditions as employed in adults. Depending on why the metabolic rate is being measured, longer periods of observation (i.e., 3 to 6 hours) are required.[9,10]

Standard Metabolic Rate in Relation to Body Mass and Age

Total heat production is related to body size; for example, the overall metabolic rate of sheep is higher than that of rabbits. Because body temperatures of homeothermic species are close to one another at similar preferred environmental temperatures, it can also be anticipated[11] that the metabolic rate/kilogram body mass (m) will be larger in the rabbit than in the sheep. In fact, the correlation between the logarithm of body weight and the logarithm of resting metabolic rate (oxygen consumption) is close and has a slope of 0.75 for adult animals of various sizes. This means that the metabolic rate per $kg^{3/4}$ of resting animals of different sizes, including adult humans, is independent of body size. This relationship has been termed the *law of metabolic reduction* by Kleiber and has been found useful by some observers for cross-species comparisons of the physiology of metabolism.

Although the Kleiber equation can be useful for predicting metabolic rates when comparing different species, attempts to predict metabolic rates for a group of individual organisms within the same species but of different body sizes reveals its limited applicability. Several deviations from the law of metabolic reduction must be introduced. Age, gender, body shape, and body composition all affect metabolic rate. The age dependency of metabolic rate makes it impossible to predict the metabolic rates of neonates and adults from an individual species with a single exponential function of weight, even if a higher exponent than Kleiber's is used.[1]

As illustrated in Figure 56–2, newborn infants up to 1 week of age have an SMR that is lower than that predicted by Kleiber's equation; that is, the SMR is lower in a 3-kg human newborn than in a 3-kg rabbit. Conversely, in the weight range of 5 to 20 kg, the SMR is higher in human infants than in adult animals of the same weight. During this period of growth, the SMR demonstrates a nearly linear relationship to body weight. Mathematically, this relationship can be expressed by an exponent of b = 1 in the equation SMR = a × m^b. During the period that corresponds to the weight range of 20 to 70 kg, the SMR approaches data in Kleiber's curve.

An exponent close to 1, or somewhat larger than 1, should also be used to calculate the SMR for infants weighing between 1 and 4 kg. This means that during the neonatal period, the SMR/body mass unit is almost independent of weight, whereas a decrease would be expected with increasing weight according to Kleiber's equation (see Fig. 56–2). These SMR values demonstrate a relatively large amount of scatter during the first day of life. A survey of these data and a discussion of the possible reasons for the scattering may be found in the references.[7,12] Given these limitations, it seems worthwhile to avoid attempts to refer observations of the metabolism of the human neonate to standards derived for other mammals.

Certain quantitative changes in the SMR during early postnatal development are worth keeping in mind:

1. Immediately after birth, the SMR/kg body mass is lower in human infants than in adult animals of the same weight (see Fig. 56–2).
2. After birth, the SMR/kg body weight increases and eventually attains a value that is up to 50% higher in infants than in adult animals of the same body mass. The time course of this process appears to be variable. It may take anywhere from 2 days to a few weeks (particularly in premature infants) to attain values that are characteristic of the post-neonatal period.[7,12]

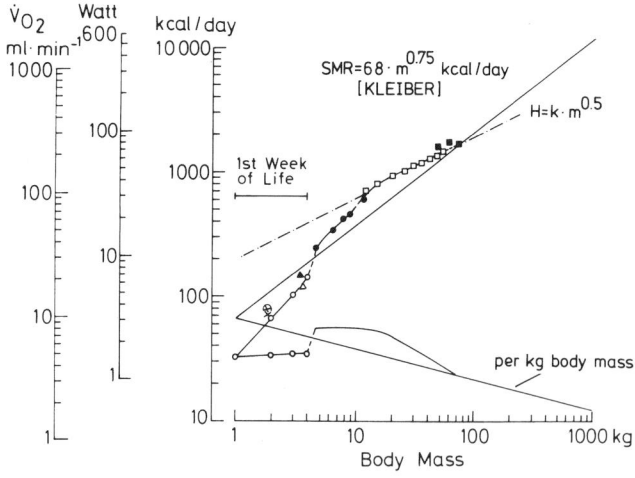

Figure 56–2. Relationship of standard metabolic rate (SMR) to body mass and age. *Top curve,* SMR and the corresponding $\dot{V}O_2$ in relationship to body mass. *Bottom curve,* The same data but expressed in relation to unit of body mass. — = SMR according to Kleiber's equation; —•— = heat production that would yield equal temperature differences between body core and environment. (See text for further discussion.) O = first week of life;[1] Δ = 0–6 h;[111] $\blacktriangle$ = 18–30 h;[111] $\times$ = 4–12 h;[97] $\otimes$ = 1–2 d;[97] $\bullet$ = 1–36 mo;[112] $\square$ = 3–15 yr;[113] $\blacksquare$ = 14–30 y.[114] (Adapted from Brück K: *In* Stave U [ed]: Perinatal Physiology. New York, Plenum Publishing, 1978, p 455.)

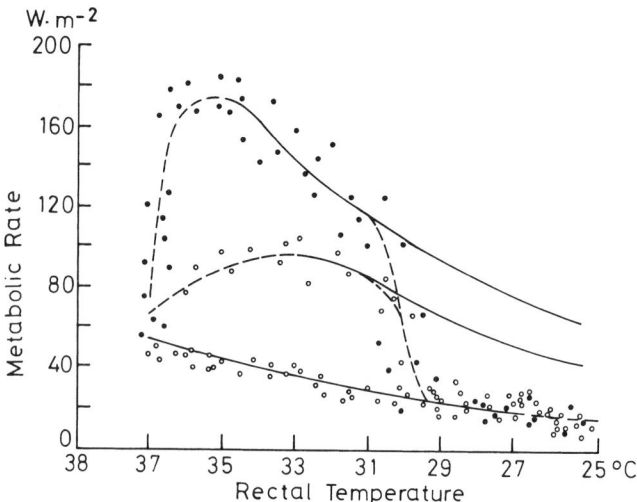

Figure 56–3. Relationship between metabolic rate and rectal temperature in anesthetized dogs the body temperatures of which were manipulated by intravascular heat exchangers. *Top curve,* Light anesthesia; hence, there is a marked cold-induced increase in heat production with decreasing body temperature. *Middle curve,* Moderate anesthesia; the response of heat production to cooling is reduced. *Lower curve,* Deep anesthesia; no cold defense reaction. After having reached a maximum, thermoregulatory heat production follows van't Hoff's law. Note that the upper and middle curves tend to approach the lower curve as soon as the rectal temperature drops below a critical temperature (about 30°C). (From Behmann FW, Bontke E: Pflügers Arch *266*:408, 1958.)

The seeming violation of the law of metabolic reduction (see Fig. 56-2) during the early neonatal period may be only a fictitious problem if one takes into account the considerable change in extracellular water content (extracellular fluid, ECF) that occurs from the early fetal to the adult stage. Sinclair and co-workers[13] have suggested using body weight minus ECF as the reference value in metabolic reference standards. According to their calculations, ECF composes as much as 44% of body weight in a 4000-g newborn infant and 58% in a 1000-g premature neonate. The corresponding average value for ECF in the adult is only 20%. Because the ECF does not participate in oxidative metabolism, the expression "body weight minus ECF" may be considered representative of the active tissue mass. Thus, it seems theoretically justified to relate metabolic rate to this active tissue mass rather than to total body weight. In contrast, the lean body mass (i.e., total body mass minus fat mass) has not been found to be a suitable reference value.

One can also relate metabolic rate in the neonate to the expression "active tissue mass plus adult ECF," that is, to a body mass that corresponds in composition to that of the adult organism. Metabolic rates related to this calculated value closely approximate Kleiber's curve, whereas the metabolic rate related to the actual body weight remains less than the predicted values.[7]

Metabolic Rate in Relationship to Body Temperature

All chemical reactions in an organism are temperature dependent and obey van't Hoff's law. According to this law, oxygen uptake and body temperature of a poikilothermic animal are expected to decrease with falling environmental temperature. This decrease has, in fact, been demonstrated in frogs, reptiles, and other poikilothermic animals without exception. The ratio of the reaction rates at temperatures differing by 10°C is called the Q_{10}. In general, the Q_{10} for the metabolic rate in poikilothermics is about 2 to 3. van't Hoff's law applies to homeotherms in the same way but is masked by regulatory processes.

Thus, in the intact homeothermic organism, the metabolic rate increases initially with decreasing body temperature (Fig. 56-3). This *regulatory metabolic rise* can be prevented by pharmacologic intervention, in particular by deep general anesthesia. As shown in Figure 56-3 (which illustrates the relationship between metabolic rate and rectal temperature in anesthetized dogs), metabolic rate decreases with falling body temperature under both cold-induced and basal conditions (bottom curve in figure). In other words, van't Hoff's law is obeyed. The slope of the curve corresponds to a Q_{10} of 2 to 3. At body temperatures below 30°C, the metabolic rate may drop steeply to the basal curve (*dashed line* in Fig. 56-3), as the thermoregulatory drive generated in the thermointegrative areas of the central nervous system vanishes with increasing hypothermia. The body temperature range at which this reduction occurs may be species dependent.

Before describing the response of the integrated system to changes in environmental temperature, we review what is known about the individual components of the biocybernetic model.

THERMAL SENSORS: THERMORECEPTIVE STRUCTURES AND THE THERMOAFFERENT SYSTEM

Location and Properties of Cutaneous Thermal Receptors

The cutaneous thermal receptors are a group of structures that function as temperature sensors in the temperature control system (the term *sensor* is gaining preference to *receptor* to avoid confusion with chemical structures reacting with specific substances. Both terms are used interchangeably within this section). It is generally agreed that the cutaneous thermosensors in the thermoregulatory system are identical with those mediating thermal sensation. The distribution of the cutaneous thermoreceptors can thus be studied in adult humans by stimulation

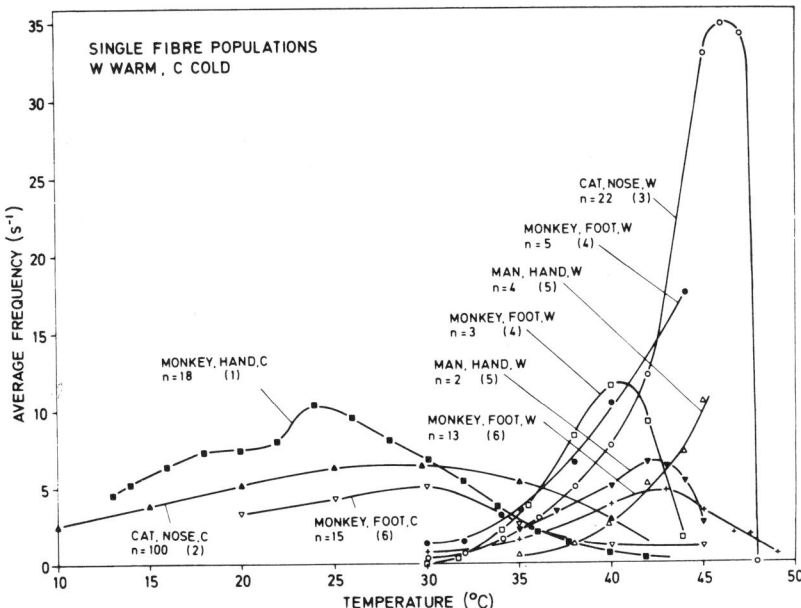

Figure 56–4. Average static discharge frequency of populations of cutaneous cold and warm receptors as a function of skin temperature obtained from various species and body sites by several authors. (From Hensel H: Thermoreception and Temperature Regulation. New York, Academic Press, 1981.)

of so-called warm and cold spots using fine temperature probes. There is scarcely any area of the skin that does not respond to cold stimulation, although the number of cold spots/cm² may vary between one and five on the palm of the hand and more than 15 on the face. The number of warm spots/cm² is much less in all skin areas (0.3–1.7). This agrees with the better spatial resolution of cold stimuli, but it does not mean that cutaneous warm sensitivity is any less developed than is cold sensitivity. In fact, with larger stimulus areas (using thermodes of 10- to 100-cm² contact areas), warm sensitivity can be demonstrated on all skin areas with few exceptions (cornea, glans penis).[14] Employing electrophysiologic methods (recording single-receptor activity from nerves), warm as well as cold receptors have been demonstrated on the faces of cats and other species and on the lower arms and legs of monkeys.[14] By inserting fine metal electrodes through the intact skin into a branch of the radial nerve, it has even been possible to record the activity of single warm and cold receptors in humans in response to thermal stimulation on the skin of the back of the hand.[15]

The morphologic correlate of cold sensors is the fine unmyelinated nerve endings penetrating into the basal layer of the epidermis.[16] These endings contain numerous mitochondria, providing energy for a temperature-sensitive Na^+,K^+ pump, which seems to be part of the transduction of the cold stimulus into an electrical signal.[17]

Figure 56-4 illustrates the average response characteristics of cold and warm receptors from different species (including humans) under static conditions (i.e., after the temperature of the skin had been constant for several minutes). There is minimum activity at a skin temperature of 35°C. The maximum discharge frequency of cold receptors is found between 35° and 20°C and that of warm receptors takes place between 40° and 45°C. At temperatures greater than 45°C, warm-receptor activity decreases. At temperatures lower than about 25°C, the activity of cold receptors may also be reduced.

Sensor activity during temperature changes is noteworthy in that receptor discharges may reach frequencies that are two- to threefold higher than under static conditions. Irrespective of the initial temperature, a warm receptor will always show an overshoot of its discharge on sudden warming and a transient inhibition on cooling, whereas a cold receptor will respond in the opposite way (with an inhibition on warming and an overshoot on cooling). Correspondingly, sensitivity to temperature changes

is also amplified and increases with the size of the exposed area. With exposure of larger areas (e.g., the whole hand), a temperature change of less than 0.01°C/second may evoke a thermal sensation[18] and probably a regulatory reaction.

In summary, thermoregulatory responses elicited through cutaneous thermoreceptors are determined by the average skin temperature (Ts), the rate and direction of temperature change (dTs/dt), and the size of the stimulated area.[14,18] Because of their temperature discharge characteristics (see Fig. 56-4), warm receptors may contribute to the stimulation of heat dissipation actions only when mean skin temperature is considerably increased above normal levels.

Location and Properties of Internal Thermosensitive Structures

Evidence for the existence of deep body thermosensors has been obtained in three ways: (1) by demonstrating that there is poor correlation between body temperature and the action of the final control elements if only skin temperature is taken into consideration,[19] (2) by observing thermoregulatory actions following heating and cooling of circumscribed areas within the body using implanted thermodes and vascular heat exchangers,[20] and (3) by recording the activity of single units of the central nervous system and relating these responses to their own local temperatures.[21]

Hypothalamus

According to thermal stimulation studies (using thermodes implanted on a long-term basis), deep body thermosensors are located in the preoptic area and the anterior hypothalamus. Local warming of this region stimulates heat-dissipating mechanisms (i.e., vasodilation, panting, sweating), whereas it inhibits heat production (i.e., metabolic reactions [Fig. 56–5] and vasoconstriction). Inversely, cooling evokes heat production and vasoconstriction, whereas heat dissipation mechanisms are inhibited.

Thermal stimulation does not permit discrimination between internal cold and warm receptors (e.g., the effects of local cooling might be ascribed to actuation of central cold receptors as well as to the inhibition of central warm receptors). Here further clarification is obtained from single-unit studies.[21] As is shown in Figure 56-6, warming of the preoptic area results in markedly increased activity of one single unit and leads to an

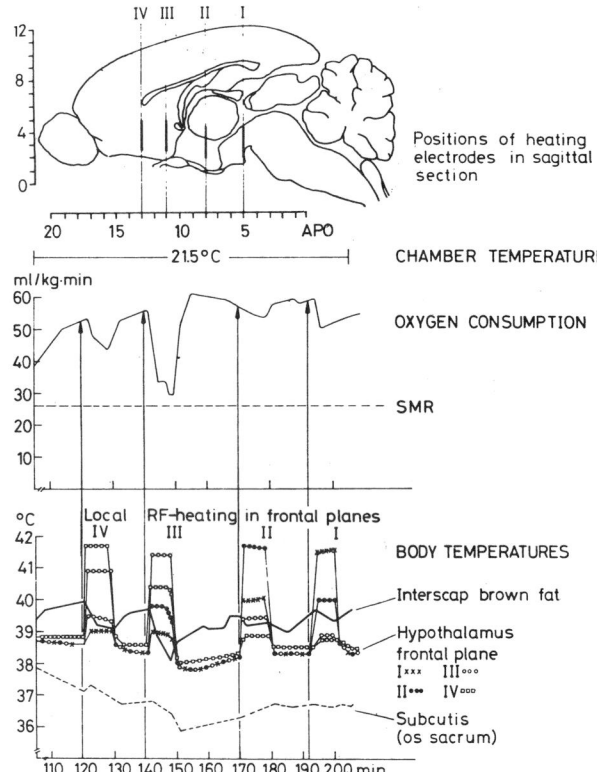

Figure 56–5. Effect of local radio frequency (*RF*) heating in different frontal planes of the hypothalamus on nonshivering thermogenesis (NST) induced by external cooling in a newborn guinea pig (for these small animals, an ambient temperature of 21.5°C is below neutral temperature). The upper part of the figure shows the projection of the four implanted electrodes on the sagittal section of the brain. The different frontal planes were locally heated in succession. Only heating of plane III, corresponding to the preoptic area and anterior hypothalamus, resulted in an almost complete suppression of the cold-induced NST (note reduction of the temperature within the interscapular brown fat). SMR = oxygen uptake corresponding to standard metabolic rate. (From Zeisberger E, et al: *In* Jansky L [ed]: Depressed Metabolism and Cold Thermogenesis. Prague, Charles University, 1977, pp 182–187.)

increase in respiratory frequency (panting). Units like this are considered to be warm sensors.

In vitro studies of hypothalamic slices[22] and of cell cultures[23] have addressed the question of whether hypothalamic thermosensitivity is tied to individual thermosensitive ganglion cells or is based on the temperature dependence of synaptic transmission between afferent and efferent neurons (Fig. 56–7). After synaptic transmission is blocked by electrolyte solutions with a low Ca^{2+} content and a high Mg^{2+} content, the structures in question remain sensitive to thermal stimuli. This implies the existence of thermosensitive cells within the preoptic region and anterior hypothalamus. Both these areas contain not only warm-sensitive cells but also thermosensitive and cold-sensitive cells, the latter two being less numerous than the warm-sensitive cells.

Lower Brain Stem and Spinal Cord

Thermosensitive structures have also been demonstrated in the lower brain stem (midbrain and medulla oblongata), and thermoregulatory reactions can be initiated by local warming of these areas.[24] However, the thermosensitivity of this region is distinctly less than in the preoptic region and anterior

hypothalamus.[20] In contrast, the spinal cord is extremely thermosensitive. When the temperature of the spinal cord is raised only a few tenths of a degree along its entire length in dogs and other animals, the results include panting, vasodilation, and inhibition of thermogenesis.[20, 25] Cooling of the spinal cord elicits shivering, but in this case a greater temperature change is required. In newborn and young guinea pigs, a local temperature change in the region of the cervical cord suffices to trigger thermoregulatory reactions.[3]

Other Thermosensors

Quantitative considerations suggest the existence of thermoreceptive structures outside the central nervous system and the skin.[20] There is experimental evidence for the presence of thermosensors in the region of the dorsal wall of the abdominal cavity and in the musculature. Evidence for the existence of subcutaneous thermosensors has also been confirmed.[26]

Afferent Thermosensitive Pathways

The cutaneous thermoreceptors are served by thin myelinated and unmyelinated axons belonging to the slowly conducting Group III and Group IV nerves. Warm fibers are mostly unmyelinated (Group IV). The axons run within the afferent cutaneous nerve bundles, and they enter the spinal cord through the segmental dorsal root ganglia. Those axons cross over to the contralateral side and ascend within the spinothalamic tract in the anterolateral section of the spinal cord. On their way to the thalamus, the ascending thermal fibers join the medial lemniscus and are accompanied by the afferents coming from the trigeminal region. From the medial lemniscus, collaterals diverge and project to the hypothalamus through a pathway not definitively described. Evidence has been obtained that part of the cutaneous thermal input is conveyed through the spinoreticular pathway to the reticular formation; from there, it is projected to the hypothalamus through the raphe nuclei and the ventral noradrenergic system, which passes the subcerulean area.[24, 27-29]

The spinal cord thermal sensors are connected to the posterior hypothalamus through axons running in an anterolateral pathway of the spinal cord, as has been shown in the young guinea pig[30] and in the cat.[31,32] The thermosensors of the preoptic area also end in the posterior hypothalamus; however, these short pathways have not yet been identified.

INTEGRATION OF THERMAL INPUTS

Integration of Multiple Thermal Inputs

The theoretical concepts of thermoregulation require the demonstration of some elements that "process" the thermal information originating at the receptors in various sites of the body (multiple-input system) and that transform these inputs from the sensors into effector outputs.

There are many experimental studies implicating the hypothalamus (especially the posterior hypothalamic area, which has no appreciable thermosensitivity) as an integration center for thermoregulation. This premise is further supported by electrophysiologic findings. For example, there are neurons in the posterior hypothalamic area the activity of which (discharge rate) is influenced by local thermal stimulation in either the preoptic region or the cervicothoracic part of the spinal cord.[33] At the boundary between the anterior and posterior hypothalamus, neurons have been found that respond to changes in the skin temperature on the limbs and trunk.[24] The posterior hypothalamus, therefore, is characterized by the presence of thermoresponsive cells (i.e., cells that respond to changes in the temperature of distant structures but are not sensitive to changes in their own temperature). However, there is no absolute spatial

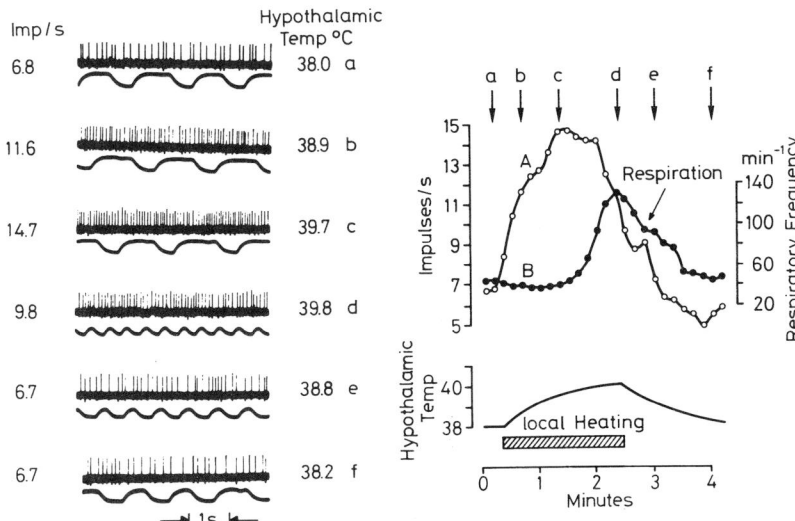

Figure 56–6. *Left panel,* Sections of original records of impulse frequency of a hypothalamic neuron and respiratory rate in relation to hypothalamic temperature. *Right panel,* Discharge of a warm-sensitive neuron in the preoptic region *(curve A)* and simultaneous record of respiratory rate during local heating of the hypothalamus. Arrows marked with lowercase letters designate time at which the original record *(left)* was taken. (From Nakayama T, et al: Am J Physiol *204*:1122, 1963.)

separation of receptive and integrative functions. In the preoptic region and anterior hypothalamus, cells shown to be thermosensitive have also been found to be affected by skin temperature changes and hence are simultaneously thermoresponsive.[4,34]

A special feature of biologic thermoregulation (as compared with the familiar simple technical system) is that two kinds of sensors in different locations (the cold and warm receptors) interact antagonistically. The cutaneous cold receptors are activated when the temperature falls to less than the lower limit of the thermoneutral zone. This reaction is counteracted by heat-activated internal thermosensors when the body temperature rises as a result of overshooting cold-protective mechanisms or after bodily activity. This circuitry enables the protective mechanisms to be set in motion rapidly in case of external cooling, long before the core temperature has begun to fall and internal thermoreceptors can be influenced.

Conversely, heat dissipation processes (vasodilation, sweating) may be activated by internal warm receptors, which are primarily stimulated when body core temperature increases. This effect is counteracted by cold activation of the cutaneous cold receptors. When the body is heated externally, sweat secretion is stimulated by the combined action of cutaneous and internal warm receptors.

Figure 56–8 shows a simplified model of the neuronal circuitry underlying the central nervous system integrative processes. Three kinds of neuronal elements are distinguished: (1) efferent neurons located in the hypothalamus, the axons of which activate the peripheral controlling elements (Fig. 56–9) either directly or, more probably, by way of a chain of interneurons; (2) facilitative and inhibitory interneurons within the hypothalamus; and (3) thermal afferents, arising in part from the cutaneous thermoreceptors and in part from internal receptors (e.g., those of the preoptic region).

Cold receptors directly activate the effectors for thermogenesis. Their inhibitory action on the efferents to heat loss effectors is exerted through interneurons. Activation of warm receptors excites the efferents to the heat loss effectors, simultaneously inhibiting (through interneurons) the efferents to the effectors for heat production. The various effector neurons may receive different combinations of thermal afferents. Thus, as shown in studies in the newborn guinea pig, nonshivering thermogenesis is driven by cutaneous cold receptors and is inhibited by hypothalamic warm receptors, whereas the inhibitory influence of shivering is exerted mainly by spinal cord warm-receptive structures (Fig. 56–10). The cervical spinal cord is the region that preferentially receives (through vascular connections) the heat that is generated in the interscapular brown adipose tissue.[3,7,35] As a result of this "meshed control" of the two heat-generation mechanisms, shivering remains suppressed in the neonate so long as sufficient heat is supplied from the interscapular brown adipose tissue to the spinal cord warm-sensitive structures and to intrathoracic organs.

Principles Guiding the Actions of the Integrator

Given that the thermosensitive structures are distributed over the entire body, the thermoregulatory effector actions (see Fig. 56–9) cannot be described as a function of a single local temperature (e.g., the rectal temperature). Thus, the goal of thermophysiology is to describe thermoregulatory actions as a function

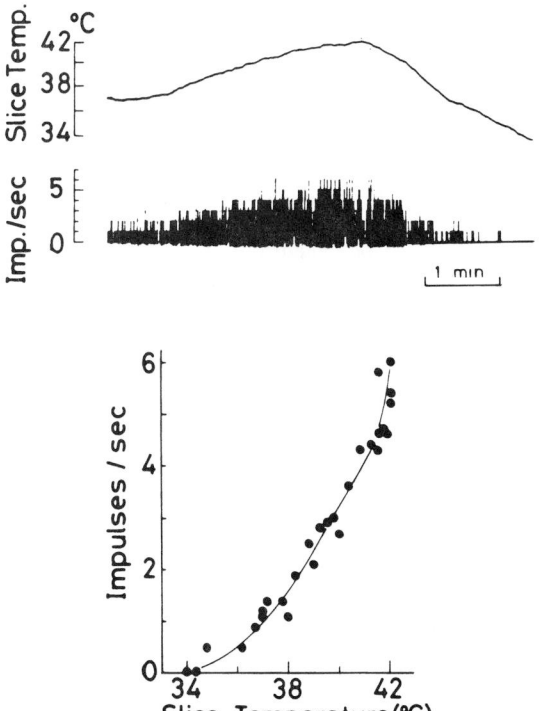

Figure 56–7. *Top,* Original record of a single warm-sensitive unit. *Bottom,* Thermal response curve of the same warm-sensitive unit located in the preoptic area of a slice preparation of the rat hypothalamus. (From Hori T, et al: Brain Res *186*:203, 1980.)

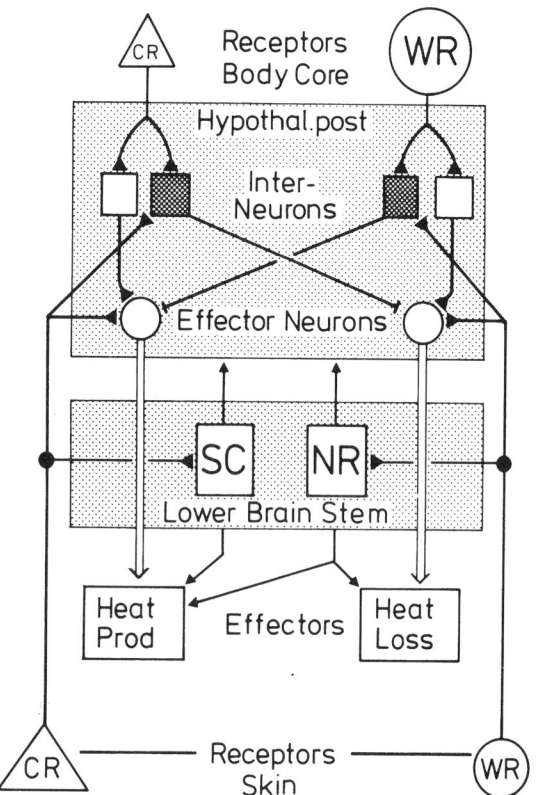

Figure 56–8. Highly simplified model of the connections between thermal afferents and the efferent neuronal networks that control the thermoregulatory effector elements. *Shaded areas* represent the thermointegrative regions of the hypothalamus (mainly the posterior hypothalamus) and the lower brain stem, which contain crucial structures for the processing of thermal information from the skin (RN = raphe nuclei; SC = subceruleus region). The inhibitory neurons shown *(crosshatched squares)* mediate the reciprocal inhibition of the heat-losing and heat-generating processes. CR = cold receptors; WR = warm receptors (size of the symbols indicates roughly the difference in numbers); –◄ = activating, –| = inhibitory synaptic connections. The symbols for neurons represent not single neurons but neuron pools. Some details of the connections among the SC, RN, and hypothalamus are known but are not within the scope of this diagram. The arrows pointing down from the lower brain stem represent pathways to mononeurons and dorsal horn neurons in the spinal cord; the latter can suppress input from the warm afferents. (Data from ref. 24.)

of as many as possible of the temperatures associated with the various thermosensitive parts of the body. Systems of equations with several variables are required for such a description. The data must be collected by experiments on animals in which spatially circumscribed temperature changes are produced by means of thermodes and heat exchangers[20]; in humans, there is only limited opportunity for experimental manipulation of local temperature while the temperature of the rest of the body is kept constant. Only an approximate description is possible, in which the thermoregulatory parameters are presented as a function of two temperatures, the temperature of the interior of the body (measured at a representative site) and the mean skin temperature.[2,28,36] Shivering and sweating threshold temperatures, as well as the temperature pairs yielding equal magnitudes of shivering and sweating, are represented by contour lines in a coordinate system with mean skin temperature and core tem-

perature as the coordinates (Fig. 56–11). Blood flow through the skin follows similar contour lines located between shivering and sweating threshold lines.[37] The contour plots portrayed in Figures 56–11 and 56–12, although involving only two temperatures, are good semiquantitative illustrations of the performance of the multiple input control system. Note that the relative impact of the sensors increases as temperatures become increasingly "out of range," and that the whole contour plot depends on other attributes such as the warm/cold adapted state of the animal. Within a certain range of temperatures (i.e., near the set point), at which the contour lines can be approximated by straight lines, it is possible to express the effector responses as well as the threshold temperature conditions for the elicitation of effector responses in terms of a weighted mean body temperature, T_b, calculated from the following linear equation:

$$T_b = a \times T_{core} + b \times T_{skin}$$

Data from the human adult can be best fitted if values of about 0.9 and 0.1 are chosen for the coefficients a and b, respectively.[28] Figure 56–12 compares the shivering threshold contour lines of adult humans, rabbit, goat, and the young (4-week-old) guinea pig. In addition, the threshold contour line for nonshivering thermogenesis in the newborn guinea pig is given. The curvilinear contour lines in small animals do not allow the use of arithmetic mean body temperature except for small sections of the temperature ranges that may be approximated by straight lines.

SET POINT AND NORMAL BODY TEMPERATURE

In a multiple-input system, the control actions of the thermoregulatory system can be ineffective at various combinations of temperatures. For instance, shivering remains suppressed so long as the combination of body surface and body core temperatures stays at or above the threshold contour line (see Figs. 56–11 and 56–12). Conversely, heat dissipation actions will be ineffective so long as the combination of surface and internal temperature values remains below the heat dissipation threshold hyperbola (see Fig. 56–11).

Under environmental conditions that allow the control actions to reach ineffective levels, the deep body temperature will stabilize at a value typical for the species (if enough time is allowed to attain steady-state heat flow). This temperature, whether measured within the tympanic canal, the rectum, the esophagus, or elsewhere, may then be called the *normal body temperature*. Deviations of such a representative temperature from an empirically attained normal value may be described as a set-point displacement or, more specifically, as a deviation of the threshold temperatures for the respective control actions.

EFFECTOR RESPONSES OF THE THERMOREGULATORY SYSTEM

The effector outputs of the thermoregulatory controller restore the system to the desired set point by regulating both heat production and heat loss. Following a brief review of the relationship between metabolic rate and environmental temperature, control of heat production and heat loss are discussed separately.

Metabolic Rate and Environmental Temperature

The cold-induced increase in metabolic rate (see Fig. 56–3) is the most characteristic feature of homeothermic organisms. In the neonates of all homeothermic species studied thus far (except for the ground squirrel and golden hamster, which are hibernators), a cold-induced increase in metabolic rate has been demonstrated immediately after birth. Although this response may be

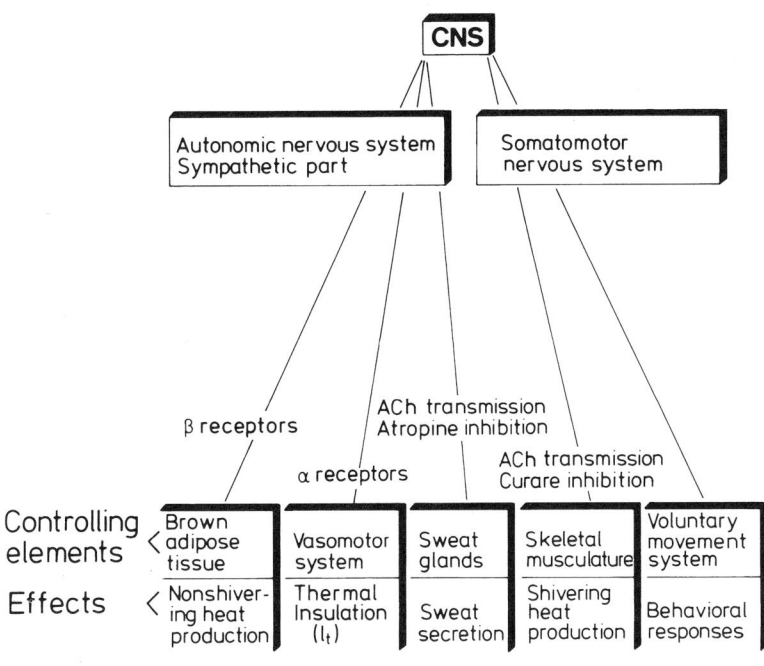

Figure 56–9. Schematic representation of the neural control of the thermoregulatory effector systems. (From Brück K: *In* Schmidt RF, Thews G [eds]: Human Physiology. Berlin, Springer-Verlag, 1983, pp 531–547.)

small during the first hours of life, the neonate should not be considered poikilothermic.

The influence of postnatal age on cold-induced thermogenesis is shown in Figure 56-13. As demonstrated by several investigators, oxygen uptake (directly proportional to thermogenesis) is distinctly higher at 28°C ambient temperature than at 32° to 35°C, even during the first few hours of life. At an ambient temperature of 23°C, oxygen consumption is even greater. Depending on the species, this cold-induced metabolic response increases to a greater or lesser extent during the first week of life. Preterm and small for date infants also increase their metabolic rate with cooling, and on average their response is not much lower than that in full-term infants (see Fig. 56-13). Oxygen uptake values of 15 mL/kg/minute measured at an ambient temperature of 23°C[1] and of 16.8 mL/kg per minute measured at 26°C[38] appear to represent the maximum (summit) metabolic response to cold in 1-week-old full-term infants. For

comparison, in the well-trained young adult, summit oxygen consumption may increase to five times the resting level, that is, to 17 to 20 mL/kg per minute, when the environmental temperature is maintained at 0° to 5°C.

The maintenance of a constant body temperature requires that heat loss and heat production be equal in the steady state. Figure 56-14 illustrates the possible ways in which body temperature can be kept constant when the environmental temperature changes. According to Newton's law, dry (nonevaporative) heat loss is proportional to the temperature difference between the body core and the surroundings. Therefore, in humans, heat loss should be nonexistent at an ambient temperature of 37°C, and it should increase linearly with falling ambient temperature. Because heat loss also depends on heat conduction and convection within the body, and thus on peripheral blood flow, two heat loss curves may be generated (see Fig. 56-14), one for peripheral vasodilation and another for vasoconstriction. Within the thermoneutral zone, heat production (corresponding to the resting [basal] metabolic rate) is in equilibrium with heat loss only if skin blood flow is progressively reduced as the temperature falls from the upper end of the thermoneutral zone (T_3) to its lower end (T_2). At temperatures lower than T_2, body temperature can be kept constant only if heat loss is exactly compensated for by increasing thermoregulatory heat production (cold-induced thermogenesis). The maximum thermogenesis (which amounts to three to five times the BMR in the adult but only two to three times the SMR in the neonate) determines the lower limit of the thermoregulatory range (T_1 in Fig. 56-14). The value for T_1 is about 5°C in the adult and 23°C in the full-term neonate.[1] When this limit is exceeded, hypothermia ensues.

At temperatures above T_3, thermal equilibrium can be achieved only by an additional heat loss mechanism, the secretion and evaporation of sweat. It is not possible for the organism to down-regulate basal metabolic rate. In Figure 56-14, point T_4 indicates the upper limit of the range of regulation, which is determined by the sweat rate capacity. Between points T_3 and T_4, body temperature inevitably increases because of a load error typical for a proportional control system, resulting in an increasing metabolic rate according to van't Hoff's rule.

The term *thermoneutral zone* was originally defined solely with respect to metabolic rate, and some problems arose concerning its use in perinatal physiology.[39] The thermoneutral

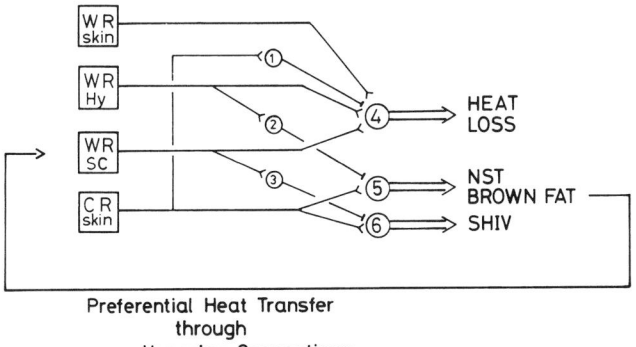

Preferential Heat Transfer
through
Vascular Connections

Figure 56–10. Schematic representation of the presumed neuronal circuitry underlying the control of heat loss and thermogenesis. Note that nonshivering thermogenesis (*NST*) and shivering (*SHIV*) are differentially controlled. CR = cold receptors; WR = warm receptors; SC = spinal cord; Hy = hypothalamus; 1, 2, 3 = inhibitory interneurons; 4, 5, 6 = effector neurons. It must be inferred from experimental evidence that with increasing age, connections are being formed between WR_{Hy} and the no. 6 effector neurons.

zone is now defined as "the range of ambient temperature at which metabolic rate is at a minimum, and within which the temperature regulation is achieved only by control of sensible ("dry" or "nonevaporative") heat loss, that is, without regulatory changes in metabolic heat production or evaporative heat loss."[8] This range is delineated by the symbols T_2 and T_3 in Figure 56-14. In the unclothed resting adult, the lower range limit of the thermoneutral zone (T_2) is 26° to 28°C (50% relative humidity, still air); however, it is 32° to 35°C (operative temperature, 50% relative humidity, still air) in the naked full-term newborn infant.[1, 39] This difference is of great importance, because it shows that environmental temperature conditions that do not require any thermoregulatory effort in the adult may seriously overtax the metabolic thermoregulatory system of the neonate.

In small premature infants (1 kg), the lower limit of the thermoneutral zone may be as high as 35°C.[39] The lower end of the thermoneutral zone may change with postnatal development as body size increases[39] and as small changes in the sensitivity of the thermoregulatory system occur. It is thus extremely difficult to provide exact standard values for the thermoneutral zone in the neonate.

CONTROL OF HEAT PRODUCTION

Modes of Extra Heat Production

The ability to produce extra heat in a cool environment is one of the characteristic features of homeothermy. There are three principal modes of heat production that are responsible for the increase of heat production with decreasing environmental temperature: (1) voluntary muscle activity, (2) involuntary tonic or rhythmic muscle activity (the latter may be manifest as shivering or may be invisible and detectable only by electromyography), and (3) nonshivering thermogenesis. The existence of nonshivering thermogenesis was originally evidenced by the demonstration of a cold-induced increase in oxygen uptake that persisted after neuromuscular blockade with curare.

Shivering and Nonshivering Thermogenesis

In adult humans and in larger adult mammals, shivering is quantitatively the most important involuntary mechanism of thermoregulatory heat production. In contrast, nonshivering thermogenesis is an important and effective mechanism of heat production in the neonates of many mammalian species, including the human infant. In comparison with nonshivering thermogenesis, shivering is a less economical form of heat production in that it inevitably increases convective heat loss because of the body oscillations. Moreover, shivering interferes with body movement. This economical aspect becomes more important in smaller organisms (high surface:mass ratio) with poorer thermal insulation. Thus it is satisfying, from a teleologic point of view, to find that the maximum extent of nonshivering thermogenesis available in one species is inversely related to its order of body size (Fig. 56-15). Extrapolating the regression line in Figure 56-15, one can conclude that subjects with body

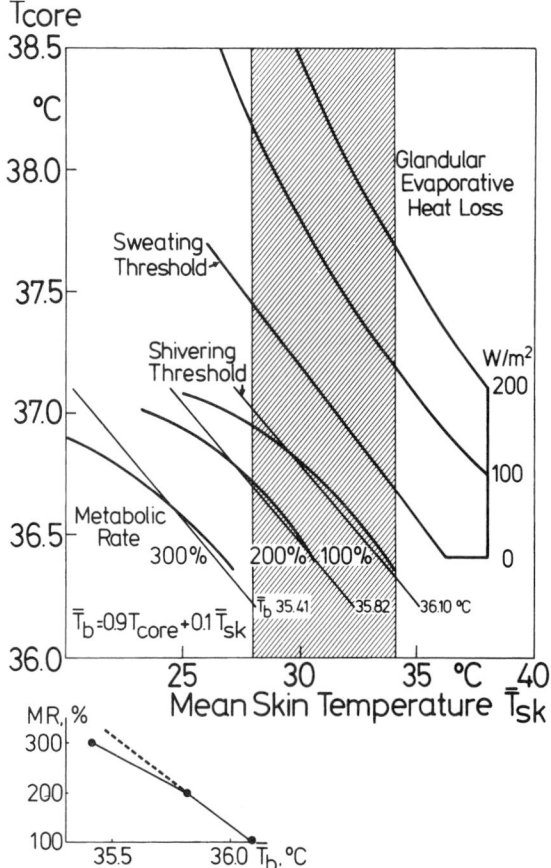

Figure 56–11. Contour plot of metabolic rate and sweat rate (glandular evaporative heat loss) as a function of core temperature and mean skin temperature. The curved lines for metabolic rate were approximated by straight lines (and so might be the 100 and 200 W curves for evaporative heat loss). Each straight line represents all pairs of core and skin temperature with equal $\overline{T}_b$ calculated from the inset equation. Hatched area indicates range of mean skin temperatures relevant for the comparison of shivering threshold values. Percentage metabolic rate *(MR)* in relation to $\overline{T}_b$ is shown at the bottom of the figure. (Data from human adults given in refs. 19 and 36.)

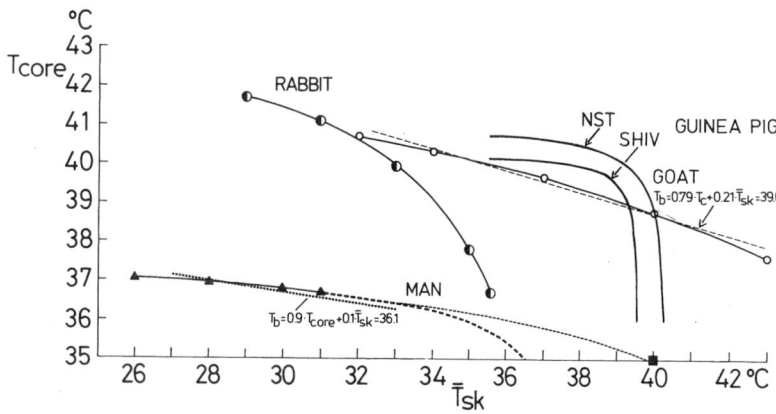

Figure 56–12. Thresholds for shivering (SHIV) and nonshivering thermogenesis (NST) as a function of core (T_{core}) and mean skin temperature ($\overline{T}_{sk}$). Compared are the shivering threshold contour lines from adult humans, rabbit,[116] goat,[20] and 4-week-old guinea pigs[3] as well as the contour line representing threshold conditions for NST in the newborn guinea pig.[117] Note that core temperature is the local hypothalamus temperature in the case of the rabbit and newborn guinea pig and the spinal cord temperature in the case of 4-week-old guinea pigs. The stippled and dashed straight lines represent all pairs of T_{core} and $\overline{T}_{sk}$ with equal $\overline{T}_b$, 36.1 and 39, as calculated from the respective inset equations. (- - - = data from ref. 19 and ···· = data from ref. 115)

weights heavier than 10 kg lack the capacity for nonshivering thermogenesis.

Loss of Nonshivering Thermogenesis

In relatively mature newborns, such as the guinea pig, the extent of nonshivering thermogenesis is greatest at the time of birth and it vanishes within a few weeks (Fig. 56–16). This involution of nonshivering thermogenesis can be retarded and partly inhibited by rearing the animals in a cold environment. After nonshivering thermogenesis has been extinguished through exposure to a warm environment, it can again be evoked by exposing the older guinea pig to a cool environment. In the human neonate, no experimental data are available to document the process of the disappearance of nonshivering thermogenesis. It may be assumed that nonshivering thermogenesis is the prevailing mechanism of thermoregulatory heat production during the first 3 to 6 months of life.[12] By contrast, in the rat, the extent of nonshivering thermogenesis increases during the postnatal period.[40, 41] Such behavior may be expected to occur in other altricious neonates that, like the rat, are born in a relatively immature stage. This would explain the gradual increase in the maximum cold-induced heat production that can be observed during the first few weeks of life in premature infants.[1]

Lack of Nonshivering Thermogenesis

There is at least one example of a species in which the neonates, although small, do not possess nonshivering thermogenesis—the pig. Thus, the piglet shivers vigorously when it is exposed to cold, even on the first day of life.[42] Miniature piglets have no demonstrable nonshivering thermogenesis even when they are reared for a few weeks in a cold environment.[43] In agreement with the data depicted in Figure 56–15, the calf (a larger neonate) has no metabolic response to norepinephrine, indicating the lack of nonshivering thermogenesis.[44]

Sites of Nonshivering Thermogenesis

For many decades, the liver, other intestinal organs, white subcutaneous adipose tissue, and the skeletal musculature were suggested as sites of nonshivering thermogenesis. During the early 1960s it was suggested that brown adipose tissue was the primary site of nonshivering thermogenesis.[40, 45-47]

Shivering

Newborn animals and the newborn infant are rarely seen to shiver in response to cooling, although the metabolic rate is considerably increased. As shown in Figure 56–17, there is no muscle activity demonstrable by electromyography on day 2 of life in the cold-stressed guinea pig. In contrast, on day 12 of life, exposure to the same ambient temperatures (16° and 8°C) evokes bursts of electrical muscle activity that are accompanied by visible muscle oscillations. This does not mean, however, that the shivering mechanism is not developed in the immediate postnatal period.

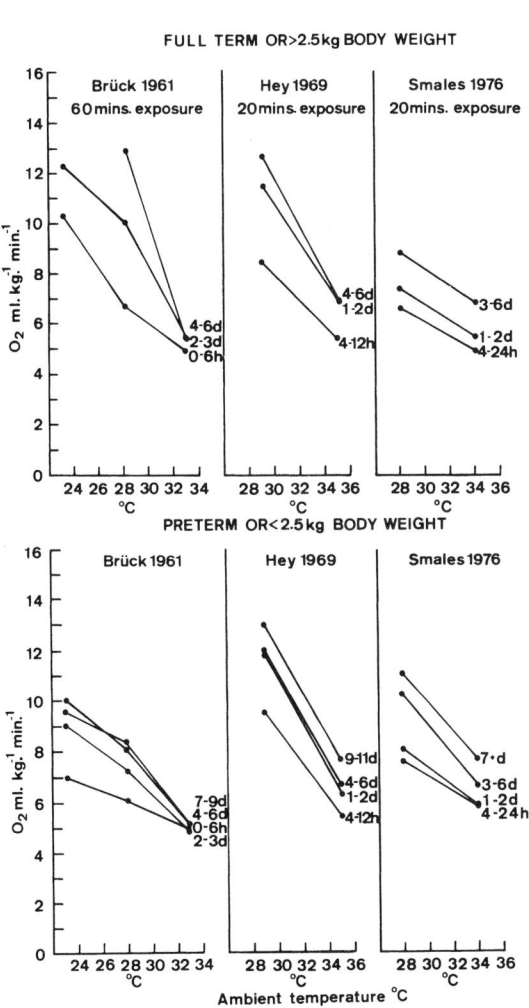

Figure 56–13. Average rates of oxygen consumption of mature infants *(top panels)* and premature infants *(bottom panels)* at different ages and different ambient temperatures as measured by Brück,[1] Hey,[38] and Smales.[118] (From Hull D, Smales ORC: *In* Sinclair JC [ed]: Temperature Regulation and Energy Metabolism in the Newborn. New York, Grune & Stratton, 1978, pp 129-156.)

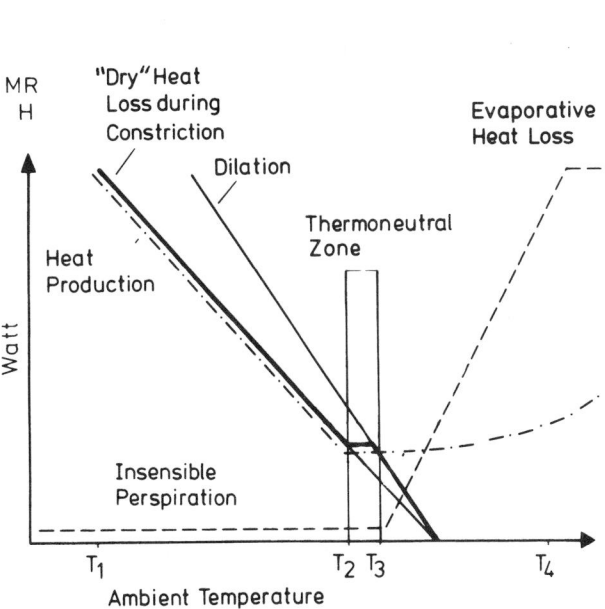

Figure 56–14. Schematic representation of thermal balance in a homeothermic organism. In the range between T_1 and T_3, heat loss is matched by heat production; between T_3 and T_4, evaporative heat loss matches heat production plus heat gain from the environment. In the range T_2-T_3 (thermoneutral zone), heat loss can be matched to resting heat production by vasomotor adjustments. Below T_1, heat loss exceeds the thermogenetic capacity. Above T_4, the production and influx of heat exceed the capacity for evaporative heat loss. MR = metabolic rate; H = heat loss. (For further discussion, see text.)

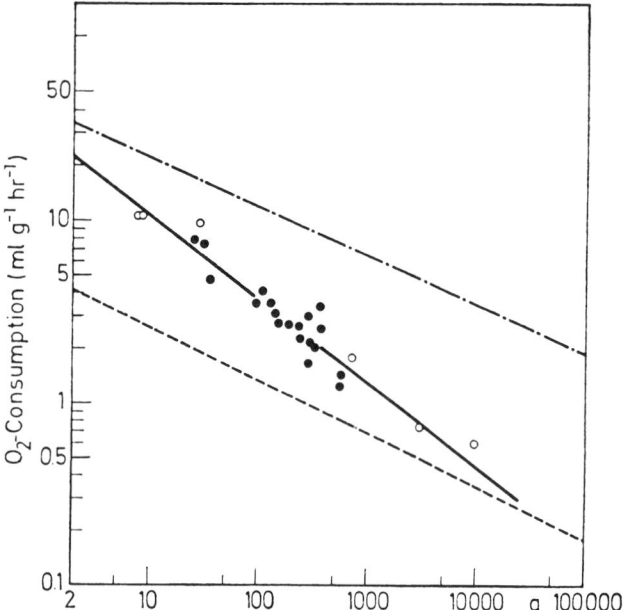

Figure 56–15. Maximum amount of nonshivering thermogenesis, measured as increase in O_2 uptake following norepinephrine injection, in relation to body mass (various species in the adult age). - - - = Minimum O_2 uptake at neutral temperature; - · - = calculated maximum O_2 uptake for exercise. • = rodents; ○ = other mammals. (From Heldmaier G: Z Vergl Physiol *73*:222, 1971.)

To the contrary, it has been shown that shivering can be elicited in the guinea pig on the first day of life when nonshivering thermogenesis is blocked by a β-receptor blocker (Fig. 56–18) and body temperature is thereby allowed to fall. One may conclude, therefore, that the shivering mechanism is well developed at the

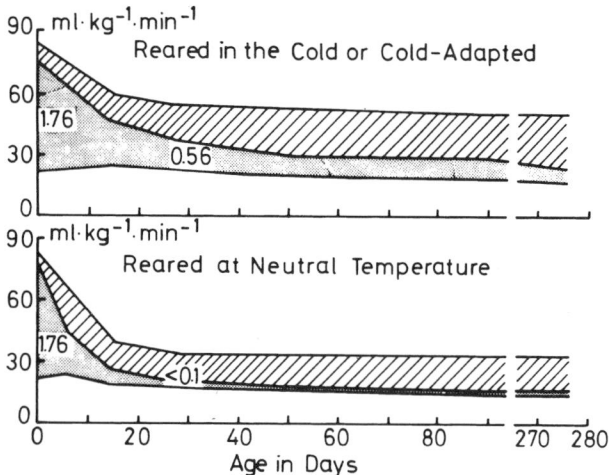

Figure 56–16. Reduction of the maximum extent of nonshivering thermogenesis (NST) with increasing age and the dependence of this process on the environmental temperature at which the guinea pigs were reared. *White area*, minimal oxygen consumption; *shaded area*, NST; *striped area*, shivering. The inset figures indicate the percentage mass of interscapular brown adipose tissue, which is closely related to the maximum extent of NST. Based on data from Zeisberger, et al.[119] (From Brück K: *In* Stave U [ed]: Perinatal Physiology. New York, Plenum Publishing, 1978, pp 455–498.)

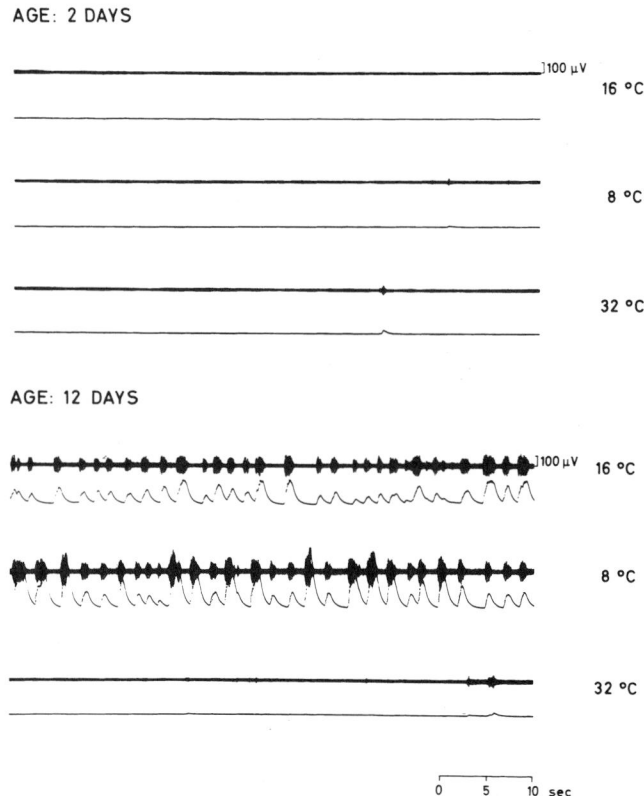

Figure 56–17. Electromyograms from a guinea pig examined on days 2 and 12 postnatally at three different environmental temperatures (indicated on the right side). The lower traces on each record represent the integrated electrical muscle activity. Note that no shivering occurred on day 2 (although oxygen uptake was increased to three times standard metabolic rate). (From Brück K: *In* Linneweh F [ed]: Fortschritte der Pädologie. Berlin, Springer-Verlag, 1965, pp 96-108.)

time of birth but is normally suppressed by nonshivering thermogenesis. Shivering has also been observed in the human neonate with severe hypothermia after birth. It has thus been concluded that the shivering threshold is displaced in the neonate to a lower body temperature in comparison with the adult.

The control of the thermoregulatory effector responses (thermogenesis, skin blood flow changes, sweat secretion, and behavioral responses) is predominantly exerted by the nervous system (see Fig. 56–9); hormonal transmission has a role only in long-term modifications of the thermoregulatory system. Two neuronal systems participate in thermoregulation: (1) the somatomotor system and (2) the sympathetic system.

Metabolic Responses: Neural Control of Shivering and Nonshivering Thermogenesis

Shivering is controlled by means of the somatomotor system. The descending axons of the central shivering pathway project from the posterior hypothalamus to the reticular formation of the midbrain and pons. There they contact the supraspinal pathways and descend to the motor neurons in the anterior horns of the spinal cord. From there the musculature is rhythmically actuated through the motor nerves that leave through the anterior roots.

Nonshivering thermogenesis is controlled from the hypothalamic ventromedial nucleus[48] through the sympathetic nervous system. The transmitter in the target system (in particular, brown adipose tissue) is norepinephrine, which acts on adrenergic

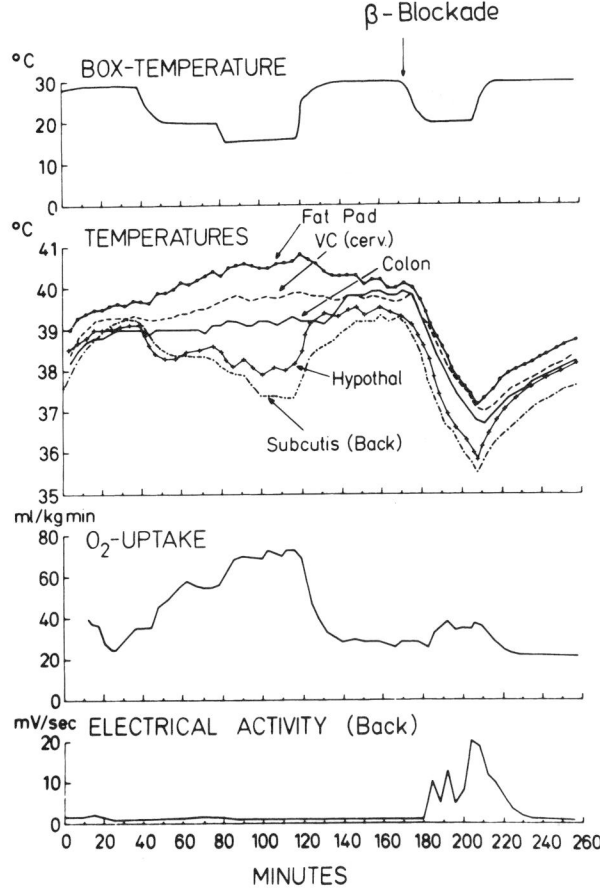

Figure 56–18. Demonstration of shivering and nonshivering thermogenesis (NST) in a newborn guinea pig, age 0 days, body mass 101 g. In the first part of the experiment, only NST occurs during cold exposure. After blockade of NST following administration of a β-receptor blocker, shivering takes place and can be recognized by the increased electrical activity of the bac‹ muscles. Note: Increasing temperature in the area of the interscapular adipose tissue *(Fat Pad)* and in the cervical part of the vertebral canal *(VC [cerv])* occurs before, but parallel decrease of all temperatures occurs after blockade of NST. (For further explanation, see text.) (Adapted from Brück K, Wünnenberg W: Pflügers Arch *290*:167, 1966.)

β-receptors located in the cell membranes. Nonshivering thermogenesis can thus be blocked by β-receptor–blocking agents (see Fig. 56–18). The norepinephrine released at the nerve endings liberates free fatty acids from the lipid droplets and stimulates their subsequent oxidation.

CONTROL OF HEAT LOSS

Vasomotor Responses

Thermoregulatory control of blood flow varies regionally.[49] At least three functionally different regions can be distinguished: (1) acral areas (e.g., fingers, hands, ears, lips, nose), (2) trunk and proximal limbs, and (3) head and brow. Blood flow through the acral areas is controlled exclusively through noradrenergic sympathetic nerves. An increase in sympathetic tone causes vasoconstriction, and a decrease in tone results in vasodilation. In contrast to the distal extremities, heat-induced reflex vasodilation in the trunk and proximal limbs results in a much larger blood flow than that observed after sympathectomy.[50] It has

been suggested that in these areas there are specific vasodilator nerves that inhibit the vascular smooth muscles (active vasodilation).[50] Conversely, additional vasodilation has been ascribed to an enzyme secreted in sweat that catalyzes the formation of a vasoactive mediator, possibly bradykinin. The latter concept is supported by the frequent occurrence of a second phase of vasodilation coinciding with the onset of sweat secretion in the forearm (Fig. 56–19) and by the observed lack of substantial vasodilation in people congenitally lacking sweat glands.[45] Vasomotor nerves exert only a slight effect on the forehead, and there is practically no vasoconstriction in response to cold stress; however, vasodilation does occur in these regions along with sweat secretion in response to heat stress.

Well-developed vasomotor responses to environmental temperature changes have been demonstrated in full-term and premature newborn infants.[7]

Sweat Secretion

Apocrine sweat glands, as found in various mammals such as the Bovidae and Equidae, are controlled by an adrenergic sympathetic mechanism. However, in humans, apocrine sweat glands are controlled by cholinergic sympathetic fibers.[51,52] Consequently, sweat secretion can be inhibited by atropine. Acetylcholine, pilocarpine, and other parasympathetic drugs evoke sweat secretion.

Behavioral Regulation

Behavioral measures must not be neglected in considering the constancy of body temperature. In adults of various species, particularly humans, behavioral measures may have a more important part in temperature constancy than do the autonomic reactions, and under some circumstances they may be the only way to maintain thermal comfort. A civilized human is rarely seen to shiver; he or she would rather increase the set temperature of the air conditioning system or decrease it before perspiration begins.

Behavioral regulation has been generally looked on as a highly developed type of thermoregulation in comparison with the autonomic regulatory measures described previously. More recent studies, however, have shown that behavioral regulation is, from a phylogenetic point of view, the more primitive state of thermoregulation. Behavioral thermoregulatory actions may even be manifested in a species that is not at all able to respond by autonomic effector actions. Thus numerous fish species have been shown to seek out a preferred water temperature when they are given a choice, thereby stabilizing body temperature at a certain level. The "sunbathing" of reptiles is another well-known behavioral thermoregulatory response by which the body temperature is increased to, and precisely maintained at, a level comparable with that of homeothermic animals.[53]

Neonates also make considerable use of behavioral measures. Both piglets and newborn rabbits[54] reduce heat loss by huddling together. Moreover, when newborn rabbits are put into a temperature-gradient environment (a tube with steadily increasing temperature from one end to the other), they will move to a section of the tube warm enough to cause their body temperatures to stabilize near the adult level.[55–57]

In human neonates, postural reactions against overheating have been described.[58] Moreover, babies may cry to signal "thermal discomfort." This would represent another type of behavioral thermoregulation, namely, one mediated by the parents.

ADAPTIVE AND DEVELOPMENTAL CHANGES IN THERMOREGULATION

Unlike engineered physical regulatory systems, thermoregulation by living organisms is not invariant; its properties are influenced by thermal loading itself—its duration, frequency, and

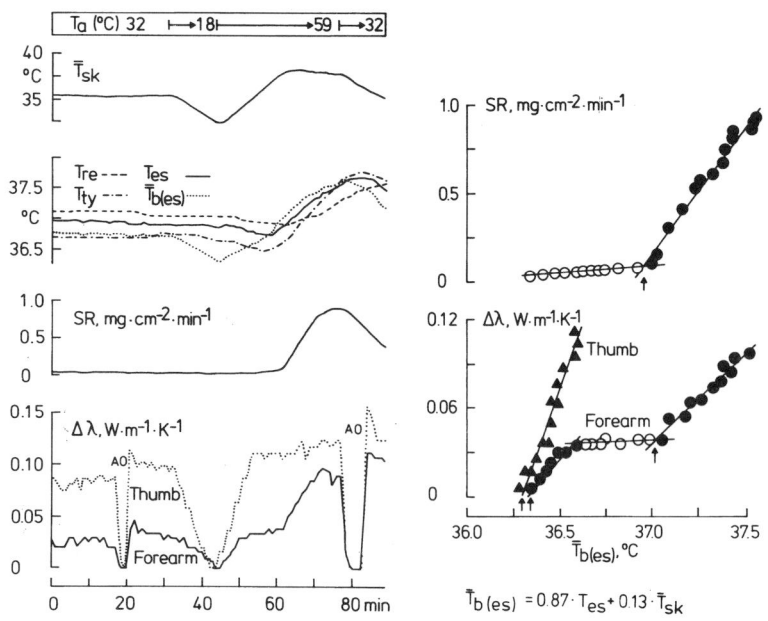

Figure 56–19. Temperature-induced changes in skin blood flow and local sweat secretion (chest) in an adult. *Left,* Before body heating, ambient temperature (T_a) was lowered from 32° to 18°C for establishing initial skin vasoconstriction (skin blood flow estimated from heat conductivity increment [$\Delta\lambda$]); thereafter, T_a was raised to 59°C. *Right,* Skin blood flow and sweat secretion in relation to mean body temperature, $T_{b(es)}$. Note second vasodilation on forearm *(arrow)* coinciding with onset of sweat secretion. $\overline{T}_{sk}$ = mean skin temperature; T_{re} = rectal temperature, T_{es} = esophageal temperature, T_{ty} = tympanic temperature; $\overline{T}_{b(es)}$ = mean weighted body temperature; SR = local sweat rate (chest); AO = arterial occlusion at upper arm. (Adapted from Hessemer V, Brück K: J Appl Physiol *59*:1902, 1985.)

intensity. Some of the so-called long-term thermoadaptive phenomena may be traced to changes in the thermoregulatory system. As for the "passive system" (see Fig. 56-1), heat insulation may change with development because of an increase in the size of the subcutaneous fat layer or growth of a fur coat. The capacity of the effector systems (nonshivering and shivering thermogenesis) and some regulatory characteristics (namely, alterations in the threshold and gain of the relationship between effector response and body temperature)[28, 59] can also undergo changes with development. As a consequence of these thermoadaptive modifications, the range of regulation (see Fig. 56-14) may increase, and the thermal discomfort evoked by thermal stress may be relieved.

Acclimation Versus Maturation

So long as the neonatal temperature control system was considered merely as deficient, it was thought that thermal acclimation, in addition to maturational processes, improved this system postnatally. With regard to nonshivering thermogenesis, however, the capacity of this cold defense mechanism is already maximized at birth in some species (see Fig. 56-16). There is only a narrow margin for improving cold resistance by adaptive modifications in the metabolic system during the neonatal period.

In neonates born in a less mature state, development of nonshivering thermogenesis and brown adipose tissue may proceed postnatally (even at thermoneutral conditions) and contribute to an improvement in temperature regulation. Thus, the increasing summit metabolic rate in response to cold during the first few days of life in full-term and premature infants (see Fig. 56-13) may be due to postnatal development of nonshivering thermogenesis and an increase in brown adipose tissue. In hamsters and rats, which are born in a rather immature state, guanosine diphosphate binding (as a measure of the thermogenic concentration) has also been shown to increase postnatally (altricious animals).[41,60]

Long-Term Threshold Temperature Displacement

Modifications in the threshold temperature for the elicitation of thermoregulatory effector actions have been demonstrated in animals other than humans. In guinea pigs reared in the cold, the shivering threshold is shifted to a temperature level about 1°C lower than in controls reared at neutral temperature (Fig. 56-20).[28,59] This shift enables these animals to make full use

of nonshivering thermogenesis before the less economical shivering mechanism is evoked. A similar shift in the shivering threshold can be produced in adult humans by repeated short-term cold exposure (Fig. 56-21). Linked with the change in shivering threshold in humans is a shift in the threshold temperature

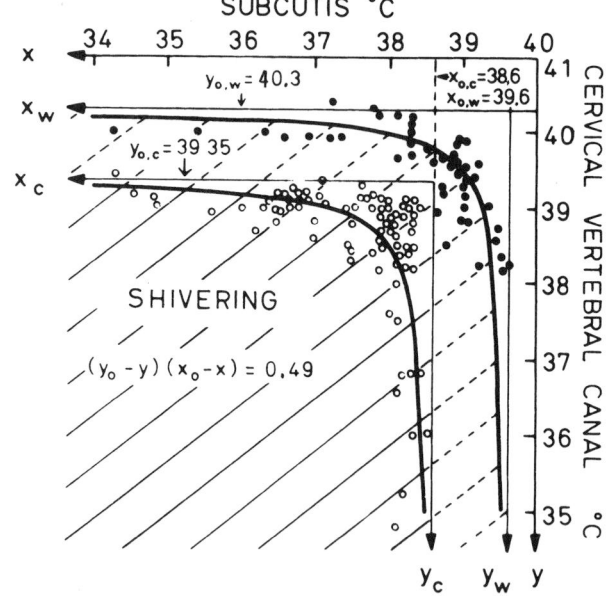

Figure 56–20. Shivering threshold curves for two groups of guinea pigs (aged 4-8 weeks) reared at different environmental temperatures. The values were obtained by independent changes of the body surface temperature and the temperature in the cervical vertebral canal. The diagram shows, for instance, that at a certain body surface temperature, which corresponds to a subcutaneous temperature of 37°C, shivering begins in warm-adapted animals (•) when the hypothalamic temperature drops below 40°C. In the cold-adapted animals (small circle), however, shivering does not occur until the hypothalamic temperature has reached a value slightly below 39°C. (From Brück K, Wünnenberg W: *In* Hardy JD, et al [eds]: Physiological and Behavioral Temperature Regulation. Courtesy of Charles C Thomas, Springfield, IL, 1970, pp 562-580.)

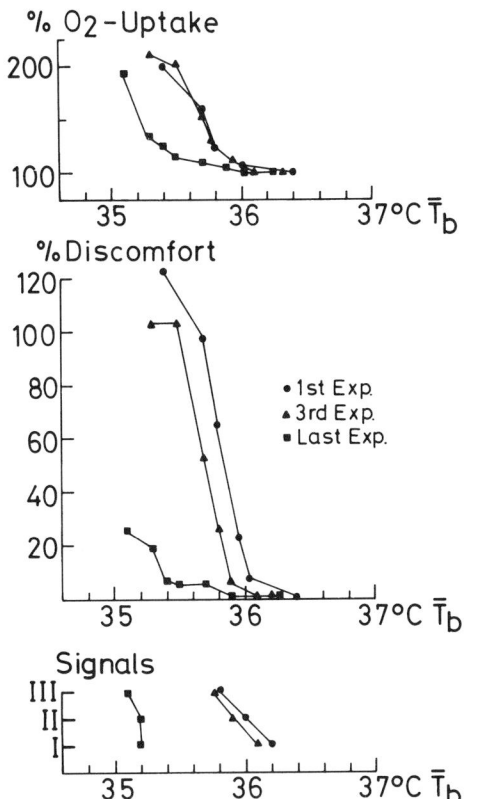

Figure 56-21. Responses of a young man wearing only shorts on exposure to cold (ambient temperature falling from 28°C to 5°C in 45 min) in the course of an acclimatization series. Note that shivering threshold (onset of increase in VO₂) and discomfort threshold were shifted to lower mean body temperatures at the last (sixth day of the acclimatization period) exposure. Signals indicate subjective rating of cold sensation: I = cool; II = cold; III = very cold. (From Brück K, et al: Pflügers Arch *363*:125, 1976.)

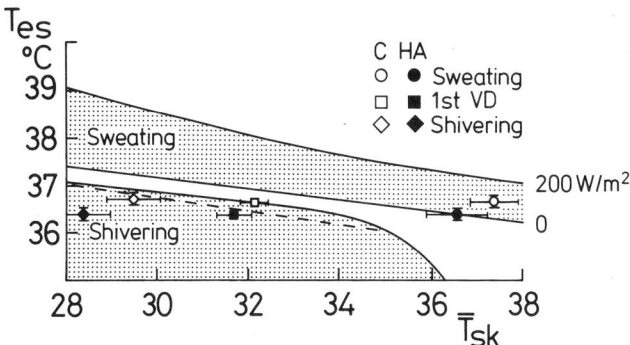

Figure 56-22. Concurrent shift of the threshold temperatures of all autonomic thermoregulatory effectors to lower body temperatures in the course of a 5-day heat adaptation series. Means of seven subjects. Each subject was exposed to heat for about 90 minutes daily. Shivering threshold was determined 1 day before and 1 day after the 5 heat exposure days. (For explanation of lines, see Fig. 56-12.) C = control studies before acclimation; HA = after heat acclimation; 1st VD = first vasodilation (see text). (Data from ref. 62.)

for the experience of thermal discomfort, estimated by the subjects being studied on the basis of a subjective rating scale.[61] This type of adaptation has been called *tolerance adaptation*, that is, larger deviations in body temperature are tolerated before actuation of the appropriate thermoregulatory effectors occurs. In other words, the precision in temperature regulation is reduced, but at the same time cold discomfort is diminished.

Repeated heat exposure has been known to decrease the sweating threshold, that is, there occurs a sensitization in the course of repeated heat exposure rather than development of tolerance. The load error of the thermoregulatory system is thereby diminished, that is, there is a tendency to keep body temperature at less than a critical level. The sweating threshold shift as it occurs during heat adaptation is accompanied by similar changes in the threshold temperatures for shivering and vasodilation (Fig. 56-22). Such concurrent shift of the thresholds for all autonomic effector systems corresponds to a resetting of the set point of the thermoregulatory control system.[28, 62] In some instances the threshold deviation may be accompanied by alterations in the gain of the temperature-response relationship.

Short-Term Threshold Temperature Displacement

In addition to the described threshold changes that occur during repeated or continuous cold-heat exposures for several days or weeks, threshold deviations developing on the order of minutes

have been demonstrated in humans as well as in animals. Short-term shivering threshold displacement in men exposed twice to a low climatic chamber temperature with an interposed 20-minute rewarming period has been observed. During the second cooling phase, shivering occurred at a 0.4°C lower mean body temperature, whereas the slope of the temperature-response relationship was unchanged. In addition, the thresholds for skin blood flow as well as for sweating were shifted to lower values when the subjects were exposed to cold before they started an exercise test; this shift led to vasodilation and sweating . Hence, a short cooling period causes a concurrent displacement of the threshold temperatures for all autonomic thermoregulatory responses in adult humans. In animals adapted to normal room temperature (21°C), this phenomenon of short-term acclimation is even more pronounced.

Previous observations in premature infants who were maintained at ambient temperatures so low as to yield steady-state body core temperatures near 35°C without arousing any cold defense have been ascribed to such short-term acclimation. In a subsequent study on a group of premature infants (i.e., those weighing less than 1500 g), minimal oxygen uptake was compatible with rectal temperatures in the range of 35° to 36°C. As judged from the time spent in quiet sleep, these babies did not show any signs of thermal discomfort.[63] Thus, the discomfort threshold can also shift to a lower level of body temperature. Moreover, the infants in that study exhibited a slight tendency toward vasodilation, indicating a decreased threshold for vasomotor responses. However, these effects may be related to postnatal maturation.

Maturation

Although the control system (passive system, see Fig. 56-1) undergoes considerable alteration during ontogenesis, the thermoregulatory system tends to maintain deep body temperature from birth onward at a value typical for the species. This maintenance requires a number of adjustments by the thermoregulatory system to the smaller body size of the neonate. These adjustments may be mediated by an increased thermogenic capacity, an additional heat production mechanism (nonshivering thermogenesis), and special changes in threshold conditions for eliciting effector responses. Conversely, modifications developing during thermal adaptation may consist of intrinsic

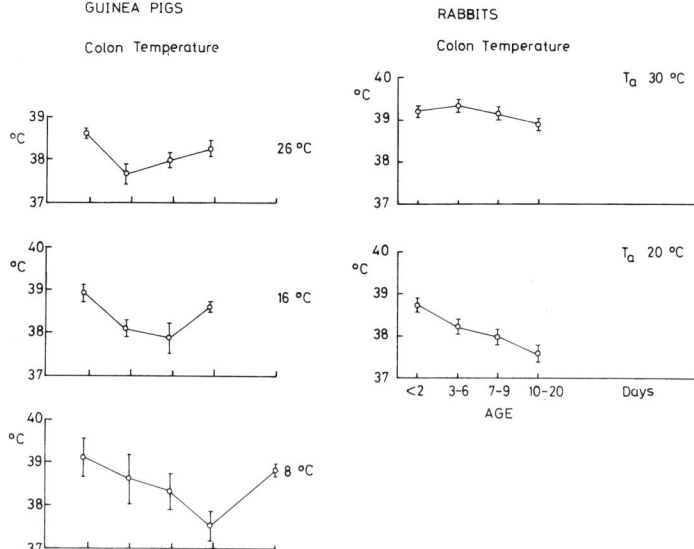

Figure 56–23. Colon temperatures in guinea pigs and rabbits in relationship to age and ambient temperature (T_a). (Data from refs. 69 and 120.)

mechanisms functioning in a neonatal organism that has not been stimulated by any environmental factor. These same mechanisms may serve to adjust the regulatory system either to body size or to special environmental conditions.

Stability of Deep Body (Core) Temperature During Ontogenesis

As shown in Figure 56-23, colon temperature in the newborn guinea pig or rabbit is maintained very close to the adult level, even during severe cold exposure. Remarkably, thermostability seems to be even greater during the first few days of life than it is later on. In the guinea pig, this enhanced stability can be accounted for by a greater metabolic response in the younger and smaller animal (Fig. 56-24). As shown in Figure 56-16, the newborn guinea pig maintains body temperature mainly by non-shivering thermogenesis. In other species, for example, the pig or miniature pig, nonshivering thermogenesis does not occur. In these species, shivering supplies the extra heat for stabilizing body temperature at ambient temperatures as low as 20°C in the neonate.[43] In the human neonate exposed to ambient temperatures of 33° to 23°C, the thermoregulatory effort is much larger

than in the adult for a given ambient temperature (Fig. 56-25). The metabolic increase is mainly due to nonshivering thermogenesis.

Changes in the Passive System

The neonatal passive system is characterized by a large body surface area:volume ratio and by decreased heat insulation resulting from the smaller absolute thickness of the body shell. With growth, the surface area:volume ratio decreases by a factor of 2.7. Comparison of data from neonates[64] and adults[65] indicates that overall insulation (I_{a+t}) (Fig. 56-26) increases by a factor of 1.8 as body mass increases from 3.5 to 70 kg. In a cool environment, maximum tissue insulation (I_t) changes by a factor of 3, and air insulation (I_a) increases by a factor of 1.2 because of the change in the curvature radii of the trunk and extremities.

The heat production, H, required for equilibrium heat flow at any given overall temperature difference would therefore have to be nearly five times as large in the neonate as in the adult (per unit of body mass). From the preceding data, an equation is derived that predicts heat loss in relation to body mass (m) at a given temperature difference between body core and environment (see Fig. 56-2):

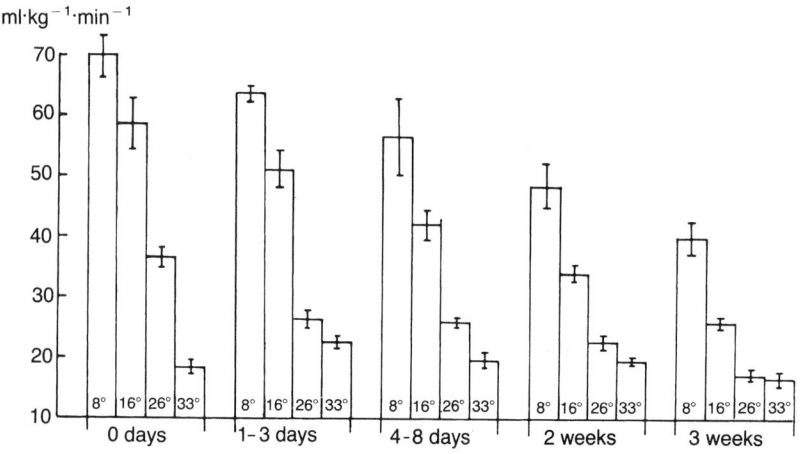

Figure 56–24. Heat production (expressed as oxygen uptake) in relationship to ambient temperature and age in the guinea pig. (From Brück K, Wünnenberg B: Pflügers Arch *282*:362, 1965.)

$$H = k \times m^{0.5}$$

The SMR is actually lower in the neonates of various species than heat loss predicted from the preceding equation. It even falls short of Kleiber's equation in which metabolic rate is related to body mass to the 0.75th power (see Fig. 56-2). In humans, beginning with the second year of life (corresponding to a body mass of more than 10 kg), the SMR is a function of the body mass to the 0.5th power. In the first year of life (especially during the first week of life), the SMR in relation to body mass is only 1.5 to 2 times larger than in the adult. This means the overall temperature difference (ΔT) that can be maintained in the full-term neonate under the condition of SMR is less than half that of the adult (and even less in the premature infant) (Fig. 56-27). At an ambient temperature less than 33°C, deep body temperature will drop unless heat production is increased. In fact, metabolic rate is increased at such high ambient temperature that the lower limit of the neutral temperature range is shifted to a higher level of ambient temperature.

Adjustment of Effector Threshold Temperatures

Because of the small amount of tissue insulation, the difference between core and mean skin temperature is considerably smaller in the neonate than in the adult. Thus cold defense reactions should be elicited at higher mean skin temperatures than in the adult to maintain core temperature at the adult level (Fig. 56-28). In other words, the threshold for increasing vasoconstrictor tone and for the metabolic reactions is shifted to a higher level in the

neonate, thereby adjusting the thermoregulatory system to the smaller body size.

The displacement of the neonatal threshold temperature can be explained in two ways. First, because of the increased body surface area to body mass quotient, the number of cutaneous cold receptors/unit body mass is increased (assuming that the density of the distribution of cold receptors is the same in adults and neonates). Second, the central processing of thermal input signals (see Figs. 56-1 and 56-8) in the neonate is different from that noted in the adult. In any case, the increased cutaneous sensitivity is a prerequisite for enabling the newborn infant to maintain core temperature (within a limited range of environmental temperature) at the same level and with the same accuracy as occurs in the adult.

Stage of Maturity of the Thermoregulatory System at Birth

Temperature regulation is frequently referred to as immature at the time of birth. However, one should be cautious in asserting immaturity of the thermoregulatory mechanisms even though the neonate shows a greater fluctuation in body temperature than does the adult. Greater fluctuations of body temperature are to be expected in smaller organisms because of their large surface area:volume ratio, the relatively small insulating body shell, and the smaller body mass that acts as a heat buffer in large organisms. Because of these peculiarities in body size and shape, a reduced range of regulation (see Fig. 56-14) should be expected in the neonate.

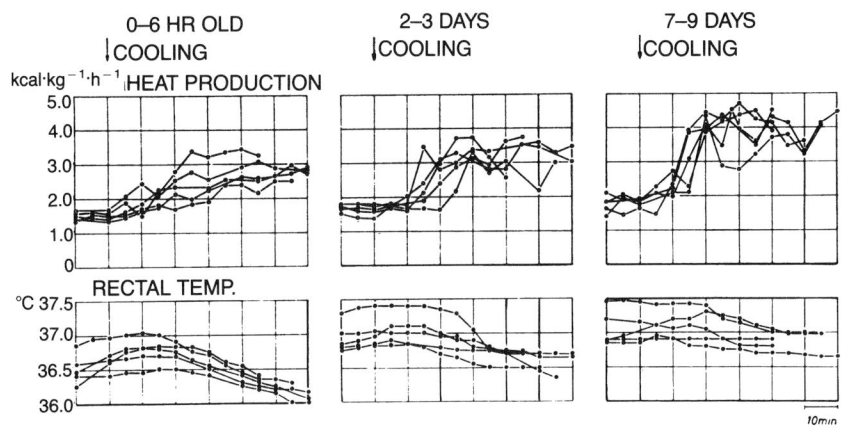

Figure 56–25. Course of rectal temperatures and heat production in full-term newborn infants. Ambient temperature to the left of downward-pointing arrow 33°C, then quick drop to 23°C. (From Brück K: Biol Neonate *3*:65, 1961. S Karger AG, Basel.)

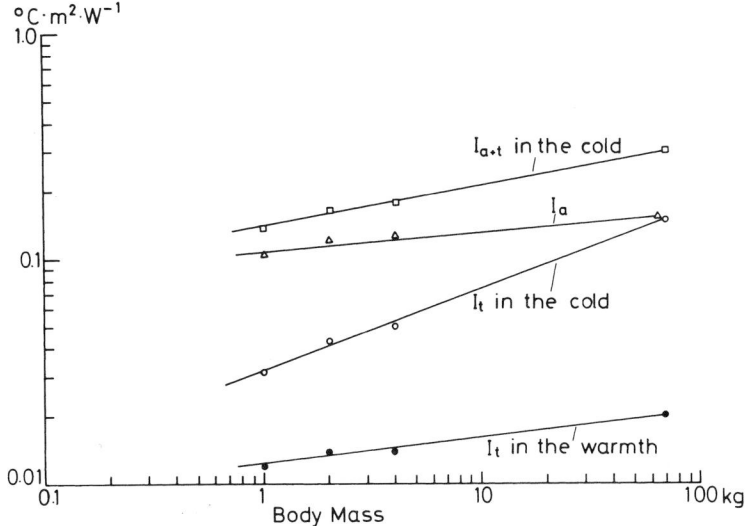

Figure 56–26. Tissue insulation (I_t) under cold and warm environmental conditions, ambient insulation (I_a), and total insulation (I_{a+t}) in relation to body mass in humans. (From Brück K: *In* Stave U [ed]: Perinatal Physiology. New York, Plenum Publishing, 1978, pp 455–498.) (Based on data from refs. 64 and 65.)

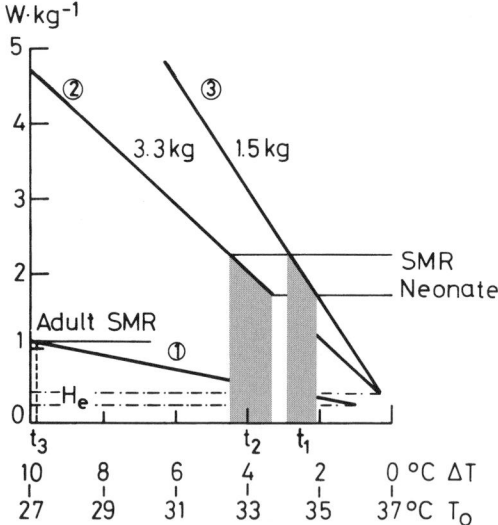

Figure 56–27. Schematic representation (based on data given in Figs. 56-2 and 56-26) of heat production/unit body mass required to maintain the temperature differences (ΔT) between body core (37°C) and environment (operative temperature, T_O = weighted mean of air and radiation temperature) in the adult (1) and in a 3.3-kg (2) and a 1.5-kg (3) infant (with maximum vasoconstriction). With the actual standard metabolic rate (SMR) given, the temperature differences t_1, t_2, and t_3 can be maintained under conditions of thermal neutrality; conversely, the neonates require an environmental temperature of about 33°C (2) or even 34° to 35°C (3) to maintain a deep body temperature of 37°C, whereas this level is much lower in the adult, 27°C (T_3). H_e = minimum evaporative heat loss. (From Brück K: *In* Stave U [ed]: Perinatal Physiology. New York, Plenum Publishing, 1978, pp 455-498.)

The degree of maturity of the thermoregulatory system should be evaluated according to the following three criteria:

1. What is the capacity of the effector system (a) in comparison with the adult and (b) in relation to body size?
2. What is the qualitative and quantitative (threshold, gain) responsiveness of the effector systems to thermal stimuli?
3. Are there qualitative or quantitative differences in the central thermointegrating system between the adult and the neonate?

With regard to the first criterion, the capacity of the metabolic system in full-sized human neonates is comparable with that of an adult system when the metabolic rate is related to body mass, but it is too small to compensate for heat loss in as wide a range of ambient temperatures as in the adult. Therefore, the tolerated ambient temperature range (range of regulation) (see Fig. 56-14) is reduced. The full-term neonate is, at best, able to maintain a stable body temperature at an ambient temperature as low as 23°C (Fig. 56-29), at which point maximum thermogenesis is required for thermal balance. In the adult, by contrast, maximum thermogenesis (although smaller/unit body weight) is sufficient to balance heat loss at an ambient temperature as low as 0° to 5°C. It is notable that the adult as well as the neonate can maintain thermal balance under these extreme conditions only for restricted periods (30-60 minutes). More extended exposure results in exhaustion of the metabolic system and hypothermia. In the neonate born at term gestation, the lower limit of the range of regulation (see Fig. 56-14, T_1) comes closer to that of the adult than it does in the preterm neonate.

With regard to the second criterion, the threshold and gain for the metabolic reactions are adjusted to the smaller body size of

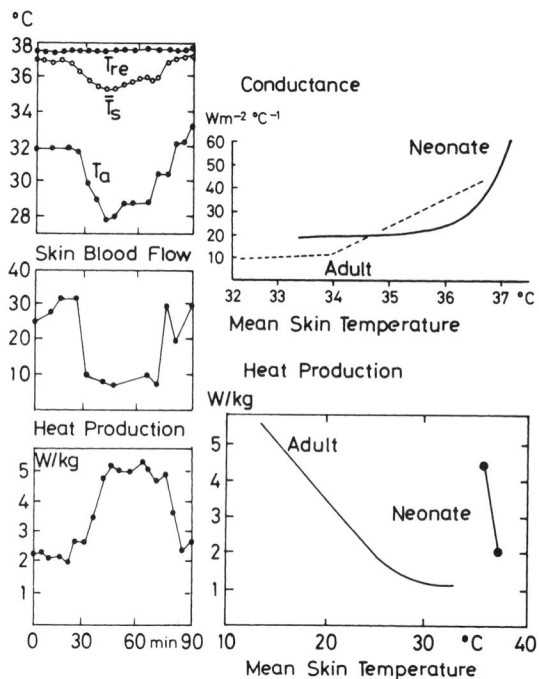

Figure 56–28. *Left,* Simultaneous response of skin blood flow (heel) and heat production to a slight drop in mean skin temperature ($\check{T}_s$) evoked by a decrease in ambient temperature (T_a) from 32° to 28°C. Study in a 7-day-old infant, 3290 g. *Right,* Relationship between $\overline{T}_s$ and heat production in adults[121] and newborn infants[1] and thermal conductance (peripheral blood flow) in relationship to mean skin temperature in neonates[122] and adults.[123] Note onset of responses at higher body temperatures in the neonate. (From Brück K: *In* Stave U [ed]: Perinatal Physiology. New York, Plenum Publishing, 1978, pp 455-498.)

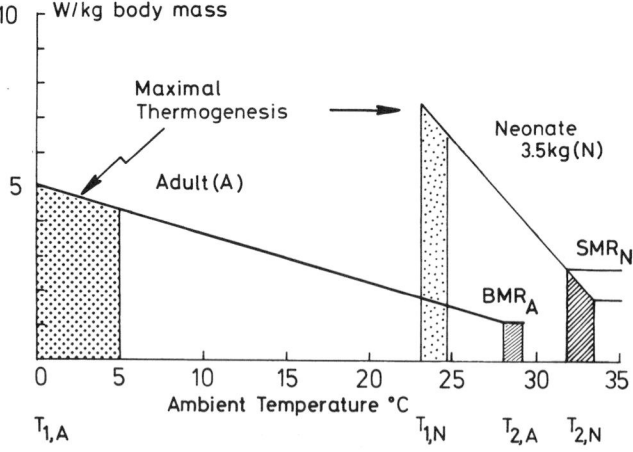

Figure 56–29. Minimal (basal or standard) and maximum metabolic rate in relation to ambient temperature in the neonate (*N*) and the adult (*A*). The inflection point of each curve marks the lower limit of the thermoneutral zone (T_2), which is shifted to a higher temperature in the neonate because of the relatively low standard metabolic rate (SMR). As the SMR rises during the first few days of life, $T_{2,N}$ shifts to lower ambient temperature. The lower limit of the range of regulation, T_1 (compare Fig. 56-14), is determined by the maximal rate of heat production and is about 23°C in the newborn and 0° to 5°C in the adult. (Data from ref. 7.)

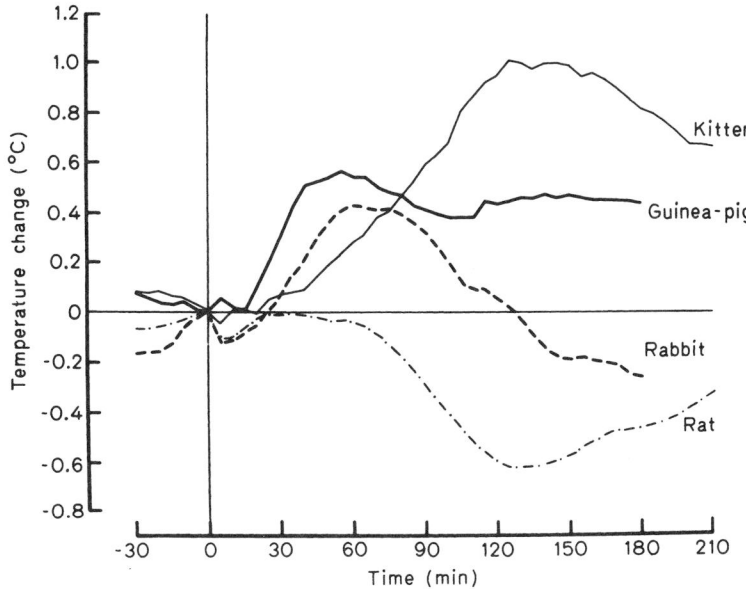

Figure 56–30. Average body temperature changes in the newborn of four species after two intraperitoneal injections of 20 µg/kg *Escherichia coli* endotoxin at the individual thermoneutral ambient temperature. (From Szeákely M, Szeleányi Z: *In* Milton AS [ed]: Pyretics and Antipyretics. Berlin, Springer-Verlag, 1982, pp 479-528.)

the neonate (see Fig. 56-28). The sweating threshold is comparable with that in the adult, except in premature and small for gestational age neonates[66] in whom the threshold is shifted upward. Even in the very small premature infant, metabolic and vasomotor control responses are developed at birth,[1,67] although the threshold for elicitation of these responses may not be appropriately adjusted to body size. In addition, the capacities of the effector systems may be smaller than in the adult. In the neonate, maximum evaporative heat loss is in the range of the SMR,[66,68] whereas in the adult it is five times the SMR.

As for the third criterion, no substantial neuronal or hormonal differences have yet been described between the neonatal and adult thermoregulatory systems.

According to these criteria, one may distinguish three groups of mammals with respect to their functional stage of temperature regulation immediately after birth. The first group exhibits a thermoregulatory system more or less completely adjusted to a smaller body size. The body temperature is stable within a certain control range. This range is narrower, however, than in the adult. Members of this group include the full-term human neonate, the guinea pig,[69] the pig,[42] the miniature pig,[43] the lamb,[70] and larger mammals such as the calf.[71]

The second group of mammals has the following characteristics: thermoregulatory responses can be evoked at birth, but either the capacity of the effector systems or the threshold temperatures, or both, are not sufficiently adjusted to the smaller body size. Body temperature drops on exposure to environmental temperatures slightly less than thermal neutrality. Mammals in this group include the low birth weight human newborn,[1] the kitten, the rabbit,[72] the puppy,[73] and the rat.[74]

In the third group, thermoregulatory responses are not evocable, and oxygen uptake does not increase with decreasing environmental temperatures, but follows van't Hoff's law (see Fig. 56-3). These animals (e.g., the ground squirrel[73] and the golden hamster[60,75]) behave as poikilothermic animals do. This group is presumably restricted to the neonates of hibernators.

PATHOPHYSIOLOGY

Sudden Infant Death Syndrome

A possible role for hyperthermia in sudden infant death syndrome (SIDS) has been hypothesized because some victims are found in unusually warm environments, are warm and sweating

when found dead, are wrapped tightly in clothing or bedding, have a history of febrile illness before death, or have high rectal temperatures at examination or autopsy.[76,77] Given the association between SIDS and another important risk factor, prone body positioning,[78] investigators have recently begun to examine the relationships among body position, body temperature, state of sleep, and cardiorespiratory activity. Infants sleeping prone have a higher peripheral skin temperature.[79,80] The heat loss is lower in infants sleeping prone than in those sleeping supine, perhaps because of less heat loss from the head. Thus, it takes prone infants longer than supine infants to reach the lower rectal temperature that occurs after the onset of sleep and rectal temperature remains higher during sleep.[81,82] The weight of evidence obtained from term and low birth weight infants and infants a few months old also suggests that prone positioning is associated with reduced heat production. Even so, heart rate,[83,84] blood pressure,[85] and absolute skin temperatures[79,80] are higher and temperature gradients from central to peripheral skin are narrower.[86] Taken together, these data suggest that despite attempts to eliminate heat through adjustments in the peripheral circulation (narrowing central-peripheral gradients) infants are unable to maintain set-point temperature(s). Alternatively, the prone position may be linked to an elevation in the set point. Either way, the evidence points toward probable differences in autonomic control of metabolism and cardiorespiratory function in the prone versus the supine position.

Fever

It is well known that newborn infants may suffer severe infection without increased body temperature. In contrast, there are clinical reports of body temperature elevations higher than 38° to 39°C in newborn infants with septicemia, purulent meningitis, and pneumonia.[87] Experimental studies suggest that some peculiarities of fever mechanisms exist during the neonatal period. Newborn lambs fail to respond with fever following the administration of bacterial pyrogen or leukocyte pyrogen during the first few days of life.[88] Newborn guinea pigs have been shown to react to adult doses of pyrogen no sooner than a few days after birth, but they do respond with fever immediately after birth when this pyrogen is administered at much higher doses than in the adult.[87] If one takes certain precautions (e.g., providing an ambient temperature that does not overwhelm thermogenesis, sufficient nutrition, and so on), a pyrogen fever comparable to that of the adult may be

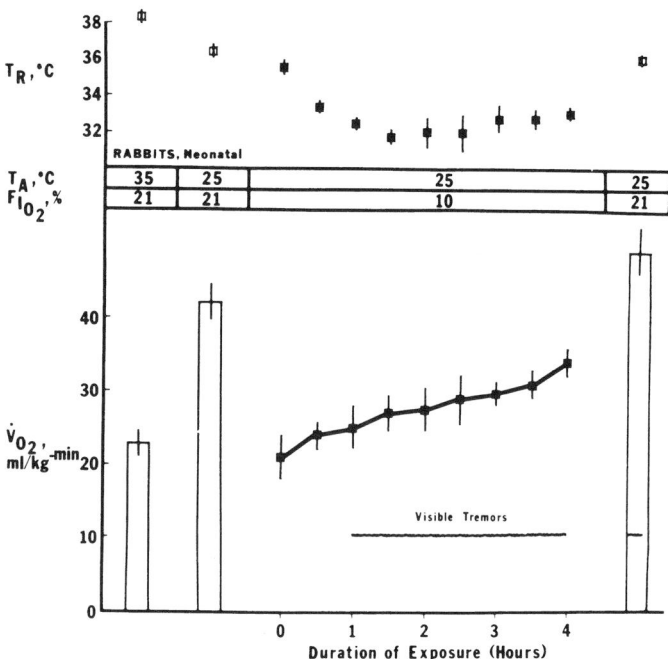

Figure 56-31. Effect of cold and hypoxia on the oxygen consumption and colonic temperature of unanesthetized newborn rabbits. Exposure to 25°C in air caused a rise in oxygen consumption, which was produced without shivering. This rise was abruptly abolished when the inspired oxygen content was lowered to 10%. During the next 4 hours, oxygen consumption gradually increased. Visible shivering developed after 1 hour and persisted into the posthypoxic period. (From Blatteis CM: *In* Smith RE [ed]: Bioenergetics. Proceedings of the International Symposium on Environmental Physiology. Bethesda, MD, 1988, pp 151-160.)

evoked in the neonates of many species. There are, however, many species-related differences in the pattern of the febrile response. For example, the newborn guinea pig demonstrates a biphasic response when endotoxin is administered intraperitoneally (Fig. 56-30). In contrast, 0- to 3-day-old rabbits exhibit a short-lasting monophasic fever, and 3- to 6-day-old kittens show a more sustained monophasic fever. A hypothermic response is commonly observed in 8- to 10-day-old rats.[87] In most cases, pyrogen administration causes heat production to increase; as in thermoregulation, nonshivering thermogenesis is a prevailing mechanism of extra heat production during febrile response.

Mechanism of Fever

Set Point Displacement. Fever develops as a result of an activation of cold defense reactions as they normally occur when an organism is exposed to cold. Generally the process begins with peripheral vasoconstriction and is followed by enhanced thermogenesis. In the adult, the latter response is accompanied by shivering, whereas in the neonate, nonshivering thermogenesis prevails. With increasing body temperature, these thermoregulatory effector actions, thermogenesis and vasoconstriction, are diminished just as if the organism aimed to reach a new target temperature. Recovery from the fever is induced by the activation of heat dissipation mechanisms—vasodilation and sweating. During the constant fever phase, thermal disturbances (see Fig. 56-1) are compensated for by the appropriate control processes. It appears from this description that the thermoregulatory effector system remains completely functional but that the organism aims to assume and sustain a higher body temperature during fever. This phenomenon has been termed *set-point displacement*, thereby excluding other conceivable interpretations, for example, a toxic effect on one or more effector systems (see Fig. 56-9). Current fever research is focusing on the question of how bacterial and viral toxins (exogenous pyrogens) act to finally affect the thermointegrative system (see Fig. 56-8) in such a way that the body temperature is shifted to a higher level.

Pathogenesis of Fever

Fever is considered an immunoreactive process.[89, 90] Certain fever-producing substances of external origin (e.g., exogenous

pyrogens), such as the heat-stable lipopolysaccharides of bacterial membranes (endotoxins), stimulate granulocytes and macrophages of the reticuloendothelial system to produce a heat-labile peptide called *endogenous pyrogen*. Endogenous pyrogen is identical to the cytokine interleukin-1. Microinjection of endogenous pyrogen into small regions of the hypothalamus triggers typical fever reactions that are not observed when it is injected into other parts of the brain. Endogenous pyrogen initiates a cascade of processes by activating phospholipase A_2, which then converts phospholipids in cell membranes to arachidonic acid. This compound may then be converted to prostaglandins.

One of the prostaglandins, prostaglandin E_2 (PGE_2), has a pyrogenic action when injected into the hypothalamus in minute amounts.[91] PGE_2 produces the set-point shift already described by interacting with thermosensitive or integrative structures (see interneurons, Fig. 56-8), or both, in the hypothalamus. Antipyretics (e.g., acetylsalicylic acid) inhibit cyclooxygenase activity and hence prostaglandin formation. However, PGE_2 is not the only fever mediator, because specific PGE_2 antagonists do not prevent pyrogen-initiated fever.[92] Evidence suggests that endogenous pyrogen may penetrate, in minute amounts, into the hypothalamus through a special transport system located in the organon vasculosum of the upper brain stem,[91] which belongs to the so-called circumventricular system. Based on evidence that PGE_2 appears before the increase in plasma cytokine concentration and the increases in related enzymatic activity, it has been suggested that rapid neural pathways may be involved in the pyrogenic sensing and signaling.[93] A more complex model for the genesis of fever is warranted and a search is under way for other fever mediators, particularly circulating products of oxidative stress and their interactions with nitric oxide and the thermointegrative networks.[94] There is expanding interest in the role of nitric oxide in body temperature control. This ubiquitous molecule appears to mediate both peripheral (vasomotor tone and brown fat metabolism) and central (set-point) responses of the thermal control system to a variety of stimuli, including exogenous pyrogens, psychological stress, and exercise.[95] The results of studies to date are too contradictory to allow secure generalizations about the role of nitric oxide in thermoregulation at this

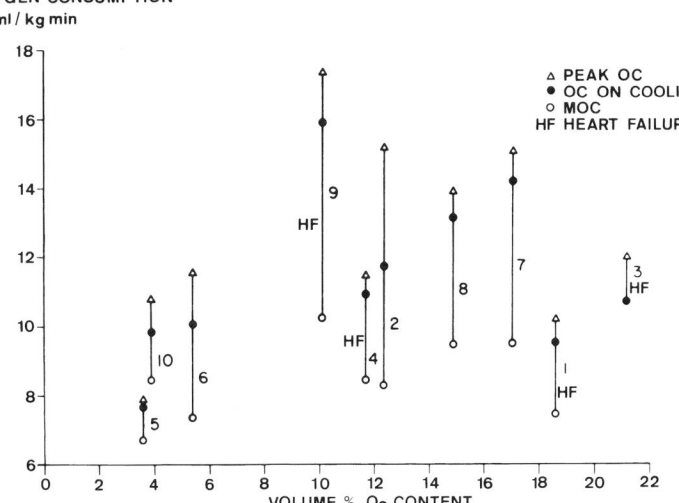

OXYGEN CONSUMPTION
ml / kg min

△ PEAK OC
● OC ON COOLING
○ MOC
HF HEART FAILURE

VOLUME % O_2 CONTENT

Figure 56–32. Responses of oxygen consumption on cold exposure (ambient temperature drop from 32° to 28°C) in relation to arterial oxygen content. small open circle = minimal oxygen consumption (mα) at neutral temperature; ● = average oxygen consumption during cooling period; △ = peak oxygen consumption during cooling period. Three infants designated with heart failure (HF) had suffered severe heart failure. Note that oxygen consumption increased on cooling even in infants with arterial oxygen content as low as 5 Vol %. (From Brück K, et al: Pediatrics 30:350, 1962.)

time,[96] but students of thermoregulation will want to follow developments in this area closely.

Behavioral Fever

In newborn rabbits, which are born in a very immature state, the thermogenic response to a standard pyrogen dose may be weak or even lacking. Nevertheless, these animals have been shown to experience fever when they are put into a temperature-gradient tube in which they are able to move to an area so hot as to cause their body temperatures to rise.[56] This response has been termed *behavioral fever* in contrast to the fever produced by the activity of the autonomous thermoregulatory effectors (see Fig. 56-9).

Hypoxia

Acute and Chronic Hypoxia

Considerable impairment of temperature regulation should be anticipated if the oxygen supply is critically reduced to the tissues subserving thermoregulatory heat production (skeletal tissues, musculature, and brown adipose tissue). Anaerobic metabolic processes are quantitatively insufficient to provide enough heat for thermoregulation. In fact, a reduction of oxygen content in the inspired gas to 10% has been shown to completely block thermogenesis in newborn kittens exposed to an ambient temperature that is lower than neutral.[97,98] As a result, body core temperature drops. Remarkably, the resting metabolic rate as measured at neutral temperature remains unaffected by this degree of hypoxia. Similar results have been obtained in the newborn lamb,[99] rhesus monkey,[100] guinea pig,[97] and rabbit.[101] By contrast, in larger adult organisms that do not possess nonshivering thermogenesis (e.g., adult humans[102] and the dog[103]), cold-induced thermogenesis (shivering) is only transiently reduced by hypoxia. With sustained hypoxia, shivering thermogenesis appears to be almost unimpaired. Thus, nonshivering thermogenesis appears to be more vulnerable to the effect of hypoxia.

This view is supported by a study in newborn rabbits.[101] As shown in Figure 56-31, oxygen uptake increases on cold exposure without shivering. Offering a 10% oxygen gas mixture immediately abolishes the cold-induced nonshivering thermogenic response. In the following hours, however, oxygen uptake steadily increases and is accompanied by shivering. Because the interscapular brown adipose tissue is a major site of thermogenesis and the heat produced in this organ inhibits shivering through cervicospinal warm-sensitive structures, the appearance

of shivering during hypoxic blockade of nonshivering thermogenesis is understandable. With prolonged hypoxia, the capacity for nonshivering thermogenesis may more or less recover. Normal thermogenic responses without obvious shivering have been observed in some neonates and infants with cyanotic congenital heart disease whose arterial oxygen contents range between 10 and 20 mL/dL (Fig. 56-32). Even with arterial oxygen content as low as 5 mL/dL, thermogenic responses can be evoked, although they are reduced in magnitude. These results suggest that in chronic hypoxia, adjustments take place that restore the capacity for nonshivering thermogenesis.

As for the mechanism of the hypoxic reduction of cold-inducible thermogenesis, two possibilities have been suggested: (1) reduced oxidative capacity from the lowered oxygen tension at the level of mitochondria in the organs involved in thermogenesis (brown adipose tissue, skeletal musculature) and (2) central inhibition of the effector systems. As shown by Blatteis,[101] the effect of norepinephrine infusion on nonshivering thermogenesis is abolished or grossly reduced during hypoxia. This would support the first hypothesis.

In hibernators, hypoxia and hypercapnia have been shown to displace the threshold for the elicitation of cold defense reactions to a lower body temperature level through a central action.[104,105] In a study in conscious adult cats,[106] hypoxia caused by inspiration of 11% oxygen reduced shivering. This suppression of shivering was partially reversed, however, when the end-tidal carbon dioxide concentration was returned to normal by addition of carbon dioxide to the inspired gas. These data would argue against the first possibility at least with regard to moderate grades of hypoxia. Thus, those authors concluded that "brain hypoxia lowers the regulated body temperature during cold stress." More recent observations suggest that, as in the case of fever, molecular mediators of the central effector response are likely to be important. Murine hypoxic hypometabolism and associated hypoventilation have been ameliorated by inhibitors of nitric oxide synthase.[107] Depending on the experimental design and species under study, various, often contradictory effects of nitric oxide have been reported. Overall, the evidence points toward a fundamental, but complex, role for nitric oxide in the control of metabolism, cardiorespiratory function, and temperature during hypoxia.

Effects of Fetal Hypoxia on the Neonate

Fetal hypoxia has been shown to increase the plasma norepinephrine concentration. This, in turn, results in peripheral vasoconstriction and circulatory centralization of cardiac output.[108] Moreover, increased norepinephrine levels have been shown in the guinea pig to cause a downward displacement of the shivering threshold temperature.[109, 110] Neonates who have suffered fetal asphyxia may thus display a delayed metabolic response to cold exposure as well as a delayed cutaneous vasodilation on heat exposure. This has been demonstrated in neonates who have undergone severe asphyxiation during delivery.[1]

REFERENCES

1. Brück K: Temperature regulation in the newborn infant. Biol Neonate 3:65, 1961.
2. Brown AC, Brengelmann GL: The temperature regulation control system. In Hardy JD, et al (eds): Physiological and Behavioral Temperature Regulation. Springfield, IL, Charles C Thomas, 1970, pp 684-702.
3. Brück K, Wünnenberg W: Meshed control of two effector systems: non-shivering and shivering thermogenesis. In Hardy JD, et al (eds): Physiological and Behavioral Temperature Regulation. Springfield, IL, Charles C Thomas, 1970, pp 562-580.
4. Hensel H, et al: Homeothermic organisms. In Precht J, et al (eds): Temperature and Life. Berlin, Springer-Verlag, 1973, pp 503-761.
5. Stolwijk JAJ, Hardy JD: Temperature regulation in man—a theoretical study. Pflügers Arch 291:129, 1966.
6. McCance RA, Strangeways WMB: Protein catabolism and oxygen consumption during starvation in infants, young adults and old men. Br J Nutr 8:21, 1954.
7. Brück K: Heat production and temperature regulation. In Stave U (ed): Perinatal Physiology. New York, Plenum Publishing, 1978, pp 455-498.
8. Bligh J, et al: Glossary of terms for thermal physiology. 2nd ed. Simon E (ed): Pflügers Arch 410:567, 1987.
9. Schulze K, et al: An analysis of the variability in estimates of bioenergetic variables in preterm infants. Pediatr Res 20:422, 1986.
10. Bell EF, et al: Estimation of 24-hour energy expenditure from shorter measurement periods in premature infants. Pediatr Res 20:646, 1986.
11. Kleiber M: The Fire of Life: An Introduction to Animal Energetics. New York, John Wiley & Sons, 1961.
12. Hull D, Smales ORC: Heat production in the newborn. In Sinclair JC (ed): Temperature Regulation and Energy Metabolism in the Newborn. New York, Grune & Stratton, 1978, pp 129-156.
13. Sinclair JC, et al: Metabolic reference standards for the neonate. Pediatrics 39:724, 1967.
14. Hensel H: Thermal Sensations and Thermoreceptors in Man. Springfield, IL, Charles C Thomas, 1982.
15. Konietzny F, Hensel H: The neural basis of the sensory quality of warmth. In Kenshalo DR (ed): Sensory Functions of the Skin of Humans. New York, Plenum Press, 1979, pp 241-259
16. Hensel H, et al: Structure and function of cold receptors. Pflügers Arch 352:1, 1974.
17. Schäfer K, et al: Temperature transduction in the skin. In Hales JRS (ed): Thermal Physiology. New York, Raven Press, 1984, pp 1-11.
18. Hensel H: Die intracutane Temperaturbewegung bei Einwirkung äußere Temperaturreize. Pflügers Arch 252:146, 1950.
19. Benzinger TH: Heat regulation: homeostasis of central temperature in man. Physiol Rev 49:671, 1969.
20. Jessen C: Thermal afferents in the control of body temperature. Pharmacol Ther 28:107, 1985.
21. Nakayama T, et al: Thermal stimulation of electrical activity of single units of the preoptic region. Am J Physiol 204:1122, 1963.
22. Kelso SR, Boulant JA: Effect of synaptic blockade on thermosensitive neurons in hypothalamic tissue slices. Am J Physiol 243:R480, 1982.
23. Baldino F, Geller HM: Electrophysiological analysis of neuronal thermosensitivity in rat preoptic and hypothalamic tissue cultures. J Physiol 327:173, 1982.
24. Brück K, Hinckel P: Thermoafferent systems and their adaptive modifications. Pharmacol Ther 17:357, 1982.
25. Simon E, et al: Central and peripheral thermal control of effectors in homeothermic temperature regulation. Physiol Rev 66:235, 1986.
26. Ivanov K, et al: Thermoreceptor localization in the deep and surface skin layers. J Therm Biol 7:75, 1982.
27. Brück K, Hinckel P: Thermal afferents to the hypothalamus and thermal adaptation. J Therm Biol 9:7, 1984.
28. Brück K, Zeisberger E: Adaptive changes in thermoregulation and their neurophysiological basis. Pharmacol Ther 35:163, 1987.
29. Hinckel P, Schröder-Rosenstock K: Central thermal adaptation of lower brain stem units in the guinea-pig. Pflügers Arch 395:344, 1982.
30. Wünnenberg W, Brück K: Studies on the ascending pathways from the thermosensitive region of the spinal cord. Pflügers Arch 321:233, 1970.
31. Simon E: Temperature regulation: The spinal cord as a site of extrahypothalamic thermoregulatory functions. Rev Physiol Biochem Pharmacol 71:1, 1974.
32. Simon E, Iriki M: Sensory transmission of spinal heat and cold sensitivity in ascending spinal neurons. Pflügers Arch 328:103, 1971.
33. Wünnenberg W, Hardy JD: Response of single units of the posterior hypothalamus to thermal stimulation. J Appl Physiol 33:547, 1972.
34. Hensel H: Thermoreception and Temperature Regulation. New York, Academic Press, 1981.
35. Brück K: Non-shivering thermogenesis and brown adipose tissue in relation to age, and their integration in the thermoregulatory system. In Lindberg O (ed): Brown Adipose Tissue. New York, American Elsevier Publishing, 1970, pp 117-154.
36. Nadel ER, et al: Importance of skin temperature in the regulation of sweating. J Appl Physiol 31:80, 1971.
37. Wenger CB, et al: Thermoregulatory control of finger blood flow. J Appl Physiol 38:1078, 1975.
38. Hey EN: The relation between environmental temperature and oxygen consumption in the new-born baby. J Physiol 200:589, 1969.
39. Hey EN: Thermal neutrality. Br Med Bull 31:69, 1975.
40. Jansky L: Non-shivering thermogenesis and its thermoregulatory significance. Biol Rev 48:85, 1973.
41. Sundin U, Cannon B: GDP-binding to the brown fat mitochondria of developing and cold-adapted rats. Comp Biochem Physiol 65B:463, 1980.
42. Mount LE: The Climatic Physiology of the Pig. London, Edward Arnold, 1968.
43. Brück K, et al: Comparison of cold-adaptive metabolic modifications in different species with special reference to the miniature pig. Fed Proc Am Soc Exp Biol 28:1035, 1968.
44. Jenkinson DM, et al: Adipose tissue and heat production in the newborn ox (Bos taurus). J Physiol 195:639, 1968.
45. Brück K: Non-shivering thermogenesis and brown adipose tissue in relation to age, and their integration in the thermoregulatory system. In Lindberg O (ed): Brown Adipose Tissue. New York, American Elsevier Publishing, 1970, pp 117-154.
46. Dawkins MJR, Hull D: Brown adipose tissue and the response of newborn rabbit to cold. J Physiol 172:216, 1964.
47. Smith RE, Horwitz BA: Brown fat and thermogenesis. Physiol Rev 49:330, 1969.
48. Perkins MN, et al: Activation of brown adipose tissue thermogenesis by the ventromedial hypothalamus. Nature 289:401, 1981.
49. Fox RH, et al: Cutaneous vasomotor control in the human head, neck and upper chest. J Physiol 161:298, 1962.
50. Roddie IC: Circulation to skin and adipose tissue. In Shepherd JT, Abboud FM (eds): Handbook of Physiology, Section 2: The Cardiovascular System. Vol 3: Peripheral Circulation, Part 1. Bethesda, American Physiologic Society, 1983, pp 285-318.
51. Dale HH, Feldberg W: The chemical transmission of secretory impulses to the sweat glands of the cat. J Physiol 82:121, 1934.
52. Ikai K, Hasigawa Y: Adrenaline sweating. In Itoh S, et al (eds): Advances in Climatic Physiology. Tokyo, Igaku Shoin, Berlin, Springer-Verlag, 1972, pp 109-121.
53. Crawshaw LI: Temperature regulation in vertebates. Ann Rev Physiol 42:473, 1980.
54. Hull J, Hull D: Behavioral thermoregulation in newborn rabbits. J Comp Physiol Psychol 96:143, 1982.
55. Hull D, et al: The preferred environmental temperature of newborn rabbits. Biol Neonate 50:323, 1986.
56. Satinoff V, et al: Behavioral fever in newborn rabbits. Science 193:1139, 1976.
57. Szeleányi Z, Szeákely M: Behavioural and autonomic responses to pyrogen in newborn rabbits. In Szeleányi Z, Szeákely M (eds): Advances in Physiological Sciences. Vol 32, Contributions to Thermal Physiology. Oxford and New York, Pergamon Press, 1981, pp 177-179.
58. Harpin VA, et al: Responses of the newborn infant to overheating. Biol Neonate 44:65, 1983.
59. Brück K: Basic mechanisms in thermal long-term and short-term adaptation. J Therm Biol 11:73, 1986.
60. Sundin U, et al: Brown fat thermoregulation in developing hamsters (Mesocricetus auratus). A GDP-binding study. Biol Neonate 39:141, 1981.
61. Brück K, et al: Cold adaptive modifications in man induced by repeated short-term cold-exposures and during a 10-day and -night cold-exposure. Pflügers Arch 363:125, 1976.
62. Hessemer V, et al: Effects of passive heat adaptation and moderate sweatless conditioning on responses to cold and heat. Eur J Appl Physiol 55:281, 1986.
63. Brück K, et al: Neutral temperature range and range of "thermal comfort" in premature infants. Biol Neonate 4:32, 1962.
64. Hey EN, et al: The total thermal insulation of the new-born baby. J Physiol 207:638, 1970.
65. Hardy JD: Physiology of temperature regulation. Physiol Rev 41:521, 1961.
66. Sulyok E, et al: Thermal balance of the newborn infant in a heat-gaining environment. Pediatr Res 7:888, 1973.
67. Brück K, Brück M: Der Energieumsatz hypothermer Frühgeborener. Klin Wochenschr 38:1125, 1960.

68. Hey EN, Katz G: Evaporative water loss in the new-born baby. J Physiol *200*:605, 1969.
69. Brück K, Wünnenberg B: Über die Modi der Thermogenese beim neugeborenen Warmblüter. Untersuchungen am Meerschweinchen. Pflügers Arch *282*:362, 1965.
70. Alexander G: Body temperature control in mammalian young. Br Med Bull *31*:62, 1975.
71. Bianca W: Animal response to meteorological stress as a function of age. Int J Biometeorol *14*:119, 1970.
72. Hull D: Oxygen consumption and body temperature of newborn rabbits and kittens exposed to cold. J Physiol *177*:192, 1965.
73. Gelineo S: Développement ontogénétique de la thermorégulation chez le chien. Bull Acad Serbe Sci *18*:97, 1957.
74. Taylor PM: Oxygen consumption in newborn rats. J Physiol *154*:153, 1960.
75. Hissa R: Postnatal development of thermoregulation in the Norwegian lemming and the golden hamster. Ann Zool *5*:345, 1968.
76. Stanton AN: Sudden infant death. Overheating and cot death. Lancet *2*;1199, 1984.
77. Kleemann WJ, et al: Hyperthermia in sudden infant death. Int J Legal Med *109*:139, 1996.
78. Ponsonby A-L, et al: Factors potentiating the risk of sudden infant sdeath syndrome associated with the prone position. N Engl J Med *39*:376, 1993.
79. Skadberg BT, Markestad T: Behaviour and physiological responses during prone and supine sleep in early infancy. Arch Dis Child *76*:320, 1997.
80. Sahni R, et al: The effects of prone vs. supine body position on thermal measurements in growing low birth weight infants. Pediatr Res *43*;296A, 1998.
81. North RG, et al: Lower body temperature in sleeping supine infants. Arch Dis Child *72*;340, 1995.
82. Tufnell CS, et al: Prone sleeping infants have a reduced ability to lose heat. Early Hum Dev *43*;109, 1995.
83. Amemiya F, et al: Effects of prone and supine position on heart rate, respiratory rate and motor activity in fullterm newborn infants. Brain Dev 13;148, 1991.
84. Sahni R, et al: Body position, sleep states, and cardiorespiratory activity in developing low birth weight infants. Early Hum Dev *54*;197, 1999.
85. Chong A, et al: Effect of prone sleeping on circulatory control in infants. Arch Dis Child. *82*;253, 2000.
86. Ammari A, et al: Prone and supine body positions, surface temperature profiles and thermal gradients in low birth weight infants. Pediatr Res *51*; 378A, 2002.
87. Székely M, Szeleányi Z: The pathophysiology of fever in the neonate. *In* Milton AS (ed): Handbook of Experimental Pharmacology. Berlin, Springer-Verlag, 1982, pp 479-528.
88. Cooper KE, et al: Observations on the development of the "fever" mechanism in the fetus and newborn. Temperature regulation and drug action. *In* Proceedings of a Symposium. Paris, 1974. Basel, S Karger, 1974, pp 43-50.
89. Hellon R, Townsend Y: Mechanisms of fever. Pharmacol Ther *19*:211, 1983.
90. Kluger MJ: Fever, Its Biology, Evolution and Function. Princeton, Princeton University Press, 1979.
91. Stitt JT: Prostaglandin E as the neural mediator of the febrile response. Yale J Biol Med *59*:137, 1986.
92. Mitchell D, et al: Is prostaglandin E the neural mediator of the febrile response? The case against a proven obligatory role. Yale J Biol Med *59*:159, 1986.
93. Blatteis CM, Sehic E, Li S: Pyrogen sensing and signaling: old views and new concepts. Clin Infect Dis. *31*;S168, 2000.
94. Riedel W, Maulik G Fever: an integrated response of the central nervous system to oxidative stress. Mol Cell Biochem *196*;125, 1999.
95. Simon E: Nitric oxide as a peripheral and central mediator in temperature regulation Amino Acids *14*; 87, 1998.
96. Gerstberger R: Nitric oxide and body temperature control News Physiolog Sci *14*;30, 1999.
97. Hill JR: The oxygen consumption of newborn and adult mammals: its dependence on the oxygen tension in the inspired air and on the environmental temperature. J Physiol *149*:346, 1959.
98. Moore RE: Oxygen consumption and body temperature in newborn kittens subjected to hypoxia and reoxygenation. J Physiol *149*:500, 1959.
99. Cross KW, et al: Anoxia, oxygen consumption and cardial output in newborn lambs and adult sheep. J Physiol *146*:316, 1959.
100. Dawes GS, et al: Some observations on foetal and newborn rhesus monkeys. J Physiol *152*:271, 1960.
101. Blatteis CM: Shivering and nonshivering thermogenesis during hypoxia. *In* Smith RE (ed): Bioenergetics, Proceedings of the International Symposium on Environmental Physiology. Bethesda, 1972, pp 151-160.
102. Wezler K, Frank E: Chemische Wärmeregulation gegen Kälte und Hitze im Sauerstoffmangel. Pflügers Arch *250*:439, 1948.
103. Hemingway A, Nahas GG: Effect of hypoxia on the metabolic response to cold. J Appl Physiol *5*:267, 1952.
104. Schaefer KE, Wünnenberg W: Threshold temperatures for shivering in acute and chronic hypercapnia. J Appl Physiol *41*:67, 1976.
105. Wünnenberg W, et al: CNS regulation of body temperature in hibernators and nonhibernators. *In* Heller HC, et al (eds): Living in the Cold. New York, Elsevier, 1986, pp 185-192.
106. Gautier H, et al: Hypoxia-induced changes in shivering and body temperature. J Appl Physiol *62*:2477, 1987.
107. Gautier H, Murariu C: Role of nitric oxide in hypoxic hypometabolism J Appl Physiol 87;104, 1999.
108. Jensen A, et al: Repetitive reduction of uterine blood flow and its influence on fetal transcutaneous PO2 and cardiovascular variables. J Dev Physiol 7;75, 1985.
109. Roth J, et al: Influence of increased catecholamine levels in blood plasma during cold-adaptation and intramuscular infusion on thresholds of thermoregulatory reactions in guinea-pigs. J Comp Physiol B *157*:855, 1988.
110. Zeisberger E: The role of noradrenergic systems in thermal adaptation. *In* Hildebrandt G, Hensel H (eds): Biological Adaptation. International Symposium Marburg/Lahn. Stuttgart, Thieme-Verlag, 1982, pp 140-147.
111. Hill JR, Rahimtulla KA: Heat balance and the metabolic rate of newborn babies in relation to environmental temperature, and the effect of age and of weight on basal metabolic rate. J Physiol *180*:239, 1965.
112. Lee VA, Iliff A: The energy metabolism of infants and young children during postprandial sleep. Pediatrics *18*:739, 1956.
113. Lewis RC, et al: Standards for the basal metabolism of children from 2 to 15 years of age, inclusive. J Pediatr *23*:1, 1943.
114. Boothby WM, et al: Studies of the energy of metabolism of normal individuals: a standard for basal metabolism, with nomogram for clinical application. Am J Physiol *116*:468, 1936.
115. Hayward JS, et al: Thermoregulatory heat production in man: prediction equation based on skin and core temperatures. J Appl Physiol *42*:377, 1977.
116. Stitt JT: Variable open-loop gain in the control of thermogenesis in cold exposed rabbits. J Appl Physiol *48*:494, 1980.
117. Brück K, Schwennicke HP: Interaction of superficial and hypothalamic thermosensitive structures in the control of nonshivering thermogenesis. Int J Biometeorol *15*:156, 1971.
118. Smales ORC: Simple method for measuring oxygen consumption in babies. Arch Dis Child *53*:53, 1978.
119. Zeisberger E, et al: Das Ausmass der zitterfreien Thermogenese des Meerschweinchens in Abhängigkeit vom Lebensalter. Pflügers Arch *296*:276, 1967.
120. Varnai I, et al: Thermoregulatory heat production and the regulation of body temperature in the new-born rabbit. Acta Physiol Hung *38*:299, 1970.
121. Adolph EF, Molnar GW: Exchanges of heat and tolerances to cold in men exposed to out-door weather. Am J Physiol *146*:507, 1946.
122. Ryser G, Jéáquier: Study by direct calorimetry of thermal balance on the first day of life. Eur J Clin Invest *2*:176, 1972.
123. Hardy JD, et al: Man. *In* Comparative Physiology of Thermoregulation. New York, Academic Press, 1971, pp 327-380.

57

Physics and Physiology of Human Neonatal Incubation

During fetal life, water and electrolytes are exchanged between the mother and the fetus through the placental circulation. The fetus contributes to the formation of amniotic fluid with urine[1] and with water transported through the respiratory epithelium and the airways.[2-5] During gestation, there is a gradual decrease in body water, and extracellular water and the contents of sodium and chloride decrease proportionally. The water content of a full-term newborn infant is about 77% of the body weight.[6] In preterm infants, the total body water at birth is higher, namely, 82% at 32 weeks of gestation and 86% at 24 weeks.[6] Heat produced by the fetus results in a fetal temperature that is about 0.5°C higher than the maternal temperature and results in a transfer of heat from the fetus to the mother through the placental circulation and through the amniotic fluid and fetal membranes.[7,8]

Immediately after birth, the skin of the infant is covered with amniotic fluid and usually vernix caseosa. Evaporation from the body surface of amniotic fluid[9] and of water in amniotic fluid[10] causes a loss of heat. At the same time, the infant is exposed to a colder temperature than it has experienced *in utero*. The body temperature will then be lowered, a change that is at least partially physiologic, because the body temperature at birth is higher than that in subsequent life. To make it possible for a newborn infant to maintain an almost constant body temperature, heat production and heat exchange with the environment have to balance each other. Exposure to cold may give rise to thermogenic responses that will increase basal heat production,[11-18] and the skin circulation may decrease to lower the heat losses.[19] Seriously ill and very preterm infants are usually nursed in an environment in which a normal body temperature can be maintained, either in an incubator at an ambient temperature within the thermoneutral zone[14,15,20] or under a radiant heater. Heat balance in newborn infants is not, however, solely dependent on the ambient temperature and the radiant energy, but also on many other factors that determine the heat transfer between the infant and the environment.[9,11,12,14-16,20-32] One of these factors is water exchange between the infant and the environment.[9,10,15,16,19,24-26,29,31,33-57] With every gram of water evaporated from the body surface or the respiratory tract, the infant will lose heat because of the latent heat of evaporation.

ROUTES OF WATER EXCHANGE

The newborn infant loses water insensibly through the skin and respiratory tract and sensibly with the urine and stools.[10,15,29,31,34,36-41,43-45,48,49,54,58-66] Water is gained by the body through the intake of fluids and food and as a result of metabolism.

Water loss from the skin surface involves two processes: continuous diffusion of water vapor through the epidermis and losses from the sweat glands in term and near-term infants. In the absence of forced convection, that is, with airflow velocity lower than 0.2 m/second, the human body is surrounded by a boundary layer of water vapor,[67] which constitutes a transition zone for transportation of moisture and heat from the body to the ambient air. In this zone of diffusion, there is a linear relationship between the water vapor pressure and the distance from the evaporating surface.[68] Evaporation of water from the skin and from the respiratory tract implies transfer of mass and of energy.[16,24] Insensible water loss (IWL) has been studied by

gravimetric methods[33,46,54,57,58,59,61,62,69,70] and with the ventilated chamber technique.[15,51,63] Hey and Katz[15] found that the IWL from the skin (IWL_s) in term infants comprised about 75% of the total IWL.[15] It has also been shown that the IWL is influenced by the ambient humidity[15,31,51,63] and is high in low birth weight infants.[62] Techniques for determining water loss from the skin[36,47,71] and from the respiratory tract[42,49] have made it possible to determine the relative contributions of these two routes of water loss to the total IWL in infants of different gestational ages[29,36-41,49,50,65] (under different conditions) and to calculate the different modes of heat exchange.[9,25,26,53,72]

Determination of Water Loss from the Skin

In the absence of forced convection, and if the effect of thermal diffusion is disregarded, the process of water exchange through a stationary water-permeable surface can be expressed in terms of the vapor-pressure gradient immediately adjacent to the surface, as

$$\text{water exchange} = -D' \frac{\delta \rho}{\delta \chi}$$

where D' is the diffusion coefficient and $\delta \rho / \delta \chi$ is the gradient.

This expression includes both a diffusive mass flow caused by a vapor-concentration gradient and a convective mass flow caused by a temperature gradient.

D' varies with the temperature (T) and the atmospheric pressure (P_{atm}), as follows:[73]

$$D' = \frac{DM}{RT} \frac{T^{1.75}}{300} \frac{101 \times 10^3}{P_{atm}}$$

where M is the molecular weight and R the gas constant (8.314 J/mol-K).

Within the ranges of temperatures and atmospheric pressures in question, the maximal variation in D' is limited. D' can then be approximated by a constant given the value 0.670×10^{-3} g/mhPa, which is valid for the water vapor pressure at a temperature of 300K and an atmospheric pressure of 101 kPa.

The evaporation rate (ER; g/m²h) can thus be determined by a method based on calculation of the water vapor pressure in the layer of air immediately adjacent to the skin surface. In this zone, there is a linear relationship between the vapor pressure and the distance from the evaporating surface.[68] If the gradient in this layer is known, the amount of water evaporated per unit time can be calculated according to the following equation:[47,71]

$$\frac{I}{A} \frac{dm}{dt} = D' \frac{dp}{dx} \quad \text{(g/m}^2\text{h)}$$

where A is the area.

The gradient method (Evaporimeter, Servomed AB, Kinna, Sweden) allows measurements of free evaporation and quick measurements without disturbing the infant.[36,47] Transepidermal water loss (TEWL; g/m²), which is a mean value of cutaneous water loss, can be calculated according to the following equation:

$$\text{TEWL} = 0.92 \cdot \text{ER}_{(a,b,c)} + 1.37$$

where $ER_{(a,b,c)}$ is the arithmetic mean of ER measured from the chest, an interscapular area, and a buttock.[36]

Measurements of Respiratory Water Loss

Respiratory water loss (RWL) is usually included in the measurements of total IWL when measurements are made with ventilated chambers, but in a few studies it has been estimated separately.[15, 31, 63] These authors all found that the RWL was higher at low ambient humidity than at high humidity.

In most of the more recent studies of RWL, an open flow-through system has been used with a mass spectrometer to measure the gas concentrations.[42] Ambient air is then sucked through a specially constructed Teflon funnel attached to the infant (or the lamb), so all expired air is collected without inclusion of evaporation from the surrounding skin.[42, 49] This system provides data on RWL, oxygen consumption, and carbon dioxide (CO_2) production.[19, 29, 30, 42, 49, 50, 65, 74-78]

ROUTES OF HEAT EXCHANGE

Heat exchange between the infant and the environment occurs through the skin and to some extent through the respiratory tract. Heat exchange through the skin takes place through conduction (H_{cond}), evaporation (H_{evap}), radiation (H_{rad}), and convection (H_{conv}). Its magnitude depends on the body surface area of the infant and the proportions of the body surface in direct contact with the mattress or clothing and exposure to the air and surrounding surfaces. To determine the heat exchange between the infant and the environment, it is thus necessary to know the heat loss from the skin per unit surface area, the total body surface area, and the proportion of the surface area participating in the different modes of heat exchange.[9, 25-27, 32, 35, 48, 71]

Calculation of Heat Exchange Between the Infant's Body Surface and the Environment

Heat exchange through conduction, evaporation, radiation, and convection can be calculated with knowledge of the TEWL, the temperature of the material on which the infant is placed (T_{bed}), the temperature of the infant's skin (T_{skin}), the temperature of the ambient air (T_{amb}), the temperature of the walls facing the infant (T_{wall}), and characteristics of the material in the infant's environment, using the following equations:[9, 25]

Heat exchange through conduction:

$$H_{cond} = k_0 (T_{skin} - T_{bed}) \qquad (W/m^2)$$

where k_0 is the conductive heat transfer coefficient. H_{cond} is dependent on the thermal characteristics of the skin, but even more on those of the mattress. T_{skin} is the temperature of the skin (K), and T_{bed} (K) is the temperature of the bed (mattress). With the thermal conductivity characteristics of most regular mattresses, the heat loss through conduction in incubators and under radiant heaters is very low.

Heat exchange through evaporation:

$$H_{evap} = k_1 \cdot TEWL (3.6 \times 10^3)^{-1} \qquad (W/m^2)$$

where k_1 is the latent heat of evaporation ($2.4 \cdot 10^3$ J/g), TEWL is the transepidermal water loss (g/m²h), and $3.6 \cdot 10^3$ is the correction factor for time (seconds). TEWL is a mean value of evaporation of water from the skin surface measured with the gradient method.[30, 36-41, 52, 53, 77, 78]

Heat exchange through radiation:

$$H_{rad} = S_0 \cdot e_1 \cdot e_2 \cdot (T^4_1 - T^4_2) \qquad (W/m^2)$$

In this equation, S_0 is Stefan-Boltzman's constant ($5.7 \cdot 10^{-8}$ W/m²K⁴), e_1 is the emissivity of the skin, e_2 is the emissivity of the surrounding walls (0.97), T_1 is the mean temperature of the skin (K), and T_2 is the mean temperature of the surrounding wall (K).

Heat exchange through convection can be calculated as follows:

$$H_{conv} = k_2 (T_1 - T_3) \qquad (W/m^2)$$

where k_2 is the convection coefficient (2.7 W/m²K), T_1 is the mean temperature of the skin (K), and T_3 is the mean temperature of the ambient air (K). This calculation does not include fast convections, which in adults occur at air velocities greater than 0.27 m/second.[24] The coefficient for convection given earlier and used in many studies referred to in this chapter has usually been determined in measurements on adult human skin. A convection coefficient suggested to be more valid for newborn infants[79] can be used; however, H_{conv} will then be 48% higher.

The extent of heat exchange between the body surface area and the environment depends on the type of heat exchange, on the position and geometry of the body, and on the magnitude and frequency of body movements. Because the different modes of heat exchange are unequally influenced by a change of body position, the relative contributions of the different modes of heat exchange may vary with time. When heat exchange is compared among different environmental conditions and among infants of different gestational and postnatal ages, it is often presented as heat exchange per unit area of body surface exposed to the ambient air or facing the walls of the incubator.

Heat Exchange Through the Respiratory Tract

The expired air is usually more humid (i.e., it has a higher water vapor pressure) than the inspired air. This implies an evaporative loss of water and of heat from the respiratory tract. A usually low degree of convective heat transfer also takes place in the respiratory tract. Often, these two processes are considered together.[16] In the newborn, heat may also be gained through the respiratory tract if the infant inspires warm air with a high humidity.

Because of the alternating displacement of air during the respiratory cycle, convective and evaporative heat transfer in the respiratory tract is complex. When ambient air, which is cooler than the body, passes along the mucosa during inspiration, it gains heat by convection and gains water vapor by evaporation from the mucosa. On reaching the alveoli, the air is at thermal equilibrium with the central body temperature and is saturated with water. During expiration, the expired air may become a little cooler than the body temperature before it leaves the infant.

Calculation of Heat Exchange from the Infant's Respiratory Tract and the Environment

The exchange of heat through convection in the respiratory tract, H_{conv-r}, is calculated from the air volume ventilated per unit time (V = ventilation volume) and from the temperature difference between expired and inspired air ($T_E - T_I$) according to the following relationship:

$$H_{conv-r} = V \cdot \rho \cdot c (T_E - T_I) m^{-1} \qquad (W/kg)$$

where V is the ventilation volume per unit time, ρ is the density of the air (1 g = 0.880 L), c is the specific heat (1 J/g/°C), m is the body weight (kg), and T_E and T_I are the temperatures of the expired and inspired air.[16]

Because of the alternating inspiratory warming and expiratory cooling of the air, the convective heat exchange in the respiratory tract depends mainly on the temperature of the inspired air. In human infants nursed in incubators, there is only a small difference between the temperatures of the inspired and expired air, and convective losses are therefore small.

Evaporative heat exchange from the airway (H_{evap-r}) depends on the difference in water content between expired and inspired air. This is the RWL.[29, 42, 49, 50, 65] Because the formation of water vapor in the respiratory tract requires thermal energy, the amount of heat exchange by evaporation per unit time will be as follows:

$$H_{evap-r} = k_1 \cdot RWL \, (3.6 \cdot 10^3)^{-1} \qquad (W/kg)$$

where k_1 is the latent heat of evaporation of water ($2.4 \cdot 10^3$ J/g), RWL is the respiratory water loss (mg/kg minute), and $(3.6 \cdot 10^3)^{-1}$ is the correction factor for time.

Heat Exchange in Incubators, Under Radiant Heaters, and in Heated Beds

Incubators

The first incubators were constructed when it was realized that a good thermal environment increases the chances of survival of newborn infants. Budin[80] found higher survival in infants whose temperature had never been lower than 32°C. Later studies by Silverman and co-workers,[81,82] Hey and Mount,[27] Hey[14] Hey and Katz,[15, 28] and Dahm and James[83] widened the knowledge concerning the influence of T_{amb} on the survival rate, oxygen consumption, and respiration of newborn infants.

In a convectively heated incubator, the warm air supplied is usually directed so both the air temperature of the incubator and the incubator walls are kept warm. If the airflow velocity close to the infant is less than 0.2 m/second, there will be a normal convective pattern around the infant, and at an airflow velocity lower than 0.1 m/second, the convective heat transfer will depend on the gradient between the skin and the air temperature. In this condition, the vapor-pressure gradient close to the skin surface will also be maintained, avoiding increased evaporative water loss resulting from airflow velocity.[16,24,35,48,79, 84] In incubators available today, both the airflow velocities and the humidification capacity vary markedly.[85] The wall temperatures also vary among different incubators.[85] It is therefore necessary to determine airflow velocities, humidity, and wall temperatures carefully before calculations of heat exchange are performed.

Radiant Heaters

Infrared radiation energy was first used by Agate and Silverman[86] to control the body temperature of small newborn infants and has since become widely used in neonatal intensive care. The radiant warmer placed over an open bed platform provides a good accessibility and visibility for the care of the newborn infant. When nursed under a radiant heater, the infant gains heat but may also have extensive heat losses through evaporation and convection and, from some surfaces, through radiation.[14,46,54,57,70] It is thus difficult to estimate the relative contributions of different modes of heat exchange when the infant is nursed under a radiant heater. Because there may be free air movements above the body surface of the infant, both evaporative and convective heat loss may increase as a result of a high air velocity. Williams and Oh[57] and Bell and Oh[60] suggested that the vapor pressure of the ambient air may be lower under a radiant heater than in an incubator, and that this could result in higher insensible loss of water from the skin or the respiratory tract. Baumgart[22] considered convective heat loss to be the major component of net heat loss under a radiant heater. It was also found that in cri-

tically ill preterm infants nursed under a radiant heater the IWL increased when the radiant power density was increased to the level required by these small infants.[33] In addition, it was pointed out by Baumgart and co-workers that convective air currents under the radiant heater could cause an increase in evaporative water loss and heat exchange.[21, 33, 34] Determinations of heat exchange in infants nursed under a radiant heater are difficult to perform because of the variations in humidity and air velocities and in the proportion of the body surface facing the walls of the nursery.

Heated Beds

Sarman and co-workers showed that infants weighing 1000 to 2000 g can be kept warm by placing them on a heated water-filled mattress.[87] In infants with a low body temperature, heat can be gained by conduction. By covering most parts of the body except the head, direct heat exchange between the infant's skin and the environment through other modes will be almost eliminated for a large proportion of the body surface. The water and heat exchange through the respiratory tract will depend on the temperature and humidity of room air.

WATER AND HEAT EXCHANGE BETWEEN THE SKIN AND THE ENVIRONMENT

Water evaporation from the skin surface of infants nursed in incubators has been determined by use of the gradient method[10, 36–41, 43, 45, 52, 53, 55, 56] (Evaporimeter, ServoMed AB, Stockholm, Sweden). TEWL[36–38, 40, 41, 53] and heat exchange[9, 25, 26] have also been calculated. In these studies, the body temperature has been maintained at 36° to 37°C, except when the effect of warming has been investigated, and the ambient humidity has been kept at 50%, except when the effects of different humidities have been analyzed. Evaporative heat loss is usually insensible, but it may become sensible when term infants are nursed in a warm environment[59] and start to sweat.[37, 55, 56] In preterm infants, the sweat glands are nonfunctional, and no sweating occurs even when preterm infants are nursed in a warm environment.[15] Not all infants born at term and nursed in a warm environment start to sweat.[56] In infants who do, the sweating is preceded by an increase in skin blood flow, as measured with the laser Doppler technique,[55,56,88] and feeding cold glucose can then inhibit both sweating and vasodilatation.[56]

Heat Exchange During the First Hours After Birth

An enormous evaporative heat loss takes place early after birth, when the infant's skin is covered with amniotic fluid, and it gradually decreases during the first hours of postnatal life (Fig. 57-1).[9] In the delivery room, heat loss to the environment through radiation is also considerable if the infant's skin surface is exposed to the room air and faces the walls of the delivery room. This early loss of heat through evaporation, radiation, and convection can usually be kept at a moderate level even when the infant is nursed in the mother's arms,[9] provided adequate precautions are taken to prevent excessive loss of heat, such as by gently wiping the infant's skin[10] and covering the infant with warm towels.[9]

Transepidermal Water Loss During the First Day After Birth and During the First 4 Postnatal Weeks

The TEWL from the skin surface of the newborn infant depends on certain factors, such as the gestational age at birth,[38] the postnatal age,[40, 41] and being small[39] or appropriate for gestational age.[38,39,41,53] TEWL is also dependent on ambient factors such as the air temperature and humidity.[36, 38–40, 52, 53] TEWL is 15 times

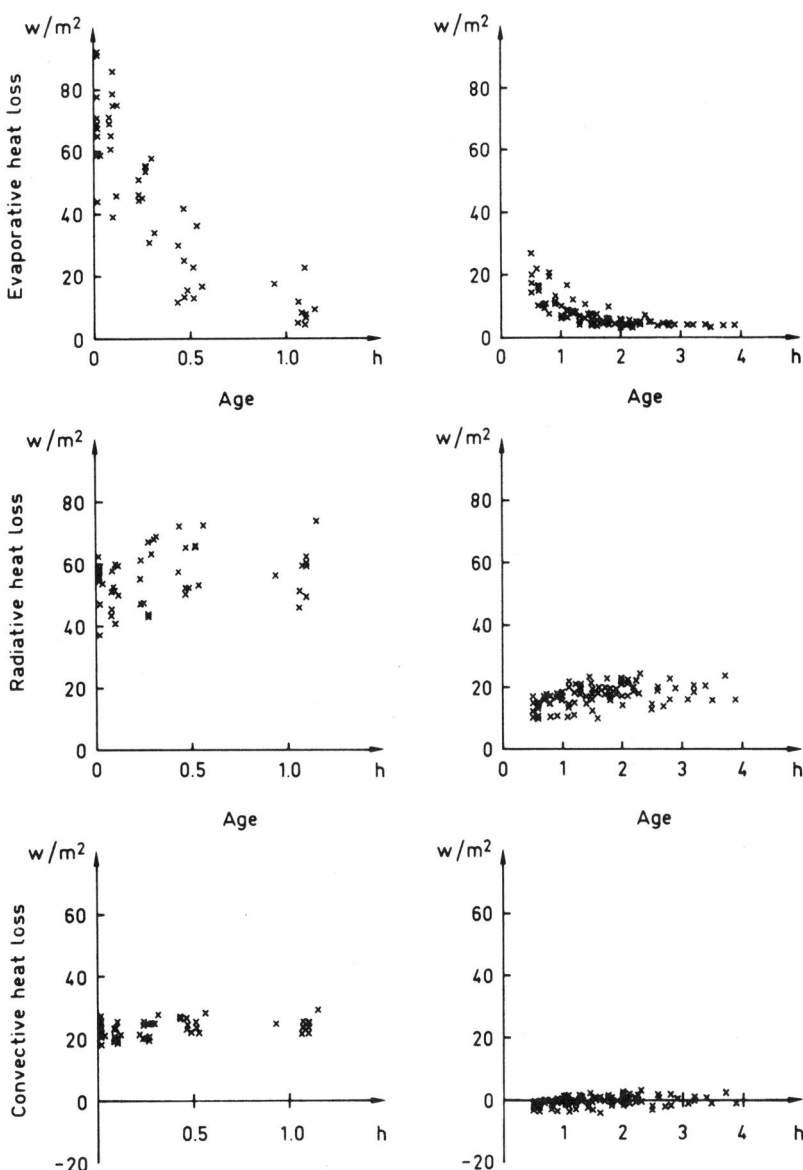

Figure 57–1. Heat exchange between the skin of full-term infants and the environment immediately after birth and during the first 1 to 4 hours postnatally. Data presented in the *left-hand scatter diagrams* are based on measurements in infants who were not washed or wiped. After the measurements at 1 and 5 minutes after birth, the infants were covered with a towel between the measurements. Data in the *right-hand diagrams* are based on measurements in infants who after birth were covered with a towel until they were placed in an incubator. (From Hammarlund K, et al: Acta Paediatr Scand *69*:385, 1980.)

higher in infants born at 25 weeks of gestation than in term infants. There is an exponential relationship between TEWL and gestational age when measurements are made during the first day after birth.[38] This type of relationship prevails over the first 4 weeks after birth (Fig. 57-2),[41] even though the difference in TEWL between the most preterm and full-term appropriate for gestational age infants gradually diminishes with age. However, at a postnatal age of 4 weeks, TEWL is still twice as high in the former as in the latter (see Fig. 57-2). The loss of water from the skin surface also depends to a higher degree on the ambient relative humidity, with much higher losses at a low humidity than at a high humidity (Fig. 57-3).[38] This relationship seems to be valid for all gestational ages and all postnatal ages studied.[36,38-40,52,53]

In very preterm infants, at an ambient humidity of 50%, water loss through the skin (Table 57-1) is the most important route early after birth. As seen in Table 57-1,[41] in infants born at 25 to 27 weeks of gestation, the water loss amounted to 129 g/kg body weight per 24 hours during the first day after birth, after which there was a gradual decrease, which was most marked during the first 7 days. These losses, however, depended on the ambient

humidity, which meant that the IWL[S] during the first day after birth in infants born at 25 to 27 weeks of gestation was 205 g/kg per 24 hours at an ambient humidity of 20% and only 53 g/kg at an ambient humidity of 80% (Table 57-2). Therefore, water balance in very preterm and in extremely preterm infants is best maintained if excessive evaporative losses of water are prevented by nursing the infants in a humid environment.[66]

Heat Exchange During the First Day After Birth

Because the evaporative heat exchange between the infant's skin and the environment during the first day after birth is directly proportional to the amount of water evaporated from the infant's skin, evaporative heat loss shows the same kind of relationship with gestational age as TEWL (Fig. 57-4). In the most preterm infants, the evaporative heat exchange may reach 50 W/m[2] of the body surface area,[25] whereas in term infants it is close to 5 W/m.[2] Because of the high evaporative heat loss in very preterm infants, a high T_{amb} is needed to maintain a normal body temperature of between 36.0° and 37.0°C. To keep the infant's thermal balance at steady state, the servocontrol system

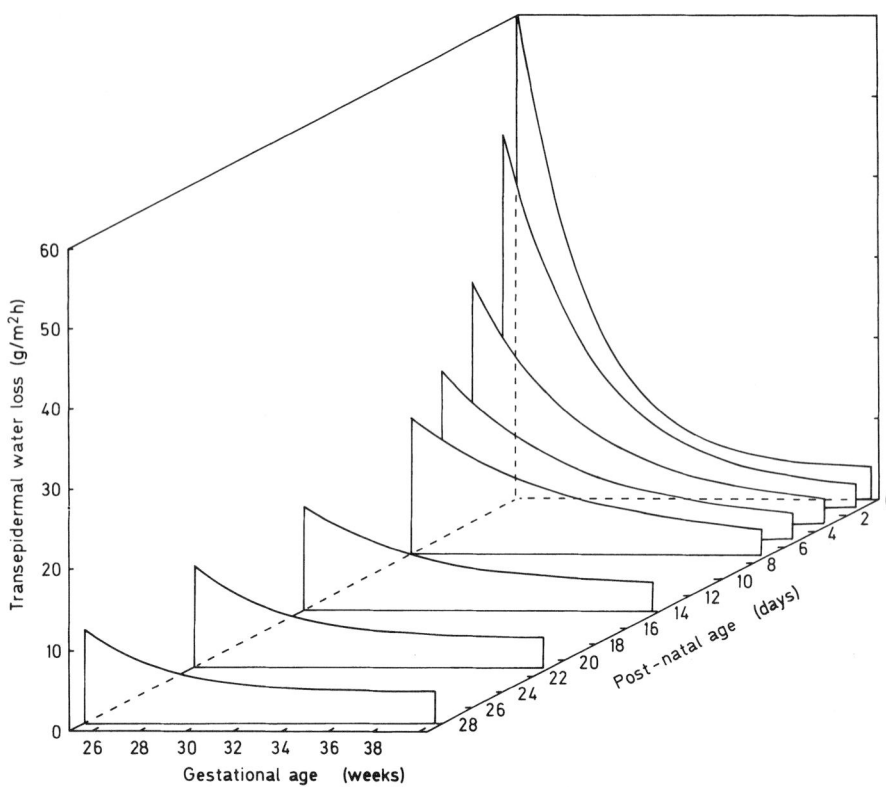

Figure 57–2. The regression of trans-epidermal water loss on gestational age at birth at different postnatal ages in appropriate for gestational age infants. (From Hammarlund K, et al: Acta Paediatr Scand 72:721, 1983.)

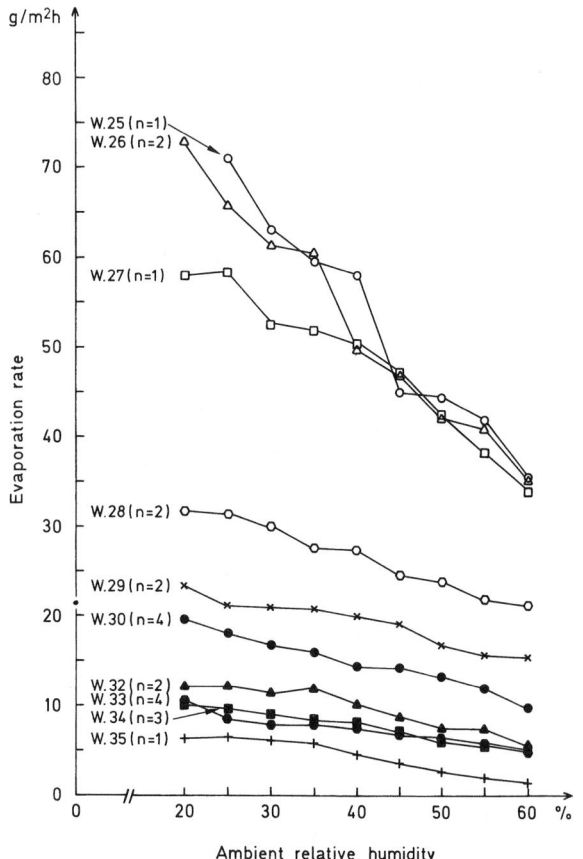

Figure 57–3. The relation between evaporation rate and ambient relative humidity in preterm appropriate for gestational age newborn infants in different gestational age groups on the first day after birth. W. = completed weeks of gestation. (From Hammarlund K, Sedin G: Acta Paediatr Scand 68:795, 1979.)

of the incubator, which controls the skin temperature, increases the temperature of the air, which leads to an increase in the temperature of the incubator walls. Thus, the loss of heat to the environment through convection and radiation decreases, and the most preterm infants can even gain heat through these modes of heat exchange (see Fig. 57–4). Because these data were obtained while the infants were being nursed in an incubator with a relative humidity of 50%, the preterm infants who needed a higher T_{amb} were nursed at a higher ambient vapor pressure than more mature infants. The difference in evaporative heat exchange between very preterm and term infants would have been even greater if the comparison had been made at equal ambient vapor pressures instead of equal ambient humidities. Infants born at a gestational age of less than 28 weeks need a T_{amb} of around 40°C to maintain a normal body temperature at an ambient humidity as low as 20%, whereas full-term infants need a T_{amb} of around 34°C at this ambient humidity (Fig. 57–5). At a higher ambient humidity, a somewhat lower T_{amb} is required to maintain a normal body temperature in the most immature infants.[25]

When calculations of heat exchange are made for three different ambient humidities, it is found that the evaporative heat exchange between the skin of very preterm infants and the environment is highest at a low humidity.[25] At a relative ambient humidity of 60%, the heat exchange through evaporation in these infants is only 50% of that at a relative ambient humidity of 20% (Fig. 57–6). Other modes of heat exchange are also influenced by the ambient humidity (see Fig. 57–6). Because the evaporative heat exchange is highest at a low humidity, the T_{amb} has to be kept high, and the infant will gain heat both through radiation and through convection. At higher ambient humidities, the evaporative heat exchange will be lower, especially in preterm infants, and if the body temperature is kept constant, radiative heat loss will be higher and heat gain through convection will be somewhat lower.[25]

If the different modes of heat exchange from the skin surface are added together, the sum will be fairly constant throughout the gestational age groups. The total heat loss cannot, however, be calculated in this way, because the proportions of the body

TABLE 57-1

Mean Insensible Water Loss from the Skin (g/kg body weight/24 h) in 68 Newborn Appropriate for Gestational Age Infants, at an Ambient Humidity of 50%

Gestational Age (wk)	No. of Infants	Mean Birth Weight (g)	*<1*	*3*	*7*	*14*	*21*	*28*
			\multicolumn{6}{c}{Postnatal Age (d)}					
25–27	9	860	129	71	43	32	28	24
28–30	13	1340	42	32	24	18	15	15
31–36	22	2110	12	12	12	9	8	7
37–41	24	3600	7	6	6	6	6	7

From Hammarlund K, et al: Acta Paediatr Scand 72:721, 1983.

surface area exchanging heat in different ways are not exactly known.

Heat Exchange During the First Weeks After Birth

During the first weeks after birth, the temperature of the incubator air can gradually be lowered both for preterm and term infants.[26] The high evaporative losses of heat from the infant's skin on the first days after birth will gradually decrease with increasing postnatal age (Fig. 57-7).[26] Heat loss through radiation, which is low early after birth in the most preterm infants born at 25 to 27 weeks of gestation, will be the most important mode of heat exchange after the first postnatal week. In infants born at more than 28 weeks, radiative heat exchange is the most important mode of heat exchange from birth. The heat loss through radiation will gradually increase with age. The smallest preterm infants will gain heat through convection over the first 10 days, after which there will be a low loss of heat through convection.

During the first weeks after birth, the relative magnitude of the different modes of heat exchange will depend on the ambient humidity (Fig. 57-8). In a dry environment, in infants born at 25 to 27 weeks of gestation, evaporative heat exchange will be the most important mode of heat exchange for more than 10 days, whereas at an ambient humidity of 60%, this mode of exchange will be much lower and will be exceeded by heat exchange through radiation from the fifth day after birth.[26]

Total Heat Exchange Between the Infant's Skin and the Environment

To calculate the total heat exchange between the infant's skin and the environment, the body surface area of the infant and the fractions of this area that participate in each mode of heat

TABLE 57-2

Mean Insensible Water Loss Through the Skin (g/kg body weight/24 h) at Different Ambient Humidities in Appropriate for Gestational Age Infants Born at 25 to 27 Weeks of Gestation

Ambient Humidity (%)	*<1*	*2*	*3*	*5*	*7*
	\multicolumn{5}{c}{Postnatal Age (d)}				
20	205	171	105	75	63
80	53	43	26	19	15

Based on data in references 38 and 41
Data from refs. 16 and 44.

exchange must be calculated. With the available methods, it is difficult to determine how different fractions of heat exchange vary over a longer period.[26] The total heat exchange is basically dependent on the metabolic rate.

Nonionizing Radiation and Evaporative Water and Heat Exchange Between the Infant's Skin and the Environment

Radiant Heaters

In studies of the ER in term, moderately preterm, and very preterm infants nursed in incubators with 50% ambient humidity and under a radiant heater, it was found that the ER from the skin surface of full-term infants was significantly higher under the radiant heater than in the incubator.[45] Preterm infants were studied both at 50% ambient humidity and at a lower ambient humidity of 30 to 40% in the incubator and then under a radiant heater. No significant difference was found between ER values obtained in the incubator at the lower ambient humidity and ER measured under the radiant heater. When using the measured values of ER and water vapor pressure in the incubator and the theoretical values of ER = 0 and the water vapor pressure in the incubator at a relative ambient humidity of 100% at incubator air temperature, the highest possible ER was calculated from the linear regression line for the value water vapor pressure = 0 (Fig. 57-9). A calculated value for ER during care under a radiant heater could then be obtained on the line between the maximum ER value at water vapor pressure = 0 and ER = 0, that is, at the saturated vapor pressure for the air temperature under the radiant heater (see Fig. 57-9).[45] The calculated values were for ER determined in this fashion were always higher than the measured values, a finding that suggests that even if the measured ER under the radiant heater is higher than the ER in the incubator on account of the higher humidity in the latter, there is no indication of an increased water loss resulting from a direct effect of nonionizing radiation on the barrier function of the infant's skin,[45] as suggested previously.[89]

In investigations of the effects of nonionizing radiation in an incubator equipped with a radiant hood warmer, a device that heats the incubator roof and ceiling independently of the incubator's main heat source, no change in TEWL in term and preterm infants was observed with use of this device.[30, 78] This finding further supports the view that an isolated change in radiative heat exchange does not influence the evaporative water and heat exchange if the ambient air temperature and ambient humidity (i.e., the vapor pressure) are unaltered.

Phototherapy

An increase in the IWL during phototherapy was reported in several publications.[58, 60, 61, 64, 70] This could be caused either by increased water loss from the skin as a result of altered barrier properties or by increased RWL. In thermally stable term and

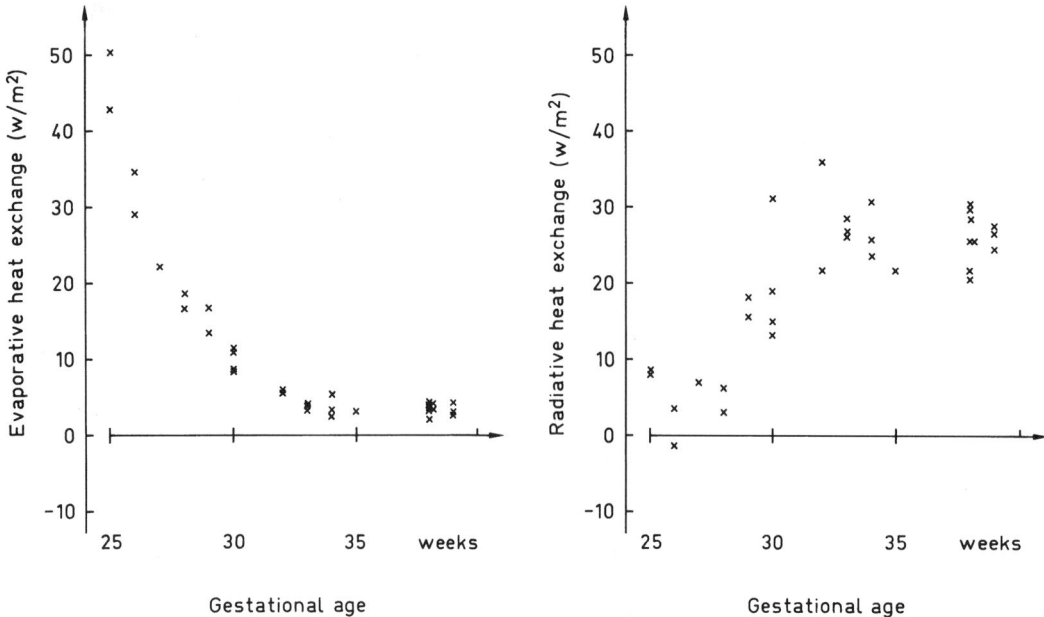

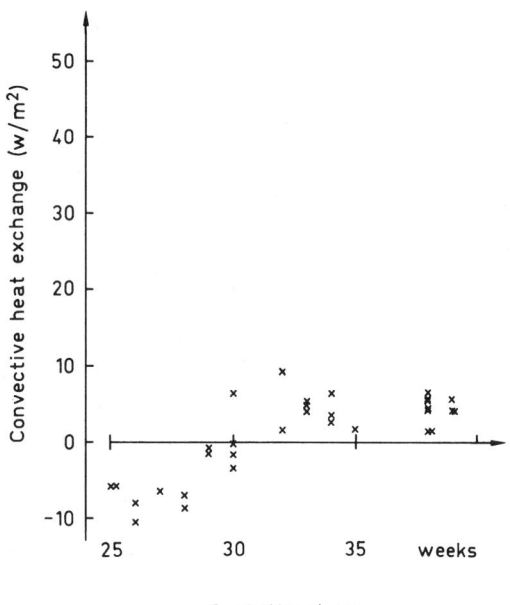

Figure 57–4. Heat exchange through evaporation, radiation, and convection at an ambient humidity of 50% in relation to gestational age. Measurements were made during the first 24 hours after birth in preterm infants and during the first 30 hours in term infants. (From Hammarlund K, Sedin G: Acta Paediatr Scand 71:191, 1982.)

preterm infants,[43] no increase in the ER from the skin surface was found during phototherapy. In that study, there was a significant increase in the temperature of the ceiling of the incubator. T_{body}, T_{skin}, heart rate, and respiratory rate were unchanged in term and preterm infants. T_{amb} was unchanged during the studies in term infants, whereas T_{amb} sometimes had to be lowered in preterm infants to avoid heat stress.[43]

WATER AND HEAT EXCHANGE BETWEEN THE RESPIRATORY TRACT AND ENVIRONMENT

Water and Heat Loss from the Respiratory Tract

When an infant is nursed in room air, water is lost from the respiratory tract with each expiration. Using indirect methods for the determination of RWL, it has been shown that RWL depends the humidity of inspired air, with lower losses at a high humidity.[15,31,54,63] In a series of studies of RWL (mg/kg/minute)

using a flow-through system with a mass spectrometer for measurements of gas concentrations,[19,29,42,49,50,65] we found that in an environment with 50% ambient humidity, the evaporative heat loss from the airway will be of moderate magnitude.[49] Actually, in term appropriate for gestational age infants who are nursed in an environment with 50% ambient humidity, the IWL from the respiratory tract (IWL^R) and that from the skin (IWL^S) will be of equal magnitude.[49] Therefore, the evaporative heat loss from the respiratory tract and the evaporative heat loss from the skin will also be of equal magnitude under these conditions.

The evaporative loss of water and heat from the airway has been found to depend on the ambient humidity in both lambs[42] and infants,[49] with lower losses at higher humidity. Whereas IWL_S decreased from 9 to 2 g/kg/24 hours in term infants when the ambient humidity was increased from 20 to 80%, the corresponding change in IWL_R was much smaller, that is, from 9 to 5 g/kg/24 hours.[49] When measuring evaporative heat loss and respiratory heat loss in infants placed in a calorimeter, Sulyok

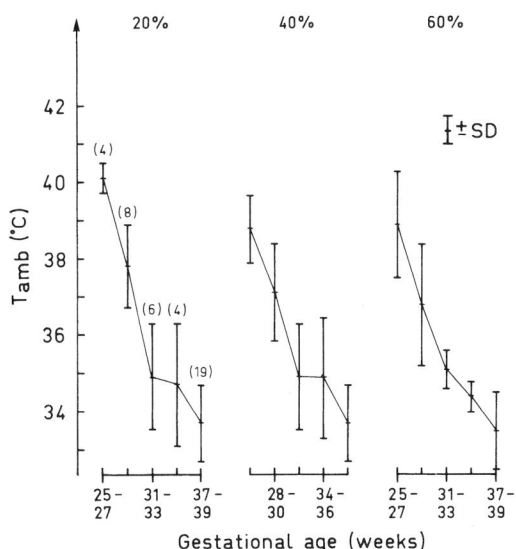

Figure 57–5. Ambient temperature (T_{amb}) in relation to gestational age at ambient relative humidity of 20%, 40%, and 60%. (From Hammarlund K, Sedin G: Acta Paediatr Scand 71:191, 1982.)

and associates[31] found that both the total evaporative heat exchange and respiratory heat exchange were related to the ambient humidity; the respiratory heat loss ranged between 0.07 and 0.22 W/kg, or 3 to 10% of the total heat production from metabolism and about 40% of the insensible heat loss. In term infants, RWL and evaporative heat loss from the respiratory tract may increase during activity by up to 140% of the values at rest.[50] In Table 57–3, data on IWL_S and IWL_R and their sum, the total IWL, are given for the hypothetical situation in which the infant spends 24 hours at the same level of activity. The oxygen consumption will also increase with higher levels of activity.[50]

Infants are able to tolerate moderate heat stress without increasing their RWL.[29] In addition, both lambs and infants can increase their RWL and evaporative heat loss without increasing their oxygen consumption and CO_2 production.[29, 75, 76] An example is given in Figure 57–10, which shows how exposure to radiant heat can alter the RWL in a lamb while leaving the oxygen consumption and CO_2 production unchanged. The RWL is directly proportional to the rate of breathing,[29, 75, 76] and this means that lambs and infants will lose more water and heat when they have a high rate of breathing (Fig. 57–11). Respiratory water and evaporative heat losses also decrease with postnatal age, at least in lambs.[42] In both lambs and infants, we observed irregular breathing during a period before a significant increase in RWL occurred.[90]

Respiratory Water and Evaporative Heat Exchange Before and After Intubation

Hammarlund and colleagues[74] studied young lambs exposed to heat stress before and after intubation. In nonintubated lambs exposed to a radiant heat source, the RWL increased from 10.5 to 33.4 mg/kg/minute, whereas the respiratory rate increased from 54 to 161 breaths/minute; oxygen consumption and CO_2 production were unaltered.[74] During exposure to the same heat source, intubated lambs increased their respiratory water loss from 8.1 to 18.7 mg/kg/minute and their rate of breathing from 46 to 125 breaths/minute. In intubated lambs, both oxygen consumption and CO_2 production increased significantly. RWL per breath did not change with intubation but increased significantly after extubation; the reason for this may be a larger tidal volume after intubation or to some extent a higher water content in the

expired air resulting from a higher body temperature after heat stress.[74]

Respiratory Water and Evaporative Heat Loss in Relation to Gestational Age

RWL was found to be highest in the most preterm infants and lower in more mature infants studied in incubators with 50% ambient relative humidity and a T_{amb} that allowed the infant to maintain a normal and stable body temperature. The infants were usually asleep during the measurements. RWL per breath (mg/kg) was almost the same at all gestational ages. Therefore, the higher RWL found in the most preterm infants as compared with the more mature infants was the result of the higher rate of breathing. As can be seen in Table 57–4, an increase in respiratory rate causes an increase in the loss of water and evaporative heat through the respiratory tract.[65]

Respiratory Water and Evaporative Heat Exchange During Phototherapy

When term and preterm infants[44] underwent phototherapy, no significant changes in RWL, oxygen consumption, CO_2 production, or rate of breathing were found (Table 57–5). In studies on term infants, the T_{amb}, T_{body}, and T_{skin} rose significantly. When preterm infants were studied, T_{amb} did not change; however, T_{roof} increased, and there was a small increase in T_{body} and T_{skin}. Thus, in the absence of heat stress, there is no increase in RWL, oxygen consumption, or CO_2 production during phototherapy in term or moderately preterm newborn infants.[44]

Respiratory Water and Heat Exchange During Mechanical Ventilation

In clinical neonatal care with a warm and humid environment or with warm and humidified gas supplied from a respirator, heat exchange through evaporation and convection between the respiratory tract and the environment will be low.[31, 42, 49] Infants who inspire cold air with a low water vapor pressure will have high evaporative loss from the respiratory tract and will also lose heat through convection. These losses may become clinically significant, for instance, during transport in a cold climate. Under these conditions, the total heat loss from the respiratory tract may increase to up to 20% of the total heat production of the infant.[72]

Skin-to-Skin Care and Heat Exchange

In skin-to-skin care, infants are placed lying naked, except for a diaper, on the mother's or father's chest, and they are covered with the parent's clothing or a blanket.[91-93] Only the head or parts of the head are exposed to the environmental air.[92-94] Several studies have shown that preterm infants can maintain a normal body temperature during skin-to-skin care even if there is no heat gain by conduction. In an infant in a thermoneutral state, skin-to-skin care should cause loss of heat.[94] Covering the infant's trunk and extremities with a blanket will eliminate convective and radiative heat losses from these parts of the body. Little is known about the evaporative heat exchange between the infant and the environment under these conditions. The heat exchange between the infant's head and the environment can be reduced by using a cap or by partly covering the head, but from areas of the head that are exposed to the environmental air there will be significant heat losses through radiation, evaporation, and convection.

Studies of body and skin temperatures and oxygen consumption in infants have revealed that preterm infants with a weight less than 1500 g and at an postnatal age less than 1 week and

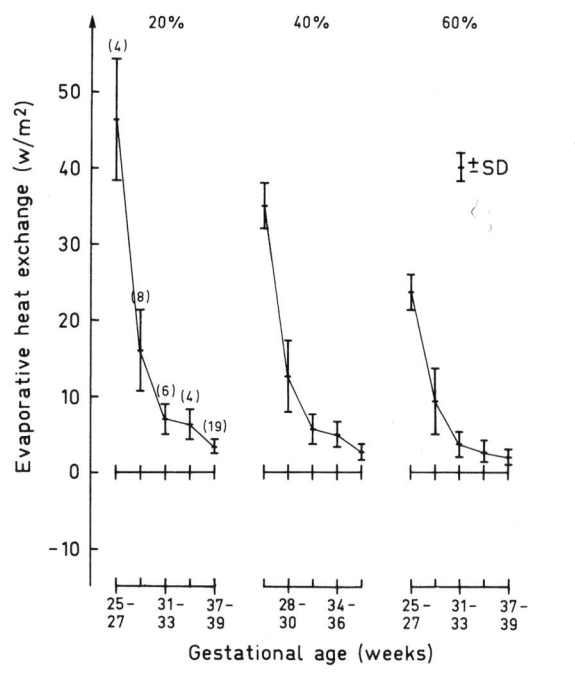

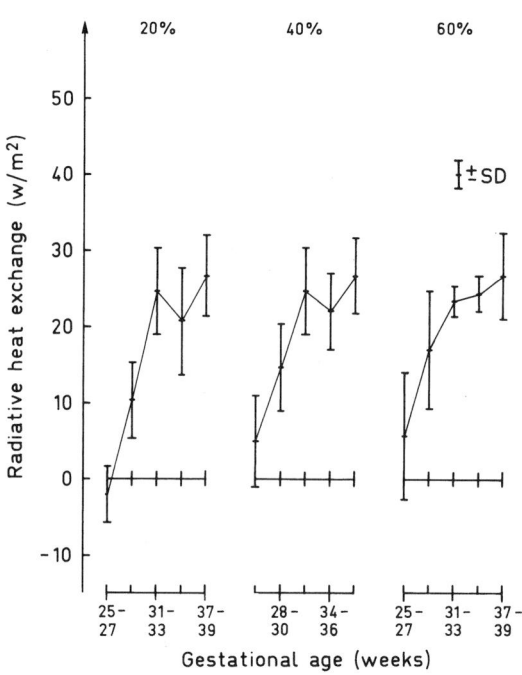

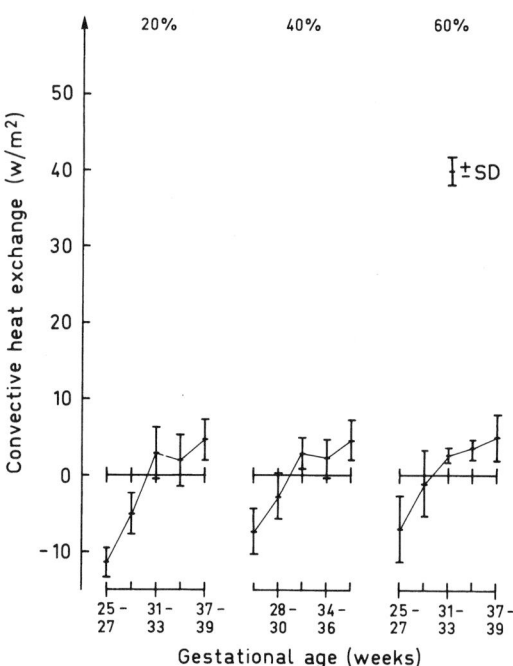

Figure 57–6. Heat exchange through evaporation, radiation, and convection in relation to gestational age at relative ambient humidities of 20%, 40%, and 60%. (From Hammarlund K, Sedin G: Acta Paediatr Scand *71*:191, 1982.)

who are nursed in incubators increase their rectal and skin temperatures during 1 hour of skin-to-skin care with no increase in oxygen consumption.[95] In a later study, Bauer and colleagues[96] also found that infants born at 28 to 30 weeks of gestation studied during the first and second week after birth increase their body temperature during 1 hour of skin-to-skin contact with no significant change in oxygen consumption. More immature infants (25 to 27 weeks of gestation) showed no increase in oxygen consumption but a decrease in rectal temperature during the same duration of skin-to-skin contact during the first week after birth. During the second postnatal week, the body temperature did not change in infants born at 25 to 27 weeks of gestation during skin-to-skin care.[96] The authors

suggested that infants born at 25 to 27 weeks of gestation may have a high evaporative heat loss during the first week after birth,[41] thus causing cold stress. Further studies on the different modes of heat exchange and oxygen consumption are needed to clarify the physiology of very preterm infants during skin-to-skin care.

SUMMARY AND CONCLUSION

The exchange of heat between the infant's skin and the environment is influenced by the insulation provided by the skin, the permeability of the skin, and environmental factors such as the T_{amb} and humidity, airflow velocity, and the temperature and

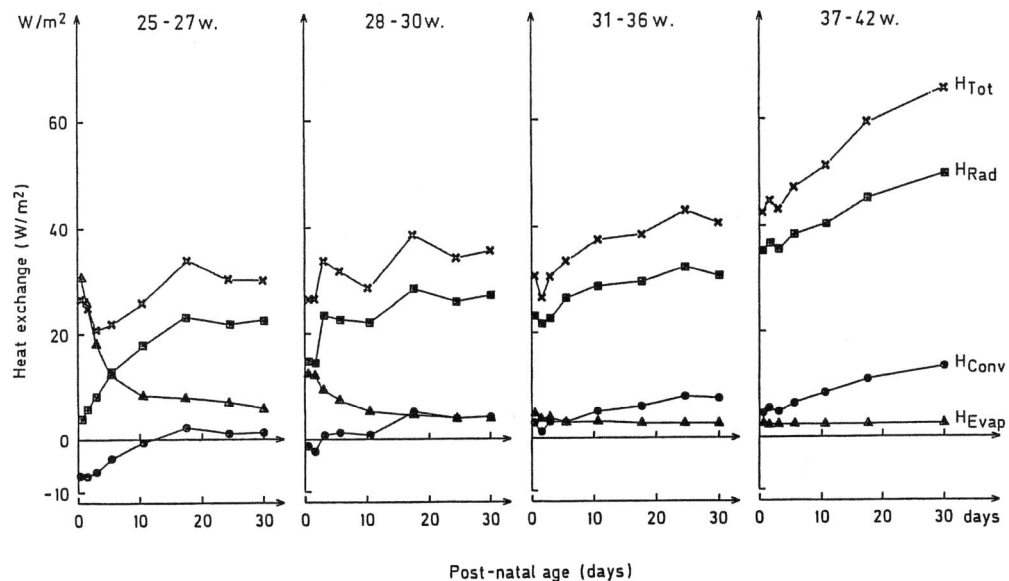

Figure 57–7. Heat exchange between the infant and the environment per square meter body surface area in relation to postnatal age in different gestational age groups at an ambient humidity of 50%. (From Hammarlund K, et al: Biol Neonate *50*:1, 1986.)

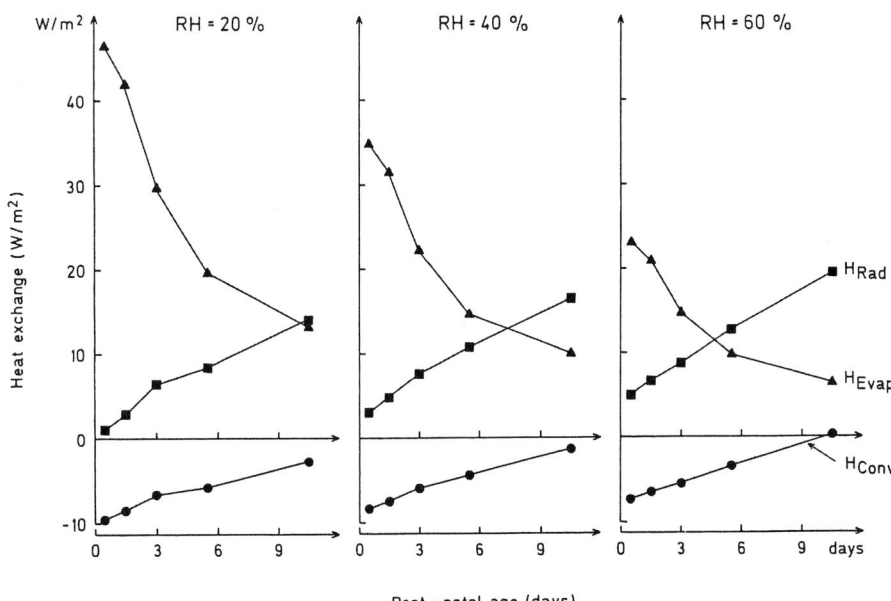

Figure 57–8. Heat exchange between the infant and the environment in relation to postnatal age at relative ambient humidity (RH) of 20%, 40%, and 60% in infants born at 25 to 27 weeks of gestation. (From Hammarlund K, et al: Biol Neonate *50*:1, 1986.)

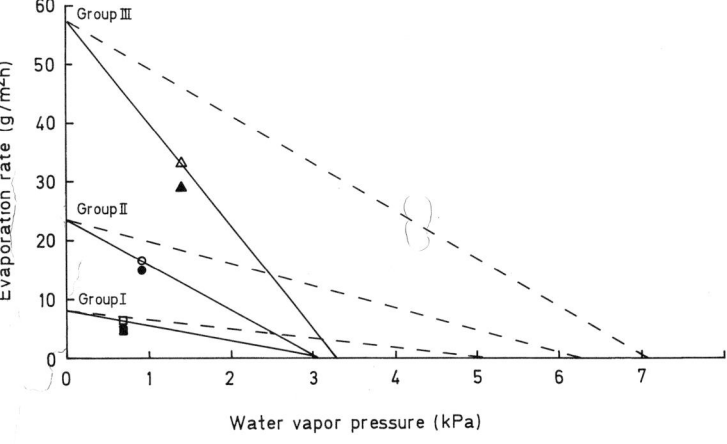

Figure 57–9. The calculated (*open symbols*) and measured (*filled symbols*) values for evaporation rate during care under a radiant heater together with corresponding regression lines for evaporation rate on water vapor pressure at the air temperatures of the incubator and the radiant heater in three infants, one from each of the studied groups: term infants (Group I; n = 12), preterm infants born at 30 to 34 weeks (Group II; n = 8), and very preterm infants born at 25 to 29 weeks (Group III; n = 8). (From Kjartansson S, et al: Pediatr Res *37*:233, 1995.)

TABLE 57-3

Insensible Water Loss from the Skin and from the Respiratory Tract and Their Sum in (g/kg/24 h) and Oxygen Consumption; L/kg/24 h), in Term Appropriate for Gestational Age Infants at Different Levels of Activity

Activity Level	IWL_S	IWL_R	IWL_T	$\dot{V}_{O_2}$
0	6	6	12	8
1	—	8	—	9
2	—	9	—	10
3	—	10	—	11
4	—	12	—	12
5	7	16	23	13

IWL_R = insensible water loss from the respiratory tract; IWL_S = insensible water loss from the skin; IWL_T = total insensible water loss; $\dot{V}_{O_2}$ = oxygen consumption. From Riesenfeld T, et al: Acta Paediatr Scand 76:889, 1987.

characteristics of the incubator surfaces facing the infant. Evaporative heat loss from the skin is the major component of heat exchange in the most preterm infants early after birth. Infants gain heat through convection and, in a very dry environment, possibly also through radiation when they are nursed in incubators. As the water loss from the skin surface of these most preterm infants decreases with postnatal age, the heat loss through evaporation will also decrease. Concurrently, the need for a high T_{amb} diminishes, and with the lower temperature of the incubator walls, the heat loss through radiation will increase, and the heat gain by convection will change to a low loss of heat during the first weeks after birth. In infants nursed under a radiant heater, heat is gained through radiation, and as a result of the low ambient humidity, evaporative loss of water and heat may be high in very preterm infants. The loss of heat through convection greatly depends on how the infant is protected from high air velocities by arrangements made under the radiant heater and also on the magnitude of air movements in the nursery.

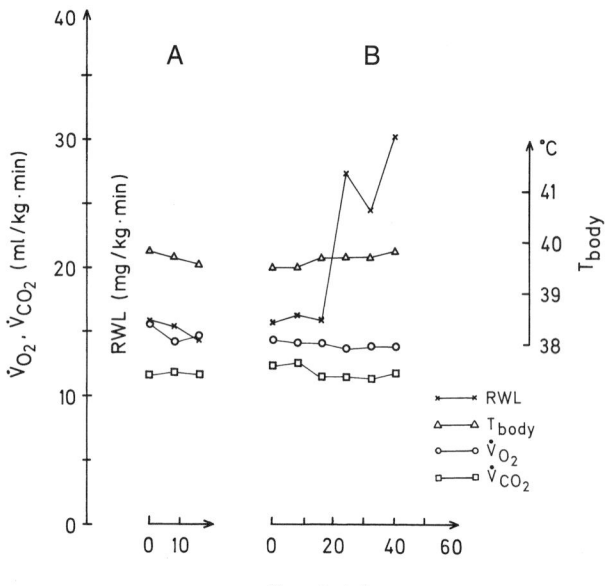

Figure 57-10. Respiratory water loss (RWL), body temperature (T_{body}), oxygen consumption ($\dot{V}_{O_2}$), and carbon monoxide production ($\dot{V}_{CO_2}$) in a 6-day-old lamb before (**A**) and during (**B**) heat stress. (From Riesenfeld T, et al: Biol Neonat 53:290, 1988.)

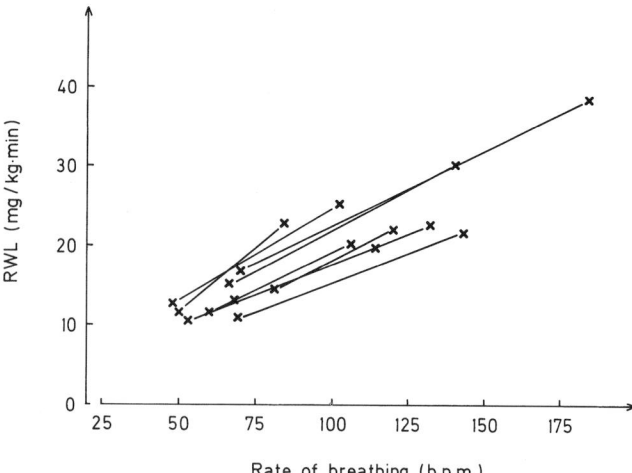

Figure 57-11. Respiratory water loss (RWL) in relation to rate of breathing before and during moderate radiant heat stress in lambs. For each lamb, the value before heat stress and the highest value during heat stress are joined. (From Riesenfeld T, et al: Biol Neonat 53:290, 1988.)

In term infants nursed in incubators with an ambient humidity of 50%, the evaporative water and heat loss from the respiratory tract and that from the skin will be of about the same magnitude. Therefore, respiratory water and evaporative heat losses are low in term infants. The respiratory evaporative water and heat loss per breath (mg/kg) is of about same magnitude in calm preterm and term infants. In preterm infants, evaporative heat losses from the skin are much greater than such heat losses from the respiratory tract. The evaporative heat loss from the airway may be considered important only in infants with high motor activity or with tachypnea, especially if they are nursed in a very dry environment. Mechanical ventilation with dry and cold air will also result in a high loss of heat from the respiratory tract through evaporation and convection. Exposure to nonionizing radiation does not increase evaporative water or heat loss from the skin or the respiratory tract. Intubated lambs have a lower ability to increase respiratory water and evaporative heat loss during heat stress than nonintubated lambs.

ACKNOWLEDGMENT

This chapter is based on studies supported by the Swedish Research Council (project 72x-04998).

REFERENCES

1. Needham J: Chemical Embryology, Vol 1. London, Cambridge University Press, 1931.
2. Adams FH, et al: The nature and origin of the fluid in fetal lamb lung. J Pediatr 63:881, 1963.
3. Bland RD, Chapman DL: Absorption of liquid from the lungs at birth: fluid and solute transport in the airspaces of the lungs. In Effros RM, Chang HK (eds): Lung Biology in Health and Disease, vol 70. New York, Marcel Dekker, 1994, pp 303–322.
4. Jost A, Policard A: Contribution experimentale à l'étude du développement prénatal du poumon chèz le lapin. Arch Anat Microsc Morphol Exp 37:323, 1948.
5. Olver RE, Strang LB: Ion fluxes across the pulmonary epithelium and the secretion of lung liquid in the foetal lamb. J Physiol (Lond) 241:327, 1974.
6. Fries-Hansen B: Changes in body water compartments during growth. Acta Paediatr Scand Suppl 110:110, 1956.
7. Morishima HO, et al: Temperature gradient between fetus and mother as an index for assessing intratuterine fetal condition. Am J Obstet Gynecol 129:443, 1977.
8. Rooth G, et al: Fetal-maternal temperature differences during labour. Contrib Gynecol Obstet 3:54, 1977.
9. Hammarlund K, et al: Transepidermal water loss in newborn infants. V. Evaporation from the skin and heat exchange during the first hours of life. Acta Paediatr Scand 69:385, 1980.

TABLE 57-4

Mean Respiratory Water Loss (Mean Values ± SD) in Preterm and Term Infants on the First Day After Birth at an Ambient Relative Humidity of 50%

GA (wk)	RWL/breath (mg)	RWL/breath (mg/kg)	RWL/min (mg/kg)		RWL/24 h (g/kg)	
			RR 40	*RR 100*	*RR 40*	*RR 100*
27–30	0.13±0.05	0.12±0.04	4.8	12	6.9	17
31–36	0.24±0.12	0.11±0.05	4.4	11	6.3	16
37–41	0.36±0.06	0.10±0.02	4.0	10	5.8	14

GA = gestational age; RR = respiratory rate; RWL = respiratory water loss.
From Riesenfeld T, et al: Acta Paediatr 84:1056, 1995.

TABLE 57-5

Respiratory Water Loss, Oxygen Consumption, and Carbon Dioxide Production (mean ± SD) in Term Infants Before, During, and After 60 Minutes of Phototherapy

	n	RWL (mg/kg/min)	$\dot{V}_{O_2}$ (ml/kg/min)	$\dot{V}_{CO_2}$ (ml/kg/min)	RR (breaths/min)
Before	11	4.4±0.7	5.9±0.9	4.0±0.7	48±7
12 min	11	4.4±0.6	5.9±1.0	3.9±0.6	
24 min	10	4.1±0.8	5.5±1.1	3.8±0.7	
36 min	9	4.2±1.0	5.4±1.0	3.6±0.6	
48 min	11	4.4±0.7	5.9±1.1	3.9±0.7	51±11
60 min	9	4.6±0.9	5.9±1.1	4.1±0.8	
After	9	4.8±0.8	6.1±0.9	4.1±0.4	

RR = respiratory rate; RWL = respiratory water loss; $\dot{V}_{CO_2}$ = Carbon dioxide production; $\dot{V}_{O_2}$ = oxygen consumption.
From Kjartansson S, et al: Acta Paediatr 81:769, 1992.

10. Riesenfeld T, et al: The influence of vernix caseosa on water transport through semipermeable membranes and the skin of full-term infants. *In* Rolfe P (ed): Neonatal Physiological Measurements. London, Butterworth, 1986, pp 3-6.
11. Brück K: Temperature regulation in the newborn infant. Biol Neonate 3:65, 1961.
12. Brück K: Heat production and temperature regulation. In Stave U (ed): Perinatal Physiology, vol 21. New York, Plenum Publishing, 1978, pp 455-521.
13. Gandy GM, et al: Thermal environments and acid-base homeostasis in human infants during the first few hours of life. J Clin Invest 43:751, 1964.
14. Hey EN: The relation between environmental temperature and oxygen consumption in the newborn baby. J Physiol (Lond) 200:589, 1969.
15. Hey EN, Katz G: Evaporative water loss in the newborn baby. J Physiol (Lond) 200:605, 1969.
16. Houdas Y, Ring EFJ: Human Body Temperature: Its Measurement and Regulation. New York, Plenum Publishing, 1982.
17. Smales ORC, Hull D: Metabolic response to cold in the newborn. Arch Dis Child 53:407, 1976.
18. Tunell R: The influence of different environmental temperatures on pulmonary gas exchange and blood gas changes after birth. Acta Paediatr Scand 64:57, 1975.
19. Sjörs G, et al: Respiratory water loss and oxygen consumption in fullterm infants exposed to cold air on the first day after birth. Acta Paediatr 83:802, 1994.
20. Sauer PJJ, et al: New standards for neutral thermal environment of healthy very low birthweight infants in week one of life. Arch Dis Child 59:18, 1984.
21. Baumgart S, et al: Physiology implications of two different heat shields for infants under radiant warmers. J Pediatr 100:787, 1982.
22. Baumgart S: Partitioning of heat losses and gains in premature newborn infants under radiant warmers. Pediatrics 75:89, 1985.
23. Bell EF, et al: Heat balance in premature infants: comparative effects of convectively heated incubator and radiant warmer, with and without plastic heat shield. J Pediatr 96:460, 1980.
24. Cooney DO: Biomedical Engineering Principles: An Introduction to Fluid, Heat, and Mass Transport Processes. New York, Marcel Dekker, 1976, pp 93-155.
25. Hammarlund K, Sedin G: Transepidermal water loss in newborn infants. VI. Heat exchange with the environment in relation to gestational age. Acta Paediatr Scand 71:191, 1982.
26 Hammarlund K, et al: Heat loss from the skin of preterm and fullterm newborn infants during the first weeks after birth. Biol Neonate 50:1, 1986.
27. Hey EN, Mount LE: Heat losses from babies in incubators. Arch Dis Child 42:75, 1967.
28. Hey EN, Katz G: The optimum thermal environment for naked babies. Arch Dis Child 45:328, 1970.

29. Riesenfeld T, et al: The effect of a warm environment on respiratory water loss in fulterm newborn infants on their first day after birth. Acta Pediatr Scand 79:893, 1990.
30. Sjörs G, et al: Thermal balance in term and preterm infants nursed in an incubator with a radiant heat source. Acta Paediatr 86:403, 1997.
31. Sulyok E, et al: Respiratory contribution to the thermal balance of the newborn infant under various ambient conditions. Pediatrics 51:641, 1973.
32. Swyer PR: Heat loss after birth. *In* Sinclair JC (ed): Temperature Regulation in Energy Metabolism in the Newborn. New York, Grune and Stratton, 1978.
33. Baumgart S, et al: Radiant warmer power and body size as determinants of insensible water loss in the critically ill neonate. Paediatr Res 15:1495, 1981.
34. Baumgart S: Radiant energy and insensible water loss in the premature newborn infant nursed under a radiant warmer. Clin Perinatol 9:483, 1982.
35. Colin J, Houdas Y: Experimental determination of coefficient of heat exchanges by convection of human body. J Appl Physiol 22:31, 1967.
36. Hammarlund K, et al: Transepidermal water loss in newborn infants. I. Relation to ambient humidity and site of measurement and estimation of total transepidermal water loss. Acta Paediatr Scand 66:553, 1977.
37. Hammarlund K, et al: Transepidermal water loss in newborn infants. II. Relation to activity and body temperature. Acta Paediatr Scand 68:371, 1979.
38. Hammarlund K, Sedin G: Transepidermal water loss in newborn infants. III. Relation to gestational age. Acta Paediatr Scand 68:795, 1979.
39. Hammarlund K, Sedin G: Transepidermal water loss in newborn infants. IV. Small for gestational age infants. Acta Paediatr Scand 69:377, 1980.
40. Hammarlund K, et al: Transepidermal water loss in newborn infants. VII. Relation to postnatal age in very pre-term and full-term appropriate for gestational age infants. Acta Paediatr Scand 71:369, 1982.
41. Hammarlund K, et al: Transepidermal water loss in newborn infants. VIII. Relation to gestational age and post-natal age in appropriate and small for gestational age infants. Acta Paediatr Scand 72:721, 1983.
42. Hammarlund K, et al: Measurement of respiratory water loss in newborn lambs. Acta Physiol Scand 127:61, 1986.
43. Kjartansson S, et al: Insensible water loss from the skin during phototherpy in term and preterm infants. Acta Paediatr 81:764, 1992.
44. Kjartansson S, et al: Respiratory water loss and oxygen consumption in newborn infants during phototherapy. Acta Paediatr 81:769, 1992.
45. Kjartansson S, et al: Water loss from the skin of term and preterm infants nursed under a radiant heater. Pediatr Res 37:233, 1995.
46. Marks KH, et al: Oxygen consumption and insensible water loss in premature infants under radiant heaters. Pediatrics 66:228, 1980.
47. Nilssons G: Measurement of water exchange through skin. Med Biol Eng Comput 15:209, 1977.

48. Okken A, et al: Effects of forced convection of heated air on insensible water loss and heat loss in preterm infants in incubators. J Pediatr *101*:108, 1982.

49. Riesenfeld T, et al: Respiratory water loss in fullterm infants on their first day after birth. Acta Paediatr Scand 76:647, 1987.

50. Riesenfeld T, et al: Respiratory water loss in relation to activity in fullterm infants on their first day after birth. Acta Pediatr Scand 76:889, 1987.

51. Sauer PJJ, et al: Influence of variations in ambient humidity on insensible water loss and thermoneutral environment of low birth weight infants. Acta Paediatr Scand 73:615, 1984.

52. Sedin G, et al: Transepidermal water loss in full-term and preterm infants. Acta Paediatr Scand Suppl 305:27, 1983.

53. Sedin G, et al: Measurements of transepidermal water loss in newborn infants. Clin Perinatol 12:79, 1985.

54. Sosulski R, et al: Respiratory water loss and heat balance in intubated infants receiving humidified air. J Pediatr *103*:307, 1983.

55. Strömberg B, et al: Transepidermal water loss in newborn infants. IX. The relationship between skin blood flow and evaporation rate in fullterm infants nursed in a warm environment. Acta Paediatr Scand 72:729, 1983.

56. Strömberg B, et al: Transepidermal water loss in newborn infants. X. Effects of central cold-stimulation on evaporation rate and skin blood flow. Acta Paediatr Scand 72:735, 1983.

57. Williams PR, Oh W: Effects of radiant warmer on insensible water loss in newborn infants. Am J Dis Child *128*:511, 1974.

58. Bell EF, et al: Combined effect of radiant warmer and phototherapy on insensible water loss in low-birth-weight infants. J Pediatr *94*:810, 1979.

59. Bell EF, et al: The effects of thermal environment on heat balance and insensible water loss in low-birth-weight infants. Pediatrics *96*:452, 1980.

60. Bell EF, Oh W: Fluid and electrolyte management. *In* Avery GB (ed) Neonatology, Pathophysiology and Management of the Newborn, 3rd ed. Philadelphia, JB Lippincott, 1987, pp 778–779.

61. Engle WD, et al: Insensible water loss in the critically ill neonate. Combined effect or radiant-warmer power and phototherapy. Am J Dis Child *135*:516, 1981.

62. Fanaroff AA, et al: Insensible water loss in low birth weight infants. Pediatrics *50*:236, 1972.

63. O'Brien D, et al: Effect of supersaturated atmospheres on insensible water loss in the newborn infant. Pediatrics 13:126, 1954.

64. Oh W, Karecki H: Phototherpay and insensible water loss in the newborn infants. Am J Dis Child *124*:230, 1972.

65. Riesenfeld T, et al: Respiratory water loss in relation to gestational age in infants on their first day after birth. Acta Paediatr *84*:1056, 1995.

66. Sedin G: Fluid management in the extremely preterm infant. *In* Hansen TH, McIntosh N (eds): Current Topics in Neonatology. Philadelphia, WB Saunders Co, 1996 pp 50–66.

67. Gates DM: The measurement of water vapor boundary layers in biological systems with a radiorefractometer. *In* Wexler A, Amdur EJ (eds): Humidity and Moisture, vol 2. New York, Reinhold, 1965, p 33.

68. Ueda M: Measurements of the gradient of water vapour pressure and the diffusion coefficient. J Appl Phys 25:144, 1956.

69. Levine SZ, et al: The insensible perspiration in infancy and in childhood. II. Proposed basal standards for infants. Am J Dis Child *39*:917, 1930.

70. Wu PYK, Hodgman JE: Insensible water loss in preterm infants: changes with postnatal development and non-ionizing radiant energy. Pediatrics 54:704, 1974.

71. Nilsson GE, et al: A transducer for measurement of evaporation from the skin. *In* Proceedings of the International Conference on Biomedical Transducers, Paris, 1975, part II, p 71.

72. Sedin G: Heat loss from the respiratory tract of newborn infants ventilated during transport. *In* XVth European Congress of Perinatal Medicine, Glasgow, 1996, p 511.

73. Roberts RC: Molecular diffusion of gases. *In* Gray DE (ed): American Institute of Physics Handbook, 2nd ed. New York: McGraw-Hill, 1963, pp 2-234–2-237.

74. Hammarlund K, et al: Endotracheal intubation influences respiratory water loss during heat stress in young lambs. J Appl Physiol 79:801, 1995.

75. Riesenfeld T, et al: Influence of radiant heat stress on respiratory water loss in new-born lambs. Biol Neonat 53:290, 1988.

76. Riesenfeld T, et al: The temperature of inspired air influences respiratory water loss in young lambs. Biol Neonat 65:326, 1994.

77. Sjörs G, et al: Thermal balance in term infants nursed in an incubator with a radiative heat source. Pediatr Res *32*:631, 1992.

78. Sjörs G, et al: Thermal balance in preterm infants nursed in an incubator with a radiative heat source (abstract). Pediatr Res *35*:278, 1994.

79. Wheldon AE: Energy balance in the newborn baby: use of a manikin to estimate radiant and convective heat loss. Phys Med Biol 27:285, 1982.

80. Budin P: Le Nourrison. Paris, Dion, 1900.

81. Silverman WA, et al: The influence of the thermal environment upon the survival of the newly born premature infant. Pediatrics *22*:876, 1958.

82. Silverman WA, et al: The oxygen cost of minor changes in heat balance of small newborn infants. Acta Pediatr Scand 55:294, 1966.

83. Dahm LS, James LS: Newborn temperature and calculated heat loss in the delivery room. Pediatrics *49*:504, 1972.

84. Thompson MH, et al: Weight and water loss in the neonate in natural and forced convection. Arch Dis Child 59:951, 1984.

85. Sjörs G, et al: An evaluation of environment and climate control in seven infant incubators. Biomed Instrum Technol 26:294, 1992.

86. Agate FJ, Silverman WA: The control of body temperature in the small newborn infant by low-energy infra-red radiation. Pediatrics *31*:725, 1963.

87. Sarman I, et al: Rewarming preterm infant on a heated, water filled mattress. Arch Dis Child *64*:687, 1989.

88. Nilsson G E, et al: A new instrument for continuous measurement of tissue blood flow by light beating spectroscopy. IEEE Trans Biomed Eng 27:12, 1980.

89. Wheldon AE, Rutter N: The heat balance of small babies nursed in incubators and under radiant warmers. Early Hum Dev 6:131:143, 1982.

90. Riesenfeld T, et al: Irregular breathing in young lambs and newborn infants during heat stress. Acta Paediatr 85:467, 1996.

91. Rey Sanabria E, Martinez Gomes H: Manejo racional del nino prematuro (Rational management of the premature infant) *In* Curso de medicina fetal y neonatal. Bogotá, Colombia, Fundacion Vivir, 1983, pp 137–151.

92. Whitelaw A, Sleath K: Myth of the marsupial mother: Home care of very low birth weight babies in Bogota, Colombia. Lancet *1*:8439:1206, 1985.

93. Whitelaw A, et al: Skin to skin contact for very low birthweight infants and their mothers. Arch Dis Child *63*:1377, 1988.

94. Sinclair JC: Management of the thermal environment. *In* Sinclair JC, Bracken MB (eds): Effective Care of the Newborn Infant. Oxford, Oxford University Press, 1992, pp 40–58.

95. Bauer K, et al: Body temperatures and oxygen consumption during skin-to-skin (kangaroo) care in stable preterm infants weighing less than 1500 grams. J Pediatr *130*:240, 1997.

96. Bauer K, et al: Effects of gestational and postnatal age on body temperature, oxygen consumption, and activity during early skin-to-skin contact between preterm infants of 25–30-week gestation and their mothers. Pediatr Res *44*:247, 1998.

Alistair J. Gunn and Laura Bennet

58

Responses of the Fetus and Neonate to Hypothermia

Moderate to severe hypoxic-ischemic encephalopathy continues to be a significant cause of acute neurologic injury at birth, occurring in approximately 1 to 2 cases per 1000 term live births. The possibility that hypothermia may be able to prevent or lessen asphyxial brain injury is a "dream revisited." Early experimental studies, mainly in precocial animals such as kittens, demonstrated that hypothermia greatly extended the "time to last gasp." This finding led to a series of small, uncontrolled studies in the 1950s and 1960s in which infants who were not breathing spontaneously at 5 minutes were immersed in cold water until respiration began.[1-3] Although outcomes were said to be better than for historical controls, this experimental approach was overtaken by two major developments: the introduction of active ventilation and resuscitation of infants exposed to asphyxia and the recognition that even mild hypothermia is associated with a wide range of potential adverse effects,[4] including increased oxygen requirements and greater mortality in the premature newborn.[5] Thus, resuscitation guidelines for the newborn exposed to asphyxia have, until recently, simply emphasized keeping the newly born warm, that is, avoiding hypothermia.

The early experimental studies noted earlier focused entirely on the effects of cooling *during* severe hypoxia, which is well known to be associated with potent, dose-related, long-lasting neuroprotection.[6] The central clinical question, of course, is whether cooling *after* asphyxial or hypoxic-ischemic injury is beneficial. This chapter reviews recent developments that helped to delineate many of the experimental parameters that are likely required for successful postresuscitation cooling.

PATHOPHYSIOLOGIC PHASES OF CEREBRAL INJURY

The critical advance has been the clinical and experimental observation in term fetuses, in newborns, and in adults that injury to the brain is not a single "event" occurring at, or just after, an insult, but rather an evolving process that leads to cell death well after the initial insult.[7,8] This observed delay between insult and injury raises the tantalizing possibility that asphyxial cell death may be prevented even well after reperfusion.

Pathophysiologically, several phases have been identified, as illustrated in Figures 58-1 and 58-2. The actual period of hypoxia and ischemia is the *primary* phase of cell injury. During this phase, there is progressive hypoxic depolarization of cells, leading to severe cytotoxic edema, with failure of reuptake, leading to extracellular accumulation of excitatory amino acids (*excitotoxins*). Excessive levels of excitatory amino acids cause activation of their ion channels and promote further excessive entry of salt, water, and calcium into the cells. After reperfusion (see Fig. 58-2) or return of cerebral circulation during resuscitation from an asphyxial insult, the initial hypoxia-induced cytotoxic edema may transiently resolve over approximately 30 to 60 minutes, with at least partial recovery of cerebral oxidative metabolism (*latent phase*). This is followed by a secondary phase of deterioration (~6 to 15 hours later) that may extend over many days.[9,10] At term gestation, this so-called *secondary phase* is marked by the delayed onset of seizures, secondary cytotoxic edema (see Fig. 58-1),[11] accumulation of excitotoxins,[12] failure of cerebral oxidative energy metabolism,[9,10] and ultimately neuronal death. In asphyxiated infants, there is a close correlation between the degree of delayed energy failure and neurodevelopmental impairment at 1 and 4 years of age.[9]

The studies discussed in this chapter strongly suggest that the latent phase represents the key window of opportunity for intervention.

FACTORS DETERMINING EFFECTIVE NEUROPROTECTION WITH HYPOTHERMIA

Experimentally, the efficacy of hypothermia is highly dependent on certain factors, including the timing of initiation of cooling, its duration, and its depth.

Cooling During Resuscitation and Reperfusion

Brief hypothermia, for 1 to 2 hours, during acute reperfusion appears to be modestly neuroprotective, provided it is initiated immediately. For example, after 15 minutes of reversible ischemia in the piglet, mild hypothermia (2° to 3°C) for 1 hour significantly improved recovery and reduced neuronal loss 3 days later.[13] However, this protection was lost when hypothermia was initiated 30 minutes after ischemia.[14] Similar data have been reported in the neonatal rat and adult dog.[15-17] Critically, protection appears to be lost if brief hypothermia is delayed by as little as 15 to 45 minutes after the primary insult.[17-19] This extreme sensitivity to delay is consistent with the hypothesis that resuscitative hypothermia can suppress damage secondary to oxygen free radical production during reperfusion.[20] Alternatively, however, this strategy may merely represent intervention at the end of the primary phase, when cerebrovascular perfusion is being reestablished, cell function is just starting to recover, and levels of excitatory amino acids are still high.[11,12]

Even if such immediate cooling during resuscitation were consistently effective, it would be almost impossible to test in

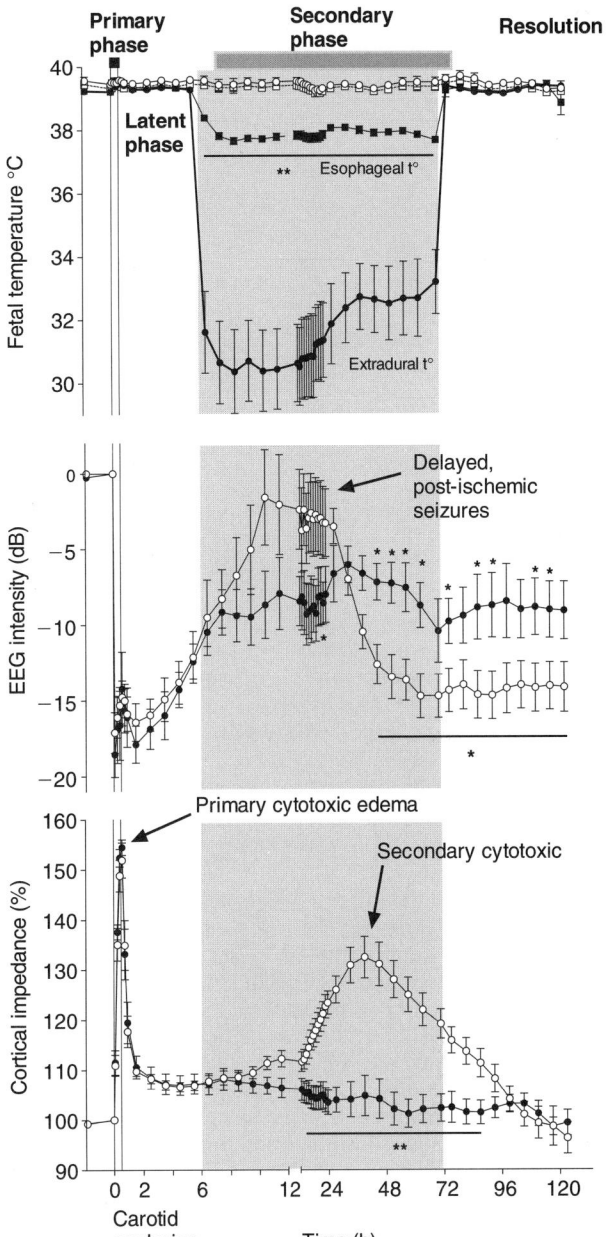

Figure 58–1. The effect of hypothermia started 5.5 hours after reperfusion from a 30 minute of cerebral ischemia in near-term fetal sheep. The period of ischemia is shown by *dotted lines*, whereas cooling is shown by the *bar*. The *top panel* shows changes in extradural (*solid circles*) and esophageal (*solid squares*) temperature in the hypothermia group and extradural (*open circles*) and esophageal (*open squares*) temperature in the sham-cooled group. The *lower two panels* show changes in electroencephalographic (EEG) intensity and cortical impedance (expressed as percentage of baseline) in the hypothermia (*solid circles*) and sham-cooled (*open circles*) groups. Impedance is a measure of cytotoxic edema (cell swelling). The hypothermia group shows greater recovery of EEG intensity after resolution of delayed seizures and complete suppression of the secondary rise in impedance. Mean ± SEM, *$p < .05$, **$p < .001$ hypothermia versus sham-cooled fetuses. (Data from Gunn AJ, et al: Pediatrics, 1998.)

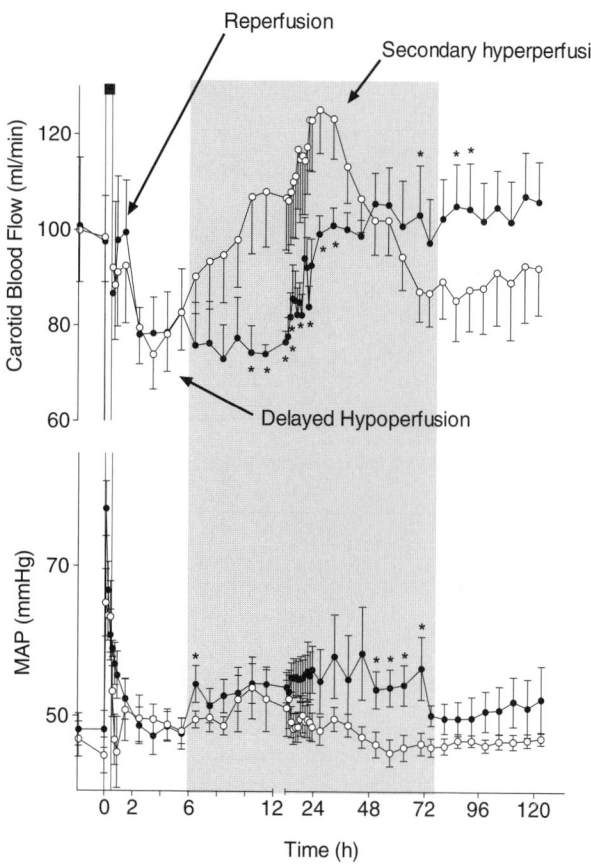

Figure 58–2. The effect of hypothermia started 5.5 hours after reperfusion from 30 minutes of cerebral ischemia in near-term fetal sheep on carotid blood flow and mean arterial blood pressure (MAP) in the hypothermia (*solid circles*) and sham-cooled (*open circles*) groups. Cerebral ischemia is shown by the *solid bar at the top* of the graph, whereas cooling is shown by the *highlighted region*. There was a significant increase in blood pressure during cooling that rapidly resolved with rewarming. Both groups show a significant phase of secondary hypoperfusion that was beginning to resolve at 6 hours; hypothermia prolonged this phase and prevented the phase of secondary hyperperfusion such that carotid blood flow was significantly reduced in the hypothermia group between 10 and 36 hours. Mean ± SEM, *p < .05 versus sham cooling. (Data from Gunn AJ, et al: Pediatrics, 1998.)

practice. It is simply not possible at present to identify reliably (until some hours after birth) the few infants requiring resuscitation who will go on to develop significant encephalopathy.

Prolonged Cooling

A more recent approach has been to try to suppress the secondary encephalopathic processes by maintaining hypothermia throughout the course of the secondary phase. Such extended periods of cooling of between 5 and 72 hours appear to be more consistently effective.[21-23] After brief global ischemia in the gerbil, extending the duration of moderate cooling from 0.5 to 6 hours after reperfusion progressively improved neuroprotection.[21] Even longer periods of cooling may be more beneficial. In a study of reversible middle cerebral artery occlusion in the adult rat, 21 hours, but not 1 hour, of mild hypothermia reduced the area of infarction after 48 hours recovery.[24] After severe global ischemia in the adult gerbil, 12 hours of mild hypothermia was ineffective, whereas extending the interval to 24 hours did afford protection.[22]

More limited reports in the perinatal brain are consistent with these data. In unanesthetized infant rats subjected to moderate hypoxia-ischemia, mild hypothermia (2° to 3°C of cerebral cooling) for 72 hours from the end of hypoxia prevented cortical infarction, whereas 6 hours of cooling only had intermediate, nonsignificant results.[25] Finally, in the anesthetized piglet exposed either to hypoxia with bilateral carotid ligation or to hypoxia with hypotension, 12 hours of moderate whole body hypothermia or 24 hours of head cooling with mild systemic hypothermia (started immediately after hypoxia) prevented delayed energy failure, reduced neuronal loss,[23, 26, 27] and suppressed posthypoxic seizures.[27]

A Window of Opportunity for Treatment? Recent Evidence

At present, the window of opportunity for any particular therapy can only be determined empirically. It is clear that initiation of neuronal degeneration is accelerated by more severe insults. For example, DNA fragmentation in the hippocampus can be detected as early as 10 hours after a 60-minute hypoxic-ischemic injury in the rat, whereas DNA fragmentation in the hippocampus is only detectable 3 to 5 days after a 15-minute hypoxic-ischemic injury.[28] However, the appearance of DNA fragmentation and classic ischemic cell change represent only the terminal events of this cascade and are thus not a good guide to determining when cell death may still be reversible. *In vitro* studies have distinguished *latent* and active or *execution* phases during the process of programmed or apoptotic cell death.[29] Whereas the active phase involves downstream factors that could induce DNA fragmentation and chromatin condensation within previously normal nuclei, the preceding latent phase is characterized by caspase activation (a large family of enzymes that mediate and amplify apoptosis)[30] confined to the cytoplasm, without downstream factors. These data suggest that activation of the downstream, intranuclear factors is the critical event that occurs at the transition from the latent to the execution phases of programmed neuronal death. Thus, in principle, it seems far more likely that intervention would be protective if applied during the initial, latent phase of programmed cell death rather than during the execution phase, even though the latter still precedes DNA fragmentation and cell death.[29]

Systematic *in vivo* studies support the central role of the latent phase. In the near-term fetal sheep, moderate hypothermia induced 90 minutes after reperfusion (i.e., in the early latent phase) and continued until 72 hours after ischemia prevented secondary cytotoxic edema and improved electroencephalographic recovery.[11] There was a concomitant, substantial reduction in parasagittal cortical infarction and improvement in neuronal loss scores in all regions. When the start of hypothermia was delayed in this paradigm until just before the onset of secondary seizures, 5.5 hours after reperfusion, partial protection was seen (Fig. 58-3; see Fig. 58-1).[31] With further delay (until after seizures were established 8.5 hours after reperfusion), there was no electrophysiologic or overall histologic protection with cooling (see Fig. 58-3).[32]

Data from adult models are consistent with this model. Thus, 5 hours of moderate hypothermia (32.5°C) initiated under anesthesia in adult rats reduced selective neuronal loss when it was started up to 12 hours after brief global ischemia, although the degree and extent of neuroprotection markedly declined as the start of cooling was delayed beyond 2 hours.[33] Similarly, in adult gerbils, 6 to 12 hours of moderate hypothermia reduced selective neuronal loss when it was started within 1 hour of global ischemia,[21, 22] whereas a period of 6 hours of hypothermia, begun 3 hours after onset of global ischemia, was not effective.[21]

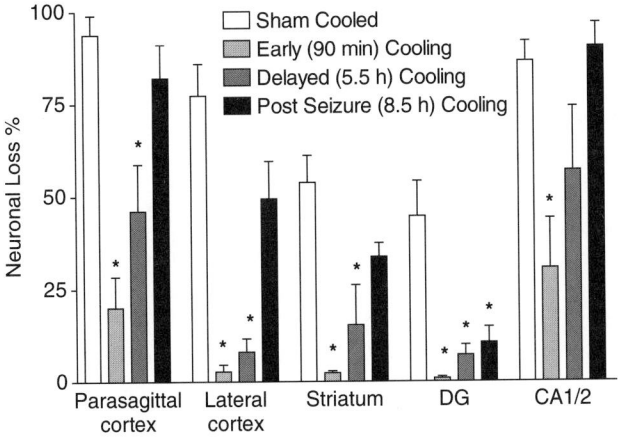

Figure 58–3. Comparison of the effect of cerebral cooling in the fetal sheep started at different times after reperfusion and continued until 72 hours on microscopically assessed neuronal loss in the neuronal regions of cortex after 5 days' recovery from 30 minutes of cerebral ischemia. Compared with the sham-cooled group (n = 13), cooling that was started 90 minutes after reperfusion (n = 7) or just before the end of the latent phase (5.5 hours after reperfusion, n = 11) was protective, whereas cooling started shortly after the start of the secondary phase (8.5 hours after reperfusion, n = 5) was not. Only cooled fetuses in which the extradural temperature was successfully maintained at less than 34°C have been included. DG = dentate gyrus. *$p < .005$ compared with sham-cooled (control) fetuses, Mann Whitney U test. Mean ± SEM. (Data from refs. 11, 31, and 32.)

How Long Is Long Enough?

There is evidence that optimal protection with delayed initiation of hypothermia requires periods of cooling longer than 12 hours. Critically, Colbourne and Corbett found in the adult gerbil that, with a slightly more severe insult (5 minutes of global ischemia compared with 3 minutes), the duration of moderate hypothermia had to be extended from 12 to 24 hours to provide neuroprotection.[22] When the delay before initiating the 24-hour period of cooling was increased from 1 to 4 hours, neuroprotection in the CA1 field of the hippocampus after 6 months of recovery fell from 70 to 12%.[34] Subsequent studies using models of both focal and global cerebral ischemia in adult rodents demonstrated that this chronic loss could be prevented by extending the duration of moderate (32° to 34°C) hypothermia to 48 hours or more, even when the start of cooling was delayed until 6 hours after reperfusion.[35, 36]

Is Neuroprotection Maintained Long Term?

Some reports have indicated that hypothermia only delays, rather than prevents, neuronal degeneration after global ischemia in the adult rat[37-39] and severe hypoxia-ischemia in the 7-day-old rat.[40] This finding may be related to two factors. First, rebound hyperthermia in the secondary phase can occur after ischemia. Even short periods of hyperthermia, 24 hours after either global or brief focal ischemia in the adult rat, exacerbates injury.[41, 42] When moderate hypothermia 2 to 9 hours after global ischemia in the rat was combined with prevention of spontaneous delayed pyrexia with antipyretics, histologic protection was seen after 2 months of recovery.[39] Each intervention alone had essentially short-term benefit only. Whether mild hypothermia could have had additional benefit com-

pared with normothermia in this late interval is, regrettably, unknown.

An alternative explanation may be that the duration of hypothermia was inadequate in relation to the severity of injury. Whereas a 72-hour period of very mild cooling in the infant rat was associated with long-term improvement, a 6-hour period was not.[25] Extensive studies in young adult and geriatric gerbils showed persistent behavioral and histologic neuroprotection with prolonged (≥48-hour) moderate (32°C) cooling, initiated up to 6 hours after ischemia.[35,36] Consistent with the postulate that an inadequate duration of hypothermia merely delays injury, in pilot studies we observed substantial rebound epileptiform activity when cerebral cooling was stopped after intervals shorter than 72 hours in the fetal lamb.[11]

If Some Is Good, Is More Better?

There appears to be a critical depth of cerebral hypothermia between 32° and 34°C required for effective neuronal rescue. In the fetal sheep cooled from 90 minutes after ischemia, substantial neuroprotection was seen only in fetuses that had a sustained fall of the extradural temperature to less than 34°C (normal temperature in the fetal sheep is 39.5°C).[11] In the adult gerbil, cooling to a rectal temperature of 32°C was associated with greater behavioral and histologic neuroprotection than 34°C.[43] Although we do not know the optimal degree of cerebral cooling in newborns, the first controlled trials of hypothermia after cardiac arrest in adults strongly support this target range, with improved neurologic outcome in patients cooled to between 32° and 34°C.[44,45]

There is a clear trade-off between the adverse systemic effects of cooling, which increase markedly below a core temperature of approximately 34°C,[4] and the potential cerebral benefit. For example, in the adult dog, deep hypothermia (15°C) after cardiac arrest was detrimental,[46] with worse cerebral and cardiac outcomes than in dogs maintained at normothermia, whereas mild hypothermia (34° to 36°C), from 10 minutes until 12 hours after cardiac arrest, was beneficial.[47] The adverse systemic effects accounting for the impaired effectiveness of greater levels of cooling are not known. However, they are likely to involve impaired cardiac contractility, leading to decreased cardiac output, arterial hypotension, and compromised perfusion.[48]

Is It Possible to Cool the Head "Selectively"?

To provide adequate neuroprotection with minimal risk of systemic adverse effects in sick, unstable neonates, ideally only the brain would be cooled. Although this has been demonstrated experimentally using cardiac bypass procedures,[49] it is clearly impractical in routine practice. More pragmatically, partially selective cerebral cooling can be obtained using a cooling cap applied to the scalp while the body is warmed by some method such as an overhead heater to limit the degree of systemic hypothermia.[50,51] In practice, mild (~34.5°C) systemic hypothermia is desirable during head cooling, first to limit the steepness of the intracerebral gradient that would otherwise be needed (avoiding excessively cold cap temperatures) and second to provide greater cooling of the brain stem. This approach was demonstrated in studies in the piglet, with a substantial (median, 5.3°C) sustained decrease in deep intracerebral temperature at the level of the basal ganglia compared with the rectal temperature.[52] Similar results from studies of brief head cooling have been reported in the young adult cat,[53] the newborn rat,[54] and the piglet.[55] Although direct temperature measurements are not feasible in asphyxiated newborns, head cooling has been shown to increase the gradient between nasopharyngeal and rectal temperature by nearly 1°C.[50]

In many ways, this approach is an extension of normal physiology. Even in the healthy neonate, there is no single cerebral temperature, but a gradient from the warmer deep regions to the cooler surface.[56,57] The head represents more than 70% of heat production,[58] and it is cooled by a combination of surface radiation and blood flow convection. Thus, the deep brain temperature is approximately 1° to 2°C higher than the surface of the head,[56] and it is 0.7°C higher than core body temperature.[57] Deep brain temperature is increased by conditions of reduced perfusion,[57] such as seen after severe asphyxia.[59,60]

MECHANISMS OF ACTION OF HYPOTHERMIA

Although the precise mechanism of hypothermic neuroprotection is not known, it suppresses many of the pathways leading to delayed cell death. Hypothermia may be helpful by (1) reducing cellular metabolic demands, (2) reducing excessive accumulation of cytotoxins such as glutamate and oxygen free radicals, (3) suppressing the postischemic inflammatory reaction, and (4) suppressing the intracellular pathways leading to programmed (i.e., apoptosis-like) cell death.

Cerebral Metabolism, Excitotoxins, and Free Radicals During the Primary and Reperfusion Phases

The combination of hypoxic depolarization and extracellular excitotoxin accumulation are key factors in the initiation of neuronal injury in the primary phase. Hypothermia produces a graded reduction in cerebral metabolism of about 5% for every degree of temperature reduction,[61] and this delays the onset of anoxic cell depolarization. However, the protective effects of hypothermia even in this phase are not simply the result of reduced metabolism, because cooling improves outcome even when the absolute duration of depolarization is controlled.[62] Cooling potently reduces postdepolarization release of numerous toxins including excitatory amino acids,[63] nitric oxide,[64] and other free radicals.[20,65] Similarly, cooling begun during reperfusion in adult species suppresses oxygen free radicals,[20,66] and it reduces levels of extracellular excitatory amino acids and nitric oxide production in the piglet.[67] However, these mechanisms are not active during the latent phase and thus cannot readily account for the protective effects of delayed cooling.

Intracellular Pathways in the Latent Phase

There is evidence that hypothermia acts on pathways distal to cell membrane ion channels. For example, intrainsult hypothermia did not prevent intracellular accumulation of calcium during cardiac arrest *in vivo*[68] or during glutamate exposure *in vitro*.[69] In contrast, *in vitro* neuronal degeneration was prevented by cooling initiated after washout of the excitotoxins.[69,70] Indeed, there is evidence in the adult rat that the apparent neuroprotective effect of NBQX, a glutamate antagonist, administered from 1 hour after mild ischemia, was actually mediated by mild hypothermia.[38] Thus, the ability of hypothermia to reduce release of excitotoxins does not appear to be central to its postinsult neuroprotective effects; rather, these data suggest that the critical effect of hypothermia is to block the intracellular consequences of excitotoxin exposure. Further, cooling prevents intracellular ion and water entry and the consequent osmotic cell swelling even if the adenosine triphosphate–dependent sodium-potassium pump is inhibited by ouabain.[71] This mechanism is likely to underlie the action of hypothermia to prevent secondary cytotoxic edema.[11]

Suppression of Inflammatory Second Messengers

Brain injury leads to induction of the inflammatory cascade with increased release of cytokines and interleukins.[72] These compounds are believed to exacerbate delayed injury, either by direct neurotoxicity and induction of apoptosis[72] or by promoting stimulation of capillary endothelial cell proinflammatory responses and leukocyte adhesion and infiltration into the ischemic brain.[73] There is good evidence that cooling can suppress this inflammatory reaction. *In vitro*, hypothermia potently inhibits proliferation, superoxide production, and nitric oxide production by cultured microglial cells.[74] In the adult rat, hypothermia suppresses the posttraumatic release of interleukin-1β,[75] as well as the accumulation of polymorphonuclear leukocytes.[76] Similarly, postischemic hypothermia delays neutrophil accumulation and microglial activation after transient focal ischemia.[77] Thus, these data suggest that the hypothermic protection against postischemic neuronal damage may be, in part, the result of suppression of microglial activation.

Does Hypothermia Specifically Prevent or Suppress Apoptosis (Programmed Cell Death)?

Some studies, particularly in adult species, show that hypothermia can prevent delayed necrotic cell death.[78] However, increasing data suggest that hypothermia has a particular role in suppressing apoptotic processes, particularly in the developing brain. In the piglet, hypothermia begun after severe hypoxia-ischemia reduced apoptotic cell death but not necrotic cell death.[26] Similarly, moderate hypothermia showed specific effect on inhibition of apoptotic cell death and cellular DNA fragmentation after cold-induced brain injury in rats.[79] In the adult rodent, postischemic hypothermia reduced both the number of TUNEL-positive cells and expression of the proapoptotic factor, Bax.[80] These data are consistent with *in vitro* studies of hypothermia after severe hypoxia in developing rat neurons. In the neuronal culture system noted earlier, preconditioning using a brief period of hypoxia activated a program that stimulated the expression of antiapoptotic gene products and regulatory components of the cell cycle; however, hypothermia did not trigger active processes, but it depressed cell activity and abolished hypoxia-associated protein synthesis.[81] Therefore, the specific mechanisms mediating suppression apoptosis by hypothermia could include reducing cytokine release, as described earlier, inhibiting the Fas (CD95) cell death–inducing complex that is a key cellular step in triggering this cascade,[82] or inhibiting the activation of the caspases.[30,83]

SYSTEMIC EFFECTS OF HYPOTHERMIA

Small controlled trials of head cooling with mild hypothermia[50,84] and of whole body cooling[85] in asphyxiated newborns have been reported, in addition to several case series.[86,87] The full range of potential adverse effects associated with moderate to deep hypothermia is beyond the scope of this chapter and has been reviewed in the literature.[4] Although the foregoing studies have suggested that mild hypothermia is generally safe, they have highlighted the importance of understanding the physiologic effects of hypothermia.

Cardiovascular Adaptation

Consistent with the known electrocardiographic effects of hypothermia to slow the atrial pacemaker and intracardiac conduction, hypothermia to less than approximately 35.5°C is associated with sustained sinus bradycardia in most infants.[84,85] Electrocardiograms done in infants with sustained heart rates of less than 90 beats per minute confirmed that a markedly prolonged QT duration above the 98th percentile corrected for age and heart rate, without arrhythmia, that resolved on rewarming. Although such a prolonged QT interval in the absence of ventricular arrhythmia may be safe, close monitoring is clearly essential, and other therapies that lengthen the QT interval (such as macrolide antibiotics) should be avoided.

As illustrated in Figure 58-2, initiation of cooling is associated with a significant increase in blood pressure both experimentally[31] and clinically.[86] This rise is mediated by rapid peripheral vasoconstriction, that is, centralization of blood flow.[88] Figure 58-2 also shows that cooling results in a marked reduction in carotid blood flow compared with sham-cooled fetuses, with prolongation of secondary hypoperfusion and abolition of hyperperfusion during delayed seizures. This relative reduction is mediated by reduced metabolism and not by nonspecific peripheral vasoconstriction; many studies, mostly in the infant pig, have shown that even during deep hypothermia, cerebral blood flow and metabolism remain closely coupled.[89]

Respiratory Management

Persistent pulmonary hypertension is a frequent association with perinatal asphyxia, while at the same time experimentally, moderate hypothermia ($31\pm0.4°C$) increased pulmonary vascular resistance.[90] One case series suggested that hypothermia was associated with a modest but consistent increase in inspired oxygen fraction.[86] In contrast, other controlled studies found no apparent change in the oxygen or ventilatory requirements of infants with persistent pulmonary hypertension of the newborn during induction of hypothermia or rewarming.[84,85] An important technical point is that the partial pressure of oxygen (and of carbon dioxide) is reduced by hypothermia. Thus, the measured level will be artifactually increased if the blood gas from a cooled infant is analyzed at $37°C$.

Nonshivering Thermogenesis

As discussed elsewhere in this book, unlike adults, infants respond to cooling with intense nonshivering thermogenesis during cooling. Active cooling exposes underlying changes in this endogenous heat production that are normally masked by the routine use of servocontrolled warming. Thus, for example, hypoxia or sedative therapy, both of which potently inhibit thermogenesis, will lead to a fall in temperature.[84,86] In contrast, seizures, which increase peripheral heat production, and ventilation with warmed gases can increase body temperature.[50,84,86] It is important to anticipate the potential for these changes, to avoid large swings in temperature. During head cooling with mild systemic hypothermia, keeping the overhead heater usually on maximum during cooling is one way to minimize the contribution of these changes in endogenous heat production and thus to keep a more stable balance over time.

Metabolic Effects

Hypokalemia and mild metabolic acidosis may occur in infants cooled to less than $34°C$. Hypokalemia occurs in animal models during deep hypothermia, but it corrects spontaneously during rewarming, a finding suggesting that this change results from intracellular redistribution.[91] Consistent with this finding, a mild fall in serum potassium was reported in the series of infants cooled to between $33°$ and $34°C$,[87] whereas no change was found in studies using milder systemic cooling.[84,85] Maintenance potassium administration during cooling must be used cautiously. There is evidence that it may actually help to protect against potassium cardiotoxicity,[91] and overcorrection of the reversible hypokalemia during hypothermia may lead to rebound hyperkalemia on rewarming.[92] Experimental hypothermia leads to transient increases in plasma glucose and lactate concentrations, likely related to increased circulating catecholamine levels.[11] In the clinic, such mild metabolic acidosis has only been suggested in infants cooled to less than $34°C$.[87] pH measurements are also markedly affected by hypothermia and must be adjusted by the patient's temperature.

CONCLUSION

There is now good experimental evidence that moderate post-asphyxial cerebral cooling can be associated with long-term neuroprotection. The key requirements are that hypothermia be initiated as soon as possible in the latent phase, before secondary deterioration, and that it be continued for a sufficient period in relation to the evolution of delayed encephalopathic processes, typically 48 hours or more. Although experimental studies suggest that cooling can be effective if started up to 6 hours after relatively short insults, it is clear that cooling started as soon as possible, within at most a few hours of birth, is most likely to be effective.

Preliminary studies of both whole body cooling and head cooling combined with mild systemic hypothermia support the general safety of selective hypothermia even in sick asphyxiated infants, but these data should not be overinterpreted. These studies are too small, and they were not designed either to test the efficacy of treatment or to detect uncommon adverse events. This issue is being addressed by large multicenter trials of different cooling strategies, with adequate power to assess longer-term outcome. Until definitive evidence of clinical benefit is shown, hypothermia must remain an investigatory technique.

ACKNOWLEDGMENTS

Our work reported in this chapter is supported by National Institutes of Health grant RO-1 HD32752 and by grants from the Health Research Council of New Zealand, the Lottery Health Board of New Zealand, and the Auckland Medical Research Foundation.

REFERENCES

1. Westin B, et al: Neonatal asphyxia pallida treated with hypothermia alone or with hypothermia and transfusion of oxygenated blood. Surgery 45:868, 1959.
2. Miller JA, et al: Hypothermia in the treatment of asphyxia neonatorum. Biol Neonate 6:148, 1964.
3. Cordey R: Hypothermia in resuscitating newborns in white asphyxia: a report of 14 cases. Obstet Gynecol 24:760, 1964.
4. Schubert A: Side effects of mild hypothermia. J Neurosurg Anesthesiol 7:139, 1995.
5. Silverman WA, et al: The influence of the thermal environment upon the survival of newly born premature infants. Pediatrics 31:876, 1958.
6. Nurse S, Corbett D: Direct measurement of brain temperature during and after intraischemic hypothermia: correlation with behavioral, physiological, and histological endpoints. J Neurosci 14:7726, 1994.
7. Kirino T: Delayed neuronal death. Neuropathology 20(Suppl):S95, 2000.
8. Banasiak KJ, et al: Mechanisms underlying hypoxia-induced neuronal apoptosis. Prog Neurobiol 62:215, 2000.
9. Roth SC, et al: Relation of deranged neonatal cerebral oxidative metabolism with neurodevelopmental outcome and head circumference at 4 years. Dev Med Child Neurol 39:718, 1997.
10. Lorek A, et al: Delayed ("secondary") cerebral energy failure after acute hypoxia-ischemia in the newborn piglet: continuous 48-hour studies by phosphorus magnetic resonance spectroscopy. Pediatr Res 36:699, 1994.
11. Gunn AJ, et al: Dramatic neuronal rescue with prolonged selective head cooling after ischemia in fetal lambs. J Clin Invest 99:248, 1997.
12. Tan WK, et al: Accumulation of cytotoxins during the development of seizures and edema after hypoxic-ischemic injury in late gestation fetal sheep. Pediatr Res 39:791, 1996.
13. Laptook AR, et al: Modest hypothermia provides partial neuroprotection when used for immediate resuscitation after brain ischemia. Pediatr Res 42:17, 1997.
14. Laptook AR, et al: A limited interval of delayed modest hypothermia for ischemic brain resuscitation is not beneficial in neonatal swine. Pediatr Res 46:383, 1999.
15. Yager J, et al: Influence of mild hypothermia on hypoxic-ischemic brain damage in the immature rat. Pediatr Res 34:525, 1993.
16. Bona E, et al: Sensorimotor function and neuropathology five to six weeks after hypoxia-ischemia in seven-day-old rats. Pediatr Res 42:678, 1997.
17. Kuboyama K, et al: Delay in cooling negates the beneficial effect of mild resuscitative cerebral hypothermia after cardiac arrest in dogs: a prospective, randomized study. Crit Care Med 21:1348, 1993.
18. Shuaib A, et al: The effect of post-ischemic hypothermia following repetitive cerebral ischemia in gerbils. Neurosci Lett 186:165, 1995.
19. Busto R, et al: Postischemic moderate hypothermia inhibits CA1 hippocampal ischemic neuronal injury. Neurosci Lett 101:299, 1989.
20. Zhao W, et al: Neuroprotective effects of hypothermia and U-78517f in cerebral ischemia are due to reducing oxygen-based free radicals: an electron paramagnetic resonance study with gerbils. J Neurosci Res 45:282, 1996.

21. Carroll M, Beek O: Protection against hippocampal CA1 cell loss by post-ischemic hypothermia is dependent on delay of initiation and duration. Metab Brain Dis 7:45, 1992.

22. Colbourne F, Corbett D: Delayed and prolonged post-ischemic hypothermia is neuroprotective in the gerbil. Brain Res 654:265, 1994.

23. Thoresen M, et al: Mild hypothermia after severe transient hypoxia-ischemia ameliorates delayed cerebral energy failure in the newborn piglet. Pediatr Res 37:667, 1995.

24. Yanamoto H, et al: Mild postischemic hypothermia limits cerebral injury following transient focal ischemia in rat neocortex. Brain Res 718:207, 1996.

25. Sirimanne ES, et al: The effect of prolonged modification of cerebral temperature on outcome after hypoxic-ischemic brain injury in the infant rat. Pediatr Res 39:591, 1996.

26. Edwards AD, et al: Specific inhibition of apoptosis after cerebral hypoxia-ischaemia by moderate post-insult hypothermia. Biochem Biophys Res Commun 217:1193, 1995.

27. Tooley JR, et al: Head cooling with mild systemic hypothermia in anesthetized piglets is neuroprotective. Ann Neurol 53:65, 2003.

28. Beilharz EJ, et al: Mechanisms of delayed cell death following hypoxic-ischemic injury in the immature rat: evidence for apoptosis during selective neuronal loss. Brain Res 29:1, 1995.

29. Samejima K, et al: Transition from caspase-dependent to caspase-independent mechanisms at the onset of apoptotic execution. J Cell Biol 143:225, 1998.

30. Gottron FJ, et al: Caspase inhibition selectively reduces the apoptotic component of oxygen-glucose deprivation-induced cortical neuronal cell death. Mol Cell Neurosci 9:159, 1997.

31. Gunn AJ, et al: Neuroprotection with prolonged head cooling started before postischemic seizures in fetal sheep. Pediatrics 102:1098, 1998.

32. Gunn AJ, et al: Cerebral hypothermia is not neuroprotective when started after postischemic seizures in fetal sheep. Pediatr Res 46:274, 1999.

33. Coimbra C, Wieloch T: Moderate hypothermia mitigates neuronal damage in the rat brain when initiated several hours following transient cerebral ischemia. Acta Neuropathol (Berl) 87:325, 1994.

34. Colbourne F, Corbett D: Delayed postischemic hypothermia: a six month survival study using behavioral and histological assessments of neuroprotection. J Neurosci 15:7250, 1995.

35. Colbourne F, et al: Prolonged but delayed postischemic hypothermia: a long-term outcome study in the rat middle cerebral artery occlusion model. J Cereb Blood Flow Metab 20:1702, 2000.

36. Colbourne F, et al: Indefatigable CA1 sector neuroprotection with mild hypothermia induced 6 hours after severe forebrain ischemia in rats. J Cereb Blood Flow Metab 19:742, 1999.

37. Dietrich WD, et al: Intraischemic but not postischemic brain hypothermia protects chronically following global forebrain ischemia in rats. J Cereb Blood Flow Metab 13:541, 1993.

38. Nurse S, Corbett D: Neuroprotection after several days of mild, drug-induced hypothermia. J Cereb Blood Flow Metab 16:474, 1996.

39. Coimbra C, et al: Long-lasting neuroprotective effect of postischemic hypothermia and treatment with an anti-inflammatory/antipyretic drug: evidence for chronic encephalopathic processes following ischemia. Stroke 27:1578, 1996.

40. Trescher WH, et al: Brief post-hypoxic-ischemic hypothermia markedly delays neonatal brain injury. Brain Dev 19:326, 1997.

41. Baena RC, et al: Hyperthermia delayed by 24 hours aggravates neuronal damage in rat hippocampus following global ischemia. Neurology 48:768, 1997.

42. Kim Y, et al: Delayed postischemic hyperthermia in awake rats worsens the histopathological outcome of transient focal cerebral ischemia. Stroke 27:2274, 1996.

43. Colbourne F, et al: Characterization of postischemic behavioral deficits in gerbils with and without hypothermic neuroprotection. Brain Res 803:69, 1998.

44. Bernard SA, et al: Treatment of comatose survivors of out-of-hospital cardiac arrest with induced hypothermia. N Engl J Med 346:557, 2002.

45. Hypothermia after Cardiac Arrest Study Group: Mild therapeutic hypothermia to improve the neurologic outcome after cardiac arrest. N Engl J Med 346:549, 2002.

46. Weinrauch V, et al: Beneficial effect of mild hypothermia and detrimental effect of deep hypothermia after cardiac arrest in dogs. Stroke 23:1454, 1992.

47. Safar P, et al: Improved cerebral resuscitation from cardiac arrest in dogs with mild hypothermia plus blood flow promotion. Stroke 27:105, 1996.

48. Dudgeon DL, et al: Mild hypothermia: its effect on cardiac output and regional perfusion in the neonatal piglet. J Pediatr Surg 15:805, 1980.

49. Wass CT, et al: Selective convective brain cooling during normothermic cardiopulmonary bypass in dogs. J Thorac Cardiovasc Surg 115:1350, 1998.

50. Gunn AJ, et al: Selective head cooling in newborn infants after perinatal asphyxia: a safety study. Pediatrics 102:885, 1998.

51. Simbruner G, et al: Induced brain hypothermia in asphyxiated human newborn infants: a retrospective chart analysis of physiological and adverse effects. Intensive Care Med 25:1111, 1999.

52. Thoresen M, et al: Effective selective head cooling during posthypoxic hypothermia in newborn piglets. Pediatr Res 49:594, 2001.

53. Sefrin P, Horn M: Selective cerebral hypothermia following cardiac arrest in the cat. Anaesthesist 40:397, 1991.

54. Towfighi J, et al: The effect of focal cerebral cooling on perinatal hypoxic-ischemic brain damage. Acta Neuropathol (Berl) 87:598, 1994.

55. Gelman B, et al: Selective brain cooling in infant piglets after cardiac arrest and resuscitation. Crit Care Med 24:1009, 1996.

56. Gunn AJ, Gunn TR: Effect of radiant heat on head temperature gradient in term infants. Arch Dis Child 74:F200, 1996.

57. Simbruner G, et al: Brain temperature discriminates between neonates with damaged, hypoperfused, and normal brains. Am J Perinatol 11:137, 1994.

58. Hull D: Temperature regulation and disturbance in the newborn infant. Clin Endocrinol Metab 5:39, 1976.

59. Rumana CS, et al: Brain temperature exceeds systemic temperature in head-injured patients. Crit Care Med 26:562, 1998.

60. Van Bel F, et al: Changes in cerebral hemodynamics and oxygenation in the first 24 hours after birth asphyxia. Pediatrics 92:365, 1993.

61. Laptook AR, et al: Quantitative relationship between brain temperature and energy utilization rate measured in vivo using ^{31}P and ^{1}H magnetic resonance spectroscopy. Pediatr Res 38:919, 1995.

62. Bart RD, et al: Interactions between hypothermia and the latency to ischemic depolarization: implications for neuroprotection. Anesthesiology 88:1266, 1998.

63. Nakashima K, Todd MM: Effects of hypothermia, pentobarbital, and isoflurane on postdepolarization amino acid release during complete global cerebral ischemia. Anesthesiology 85:161, 1996.

64. Kader A, et al: Effect of mild hypothermia on nitric oxide synthesis during focal cerebral ischemia. Neurosurgery 35:272, 1994.

65. Lei BP, et al: The effect of hypothermia on H_2O_2 production during ischemia and reperfusion: a microdialysis study in the gerbil hippocampus. Neurosci Lett 222:91, 1997.

66. Lei B, et al: Effect of moderate hypothermia on lipid peroxidation in canine brain tissue after cardiac arrest and resuscitation. Stroke 25:147, 1994.

67. Thoresen M, et al: Post-hypoxic hypothermia reduces cerebrocortical release of NO and excitotoxins. Neuroreport 8:3359, 1997.

68. Kristian T, et al: The influence of moderate hypothermia on cellular calcium uptake in complete ischaemia: implications for the excitotoxic hypothesis. Acta Physiol Scand 146:531, 1992.

69. Bruno VMG, et al: Neuroprotective effect of hypothermia in cortical cultures exposed to oxygen-glucose deprivation or excitatory amino acids. J Neurochem 63:1398, 1994.

70. Shuaib A, et al: Hypothermia protects astrocytes during ischemia in cell culture. Neurosci Lett 146:69, 1992.

71. Zeevalk GD, Nicklas WJ: Hypothermia and metabolic stress: narrowing the cellular site of early neuroprotection. J Pharmacol Exp Ther 279:332, 1996.

72. Rothwell NJ, Strijbos PJLM: Cytokines in neurodegeneration and repair. Int J Dev Neurosci 13:179, 1995.

73. Silverstein FS, et al: Cytokines and perinatal brain injury. Neurochem Int 30:375, 1997.

74. Si QS, et al: Hypothermic suppression of microglial activation in culture: inhibition of cell proliferation and production of nitric oxide and superoxide. Neuroscience 81:223, 1997.

75. Goss JR, et al: Hypothermia attenuates the normal increase in interleukin 1 beta RNA and nerve growth factor following traumatic brain injury in the rat. J Neurotrauma 12:159, 1995.

76. Chatzipanteli K, et al: Posttraumatic hypothermia reduces polymorphonuclear leukocyte accumulation following spinal cord injury in rats. J Neurotrauma 17:321, 2000.

77. Inamasu J, et al: Post-ischemic hypothermia delayed neutrophil accumulation and microglial activation following transient focal ischemia in rats. J Neuroimmunol 109:66, 2000.

78. Colbourne F, et al: Electron microscopic evidence against apoptosis as the mechanism of neuronal death in global ischemia. J Neurosci 19:4200, 1999.

79. Xu RX, et al: Specific inhibition of apoptosis after cold-induced brain injury by moderate postinjury hypothermia. Neurosurgery 43:107, 1998.

80. Inamasu J, et al: Postischemic hypothermia attenuates apoptotic cell death in transient focal ischemia in rats. Acta Neurochir Suppl (Wien) 76:525, 2000.

81. Bossenmeyer-Pourie C, et al: Effects of hypothermia on hypoxia-induced apoptosis in cultured neurons from developing rat forebrain: comparison with preconditioning. Pediatr Res 47:385, 2000.

82. Nagata S: Fas-mediated apoptosis. Adv Exp Med Biol 406:119, 1996.

83. Schwartz LM, Milligan CE: Cold thoughts of death: the role of ICE proteases in neuronal cell death. Trends Neurosci 19:555, 1996.

84. Battin MR, et al: Treatment of term infants with head cooling and mild systemic hypothermia (35.0 degrees C and 34.5 degrees C) after perinatal asphyxia. Pediatrics 111:244, 2003.

85. Shankaran S, et al: Whole-body hypothermia for neonatal encephalopathy: animal observations as a basis for a randomized, controlled pilot study in term infants. Pediatrics 110:377, 2002.

86. Thoresen M, Whitelaw A: Cardiovascular changes during mild therapeutic hypothermia and rewarming in infants with hypoxic-ischaemic encephalopathy. Pediatrics 106:92, 2000.

87. Azzopardi D, et al: Pilot study of treatment with whole body hypothermia for neonatal encephalopathy. Pediatrics 106:684, 2000.

88. Gordon CJ, Heath JE: Integration and central processing in temperature regulation. Annu Rev Physiol 48:595, 1986.

89. Walter B, et al: Coupling of cerebral blood flow and oxygen metabolism in infant pigs during selective brain hypothermia. J Cereb Blood Flow Metab 20:1215, 2000.

90. Benumof JL, Wahrenbrock EA: Dependency of hypoxic pulmonary vasoconstriction on temperature. J Appl Physiol 42:56, 1977.

91. Sprung J, et al: The effect of acute hypothermia and serum potassium concentration on potassium cardiotoxicity in anesthetized rats. Acta Anaesthesiol Scand 36:825, 1992.

92. Zydlewski AW, Hasbargen JA: Hypothermia-induced hypokalemia. Mil Med 163:719, 1998.

Skin

59

David H. Chu and Cynthia A. Loomis

Structure and Development of the Skin and Cutaneous Appendages

OVERVIEW

Skin is a complex organ that comprises many different cells and cell types; it forms a critical physical barrier that protects the body and maintains fluid homeostasis, temperature regulation, and sensation. Skin cells derive from both embryonic mesoderm and ectoderm, and development from these precursors is tightly regulated. Perturbations in the developmental process, either from genetic anomalies or as a result of exogenous (e.g., teratogenic) agents, can result in severe abnormalities that have important consequences in the care of infants. Understanding the normal progression of molecular and cellular events that underlie the development and differentiation of skin allows for a more rational approach to infants who have defects in these processes. For the clinician, this knowledge will direct diagnosis, therapy, and parental counseling necessary for care of the patient.

Organogenesis of the skin proceeds, as with all organs, through three distinct but overlapping stages, from early embryonic through fetal and neonatal development.[1,2] These stages are as follows: *specification,* in which portions of superficial ectoderm and lateral plate mesoderm become distinct from other portions of the body wall; *morphogenesis,* in which the specific structural and biochemical characteristics of skin begin to appear; and *differentiation,* in which the skin tissue further develops to take on its mature form.

For the sake of clarity, we have organized the discussion of the developmental progression of the skin to follow each component sequentially, first with a discussion of the epidermis, followed by the dermis and subcutaneous tissue, the dermal-epidermal junction (DEJ), and, finally, epidermal appendages. Each of these sections discusses the structural and biochemical changes that are occurring during the particular stage of development, followed by a discussion of related clinical syndromes and genetic disorders that are related to defects in this developmental progression.[3] However, all these tissues of the skin are, in fact, developing in parallel, and in some cases they require interaction with adjacent tissues for development. A timeline is included to illustrate the sequence of events that are occurring simultaneously (Fig. 59-1).

EPIDERMIS

Overview

The mature adult *epidermis* is a stratified squamous epithelium that develops from the ectoderm. Keratinocytes form 80% of the cellular composition. The germinative keratinocytes reside in the deepest portion of the epidermis, known as the basal layer, and these cells are known as basal cells. As differentiation of the basal cells proceeds, these cells migrate to more superficial cell layers and become progressively flattened; they also begin to express large insoluble proteins that ultimately become cross-linked along the exterior of the cell to form an insoluble shell or brick, known as the cornified cell envelope.

Above the basal cell layer rests the spinous layer, or stratum spinosum. The "spines" seen in this layer result from the abundance of desmosomes, specialized regions of the keratinocyte cell surface that promote adhesion between these cells in a calcium-dependent manner. Desomosomal proteins include plakoglobin, desmoplakins I and II, keratocalmin, desmoyokin, band 6 protein, and the cadherins—desmogleins 1 and 3 and desmocollins I and II.[4]

The cell layer superficial to the stratum spinosum is the stratum granulosum. Granular cells begin to express some of the components that will contribute to the cornified cell envelope, a protein-lipid polymer that is found on the outer boundary of terminally differentiated keratinocytes.[5] The cornified cell envelope serves a critical role in the barrier function of the epidermis. Keratohyaline granules, found within the granular cells, are principally composed of two proteins, loricrin and profilaggrin. Profilaggrin undergoes sequential proteolytic cleavage into filaggrin oligomers and finally monomers, as well as desphosphorylation, during its processing. This process is initiated at the time of formation of the granular layer and continues even after its eventual extrusion from the cornified cell. Loricrin, another major component of the cornified envelope, is also initially localized to the keratohyaline granules. Lamellar granules, which are also abundant in the granular cell layer, contain the lipid components that will be extruded from the cells and cross-linked to the cornified cell envelope. Other proteins that contribute to the cornified envelope include involucrin, small proline-rich proteins, annexin, elafin, desmoplakin, envoplakin, periplakin, repetin, and trichohyalin. Modifying enzymes such as transglutaminases are important in the final cross-linking of the cornified envelope components. As described later, mutations in either the structural proteins or the enzymes involved in protein cross-linking and lipid and steroid metabolism can have clinically significant outcomes in genetic skin disease.

The stratum corneum contains the terminally differentiated keratinocytes, flattened dead "squames" that lack nuclei and other organelles. These cells are composed primarily of keratin filaments, tightly packed within the cross-linked cornified envelopes. Some specialized components present within the epidermis maintain its architecture. Keratins are some of the most important structural proteins within the epidermal cells. They

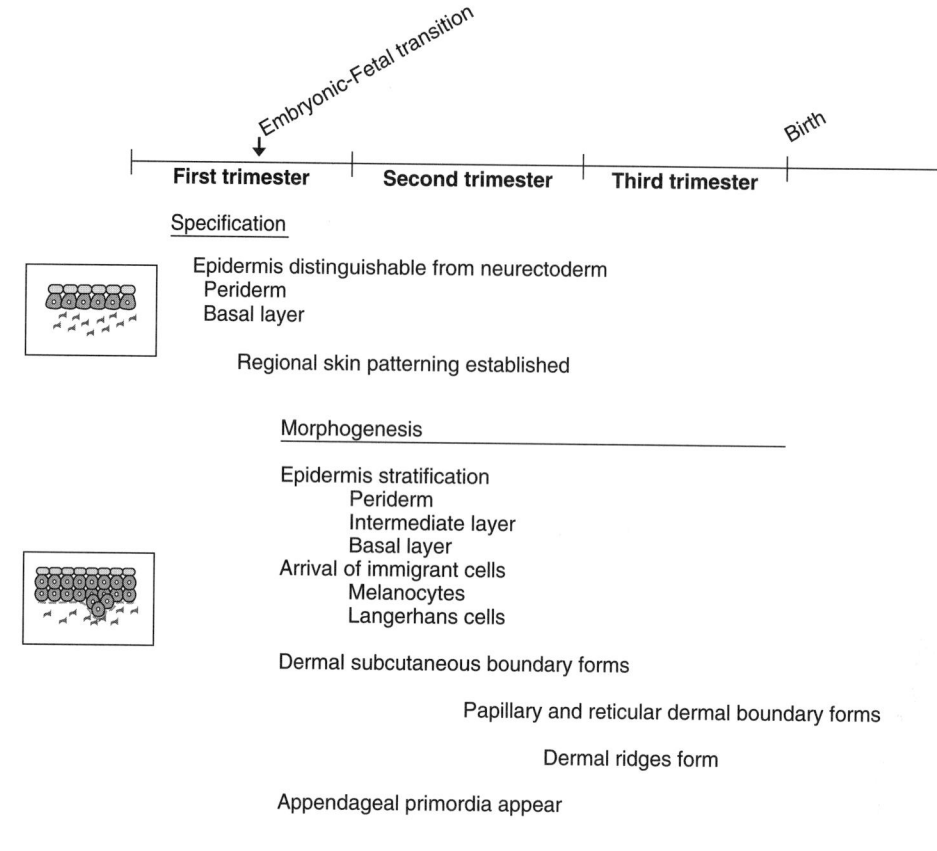

Specification

Epidermis distinguishable from neurectoderm
    Periderm
    Basal layer

Regional skin patterning established

Morphogenesis

Epidermis stratification
    Periderm
    Intermediate layer
    Basal layer
Arrival of immigrant cells
    Melanocytes
    Langerhans cells

Dermal subcutaneous boundary forms

Papillary and reticular dermal boundary forms

Dermal ridges form

Appendageal primordia appear

Differentiation

Periderm sloughs
Interfollicular keratinization:
    Stratum corneum
    Granular layer
    Basal layer

Hair shafts, nail plates produced
Glands mature

Increased fibrillogenesis of dermis

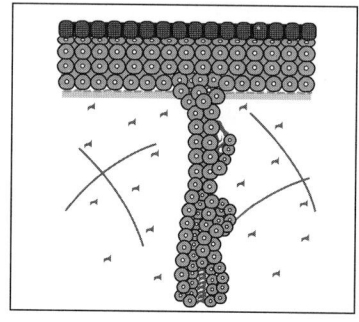

Figure 59–1. Timeline for the development of skin tissue. (Adapted from Loomis CA, Koss T: Embryology. *In* Bolognia JL, Jorizzo JL, Rapini RP (eds): Dermatology. Philadelphia: Elsevier, 2003.)

assemble as filaments composed of "basic" and "acidic" keratin peptides, which form *obligate heterodimers*; that is, different keratins are found to associate with a limited number of partners.[6, 7] Their expression is regulated in a tissue-specific and developmentally selective manner. Mutations in these genes often exhibit clinical phenotypes that reflect the tissue expression of the specific keratin gene. For example, whereas basal cells express K5 and K14, suprabasilar keratinocytes express K1 and K10 (K1 and K9 in palmoplantar epidermis).

Other critical structural elements of the epidermis are the cell-cell and cell-matrix adhesion systems. The major cell-cell adhesion junctions of the epidermis are desmosomes. The proteins in these complexes include specialized adhesion proteins (cadherins, calcium-dependent adhesion molecules) as well as intracellular plaque and adaptor proteins. An analogous adhesion structure, the hemidesmosome, attaches basal cells to the basement membrane at the DEJ. Although the proteins in the hemidesmosome are distinct from those of the desmosome, the plaque proteins have similar amino acid sequences, and both are tightly associated with the keratin filament network. Gap junctions form important intercellular bridges that allow small molecules to pass from one keratinocyte to another. These specialized junctions are formed by proteins known as connexins. Mutations in any of these molecules have effects on the normal formation of the epidermis that can result in certain genodermatoses, many of which have manifestations from birth.

Specification

Gastrulation of the embryo occurs during the third week after fertilization. This is a critical process that results in the generation of the three primary embryonic germ layers: endoderm, mesoderm, and ectoderm. The ectoderm then is further divided into the neuroectoderm and the presumptive epidermis. The epidermis is then subsequently specified into distinct regional domains, such as palmoplantar skin, scalp skin, and mammary skin.

The earliest presumptive epidermis consists of a basal cell layer, which covers the embryo.[8,9] By 6 weeks' estimated gestational age (EGA), the surface ectoderm consists of two layers: basal cells and more superficial periderm cells. The periderm layer does not give rise to any portion of the definitive epidermis, and as such it serves as a transient embryonic covering. This layer is ultimately sloughed during late gestation and contributes to the vernix caseosa, which covers the newborn.

Morphogenesis

The process of *morphogenesis* begins at approximately 8 weeks' EGA, the classic transition between embryonic and fetal development, when hemopoietic production shifts to the bone marrow. At this point, the epidermis begins its process of stratification, by forming an intermediate layer between the basal cell and the periderm layers. This intermediate layer remains highly proliferative, and more layers are added as development proceeds over the next several weeks. In mice, it has been shown that this process of epidermal stratification requires the *p63* and *Dlx-3* genes.[10-12] In humans, partial loss of function mutations in *p63* has been seen in various ectodermal dysplasias, as discussed later.

Differentiation

Maturation of the epidermal layers includes keratinization, which results in the *differentiation* of granular and stratum corneal layers and the formation of a water-impermeable barrier. Accompanying this stage of development is the sloughing of the periderm. Keratinization occurs first in the skin appendages between 11 and 15 weeks' EGA, followed by the interfollicular epidermis between 22 and 24 weeks' EGA.[13,14]

The process of keratinization involves the production of certain proteins, including filaggrin and loricrin. Posttranslational modification of the cross-linked proteins and production of specialized lipid and steroid components contribute to the water-impermeable matrix formed in the mature cornified layer. Structurally, the third trimester stratum corneum is similar to that of an adult, but functional studies have shown that it is much less effective at preventing water loss and is more permeable than the mature epidermis. It is actually not until the third week of life that the barrier function of a newborn's stratum corneum is comparable to that of an adult. Emollient use is of therapeutic benefit in many of these patients with defective epidermal barriers, because the stratum corneum is insufficiently differentiated in very low birth weight preterm infants.[15]

Clinical Relevance

Human mutations that inhibit the process of specification in the epidermis have not been reported, most likely because such mutations would be incompatible with further development of the embryo. However, experiments in animals have suggested that a group of proteins, the bone morphogenetic proteins (BMPs), as well as the Engrailed-1 (*En-1*) gene, may play an important early role in these processes.[16-18] Similarly, few mutations in humans have been found that affect epidermal morphogenesis although, as mentioned earlier, *p63* and *Dlx-3* have been implicated in the process of epidermal stratification based on studies in mouse models.

In contrast to the relative lack of mutations that affect epidermal specification and morphogenesis, mutations that have an important impact on epidermal differentiation are quite numerous. In general, these genes are not required for development *in utero*, but they become critical for effective barrier function of the epidermis after birth. Thus, defects in these genes can often cause significant postnatal morbidity.

Two groups of such diseases include the palmoplantar keratodermas and ichthyoses. The *palmoplantar keratodermas* are a diverse group of disorders that share a common presentation of hyperkeratosis of the palms and soles. These disorders commonly are also associated with other cutaneous as well as noncutaneous findings. The genetic bases of many of these disorders have been discovered, and they include defects in connexins, differentiation keratins, and desmosomal components.[19]

The *ichthyoses* are another diverse group of diseases that often present around birth with diffuse scaly skin and defective epidermal barrier function.[20,21] These conditions differ in both pattern and morphology of scaling, as well as extracutaneous features. Ichthyosis vulgaris, lamellar ichthyosis, and X-linked ichthyosis have phenotypes predominantly restricted to the skin. Ichthyoses can also be a cause of erythroderma (e.g., in bullous and nonbullous congenital ichthyosiform erythroderma). Neurologic abnormalities can be associated with the skin condition, as in Sjögren-Larsson syndrome, Refsum syndrome, or Tay syndrome (IBIDS: ichthyosis, brittle hair, intellectual deficit, decreased fertility, and short stature). In X-linked dominant ichthyoses, female children inheriting the relevant mutation can develop asymmetry of limbs, as in CHILD syndrome (congenital hemidysplasia with ichthyosiform erythroderma and limb defects) or chondrodysplasia punctata (Conradi-Hünermann disease).

One of the earliest phenotypic presentations of a group of these disorders is known as the *collodion baby,* in which the infant is born encased in a parchment-like membrane. Over the next few days to weeks, the membrane is shed, eventuating in lamellar ichthyosis, nonbullous congenital ichthyosiform erythroderma (NBCIE), Netherton syndrome, Tay syndrome (IBIDS), Conradi-Hünermann disease, and occasionally, a normal baby.[3,20]

In contrast to the relatively benign outcome for collodion babies, the so-called *harlequin fetus* usually dies soon after birth. These babies are born encased in restrictive plates of thick, armor-like scale that have extremely poor barrier function, often resulting in fluid derangements, infections, sepsis, and death.

Nonkeratinocytes in the Epidermis

Melanocytes

Although keratinocytes are the most abundant cell type that makes up the epidermis, other cell types also migrate there early in development. Among these are the melanocytes, neural crest–derived dendritic cells that synthesize and distribute pigment to the epidermis. Melanocyte precursors exit the dorsal region of the neural tube, migrate through the superficial mesenchyme, and ultimately come to reside in the epidermis by 7 weeks' EGA.

Langerhans Cells

Langerhans cells are another migratory cell population that enters the epidermis before the embryonic-fetal transition. They are bone marrow–derived cells that, when mature, are important for antigen presentation within the skin. They remain relatively undifferentiated until the embryonic-fetal transition, at which time they begin to express CD1 on their cell surface and begin to produce their characteristic Birbeck granules, tennis racket–shaped intracellular vesicles that form during the processing of membrane-bound antigens. The density of Langerhans cells remains low until the third trimester, when it increases to those of a typical adult.

Merkel Cells

The third type of specialized cell within the epidermis is the Merkel cell, a highly innervated neuroendocrine cell type involved in mechanoreception. These cells are first detectable around 8 to 12 weeks in volar skin and slightly later in interfollicular skin. They are often associated with skin appendages. Merkel cells express both neural-specific markers and epithelial-specific proteins, such as keratins.

Clinical Relevance

Many mutations have been identified that are critical for melanoblast migration and survival, as well as for melanocyte differentiation and function (summarized in Table 59-1). Defects in these genes result in disorders of pigmentation, which can be detected at an early age.

One of the most common abnormalities is that of albinism. There are variations in severity of depigmentation as well as associated abnormalities. These differences depend on the particular gene affected and its global function.

TABLE 59-1

Disorders of Pigmentation

Disorder	Mutant Gene	Defective Protein/Function
Melanocyte specification, migration, or survival		
Piebaldism	c-KIT	Growth factor receptor, proto-oncogene
Waardenburg syndrome		
Types 1 and 3	HuP2	Pax3 transcription factor
Type 2	MITF	Transcription factor
Type 4	EDNRB	Endothelin receptor B
	EDN3	Endothelin 3
	Sox 10	Sox 10 transcription factor
Melanin biosynthesis		
Oculocutaneous albinism		
Type 1	Tyrosinase, null alleles	Rate-limiting enzyme of pigment production
Type 1b	Tyrosinase, partially functional alleles	Rate-limiting enzyme of pigment production
Type 2	P gene	Putative tyrosine transporter
Type 3	TRP-1	Tyrosinase-related protein-1
Melanosome production		
Hermansky-Pudlak syndrome	HPS1	Putative membrane component of various organelles
	AP3	Putative component of endocytic protein trafficking pathway
Chédiak-Higashi syndrome	LYST	Putative involvement in protein trafficking
Griscelli syndrome	RAB27A	Guanosine triphosphate–binding protein involved in membrane fusion and protein trafficking

Defects in melanin synthesis result in oculocutaneous albinism (OCA), a set of disorders characterized by absent pigment in the skin, hair, and eyes at birth. Often associated with the skin findings are neurologic and ophthalmologic findings of nystagmus, photophobia, and visual disturbances, reflecting the neuroectodermal derivation of melanocytes. In OCA Type 1, mutations in the enzyme tyrosinase, critical for the conversion of tyrosine to melanin (either null or partial loss of function alleles), are responsible. In OCA Type 2, tyrosinase functions normally (tyrosinase-positive albinism), but the P gene, a putative tyrosine transporter, is defective. This subtype can be distinguished from OCA Type 1 because the child's skin and eyes begin to darken with age. Such children usually have white, yellow, or red hair. OCA Type 3 results from defects in tyrosinase-related protein-1. This condition is also known as *brown OCA*, featuring minimal to light brown skin pigmentation in some persons of African descent.[22]

Other genes result in a more patchy distribution of pigmentation defects, as in the white forelock (poliosis) seen in both piebaldism and Waardenburg syndrome. These diseases occur as a result of defective melanocyte specification, migration, or survival. The gene responsible for piebaldism is c-*KIT*, a growth factor receptor and proto-oncogene.[23] Waardenburg syndrome subtypes can be caused by defects in transcription factors Pax3, Sox10, MITF as well as in endothelin receptor B and endothelin 3 ligand. In Waardenburg syndrome, depending on the subtype, neural tube defects, heterochromia iridis, deafness, and Hirschsprung disease may be associated with depigmentation.[24]

Finally, defects in melanosome production result in the entities Hermansky-Pudlak, Chédiak-Higashi, and Griscelli syndromes. Patients with Hermansky-Pudlak syndrome have mutations in the HPS1 gene, which is a putative transmembrane component of a number of cytoplasmic organelles, or the AP3 gene, which is a protein subunit involved in the sorting of proteins in the exocytic/endocytic pathway. These patients present with creamy, light skin tones, dysfunctional platelets (prolonged bleeding time), pulmonary fibrosis, granulomatous colitis, and ceroid lipofuscinosis in phagocytic cells.[25] Chédiak-Higashi syndrome is characterized by nystagmus, decreased visual acuity, skin and respiratory infections, light skin tones, and silvery

yellow to brown hair. Giant melanosomes are found in white blood cell smears and hair, and giant lysosomal inclusion granules are found in all leukocytes. The defect is in LYST, a protein proposed to be important in intercellular protein trafficking.[26] Griscelli syndrome also features hair shafts with large pigment granules and hypopigmentation with silver-gray hair. These patients have hemophagocytic syndrome and experience episodes of massive lymphocyte and leukocyte activation and organ infiltration. Polymorphonuclear leukocytes are morphologically normal, unlike in Chédiak-Higashi syndrome. The defect is in a guanosine triphosphate–binding protein involved in vesicular fusion and trafficking, RAB27A.[27]

DERMIS AND SUBCUTIS

Overview

Unlike the epidermis, which is derived exclusively from ectoderm, the *dermis* originates from different tissues depending on the specific body site. Dermal mesenchyme of the face and anterior scalp comes from neural crest ectoderm, whereas that of the back is derived from the dermomyotome of the embryonic somite. Dermal mesenchyme of the limbs and ventral trunk, conversely, is likely derived from the lateral plate mesoderm.

Early fetal mesenchyme is highly cellular, containing few fibrillar elements. These fetal mesenchymal cells are thought to be pluripotent, able to give rise to adipose tissue, cartilage, and dermal fibroblasts. The superficial mesenchyme becomes visibly distinct from underlying skeletal elements by 60 days' EGA. By 12 to 15 weeks, the different characteristics of the dermis can first be observed—the papillary dermis has a finer weave than the thicker reticular dermis. Collagen and elastic fibers begin to be assembled in the latter half of pregnancy, and a more rigid, fibrillar meshwork gradually forms.

Dermal repair shifts from nonscarring to scarring by the end of the second trimester. At birth, the dermis is thick and well organized but is still more cellular than in the adult.

A distinct region identifiable as the subcutis can be seen by 50 to 60 days' EGA. It is separated from the dermis by a plane of thin-walled vessels. By the end of the first trimester, the distinc-

TABLE 59-2

Ehlers-Danlos Syndrome Classification

Type	Clinical Findings	Inheritance	Gene Defect(s)
Classic (I/II)	Skin and joint hypermobility, atrophic scars, easy bruising	AD	COL5A1, COL5A2
Hypermobility (III)	Joint hypermobility, pain, dislocations	AD	COL3A1
Vascular (IV)	Thin skin, arterial or uterine rupture, easy bruising, small joint hyperextensibility	AD	COL3A1
Kyphoscoliosis (VI)	Scoliosis, joint laxity, ocular fragility and retinal detachment, skin laxity, muscle hypotonia	AR	Lysyl hydroxylase
Arthrochalasia (VIIA, VIIB)	Joint hypermobility, mild skin laxity, bruising, scoliosis	AD	COL1A1, COL1A2
Dermatosparaxis (VIIC)	Severe skin fragility, cutis laxa, bruising	AR	ADAMTS2 (procollagen N-peptidase)
Other			
X-linked EDS (V)	Skin laxity, bruising	XL	Lysyl oxidase
Periodontitis (VIII)	Periodontitis, blue sclerae, atrophic scarring, bruisability	AD	?
Fibronectin-deficient (X)	Striae distensae, joint laxity, skin laxity, scarring, bruisability, bleeding (platelet) disorder (petechiae)	?	?
Familial hypermobility (XI)	Recurrent joint dislocation, joint laxity	AD	
Progeroid	Progeroid facies, short stature, osteopenia, skin laxity, atrophic scarring, hypermobile joints	?	XGPT-1

AD = autosomal dominant; AR = autosomal recessive; XL = X-linked.

tion between the fibrous dermis and the sparse matrix of the subcutis can be seen. Preadipocytes arising from the undifferentiated mesenchyme begin to mature and accumulate lipids by the second trimester. By the third trimester, the more differentiated adipocytes begin to aggregate into lobules separated by fibrous septa. Although the initial events leading to the commitment of mesenchymal cells to become adipocytes are not well understood, numerous regulators of later preadipocyte-adipocyte differentiation have been identified, including the hormone leptin.[28]

Blood Vessels, Lymphatics, and Nerves

Blood vessels and lymphatics begin to develop early in gestation but do not evolve into those of the adult until a few months after birth. Initially, these vessels form horizontal plexuses within the subpapillary and deep reticular dermis, which are interconnected by groups of vertical vessels. This vascular framework has been shown to be in place by 45 to 50 days' EGA. By the fifth month of EGA, arterioles and venules are able to be distinguished. Capillary loops, which supply the developing epidermal appendages and maintain thermoregulation, are established at the time of rete ridge formation at the DEJ. During the period of embryonic and fetal development, this framework changes constantly, depending on many factors, including site of the body and presence of associated adnexal structures.

Accumulating evidence suggests that lymphatics originate from endothelial cells that bud from veins, and the pattern of embryonic lymphatic vessel development parallels that of blood vessels. Studies using newly discovered molecular markers specific for lymphatics have allowed a more detailed understanding of lymphatogenesis. As described later, defects in some of the genes encoding some of these proteins have been found to result in congenital disorders of the lymphatic system.

Nerves, like blood vessels and lymphatics, are also present in early embryonic skin and continue to develop after birth. Nerves begin as large trunks at the dermal-subcutaneous boundary that branch into fibers and extend into the dermis. They form networks distinct from the cutaneous vasculature, although they become more closely juxtaposed in the fetal dermis. At 70 days' EGA, an arrangement of nerves that is similar to the adult configuration can

be detected, although the density and final distribution of fibers continue to be modified until after birth. Sensory receptors such as the Pacinian and Meissner corpuscles begin to develop in the fourth month of EGA. Whereas Meissner corpuscles are fully developed only after birth, Pacinian corpuscles are completed and are found in plantar and palmar skin in neonates.

Clinical Relevance

Few human mutations have been identified that result in defective dermal specification and differentiation, most likely because such mutations would be incompatible with life. However, experiments in animal model systems have suggested that the genes *Lmx-1B*, *Wnt 7a*, and *Engrailed-1* may be important in specifying dorsal and ventral (palmoplantar) mesenchyme as distinct tissues.

Restrictive dermopathy is a clinical entity in which the dermis is universally abnormal.[29] Some mosaic conditions also show localized defects in dermal development, most notably focal dermal hypoplasia (Goltz syndrome), as well as Proteus syndrome. In Goltz syndrome, dermal hypoplasia exists in Blaschkoid patterns.[30] Proteus syndrome is characterized by subcutaneous masses, lipomas, capillary malformations, plantar and palmar hyperplasia, varicose veins, and asymmetric soft tissue and bony hypertrophy of the hands, feet, and limbs.[31]

Connective tissue disorders are caused by mutations in genes encoding differentiation products of mature dermal fibroblasts and other mesenchymal cells. Ehlers-Danlos syndrome has many clinical subtypes, caused by a variety of mutations in genes affecting collagen Types I, III, and V, collagen-modifying enzymes, and other important structural proteins (Table 59-2).[32,33] Elastin mutations can result in cutis laxa, characterized by loose, redundant skin, a syndrome that can be complicated by lung hypoplasia, diaphragmatic hernias, gastrointestinal diverticula, bladder diverticula, and emphysema.[34] Osteogenesis imperfecta, characterized by multiple fractures *in utero*, beaded ribs, crumpled humeri and femora, limb avulsion during delivery, kyphoscoliosis, blue sclerae, and easily bruisable skin, has been found to result from defects in collagen Type I.[35] Marfan syndrome results from mutations in fibrillin, which codes for a vital component of the microfibrillar elastic tissue network, resulting in defects in ocular, cardiovascular, and musculoskeletal systems.[36]

Defects in angiogenesis have also been identified. Hereditary hemorrhagic telangiectasia (Osler-Weber-Rendu syndrome) is a vascular dysplasia that leads to telangiectases and arteriovenous malformations of skin, mucosa, and viscera. Mucosal involvement often results in epistaxis and gastrointestinal bleeding. Visceral involvement includes that of the lung, liver, and brain. Mutations in endgolin, as well as activin receptor-like kinase 1 have been shown to cause this disease.[37,38] TIE-2 is a tyrosine kinase, mutations in which have been shown to result in a dominantly inherited syndrome of venous malformations.[39,40]

Work on lymphangiogenesis has uncovered genetic mutations in some forms of hereditary lymphedema. The most common form of primary hereditary lymphedema, Milroy disease, is caused by mutations in vascular endothelial growth factor receptor 3. This disease is characterized by severe edema, especially below the waist.[41] Mutations in MFH1 (FOXC2), a transcription factor, have been implicated in lymphedema-distichiasis syndrome, featuring late-onset lymphedema and a double row of eyelashes (distichiasis).[42]

DERMAL-EPIDERMAL JUNCTION

The DEJ is a key interface for inductive interactions during early skin organogenesis. Defects in this region are also responsible for many well-studied congenital blistering diseases, the group of diseases known as epidermolysis bullosa (EB). This zone includes the adhesive structural elements along the basal surface of the basal keratinocyte plasma membrane, as well as the extracellular matrix proteins of the basal lamina and the most superficial fibrillar structures of the papillary dermis.

The most primitive form of the DEJ can be seen between the epidermis and the dermis by 8 weeks' EGA. Laminin, collagen Type IV, heparan sulfate, and proteoglycans, components common to all basal lamina, can be found at this stage. The more specific molecules that make up the basal lamina of stratified epithelia, such as hemidesmosomal components, begin to be detected at the time when the presumptive epidermis begins to stratify. It is at this time that such proteins as integrins (α_6 and β_4) become properly localized to the DEJ, even though the expression of some can be detected at earlier times.

Clinical Relevance

As alluded to earlier, several congenital disorders characterized by severe blistering occur as a result of mutations in the genes encoding the components of this region (Table 59-3).[43] The severity of the disorder, the plane of tissue separation, and the involvement of noncutaneous tissues depend on the specific proteins affected by the mutations. These diseases carry with them a high degree of morbidity and mortality, and as such they are frequent candidates for prenatal testing.

The most superficial of these phenotypes is EB simplex. Keratins 5 and 14, the proteins defective in this disease subtype, are expressed by basal keratinocytes. Because of loss of adhesion at the level of the basal keratinocyte, the epidermis is fragile, and bullae develop. Depending on the particular mutation, the blistering phenotype can be more or less severe. These blisters can involve the mucous membranes and can result in a hoarse voice. One specific subtype of EB simplex is associated with muscular dystrophy. The mutation for this disease is within a protein called plectin, involved in adhesion within the hemidesmosome.

Junctional EB variants form bullae within the lamina lucida, the superficial portion of the DEJ. These patients have been found to have defects in laminin 5. One form of junctional EB, the Herlitz variant, is more severe: in addition to blistering, laryngeal and respiratory edema can be associated with the disorder, as well as anemia and hypoproteinemia. The non-Herlitz variant is less life-threatening, although, in this case, bullae heal with atrophic scarring. Nails and hair can also be affected. Another subtype is associated with pyloric atresia, which is caused by mutations in the $\alpha_6\beta_4$-integrin.

The most disfiguring form of EB is termed dystrophic EB. Because the blisters in this variant affect the superficial dermis, with defects in collagen Type VII, they heal with scarring. In the more severe forms, extensive scarring can lead to digital fusions and so-called "mitten" deformities of the hands and feet, flexion contractures, mucous membrane scarring, dental abnormalities, and hematologic disorders.

SKIN APPENDAGES

Skin appendages include hair, nails, and sweat and mammary glands. These structures are derived from both an epidermal component and a dermal component. The epidermis contributes the physical structure of the unit, whereas the dermis provides signals for the unit's differentiation. During embryogenesis, interactions between the dermis and the epidermis are critical for normal development of these structures, disruption of which often result in defects in the formation of skin appendages.

Hair

Between 75 and 80 days' EGA, dermal signals instruct the basal cells of the scalp epidermis to cluster together at regularly spaced intervals. This initial group is known as the follicular placode or anlage.[44] Although the specific mediators of this first "dermal signal" are not definitively identified, β-catenin has been implicated as a candidate gene, based on its molecular localization.

From the scalp, the follicular placodes develop ventrally and caudally and eventually cover the skin. The epidermal placodes then signal back to the underlying dermis to form a dermal condensate, which occurs at 12 to 14 weeks' EGA. The communication between the epidermis and dermis at this stage and the morphogenetic development are considered to be a balance between placode promoters and placode inhibitors.[44] Wnt family signaling molecules are proposed to mediate placode

---

TABLE 59-3

Disorders of the Dermal-Epidermal Junction

Location	Disorder	Defective Protein(s)
Basal cell adhesion complex	EB simplex	K5, K14
	EB with muscular dystrophy	Plectin
Basal lamina	Generalized atrophic benign EB	BPAG2 (collagen XVII)
	EB with pyloric atresia	β_4 subunit of $\alpha_6\beta_4$ integrin
	Junctional EB, lethal and less severe forms	Laminin 5 subunits
Superficial dermis	Dystrophic EB (dominant and recessive)	Collagen Type VII

EB = epidermolysis bullosa.

promoting effects via the molecules LEF and β-catenin, as well as fibroblast growth factor, transforming growth factor-β_2, Msx1 and 2, and ectodysplasin A (EDA) and EDA receptor (EDAR). BMP family molecules, conversely, act as inhibitors of follicle formation. In model systems, ectopic expression of this family of molecules tends to suppress the formation of follicles. In mice, EDAR and β-catenin expression are required for expression of BMP4 and sonic hedgehog (Shh), a finding implicating these molecules in early follicular morphogenesis. Furthermore, EDAR may be important for lateral inhibition of cells surrounding the follicles.

The dermal papilla is thought to be formed as a result of epithelial cell instructions transmitted to the underlying mesenchyme. Molecular candidates for this signal include platelet-derived growth factor and Shh. The dermal cells, in turn, instruct the epidermal cells to proliferate and invade the dermis. The dermal cells differentiate into the dermal papilla, whereas the involved epithelial cells become the inner root sheath and hair shaft of the mature follicle.

In addition to the widened bulge at the base of the mature hair follicle, two other bulges form along the length of the developing follicle. The uppermost bulge is the presumptive sebaceous gland, whereas the middle bulge serves as the site for insertion of the arrector pili muscle. Accumulating evidence also suggests that hair stem cells reside in the middle follicular bulge. These important multipotent cells are able to differentiate into any of the cells of the hair follicle, as well as to reconstitute the entire epidermis, as has been reported in cases of extensive surface wounds or burns.

By 19 to 21 weeks' EGA, the hair canal has completely formed, and fetal scalp hair becomes visible. These hairs continue to lengthen until 24 to 28 weeks, at which time they shift from the active growth (anagen) phase to the degenerative phase (catagen), then to the resting phase (telogen), thus completing the first hair cycle. With subsequent hair cycles, hairs increase in diameter and coarseness. During adolescence, vellus hairs of androgen-sensitive areas mature to terminal-type hair follicles.

Sebaceous Glands

Sebaceous glands, as mentioned earlier, mature during the course of follicular differentiation, beginning between 13 and 16 weeks' EGA.[45] At this time, the presumptive sebaceous gland is the most superficial bulge in the developing hair follicle. As the sebaceous gland develops further, the outer cells differentiate and proliferate, giving rise to cells that accumulate lipids and sebum.[46, 47] These differentiated cells ultimately disintegrate to release their contents into the upper portion of the hair canal. The production of sebum is responsive to hormonal influences, including maternal steroids during the second and third trimesters, and then again at adolescence, a finding suggesting a factor contributing to the increased incidence of acne at this age.[48]

Nail Development

The earliest nail structures begin to appear on the dorsal digit tip at 8 to 10 weeks' EGA, slightly earlier than the initiation of hair follicle development.[49] The first sign is the delineation of the flat surface of the future nail bed. The proximal nail fold is formed from a portion of ectoderm that buds inward at the proximal boundary of the early nail field. The presumptive nail matrix cells ultimately differentiate to become the nail plate; these cells are present on the ventral side of the proximal invagination. At 11 weeks' EGA, the dorsal nail bed surface begins to keratinize. By the fourth month of gestation, the nail plate grows out from the proximal nail fold and completely covers the nail bed by the fifth month.[50]

Eccrine and Apocrine Sweat Gland Development

Eccrine glands begin to develop on the volar surfaces of the hands and feet, beginning as mesenchymal pads between 55 and 65 days' EGA. By 12 to 14 weeks' EGA, parallel ectodermal ridges overly these mesenchymal pads. The eccrine glands arise from the ectodermal ridge. By 16 weeks' EGA, the secretory portion of the gland becomes detectable. The dermal duct is complete by this time, but the epidermal portion of the duct is not canalized until 22 weeks' EGA. Dermatoglyphics are formed by the curvilinear patterns of the epidermal ridges, and these become visible on the volar surfaces of the digits by 5 months' EGA.

Interfollicular eccrine and apocrine glands, in contrast to volar glands, do not begin to bud until the fifth month of gestation. Apocrine sweat glands usually bud from the upper portion of the hair follicle. By 7 months' EGA, the cells of the apocrine glands become distinguishable, composed of both clear cells and mucin-secreting dark cells. Apocrine glands become transiently functional during the third trimester, but eccrine glands are not functional until the postnatal period.

Although not much is known with regard to the molecular signals responsible for the differentiation of these structures, it has been suggested that the EDA, EDAR, En1, and Wnt10b genes are involved.

Clinical Relevance

As has been described in some of the genetic diseases affecting development of the skin, genes that affect cutaneous appendage formation can also have effects on noncutaneous tissues; findings suggest an early role for these factors or a more global role in development and differentiation.

Certain genetic syndromes with prominent hair defects, often associated with other ectodermal appendageal abnormalities, have been identified; some of the responsible genes have been cloned. Menkes kinky hair syndrome is an X-linked recessive syndrome featuring pili torti (twisted hair) that is sparse and brittle with a "steel wool" quality. The skin is doughy, and patients have skeletal abnormalities and general failure to thrive. The defect for this disease is an adenosine triphosphate–dependent copper transporter, ATP7A. Argininosuccinic aciduria is an autosomal recessive disorder, resulting from defective argininosuccinate lyase, that may present neonatally with trichorrhexis nodosa and short, broken scalp hairs, neurologic deficits including lethargy and mental retardation, hepatomegaly, and failure to thrive. The mechanism responsible for the hair defects is not known.

Other defects occur in the structural proteins of hair, such as hair keratins. Monilethrix is caused by defects in hair cortex keratins 1 and 6 (HB1, HB6), which result in beaded hair and brittle nails. Diseases such as pachyonychia congenita present primarily with cutaneous and ectodermal appendageal defects, including hyperkeratotic nails, palmoplantar keratoderma, follicular hyperkeratosis, and steatocystoma multiplex. These defects have been found to be mutations in typical "soft" keratin genes: K6a, K6b, K16, and K17. Trichothiodystrophy, or Tay syndrome, presents as short, brittle hair with alternating dark and light "tiger-tail" bands as well as trichoschisis. Nails are dystrophic, skin is ichthyotic, and patients exhibit photosensitivity, short stature, intellectual impairment, and decreased fertility. Two genes have been identified, both involved in DNA repair and identical to the genes mutated in the xeroderma pigmentosum complementation groups B and D. The reasons for the cutaneous manifestations of this disease are not clear, but the hair and nail phenotypes have been proposed to be a result of low cysteine content.

Mutations in critical developmental regulatory genes, such as those encoding DNA binding proteins and growth factors, have also been found in congenital syndromes affecting skin appendage formation.[1, 44] Hypohidrotic ectodermal dysplasia, a defect in either EDA or EDAR, features sparse hair, nail dystrophy, as well as hypohidrosis or anhidrosis, which can lead to poor thermoregulation. In contrast, hidrotic ectodermal dysplasia, which presents with sparse hair, dystrophic nails, palmoplantar keratoderma, and tufting of terminal phalanges, is associated with defects in connexin 30. Mutations in p63 affect nail development in syndromes such as AEC (ankyloblepharon, ectodermal defects, and cleft lip) and EEC (ectrodactyly-ectodermal dysplasia clefting).[51] Functional p63 is required for the formation and maintenance of the apical ectodermal ridge, an embryonic signaling center essential for limb outgrowth and hand plate formation. The secreted factor Wnt7a and the transcription factor Lmx1b are important for dorsal limb patterning, including nail formation. Nail-patella syndrome results from mutations in LMX-1b. In contrast, the transcription factor En1 is required for ventral limb patterning and eccrine gland formation. Other regulatory molecules important in appendage development include the secreted factor Shh, which is required for hair follicle formation but not nail plate formation, and the transcription factor MSX1, which is required for tooth and nail formation. *Hoxc13* is an important homeodomain-containing gene for later stages of follicular and nail differentiation, at least in murine models.

PRENATAL DIAGNOSIS

Identification of the genes involved in early cutaneous development and determination of associated mutations responsible for disease have allowed prenatal diagnosis of life-threatening or debilitating cutaneous disease.[52] Some techniques have been devised for such testing, such as chorionic villous sampling, which can be performed at 8 to 10 weeks' EGA, or amniocentesis, which can be done at 16 to 18 weeks' EGA. These diagnostic procedures can be performed earlier and are associated with less fetal morbidity and mortality than the only previously available technique, fetal skin biopsy, performed between 19 and 22 weeks' EGA. Even though chorionic villous sampling and amniocentesis are less invasive, certain diseases, such as harlequin fetus, still require fetal biopsy for diagnosis, because no definitive genetic mutations have yet been identified. Candidates for prenatal testing include fetuses with an affected sibling or family member.

REFERENCES

1. Loomis CA: Development and morphogenesis of the skin. Adv Dermatol 17:183, 2001.
2. Holbrook KA: Structure and function of the developing human skin. *In* Goldsmith LA (ed): Physiology, Biochemistry, and Molecular Biology of the Skin. New York, Oxford University Press, 1991, pp 63–110.
3. Online Mendelian Inheritance in Man (OMIM): McKusick-Nathans Institute for Genetic Medicine, Johns Hopkins University (Baltimore, MD) and National Center for Biotechnology Information, National Library of Medicine (Bethesda, MD). 2000.
4. Kowalczyk AP, et al: Desmosomes: intercellular adhesive junctions specialized for attachment of intermediate filaments. Int Rev Cytol 185:237, 1999.
5. Kalinin AE, et al: Epithelial barrier function: assembly and structural features of the cornified cell envelope. Bioessays 24:789, 2002.
6. Fuchs E, Cleveland DW: A structural scaffolding of intermediate filaments in health and disease. Science 279:514, 1998.
7. Freedberg IM, et al: Keratins and the keratinocyte activation cycle. J Invest Dermatol 116:633, 2001.
8. Breathnach AS, Robins J: Ultrastructural features of epidermis of a 14 mm. (6 weeks) human embryo. Br J Dermatol 81:504, 1969.
9. Holbrook KA, Odland GF: Regional development of the human epidermis in the first trimester embryo and the second trimester fetus (ages related to the timing of amniocentesis and fetal biopsy). J Invest Dermatol 74:161, 1980.
10. Mills A, et al: p63 is a p53 homologue required for limb and epidermal morphogenesis. Nature 398:708, 1999.
11. Morasso MI, et al: Regulation of epidermal differentiation by a distal-less homeodomain gene. J Cell Biol 135:1879, 1996.
12. Yang Å, et al: p63 is essential for regenerative proliferation in limb, craniofacial and epithelial development. Nature 398:714, 1999.
13. Dale BA, et al: Expression of epidermal keratins and filaggrin during human fetal skin development. J Cell Biol 101:1257, 1985.
14. Evans NJ, Rutter N: Development of the epidermis in the newborn. Biol Neonate 49:74, 1986.
15. Hoath SB, Narendran V: Adhesives and emollients in the preterm infant. Semin Neonatol 5:289, 2000.
16. Loomis CA, et al: The mouse engrailed-1 gene and ventral limb patterning. Nature 382:360, 1996.
17. Pizette S, Niswander L: Early steps in limb patterning and chondrogenesis. Novartis Found Symp 232:23; discussion 36, 2001.
18. Ahn K, et al: Bmpr-Ia signaling is required for the formation of the apical ectodermal ridge and dorsal-ventral patterning of the limb. Development 128:4449, 2001.
19. Kimyai-Asadi A, et al: The molecular basis of hereditary palmoplantar keratodermas. J Am Acad Dermatol 47:327; quiz 344, 2002.
20. Moss C: Genetic skin disorders. Semin Neonatol 5:311, 2000.
21. Shwayder T: Ichthyosis in a nutshell. Pediatr Rev 20:5, 1999.
22. Oetting WS: Albinism. Curr Opin Pediatr 11:565, 1999.
23. Ezoe K, et al: Novel mutations and deletions of the kit (steel factor receptor) gene in human piebaldism. Am J Hum Genet 56:58, 1995.
24. Dourmishev AL, et al: Waardenburg syndrome. Int J Dermatol 38:656, 1999.
25. Dimson O, et al: Hermansky-Pudlak syndrome. Pediatr Dermatol 16:475, 1999.
26. Introne W, et al: Clinical, molecular, and cell biological aspects of Chédiak-Higashi syndrome. Mol Genet Metab 68:283, 1999.
27. Seabra MC, et al: Rab GTPases, intracellular traffic and disease. Trends Mol Med 8:23, 2002.
28. Fajas L, et al: Transcriptional control of adipogenesis. Curr Opin Cell Biol 10:165, 1998.
29. Smitt JH, et al: Restrictive dermopathy: report of 12 cases. Dutch task force on genodermatology. Arch Dermatol 134:577, 1998.
30. Hardman CM, et al: Focal dermal hypoplasia: report of a case with cutaneous and skeletal manifestations. Clin Exp Dermatol 23:281, 1998.
31. Hamm H: Cutaneous mosaicism of lethal mutations. Am J Med Genet 85:342, 1999.
32. Mao JR, Bristow J: The Ehlers-Danlos syndrome: on beyond collagens. J Clin Invest 107:1063, 2001.
33. Beighton P, et al: Ehlers-Danlos syndromes: revised nosology, Villefranche, 1997. Ehlers-Danlos National Foundation (USA) and Ehlers-Danlos Support Group (UK). Am J Med Genet 77:31, 1998.
34. Milewicz DM, et al: Genetic disorders of the elastic fiber system. Matrix Biol 19:471, 2000.
35. Cohen MM Jr: Some chondrodysplasias with short limbs: molecular perspectives. Am J Med Genet 112:304, 2002.
36. Pyeritz RE: The Marfan syndrome. Annu Rev Med 51:481, 2000.
37. Guttmacher AE, et al: Hereditary hemorrhagic telangiectasia. N Engl J Med 333:918, 1995.
38. Kjeldsen AD, et al: Mutations in the alk-1 gene and the phenotype of hereditary hemorrhagic telangiectasia in two large Danish families. Am J Med Genet 98:298, 2001.
39. Vikkula M, et al: Vascular dysmorphogenesis caused by an activating mutation in the receptor tyrosine kinase tie2. Cell 87:1181, 1996.
40. Calvert JT, et al: Allelic and locus heterogeneity in inherited venous malformations. Hum Mol Genet 8:1279, 1999.
41. Holberg CJ, et al: Segregation analyses and a genome-wide linkage search confirm genetic heterogeneity and suggest oligogenic inheritance in some Milroy congenital primary lymphedema families. Am J Med Genet 98:303, 2001.
42. Erickson RP, et al: Clinical heterogeneity in lymphedema-distichiasis with foxc2 truncating mutations. J Med Genet 38:761, 2001.
43. Ghohestani RF, et al: Molecular organization of the cutaneous basement membrane zone. Clin Dermatol 19:551, 2001.
44. Millar SE: Molecular mechanisms regulating hair follicle development. J Invest Dermatol 118:216, 2002.
45. Serri F, Huber MW: The development of sebaceous glands in man. *In* Montagna W, et al (eds): Advances in Biology of Skin: The Sebaceous Glands. Oxford, Pergamon Press, 1963, pp 1–18.
46. Fujita H: Ultrastructural study of embryonic sebaceous cells, especially of their droplet formation. Acta Dermatol Venereol 52:99, 1972.
47. Williams ML, et al: Skin lipid content during early fetal development. J Invest Dermatol 91:263, 1988.
48. Pochi PE, et al: Age-related changes in sebaceous gland activity. J Invest Dermatol 73:108, 1979.
49. Hashimoto K, et al: The ultrastructure of human embryo skin. II. The formation of intradermal portion of the eccrine sweat duct and of the secretory segment during the first half of embryonic life. J Invest Dermatol 46:205, 1966.
50. Lewis BL: Microscopic studies, fetal and mature nail and surrounding soft tissue. Arch Dermatol 70:732, 1954.
51. Brunner HG, et al: p63 gene mutations and human developmental syndromes. Am J Med Genet 112:284, 2002.
52. Ashton GH, et al: Prenatal diagnosis for inherited skin diseases. Clin Dermatol 18:643, 2000.

Steven B. Hoath

Physiologic Development of the Skin

Human skin is a complex structure with unusual functional diversity.[1] Topologically, the skin is continuous with the lung and intestinal epithelia. Whereas the lung and gut are commonly viewed as exchange surfaces for gases and nutrients, the skin is more commonly considered a barrier.[2-7] The concept of an integumental barrier emphasizes the role of the skin as a protective boundary between the organism and a potentially hostile environment. This protective role is evident at birth as the fetus abruptly transitions from a warm, wet, sterile, protected milieu to a cold, dry, microbe-laden world filled with physical, chemical, and mechanical dangers. Focusing only on the barrier properties of the skin, however, de-emphasizes the important role of the skin in social communication, perception, and behavioral interactions. The skin, as the surface of the organism, is both a cellular and molecular structure as well as a perceptual and psychological interface.[8] This dual functionality befits a true boundary and must be kept in mind to fully appreciate the dynamic organization of the skin and its close kinship with the nervous system.

The skin also provides the physical scaffold that defines the form of the animal.[9] Due to the action of the somatic musculature, a vertebrate's body continually changes shape, which is difficult in a dry, terrestrial environment. A wide variety of strategies have been devised by different animals to cope with the exigencies of different habitats (Table 60-1).[10] Arthropods have a largely inflexible body surface, covered with an exoskeleton. Many vertebrates, such as amphibians, live on land but are confined to humid or wet microhabitats. Reptiles and fish have a skin surface covered predominantly with scales; birds have evolved feathers; and most mammals are covered with a protective mantle of fur. Among primates, humans are unique in possessing a nonfurred skin with a thick stratified interfollicular epidermis and a well-developed stratum corneum.[9,11]

The question of the presumptive advantage of losing a protective and insulating coat of fur has long intrigued evolutionary biologists and physical anthropologists.[12] Three of the most distinctive physical features distinguishing human beings are

(1) a nonfurred skin surface; (2) a large, versatile, highly organized brain; and (3) opposable thumbs. The close embryologic connection between the epidermis and the brain (both are ectodermal derivatives) supports the contention that these peculiar structural aspects of human development have co-evolved. We often overlook the direct participation of the skin in higher level functions such as perception and behavioral interactions.[8,13] Cutaneous attributes form the basis for many readily observed biologic distinctions (age, race, gender) as well as multiple, overlapping sociocultural characteristics (tattooing, cosmetics, tanning). In healthcare environments, the skin forms an important component of caregiver/patient interactions.

In this review, specific aspects of the physiologic development of fetal and neonatal skin are highlighted, focusing particularly on the development of the epidermal barrier and the functions subserved by the outermost layer of the skin, the stratum corneum. Where possible, new areas of skin biology pertinent to the fetus and the newborn are emphasized. Areas of active research and unanswered questions will be identified in hopes of spurring new investigation of this highly accessible but extraordinarily complex interface.

DEVELOPMENT OF THE EPIDERMAL BARRIER

Human epidermis consists of a number of renewing structures, including the interfollicular epidermis, the hair follicle, the sweat gland, and the sebaceous gland.[14] The bulk of human skin is composed of the dermis and consists of collagen and elastin fibers embedded in a hydrated matrix of glycosaminoglycans. Blood vessels and the majority of cutaneous nerve endings are present in the dermis. The cells of the dermis and subcutaneous fat derive from the embryonic mesoderm. In contrast, epidermal appendages, such as hair follicles, sweat glands, and sebaceous glands, as well as the interfollicular epidermis, derive from embryonic ectoderm.

The epidermis is a composite tissue containing multiple cell types, including keratinocytes, melanocytes, Merkel cells, and Langerhans cells. Only the antigen-presenting Langerhans cells are of mesodermal origin. The epidermis is traditionally segmented into four separate structural and functional compartments:[15] (1) the stratum basale, responsible for keratinocyte proliferation and epidermal renewal, (2) the stratum spinosum, consisting of tightly packed keratinocytes linked via desmosomal connections, (3) the stratum granulosum, responsible for barrier lipid synthesis and corneocyte production via programmed cell death, and (4) the stratum corneum, the anucleated outermost layer, which forms the physical interface with the environment. The stratum corneum is markedly deficient in preterm human infants. Protective functions of the stratum corneum are listed in Table 60-2.

Cornified Envelope and Epidermal Lamellar Body

During the latter part of gestation, epithelial surfaces at environmental interfaces undergo structural and functional changes, including synthesis of complex, proteolipid materials. These events are highly coordinated and can be influenced by prenatal

TABLE 60-1

Animal Body Covering

Type	Biologic Example
Simple membrane	Earthworm
Simple stratified epidermis, often mucus-secreting	Frog, toad
Exoskeleton	Insects, crustaceans
Scales	Reptiles, fish
Feathers	Birds
Fur	Most mammals (including all primates except humans)
Complex stratified epidermis, nonfurred	
Thick interfollicular epidermis, separate functional strata, well-developed stratum corneum	Humans
Lipid droplets in stratum corneum	Dolphins

TABLE 60-2

Protective Functions of the Stratum Corneum

Functions	Structural Basis	Biochemical Mechanisms
Mechanical integrity/resilience	Cornified envelope, cytosolic filaments	Cross-linked peptides; e.g., loricrin; keratin filaments
Xenobiote defense	Lamellar bilayers, extracellular matrix	Acidic pH; free fatty acids; antimicrobial peptides
Antioxidant defense	Corneocytes and extracellular matrix	Keratins; sebaceous gland–derived vitamin E and other antioxidants
Cytokine signaling	Corneocyte cytosol	Storage and release of interleukins; serine proteases
Permeability barrier	Lamellar bilayers	Hydrophobic lipids
Hydration	Lamellar bilayers	Sebaceous gland-derived glycerol; filaggrin breakdown
	Corneocyte cytosolic matrix	products (NMFs)
Waterproofing/repellency	Lamellar bilayers	Keratinocyte and sebum-derived lipids
Cohesion/desquamation	Corneodesmosomes	Acidic pH serine proteases
UV protection	Corneocyte cytosol	Structural proteins; urocanic acid; light scattering/absorption

Modified from Chuong CM, et al: Exp Dermatol *11*:159, 2002.[9]

hormone exposure, such as glucocorticoids given to the mother.[5,16-20] Skin development in the human fetus is separated into three stages that correlate with the major events in epidermal differentiation: stratification, follicular keratinization, and keratinization of the interfollicular epidermis.[14] The stratum corneum is generally formed after 23 to 24 weeks of gestation. The formation of a barrier to water loss and infection is a sine qua non for survival in the extrauterine environment. Figure 60–1 illustrates the complex stages in the assembly of the cornified envelope in human stratum corneum.[21] Of note, synthesis and secretion of epidermal barrier lipids occurs in the form of lamellar bodies. This process is similar to that occurring over a parallel time frame in the developing lung.[5] Fusion of the intracellular lamellar body with the limiting plasma membrane

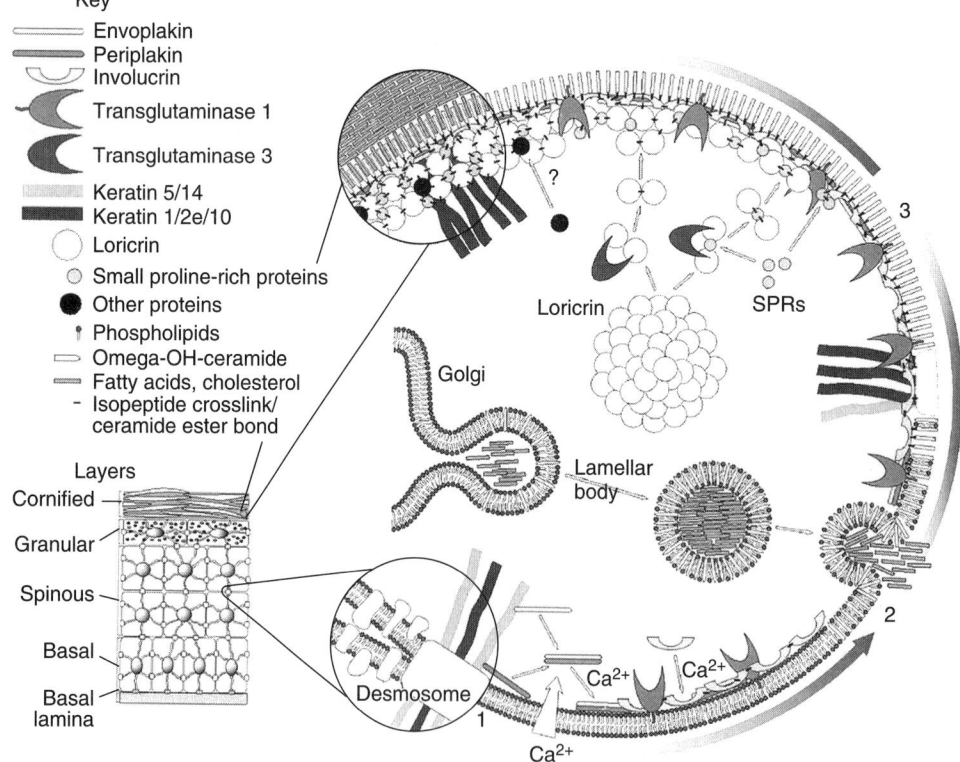

Figure 60–1. Stages in the assembly of the cornified envelope in human stratum corneum. (1) In the upper layers of the epidermis, rising levels of intracellular Ca^{2+} lead to expression of envoplakin, periplakin, and involucrin, as well as transglutaminase 1 with subsequent covalent cross-linking of the structural proteins along the inner surface of the plasma membrane. (2) Synthesis, packaging, and extrusion of barrier lipids (free fatty acids, cholesterol, ceramides) in the form of lamellar bodies are accompanied by replacement of the plasma membrane with covalently bound ceramides that serve to interdigitate with and organize the extracellular lipids into the characteristic lamellar pattern. (3) Covalent cross-linking of intracorneocyte proteins, including keratins, loricrin, and small proline-rich peptides, occurs via mediation of transglutaminase 1 and 3. The end product is the transformation of nucleated keratinocytes in the uppermost granular layer of the epidermis into a network of interlinked, terminally differentiated corneocytes embedded in a matrix of structured lipid lamellae, collectively called the stratum corneum. The stratum corneum provides the vital barrier to water loss and infection necessary for life after birth. (Modified from Kalinin A, et al: J Cell Sci *114*(Pt 17); 3069, 2001.[21])

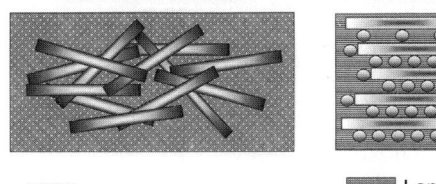
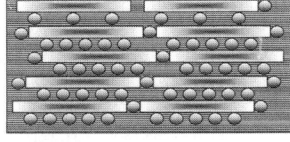

VERNIX CASEOSA   STRATUM CORNEUM

☐ Non-lamellar lipid matrix   ☐ Lamellar lipid matrix
▬ Fetal corneocyte   ○ Desmosome
                                 ▭ Mature corneocyte

Figure 60–2. Comparison of cellular architectures of vernix caseosa and stratum corneum. Vernix consists of thin, hydrated, polygonal, terminally differentiated, fetal corneocytes embedded in a nonlamellar lipid matrix. In intact stratum corneum, mature corneocytes (bricks) are embedded in a lamellar lipid matrix (mortar). The lipids provide the primary barrier to transepidermal water loss. In the stratum corneum, the corneocytes are interconnected by molecular complexes called desmosomes, which allow the stratum corneum to function as a coherent mechanical sheet. By contrast, corneocytes in vernix have few intercellular connections, which results in a viscous, creamlike mobility compared with the more rigid "brick and mortar" model of stratum corneum. (Modified from Hoath SB, Pickens W: *In* Hoath SB, Maibach H (eds): Neonatal Skin Structure and Function. New York, Marcel Dekker, 2003, p. 193.[26])

results in extrusion of barrier lipids, which subsequently undergo extracellular organization providing the primary barrier to transepidermal water loss. The barrier lipids in the epidermis, unlike the lung, are generally devoid of phospholipids and consist primarily of free fatty acids, cholesterol, and ceramides.[3]

Covalent cross-linking of structural proteins and ceramides results in formation of a highly insoluble cornified envelope, typical of the mature mammalian stratum corneum.[21] Each corneocyte consists of a covalently cross-linked envelope, linked internally to structural proteins such as keratins and externally to other corneocytes via desmosomes, resulting in the assembly of a huge macromolecule. The complexity and redundancy of the cornified envelope provide evidence for a highly organized and conserved molecular structure.[22,23] The cornified envelope, while only 10 nanometers thick and of uniform density, is highly insoluble, secondary to cross-linking by intracellular transglutaminases.[24] The isopeptide bond formed by these enzymes cannot be cleaved in vertebrate cells, therefore the resulting macromolecular protein complex is stable and essentially insoluble. This cross-linked assembly forms the scaffolding for the highly ordered lamellar lipid matrix. The very low birth weight preterm infant lacks an effective epidermal barrier.[4,5] A better understanding of the mechanisms by which the stratum corneum forms *in utero* may offer insights and direction to therapeutic regimens aimed at epidermal barrier formation postnatally (Fig. 60-2).

The Biology of Vernix

Scientifically, the development of epidermal barrier function has many similarities to surfactant production and lung development (Table 60-3.) Both the epidermal keratinocyte and the Type 2 alveolar cell are lipid-synthesizing cells that secrete barrier lipids in the form of lamellar bodies. Both interface with a gaseous environment under similar hormonal control at similar periods of development. There is a clear analogy between the mechanisms by which the lung develops a functionally mature epithelial surface ready for air adaptation and those by which the skin surface matures under total aqueous conditions for terrestrial adaptation to a dry environment. An unanswered question in epidermal biology, however, is by which mechanism the epidermal barrier forms under conditions of total aqueous immersion.

Prolonged exposure of the skin surface to water in adults is harmful.[25] Growing evidence indicates that vernix interacts with the developing epidermis and facilitates the *in utero* formation of the stratum corneum.[26,27]

Recent studies in rodent and fetal human skin using the technique of methylene blue dye exclusion,[28,29] have demonstrated the development of the epidermal barrier. Cellular tissue exposed to this dye turns blue, whereas an intervening cornified barrier prevents tissue staining. This technique offers a relatively straightforward method of determining the pattern and timing of permeability barrier formation. In rodents, epidermal barrier development begins dorsally and extends in a ventral direction over the course of the 16th and 19th days of gestation in mice and rats, respectively.[29] This process leads to a slightly thicker stratum corneum over the back than the front in the late-gestation fetal rat.[30] Stratum corneum formation in the rat at birth requires approximately 3 cells/cm²/second to undergo programmed cell death.[30] Corneocyte formation rate in humans has not been measured.

In humans, unlike rodents which lack body hair at birth, the permeability barrier forms initially in the region of the pilosebaceous apparatus.[28] This finding strongly supports the hypothesis that vernix caseosa (a product of sebaceous secretions) participates in "water-proofing" the skin surface, thereby allowing cornification to occur initially in the area of the hair follicles and then over the interfollicular skin.[31] Standard skin culture systems are organizationally simpler than fetal skin and notably lack skin appendages. Such systems must be raised to an air-liquid interface to obtain adequate cornification.[32] A better understanding of vernix caseosa and fetal sebaceous gland physiology is biologically relevant and may be applicable to clinical situations in which the epidermal surface is inadequately developed, burned, or traumatized.

Sebaceous glands are found in the skin of all mammals except whales and porpoises.[33] Their primary function is the excretion of sebum, which is a complex mixture of relatively nonpolar lipids, most of which are synthesized *de novo* by the glands.[34] Sebum provides a hydrophobic coating for the fur of mammals, which protects against overwetting. Sebaceous glands are multi-acinar, holocrine-secreting structures that occur in all areas of the skin except the palms and soles and only sparsely on the dorsal surfaces of the hand and foot.[35] The development of the sebaceous glands is closely related to the differentiation of hair follicles in the epidermis. In newborn infants, sebaceous glands are well formed, hyperplastic, and macroscopically visible over certain body areas, such as the nose. The close connection of vernix production *in utero* with the developing pilosebaceous apparatus supports a mechanism by which the surge in sebaceous gland activity during the last trimester of pregnancy leads to production of a thick, lipid-rich, hydrophobic film (the vernix caseosa) overlying the developing stratum corneum.[26,34] The hyperplasia of the sebaceous glands in term infants is putatively secondary to androgenic stimulation from the equally hyperplastic adrenal glands.[26] This hypothesis provides a working model that remains to be fully tested. It has the advantage of functionally integrating two disconnected facts; i.e., the mutual hyperplasia during the latter half of gestation of the sebaceous gland and the adrenal gland in the human fetus.

Other clinical observations are also explicable under this hypothesis. Obstetricians have long observed that the amniotic fluid becomes turbid during the last trimester of pregnancy.[36] *In vitro*, the addition of physiologically relevant amounts of pulmonary surfactant leads to emulsification and release of immobilized vernix. This finding is consistent with a mechanism by which vernix is progressively released from the skin surface after formation of an intact stratum corneum under the influence of lung-derived surfactant within the amniotic fluid.[36] The fetus subsequently swallows the detached vernix (Fig. 60-3). Measurements of the amino acids of vernix have demonstrated that it

TABLE 60-3

Comparison of Lamellar Bodies of Epidermal and Pulmonary Origins

	Epidermis	Lung
Cell type	Spinous and granular keratinocytes	Type II alveolar cell
Size/structure	Ovoid (0.25–0.5 micron)	Spheroid (1.2–1.6 microns)
	Disklike lamellations	Lamellated sacs with amorphous core
Lipid content	40% phospholipids	85% phospholipids
	20% glycosphingolipids	10% free sterols
	20% free sterols	5% other neutral lipids
	20% other neutral lipids	
Protein content	Acid phosphatase	Acid phosphatase
	Glycosidases	Proteases
	Proteases	Glycosidases
	Lipases	Surfactant apoproteins
Function	Delivery of lipids to form extracellular matrix of stratum corneum	Delivery of surfactant lipid to alveolar spaces
	Skin permeability barrier	Lower alveolar surface tension

is rich in glutamine, a known trophic factor for the developing gut.[37, 38] Further work is required to establish the degree to which epithelial surfaces "cross-talk" in preparation for birth. What emerges from the available data, however, is a coherent and intriguing glimpse of a new area in perinatal biology.

TRANSITION AT BIRTH

Few events in mammalian life are as physiologically abrupt as birth. As with other epithelial surfaces that interface with the environment after birth (lung, gut, and kidney), the skin must immediately perform multiple functions vital to the survival of the organism (Table 60-4).[7] Many of these functions, such as thermoregulation, were unnecessary prior to birth and largely performed by the placenta. Birth, however, marks a transition to

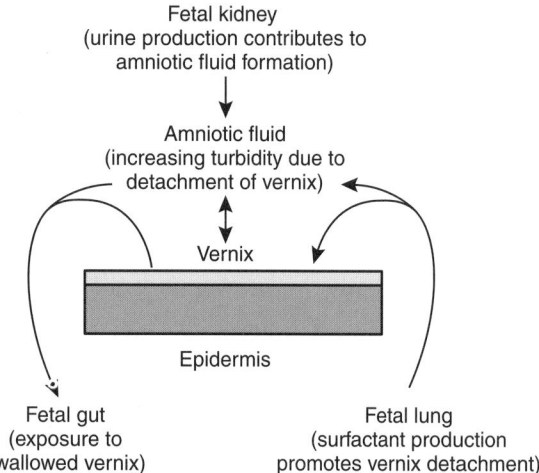

Figure 60–3. Proposed mechanism for pulmonary surfactant–mediated vernix detachment. The fetal kidney contributes significantly to amniotic fluid production. During the third trimester, vernix covers the developing epidermis and the fetal lung produces and secretes increasing amounts of pulmonary surfactant into the amniotic fluid. Vernix on the skin surface builds up and detaches into the surrounding milieu, leading to amniotic fluid turbidity.[36] Vernix within the amniotic fluid is subsequently swallowed by the fetus with potential effects on the fetal foregut and/or systemic absorption of vernix components. (Adapted and expanded from Hoath S, Pickens W: *In* Hoath SB, Maibach H (eds): Neonatal Skin: Structure and Function. New York, Marcel Dekker, 2003.[26]

a cold, nonsterile environment that includes high oxidative stress and exposure to ultraviolet light.

Physiologic mechanisms in the epidermis that contribute to formation of an adaptive environmental interface include activation of eccrine sweating, which is important for thermoregulation and bacterial homeostasis, and sebum production by hyperplastic sebaceous glands.[39] At birth, the epidermal barrier is essentially pH neutral, but it rapidly develops an acid mantle via mechanisms distinct from simple bacterial colonization.[40] Physiologically, the epidermis and its ultimate differentiation product, the stratum corneum, remain in balance by the dual properties of renewability and self-cleaning, which reflect the distinct but tightly coupled processes of cornification and desquamation.[41] Recent data have indicated that transepidermal water flux is an important regulator of both DNA and lipid synthesis within the epidermis.[42-44] Environmental humidity and maintenance of stratum corneum hydration are necessary for normal desquamation.[45, 46] The preterm infant is vulnerable to disruption of all these physiologic mechanisms.

Prenatally, lipid synthesis is necessary for both production of the vernix caseosa and formation of the interfollicular barrier lipids of the epidermis, which are required for successful postnatal adaptation. Postnatally, lipid synthesis and metabolism continue to subserve multiple functions (Table 60-5). Thus, specific barrier lipids in the stratum corneum form the primary structural basis for the postnatal epidermal permeability barrier. The epidermis and the brain both contain unusually high concentrations of ceramides.[47-49] This fact deserves further examination given the close embryologic and functional connection between these two ectodermal derivatives. Other skin lipids include sebum, and triglycerides in adipose tissue. The latter functions primarily as a systemic energy reservoir in addition to providing cushioning and biomechanical support.

TABLE 60-4

Multiple Physiologic Roles of the Skin at Birth

Barrier to water loss
Thermoregulation
Infection control
Immunosurveillance
Acid mantle formation
Antioxidant function
UV light photoprotection
Barrier to chemicals
Tactile discrimination
Attraction to caregiver

TABLE 60-5

Sources, Composition, and Presumed Functions of Skin Lipids in the Neonate

Source	Composition	Functions
Stratum corneum	Ceramides, cholesterol sulfate, neutral lipids (free and esterified sterols, free fatty acids, triglycerides)	Permeability barrier Cohesion/ desquamation Antibacterial
Sebaceous glands	Triglyceride, wax/sterol esters/squalene	Antibacterial Moisturization
Adipose tissue	Triglyceride	Systemic energy reservoir

Water Loss, Temperature Control, and Blood Flow

Life in a dry, terrestrial environment necessitates protection against the constant dehydrating effects of air exposure. The formation of a barrier against transepidermal water loss is well known to be a direct function of gestational age.[50,51] As shown in Figure 60-4, transepidermal water loss decreases dramatically as term approaches, with levels in the near term infant equal to or less than adult values. This critical and vital postnatal function resides almost entirely in the outermost 20 microns of the skin surface; i.e., in the stratum corneum.[2] Heat exchange between the skin of an infant and the surrounding environment occurs via evaporation, radiation, conduction, and convection.[52] Of these, evaporative heat loss is the primary mode of temperature instability in very low birth weight preterm infants and is the primary mode of heat loss in all infants at the time of birth. It is important to distinguish between evaporative heat loss from standing water or amniotic fluid on the skin surface and evaporative heat loss secondary to a poor epidermal barrier, as occurs after delivery in very low birth weight preterm infants. The second mode of heat and fluid loss is ongoing and is exacerbated in nonhumidified, radiant heating environments.

Given the critical importance of limiting evaporative water and heat loss in temperature control, it is surprising how little attention is given to the role of the stratum corneum in thermoregulation. Most reviews of body temperature control assume the presence of this water-retentive envelope. As with many other functions, the strategic position of the stratum corneum is taken for granted and focus is placed on more central mechanisms. In the newborn infant, however, it is important to continually bear in mind the role of peripheral mechanisms in organizing, maintaining, and guiding central nervous system development. The classic study by Adamsons and associates on the regulation of systemic oxygen consumption in term infants shortly following birth, provides an example of the importance of the periphery in temperature control in newly born infants (Fig. 60-5).[53]

Thus, oxygen consumption, measured in term infants 4 hours following birth, is not a function of central body temperature, as might be expected with warm-blooded endothermic organisms.[53] Systemic oxygen consumption is, rather, a function of heat exchange at the skin-environment interface. Central homeothermic mechanisms are not well developed at birth. A basic knowledge of skin-environment interactions, therefore, is key for the infant caregiver. Preterm infants exhibit even more vulnerability to the environment owing to higher surface area to mass ratios, lower endogenous sources of heat generation such as brown adipose tissue, an incompetent epidermal barrier, and the inability to self-regulate with flexural positioning.[54]

The central control of body temperature also requires mechanisms such as eccrine sweating and vasodilatation/vasoconstric-

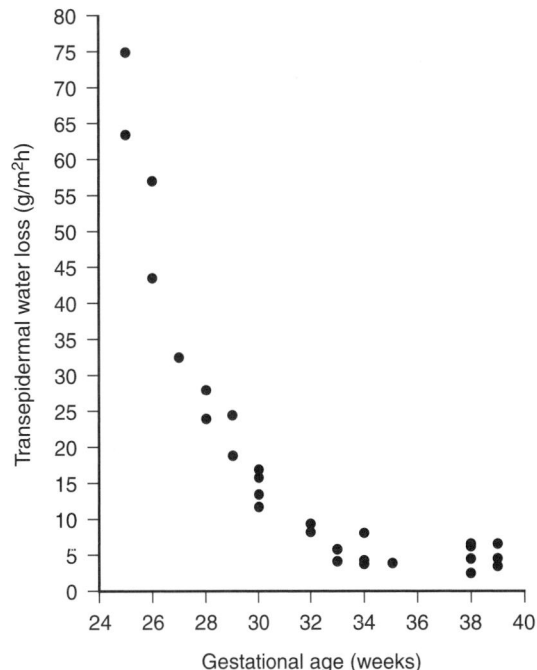

Figure 60-4. Transepidermal water loss as a function of gestational age. These data demonstrate the inverse relationship between transepidermal water loss (TEWL) and gestational age. Very low birth weight preterm infants have extraordinarily high TEWL in the range of 50 to 70 g/m²/hour. Term infants have low TEWL, in the range of 5 g/m²/hour, which is comparable with or lower than adult values. (After Hammarlund K, Sedin G: Acta Paediatr Scand 68:795, 1979.[50])

tion, which are under autonomic nervous system control.[55] These mechanisms are generally not well established at birth. Newborn infants may exhibit vasoconstriction of the extremities (acrocyanosis) and may have wide fluctuations in red blood cell content (hematocrit) as well as blood volume. Peripheral cooling results in increased blood viscosity and decreased blood flow. After birth, there is considerable reorganization of the cutaneous vascular bed, with development of a subpapillary plexus over the first 3 months of life (Fig. 60-6). The formation of a superficial vascular plexus is also associated with increased convolution of the undersurface of the epidermis (rete peg formation), which is a hallmark of the mature human epidermis. The development of the cutaneous vasculature and the role of growth factors, such as vascular endothelial growth factor (VEGF) have been reviewed elsewhere.[56]

Development of the Acid Mantle

A number of physiologic mechanisms are triggered at the time of birth, which persist into later life. Human skin, for example, is characterized by an acidic skin surface, the so-called "acid mantle." At birth, the skin surface pH is relatively neutral and gradually becomes more acidic over the first few postnatal weeks (Fig. 60-7). The first measurements of infant skin pH were performed by Taddei in 1935, who reported surface skin pH in the range of 6.5 at birth.[57] The use of alkaline soaps for infant bathing can markedly alter the development of the acid mantle, as can the local environment.[58] Acid mantle development is delayed in very low birth weight preterm infants.[59] Surface skin pH measurements are generally higher under occluded sites, such as the diaper region.[60] Site-dependent differences in surface pH have also been reported in the neonate.[61]

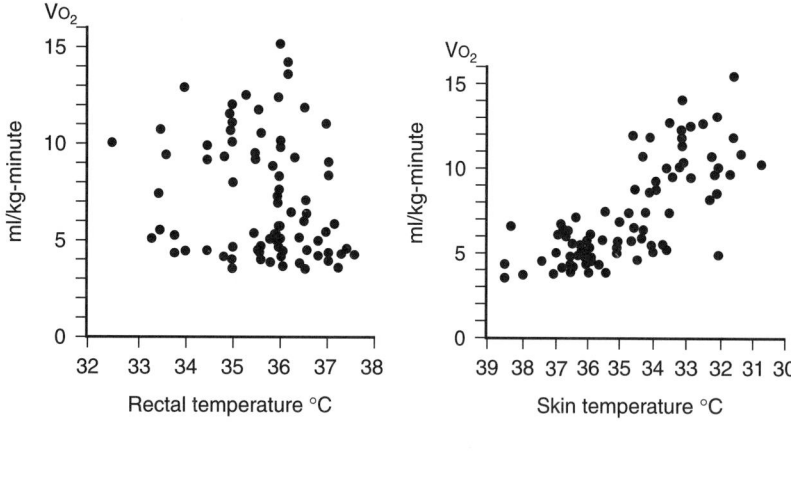

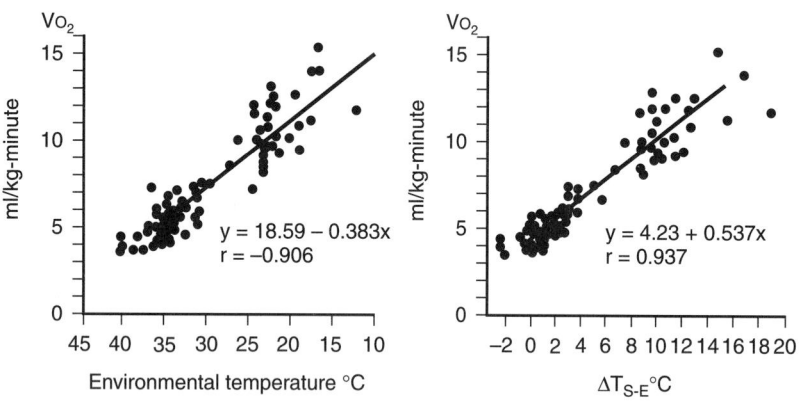

Figure 60–5. Oxygen consumption of term newborn human infants approximately 4 hours after birth. Systemic oxygen consumption correlates best with the skin-environment gradient, indicating the importance of peripheral heat flux in regulating body temperature in the neonate. (From Adamsons K, et al: J Pediatr *66*:495, 1965.[53])

A number of different mechanisms for establishing the acid mantle have been proposed, including endogenous factors such as lactic acid from sweat, free fatty acid generation from metabolism of triglycerides in sebum, and metabolic by products of bacterial colonization.[40] Endogenous factors include the formation of lactic acid from epidermal cell metabolism and free fatty acid generation from phospholipid breakdown within the stratum corneum. Active proton pump mechanisms also have been proposed, as well as the controlled degradation of structural proteins such as filaggrin to form acidic byproducts such as urocanic acid.[40]

The presence of an acidic skin surface has advantages.[40] Proposed functions of the acid mantle include antimicrobial defense and maintenance of epidermal barrier integrity.[62] Enzymes involved in stratum corneum desquamation, which are pH sensitive, include cathepsin D, chymotryptic serine protease, and tryptic serine protease. Extracellular lipids involved in formation of the epidermal barrier are also processed via pH-sensitive enzymes, including beta-glucocerebrosidase. Thus, the acid mantle is derived from multiple redundant sources and may regulate a number of processes essential for maintenance of a competent epidermal barrier. The newborn infant offers an exciting and accessible area for studying these multiple etiologic mechanisms and functions.

Bacterial Colonization and Skin Cleansing

Paramount among the many functions served by the skin is the prevention of infection. Prior to birth, the fetus resides in a sterile environment. Colonization of newborn skin begins upon first exposure to the external world. Infants born vaginally become colonized during passage through the birth canal, whereas infants born by cesarean section are typically sterile if the amniotic membranes were not ruptured prior to the onset of labor.[63] A list of the common skin-colonizing bacterial flora is given in Table 60-6.

Staphylococcus epidermidis, one of 13 species of coagulase-negative staphylococci, is the most common vaginal organism prior to birth and is ubiquitous in the environment. This organism rapidly colonizes the skin surface and is the predominate organism on the skin of most neonates.[64-68] Under normal conditions, the resident flora of the neonate resembles that of adults after the first few weeks of life. These skin-colonizing flora are generally nonvirulent, stable in number, and only infrequently pathogenic given a normal epidermal barrier and immune properties.[69] In the very low birth weight preterm infant, however, *Staphylococcus epidermidis* is the most common cause of sepsis.[69] This fact complicates greatly the choice of appropriate skin care procedures and practices. Normally, commensal bacterial flora play a protective role, and recent evidence suggests that organisms such as *Staphylococcus epidermidis* may up-regulate expression of antimicrobial peptides, such as human beta-defensin 2.[70,71]

The mechanisms leading to colonization of the skin are incompletely understood and involve a complex interplay between rapid growth of commensal organisms, the development of the acid mantle, local microenvironmental factors such as occlusion and humidity, and the choice of exogenous soaps and skin care practices.[70] There is a surprising lack of standard guidelines regarding optimal skin care in the neonate.[72,73] Specific aspects of care include hand washing procedures, bathing and choice of surfactants, regional skin care including the umbilical cord stump, and preparation of the skin prior to invasive procedures such as venipuncture.[72] Recently, the use of alcohol-based disin-

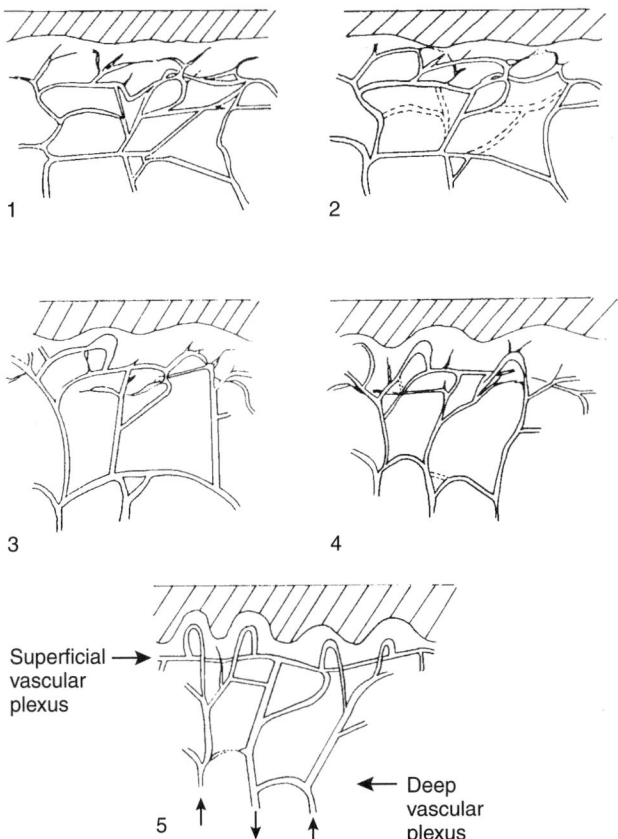

Figure 60–6. Diagrammatic representation of the blood supply at birth (*1*), the gradual development of papillary buds and organization of the subpapillary plexus from birth to 3 months of age (*2-4*), and the vascular pattern at 3 months of age (*5*). The arrows (*5*) show the direction of blood flow for arteriolar and venous systems. (Modified from Perera P, et al: Br J Dermatol *82*(Suppl 5):86, 1970.[145]

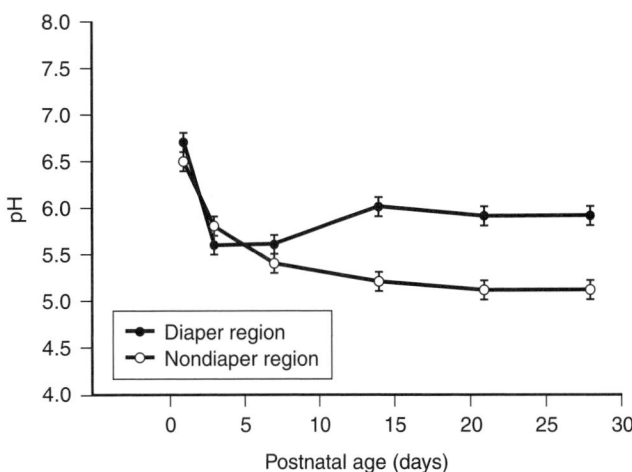

Figure 60–7. Postnatal development of the acid mantle in term newborn infants—effect of body site. Skin pH was measured using a flat surface electrode (Courage and Khazaka pH meter, model 900, Cologne, Germany) in male and female infants born between 37 and 42 weeks of gestation. Values are means ± SE. (Data from Visscher M, et al: Pediatr Dermatol *17*:45, 2000.[60])

fectants has been promoted as an alternative to routine hand washing.[74,75] It is important to recognize that such disinfectants have no cleansing function and will not remove soils on the skin surface. Recently, vernix caseosa has been reported to function as an endogenous skin cleanser that readily removes topical soils, such as carbon particles.[76] This finding is consistent with the view that the surface of the newly born infant possesses endogenous skin cleansing mechanisms (vernix, stratum corneum desquamation). These natural functions should be incorporated into the design of exogenous skin cleansing regimens.

Cutaneous Immunosurveillance

Given the plethora of bacteria and the multiple opportunities for superficial trauma, it is not surprising that the skin has a well-developed immune system.[9] There is increasing evidence that innate immune function in term infants may be well developed, whereas such function in the preterm infant is poor.[77] Once pathogenic bacteria or fungi have established adherence to the skin, a number of cutaneous mechanisms of host defense are called into play, including (1) the role of the stratum corneum as a mechanical barrier, (2) the establishment of an acid environment inhospitable for bacterial growth, and (3) the presence of metabolic products within the stratum corneum itself with antimicrobial activity.[78,79] Commensal organisms, such as the lipophilic corynebacteria, have been reported to contribute to

host defense by liberating antibacterial fatty acids from the triglycerides of sebum.[80] Cationic peptides may be elaborated in the skin with direct antimicrobial effects on the bacterial side of the cytoplasmic membrane.[81] A list of potential antimicrobial peptides in human epidermis is given in Table 60–7.

Specific cell types within the epidermis play critical roles in host defense. In addition to terminal differentiation and formation of the stratum corneum, keratinocytes have been reported to internalize bacteria, leading to bacterial death and containment of infection.[82,83] The epidermis also contains migratory dendritic cells associated with antigen presentation.[84] These Langerhans cells are derived from the bone marrow and are located in the mid-to-lower epidermis, where they maintain a

---

TABLE 60–6

Common Skin Flora Colonizing Newborn Skin

Micrococcaceae

Coagulase-negative staphylococci
Staphylococcus epidermidis
Staphylococcus hominis
Staphylococcus saprophyticus (perineum)
Staphylococcus capitis (sebum-rich areas)
Staphylococcus auricularis (ear canal)
Peptococcus species
Micrococcus species

Diphtheroids

Corynebacterium (moist intertriginous areas)
Brevibacterium (toe webs)
Propionibacterium (hair follicles, sebaceous glands)

Gram-negative rods

Acinetobacter (moist, intertriginous areas, perineum)
Rarely *Klebsiella, Enterobacter, Proteus*

Yeast

Malassezia species

Modified from Sidbury R, Darmstadt G: *In* Hoath SB, Maibach H (eds): Neonatal Skin: Structure and Function. New York, Marcel Dekker, 2003[70]; and Darmstadt G: *In* Harahap M (ed): Diagnosis and Treatment of Skin Infections, Oxford, Blackwell Scientific Publications, 1997.[69]

TABLE 60-7

Antimicrobial Agents Produced in the Epidermis

Complement
Defensins
Cathelicidins
Cytokines
Chemokines
Reactive oxygen species

Modified from Chuong CM, et al: Exp Dermatol *11*:159, 2002.[9]

strategic position for immunosurveillance (Fig. 60-8). Breach of the epidermal barrier leads to exposure of Langerhans cells to microorganisms and other potentially pathogenic material. Following exposure, Langerhans cells migrate to regional lymph nodes. Their density and function within preterm epidermis have not been explored.

PROBLEMS OF THE VERY LOW BIRTH WEIGHT INFANT

Ineffective Barrier

Without the prevention of water and heat loss provided by the stratum corneum, life in a terrestrial environment is impossible. Immaturity of the dermis and the cutaneous appendages poses problems of lesser magnitude for the very low birth weight infant. Exposure to air following birth, in conjunction with other unknown stimulatory factors, results in marked acceleration of barrier maturation (Fig. 60-9). This effect is thought to be secondary to xeric stress imposed by the dry environment.[43, 44] Similar effects are observed in cultured human skin, where lifting the culture system to an air-liquid interface is required for adequate barrier formation *in vitro*.[32] Following preterm delivery, the normal slow intrauterine rate of epidermal barrier maturation is forgone. Birth of the very low birth weight infant triggers immediate lipid and DNA synthesis, with subsequent cornification of the nucleated epidermal keratinocytes. The rapid transition from the sticky, wet, translucent skin surface of the

very low birth weight infant to the dry, opaque stratum corneum of the older preterm infant is familiar to infant caregivers. Such rapid formation of the stratum corneum often results in excessive desquamation and scaling several weeks following preterm birth. Measurements of transepidermal water loss and surface electrical capacitance have been used to track the rate of barrier formation following preterm birth.[51, 85] As shown in Figure 60-10, transepidermal water loss in immature 24- to 25-week gestation infants decreases during the first few days after birth, but still remains elevated on the 28th postnatal day, compared with expected levels of 5 to 10 g/m²/hr in term infants (see Fig. 60-4). The etiology of the poor stratum corneum barrier in these infants is unclear, but may relate to the extreme rapidity of barrier formation in this vulnerable population. Other skin conditions characterized by rapid epidermal turnover, such as atopic dermatitis and psoriasis, have similar high water loss rates.

The immature epidermal barrier of the very low birth weight infant is permeable to substances other than water. Care must be exercised to avoid toxic substances, which can enter the body via a transdermal route.[86, 87] Respiratory gases can also move across the epidermal barrier under normal conditions. The immature barrier of the preterm infant, for example, allows the efflux of carbon dioxide[88] and the influx of oxygen[89] in a manner similar to that of water vapor. These findings support the contention that increasing ambient oxygen in a conductive incubator during the first few postnatal days may lead to an appreciable augmentation of systemic oxygen. The rapid development of the stratum corneum, however, precludes long-term utility of this novel therapeutic approach.

Strategies for Epidermal Barrier Maturation/Repair

Therapeutic strategies for facilitating epidermal barrier development and protection of the preterm infant are shown in Table 60-8. Prematurity and infection are leading worldwide causes of neonatal morbidity and mortality.[90,91] Preterm infants are vulnerable to infection because of a poorly developed epidermal barrier combined with developmentally immature host defense mechanisms. The first week of life is a vulnerable period, particu-

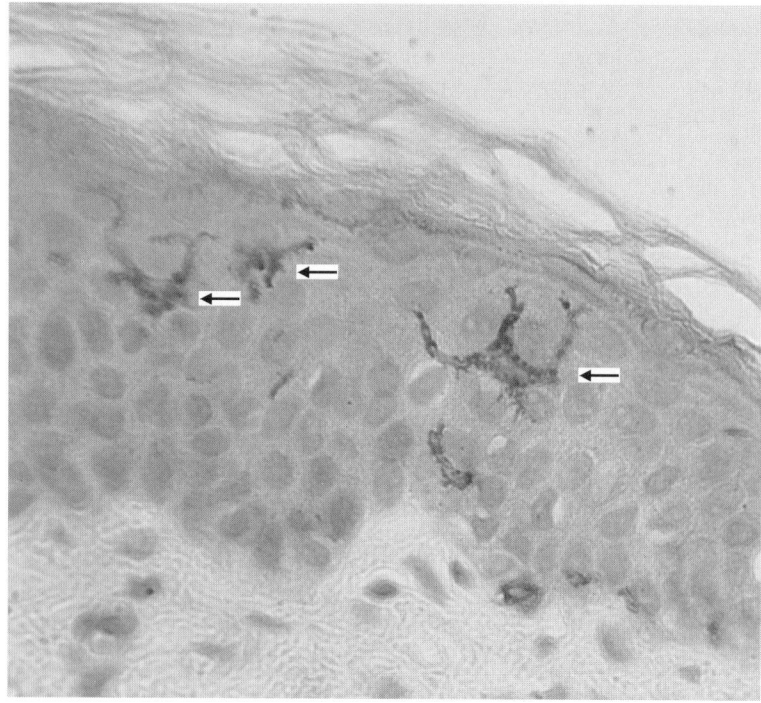

Figure 60-8. Immunolocalization of Langerhans cells in premature human epidermis (foreskin) by CD1a antibody staining (*arrows*). Langerhans cells are dendritic, antigen-presenting cells derived from the fetal bone marrow. They are typically located within the epidermis and function as a major component of the skin immune system. Skin specimen is from an approximately 32-week premature infant circumcised 1 month after birth.

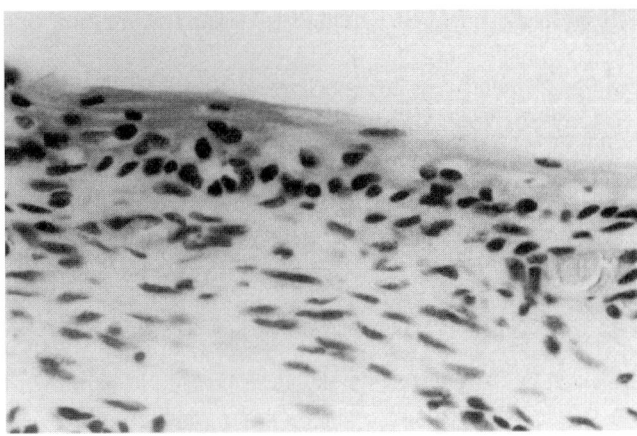

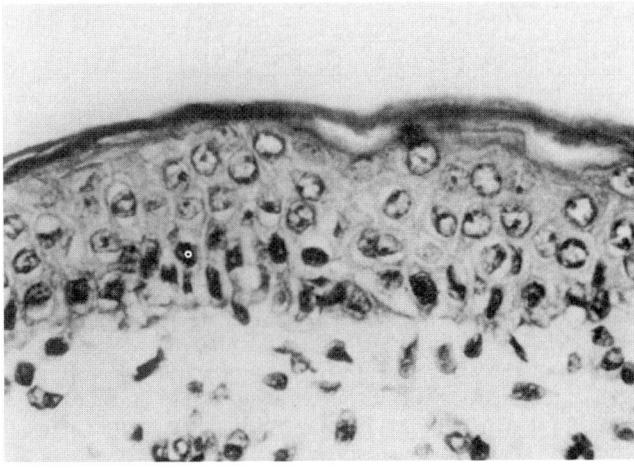

Figure 60–9. Rapid development of the epidermal barrier following exposure to the ambient environment (xeric stress) in the very low birth weight preterm infant. The top panel shows the epidermis of a 26-week infant on day 1 of life. There is no stratum corneum and the nucleated epidermis is thin. The lower panel shows the epidermis of a 26-week infant on postnatal day 10. (Reproduced from Rutter N: Clin Perinatol *14*:911, 1987.[146]

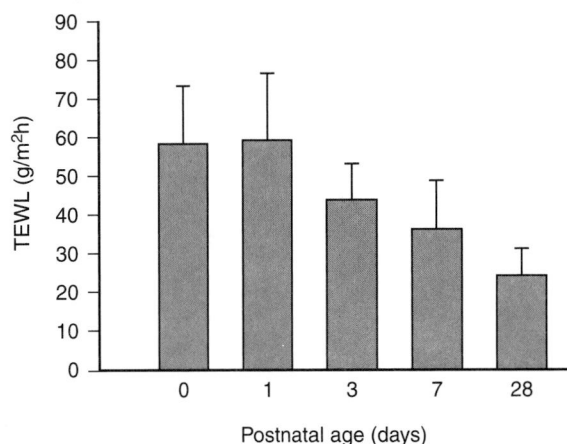

Figure 60–10. Transepidermal water loss as a function of postnatal age in very low birth weight preterm infants. (After Agren J, et al: Acta Paediatr Scand *87*:1185, 1998.[51])

larly in developing countries, when 50% to 70% of fatal and life-threatening neonatal illnesses occur, many of which are infectious complications associated with low birth weight infants.[72] Because the consequences of systemic infections are so devastating in premature and low birth weight infants, therapeutic options for preventing bacterial and fungal infections assume high priority as a means for improving neonatal outcomes.[91]

One of the earliest methods of improving outcome in the preterm infant was the provision of a thermal neutral environment with increased ambient humidity.[92-94] Ambient humidity is inversely related to transepidermal water loss as a function of gestational age.[95] Increasing the humidity within a convective

incubator, for example, creates a microenvironment in which transepidermal water loss is lessened. A similar microenvironment can be created under semipermeable membranes with the infant lying beneath radiant warming devices. High humidities, however, may result in "rain-out" with obscuration of the infant. Warm, wet environments are also associated with an increased risk of infection. Radiant warming devices increase transepidermal water loss and require a concomitant increase in fluid replacement rates. Recent studies have demonstrated that the increase in transepidermal water loss with infrared warmers is due entirely to the low humidity of the overlying air rather than any direct drying effect of the infrared radiation.[96]

Evaporation of amniotic fluid at the time of delivery, coupled with an incompetent epidermal barrier, may create severe fluid imbalances and heat loss in the newborn infant. Vohra and associates studied the use of polyethylene films on premature infants in the delivery room.[97] This study reported better temperature stability and a significant decrease in mortality in extremely low birth weight infants treated with vapor-reducing occlusive membranes at birth. This approach highlights the "golden hour" concept of care originally developed for treatment of adult stroke and myocardial infarction patients.[98] Unlike the latter events, however, the birth of a preterm infant often can be anticipated and prepared for with emergency personnel and equipment. Attention to environmental temperature, humidity, adhesive application, and the presence or absence of surface biomaterials such as vernix, all play a role in delivery room management. Therapeutic regimens should be tailored to begin in the delivery room with extension to the neonatal intensive care unit.

One innovative approach for enhancing epidermal barrier function is application of topical lipid-rich emollients to the skin surface.[99] These agents may contain a mixture of non-physiologic lipids, such as petrolatum or a mixture of physiologic lipids, such as ceramides, cholesterol, and free fatty acids.[100] In addition to their ability to decrease transepidermal water loss and form a

---

TABLE 60–8

Epidermal Barrier Repair Strategies

Topical application of one or more nonphysiologic lipids (e.g., petrolatum)
Topical application of mixtures of physiologic lipids (ceramides, cholesterol, free fatty acids) in appropriate molar ratios
Topical dressings
    Vapor-permeable: allow metabolic (repair) processes to continue in the underlying epidermis
    Vapor-impermeable (occlusive): delay metabolic responses in the underlying epidermis

Modified from Chuong, CM, et al: Exp Dermatol *11*:159, 2002.[9]

mechanical barrier to bacteria, the components of the emollient may serve as a source of material for active lipid metabolism in the epidermis.[101] In moderately preterm infants, petrolatum application to the skin surface has been reported to improve barrier function with concomitant reduction of the rate of nosocomial infections.[102] Recently, a large study of more than 1200 low birth weight preterm infants demonstrated an increase in late-onset nosocomial infections secondary to coagulase-negative staphylococci in extremely low birth weight infants (500 to 750 g birth weight).[103] More therapeutic strategies involving topical emollient application intended to facilitate epidermal barrier development are needed.

In many developing countries, natural oils are applied topically after birth as part of a traditional oil massage regimen. A recent study by Darmstadt and colleagues examined the effects of a variety of naturally occurring vegetable oils on the skin barrier.[104] The goal was to identify safe, inexpensive vegetable oils available in developing countries that might improve epidermal barrier function in very low birth weight infants. When vegetable oils were applied to barrier-compromised skin of adult hairless mice, oils rich in linoleic acid enhanced epidermal barrier formation. In contrast, mustard oil, a topical emollient used routinely in newborn care throughout South Asia, had toxic effects on the epidermal barrier. The investigators noted that emollients containing a physiologic balance of epidermal lipids (3:1:1 molar ratio of cholesterol, ceramide, palmitate and linoleate) may be optimal for barrier repair.[100] Vegetable oils are readily available worldwide. Such oils provide a simple, inexpensive, and effective alternative for topical use. Clearly, this is a research area requiring further investigation.

Visscher and associates, studied the effects of semipermeable films on human skin following a standardized superficial wound (removal of the stratum corneum by tape stripping), which mimics the immature epidermal barrier of the premature infant.[105] Transepidermal water loss, skin hydration, rate of moisture accumulation, and erythema were measured. Wounds treated with semipermeable films had more rapid barrier recovery than either nonoccluded wounds or wounds under complete occlusion. This finding is consistent with a role for vapor permeability to regulate epidermal barrier formation.

Therapeutic strategies may result from a combination of individual methods optimized for a specific infant.[54] Prenatal steroid administration coupled with optimal delivery room management and a seamless transition to a controlled NICU environment with use of physiologic emollients and minimal adhesive injury may provide the optimal therapeutic interface between the preterm infant and the care environment.

Many questions remain unanswered at the present time. For example, the efficacy of prenatal glucocorticoid therapy to accelerate epidermal barrier maturation is well documented for rodent skin as well as for fetal lung maturation.[16, 18-20, 106] Studies in the neonatal clinical literature provide conflicting reports on the efficacy of steroids in mature fetal epidermis.[20] Similarly, the use of topical emollients has been questioned for the very low birth weight preterm infant.[103] Work thus far suggests that provision of a semipermeable membrane or dressing may be optimal for promoting epidermal maturation.[105] In contrast to Aquaphor, vernix is highly vapor permeable and may provide a more physiologically relevant prototype for development of a natural wound dressing for use in the low birth weight preterm infant. "Smart fabrics" with heat- and motion-activated transfer of topical emollients and wound-healing ointments to the skin surface have been developed for treatment of diaper rash.[107, 108] An attractive concept is that clothing or bedding material, in addition to wound dressings, may contain physiologic emollients and growth factors for facilitation of epidermal barrier development. All these therapies draw attention to the role of the skin in environmental coupling and the close interconnection between the human skin surface and the caregiver.

THE SKIN AS A NEURODEVELOPMENTAL INTERFACE

In all vertebrates, touch is the first sense to develop, followed closely by vestibular or position sensing.[109] The human neonate, compared with neonates of other species, is relatively helpless in motor capabilities and relatively precocious in sensory capabilities.[110] Sensory and affective information is necessary for body orientation and the spatial organization required for proper motor output. Evaluation of sensory competency is difficult, however, and neonatal outcome studies typically utilize developmental scoring systems, which rely heavily upon tests of motor skills or behavior. The idea that the sensory system is precocious in early human development places the skin in a strategic location to affect subsequent development.[8] As an interface between the body and the environment, the skin links to the developing brain, on the one hand, and to external factors including light, heat, fabrics, and the interactions of caregivers and parents, on the other hand. Neonatal animals such as the kitten and the rodent have proved to be useful models to study the effect of sensory inputs on central nervous system development.[111-115] These models clearly suggest that sensory signals are required during critical developmental windows for proper central nervous system maturation. In humans, clinical studies have demonstrated various effects of tactile stimulation during infancy. Field and associates have shown that tactile stimulation of hospitalized preterm infants results in greater weight gain and higher behavorial scores.[116]

Cutaneous Receptors and Electrical Maturation

A useful concept for interpreting the functional role of the skin surface is the idea (derived from the engineering sciences) of a "smart material" interface.[117, 118] The outermost layer of the epidermis, the stratum corneum, has many of the attributes of a smart material.[8, 15] It is strategically positioned as part of a larger functional system and adapts readily to changes in the environment. This material is self-cleaning and self-assembling and possesses sensing and actuating properties possibly secondary to the piezoelectric and piezomechanical properties of the contained keratin filaments.[119] In its role as the limiting surface of the body, the stratum corneum simultaneously forms both the perceived surface of the organism and the biologic boundary with the environment. Thus, the stratum corneum and, by extension, the skin in general, corresponds in a simple manner to the distinction between subject and object.[8]

Most textbooks on neurophysiology consider sensory signal processing to be mediated initially by specialized nerve endings (Fig. 60-11). Nerve endings, however, never directly touch the environment. Interfacing with the environment is a function of the material in which the nerve endings are embedded.[8] This perspective applies an engineering view to the material properties of the skin surface[117] and is important for understanding innovative approaches to skin–central nervous system interactions as put forth by Ansel and colleagues.[120] Thus, the stratum corneum and the epidermal/dermal matrix are potential mediators of sensory signal processing. Following birth, the physical properties of the epidermis change rapidly during adaptation to a gaseous environment.[85] Biophysical properties of the skin can be easily measured with noninvasive instrumentation.[121] These properties include skin viscoelasticity, hydrophobicity, thermal conductivity, color, transepidermal water loss, and pH. In particular, the study of the electrical properties of the skin may be relevant for the very low birth weight preterm infant.[85] Table 60-9 shows the measured electrical resistance to direct current in human skin (adult) and various commonly used animal models.[122] Only the newborn rat has an electrical resistance comparable with that seen in adult humans. By contrast, the electrical resistance of the epidermal barrier in the very low birth weight preterm infant is likely to be low owing to relative deficiency of both vernix and stratum corneum.

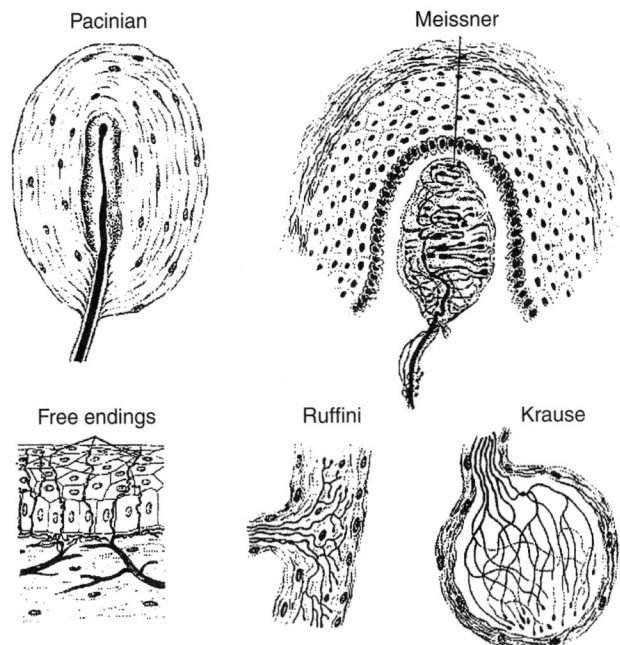

Figure 60–11. Types of cutaneous nerve endings. Pacinian corpuscles are deep cutaneous receptors for crude touch and vibration over both hairy and glabrous skin. Meissner's corpuscles are superficially located, rapidly adapting nerve endings modulating light touch and vibration over primarily glabrous skin. Free nerve endings are associated with crude touch, tickle, and itch sensations. Ruffini organs are deep, slowly adapting structures for pressure sensing. The Krause end bulb is particularly associated with the perception of cold. Nerve endings typically are embedded in a material biomatrix and never touch the environment. The biomatrix surrounding the nerve endings directly contacts the environment.

Recently, Wakai and associates demonstrated the development of a high electrical impedance barrier *in utero* during the last trimester of pregnancy.[123] During the first half of gestation, the amplitude of the fetal electrocardiogram can be measured directly from the surface of the maternal abdomen. After 26 to 27 weeks' gestation, the amplitude gradually disappears, concomitant with the intrauterine development of an epidermal barrier consisting of vernix caseosa and the stratum corneum. Thus, the gradual disappearance of the fetal electrocardiogram from the maternal skin surface is secondary to a film of high electrical impedance developing between the fetus and the amniotic fluid. This process presumably reflects electrical isolation of the fetus from the mother with growing fetal autonomy.

Following birth, the electrical resistance of the skin of the term newborn is relatively high.[124] Surface electrical measurements are a common form of noninvasive monitoring in newborn intensive care units. New advances in monitoring, such as evoked potential

TABLE 60–9

Electrical Resistance to Direct Current in Skin

Skin Specimens	Effective Resistance (kOhms/cm^2)
Excised human skin	135 ± 54.0 (n = 40)
Newborn rat (day 0)	124 ± 24.2 (n = 18)
Infant rat (day 6)	27.7 ± 8.9 (n = 9)
Adult rat	28.3 ± 6.8 (n = 4)
Hairless mouse	9.3 ± 5.3 (n = 10)

Data from Shivanand P, PhD thesis, University of Cincinnati, 1995.[122]

testing of the brain, hold great promise for the assessment of multiple clinical conditions such as birth asphyxia.[125, 126] In contrast to commonly performed electrocardiographic measurements, however, evoked potential testing of the electrical activity of the brain requires measurement of low amplitude voltages (microvolts versus millivolts), which are greatly affected by the skin-electrode contact surface.[122] It is common practice for electrical signals to be obtained after abrading the skin surface with a gritty contact paste. From a practical standpoint, the field of evoked potential testing in newborns could be improved by focus on the electrode/skin interface and the development of a seamless electrical contact, which avoids wounding the skin.

Skin as an Information-Rich Surface

Development of the immature central nervous system depends on sensory input during the immediate postnatal period. Experimental interference with several sensory modalities, such as vision, touch, and hearing, results in profound anatomic, functional, and biochemical impairment to the central nervous system structures that regulate such modalities. In newborn rats, tactile stimulation is an important regulator of somatic growth. Schanberg and associates have studied the link between tactile stimulation and the molecular regulation of internal cellular growth promoting enzymes, such as ornithine decarboxylase (ODC).[111-113] ODC is a sensitive index of the maturation and growth of internal organs like the heart, liver, and brain. Brain, liver, and heart ODC levels are decreased by 35%, 81%, and 53%, respectively, when rat pups are removed from their mothers for periods as short as 1 hour. Restoration of the pups to the litters rapidly normalizes enzyme activity. This normalization is specific for touch. Other potential mediators, such as nutrition, have no effect.

In other work, tactile stimulation of the neonate influences circulating levels of lactate, an important energy substrate for brain metabolism.[114] In both newborn rats and human infants, lactate levels are high immediately following birth and fall rapidly after the first few hours of age.[114, 127] When newborn rat pups are removed from maternal contact and receive light tactile stimulation by means of rostral-caudal stroking with a camel hair brush (similar to the methodology established by Schanberg), lactate levels rise significantly and the elevations persist for up to 30 minutes following cessation of the tactile stimulus. These same stimuli fail to elicit an increase in serum lactate at 1 week of age. These results are noteworthy since the brain of the early suckling rat uses lactate in preference to other metabolic fuels like glucose and 3-hydroxybutyrate.[128] Moreover, lactate levels increase without development of hypoxic metabolic acidosis. This experiment demonstrates, in an animal model, that sensory interaction between the organism and the environment is a potential regulator of the availability of cerebral energy substrates. Such studies have yet to be performed in humans.

The concept that the human newborn infant is precocious in terms of sensory capabilities and relatively helpless in terms of motor capabilities[110] provides a conceptual framework within which to investigate the complex maturation of sensorimotor feedback loops. Preterm infants exhibit an age-dependent neurophysiologic response pattern similar to newborn rats insofar as the threshold for eliciting a motor response (flexor withdrawal) progressively increases with advancing gestational age (Fig. 60-12).[129] This finding is usually attributed to increased inhibition of the reflex arc by central nervous system structures. The cutaneous flexor response is elicited by stimulation of the foot with nylon filaments (von Frey hairs) of graded thickness. In addition to maturation of central nervous system structures, the material properties of the interface (dermis, epidermis/stratum corneum) are changing concomitantly and may contribute to the effect observed in Figure 60-12. The accessibility of the skin surface and the availability of multiple biomedical instruments for noninvasive measurement[121] provide an open area for

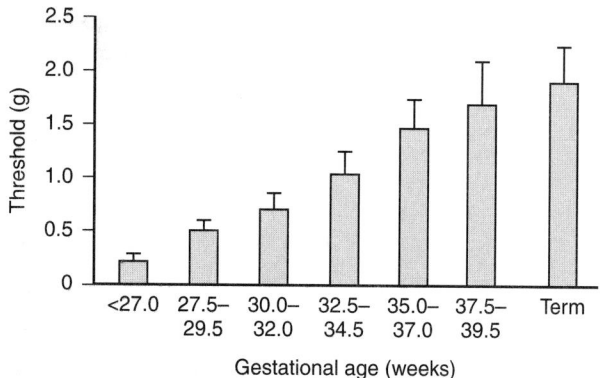

Figure 60–12. Threshold stimulus for eliciting flexor withdrawal in neonates of varying gestational age. Flexor withdrawal is elicited by stimulation of the foot with nylon filaments (von Frey hairs) of graded thickness. Preterm infants exhibit progressively lower thresholds for withdrawal than term infants. (Data from Fitzgerald M, et al: Dev Med Child Neurol 30:520, 1988.[129])

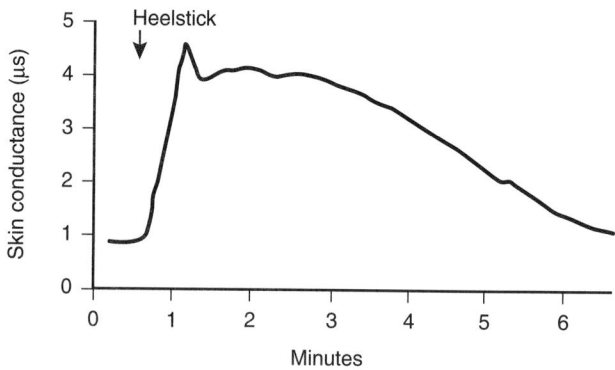

Figure 60–13. Effect of painful stimulus on skin conductance measurements in a term newborn infant. Skin conductance measured on the sole of the foot shows a sharp increase over the first minute in response to a heel prick on the other side. Values are in microsiemens (µS). (From Gladman G and Chiswick ML: Arch Dis Child 65:1063, 1990.[131])

skin-based research in neonatology, with potential relevance for central nervous system organization and control. The concept of a smart material interface presumes that changes in the biophysical properties of the skin surface will have a direct influence on adaptive environmental interfacing and sensorimotor response loops.[8,13,118]

An area in which noninvasive monitoring of the skin surface may reveal important information on central nervous system response and behavioral state involves skin conductance measurements in the newborn infant associated with eccrine (emotional/nonthermal) sweating.[55] Sweating is commonly viewed as secondary to the need for thermoregulation and evaporative cooling. It also occurs in response to arousal and pain, rather than temperature. This "emotional" sweating is easily measured from the palm or sole using a skin evaporimeter[130] but is usually estimated indirectly by measuring skin electrical conductance or resistance.[131] The presence of sweat within the eccrine ducts of the epidermis, and, to a lesser extent, the circumferential hydration of the stratum corneum surrounding the sweat glands, lowers the electrical resistance of the skin and raises its electrical conductance. Various instruments are now available for directly, simply, and noninvasively measuring skin surface conductance at the bedside. This technique has been widely used in psychological research for many years but has yet to be systematically applied in neonatology.

Figure 60-13 shows the rise in skin conductance following a painful stimulus.[131] In this case, a heel prick was administered to the foot followed by skin conductance measurement over the sole of the other foot. Peak values are reached at approximately 1 minute after the heel prick. This response is characteristic of the change in skin conductance caused by arousal in the neonate. Confirmatory measurements also can be made using different techniques, such as transepidermal water loss. Figure 60-14 shows palmar water loss in crying infants ranging from 25 to 41 weeks' gestational age.[55,132] Of note, the profile for palmar water loss is inversely related to transepidermal water loss over the same age range (see Fig. 60-4). This inverse relationship deserves further investigation. Recently, Storm and Fremming utilized conductance measurements of the skin surface to study behavioral state changes and developmental effects.[133-135] This skin-based method, combined with sensory evoked potential testing, offers new techniques for assessment of central nervous system functioning in the developing preterm infant.

Studies of epidermal barrier function may exhibit not only short-term responses secondary to autonomic nervous system

activation of eccrine sweating, but also long-term consequences related to stress and glucocorticoid secretion. Denda and colleagues have shown that stressful events such as immobilization, overcrowding, and abrupt change in physical environment can result in impaired epidermal barrier function in murine skin.[136,137] Similarly, Garg and associates demonstrated a delay in recovery of epidermal barrier function following induced

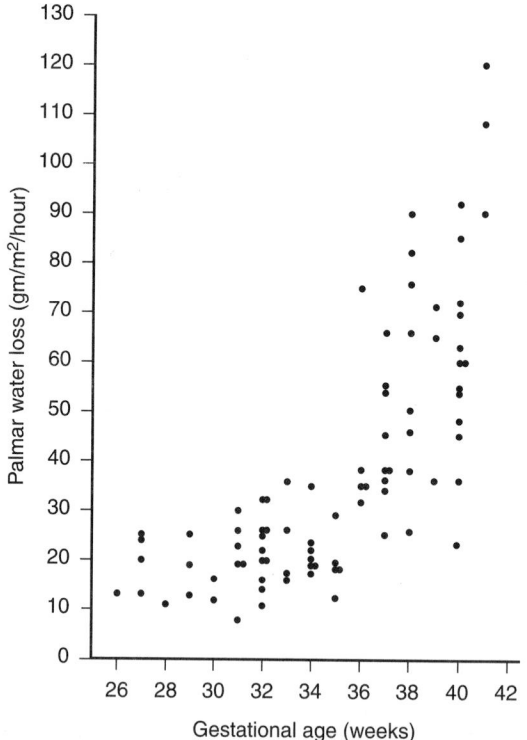

Figure 60–14. Palmar water loss in infants ranging from 25 to 41 weeks' gestation showing values at maximal arousal (vigorous crying). Results are displayed according to equivalent gestational age (gestation plus postnatal age). Values are 10 to 30 g/m²/hour until the equivalent gestational age of 36 weeks is reached. Values then increase abruptly to 30 to 100 g/m²/hour. (From Rutter N: *In* Hoath SB, Maibach H (eds): Neonatal Skin: Structure and Function. New York, Marcel Dekker, 2003[55]; as modified from Harpin V: Dissertation, University of Cambridge, 1986.[132])

Aspects of the Skin as a Primary Care Interface

- Surface of interaction with soaps, surfactants, disinfectants, and bacteria
- Support for tapes and other adhesives
- Interface for bedding, clothing, and the environment
- Site of action of topical anesthetics and analgesics
- Surface for wound and ostomy care
- Barrier for transdermal drug delivery
- Site of most laboratory blood drawing
- Platform for percutaneous catheters
- Boundary for noninvasive monitoring and skin-based sensing techniques
- Medium of interaction in kangaroo care and massage therapy
- Basis for initial clinical evaluation of patient well-being (appearance)

Modified from Hoath S, Narendran V: NeoReviews 2: e269, 2001.[41]

trauma in a group of psychologically stressed graduate students.[138] These studies indicate a link between physiologic stress of the organism and epidermal barrier function. As presented earlier, the very low birth weight preterm infant exhibits compromised barrier function up to 28 days following delivery (see Fig. 60-10).[51] Whether this increased transepidermal water loss is secondary to stress-related events is unclear but worthy of further investigation.

The idea of the skin as an information-rich surface can be extended to the intensive care or emergency room setting.[139,140] Indeed, cardiorespiratory and thermal monitoring, as well as transcutaneous blood gas measurements, are all skin-based systems of clinical data retrieval. Given the ready accessibility of the skin surface and the plethora of noninvasive measurement techniques that have yet to be applied to the study of newborn physiology,[121] it seems reasonable to assume that a number of innovative and useful skin-based sensing systems will be designed for clinical decision making in the future. This concept extends Kligman's idea of "invisible dermatology"[141] to the NICU bedside: early, objectively measured changes in the physical properties of the skin may herald illness in the term or preterm infant *before* such illness is apparent to the caregiver. De Felice and colleagues, for example, recently used skin colorimetry to provide a significant quantitative predictor of illness severity in hospitalized newborns.[142] This work supports the hypothesis that noninvasive measurements of skin physical properties directly reflect the pathophysiologic state of the infant. Such measurements can be used as objective adjuncts to clinical decision making and bedside subjective assessment.

FUTURE DIRECTIONS

A better understanding of fetal and neonatal skin physiology and the use of quantitative measures of skin structure and function is a goal for perinatal medicine,[41] with implications for care delivery beyond the newborn period. Table 60-10 lists a number of roles of the skin in the provision of primary health care. These functions are disease-independent but essential for the delivery of high quality care, whether the health care environment is hospital based or home based.

Recognition of the skin as a primary care interface for patient care and parental satisfaction creates an opportunity for collaborative practice between nursing and medicine.[143] The provision of many of the functions listed in Table 60-10 falls largely in the domain of nursing. The coupling of the infant and the care environment is often an assumption of fields such as developmental care.[144] The dual nature of the skin as a boundary interfacing cellular and molecular domains with psychological and perceptual domains is consistent with this approach. A better understanding

of skin development, especially the role of the epidermal barrier and infection control, has implications for improving infant care in developing countries.[91,104]

REFERENCES

1. Goldsmith L (ed): Physiology, Biochemistry, and Molecular Biology of the Skin. Oxford, Oxford University Press, 1991.
2. Elias P: The stratum corneum revisited. Journal of Dermatology 23:756, 1996.
3. Elias PM, Feingold KR: Coordinate regulation of epidermal differentiation and barrier homeostasis. Skin Pharmacol Appl Skin Physiol 14(Suppl 1):28, 2001.
4. Williams M, Feingold K: Barrier function of neonatal skin. Journal of Pediatrics 133:467, 1998.
5. Williams M, Hanley K, Elias P, et al: Ontogeny of the epidermal permeability barrier. Journal of Investigative Dermatology: Symposium Proceedings 3:75, 1998.
6. Scheuplein R: The skin as a barrier, in Jarrett A (ed): The Physiology and Pathophysiology of the Skin, vol 5, pp 1669-1692. London-New York-San Francisco, Academic Press, 1978.
7. Rutter N: The immature skin. European Journal of Pediatrics 155 Suppl 2(Aug):S18, 1996.
8. Hoath S, Visscher M, Heaton C, et al: Skin science and the future of dermatology. Journal of Cutaneous Medicine and Surgery 3:2, 1998.
9. Chuong CM, Nickoloff BJ, Elias PM, et al: What is the 'true' function of skin? Exp Dermatol 11:159, 2002.
10. Bereiter-Han J, Matoltsy A, Sylvia Richards K (eds): Biology of the Integument: Vertebrates. Berlin, Springer Verlag, 1986.
11. Kligman A: The biology of the stratum corneum, in Montagna W, Lobitz W (eds): The Epidermis, pp 387-433. New York, Academic Press, 1964.
12. Morris D: The Naked Ape: A Zoologist's Study of the Human Animal. New York, Random House, Incorporated, 1999 (paperback edition).
13. Hoath S: The skin as a neurodevelopmental interface. NeoReviews 2:e292, 2001.
14. Holbrook K: Structure and function of the developing human skin, in Goldsmith L (ed): Physiology, Biochemistry, and Molecular Biology of the Skin, pp 63-110. Oxford, Oxford University Press, 1991.
15. Hoath S, Leahy D: Formation and function of the stratum corneum, in Marks E, Leveque J-L, Voegeli R (eds): The Essential Stratum Corneum, pp 31-40. London, Martin Dunitz, Ltd, 2002.
16. Patrias K, Wright LL, Merenstein G: Effect of Corticosteroids for Fetal Maturation on Perinatal Outcomes, in Patrias K (ed): NIH Current Bibliographies in Medicine. National Library of Medicine's Literature Search Series., vol 94-1, National Institutes of Health, 1994.
17. Hanley K, Feingold K, Komuves L, et al: Glucocorticoid deficiency delays stratum corneum maturation in the fetal mouse. Journal of Investigative Dermatology 111:440, 1998.
18. Hanley K, Rassner U, Elias P, et al: Epidermal barrier ontogenesis: maturation in serum-free media and acceleration by glucocorticoids and thyroid hormone but not selected growth factors. Journal of Investigative Dermatology 106:404, 1996.
19. Okah F, Pickens W, Hoath S: Effect of prenatal steroids on skin surface hydrophobicity in the premature rat. Pediatric Research 37:402, 1995.
20. Jain A, Rutter N, Cartlidge PH: Influence of antenatal steroids and sex on maturation of the epidermal barrier in the preterm infant. Arch Dis Child Fetal Neonatal Ed 83:F112, 2000.
21. Kalinin A, Marekov LN, Steinert PM: Assembly of the epidermal cornified cell envelope. J Cell Sci 114(Pt 17):3069, 2001.
22. Steinert PM: The complexity and redundancy of epithelial barrier function. J Cell Biol 151:F5, 2000.
23. Kalinin AE, Kajava AV, Steinert PM: Epithelial barrier function: assembly and structural features of the cornified cell envelope. Bioessays 24:789, 2002.
24. Kim SY, Jeitner TM, Steinert PM: Transglutaminases in disease. Neurochem Int 40:85, 2002.
25. Warner RR, Boissy YL, Lilly NA, et al: Water disrupts stratum corneum lipid lamellae: damage is similar to surfactants. J Invest Dermatol 113:960, 1999.
26. Hoath S, Pickens W: The Biology of Vernix, in Hoath SB, Maibach H (eds): Neonatal Skin: Structure and Function. New York, Marcel Dekker, 2003, pp 193-210.
27. Pickens W, Warner R, Boissy R, et al: Characterization of human vernix: Water content morphology and elemental analysis. Journal of Investigative Dermatology 115:875, 2000.
28. Hardman MJ, Moore L, Ferguson MW, et al: Barrier formation in the human fetus is patterned. J Invest Dermatol 113:1106, 1999.
29. Hardman MJ, Sisi P, Banbury DN, et al: Patterned acquisition of skin barrier function during development. Development 125:1541, 1998.
30. Hoath S, Tanaka R, Boyce S: Rate of stratum corneum formation in the perinatal rat. Journal of Investigative Dermatology 100:400, 1993.
31. Youssef W, Wickett R, Hoath S: Surface free energy characterization of vernix caseosa: Role in waterproofing the newborn infant. Skin Research and Technology 7:10, 2001.
32. Supp A, Wickett R, Swope V, et al: Incubation of cultured skin substitutes in reduced humidity promotes cornification in vitro and stable engraftment in athymic mice. Wound Repair and Regeneration 7:226, 1999.

33. Montagna W: Comparative aspects of sebaceous glands, in Montagna W, Ellis R, Silver A (eds): Advances in the Biology of the Skin., vol IV. The Sebaceous Glands, pp 32–45. Oxford, Pergamon Press, 1963.

34. Zouboulis C, Fimmel S, Ortmann J, et al: Sebaceous Glands, in Hoath SB, Maibach H (eds): Neonatal Skin: Structure and Function, pp 59–88. New York, Marcel Dekker, 2003.

35. Pochi P: The Sebaceous Gland, in Maibach H, Berardesca E (eds): Neonatal Skin, pp 67–80. New York, Marcel Dekker, 1982.

36. Narendran V, Pickens W, Wickett R, et al: Interaction between pulmonary surfactant and vernix: A potential mechanism for induction of amniotic fluid turbidity. Pediatric Research 48:120, 2000.

37. Baker SM, Balo NN, Abdel Aziz FT: Is vernix a protective material to the newborn? A biochemical approach. Indian Journal of Pediatrics 62:237, 1995.

38. Buchman AL: Glutamine: Is it conditionally required nutrient for the human gastrointestinal system? Journal of the American College of Nutrition 15:199, 1996. 1996.

39. Hoath SB, Maibach H (eds): Neonatal Skin: Structure and Function. New York, Marcel Dekker, 2003.

40. Mauro T, Behne M: Acid mantle, in Hoath SB, Maibach H (eds): Neonatal Skin: Structure and Function, pp 47–58. New York, Marcel Dekker, 2003.

41. Hoath S, Narendran V: Development of the epidermal barrier. NeoReviews 2:e269, 2001.

42. Proksch E, Holleran W, Menon G, et al: Barrier function regulates epidermal lipid and DNA synthesis. British Journal of Dermatology 128:473, 1993.

43. Denda M, Sato J, Tsuchiya T, et al: Low humidity stimulates epidermal DNA synthesis and amplifies the hyperproliferative response to barrier disruption: implication for seasonal exacerbations of inflammatory dermatoses. Journal of Investigative Dermatology 111:873, 1998.

44. Denda M, Sato J, Masuda Y, et al: Exposure to a dry environment enhances epidermal permeability barrier function. Journal of Investigative Dermatology 111:858, 1998. 1998.

45. Rawlings A, Harding C, Watkinson A, et al: The effect of glycerol and humidity on desmosome degradation in stratum corneum. Archives of Dermatological Research 287:457, 1995.

46. Rawlings A, Scott I, Harding C, et al: Stratum corneum moisturization at the molecular level. Journal of Investigative Dermatology 103:731, 1994.

47. Bouwstra JA, Thewalt J, Gooris GS, et al: A model membrane approach to the epidermal permeability barrier: an X-ray diffraction study. Biochemistry 36:7717, 1997.

48. Hoeger PH, Schreiner V, Klaassen IA, et al: Epidermal barrier lipids in human vernix caseosa: corresponding ceramide pattern in vernix and fetal skin. Br J Dermatol 146:194, 2002.

49. Vielhaber G, Pfeiffer S, Brade L, et al: Localization of ceramide and glucosylceramide in human epidermis by immunogold electron microscopy. J Invest Dermatol 117:1126, 2001.

50. Hammarlund K, Sedin G: Transepidermal water loss in newborn infants. III. Relation to gestational age. Acta Paediatr Scand 68:795, 1979.

51. Agren J, Sjors G, Sedin G: Transepidermal water loss in infants born at 24 and 25 weeks of gestation. Acta Paediatr Scand 87:1185, 1998.

52. Dollberg S, Hoath S: Temperature regulation in preterm infants: Role of the skin-environment interface. NeoReviews 2:e282, 2001.

53. Adamsons K, Gandy G, James L: The influence of thermal factors upon oxygen consumption of the newborn human infant. J Pediatr 66:495, 1965.

54. Hoath S, Rutter N: Prematurity, in Hoath SB, Maibach H (eds): Neonatal Skin: Structure and Function, pp 153–178. New York, Marcel Dekker, 2003.

55. Rutter N: Eccrine Sweating in the Newborn, in Hoath SB, Maibach H (eds): Neonatal Skin: Structure and Function. New York, Marcel Dekker, 2003, pp 109–124.

56. Ryan T: The cutaneous vasculature in normal and wounded neonatal skin, in Hoath SB, Maibach H (eds): Neonatal Skin: Structure and Function. New York, Marcel Dekker, 2003, pp 125–152.

57. Taddei A: Ricerche, mediante indicatori, sullar reazione attuale della cute nel neonato. Riv Ital Ginec 18:496, 1935.

58. Lund C, Kuller J, Lane A, et al: Neonatal skin care: the scientific basis for practice. Neonatal Network 18:15, 1999.

59. Fox C, Nelson D, Wareham J: The timing of skin acidification in very low birth weight infants. J Perinatol 18:272, 1998.

60. Visscher M, Munson K, Pickens W, et al: Changes in diapered and nondiapered infant skin over the first month of life. Pediatric Dermatology 17:45, 2000.

61. Yosipovitch G, Maayan-Metzger A, Merlob P, et al: Skin barrier properties in different body areas in neonates. Pediatrics 106(1 Pt 1):105, 2000.

62. Bouwstra JA, Gooris GS, Cheng K, et al: Phase behavior of isolated skin lipids. J Lipid Res 37:999, 1996.

63. Sarkany I, Gaylarde CC: Bacterial colonisation of the skin of the newborn. J Pathol Bacteriol 95:115, 1968.

64. Evans HE, Akpata SO, Baki A: Factors influencing the establishment of the neonatal bacterial flora. II. The role of environmental factors. Arch Environ Health 21:643, 1970.

65. Evans HE, Akpata SO, Baki A: Factors influencing the establishment of the neonatal bacterial flora. I. The role of host factors. Arch Environ Health 21:514, 1970.

66. D'Angio CT, McGowan KL, Baumgart S, et al: Surface colonization with coagulase-negative staphylococci in premature neonates. J Pediatr 114:1029, 1989.

67. Rotimi VO, Duerden BI: The development of the bacterial flora in normal neonates. J Med Microbiol 14:51, 1981.

68. Rotimi VO, Olowe SA, Ahmed I: The development of bacterial flora of premature neonates. J Hyg (Lond) 94:309, 1985.

69. Darmstadt G: Staphylococcal and streptococcal skin infections., in Harahap M (ed): Diagnosis and Treatment of Skin Infections. Oxford, Blackwell Scientific Publications, 1997, pp 7–115.

70. Sidbury R, Darmstadt G: Microbiology, in Hoath SB, Maibach H (eds): Neonatal Skin: Structure and Function. New York, Marcel Dekker, 2003.

71. Krisanaprakornkit S, Kimball JR, Weinberg A, et al: Inducible expression of human beta-defensin 2 by Fusobacterium nucleatum in oral epithelial cells: multiple signaling pathways and role of commensal bacteria in innate immunity and the epithelial barrier. Infect Immun 68:2907, 2000.

72. Darmstadt G, Dinulos J: Neonatal skin care. Pediatric Clinics of North America 47:757, 2000.

73. Lund CH, Kuller J, Lane AT, et al: Neonatal skin care: evaluation of the AWHONN/NANN research-based practice project on knowledge and skin care practices. Association of Women's Health, Obstetric and Neonatal Nurses/National Association of Neonatal Nurses. J Obstet Gynecol Neonatal Nurs 30:30, 2001.

74. Pittet D, Kramer A: Alcohol-based hand gels and hand hygiene in hospitals. Lancet 360:1511, 2002.

75. Boyce JM, Pittet D: Guideline for Hand Hygiene in Health-Care Settings. Recommendations of the Healthcare Infection Control Practices Advisory Committee and the HICPAC/SHEA/APIC/IDSA Hand Hygiene Task Force. Society for Healthcare Epidemiology of America/Association for Professionals in Infection Control/Infectious Diseases Society of America. MMWR Recomm Rep 51(RR-16):1, 2002, quiz CE1–4.

76. Pickens W, Narendran V, Moraille R, et al: Does vernix caseosa function as an endogenous cleanser? Pediatr Res 51:371A, 2002.

77. Quie PG: Antimicrobial defenses in the neonate. Semin Perinatol 14(4 Suppl 1):2, 1990.

78. Miller SJ, Aly R, Shinefeld HR, et al: In vitro and in vivo antistaphylococcal activity of human stratum corneum lipids. Arch Dermatol 124:209, 1988.

79. Bibel DJ, Miller SJ, Brown BE, et al: Antimicrobial activity of stratum corneum lipids from normal and essential fatty acid-deficient mice. J Invest Dermatol 92:632, 1989.

80. Ushijima T, Takahashi M, Ozaki Y: Acetic, propionic, and oleic acid as the possible factors influencing the predominant residence of some species of Propionibacterium and coagulase-negative Staphylococcus on normal human skin. Can J Microbiol 30:647, 1984.

81. Gallo RL, Huttner KM: Antimicrobial peptides: an emerging concept in cutaneous biology. J Invest Dermatol 111:739, 1998.

82. Jonas M, Darmstadt G, Rubens C, et al: Ultrastructure of invasion of group A streptococcus into human keratinocytes: 14th International Congress of Electron Microscopy, 1998, vol 4, pp 375–376.

83. Darmstadt GL, Fleckman P, Jonas M, et al: Differentiation of cultured keratinocytes promotes the adherence of Streptococcus pyogenes. J Clin Invest 101:128, 1998.

84. Sallusto F: Origin and migratory properties of dendritic cells in the skin. Curr Opin Allergy Clin Immunol 1:441, 2001.

85. Okah F, Wickett R, Pickens W, et al: Surface electrical capacitance as a noninvasive bedside measure of epidermal barrier maturation in the newborn infant. Pediatrics 96:688, 1995.

86. Dourson M, Charnley G, Scheuplein R: Differential sensitivity of children and adults to chemical toxicity. II. Risk and regulation. Regul Toxicol Pharmacol 35:448, 2002.

87. Scheuplein R, Charnley G, Dourson M: Differential sensitivity of children and adults to chemical toxicity. I. Biological basis. Regul Toxicol Pharmacol 35:429, 2002.

88. Cartlidge PH, Rutter N: Percutaneous carbon dioxide excretion in the newborn infant. Early Hum Dev 21:93, 1990.

89. Cartlidge PH, Rutter N: Percutaneous oxygen delivery to the preterm infant. Lancet 1:315, 1988.

90. Stoll BJ, Hansen N, Fanaroff AA, et al: Late-onset sepsis in very low birth weight neonates: the experience of the NICHD Neonatal Research Network. Pediatrics 110(2 Pt 1):285, 2002.

91. Darmstadt G, Black R, Santosham M: Research priorities and postpartum care strategies for the prevention and optimal management of neonatal infections in less developed countries. Pediatric Infectious Disease Journal 19:739, 2000.

92. Silverman WA, Sinclair JC: Temperature regulation in the newborn infant. N Engl J Med 274:146-148, 1966.

93. Silverman WA, Sinclair JC: Temperature regulation in the newborn infant. N Engl J Med 274:92-94, 1966.

94. Silverman W, Fertig J, Berger A: The influence of thermal enviroment upon the survival of newly born premature infants. Pediatrics 22:876, 1958.

95. Hammarlund K, Nilsson G, Oberg P, et al: Transepidermal water loss in newborn infants. I. Relation to ambient humidity and site of measurement and estimation of total transepidermal water loss. Acta Paediatr Scand 66:553, 1977.

96. Kjartansson S, Arsan S, Hammarlund K, et al: Water loss from the skin of term and preterm infants nursed under a radiant heater. Pediatr Res 37:233, 1995.

97. Vohra S, Frent G, Campbell V, et al: Effect of polyethylene occlusive skin wrapping on heat loss in very low birth weight infants at delivery: a randomized trial. Journal of Pediatrics 134:547, 1999.

98. Narendran V, Hoath SB: Thermal management of the low birth weight infant: a cornerstone of neonatology. J Pediatr *134*:529, 1999.
99. Lane AT, Drost SS: Effects of repeated application of emollient cream to premature neonates' skin. Pediatrics *92*:415, 1993.
100. Man MM, Feingold KR, Thornfeldt CR, et al: Optimization of physiological lipid mixtures for barrier repair. J Invest Dermatol *106*:1096, 1996.
101. Elias P, Mao-Quiang M, Thornfeldt C, et al: The epidermal permeability barrier: effects of physiologic and nonphysiologic lipids, in Hoppe U (ed): The Lanolin Book, pp 253–279. Hamburg, Beiersdorf AG, 1999.
102. Nopper A, Horii K, S. S-D, et al: Topical ointment therapy benefits premature infants. Journal of Pediatrics *128*:660, 1996.
103. Edwards WH, Conner JM, Soll RF: The effect of Aquaphor® original emollient ointment on nosocomial sepsis rates and skin integrity in infants of birth weight 501 to 1000 grams. Pediatric Research *49*:388A, 2001.
104. Darmstadt GL, Mao-Qiang M, Chi E, et al: Impact of topical oils on the skin barrier: possible implications for neonatal health in developing countries. Acta Paediatr *91*:546, 2002.
105. Visscher M, Hoath SB, Conroy E, et al: Effect of semipermeable membranes on skin barrier repair following tape stripping. Archives of Dermatological Research *293*:491, 2001.
106. Hanley K, Jiang Y, Elias PM, et al: Acceleration of barrier ontogenesis *in vitro* through air exposure. Pediatric Research *41*:293, 1997.
107. Odio M, Abbinante-Nissen J, Neihaus D, et al: Improved condition of infant skin with use of a novel diaper designed for sustained, low level topical delivery of a petrolatum-based formulation. The Procter & Gamble Co., Cincinnati, OH. 1999.
108. Odio M, Haines S, Baldwin S, et al: A petrolatum-based formulation delivered topically during use of a novel disposable diaper penetrates the superficial layers of the stratum corneum.: Society of Pediatric Dermatology Annual Meeting, 1998.
109. Montagu A: Touching: The Human Significance of the Skin, Harper and Row, 1986.
110. Brazelton T: Behavioral competence, in Avery G, Fletcher M, MacDonald M (eds): Neonatology: Pathophysiology and Management of the Newborn, pp 289–300. Philadelphia, JB Lippincott Company, 1994.
111. Schanberg SM, Field TM: Sensory deprivation stress and supplemental stimulation in the rat pup and preterm human neonate. Child Dev *58*:1431, 1987.
112. Schanberg S, Evoniuk G, Kuhn C: Tactile and nutritional aspects of maternal care: Specific regulators of neuroendocrine function and cellular development. Proceedings of the Society of Experimental Biology and Medicine *175*:135, 1984.
113. Wang S, Bartolome JV, Schanberg SM: Neonatal deprivation of maternal touch may suppress ornithine decarboxylase via downregulation of the proto-oncogenes c-myc and max. J Neurosci *16*:836, 1996.
114. Alasmi M, Pickens W, Hoath S: Effect of tactile stimulation on serum lactate in the newborn rat. Pediatric Research *41*:857, 1997.
115. Blakemore C, Cooper GF: Development of the brain depends on the visual environment. Nature *228*:477, 1970.
116. Field T, Schanberg S, Scafidi F, et al: Tactile/kinesthetic stimulation effects on preterm neonates. Pediatrics *77*:654, 1986.
117. Bhansali S, Henderson T, Hoath S: Probing human skin as an information-rich smart biological interface using MEMS-sensors. Microelectronics Journal *33*:121, 2002.
118. Hoath S, Donnelly M, Boissy R: Sensory transduction and the mammalian epidermis. Biosensors and Bioelectronics *5*:351, 1990.
119. Athenstaedt H, Claussen H, Schaper D: Epidermis of human skin: pyroelectric and piezoelectric sensor layer. Science *216*:1018, 1982.
120. Ansel J, Kaynard A, Armstrong C: Skin-nervous system interactions. Journal of Investigative Dermatology *106*:198, 1996.
121. Serup J, Jemec G (eds): Handbook of Noninvasive Methods and the Skin. Boca Raton, FL, CRC Press, 1995.
122. Shivanand P: Electrical and transport properties of neonatal rat skin; PhD Thesis, University of Cincinnati, 1995.
123. Wakai R, Lengle J, Leuthold A: Transmission of electric and magnetic foetal cardiac signals in a case of ectopia cordis: the dominant role of the vernix caseosa. Phys Med Biol. *45*:1989, 2000.
124. Tagami H, Kikuchi K, Kobayashi H, et al: Electrical properties of newborn skin, in Hoath SB, Maibach H (eds): Neonatal Skin: Structure and Function. New York, Marcel Dekker, 2003, pp 179–192.
125. Scher M: Perinatal asphyxia: timing and mechanisms of injury in neonatal encephalopathy. Curr Neurol Neurosci Rep *1*:175, 2001.
126. Zeinstra E, Fock JM, Begeer JH, et al: The prognostic value of serial EEG recordings following acute neonatal asphyxia in full-term infants. Eur J Paediatr Neurol *5*:155, 2001.
127. Lorenz JM, Kleinman LI, Markarian K, et al: Serum anion gap in the differential diagnosis of metabolic acidosis in critically ill newborns. J Pediatr *135*:751, 1999.
128. Dombrowski GJ, Jr., Swiatek KR, Chao KL: Lactate, 3-hydroxybutyrate, and glucose as substrates for the early postnatal rat brain. Neurochem Res *14*:667, 1989.
129. Fitzgerald M, Shaw A, MacIntosh N: Postnatal development of the cutaneous flexor reflex: comparative study of preterm infants and newborn rat pups. Dev Med Child Neurol *30*:520, 1988.
130. Rutter N: The evaporimeter and emotional sweating in the neonate. Clin Perinatol *12*:63, 1985.
131. Gladman G, Chiswick ML: Skin conductance and arousal in the newborn. Arch Dis Child *65*(10 Spec No):1063, 1990.
132. Harpin V: The functional maturation of the skin; Dissertation, University of Cambridge, 1986.
133. Storm H: Skin conductance and the stress response from heel stick in preterm infants. Arch Dis Child Fetal Neonatal Ed *83*:F143, 2000.
134. Storm H: Development of emotional sweating in preterms measured by skin conductance changes. Early Hum Dev *62*:149, 2001.
135. Storm H, Fremming A: Food intake and oral sucrose in preterms prior to heel prick. Acta Paediatr *91*:555, 2002.
136. Denda M, Tsuchiya T, Elias PM, et al: Stress alters cutaneous permeability barrier homeostasis. Am J Physiol Regul Integr Comp Physiol *278*:R367, 2000.
137. Denda M, Tsuchiya T, Hosoi J, et al: Immobilization-induced and crowded environment-induced stress delay barrier recovery in murine skin. Br J Dermatol *138*:780, 1998.
138. Garg A, Chren MM, Sands LP, et al: Psychological stress perturbs epidermal permeability barrier homeostasis: implications for the pathogenesis of stress-associated skin disorders. Arch Dermatol *137*:53, 2001.
139. Tatevossian RG, Wo CC, Velmahos GC, et al: Transcutaneous oxygen and CO2 as early warning of tissue hypoxia and hemodynamic shock in critically ill emergency patients. Crit Care Med *28*:2248, 2000.
140. Velmahos GC, Wo CC, Demetriades D, et al: Invasive and non-invasive physiological monitoring of blunt trauma patients in the early period after emergency admission. Int Surg *84*:354, 1999.
141. Kligman AM: The invisible dermatoses. Arch Dermatol *127*:1375, 1991.
142. De Felice C, Flori ML, Pellegrino M, et al: Predictive value of skin color for illness severity in the high-risk newborn. Pediatr Res *51*:100, 2002.
143. Horbar JD: The Vermont Oxford Network: evidence-based quality improvement for neonatology. Pediatrics *103*(1 Suppl E):350, 1999.
144. Jacobs SE, Sokol J, Ohlsson A: The Newborn Individualized Developmental Care and Assessment Program is not supported by meta-analyses of the data. J Pediatr *140*:699, 2002.
145. Perera P, Kurban A, Ryan T: The development of the cutaneous microvascular system in the newborn. British Journal of Dermatology *82*(Supplement 5):86, 1970.
146. Rutter N: Percutaneous drug absorption in the newborn: hazards and uses. Clin Perinatol *14*:911, 1987.

Fetal and Neonatal Cardiovascular Physiology

Margaret L. Kirby

61

Development of the Fetal Heart

The heart develops from a simple tube whose precursors reside in bilaterally paired primary heart fields (Fig. 61-1). The bilateral heart primordia fuse in the ventral midline as the foregut pocket closes, to form a myocardial sleeve enveloping an endocardial tube.[1] Although most of the myocardium and endocardium of the adult heart are products of this tube, several extracardiac sources of cells are essential to provide all the cells of the mature heart (see Fig. 61-1). These include derivation of the myocardium of the outflow tract from a secondary heart field,[2-4] formation of the outflow septum by derivatives of the neural crest,[5] involvement of the vestibular spine in formation of the atrial septum,[6, 7] and development of the epicardium from the proepicardium.[8, 9] The epicardium generates all the coronary vasculature and cardiac fibroblasts.[10]

The heart begins to beat long before it attains its mature form. It continues to maintain adequate cardiac output and pressure to sustain the growing embryo even while it undergoes major morphologic changes. The processes involved in forming a simple heart such as that in zebrafish, or a multichambered heart as seen in oxygen-breathing vertebrates, follows similar principles in all vertebrates. The chick embryo, because of its easy accessibility, has been used extensively to elucidate many of the mechanisms involved in heart development, and much of our current working knowledge of heart development is derived from studies of chick heart development. However, the advent of techniques to alter single gene expression in zebrafish and mouse embryos has brought a wealth of new knowledge about heart development from these animals.

PRECURSORS OF HEART DEVELOPMENT

Primary Heart Fields

In the primitive streak stage chick embryo, heart-forming cells can be found in the epiblast about midway along the length of the streak. The cells extend laterally from the midline about halfway to the edge of the area pellucida,[11] and they migrate medially to and through the streak to form mesoderm. It was thought from early marking experiments that there was a spatial order in which the cells migrated through the primitive streak;[12] however, more recent experiments have not found a one-to-one spatial order in which the cells are invaginated.[13] These cells migrate in the mesodermal germ layer to a craniolateral position to form bilaterally paired primary heart-forming regions.[14] The heart-forming regions were once thought to form a horseshoe-shaped region that was joined cranial to the head, but more recent data from chick studies indicate that the heart-forming regions are not connected across the midline until they are

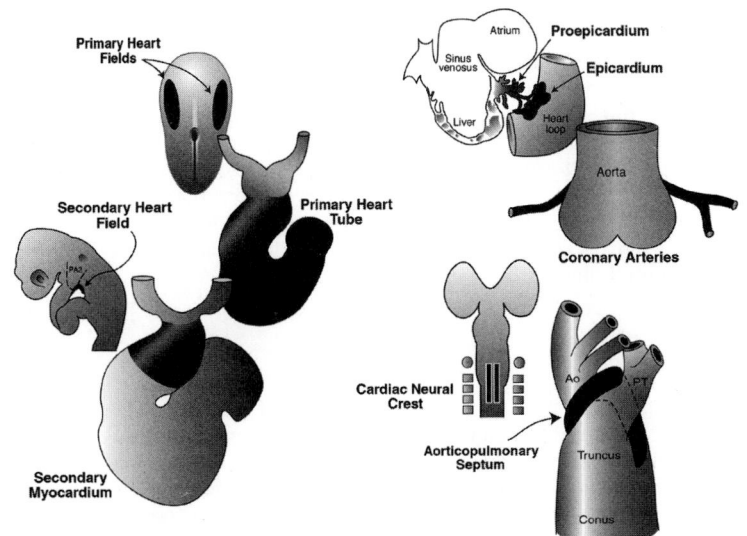

Figure 61-1. Drawing illustrating the derivation of the various components of the heart derived from the primary and secondary heart fields and extracardiac sources. The initial heart tube composed of endocardium and myocardium forms from bilateral cardiogenic mesenchyme in the heart fields. The outflow myocardium is added secondarily from the secondary heart field. Other cells needed for normal development are extracardiac and include neural crest cells needed for outflow septation and proepicardial cells from liver mesenchyme that form the epicardium and coronary vasculature.

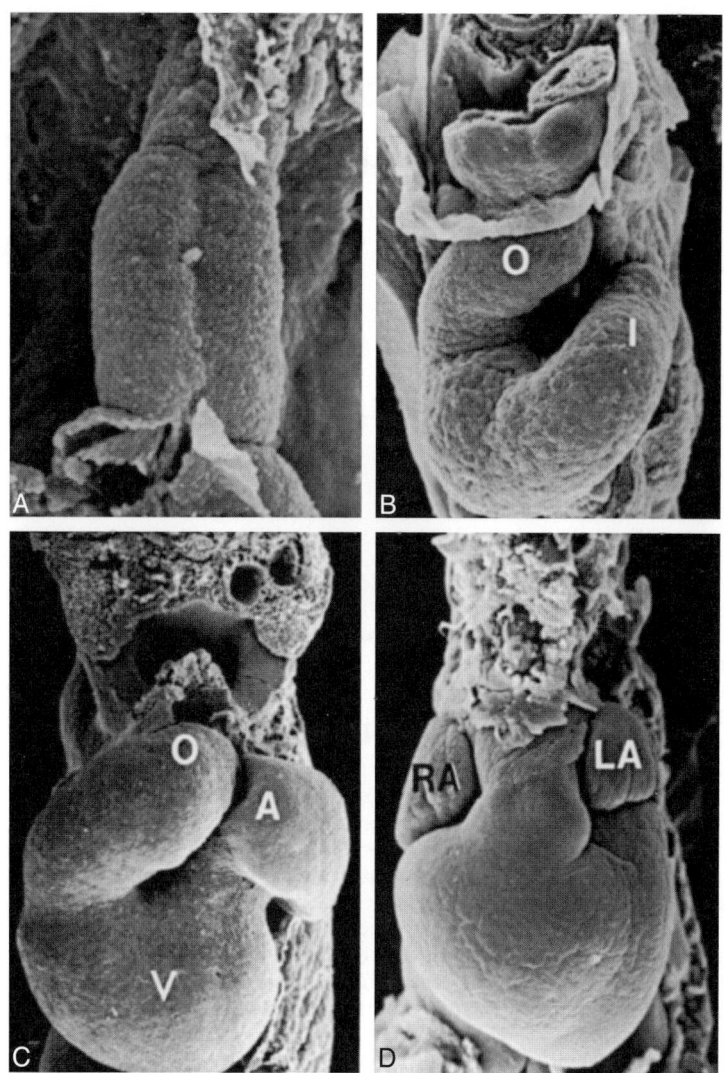

Figure 61–2. Scanning electron micrographs of normal chick hearts. **A,** From a stage 12 embryo showing the simple tubular heart. **B,** Stage 16 shows the looped heart tube. **C,** At stage 18, the common atrium and ventricle can be distinguished. **D,** By stage 19, features of the adult heart have become discernible. A = atrium; I = inflow tract; LA = left atrium; O = outflow tract; RA = right atrium; V = presumptive ventricles. (×80.) (From Bockman DE, et al: Am J Anat *180*:332, 1987. Reprinted by permission of Wiley-Liss, a division of John Wiley & Sons, Inc. © Copyright 1987.)

brought to the ventral midline during formation of the foregut.[14] It is still not known whether the bilateral primary heart fields are independent in mammals or are connected across the midline cranially.

Secondary Heart Field

Formerly, it was thought that the primary heart fields contained all the myocardial cells that would be found in the mature heart,[12, 15] but a secondary heart field has been recognized in both chick and mouse (Fig. 61–2).[2-4] Thus, the primary heart fields appear to form the sinus venosus, atria, atrioventricular canal, and ventricles but not the definitive outflow tract. The myocardium of the definitive outflow tract or conotruncus is formed from a secondary heart field located in the mesenchyme of the ventral pharynx.

Vestibular Spine

The origin, exact location, and importance of the vestibular spine are still contentious. The vestibular spine, first described by His,[16] is considered by some authors to be a cap of mesenchyme located on the leading edge of the primary atrial septum,[6] which may be important in fusion of the primary atrial septum with the atrioventricular endocardial cushions. The vestibular spine extends from the splanchnic mesoderm ventral to the foregut

into the right pulmonary ridge and is discussed further in the section on atrial septation.[17]

Neural Crest

The neural crest develops in the dorsalmost part of the neural folds, which are located at the junction of the neural plate with the nonneural ectoderm.[18] As the neural plate closes to form the neural tube, the neural crest cells are released from the neural folds. The neural crest is divided into two regions based on its potential for formation of ectomesenchyme (neural crest-derived mesenchyme is referred to as ectomesenchyme because of its unique origin from the ectoderm). The cranial neural crest extends from the mid-diencephalon to the caudal limit of somite 5, whereas the trunk neural crest begins at somite 5 and extends caudally into the tail. Neural crest cells derived from the cranial region can differentiate into ectomesenchyme. This ectomesenchyme is important in development of the face, pharyngeal apparatus, glands of the neck, great arteries, and cardiac outflow septation. The same region of neural crest provides the autonomic and a majority of the sensory innervation to the head and heart. Trunk neural crest, conversely, differentiates into neurons, neuron-supporting cells, and melanocytes, but it is unable to differentiate into ectomesenchyme.

The region of the cranial neural crest that participates in outflow tract development is called *cardiac neural crest* (see

Fig. 61-1).[19] It extends from the level of the midotic placode to the caudal limit of somite 3 (rhombomeres 6, 7, and 8). The cardiac neural crest migrates into pharyngeal arches 3, 4, and 6.[20] In the pharyngeal arches, the crest cells provide support for repatterning of the bilaterally symmetric aortic arch arteries to the great arteries.[21] Some of these cells continue their migration into the cardiac outflow tract, where they participate in and direct outflow septation.[22, 23] Cells from this area also seed the cardiac ganglia that provide parasympathetic innervation to the heart.[24]

Epicardium

The *epicardium* grows over the heart from the liver mesenchyme, although the precise region of origin is not known. Growth of the epicardium begins as addition of the definitive outflow tract is completed.[8, 9, 25, 26] The epicardium is the source of all the visceral pericardium, the subepicardial connective tissue, myocardial fibroblasts, and all the elements of the coronary vascular system (see Fig. 61-1).[10, 27]

CARDIAC TUBE FORMATION AND LOOPING

The cells in the paired heart-forming lateral plate mesoderm are brought to the ventral midline during foregut closure. The bilateral primordia composed of endothelial tubes partially enclosed in myocardial precursor cells fuse to form a single endothelial tube that is at first incompletely invested in myocardium in a sort of trough that is open toward the pharyngeal endoderm (see Fig. 61-2).[1] The trough closes dorsally to form a complete myocardial sleeve for the endocardium. The wall of the tubular heart is composed of loosely organized myocardium that is several cells thick and is separated from the endocardium by a layer called the *cardiac jelly.* The epicardium is added later. Weak myocardial contractions begin as the tube becomes complete. Growth and differentiation of the tube cause it to bend to the right and ventrally until it assumes an S shape. Looping occurs independently of function.[28] In the absence of the sodium-calcium exchanger, the heart fails to beat, but even so, it loops correctly. Hence, the early events in cardiac morphogenesis do not depend on cardiac function.

Two things happen during the early process of looping. First, the tube is elongated by the addition of the definitive outflow tract to the cranial end of the tube. Second, the cardiac tube continues to mature by continued expansion of the atrium and the development of trabeculae in the presumptive ventricular regions. During the process, the chamber identity is established.

The extended process of looping involves convergence of the outflow and inflow tracts.[29] After convergence, a new period of outflow tract adjustment begins, in which the outflow tract moves leftward, accompanied by a rotation of the aortic side of the truncus posteriorly, to be nestled between the mitral and tricuspid valves. This process, called *wedging,* brings the left ventricle into continuity with the aortic outflow tract. Wedging and sepation of the outflow tract occur simultaneously, so as wedging is completed, the outflow septum is in proper alignment for merger with the ventricular and atrioventricular septa, thus completing the separation of the ventricular outflow tracts. If looping and convergence do not occur normally, wedging cannot occur, and a malalignment of the outflow tract can result.

ELECTRICAL ACTIVITY AND CONTRACTILITY

Electrical activity begins before the contractile apparatus differentiates. Action potentials appear in the caudal part of the cardiac tube and are conducted to the rostral end.[30,31] It has long been a point of fascination that when union of the two half hearts is prevented, two independently beating hearts develop.[32]

Visible contractile activity proceeds quickly after electrical activity begins. The contractions are initially in different parts of the tube and are uncoordinated, but they quickly assume a peristaltic character.[33] Because the electrical activation of the tubular heart is base to apex, whereas that of the four-chambered heart is apex to base, differentiation and maturation of the His-Purkinje system are required shortly before closure of the ventricular septum.[34] This ensures that the activation sequence is appropriate for the septated heart at the correct time.

Contractile Proteins

Before the onset of contractions, the myocardium does not contain any demonstrable cytoplasmic filaments. The sarcomeric proteins for myofibrillar assembly are synthesized before myofibrillar assembly, which is a prerequisite for initiation of contractions.[35] The outer surface layer of myocardium remains the proliferative or stem cell population and generates more myocardial cells, whereas the inner trabecular myocardium establishes mature myofibrils.[36] Chamber specification occurs through distinct transcriptional programs that govern myocardial identity at various stages of specialization in the forming heart. Thus, distinct myosin heavy chains are found in the atria, ventricles, and conducting system of the heart as chamber identity is established.[37, 38] The ventricular chambers develop by ballooning from the outer curvature.[39] Whereas the ballooning chamber myocardium in the outer curvature assumes a new molecular profile that is specific for each chamber, the myocardium of the inner curvature, inflow tract, atrioventricular canal, and outflow tract retains the molecular profile originally found in the primary myocardium.[39] The subject of molecular identity in establishing the cardiac chambers is too extensive and transitory for this overview, but excellent reviews are available.[39-42]

DEVELOPMENT OF THE EPICARDIUM AND CORONARY CIRCULATION

The myocardium initially contains only myocytes. The epicardium, blood vessels, and fibroblasts found in the mature heart originate from the epicardium, which develops from the proepicardium. The proepicardium, derived from liver mesenchyme, is first identified as mesothelial protrusions near the sinus venosus.[25] The protrusions touch the dorsal wall of the atrioventricular groove, adhere, and begin to form a single cell layer investment of epicardium that ultimately covers the entire myocardium. The epicardium seeds the mesenchymal cells that form the cardiac vascular plexus (i.e., endothelial and smooth muscle cells), which ultimately becomes the adult coronary vasculature, by epithelial-to-mesenchymal transformation.[43]

During early development, the myocardium is nourished via the intertrabecular sinusoids. This gradually shifts to a system in which the myocardium is nourished by coronary vessels. Ultimately, each myocardial cell is in contact with a capillary. Development of the cardiac veins precedes development of the coronary arteries. A well-established capillary network develops that extends endothelial channels into the base of the aorta. These endothelial channels become the stems of the coronary arteries.[44, 45]

SEPTATION

Septation of the tubular heart begins in the atrioventricular canal and outflow areas. Initially, two opposing masses or swellings called *endocardial cushions* appear. The endocardial cushions are formed in the cardiac jelly by local epithelial-to-mesenchymal conversion of the endocardial cells that populate the cardiac jelly.[46]

Endocardial Cushions

The primary heart tube consists of two cellular layers, the myocardium and endocardium, separated by a thick, initially acellular layer called the cardiac jelly. The cardiac jelly consists of various proteinaceous components secreted by the myocardium.[47] The composition of the proteinaceous components resembles that of basement membranes.[48] Endocardial cushion tissue is formed only in the atrioventricular canal and proximal outflow tract. This tissue ultimately forms the atrioventricular and semilunar valves and parts of the atrial and outflow tract septa. The formation of endocardial cushion tissue occurs via the process of epithelial-to-mesenchymal transformation in which cells in the endocardium delaminate and migrate into the cardiac jelly.[46] The other regions of the endocardium do not seed the cardiac jelly with mesenchyme, a finding implying that only myocardium at the atrioventricular canal and conus is able to release inductive factors for this process.[46] Bone morphogenetic protein and transforming growth factor family members are required for the process, although the details of the conversion are not completely known.[49-51] Once this mesenchyme is formed, the atrioventricular canal is divided into right and left atrioventricular canals by apposition of the cushions followed by fusion.

Septation of the Atrioventricular Canal and Atria

The atrial chamber of the heart tube, which receives blood from the sinus venosus (systemic venous sinus), communicates with the ventricular loop via the atrioventricular canal.[7] A persisting connection with the body dorsally allows continuity of the myocardium with mesenchyme of the developing mediastinum and growth of the pulmonary veins. The venous return to the atria is asymmetric even from it earliest development, because the developing left horn of the sinus venosus is incorporated into the developing left atrioventricular junction. This left horn diminishes in size to become incorporated as the coronary sinus. This brings the venous drainage entirely to the right side of the common atrial chamber.[7] The atrial appendages form and the primary pulmonary vein develops in the dorsal mesocardium, which connects the mediastinum and dorsal wall of the atrium. A ridge to the right of the mouth of the pulmonary vein enlarges as the spina vestibuli.[16] These events set the stage for atrial septation.

Development of the atrioventricular and atrial septation is complex and requires more elements than are usually recognized.[17] These include generation of the cardiac cushion tissue, remodeling of the inner heart curvature, rotation of the horns of the systemic venous sinus around the pulmonary portal, expansion of the right atrioventricular junction, formation of the muscular atrial and ventricular septa, bridging by the dextrodorsal outflow ridge and the superior endocardial cushion, fusion with the inferior margins of the venous valves, and formation of the mouth of the coronary sinus from the cranial muscular wall of the left sinus horn. Several cell populations including the mesenchyme on the leading edge of the primary atrial septum, the atrioventricular endocardial cushions, and the cap of mesenchyme on the spina vestibuli contribute to the central mesenchymal mass. Fusion of these components closes the foramen primum.[17]

Before atrial septation occurs, the common atrium is externally demarcated into left and right atria by a furrow lying in the plane of the truncus arteriosus. The initial atrial septum forms inside the common atrial chamber as a crescentic ridge.[7] This is called the *septum primum* and appears during the sixth week of gestation. The free edge of the septum primum provides the superior border of the foramen primum. The foramen primum becomes progressively smaller as the septum primum grows

toward the atrioventricular endocardial cushions. The septum primum fuses with the endocardial cushions and obliterates the foramen primum. The septum primum then becomes perforated to create the foramen secundum as the septum secundum grows from the dorsocranial wall of the atrium to the right of the septum primum. This septum acts as a flap over the foramen secundum, and the flap and foramen are known as the *foramen ovale*. The mechanism for foramen secundum formation is not known. Several mechanisms have been proposed, including rupture of the septum primum as a result of increased right atrial pressure, incomplete growth of the septum primum, and programmed cell death. Initial closure of the foramen ovale in the human heart occurs at birth because of decreased pulmonary resistance and increased flow into the left atrium, which functionally close the septum. The spina vestibuli has a mesodermal core, which contributes to the muscularization of the lower margin of the oval fossa. This contrasts with the formation of the upper rim, which is formed by the septum secundum.[17]

Outflow Tract

The mesenchyme of the endocardial cushions of the outflow tract is derived from at least three sources. One population of mesenchymal cells in the proximal outflow tract or conus is delaminated from the endocardium in a manner similar to that of the atrioventricular cushion tissue mesenchyme.[46] A second source of mesenchyme is from the pharyngeal arches and is a non–neural crest–derived mesenchymal cell population probably originating from the splanchnic mesoderm.[52] The third source of mesenchyme is derived from the neural crest that has migrated through the caudal pharyngeal arches (Fig. 61-3) and

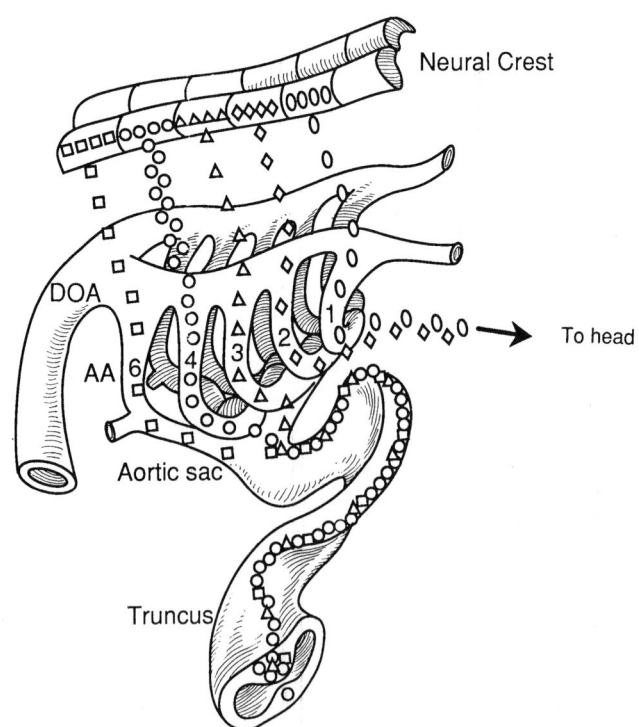

Figure 61–3. Diagram illustrating the neural crest seeding pharyngeal arches 1, 2, 3, 4, and 6. Ectomesenchyme provides the support for the aortic arch (*AA*) arteries that traverse the pharyngeal arches. Neural crest from arches 3 to 6 migrates into the outflow region of the heart, initiating closure of the outflow septation. DOA = dorsa aorta. (From Kirby ML, Walko KL: Circulation *82*:332, 1990.)

arrives in the outflow tract after the non-neural crest-derived mesenchyme.[5]

Septation of the outflow tract lumen occurs by three different processes, all of which involve neural crest cells (Fig. 61-4). The aortic sac is divided by a shelflike partition located between arch arteries 4 and 6, which represent systemic and pulmonary circulations, respectively. The shelf is connected to two prongs of condensed neural crest cells that are located in the cushions of the truncus. The shelf elongates into the truncus at the expense of the prongs, which become progressively shorter. After the prongs are used in building the truncal portion of the septum,

the conal septum closes as a zipper from the former truncus to the ventricles. This occurs as the conal cushions are myocardialized by ingrowing myocardial cells, thus causing them to bulge into the conal lumen. The endocardium breaks down, fusing the opposing cushions to form the septum.[22, 23]

Removal of the cardiac neural crest before its migration results in various outflow tract anomalies, depending to some extent on the amount of premigratory neural crest that is removed (Fig. 61-5).[53] The cardiac malformations that occur after ablation of the premigratory cardiac neural crest can be classified into two major categories: absence of outflow septation and

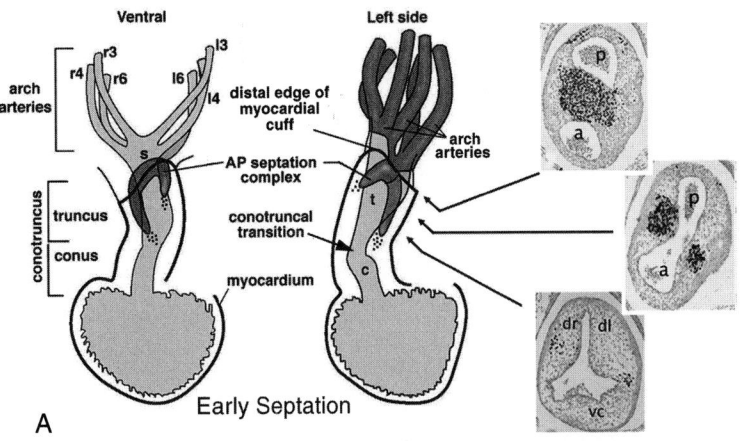

A   Early Septation

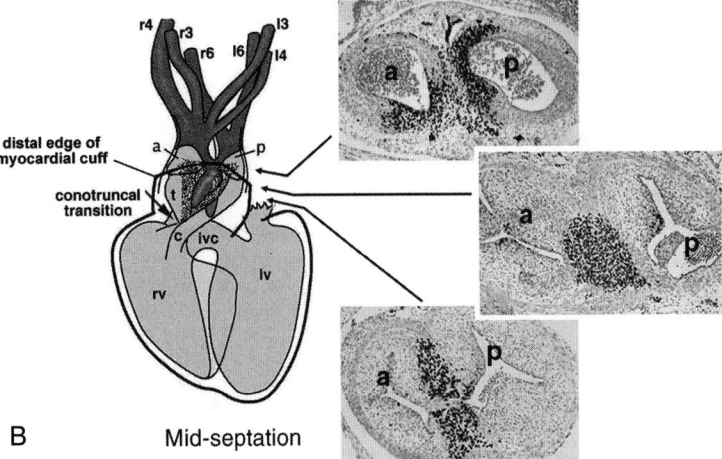

Figure 61–4. Diagram showing the contribution of cardiac neural crest to outflow septation. **A,** Early septation. Neural crest-derived mesenchyme forms an inverted U. The dorsal and ventral prongs extend into the cardiac jelly. The bridging part of the U crosses the aortic sac between the origins of the fourth (systemic) and sixth (pulmonary) aortic arch arteries. The neural crest-derived mesenchyme surrounding the arch arteries is in continuity with the condensed mesenchyme of the outflow septation complex. **B,** Midseptation. The aortic sac and truncus have been divided by the elongating aorticopulmonary septation complex. The prongs shorten, whereas the septum lengthens. **C,** Final events in outflow septation. The conus is divided by fusion of the conal ridges. The aortic vestibule and pulmonary infundibulum direct blood from left and right ventricles into their own outflow vessels through separate semilunar valves. a = aorta or aortic side; AP = aorticopulmonary; c = conus cordis; dl = dorsal left truncal cushion; dr = dorsal right truncal cushion; ivc = primary interventricular connection; 13, 14, 16 = left third, fourth, and sixth arch arteries; lavc = left atrioventricular canal; lv = left ventricle; p = pulmonary trunk or pulmonary side; pi = pulmonary infundibulum; r3, r4, r6 = right third, fourth, and sixth arch arteries; rv = right ventricle; ravc = right atrioventricular canal; t = truncus arteriosus; vc = ventral cushion. (From Waldo KL, et al: Dev Biol 186:129, 1998.)

B   Mid-septation

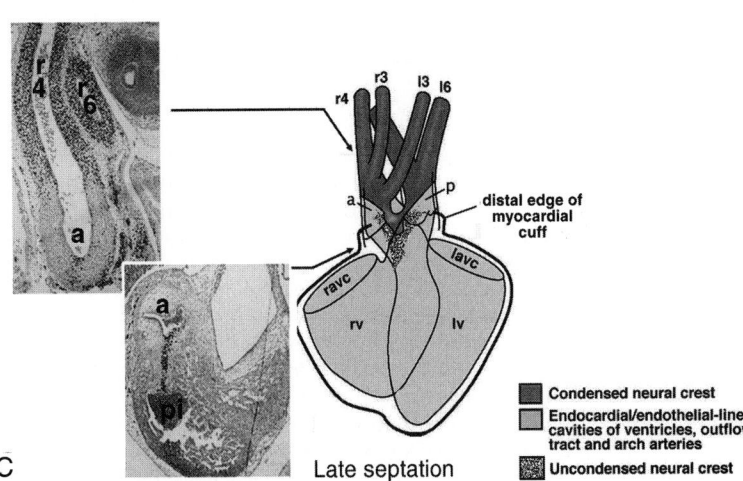

C   Late septation

- ■ Condensed neural crest
- ▨ Endocardial/endothelial-lined cavities of ventricles, outflow tract and arch arteries
- ▨ Uncondensed neural crest

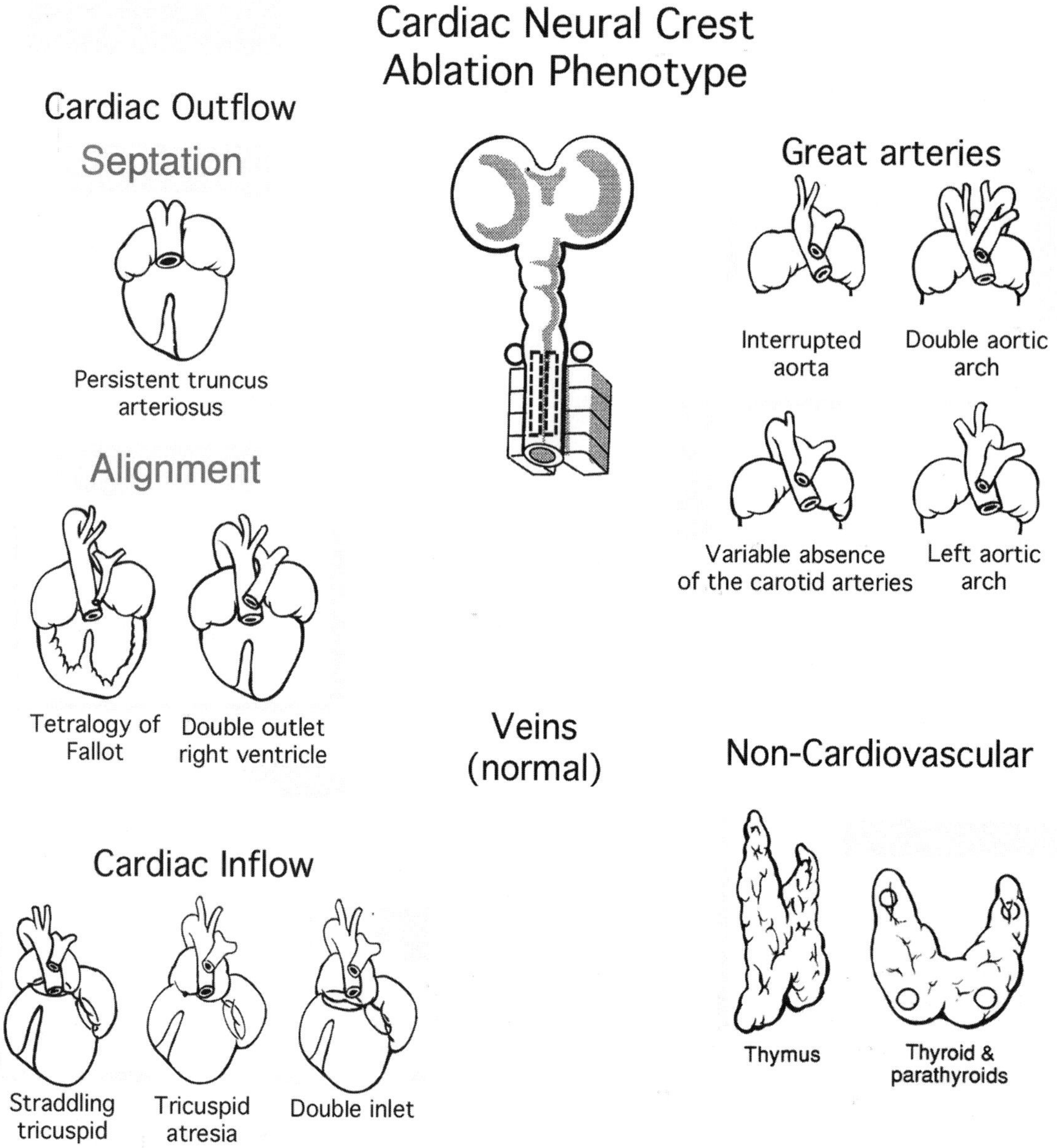

Figure 61–5. Diagram illustrating the phenotypes produced by ablation of the cardiac neural crest. (Adapted from Kirby ML: Trends Cardiovasc Med *3*:18, 1993.)

malalignment of the septum. The most severe defect is *persistent truncus arteriosus,* in which the outflow septum fails to form altogether. Outflow septation fails when the number of neural crest cells reaching the aortic sac and conotruncal ridges is less than a critical number required for septation or when the neural crest cells reaching the outflow tract are incompetent. Alternatively, signals from the endocardium, myocardium, or mesenchyme in the outflow cushions are apparently needed for neural crest cells to form a competent outflow septation complex. Although the details of these signals are not known, semaphorin/plexinA2 signaling is a required component.[54,55]

The second type of defect includes a spectrum ranging from double-outlet right ventricle to ventricular septal defect. In these malformations, a robust outflow septum is present, but it is malaligned with respect to the ventricular outlets. This results in the aorta's overriding the ventricular septum and arising at least partially from the right ventricle. Another manifestation of abnormal torsion in hearts with outflow abnormalities is the potential for coexistence of inflow anomalies, including double-inlet left

ventricle, straddling tricuspid valve, and tricuspid atresia. After neural crest ablation, the myocardium is not added appropriately from the secondary heart field to lengthen the heart tube.[56] This causes a shorter outflow tract than normal, which disturbs the relationship of the inflow and outflow ultimately resulting in malalignment defects of the outflow tract.

Alignment abnormalities of the outflow tract associated with neural crest ablation can be predicted very early in heart development from the configuration of the looped tube.[57] Neural crest cells, which have migrated to the pharyngeal arches, regulate the availability of growth factors that control the conversion of cells in the secondary heart field to outflow myocardium.[16,58] In the absence of cardiac neural crest cells in the pharynx, myocardium of the secondary heart field fails to be added to the outflow tract during lengthening of the tubular heart.

The neural crest that populates the pharyngeal arches also participates in development of the face and the glands of the neck and thorax (e.g., thyroid, parathyroids, and thymus).[59] In the case of the thymus, the neural crest–derived ectomesenchyme inter-

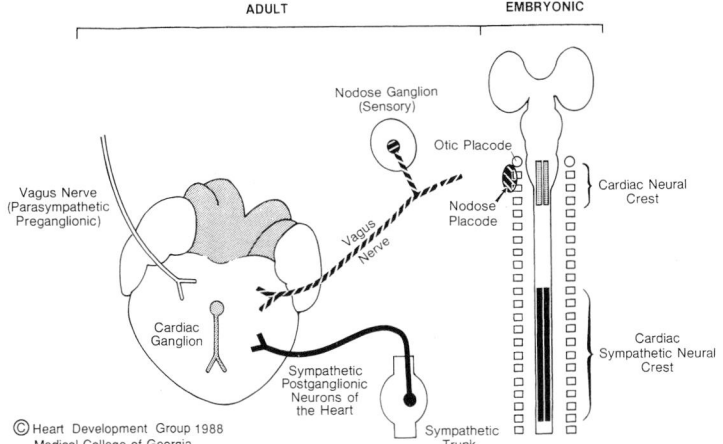

Figure 61–6. Illustration of the relationship of cardiac innervation and its derivation. The parasympathetic (cardiac ganglia) postganglionic neurons are derived from neural crest extending from the midotic placode to the caudal limit of somite 3 (cardiac neural crest). The cardiac sympathetic postganglionic neurons (sympathetic trunk) arise from trunk neural crest adjacent to somites 10 to 20. Sensory innervation of the heart is primarily from neurons in the nodose ganglion of the vagus, which arises from the nodose placode with support cells derived from the cardiac neural crest. (From Kirby ML: Pediatr Res *21*:219, 1987.)

acts with the endothelium of pharyngeal pouches 3 and 4 to produce the thymic primordium, which attracts circulating lymphocytes. Thus, in addition to cardiac anomalies, abnormal development of the cranial neural crest has the potential to result in various anomalies of the face and glands of the neck and thorax. About 50% of persons with conotruncal anomalies have been found to have a hemizygous interstitial deletion in chromosome 22.[60] Patients with persistent truncus arteriosus, tetralogy of Fallot, or interrupted arch frequently also show absent or hypoplastic thymus, parathyroid, or thyroid glands, and abnormal facies (i.e., low-set ears and hypertelorism). This sequence of anomalies, which has been traditionally called *DiGeorge or velocardiofacial syndrome,* is also known by the name Catch-22. The sequence does occur with microdeletions on chromosomes other than 22 in lower frequency. Many of the components of the sequence are present in Tbx-1 homozygous null mice.[61-63] Tbx-1 is a T-box type transcription factor that is located in the commonly microdeleted region of chromosome 22.

Ventricular Septation

The earliest sign of ventricular septation is the bulboventricular septum, which separates the presumptive right ventricle from the presumptive left ventricle. Its appearance is caused by differential growth of the prospective right and left ventricular cavities on either side.[64] The connection between the prospective right and left ventricles is through the primary interventricular foramen. At this stage, the atrioventricular canal leads exclusively into the presumptive left ventricle.[65] During early development of the heart, the presumptive left and right ventricles enlarge by centrifugal growth of the myocardium and become trabeculated, with the trabeculae oriented dorsoventrally. In the chick, the trabecular sheets begin to coalesce at stage 26 in the area of the bulboventricular septum and then proceed toward the floor of the ventricle. This fusion results in a ventricular septum that divides the presumptive right and left ventricles. Growth of the ventricular septum occurs with continued fusion of adjacent trabecular sheets.[66] This process is similar in mammals, in which the bulboventricular fold provides the anchor for accumulation of the ventricular trabeculations to form a concrete ridge. The primary interventricular foramen never closes, and in the adult heart, it gives left ventricular access to the aortic infundibulum.[65] The ventricular septum, atrioventricular endocardial cushions, and truncal cushions coalesce to complete the closure of the ventricular septum. As the outflow septum is completed, the originally large interventricular foramen becomes smaller, to form a secondary interventricular foramen. This secondary interventricular foramen is bordered by the conal cushions, the cranialmost part of the muscular interventricular septum, and the

atrioventricular endocardial cushions. These three structures coalesce to effect the final closure of the secondary interventricular foramen. In humans, the area of the atrioventricular endocardial cushion contributing to this closure becomes thinner, to form the membranous septum. The bifurcation of the ventricular conduction system is the landmark that separates the contribution of the atrioventricular cushions from that of the outflow tract ridges to the septum.[67]

HEMODYNAMICS

Although early morphogenetic events in heart development appear to be independent of function,[28] this is probably not the case with later development. During the first few hours after circulation begins, it is not possible to record blood pressure.[68, 69] By about 2 days of development, a nonpulsatile pressure of 0.3 mm Hg can be recorded in the chick.[70] Pulsatile pressure is seen slightly later and coincides with embryo turning. The pressure increases over the next 24 hours and continues to increase, slowly at first and then more rapidly.[71] In the chick, the ventricular pressure is nearly zero at the time the outflow tract is added, and by the time septation is almost complete, the pressure is about 3.5 mm Hg.[72] Maximum systolic and minimum diastolic intramyocardial pressures tend to be greater in the dorsal wall than in the ventral wall, whereas peak active intramyocardial pressure near the midwall is similar to peak active ventricular pressure.[73]

INNERVATION

The heart is innervated by three different sets of nerves (Fig. 61-6). Sympathetic innervation is via the cervical and first thoracic ganglia in the sympathetic trunks. These ganglia are derived entirely from the trunk neural crest.[74] Although sympathetic nerves are present rather early after septation is complete, sympathetic stimulation does not elicit positive chronotropism until much later.[75-77]

Parasympathetic innervation of the heart originates from cardiac ganglia located on the surface of the heart and near the outflow tract. These cardiac ganglia are derived from the cardiac neural crest, the same area that provides ectomesenchyme to the outflow tract.[24]

Sensory innervation originates from the distal ganglia of the vagus nerves. The neurons of these ganglia arise from the nodose placodes located lateral to the cardiac neural crest.[78] Other sensory innervation is probably present in the sympathetic cardiac nerves, but the extent of this innervation is not known. It is also not known when the cardiac sensory innervation begins to function.

REFERENCES

1. de la Cruz MV, Markwald RR (eds): Living Morphogenesis of the Heart. Boston, Birkhäuser, 1999.
2. Waldo KL, et al: Conotruncal myocardium arises from a secondary heart field. Development 128:3179, 2001.
3. Kelly RG, et al: The arterial pole of the mouse heart forms from Fgf10-expressing cells in pharyngeal mesoderm. Dev Cell 1:435, 2001.
4. Mjaatvedt CH, et al: The outflow tract of the heart is recruited from a novel heart-forming field. Dev Biol 238:97, 2001.
5. Kirby ML, et al: Neural crest cells contribute to normal aorticopulmonary septation. Science 220:1059, 1983.
6. Kim JS, et al: Development of the myocardium of the atrioventricular canal and the vestibular spine in the human heart. Circ Res 88:395, 2001.
7. Anderson RH, et al: Development and structure of the atrial septum. Heart 88:104, 2002.
8. Manasek FJ: Histogenesis of the embryonic myocardium. Am J Cardiol 25:249, 1970.
9. Ho E, Shimada Y: Formation of the epicardium studied with the scanning electron microscope. Dev Biol 66:579, 1978.
10. Virágh SZ, Challice CE: The origin of the epicardium and the embryonic myocardial circulation in the mouse. Anat Rec 201:157, 1981.
11. Rosenquist GC: Location and movements of cardiogenic cells in the chick embryo: the heart-forming portion of the primitive streak. Dev Biol 22:461, 1970.
12. Rosenquist GC, DeHaan RL: Migration of precardiac cells in the chick embryo: a radioautographic study. Carnegie Institute Washington publication 625. Contrib Embryol 38:111, 1966.
13. Redkar A, et al: Fate map of early avian cardiac progenitor cells. Development 128:2269, 2001.
14. Colas JF, et al: Evidence that translation of smooth muscle alpha-actin mRNA is delayed in the chick premyocardium until fusion of the bilateral heart-forming regions. Dev Dyn 218:316, 2000.
15. Schoenwolf GC, Garcia-Martinez V: Primitive-streak origin and state of commitment of cells of the cardiovascular system in avian and mammalian embryos. Cell Mol Biol Res 41:233, 1995.
16. His W: Die Area interposita, die Eustachi'sche Klappe und die Spina vestibuli. In Anatomie Menschlicher Embryonen. Leipzig, von FCW Vogel, 1880, pp 49–152.
17. Webb S, et al: Formation of the atrioventricular septal structures in the normal mouse. Circ Res 82:645, 1998.
18. Le Douarin NM, Kalcheim C: The Neural Crest, 2nd ed. Cambridge, Cambridge University Press, 1999.
19. Kirby ML, et al: Characterization of conotruncal malformations following ablation of "cardiac" neural crest. Anat Rec 213:87, 1985.
20. Miyagawa-Tomita S, et al: Temporospatial study of the migration and distribution of cardiac neural crest in quail-chick chimeras. Am J Anat 192:79, 1991.
21. Waldo KL, et al: Cardiac neural crest is essential for the persistence rather than the formation of an arch artery. Dev Dyn 205:281, 1996.
22. Waldo K, et al: Cardiac neural crest cells provide new insight into septation of the cardiac outflow tract: aortic sac to ventricular septal closure. Dev Biol 196:129, 1998.
23. Waldo KL, et al: Connexin 43 expression reflects neural crest patterns during cardiovascular development. Dev Biol 208:307, 1999.
24. Kirby ML, Stewart DE: Neural crest origin of cardiac ganglion cells in the chick embryo: identification and extirpation. Dev Biol 97:433, 1983.
25. Hiruma T, Hirakow R: Epicardium formation of chick embryonic heart: computer-aided reconstruction, scanning, and transmission electron microscopic studies. Am J Anat 184:129, 1989.
26. Komiyama M, et al: Origin and development of epicardium in the mouse embryo. Anat Embryol 176:183, 1996.
27. Männer J, et al: The origin, formation and developmental significance of the epicardium: a review. Cells Tissues Organs 169:89, 2001.
28. Koushik SV, et al: Targeted inactivation of the sodium-calcium exchanger (Ncx1) results in the lack of a heartbeat and abnormal myofibrillar organization. FASEB J 15:1209, 2001.
29. Kirby ML, Waldo KL: Neural crest and cardiovascular patterning. Circ Res 77:211, 1995.
30. Kamino K, et al: Localization of pacemaking activity in early embryonic heart monitored using voltage sensitive dye. Nature 190:595, 1981.
31. Van Mierop LHS: Location of pacemaker in chick embryo heart at the time of initiation of heartbeat. Am J Physiol 212:407, 1967.
32. Warynski S (cited by Romanoff): Rec Zool Suisse 3:261, 1886.
33. Patten BM, Kramer TC: The initiation of contraction in the embryonic chick heart. Am J Anat 53:349, 1933.
34. Chuck ET, et al: Changing activation sequence in the embryonic chick heart: implications for the development of the His-Purkinje system. Circ Res 81:470, 1997.
35. Ehler E, et al: Myofibrillogenesis in the developing chicken heart: assembly of Z-disk, M-line and the thick filaments. J Cell Sci 112:1529, 1999.
36. Sedmera D, et al: Cellular changes in experimental left heart hypoplasia. Anat Rec 267:137, 2002.
37. Gonzalez-Sanchez A, Bader D: Immunochemical analysis of myosin heavy chains in the developing chicken heart. Dev Biol 103:151, 1984.
38. Sweeney LJ, et al: Transitions in cardiac isomyosin expression during differentiation of the embryonic chick heart. Circ Res 61:287, 1987.
39. Christoffels VM, et al: Chamber formation and morphogenesis in the developing mammalian heart. Dev Biol 223:266, 2000.
40. Harvey RP: Organogenesis: patterning the vertebrate heart. Nat Rev Genet 3:544, 2002.
41. Nemer G, Nemer M: Regulation of heart development and function through combinatorial interactions of transcription factors. Ann Med 33:604, 2001.
42. Cripps RM, Olson EN: Control of cardiac development by an evolutionarily conserved transcriptional network. Dev Biol 246:14, 2002.
43. Morabito CJ, et al: Positive and negative regulation of epicardial-mesenchymal transformation during avian heart development. Dev Biol 234:204, 2001.
44. Bogers AJ, et al: Development of the origin of the coronary arteries: a matter of ingrowth or outgrowth? Anat Embryol (Berl) 180:437, 1989.
45. Waldo KL, et al: Origin of the proximal coronary artery stems and a review of ventricular vascularization in the chick embryo. Am J Anat 188:109, 1990.
46. Eisenberg LM, Markwald RR: Molecular regulation of atrioventricular valvuloseptal morphogenesis. Circ Res 77:1, 1995.
47. Krug EL, et al: Protein extracts from early embryonic hearts initiate cardiac endothelial cytodifferentiation. Dev Biol 112:414, 1985.
48. Markwald RR, et al: Proteins in cardiac jelly which induce mesenchyme formation. In Ferrans CVJ, et al (eds): Cardiac Morphogenesis. New York, Elsevier, 1985, pp 60–69.
49. Nakajima Y, et al: Mechanisms involved in valvuloseptal endocardial cushion formation in early cardiogenesis: roles of transforming growth factor (TGF)-beta and bone morphogenetic protein (BMP). Anat Rec 258:119, 2000.
50. Boyer AS, et al: TGFbeta2 and TGFbeta3 have separate and sequential activities during epithelial-mesenchymal cell transformation in the embryonic heart. Dev Biol 208:530, 1999.
51. Romano LA, Runyan RB: Slug is an essential target of TGFbeta2 signaling in the developing chicken heart. Dev Biol 223:91, 2000.
52. Thompson RP, Fitzharris TP: Morphogenesis of the truncus arteriosus of the chick embryo heart: tissue reorganization during septation. Am J Anat 156:251, 1979.
53. Nishibatake M, et al: Pathogenesis of persistent truncus arteriosus and dextroposed aorta in the chick embryo after neural crest ablation. Circulation 75:255, 1987.
54. Feiner L, et al: Targeted disruption of semaphorin 3C leads to persistent truncus arteriosus and aortic arch interruption. Development 128:3061, 2001.
55. Brown CB, et al: PlexinA2 and semaphorin signaling during cardiac neural crest development. Development 128:3071, 2001.
56. Yelbuz TM, et al: Shortened outflow tract leads to altered cardiac looping after neural crest ablation. Circulation 106:504, 2002.
57. Tomita H, et al: Relation of early hemodynamic changes to final cardiac phenotype and survival after neural crest ablation in chick embryos. Circulation 84:1289, 1991.
58. Farrell MJ, et al: FGF-8 in the ventral pharynx alters development of myocardial calcium transients after neural crest ablation. J Clin Invest 107:1509, 2001.
59. Bockman DE, Kirby ML: Dependence of thymus development on derivatives of the neural crest. Science 223:498, 1984.
60. Funke B, et al: Der(22) syndrome and velo-cardio-facial syndrome/DiGeorge syndrome share a 1.5-Mb region of overlap on chromosome 22q11. Am J Hum Genet 64:747, 1999.
61. Merscher S, et al: TBX1 is responsible for cardiovascular defects in velo-cardio-facial/DiGeorge syndrome. Cell 104:619, 2001.
62. Jerome LA, Papaioannou VE: DiGeorge syndrome phenotype in mice mutant for the T-box gene, Tbx1. Nat Genet 27:286, 2001.
63. Lindsay EA, et al: Tbx1 haploinsufficiency in the DiGeorge syndrome region causes aortic arch defects in mice. Nature 410:97, 2001.
64. Wenink ACG: Development of the ventricular septum. In Wenink ACG, et al (eds): The Ventricular Septum of the Heart. The Hague, Leiden University Press, 1981, pp 23–34.
65. Van Mierop LHS: Morphological development of the heart. In Berne RM (ed): Handbook of Physiology. Bethesda, MD, American Physiologic Society, 1979, pp 1–28.
66. Ben-Shachar G, et al: Ventricular trabeculations in the chick embryo heart and their contribution to ventricular and muscular septal development. Circ Res 57:759, 1985.
67. Lamers WH, Moorman AF: Cardiac septation: a late contribution of the embryonic primary myocardium to heart morphogenesis. Circ Res 91:93, 2002.
68. Van Mierop LHS, Bertuch CJ Jr: Development of arterial blood pressure in the chick embryo. Am J Physiol 212:42, 1967.
69. Nakazawa M, et al: Hemodynamics and ventricular function in the day-12 rat embryo: basic characteristics and the responses to cardiovascular drugs. Pediatr Res 37:117, 1995.
70. Van Mierop LHS: Morphological and functional development of the chick cardiovascular system during the first week of incubation. In Jaffee OC (ed): Cardiac Development with Special Reference to Congenital Heart Disease. Dayton, OH, University of Dayton Press, 1970, pp 57–66.
71. Hu N, Clark EB: Hemodynamics of the stage 12 to stage 29 chick embryo. Circ Res 65:1665, 1989.
72. Clark EB, et al: Ventricular function and morphology in the chick embryo stage 18 to 29. Am J Physiol 250:H407, 1989.

73. Chabert S, Taber LA: Intramyocardial pressure measurements in the stage 18 embryonic chick heart. Am J Physiol *282*:H1248, 2002.

74. Kirby M, Stewart D: Adrenergic innervation of the developing chick heart: neural crest ablations to produce sympathetically aneural hearts. Am J Anat *171*:295, 1984.

75. Higgins D, Pappano AJ: A histochemical study of the ontogeny of catecholamine-containing axons in the chick embryo heart. J Mol Cell Cardiol *11*:661, 1979.

76. Kirby ML, et al: Developing innervation of the chick heart: a histofluorescence and light microscopic study of sympathetic innervation. Anat Rec *196*:333, 1980.

77. Higgins D, Pappano AJ: Development of transmitter secretory mechanisms by adrenergic neurons in the embryonic chick heart ventricle. Dev Biol *87*:148, 1981.

78. D'Amico-Martel A, Noden DM: Contributions of placodal and neural crest cells to avian cranial peripheral ganglia. Am J Anat *166*:445, 1983.

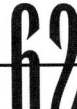

H. Scott Baldwin and Justin C. Grindley

62 Molecular Determinants of Embryonic Vascular Development

The establishment of the cardiovascular system represents an early, critical event essential for normal embryonic development. Although much of the attention to date has focused on factors involved in key events in cardiac development, such as myocardial differentiation and neural crest migration, the importance of normal vascular morphogenesis has recently become a central focus of cardiovascular research. Considerable new information has accumulated concerning the pivotal role of endothelial differentiation in establishment of the vascular tree. The purpose of this chapter is to review the general mechanisms of vascular development in light of some of the new information on critical molecular interactions that has recently been delineated. Specifically, this chapter focuses on (1) initial differentiation of the endothelium and formation of the primary vascular plexus; (2) vascular heterogeneity and remodeling; and (3) epigenetic factors that play a primary role in vascular ontogeny. Finally, we review some of the recent data that demonstrate how all these factors are involved in regulation of pulmonary vascular development.

ORIGIN OF ENDOTHELIAL CELLS

Early observers noted the initial formation of blood vessels outside the embryo in the blood islands of the yolk sac, which preceded intraembryonic vascular development. This led to the conclusion that all vessels within the embryo resulted from a direct extension of extraembryonic vessels.[1] This hypothesis was quickly refuted when parts of the embryo, separated from the yolk sac before vascular invasion, were shown subsequently to develop vascular channels.[2] This suggested the possibility of endothelial cell (EC) precursors intrinsic to the embryo. Perhaps the most significant breakthrough in the study of endothelial ontogeny came with the development of monoclonal antibodies that recognized a species-specific epitope on the cell membrane of quail endothelial cells. For the first time, this antibody allowed definitive identification of ECs independent of potentially ambiguous morphologic criteria. Utilizing one of these antibodies, QH1, several investigators have been able to demonstrate that vascular development commences in the embryo proper shortly after gastrulation, as individual presumptive ECs, or angioblasts, differentiate from the mesoderm. These cells soon connect into a vascular plexus that matures into the major vessels of the adult (see later). These studies have documented that most mesodermal tissues contain endothelial precursors and thus have the capacity for vascular formation.[3, 4] Similar studies utilizing a battery of endothelial specific antibodies have

defined a similar pattern of endothelial differentiation and vascular development in the mouse.[5]

For more than 70 years, a central question in vascular development has been whether endothelial cells and hematopoietic cells (HCs) share a common origin. In the yolk sac blood islands, and at certain sites within the embryo such as the developing aorta, hematopoiesis and EC differentiation occur side-by-side. Early observation of simultaneous HC and EC differentiation[6, 7] led to the hypothesis that HCs and EC precursors (angioblasts) are derived from the same progenitor cell, the hemangioblast (reviewed in Refs 8 to 10). Again, this question has been answered by the identification of molecular markers that define specific stages of mesodermal differentiation, most notably the vascular endothelial growth factor (VEGF) receptor 2 (VEGFR2). VEGFR2-deficient mice do not develop blood vessels or yolk sac blood islands[11, 12] and thus lack both endothelial and hematopoietic components. The combined EC and HC defects are consistent with a common molecular pathway governing EC and HC differentiation and support a direct lineage association between blood and endothelium. However, the combined defects could merely reflect a developmental arrest, since loss of VEGFR2 function results in a relatively early embryonic demise.

To separate embryonic survival from the equation, VEGFR2–deficient embryonic stem cells have been used in both chimera and *in vitro* differentiation studies. These approaches have demonstrated that a single VEGFR2+ cell can give rise to both endothelial and hematopoietic cells, and further suggest a requirement for VEGF/VEGFR2 signaling in hemangioblast survival, proliferation, or migration, as well as in differentiation.[8, 12] Similar knock-out, chimera, and *in vitro* studies suggest that the basic helix-loop-helix transcription factor TAL1/SCL (T-cell acute leukemia/stem cell leukemia) might play a concomitant role in differentiation of both the hematopoietic and endothelial cell lineages. TAL1/SCL-deficient animals have defective hematopoiesis, and TAL1/SCL-deficient cells fail to contribute to vascular remodeling. TAL1/SCL deficiency in embryoid bodies (differentiating cultures of embryonic stem cells) leads to defective hematopoiesis, accompanied by an increase in the percentage of cells expressing endothelial markers. Thus, it was hypothesized that TAL1/SCL might have a biphasic action, acting in a common precursor to promote formation of hematopoietic cells, but also acting within the endothelial lineage during angiogenesis.[8] TAL1/SCL is not expressed in VEGFR2-deficient embryos, suggesting a pathway in which expression of this transcription factor is downstream of a VEGF signal through VEGFR2.[13]

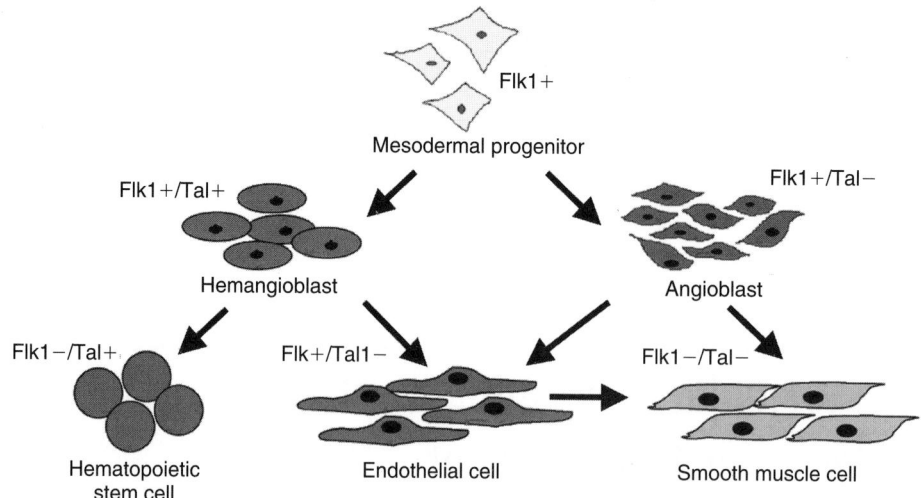

Figure 62–1. The common origins of endothelial and hematopoietic cells. Endothelial cells (ECs) and hematopoietic cells (HCs) both derive from mesodermal progenitor cells that express the VEGF receptor VEGFR2 (Flk1). The hemangioblast is a Flk1+ cell that also expresses the transcription factor TAL1/SCL (Flk1+/Tal1+) and can give rise to both HCs (down-regulating Flk1) or to ECs (down-regulating Tal1). ECs can also be derived from the angioblast, a precursor cell that, like the ECs themselves, is Flk1+ but Tal1–. An additional cell-fate choice important for blood vessel formation is the production of smooth muscle cells (SMCs) versus ECs. Recent data suggest that both angioblasts and mature ECs can give rise to SMCs, which are Flk1–/Tal1–. (Adapted from Ema M, et al: Genes Dev *17*:380, 2003.)

In an elegant series of experiments, Ema and colleagues[13] delineated a combinatorial role for VEGFR2 and TAL1/SCL in vascular and hematopoietic development. By knocking-in TAL1/SCL into the VEGFR2 locus, they could separate TAL1/SCL activation from additional downstream effects of VEGFR2 action. They showed that TAL1/SCL partially rescues the *in vivo* endothelial defects seen in VEGFR2-null mutants but significantly improves hematopoietic differentiation *in vitro* and *in vivo*. This study (summarized in Fig. 62-1) was able definitely to identify the hemangioblast as expressing TAL1/SCL (Tal1+) and the angioblast as nonexpressing (Tal1–). It was also able to confirm that angioblasts and definitive endothelial cells could both give rise to smooth muscle cells (SMCs), as had been previously suggested by others.[14] Thus, ECs, HCs, and SMCs have a common lineage in which cell-fate choices are governed in part by the combinatorial action of VEGFR2 and TAL1/SCL.

The Two Mechanisms of New Blood Vessel Formation

Following the differentiation and development of the EC populations, as just described, there must be a subsequent organization of these endothelial cells into a complex but highly regulated system of arteries, capillaries, and veins. Two different processes are thought to be involved in new blood vessel formation (Fig. 62-2): *vasculogenesis*, which is the *de novo* organization of blood vessels by *in situ* differentiation of endothelial cells from mesoderm; and *angiogenesis*, the budding and branching of vessels from preexisting vessels.[15-17]

Angiogenesis is the characteristic vascularization process for organs such as the brain and kidney; vasculogenesis is more prominent in the formation of the larger vascular network, including the dorsal aorta, blood islands, endocardium of the heart, and cardinal and vitelline vessels, as well as the liver. In some instances, vascular development may occur by simultaneous angiogenesis and vasculogenesis, which is characteristic of the developing lung.[18, 19] Although angiogenesis can occur in both the embryo and the adult (e.g., wound healing, tumor vasculogenesis[20, 21]), vasculogenesis is usually considered to be restricted to embryonic development. However, recently identified circulating ECs and EC precursors that can contribute

to new blood vessel formation may represent exceptions to this temporal limit on vasculogenesis.[22] Despite this distinction between these two processes, the tasks that ECs subsequently perform in forming a new vessel are similar in both. Thus, vasculogenesis and angiogenesis likely share many molecular components involved in cell-cell or cell-matrix signaling or in coordinated cell movement, organization, and adhesion.

Formation of a Primary Vascular Plexus

In vasculogenesis, ECs first assemble into vessel primordia, which lack a lumen, and then rearrange into endothelial tubes of polarized cells. Many such tubes then are joined into a polygonal array generating the primary vascular network. Recent work has identified key molecules involved in vessel assembly and morphogenesis. An early role for VEGF signaling is revealed by VEGFR1-deficient mice, which form angioblasts but fail to properly assemble endothelial cells into tubes.[23] Inhibition of VEGF signaling using soluble VEGFR1 in quail embryos supports the requirement for VEGF signaling in this phase of vessel assembly.[24] Normally, the polygonal array of vessels is formed through the protrusive behavior of individual ECs, which adopt a bipolar shape and extend processes to link with neighboring ECs. In embryos injected with soluble VEGFR1, normal numbers of ECs are present, but they fail to exhibit protrusive behavior, resulting in a profound deficiency of vessels.[24]

As well as signaling molecules, cell–cell contact and cell–extracellular matrix (ECM) interactions are important for early vascular morphogenesis. After the formation of vessel primordia, cells rearrange into tubes with lumens. Integrins, the best-characterized group of cell–ECM adhesion molecules, have been implicated in this phase of vasculogenesis, as well as in angiogenesis and vessel maintenance. Integrins are heterodimeric proteins that consist of an α-subunit noncovalently associated with a β-subunit. Currently, 8 different β- and 18 different α-subunits have been identified; however, members of the β_1 and β_3 family of integrin receptors, together with other cell adhesion family members, are thought to be particularly important in both vasculogenesis and angiogenesis.[25] The combination of specific α- and β-subunits determines ligand-binding specificity. For

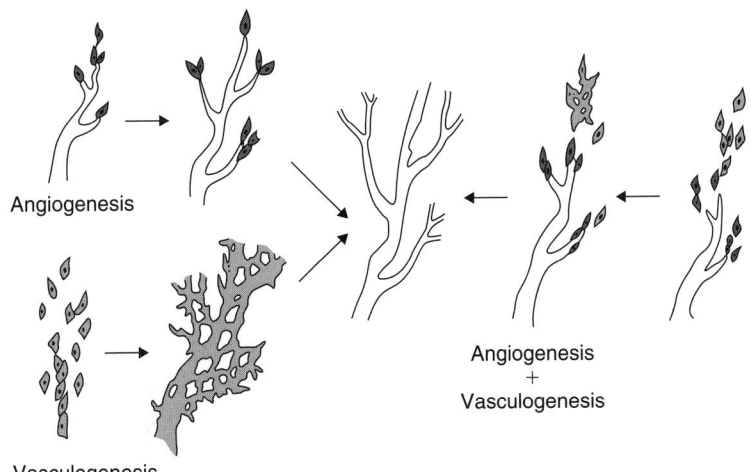

Figure 62–2. The basic mechanisms of vascular development in the embryo. *Angiogenesis* is the sprouting of new vessels from existing vessels, and *vasculogenesis* is the *de novo* differentiation of angioblasts from mesoderm and organization into a vascular plexus with remodeling into a definitive vessel. A third process may involve congruent angiogenesis and vasculogenesis.

example, β_1 in combination with α_5 functions exclusively as a fibronectin receptor, whereas β_1 in combination with α_6 serves as a laminin receptor. Thus the ability of a cell to modulate adhesive characteristics is determined by both the types of integrins expressed and the absolute number of any given integrin.

Utilizing the monoclonal antibody CSAT, which interferes with ligand binding to the β_1 integrins, Drake and colleagues were able to block formation of the lumen of the dorsal aorta in the early chick embryo.[26] It is interesting that in these experiments, the early stages of vasculogenesis were not obviously affected in that angioblast differentiation and spatial organization into cords appeared normal. Only the final stages of tube formation were inhibited, suggesting that although β_1 integrins are critical for final development of an endothelial tube, they are not involved in the initial commitment of mesoderm to EC lineage or in initial spatial organization. In results similar to those seen for injection of β_1 antagonists, $\alpha_v\beta_3$-blocking agents prevented lumen formation but not differentiation or spatial organization of the ECs.[27]

To assign roles in vascular development to specific subunits, integrins, or their ECM ligands requires much additional work, and it should be noted that inhibitor studies and gene inactivation studies have not always produced concordant results. The majority of α_v-knock-out mouse embryos die by midgestation, probably due to placental defects, but around one fifth of the embryos survive until birth.[28] These embryos have vascular abnormalities and hemorrhaging that are unexpectedly restricted to intracerebral and intestinal vessels.[28] Similarly, β_3-knock-out mice are viable and fertile but have defects characteristic of the human bleeding disorder Glanzmann thrombasthenia, including cutaneous and gastrointestinal bleeding.[29] Thus, although both the α_v and β_3 gene-inactivations in mice have vascular defects, neither recapitulates the defects seen in avians in response to a specific $\alpha_v\beta_3$ inhibitor.

ANGIOGENESIS, REMODELING, AND VESSEL MATURATION

To generate a fully functional, arborized vascular tree, the primary vascular plexus must be extended and modified, and vessel maturation must occur. Angiogenesis generates new vessels from existing ones either by a sprouting mechanism or by a nonsprouting (intussusception) mechanism in which columns of interstitial tissue are inserted inside the lumen of an existing vessel, dividing it into two or more new vessels.[30]

During angiogenesis, the preexisting network of vessels with relatively uniform diameters is also extensively remodeled to generate a hierarchic arrangement of large and small vessels. These changes are accompanied by vessel maturation and stabilization, which depend upon the recruitment from mesenchyme of periendothelial mural cells, including pericytes and smooth muscle cells, as well as on the deposition of basement membrane. Interactions with periendothelial mural cells established during angiogenesis are critical for proper functioning of the vascular network. In particular, blood vessels located in different parts of the vascular tree, such as the elastic vessels, muscular arteries, resistance vessels, veins and lymphatics, each require different physical properties. Many of these distinctions between vessels stem from local variation in extracellular matrix production by the mural cells.

In the last few years, considerable progress has been made in uncovering the molecular signals controlling angiogenesis, vessel remodeling, and maturation. This work has highlighted the involvement of several families of receptor tyrosine kinases (RTKs) and their ligands, shown schematically in Fig. 62–3. The functions of selected RTKs and ligands in vascular development are illustrated in Fig. 62–4. As well as functioning during vasculogenesis, signaling by VEGF ligands and VEGF receptors is important for angiogenesis and regulates endothelial cell sprouting and survival (reviewed in Ref 31). Vascular development is particularly sensitive to VEGF dosage. Heterozygosity for a null mutation in the VEGF gene leads to multiple cardiovascular defects and embryonic lethality.[32, 33] Consistent with a role in vessel sprouting, there are deficiencies in intersomitic vessels, in vessel in-growth to the neuroepithelium, and in the sprouting of head mesenchyme vessels. The vitelline vessels fail to fuse with the yolk sac, and an irregular primary plexus within the yolk sac is not remodeled to generate larger vessels.[32,33]

Specific inhibition of VEGF signaling with a soluble receptor and a conditional knock-out of VEGF in which the gene is excised only in newborn mice further highlights the dependence on VEGF of vessels that form by angiogenesis.[34] In these animals, there is growth retardation and hypoplasia of multiple organs, which is associated with dramatic reductions in organ vascularization. As well as reducing postnatal angiogenesis, the inhibition of VEGF signaling appears to cause loss of existing vessels, since animals treated with soluble receptor exhibit a marked increase in EC apoptosis. Therefore, VEGF acts as a survival factor for ECs in immature vessels. This survival function observed in the perinatal period does not appear to extend to

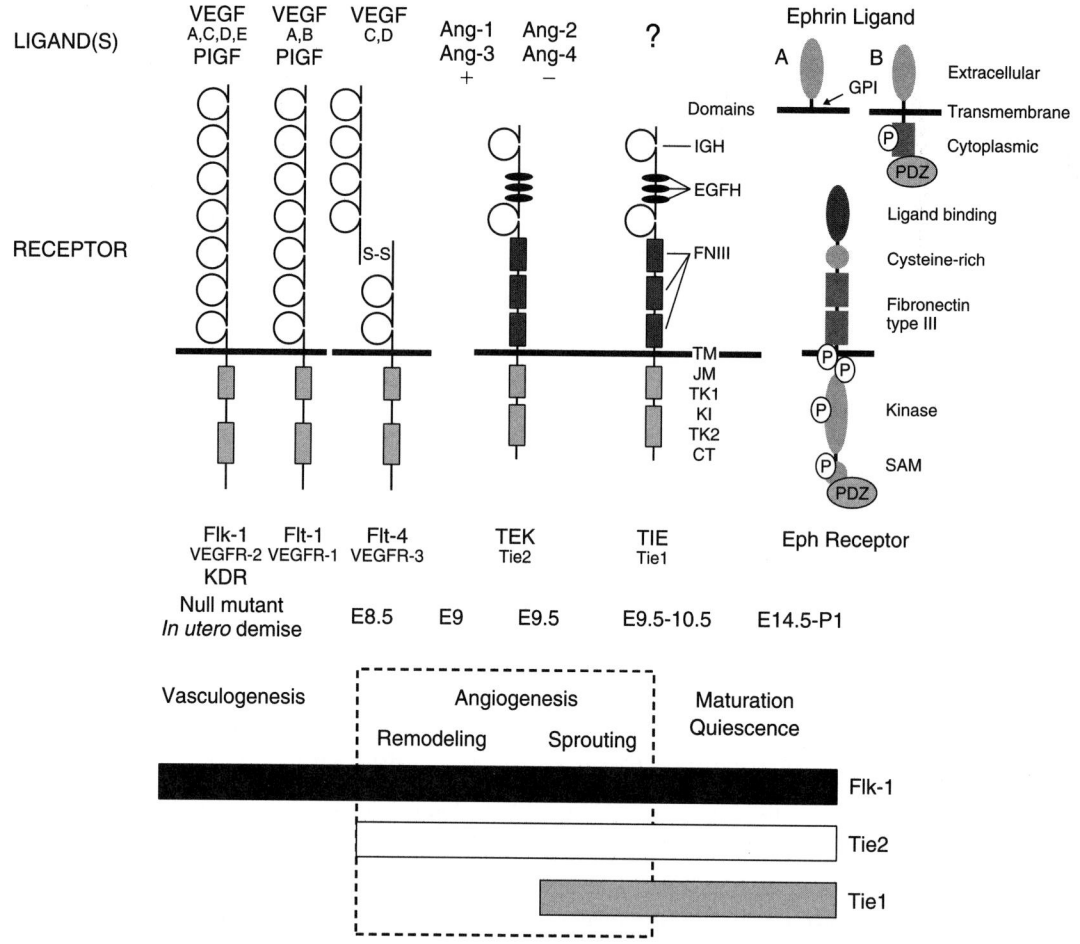

Figure 62–3. Major EC receptor tyrosine kinases (RTKs) and growth factor ligands involved in vascular development. The structures of the receptors are shown schematically, and major protein domains have been indicated. (Ang = angiopoietin; IGH = immunoglobulin homology domain; EGFH = epidermal growth factor homology domain; FNIII = fibronectin type III homology domain; TM = transmembrane domain; JM = juxtamembrane domain; TK1 and TK2 = tyrosine kinase catalytic domains; KI = kinase insert; CT = carboxyl terminal tail; S-S = disulfide bridge; P = phosphorylation site; GPI = glycosylphosphatidyl inositol anchor; PDZ = site of interaction with the PSD-95/Discs Large/ZO-1 (PDZ) class signaling proteins; PlGF = placental growth factor; SAM = domain that forms homodimers and may regulate receptor dimerization; PDZ = site of interaction with the PSD-95/Discs Large/ZO-1 (PDZ) class of signaling proteins; SAM = domain that forms homodimers and may regulate receptor dimerization; Ang-1, Ang-2, Ang-3 and Ang-4 = The angiopoietin family of Tie2 ligands; PlGF = placenta growth factor.) Also shown are the requirements for three RTKs relative to mouse gestation and phases of blood vessel development. Animals deficient in VEGFR2 (Flk1) fail to undergo vasculogenesis, indicating a very early requirement for this receptor. In contrast, Tie2 is not required for vasculogenesis but is necessary for subsequent angiogenesis. Tie1 appears to act later still, mainly in vessel maturation and vessel stability (quiescence).

mature vessels, since treated adult animals did not exhibit organ abnormalities.

Whereas VEGF receptors such as VEGFR2 are expressed by the earliest EC precursors, other endothelium-specific RTKs are most prominently expressed at later phases of vessel development and are believed to act once initial vessel formation has occurred. Tie1 (tyrosine kinase with Ig-like loops and epidermal growth factor homology domains) and Tie2 are closely related endothelium-specific RTKs that are involved in angiogenesis and vessel maintenance. Tie2-deficient animals exhibit normal vasculogenesis but fail to remodel the primary vascular plexus correctly and are deficient in vessels that normally form by angiogenic mechanisms. A key defect is in the generation of small vessels from large ones by intussusception. Folds of interstitial tissue that normally invade vessels collapse to produce irregular, abnormally spaced vessel patterns.[35] The failure of proper tissue-fold formation apparently stems from a striking inability of Tie2-null vessels to recruit periendothelial cells to the vessel walls and into the tissue folds. The ECs themselves also exhibit abnormal morphology, being rounder than normal and often projecting into the vessel lumen.[35]

Ang-1 and Ang-2 (see Fig. 62–3) are two members of a family of four structurally related Tie2 ligands (in Ref 36). Ang-1 null mice have a similar phenotype to Tie2 mutants, suggesting that this molecule is the main agonist ligand. Ang-1 is not expressed in EC cells but rather is produced in tissue adjacent to vessels in areas of angiogenesis, implying that the signals mediated by Ang-1/Tie2 are directed to ECs from their environment. The effect on mural cells indicates a critical place of Ang-1/Tie2 in reciprocal signaling between ECs and their surroundings, since it suggests that the loss of Tie2 activity causes a disruption of some further signal produced by the EC cells. Ang-2, identified by its sequence similarity to Ang-1, was found *in vitro* to antagonize Ang-1 activation of Tie2, a role supported by *in vivo* overexpression studies that generated a phenotype similar to loss of function of Ang-1 or Tie2.[37] In vitro data and gene knock-out experiments suggest a more complex picture, in which Ang-2's function is context-dependent and may be modulated by the bioavailability of VEGF.[38-40] Ang-2 appears to induce vessel regression in the absence of VEGF, but it can promote sprouting in the presence of VEGF.[41] In blood vessels, Ang-2 functions in vessel

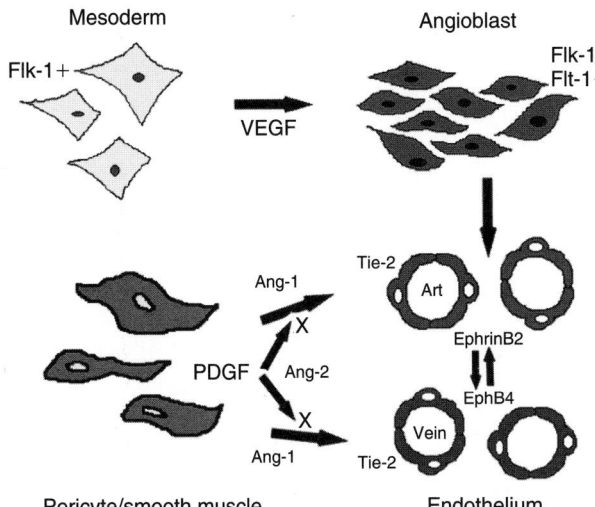

Figure 62–4. Key signals in the production of a vascular tree.
Schematic of the cell types contributing to blood vessels, illustrating the action of selected signaling molecules. VEGF signals are involved in the differentiation of endothelial precursor cells (angioblasts) from mesoderm that contains progenitor cells that express VEGFR2 (Flk1). Angioblasts require VEGFR1 (Flt1) to assemble into endothelial tubes. The endothelium is patterned and remodeled. Patterning of vessels includes the expression of ephrin-B2 on arteries (Art) and Eph-B4 on veins. The Tie2 receptor, expressed on ECs, and its ligand Ang-1, expressed in adjacent tissues, are required for vessel remodeling and formation of new vessels by angiogenic mechanisms. Ang-2 can act as a negative regulator of these signals. Platelet-derived growth factor B (PDGF) is involved in the recruitment of periendothelial mural cells to vessels, which is necessary for vessel maturation and stability. art = artery.

regression, as revealed by the failure of the normal programmed regression of the hyaloid vasculature of the eye in Ang-2-deficient mice. Conversely, the effect of Ang-2 on intestinal and dermal lymphatic ECs is proangiogenic, and loss of Ang-2 results in hypoplasia of these vessels.[38]

A necessary starting point for vessel regression (pruning of the vascular tree), sprouting (generating new branches), and intussusception (dividing vessels) is the destabilization of existing blood vessels. Work with additional RTKs and their ligands reveals the existence of mechanisms that stabilize ECs and highlights the importance of mural cells in vessel maintenance. Tie1 is an endothelium-specific orphan receptor (a receptor with no known ligand) closely related to Tie2. Tie1 is expressed in ECs and their precursors during development but is also expressed in most non-proliferating adult endothelium. Mice homozygous for null Tie1 mutations exhibit normal vascular development until midgestation. They then appear to suffer a loss of the microvasculature, accompanied by hemorrhage.[42] More detailed analysis of these animals suggests that the vascular density is actually higher than normal in many tissues because intussusception occurs more frequently.[35] This change appears due to the "hyperactive" behavior of Tie1-deficient ECs, which also compromises vessel integrity. Individual Tie1-null ECs project numerous extensions and filopodia and frequently have other defects in morphology, such as frequent intra- and transcellular holes. Periendothelial mural cells associated with these defective vessels also exhibit a "hyperactive" phenotype.[35] Together, these studies suggest that the normal function of Tie1 activity is to suppress the exploratory behavior of EC cells and their associated mural cells, thereby stabilizing vessels and preventing further vessel division.

Recruitment of periendothelial mural cells to new blood vessels is mediated by EC expression of platelet-derived growth factor B (PDGF-B), acting through its receptor PDGFR-β, which is expressed in the adjacent mesenchyme (reviewed in Ref 43). Inactivation of either the PDGF-B or PDGFR-β genes in the mouse results in death in late gestation that is associated with dilation of the heart and blood vessels, rupture of capillaries, and widespread edema and hemorrhage.[44-47] Deficiencies in vascular smooth muscle cell and pericytes occur in many tissues, with the extent of deficiency correlating with the occurrence of vessel dilation and microaneurysms.[47] Absence of pericytes is linked to EC hyperplasia, with the walls of dilated vessels containing a higher than normal density of ECs. In the pericyte-deficient vessels of PDGF-B, null mice ECs exhibit a "hyperactive" morphology that is reminiscent of the Tie1-null phenotype, with the most extreme disorganization of ECs occurring in microaneurysms.[48] Thus the recruitment of periendothelial cells mediated by PDGF-B and PDGFR-β appears to be a critical part of stabilizing both EC number and organization (see Fig. 62–4).

Vascular Patterning—Not All Endothelial Cells Are Created Equal

Many differences between classes of vessels involve the vessel wall and stem from differential extracellular matrix production by the mural cells. It has long been postulated that the ECs themselves also form very distinct populations, with unique characteristics and perhaps unique origins. However, strong molecular evidence for such distinctions has only recently been obtained, when localized expression of regulatory molecules, such as transcription factors, receptors, and ligands, revealed multiple levels of EC heterogeneity. In particular, distinct molecular signatures for ECs are located within arteries, veins, and lymphatic vessels and in the endocardium of the heart.[49-54]

The functional significance of such distinctions is exemplified by differences in the venous and arterial expression patterns of the RTK Eph-B4 and its transmembrane ligand ephrin-B2.[49, 51] The Eph receptors, the largest described family of RTKs, bind membrane-bound ephrin family ligands. Members of the ephrin-B family of ligands can autophosphorylate upon receptor binding, thereby allowing bidirectional signaling during cell–cell interactions.[55] During embryogenesis, the Eph-B4 receptor is specifically expressed in ECs almost exclusively in developing veins, whereas its only known specific ligand, ephrin-B2, is expressed in ECs in arteries.[49-51] Homozygosity for null mutations in either ephrin-B2 or Eph-B4 results in defects in angiogenesis, but not in vasculogenesis, both in the yolk sac and in the embryo. In both cases, the primary vascular plexi are established, but there are abnormalities in remodeling that have an impact on both arteries and veins. Although both classes of vessels are disrupted, the venous system is more strongly affected in the Eph-B4 null embryos, and, conversely, the loss of ephrin-B2 has a greater impact on the arterial system.[49,51] The venous and arterial expression of this receptor-ligand pair is suggestive of a role in mediating interactions between the two classes of vessels. Consistent with this idea, normal intercalation between arteries and veins fails to occur in yolk sacs of ephrin-B2–deficient embryos.[49] Together with other data on the expression and function of Eph family members,[50] these results demonstrate that molecular differences between the arterial and venous ECs are established early in development. Moreover, these molecules are essential for the normal development of the vascular tree, likely mediating cell–cell interactions specific for subsets of the endothelium (see Fig. 62–4).

The patterns of expression and localized functions of certain transcription factor genes reveal further levels of EC heterogeneity. Notably, the transcription factor gene, nuclear factor of activated T cells-1 (NFATc1), is expressed in the endothelial lining of the heart and the endocardium but not in other EC populations. In valve formation, ECs in the valve-forming region undergo an epithelial-mesenchymal transition, delaminating and entering the underlying endocardial cushion. During development, NFATc1 expression becomes restricted to the valve-forming regions of the endocardium. Thus NFATc1 expression defines an endothelial subpopulation with unique properties. A functional requirement for NFATc1 activity in endocardium is demonstrated by targeted disruption of the NFATc1 gene. Mouse embryos homozygous for NFATc1 mutations die *in utero* with congestive heart failure associated with the absence of aortic and pulmonary valve formation, as well as ventricular septal defects.[53,54]

The ECs of the lymphatic system are also distinct from other ECs at the molecular level. They exhibit higher levels of expression of several markers, including the transcription factor gene Prox1, the VEGF receptor VEGFR3, and the lymphatic endothelial hyaluronan receptor LYVE-1.[52,56,57] (reviewed in Refs 58 and 59). The lymphatic system appears to develop through budding of the preexisting venous system.[60, 61] Prox1 is expressed at sites where lymphatic vessels bud from veins, and its expression is subsequently restricted to the lymphatic system.[52] In Prox1-deficient mice, the early budding of the future lymphatic vessels from the cardinal vein occurs normally, but this process arrests in such a way that the animals lack lymphatic ECs.[52] Failure of budding cells to express high levels of VEGFR3 or LYVE-1 suggests that Prox1 controls a program of lymphatic EC differentiation, as well as being required to maintain the budding process.[52,58]

Our understanding of endothelial heterogeneity is extremely limited, and much remains to be discovered about the extent of such heterogeneity, its significance, and the cellular and molecular mechanisms by which it is acquired. A key question is, "How does such EC heterogeneity arise?" For example, do such differences reflect variation in the origin of ECs, or are they acquired by naive ECs through local environmental cues? Since localized expression of genes within the EC has only recently been described, few experiments have yet addressed this issue. A recent study of vessels in the skin, however, indicates that the arterial-venous identity of smaller vessels is defined at the time of vessel remodeling through local cues.

It has long been recognized that in peripheral tissues, nerves often run along blood vessels. The vascular system and peripheral nervous system are both complex branched structures, so this intimate association raised the question of whether one branched pattern determined the other, or whether they are independently responding to common cues from their surroundings (reviewed in Ref 62). In the embryonic chick skin, only some vessels are co-localized with nerves. Using the arterial and venous markers ephrin-B2 and Eph-B4 (described earlier), Mukouyama and co-workers[63] found that arteries but not veins ran along nerves (Fig. 62–5). Mutations that eliminate or alter the patterns of peripheral sensory nerves caused corresponding alterations in arterial patterning, particularly in small-diameter vessels. Thus, the pattern of small arteries appears to follow that of the sensory nerves. Expression of the arterial marker ephrin-B2 was found to be acquired during remodeling of the vascular plexus, around the time at which the patterns of vessels and nerves begin to correlate, suggesting that nerves might influence both arterial identity and vessel remodeling. Nerves and their associated Schwann cells are local sources of VEGF, and this factor can account for the ability of both neurons and Schwann cells to induce expression of the ephrin-B2 arterial marker from cultures of ephrin-B2–negative ECs. A specific marker of arterial identity thus appears to be induced by a local VEGF signal from sensory nerves. However, in these experiments the percentage of ECs that could be induced to express ephrin-B2 was never greater than 50, perhaps also suggesting that only certain ECs are able to respond to this signal.[63]

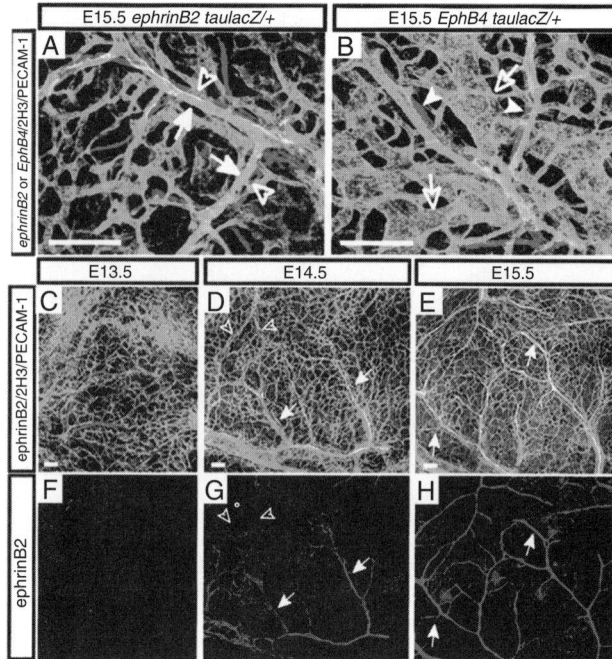

Figure 62–5. Peripheral nerves provide a template for arterio-genesis in the skin (see also color plates). Whole-mount triple immunofluorescence confocal microscopy was used to follow the differentiation of arteries (during embryogenesis; e.g., E15.5 = embryonic day 15.5) by ephrin-B2 in red (**A, C, D**), of veins by Eph-B4 immunolocalization in red (**B**), of nerves with 2H3 localization in green, and of endothelial cells with PECAM11/CD31 localization in blue. Arteries (arrows) are specifically aligned with peripheral nerves (arrowheads) (**A**), whereas veins (open arrows) show a more random distribution (**B**). In parts **C** to **H**, a time-course from mouse embryonic ages 13.5 days to 15.5 days (E13.5–E15.5), it is apparent that nerve innervation of the skin (green) precedes arterial differentiation (red) of the primary vascular plexus (blue). (Adapted from Mukouyama YS, et al: Cell *109*:693, 2002.)

Epigenetic Factors Driving Vascular Development and Morphogenesis

In the mature vascular system, the extent of vascularization is exquisitely matched to the physiologic needs of the tissue. Moreover, at different points in the vascular tree the properties of blood vessels, such as their number, diameter, and wall thickness, are all matched to the flows and pressures in that part of the circulatory system. These relationships between vascular system structure and physiology are not the result of a rigid genetic program that predetermines the genesis and final properties of every blood vessel. Instead, physiologic (epigenetic) factors exert a major influence over the form of the cardiovascular system. Epigenetic factors help explain some key questions that have arisen from observation of normal blood vessel morphogenesis and play important roles in cardiovascular malformations and disease. As discussed earlier, remodeling results in large vessels being created from a relatively uniform plexus of small vessels. What makes some vessels increase in size while others do not? Extensive vessel regression also occurs, so only a fraction of the original capillaries within a primary plexus is present in the mature vascular network. What determines which vessels survive? Equally, new vessels are generated in angiogenesis by sprouting and intussusception. Why do new vessels form in one location and not another? What determines how many new vessels should be formed? Two epigenetic factors that play significant roles in vascular development are hemodynamic forces and hypoxia.

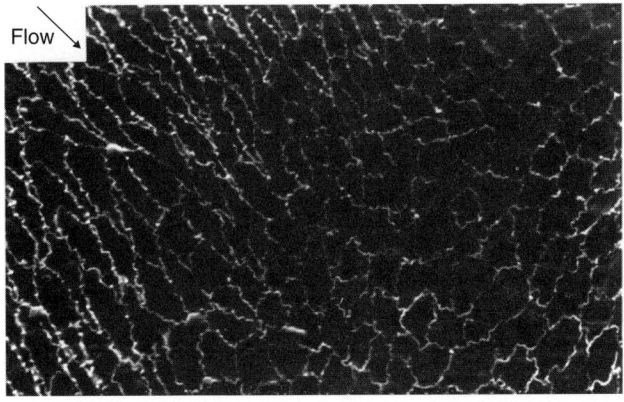

A

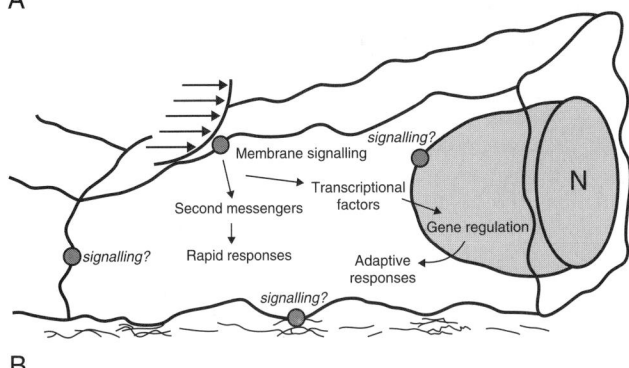

B

Figure 62–6. Shear stress is a major epigenetic determinant of vascular morphogenesis. A, ECs align themselves with direction of flow. **B,** Endothelial response to flow results in numerous alterations at the cell membrane, intercellular junctions, and basal lamina, which result in both primary and secondary alterations in gene regulation. Thus, the EC serves as a "mechanotransducer" for flow within the cardiovascular system. N = nucleus. (Adapted from Davies PF: Physiol Rev 75:519, 1995.)

Hemodynamic Forces

The forces acting on a blood vessel due to blood flow can be resolved into at least two components (reviewed in Ref 64). Blood pressure acts perpendicular to the lumen surface, so changes in pressure stretch all components of the vessel wall (endothelium, smooth muscle, and extracellular matrix). Tangential to the lumen surface, the flowing blood generates a frictional force. This produces a shear stress, which mainly has an impact on the endothelium, since these are the cells in contact with the fluid.[64] ECs *in vivo* are aligned in the direction of blood flow, and *in vivo* and *in vitro* experiments demonstrate that flow can cause ECs to alter their morphology to adopt this alignment (Fig. 62–6). In fact, ECs exhibit numerous responses to shear stresses, including alterations in morphology, mechanical properties, and gene expression (reviewed in Refs 64 and 65).

In model organisms, the manipulation of blood flow patterns can have a profound impact on cardiovascular development. For example, the vitelline veins in the avian yolk sac have been ligated to alter the hemodynamics of the developing embryo. Vitelline vein ligation alters the path through the heart adopted by blood flow originating from each region of the yolk sac.[66] Heart rate is also decreased, but there is a compensatory increase in cardiac output.[67] Although the ligation occurs at a site distant from the heart, these altered hemodynamics produce changes in cardiac morphology and disruption of the remodeling of the pharyngeal arch arteries (PAAs). Typical outcomes include ventricular septal defects, semilunar valve malformations, and PAA abnormalities.[66,67] Most recently, experiments in the zebrafish[68]

further demonstrate that hemodynamic forces are epigenetic factors required for normal heart morphogenesis. Blocking either inflow or outflow to the heart results in similar malformed, hypoplastic hearts with poor differentiation of the valves. The similarity between these phenotypes suggests that shear stress, rather than blood pressure, is the main morphogenetic influence, since obstructed inflow and outflow will both result in a reduced flow but are expected to have opposite effects on intracardiac pressure.[68]

During angiogenesis, local variation in hemodynamic forces likely exerts a major influence upon the remodeling of embryonic vessels,[30,69] particularly in determining which vessels are to be enlarged and in controlling the size they attain. For example, it is notable that the large yolk sac vessels develop only after there is significant flow when the connection with the intraembryonic vessels has been established. Defects in this connection are often associated with a failure of subsequent yolk sac remodeling.[32,33,70] Moreover, the vitelline vein ligation experiments just described lead to altered remodeling of the capillary plexus, producing a new vein that bypasses the ligation.[66] Thus, local changes of blood flow lead to alterations in the pattern of vessel remodeling.

The molecular basis of shear stress responses has yet to be fully characterized, but the wide variety of cellular and molecular responses observed is consistent with multiple structures acting as mechanosensors (see Fig. 62–6) and consequently with a diversity of molecules acting in shear stress signal transduction.[64] Because the EC layer provides an "interface" between blood and tissue, it serves as the primary mechanotransducer. Variations in flow result in altered levels of many vasoconstrictive and vasodilatory factors, including endothelin-1, prostacyclin, and nitric oxide.[64,69] These can certainly modulate vascular tone in response to hemodynamics, but such effects probably play roles late in vascular differentiation.[64,69]

Less is known about flow-responsive pathways in earlier vascular morphogenesis, but some key molecules in vascular development are also implicated in shear stress responses. For example, altered flow changes the EC cytoskeleton and the pattern of focal adhesions, the points of contact between ECs and extracellular matrix. Transmembrane integrins are prominent components of focal adhesions, where they bind extracellular adhesion proteins and link the extracellular matrix (ECM) to the actin filaments of the cytoskeleton. New integrin binding to the ECM activates the small GTPase Rac1. Rac1 activation mediates cell alignment and orientation of filamentous actin (F-actin) stress fibers, as well as flow-induced stimulation of the transcription factor nuclear factor kappa B (NF-kappaB).[71] Thus, EC integrins, important for vascular morphogenesis, also play a role in sensing shear stress.

One key transcriptional target of shear stress in ECs is PDGF-B, which is up-regulated by shear stress.[72] The up-regulation of the PDGF-B promoter is mediated by a shear stress–responsive element (SSRE) that is bound by NF-kappaB.[73] Since PDGF-B mediates recruitment of perivascular mural cells,[47] regulation of its expression by shear stress could link flow to stabilization of vessels during vascular development.

Hypoxia

In healthy adults, angiogenesis is primarily limited to select sites such as the female reproductive system, but extensive angiogenic responses (neovascularization) can accompany disruptions in oxygen homeostasis, such as those that occur during tumor growth or in tissue ischemia.[21] Evidence for oxygen tension governing angiogenic processes in disease states has led to investigation of whether such mechanisms operate during the normal vascular development *in utero*. Consistent with this idea, multiple components of the signaling systems responsible for normal vascular development are regulated by hypoxia. Notably, VEGF and VEGF receptor 2 are both up-regulated in hypoxic

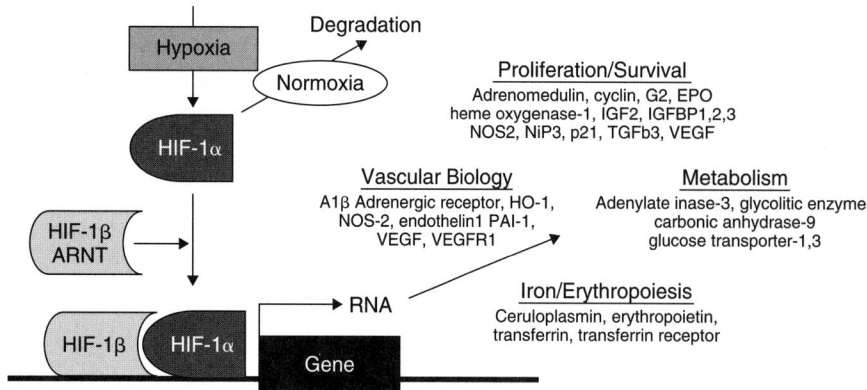

Proliferation/Survival
Adrenomedulin, cyclin, G2, EPO
heme oxygenase-1, IGF2, IGFBP1,2,3
NOS2, NiP3, p21, TGFb3, VEGF

Vascular Biology
A1β Adrenergic receptor, HO-1,
NOS-2, endothelin1 PAI-1,
VEGF, VEGFR1

Metabolism
Adenylate inase-3, glycolitic enzymes
carbonic anhydrase-9
glucose transporter-1,3

Iron/Erythropoiesis
Ceruloplasmin, erythropoietin,
transferrin, transferrin receptor

Figure 62–7. Hypoxia-mediated gene regulation through HIF-1α and HIF-1β. The level of HIF-1α is determined by the balance between hypoxia, which drives increased expression, and normoxia, which accentuates expression of signaling cascades, that result in degradation of HIF-1α. Under hypoxic conditions, HIF-1α and HIF-1β dimerize and then bind the hypoxia response element (HRE) in the regulatory region of several genes, resulting in transcription of numerous gene products.

conditions,[74,75] potentially enabling enhanced VEGF signaling to promote new blood vessel formation and/or promote survival of existing vessels. Additional hypoxia-responsive genes important for vascular morphogenesis include *Tie1*,[76] the angiopoietins *Ang-1* and *Ang-2*[77,78] and *PDGF-B*.[79] Many of these responses occur at the transcriptional level and are mediated by the hypoxia-induced transcription factor HIF-1, discussed later. However, hypoxia also affects expression by other mechanisms, such as specific increases in VEGF messenger RNA stability.[80]

Recently, some critical components of the oxygen-sensing pathways have been identified. Central to hypoxia-mediated control of gene expression is the hypoxia-inducible transcription factor HIF-1. HIF-1 target genes up-regulated in hypoxia are involved in increasing O_2 delivery (via erythropoiesis, vascularization, or vasodilation) or are involved in metabolic adaptation to limited O_2 (principally glycolysis) (reviewed in Ref 81). The HIF-1 factor is a heterodimeric complex,[82] consisting of a regulatory α subunit and a constitutive β subunit, both of which are helix-loop-helix PAS domain proteins (Fig. 62–7). The α subunits, Hif-1α and Hif-2α, confer the hypoxia responsiveness of the complex. Expression of HIF-1 increases exponentially with decreasing oxygen tension.[83] It is interesting that the majority of this up-regulation is achieved not through an increase in HIF-1α production in response to hypoxia, but rather through increased protein stability of the Hif-α subunits and diversion from the normal pathway of rapid protein degradation (reviewed in Refs 84 and 85).

With the exception of structures in direct contact with the atmosphere, such as the respiratory epithelium and outer layers of skin, the normal environment for most mammalian tissues is an O_2 concentration of around 3% to 5%, making the tissues "hypoxic" relative to the 20% atmospheric O_2 concentration. The intrauterine environment is likely at a similar low oxygen tension since the optimum O_2 concentration for *in vitro* culture of early mammalian embryos is 5%, not 20%.[86] Embryonic tissues are thus generally developing at low oxygen tensions but also appear to contain regions of significant hypoxia. Using the hypoxia marker pimonidazole hydrochloride, Lee and co-workers examined the spatiotemporal distribution of tissue hypoxia in the developing mouse embryo.[87] They found multiple domains of local hypoxia that were not only closely correlated with the Hif-1α and VEGF immunoreactivity but also were mapped to locations where angiogenesis is known to occur, including the extraembryonic tissues, neural tissue, intersomitic regions, and ventricles of the heart.[87] These data support the idea that during embryogenesis there is local tissue hypoxia that could modulate blood vessel morphogenesis through induction of VEGF or other HIF-1 responsive genes.

The existence of embryonic tissue hypoxia, together with the oxygen-tension effects on regulators of vascular morphogenesis, has led to the idea that the proper morphogenesis of the vascular system *depends* upon the relatively hypoxic state of tissues *in*

utero. Explant organ-culture models appear to confirm this idea, since EC survival and development of the vasculature are sensitive to oxygen tension.[88] Additional evidence supporting an important role for hypoxia in the regulation of vascular development comes from analysis of animals with targeted deficiencies in the HIF-1 regulatory cascade. Mice homozygous for null mutations in the Hif-1α gene die at midgestation with pericardial effusion and myocardial hyperplasia. There are vascular malformations, including defects in yolk sac remodeling, interruptions in the intersomitic vessels, and a marked deficiency of cephalic vessels, accompanied by dramatic cephalic vessel dilation.[89,90] It is surprising, however, that the defective remodeling and vascular regression do not appear to be related to a deficiency in VEGF; they may instead by a consequence of extensive cell death in mesenchyme, probably of neural crest origin.[91] These studies also found that glucose deprivation was able to stimulate VEGF expression independently of HIF-1. Therefore, in regions of vascular insufficiency, VEGF up-regulation may be achieved either by a response to inadequate glucose supply or by a response to hypoxia through HIF-1.[91]

Another member of the hypoxia-inducible factor family, Hif-2α (also known as hypoxia-inducible factor-like [HIFL]/endothelial PAS domain protein 1[EPAS1]), which is 48% similar to Hif-1α at the amino acid sequence level, can modulate expression of genes important for vascular development, including Tie2.[92] Mice deficient in Hif-2α die *in utero* and either exhibit a failure of vascular remodeling[93] or exhibit defects of catecholamine homeostasis coupled with heart failure.[94] Mice homozygous for a hypomorphic allele of Hif-2α are viable and apparently develop normally, but they exhibit a diminished response to changes in oxygen tension.[95] In a mouse model of retinopathy of prematurity, exposure of young animals to 75% O_2 for 5 days causes obliteration of retinal vessels, which is followed by neovascularization when the animals are returned to room air and the retina experiences hypoxia due to vascular insufficiency. Following the transfer to room air, Hif-2α expression levels in the eye are around 20% of normal in the hypomorphic Hif-2α mutants, and erythropoietin (Epo) levels are similarly reduced. The retinas of these animals do not undergo neovascularization and instead undergo retinal degeneration. Recombinant Epo restores neovascularization in mutant retinas, suggesting overlap between Hif-2α functions in regulating oxygen delivery and in hypoxia-induced neovascularization.[95]

Two other components of the HIF-1 pathway, Hif-1β (also known as aryl hydrocarbon receptor nuclear translocator, ARNT) and VHL (von Hippel–Lindau syndrome tumor suppressor), also have been studied in the mouse by targeted gene disruption experiments. Deficiencies in these factors have been shown to have profound impacts on vascular development, generating defects that ultimately result in embryonic lethality.[96-100] Animals deficient for Hif-1β also have defective angiogenesis in yolk sac and branchial arch arteries.[97] Defects are also seen in the placenta, where there is a failure of the labyrinth to vascularize.[98,100] The mechanism by which Hif-1β deficiency disrupts placental vascular development has not yet been established, but there has been considerable progress toward identifying the specific cell types and molecules involved.

Studies in which Hif-1β null ES cells are combined with wild-type cells, in chimeric embryos or with tetraploid embryos, demonstrate that Hif-1β function is required in the trophoblast cells rather than in the embryonic endothelial component of the placenta.[100] Placental levels of VEGF are unaltered in Hif-1β null embryos, but VEGFR2 is significantly lower in the labyrinth endothelial, trophoblast, and giant cells.[99] Deficiency for VHL, which normally serves to "mark" the Hif-1α subunits for degradation, also results in embryonic lethality from defects in the development of the placental vasculature. On the maternal side, the capillary networks of the placenta form by angiogenesis, whereas on the embryonic side, the first capillaries develop in the allantois by vasculogenesis.[101] In VHL-deficient embryos, there is a lack of embryonic blood vessels within the placental labyrinth, which leads to the formation of a severely disrupted, hemorrhagic placental site.[96]

Certainly, VHL and Hif-1β may each have functions besides their contributions to HIF-1 action; nevertheless, the embryonic and placental defects observed in mice with deficiencies in four separate components of the HIF-1 hypoxia-response cascade (Hif-1α, Hif-2α, Hif-1β, and VHL) collectively provide strong genetic evidence for oxygen tension acting as a regulator of cardiovascular development *in utero*. For the future, examining how the cellular sensing of oxygen tension is integrated with vascular morphogenesis can be expected to offer significant insight into how the developing vascular system is matched to the metabolic needs of embryonic tissues.

Development of Pulmonary Vessels

Although treatment of airway immaturity in the premature lung is a significant focus of clinical effort in neonatal intensive care units, the pathology associated with abnormal development of the pulmonary vascular bed has been one of the least-studied areas in cardiovascular biology. Establishment of a dual blood supply, considerable development after birth, and an apparent dependence on airway formation all combine to make pulmonary vascular ontogeny an extremely challenging area of research. Much of what is known is currently descriptive in nature. Nevertheless, a renewed interest in this vascular bed,[102-106] accompanied by the use of new molecular-genetic tools, cellular markers, and culture models,[103,105,107-109] is beginning to provide answers to some long-standing questions and may provide novel strategies for therapeutic intervention.

Based primarily on epithelial processes, lung development has been divided into four or five stages (Fig. 62–8).[110,111] The embryonic stage (26 days to 6 weeks in humans) begins with the first appearance of lung buds as outpocketings of the foregut endoderm, surrounded by splanchnic mesoderm. The pseudoglandular stage (6 to 16 weeks) is characterized by rapid and extensive epithelial branching so that by the end of this stage, all preacinar airways are present. During the canalicular stage (16 to 28 weeks), the airways continue to branch, the mesenchyme thins, capillaries come to underlie the epithelium, and effective blood-gas barriers are first formed. The epithelium differentiates into type I and type II pneumocytes, and surfactant production begins. The saccular stage (26 to 36 weeks) features division of distal air spaces into smooth-walled structures known as saccules. In the alveolar stage (36 weeks onward), the saccules are remodeled into alveoli.

The lung epithelium is closely associated with developing vasculature from the earliest stage. Differentiation of a ventral vascular plexus into which a bud of foregut endoderm protrudes was first described in 1931 by Chang[112] and has since been

observed by numerous investigators using a variety of animal models.[113] The arterial system of the lung is ultimately connected through the sixth pharyngeal arch, which becomes the pulmonary artery. The venous system of the lung connects directly to the left atrium. A major issue in past decades has been whether the early vascularization of the lung and its connection to the arterial and venous systems involves vasculogenesis, angiogenesis, or some combination of the two. Incorporated in this question is the origin of the ECs in the pulmonary vessels. Are their precursors endogenous to the lung, or do they immigrate into the lung from elsewhere?

Some of the debate over the relative contributions of angiogenesis or vasculogenesis in pulmonary vascular development may reflect the limitations of the individual techniques employed. Classic histologic analysis and methods that rely on the presence of a patent lumen, such as India ink injections and Mercox casts, tend to suggest penetration of the lung primordia by angiogenic mechanisms arising from major pharyngeal arch arteries.[18] On the other hand, using marker gene expression to identify individual ECs or precursors reveals more cell behavior that is not associated with a definitive vessel, behavior characterized as vasculogenesis.[103-105,113] Figure 62–9A shows a reconstruction[105] of thorax sections from a 34-day-old human embryo, illustrating the early vascular network of the lung primordia in relation to the heart and major vessels. The presumptive pulmonary arteries and pulmonary veins are already present and associate through a capillary plexus. Sections from transgenic mice expressing β-galactosidase in all ECs (Fig. 62–9B) reveal a similar continuity between the future arterial, venous, and capillary vessels.[103] In the periphery of the developing pseudoglandular-stage human or mouse lung, ECs assemble into local networks before the anastomosis with the intrapulmonary arteries.[18,106] Thus, vasculogenesis is responsible for much of the early lung vascular development.[106]

At this stage, two classes of ECs can already be identified: those associated with smooth muscle actin (SMA)-positive mural cells, and those that are not.[106] These differences reflect distinctions between capillaries and major vessels, suggesting that extensive differentiation of the lung vasculature begins very early in lung morphogenesis. Allografts of early pseudoglandular-stage mouse lungs under the kidney capsule have been shown to allow for extensive lung development and maturation to the saccular stage, including formation of appropriate vasculature.[108] Genetic marking of host ECs revealed that all vessels within the lung were derived from the graft. Therefore, at the time of grafting the explant contained all the ECs and angioblasts required for production of the complete saccular-stage vascular tree, independent of angiogenic contributions from the extrapulmonary vasculature. Connections with the host circulation were made, but host vessels never penetrated the graft (host to graft), implying that the lung tissue prevents other vessels from entering it while maintaining the intrinsic ability to establish angiogenic connections (graft to host) with the circulatory system.

It was previously thought that the canalicular stage represented a burst of vascular growth/differentiation, but recent studies relating EC number to lung protein content (lung size) refute this idea. It now appears that the pulmonary vasculature expands smoothly, rather than in a burst, so that the increase in the vasculature with gestation age largely mirrors the total growth of the lung.[103] Of importance in this period, however, is an apparent transition from vasculogenesis to angiogenesis. In particular, whereas undifferentiated mesenchyme in the early pseudoglandular lung is highly proliferative, the endothelium now exhibits a greater proliferative rate than the remaining mesenchyme, suggesting that the vascular network may be growing by angiogenesis as well.[105]

Lung vasculature development parallels the branching morphogensis of the lung epithelium (reviewed in Ref 114), which suggests that epithelial and vascular development are somehow

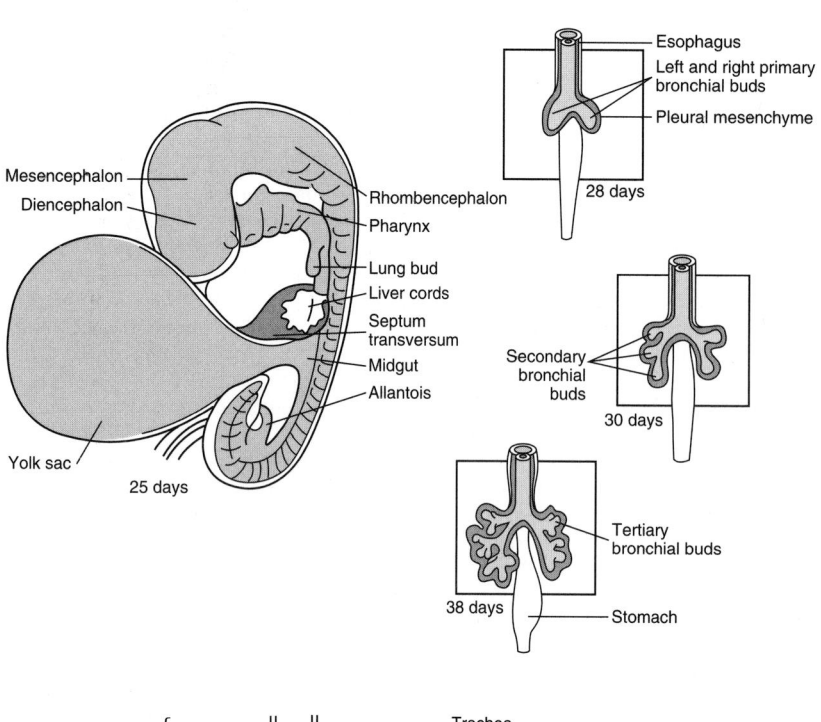

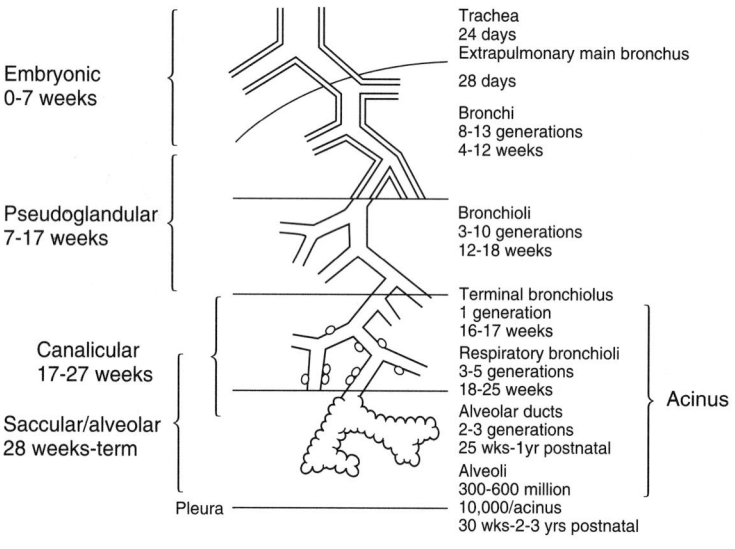

Stage	Mouse	Human
Embryonic	E9-14.2	3-7 wk
Pseudoglandular	E14.2-16.6	7-17 wk
Canalicular	E16-17.5	17-27 wk
Saccular	E17.5-5d p.c.	24-38 wk
Alveolar	5-30 p.c.	36.5 yrs p.c.

Figure 62–8. The critical stages of lung development, with a comparison of equivalent developmental stages in both mouse and human embryos. These stages are based on branching morphogenesis and relation to alveolar development. Comparative stages in vascular development have not yet been fully defined. (Adapted from Larsen WJ (ed): Human Embryology, 2nd ed. New York, Churchill Livingstone, 1997, p 138; and Hislop AA: J Anat *201*:325, 2002.)

coordinated. This would likely demand active signaling between epithelium and ECs. Tissue recombination experiments with embryonic lung mesenchyme and epithelium confirm that the lung epithelium produces some factor(s) that promotes or maintains normal vascular development in lung mesenchyme.[109] Separating the lung mesenchyme and epithelium disrupts the normal spatial relationship between epithelium and endothelium, but recombining the separated epithelium and mesenchyme and culturing them together generates new EC patterns in appropriate positions relative to the epithelium. Furthermore, culturing lung mesenchyme in the absence of epithelium results in decreased mesenchymal proliferation and increased apoptosis, as well as a marked reduction in the number of ECs.[109]

The pulmonary ECs express VEGF receptors 1 and 2. These likely mediate signals from the nearby epithelium, which expressed VEGF ligand.[106, 115-118] Early lethality of VEGF-null mutations has precluded use of these mice to study the dependence

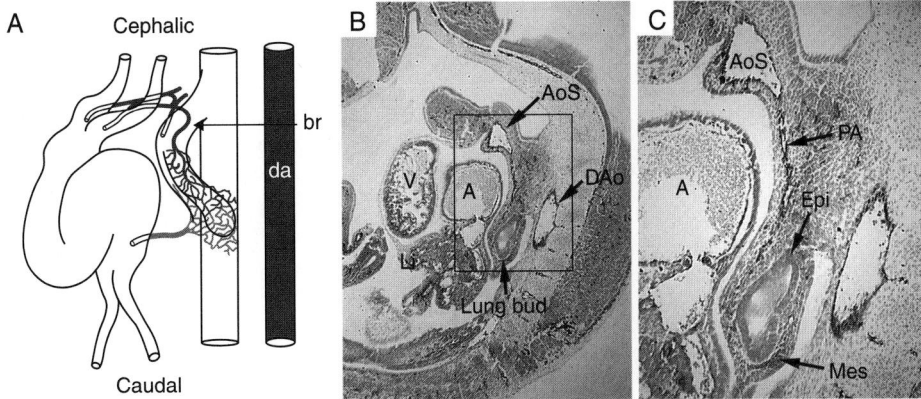

Figure 62–9. A, Diagram produced from a serial reconstruction of a 34-day human embryo, showing continuity of the lung bud capillary network with central vascular structures from the onset of lung development. **B,** Low-power and **C,** high-power magnification of a sagittal section through an embryonic day 10.5 mouse embryo of similar gestational age to that of the human embryo in **A.** ECs can be identified by β-galactosidase activity resulting from lacZ inserted into the Flk1 locus. The pulmonary artery (PA) can be seen connecting the aortic sac (AoS) and lung mesoderm (Mes). These examples document that in both human and mouse, development of the pulmonary vascular bed occurs in continuity with the major vascular structures of the embryo. br = bronchus; da = dorsal aorta; V = ventricle of the heart; A = atrium of the heart; DAo = dorsal aorta; Li = liver; and Epi = epithelium of the lung bud. (Adapted from Hall SM, et al: Am J Respir Cell Mol Biol *26*:333, 2002; and Schachtner SK, et al: Am J Respir Cell Mol Biol *22*:157, 2000.)

of pulmonary vascular development on VEGF, but other approaches have recently revealed the importance and complexity of VEGF signaling in the lung. Through alternative splicing, the VEGF gene produces multiple protein isoforms that differ in their abilities to bind cell-surface and ECM-associated heparan sulfate proteoglycans and the VEGF receptors (reviewed in Ref 119).

In the mouse, there are at least three such isoforms: $VEGF_{120}$, $VEGF_{164}$, and $VEGF_{188}$, of which only $VEGF_{164}$ and $VEGF_{188}$ can bind heparan sulfate. These heparan sulfate-binding VEGFs are the predominant isoforms expressed in the developing lung.[117, 118] Upon synthesis by the epithelium, VEGFs are localized to the subepithelial matrix. Heparin-bound $VEGF_{164}$ on beads implanted into pseudoglandular-stage lung explants induces neovascularization around the bead, suggesting that VEGF localized close to the distal epithelium helps direct the pattern of new blood vessel formation, linking epithelial and vascular morphogenesis.[117] Isoform-specific gene knock-out experiments support this idea but also suggest that the heparan-binding VEGF isoforms may be uniquely required only for the microvessels of the pulmonary vascular tree. Mice engineered to produce $VEGF_{120}$, but not $VEGF_{164}$ or $VEGF_{188}$, survive to birth but exhibit pulmonary hypoplasia, with reductions in air spaces and multiple defects in pulmonary vasculature.[120] The diameter and branching patterns of the preacinar vessels are relatively unaffected, but animals producing only $VEGF_{120}$ have dramatically fewer small, but dilated, peripheral vessels (Fig. 62–10). Blood-gas barriers are reduced in number, and intervening cells aberrantly separate the capillaries from the air space.[120] These data point to a requirement for epithelium-derived matrix-binding VEGF isoforms in the generation and proper juxtaposition of capillaries with alveolar type I cells.

Pulmonary vascular development depends upon the combinatorial action of multiple signals from the lung epithelium as well as inputs from other cell types, and the repertoire of signals is not limited to the VEGF signaling cascade. During branching morphogenesis, distal lung epithelium expresses high levels of the Wnt7b gene,[121] a member of the Wnt family of at least 19 mammalian growth factor genes (reviewed in Refs 122 and 123). Wnt7b-deficient mice die at birth from respiratory failure associated with hypoplastic lungs that exhibit pulmonary hemorrhage. There are deficiencies in the integrity of the vascular

smooth muscle, including both vascular smooth muscle cell (VSMC) hypertrophy and apoptosis.[121] These observations suggest that a Wnt7b signal from the lung epithelium promotes mesenchymal proliferation in the early lung and later supports VSMC differentiation and/or survival. Together, the studies on the actions of VEGFs and Wnt7b indicate that the epithelium produces factors controlling and supporting pulmonary vascular development at many levels that include:

1. Promoting and localizing neovascularization;
2. Regulating vessel size;
3. Enabling proper association between capillaries and epithelium; and
4. Regulating the behavior of VSMC on larger vessels.

Conversely, reciprocal signaling likely occurs from the vessels to the lung epithelium since pulmonary vasculature influences epithelial morphogenesis. Interfering with VEGF signaling in the neonatal animal, normally a time of significant alveolargenesis, provides an example of this phenomenon. Mice in which VEGF signaling has been blocked for the first 5 days of life have lungs that appear immature and exhibit a less complex alveolar pattern than normal, establishing that ongoing VEGF-mediated development or function or both of the vasculature is essential for normal alveolar morphogenesis.[34]

Epigenetic factors like hypoxia and shear stress are almost certain to be important for pulmonary vascular development. An example from our own work on the role of oxygen tension in pulmonary vascular development is shown in Fig. 62–11. Mouse lung explants cultured in 3% O_2 and 19% O_2 exhibit very different patterns of EC localization (revealed by whole-mount immunohistochemisty for the EC-specific adhesion molecule PECAM/CD31). In low-oxygen tension, comparable to that detected *in utero*, many PECAM-positive cells are present, and an extensive vascular network, including major vessels, is apparent. In contrast, the lungs cultured in 19% O_2 exhibit much lower levels of PECAM immunoreactivity, with most ECs present being located in clusters of small vessels near the periphery of the explant. Thus, variation in oxygen tension profoundly alters EC survival and vascular patterning in developing lungs.

The relationship between oxygen tension and lung development has yet to be extensively studied at the molecular level, but recent genetic evidence suggests that the hypoxia-inducible

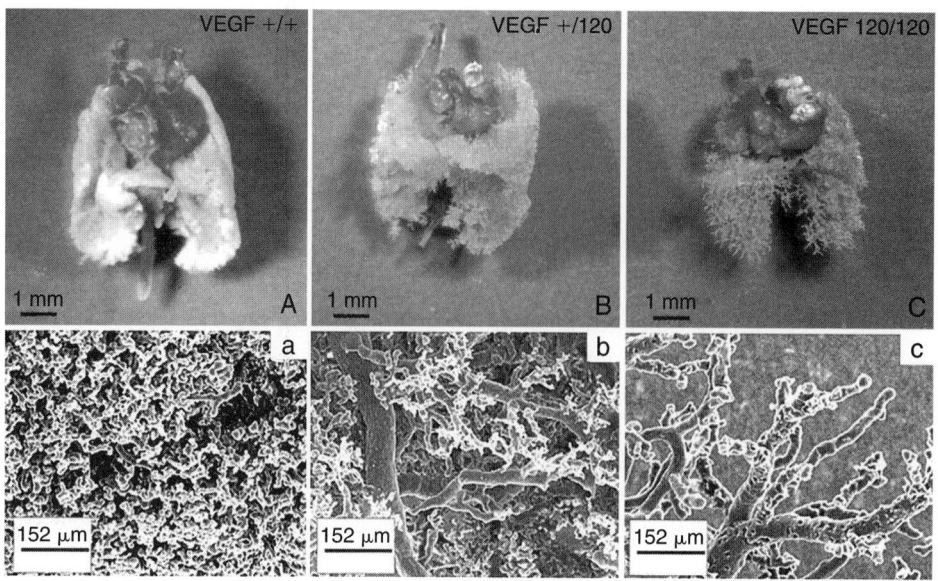

Figure 62–10. The impact of altered VEGF signaling on pulmonary vascular development. Lung Mercox casts (**A–C**) and scanning electron micrographs (**a–c**) from E17 wildtype (**A, a**), heterozygous $VEGF_{120/+}$ (**B, b**), or homozygous $VEGF_{120/120}$ mice (**C, c**). Replacement of all VEGF isoforms with $VEGF_{120}$ alone results in a marked, "dose-dependent" reduction in the number of small peripheral vessels without a noticeable impact on the preacinar vessels. (Adapted from Galambos C, et al: Am J Respir Cell Mol Biol 27:194, 2002.)

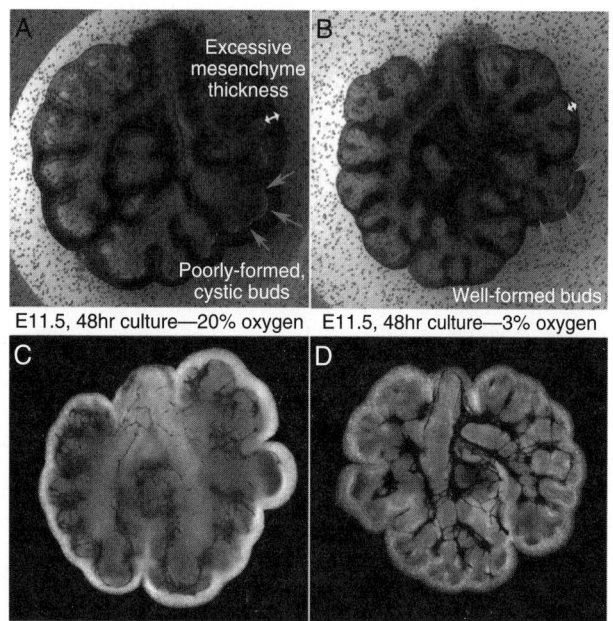

Figure 62–11. A comparison of E11.5 mouse lung buds grown under normoxia (**A, C**) or hypoxia (**B, D**). In normoxia, branching morphogenesis is diminished, with development of poorly formed cystic buds and excessive mesenchymal thickening when compared with that seen in hypoxia. **C** and **D**, Whole-mount immunohistochemical staining with anti-PECAM/CD31 antibody to delineate vascular development. Under hypoxic conditions there is a marked accentuation in larger vessel development (in the regions surrounding the main bronchi), combined with an attenuation of endothelial differentiation surrounding the distal epithelial buds. These data suggest that hypoxia may not only affect endothelial proliferation and survival but also play a critical role in promoting the vascular remodeling required for more proximal large vessel formation.

factor Hif-2α regulates VEGF, which in turn is required for proper lung maturation, including the production of surfactant.[124] Hif-2α-deficient animals that do not die *in utero* breathe irregularly at birth, are cyanotic, and succumb to severe respiratory failure within a few hours. Analysis of lung morphogenesis in these animals reveals that Hif-2α is required both before and after birth to establish an adequate lung microvasculature, to thin the alveolar septa, and to remodel the vessels juxtaposing the endothelium and type 1 pneumocytes. The lung epithelium is immature, and there is abnormally low production of surfactant phospholipids and surfactant proteins A, B, and D. The normal rise in pulmonary VEGF levels during late gestation fails to occur in Hif-2α-deficient animals, which suggests the possible involvement of VEGF in their lung pathology. Consistent with this idea, inhibiting prenatal VEGF signaling by intra-amniotic injection of neutralizing antibodies to VEGFR2 results in a comparable level of lung immaturity. Conversely, respiratory distress resulting from premature delivery of mice can be alleviated by *in utero* or intra-tracheal administration of VEGF, which results in thinner alveolar septa and increased surfactant production.[124] Studies such as these reveal components of the complex interactions among oxygen tension, lung vascular development, and maturation of the lung epithelium, which may be disrupted by premature birth or oxygen therapy. Understanding such interactions has important clinical implications, since disruption of the lung vasculature may contribute to poor outcomes in bronchopulmonary dysplasia, a chronic lung disease in infants that is typically associated with both premature birth and oxygen therapy for acute respiratory failure.[125]

Likewise, flow and resultant shear stress may play a significant role in pulmonary vascular development. Previous work utilizing *in utero* sheep models suggested that pulmonary blood flow represented only a small percentage of combined cardiac output (3.7% to 7%), with no significant increase in flow despite a dramatic increase in vascular density during the last trimester.[126] Therefore, blood flow was not thought to be a primary modulator of pulmonary vascular growth. However, more recent studies on human fetuses suggest that at least 11% of the combined cardiac output from 11 to 41 weeks of gestation is directed to the lung.[127] Additional studies report a gestational increase in pulmonary blood flow from 13% to 25% of combined cardiac output by the 30th week of gestation.[128] Similarly, *in vitro* studies suggest that flow to the pulmonary vascular bed may increase vascular morphogenesis.[129] Although the exact role of flow in pulmonary vascular development remains to be defined, it will likely play a significant role in defining optimal pulmonary development.

CONCLUSIONS AND FUTURE PROSPECTS

There has been an explosion of new information concerning the molecular regulation of vascular development. However, future efforts to characterize the molecular genetic pathways governing vascular morphogenesis in the lung and elsewhere will need to go beyond molecular characterization and examine the interplay of developmental genetics with shear stress, hypoxia, and other epigenetic phenomena during critical periods of development. In this review, we have highlighted just a few of the molecular players that are involved in the production of the vascular system. Many more await discovery. The challenge ahead is not only to identify the interactions among molecules, cells, and environment that govern vessel morphogenesis, but also to build the growing knowledge of these interactions into useful models of vascular development that can help us understand vascular system defects and direct future therapeutic interventions.

REFERENCES

1. His W: Lecithoblast und Angioblast der Wirbeltiere. Ahandl math-phys CI sachs Ges 26:171, 1900.
2. Reagan FP: Vascularization phenomena in fragments of embryonic bodies completely isolated from yolk sac entoderm. Anat Rec 9:329, 1915.
3. Pardanaud L, et al: Vasculogenesis in the early quail blastodisc as studied with a monoclonal antibody recognizing endothelial cells. Development 100:339, 1987.
4. Coffin JD, Poole TJ: Embryonic vascular development: immunohistochemical identification of the origin and subsequent morphogenesis of the major vessel primordia in quail embryos. Development 102:735, 1988.
5. Drake CJ, Fleming PA: Vasculogenesis in the day 6.5 to 9.5 mouse embryo. Blood 95:1671, 2000.
6. Sabin FR: Studies on the origin of blood vessels and of red corpuscles as seen in the living blastoderm of the chick during the second day of incubation. Contrib Embryol 9:213, 1920.
7. Murray PDF: The development in vitro of the blood of the early chick embryo. Proc R Soc (Lond) B 111:497, 1932.
8. Choi K: The hemangioblast: a common progenitor of hematopoietic and endothelial cells. J Hematother Stem Cell Res 11:91, 2002.
9. Eichmann A, et al: Vasculogenesis and the search for the hemangioblast. J Hematother Stem Cell Res 11:207, 2002.
10. Kubo H, Alitalo K: The bloody fate of endothelial stem cells. Genes Dev 17:322, 2003.
11. Shalaby F, et al: Failure of blood-island formation and vasculogenesis in Flk-1-deficient mice. Nature 376:62, 1995.
12. Shalaby F, et al: A requirement for Flk1 in primitive and definitive hematopoiesis and vasculogenesis. Cell 89:981, 1997.
13. Ema M, et al: Combinatorial effects of Flk1 and Tal1 on vascular and hematopoietic development in the mouse. Genes Dev 17:380, 2003.
14. DeRuiter MC, et al: Embryonic endothelial cells transdifferentiate into mesenchymal cells expressing smooth muscle actins in vivo and in vitro. Circ Res 80:444, 1997.
15. Noden DW: Embryonic origins and assembly of blood vessels. Am Rev Respir Dis 140:1097, 1989.
16. Poole TJ, Coffin JD: Vasculogenesis and angiogenesis: two distinct morphogenetic mechanisms establish embryonic vascular patterns. J Exp Zool 251:21, 1989.
17. Risau W: Vasculogenesis, angiogenesis and endothelial cell differentiation during embryonic development. In Feinberg RN, et al (eds): The Development of the Vascular System, Vol 14. Basel, Karger, 1991, pp 27–31.
18. deMello DE, et al: Early fetal development of lung vasculature. Am J Respir Cell Mol Biol 16:568, 1997.
19. deMello DE, Reid LM: Embryonic and early fetal development of human lung vasculature and its functional implications. Pediatr Dev Pathol 3:439, 2000.
20. Folkman J: Angiogenesis in cancer, vascular, rheumatoid and other diseases. Nat Med 1:27, 1995.
21. Timar J, et al: Angiogenesis-dependent diseases and angiogenesis therapy. Pathol Oncol Res 7:85, 2001.
22. Ribatti D, et al: Postnatal vasculogenesis. Mech Dev 100:157, 2001.
23. Fong GH, et al: Role of the Flt-1 receptor tyrosine kinase in regulating the assembly of vascular endothelium. Nature 376:66, 1995.
24. Drake CJ, et al: VEGF regulates cell behavior during vasculogenesis. Dev Biol 224:178, 2000.
25. Rupp PA, Little CD: Integrins in vascular development. Circ Res 89:566, 2001.
26. Drake CJ, et al: Antibodies to β1 integrins cause alterations of aortic vasculogenesis, in vivo. Dev Dyn 193:83, 1992.
27. Drake CJ, et al: An antagonist of integrin alpha v beta-3 prevents maturation of blood vessels during embryonic neovascularization. J Cell Sci 108:2655, 1995.
28. Bader BL, et al: Extensive vasculogenesis, angiogenesis, and organogenesis precede lethality in mice lacking all alpha v integrins. Cell 95:507, 1998.
29. Hodivala-Dilke KM, et al: Beta3-integrin-deficient mice are a model for Glanzmann thrombasthenia showing placental defects and reduced survival. J Clin Invest 103:229, 1999.
30. Risau W: Mechanisms of angiogenesis. Nature 386:671, 1997.
31. Carmeliet P, Collen D: Molecular basis of angiogenesis. Role of VEGF and VE-cadherin. Ann N Y Acad Sci 902:249, 2000.
32. Ferrara N: Heterozygous embryonic lethality induced by targeted inactivation of the VEGF gene. Nature 380:439, 1996.
33. Carmeliet P, et al: Abnormal blood vessel development and lethality in embryos lacking a single VEGF allele. Nature 380:435, 1996.
34. Gerber HP, et al: VEGF is required for growth and survival in neonatal mice. Development 126:1149, 1999.
35. Patan S: TIE1 and TIE2 receptor tyrosine kinases inversely regulate embryonic angiogenesis by the mechanism of intussusceptive microvascular growth. Microvasc Res 56:1, 1998.
36. Ward NL, Dumont DJ: The angiopoietins and Tie2/Tek: adding to the complexity of cardiovascular development. Semin Cell Dev Biol 13:19, 2002.
37. Maisonpierre PC, et al: Angiopoietin-2, a natural antagonist for Tie2 that disrupts in vivo angiogenesis. Science 277:55, 1997.
38. Gale NW, et al: Angiopoietin-2 is required for postnatal angiogenesis and lymphatic patterning, and only the latter role is rescued by angiopoietin-1. Dev Cell 3:411, 2002.
39. Veikkola T, Alitalo K: Dual role of Ang2 in postnatal angiogenesis and lymphangiogenesis. Dev Cell 3:302, 2002.
40. Ramsauer M, D'Amore PA: Getting Tie(2) up in angiogenesis. J Clin Invest 110:1615, 2002.
41. Lobov IB, et al: Angiopoietin-2 displays VEGF-dependent modulation of capillary structure and endothelial cell survival in vivo. Proc Natl Acad Sci U S A 99:11205, 2002.
42. Puri MC, et al: The receptor tyrosine kinase TIE is required for integrity and survival of vascular endothelial cells. EMBO J 14:5884, 1995.
43. Betsholtz C, et al: Developmental roles of platelet-derived growth factors. Bioessays 23:494, 2001.
44. Leveen P, et al: Mice deficient for PDGF-B show renal, cardiovascular, and hematological abnormalities. Genes Dev 8:1875, 1994.
45. Soriano P: Abnormal kidney development and hematological disorders in PDGF beta-receptor mutant mice. Genes Dev 8:1888, 1994.
46. Lindahl P: Pericyte loss and microaneurysm formation in PDGF-B-deficient mice. Science 277:242, 1997.
47. Hellström M, et al: Role of PDGF-B and PDGFR-beta in recruitment of vascular smooth muscle cells and pericytes during embryonic blood vessel formation in the mouse. Development 126:3047, 1999.
48. Hellström M, et al: Lack of pericytes leads to endothelial hyperplasia and abnormal vascular morphogenesis. J Cell Biol 153:543, 2001.
49. Wang HU, et al: Molecular distinction and angiogenic interaction between embryonic arteries and veins revealed by ephrin-B2 and its receptor Eph-B4. Cell 93:741, 1998.
50. Adams RH, et al: Roles of ephrin-B ligands and Eph-B receptors in cardiovascular development: demarcation of arterial/venous domains, vascular morphogenesis, and sprouting angiogenesis. Genes Dev 13:295, 1999.
51. Gerety SS, et al: Symmetrical mutant phenotypes of the receptor Eph-B4 and its specific transmembrane ligand ephrin-B2 in cardiovascular development. Mol Cell 4:403, 1999.
52. Wigel JT, Oliver G: Prox1 function is required for the development of the murine lymphatic system. Cell 98:769, 1999.
53. de la Pompa JL, et al: Role of the NF-ATc transcription factor in morphogenesis of cardiac valves and septum. Nature 392:182, 1998.
54. Ranger AM, et al: The transcription factor NF-ATc is essential for cardiac valve formation. Nature 392:186, 1998.
55. Holland SJ, et al: Bidirectional signalling through the EPH-family receptor Nuk and its transmembrane ligands. Nature 383:722, 1996.
56. Kaipainen A, et al: Expression of the fms-like tyrosine kinase 4 gene becomes restricted to lymphatic endothelium during development. Proc Natl Acad Sci U S A 92:3566, 1995.
57. Banerji S, et al: LYVE-1, a new homologue of the CD44 glycoprotein, is a lymph-specific receptor for hyaluronan. J Cell Biol 144:789, 1999.
58. Oliver G, Harvey N: A stepwide model of the development of lymphatic vasculature. Ann NY Acad Sci 979:159, 2002.
59. Baldwin M, et al: Molecular control of lymphangiogenesis. BioEssays 24:1030, 2002.
60. Sabin FR: On the origin of the lymphatic system from the veins, and the development of the lymph hearts and thoracic duct in the pig. Am J Anat 1:367, 1902.

61. Sabin FR: On the development of the superficial lymphatics in the skin of the pig. Am J Anat 3:183, 1904.

62. Shima DT, Mailhos C: Vascular developmental biology: getting nervous. Curr Opin Genet Dev 10:536, 2000.

63. Mukouyama YS, et al: Sensory nerves determine the pattern of arterial differentiation and blood vessel branching in the skin. Cell 109:693, 2002.

64. Davies PF: Flow-mediated endothelial mechanotransduction. Physiol Rev 75:519, 1995.

65. Topper JN, Gimbrone MA Jr: Blood flow and vascular gene expression: fluid shear stress as a modulator of endothelial phenotype. Mol Med Today 5:40, 1999.

66. Hogers B, et al: Extraembryonic venous obstructions lead to cardiovascular malformations and can be embryolethal. Cardiovasc Res 41:87, 1999.

67. Broekhuizen MLA, et al: Altered hemodynamics in chick embryos after extraembryonic venous obstruction. Ultrasound Obstet Gynecol 13:437, 1999.

68. Hove JR, et al: Intracardiac fluid forces are an essential epigenetic factor for embryonic cardiogenesis. Nature 421:172, 2003.

69. Risau W, Flamme I: Vasculogenesis. Annu Rev Cell Dev Biol 11:73, 1995.

70. Heine UI, et al: Effects of retinoid deficiency on the development of the heart and vascular system of the quail embryo. Virchows Arch B Cell Pathol Mol Pathol 50:135, 1985.

71. Tzima E, et al: Activation of Rac1 by shear stress in endothelial cells mediates both cytoskeletal reorganization and effects on gene expression. EMBO J 21:6791, 2002.

72. Resnick N, et al: Platelet-derived growth factor B chain promoter contains a cis-acting fluid shear-stress-responsive element. Proc Natl Acad Sci U S A 90:4591, 1993.

73. Khachigian LM, et al: Nuclear factor-kappa B interacts functionally with the platelet-derived growth factor B-chain shear-stress response element in vascular endothelial cells exposed to fluid shear stress. J Clin Invest 96:1169, 1995.

74. Shweiki D, et al: Vascular endothelial growth factor induced by hypoxia may mediate hypoxia-initiated angiogenesis. Nature 359:843, 1992.

75. Waltenberger J, et al: Functional upregulation of the vascular endothelial growth factor receptor KDR by hypoxia. Circulation 94:1647, 1996.

76. McCarthy MJ, et al: The endothelial receptor tyrosine kinase tie-1 is upregulated by hypoxia and vascular endothelial growth factor. FEBS Lett 423:334, 1998.

77. Enholm B, et al: Comparison of VEGF, VEGF-B, VEGF-C and Ang-1 mRNA regulation by serum, growth factors, oncoproteins and hypoxia. Oncogene 14:2475, 1997.

78. Mandriota SJ, Pepper MS: Regulation of angiopoietin-2 mRNA levels in bovine microvascular endothelial cells by cytokines and hypoxia. Circ Res 83:852, 1998.

79. Kourembanas S, et al: Oxygen tension regulates the expression of the platelet-derived growth factor-B chain gene in human endothelial cells. J Clin Invest 86:670, 1990.

80. Semenza GL, et al: Regulation of cardiovascular development and physiology by hypoxia-inducible factor 1. Ann N Y Acad Sci 874:262, 1999.

81. Ikeda E, et al: Hypoxia-induced transcriptional activation and increased mRNA stability of vascular endothelial growth factor in C6 glioma cells. J Biol Chem 270:19761, 1995.

82. Wang GL, et al: Hypoxia-inducible factor 1 is a basic-helix-loop-helix-PAS heterodimer regulated by cellular O₂ tension. Proc Natl Acad Sci U S A 92:5510, 1995.

83. Jiang BH, et al: Hypoxia-inducible factor 1 levels vary exponentially over a physiologically relevant range of O₂ tension. Am J Physiol 271:C1172, 1996.

84. Lando D, et al: Oxygen-dependent regulation of hypoxia-inducible factors by prolyl and asparaginyl hydroxylation. Eur J Biochem 270:781, 2003.

85. Maxwell PH, Ratcliffe PJ: Oxygen sensors and angiogenesis. Semin Cell Dev Biol 13:29, 2002.

86. Maltepe E, Simon MC: Oxygen, genes, and development: an analysis of the role of hypoxic gene regulation during murine vascular development. J Mol Med 76:391, 1998.

87. Lee YM, et al: Determination of hypoxic region by hypoxia marker in developing mouse embryos in vivo: a possible signal for vessel development. Dev Dyn 220:175, 2001.

88. Loughna S, et al: Effects of oxygen on vascular patterning in Tie1/LacZ metanephric kidneys in vitro. Biochem Biophys Res Comm 247:361, 1998.

89. Iyer NV, et al: Cellular and developmental control of O₂ homeostasis by hypoxia-inducible factor 1α. Genes Dev 12:149, 1998.

90. Ryan HE, et al: HIF-1alpha is required for solid tumor formation and embryonic vascularization. EMBO J 17:3005, 1998.

91. Kotch LE, et al: Defective vascularization of HIF-1α-null embryos is not associated with VEGF deficiency but with mesenchymal cell death. Dev Biol 209:254, 1999.

92. Tian H, et al: Endothelial PAS domain protein 1 (EPAS1), a transcription factor selectively expressed in endothelial cells. Genes Dev 11:72, 1997.

93. Peng J, et al: The transcription factor EPAS-1/hypoxia-inducible factor 2 plays an important role in vascular remodeling. Proc Natl Acad Sci U S A 97:8386, 2000.

94. Tian H, et al: The hypoxia-responsive transcription factor EPAS1 is essential for catecholamine homeostasis and protection against heart failure during embryonic development. Genes Dev 12:3320, 1998.

95. Morita T, et al: HLF/HIF-2α is a key factor in retinopathy of prematurity in association with erythropoietin. EMBO J 22:1134, 2003.

96. Gnarra JR, et al: Defective placental vasculogenesis causes embryonic lethality in VHL-deficient mice. Proc Natl Acad Sci U S A 94:9102, 1997.

97. Maltepe E, et al: Abnormal angiogenesis and responses to glucose and oxygen deprivation in mice lacking the protein ARNT. Nature 386:403, 1997.

98. Kozak KR, et al: ARNT-deficient mice and placental differentiation. Dev Biol 191:297, 1997.

99. Abbott BD, Buckalew AR: Placental defects in ARNT-knockout conceptus correlate with localized decreases in VEGF-R2, Ang-1, and Tie-2. Dev Dyn 219:526, 2000.

100. Adelman DM, et al: Placental cell fates are regulated in vivo by HIF-mediated hypoxia responses. Genes Dev 14:3191, 2000.

101. Downs KM, et al: Vascularization in the murine allantois occurs by vasculogenesis without accompanying erythropoiesis. Development 25:4507, 1998.

102. deMello DE, Reid LM: Embryonic and early fetal development of human lung vasculature and its functional implications. Pediatr Dev Pathol 3:439, 2000.

103. Schachtner SK, et al: Qualitative and quantitative analysis of embryonic pulmonary vessel formation. Am J Respir Cell Mol Biol 22:157, 2000.

104. Hall SM, et al: Prenatal origins of human intrapulmonary arteries: formation and smooth muscle maturation. Am J Respir Cell Mol Biol 23:194, 2000.

105. Hall SM, et al: Origin, differentiation, and maturation of human pulmonary veins. Am J Respir Cell Mol Biol 26:333, 2002.

106. Maeda S, et al: Analysis of intrapulmonary vessels and epithelial-endothelial interactions in the human developing lung. Lab Invest 82:293, 2002.

107. Schwarz MA, et al: Angiogenesis and morphogenesis of murine fetal distal lung in an allograft model. Am J Physiol Lung Cell Mol Physiol 278:L1000, 2000.

108. Vu TH, et al: New insights into saccular development and vascular formation in lung allografts under the renal capsule. Mech Dev 120:305, 2003.

109. Gebb SA, Shannon JM: Tissue interactions mediate early events in pulmonary vasculogenesis. Dev Dyn 217:159, 2000.

110. Ten Have-Opbroek AA: Lung development in the mouse embryo. Exp Lung Res 17:111, 1991.

111. Burri PH: Fetal and postnatal development of the lung. Annu Rev Physiol 46:617, 1984.

112. Chang C: On the origin of the pulmonary vein. Anat Rec 50:1, 1931.

113. DeRuiter MC, et al: Development of the pharyngeal arch system related to the pulmonary and bronchial vessels in the avian embryo. With a concept on systemic-pulmonary collateral artery formation. Circulation 87:1306, 1993.

114. Hislop AA: Airway and blood vessel interaction during lung development. J Anat 201:325, 2002.

115. Kaipainen A, et al: The related FLT4, FLT1, and KDR receptor tyrosine kinases show distinct expression patterns in human fetal endothelial cells. J Exp Med 178:2077, 1993.

116. Miquerol L, et al: Multiple developmental roles of VEGF suggested by a LacZ-tagged allele. Dev Biol 212:307, 1999.

117. Healy AM, et al: VEGF is deposited in the subepithelial matrix at the leading edge of branching airways and stimulates neovascularization in the murine embryonic lung. Dev Dyn 219:341, 2000.

118. Ng YS, et al: Differential expression of VEGF isoforms in mouse during development and in the adult. Dev Dyn 220:112, 2001.

119. Neufeld G, et al: Vascular endothelial growth factor (VEGF) and its receptors. FASEB J 13:9, 1999.

120. Galambos C, et al: Defective pulmonary development in the absence of heparin-binding vascular endothelial growth factor isoforms. Am J Respir Cell Mol Biol 27:194, 2002.

121. Shu W, et al: Wnt7b regulates mesenchymal proliferation and vascular development in the lung. Development 129:4831, 2002.

122. Moon RT, et al: WNTs modulate cell fate and behavior during vertebrate development. Trends Genet 13:157, 1997.

123. Wodarz A, Nusse R: Mechanisms of wnt signaling in development. Annu Rev Cell Dev Biol 14:59, 1998.

124. Compernolle V, et al: Loss of HIF-2alpha and inhibition of VEGF impair fetal lung maturation, whereas treatment with VEGF prevents fatal respiratory distress in premature mice. Nat Med 8:702, 2002.

125. Abman SH: Bronchopulmonary dysplasia: "a vascular hypothesis." Am J Respir Crit Care Med 164:1755, 2001.

126. Morin FC 3rd, Egan EA: Pulmonary hemodynamics in fetal lambs during development at normal and increased oxygen tension. J Appl Physiol 73:213, 1992.

127. Mielke G, Benda N: Cardiac output and central distribution of blood flow in the human fetus. Circulation 103:1662, 2001.

128. Rasanen J, et al: Role of the pulmonary circulation in the distribution of human fetal cardiac output during the second half of pregnancy. Circulation 94:1068, 1996.

129. Zgleszewski SE, et al: Maintenance of fetal murine pulmonary microvasculature in heart-lung end bloc whole organ culture. J Pediatr Surg 32:1171, 1997.

Page A. W. Anderson, Charles S. Kleinman, George Lister, and Norman S. Talner

63

Cardiovascular Function During Development and the Response to Hypoxia

This chapter reviews developmental changes in cardiovascular function in the fetus and newborn during normal and pathologic conditions. We discuss the biologic bases for differences in fetal and neonatal ventricular performance, the effects of hypoxia on cardiovascular function, and the implications of perinatal stress on the transition from fetal to neonatal life. Finally, illustrative paradigms are presented to place these basic observations into an applied clinical perspective.

THE BASIS OF CONTRACTION

The ability of the fetal and adult myocardium to contract and relax depends on similar structures and mechanisms that regulate cytosolic calcium concentration and the response of myofilaments to changes in calcium content. The membrane systems that control cell calcium flux and the sarcomeres that make up the myofibrils are present in both the fetal and the adult heart. However, the components of each system undergo qualitative and quantitative changes during development.

Myofilament and Cell Structure

The sarcomere is the basic force-generating unit of the myofilament.[1] At physiologic lengths, the sarcomere consists of interdigitating thick and thin filaments whose interaction causes force development and shortening. The order and arrangement of these filaments result in the typical microscopic appearance of the sarcomere: a central A-band with flanking I-bands that are divided by Z-lines or Z-disks (Fig. 63–1). The myosin-containing thick filaments give the A-band its appearance, while the thin filaments, which contain actin and regulatory proteins, produce the isotropic properties of the I-band. The thin filaments are attached to the Z-disk, which is in the center of the I-band, and they extend into the A-band. The A-band has a centrally located M-band that is made up of an M-protein–containing structure.

The translation of force development by the myofibrils into the systolic pressure waveform of the ventricle depends on the cell cytoskeleton, a complex intracellular meshwork made up of structural proteins (including titin, desmin, and spectrin)[1-7] and the extracellular matrix. The cytoskeleton also provides shape and organization to the cardiac cell. The cytoskeletal scaffolding of microtubules, intermediate filaments, and costameres connects the Z-disks of one myofibril to those of other myofibrils and to the T tubules, mitochondria, nuclei, and sarcolemma (Fig. 63–2). This scaffolding results in an integrated movement of the contractile apparatus and sarcolemma during contraction and relaxation. Integrins serve as sarcolemmal binding sites of the cytoskeleton and provide sites for collagen strut formation on the cell surface.[8-11] This co-localization of the extracellular matrix with the cytoskeleton promotes efficient transduction of sarcomere dynamics into myocardial force development.[2,10,12]

Sarcomeres in striated muscle are found in a striking repetitive order within the myofibrillar array. This sarcomeric order is a product of the cytoskeletal matrix. The thick and thin filaments are arranged within the sarcomere so that each thick filament is surrounded by a hexagonal array of thin filaments. The thick filaments of the cardiac sarcomere are kept directly centered between the Z-disks by filaments that are made of the extremely large protein titin (M_r in excess of 1 million daltons).[13,14] Titin filaments extend from the Z-disks (independently of the thin filaments) to attach to the thick filaments and continue along the thick filaments to the M-line.

The titin filaments predominantly and the other components of the cytoskeletal matrix to a lesser extent[7] (e.g., the desmin-containing intermediate filaments, the vinculin-containing costameres, and the microtubules) produce the passive properties of the cardiomyocyte, as described later (Figs. 63–2 and 63–3). The developmental increase in ventricular compliance[15,16] is partly due to changes in the organization of the cytoskeleton within the cardiac cell.

Sarcomere Proteins and Active Force Development

Myosin is composed of two heavy chains and four light chains (a pair of regulatory light chains and a pair of essential light chains).[17,18] The myosin heavy-chain monomer consists of a large globular head joined by a flexible joint to a rodlike body. The energy-transducing myosin head contains the enzymatic portion of the myosin molecule and its adenosine triphosphatase (ATPase) activity.[19] It catalyzes the conversion of a portion of the chemical energy of the adenosine triphosphate (ATP) into mechanical work. The rods are coiled around each other to form a myosin dimer. C-protein, another thick filament protein, contributes, in a yet to be defined manner, to binding the dimers into the thick filament and modulating cross-bridge function.[20] The myosin dimer is oriented within the thick filament so that the rod ends are nearest the center of the thick filament, leaving a central portion of the thick filament bare of myosin heads. The pair of globular heads for each dimer rests in a different plane than those of the neighboring pairs of heads within the thick filament. This arrangement ensures optimal relationships between the myosin heads and the actin monomers within the thin filaments arrayed around each thick filament.

Each thin filament is made up of a coiled coil of F-actin, a filament of actin monomers capped by tropomodulin, wrapped by a coil of tropomyosin molecules, to which troponin complexes are bound at regular intervals.[21,22] Troponins and tropomyosin constitute the thin filament regulatory proteins, which regulate the calcium-concentration–dependent force development of the myofilaments. The troponin complex is made up of three proteins: troponin T, troponin I, and troponin C.[21,22] Troponin T binds the troponin complex to tropomyosin. Troponins I and C are located at the troponin T carboxyl terminus. The amino terminus of the troponin T molecule overlaps the junction of the head of one tropomyosin molecule with the tail of the next tropomyosin in the filament. The highly ordered nature of the thin filaments and their interaction is demonstrated by the thin filaments containing a fixed stoichiometry of 7 actin monomers, 1 tropomyosin molecule, and 1 troponin complex containing 1 molecule each of troponins T, I, and C.

Force Development

Muscle contraction is an energy-dependent process that requires ATP, calcium, and the ATPase located in the myosin head. The production of force and cell shortening occurs through the binding

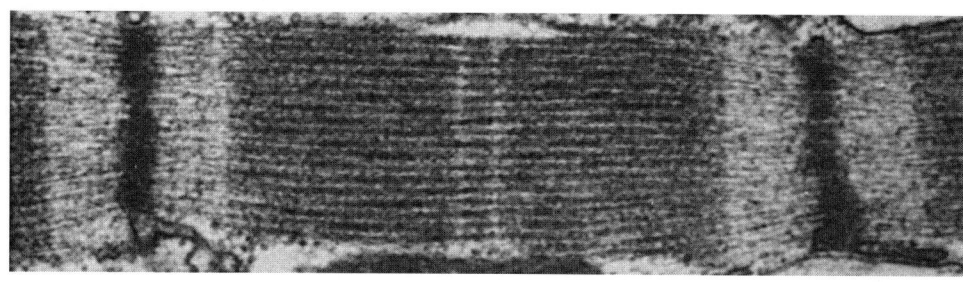

Figure 63–1. Electron micrograph of a cardiac sarcomere. The central dark A-band is flanked by two I-bands that are divided by Z-bands. The line in the middle of the A-band is the M-band.

of myosin heads to actin.[22-24] Based on the sliding filament theory,[25,26] the making and breaking of these force-generating cross-bridges depend on the availability of ATP. In addition, the thin filament regulatory proteins (tropomyosin and troponin complex) modulate the number of cross-bridge attachments and force development through a calcium-concentration–dependent process.[21-23,27] Troponin I inhibits cross-bridge formation, in part through a strong interaction with actin. This inhibitory effect is removed when troponin C binds calcium; the strength of the troponin I-actin interaction subsequently decreases, allowing troponins I and C to interact more strongly. When the calcium concentration increases, the calcium-sensitive tropomyosin binding site of troponin T also moves away from tropomyosin, altering the spatial relation of tropomyosin and actin. These structural changes facilitate the interaction of the myosin heads and actin. The description of the three-dimensional structure of the myosin head has provided a model for the interaction of ATP, adenosine diphosphate (ADP), actin, and myosin.[28,29] In the

absence of the troponin complex, calcium is not necessary for actin-myosin interactions and maximal ATPase activity. However, when troponins T, I, and C are all present, force development and ATPase activity demonstrate a graded sensitivity to calcium (Fig. 63–4). A sigmoidal relationship between force development and calcium concentration is found in fetal and adult myocardium of all species, but the sensitivity of myofilaments to calcium changes with development.[30-32]

Effect of Length/Preload

The Frank-Starling relationship, characterized by the positive relation between ventricular end-diastolic volume and the ability of the heart to develop pressure and eject blood, and the dependence of myocardial force development on muscle length, is found in fetal, neonatal, and adult mammalian hearts and myocardium.[15,41-46] The Frank-Starling relationship has also been described in the embryonic heart.[47] The basis of the Frank-

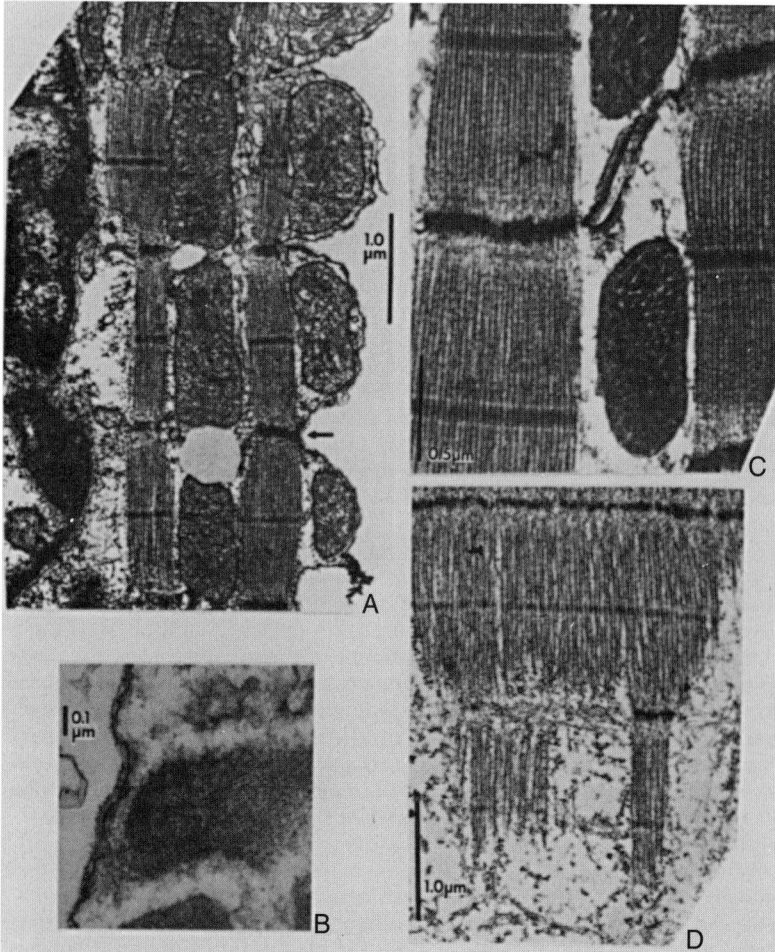

Figure 63–2. Composite of several electron micrographs, illustrating components of the cytoskeleton and the relationship of the Z-band to the sarcolemma and the intermediate filaments. **A,** Longitudinal section of a cell isolated from an adult rabbit heart shows two rows of myofibrils and mitochondria. The sarcolemma is on the right, and a nucleus is at the left. The sarcolemma appears fused with the Z–I area of the sarcomere at the arrow. **B,** A cross-section of a comparable area of another adult cell. The density between the sarcolemma and the Z–I-band area is likely to be vinculin. **C,** Attachment of the T tubule to the Z-lines by intermediate filaments is suggested by this image in which the T-tubule profile maintains a proximity to two Z-lines that are out of register. The section crosses part of a triad, consisting of the specialized region of the sarcoplasmic reticulum, the junctional SR, and the T tubule. **D,** Slightly oblique longitudinal section of a myocyte from a 3-week postnatal rabbit illustrates the ring of intermediate filaments surrounding the Z-line. (From Nassar R, et al: Circ Res *61*:465, 1987, by permission of the American Heart Association, Inc.)

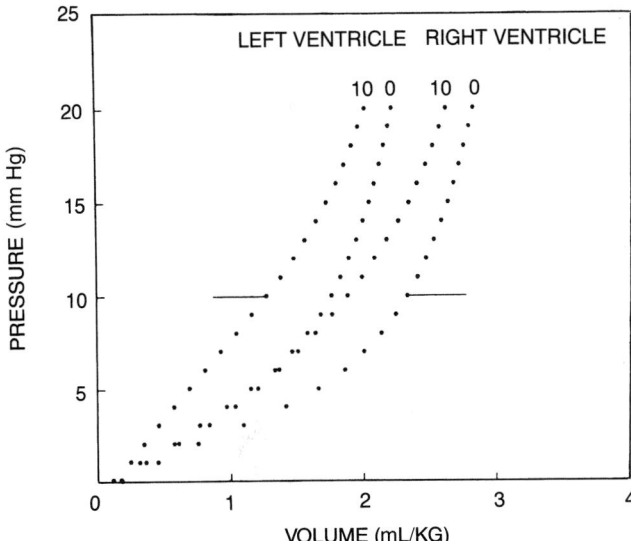

Figure 63–3. The passive pressure-volume relations of eight fetal lamb ventricles *in vitro* are shown during changes in contralateral ventricular pressure with the pericardium in place. The pressure-volume curves of the right and left ventricles were determined with the pericardium in place and the opposite ventricle at 0 or 10 mm Hg. The horizontal lines at 10 mm Hg are two standard errors of the mean. Note that the right ventricular volume is larger than that of the left ventricle, consistent with the different contributions of these ventricles to the fetal cardiac output. Increased pressure in the contralateral ventricle shifts the ipsilateral pressure-volume relation to the left—that is, in the *in situ* heart, the higher right ventricular end-diastolic pressure, the less a given filling pressure is able to fill the left ventricle. This effect of the right ventricle on left ventricular filling is greater in the immature than in the adult heart. Changes in left ventricular end-diastolic pressure affect right ventricular filling in a similar manner. (From Pinson CW, et al: J Dev Physiol *9*:253, 1987.)

Starling relationship (Fig. 63-5) rests on the general relations between sarcomere length, cross-bridge attachments, and force. Sarcomere length, the extent of overlap of the thin and thick filaments, is crucial to the process of force development and sarcomere shortening.[33-38] For any given calcium concentration, developed force depends on the number of cross-bridges, and sarcomere length affects the number of cross-bridge attachments. The effect of thick and thin filament overlap can be demonstrated by stretching the sarcomeres within a muscle to a length that ensures no overlap.[34] At that length, cross-bridge attachments cannot be made, and no force is generated regardless of the calcium concentration. When sarcomere length permits the maximum number of cross-bridge attachments, peak force will be developed at saturating calcium concentrations. At this length, all the myosin heads can interact with actin. Furthermore, at the optimal sarcomere length, thin filaments do not cross through the M-line, interfering with cross-bridge formation through thick-thin filament double overlap.[35] The optimum sarcomere length in many forms of striated muscle is 2 to 2.2 μm (this corresponds to a thin filament length of approximately 1 μm).

Sarcomere length also affects the sensitivity of myofilaments to calcium (as described by the calcium concentration that generates half-maximal force; see Fig. 63-4).[39,40] At shorter sarcomere lengths, myofilaments are less sensitive to calcium; that is, a higher calcium concentration is required to achieve half-maximal activation. This length dependency of myofilament

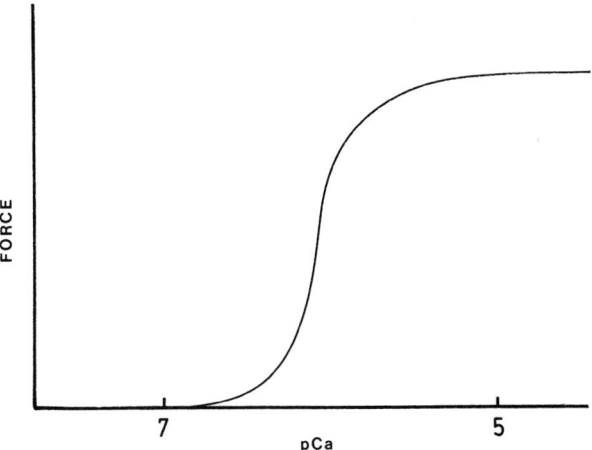

Figure 63–4. This representation of the effect of calcium concentration bathing the myofibrils on the force generated by the myofibrils is common to fetal, neonatal, and adult myocardium (pCa, negative log of the calcium concentration). At any given stage of development, the relationship is affected by pharmacologic stimulation, either directly or indirectly. The latter is exemplified by the rightward shift of the relationship (a decreased sensitivity of the myofilaments to calcium) that follows cyclic AMP-dependent phosphorylation of cardiac troponin I (an effect of sympathomimetic stimulation). Acidosis also shifts the relationship to the right, decreasing the sensitivity of the myofilaments to calcium, with adult myofibrils being more affected by respiratory acidosis than are fetal or neonatal myofibrils.

responsiveness to calcium provides another basis for the Frank-Starling relationship (see Fig. 63-5), in addition to one based on the number of myosin heads found in the portion of the thick filament that overlaps the thin filament.

Quantitative changes in force development and the Frank-Starling relationship are also due to changes in the expression of different isoforms of thin filament proteins, which may affect changes in myofilament sensitivity to calcium with development.[30,48] Post-translational modification of the myofilament proteins also affects actin-myosin interactions. Phosphorylation of the regulatory myosin light chain increases the sensitivity of

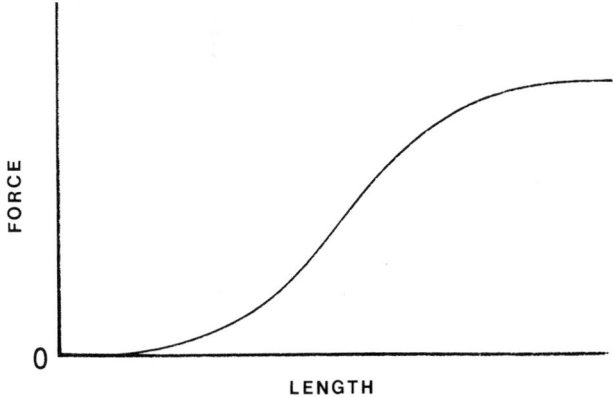

Figure 63–5. The Frank-Starling relationship in isolated cardiac muscle. With increasing muscle length, the myocardium develops greater force. This length-dependent enhancement has been related to sarcomere length, through changes in thick and thin filament overlap, the sensitivity of the myofilaments to calcium, and membrane properties.

myofibrillar ATPase activity to calcium.[49] On the other hand, cyclic adenosine monophosphate (cAMP)–dependent phosphorylation of troponin I decreases cardiac myofilament sensitivity to calcium (as measured by ATPase activity or force) and leaves maximal ATPase activity unaffected.[32,50,51] This decrease in myofilament sensitivity contributes to the β-agonist–induced shortening of the cardiac contraction that occurs in association with β-agonist–induced increase in contractility. In contrast to protein kinase A phosphorylation, protein kinase C–mediated phosphorylation of troponin I decreases maximal ATPase activity.[50,51] The physiologic significance of the *in vivo* phosphorylation of the contractile proteins and how these modifications may alter myocardial function and the Frank-Starling relationship at different stages of development continue to be explored.

Effect of Afterload

Throughout development, the ventricular wall must be able to develop tensions that generate ventricular pressures that open the semilunar valves and allow ventricular ejection. Arterial pressure is the major component of afterload, the load that the sarcomere bears during contraction. The level of the afterload modulates the ability of the myocardium to shorten and the ventricle to eject blood.[15,45,46,52,53] The higher the afterload, the slower is the rate of sarcomere and, therefore, muscle shortening. If the load is sufficiently high, muscle shortening is prevented. The greatest velocity of sarcomere shortening occurs when the afterload is zero (i.e., when the sarcomere is unloaded and shortens against no load) and is considered to be independent of sarcomere length (until sarcomere shortening causes double overlap of the thin filaments).[25,35] Given this independence of sarcomere length, unloaded sarcomere shortening is controlled by the rate of cross-bridge cycling and not by the number of cross-bridge attachments. The rate of cross-bridge detachment depends on the ATPase activity of the myosin head: the higher the activity, the more rapidly ATP is hydrolyzed, the faster the actinomyosin cross-bridges are broken, and the more rapidly the sarcomere shortens.

Cytosolic Calcium and Contraction

Membrane systems that control cytosolic calcium are central to mechanisms of contraction and relaxation that result in ventricular ejection and filling. With activation, the calcium concentration bathing the myofilaments rises to a level that allows cross-bridge formation and force development. Intracellular calcium concentration depends on the shift of extracellular calcium, trans-sarcolemmal movement of calcium, intracellular calcium stores, the uptake or release of calcium from intracellular compartments, and the intra- and extracellular concentrations of ions that affect trans-sarcolemmal movement of calcium and cell calcium content. The sarcolemma contains pumps, channels, and exchangers that modify cytosolic calcium and cell calcium. These include the dihydropyridine (DHP)-sensitive L-type calcium channel; Na^+,K^+-ATPase; the sarcolemmal Ca^{2+}-ATPase; and the Na^+-Ca^{2+} exchanger.[63-66] Changes in hydrogen, sodium, and potassium extracellular concentrations also affect intracellular calcium stores through their effects on these and other components of the sarcolemma. The function of these membrane-bound systems is modulated by phosphorylation, a consequence of the adrenoceptors and other ligand receptors and their signaling proteins.

Within the cardiac cell, the sarcoplasmic reticulum (SR) is the most important structure for controlling cytosolic calcium concentration during contraction.[67-71] The SR releases calcium into the cytosol through the ryanodine receptor, or the SR calcium release channel, in response to increases in cytosolic calcium concentration due to the calcium current through the L-type channel.[70-75] The SR removes calcium from the cytosol through its calcium ATPase and stores the calcium for release during sub-

sequent contractions.[70,72,73,76-78] Junctional SR, a region of SR that has a close, specialized relationship with the sarcolemma, and the corbular SR contain the SR calcium release channels. The lumen of these specialized components of the SR contains calsequestrin, a calcium-binding protein.[77] The rapidity with which the SR removes calcium from the cytosol depends on SR calcium ATPase activity.[32] This activity depends, in turn, on the cytosolic calcium concentration: the higher the cytosolic concentration, the higher the ATPase activity. SR calcium ATPase is inhibited by phospholamban, a closely associated SR protein. Phosphorylation of phospholamban (e.g., through β-receptor stimulation) removes its inhibitory effects and enhances ATPase activity.[78-80] The net result of β-agonist stimulation on this aspect of SR function is an increase in the rate of relaxation of the contraction and an increase in the amount of calcium available for SR release during the next contraction. Interactions between the sarcolemmal and SR systems and their control of cytosolic calcium remain under investigation. As described later, maturational changes in these systems have been identified, and they likely explain key functional differences during development.

Excitation-Contraction Coupling

The process that activates the myocardium from its diastolic resting state and initiates contraction has been termed *excitation-contraction coupling*.[70,81-85] With activation and depolarization of the cell, calcium moves across the sarcolemma through voltage-dependent, DHP-sensitive channels.[63] It has been suggested that, when calcium enters the cell through the L-type channel, the SR calcium release channel binds this calcium, opens, and releases a graded amount of calcium from SR stores (calcium-induced calcium release [CICR]).[73,84,85] Calcium release is dependent on the local cytosolic calcium concentration, which is the product of the calcium channel current. Unlike skeletal muscle, cardiac muscle quickly stops contracting when the extracellular calcium concentration is brought to very low levels,[86] demonstrating the crucial role of trans-sarcolemmal calcium movement in the process of excitation-contraction coupling in cardiac muscle.

In addition to the L-type Ca^{2+} channel, the trans-sarcolemmal movement of calcium also depends on the Na^--Ca^{2+} exchanger and the sarcolemmal calcium ATPase which can lower cell calcium content.[64,65] The Na-Ca exchanger is usually thought of as a mechanism for removing calcium from the cell in exchange for sodium. However, when the reversal potential of the Na^+-Ca^{2+} exchanger exceeds depolarization and the potential becomes more positive, the exchanger works in the opposite mode.[87-89] The Na^+-Ca^{2+} exchanger then introduces calcium into the cell, increasing the cytosolic calcium concentration. During repolarization and the fall of the transmembrane potential, the Na^+-Ca^{2+} exchanger again reverses the direction in which it moves calcium, and calcium is extruded from the cell.

In the mammal, the amount of calcium that enters the cardiac cell through the L-type calcium channel appears to be insufficient to produce a maximal contraction. This calcium may primarily serve as a trigger for CICR, never becoming available to the myofilaments during a given contraction. In the mammalian heart, trans-sarcolemmal movement of calcium may be of prime importance in inducing SR calcium release during a given contraction and for maintaining SR calcium stores.[82,84,85,89,90]

Although excitation is all or none in the heart, the amount of force developed can be altered from beat to beat. CICR is thought to be the basis for the cardiac cell's ability to vary the cytosolic calcium concentration from one contraction to another. This ability to change the strength or forcefulness of the contraction in response to varying the rate and pattern of stimulation is a basic property of the mammalian heart.[91] This property has been termed the force-interval or force-frequency relationship. This relationship allows the heart to respond rapidly to changes in workload and to alter cardiac output. The underlying basis of this relationship is the beat-to-beat modulation of cytosolic calcium concentration. For example, potentiation in the force of a post-extrasystolic contraction is the result of the cytosolic calcium concentration exceeding levels achieved during contraction at the basic rate.[92] The source of this calcium is most likely the SR. In addition to the amount of calcium within the SR, SR calcium release depends on the initial increase in cytosolic calcium concentration, the rate of its increase, and the time following the previous release of calcium.[84,85,91,93,94] These dependencies may arise from the properties of the SR calcium release channel. Four apparent calcium-binding sites and those for calmodulin and ATP are present on the calcium release channel tetramer.[95] This configuration supports the possibility that different calcium levels will variably alter the release channel configuration (and its release of calcium), and that these properties will be modified by binding of other ligands.

The importance of SR calcium release in the activation-induced increase in the cytosolic calcium contraction is demonstrated by modification of the force-interval relationship by ryanodine.[75,92] Ryanodine, which binds to the SR calcium release channel and interferes with SR calcium storage and release, abolishes the post-extrasystolic potentiation of cytosolic calcium concentration and force. This suggests that the normal post-extrasystolic increment in calcium is released from the SR.[92]

Changes in the cytosolic calcium concentration from one contraction to another have also been attributed to variations in the amount of calcium crossing the sarcolemma (see earlier discussion of CICR). The quantity of calcium entering the cell depends to some extent on the extracellular calcium concentration.[81,82,86,87] In some species, beat-to-beat increases in force following the initiation of pacing are accompanied by beat-to-beat transient decreases in the extracellular calcium concentration when measured close to the sarcolemma.[84] Although calcium movement through the DHP-sensitive calcium channel can be enhanced (e.g., as a consequence of β-agonist–induced phosphorylation),[63] the beat-to-beat modulation of trans-sarcolemmal calcium movement has been attributed to the Na^+-Ca^{2+} exchanger.[82,87,88]

As described previously, the SR is an important contributor to the beat-to-beat modulation of cytosolic calcium. This modulation follows, in part, from the ability of the SR to remove calcium from the cytosol,[72] by the effects of the Na^+-Ca^{2+} exchanger,[64] and possibly the sarcolemmal Ca^{2+}-ATPase on the cell calcium content[65] and from the release of calcium from the SR,[84,85] which are all intertwined.[32,64,65,93] The greater the amount of calcium taken up by the SR, the smaller will be the amount of calcium extruded from the cell through the Na^+-Ca^{2+} exchanger. Consequently, more calcium will be available for release from this intracellular store during subsequent contractions.

In summary, the ability of the myocardium to contract and relax depends on the interaction of systems that control cytosolic ionic concentrations. These dependencies include the organization of the cell membranes, the membrane proteins that control the intracellular ionic environment, cell coupling through connexins,[95,96] and the alteration of their function through pharmacologic agents, receptor stimulation, biophysical stimuli, isoform expression, extracellular ionic concentrations, and the pattern of activation. The force of the contraction generated in response to the increase in the calcium concentration bathing the myofilaments depends on cell shape, myofibril organization, cell myofibril content, cytoskeletal organization, number of cells/myocardial volume, sarcomere length, sensitivity of the myofilaments to calcium, concentrations of hydrogen and other cytosolic ions,[97] the contractile protein isoforms (see Refs 98 and 99), post-translational modifications of these proteins,[32,50,100] and the direct effects of pharmacologic agents.[101-103] It is not surprising that development affects many of these factors or dependencies, while the effects on others remain to be characterized.

MATURATION AND CARDIAC FUNCTION

A maturational increase in the ability of the myocardium to develop force and to contract against a load has been observed in a wide range of preparations.[15,104-108] A clinical manifestation of the decreased strength of contraction of immature myocardium is the inability of the heart of the preterm infant to sustain an adequate cardiac output when ejecting against arterial pressures that are easily supported by the adult heart. The failure of the preterm heart can be explained by its relatively smaller myocardial mass and thinner left ventricular wall, which are unable to generate the wall stresses needed to eject blood in the face of such arterial pressures. In addition, when force is measured as a function of cross-sectional area (i.e., stress) in isolated muscle experiments, contraction of the immature myocardium is weaker than that of adult myocardium.

A major basis for the developmental increase in contractility rests in the cardiac myocyte. In isolated, single ventricular myocytes, the velocity and amount of sarcomere shortening are lower in the immature myocyte than in the adult myocyte[94] (Fig. 63-6). Thus, when the ventricular myocyte contracts free of the loads imposed by the extracellular matrix, arterial pressure, and cell-to-cell connections, myocardial contractility is found to increase with maturation. The following sections explore the bases for the maturational increase in myocardial contractility.

Structure

Hyperplasia and Physiologic Hypertrophy

The myocardium undergoes many structural changes during development that affect a wide range of components, including the proteins that make up the membranes, the contractile apparatus, the extracellular matrix, and cell and myocardial organization and content. Remarkably, many of these structural changes and the process of cell division occur while the myocytes are contracting and relaxing. By themselves, these variables would seem to be major reasons for the decreased ability of the immature cell to contract and develop force. However, other components appear to be directly related to the developmental increase in contractility. For example, the myofibril content of the myocyte increases with development,[15,109-111] providing the potential for more cross-bridge attachments per cell cross-sectional area. In addition, maturational changes in cell shape and myofibril order and orientation would be expected to improve the mechanical advantage of the myofibril in the generation of force.[94,110,112,113]

Ventricular mass increases during development *in utero*.[109,114] In the postnatal period, there is differential growth of the right and left ventricular myocardium.[109] Left ventricular weight and wall thickness increase relative to body weight, whereas the ratio of right ventricular weight to body weight and wall thickness remains the same or decreases.[109,114,115] These differences appear to be in response to the birth-associated changes in ventricular work. During fetal life, the right ventricle performs the majority of ventricular work, although the relative amounts of right and left ventricular work may be similar in the human fetus.[116-123] Immediately following birth, work performed by the right ventricle and the left ventricle undergoes large and opposite changes; left ventricular work increases because of the increase in left ventricular stroke volume, systolic pressure, and wall tension, whereas right ventricular work falls in association with the fall in pulmonary artery pressure.[118,124] The relations between ventricular work, mass, and protein expression and

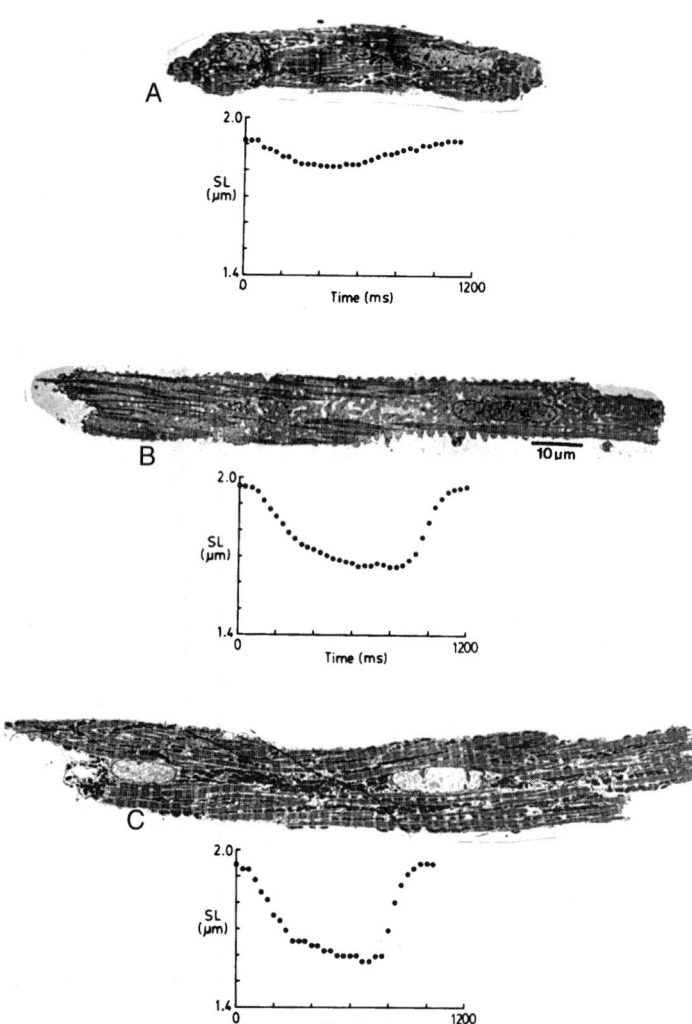

Figure 63–6. Longitudinal sections through the near-central region of three myocytes isolated from rabbit ventricular myocardium. Sarcomere dynamics of the cells were studied, and the cells were then prepared for electron microscopy. The contraction waveform of each cell appears beneath its electron micrograph. Sarcomere length (SL) is plotted as a function of time (1 mM extracellular calcium). All cells in the figure are shown at identical magnification. **A,** An average-sized myocyte from a 3-week-old rabbit. **B,** A small-sized myocyte from an adult rabbit. Even this relatively small adult cell has a faster and greater amount of sarcomere shortening than that of the immature cell. **C,** An average-sized cell from an adult heart. (From Nassar R, et al: Circ Res *61*:465, 1987, by permission of the American Heart Association, Inc.)

how they are affected by development are exemplified in the infant and the young adult with transposition of the great vessels. Banding the pulmonary artery to prepare the left ventricle for a physiologic anatomic correction (the arterial switch operation) results in a marked increase in ventricular messenger RNA (mRNA) and myocardial mass within days of the surgically imposed increase in left ventricular afterload.[125] In contrast, the increase in left ventricular mass, in response to pulmonary artery banding, appears to occur more slowly in young adults.[126]

Cell division is a major contributor to the increase in myocardial mass of the fetus and the neonate.[109,114] The pre- and postnatal increase in ventricular mass is a function of both the number and size of the ventricular myocytes. During neonatal life, the left ventricular myocyte population increases more rapidly than does that of the right ventricle.[109] The stimulus for the differential increase in cell population size also may contribute to the ventricular differences in cell volume and length.[110,111] By the second postnatal month, cell division is thought to have ceased, and physiologic hypertrophy (i.e., the normal developmental increase in cell size) becomes the dominant process through which ventricular mass increases.[109,114] It is interesting that the finding of a larger number of relatively small myocytes in the aging human heart has suggested that cell division may begin again in response to the loss of myocytes with aging.[127]

During fetal and neonatal life, the ventricular myocyte undergoes prominent changes in size and shape (Figs. 63–6 and 63–7).[94,110,113,128,129] For example, myocytes of the 1-week-old rabbit heart are typically about 40 μm long and 5 μm in width,

while the average adult ventricular myocyte is well over 100 μm in length and more than 25 μm in width in the central portion of the cell.[94] The maturational increase in cell dimensions is associated with a change in cell shape (see Fig. 63–6). The very immature myocyte is spheroidal. As cell length increases, the cell initially maintains an overall smooth shape with tapered ends. In the adult, step-changes in cell width and thickness are marked by the intercalated disks,[1] making the two-dimensional profiles of the myocyte rectangular in appearance. Serial sectioning of myocytes demonstrates that, in contrast to the immature myocyte, the adult cell surface often has a complex three-dimensional shape.[94] The rate at which the maturational shape changes occur differs within the two ventricles.[109,110,128,129] In comparison with left ventricular myocytes, those in the right ventricle undergo these shape changes at a slower rate. All these changes in shape help adapt the myocyte into becoming a more efficient force development machine.

Multiple mechanisms that regulate myocyte hypertrophy are uncertain; however, α-agonist stimulation may play a key role.[130-132] In addition, transforming growth factors, which are expressed by ventricular myocytes, may serve as paracrine or autocrine stimuli to induce differentiation and hypertrophy.[133] The increase in expression and fall in expression of proto-oncogenes also may be important signals that initiate and maintain the processes of differentiation and hypertrophy.[134-136] However, stimuli that commit progenitor cells to become cardiac cells and the process that turns off cell division remain under intense investigation.

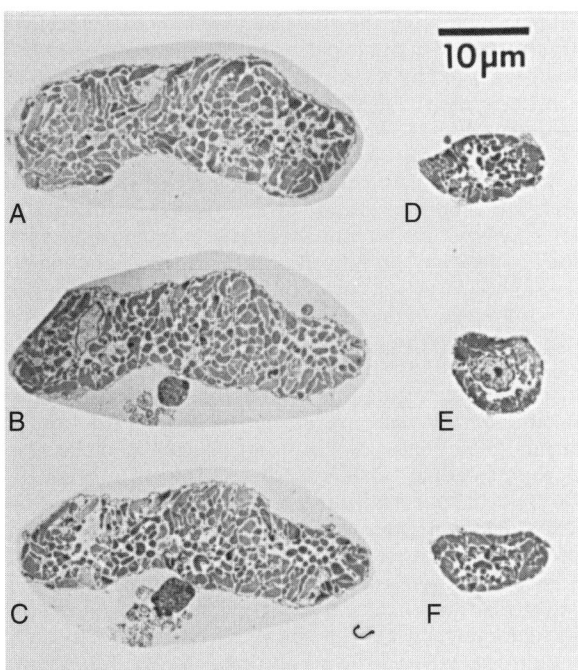

Figure 63–7. Cross-sections through widely separated levels of a ventricular myocyte isolated from an adult heart (**A, B, C**) and of a myocyte from a 3-week postnatal rabbit (**D, E, F**). The striking differences in size and shape between the adult and the immature cell exemplify the marked increase in size that occurs with physiologic hypertrophy. (From Nassar R, et al: Circ Res *61*:465, 1987, by permission of the American Heart Association, Inc.)

Myofibrillar Structure

Sarcomeres, the basic contractile units of the myofilament, undergo prominent changes in architecture during fetal and postnatal life.[94,109,110,113,128,129] In the immature myocyte, myofibrils appear chaotic, with no given direction of orientation. In contrast, myofibrils are arranged in long parallel rows from one side of the cell to the other in the adult myocyte. These rows of myofibrils extend the length of the cell from intercalated disk to intercalated disk. Furthermore, they are wrapped by the SR and interspersed with rows of mitochondira. Before achieving these adult morphologic characteristics and organization, the myofibril orientation initially goes from being haphazardly arranged to being oriented with the longitudinal axis of the cell. Initially, these longitudinally oriented myofibrils are localized to a subsarcolemmal shell, which may be only one or two myofibrils deep.[94] This thin layer of myofibrils surrounds a large central mass of nuclei and mitochondria. Because trans-sarcolemmal movement of calcium is thought to be more important than intracellular calcium release in supporting the contraction of the immature myocyte, this localization of the myofibrils to a subsarcolemmal shell has been proposed to result teleologically in a more efficient response to this trans-sarcolemmal calcium movement.[94] With time the layers of myofibrils extend through the thickness of the cell. The time course of these maturational changes in ultrastructure differs among species.[15,109,110]

Temporal differences in myocyte maturation between species appear to be related to the general maturational level of the neonate. For example, myocytes of the sheep and guinea pig (the guinea pig is ready to flee the nest at birth and the lamb runs after its mother) appear mature at birth in comparison with those of the dog and rat (recall the helpless puppy and the hairless rat pup). Variation in the maturational level of cell architec-

ture also has been found even within the same ventricle.[94,110] For example, occasional cells, isolated from hearts of 3-week-old rabbits, have the dimensions and ultrastructural appearance of a typical adult ventricular myocyte.[94]

Expression of the sarcomeric contractile proteins is basic to the process of myofibrillogenesis.[139,140] The importance of myosin, actin, and thin filament regulatory protein expression was first established in nonvertebrate muscle.[139,140] Failure to express actin results in nonfunctional flight muscles in *Drosophila* that contain thick filaments but no thin filaments. Abnormalities in the primary structure of the thin filament regulatory proteins troponin T and troponin I also result in disorders of myofilament structure, abnormal levels of expression of the nonmutated contractile proteins, and decreased myofibril size.[140] The effects of very modest alterations in protein expression have been assessed using site-directed mutation. Single residue changes in thin filament proteins can affect myofibril function and the incorporation of the thick filament into the sarcomere. For example, changes in two amino acids in sarcomeric actin have been shown to have a devastating effect on function and to cause the thick and thin filaments in the myofibril periphery to be misregistered and unincorporated into the Z-lines.[139] In those peripheral regions, thick filaments are flanked by thin filaments that have apparently opposite polarity. Thus, the organization of the sarcomere and the myofibril depends on the coordinated expression of the contractile proteins and the preservation of structural domains within those proteins.

The general importance of mutations in sarcomeric proteins on cardiac myofibril structure has been established in humans. Mutations in β-myosin heavy chain, α-tropomyosin, troponin T, and C-protein genes have been found in affected members of families with hypertrophic cardiomyopathy.[141-143] In a manner that remains to be understood, these mutations result in marked myofibril disorder, myocardial hypertrophy, and sudden death in affected patients. The β-myosin heavy-chain gene expressed in the heart is also expressed in slow skeletal muscle. This expression pattern has allowed abnormalities in myofibril function to be related to the presence of missense mutations in the β-myosin heavy chain isolated from soleus muscle biopsies of affected patients.[144] Similarly, a mutant cardiac troponin T found in individuals with hypertrophic cardiomyopathy has been shown to result in faster motility of thin filaments in vitro.[145] These abnormalities in function may induce abnormal myofibrillogenesis and hypertrophy. On the other hand, abnormalities in the normally fixed stoichiometry of sarcomeric protein expression may be a product of these mutations. For example, in flight muscle, troponin T mutations alter mRNA and protein stability and produce abnormal myofibril structure.[140]

Contractile Proteins

A large number of isoforms of the sarcomeric proteins have been found.[17,18,55,56,58,62,146-160] The isoforms of each protein differ somewhat in structure; such differences probably modulate the basic function of each protein. For example, the ATPase activity of the α-myosin homodimer is significantly greater than that of the β-myosin homodimer.[18] Functional differences have yet to be established for all isoforms. Some isoforms are products of a multigene family, whereas others are the product of alternative splicing of the primary transcript of a single gene. For example, the α- and β-myosin heavy chains arise from two genes,[17] whereas isoforms of cardiac troponin T arise from a single gene.[156,161] The isoforms, including those of the myosin light chains, tropomyosin, troponin T, troponin I, actin, and the myosin heavy chain, are expressed in complex temporal and chamber-specific patterns.* Although stimuli that affect these patterns of expression have

---

* Refs 18,58,62,148-153,156,158-160,162-164.

been found, the *cis*- and *trans*-acting factors that determine the developmental and regional pattern of isoform expression in cardiac muscle remain to be established.[130,131,133-135]

Studies of the myosin heavy chain isozymes have demonstrated that (1) myosin ATPase activity has been related to the rate of cross-bridge attachment and detachment[19,54]; (2) myocardium with a lower myosin ATPase activity appears to work more efficiently[165]; and (3) the peak unloaded velocity of myocardial shortening depends on myosin ATPase activity. Myocardial shortening velocity has been shown to increase with maturation[15] and in some species might result from changes in myosin isozyme expression.

Species differences exist in the developmental expression of myosin isoenzymes.[18,58,59,62,160] In rodents, α-myosin heavy chain is most commonly expressed in the adult, whereas in larger animals, including humans, β-myosin heavy chain is the dominant adult isozyme. In the rat, development affects myosin isozyme expression in the following manner: β-myosin heavy chain is predominantly expressed in the fetal and neonatal heart, α-myosin heavy chain is predominantly expressed in the adult heart, and, with senescence, β-myosin heavy chain is re-expressed. In contrast, in the rabbit, myosin expression changes with development in the opposite manner. The neonatal rabbit myocardium predominantly expresses α-myosin heavy chain, whereas the adult rabbit myocardium predominantly expresses β-myosin heavy chain. In the human, β-myosin heavy chain is predominantly expressed in the ventricle from late fetal life throughout adult life. This pattern of expression is not altered in the cardiomyopathic, hypertrophied, or failing heart.[59-62] Heterogeneity in the cardiac β-myosin heavy chain has been observed in pressure-overloaded nonhuman primate heart.[55] The molecular basis of this heterogeneity, its presence in humans, and its functional importance remain to be determined.

In humans, the effects of maturation on the isoform expression of cardiac contractile proteins other than myosin heavy chain are more dynamic. The tissue-specific expression of these other genes has been examined in several species and found to be affected by a number of factors, including maturation, workload, and hormonal and α-adrenoceptor stimulation.[155,159,162,166-171] In the rat heart, cardiac α-actin is expressed in the adult, whereas the skeletal α-actin gene is expressed in the embryonic and fetal heart. When a pressure overload is imposed on the adult rat heart, skeletal α-actin expression is reinduced transiently. Similarly, in neonatal rat myocytes, α-adrenoceptor stimulation will induce expression of the skeletal actin gene. The transient reversal of isoform expression in the adult rat heart exposed to pressure overload has been considered a general and basic response of the heart to stresses that induce hypertrophy. In humans, cardiac α-actin is predominantly expressed in the fetus, whereas after birth, skeletal α-actin becomes the predominantly expressed isoform. This pattern of expression is opposite to what is seen in the rat and other species.[163] Furthermore, unlike that of the rat heart, human cardiac hypertrophy is not associated with a switch in actin isoform expression. Perinatal changes in α-actin isoform expression in the human heart may have functional significance. In a murine model, in which skeletal α-actin isoform expression was increased in the adult heart, the higher expression of skeletal α-actin was accompanied by an increase in contractility.[172] This finding suggests that in the postnatal human heart the maturational increase in expression of skeletal α-actin will have a positive effect on cardiac contractility.

The myosin light chains, which consist of the essential light chain, or LC1, and the regulatory light chain, LC2, have different isoforms.[149,153,154,157,173] In human hypertrophied myocardium, a change in MLC1 isoform expression has been correlated to a change in myofibril function.[171] The expression of these isoforms follows a temporal and chamber-specific pattern and is affected by pressure overload. For example, in humans, an LC1 isoform

indistinguishable from the atrial light chain is expressed in the fetal ventricle and is not expressed in the postnatal heart.[149]

Multiple myosin light chain isoforms are associated with functionally specialized muscle, whose expression is affected by physiologic state and development. This suggests that these isoforms are important in modulating muscle function. Phosphorylation of the light chains may alter their functional effects differentially. Phosphorylation of the regulatory myosin light chain increases myofilament sensitivity to calcium in striated muscle.[49] However, the full role of the myosin light chain isoforms in cardiac muscle function is still being defined. Unlike other contractile proteins, troponin C expression does not change during development.[174,175]

Tropomyosin, the thin filament protein to which the regulatory complex of troponin is bound, has two major isoforms, alpha and beta, which are assembled into homo- and heterodimers.[18,21,176] These isoforms are present in different proportions, depending on the species and developmental stage of the myocardium. The α-tropomyosin gene in the rat is responsible (through alternative splicing) for the expression of α-tropomyosin isoforms in cardiac, smooth, and skeletal muscle cells.[147] In small animals, only α-tropomyosin is expressed in the normal adult heart, whereas fetal and hypertrophied myocardium contain both α- and β-tropomyosin.[176] In humans and other large animals, the proportion of α- and β-tropomyosin changes with development so that the α-isoform is expressed predominantly in the adult.[159] The functional importance of these cardiac isoforms is suggested by data indicating that the binding of tropomyosin to troponin T is affected by the tropomyosin isoform, and that higher levels of β-tropomyosin (as found in skeletal muscle fibers) have slower contraction speeds. Using a transgenic mouse model, β-tropomyosin overexpression has been shown to slow ventricular diastolic relaxation.[176] α-Tropomyosin, which allows more rapid relaxation, is the predominant isoform in hearts with faster rates.

Development affects the cardiac expression of the cardiac and slow skeletal muscle genes of troponin I.[150,159,170] Each gene expresses a single isoform. In human, chicken, and rat myocardium, the expression of the two isoforms is developmentally controlled, with the cardiac isoform being expressed in the adult heart. These isoforms confer the myocardium with different functional responses to hormonal stimulation and acidosis.[31,177,178] For example, slow skeletal muscle troponin I is a major contributor to the immature myocardium's resistance to acidosis.[31,178] Consequently, respiratory acidosis depresses myocardial contractility more in the adult heart (which expresses only cardiac troponin I) than in the fetal and neonatal heart (in which slow skeletal muscle troponin I is highly expressed). The finding that the neonatal human heart expresses slow skeletal muscle troponin I at much higher levels than cardiac troponin I[170] suggests a selective maturational regulation of gene expression that recognizes the need for resistance to respiratory acidosis during perinatal development. Indeed, a high level of slow skeletal muscle troponin I expression is still found in the 2-year-old toddler.

The developmental differences in expression of these troponin I isoforms also affect the response of the myocardium to sympathetic stimulation. The cardiac isoform is phosphorylated as a consequence of β-adrenoceptor stimulation, while the slow skeletal muscle isoform is not. This cAMP-dependent phosphorylation decreases the sensitivity of the myofibrils to calcium,[50,51,177] apparently contributing to the more rapid relaxation of ventricular pressure that is induced by β-agonists. Protein kinase C, which may be activated by α-agonist stimulation, also phosphorylates cardiac troponin I, decreasing maximal ATPase activity.[50,51] The presence of a β-agonist–induced enhancement in SR uptake and release of calcium in the immature heart, and the absence of a contemporaneous change in

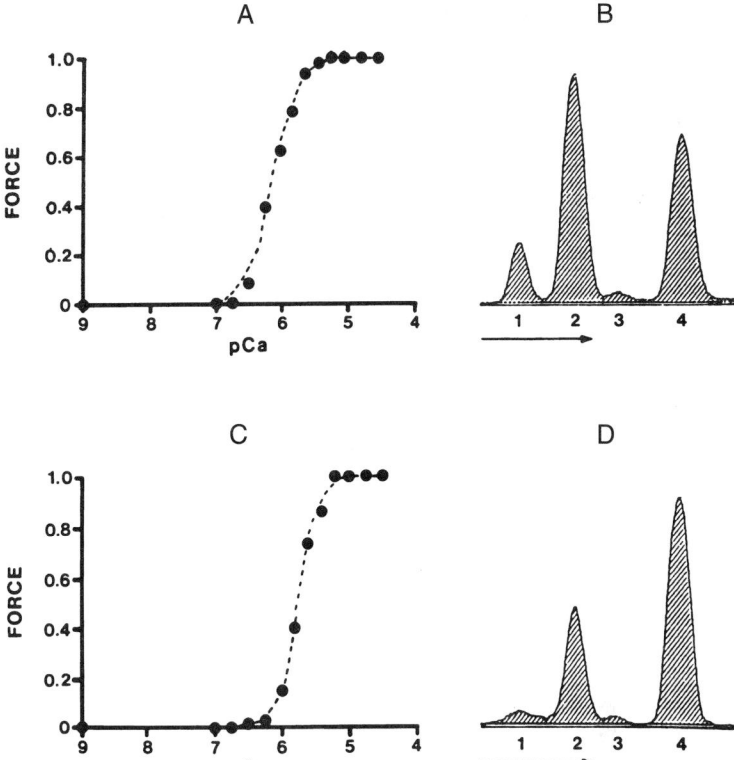

Figure 63–8. The force-pCa relations of two neonatal rabbit ventricular strands and the densitometric scans of the Western blots of these two strands probed with a cardiac troponin T–specific monoclonal antibody. The proteins were transblotted from 7.5% polyacrylamide gels. Force shown is normalized with respect to that generated at maximum activation. The force-pCa curve in **A** is shifted to the left relative to the curve shown in **C**, implying that the myofilaments of the strand that provided the force-pCa data in **A** and the Western blot in **B** were more sensitive to calcium. The densitometric scans of the Western blots show that the strand that was more sensitive to calcium (**A**) had a greater proportion of the isoform TnT_2 (**B**) than did the other strand (**D**). The arrows indicate the direction of electrophoresis. The troponin T isoforms TnT_1, TnT_2, TnT_3, and TnT_4, are numbered. (From Nassar R, et al: Circ Res 69:1470, 1991.)

myofilament function, may have an undefined negative effect on diastolic function in the immature heart.

Multiple isoforms of cardiac troponin T are expressed in mammalian myocardium through a developmentally controlled process.[151,152,179,180] As found in rabbit, dog, pig, and rat hearts, the human heart expresses at least four cardiac troponin T isoforms.[99,146] The larger isoforms are expressed more highly in the fetal heart. Tropinin T isoforms are products of combinatorial alternative splicing of the primary transcript.[99,161] Their expression in the adult heart is altered by severe heart failure, with a fetal isoform being re-expressed.[99,146] Troponin T isoforms appear to have different functional effects (Fig. 63–8). In fast skeletal muscle, the sensitivity of the myofilaments to calcium is related to myofilament troponin T and tropomyosin isoform content.[98] Furthermore, cardiac troponin T isoform expression has been correlated with the sensitivity of myofilaments to calcium as assessed by force development and myofibrillar ATPase activity, cardiac myofibril binding of calcium in the normal heart, and sarcomere length–dependence of myofilament sensitivity to calcium in the diabetic rat heart.[48,146,181-183] These functional effects would follow from the inclusion or exclusion of short amino-terminal peptides in troponin T, and they suggest that enhanced expression of specific cardiac troponin T isoforms could be used as a therapeutic intervention in the failing heart.

The presence of thin filament regulatory protein isoforms and a variety of biophysical and biochemical observations suggest that the complex developmental variation in contractile protein expression modulates the force of cardiac contraction and its rate of contraction and relaxation directly, and through post-translational modifications of the proteins. In large animals, myofibrillar ATPase activity increases with development from the neonate to the adult, although myosin ATPase activity is unchanged or decreases with development.[106,160] This increase in myofibrillar ATPase activity may result from changes in thin filament isoform expression and their post-translational modifications. For example, phosphorylation of tropomyosin

increases ATPase activity,[184] and the amino-terminal region differences among the troponin T isoforms (whose expression are changed by development) have been shown to affect the ATPase activity–pCa relationship in actinomyosin systems.[182] An interesting corollary to the different effects of maturation on myosin and myofibrillar ATPase is the effect of human heart disease. Myosin ATPase activities of ventricular myocardium from normal and severely frail human hearts do not differ, whereas myofibrillar ATPase activity is depressed in the failing heart.[185,186] Of note, the heart failure–associated increase in the expression of a cardiac troponin T isoform, expressed in the fetal heart, correlates with the disease-associated fall in myofibrillar ATPase activity.

The effects of development and disease on the complex combinations of expression and post-translational modifications of the contractile proteins suggest that pharmacologic agents, which alter the sensitivity of the myofilaments to calcium,[101-103] will have different physiologic effects in hearts at different stages of development, and in different physiologic and pathophysiologic states.

The Cytoskeleton, Extracellular Matrix, and Maturation

The cytoskeleton and extracellular matrix provide mechanical support that transduces sarcomere motion into ventricular systolic pressure and ventricular filling into diastolic pressure[7,10-14,187] (see Fig. 63-3). The developmental increase in myocardial contractility and the decrease in myocardial compliance must be, in part, related to these changes in the cytoskeleton and the extracellular matrix.[15] In addition to general organizational changes, the distribution of the cytoskeletal proteins within the cell is affected by development.[6,94,187-189] For example, in the neonatal myocyte, desmin appears to be diffusely localized to a subsarcolemmal shell. The mass of nuclei and mitochondria in the center of the cell appears to prevent the desmin-containing intermediate filaments from linking the Z-disks of myofibrils on one side of the cell to those on the other. With increasing development, desmin-containing intermediate filaments are seen to divide the adult cell into many compartments while connecting the myofibrils, membranous system, and mitochondria. From a functional standpoint, the central mass of nuclei and mitochondria in the immature cell appears to provide a large internal load that opposes sarcomere shortening. This structure contrasts with the mechanically more efficient cytoskeletal defined organization of the adult myocyte. Passive properties also may be affected by the developmental changes in myocyte organization. The organization found in the immature myocyte may impose a greater restraining load on the resting sarcomere and produce the shorter sarcomere length found in the immature ventricular myocyte.[94]

Integrins[8] are localized to the cell surface and recognize, attach to extracellular matrix proteins (e.g., fibronectin, laminin, and collagen), and change distribution with age.[191,192] In neonatal myocytes, these sites of attachment are well developed. In the adult, the ends of the cell and the sarcolemmal regions near the Z-disk contain sites of attachment. Maturational differences in the site of extracellular matrix attachment to the cell and the intracellular cytoskeletal and myofibril organization should affect the generation of force through alterations in the coupling of sarcomere shortening to the extracellular matrix.

Components of the extracellular matrix change with development.[129,193-195] A quantitative increase occurs during fetal and neonatal growth. At birth, the left ventricular free wall of the rodent demonstrates little organized collagen, whereas the numerous fibroblasts that form the collagen struts on the myocyte surface are closely associated with the ventricular cells. The neonatal formation of the collagen network parallels the development and distribution of fibronectin. This extracellular matrix protein can be found in largest amounts at the locations in which the connective tissue network is being formed. In the human heart, the ratio of collagen to total myocardial protein falls with perinatal development toward the lower ratio of the adult heart,[196] in a direction correlating with a maturational increase in myocardial compliance. The effect of development on the proportion of the collagen types that compose the cardiac extracellular matrix is still being characterized. A decrease in the ratio of type I to type III collagen has been described in the human heart during fetal and neonatal life.[196,197] Type III collagen is thought to provide elasticity. Altogether, these alterations in ratios and collagen expression are likely to affect myocardial compliance and contribute to the developmental changes in myocardial passive properties.[15,16,111]

In humans, within weeks of birth, the extracellular matrix has acquired the properties of the adult myocardium. The resulting extracellular matrix three-dimensional structure is composed of a weave that surrounds groups of myocytes, bundles of collagen that connect myocytes to myocytes and myocytes to capillaries, and microthreads that interact with the collagen bundles.[10,195] Collagen, elastin, glycoproteins, proteoglycans, and cell surface components make up the interconnected components of this system.[9,194] These components, which change during development, also change with aging and in the adult heart in response to stress (e.g., pressure overload).[197]

Passive Mechanical Properties and Maturation

The immature myocardium is less compliant than that of the older animal.[15,16] The maturational increase in compliance is likely to arise from differences in both the extracellular matrix and the cytoskeleton. Because of the relative stiffness of the immature myocardium, an increase in ventricular preload (end-diastolic volume) in the fetal and neonatal heart is likely to have a greater effect on properties of the contralateral ventricle than a comparable increase in preload in the adult heart.[16,115,198-201] In the developing heart, in vitro increases in right ventricular volume have a greater effect on the left ventricular passive pres-

sure-volume relationship than in the adult heart.[16] The consequence is that the same filling pressure achieves a relatively smaller left ventricular volume in the fetus than in the adult.[16] These effects may be, related in part, to the relatively larger right ventricle of the immature heart and thicker right ventricular free wall.[115,202] However, as a corollary to the effects of the right ventricle on left ventricular properties, increases in left ventricular volume have a greater effect on the passive filling properties of the immature right ventricle than that of the adult.

Maturational changes in ventricular compliance, volume, and geometry make ventricular function in the immature heart more susceptible to changes in systolic pressure and diastolic volume of the contralateral ventricle. For example, if right ventricular afterload is increased and right ventricular ejection decreases, the resulting increase in right ventricular volume will have a greater negative effect on left ventricular filling and ejection in the fetal and neonatal heart than in the adult. Similarly, if pulmonary arterial pressure is elevated in the neonate, left ventricular filling and stroke volume will be compromised (see Fig. 63-3). In addition, any increase in right ventricular preload in the neonate (e.g., secondary to tricuspid papillary muscle dysfunction) will also reduce left ventricular end-diastolic volume and thus decrease left ventricular stroke volume.

Maturation and Membrane Systems

In addition to maturational changes in the mechanical components that result in force development, developmental changes also occur in cell membranes, which are important in the process of activation and the modulation of cytosolic calcium concentration. Currently, it is not known whether coordinated expression of membrane and contractile proteins occurs in the heart. It is of interest that maturational and regional changes in the atrial transmembrane action potential have been correlated with maturational and regional changes in troponin T isoform expression. This suggests that the expression of the proteins that control the action potential configuration and intracellular ionic concentrations, and of the proteins that make up the sarcomere and respond to these ionic concentrations, is coordinately expressed.[164] Many ultrastructural and biochemical studies of the cardiac membrane systems indicate that these systems undergo prominent qualitative and quantitative changes in organization, amount, and function with maturation. However, in comparison with the contractile proteins, less is known about the maturational changes in the expression of membrane proteins and the existence of isoforms.

The time course of restitution of contractility is abbreviated in the immature myocardium.[94,207] In the isolated myocyte from the neonatal heart, sarcomere shortening in the most premature extrasystole equals that in the steady-state contraction.[94] In contrast, restitution of sarcomere shortening is observed in the adult myocyte; that is, the extrasystolic amount and velocity of sarcomere shortening gradually increase as the extrasystole is applied at longer intervals following the previous contraction. These differences in the restitution of contractility are the consequence of maturational changes in SR function.[92] Post-extrasystolic potentiation also increases with maturation,[104] which is consistent with a maturational increase in the ability of the myocyte to modulate cytosolic calcium concentration over a wider range and to higher levels.[104] The near-abolishment of post-extrasystolic potentiation in adult myocardium by ryanodine suggests that the maturational increase in potentiation is based on the increased availability or increased release of calcium from intracellular stores, specifically the SR (Fig. 63-9).

The distribution and number of the specialized connections between the junctional SR and sarcolemma (peripheral and internal couplings or dyads and triads; see Fig. 63-2) change and increase with maturation.[210,211] These couplings contain the SR

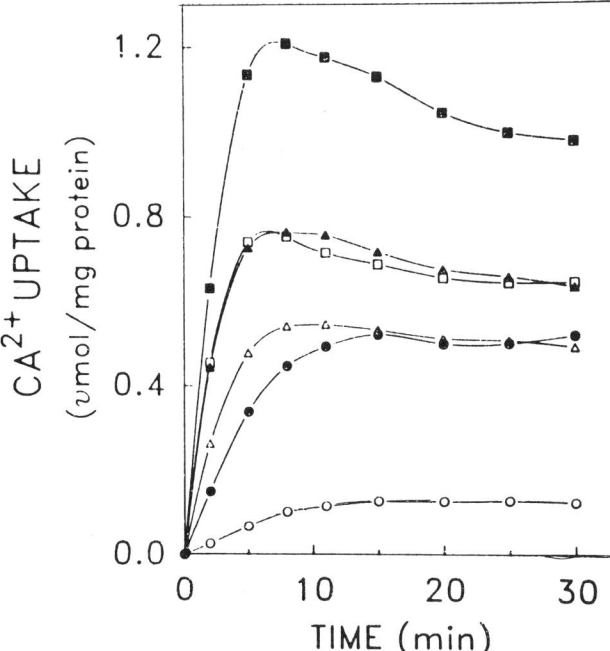

Figure 63–9. Time course for Ca²⁺ uptake by cardiac sarcoplasmic reticulum (SR) vesicles. Cardiac SR vesicles were isolated from Gp I (*white* ○), Gp II (*black* ●), Gp III (*white* △), Gp IV (*black* ▲), Gp V (*white* □), and Gp VI (*black* ■) sheep. Gp I = 100 to 105 days' gestation; Gp II = 128 to 132 days' gestation; Gp III = postnatal, 0 to 3 days; Gp IV = postnatal, 4 weeks; Gp V = postnatal, 8 weeks; Gp VI = maternal sheep. Ca²⁺ uptake was measured at 37°C. The initial velocity of Ca²⁺ uptake and maximal Ca²⁺ uptake measured in vesicles from Gp I to Gp V was significantly less ($p < .01$) than that measured in Gp IV vesicles. (From Mahoney L: Pediatr Res *24*:639, 1988.)

calcium release channel. Peripheral couplings are present before the acquisition of the transverse tubular system, and, with its acquisition (see further on), internal couplings within the transverse tubular system (T-system) are formed. Couplings are not distributed uniformly on the adult myocyte cell surface. Internal couplings are many times more frequent. Thus, the couplings that are acquired with development are located primarily in the T-system. The ratio of junctional SR membrane area to myofibrillar volume in the rabbit increases during late gestation and then appears to remain constant from neonatal to adult life. Given the importance of this structure in SR calcium release, the changes in this proportion may contribute to the maturational increase in the sensitivity of the calcium-induced calcium release process (CICR; see earlier).[84] These findings are consistent with the maturational quantitative increase in post-extrasystolic potentiation and changes in the restitution of contractility.

The T-system is acquired with maturation.[1,94] This system is made up of invaginations of the sarcolemma and its associated cell coat into the cell, and it allows the extracellular environment to extend deeply within the cell (yet remain extracellular).[212] The rate of T-system acquisition with development varies among species and appears to be related to the general rate of physiologic maturation. For example, the T-system is present as a well-organized system in the late-gestation fetal lamb and guinea pig, is found in the human fetus, and is acquired during neonatal life in the mouse, rat, rabbit, and dog.[94,110,129,211] The T-system has been related to qualitative changes in cell physiology. However, the T-system is not necessary for the modulation of cytosolic calcium with activation. For example, mammalian myocardium contains a T-system and avian myocardium does not, but post-

extrasystolic potentiation and restitution of contractility are present in both.[212] Attempts to define functional differences between free and T-tubule sarcolemma are continuing; however, the sarcolemma of the T-tubule in cardiac muscle does not appear to differ from that of free sarcolemma. The DHP-sensitive calcium channels may be found in greater density in the T-system.[213]

The marked increase in cardiac myocyte size that occurs with maturation would result in a large decrease in the cell surface-to-volume ratio if it were not for the acquisition of the T-system. In species in which adult myocytes are markedly wider, thicker, and longer than immature myocytes, morphometric analysis of the cell surface-to-volume ratio has demonstrated that the acquisition of the T-system is a normal part of development.[1] Although some difference of opinion exists as to whether the cell surface-to-volume ratio changes with cell growth,[1,128] it is generally agreed that the cardiac cell surface-to-volume ratio remains constant during the acquisition of the T-system. Consequently, acquisition of the T-system in cardiac muscle is important in maintaining this ratio. This conclusion is supported in part by the observation that just as left ventricular cells increase in size more rapidly following birth, the left ventricular myocytes also acquire a T-system more rapidly than right ventricular cells. The T-tubules would appear to provide a means for avoiding intracellular ionic gradients that would be expected to occur if the extracellular media could not be brought deep within the large, complexly shaped adult myocyte. However, some differences in the temporal acquisition of the T-system and maturation of physiologic properties suggest the importance of other membrane systems in calcium flux and illustrate the difficulty in establishing structure-function relationships.

Sarcolemmal Function

Na⁺,K⁺-ATPase undergoes developmental changes in isoform expression and in ATPase activity from fetal to adult life.[66,214,215] This ATPase is important in maintaining the cytosolic sodium and calcium concentrations and cell calcium content. The enzyme, which is the digitalis receptor site, is found in increasing numbers with development.[214] In addition, maturational changes in ATPase activity have been related to the maturational changes in myocardial sensitivity to cardiac glycosides.[216,217] In general, the myocardium of the neonatal mammal (the rat being the major exception[217]) is less sensitive than is adult myocardium to the inotropic effects of digoxin. The observed differences in cardiac glycoside sensitivity from one stage of development to another may result, in part, from differences in the control state (e.g., the enhanced inotropic state of the neonatal heart *in situ* is less likely to be further enhanced by cardiac glycosides or the level of sympathetic stimulation).[218] Although the basis of species-to-species variation in sensitivity to digoxin remains uncertain, in humans the young patient does respond to digoxin with an enhancement in contractility.[219,220]

The inhibition of Na⁺,K⁺-ATPase caused by digitalis intoxication results in an increase in extracellular potassium concentration.[221] The associated higher intracellular sodium activity will increase cell calcium content through sodium-calcium exchange. When this effect is potentiated by increasing extracellular calcium, for example, by an intravenous infusion of calcium, digitalis-induced dysrhythmias are increased in frequency and severity.

The expression and activity of the α-subunit isoforms of Na⁺,K⁺-ATPase (its catalytic subunit) have been studied in the rat and found to undergo a tissue-specific, developmentally regulated expression that is accompanied by changes in ATPase activity.[66,215] A family of genes produces three α-subunit isoforms that have different Na⁺,K⁺-ATPase activities and different sensitivities and binding affinities to the cardiac glycosides.

Maturational changes in the effects of cardiac glycosides in other species suggest that developmental changes in Na+,K+-ATPase isoform expression are a general property of mammalian myocardium. The differential expression of these isoforms and their responses to hormones and other cell ligands may contribute to differences in the cellular response to a range of pharmacologic agents.

Cardiac muscle demonstrates two calcium currents that have been characterized by their electrophysiologic properties as being T-type (transient) or L-type (long) dihydropyridine (DHP)-sensitive calcium channels.[63] The T-type current is affected primarily by inorganic calcium channel blockers, whereas the L-type slow calcium channel is sensitive to organic blockers. At early stages of development, the net calcium channel current is more sensitive to inorganic blockers, indicating that the majority of the current is carried through T-type channels. For example, embryonic chick heart cells have been described as having a greater T-type channel density than do adult cells, whereas in the adult, the DHP-sensitive L-type channel current is the dominant calcium current.[222]

The density of the slow calcium channel current increases during neonatal life in the rabbit heart and during fetal life in the mouse.[223-225] Conversely, an embryonic decrease in the L-type current occurs in the bird,[226] and a neonatal decrease in current density occurs in the rat,[227] which are associated with changes in transcription.[228] These apparently conflicting results do not provide a straightforward explanation for the immature myocardial contraction being apparently more dependent on extracellular calcium.

Based on variations in the effects of the organic calcium channel antagonists on preparations from different stages of development, the properties of the calcium channel and its associated proteins change with maturation.[229] The multiple large subunits of this channel (estimated M_r 175, 170, 52, and 32 kDa) and their associated proteins make isoforms, whose likely expression changes with maturation. Cardiac complementary DNA (cDNA) analysis provides evidence for alternative splicing of the primary transcript as the basis of α_1- and β-isoforms.[230,231] The presence of additional isoforms is suggested by the different effects of calcium channel antagonists on various tissues.[63] Additional explanations for these various effects include developmental and/or tissue-specific expression of different guanine-binding proteins that modulate the effect of ligand binding on calcium channel function.

An alternate source for providing calcium to support the cardiac contraction is the Na+-Ca2+ exchanger. As discussed previously, when the cell depolarizes sufficiently and its equilibrium potential is passed, the direction of the Na+-Ca2+ exchange is reversed, so that calcium enters the cell during the contraction.[87-89] This calcium could contribute directly to the calcium transient producing strong cross-bridge formation, or it could only elicit SR calcium release.[88] In adult myocardium and in neonatal myocardium of species that are mature at birth (e.g., guinea pig), this mechanism appears to have little functional consequence in that the neonatal Na+-Ca2+ exchanger current density is low.[232] In contrast, in species in which the expression of the exchanger is highest during perinatal life, falling with postnatal development to low levels in the adult heart,[233,234] the Na+-Ca2+ exchanger current density is higher in neonatal myocytes than in adult myocytes.[232,235] These findings suggest a mechanism that would make the immature myocyte more dependent on extracellular calcium than that of the adult heart. Given the relative immaturity of the human at birth (similar to the rat and rabbit) the Na+-Ca2+ exchanger is likely to contribute to the marked sensitivity of the neonatal human heart to a fall in extracellular calcium concentration observed during the postoperative period.[236]

Developmental changes in the sarcolemmal properties that are a consequence of the observed and likely changes in Na+,K+-ATPase, the DHP-sensitive calcium channel, the Na+-Ca2+ exchanger, and other sarcolemmal systems should contribute to changes in cardiac contractility. It remains to be established, however, how their interactions in the immature myocardium blunt the contractile response to a perturbation in the pattern of stimulation while yielding a greater increase in contractility in response to an increase in extracellular calcium concentration.

Myocardial Sympathetic Nervous System

The sympathetic nervous system is important in multiple cell processes, including cell growth and differentiation, the control of cytosolic calcium concentration, and the responses of the contractile and membrane proteins to calcium. The components of this system undergo extensive developmental changes. For example, the innervation of the myocardium and the local availability of neurotransmitters increase with maturation.[237-241] At the level of the myocyte, the number and proportion of adrenoceptors and the membrane-coupled and intracellular systems that transduce sympathetic stimulation also change.[242-244]

The sympathetic nervous system has a major role in the adaptation of the cardiovascular system to changes imposed by birth.[245-247] Circulating catecholamine concentrations increase during labor and following birth in humans. These levels are markedly increased in the severely stressed neonate. The importance of these elevated levels of catecholamines in opposing the negative inotropic effects of perinatal acidosis, and for enhancing contractility in response to stress, is revealed by the lethal effect of β-adrenoceptor blockade in the stressed neonate.[248]

The time-course of cardiac innervation varies across species. In the lamb, it appears during fetal life, whereas in other species it does not begin until postnatal life.[237-241] Myocardial innervation is first seen around the large coronary vessels before the nerves extend into the cardiac muscle bundles and adrenergic plexuses are seen. The adrenergic plexus density increases until an adult pattern is achieved. The intramyocardial availability of norepinephrine depends on this innervation and the storage of neurotransmitter in the synaptic vesicles.[249,250] The maturational increase in myocardial norepinephrine concentration is accompanied by changes in the response to tyramine (a norepinephrine-release agent). For example, tyramine increases heart rate in the puppy much less than in the adult dog, and tyramine or field stimulation of intramyocardial nerves in the rat evokes little contractile response during the first few postnatal weeks when compared with the adult.[251] During gestation in humans, there is a developmental increase in norepinephrine stores, which suggests that endogenous cardiac norepinephrine levels are decreased in the preterm infant.[252]

The response of the myocardium to β- and α-agonists precedes the acquisition of myocardial innervation.[238] The developmental changes in the response to exogenous catecholamines vary across species and from study to study.[238,251,253-255] The myocardium of the fetal and neonatal lamb and the neonatal rat are more sensitive to norepinephrine than are those of the older neonate or the adult. Similarly, the heart rate of the neonatal puppy is more sensitive to exogenous norepinephrine. This supersensitivity of the immature myocardium to norepinephrine has been characterized as being comparable to denervation hypersensitivity.

It is of interest that despite the changes in the response to norepinephrine, there is no developmental change in the response to isoproterenol in the sheep myocardium. This maturational difference has been attributed to the relative lack of the adrenergic plexus system in the immature myocardium. The plexus serves as an intramyocardial uptake and release site for norepinephrine, but it does not take up isoproterenol.

Responsiveness of the immature myocardium to sympathomimetic agents indicates that adrenoceptors are present in fetal and neonatal myocardium. Maturational differences observed in the number and proportion of α- and β-adrenoceptors may contribute to the maturational differences in the sensitivity to norepinephrine and isoproterenol. The process of innervation may also modify the responses to sympathomimetic agents. For example, the presence of sympathetic nerves alters the responses of the ventricular myocyte to α-adrenoceptor stimulation.[256] Signal transduction is altered by the expression of different isoforms of the α-adrenoceptor–linked guanine-protein (G-protein) binding regulatory protein.[257,258] An example of developmental changes in G-protein isoform expression is the increase in the rate of beating of immature myocytes when they are exposed to phenylephrine; the opposite effect is observed in adult myocytes (i.e., a decrease in the spontaneous beating rate).[259]

Developmental changes in β-adrenoceptor number have been observed, including an increase in the number of β-receptors per cell.[260-263] In one study, the proportion of β1- to β2-receptors was found not to differ with development. Moreover the developmental changes in β3-receptor expression, whose stimulation results in a negative inotropic effect, remain unknown.[264] The maturational changes in the α-adrenoceptor number differ substantially in direction from those of the β-receptor.[265-267] In the sheep, the highest level of expression of the α-adrenoceptor occurs during late gestation and early postnatal life. In the adult myocardium of the dog and sheep, very low levels of α-adrenoceptors are common. This developmental decrease in the number of α-adrenoceptors is opposite to the developmental increase in β-adrenoceptors.

The developmental differences in the amount and density of α- and β-adrenoceptors may be important in bringing about the physiologic hypertrophy in neonatal myocytes.[130-132] Cultured immature myocytes respond to α1-agonist stimulation by increasing their size and protein content. The agonist-induced increase in protein synthesis in the immature myocyte is prevented by α1-blockade. β1-Stimulation, in contrast, does not induce hypertrophy but does increase the frequency of beating. In contrast, adult myocytes that have low levels of α-adrenoceptors do not hypertrophy in response to α-agonists. The maturational decrease in responsiveness to this stimulation may be a consequence of the decrease in the number of α1-adrenoceptors already noted or secondary to changes in the transduction of α1-adrenergic stimulation and the intracellular effector.[268-272]

The developmental changes in the myocardial contractile responses to autonomic agents may result from differences in the components of the system that transduce cholinergic and sympathetic stimulation into alterations in cytosolic ionic concentrations and contractility. In that regard, maturational changes in the expression of isoforms of the catalytic subunit of the G-proteins have been described.[257,258] Against a background of β-stimulation at a physiologic level, carbachol (a cholinergic agonist) has a greater positive effect on the L-type calcium current density in the neonatal rabbit myocyte, compared with the adult.[243] This maturational change in the effect of cholinergic stimulation on the calcium current may be related to G-protein isoform expression. Adenylate cyclase, the enzyme system stimulated by β-agonists, is found to undergo a wide range of developmental changes that may alter cell functions.[271,273] Adenylate cyclase activity has been found to increase during development, perhaps in relation to the maturational increase in endogenous catecholamines and their stimulatory effects. The coupling of adenylate cyclase activity and force development may change with development. In fetal myocardium the production of cAMP has been found to be out of proportion to the catecholamine-induced increase in force.[274]

Maturational changes in the multiple components of the sympathetic nervous system should modulate the functional effects of the membrane and contractile proteins on heart rate and contractility. α-Adrenoceptor and β-adrenoceptor stimulation and

the ingrowth of sympathetic and cholinergic nerves into the myocardium also alter contractile protein expression. Post-translational modifications of these proteins follow from adrenoceptor stimulation and are physiologically important. For example, cAMP-dependent phosphorylation of the calcium channel increases the calcium current,[63] phosphorylation of phospholamban (the SR calcium ATPase-inhibitory protein) increases SR calcium uptake and ATPase activity,[32,78,80] and phosphorylation of cardiac troponin I decreases the sensitivity of the myofibrils to calcium.[32,50,100] The myosin ATPase isoforms are also differentially affected by adrenoceptor stimulation; myosin V1 is more sensitive to β stimulation.[275] Given the functional changes in these proteins with agonist stimulation and their changes in expression with development, the effects of the sympathetic system on myocardial function will differ from one stage of development to another.

VENTRICULAR FUNCTION OF THE IMMATURE HEART

The output of the fetal heart and its ability to contract are modulated by changes in end-diastolic volume (preload), heart rate, and arterial pressure (afterload) and many forms of inotropic interventions (i.e., stimuli that change cytosolic calcium concentration and myofilament response to calcium).* Many of these responses are qualitatively similar to those of the adult heart.[53,277-280] The similarity of these effects on ventricular function is not surprising, considering that these variables exert similar effects on force development and shortening in myocardium isolated from fetal and adult hearts. Specifically, increasing muscle length, rate of stimulation, or inotropic state enhances the ability of myocardium, isolated from either the adult or the immature heart, to generate tension, whereas increasing afterload decreases the velocity of myocardial shortening at all stages of development. It must be remembered, however, that a physiologic perturbation that enhances contractility in the isolated myocardium can have a negative effect on *in vivo* ventricular function, a consequence of the interaction of venous return, heart rate, diastolic volume, inotropic state, and afterload. For example, an increase in the pacing rate of the *in situ* heart leads to a fall in stroke volume through the concomitant decrease in end-diastolic volume, whereas an increase in the pacing rate of isolated myocardium increases the force of contraction.[42,116,117,281] In the isolated myocardium, in contrast to the *in vivo* heart, the experimental parameters—muscle length, afterload, inotropic state, and rate of stimulation—can be easily controlled, allowing the effects of various perturbations to be clearly revealed.

Some effects of maturation on the function of the intact in vivo heart can be explained by differences in the *in utero* and postnatal circulations and the relative differences in the right and left ventricular outputs and workloads at various stages of development. For example, fetal right ventricular output is higher than that of the left ventricle,[282] and neonatal ventricular output per body weight is much greater than that of the adult ventricle.[119] Additional reasons for apparent maturational differences in ventricular function can be attributed to variations among experimental protocols and the mechanisms used to alter specific parameters. For example, the site of atrial pacing will determine the effect of heart rate on fetal ventricular function.[41,116,117,119,281]

The experimental complexities imposed by studying the intact *in utero* fetus have resulted in relatively few fetal studies being performed in which the fetus was given days to recover from the acute effects of surgery and instrumentation. The following sections focus on such studies in the chronically

---

* Refs 32,41–43,45,46,52,104,116–119,276.

instrumented *in utero* animal and contrast them to studies of the neonate and the adult.

Heart Rate

The heart was once thought to undergo a development change in its response to rate, until it was recognized that the effects of spontaneous changes in heart rate must be considered separately from those induced by pacing.[116,117,119] In fact, apparent maturational changes in the response of the *in vivo* heart to changes in heart rate can be explained by experimental differences between studies. The consequent conclusion is that heart rate affects the function of the embryonic, fetal, and adult heart in a similar manner.

In the fetus, the maximum rate of rise of left ventricular pressure, dP/dt_{max}, is affected positively by an increase in rate (Fig. 63–10), in a fashion similar to that observed in the neonate and the adult.[41,42,277,281,283] This rate-induced increase in dP/dt_{max} occurs over a wide range of rates despite a rate-induced fall in ventricular end-diastolic volume (see Fig. 63–10). When end-diastolic volume is held constant, the heart rate–induced increase in dP/dt_{max} is even greater. The same relationships are found in the adult heart. Thus, if dP/dt_{max} is used to measure ventricular function, maturation has no effect on the ventricular response to heart rate. An increase in rate through atrial pacing usually decreases fetal ventricular ejection. For example, stroke volume falls with an increase in heart rate[116,117] (Fig. 63–11). When atrial pacing is used to alter rate, the negative effect on stroke volume is driven by the heart rate–induced fall in end-

diastolic volume consequent to a decrease in diastolic filling time. These findings are the same as those of atrial pacing studies in the intact adult animal and human.[249,280] Thus, when atrially induced changes in heart rate are used to characterize the effects of heart rate on ventricular function, no maturational differences in the effects of heart rate on ventricular function are observed.

The effect of rate on end-diastolic volume in the *in vivo* heart can be circumvented by interpolating infrequently longer-paced intervals into the paced rate to allow the ventricle to eject from the same end-diastolic volume at overall different rates (Fig. 63–12). By avoiding the usual rate-induced fall in ventricular volume, heart rate can be shown in the fetal and adult heart to exert a positive inotropic effect on stroke volume.

A spontaneous change in heart rate, which by definition is induced by endogenous stimuli, is accompanied by hemodynamic effects secondary to factors other than rate.[116,117,119] The stimuli that induce a spontaneous increase in cardiac rate often enhance inotropy and increase venous return while having little or no effect on arterial pressure. The positive effect on inotropy can enhance stroke volume even if end-diastolic volume falls. At other times, venous return is augmented, producing a greater rate of ventricular filling so that despite the heart rate–associated shortening of diastolic filling time, end-diastolic volume is maintained. Consequently, in contrast to the absence of an effect or a negative effect of an atrial pacing–induced increase in heart rate on fetal ventricular output, a spontaneous increase in heart rate usually has a positive effect on ventricular output: fetal right and left ventricular outputs both increase. However, exceptions to the positive effects of spontaneous increase in heart rate are

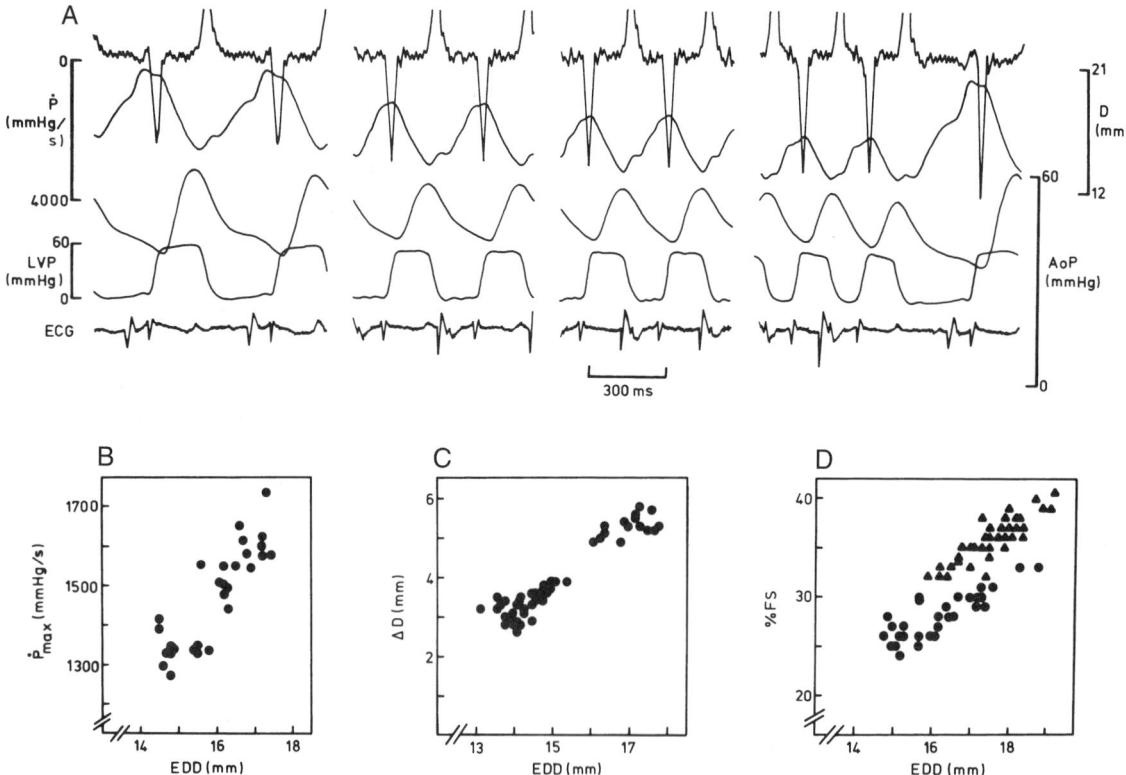

Figure 63–10. A, The effect of heart rate on a fetal lamb's left ventricular peak first derivative of pressure ($\dot{P}$), minor axis dimension (D), pressure (LVP), and aortic pressure (AoP); ECG = electrocardiogram. The groups of data were obtained during spontaneous (cycle interval of 430 ms) and paced rhythm (t_0 = 350, 300, and 250 ms). The data at the far right include a pause in pacing. **B, C,** and **D,** The effect of end-diastolic dimension (EDD) on the maximum rate of rise in left ventricular pressure (**B,** $\dot{P}_{max}$), systolic shortening (**C,** EDD; $\triangle$D), and percentage of fractional shortening ($\triangle$D $\div$ EDD × 100%), (**D,** %FS) in a fetal lamb (basic pacing interval, 300 ms). The %FS data were obtained at two infusion rates of isoproterenol: 0.006 µg/kg/min (*black* ●) and 0.024 µg/kg/min (*black* ▲). Note the inotropic effect of isoproterenol. At the higher infusion rate, a greater percent fractional shortening is achieved for equal end-diastolic dimensions. (From Anderson PAW, et al: Am J Obstet Gynecol *143*:195, 1982.)

occasionally seen. In some instances they can be explained by an increase in arterial pressure: an increase in afterload negatively affects ventricular output.[45,46]

In general, however, spontaneous increases in rate usually enhance fetal cardiac output. In the adult heart, spontaneous increases in rate also generally increase ventricular output. Thus, the effects on ventricular function of an increase in heart rate induced by atrial pacing or by endogenous stimuli do not differ between the fetal and the adult heart. In summary, throughout maturation, the effects of heart rate on ventricular ejection and pressure development depend on the interaction of diastolic filling time, venous return, inotropic state, and afterload.

Preload

The Frank-Starling relationship is present in the right and left ventricles of the *in vivo* fetal heart and isolated fetal myocardium[15,41-46] (see Fig. 63-12). Conflicting opinions exist regarding the importance of ventricular end-diastolic volume on ventricular function in the intact fetus and neonate.[43-46,104,116,117,119,284-286] When dP/dt$_{max}$ is used to assess the effects of end-diastolic volume, an increase in end-diastolic volume is found to have a positive effect on fetal ventricular function (i.e., dP/dt$_{max}$ increases).[41,42] When ejection measures of fetal ventricular function are used, different conclusions have been reached about the relation between end-diastolic volume and ventricular function in the fetal heart. For example, when fetal ventricular output has been used to assess the effect of volume infusions, some investigators have found that at nonphysiologically high atrial filling pressures, the fetal heart has little functional reserve in the Frank-Starling relationship[43,45,46] (Figs. 63-13 and 63-14). However, a fall in atrial pressure produced by blood withdrawal decreases ventricular output. In these latter experiments, the major difference between the responses of the fetal right and left ventricle is that the maximum right ventricular output is greater than that of the left ventricle (Fig. 63-15; see also Fig. 63-14).

It is of importance to note that a volume-induced increase in fetal arterial pressure has to be avoided when performing these kinds of experiments (compare the fetal right ventricular function curves obtained in the presence of nitroprusside and phenylephrine; see Fig. 63-13). The immature cardiovascular system appears to respond to volume loading with a greater increase in afterload than does the mature system. This developmental difference in the effect of increasing blood volume can explain, in part, a maturational acquisition of a greater reserve in the Frank-Starling relationship.[287]

Previous studies have suggested that the Frank-Starling relationship provides little functional reserve for the fetal heart; however, these studies have characterized the effect of preload on function by using indirect measures of ventricular volume, such as mean atrial pressure. These approaches can be misleading. When a change in atrial pressure is used to measure a change in ventricular end-diastolic volume, the extent of the change in ventricular volume is unknown. In the adult heart, for example, when the left ventricular filling pressure is high and filling pressure is increased further, only a small increment in end-diastolic volume occurs. Because the fetal myocardium has a relatively low compliance, that is, is stiffer than adult myocardium,[15,16] increments in atrial pressure from levels that might be considered low in the normal adult heart will result in trivial increases in end-diastolic volume (see Fig. 63-3). Indeed, some studies have suggested that the development acquisition of the Frank-Starling relationship is only apparent and not real, being a consequence of the maturational increase in myocardial compliance and developmental differences in the extent to which an increase in filling pressure increases end-diastolic volume.

To measure the effects of preload on ventricular function more directly, ventricular ultrasonic dimension transducers have been used to examine the relationship between ventricular end-diastolic volume and stroke volume in the fetal right and left ventricles.[44,116,117,288] An increase in fetal left ventricular end-diastolic dimension is accompanied by an increase in systolic minor axis shortening (see Fig. 63-10). When aortic and pulmonary

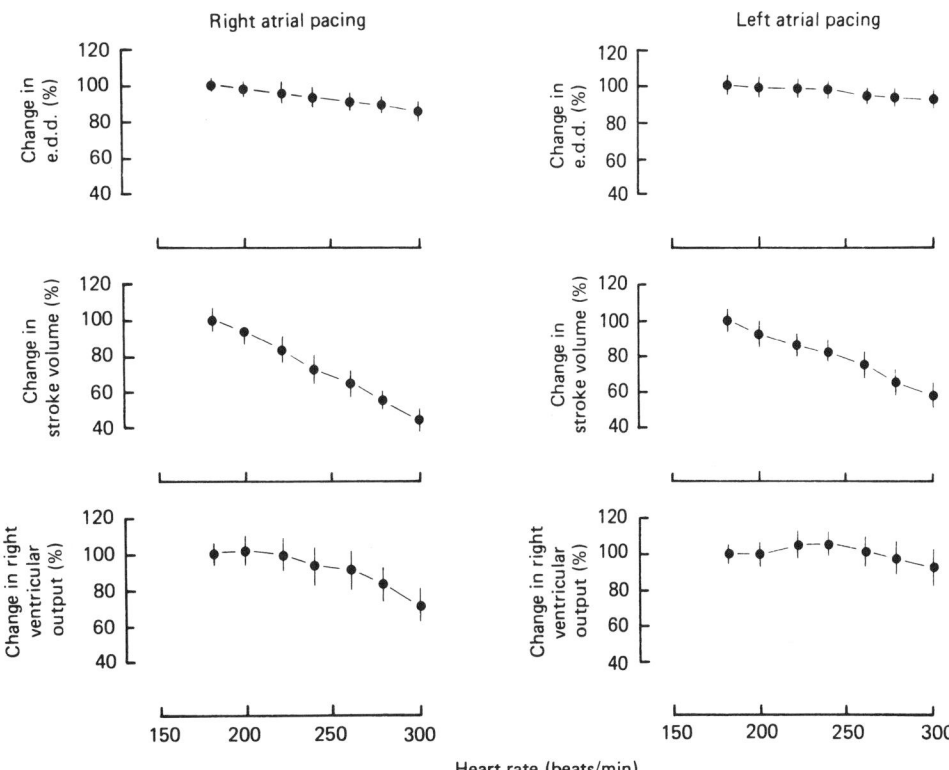

Figure 63–11. The effects of right atrial pacing and left atrial pacing on right ventricular filling and ejection in a group of chronically instrumented fetal lambs. Values are normalized and expressed as percentages; 100% represents data at the slowest rate. Percentage changes in right ventricular end-diastolic dimension (right ventricular free wall endocardium to ventricular septum) % e.d.d. The paced rates range from 182 to 300 beats/min. The vertical bars represent two standard deviations about the mean. Right ventricular output fell with an increase in right atrial pacing rate, whereas output was unaffected by increasing left atrial pacing rate. (From Anderson PAW et al: J Physiol [Lond] *387*:297, 1987.)

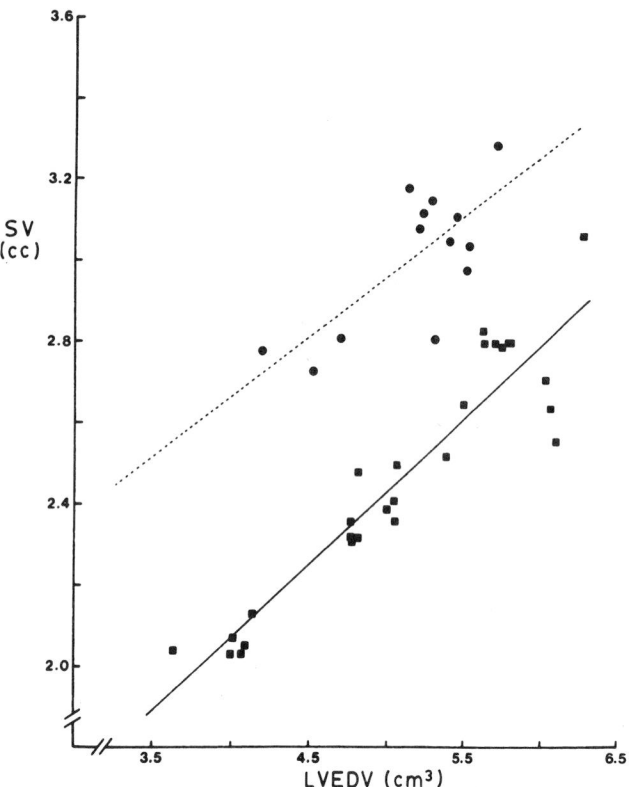

Figure 63–12. Relationship between fetal left ventricular stroke volume (SV) and end-diastolic volume (LVEDV) in a chronically instrumented fetal lamb. By altering cardiac rate through atrial pacing, a range of left ventricular end-diastolic volume is obtained during a control state (■) and during an infusion of isoproterenol (●). Stroke depends on end-diastolic volume and inotropic state. For a given end-diastolic volume, the stroke volume is larger in the presence of isoproterenol. Left ventricular end-diastolic volume is computed by measuring sonomicrometrically three left ventricular dimensions, two minor axes, and one major axis.

artery systolic flows are measured, the fetal right and left ventricle demonstrate a Frank-Starling relationship: over a physiologic range of filling pressures, an increase in end-diastolic volume is accompanied by an increase in ventricualr stroke volume (see Figs. 63–10 and 63–12). Thus, the fetal heart does exhibit a functionally important Frank-Starling relationship.

Maturational changes in ventricular size, compliance, and interaction may contribute to quantitative differences between the fetal and adult heart.[15,16,115,120,121,200,202] For example, the marked and immediate increase in left ventricular volume with birth[42,104,120,121] may transiently expend most of the immature heart's Frank-Starling reserve, so the neonatal heart might be expected to respond less well to volume loading than does the older heart. However, this conclusion must be considered in light of the ability of the preterm infant's heart to respond with a large increase in stroke volume to the ventricular volume loading that accompanies a patent ductus arteriosus.[284,285,289]

Afterload

Fetal ventricular function is affected by afterload in a manner similar to that of the adult: as aortic or pulmonary artery pressure rises, left or right ventricular stroke volume falls[43,45,46,53,198] (Fig. 63–16; see also Figs. 63–13 and 63–15). Thus, an increase in afterload decreases systolic function. The study of isolated muscle provides a corollary: an increase in afterload decreases the velocity and amount of muscle shortening for both fetal and adult myocardial preparations.[15]

Developmental changes in the quantitative relationship between afterload and myocardial function exist. When shortening against the same load, the immature myocardium shortens more slowly and by a smaller amount than does the adult myocardium. Similarly, in the intact animal, fetal and neonatal ventricular function is profoundly and negatively affected by arterial pressures that the adult ventricle is able to support easily. These quantitative differences probably have their basis in the structural differences in the ventricular myocardium described earlier.

In the intact fetus, the right and left ventricles appear to be affected in a quantitatively different manner by afterload[45,46] (see Fig. 63–16). The following provides a basis for the greater after-

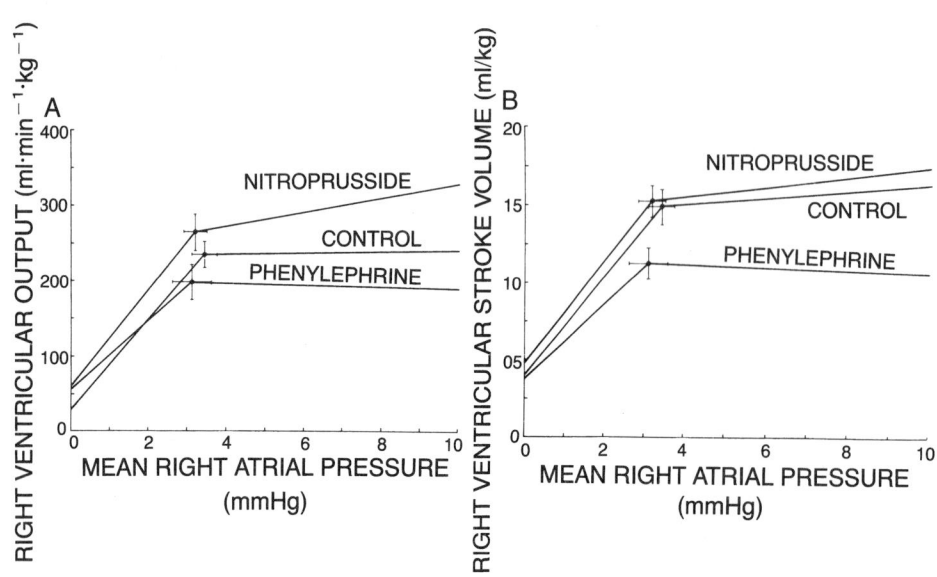

Figure 63–13. A, Composite curves of right ventricular output as a function of mean right atrial pressure for a group of chronically instrumented *in utero* fetal lambs. Experiments performed during nitroprusside (NP) infusion produced lower arterial pressures than control; arterial pressure was higher during the phenylephrine infusion. Curves from experiments with increased fetal arterial blood pressure (phenylephrine infusion) showed a decreased ascending limb and plateau slopes. **B,** Right ventricular stroke volume as a function of mean atrial pressure for NP, control, and phenylephrine. The plateau slopes for normal, reduced, and elevated arterial pressures were not different from zero. (From Thornburg KL, Morton MJ: Am J Physiol *244*:H656, 1983.)

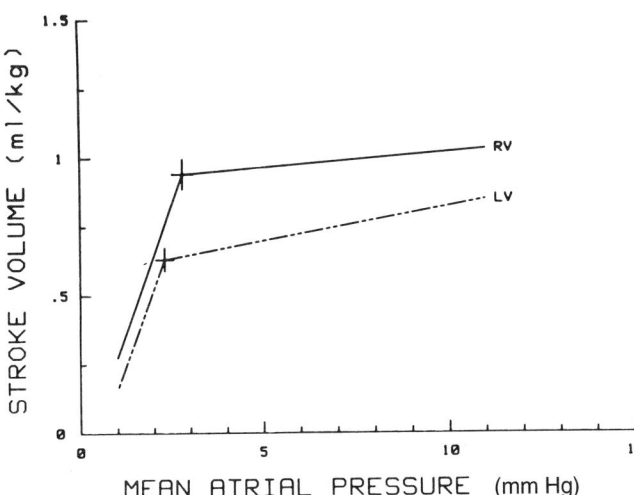

Figure 63–14. The average simultaneous ventricular function curves for 12 fetal lambs were determined for the right and left ventricle. The right ventricular function curve (*RV*) has a steep ascending limb similar to that of the left ventricular function curve (*LV*). The plateaus differ significantly. (From Reller MD, et al: Pediatr Res *22*:621, 1987.)

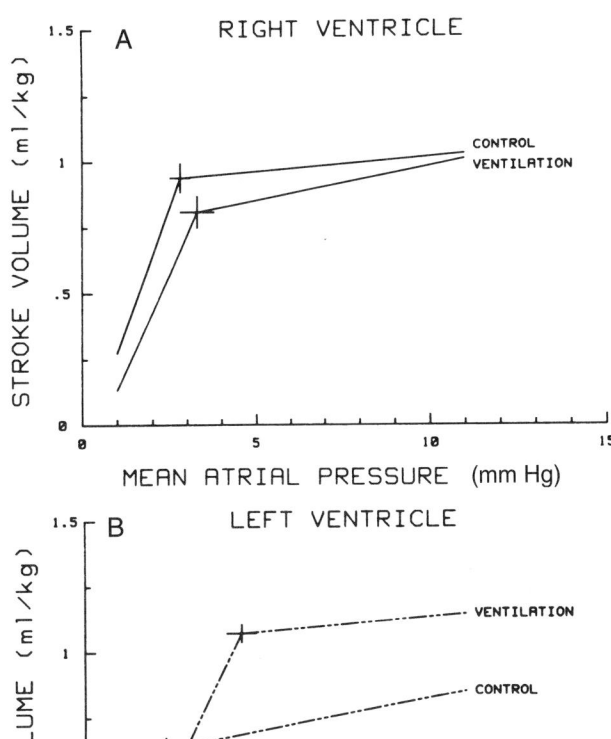

Figure 63–15. Average function curves for the right and left ventricle of a group of fetal lambs before and during *in utero* ventilation (n = 8). **A,** The right ventricular function curve was depressed by *in utero* ventilation. **B,** The left ventricular function curve was shifted upward during *in utero* ventilation. (From Reller MD, et al: Pediatr Res *22*:621, 1987.)

load effect on the fetal right ventricle: The fetal right ventricular stroke work is greater than that of the left ventricle[116,117,119,202,282] (see Figs. 63-14 and 63-15). In addition, fetal right ventricular end-diastolic volume is greater than that of the left ventricle, right ventricular dimensions are larger, and the curvature of the right ventricle free wall is greater.[117,120,121,202] Consequently, in the presence of similar aortic and pulmonary artery pressures (and they usually are similar until late gestation when mild ductal constriction may be present), right ventricular systolic wall stress is greater than that of the left ventricle.[202] Thus, when afterload is increased, fetal right ventricular wall stress increases by a greater amount and to a higher level than does that of the left ventricle. The result will be a greater sensitivity of the right ventricle to afterload.

Inotropy

The response of the fetal heart to inotropic stimulation depends on the stimulus and the measure of ventricular function. Norepinephrine does not increase cardiac output in the intact *in utero* fetal lamb,[290] yet isolated fetal myocardium is very sensitive to norepinephrine.[15] The differences between the responses of the *in vivo* heart and the isolated myocardium can be explained by the norepinephrine-induced increase in afterload and decrease in heart rate. These changes will oppose any intrinsic positive inotropic effect of norepinephrine. When isoproterenol is infused into the fetal lamb, cardiac output is enhanced[291] (see Figs. 63-10 and 63-12). This effect is augmented by volume loading.[52] Isoproterenol increases fetal left ventricular output because of the positive effects of isoproterenol on inotropy and heart rate, and the absence of the increase in systolic pressure that occurs with norepinephrine. Isoproterenol also increases dP/dt$_{max}$, a measure of inotropy.[41] Thus, like the effects of positive inotropic stimulation on adult heart function,[277] fetal ventricular function is enhanced by positive inotropic stimulation.

Post-extrasystolic potentiation is another measure of inotropy that can be used to assess the responses of myocardial and ventricular function to inotropic interventions. Post-extrasystolic potentiation is independent of muscle length and ventricular volume in the developing heart and in the adult.[41,277] For example, isoproterenol increases dP/dt$_{max}$ of the systole at the

basic heart rate more than it increases dP/dt$_{max}$ of the post-extrasystolic systole, so that this positive inotropic agent decreases post-extrasystolic potentiation. This effect is present in the adult and fetal heart.[41,277] The sensitivity of post-extrasystolic potentiation to the inotropic state and the lack of an effect of preload form the basis for using post-extrasystolic potentiation to measure changes in ventricular function during maturation.

The assessment of the effects of maturation on ventricular function depends on the measures used to characterize this process. For example, stroke volume increases with maturation. However, this is accompanied by a marked increase in ventricular size, obscuring changes in intrinsic inotropic state. When dP/dt$_{max}$ is used to characterize maturational changes, the fetal and adult heart are functionally the same, that is, dP/dt$_{max}$ of fetal, child, and adult hearts *in vivo* usually ranges between 1500 and 3000 mm Hg per second, depending on the state of the individual.[41,42,104,277,283,288] When systolic pressure is used to assess ventricular function, maturation exerts both a positive effect (left ventricular systolic pressure increases) and a negative effect (right ventricular systolic pressure decreases) during the transition to postnatal life.[119,124] These discrepant conclusions result from using measures that are affected by maturational changes in ventricular volume and vascular resistance.

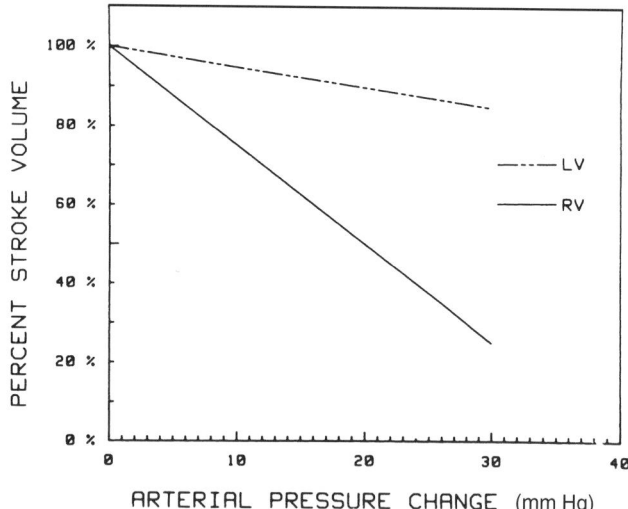

Figure 63–16. The simultaneous average responses of the right and left ventricle to increased arterial pressure are shown for 9 fetal lambs. Stroke volume is expressed as a percentage of control value, and arterial pressure as the increment above control. The linear regression coefficient for each ventricle was calculated, the average slope forced through 100% on the y axis, and the lines extended through the pressure range studied. The right ventricular pressure sensitivity was more than five times the left ventricular pressure sensitivity. (From Reller MD, et al: Pediatr Res *22*:621, 1987.)

Quantitative changes in post-extrasystolic potentiation provide another measure to assess the effects of maturation on ventricular function. The fetal heart *in vivo* demonstrates post-extrasystolic potentiation, the same basic property found in the adult heart.[41,42,104,277] During the last portion of gestation, there is an increase in post-extrasystolic potentiation in the *in utero* lamb.[104] This increase is similar to that observed in isolated myocardium from the same gestational period.[104,205] The quantitative increase in post-extrasystolic potentiation indicates a maturational increase in the range over which cytosolic calcium concentration is modulated. These findings illustrate the *in vivo* effects of the maturational increase in SR amount and organization and the resulting increased availability of calcium from intracellular stores (see later, Maturation and the Membrane Systems). Thus, in the *in vivo* heart, maturation enhances the level to which inotropy can be increased, as measured by the effects of cytosolic calcium concentration and myofilament responsiveness to calcium on post-extrasystolic potentiation.

Effects of Birth on Myocardial Function

With birth, left ventricular output is markedly enhanced, and right ventricular output is increased to a smaller extent.[42,104,119,282] The neonatal enhancement in left ventricular output can be attributed to the combined effects of the neonatal increase in heart rate, venous return, end-diastolic volume, and inotropy, in association with the effects of birth on right and left ventricular interaction.[42,104] The increase in right ventricular output results in part from a fall in pulmonary artery pressure. The increase in intropy in the newborn infant is reflected in the increase in left ventricular dP/dt$_{max}$ with birth (or the decrease in post-extrasystolic potentiation), which is similar to the effects of isoproterenol in the fetus.

Recall that an increase in heart rate in the fetus leads to a fall in end-diastolic volume and stroke volume unless ventricular diastolic filling is maintained. When end-diastolic volume is main-

tained, stroke volume and ventricular output increase in response to an increase in heart rate and to a positive inotropic stimulus (e.g., an isoproterenol infusion leads to an enhanced fetal stroke volume and increased ventricular output.[291] Consequently, the increases in heart rate, left ventricular venous return, and inotropy will combine to enhance left ventricular output.

The rearrangement of the circulation with birth should contribute significantly to the postnatal increase in left ventricular end-diastolic volume and thus, stroke volume. For example, ventilation with oxygen *in utero* decreases pulmonary vascular resistance. As a result, fetal right ventricular output flows through the pulmonary arteries, with reversal of shunting from right-to-left to left-to-right through the ductus arteriosus.[118,282,292] The large rise in pulmonary blood flow increases left atrial pressure and left ventricular output (Fig. 63–17; see also Fig. 63–15).

The effects of *in utero* ventilation on pulmonary vascular resistance, pulmonary venous return and left ventricular filling, stroke volume, and output have been proposed to mimic those associated with birth. Birth has a dramatic effect on the relationship between ventricular filling pressure and ventricular output. In the neonatal lamb, studied with its chest open, ventricular stroke volume and output are markedly increased by left atrial pressures that have much more modest effects on fetal cardiac output in the intact state.[45,293] The differences between the fetal and the neonatal ventricular responses may be a consequence of the removal of the ventricular filling constraints imposed by the intact chest, the pericardium, and the nonaerated lungs.[294] Consistent with those findings is the observation that the effects of increasing blood volume and left atrial pressure on left ventricular output in the presence of *in utero* ventilation with liquid are less than occurs with *in utero* ventilation with oxygen and similar volume-induced increases in left atrial pressure[118,282,292] (see Figs. 63–15 and 63–17).

Studies performed on intact postnatal animals have been interpreted to indicate that with increasing postnatal age the Frank-Starling relationship exerts a greater effect on ventricular function:[286] in response to a volume infusion, cardiac output in the older lamb increases by a greater percentage than does that of the newborn lamb. These findings suggest either that birth depletes the Frank-Starling reserves or that this relationship is acquired with maturation. However, when the size of the increases in volume are compared instead of the percentage changes, the 1-week-old newborn lamb increases its cardiac output by a greater amount than does the older lamb. Regardless of the presentation of these results, the crucial observation is that the newborn lamb is able to increase its output in response to a volume infusion.[284,286]

An increase in left ventricular inotropy also may enhance cardiac output at birth. In the fetal lamb, isoproterenol increases left ventricular dP/dt$_{max}$ and decreases post-extrasystolic potentiation.[41,42] Birth has a similar effect on ventricular function: left ventricular dP/dt$_{max}$ increases, and post-extrasystolic potentiation decreases.[42,104] However, these changes in the neonate occur spontaneously without the need for an exogenous inotropic agent. Circulating catecholamine levels are elevated in the neonate, and the neonatal cardiovascular system appears to be more dependent on sympathetic stimulation than that of the adult.[245,246,295] The response of the newborn heart to exogenous inotropic stimulation has been thought to be limited because of this stimulation by endogenous catecholamines. However, even stressed neonates respond well to exogenous administration of inotropic agents. For example, newborn lambs that are made hypoxemic (to induce an elevation of circulating catecholamines) respond to isoproterenol and dobutamine administration with a significant enhancement in cardiac output.[296] Furthermore, the increase in left ventricular stroke volume in the prematurely delivered animal with a patent ductus

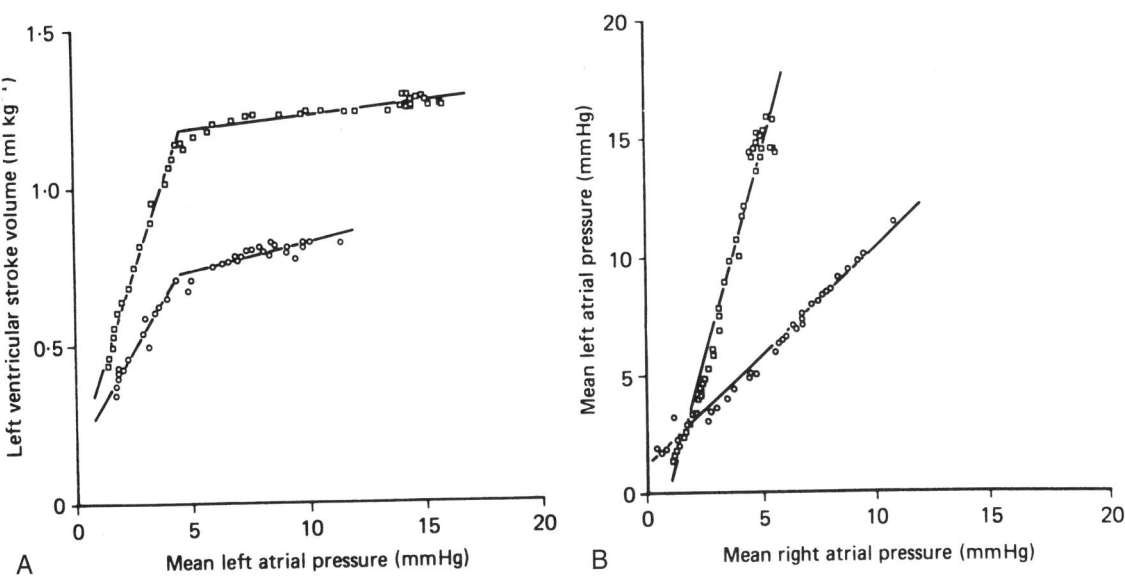

Figure 63–17. Chronically instrumented fetal lamb, body weight 3.0 kg. **A,** Left ventricular function curves before (○) and during (□) *in utero* oxygen ventilation obtained by changing blood volume (left ventricular stroke volume as a function of filling pressure, left atrial mean pressure). Best-fit regression lines are illustrated. For any given mean left atrial pressure, stroke volume was greater during oxygen ventilation. The normal operating mean filling pressure in this fetus was approximately 4 mm Hg before ventilation and approximately 14 mm Hg during ventilation. **B,** Mean left atrial pressure versus right atrial pressure during control (○) and oxygen ventilation (□). Best-fit line under control conditions was $P_{l.a} = 0.93\ P_{r.a} + 1.1$, $r = 1.0$, and during oxygen ventilation was $P_{l.a} = 0.35\ P_{r.a} - 3.0$, $r = 0.99$, where $P_{l.a}$ and $P_{r.a}$ are mean left and right atrial pressures (mm Hg). (From Morton MJ, et al: J Physiol *383*:413, 1987.)

arteriosus can be blunted by β-adrenoceptor blockade.[285] Taken together, these data suggest that (1) inotropy increases with birth, and (2) sympathetic stimulation is an important contributor to the enhancement of ventricular function in the neonate.

A surge in endocrine activity also occurs with birth. Enhanced thyroid function may contribute to increased ventricular function in the neonate, although thyroidectomy at birth does not blunt the enhancement of cardiac output.[297] The importance of circulating tropic agents and catecholamines is evidenced by the differences in post-extrasystolic potentiation in the intact neonatal heart in vivo and in myocardium isolated from the newborn heart. A fall in post-extrasystolic potentiation is observed in the neonatal heart *in vivo*, but no fall is observed in isolated myocardium.[104] That is, an essentially monotonic developmental increase in post-extrasystolic potentiation is observed when isolated myocardium is studied,[104,205] whereas *in vivo*, a fall in potentiation occurs during the postnatal period.[42,104] The fall in potentiation *in vivo* reflects the effects of circulating endogenous inotropic agents and *in situ* neural input on ventricular function, which are both lost when the myocardium is placed in a tissue bath.

The functional effects of the interaction of the right and left ventricles also may contribute to the increase in cardiac output in the newborn infant. Increases in right ventricular afterload and end-diastolic volume adversely affect left ventricular filling and ejection[16,115,199,201] (see Fig. 63–3). Consequently, the ventilation-induced fall in right ventricular afterload in the neonate may increase left ventricular output: when right ventricular systolic pressure and end-diastolic volume fall with birth, the left ventricle is able to fill to a larger end-diastolic volume and contract more forcefully. These effects of ventricular interaction provide an explanation as to why neonatal diseases that increase right ventricular end-diastolic volume and pulmonary artery pressure decrease left ventricular output.

In summary, the increase in left ventricular output in the newborn infant is due to increases in venous return and heart rate, by sympathetic stimulation that enhances inotropy, and by decreases in right ventricular systolic and diastolic load. Although the prematurely delivered fetal lamb is able to increase left ventricular output in response to volume loading and catecholamine infusions,[284,285] the marked increase in left ventricular output with birth suggests that the heart of the neonate has used much of its reserves for increasing output. Consequently, the neonate will not tolerate states that require further increases in output or diseases that blunt the effectiveness of these mechanisms.

In the days following birth, cardiac output (corrected for body weight) gradually falls,[286] and dP/dt$_{max}$ returns to fetal levels (which is to the same level measured in the adult left ventricle).[104] Heart rate decreases,[104] post-extrasystolic potentiation increases to equal or exceed late-gestational levels,[104] and the inotropic response to catecholamine stimulation increases.[119] These postnatal changes suggest that the heart is acquiring greater functional reserves during the early postnatal period, which may enable the heart to respond better to stress and to meet increased workload demands imposed by cardiac defects during the weeks and months following birth.

RESPONSE TO HYPOXIC STRESS

During normal development, cardiovascular function and circulatory function progress from fetal life through the transition at birth, and the fetus is clearly able to develop and thrive despite its "hypoxic" environment. Moreover, due to adaptive responses of the cardiovascular system, relatively severe intrauterine stress may be tolerated and permit the fetus to have relatively normal somatic growth. However, hypoxic stress *in utero* can be severe enough to cause compromised circulatory function and threaten survival. Moreover, at the time of transition, signs of depressed circulatory function may become more apparent owing to the increase in metabolic demands at birth and the loss of gas exchange via the placenta. Using examples from both experimental work and clinical observations, the subsequent sections address the response of the circulation to hypoxic stress and the manifestations of these responses in the fetus and neonate.

Effects of Hypoxia and Acidosis on Cardiac Function

The combined effects of hypoxemia and acidemia on myocardial performance have been studied in several experimental models. Acidosis decreases contractility of isolated papillary muscle.[298] In the intact newborn lamb heart studied *in situ*, under conditions in which heart rate and afterload were controlled and sympathoadrenal function was intact, acute hypoxia (PO_2 < 25 mm Hg) with a normal pH did not depress ventricular contractility.[299,300] In addition, severe acidosis (pH < 6.8; due to acid infusion or hypercapnia) did not impair ventricular performance during normoxia, as long as adrenergic support was available.[301,302] However, the combination of acidemia and hypoxemia depressed ventricular function, even with intact sympathoadrenal mechanisms.[300] Disruption of the central nervous system circulation or blockade of calcium influx depressed ventricular contractility during hypoxemia or acidemia alone.[303] These data suggest that the adrenergic nervous system and calcium ions play key roles in cardiac adaptation to acute asphyxia. It is interesting that studies performed in intact, unanesthetized newborn lambs suggest that acidemia alone impairs ventricular function.[304] The reasons for the discrepancy between these findings and those described in the more invasive preparation are unclear. An important factor influencing the myocardial contractile response to acidemia may be the decrease or maintenance of intracellular pH and secondary effects on calcium ion activity.[305,306] A decrease in intracellular pH with the accumulation of lactate may depress the contractile process through inhibition of the interaction between calcium and troponin, whereas maintenance of normal intracellular hydrogen ion concentration may preserve myocardial function.

The fetal and neonatal myocardium seems to be more resistant to hypoxia than the adult myocardium.[307-311] Contractility of the adult heart decreases markedly during oxygen deprivation, whereas the fetal or neonatal myocardium has a greater ability to withstand the effects of hypoxemia. This resistance is demonstrated by the immature myocardium's ability to sustain mechanical function during periods of marked oxygen deprivation.

This greater resistance of the immature myocardium may be the result of higher rates of anaerobic glycolysis. Glucose ameliorates the effects of prolonged hypoxia in the fetal heart and the adult heart.[309,311] Therefore, the ability of the neonatal myocardium to tolerate hypoxia *in vitro* also may be related to greater myocardial glycogen stores.[309,312-315] Whatever the biochemical basis, this relative resistance of the immature myocardium to hypoxemia and respiratory acidosis is an important and useful attribute, given the occurrence of transient hypoxia and hypercapnia during labor and delivery and the early neonatal period.

In contrast with hypoxemia, myocardial substrate delivery and the efflux of metabolic products are inhibited during ischemia. As a result, the ability to contract is depressed, while diastolic pressure is increased. Following the reversal of short periods of ischemia, the immature heart can work almost as effectively as before the ischemic insult, whereas the function of the adult heart is usually prominently depressed.[315-317] Irreversible myocardial damage and cell death ultimately occur with persistent ischemia, but cell death in response to similar periods of ischemia is greater in the adult heart. The relatively greater resistance of the immature myocardium to ischemia is reassuring when considered in the light of surgical approaches to the repair of congenital cardiac defects and resuscitation of the neonate.

EFFECTS OF HYPOXIA ON THE CIRCULATION

Local Response

The heart and circulation regulate oxygen transport to the various regional organ systems. After birth, the local circulation to each organ (except the lungs) is exposed to the same pressure, but each has unique functional demands for oxygen and other nutrients. For any given cardiac output and arterial pressure, blood flow may be redistributed by altering local vascular resistance. Organs that increase vascular resistance receive less blood flow; however, in some settings, modulation of flow to any one organ may influence flow to the other organs as well. In general, perfusion of an organ system matches the metabolic needs of that organ, with some notable exceptions, such as the kidneys and skin.[318,319] Excessive blood flow to the kidneys is required to ensure proper filtering and excretory function, whereas skin blood flow is a determinant of heat transfer vital for the regulation of body temperature. Overall, however, the metabolic activity of most organs determines organ blood flow.[320]

The various local metabolic responses, as well as adaptations to low perfusion states during development, have been reviewed and are summarized here.[321] When organ-specific perfusion pressure is altered, the vascular resistance changes in response, thereby maintaining constant levels of blood flow, a vascular response defined as *autoregulation*, due in part to the *myogenic response*. The myogenic response is defined by the direct effects of intraluminal pressure on vascular tone, in which high or low pressure causes vasoconstriction or vasodilation, respectively. The capacity of organs to sustain perfusion when cardiac output is disturbed depends on the capacity for autoregulation and the response to neural and humoral stimulati. Although the precise mechanism for this myogenic response is not resolved, it is well recognized that organs vary in their ability to autoregulate; the heart, brain, and kidney are efficient at autoregulation and can maintain their blood flow over a wide range of perfusion pressures, whereas the skin and muscle have poor autoregulatory capabilities. Furthermore, skin, muscle, splanchnic organs, and kidneys have extensive autonomic innervation and blood flow regulated via neural and humoral input. Thus, organ resistance may vary consequent to its intrinsic properties and in response to systemic influences.

Local adjustments in vascular tone in the microcirculation of various organs may improve utilization of oxygen and other nutrients in the face of a limited perfusion.[318,322] As organ blood flow diminishes, previously closed capillaries are opened, probably by metabolically controlled sphincter dilation. This allows the tissues to extract more of the available oxygen by (1) increasing the surface area available for diffusion of oxygen from blood to tissue cells, (2) decreasing the distances between blood and tissue cells, and (3) increasing the cross-sectional area available for blood flow, thus slowing the flow of blood through the capillaries and allowing a longer time for the diffusion of oxygen. The net effect of these responses is to allow very high levels of tissue oxygen extraction, which permits maintenance of tissue oxygen consumption at near-normal levels over a wide range of oxygen delivery.

Hematologic Adjustments

Regional perfusion is also modulated by local metabolic changes that may help enhance regional oxygen extraction by decreasing the affinity of hemoglobin for oxygen and increasing the unloading of oxygen from venous blood. Acutely, local pH decreases when perfusion falls, and lactic acid production is increased; this shifts the hemoglobin oxygen dissociation curve to the right (decreased affinity).[319] Chronically, there may be an increase in red blood cell production of 2,3-diphosphoglycerate (2,3-DPG), which also decreases hemoglobin oxygen affinity. However, two factors can limit the utility of this chronic mechanism:[321,323,324] (1) 2,3-DPG synthesis is regulated by intracellular pH, and if the red cell remains acidotic, the synthesis may not be stimulated. It is important to note that red blood cell pH may not vary in parallel with plasma pH, because the proportion of deoxyhemoglobin in venous blood, which is increased when oxygen extraction is increased, influences red cell buffering. (2) For neonates and infants, fetal hemoglobin binds 2,3-DPG much less effectively than does adult hemoglobin, which explains why fetal hemoglobin has a relatively low P50 (or, high affinity for oxygen) *in vivo*. The reduced binding to hemoglobin causes end-product inhibition of 2,3-DPG synthesis. Therefore, a shift in the oxygen dissociation curve cannot be employed as a significant mechanism by young infants in response to impaired oxygen delivery. The proportion of fetal hemoglobin decreases from about 77% at birth to less than 2% by 8 months of age, and the concentration of 2,3-DPG increases during this time period. As a result, the P50 progressively increases in the normal infant (from 20 to 30 mm Hg) and the capacity to respond by altering hemoglobin oxygen affinity improves later in childhood.

Persistent hypoxemia usually increases hemoglobin synthesis due to enhanced erythropoietin production. In the fetus, the liver is the predominant source for erythropoietin, whereas the kidney plays a major role in the adult. The time of the switch from liver to kidney as the major site in the human is uncertain. It is interesting that low amounts of erthyropoietin mRNA also have been detected in other tissues (e.g., brain, lung) during hypoxia.[325] It has been well demonstrated that a decrease in renal venous PO2 can stimulate production of erythropoietin, and oxygen sensing appears to occur in the peritubular cells. Hypoxia-inducible factor-1 (HIF-1) is a transcription factor that is increased by low cellular oxygen tension, and it appears to be essential for the transcription of the erythropoietin gene and the subsequent enhancement red blood cell production in the face of lowered oxygen tension.[326,327] HIF-1 activity can be induced in diverse cell types, and genes that encode for glycolytic enzymes are transcriptionally activated in hypoxic cells via a similar mechanism. Clearly, several molecular mechanisms, including those that increase erthyropoietin transcription, also control the expression of multiple genes that are responsible for cellular and systemic homeostasis during adaptation to hypoxia.

Although the increase in hemoglobin mass will augment the arterial oxygen content (for any given per cent oxyhemoglobin [HbO2]), the increase in viscosity also can impede blood flow; thus, the adaptive value of polycythemia is limited, and a high hematocrit can reduce blood oxygen transport in the fetus or neonate. It is important to note that low cardiac output alone (i.e., without hypoxemia) does not seem to be a stimulus for erythropoietin production, even though it might be predicted that renal venous PO2 would be low under these conditions.[328] It has been suggested, however, that with low renal blood flow, there also would be a decrease in real oxygen consumption, thereby restoring venous levels of PO2 toward normal.[329]

Reflex Responses

Several cardiovascular neurohumoral reflexes are stimulated by low cardiac output. Afferent limbs of these reflexes arise from cardiopulmonary receptors, notably atrial receptors and arterial baroreceptors.[330] The afferent input from these receptors is processed in the medullary cardiac and vasomotor centers and results in increased adrenergic discharge from cardiac sympathetic nerves and vasoconstrictor fibers concerned with blood vessel tone in different organ system. Increased sympathetic input to the heart augments heart rate and increases contractility. Vasoconstriction of regional vascular beds diminishes vascular capacitance and may increase ventricular preload and afterload. Neurally mediated vasoconstriction of regional vascular beds in response to hypoxia is present in the developing lamb by at least 90 days of gestation and can be abolished by α-adrenergic blockade.[331,332]

Studies in the instrumented fetal lamb indicate that the heart rate responses to acute hypoxemia are mediated primarily by the peripheral chemoreceptors located in the carotid body.[333,334] Accordingly, denervation of the chemoreceptors abolishes hypoxia-induced bradycardia and peripheral vasoconstriction in the fetus.[335] On the other hand, the vascular response to hypoxemia in the brain, heart, and adrenal gland is not mediated by arterial chemoreceptors, but rather by local mechanisms.[336,337] This local response permits the fetus to maintain a constant delivery of oxygen to these organs. Thus, the role of the chemoreceptors in response to fetal hypoxemia involves peripheral vasoconstriction with preservation of umbilical-placental blood flow.

Humoral Responses

In addition to neurally mediated release of catecholamines and the release of circulating catecholamines from the adrenal medulla, other humoral agents modulate systemic vascular resistance. For example, renal vasoconstriction via sympathetic stimulation increases renin release from the kidney and activates the renin-angiotensin-aldosterone cascade. Angiotensin II, derived from the conversion of angiotensin I in the pulmonary vascular bed or from local sources, has potent vasoconstrictor effects and stimulates aldosterone release. Angiotensin II and renin can cross the blood-brain barrier and alter medullary cardiovascular centers that control blood pressure and blood volume. Arginine vasopressin is released centrally and results in further vasoconstriction, whereas increased aldosterone and vasopressin levels stimulate increased sodium and water reabsorption by the kidney, which tends to restore blood volume.[338]

Many local factors contribute to control of vascular smooth muscle tone, two of which in the fetus and neonate have received much attention. The so-called endothelial-derived relaxing factor (EDRF) is derived from endothelium from L-arginine. Nitric oxide (NO) has been identified as the EDRF, and it stimulates guanylate cyclase to produce cyclic guanosine monophosphate (cGMP), which causes vasodilation.[339] Nitric oxide has been shown to induce dilation of the coronary and cerebral vascular beds in response to hypoxemia.[336,337] On the other hand, a 21-amino acid peptide, endothelin-1 (ET-1), induces vasoconstriction when released from endothelium. This agent stimulates the formation of inositol triphosphate, which acts intracellularly to stimulate Ca2+ release.[340,341] NO and ET-1 have been shown to play critical roles in normal cardiovascular regulation throughout fetal life, and in the transition of the circulation at birth.

Thus, multiple neural, humoral, and local mechanisms act in a complementary fashion to maintain perfusion pressure and to redistribute a marginal cardiac output and oxygen supply to the brain, heart, and adrenal glands. This helps improve the matching of oxygen delivery to oxygen needs during the time when oxygen supply is limited. Under nonstress conditions, the kidneys, skin, and splanchnic vascular beds have high blood flows in relation to their oxygen requirement and thus exhibit low extraction ratios. By decreasing blood flow to such organ systems while maintaining flow to higher extraction systems, such as the brain and myocardium, the redistribution of cardiac output permits a more efficient use of oxygen in an attempt to preserve vital tissue metabolism.

Flow Redistribution

Studies in the fetal and newborn lamb during hypoxemia and acidemia have shown striking changes in the proportion of the combined ventricular output distributed to the various fetal vascular beds.[342-348] The proportion of combined ventricular output distributed to the gut, spleen, and carcass is reduced, whereas the percentage of combined ventricular output distributed to the brain, heart, placenta, and adrenal glands markedly increases during hypoxemia. Reducing the arterial PO_2 to 12 to 14 mm Hg in the fetal lamb increases myocardial blood flow by four- to sevenfold without a fall in oxygen consumption or evidence of myocardial ischemia. Myocardial performance appears to be sustained by increased sympathoadrenal activity and augmentation of coronary blood flow.[349-351]

Impaired fetal oxygen supply due to disruption of the fetal umbilical-placental circulation causes the redistribution of cardiac output, as with hypoxemia and acidemia. However, reduced uterine blood flow also results in a redistribution of fetal oxygen delivery and flow patterns that differ from those observed during graded umbilical cord occlusion.[352] With reduction of uterine flow, umbilical flow remains constant, but umbilical venous oxygen content is reduced proportionally. Peripheral blood flow can markedly decrease, thereby dramatically interfering with peripheral oxygen delivery. When umbilical flow is decreased, the umbilical venous oxygen content is unchanged, and peripheral blood flow may remain constant or even increase. Under all conditions that cause fetal or neonatal hypoxemia, stimulation of the medullary vasomotor center and carotid chemoreceptor serves to redistribute blood flow and maintain perfusion of critical regional circulations, a major adaptive response to the hypoxic event.

Metabolism

When organ blood flow and oxygen delivery are severely compromised, increased tissue oxygen extraction cannot fully compensate for the decreased oxygen delivery, and if tissue oxygen demands remain the same, organ oxygen consumption will decline as a direct consequence of inadequate delivery.[353,354] As oxygen delivery falls below this critical level, tissues must utilize anaerobic metabolism (glycolysis) to maintain cellular energy stores. This is accompanied by accumulation of lactic acid and impairment of organ function.

As has been stated, the fetus and neonate are reputedly better able to tolerate hypoxic events than are older subjects and adults. For example, for comparable decreases in cardiac output and whole body oxygen consumption, 2-week-old lambs accumulate lactate at slower rates and repay less of the accumulated oxygen deficit when compared with 8-week-old lambs.[355] A potential explanation for the tolerance of the young subjects is that a large proportion of the oxygen demand is facultative or nonessential. In theory, *facultative metabolism* is a part of normal metabolism that requires oxygen but is not essential for survival. Metabolism used for growth, other anabolic processes, and thermoregulation are examples of facultative metabolism. It has been estimated that the late-gestation fetal lamb uses 30% to 40% of its oxygen consumption for growth, and in the term newborn lamb, growth represents approximately 30% of total oxygen consumption.[356,357] Therefore, decreasing organ oxygen consumption through the loss of facultative metabolism during limited oxygen delivery might preserve normal organ function, at least over the short term, by matching demand to supply. This adaptation would be expected to be much more important in the neonate, than in the adult. Parer,[358] for example, has reported that the fetal lamb tolerates a 50% reduction in oxygen consumption during maternal hypoxemia without developing a metabolic acidosis. The precise mechanism of adaptation at the cellular level that results in metabolic depression remains speculative. Hochachka[359] has advanced the concept that hypoxia-tolerant cell systems avoid calcium-mediated pathogenic processes by maintaining low-permeability membranes, resulting in a lower density of ion-specific channels. This would achieve a matching of the energy costs of ion pumping to that of decreased ATP synthesis under the metabolically depressed conditions of hypoxia. In organs with high metabolic activity, such as the heart and brain, the amount of oxygen expended for growth is a very small percentage of the total oxygen requirement.

The fetal cardiac response to acute pressure loading does not appear to be associated with a limitation in myocardial blood flow, indicating a remarkable flow reserve.[360,361] The heart, therefore, depends on the maintenance of an increased blood supply during hypoxic stress in order to maintain normal function.[362] This can take place only if the other organs can decrease metabolic demands and increase oxygen extraction by previously described mechanisms (flow and extraction). When these mechanisms cannot fully compensate, the heart becomes ischemic as well, and the following biochemical and pathologic myocardial changes take place.

MALADAPTATION TO HYPOXIC STRESS

Chronic adaptation of the heart to pressure/volume loading is achieved by stimulation of myocardial growth (hypertorphy or hyperplasia), which in the fetus and neonate primarily involves a hyperplastic response. The hypertrophic or hyperplastic response tends to restore wall stress (force per unit area) to normal and is typical of situations in which the major functional component has been an increase in afterload.[363] The hemodynamic overload increases protein synthesis by stimulating myocardial stretch receptors that respond to cellular deformation and set in motion a chain of molecular events that increases muscle mass. These steps involve increased activation of proto-oncogenes, gene expression of new types of protein such as myosin isoenzymes, and creatine kinase isoforms.[364] It appears that angiotensin-II is a growth factor helping regulate the early stages of protein synthesis and is important in myocardial remodeling.[365]

In addition to the influence on the myocardial response, there also may be hypertrophy or hyperplasia of conduit and resistance vessels.[366] These actions are partly mediated through angiotensin-II receptors that activate G-protein, phospholipase C, diacylglycerol, and the phosphatidylinositol triphosphate pathway, which can increase expression of certain proto-oncogenes. There is also an increase in the number of cells surrounding the myocardial capillaries and in interstitial material, although capillary growth may not match the amount of muscular hypertrophy and hyperplasia that has taken place. The latter, therefore, can establish a condition in which oxygen supply may not match demand, particularly in the vulnerable subendocardial regions of the myocardium. With an increased ratio of myofibrils to mitochondria, the energy-consuming myofibrils must be supplied with adenosine triphosphate (ATP) from relatively fewer mitochondria.[367] In addition, myocardial connective tissue proliferation causes accumulation of type I collagen and the production of high tensile-strength scar tissue.[368] Therefore, although the hypertrophic or hyperplastic response is an adaptive mechanism, portions of the overall growth response may become maladaptive over time.

The increase in neurohumoral activity with hypoxia also may be maladaptive in the chronic situation. The vasoconstrictive process responsible for the redistribution of cardiac output increases the afterload on the myocardium α-adrenergic response), further reducing cardiac output and increasing myocardial energy demands. Furthermore, myocardial cells lose their ability to respond to β-agonists with chronic stimulation, a process known as *desensitization*.[369] Desensitization results in a decrease in β-receptors, thus blunting the inotropic response of the hypoxic heart to sympathetic stimulation.

FAILURE OF ADAPTATION TO STRESS

When the oxygen and blood supply to the developing myocardium are severely limited, irrespective of etiology, a decreased rate of ATP production occurs that can lead to cell membrane depolarization, potassium and sodium efflux, and calcium influx into the cell. With the collapse of mitochondrial membrane potential, calcium influx takes place or is released from the sarcoplasmic reticulum as the activity of calcium-dependent ATP decreases and the sodium-calcium ion exchange mechanism becomes impaired.[370,371] The net result is a dramatic increase in cytosolic calcium ion concentration that leads to activation of phospholipases A_1, A_2, and C. The stage is then set for increased membrane phospholipid hydrolysis, accumulation of free fatty acids, and an increase in cell and mitochondrial membrane permeability.[372] The final common pathway, as these alterations take place, is myocardial cell injury and eventually cell death. There are no apparent differences from the pathologic process that takes place in adult myocardial cells subjected to ischemic injury.

The principal pathologic changes associated with myocardial hypoxia in the fetus and neonate have been documented most commonly with severe asphyxia but could be expected under any analogous circumstance in which myocardial perfusion and oxygenation are threatened. The subendocardial regions of the papillary muscles, particularly the septal papillary muscle of the tricuspid valve, are particularly vulnerable and represent the sites of predilection for severe hypoxic insults.[373,374] Medial necrosis of the coronary arteries has been observed in cases with severe asphyxia and has resulted in widespread areas of hemorrhagic myocardial infarction.[375,376] The conduction tissue also may be injured by the hypoxic process. Such damage may therefore be responsible for fixed slow heart rates, atrioventricular block, and tachyarrhythmias.

Changes in myocardial cell structure and metabolism secondary to severe hypoxia have been observed during development in a number of species. The release of creatine kinase in the anoxic myocardium is associated with massive cellular swelling, clumping of nuclear chromatin, and prominent disruption of plasma membranes.[373,377] With the conversion to anaerobic glycolysis, glycogen and cellular stores of phosphocreatine and ATP are rapidly depleted, and the heart eventually ceases to contract.[309,378,379] Although the discussion thus far has focused on the role of hypoxia in producing myocardial necrosis, programmed cell death (apoptosis), which is a central feature of normal tissue development in the fetus and of cell replacement in certain adult tissues, has recently received considerable attention. Abnormal levels of resting oxygen tension appear to be associated with activation of the apoptosis process and with reduction in mechanical performance and myocardial remodeling.[380,381]

MANIFESTATIONS OF IMPAIRED VENTRICULAR FUNCTION IN THE FETUS AND NEONATE

Fetal Blood Flow Patterns with Congenital Malformation of the Heart

With some exceptions, congenital malformations of the heart do not generally disturb fetal oxygenation or cardiac performance.[382-384] However, fetal echocardiographic and Doppler flow measurements have shown that the fetal flow pathways play critical roles in the adaptation to many types of congential cardiac malformations.[385,386] When the right side of the heart is underdeveloped (e.g., with absent right atrioventricular connection and right ventricular hypoplasia; or when there is severe right ventricular outflow obstruction, e.g., with critical pulmonary stenosis or atresia), patency of an in utero flow pathway permits fetal survival (Fig. 63-18). In such situations, the magnitude of flow across the foramen ovale and its size are greater than normal.[387,388] In addition, although right ventricular volume is diminished due to decreased venous filling, the left ventricular internal diameter usually greatly exceeds that of the right ventricle. This reflects a redistribution of diastolic return, allowing for normalization of the combined stroke volume of the ventricles.

With obstruction of the left side of the heart, the fetal right ventricle and pulmonary artery are much larger than usual; this reflects redistribution of flow and allows normal or near-normal combined ventricular stroke volume (Figs. 63-19 and 63-20). In most cases the foramen ovale and left atrium are smaller than usual.[387,388] It is unclear whether there is a cause-and-effect relationship between the small foramen ovale and left ventricular hypoplasia, or whether an intrinsic abnormality in left ventricular filling and emptying reduces flow to the foramen ovale, thereby preventing its normal growth throughout gestation. Serial observations of the fetal heart have demonstrated that there is a spectrum of left ventricular hypoplasia that varies from mild left ventricular underdevelopment (e.g., with a bicuspid aortic valve and/or mild abnormalities of mitral valve architecture) through moderate degrees of left ventricular hypoplasia and relative right ventricular dilation (e.g., with aortic coarctation) to more florid examples of mitral hypoplasia and atresia (e.g., with severe forms of left ventricular hypoplasia, fibroelastosis, and aortic atresia/hypoplasia).[389]

Hutchins[390] postulated that, in situations in which right ventricular outflow exceeds that found in the normal fetal circulation, flow via the ductus arteriosus may proceed both to the lower fetal body and placenta (as in the normal circulation) and to the left arm and perhaps to the neck and head, with the division of the ductal stream representing a branch point in the arterial flow. Of import, this branch point may then serve as a site for obstruction following postnatal closure of the ductus arteriosus. In most severe forms of left ventricular inflow or outflow obstruction, color-Doppler and pulsed-Doppler flow studies demonstrate the presence of left-to-right shunting across the fetal foramen ovale.

The presence of marked dilation of the right ventricle and right atrium and tricuspid valve regurgitation has been described in association with placental insufficiency and fetal growth failure.[385] Doppler-flow studies have demonstrated umbilical arterial flow waveforms compatible with high resistance in the usually low-resistance placental vascular bed, with or without flow redistribution to the fetal brain.[391,392] Increases in placental resistance due to vasoconstriction of resistance vessels or, more likely, in the low volume of placenta, result in an acute afterload mismatch similar to that seen with acute ductal constriction.[393] Regional flow studies in such cases have suggested that increased placental vascular resistance may be associated with high systolic and end-diastolic flow velocities in the fetal middle cerebral arteries, consistent with a dramatic decrease in arterial resistance in the fetal cerebrovascular bed. These changes may represent evidence of autoregulation of systemic arterial flow distribution and may explain the well-described phenomenon of relative "head sparing" in many cases of intrauterine growth retardation.

Circulatory Failure in the Fetus

Nonimmune hydrops fetalis, a manifestation of fetal congestive heart failure, has been observed in fetuses with abnormal cardiac structure and/or sustained arrhythmias[394] (Fig. 63-21). Similarly, hydrops has been produced in fetal lambs by rapid atrial pacing.[395,396] Fetal cardiac diagnostic ultrasound studies have demonstrated a 20% to 30% incidence of fetal cardiovascular disease as the underlying explanation for nonimmune hydrops.[397]

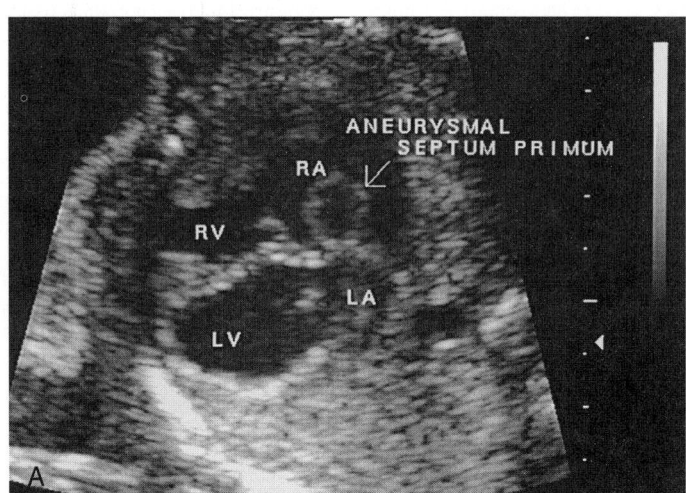

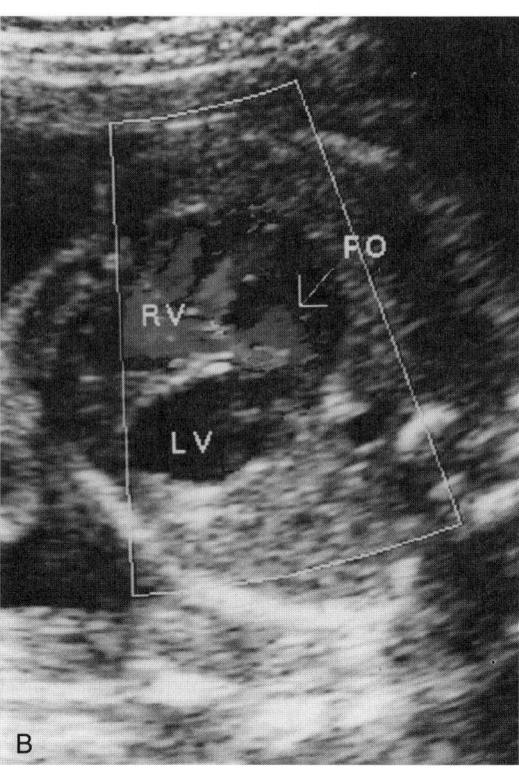

Figure 63–18. A, Four-chamber view of an abnormal fetal heart at 27 weeks of gestation. Note that there is a disproportion in the size of the two fetal ventricles, with the left ventricle (LV) appearing relatively dilated. In addition, the immediate subendocardial surface of the left ventricle is relatively echogenic, suggesting the presence of endocardial fibroelastosis. In addition, the atrial septum primum is aneurysmally dilated and prolapsed into the right atrial cavity. This fetus was demonstrating the poor myocardial reserve that exists in the face of increased afterload. Although not visualized in this view, the primary pathology related to a unicuspid, critically stenotic aortic valve. **B,** This is a color-flow–encoded Doppler study of the same heart, positioned in the same fashion. Note the absence of significant flow into the left ventricle, whereas there is plentiful color flow within the right ventricle. In addition, the flow across the foramen ovale represents left-to-right shunting across the foramen ovale. This reversal of flow direction across the interatrial septum suggests the decreased compliance of the fibrotic left ventricular cavity and furthermore is suggestive that the size of the left ventricle will ultimately be determined by the degree of mitral insufficiency and small amount of pulmonary venous return that enters the left ventricle rather than shunts across the foramen ovale. RV = right ventricle; RA = right atrium; LA = left atrium; FO = foramen ovale.

The propensity of the fetus to develop hydrops in response to systolic pump failure is different from the usual presentation of systolic pump failure postnatally and may result from several factors[398,399]: (1) the increased capillary filtration coefficient increases water flux for any given driving force; (2) the high compliance of the interstitial space permits retention of more water for any given perivascular hydraulic pressure; and (3) the increased permeability of fetal capillaries to protein (lower reflection coefficient) causes less fluid to move from the interstitium to the capillary. Furthermore, if central venous pressure is increased, (4) capillary colloid oncotic pressure decreases from impaired hepatic function, and this reduces fluid reabsorption from the interstitium, and (5) because limitation of lymphatic flow occurs at a lower central venous pressure than in adults, there is reduced clearance of the interstitial edema (Fig. 63–22).

Elevation of systemic venous pressure leading to hydrops may arise from disorders involving either the right or left ventricle in the fetus. Due to the presence of the parallel fetal flow circuitry, left ventricular inflow is provided in major part by venous return from the inferior vena cava and directed across the foramen ovale. Pulmonary venous return to the left ventricle reflects only a small proportion of combined ventricular output that is directed into the fetal pulmonary arteries.[384] There is marked diastolic interdependence between the two fetal ventricular cavities. Any acute increase in right ventricular filling pressure

results in an increased systemic venous hydrostatic pressure. Likewise, in the fetus, an acute or chronic increase in left ventricular filling pressure alters the pressure relationship across the foramen ovale. This results in an increase in right atrial and systemic venous hydrostatic pressure, again favoring the development of fetal edema.

Pulsed-Doppler flow analysis has demonstrated the frequent association of atrioventricular valve regurgitation with congenital cardiac malformations and nonimmune hydrops fetalis.[400] The presence of significant atrioventricular valve regurgitation imparts an increase in atrial pressure related both to the regurgitant v-wave in the atrial pressure trace, and to the subsequent increment in the diastolic filling volume presented to the fetal ventricle. The latter results in a marked increase in filling pressure in the presence of the "restrictive" ventricular myocardium of the fetus.[401]

These flow studies of ventricular diastolic filling also have suggested that the fetal ventricle fills primarily during atrial contraction.[402] This filling pattern is reminiscent of that seen postnatally in the presence of a restrictive cardiomyopathy and suggests relative restriction to myocardial filling in the normal human fetus. At the very least, it suggests a dependence of the fetal ventricle on active, rather than passive, diastolic filling. This, in conjunction with the limited compliance of fetal ventricular myocardium and the marked interdependence of the two fetal

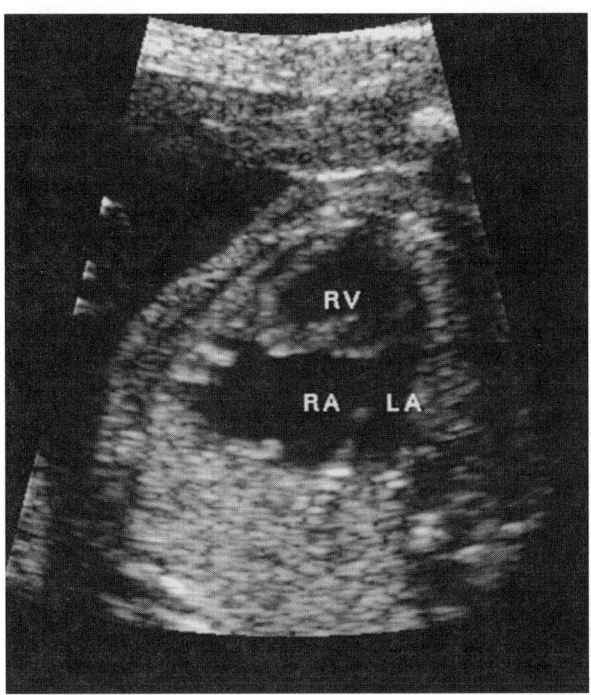

Figure 63–19. Four-chamber view of an abnormal fetal heart at 22 weeks' gestation. The heart is oriented with the apex to the right of the frame. Note the extremely large right atrium (*RA*) and right ventricle (*RV*), the relatively small left atrium (*LA*), and the absence of an identifiable left ventricular cavity. This fetus had mitral-aortic atresia and hypoplastic left heart syndrome. The right ventricle is approximately twice normal in size, accounting for a normal "combined ventricular output" and normal growth of the fetus, despite the severe congenital cardiac malformation.

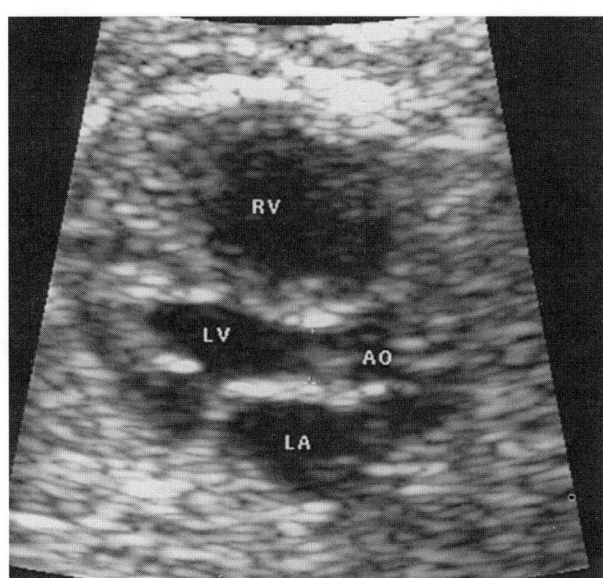

Figure 63–20. Four-chamber view of an abnormal fetal heart at 32 weeks' gestation. The heart is oriented with the apex to the left of the frame. Note the marked disproportion between the left (*LV*) and right ventricles (*RV*), implying a relatively smaller flow into and out of the fetal left ventricle. Combined ventricular output was normal, as were other fetal growth parameters, except for marked fetal limb edema and prominent nuchal folds. This four-chamber view is characteristic of what one would expect in a fetus with a severe aortic coarctation, with a significant shift of cardiac output via the right, rather than the left, ventricle. Genetic amniocentesis confirmed the clinical impression of Turner syndrome. LA = left atrium; AO = aorta.

ventricles, explains the frequent association between volume overloading of either ventricle (either mitral or tricuspid regurgitation) and marked fetal systemic edema.

Sustained supraventricular tachyarrhythmias, including supraventricular tachycardia and atrial flutter, have been shown to predispose the fetus to the development of hydrops fetalis.[397,403] It is now believed that the site of initial atrial depolarization may determine which fetuses become hydropic in the face of supraventricular tachycardia, and why some fetuses seem to tolerate the arrhythmia better than others. When the supraventricular tachycardia has its origin in the left atrium (by depolarizing the left atrium before the right), both right-to-left shunting across the foramen and left ventricular output diminish. By "trapping" venous return on the right side of the fetal circulation, subsequent venous hypertension results in fetal edema (C. S. Kleinman, personal observations). Fetuses with sustained atrial flutter often have associated congenital heart disease. Atrioventricular valve regurgitation results in marked atrial dilation, which appears to predispose the fetus to the development of atrial flutter.[403]

The development of hepatic venous congestion, in association with the supraventricular tachyarrhythmia, ultimately leads to hepatic dysfunction and hypoalbuminemia.[395] The latter results in a decreased plasma oncotic pressure, further disposing the fetal circulation toward the development of systemic edema.

Nonimmune hydrops fetalis also has been encountered in the presence of complete heart block.[404] Approximately half the cases of complete heart block have been associated with a high maternal anti-Ro or anti-La antibody titer.[394] It has been suggested that the development of heart block in these fetuses is related to

an antibody-mediated inflammatory process of conduction tissue to which maternal autoantibodies cross-react. The development of edema is thought to relate to the presence of a cardiomyopathy and of atrioventricular disassociation with cannon a-waves, resulting in a persistently elevated mean atrial pressure (already high in the presence of bradycardia and a relatively restrictive fetal ventricular myocardium). Approximately 50% of cases with complete heart block have associated congenital cardiac malformations with no evidence of maternal autoantibody. The most frequently associated cardiac malformation has been complete atrioventricular septal defect in the presence of left atrial isomerism and atrioventricular valve regurgitation.[394]

Fetal Cardiomegaly

Fetuses with cardiomegaly commonly have right and left atrial dilation secondary to severe atrioventricular valve regurgitation and/or ventricular dilation secondary to severe congestive cardiomyopathy. Severe cardiomegaly in the fetus during the early to midportion of the second trimester also has been associated with lung hypoplasia, which may be due to the mass effect of the heart occupying an inappropriately large proportion of the intrathoracic volume.[405] This has been well demonstrated in the presence of fetal diaphragmatic hernia. The associated presence of cardiomegaly, hydrothorax, and pericardial effusion probably accounts for the high incidence of pulmonary hypoplasia that has been reported in neonates with hydrops fetalis.

Impaired Ventricular Function in the Neonate

A number of clinical syndromes have been observed in neonates subjected to a perinatal hypoxic event. These include (1) a low

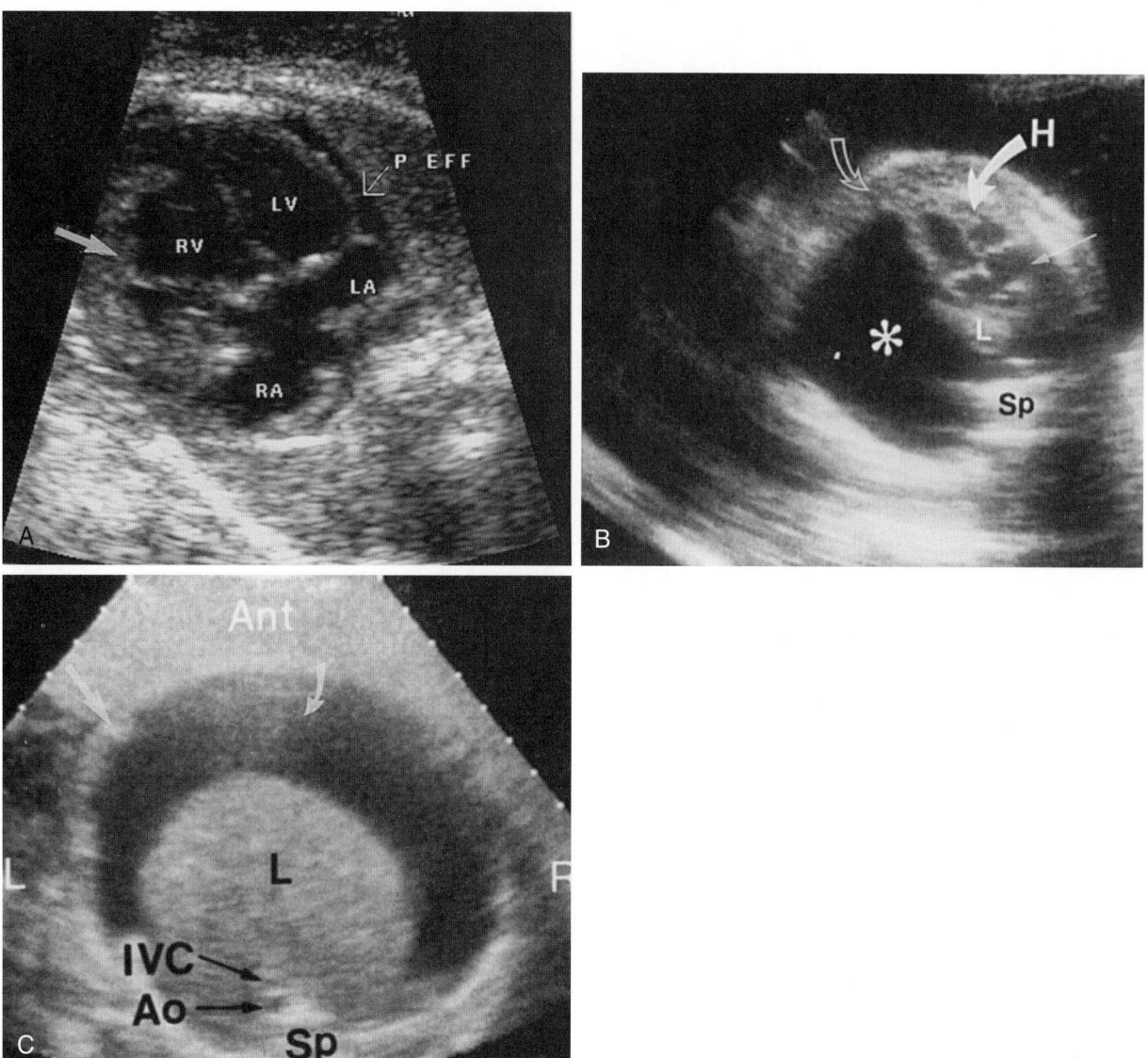

Figure 63–21. A, Four-chamber view of an abnormal fetal heart at 34 weeks' gestation. Note the disproportionately enlarged fetal right ventricle (RV) and right atrium (RA). The right ventricular wall (*arrow*) is quite hypertrophic, and Doppler echocardiography confirmed the presence of tricuspid valve insufficiency. The pericardial effusion (P EFF) is an early sign of fetal heart failure, which later became associated with hydrops fetalis (systemic edema, placental edema, and polyhydramnios) secondary to high central venous pressure, which in turn is related to the high right ventricular filling volume and the poor right ventricular diastolic compliance. Although not seen in this view, the primary problem was related to premature partial closure of the ductus arteriosus. The mother had been receiving high doses of nonsteroidal anti-inflammatory agents for a variety of joint complaints. LV = left ventricle; LA = left atrium. **B,** Transverse scan of the chest of the thorax in a fetus with a hypertrophic right ventricle (*curved white arrow*), secondary to severe pulmonic stenosis and dilated right atrium (*straight arrow*), secondary to tricuspid regurgitation. Note the large pleural effusion (*), the hypoplastic left lung (L), and the chest wall edema (*open arrow*). Fetal spine (Sp) denotes the posterior pole of the chest. **C,** Transverse scan of the upper abdomen in a fetus with right atrial isomerism (asplenia syndrome), with complex atrioventricular septal defect, severe atrioventricular valve regurgitation, and nonimmune hydrops (congestive heart failure). Posterior to the centrally located liver (L), the abdominal aorta (Ao) and inferior vena cava (IVC) are on the same side of the fetal spine (Sp). This is a characteristic finding in this syndrome. A large layer of ascitic fluid is seen (*curved arrow*) anteriorly (Ant) and to the right (R) and left (L) sides of the fetal liver. There is also abdominal wall edema (*straight arrows*).

systemic perfusion state in which global myocardial ischemia appears to be responsible for the clinical picture of "cardiogenic" shock; (2) massive tricuspid valve regurgitation secondary to papillary muscle necrosis, with the clinical presentation dominated by right-to-left shunting across the foramen ovale; and (3) persistent pulmonary hypertension, with hypoxemia secondary to high pulmonary vascular resistance and right-to-left shunting across the ductus arteriosus and foramen ovale. The first two syndromes, which relate to the effects of hypoxia on the myocardium, are now discussed in detail. The third syndrome is discussed only when the pulmonary vascular bed has an impact on the other clinical areas. Although we describe two separate clinical entities, it is important to recognize that the distinction may not always be clear and that there is much overlap in the pathogenesis.

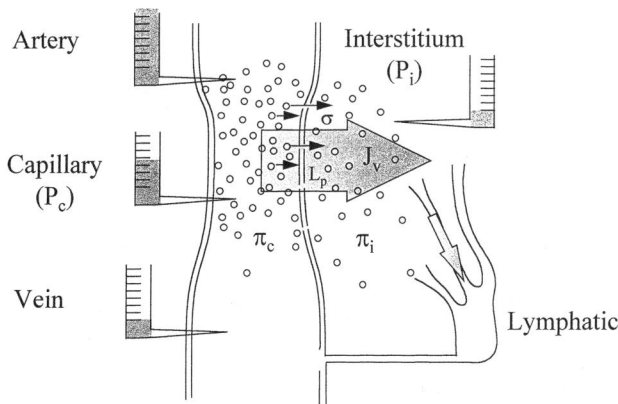

Figure 63–22. Interstitial fluid balance. Interstitial fluid is formed by ultrafiltration of plasma at the capillary. Capillary ultrafiltration is driven by the difference between capillary (P_c) and interstitial (P_i) hydrostatic pressures. Fluid reabsorption by the capillary is driven by the difference between the capillary (π_c) and the interstitial (π_i) colloid oncotic pressures. Measures of the concentrations of oncotically active molecules, σ, the reflection coefficient, and L_p, the hydraulic permeability, are intrinsic properties of the capillary wall that characterize the efficacy of such driving forces to produce water flux (J_v). Interstitial fluid is returned to the circulation via the lymphatic system. The outflow pressure of the lymphatic pressure is the venous pressure. The "manometers" indicate the relative pressures in each compartment. Thus, overall fluid flux is described by the following equation:

$$J_v = CFC \left[(P_c - P_i) - \sigma (\pi_c - \pi_i) \right]$$

where CFC, the capillary filtration coefficient, is a measure of the fluid volume filtered per unit time per driving pressure.

Low Systemic Perfusion State

The possibility of myocardial failure after undue asphyxia at birth was first reported in 1961 by Burnard and James.[406] These investigators described a group of asphyxiated newborn infants with left ventricular failure that occurred within the first 24 hours of life. This report was followed a decade later by the report of Rowe and Hoffman,[407] who described three term newborn infants with a syndrome of acute left ventricular failure accompanied by cyanosis and pulmonary and systemic venous congestion. The clinical presentation mimicked severe congenital heart disease; the weak arterial pulses, liver enlargement, and right-sided heart dominance on the electrocardiogram suggested the diagnosis of hypoplastic left ventricle. These investigation hypothesized that this disorder arose from impaired coronary perfusion to the right and left ventricles in the presence of an increased afterload produced by the elevated pulmonary and systemic vascular resistances accompanying hypoxia. Angiographic studies on these infants showed striking decreases in left ventricular contractility. ST-T wave alterations on the electrocardiogram provided evidence for myocardial ischemia. These infants survived, and signs of myocardial involvement abated; thus, the syndrome was labeled transient myocardial ischemia. Although this is the usual clinical course, we have encountered newborn infants who experienced myocardial infarction secondary to a severe asphyxial event and who expired in a low-cardiac-output state despite vigorous medical management. At postmortem examination, diffuse necrosis of the left ventricle was noted.

Cabal and co-workers[408] reported a similar clinical picture of cardiogenic shock in preterm infants in whom fetal distress was

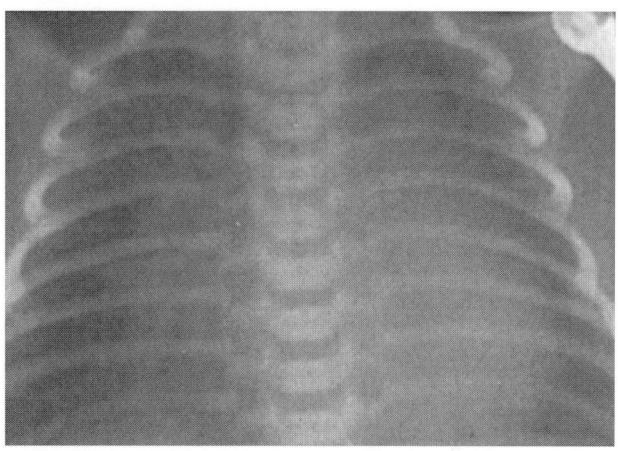

Figure 63–23. Chest film obtained on an 18-hour-old male infant who had an Apgar score of 4 at 5 minutes, clinical signs of low perfusion, and ischemic changes on the electrocardiogram. Of note is the presence of cardiac enlargement and pulmonary venous congestion, which are secondary to decreased systolic function of the left ventricle, with accompanying pulmonary edema.

documented by the presence of severe late and variable decelerations associated with decreased fetal heart rate variability. At birth, Apgar scores were less than 5, with signs of respiratory distress. A diagnosis of cardiac failure was established on the basis of cardiomegaly, hepatomegaly, echocardiographic evidence of decreased ventricular contractility, elevated central venous pressure, and the presence of lactic acidosis. Rapid clinical improvement took place following the administration of inotropic agents, with restoration of systemic perfusion.

This low perfusion state usually involves term infants, although it has been described in the preterm infant as well. There is a history of perinatal asphyxia, and infants may be cyanotic, but the clinical picture is usually dominated by signs of shock and circulatory congestion. There are diminished arterial pulsations, pallor, poor capillary refill, and hypothermia. In addition, the breathing pattern is generally rapid and shallow (tachypnea). The heart sounds may be distant, although the pulmonary closure sound can be prominent. Occasionally, murmurs of mitral or tricuspid regurgitation may be present, with tricuspid insufficiency more likely. The finding of atrioventricular valve regurgitation will tend to obscure the distinction between this syndrome and that of myocardial ischemia associated with tricuspid regurgitation and hypoxemia (see later). The edge of the liver is usually palpable and may, on occasion, pulsate in systole. The chest x-ray film shows cardiac enlargement with accompanying evidence of pulmonary venous engorgement, which steadily improves with recovery (Fig. 63-23). The initial electrocardiogram (less than 24 hours after birth) shows right ventricular dominance with accompanying ST-T wave changes suggesting myocardial ischemia, or rarely, a true infarct pattern with Q waves may be seen. In addition, there may be conduction abnormalities such as ventricular ectopy, interventricular conduction delay, and first- and second-degree heart block. These infants will usually have a metabolic acidosis, which can be severe (pH 6.8 to 7.1), with variable levels of Pa_{O_2}. Although hemoglobin and hematocrit values are usually normal, polycythemia may be present, so that viscosity can further impair perfusion. Blood glucose and calcium levels may be low and require correction. The creatine kinase MB fraction has been a useful test to assess for the possible presence of myocardial necrosis.[409]

Ultrasound evaluation of the heart is mandatory in the evaluation of these infants. The possibility of structural cardiac

FLOW PATTERNS
MYOCARDIAL ISCHEMIA OF THE NEWBORN

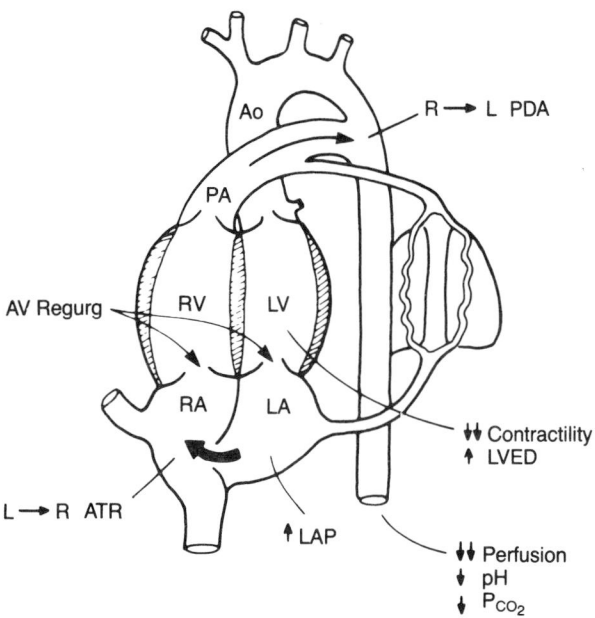

Figure 63–24. Schematic diagram of the blood flow patterns in a newborn infant with low systemic perfusion as a result of myocardial ischemia. The myocardial insult results in diminished left ventricular contractility ($\downarrow\downarrow$*Contractility*) and increase in end-diastolic pressure ($\uparrow$*LVED*), with an acute decrease in cardiac output ($\downarrow\downarrow$*Perfusion*). The increased left-sided filling pressures ($\uparrow$*LAP*) produce pulmonary edema and a left-to-right atrial shunt (*L→R ATR*) through an incompetent foramen ovale. With compromised systemic perfusion, metabolic acidemia develops ($\downarrow pH$, $\downarrow Pco_2$). Atrioventricular valve regurgitation (*AV Regurg*) may be present, whereas right-to-left shunting may take place via the ductus arteriosus (*R→L PDA*).

problems, particularly hypoplastic left heart syndrome, must be ruled out. It is of equal importance that the atrioventricular valves be evaluated for regurgitation by Doppler interrogation, as well as the presence and direction of shunting across the foramen ovale and ductus arteriosus. Ventricular systolic function, as determined by calculation of the shortening or ejection fraction, is decreased if global ischemia is present.[410] The echocardiogram is also important as a noninvasive means to assess the response to therapeutic interventions. When performed, radionuclide imaging has shown a decrease in the uptake of isotope, which can reflect global or segmental ischemia.[411]

Cardiac catheterizations have shown elevated ventricular filling pressures, low mixed venous oxygen saturations, and a decreased arterial pulse pressure in this setting. Pulmonary artery pressure can be elevated to systemic levels, with right-to-left shunting across the ductus arteriosus almost always present. In addition, left-to-right atrial shunting also can be seen secondary to elevated left-sided filling pressures.[407,412] Left ventricular angiography has demonstrated dilatation of the left atrium and left ventricle, a decrease in left ventricular contractility, and, on occasion, mitral or tricuspid valve regurgitation. The clinical picture described with myocardial ischemia is often confused with the low-output states associated with the hypoplastic left heart syndrome, critical aortic stenosis, interruption of the aortic arch, coarctation, and primary disorders of cardiac muscle function such as myocarditis, or certain biochemical defects affecting systolic function. Salient physiologic findings in the low-perfusion state are shown in Figure 63–24.

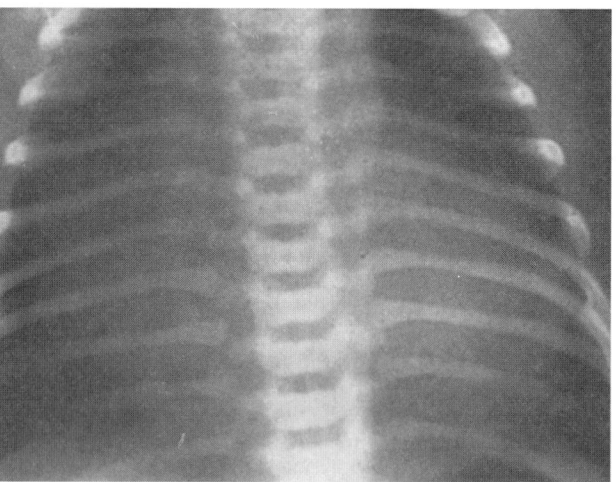

Figure 63–25. Chest roentgenogram in a newborn infant who had an Apgar score of 4 and presented with cyanosis and the murmur of tricuspid valve regurgitation. There is cardiomegaly, with a decrease in pulmonary vascular markings. The decrease in lung perfusion contrasts with the congested lung observed in the infant with a low systemic perfusion state (see Fig. 63–23).

Myocardial Ischemia Associated with Tricuspid Regurgitation and Hypoxemia

In contrast to the stressed infant who presents with low systemic perfusion, hypoxemia often dominates the clinical picture of the infant with tricuspid regurgitation. Attention was first focused on this entity by Bucciarelli and associates,[413] who described 14 term infants with tricuspid regurgitation associated with significant perinatal hypoxic stress. Cardiac catheterization and angiography performed in 5 of these infants showed massive regurgitation across a normally inserted tricuspid valve. In 12 of the 14 infants, all clinical and laboratory findings resolved. Two patients died and had histopathologic evidence of necrosis of the anterior papillary muscle of the tricuspid valve. In a retrospective histologic study of term infants who died within 7 days of birth and in whom congenital heart disease, erythroblastosis, intrauterine viral infections, and multiple major malformations had been excluded, 31 of 82 infants had at least one site of ischemic myocardial necrosis.[378,379] The pathologic lesions were approximately evenly distributed between the right and left ventricles, with some having bilateral lesions. The apical region of the anterior papillary muscle of the right ventricle was the most common site.

The severity of the clinical picture of tricuspid regurgitation in the stressed newborn relates to the high pulmonary vascular resistance, increased right ventricular afterload, and hypoxemia secondary to right-to-left shunting across the foramen ovale. Volume loading of the right ventricle might also impair filling of the left ventricle because of ventricular interdependence. A confounding problem in some of these infants may be premature closure of the ductus arteriosus with pressure and volume loading of the right ventricle. This might occur in situations in which there has been maternal intake of prostaglandin synthetase inhibitors, such as salicylates or nonsteroidal anti-inflammatory agents. The presence of a holosystolic murmur along the lower left sternal border within the first 24 hours of life in a postasphyxiated infant who is hypoxemic should raise the suspicion of this entity. A supporting history of the ingestion of salicylates or nonsteroidal anti-inflammatory agents should heighten suspicion. The liver is usually enlarged and may pulsate with systole. The presence of significant tricuspid regurgitation results in right-sided cardiac enlargement with cardiomegaly and

MYOCARDIAL ISCHEMIA OF THE NEWBORN
Tricuspid Regurgitation with R → L Atrial Shunting

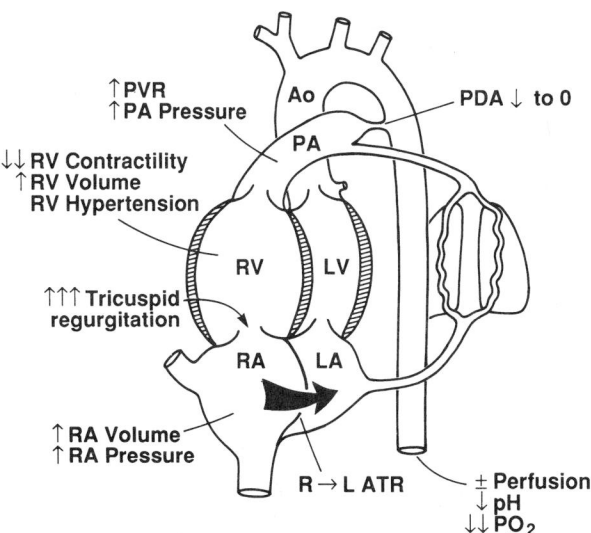

Figure 63–26. Blood flow patterns in the infant with hypoxemia and tricuspid valve regurgitation. With a perinatal asphyxial event, the papillary muscles of the tricuspid valve apparatus, particularly the anterior leaflet, may receive an ischemic insult. This results in the development of tricuspid valve regurgitation (↑↑↑*Tricuspid regurgitation*). The volume of regurgitation is enhanced by the presence of an elevated pulmonary artery pressure (↑*PA pressure*) and pulmonary vascular resistance (↑*PVR*). Premature constriction or closure of the ductus arteriosus (*PDA↓to 0*) also tends to foster a high pulmonary vascular resistance (↑*PVR*), with the latter increasing the afterload on the right ventricle. The pressure and volume-loaded right ventricle dilates (*RV Hypertension*, ↑*RV Volume*, ↓↓*RV Contractility*), and right atrial pressure and volume (↑*RA Volume*, ↑*RA Pressure*) rises. The elevated right atrial pressure favors right-to-left shunting (*R→L ATR*) across the foramen ovale and the development of significant hypoxemia (↓↓*Po₂*) and metabolic acidemia (↓*pH*). Systemic perfusion is usually maintained (± *Perfusion*).

decreased pulmonary vascular markings secondary to low right ventricular output and bypass of the pulmonary circulation via the right-to-left shunt across the foramen ovale (Fig. 63–25). Arterial blood gas and pH determinations in these patients show low arterial oxygen tension (25 to 40 mm Hg) without significant hypercapnia; the pH is either normal or low, depending on the severity of the hypoxemia. Two-dimensional ultrasound imaging with color flow mapping shows a normally inserted tricuspid valve with tricuspid valve regurgitation. Right atrial and right ventricular volumes are increased. The atrial septum bows to the left, and a right-to-left atrial shunt can be demonstrated.

In the few patients who have had cardiac catheterization, elevation of right-sided filling pressures and right ventricular and pulmonary artery hypertension have been noted.[413] Angiography has demonstrated the presence of tricuspid valve regurgitation at the site of a normally inserted tricuspid valve. The foramen ovale has been noted to be patent, and right-to-left shunting is usually apparent. Imaging of the aortic arch has failed to show a patent ductus arteriosus in a few instances, suggesting the possibility of premature closure of the ductus arteriosus.

Structural cardiac disease, particularly the Ebstein malformation of the tricuspid valve, atrioventricular canal defects, pulmonary atresia with intact ventricular septum, critical pul-

monary valve stenosis, and primary and secondary pulmonary hypertension, must be ruled out, usually by echocardiographic studies. Rarely, the tricuspid valve may insert normally and be regurgitant when there is primary hypoplasia of the septal leaflet of the tricuspid valve with short chordae tendineae. The principal physiologic findings in infants with tricuspid regurgitation and hypoxemia are depicted in Figure 63–26.

REFERENCES

1. Sommer JR, Johnson EA: Ultrastructure of cardiac muscle. *In* Berne RM, et al (eds): Handbook of Physiology, Vol 1. Bethesda, MD, American Physiological Society, 1979, pp 113–186.
2. Craig SW, Pardo JV: Gamma actin, spectrin, and intermediate filament proteins co-localize with vinculin at costameres, myofibril-to-sarcolemma attachment sites. Cell Motil *3*:449, 1983.
3. Messina DA, Lemanski LF: Immunocytochemical studies of spectrin in hamster cardiac tissue. Cell Motil Cytoskel *12*:139, 1989.
4. Pardo JV, et al: Vinculin is a component of an extensive network of myofibril-sarcolemma attachment regions in cardiac muscle fibers. J Cell Biol *97*:1081, 1983.
5. Price MG, Sanger JW: Intermediate filaments in striated muscle: a review of structural studies in embryonic and adult skeletal and cardiac muscle. *In* Dowben RM, Shay JW (eds): Cell and Muscle Motility, Vol 3. New York, Plenum Press, 1983, pp 1–40.
6. Traub P: Intermediate Filaments: A Review. Berlin, Springer-Verlag, 1985, pp 150–163.
7. Granzier HL, Irving TC: Passive tension in cardiac muscle: contribution of collagen, titin, microtubules, and intermediate filaments. Biophys J *68*:1027, 1995.
8. Hynes RO: Integrins, a family of cell surface receptors. Cell *48*:549, 1987.
9. Robinson TF, et al: Skeletal framework of mammalian heart muscle: arrangement of inter- and pericellular connective tissue structures. Lab Invest *49*:482, 1983.
10. Robinson TF, et al: Morphology, composition, and function of struts between cardiac myocytes of rat and hamster. Cell Tissue Res *249*:247, 1987.
11. Terracio L, et al: Expression of collagen adhesion proteins and their association with the cytoskeleton in cardiac myocytes. Anat Rec *223*:62, 1989.
12. Ohayon J, Chadwick RS: Effects of collagen microstructure on the mechanics of the left ventricle. Biophys J *54*:1077, 1988.
13. Kolmerer B, et al: Genomic organization of M line titin and its tissue-specific expression in two distinct isoforms. J Mol Biol *256*:556, 1996.
14. Trombitas K, et al: The mechanically active domain of titin in cardiac muscle. Circ Res *77*:856, 1995.
15. Friedman WF: The intrinsic physiologic properties of the developing heart. Prog Cardiovasc Dis *15*:87, 1972.
16. Romero T, et al: A comparison of pressure-volume relations of the fetal, newborn and adult heart. Am J Physiol *222*:1285, 1972.
17. Mahdavi V, et al: Molecular characterization and expression of the cardiac α- and β-myosin heavy chain genes. *In* Ferrans VJ, et al (eds): Cardiac Morphogenesis. New York, Elsevier, 1985, pp 2–9.
18. Zak R, Galhotra SS: Contractile and regulatory proteins. *In* Drake-Holland AJ, Noble MIM (eds): Cardiac Metabolism. New York, John Wiley & Sons, 1983, pp 339–364.
19. Barany M: ATPase activity of myosin correlated with speed of muscle shortening. J Gen Physiol *50*:197, 1967.
20. Yamamoto K, Moos C: The C-proteins of rabbit, red, white and cardiac muscles. J Biol Chem *258*:8395, 1983.
21. Leavis PC, Gergely J: Thin filament proteins and thin filament-linked regulation of vertebrate muscle contraction. CRC Crit Rev Biochem *16*:235, 1984.
22. Zot AS, Potter JD: Structural aspects of troponin-tropomyosin regulation of skeletal muscle contraction. Annu Rev Biophys Chem *16*:535, 1987.
23. Weber A, Murray JM: Molecular control mechanisms in muscle contraction. Physiol Rev *53*:612, 1973.
24. Lehman W, et al: Steric-blocking by tropomyosin visualized in relaxed vertebrate muscle thin filaments. J Mol Biol *251*:191, 1995.
25. Huxley AF: The activation of striated muscle and its mechanical response. The Croonian Lecture, 1967. Proc R Soc Lond (Biol) *178*:1, 1971.
26. Huxley HE: Molecular basis of contraction in cross-striated muscles. *In* Bourne GH (ed): The Structure and Function of Muscle, 2nd ed, Vol 1. New York, Academic Press, 1972, pp 301–387.
27. Ebashi S: Ca²⁺ and the contractile proteins. J Mol Cell Cardiol *16*:129, 1984.
28. Rayment I, et al: Three-dimensional structure of myosin subfragment-1: a molecular motor. Science *261*:50, 1993.
29. Rayment I, et al: Structure of the actin-myosin complex and its implications for muscle contraction. Science *261*:58, 1993.
30. Godt RE, et al: Changes in force and calcium sensitivity in the developing avian heart. Can J Physiol Pharmacol *69*:1692, 1991.
31. Solaro RJ, et al: Differential effects of pH on calcium activation and myofilaments of adult and perinatal dog hearts: evidence for developmental differences in thin filament regulation. Circ Res *58*:721, 1986.

32. Kranias EG, et al: Phosphorylation and functional modifications of sarcoplasmic reticulum and myofibrils in isolated rabbit hearts stimulated with isoprenaline. Biochem J 226:113, 1985.

33. Gordon AM, et al: The variation in isometric tension with sarcomere length in vertebrate muscle fibres. J Physiol (Lond) 184:170, 1966.

34. Gordon AM, et al: Tension development in highly stretched vertebrate muscle fibres. J Physiol (Lond) 184:143, 1966.

35. Robinson TF, Winegrad S: The measurement and dynamic implications of thin filament lengths in heart muscle. J Physiol (Lond) 286:607, 1979.

36. Nassar R, et al: Light diffraction of cardiac muscle: sarcomere motion during contraction. In Porter R, Fitzsimons DW (eds): Physiological Basis of Starling's Law of the Heart. Ciba Foundation Symposium 24. Amsterdam, Elsevier, 1974, pp 57–91.

37. Wang Y-P, Fuchs F: Osmotic compression of skinned cardiac and skeletal muscle bundles: effects on force generation, Ca²⁺ sensitivity and Ca²⁺ binding. J Mol Cell Cardiol 27:1235, 1995.

38. McDonald KS, Moss RL: Osmotic compression of single cardiac myocytes eliminates the reduction in Ca²⁺ sensitivity of tension at short sarcomere length. Circ Res 77:199, 1995.

39. Babu A, et al: Molecular basis for the influence of muscle length on myocardial performance. Science 240:74, 1988.

40. Hibberd MG, Jewell BR: Calcium- and length-dependent force production in rat ventricular muscle. J Physiol (Lond) 329:527, 1982.

41. Anderson PAW, et al: Biophysics of the developing heart, II: The interaction of the force-interval relationship with inotropic state and muscle length (preload). Am J Obstet Gynecol 138:44, 1980.

42. Anderson PAW, et al: Biophysics of the developing heart, III: A comparison of the left ventricular dynamics of the fetal and neonatal lamb heart. Am J Obstet Gynecol 143:195, 1982.

43. Gilbert RD: Control of fetal cardiac output during changes in blood volume. Am J Physiol 238:H80, 1980.

44. Kirkpatrick SE, et al: Frank-Starling relationship as an important determinant of fetal cardiac output. Am J Physiol 231:495, 1976.

45. Thornburg KL, Morton MJ: Filling and arterial pressures as determinants of left ventricular stroke volume in fetal lambs. Am J Physiol 251:H961, 1986.

46. Thornburg KL, Morton MJ: Filling and arterial pressures as determinants of RV stroke volume in the sheep fetus. Am J Physiol 244:H656, 1983.

47. Wagman A, et al: Evidence for the Frank-Starling relationship in the stage 24 chick embryo. Circulation 70(Suppl II):11, 1984.

48. Nassar R, et al: Force-pCa relation and troponin T isoforms of rabbit myocardium. Circ Res 69:1470, 1991.

49. Sweeney HL, et al: Myosin light chain phosphorylation in vertebrate striated muscle: regulation and function. Am J Physiol 264:C10085, 1993.

50. Venema RC, Kuo JF: Protein kinase C–mediated phosphorylation of troponin I and C-protein in isolated myocardial cells is associated with inhibition of myofibrillar actomyosin MgATPase. J Biol Chem 268:2705, 1993.

51. Noland TA Jr, et al: Cardiac troponin I mutants: phosphorylation by protein kinases C and A and regulation of Ca²⁺-stimulated MgATPase of reconstituted actomyosin S-1. J Biol Chem 270:25445, 1995.

52. Gilbert RD: Effects of afterload and baroreceptors on cardiac function in fetal sheep. J Dev Physiol 4:299, 1982.

53. MacGregor DC, et al: Relations between afterload, stroke volume, and descending limb of Starling's curve. Am J Physiol 227:884, 1974.

54. Pagani ED, Julian FJ: Rabbit papillary muscle myosin isozymes and the velocity of muscle shortening. Circ Res 54:586, 1984.

55. Henkel RD, et al: Cardiac beta myosin heavy chain diversity in normal and chronically hypertensive baboons. J Clin Invest 83:1487, 1989.

56. Tsuchimochi H, et al: Heterogeneity of β-type myosin isozymes in the human heart and regulational mechanisms in their expression: immunohistochemical study using monoclonal antibodies. J Clin Invest 31:110, 1988.

57. Mahdavi V, et al: Developmental and hormonal regulation of sarcomeric myosin heavy chain gene family. Circ Res 60:804, 1987.

58. Lompre AM, et al: Species- and age-dependent changes in the relative amounts of cardiac myosin isoenzymes in mammals. Dev Biol 84:286, 1981.

59. Schwartz K, et al: Left ventricular isomyosins in normal and hypertrophied rat and human hearts. Eur Heart J 5(Suppl F):77, 1984.

60. Mercadier J-J, et al: Myosin isoenzymes in normal and hypertrophied human ventricular myocardium. Circ Res 53:52, 1983.

61. Bouvagnet P, et al: Distribution pattern of α- and β-myosin in normal and diseased human ventricular myocardium. Basic Res Cardiol 84:91, 1989.

62. Cummins P, Lambert SJ: Myosin transitions in the bovine and human heart: a developmental and anatomical study of heavy and light chain subunits in the atrium and ventricle. Circ Res 58:846, 1986.

63. Hille B: Calcium channels. In Ionic Channels of Excitable Membranes, 2nd ed. Sunderland, MA, Sinauer Associates, 1991, pp 83–114, 175–178, 250–252.

64. Barcenas-Ruiz L, et al: Sodium-calcium exchange in heart: membrane currents and changes in [Ca²⁺]. Science 238:1720, 1987.

65. Bassani RA, et al: Relaxation in ferret ventricular myocytes: role of the sarcolemmal Ca ATPase. Pflugers Arch 430:573, 1995.

66. Herrera VLM, et al: Three differentially expressed Na, K-ATPase α-subunit isoforms: structural and functional implications. J Cell Biol 105:1855, 1987.

67. Jorgensen AO, et al: Two structurally distinct calcium storage sites in rat cardiac sarcoplasmic reticulum: an electron microprobe analysis study. Circ Res 63:1060, 1988.

68. Mahony L: Maturation of calcium transport in cardiac sarcoplasmic reticulum. Pediatr Res 24:639, 1988.

69. Mahony L, Jones LR: Developmental changes in cardiac sarcoplasmic reticulum in sheep. J Biol Chem 261:15257, 1986.

70. Fabiato A: Appraisal of the physiological relevance of two hypotheses for the mechanisms of calcium release from the mammalian cardiac sarcoplasmic reticulum: calcium-induced release versus charge-coupled release. Mol Cell Biochem 89:135, 1989.

71. Beuckelmann DJ, Wier WG: Mechanism of release of calcium from sarcoplasmic reticulum of guinea-pig cardiac cells. J Physiol 405:233, 1988.

72. Lai FA, et al: Purification and reconstitution of the calcium release channel from skeletal muscle. Nature 331:315, 1988.

73. Takeshima H, et al: Primary structure and expression from complementary DNA of skeletal muscle ryanodine receptor. Nature 339:439, 1989.

74. Wagenknecht T, et al: Three-dimensional architecture of the calcium channel/foot structure of sarcoplasmic reticulum. Nature 338:167, 1989.

75. Meissner G: Ryanodine activation and inhibition of the Ca²⁺ release channel of sarcoplasmic reticulum. J Biol Chem 261:6300, 1986.

76. Clarke DM, et al: Location of high affinity Ca²⁺ binding sites within the predicted transmembrane domain of the sarcoplasmic reticulum Ca²⁺ ATPase. Nature 339:476, 1989.

77. Jorgensen AO, et al: Ultrastructural localization of calsequestrin in adult rat atrial and ventricular muscle cells. J Cell Biol 101:257, 1985.

78. Katz AM: Role of phosphorylation of the sarcoplasmic reticulum in the cardiac response to catecholamines. Eur Heart J 1(Suppl A):29, 1980.

79. Kadambi VJ, et al: Cardiac-specific overexpression of phospholamban alters calcium kinetics and resultant cardiomyocyte mechanics in transgenic mice. J Clin Invest 97:533, 1996.

80. Kranias EG, Solaro RJ: Phosphorylation of troponin I and phospholamban during catecholamine stimulation of rabbit heart. Nature 298:182, 1982.

81. Chapman RA: Control of cardiac contractility at the cellular level. Am J Physiol 245:H535, 1983.

82. Hilgemann DW, Noble D: Excitation-contraction coupling and extracellular calcium transients in rabbit atrium: reconstruction of basic cellular mechanisms. Proc R Soc [Lond] B Biol Sci 230:163, 1987.

83. Morad M, Goldman Y: Excitation-contraction coupling in heart muscle: membrane control of development of tension. In Butler JAV, Noble D (eds): Progress in Biophysics and Molecular Biology, Vol 27. Oxford, United Kingdom, Pergamon, 1973, pp 257–313.

84. Fabiato A, Fabiato F: Calcium-induced release of calcium from the sarcoplasmic reticulum of skinned cells from adult human, dog, cat, rabbit, rat and frog hearts and from fetal and newborn rat ventricles. Ann N Y Acad Sci 307:491, 1978.

85. Fabiato A: Myoplasmic free calcium concentration reached during the twitch of an intact isolated cardiac cell during calcium-induced release of calcium from the sarcoplasmic reticulum of a skinned cardiac cell from the adult rat or rabbit ventricle. J Gen Physiol 78:457, 1981.

86. Nabauer M, et al: Regulation of calcium release is gated by calcium current, not gating charge, in cardiac myocytes. Science 244:800, 1989.

87. Levesque PC, et al: Role of reverse-mode Na⁺-Ca²⁺ exchange in excitation-contraction coupling in the heart. Ann N Y Acad Sci 639:386, 1991.

88. Leblanc PC, Hume JR: Sodium current–induced release of calcium from cardiac sarcoplasmic reticulum. Science 248:850, 1990.

89. Beuckelmann DJ, Wier WG: Sodium-calcium exchange in guinea-pig cardiac cells: exchange current and changes in intracellular Ca²⁺. J Physiol 414:499, 1989.

90. Cleemann L, Morad M: Role of Ca²⁺ channel in cardiac excitation-contraction coupling in the rat: evidence from Ca²⁺ transients and contraction. J Physiol 432:283, 1991.

91. Johnson EA: Force-interval relationship of cardiac muscle. In Berne RM, et al (eds): Handbook of Physiology, Vol 1. Bethesda, MD, American Physiological Society, 1979, pp 475–496.

92. Weir WG, Yue DT: Intracellular calcium transients underlying the short-term force-interval relationship in ferret ventricular myocardium. J Physiol (Lond) 376:507, 1986.

93. Meissner G, Henderson JS: Rapid calcium release from cardiac sarcoplasmic reticulum vesicles is dependent on Ca²⁺ and is modulated by Mg²⁺ adenine nucleotide, and calmodulin. J Biol Chem 262:3065, 1987.

94. Nassar R, et al: Developmental changes in the ultrastructure and sarcomere shortening of the isolated rabbit ventricular myocyte. Circ Res 61:465, 1987.

95. Beyer EC, et al: Connexin family of gap junction proteins. J Membr Biol 116:187, 1990.

96. Veenstra RD, et al: Multiple connexins confer distinct regulatory and conductance properties of gap junctions in developing heart. Circ Res 71:1277, 1992.

97. Blanchard EM, Solaro RJ: Inhibition of the activation and troponin calcium binding of dog cardiac myofibrils by acidic pH. Circ Res 55:382, 1984.

98. Schachat FH, et al: Effect of different troponin T-tropomyosin combinations on thin filament activation. J Mol Biol 198:551, 1987.

99. Anderson PAW, et al: Molecular basis of human cardiac troponin T isoforms expressed in developing, adult and failing heart. Circ Res 76:681, 1995.

100. Robertson SP, et al: The effect of troponin I phosphorylation on the Ca²⁺-binding properties of the Ca²⁺-regulatory site of bovine cardiac troponin. J Biol Chem 257:260, 1982.

101. Van Meel JCA, et al: Increase in calcium sensitivity of cardiac myofibrils contributes to the cardiotonic action of sulmazole. Biochem Pharmacol 37:213, 1988.

102. Solaro R, et al: Stimulation of cardiac myofilament force, ATPase activity and troponin C Ca-binding by bepridil. J Pharmacol Exp Ther 238:502, 1986.

103. Fujino K, et al: Sensitization of dog and guinea pig heart myofilaments to Ca²⁺ activation and the inotropic effect of pimobendan: comparison with milrinone. Circ Res 63:911, 1988.

104. Anderson PAW, et al: Developmental changes in cardiac contractility in fetal and postnatal sheep: in vitro and in vivo. Am J Physiol 247:H371, 1984.

105. Davies P, et al: Post-natal developmental changes in the length-tension relationship of cat papillary muscles. J Physiol (Lond) 253:95, 1975.

106. Nakanishi T, Jarmakani JM: Developmental changes in myocardial mechanical function and subcellular organelles. Am J Physiol 246:H615, 1984.

107. Nishioka K, et al: The effect of calcium on the inotropy of catecholamine and paired electrical stimulation in the newborn and adult myocardium. J Mol Cell Cardiol 13:511, 1981.

108. Urthaler F, et al: Canine atrial and ventricular muscle mechanics studied as a function of age. Circ Res 42:703, 1978.

109. Anversa P, et al: Morphometric study of early postnatal development in the left and right ventricular myocardium of the rat. I: Hypertrophy, hyperplasia, and binucleation of myocytes. Circ Res 46:495, 1980.

110. Legato MJ: Cellular mechanisms of normal growth in the mammalian heart, II: A quantitative and qualitative comparison between the right and left ventricular myocytes in the dog from birth to five months of age. Circ Res 44:263, 1979.

111. Sheridan DJ, et al: Qualitative and quantitative observations on ultrastructural changes during postnatal development in the cat myocardium. J Mol Cell Cardiol 11:1173, 1979.

112. Legato MJ: Sarcomerogenesis in human myocardium. J Mol Cell Cardiol 1:425, 1970.

113. Markwald RR: Distribution and relationship of precursor Z material to organizing myofibrillar bundles in embryonic rat and hamster ventricular myocytes. J Mol Cell Cardiol 5:341, 1973.

114. Korecky B, Rakusan K: Normal and hypertrophic growth of the rat heart: changes in cell dimensions and number. Am J Physiol 234:H123, 1978.

115. Versprille A, et al: Functional interaction of both ventricles at birth and the changes during the neonatal period in relation to the changes of geometry. In Longo LD, Reneau DD (eds): Fetal and Newborn Cardiovascular Physiology, Vol 1. New York, Garland, 1976, pp 399–413.

116. Anderson PAW, et al: The effect of heart rate on in utero left ventricular output in the fetal sheep. J Physiol (Lond) 372:557, 1986.

117. Anderson PAW, et al: In utero right ventricular output in the fetal lamb: the effect of heart rate. J Physiol (Lond) 387:297, 1987.

118. Morton MJ, et al: In utero ventilation with oxygen augments left ventricular stroke volume in lambs. J Physiol (Lond) 383:413, 1987.

119. Rudolph AM: Distribution and regulation of blood flow in the fetal and neonatal lamb. Circ Res 57:811, 1985.

120. Sahn DJ, et al: Quantitative real-time cross-sectional echocardiography in the developing normal human fetus and newborn. Circulation 62:588, 1980.

121. Veille JC, et al: Accuracy of echocardiography measurements in the fetal lamb. Am J Obstet Gynecol 158:1225, 1988.

122. Kim HD, et al: Human fetal heart development after mid-term: morphometry and ultrastructural study. J Mol Cell Cardiol 24:949, 1992.

123. Kenny JF, et al: Changes in intracardiac blood flow velocities and right and left ventricular stroke volumes with gestational age in the normal human fetus: a prospective Doppler echocardiographic study. Circulation 74:1208, 1986.

124. Dawes GS: Changes in the circulation after birth. In Foetal and Neonatal Physiology: A Comparative Study of the Changes at Birth. Chicago, Year Book Medical Publishers, 1968, pp 160–176.

125. Jonas RA, et al: Rapid two-stage arterial switch for TGA and intact septum beyond the neonatal period. Circulation 78(Suppl II): 11, 1988.

126. Cochrane AD, et al: Staged conversion to arterial switch for late failure of the systemic right ventricle. Ann Thorac Surg 56:854, 1993.

127. Anserva P, et al: Myocyte cell loss and myocyte cellular hyperplasia in the hypertrophied aging rat heart. Circ Res 67:871, 1990.

128. Hoerter J, et al: Perinatal growth of the rabbit cardiac cell: possible implications for the mechanism of relaxation. J Mol Cell Cardiol 13:725, 1981.

129. Olivetti G, et al: Morphometric study of early postnatal development in the left and right ventricular myocardium of the rat, II: Tissue composition, capillary growth, and sarcoplasmic alterations. Circ Res 46:503, 1980.

130. Simpson P: Norepinephrine-stimulated hypertrophy of cultured rat myocardial cells is an alpha₁-adrenergic response. J Clin Invest 72:732, 1983.

131. Simpson P: Stimulation of hypertrophy of cultured neonatal-rat heart cells through an α1-adrenergic receptor and induction of beating through an α₁- and β₁-adrenergic receptor interaction: evidence for independent regulation of growth and beating. Circ Res 56:884, 1985.

132. Simpson P, et al: Myocyte hypertrophy in neonatal rat heart cultures and its regulation by serum and by catecholamines. Circ Res 51:787, 1982.

133. Weiner HL, Swain JL: Acidic fibroblast growth factor mRNA is expressed by cardiac myocytes in culture and the protein is localized to the extracellular matrix. Proc Natl Acad Sci U S A 86:2683, 1989.

134. Izumo S, et al: Protooncogene induction and reprogramming of cardiac gene expression produced by pressure overload. Proc Natl Acad Sci U S A 85:339, 1988.

135. Komuro I, et al: Expression of cellular oncogenes in the myocardium during the developmental stage and pressure-overload hypertrophy of the rat heart. Circ Res 62:1075, 1988.

136. Pasumarthi KBS, et al: High and low molecular weight fibroblast growth factor-2 increase proliferation of neonatal rat cardiac myocytes but have differential effects on binucleation and nuclear morphology: evidence for both paracrine and intracrine actions of fibroblast growth factor-2. Circ Res 78:126, 1996.

137. Tokuyasu KT: Immunocytochemical studies of cardiac myofibrillogenesis in early chick embryos. III: Generation of fasciae adherentes and costameres. J Cell Biol 108:43, 1989.

138. Wang S-M, et al: Studies on cardiac myofibrillogenesis with antibodies to titin, actin, tropomyosin, and myosin. J Cell Biol 107:1075, 1988.

139. Reedy MC, et al: Formation of reverse rigor chevrons by myosin heads. Nature 339:481, 1989.

140. Fyrberg E, et al: Drosophila melanogaster troponin-T mutations engender three distinct syndromes of myofibrillar abnormalities. J Mol Biol 216:657, 1990.

141. Thierfelder L, et al: α-Tropomyosin and cardiac troponin T mutations cause familial hypertrophic cardiomyopathy: a disease of the sarcomere. Cell 77:701, 1994.

142. Watkins H, et al: Mutations in the genes for cardiac troponin T and α-tropomyosin in hypertrophic cardiomyopathy. N Engl J Med 332:1058, 1995.

143. Watkins H, et al: Characteristics and prognostic implications of myosin missense mutations in familial hypertrophic cardiomyopathy. N Engl J Med 326:1108, 1992.

144. Cuda G, et al: Skeletal muscle expression and abnormal function of β-myosin in hypertrophic cardiomyopathy. J Clin Invest 91:2861, 1993.

145. Lin D, et al: Altered cardiac troponin T in vitro function in the presence of a mutation implicated in familial hypertrophic cardiomyopathy. J Clin Invest 97:2842, 1996.

146. Anderson PAW, et al: Troponin T isoform expression in humans: a comparison among normal and failing adult heart, fetal heart, and adult and fetal skeletal muscle. Circ Res 69:1226, 1991.

147. Wieczorek DF, et al: The rat α-tropomyosin gene generates a minimum of six different mRNAs coding for striated, smooth, and nonmuscle isoforms by alternative splicing. Mol Cell Biol 8:679, 1988.

148. Schiaffino S, et al: Developmental and adaptive changes of atrial isomyosins. In Legato MJ (ed): The Developing Heart. Boston, Martinus Nijhoff, 1984, pp 173–189.

149. Price KM, et al: Human atrial and ventricular myosin light-chain subunits in the adult and during development. Biochem J 191:571, 1980.

150. Sabry MA, Dhoot GK: Identification and pattern of expression of a developmental isoform of troponin I in chicken and rat cardiac muscle. J Muscle Res Cell Motil 10:85, 1989.

151. Anderson PAW, et al: Developmental changes in the expression of rabbit left ventricular troponin T. Circ Res 63:742, 1988.

152. Anderson PAW, Oakeley AE: Immunological identification of five troponin T isoforms reveals an elaborate maturational troponin T profile in rabbit myocardium. Circ Res 65:1087, 1989.

153. Arnold H-H, et al: A novel human myosin alkali light chain is developmentally regulated: expression in fetal cardiac and skeletal muscle and in adult atria. Eur J Biochem 178:53, 1988.

154. Barton PJR, Buckingham ME: The myosin alkali light chain proteins and their genes. Biochem J 231:249, 1985.

155. Bishopric NH, et al: Induction of the skeletal α-actin gene in α₁-adrenoceptor–mediated hypertrophy of rat cardiac myocytes. J Clin Invest 80:1194, 1987.

156. Cooper TA, Ordahl CP: A single cardiac troponin T gene generates embryonic and adult isoforms via developmentally regulated alternate splicing. J Biol Chem 260:11140, 1985.

157. Fodor WL, et al: Human ventricular/slow twitch myosin alkali light chain gene characterization, sequence, and chromosomal location. J Biol Chem 264:2143, 1989.

158. Gorza L, et al: An embryonic-like myosin heavy chain is transiently expressed in nodal conduction tissue of the rat heart. J Mol Cell Cardiol 20:931, 1988.

159. Humphreys JE, Cummins P: Regulatory proteins of the myocardium: atrial and ventricular tropomyosin and troponin-I in the developing and adult bovine and human heart. J Mol Cell Cardiol 16:643, 1984.

160. Litten RZ, et al: Heterogeneity of myosin isozyme content of rabbit heart. Circ Res 57:406, 1985.

161. Greig A, et al: Molecular basis of cardiac troponin T isoform heterogeneity in rabbit heart. Circ Res 74:41, 1994.

162. Boheler KR, et al: Skeletal actin mRNA increases in the human heart during ontogenic development and is the major isoform of control and failing adult hearts. J Clin Invest 88:323, 1991.

163. Ruzicka DL, Schwartz RJ: Sequential activation of α-actin genes during avian cardiogenesis: vascular smooth muscle α-actin gene transcripts mark the onset of cardiomyocyte differentiation. J Cell Biol 107:2575, 1988.

164. Spach MS, et al: Multiple regional differences in cellular properties that regulate repolarization and contraction in the right atrium of adult and newborn dogs. Circ Res 66:1594, 1989.

165. Wikman-Coffelt J, et al: Influence of myocardial isomyosins on cardiac performance and oxygen consumption. Biochem Biophys Res Commun 130:1314, 1985.

166. Claycomb WC: Atrial natriuretic-factor mRNA is developmentally regulated in heart ventricles and actively expressed in cultured ventricular cardiac muscle cells of rat and human. Biochem J 255:617, 1988.

167. Gustafson TA, et al: Hormonal regulation of myosin heavy chain and α-actin gene expression in cultured fetal rat heart myocytes. J Biol Chem 262:13316, 1987.

168. Ordahl CP, et al: Structure and expression of the chick skeletal muscle alpha-actin gene. Exp Biol Med 9:211, 1984.

169. Zeller R, et al: Localized expression of the atrial natriuretic factor gene during cardiac embryogenesis. Gene Dev 1:693, 1987.

170. Hunkeler NM, et al: Troponin I isoform expression in human heart. Circ Res 69:1409, 1991.

171. Morano M, et al: Regulation of human heart contractility by essential myosin light chain isoforms. J Clin Invest 98:467, 1996.

172. Hewett TE, et al: Alpha-skeletal actin is associated with increased contractility in the mouse heart. Circ Res 74:740, 1994.

173. Kumar CC, et al: Heart myosin light chain 2 gene: nucleotide sequence of full length cDNA and expression in normal and hypertensive rat. J Biol Chem 261:2866, 1986.

174. Wilkinson JM: Troponin C from rabbit slow skeletal and cardiac muscle is the product of a single gene. Eur J Biochem 103:179, 1980.

175. Toyota N, et al: Molecular cloning and expression of chicken cardiac troponin C. Circ Res 37:531, 1989.

176. Muthuchamy M, et al: Molecular and physiological effects of overexpressing striated muscle β-tropomyosin in the adult murine heart. J Biol Chem 270:30593, 1995.

177. Wattanapermpool J, et al: The unique amino-terminal peptide of cardiac troponin I regulates myofibrillar activity only when it is phosphorylated. J Mol Cell Cardiol 27:1383, 1995.

178. Solaro RJ, et al: Effects of acidosis on ventricular muscle from adult and neonatal rats. Circ Res 63:779, 1988.

179. Malouf NN, et al: A cardiac troponin T epitope conserved across phyla. J Biol Chem 67:9269, 1992.

180. Jin J-P, Lin JJ-C: Rapid purification of mammalian cardiac troponin T and its isoform switching in rat hearts during development. J Biol Chem 263:7309, 1988.

181. McAuliffe JJ, et al: Changes in myofibrillar activation and troponin C Ca²⁺ binding associated with troponin T isoform switching in developing rabbit heart. Circ Res 66:1204, 1990.

182. Tobacman LS, Lee R: Isolation and functional comparison of bovine cardiac troponin I isoforms. J Biol Chem 226:12432, 1987.

183. Akella AB, et al: Diminished Ca²⁺ sensitivity of skinned cardiac muscle contractility coincident with troponin T-band shifts in the diabetic rat. Circ Res 76:600, 1995.

184. Heeley DH, et al: Effect of phosphorylation on the interaction and functional properties of rabbit striated muscle α tropomyosin. J Biol Chem 264:2424, 1989.

185. Alpert NR, Gordon MS: Myofibrillar adenosine triphosphatase activity in congestive heart failure. Am J Physiol 202:940, 1962.

186. Pagani ED, et al: Changes in myofibrillar content and Mg-ATPase activity in ventricular tissues from patients with heart failure caused by coronary artery disease, cardiomyopathy, or mitral valve insufficiency. Circ Res 63:380, 1988.

187. DeTombe PP, Ter Keurs HEDJ: An internal viscous element limits unloaded velocity of sarcomere shortening in rat myocardium. J Physiol (Lond) 454:619, 1992.

188. Fischman DA, Danto SI: Monoclonal antibodies to desmin: evidence for stage-dependent intermediate filament immunoreactivity during cardiac and skeletal muscle development. Ann N Y Acad Sci 455:167, 1985.

189. van der Loop FTL, et al: Rearrangement of intercellular junctions and cytoskeletal proteins during rabbit myocardium development. Eur J Cell Biol 68:62, 1995.

190. Schachat FH, et al: The presence of two skeletal muscle α-actinins correlates with troponin-tropomyosin expression and Z-line width. J Cell Biol 101:1001, 1985.

191. Borg TK, et al: Recognition of extracellular matrix components by neonatal and adult cardiac myocytes. Dev Biol 104:86, 1984.

192. Rubin K, et al: Interactions of mammalian cells with collagen. Ciba Found Symp 108:93, 1984.

193. Borg TK, et al: Changes in the distribution of fibronectin and collagen during development of the neonatal rat heart. Coll Relat Res 2:211, 1982.

194. Borg TK, et al: Connective tissue of the myocardium. In Ferrans VJ, et al (eds): Cardiac Morphogenesis. New York, Elsevier, 1985, pp 69–77.

195. Caulfield JB, Borg TK: The collagen network of the heart. Lab Invest 40:364, 1979.

196. Marijanowski M, et al: The neonatal heart has a relatively high content of total collagen and type I collagen, a condition that may explain the less compliant state. J Am Coll Cardiol 23:1204, 1994.

197. Mays PK, et al: Age-related changes in the proportion of types I and III collagen. Mech Aging Dev 45:203, 1988.

198. Badke FR: Left ventricular dimensions and function during right ventricular pressure overload. Am J Physiol 242:H611, 1982.

199. Bove AA, Santamore WP: Ventricular interdependence. Prog Cardiovasc Dis 23:365, 1981.

200. Minczak BM, et al: Developmental changes in diastolic ventricular interaction. Pediatr Res 23:466, 1988.

201. Slinker BK, Glantz SA: End-systolic and end-diastolic ventricular interaction. Am J Physiol 251:H1062, 1986.

202. Pinson CW, et al: An anatomic basis for fetal right ventricular dominance and arterial pressure sensitivity. J Dev Physiol 9:253, 1987.

203. Langer GA, Jarmakani JM: Calcium exchange in the developing myocardium. In Legato MJ (ed): The Developing Heart. Boston, Martinus Nijhoff, 1984, pp 95–111.

204. Chin TK, et al: Developmental changes in cardiac myocyte calcium regulation. Circ Res 67:574, 1990.

205. Nakanishi T, et al: Development of myocardial contractile system in the fetal rabbit. Pediatr Res 22:201, 1987.

206. Penefsky ZJ: Studies on mechanism of inhibition of cardiac muscle contractile tension by ryanodine: mechanical response. Pflugers Arch 347:173, 1974.

207. Maylie JG: Excitation-contraction coupling in neonatal and adult myocardium of cat. Am J Physiol 242:H834, 1982.

208. Nayler WG, Fassold E: Calcium accumulating and ATPase activity of cardiac sarcoplasmic reticulum before and after birth. Cardiovasc Res 11:231, 1977.

209. Anger M, et al: In situ mRNA distribution of sarco(endo)plasmic reticulum Ca²⁺-ATPase isoforms during ontogeny in the rat. J Mol Cell Cardiol 26:539, 1994.

210. Page E, Surdyk-Droske M: Distribution, surface density, and membrane area of dyadic junctional contacts between plasma membrane and terminal cistern in mammalian ventricle. Circ Res 45:260, 1979.

211. Page E, Buecker JL: Development of dyadic junctional complexes between sarcoplasmic reticulum and plasmalemma in rabbit left ventricular myocardial cells: morphometric analysis. Circ Res 48:519, 1981.

212. Anderson PAW, et al: Cardiac muscle: an attempt to relate structure to function. J Mol Cell Cardiol 8:123, 1976.

213. Iwata Y, et al: Ca²⁺-ATPase distributes differently in cardiac sarcolemma than dihydropyridine receptor alpha 1 subunit and Na⁺/Ca²⁺ exchanger. FEBS Lett 355:65, 1994.

214. Khatter JC, Hoeschen RJ: Developmental increase of digitalis receptors in guinea pig heart. Cardiovasc Res 16:80, 1982.

215. Orlowski J, Lingrel JB: Tissue-specific and developmental regulation of rat Na, K-ATPase catalytic α isoform and β subunit mRNAs. J Biol Chem 263:10436, 1988.

216. Hougen TJ, Friedman WF: Age-related effects of digoxin on myocardial contractility and Na-K pump in sheep. Am J Physiol 243:H517, 1982.

217. Langer GA, et al: Correlation of the glycoside response, the force-staircase, and the action potential configuration in the neonatal rat heart. Circ Res 36:744, 1975.

218. Nagai K, et al: Digoxin reduces β-adrenergic contractile response in rabbit hearts: Ca²⁺ dependent inhibition of adenylyl cyclase activity via Na⁺/Ca²⁺ exchange. J Clin Invest 97:6, 1996.

219. Hofstetter R, et al: Effect of digoxin on left ventricular contractility in newborns and infants estimated by echocardiography. Eur J Cardiol 9:1, 1979.

220. Pinsky WW, et al: Dosage of digoxin in premature infants. J Pediatr 96:639, 1979.

221. Akera T, Brody TM: The role of Na,⁺ K⁺-ATPase in the inotropic action of digitalis. Pharmacol Rev 29:187, 1978.

222. Kawano S, DeHaan RL: Low-threshold current is major calcium current in chick ventricle cells. Am J Physiol 256:H1505, 1989.

223. Huynh TV, et al: Developmental changes in membrane Ca²⁺ and K⁺ currents in fetal, neonatal, and adult rabbit ventricular myocytes. Circ Res 70:508, 1992.

224. Osaka T, Joyner RW: Developmental changes in calcium currents of rabbit ventricular cells. Circ Res 68:788, 1991.

225. Davies MP, et al: Developmental changes in ionic channel activity in the embryonic murine heart. Circ Res 78:15, 1996.

226. Toshe N, et al: Developmental changes in long-opening behavior of L-type Ca²⁺ channels in embryonic chick heart cells. Circ Res 71:376, 1992.

227. Cohen NM, Lederer WJ: Changes in the calcium current of rat heart ventricular myocytes during development. J Physiol 406:115, 1988.

228. Brillantes A-MB, et al: Developmental and tissue-specific regulation of rabbit skeletal and cardiac muscle calcium channels involved in excitation-contraction coupling. Circ Res 75:503, 1994.

229. Boucek RJ Jr, et al: Comparative effects of verapamil, nifedipine, and diltiazem on contractile function in the isolated immature and adult rabbit heart. Pediatr Res 18:948, 1984.

230. Collin T, et al: Molecular cloning of three isoforms of the L-type voltage-dependent calcium channel β subunit from normal human heart. Circ Res 72:1337, 1993.

231. Diebold RJ, et al: Mutually exclusive exon splicing of the cardiac calcium channel α₁ subunit gene generates developmentally regulated isoforms in the rat heart. Proc Natl Acad Sci U S A 89:1497, 1992.

232. Artman M, et al: Na⁺-Ca²⁺ exchange current density in cardiac myocytes from rabbit and guinea pigs during postnatal development. Am J Physiol 268:H1714, 1995.

233. Artman M: Sarcolemmal Na/Ca exchange activity and exchanger immunoreactivity in developing rabbit hearts. Am J Physiol 263:H1506, 1992.

234. Boerth SR, et al: Steady-state mRNA levels of the sarcolemmal Na⁺-Ca²⁺ exchanger peak near birth in developing rabbit and rat hearts. Circ Res 74:354, 1994.

235. Katsube Y, et al: Functional activity of the Na-Ca exchanger estimated from whole-cell current in the developing rabbit ventricular cells. Circulation *90*:1, 1994.

236. Sham JS, et al: Species differences in the activity of the Na$^+$-Ca^{2+} exchanges in mammalian cardiac myocytes. J Physiol (Lond) *488*(Pt 3):623, 1995.

237. DeChamplain J, et al: Ontogenesis of peripheral adrenergic neurons in the rat: pre- and postnatal observations. Acta Physiol Scand *80*:276, 1970.

238. Friedman WF: Neuropharmacologic studies of perinatal myocardium. Cardiovasc Clin *4*:43, 1972.

239. Hoar RM, Hall JL: The early pattern of cardiac innervation in the fetal guinea-pig. Am J Anat *128*:499, 1970.

240. Lebowitz EA, et al: Development of myocardial sympathetic innervation in the fetal lamb. Pediatr Res *6*:887, 1972.

241. Papka RE: Development of innervation to the ventricular myocardium of the rabbit. J Mol Cell Cardiol *13*:217, 1981.

242. Osaka T, Joyner RW: Developmental changes in the β-adrenergic modulation of calcium currents of rabbit ventricular cells. Circ Res *70*:104, 1992.

243. Osaka T, et al: Postnatal decrease in muscarinic cholinergic influence on Ca^{2+} currents of rabbit ventricular cells. Am J Physiol *264*(6 Pt 2):H1916, 1993.

244. Akita T, et al: Developmental changes in modulation of calcium currents of rabbit ventricular cells by phosphodiesterase inhibitors. Circulation *90*:469, 1994.

245. Eliot RJ, et al: Plasma catecholamine concentrations in infants at birth and during the first 48 hours of life. J Pediatr *96*:311, 1980.

246. Erath HG Jr, et al: Functional significance of reduced cardiac sympathetic innervation in the newborn dog. Am J Physiol *243*:H20, 1982.

247. Padbury JF, et al: Neonatal adaptation: sympatho-adrenal response to umbilical cord cutting. Pediatr Res *15*:1483, 1981.

248. Dagbjartsson A, et al: Acute blockade of β$_1$-receptors in the asphyxiated sheep fetus. Acta Physiol Scand *130*:381, 1987.

249. Padbury JF, et al: Ontogenesis of tissue catecholamines in fetal and neonatal rabbits. J Dev Physiol *3*:297, 1981.

250. Tynan M, et al: Postnatal maturation of noradrenaline uptake and release in cat papillary muscles. Cardiovasc Res *11*:206, 1977.

251. Mackenzie E, Standen NB: The postnatal development of adrenoceptor responses in isolated papillary muscles from rat. Pflugers Arch *383*:185, 1980.

252. Saarikoski S: Functional development of adrenergic uptake mechanisms in the human fetal heart. Biol Neonate *43*:158, 1983.

253. Anderson PAW: Biophysics of the developing heart. *In* Elkayam U, Gleicher N (eds): Cardiac Problems in Pregnancy. New York, Alan R Liss, 1990, pp 485–518.

254. Buckley NM, et al: Age-related cardiovascular effects of catecholamines in anesthetized piglets. Circ Res *45*:282, 1979.

255. Rockson SG, et al: Cellular mechanisms of impaired adrenergic responsiveness in neonatal dogs. J Clin Invest *67*:319, 1981.

256. Lee JC, et al: Myocardial responses to α-adrenoceptor stimulation with methoxamine hydrochloride in lambs. Am J Physiol *242*:H405, 1982.

257. Steinberg SF, et al: Acquisition by innervated cardiac myocytes of a pertussis toxin–specific regulatory protein linked to the α$_1$-receptor. Science *230*:186, 1985.

258. Robinson RB: Review: autonomic receptor-effector coupling during postnatal development. Cardiovasc Res *31*:E68, 1996.

259. Drugge ED, et al: Neuronal regulation of the development of the α-adrenergic chronotropic response in the rat heart. Circ Res *57*:415, 1985.

260. Baker SP, Potter LT: Cardiac β-adrenoreceptors during normal growth of male and female rats. Br J Pharmacol *68*:65, 1980.

261. Chen F-CM, et al: Ontogeny of mammalian myocardial β-receptors. Eur J Pharmacol *58*:255, 1979.

262. Schumacher W, et al: Biological maturation and β-adrenergic effectors: development of β-adrenergic receptors in rabbit heart. Mol Cell Biochem *58*:173, 1984.

263. Whitsett JA, Darovec-Beckerman C: Developmental aspects of β-adrenergic receptors and catecholamine-sensitive adenylate cyclase in rat myocardium. Pediatr Res *15*:1363, 1981.

264. Gauthier C, et al: Functional β$_3$ adrenoceptor in the human heart. J Clin Invest *98*:556, 1996.

265. Felder RA, et al: Ontogeny of myocardial adrenoceptors. II: Alpha adrenoceptors. Pediatr Res *16*:340, 1982.

266. Wei JW, Sulakhe PV: Regional and subcellular distribution of β- and α-adrenergic receptors in the myocardium of different species. Gen Pharmacol *10*:263, 1979.

267. Yamada S, et al: Ontogeny of mammalian cardiac α$_1$-adrenergic receptors. Eur J Pharmacol *68*:217, 1980.

268. Luetje CW, et al: Differential tissue expression and developmental regulation of guanine nucleotide binding regulatory proteins and their messenger RNAs in rat heart. J Biol Chem *263*:13357, 1988.

269. Moschella MC, Marks AR: Inositol 1,4,5,-trisphosphate receptor expression in cardiac myocytes. J Cell Biol *120*:1137, 1993.

270. Su Y, et al: Regulatory subunit of protein kinase A: structure of deletion mutant with cAMP binding domains. Science *269*:807, 1995.

271. Cooper DMF, et al: Adenylyl cyclases and the interaction between calcium and cAMP signalling. Nature *374*:421, 1995.

272. Clerk A, et al: Expression of protein kinase C isoforms during cardiac ventricular development. Am J Physiol *269*:H1087, 1995.

273. Schumacher WA, et al: Biological maturation and beta-adrenergic effectors: pre- and postnatal development of the adenylate cyclase system in the rabbit heart. J Pharmacol Exp Ther *223*:587, 1982.

274. Okuda H, et al: Effect of isoproterenol on myocardial mechanical function and cyclic AMP content in the fetal rabbit. J Mol Cell Cardiol *19*:151, 1987.

275. Winegrad S, Weisberg A: Isozyme specific modification of myosin ATPase by cAMP in rat heart. Circ Res *60*:384, 1987.

276. Gilbert RD: Venous return and control of fetal cardiac output. *In* Longo LD, Reneau DD (eds): Fetal and Newborn Cardiovascular Physiology, Vol 1. New York, Garland, 1978, pp 299–316.

277. Anderson PAW, et al: Evaluation of the force-frequency relationship as a descriptor of the inotropic state of canine left ventricular myocardium. Circ Res *39*:832, 1976.

278. Arentzen CE, et al: Force-frequency characteristics of the left ventricle in the conscious dog. Circ Res *42*:64, 1978.

279. Ross J Jr, et al: Effects of changing heart rate in man by electrical stimulation of the right atrium: studied at rest, during exercise, and with isoproterenol. Circulation *32*:549, 1965.

280. Sugimoto T, et al: Effect of tachycardia on cardiac output during normal and increased venous return. Am J Physiol *211*:288, 1966.

281. Kirkpatrick SE, et al: Influence of poststimulation potentiation and heart rate on the fetal lamb heart. Am J Physiol *229*:318, 1975.

282. Reller MD, et al: Fetal lamb ventricles respond differently to filling and arterial pressures and to in utero ventilation. Pediatr Res *22*:621, 1987.

283. Anderson PAW, et al: The force-interval relationship of the human left ventricle. Circulation *60*:334, 1979.

284. Clyman RI, et al: Cardiovascular effects of patent ductus arteriosus in preterm lambs with respiratory distress. Am J Physiol *111*:579, 1987.

285. Clyman RI, et al: The role of β-adrenoreceptor stimulation and contractile state in the preterm lamb's response to altered ductus arteriosus patency. Pediatr Res *23*:316, 1988.

286. Klopfenstein HS, Rudolph AM: Postnatal changes in the circulation and responses to volume loading in sheep. Circ Res *42*:839, 1978.

287. Romero TE, Friedman WF: Limited left ventricular response to volume overload in the neonatal period: a comparative study with the adult animal. Pediatr Res *13*:910, 1979.

288. Kirkpatrick SE, et al: A new technique for the continuous assessment of fetal and neonatal cardiac performance. Am J Obstet Gynecol *116*:963, 1973.

289. Shimada E, et al: Effects of patent ductus arteriosus on left ventricular output and organ blood flows in preterm infants with respiratory distress syndrome treated with surfactant. J Pediatr *125*:270, 1994.

290. Lorijn RHW, Longo LD: Norepinephrine elevation in the fetal lamb: oxygen consumption and cardiac output. Am J Physiol *239*:R115, 1980.

291. Anderson PAW, et al: The in utero left ventricle of the fetal sheep: the effects of isoprenaline. J Physiol (Lond) *430*:441, 1990.

292. Teitel DF, et al: In utero ventilation augments the left ventricular response to isoproterenol and volume loading in fetal sheep. Pediatr Res *29*:466, 1991.

293. Downing SE, et al: Ventricular function in the newborn lamb. Am J Physiol *208*:931, 1965.

294. Grant DA, et al: Changes in pericardial pressure during the perinatal period. Circulation *86*:1615, 1992.

295. Geis WP, et al: Factors influencing neurohumoral control of the heart in the newborn dog. Am J Physiol *228*:1685, 1975.

296. O'Laughlin MP, et al: Augmentation of cardiac output with intravenous catecholamines in unanesthetized hypoxemic newborn lambs. Pediatr Res *22*:667, 1987.

297. Breall JA, et al: Role of thyroid hormone in postnatal circulatory and metabolic adjustments. J Clin Invest *73*:1418, 1984.

298. Su JY, Friedman WF: Comparison of the responses of fetal and adult cardiac muscle to hypoxia. Am J Physiol *224*:1249, 1973.

299. Downing SE, et al: Influences of hypoxemia and acidemia on left ventricular function. Am J Physiol *210*:1327, 1966.

300. Downing SE, et al: Influences of arterial oxygen tension and pH on cardiac function in the newborn lamb. Am J Physiol *211*:1203, 1966.

301. Downing SE, et al: Influences of hypercapnia on cardiac function in the newborn lamb. Yale J Biol Med *38*:242, 1971.

302. Talner NS, et al: Influence of acidemia on left ventricular function in the newborn lamb. Pediatrics *38*:457, 1966.

303. Downing SE: Potentiation by calcium channel blockade of hypoxic myocardial depression in the neonate. Am Heart J *110*:395, 1985.

304. Fisher DJ: Acidaemia reduces cardiac output and left ventricular contractility in conscious lambs. J Dev Physiol *8*:23, 1986.

305. Katz AM, Hecht HH: The early pump failure of the ischemic heart. Am J Med *47*:497, 1969.

306. Nakanishi T, et al: Effect of acidosis on contractile function in the newborn rabbit heart. Pediatr Res *19*:482, 1985.

307. Fisher DJ: Left ventricular oxygen consumption and function in hypoxemia in conscious lambs. Am J Physiol *244*:H664, 1983.

308. Hoerter JA: Changes in the sensitivity to hypoxia and glucose deprivation in the isolated perfused rabbit heart during peri-natal development. Pflugers Arch *363*:1, 1976.

309. Jarmakani JM, et al: Effect of hypoxia on mechanical function on the neonatal mammalian heart. Am J Physiol *235*:H469, 1978.

310. Lee JC, et al: Coronary flow and myocardial metabolism in newborn lambs: effects of hypoxia and acidemia. Am J Physiol *224*:1381, 1973.

311. Penney DG, Cascarano J: Anaerobic rat heart: effects of glucose and tricarboxylic acid–cycle metabolites on metabolism and physiological performance. Biochem J *118*:221, 1970.

312. Hoerter JA, Opie LH: Perinatal changes in glycolytic function in response to hypoxia in the incubated or perfused rat heart. Biol Neonate *33*:144, 1978.

313. Jones CT, Rolph TP: Metabolism during fetal life: a functional assessment of metabolic development. Physiol Rev *65*:357, 1985.

314. Rolph TP, et al: Ultrastructural and enzymatic development of fetal guinea pig heart. Am J Physiol *243*:H87, 1982.

315. Abd-Elfattah AS, et al: Biochemical bases for tolerance of the newborn heart to ischemic injury; developmental differences in adenine nucleotide degradation between ischemic immature and adult myocardium: a possible role of sarcolemmal 5-nucleotidase. Pediatr Res *19*:122A, 1985.

316. Bove EL, Stammers AH: Recovery of left ventricular function after hypothermic global ischemia. J Thorac Cardiovasc Surg *91*:115, 1986.

317. Yee ES, Ebert PA: Effect of ischemia on ventricular function, compliance, and edema in immature and adult canine hearts. Surg Forum *30*:250, 1979.

318. Robin ED: Of men and mitochondria: coping with hypoxic dysoxia. Am Rev Respir Dis *122*:517, 1980.

319. Robin ED: Overview: Dysoxia abnormalities of tissue oxygen use. *In* Lenfant C (ed): Extrapulmonary Manifestations of Respiratory Disease. New York, Marcel Dekker, 1978, pp 3–12.

320. Granger HJ, et al: Metabolic models of microcirculatory regulation. Fed Proc *34*:2025, 1975.

321. Fahey JT, Lister G: Oxygen transport in low cardiac output states. J Crit Care *2*:288, 1987.

322. Haddy FJ, Scott JB: Metabolic factors in peripheral circulatory regulation. Fed Proc *34*:2006, 1975.

323. Lister G, et al: Oxygen delivery in lambs: cardiovascular and hematologic development Am J Physiol *237*:H668, 1979.

324. Lister G, et al: Effects of alterations of oxygen transport on the neonate. Semin Perinatol *8*:192, 1984.

325. Tam CC, et al: Feedback modulation of renal and hepatic erythropoietin mRNA in response to graded anemia and hypoxia. Am J Physiol *263*:F474, 1992.

326. Semenza GL: Review: Regulation of erythropoietin production: new insights into molecular mechanisms of oxygen homeostasis. Hematol Oncol Clin North Am *8*:863, 1994.

327. Wang GL, et al: Hypoxia-inducible factor-1 is a basic helix-loop-helix-PAS heterodimer regulated by cellular oxygen tension. Proc Natl Acad Sci USA *92*:5510, 1995.

328. Jelkmann W: Renal erythropoietin L properties and production. Rev Physiol Biochem Pharmacol *104*:140, 1986.

329. Bauer CM, et al: Factors governing the O_2 affinity of human and foetal blood. Respir Physiol *7*:272, 1969.

330. Abboud FM, et al: Reflex control of the peripheral circulation. Prog Cardiovasc Dis *28*:371, 1976.

331. Dawes GS, et al: Vasomotor responses in the hind limbs of foetal and newborn lambs to asphyxia and aortic chemoreceptor stimulation. J Physiol *195*:55, 1968.

332. Paulick RP, et al: Hemodynamic responses to alpha-adrenergic blockade during hypoxemia in the fetal lamb. J Dev Physiol *16*:63, 1991.

333. Baan J Jr, et al: Heart rate fall during acute hypoxemia: a measure of chemoreceptor response in fetal sheep. J Dev Physiol *19*:105, 1993.

334. Bartelds V, et al: Carotid, not aortic, chemoreceptors mediate the fetal cardiovascular response to acute hypoxemia in lambs. Pediatr Res *34*:51, 1993.

335. Itskovitz J, et al: Cardiovascular responses to hypoxemia in sinoaortic-denervated fetal sheep. Pediatr Res *30*:381, 1991.

336. Van Bel F, et al: Role of nitric oxide in the regulation of the cerebral circulation in the lamb fetus during normoxemia and hypoxemia. Biol Neonate *68*:200, 1995.

337. Reller MD, et al: Nitric oxide is an important determinant of coronary flow at rest and during hypoxemic stress in fetal lambs. Am J Physiol *269*(6 Pt 2):H2074, 1995.

338. Share L: Interactions between vasopressin and the renin-angiotensin system. Fed Proc *38*:2267, 1979.

339. Ignarro LJ: Biosynthesis and metabolism of endothelium-derived nitric oxide. Annu Rev Pharmacol Toxicol *30*:535, 1990.

340. Berridge MJ, Irvine RF: Inositol phosphates and cell signaling. Nature *341*:197, 1989.

341. Yanagisawa M, et al: A novel potent vasoconstrictor peptide produced by vascular endothelial cells. Nature *332*:411, 1988.

342. Cohn HE, et al: Cardiovascular responses to hypoxemia and acidemia in fetal lambs. Am J Obstet Gynecol *120*:817, 1974.

343. Edelstone DI: Fetal compensatory responses to reduced oxygen delivery. Semin Perinatol *8*:184, 1984.

344. Fisher DJ: Cardiac output and regional blood flows during hypoxemia in unanesthetized newborn lambs. J Dev Physiol *6*:485, 1984.

345. Fisher DJ: Increased regional myocardial blood flows and oxygen delivery during hypoxemia in lambs. Pediatr Res *18*:602, 1984.

346. Jensen A, et al: Dynamic changes in organ blood flow and oxygen consumption during acute asphyxia in fetal sheep. J Dev Physiol *9*:543, 1987.

347. Rudolph AM, et al: Fetal cardiovascular responses to stress. Semin Perinatol *5*:109, 1981.

348. Rudolph AM: Distribution and regulation of blood flow in the fetal and neonatal lamb. Circ Res *57*:811, 1985.

349. Fisher DJ, et al: Fetal myocardial oxygen and carbohydrate consumption during acutely induced hypoxemia. Am J Physiol *242*:H657, 1982.

350. Fisher DJ, et al: Fetal myocardial oxygen and carbohydrate metabolism in sustained hypoxemia in utero. Am J Physiol *243*:H959, 1982.

351. Behrman RE, et al: Distribution of the circulation in the normal and asphyxiated fetal primate. Am J Obstet Gynecol *108*:956, 1970.

352. Jensen A, et al: Effects of reducing uterine blood flow on fetal blood flow distribution and oxygen delivery. J Dev Physiol *15*:301, 1991.

353. Adams RP, Cain JM: Total and hindlimb oxygen deficit and "repayment" in hypoxic anesthetized dogs. J Appl Physiol *55*:913, 1983.

354. Cain SM: Oxygen deficit incurred during hypoxia and its relation to lactate and excess lactate. Am J Physiol *213*:57, 1967.

355. Fahey JT, Lister G: Response to low cardiac output: developmental differences in metabolism during oxygen deficit and recovery in lambs. Pediatr Res *26*:180, 1989.

356. Sidi D, et al: Developmental changes in oxygenation and circulatory response to hypoxemia in lambs. Am J Physiol *254*:H674, 1983.

357. Teitel D, Rudolph AM: Perinatal oxygen delivery and cardiac function. Adv Pediatr *32*:321, 1985.

358. Parer JT: The effect of acute maternal hypoxia on fetal oxygenation and the umbilical circulation in the sheep. Eur J Obstet Gynecol Reprod Biol *10*:125, 1980.

359. Hochachka PW: Defense strategies against hypoxia. Science *231*:234, 1986.

360. Reller MD, et al: Maximal myocardial blood flow is enhanced by chronic hypoxemia in late gestation fetal sheep. Am J Physiol *263*(4 Pt 2):H1327, 1992.

361. Reller MD, et al: Severe right ventricular pressure loading in fetal sheep augments global myocardial blood flow to submaximal levels. Circulation *86*:581, 1992.

362. Teitel D, et al: Developmental changes in myocardial contractile reserve. Pediatr Res *19*:948, 1985.

363. Morgan HE, Baker KM: Cardiac hypertrophy: mechanical, neural and endocrine dependence. Circulation *83*:13, 1991.

364. Kimuro I, et al: Stretching cardiac myocytes stimulates protooncogene expression. J Biol Chem *265*:3595, 1990.

365. Katz AM: Angiotensin II: hemodynamic regulator or growth factor? J Mol Cell Cardiol *22*:739, 1990.

366. Griendling KK, et al: Angiotensin II stimulation of vascular smooth muscle. J Cardiovasc Pharm *14*(Suppl 6):S27, 1989.

367. Anversa P, et al: Stereological measurement of cellular and sub-cellular hypertrophy and hyperplasia in the papillary muscle of the adult rat. J Mol Cell Cardiol *12*:781, 1980.

368. Weber KT, et al: Collagen remodeling of the pressure overloaded hypertrophied nonhuman primate myocardium. Circ Res *62*:757, 1988.

369. Bristow MR, et al: β-Adrenergic function in heart muscle disease and heart failure. J Mol Cell Cardiol *17*(Suppl 2):41, 1985.

370. Maenpaa PH, Raiha NCR: Effects of anoxia on energy-rich phosphates, glycogen, lactate and pyruvate in the brain, heart and liver of the developing rat. Ann Med Exp Fenn *46*:306, 1968.

371. Tagawa K, et al: Mechanism of anoxic damage of mitochondria: depletion of mitochondrial ATP and concomitant release of free Ca^{2+}. Mol Physiol *8*:55, 1985.

372. Matthys E, et al: Lipid alterations induced by renal ischemia: pathogenesis factor in membrane damage. Kidney Int *26*:153, 1984.

373. Donnelly WH, et al: Ischemic papillary muscle necrosis in stressed newborn infants. J Pediatr *96*:295, 1980.

374. Setzer E, et al: Papillary muscle necrosis in a neonatal autopsy population: incidence and associated clinical manifestations. J Pediatr *96*:289, 1980.

375. Berry CL: Myocardial ischemia in infancy and childhood. J Clin Pathol *20*:38, 1967.

376. Esterly JR, Oppenheimer EH: Some aspects of cardiac pathology in infancy and childhood. 1: Neonatal myocardial necrosis. Bull Johns Hopkins Hosp *119*:191, 1966.

377. David H, et al: Postnatal development of myocardial cells after oxygen deficiency in utero. Pathol Res Pract *179*:370, 1985.

378. Jarmakani JM, et al: Effect of hypoxia on myocardial high energy phosphates in the neonatal mammalian heart. Am J Physiol *25*:H475, 1978.

379. Nishioka K, Jarmakani JM: Effect of ischemia on mechanical function and high energy phosphates in rabbit myocardium. Am J Physiol *242*:H1077, 1982.

380. Cheng W, et al: Stretch-induced programmed myocyte cell death. J Clin Invest *96*:2247, 2259, 1995.

381. Tanaka M, et al: Hypoxia induces apoptosis with enhanced expression of fas antigen messenger RNA in cultured neonatal rat cardiomyocytes. Circ Res *75*:426, 1994.

382. Heymann MA, Rudolph AM: Effects of congenital heart disease on fetal and neonatal circulation. Prog Cardiovasc Dis *15*:115, 1972.

383. Rudolph AM, Heymann MA: Fetal and neonatal circulation and respiration. Am Rev Physiol *36*:187, 1974.

384. Rudolph AM: Congenital Diseases of the Heart. Chicago, Year Book Medical Publishers, 1974.

385. Kleinman CS, Donnerstein RL: Ultrasonic assessment of cardiac function in the intact fetus. J Am Coll Cardiol *5*:(Suppl 1):845, 1985.

386. Berman W, et al: Pulsed Doppler evaluation of the fetal circulation. In Altobelli SA (ed): Cardiovascular Ultrasonic Flowmetry. New York, Elsevier, 1985, pp 411–430.

387. Atkins D, et al: Foramen ovale/atrial septum ratio: a marker of transatrial flow. Circulation 66:281, 1982.

388. Feit LR, et al: Foramen ovale size in the human fetal heart: an indicator of transatrial flow physiology. Ultrasound Obstet Gynecol 1:313, 1991.

389. Hornberger LK, et al: Antenatal diagnosis of coarctation of the aorta: a multicenter experience. J Am Coll Cardiol 21:417, 1994.

390. Hutchins GM: Coarctation of the aorta as explained as a branch point of the ductus arteriosus. Am J Pathol 63:203, 1971.

391. Groenenberg IAL, et al: Fetal cardiac and peripheral arterial flow velocity waveforms in intrauterine growth retardation. Circulation 89:1711, 1989.

392. Mari G, Deter RL: Middle cerebral artery flow velocity waveforms in normal and small-for-gestational-age fetuses. Am J Obstet Gynecol 166:1262, 1992.

393. Huhta JC, et al: Detection and quantitation of constriction of the fetal ductus arteriosus by Doppler echocardiography. Circulation 75:406, 1987.

394. Schmidt KG, et al: Perinatal outcome of fetal complete atrioventricular block: a multicenter experience. J Am Coll Cardiol 17:1360, 1991.

395. Nimrod C, et al: Ultrasound evaluation of tachycardia-induced hydrops in the fetal lamb. Am J Obstet Gynecol 157:655, 1987.

396. Stevens DC, et al: Supraventricular tachycardia with edema, ascites and hydrops in fetal sheep. Am J Obstet Gynecol 142:316, 1982.

397. Kleinman CS, et al: Fetal echocardiography for evaluation of in utero congestive heart failure. N Engl J Med 306:568, 1982.

398. Apkon M: Pathophysiology of hydrops fetalis. Semin Perinatol 19:437, 1995.

399. Hutchison AA: Pathophysiology of hydrops fetalis. In Long WA (ed): Fetal and Neonatal Cardiology. Philadelphia, WB Saunders, 1990, pp 197–210.

400. Silverman NS, et al: Fetal atrioventricular valve insufficiency associated with nonimmune hydrops: a two-dimensional echocardiographic and pulsed Doppler ultrasound study. Circulation 72:825, 1985.

401. Friedman WF: The intrinsic physiologic properties of the developing heart. In Friedman WF, et al (eds): Neonatal Heart Disease. New York, Grune & Stratton, 1973.

402. Reed KL, et al: Doppler echocardiographic studies of diastolic function in the human fetal heart: changes during gestation. J Am Coll Cardiol 8:391, 1986.

403. Kleinman CS, et al: In utero diagnosis and treatment of fetal supraventricular tachycardia. Semin Perinatol 9:113, 1985.

404. Buyon JP, et al: In utero identification and therapy of congenital heart block. Lupus 41:116, 1995.

405. Hornberger LK, et al: Tricuspid valve disease with significant tricuspid insufficiency in the fetus: diagnosis and outcome. J Am Coll Cardiol 17:167, 1991.

406. Burnard ED, James LS: Failure of the heart after cardiac asphyxia at birth. Pediatrics 28:545, 1961.

407. Rowe RD, Hoffman T: Transient myocardial ischemia of the newborn infant: a form of severe cardiorespiratory distress in full-term infants. J Pediatr 81:243, 1972.

408. Cabal LA, et al: Cardiogenic shock associated with perinatal asphyxia in preterm infants. J Pediatr 96:705, 1980.

409. Nelson RM, et al: Serum creatinine phosphokinase MB fraction in newborns with transient tricuspid insufficiency. N Engl J Med 298:146, 1978.

410. Walther FJ, et al: Cardiac output in newborn infants with transient myocardial dysfunction. J Pediatr 107:781, 1985.

411. Finley JP, et al: Transient myocardial ischemia of the newborn infant demonstrated by thallium-201 myocardial imaging. J Pediatr 94:263, 1979.

412. Guller B, Gozic C: Right-to-left shunting through a patent ductus arteriosus in a newborn with myocardial infarction. Cardiology 37:348, 1972.

413. Bucciarelli R, et al: Transient tricuspid insufficiency of the newborn: a form of myocardial dysfunction in stressed newborns. Pediatrics 59:330, 1977.

64

Arthur S. Pickoff

Developmental Electrophysiology in the Fetus and Neonate

In this chapter the physiology of both impulse formation and conduction within the developing heart is discussed. Growing numbers of electrophysiologic, morphologic, and immunohistochemical studies of the developing heart have clearly shown that there are significant age-related changes in the ionic currents responsible for the generation of the cardiac action potential, as well as changes in the microscopic and macroscopic anatomic and neural substrates that govern the physiology of intracardiac conduction.

THE CARDIAC ACTION POTENTIAL

The cardiac action potential is the electrical event responsible for the generation of the cardiac impulse and conduction of the electrical impulse through the myocardium and specialized cardiac conduction system. It is based on a complex series of transmembrane ion fluxes that result in a net flow of electrical current across the cell membrane.[1,2] The cell membrane is a lipid bilayer and is thus highly impermeable to charged ions. The cardiac action potential is generated as a result of two important conditions. The first is an unequal distribution of electrically charged ions, most importantly sodium, potassium, and calcium ions, across the cell membrane (Table 64-1). These ion gradients are established and maintained largely as a result of the activity of energy-expending membrane ion pumps (sodium-potassium adenosine triphosphatase [ATPase]) and ion exchange complexes (the sodium-calcium exchanger). The second critical factor in the generation of the action potential is that under appropriate biophysical conditions, complex polypeptide pores known as *ion channels*, embedded within the cell membrane, are open, thereby allowing the passage of charged ions through the cell membrane. The detailed molecular structure of many of these ion channels is now understood (Fig. 64-1A–C).[3,4] The direction and magnitude of ion flow through these channels are determined by both ion concentration and electrical gradients, and also, in part, by physical properties inherent to the specific ion channel.

It is useful to consider the ionic events that determine the cardiac action potential before considering the influence of development on this process. The descriptions that follow are derived in part from intracellular microelectrode recordings of changes in the cellular transmembrane potential and also from voltage-clamp studies. At rest, the interior of the typical cardiac cell exhibits a negative electrical potential with respect to the extracellular space. For Purkinje fibers and atrial and ventricular myocytes, this transmembrane potential is approximately −90 mV. In the sinoatrial and atrioventricular (AV) nodes, the interior of the cell is somewhat less negative, approximately −60 mV (Table 64-2). This negative resting membrane potential is generated in part by the

TABLE 64-1

Intracellular and Extracellular Ion Distribution in the Cardiac Cell

	Na⁺	K⁺	Cl⁻	Ca²⁺
Extracellular	145 mM	4 mM	120 mM	2 mM
		cell membrane		
Intracellular	15 mM	145 mM	5 mM	10^{-4} mM

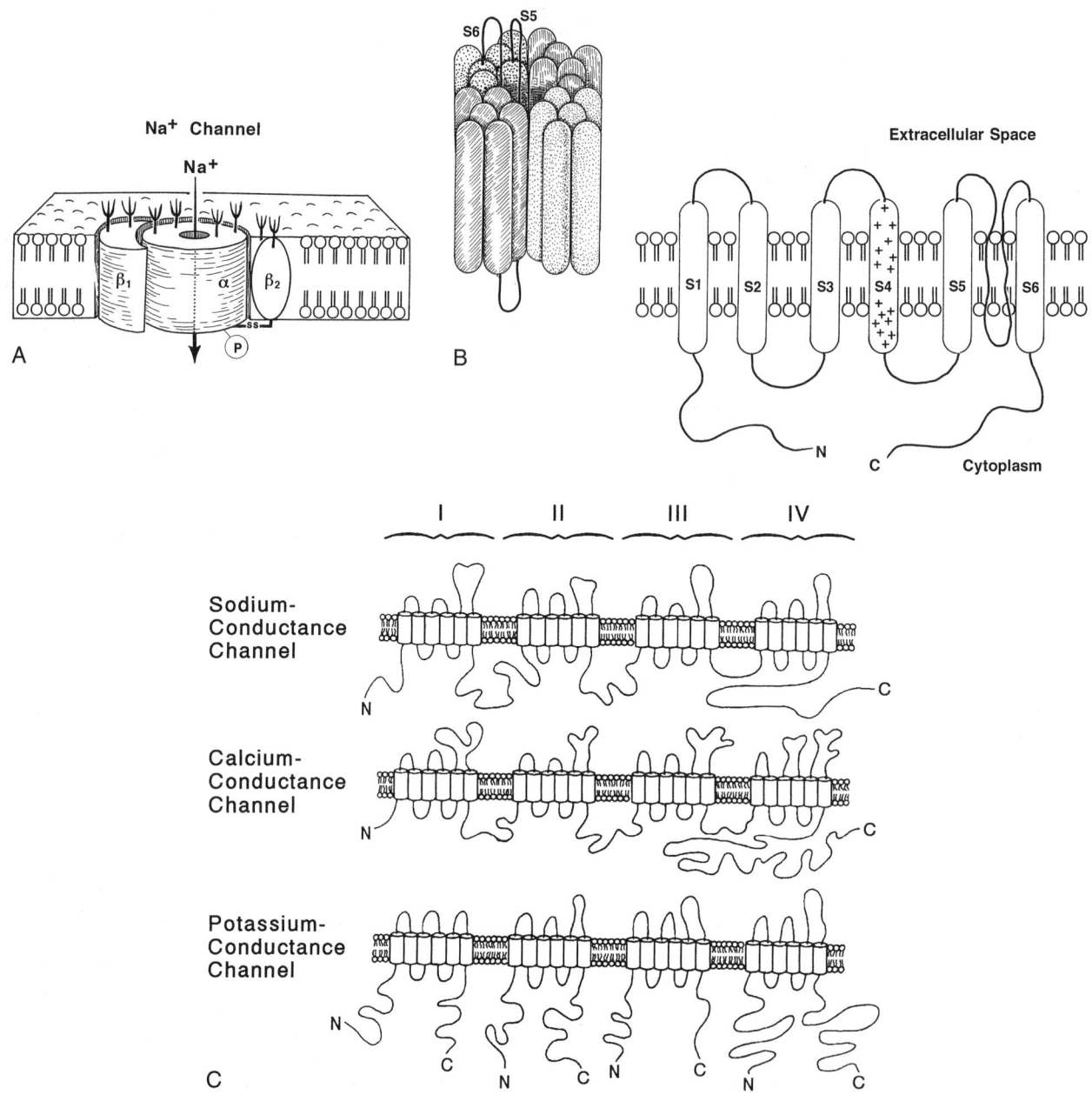

Figure 64–1. A, Three-dimensional representation of a sodium channel from mammalian brain. The ion channel consists of the α subunit, with two smaller protein subunits (β₁ and β₂) associated with the main channel. The β₁ subunit is found only in cardiac sodium channels and is thought to stabilize the channel. S S = disulfide bond, P = phosphorylation sites, and the treelike (cactuslike) structures = glycosylation sites. (Adapted from Shih H-T: Texas Heart Inst J *21*:30, 1994.) **B,** The ion channel is composed of four domains of a protein complex that consists of six separate transmembrane segments (S1–S6). The topographic arrangement of one such domain is shown on the left. The peptide loops between S5 and S6 are thought to represent the central pore of the channel. Subunit S4 is a highly charged protein segment that is believed to serve as the voltage sensor of the ion channel. (Reproduced with permission from Brown AM: Ion channels in action potential generation. Hosp Pract [Off Ed] *27*:129, 1992. Illustration by Alan D. Iselin). **C,** Diagrammatic representation of the sodium channel, calcium channel, and potassium channel. In sodium and calcium channels, there is covalent linkage of the four domains (I–IV). (Each domain consists of the six transmembrane segments S1–S6 already described.) Potassium channels consist of single domains. There is no covalent linkage between domains. (Modified with permission from Catterall WA: Science *242*:50, 1988. Copyright 1988 American Association for the Advancement of Science.)

activity of the sodium-potassium ATPase pump. This energy-requiring pump maintains a high intracellular concentration of potassium ions and low intracellular sodium concentration relative to the extracellular space, by pumping two potassium ions into the cell for every three sodium ions extruded into the extracellular space. This unequal exchange rate of positive ions results in a net negative charge of the intracellular space. The most important factor responsible for the negative resting membrane potential of the cardiac cell is the relatively high permeability of the resting cell membrane to the potassium ion. This high permeability permits the movement of potassium ions down their concentration gradient (from the intracellular space into the

TABLE 64-2

Action Potential Characteristics in Cardiac Cells

	SA Node	Atrium	AV Node	His-Purkinje	Ventricle
Resting potential (mV)	−50−−60	−80−−90	−60−−70	−90−−95	−80−−90
Action potential					
Amplitude (mV)	60-70	110-120	70-80	120	110-120
Overshoot (mV)	0-10	30	5-15	30	30
Duration (msec)	100-300	100-300	100-300	300-500	100-200
$\dot{V}_{max}$ (V/sec)	1-10	100-200	5-15	500-700	100-200
Conduction velocity (M/sec)	<0.05	0.3-0.4	0.1	2-3	0.3-0.4

SA = sinoatrial; AV = atrioventricular; mV = millivolts; msec = milliseconds; $\dot{V}_{max}$ = maximum rate of rise of the action potential phase 0 in volts per second (V/sec); M/sec = meters per second.

(Modified from Sperelakis N: Origin of the cardiac resting potential. *In* Berne RM, Sperelakis N (eds): Handbook of Physiology, Vol 1. The Cardiovascular System. Bethesda, MD, American Physiological Society, 1979, pp. 187-267.)

extracellular space), thereby rendering the interior of the cell more negative with respect to the exterior. The relationship of resting membrane potential to the intracellular-extracellular potassium concentration gradient is described by the Nernst equation:

$$E = (RT/F) \log(K^+_{in}/K^+_{out})$$

where E is the membrane potential, R is the gas constant, T is the temperature, F is the Faraday constant, and K^+_{in} and K^+_{out} represent the concentrations of potassium ion inside and outside of the cell.

When the resting potential of the cardiac cell is made less negative, either as a result of the cell's exhibiting spontaneous depolarization (automaticity), or as a result of an advancing wave of electrical current, the cell reaches a level of depolarization, called the *activation potential*. At that point, there is a sudden and rapid influx of positively charged sodium ions (in the case of atrial and ventricular myocytes and Purkinje fibers). This rapid influx of positively charged sodium ions rapidly depolarizes the cell to potentials close to +20 to +30 mV. This rapid phase of depolarization is commonly referred to as *phase 0 of the action potential* (Fig. 64-2). The maximum rate of rise of the action potential phase 0, $\dot{V}_{max}$, in ventricular and atrial muscle approaches 200 volts (V)/sec; in Purkinje fibers, even higher rates of change in membrane potential are observed ($\dot{V}_{max}$ of approximately 500 V/sec) (see Table 64-2). The amplitude and rate of rise of phase 0 of the action potential are key determinants of conduction velocity in the myocardium and specialized conduction system, with greater conduction velocities resulting from action potentials of greater amplitude and greater $\dot{V}_{max}$. The sudden influx of sodium ions, triggered by the change in membrane potential, results from the sodium channel's changing from a conformationally specific "rested" state to an active or "open" channel configuration[3] (Fig. 64-3). A highly charged protein subunit (subunit S4; see Fig. 64-2B) of the sodium channel serves as the so-called voltage sensor. After the activation potential has been reached, the voltage sensor moves within the membrane, inducing a conformational change in the sodium channel and resulting in the opening of an "m" or activation gate. This, in turn, allows free passage of sodium ions. As the membrane potential becomes more positive, the sodium channel enters into a third distinct conformational state, the inactivated state, which results from closure of an "h," or inactivation, gate (see Fig. 64-3). This inactivation gate may correspond to one of the intracellular peptide loops of the cardiac ion channel.[5, 6] Activation and inactivation of the sodium channel occur rapidly, within a time course of a few milliseconds. Allowing for significant differences in the kinetics of channel activation and inactivation, other voltage-gated ion channels, such as calcium

and potassium channels, are believed to function in a similar state-dependent fashion (Table 64-3).

After the completion of phase 0, there is often a short, rapid repolarization phase, which creates a notch in the action potential. This notch, which comprises phase 1 of the action potential, and the resulting spike-and-dome appearance of the initial portion of the action potential plateau, are most notable in epicardial ventricular muscle cells and in Purkinje fibers (Fig. 64-4A). There are two principal charge carriers responsible for this phase 1 notch. One is a transiently activated outward potassium current, referred to as I_{to}, and the second is an inward chloride current (I_{to2}).[7] The transient outward current is markedly reduced or absent in ventricular endocardium. It exhibits significant rate-dependent behavior (except possibly in the human) (see Fig. 64-4B).

The plateau of the action potential, phase 2 (see Fig. 64-1), can persist for hundreds of milliseconds and reflects the delicate balance of both inward and outward currents on a high-resistance membrane. The most important of the inward currents during the action potential plateau is the inward calcium current. L-type ("long lasting," "large"), and T-type ("tiny," "transient") calcium channels predominate in the heart.[8] The L-type calcium current (I_{Ca-L}) activates at membrane potentials of −55 to −30 mV and is the main charge carrier responsible for maintaining the action potential plateau during phase 2. Activation of I_{Ca-L} is also highly dependent upon intracellular calcium concentration.[9] T-type calcium channels, which activate at potentials more negative than those of the L-type channels, may primarily contribute to pacemaker activity in the heart.[8] The magnitude of I_{Ca-L} is nearly 10-fold less than that of the sodium current. Activation and inactivation kinetics of I_{Ca-L} are also an order of magnitude slower than those of the sodium channel (see Table 64-3).[10] The slow inward current, I_{Ca-L}, also represents the major current responsible for phase 0 of the action potential in the sinus and AV nodes (see Fig. 64-1, *right side*) and is characterized by a very slow $\dot{V}_{max}$ of approximately 10 V/sec. The action potentials recorded from these regions are, therefore, referred to as *slow response* action potentials. A small inward sodium current is also present during phase 2 of the action potential, termed the *window current*.

Balancing the inward depolarizing plateau currents is a family of repolarization currents, largely outward potassium currents, that drive the membrane potential back toward the resting potential (see Fig. 64-1). Experiments with cloned pore-forming (α) and accessory (β) subunits of potassium channels have provided new insights into the relationships between molecular assembly and the functional expression of the major repolarization currents (I_K, I_{Kr}, I_{Ks}, I_{Kur}) in the mammalian heart.[11] The first major repolarizing current is referred to as the *delayed rectifier*, I_K. This large outward potassium current is termed *delayed* because of its slow time course of activation. I_K begins to activate relatively late during the action potential plateau, as the time-dependent slow calcium

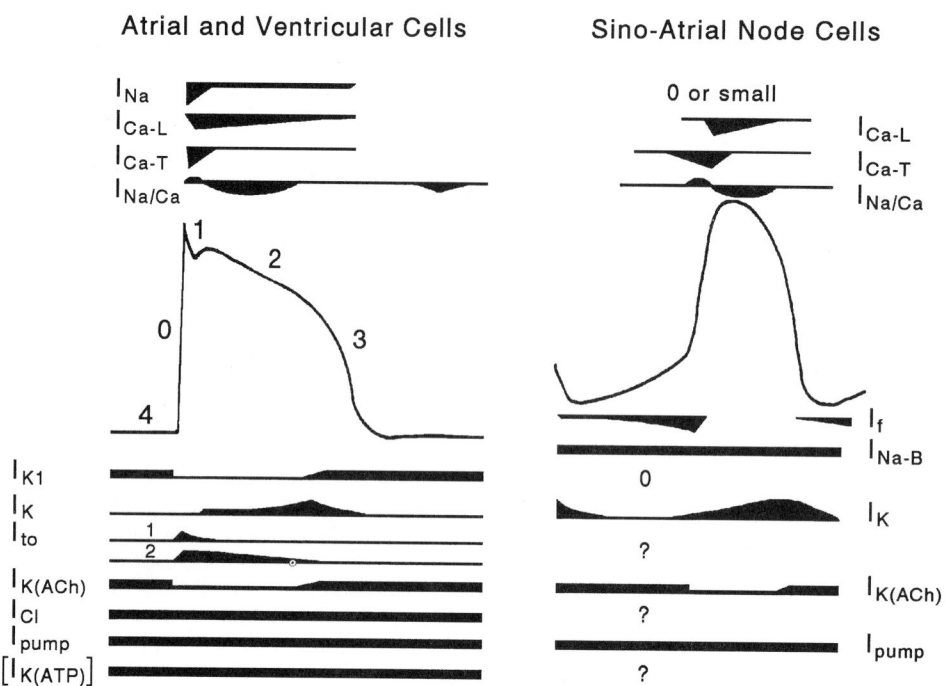

Figure 64–2. Diagrammatic representation of the atrial and ventricular action potential (*left*) and sinus node action potential (*right*). The major ion currents and ion pumps involved in the generation of the action potentials are depicted. For each of the currents, the direction of current flow is indicated (downward indicating an inward current, upward indicating an outward current) as well as the approximate time course of activation and inactivation. Relative current amplitudes are *not* depicted. I_{Na} represents the inward sodium current; I_{Ca-L}, the large, long-lasting slow inward calcium current; I_{Ca-T}, the tiny, transient calcium current; and $I_{Na/Ca}$, the current generated by the action of the sodium-calcium exchanger. Outward potassium currents depicted include I_{K1}, the inward rectifier current; I_K, the delayed rectifier current; and I_{to}, the transient outward current (of which there are two components). In atrial cells there is an additional outward potassium current, I_{Kur}, that is not shown in the figure. In the sinus node, I_f represents the "funny" pacemaker current, a current carried by both sodium and potassium. $I_{K(ACh)}$ represents the receptor-activated potassium channel (activated by acetylcholine and adenosine) and $I_{K(ATP)}$ the outward potassium current activated by falling levels of intracellular adenosine triphosphate (the bracket indicates that this current is activated under pathophysiologic conditions). All these currents are discussed further in the text. Not discussed but presented here for completeness are I_{Cl} a chloride current; I_{pump}, an ion pump current; and I_{Na-B}, an inward background current thought to be present in sinus node cells. (Modified from Task Force of the Working Group on Arrhythmias of the European Society of Cardiology: Circulation *84*:1831, 1991, by permission of the American Heart Association, Inc.)

current I_{Ca-L} begins to inactivate. In some species, including the human, there are two principal components of the delayed rectifier potassium current, a fast (I_{Kr}) and a slow (I_{Ks}) component.[12] Phase 3 of the action potential represents the phase of rapid repolarization of the cell toward the resting membrane potential. Phase 3 occurs as the result of decay in the inward calcium current and the activation of (several) outward potassium currents. The ion current responsible for the terminal portion of this phase of the action potential, as well as the current responsible for maintaining the resting potential, is an outward potassium current activated at negative membrane potentials, referred to as the *inward rectifier*, or I_{K1}.[13] An additional outward potassium repolarization current called I_{Kur} ('ur' for 'ultrarapid') is identified in the human atrium. This atrial current is a rapidly activating, non-inactivating potassium current.[14]

The repolarizing outward potassium currents described are the *major* currents involved in cardiac repolarization. There are other outward potassium currents that have been described that can become important under specific conditions. For example, the ATP-dependent potassium current, $I_{K(ATP)}$, is an outward current that is small under normal conditions; however, it activates strongly under conditions of depleted intracellular stores of ATP.[15] This outward current may become important under hypoxic conditions. The receptor-activated potassium channel, $I_{K(ACh)}$, is activated by exposure to either the parasympathetic

agonist acetylcholine or to adenosine.[13] Other potassium channels that have been described include one that activates in response to elevated intracellular calcium concentrations ($I_{K(Ca)}$), and another that activates in response to increased intracellular sodium concentrations ($I_{K(Na)}$).[2]

Under normal conditions spontaneous automaticity is generally confined to the pacemaker cells of the sinus node. In these cells, microelectrode recordings reveal a slow depolarization of the membrane potential during phase 4 of the action potential, from the maximum diastolic potential (MDP) toward the activation, or threshold potential (Fig. 64–5). Atrial myocytes, atrioventricular junctional cells, and His-Purkinje cells can all exhibit spontaneous diastolic depolarization, although at significantly slower rates than the sinus node. The precise currents responsible for pacemaker activity are still not completely delineated and may vary from site to site. A decline in an outward potassium current (referred to originally as I_{K2}) was initially proposed as the major depolarizing force resulting in spontaneous automaticity. It is now believed that spontaneous automaticity may result from a combination of factors, including a decline in an outward potassium current (possibly a decline in I_K or, in AV nodal cells, I_{K1}), increases in both L- and T-type calcium currents, as well as in a transient and background Na+ current.[16,17] Another inward current, carried partly by potassium and partly by sodium and termed I_f ('f' for 'funny'), has been described and is believed to be an important pacemaker

CARDIAC ACTION POTENTIAL

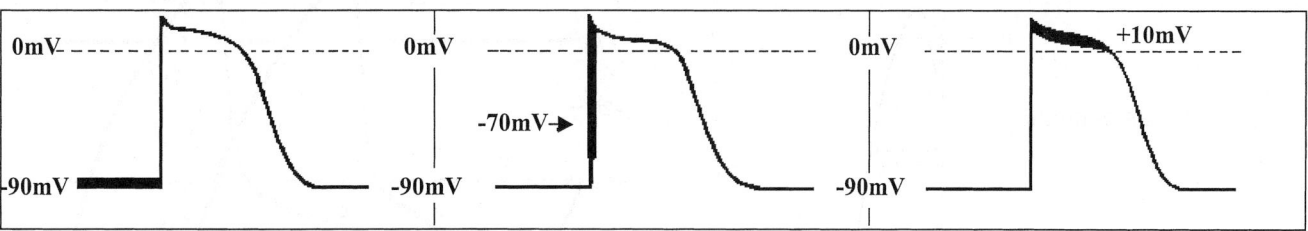

SODIUM CHANNEL

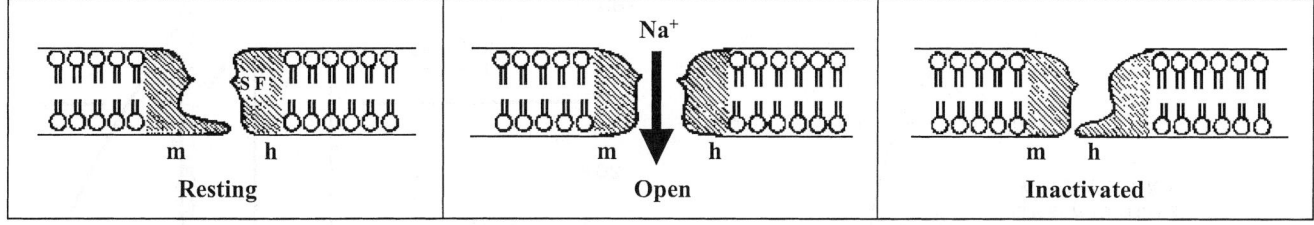

SODIUM CURRENT

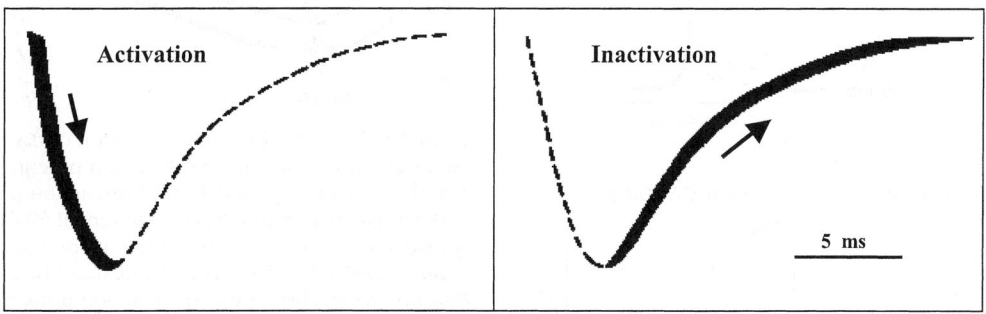

Figure 64–3. Three conformation states of the sodium channel. Illustration of the changes in transmembrane action potential (*top three diagrams*), changes in the conformational state of the sodium channel (*middle diagrams*), and corresponding activation and inactivation of the sodium current (*lower diagrams*). At rest, the membrane potential is approximately –90 mV (*left*). At this membrane potential, the sodium channel exists primarily in the rested state. The *m* gate of the sodium channel is closed. (*SF* denotes the selectivity filter of the ion channel.) As the cell membrane depolarizes (phase 0 of the action potential), the sodium channel changes to the open conformation, associated with opening of the *m* gate (*middle*). The sodium current rapidly activates because sodium ions can now pass through the ion channel. As the membrane potential becomes more positive, the sodium channel enters into its third conformational state, the inactivated state. This occurs as a result of closure of the inactivation gate *h* (*right*). The sodium current rapidly inactivates, or decays, back toward zero current.

TABLE 64-3

Comparison of Functional Characteristics of Three Different Ion Channels in Cardiac Tissue

	I_{Na}	I_{Ca-L}	I_K
Charge carrier	Sodium	Calcium	Potassium
Activation threshold (mV)	$-70--55$	$-55--30$	-20
Magnitude (mA/cm²)	0.9-1.8	0.035-0.1	0.003
Time constraint (T, msec)			
Activation	<1	<10	400-2400
Inactivation	<1	10-100	—

I_{Na} = sodium channel; I_{Ca-L} = L-type calcium channel; I_K = delayed rectifier current (the "s" or slow component); mV = millivolts; msec = milliseconds; mA/cm² = milliamperes per squared centimeter.
(Adapted from Table 22–3 in Zipes DP: Genesis of cardiac arrhythmias: seen in electrophysiological considerations. *In* Braunwald E (ed): Heart Disease. A Textbook of Cardiovascular Medicine, 4th ed. Philadelphia, WB Saunders Co. 1992: 599; Moak JP: Cardiac electrophysiology. *In* Garson A Jr, et al. (eds): The Science and Practice of Pediatric Cardiology. Philadelphia, PA, Lea & Febiger, 1990: 294–317; Isenberg G, Klockner U: Pflugers Arch *395*: 30, 1982; *and* Sanguinetti MC, Jurkiewicz NK: J Gen Physiol *96*:195, 1990.)

current in relatively hyperpolarized cells.[18] It is not clear whether I_f has a significant role in mediating pacemaker automaticity under normal conditions in the sinus node, where maximum diastolic potentials of only –50 to –60 mV are achieved.

DEVELOPMENTAL CHANGES IN ACTION POTENTIAL MORPHOLOGY AND TRANSMEMBRANE ION CURRENTS

Changes in action potential morphology and corresponding changes in ion current physiology occur throughout the course of development, beginning in early embryonic life, in both mammalian and nonmammalian species. Although important species-related differences do exist, increases in membrane resting potential, action potential amplitude, $\dot{V}_{max}$, and action potential duration are most often noted during the course of development.

Resting Membrane Potential

Increases in the resting membrane potential during development have been reported in several species. The resting membrane potential in the chick embryo doubles from –35 mV to

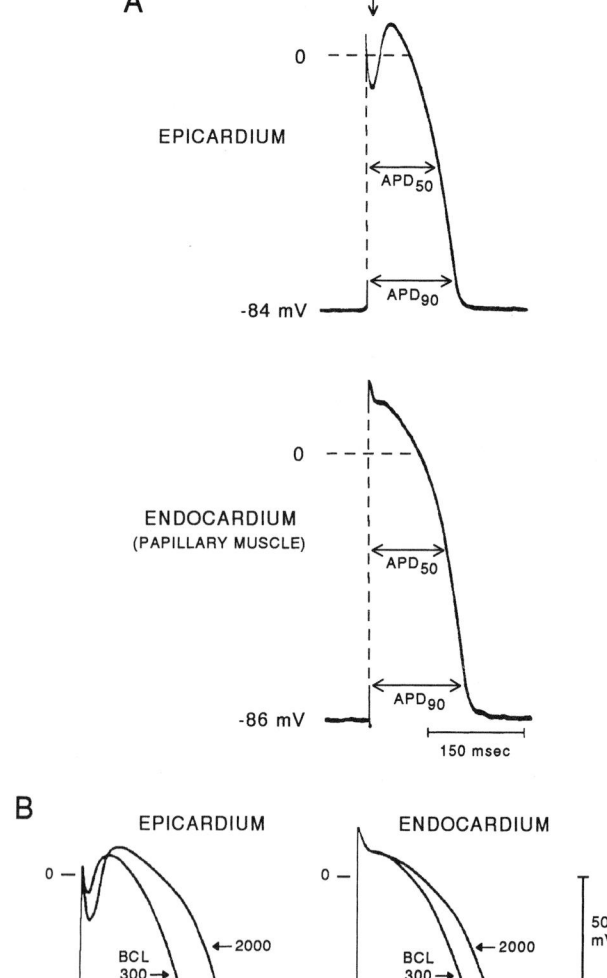

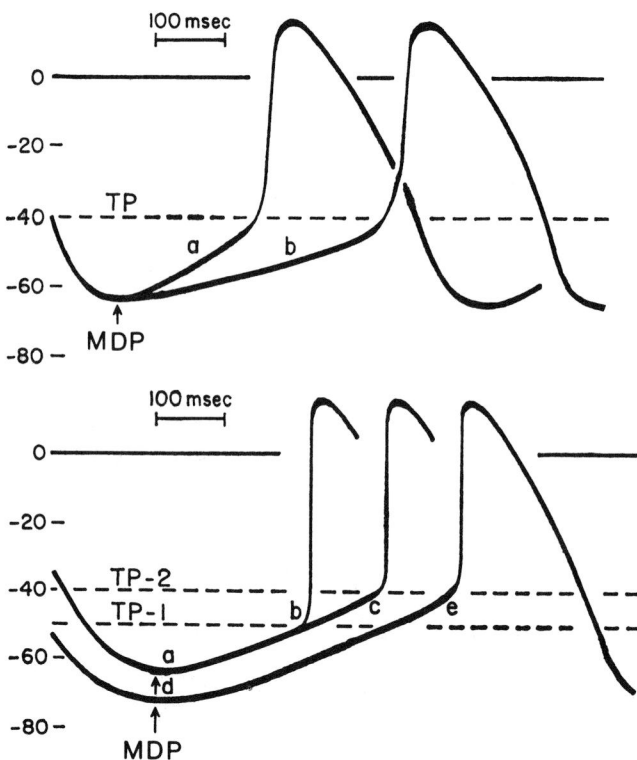

Figure 64–4. A, Representative action potentials from ventricular endocardium and epicardium. In the epicardium, there is a prominent spike and dome appearance of the action potential plateau (*arrow*). This spike and dome appearance is the result of a prominent transient outward current, carried by potassium, which is present in the epicardium and separates phases 1 and 2 of the action potential. This is much less pronounced in action potentials recorded from the endocardium. (Modified from Litovsky SH, Antzelevitch C: Circ Res *62*:116, 1988, by permission of the American Heart Association, Inc.) **B,** Demonstration of the rate-dependent behavior of the transient outward current in canine ventricular myocardium. In epicardium, decreasing basic cycle length (BCL) (i.e., increasing heart rate) from 2000 to 300 msec markedly diminishes the spike and dome appearance of the action potential plateau and causes marked shortening of action potential duration. This is due to rate-dependent reduction of the transient outward current at faster heart rates (due to incomplete recovery from inactivation). This is not seen in endocardium, where I_{to} is negligible, resulting in little or no change in action potential duration in response to increases in heart rate. (*Note:* The effects of the rate-dependent decreases in I_{to} on action potential duration are variable. In some species and preparations, action potential increases; in others, it decreases.) (From Litovsky SH, Antzelevitch C: J Am Coll Cardiol *14*:1053, 1989. Reprinted with permission from the American College of Cardiology.)

Figure 64–5. Mechanisms of modulation of cardiac pacemaker rate. *Top panel,* Two sinus node action potentials are illustrated. The threshold potential (TP) for both action potentials is –40 mV. The maximum diastolic potential (MDP) is approximately –60 mV. If the slope of spontaneous depolarization decreases (*b*), pacemaker firing rate is delayed. *Bottom panel,* Three sinus node action potentials are shown. A decrease in the threshold potential (i.e., less negative, TP-1 to TP-2) results in a delay in firing rate (*c* versus *b*). Pacemaker firing rate can also be delayed (*e* versus *c*) by an increase in the maximum diastolic potential (i.e., a more negative diastolic potential) (*a* versus *d*), with the slope of spontaneous depolarization and the threshold potential remaining constant. (From Hoffman BF, Cranefield PF: Electrophysiology of the Heart. New York, McGraw-Hill, 1960, p 109.)

approximately –70 mV from day 2 to day 18.[19] Similar increases in resting membrane potential have been reported in fetal rat, dog, and guinea pig hearts.[20-22] In rat and dog hearts, further increases in the resting membrane potential occur postnatally. There are several likely mechanisms responsible for the increasing resting membrane potential noted with development. Increases in activity of the sodium-potassium ATPase pump have been reported with maturation. In the chick heart, a threefold increase in the activity of sodium-potassium ATPase has been reported between day 6 and day 20 of incubation.[23] Similar increases in sodium-potassium ATPase have been observed in guinea pig myocardium from fetal day 45 to neonatal days 21 to 25.[24] The increase in sodium-potassium ATPase activity noted during development may in part result from expression of different isoforms of the sodium-potassium ATPase pump.[25] Increased activity of the sodium-potassium ATPase pump increases the concentration of potassium intracellularly and decreases the concentration of sodium. This results in a more strongly negative resting membrane potential, as discussed earlier in this chapter.

An increase in membrane permeability to potassium with development also contributes to the more negative resting potential observed with maturation. Specific increases in the current density of the inward rectifier current, I_{K1}, the main outward potassium current responsible for maintenance of the resting membrane potential, have been reported in the chick embryo, and in fetal and newborn rat and rabbit ventricular myocytes.[26-31] In the rat, the increase in I_{K1} may occur as a result of acquisition of a high-conductance potassium channel, one that is absent in the neonate.[31] In the human fetus, resting membrane potentials at midgestation (about 20 weeks) are similar to values reported in adult mammalian tissue.[32] In studies performed in atrial myocytes isolated from young infants (more than 2 months) undergoing heart surgery, the resting membrane potential is similar to that of the adult.[33] These studies suggest that in the human, developmental increases in resting membrane potential are not evident after midterm gestation. This does not preclude the possibility that increases in resting membrane potential might occur earlier in gestation.

Action Potential Upstroke, Phase 0

An increase in action potential phase 0 amplitude and $\dot{V}_{max}$ with maturation has been documented in several species. In the chick heart, $\dot{V}_{max}$ increases from 20 V/sec at day 2 to more than 250 V/sec at day 18.[19] In the rat, $\dot{V}_{max}$ increases 10-fold from day 10 of gestation to day 21 (term).[20] A threefold increase in $\dot{V}_{max}$ (200-550 V/sec) occurs in the canine fetus Purkinje fiber action potential, from early fetal life to near term.[21] Similar trends are noted in guinea pig atrium and ventricle.[22] These increases in action potential amplitude and $\dot{V}_{max}$ are only partly the result of the increases in the resting membrane potential already described. Developmental changes in the structure and/or function of the ion channel or channels responsible for the upstroke of the action potential appear to contribute importantly to the developmental changes noted in the rate of rise of phase 0 of the action potential in the young embryo and fetus. In the early embryonic chick heart (before day 5), phase 0 of the action potential appears to depend on an ion channel that is not sensitive to the potent sodium channel blocker tetrodotoxin. Through day 8 of incubation, as $\dot{V}_{max}$ increases, a marked increase is noted in the sensitivity of phase 0 of the action potential to tetrodotoxin.[19] This suggests that in the early embryonic phase, the current responsible for the upstroke of the action potential is an embryonic sodium channel, one with slow kinetics, and one that is insensitive to tetrodotoxin. With maturation an apparent switch occurs, with increased expression of a fast, tetrodotoxin-sensitive sodium channel. (Phase 0 of the action potential in the early chick embryonic heart is inhibited by calcium channel blockers, but sodium is still believed to be the dominant charge carrier.) An increasing sensitivity with maturation of phase 0 of the action potential to tetrodotoxin has also been reported in the fetal rat heart.[20] In the fetal mouse heart (fewer than 13 days' gestation) L-type calcium currents appear to play the dominant role in cardiac excitation, with sodium channel expression increasing only just before birth.[134] In contrast, in the canine heart, although increases in action potential amplitude and $\dot{V}_{max}$ also occur during fetal life, there appears to be no change in the apparent sensitivity of phase 0 to tetrodotoxin.[21] In summary, substantial increases in the amplitude and rate of rise of phase 0 of the action potential occur during avian embryonic and mammalian fetal life. Although increases in resting membrane potential undoubtedly contribute to this increase, developmental changes in the structure and function of cardiac ion channels, including the expression or function of accessory protein subunits, or changes in posttranslational modification of channel function, also likely contribute to the observed differences.

Phase 1 of the Action Potential

Developmental increases in the transient outward current, the outward current responsible for the spike-and-dome appearance of the action potential, have been described in several species. In rabbit ventricular cells, the current density of I_{to} in the neonate is about half that recorded in adult tissue.[29] The rate of inactivation and the rate of recovery from inactivation of I_{to} are both significantly faster (5-10×) in neonatal cells. Because I_{to} displays rate-dependent behavior (decreasing as rate increases), developmental changes are observed in the response of action potential duration to pacing. In the adult rabbit, action potential duration increases whereas in neonatal cells little change in action potential duration is observed.[29, 35] In rat ventricular myocytes, I_{to} appears to be absent in newborn myocytes and increases slightly between days 1 and 8. The most significant increases occur between 1 week of age and adulthood.[36] In canine ventricular myocytes, neither a notch nor spike-and-dome appearance in the action potential plateau is observed in epicardial myocytes until 2 months of age.[37] In human atrial cells, an absence of the typical spike-and-dome shape of the action potential has been reported in infant tissue, believed to reflect an absence of the transient outward current (Fig. 64-6A).[33] Although I_{to} has subsequently been identified in

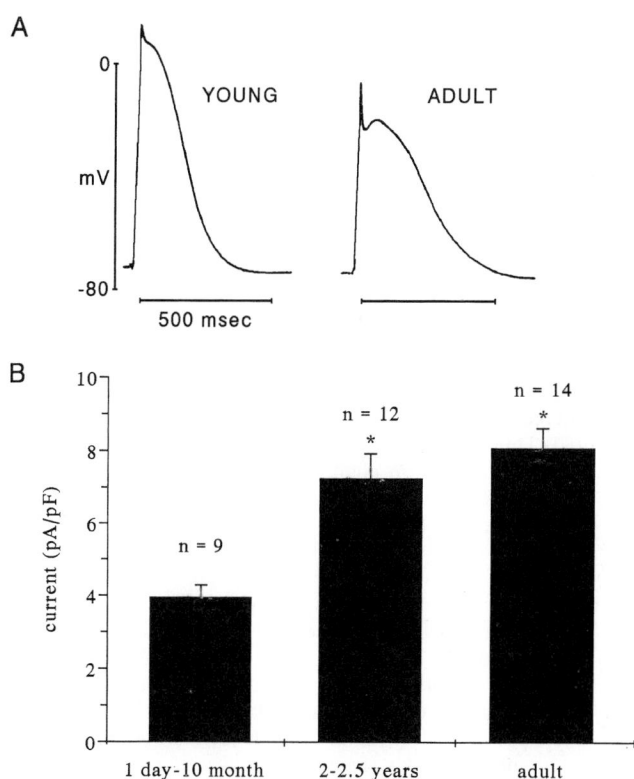

Figure 64-6. A, Comparison of human atrial action potentials. Note that in the adult atrial action potential, there is a prominent spike-and-dome appearance to the plateau phase of the action potential. This is presumed to reflect a prominent transient outward current (I_{to}) in the adult. This spike-and-dome shape of the atrial action potential is absent in the recording from a young infant. (From Escande D, et al: Am J Physiol *249*:H843, 1985.) **B,** Relationship between age and transient outward current amplitude (I_{to}) in human atrial myocytes. Note that the transient outward current amplitude (pA/pF) is significantly less (* = $p < 0.05$) in atrial cells isolated from infants less than 2 years of age. (From Crumb WJ Jr, et al: Am J Physiol *268*:H1335, 1995.)

some cells isolated from young infants undergoing heart surgery,[38, 39] a twofold increase in both the current density and in recovery kinetics has been reported with maturation (see Fig. 64-6B).[39] Thus, there appear to be consistent age-related increases in I_{to}, the transient outward current. The functional significance of this increase in the transient outward current is not fully understood, nor are the mechanisms that lead to the increased expression of the transient outward current in postnatal life, though augmentation in I_{to} may be linked to postnatal increases in oxygen tension.[40]

The Action Potential Plateau and Repolarization, Phases 2 and 3

The slow inward calcium current (I_{Ca-L}) contributes importantly to the sustained depolarization that constitutes the action potential plateau. In the chick heart, nitrendipine (a calcium channel blocker) binding sites increase in number, beginning from day 3 of incubation, but channel affinity appears to be similar throughout development.[41] In day 11 chick embryos, calcium channels detected by nitrendipine binding studies are 100-fold more numerous than calcium channels determined by voltage-clamp studies.[42] These so-called silent calcium channels (present in ligand binding studies, absent from electrophysiologic studies) appear to become electrically active with further development. Kinetic changes in the behavior of the calcium channel have also been described in the chick heart with maturation. In voltage-clamp studies of very young (i.e., 3-day-old) chick embryos, the L-type calcium channel exhibits two distinct modes of firing, a bursting, transient mode and a long-lasting mode. With maturation, a significant decrease occurs in the long-lasting firing mode, and there is an increase in the bursting mode.[43] This *loss* of the long-lasting firing mode may contribute to the decrease in calcium current density that has been observed during chick embryonic development, despite an increasing number of calcium channels.[43, 44] In mammalian hearts, increases in nitrendipine binding sites have been described in fetal rat and mouse hearts.[45, 46] In the fetal rat heart (18 days), novel non-L, non-T-type calcium channels have been described.[47] These novel channels inactivate faster than the typical L-type calcium channel, and they have a different steady-state inactivation curve (percentage of channels inactivated as a function of membrane potential). Thus, as in the chick heart, there appears to be a functionally different calcium channel present in the rat fetus, one that is less expressed with further development. Calcium current density in the rat heart is fivefold larger in cells isolated from neonates compared with those from adults.[48] In addition to the inward calcium current, an inward sodium current (the window current) appears to play a relatively greater role in maintaining the action potential plateau in the fetal rat myocyte.[49]

In contrast to the developing chick and rat heart, in which calcium current densities tend to decrease with maturation, in the rabbit progressive increases in myocardial calcium current density have been described from fetal to adult life.[27] In addition to an increase in current density, significant changes in calcium channel kinetics also occur during development in the rabbit.[50] Inactivation of the calcium current occurs at less-negative membrane potentials in fetal myocytes compared to adult myocytes. In addition, recovery from inactivation occurs over a longer time course in immature cells. Because of the more prolonged time course of recovery from inactivation in immature cells, the calcium current becomes inhibited to a greater extent at faster stimulation frequencies in the fetus and newborn. This inhibition of the calcium current at faster heart rates may place the immature heart at a potential disadvantage for excitation-contraction coupling (a process that is dependent on transsarcolemmal calcium transport).[51] Finally, it has been reported that calcium current density is equivalent in atrial myocytes of newborn and adult humans.[52]

Concerning repolarization, it is the gradual activation of outward potassium currents during phases 2 and 3 that initiates and then drives the repolarization process. Marked developmental changes have been reported in the densities and distribution of the various K^+ repolarization currents over the course of development (Table 64-4).[11, 53] In the rat, rabbit, and mouse, significant increases in I_K have been described from the fetal to neonatal period. In the rabbit, current density of I_K doubles postnatally through adulthood.[29] Interestingly, functional expression of I_{Kr} and I_{Ks}, the two main components of I_K, are only detectable in fetal or neonatal mouse hearts, and not in those of the adult.[54] I_{Kur}, the ultrarapid component of the delayed rectifier I_K, which is detected only in the atrium of the adult dog, rat, and human heart, is also detected in neonatal rat ventricular myocytes.[55] Finally, an outward repolarization current unique to the newborn heart has been described in canine epicardial ventricular myocytes.[37] In neonatal myocytes, but not adult myocytes, an outward current is present (probably a potassium current) that rapidly activates with depolarization and shows little decay as a function of time, features qualitatively similar to I_{Kur} (Fig. 64-7).

In summary, substantial changes have been described with maturation in action potential morphology and in the kinetics and densities of the individual ion currents that constitute the action potential. Allowing for some significant species-related and tissue site differences, increases in (1) the resting membrane potential; (2) the major inward cationic currents responsible for the upstroke of the action potential; (3) the plateau currents; and (4) many outward repolarization currents have been observed from early embryonic or fetal life. These maturational changes undoubtedly contribute to some important functional differences in impulse formation, conduction, and myocardial refractoriness that have been noted with development.

IMPULSE FORMATION AND INTRA-ATRIAL AND ATRIOVENTRICULAR CONDUCTION IN THE EMBRYO, FETUS, AND NEONATE: MORPHOLOGIC AND PHYSIOLOGIC CONSIDERATIONS

In the chick embryo, spontaneous cardiac electrical depolarizations can be detected by voltage-sensitive dyes at about the seventh somite stage, well before contractions become evident.[56] These studies, as well as direct microelectrode recordings,[57] have demonstrated that, although contraction is first noted in the primitive ventricle of the chick embryo (somite stage 10), pacemaker activity evolves simultaneously in both

TABLE 64-4

Developmental Variations in Voltage-Gated K^+ Currents in Mammalian Ventricular Myocytes

Current	Fetal	Neonatal	Adult	Species
I_{to}	ND	−	++++	Dog
		+	++++	Human
	+	+++	++++	Mouse
	ND	++	+++	Rabbit*
	+	++	++++	Rat
I_{Kr}	++	++	−	Mouse
	ND	+	+	Rat
I_{Ks}	−	++	−	Mouse
	ND	−	−	Rat
I_K	+	++	++	Mouse
	+	++	++	Rat
I_{Kur}	ND	+	−	Rat

* Properties of rabbit I_{to} also change with age (Sánchez-Chapula et al., 1994).
+ = detectable; ++ = moderate density; ++++ = high density; − = not detected; ND = not determined.
(From Nerbonne JM: J Neurobiol 37:37, 1998.)

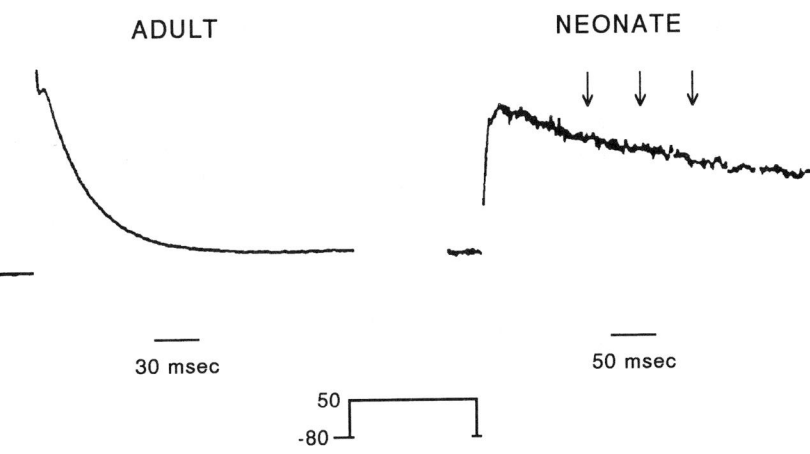

Figure 64–7. Comparison of outward currents recorded from ventricular myocytes isolated from adult and neonatal dogs. On the left, the transient outward current (I_{to}) is elicited in the adult myocyte in response to changing membrane voltage from −80 mV to +50 mV. The transient outward current is not recorded in neonatal cells. In the neonate, a unique outward current is elicited that rapidly activates and shows little decay over time. This current is not observed in adult myocytes. (Modified from Jeck CD, Boyden PA: Circ Res *71*:1390, 1992, by permission of the American Heart Association, Inc.)

atrial and ventricular sites. With subsequent development, pacemaker activity becomes confined to atrial sites. There is little information concerning the specific ion currents responsible for cardiac automaticity during development. It has been suggested that the so-called funny inward pacemaker current, I_f, which normally activates at hyperpolarized membrane potentials, may contribute importantly to cardiac automaticity in very early embryonic life.[58] I_f is prominent in ventricular cells of 3-day-old chick embryos and is virtually absent from cells isolated from 17-day-old embryos. In the newborn rabbit, sinus node automaticity can be shown to be due in part to a small, slowly inactivating, tetrodotoxin sensitive inward sodium current. This current completely disappears shortly after birth.[59, 60] Postnatal differences in sinus node L-type (but not T-type) calcium current density and kinetics have also been identified.[61]

The genetic and environmental factors that contribute to pacemaker formation are largely unknown. It is known that cardiac mesenchymal tissues that are destined to form specific regions of the embryonic heart beat at predetermined, characteristic rates.[62] Tissue explanted from regions destined to form the sinoatrial region beats at a faster intrinsic rate than tissue destined to form the primitive ventricle.[63] Genetically determined differences in ion channel populations and kinetics of ion channel function are believed to be important in determining these programmed beating rates. That environmental cues can also modulate pacemaker development and function is demonstrable, in that transplanting mesenchymal tissue from "fast" sinoatrial regions into "slow" regions results in a gradual decrease in the rate of spontaneous firing of the transplanted tissue.[64] Physical contact between myocardial cells and nonmyocardial elements also may contribute to the induction of pacemaker cell aggregates.[65] *In vivo*, looping of the heart may bring the sinoatrial region of the heart into close contact with nonmyocardial mesenchyme and thereby induce formation of the sinoatrial pacemaker. In the human embryo, a sinus node is first identified shortly after the looping process is completed. The sinus node is an epicardial structure; it is positioned at the junction of the superior vena cava and the right atrium. It is relatively larger in the fetus than in the adult and is horseshoe shaped rather than having the spindle shape observed in the adult.[66]

Conduction of the Impulse from Sinus Node to Atrioventricular Node

The existence of specialized "internodal" conduction pathways within the right atrium, linking the sinus and AV nodes, has been proposed.[67] These putative specialized conduction pathways are located laterally, along the terminal crest of the right atrium, and medially, along the posterior and anterior rims of the fossa ovalis.

Although such internodal pathways have been demonstrated histologically and by immunochemistry (including in the developing heart,[68, 69]) a lack of true specialized cell types and lack of insulation from surrounding myocardium have been cited by some researchers as evidence against true specialized internodal conduction pathways.[70] Published studies of HNK-1 (Leu-7) antigen expression patterns in the embryonic rat heart provide evidence that connections between the sinus and AV nodes do exist, that they are derived from the embryonic sinoatrial junction, and will, by necessity, join the sinus and AV nodes in anatomic proximity to the putative special internodal tracks.[71] Electrophysiologic studies of intra-atrial conduction have also yielded conflicting results. In the dog and rabbit atrium, Spach and colleagues[72] were unable to find electrophysiologic evidence of specialized internodal conduction pathways. More recent studies in the canine atrium, however, have identified three bundles of myocardium that appear to serve as specialized inputs to the canine AV node. These myocardial fibers are electrically active even when atrial contractility is abolished by exposure to high levels of extracellular potassium, and they fire at the same rate as the sinus node.[73]

Whether or not true specialized internodal pathways exist, intra-atrial conduction tends to propagate as waves of excitation within the atrium along directions that roughly follow the anatomic courses of the putative internodal pathways. This preferential conduction, along the terminal crest and the anterior and posterior interatrial septum, may be the result of a more uniform, longitudinal alignment of atrial myocytes in these anatomic locations, rather than being the result of specialized conduction pathways.[74]

Electrophysiologic differences in atrial action potential morphology and intra-atrial conduction have been described during the course of development. In the adult dog, atrial action potential durations tend to decrease as recordings are made at sites more distal to the sinus node. Action potential durations in the newborn, in contrast, tend to be much more uniform throughout the atrium.[75] Atrial action potential durations also tend to be significantly shorter in the newborn rat, dog, and human compared to the adult (Fig. 64-8A).[33, 75, 76] Shorter action potential durations result in shorter refractory periods in the neonatal atrium compared with in the adult, which may facilitate the development of intra-atrial reentry (see Fig. 64-8B).[77, 78] It is possible that the occurrence of "benign" atrial flutter, observed at times in the fetus and newborn with an otherwise structurally normal heart, results in part from these shorter atrial refractory periods.[77, 79] Finally, in addition to developmental changes in the electrophysiology of the developing atrial myocyte, growth of nonmyocardial elements within the atrium is believed to contribute to developmental differences noted in propagation

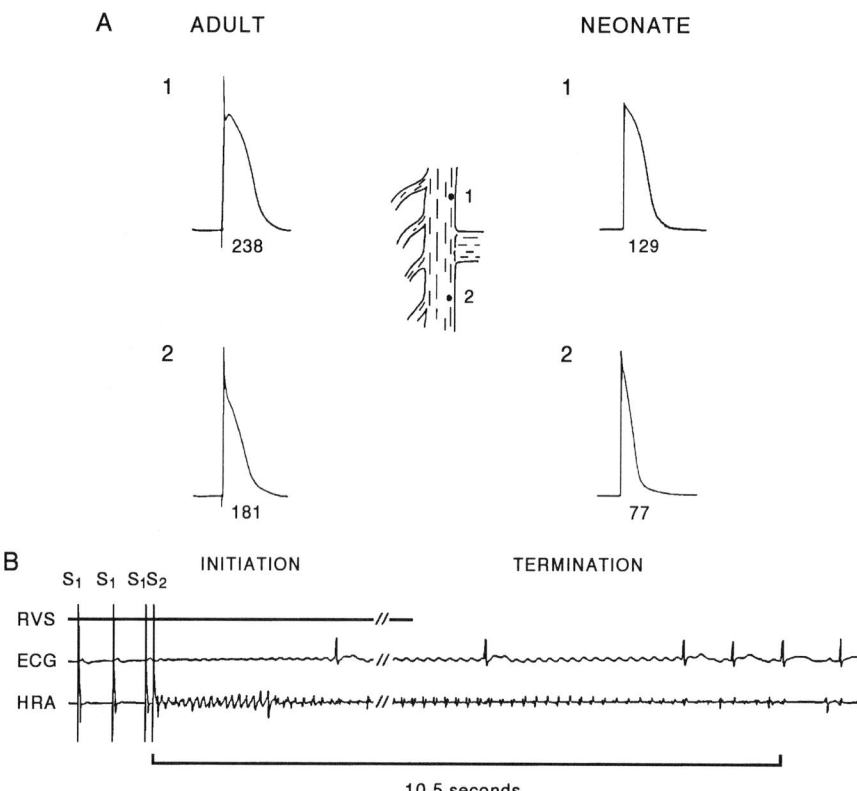

Figure 64–8. A, Atrial action potentials recorded from roughly similar locations along the terminal crest in adult and newborn dogs. Note that neonatal action potentials are characterized by little or no action potential plateau and shorter action potential durations (indicated beneath each action potential, in milliseconds) when compared to the adult. (Modified from Spach MS, et al: Circ Res 65:1594, 1989, by permission of the American Heart Association, Inc.) **B,** The effect of premature atrial simulation during vagal stimulation in the newborn dog. RVS indicates the period of stimulation of the right vagus nerve. S_1 refers to a basic paced drive train; S_2 refers to a single premature atrial paced beat. Surface ECG lead II and intracardiac recordings of atrial activity from the right atrium (HRA) are shown. Note that with the introduction of the premature beat (S_2), a long train of atrial fibrillation-flutter is induced. (Similar but shorter runs of atrial fibrillation-flutter are induced in the atrium of the newborn in the absence of vagal stimulation.) (Modified from Pickoff AS, Stolfi A: Am J Physiol 258:H38, 1990.)

patterns within the atrium. For example, in the neonatal heart, impulses conduct directly from the superior rim of the terminal crest to the adjacent atrial myocardium, whereas in the adult, atrial conduction proceeds inferiorly first, before activation of the myocardium adjacent to the superior terminal crest.[75]

Atrioventricular Conduction Before the Formation of the Specialized Atrioventricular Conduction System

Delay between contraction of the chick atrium and contraction of the ventricle is first noted 50 hours after conception (20th somite stage).[80,81] This emulation of AV nodal function occurs before the development of the AV conduction system. Microcellular recordings from the AV canal region at this stage of development demonstrate the presence of slow response-type action potentials. The slow rate of rise of the action potential upstroke functionally corresponds to this zone of slow conduction. It is likely that AV canal cells are the mediators of atrioventricular delay in the early chick embryo.[82] These cells, however, can be shown *not* to contribute to the formation of the definitive AV node in later development.[83] Similar findings have been reported in mammalian hearts. In the prelooped, preinnervated rat heart, AV delay also appears to originate in cell populations corresponding to the endocardial cushions or AV canal.[84] Although the endocardial cushions stain positive for acetylcholinesterase in these preinnervated hearts (and adjacent myocardium lacks this cholinergic enzyme),[85] it is not clear that this intrinsic cholinergic system contributes to the observed AV delay. Finally, in the rat embryo, simulation of His-Purkinje system function is also observed before formation of the true AV conduction system. Shortly after looping, a synchronization of ventricular wall motion is observed, coupled with a 10-fold increase in conduction velocity.[84] These changes are highly correlated with expression of the major gap junction protein, connexin43.[86] Gap junctions are the specialized protein channels that connect adjacent myocytes (Fig. 64-9A–C).[87] These channels allow not only the passage of electrical current through

a low-resistance pathway from cell to cell, but also the exchange of larger molecules between cells. The expression of different isoforms of the connexin proteins form gap junctions with different functional characteristics. Expression of connexin isoforms is highly regulated throughout cardiac development.[88] In the mouse heart, connexin40 is diffusely up-regulated through embryonic day 14, at which time its expression becomes largely confined to the atrium, whereas connexin43 becomes the dominant isoform expressed in the ventricular myocardium.[86, 89] Expression of a third isoform, connexin45, is largely confined to the specialized cardiac conduction system (see Fig. 64-9D). The critical role of connexins for normal cardiac conduction, as well as normal cardiac development, is demonstrated by reports of abnormal, sometimes lethal, intracardiac cardiac conduction abnormalities, and of abnormal anatomic development, in hearts of mice with absent or diminished expression of specific connexins.[90,91]

Formation of the Specialized Atrioventricular Conduction System

The true specialized AV conduction system, including the AV node, bundle of His, and right and left bundle branches, forms after the looping process is completed. Multiple immunohistochemical markers have been employed to delineate and track the development of the specialized conduction system, including in the human heart (Table 64-5). Although many of these molecular markers are also markers of neural tissue (e.g., ganglion nodosum [GLN], HNK-1), the conduction system is not derived from neural (i.e., ectodermal) precursors. Rather, the conduction system is derived from multipotential mesenchymal precursors. Recruitment of mesenchymal tissue into the specialized cardiac conduction system may involve induction by paracrine cues, originating from nearby developing coronary vasculature.[92] With differentiation, the specialized conduction system expresses a molecular pattern that is distinct from the surrounding atrial or ventricular myocardium.[93-95]

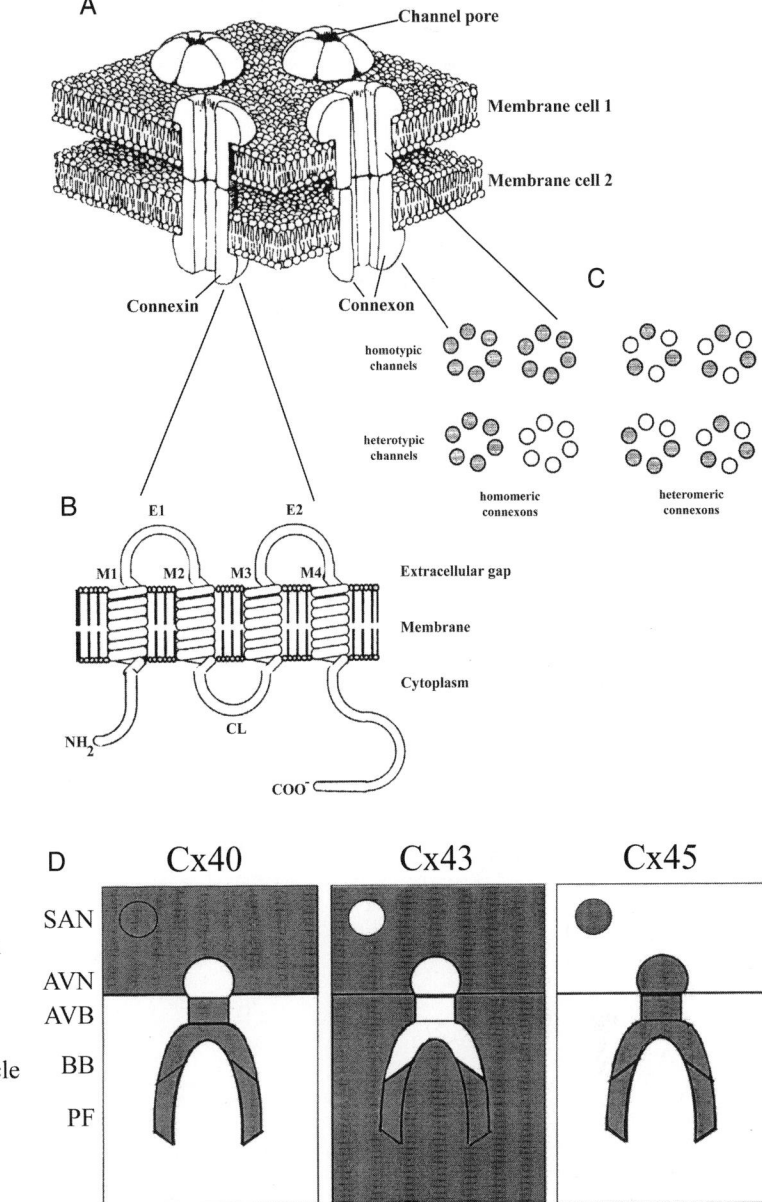

Figure 64–9. Ultrastructure of cardiac gap junctions. Gap junctions occur as "plaques" of multiple intercellular channels. **A,** Portion of a gap junction plaque demonstrating the structure of the intercellular channels, which join cell membranes from two adjacent cardiac myocytes (membrane cell 1, membrane cell 2). Each cell membrane contributes half of the channel structure, called a connexon. Each connexon consists of 6 connexin proteins. **B,** Secondary structure of a single connexin protein. **C,** Connexons formed from identical sets of connexins are termed homomeric connexons. Those formed from dissimilar connexin isoforms are termed hetero-meric connexons. These then combine to form either homotypic or heterotypic intercellular channels. **D,** Expression of the major connexin isoforms, Cx40, Cx43, and Cx45, in the mammalian myocardium and specialized conduction system. SAN = sinoatrial node; AVN = atrio-ventricular node; AVB = His-bundle; BB = bundle branches; PF = Purkinje fibers. (From van Veen TA, et al: Cardiovasc Res *51*:217, 2001, with permission.)

In the human, recent immunohistochemical studies have demonstrated that the entire AV conduction system forms from a single ring of specialized tissue. This ring of tissue can be identified by its binding of a specific monoclonal antibody raised against chicken GLN antigen (Fig. 64-10*A*). The region can be tracked throughout the development of the AV conduction system.[96] In the human embryo (Carnegie stage 14), the original GLN ring surrounds the interventricular foramen, which connects the primitive left and right ventricles (see Fig. 64-10*B*). At this early stage of development, just after looping of the heart has occurred, the atrium is connected only with the left ventricle. With further development (Carnegie stages 15-17) rightward expansion of the GLN ring is observed, as the atrium expands rightward to form the tricuspid orifice (see Fig. 64-10*C*). Thus, the GLN ring always outlines the pathways of blood that flow into the primitive right ventricle. As development of the interventricular septum proceeds (Carnegie stages 18-23), the lower rim of the original GLN ring is raised superiorly. Following contact

between the rising interventricular septum and the lesser curve of the looped heart, the AV node and proximal bundle of His are formed at the medial posterior aspect of the rightward expansion of the GLN ring, with the bundle of His in continuity with the right and left bundle branches (see Fig. 64-10*D*).

In the normal heart, the AV node is positioned anatomically within the triangle of Koch. This triangle is formed by the septal leaflet of the tricuspid valve and the tendon of Todoro, forming two arms of the triangle, and the coronary sinus orifice, defining the base of the triangle. The AV node is positioned at the apex of the triangle. Histologically, the node consists of a loose or transitional zone and a compact region.[97] In hearts from some neonates, extensions from the compact zone of the AV node have been observed and in the past have been considered by some as possible substrates of electrical instability and a possible cause of sudden death.[98] These extensions are now believed to more likely represent normal variants.[99] From the compact node, the AV bundle arises, piercing the central fibrous body of the heart and branching

Expression of Selected Genetic Markers in the Conduction System of the Human Heart

	Sinoatrial Node	Atrioventricular Node	His Bundle	Bundle Branches
Connexin 40/42	−/+*	−/−	−/+	−/−
Connexin 43	−/−	−/−	−/+	−/+
Co-expression of α and β myosin isoforms	+/+	+/+	+/+	+/+
Nodal myosin	?/?	?/?	?/?	?/?
Troponin I	?/?	?/?	?/?	?/?
Desmin	?/?	?/?	?/?	?/?
Leu-7/HNK-1	+/−	+/−	+/−	+/−
GIN2 (GLN)	?/−	+/−	+/−	+/−
Polysialytic NCAM	?/?	?/?	?/?	?/?
Slow tonic MHC	−/−	−/−	−/−	−/−
ANF	?/?	?/?	+/+	+/+
Creatine kinase M	−/?	−/?	+/?	+/?

* Fetal Heart/Adult Heart: +, expressed; −, not expressed; ?, not known.
Connexin 40/42, 43, gap junction proteins; myosin, nodal myosin, troponin I, contractile proteins; desmin, cytoskeletal protein (major component of intermediate filaments of Purkinje fibers); Leu-7/HNK-1, antibody markers for the chick neural crest that also delineate the developing conduction system (neural crest cells do not contribute to the formation of the conduction system); GIN2 (GLN), antibody raised against chick ganglion nodosum that delineates the developing conduction system; polysialytic NCAM, polysialyted form of neural cell adhesion molecule, which may play a role in "insulation" of the conduction system; slow tonic MHC, slow tonic myosin heavy chain; ANF, atrial natriuretic factor; creatine kinase M, muscle isoform of creatine kinase.
(From Pickoff AS. Development and function of the cardiac conduction System. *In* Allen HD, et al (eds): Moss and Adams' Heart Disease in Infants, Children, and Adolescents: Including the Fetus and Young Adult, 6th ed. Philadelphia, Lippincott Williams & Wilkins, 2001, p 419.)

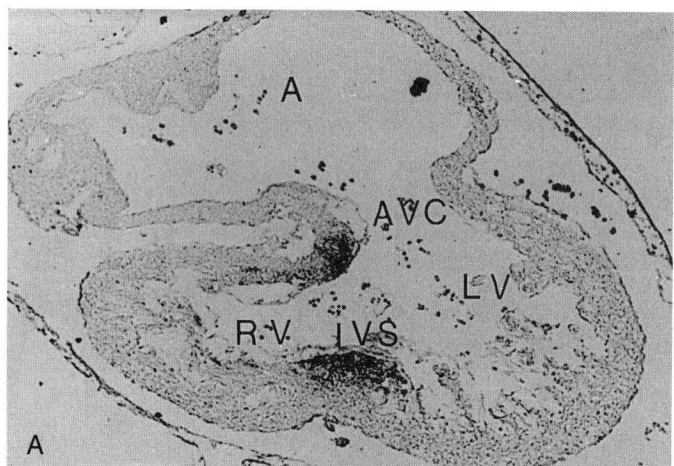

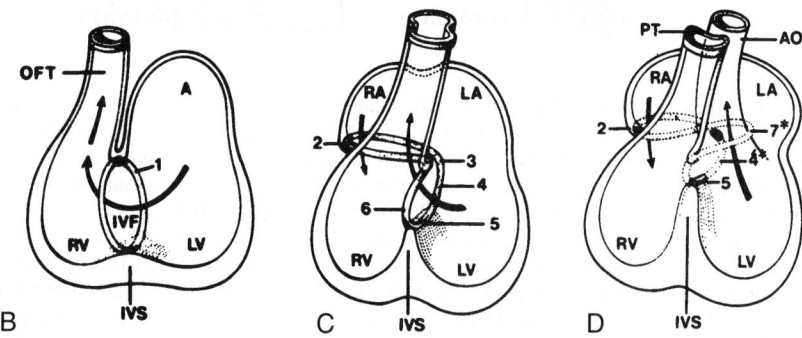

Figure 64–10. A, Immunohistochemical staining of the embryonic precursor of the atrioventricular (AV) conduction system in the human heart (Carnegie stage 14). A single ring of tissue, stained for the ganglion nodosum (GLN) antigen, is seen surrounding the interventricular foramen. It is from this single ring of tissue that the entire AV conduction system forms. This includes the AV node, His bundle, and right and left bundle branches. AVC = atrioventricular canal. **B** through **D,** Formation of the AV conduction system. **B,** The single GLN ring surrounds the interventricular foramen (IVF) in the looped heart (Carnegie stage 14). At this stage of development, the primitive atrium connects solely with the left ventricle (LV). **C,** At Carnegie stages 15–17, there is rightward expansion of the GLN ring, as the right atrium (RA) and tricuspid orifice form over the right ventricle (RV). Note the interventricular septum (IVS) rising from the floor of the ventricles. The AV node forms at position 3, the His bundle at position 4, and the bundle branches at position 5. **D,** At Carnegie stages 18–23, there is further development of the IVS. Involution of much of the original GLN ring now occurs, leaving the newly formed AV conduction system. (From Wessels A, et al: Anat Rec *232*:97, 1992, by permission of Wiley-Liss, Inc., a subsidiary of John Wiley & Sons, Inc.)

into the right and left bundle branches. The left bundle branch is located in a subendocardial position and spreads in a fanlike fashion over the left ventricular septal surface. The right bundle branch runs an intramyocardial course within the right septal surface, is more cordlike, and emerges onto the endocardial surface of the right ventricle beneath the medial papillary muscle, descending to the apex of the right ventricle along the moderator band.

Physiology of Atrioventricular Conduction

Earlier studies of AV conduction in the developing mammal suggested that the AV node and specialized conduction system of the younger animal offered little or no protection for the ventricles against rapid atrial rates. In young goats, pigs, and puppies, it was reported that the refractory period of the AV conduction system (which determines how closely two impulses can be conducted) was shorter than the refractory period of the ventricle. Thus, rapid atrial rates were reported to conduct down the specialized conduction system to the ventricles causing ventricular fibrillation in young goats and pigs.[100,101] In newborn calves, little or no increase in AV nodal conduction time was noted during closely coupled electrical stimulation of the atrium.[102] Collectively, these studies suggested that the neonatal AV node was ineffective as a filter.

More recent studies have challenged these conclusions. In the intact, anesthetized newborn dog, intracardiac electrographic recordings have demonstrated that, when corrected for inherent differences in heart rate, the neonatal AV node does in fact act as an effective filter.[103] The refractory period of the AV node in the neonate was found to be significantly longer than the ventricular refractory period and the AV node served as the primary site of conduction slowing in both neonates and adult animals. Microelectrode recordings within the neonatal and adult rabbit AV node have also demonstrated little developmental difference in the electrophysiologic characteristics of the AV node.[104] Normal AV conduction delay has been demonstrated in fetal sheep and in human fetuses of more than 20 weeks' gestation.[105, 106] In the human, there are few differences in the AV nodal conduction times

of young infants and adults.[107] Thus, the neonatal AV node may act as more of an effective filter than was suggested by earlier studies.

In the dog, the electrophysiology of the specialized conduction system has been studied from the time of implantation to birth.[21] Conduction velocities increase during the course of development. This increase in conduction velocity is due in part to maturational changes in Purkinje fiber action potential characteristics (increases in resting membrane potential and increases in amplitude and $\dot{V}_{max}$). Changes in the architecture of the developing Purkinje fiber, however, likely contribute to the increase in conduction velocity as well. Increases in Purkinje fiber diameter and cell-to-cell contacts have been described in the developing canine conduction system.[108] In addition to an increase in cell size, gap junctions "redistribute" with maturation. In newborn ventricular myocytes, gap junctions are located over the entire cell surface (ends and sides), where in the adult an end-to-end arrangement is observed (Fig. 64–11). Both the increase in cell size and the redistribution of gap junctions contribute to the significant increase in $\dot{V}_{max}$ observed in conduction along the transverse (but not longitudinal) direction in the adult heart.[109]

Maturational changes in His-Purkinje conduction characteristics other than conduction velocity have also been described in the canine conduction system. In the newborn dog, the initial

A. Myocytes

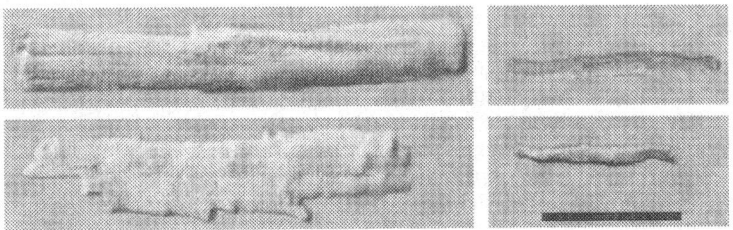

B. Adult model

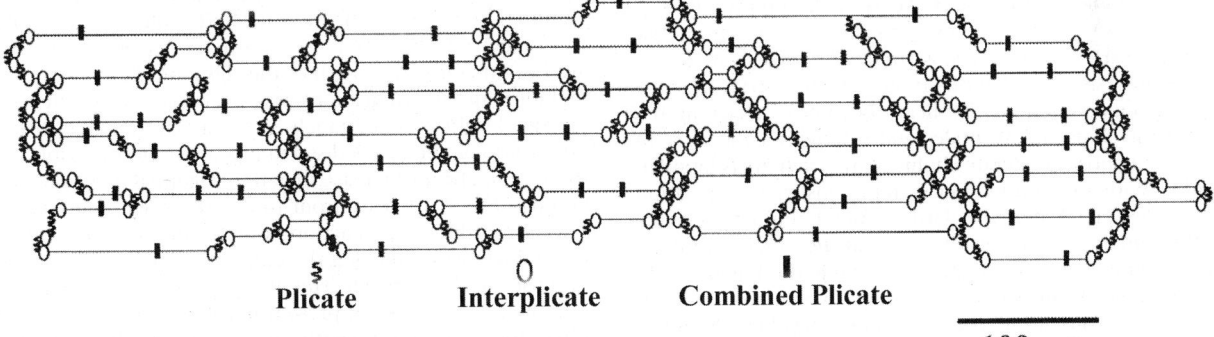

C. Neonatal model

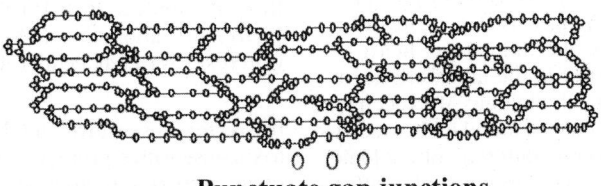

Punctuate gap junctions

Figure 64–11. Ventricular myocyte dimensions and gap junction distributions in the adult and newborn dog. **A,** Relative size of adult compared with newborn ventricular myocytes. Adult myocytes are significantly larger than newborn myocytes. (Bar measurement = 50 µm). **B,** Two-dimensional multicellular model of adult ventricular myocytes. Three different gap junction morphologies are illustrated (plicate, interplicate, and combined plicate). Note that the location of most gap junctions in the adult (all of the plicate and interplicate types) are confined to the ends of the ventricular myocytes. **C,** Two-dimensional multicellular model of neonatal ventricular myocytes. A diffuse end and side distribution of gap junctions is illustrated. (From Spach MS, et al: Circ Res *86*:302, 2000, by permission of the American Heart Association.)

site of activation of the ventricles appears to be a right ventricular site rather than the left aspect of the interventricular septum, as in the adult.[110] Retrograde conduction, the ability to conduct an impulse from the ventricle to the atrium, appears more common in the neonatal heart.[111] Finally, action potential durations along the His-Purkinje system are more uniform in the neonate than in the adult in whom there is an abrupt increase distally in the action potential duration of the Purkinje fiber, at the level of the distal false tendon.[112] This abrupt increase in action potential duration at the site of insertion of the Purkinje fiber into the ventricular muscle has been interpreted as functioning as a "physiologic gate," serving as a protector against closely coupled, rapid impulses.[112, 113] This physiologic gate appears to be absent in the neonatal heart, rendering the neonatal ventricle *potentially* susceptible to the rapid conduction of supraventricular impulses (Fig. 64–12).

Autonomic Innervation-Modulation of Cardiac Automaticity and Conduction

In considering developmental cardiac electrophysiology, it is also necessary to consider maturation of the autonomic nervous system and its effect on the electrophysiologic properties of the heart. Changes in autonomic tone profoundly affect pacemaker impulse generation, as well as AV conduction and myocardial refractoriness.

The Parasympathetic Nervous System

In the chick heart, evidence of cholinergic innervation, assessed by the histochemical detection of choline acetyltransferase (CAT) (the enzyme responsible for the synthesis of acetylcholine), is first noted about 3 days after fertilization. Progressive increases in CAT, and in the uptake of the parasympathetic neurotransmitter precursor choline, occur with further development. Choline uptake peaks at approximately 10 days after fertilization, just before the onset of ganglionic transmission.[114] In the mammalian heart, muscarinic receptors are present before actual innervation of the heart. Acetylcholinesterase is also demonstrable before innervation in the developing rat, rabbit, and human heart.[115] Progressive age-related increases in acetylcholine synthesis are demonstrable in the atria of rats. Cholinergic innervation of the heart becomes denser in the regions of the sinus and AV nodes and throughout the atria. In the human newborn, moderate cholinesterase activity is found in association with the conduction system, mostly in association with the sinus and AV nodes.[116] Little or no cholinesterase staining of the bundle branches is observed in the newborn infant. Postnatal maturation of innervation to include the remainder of the conduction system occurs, reaching a maximum density in childhood.[117, 118] Muscarinic receptor density has been found to be significantly higher in the myocardium of fetal rat and sheep hearts compared with in the adult. The production of phosphoinositol (a secondary muscarinic messenger) is also greater after muscarinic receptor activation in the immature heart.[119] Muscarinic receptor subtypes may differ in the immature heart. In addition to the dominant cardiac cholinergic M2 receptor found in the adult heart, M1 subtypes may be found in the neonatal heart. These receptors may subserve different physiologic responses to acetylcholine stimulation. The presence of a different subpopulation of muscarinic receptors in the neonate may explain the paradoxical increase in automaticity observed in neonatal ventricular cells in response to low concentrations of acetylcholine, a response not seen in adult cells.[120]

The primary actions of acetylcholine on cardiac ion channels include an increase in outward potassium currents ($I_{K(ACh)}$ and I_{K1}) and an inhibition of the inward calcium current, I_{Ca-L}.[120–123] These primary effects are mediated through a membrane-bound, per-

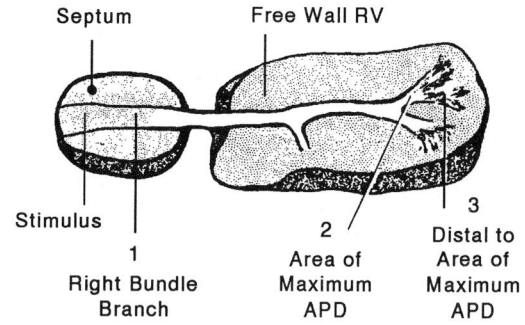

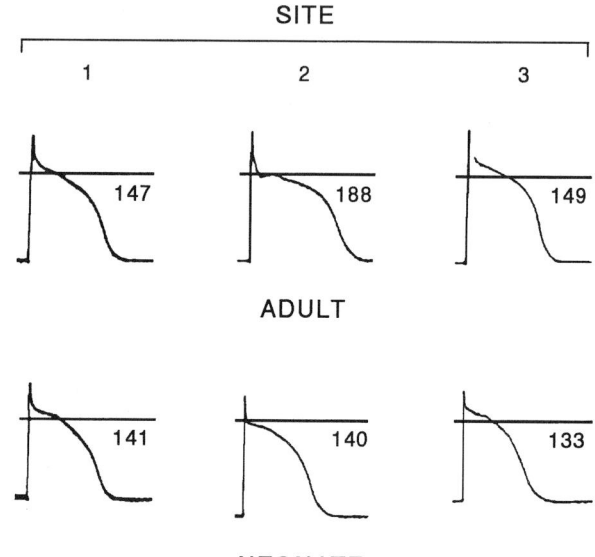

Figure 64–12. Physiology of the specialized ventricular conduction system in the neonatal and adult dog. Intracellular microelectrode recordings of transmembrane action potentials are shown along the length of the right bundle branch, including distal ramifications. Site 1 corresponds to the proximal right bundle branch, Site 2 just proximal to distal ramifications, and Site 3 distal ramifications. In the adult dog, there is an abrupt increase in action potential duration (APD) noted at Site 2 (increase from 147 to 188 msec, Site 1 to Site 2). This abrupt increase in action potential duration functions as a physiologic gate, blocking the conduction of closely coupled impulses to the ventricle. This abrupt increase in action potential duration is not present in the neonate. Therefore, the physiologic gate is inoperative in the neonate. (Diagram of right bundle branch and right ventricle free wall is from Myerburg RJ, et al: Circ Res *26*:361, 1970, by permission of the American Heart Association, Inc. Action potentials are modified from Untereker WJ, et al: Pediatr Res *18*:53, 1984.)

tussis toxin–sensitive, inhibitory G_i protein and a pertussis toxin–insensitive protein, G_q (Fig. 64–13*A*). In sinus and AV nodal tissue, increases in outward potassium currents result in hyperpolarization of the cell. This increase in membrane potential, coupled with muscarinic inhibition of the inward calcium current, accounts for the slowing of the cardiac pacemaker rate that is characteristic of muscarinic stimulation. It has also been shown that acetylcholine inhibits I_f, the funny pacemaker current, which also contributes to cardiac pacemaker slowing by acetylcholine.[124] Increases in outward potassium currents account for the marked shortening of atrial action potential duration and the marked

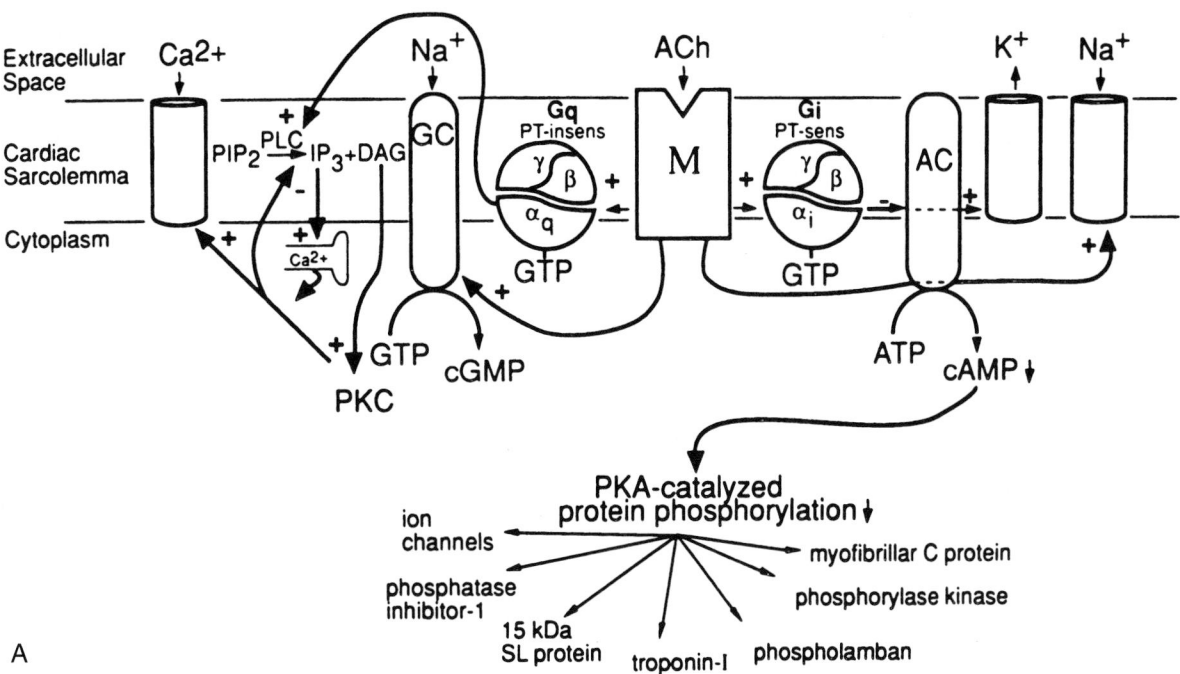

A

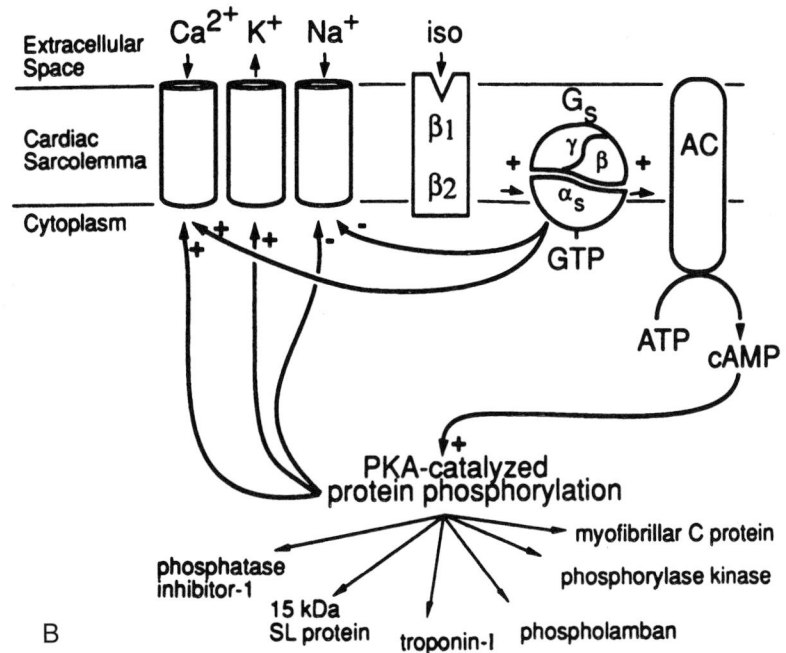

B

Figure 64–13. A, Schematic of cholinergic receptor-effector coupling. The muscarinic receptor is coupled to a pertussis toxin-sensitive inhibitory G protein (G_i). When activated, the α_i-subunit of the G protein dissociates and causes an inhibition of adenylate cyclase (AC) and a fall in intracellular cyclic adenosine monophosphate (cAMP) levels, with a resultant decrease in protein kinase A (PKA) phosphorylation of cellular proteins, including cardiac ion channels. It is by this mechanism that muscarinic stimulation decreases the inward calcium current. Direct activation of potassium channels by the G protein is also known to occur. There is also a pertussis toxin-insensitive G protein (G_q) that is linked to the muscarinic receptor. This G protein stimulates phospholipase C production, which stimulates the production of diacylglycerol (DAG) and 1,4,5-trisphosphate (IP_3). DAG stimulates protein kinase C (PKC), which phosphorylates and stimulates sarcoplasmic reticulum receptors causing intracellular release of calcium. IP_3 directly stimulates release of calcium from the sarcoplasmic reticulum. **B,** Schematic of β-adrenergic receptor-effector coupling. The β-adrenergic receptor is coupled to the stimulatory trimeric G protein, G_s. In the presence of GTP, this G protein dissociates, and the α_s subunit results in direct activation of adenylate cyclase (AC). This increases intracellular cAMP and stimulates protein kinase A. This enhances phosphorylation of cellular proteins, including cardiac ion channels. (From Fleming JW, et al: Circulation 85:420, 1992, by permission of the American Heart Association, Inc.)

shortening of atrial refractoriness observed with muscarinic stimulation in atrial tissue. In the rat atrium, acetylcholine-induced outward potassium current density progressively increases from 12 days' gestation to 20 days postnatally (and then decreases in adulthood as cell capacitance [i.e., cell size] increases).[125] Inhibition of the inward calcium current, primarily within the nodal or N region of the AV node, reduces the amplitude and rate of rise of the slow response AV nodal action potential. This accounts for the slowing of conduction through the AV node. The refractoriness of the AV node is also markedly increased by muscarinic stimulation. In ventricular myocardium, a slight but significant increase in ventricular refractory periods occurs with vagal stimulation. Evidence is increasing that this is a direct effect of acetylcholine.[126] The precise ionic basis for this effect is not well understood.

Maturation of parasympathetic control of cardiac electrophysiology is evident from studies of the effects of muscarinic blockade, vagus nerve transection, and vagal nerve stimulation in the developing animal. In the human fetus, the increase in heart rate observed in response to a maternal dose of atropine increases with advancing gestation.[127] In the fetal rabbit, cutting the vagus nerve causes a smaller increase in heart rate than is observed in the adult.[128] In the fetal lamb, vagal stimulation causes a greater slowing of the heart rate as gestation progresses.[129] Continued maturation of parasympathetic responses is evident in many species postnatally. In the puppy, the magnitude of the response of heart rate to long trains of vagal nerve stimulation increases postnatally.[130] The response to brief trains of vagal stimuli, which experimentally mimics how the vagus actually fires *in vivo*, also changes with development. In the adult, the degree of prolonga-

tion of sinus cycle length (as well as the degree of prolongation of AV nodal conduction) progressively *increases* as a brief vagal train is delivered progressively later in the cardiac cycle. This typical phase-response relationship is not observed in the newborn (Fig. 64–14). Full maturation of the response to brief vagal stimuli is not observed until approximately 1 to 2 months of age.[131, 132] Thus, although parasympathetic responses and reflexes are clearly present *in utero* and in the preterm infant, it is incorrect to consider the parasympathetic nervous system as being fully mature at birth. Significant maturation occurs in both the magnitude and type of responses elicited by parasympathetic stimulation in postnatal life.

The Sympathetic Nervous System

Evidence of functional β-adrenergic receptor modulation of calcium channel currents is observed in the early mammalian heart, before the time of sympathetic innervation.[133] However, in many mammalian species, including the human, rat, and dog, it is believed that the sympathetic nervous system is not as well developed as the parasympathetic nervous system at the time of birth. Rapid maturation occurs within the first postnatal months. Immunohistochemical studies of the specialized cardiac conduction system of the newborn human and dog heart have demonstrated nerve fibers reactive to dopamine β-hydroxylase (putative sympathetic neurons) mostly in the sinus and AV nodes, principally in association with small blood vessels, and only in small numbers.[116, 134] Evidence of sympathetic innervation of the atrium, sinus, and AV nodes, as well as the ventricular epicardium, is first observed at midgestation and progressively

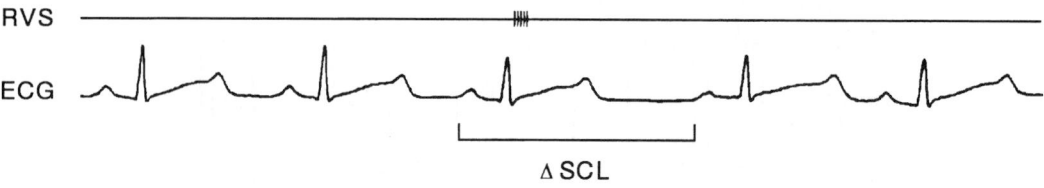

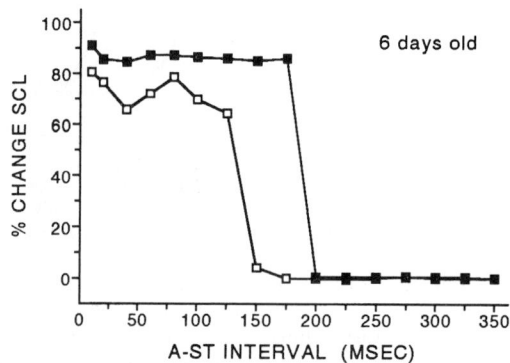

Figure 64–14. The response of heart rate to brief vagal stimulation. A short train of vagal stimulation is delivered once, at varying times, within the cardiac cycle. The effect of each brief, critically timed vagal train on sinus cycle length is determined, and a phase-response curve is generated. On the left, a typical adult-type vagal phase response curve is shown, obtained in experiments performed on a 2-month-old puppy. As the vagal train is delivered at progressively later times after the last atrial depolarization (A-ST interval), the change in sinus cycle length (percentage change of sinus cycle length [SCL]) evoked by that vagal stimulation train progressively increases. Eventually the vagal train is delivered too late in the cardiac cycle to affect sinus cycle length. On the right, a typical phase response curve in a newborn is shown. In contrast to in the older puppy, in the neonate, the vagal response remains flat as the vagal train is advanced through the cardiac cycle. Closed squares = right vagal stimulation (RVS); open squares = left vagal stimulation (LVS). (Phase response curves are from Pickoff AS, et al: Pediatr Res *35*:55, 1994.)

increases, reaching full maturity only after 2 months of age. In the dog, there is no sympathetic innervation of the AV bundle noted at birth, but this region also is fully innervated by 2 months of age. These histochemical studies of the mammalian cardiac conduction system complement earlier reports of increasing catecholamine content with maturation in the hearts of fetal and newborn dogs, as well as other mammalian species.[135-137]

Maturation of sympathetic innervation is associated with profound changes in the electrophysiologic responses of the developing heart to catecholamine stimulation. In Purkinje fibers of neonatal dogs, exposure to the α-adrenergic agonist phenylephrine increases the rate of spontaneous firing in a dose-dependent fashion.[138] This α-adrenergic–mediated *increase* in automaticity is not observed in Purkinje fibers from adult animals in whom α-adrenergic stimulation *decreases* automaticity. It has been shown that the conversion of the chronotropic response to α-adrenergic stimulation from the neonatal response (increase in automaticity) to the adult response (decrease in automaticity) is contingent on the process of sympathetic innervation. In rat myocytes that are co-cultured with sympathetic nerves, it can be shown that a specific pertussis toxin-sensitive 41-kDa guanosine triphosphate–binding protein is acquired that links the α-adrenergic receptor to the sodium-potassium pump, increasing maximum diastolic potential and thus causing a corresponding decrease in automaticity.[139, 140] Two separate subtypes of α_1-adrenergic receptors appear to mediate the positive and negative chronotropic responses. One subtype is antagonized by an analogue of clonidine and is linked to the neonatal positive chronotropic response. The other subtype is linked to the adult negative chronotropic response.[141] In the neonatal rat, α_1-adrenergic activation increases the L-type calcium current, I_{Ca-L}, one of the currents responsible for automaticity. This α_1-adrenergic mediated increase in calcium current is not observed in the adult heart. This suggests that there is also a developmentally determined switching of the coupling of α_1-adrenergic receptors with respect to calcium channels during development.[142]

In contrast to the cardiac electrophysiologic effects of parasympathetic stimulation, which exhibit rapid kinetics, the kinetics of sympathetic stimulation are more prolonged. The maximal effects of adrenergic stimulation on heart rate, myocardial refractoriness, and conduction tend to develop over several seconds, in contrast to the nearly instantaneous effects of vagal stimulation. The dominant electrophysiologic actions of sympathetic stimulation in the heart are mediated by the β_1 receptor, although β_2 receptors do coexist on the cardiac myocyte. The main electrophysiologic effects of β-adrenergic stimulation include an increase in sinus node automaticity, which is in part mediated by an increase in the rate of diastolic depolarization (phase 4 of the action potential). There is also an increase in the maximum diastolic potential of the sinus node, which serves to increase the activity of the I_f pacemaker current. In the AV node, conduction velocities are increased and refractory periods are shortened; the increases in AV nodal action potential amplitude and $\dot{V}_{max}$ account for the increase in conduction velocity. In the myocardium, β-adrenergic stimulation increases the height of the action potential plateau by increasing the inward calcium current; it also increases the speed of repolarization by increasing outward potassium currents. Overall, these effects tend to shorten myocardial refractoriness. The increase in maximum diastolic potential, observed in the sinus node and in the working myocardium, is likely caused by an adrenergic mediated increase in the activity of the sodium-potassium pump. These primary effects of β-adrenergic stimulation are mediated through a membrane-bound stimulatory guanine nucleotide binding protein, G_s (see Fig. 64-13*B*). The effects of sympathetic stimulation on the heart of the newborn and young infant are qualitatively similar to those in the adult. The degree of change in heart rate with sympathetic stimulation, however, is considerably less in the young puppy compared with the adult.[130] The increase in

response to sympathetic stimulation with maturation is probably multifactorial. As was mentioned previously, the density of sympathetic innervation continues to increase in many species postnatally. Furthermore, the stimulatory effect of β-agonists on adenylate cyclase increases postnatally in many mammalian species.[143-146] In rabbit ventricular cells, it has been reported that the postnatal increase in β-adrenergic stimulated cyclic adenosine monophosphate is more related to a reduction in inhibition of adenylate cyclase by the inhibitory G protein, G_i, with maturation, rather than to a change in the β receptor-adenylate cyclase complex.[146]

Several complex interactions between the two branches of the autonomic nervous system have been described.[147] These interactions involve complex pre- and postsynaptic mechanisms that allow for fine regulation of autonomic modulation of the electrophysiologic and mechanical properties of the heart. One classic interaction is the "accentuated antagonism" interaction between the sympathetic and parasympathetic nervous systems. With respect to heart rate and contractility, the effect of a given vagal stimulus becomes progressively greater as the level of background sympathetic tone increases.[147, 148] At the presynaptic level, it is believed that a cholinergic inhibition of norepinephrine release from sympathetic nerve endings contributes to the antagonism of sympathetic effects. At the postsynaptic level, the precise basis for interaction between the sympathetic and parasympathetic nervous systems is still somewhat speculative but may involve a muscarinic-mediated stimulation of phosphatases (enzymes), which results in a reversal of the adrenergic-stimulated phosphorylation of key intracellular proteins, such as the calcium channel.[149] Nitric oxide, a derivative of L-arginine, has also been implicated as a mediator of the cholinergic inhibition of β-adrenergic responses.[150, 151]

There have been few studies of the effects of development on autonomic interactions. In isolated canine Purkinje fibers, Moak and colleagues[152] reported that acetylcholine attenuated the isoproterenol-induced shortening of action potential duration in adult cells. In neonatal (i.e., 1-10 days old) Purkinje cells, in contrast, action potential duration lengthened after exposure to isoproterenol. Furthermore, this effect was not modified by exposure to acetylcholine. This was interpreted to indicate that accentuated antagonism is not present in the neonate. In somewhat older (e.g., 35 days) animals, however, prominent sympathetic-vagal interactions in the control of heart rate can be demonstrated, with sympathetic effects becoming more attenuated with higher levels of background vagal stimulation.[153] With respect to AV nodal conduction, Urthaler and associates[154] have demonstrated an interaction between the sympathetic and parasympathetic nervous systems in young puppies, but one with dominance of the sympathetic, not parasympathetic, nervous system. Further studies characterizing interactions between the branches of the autonomic nervous system in the developing heart are needed.

It is now known that in addition to the classic autonomic neurotransmitters, acetylcholine and norepinephrine, there exists a family of neuropeptides that histochemically appear to innervate the human heart. These peptides include neuropeptide Y, vasoactive intestinal peptide, calcitonin gene–related peptide, somatostatin, and substance P.[155] These neuropeptides exist, either co-localized with the classic neurotransmitters within neurons of the sympathetic or parasympathetic nervous system, or confined to neurons that appear to be separate from the two major branches of the autonomic nervous system. In the fetal heart, peptide immunoreactive nerves first appear at approximately 10 weeks' gestation, or 3 weeks after the appearance of cardiac ganglia and nerves.[156] Neuropeptide Y–containing nerves are the dominant peptide-containing nerves in the heart.[157] In the early fetal heart, neuropeptide Y is initially localized within the atria. With further development, innervation of the ventricles becomes evident. Vasoactive intestinal peptide and somatostatin appear localized primarily within the atrium and are first observed at 10- to 12-weeks' gestation. Substance P and calcitonin gene–related peptide do not appear in the fetal heart until somewhat later, at 18- to 24-weeks' gestation. In the newborn canine heart, neuropeptide Y and vasoactive intestinal peptide are both found in higher concentrations in the atria than ventricles, and for both peptides, concentrations in the first weeks after birth are higher than in the adult.[158]

Although the precise function and mechanisms of action of this peptidergic neurotransmission system remain to be fully elucidated, it is clear that at least two of these peptides, vasoactive intestinal peptide and neuropeptide Y, may exert significant direct or indirect (or combined) effects on cardiac automaticity and conduction. Vasoactive intestinal peptide can be shown to increase sinus node automaticity directly and to enhance AV nodal conduction in both the adult dog[159, 160] and the newborn.[161] In the adult dog, vasoactive intestinal peptide shortens atrial refractoriness,[160] an effect not observed in the neonatal atrium.[161] Vasoactive intestinal peptide may be responsible for the acceleration in heart rate observed with vagal stimulation in the presence of autonomic blockade.[162] Neuropeptide Y appears to function as

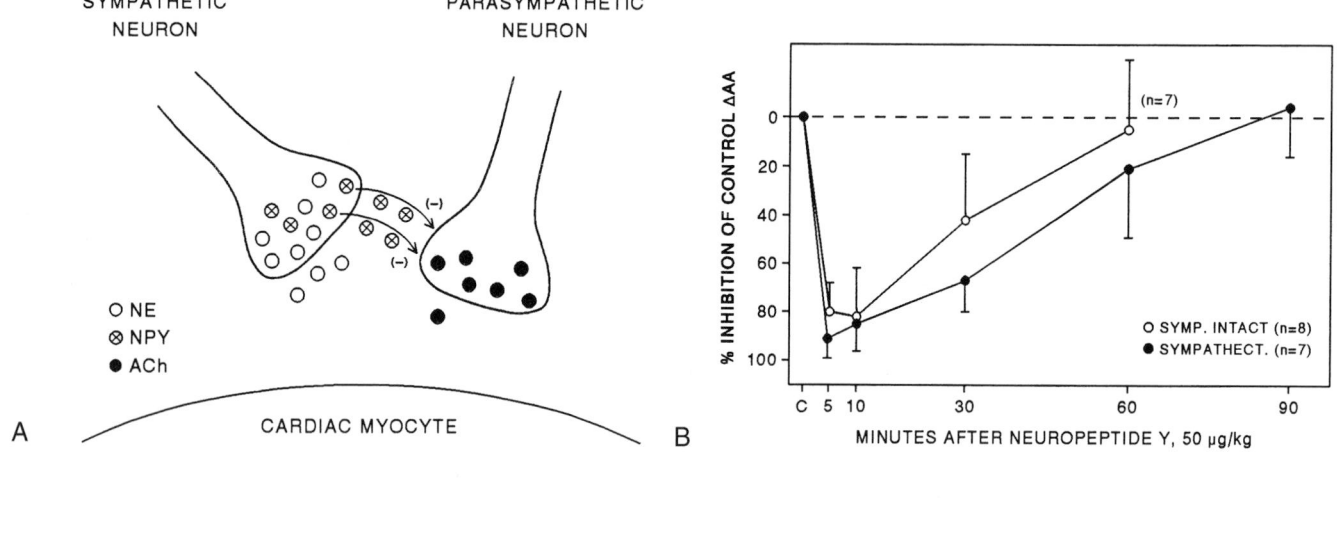

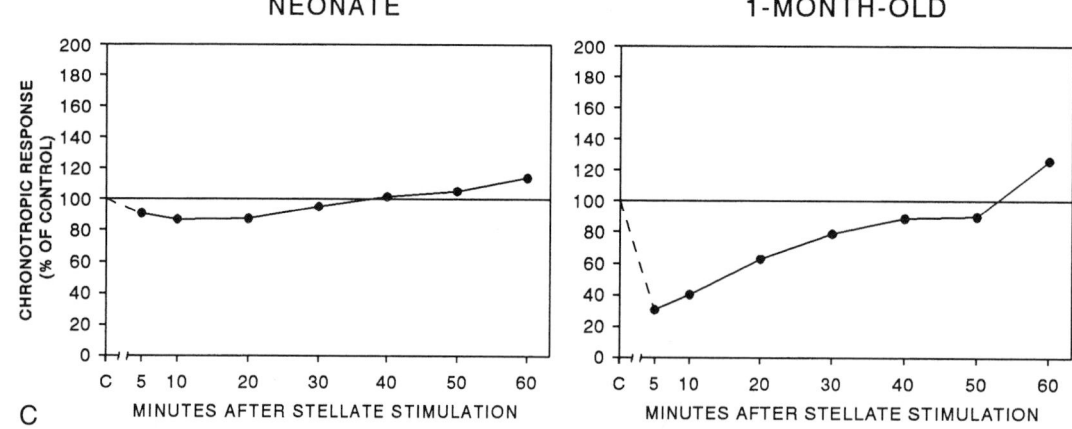

Figure 64–15. **A,** Illustration of the neuropeptide Y (NPY)-mediated sympathetic-parasympathetic interaction. NPY is stored within neuronal vesicles, along with norepinephrine (NE), in sympathetic nerve endings. When released, NPY can bind to receptors on the parasympathetic nerve terminals and inhibit the release of acetylcholine (ACh). (From Rios R, et al: Cardiovasc Res *31*:E96, 1996, with kind permission of Elsevier Science-NL.) **B,** The effects of an intravenous injection of NPY (50 μg/kg) on the vagal response of heart rate to vagal stimulation in sympathetically intact and sympathectomized newborn dogs. In both groups, NPY causes a profound (nearly 100%) and long-lasting (nearly 60 minutes) inhibition of the change in sinus cycle length caused by vagal stimulation (percentage inhibition of control ΔAA). C = control (pre-NPY administration). (From Yamasaki S, et al: Circ Res *69*:406, 1991, by permission of the American Heart Association, Inc.) **C,** The effects of right stellate ganglion stimulation (10 Hz, 5 minutes) on cardiac vagal chronotropic responses in young puppies. In these graphs, 100% represents the control (i.e., prestellate stimulation) vagal response. In the neonate (*left*), stellate stimulation causes little change in the magnitude of elicited vagal responses. In contrast, in the 1-month-old puppy, 5 minutes of stellate stimulation causes a profound, long-lasting inhibition of the cardiac vagal response. This occurs, presumably, as a result of the release of NPY during stellate stimulation. (Neonate graph from Rios R, et al: Cardiovasc Res *31*:E96, 1996, with kind permission of Elsevier Science-NL.)

a sympathetic co-transmitter, being localized with norepinephrine within adrenergic neurons.[163, 164] Neuropeptide Y release from sympathetic nerves is believed to inhibit release of acetylcholine from adjacent parasympathetic nerve endings, thus representing another type of autonomic sympathetic-parasympathetic interaction (Fig. 64-15, *top*). This interaction is believed to explain the profound and prolonged attenuation of vagal responses that is observed after a period of antecedent stellate ganglion stimulation in the adult dog.[165] In the neonatal dog, intravenous neuropeptide Y causes a profound and long-lasting inhibition of cardiac vagal response (see Fig. 64-15, *middle*).[166] Stellate stimulation, however, causes only a small inhibition of cardiac vagal response in the neonate, suggesting that the neuropeptide Y–sympathetic-parasympathetic autonomic interaction is immature at birth. The magnitude of the neuropeptide Y-autonomic interaction increases dramatically within the first postnatal month, probably as a result of the general postnatal maturation of adrenergic innervation (see Fig. 64-15, *bottom*).[167] Further research is warranted to elucidate the role of peptidergic transmission in the modulation of cardiac electrophysiology throughout development.

REFERENCES

1. Shih H-T: Anatomy of the action potential in the heart. Tex Heart Inst J *21*:30, 1994.
2. Task Force of the Working Group on Arrhythmias of the European Society of Cardiology: The Sicilian gambit. A new approach to the classification of anti-arrhythmic drugs based on their actions on arrhythmogenic mechanisms. Circulation *84*:1831, 1991.
3. Katz AM: Cardiac ion channels. N Engl J Med *328*:1244, 1993.
4. Roden DM, et al: Cardiac ion channels. Annu Rev Physiol *64*:431, 2002.
5. Stuhmer W, et al: Structural parts involved in activation and inactivation of the sodium channel. Nature *339*:597, 1989.
6. Balser JR: The cardiac sodium channel: Gating function and molecular pharmacology. J Mol Cell Cardiol *33*:599, 2001.
7. Tseng G-N, Hoffman BF: Two components of transient outward current in canine ventricular myocytes. Circ Res *64*:633, 1989.
8. Hess P: Cardiac calcium channels. *In* Zipes DP, Jalife J (eds): Cardiac Electrophysiology. From Cell to Bedside. Philadelphia, WB Saunders Co, 1990, pp 10-17.
9. Anderson ME: Ca^{2+}-dependent regulation of cardiac L-type channels: is a unifying mechanism at hand? J Mol Cell Cardiol *33*:639, 2001.
10. Zipes DP: Genesis of cardiac arrhythmias: electrophysiological considerations. *In* Braunwald E (ed): Heart Disease. A Textbook of Cardiovascular Medicine. Philadelphia, WB Saunders Co, 1992, pp 588-627.
11. Nerbonne JM: Regulation of voltage-gated K^+ channel expression in the developing mammalian myocardium. J Neurobiol *37*:37, 1998.
12. Wang Z, et al: Rapid and slow components of delayed rectifier current in human atrial myocytes. Cardiovasc Res *28*:1540, 1994.
13. Pennefather P, Cohen IS: Molecular mechanisms of cardiac K^+-channel regulation. *In* Zipes DP, Jalife J (eds): Cardiac Electrophysiology. From Cell to Bedside. Philadelphia, WB Saunders Co, 1990, pp 17-28.
14. Wang Z, et al: Sustained depolarization-induced outward current in human atrial myocytes: evidence for a novel delayed rectifier K^+ current similar to Kv1.5 cloned channel current. Circ Res *73*:1061, 1993.
15. Rorsman P, Trube G: Biophysics and physiology of ATP-regulated K^+ channels (K_{ATP}). *In* Cook NS (ed): Potassium Channels. Structure, Classification, Function and Therapeutic Potential. Chichester (UK), Halstead Press, 1990, pp 96-116.
16. Noble D: Ionic mechanisms in normal cardiac activity. *In* Zipes DP, Jalife J (eds): Cardiac Electrophysiology. From Cell to Bedside. Philadelphia, WB Saunders Co, 1990, pp 163-171.
17. Kodama I et al: Regional differences in the role of Ca 2+ and Na+ currents in pacemaker activity in the sinoatrial node. Am J Physiol *272*:H2793, 1997.
18. DiFrancesco D: Current i_f and the neuronal modulation of heart rate. *In* Zipes DP, Jalife J (eds): Cardiac Electrophysiology. From Cell to Bedside. Philadelphia, WB Saunders Co, 1990, pp 28-35.
19. Sperelakis N: Developmental changes in membrane electrical properties of the heart. *In* Sperelakis N (ed): Physiology and Pathophysiology of the Heart. 2nd ed. Boston, Kluwer Academic Publishers, 1989, pp 595-623.
20. Bernard C: Establishment of ionic permeabilities of the myocardial membrane during embryonic development of the rat. *In* Lieberman M, Sano T (eds): Developmental and Physiological Correlates of Cardiac Muscle. New York, Raven Press, 1975, pp 169-184.
21. Danilo P Jr, et al: Fetal canine cardiac Purkinje fibers: electrophysiology and ultrastructure. Am J Physiol *246*:H250, 1984.
22. Agata N, et al: Developmental changes in action potential properties of the guinea-pig myocardium. Acta Physiol Scand *149*:331, 1993.
23. Sperelakis N, Pappano AJ: Physiology and pharmacology of developing heart cells. Pharmacol Ther *22*:1, 1983.
24. Khatter JC, Hoeschen RJ: Developmental increase of digitalis receptors in guinea pig heart. Cardiovasc Res *16*:80, 1982.
25. Ng Y-C, Akera T: Relative abundance of two molecular forms of Na^+, K^+-ATPase in the ferret heart: developmental changes and associated alterations of digitalis sensitivity. Mol Pharmacol *32*:201, 1987.
26. Josephson IR, Sperelakis N: Developmental increases in the inwardly rectifying K^+ current of embryonic chick ventricular myocytes. Biochim Biophys Acta *1052*:123, 1990.
27. Huynh TV, et al: Developmental changes in membrane Ca^{2+} and K^+ currents in fetal, neonatal, and adult rabbit ventricular myocytes. Circ Res *70*:508, 1992.
28. Chen F, et al: Single-channel recording of inwardly rectifying potassium currents in developing myocardium. J Mol Cell Cardiol *23*:259, 1991.
29. Sanchez-Chapula J, et al: Differences in outward currents between neonatal and adult rabbit ventricular cells. Am J Physiol *266*:H1184, 1994.
30. Wahler GM: Developmental increases in the inwardly rectifying potassium current of rat ventricular myocytes. Am J Physiol *262*:C1266, 1992.
31. Masuda H, Sperelakis N: Inwardly rectifying potassium current in rat fetal and neonatal ventricular cardiomyocytes. Am J Physiol *265*:H1107, 1993.
32. Gennser G, Nilsson E: Excitation and impulse conduction in the human fetal heart. Acta Physiol Scand *79*:305, 1970.
33. Escande D, et al: Age-related changes of action potential plateau shape in isolated human atrial fibers. Am J Physiol *249*:H843, 1985.
34. Davies MP, et al: Developmental changes in ionic channel activity in the embryonic murine heart. Circ Res *78*:15, 1996.
35. Saxon ME, Safronova VG: The rest-dependent depression of action potential duration in rabbit myocardium and the possible role of the transient outward current. A pharmacological analysis. J Physiol Paris *78*:461, 1982.
36. Wahler GM, et al: Time course of postnatal changes in rat heart action potential and in transient outward current is different. Am J Physiol *267*:H1157, 1994.
37. Jeck CD, Boyden PA: Age-related appearance of outward currents may contribute to developmental differences in ventricular repolarization. Circ Res *71*:1390, 1992.
38. Gross GJ, et al: Characterisation of transient outward current in young human atrial myocytes. Cardiovasc Res *29*:112, 1995.
39. Crumb WJ Jr, et al: Comparison of I_{to} in young and adult human atrial myocytes: evidence for developmental changes. Am J Physiol *268*:H1335, 1995.
40. Kamiya K, et al: Hypoxia inhibits the changes in action potentials and ion channels during primary culture of neonatal rat ventricular myocytes. J Mol Cell Cardiol *31*:1591, 1999.
41. Renaud J-F, et al: Differentiation of receptor sites for [^{3}H] nitrendipine in chick hearts and physiological relation to the slow Ca^{2+} channel and to excitation-contraction coupling. Eur J Biochem *139*:673, 1984.
42. Aiba S, Creazzo TL: Comparison of the number of dihydropyridine receptors with the number of functional L-type calcium channels in embryonic heart. Circ Res *72*:396, 1993.
43. Tohse N, et al: Developmental changes in long-opening behavior of L-type Ca^{2+} channels in embryonic chick heart cells. Circ Res *71*:376, 1992.
44. Kawano S, DeHaan RL: Developmental changes in the calcium currents in embryonic chick ventricular myocytes. J Membr Biol *120*:191, 1991.
45. Kojima M, et al: Developmental changes in β-adrenoceptors, muscarinic cholinoceptors and Ca^{2+} channels in rat ventricular muscles. Br J Pharmacol *99*:334, 1990.
46. Erman RD, et al: The ontogeny of specific binding sites for calcium channel antagonist, nitrendipine, in mouse heart and brain. Brain Res *278*:327, 1983.
47. Tohse N, et al: Novel isoform of Ca^{2+} channel in rat fetal cardiomyocytes. J Physiol (Lond) *451*:295, 1992.
48. Cohen NM, Lederer WJ: Changes in the calcium current of rat heart ventricular myocytes during development. J Physiol (Lond) *406*:115, 1988.
49. Conforti L, et al: Tetrodotoxin-sensitive sodium current in rat fetal ventricular myocytes—contribution to the plateau phase of action potential. J Mol Cell Cardiol *25*:159, 1993.
50. Wetzel GT, et al: Ca^{2+} channel kinetics in acutely isolated fetal, neonatal, and adult rabbit cardiac myocytes. Circ Res *72*:1065, 1993.
51. Chin TK, et al: Developmental changes in cardiac myocyte calcium regulation. Circ Res *67*:574, 1990.
52. Roca TP, et al: L-type calcium current in pediatric and adult human atrial myocytes: evidence for developmental changes in channel inactivation. Pediatric Res *40*:462, 1996.
53. Franco D, et al: Divergent expression of delayed rectifier K(+) channel subunits during mouse heart development. Cardiovasc Res *52*:65, 2001.
54. Wang L, et al: Developmental changes in the delayed rectifier K+ channels in mouse heart. Circ Res *79*:79, 1996.
55. Guo W, et al: Developmental changes in the ultrarapid delayed rectifier K^+ current in rat ventricular myocytes. Pflügers Arch *433*:442, 1997.
56. Kamino K, et al: Localization of pacemaking activity in early embryonic heart monitored using voltage-sensitive dye. Nature *290*:595, 1981.
57. Van Mierop LHS: Location of pacemaker in chick embryo heart at the time of initiation of heartbeat. Am J Physiol *212*:407, 1967.
58. Satoh H, Sperelakis N: Hyperpolarization-activated inward current in embryonic chick cardiac myocytes: developmental changes and modulation by isoproterenol and carbachol. Eur J Pharmacol *240*:283, 1993.
59. Baruscotti M, et al: Na(+) current contribution to the diastolic depolarization in newborn rabbit SA node cells. Am J Physiol *279*:H2303, 2000.
60. Baruscotti M, et al: Single-channel properties of the sinoatrial node Na+ current in the newborn rabbit. Pflügers Arch *442*:192, 2001.

61. Protas L, et al: L-type but not T-type calcium current changes during postnatal development in rabbit sinoatrial node. Am J Physiol 281:H1252, 2001.

62. Sakai T, et al: A regional gradient of cardiac intrinsic rhythmicity depicted in embryonic cultured multiple hearts. Pflügers Arch 437:61, 1998.

63. DeHaan RL: Regional organization of pre-pacemaker cells in the cardiac primordia of the early chick embryo. J Embryol Exp Morphol 11:65, 1963.

64. Satin J, et al: Development of cardiac heart rate in early chick embryos is regulated by regional cues. Dev Biol 129:103, 1988.

65. Tucker DC, et al: Pacemaker development in embryonic rat heart cultured in oculo. Pediatr Res 23:637, 1988.

66. Anderson RH, et al: The development of the sinoatrial node. In Bonke FIM (ed): The Sinus Node. Structure, Function and Clinical Relevance. The Hague, Martinus Nijhoff, 1978, pp 166–182.

67. James TN: The connecting pathways between the sinus node and A-V node and between the right and the left atrium in the human heart. Am Heart J 66:498, 1963.

68. Gittenberger-de Groot AC, Wenink ACG: The specialized myocardium in the foetal heart. In Van Mierop LHS, et al (eds): Embryology and Teratology of the Heart and the Great Arteries. The Hague, Leiden University Press, 1978, pp 15–24.

69. Obrucnik M, et al: Development of the conduction system of human embryonic and fetal heart: differentiation of internodal connection. Acta Univ Palacki Olomuc Fac Med 102:39, 1982.

70. Anderson RH, et al: The internodal atrial myocardium. Anat Rec 201:75, 1981.

71. Wenink AC, et al: HNK-1 expression patterns in the embryonic rat heart distinguish between sinuatrial and atrial myocardium. Anat Embryol 201:39, 2000.

72. Spach MS, et al: Excitation sequences of the atrial septum and the AV node in isolated hearts of the dog and rabbit. Circ Res 29:156, 1971.

73. Racker DK: Sinoventricular transmission in 10 mM K+ by canine atrioventricular nodal inputs. Superior atrionodal bundle and proximal atrioventricular bundle. Circulation 83:1738, 1991.

74. Spach MS, et al: Electrophysiology of the internodal pathways: determining the difference between anisotropic cardiac muscle and a specialized tract system. In Little RC (ed): Physiology of Atrial Pacemakers and Conductive Tissues. Mt. Kisco, NY, Futura Publishing Co, 1980, pp 367–380.

75. Spach MS, et al: Multiple regional differences in cellular properties that regulate repolarization and contraction in the right atrium of adult and newborn dogs. Circ Res 65:1594, 1989.

76. Cavoto FV, et al: Electrophysiological changes in the rat atrium with age. Am J Physiol 226:1293, 1974.

77. Pickoff AS, et al: Atrial vulnerability in the immature canine heart. Am J Cardiol 55:1402, 1985.

78. Pickoff AS, Stolfi A: Modulation of electrophysiological properties of neonatal canine heart by tonic parasympathetic stimulation. Am J Physiol 258:H38, 1990.

79. Mendelsohn A, et al: Natural history of isolated atrial flutter in infancy. J Pediatr 119:386, 1991.

80. Hoff EC, et al: The development of the electrocardiogram of the embryonic heart. Am Heart J 17:470, 1939.

81. Patten BM: The development of the sinoventricular conduction system. Univ Mich Med Bull 22:1, 1956.

82. Arguello C, et al: Electrophysiological and ultrastructural study of the atrioventricular canal during the development of the chick embryo. J Mol Cell Cardiol 18:499, 1986.

83. Arguello C, et al: The early development of the atrioventricular node and bundle of His in the embryonic chick heart. An electrophysiological and morphological study. Development 102:623, 1988.

84. Lloyd TR, Baldwin HS: Emulation of conduction system functions in the hearts of early mammalian embryos. Pediatr Res 28:425, 1990.

85. Lamers WH, et al: Acetylcholinesterase in prenatal rat heart: a marker for the early development of the cardiac conductive tissue? Anat Rec 217:361, 1987.

86. van Kempen MJA, et al: Spatial distribution of connexin43, the major cardiac gap junction protein, in the developing and adult rat heart. Circ Res 68:1638, 1991.

87. van Veen TA, et al: Cardiac gap junction channels: modulation of expression and channel properties. Cardiovasc Res 51:217, 2001.

88. Veenstra RD, et al: Multiple connexins confer distinct regulatory and conductance properties of gap junctions in developing heart. Circ Res 71:1277, 1992.

89. Gourdie RG, et al: Immunolabelling patterns of gap junction connexins in the developing and mature rat heart. Anat Embryol 185:363, 1992.

90. Kirchhoff S, et al: Abnormal cardiac conduction and morphogenesis in connexin40 and connexin43 double deficient mice. Circ Res 87:399, 2000.

91. Gutstein DE, et al: Conduction slowing and sudden arrhythmic death in mice with cardiac-restricted inactivation of connexin43. Circ Res 88:333, 2001.

92. Cheng G, et al: Development of the cardiac conduction system involves recruitment within a multipotent cardiomyogenic lineage. Development 126:5041, 1999.

93. Takebayashi-Suzuki K, et al: Purkinje fibers of the avian heart express a myogenic transcription factor program distinct from cardiac and skeletal muscle. Dev Biol 234:390, 2001.

94. Franco D, Icardo JM: Molecular characterization of the ventricular conduction system in the developing mouse heart: topographical correlation in normal and congenitally malformed hearts. Cardiovasc Res 49:417, 2001.

95. Thomas PS, et al: Elevated expression of Nkx-2.5 in developing myocardial conduction cells. Anat Rec 263:307, 2001.

96. Wessels A, et al: Spatial distribution of "tissue-specific" antigens in the developing human heart and skeletal muscle. III. An immunohistochemical analysis of the distribution of the neural tissue antigen G1N2 in the embryonic heart; implications for the development of the atrioventricular conduction system. Anat Rec 232:97, 1992.

97. Anderson RH, Ho SY: Cardiac conduction system in normal and abnormal hearts. In Roberts NK, Gelband H (eds): Cardiac Arrhythmias in the Neonate, Infant, and Child. 2nd ed. Norwalk, CT, Appleton-Century-Crofts, 1983, pp 1–35.

98. James TN: Sudden death in babies: new observations in the heart. Am J Cardiol 22:479, 1968.

99. Suarez-Mier MP, Gamallo C: Atrioventricular node fetal dispersion and His bundle fragmentation of the cardiac conduction system in sudden cardiac death. J Am Coll Cardiol 32:1885, 1998.

100. Preston JB, et al: Atrioventricular transmission in young mammals. Am J Physiol 197:236, 1959.

101. Gough WB, Moore EN: The differences in atrioventricular conduction of premature beats in young and adult goats. Circ Res 37:48, 1975.

102. Moore EN: Atrioventricular transmission in newborn calves. Ann NY Acad Sci 127:113, 1965.

103. McCormack J, et al: Atrioventricular nodal function in the immature canine heart. Pediatr Res 23:99, 1988.

104. Hewett KW, et al: Cellular electrophysiology of neonatal and adult rabbit atrioventricular node. Am J Physiol 260:H1674, 1991.

105. Kirchhof P, et al: Simultaneous in utero assessment of AV nodal and ventricular electrophysiologic parameters in the fetal sheep heart. Basic Res Cardiol 96:251, 2001.

106. Horigome H, et al: Magnetocardiographic determination of the developmental changes in PQ, QRS and QT intervals in the foetus. Acta Paediatr 89:64, 2000.

107. Gillette PC, et al: Intracardiac electrography in children and young adults. Am Heart J 89:36, 1975.

108. Legato MJ, et al: The morphology of the developing canine conducting system: bundle branch and Purkinje cell architecture from birth to week 12 of life. J Mol Cell Cardiol 23:1063, 1991.

109. Spach MS, et al: Changes in anisotropic conduction caused by remodeling cell size and the cellular distribution of gap junctions and Na(+) channels. J Electrocardiol 34(Suppl):69, 2001.

110. Myerburg RJ, et al: Physiology of the ventricular specialized conduction system. In Roberts NK, Gelband H (eds): Cardiac Arrhythmias in the Neonate, Infant, and Child. New York, Appleton-Century-Crofts, 1977, pp 55–90.

111. Pickoff AS, et al: Maturational changes in ventriculoatrial conduction in the intact canine heart. J Am Coll Cardiol 3:162, 1984.

112. Untereker WJ, et al: Developmental changes in action potential duration, refractoriness, and conduction in the canine ventricular conducting system. Pediatr Res 18:53, 1984.

113. Myerburg RJ, et al: Functional characteristics of the gating mechanism in the canine A-V conducting system. Circ Res 28:136, 1971.

114. Kirby ML, Stewart DE: Development of ANS innervation to the avian heart. In Gootman PM (ed): Developmental Neurobiology of the Autonomic Nervous System. Clifton, NJ, Humana Press, 1986, pp 135–158.

115. Cohen HL: Development of autonomic innervation in mammalian myocardium. In Gootman PM (ed): Developmental Neurobiology of the Autonomic Nervous System. Clifton, NJ, Humana Press, 1986, pp 159–191.

116. Chow LT, et al: Innervation of the human cardiac conduction system at birth. Br Heart J 69:430, 1993.

117. Chow LT, et al: Autonomic innervation of the human cardiac conduction system: changes from infancy to senility—an immunohistochemical and histochemical analysis. Anat Rec 264:169, 2001.

118. Kent KM, et al: Cholinergic innervation of the canine and human ventricular conducting system. Anatomic and electrophysiologic correlations. Circulation 50:948, 1974.

119. Birk E, Riemer RK: Myocardial cholinergic signaling changes with age. Pediatr Res 31:601, 1992.

120. Danilo P Jr, et al: Effects of acetylcholine on the ventricular specialized conducting system of neonatal and adult dogs. Circ Res 43:777, 1978.

121. Jalife J, Michaels DC: Neural control of sinoatrial pacemaker activity. In Levy MN, Schwartz PJ (eds): Vagal Control of the Heart: Experimental Basis and Clinical Implications. Armonk, NY, Futura Publishing Co, 1994, pp 173–205.

122. Martin P: Vagal control of atrioventricular conduction. In Levy MN, Schwartz PJ (eds): Vagal Control of the Heart: Experimental Basis and Clinical Implications. Armonk, NY, Futura Publishing Co, 1994, pp 221–239.

123. Brown AM: Coupling of G-proteins to cardiac ion channels. In Levy MN, Schwartz PJ (eds): Vagal Control of the Heart: Experimental Basis and Clinical Implications. Armonk, NY, Futura Publishing Co, 1994, pp 133–146.

124. DiFrancesco D: Regulation of the pacemaker current by acetylcholine. In Levy MN, Schwartz PJ (eds): Vagal Control of the Heart: Experimental Basis and Clinical Implications. Armonk, NY, Futura Publishing Co, 1994, pp 207–220.

125. Takano M, Noma A: Development of muscarinic potassium current in fetal and neonatal rat heart. Am J Physiol 272:H1133, 1997.

126. Prystowsky EN, et al: Effect of autonomic blockade on ventricular refractoriness and atrioventricular nodal conduction in humans. Evidence supporting a direct cholinergic action on ventricular muscle refractoriness. Circ Res 49:511, 1981.

127. Schifferli P-Y, Caldeyro-Barcia R: Effects of atropine and beta-adrenergic drugs on the heart rate of the human fetus. *In* Boreus L (ed): Fetal Pharmacology. New York, Raven Press, 1973, pp 259–279.

128. Dawes GS, et al: Some cardiovascular responses in foetal, new-born and adult rabbits. J Physiol (Lond) *139*:123, 1957.

129. Born GVR, et al: Oxygen lack and autonomic nervous control of the foetal circulation in the lamb. J Physiol (Lond) *134*:149, 1956.

130. Mace SE, Levy MN: Neural control of heart rate: a comparison between puppies and adult animals. Pediatr Res *17*:491, 1983.

131. Yamasaki S, et al: Characterization of responses of neonatal sinus and AV nodes to critically timed, brief vagal stimuli. Am J Physiol *260*:H459, 1991.

132. Pickoff AS, et al: Postnatal maturation of the response of the canine sinus node to critically timed, brief vagal stimulation. Pediatr Res *35*:55, 1994.

133. Liu W, et al: β-adrenergic modulation of L-type Ca^{2+}-channel currents in early-stage embryonic mouse heart. Am J Physiol *276*:H608, 1999.

134. Ursell PC, et al: Anatomic distribution of autonomic neural tissue in the developing dog heart: I. Sympathetic innervation. Anat Rec *226*:71, 1990.

135. Danilo P Jr, et al: Developmental changes in cellular electrophysiologic characteristics and catecholamine content of fetal hearts. Circulation *59-60*(Suppl II):II-50, 1979.

136. Friedman WF, et al: Sympathetic innervation of the developing rabbit heart. Biochemical and histochemical comparisons of fetal, neonatal, and adult myocardium. Circ Res *23*:25, 1968.

137. Lebowitz EA, et al: Development of myocardial sympathetic innervation in the fetal lamb. Pediatr Res *6*:887, 1972.

138. Reder RF, et al: Developmental changes in alpha adrenergic effects on canine Purkinje fiber automaticity. Dev Pharmacol Ther *7*:94, 1984.

139. Steinberg SF, et al: Acquisition by innervated cardiac myocytes of a pertussis toxin-specific regulatory protein linked to the α_1-receptor. Science *230*:186, 1985.

140. Shah A, et al: Stimulation of cardiac alpha receptors increases Na/K pump current and decreases g_K via a pertussis toxin-sensitive pathway. Biophys J *54*:219, 1988.

141. del Balzo U, et al: Specific α_1-adrenergic receptor subtypes modulate catecholamine-induced increases and decreases in ventricular automaticity. Circ Res *67*:1535, 1990.

142. Liu Q-Y, et al: Changes in α_1-adrenoceptor coupling to Ca^{2+} channels during development in rat heart. FEBS Lett *338*:234, 1994.

143. Whitsett JA, Darovec-Beckerman C: Developmental aspects of β-adrenergic receptors and catecholamine-sensitive adenylate cyclase in rat myocardium. Pediatr Res *15*:1363, 1981.

144. Schumacher WA, et al: Biological maturation and beta-adrenergic effectors: pre- and postnatal development of the adenylate cyclase system in the rabbit heart. J Pharmacol Exp Ther *223*:587, 1982.

145. Vulliemoz Y, et al: Developmental changes in adenylate cyclase activity in canine myocardium. Dev Pharmacol Ther *7*:409, 1984.

146. Osaka T, Joyner RW: Developmental changes in the β-adrenergic modulation of calcium currents in rabbit ventricular cells. Circ Res *70*:104, 1992.

147. Levy MN: Sympathetic-vagal interactions in the sinus and atrioventricular nodes. Prog Clin Biol Res *275*:187, 1988.

148. Levy MN, Martin P: Parasympathetic control of the heart. *In* Randall WC (ed): Nervous Control of Cardiovascular Function. New York, Oxford University Press, 1984, pp 68–94.

149. Neumann J, et al: Biochemical basis of cardiac sympathetic-parasympathetic interaction. *In* Levy MN, Schwartz PJ (eds): Vagal Control of the Heart: Experimental Basis and Clinical Implications. Armonk, NY, Futura Publishing Co, 1994, pp 161–170.

150. Hare JM, et al: Role of nitric oxide in parasympathetic modulation of β-adrenergic myocardial contractility in normal dogs. J Clin Invest *95*:360, 1995.

151. Han X, et al: An obligatory role for nitric oxide in autonomic control of mammalian heart rate. J Physiol (Lond) *476*:309, 1994.

152. Moak JP, et al: Developmental changes in the interactions of cholinergic and β-adrenergic agonists on electrophysiologic properties of canine cardiac Purkinje fibers. Pediatr Res *20*:613, 1986.

153. Mace SE, Levy MN: Autonomic nervous control of heart rate: sympathetic-parasympathetic interactions and age related differences. Cardiovasc Res *17*:547, 1983.

154. Urthaler F, et al: Differential sympathetic-parasympathetic interactions in sinus node and AV junction. Am J Physiol *250*:H43, 1986.

155. Corr L: Neuropeptides and the conduction system of the heart. Int J Cardiol *35*:1, 1992.

156. Gordon L, et al: Development of the peptidergic innervation of human heart. J Anat *183*:131, 1993.

157. Crick SJ, et al: Innervation of the human cardiac conduction system. A quantitative immunohistochemical and histochemical study. Circulation *89*:1697, 1994.

158. Kralios FA, et al: Postnatal development of peptidergic innervation of the canine heart. J Mol Cell Cardiol *31*: 215, 1999.

159. Rigel DF, Lathrop DA: Vasoactive intestinal polypeptide enhances automaticity of supraventricular pacemakers in anesthetized dogs. Am J Physiol *261*:H463, 1991.

160. Rigel DF, Lathrop DA: Vasoactive intestinal polypeptide facilitates atrioventricular nodal conduction and shortens atrial and ventricular refractory periods in conscious and anesthetized dogs. Circ Res *67*:1323, 1990.

161. Pickoff AS, et al: Vasoactive intestinal peptide: electrophysiologic activity in the newborn heart. Pediatr Res *35*:244, 1994.

162. Henning RJ: Vagal stimulation during muscarinic and β-adrenergic blockade increases atrial contractility and heart rate. J Auton Nerv Syst *40*:121, 1992.

163. Allen JM, et al: Studies on cardiac distribution and function of neuropeptide Y. Acta Physiol Scand *126*:405, 1986.

164. Dalsgaard C-J, et al: Distribution and origin of substance P- and neuropeptide Y-immunoreactive nerves in the guinea-pig heart. Cell Tissue Res *243*:477, 1986.

165. Potter EK: Effects of neuropeptides on the vagal neuroeffector junction. *In* Levy MN, Schwartz PJ (eds): Vagal Control of the Heart: Experimental Basis and Clinical Implications. NY, New York, Futura Publishing Co, 1994, pp 289–303.

166. Yamasaki S, et al: Rapid attenuation ("fade") of the chronotropic response during vagal stimulation in the canine newborn. Evidence for a prominent neuropeptide Y effect. Circ Res *69*:406, 1991.

167. Rios R, et al: Postnatal maturation of the neuropeptide Y (NPY) type sympathetic-parasympathetic autonomic interaction in the young canine. Am J Cardiol *70*:560, 1992.

65

Developmental Biology of the Pulmonary Vasculature

This chapter discusses the fetal, neonatal, and postnatal changing morphology of the developing pulmonary vascular bed. Studies have focused on structural and functional alterations in endothelial cells during postnatal development and have addressed the phenotypic heterogeneity of the vascular smooth muscle cells in the perinatal period. There are new insights into mechanisms regulating endothelial migration and angiogenesis, smooth muscle cell proliferation, hypertrophy, and migration. These studies have also provided novel therapeutic targets whereby progression of pulmonary vascular disease may be retarded or prevented and regression induced.

MORPHOLOGY OF THE DEVELOPING PULMONARY CIRCULATION IN THE FETUS

Early embryologic studies have shown that in the 5-week human embryo there are primitive pulmonary vessels from the sixth aortic arch. These vessels supply the upper poles of the right and left lung. The lower poles are supplied by a pair of intersegmental arteries arising from the dorsal aorta that penetrate upward through the diaphragm. At this stage, the developing lung parenchymal blood vessels are largely localized to the interlobular septa. Between 5 and 8 weeks of gestation, it is likely that numerous paired dorsal intersegmental arteries supply the emerging blood vessels that are developing alongside the branching bronchi in the lung parenchyma. As the true central pulmonary arteries form from the aortopulmonary trunk and anastomose with the intrapulmonary arteries, the primitive pulmonary arteries arising from the

aorta as well as the primitive intersegmental arteries involute. By 9 weeks of gestation, the bronchial system has formed. With each airway generation, there is an accompanying artery, in addition to numerous supernumerary arteries that are also produced. By 16 weeks of gestation, the number of preacinar airways and accompanying arteries is complete. Thereafter, as the acini develop (terminal bronchioli, respiratory bronchioli, alveolar ducts, and alveoli), so do the accompanying and supernumerary arteries.[1,2]

Abnormal maturation or maturational arrest in pulmonary arterial development is reflected in functional derangement that can appear in the newborn period. For example, persistent pulmonary hypertension of the neonate has been reported in association with pulmonary arterial maturational arrest at the fifth-week gestational time point (Fig. 65-1).[3] Infants with pulmonary atresia and ventricular septal defect frequently have persistence of the intersegmental arteries (aortopulmonary collaterals) (Fig. 65-2).[4] These vessels can serve as the sole source of blood supply to a lobe or lobar segment. Alternatively, there is a dual circulation with intersegmental arteries anastomosing to arteries that can be traced back to a central pulmonary artery origin. In these infants, there can also be multiple indirect aortopulmonary collaterals arising from branches of aortic branches (e.g., from subclavian, intercostals, coronary arteries). Because these indirect collaterals can be observed in the absence of direct collaterals, they probably represent the sequelae of pulmonary atresia when it occurs later in development. Finally, in some cases of pulmonary atresia, there is supply by anastomotic vessels, which arise from true bronchial arteries.

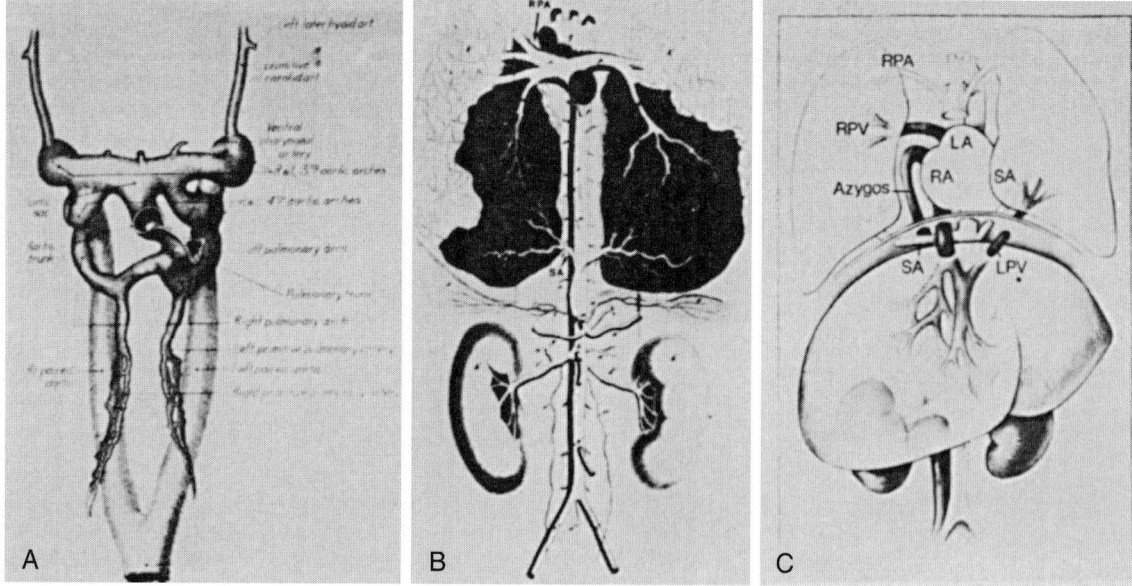

Figure 65–1. A, Early embryologic development shows normal disparity between the large main pulmonary artery and narrow right and left branch pulmonary arteries at 5 weeks. (From Congdon ED: Contrib Embryol *14*:47, 1922.) **B,** Only the arterial system is shown. The bilateral systemic arteries arising from a single trunk supply the lower lobes. (From Maugars A: J Med Chir Pharm Paris *3*:453, 1802.) **C,** An infant with persistent pulmonary hypertension and developmental arrest at 5 weeks' gestation. LA = left atrium; LPV = left pulmonary vein; RA = right atrium; RPA = right pulmonary artery; RPV = right pulmonary vein; SA = systemic arteries. (Reprinted by permission of the publisher from Goldstein JD, et al: Am J Cardiol *43*:962, 1979. Copyright 1979 by Excerpta Medica, Inc.)

Another morphologic pulmonary vascular abnormality is observed with absence of the pulmonary valve.[5] In those patients who present with severe respiratory problems from birth, abnormal branching of the vessels has been observed. Tufts of intersegmental pulmonary arteries are seen arising in weeping willow or squidlike fashion, encircling and compressing the intrapulmonary airways (Fig. 65-3).

Microscopic Features

The normal morphologic development of the pulmonary circulation has also been studied at the microscopic level. In the fetus, the preacinar arteries and those at the terminal bronchiolus level are muscular, whereas the intra-acinar arteries (i.e., those accompanying respiratory bronchioli) are partially muscular (surrounded by a spiral of muscle) or nonmuscular. Arteries at alveolar duct and alveolar wall levels are nonmuscular. The preacinar arteries are thick walled and change little in wall thickness relative to external diameter throughout the fetal period. Experimental studies[6] suggest that the immediate postnatal period is characterized by rapid recruitment of small alveolar duct and wall vessels, which appear to be functionally and structurally closed in the prenatal period. There is also progressive dilation of muscular arteries. Within a few days, the smallest muscular arteries (<250 μm) dilate, and their walls thin to adult levels; by 4 months of age, this process has included the largest pulmonary arteries at the hilum. As intra-acinar arteries at the various airway levels increase in external diameter, muscle is said to extend peripherally (i.e., it is observed in arteries located more peripherally within the acinus). At first, nonmuscular arteries become partially muscular, and later they become fully muscularized. For example, in infancy, vessels at

alveolar duct level are still largely nonmuscular, but, in childhood, they become partially muscularized, and, in the adult, they are fully muscularized.[7] Alveolar wall arteries remain largely nonmuscular, even in the adult.

Clinical as well as experimental studies have suggested that the muscularization of these peripheral pulmonary arteries may be related to the differentiation of pericytes as well as to the recruitment of fibroblasts.[8, 9] Arteries proliferate through the neonatal period and early infancy, accompanying the proliferation of alveoli; the alveoli/arteries ratio can therefore be used as a measure of numerical arterial growth. The alveoli/arteries ratio actually decreases from the newborn value of 20:1 to the value of 8:1, which is achieved first in early childhood and persists (Fig. 65-4). The growth and development of the pulmonary circulation is also likely influenced by the trophic effects of neuropeptides[10] released from nerve endings, as well as from neuroendocrine bodies[11] associated with accompanying airways (Fig. 65-5).

Experimental studies have indicated how changes in connective tissue, especially elastin and collagen,[12, 13] and cellular arrangement[14] govern the normal adaptation to postnatal life. The endothelial cells begin to flatten as there is increased deposition of elastin in peripheral arteries, forming an intact elastic lamina. In the central pulmonary arteries, similar changes occur, and elastin remodeling is prominent in the subendothelium in the early neonatal period,[13] whereas elastin synthesis, as judged by mRNA levels, appears to be less prominent in the outer media and adventitia (Fig. 65-6). It has also been shown experimentally that there are smooth muscle cells with differing proliferative potentials and that, in the neonatal period, the specialized functions of selective subgroups of smooth muscle cells, characterized by

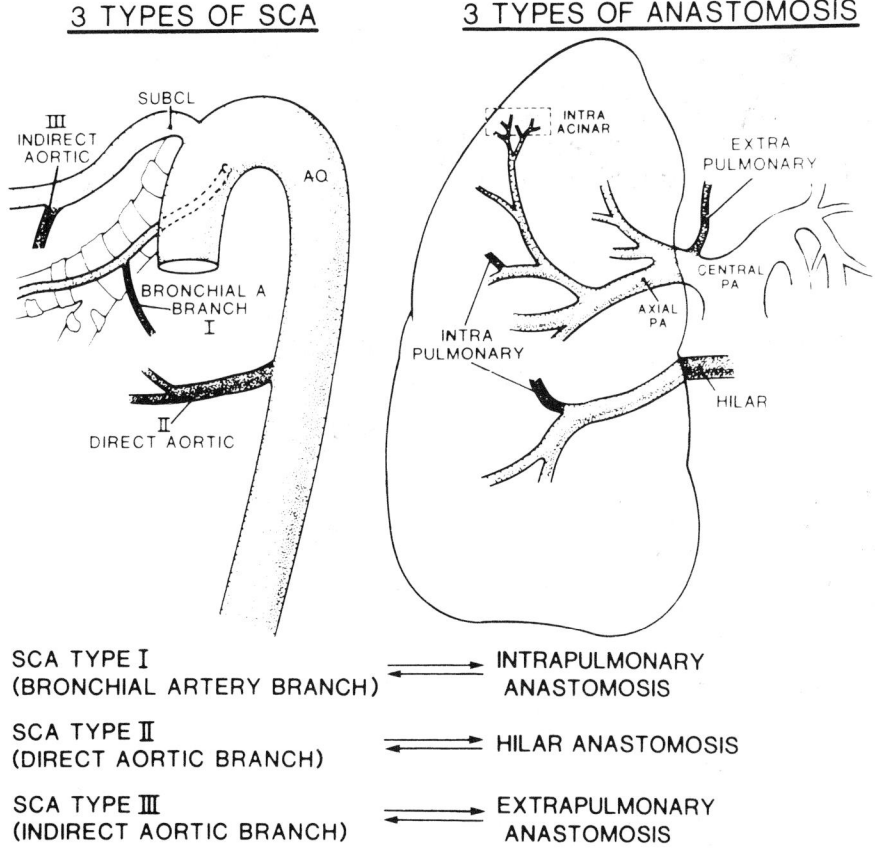

Figure 65–2. The three types of systemic collateral artery (SCA) and the three types of anastomosis with the pulmonary artery (PA). The characteristic pattern of anastomosis for each type of SCA is given. SUBCL = subclavian; AO = aorta. (From Rabinovitch M, et al: Circulation 64:1234, 1981.)

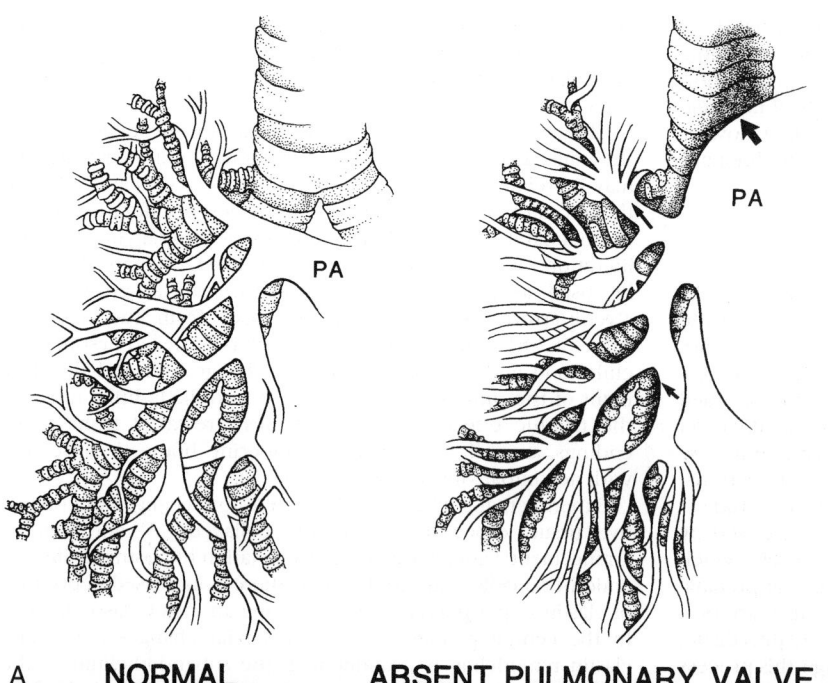

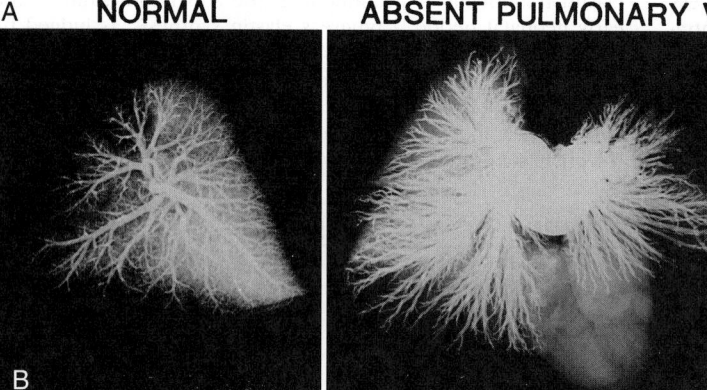

A   **NORMAL**   **ABSENT PULMONARY VALVE**

B

Figure 65–3. A, Diagrammatic representation of normal pulmonary artery (PA) branching and the abnormal pattern seen in cases of absent pulmonary valve syndrome—tufts of vessels emerging at the segmental artery level that entwine the bronchi. *Arrows* denote large right pulmonary artery compressing right main stem bronchus. **B,** Postmortem arteriograms from a 4-day-old normal infant (*left*) and from a 4-day-old patient with absent pulmonary valve syndrome associated with a ventricular septal defect and D-transposition of the great arteries (*right*), showing tufts of vessels in both lungs. (Reprinted by permission of the publisher from Rabinovitch M, et al: Am J Cardiol *50*:804, 1982. Copyright 1982 by Excerpta Medica, Inc.)

expression of cytoskeletal proteins, become even better defined.[15] The metavinculin positive smooth muscle cells are relatively resistant to proliferation. Moreover, the high proliferative potential demonstrated in neonatal bovine pulmonary artery smooth muscle cells is reflective of a difference in activation of protein kinase C.[16]

Cellular Mechanisms

The cellular and molecular mechanisms that regulate fetal growth and development of the vasculature are currently being studied by a number of groups.[17] There has been extensive investigation into the expression in early vascular development of cell adhesion molecules, such as V-CAM-1[18] and PECAM[19] (Fig. 65–7) in addition to the β_1[20] and, more recently, the β_3 family of integrin receptors, especially $\alpha_v\beta_3$.[21] These molecules appear to direct interactions between endothelial and smooth muscle cells, and the extracellular matrix and perturbations of these interactions lead to malformation of the pulmonary and systemic arteries. The β_1 family of integrins bind fibronectin, and the β_3 family also bind fibronectin as well as a host of matrix molecules, but especially tenascin, osteopontin, and vitronectin, some of which have been shown to govern vascular cell migration (e.g., fibronectin)[22-25] and proliferation (e.g., tenascin).[26] In addition, a variety of growth factors also appear to be responsible for the orderly growth and branching morphogenesis of blood vessels. These include vascular endothelial growth factor (VEGF),[27] particularly VEGF A and D,[28] and angiopoietin,[29] as well as acidic and basic fibroblast growth factor (FGF-1 and FGF-2).[30] Recently, it has been suggested that these growth factors promote the induction of stromal derived factor-1,[31] a chemokine for endothelial cells bearing the receptor CXCR4, which is also induced.

Growth and matrix (especially elastin and collagen) production in blood vessels is regulated by insulin-like growth factor-1[32, 33] and transforming growth factor (TGF)-β.[34] Insulin-like growth factor-1 and its receptor act in concert with VEGF to stimulate fetal vascular growth through the same intracellular signaling pathways.[33] Platelet-derived growth factor contributes to aberrant vascular development in response to hypoxia.[35] Growth factors are regulated in their function by specific tyrosine kinase receptors, such as flt-1 and flk-1, tek, and tie,[36-38] as well as the activin receptor-like kinase (Alk)-1[39] and bone morphogenetic protein receptor II. Alk-1 has been implicated in the later stages of vasculogenesis, and a mutation is associated with hereditary hemorrhagic telangiectasia,[40] whereas BMPR II mutations are found in primary pulmonary hypertension.[41] Using a flk-1 reporter construct, Schachtner and colleagues[42] found lung vascular development at all stages of lung growth. Notch and Jagged1 interaction are associated with early stages of lung vascular development.[43]

The regulation of growth factor interaction with cell surface molecules is also determined by the balance between proteases and antiproteinases. Plasmin, thrombin,[44,45] and elastases, including

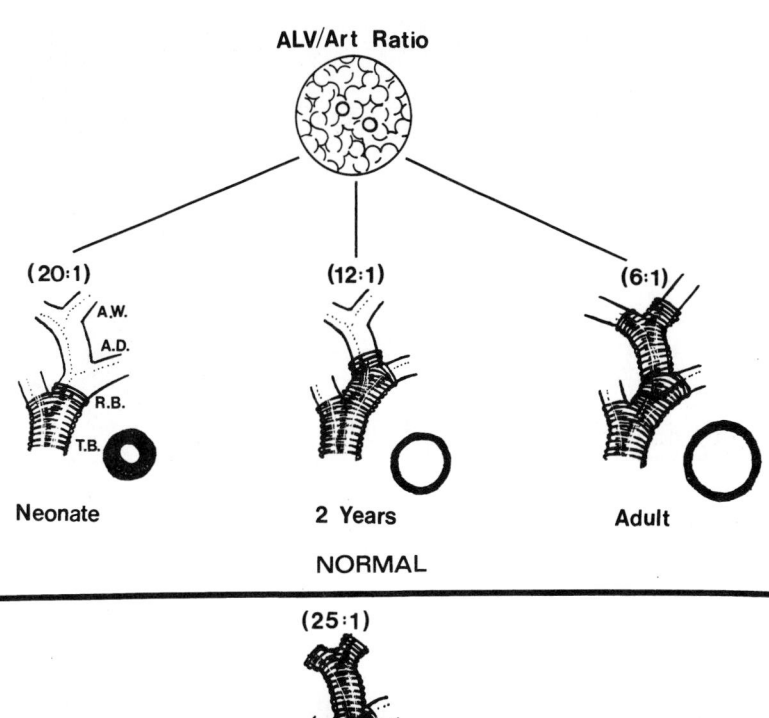

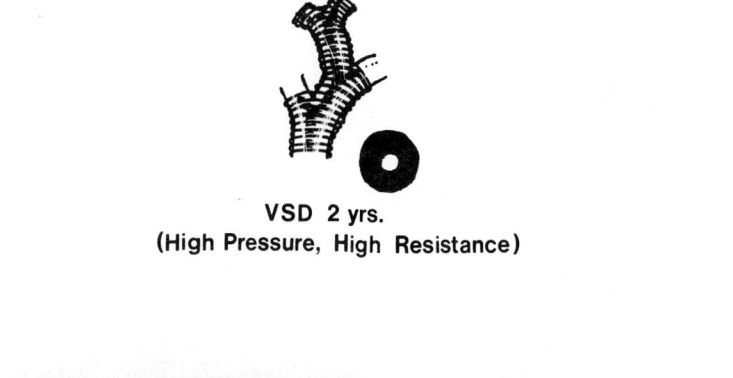

Figure 65–4. Schema showing peripheral pulmonary arterial development through morphometric changes: extension of muscle into peripheral arteries, percent wall thickness, and artery number (alveolar/arterial ratio), as they relate to age. *Upper panel*, Normal development. *Bottom panel*, Abnormalities in all three features in a 2-year-old child with a hypertensive ventricular septal defect (VSD). T.B. = artery accompanying a terminal bronchiolus; R.B. = artery accompanying a respiratory bronchiolus; A.D. = artery accompanying an alveolar duct; A.W. = artery accompanying an alveolar wall; ALV/Art = alveolar-arterial. (From Rabinovitch M, et al: Circulation *58*:1107, 1978.)

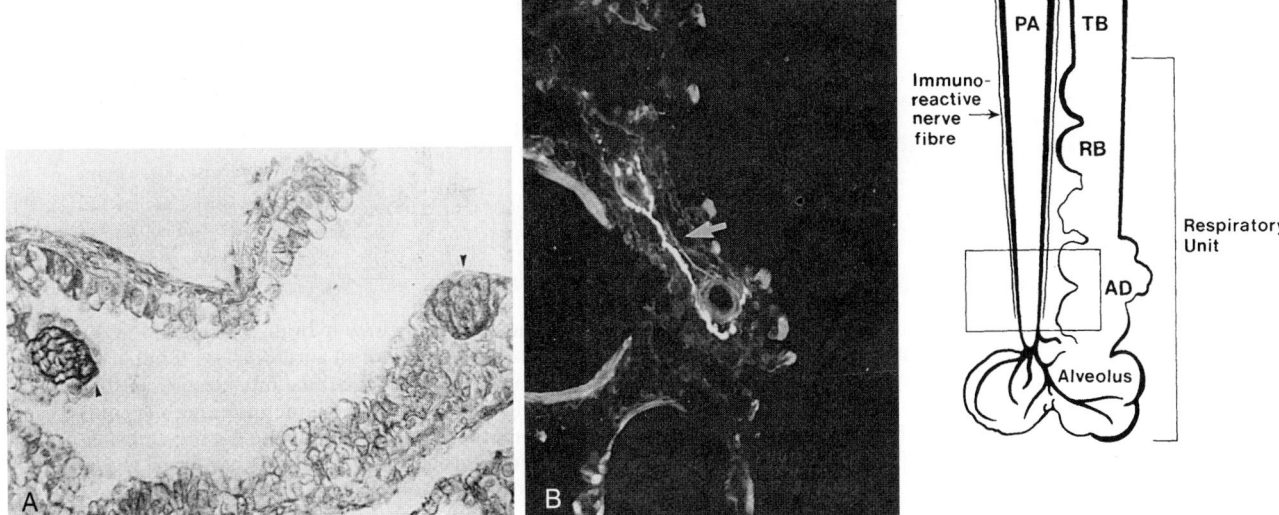

Figure 65–5. A, Neuroepithelial bodies (*arrowheads*) are seen as dark-staining regions (immunoreactive for serotonin) in the airway of a newborn infant. (From Rabinovitch M: Pathophysiology of pulmonary hypertension. *In* Emmanouilides GC, et al [eds]: Moss and Adams Heart Disease in Infants, Children, and Adolescents Including the Fetus and Young Adult. Baltimore, Williams & Wilkins, 1995, pp 1659–1695. Original supplied by E. Cutz, Hospital for Sick Children.) **B,** Tyrosine hydroxylase immunoreactive perivascular nerve fibers (*arrow*) at the advential-medial border of an alveolar duct artery in a child aged 2.5 years. Diagram on the right shows terminal bronchiolus (*TB*) and airways of respiratory unit accompanied by an innervated pulmonary artery (*PA*). RB = respiratory bronchiolus; AD = alveolar duct. Square indicates area shown in **B.** (From Allen KM, et al: Br Heart J *62*:353, 1989.)

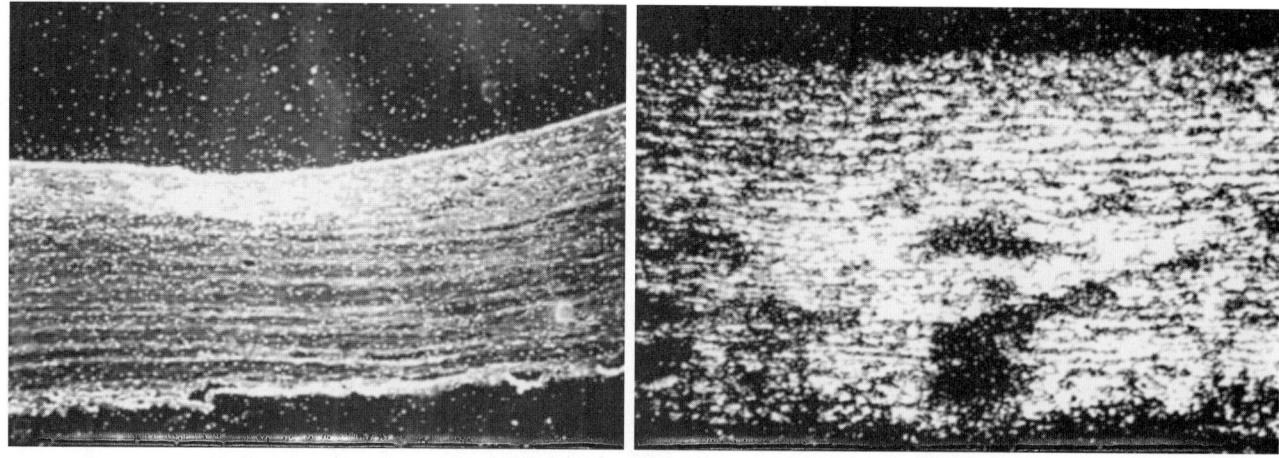

Figure 65–6. *In situ* hybridization localization of tropoelastin mRNA in control and hypertensive vessels from neonatal calves. White staining over areas indicates tropoelastin mRNA labeling. In normotensive vessels (*left*), labeled cells (^{35}S-labeled T66-T7) were confined to the inner media. Minimal signal is noted in the outer vessel wall. In vessels from hypertensive animals (14 days of hypoxia) (*right*), intense autoradiographic signal was observed throughout the media, albeit in a patchy distribution. (From Prosser IW, et al: Am J Pathol *135*:1073, 1989.)

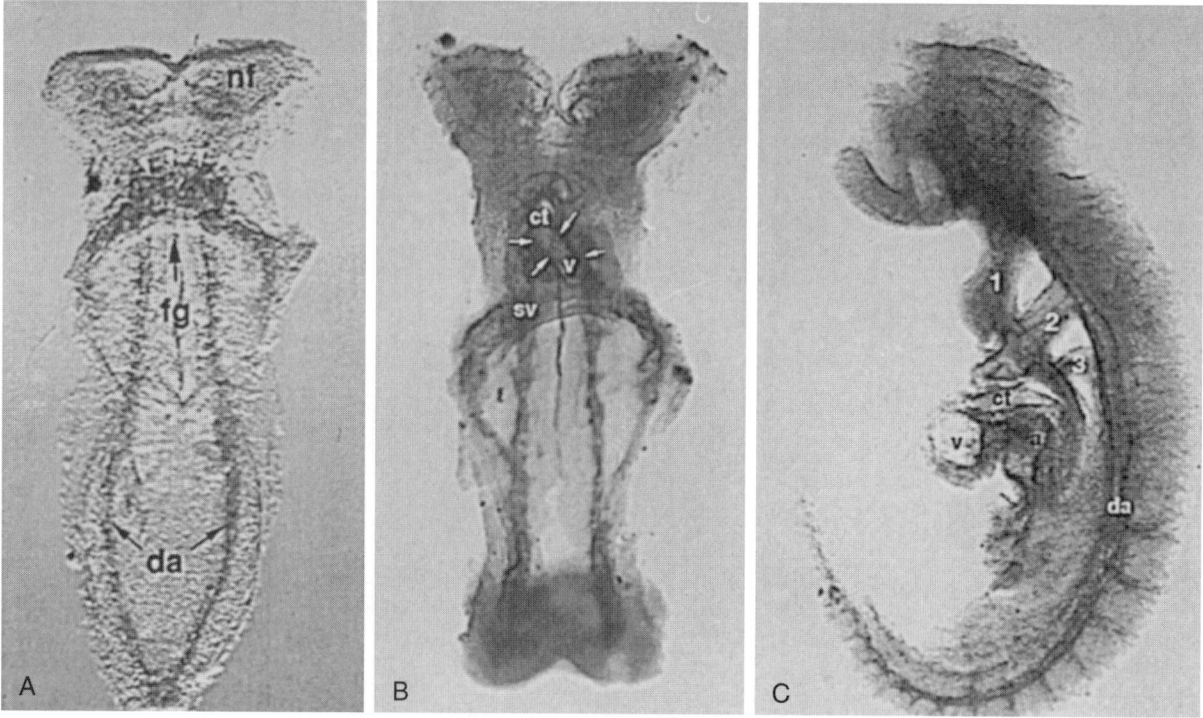

Figure 65–7. Early vascular development in the mouse embryo as defined by whole-mount *in situ* hybridization with PECAM-1 (CD31) riboprobes. **A,** Day 7.5 mouse embryo (four somites) showing an organized bilateral dorsal aorta (*da*) with initial formation of a vascular plexus in the cardiogenic crescent just cranial to the developing foregut (*fg*). **B,** Sequential organization of the endocardial cell of the vascular plexus (*arrows*) in the 8.5-day embryo (six to eight somites) into a lumen forming the sinus (*sv*), ventricle (*v*), and conotruncus (*ct*). **C,** Definitive organization of endothelial cells into the vascular template for the embryo, including clearly defined endocardium of the atrium (*a*), ventricle (*v*), and conotruncus (*ct*) as well as the pharyngeal arches 1 to 3 and dorsal aorta (*da*). (From Baldwin HS: Cardiovasc Res *31*:E34, 1996, with kind permission of Elsevier Science-NL.)

leukocyte and endogenous vascular elastase,[46] have all been shown to release growth factors from storage sites in the extracellular matrix in an active form. In addition, a variety of endogenously expressed inhibitors of proteinases and elastases, such as plasminogen activator inhibitor[47] and elafin,[48] control growth and development, and other classes of molecules are known to control

angiogenesis, such as angiostatin, a molecule that appears to be derived from plasminogen.[49]

The expression of vasoactive peptides in the lung during development also may play a role in the development of the pulmonary vasculature. Endothelin has been associated with cell proliferation and nitric oxide with the suppression of smooth

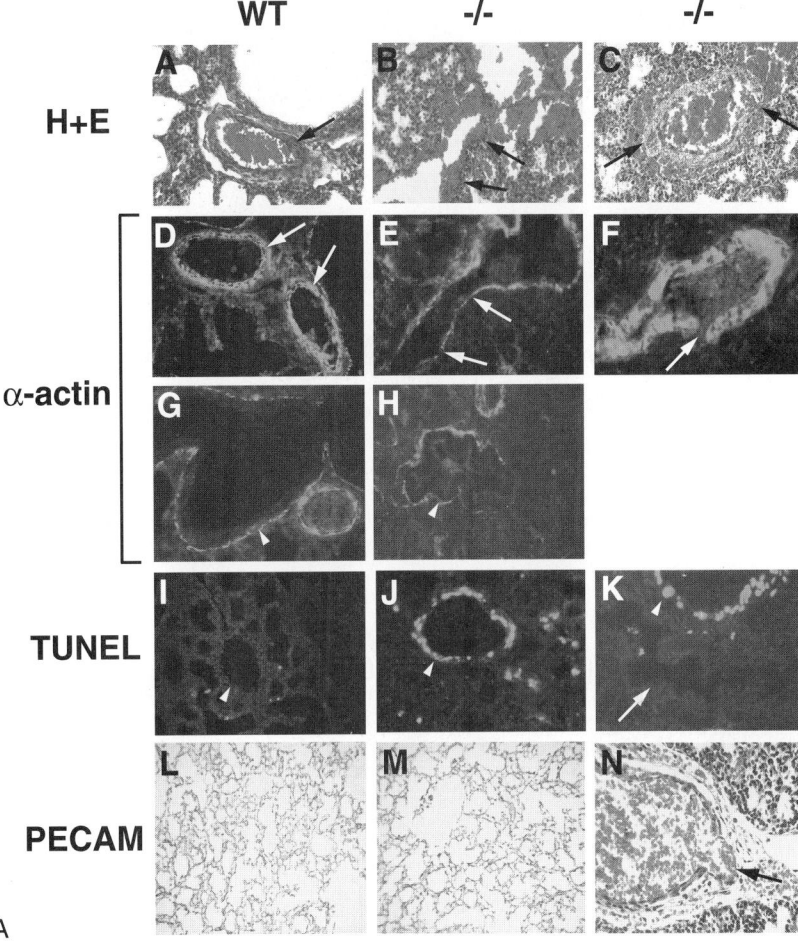

WT -/- -/-

H+E

α-actin

TUNEL

PECAM

Figure 65–8. A, **Defective smooth muscle integrity in** *Wnt7b^{lacZ}-/-* **embryos and mice** (see also color plates). Close examination of blood vessels in wild-type (*A, arrow*) and *Wnt7b^{lacZ}-/-* P0 neonates (*B, C*) reveals several breaches in the vessel wall in *Wnt7b^{lacZ}-/-* mice. In some instances, very little of the structure of the wall is left (*B, arrows*), while in others a thicker vessel wall with several ruptures is observed (*C, arrows*). Staining of sections with an antibody against smooth muscle α-actin shows robust staining surrounding blood vessels in wild-type neonates (*D, arrows*). Smooth muscle α-actin staining shows reduced staining, suggesting degradation of smooth muscle surrounding some vessels in *Wnt7b^{lacZ}-/-* neonates (*E, arrows*), while other vessels show frank breaches in the hypertrophic vessel wall (*F*). Bronchial smooth muscle appears normal in both wild-type (*G, arrowhead*) and *Wnt7b^{lacZ}-/-* neonates (*H, arrowhead*). TUNEL staining shows an increase in TUNEL-positive cells in the smooth muscle of the blood vessel wall in *Wnt7b^{lacZ}-/-* neonates (*J, arrowhead*) but not in bronchial smooth muscle (*K, arrow*). This is not observed in wild-type littermates (*I, arrow*). PECAM staining reveals a normal endothelial network in wild-type (*L*) and *Wnt7b^{lacZ}-/-* neonates (*M*). Many large blood vessels showed rupture of the smooth muscle layer, with herniation of the intact endothelial cell layer (*N, arrow*).

A

muscle cell growth,[50] and the early expression of nitric oxide synthase,[51] and it likely regulates vasculogenesis in addition to vascular tone. Work on transcription factors that control vascular smooth muscle cell differentiation should shed light on the genes that are programmed at various stages of development to control pulmonary vascular morphogenesis. A variety of transcription factors have been implicated in vascular development; these include Wnt7b,[52] which regulates investment of smooth muscle cells around the endothelial framework (Fig. 65-8), as well as TAL1[53] and Foxp,[54] which are implicated in vasculogenesis from precursor cells of the hematopoietic lineage.

ABNORMAL LUNG GROWTH

Underdevelopment of the lung parenchyma and associated pulmonary vasculature[1] is associated with congenital diaphragmatic hernia,[55] hypoplastic or dysplastic lungs, scimitar syndrome, and oligohydramnios secondary to renal agenesis and dysplasia. Pulmonary hypoplasia is also a feature of prematurity, absence of the phrenic nerve, asphyxiating thoracic dystrophy, rhesus isoimmunization, and, experimentally, amniocentesis[56] and smoking.[57]

Reversible or irreversible pulmonary artery hypertension and right-to-left shunting from birth can be a direct result of derangement or hypoplasia of the pulmonary vascular bed, or both. In addition to the structural changes in the vessels, heightened pulmonary vascular resistance also can be attributed to impaired gas exchange (hypoxia, hypercapnia). In infants with congenital diaphragmatic hernia, reversal of pulmonary hypertension has been achieved with the use of vasodilators,[58] extracorporeal membrane oxygenation (ECMO) (or high-frequency oscilla-

tion),[59] and nitric oxide alone or in combination with phosphodiesterase inhibitors.[60] Infants with hypoplastic lungs that had been refractory to nitric oxide before ECMO have demonstrated a beneficial effect from nitric oxide after ECMO. The expectation is that the reduction in pulmonary artery resistance will stimulate regression of vascular changes and maturation in growth of the pulmonary arteries.

Although the degree of arterial muscularity may predict whether the pulmonary vascular bed will be reactive, in studies of infants who succumbed after attempt at repair of congenital diaphragmatic hernia, a striking decrease in the number of alveoli and associated arteries was the major determinant of mortality (Fig. 65-9). This is probably why attempts to reverse severe pulmonary hypertension with nitric oxide have been less successful in this group of patients. Recent studies in experimental models of diaphragmatic hernia in lambs have indicated that endothelin A receptor blockade and endothelin B receptor-stimulated might reverse pulmonary hypertension[61] and that soluble guanylate cyclase activity is reduced.[62] It was also shown that vitamin A might stimulate lung maturation in a nitrofen-induced model of congenital diaphragmatic hernia.[63] Inflation of the lungs *in utero* via occlusion of the trachea has been proposed to help mature the lung.[64,65] Future strategies to improve lung growth may come from understanding underlying transcription factor pathways that are repressed, such as the sonic hedgehog pathway.[66]

In lungs studied at postmortem from infants with pulmonary hypoplasia or dysplasia, a reduced number of arteries is observed, appropriate to the reduced number of airways (see Fig. 65-9). The arteries are also generally small but not incompatible with the

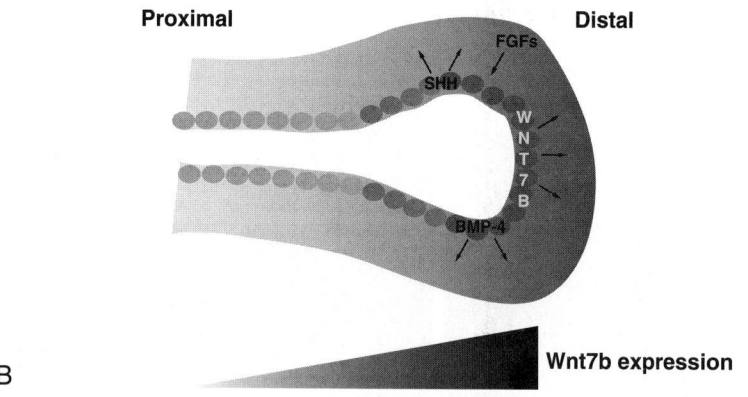

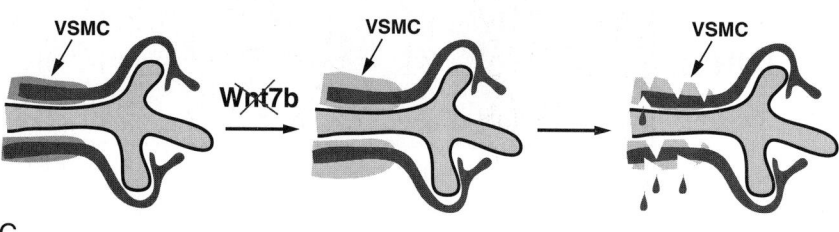

Figure 65–8—cont'd. B, A model for the role of *Wnt7b* in lung development (see also color plates). **B,** *Wnt7b* is expressed at the distal tips of the airway epithelium in a pattern similar to that observed with BMP4 and overlapping that of SHH. In addition, *Wnt7b* is expressed in an increasing gradient from the proximal-to-distal airway epithelium. FGFs are expressed in the mesenchyme and are known to regulate epithelia branching and proliferation. However, because BMP-4 and SHH expression are unchanged in *Wnt7b^lacZ-/-* embryos and *Wnt7b* expression is unchanged in *Shh*-null mice, *Wnt7b* regulates mesenchymal proliferation and differentiation through a unique pathway. **C,** Lung vasculature is composed of both endothelium (red) and vascular smooth muscle (VSMC, blue), and develops in parallel with the airways (green). Loss of *Wnt7b* function results in defects in vascular smooth muscle differentiation and/or survival, leading to a hypertrophic response (change from dark blue to light blue), degradation of the vessel wall, and eventual rupture of the weakened vessels. (FBFs = fibroblast growth factors; BMP = bone morphogenetic protein.) (From Shu W, et al: Development *129*:4831, 2002.)

size of the lung. Also, although the arteries, both centrally and peripherally, may be more muscular than normal, as in congenital diaphragmatic hernia, there may be hypoplasia of the pulmonary musculature, as in renal agenesis. Dysplasias of the lung associated with persistent pulmonary hypertension of the newborn (e.g., alveolar capillary dysplasia) (Fig. 65–10)[67] are currently so refractory to treatment that a biopsy should probably be done to guide clinical management.

Experimental studies carried out in newborn lambs and rabbits have shown that heparin can stimulate remodeling of the pulmonary circulation.[68] Accelerated maturation of the pulmonary circulation was achieved by inducing an increase in the number of peripheral pulmonary arteries relative to alveoli. This therapeutic strategy might prove clinically useful in inducing the growth of peripheral arteries and thereby reducing pulmonary vascular resistance.

FAILURE TO REVERSE ELEVATED PULMONARY VASCULAR RESISTANCE

Perinatal stress (e.g., hemorrhage, hypoglycemia, aspiration, or hypoxia) may result in failure of dilation of normally muscular vessels and left ventricular dysfunction, both contributing to persistent pulmonary hypertension. The use of inhaled nitric oxide in clinical studies,[69] L-arginine in experimental studies,[70] as well as gene transfer of endothelial nitric oxide synthase[71] and strategies to maximize dilator effects owing to cyclic guanosine monophosphate (GMP) by inhibiting phosphodiesterases[72] have all proved effective in lowering pulmonary artery pressure.

Because increased production of endothelin may underlie the pathophysiology of persistent pulmonary hypertension of the newborn,[73] the use of endothelin receptor blockade or endothelial converting-enzyme inhibition[74] may prove beneficial, especially if specificity could be controlled to maximize dilatory activity.[75]

That is, endothelin A receptors and endothelin B constrictor (as opposed to endothelin B dilator) receptors should be targeted.

INDUCTION OF VASCULAR ABNORMALITIES

In Utero

Structural studies of the lung at postmortem in fatal cases of meconium aspiration suggest that there were antecedent pulmonary vascular abnormalities that exacerbated the postnatal pulmonary hypertension.[76] The most striking feature is the presence of muscle in arteries small and peripheral in location and normally nonmuscular. The muscle cells are surrounded by darkly stained elastic laminae, suggesting that they formed several weeks before death and therefore *in utero*. Clinical studies have suggested a relationship between maternal ingestion of prostaglandin synthetase inhibitors and subsequent persistent pulmonary hypertension.[77] There is, however, a large population of women who take aspirin or indomethacin during pregnancy, and a low incidence of persistent pulmonary hypertension occurs in their newborn infants. Conversely, in the majority of infants with persistent pulmonary hypertension, no history of maternal ingestion of these compounds can be documented. Experimental studies in lambs have shown that prostaglandin synthetase inhibitors constrict the ductus arteriosus *in utero*. Chronic indomethacin treatment in pregnant rats produces structural changes in the pulmonary vascular bed of the newborn.[78] Thus, it seems likely that, in an occasional susceptible human fetus, there may be a relationship between prostaglandin synthetase inhibitors and persistent pulmonary hypertension.

Chronic maternal hypoxemia in experimental guinea pigs has not reproduced the structural and physiologic changes of pulmonary hypertension.[79] In lambs, the clinical syndrome has been produced by administration of a cytokine associated with

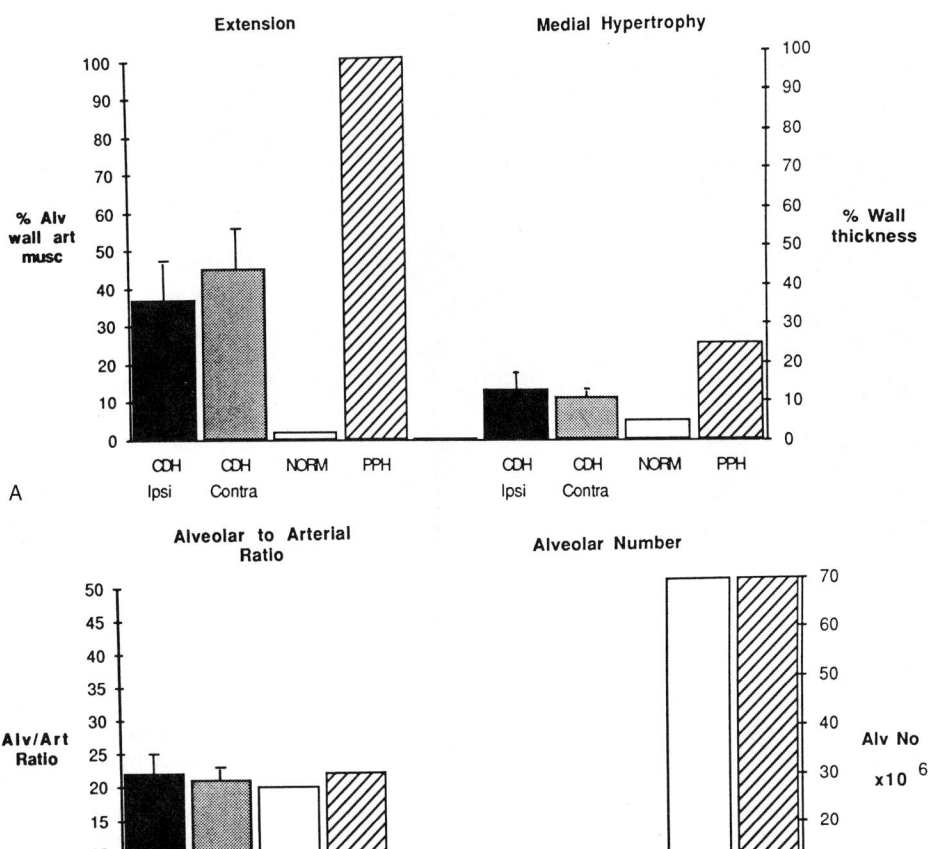

Figure 65–9. A, Morphometric data from nine patients with congenital diaphragmatic hernia (CDH), compared with published values in normal neonates and in infants with idiopathic persistent pulmonary hypertension of the newborn (PPH). Infants with CDH had greater smooth muscle extension into peripheral arteries and increased medial hypertrophy than normal infants but less than infants with PPH. **B,** Morphometric data from 6 infants with CDH compared with normal neonates and infants with PPH. Alveolar/arterial ratio was similar to that in normal infants, but total alveolar number was severely reduced in both ipsilateral and contralateral lungs. (From Bohn D, et al: J Pediatr *111*:423, 1987.)

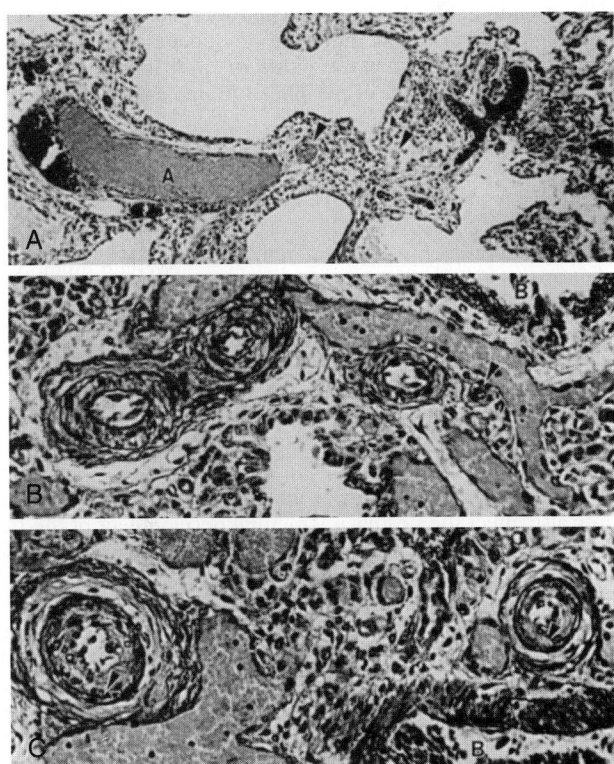

Figure 65–10. Lung micrographs from the left (**A**) and right (**B, C**) lungs of a patient with alveolar capillary dysplasia. **A,** Barium distends the lumen of a preacinar artery (*A*) but does not enter the anomalous vein to the left of the artery. Intra-acinar arterial branches that contain barium are identified (*arrowheads*), but intra-acinar veins and venules are distended with red blood cells, presumably forced ahead of the barium by the postmortem angiogram. Air spaces are lined by cuboidal epithelium, and no luminal capillaries are seen, all vessels lying centrally in the air space walls. (Hematoxylin and eosin, ×90.) **B,** Intra-acinar pulmonary arteries showing medial muscular thickening that forms a continuous layer even in the smallest branch (*arrowhead*), which is 20 μm in external diameter. Media is demarcated by external and internal elastic laminae, stained black in this elastic stain. A bronchiole is identified (*B*). (Elastic–van Gieson, ×220.) **C,** Intra-acinar arteries, the smaller measuring 60 μm in external diameter, with concentric intimal fibrosis; the latter is overlaid by *arrowheads* that mark the internal elastic laminae. The media is narrow in these branches, but note that the lumen (containing festooned endothelial cells) is the same size as in the similar-sized arteries seen in *B*. (Elastic–van Gieson, ×220.) (From Cullinane C, et al: Pediatr Pathol *12*:499, 1992. Reproduced with permission. All rights reserved.)

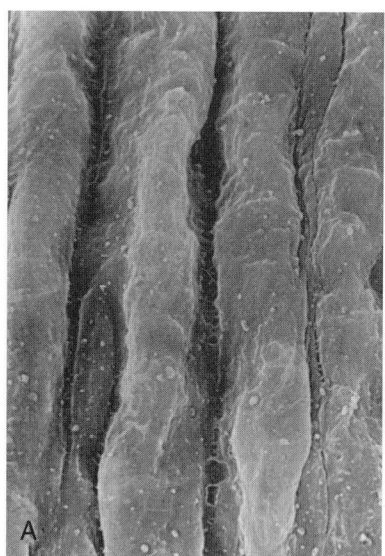
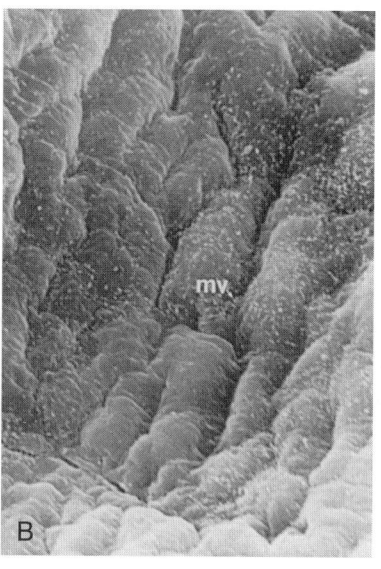

Figure 65–11. Scanning electron photomicrographs of pulmonary artery endothelium. A, Normal pulmonary artery shows corduroy pattern, closely aligned ridges. **B,** Hypertensive pulmonary artery shows cable pattern, deep knotted ridges, and numerous microvilli (*mv*) (×810). (From Rabinovitch M, et al: Lab Invest 55:632, 1986.)

inflammation (i.e., tumor necrosis factor-α).[80] Relatively short periods of hypoxia in the fetal lamb result in sustained elevation of pulmonary artery pressure and structural changes in the pulmonary arteries. *In utero* closure or constriction of the ductus arteriosus has proved to simulate the structural changes and the initial hemodynamic profile of persistent pulmonary hypertension.[81,82] Recently, an intriguing observation between increased superoxide generation and pulmonary hypertension has been established in this model,[83] suggesting a potential for treatment with superoxide dismutase.[84] This would also help explain the refractoriness of this particular group of patients to nitric oxide[85] and would be in keeping with the elevated levels of soluble guanylate cyclase and phosphodiesterase.[86]

Although the mechanism is not established, changes in the regulation of production of vasodilators and vasoconstrictors may be pertinent. That is, because nitric oxide can induce angiogenesis and endothelin may be a mitogen for smooth muscle cells, one might speculate that increased production of endothelin or reduced production of nitric oxide *in utero* might lead to an increase in muscularity of peripheral pulmonary arteries and a reduction in their number.

As previously discussed, smooth muscle cells with differences in potential for proliferation and for production and accumulation of extracellular matrix connective tissue components may also be differentially responsive to stimuli that perturb the pulmonary vasculature. Conversely, structural remodeling of the pulmonary circulation affects the responsivity to vasodilator stimuli. For example, increased adventitial thickening, as observed in hypoxia-induced neonatal pulmonary hypertension, may prevent the access of nitric oxide to the vascular smooth muscle cells.[87]

ALTERED POSTNATAL PULMONARY VASCULAR DEVELOPMENT

Hypoxia, hyperoxia, toxins, or alterations in pulmonary blood flow also affect the postnatal structural development of the pulmonary vascular bed in infancy and childhood. We have shown in clinical studies that high flow and pressure induce increasing pulmonary hypertension in association with progressive vascular abnormalities.[88] First, there is extension of muscle into peripheral, normally nonmuscular arteries (morphometric grade A). This is followed by medial hypertrophy of muscular arteries (grade B = Heath Edwards Grade I)[89] and reduced arterial concentration (morphometric grade C), associated with increased pulmonary artery pressure and resistance.[88] There is also the

concomitant development of neointimal formation. This is initiated by cellular changes (Heath Edwards Grade II), which further progress to occlusive fibroproliferative lesions (Grade III) and culminate in plexiform networks of obstructed and dilated vessels (Grade IV). The potential for reversibility of these changes is dictated by their severity; for example, Grade I-B almost always regresses following removal of the abnormal hemodynamic stimulus, whereas the loss of arteries (grade C) and the higher Heath Edwards grades generally regress or remain functionally insignificant only if the hemodynamic insult is relieved in early infancy (first 8 months of life).[90]

To investigate the cellular mechanisms that control the pulmonary vascular abnormalities in congenital heart defects, we applied electron microscopy to the study of lung biopsy tissue. Endothelial changes were observed on scanning and transmission electron microscopy, suggesting a potential for altered interaction with circulating blood elements, such as platelets and leukocytes (Fig. 65–11).[91] There were also functional abnormalities reflected in increased production of von Willebrand factor.[92,93] In addition, alterations in the subendothelium, reflected in fragmentation of elastin, suggested that an elastolytic enzyme might be stimulating the remodeling process.[91]

EXPERIMENTAL PATHOPHYSIOLOGY OF PULMONARY HYPERTENSION

We have shown experimentally in infant rats that exposure to low oxygen (equivalent to 10% $F_{I_{O_2}}$) or hyperoxia (80% to 100% $F_{I_{O_2}}$), or to the toxin monocrotaline induces abnormal muscularization of peripheral arteries, medial hypertrophy of muscular arteries, and reduced arterial relative to alveolar density.[1] Although the pulmonary vascular abnormalities induced by changes in ambient oxygen may be largely reversible, monocrotaline-induced changes progress in the adult animal but not in the infant. Hyperoxia is especially associated with a failure of normal lung compliance and growth, whereas monocrotaline induces only alveolar abnormalities when given to neonatal rats.

Experimentally, we have related the induction of structural changes in pulmonary arteries to the increased activity of the endogenous vascular elastase (EVE).[94,95] Increased EVE is observed in rat pulmonary arteries several days after exposure to hypoxia or injection of monocrotaline. A second increase in elastase activity is seen in adult animals injected with monocrotaline but not in infant rats or adult or infant hypoxic rats in which there is potential for regression. A cause-and-effect relationship

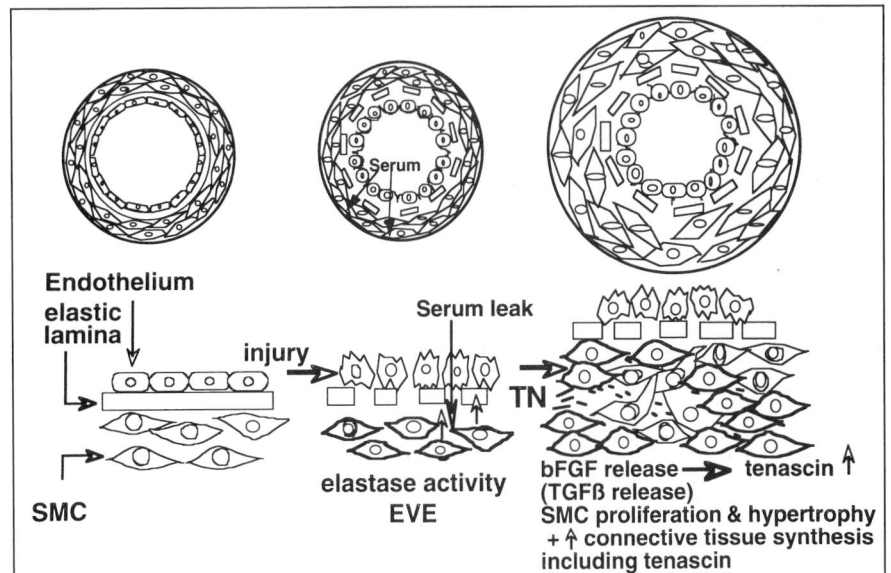

Figure 65–12. Schema describing relationship of elastase to pulmonary vascular disease. SMC = smooth muscle cell; TN = tenascin; EVE = endogenous vascular elastase; bFGF = basic fibroblast growth factor; TGFβ = transforming growth factor-beta. (From Rabinovitch M: *In* Emmanouilides GC, et al [eds]: Moss and Adams Heart Disease in Infants, Children, and Adolescents, Including the Fetus and Young Adult. Baltimore, Williams & Wilkins, 1995, pp 1659-1695.)

between elastase and the pathophysiology of pulmonary arterial changes and hypertension is further demonstrated in studies in which a variety of serine elastase inhibitors proved effective in preventing development or progression of pulmonary vascular changes and pulmonary hypertension (Fig. 65-12).[95,96]

The induction of elastase activity appears to be related to the functional changes associated with the perturbed endothelium, which result in loss of the barrier function. We speculated and subsequently showed *in vitro* that serum factors or endothelial factors that might gain access to the subendothelium when the barrier is lost can induce release of a serine elastase from pulmonary vascular smooth muscle cells.[97] This elastase can liberate biologically active smooth muscle cell mitogens, such as basic fibroblast growth factor (FGF) (FGF-2), from extracellular matrix stores.[46]

The resulting smooth muscle cell hyperplasia contributes to the hypertrophy of the arterial wall. Release of other growth factors, such as transforming growth factor-β (TGF-β), which can induce increased synthesis of elastin and collagen, might also add to the thickening. We have shown further that there is also induction of the matrix glycoprotein tenascin,[98] which interacts cooperatively with growth factors, such as epidermal growth factor and basic FGF, in inducing the proliferative response in the vessel wall. Having shown that hyperoxia-induced pulmonary hypertension and altered lung compliance in newborn rats could also be largely prevented with the use of elastase inhibitors,[99] we initiated a clinical trial with promising results in preventing and reducing the severity of bronchopulmonary dysplasia in premature infants.[100]

DECREASED GROWTH OF THE PULMONARY VASCULAR BED

Reduced pulmonary blood flow and pressure may also result in reduced growth of the pulmonary vascular bed with relative hypomuscularity of vessels that are decreased in size and number. This can be further aggravated by suppressed growth of the lung parenchyma, which can also be a feature of low pulmonary blood supply.[4]

PULMONARY VENOUS ABNORMALITIES

Pulmonary venous abnormalities are among the least likely to regress with surgical or interventional cardiologic approaches. We created a neonatal piglet model of progressive pulmonary venous obstruction and showed that there was altered compliance of the veins, which was reflected in an increase in pulmonary arterial pressure.[101] This preceded the elevation in pulmonary venous pressure, which occurred later when there was evidence of some compromise of the vessel lumen by the intimal lesion. At this stage, there was a disproportionate increase in collagen in the vessel wall, which likely further contributed to the hemodynamic abnormality and the resistance to successful intervention.

CLINICAL IMPLICATIONS

The reduced growth of the pulmonary circulation may pose a contraindication for surgery using the Fontan principle.[102] Also, consideration of patients for cavopulmonary anastomoses in preparation for a final-stage Norwood operation must take into account the left-sided obstructive lesion–induced vascular changes, consisting of increased muscularity of pulmonary arteries and veins, because these are associated with heightened pulmonary vascular reactivity. Studies from our group aimed at accelerating the structural maturation of the lung through the use of heparin have shown that both dilation and recruitment of small vessels can be affected, and this may prove of benefit in allowing surgical correction of complex congenital heart disease in the newborn infant.

CONCLUSION

Increasing knowledge of the genes that control vascular cell phenotype and differentiation and their regulation in development will lead to new and fruitful directions in preventing or reversing abnormal structural development of the lung.

REFERENCES

1. Rabinovitch M: Pathophysiology of pulmonary hypertension. *In* Emmanouilides GC, et al (eds): Moss and Adams Heart Disease in Infants, Children, and Adolescents, Including the Fetus and Young Adult. Baltimore, Williams & Wilkins, 1995, pp 1659-1695.
2. Hislop A, Reid L: Intrapulmonary arterial development during fetal life. Branching pattern and structure. J Anat *113*:35, 1972.
3. Goldstein J, et al: Unusual vascular anomalies causing persistent pulmonary hypertension in a newborn. Am J Cardiol *43*:962, 1979.
4. Rabinovitch M, et al: Growth and development of the pulmonary vascular bed in patients with tetralogy of Fallot with and without pulmonary atresia. Circulation *64*:1234, 1981.

5. Rabinovitch M, et al: Compression of intrapulmonary bronchi by abnormally branching pulmonary arteries associated with absent pulmonary valves. Am J Cardiol 50:804, 1982.

6. Hall SM, Haworth SG: Normal adaptation of pulmonary arterial intima to extrauterine life in the pig: ultrastructural study. J Pathol 149:55, 1986.

7. Hislop A, Reid L: Pulmonary arterial development during childhood: branching pattern and structure. Thorax 28:129, 1973.

8. Meyrick B, Reid L: Ultrastructural findings in lung biopsy material from children with congenital heart defects. Am J Pathol 101:527, 1980.

9. Jones R: Ultrastructural analysis of contractile cell development in lung microvessels in hyperoxic pulmonary hypertension: fibroblasts and intermediate cells selectively reorganize nonmuscluar segments. Am J Pathol 141:1491, 1993.

10. Allen KM, et al: A study of nerves containing peptides in the pulmonary vasculature of healthy infants and children and of those with pulmonary hypertension. Br Heart J 62:353, 1989.

11. Cutz E, et al: Pulmonary neuroendocrine cells in normal human lung and in pulmonary hypertension. Lab Invest 54:14A, 1986.

12. Prosser I, et al: Regional heterogeneity of elastin and collagen gene expression in intralobar arteries in response to hypoxic pulmonary hypertension as demonstrated by in situ hybridization. Am J Pathol 135:1073, 1989.

13. Durmowicz A, et al: Persistence, re-expression and induction of pulmonary arterial fibronectin, tropoelastin, and type I procollagen mRNA expression in neonatal hypoxic pulmonary hypertension. Am J Pathol 145:1411, 1994.

14. Allen K, Haworth S: Human postnatal pulmonary arterial remodeling: ultrastructural studies of smooth muscle cell and connective tissue maturation. Lab Invest 48:702, 1988.

15. Frid MG, et al: Multiple phenotypically distinct smooth muscle cell populations exist in the adult and developing bovine pulmonary arterial media in vivo. Circ Res 75:669, 1994.

16. Das M, et al: Enhanced growth factor of fetal and neonatal pulmonary artery adventitial fibroblasts is dependent on protein kinase C. Am J Physiol 269:L660, 1995.

17. Baldwin HS: Early embryonic vascular development. Cardiovasc Res 31:E34, 1996.

18. Kwee L, et al: Defective development of the embryonic and extraembryonic circulatory systems in vascular cell adhesion molecule (VCAM-1) deficient mice. Development 121:489, 1995.

19. Baldwin H, et al: Platelet endothelial cell adhesion molecule-1 (PECAM-1/CD31): alternatively spliced, functionally distinct isoforms expressed during mammalian cardiovascular development. Development 120:2539, 1994.

20. Drake C, et al: Antibodies to beta 1-integrins cause alterations of aortic vasculogenesis, in vivo. Dev Dyn 193:83, 1992.

21. Drake C, et al: An antagonist of integrin alpha v beta 3 prevents maturation of blood vessels during embryonic neovascularization. J Cell Sci 108:2655, 1995.

22. Drake C, et al: Avian vasculogenesis and the distribution of collagens, I, IV, laminin, and fibronectin in the heart primordia. J Exp Zool 155:309, 1990.

23. Roman J, McDonald J: Expression of fibronectin, the integrin alpha 5, and alpha-smooth muscle actin in lung and heart development. Am J Respir Cell Mol Biol 6:472, 1992.

24. French F, et al: Patterns of fibronectin gene expression and splicing during cell migration in chicken embroys. Development 104:369, 1989.

25. Boudreau N, et al: Fibronectin, hyaluronan and a hyaluronan-binding protein contribute to increased ductus arteriosus smooth muscle cell migration. Dev Biol 143:235, 1991.

26. Jones PL, Rabinovitch M: Tenascin-C is induced with progressive pulmonary vascular disease in rats and is functionally related to increased smooth muscle cell proliferation. Circ Res 79:1131, 1996.

27. Drake CJ, Little CD: Exogenous vascular endothelial growth factor induces malformed and hyperfused vessels during embryonic neovascularization. Proc Natl Acad Sci U S A 92:7657, 1995.

28. Greenberg JM, et al: Mesenchymal expression of vascular endothelial growth factors D and A defines vascular patterning in developing lung. Dev Dyn 224:144, 2002.

29. Chinoy MR, et al: Angiopoietin-1 and VEGF in vascular development and angiogenesis in hypoplastic lungs. Am J Physiol Lung Cell Mol Physiol 283:L60, 2002.

30. Klein S, et al: Basic fibroblast growth factor modulates integrin expression in microvascular endothelial cells. Mol Biol Cell 4:973, 1993.

31. Salcedo R, et al: Vascular endothelial growth factor and basic fibroblast growth factor induce expression of CXCR4 on human endothelial cells: in vivo neovascularization induced by stromal-derived factor-1alpha. Am J Pathol 154:1125, 1999.

32. Wolfe BL, et al: Insulin-like growth factor-I regulates transcription of the elastin gene. J Biol Chem 268:12418, 1993.

33. Han RN, et al: Insulin-like growth factor-I receptor-mediated vasculogenesis/angiogenesis in human lung development. Am J Respir Cell Mol Biol 28:159, 2003.

34. Liu J, Davidson JM: The elastogenic effect of recombinant transforming growth factor-beta on porcine aortic smooth muscle cells. Biochem Biophys Res Commun 154:895, 1988.

35. Balasubramaniam V, et al: Role of platelet-derived growth factor in vascular remodeling during pulmonary hypertension in the ovine fetus. Am J Physiol Lung Cell Mol Physiol 284:L964,. 2003.

36. Dumont DJ, et al: Vascularization of the mouse embryo: a study of flk-1, tek, tie, and vascular endothelial growth factor expression during development. Dev Dyn 203:80, 1995.

37. Shalaby F, et al: Failure of blood-island formation and vasculogenesis in FLK-1 deficient mice. Nature 376:62, 1995.

38. Fong GH, et al: Role of the Flt-1 receptor tyrosine kinase in regulating the assembly of vascular endothelium. Nature 376:66, 1995.

39. Lamouille S, et al: Activin receptor-like kinase 1 is implicated in the maturation phase of angiogenesis. Blood 100:4495, 2002.

40. Trembath RC, Harrison R: Insights into the genetic and molecular basis of primary pulmonary hypertension. Pediatr Res 53:883, 2003.

41. Thomson JR, et al: Sporadic primary pulmonary hypertension is associated with germline mutations of the gene encoding BMPR-II, a receptor member of the TGF-beta family. J Med Genet 37:741, 2000.

42. Schachtner SK, et al: Qualitative and quantitative analysis of embryonic pulmonary vessel formation. Am J Respir Cell Mol Biol 22:157, 2000.

43. Taichman DB, et al: Notch1 and Jagged1 expression by the developing pulmonary vasculature. Dev Dyn 225:166, 2002.

44. Taipale J, et al: Human mast cell chymase and leukocyte elastase release latent transforming growth factor-β1 from the extracellular matrix of cultured human epithelial and endothelial cells. J Biol Chem 270:4689, 1995.

45. Saksela O, Rifkin DB: Release of basic fibroblast growth factor-heparan sulfate complexes from endothelial cells by plasminogen activator-mediated proteolytic degradation. J Cell Biol 107:743, 1990.

46. Thompson K, Rabinovitch M: Exogenous leukocyte and endogenous elastases can mediate mitogenic activity in pulmonary artery smooth muscle cells by release of extracellular matrix-bound basic fibroblast growth factor. J Cell Physiol 166:495, 1995.

47. Lee E, et al: Regulation of matrix metalloproteinases and plasminogen activator inhibitor-1 synthesis by plasminogen in cultured human vascular smooth muscle cells. Circ Res 78:44, 1996.

48. Sallenave JM, et al: Regulation of secretory leukocyte proteinase inhibitor (SLPI) and elastase-specific inhibitor (ESI/elafin) in human airway epithelial cells by cytokines and neutrophilic enzymes. Am J Respir Cell Mol Biol 1:733, 1994.

49. O'Reilly MS, et al: Angiostatin: a novel angiogenesis inhibitor that mediates the suppression of metastases by a Lewis lung carcinoma. Cell 79:315, 1994.

50. Ziegler JW, et al: The role of nitric oxide, endothelin, and prostaglandins in the transition of the pulmonary circulation (review). Clin Perinatol 22:387, 1995.

51. Halbower AC, et al: Maturation-related changes in endothelial nitric oxide synthase immunolocalization in developing ovine lung. Am J Physiol 267:L585, 1994.

52. Shu W, et al: Wnt7b regulates mesenchymal proliferation and vascular development in the lung. Development 129:4831, 2002.

53. Drake CJ, et al: TAL1/SCL is expressed in endothelial progenitor cells/angioblasts and defines a dorsal-to-ventral gradient of vasculogenesis. Dev Biol 192:17, 1997.

54. Lu MM, et al: Foxp4: a novel member of the Foxp subfamily of winged-helix genes co-expressed with Foxp1 and Foxp2 in pulmonary and gut tissues. Gene Expr Patterns 2:223, 2002.

55. Bohn D, et al: Ventilatory predictors of pulmonary hypoplasia in congenital diaphragmatic hernia confirmed by morphometric assessment. J Pediatr 111:423, 1987.

56. Hislop A, et al: The effect of amniocentesis and drainage of amniotic fluid on lung development in Macaca fascicularis. Br J Obstet Gynaecol 91:835, 1984.

57. Collins MH, et al: Fetal lung hypoplasia associated with maternal smoking: a morphometric analysis. Pediatr Res 19:408, 1989.

58. Karamanoukian HL, et al: Inhaled nitric oxide in congenital hypoplasia of the lungs due to diaphragmatic hernia or oligohydramnios. Pediatrics 94:715, 1994.

59. Schranz D, et al: Norepinephrine, enoximone and nitric oxide for treatment of myocardial stunning and pulmonary hypertension in a newborn with diaphragmatic hernia. J Pediatr 111:423, 1995.

60. Steinhorn RH, et al: Persistent pulmonary hypertension of the newborn: role of nitric oxide and endothelin in pathophysiology and treatment (review). Clin Perinatol 22:405, 1995.

61. Thebaud B, et al: ET(A)-receptor blockade and ET(B)-receptor stimulation in experimental congenital diaphragmatic hernia. Am J Physiol Lung Cell Mol Physiol 278:L923, 2000.

62. Thebaud B, et al: Altered guanylyl-cyclase activity in vitro of pulmonary arteries from fetal lambs with congenital diaphragmatic hernia. Am J Respir Cell Mol Biol 27:42, 2002.

63. Thebaud B, et al: Restoring effects of vitamin A on surfactant synthesis in nitrofen-induced congenital diaphragmatic hernia in rats. Am J Respir Crit Care Med 164:1083, 2001.

64. Davey MG, et al: Temporary tracheal occlusion in fetal sheep with lung hypoplasia does not improve postnatal lung function. J Appl Physiol 94:1054, 2003.

65. Chiba T, et al: Balloon tracheal occlusion for congenital diaphragmatic hernia: experimental studies. J Pediatr Surg 35:1566, 2000.

66. Unger S, et al: Down-regulation of sonic hedgehog expression in pulmonary hypoplasia is associated with congenital diaphragmatic hernia. Am J Pathol 162:547, 2003.

67. Cullinane C, et al: Persistent pulmonary hypertension of the newborn due to alveolar capillary dysplasia. Pediatr Pathol 12:499, 1992.

68. O'Blenes S, et al: Low molecular weight heparin and unfractionated heparin are both effective at accelerating pulmonary vascular maturation in neonatal rabbits. Circulation (submitted).
69. Kinsella JP, Abman SH: Recent developments in the pathophysiology and treatment of persistent pulmonary hypertension of the newborn. J Pediatr 126:853, 1995.
70. Cornfield DN, et al: Effects of birth-related stimuli on L-arginine-dependent pulmonary vasodilation in ovine fetus. Am J Physiol 262:H1474, 1992.
71. Aschner JL, et al: Endothelial nitric oxide synthase gene transfer enhances dilation of newborn piglet pulmonary arteries. Am J Physiol 277:H371, 1999.
72. Thusu KG, et al: The cGMP phosphodiesterase inhibitor zaprinast enhances the effect of nitric oxide. Am J Respir Crit Care Med 152:1605, 1995.
73. Rosenberg AA, et al: Elevated immunoreactive endothelin-1 levels in newborn infants with persistent pulmonary hypertension (see comments). J Pediatr 123:109, 1993.
74. Kirshbom PM, et al: Blockade of endothelin-converting enzyme reduces pulmonary hypertension after cardiopulmonary bypass and circulatory arrest. Surgery 118:440, 1995.
75. Perreault T, De Marte J: Endothelin-1 has a dilator effect on neonatal pit pulmonary vasculature. J Cardiovasc Pharmacol 18:43, 1991.
76. Murphy JD, et al: The structural basis of persistent pulmonary hypertension of the newborn infant. J Pediatr 98:962, 1981.
77. Manchester D, et al: Possible association between maternal indomethacin therapy and primary pulmonary hypertension of the newborn. Am J Obstet Gynecol 126:467, 1976.
78. Harker L, et al: Effects of indomethacin on the fetal rat lungs: a possible cause of persistent fetal circulation. Pediatr Res 15:147, 1981.
79. Murphy JD, et al: Effects of chronic in utero hypoxia on the pulmonary vasculature of the newborn guinea pig. Pediatr Res 20:292, 1986.
80. Truog WE, et al: Tumor necrosis factor–induced neonatal pulmonary hypertension: effect of dizmagral pretreatment. Pediatr Res 27:166, 1990.
81. McQueston JA, et al: Chronic pulmonary hypertension in utero impairs endothelium-dependent vasodilation. Am J Physiol 268:H288, 1995.
82. Zayek M, et al: Treatment of persistent pulmonary hypertension in the newborn lamb by inhaled nitric oxide. J Pediatr 122:743, 1993.
83. Brennan LA, et al: Increased superoxide generation is associated with pulmonary hypertension in fetal lambs. A role for NADPH oxidase. Circ Res 92:683, 2003.
84. Steinhorn RH, et al: Recombinant human superoxide dismutase enhances the effect of inhaled nitric oxide in persistent pulmonary hypertension. Am J Respir Crit Care Med 164:834, 2001.
85. Kelly LK, et al: Inhaled prostacyclin for term infants with persistent pulmonary hypertension refractory to inhaled nitric oxide. J Pediatr 141:830, 2002.
86. Black SM, et al: sGC and PDE5 are elevated in lambs with increased pulmonary blood flow and pulmonary hypertension. Am J Physiol Lung Cell Mol Physiol 281:L1051, 2001.
87. Steinhorn RH, et al: The adventitia may be a barrier specific to nitric oxide in rabbit pulmonary artery. J Clin Invest 94:1883, 1993.
88. Rabinovitch M, et al: Lung biopsy in congenital heart disease: a morphometric approach to pulmonary vascular disease. Circulation 58:1107, 1978.
89. Heath D, Edwards J: The pathology of hypertensive pulmonary vascular disease. Circulation 18:533, 1958.
90. Rabinovitch M, et al: Vascular structure in lung biopsy tissue correlated with pulmonary hemodynamic findings after repair of congenital heart defects. Circulation 69:655, 1984.
91. Rabinovitch M, et al: Pulmonary artery endothelial abnormalities in patients with congenital heart defects and pulmonary hypertension: a correlation of light with scanning electron microscopy and transmission electron microscopy. Lab Invest 55:632, 1986.
92. Rabinovitch M, et al: Abnormal endothelial factor VIII associated with pulmonary hypertension and congenital heart defects. Circulation 76:1043, 1987.
93. Turner-Gomes SO, et al: Abnormalities in von Willebrand factor and antithrombin III after cardiopulmonary bypass operations for congenital heart disease. Thorac Cardiovasc Surg 103:87, 1992.
94. Todorovich-Hunter L, et al: Increased pulmonary artery elastolytic activity in adult rats with monocrotaline-induced progressive hypertensive pulmonary vascular disease compared with infant rats with nonprogressive disease. Am Rev Respir Dis 146:213, 1992.
95. Maruyama K, et al: Chronic hypoxic pulmonary hypertension in rats and increased elastolytic activity. Am J Physiol 261:H1716, 1991.
96. Ye C, Rabinovitch M: Inhibition of elastolysis by SC-37698 reduces development and progression of monocrotaline pulmonary hypertension. Am J Physiol 261:H1255, 1991.
97. Jones PL, et al: Regulation of tenascin-C, a vascular smooth muscle cell survival factor that interacts with the $\alpha v \beta 3$ integrin to promote epidermal growth factor receptor phosphorylation and growth. J Cell Biol 139:279, 1997.
98. Kobayashi J, et al: Serum-induced vascular smooth muscle cell elastolytic activity through tyrosine kinase intracellular signalling. J Cell Physiol 160:121, 1994.
99. Koppel R, et al: α_1-Antitrypsin protects neonatal rats from pulmonary vascular and parenchymal effects of oxygen toxicity. Pediatr Res 36:763, 1994.
100. Stiskal J, et al: Alpha1-proteinase inhibitor (A1PI) therapy for the prevention of bronchopulmonary dysplasia (BPD) in premature infants. Pediatr Res 39:247a, 1996.
101. LaBourene JI, et al: Alterations in elastin and collagen related to the mechanism of progressive pulmonary venous obstruction in a piglet model: a hemodynamic, ultrastructural, and biochemical study. Circ Res 66:438, 1990.
102. Haworth SG, Reid L: Quantitative structural study of pulmonary circulation on the newborn with aortic atresia, stenosis or coarctation. Thorax 32:121, 1977.

David A. Clark and Upender K. Munshi

66

Development of the Gastrointestinal Circulation in the Fetus and Newborn

The rapid cellular growth of the intestine in fetal life requires sufficient substrate for energy and a way to clear metabolic waste. This is accomplished by a rapid and proportionate growth of the intestinal circulation. Although anatomic and histologic studies have been performed on salvaged human fetal intestines, lack of availability of samples and autolysis have precluded detailed and systematic studies of the physiology of the developing gastrointestinal circulation. Therefore, much of the information presented in this chapter is derived from controlled studies in animals. In addition, the most reliable data involve only that portion of the alimentary tract below the diaphragm, namely, the gastrointestinal and colonic circulations.

There are several principles of gut development that have an impact on intestinal blood flow. The cephalic portion of the embryonic intestinal tract develops and matures more rapidly than caudal areas.[1] As the gut intestinal lining rapidly multiplies, the embryonic ileum is obliterated and eventually recanalizes.

Although the intestine begins as a straight tube, differential growth rates result in the contrasting calibers of various gut segments and in the rotation and final positioning of various components.[2]

The arterial supply to the intestine does not develop in isolation but forms in response to the rapid growth of this organ. Most intestinal tract mucosa, along with the liver parenchyma and pancreas, is derived from endoderm. However, the connective tissue and muscular components are derived from splanchnopleuric mesoderm. Oral and anal epithelium are derived from the ectoderm of the stomatodeum and proctodeum, respectively. Progressing from the germ cell stage, the intestine is divided into three primary portions: the foregut, midgut, and hindgut.[2-4] The foregut includes all structures distal to the tracheal diverticulum from the esophagus through the first half of the duodenum. The midgut is composed of structures distal to the second portion of the duodenum, including the jejunum, ileum, and proximal two-thirds of the transverse colon. The hindgut consists of the distal transverse colon and the proximal two-thirds of the anal canal.

DEVELOPMENT OF INTESTINAL CIRCULATION

Early somite embryos have an extensive vascular network within the yolk sac. In the process of vasculogenesis, vascular endothelial precursor cells (angioblasts) migrate to the location of future vessels, coalesce into cords, differentiate into endothelial cells, and ultimately form patent vessels. Vascular endothelial growth factors and their receptors have been identified. Erythropoietin has been shown to stimulate vasculogenesis in neonatal rat mesenteric microvascular endothelial cells.[5] Unpaired ventral branches of the dorsal aorta (vitelline arteries) pass to the yolk sac, allantois, and chorion. The network drains by way of the vitelline veins to the heart. During the fourth week, the primitive gut is formed as the dorsal portion of the yolk sac is incorporated into the embryo. Three vitelline arteries persist to supply the foregut (celiac artery), midgut (superior mesenteric artery), and hindgut (inferior mesenteric artery).[2]

The vessels distributed to the foregut fuse and form a single vessel, the celiac artery. With a downward migration of the viscera, the aortic attachment of the celiac artery moves caudally. It divides into the hepatic artery, splenic artery, and left gastric branches to supply the stomach and duodenum. The liver, pancreas, and related mesodermal spleen receive their blood supply from these branches. At the vascular division between the foregut and midgut is the anastomosis between the superior pancreaticoduodenal and the inferior pancreaticoduodenal arteries.[4]

The embryonic vitelline arteries fuse to form a superior mesenteric trunk, which reaches the midgut by passing through the mesentery. Terminal branches of this trunk supply the yolk sac. The various branches distal to the intestine are obliterated when the ileum separates from the yolk sac and vitelline stalk. However, the superior mesenteric artery remains and supplies the intestinal circulation from the second part of the duodenum through the proximal two-thirds of the transverse colon.[3,4]

The ventral branches of the aorta supplying the hindgut fuse to form a single inferior mesenteric trunk. Its final distribution includes the distal one-third of the transverse colon and the entire descending colon and sigmoid. The inferior mesenteric trunk anastomoses with the middle colic artery, which is a branch of the superior mesenteric artery. Furthermore, distal to this, there is an anastomosis to branches of the inferior and middle rectal arteries from the internal iliac trunk.[2,3]

VENOUS DRAINAGE OF THE GASTROINTESTINAL TRACT

Venous drainage of the intestine is much more variable than arterial blood supply. The low-pressure venous drainage in the embryo is plexiform, and therefore patency is based somewhat on blood flow. In addition, blood has a tendency to seek the most direct route of flow because of hydrodynamic factors.

The vitelline veins initially pass along each side of the anterior intestinal portal vein. They form an anastomosing plexus around the developing duodenal loop in the substance of the septum transversum. Cords of liver cells extend into the septum transversum and divide the vitelline plexus into the primitive hepatic sinusoids. Anterior stems of the vitelline veins enter the primitive sinus venosus. As the stomach, duodenum, and small intestine elongate and rotate from their original midsagittal position to an adult position, blood flow develops along the most direct route to the liver, cutting from one vitelline vein to another through the connecting plexus. Thus, the portal venous system does not develop in a spiral fashion around the developing intestine but instead evolves in a short and straight fashion with the duodenum and intestine around it.[2,3]

In embryos of less than 5-mm crown-rump length (<5 weeks), blood from the paired umbilical veins passes into the liver at which point it communicates with the vitelline sinusoids. At a 7-mm crown-rump length (33–34 days), the right umbilical vein atrophies and disappears.[2] As a result, all placental blood entering the embryo enters through the left umbilical vein and empties into the hepatic sinusoids. As the right side of the sinus venosus elaborates, an enlargement of the hepatic sinusoidal communication occurs between the right hepatocardiac channel and the left umbilical vein to form the ductus venosus.[4] Thus, blood entering from either the umbilical or vitelline systems can pass by way of the ductus venosus to the right atrium or into the liver sinusoids. The venae advehentes, connecting the umbilical and vitelline systems to the hepatic sinusoids, become the branches of the portal vein in the liver. In addition, the venae revehentes connecting the sinusoids to the right hepatocardiac channel become the tributaries to the hepatic veins. After birth, the left umbilical vein and the ductus venosus are obliterated and become the ligamentum teres and the ligamentum venosum, respectively.[3]

THE INTESTINAL MICROCIRCULATION

The microscopic anatomy of the intestinal circulation varies from species to species. In rabbits and humans, villous arterioles ascend from the submucosal arterioles into the villus. As the arteriole reaches the villus tip, it divides into a diffused capillary network, which then drains into a centrally located villus venule originating in the distal one-third of the villus.[6] In most mammals, the capillaries of the intestinal villus are fenestrated. Just as the villus and the microvillus are exposed to a large solute and water load, so the villus capillaries must be capable of handling these absorbed materials. The endothelium of the capillary facing the epithelium is thin and usually contains fenestrae, with the greatest number at the villus tips and in the crypts.

Water and solutes are transported into the capillary by various different pathways (Fig. 66–1). Low molecular weight nonpolar substances and lipid-soluble substances such as oxygen and carbon dioxide may cross directly through the cell membrane. The bulk of absorbed materials passes through fenestrae, which are numerous circular openings of up to 30 nm in the capillary endothelium and may be either open or have a diaphragm.[6] At least 60% of the fenestrae have a diaphragm. Although the porosity is not known, these diaphragms limit the movement of molecules. Much less commonly, water and solutes move slowly by pinocytosis. In this process, vesicles are formed that move through the cell to the opposing side before releasing their contents. On rare occasions, transendothelial channels may be formed when several vesicles simultaneously open and bridge the cell. These occurrences are relatively infrequent and do not produce any major impact on total absorptive capacity. Intercellular junctions are impermeable to solutes of up to 2 nm diameter in the arteriole and capillary but may play a limited role in venule absorption.

CONTROL OF BLOOD FLOW

Numerous factors affect the maintenance of intestinal blood flow. They can be grouped into at least four major categories: cardiovascular status, neural control, humoral substances, and local control.[7-9] Although not many specific data are available about the fetal intestine in these areas, certain principles can be inferred as operative in the fetus.

Cardiovascular Function

Adequate perfusion of any tissue in the body depends on the maintenance of sufficient cardiac output and mean arterial pressure. Reduction in cardiac output or systemic arterial pressure

**VASCULAR
LUMEN**

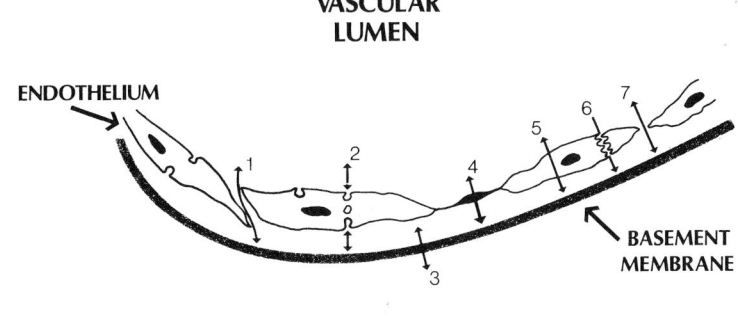

Figure 66–1. Transport pathways in intestinal capillaries. Arrows represent potential direction of movement of fluid and solutes. *(1)* Intercellular junction, *(2)* pinocytosis, *(3)* basement membrane, *(4)* fenestrae with diaphragms, *(5)* cell membrane, *(6)* transendothelial channel, and *(7)* open fenestrae.

EPITHELIUM

within the physiologic range leads to compensatory vasodilation of the regional circulation to keep the tissue blood flow relatively constant. The process is termed *pressure-flow autoregulation*. The autoregulation of intestinal blood flow guarantees the preservation of continuous blood flow to the intestine while large fluctuations are occurring in the arterial perfusion pressure.[8,10] Although superior mesenteric circulation autoregulation has been well established in canine, porcine, and feline circulation, the mechanism for this regulation is controversial.[11] The capacity to autoregulate intestinal blood flow is a function of gestational maturation. However, in the presence of profound hypotension, net vasoconstriction and decrease in intestinal blood flow are seen to exist. In newborn swine, moderate systemic arterial hypoxemia causes vasodilation and increase in gut perfusion whereas severe hypoxemia (i.e., Po_2 < 40 mm Hg) causes vasoconstriction and gut ischemia.[12] Intestinal perfusion and oxygenation are profoundly reduced in puppies made polycythemic by exchange transfusion. Fortunately, few infants have polycythemia and most escape intestinal damage. Both these factors are influenced by blood volume. The proportion of cardiac output destined for the intestine is altered in newborns with cyanotic congenital heart disease and vascular malformations such as coarctation of the aorta, which limits blood flow to the intestinal tract. In the fetus, systemic circulatory needs are maintained even with severe left ventricular obstruction. However, fetal asphyxia and other fetal problems may be associated with reduced myocardial contractility and tricuspid regurgitation, thus limiting cardiac output and consequently reducing intestinal flow.

Intestinal oxygen uptake and blood flow increase dramatically after birth to sustain rapid growth of the mucosa and oxidative demands of enteral nutrition (secretion, absorption, motility).[10] Postnatally, splanchnic circulation accounts for 20% of cardiac output; however, splanchnic blood flow increases 30 to 130% after a meal, termed *postprandial hyperemia*.[10] Glucose and solubilized long-chain fatty acids increase jejunal blood flow. Bile and bile salts may double ileal blood flow. Volatile fatty acids (e.g., acetic, butyric, propionic), which are derived from fermentation of undigested carbohydrates by microflora, increase colonic blood flow and serve as a metabolic substrate for colonic enterocytes.[8]

Neural Controls

The gastrointestinal tract is extensively innervated by the autonomic and enteric nervous systems.[7,10] Enhanced sympathetic tone elicits arterial smooth muscle contraction, thereby raising intestinal vascular resistance and decreasing blood flow. This effect is mediated through the α-adrenergic receptors in the vascular smooth muscle. However, this vasoconstrictor response is short lived, and decreased vascular resistance and improved blood flow rapidly return by stimulation of β-adrenergic receptors.[13] Thus, sympathetic stimulation may produce a variable response (Table 66-1).[10] Although acetylcholine causes vasodilation through an endothelium-dependent mechanism,[14-16] the effects of acetylcholine on intestinal blood flow are also variable. Acetylcholine has the ability to initiate intestinal smooth muscle contraction, which can impede blood flow by increasing transmural pressure.

Marginal tissue oxygenation antagonizes the sympathetic response by inducing vasodilation. Furthermore, intestinal wall relaxation resulting from sympathetic stimulation decreases the resistance of the vessels and allows increased blood flow to the stomach and intestines. The adrenal medullary catecholamines and angiotensin II, formed locally in response to renal renin, combine to constrict vascular smooth muscle in the gastrointestinal circulation and therefore decrease local blood flow.[17,18] This effect may be temporary, however, and can be readily overridden by local metabolic control.

Most extrinsic nerves innervating the intestine are afferent types. They contain two important polypeptides, substance P and calcitonin gene-related peptide (CGRP), which are released by noxious chemical and mechanical stimulation. These agents induce local vasodilation and contribute to neurogenic inflammation by mast cell degranulation and altering vascular permeability.[19]

Humoral Controls

Numerous humoral substances have been shown to alter gastrointestinal blood flow in experimental animals. Some are circulating substances, whereas others are released locally. Tables 66-1 and 66-2 summarize the agents that have been well demonstrated to increase or decrease intestinal blood flow. Gastrointestinal hormones released during various phases of digestion may dilate the

TABLE 66-1

Agents That Increase Intestinal Blood Flow

Acetylcholine[15,18,20,41]	Nitric oxide[14,25,26,45]
Adenosine[8]	Peptide hormones
Adrenergics[17]	Cholecystokinin[20-22]
Isoproterenol	Gastrin[20-22]
Salbutamol	Glucagon[44,46]
Aminophylline[1]	Vasoactive intestinal polypeptide[47]
Bradykinin[23,42]	Platelet-activating factor (directly)[16,40]
Calcium antagonists[43]	Potassium-low dose[17,21,24]
Carbon dioxide[15]	Prostaglandins[8,42,48]
Histamine[18,44]	PGD$_2$
Magnesium[17,24]	PGE$_1$
Methionine-enkephalin[47]	PGE$_2$
Motilin[8,10,21]	Serotonin[8]
Neurotensin[10]	Substance P[19]

TABLE 66-2

Agents That Decrease Intestinal Blood Flow

Adrenergics[8,17]	Methacholine[46]
Dopamine	Peptide hormones
Epinephrine	Angiotensin II[8]
Methoxamine	Vasopressin[22,49]
Norepinephrine	Physostigmine[8]
Phenylephrine	Potassium-high dose[17,21]
Calcium[17,24,43]	Prostaglandin F_{2a}[41]
Endothelin[35]	Somatostatin[50]
5-Hydroxytryptamine[1]	Thromboxane A_2[48]
Leukotriene D_4[38,39]	Tyramine[1]

gastrointestinal circulation. Glucagon and cholecystokinin increase both intestinal blood flow and pancreatic flow.[20–22] Gastrin specifically increases blood flow to the gastric mucosa.[20,21]

Local Controls

The local extracellular environment is altered by the increased metabolic activity of the gastrointestinal parenchymal cells, for example, during digestion.[11] An increased metabolic demand may lead to relative tissue hypoxia and consequently the release of many vasodilators, for example, K^+, Mg^{2+}, histamine, polypeptides (e.g., bradykinin, vasoactive intestinal polypeptide), prostaglandins, CO_2, and adenosine.[8,15,17,18,23,24] Cells with an increased metabolic rate are likely to produce greater quantities of dilator metabolites, which ensure the provision of more substrate by increasing blood flow.

Role of Nitric Oxide

Basal vascular resistance, which determines the regional gastrointestinal blood flow, depends on a delicate balance between the constrictor and dilator forces that are acting on vascular smooth muscle. Nitric oxide is the major dilator that counterbalances the constrictive effect of endothelin 1 and the intrinsic contractile response of smooth vascular muscle. Under basal conditions, nitric oxide is continuously produced by endothelial cells in presence of nitric oxide synthase (constitutive isoform) derived from L-arginine. It relaxes vascular smooth muscle by decreasing cytosolic free calcium via increased cGMP.[25,26] In rats, acute administration of a nitric oxide synthase inhibitor (L-NNA) reduces basal intestinal blood flow.[27] The rate of nitric oxide production can increase markedly following chemical or mechanical stimulation of nitric oxide synthase (induced or stimulated isoform). Methylene blue, a guanylate cyclase inhibitor, abolishes intestinal vasodilation resulting from administration of sodium nitroprusside, a nitric oxide donor.[14] Following ischemia with reperfusion, exogenous nitric oxide sources (SIN-1, CAS-754, and nitroprusside) and L-arginine reduce mucosal barrier dysfunction without improving intestinal blood flow.[28]

Fetal circulation has an increased basal production of nitric oxide compared with findings in the adult.[29] In late gestation ovine fetus, nitric oxide plays an important role in contributing to low vascular resistance and increased blood flow throughout the gastrointestinal tract, as well as in redistribution of intestinal blood flow between intestinal segments.[30] Inhibition of endogenous nitric oxide in midestation fetal sheep results in substantial blood flow reduction across all segments of the fetal gastrointestinal tract, which implies that nitric oxide plays a major vasodilator role at an early stage of development of gastrointestinal circulation.[31] Sustained inhibition of nitric oxide synthase *in utero* results in vasoconstriction of fetal blood vessels, but there is no evidence of injury to the gastrointestinal tract.[32] A lack of nitric oxide synthesis appears to be causative in neonatal hypertrophic pyloric stenosis,[33] but this effect is mediated by

the neuronal not the endothelial isoform of nitric oxide synthase based on gene knockout studies.[34]

Endothelin 1

Endothelin 1 is a vasoactive and mitogenic polypeptide synthesized and secreted by endothelial cells.[16] It acts on specific receptor ET_A on vascular smooth muscle to cause sustained powerful vasoconstriction, whereas binding to ET_B receptor on endothelial cell causes release of nitric oxide with resultant vascular relaxation. Although cord blood levels are higher than any other values reported in humans, limited information is available about its role in the splanchnic circulation of the fetus and newborn.[35] Hypoxia and shear stress stimulate endothelian 1 secretion.[36] Preterm neonates born to mothers with pre-eclampsia have increased circulating levels of endothelin-1 and reduced superior mesenteric artery blood flow velocity, possibly due to fetal hypoxia.[37]

Local Inflammatory Mediators. Systemic or local activation of polymorphonuclear cells has been demonstrated to be a component of the pathophysiology of various altered blood flow states. Activated neutrophils adhere to vascular endothelium and may damage or occlude them. Secondary release of vasoconstrictors (e.g., leukotrienes) and substances that increase permeability (e.g., platelet-activating factor [PAF], leukotrienes) may further compromise tissue perfusion.[38,39]

PAF is a phospholipid synthesized by many types of cells including those in endothelium, as well as macrophages and granulocytes.[14] Although PAF is a vasodilator, it may cause paradoxical vasoconstriction and ischemic injury to the intestine as a consequence of its ability to activate leukocytes. PAF-activated leukocytes may plug postcapillary venules and release vasoconstrictors, for example, leukotriene C_4.[39]

CLINICAL CONSIDERATIONS

Virtually no study has examined the human fetal and neonatal intestinal blood flow *in vivo*. It may be inferred from various animal models that some clinical conditions encountered in critically ill neonates may result from compromise of the gastrointestinal circulation.[7] Limitation of blood flow as local tissue metabolism increases may result in malabsorption. The early-onset form of necrotizing enterocolitis (in the first week of life) is often associated with perinatal asphyxia, arterial catheterization, or the polycythemia-hyperviscosity syndrome.[40] In each of these conditions, poor tissue perfusion may result in ischemic necrosis of the intestine.

With gene expression techniques, it may be possible to trace the ontogeny of systems regulating gastrointestinal circulation (neural and humoral) in the developing human and experimental animals. These approaches may circumvent the technical problems of directly assessing the splanchnic circulation in the perinatal period. Insights drawn from these molecular approaches may help guide improvements in therapeutic management of the fetus and newborn.

REFERENCES

1. Edelstone DI, Holzman IR: Fetal and neonatal circulations. *In* Shepard AP, Granger DN (eds): Physiology of the Intestinal Circulation. New York, Raven Press, 1984, pp 179–190.
2. Moore KL, Persaud TVN: The Developing Human. Philadelphia, WB Saunders Co, 1993.
3. Hamilton WJ, et al: Human Embryology. 3rd ed. Baltimore, Williams & Wilkins, 1962, pp 189–266.
4. Langman J: Medical Embryology. 4th ed. Baltimore, Williams & Wilkins, 1981.
5. Ashley RA, et al: Erythropoietin stimulates vasculogenesis in neonatal rat mesenteric microvascular endothelial cells. Pediatr Res *51*:472–478, 2002.
6. Granger DN, et al: The microcirculation and intestinal transport. *In* Johnson LR (ed): Physiology of the Gastrointestinal Tract. 2nd ed. New York, Raven Press, 1987, pp 1671–1697.
7. Crissinger KD, Granger DN: Characterization of intestinal collateral blood flow in the developing piglet. Pediatric Res *24*:473, 1988.

8. Jacobson ED: The splanchnic circulation. *In* Johnson LR (ed): Gastrointestinal Physiology. 4th ed. St. Louis, Mosby-Year Book, 1991.

9. Parks DA, Jacobson ED: Mesenteric circulation. *In* Johnson LR (ed): Physiology of the Gastrointestinal Tract. New York, Raven Press, 1987, pp 1649-1670.

10. Perry MA, et al: Physiology of the splanchnic circulation. *In* Kvietys PR, et al (eds): Pathophysiology of the Splanchnic Circulation. Vol 1. Boca Raton, CRC Press, 1987, pp 1-56.

11. Svanik J, Laudgren O: Gastrointestinal circulation. *In* Crane R (ed): International Review of Physiology. Vol 12: Gastrointestinal Physiology II. Baltimore, University Park Press, 1972, pp 1-34.

12. Reber KM, et al: Newborn intestinal circulation, physiology and pathology. Clin Perinatol 29:23, 2002.

13. Mellander S, Johansson B: Control of resistance, exchange and capacitance functions in the peripheral circulation. Pharmacol Rev 20:117, 1968.

14. Andriantsitohaina R, Suprenant A: Acetylcholine released from guinea-pig submucosal neurons dilates arterioles by releasing nitric oxide from endothelium. J Physiol (Lond) 453:493, 1992.

15. Bean JW, Sidky MM: Intestinal blood flow as influenced by vascular and motor reactions to acetylcholine and carbon dioxide. Am J Physiol 194:512, 1988.

16. Caplan MS, Mackendrick W: Inflammatory mediators and intestinal injury. Clin Perinatol 21:235, 1994.

17. Chou CC, Gallavan RH: Blood flow and intestinal motility. Fed Proc 41:2090, 1982.

18. Jacobson ED, et al: Intestinal motor activity and blood flow. Gastroenterology 58:575, 1970.

19. Sharkey KA, Parr EJ: The enteric nervous system in intestinal inflammation. *In* Sutherland LR et al (eds): Inflammatory Bowel Disease: Basic Research Clinical Implications and Trends in Therapy. Boston, Kluwer Academic Publishers, 1994, pp 40-60.

20. Bowen JC, et al: Pharmacologic effects of gastrointestinal hormones on intestinal oxygen consumption and blood flow. Surgery 78:516, 1975.

21. Fasth S, et al: The effect of the gastrointestinal hormones on small intestinal motility and blood flow. Experientia 29:1447, 1973.

22. Schuurkes JAJ, Charbon GA: Motility and hemodynamics of the canine gastrointestinal tract: stimulation by pentagastrin, cholecystokinin and vasopressin. Arch Int Pharmacodyn Ther 236:214, 1978.

23. Chou CC, Grasmick B: Motility and blood flow distribution within the wall of the gastrointestinal tract. Am J Physiol 235:H34, 1978.

24. Dabney JM, et al: Effects of cations on ileal compliance and blood flow. Am J Physiol 212:835, 1967.

25. Alemayehu A, et al: L-NAME, nitric oxide and jejunal motility, blood flow and oxygen uptake in dogs. Br J Pharm 111:205, 1994.

26. Ignarro L: Biologic actions and properties of endothelium-derived nitric oxide formed and released from artery and vein. Circ Res 65:1, 1989.

27. Pawlik WW, et al: Microcirculatory and motor effects of endogenous nitric oxide in the rat gut. J Physiol Pharmacol 44:139, 1993.

28. Kubes P, Granger D: Nitric oxide modulates microvascular permeability. Am J Physiol 262:H611, 1992.

29. Pierce RL, et al: Endothelium dependent limb reduction defects following prenatal inhibition of nitric oxide synthase in rats. Circulation 94:1948, 1996.

30. Fan WQ, et al: Nitric oxide modulates the regional blood flow differences in the fetal gastrointestinal tract. Am J Physiol 271:G598-604, 1996.

31. Fan WQ, et al: Major vasodilator role for nitric oxide in the gastrointestinal circulation of the mid-gestation fetal lambs. Pediatr Res 44:344-350, 1998.

32. Bustamante SA, et al: Inducible nitric oxide synthase and the regulation of central vessel caliber in the fetal rat. Circulation 94:1948, 1996.

33. Voelker CA, et al: Perinatal nitric oxide synthase inhibition retards fetal and neonatal growth in rats. Pediatr Res 38:768, 1995.

34. Huang PL, et al: Targeted disruption of the neuronal nitric oxide synthase gene. Cell 75:1273, 1993.

35. Ekblad H, et al: Plasma endothelin-1 concentrations at different ages during infancy and childhood. Acta Paediatr 82:302, 1993.

36. Masaki T: Possible role of endothelin-1 in endothelin regulation of vascular tone. Annu Rev Pharmacol Toxicol 35:235, 1995.

37. Weir FJ, et al: Does endothelin-1 reduce superior mesenteric artery blood flow velocity in perterm neonates? Arch Dis Child FN Ed 80:F123-127, 1999.

38. Pawlik WW, et al: Vasoactive and metabolic effects of leukotriene C_4 and D_4 in the intestine. Hepatogastroenterology 35:87, 1988.

39. Wallace JL, MacNaughton WK: Gastrointestinal damage induced by platelet-activating factor: role of leukotrienes. Eur J Pharmacol 151:43, 1988.

40. Oh W: Neonatal polycythemia and hyperviscosity. Pediatr Clin North Am 33:523, 1986.

41. Walus KM, et al: Hemodynamic and metabolic changes during stimulation of ileal motility. Dig Dis Sci 26:1069, 1981.

42. Fasth S, Hulten L: The effect of bradykinin on intestinal motility and blood flow. Acta Chir Scand 139:699, 1973.

43. Walus KM, et al: Effects of calcium and its antagonists on the canine mesenteric circulation. Circ Res 48:692, 1981.

44. Schwaiger MM, et al: Effects of glucagon, histamine and perhexiline on the ischemic canine mesenteric circulation. Gastroenterology 77:730, 1979.

45. Stark ME, Szurszewski JH: Role of nitric oxide in gastrointestinal and hepatic function and disease. Gastroenterology 103:1928, 1992.

46. Walus KM, Jacobson ED: Relation between intestinal motility and circulation. Am J Physiol 241:G1, 1981.

47. Eklund S, et al: Effects of vasoactive intestinal polypeptide on blood flow, motility and fluid transport in the gastrointestinal tract of the cat. Acta Physiol Scand 105:461, 1979.

48. Zipser RD, et al: Hypersensitive prostaglandin and thromboxane response to hormones in rabbit colitis. Am J Physiol 249:G457, 1985.

49. Shapiro H, Britt LG: The action of vasopressin on the gastrointestinal tract: a review of the literature. Am J Dig Dis 17:649, 1972.

50. Kontorek SJ, et al: Pharmacology of somatostatin. *In* Gloom SR (ed): Gut Hormones. Edinburgh, Churchill Livingstone, 1986.

67

Thomas J. Kulik

Physiology of Congenital Heart Disease in the Neonate

If one juxtaposes a line drawing of the heart and great arteries—four chambers and a few large blood vessels—with a depiction of the cascade of biochemical events that follow, say, a growth factor binding to its receptor, it may seem that the physiology of congenital heart disease ought to be child's play. It is not, for several reasons key to understanding the physiologic responses to congenital heart lesions.

A comprehensive understanding of the cardiovascular physiology of a neonate with a cardiac lesion requires consideration of *many factors*. The first factor pertains to key *hemodynamic* variables (myocardial function, intravascular volume, cardiac and vascular transmural pressures, flows, and compliances, and pulmonary venous oxygen [O_2] content)[1] sufficient to describe the physiology of a neonate with a cardiac lesion. However, any description taking into account only these variables, although complex, would be incomplete because cardiac lesions affect somatic physiology in various ways (e.g., sympathetic nervous system activation) that cannot be specified from these hemodynamic variables alone. Indeed, alterations in somatic physiology linked to altered hemodynamics account for many of the clinical manifestations of cardiac lesions.[2, 3] Hence, the net physiology observed is caused by the interaction of many elements: (1) cardiac and vascular anatomy, (2) hemodynamic variables related to cardiovascular function as noted earlier, (3) pulmonary function, (4) O_2 carrying capacity and O_2 release from the blood, and (5) myriad other factors, such as O_2 consumption (V_{O_2}), autonomic nervous system, endocrine, lymphatic, and other organ system function.

The physiology of such lesions is complex for other reasons as well. With cardiac structural anomalies, *more than one type* of physiologic derangement will often be operative. For example, with a large patent ductus arteriosus (PDA), the left ventricle (LV) may have both an increased volume load and reduced myocardial perfusion, the latter resulting from decreased aortic diastolic pressure. In addition, the consequences of multiple anatomic cardiac abnormalities may be *additive, or,* conversely, *they may balance each other*. Finally, subtle differences in physiology may result in very different clinical phenotypes in anatomically identical patients. For example, the arterial O_2 saturation in neonates with D-transposition of the great arteries after balloon atrial septostomy is variable and unpredictable, related to subtle differences in physiology.[4]

The second factor to consider in understanding the cardiovascular physiology of a neonate with a cardiac lesion pertains to physiologic changes. Some factors that affect cardiovascular physiology may change over months (especially those related to anatomic changes, e.g., pressure-related remodeling of pulmonary blood vessels), whereas others may vary significantly over seconds or minutes (e.g., alteration in pulmonary vascular tone resulting from various perturbations). The physiology that attends a given cardiac defect may actually be a spectrum of physiologic features.

Finally, there are patient factors that must be considered. The precise elucidation of a given patient's hemodynamics may be difficult or impossible, even with "simple" anatomic lesions. Measurement of relevant pressures and blood flows and of human ventricular function is often not feasible, especially when invasive studies are not warranted. Fortunately, information derived from noninvasive evaluation and clinical acumen are usually sufficient for design of therapy. There are situations, however, in which important information is difficult or impossible to obtain. For example, in patients with reduced pulmonary blood flow (Qp) and an anatomic restriction to flow, it can be difficult to determine to what extent flow is limited by the anatomic restriction versus increased pulmonary vascular resistance (PVR).

This chapter focuses on congenital cardiovascular *anatomic* lesions; nonanatomic abnormalities (e.g., arrhythmia, infection, intrinsic myocardial muscle dysfunction) are not discussed. It is also beyond the scope of this chapter (and authorial competence) to examine the biology of specific elements related to cardiovascular function (e.g., cardiac mechanics) or to discuss structural alterations caused by cardiac lesions (e.g., ventricular hypertrophy with pressure overload). Essential to understanding of congenital cardiac malformations is an appreciation of normal fetal and neonatal physiology,[5,6] the physiology and pharmacology of the pulmonary circulation,[7-9] the general principles of cardiac hemodynamics,[10] and the anatomy of congenital cardiac lesions (found in most any standard text).

HOW CONGENITAL HEART LESIONS ALTER THE CLINICAL PHENOTYPE OF THE NEONATE

A description of the hemodynamic characteristics of an anatomic cardiac lesion is only characters on a page unless the impact of the abnormal hemodynamics on the greater physiology of the organism is considered. Leaving aside that a congenital heart lesion may occasion the need for neonatal surgery, and ignoring the important issue of the impact of abnormal hemodynamics on cardiovascular growth and remodeling, a congenital anatomic lesion may affect a neonate in three ways, as described in the following sections.

No Appreciable Effect

An anatomic lesion may be such a minor perturbation of normal structure (e.g., a small ventricular septal defect [VSD]) that it may *never* have any appreciable physiologic consequences. In other cases, a lesion destined to later have significant impact may have few manifestations in the neonate, owing to the physiologic characteristics of the newborn. The classic example is that of a large VSD, which may have little effect initially but causes congestive heart failure (CHF) a few weeks later. The clinical phenotype changes partly because the relatively high neonatal PVR falls over time, increasing left-to-right shunting through the VSD

and hence the LV volume pumped[11] and partly because of the normal postnatal decline in hematocrit[12] (along with even more possible variables). Lesions that cause higher than normal right ventricular (RV) pressure (e.g., pulmonary stenosis) usually have little impact on ventricular function in the newborn, because the neonate's RV is well adapted to pumping at systemic pressure.[6] Ductal-dependent left-sided obstructive lesions (e.g., severe coarctation of the aorta) may also have only subtle manifestations in the first few days of life if the ductus remains widely patent.

Reduction of Oxygen Transport

Congenital cardiac lesions may reduce systemic arterial blood O_2 tension (*hypoxemia*) or *systemic blood flow* (Qs) and thus decrease systemic O_2 transport (systemic O_2 transport = arterial O_2 content × Qs).[13]

Reduction of Oxygen Transport Resulting from Hypoxemia

Hypoxemia may be the only manifestation of some lesions (e.g., tetralogy of Fallot), or it may be present with defects that also cause reduced Qs (e.g., severe Ebstein anomaly). It appears that the neonate can tolerate low Po_2 better than the mature organism,[14] and moderate hypoxemia, as an isolated abnormality, generally has little obvious physiologic effect on the neonate. Increased O_2 extraction, redistribution of blood flow to organs of high O_2 need, and perhaps increased Qs help to maintain systemic Vo_2 with hypoxemia.[15,16] For example, when conscious lambs less than 1 week old were submitted to acute alveolar hypoxia (fraction of inspired O_2 [Fio_2] = 0.12; arterial Po_2 = 35 mm Hg) there was neither a fall in Vo_2 nor acidosis.[16] More severe hypoxia (Fio_2 <0.10; arterial Po_2 ~25 mm Hg) caused Vo_2 to fall, but it was not associated with much acidosis in conscious newborn lambs.[15,16] Thus, multiple variables (e.g., hematocrit, half-saturation O_2 pressure [P_{50}] of hemoglobin, environmental temperature, Qs, Vo_2, and whether the organism is spontaneously ventilating) determine the physiologic impact of hypoxemia.[13-16]

The quantitative relationship between hypoxemia and organ dysfunction or damage in the *human* neonate is unknown. One study found an Fio_2 of 0.15 to cause Vo_2 to fall significantly in human infants, albeit without obvious detrimental effect.[17] Perhaps the clearest evidence that neonates can tolerate substantial hypoxemia with modest or no long-term consequences comes from experience treating infants with D-transposition of the great arteries, a lesion that almost always causes considerable hypoxemia, especially before balloon septostomy can be performed. One hundred twenty-nine neonates with this lesion were operated on in the first week of life at the Children's Hospital in Boston; the mean lowest preoperative arterial Po_2 was approximately 24 mm Hg. Even though these infants had undergone a period of substantial hypoxemia (before operation), the hospital survival rate for these patients was more than 98%.[18] Neurologic evaluation at 4 years of age revealed that only 4% of these patients had moderate or severe neurologic abnormalities; average intelligence quotient scores were lower than average, but not terribly so (94 versus 100).[19] Furthermore, it is likely that some or all of the observed decrement in neurologic function was related to aspects of the patient's treatment and clinical course distinct from the hypoxemia.

Reduction of Oxygen Transport Resulting from Reduction of Systemic Blood Flow

Congenital heart lesions may also decrease systemic O_2 transport by decreasing Qs. As is the case for hypoxemia, modest reductions of Qs may not affect tissue oxygenation. For example, Fahey and Lister[20] found that Qs could be reduced to approximately 42% of the resting value before Vo_2 fell in the conscious 2-week-old lamb; increased fractional extraction of O_2 from the blood maintained O_2 delivery with decreased Qs. Most congenital cardiac lesions that reduce Qs do so by one or more of three mechanisms: (1) abnormally low systemic ventricular output, (2) abnormal arterial connection between the heart and peripheral tissues, and (3) recirculation of previously oxygenated blood to the lungs (see later). Few quantitative data regarding Qs in the neonate with heart disease are available, at least in part because of the difficulty in measuring this variable.

Duration of Effects of Heart Lesions

Symptoms can occur in infants with many different heart lesions without a significant reduction in systemic O_2 transport. For example, infants with CHF resulting from a large VSD generally have Qs within the normal range[11,21,22]; but see references 12 and 23. However, cardiac lesions can trigger a complex *neurohumoral* response that affects overall patient physiology.[2, 3, 24] Furthermore, the symptoms of "CHF" are often a direct consequence of these neurohumoral alterations, not altered O_2 transport. These alterations help to maintain adequate blood pressure and tissue perfusion in part by augmenting myocardial contractility (sympathetic nervous system activation)[25, 25] and by increasing systemic vascular resistance (SVR; activation of the sympathetic nervous system, the renin-angiotensin-aldosterone system,[24, 27, 28] and release of vasopressin). Ventricular output is also increased (via the Frank-Starling principle) through fluid retention caused by activation of the renin-angiotensin-aldosterone system and other variables.[2,3,24]

These factors help to maintain adequate O_2 transport, but they also have *unfavorable consequences.* For example, increased circulating catecholamine levels raise SVR and therefore ventricular afterload; the clinical result is decreased peripheral perfusion. Increased catecholamines also contribute to failure to thrive by increasing Vo_2.[29] Fluid retention causes systemic edema,[30] and it increases lung water and the work of breathing. It is these secondary manifestations of abnormal cardiovascular function, rather than critically reduced systemic O_2 transport, that most commonly affect infants with congenital cardiac lesions.

PHYSIOLOGY OF SHUNTING AND SINGLE VENTRICLE PHYSIOLOGY

Key Concepts

Multiple formulas are useful for calculating flows and resistances relevant to understanding intracardiac shunting, but because space constraints prohibit delineation and derivation of most of them here, the reader is referred to the literature.[10] However, a few concepts are especially important and are briefly covered.

Pulmonary Vascular Resistance

The *resistance to blood flow through the lungs* is an important determinant of the physiologic effects (ventricular work and systemic O_2 saturation) of many cardiac lesions. A useful, but simplified,[31] way to conceive of PVR is: PVR = (PAP – LAP)/Qp, where PAP is mean pulmonary arterial pressure (mm Hg), LAP is mean left atrial pressure (mm Hg), and Qp is pulmonary blood flow (which, for pediatric patients, is usually indexed—L/min/m²). SVR is calculated in an analogous way. Because PVR is primarily a reflection of resistance to flow through the pulmonary microcirculation, it is sometimes referred to as pulmonary *arteriolar* resistance. The calculated PVR can be low, but total resistance to flow through the lungs and into the heart can be high, if the patient has obstruction to systemic ventricular inflow or poor ventricular compliance. The concept of *total pulmonary resistance* (total pulmonary resistance = mean PAP/Qp) takes into account all resistance to flow from the central pulmonary arteries to the ventricle,

but the term is misleading because some of the resistance to flow resides outside the lungs.

PVR is much higher than SVR in the fetus,[8,32] but PAP normally decreases to approximately one-half systemic arterial pressure in the first 24 hours of life (presuming the ductus does not remain widely patent), and it is at essentially mature levels by 1 to 2 weeks after birth.[33] The postnatal decline in PVR is considerably slower with cardiac lesions (e.g., a large VSD) that maintain elevated PAP, although PVR often falls much more rapidly in premature infants than in term infants with such lesions.[32]

Ratio of Pulmonary to Systemic Blood Flow

The *Qp/Qs ratio* provides an estimate of the volume pumped by the ventricles and an estimate of the Qp (and hence of PVR if the PAP is known). It can be calculated using blood oximetry values:

$$Qp/Qs = Sao_2 - Mvo_2 / Pvo_2 - Pao_2$$

where Sao_2 is the systemic arterial O_2 saturation, Mvo_2 is the mixed venous O_2 saturation, Pvo_2 is the pulmonary venous O_2 saturation, and Pao_2 is the pulmonary arterial O_2 saturation. The superior vena caval O_2 saturation is generally taken as representative of the Mvo_2 when there is left-to-right shunting. This formula can be used to calculate Qp/Qs with any sort of lesion, presuming that the relevant O_2 saturations can be measured. It cannot be used when multiple sources of pulmonary or systemic flow are present, with each source having a different O_2 saturation. For example, with right-to-left ductal shunting, O_2 saturations in the ascending aorta or transverse arch and descending aorta will differ, making the calculation of Qp/Qs impossible.

Effective Versus Ineffective Blood Flow

Left-to-right shunting occurs when blood that has traversed the lungs is recirculated to them without having first crossed the systemic capillary bed. Such pulmonary flow is sometimes termed *ineffective,* because little additional O_2 is picked up with more than one passage through the lungs. Pulmonary flow composed of systemic venous blood is *effective* pulmonary flow. Ineffective Qp represents volume pumped by the heart to no useful end, at least as far as systemic O_2 transport is concerned (see later). In an analogous fashion, blood that has traversed the lungs before being pumped to the systemic circulation is considered *effective* Qs, whereas systemic venous blood that enters the systemic arterial circulation without passage through the lungs (right-to-left shunting) is *ineffective* Qs. The concepts of effective and ineffective blood flow are useful because they help in thinking about complex cardiac physiology, such as that observed with D-transposition of the great arteries (see later).

Left-to-Right Shunting at the Ventricular or Great Artery Level

Because the ventricle pumps only blood that enters it during diastole, left-to-right shunting at the ventricular or great artery level imposes a volume load on the *systemic* ventricle (LV in an otherwise normal heart). Actually, with a large VSD, because some pulmonary venous blood enters the RV during diastole, the RV volume pumped is also somewhat increased.[34,35]

If the connection between the systemic and pulmonary circulations (e.g., VSD or PDA) is large enough so the systolic pressure in the two circuits is equal, the communication is said to be *unrestrictive.* With an unrestrictive defect, the *Qp/Qs is primarily determined by the ratio of total pulmonary resistance to SVR.* (With a small defect, the pressure difference between the two ventricles and the size of the communication are usually the primary determinants of the shunt magnitude.) However, not only PVR, but also *all* resistances to flow affect Qp/Qs; that is, relevant variables include not only the cross-sectional area of the pulmonary microcirculation but also the size of the central pulmonary arteries and large pulmonary veins, any impediment to ventricular filling (such as obstruction to ventricular inflow), and the compliance of the ventricle. For example, with mitral stenosis, the calculated PVR may be normal or even low, but total pulmonary resistance is high. Because the systemic and pulmonary microvascular resistance can change substantially with physiologic, pharmacologic, and other perturbations,[8,36] the Qp/Qs can vary considerably (Fig. 67–1).

Other factors also influence cardiovascular physiology with ventricular or great artery level shunting lesions. For example, Jarmakani and colleagues[37] demonstrated that infants less than 2 years old with a PDA had greater LV end-diastolic pressure and end-diastolic wall stress than patients with a VSD and comparable magnitude of shunt. The reason for this is unclear, but it may be related to differences in LV stroke work with the two lesions.[37] *Diastolic runoff* into the pulmonary arteries with connections between the aorta and pulmonary artery may decrease aortic diastolic pressure and hence may reduce coronary perfusion.[38] *Streaming* of blood can affect whether pulmonary venous blood ends up in the aorta or in the pulmonary artery. For example, with double-outlet RV, the location of the VSD (subpulmonary versus subaortic) will influence the volume of *effective* Qp (with a subpulmonary VSD, pulmonary venous blood tends to be recirculated to the lungs rather than find its way into the aorta).[39] Left-to-right shunting from the *LV to the right atrium* can occur, mostly with atrioventricular canal defects. The shunt magnitude is primarily determined by the effective size of the LV–right atrial communication; PVR and right atrial pressure have no appreciable role.

Pressure Transmission and Pulmonary Hemodynamics

In an anatomically normal heart, PAP is a function of Qp and total pulmonary resistance. However, the *systolic PAP will always be essentially the same as the ventricle or artery to which it is connected* (assuming that the connection is unobstructed), regardless of the volume of flow through the lungs or the resistance to flow. Therefore, with an unrestrictive VSD or PDA, systolic PAP will be essentially the same as aortic pressure regardless of the magnitude of flow or PVR. Neonates with unrestrictive ventricular or great vessel communications generally develop large shunts as their PVR falls postnatally, but the systolic PA pressure remains elevated. High PVR with unrestrictive communications is reflected by a low Qp/Qs, not the pulmonary arterial systolic pressure per se. Thus, pulmonary hypertension and increased PVR are related but distinct concepts (see Fig. 67–1).

Left-to-Right Shunting at the Atrial Level

Left-to-right shunts across an atrial septal opening increase the volume of blood pumped by the pulmonary ventricle (the RV in an otherwise normal heart). With a small defect, left atrial mean pressure is usually substantially different from that of the right atrium, and shunting is primarily the result of this pressure difference. Given a large defect (in which the mean atrial pressures are essentially the same), the magnitude of shunting is generally ascribed to the relative compliances of the left atrium/pulmonary veins/LV, and the right atrium/vena cava/RV: blood tends to flow into the venous chamber/ventricle that most readily accepts it (see Fig. 67–1).[40] This finding explains the presence of left-to-right shunting in older patients, because the RV is thinner than the LV and is more compliant. Because substantial atrial shunting can occur in the neonate,[41,42] whose RV and LV presumably have similar compliances, Rudolph[43] proposed that such shunting may be a function of *differential ejection* of blood from the two ventricles, given that RV afterload is less than that of the LV. Left-to-right atrial shunting also occurs *with partial anomalous pulmonary venous connection* to the right side of

the circulation. Assuming that there is no defect in the atrial septum, the shunt magnitude is determined by the fraction of Qp that goes to the lobes of the lungs drained by the anomalously connected veins, a function of the total resistance to blood flow through those lobes relative to lobes normally connected to the heart. It is unusual for atrial level shunts in *children*—even if the Qp is very large—to be associated with significant pulmonary hypertension. However, in the neonate, the capacity for flow-related dilation or recruitment in the pulmonary vascular bed is apparently limited, and large *atrial* level shunts (e.g., unobstructed total anomalous pulmonary venous connection) are often accompanied by *considerably* increased PAP.[44-47]

Right-to-Left Shunting

Right-to-left shunting occurs when systemic venous blood enters the systemic arterial circulation without having passed through the pulmonary microcirculation. Isolated right-to-left shunting is unusual, and in most congenital heart defects associated with right-to-left shunting, there is also a left-to-right shunt.

Determinants of Systemic Arterial Oxygen Saturation with Right-to-Left Shunting

Whenever there is right-to-left shunting, *systemic arterial O_2 saturation* is a function of four major variables:

1. The *fraction of systemic arterial blood composed of systemic venous blood.* No matter how complex the pattern of intracardiac shunting is, a certain fraction of the aortic blood will not have crossed the lungs, and this results in a reduced systemic O_2 saturation. For any given amount of systemic and pulmonary flow, the systemic arterial saturation varies and depends on the shunting pattern (isolated right-to-left, right-to-left with coexisting left-to-right shunting or with complete admixture of systemic and pulmonary venous blood) (Fig. 67–2).

2. *Mixed* venous O_2 saturation. The O_2 saturation of venous blood that reaches the aorta will obviously affect the O_2 saturation of the aortic blood. Because the mixed venous O_2 saturation reflects what O_2 is left in the blood after it has crossed the systemic capillary bed, this value is influenced by the following:
   a. Hematocrit. The greater the O_2 carrying capacity of the blood, the better the O_2 transport will be, and given a fixed quantity of O_2 unloaded to the tissue, the greater the venous O_2 saturation.
   b. Qs. Given a fixed amount of O_2 unloaded into the tissues, the greater the quantity of O_2 transported, the greater the venous O_2 saturation will be.
   c. V_{O_2}. The greater the quantity of O_2 consumed, given a fixed amount transported, the lower the venous O_2 saturation will be.

3. *Pulmonary venous O_2 saturation.* For obvious reasons, the lower the pulmonary venous O_2 saturation, the lower the systemic arterial O_2 saturation will be.

4. *The O_2 dissociation characteristics of hemoglobin.* With a leftward shift of the O_2 dissociation curve, *less* O_2 is unloaded from hemoglobin at any given P_{O_2}. Therefore, for any given end capillary P_{O_2}, the mixed venous saturation will be a function of the P_{50} of the hemoglobin. With a right-to-left shunt, a leftward shift of the curve will increase the mixed venous O_2 saturation and therefore will *increase* the systemic arterial saturation.

Systemic Oxygen Delivery with Right-to-Left Shunting

Systemic O_2 transport and O_2 delivery to the tissues are not necessarily proportional to arterial O_2 saturation with *right-to-left* shunting lesions. For example, a leftward shift in the hemoglobin

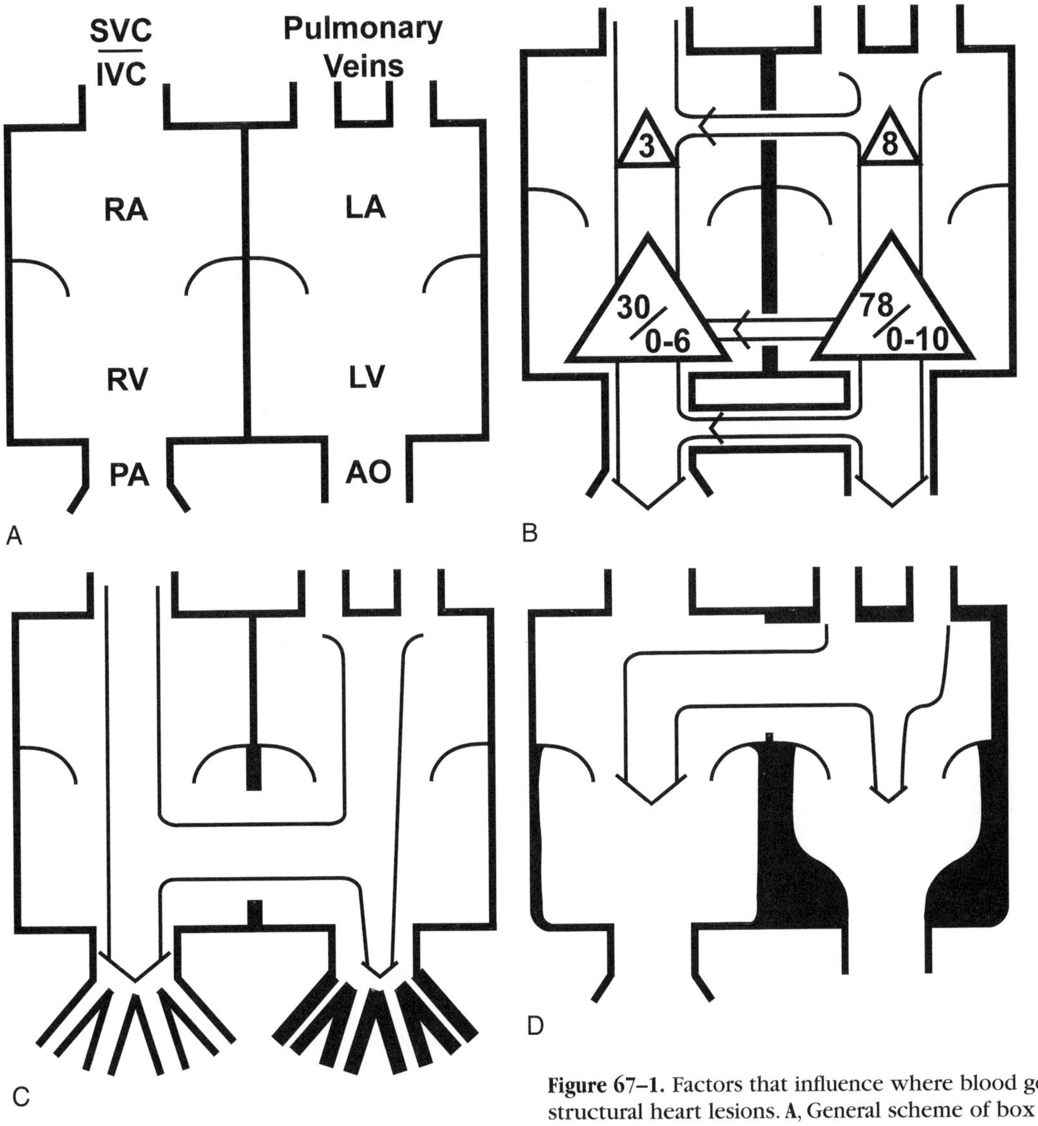

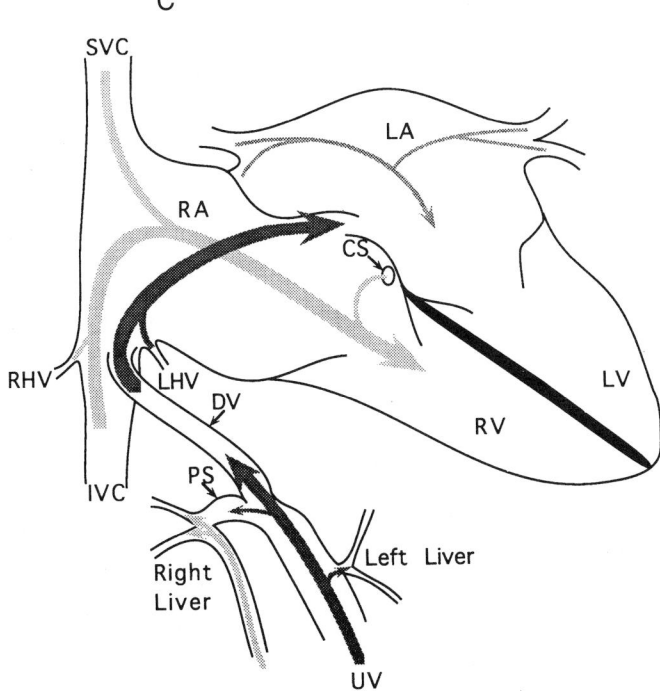

A

SVC
⎯⎯
IVC

Pulmonary
Veins

RA   LA

RV   LV

PA   AO

B

△3   △8

△30/0-6   △78/0-10

C

D

E

SVC

LA

RA

CS

RHV

LHV

DV

IVC

PS

Right Liver

Left Liver

LV

RV

UV

Figure 67–1. Factors that influence where blood goes with structural heart lesions. **A,** General scheme of box diagrams. **B,** Blood moves from high pressure to low. Shunting at the atrial, ventricular, and great vessel levels can result from a pressure gradient between communicating structures. **C,** When two vascular beds differing in resistance to flow are connected to a source of flow, more blood finds its way into the lower than into the higher resistance circuit. With an unrestrictive ventricular septal defect and low pulmonary vascular resistance, systolic pressures are essentially the same in both the aorta and the pulmonary artery, yet there is more flow to the pulmonary artery. **D,** When two chambers differing in resistance to filling (compliance) are connected to a source of flow, more blood finds its way into the chamber with the greater compliance. **E,** Streaming can influence the chamber or vessel to which the blood flows. As depicted here, in the fetus, umbilical venous blood preferentially crosses the tricuspid valve and tends to match the most highly oxygenated blood with organs of greatest need. Streaming can also take place at the ventricular and great vessel level. AO = aorta; CS = coronary sinus; DV = ductus venosus; IVC = inferior vena cava; LA = left atrium; LHV = left hepatic vein; LV = left ventricle; PA = pulmonary artery; PS = portal sinus; RA = right atrium; RHV = right hepatic vein; RV = right ventricle; SVC = superior vena cava; UV = umbilical vein; numbers in *triangles* indicate pressure. (*E*, From Teitel DF, et al: Moss and Adams: Heart Disease in Infants, Children, and Adolescents, Vol 1, 5th ed. Baltimore, Williams & Wilkins, 1995, p 49.)

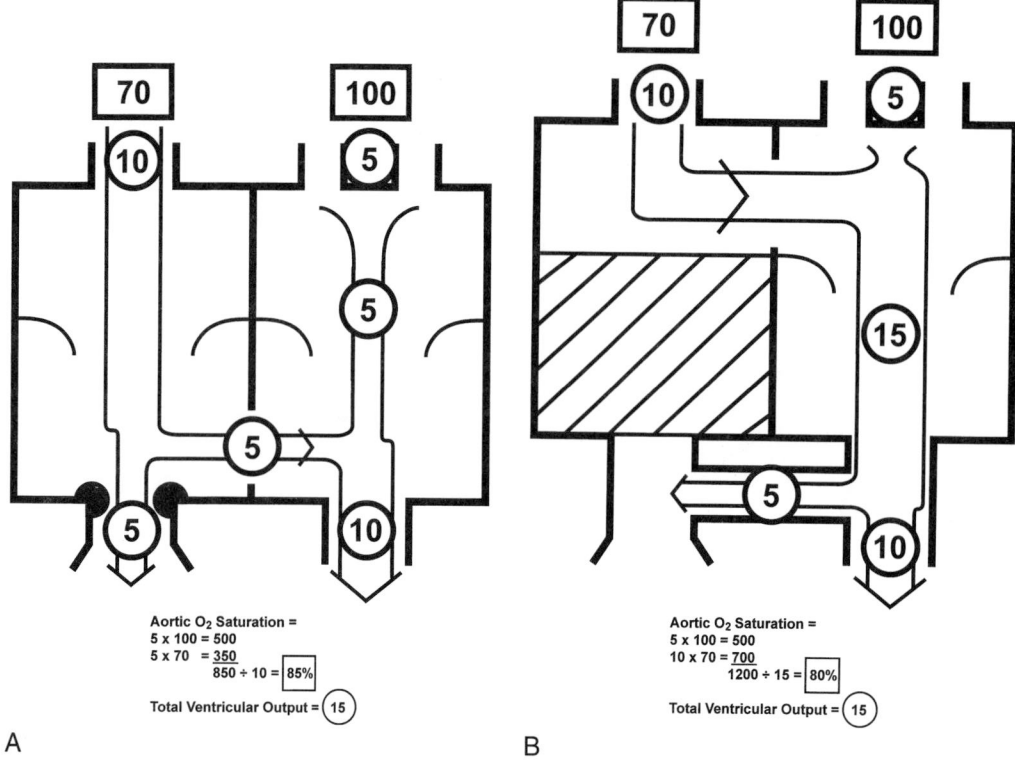

Aortic O₂ Saturation =
5 x 100 = 500
5 x 70 = 350
        850 ÷ 10 = 85%

Total Ventricular Output = 15

A

Aortic O₂ Saturation =
5 x 100 = 500
10 x 70 = 700
        1200 ÷ 15 = 80%

Total Ventricular Output = 15

B

Figure 67–2. Patterns of intracardiac blood flow and ventricular output with right-to-left shunting. This illustration aims to provide a conceptual understanding of the relationship among intracardiac shunting, ventricular output, and oxygen saturation, but it is a simplified view relative to cardiac physiology; for example, given a fixed oxygen consumption, it would be unrealistic to expect systemic venous saturation to remain constant because systemic oxygen transport varies. Numbers in *boxes* indicate blood oxygen saturation; numbers in *circles* indicate the relative amount of blood flow. **A,** With an isolated right-to-left shunt (e.g., tetralogy of Fallot), all pulmonary blood flow is effective, and combined ventricular output is less than normal. **B,** With admixture physiology, there is ineffective pulmonary blood flow, and therefore systemic arterial saturation is less, for a given amount of ventricular output, than for a lesion with isolated right-to-left shunting.

O_2 dissociation curve will increase the arterial O_2 saturation with right-to-left shunting lesions; however, this increase in saturation does not imply an increase in O_2 delivery to the tissue, because less O_2 is released at any given tissue Po_2. In addition, with admixture lesions, systemic O_2 transport actually *declines* as arterial O_2 saturation increases beyond a certain point (see later). *Maximum* Vo_2 = maximum O_2 uptake in the lungs, which is a function of effective Qp, pulmonary arterial O_2 saturation, and the O_2 capacity of the blood. Hence, if effective Qp is severely reduced, O_2 delivery will be compromised, regardless of Qs or other factors.

Isolated Right-to-Left Shunting

Isolated right-to-left shunting occurs at the *ventricular level* when a VSD is present and resistance to Qp (resulting from obstruction at the level of the RV outflow tract or points beyond) is greater than resistance to flow into the systemic vascular bed, thus causing a shunt of desaturated (RV) blood into the aorta. Right-to-left *ductal* shunting occurs when total pulmonary resistance is greater than SVR, which is most often the result of increased PVR but can also be caused by pulmonary venous or left atrial hypertension. There is also right-to-left ductal shunting when the descending aorta is mostly or entirely supplied by the RV, such as severe coarctation of the aorta. In such cases, however, there is always a component of left-to-right shunting—at the atrial or ventricular level—as well. The magnitude of right-to-left shunting with ventricular or arterial communications is determined by the ratio of resistance to flow into and through the pulmonary circuit relative to the systemic circuit. Because

SVR and PVR (and sometimes even the degree of RV outflow tract obstruction, as in tetralogy of Fallot) may fluctuate with time, the magnitude of right-to-left shunting may be variable. Right-to-left shunting across an atrial defect most commonly results from a reduction in RV compliance, usually because of RV hypertrophy or hypertension (see Fig. 67–2).

Bidirectional Shunting

Both left-to-right shunting and right-to-left shunting are present in various cardiac lesions. For example, a patient with severe aortic stenosis (and severely reduced LV ejection) with an open ductus arteriosus will often have a left-to-right atrial shunt, as well as a right-to-left shunt across the ductus to the aorta. Right-to-left atrial shunting can also occur simultaneously with a left-to-right ventricular shunt (e.g., with an atrioventricular septal defect).

With total anomalous connection of the pulmonary veins, all pulmonary veins connect to the systemic veins or right atrium; therefore, a fraction of both the pulmonary and systemic venous return must cross the atrial septum to supply the LV. The variables that influence Qp (the mixture of systemic and pulmonary venous blood that finds its way into the RV) and Qs (the mixture of systemic and pulmonary venous blood entering the LV) likely include the size of the atrial opening,[47] the relative ventricular compliances, and possibly any preferential streaming of venous blood. Whether streaming of venous blood actually affects Qp per se is unclear, but it can affect the *effective* Qp,[44,47] because pulmonary venous return from the inferior vena cava can preferentially stream across the foramen ovale into the left atrium.

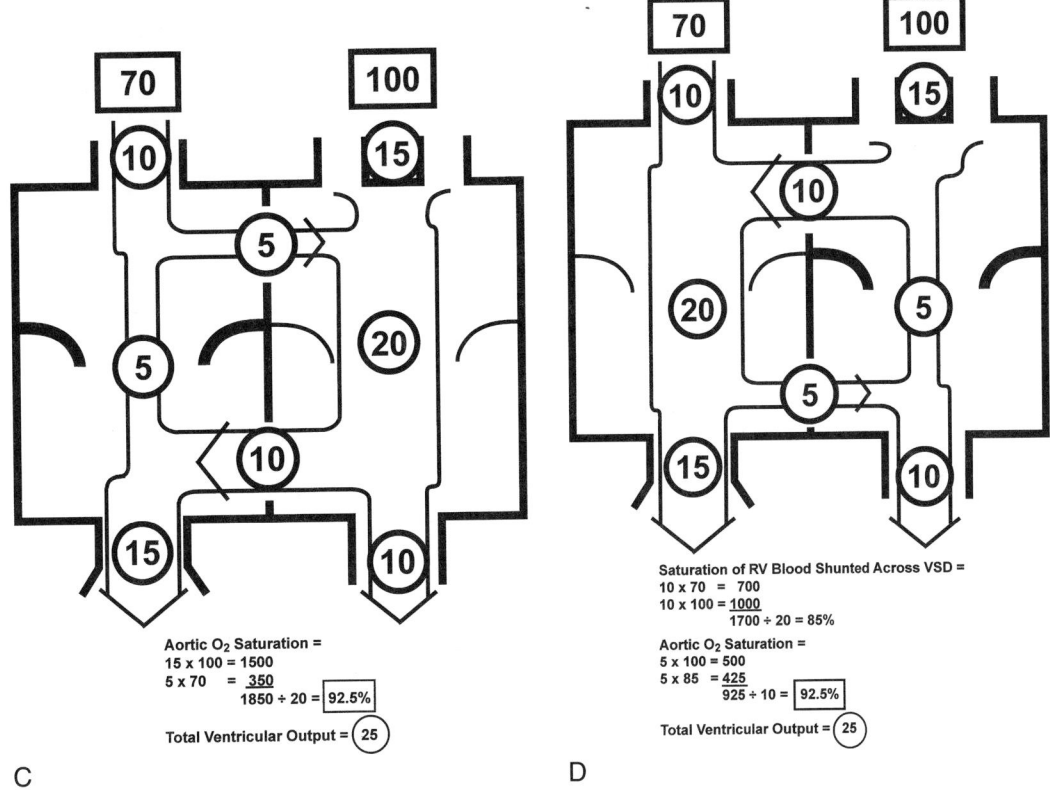

Figure 67–2—cont'd. C and **D,** With bidirectional shunting, equal volumes of right-to-left shunting at either the atrial or ventricular level will result in equal systemic arterial oxygen saturation and equal ventricular output. The relationship between systemic arterial oxygen saturation and ventricular output depends on the volume of ineffective pulmonary blood flow (left-to-right shunt). RV = right ventricular; VSD = ventricular septal defect.

With a total anomalous pulmonary venous connection (assuming no other communication between the pulmonary and systemic arterial circuits), PVR only affects the pattern of intracardiac shunting insofar as it influences RV pressure and therefore RV compliance and systolic function. However, because PAP may be at or above systemic levels, especially if the veins are obstructed, there can be considerable reduction of Qp resulting from reduced RV compliance and output. In addition, pulmonary venous hypertension causes pulmonary edema, which interferes with gas exchange and reduces lung compliance. The shunting physiology with cerebral arteriovenous malformations is similar in many ways[46] (see Fig. 67–2).

Admixture Lesions and the Physiology of the Single Ventricle

Cardiac lesions that cause complete mixing of systemic and pulmonary venous blood are sometimes termed *admixture lesions.* All malformations with a single functional ventricle (e.g., hypoplastic left heart syndrome, tricuspid atresia) have this physiology, as well as some two-ventricle defects (e.g., tetralogy of Fallot with pulmonary atresia). Actually, there can be preferential streaming of pulmonary or systemic venous blood into one or the other great artery in some lesions with substantial mixing of pulmonary and systemic venous blood (e.g., truncus arteriosus), but unless the quantity of "streamed" blood is significant, the physiology is perhaps best understood as admixture.

Determinants of Systemic Arterial Oxygen Saturation with Admixture Lesions

With admixture lesions, systemic arterial O_2 saturation is a function of all the variables outlined earlier. The fraction of aortic blood composed of pulmonary venous blood is determined by the *Qp/Qs:* because pulmonary venous blood mixes with systemic venous blood, the ratio of "blue" and "pink" blood will influence aortic O_2 saturation. For lesions in which the systemic and pulmonary arterial circuits are in unrestricted communication, the Qp/Qs is primarily determined by the ratio of SVR to total pulmonary resistance. When mixing of venous blood occurs at the atrial level and systemic and pulmonary arterial circulations are separate (e.g., total anomalous pulmonary venous connection), Qp/Qs may be largely determined by other factors (see earlier) (see Fig. 67–2).

Systemic Arterial Oxygen Saturation Versus Systemic Oxygen Transport in Admixture Lesions

The variables that determine systemic arterial O_2 *transport* in admixture lesions (usually more relevant to tissue oxygenation than arterial saturation per se) are more complex. At any given ventricular output (from either a single ventricle or two ventricles), every milliliter of blood pumped to the lungs is one less milliliter that goes to the systemic circulation. Therefore, as the Qp/Qs (and systemic arterial O_2 saturation) *increases*, Qs *falls*. Systemic O_2 transport is therefore a function of total ventricular output, hematocrit, pulmonary venous O_2 saturation, Vo₂, and Qp/Qs; the relationship between Qp/Qs and systemic O_2 transport is sigmoidal[48-50] (Fig. 67–3).

"Single-Ventricle" Physiology

Multiple factors affect the physiology of neonates with complete mixing of systemic and pulmonary venous blood and communication at the level of the ventricle or great arteries (sometimes referred to as *single-ventricle physiology*). This physiology actually pertains to some lesions with two ventricles

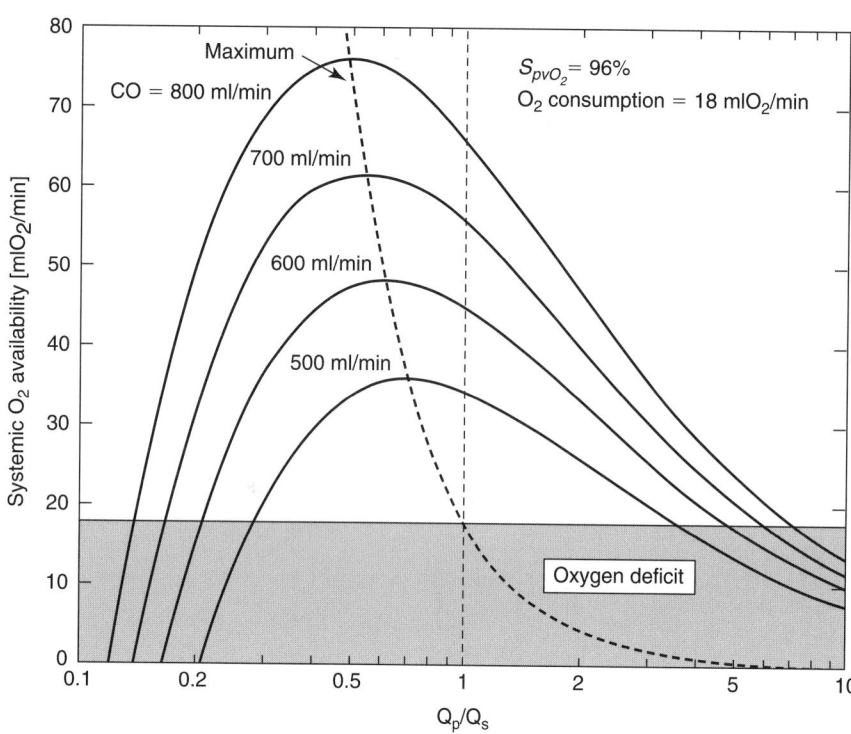

Figure 67–3. The relationship between systemic oxygen availability (transport) and the ratio of pulmonary to systemic blood flow (Q_p/Q_s) with cardiac admixture lesions. Barnea and colleagues[48] used a mathematical model to determine systemic oxygen transport for a patient with a single ventricle, with the aorta and pulmonary artery in communication, assuming the oxygen capacity of the blood to be 22 mL oxygen/dL, pulmonary venous oxygen saturation (Spv_{O_2}) to be 96%, and oxygen consumption to be 18 mL oxygen/minute (the normal mean value for a 3-kg neonate). Systemic oxygen transport is a function of both cardiac output and the ratio of pulmonary to systemic blood flow. Maximum systemic oxygen transport occurs with a ratio of less than 1, a value lower than that typical of most patients with hypoplastic left heart syndrome[86] and probably most patients with a "single ventricle" lesion. (From Barnea O, et al: Balancing the circulation: theoretic optimization of pulmonary/systemic flow ratio in hypoplastic left heart syndrome. J Am Coll Cardiol *24*:1376, 1994.)

(e.g., truncus arteriosus or tetralogy of Fallot with pulmonary atresia), as well as with as the single ventricle. It is unclear whether the number of ventricles materially affects the physiology, at least in the neonate. It may seem that two separate pumping chambers would be better than one at providing systemic O_2 transport in this context, but there are no relevant data in this regard.

1. With single-ventricle physiology (and ineffective Qp), there is increased volume work for the ventricle, which can be considerable (see later and Fig. 67-2).
2. In patients with a left-sided obstructive lesion and an unrestrictive PDA (e.g., hypoplastic left heart syndrome), there is a marked tendency for Qp to be large, especially as PVR falls in the perinatal period, and hence for *Qs to be reduced*, as detailed earlier. This is less the case for right-sided obstructive ductal dependent lesions (e.g., pulmonary atresia with intact ventricular septum) because the ductus is usually restrictive.
3. With single-ventricle physiology, *arterial O_2 saturation is less* than normal, also contributing to a tendency to reduced systemic O_2 transport.
4. Lesions with aortic diastolic runoff into the pulmonary circuit can have *decreased diastolic perfusion pressure* and therefore decreased myocardial perfusion.[38] Diastolic retrograde flow from the mesenteric arteries, perhaps in combination with reduced O_2 transport for the reasons noted earlier, also appears to increase the risk of necrotizing enterocolitis.[51]

The concurrence of the foregoing factors, especially in infants with high Qp, often leads to CHF and sometimes even frank hemodynamic compromise. For example, many babies with truncus arteriosus develop severe CHF and even die in the neonatal period,[52] presumably because of the combination of large ventricular volume load, cyanosis, and reduced myocardial perfusion.

Transposition Physiology

With D-transposition of the great arteries, the aorta arises from the RV, and the pulmonary artery arises from the LV. Because systemic and pulmonary venous blood enters the right and left atria, respectively, the systemic and pulmonary circulations function in parallel, rather than in series. Systemic venous blood, largely depleted of O_2, entering the RV is pumped out again to the body, whereas oxygenated pulmonary venous blood is ejected into the lungs.[53] Without any communication between the two circuits, all blood flow would be ineffective, and life would cease shortly after the gas-exchanging organ (the placenta) was disconnected from the systemic circulation. As it happens, communications between the systemic and pulmonary circuits usually exist at one or more levels (atrial septum, ventricular septum, ductus arteriosus, aorticopulmonary connections), and, if of sufficient size, they usually allow for enough *mixing* of systemic and pulmonary venous blood for adequate systemic arterial O_2 saturation (Fig. 67-4).

The essence of mixing is that for every milliliter of systemic venous blood that crosses from the right side of the heart, or the aorta, into the left side of the heart or pulmonary artery (and then into the lungs, constituting effective Qp), one milliliter of pulmonary venous blood must cross from the left heart into the right heart and into the aorta (becoming effective Qs). Were more blood to flow in one direction than the other, one of the two circulations would become depleted of blood. That is not to say that the volumes of blood pumped by the LV and RV need be equal, just that the average amount of blood crossing from left to right must equal the amount moving from right to left.[53] Indeed, whereas in the neonate with this lesion the LV volume pumped is similar to that of a normal neonate, by approximately 6 months of age it is considerably greater than normal.[54,55]

Echocardiographic studies have shown that infants with D-transposition and an atrial septal opening have shunting from the left atrium to the right atrium during systole, and right-to-left

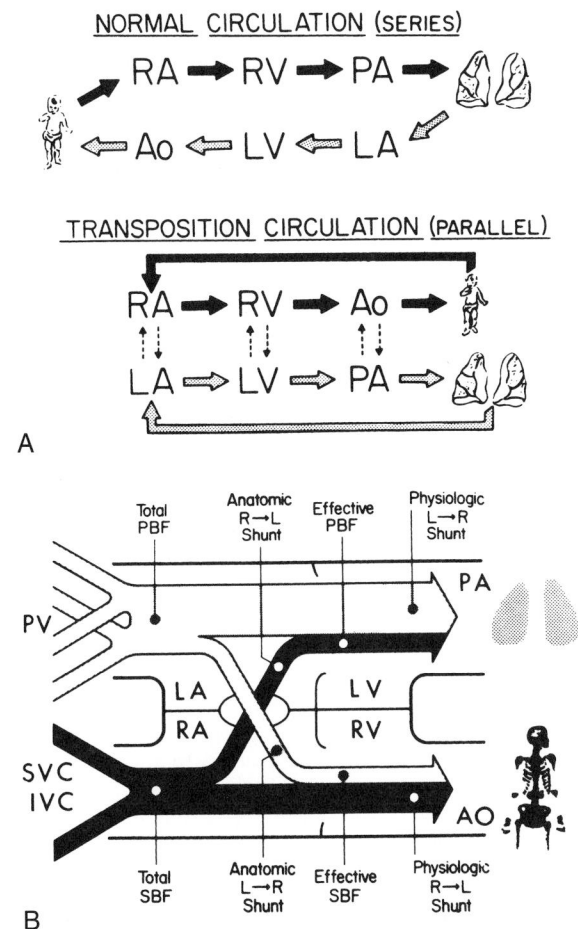

A

B

Figure 67–4. A and **B,** Intracardiac blood flow with D-transposition of the great arteries. Most pulmonary and systemic blood flow is ineffective. Systemic oxygen delivery depends on the passage of blood from the right side of the heart into the lungs (effective pulmonary blood flow) and the passage of an equal amount from the left side of the heart to the aorta (effective systemic blood flow). AO = aorta; IVC = inferior vena cava; LA = left atrium; LV = left ventricle; PV = pulmonary vein; RA = right atrium; RV = right ventricle; SBF = systemic blood flow; SVC = superior vena cava. (From Paul MH, et al: Moss and Adams: Heart Disease in Infants, Children, and Adolescents, Vol 2, 5th ed. Baltimore, Williams & Wilkins, 1995, pp 1166–1170.)

blood flow during diastole.[56] One way of explaining this pattern of blood flow is as follows: if the LV *compliance* is greater than that of the RV, there will be right-to-left shunting during ventricular filling, but greater *capacitance* on the systemic venous than the pulmonary venous side will result in left-to-right shunting when the atrioventricular valves are closed. The factors determining mixing have not been precisely determined, although it is clear that Qp is strongly positively related to the aortic O$_2$ saturation.[57] Thus, the presence of a PDA increases mixing by increasing Qp.[58] Conversely, increased PVR in neonates with D-transposition can markedly reduce the aortic saturation.[59] The number of sites of mixing also plays a role, with arterial saturation increasing with the number of mixing sites.[57]

Whereas cyanosis is usually the key physiologic feature of the newborn with this lesion (although some neonates with D-transposition and a large VSD may not be obviously cyanotic), CHF

can develop even in the neonate with a large PDA or VSD.[58,60] With a large VSD, the pattern of blood flow has not been fully elucidated, but there appears to be increased volume pumped by both ventricles.[61]

HOW CONGENITAL HEART LESIONS AFFECT CARDIOVASCULAR PHYSIOLOGY IN THE NEONATE: GENERAL MECHANISMS

Because one's ultimate aim is not to understand general principles of physiology, but rather individual patients, it is necessary to link these general principles with specific cardiac lesions. However, given the large number of distinct malformations, it is not feasible to describe the physiologic characteristics of each one. Even describing various classes of lesions (e.g., defects with left-to-right shunting) is unsatisfactory, because lesions within a class vary significantly in physiologic detail. The approach taken here is to describe several *characteristics of the efficient cardiovascular system* and to indicate how selected cardiac malformations *lack* one or more of these characteristics resulting in physiologic consequences.

Adequate Capacity to Pump Blood to the Lungs and Body

The capacity to supply blood requires one or two pumping chambers of adequate size, with acceptable rhythm, and systolic and diastolic function, in communication with the greater and lesser circulations. Only a single ventricle is required for fetal development and postnatal survival, and inadequate pumping capacity resulting from a lack of ventricular capacity is rare in neonates with congenital heart disease. Far more commonly, an adequate pump is not connected to the systemic (e.g., the RV in hypoplastic left heart syndrome with ductal closure) or pulmonary circulation (e.g., the LV in pulmonary atresia with intact ventricular septum with ductal closure). Whereas modest degrees of ventricular dysfunction are not uncommon in neonates with cardiac lesions (especially those who suffer severe hypoxia or ischemia), frankly inadequate systolic or diastolic ventricular function resulting from intrinsic abnormality of the myocardium is rare. The rare infants with a coronary artery anomaly, such as anomalous origin of the left coronary artery,[62] or pulmonary atresia with intact ventricular septum and coronary artery stenoses,[63] can develop ventricular dysfunction resulting from myocardial ischemia.

Effect of Increased Afterload on Cardiovascular Physiology

The amount of blood ejected by the ventricle is inversely related to the magnitude of afterload against which it ejects.[64, 65] Although the normal heart can to some extent maintain its output in the presence of *acutely* increased afterload,[65, 66] this reserve is limited, especially for a dysfunctional ventricle. Because the neonatal heart has less contractile reserve than the more mature one,[67] this is especially pertinent. Furthermore, because the major determinant of myocardial Vo$_2$ is pressure work,[68,69] the ventricle's ability to respond to an increase in afterload is crucially dependent on coronary perfusion pressure;[70] when increased afterload occurs with normal or decreased aortic pressure (e.g., severe valvar aortic stenosis), myocardial O$_2$ supply may be inadequate.

More relevant to the neonate is *chronically* increased afterload, which, if severe enough, causes a reduction in ventricular systolic and diastolic function. Chronically increased afterload also causes myocardial hypertrophy. Whereas hypertrophy is an adaptive response insofar as it normalizes wall stress,[71] *ventricular compliance* can be reduced by hypertrophy, manifested in *increased atrial pressure.* Left atrial hypertension can cause pulmonary edema, or left-to-right shunting if there is an atrial opening, and "reflex" pulmonary vasoconstriction,[72, 73] thereby increasing PAP beyond that accounted for by the elevation in LAP alone. Pressure overload of the RV can also cause increased right atrial pressure and systemic venous congestion. However, because the foramen ovale is usually nonrestrictive to right-to-left flow in the neonate, a reduction in RV filling is usually reflected by a right-to-left atrial shunt, rather than by systemic venous hypertension. Finally, *subendocardial ischemia* from severe chronic pressure overload can lead to endocardial fibrosis and to papillary muscle dysfunction or infarction and hence mitral regurgitation.[74]

Congenital Cardiac Lesions Causing Increased Afterload

The effects of increased afterload are clearly manifest in neonates with severe valvar *aortic stenosis*.[74] LV output is reduced,[75] sometimes so much so that adequate systemic perfusion can be maintained only by maintaining patency of the ductus to allow the RV to contribute to Qs. Left atrial hypertension often causes a considerable left-to-right atrial shunt, pulmonary edema, and pulmonary arterial hypertension. Whereas relief of the increased afterload by balloon dilation of the aortic valve results in an immediate decrease in (but not normalization of) LAP,[76, 77] LV systolic function remains abnormal for some time—at least days and probably weeks—after dilation.[78] *Severe coarctation of the aorta* in the neonate also causes reduction in LV systolic and diastolic function and output, as well as left-to-right atrial shunting. PAP is markedly increased, largely resulting from left atrial hypertension.[79]

Because the fetal RV operated at (and is therefore well-adapted to) systemic pressure,[6] *increased RV pressure* does not appear to have a measurable impact on RV systolic performance in a neonate, as long as it is approximately at or lower than systemic blood pressure. However, neonates with *severe valvar pulmonary stenosis* with suprasystemic RV pressure will have a reduction in RV output and a large atrial right-to-left shunt.[80] Right-to-left atrial shunting, often enough to cause substantial arterial desaturation, may persist for weeks after reduction of RV afterload by balloon dilation, a reflection of the relatively slow pace of normalization of RV compliance.[81]

Effect of Decreased Afterload on Cardiovascular Physiology

Because pressure is a function of vascular resistance and flow, inappropriately *low* SVR will cause hypotension unless blood flow is increased. Lower than normal SVR (resulting from dilation of systemic arterioles) occurs in some settings (e.g., with sepsis), but it does not seem to be an inherent feature of congenital cardiac malformations. In lesions in which the systemic circulation is in unrestricted communication with the venous (e.g., arteriovenous malformation)[46] or pulmonary (e.g., large VSD or PDA) circulation, outflow resistance to systemic ventricular ejection is reduced (at least if PVR is lower than SVR, in the case of the latter). This does not generally have a clinically significant impact on blood pressure because total blood flow into the systemic and pulmonary circuits is usually sufficient to maintain normal blood pressure. However, the relatively low blood pressure associated with a large PDA in the premature infant[82, 83] suggests that, in these cases, total (systemic plus pulmonary) flow is insufficient to compensate for the low total vascular resistance, owing to inclusion of the pulmonary circuit (see later).

ALL THE BLOOD PUMPED BY THE VENTRICLES MOVES DIRECTLY TOWARD THE APPROPRIATE CAPILLARY BED

In other words, the valves do not leak, and there is no left-to-right shunt. Valvar regurgitation and left-to-right shunting result in an inefficient circulation because the heart pumps volume that does not participate in gas exchange or O_2 transport. Lumping together these multiple causes of volume overload is in one sense a crude approach, because these lesions perturb cardiac mechanics and biology differently. For example, acute mitral regurgitation increases LV systolic and diastolic wall tension much less than aortic regurgitation.[84] Furthermore, as noted previously, left-to-right shunting at the ventricular level affects the LV differently than ductal level shunting. The virtue of considering these defects together is that their physiologic impact is in many ways very similar (increased ventricular volume load with consequent ventricular dilation; CHF).

Effect of Valve Regurgitation on Cardiovascular Physiology

Regurgitation of either the semilunar valves or the atrioventricular valves increases the volume pumped by the relevant ventricle. The magnitude of semilunar valve regurgitation is influenced by the degree of valve deformity, the heart rate, and the vascular resistance of the relevant circulation. Atrioventricular valve regurgitation is also influenced by the anatomy of the valve and by resistance to ventricular ejection. Mild regurgitation has minimal effects on patient physiology, but more severe volume overload may be attended by symptoms of CHF, increased atrial pressure, and even reduced Qs. *Aortic valve regurgitation*, by reducing coronary perfusion pressure, may also compromise myocardial perfusion.[38] *Pulmonary valve* regurgitation may be more pernicious in the neonate relative to the older patient because PVR is likely to be higher in the newborn.

Effect of Left-to-Right Shunting on Cardiovascular Physiology

As with valve regurgitation, left-to-right shunts of sufficient size cause symptoms of CHF. Profound reduction in Qs, as may be seen with severe aortic stenosis, is unusual with left-to-right shunting lesions. More modest compromise in Qs may occur with a large left-to-right shunt, although there are few quantitative data regarding neonates.

Other physiologic perturbations, although not a direct consequence of the shunting per se, may attend lesions that cause left-to-right shunting: (1) with a large communication between the aorta and pulmonary artery, diastolic pressure and hence myocardial perfusion may be reduced;[38] and (2) shunting lesions attended by increased PAP are associated with decreased lung compliance.[85]

How Much Volume Reserve Does the Neonatal Heart Have?

The neonatal ventricle is capable of pumping considerably more blood than normal under certain circumstances. For example, Tabbutt and co-workers[86] measured the Qp/Qs in 10 anesthetized and hemodynamically stable neonates with hypoplastic left heart syndrome; they found the mean Qp/Qs was approximately 3.4:1. Neither actual Qp nor actual Qs was measured, so the output from the (single) RV could not be determined. However, if one assumes that Qs was only 50% of usual (likely an underestimate), the single ventricle (RV) in these patients pumped 2.2 times as much blood as normal.

Data from animals are conflicting regarding how much extra volume can be pumped without significantly compromising Qs. In one study of mechanically ventilated preterm newborn lambs, relevant blood flows were measured with the ductus arteriosus open and closed; an approximately 60% increase in LV output resulting from opening the ductus was associated with a significant fall in Qs.[87] A similar study, however, showed no significant fall in Qs even with a 100% increase in LV output with opening of the ductus arteriosus.[88] Both studies were conducted over an hour or two and may not be reflective of long-term physiology. The newborn *human* with a PDA can have an LV output greater than 150% of normal,[89–92] but information regarding Qs in these neonates is very limited. Data from a few neonates with a PDA suggest that LV output of even more than three times normal may be generated with Qs greater than 3 L/m²/minute,[89, 91] although accurate measurement of Qp in this setting is very difficult. Infants (generally >1 month old) with a VSD may have a LV output of three to four times normal, assuming normal cardiac output = 4.2 ± 1.2 L/m²/minute,[93] while still maintaining Qs greater than 3 L/m²/minute.[11,21,22]

Congenital Cardiac Lesions with Valve Regurgitation

Atrioventricular valve regurgitation is uncommon in the neonate, although it can occur as an isolated lesion, with cardiac malformations,[74, 94, 95] or in association with papillary muscle dysfunction secondary to neonatal asphyxia.[96] Aortic regurgitation is exceedingly unusual (absent surgical intervention on the aortic valve). With absent pulmonary valve syndrome (tetralogy of Fallot with absent pulmonary valve), there is severe pulmonary regurgitation, but it is unclear precisely how this affects cardiac physiology because these patients also have a large VSD and RV outflow tract obstruction. With this condition, clinical phenotype is often primarily determined by large airway abnormalities.[97]

Congenital Cardiac Lesions with Left-to-Right Shunting

Most cardiac lesions in the neonate have at least a component of left-to-right shunting. An isolated *VSD* causes left-to-right shunting, although for the reasons noted earlier, symptoms of CHF usually do not develop for a few weeks. However, premature babies with a large VSD can develop symptoms within 1 to 2 weeks of age, perhaps in part because PVR declines more rapidly than in the term infant.[32] A large PDA is usually associated with a large left-to-right shunt, especially in the premature infant.

It is also unusual, but well described,[42] for left-to-right atrial level shunting through an isolated *atrial septal defect* to cause symptoms in infants. Left-to-right atrial shunting across the foramen ovale may be quite significant in neonates with left-sided obstructive lesions (e.g., aortic stenosis, coarctation).[98]

ALL SYSTEMIC VENOUS BLOOD PASSES THROUGH THE LUNGS BEFORE BEING PUMPED TO THE SYSTEMIC CIRCULATION

In other words, there is no right-to-left shunting. Actually, in the neonate, mildly to moderately reduced systemic arterial O₂ saturation may have little detectable impact on physiology; the unfavorable effects of chronic hypoxia (e.g., excessive polycythemia, brain abscess, stroke, and other neurologic symptoms) are rarely manifest in the neonate. However, it is unclear where to draw the line between mild to moderate hypoxemia (with modest if any physiologic impact) and severe hypoxemia (which threatens critical organ function) in the neonate. As previously noted, other determinants of O₂ transport (especially Qp and hematocrit) and Vo₂ undoubtedly influence what level of hypoxemia is compatible with aerobic metabolism, and there must be intraindividual variation as well. It seems clear that an arterial Po₂ in the mid-20 range (and probably even somewhat lower) can be tolerated for at least hours or days in most patients, presuming that other factors influencing systemic O₂ transport are acceptable. A lack of metabolic acidosis is often taken as an indication that systemic O₂ transport (and hence Po₂) is acceptable, but whether a lack of acidosis with hypoxemia correlates with a lack of long-term sequelae (especially central nervous system dysfunction) has not been clearly established.

Congenital Cardiac Lesions with Right-to-Left Shunting

Hypoxemia is usually the primary or sole physiologic manifestation of most lesions with *reduced Qp* (e.g., tetralogy of Fallot or severe valvar pulmonary stenosis). When some or all Qp is provided by a ductus in a patient with a right-sided obstructive lesion, there will be ineffective Qp and therefore increased volume pumped by the ventricle, but this volume load is usually modest, presumably because the ductus is somewhat restrictive with those lesions. Patients with lesions with *admixture physiology* and an unrestictive communication between the systemic and pulmonary circulations (e.g., truncus arteriosus, single-ventricle lesions without significant pulmonary stenosis, hypoplastic left heart syndrome, and PDA) usually have only mild hypoxemia (presuming that PVR falls normally in the postnatal period), but they commonly manifest CHF resulting from increased ventricular volume load. Single-ventricle lesions with some limitation of Qp resulting from increased PVR or anatomic restriction (e.g., tricuspid atresia with a restrictive VSD) can be well balanced and may have adequate arterial O₂ saturation but not CHF.

SYSTEMIC AND PULMONARY VENOUS BLOOD READILY ENTERS THE VENTRICLES

Under these conditions, there is no anatomic obstruction to ventricular filling. Rarely, a massively enlarged ventricle can encroach on the other and inhibit ventricular filling, such as LV encroachment by the right atrium/RV with a severe Ebstein anomaly[95] (Fig. 67–5). There are other impediments to ventricular filling, such as pericardial effusion, which are not congenital malformations per se. The physiologic consequences of obstruction to ventricular inflow are discussed earlier.

Congenital Cardiac Lesions with Restriction of Ventricular Filling

Isolated obstruction to ventricular inflow is very unusual in the neonate; when the tricuspid or mitral valve is small, the corresponding ventricle is usually reduced in volume. When filling of the RV is impeded (e.g., pulmonary atresia with intact ventricular septum), right-to-left flow across the foramen ovale is rarely obstructed; hence right atrial pressure is usually normal. With

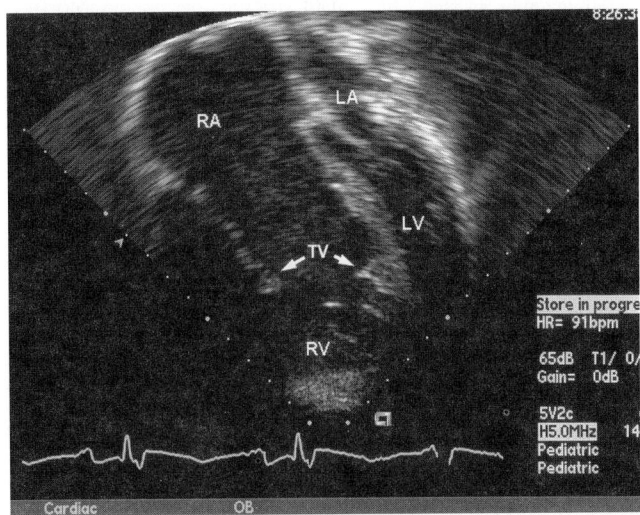

Figure 67–5. A cardiac ultrasound scan of a patient with Ebstein's anomaly. The dilated right-sided structures impinge on the much smaller left ventricle (LV). LA = left atrium; RA = right atrium; RV = right ventricle; TV = tricuspid valve.

mitral stenosis or atresia and hypoplasia of the LV (hypoplastic left heart syndrome), the atrial septal opening is usually large enough so pulmonary venous return is not significantly obstructed, although the size of the opening often becomes smaller over the first few weeks of life. Occasionally, the atrial septal opening is small, and the patient has left atrial hypertension and increased total pulmonary resistance, causing a reduction in Qp. Pulmonary edema further reduces systemic arterial saturation by interfering with gas exchange and by reducing lung compliance. Qs, however, is not reduced and may be increased, because systemic venous return to the RV is not obstructed, and the increased total pulmonary resistance reduces the fraction of RV output that goes to the lungs.

Mitral stenosis with adequate LV size is rare in the neonate, and it almost always occurs with other cardiac lesions.[99] Obstruction to pulmonary venous return can occur with *total anomalous pulmonary venous connection,* cor triatriatum, and stenosis of the individual pulmonary veins, the latter two being very rare. Pulmonary arterial hypertension, a reduction of RV compliance and output, and pulmonary edema are the primary physiologic manifestations.

REFERENCES

1. Sylvester JT, et al: The role of the vasculature in the regulation of cardiac output. Clin Chest Med 4:111, 1983.
2. Packer M: Pathophysiology of chronic heart failure. Lancet 340:88, 1992.
3. Schrier RW, Abraham WT: Hormones and hemodynamics in heart failure. N Engl J Med 341:577, 1999.
4. Turley K, Ebert PA: Transposition of the great arteries in the neonate: failed balloon septostomy. J Cardiovasc Surg 26:564, 1985.
5. Anderson P: Cardiovascular function during normal fetal and neonatal development and with hypoxic stress. In Polin RA, et al (eds): Fetal and Neonatal Physiology, 3rd ed. Philadelphia, Elsevier Science, 2003.
6. Rudolph AM: Fetal circulation and postnatal adaptation. In Rudolph AM (ed): Congenital Diseases of the Heart: Clinical-Physiological Considerations, 2nd ed. Armonk, NY, Futura Publishing, 2001, pp 3–44.
7. Fineman JR, et al: Regulation of pulmonary vascular tone in the perinatal period. Annu Rev Physiol 57:115, 1995.
8. Abman SH, Stevens T: Perinatal pulmonary vasoregulation: implications for the pathophysiology and treatment of neonatal pulmonary hypertension. In Haddad GG, Lister G (eds): Tissue Oxygen Deprivation: From Molecular to Integrated Function. New York, Marcel Dekker, 1996, pp 367–432.
9. Rabinovitch M: Developmental biology of the pulmonary vasculature. In Polin RA, et al (eds): Fetal and Neonatal Physiology, 3rd ed. Philadelphia, Elsevier Science, 2003.
10. Vargo TA: Cardiac catheterization: Hemodynamic measurements. In Garson A Jr, et al (eds): The Science and Practice of Pediatric Cardiology, 2nd ed. Baltimore, Williams & Wilkins, 1998, pp 961–993.
11. Hoffman JIE, Rudolph AM: The natural history of ventricular septal defects in infancy. Am J Cardiol 16:634, 1965.
12. Lister G, et al: Physiologic effects of increasing hemoglobin concentration in left-to-right shunting in infants with ventricular septal defects. N Engl J Med 306:502, 1982.
13. Lister G, et al: Effects of alterations of oxygen transport on the neonate. Semin Perinatol 8:192, 1984.
14. Rudolph AM: Hypoxia: historical and unresolved issues. In Haddad GG, Lister G (eds): Tissue Oxygen Deprivation: From Molecular to Integrated Function. New York, Marcel Dekker, 1996, pp 5–11.
15. Sidi D, et al: Developmental changes in oxygenation and circulatory responses to hypoxia in lambs. Am J Physiol 245:H674, 1983.
16. Moss M, et al: Oxygen transport and metabolism in the conscious lamb: the effects of hypoxia. Pediatr Res 22:177, 1987.
17. Cross KW, et al: The gaseous metabolism of the new-born infant breathing 15% oxygen. Acta Paediatr 47:217, 1958.
18. Newburger JW, et al: A comparison of the perioperative neurologic effects of hypothermic circulatory arrest versus low-flow cardiopulmonary bypass in infant heart surgery. N Engl J Med 329:1057, 1993.
19. Bellinger DC, et al: Developmental and neurological status of children at 4 years of age after heart surgery with hypothermic circulatory arrest of low-flow cardiopulmonary bypass. Circulation 100:526, 1999.
20. Fahey JT, Lister G: Postnatal changes in critical cardiac output and oxygen transport in conscious lambs. Am J Physiol 253:H100, 1987.
21. Beekman RH, et al: Hemodynamic effects of nitroprusside in infants with a large ventricular septal defect. Circulation 64:553, 1981.
22. Beekman RH, et al: Hemodynamic effects of hydralazine in infants with a large ventricular defect. Circulation 65:523, 1982.
23. Berman W Jr, et al: Effects of digoxin in infants with a congested circulatory state due to a ventricular septal defect. N Engl J Med 308:363, 1983.
24. Weber KT: Aldosterone in congestive heart failure. N Engl J Med 345:1689, 2001.
25. Lees MH: Catecholamine metabolite excretion of infants with heart failure. J Pediatr 69:259, 1966.
26. Ross RD, et al: Plasma norepinephrine levels in infants and children with congestive heart failure. Am J Cardiol 59:911, 1987.
27. Baylen BG, et al: The occurrence of hyperaldosteronism in infants with congestive heart failure. Am J Cardiol 45:305, 1980.
28. Scammell AM, Diver MJ: Plasma renin activity in infants with congenital heart disease. Arch Dis Child 62:1136, 1987.
29. Barrington K, Chan W: The circulatory effects of epinephrine infusion in the anesthetized piglet. Pediatr Res 33:190, 1993.
30. Brace RA: Fluid distribution in the fetus and neonate. In Polin RA, Fox WW (eds): Fetal and Neonatal Physiology, 2nd ed. Philadelphia, WB Saunders Co, 1998, p 1711.
31. Mitzner W: Resistance of the pulmonary circulation. Clin Chest Med 4:127, 1983.
32. Rudolph AM: Prenatal and postnatal pulmonary circulation. In Rudolph AM (ed): Congenital Diseases of the Heart: Clinical-Physiological Considerations, 2nd ed. Armonk, NY, Futura Publishing, 2001, pp 121–152.
33. Dawes GS: Sudden death in babies: physiology of the fetus and newborn. Am J Cardiol 22:469, 1968.
34. Levin AR, et al: Intracardiac pressure-flow dynamics in isolated ventricular septal defects. Circulation 35:430, 1967.
35. Graham TP Jr, et al: Right ventricular volume overload characteristics in ventricular septal defect. Circulation 54:800, 1976.
36. Reddy VM, et al: Fetal model of single ventricle physiology: hemodynamic effects of oxygen, nitric oxide, carbon dioxide, and hypoxia in the early postnatal period. J Thorac Cardiovasc Surg 112:437, 1996.
37. Jarmakani MM, et al: Effect of site of shunt on left heart-volume characteristics in children with ventricular septal defect and patent ductus arteriosus. Circulation 40:411, 1969.
38. Hoffman JIE: Transmural myocardial perfusion. Prog Cardiovasc Dis 29:429, 1987.
39. Bernhard WF, et al: The palliative Mustard operation for double outlet right ventricle or transposition of the great arteries associated with ventricular septal defect, pulmonary arterial hypertension, and pulmonary vascular obstructive disease. Circulation 54:810, 1976.
40. Levin AR, et al: Atrial pressure-flow dynamics in atrial septal defects (secundum type). Circulation 37:476, 1968.
41. Hoffman JIE, et al: Left to right atrial shunts in infants. Am J Cardiol 30:868, 1972.
42. Hunt CE, Lucas RV: Symptomatic atrial septal defect in infancy. Circulation 67:1042, 1973.
43. Rudolph AM: Atrial septal defect: partial anomalous drainage of pulmonary veins. In Rudolph AM (ed): Congenital Diseases of the Heart: Clinical-Physiological Considerations, 2nd ed. Armonk, NY, Futura Publishing, 2001, pp 253–254.
44. Gathman GE, Nadas AS: Total anomalous pulmonary venous connection: clinical and physiologic observations of 75 pediatric patients. Circulation 62:143, 1970.
45. Delisle G, et al: Total anomalous pulmonary venous connection: report of 93 autopsied cases with emphasis on diagnostic and surgical considerations. Am Heart J 91:99, 1976.
46. Cumming GR: Circulation in neonates with intracranial arteriovenous fistula and cardiac failure. Am J Cardiol 45:1019, 1980.
47. Ward KE, et al: Restrictive interatrial communication in total anomalous pulmonary venous connection. Am J Cardiol 57:1131, 1986.
48. Barnea O, et al: Balancing the circulation: theoretic optimization of pulmonary/systemic flow ratio in hypoplastic left heart syndrome. J Am Coll Cardiol 24:1376, 1994.
49. Barnea O, et al: Estimation of oxygen delivery in newborns with a univentricular circulation. Circulation 98:1407, 1998.
50. Migliavacca F, et al: Modeling of the Norwood circulation: effect of shunt size, vascular resistances, and heart rate. Am J Physiol 280:H2071, 2001.
51. McElhinney DB, et al: Necrotizing enterocolitis in neonates with congenital heart disease: risk factors and outcomes. Pediatrics 106:1080, 2000.
52. Williams JM, et al: Factors associated with outcomes of persistent truncus arteriosus. J Am Coll Cardiol 34:545, 1999.
53. Paul MH: Moss and Adams: Heart Disease in Infants, Children, and Adolescents, Vol 2, 5th ed. Baltimore, Williams & Wilkins, 1995, pp 1166–1170.
54. Graham TP Jr, et al: Quantification of left heart volume and systolic output in transposition of the great arteries. Circulation 44:899, 1971.
55. Keane JF, et al: Pulmonary blood flow and left ventricular volumes in transposition of the great arteries and intact ventricular septum. Br Heart J 35:521, 1973.
56. Satomi G, et al: Blood flow pattern of the interatrial communication in patients with complete transposition of the great arteries: a pulsed Doppler echocardiographic study. Circulation 73:95, 1986.
57. Mair DD, Ritter DG: Factors influencing intercirculatory mixing in patients with complete transposition of the great arteries. Am J Cardiol 30:653, 1972.
58. Waldman JD: Transposition of the great arteries with intact ventricular septum and patent ductus arteriosus. Am J Cardiol 39:232, 1977.
59. Chang AC, et al: Management of the neonate with transposition of the great arteries and persistent pulmonary hypertension. Am J Cardiol 68:1253, 1991.

60. Plauth WH Jr, et al: Changing hemodynamics in patients with transposition of the great arteries. Circulation *42*:131, 1970.
61. Graham TP Jr, et al: Right heart volume characteristics in transposition of the great arteries. Circulation *51*:881, 1975.
62. Shivalkar B, et al: ALCAPA syndrome: an example of chronic myocardial hypoperfusion? J Am Coll Cardiol *23*:772, 1994.
63. Giglia TM, et al: Diagnosis and management of right-ventricle-dependent coronary circulation in pulmonary atresia with intact ventricular septum. Circulation *86*:1516, 1992.
64. Van Hare GF, et al: The effects of increasing mean arterial pressure on left ventricular output in newborn lambs. Circ Res *67*:78, 1990.
65. Braunwald E, et al: Normal and abnormal circulatory function. *In* Braunwald E (ed): Heart Disease: A Textbook of Cardiovascular Medicine, 4th ed. Philadelphia, WB Saunders Co, 1992, pp 379–380.
66. Klautz RJ, et al: Interaction between afterload and contractility in the newborn heart: evidence of homeometric autoregulation in the intact circulation. J Am Coll Cardiol *25*:1428, 1995.
67. Teitel DF, et al: Developmental changes in myocardial contractile reserve in the lamb. Pediatr Res *19*:948, 1985.
68. Shaddy RE, et al: The effects of changes in heart rate and aortic systolic pressure on left ventricular myocardial oxygen consumption in lambs. J Dev Physiol *11*:213, 1989.
69. Braunwald E, Sobel BE: Coronary blood flow and myocardial ischemia. *In* Braunwald E (ed): Heart Disease: A Textbook of Cardiovascular Medicine, 4th ed. Philadelphia, WB Saunders Co, 1992, pp 1162–1163.
70. Vlahakes GJ, et al: The pathophysiology of failure in acute right ventricular hypertension: hemodynamic and biochemical correlations. Circulation *63*:87, 1981.
71. Perloff JK: Development and regression of increased ventricular mass. Am J Cardiol *50*:605, 1982.
72. Belik J: Myogenic response in large pulmonary arteries and its ontogenesis. Pediatr Res *36*:34, 1994.
73. Storme L, et al: In vivo evidence for a myogenic response in the fetal pulmonary circulation. Pediatr Res *45*:425, 1999.
74. Hoffman JIE: Aortic stenosis. *In* Moller JH, Neal WA (eds): Fetal, Neonatal, and Infant Cardiac Disease. Norwalk, CT, Appleton & Lange, 1990, pp 451–473.
75. Lakier JB, et al: Isolated aortic stenosis in the neonate. Circulation *50*:801, 1974.
76. Beekman RH, et al: Balloon valvuloplasty for critical aortic stenosis in the newborn: influence of new catheter technology. J Am Coll Cardiol *17*:1172, 1991.
77. Egito EST, et al: Transvascular balloon dilation for neonatal critical aortic stenosis: early and midterm results. J Am Coll Cardiol *29*:442, 1997.
78. Magee AG, et al: Balloon dilation of severe aortic stenosis in the neonate: comparison of antegrade and retrograde catheter approaches. J Am Coll Cardiol *30*:1061, 1997.
79. Graham TP Jr, et al: Right and left heart size and function in infants with symptomatic coarctation. Circulation *56*:641, 1977.
80. Sommer RJ, et al: Physiology of critical pulmonary valve obstruction in the neonate. Cathet Cardiovasc Intervent *50*:473, 2000.
81. Rome JJ: Balloon pulmonary valvuloplasty. Pediatr Cardiol *19*:18, 1998.
82. Evans N, Moorcraft J: Effect of patency of the ductus arteriosus on blood pressure in very preterm infants. Arch Dis Child *67*:1169, 1992.
83. Pladys P, et al: Left ventricular output and mean arterial pressure in preterm infants during 1st day of life. Eur J Pediatr *158*:817, 1999.
84. Braunwald E: Valvular heart disease. *In* Braunwald E (ed): Heart Disease: A Textbook of Cardiovascular Medicine, 4th ed. Philadelphia, WB Saunders Co, 1992, pp 1020–1048.
85. Bancalari E, et al: Lung mechanics in congenital heart disease with increased and decreased pulmonary blood flow. J Pediatr *90*:192, 1977.
86. Tabbutt S, et al: Impact of inspired gas mixtures on preoperative infants with hypoplastic left heart syndrome during controlled ventilation. Circulation *104*(Suppl I):I-159, 2001.
87. Clyman RI, et al: Cardiovascular effects of patent ductus arteriosus in preterm lambs with respiratory distress. J Pediatr *111*:579, 1987.
88. Baylen BG, et al: The contractility and performance of the preterm left ventricle before and after early patent ductus arteriosus occlusion in surfactant-treated lambs. Pediatr Res *19*:1053, 1985.
89. Rudolph AM, et al: Patent ductus arteriosus: a clinical and hemodynamic study of 23 patients in the first year of life. Pediatrics *22*:892, 1958.
90. Burnard ED, et al: Cardiac output in the newborn infant. Clin Sci *31*:121, 1966.
91. Danilowicz D, et al: Delayed closure of the ductus arteriosus in premature infants. Pediatrics *37*:74, 1966.
92. Lindner W, et al: Stroke volume and left ventricular output in preterm infants with patent ductus arteriosus. Pediatr Res *27*:278, 1990.
93. Jegier W, et al: The relation between cardiac and body size. Br Heart J *25*:425, 1963.
94. Barber G, et al: The significance of tricuspid regurgitation in hypoplastic left heart syndrome. Am Heart J *116*:1563, 1988.
95. Robertson DA, Silverman NH: Ebstein's anomaly: echocardiographic and clinical features in the fetus and neonate. J Am Coll Cardiol *14*:1300, 1989.
96. Bucciarelli RL, et al: Transient tricuspid insufficiency of the newborn: a form of myocardial dysfunction in stressed newborns. Pediatrics *59*:330, 1977.
97. Pinsky WW, et al: The absent pulmonary valve syndrome: considerations of management. Circulation *57*:159, 1978.
98. Graham TP, et al: Absence of left ventricular volume loading in infants with coarctation of the aorta and a large ventricular septal defect. J Am Coll Cardiol *14*:1545, 1989.
99. Moore P, et al: Severe congenital mitral stenosis in infants. Circulation *89*:2099, 1994.
100. Teitel DF, et al: Moss and Adams: Heart Disease in Infants, Children, and Adolescents, Vol 1, 5th ed. Baltimore, Williams & Wilkins, 1995, p 49.

Jeffrey L. Segar

68

Neural Regulation of Blood Pressure During Fetal and Newborn Life

Control of circulatory function is mediated through interacting neural, hormonal, and metabolic mechanisms acting at both central and local levels. The role of the central nervous system, in particular, is critical for cardiovascular homeostasis, including the maintenance of blood pressure within normal limits.[1,2] Sympathetic outflow to the heart and blood vessels is continuously modulated by an array of peripheral sensors, including arterial baroreceptors and chemoreceptors located in the aortic arch and carotid sinus, as well as mechanoreceptors located in the heart and lungs.[3] Cardiovascular centers within the brain, inserted between afferent and efferent pathways of the reflex arc, integrate a variety of visceral and behavioral sensations, allowing for a wide range of modulation of specific autonomic, cardiovascular, and endocrine responses. Although these basic mechanisms likely exist in the fetus and newborn, differential rates of maturation of these systems influence the ability of the developing animal to maintain adequate blood pressure and organ blood flow.

NEURAL MODULATION OF THE BASAL HEMODYNAMIC STATE

Tonic discharge of spinal vasoconstrictor neurons is an important regulator of vasomotor tone and, ultimately, the maintenance of arterial pressure within its physiologic range.[4] The contribution of the autonomic nervous system on cardiovascular homeostasis clearly changes during development. Both α-adrenergic and ganglionic blockades produce greater decreases in blood pressure in term than in preterm fetal lambs.[5,6] The hypotensive effect following α-adrenergic and ganglionic blockade is less in newborn lambs than in term fetuses and continues to decline with postnatal development.[7] These findings suggest that sympathetic tone is higher late in fetal life and is important in the maintenance of fetal arterial pressure. The influence of the parasympathetic system on resting heart rate appears to increase with maturation.[8] Cholinergic blockade produces no consistent effect of heart rate in premature fetal sheep, a slight increase in heart rate in term fetuses, and the greatest effect in lambs beyond the first week of life.[5,7]

Within a physiologic range, arterial pressure displays a naturally occurring variability, the degree of which is similar in fetal and postnatal life.[9-12] In the adult rat, ganglionic blockade increases arterial pressure variability,[11,13] suggesting that a component of arterial pressure lability is peripheral or humoral in origin and is buffered by autonomic functions. In contrast, ganglionic blockade in term fetal sheep significantly attenuates heart rate and arterial pressure variability.[10] Changes in sympathetic tone, as recorded from the renal sympathetic nerve have been shown to be positively correlated with fluctuations in heart rate and arterial pressure.[10] Therefore, fluctuations in basal sympathetic tone appear to play a more significant role in the generation of blood pressure variability during fetal than during postnatal life. Oscillations in basal sympathetic tone appears to be related to changes in the behavior state of the fetus.[14-16] Although fetal electrocortical and sympathetic activity has not been recorded simultaneously, electrocortical activity appears to mediate changes in both sympathetic and parasympathetic tone.[15,17] Basal heart rate, arterial pressure, and catecholamine levels are highest during periods of high-voltage low-frequency electrocortical activity.[14,18-20] Other physiologic parameters, including organ blood flows, regional vascular resistances, and cerebral oxygen consumption also depend on electrocortical state and likely reflect changes in autonomic activity.[19,21,22]

Short-term changes in vascular stretch related to arterial pressure modify the discharge of afferent baroreceptors fibers located in the carotid sinus and aortic arch.[1] This, in turn, produces alterations in parasympathetic and sympathetic nerve activities that influence heart rate and peripheral vascular resistance and serve to buffer changes in arterial pressure.[23,24] Results of studies in sheep, which have to date been the most common model for studying integrative developmental cardiovascular physiology, demonstrate the arterial baroreflex is functional during fetal and postnatal life.[8,9,25,26] Investigators disagree, however, about the magnitude of the baroreflex early in development and the influence of these reflexes on controlling heart rate and arterial pressure. Results of earlier studies indicated that the threshold for baroreceptor activity is above the normal range of arterial pressure during fetal and neonatal life, and that baroreceptors may not be loaded during fetal life.[27,28] Other studies in fetal sheep demonstrate that sinoaortic denervation produces marked fluctuations in fetal arterial pressure and heart rate,[9,25] suggesting that the arterial baroreflex plays an important role in maintaining cardiovascular homeostasis. Evidence for the presence of functional baroreceptors in the immature animal is provided by single fiber recordings of baroreceptor afferents in the carotid sinus and aortic depressor nerves.[29-33] In fetal and newborn animals, carotid sinus nerve activity is phasic and pulse synchronous, whereas activity increases with a rise in arterial or carotid sinus pressure.[29,31,33] Basal discharge of baroreceptor afferents does not change during fetal and postnatal maturation, despite a considerable increase in mean arterial pressure during this time.[29] These findings are consistent with those demonstrated in developing rabbits[30] and indicate that baroreceptors reset during development, such that they continue to function within the physiologic range for arterial pressure. Furthermore the response of carotid baroreceptor activity to increases in carotid sinus pressure is greater in fetal than in newborn and 1 month old lambs.[29] The threshold for carotid baroreceptor discharge is lower, and the sensitivity of the baroreceptor is also greater in newborns than in adult rabbits.[30] Although parasym-

pathetic influence on heart rate early during development is limited,[26,34-37] results obtained from direct recording of baroreceptor afferents[29,30] demonstrate that the sensitivity of the baroreceptors is greater early during development and resets at a lower level as arterial pressure increases during fetal and postnatal life. These findings suggest that reduced heart rate responses to changes in arterial pressure during fetal life are not due to underdeveloped afferent activity of baroreceptors but to differences in central integration and efferent parasympathetic nerve activity.

The mechanisms regulating the changes in sensitivity of the baroreceptors early in development have not been investigated but may be similar to those proposed in the adult.[38-40] In younger animals, the carotid sinus is more distensible, increasing the degree of mechanical deformation of nerve endings and ultimately producing a greater strain sensitivity.[40] Alternatively, ionic mechanisms,[38,41] such as activation of the sodium pump that may operate at the receptor membrane to cause hyperpolarization of the endings, and substances released from the endothelium including prostacyclin,[42] and nitric oxide[43-45] may modulate baroreceptor activity during development. Blockade of cyclooxygenase with indomethacin reduces carotid baroreceptor sensitivity in newborn but not adult sheep.[46] Along these lines, prostaglandin E_2 and I_2 levels within carotid sinus tissues are sixfold higher in newborn than adult sheep.[46] Whether such influences on baroreceptor activity are present during fetal development has not been investigated.

Arterial baroreflex function and sensitivity are equally dependent on the efferent limb of the reflex—including sympathetic and parasympathetic nerve activity and end-organ neuroeffector responsiveness. The arterial baroreflex during fetal and postnatal maturation has primarily been investigated by examining the relationship between the increase in arterial pressure and the fall in heart rate.[25,28,36,47,48] Baroreflex control of fetal heart rate is dominated by changes in cardiac vagal tone, although integrity of the reflex depends on both sympathetic and parasympathetic pathways.[49] Results of several studies have described a relatively reduced heart rate response to alterations in arterial pressure in fetal and newborn animals and in human infants.[28,34,35,50] Using reflex bradycardia in response to increased blood pressure by balloon inflation, Shinebourne and colleagues[34] found that baroreflex activity is present as early as 0.6 of gestation in fetal lambs, and that the sensitivity of the reflex increased up to term. Additional studies in sheep[35] and other species[51,52] have similarly found increasing baroreflex sensitivity with postnatal age. For example, reflex bradycardia in response to carotid sinus stimulation is absent during the first week of life in the piglet, although vagal efferents exert a tonic action on the heart at this stage of development.[52] Age-related changes in heart rate in response to phenylephrine are also greater in 2-month-old piglets than in 1-day-old animals.[51]

Other studies suggest that the sensitivity of the cardiac baroreflex is in fact greater in the fetus than in the newborn and decreases with maturation.[48,53] More recently, the developmental changes in heart rate and efferent renal sympathetic nerve activity (RSNA) in response to increases and decreases in blood pressure in fetal, newborn and 4- to 6-week-old sheep have been examined.[54] These studies demonstrate that baroreceptor activity regulates sympathetic outflow as well as heart rate during fetal life, that functional baroreflex control of RSNA and heart rate shifts toward higher pressures during development, and that the sensitivity of the RSNA baroreflex function curve is greater early in development and decreases following the transition from fetal to newborn life (Fig. 68–1). Interestingly, studies during postnatal life have shown that baroreflex control heart rate and sympathetic nerve activity are impaired with senescence,[55] an effect that may contribute to the development of hypertension.

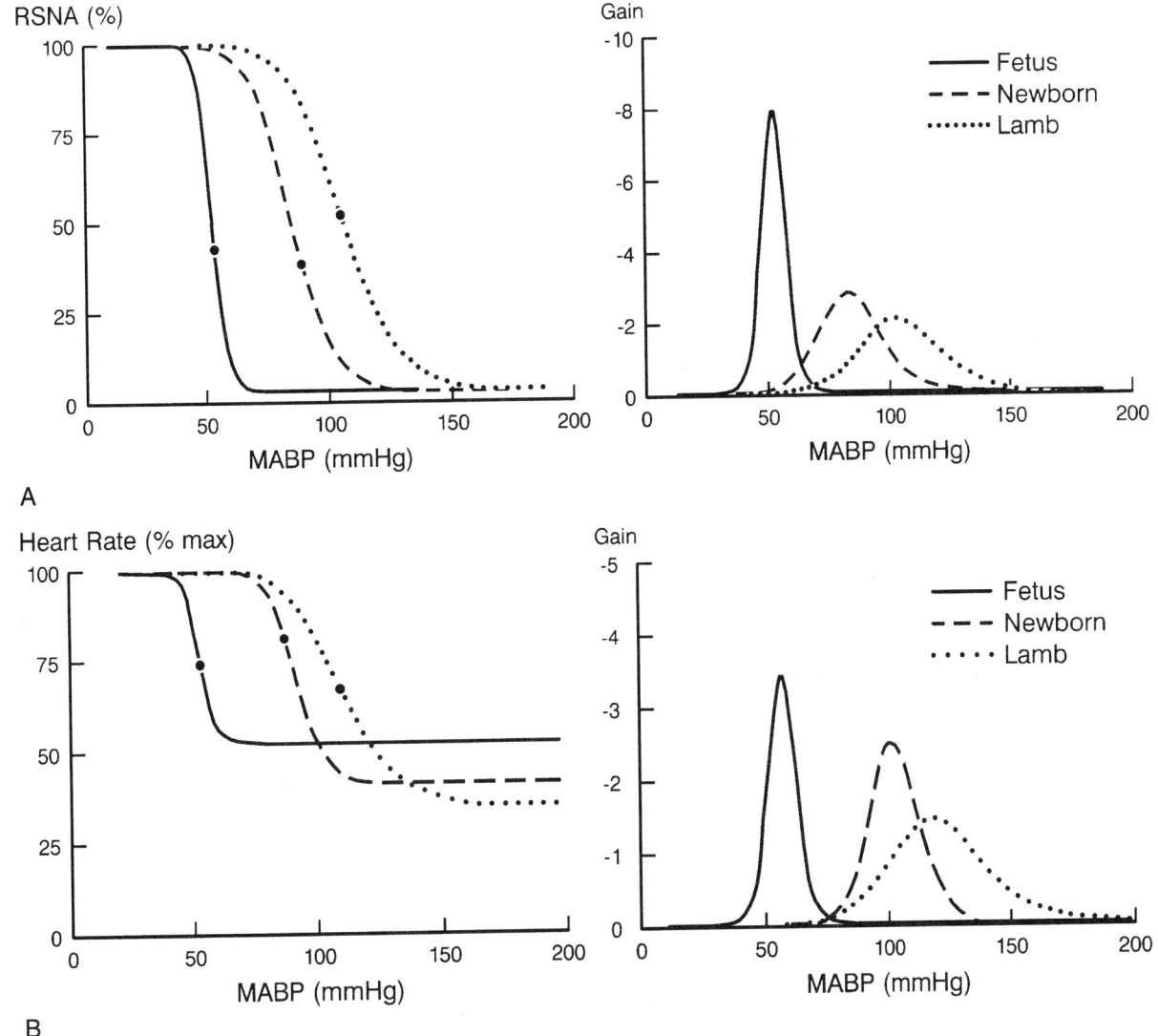

Figure 68–1. Baroreflex function relating renal sympathetic nerve activity (RSNA) **(A)** or heart rate **(B)** and mean arterial blood pressure (MABP) in near-term fetal, newborn (7 days old), and 4- to 6-week old lambs. RSNA and heart rate are expressed as percentages of maximum response. • = point on curves representing basal values. (From Segar JL, et al: Am J Physiol 263:H1819, 1992.)

Several reasons for reported differences in the sensitivity of baroreflex function early in development are apparent. First, interspecies variability in the maturation of sympathetic and parasympathetic activity and function, including maturity of the central and efferent components of the reflex exist.[51] For example, a functional baroreflex is not present in rats until 3 weeks of age,[56] whereas baroreceptor sensitivity in newborn pigs and dogs is low and increases with postnatal age.[35, 51] Second, some investigators have examined the heart rate response to a rise in blood pressure using either phenylephrine[25, 48] or aortic balloon inflation,[34, 48] whereas others derived complete sigmoidal baroreflex curves for heart rate and efferent sympathetic activity.[54] Third, use of anesthesia in several studies might also have altered baroreflex mediated responses, as previously suggested in adults.[57]

Resetting of the Arterial Baroreflex

Resetting of the arterial baroreflex is defined as a change in the relationship between arterial pressure and heart rate or between pressure and sympathetic and parasympathetic nerve activities.[38, 39] Results of several studies demonstrate that the sensitivity of the baroreflex changes with maturation and shifts,

or resets, toward higher pressures.[54, 55, 58] This shift occurs during fetal life, is present immediately after birth, and continues with postnatal maturation, paralleling the naturally occurring increase in blood pressure.[59] The mechanisms regulating developmental changes in baroreflex sensitivity and controlling resetting of the baroreflex are poorly understood. Changes in the relationship between arterial pressure and sympathetic activity or heart rate occur at the level of the baroreceptor itself (peripheral resetting), as discussed earlier, and from altered coupling within the central nervous system of afferent impulses from baroreceptors to efferent sympathetic or parasympathetic activities (central resetting).[38] Endogenous nitric oxide may contribute to the maturational alterations in the arterial baroreflex as pharmacologic blockade of nitric oxide synthase abolishes age-related differences in baroreflex control of heart rate in 1- and 6-week-old lambs.[45] This site of this effect has not been investigated. Changes in the levels of circulating hormones and neuropeptides, such as angiotensin II (ANG II), vasopressin (AVP), and serotonin; changes in basal autonomic neural activity; and activation of additional neural reflex pathways are other factors that may modulate the changes in arterial baroreflex during development.[38, 60, 61]

In adults, adaptation or resetting of the baroreflex during acute or chronic increases in arterial pressure is modulated by both peripheral and central mechanisms.[38] Early in development, however, short-term increases in blood pressure do not alter the arterial baroreflex.[54] This failure of resetting results in part from the absence of the arterial pressure–baroreceptor activity in relationship to adaptation to increased pressure (personal observation). With a sustained increase in arterial pressure, activity of the aortic depressor nerve, which contains afferent fibers from aortic arch baroreceptors remains elevated, and fails to decrease or "escape" from constant baroreceptor stimulation. These findings suggest that factors other than the maturational increase in blood pressure influence ontogenic changes in the arterial baroreflex.

Humoral Interactions on Baroreflex Function

The arterial baroreflex not only modulates heart rate and the peripheral vascular tone by altering autonomic activity, it also regulates the release of vasoactive hormones, such as ANG II and AVP.[61,62] Changes in the levels of these circulating hormones, in turn, influence neural regulation of cardiovascular function by acting at several sites along the reflex arc.[61] In the adult, ANG II facilitates activation of sympathetic ganglia and enhances the release and response of norepinephrine at the neuroeffector junction.[63] Within the central nervous system, ANG II stimulates sympathetic outflow and alters baroreceptor reflexes by acting on ANG II type 1 (AT_1) receptors located within the hypothalamus, medulla, and circumventricular organs.[64-66]

The effects of exogenous ANG II on reflex control of fetal heart rate have been studied. In the sheep fetus a rise in arterial blood pressure produced by ANG II administration produces little or no cardiac slowing,[67,68] although other researchers have reported dose-dependent decreases in heart rate.[36,53] The bradycardic and sympathoinhibitory responses to any given increase in blood pressure is less for ANG II than that produced by other vasoconstrictor agents.[60] ANG II acts centrally (primarily within the area postrema) to interfere with the cardiac baroreflex through suppression of vagal efferents.[36,69,70]

Endogenous ANG II participates in regulating arterial baroreflex responses early during development. The absence of rebound tachycardia after reduction in blood pressure by angiotensin-converting enzyme (ACE) inhibitors is well described in fetal and postnatal animals,[71] as well in human adults and infants.[72] In the newborn lamb, ACE inhibition or AT_1-receptor blockade decreases RSNA and heart rate, and resets the baroreflex toward lower pressure.[60,73] Resetting of the reflex is independent of changes in prevailing blood pressure. Lateral ventricle administration of an AT_1, but not AT_2, receptor antagonist also lowers blood pressure and reset the baroreflex toward lower pressure in newborn and 8-week-old sheep at doses that have no effect when given systemically.[73] Converting enzyme inhibition has no effect on baroreflex control of RSNA in fetal sheep.[60] However, when enalapril is administered to the fetus immediately before delivery, baroreflex control of RSNA and heart rate is shifted toward lower pressures.[60] In newborn lambs, plasma levels of ANG II are two- to fourfold higher than in fetal or adult sheep.[68] Thus the elevated endogenous levels of ANG II during the newborn period may help explain the observation that inhibition of ANG II during this time alters reflex control of HR and RSNA, whereas little effect is seen in the fetus.

In several adult species, vasopressin modulates parasympathetic and sympathetic tone and ultimately regulates cardiovascular and baroreflex function.[61,74] Administration of AVP evokes are greater sympathoinhibition and bradycardia than other vasoconstrictors for a comparable increase in blood pressure.[61,75] This modulation of the baroreflex has been attributed to AVP's enhancing the gain of the reflex as well as resetting the reflex to

a lower pressure.[61,75] There is disagreement, however, regarding the type of vasopressin receptor that mediates the action of the peptide on the baroreflex. Several studies suggest that activation of AVP type 1 (V_1) receptor enhances the inhibitory effect of the arterial baroreflex on heart rate and sympathetic outflow, whereas others conclude that V_2 receptors are involved.[75,76]

Studies during fetal and newborn life demonstrate that AVP secretory mechanisms are well developed early in life, and that AVP increases fetal arterial pressure and decreases heart rate in a dose-dependent manner.[77,78] However, sequential increases in plasma AVP in fetal and newborn sheep does not alter baroreflex control of RSNA and heart rate in response to acute changes in blood pressure.[79] In contrast in adult sheep, increased plasma AVP caused significant bradycardia and sympathoinhibition without any change in resting blood pressure, along with resetting of heart rate and RSNA baroreflex curves toward lower pressures.[80]

Circulating endogenous AVP also appears to have little effect on baroreflex function early during development. Administration of a V_1-receptor antagonist has no measurable effects on resting hemodynamics in fetal sheep or on basal arterial blood pressure,[81] heart rate, RSNA, or baroreflex response in newborn lambs.[79] Taken together, these results indicate that the effect of AVP on the arterial baroreceptor is developmentally regulated, with little effect observed during fetal and newborn life. This lack of baroreflex modulation by AVP may therefore facilitate the pressor response to AVP in fetuses and newborns during stressful situations (e.g., hypoxia and hemorrhage). In this way, AVP could play a particularly important role in maintaining arterial pressures during these states early in development.

Vasopressin and specific AVP receptors have been localized in areas of the brain known to be involved in autonomic and cardiovascular regulation, suggesting that central AVP plays a role in the control of blood pressure and heart rate.[74,76] In some adult species, intracerebroventricular injection of AVP increases blood pressure and heart rate.[74,76] These effects are primarily mediated by stimulation of sympathetic vasomotor activity and are blocked by central but not peripheral administration of V_1 receptor antagonists.[74,82] The influence of central AVP on baroreflex function appears to differ among species. In rabbits and dogs, central AVP facilitates the effect of the arterial baroreflex-mediated changes on heart rate and sympathetic outflow, whereas work done in rats and cats has shown that AVP may exert on inhibitory influence on the reflex.[82]

The role of central vasopressin in maintaining hemodynamic homeostasis in the developing animal has not been extensively studied. The fact that under basal conditions fetal AVP levels are 10-fold higher in cerebrospinal fluid than in plasma suggests that AVP may contribute to central regulation of autonomic function.[83] Intracerebroventricular infusion of AVP produces significant decreases in mean arterial blood pressure and heart rate in newborn lambs although no reflex changes in RSNA are seen.[84] The changes in blood pressure and heart rate are completely inhibited by administration of a V_1 antagonist, suggesting the central cardiovascular effects of AVP are mediated by V_1 receptors, as has been reported in mature animals.[82] Intracerebroventricular administration of AVP increases RSNA in 8-week-old sheep, suggesting that the role of AVP receptors within the CNS in regulation of autonomic function is developmentally regulated.[84]

Endogenous production of cortisol is important for the resetting of the baroreflex that occurs with normal maturational increases in blood pressure. In adrenalectomized fetal sheep, restoring circulating cortisol levels to the prepartum physiologic range shifts the fetal and neonatal heart rate and RSNA baroreflex curves toward higher pressure without altering the slope of the curves.[85] In a similar manner, elevation of corticosterone levels in adult rats resets baroreflex control of heart rate and RSNA and reduces the gain of the responses.[86,87] Antenatal administration of betamethasone decreases the sensitivity of baroreflex-mediated changes in heart rate in preterm fetuses and premature lambs.[88] Taken together, these studies suggest glucocorticoids influence baroreflex function before and after birth.

BAROREFLEX FUNCTION IN THE HUMAN NEONATE

In the human neonate, neural control of the circulation has been assessed most commonly by recording alterations in the heart rate in response to postural changes. Several studies have demonstrated in healthy term and preterm infants that head-up tilting (to unload arterial baroreceptors) produces a significant heart rate response[89, 90] and that the magnitude of the response is proportional to the degree of tilting.[90] In contrast, other investigators have been unable to demonstrate a consistent response of heart rate to tilting and concluded that the heart rate component of the baroreflex is poorly developed during the neonatal period.[91] Using venous occlusion plethysmography, Waldman and colleagues[91] found in otherwise healthy preterm and term infants that 45° head-up tilting produced on average a 25% decrease in limb blood flow, suggestive of an increase in peripheral vascular resistance, although no significant tachycardia was observed.

Power spectral analysis (PSA), a computer-assisted technique that quantifies the small spontaneous beat-by-beat variations in heart rate, has been used in human adults,[92] infants[93, 94] and fetuses[95] to evaluate the contribution of the autonomic nervous system in maintaining cardiovascular homeostasis and determine the sympathovagal interactions regulating heart rate during resting conditions and following postural changes. Studies of fetal electrocardiogram tracings have shown that younger fetuses have a greater total energy of the power spectrum compared with more mature fetuses, consistent with the evolution of a stable and mature autonomic nervous system.[95] Maturational changes in the power spectra of HR variability have also been shown by comparing preterm with term infants.[93, 94] There is a progressive decline in the low-frequency:high-frequency (LF:HF) power ratio associated with both increasing postnatal and gestational age, indicating an increase in parasympathetic contribution to control of resting HR with maturation. Clairambault et al.[94] found that changes in the HF component of the spectrum were greater at 37 to 38 weeks, suggesting a steep increase in vagal tone at this age.

PSA has also been used to characterize developmental changes in sympathovagal balance in response to arterial baroreceptor unloading in preterm infants beginning at 28 to 30 weeks' post-conceptional age.[96] By longitudinally examining changes in heart rate power spectrum on a weekly basis, Mazursky and coworkers[96] found that in infants at 28 to 30 weeks the LF:HF ratio did not change with head-up postural change, whereas with increasing postnatal age, the LF component of the spectrum increases with head-up tilt. These findings suggest that neural regulation of cardiac function undergoes changes with maturation, becoming more functional with postnatal development.

CARDIOPULMONARY REFLEXES DURING DEVELOPMENT

In the adult, extracellular fluid (ECF) volume remains remarkably constant despite day-to-day variations in dietary intake of salt and water.[97] The integrity of this system is essential to preserve circulatory performance and to ensure appropriate fluid and electrolyte homeostasis. Contrary to the steady-state condition of ECF volume in the adult, significant changes in total body water and in the partition of body water between intracellular and extracellular compartments occur during fetal and postnatal development.[98, 99] It is likely that the changes in body water during development are, in part, linked to ontogenic changes in the sensing and effector mechanisms regulating ECF volume, including the cardiopulmonary baroreflex. Cardiopulmonary

receptors are sensory endings located in the four cardiac chambers, in the great veins and in the lungs.[100] In the adult, the volume sensors' mediating reflex changes in cardiovascular and renal function are believed to be primarily those residing in the atria[101, 102] and the ventricles,[100] with the ventricular receptors being of utmost importance during decreases in cardiopulmonary pressures.[100,103,104] Most ventricular receptor vagal afferents are unmyelinated C-fibers that can be activated by exposure to chemical irritants (chemosensitive) and changes in pressure or strength (mechanosensitive receptors).[105, 106] These receptors have a low basal discharge rate that exerts a tonic inhibitory influence on sympathetic outflow and vascular resistance[100] and regulates plasma AVP concentration.[107] Interruption of this basal activity results in increases in heart rate, blood pressure, and sympathetic nerve activity, whereas activation of cardiopulmonary receptors results in reflex bradycardia, vasodilation, and sympathoinhibition.[100]

Characterization of the cardiopulmonary reflex during the perinatal and neonatal periods was initially performed by stimulation of chemosensitive cardiopulmonary receptors.[51, 108, 109] These studies[108, 109] demonstrate that the heart rate, blood pressure, and regional blood flow responses to stimulation of chemosensitive cardiac receptors are smaller early in development than later in life and are in fact absent in premature fetal lambs[109] and in piglets younger than 1 week old.[108]

Indirect evidence suggests that cardiopulmonary mechanoreceptors are functional early during development and respond to changes in blood volume by eliciting reflexes that influence both renal and cardiac function. Inhibition of vagal afferents during slow and nonhypotensive hemorrhage blocks the normal rise in plasma vasopressin but does not alter the rise in plasma renin activity in near-term fetal sheep.[110] Fetal heart rate also increases in response to nonhypotensive hemorrhage[111] or to a decline in central venous pressure following furosemide administration.[112] With direct recording of renal sympathetic activity in fetal and newborn sheep, the role of cardiac mechanoreceptors in modulating sympathetic outflow and circulatory function during development has been more clearly defined. Stimulation of cardiopulmonary receptors with volume expansion has no effect on basal renal nerve activity in the fetus, but significantly reduces RSNA in newborn and 8-week-old sheep.[113,114] However, in these studies, stimulation of carotid sinus and aortic arterial baroreceptors may have contributed to the sympathoinhibitory and natriuretic responses observed during volume expansion. To clarify this issue, studies were repeated in newborn and 6- to 8-week-old sheep following sinoaortic denervation (SAD).[115] The decrease in RSNA in response to volume expansion was totally abolished in SAD newborn lambs but was not affected by SAD in 6- to 8-week-old sheep. These results indicate that cardiopulmonary reflexes are not fully mature early in life, and that stimulation of sinoaortic baroreceptors plays a greater role than cardiopulmonary mechanoreceptors in regulating changes in RSNA in response to changes in vascular volume early during development.

Developmental changes in cardiovascular and autonomic responses to blood volume reduction also exist. Gomez and associates[111] found that the systemic hemodynamic responses to fetal hemorrhage were dependent on the maturational state of the animal. Hemorrhage produced a significant decrease in arterial blood pressure without accompanying changes in heart rate in fetuses of less than 120 days' gestation, whereas blood pressure remained stable and heart rate increased in near-term fetuses. However, other investigators[110, 116] found the hemodynamic response to hemorrhage to be similar in immature and near-term fetuses, this being reductions in both heart rate and blood pressure. In newborn lambs, cardiovascular responses to hemorrhage are dependent on intact renal nerves that in turn modulate release of AVP.[117]

When input from cardiopulmonary receptors is removed by section of the cervical vagosympathetic trunks, the decrease in fetal blood pressure in response to hemorrhage is similar to that in intact fetuses,[118] whereas vagotomy with SAD enhance the decrease in blood pressure.[110] Therefore, it is likely that activation of fibers from the carotid sinus (arterial baroreceptors and chemoreceptors) but not vagal afferents (cardiopulmonary baroreceptors and chemoreceptors) are involved in the maintenance of blood pressure homeostasis during fetal hemorrhage. Cardiopulmonary receptors also appear to have a diminished role in early postnatal life. O'Mara and colleagues[119] demonstrated that reflex changes in newborn lamb RSNA during nonhypotensive and hypotensive hemorrhage are dependent on the integrity of arterial baroreceptors but not cardiopulmonary receptors. Factors responsible for the decreased sensitivity of the cardiopulmonary reflex early in development may involve maturational changes in the mechanoreceptor organ itself, the mechanical properties of the tissue in which the baroreceptor is located, the vagal afferent fibers, the central neural processing of afferent input, or efferent sympathetic fibers. In addition, alterations in neuroendocrine control of cardiopulmonary reflex activity may contribute to the attenuated sympathetic and cardiovascular responses to volume expansion in SAD newborn lambs. Indirect evidence suggests that atrial natriuretic peptide (ANP) plays an important role in the regulation of the autonomic nervous system during fetal life and that its role changes with maturation.[120] The sympathoinhibition seen in older lambs but not newborn SAD lambs may therefore be due to either a greater sensitivity to the central actions of ANP or a consequence of the larger increase in circulating ANP concentration in older lambs,[115] or both.

The RSNA responses to vagal afferent nerve stimulation are similar in sinoaortic denervated fetal and postnatal lambs,[121] suggesting that delayed maturation of the cardiopulmonary reflex is not secondary to incomplete central integration of vagal afferent input. Conversely, decreased sensitivity of the cardiopulmonary reflex early in development in the face of a hypersensitive arterial baroreflex response (as outlined earlier in this chapter) is intriguing. One may suggest that there is an occlusive interaction between these two reflexes during development. In support of this hypothesis, studies in adults[122,123] have shown that activation of arterial baroreceptors may impair the reflex responses to activation of cardiopulmonary receptors.

CHEMOREFLEX RESPONSES DURING DEVELOPMENT

Peripheral chemoreceptors located in the aortic arch and carotid bodies are functional during fetal life and participate in cardiovascular regulation.[124-126] Acute hypoxemia evokes integrated cardiovascular, metabolic, and endocrine responses that likely facilitate fetal survival. The fetal cardiovascular responses include transient bradycardia, an increase in arterial blood pressure, and an increase in peripheral vascular resistance.[125,127] The bradycardia is mediated by parasympathetic efferents whereas initial vasoconstriction results from increased sympathetic tone.[126,128] In fetal lambs, the cardiovascular responses to acute hypoxemia are eliminated by carotid but not aortic chemodenervation.[129] Several investigators have studied the relative sensitivity and contribution of these receptors to cardiovascular and respiratory control, although differences in experimental preparations make conclusions difficult. Although chemoreceptors are active and responsive in the fetus and newborn, studies in sheep and human infants suggest that chemoreceptor sensitivity and activity is reduced immediately after birth.[124,130] This decreased sensitivity persists for several days until the chemoreceptors adapt and reset their sensitivity from the low oxygen tension of the fetus to that seen postnatally.[130,131] The mechanisms involved

with this resetting are not known, although the postnatal rise in Pao_2 appears crucial as raising fetal Pao_2 produces a rightward shift in the response curve of carotid baroreceptors to differing oxygen tension.[132] Holgert and associates[133] hypothesized that developmental changes in dopamine turnover within the carotid body contribute to the postnatal resetting of the arterial chemoreceptors. Studies of carotid chemoreceptor cells isolated from neonatal and adult rabbits suggest differences in intracellular calcium mobilization during hypoxia may be an important component of chemoreceptor maturation.[134]

The purine nucleoside adenosine appears to play an important role in chemoreceptor-mediated responses as adenosine receptor blockade abolishes hypoxia-induced bradycardia and hypertension in fetal sheep.[135,136] Treatment with an adenosine-receptor antagonist or carotid sinus denervation before acute fetal hypoxia also prevents an increase in plasma epinephrine and markedly reduces any increase in plasma norepinephrine.[137,138] Thus, adenosine receptor blockade may act through chemoreceptor-dependent mechanisms to abolish circulatory and adrenergic responses to acute hypoxemia in fetal sheep, although chemoreflex-independent mechanisms also likely exist. In postnatal animals adenosine increases the carotid bodies' afferent discharge, whereas hypoxia-induced increases in afferent activity are attenuated by adenosine receptor antagonists.[139] The adenosine A_{2A} receptor gene is also expressed in the carotid body, suggesting receptors in this location may regulate chemoreceptor responses to hypoxia.[140]

The cardiovascular response to acute fetal hypoxemia depends on the prevailing intrauterine condition.[127,141] Gardner and partners[127] studied chronically instrumented fetal sheep grouped according to postsurgical PaO_2. Chronically hypoxic fetuses (baseline PaO_2 17.3 ± 0.5 mm Hg) display greater increases in arterial blood pressure and femoral vascular resistance than control fetuses (baseline PaO_2 22.9 ± 1.0 mm Hg) in response to acute hypoxia. Functional chemoreflex analysis during early hypoxemia, performed by plotting the change in PaO_2 against the change in heart rate and femoral vascular resistance demonstrated that the slopes of the cardiac and vasoconstrictor chemoreflex curves were enhanced in hypoxic fetuses relative to those in controls. Additional evidence suggests exposure to hypoxia for a limited period of time (i.e., hours to days) has a sensitizing effect on the chemoreflex, whereas sustained hypoxia (days to weeks) may have a desensitization effect.[141] The mechanisms responsible for this switch in effect remain unclear. In the chick embryo, hypoxia increases sympathetic nerve fiber density and neuronal capacity for norepinephrine synthesis.[142] Thus, augmented efferent pathways may contribute to the enhanced responses. Conversely, recordings from carotid chemoreceptors in chronically hypoxic kittens demonstrate blunted responses to acute decreases in PaO_2 relative to control animals.[143] It is therefore possible that with long-term hypoxia blunting of the chemoreflex responses may be related to afferent mechanisms.

SYMPATHETIC ACTIVITY AT BIRTH

The transition from fetal to newborn life is associated with numerous hemodynamic adjustments, including changes in heart rate and peripheral vascular resistance, and a redistribution of blood flow.[144,145] Although the mechanisms regulating these changes are not fully understood, the striking increases in circulating catecholamine levels at birth[146,147] have led investigators to suggest that activation of the sympathetic nervous system is vital for cardiovascular adaptation at birth.[145] In sheep, arterial pressure and cardiac function (including heart rate and cardiac output) are depressed by ganglionic blockade in newborn (1–3 days) but not older lambs,[148] suggesting that sympathetic tone is high during the immediate postnatal period. In support of this hypothesis, RSNA

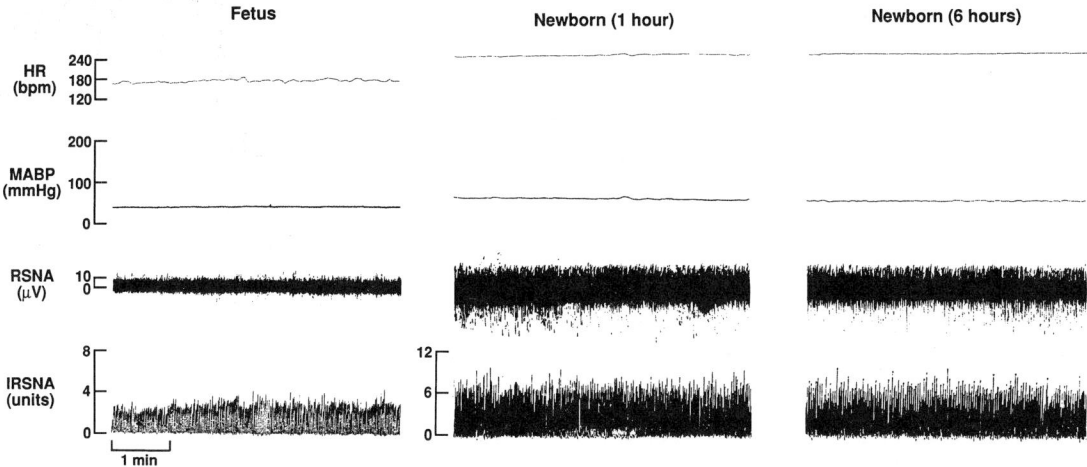

Figure 68–2. Recordings from a single lamb illustrating the effects of delivery on heart rate (HR), mean arterial blood pressure (MABP), renal sympathetic nerve activity (RSNA), and integrated RSNA (IRSNA). Note change in scale for IRSNA for newborns. (From Segar JL, et al:Am J Physiol 267:H1824, 1994.)

increases nearly 250% following delivery of term fetal sheep by cesarean section and parallels the rise in arterial pressure and heart rate (Fig. 68-2).[59] This increase in sympathetic outflow is sustained for at least 6 hours after birth, significantly longer than catecholamine levels are.[59] Delivery appears to produce near maximal stimulation of renal sympathetic outflow, because further increases cannot be elicited by small decreases in blood pressure.[59] This finding may help explain the inability of the newborn to increase cardiac output further in response to decreases in blood pressure.[149, 150] Furthermore, reflex inhibition of this increase in RSNA could not be achieved by arterial baroreceptor stimulation, as seen in fetal and 3- to 7-day-old lambs,[54] suggesting that central influences exist that override arterial baroreflex and that maintenance of a high sympathetic tone is vital during this transition period. A similar pattern of baroreceptor reflex inhibition has been well described in adult animals as part of the defense reaction.[151] The cardiovascular component of this group of behavioral responses, characterized by sympathetic nerve–mediated tachycardia, increased cardiac contractile force, vasoconstriction, and hypertension mimics the physiologic changes that occur at birth.[152]

The factors mediating the large increase in sympathetic outflow at birth are unclear. Removal of the placental circulation, the onset of spontaneous respiration, and exposure to ambient cold, are factors occurring at birth that may stimulate changes in sympathetic activity.[153, 154] *In utero* ventilation studies of fetal sheep have shown that rhythmic lung inflation increases plasma catecholamine concentrations,[154, 155] although there are no consistent effects on blood pressure and heart rate. Fetal RSNA increases only 50% during *in utero* ventilation, whereas oxygenation and removal of the placental circulation by umbilical cord occlusion produce no additional effect.[156] Such studies demonstrate that lung inflation and an increase in arterial oxygen tension contribute little to the sympathoexcitation process at birth. The increases in heart rate, mean arterial blood pressure, and RSNA following delivery are similar in intact and sinoaortic denervated plus vagotomized fetal lambs,[157] suggesting that afferent input from peripheral chemoreceptors and mechanoreceptors contribute little to the hemodynamic and sympathetic responses at delivery.

The change in environmental temperature at birth may play an important role in the sympathoexcitatory response at birth. Cooling of the near-term fetus both *in utero* and in exteriorized preparations results in an increase in heart rate, blood pressure,

and norepinephrine concentrations, consistent with sympathoexcitation.[153, 158] However, exteriorization of the near-term lamb fetus into a warm water bath does not produce the alterations in systemic hemodynamics or catecholamine values typically seen at birth.[153] Fetal cooling, but not ventilation or umbilical cord occlusion, initiates nonshivering thermogenesis through neurally mediated sympathetic stimulation of brown adipose tissue.[159] *In utero* cooling of fetal lambs also produces an increase in RSNA of similar magnitude to that at delivery by cesarean section,[91] suggesting that cold stress plays a role in the activation of the sympathetic nervous system at birth. These changes occur before a decrease in core temperature and are reversible with rewarming. Taken together, these results suggest that the increase in sympathetic nerve activity seen with cooling is neurally mediated by sensory input from cutaneous cold-sensitive thermoreceptors rather than in response to a change in core temperature.

Studies in adults suggest that multiple brain centers are involved in autonomic control of the systemic circulation. Sympathetic outflow is controlled not only by the medulla oblongata,[4] as well described previously, but also by higher centers, especially the hypothalamus,[152, 160] allowing for a wide range of modulation. Neuroanatomic studies have shown that nuclei within the hypothalamus project directly to a number of areas in the hindbrain containing preganglionic sympathetic and parasympathetic neurons, including the rostral and caudal ventrolateral medulla, the intermediolateral cell column, and the dorsal motor nucleus of the vagus.[152, 161, 162] There is no clear understanding of the role supramedullary regions play in influencing cardiovascular function in developing animals. In fetal sheep, electrical stimulation of the hypothalamus evokes tachycardia and a pressor response that are attenuated by α-adrenoceptor blockade.[163] Stimulation of the dorsolateral medulla and lateral hypothalamus in the newborn piglet similarly increases blood pressure and femoral blood flow.[51] Given that the responses to hypothalamic stimulation are lost during stress (e.g., hypoxia, hypercapnia, hemorrhage) whereas those elicited from the medulla are not, some investigators have proposed that the hypothalamus exerts little influence of cardiovascular function until later in postnatal development.[51] However, other studies suggest forebrain structures are vital for normal physiologic adaptation following the transition from fetal to newborn life.[156] The increases in heart rate, mean arterial blood pressure, and RSNA that normally occur at birth are absent in animals subjected to transection of the brain stem at the level of the rostral pons before delivery. These data suggest that supramedullary structures are involved in mediating the sympathoexcitation seen at birth. Preliminary studies, also in fetal sheep, demonstrate the paraventricular nucleus of the hypothalamus plays a vital role in regulating postnatal increases in sympathetic outflow and baroreflex function.[164] Given the known role of the hypothalamus in temperature and cardiovascular regulation,[160] one may suggest that this structure is intimately involved in the regulation of circulatory and autonomic functions during the transition from fetal to newborn life.

The hemodynamic and sympathetic responses at birth are markedly different in prematurely delivered lambs (0.85 of gestation) compared with those delivered at term.[88] Postnatal increases in heart rate and blood pressure are attenuated, and the sympathoexcitatory response, as measured by RSNA is absent (Fig. 68–3).[88] This impaired response occurs despite the fact the descending pathways of the sympathetic nervous system are intact and functional at this stage of development, as demonstrated by a large pressor and sympathoexcitatory response to *in utero* cooling.[88] Antenatal administration of glucocorticoids, which has been shown to improve postnatal cardiovascular as well as pulmonary function, augments sympathetic activity at birth in premature lambs, and decreases the sensitivity of the cardiac baroreflex.[88] The mechanisms responsible for this augmentation of cardiovascular and sympathetic responses at birth are unclear, although stimulation of the peripheral renin-angiotensin system and activation of systemically accessible AT_1 receptors are not involved.[165]

Understanding the mechanisms regulating sympathetic tone and baroreflex function is of particular significance to fetal and neonatal development. Evidence suggests that autonomic reflexes and the sympathetic activity are important regulators of blood pressure and circulatory function in the developing fetus and infant and the physiologic changes occurring at birth. To date, most work in this area has focused primarily on demonstrating function of these reflexes early during development and characterizing how these reflexes are altered with maturation. Further work is needed to determine the role of the sympathetic nervous system during relevant pathophysiologic conditions. Continued investigation of sympathetic function and the factors influencing autonomic control of circulatory function, particularly as they relate many of the physiologic adaptations occurring with the transition from fetal to newborn life, is of significant importance. Failure to regulate arterial pressure, peripheral resistance, and blood volume may lead to significant variations in organ blood flow and substrate delivery, resulting in ischemic or hemorrhagic complications. A more complete understanding of neural control of cardiovascular function early in life could potentially result in the development of new therapeutic strategies to prevent complications during the perinatal period that are thought to be associated with alterations in blood pressure.

REFERENCES

1. Persson P: Cardiopulmonary receptors and "neurogenic hypertension." Acta Physiol Scand 1988;570:1–53.
2. Kirscheim HR: Systemic arterial baroreceptor reflexes. Physiol Rev 1976;56:100–77.
3. Spyer KM: Central nervous mechanisms contributing to cardiovascular control. J Physiol 1994;474:1–19.
4. Calaresu FR, Yardley CP: Medullary basal sympathetic tone. Ann Rev Physiol 1988;50:511–24.
5. Woods JR, et al: Autonomic control of cardiovascular functions during neonatal development and in adult sheep. Circ Res 1977;40:401–7.
6. Nuwayhid B, et al: Development of autonomic control of fetal circulation. Am J Physiol 1975;228:237–344.
7. Vapaavouri EK, et al: Development of cardiovascular responses to autonomic blockade in intact fetal and neonatal lambs. Biol Neonate 1973;22:177–88.
8. Walker AM, et al: Sympathetic and parasympathetic control of heart rate in unanaesthetized fetal and newborn lambs. Biol Neonate 1978;33:135–43.
9. Yardly RW, et al: Increased arterial pressure variability after arterial baroceptor denervation in fetal lambs. Circ Res 1983;52:580–8.
10. Segar JL, et al: Role of sympathetic activity in the generation of heart rate and arterial pressure variability in fetal sheep. Pediatr Res 1994;35:250–4.
11. Alper RH, et al: Regulation of arterial pressure lability in rats with chronic sinoaortic deafferentation. Am J Physiol 1987;253:H466–74.
12. Barres C, et al: Arterial pressure lability and renal sympathetic nerve activity are disassociated in SAD rats. Am J Physiol 1992;263:R639–46.
13. Robillard JE, et al: Effects of renal denervation on renal responses to hypoxemia in fetal lambs. Am J Physiol 1986;250:F294–301.
14. Mann LI, et al: Fetal EEG sleep stages and physiologic variability. Am J Obstet Gynecol 1974;119:533–8.
15. Zhu Y, Szeto HH: Cyclic variation in fetal heart rate and sympathetic activity. Am J Obstet Gynecol 1987;156:1001–5.
16. Davidson SR, et al: Fetal heart rate variability and behavioral state: analysis by power spectrum. Am J Obstet Gynecol 1992;167:712–7.
17. Walker AM: Development of reflex control of the fetal circulation. *In* Künzel W, Jensen A (eds): The Endocrine Control of the Fetus. Berlin, Springer-Verlag, 1988, pp. 108–20.
18. Wakatsuki A, et al: Physiologic baroreceptor activity in the fetal lamb. Am J Obstet Gynecol 1992;167:820–7.
19. Clapp JF, et al: Physiologic variability and fetal electrocortical activity. Am J Obstet Gynecol 1980;136:1045–50.
20. Reid DL, et al: Relationship between plasma catecholamine levels and electrocortical state in the mature fetal lamb. J Dev Physiol 1990;13:75–9.
21. Jensen A, et al: Changes in organ blood flow between high and low voltage electrocortical activity in fetal sheep. J Dev Physiol 1986;8:187–94.
22. Richardson BS, et al: Cerebral oxidative metabolism in the fetal lamb: relationship to electrocortical state. Am J Obstet Gynecol 1985;153:426–31.
23. Abboud F, Thames M: Interaction of cardiovascular reflexes in circulatory control. *In* Shepherd JT, Abboud FM (eds): Handbook of Physiology. Sect 2, Vol III, Part 2. Bethesda, MD, American Physiological Society, 1983, pp. 675–753.
24. Persson PB, et al: Cardiopulmonary-arterial baroreceptor interaction in control of blood pressure. News Physiol Sci 1989;4:56–9.
25. Itskovitz J, et al: Baroreflex control of the circulation in chronically instrumented fetal lambs. Circ Res 1983;52:589–96.
26. Brinkman CRI, et al: Baroreceptor functions in the fetal lamb. Am J Physiol 1969;217:1346–51.
27. Bauer DJ: Vagal reflexes appearing in the rabbit at different ages. J Physiol 1939;95:187–202.
28. Dawes GS, Johnston BM, Walker DW: Relationship of arterial pressure and heart rate in fetal, new-born and adult sheep. J Physiol 1980;309:405–17.
29. Blanco CE, et al: Carotid baroreceptors in fetal and newborn sheep. Pediatr Res 1988;24:342–6.
30. Tomomatsu E, Nishi K: Comparison of carotid sinus baroreceptor sensitivity in newborn and adult rabbits. Am J Physiol 1982;243:H546–50.
31. Downing SE: Baroreceptor reflexes in new-born rabbits. J Physiol 1960;150:201–13.

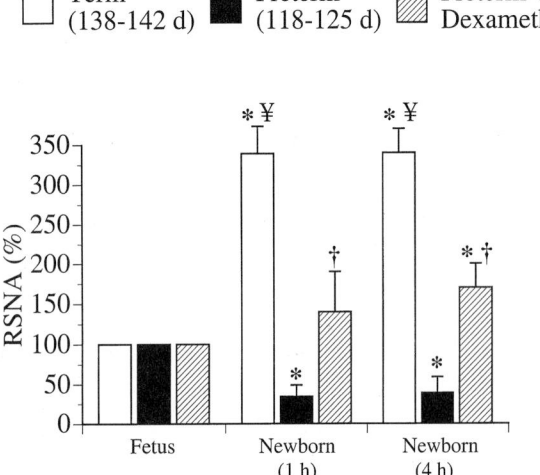

Term (138–142 d) ☐ Preterm (118–125 d) ■ Preterm + Dexamethasone ▨

Figure 68–3. Changes in renal sympathetic nerve activity (RSNA) at birth in term, preterm, and dexamethasone (Dex)-treated preterm lambs delivered by cesarean section. Bpm = beats/min; d, days. *p <0.05 compared with fetus in same group; †p <0.05 compared with preterm at similar chronologic age; ¥p <0.05 compared with other groups of similar chronologic age. (From Segar JL, et al: Am J Physiol 274:R160, 1998.)

32. Biscoe TJ, Purves MJ, Sampson SR: Types of nervous activity which may be recorded from the carotid sinus nerve in the sheep foetus. J Physiol 1969;202:1-23.

33. Ponte J, Purves MJ: Types of afferent nervous activity which may be measured in the vagus nerve of the sheep foetus. J Physiol 1973;229:51-76.

34. Shinebourne EA, et al: Development of baroreflex activity in unanesthetized fetal and neonatal lambs. Circ Res 1972;31:710-18.

35. Vatner SF, Manders WT: Depressed responsiveness of the carotid sinus reflex in conscious newborn animals. Am J Physiol 1979;237:H40-3.

36. Ismay MJ, et al: The action of angiotensin II on the baroreflex response of the conscious ewe and the conscious fetus. J Physiol 1979;288:467-79.

37. Gootman PM, et al: Postnatal maturation of neural control of the circulation. In Scarpelli EM, Cosmi EV (eds): Reviews in Perinatal Medicine. Vol 3. New York: Raven Press; 1979, p. 1.

38. Chapleau MW, et al: Mechanisms of resetting of arterial baroreceptors: an overview. Am J Med Sci 1988;295:327-34.

39. Chapleau MW, et al: Resetting of the arterial baroreflex: Peripheral and central mechanisms. In Zucker IH, Gilmore JP (eds): Reflex Control of the Circulation. Boca Raton, CRC Press, 1991, pp. 165-94.

40. Andresen MC: Short and long-term determinants of baroreceptor function in aged normotensive and spontaneously hypertensive rats. Circ Res 1984;54:750-9.

41. Heesch CM, et al: Acute resetting of carotid sinus baroreceptors. II. Possible involvement of electrogenic Na+ pump. Am J Physiol 1984;247:H833-9.

42. McDowell TS, et al: Prostaglandins in carotid sinus enhance baroreflex in rabbits. Am J Physiol 1989;257:R445-50.

43. Matsuda T, et al: Modulation of baroreceptor activity by nitric oxide and S-nitrocysteine. Circ Res 1995;76:426-33.

44. Jimbo M, et al: Role of nitric oxide in regulation of baroreceptor reflex. J Auton Nerv Syst 1994;50:209-19.

45. Sener A, Smith FG: Nitric oxide modulates arterial baroreflex control of heart rate in conscious lambs in an age-dependent manner. Am J Physiol 2001;280:H2255-H2263.

46. Nuyt A-M, et al: Role of endogenous prostaglandins in the regulation of arterial baroreceptor activity during development. 1996; 39:234A.

47. Abboud FM, Thames MD: Interaction of cardiovascular reflexes in circulatory control. In Shepherd JT, Abboud FM (eds): Handbook of Physiology. Sect 2, Vol III, Part 2. Bethesda, MD: American Physiological Society; 1983, p. 675.

48. Maloney JE, et al: Baroreflex activity in conscious fetal and newborn lambs. Biol Neonate 1977;31:340-50.

49. Yu ZY, Lumbers ER: Measurement of baroreceptor-mediated effects on heart rate variability in fetal sheep. Pediatr Res 2000;47:233-9.

50. Young M: Responses of the systemic circulation of the new-born infant. Br Med Bull 1966;22:70-2.

51. Gootman PM: Developmental aspects of reflex control of the circulation. In Zucker IH, Gilmore JP (eds): Reflex Control of the Circulation. Boca Raton, CRC Press, 1991, pp. 965-1027.

52. Buckley NM, et al: Age-dependent cardiovascular effects of afferent stimulation in neonatal pigs. Biol Neonate 1976;30:268-79.

53. Scroop GC, et al: Angiotensin I and II in the assessment of baroreceptor function in fetal and neonatal sheep. J Dev Physiol 1986;8:123-37.

54. Segar JL, et al: Ontogeny of baroreflex control of renal sympathetic nerve activity and heart rate. Am J Physiol 1992;263:H1819-26.

55. Hajduczok G, et al: Increase in sympathetic activity with age. I. Role of impairment of arterial baroreflexes. Am J Physiol 1991;260:H1113-20.

56. Bartolome J, Mills E, Lau C, et al: Maturation of sympathetic neurotransmission in the rat heart. J Pharmacol Exp Ther 1980;215:596-600.

57. Dorward PK, et al: The renal sympathetic baroreflex in the rabbit. Arterial and cardiac baroreceptor influences, resetting, and effect of anesthesia. Circ Res 1985;57:618-33.

58. Palmisano BW, et al: Development of baroreflex control of heart rate in swine. Pediatr Res 1989;27:148-52.

59. Segar JL, et al: Changes in ovine renal sympathetic nerve activity and baroreflex function at birth. Am J Physiol 1994;267:H1824-32.

60. Segar JL, et al: Role of endogenous angiotensin II on resetting of the arterial baroreflex during development. Am J Physiol 1994;266:H52-9.

61. Bishop VS, Haywood JR: Hormonal control of cardiovascular reflexes. In Zucker IH, Gilmore JP (eds): Reflex Control of the Circulation. Boca Raton, CRC Press, 1991, pp. 253-71.

62. Wood CE: Baroreflex and chemoreflex control of fetal hormone secretion. Reproduct Fertil Dev 1995;7:479-89.

63. Reid IA: Interactions between ANG II, sympathetic nervous system and baroreceptor reflex in regulation of blood pressure. Am J Physiol 1992;262:E763-E778.

64. Bunnemann B, et al: The renin-angiotensin system in the brain: an update 1993. Reg Peptides 1993;46:487-509.

65. Toney GM, Porter JP: Effects of blockade of AT1 and AT2 receptors in brain on the central angiotensin II pressor response in conscious spontaneously hypertensive rats. Neuropharmacology 1993;32:581-9.

66. Head GA, Mayorov DN: Central angiotensin and baroreceptor control of circulation. Ann NY Acad Sci 2001;940:361-79.

67. Jones III OW, et al: Dose-dependent effects of angiotensin II on the ovine fetal cardiovascular system. Am J Obstet Gynecol 1991;165:1524-33.

68. Robillard JE, et al: Comparison of the adrenal and renal responses to angiotensin II in fetal lambs and adult sheep. Circ Res 1982;50:140-7.

69. Lumbers ER, et al: Inhibition by angiotensin II of baroreceptor-evoked activity in cardiac vagal efferent nerves in the dog. J Physiol 1979;294:69-80.

70. Bishop VS, Sanderford MG: Angiotensin II modulation of the arterial baroreflex: role of the area postrema. Clin Exp Pharmacol Physiol 2000;27:428-31.

71. Robillard JE, et al: Renal and adrenal responses to converting-enzyme inhibition in fetal and newborn life. Am J Physiol 1983;244:R249-R256.

72. Wells TG, et al: Treatment of neonatal hypertension with enalaprilat. J Pediatr 1990;117:664-7.

73. Segar JL, et al: Role of endogenous ANG II and AT1 receptors in regulating arterial baroreflex responses in newborn lambs. Am J Physiol 1997;272:R1862-73.

74. Berecek KH, Swords BH: Central role for vasopressin in cardiovascular regulation and the pathogenesis of hypertension. Hypertension 1990;16:213-24.

75. Luk J, et al: Role of V1 receptors in the action of vasopressin on the baroreflex control of heart rate. Am J Physiol 1993;265:R524-9.

76. Unger T, et al: Differential modulation of the baroreceptor reflex by brain and plasma vasopressin. Hypertension 1986;8:II-157-62.

77. Tomita H, et al: Vasopressin dose-response effects on fetal vascular pressures, heart rate, and blood volume. Am J Physiol 1985;249:H974-H980.

78. Miyake Y, et al: Cardiovascular responses to norepinephrine and arginine vasopressin infusion in chronically catheterized fetal lambs. J Reproduct Med 1991;36:735-40.

79. Nuyt A-M, et al: Arginine vasopressin modulation of arterial baroreflex responses in fetal and newborn sheep. Am J Physiol 1996;271:R1643-53.

80. Drummond HA, Seagard JL: Acute baroreflex resetting. Differential control of pressure and nerve activity. Hypertension 1996;27:442-8.

81. Ervin MG, et al: V1- and V2-receptor contributions to ovine fetal renal and cardiovascular responses to vasopressin. Am J Physiol 1992;262:R636-43.

82. Unger T, et al: Opposing cardiovascular effects of brain and plasma AVP: Role of V1- and V2-AVP receptors. In Buckley JP, Ferrario CM (eds): Brain Peptides and Catecholamines in Cardiovascular Regulation. New York, Raven Press, 1987, pp. 393-401.

83. Stark RI, et al: Cerebrospinal fluid and plasma vasopressin in the fetal lamb: basal concentration and the effect of hypoxia. Endocrinology 1985;116:65-72.

84. Segar JL, et al: Developmental changes in central vasopressin regulation of cardiovascular function. 1995;37:34A.

85. Segar JL, et al: Effects of fetal ovine adrenalectomy on sympathetic and baroreflex responses at birth. Am J Physiol 2002;283:R460-R467.

86. Scheuer DA, Bechtold AG: Glucocorticoids modulate baroreflex control of heart rate in conscious normotensive rats. Am J Physiol 2001;282:R475-83.

87. Scheuer DA, Mifflin SW: Glucocorticoids modulate baroreflex control of renal sympathetic nerve activity. Am J Physiol 2001;280:R1440-49.

88. Segar JL, et al: Effect of antenatal glucocorticoids on sympathetic nerve activity at birth in preterm sheep. Am J Physiol 1998;274:R160-7.

89. Picton-Warlow CG, Mayer FE: Cardiovascular responses to postural changes in the neonate. Arch Dis Child 1970;45:354-9.

90. Thoresen M, et al: Cardiovascular responses to tilting in healthy newborn babies. Early Human Dev 1991;26:213-22.

91. Waldman S, et al: Baroreceptors in preterm infants: their relationship to maturity and disease. Dev Med Child Neurol 1979;21:714-22.

92. Malliani A, et al: Clinical and experimental evaluation of sympatho-vagal interaction: Power spectral analysis of heart rate and arterial pressure variabilities. In Zucker IH, Gilmore JP (eds): Reflex Control of the Circulation. Boca Raton, CRC Press, 1991, pp. 937-64.

93. Chatow U, et al: Development and maturation of the autonomic nervous system in premature and full-term infants using spectral analysis of heart rate fluctuations. Pediatr Res 1995;37:294-302.

94. Clairambault J, et al: Heart rate variability in normal sleeping full-term and preterm neonates. Early Human Dev 1992;28:169-83.

95. Karin J, et al: An estimate of fetal autonomic state by spectral analysis of fetal heart rate fluctuations. Pediatr Res 1993;34:134-8.

96. Mazursky JE, et al: Development of baroreflex influences on heart rate variability in preterm infants. Early Hum Dev 1998;53:37-52.

97. Moe GW, et al: Control of extracellular fluid volume and pathophysiology of edema formation. In Brenner BM, Rector FC Jr. (eds): The Kidney. Philadelphia: W.B. Saunders Company; 1991, p. 623.

98. Friis-Hansen B: Body water compartments in children: Changes during growth and related changes in body composition. Pediatrics 1961;28:169.

99. Oh W: Transitional changes of body fluid and blood volume during the perinatal period. In Brace RA, et al (eds): Fetal and Neonatal Body Fluids. Vol XI. Ithaca, NY: Perinatology Press; 1989, p. 293.

100. Minisi AJ, Thames MD: Reflexes from ventricular receptors with vagal afferents. In Zucker IH, Gilmore JP (eds): Reflex Control of the Circulation. Boca Raton: CRC Press; 1991, p. 359.

101. Goetz KL: Atrial receptors: Reflex effects in quadripeds. Reflex Control of the Circulation. Boca Raton: CRC Press; 1991, p. 291.

102. Hainsworth R: Reflexes from the heart. Physiol Rev 1991;71:617-58.

103. Victor RG, et al: Differential control of adrenal and renal sympathetic nerve activity during hemorrhagic hypertension in rats. Circ Res 1989;64:686-94.

104. Togashi H, et al: Differential effects of hemorrhage on adrenal and renal nerve activity in anesthetized rats. Am J Physiol 1990;259:H1134-41.

105. Baker DG, et al: Vagal afferent C fibers from the ventricle. In Hainsworth R, et al (eds): Cardiac Receptors. Cambridge: Cambridge University Press; 1979, p. 117.

106. Gupta BN, Thames MD: Behavior of left ventricular mechanoreceptors with myelinated and nonmyelinated afferent vagal fibers in cats. Circ Res 1983;52:291–301.
107. Thames MD, et al: Stimulation of cardiac receptors with Veratrum alkaloids inhibits ADH secretion. Am J Physiol 1980;239:H784–8.
108. Gootman PM, et al: Age-related responses to stimulation of cardiopulmonary receptors in swine. Am J Physiol 1986;251:H748–55.
109. Assali NS, Briet al: Ontogenesis of the autonomic control of cardiovascular function in the sheep. In Longo LD, Reneau DD (eds): Fetal and Newborn Cardiovascular Physiology. New York, Garland STPM Press, 1978, pp. 47–91.
110. Chen HG, Wood CE: Reflex control of fetal arterial pressure and hormonal responses to slow hemorrhage. Am J Physiol 1992;262:H225–H233.
111. Gomez RA, et al: Developmental aspects of the renal response to hemorrhage during fetal life. Pediatr Res 1984;18:40–6.
112. Kelly TF, et al: Hemodynamic and fluid responses to furosemide infusion in the ovine fetus. Am J Obstet Gynecol 1993;168:260–8.
113. Smith F, et al: Effects on volume expansion on renal sympathetic nerve activity and cardiovascular and renal function in lambs. Am J Physiol 1992;262:R2651–8.
114. Merrill DC, et al: Cardiopulmonary and arterial baroreflex responses to acute volume expansion during fetal and postnatal development. Am J Physiol 1994;267:H1467–75.
115. Merrill DC, et al: Impairment of cardiopulmonary baroreflexes during the newborn period. Am J Physiol 1995;268:H134–51.
116. Toubas PL, et al: Cardiovascular effects of acute hemorrhage in fetal lambs. Am J Physiol 1981;240:H45–8.
117. Smith FG, Abu-Amarah I: Renal denervation alters cardiovascular and endocrine responses to hemorrhage in conscious newborn lambs. Am J Physiol 1998;275:H285–91.
118. Wood CE: Role of vagosympathetic fibers in the control of adrenocorticotropic hormone, vasopressin, and renin responses to hemorrhage in fetal sheep. Circ Res 1989;64:515–23.
119. O'Mara MS, et al: Ontogeny and regulation of arterial and cardiopulmonary baroreflex control of renal sympathetic nerve activity (RSNA) in response to hypotensive (NH) and hypotensive hemorrhage (HH) postnatally. Pediatr Res 1995;37:31A.
120. Cheung CY: Autonomic and arginine vasopressin modulation of the hypoxia-induced atrial natriuretic factor release in immature and mature ovine fetuses. Am J Obstet Gynecol 1992;167:1443–53.
121. Merrill DC, et al: Sympathetic responses to cardiopulmonary vagal afferent stimulation during development. Am J Physiol 1999;277:H1311–16.
122. Cornish KG, et al: Volume expansion attenuates baroreflex sensitivity in the conscious nonhuman primate. Am J Physiol 1989;257:R595–R598.
123. Hajduczok G, et al: Increase in sympathetic activity with age: I. Role of impairment of cardiopulmonary baroreflexes. Am J Physiol 1991;260:H1121–7.
124. Blanco CE, et al: The response to hypoxia of arterial chemoreceptors in fetal sheep and newborn lambs. J Physiol 1984;351:25–37.
125. Giussani DA, et al: Fetal cardiovascular reflex responses to hypoxaemia. 1994;6:17–37.
126. Giussani DA, et al: Afferent and efferent components of the cardiovascular reflex responses to acute hypoxia in term fetal sheep. J Physiol 1993;461:431–49.
127. Gardner DS, et al: Effects of prevailing hypoxaemia, acidaemia or hypoglycaemia upon the cardiovascular, endocrine and metabolic responses to acute hypoxaemia in the ovine fetus. J Physiol 2002;540:351–66.
128. Iwamota HS, et al: Circulatory and humoral responses of sympathectomized fetal sheep to hypoxemia. Am J Physiol 1983;245:H267–72.
129. Bartelds B, et al: Carotid, not aortic, chemoreceptors mediate the fetal cardiovascular response to acute hypoxemia in lambs. Pediatr Res 1993;34:51–5.
130. Hertzberg T, Lagercrantz H: Postnatal sensitivity of the peripheral chemoreceptors in newborn infants. Arch Dis Child 1987;62:1238–41.
131. Kumar P, Hanson MA: Re-setting of the hypoxic sensitivity of aortic chemoreceptors in the new-born lamb. J Dev Physiol 1989;11:199–206.
132. Blanco CE, et al: Effectds on carotid chemoreceptor resetting of pulmonary ventilation in the fetal lamb in utero. J Dev Physiol 1988;10:167–174.
133. Holgert H, et al: Neurochemical and molecular biological aspects on the resetting of the arterial chemoreceptors in the newborn rat. Adv Exp Med Biol 1993;337:165–170.
134. Sterni LM, et al: Developmental changes in intracellular Ca^{2+} response of carotid chemoreceptor cells to hypoxia. Am J Physiol 1995;268:L801–8.
135. Koos BJ, et al: Adenosine mediates metabolic and cardiovascular responses to hypoxia in fetal sheep. J Physiol (Lond) 1995;488:761–6.
136. Koos BJ, Maeda T: Adenosine A_{2A} receptors mediate cardiovascular responses to hypoxia in fetal sheep. Am J Physiol 2001;280:H83–9.
137. Giussani DA, et al: Purinergic contribution to circulatory, metabolic, and adrenergic responses to acute hypoxemia in fetal sheep. Am J Physiol 2001;280:R678–85.
138. Jensen A, Hanson MA: Circulatory response to acute asphyxia in intact and chemodenervated fetal sheep near term. Reprod Fertil Dev 1995;7:1351–9.
139. McQueen DS, Ribeiro JA: Pharmacological characterization of the receptor involved in chemoexcitation induced by adenosine. Br J Pharmacol 1986;88:615–20.
140. Kaelin-Lang A, et al: Expression of adenosine A_{2a} receptor gene in rat dorsal root and autonomic ganglia. Neurosci Lett 1998;246:21–4.
141. Hanson MA: Role of chemoreceptors in effects of chronic hypoxia. Comp Biochem Physiol 1997;119A:695–703.
142. Ruijtenbeek K, et al: Chronic hypoxia stimulates periarterial sympathetic nerve development in chicken embryo. Circulation 2000;102:2892–7.
143. Hanson MA, et al: Peripheral chemoreceptors and other O_2 sensors in the fetus and newborn. New York, Oxford University Press, 1989, pp. 113–20.
144. Dawes GS: Changes in the circulation at birth. Br Med Bull 1961;17:148–53.
145. Padbury JF, Martinez AM: Sympathoadrenal system activity at birth: integration of postnatal adaptation. Semin Perinatal 1988;12:163–72.
146. Lagercrantz H, Bistoletti P: Catecholamine release in the newborn at birth. Pediatr Res 1973;11:889–93.
147. Padbury JF, et al: Neonatal adaptation: sympatho-adrenal response to umbilical cord cutting. Pediatr Res 1981;15:1483–7.
148. Minoura S, Gilbert RD: Postnatal changes of cardiac function in lambs: effects of ganglionic block and afterload. J Dev Physiol 1986;9:123–35.
149. Teitel DF, et al: Developmental changes in myocardial contractile reserve in the lamb. Pediatr Res 1985;19:948–55.
150. Teitel DF, et al: The end-systolic pressure-volume relationship in the newborn lamb: effects of loading and inotropic interventions. Pediatr Res 1991;29:473–82.
151. Hilton SM: The defense-arousal system and its relevance for circulatory and respiratory control. J Exp Biol 1982;100:159–74.
152. Gebber GL: Central determinants of sympathetic nerve discharge. In Loewy AD, Spyer KM (eds): Central Regulation of Autonomic Function. New York, Oxford University Press, 1990, pp. 126–44.
153. Van Bel F, et al: Sympathoadrenal, metabolic, and regional blood flow responses to cold in fetal sheep. Pediatr Res 1993;34:47–50.
154. Ogundipe OA, et al: Fetal endocrine and renal responses to in utero ventilation and umbilical cord occlusion. Am J Obstet Gynecol 1993;169:1479–86.
155. Smith FG, et al: Endocrine effects of ventilation, oxygenation and cord occlusion in near-term fetal sheep. J Dev Physiol 1991;15:133–8.
156. Mazursky JE, et al: Regulation of renal sympathetic nerve activity at birth. Am J Physiol 1996;270:R86–93.
157. Segar JL, et al: Mechano- and chemoreceptor modulation of renal sympathetic nerve activity at birth in fetal sheep. Am J Physiol 1999;276:R1295–1301.
158. Gunn TR, et al: Haemodynamic and catecholamine responses to hypothermia in the fetal sheep in utero. J Dev Physiol 1985;7:241–9.
159. Gunn TR, et al: Factors influencing the initiation of nonshivering thermogenesis. Am J Obstet Gynecol 1991;164:210–17.
160. Loewy AD: Central autonomic pathways. In Loewy AD, Spyer KM (eds): Central Regulation of Autonomic Functions. New York, Oxford University Press, 1990, pp. 88–103.
161. Swanson LW, Sawchenko PE: Hypothalamic integration: organization of the paraventricular and supraoptic nuclei. Ann Rev Neurosci 1983;6:269–324.
162. Strack AM, et al: CNS cell groups regulating the sympathetic outflow to adrenal gland as revealed by transneuronal cell body labeling with pseudorabies virus. Brain Res 1989;491:274–96.
163. Williams RL, et al: Cardiovascular effects of electrical stimulation of the forebrain in the fetal lamb. Pediatr Res 1976;10:40–5.
164. Ellsbury DL, et al: Ablation of the paraventricular nucleus attenuates sympathoexcitation at birth. Pediatr Res 2000;47:397A.
165. Segar JL, et al: Glucocorticoid modulation of cardiovascular and autonomic function in preterm lambs: role of ANG II. Am J Physiol 2001;280:R646–54.

69 Programming of the Fetal Circulation

The fetus depends on its cardiovascular system for growth and development. Of necessity, vascular growth must be closely linked to tissue growth, and the fetal heart must develop in relation to the venous return (preload), primarily from the umbilical vein, and the similar arterial pressures in the pulmonary trunk and the aortic arch (afterload). This matching of cardiovascular function to growth is particularly important in late gestation when cardiovascular redistribution, as well as changes in tissue metabolism, occurs in response to placental insufficiency (see reviews in Refs 1 and 2). Whether such processes operate in early gestation is not known.

Current knowledge of late-gestation fetal cardiovascular control is based on the concept that the mechanisms of such control will be best revealed when the system is challenged with a stimulus and the resulting response measured. The stimulus most widely employed is hypoxia, and this has permitted a fairly complete picture of a temporal and functional hierarchy of reflex, endocrine, and local mechanisms operating during acute hypoxia.[3] Such mechanisms change in the face of repeated acute or sustained hypoxia[4-6] and in species adapted to life in the hypoxia of altitude.[7-10] However, whether such mechanisms operate in response to changes in fetal nutrition (e.g., glucose, amino acid, or micronutrient provision) is unknown. In this review, we address this question in the context of what is known of the programming effects of prenatal nutrition on cardiovascular development and fetal circulatory control mechanisms.

EPIDEMIOLOGIC OBSERVATIONS

There is now considerable evidence from a variety of studies that small or disproportionate size at birth is associated with increased risk of cardiovascular disease. The studies of Barker and colleagues[11] on adult men and women showed that the standardized mortality ratio for coronary heart disease increased in a graded manner across the normal birth weight range. There are now numerous studies linking low birth weight to the metabolic syndrome[12] or to components of the syndrome (defined as fasting plasma glucose more than 6 mmol/L; blood pressure more than 130/85 mm Hg; fasting plasma triglyceride more than 1.7 mmol/L; plasma high-density lipoprotein–cell surface (HDLc) less than 1.1 mmol/L; [in men] waist measurement > 102 cm). Meta-analysis of the blood pressure effect suggests that a 1-kg increase in birth weight is associated with a fall of 2 mm Hg in systolic blood pressure in later life.[13] Inevitably, the size and nature of these studies vary enormously, and the effect of study size has recently been questioned,[14] since larger studies (in which birth weight is more likely to have been self-reported than actually measured) show weaker associations between birth weight and blood pressure than smaller studies. Nonetheless, the direction of the effect (small size at birth predicting higher blood pressure in later life) is not under question even if the magnitude of the effect is debated.

Birth weight is a poor proxy for fetal growth, and of course blood pressure is a poor proxy for cardiovascular function or tissue perfusion. For these reasons it is vital that physiologic studies are conducted to understand the mechanisms underlying programming of cardiovascular function by life events *in utero*. Moreover, it is highly unlikely that appropriate intervention measures to prevent the progression to disease (i.e., the metabolic syndrome) in susceptible individuals can be developed

without an understanding of the mechanisms underlying the development of the disease. The exercise may have enormous implications for public health, since calculations based on the epidemiologic studies conducted in Finland[15] suggest that if all male offspring could have been prevented from being thin at birth and thin and short at 1 year of age, then the incidence of coronary heart disease would have been halved. Indeed, since the phenomenon exists in developing societies, across the normal birth weight range which averages 1 kg less than in developed societies,[16] the implications are not confined to developed societies. Probably those at greatest risk throughout the world belong to transitional societies where, for example, children from agrarian societies in the developing world move to cities as adolescents. These considerations may explain the epidemic in coronary heart disease and in type 2 diabetes, developing, for example, in the Indian subcontinent.[17]

GENE VERSUS ENVIRONMENT

There are many reasons for believing that the effects just described are not purely genetic in origin, the most obvious being that changes in the incidence of the metabolic syndrome within a generation cannot be purely due to genetic (heritable) traits. Moreover, the maternal and paternal genetic contribution to fetal growth (see later), and to outcome measures such as systolic blood pressure in adulthood, is highly dissimilar. In a study of adults in Preston, United Kingdom, systolic pressure was inversely related to maternal but not to paternal birthweight.[18] In pursuing the mechanisms underlying programming of cardiovascular function, it is therefore important to consider the interaction between the genome and the early environment in determining a phenotype that is susceptible to disease. This argument is substantiated by the discovery of numerous processes that modify genomic DNA, gene expression, and hence the production of the proteins that confer the phenotype. These include not only single nucleotide polymorphisms (SNPs), DNA methylation that alters gene expression, but also the many transcription factors that act to modify gene transcription and the processes that control the half-life of mRNA.

A good example of the interaction between genotype and the early environment is provided by studying peroxisome proliferator-activated receptor gamma (PPAR-γ), a nuclear hormone receptor that mediates the effect of synthetic and endogenous ligands on the modulation of gene expression. Polymorphisms in the PPAR-γ2 gene are associated with type 2 diabetes. Moreover, the well-documented link between low birth weight and insulin resistance is seen only in subjects with *PPAR-γ* gene polymorphism.[19] Dennison and colleagues[20] have shown a similar relationship between the programming of osteoporosis, known to be inversely related to birth weight, and a polymorphism in the vitamin D receptor gene.

The processes most likely to be involved in mediating the maternal versus paternal genomic effects on development involve imprinting. Of the range of genes that are imprinted, the H19/IGF2 cluster has received particular attention[21]: the IGF-II peptide has been shown to be paternally expressed while the IGF-II receptor is maternally expressed. As IGF-II is a potent stimulator of fetal cell division and differentiation, this shows how the paternal genome drives growth in various key tissues such as the fetal liver. However, as the IGF-II receptor is a clearance receptor, which modulates IGF-II peptide action in the tissues, the maternal genome can down-regulate growth to be appropriate for maternal body habitus. This is consistent with the concept of maternal constraint on fetal growth that was highlighted by the pioneering studies of Walton and Hammond, in which Shire horses were crossed with Shetland ponies.[22]

A recent development in this story has been the demonstration that the IGF2 gene variant IGF2P0, which is expressed in the placenta of the rodent, is paternally expressed.[23] Hence the paternal genome drives fetal growth not only via a direct effect at the tissues but also via increased placental growth and nutrient transport. It is therefore clear that the trajectory of growth in early life is determined by maternal and environmental factors acting to regulate the gene expression of the early embryo. First trimester growth in the human sets the trajectory for later fetal growth and predicts risk of low birth weight.[24]

ENVIRONMENTAL STIMULI

Timing

In investigating the interaction between gene and environment, it is important to take a life span perspective in considering the influence of maternal diet, body composition, social status, smoking, and so on; the effect of the tubal and uterine fluid environment on the early embryo; the development of the placenta; fetal adaptations; and postnatal effects that may exacerbate the problem. One of the animal models most widely used for studying programming phenomena is the rat to which a low protein diet is given during pregnancy (reviewed in Ref 25). Most previous studies with this model involved administration of the diet for the whole of pregnancy (about 21 days). However, recently Kwong and associates[26] have shown that administration of the low protein diet to rat dams in the first 4 days of gestation, i.e., preimplantation, produces blastocysts that have altered allocation of cells to the trophectoderm and inner cell mass and to offspring, with permanently increased blood pressure in adult life. Further observations in the mouse have been made by Watkins and colleagues,[27] who showed that embryos transferred to recipient females developed elevated blood pressure in adult life. Apart from demonstrating the importance of the early preimplantation embryonic environment in the programming of subsequent phenotype, these studies raise important questions about the long-term effects of reproductive technologies increasingly used in humans.

Nutrients

The relative contribution of specific macro- or micronutrients in determining the balance between supply and demand during fetal growth has not yet been resolved. Recent attention has focused on the amino acid glycine, for which the fetal requirements in late gestation are greater than any other amino acid, even though this amino acid is not normally considered to be essential. Glycine provision, along with the availability of the micronutrient co-factor folate, is important in a range of biologic processes that may alter cardiovascular function (Fig. 69–1). Firstly, it is involved in the synthesis of DNA and RNA, important for cell growth and differentiation. In addition, it provides a source of methyl groups for the methylation processes that affect gene silencing, and hence the transition from genotype to phenotype. An example of such methylated genes with an important role in the pathogenesis of cardiovascular disease is the ER alpha receptor, which is linked to risk of atherosclerosis. Finally, glycine is important in the interconversion of homocysteine to methionine, such that its deficiency (or that of vitamin B_{12}) leads to accumulation of homocysteine in the plasma and associated

vascular damage. The offspring of low protein–fed rat dams show elevated plasma homocystine levels. In rats, the addition of glycine, or indeed folate, to the low protein diet prevents the elevation of blood pressure in the offspring, and also the development of vascular dysfunction in these offspring.[28] There have now been a range of studies showing that offspring of rats fed the low protein diet during pregnancy have altered endothelial function, e.g., the degree of relaxation to the endothelium-dependent vasodilator to acetylcholine (Fig. 69–2).

The major provision of fetal glycine is from placental glycine production from the conversion of serine by the serine hydroxymethyltransferase. The serine itself enters the placenta from the maternal and fetal circulation via system A and ASC amino acid transporter systems.[29,30] It is known that placental size relates not only to fetal growth but also to blood pressure in later life.[31] However, relatively few studies have been performed of placental transport function in relation to fetal growth and outcome. It is of interest that placental system A activity increases with reductions in birth weight in the normal range,[32] although there is also an association between reduced system A activity and intrauterine growth restriction (IUGR).[33]

FETAL ADAPTATIONS

Studies of the fetal adaptations to perturbed nutrition are just now beginning. The well-established "brain-sparing" cardiovascular phenomenon, in which a higher percentage of the combined ventricular output is directed to the brain at the expense of the developing fetal carcass, has been demonstrated extensively in hypoxic fetuses. In addition, it is associated in the human fetus with late-gestation asymmetrical growth retardation. The supposition has been that, if such fetuses are not hypoxic, then the response is to reduced nutrition. However, such an idea has not been tested directly. The rapid phase of the vasoconstrictor component of the response to hypoxia is mediated by the carotic bodies, and it is therefore of great interest that these chemoreceptors have recently been shown to be also responsive to a reduction in plasma glucose.[34]

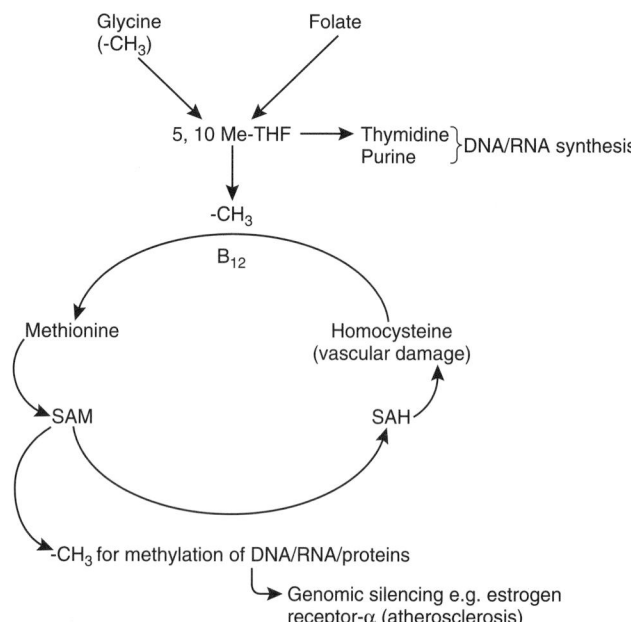

Figure 69–1. Diagram to illustrate the importance of glycine and folate in the processes that may underlie atherosclerosis. Me-THF, methyl tetrahydrofolate; —CH_3, methyl group; B_{12}, vitamin B_{12}; SAM, S-adenosyl-L-methionine; SAH, S-adenosyl-L-homocysteine.

Figure 69–2. The effect of maternal low protein (casein) diet during pregnancy on vasorelaxation to acetylcholine (ACh) in mesenteric arteries from male offspring aged (**A**) day 87: 18% casein (open circle, $n = 8$); 9% casein (closed circle, $n = 9$), ***$p < 0.001$ vs. control pEC_{50} value (t-test). Control vs. protein-restricted overall relaxation (two-way ANOVA) was $p < 0.001$ or (**B**) day 164: 18% casein (open square, $n = 9$); 9% casein (closed square, $n = 8$) groups, *$p < 0.05$ vs. control maximum relaxation (t-test). Control vs. protein-restricted overall relaxation (two-way ANOVA) was $p < 0.001$. (From Brawley L, Itoh S, Torrens C, et al: Dietary protein restriction in pregnancy induces hypertension and vascular defects in rat male offspring. Pediatr Res 54:1–7, 2003.)

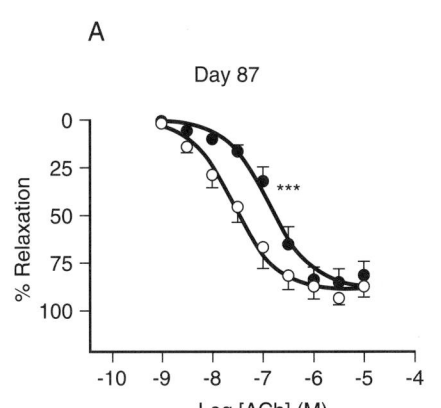

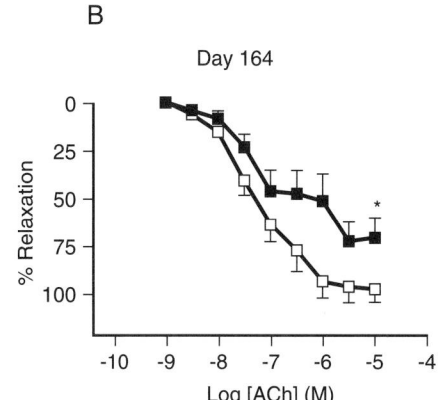

Understanding of the fetal redistribution requires consideration of effects on individual organs, and one of particular interest is the developing fetal liver. Blood supply to the liver comes from a range of sources, primarily the oxygenated and highly nutritious blood from the umbilical vein. However, this blood entirely supplies the left lobe of the liver and to a lesser extent the right lobe, as the latter in addition receives blood from the hepatic portal veins and the hepatic arteries (which is less well-oxygenated and nutritious). A proportion of oxygenated umbilical blood is shunted through the ductus venosus toward the foramen ovale and through into the left atrium. The degree of shunting of this blood changes during gestation and is altered by challenges such as acute hypoxemia.[35] We have recently shown that the degree of shunting is also increased in late-gestation fetuses of mothers who had a high body mass index (BMI) or skinfold thickness prepregnancy.[36] This therefore fits with the notion that women with greater fat stores, or with altered endocrine status leading to increased body fat mass, produce fetuses with a more rapid trajectory of growth, at least in early gestation. If this growth imposes demands on the developing placenta that cannot be met, then fetal cardiovascular redistributions must come into play.

Sheep are widely used as an animal model for studying programming phenomena during fetal life. They share similarities with humans in that the full complement of cardiomyocytes and renal glomeruli are formed prenatally. Moreover, the incidence of singleton pregnancies in sheep allows the comparison of fetal growth patterns with human pregnancies, and their size and tolerance to surgery permits cardiovascular and growth measurements to be made over several weeks of gestation. However, the extent to which concomitant changes in cardiovascular control and growth result from perturbations in the fetal nutrient supply line is unclear. The normal developmental rise in arterial pressure over late gestation in sheep is perturbed in small fetuses.[38] Restricted fetal nutrient supply by removal of placental caruncles before conception perturbs cardiovascular development and function in late-gestation fetuses—with or without growth restriction.[39] Moreover, mild to moderate (15 to 30%) reduction in maternal nutrient intake for the first half of gestation lowered blood pressure in late-gestation fetuses[40] and impaired vascular function in vitro,[41] with no change in fetal organ or body weight. Preliminary data in these fetuses indicate a redistribution of combined ventricular output in late gestation, since baseline femoral blood flow tended to be lower, and carotid blood flow tends to be elevated (unpublished observations). Specific early-gestation moderate (30%) reduction of maternal protein intake markedly exacerbated the vascular dysfunction of isolated fetal resistance vessels,[42] indicating the importance of nutrient balance (see earlier).

Taken as a whole, these observations suggest that cardiovascular adaptations may be able to buffer changes in growth when faced with an altered nutrient supply, but it may be that once the upper limit in this buffering capacity has been reached, a change in growth will result. Indeed we have recently observed that 50% maternal nutrient restriction for 30 days at conception or in early gestation decreases fetal liver and thyroid weight at midgestation (unpublished observations). This concept fits with the epidemiologic observations that adult blood pressure is inversely related in a graded manner across the normal birth weight range[13] (see earlier). Moreover, the growth response of the fetus to a late-gestation severe undernutrition insult depends on the rate at which it is growing: the growth of a rapidly growing fetus is slowed, whereas slow-growing fetuses fail to respond.[43] Such fetuses may have adapted to an earlier gestation insult, such as periconceptual undernutrition, thereby protecting them from a subsequent late-gestation challenge. Thus fetal adaptations, in the face of altered partitioning of nutrients between the maternal body, the placenta, and the fetus, may be beneficial in customizing fetal growth and development to the supply of oxygen and nutrients, but they may have long-term sequelae postnatally. Indeed, early-gestation nutrient restriction alters cardiovascular function in young adult sheep.[44]

POSTNATAL ADAPTATIONS

The window of opportunity for programming of cardiovascular function in early life does not stop at birth. The Helsinki Study[45] showed that the effect of low ponderal index at birth on the risk of coronary heart disease in adulthood in men was amplified by increasing BMI during the first 12 years of life. There is now considerable interest in the effects of obesity in childhood (which in Western societies may affect 20% of children under the age of 12 years) on risk of later disease. In addition, animal studies show that severe undernutrition during fetal life results in offspring that are hyperphagic, obese, and insulin resistant and demonstrate reduced physical activity.[46,47] This is suggestive of a compounding of fetal programming effects by postnatal adaptations. Our recent observations in sheep are consistent with this notion, since the detrimental effect of low birth weight on adult glucose tolerance is less in animals that were nutritionally restricted (12 weeks of moderate restriction) in early postnatal life.[48] In addition, this acute (12-week) restriction of dietary intake during early postnatal life decreased baroreflex sensitivity in young adulthood,[49] indicative of altered autonomic function, which could predispose offspring to hypertension in later life. These postnatally challenged offspring also demonstrate an enhanced blood pressure response to activation of the renin-angiotensin system by frusemide, but this effect was blunted by prior exposure to a poor nutritional environment in early gestation.[50]

Current postnatal studies in animals focus on the mechanisms by which programming alters peripheral vascular function. The observation that small-resistance-vessel responses to endothelium-dependent vasodilators, such as acetylcholine and bradykinin, are impaired in offspring of rat dams fed a low-protein diet during gestation[51,52] are supported by our finding that both basal and acetylcholine-stimulated nitric oxide release is reduced in the mesenteric arteries of such offspring.[25] Using global undernutrition during pregnancy, rather than the low protein diet, Franco and colleagues[53] have shown that the adult offspring have reduced endothelial nitric oxide synthase (eNOS) activity and mRNA in the aorta. Endothelial responsiveness mediates flow-mediated vasodilatation in many vascular beds, and this can be studied in humans by techniques such as forearm plethysmography.[54] Such methods have demonstrated reduced flow-mediated vasodilatation with lower birth weight in adults[55] and an effect comparable in size to that of smoking. Similarly, endothelium-dependent vasodilator responses in the leg are reduced in obese type II diabetic subjects compared with controls.[56] Disorders of endothelial function predispose to atherosclerosis as well as hypertension.

MATERNAL ADAPTATIONS

Cardiovascular adaptations of the mother to pregnancy provide another potential route by which dietary/endocrine stressors may be transmitted to her fetus. The increase in blood volume and cardiac output during pregnancy[57] involves a redistribution of cardiac output in favor of the reproductive tract. In humans this is mediated primarily by a dramatic fall in resistance in the spiral arteries supplying the endometrium, but there is an additional component of vasodilatation in the uterine bed provided by vascular endothelial growth factor (VEGF)/nitric oxide mechanisms.[58] Ahokas and associates[59] observed that dietary restriction of the rat dam (50%) resulted in maintained maternal liver blood flow at the expense of the pregnant uterus.[59] In the low-protein rat model, we found an impaired vasodilator response to VEGF in late pregnancy uterine arteries in vitro.[60] Innes and colleagues[61] recently reported a negative association between women's birth weight and the risk of gestational diabetes mellitus. This effect persists after adjusting for gestational age and current BMI. Similarly, in hypertensive rat offspring of protein-restricted dams, we found a blunting of mesenteric vasodilator responses to acetylcholine.[62] This effect clearly persists in the female offspring when they become pregnant despite their adaptations to pregnancy and even though they had not been exposed to any dietary challenge during postnatal life or pregnancy itself (unlike their mothers).

Of even greater importance may be the observation that the F2 generation (i.e., the grandchildren of the mothers exposed to a dietary impairment during pregnancy) also show impaired vasodilator function.[63] This may depend more on endothelium-derived hyperpolarizing factor (EDHF) than on nitric oxide (NO) mediated mechanisms, and in this respect is similar to other models of hypertension in the rat.[64] This is potentially an extremely important observation as it demonstrates that programmed effects on vascular function can be passed in a transgenerational fashion, even in the absence of additional dietary or other stressors. Recently, similar transgenerational programming of risk for diabetes has been demonstrated for the male lineage.[65] The mechanisms underlying such transmission are not known, although it is of interest that the DNA methylation processes that mediate imprinting are known to be passed at least from mother to offspring.[66] The implications of such findings to medicine are extensive, not least for the use of family linkage analysis in tracing the origins of diseases such as coronary heart disease.

TRANSDUCTION OF ENVIRONMENTAL STIMULI

The carotid chemoreceptors, which mediate rapid fetal cardiovascular adaptations to hypoxia, are responsive to reductions in circulating plasma glucose.[34,67] Thus common mechanisms of detection of changes in substrate (e.g., glucose) and oxygen may exist. There is evidence in cultured rat hepatocytes that regulation of glucagon receptor, insulin receptor, and L-type pyruvate kinase gene expression by glucose and oxygen may be due to cross-talk between hypoxia-inducible factor-1 (HIF-1) and glucose-responsive transcription factors at the glucose response element and hypoxia response element.[68]

Considerable work has now been conducted into the mechanisms by which dietary imbalance in pregnancy may be transmitted to the fetus. Unraveling the relative contribution of the key mechanisms is likely to be complicated. At the most basic level, a change in the quantity of a dietary component may have direct implications on the amount of substrate that is available for fetal metabolism, but maternal body composition (see earlier) and maternal metabolic demands, as well as placental metabolic demands, have to be taken into account. An additional consideration is of the multiple genes/proteins that may respond simultaneously to altered nutrition—analogous to the 14-protein "stimulon" induced by glucose depletion in *Escherichia coli*.[69] There is evidence that the expression of a variety of genes, implicated in cardiovascular control and growth during fetal life, can be modulated by the direct action of nutrients: for example, insulin-like growth factor-II gene expression in cultured beta cells is regulated by glucose.[70] During fetal life, glucose appears to regulate IGF-II directly but its effect on IGF-I is likely to be mediated by insulin.[71] Glucose activation of plasminogen activator inhibitor-1 gene expression in cultured rat vascular smooth muscle cells,[72] and of the osteopontin gene,[73] may be of relevance to vascular complications in diabetic patients. High glucose stimulates angiotensinogen gene expression in rat kidney proximal tubular cells, mediated in part by the generation of reactive oxygen species.[74]

Currently there is much interest in fetal exposure to increased levels of glucocorticoid from the viewpoint of the clinical use of steroids in pregnancy, but also to the potential "stress" experienced concomitant with altered nutrition. Glucocorticoids reduce fetal growth[75] and have an impact on the hypothalamic-pituitary-adrenal (HPA) axis of the developing fetus itself.[76] Glucocorticoids may mediate effects of altered maternal nutrition, including via interaction with the expression of other genes,[77,78] NO signaling pathways,[79] and effects on DNA methylation.[80] Although there is some evidence that nutrient restriction in guinea pigs elevates maternal plasma cortisol,[81] and a high-fat diet in rats is associated with stimulation of the HPA axis,[82] it has not been shown unequivocally in animals that altered maternal nutritional balance alters the level of plasma glucocorticoid in fetal life.[83,84] Even in the absence of such an elevation in maternal glucocorticoid, the fetus may be exposed to greater levels of steroid as a result of a reduction in placental 11-beta hydroxysteroid dehydrogenase type 2 (11-βHSD2).[85] In addition, at least in the hypertensive offspring of rat dams fed a low-protein diet, the tissue levels of glucocorticoid receptors (GR) are elevated and 11-βHSD2 activity is reduced, thereby exposing the tissues to greater levels of active steroid. Corresponding effects on 11-βHSD1 are not seen (see review in Ref 86). Finally, evidence for increased action of glucocorticoid tissues comes from the observation that glucorticoid-responsive gene expression (e.g., $Na^+,K^+,ATPase$) is altered in programmed offspring.[86]

The effects of gestational protein restriction on GR protein expression are greatest in the kidney, and this develops postnatally from 2 to 12 weeks, with similar effects being seen in the liver and lung, but not in the heart. In addition, despite no evidence of elevated late-gestation fetal cortisol levels (at least in the sheep), fetal HPA axis responsiveness is altered following early-gestation maternal nutrient restriction, although it is reduced rather than being enhanced, as predicted.[87] However, these observations are coupled to a reduction in GR messenger RNA in the pituitary in the "programmed" late-gestation sheep fetuses,[88] and the implied reduction in feedback inhibition of the HPA axis is consistent with the hyper-responsiveness of the HPA axis seen in offspring from this sheep cohort at 3 months of age,[87] and in adult men who were of a low birth weight studied in the Hertfordshire cohort.[89] Recent data show that once lambs have reached young adulthood (16 to 20 months), HPA axis responsiveness changes again, possibly involving altered peripheral tissue GR levels.[44]

Several decades of work have now contributed to our understanding of the mechanisms that underlie fetal cardiovascular control and growth under baseline conditions and during hypoxemia, which include carotid chemoreflex mechanisms, hormonal factors (e.g., catecholamines, arginine vasopressin, ACTH, cortisol, angiotensin, and the insulin-like growth factor system), and local mechansims such as nitric oxide and endothelin-1.[3] The extent to which similar mechanisms mediate the fetal response to altered nutrition has not yet been fully elucidated. Likely candidates include components of the HPA axis, renin-angiotensin system (RAS), and IGF axis. As for the HPA axis (discussed earlier), there is evidence that the fetal and postnatal RAS[90-93] and IGF axis[94] are programmable by altered substrate supply during pregnancy. Moreover, as discussed earlier, fetal cardiovascular control and growth may be related in a graded manner in the face of altered nutrient supply. It is therefore conceivable that common mechanisms are integrating their control—a concept that is consistent with the dual roles for substances like Ang-II, IGF-I, and cortisol in cardiovascular control and growth.[3]

CONCLUSION

The formation of the Fetal Origins of Adult Disease hypothesis has made it necessary to take a new perspective of the mechanisms underlying fetal cardiovascular control. Moreover, repeated demonstration of the association between size at birth and adult cardiovascular disease necessitates looking more closely at the link between cardiovascular control and growth during fetal life. A number of candidate mechanisms have been suggested from work in the field of fetal hypoxia, and in fact certain components of the RAS, HPA axis, and IGF system share physiologic end-points in the regulation of cardiovascular control and growth. Determining whether fetal growth and cardiovascular control are related in a graded fashion in the face of altered nutrition is likely to be crucial to our understanding of fetal programming, and to the development of future intervention strategies to prevent disease in later life.

ACKNOWLEDGMENT

Supported by the British Heart Foundation.

REFERENCES

1. Newman J, et al: Oxygen sensing in fetal hypoxia. *In* Lahiri S, et al (eds): Lung Biology in Health and Disease. New York, Marcel Dekker, 2002, pp.209–234.
2. Hanson MA: *In* Hanson MA, et al: (eds): The Circulation, vol 1. Cambridge, UK, Cambridge University Press, 1993, pp 1–22.
3. Green LR: Programming of endocrine mechanisms of cardiovascular control. J Soc Gynecol Invest 8:57, 2001.
4. Green LR, et al: Adaptation of cardiovascular responses to repetitive umbilical cord occlusion in the late gestation ovine fetus. J Physiol 535:879, 2001.
5. Stein P, et al: Altered fetal cardiovascular responses to prolonged hypoxia after sinoaortic denervation. Am J Physiol 276:R340, 1999.
6. Gardner DS, et al: Effects of prevailing hypoxaemia, acidaemia or hypoglycaemia upon the cardiovascular, endocrine and metabolic responses to acute hypoxaemia in the ovine fetus. J Physiol 540:351, 2002.
7. Giussani DA, et al: Chemoreflex and endocrine components of cardiovascular responses to acute hypoxia in the llama fetus. Am J Physiol 271:R73, 1996.
8. Giussani DA, et al: Adrenergic and vasopressinergic contributions to the cardiovascular response to acute hypoxaemia in the llama fetus. J Physiol 515 (Pt 1):233, 1999.
9. Llanos AJ, et al: Regional brain blood flow and cerebral hemispheric oxygen consumption during acute hypoxaemia in the llama fetus. J Physiol 538:975, 2002.
10. Riquelme RA, et al: Chemoreflex contribution to adrenocortical function during acute hypoxemia in the llama fetus at 0.6 to 0.7 of gestation. Endocrinology 139:2564, 1998.
11. Barker DJ, et al: The relation of small head circumference and thinness at birth to death from cardiovascular disease in adult life. BMJ 306:422, 1993.
12. Hales CN, Barker DJ: The thrifty phenotype hypothesis. Br Med Bull 60:5, 2001.
13. Huxley RR, et al: The role of size at birth and postnatal catch-up growth in determining systolic blood pressure: a systematic review of the literature. J Hypertens 18:815, 2000.
14. Huxley R, et al: Unravelling the fetal origins hypothesis: is there really an inverse association between birthweight and subsequent blood pressure? Lancet 360:659, 2002.
15. Eriksson JG, et al: Early growth and coronary heart disease in later life: longitudinal study. BMJ 322:949, 2001.
16. Stein CE, et al: Fetal growth and coronary heart disease in south India. Lancet 348:1269, 1996.
17. Fall CH, et al: Size at birth, maternal weight, and type 2 diabetes in South India. Diabet Med 15:220, 1998.
18. Barker DJ, et al: Growth in utero and blood pressure levels in the next generation. J Hypertens 18:843, 2000.
19. Eriksson JG, et al: The effects of the Pro12Ala polymorphism of the peroxisome proliferator–activated receptor-γ2 gene on insulin sensitivity and insulin metabolism interact with size at birth. Diabetes 51:2321, 2002.
20. Dennison EM, et al: Birthweight, vitamin D receptor genotype, and the programming of osteoporosis. Paediatr Perinat Epidemiol 15:211, 2001.
21. Reik W, Murrell A: Genomic imprinting. Silence across the border. Nature 405:408, 2000.
22. Hammond J: Physiological factors affecting birth weight. Proce Nutr Soc 2:8, 1944.
23. Constancia M, et al: Placental-specific IGF-II is a major modulator of placental and fetal growth. Nature 417:945, 2002.
24. Smith GC, et al: First-trimester growth and the risk of low birth weight. N Engl J Med 339:1817, 1998.
25. Brawley L, et al: Mechanisms underlying the programming of small artery dysfunction: review of the model using low protein diet in pregnancy in the rat. Arch Physiol Biochem 111:23, 2003.
26. Kwong WY, et al: Maternal undernutrition during the preimplantation period of rat development causes blastocyst abnormalities and programming of postnatal hypertension. Development 127:4195, 2000.
27. Watkins A, et al: Factors influencing the relative size of mouse blastocyst cell lineages and their impact on later development. Ceska Gynekol 67(suppl 3):40, 2003.
28. Jackson AA, et al: Increased systolic blood pressure in rats induced by a maternal low-protein diet is reversed by dietary supplementation with glycine. Clin Sci (Lond) 103:633, 2002.
29. Battaglia FC, Regnault TR: Placental transport and metabolism of amino acids. Placenta 22:145, 2001.
30. Cetin I: Amino acid interconversions in the fetal-placental unit: the animal model and human studies in vivo. Pediatr Res 49:148, 2001.
31. Thame M, et al: Blood pressure is related to placental volume and birth weight. Hypertension 35:662, 2000.

32. Godfrey KM, et al: Neutral amino acid uptake by the microvillous plasma membrane of the human placenta is inversely related to fetal size at birth in normal pregnancy. J Clin Endocrinol Metab *83*:3320, 1998.

33. Glazier JD, et al: Association between the activity of the system A amino acid transporter in the microvillous plasma membrane of the human placenta and severity of fetal compromise in intrauterine growth restriction. Pediatr Res *42*:514, 1997.

34. Pardal R, Lopez-Barneo J: Low glucose-sensing cells in the carotid body. Nat Neurosci *5*:197, 2002.

35. Kiserud T, et al: Circulatory responses to maternal hyperoxaemia and hypoxaemia assessed non-invasively in fetal sheep at 0.3–0.5 gestation in acute experiments. Br J Obstet Gynecol *108*:359, 2001.

36. Haugen G, et al: Relation of maternal body composition before pregnancy to fetal liver blood flow in late gestation. Czech Gynecol *67*(suppl 3):2, 2002.

37. Crowe C, et al: Nutritional plane in early pregnancy and fetal cardiovascular development in sheep. Society for the Study of Fetal Physiology, 1995.

38. Crowe C, et al: Blood pressure and cardiovascular reflex development in fetal sheep. Relation to hypoxaemia, weight, and blood glucose. Reprod Fertil Dev *7*:553, 1995.

39. Robinson JS, et al: Studies on experimental growth retardation in sheep. The effects of maternal hypoxaemia. J Dev Physiol *5*:89, 1983.

40. Hawkins P, et al: Effect of maternal undernutrition in early gestation on ovine fetal blood pressure and cardiovascular reflexes. Am J Physiol Regul Integr Comp Physiol *279*:R340, 2000.

41. Ozaki T, et al: Effects of undernutrition in early pregnancy on systemic small artery function in late-gestation fetal sheep. Am J Obstet Gynecol *183*:1301, 2000.

42. Nishina H, et al: Effect of nutritional restriction in early pregnancy on isolated systemic small artery function in mid gestation fetal sheep. J Soc Gynecol Invest *7*:101A, 2000.

43. Harding J, et al: Intrauterine feeding of the growth retarded fetus: can we help? Early Hum Dev *29*:193, 1992.

44. Green LR, et al: Programming of cardiovascular and hypothalamo-piuitary-adrenal (HPA) axis responses in young adult sheep following mild early gestation nutrient restriction. J Soc Gynecol Invest *9*:128A, 198, 2002.

45. Eriksson JG, et al: Early growth and coronary heart disease in later life: longitudinal study. BMJ *322*:949, 2001.

46. Vickers MH, et al: Dysregulation of the adipoinsular axis—a mechanism for the pathogenesis of hyperleptinemia and adipogenic diabetes induced by fetal programming. J Endocrinol *170*:323, 2001.

47. Vickers MH, et al: Fetal origins of hyperphagia, obesity, and hypertension and postnatal amplification by hypercaloric nutrition. Am J Physiol Endocrinol Metab *279*:E83, 2000.

48. Poore KR, et al: Glucose tolerance in young adult sheep following moderate postconceptual undernutrition and undernutrition in early postnatal life. Pediatr Res *53*:12A, 11A.4, 2003.

49. Newman JM, et al: Baroreflexes in young adult sheep following moderate postconceptual undernutrition and undernutrition in early postnatal life. Pediatr Res *53*:18A, 148, 2003.

50. Cleal J, et al: The effect of early gestation nutrient restriction on ovine fetal growth and the development of the renin-angiotensin system. Ceska Gynekol *67*: (Suppl 3):22, 2002.

51, 52. Brawley L, et al: Dietary protein restriction in pregnancy induces hypertension and vascular defects in rat adult offspring. Pediatr Res *54*:83, 2003.

53. Franco MC, et al: Intrauterine undernutrition: expression and activity of the endothelial nitric oxide synthase in male and female adult offspring. Cardiovasc Res *56*:145, 2002.

54. Leeson P, et al: Non-invasive measurement of endothelial function: effect on brachial artery dilatation of graded endothelial dependent and independent stimuli. Heart *78*:22, 1997.

55. Leson CP, et al: Flow-mediated dilation in 9- to 11-year-old children: the influence of intrauterine and childhood factors. Circulation *96*:2233, 1997.

56. Steinberg HO, et al: Obesity/insulin resistance is associated with endothelial dysfunction. Implications for the syndrome of insulin resistance. J Clin Invest *97*:2601, 1996.

57. Thornburg KL, et al: Hemodynamic changes in pregnancy. Semin Perinatol *24*:11, 2000.

58. Ni Y, et al: Pregnancy augments uteroplacental vascular endothelial growth factor gene expression and vasodilator effects. Am J Physiol *273*:H938, 1997.

59. Ahokas RA, et al: Maternal organ distribution of cardiac output in the diet-restricted pregnant rat. J Nutr *114*:2262, 1984.

60. Itoh S, et al: Vasodilation to vascular endothelial growth factor in the uterine artery of the pregnant rat is blunted by low dietary protein intake. Pediatr Res *51*:485, 2002.

61. Innes KE, et al: Association of a woman's own birth weight with subsequent risk for gestational diabetes. JAMA *287*:2534, 2002.

62. Torrens C, et al: Maternal protein restriction in the rat impairs resistance artery but not conduit artery function in pregnant offspring. J Physiol *547*:77, 2003.

63. Torrens C, et al: Transgenerational programming of vascular function in the rat protein restriction model. Ceska Gynekol *67*:1, 2003.

64. Sofola OA, et al: Change in endothelial function in mesenteric arteries of Sprague-Dawley rats fed a high salt diet. J Physiol *543*:255, 2002.

65. Kaati G, et al: Cardiovascular and diabetes mortality determined by nutrition during parents' and grandparents' slow growth period. Eur J Hum Genet *10*:682, 2002.

66. Lane N, et al: Resistance of IAPs to methylation reprogramming may provide a mechanism for epigenetic inheritance in the mouse. Genesis *35*:88, 2003.

67. Hamon MH, Heap RB: Progesterone and oestrogen concentrations in plasma of Barbary sheep (aoudad, *Ammotragus lervia*) compared with those of domestic sheep and goats during pregnancy. J Reprod Fertil *90*:207, 1990.

68. Kietzmann T, et al: Signaling cross-talk between hypoxia and glucose via hypoxia-inducible factor 1 and glucose response elements. Biochem Pharmacol *64*:903, 2002.

69. Nystrom T: Glucose starvation stimulon of *Escherichia coli*: role of integration host factor in starvation survival and growth phase–dependent protein synthesis. J Bacteriol *177*:5707, 1995.

70. Asfari M, et al: Insulin-like growth factor-II gene expression in a rat insulin-producing beta-cell line (INS-1) is regulated by glucose. Diabetologia *38*:927, 1995.

71. Oliver MH, et al: Fetal insulin-like growth factor (IGF)-I and IGF-II are regulated differently by glucose or insulin in the sheep fetus. Reprod Fertil Dev *8*:167, 1996.

72. Suzuki M, et al: Glucose upregulates plasminogen activator inhibitor-1 gene expression in vascular smooth muscle cells. Life Sci *72*:59, 2002.

73. Asaumi S, et al: Identification and characterization of high glucose and glucosamine responsive element in the rat osteopontin promoter. J Diabetes Complications *17*:34, 2003.

74. Hsieh TJ, et al: High glucose stimulates angiotensinogen gene expression via reactive oxygen species generation in rat kidney proximal tubular cells. Endocrinology *143*:2975, 2002.

75. Moss TJ, et al: Programming effects in sheep of prenatal growth restriction and glucocorticoid exposure. Am J Physiol Regul Integr Comp Physiol *281*:R960, 2001.

76. McCabe L, et al: Repeated antenatal glucocorticoid treatment decreases hypothalamic corticotropin-releasing hormone mRNA but not corticosteroid receptor mRNA expression in the fetal guinea-pig brain. J Neuroendocrinol *13*:425, 2001.

77. Li J, et al: Transcriptional regulation of insulin-like growth factor-II gene expression by cortisol in fetal sheep during late gestation. J Biol Chem *273*:10586, 1998.

78. Forhead AJ, et al: Effect of cortisol on blood pressure and the renin-angiotensin system in fetal sheep during late gestation. J Physiol *526*:167, 2000.

79. Radomski MW, et al: Glucocorticoids inhibit the expression of an inducible, but not the constitutive, nitric oxide synthase in vascular endothelial cells. Proc Natl Acad Sci USA *87*:10043, 1990.

80. Thomassin H, et al: Glucocorticoid-induced DNA demethylation and gene memory during development. EMBO J *20*:1974, 2001.

81. Lingas R, et al: Maternal nutrient restriction (48 h) modifies brain corticosteroid receptor expression and endocrine function in the fetal guinea pig. Brain Res *846*:236, 1999.

82. Tannenbaum BM, et al: High-fat feeding alters both basal and stress-induced hypothalamic-pituitary-adrenal activity in the rat. Am J Physiol *273*:E1168, 1997.

83. Hawkins P, et al: Effect of maternal nutrient restriction in early gestation on development of the hypothalamic-pituitary-adrenal axis in fetal sheep at 0.8–0.9 of gestation. J Endocrinol *163*:553, 1999.

84. Hawkins P, et al: Effect of maternal nutrient restriction in early gestation on responses of the hypothalamic-pituitary-adrenal axis to acute isocapnic hypoxaemia in late gestation fetal sheep. Exp Physiol *85*:85, 2000.

85. Whorwood CB, et al: Maternal undernutrition during early to midgestation programs tissue-specific alterations in the expression of the glucocorticoid receptor, 11 beta-hydroxysteroid dehydrogenase isoforms, and type 1 angiotensin II receptor in neonatal sheep. Endocrinology *142*:2854, 2001.

86. Bertram CE, Hanson MA: Prenatal programming of postnatal endocrine responses by glucocorticoids. Reproduction *124*:459, 2002.

87. Hawkins P, et al: Cardiovascular and hypothalamic-pituitary-adrenal axis development in late gestation fetal sheep and young lambs following modest maternal nutrient restriction in early gestation. Reprod Fertil Dev *12*:443, 2000.

88. Hawkins P, et al: Maternal undernutrition in early gestation alters molecular regulation of the hypothalamic-pituitary-adrenal axis in the ovine fetus. J Neuroendocrinol *13*:855, 2001.

89. Reynolds RM, et al: Altered control of cortisol secretion in adult men with low birth weight and cardiovascular risk factors. J Clin Endocrinol Metab *86*:245, 2001.

90. Edwards LJ, et al: Restriction of placental and fetal growth in sheep alters fetal blood pressure responses to angiotensin II and captopril. J Physiol (Lond) *515*(Pt 3):897, 1999.

91. Edwards LJ, McMillen IC: Periconceptional nutrition programs development of the cardiovascular system in the fetal sheep. Am J Physiol Regul Integr Comp Physiol *283*:R669, 2002.

92. Green LR, et al: Effect of maternal nutrient restriction in early gestation on the plasma angiotensin II and arginine vasopressin responses during acute hypoxaemia in late gestation fetal sheep. Pediatr Res *50*:24A, 2001.

93. Trowern AR, et al: The intrauterine environment programmes hypertension in later life through increased expression of renal type 1 angiotensin II receptor. Pediatr Res *50*:42A, 2001.

94. Gallaher BW, et al: Fetal programming of insulin-like growth factor (IGF)-I and IGF-binding protein-3: evidence for an altered response to undernutrition in late gestation following exposure to periconceptual undernutrition in the sheep. J Endocrinol *159*:501, 1998.

Physiology of Nitric Oxide in the Developing Lung

Since its recognition as an important endogenous mediator of vasorelaxation in 1987,[1, 2] the role of nitric oxide (NO) in the regulation of pulmonary vasomotor tone has been intensively investigated. The successful transition from fetal placental dependence to survival at birth requires that pulmonary vascular resistance (PVR) rapidly declines and pulmonary blood flow increases.[3-6] Therefore, the role of endogenous NO production in the transitional circulation has received considerable attention. In particular, the physiology of NO-mediated vasoregulation in the fetal and neonatal lung has been of keen interest to developmental lung biologists because of the life-threatening clinical disorder of persistent pulmonary hypertension of the newborn (PPHN). In this chapter, we review the physiologic role of endogenous NO production in the fetal and transitional pulmonary circulation, the normal ontogeny of NO synthase (NOS) isoform expression in the fetal lung and alterations observed in animal models of PPHN, the effects of inhaled NO (iNO) on the pulmonary circulation of the term and preterm newborn, and the current clinical role of iNO.

ENDOGENOUS NITRIC OXIDE: FETAL AND TRANSITIONAL VASOREGULATION

Vasomotor tone in the fetus is modulated by both vasoconstrictor and vasodilator substances. The role of vasodilator substances such as NO has been of particular interest because of their part in the pulmonary vasorelaxation that must occur at birth to ensure a successful transition from fetal to neonatal life. NO was recognized as a potent vasodilator as early as 1979,[7] and in 1980, Furchgott and Zawadzki reported that acetylcholine-induced vasorelaxation was dependent on an intact endothelium through the elaboration of an endothelial-derived relaxing factor (EDRF) that diffused to the subjacent vascular smooth muscle.[1] In 1987, investigators from two separate laboratories reported that the biologic activity of EDRF was identical to that of NO or an NO-containing substance. Palmer and colleagues[1] induced the release of EDRF from porcine aortic endothelial cells in culture and compared the effects on superfused aortic strips with that of NO in solution. They found that the effects of EDRF were indistinguishable from those of NO. Ignarro and colleagues[8] used a bioassay cascade superfusion technique with intrapulmonary arteries and veins, identified EDRF pharmacologically and chemically as NO, and found that EDRF and NO produced similar vasorelaxation and were inhibited by common antagonists. Ignarro and associates also recognized that NO was inactivated by combining with hemoproteins, and they speculated that hemoglobin could trap endogenously produced NO that diffused into the vascular lumen, thus preventing any downstream vasorelaxation by this paracrine mediator.

In mammalian cells, NO is produced from the terminal guanidino nitrogen of L-arginine on its conversion to L-citrulline by the enzyme NOS in a reaction that requires molecular oxygen.[9] NOS is a family of enzymes that includes three major isoforms known as neuronal NOS (nNOS), inducible NOS (iNOS), and endothelial NOS (eNOS).[10-16] The three isoforms—nNOS, iNOS, and eNOS—are also referred to as NOS-I, NOS-II, and NOS-III. The activity of nNOS and eNOS is calcium dependent, whereas the activity of iNOS is calcium independent.[11] nNOS and iNOS are primarily found in the soluble fraction, whereas eNOS is primarily in the membrane fraction, particularly in specialized signaling micro-domains on the plasma membrane called *caveolae*.[17] All NOS isoforms are homodimers of subunits that range between 130 and 160 kDa.[18] nNOS and eNOS expression was first believed to be primarily constitutive in nature, whereas the expression of iNOS is inducible by cytokines.[11, 19]

The recognition that the endogenous production of this EDRF/NO mediator could be competitively blocked by modified L-arginine analogues prompted early experiments into the effects of NO in the fetal and transitional pulmonary circulation. The earliest studies were performed in fetal lambs because the relatively large size of the ovine fetus allows for instrumentation with catheters to monitor vascular pressure and electromagnetic or ultrasound probes to monitor blood flow. Moreover, the ovine fetus is a suitable candidate for such experiments because operating on the fetus does not induce parturition, as commonly occurs in primate models. Abman and colleagues[20] performed the first experiments on the role of EDRF in the ovine model and demonstrated that endogenous EDRF/NO production modulates basal pulmonary vascular tone in the late-gestation fetus and pharmacologic NO blockade inhibits endothelium-dependent pulmonary vasodilation.[20] These investigators also showed that pharmacologic NO blockade attenuates the rise in pulmonary blood flow at delivery, thus implicating endogenous NO formation in postnatal adaptation after birth and linking this laboratory observation to the life-threatening clinical condition of PPHN (Fig. 70-1). Further, experiments demonstrated that increased fetal oxygen tension augments endogenous NO release,[21, 22] and increases in pulmonary blood flow in response to rhythmic distention of the lung and high inspired oxygen concentrations are mediated in part by endogenous NO elaboration.[23]

The major NOS isoform responsible for modulation of basal pulmonary vascular tone in the fetus and pulmonary vasodilation at birth may not be eNOS. Studies have shown that the iNOS is expressed in airway epithelium and vascular smooth muscle in the late-gestation ovine fetus.[24] Moreover, in the late-gestation ovine fetus, selective inhibition of iNOS increases basal PVR, reduces shear stress–induced pulmonary vasodilation, and attenuates NO-mediated pulmonary vasodilation at birth.[25-27]

In contrast to the mature fetus, there is indirect evidence that *endothelium-dependent* pulmonary vasodilation in pulmonary circulation of the preterm fetus is diminished until late in gestation. Acetylcholine and increased oxygen tension cause marked pulmonary vasodilation in the late-gestation ovine fetus, but dilator responses to these stimuli are decreased in the premature fetus.[28-30] Because acetylcholine- and oxygen-induced fetal pulmonary vasodilation are partly mediated by endogenous NO formation, it appears that endogenous NO activity increases with advancing gestational age.[31-33] Similarly, maturational changes in vasorelaxation of ovine pulmonary artery rings were observed with endothelium-dependent vasodilators, but no differences were found in relaxation of ovine fetal pulmonary artery rings compared with adult rings when both were exposed to an endothelium-independent vasodilator (sodium nitroprusside).[34]

NITRIC OXIDE SYNTHASES IN THE DEVELOPING LUNG

The cellular distribution of the three NOS isoforms has been evaluated in parallel, isoform-specific immunohistochemical analyses in developing ovine lung. In third trimester fetal lung,

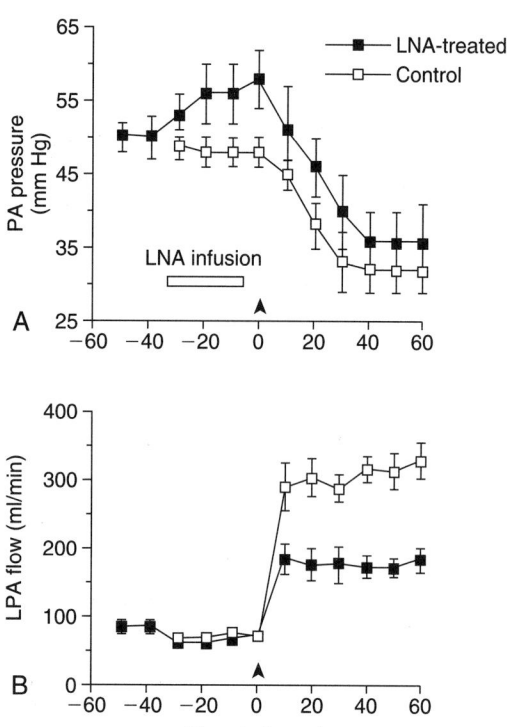

Figure 70–1. A and **B,** Inhibition of endogenous nitric oxide production attenuates the decline in pulmonary vascular resistance associated with birth-related events. LPA = left pulmonary artery; PA = pulmonary artery. (From Abman SH, et al: Am J Physiol 1990;259:H1921.)

eNOS was found in vascular endothelium as expected, but it was also markedly abundant in bronchial and proximal bronchiolar epithelium. eNOS was not detected in terminal or respiratory bronchiolar epithelium or in alveolar epithelium. Similar to eNOS, iNOS protein was detected in bronchial and proximal bronchiolar epithelium but not in alveolar epithelium. However, iNOS was also expressed in terminal and respiratory bronchioles. nNOS protein was found in epithelium at all levels including the alveolar wall. In addition, there was positive immunostaining for iNOS and nNOS in airway and vascular smooth muscle. The cellular distribution of all three isoforms was similar in fetal, newborn, and adult ovine lung, and the observations made in the epithelium by immunohistochemistry were confirmed by isoform-specific reverse transcription–polymerase chain reaction (RT-PCR) assays and reduced nicotinamide-adenine dinucleotide phosphate diaphorase histochemistry.[26] More recent studies in lungs from late-gestation fetal baboons have yielded similar findings, demonstrating that nNOS, eNOS, and iNOS are primarily expressed in the airway epithelium in the fetal primate.[35] Thus, the three NOS isoforms are abundant and commonly expressed in proximal lung epithelium, and they are differentially expressed in distal lung epithelium. All three isoforms may be important sources of pulmonary NO throughout lung development.

Maturational changes in NOS isoform expression in the lung have also been delineated. The ontogeny of eNOS and nNOS expression was first determined in lungs from fetal and newborn rats. Both eNOS and nNOS proteins were detectable in 16-day fetal lung; they increased fourfold and threefold, respectively, to reach maximal levels at 20 days' gestation (term = 22 days), and they fell postnatally (1 to 5 days). In parallel with the findings for eNOS protein, eNOS mRNA levels assessed using semiquantitative RT-PCR increased from 16 to 20 days' gestation and fell after birth. In

contrast, nNOS mRNA abundance declined during late fetal life and rose postnatally. These observations indicate that eNOS and nNOS gene expression is developmentally regulated in rat lung, with maximal eNOS and nNOS protein expression near term. Furthermore, the regulation of pulmonary eNOS may primarily involve alterations in transcription or mRNA stability, whereas nNOS expression in the maturing lung may also be mediated by additional posttranscriptional processes.[36] The developmental regulation of eNOS expression has also been discerned in ovine fetal lung. eNOS is present in the pulmonary vasculature of the premature ovine fetus as early as 43 days' gestation (29% of term gestation),[37] with maximal eNOS mRNA and protein expression observed early in the third trimester.[38] Differences in the timing of eNOS up-regulation in the sheep and rat may be related to the temporal features of lung development in the two species, with a greater proportion of maturation occurring postnatally in the rat.[39]

To understand the regulation of pulmonary NO production in the developing primate better, maturational changes in NOS isoform expression and action have been determined in the proximal lung of third trimester fetal baboons from 125 to 175 days' gestation (term = 185 days) (Fig. 70-2). There was a marked increase in total NOS enzymatic activity from 125 to 140 days' gestation because of elevations in nNOS and eNOS expression, whereas iNOS expression and activity were minimal. Total NOS activity was constant from 140 to 175 days' gestation, and during the latter stages (160 to 175 days' gestation), a dramatic fall in nNOS and eNOS was replaced by a rise in iNOS. Studies done within 1 hour of delivery at 125 or 140 days' gestation revealed that the principal increase in NOS during the third trimester is associated with an elevation in exhaled NO levels, a decline in expiratory resistance, and greater pulmonary compliance.[19] These cumulative observations indicate that normal developmental increases in pulmonary NO expression and NO production during the third trimester may serve to optimize not only pulmonary vascular tone, but also airway and parenchymal function in the immediate postnatal period.

Alterations in NO production and NOS expression have been evaluated in animal models of perinatal pulmonary vascular disease, with particular emphasis on eNOS action and expression. Chronic hypoxia is an important causal factor in the development of pulmonary hypertension in the perinatal period, and in newborn piglets, chronic hypoxia attenuates acetylcholine-stimulated (eNOS-dependent) pulmonary vasodilation. There is marked diminution in both basal and acetylcholine-stimulated pulmonary NO production, and eNOS expression is attenuated.[40–42] In studies of the direct effects of varying oxygen exposure on isolated ovine fetal pulmonary artery endothelial cells, eNOS mRNA and protein expression were both attenuated (by threefold) with hypoxia.[43] These findings suggest that decreased eNOS expression and resultant diminution in pulmonary NO production may contribute to the pathogenesis of hypoxic pulmonary hypertension in the newborn.

NOS expression has also been evaluated in a rat model of congenital diaphragmatic hernia. The development of congenital diaphragmatic hernia can be induced in approximately 50 to 60% of rat fetuses after maternal ingestion of the herbicide nitrofen early in gestation. Studies of this model revealed that eNOS protein abundance is decreased by 42% in the lung ipsilateral to the hernia compared with lungs from control fetuses exposed to nitrofen but lacking congenital diaphragmatic hernia. Immunoblots for Factor VIII–related antigen indicate that this is not related to alterations in endothelial cell density, and studies of nNOS protein reveal that this finding is unique to the endothelial isoform of NOS. eNOS mRNA abundance evaluated by RT-PCR assay is also decreased in lung in congenital diaphragmatic hernia, and it falls to 22% of control levels.[44] These observations indicate that attenuated eNOS expression may contribute to PPHN in infants with congenital diaphragmatic hernia.

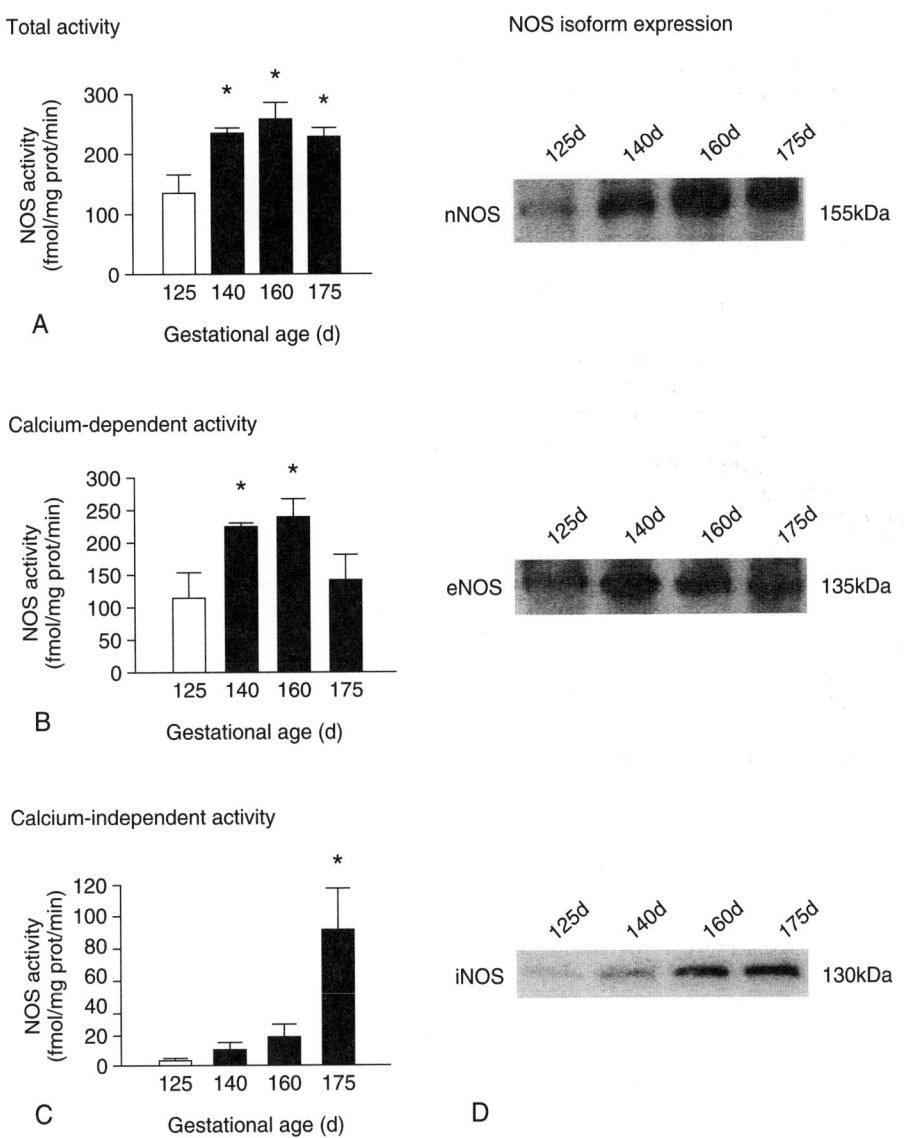

Figure 70–2. **A** to **D**, Nitric oxide synthase (NOS) enzymatic activity and NOS isoform expression in proximal baboon lung are developmentally regulated during the third trimester. eNOS = endothelial NOS; iNOS = inducible NOS; nNOS = neuronal NOS. (From Shaul PW, et al:Am J Physiol 2002;283:1192.)

Potentially important observations have also been made in a lamb model of neonatal pulmonary hypertension created by ligation of the fetal ductus arteriosus 10 to 20 days before delivery. NO-dependent relaxation is attenuated in intrapulmonary arteries from these animals.[45] In parallel, eNOS protein expression is decreased by one-half in the hypertensive lung, and nNOS expression is unaltered. Similarly, NOS enzymatic activity is decreased 45 to 75% in the hypertensive lung. Paralleling the declines in eNOS protein and NOS enzymatic activity, eNOS mRNA abundance is decreased in the hypertensive lung.[46, 47] Thus, pulmonary eNOS gene expression is attenuated in the lamb model of neonatal pulmonary hypertension. As such, there is evidence of diminished NOS function in multiple models of PPHN in multiple species.

EXOGENOUS (INHALED) NITRIC OXIDE AS A SELECTIVE PULMONARY VASODILATOR

In its natural form, NO exists as a gas, prompting its application to clinical medicine. The first clinical experiments with iNO gas were unrelated to its effects on pulmonary vasodilation. Based on the finding that iNO gas diffuses into the pulmonary circulation much faster than carbon monoxide, Borland, Chamberlain, and Higenbottam[48] tested the hypothesis that iNO could serve as a measure of diffusing capacity of the alveolar-capillary membrane in 1983. After the discovery that EDRF was actually NO, Higenbottam and associates studied the effects of iNO on pulmonary vasodilation in adults with primary pulmonary hypertension in the cardiac catheterization laboratory. At a platform presentation during the American Thoracic Society meeting in 1988, these investigators reported that, compared with prostacyclin, iNO caused equivalent reductions in PVR, but without systemic vascular effects.[49]

These observations captured the interest of physiologists studying the newborn pulmonary circulation because, after birth (with the initiation of air breathing), PVR rapidly declines and pulmonary blood flow markedly increases. These changes are essential for the normal transition to extrauterine life, and the potential of a selective pulmonary vasodilator was appealing, because available alternatives for the treatment of PPHN caused adverse systemic vascular effects.

In 1991, prompted by the observations of Higenbottam and associates, investigators commissioned an industrial gas manufacturer to combine NO with nitrogen to yield an NO concentration of 450 ppm, based on calculations designed to deliver 20 ppm NO within a continuous-flow, time-cycled, pressure-limited neonatal ventilator with a bias gas flow rate of 10 L/minute. The concentration of 450 ppm was chosen to balance environmental risk from sudden, complete tank evacuation against the obligate decrease in inspired oxygen concentration within the ventilator circuit during the administration of iNO. The first experiments of iNO in the late-gestation newborn lamb tested the effects at doses of 5, 10, and 20 ppm (based on the chronic ambient levels considered to be safe for adults by regulatory agencies in the United States[50]). Using vascular flow probes and radiolabeled microspheres to measure pulmonary and systemic blood flow, these investigators found that iNO caused potent, selective, and sustained pulmonary vasodilation in the late-gestation newborn lamb (Fig. 70–3).[51] Moreover, cerebral blood flow and cerebral metabolic rate for oxygen were not affected by NO inhalation.[52] Frostell and colleagues[53] showed that iNO caused pulmonary vasodilation in adult animals during acute hypoxia and during pharmacologically induced pulmonary hypertension (U46619), and Roberts and associates[54] demonstrated that iNO reversed hypoxic pulmonary vasoconstriction in the juvenile lamb with respiratory acidosis. Corroborating studies in other animal models supported the observations that iNO is a selective pulmonary vasodilator at low doses (<20 ppm),[55-58] and studies using a model of PPHN in which marked structural pulmonary vascular changes were induced by prolonged fetal ductus arteriosus compression demonstrated that, despite the loss of endothelium-dependent vasodilation, the response to iNO remained intact.[59,60]

The effects of iNO in the premature subject have also been of interest to translational physiologists. However, the premature fetus is characterized by both structural and functional pulmonary parenchymal and vascular immaturity. Thus, separating the relative effects of pulmonary immaturity from its effects on lung inflation has been difficult because the pulmonary vascular, parenchymal, and airway responses of the premature lung to mechanical ventilation are different from those in the term subject. For example, surfactant deficiency compromises the normal increase in lung volume caused by tidal volume ventilation in extremely premature lambs. Although changes in PVR after delivery are mediated in part through the elaboration of vasoactive mediators by the pulmonary vascular endothelium, decreased lung volume exerts mechanical effects on the pulmonary circulation that increase pulmonary vascular tone. The early observations of Dawes and partners[61] predicated the notion that dilation of the premature pulmonary vascular bed was insufficient at birth, and this suboptimal vasodilation contributed to respiratory distress syndrome (RDS). Dawes and colleagues delivered four extremely premature lambs (76 to 83% of term gestation) and noted that the most immature animals had minimal reduction in PVR during tidal volume ventilation for 2 minutes after delivery, in contrast to the marked decrease in PVR noted in term animals. Indeed, pulmonary hypoperfusion was implicated in the evolution of "idiopathic" RDS.[62] However, after the seminal observations of Avery and Mead[63] and of Fujiwara and associates,[64] the contribution of surfactant deficiency to respiratory failure in the premature newborn became the pivotal pathophysiologic focus.

Surfactant therapy has dramatically improved the outcome of infants born prematurely. However, surfactant treatment alone does not consistently cause sustained improvement in oxygenation in extremely premature lambs. Jobe and associates[65] found only transient improvement in oxygenation in response to exogenous surfactant in lambs delivered at 120 days' gestation (82% of term), and repeated doses were less predictably effective. Walther and partners[66] showed that repeated doses of

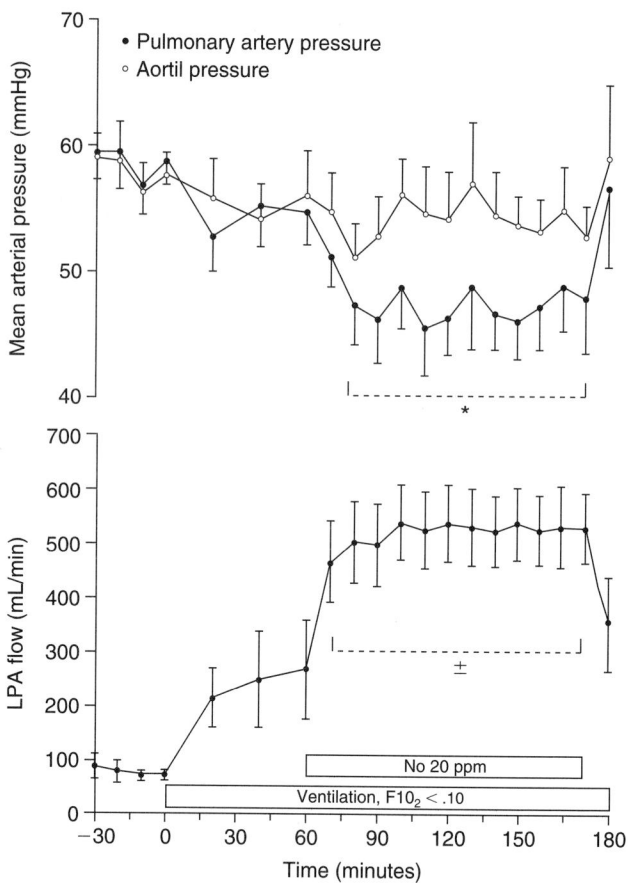

Figure 70–3. Inhaled nitric oxide causes potent, selective, and sustained pulmonary vasodilation in the term newborn lamb. (From Kinsella JP, et al: Am J Physiol 1992;262:H875.)

exogenous surfactant caused sustained improvement in oxygenation in lambs at 128 days' gestation (87% of term), but serial surfactant replacement in more immature lambs at 118 days' gestation (80% of term) did not modify the course of respiratory deterioration. These observations support the suggestion that other problems of prematurity (e.g., structural lung immaturity or altered vascular responses to dilator stimuli) contribute to respiratory failure in RDS. It is possible that persistent hypoxemia after surfactant replacement in the most immature subject is caused by pulmonary hypertension associated with decreased endogenous pulmonary vasodilator production.

After delivery, the fall in PVR in the premature lamb in response to birth-related events (rhythmic lung distention and increased inspired oxygen) is maximal with tidal volume mechanical ventilation and lung inflation alone, and there is little pulmonary hemodynamic response to high inspired oxygen.[67] However, when endogenous NO production is blocked during delivery of the premature lamb, the normal increase in pulmonary blood flow associated with mechanical ventilation and lung inflation is markedly attenuated, and subsequent treatment with iNO increases pulmonary blood flow to the same level as in control animals (Fig. 70–4).

The premature lamb has been extensively studied as a model of severe RDS.[68] Survival with exogenous surfactant treatment and mechanical ventilation at delivery varies, depending on the gestational age of the lamb and the type of surfactant given.[69,70] In very immature lambs (115 days' gestation), gas exchange worsens, and PVR increases during mechanical ventilation beyond 60 to 90 minutes after birth, despite treatment with exogenous surfactant at delivery.

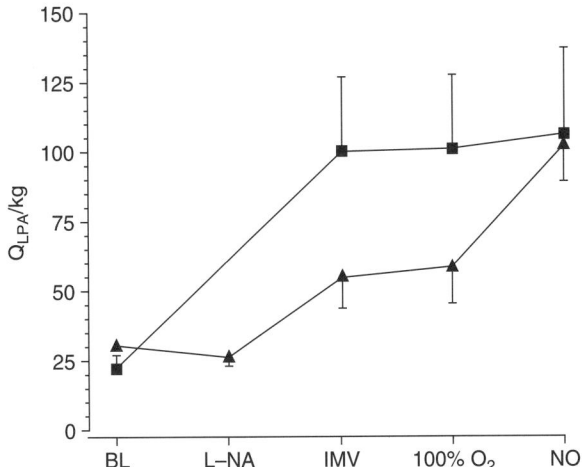

Figure 70–4. Inhibition of endogenous nitric oxide (NO) production in the premature lamb attenuates the increase in blood flow associated with birth-related events. Low-dose inhaled NO increases pulmonary blood flow to normal levels. BL = baseline; IMV = intermittent mandatory ventilation; L-NA = nitro-L-arginine; Q_{LPA} = left pulmonary artery flow. (From Kinsella JP, et al: Am J Physiol 1994;267:H1955.)

Several studies have examined the effects of iNO in the premature lamb with hyaline membrane disease. Skimming and colleagues[71] treated premature lambs (126 to 127 days' gestation) with iNO at 5 and 20 ppm for brief periods and showed improvement in oxygenation and PVR. In another study, intermittent mandatory ventilation over 2 hours in the extremely premature ovine fetus (115 days' gestation, 78% of term) resulted in progressive worsening of gas exchange and increased PVR. After 2 hours of ventilation, brief NO treatment lowered PVR and improved gas exchange.[72] Moreover, early and continuous treatment with iNO (20 ppm) caused sustained improvement in gas exchange and pulmonary hemodynamics over 3 hours of mechanical ventilation in the extremely premature lamb. Lung recruitment strategies employing high-frequency oscillatory ventilation (HFOV) have been shown to augment the response to low-dose iNO in premature lambs with RDS, a finding emphasizing the critical role of adequate lung inflation during inhalational vasodilator therapy.[73]

In addition to the effects of iNO on pulmonary hemodynamics and gas exchange, endogenous NO has been shown to regulate vascular permeability and neutrophil adhesion in the microcirculation.[74] Although some reports suggest that iNO may decrease capillary permeability in acute lung injury,[75, 76] the immature lung is particularly susceptible to lung protein leak during mechanical ventilation.[77] This proteinaceous pulmonary edema causes atelectasis and ventilation/perfusion abnormalities, thus worsening gas exchange and PVR. Increasing pulmonary blood flow with iNO in the premature subject could also have potential adverse effects. For example, conditions associated with increased pulmonary blood flow in the premature infant (patent ductus arteriosus) increase lung neutrophil accumulation.[78] The effects of iNO on pulmonary vascular permeability and lung leukosequestration in premature lambs with RDS were reported.[79] In premature lambs delivered at 78% of term, low-dose iNO (5 ppm) increased pulmonary blood flow and improved gas exchange (without increasing pulmonary edema) and decreased lung neutrophil accumulation (Fig. 70-5). Sequestration of neutrophils in the lung is an early step in a complex inflammatory response mediated through the elaboration of oxyradicals, proteases, phospholipases, and lipid compounds.[80] Therapies that reduce neutrophil accumulation in the lung in hyaline membrane disease could potentially modify the early inflammatory process that amplifies acute lung injury and contributes to the development of chronic lung disease.[81]

CLINICAL EFFECTS OF INHALED NITRIC OXIDE IN THE TERM NEWBORN WITH PERSISTENT PULMONARY HYPERTENSION OF THE NEWBORN

Early studies showed that iNO therapy caused marked improvement in oxygenation in term newborns with PPHN.[82-87] Multicenter randomized clinical studies subsequently confirmed that iNO therapy reduces the need for extracorporeal membrane oxygenation treatment in term neonates with hypoxemic respiratory failure.[88, 89] Extensive supportive data have demonstrated its overall safety and efficacy, as evidenced by the approval of this technique by the United States Food and Drug Administration.

PPHN[90] is a syndrome associated with diverse neonatal cardiac and pulmonary disorders that are characterized by high PVR causing extrapulmonary right-to-left shunting of blood across the ductus arteriosus or foramen ovale.[91] Extrapulmonary shunting resulting from high PVR in severe PPHN can cause critical hypoxemia that is poorly responsive to inspired oxygen or pharmacologic vasodilation. Vasodilator drugs administered intravenously, such as tolazoline and sodium nitroprusside, are often unsuccessful because of systemic hypotension and an inability to achieve or sustain pulmonary vasodilation.[92, 93] Thus, the ability of iNO therapy selectively to lower PVR and to decrease extrapulmonary venoarterial admixture accounts for the acute improvement in oxygenation observed in newborns with PPHN.[94]

The first studies of iNO treatment in term newborns reported initial doses that ranged from 80 ppm[82] to 6 to 20 ppm[83] (Fig. 70-6). The rationale for doses used in these clinical trials was based on concentrations that had previously been found to be effective in animal experiments by the same investigators.[51, 54] Roberts and partners[82] reported that brief (30 minutes) inhalation of NO at 80 ppm improved oxygenation in patients with PPHN, but this response was sustained in only one patient after NO was discontinued. In the second report, rapid improvement in oxygenation in neonates with severe PPHN was also demonstrated, but this was achieved at lower doses (20 ppm) for 4 hours.[83] This study also reported that decreasing the iNO dose to 6 ppm for the duration of treatment provided sustained improvement in oxygenation. The relative effectiveness of low-dose iNO in improving oxygenation in patients with severe PPHN was corroborated in a study by Finer and colleagues.[95] Acute improvement in oxygenation during treatment was not different with doses of iNO ranging from 5 to 80 ppm.

Because of its selective pulmonary vasodilator effects, iNO therapy is an important adjunct to available treatments for term newborns with hypoxemic respiratory failure. However, hypoxemic respiratory failure in the term newborn represents a heterogeneous group of disorders, and disease-specific responses have clearly been described. For example, patients with extrapulmonary right-to-left shunting (PPHN) show acute improvement in oxygenation when PVR becomes subsystemic during iNO therapy; however, patients with predominantly intrapulmonary shunting (e.g., RDS) have less dramatic responses[90] (Fig. 70-7).

Several pathophysiologic disturbances contribute to hypoxemia in the newborn infant, including cardiac dysfunction, airway and pulmonary parenchymal abnormalities, and pulmonary vascular disorders. In some newborns with hypoxemic respiratory failure, a single mechanism predominates (e.g., extrapulmonary right-to-left shunting in idiopathic PPHN), but more commonly, several of these mechanisms contribute to hypoxemia. For example, in a newborn with meconium aspiration syndrome, meconium may obstruct some airways, thus decreasing ventilation/perfusion ratios and increasing intrapulmonary

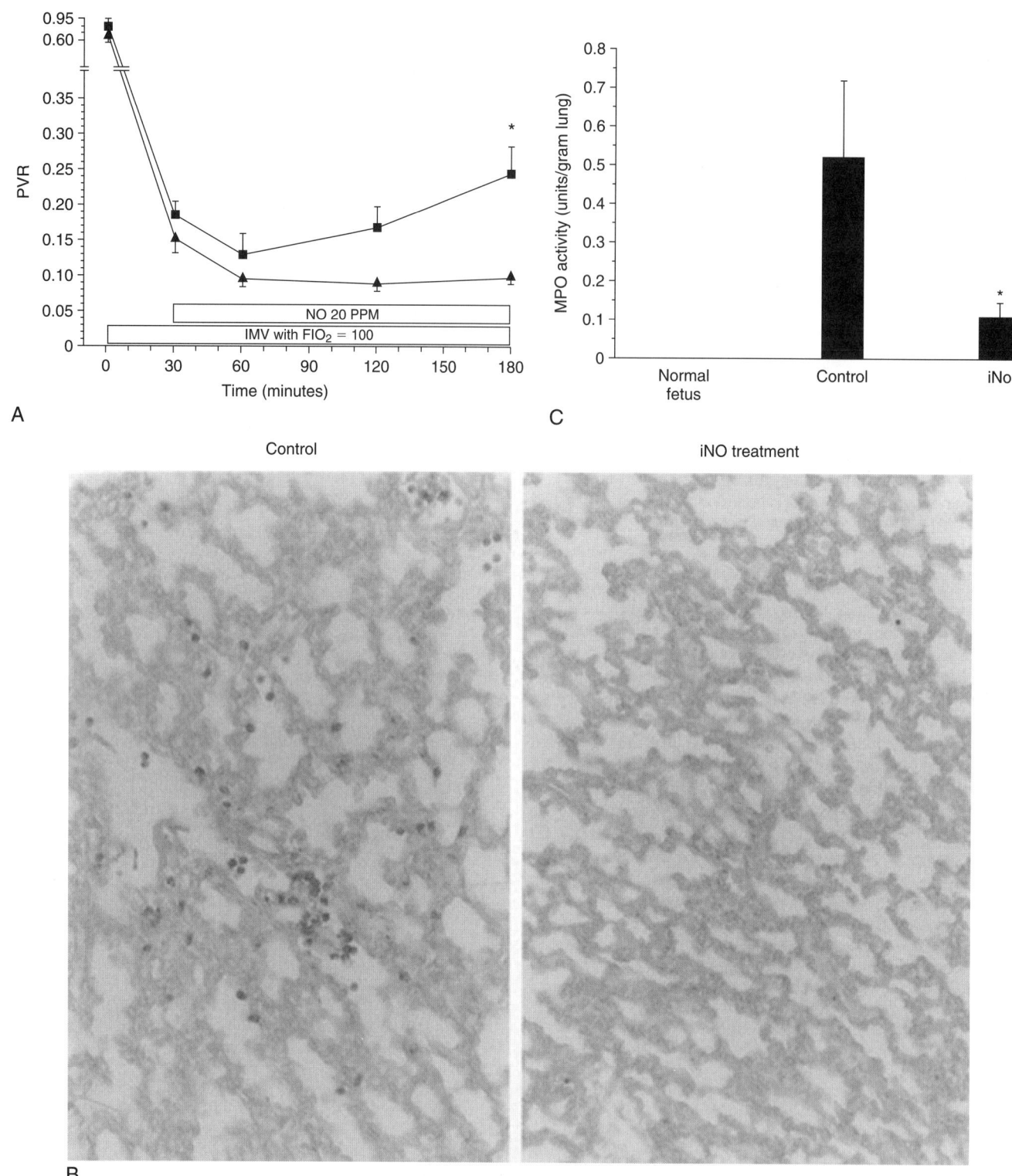

A

C

Control

iNO treatment

B

Figure 70–5. A, Low-dose inhaled nitric oxide causes sustained pulmonary vasodilation in mechanically ventilated premature lambs with RDS. PVR = pulmonary vascular resistance. **B,** Histologic features in control group (*left*) and those treated with inhaled nitric oxide (iNO; *right*). **C,** Low-dose iNO decreases lung neutrophil accumulation in the premature lamb with respiratory distress syndrome. MPO = myeloperoxidase. (*A,* From Kinsella JP, et al: Pediatr Res 1997;41:457.)

shunting. Other lung segments may be overventilated relative to perfusion and may cause increased physiologic dead space. Moreover, the same patient may have severe pulmonary hypertension with extrapulmonary right-to-left shunting at the ductus

arteriosus and foramen ovale. Not only does the overlap of these mechanisms complicate the clinical management, but also the tendency for time-dependent changes in the relative contribution of each mechanism to hypoxemia requires continued

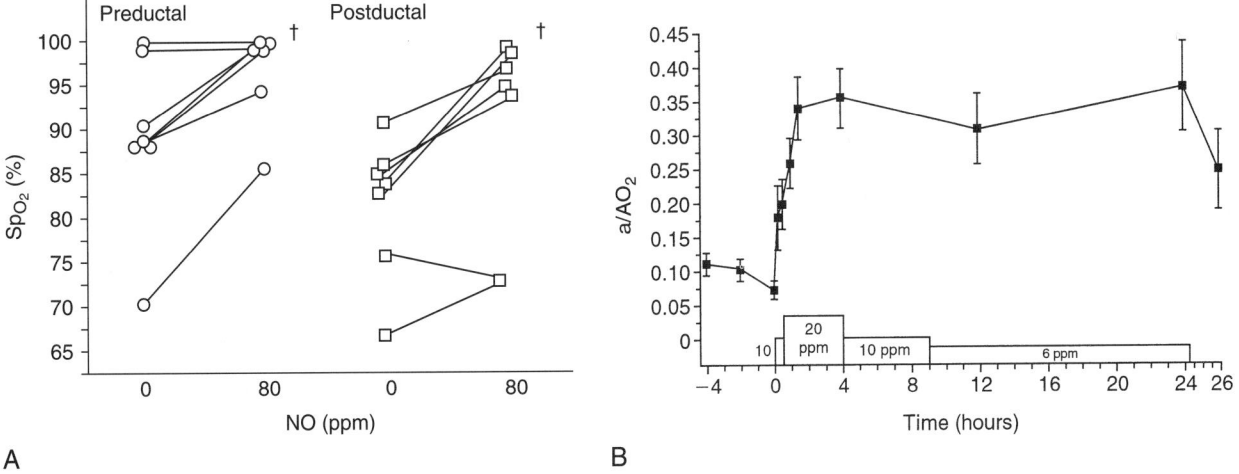

Figure 70–6. A, Brief treatment with 80 ppm inhaled nitric oxide (NO) caused acute improvement in newborns with persistent pulmonary hypertension of the newborn (PPHN). **B,** Treatment with low-dose inhaled NO for 24 hours caused sustained improvement in oxygenation in newborns with PPHN. (*A,* From Roberts JD, et al: Lancet 1992;340:818; *B,* from Kinsella JP, et al: Lancet 1992;340:819.)

vigilance as the disease progresses. Therefore, understanding the relative contribution of these different causes of hypoxemia becomes critically important as the inventory of therapeutic options expands.

Considering the important role of parenchymal lung disease in many cases of PPHN, pharmacologic pulmonary vasodilation alone would not be expected to cause sustained clinical improvement. The effects of iNO may be suboptimal when lung volume is decreased in association with pulmonary parenchymal disease.[96] Atelectasis and air space disease (pneumonia, pulmonary edema) will decrease effective delivery of iNO to its site of action in terminal lung units. In PPHN associated with heterogeneous (patchy) parenchymal lung disease, iNO may be effective in optimizing ventilation/perfusion matching by preferentially causing vasodilation in lung units that are well ventilated. The effects of iNO on ventilation/perfusion matching appear to be optimal at low doses (<20 ppm).[97] However, in cases complicated by homogeneous (diffuse) parenchymal lung disease and underinflation, pulmonary hypertension may be exacerbated because of the adverse mechanical effects of underinflation on PVR. In this setting, effective treat-

ment of the underlying lung disease is essential (and sometimes sufficient) to cause resolution of the accompanying pulmonary hypertension.

Along with iNO treatment, other therapeutic strategies have emerged for the management of the term infant with hypoxemic respiratory failure. Considering the important role of parenchymal lung disease in specific disorders included in the syndrome of PPHN, pharmacologic pulmonary vasodilation alone should not be expected to cause sustained clinical improvement in many cases.[98] Moreover, patients not responding to iNO can show marked improvement in oxygenation with adequate lung inflation alone.[84] High success rates in early studies were achieved by withholding iNO treatment until aggressive attempts were made to optimize ventilation and lung inflation with mechanical ventilation. These early studies demonstrated that the effects of iNO may be suboptimal when lung volume is decreased in association with pulmonary parenchymal disease, for several reasons. First, atelectasis and air space disease (pneumonia, pulmonary edema) may decrease the effective delivery of iNO to its site of action in terminal lung units. Second, in cases complicated by severe lung disease and underinflation, pulmonary hypertension may be exacerbated because of the adverse mechanical effects of underinflation on PVR. Third, attention must be given to minimize overinflation, to avoid inadvertent positive end-expiratory pressure and gas trapping that may elevate PVR from vascular compression. This commonly complicates the management of infants with asymmetric lung disease or airways obstruction, as observed in meconium aspiration syndrome.

In newborns with severe lung disease, HFOV is frequently used to optimize lung inflation and minimize lung injury.[99] In clinical pilot studies using iNO, the combination of HFOV and iNO caused the greatest improvement in oxygenation in newborns who had severe PPHN complicated by diffuse parenchymal lung disease and underinflation (e.g., RDS, pneumonia).[100,101] A randomized, multicenter trial demonstrated that treatment with HFOV and iNO was often successful in patients who failed to respond to HFOV or iNO alone in severe PPHN, and differences in responses were related to the specific disease associated with the complex disorders of PPHN[84] (Fig. 70–8). For patients with PPHN complicated by severe lung disease, response rates for HFOV and iNO were better than with HFOV alone or with iNO with conventional ventilation. In contrast, for patients without significant parenchymal lung disease, both iNO

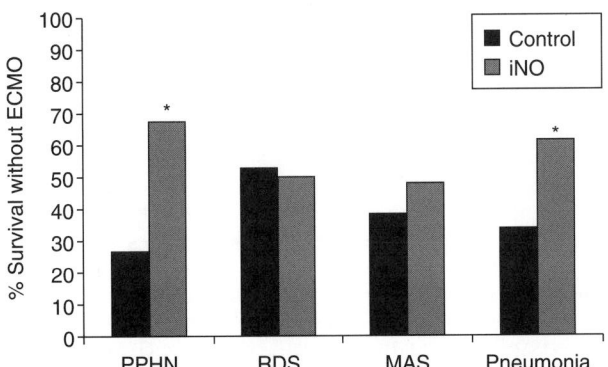

Figure 70–7. Marked improvement in survival without extracorporeal membrane oxygenation (ECMO) in newborns with persistent pulmonary hypertension of the newborn (PPHN). INO = inhaled nitric oxide; MAS = meconium aspiration syndrome; RDS = respiratory distress syndrome. (From Neonatal Inhaled Nitric Oxide Study Group: N Engl J Med 1997;336:597.)

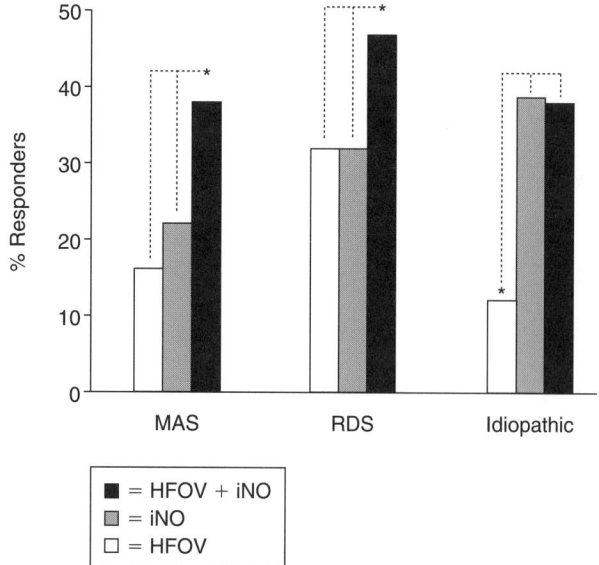

Figure 70–8. Lung recruitment with high-frequency oscillatory ventilation (HFOV) augments the response to inhaled nitric oxide (iNO) in patients with severe parenchymal lung disease. MAS = meconium aspiration syndrome; RDS = respiratory distress syndrome. (From Kinsella JP, et al: J Pediatr 1997;131:55.)

and HFOV and iNO were more effective than HFOV alone. This response to combined treatment with HFOV and iNO likely reflects both improvement in intrapulmonary shunting in patients with severe lung disease and PPHN (using a strategy designed to recruit and sustain lung volume, rather than to hyperventilate) and augmented NO delivery to its site of action. Although iNO may be an effective treatment for PPHN, it should be considered only as part of an overall clinical strategy that cautiously manages parenchymal lung disease, cardiac performance, and systemic hemodynamics.

Pharmacologic augmentation of the iNO response may also prove to be effective in some patients with PPHN. iNO causes pulmonary vasodilation by stimulating soluble guanylate cyclase and increasing cyclic guanosine monophosphate (cGMP) content in vascular smooth muscle. Smooth muscle cGMP content is further regulated by cGMP-specific phosphodiesterase-5, which inactivates cGMP by hydrolysis.[102] Whether the inability to sustain cGMP contributes to the failure of some patients with PPHN to respond or to sustain improved oxygenation during iNO therapy is uncertain. Early clinical experience with dipyridamole, which has PDE5 inhibitory activity, has been variable. Although dipyridamole may enhance the response to iNO in some patients,[103] its effects are variable and are not selective for the pulmonary circulation.[104] Further studies with more selective PDE5 antagonists (such as sildenafil) may lead to novel clinical strategies to enhance the treatment of pulmonary hypertension with iNO.

INHALED NITRIC OXIDE IN PREMATURE NEWBORNS

In the premature human neonate, severe respiratory failure is often the result of surfactant deficiency, and treatment with exogenous surfactant can cause dramatic improvements in oxygenation.[105] However, surfactant therapy results in suboptimal responses in up to 50% of human newborns with RDS.[106] Echocardiographic studies in human premature infants with RDS have shown that pulmonary hypertension may complicate the course of severe RDS.[107-111] Other studies have also shown that

the association of pulmonary hypertension with severe RDS leads to increased mortality despite surfactant therapy.[112] Walther and associates[112] performed echocardiographic studies on premature neonates with fatal RDS and found that severe pulmonary hypertension was an early and consistent finding in premature neonates who subsequently died. The frequency of severe pulmonary hypertension complicating RDS in premature neonates is unknown. However, the National Institute of Child Health and Human Development (NICHD) Neonatal Research Network reported that respiratory causes of early death in premature neonates remained a significant problem despite the availability of surfactant therapy.[113] Among 2867 infants with birth weights lower than 1500 g who were born between March 1993 and February 1994, a mortality rate of 19% (553) was reported. For 26% (146) of these premature neonates, the major cause of death was pulmonary (RDS, chronic lung disease).

These observations suggest that factors other than surfactant deficiency may contribute to the cardiopulmonary failure associated with prematurity. The occurrence of pulmonary hypertension in the preterm infant has many possible causes, including the production of pulmonary vasoconstrictor agents or diminished endogenous vasodilator formation causing increased PVR and extrapulmonary right-to-left shunting of blood across the ductus arteriosus and foramen ovale. Surfactant inactivation may also occur in severe RDS, caused by alveolar-capillary leak and pulmonary edema.[114, 115] Surfactant inactivation results in atelectasis, disturbances in ventilation/perfusion matching, and intrapulmonary shunting.

Treatment of pulmonary hypertension and ventilation/perfusion mismatching in newborn infants has been limited by the lack of a selective pulmonary vasodilator. Nonselective pulmonary vasodilators have been used in RDS complicated by pulmonary hypertension, but their use has been marked by lack of responsiveness and inability to sustain vasodilation. In addition, adverse systemic vascular effects may occur, and the risks of systemic hypotension are of particular concern in premature subjects, owing to markedly reduced cerebral blood flow in the first days after delivery.[116, 117] Moreover, vasodilators delivered to the lung by intravenous administration may worsen ventilation/perfusion matching by increasing blood flow to both well-ventilated and poorly ventilated areas of the lung.[118]

As described earlier, there is now convincing evidence that low-dose (<20 ppm) iNO delivered directly to the pulmonary circulation by inhalation causes potent, selective, and sustained pulmonary vasodilation in premature animals. Because of the inhalational route of delivery, low-dose iNO also improves matching of ventilation with perfusion within the lung by vasodilating vessels associated with well-ventilated lung units.

Preliminary studies in human premature neonates with severe hypoxemic respiratory failure support the potential role of low-dose iNO as adjuvant therapy. Low-dose iNO caused marked improvement in oxygenation in a premature neonate with group B streptococcal sepsis and severe pulmonary hypertension, and it allowed a reduction in ventilator pressure and inspired oxygen concentration, with complete clinical recovery.[119] Peliowski and associates[120] studied eight premature neonates with severe hypoxemia associated with prolonged oligohydramnios and suspected pulmonary hypoplasia who showed marked improvement in response to iNO therapy. Five patients survived in this trial, three with severe intracranial hemorrhage (ICH). Skimming and colleagues[121] also reported a dose-response study in premature infants and concluded that 5 ppm was as effective as 20 ppm in improving oxygenation. In a small, unmasked, randomized trial of iNO (20 ppm) and dexamethasone treatment, no differences were found in survival, chronic lung disease, or intracranial hemorrhage between iNO-treated infants and controls.[122] In another report, Van Meurs and associates[123] described a dose-response study of iNO in 11 premature newborns and

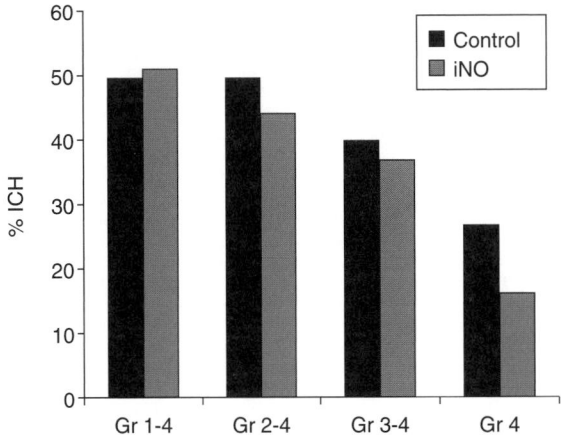

Figure 70–9. Low-dose inhaled nitric oxide (iNO) does not increase the incidence of intracranial hemorrhage (ICH) in premature newborns with severe hypoxemic respiratory failure. (From Kinsella JP, et al: Lancet 1999;354:1061.)

noted that 5 ppm was as effective as 20 ppm. Seven (64%) of these infants had ICH, and five (45%) had ICH of Grade 3 to 4. However, when the authors compared these results with the NICHD Neonatal Network database (for historical controls matched for severity of illness), the incidence of ICH in premature newborns not treated with iNO was identical (64%). One of the most concerning potential risks of iNO treatment for premature neonates is the prolongation in bleeding time described at NO doses of 30 to 300 ppm.[124] Endogenous NO inhibits platelet adhesion to the vascular endothelium, and this effect may be related to the formation of stable *S*-nitroso-proteins.[125, 126] However, in a small study of premature infants treated with iNO, no change in bleeding time occurred.[127] These observations illustrate the limitations of toxicity determinations without appropriately designed clinical trials. One randomized controlled trial of iNO in premature newborns with severe hypoxemic respiratory failure found no difference in the incidence or severity of ICH[128] (Fig. 70–9).

The effects of iNO on surfactant function was also reviewed by Hallman and Bry.[129] Although high doses of iNO may have adverse effects on surfactant function, doses relevant to clinical application do not appear to compromise surfactant activity. Indeed, the antioxidant activity of low-dose iNO may have a beneficial effect on endogenously produced surfactant.

REFERENCES

1. Palmer RMJ, et al: Nitric oxide release accounts for the biological activity of endothelium-derived relaxing factor. Nature 1987;327:524.
2. Ignarro LJ, et al: Endothelium-derived relaxing factor produced and released from artery and vein in nitric oxide. Proc Natl Acad Sci USA 1987;84:9265.
3. Dawes GS, et al: Changes in the lungs of the newborn lamb. J Physiol (Lond) 1953;121:141.
4. Cassin S, et al: The vascular resistance of the fetal and newly-ventilated lung of the lamb. J Physiol (Lond) 1964;171:61.
5. Cassin S, et al: Pulmonary blood flow and vascular resistance in immature fetal lambs. J Physiol (Lond) 1964;171:80.
6. Fineman JR, et al: The role of pulmonary vascular endothelium in perinatal pulmonary circulatory regulation. Semin Perinatol 1991;15:58.
7. Gruetter CA, et al: Relaxation of bovine coronary artery and activation of coronary arterial guanylate cyclase by nitric oxide, nitroprusside and a carcinogenic nitrosoamine. J Cyclic Nucleotide Res 1979;5:211.
8. Ignarro LJ, et al: Endothelium-derived relaxing factor produced and released from artery and vein in nitric oxide. Proc Natl Acad Sci USA 1987;84:9265.
9. Schmidt HHHW, et al: The nitric oxide and cGMP signal transduction system: regulation and mechanism of action. Biochim Biophys Acta 1993;1178:153.
10. Bredt DS, et al: Cloned and expressed nitric oxide synthase structurally resembles cytochrome P-450 reductase. Nature 1991;351:714.
11. Lyons CR, et al: Molecular cloning and functional expression of an inducible nitric oxide synthase from a murine macrophage cell line. J Biol Chem 1992;267:6370.
12. Xie Q, et al: Cloning and characterization of inducible nitric oxide synthase from mouse macrophages. Science 1992;256:225.
13. Lamas S, et al: Endothelial nitric oxide synthase: molecular cloning and characterization of a distinct constitutive enzyme isoform. Proc Natl Acad Sci USA 1992;89:6348.
14. Sessa WC, et al: Molecular cloning and expression of a cDNA encoding endothelial cell nitric oxide synthase. J Biol Chem 1992;267:15274.
15. Marsden PA, et al: Molecular cloning and characterization of human endothelial nitric oxide synthase. FEBS Lett 1992;307:287.
16. Nishida K, et al: Molecular cloning and characterization of the constitutive bovine aortic endothelial cell nitric oxide synthase. J Clin Invest 1992;90:2092.
17. Shaul PW: Regulation of endothelial nitric oxide synthase: location, location, location. Annu Rev Physiol 2002;64:749.
18. Lowenstein CJ, Snyder SH: Nitric oxide, a novel biologic messenger. Cell 1992;70:705.
19. Nunokawa Y, et al: Promoter analysis of human inducible nitric oxide synthase gene associated with cardiovascular homeostasis. Biochem Biophys Res Commun 1994;200:802.
20. Abman SH, et al: Role of endothelium-derived relaxing factor activity during transition of pulmonary circulation at birth. Am J Physiol 1990;259:H1921.
21. McQueston JA, et al: Effects of oxygen and exogenous L-arginine on EDRF activity in fetal pulmonary circulation. Am J Physiol 1993;264:865.
22. Tiktinsky MH, Morin FC: Increasing oxygen tension dilates fetal pulmonary circulation via endothelium-derived relaxing factor. Am J Physiol 1993;265:H376.
23. Cornfield DN, et al: Effects of birth related stimuli on L-arginine–dependent vasodilation. Am J Physiol 1992;262:H1474.
24. Sherman TS, et al: Nitric oxide synthase isoform expression in the developing lung epithelium. Am J Physiol 1999;276:L383.
25. Rairigh RL, et al: Role of inducible nitric oxide synthase in regulation of pulmonary vascular tone in the late-gestation ovine fetus. J Clin Invest 1998;101:15.
26. Rairigh RL, et al: Inducible NO synthase inhibition attenuates shear stress-induced pulmonary vasodilation in the ovine fetus. Am J Physiol 1999;276:513.
27. Rairigh RL, et al: Role of inducible nitric oxide synthase in the pulmonary vascular response to birth-related stimuli in the ovine fetus. Circ Res 2001;88:721.
28. Accurso FJ, et al: Time-dependent response of fetal pulmonary blood flow to an increase in fetal oxygen tension. Respir Physiol 1986;63:43.
29. Lewis AB, et al: Gestational changes in pulmonary vascular responses in fetal lambs in utero. Circ Res 1977;39:536.
30. Morin FC, et al: Development of pulmonary vascular response to oxygen. Am J Physiol 1988;254:H542.
31. Cornfield DN, et al: Effects of birth-related stimuli on L-arginine-dependent vasodilation in ovine fetus. Am J Physiol 1992;262:H1474.
32. McQueston JA, et al: Effects of oxygen and exogenous L-arginine on endothelium-derived relaxing factor activity in the fetal pulmonary circulation. Am J Physiol 1993;264:H865.
33. Tiktinsky MH, Morin FC: Increasing oxygen tension dilates fetal pulmonary circulation via endothelium-derived relaxing factor. Am J Physiol 1993;265:H376.
34. Abman SH, et al: Maturational changes in endothelium-derived relaxing factor activity of ovine pulmonary arteries in vitro. Am J Physiol 1991;260:L280.
35. Shaul PW, et al: Developmental changes in nitric oxide synthase isoform expression and nitric oxide production in fetal baboon lung. Am J Physiol 2002;283:1192.
36. North AJ, et al: Nitric oxide synthase Type I and Type III gene expression is developmentally regulated in rat lung. Am J Physiol 1994;266:L635.
37. Halbower AC, et al: Maturation-related changes in endothelial nitric oxide synthase immunolocalization in developing bovine lung. Am J Physiol 1994;266:L585.
38. Parker TA, et al: Developmental changes in endothelial nitric oxide synthase expression and activity in ovine fetal lung. Am J Physiol 2000;278:L202.
39. Davies P, et al: Postnatal growth of the sheep lung: a morphometric study. Anat Rec 1988;220:281.
40. Fike CD, Kaplowitz MR: Chronic hypoxia alters nitric oxide-dependent pulmonary vascular responses in lungs of newborn pigs. J Appl Physiol 1996;81:2078.
41. Tulloh RMR, et al: Chronic hypoxia inhibits the postnatal maturation of porcine intrapulmonary artery relaxation. Am J Physiol 1997;272:H2436.
42. Fike CD, et al: Chronic hypoxia decreases nitric oxide production and endothelial nitric oxide synthase in newborn pig lungs. Am J Physiol 1998;274:L517.
43. North AJ, et al: Oxygen upregulates nitric oxide synthase gene expression in ovine fetal pulmonary artery endothelial cells. Am J Physiol 1996;270:L643.
44. North AJ, et al: Pulmonary endothelial nitric oxide synthase gene expression is decreased in a rat model of congenital diaphragmatic hernia. Am J Respir Cell Mol Biol 1995;13:676.
45. Steinhorn RH, et al: Disruption of cGMP production in pulmonary arteries isolated from fetal lambs with pulmonary hypertension. Am J Physiol 1995;268:H1483.

46. Shaul PW, et al: Pulmonary endothelial nitric oxide synthase gene expression is decreased in fetal lambs with pulmonary hypertension. Am J Physiol 1997;272:L1005.

47. Villamor E, et al: Chronic intrauterine pulmonary hypertension impairs endothelial nitric oxide synthase in the ovine fetus. Am J Physiol 1997;272:L1013.

48. Borland C, et al: The fate of inhaled nitric oxide. Clin Sci 1983;65:37.

49. Higenbottam T, et al: Inhaled "endothelium derived relaxing factor" in primary hypertension. Am Rev Respir Dis 1988;137:A107.

50. Centers for Disease Control: Recommendations for occupational safety and health standards. MMWR Morb Mortal Wkly Rep 1988;37:S7.

51. Kinsella JP, et al: Hemodynamic effects of exogenous nitric oxide in ovine transitional pulmonary circulation. Am J Physiol 1992;262:H875.

52. Rosenberg AA, et al: Cerebral hemodynamics and distribution of systemic blood flow during inhalation of nitric oxide. Crit Care Med 1995;3:1391.

53. Frostell C, et al: Inhaled nitric oxide: a selective pulmonary vasodilator reversing hypoxic pulmonary vasoconstriction. Circulation 1991;83:2038.

54. Roberts JD, et al: Inhaled nitric oxide reverses pulmonary vasoconstriction in the hypoxic and acidotic newborn lamb. Circ Res 1993;72:246.

55. Berger JI, et al: Effect of inhaled nitric oxide during group B streptococcal sepsis in piglets. Am Rev Respir Dis 1993;147:1080.

56. Zayek M, et al: Effect of nitric oxide on the survival rate and incidence of lung injury in newborn lambs with persistent pulmonary hypertension. J Pediatr 1993;123:947.

57. Etches PC, et al: Nitric oxide reverses acute hypoxic pulmonary hypertension in the newborn piglet. Pediatr Res 1994;35:15.

58. Nelin LD, et al: The effect of inhaled nitric oxide on the pulmonary circulation of the neonatal pig. Pediatr Res 1994;35:20.

59. McQueston JA, et al: Chronic pulmonary hypertension in utero impairs endothelium-dependent vasodilation. Am J Physiol 1995;268:H288.

60. Zayek M, et al: Treatment of persistent pulmonary hypertension in the newborn lamb by inhaled nitric oxide. J Pediatr 1993;122:743.

61. Dawes GS, et al: Changes in the lungs of the newborn lamb. J Physiol 1953;121:141.

62. Chu J, et al: Neonatal pulmonary ischemia. I. Clinical and physiological studies. Pediatrics 1967;409(Suppl):709.

63. Avery ME, Mead J: Surface properties in relation to atelectasis and hyaline membrane disease. Am J Dis Child 1959;97:517.

64. Fujiwara T, et al: Artificial surfactant therapy in hyaline membrane disease. Lancet 1980;1:55.

65. Jobe A, et al: Duration and characteristics of treatment of premature lambs with natural surfactant. J Clin Invest 1981;67:370.

66. Walther FJ, et al: Single versus repetitive doses of natural surfactant as treatment of respiratory distress syndrome in premature lambs. Pediatr Res 1985;19:224.

67. Kinsella JP, et al: Ontogeny of NO activity and response to inhaled NO in the developing ovine pulmonary circulation. Am J Physiol 1994;267:H1955.

68. Jobe A, Ikegami M: The prematurely delivered lamb as a model for studies of neonatal adaptation. In: Nathanielsz PW (ed): Animal Models in Fetal Medicine. Ithaca, NY, Perinatology Press, 1984, pp 1–30.

69. Jobe A, et al: The duration and characteristics of treatment of premature lambs with natural surfactant. J Clin Invest 1981;67:370.

70. Cummings JJ, et al: A controlled clinical comparison of four different surfactant preparations in surfactant-deficient preterm lambs. Am Rev Respir Dis 1992;145:999.

71. Skimming JW, et al: The effects of nitric oxide inhalation on the pulmonary circulation of preterm lambs. Pediatr Res 1995;37:35.

72. Kinsella JP, et al: Inhaled nitric oxide lowers pulmonary: vascular resistance and improves gas exchange in severe experimental hyaline membrane disease. Pediatr Res 1994;36:402.

73. Kinsella JP, et al: Independent and combined effects of inhaled nitric oxide, liquid perflurochemical, and high frequency oscillatory ventilation in premature lambs with respiratory distress syndrome. Am J Respir Crit Care Med 1999;159:1220.

74. Kanwar S, Kubes P: Nitric oxide is an antiadhesive molecule for leukocytes. New Horizons 1995;3:93.

75. Kavanagh BP, et al: Effects of inhaled NO and inhibition of endogenous NO synthesis in oxidant-induced acute lung injury. J Appl Physiol 1994;76:1324.

76. Kurose I, et al: Inhibition of nitric oxide production: mechanisms of vascular albumin leakage. Circ Res 1993;73:164.

77. Jobe A, et al: Lung protein leaks in ventilated lambs: effect of gestational age. J Appl Physiol 1985;58:1246.

78. Varsila E, et al: Closure of patent ductus arteriosus decreases pulmonary myeloperoxidase in premature infants with respiratory distress syndrome. Biol Neonate 1995;67:167.

79. Kinsella JP, et al: Effects of inhaled nitric oxide on pulmonary edema and lung neutrophil accumulation in severe experimental hyaline membrane disease. Pediatr Res 1997;41:457.

80. Zimmerman JJ: Bronchoalveolar inflammatory pathophysiology of bronchopulmonary dysplasia. Clin Perinatol 1995;22:429.

81. Sugiura M, et al: Ventilator pattern influences neutrophil influx and activation in atelectasis-prone rabbit lung. J Appl Physiol 1994;77:1355.

82. Roberts JD, et al: Inhaled nitric oxide in persistent pulmonary hypertension of the newborn. Lancet 1992;340:818.

83. Kinsella JP, et al: Low-dose inhalational nitric oxide in persistent pulmonary hypertension of the newborn. Lancet 1992;340:819.

84. Kinsella JP, et al: Randomized, multicenter trial of inhaled nitric oxide and high frequency oscillatory ventilation in severe persistent pulmonary hypertension of the newborn. J Pediatr 1997;131:55.

85. Roberts JD, et al: Inhaled nitric oxide and persistent pulmonary hypertension of the newborn. N Engl J Med 1997;336:605.

86. Wessel DL, et al: Improved oxygenation in a randomized trial of inhaled nitric oxide for persistent pulmonary hypertension of the newborn. Pediatrics 1997;100:7.

87. Davidson D, et al: Inhaled nitric oxide for the early treatment of persistent pulmonary hypertension of the term newborn: a randomized, double-masked, placebo-controlled, dose-response, multicenter study. Pediatrics 1998;101:325.

88. Neonatal Inhaled Nitric Oxide Study Group: Inhaled nitric oxide in full-term and nearly full-term infants with hypoxic respiratory failure. N Engl J Med 1997;336:597.

89. Clark RH, et al: Low-dose nitric oxide therapy for persistent pulmonary hypertension of the newborn. N Engl J Med 2000;342:469.

90. Levin DL, et al: Persistent pulmonary hypertension of the newborn. J Pediatr 1976;89:626.

91. Gersony WM: Neonatal pulmonary hypertension: pathophysiology, classification and etiology. Clin Perinatol 1984;11:517.

92. Stevenson DK, et al: Refractory hypoxemia associated with neonatal pulmonary disease: the use and limitations of tolazoline. J Pediatr 1979;95:595.

93. Drummond WH, et al: The independent effects of hyperventilation, tolazoline, and dopamine on infants with persistent pulmonary hypertension. J Pediatr 1981;98:603.

94. Kinsella JP, et al: Clinical responses to prolonged treatment of persistent pulmonary hypertension of the newborn with low doses of inhaled nitric oxide. J Pediatr 1993;123:103.

95. Finer NN, et al: Inhaled nitric oxide in infants referred for extracorporeal membrane oxygenation: dose response. J Pediatr 1994;124:302.

96. Antunes MJ, et al: Assessment of lung function pre-nitric oxide therapy: a predictor of response? Pediatr Res 1994;35:212A.

97. Gerlach H, et al: Time-course and dose-response of nitric oxide inhalation for systemic oxygenation and pulmonary hypertension in patients with adult respiratory distress syndrome. Eur J Clin Invest 1993;23:499.

98. Kinsella JP, Abman SH: Recent developments in the pathophysiology and treatment of persistent pulmonary hypertension of the newborn. J Pediatr 1995;126:853.

99. Clark RH: High-frequency ventilation. J Pediatr 1994;124:661.

100. Kinsella JP, Abman SH: Efficacy of inhalational nitric oxide therapy in the clinical management of persistent pulmonary hypertension of the newborn. Chest 1994;105:S92.

101. Kinsella JP, Abman SH: Clinical approach to the use of high frequency oscillatory ventilation in neonatal respiratory failure. J Perinatol 1996;16:S52.

102. Braner DA, et al: M&B 22948, a cGMP phosphodiesterase inhibitor, is a pulmonary vasodilator in lambs. Am J Physiol 1993;264:H252.

103. Kinsella JP, et al: Dipyridamole augmentation of response to NO. Lancet 1995;346:647.

104. Ziegler JW, et al: Effects of dipyridamole and inhaled nitric oxide in pediatric patients with pulmonary hypertension. Am J Respir Crit Care Med 1998;158:1388.

105. Jobe AH: Pulmonary surfactant therapy. N Engl J Med 1993;328:861.

106. Jobe AH: Surfactant in the perinatal period. Early Hum Dev 1992;29:57.

107. Halliday HL, et al: Respiratory distress syndrome: echocardiographic assessment of cardiovascular function and pulmonary vascular resistance. Pediatrics 1977;60:444.

108. Chu J, et al: Neonatal pulmonary ischemia. I. Clinical and physiological studies. Pediatrics 1967;40:109.

109. Stahlman M, et al: Circulatory studies in clinical hyaline membrane disease. Biol Neonate 1972;20:300.

110. Evans NJ, Archer LNJ: Doppler assessment of pulmonary artery pressure and extrapulmonary shunting in the acute phase of hyaline membrane disease. Arch Dis Child 1991;66:6.

111. Skinner JR, et al: Pulmonary and systemic arterial pressure in hyaline membrane disease. Arch Dis Child 1992;67:366.

112. Walther FJ, et al: Persistent pulmonary hypertension in premature neonates with severe respiratory distress syndrome. Pediatrics 1992;90:899.

113. Shankaran S, et al: Characteristics of early (<12 HR) death among VLBW neonates. Ped Res 1995;37:236A.

114. Said SI, et al: Pulmonary surface activity in induced pulmonary edema. J Clin Invest 1965;44:458.

115. Ikegami M, et al: Surfactant function in respiratory distress syndrome. J Pediatr 1983;102:443.

116. Kinsella JP, et al: Circulatory changes following premature delivery in a baboon model of hyaline membrane disease. Am J Physiol 1991;261:H1148.

117. Altman DI, et al: Cerebral blood flow requirement for brain viability in newborn infants is lower than in adults. Ann Neurol 1988;24:218.

118. Gerlach H, et al: Time course and dose-response of NO inhalation for systemic oxygenation and pulmonary hypertension in patients with adult respiratory distress syndrome. Eur J Clin Invest 1993;23:499.

119. Abman SH, et al: Inhaled nitric oxide in the management of a premature newborn with severe respiratory distress and pulmonary hypertension. Pediatrics 1993;92:606.

120. Peliowski A, et al: Inhaled nitric oxide for premature infants after prolonged rupture of the membranes. J Pediatr 1995;126:450.

121. Skimming JW, et al: Nitric oxide inhalation in infants with respiratory failure. J Pediatr 1997;130:225.

122. Subhedar NV, et al: Open randomised controlled trial of inhaled nitric oxide and early dexamethasone in high risk preterm infants. Arch Dis Child 1997;77:F185.

123. Van Meurs KP, et al: Response of premature infants with severe respiratory to inhaled nitric oxide. Pediatr Pulmonol 1997;24:319.

124. Hogman M, et al: Bleeding time prolongation and NO inhalation. Lancet 1993;341:1664.

125. Radomski MW, et al: Endogenous nitric oxide inhibits platelet adhesion to vascular endothelium. Lancet 1987;2:1057.

126. Simon DI, et al: Antiplatelet properties of protein S-nitrosothiols derived from nitric oxide and endothelium-derived relaxing factor. Arterioc Thromb 1993;13:791.

127. Ahluwalia J, et al: Nitric oxide improves oxygenation in neonates with respiratory distress syndrome and pulmonary hypertension. Pediatr Res 1994;36:3A.

128. Kinsella JP, et al: Inhaled nitric oxide in premature neonates with severe hypoxaemic respiratory failure: a randomised controlled trial. Lancet 1999;354:1061.

129. Hallman M, Bry K: Nitric oxide and lung surfactant. Semin Perinatol 1996;20:173.

71

Ronald I. Clyman

Mechanisms Regulating Closure of the Ductus Arteriosus

The ductus arteriosus is an extension of the terminal portion of the sixth branchial arch. During fetal life, the ductus arteriosus serves to divert blood away from the fluid-filled lungs toward the descending aorta and placenta. After birth, constriction of the ductus arteriosus and obliteration of its lumen separates the pulmonary and systemic circulations. In full-term infants, obliteration of the ductus arteriosus takes place through a process of vasoconstriction and anatomic remodeling. In the preterm infant, the ductus arteriosus frequently fails to close. The clinical consequences of a patent ductus arteriosus (PDA) are related to the degree of left-to-right shunt through the PDA with its associated change in blood flow to the lungs, kidneys, and intestine.

INCIDENCE

Pulsed Doppler echocardiographic assessments of full-term infants indicate that functional closure of the ductus has occurred in almost 50% by 24 hours, in 90% by 48 hours, and in all by 72 hours. The rate of ductus closure is delayed in preterm infants; however, essentially all healthy preterm infants of 30 weeks' or longer gestation will have closed their ductus by the fourth day after birth. Respiratory distress syndrome (RDS) delays ductus closure; however, in most infants who are 30 weeks' (or longer) gestation, the actual impact of RDS on ductal shunting may be less than commonly assumed (only 11% remain open after 4 days). Conversely, preterm infants of less than 30 weeks' gestation with severe respiratory distress have a 65% incidence of persistent PDA.

The recent introduction of exogenous surfactant therapy has altered both the incidence and the presentation of PDA. Although surfactant has no effect on the contractile behavior of the ductus, its effects on pulmonary vascular resistance lead to an earlier clinical presentation of the left-to-right shunt in preterm animals[1,2] and humans.[3-6] Infants who receive excessive fluid administration during the first days of life also are more likely to develop a clinically symptomatic PDA.[7]

REGULATION OF DUCTUS ARTERIOSUS PATENCY

In the full-term infant, closure of the ductus arteriosus occurs in two phases: (1) "functional" closure of the lumen within the first hours after birth by smooth muscle constriction, and (2) "anatomic" occlusion of the lumen over the next several days due to extensive neointimal thickening and loss of smooth muscle cells from the inner muscle media.

Balance Between Vasoconstriction and Vasorelaxation

Patency of the fetal ductus arteriosus is regulated by both dilating and contracting factors. The ductus normally has a high level of intrinsic tone during fetal life.[8] The factors that promote ductus constriction in the fetus have yet to be identified. The intrinsic ductus tone results from components that are both dependent on and independent of extracellular calcium.[8] Permeabilized smooth muscle from the fetal ductus is significantly more sensitive to the contractile effects of calcium than is smooth muscle from the aorta and the pulmonary artery.[9] Endothelin-1 also appears to play a role in producing the basal tone of the ductus.[10]

The factors that oppose ductus arteriosus constriction *in utero* are better understood. The elevated vascular pressure within the ductus lumen (due to the constricted pulmonary vascular bed) plays an important role in opposing ductus constriction.[11] The fetal ductus also produces several vasodilators that oppose the ability of the intrinsic ductus tone to constrict the vessel. Vasodilator prostaglandins (PGs) appear to be the dominant vasodilators that oppose ductus constriction in the later part of gestation.[12] Inhibitors of PG synthesis constrict the fetal ductus both *in vitro* and *in vivo*. PGE_2 is the most potent PG produced by the ductus[13, 14] and appears to be the most important prostanoid to regulate ductus patency. The response of the ductus to PGE_2 is unique among blood vessels in that it is extraordinarily sensitive to this vasodilating substance. PGE_2 produces ductus relaxation by interacting with several of the PGE receptors (EP_2, EP_3, and EP_4).[15] In the ductus, all three EP receptors participate in vasodilation by activating adenylate cyclase.[15] The increased intracellular concentrations of cyclic adenosine monophosphate (cAMP) inhibit the sensitivity of the ductus' contractile proteins to calcium.[9] In addition, one of the EP receptors (EP_3) also relaxes the ductus smooth muscle by opening potassium adenosine triphosphatase (K^+-ATP) channels that hyperpolarize the muscle and inhibit ductus tone.[15]

Both isoforms of the enzyme responsible for synthesizing PGs (cyclooxygenase [COX]-1 and COX-2), are expressed in the fetal ductus.[16] Depending on the species, both nonselective (e.g., indomethacin) and selective COX inhibitors constrict the ductus. In the fetal mouse, COX-2 appears to be primarily responsible for the PGs that dilate the ductus[17]; whereas in the fetal sheep, both COX-1 and COX-2 play a role in ductus patency.[16]

In addition to the PGs that are made within the ductus, the fetal ductus is also under the influence of circulating concentrations of PGE_2. Circulating concentrations of PGE_2 appear to be of placental origin.[18] Circulating concentrations of PGE_2 (1–2 nM) in the late gestation fetal lamb are close to those that produce maximal relaxation of the ductus.[19] PGE_2 concentrations are particularly high in the fetus because of the reduced pulmonary clearance of circulating PGs due to the low fetal pulmonary blood flow.[20]

Nitric oxide (NO) is made by the fetal ductus arteriosus and appears to play an important role in maintaining ductus patency in rodent fetuses early in gestation.[12] Although NO is also made in the ductus of larger species, its importance in maintaining ductus patency under normal *in utero* conditions has not been conclusively demonstrated[21] (see later discussion for the role of NO in fetuses exposed to indomethacin tocolysis and in premature newborns).

Carbon monoxide relaxes the ductus arteriosus and both hemoxygenase-1 and -2 (the enzymes that compose carbon monoxide) are found within the endothelial and smooth muscle cells of the ductus. Under physiologic conditions, the amount of carbon monoxide made by the ductus does not seem to affect ductus tone; however, in circumstances where its synthesis is up-regulated, for instance, in endotoxinemia, it may exert a relaxing influence on the ductus.[22] There is little evidence to suggest that adenosine or β-adrenergic stimulation plays a significant role in ductus patency.[23]

Although pharmacologic inhibition of PG synthesis produces ductus constriction, *in utero*, genetic interruption of either PG synthesis (i.e., homozygous combined COX-1 and COX-2 null mice)[17] or PG signaling (i.e., homozygous EP4 receptor null mice)[24] does not produce ductus closure *in utero*. In contrast to what would be expected from the pharmacologic inhibition studies, both genetic interruptions produce newborn mice that fail to close their ductus after birth.[17,24] The mechanisms through which the absence of PG stimulation alters the normal balance of other vasoactive factors in the ductus have yet to be elucidated. Pharmacologic inhibition of PG synthesis in human is also associated with an increased incidence of PDA after birth.[25] However, this appears to be due to indomethacin's ability to produce ductus constriction *in utero*. Ductus constriction *in utero* produces ischemic hypoxia, increased NO production, and smooth muscle cell death within the ductus wall. These factors prevent the ductus from constricting after birth and make it resistant to the constrictive effects of postnatal indomethacin.[26,27]

After delivery, several events promote ductus constriction in the full-term newborn: (1) an increase in arterial partial pressure of oxygen (Pao_2), (2) a decrease in blood pressure within the ductus lumen (due to the postnatal decrease in pulmonary vascular resistance), (3) a decrease in circulating PGE_2 (due to the loss of placental PG production and the increase in PG removal by the lung), and (4) a decrease in the number of PGE_2 receptors in the ductus wall.[15] Although the newborn ductus continues to be sensitive to the vasodilating effects of NO, it loses its ability to respond to PGE_2.[28,29] All these factors promote ductus constriction after birth.

The postnatal increase in Pao_2 plays an important role in ductus constriction. Oxygen's mechanism of action is still unknown. Although neural and hormonal factors possibly contribute to ductus closure under physiologic conditions, they do not mediate oxygen-induced vessel closure. Oxygen appears to constrict the ductus arteriosus by a mechanism that involves smooth muscle membrane depolarization and by a mechanism that is independent of membrane potential.[30]

A cytochrome P450 hemoprotein, which is located in the plasma membrane of the vascular smooth muscle cells, appears to act as a receptor for the oxygen-induced events in the ductus.[31,32] Oxygen inhibits potassium channels.[33,34] This is associated with membrane depolarization, an increase in smooth muscle intracellular calcium,[35] and formation of the potent vasoconstrictor, endothelin-1.[36] However, the role of endothelin-1 in postnatal ductus closure has recently been questioned[10,34,37] and the pathways through which oxygen alters membrane potential are still unclear.[33,38]

In contrast with the full-term ductus, the premature ductus is less likely to constrict after birth. This is due to several mechanisms. The intrinsic tone of the extremely immature ductus (less than 70% of gestation) is decreased compared with that of the ductus at term.[8] This may be due in part to the presence of smooth muscle myosin isoforms with a weaker contractile capacity in the immature ductus.[39-41] In addition, the potassium channels that promote ductus relaxation change during gestation from K_{Ca} channels (which are not regulated by the postnatal increase in oxygen tension) to K_{DR} channels (which can be inhibited by oxygen).[42] Premature infants have elevated circulating concentrations of PGE_2, which may play a significant role in maintaining ductus patency during the first days after birth. This is due to the decreased ability of the premature lung to clear circulating PGE_2.[20] In addition, during episodes of bacteremia and necrotizing enterocolitis, circulating concentrations of PGE_2 reach the pharmacologic range and are often associated with reopening of the ductus arteriosus.[43] The most important mechanism that prevents the preterm ductus from constricting after birth is its increased sensitivity to the vasodilating effects of PGE_2 and NO.[44] The increased sensitivity is not due to an increased number of PGE_2 receptors but rather to enhanced coupling between the receptors and the downstream signaling pathways. As a result, inhibitors of PG production (e.g., indomethacin, ibuprofen, and mefanamic acid) are usually effective agents in promoting ductus closure in the premature infant. It follows that drugs interfering with NO synthesis or function also could become useful adjuncts, especially in situations in which indomethacin has proven to be ineffective.[45]

The endogenous factors that alter the ability of the preterm ductus to constrict with advancing gestation are unknown. Recently, prenatal administration of vitamin A has been shown to increase both the intracellular calcium response and the contractile response of the preterm ductus to oxygen.[46] During normal fetal development, there is an increase in circulating cortisol that occurs near the end of gestation. Elevated cortisol concentrations in the fetus have been found to decrease the sensitivity of the ductus to the vasodilating effects of PGE_2[47]; consistent with these findings, prenatal administration of glucocorticoids causes a significant reduction in the incidence of PDA in premature humans and animals Collaborative Group on Antenatal Steroid Therapy.[47-52] The postnatal administration of glucocorticoids also has been shown to reduce the incidence of PDA.[53] However, postnatal glucocorticoid treatment also seems to increase the incidence of several of the other neonatal morbidities.[53]

Anatomic Closure: Histologic Changes

In normal, full-term animals, loss of responsiveness to PGE_2 shortly after birth prevents the ductus arteriosus from reopening after it has constricted.[28,29] This is due, in part, to the decreased synthesis of PGE_2 receptors in the ductus. The loss of responsiveness is accompanied by rapid histologic changes that ultimately lead to obliteration of the vessel's lumen and loss of smooth muscle cells from the inner muscle media.

In the full-term newborn, there is progressive intimal thickening and fragmentation of the internal elastic lamina after delivery. As the intima increases in size, it ultimately forms mounds that occlude the already constricted lumen. The increase in intimal thickening is due (1) to migration of smooth muscle cells from the muscle media into the intima and (2) to proliferation of luminal endothelial cells. The process of intimal cushion formation starts with the accumulation of hyaluron (HA) below the luminal endothelial cells. This is accompanied by the loss of laminin and collagen IV from the basement membrane of the endothelial cells and their subsequent separation from the internal elastic lamina. Laminin and collagen IV ultimately reform under the detached endothelial cells but HA continues to accumulate in the subendothelial space. The hygroscopic properties of HA cause an influx of water and widening of the subendothelial space; this creates an environment well suited for cell migration. Accompanying the increase in HA is an increase in fibronectin (FN) and chondroitin sulfate (CS) in the neointimal space.[54] The endothelial and smooth muscle cells of the ductus arteriosus differ from those of the adjacent vessels in their ability to form neointimal cushions. Isolated endothelial cells of the ductus arteriosus have an increased rate of HA accumulation compared with those of the aorta or pulmonary artery; this increase appears to be due to transforming growth factor β (TGFβ).[55] Following delivery, there is a marked increase in ductus arteriosus TGFβ expression, which accentuates the accumulation of HA within the neointima.

HA makes ductus smooth muscle cells migrate faster than aortic smooth muscle cells. The potentiating effect of HA on ductus smooth muscle cells is mediated through a hyaluron binding protein (RHAMM). Ductus smooth muscle cells synthesize more RHAMM than aortic smooth muscle cells and concentrate it at the leading edges of the cells. Antibodies against RHAMM will reduce the migration of ductus smooth muscle cells to the level found in aortic smooth muscle cells.[56]

Ductus smooth muscle cells also secrete more FN and CS than those of the aorta or pulmonary artery.[57] This does not appear to be due to TGFβ. Fibronectin plays an important role in facilitating ductus smooth muscle cell migration. When fibronectin production in the ductus is inhibited, intimal cushion formation is blocked.[58] Conversely, fibronectin has no effect on the migration of aortic smooth muscle cells. The increased production of CS, however, appears to have no direct effect on either ductus or aortic smooth muscle cell migration.[59]

Ductus arteriosus smooth muscle cells use a family of cell surface receptors, called *integrins*, to interact with, adhere to, and migrate through the extracellular matrix that surrounds them. When smooth muscle cells of the ductus are in a quiescent, contractile state, they express the same integrins on their cell surface as smooth muscle cells of the aorta. However, when ductus smooth muscle cells of the inner muscle media begin to migrate into the subendothelial space, two new integrin complexes appear on their cell surface: the αvβ3 and the α5β1 receptors. The αvβ3 integrin is a promiscuous receptor that interacts with most extracellular matrix glycoproteins and is essential for migration of ductus smooth muscle cells *in vitro*. The α5β1 integrin binds exclusively to fibronectin and mediates the potentiating effects of fibronectin on ductus smooth muscle cell migration. During the process of migration, ductus smooth muscle cells secrete laminin, which also has an important promigratory role. Laminin facilitates smooth muscle cell migration by destabilizing the interactions of the cell's integrin receptors with other matrix glycoproteins. Because strong adhesion between a cell and its surrounding matrix renders a cell ill suited for migration, this antiadhesive property of laminin allows the cell to make and break contacts with the surrounding matrix, thus promoting locomotion. Antibodies against laminin will inhibit ductus smooth muscle cell migration.

Intimal cushion formation in the ductus is also associated with striking alterations in elastin fiber assembly. In contrast to the aorta, where formation of well developed elastic laminae are seen between layers of muscle cells, smooth muscle cells of the ductus muscle media are surrounded by thin and fragmented elastin fibers. Smooth muscle cells in the neointima are surrounded by even fewer elastin fibers.[60] Disruption of normal elastin fiber assembly in the ductus does not appear to be due to increased elastase activity or decreased tropoelastin production. Rather, it appears to be due to a developmental mechanism that reduces insolubilization of elastin and prevents formation of intact elastic laminae. Vascular smooth muscle cells synthesize a 67-kD elastin-binding protein (EBP) that is central to the assembly of soluble tropoelastin molecules into a mature matrix of insoluble elastic fibers. The 67-kD EBP appears to be an alternatively spliced, catalytically inactive variant of β-galactosidase.[61] It has three separate binding sites: one for the VGVAPG hydrophobic region of tropoelastin, one for the cell membrane, and one for galactosugars.[62] The 67-kD EBP binds the hydrophobic tropoelastin molecule intracellularly and escorts it through the smooth muscle cell's secretory pathways, protecting it from premature aggregation and premature proteolytic degradation. Tropoelastin is secreted, with the 67-kD EBP, as a complex. The 67-kD EBP attaches the tropoelastin molecule to the cell's surface. When galactosugars come in contact with the lectin-binding site of the 67-kD EBP, the affinity for both tropoelastin and the cell binding site is lowered. As a result, bound tropoelastin is released and the 67-kD EBP dissociates from the cell membrane. Coordinated presentation of galactosugars, contained within the growing elastin microfibrillar scaffold, may regulate the orientation and proper alignment of tropoelastin for cross-linking during normal elastin fiber assembly. Conversely, excess galactosugars, from other matrix elements, may compete with this process and lead to abnormal assembly.[63]

Ductus smooth muscle cells have less 67-kD EBP on their cell surface when compared with aortic smooth muscle cells.[64] As a result, ductus smooth muscle cells deposit little insoluble elastin compared with the action of aortic smooth muscle cells. They also secrete large amounts of a truncated form of tropoelastin, which appears to be due to proteolytic intracellular degradation caused by the 67-kD EBP deficiency. This truncated tropoelastin lacks the C-terminus of the molecule and is impaired in its ability to align on microfibrils and cross-link.[65, 66] As already noted, ductus smooth muscle cells secrete increased amounts of chondroitin sulfate compared with aortic smooth muscle cells. Chondroitin sulfate, through its galactosugar side chains, removes the 67-kD EBP from smooth muscle cell surfaces, which further interferes with elastin fiber assembly.[64]

The exact relationship between impaired elastin assembly and smooth muscle migration into the neointima is still open for speculation. Impaired assembly of thick elastic laminae might facilitate smooth muscle cell migration by removing a physical barrier to which they might attach. Ductus smooth muscle cells are able to migrate through elastin membranes that restrain aortic smooth muscle cell migration. Treatment of aortic smooth muscle cells with chondroitin sulfate causes the release of the 67-kD EBP from the aortic cell's surface and enables them to migrate through elastin membranes at the same rate as ductus smooth muscle cells.[67] Finally, accumulation of a relatively stable, soluble, truncated tropoelastin may act as a chemoattractant for smooth muscle cells.[68] Thus, there appear to be mechanisms that link elastin fragmentation with formation of ductus intimal cushions. Conversely, in some genetic forms of PDA, the elastic laminae of the ductus appear abnormally well developed and similar to those in the aorta; when this occurs, intimal cushions fail to develop.[60]

Relationship Between Vasoconstriction and Anatomic Closure

The process that initiates the permanent closure of the ductus has just recently been elucidated. Both the loss of vasodilator regulation and the anatomic events that lead to permanent closure appear to be controlled by the degree of ductus smooth muscle constriction. Experimental models that alter the ability of the ductus to constrict at term also prevent the normal histologic changes that occur after birth.[11, 17, 24, 58, 69, 70] Constriction produces ischemic hypoxia of the vessel wall.[71] In the full-term newborn's ductus, the ischemic hypoxia that accompanies constriction occurs even before luminal flow has been eliminated and depends on the presence of intramural vasa vasorum.[72] With advancing gestation, the thickness of the ductus wall increases in size to a dimension that requires the presence of intramural vasa vasorum to provide nutrients to its outer half. These collapsible, intramural vasa vasorum provide the ductus with a unique mechanism for controlling the maximal diffusion distance for oxygen and nutrients across its wall. In the full-term newborn, ductus constriction obliterates vasa vasorum flow to the outer muscle media, which turns the entire thickness of the muscle media into a virtual avascular zone. The profound ischemic hypoxia that follows the compression of the vasa vasorum inhibits local production of PGE_2 and NO, induces local production of growth factors (e.g., TGF_β and vascular endothelial growth factor [VEGF]), and produces smooth muscle apoptosis in the ductus wall. VEGF plays a critical role in the migration of the ductus smooth muscle cells into the neointima and in the proliferation of intramural vasa vasorum.[73]

In preterm infants, the ductus frequently remains open for many days after birth. Even when it does constrict, the premature ductus frequently fails to develop profound hypoxia and anatomic remodeling. The preterm infant seems to require a greater degree of ductal constriction than the full-term infant, in order to develop a comparable degree of hypoxia. In contrast with the full-term ductus, the thinner-walled preterm ductus does not depend on intramural vasa vasorum to provide oxygen and nutrients to its wall. The absence of intramural vasa vasorum leaves the preterm ductus without a mechanism to increase the diffusion distance across its wall during postnatal constriction. If any degree of luminal patency remains, the thin-walled preterm ductus fails to become profoundly hypoxic and fails to undergo anatomic remodeling after birth. As a result, the preterm ductus requires that there be complete cessation of luminal flow before it can develop the same degree of hypoxia as found in term infants. If this degree of hypoxic ischemia can be induced in the preterm ductus, then most of the anatomic changes seen at term will occur.[8, 45] If the premature ductus does not develop the degree of ischemic hypoxia necessary to induce anatomic remodeling and smooth muscle death, it remains essentially fetal in appearance and is still susceptible to vessel reopening.

In contrast with the full-term newborn ductus, the preterm newborn ductus continues to respond to PGE_2 after birth. In addition to its persistent responsiveness to PGE_2, the premature ductus produces an increased amount of NO after birth. This is due to the ingrowth of new intramural vasa vasorum that expressly synthesize NO.[73] As a result, there is a change in the relative balance of the vasodilators that maintain ductus patency after birth. Ductus patency becomes less dependent on PG generation and more dependent on other vasodilators during the first weeks after birth. This could explain why the effectiveness of indomethacin wanes with increasing postnatal age.[74, 75] In premature baboons, the combined use of a NO synthase-inhibitor and indomethacin produces a much greater degree of ductus constriction than indomethacin alone.[45] It follows that drugs that interfere with NO synthesis could become a useful adjunct, especially in situations in which indomethacin has been found to be ineffective.

HEMODYNAMIC AND PULMONARY ALTERATIONS

The pathophysiologic features of PDA depend both on the magnitude of the left-to-right shunt and on the cardiac and pulmonary responses to the shunt. There are important differences between immature and mature infants in the heart's ability to handle a volume load. Immature infants have less cardiac sympathetic innervation. Before term, the myocardium has more water and less contractile mass. Therefore, in the immature fetus the ventricles are less distensible than at term and also generate less force per gram of myocardium (even though they have the same ability to generate force per sarcomere).[76] The relative lack of left ventricular distensibility in immature infants is more a function of the ventricle's tissue constituents than of poor muscle function. As a result, left ventricular distention secondary to a large left-to-right PDA shunt may produce a higher left ventricular end-diastolic pressure at smaller ventricular volumes. The increase in left ventricular pressure increases pulmonary venous pressure and causes pulmonary congestion.

Studies in preterm lamb and human newborns[77,78] have shown that despite these limitations, preterm newborns are able to increase left ventricular output, and maintain their "effective" systemic blood flow, even with left-to-right PDA shunts equal to 50% of left ventricular output. With shunts greater than 50% of left ventricular output, "effective" systemic blood flow falls, despite a continued increase in left ventricular output. The increase in left ventricular output associated with a PDA is accomplished not by an increase in heart rate, but by an increase in stroke volume.[77,78] Stroke volume increases primarily as a result of the simultaneous decrease in afterload resistance on the heart and the increase in left ventricular preload. Despite the ability of the left ventricle to increase its output in the face of a left-to-right ductus shunt, blood flow distribution is significantly rearranged. This redistribution of systemic blood flow occurs even with small shunts.[77] Blood flow to the skin, bone, and skeletal muscle is most likely to be affected by the left-to-right ductus shunt. The next most likely organs to be affected are the gastrointestinal tract and kidneys. These organs receive decreased blood flow due to a combination of decreased perfusion pressure (due to a drop in diastolic pressure) and localized vasoconstriction. These organs may experience significant hypoperfusion before there are any signs of left ventricular compromise.[78,79] This decrease in organ perfusion contributes to some of the morbidities caused by a patent ductus arteriosus: necrotizing enterocolitis and decreased glomerular filtration rate.[74,80]

The decreased ability of the preterm infant to maintain active pulmonary vasoconstriction[81] may be responsible in part for the earlier presentation of a "large" left-to-right PDA shunt.[82,83] In addition, therapeutic maneuvers (e.g., surfactant replacement) that lead to a more rapid drop in pulmonary vascular resistance can exacerbate the amount of left-to-right shunt in preterm infants with RDS and lead to pulmonary hemorrhage.[6, 84] Although the mechanisms responsible for pulmonary hemorrhage after surfactant remain uncertain, a retrospective cohort study found that a clinically detectable PDA was associated with the onset of the hemorrhage.[85] Early ductus closure has been shown to decrease the incidence of significant pulmonary hemorrhage.[74,86]

The factors responsible for preventing plasma fluid and protein from moving into the lung interstitium and from the interstitium into the air spaces have been described elsewhere. With a wide-open PDA, the pulmonary vasculature is exposed to systemic blood pressure and increased pulmonary blood flow. Because the premature infant, with respiratory distress syndrome, frequently has low plasma oncotic pressure and increased capillary permeability, increases in microvascular perfusion pressure, that result from a PDA, may increase interstitial and alveolar lung fluid. Leakage of plasma proteins into the alveolar space inhibits surfactant function and increases surface tension in the immature air sacs,[87] which are already compromised by surfactant deficiency. The increased fraction of inspired oxygen and mean airway pressures required to overcome these early changes in compliance may be important factors in the association of PDA with chronic lung disease.[74, 88, 89] However, these changes in pulmonary mechanics appear to occur only after several days of exposure to a PDA. Although it is true that preterm animals with a PDA have increased fluid and protein clearance into the lung interstitium, due to an increase in pulmonary microvascular filtration pressure, a simultaneous increase in lung lymph flow appears to eliminate the excess fluid and protein from the lung. This compensatory increase in lung lymph acts as a so-called edema safety factor, inhibiting fluid accumulation in the lungs. As a result, there is no net increase in water or protein accumulation in the lung and there is no change in pulmonary mechanics.[1, 74, 90-92] This delicate balance between the PDA-induced fluid filtration and lymphatic reabsorption is consistent with the observation, made in human infants, that closure of the ductus arteriosus, within the first 24 hours after birth, has no effect on the course of the newborn's hyaline membrane disease. However, if lung lymphatic drainage is impaired, as it is in the presence of pulmonary interstitial emphysema or fibrosis, the likelihood of edema increases dramatically. After several days of lung disease and mechanical ventilation, the residual functioning lymphatics are more easily overwhelmed by the same size ductus shunt that could be accommodated on the first day after delivery. As a result, it is not uncommon for infants with a persistent PDA to develop pulmonary edema and alterations in pulmonary mechanics at 7 to 10 days after birth. In these infants, improvement in lung compliance occurs following closure of the PDA.[74, 93-97]

Not all the changes associated with a PDA are necessarily detrimental to the immature infant with respiratory distress syndrome. Persistence of the left-to-right shunt maintains an elevated Pao_2 in the presence of atelectasis. Decreases in systemic arterial O_2 content have been observed following PDA closure, despite the absence of any alterations in pulmonary mechanics. This phenomenon is due to recirculation of oxygenated arterial blood through lungs that are not fully expanded.[77, 98]

REFERENCES

1. Shimada S, et al: Treatment of patent ductus arteriosus after exogenous surfactant in baboons with hyaline membrane disease. Pediatr Res 26:565, 1989.
2. Clyman RI, et al: Increased shunt through the patent ductus arteriosus after surfactant replacement therapy. J Pediatr 100:101, 1982.
3. Kaapa P, et al: Pulmonary hemodynamics after synthetic surfactant replacement in neonatal respiratory distress syndrome. J Pediatr 123:115, 1993.
4. Reller MD, et al: Ductal patency in neonates with respiratory distress syndrome. A randomized surfactant trial. Am J Dis Child 145:1017, 1991.
5. Reller MD, et al: Review of studies evaluating ductal patency in the premature infant. J Pediatr 122:S59, 1993.
6. Alpan G, Clyman RI: Cardiovascular effects of surfactant replacement with special reference to the patent ductus arteriosus. In Robertson B, Taeusch HW (eds): Surfactant Therapy for Lung Disease: Lung Biology in Health and Disease. Vol 84. New York, Marcel Dekker, 1995, 531-545.
7. Bell EF, Acarregui MJ: Restricted versus liberal water intake for preventing morbidity and mortality in preterm infants (Cochrane Review). Cochrane Database Syst Rev. 2001;3.
8. Kajino H, et al: Factors that increase the contractile tone of the ductus arteriosus also regulate its anatomic remodeling. Am J Physiol 281:R291, 2001.
9. Crichton CA, et al: α-Toxin-permeabilised rabbit fetal ductus arteriosus is more sensitive to Ca^{2+} than aorta or main pulmonary artery. Cardiovasc Res 33:223, 1997.
10. Coceani F, et al: Endothelin A receptor is necessary for O(2) constriction but not closure of ductus arteriosus. Am J Physiol 1999;277(4 Pt 2):H1521-31.
11. Clyman RI, et al: Influence of increased pulmonary vascular pressures on the closure of the ductus arteriosus in newborn lambs. Pediatr Res 25:136, 1989.
12. Momma K, Toyono M: The role of nitric oxide in dilating the fetal ductus arteriosus in rats. Pediatr Res 46:311, 1999.
13. Clyman RI, et al: PGE_2 is a more potent vasodilator of the lamb ductus arteriosus than either PGI_2 or 6 keto PGF_{1a}. Prostaglandins 16:259, 1978.
14. Coceani F, et al: Prostaglandin I_2 is less relaxant than prostaglandin E_2 on the lamb ductus arteriosus. Prostaglandins 15:551, 1978.
15. Bouayad A, et al: Characterization of PGE(2) receptors in fetal and newborn lamb ductus arteriosus. Am J Physiol Heart Circ Physiol 280:H2342, 2001.

16. Takahashi Y, et al: Cyclooxygenase-2 inhibitors constrict the fetal lamb ductus arteriosus both in vitro and in vivo. Am J Physiol Regul Integr Comp Physiol 278:R1496, 2000.
17. Loftin CD, et al: Failure of ductus arteriosus closure and remodeling in neonatal mice deficient in cyclooxygenase-1 and cyclooxygenase-2. Proc Natl Acad Sci USA 98:1059, 2001.
18. Thorburn G (ed): The placenta, PGE2 and parturition. Amsterdam, Elsevier, 1992.
19. Clyman RI, et al: Circulating prostaglandin E_2 concentrations and patent ductus arteriosus in fetal and neonatal lambs. J Pediatr 97:455, 1980.
20. Clyman RI, et al: Effect of gestational age on pulmonary metabolism of prostaglandin E1 & E2. Prostaglandins 21:505, 1981.
21. Fox JJ, et al: Role of nitric oxide and cGMP system in regulation of ductus arteriosus tone in ovine fetus. Am J Physiol 271:H2638, 1996.
22. Coceani F, et al: Carbon monoxide formation in the ductus arteriosus in the lamb: implications for the regulation of muscle tone. Br J Pharmacol 120:599, 1997.
23. Friedman WF, et al: The vasoactivity of the fetal lamb ductus arteriosus studied in utero. Pediatr Res 17:331, 1983.
24. Nguyen M, et al: The prostaglandin receptor EP4 triggers remodelling of the cardiovascular system at birth. Nature 390:78, 1997.
25. Norton ME, et al: Neonatal complications after the administration of indomethacin for preterm labor. N Engl J Med 329:1602, 1993.
26. Goldbarg SH, et al: In utero indomethacin alters O_2 delivery to the fetal ductus arteriosus: implications for postnatal patency. Am J Physiol Regul Integr Comp Physiol 282:R184, 2002.
27. Clyman RI, et al: In utero remodeling of the fetal lamb ductus arteriosus: the role of antenatal indomethacin and avascular zone thickness on vasa vasorum proliferation, neointima formation, and cell death. Circulation 103:1806, 2001.
28. Abrams SE, et al: Responses of the post-term arterial duct to oxygen, prostaglandin E2, and the nitric oxide donor, 3-morpholinosydnoneimine, in lambs and their clinical implications. Br Heart J 73:177, 1995.
29. Clyman RI, et al: Factors determining the loss of ductus arteriosus responsiveness to prostaglandin E_2. Circulation 68:433, 1983.
30. Roulet MJ, Coburn RF: Oxygen-induced contraction in the guinea pig neonatal ductus arteriosus. Circ Res 49:997, 1981.
31. Coceani F, et al: Ductus arteriosus: involvement of a sarcolemmal cytochrome P-450 in O_2 constriction? Can J Physiol Pharmacol 67:1448, 1989.
32. Coceani F, et al: Cytochrome P450 during ontogenic development: occurrence in the ductus arteriosus and other tissues. Can J Physiol Pharmacol 72:217, 1994.
33. Reeve HL, et al: Redox control of oxygen sensing in the rabbit ductus arteriosus. J Physiol 533:253, 2001.
34. Michelakis E, et al: Voltage-gated potassium channels in human ductus arteriosus. Lancet 356:134, 2000.
35. Nakanishi T, et al: Mechanisms of oxygen-induced contraction of ductus arteriosus isolated from the fetal rabbit. Circ Res 72:1218, 1993.
36. Coceani F, et al: Endothelin is a potent constrictor of the lamb ductus arteriosus. Can J Physiol Pharmacol 67:902, 1989.
37. Fineman JR, et al: Endothelin-receptor blockade does not alter closure of the ductus arteriosus. Am J Physiol 275:H1620, 1998.
38. Clyman RI, et al: Oxygen metabolites stimulate prostaglandin E_2 production and relaxation of the ductus arteriosus. Clin Res Vol 36:228A, 1988.
39. Brown S, et al: Differential maturation in ductus arteriosus and umbilical artery smooth muscle during ovine development. Pediatric Research 51:34A, 2002.
40. Sakurai H, et al: Expression of four myosin heavy chain genes in developing blood vessels and other smooth muscle organs in rabbits. Eur J Cell Biol 69:166, 1996.
41. Colbert MC, et al: Endogenous retinoic acid signaling colocalizes with advanced expression of the adult smooth muscle myosin heavy chain isoform during development of the ductus arteriosus. Circ Res 78:790, 1996.
42. Reeve H, et al: Developmental changes in K+ channel expression may determine the O2 response of the ductus arteriosus. FASEB J 11:420A, 1997.
43. Gonzalez A, et al: Influence of infection on patent ductus arteriosus and chronic lung disease in premature infants weighing 1000 grams or less. J Pediatr 128:470, 1996.
44. Clyman RI, et al: Regulation of ductus arteriosus patency by nitric oxide in fetal lambs. The role of gestation, oxygen tension and vasa vasorum. Pediatr Res 43:633, 1998.
45. Seidner SR, et al: Combined prostaglandin and nitric oxide inhibition produces anatomic remodeling and closure of the ductus arteriosus in the premature newborn baboon. Pediatr Res 50:365, 2001.
46. Wu GR, et al: The effect of vitamin A on contraction of the ductus arteriosus in fetal rat. Pediatr Res 49:747, 2001.
47. Clyman RI, et al: Effects of antenatal glucocorticoid administration on the ductus arteriosus of preterm lambs. Am J Physiol 241:H415, 1981.
48. Collaborative Group on Antenatal Steroid Therapy: Prevention of respiratory distress syndrome: effect of antenatal dexamethasone administration. (Publication No 85-2695) Bethesda, National Institutes of Health, 1985, p 44.
49. Clyman RI, et al: Prenatal administration of betamethasone for prevention of patent ductus arteriosus. J Pediatr 98:123, 1981.
50. Momma K, et al: Constriction of the fetal ductus arteriosus by glucocorticoid hormones. Pediatr Res 15:19, 1981.
51. Thibeault DW, et al: Pulmonary and circulatory function in preterm lambs treated with hydrocortisone in utero. Biol Neonate 34:238, 1978.

52. Waffarn F, et al: Effect of antenatal glucocorticoids on clinical closure of the ductus arteriosus. Am J Dis Child *137*:336, 1983.

53. Early postnatal dexamethasone therapy for the prevention of chronic lung disease. Pediatrics *108*:741, 2001.

54. de Reeder EG, et al: Hyaluronic acid accumulation and endothelial cell detachment in intimal thickening of the vessel wall. The normal and genetically defective ductus arteriosus. Am J Pathol *132*:574, 1988.

55. Boudreau N, et al: Transforming growth factor-beta regulates increased ductus arteriosus endothelial glycosaminoglycan synthesis and a post-transcriptional mechanism controls increased smooth muscle fibronectin, features associated with intimal proliferation. Lab Invest *67*:350, 1992.

56. Boudreau N, et al: Fibronectin, hyaluron and a hyaluron binding protein contribute to increased ductus arteriosus smooth muscle cell migration. Dev Biol *143*:235, 1991.

57. Boudreau N, Rabinovitch M: Developmentally regulated changes in extracellular matrix in endothelial and smooth muscle cells in the ductus arteriosus may be related to intimal proliferation. Lab Invest *64*:187, 1991.

58. Mason CA, et al: Gene transfer in utero biologically engineers a patent ductus arteriosus in lambs by arresting fibronectin-dependent neointimal formation. Nat Med *5*:176, 1999.

59. Boudreau N, Rabinovitch M: Fibronectin, hyaluronic acid and a hyaluronic acid binding protein contribute to increased smooth muscle cell migration in the ductus arteriosus. J Cell Biochem *14A*(Suppl):150, 1990.

60. de Reeder EG, et al: Changes in distribution of elastin and elastin receptor during intimal cushion formation in the ductus arteriosus. Anat Embryol *182*:473, 1990.

61. Hinek A, et al: The 67-kD elastin/laminin-binding protein is related to an enzymatically inactive, alternatively spliced form of beta-galactosidase. J Clin Invest *91*:1198, 1993.

62. Mecham RP, Heuser J: The elastic fiber. *In* Hay E (ed): Cell Biology of Extracellular Matrix. 2nd ed. New York, Plenum Publishing, 1991, 79–109.

63. Hinek A, Rabinovitch M: 67-kD elastin-binding protein is a protective "companion" of extracellular insoluble elastin and intracellular tropoelastin. J Cell Biol *126*:563, 1994.

64. Hinek A, et al: Impaired elastin fiber assembly related to reduced 67-kD elastin-binding protein in fetal lamb ductus arteriosus and in cultured aortic smooth muscle cells treated with chondroitin sulfate. J Clin Invest *88*:2083, 1991.

65. Hinek A, Rabinovitch M: The ductus arteriosus migratory smooth muscle cell phenotype processes tropoelastin to a 52-kDa product associated with impaired assembly of elastic laminae. J Biol Chem *268*:1405, 1993.

66. Zhu L, et al: A developmentally regulated program restricting insolubilization of elastin and formation of laminae in the fetal lamb ductus arteriosus. Lab Invest *68*:321, 1993.

67. Hinek A, et al: Vascular smooth muscle cell detachment from elastin and migration through elastic laminae is promoted by chondroitin sulfate-induced "shedding" of the 67-kDa cell surface elastin binding protein. Exp Cell Res *203*:344, 1992.

68. Mecham RP, et al: Appearance of chemotactic responsiveness to elastin peptides by developing fetal bovine ligament fibroblasts parallels the onset of elastin production. J Cell Biol *98*:1813, 1984.

69. Jarkovska D, et al: Effect of prostaglandin E2 on the ductus arteriosus in the newborn rat. An ultrastructural study. Physiol Res *41*:323, 1992.

70. Fay FS, Cooke PH: Guinea pig ductus arteriosus. II. Irreversible closure after birth. Am J Physiol *222*:841, 1972.

71. Clyman RI, et al: Permanent anatomic closure of the ductus arteriosus in newborn baboons: the roles of postnatal constriction, hypoxia, and gestation. Pediatr Res *45*:19, 1999.

72. Kajino H, et al: Vasa vasorum hypoperfusion is responsible for medial hypoxia and anatomic remodeling in the newborn lamb ductus arteriosus. Pediatr Res *51*:228, 2002.

73. Clyman RI, et al: VEGF regulates remodeling during permanent anatomic closure of the ductus arteriosus. Am J Physiol Regul Integr Comp Physiol. *282*:R199, 2002.

74. Clyman RI: Commentary: Recommendations for the postnatal use of indomethacin. An analysis of four separate treatment strategies. J Pediatr *128*:601, 1996.

75. Schmidt B, et al: Long-term effects of indomethacin prophylaxis in extremely-low-birth-weight infants. N Engl J Med *344*:1966, 2001.

76. Friedman WF: The intrinsic physiologic properties of the developing heart. *In* Friedman WF et al (eds): Neonatal Heart Disease. New York, Grune and Stratton, 1972, 21–49.

77. Clyman RI, et al: Cardiovascular effects of a patent ductus arteriosus in preterm lambs with respiratory distress. J Pediatr *111*:579, 1987.

78. Shimada S, et al: Effects of patent ductus arteriosus on left ventricular output and organ blood flows in preterm infants with respiratory distress syndrome treated with surfactant. J Pediatr *125*:270, 1994.

79. Meyers R, et al: Effect of patent ductus arteriosus and indomethacin on intestinal blood flow in the newborn lamb. Pediatr Res *27*:216A, 1990.

80. Cassady G, et al: A randomized, controlled trial of very early prophylactic ligation of the ductus arteriosus in babies who weighed 1000 g or less at birth. N Engl J Med *320*:1511, 1989.

81. Lewis AB, et al: Gestational changes in pulmonary vascular responses in fetal lambs in utero. Circ Res *39*:536, 1976.

82. Jacob J, et al: The contribution of PDA in the neonate with severe RDS. J Pediatr *96*:79, 1980.

83. Gersony WM, et al: Effects of indomethacin in premature infants with patent ductus arteriosus: results of a national collaborative study. J Pediatr *102*:895, 1983.

84. Raju TNK, Langenberg P: Pulmonary hemorrhage and exogenous surfactant therapy—a metaanalysis. J Pediatr *123*:603, 1993.

85. Garland J, et al: Pulmonary hemorrhage risk in infants with a clinically diagnosed patent ductus arteriosus: a retrospective cohort study. Pediatrics *94*:719, 1994.

86. Domanico RS, et al: Prophylactic indomethacin reduces the incidence of pulmonary hemorrhage and patent ductus arteriosus in surfactant treated infants <1250 grams. Pediatr Res *35*:331A, 1994.

87. Ikegami M, et al: Surfactant function in respiratory distress syndrome. J Pediatr *102*:443, 1983.

88. Brown E: Increased risk of bronchopulmonary dysplasia in infants with patent ductus arteriosus. J Pediatr *95*:865, 1979.

89. Cotton RB, et al: Randomized trial of early closure of symptomatic patent ductus arteriosus in small preterm infants. J Pediatr *93*:647, 1978.

90. Krauss AN, et al: Pulmonary function in preterm infants following treatment with intravenous indomethacin. Am J Dis Child *143*:78, 1989.

91. Alpan G, et al: Effect of patent ductus arteriosus on water accumulation and protein permeability in the premature lungs of mechanically ventilated premature lambs. Pediatr Res *26*:570, 1989.

92. Pérez Fontán JJ, et al: Respiratory effects of a patent ductus arteriosus in premature newborn lambs. J Appl Physiol *63*:2315, 1987.

93. Gerhardt T, Bancalari E: Lung compliance in newborns with patent ductus arteriosus before and after surgical ligation. Biol Neonate *38*:96, 1980.

94. Johnson DS, et al: The physiologic consequences of the ductus arteriosus in the extremely immature newborn. Clin Res *26*:826A, 1978.

95. Naulty CM, et al: Improved lung compliance after ligation of patent ductus arteriosus in hyaline membrane disease. J Pediatr *93*:682, 1978.

96. Stefano JL, et al: Closure of the ductus arteriosus with indomethacin in ventilated neonates with respiratory distress syndrome. Effects of pulmonary compliance and ventilation. Am Rev Respir Dis *143*:236, 1991.

97. Yeh TF, et al: Improved lung compliance following indomethacin therapy in premature infants with persistent ductus arteriosus. Chest *80*:698, 1981.

98. Dawes GS, et al: The patency of the ductus arteriosus in newborn lambs and its physiological consequences. J Physiol *128*:361, 1955.

S. Lee Adamson, Leslie Myatt, and Bridgette M. P. Byrne

72 Regulation of Umbilical Blood Flow

OVERVIEW

Oxygen, carbon dioxide, nutrients, metabolic wastes, and hormones are transported by blood flowing between the placenta and the fetal body in the umbilical cord. Normal fetal growth and development depend on ever-increasing umbilical blood flows to meet the growing demand for exchange with the maternal circulation. Growth of the placenta and the creation of new vascular channels provides an important mechanism for the long-term regulation of umbilical blood flow.[1,2] However, the focus of this chapter is the vasoactive regulation of umbilical blood flow, which is accomplished by numerous mediators that influence vascular resistance in umbilicoplacental circulation. Umbilical blood flow regulation plays a role in maintaining fetal growth and central arterial pressure, in perfusion-perfusion matching within the placenta, and in the closure of the umbilical vessels at birth.

The umbilicoplacental circulation is critically important for the normal growth and development of the fetus. This interesting vascular bed has many unique features. For instance, the umbilical artery and vein are extremely long and muscular, and the resistance of the placental microcirculation is low. This means that a significant proportion of the total vascular resistance in this circulation resides in the umbilical vessels themselves. Under normal *in utero* conditions, the umbilicoplacental circulation appears to be nearly maximally dilated, yet the umbilical vessels are highly vasoactive and, unlike most large vessels, are capable of constricting so vigorously that the lumen is obliterated (e.g., at birth). The umbilical artery is sensitive to many circulating vasoconstrictors but has the unusual feature of being refractory to active vasorelaxation by the cyclic adenosine monophosphate (cAMP) and cyclic guanosine monophosphate (cGMP) pathways.[3, 4] Perhaps the absence of active relaxation contributes to the vasospasm of the umbilical vasculature after birth. How the umbilical vessels are maintained in a nearly fully relaxed state throughout pregnancy is an interesting unanswered question.

In this chapter, we briefly describe the anatomy of the umbilicoplacental circulation and the sites of blood flow regulation in this bed. The important functions of blood flow regulation, and the factors involved are presented after a brief outline of the major experimental methods that have been used to obtain this information. Finally, we end by describing abnormalities in umbilical blood flow regulation in intrauterine growth restriction, a common and serious cause of mortality and morbidity in human pregnancy.

ANATOMY OF THE HUMAN UMBILICO-PLACENTAL CIRCULATION

The umbilical arteries in the human arise from the internal iliac arteries (Fig. 72-1) then curve upward along either side of the bladder. At the umbilicus, they enter the umbilical cord where the arteries form a loose spiral around a single umbilical vein. The umbilical vessels are embedded in Wharton jelly within the umbilical cord which is about 60 cm long at term.[5, 6] The umbilical arterial wall is atypical because it has a high wall thickness relative to its lumen diameter, the vascular smooth muscle cells form several layers that differ in cellular orientation from circular near the outside to longitudinal near the lumen, and there is no internal elastic lamina separating the smooth muscle from the endothelial cells lining the lumen of the vessel.[7, 8] The thick arterial muscle wall is sparsely supplied by vasa vasorum.[8, 9] The umbilical arteries are joined by Hyrtl anastomosis near the surface of most (approximately 96%) placentas so that arterial pressure is equalized near the placental surface.[5, 6]

The umbilical arteries branch at the fetal surface of the discoid human placenta to form many radially oriented chorionic arteries located on the surface of the chorionic plate. Distal branches of the chorionic arteries penetrate the fetal surface of the human placenta to supply 60 to 70 villous arteries that supply 10 to 40 cotyledons.[10] Cotyledonary units are separated by decidual septa arising from maternal tissue. Within the villous trees, the arteries continue branching to ultimately form arterioles within the intermediate villi. Exchange with maternal blood in the intervillous space of the cotyledons occurs primarily across the fetal capillaries of the terminal villi.

Veins within the villi merge progressively to return blood from the placenta to the chorionic veins on the fetoplacental surface. Blood then enters a single umbilical vein. The wall of the umbilical vein is highly muscular with circularly oriented smooth

Figure 72-1. A simplified scheme of the human umbilicoplacental circulation. The umbilical arteries arise from the internal iliac arteries, then curve upward to the umbilicus on either side of the bladder. After emerging from the umbilicus, the arteries form a spiral around the umbilical vein before branching into the chorionic arteries on the surface of the placenta. Villous arteries penetrate the surface of the placenta then branch further ultimately reaching the gas exchange surfaces in the terminal placental villi. Villous veins return blood from the placenta to the chorionic veins, visible on the surface of the placenta; blood then enters the umbilical vein in the umbilical cord. Within the abdomen, the umbilical vein enters the liver, where flow passes to the inferior vena cava either through the ductus venosus or the hepatic circulation. Not drawn to scale. (Modified from Moore KL, Persaud TVN: The Developing Human. 5th ed. Philadelphia, WB Saunders Co, 1993, p 344.)

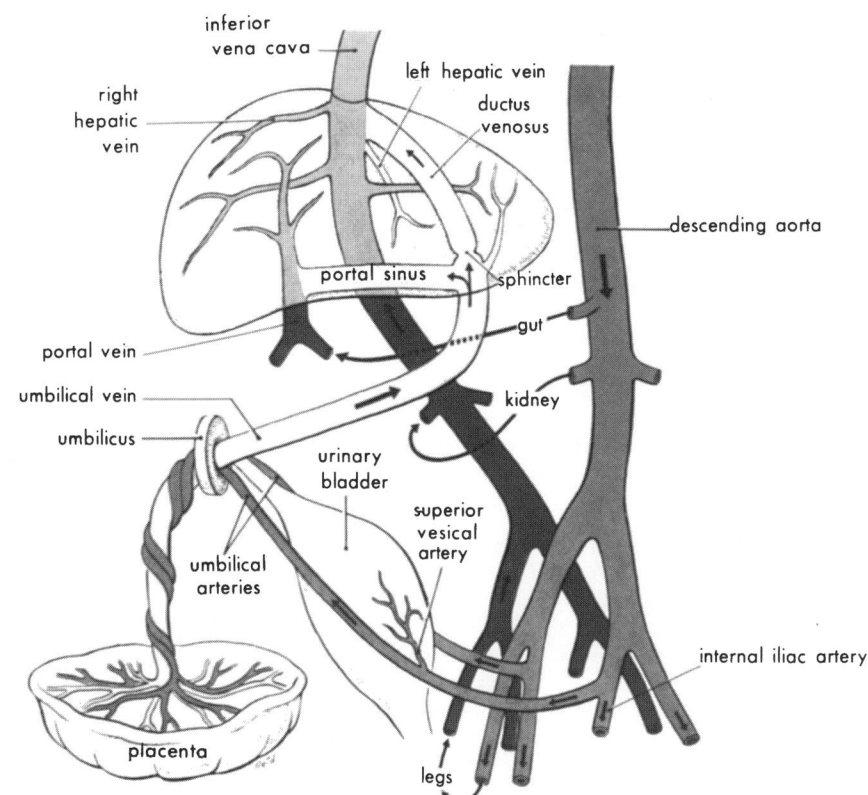

muscle cells arranged in concentric sheets loosely connected by ground substance.[7,8] Venous blood is then returned to the fetal inferior vena cava through the parallel arrangement of the ductus venosus and the hepatic vessels. The percentage of umbilical blood flow bypassing the hepatic circulation through the ductus venosus decreases from about 30 to 40% at midgestation to between 15 and 20% at term.[11,12]

HEMODYNAMICS OF UMBILICAL BLOOD FLOW

Umbilical arterial blood flow can be thought of as consisting of a mean blood flow component (i.e., the mean flow over the cardiac cycle) with a superimposed pulsatile component (i.e., the phasic flow within a cardiac cycle). In terms of the net transport of substances to and from the placenta, it is the mean blood flow component that is of primary importance. The sites and mechanisms regulating these two components of arterial blood flow differ; for this reason they are considered in separate sections of this chapter.

Mean Blood Flow

Mean umbilical blood flow (Q_{Um}) depends on the pressure gradient that drives flow from the iliac artery in humans (BP_A) to the inferior vena cava (BP_{IVC}), and on the total vascular resistance of the serially arranged segments of the umbilicoplacental pathway (R_{tot}). Total vascular resistance represents the sum of the resistances in the umbilical artery and its branches (R_{UmA}), in the placental microcirculation (R_{Pl}), in the umbilical vein and its branches (R_{Umv}) and the parallel arrangement of the ductus venosus (R_{DV}) and hepatic circulation (R_H). Each of these segments is a potential site for regulation of mean blood flow through this bed.

$$Q_{Um} = (BP_A - BP_{IVC})/R_{tot}$$

$$R_{tot} = R_{UmA} + R_{Pl} + R_{Umv} + (1/R_{DV} + 1/R_H)^{-1}$$

In most systemic vascular beds, large arteries and veins contribute little to the total vascular resistance of the circulation and therefore are not important regulators of organ blood flow. However, the umbilicoplacental circulation is unusual in that the umbilical artery and vein are extremely long and muscular, and the resistance of the placental microcirculation is very low. In sheep, although the largest fraction of the total vascular resistance resides in the placental microcirculation (around 55%), almost half the total resistance resides in the umbilical vessels and their major branches, and in the ductus venosus-hepatic circulation (Fig. 72-2).[13,14] Human umbilical vessels are perhaps four times longer than in sheep so it is possible that the human umbilical vessels make an even larger contribution to total umbilicoplacental vascular resistance. The greater prevalence of Hyrtl anastamoses in humans (about 96%) than sheep (about 50%) may be caused by the greater need for pressure equalization at the placenta as a result of the much greater length of the umbilical artery in humans.

Pulsatile Blood Flow

The pulsatile component of umbilical arterial blood flow is driven by the pulsatile component of pressure at the entrance to the umbilical artery. The pulse amplitude of umbilical arterial flow depends on the pulse amplitude of arterial pressure and on the so-called vascular input impedance that is primarily dependent on the attributes of the umbilical artery, its radius, wall thickness, and wall stiffness.[15] Umbilical input impedance is also influenced by the properties of the chorionic and stem arteries, but it is entirely independent of the properties of the vessels past the point where all pulsations generated by the heart have been attenuated (e.g., past the arterioles). The pulsatile component of flow is not important for transport because there is no net motion when it is averaged over the cardiac cycle; even so, this pulsatility may be important in promoting endothelial nitric oxide production and maintaining low placental vascular resistance as suggested by bypass experiments in fetal sheep.[16] It is also of interest clinically because the pulse amplitude of the flow velocity waveform in the umbilical artery is the numerator in the so-called pulsatility index as well as being an important factor in other indices of pulsatility. Indices of pulsatility are elevated in the umbilical artery of intrauterine growth restricted fetuses that are at highest risk of poor outcome.[17] The pulse amplitude of umbilical arterial flow tends to decrease with distance along the umbilical cord due to viscous losses in the blood and vessel wall. This attenuation results in a progressive decrease in indices of pulsatility when blood velocity waveforms are obtained at more distant sites along the cord.[18]

Atrial contraction of the heart generates pulse waves that are transmitted away from the heart into the venous system causing brief negative deflections in the predominantly forward-moving blood in the veins in association with the cardiac cycle. This effect can cause pulsatility in the blood velocity waveform of the umbilical vein and ductus venosus. Although such pulsatility is normal in early human pregnancy when propagation distances are short, pulsatility in the umbilical vein and ductus venosus is not normally observed in late pregnancy unless the fetus has cardiovascular pathologies that augment the strength of atrial contraction or the efficiency of pulse wave propagation in the venous system.[12] Wave propagation into the umbilical vein and ductus venosus is increased by dilation of the ductus venosus alone or in combination with constriction of the umbilical vein, such as may occur during fetal hypoxia or hemorrhage.[12]

METHODS USED TO STUDY UMBILICAL BLOOD FLOW REGULATION

Ultrasound

Pulsed Doppler ultrasound provides a sensitive and noninvasive means of detecting the velocity of red blood cells in the umbilical artery or vein in humans[19] and other species including sheep,[19] guinea pigs,[20] and mice (Fig. 72-3).[21] The shift in the frequency of the echo relative to the transmitted Doppler sound wave, is directly proportional to the velocity of the red blood

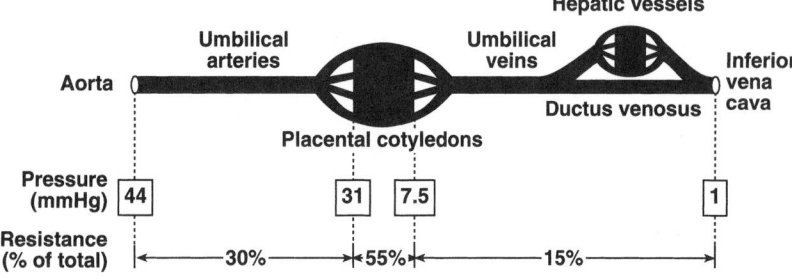

Figure 72–2. Distribution of blood pressures and vascular resistances within the sheep umbilicoplacental circulation near term (128-days' gestation). Flow through this circulation is approximately 200 mL/min/kg. (Data from Adamson SL, et al: Circ Res 70:761, 1992.)

cells that generate the echo. For accurate velocity determination, angle correction is required if the angle between the transmitted wave and the direction of red blood cell motion exceeds about 20°. This can be a problem in the umbilical artery because of the spiral path of this vessel, but this angle can be measured with some accuracy in the much straighter intra-abdominal umbilical vein. Blood velocity can be used to calculate blood flow by multiplying by vessel cross-sectional area determined from blood vessel diameter measurements. Flow per kg fetal body weight can be calculated using an estimate of fetal body weight determined from ultrasound measurements of fetal abdominal and head circumferences.[22-24]

Perfused Placenta *in Vitro*

Early studies investigated the vasoactivity of the human umbilicoplacental circulation by perfusing the entire placenta through the umbilical cord after delivery at a fixed flow rate and then recording the change in perfusion pressure induced by vasoactive agents delivered into the umbilical artery.[25] However obtaining a completely undamaged (i.e., leak-free) placenta was difficult so that most current work perfuses a single peripheral placental cotyledon through cannulas inserted into a chorionic artery and vein on the fetal placental surface, and through two or more cannulae inserted into the corresponding intervillous space through the maternal placental surface. This method, originally developed to study placental transfer,[26] has been used to investigate vasoactivity. The cotyledon is perfused at a fixed flow rate so that an increase in perfusion pressure in the fetal chorionic artery indicates an increase in fetoplacental vascular resistance. The preparation is viable for 12 hours or more of perfusion.[27]

Umbilicoplacental Vessels *in Vitro*

The vasoactivity of segments, rings, or strips of larger vessels in the human umbilicoplacental circulation have been extensively studied *in vitro*. In early studies, endothelial cell damage may have occurred before the importance of the endothelium in regulation of smooth muscle tone was recognized. The vasoactivity of vessel strips or rings is studied by recording muscle tension with a strain gauge whereas the vasoactivity of a vessel segment is detected by perfusing the segment at a constant rate and recording changes in perfusion pressure.[28] The vasoactivity of umbilical and chorionic vessels, as well as stem villous arteries, and their second and third order branches have been studied using these methods.[29] The production of vasoactive substances by placental vessels can be studied by determining the effect of placental vessel effluent on a strip of isolated smooth muscle used as a detector tissue. The degree of contraction or relaxation of the detector muscle provides a bioassay for vasoactive substances.[30] Differences in vasoactivity between different segments of the umbilicoplacental circulation have been observed (Table 72–1).[31,32]

Implanted Instrumentation

Fetal sheep are most commonly used for studies requiring implanted instrumentation, although similar studies are possible in other species such as goats and baboons. For studies on the umbilicoplacental circulation, chronic instrumentation is preferred to avoid the elevated umbilicoplacental vascular resistances observed in acutely instrumented fetal sheep under halothane anesthesia (about a 2.5-fold increase).[13,33] Mean blood pressure is measured using fluid-filled catheters implanted in arteries or veins that are coupled to strain-gauge pressure transducers outside the animal. Most studies measure only the total pressure gradient across the umbilicoplacental circulation (aorta to inferior vena cava) so that only total vascular resistance is determined. However, several studies have measured pressure gradients across individual segments of the umbilicoplacental circulation enabling determination of segmental vascular resistance.[13,33-35] These studies have revealed large differences in vasoactivity among the umbilical arteries, veins, microcirculation, ductus venosus, and hepatic circulation in fetal sheep. Mean blood flow is measured using electromagnetic transducers or ultrasound transit-time transducers implanted around the common umbilical artery or vein,[36,37] or by using labeled microspheres,[38] dye dilution methods,[41] or Fick's principle (e.g., with antipyrine).[39,40] It is now recognized that antipyrine is not an ideal tracer for flow studies because it inhibits prostaglandin (PG) synthesis and has measurable physiologic effects in fetal sheep.[42]

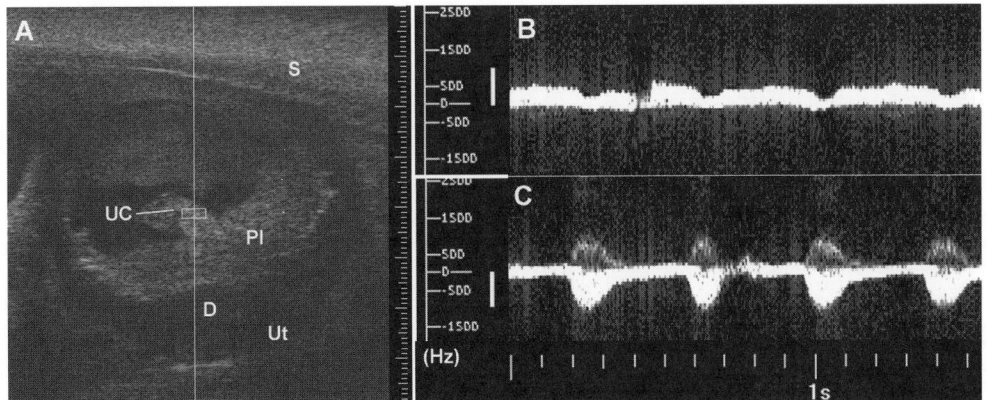

Figure 72–3. High frequency ultrasound technology permits Doppler blood velocity measurements in the umbilical cord throughout embryonic and fetal development in the mouse. This combined with the potential for exploring gene function in genetically modified mice, make it an attractive new model for future research. **A,** The placenta (Pl) and umbilical cord (UC) of a mouse embryo at day 10.5 of gestation. The anesthetized pregnant mouse was imaged transcutaneously using 40 MHz ultrasound. The location of the maternal skin (S), decidua (D), and uterus (Ut) are indicated. The box shows the location of the Doppler sample volume on the umbilical cord. By moving the sample volume slightly, the Doppler blood velocity waveform was obtained separately in the **(B)** umbilical vein, and **(C)** umbilical artery of the embryo. The smallest division on the scale bar in **A** is 100 μm. The vertical white bar along the y-axis in **(B)** and **(C)** shows a Doppler shift frequency of 0 to 1000 Hz. (Zhou YQ and Adamson SL, unpublished data).

TABLE 72-1

Vasoactive Mediators of the Human Umbilical-Placental Circulation

Mediator	Detected in Cord Blood	Receptor Localization Sites	Local Production Sites	Vasoactivity						References
				Umbilical Artery	Chorionic Artery	Stem Artery/Arteriole	Perfused Cotyledon	Chorionic Vein	Umbilical Vein	
Acetylcholine[1]			PI	+		0	0			(29,30,74,122–124)
Adenosine				–			–			(125–127)
Adrenomedullin		PI	PI			–	–			(128–131)
Angiotensin II[2]		PI	PI	+/0	+	+	+			(32,74,114,132–134)
ANP[3]		PI		–			–			(135–140)
BNP[3]			Amnion							(136,141)
Bradykinin			PI	+	+	+	+/0			(32,74,76,123,142,143)
Carbon monoxide							–			(116,144–147)
CGRP[4]					–					(148,149)
CRH[5]			PI		–					(80,81,106,150–152)
Cortisol							0			(153)
Endothelin-1[6]		UmA, PI	PI	+	+	+	+			(31,79,154–162)
Histamine[7]			Mast cells, basophils	+			–	+	+	(74,123,163)
Leukotrienes							+			(143,164)
Nitric oxide			UmA,UmV,PI, ChA,SA	0/–			–			(3,30,89,165–169)
Norepinephrine				+			+/0		+	(74,127,139,143, 170–172)
Neuropeptide Y[8]				+/0						(74,159)
Oxytocin			UmA,PI	+	+	+		+	+	(74,172–174)
PGE2 and PGF2α			PI,UmA,UmV, ChV,ChA	+			+			(74,134,143,175–177)
PGI2[9]				–	–	–	–	–	–	(143,171,178–182)
PTH[10]			C				–			(149,183)
PTHrP[10]		PI								(149,183)
Serotonin			Platelets	+	+	+	+/0		+	(29,31,32,74,76, 134,143,171)
Substance P						–				(185)
Thromboxane[11]		PI	UmA,UmV,PI	+	+	+	+		+	(125,134,143,180, 182,186)
Urotensin-1							–			(152)
Urocortin			D,PI				–			(152,187–189)
Vasopressin				+	+	+		+		(74,172–174)
VIP[12]					–	–				(179,185)

[1] Acetylcholine does not stimulate release of nitric oxide from umbilical artery or umbilical vein segments (reference 30).

[2] Angiotensin II response is likely mediated by AT_1 receptors in the placenta because the AT_2 subtype is not detectable (reference 114). Vasoconstrictive response is greatest in villous stem arterioles, moderate in chorionic arteries, and nearly absent in umbilical artery near term (references 32, 74, 134). Preterm umbilical arteries (<35 wk) do not vasoconstrict to angiotensin II (reference 74).

[3] BNP (brain natriuretic peptide) is a more potent vasodilator of perfused cotyledons than ANP (atrial natriuretic peptide) (reference 136).

[4] CGRP (calcitonin gene-related peptide) mediated vasodilation in the perfused cotyledon appears to be independent of nitric oxide synthesis and mediated by both CGRP-1 and CGRP-2 receptors (reference 149).

[5] CRH (corticotropin releasing hormone) acts via nitric oxide/cGMP pathway (reference 106) and vasodilates the placenta cotyledon at physiologic concentrations (reference 151).

[6] Subthreshold doses of endothelin-1 increase the sensitivity of the umbilical artery to other vasoconstrictors (reference 190). Bolus doses cause prolonged vasoconstrictive responses (45–60 min) in the perfused cotyledon (reference 160).

[7] Histamine's vasodilator effects may be mediated, at least in part, by endothelial cell-derived relaxing factor (presumably nitric oxide) (reference 30).

[8] Neuropeptide Y constricts umbilical arteries collected at term but not when collected preterm (references 74, 159).

[9] PGI_2 release by the perfused cotyledon is increased during angiotensin II-mediated vasoconstriction (reference 182), thereby attenuating the vasoconstrictive response to angiotensin II (reference 178).

[10] PTHrP (parathyroid hormone–related peptide) is ~100 × more potent than PTH (parathyroid hormone) as a vasodilator of the perfused placental cotyledon.

[11] Or the thromboxane analog, U46619.

[12] VIP (vasoactive intestinal peptide).

Ch, chorionic vein; ChA, chorionic artery; D, decidua; PGE, prostaglandin E; PGF, prostaglandin F; PI, placenta; SA, stem artery; UmA, umbilical artery; UmV, umbilical vein; +, construction; –, relaxation; +/0, little or no construction; 0/–, little or no relaxation.

IMPORTANCE OF UMBILICAL BLOOD FLOW REGULATION

The umbilicoplacental circulation is nearly maximally dilated[35] and the fetal biventricular cardiac output is near maximal under basal conditions in the near-term fetal sheep.[43] Thus, umbilical blood flow can be increased little by further dilating this vascular bed to reduce the resistance to flow or by increasing the driving pressure for flow by increasing cardiac output (hence mean arterial pressure). Nevertheless, umbilical blood flow can be increased by increasing vascular resistance in the fetal body to increase mean arterial pressure and thereby directing a larger proportion of the biventricular cardiac output to the placenta. In practice, however, umbilical blood flow is remarkably constant. During episodes of breathing activity in fetal sheep, fetal oxygen consumption increases and PaO_2 decreases significantly, yet umbilical blood flow and mean arterial pressure remain essentially constant.[44] Umbilical blood flow also changes little when the fetal sheep changes sleep state.[45] Even when the sheep fetus is made hypoxemic, umbilical blood flow remains nearly constant in fetuses near term.[46] This has led to the impression that the umbilicoplacental circulation is passive. Nevertheless, short-term regulation of vascular resistance does occur in this vascular bed and it plays important physiologic roles in optimizing placental exchange by matching regional maternal and fetal blood flows, in maintaining mean arterial blood pressure during hemorrhage, and in causing complete closure of this vascular bed at birth. In addition, abnormalities in vasoactive control of the umbilicoplacental circulation may contribute to the etiology of intrauterine growth restriction (IUGR). Each of these roles is described in detail later in this chapter.

Support Fetal Growth

Umbilical blood flow gradually increases as the fetus grows and placental exchange requirements increase. In humans, umbilical blood flow increases in direct proportion to the increase in fetal body weight so that flow expressed relative to fetal weight remains approximately constant at 110 to 125 mL min^{-1} kg^{-1} over the last third of pregnancy.[23,47-49] Human fetal biventricular cardiac output is about 450 mL/min^{-1} kg^{-1} and it also remains approximately constant over this gestational age range.[24,50] Thus, umbilical blood flow represents about 30% of fetal biventricular cardiac output.[24]

In IUGR, fetuses fail to achieve their full growth potential for a wide variety of reasons including infection, drug abuse, maternal malnutrition, and placental insufficiency due to increased umbilicoplacental resistance or unknown etiology. The fetus appears to respond to inadequate placental transfer of nutrients or oxygen by restricting growth to conserve limited resources for more essential functions thereby maintaining viability. Umbilical blood flow and umbilical blood flow per kg estimated fetal body weight are lower than normal in growth-restricted fetuses.[49,51] Early work suggested that umbilical blood flow in the sheep fetus normally exceeds that required so that there is a margin of safety in umbilical flow. This was based on evidence that acute reductions in umbilical blood flow caused an increase in oxygen extraction and no change in fetal oxygen consumption until flow was reduced by more than 40 to 50%.[52,53] However, a 30 to 40% reduction in umbilical blood flow that was maintained for 10 to 14 days reduced fetal growth and oxygen consumption suggesting that there is little margin of safety in umbilical blood flow with respect to fetal growth.[54,55]

Perfusion/Perfusion Matching to Optimize Maternal/Fetal Exchange

To maximize exchange, highly perfused regions on the maternal side of the placenta should be matched with well-perfused regions on the fetal side. This matching, analogous to ventilation-

perfusion matching in the lung, makes teleologic sense and there is evidence to support this mechanism from experiments in the perfused human placental cotyledon and in fetal sheep. Human cotyledons *in vitro* are usually perfused through the maternal intervillous space with media that have been equilibrated with 95% O_2 and 5% CO_2, which results in a perfusate pO_2 that exceeds 500 mm Hg. A large reduction in maternal perfusate pO_2 (to about 25 mm Hg) results in a rapid vasoconstrictive response in the fetal placental vasculature; an effect that is rapidly reversed by increasing maternal perfusate pO_2.[56] Hypoxic vasoconstriction of the fetal placental microcirculation has been postulated to mediate perfusion–perfusion matching in the human placenta[56] and it appears to be mediated by an hypoxia-induced decrease in nitric oxide production.[57]

In sheep, regional maternal and fetal blood flows measured using radioactive microspheres within cotyledons are correlated under baseline conditions.[58] When maternal blood flow to a placental region is reduced (e.g., by ligating maternal vessels or by embolizing with microspheres) fetal blood flow to the corresponding region decreases within 24 hours.[59] The mechanisms that increase umbilicoplacental vascular resistance in response to a decrease in maternal placental blood flow in sheep are not fully understood. However, they may be mediated by hypoxic vasoconstriction as occurs in ventilation-perfusion matching in the lung. In the fetal sheep near term, fetal hypoxia induced by maternal inhalation of a low oxygen mixture causes only a small increase in umbilicoplacental vascular resistance (e.g., 20%).[14,60] It is possible that hypoxic vasoconstriction in the placenta is reversed by enhanced β-adrenergic activity caused by fetal hypoxia.[61] The small increase in umbilicoplacental resistance during fetal hypoxia is caused specifically by a more than 100% increase in resistance of the umbilical vein and hepatic circulation, which is mediated by the α-adrenergic system.[14,60,62] In preterm fetal sheep (at approximately 95-days' gestation), fetal hypoxia causes a larger (e.g., 50%) increase in umbilicoplacental resistance.[63] The site and the mechanism of vasoconstriction in these preterm fetuses are not known. Possibly locally mediated hypoxic vasoconstriction within the placenta is not so effectively reversed by systemic hypoxic responses in preterm fetuses.

Maintenance of Fetal Arterial Blood Pressure

The umbilicoplacental circulation appears to play a role in maintaining central arterial blood pressure during hemorrhage in fetal sheep. During mild hemorrhage (about 15% loss of fetal blood volume), vascular resistance of the umbilicoplacental circulation increases to a similar extent as the fetal body (20%) so that the proportion of biventricular cardiac output directed toward the placenta remains unchanged.[64] However, during life-threatening, severe hemorrhage (around 40% loss of fetal blood volume) vascular resistance in the umbilicoplacental circulation increases 260%, thereby helping to maintain central arterial pressure.[65] Resistance increases significantly in all segments; the umbilical arteries and placenta (+250%), the umbilical veins (+390%), and the hepatic circulation (+540%) and nonsignificantly in the ductus venosus (+190%).[65] Umbilicoplacental vasoconstriction may be mediated by increased circulating concentrations of catecholamines, angiotensin II, and vasopressin, individually or in combination.[65-68]

Factors affecting the exchange of water between the maternal and fetal circulations at the placental interface could influence fetal blood volume and hence play a role in maintaining fetal arterial blood pressure. The net transfer of water across the placenta is presumably controlled by the balance of osmotic and hydrostatic pressures across placental capillary walls as in other microcirculatory beds. It has been proposed that a decrease in placental capillary blood pressure could promote the movement of water from the maternal to the fetal circulation, thereby increasing fetal blood volume and, thus, fetal arterial blood pressure.[69] However, when pressure in the umbilicoplacental circulation was decreased 33% by partially occluding the fetal distal aorta for 2 weeks, there was no decrease in hematocrit suggesting that there was no increase in plasma volume nor was there an increase in central arterial blood pressure in the sheep fetus.[54] Thus, it remains unknown whether alterations in water transport caused by physiologic alterations in placental capillary pressure play an important role in maintaining fetal arterial blood pressure.

Closure of Umbilicoplacental Circulation at Birth

In humans, umbilical blood flow rapidly decreases after delivery of the fetus to less than 20% of the normal fetal value[23] by 40 to 60 seconds after delivery.[70,71] This is accompanied by significant decreases in umbilical artery and vein diameters within 120 seconds.[72] The factors responsible for the rapid constriction of the umbilical vessels and the rapid increase in umbilicoplacental vascular resistance at birth are poorly understood.

It is possible that the sudden exposure of the umbilical cord after birth to a cool, more highly oxygenated room air environment plays a role. Cooling human umbilical vein segments from 37°C to 20°C caused vasoconstriction mediated by increased prostaglandin and thromboxane synthesis.[73] Cooling over this temperature range also caused constriction of human umbilical artery rings, but the contraction was transient, lasting less than 5 to 10 minutes,[74] which suggests this mechanism may not be important in the sustained closure of umbilical vessels at birth. Similarly, an increase in oxygen tension elicits a transient vasoconstriction of the umbilical artery, which is mediated by increased thromboxane synthesis.[74-76] An increase in oxygenation also enhances the contractile effects of bradykinin and serotonin[28,75,76] but not endothelin-1[31] on the human umbilical artery. Nevertheless, umbilical artery and vein diameters decrease markedly within 2 minutes after delivery despite no significant increase in arterial or venous pO_2.[72] Thus factors other than an increase in oxygenation (contraction precedes it) and cooling (contraction is transient) are likely involved in the rapid constriction of the umbilical vasculature at birth.

Local mediators produced by cells in the vicinity of the umbilical vessels may be the primary source of vasoactive agents that effect closure of these vessels after birth.[74] Serotonin in particular, may have sufficient potency and efficacy, and a sufficiently long duration of action (longer than 2.5 hours) to effect cord closure.[74] Alternatively vasoconstriction may be stimulated by mechanical stretch of the cord.[77] Umbilical vessels may be prone to vasospasm due to the absence of active vasodilation by cAMP or cGMP pathways.[3,4]

FACTORS THAT REGULATE UMBILICAL BLOOD FLOW

Mean blood flow through the umbilicoplacental circulation depends on the total pressure gradient driving flow, and the sum of the resistances in each segment of this vascular bed (see Fig. 72-2). Vasoactive factors, as well as changes in heart rate, can

indirectly affect umbilical blood flow by altering the central blood pressures that drive flow through this circulation. However, umbilical flow can be affected more directly by alterations in vascular resistance within the umbilico-placental vascular bed.

Vasoactive Mediators

The effects of numerous vasoactive mediators on different segments of the human umbilicoplacental vasculature are shown in Table 72-1. Note that vasodilator activity is normally evaluated in vessels that have been preconstricted with substances such as angiotensin II, $PGF_{2\alpha}$, or thromboxane. The mediators are listed in alphabetical order in the table because it is difficult to divide vasoactive substances into extrinsic (humoral) or intrinsic (local, paracrine/autocrine) categories; substances that act locally postnatally (e.g., PGE_2, endothelin) circulate in relatively high concentrations in the fetus[78,79] and therefore may have humoral effects. Similarly, other classic hormones (e.g., corticotropin-releasing hormone [CRH]) are produced in the placenta[80,81] and therefore may have local effects. It is also difficult to divide them into dilators and constrictors because some mediators may cause vasoconstriction in one segment but vasodilation in another (e.g., histamine), and others usually considered vasodilators cause vasoconstriction in this bed (e.g., acetylcholine, bradykinin).

Table 72-1 summarizes the vasoactive effect observed when exogenous mediators are applied. However, this does not necessarily mean that the mediator has an important physiologic role in controlling placental perfusion. Further evidence for a role includes detection of the mediator in cord blood and/or the presence of local sites of synthesis within the umbilicoplacental circulation, as well as the presence of receptors. Thus, this information has also been included in Table 72-1. A role for endogenous production of a mediator can also be shown by blocking its synthesis or receptors and showing that this elicits a change in vascular resistance. Studies that have taken this approach are summarized on Table 72-2.

The effects of vasoactive mediators on the human umbilicoplacental vasculature are usually studied using isolated tissues *in vitro* that were collected following delivery at term. However, it is important to keep in mind that responses may differ from those observed *in vivo* (umbilical arteries, for example, may not fully relax *in vitro*[82]), and that responses may also change during gestation. For example, relative to umbilical arteries collected following preterm delivery (less than 35 weeks), arteries collected following delivery at term (38 weeks and beyond) constrict much less vigorously to angiotensin II, but more vigorously to vasopressin, norepinephrine, and PGE_2.[74]

Innervation

There are no detectable adrenergic or cholinergic nerve fibers in the human placenta nor in human or sheep umbilical cord vessels except in the immediate vicinity of the umbilicus.[5,8] In contrast, the intrafetal portion of the human umbilical artery is

TABLE 72-2

Effect of Inhibitors of Vasoactive Mediators on the Human Umbilical-Placental Circulation

Substance	Inhibitor	Response
Cyclooxygenase	Indomethacin	No effect on basal tone of umbilical vein, perfused placental cotyledon, or stem Villous arterioles (references 29, 143, 178, 191)
Nitric oxide synthase	L-NAME	Increases basal tone and sensitivity to vasoconstrictors in perfused placental cotyledons (references 123, 192)
Angiotensin II	Saralasin	Inhibits angiotensin II constriction of perfused placental cotyledons (references 132, 133)
Heme oxygenase	Zinc protoporphyrin	Increases basal tone in perfused placental cotyledons (reference 147)

innervated[5] as is the ductus venosus in sheep.[83] This innervation apparently exerts little influence over ductus venosus blood flow under basal conditions[83] or during increased α-adrenergic activity induced by hypoxia in fetal sheep[62,84] so the function of this innervation is unknown. Similarly, a significant neural role in control of the intrafetal portion of the umbilical artery has not been demonstrated to date. The absence of innervation of extrafetal umbilical cord vessels and the placenta indicates that these vessels are not under neural control.

Wall Shear Stress

Changes in the flow rate or viscosity of fluid moving through a vessel alters the wall shear stress (i.e., viscous drag) imposed on the endothelial cells lining the vessel lumen. Shear stress is an important stimulus for the tonic secretion of vasodilators such as nitric oxide from endothelial cells.[85,86] In the perfused human cotyledon, alterations in endothelial shear stress effected by alterations in flow appear to alter endothelial nitric oxide release.[87] Furthermore, in small placental arteries, flow-induced vasodilation is observed and this effect is blocked by nitric oxide synthase inhibitors.[88] Flow-induced vasodilation may not occur in umbilical arteries, however, because the smooth muscle cells of these vessels exhibit little or no relaxation response to nitric oxide.[3,89] Alternatively, other mediators could regulate this response.[86]

UMBILICAL BLOOD FLOW IN INTRAUTERINE GROWTH RESTRICTION

Umbilical blood flow and umbilical blood flow per kg of estimated fetal body weight are lower than normal in human IUGR fetuses.[49,51] indicating that either the vascular resistance of the umbilicoplacental circulation is high or the driving pressure for flow is low. In addition, many fetuses with IUGR have umbilical arterial blood velocity waveforms that are highly pulsatile.[49,90] Diastolic blood velocity in these fetuses may be reduced, absent or even reversed (i.e., blood returns toward the heart) compared with the normally high diastolic velocities recorded in the umbilical artery in latter part of normal pregnancy.[91]

IUGR fetuses, especially those with highly pulsatile umbilical arterial velocity waveforms, are often hypoxemic[92,93] but hypoxemia itself does not increase blood flow pulsatility in the umbilical artery when induced experimentally in fetal sheep.[94,95] High pulsatility can be induced, however, by increasing the vascular resistance of the placental microcirculation.[96-98] In IUGR, elevated placental vascular resistance may be caused by structural abnormalities of the fetoplacental vasculature[99-103] or by abnormalities in placental vasoconstrictor tone.[104,105] Interestingly, perfused cotyledons of such fetuses do not require significantly higher pressures to achieve the same perfusion rate, indicating that their vascular resistances are near normal in vitro.[106,107] Therefore, if elevated pulsatility of umbilical arterial velocity waveforms in these fetuses is caused by elevated resistance in vivo, then elevated vascular resistance appears to be mediated by vasoactive factors or by a site not represented in the perfused cotyledon in vitro.[15,107] The possibility that resistance is elevated within the umbilical cord, hepatic circulation, or ductus venosus in at least some cases of IUGR warrants further consideration.[108]

Pulsatility of umbilical arterial velocity waveforms can be improved by bed rest,[109,110] maternal hydration[110] or oxygen administration[111] further suggesting that, at least in some cases, altered vasoactive tone rather than anatomic abnormalities of the umbilicoplacental circulation is involved. Some evidence does support abnormalities in vasoactive mediators in IUGR pregnancies. For instance, vasoconstriction of the placental vasculature may be augmented by angiotensin II, endothelin-1, or by the proinflammatory cytokine, tumor necrosis factor-α, all of which are elevated in umbilical cord blood of IUGR fetuses.[104,112,113]

Alternatively, high circulating angiotensin II levels may be offset by reduced protein level, binding capacity, and affinity of the AT_1 receptor in IUGR placentas.[114,115] Vasoconstriction may also be enhanced by decreased expression of heme oxygenase-2 and thus reduced production of the vasodilator, carbon monoxide, by the endothelium in IUGR placentas.[116] Thromboxane and vasoconstrictor PGs do not appear to be involved as production of these mediators is not enhanced in perfused placental cotyledons from IUGR fetuses.[117] Vasoconstrictive influences may be offset, at least in part, by a fourfold increase in cord blood concentrations of the vasodilator corticotropin-releasing hormone[118-120] the activity of which is mediated by nitric oxide,[106] and by increased expression of endothelial nitric oxide synthase in placental villous vessels.[121]

SUMMARY/CONCLUSIONS

There are many potentially important mechanisms regulating umbilicoplacental vascular resistance in vivo. Of these, evidence supports an important physiological role for the local production of CRH and nitric oxide in promoting the normally low vascular resistance of the umbilicoplacental circulation. There are also many factors capable of vasoconstricting the umbilicoplacental circulation; endothelin-1 and thromboxane are among the most potent. Local alterations in resistance in the placental microcirculation may play a physiologic role matching flow with the corresponding flow on the maternal side of the placenta. In addition, vasoconstrictors may play a critical physiologic role in the closure of the umbilicoplacental circulation after birth. In IUGR fetuses, abnormalities in levels or in responsiveness to vasoactive factors may increase umbilicoplacental vascular resistance thereby reducing umbilical blood flow resulting in impaired fetal growth.

REFERENCES

1. Challier J-C, et al: Ontogenesis of Villi and Fetal Vessels in the Human Placenta. Fetal Diagn Ther 2001;16: 218.
2. Reynolds LP, Redmer DA. Angiogenesis in the Placenta. Biol Reprod 2001;64: 1033.
3. Bergh CM, et al: Impaired Cyclic Nucleotide-Dependent Vasorelaxation in Human Umbilical Artery Smooth Muscle. Am J Physiol 1995;268: H202.
4. Brophy CM, et al: Heat Shock Protein Expression in Umbilical Artery Smooth Muscle. J Reprod Fertil 1998;114: 351.
5. Benirschke K, Kaufmann P: Umbilical cord and major fetal vessels. In Benirschke K, Kaufmann P (eds): Pathology of the Human Placenta. 2nd ed. New York, Springer-Verlag, 1990, pp 180–243.
6. Raio L, et al: In-utero characterization of the blood flow in the Hyrtl anastomosis. Placenta 2001;22: 597.
7. Meyer WW, et al: Functional morphology of human arteries during fetal and postnatal development. In Schwartz CJ, et al (eds): Structure and Function of the Circulation. New York, Plenum Press, 1980, pp 95–379.
8. Sheppard BL, Bishop AJ: Electron microscopical observations on sheep umbilical vessels. Q J Exp Physiol Cogn Med Sci 1973;58: 39.
9. Roach MR: A biophysical look at the relationship of structure and function in the umbilical artery. Proceedings of the Barcroft Symposium. Cambridge, U.K., Cambridge University Press, 1972, pp 141–163.
10. King BF: The functional anatomy of the placental vasculature. In Rosenfeld CR (ed): Reproductive and Perinatal Medicine; The Uterine Circulation. Ithaca, NY, Perinatology Press, 1989, pp 17–33.
11. Bellotti M, et al: Role of ductus venosus in distribution of umbilical blood flow in human fetuses during second half of pregnancy. Am J Physiol Heart Circ Physiol 2000;279: H1256.
12. Kiserud T: The ductus venosus. Semin Perinatol 2001;25: 11.
13. Adamson SL, et al: Pulsatile pressure—flow relations and pulse-wave propagation in the umbilical circulation of fetal sheep. Circ Res 1992;70: 761.
14. Paulick RP, et al: Venous responses to hypoxemia in the fetal lamb. J Dev Physiol 1990;14: 81.
15. Adamson SL: Arterial pressure, vascular input impedance, and resistance as determinants of pulsatile blood flow in the umbilical artery. Eur J Obstet Gynecol Reprod Biol 1999;84: 119.
16. Vedrinne C, et al: Better preservation of endothelial function and decreased activation of the fetal renin-angiotensin pathway with the use of pulsatile flow during experimental fetal bypass. J Thorac Cardiovasc Surg 2000;120: 770.
17. Baschat AA, Weiner CP: Umbilical artery doppler screening for detection of the small fetus in need of antepartum surveillance. Am J Obstet Gynecol 2000;182: 154.

18. Sonesson S-E, et al: Reference values for doppler velocimetric indices from the fetal and placental ends of the umbilical artery during normal pregnancy. J Clin Ultrasound 1993;21: 317.

19. Barbera A, et al: Relationship of umbilical vein blood flow to growth parameters in the human fetus. Am J Obstet Gynecol 1999;181: 174.

20. Turner AJ, Trudinger BJ: Ultrasound measurement of biparietal diameter and umbilical artery blood flow in the normal fetal guinea pig. Comp Med 2000;50: 379.

21. Phoon CKL, et al: 40 MHz Doppler characterization of umbilical and dorsal aortic blood flow in the early mouse embryo. Ultrasound Med Biol 2000;26: 1275.

22. Gill RW: Pulsed Doppler with B-mode imaging for quantitative blood flow measurement. Ultrasound Med Biol 1979;5: 223.

23. Gill RW, et al: Fetal umbilical venous flow measured in utero by pulsed Doppler and B-mode ultrasound. I. Normal pregnancies. Am J Obstet Gynecol 1981;139: 720.

24. St. John Sutton MG, et al: Relationship between placental blood flow and combined ventricular output with gestational age in normal human fetus. Cardiovasc Res 1991;25: 603.

25. Krantz KE, et al: Physiology of maternal-fetal relationship through the extracorporeal circulation of the human placenta. Am J Obstet Gynecol 1962;83: 1214.

26. Schneider H, et al: Transfer across the perfused human placenta of antipyrine, sodium and leucine. Am J Obstet Gynecol 1972;114: 822.

27. Miller RK, et al: Human placenta in vitro: characterization during 12 h of dual perfusion. Contrib Gynecol Obstet 1985;13: 77.

28. McGrath JC, et al: Comparison of the effects of oxygen, 5-hydroxytryptamine, bradykinin and adrenaline in isolated human umbilical artery smooth muscle. Q J Exp Physiol 1988;73: 547.

29. McCarthy AL, et al: Functional characteristics of small placental arteries. Am J Obstet Gynecol 1994;170: 945.

30. Van de Voorde J, et al: Release of endothelium-derived relaxing factor from human umbilical vessels. Circ Res 1987;60: 517.

31. MacLean MR, et al: The influence of endothelin-1 on human foeto-placental blood vessels: a comparison with 5-hydroxytryptamine. Br J Pharmacol 1992;106: 937.

32. Tulenko TN: Regional sensitivity to vasoactive polypeptides in the human umbilicoplacental vasculature. Am J Obstet Gynecol 1979;135: 629.

33. Adamson SL, et al: Vasomotor responses of the umbilical circulation in fetal sheep. Am J Physiol 1989;256: R1056.

34. Paulick RP, et al: Umbilical and hepatic venous responses to circulating vasoconstrictive hormones in fetal lamb. Am J Physiol 1991;260: H1205.

35. Paulick RP, et al: Vascular responses of umbilical-placental circulation to vasodilators in fetal lambs. Am J Physiol 1991;261: H9.

36. Oakes GK, et al: Effect of propranolol infusion on the umbilical and uterine circulations of pregnant sheep. Am J Obstet Gynecol 1976;126: 1038.

37. Berman W, Jr, et al: Measurement of umbilical blood flow in fetal lambs in utero. J Appl Physiol 1975;39: 1056.

38. Heymann MA, et al: Blood flow measurements with radionuclide-labeled particles. Prog Cardiovasc Dis 1977;20: 55.

39. Meschia G, et al: Simultaneous measurement of uterine and umbilical blood flows and oxygen uptakes. Q J Exp Physiol 1966;52: 1.

40. Rudolph AM, Heymann MA: Validation of the antipyrine method for measuring fetal umbilical blood flow. Circ Res 1967;21: 185.

41. Novy MJ, Metcalfe J: Measurements of umbilical blood flow and vascular volume by dye dilution. Am J Obstet Gynecol 1970;106: 899.

42. Gull I, Charlton V: Effects of antipyrine on umbilical and regional metabolism in late gestation in the fetal lamb. Am J Obstet Gynecol 1993;168: 706.

43. Rudolph AM, Heymann MA: Fetal and neonatal circulation and respiration. Annu Rev Physiol 1974;36: 187.

44. Rurak DW, Gruber NC: Increased oxygen consumption associated with breathing activity in fetal lambs. J Appl Physiol 1983;54: 701.

45. Slotten P, et al: Relationship between fetal electrocorticographic changes and umbilical blood flow in the near-term sheep fetus. J Dev Physiol 1989;11: 19.

46. Cohn HE, et al: Cardiovascular responses to hypoxemia and acidemia in fetal lambs. Am J Obstet Gynecol 1974;120: 817.

47. St. John Sutton MS, et al: Changes in placental blood flow in the normal human fetus with gestational age. Pediatr Res 1990;28: 383.

48. Erskine RLA, Ritchie JWK: Quantitative measurement of fetal blood flow using doppler ultrasound. Br J Obstet Gynaecol 1985;92: 600.

49. Ferrazzi E, et al: Doppler investigation in intrauterine growth restriction—from qualitative indices to flow measurements. A review of the experience of a collaborative group. Ann NY Acad Sci 2001;943: 316.

50. Kenny JF, et al: Changes in intracardiac blood flow velocities and right and left ventricular stroke volumes with gestational age in the normal human fetus: a prospective doppler echocardiographic study. Circulation 1986;74: 1208.

51. Gill RW, et al: Umbilical venous flow in normal and complicated pregnancy. Ultrasound Med Biol 1984;10: 349.

52. Itskovitz J, et al: The effect of reducing umbilical blood flow on fetal oxygenation. Am J Obstet Gynecol 1983;145: 813.

53. Meschia G: Safety margin of fetal oxygenation. J Reprod Med 1985;30: 308.

54. Anderson DF, Faber JJ: Regulation of fetal placental blood flow in the lamb. Am J Physiol 1984;247: R567.

55. Anderson DF, et al: Fetal O2 consumption in sheep during controlled long-term reductions in umbilical blood flow. Am J Physiol 1986;250: H1037.

56. Howard RB, et al: Hypoxia-induced fetoplacental vasoconstriction in perfused human placental cotyledons. Am J Obstet Gynecol 1987;157: 1261.

57. Byrne BM, et al: Role of the L-arginine nitric oxide pathway in hypoxic fetoplacental vasoconstriction. Placenta 1997;18: 627.

58. Rankin J, et al: Macroscopic distribution of blood flow in the sheep placenta. Am J Physiol 1970;219: 9.

59. Stock MK, et al: Vascular response of the fetal placenta to local occlusion of the maternal placental vasculature. J Dev Physiol 1980;2: 339.

60. Reuss ML, et al: Hemodynamic effects of alpha-adrenergic blockade during hypoxia in fetal sheep. Am J Obstet Gynecol 1982;142: 410.

61. Cohn HE, et al: The effect of β-adrenergic stimulation on fetal cardiovascular function during hypoxemia. Am J Obstet Gynecol 1982;142: 810.

62. Paulick RP, et al: Hemodynamic responses to alpha-adrenergic blockade during hypoxemia in the fetal lamb. J Dev Physiol 1991;16(2): 63.

63. Iwamoto HS, et al: Responses to acute hypoxemia in fetal sheep at 0.6–0.7 gestation. Am J Physiol 1989;256: H613.

64. Toubas PL, et al: Cardiovascular effects of acute hemorrhage in fetal lambs. Am J Physiol 1981;240: H45.

65. Meyers RL, et al: Cardiovascular responses to acute, severe haemorrhage in fetal sheep. J Dev Physiol 1991;15: 189.

66. Gomez RA, et al: Developmental aspects of the renal response to hemorrhage during fetal life. Pediatr Res 1984;18: 40.

67. Iwamoto HS, Rudolph AM: Role of renin-angiotensin system in response to hemorrhage in fetal sheep. Am J Physiol 1981;240: H848.

68. Jones CM, et al: Catecholamine responses in fetal lambs subjected to hemorrhage. Am J Obstet Gynecol 1985;151: 475.

69. Faber JJ, et al: Fetal blood volume and fetal placental blood flow in lambs. Proc Soc Exp Biol Med 1973;142: 340.

70. Yao AC, Lind J: Blood flow in the umbilical vessels during the third stage of labour. Biol Neonate 1974;25: 186.

71. McCallum WD: Thermodilution measurement of human umbilical blood flow at delivery. Am J Obstet Gynecol 1977;127: 491.

72. McCallum WD, McAreavey DRM: Human umbilical vessel diameters and blood gas tensions in the first two minutes after delivery. Gynecol Invest 1976;7: 201.

73. Boura AL, et al: Release of prostaglandins during contraction of the human umbilical vein on reduction of temperature. Br J Pharmacol 1979;65: 360.

74. White RP: Pharmacodynamic study of maturation and closure of human umbilical arteries. Am J Obstet Gynecol 1989;160: 229.

75. Templeton AGB, et al: The role of endogenous thromboxane in contractions to U46619, oxygen, 5-HT and 5-CT in the human isolated umbilical artery. Br J Pharmacol 1991;103: 1079.

76. Eltherington LG, et al: Constriction of human umbilical arteries: interaction between oxygen and bradykinin. Circ Res 1968;22: 747.

77. Silva de Sá MF, Meirelles RS: Estriol reduces the reactivity of the human umbilical artery to mechanical stimuli. Gynecol Obstet Invest 1989;27: 188.

78. Jones SA, et al: Eicosanoids in third ventricular cerebrospinal fluid of fetal and newborn sheep. Am J Physiol 1993;264: R135.

79. Nakamura T, et al: Immunoreactive endothelin concentrations in maternal and fetal blood. Life Sci 1990;46: 1045.

80. Jones SA, Challis JRG: Local stimulation of prostaglandin production by corticotrophin-releasing hormone in human fetal membranes and placenta. Biochem Biophys Res Commun 1989;159: 192.

81. Riley SC, et al: The localization and distribution of corticotropin-releasing hormone in the human placenta and fetal membranes throughout gestation. J Clin Endocrinol Metab 1991;72: 1001.

82. Bjoro K, Stray-Pedersen S: In vitro perfusion studies on human umbilical arteries: vasoactive effects of serotonin, PGF2α and PGE2. Acta Obstet Gynecol Scand 1986;65: 351.

83. Edelstone DI: Regulation of blood flow through the ductus venosus. J Dev Physiol 1980;2: 219.

84. Edelstone DI, et al: Effects of hypoxemia and decreasing umbilical flow on liver and ductus venosus blood flows in fetal lambs. Am J Physiol 1980;238: H656.

85. Rubanyi GM, et al: Flow-induced release of endothelium-derived relaxing factor. Am J Physiol 1986;250: H1145.

86. Melkumyants AM, et al: Control of arterial lumen by shear stress on endothelium. News Physiol Sci 1995;10: 204.

87. Wieczorek KM, et al: Shear stress may stimulate release and action of nitric oxide in the human fetal-placental vasculature. Am J Obstet Gynecol 1995;173: 708.

88. Learmont JG, et al: Flow induced dilatation is modulated by nitric oxide in isolated human small fetoplacental arteries. J Vasc Res 1994; 31(Suppl. 1), 26.

89. Chaudhuri G, et al: Characterization and actions of human umbilical endothelium derived relaxing factor. Br J Pharmacol 1991;102: 331.

90. Fleischer A, et al: Umbilical artery velocity waveforms and intrauterine growth retardation. Am J Obstet Gynecol 1985;151: 502.

91. McCowan LM, et al: Umbilical artery doppler blood flow studies in the preterm, small for gestational age fetus. Am J Obstet Gynecol 1987;156: 655.

92. Weiner CP: The relationship between the umbilical artery systolic/diastolic ratio and umbilical blood gas measurements in specimens obtained by cordocentesis. Am J Obstet Gynecol 1990;162(5): 1198.

93. Nicolaides KH, et al: Blood gases, PH, and lactate in appropriate- and small-for-gestational-age fetuses. Am J Obstet Gynecol 1989;161: 996.

94. Morrow RJ, et al: Acute hypoxemia does not affect the umbilical artery flow velocity waveform in fetal sheep. Obstet Gynecol 1990;75: 590.

95. Morrow RJ, et al: Hypoxic acidemia, hyperviscosity, and maternal hypertension do not affect the umbilical arterial velocity waveform in fetal sheep. Am J Obstet Gynecol 1990;163: 1313.

96. Trudinger BJ, et al: Umbilical artery flow velocity waveforms and placental resistance: the effects of embolization of the umbilical circulation. Am J Obstet Gynecol 1987;157: 1443.

97. Morrow RJ, et al: Effect of placental embolization on the umbilical arterial velocity waveform in fetal sheep. Am J Obstet Gynecol 1989;161: 1055.

98. Norton JL, et al: Prostaglandin-H synthase-1 (PGHS-1) gene is expressed in specific neurons of the brain of the late gestation ovine fetus. Brain Res Dev Brain Res 1996;95: 79.

99. Jackson MR, et al: Reduced placental villous tree elaboration in small-for-gestational-age pregnancies: relationship with umbilical artery doppler waveforms. Am J Obstet Gynecol 1995;172: 518.

100. Arabin B, et al: Relationship of utero- and fetoplacental blood flow velocity wave forms with pathomorphological placental findings. Fetal Diagn Ther 1992;7: 173.

101. Giles WB, et al: Fetal umbilical artery flow velocity waveforms and placental resistance: pathological correlation. Br J Obstet Gynaecol 1985;92: 31.

102. McCowan LM, et al: Umbilical artery flow velocity waveforms and the placental vascular bed. Am J Obstet Gynecol 1987;157: 900.

103. Todros T, et al: Umbilical Doppler waveforms and placental villous angiogenesis in pregnancies complicated by fetal growth restriction. Obstet Gynecol 1999;93: 499.

104. Kingdom JCP, et al: Fetal angiotensin II levels and vascular (type I) angiotensin receptors in pregnancies complicated by intrauterine growth retardation. Br J Obstet Gynaecol 1993;100: 476.

105. McQueen J, et al: Fetal endothelin levels and placental vascular endothelin receptors in intrauterine growth retardation. Obstet Gynecol 1993;82: 992.

106. Clifton VL, et al: Corticotropin-releasing hormone-induced vasodilation in the human fetal-placental circulation involvement of the nitric oxide-cyclic guanosine 3′,5′-monophosphate-mediated pathway. J Clin Endocrinol Metab 1995;80: 2888.

107. Challis DE: Glucose metabolism is elevated and vascular resistance and maternofetal transfer is normal in perfused placental cotyledons from severely growth-restricted fetuses. Pediatr Res 2000;47: 309.

108. Todros T, et al: Umbilical cord and fetal growth—a workshop report. Placenta 2002;23(Suppl A): S130.

109. Brar HS, Platt LD: Antepartum improvement of abnormal umbilical artery velocimetry: does it occur? Am J Obstet Gynecol 1989;160: 36.

110. Bell JG, et al: The effect of improvement of umbilical artery absent end-diastolic velocity on perinatal outcome. Am J Obstet Gynecol 1992;167: 1015.

111. Nicolaides KH, et al: Maternal oxygen therapy for intrauterine growth retardation. Lancet 1987;1(8539): 942.

112. Harvey-Wilkes KB, et al: Elevated endothelin levels are associated with increased placental resistance. Am J Obstet Gynecol 1996;174: 1599.

113. Holcberg G, et al: Increased production of tumor necrosis factor-alpha (TNF-alpha) by IUGR human placentae. Eur J Obstet Gynecol Reprod Biol 2001;94: 69.

114. Knock GA, et al: Angiotensin II (AT$_1$) vascular binding sites in human placentae from normal-term, preeclamptic and growth retarded pregnancies. J Pharmacol Exp Ther 1994;271: 1007.

115. Li X, et al: Cellular localization of AT$_1$ receptor MRNA and protein in normal placenta and its reduced expression in intrauterine growth restriction: angiotensin ii stimulates the release of vasorelaxants. J Clin Invest 1998;101: 442.

116. Barber A, et al: Heme oxygenase expression in human placenta and placental bed: reduced expression of placenta endothelial HO-2 in preeclampsia and fetal growth restriction. FASEB J 2001;15: 1158.

117. Sorem KA, Siler-Khodr TM: Placental prostanoid release in severe intrauterine growth retardation. Placenta 1995;16: 503.

118. Lyall F, et al: Nitric oxide concentrations are increased in the feto-placental circulation in intrauterine growth restriction. Placenta 1996;17: 165.

119. Goland RS, et al: Elevated levels of umbilical cord plasma corticotropin-releasing hormone in growth-retarded fetuses. J Clin Endocrinol Metab 1993;77: 1174.

120. Giles WB, et al: Abnormal umbilical artery doppler waveforms and cord blood corticotropin-releasing hormone. Obstet Gynecol 1996;87: 107.

121. Myatt L, et al: Endothelial nitric oxide synthase in placental villous tissue from normal, pre-eclamptic and intrauterine growth restricted pregnancies. Hum Reprod 1997;12: 167.

122. Brennecke SP, et al: Human placental acetylcholine content and release at parturition. Clin Exp Pharmacol Physiol 1988;15: 715.

123. Myatt L, et al: Attenuation of the vasoconstrictor effects of thromboxane and endothelin by nitric oxide in the human fetal-placental circulation. Am J Obstet Gynecol 1992;166: 224.

124. Lewis BV: The response of isolated sheep and human umbilical arteries to oxygen and drugs. J Obstet Gynaecol Br Commonw 1968;75: 87.

125. Di Grande A, et al: Modulation by adenosine of thromboxane a$_2$ receptor-mediated constriction in the human umbilical artery. Int J Clin Pharmacol Ther 1994;32: 344.

126. Read MA, et al: Vascular actions of purines in the foetal circulation of the human placenta. Br J Pharmacol 1993;110: 454.

127. Irestedt L, et al: Adenosine concentration in umbilical cord blood of newborn infants after vaginal delivery and cesarean section. Pediatr Res 1989;26: 106.

128. Moriyama T, et al: Expression of adrenomedullin by human placental cytotrophoblasts and choriocarcinoma JAr cells. J Clin Endocrinol Metab 2001;86: 3958.

129. Kanenishi K, et al: Immunohistochemical adrenomedullin expression is decreased in the placenta from pregnancies with pre-eclampsia. Pathol Int 2000;50: 536.

130. Jerat S, et al: Effect of adrenomedullin on placental arteries in normal and preeclamptic pregnancies. Hypertension 2001;37: 227.

131. Hoeldtke NJ, et al: Vasodilatory response of fetoplacental vasculature to adrenomedullin after constriction with the thromboxane sympathomimetic U46619. Am J Obstet Gynecol 2000;183: 1573.

132. Wilkes BM: Evidence for a functional renin-angiotensin system in full-term fetoplacental unit. Am J Physiol 1985;249: E366.

133. Glance DG, et al: The effects of the components of the renin-angiotensin system on the isolated perfused human placental cotyledon. Am J Obstet Gynecol 1984;149: 450.

134. Bjoro K, Stray-Pedersen S: Effects of vasoactive autacoids on different segments of human umbilicoplacental vessels. Gynecol Obstet Invest 1986;22: 1.

135. McQueen J, et al: Interaction of angiotensin ii and atrial natriuretic peptide in the human fetoplacental unit. Am J Hypertens 1990;3: 641.

136. Holcberg G, et al: The action of two natriuretic peptides (atrial natriuretic peptide and brain natriuretic peptide) in the human placental vasculature. Am J Obstet Gynecol 1995;172: 71.

137. Templeton AGB, et al: Atrial natriuretic peptide counteracts the vasoconstrictor effects of 5-hydroxytryptamine, u46619 and endothelin-1 in the human umbilical artery. Placenta 1994;15: 715.

138. McQueen J, et al: Characterization of atrial natriuretic peptide receptors in human fetoplacental vasculature. Am J Physiol 1993;264: H798.

139. Weiner CP, Robillard JE: Atrial natriuretic factor, digoxin-like immunoreactive substance, norepinephrine, epinephrine, and plasma renin activity in human fetuses and their alteration by fetal disease. Am J Obstet Gynecol 1988;159(6): 1353.

140. Lim AT, Gude NM: Atrial natriuretic factor production by the human placenta. J Clin Endocrinol Metab 1995;80: 3091.

141. Itoh H, et al: Brain natriuretic peptide is present in the human amniotic fluid and is secreted from amnion cells. J Clin Endocrinol Metab 1993;76: 907.

142. Melmon KL, et al: Kinins: possible mediators of neonatal circulatory changes in man. J Clin Invest 1968;47: 1295.

143. Mak KKW, et al: Effects of vasoactive autacoids on the human umbilical-fetal placental vasculature. Br J Obstet Gynaecol 1984;91: 99.

144. Yoshiki N, et al: Expression and localization of heme oxygenase in human placental villi. Biochem Biophys Res Commun 2000;276: 1136.

145. McLean M, et al: Expression of the heme oxygenase—carbon monoxide signalling system in human placenta. J Clin Endocrinol Metab 2000;85: 2345.

146. McLaughlin BE, et al: Endogenous carbon monoxide formation by chorionic villi of term human placenta. Placenta 2001;22: 886.

147. Lyall F, et al: Hemeoxygenase expression in human placenta and placental bed implies a role in regulation of trophoblast invasion and placental function. FASEB J 2000;14: 208.

148. Firth KF, Pipkin FB: Human α- and β-calcitonin gene-related peptides are vasodilators in human chorionic plate vasculature. Am J Obstet Gynecol 1989;161: 1318.

149. Mandsager NT, et al: Vasodilator effects of parathyroid hormone, parathyroid hormone-related protein, and calcitonin gene-related peptide in the human fetal-placental circulation. J Soc Gynecol Invest 1994;1: 19.

150. Chan E-C, et al: Plasma corticotropin-releasing hormone, B-endorphin and cortisol inter-relationships during human pregnancy. Acta Endocrinol (Copenh) 1993;128: 339.

151. Clifton VL, et al: Corticotropin-releasing hormone-induced vasodilatation in the human fetal placental circulation. J Clin Endocrinol Metab 1994;79: 666.

152. Leitch IM, et al: Vasodilator actions of urocortin and related peptides in the human perfused placenta in vitro. J Clin Endocrinol Metab 1998;83: 4510.

153. Sun K, et al: Interconversion of cortisol and cortisone by 11β-hydroxysteroid dehydrogenases type 1 and 2 in the perfused human placenta. Placenta 1999;20: 13.

154. Benigni A, et al: Human placenta expresses endothelin gene and corresponding protein is excreted in urine in increasing amounts during normal pregnancy. Am J Obstet Gynecol 1991;164: 844.

155. Haegerstrand A, et al: Endothelin: presence in human umbilical vessels, high levels in fetal blood and potent contrictor effect. Acta Physiol Scand 1989;137(4): 541.

156. Radunovic N, et al: Fetal and maternal plasma endothelin levels during the second half of pregnancy. Am J Obstet Gynecol 1995;172: 28.

157. Bodelsson G, Stjernquist M: Characterization of endothelin receptors and localization of ^{125}I-endothelin-1 binding sites in human umbilical artery. Eur J Pharmacol 1993;249: 299.

158. Robaut C, et al: Regional distribution and pharmacological characterization of [^{125}I]endothelin-1 binding sites in human fetal placental vessels. Placenta 1991;12: 55.

159. Hemsén A, et al: Characterization, localization and actions of endothelins in umbilical vessels and placenta of man. Acta Physiol Scand 1991;143: 395.

160. Myatt L, et al: Endothelin-1-induced vasoconstriction is not mediated by thromboxane release and action in the human fetal-placental circulation. Am J Obstet Gynecol 1991;165: 1717.

161. Myatt L, et al: The comparative effects of big endothelin-1, endothelin-1, and endothelin-3 in the human fetal-placental circulation. Am J Obstet Gynecol 1992;167: 1651.

162. Gude NM, et al: Endothelin: release by and potent constrictor effect on the fetal vessels of human perfused placental lobules. Reprod Fertil Dev 1991;3: 495.

163. Engberg Damsgaard TM, et al: Estimation of the total number of mast cells in the human umbilical cord: a methodological study. APMIS 1992;100: 845.

164. Thorp JA, et al: Comparison of the vasoactive effects of leukotrienes with thromboxane mimic in the perfused human placenta. Am J Obstet Gynecol 1988;159: 1376.

165. Myatt L, et al: Constitutive calcium-dependent isoform of nitric oxide synthase in the human placental villous vascular tree. Placenta 1993;14: 373.

166. Garvey EP, et al: Purification and characterization of the constitutive nitric oxide synthase from human placenta. Arch Biochem Biophys 1994;311: 235.

167. Buttery LDK, et al: Endothelial nitric oxide synthase in the human placenta: regional distribution and proposed regulatory role at the feto-maternal interface. Placenta 1994;15: 257.

168. Klockenbusch W, et al: Prostacyclin rather than nitric oxide lowers human umbilical artery tone in vitro. Eur J Obstet Gynecol Reprod Biol 1992;47: 109.

169. Myatt L, et al: The action of nitric oxide in the perfused human fetal-placental circulation. Am J Obstet Gynecol 1991;164: 687.

170. Falconer AD, Lake DM: Circumstances influencing umbilical-cord plasma catecholamines at delivery. Br J Obstet Gynaecol 1982;89: 44.

171. Maigaard S, et al: Relaxant and contractile effects of some amines and prostanoids in myometrial and vascular smooth muscle within the human uteroplacental unit. Acta Physiol Scand 1986;128: 33.

172. Allen J, et al: Effect of endogenous vasoconstrictors on maternal intramyometrial and fetal stem villous arteries in pre-eclampsia. J Hypertens 1989;7: 529.

173. Chard T, et al: Release of oxytocin and vasopressin by the human foetus during labour. Nature 1971;234: 352.

174. Maigaard S, et al: Differential effects of angiotensin, vasopressin and oxytocin on various smooth muscle tissues within the human uteroplacental unit. Acta Physiol Scand 1986;128: 23.

175. Haugen G, et al: Prostanoid production in umbilical arteries from preterm and term deliveries perfused in vitro. Early Hum Dev 1990;24: 153.

176. McCoshen JA, et al: Umbilical cord is the major source of prostaglandin e_2 in the gestational sac during term labor. Am J Obstet Gynecol 1989;160: 973.

177. Mitchell MD, et al: Prostaglandins in the human umbilical circulation at birth. Br J Obstet Gynaecol 1978;85: 114.

178. Glance DG, et al: The actions of prostaglandins and their interactions with angiotensin ii in the isolated perfused human placental cotyledon. Br J Obstet Gynaecol 1986;93: 488.

179. Maigaard S, et al: Digoxin inhibition of relaxation induced by prostacyclin and vasoactive intestinal polypeptide in small human placental arteries. Placenta 1985;6: 435.

180. Benedetto C, et al: Production of prostacyclin, 6-keto-PGF$_{1\alpha}$ and thromboxane B$_2$ by human umbilical vessels increases from the placenta towards the fetus. Br J Obstet Gynaecol 1987;94: 1165.

181. Kawano M, Mori N: Prostacyclin producing activity of human umbilical, placental and uterine vessels. Prostaglandins 1983;26: 645.

182. Glance DG, et al: Prostaglandin production and stimulation by angiotensin ii in the isolated perfused human placental cotyledon. Am J Obstet Gynecol 1985;151: 387.

183. Hellman P, et al: Parathyroid-like regulation of parathyroid-hormone-related protein release and cytoplasmic calcium in cytotrophoblast cells of human placenta. Arch Biochem Biophys 1992;293: 174.

184. Abramovich DR, et al: Effect of angiotensin ii and 5-hydroxytryptamine on the vessels of the human foetal cotyledon. Br J Pharmacol 1983;79: 53.

185. Hansen V, et al: Effects of vasoactive intestinal polypeptide and substance P on human intramyometrial arteries and stem villous arteries in term pregnancy. Placenta 1988;9: 501.

186. Hedberg A, et al: Evidence for functional thromboxane A$_2$-prostaglandin H$_2$ receptors in human placenta. Am J Physiol 1989;256: E256.

187. Petraglia F, et al: Human placenta and fetal membranes express human urocortin MRNA and peptide. J Clin Endocrinol Metab 1996;81: 3807.

188. Watanabe F, et al: Urocortin in human placenta and maternal plasma. Peptides 1999;20: 205.

189. Clifton VL, et al: Localization and characterization of urocortin during human pregnancy. Placenta 2000;21: 782.

190. Okatani Y, et al: Amplifying effect of endothelin-1 on serotonin-induced vasoconstriction of human umbilical artery. Am J Obstet Gynecol 1995;172: 1240.

191. Tulenko TN: The actions of prostaglandins and cyclo-oxygenase inhibition on the resistance vessels supplying the human fetal placenta. Prostaglandins 1981;21: 1033.

192. Gude NM, et al: Effects of eicosanoid and endothelial cell derived relaxing factor inhibition on fetal vascular tone and responsiveness in the human perfused placenta. Trophoblast Res 1993;7: 133.

73

Karel Maršál

Fetal and Placental Circulation During Labor

PHYSIOLOGIC BACKGROUND

A sufficient maternal blood supply to the placenta is of utmost importance to the fetus during pregnancy and labor. It has long been recognized that uterine contractions diminish uteroplacental blood flow. Contractions of myometrium compress the vessels traversing the uterine wall and increase intrauterine pressure, thus influencing the intervillous space pressure as well. The intrauterine pressure during labor usually ranges from 25 to 100 mm Hg. In contrast, the mean pressure in small arteries is 70 to 95 mm Hg and only 15 mm Hg at the capillary venous end. Thus, compression and even collapse of the myometrial vessels during labor is probable. Even a slight reduction in the diameter of an artery decreases flow because resistance to flow is inversely proportional to the fourth power of the vessel radius, according to the Poiseuille law. Obviously, during a contraction, the uterine veins are affected first, and the restricted venous outflow results in a reduction of the pressure gradient over the placenta. As demonstrated by the use of radioangiographic techniques in pregnant women, there is a marked decrease in maternal blood flow to the placenta during contraction.[1] Similarly, diminished arteriolar jets have also been demonstrated in the rhesus monkey.[2] Flow to the intervillous space, however, appears to remain constant.

The intermittent decrement in blood flow during myometrial contractions has been found to be inversely related to the increase in intrauterine pressure.[3-6] During uterine relaxation following a contraction, an increase in the blood flow—a reactive hyperemia—has been observed,[4, 6] which compensates for the decreased oxygen delivery during the preceding contraction.

With the progress of labor, the peak intrauterine pressure during each contraction increases, and the time-averaged blood flow in the uterine artery diminishes[7] (Fig. 73-1). Woodbury and co-workers[8] described a "maternal effective placental arterial pressure," defined as the arterial pressure minus the pressure within the uterus, which opposes the inflow of maternal blood. To ensure the perfusion of the placenta, the maternal central blood circulation responds to contractions by increasing both blood pressure and cardiac output.[9, 10]

The circulation of a healthy fetus in uncomplicated labor usually remains unaffected. The umbilical circulation is relatively unreactive and does not seem to respond to the changes in intrauterine pressure or to the short-term changes in the maternal placental blood flow during contractions. During normal labor, uterine contractions are not of sufficient magnitude to negatively affect gas exchange over the placenta. Therefore, they do not endanger the fetus. In labor with a pathologic course, in which uteroplacental blood flow is diminished, fetal hypoxemia can develop. In that

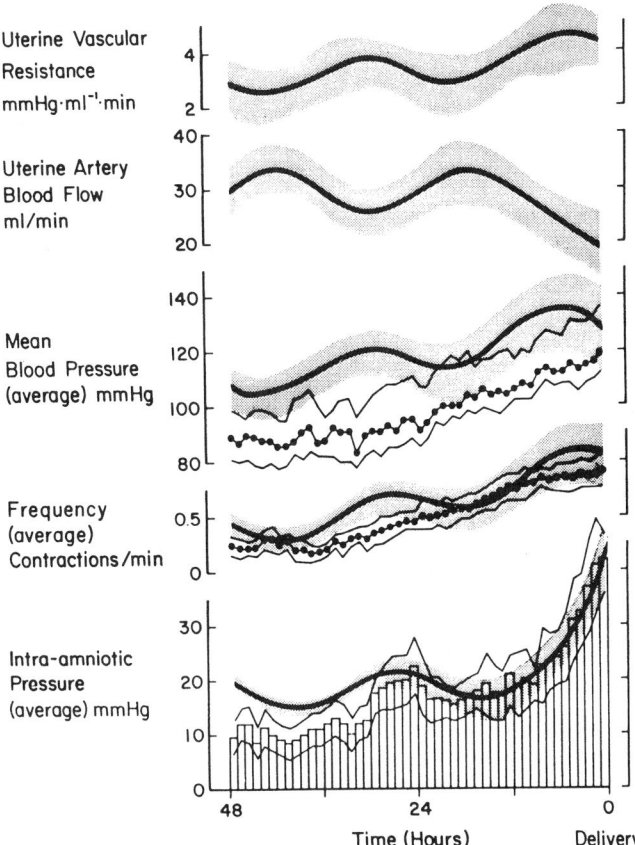

Figure 73–1. Composite drawing showing the incorporation of the circadian changes of uterine dynamics into the process of labor and delivery. The open bars of intra-amniotic pressure and the solid points depicting frequency of contractions and mean blood pressure represent data obtained from five patients monitored continuously during the last 48 hours of pregnancy. Each bar and point represent the mean of hourly average values. The thin solid lines delineate the 95% confidence intervals. The heavy solid lines of intra-amniotic pressure, frequency of contraction, mean blood pressure, uterine artery blood flow, and uterine vascular resistance were calculated from continuous recordings made in 15 monkeys during the 48 hours terminating in spontaneous labor and delivery. The shaded areas represent the 95% confidence intervals determined for individual mean values. Uterine vascular resistance was calculated by the formula: aortic blood pressure minus intra-amniotic pressure divided by uterine artery blood flow. (From Harbert GM Jr: *In* Rosenfeld CR [ed]: The Uterine Circulation, Reproductive and Perinatal Medicine, Vol X. Ithaca, NY, Perinatology Press, 1989, p 157.)

situation, the fetus reacts with changes in heart rate, blood pressure, and blood flow.[11] Uterine contractions can also cause a direct compression of the umbilical cord with restriction of the umbilical blood flow, leading to changes in the fetal circulation.

METHODS OF RECORDING HUMAN FETAL AND UTEROPLACENTAL BLOOD FLOW

Previously, most of our knowledge of uteroplacental and fetal circulation was based on animal experiments, in which invasive methods were used. In the early 1980s, a noninvasive method making use of Doppler ultrasound was introduced in the field of perinatal medicine, which has made it possible to obtain data on blood flow in human pregnancies.[12,13]

Flow Probe Techniques

Measurement of the uterine, uteroplacental, or fetal blood flow using a flow probe technique (measuring the flow in a single vessel by evaluating changes caused by the blood flow in either the electromagnetic field or the ultrasound passage time) requires an application of the probe on an exposed vessel. Only in exceptional circumstances has the electromagnetic method been used on a human uterine artery during laparotomy for hysterectomy in pregnancy.[14]

Radioangiography

The radioangiographic technique, with injection of contrast medium followed by serial x-ray exposures, has made it possible to establish the time of appearance and disappearance of contrast dye in various parts of the uteroplacental circulation.[1] However, absolute flow cannot be determined and, because of the high radiation hazard to the fetus, this method is not acceptable for use on humans.

Placenta Scintigraphy

Radioactive isotopes (^{24}Na, ^{133}Xe) can be injected into either the myometrium or the intervillous space, and the time rate of washout can then be determined by external measurement. This gives a semiquantitative measure of the maternal placental blood flow. To circumvent the disadvantage of the method's invasiveness, placenta scintigraphy has been developed that uses an intravenous injection of a radionuclide tracer (^{99m}Tc, ^{133}Xe, or ^{113m}In) and external measurement of accumulation or disappearance of radioactivity over the placenta.[15] Clinical application of this method is limited because it cannot be used for continuous measurement of the changes in placental blood flow over time, and only the anterior placenta can be examined. The most serious drawback of the method is exposure of the fetus to ionizing radiation.

Thermistor Method

The relative uterine blood flow can be evaluated by placing a preheated thermistor pearl into cervical tissue and then recording heat dispersal.[16] This method has the disadvantages of being invasive and of measuring flow in the cervix and lower segment of uterus and not directly in the placenta.

Doppler Ultrasound Method

Physical Principle

The Doppler ultrasound technique makes it possible to estimate blood velocity and blood flow in maternal and fetal vessels in a noninvasive way during late pregnancy and labor. The first report on the detection of flow signals from the umbilical artery was published in 1977 by FitzGerald and Drumm.[13] In recent years, Doppler velocimetry has become a method of choice for evaluation of the uteroplacental and fetal circulation.

According to the Doppler principle, a wave energy is reflected by a moving reflector with a wavelength (frequency) that is different from the emitted wavelength. The change in frequency (Doppler shift) is proportional to the velocity of the reflector. In the situation of blood flow measurement, ultrasound with a frequency of 1 to 10 MHz is transmitted to the tissue and reflected by the moving red cells within the vessel. The frequency of the received ultrasound is higher than the emitted frequency when the blood is moving toward the transducer, and it is lower when the blood is moving away from the transducer. The Doppler shift (f_d) is defined by the formula:

$$f_d = 2 \cdot f_o \cdot V \cdot \cos \theta / c$$

where f_o is the ultrasound frequency, V is the blood velocity, θ is the angle between the ultrasound beam and the bloodstream direction, and c is the velocity of ultrasound in tissue. The Doppler shift frequencies are within the range of audible sound. They can be analyzed, for example, by the Fast Fourier Transform and displayed as a Doppler shift spectrum (Fig. 73–2). From the spectrum, the mean and the maximum velocity can be estimated and further processed.

Doppler ultrasound can be used in three modes: continuous-wave Doppler ultrasound (CW), pulsed-wave Doppler ultrasound (PW), or color flow imaging. In the first mode, CW Doppler ultrasound is continuously transmitted by one piezo-electric crystal, and the reflected ultrasound is received by another crystal. Signals of blood flow are obtained from all vessels traversed by the ultrasound beam. The CW Doppler instruments are technically simpler than are the instruments of the other two modes and thus are usually cheaper. However, the application of CW Doppler ultrasound is limited because of the lack of range resolution.

In the PW mode, one single piezoelectric crystal is used for transmission and reception of the ultrasound bursts. By changing the time delay between the transmission and reception of signals, it is possible to determine the range within the tissue from which the Doppler-shifted signals are received. In other words, it is possible to choose a specific vessel for recording of blood velocity signals. The PW ultrasound is usually combined with imaging ultrasound (linear array or sector real-time scanner) to locate and identify the vessel of interest.

The color flow imaging enables a color coding of the received Doppler signals, usually red for the blood flow toward the transducer and blue for the flow in the opposite direction. The color signals are then superimposed on the two-dimensional real-time image. Color flow imaging facilitates detection of flow even in very small vessels, for example, fetal cerebral or renal vessels. It is often combined with PW Doppler ultrasound for quantification of flow velocity.

Volume Flow Estimation

The information on the time-averaged mean velocity (V) obtained from a specific vessel and corrected for the cosine θ can be used for calculation of the volume flow (Q) in milliliters/minute according to formula:

$$Q = V \cdot d^2 \cdot \pi/\cos \theta \cdot 4$$

This assumes that the diameter of the vessel (d) is known for the calculation of the cross-sectional area of the vessel.

The measurement of vessel diameter using the two-dimensional ultrasound image is relatively inaccurate and therefore can be performed only in vessels of large caliber (in the fetus, only in the umbilical vein or descending aorta).[17] The estimation of the volume blood flow also requires knowledge of the insonation angle and uniform insonation of the vessel for reliable estimation of the mean velocity. Because of all these possible sources of error, this method has not found wide application. Nevertheless, it can be expected that further technical development will enable reliable estimation of flow and that we will experience a revival of this method in perinatology.

Velocity Waveform Analysis

The maximum blood velocity (i.e., the envelope of the Doppler spectrum) recorded from an artery can be analyzed for its waveform and characterized by various indices (Fig. 73–3). These indices are angle-independent. The diameter of the vessel need not be known for waveform analysis, and the maximum velocity is easier to record than is the mean velocity. Thus, a number of errors involved in the estimation of blood flow are eliminated. However, this method does not directly reflect flow, and the interpretation of results is not always obvious.

The diastolic part of the flow velocity waveform is mainly influenced by the peripheral vascular resistance; an increase in the resistance lowers the diastolic velocity and, consequently, increases the values of the waveform indices described in Figure 73–3. However, the waveform and its indices are also influenced by cardiac performance, blood pressure, vessel wall properties, and the viscosity of blood.

A simple semiquantitative evaluation of the waveform recorded from the umbilical artery or fetal descending aorta with regard to the presence or lack of the end-diastolic flow (blood flow classes) has proved useful in the identification of growth-

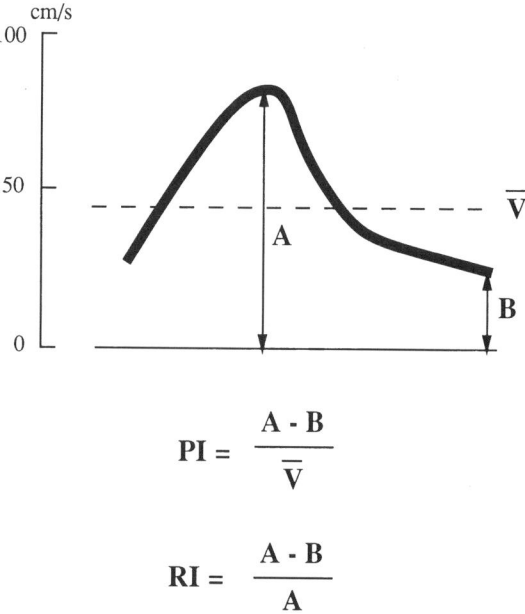

$$PI = \frac{A - B}{\overline{V}}$$

$$RI = \frac{A - B}{A}$$

A / B ratio (S / D ratio)

Figure 73–3. Schematic drawing demonstrating waveform analysis of the fetal arterial maximum blood velocity. A (S) = peak maximum velocity; B (D) = minimum diastolic velocity; $\overline{V}$ = mean velocity over the cardiac cycle; PI = pulsatility index according to ref. 87; RI = resistance index according to ref. 88; A/B ratio according to ref. 89.

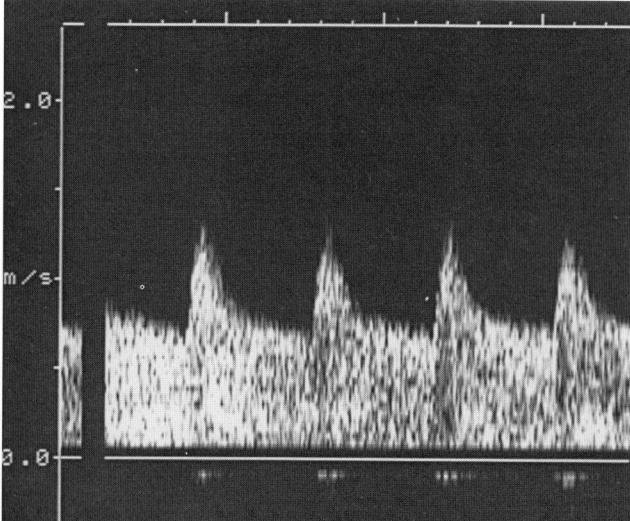

Figure 73–2. Doppler shift spectrum recorded from the uterine artery in a term pregnancy.

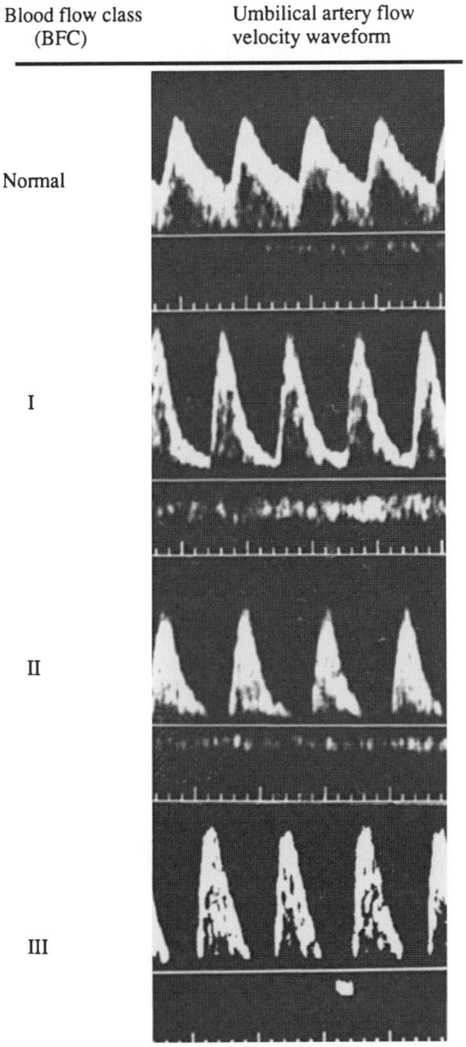

Blood flow class
(BFC)

Umbilical artery flow
velocity waveform

Normal

I

II

III

Figure 73–4. Blood flow classes of the umbilical artery flow velocity waveforms.

retarded fetuses and fetuses at risk of intrauterine asphyxia[18] (Fig. 73-4). In the cerebral vessels of hypoxic fetuses, an increase in diastolic velocity can be observed as an expression of decreased resistance in the cerebral vascular bed and redistribution of blood flow (brain-sparing phenomenon).

HUMAN UTEROPLACENTAL BLOOD FLOW DURING LABOR

PW Doppler ultrasound has been used for recording of flow velocity signals from the uteroplacental vessels in labor.[19, 20] CW Doppler ultrasound was also used for this purpose.[21, 22] All Doppler studies on uteroplacental vessels in labor have shown that during uterine contractions, both the systolic and diastolic blood velocities diminish, suggesting a decrease in blood flow. At the acme of contraction, the diastolic velocities disappear completely. An inverse linear relationship has been found between the intensity of the contraction, measured as the intrauterine amniotic pressure, and the degree of the end-diastolic flow. When intra-amniotic pressure exceeds 60 mm Hg, there is an elimination of end-diastolic flow velocity in all cases[23] (Fig. 73-5).

During the third stage of labor, PW Doppler studies of uterine arteries have shown that after a latent phase, during the contraction and detachment phase, there was a significant increase in the resistance to flow reflected by an increase in pulsatility index (PI).[24] Following placental separation, a slight uterine relaxation occurred, resulting in decreased resistance to flow in the uterine arteries. By using color flow imaging, the changes of blood flow between myometrium and placenta can be followed.[25] In cases with normal placental separation, blood flow between myometrium and placenta ceases immediately after delivery of the baby during the latent phase. In patients in whom manual removal of placenta was necessary, the blood flow continued into the placenta beyond the latent phase. Thus, color Doppler examination might be used to diagnose placenta accreta.

HUMAN FETAL BLOOD FLOW DURING LABOR

Umbilical Artery Blood Flow

According to several reports, the waveform indices of flow velocities (pulsatility index [PI] and A/B ratio; see Fig. 73-3) recorded from the umbilical artery of healthy fetuses in uncomplicated labor do not change during contractions or with the progression of labor.[21,26-28] This suggests that normal uterine activity in labor does not increase the vascular resistance on the fetal side of the placenta, which helps the fetus withstand the stress of labor. Fleischer and associates[29] found that the umbilical artery waveform did not change over a wide range of uterine pressures in

Figure 73–5. Changes of the Doppler velocity waveforms recorded from the uterine artery before, during, and after uterine contraction. (From Fendel H, et al: Z Geburtshilfe Perinatol *191*:121, 1987.)

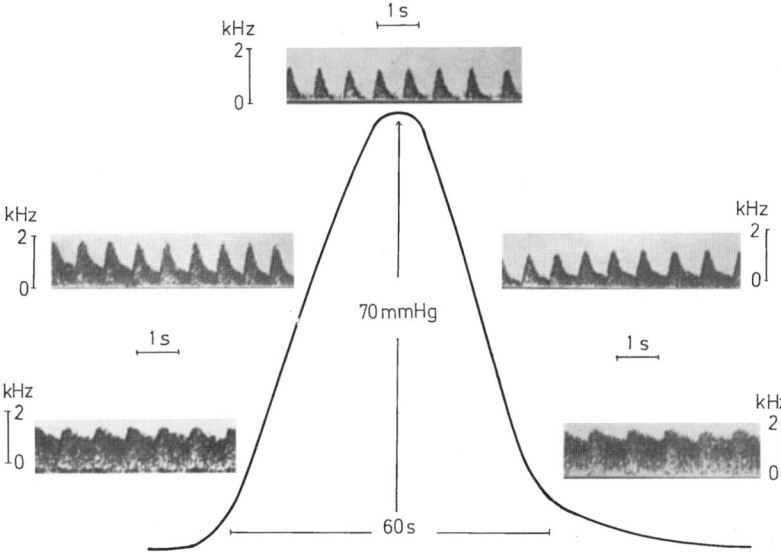

labor. Conversely, Malcus and co-workers[30] examined 575 fetuses in early labor and found a significant increase in the PI during contraction, compared with the recording taken before the onset of contraction. Nevertheless, the absolute difference in the PI was small and probably without importance for an undisturbed fetus. In fetuses with already compromised umbilical blood flow, however, such a slight increase in placental resistance might be of pathophysiologic and clinical importance. This is in agreement with the observation that fetuses that exhibit a lack of end-diastolic velocity during pregnancy often experience signs of distress in labor and frequently require operative delivery.[18, 31, 32] In a study that recorded umbilical artery waveform changes continuously through different stages of labor, a significant increase in systolic/diastolic (S/D) ratio was observed during contractions in the second stage of labor.[33] The increase in S/D ratio correlated well with a decrease in umbilical artery pH. No significant changes in the umbilical artery velocity waveform were observed during the first stage of labor.

In pregnant women with decelerations in the fetal heart rate (FHR) during contractions in labor, a concomitant increase in the PI,[26] or S/D ratio,[34] has been found. Sakai and colleagues[35] have found that the increase in the umbilical artery resistance index (RI) was particularly pronounced at downward and bottom stages of variable decelerations. During early decelerations or during contractions not associated with FHR decelerations, there were no changes in the resistance to flow. Tadmor and colleagues,[36] using computerized analysis of umbilical artery velocity waveforms, recorded an increase in S/D ratio and PI in about 50% of FHR variable decelerations. They have shown that in one group of pregnancies the increase in the resistance to flow preceded the decrease in FHR. In other cases, the deceleration was not preceded by a measurable increase in umbilical artery resistance. The investigators considered this to reflect impaired fetal oxygenation.

Operative delivery is significantly more frequent in patients with abnormal PI values. Brar and associates[37] compared the S/D ratio (see Fig. 73-3) in a group of patients with late decelerations with the S/D ratio in matched controls: The mean S/D ratio in the former group was significantly higher than that in the latter group. Among women with late decelerations, there was also a progressive increase in the incidence of adverse pregnancy outcome with increasing abnormality in the waveform. Patients with late decelerations and a normal umbilical S/D ratio had an incidence of adverse pregnancy outcome similar to that of controls. Murakami and co-workers[38] showed that the blood flow in the intra-abdominal part of the umbilical vein decreased in association with late and variable FHR decelerations. The reduction of blood flow was more pronounced with variable than late decelerations, and the blood flow change preceded the deceleration.

Feinkind and colleagues[39] performed a similar analysis of the relationships among FHR tracings and umbilical artery velocity waveform during the first stage of labor and outcome of pregnancy in 273 unselected patients. Both the umbilical A/B ratio and the FHR had similar low positive predictive values (30% and 23%, respectively). If the two methods were combined, the predictive value increased to 56%. In the study by Somerset and colleagues,[40] the positive predictive values for prediction of cesarean section for fetal distress were 31% for umbilical artery S/D ratio and 15% for admission FHR recording. The positive predictive value of the umbilical artery PI in early labor was also examined by Malcus and co-workers[30] and was found to be 19% for fetal distress and 15% for intrauterine growth retardation. Similar results have been subsequently reported by others.[41, 42] Rupture of membranes or amniotomy does not influence the umbilical velocity waveform.[28-30, 43]

Umbilical artery Doppler velocimetry has been shown to be a clinically useful test when applied for antenatal monitoring of fetal health in high-risk pregnancies.[44] However, the clinical studies on umbilical artery velocimetry in labor reviewed by Farrell and associates[45] do not seem to provide similarly convincing results. Therefore, this method has not found widespread clinical application in laboring patients.

Fetal Aortic Blood Flow

The fetal aortic volume blood flow, estimated on two occasions during the first stage of uncomplicated labor, has been shown to increase with progression of labor.[46] These measurements were performed between contractions, and the finding of increased fetal flow might be a phenomenon similar to reactive hyperemia in the uteroplacental circulation described in animals.[9] In the study by Lindblad and associates,[46] there was no change in the aortic PI with advancing labor, and there was no difference between patients with and patients without ruptured membranes. Fendel and colleagues[23] measured the mean fetal aortic velocity in labor and found a drop in the velocity during contractions. The aortic PI and resistance index (RI) remained unchanged.

Fetal Cerebral Blood Flow

The flow velocity in cerebral arteries of fetuses during uncomplicated labor has been examined using either CW[47] or PW[48] Doppler ultrasound. In both studies the transcervical access without imaging was used. Dougall and co-workers[47] did not find any change in the mean velocity or the RI of the anterior cerebral artery with advancing labor. During contractions, there was a fall in the diastolic velocities, suggesting that there might be an increase in the cerebral vascular resistance caused by head compression during contractions (assuming that the fetal cardiac output and blood pressure remain unchanged). The mean RI was 0.69 and 0.81 between and during contractions, respectively ($p < .001$). However, this finding was not confirmed by Maesel and colleagues[48] in the fetal middle cerebral artery.

More recently, several research groups have examined the fetal cerebral circulation in labor, using a combined two-dimensional real-time and PW Doppler ultrasound method. The waveforms of velocities recorded from the fetal internal carotid artery and middle cerebral artery were similar to those recorded antenatally.[49, 50] Furthermore, there was no significant difference in PI values of velocities recorded between and during uterine contractions.[50] In the late first and second stages of labor, there were lower values of PI in the middle cerebral artery, suggesting a decrease in impedance to flow in fetal cerebral circulation with progress of labor.[27, 51] It has been shown that fetal cerebral oxygenation decreases in the second stage of labor,[52] which might lead to vasodilation of the cerebral vascular bed. This has been confirmed by Sütterlin and co-workers,[53] who have measured fetal oxygen saturation simultaneously with Doppler waveforms of the fetal middle cerebral artery. They have shown that in fetuses with abnormal heart rate patterns and oxygen saturation < 30%, the PI and RI of the middle cerebral artery was significantly lower than in control fetuses. During uterine contractions in late labor, transient increases in the PI were observed in the fetal internal carotid artery[54] and middle cerebral artery[55] as an expression of higher intrauterine pressure, compared with that in early labor.

Fetal Ductus Venosus Blood Flow

Fetal ductus venosus blood flow velocity waveforms during the first stage of labor have been described by Krapp and colleagues.[56] They found that mean values of pulsatility index (PI) and peak velocity index for veins between contractions in normal term fetuses were 0.48 (SD 0.19) and 0.44 (0.18), respectively. During contractions, the mean values increased to 1.66 (0.85) and 1.46 (0.65), respectively. The investigators proposed that Doppler examinations of the ductus venosus in labor may be useful in at risk fetuses. So far, no further studies have been reported.

PHARMACOLOGIC EFFECTS ON UTEROPLACENTAL AND FETAL BLOOD FLOW IN LABOR

The possible effects on the fetal and uteroplacental circulation of drugs used in clinical obstetrics for treatment of preterm labor (tocolysis) or for obstetric analgesia in labor have been examined in a number of studies using various techniques. Ritodrine given to patients with preterm labor results in a significant decrease in the uterine and umbilical S/D ratio.[57] A concomitant increase in both the maternal heart rate and the FHR occurs, suggesting that the response of the S/D ratio might be secondary to the changes in the heart rate. In a study comparing the effects of nifedipine and ritodrine in preterm labor, no significant effect on umbilical artery Doppler velocimetry was reported for any of the two treatments.[58] On the contrary, Gokay and colleagues[59] reported a decrease in the umbilical artery PI during ritodrine infusion. In addition, they found a selective increase of left ventricular output, indicating a redistribution of fetal blood flow. Furthermore, there was an increase in PI of the fetal middle cerebral artery, which may be particularly important in the preterm fetus. In the study by Brar and co-workers,[57] magnesium sulfate tocolysis was not associated with any significant changes in the S/D ratio and maternal and fetal heart rate. Keeley and colleagues[60] observed a decrease in the uterine artery PI and an increase in the fetal middle cerebral artery PI during the administration of magnesium sulfate. They interpreted these findings as a "physiologic normalization process" related to the stressed preterm fetus during labor.

Treatment of preterm labor with indomethacin has been shown to cause a constriction of the fetal ductus arteriosus in about 50%.[61] In these cases, Doppler recordings showed very high ductal blood flow velocities. After discontinuation of the indomethacin, normal function of the ductus arteriosus usually returned. No increase in the ductal flow velocity was observed when a selective cyclooxygenase-2 inhibitor (celecoxib) was used in a comparative study by Stika and associates.[62]

Tocolysis with an oral dose of 30 mg nifedipine, followed by an additional oral dose of 20 mg after 4 hours, did not influence either fetal or uteroplacental circulation.[63] This is in agreement with the observation from a study of oral nifedipine in women with pregnancy-induced hypertension.[64]

Following epidural analgesia, there is a rapid uptake of local anesthetics in the maternal circulation and a rapid transport to the fetus. Epidural analgesia for labor uncomplicated by hypotension is, however, not associated with any alterations in placental blood flow as measured by placental scintigraphy.[65, 66] Fetal aortic blood flow in women receiving epidural analgesia during labor increases with advancing labor in a fashion similar to that in women without any obstetric analgesia. Furthermore, there are no signs of negative effects on the fetal circulation.[46] Several Doppler studies have examined umbilical and uterine artery S/D ratios in term parturients before and after establishing epidural block, and in none have any changes been found.[67-69] Similar observation was reported by Mires and co-workers[70] for women with normal pregnancy and uncomplicated labor. However, in women with pregnancy-induced hypertension, epidural analgesia led to a fall in maternal blood pressure and concomitant decrease in umbilical artery S/D ratio.[70] Oláh[71] studied the effects of an epidural top-up in labor and did not find any change in the umbilical artery PI. However, a transient increase in the uterine artery PI was observed, with a maximum at 15 minutes after the top-up. This change in uteroplacental circulation was preceded by an increase in the maternal femoral artery flow, probably causing a loss of circulating volume in the uterine circulation.

Pethidine crosses the placenta rapidly, and maximum concentrations are found in fetal scalp blood and umbilical arterial blood between 1 and 5 hours after an intramuscular injection to the mother.[72] Following the intramuscular injection of 75 to 100 mg pethidine, the fetal aortic blood flow has been shown to decrease.[46]

Considerable maternal plasma and fetal scalp concentrations of local anesthetics have been found 20 to 30 minutes after paracervical block.[73] Reduced placental flow has been proposed as the cause of the fetal bradycardia that is sometimes observed following paracervical block.[74] However, no change in the intervillous blood flow[18] or in the uterine artery PI[75] has been observed after paracervical block. As long as there was no fetal bradycardia, the umbilical artery PI remained unchanged.[75] In a recent study by Manninen and colleagues,[76] paracervical block initiated a significant increase in uterine artery PI, suggesting a vasoconstrictive effect.

FETAL HEART RATE IN LABOR

Rhythmic contractions of the fetal heart are initiated by electric stimuli generated in the pacemaker, the sinus node. The rate of cardiac contractions is subject to autonomic central nervous influences, humoral factors, and the metabolic condition of the myocardium. The main determinants of FHR are the sympathetic and parasympathetic nervous systems, which are in continuous counteraction. This interplay causes changes in beat-to-beat intervals, expressed as heart rate variability. The variability also reflects the function of the fetal central nervous system and shows cyclic changes related to fetal behavioral states. The variability changes due to fetal behavior continue even during labor.[77]

During labor, an increase in fetal blood pressure (e.g., caused by a compression of the umbilical cord) leads to bradycardia by initiating a vagal nerve reflex. Fetal hypoxemia can have a direct depressing effect on the function of the central nervous system and fetal myocardium, which can result in a decrease in, or even loss of, FHR variability. The complex effects of hypoxemia and developing acidemia on chemoreceptors of the fetus result in an increase of blood pressure and bradycardia.[78] During labor, signals of fetal heart action can be detected either transabdominally using a Doppler ultrasound transducer or, after rupture of membranes, transcervically with a fetal scalp electrode. From beat-to-beat intervals, FHR is calculated and recorded simultaneously with the signals of uterine activity as a cardiotocogram. Uterine activity is recorded either with an external tocodynamometer or with an intrauterine pressure catheter. Cardiotocography is widely used today as the preferred method for monitoring fetal health in labor.

FETAL ELECTROCARDIOGRAM IN LABOR

Fetal electrocardiogram (ECG) signals are easily obtained from the fetal scalp during labor. The early interest of researchers in revealing information on fetal myocardial function from the ECG was hampered by difficulties in obtaining signals of good quality and performing accurate waveform analysis.[79] Technologic developments have made it possible to design computerized techniques for improved isolation and analysis of fetal ECG signals.

In studies on animal fetuses, it has been shown that the ECG waveform is changed in a characteristic fashion with fetal hypoxia.[80,81] When the oxygen supply is insufficient to satisfy the energy needs of fetal myocardium, myocardial energy balance becomes negative, metabolism changes to anaerobic, and acidosis occurs. When the fetus compensates for hypoxia by additional glycogenolysis, there is an elevation in the ST segment of the waveform and an increase in the height of the T wave. This change can be quantified by calculating a ratio between the amplitude of the QRS complex and the T wave (T/QRS ratio), which in noncompromised fetuses does not exceed 0.25. In normal fetuses, there is a direct correlation between the PR interval and FHR. This relationship is inverted and the PR interval shortens[82] with fetal acidosis, which might enable distinction between FHR decelerations of various origins. The first studies on human fetuses during labor reported promising results, suggesting that changes in the fetal ECG waveform may be an early sign of fetal hypoxia.[83]

The clinical usefulness of this new method of fetal surveillance during labor has recently been demonstrated in two large randomized controlled trials.[84,85] In the Swedish trial comprising 4966 parturients, the cardiotocography plus automatic analysis of fetal ST-segment has been shown to reduce both the cord artery metabolic acidosis rate and the rate of operative delivery for fetal distress.[85] In addition, it was shown that cardiotocography plus ST-analysis provides information on intrapartum hypoxia, thus allowing for intervention in time and prevention of intrapartum asphyxia and neonatal encephalopathy.[86]

REFERENCES

1. Borell V, et al: Influence of uterine contractions on the uteroplacental circulation at term. Am J Obstet Gynecol *93*:44, 1965.
2. Ramsey EM, et al: Serial and cine-radioangiographic visualization of maternal circulation in the primate (hemochorial) placenta. Am J Obstet Gynecol *86*:213, 1963.
3. Ahlquist RP, Woodbury RA: Influence of drugs and uterine activity upon uterine blood flow. Fed Proc *6*:305, 1947.
4. Assali NS, et al: Measurement of uterine blood flow and uterine metabolism. V. Changes during spontaneous and induced labor in unanaesthetized pregnant sheep and dogs. Am J Physiol *195*:614, 1958.
5. Greiss FC Jr: Effect of labor on uterine blood flow. Observations on gravid ewes. Am J Obstet Gynecol *93*:917, 1965.
6. Lees MH, et al: Maternal placental and myometrial blood flow of the rhesus monkey during uterine contractions. Am J Obstet Gynecol *110*:68, 1971.
7. Harbert GM, Spisso KR: Biorhythms of the primate uterus (*Macaca mulatta*) during labor and delivery. Am J Obstet Gynecol *138*:686, 1980.
8. Woodbury RA, et al: Effects of posterior pituitary extract, oxytocin (pitocin) and ergonovine hydracrylate (ergotrate) on uterine, arterial, venous and maternal effective placental arterial pressures in pregnant humans. J Pharmacol Exp Ther *80*:256, 1944.
9. Hendricks CH, Quilligan EJ: Cardiac output during labor. Am J Obstet Gynecol *71*:953, 1956.
10. Ueland K, Hansen JM: Maternal cardiovascular dynamics. Am J Obstet Gynecol *103*:1, 1969.
11. Dawes GS: Fetal and Neonatal Physiology. Chicago, Year Book Medical Publishers, 1968.
12. Eik-Nes SH, et al: Ultrasonic measurement of human fetal blood flow. J Biomed Eng *4*:28, 1982.
13. FitzGerald DE, Drumm JE: Non-invasive measurement of human fetal circulation using ultrasound: a new method. BMJ *2*:1450, 1977.
14. Assali NS, et al: Measurement of uterine blood flow and uterine metabolism. VIII. Uterine and fetal blood flow and oxygen consumption in early human pregnancy. Am J Obstet Gynecol *79*:86, 1960.
15. Rekonen A, et al: Measurement of intervillous and myometrial blood flow by an intravenous ^{133}Xe method. Br J Obstet Gynaecol *83*:723, 1976.
16. Brotanek V, et al: Changes in uterine blood flow during uterine contractions. Am J Obstet Gynecol *103*:1108, 1969.
17. Eik-Nes SH, et al: Methodology and basic problems related to blood flow studies in the human fetus. Ultrasound Med Biol *10*:329, 1984.
18. Laurin J, et al: Fetal blood flow in pregnancies complicated by intrauterine growth retardation. Obstet Gynecol *69*:895, 1987.
19. Fendel H, et al: Doppleruntersuchungen des arteriellen uterinen Flows während der Wehentätigkeit. Z Geburtshilfe Perinatol *188*:64, 1984.
20. Janbu T, et al: Blood velocities in the uterine artery in humans during labour. Acta Physiol Scand *124*:153, 1985.
21. Brar HS, et al: Qualitative assessment of maternal uterine and fetal umbilical artery blood flow and resistance in laboring patients by Doppler velocimetry. Am J Obstet Gynecol *158*:952, 1988.
22. Takeuchi Y: Changes in arterial uterine blood flow velocity waveform during uterine contraction and relaxation in labor. Nippon Sanka Fujinka Gakkai Zasshi *42*:79, 1990.
23. Fendel H, et al: Doppleruntersuchungen des arteriellen uterofeto-plazentaren Blutflusses vor und während der Geburt. Z Geburtshilfe Perinatol *191*:121, 1987.
24. Maymon R, et al: Changes in uterine artery Doppler flow velocity waveforms during the third stage of labor. Gynecol Obstet Invest *40*:24, 1995.
25. Krapp M, et al: Gray scale and color Doppler sonography in the third stage of labor for early detection of failed placental separation. Ultrasound Obstet Gynecol *15*:138, 2000.
26. Fairlie FM, et al: Umbilical artery flow velocity waveforms in labour. Br J Obstet Gynaecol *96*:151, 1989.
27. Ghezzi F, et al: Doppler velocimetry of the fetal middle cerebral artery in patients with preterm labor and intact membranes. J Ultrasound Med *14*:361, 1995.
28. Stuart B, et al: Fetal blood velocity waveforms in uncomplicated labour. Br J Obstet Gynaecol *88*:865, 1981.
29. Fleischer A, et al: Uterine and umbilical artery velocimetry during normal labor. Am J Obstet Gynecol *157*:40, 1987.
30. Malcus P, et al: Umbilical artery Doppler velocimetry as a labor admission test. Obstet Gynecol *77*:10, 1991.
31. Gudmundsson S, Maršál K: Blood velocity waveforms in the fetal aorta and umbilical artery as predictors of fetal outcome—a comparison. Am J Perinatol *8*:1, 1991.
32. Rochelson B, et al: The significance of absent end-diastolic velocity in umbilical velocity waveforms. Am J Obstet Gynecol *156*:1213, 1987.
33. Abithol MM, et al: Continuous monitoring of Doppler umbilical artery waveforms in labor. J Matern Fetal Invest *2*:45, 1992.
34. Mansouri H, et al: Relationship between fetal heart rate and umbilical blood flow velocity in term human fetuses during labor. Am J Obstet Gynecol *160*:1007, 1989.
35. Sakai M, et al: Doppler blood flow velocity waveforms of the umbilical artery during variable decelerations in labor. Int J Gynecol Obstet *59*:207; 1997.
36. Tadmor O, et al: Analysis of umbilical artery flow parameters during fetal variable decelerations using computerized Doppler waveforms. Fetal Diagn Ther *14*:2, 1999.
37. Brar HS, et al: Fetal umbilical blood flow velocity waveforms using Doppler ultrasonography in patients with late decelerations. Obstet Gynecol *73*:363, 1989.
38. Murakami M, et al: Changes in the umbilical venous blood flow of human fetus in labor. Acta Obstet Gynaecol Jpn *37*:776, 1985.
39. Feinkind L, et al: Screening with Doppler velocimetry in labor. Am J Obstet Gynecol *161*:765, 1989.
40. Somerset DA, et al: Screening for fetal distress in labour using the umbilical artery blood velocity waveform. Br J Obstet Gynaecol *100*:55, 1993.
41. Chan FY, et al: Umbilical artery Doppler velocimetry compared with fetal heart rate monitoring as a labor admission test. Eur J Obstet Gynecol Reprod Biol *54*:1, 1994.
42. Chua S, et al: Search for the most predictive tests of fetal well-being in early labor. J Perinat Med *24*:199, 1996.
43. Bruner JP, Gabbe SG: Effect of amniotomy on uteroplacental and fetoplacental flow velocity waveforms. Am J Perinatol *6*:421, 1989.
44. Divon MY: Randomized controlled trials of umbilical artery Doppler velocimetry: how many are too many? Ultrasound Obstet Gynecol *6*:377, 1995.
45. Farrell T, et al: Intrapartum umbilical artery Doppler velocimetry as a predictor of adverse perinatal outcome: a systematic review. Br J Obstet Gynaecol *106*:783, 1999.
46. Lindblad A, et al: Obstetric analgesia and fetal aortic blood flow during labour. Br J Obstet Gynaecol *94*:306, 1987.
47. Dougall A, et al: Fetal anterior cerebral flow velocity waveforms during labour. *In* Gennser G, et al (eds): Fetal and Neonatal Physiological Measurements III. Malmö, Sweden, Dept Obstet Gynecol, 1989, pp 301–304.
48. Maesel A, et al: Cerebral blood flow during labour in the human fetus. Acta Obstet Gynecol Scand *69*:493, 1990.
49. Cynober E, et al: Fetal cerebral blood flow velocity during labour. Fetal Diagn Ther *7*:93, 1992.
50. Maesel A, et al: Fetal cerebral blood flow velocity during labor and the early neonatal period. Ultrasound Obstet Gynecol *4*:372, 1994.
51. Yagel S, et al: Fetal middle cerebral artery blood flow during normal active labour and in labour with variable decelerations. Br J Obstet Gynaecol *99*:483, 1992.
52. Aldrich CJ, et al: The effect of maternal pushing on fetal cerebral oxygenation and blood volume during the second stage of labour. Br J Obstet Gynaecol *102*:448, 1995.
53. Sütterlin MW, et al: Doppler ultrasonographic evidence of intrapartum brain-sparing effect in fetuses with low oxygen saturation according to pulse oximetry. Am J Obstet Gynecol *181*:216, 1999.
54. Fendel H, et al: Zerebraler Blutfluss unter der Geburt. Z Geburtsh Perinat *194*:272, 1990.
55. Ueno N: Studies on fetal middle cerebral artery blood flow velocity waveforms in the intrapartum period. Nippon Sanka Fujinka Gakkai Zasshi *44*:97, 1992.
56. Krapp M, et al: Normal values of fetal ductus venosus blood flow waveforms during the first stage of labor. Ultrasound Obstet Gynecol *19*:556, 2002.
57. Brar HS, et al: Maternal and fetal blood flow velocity waveforms in patients with preterm labor: effect of tocolytics. Obstet Gynecol *72*:209, 1988.
58. García-Velasco JA, González AG: A prospective, randomized trial of nifedipine vs. ritodrine in threatened preterm labor. Int J Gynecol Obstet *61*:239, 1998.
59. Gokay Z, et al: Changes in fetal hemodynamics with ritodrine tocolysis. Ultrasound Obstet Gynecol *18*:44, 2001.
60. Keeley MM, et al: Alterations in maternal-fetal Doppler flow velocity waveforms in preterm labor patients undergoing magnesium sulfate tocolysis. Obstet Gynecol *81*:191, 1993.
61. Moise KJ Jr, et al: Indomethacin in the treatment of premature labor. Effects on the fetal ductus arteriosus. N Engl J Med *319*:327, 1988.
62. Stika CS, et al: A prospective randomized safety trial of celecoxib for treatment of preterm labor. Am J Obstet Gynecol *187*:653, 2002.

63. Mari G, et al: Doppler assessment of the fetal and uteroplacental circulation during nifedipine therapy for preterm labor. Am J Obstet Gynecol *161*:1514, 1989.
64. Allen J, et al: Effects of nifedipine on isolated arteries and placental perfusion in the human uteroplacental unit. Clin Exper Hyper Pregn *B10*:353, 1991.
65. Husemeyer RP, Crawley JCW: Placental intervillous blood flow measured by inhaled ^{133}Xe clearance in relation to induction of epidural analgesia. Br J Obstet Gynaecol *86*:426, 1979.
66. Jouppila R, et al: Effect of segmental extradural analgesia on placental blood flow during normal labour. Br J Anaesth *50*:563, 1978.
67. Hughes AB, et al: The effects of epidural anesthesia on the Doppler velocimetry of umbilical and uterine arteries in normal term labor. Obstet Gynecol *75*:809, 1990.
68. Patton DE, et al: Maternal, uteroplacental, and fetoplacental hemodynamic and Doppler velocimetric changes during epidural anesthesia in normal labor. Obstet Gynecol *77*:17, 1991.
69. Ramos SE, et al: The effects of epidural anesthesia on the Doppler velocimetry of umbilical and uterine arteries in normal and hypertensive patients during active term labor. Obstet Gynecol *77*:20, 1991.
70. Mires GJ, et al: Epidural analgesia and its effect on umbilical artery flow velocity waveform patterns in uncomplicated labour and labour complicated by pregnancy-induced hypertension. Eur J Obstet Gynecol Reprod Biol *36*:35, 1990.
71. Oláh KSJ: Epidural analgesia—a cause of transient impairment of the uteroplacental circulation? Br J Obstet Gynaecol *98*:1174, 1991.
72. Tomson G, et al: Maternal kinetics and transplacental passage of pethidine during labour. Br J Clin Pharmacol *13*:653, 1982.
73. Puolakka J, et al: Maternal and fetal effects of low-dosage bupivacaine paracervical block. J Perinat Med *12*:75, 1984.
74. Greiss FC Jr, et al: Effects of local anesthetic agents on the uterine vasculatures and myometrium. Am J Obstet Gynecol *124*:889, 1976.
75. Räsänen J, Jouppila P: Does a paracervical block with bupivacaine change vascular resistance in uterine and umbilical arteries? J Perinat Med *22*:301, 1994.
76. Manninen T, et al: A comparison of the hemodynamic effects of paracervical block and epidural anesthesia for labor analgesia. Acta Anaesthesiol Scand *44*:441, 2000.
77. Spencer JAD, Johnson P: Fetal heart rate variability changes and fetal behavioural cycles during labour. Br J Obstet Gynaecol *93*:314, 1986.
78. Parer JT: Handbook of Fetal Heart Rate Monitoring. Philadelphia, WB Saunders, 1983.
79. Hon EH, Lee ST: The fetal electrocardiogram. I. The electrocardiogram of the dying fetus. Am J Obstet Gynecol *87*:804, 1963.
80. Greene KR, et al: Changes in the ST waveform of the fetal lamb electrocardiogram with hypoxia. Am J Obstet Gynecol *144*:950, 1982.
81. Rosén KG, et al: The relationship between circulating catecholamines and ST waveform in the fetal lamb electrocardiogram during hypoxia. Am J Obstet Gynecol *149*:190, 1984.
82. Murray HG: The fetal electrocardiogram: current clinical developments in Nottingham. J Perinat Med *14*:399, 1986.
83. Lilja H, et al: ST waveform changes of the fetal electrocardiogram during labour—a clinical study. Br J Obstet Gynaecol *92*:611, 1985.
84. Westgate J, et al: Randomised trial of cardiotocography alone or with ST waveform analysis for intrapartum monitoring. Lancet *340*:194, 1992.
85. Amer-Wahlin I, et al: Cardiotocography only versus cardiotocography plus ST analysis of fetal electrocardiogram for intrapartum fetal monitoring: a Swedish randomised controlled trial. Lancet *358*:534, 2001.
86. Norén H, et al: Fetal electrocardiography in labor and neonatal outcome: Data from the Swedish randomized controlled trial on intrapartum fetal monitoring. Am J Obstet Gynecol *188*:183, 2003.
87. Gosling RG, King DH: Arterial assessment by Doppler-shift ultrasound. Proc R Soc Med *67*:447, 1974.
88. Pourcelot L: Applications clinique de l'examen Doppler transcutane. *In* Peroneau P (ed): Velocimetric Ultrasonor Doppler. Paris, Inserm, 1974, pp 213–240.
89. Stuart B, et al: Fetal blood velocity waveforms in normal pregnancy. Br J Obstet Gynaecol *87*:780, 1980.

Ola Didrik Saugstad

74 Physiology of Resuscitation

Active resuscitation is required in 1 to 2% of newborn infants; one of five newborns requires intubation. Of the 130 million annual births globally, it has been estimated that 5 to 7 million newborn infants need some kind of intervention immediately after birth.[1-5] To perform an optimal resuscitation procedure, it is important to understand the physiologic events that occur as the fetus makes the transition from intrauterine to extrauterine life and the physiologic changes that occur during asphyxia and resuscitation.

It has been estimated that 50 to 70% of infants who require resuscitation at birth come from high-risk pregnancies, and therefore the need for resuscitation often can be predicted.[6] Nonetheless, at least 30% of babies who require resuscitation with endotracheal intubation come from apparently low-risk situations, a finding demonstrating the need for attendance by expert personnel within minutes after birth.

BASIC PHYSIOLOGIC CHANGES

Our basic knowledge of the physiologic changes during peripartum asphyxia and resuscitation comes from animal experiments in the early 1960s.[7] However, newer techniques, such as near infrared spectroscopy and proton spectroscopy, have taught us more about the sequence of biochemical and physiologic changes during and after an asphyxial event.

The classic data from Dawes and associates from experimental studies with rhesus monkeys is presented in Figure 74-1.[4, 5, 7] This well-known illustration represents the basis for our current understanding of the physiology related to asphyxia and resuscitation. These data also describe changes in pulse, respiration, and blood pressure and emphasize the difference between primary and secondary apnea.

In this model, rhesus monkeys were delivered by cesarean section, the umbilical cord was immediately tied, and the animals were prevented from breathing by immediately sealing their heads in a bag of saline. After a few shallow breathing movements, respiratory efforts stopped, and the animals developed primary apnea, which, in some cases, lasted for up to 10 minutes. However, after 1 to 2 minutes of primary apnea, gasping movements started and progressed with increasing vigor and frequency. These respiratory efforts were accompanied by thrashing movements of the extremities. In this period, spontaneous ventilation could still be induced by appropriate sensory stimuli. The heart rate decreased from 200 beats/minute in the normal fetal rhesus monkeys to 100 beats/minute. After 4 to 5 minutes, a series of spontaneous deep gasps occurred that gradually became weaker until the last gasp after approximately 8 minutes. Cardiac activity continued for 10 minutes or more before cardiac arrest. The period between the last gasp and cardiac arrest is known as secondary or terminal apnea.

Blood pressure initially increases during primary apnea, but it then abruptly decreases and reaches a plateau before declining during secondary apnea. The longer the period before the initiation of ventilation, the greater was the delay until the animal took its first spontaneous gasp. For every minute of delay in establishing assisted ventilation, the time to first gasp was delayed by 2 minutes, and the time to spontaneous rhythmic ventilation was delayed by 4 minutes (Fig. 74-2).[8]

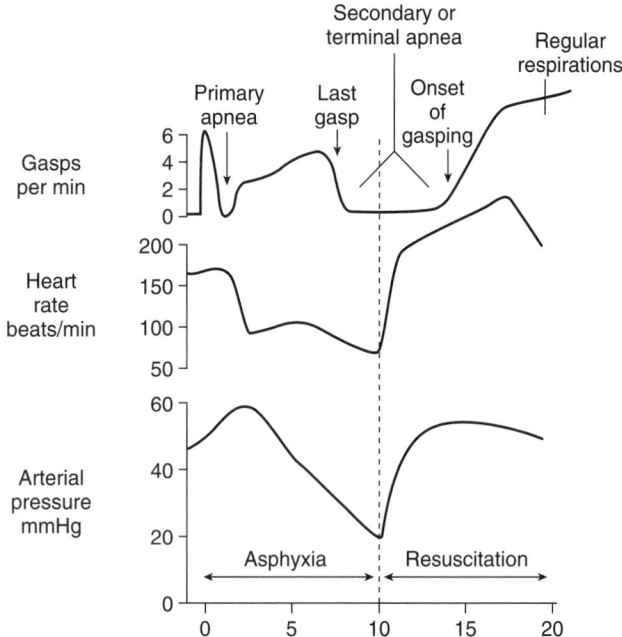

Figure 74-1. The relation between heart rate, blood pressure, and respiratory efforts in rhesus monkeys during asphyxia and resuscitation. (From Dawes GS, et al: J Physiol (Lond) *169*:167, 1963.)

During severe asphyxia, the pH drops from 7.30 to 6.80 within 5 minutes, which is primarily the result of an increase in arterial carbon dioxide tension of 10 mm Hg (1.3 kPa) per minute. By the end of secondary apnea, arterial carbon dioxide tension can exceed 100 mm Hg (>13 kPa), and serum potassium can rise to 15 mmol/L or more.[4]

The physiologic changes that occur with asphyxia and resuscitation were also assessed in a newborn piglet model in which hypoxia was induced by exposure to 8% oxygen (O_2), followed by 20 minutes of active resuscitation with different O_2 concentrations.[9-11] Although this model differs in several ways from human intrauterine asphyxia, it likely describes general principles in the physiologic response to neonatal asphyxia and reoxygenation. In this model, arterial oxygen tension (PaO_2) typically decreases to 20 to 30 mm Hg (3 to 4 kPa) within 5 minutes, with severe hypotension and lactic acidosis.[9-11]

Repetitive episodes of intrauterine hypoxia in animals cause global neuronal, cortical, midbrain, and cerebellar damage. Damage to the watershed areas between the areas of blood vessels supplying the cerebral cortex is commonly observed.[4] This is an important model because the human fetus may experience recurrent episodes of acute, total, or partial asphyxia before the start of labor, with recovery of biochemical abnormalities. Thus, severe asphyxial damage may occur without a decrease in fetal pH, and the child may have a normal Apgar score after delivery.[4]

RESPONSE TO RESUSCITATION

A newborn infant who does not breathe may have experienced birth asphyxia. However, apnea can also be caused by central nervous system depression resulting from maternal drugs, central nervous system injury, septicemia, anemia, primary muscular or neurologic disease, or congenital malformations obstructing the airways. Premature infants may not initiate respirations at birth because of muscular weakness or poorly compliant lungs.[4] These babies are often in need of immediate intervention, and there is a great need for a quick and easy way to assess the response of the resuscitative efforts.

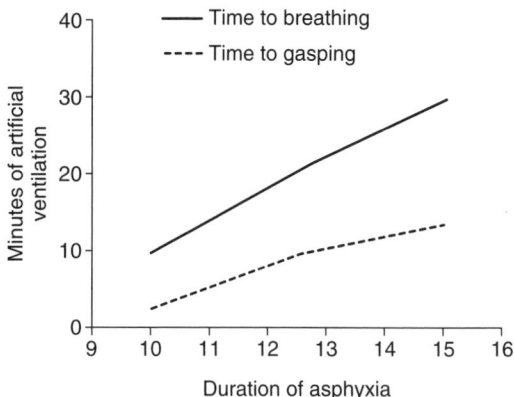

Figure 74-2. The relation between the duration of asphyxia and artificial ventilation until the first gasp and breath are detected. (Data from Adamsons K Jr, et al: J Pediatr *65*:807, 1964.)

Apgar Scoring

The Apgar scoring system is not the best means to assess the acute response of resuscitation, because it is taken first at 1 minute and then at 5 minutes. Moreover, most babies with an umbilical cord pH lower than 7.10 have normal Apgar scores; only when the pH is less than 7.00 are low Apgar scores commonly observed.[12] The five components of the Apgar scoring system (heart rate, respiration, muscle tone, reflex responsiveness, color) are indicators of different physiologic responses and therefore carry different significance. Heart rate and respiration are obviously more important than reflex responsiveness. Muscle tone represents higher cerebral function, whereas the other components, including heart rate, respiration, and reflex responsiveness, are brain stem responses.[4] Color is dependent both on respiration and heart rate. Rapid achievement of higher Apgar scores has, traditionally, been considered the hallmark of a successful resuscitation and persistent low Apgar scores may be related to poor prognosis.[13,14]

In a clinical study of 600 newborn infants who required resuscitation at birth because of bradycardia (heart rate <80 beats/minute) or apnea, the median 1-minute Apgar score increased from 4 to 8 within 10 minutes.[15] Table 74-1 shows the median Apgar scores in this population and the percentage with an Apgar score of less than 4 and less than 7, respectively. However, a controversy has arisen over whether resuscitation with room air is preferable, and in one study, the Apgar score was, in fact, higher in those resuscitated with room air compared with pure O_2.[15]

Heart Rate

The best way to assess the response to resuscitation is to count the pulse. This can be done by listening to the heart by stethoscope, or by palpating the pulse at the base of the umbilical cord. In infants with a 1-minute Apgar score higher than 6, the median heart rate at

TABLE 74-1

Changes in Apgar Scores the First 10 Minutes of Life*

1-min Apgar	5-min Apgar	10-min Apgar
4 (1-7)	7 (3-9)	8 (4-9)
40%[†]	6%[†]	3.4%[†]
94%[‡]	29%[‡]	13%[‡]

* Median (5th to 95th percentile) Apgar scores in 600 newly born infants needing resuscitation.

[†] Percentage with Apgar score < 4.

[‡] Percentage with Apgar score < 7.

Response to resuscitation—heart rates

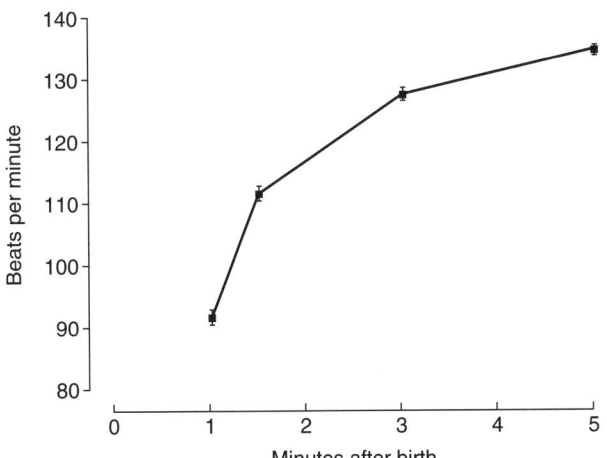

Figure 74–3. Heart rate development in newborn infants requiring resuscitation at birth. (Data from Saugstad OD, et al: Pediatrics *102*:1, 1998.)

1 minute was more than 130 beats/minute. Figure 74-3 shows heart rate responses, between 1 and 10 minutes of life, in a population of 600 newborn infants who required resuscitation.[15] Median heart rate was restored from about 90 to 114 beats/minute at age 60 to 90 seconds. From 3 minutes onward, heart rate remained stable (>130 beats/minute). The lower the Apgar score, the lower was the initial heart rate. When the Apgar score was less than 4 at 1 minute, the median heart rate was 80 beats/minute at 60 seconds and 100 beats/minute after 90 seconds. However, after 3 minutes, the median heart rate returned to a normal range. Table 74-2 shows median heart rates the first 10 minutes of life related to Apgar score at 1 minute.

In the population noted earlier, only 1.7% had a heart rate lower than 60 beats/minute after 3 minutes of resuscitation, and 1% after 5 minutes. In patients with persistent bradycardia, chest compressions are recommended, according to the current resuscitation guidelines of the American Heart Association, the American Academy of Pediatrics, and the International Liaison Committee on Resuscitation.[16, 17] In the study population

described earlier, chest compressions were performed in nearly 20% of cases, even though this approach was indicated in only 1 to 2% of the infants, a finding suggesting an inappropriate and overly aggressive approach in many cases.

Time to First Breath

The time to first breath and first cry (and to a normalization of the breathing pattern) is another simple means to assess the response to resuscitation. It has been reported that time to first breath is around 10 seconds in healthy full-term infants after vaginal delivery and 15 seconds after cesarean section.[18]

In the population of 600 infants noted previously, those with 1-minute Apgar score higher than 6 took their first breath at a median time of 42 seconds. There were no differences between term infants and preterm infants (>1000 g birth weight). Those resuscitated with ambient air took their first breath and cried significantly earlier than infants given pure O_2.[15] In term babies, median time to first breath increased to 90 seconds when the 1-minute Apgar score was less than 7 and 120 seconds if the 1-minute Apgar score was less than 4. Time to first breath was approximately three times longer when the heart rate at 1 minute was less than 60 vs 80 beats/minute. Table 74-3 shows the median time to first breath and cry related to 1-minute Apgar scores and heart rates at 1 minute. Data for room air, as well as infants resuscitated with 100% O_2, are given.

In another series of normal babies, the mean time to first audible cry was 36 seconds (with a standard deviation of 24 seconds). In asphyxiated babies needing resuscitation, first cry occurred in mean at 72 seconds with room air resuscitation and at 102 seconds for those resuscitated with pure O_2. The mean time to establish a regular, spontaneous respiratory pattern with effective respiratory movements (allowing a maintenance of heart rate and arterial O_2 saturation [SaO_2] greater than 90%) was less than 1 minute in normal, nonasphyxiated term infants, 4.6 minutes with room air resuscitation, and 6.6 minutes for infants resuscitated with 100% O_2.[19, 20] Therefore, as in studies in animals, pure O_2 inhibits respiratory activity in the newborn infant.[21, 22]

Oxygen Saturation

Another means to assess the response to resuscitation is to follow SaO_2 by pulse oximetry. Normal SaO_2 values for term infants during the first 10 minutes after birth have been reported. For infants

TABLE 74-2

Heart Rate and Arterial Oxygen Saturation in Relation to 1-minute Apgar Score*

	Min	1-min Apgar ≥7	1-min Apgar <7	1-min Apgar <4
HR	1	136 (85-156)	86 (40-140)	80 (10-131)
	1.5	140 (110-156)	110 (60-150)	100 (50-158)
	3	142 (120-167)	130 (80-163)	128 (69-160)
	5	142 (136-164)	140 (100-168)	139 (80-168)
	10	142 (120-169)	140 (110-170)	140 (100-174)
SaO_2	1	75 (57-82)	65 (40-82)	60 (40-81)
		57/79	*67/60*	*65/58*
	3	90 (65-98)	85 (59-92)	80 (41-94)
		65/90	*85/85*	*82/78*
	5	93 (84-98)	90 (68-95)	87 (62-96)
		86/95	*90/90*	*87/85*
	10	94 (88-96)	92 (80-97)	90 (72-97)
		88/95	*92/90*	*90/90*

* Median and 5th to 95th percentiles for heart rate (HR, beats/minute) and arterial oxygen saturation (SaO_2, %) according to 1-minute Apgar score the first 10 minutes after birth in 600 newborn infants requiring resuscitation at birth. Median values for SaO_2 are given separately also for *room air*/100% O_2 resuscitated, respectively.
(From Saugstad OD, et al: Pediatrics *102*: 1, 1998.)

TABLE 74-3

Time to First Breath and First Cry in Relation to 1-minute Heart Rate and Apgar Score*

	1-min HR >80	1-min HR <80	1-min HR <60	1-min Apgar >6	1-min Apgar <4
First breath	1.0 (0.25–5.0)	1.5 (0.25–27.4)	3.0 (1.0–44)	0.75 (0.25–2.1)	2.0 (0.6–30)
	1.0/1.33	*1.5/2.0*	*2.5/3.0*	*0.64/0.75*	*2.0/2.5*
First cry	2.0 (0.5–14.9)	2.1 (0.5–1032)	3.5 (1.5–>)	1.0 (0.5–2.4)	3.5 (1.0–>)
	1.5/2.0	*1.8/3.0*	*3.0/4.3*	*1.0/1.0*	*3.0/4.0*

* Median and 5th to 95th percentile time in minutes after birth to first breath and cry according to heart rate (HR, in beats/minute) at 1 minute after birth in 600 newly born infants requiring resuscitation at birth. Median values are given also for *room air*/100% O₂ resuscitated, respectively.
(From Saugstad OD, et al: Pediatrics *102*: 1, 1998.)

with a 1-minute Apgar score higher than 6, the median Sao₂ value increased from 75% (at 1 minute) to 90% after 3 minutes and to 93 and 94% after 5 and 10 minutes, respectively. When the 1-minute Apgar score was less than 4, Sao₂ values increased from 60% at 1 minute, to 80% at 3 minutes, and to 87% and 90% at 5 and 10 minutes of life, respectively (see Table 74-2). Surprisingly, the Sao₂ was identical either using room air or 100% O₂ for resuscitation—paradoxically, with a tendency to higher Sao₂ in room air–resuscitated infants. However, in children with a 1-minute Apgar score higher than 6, Sao₂ was significantly higher in those given 100% O₂ (90% versus 75% at 3 minutes and 95% versus 86% at 5 minutes, with no differences at 10 minutes). Supplemental O₂ therefore does not elevate Sao₂ faster than room air during the first 10 minutes of life in depressed infants, but it does in nondepressed infants. Table 74-4 shows the development in Sao₂ during the first 10 minutes of life according to 1-minute Apgar score. Figure 74-4 depicts the changes in Sao₂ in asphyxiated and nonasphyxiated term infants during the first 10 minutes of life.[23]

METABOLIC CHANGES

The changes in base deficit (BD) during hypoxia and reoxygenation in newborn piglets are shown in Figure 74-5.[11] The increase in BD exhibited a linear relationship with the duration of hypoxia. Hypoxia induced by the breathing of 8% O₂ results in a rise in BD of 0.4 mmol/L/minute compared with a rate rise of 0.67 mmol/L/minute when animals breathed 6% O₂. During reoxygenation, BD continues to increase or plateau during the first 5 minutes or so, most likely because of vasodilatation in peripheral tissues with release and washout of lactic acid and other metabolites. This phase is followed by a steady decrease of BD with a typical rate of approximately 0.17 mmol/L/minute

between 30 and 60 minutes and 0.12 mmol/L/minute between 60 and 90 minutes after onset of reoxygenation.[10-12] These data indicate that, depending on the severity and duration of the hypoxemia, it takes 2.5 to 4 times longer to normalize BD. A similar pattern and relationship have been observed for arterial hypoxanthine.

Figure 74-6 shows the changes in heart rate compared with BD in newborn infants requiring resuscitation.[24] The decrease of BD in human infants follows the same pattern and rate as in piglets, decreasing 6 to 7 mmol/L/hour. It can be inferred from this figure that heart rate changes represent a rapid response to successful resuscitation, whereas metabolic changes are slower indicators of the success of resuscitation.

In the brain, excitatory amino acids such as glutamate and aspartate increase in the striatum during hypoxia, and the concentrations double during the first minutes of resuscitation before a rapid decline. Normalization is reached within 15 minutes after start of resuscitation, but a secondary peak in these amino acids may be found several hours after asphyxia.[25]

The concentration of nitric oxide decreases in the brain during hypoxia and increases rapidly during reoxygenation, exceeding basal levels by approximately 40% (more so in infants resuscitated with 100% O₂ than those resuscitated with room air).[26] Hydrogen peroxide in lymphocytes in the sagittal sinus also increases during reoxygenation, although not when room air resuscitation is used.[27]

REGULATION OF BREATHING

Breathing in fetal life is controlled by several factors. It is inhibited at the brain stem level by humoral factors such as endogenous opioids, prostaglandins, and adenosine, and it is stimulated

TABLE 74-4

Changes in Arterial Oxygen Saturation According to 1-minute Heart Rate*

Min	1-min HR >80	1-min HR <80	1-min HR <60
1	70 (39–82)	60 (40–75)	45 (40–99)
3	85 (41–94)	85 (60–93)	76 (60–94)
5	90 (72–96)	90 (69–95)	80 (60–93)
10	93 (70–97)	90 (80–97)	90 (74–99)

* Median SO₂, % (5th to 95th percentiles) in the first 10 minutes of life according to heart rate (HR, in beats/minute) at 1 minute after birth in newly born infants requiring resuscitation at birth.
(From Saugstad OD, et al: Pediatrics *102*: 1, 1998.)

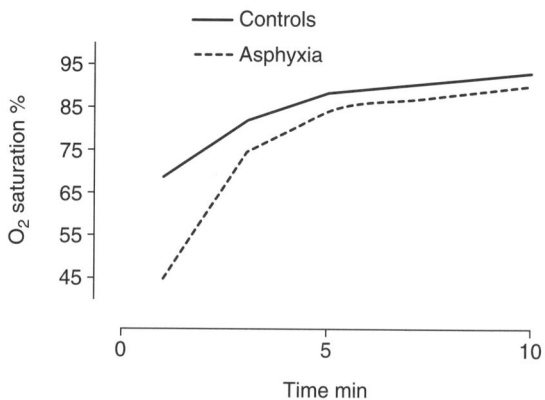

Figure 74-4. Development in arterial oxygen saturation in both asphyxiated and nonasphyxiated term infants after birth. (Data from Rao R, Ramji S: Indian Pediatr *38*:762, 2001.)

Base deficit

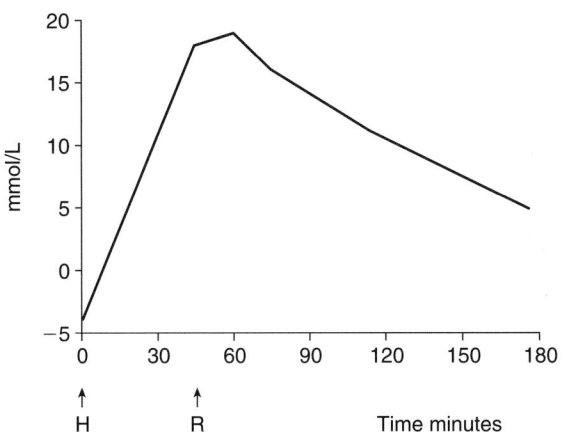

Figure 74–5. Development in base deficit in newborn piglets during hypoxemia (H; inspired oxygen fraction, 0.08) and during reoxygenation (R). (Data from Medbo S, et al: Pediatr Res *44*:843, 1998.)

Response to resuscitation: HR and BD

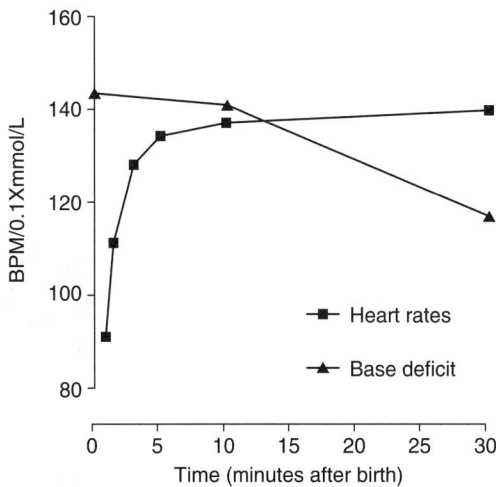

Figure 74–6. The change in heart rate (HR) compared with base deficit (BD) in newborn infants requiring resuscitation. (From Saugstad OD: Clin Perinatol *25*:741, 1998.)

by carbon dioxide, during active sleep. Hypoxemia completely inhibits breathing. During parturition, breathing movements are completely inhibited; however, severe asphyxia can induce gasping movements, resulting in the aspiration of meconium during delivery.[28]

The first breaths normally are vigorous, a finding suggesting a strong respiratory drive. Breathing is triggered by numerous mechanisms, such as removal of placental humoral inhibitory factors, cooling, catecholamine surge induction of genes encoding for substances important for breathing (e.g., substance P), and rising carbon dioxide concentrations. Because the set point for Pao_2 oxygen tension is relatively low after birth, it seems counterintuitive that a high O_2 concentration during resuscitation would delay the time to first breath. It takes 2 to 3 days until the set point of the peripheral chemoreceptors is increased to adult levels.[28]

EFFECTS OF FIRST INFLATIONS

Insufflation Pressure

The insufflation pressure needed to open the lungs after birth varies, but an opening pressure greater than 10 cm H_2O is rarely needed. In most babies, air enters the lungs as soon as the intrathoracic pressure begins to fall. In 80% of newborn infants needing artificial ventilation, this is satisfactorily achieved by bag and mask.[29]

When resuscitation is performed, one should use only the minimal pressure needed to achieve small chest wall excursions. Generally, peak intrathoracic pressures of 20 to 30 cm H_2O are required. However, an occasional infant may require pressures of 40 to 50 cm H_2O if air entry is poor.[30]

When positive pressure ventilation is applied to intubated newborn babies in need of ventilatory support immediately after birth, various reactions have been described. The most common response to lung inflation is the generation of a large positive intrathoracic (intraesophageal) pressure (≤82 mm Hg, 11 kPa). Head's paradoxical reflex is also commonly seen during bag and mask ventilation. This means that the inflation triggers an inspiratory effort, creating a negative esophageal pressure; levels up to 48 cm H_2O have been described. Such inspiratory efforts often produce a fall in inflation pressure. Occasionally, no change in esophageal pressure is observed.[31,32]

Poor Efficacy of Bag and Mask Ventilation

The efficacy of face mask respiration has been questioned. Tidal volume exchange is less than one-third of that noted with endotracheal intubation. Even when very high pressure is used, (≤40 cm H_2O) mean tidal exchange is less than in intubated babies. Face mask ventilation is helpful in establishing a functional residual capacity. Figure 74-7 shows expiratory tidal exchange with the first three breaths in infants ventilated by face mask versus those who were intubated. For the first breath, expiratory tidal exchange by face mask is only one-fifth of that measured in intubated infants.[33]

First Inflations in Premature Infants

The patterns described previously are probably not relevant for premature infants. In the smallest babies, heart rate and blood pressure quickly decline with the onset of hypoxemia. Furthermore, the response to resuscitative efforts in the preterm infant is affected by the state of surfactant sufficiency or deficiency. A few manual breaths with a high tidal volume (30 to 40 mL/kg) in premature, surfactant-deficient newborn lambs can induce lung injury. Large inflations at birth also cause an uneven surfactant distribution and may compromise the effect of surfactant. Therefore, it is extremely important to initiate ventilation gently in these babies.[34] In newborn infants less than 29 weeks' gestational age who received surfactant before the first breath, the median inspiratory pressure needed was 20 cm H_2O. Fewer than one-fifth of these infants needed more than 20 cm H_2O, and none needed more than 30 cm H_2O. The use of high inspiratory pressures may contribute to an increased risk of chronic lung disease.[34-36]

HEMODYNAMIC CHANGES

Systemic Blood Flow and Myocardial Function

Blood pressure follows a typical pattern during hypoxia and resuscitation, as described by Dawes and colleagues. In the newborn piglet model, hypoxia increases mean arterial blood pressure initially from basal levels of approximately 70 mm Hg before it starts to fall[9-11] (Fig. 74-8). During resuscitation either with room air or 100% O_2, a rapid restoration of blood pressure

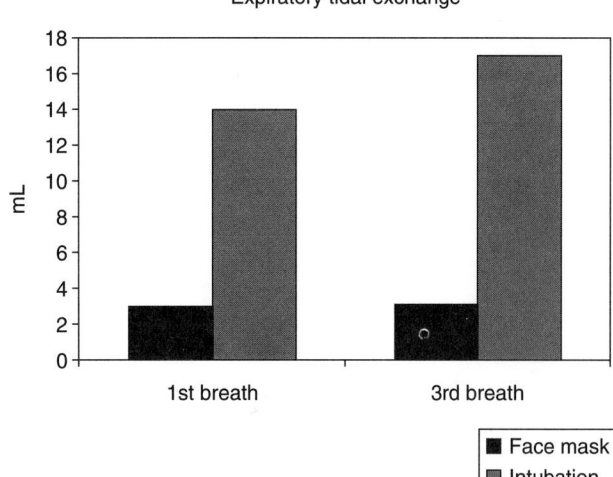

Figure 74–7. Tidal exchange in the first three breaths in term newborn infants ventilated with bag and mask versus intubated. (Data from Milner AD, et al: BMJ *289*:1563, 1984.)

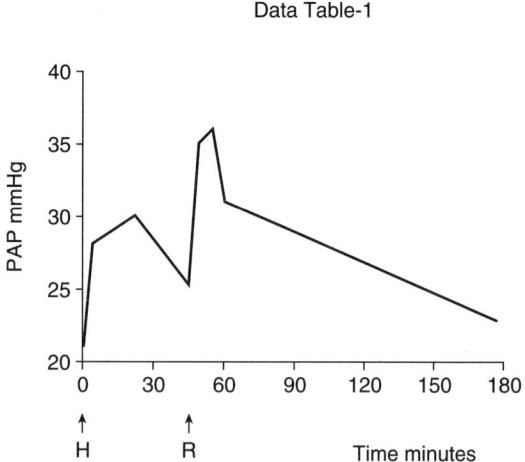

Figure 74–9. Change in pulmonary arterial blood pressure (PAP) in newborn piglets exposed to hypoxia (H) and reoxygenation (R). (Data from Medbo S, et al: Pediatr Res *44*:843, 1998.)

was observed within 5 to 10 minutes; however, there was often a secondary decline in blood pressure.[11] In this model, 2 hours after reoxygenation was initiated, some piglets needed inotropic support because of myocardial insufficiency, and markers of myocardial damage were found.[37]

Cardiac output follows a pattern similar to arterial blood pressure, with a 50 to 60% initial increase followed by a rapid decline, approximately 20 minutes after hypoxemia occurs. At the start of resuscitation, cardiac output was only about 50% of basal levels. However, resuscitation restored cardiac output quickly, and it reached levels approximately 30% higher than the basal levels (~180 mL/kg/minute). Subsequently, a relatively rapid decline was observed, to 30% lower than basal levels 2 hours after start of resuscitation. Relatively speaking, the blood pressure is maintained better than cardiac output during this period.[11] Systemic vascular resistance decreased by 25 to 50% during hypoxemia and increased to 75 to 90% of the basal level within 5 to 10 minutes after start of resuscitation.[11]

Pulmonary Blood Flow

Pulmonary artery pressure and vascular resistance also follow a biphasic pattern during hypoxia and reoxygenation, with a rapid increase in pulmonary vascular resistance during the first few minutes of hypoxemia, followed by a slower increase until a peak is reached at 50% higher than basal levels.[11] Pulmonary arterial pressure declines in parallel with cardiac output until the start of resuscitation. At that point, a rapid restoration of pulmonary arterial pressure is observed, sometimes even to higher than basal values (Fig. 74–9). Within 2 to 3, hours normalization of the pulmonary arterial pressure is found. However, in newborn infants who have inadequate responses to resuscitation, pulmonary arterial pressure may not decrease.

Pulmonary vascular resistance (Fig. 74-10) immediately rises (approximately threefold) from basal values during hypoxia, but it returns to basal levels within 5 minutes of resuscitation in piglets. In this model, the pulmonary vascular resistance does not differ whether 21 or 100% O_2 is used during resuscitation.[11]

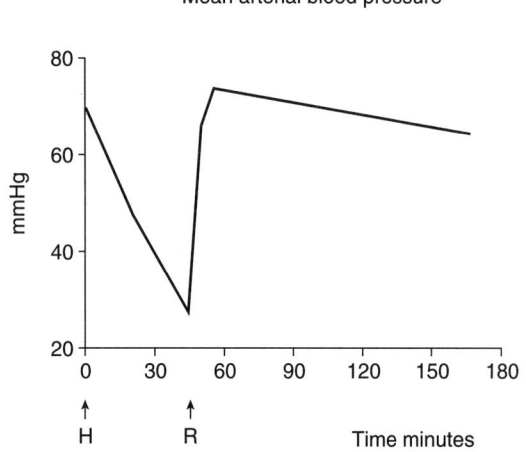

Figure 74–8. Change in blood pressure in newborn piglets exposed to hypoxia (H) and reoxygenation (R). (Data from Medbo S, et al: Pediatr Res *44*:843, 1998.)

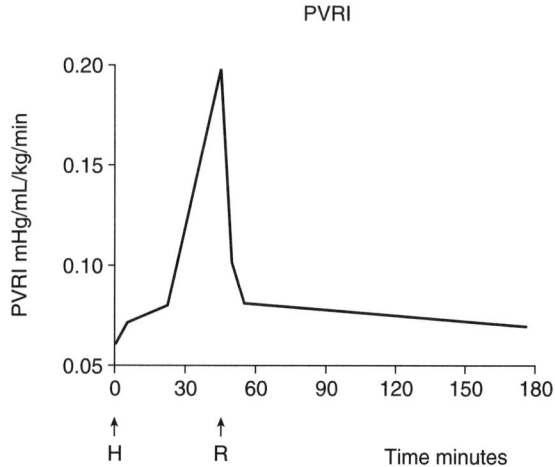

Figure 74–10. Change in pulmonary vascular resistance (PVRI) in newborn piglets exposed to hypoxia (H) and reoxygenation (R). (Data from Medbo S, et al: Pediatr Res *44*:843, 1998.)

Cerebral Blood Flow

Cerebral blood flow in newborn piglets, as measured by radio-labeled microspheres, increases initially during hypoxemia, but then it declines with persistent hypoxia. During successful resuscitation, cerebral blood flow is quickly restored.[38] Blood flow in the microcirculation quickly falls to zero both in the cortex and in the striatum of hypoxic newborn piglets.[26, 27, 39] During resuscitation, blood flow in the cerebral circulation is restored; however, it can take substantial time, and sometimes it never reaches baseline.[40] Resuscitation with 100% O_2 in piglets restored cerebral blood flow more efficiently than 21% O_2 when normocapnia was maintained. However, when resuscitation was performed in moderately hypercapnic animals, this difference was diminished.[39]

Premature infants randomized to receive either 80 or 21% O_2 a few minutes after birth experienced a 20% reduction in cerebral blood flow in 80% O_2 compared with babies breathing 21% O_2.[40] It is still unknown whether rapid or slower restoration of cerebral blood flow is best for the preterm infant. However, restoration of cerebral blood flow that is too slow obviously is not beneficial.

BRAIN OXYGENATION

Brain oxygenation can be assessed experimentally by continuous measurements with a Po_2 electrode in the brain region of interest. Clinically, near infrared spectroscopy can be used. During hypoxia, brain Po_2 quickly falls close to zero and is gradually restored during reoxygenation.

Near infrared spectroscopy measurements in newborn piglets showed that the so-called *oxygenation index* (change in oxygenated hemoglobin minus change in deoxygenated hemoglobin) rapidly declines to zero; however, 5 minutes after the start of reoxygenation, it is higher than baseline using 21 or 100% O_2. The oxygenation index is significantly higher with 100% O_2 than with room air resuscitation.[41]

After the onset of hypoxemia in newborn piglets, the Pao_2 in the sagittal sinus dropped from 40 mm Hg to zero. After reoxygenation, an overshoot was found during the first 15 to 30 minutes, more so in animals reoxygenated with 100% O_2 than in those reoxygenated with 21% O_2. Sao_2 values in the sagittal sinus also dropped to zero during hypoxemia (from an initial level of 50%) and rose to 70% and 90%, respectively, using 21% and 100% O_2 for reoxygenation.[41]

Employing near infrared spectroscopy, several investigations showed that cerebral blood volume increases markedly during hypoxia.[41, 42] The blood volume of the brain continues to increase after initiation of resuscitation, and it reaches a maximum at 5 to 10 minutes, returning to baseline values after approximately 1 to 2 hours.

CEREBRAL ELECTROPHYSIOLOGIC CHANGES

The electroencephalogram (EEG) becomes isoelectric within about 20 minutes in newborn piglets breathing 8% O_2, but variation is great, with the 25th to the 75th percentile ranging from 7 to 37 minutes. The EEG reappears during resuscitation within a median time of 2 minutes in animals resuscitated with 21% and 12 minutes if pure O_2 is used; however, those values are not significantly different. Within a 2-hour observation period, 75% of the piglets had EEG return to basal levels; of these, one-third had an abnormal pattern.[43]

Somatosensory evoked potentials also disappeared during severe hypoxia, but they reappeared in approximately 90% of the piglets during resuscitation. The amplitude increased steadily from zero at the beginning of resuscitation to approximately 25%

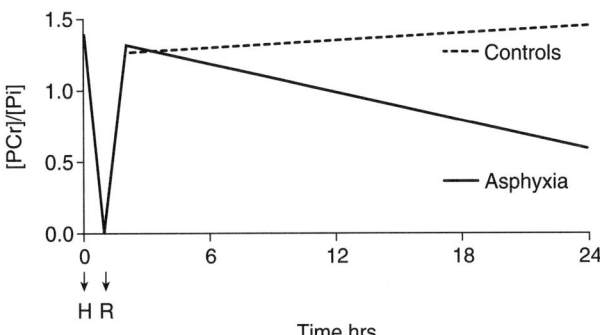

Figure 74–11. The ratio between phosphocreatinine (Pcr) and inorganic phosphate (Pi) in the newborn piglet brain assessed by proton spectroscopy during asphyxia and the postasphyxic period illustrating primary and secondary energy failure. H = hypoxia; R = reoxygenation. (Data from Lorek A, et al: Pediatr Res *36*:699, 1994.)

after 30 minutes and to 50 to 60% of baseline after 60 minutes, followed by a stable plateau. No differences were found regardless of whether 21 or 100% O_2 was used for reoxygenation.[38,43]

ENERGY STATUS IN THE BRAIN

Proton magnetic resonance spectroscopy of the newborn piglet brain revealed that pH, adenosine triphosphate, and phosphocreatinine rapidly decreased during hypoxemia.[42, 44] This is the so-called *primary energy failure*. However, during resuscitation, the energy status is quickly restored to normal levels. Typically, 8 to 36 hours later, a new gradual decline in the energy status of the brain occurs.[44, 45] This secondary energy failure is associated with irreversible brain damage (Fig. 74–11), a finding suggesting that there is a window for therapeutic options hours after restoration of the primary energy failure and before secondary failure occurs.

Using spectroscopy techniques, it has also been established that increased intracerebral lactic acid levels are detected weeks after the initial hypoxic insult. In newborn infants with brain injury after a hypoxic ischemic episode, high lactate levels persisted more than a month after birth, in contrast to those who developed normally in spite of a hypoxic insult. Further, this high lactate level has been accompanied by persistent alkalosis. Because alkalosis accelerates lactic acid production, this may be the cause of the elevated lactic acid levels detected.[46] Possible mechanisms leading to persistent cerebral lactic alkalosis are a prolonged change in redox state within neuronal cells, the presence of phagocytic cells, the proliferation of glial cells, or altered buffering mechanisms. An early (<18 hours after birth) elevation of brain lactate seems to indicate a poorer prognosis. It is now clear that brain alkalosis is a negative marker in the newborn infant with birth asphyxia, and the prognosis is best when moderate cerebral acidosis is present.[47]

REFERENCES

1. World Health Organization: Child Health and Development: Health of the Newborn. Geneva, World Health Organization, 1991.
2. World Health Organization: World Health Report. Geneva, World Health Organization, 1995.
3. World Health Organization: Basic Newborn Resuscitation: A Practical Guide. Geneva, World Health Organization, 1998.
4. Roberton NRC: Resuscitation of the newborn. *In* Rennie JM, Roberton NRC (eds): Textbook of Neonatology, 3rd ed. Edinburgh, Churchill Livingstone, 1999, p 241.
5. Bloom RS: Delivery room resuscitation of the newborn. *In* Fanaroff AA, Martin RJ (eds): Neonatal-Perinatal Medicine, 7th ed. St. Louis, CV Mosby, 2002, p 416.

6. Gupta JM, Tizard JPM: The sequence of events in neonatal apnea. Lancet 2:55, 1967.

7. Dawes GS, et al: Treatment of asphyxia in newborn lambs and monkeys. J Physiol (Lond) 169:167, 1963.

8. Adamsons K Jr, et al: Resuscitation by positive pressure ventilation and tris-hydroxymethyl-aminomethane of rhesus monkeys asphyxiated at birth. J Pediatr 65:807, 1964.

9. Rootwelt T, et al: Hypoxemia and reoxygenation with 21% or 100% oxygen in newborn pigs: changes in blood pressure, base deficit, and hypoxanthine and brain morphology. Pediatr Res 32:107, 1992.

10. Feet BA, et al: Effects of hypoxemia and reoxygenation with 21% or 100% oxygen in newborn piglets: extracellular hypoxanthine in cerebral cortex and femoral muscle. Crit Care Med 25:1384, 1997.

11. Medbo S, et al: Pulmonary hemodynamics and plasma endothelin-1 during hypoxemia and reoxygenation with room air or 100% oxygen in a piglet model. Pediatr Res 44:843, 1998.

12. Gilstrap LC, et al: Diagnosis of birth asphyxia on the basis of fetal pH, Apgar scores, and newborn cerebral dysfunction. Am J Obstet Gynecol 161:825, 1989.

13. Carter BS, et al: The definition of acute perinatal asphyxia. Clin Perinatol 20:287, 1993.

14. Nelson KB, Ellenberg JH: Apgar scores as predictors of chronic neurologic disability. Pediatrics 68:36, 1981.

15. Saugstad OD, et al: Resuscitation of asphyxiated newborn infants with room air or oxygen: an international controlled trial: the Resair 2 study. Pediatrics 102:1, 1998.

16. Kattwinkel J, et al: Resuscitation of the newly born infant: an advisory statement from the Pediatric Working Group of the International Liaison Committee on Resuscitation. Resuscitation 40:71, 1999.

17. Niermeyer S, et al: International guidelines for neonatal resuscitation: an excerpt from the guidelines 2000 for cardiopulmonary resuscitation and emergency cardiovascular care. International Consensus on Science. Pediatrics 106:29, 2000.

18. Vyas H, Milner AD, Hopkin IE: Intrathoracic pressure and volume changes during the spontaneous onset of respiration in babies born by cesarean section and by vaginal delivery. J Pediatr 99:787, 1981.

19. Vento M, et al: Resuscitation with room air instead of 100% oxygen prevents oxidative stress in moderately asphyxiated term neonates. Pediatrics 107:642, 2001.

20. Vento M, et al: Six years of experience with the use of room air for the resuscitation of asphyxiated newly born term infants. Biol Neonate 79:261, 2001.

21. Hutchinson AA: Recovery from hypoxia in preterm lambs: effects of breathing air or oxygen. Pediatr Pulmonol 3:317, 1987.

22. Mortola JP, et al: Ventilatory and metabolic responses to acute hyperoxia in newborns. Am Rev Respir Dis 146:11, 1992.

23. Rao R, Ramji S: Pulse oximetry in asphyxiated newborns in the delivery room. Indian Pediatr 38:762, 2001.

24. Saugstad OD: Resuscitation with room-air or oxygen supplementation. Clin Perinatol 25:741, 1998.

25. Feet BA, et al: Cerebral excitatory amino acids and Na^+,K^+-ATPase activity during resuscitation of severely hypoxic newborn piglets. Acta Paediatr 87:889, 1998.

26. Kutzsche S, et al: Effects of hypoxia and reoxygenation with 21% and 100% oxygen on cerebral nitric oxide concentration and microcirculation in newborn piglets. Biol Neonate 76:153, 1999.

27. Kutzsche S, et al: Hydrogen peroxide production in leukocytes during cerebral hypoxia and reoxygenation with 100% or 21% oxygen in newborn piglets. Pediatr Res 49:834, 2001.

28. Lagercrantz H, Wickstrom R: Perinatal control of respiration. In Greenough A, Milner AD (eds): Neonatal respiratory disorders, 2nd ed. London, Edward Arnolds, 2003.

29. Palme-Kilander C: Methods of resuscitation in low Apgar-score newborn infants: a national survey. Acta Paediatr 81:739, 1992.

30. Milner A: The importance of ventilation to effective resuscitation in the term and preterm infant. Semin Neonatol 6:219, 2001.

31. Boon AW, et al: Physiological responses of the newborn infant to resuscitation. Arch Dis Child 54:492, 1979.

32. Boon AW, et al: Lung expansion, tidal exchange, and formation of the functional residual capacity during resuscitation of asphyxiated neonates. J Pediatr 95:1031, 1979.

33. Milner AD, et al: Efficacy of facemask resuscitation at birth. BMJ 289:1563, 1984.

34. Bjorklund L, et al: Manual ventilation with a few large breaths at birth compromises the therapeutic effect of subsequent surfactant replacement in immature lambs. Pediatr Res 42:348, 1997.

35. Jobe AH, Ikegami M: Mechanisms initiating lung injury in the preterm. Early Hum Dev 53:81, 1998.

36. Stenson B: Resuscitation of extremely preterm infants: the influence of positive pressure, surfactant replacement and supplemental oxygen on outcome. In Hansen TN, McIntosh N (eds): Current Topics in Neonatology. London, WB Saunders Co, 2000, p 125.

37. Borke W, et al: Resuscitation with 100% O_2 does not protect the myocardium in hypoxic newborn piglets. Arch Dis Child Fetal Neonatal Ed 2003, in press.

38. Rootwelt T, et al: Cerebral blood flow and evoked potentials during reoxygenation with 21 or 100% O_2 in newborn pigs. J Appl Physiol 75:2054, 1993.

39. Sollas AB, Kalous P, Davis JM, Sangsted OD: Effects of recombinant human superoxide dismutase (rhSOD) and reoxygenation with 21% or 100% O_2 in asphyxiated newborn piglets. Pediatr Res 49:370A, 2001.

40. Lundstrom K, et al: Oxygen at birth and prolonged vasoconstriction in preterm infants. Arch Dis Child 73:F81, 1995.

41. Brun NC, et al: Near-infrared monitoring of cerebral tissue oxygen saturation and blood volume in newborn piglets. Am J Physiol 273:H682, 1997.

42. Wyatt JS, et al: Magnetic resonance and near infrared spectroscopy for investigation of perinatal hypoxic-ischaemic brain injury. Arch Dis Child 64:953, 1989.

43. Feet BA, et al: Early cerebral metabolic and electrophysiological recovery during controlled hypoxemic resuscitation in piglets. J Appl Physiol 84:1208, 1998.

44. Azzopardi D, et al: Prognosis of newborn infants with hypoxic-ischemic brain injury assessed by phosphorous magnetic resonance spectroscopy. Pediatr Res 25:445, 1989.

45. Lorek A, et al: Delayed ("secondary") cerebral energy failure after acute hypoxia-ischemia in the newborn piglet: continuous 48-hours studies by phosphorous magnetic resonance spectroscopy. Pediatr Res 36:699, 1994.

46. Amess PN, et al: Early brain proton magnetic resonance spectroscopy and neonatal neurology related to neurodevelopmental outcome at 1 year in term infants after presumed hypoxic-ischaemic brain injury. Dev Med Child Neurol 41:436, 1999.

47. Robertson NJ, Cowan FM, Cox IJ, Edwards AD: Brain alkaline intracellular pH after neonatal encephalopathy. Ann Neurol 52:732, 2002.

Shahab Noori, Philippe S. Friedlich, and Istvan Seri

75

Pathophysiology of Shock in the Fetus and Neonate

Cardiovascular compromise in the fetus and neonate often leads to severe organ injury or death, and the success of therapeutic interventions is limited by difficulties with accurate and timely detection of the condition, especially in the fetus, and the sensitivity of the developing organism to alterations in blood and oxygen (O_2) supply. Studies using animal models of fetal and neonatal shock have investigated the cause-specific pathophysiologic changes in the cardiovascular system and, although in much less detail, the cardiovascular response to therapeutic interventions. However, very little is known about the cellular effects of shock in the developing animal, and virtually no data exist for the human fetus and neonate. Extrapolation of animal data to humans must be done with caution in any case, and, because of the unpredictable impact of interspecies differences on organ development and maturational processes, extrapolation of data obtained in animal models of fetal and neonatal shock to the human fetus and neonate is even more prone to error.

CARDIOVASCULAR COMPROMISE IN THE FETUS

In the fetus, inadequate tissue O_2 delivery is most often caused by decreased blood flow to the uterus, the placenta, or the fetus. In addition, circulatory failure resulting from structural developmental abnormalities, infections, cardiac arrhythmias, and decreased O_2 carrying capacity of the blood also occurs, leading to development of hydrops and, unless intervention is successful, to fetal or neonatal demise. The studies on fetal shock have primarily employed experimental models of decreased blood flow or O_2 delivery, or both, to the fetus, and most of these studies have used the pregnant sheep model.

Developmental Changes in Fetal Gas Parameters

Under normal circumstances, hemoglobin O_2 saturation in fetal umbilical artery and vein is 50 and 75%, respectively.[1] Thus, the fetus is exposed to lower levels of oxidant stress compared with the newborn. Fetal O_2 tension (Po_2) and pH decrease and carbon dioxide tension (Pco_2) increase with advancing gestational age.[2-4] These changes are primarily driven by the increased O_2 consumption and associated CO_2 production of the growing fetus; the fall in the pH is secondary to the higher CO_2 production as gestational age progresses. Because O_2 carrying capacity also increases, total O_2 content in the fetal blood remains stable throughout gestation. However, although disputed,[4] fetal O_2 saturation has been found to decrease with advancing gestational age.[5] The decrease in fetal O_2 saturation is thought to result from the effect of decreasing pH and increasing Pco_2 on the hemoglobin-O_2 dissociation curve and a drop in Po_2.[5]

Oxygen Delivery, Oxygen Consumption, and Oxygen Extraction in the Fetus

Delivery of O_2 depends on blood O_2 content and cardiac output. In the fetus, regional O_2 delivery is unique because the O_2 content of blood flowing to the different organs varies significantly. Under physiologic conditions, despite the low fetal Po_2, O_2 delivery exceeds the metabolic demand of the tissues. The high cardiac index and hematocrit, the increased O_2 affinity of fetal hemoglobin, and the balanced distribution of cardiac output between the placenta and fetus all contribute to ensure appropriate O_2 delivery to the fetal organs.[1] In addition, the tight regulation of uterine and umbilical blood flow plays a major role in ensuring appropriate fetal O_2 uptake. However, reductions in uterine blood flow are relatively well tolerated by the fetus, and, in the sheep, decreasing uterine blood flow by as much as 50% does not adversely affect fetal blood gas parameters.[6] The increase in O_2 extraction is an immediate and effective mechanism compensating for the decrease in O_2 delivery in cases of reduced uterine blood flow.[7] O_2 extraction, defined as the ratio between O_2 consumption and O_2 delivery, is between 0.52 and 0.62 in the fetus.[5,8] Because of lower O_2 consumption in the immature compared with the more mature fetus, O_2 extraction is significantly lower during early gestation.[5,9] When O_2 consumption is increased up to 28% higher than baseline levels by the infusion of norepinephrine or thyroid hormone in the fetus, arterial or venous blood gas values remain unaffected.[10] This finding underscores that, despite the low PaO_2, the fetus is able to adapt to conditions associated with significant increases in O_2 consumption without evidence of disturbances in oxidative metabolism in the tissues.

Fetal Response to Hypoxemia

Lactic Acidosis in Fetal Hypoxemia

Under physiologic conditions, lactate level is higher in the fetal than the maternal circulation. The mild increase in fetal lactate levels is the result of enhanced placental lactate production and decreased fetal gluconeogenic utilization of lactate.[1]

Under pathologic conditions in which O_2 delivery decreases to the point at which compensatory increases in O_2 extraction and cardiac output have reached their limit to satisfy tissue O_2 demand, lactic acidosis develops. Critical O_2 delivery in fetal sheep appears to be at 12 mL/kg/minute, and decreases in O_2 delivery to less than this value are associated with impaired oxidative metabolism and the accumulation of lactic acid in the fetal tissues and blood.[11] Indeed, elevated plasma lactate has been shown to be a good indicator of fetal hypoxemia. After 4 to 5 hours of fetal hypoxemia, blood lactate reaches a plateau despite continued anaerobic metabolism. The placental clearance of lactate is responsible for this phenomenon.[7] Thus, despite the ongoing fetal anaerobic metabolism in cases of chronic and severe fetal hypoxemia, the fetal serum lactate level does not rise beyond the point of equilibrium.[7]

The fetus responds differently to various levels of severity of hypoxia. Maternal hypoxia-induced mild fetal hypoxia does not alter fetal acid-base balance when fetal arterial O_2 saturations remain in the 40% range even when the hypoxemia persists for 24 hours.[12] Conversely, when fetal hypoxia results in fetal arterial O_2 saturations of less than 30%, metabolic acidosis develops.[13] Thus, the *critical threshold of arterial O_2 saturation,* defined as the arterial O_2 saturation below which metabolic acidosis develops, is around 30% in the maternal hypoxia-induced fetal hypoxia model in the sheep. It appears that susceptibility of the fetus to hypoxia is developmentally regulated; the preterm fetus is less sensitive to the effects of maternal hypoxia than its term counterpart.[13,14] For instance, when maternal hypoxia results in fetal arterial O_2 saturations of less than 30%, the preterm ovine fetus develops metabolic acidosis at a much slower pace[14] than that described for the fetus near or at term.[14]

The fetus also appears to respond differently to various causes of hypoxia.[15] When fetal hypoxemia is induced by umbilical cord occlusion, the fetal response differs from that seen with maternal hypoxia.[16] When fetal hypoxemia is caused by umbilical cord occlusion, metabolic acidosis develops more rapidly compared with that maternal hypoxia-induced fetal hypoxia.[16] The lack of placental compensatory mechanisms in the cord occlusion model may be responsible for this difference. Finally, the fetal response to hypoxemia is also altered when hypoxia is caused by decreased uterine blood flow. In this model, the critical threshold of arterial O_2 saturation is lower than in the maternal hypoxia or cord occlusion models, and rapid lactate accumulation and fall in pH only occur when fetal O_2 saturation is in the 15 to 20% range.[17] This finding suggests that placental compensatory mechanisms remain effective when blood flow to the uterus is decreased. Because of interspecies differences, these findings obtained in the sheep should be translated to the human fetus with caution.

Endocrine Responses to Fetal Hypoxemia

In the fetus, acute hypoxemia is associated with an increase in the plasma concentration of several hormones including adrenocorticotropic hormone,[18-20] β-endorphin,[21,22] vasopressin,[23-25] glucocorticoids,[18,20] norepinephrine, and epinephrine.[17,25,26] This stress hormone response facilitates fetal adaptation to hypoxemia in part by ensuring the redistribution of blood flow to vital organs.[27]

However, the effectiveness of the fetal stress hormone response is limited by the developmentally regulated immaturity of certain endocrine organs and the cellular mechanisms of end-organ responses. For instance, although the fetal adrenal glands increase cortisol secretion in response to hypoxemic stress, the increase in the cortisol level is significantly less, whereas the increase in the catecholamine levels is similar to that seen in the mature animal.[17] In addition, expression of the cardiovascular adrenergic receptors and second-messenger systems is developmentally regulated, contributing to the observed differences in the stress response between the fetus and the mature animal.

The exact mechanisms of the 50- to 1000-fold increase in fetal catecholamine release to fetal stress remain to be clarified. One study[28] investigated the effect of metabolic acidosis on adrenal catecholamine secretion. In an effort to avoid the adrenal stimulatory effect of hypoxemia associated with acidosis-induced rightward shift in oxyhemoglobin dissociation curve, 100% O_2 was administered to the pregnant ewe during the infusion of 30% lactic acid to the fetus. Under these experimental circumstances, metabolic acidosis in the absence of hypoxia did not stimulate adrenal catecholamine secretion. Conversely, studies investigating fetal catecholamine release in the presence of hypoxemia have reported increased catecholamine and vasopressin secretion in the presence or absence of associated metabolic acidosis.[25, 29]

Cardiovascular Effects of Fetal Hypoxemia

In the fetus, the right and left ventricles work in series, and therefore the combined left and right cardiac output is considered the total cardiac output. In the fetal lamb, the combined cardiac output is 450 mL/kg/minute, to which the right and left ventricles contribute 300 and 150 mL/kg/minute, respectively.[30] Similarly, in the human fetus, the contribution of the right ventricle to the combined cardiac output is significantly higher than that of the left ventricle.

In the fetal lamb, the cardiovascular response to acute hypoxemia is characterized by the rapid development of hypertension, bradycardia, increased peripheral vascular resistance, and a 15 to 20% decrease in the cardiac output. The decrease in cardiac output is primarily the result of the increased peripheral vascular resistance (afterload), bradycardia, vagal stimulation, and myocardial depression. However, significant myocardial depression occurs only if the hypoxemia is severe or prolonged or is associated with metabolic acidosis.[27] In the fetus, adenosine may play an important modulatory role in the previously described cardiovascular "maladaptation" by influencing fetal autonomic and glycolytic responses to hypoxia. In the sheep, blockade of the adenosine receptors during fetal hypoxia significantly attenuates the development of hypertension (systemic vascular resistance increase), bradycardia, and metabolic acidosis.[31,32] The fetal cardiovascular response to prolonged hypoxemia is different from that seen in the acute hypoxemia models. In fetal sheep with sustained hypoxemia, cardiac output drops progressively to 38%, and, not unexpectedly, right ventricular output is compromised earlier than the left ventricular output.[33]

In response to fetal hypoxemia, distribution of cardiac output and venous return is altered in an effort to maintain perfusion and O_2 delivery to the vital organs such as the heart, brain, and adrenal glands.[34-36] During induced maternofetal hypoxia, the percentage of systemic venous blood recirculated to the fetal body and not sent to the placenta for oxygenation is decreased, whereas the proportion of umbilical venous blood contributing to fetal cardiac output is increased from 27 to 39%.[34] As mentioned earlier, there are differences in the fetal response including the distribution of cardiac output, venous return, and O_2 delivery among the different models of fetal hypoxia. However, regardless of the cause of hypoxia, the blood flow and O_2 delivery to the heart, brain, and adrenal glands are maintained, and the proportion of umbilical venous blood bypassing the liver via ductus venosus is increased in all cases.[34-36]

Finally, the fetal cardiovascular and endocrine response to acute hypoxemia is altered when repeated hypoxic events occur. This is important because recurrence of hypoxic insults to the fetus may not be infrequent in human pregnancies in which blood flow to the uterus, placenta, or the fetus is repeatedly compromised. It appears that prevailing hypoxemia sensitizes the cardiac and vasoconstrictor chemoreflex responses because enhanced femoral vasoconstriction and marked elevation in plasma norepinephrine and vasopressin have been demonstrated in response to acute hypoxemia in fetal sheep that were previously exposed to sustained hypoxemia.[37]

Renal Responses to Hypoxemia

Although the placentomaternal unit performs most of the effective compensatory functions,[38] the fetal kidney has the ability to contribute to the maintenance of fetal acid-base balance. For instance, ammonium excretion and hence generation of bicarbonate as well as sodium excretion increase during the recovery period from hypocapnic hypoxia in the fetal sheep.[39] The possible reason that the foregoing fetal renal compensatory changes only occur during the recovery period from acute hypocapnic hypoxia is the hypocapnia itself. Because fetal P_{CO_2} is low as a result of maternal compensatory hyperventilation to hypoxia in this model and because CO_2 is required for bicarbonate absorption in the proximal tubule, bicarbonate reabsorption and acid excretion in the fetus are delayed until hypoxemia subsides and maternal, and thus fetal, P_{CO_2} returns to normal.

In addition to the effects of hypoxemia on the renal compensatory mechanisms maintaining fetal acid-base balance, there are other changes in renal function induced by hypoxemia. Fractional excretion of sodium is increased by a decrease in proximal tubule sodium reabsorption.[39, 40] Urine osmolality also increases, and free water clearance drops secondary to increases in vasopressin release.[39, 41] Finally, like the other organs, the immature kidney is also less susceptible to hypoxemia than the mature kidney.[42] The renal response to lactic acidosis induced by acid infusion in the fetal sheep is confined to tubular adaptive responses with decreases in urine pH and increases in ammonium and titratable acid excretion without changes in glomerular filtration rate.[43]

CARDIOVASCULAR COMPROMISE IN THE NEONATE

Definition and Phases of Neonatal Shock

Shock develops when O_2 delivery to the tissues is inadequate to satisfy cellular metabolic demand. Independent of the origin, there are three phases of shock, and each phase is characterized by unique pathophysiologic changes.

In the *compensated phase*, vital organ function is maintained by intrinsic neurohormonal compensatory mechanisms resulting in distribution of organ blood flow primarily to the heart, brain, and adrenal glands and away from other "nonvital" organs. Several hormones and local factors affecting myocardial function, organ blood flow distribution, capillary integrity, systemic and pulmonary vascular resistance, and cellular metabolism are released during this phase. Stroke volume, central venous pressure, and urine output all decrease. However, blood pressure remains within normal limits because the increases in myocardial contractility and heart rate maintain cardiac output close to the normal range. Because blood pressure is the function of blood flow and systemic vascular resistance, blood pressure may not always appropriately reflect the status of organ blood flow in this phase. This observation especially concerns the nonacidotic extremely low birth weight preterm neonate with immature myocardium and compensated shock during the first postnatal day.[44, 45] In addition, the developing cerebral cortex of the extremely low birth weight preterm neonate may function as a "nonvital" organ with low-priority circulation resulting in vasoconstriction and decreased cortical perfusion in cases with low cardiac output,[46] just like the vasoconstriction that occurs to maintain blood pressure in the traditional "nonvital" organs (e.g., skin, muscle, kidney, liver, mesenterium). Thus, in these patients, blood flow to the brain stem and not to the entire brain may be maintained only during the compensated phase of shock.

If the circulatory compromise is not recognized and treated, neonatal shock will enter the *uncompensated phase,* in which failure of the intrinsic neurohormonal compensatory mechanisms results in decreased microvascular perfusion, myocardial contractility, stroke volume, and blood pressure, with ensuing significant decreases in organ blood flow and tissue perfusion and lactic acidosis. If treatment is delayed or the condition is prone to rapid deterioration, such as in fulminant sepsis, myocarditis, or asphyxia with multiorgan failure, neonatal shock will enter the final and *irreversible phase,* in which cellular damage leading to complete organ failure dominates the clinical picture, and death occurs invariably.

Factors in the Pathophysiology of Shock at the Cellular and Molecular Level

Reactive Oxygen Species

These molecules are involved in initiation and amplification of cellular injury in shock. Under normal conditions, the redox coupling reactions generate water as a result of complete O_2 reduction with only minimal (1%) univalent O_2 reduction ($O^{\bullet}_2{}^-$).[47] However in shock, $O^{\bullet}_2{}^-$ is significantly increased.[48] Ischemia and hypoxia result in accumulation of electron donor compounds such as reduced nicotinamide adenine dinucleotide secondary to impairment of oxidative phosphorylation in the mitochondria.[48] Subsequent reperfusion then leads to enhanced reactive O_2 species production by the enhanced availability of the electron acceptor O_2.

Furthermore, because anaerobic metabolism leads to inadequate production of adenosine triphosphate (ATP), hypoxanthine and xanthine accumulate. Under normal physiologic conditions, hypoxanthine is oxidized to urate by xanthine dehydrogenase and xanthine oxidase, with the latter generating $O^{\bullet}_2{}^-$ and H_2O_2 as byproducts. During ischemia-reperfusion, cellular changes favor hypoxanthine oxidation by xanthine oxidase, with a resultant significant increase in the production of reactive O_2 species. Reactive O_2 species cause cellular injury via their adverse effects on different cellular structures that lead to polysaccharide depolymerization, lipid peroxidation,[49] alterations in the primary structure of amino acids,[50] and nucleic acid oxidation.[51] These effects impair the cellular adhesion and receptor physiology, disrupt cell membrane integrity[49] and the function of many enzymes,[50] and damage DNA,[51] respectively. The fetus and neonate are prone to develop severe cellular injury during the ischemia-reperfusion cycle because they have immature antioxidant defenses.

Nitric Oxide

Under physiologic conditions, nitric oxide (NO) plays an important role in the regulation of vascular tone. However, under pathologic conditions, inducible NO synthase (iNOS) is up-regulated by endotoxin and proinflammatory cytokines, and large amounts of NO are produced.[52, 53] Overproduction of NO by iNOS has been implicated in pathogenesis of shock in pediatric patients including newborn infants.[54, 55] Excessive production of NO then leads to hypotension, decreased vascular response to vasoconstrictor hormones, and myocardial dysfunction.[52] In addition to the adverse cardiovascular effects, NO can cause direct cellular injury through formation of reactive free radicals such as peroxynitrite[56] and by inhibiting mitochondrial respiratory function.[57]

Because excess NO is involved in pathogenesis of shock, studies have focused on testing therapeutic modalities that inhibit NOS as a possible treatment strategy, especially in septic shock. However, the use of nonselective NOS inhibitors that inhibit both endothelial (e)NOS and iNOS has resulted in delete-

rious effects in immature[58] and mature animal models of shock and increased mortality in human adults with septic shock.[59, 60] In contrast, selective inhibition of iNOS improves hypotension and lactic acidosis in the mature canine endotoxic shock model.[61] However, whether selective iNOS inhibition is helpful in treatment of neonatal shock remains to be elucidated.[62]

Platelet-Activating Factor

This phospholipid mediator has been implicated in pathogenesis of shock in both animal models[63, 64] and adult subjects.[65] In animal models of septic shock, animals treated with a platelet-activating factor antagonist showed improvement in their cardiovascular status.[66, 67] Although there is no study on the role of platelet-activating factor in neonatal shock, its association with necrotizing enterocolitis is well documented.[68, 69]

Eicosanoids

In inflammation, arachidonic acid derived from cell membrane phospholipids is metabolized by cyclooxygenase or lipoxygenase to produce inflammatory mediators such as prostaglandins, thromboxanes, and leukotrienes. Although eicosanoids have been implicated in the pathogenesis of organ failure and shock, their exact role remains to be elucidated. Rats deficient in essential fatty acid, and thus unable to produce significant amounts of eicosanoids, are much less susceptible to endotoxic shock and have significantly improved survival rate compared with wild-type rats.

Eicosanoids, such as the predominantly vasodilator prostacyclin and prostaglandin E_2, and the vasoconstrictor thromboxane A_2, play an important role in the regulation of vascular tone. Some eicosanoids (thromboxane A_2) induce platelet and neutrophil aggregation and thus have significant proinflammatory effects, whereas others, such as prostaglandin E_2, also exert an antiinflammatory action by down-regulating cytokine release by macrophages and lymphocytes. Indeed, there are both animal and human data supporting the role of prostaglandins as both proinflammatory and antiinflammatory agents. In animals with hypovolemic shock, administration of prostacyclin and prostaglandin E_1 and E_2 improves cardiovascular status.[70, 71] Conversely, in the septic human and animal, inhibition of cyclooxygenase may improve both the cardiovascular status and survival.[72, 73]

Studies in animal models and humans have also shown that the levels of thromboxane B_2, a metabolite of thromboxane A_2, are increased in septic shock.[74, 75] In addition to its proinflammatory and vasoconstrictor effects, thromboxane A_2 may have a direct myocardial depressant effect, and therefore it may significantly compromise cardiac output.[74]

Other Factors

Among other factors with potential clinical importance in shock, nuclear factor-κB (NF-κB) has been suggested to have a prognostic value. In patients with septic shock, a higher peripheral mononuclear cell NF-κB activity is associated with increased mortality.[76] It is not known whether this is an association or a causative relationship.

Down-Regulation of Adrenergic Receptors

Down-regulation of the adrenergic receptors and second-messenger systems in cases of critical illness and exogenous catecholamine administration,[77] as well as a relative or absolute adrenal insufficiency,[78] have emerged as probable causative factors in adults[79] and neonates[80] for the development of pressor-resistant shock. Because expression of the cardiovascular adrenergic receptors and some components of their second-messenger systems is inducible by glucocorticoids,[81] steroid administration offers a powerful clinical tool to reverse the effects of adrenergic receptor down-regulation.[79, 80] These genomic effects of steroids resulting in the synthesis and membrane assembly of new receptor proteins require at least several hours to take place. However, improvement in cardiovascular function occurs within 1 to 2 hours after hydrocortisone administration to neonates.[80] This finding can be explained by the observations that steroids also exert certain nongenomic actions, which affect the cardiovascular system without delay. Glucocorticoids inhibit the catechol-O-methyltransferase, the rate-limiting enzyme in catecholamine metabolism, and decrease the reuptake of norepinephrine by the sympathetic nerve endings, leading to increases in the plasma concentration of catecholamines.[82] Physiologic doses of mineralocorticoids and, to a lesser degree, pharmacologic doses of glucocorticoids also instantly increase cytosolic calcium availability in myocardial and vascular smooth muscle cells by acting via putative cell membrane-bound specific steroid receptors.[82] In addition, steroids inhibit prostacyclin production and the induction of iNOS,[83] and they limit the pathologic vasodilation associated with the nonspecific or specific inflammatory response in the critically ill neonate. Finally, by improving capillary integrity, steroid administration may also increase the effective circulating blood volume in neonates with capillary leak.

Physiology of Neonatal Circulation

Cardiac Output

Under physiologic conditions, tissue perfusion is maintained by the provision of uninterrupted blood flow through the microcirculation. Normal microcirculation, in turn, depends on the organ perfusion pressure maintained by the interaction between cardiac output, preload, and afterload. *Cardiac output* is the product of stroke volume and heart rate and is determined by the amount of blood returning to the heart (preload), the strength of myocardial contractility, and the resistance against which the heart must pump (afterload). When myocardial function is intact, cardiac output depends solely on preload and afterload, according the relationships described by the Starling curve.

Normal ranges for left and right ventricular output for preterm and term neonates have been reported between 150 and 300 mL/kg/minute.[84, 85] In the transitional circulation of the newborn infant, in whom ventricular output does not consistently reflect systemic blood flow because of the shunts across the fetal channels,[85] superior vena cava blood flow can be measured and used to estimate systemic blood flow.[45] Normal values for superior vena cava blood flow in well preterm neonates range between 40 and 120 mL/kg/minute, with a median rising from 70 mL/kg/minute at 5 hours of age to 90 mL/kg/minute at 48 hours.[45]

The strength of myocardial contractility depends on the filling volume and pressure and on the maturity and integrity of the myocardium. Thus, decreases in preload (hypovolemia, cardiac arrhythmia) as well as prematurity and hypoxic and infectious insults all decrease contractility and lead to decreases in cardiac output.

If the systemic or pulmonary vascular resistance (afterload) is too high, the ability of the myocardium may become compromised to pump against the increased resistance, and cardiac output will fall.[86] In the neonate, significant increases in the afterload may occur with enhanced endogenous catecholamine release during the period of immediate postnatal adaptation as well as in hypovolemia or hypothermia, or when inappropriately high doses of vasopressors are administered to a patient with intact cardiovascular adrenoreceptor responsiveness. Depending on which circulation (systemic or pulmonary) is more severely affected, the high afterload can impair the function of either ventricle. However, by the ensuing decrease in blood return to the initially unaffected ventricle, the reduction in the output of one of the ventricles will influence the function of the other ventricle. In addition, in the immediate postnatal period, shunts through the patent ductus arteriosus or foramen ovale may com-

promise the circulation.[87] In the extremely low birth weight neonate, normal postnatal closure of these fetal channels frequently fails, and as the right-sided pressures fall, pulmonary edema may rapidly develop, further compromising the hemodynamic status of these critically ill patients.[87]

Systemic Blood Pressure

Systemic blood pressure is the product of systemic blood flow and systemic vascular resistance. The gestational and postnatal age-dependent "normal ranges" for systemic blood pressure in neonates have been described in the literature.[88, 89] Although blood pressure only weakly correlates with blood flow in the critically ill extremely low birth weight neonate during the period of immediate postnatal adaptation,[45,86] there is an association between low blood pressure and early central nervous system injury in this patient population.[90, 91] Data indicate that only when mean blood pressures in extremely low birth weight neonates are less than or equal to 20 mm Hg and greater than or equal to 40 mm Hg, blood pressure becomes a more accurate indicator of abnormal and normal systemic blood flow.[92] Thus, in the extremely preterm neonates with mean blood pressures between 20 and 40 mm Hg in the immediate postnatal period, the state of systemic blood flow is unclear, and the situation can be clarified only with ultrasonographic evaluation of cardiac function and organ blood flow. In more mature preterm and term neonates, blood pressure and organ blood flow appear to have a better correlation.

Organ Blood Flow and Its Autoregulation

Even extremely immature preterm neonates appear to be able to autoregulate their cerebral blood flow.[91, 93-95] However, organ blood flow autoregulation is impaired in some preterm neonates, especially in those with birth asphyxia, acidosis, infection, tissue ischemia, and sudden alterations in arterial P_{CO_2}, rendering these patients at higher risk for cerebral injury. As mentioned earlier, because most of the severe cerebral injuries occur in extremely low birth weight neonates during the immediate postnatal period, the cortical vessels of these patients may be regulated as low-priority vessels, and thus blood is shifted away from the immature cerebral cortex during periods of circulatory compromise as it is in other low-priority organ systems such as the kidneys, muscles, skin, and the hepatic and mesenteric circulation.[27,34-36] Because afterload abruptly increases with delivery, the immature myocardium struggles to maintain cardiac output in these subjects. Indeed, it is likely that the development of compensated shock and relative cortical ischemia is part of the transition to extrauterine life in most extremely low birth weight neonates. The cortical ischemia then sets the stage for reperfusion injury (intracranial hemorrhage or periventricular white matter injury) to occur once myocardial function and organ perfusion improve.[96]

Pathogenesis of Neonatal Shock

The clinical presentation, pathophysiology, and treatment of neonatal shock are significantly affected by the primary cause of the condition. Hypovolemia, myocardial dysfunction, and abnormal regulation of peripheral vascular tone are the primary etiologic factors leading to shock in the neonate. In the critically ill neonate, more than one of these factors may be involved. For instance, in a newborn with septic shock, the capillary leak-induced hypovolemia, direct myocardial injury, and abnormal regulation of vascular tone may all contribute to the development of the circulatory compromise.

Hypovolemia

Hypovolemia is an uncommon primary cause of neonatal shock, especially during the first postnatal days. In preterm newborns, there is no evidence that hypotensive babies as a group are hypovolemic.[97] Hypovolemia causes low cardiac output and hypotension by decreasing the preload. Hypovolemia can result from loss of circulating blood volume after hemorrhage (absolute hypovolemia) or from inappropriate increases in the capacitance of the blood vessels as in vasodilatory shock (relative hypovolemia). In addition, the positive intrathoracic pressure associated with positive pressure mechanical ventilation reduces venous return and hence preload and cardiac output in ventilated preterm and term neonates.[98]

Absolute hypovolemia in the neonate can be caused by intrapartum fetal blood loss resulting from a hemorrhage from the fetal side of the placenta or from acute fetomaternal hemorrhage or acute fetoplacental hemorrhage. The latter may occur in neonates with breech presentation or a tight nuchal cord in whom the umbilical cord comes under significant pressure.[99] Postnatal hemorrhage may occur from any site and is frequently associated with endothelial damage and disseminated intravascular coagulation induced by perinatal infections or asphyxia. Acute abdominal surgical problems and conditions associated with increased capillary leak with loss of fluid into the interstitium can also lead to significant decreases in the circulating blood volume.

Myocardial Dysfunction and Structural Heart Disease

Heart disease resulting in cardiogenic shock can be congenital or acquired. In cardiogenic shock, cardiac output and organ blood flow are compromised, and metabolic acidosis develops rapidly. As for the clinical presentation, structural heart defects that produce a ductally dependent systemic circulation (hypoplastic left heart syndrome, critical coarctation, and critical aortic stenosis) classically present as acute circulatory compromise as the duct starts closing. Acquired heart disease frequently presenting as neonatal shock includes primary cardiomyopathies and postasphyxial myocardial dysfunction.

Abnormal Peripheral Vasoregulation and Neonatal Shock with Complex Pathogenesis

Extreme Prematurity. The transitional circulatory changes in the first 12 to 24 hours after birth comprise a period of unique circulatory vulnerability for the extremely preterm infant. During the period of immediate postnatal adaptation, the left ventricle has to double its output. As described in the section on organ blood flow autoregulation, the extremely premature infant has significant difficulties to adjust to extrauterine life and is prone to develop reperfusion injury in the brain.[86,96] Under these conditions, blood pressure in the low-normal to normal range does not necessarily translate into normal organ blood flow and tissue perfusion in the extremely premature neonate.[45,86]

In the transitional circulation of the preterm infant, neither ventricular output will consistently reflect systemic blood flow because of the shunts across the ductus arteriosus and foramen ovale.[85] Consequently, measurement of either ventricular output can overestimate systemic blood flow by more than 100% in some cases.[85] As mentioned earlier, superior vena cava flow can be used as a marker of total systemic blood flow,[46] and serial measurements of superior vena cava flow have been used to describe the natural history of systemic blood flow changes in preterm neonates in the early postnatal period.[96,100] At least one-third of preterm neonates born before 30 weeks' gestation have a period of low systemic blood flow, mostly during first 12 hours of life.[45,96] Gestational age is the dominant predictor of the development of the low-flow state; 70% of babies born before 26 weeks' gestation have a period of low systemic flow compared with around 10% at 29 weeks' gestation. Thus, the development of a low-flow state with compensated neonatal shock appears to be part of the transitional adaptation process in the extremely low birth weight patient population immediately after

birth. The low-flow state can persist for up to 24 hours but usually improves after thereafter. There is a strong relationship between recovery from the low-flow state and subsequent intraventricular hemorrhage,[96] and the low-flow state itself has been identified as a significant risk factor for poor neurodevelopmental outcome.[101]

Sepsis. Endotoxin or lipopolysaccharide plays a major role in the pathophysiology of septic shock caused by gram-negative organism. Lipopolysaccharide induces the production of proinflammatory cytokines such as tumor necrosis factor-α (TNF-α) and interleukin-1. In addition to activating the inflammatory response, TNF-α induces apoptosis.[102] NF-κB, a nuclear transcriptional factor, mediates the inflammatory response induced by TNF-α.[103] TNF-α is a potent stimulator of iNOS, and overproduction of NO causes vasodilatation, systemic hypotension, and the generation of reactive free radicals such as peroxynitrite. In gram-negative septic shock, myocardial dysfunction develops, at least in part because of the effect of up-regulated TNF-α production,[104] as evidenced by improvement in cardiac function after administration of anti–TNF-α antibody.[105] Finally, TNF-α, by up-regulating tissue factor production in endothelial cells, also activates the extrinsic coagulation pathway and contributes to the generation of thrombi in the microcirculation.[106]

The triggers of inflammation and the host response in septic shock caused by gram-positive organisms are less well defined. However, cell wall components such as peptidoglycans and lipoteichoic acid as well as exotoxins have been implicated in the induction of the cytokine cascade.[107]

Although clinical evidence of circulatory compromise is a feature of many infectious processes in the newborn, the hemodynamics in neonatal septic shock has not been well studied. In older subjects, two distinct hemodynamic patterns occur. *Warm shock* is characterized by loss of vascular tone, increased systemic blood flow, and low blood pressure, and it is difficult to recognize initially unless the blood pressure is closely monitored. *Cold shock,* conversely, is characterized by increased vascular tone, low systemic blood flow, and eventually falling blood pressure, and it has been well described in the newborn.[108]

Pressor-Resistant Systemic Hypotension in Neonates

As discussed in the section on down-regulation of adrenergic receptors, pressor-resistant hypotension in preterm and term infants is now a well-recognized condition.[80,109] The underlying systemic hemodynamic changes, although not well defined, appear to be similar to those seen in adult vasodilatory shock, with normal to high systemic blood flow and possibly supranormal cardiac output.[110] Neonates with this condition are more likely to be extremely premature ($\leq$27 weeks) or to have been critically ill or suffered a degree of perinatal asphyxia. Potential mechanisms of the uncontrolled vasodilation include dysregulated cytokine release, excess NO synthesis, vasopressin deficiency, overactivation of the potassium-ATP channels in the vascular smooth muscle cell membrane in response to tissue hypoxia, and down-regulation of the cardiovascular adrenergic receptors.[80] In the neonate, the foregoing mechanisms may be exacerbated by immaturity, relative adrenal insufficiency,[78,111] or preceding asphyxia, or they may be secondary to the transitional circulatory failure of the extremely low birth weight neonate.

Treatment of Neonatal Shock

Treatment of neonatal shock must be tailored to the primary cause or pathogenesis and to the level of maturation of the critically ill neonate.[112]

Volume Administration

Because hypotensive neonates as a group are not hypovolemic,[97] because myocardial dysfunction frequently contributes to the development of neonatal hypotension,[113] because dopamine is more effective in normalizing blood pressure than is volume administration,[114, 115] and because excessive fluid administration increases morbidity especially in the preterm neonate,[116] fluid resuscitation should be minimized.

Concerning the type of fluid administration, isotonic saline has been shown to be as effective as 5% albumin in increasing the blood pressure.[117] In addition, albumin may cause an impairment of gas exchange, may induce a fluid shift from the intracellular compartment[118] and may be associated with increased mortality.[119] Therefore, the use of isotonic saline has been advocated.[112, 120] However, because of the unbalanced nature of normal saline, its administration in large amounts may worsen metabolic acidosis. If there is an identifiable volume loss, the type of fluid lost should be replaced.

Dopamine and Dobutamine

There is only indirect evidence that the use of these sympathomimetic amines improves neonatal mortality or morbidity. Studies in developing and mature animals showed significant age-dependent differences in the cardiovascular and renal effects of dopamine[121] and the cardiovascular effects of dobutamine.[122] However, owing to maturation-dependent and maturation-independent interspecies differences, interpolation of these findings to the human neonate may be misleading.[93, 120] Although a few studies examined the developmentally regulated hemodynamic effects of dopamine[93, 95, 115, 123, 124] and dobutamine[86, 110, 125] in the human neonate, there is still only limited information available on the effects of dopamine and dobutamine on tissue O_2 delivery and consumption[126] and systemic blood flow in the newborn.[86]

Hemodynamic Effects. Dopamine, an endogenous catecholamine, exerts its cardiovascular actions via the dose-dependent stimulation of the cardiovascular dopaminergic receptors and the α- and β-adrenergic receptors. In addition, by stimulating epithelial and peripheral neuronal dopaminergic and adrenergic receptors, the drug exerts significant renal and endocrine effects independent of its cardiovascular actions.[120] Although dopamine affects all three major determinants of cardiovascular function, the drug-induced increases in myocardial contractility[115, 120] and peripheral vascular resistance[115, 120, 125] are the most important factors in increasing systemic blood pressure and improving the cardiovascular status.

Animal studies on the cardiovascular effects of dopamine during development showed that the drug's positive inotropic effect and selective vasodilatory actions in the different regional circulations are maturation dependent.[127-129] However, in the human preterm neonate, clinical studies have demonstrated greater increases in stroke volume[130] and glomerular filtration rate[131, 132] in response to dopamine administration than expected from the findings of the developmental animal studies. Thus, functional cardiovascular β–adrenergic and dopaminergic receptors exist, at least beyond 23 weeks' gestation, in the heart and the renal circulation of the human neonate.[93, 95, 115, 120, 123, 124, 130] In addition, during the early phases of shock, when the cardiovascular adrenergic receptors are not yet down-regulated, dopamine increases blood pressure in preterm infants at lower doses compared with children and adults.[130-133] The increased sensitivity to the vasoconstrictive (afterload-increasing) effects of dopamine may be related to the enhanced expression of α-adrenergic receptors during early development,[134] as well as to the differences in the maturation of hepatic and renal dopamine-clearance mechanisms.[132]

The original dose range recommendation of 2 to 20 µg/kg/minute of dopamine was based on pharmacodynamic data obtained in healthy adults. However, changes in cardiovascular adrenergic receptor expression by critical illness,[82] relative or absolute adrenal insufficiency and immaturity,[78, 111] and the dysregulated production of local vasodilators during severe illness decrease the sensitivity of the cardiovascular system to dopamine

and result in the emergence of hypotension resistant to "conventional" doses of the drug.[80, 109] Thus, with the advancing disease process, increased doses of dopamine and other sympathomimetic amines may be needed to exert the same magnitude of cardiovascular response. Indeed, there is no evidence that, when required to normalize blood pressure, high-dose dopamine treatment with or without additional epinephrine administration has detrimental vasoconstrictive effects.[80, 109, 135] However, there are no data available on changes in cardiac output and organ blood flow in response to high-dose catecholamine treatment in pressor-resistant neonatal shock.

Unlike dopamine, dobutamine is a relatively cardioselective sympathomimetic amine with significant α- and β-adrenoreceptor-mediated direct inotropic effects and limited chronotropic actions.[122, 136, 137] Dobutamine administration is usually also associated with a variable decrease in total peripheral vascular resistance[137] and, at least in adults, with improved coronary blood flow and myocardial O_2 delivery.[136] Furthermore, unlike dopamine,[120] dobutamine increases myocardial contractility exclusively through the direct stimulation of the myocardial adrenergic receptors. Because myocardial norepinephrine stores are immature and are rapidly depleted in the newborn, and because dobutamine may decrease afterload, newborns with primary myocardial dysfunction and elevated peripheral vascular resistance are most likely to benefit from dobutamine treatment.[120, 137] Although addition of dobutamine to dopamine in preterm infants with respiratory distress syndrome is effective in increasing blood pressure, this approach is associated with supranormal cardiac output states and lower systemic vascular resistance.[110] Whether the benefits of supranormal cardiac output by providing adequate tissue O_2 delivery throughout the body outweigh the risks of sustained hypercontractility potentially resulting in myocardial injury remains to be investigated. Although dopamine is effective in normalizing the cardiovascular status in most neonates with hypotension,[120] neither dopamine nor dobutamine effectively improves low systemic blood flow in extremely low birth weight neonates during the first 24 hours of life.[86] This finding underscores the earlier-described complexity of the cardiovascular changes during the immediate postnatal transition of the extremely low birth weight human neonate.

The vasodilatory dopamine receptors are primarily expressed in the renal, mesenteric, and coronary circulations.[120] Dopamine has been shown to decrease renal vascular resistance selectively[93, 95] and to increase glomerular filtration rate[131, 132] in preterm infants as early as the 23rd week of gestation. However, dopamine decreases mesenteric vascular resistance in preterm infants only beyond the first postnatal day,[93, 95, 124] and the effect may be variable.[124] Similarly, there are some differences in the reported magnitude of the drug-induced increases in ventricular function, cardiac output, and systemic vascular resistance.[115, 124, 125] These findings may be best explained by differences in the intravascular volume status, the postnatal age, the developmentally regulated expression of cardiovascular adrenergic and dopaminergic receptors, and the severity of adrenergic receptor down-regulation among the different populations of critically ill preterm infants studied. None of the studies has, however, found evidence of a direct effect of dopamine on cerebral blood flow.[93, 95, 115, 124] Finally, in addition to increasing afterload, dopamine also increases pulmonary vascular resistance in preterm neonates.[138] However, because the drug-induced increases in systemic blood pressure are not associated with impaired oxygenation in most neonates,[120] there is no evidence of consistent increases in extrapulmonary right-to-left shunting during dopamine treatment. In preterm neonates, dopamine also improves right ventricular performance.[139]

There are no data available on the direct renal, cerebral, or pulmonary hemodynamic effects of dobutamine in the human newborn. However, when dobutamine increases blood pressure, it may also increase mesenteric blood flow in preterm infants.[140]

Because dobutamine does not stimulate the dopaminergic receptors, β-adrenoreceptor–induced selective vasodilation may be responsible for the observed mesenteric vasodilation.

Epithelial and Neuroendocrine Effects. Independent of the previously described cardiovascular effects, dopamine exerts direct renal[120,132] and endocrine[120] actions in the newborn. Via its direct effects on sodium, phosphorus, and water transport processes and sodium, potassium–ATPase activity[141] in the renal tubules, dopamine increases sodium, phosphorus, and free water excretion and may increase the hypoxic threshold of renal tubular cells during episodes of hypoperfusion and hypoxemia.[120] Via its renal vascular and epithelial actions, dopamine also potentiates the diuretic effects of furosemide[142] and theophylline.[143] Among its endocrine actions, the dopamine-induced decreases in plasma prolactin and thyrotropin levels[120] may be of clinical importance. The potential impact on long-term neurodevelopmental outcome and immunologic function of the drug-induced alterations in the neuroendocrine function has not been investigated in the preterm or term neonate. Because dobutamine does not directly stimulate the dopaminergic receptors, its administration is likely to be devoid of neuroendocrine effects.

Other Sympathomimetic Amines and Hormones

Although both epinephrine and norepinephrine have been used in the treatment of hypotension in preterm infants, data in peer-reviewed literature on the cardiovascular actions of epinephrine during development are available only from studies on newborn animals.[144] Studies of the cardiovascular and renal effects of these catecholamines in the human neonate have been published only in abstract form.[145-147] It is not known whether there is a difference in the cardiovascular response or side effects with the combined use of epinephrine and dopamine compared with the use of increasing doses of dopamine beyond 20 μg/kg/minute with or without dobutamine in the human neonate. In addition to sympathomimetic amines, arginine vasopressin has been reported to improve cardiovascular function in newborns with vasodilatory shock.[148]

Steroid Administration

There is emerging evidence that brief steroid treatment stabilizes the cardiovascular status and decreases the need for pressor support in the critically ill newborn with pressor-resistant hypotension.[78, 80, 109, 111, 149, 150] The potential mechanisms of steroid treatment in hypotensive preterm and term neonates on improving the cardiovascular status are described earlier, in the section on pressor-resistant hypotension. Finally, there are no data on the potential long-term neurodevelopmental side effects of the attempted physiologic supplementation with hydrocortisone or the use of low-dose dexamethasone to enhance cardiovascular stability and pulmonary function in critically ill preterm and term infants.

Supportive Measures

Maintenance of normal arterial pH and serum ionized calcium concentrations is important for optimizing the cardiovascular response to catecholamines. Because metabolic acidosis with a pH of less than 7.25 compromises myocardial function in preterm infants,[151] maintenance of the arterial pH above this range in infants with acidosis with a significant metabolic component may be warranted.[151] However, the efficacy and potential short- and long-term adverse effects of the administration of sodium bicarbonate or tromethamine have not been studied in the neonatal patient population.

SUMMARY

Treatment of hypotensive, critically ill preterm and term neonates requires the ability to monitor the most important determinants of cardiovascular function including the blood pressure and systemic and organ blood flow, a thorough understanding of the pathogenesis and pathophysiology of neonatal shock, and knowledge of the developmentally regulated mechanisms of actions, pharmacodynamics, and potential side effects of the sympathomimetic amines and other medications used in the management of neonatal shock.

REFERENCES

1. Rothstein RW, Longo LD: Respiration in the fetal-placental unit. *In* Cowett RM (ed): Principles of Perinatal-Neonatal Metabolism. New York, Springer-Verlag, 1998, p 451.
2. Nicolaides KH, et al: Blood gases, pH, and lactate in appropriate- and small-for-gestational-age fetuses. Am J Obstet Gynecol *161*:996, 1989.
3. Weiner CP, et al: The effect of fetal age upon normal fetal laboratory values and venous pressure. Obstet Gynecol *79*:713, 1992.
4. Arikan GM, et al: Low fetal oxygen saturation at birth and acidosis. Obstet Gynecol *95*:565, 2000.
5. Richardson B, et al: Fetal oxygen saturation and fractional extraction at birth and the relationship to measures of acidosis. Am J Obstet Gynecol *178*:572, 1998.
6. Ehrenkranz RA, et al: Effect of ritodrine infusion on uterine and umbilical blood flow in pregnant sheep. Am J Obstet Gynecol *126*:343, 1976.
7. Hooper SB: Fetal metabolic responses to hypoxia. Reprod Fertil Dev 7:527, 1995.
8. Rurak D, et al: Fetal oxygen extraction: comparison of the human and sheep. Am J Obstet Gynecol *156*:360, 1987.
9. Bell AW, et al: Metabolic and circulatory studies of fetal lamb at midgestation. Am J Physiol *250*:E538, 1986.
10. Lorijn RHW, Longo LD: Clinical and physiological implications of increased fetal oxygen consumption. Am J Obstet Gynecol *136*:451, 1980.
11. Eldestone DI, et al: Effects of reductions in hemoglobin-oxygen affinity and hematocrit level on oxygen consumption and acid-base state in fetal lambs. Am J Obstet Gynecol *160*:820, 1989.
12. Towell ME, et al: The effect of mild hypoxemia maintained for twenty-four hours on maternal and fetal glucose, lactate, cortisol, and arginine vasopressin in pregnant sheep at 122 to 139 days' gestation. Am J Obstet Gynecol *157*:1550, 1987.
13. Nijland R, et al: Fetus-placenta-newborn: arterial oxygen saturation in relation to metabolic acidosis in fetal lambs. Am J Obstet Gynecol *172*:810, 1995.
14. Mastuda Y, et al: Effects of sustained hypoxia on the sheep fetus at mid-gestation: endocrine, cardiovascular, and biophysical responses. Am J Obstet Gynecol *167*:53, 1992.
15. Ross MG, Gala R: Use of umbilical artery base excess: algorithm for the timing of hypoxic injury. Am J Obstet Gynecol *187*:1, 2002.
16. Ball RH, et al: Fetus-placenta-newborn: regional blood flow and metabolism in ovine fetuses during severe cord occlusion. Am J Obstet Gynecol *171*:1549, 1994.
17. Paulick R, et al: Metabolic, cardiovascular and sympathoadrenal reactions of the fetus to progressive hypoxia: animal experiment studies. Z Geburtshilfe Perinatol *191*:130, 1987.
18. Jones CT, et al: Developmental changes in the responses of the adrenal glands of fetal sheep to endogenous adrenocorticotrophin, as indicated by hormone responses to hypoxemia. J Endocrinol *72*:279, 1977.
19. Chalilis JR, et al: Plasma adrenocorticotropic hormone and cortisol and adrenal blood flow during sustained hypoxemia in fetal sheep. Am J Obstet Gynecol *155*:1332, 1986.
20. Challis JR, et al: Fetal and maternal endocrine responses to prolonged reductions in uterine blood flow in pregnant sheep. Am J Obstet Gynecol *160*:926, 1989.
21. Wardlaw SL, et al: Effects of hypoxia on β-endorphin and β-lipotropin release in fetal, newborn and maternal sheep. Endocrinology *108*:1710, 1981.
22. Skillman CA, Clark KE: Fetal beta-endorphin levels in response to reductions in uterine blood flow. Biol Neonate *51*:217, 1987.
23. Raff H, et al: Arginine vasopressin responses to hypoxia and hypercapnia in late-gestation fetal sheep. Am J Physiol *260*:R1077, 1991.
24. Stark RI, et al: Cerebrospinal fluid and plasma vasopressin in the fetal lamb: basal concentration and the effect of hypoxia. Endocrinology *116*:65, 1985.
25. Sameshima H, et al: Vasopressin and catecholamine responses to 24-hour, steady-state hypoxia in fetal goats. J Matern Fetal Med *5*:262, 1996.
26. Cohen WR, et al: Plasma catecholamines during hypoxemia in fetal lamb. Am J Physiol *243*:R520, 1982.
27. Cohn HE, et al: Cardiovascular responses to hypoxemia and acidemia in fetal lambs. Am J Obstet Gynecol *120*:817, 1974.
28. Cohn HE, et al: The adrenal secretion of catecholamines during systemic metabolic acidosis in fetal sheep. Biol Neonate *72*:125, 1997.
29. Faucher DJ, et al: Vasopressin and catecholamine secretion during metabolic acidemia in the ovine fetus. Pediatr Res *21*:38, 1987.
30. Clyman RI, et al (eds): Maternal-Fetal Medicine. Philadelphia, WB Saunders Co, 1999, p 249.
31. Koos BJ, et al: Adenosine mediates metabolic and cardiovascular responses to hypoxia in fetal sheep. J Physiol (Lond) *488*:761, 1995.

32. Koos BJ, Maeda T: Adenosine A_{2A} receptors mediate cardiovascular responses to hypoxia in fetal sheep. Am J Physiol *280*:H83, 2001.

33. Kamitomo M, et al: Cardiac function in fetal sheep during two weeks of hypoxemia. Am J Physiol *266*:R1778, 1994.

34. Reuss ML, Rudolph AM: Distribution and recirculation of umbilical and systemic venous blood flow in fetal lambs during hypoxia. J Dev Physiol *2*:71, 1980.

35. Itskovitz J, et al: Effects of cord compression on fetal blood flow distribution and O_2 delivery. Am J Physiol *252*:H100, 1987.

36. Jensen A, et al: Effects of reducing uterine blood flow on fetal blood flow distribution and oxygen delivery. J Dev Physiol *15*:309, 1991.

37. Gardner DS, et al: Effects of prevailing hypoxemia, acidemia or hypoglycemia upon the cardiovascular, endocrine and metabolic responses to acute hypoxemia in the ovine fetus. J Physiol (Lond) *540*:351, 2002.

38. Blechner JN: Maternal-fetal acid-base physiology. Clin Obstet Gynecol *36*:3, 1993.

39. Gibson KJ, et al: Renal acid-base and sodium handling in hypoxia and subsequent mild metabolic acidosis in foetal sheep. Clin Exp Pharmacol Physiol *27*:67, 2000.

40. Cock ML, et al: Alteration in fetal urine production during prolonged hypoxemia induced by reduced uterine blood flow in sheep: mechanisms. Clin Exp Pharmacol Physiol *23*:57, 1996.

41. Wintour EM, et al: Regulation of urine osmolality in fetal sheep. Q J Exp Physiol *67*:427, 1982.

42. Gaudio KM, et al: Immature tubules are tolerant of oxygen deprivation. Pediatr Nephrol *11*:757, 1997.

43. Kesby GJ, Lumbers ER: The effect of metabolic acidosis on renal function of the fetal sheep. J Physiol (Lond) *396*:65, 1988.

44. Kluckow M, Evans N: Relationship between blood pressure and cardiac output in preterm infants requiring mechanical ventilation. J Pediatr *129*:506,1996.

45. Kluckow M, Evans N: Superior vena flow in preterm infants: a novel marker of systemic blood flow. Arch Dis Child *82*:F182, 2000.

46. Wardle SP, et al: Determinants of cerebral fractional oxygen extraction using near infrared spectroscopy in preterm neonates. J Cereb Blood Flow Metab *20*:272, 2000.

47. Flowers F, Zimmerman JJ: Reactive oxygen species in the cellular pathophysiology of shock. New Horiz *6*:169, 1998.

48. Simonson SG, et al: Altered mitochondrial redox responses in gram negative septic shock in primates. Shock *43*:3, 1994.

49. Winterbourn CC, et al: Chlorohydrin formation from unsaturated fatty acids reacted with hypochlorous acid. Arch Biochem Biophys *296*:547, 1992.

50. Davies KJ, et al: Protein damage and degradation by oxygen radicals. II. Modification of amino acids. J Biol Chem *262*:9902, 1987.

51. Spragg RG: DNA strand break formation following exposure of bovine pulmonary artery and aortic endothelial cells to reactive oxygen products. Am J Respir Cell Mol Biol *4*:4, 1991.

52. Rubanyi GM: Nitric oxide and circulatory shock. Adv Exp Med Biol *454*:165, 1998.

53. Liu S, et al: Lipopolysaccharide treatment in vivo induces widespread tissue expression of inducible nitric oxide synthase mRNA. Biochem Biophys Res Commun *196*:1208, 1993.

54. Doughty L, et al: Plasma nitrite and nitrite concentrations and multiple organ failure in pediatric sepsis. Crit Care Med *26*:157, 1998.

55. Carcillo J: Nitric oxide production in neonatal and pediatric sepsis. Crit Care Med *27*:1063, 1999.

56. Beckman JS, et al: Nitric oxide and peroxynitrite in the perinatal period. Semin Perinatol *24*:37, 2000.

57. Shen W, et al: Nitric oxide: an important signaling mechanism between vascular endothelium and parenchymal cells in the regulation of oxygen consumption. Circulation *92*:3505, 1995.

58. Barrington KJ, et al: The hemodynamic effects of inhaled nitric oxide and endogenous nitric oxide synthesis blockade in newborn piglets during infusion of heat-killed group B streptococci. Crit Care Med *28*:800, 2000.

59. Mitaka C, et al: Effects of nitric oxide synthase inhibitor on hemodynamic change and O_2 delivery in septic dogs. Am J Physiol *268*:H2017, 1995.

60. Grover R, et al: Multi-center, randomized, placebo-controlled, double blind study of the nitric oxide synthase inhibitor 546C88: effect on survival in patients with septic shock. Crit Care Med *27*(Suppl):A33, 1999.

61. Mitaka C, et al: A selective inhibitor for inducible nitric oxide synthase improves hypotension and lactic acidosis in canine endotoxic shock. Crit Care Med *29*:2156, 2001.

62. Carcillo JA: Nitric oxide production in neonatal and pediatric sepsis. Crit Care Med *27*:1063 1999.

63. Doebber TW, et al: Platelet activating factor (PAF) involvement in endotoxin-induced hypotension in rats: studies with PAF-receptor antagonist kadsurenone. Biochem Biophys Res Commun *127*:799, 1985.

64. Handley DA, et al: Vascular responses of platelet-activating factor in the *Cebus apella* primate and inhibitory profiles of antagonists SRI 63–072 and SRI 63–119. Immunopharmacology *11*:175, 1986.

65. Ayala A, Chaudry IH: Platelet activating factor and its role in trauma, shock, and sepsis. New Horiz *4*:265, 1996.

66. Fletcher JR, et al: Platelet activating factor receptor antagonist improves survival and attenuates eicosanoid release in severe endotoxemia. Ann Surg *211*:312, 1990.

67. Rabinovici R, et al: Platelet activating factor (PAF) and tumor necrosis factor-alpha (TNF alpha) interactions in endotoxemic shock: studies with BN 50739, a novel PAF antagonist. J Pharmacol Exp Ther *255*:256, 1990.

68. Rabinowitz SS, et al: Platelet-activating factor in infants at risk for necrotizing enterocolitis. J Pediatr *138*:81, 2001.

69. Ewer AK: Role of platelet-activating factor in the pathophysiology of necrotizing enterocolitis. Acta Paediatr Suppl *91*:2, 2002.

70. Feuerstein G, et al: Alteration of cardiovascular, neurogenic, and humoral responses to acute hypovolemic hypotension by administered prostacyclin. J Cardiovasc Pharmacol *4*:246, 1982.

71. Machiedo GW, et al: Hemodynamic effects of prolonged infusion of prostaglandin E_1 (PGE$_1$) after hemorrhagic shock. Adv Shock Res *8*:171, 1982.

72. Fink MP: Therapeutic options directed against platelet activating factor, eicosanoids and bradykinin in sepsis. J Antimicrob Chemother *41*(Suppl A):81, 1998.

73. Arons MM, et al: Effects of ibuprofen on the physiology and survival of hypothermic sepsis. Crit Care Med *27*:699, 1999.

74. Reines HD, et al: Plasma thromboxane concentrations are raised in patients dying with septic shock. Lancet *2*:174, 1982.

75. Ball HA, et al: Role of thromboxane, prostaglandins and leukotrienes in endotoxic and septic shock. Intensive Care Med *12*:116, 1986.

76. Bohrer H, et al: Role of NFkappaB in the mortality of sepsis. J Clin Invest *100*:972, 1997.

77. Collins S, et al: Regulation of adrenergic receptor responsiveness through modulation of receptor gene expression. Annu Rev Physiol *53*:497, 1991.

78. Watterberg KL, et al: Prophylaxis against early adrenal insufficiency to prevent chronic lung disease in premature infants. Pediatrics *104*:1258, 1999.

79. Annane D, et al: Effect of treatment with low doses of hydrocortisone and fludrocortisone on mortality in patients with septic shock. JAMA *288*:862, 2002.

80. Seri I, et al: The effect of hydrocortisone on blood pressure in preterm neonates with pressor-resistant hypotension. Pediatrics *107*:1070, 2001.

81. Tseng YT, et al: Regulation of β_1-adrenoreceptors by glucocorticoids and thyroid hormones in fetal sheep. Eur J Pharmacol *289*:353, 1995.

82. Wehling M: Specific, nongenomic actions of steroid hormones. Annu Rev Physiol *59*:365, 1997.

83. Knowles RG, et al: Glucocorticoids inhibit the expression of an inducible, but not the constitutive, nitric oxide synthase in vascular endothelial cells. Proc Natl Acad Sci USA *87*:10043, 1990.

84. Walther FJ, et al: Pulsed Doppler determinant of cardiac output in neonates: normal standards for clinical use. Pediatrics *76*:829, 1985.

85. Evans N, Kluckow M: Early determinants of right and left ventricular output in ventilated preterm infants. Arch Dis Child *74*:F88, 1996.

86. Osborn D, et al: Randomised trial of dopamine and dobutamine in preterm infants with low systemic blood flow. J Pediatr *140*:183, 2002.

87. Kluckow M, Evans N: Ductal shunting, high pulmonary blood flow, and pulmonary hemorrhage. J Pediatr *137*:68, 2000.

88. Nuntarumit P, et al: Blood pressure measurements in the newborn. Clin Perinatol *26*:981, 1999.

89. Lee J, et al: Blood pressure standards for very low birthweight infants during the first day of life. Arch Dis Child *81*:F168, 1999.

90. Bada HS, et al: Mean arterial blood pressure changes in premature infants and those at risk for intraventricular haemorrhage. J Pediatr *117*:607, 1990.

91. Tsuji M, et al: Cerebral intravascular oxygenation correlates with mean arterial pressure in critically ill premature infants. Pediatrics *106*:625, 2000.

92. Osborn D, et al: Accuracy of capillary refill time and blood pressure for detecting low systemic blood flow in preterm infants. Pediatr Res *49*:376A, 2001.

93. Seri I, et al: Effect of dopamine on regional blood flows in sick preterm infants. J Pediatr *133*:728, 1998.

94. Tyszczuk L, et al: Cerebral blood flow is independent of mean arterial blood pressure in preterm infants undergoing intensive care. Pediatrics *102*:337, 1998.

95. Seri I, et al: Regional hemodynamic effects of dopamine in the indomethacin-treated preterm infant. J Perinatol *22*:300, 2002.

96. Kluckow M, Evans N: Low superior vena flow and intraventricular haemorrhage in preterm infants. Arch Dis Child *82*:F188, 2000.

97. Wright IMR, Goodhall SR: Blood pressure and blood volume in preterm infants. Arch Dis Child *70*:F230, 1994.

98. Biondi JW, et al: The effect of incremental positive end expiratory pressure on right ventricular haemodynamics and ejection fraction. Anesth Analg *67*:144, 1988.

99. Vanhaesebrouck P, et al: Tight nuchal cord and neonatal hypovolaemic shock. Arch Dis Child *62*:1276, 1987.

100. Kluckow M, Evans N: Low systemic blood flow and hyperkalemia in preterm infants. J Pediatr *139*:227, 2001.

101. Hunt R, et al: Low superior vena cava flow and neurodevelopmental outcome at 3 years. Pediatr Res *49*:336A, 2001.

102. Hsueh W, et al: The role of the complement system in shock and tissue injury induced by tumor necrosis factor and endotoxin. Immunology *70*:309, 1990.

103. Schutze S, et al: TNF-induced activation of NF-kappa B. Immunobiology *193*:193, 1995.

104. Giroir BP, et al: The tissue distribution of tumor necrosis factor biosynthesis during endotoxemia. J Clin Invest *90*:693, 1992.

105. Boekstegers P, et al: Repeated administration of a F(ab')2 fragment of an anti-tumor necrosis factor alpha monoclonal antibody in patients with severe sepsis: effects on the cardiovascular system and cytokine levels. Shock *1*:237, 1994.

106. Taylor FB Jr: Role of tissue factor and factor VIIa in the coagulant and inflammatory response to LD100 *Escherichia coli* in the baboon. Haemostasis 26(Suppl 1):83, 1996.

107. Murphy K, et al: Molecular biology of septic shock. New Horiz 6:181, 1998.

108. Meadow W, Rudinsky B: Inflammatory mediators and neonatal sepsis. Clin Perinatol 22:519, 1995.

109. Ng PC, et al: Refractory hypotension in preterm infants with adrenocortical insufficiency. Arch Dis Child 84:F122, 2001.

110. Lopez SL, et al: Supranormal cardiac output in dopamine and dobutamine dependent preterm infants. Pediatr Cardiol 18:292, 1997.

111. Watterber KL: Adrenal insufficiency and cardiac dysfunction in the preterm infant. Pediatr Res 51:422, 2002.

112. Seri I, Evans J: Controversies in the diagnosis and management of hypotension in the newborn infant. Curr Opin Pediatr 13:116, 2001.

113. Gill AB, Weindling AM: Cardiac function in the shocked very low birth weight infant. Arch Dis Child 68:17, 1993.

114. Gill AB, Weindling AM: Randomized controlled trial of plasma protein fraction versus dopamine in hypotensive very low birth weight infants. Arch Dis Child 69:284, 1993.

115. Lundstrom K, et al: The hemodynamic effects of dopamine and volume expansion in sick preterm infants. Hum Dev 57:157, 2000.

116. Kavvadia V, et al: Randomized trial of fluid restriction in ventilated very low birth weight infants. Arch Dis Child 83:F91, 2000.

117. So KW, et al: Randomized controlled trial of colloid or crystalloid in hypotensive preterm infants. Arch Dis Child 76:F43, 1997.

118. Ernest D, et al: Distribution of normal saline and 5% albumin infusions in septic patients. Crit Care Med 27:46, 1999.

119. Nadel S, et al: Albumin: saint or sinner? Arch Dis Child 79:384, 1998.

120. Seri I: Cardiovascular, renal, and endocrine actions of dopamine in neonates and children. J Pediatr 126:333, 1995.

121. Felder RA: The dopamine receptor in adult and maturing kidney. Am J Physiol 257:F315, 1989.

122. Cheung PY, et al: The hemodynamic effects of dobutamine infusion in the chronically instrumented newborn piglet. Crit Care Med 27:558, 1999.

123. Seri I, et al: The effect of dopamine on renal function, cerebral blood flow and plasma catecholamine levels in sick preterm neonates. Pediatr Res 34:742, 1993.

124. Zhang J, et al: Mechanisms of blood pressure increase induced by dopamine in hypotensive preterm neonates. Arch Dis Child 81:F99, 1999.

125. Roze JC, et al: Response to dopamine and dobutamine in hypotensive very preterm infants. Arch Dis Child 69:59, 1993.

126. Wardle SP, et al: Peripheral oxygenation in hypotensive preterm babies. Pediatr Res 45:343, 1999.

127. Driscoll DJ, et al: Inotropic response of the neonatal canine myocardium to dopamine. Pediatr Res 12:42, 1978.

128. Pelayo JC, et al: Age-dependent renal effects of intrarenal dopamine infusion. Am J Physiol 247:R212, 1984.

129. O'Laughlin MP, et al: Augmentation of cardiac output with intravenous catecholamines in unanesthetized hypoxemic newborn lambs. Pediatr Res 22:667, 1987.

130. Padbury JF, et al:. Dopamine pharmacokinetics in critically ill newborn infants. J Pediatr 110:293, 1986.

131. Seri I, et al: Cardiovascular response to dopamine in hypotensive preterm infants with severe hyaline membrane disease. Eur J Pediatr 142:3, 1984.

132. Seri I, et al: Effects of low-dose dopamine on cardiovascular and renal functions, cerebral blood flow, and plasma catecholamine levels in sick preterm neonates. Pediatr Res 34:742, 1993.

133. DiSessa TG, et al: The cardiovascular effects of dopamine in the severely asphyxiated neonate. J Pediatr 99:772, 1981.

134. Felder RA, et al: Alpha-adrenoreceptors in the developing kidney. Pediatr Res 17:177, 1983.

135. Perez CA, et al: Effect of high-dose dopamine on urine output in newborn infants. Crit Care Med 14:1045, 1986.

136. Ruffolo RR: The pharmacology of dobutamine. Am J Med Sci 294:244, 1987.

137. Martinez AM, et al: Dobutamine pharmacokinetics and cardiovascular responses in critically ill neonates. Pediatrics 89:47, 1992.

138. Liet JM, et al: Dopamine effects on pulmonary artery pressure in hypotensive preterm infants with patent ductus arteriosus. J Pediatr 140:373, 2002.

139. Clark SJ, et al: Right ventricular performance in hypotensive preterm neonates treated with dopamine. Pediatr Cardiol 23:167, 2002.

140. Hentschel R, et al: Impact on blood pressure and intestinal perfusion of dobutamine or dopamine in hypotensive preterm infants. Biol Neonate 68:18, 1995.

141. Seri I, et al: Locally formed dopamine inhibits Na+-K+-ATPase activity in rat renal cortical tubule cells. Am J Physiol 255:F666, 1988.

142. Tulassay T, Seri I: Interaction of dopamine and furosemide in acute oliguria of preterm infants with hyaline membrane disease. Acta Paediatr Scand 75:420, 1986.

143. Bell M, et al: Low-dose theophylline increases urine output in diuretic-dependent critically ill children. Intensive Care Med 24:1099, 1998.

144. Cheung PY, Barrington KJ: The effects of dopamine and epinephrine on hemodynamics and oxygen metabolism in hypoxic anesthetized piglets. Crit Care 5:158, 2001.

145. Derleth DP: Clinical experience with norepinephrine infusions in critically ill newborns. Pediatr Res 40:145A, 1997.

146. Campbell ME, Byrne PJ: Outcome after intravenous epinephrine infusion in infants <750 g birthweight. Pediatr Res 43:209A, 1998.

147. Seri I, Evans J: Addition of epinephrine to dopamine increases blood pressure and urine output in critically ill extremely low birth weight neonates with uncompensated shock. Pediatr Res 43:194A, 1998.

148. Rosenzweig EB, et al: Intravenous arginine-vasopressin in children with vasodilatory shock after cardiac surgery. Circulation 100(Suppl 2):II-182, 1999.

149. Bouchier D, Weston PJ: Randomized trial of dopamine compared with hydrocortisone for the treatment of hypotensive very low birth weight infants. Arch Dis Child 76:F174, 1997.

150. Gaissmaier RE, Pohlandt F: Single-dose dexamethasone treatment of hypotension in preterm infants. J Pediatr 134:701, 1999.

151. Fanconi S, et al: Hemodynamic effects of sodium bicarbonate in critically ill neonates. Int Care Med 19:65, 1993.

76

Susan E. Wert

Normal and Abnormal Structural Development of the Lung

The *respiratory system* is composed of the lung, its conducting airways, and the respiratory muscles of the thorax. These structures function together to provide oxygen to the organism from the external environment while removing excess carbon dioxide from the blood. The respiratory system consists of four primary groups of anatomic components: (1) the *upper airways* (nasal cavity, sinuses, nasopharynx, larynx, and trachea), which warm, moisten, and filter inspired air; (2) the *lower airways* (bronchi and bronchioles), which distribute air throughout the lung; (3) the *respiratory parenchyma* (respiratory bronchioles, alveolar ducts, and alveoli), where exchange of oxygen and carbon dioxide occurs; and (4) the *musculoelastic structures* (intercostal muscles of the thorax, muscular diaphragm, and elastic tissue in the lung), which move air in and out of the lung and across the respiratory surface. Appropriate anatomic development of these structures, along with histologic, cellular, and biochemical maturation of the lung, is critical for proper physiologic function at birth. This chapter describes the anatomic development of the lung and its conducting airways, along with a review of associated pulmonary malformations. Selected molecular mechanisms that regulate structural development of the lung and its conducting airways are also discussed briefly.

OVERVIEW OF LUNG DEVELOPMENT

Lung development can be divided into five distinct, but overlapping, chronologic stages of organogenesis, which describe the histologic changes that the lung undergoes during morphogenesis and maturation of its structural elements. These are the *embryonic, pseudoglandular, canalicular, saccular,* and *alveolar* phases of lung development, which extend throughout gestation and into the postnatal period (Table 76-1). Human lung development is initiated early in gestation as a small, saccular outgrowth, or *diverticulum,* of the ventral wall of the foregut. During subsequent embryonic and pseudoglandular stages of lung development, formation of the conducting airways, or *tracheobronchial tree,* takes place by a process called *branching morphogenesis.* This process involves rapid growth and repetitive branching of the primitive respiratory diverticulum until all the branches of the tracheobronchial tree are formed. Outgrowth, expansion, and maturation of the alveolar, or gas-exchange, regions of the lung occur later in gestation, during the canalicular, saccular, and alveolar stages of morphogenesis. The alveolar stage of lung development extends into the postnatal

period, during which millions of additional alveoli are formed and maturation of the microvasculature, or *air-blood barrier,* takes place.[1] Although definitive alveoli can be found in the human lung by 36 weeks of gestation, more than 85 to 90% of all alveoli are formed within the first 6 months of life.[2] Overall, the number of alveoli increases by about sixfold between birth and adulthood, that is, from an average of 50 million (ranging from 20 to 70 million) alveoli in the term lung to an average of 300 million (ranging from 212 to 605 million) alveoli in the adult human lung.[2-4] After the first 6 months of life, alveolar formation continues at a slower pace until about 1.5 to 2 years of age, when further growth of the lung becomes proportional to growth of the body. The gas-exchange surface area and its diffusion capacity increase linearly with body weight up to about 18 years of age.[5]

Embryonic Stage (3 to 7 Weeks Post Conception)

The lung is a derivative of the primitive foregut endoderm and the adjacent mesoderm. The *respiratory primordium* of the lung first appears on day 22 post conception (PC) as an enlargement of the caudal end of the *laryngotracheal sulcus,* which is located in the medial pharyngeal groove, an outgrowth of the ventral wall of the primitive foregut endoderm.[1,6] The *primitive respiratory diverticulum,* or lung bud, appears on day 26 PC, when the embryo is only about 3 mm long, and begins to grow ventrocaudally through the mesoderm surrounding the foregut, that is, in a position anterior and parallel to the primitive esophagus. Epithelial cells of the primitive respiratory diverticulum invade the surrounding mesoderm, or *splanchnic mesenchyme,* and they form tubules that undergo repetitive lateral and terminal (dichotomous) branching to form the proximal structures of the tracheobronchial tree. On day 28 PC, the respiratory diverticulum branches, or bifurcates, into right and left primary bronchial buds (main stem bronchi), the left bud shorter and more horizontal than the right bud. The region proximal (or cephalic) to the first bifurcation becomes the trachea and larynx. Shortly thereafter, the trachea and the esophagus begin to separate into two distinct structures. A second round of asymmetric branching occurs during the fifth week of gestation (day 33 to 41 PC) to yield three secondary bronchial buds on the right and two on the left (lobar bronchi), which become the primary lobes of the right and left lung. During the sixth week (day 41 to 44 PC), a third round of branching yields 10 tertiary bronchi on the right

TABLE 76–1

Human Lung Development and Associated Abnormalities

Stage	Major Developmental Events	Abnormalities/Syndromes
Embryonic 3–7 wk post conception	Lung bud arises from ventral foregut endoderm Branching morphogenesis initiated Main stem, lobar, segmental, and subsegmental bronchi form Trachea and esophagus separate Pulmonary arteries bud off sixth pair of aortic arches Pulmonary veins develop as outgrowths of left atrium	Laryngeal, esophageal, tracheal atresia Tracheal and bronchial stenosis Bronchogenic cysts Tracheoesophageal fistula Pulmonary agenesis/aplasia Extralobar pulmonary sequestration

Pseudoglandular
5–17 wk post conception
	Formation of tracheobronchial tree complete by 16 wk
	Pulmonary arterial development parallels airway
	   branching
	Acinar tubules and buds form in peripheral lung
	Ciliated, goblet, neuroepithelial, and basal cells
	   differentiate
	Pulmonary lymphatics appear
	Cartilage, mucous glands, and smooth muscle develop
	Pleuroperitoneal cavity closes
		Renal agenesis–pulmonary hypoplasia
		Intralobar pulmonary sequestration
		Pulmonary cysts
		Cystic adenomatoid malformation
		Pulmonary lymphangiectasia
		Tracheomalacia and bronchomalacia
		Congenital diaphragmatic hernia

Canalicular 16–26 wk post conception	Acinar tubules and buds expand Air-blood barrier and capillary network forms Alveolar Type I and Type II cells differentiate Lamellar bodies form in Type II cells	Renal dysplasia and pulmonary hypoplasia Alveolar capillary dysplasia Respiratory insufficiency Surfactant deficiency
Saccular 24–38 wk post conception	Distal air spaces continue to branch and grow Air spaces expand to form saccules Mesenchyme thins and condenses Septal walls contain double capillary network Elastin deposited at sites of secondary septal crest formation Surfactant synthesized and secreted by Type II cells Fetal lung fluid and fetal breathing	Oligohydramnios and pulmonary hypoplasia Alveolar capillary dysplasia Surfactant deficiency Respiratory distress syndrome Hyaline membrane disease Apnea of prematurity Transient tachypnea
Alveolar 36 wk post conception to 2 yr	Secondary septa form, subdividing saccules into alveoli Alveolar septal walls thin with loss of connective tissue Alveolar surface area increases Double capillary network fuses into a single network Fibroblasts differentiate Collagen, elastin, and fibronectin deposited Surfactant production increases in Type II cells	Lobar emphysema (overinflation) Pleural effusions and fetal hydrops Persistent fetal circulation Pulmonary hypertension Pneumonia Meconium aspiration syndrome Respiratory distress syndrome/hyaline membrane disease/surfactant deficiency

and eight to nine bronchi on the left, which become the bronchopulmonary segments of the mature lung. At this stage of development, the mesenchyme is composed of a loose arrangement of primitive cells that will later differentiate into progenitor cells of future blood vessels, lymphatics, smooth muscle, cartilage, and connective tissue components. The extracellular matrix (ECM) is composed primarily of fluid, hyaluronic acid, and proteoglygans. The basement membrane underlying the epithelium contains Type IV collagen and other basement membrane glycoproteins, such as laminin and fibronectin, and proteoglycans.[7] The trachea and bronchial tubules lack underlying cartilage, smooth muscle, and nerves; the pulmonary and bronchial blood vessels are not well developed; and the pseudostratified columnar epithelium is composed of relatively primitive, undifferentiated epithelial cells. At the end of this stage, the lung resembles a small tubuloacinar gland, and separation of the trachea and esophagus is complete.

Vascular connections with the right and left atria are established at the end of the embryonic stage, creating the primitive pulmonary vascular bed. The pulmonary arteries arise from the sixth pair of aortic arches and grow into the surrounding mesoderm, where they accompany the developing airways, segmenting with each bronchial subdivision, and connect to the vascular plexus forming in the pulmonary mesenchyme.[8, 9] During fetal life, the pulmonary artery is connected to the aortic arch by the ductus arteriosus, which enables the right ventricular output

from the heart to bypass the pulmonary vascular bed. The pulmonary veins develop as an outgrowth of the left atrium, which divides several times before connecting to the pulmonary vascular bed.[10]

Developmental abnormalities that arise during the embryonic stage of lung development are related to lung bud formation, separation of the trachea and esophagus, formation of the proximal conducting airways, and initial lobe formation. These abnormalities include laryngeal, esophageal, and tracheal atresia, tracheal and bronchial stenosis, tracheomalacia and bronchomalacia, tracheoesophageal fistulas, pulmonary agenesis, ectopic lobes, bronchogenic cysts, and arteriovenous malformations (see Table 76–1).

Molecular Mechanisms Regulating Early Lung Development

Experimental studies have demonstrated that dorsal-ventral, lateral, and proximal-distal patterning of the developing lung is regulated by interactions with the surrounding mesenchyme.[11, 12] These interactions involve both positive and negative signaling mechanisms that result in normal growth and organization of the lung. Furthermore, experimental removal of mesenchymal tissue from the embryonic endoderm arrests branching morphogenesis *in vitro,* which demonstrates a critical role for the mesenchyme in the initial formation of the respiratory tract.[13-15]

Molecular mechanisms that regulate the initiation of lung bud formation and early branching morphogenesis include the following: (1) expression of nuclear DNA-binding proteins, or *tran-*

scription factors, that are important for specification of the foregut endoderm and its derivatives; (2) endogenous, secreted polypeptides, or *morphogens*, that are important for pattern formation; (3) *growth and differentiation factors* that are important for cellular proliferation, migration, and cytodifferentiation; and (4) exogenous factors, such as retinoic acid (vitamin A) that functions as a morphogen and is required for early lung bud formation.[16-19]

Transcription factors that are critical for foregut development and, by extension, early lung development, include members of the FOX, GATA, and GLI families of transcription factors. FOXa2 (also called HNF-3β) is a member of a large family of nuclear transcription factors, termed the *forkhead box* (forkhead DNA-binding domain) family of transcription factors. These nuclear proteins are involved in cell commitment, cytodifferentiation, and gene transcription in various organs, including the central nervous system and derivatives of the foregut endoderm.[20-22] FOXa2 regulates regional specification of cell fate, or cell commitment, in the primitive foregut endoderm and cooperates with another transcription factor, thyroid transcription factor-1 (TTF-1, also known as T/EBP, or Nkx2.1) to determine epithelial cell lineages. FOXa2 expression is detected in the pulmonary epithelium throughout lung development, and its expression is maintained in the fully differentiated adult bronchial and alveolar epithelium.[23, 24] FOXa2 is required for formation of the foregut endoderm, as well as organogenesis and cytodifferentiation of the lung. GATA-6 is a zinc finger transcription factor that induces differentiation of the primitive foregut endoderm into respiratory cell lineages via its interactions with TTF-1 and FOXa2. GATA-6 is expressed in the foregut endoderm and in the pulmonary epithelium during lung development. Genetic ablation of *Foxa2* or *Gata6* in mice disrupts formation of the foregut endoderm and all its developmental derivatives, including the lung.[25-27] TTF-1 is a nuclear transcription factor, or homeobox protein, that is expressed in the epithelium of the lung throughout development, as well as in the adult lung.[23, 28, 29] TTF-1 is essential for branching morphogenesis, epithelial cell proliferation, development of distal lung structures, and expression of the surfactant proteins. When *Ttf1* is inactivated in gene-targeted mice, lung development is perturbed, resulting in the formation of bilateral, saclike structures that are lined with primitive epithelial cells and originate from a short, common tracheoesophageal tube.[30, 31] The absence of TTF-1 arrests dorsoventral separation of the trachea and esophagus, branching morphogenesis of the lung, and epithelial cell differentiation.

Members of the GLI family of zinc finger transcription factors—GLI1, GLI2, GLI3—are expressed in the foregut mesoderm and are downstream transducers of sonic hedgehog (SHH) signaling.[32] SHH is a secreted polypeptide that is expressed in the foregut endoderm and in the primitive epithelial cells of the lung, as well as in the notochord, the neural plate, and the brain. Its receptors, patched1 (PTCH1) and patched2 (PTCH2), are expressed in both the mesoderm (PTCH1) and the endoderm (PTCH2) of the lung. When SHH binds to its receptor, another transmembrane protein, called smoothened (SMO), is released and translocated to the nucleus, where it activates the *Gli2* and *Gli3* genes.[32] The *Gli2* and *Gli3* genes, in turn, modulate the expression of other genes that play a role in lung development, such as *Gli1*, *Ptch1*, *Foxa2*, and *Fgf10*.[16,32] Both SHH and the GLI family members are associated with induction of cellular proliferation, as well as dorsal-lateral patterning of the lung. SHH expression is found at the growing tips of the bronchial tubules, where it is thought to act as a mitogen for the adjacent, primitive, mesenchymal cells. *Shh* null mutant mice exhibit foregut abnormalities. Branching morphogenesis is severely impaired, resulting in extremely hypoplastic, rudimentary lungs that originate from a fused tracheoesophageal tube.[33] Genetic ablation of *Gli2* (*Gli2-/-*) in mice also causes foregut defects, including

esophageal and tracheal stenosis, pulmonary hypoplasia, and lobulation defects (fusion of the four right lobes into one lobe), coincident with diminished expression of *Ptch1* and the *Gli1* isoform.[34] Genetic inactivation of both *Gli2* and *Gli3* in compound, homozygous *Gli2-/-;Gli3-/-* mice results in complete pulmonary agenesis, including agenesis of both the trachea and the lung, as well as the esophagus. Esophageal atresia and tracheoesophageal fistula with fusion of the lung in the midline are found in compound *Gli2-/-;Gli3+/-* mice.[34]

Growth factors that are critical for early lung formation include members of the fibroblast growth factor family (FGF) and their receptors, FGFR1, 2, 3, and 4, which induce cellular proliferation, migration, and differentiation in the developing lung. One of the most critical events in the induction of early branching morphogenesis is the activation of FGF-10 expression in the mesoderm. FGF-10 functions as a chemoattractant, inducing growth of the bronchial buds toward regions of FGF-10 expression in the mesoderm. FGF-10 signaling is mediated by its receptor, FGFR2, which is a tyrosine kinase receptor expressed in the foregut endoderm and primitive respiratory epithelium. Disruption of *Fgf10* or *FgfR2* expression in mutant mice results in the formation of a trachea but no lungs,[35-38] whereas blockade of FGFR2 signaling in transgenic mice, by using a mutant, dominant-negative, receptor *FgfR2(IIIb)*, completely blocks branching of all the conducting airways distal to the primary bronchi.[39] More recently, excision of a single copy of the *FgfR(IIIc)* isoform (expressed in the mesenchyme) resulted in a gain of function mutation with increased expression of the *FgfR2(IIIb)* isoform in mice.[38] This mutation resulted in kidney, lung, lacrimal gland, and skeletal defects, similar to those found in the human congenital disorders, *Apert* and *Pfeiffer syndromes*, which are caused by missense mutations in the human *FGFR2* gene.[40]

Retinoic acid signaling is required for normal development of many different organs, including the lung. Retinoic acid signaling appears to be required for lung bud formation, because acute vitamin A deprivation in pregnant animals at the onset of lung development results in tracheal stenosis and pulmonary agenesis.[18] Retinoic acid activity is mediated by binding to retinoic acid receptors, RAR(α,β,γ) and RXR(α,β,γ), to form a complex that is translocated to the nucleus, where it modulates gene transcription by binding to retinoic acid response elements in noncoding regions of its target genes. These receptors have multiple isoforms that form heterodimers with each other and are widely expressed throughout the embryo, as well as in the pulmonary epithelium and surrounding mesenchyme. Genetic ablation of retinoic acid receptors in mice causes abnormalities resembling those found in vitamin A–deficient animals, including malformations of the eyes, skeleton, limbs, aortic arch, genitourinary tract, and lung. Disruption of retinoic acid signaling in compound *Rarα1-/-;Rarβ2-/-* mice results in tracheoesophageal fistula, agenesis of the left lung, and hypoplasia of the right lung.[41] Subsequent development of the lung during branching morphogenesis is associated with down-regulation of retinoic acid signaling, which increases FGF-10 expression and limits proliferation of distal epithelial structures.[42] Conversely, maintenance of retinoic acid signaling in embryonic lung cultures disrupts the formation of distal lung structures while promoting the formation of proximal structures, most likely through up-regulation of the SHH pathway, which inhibits FGF-10 signaling.[42] Retinoic acid signaling may be further mediated by interactions with the HOX family of homeodomain transcription factors, which determine anteroposterior patterning of the body axis during development. Expression of the HOX genes is regulated both spatially and temporally during lung development and is associated with branching morphogenesis. In the mouse, *Hoxb3*, *Hoxb4*, and *Hoxb5* are expressed in the foregut endoderm where the lung buds will form. Aberrant expression of HOXb5 was associated with human *bronchopulmonary sequestration*, a finding suggesting that dysregulation of the *HOXb5* gene may be involved in the development of this accessory, or extrapulmonary, lung structure.[43] In the mouse lung, *Hoxb3* and *Hoxb4* are expressed in the mesenchyme of the trachea, bronchi, and distal lung, whereas *Hoxa5, Hoxb2,* and *Hoxb5* are restricted to the distal mesenchyme.[44] Retinoic acid up-regulates *Hoxb5* in embryonic lung cultures, resulting in abnormally elongated bronchial tubes and decreased branching,[45] whereas inhibition of *Hoxb5* expression results in short primary branches with decreased secondary branching.[45] Targeted deletion of the *Hoxa5* gene in mice results in laryngotracheal malformation, reduced number of cartilaginous, tracheal, and bronchial rings, tracheal stenosis, impaired branching morphogenesis, and thickened alveolar walls.[46] Loss of HOXa5 was also associated with decreased expression of TTF-1 and FOXa2, as well as their target genes, the surfactant proteins, in this experimental model.[46] Expression of N-*myc*, a proto-oncogene involved in cellular proliferation and branching morphogenesis in the lung,[47] was enhanced.[46]

Congenital Disorders and Mutations Associated with Early Pulmonary Malformations

Pulmonary agenesis, lung lobulation defects, tracheal stenosis (dysplastic tracheal cartilage), and tracheoesophageal fistula have been observed in some patients with *Pallister-Hall syndrome*, which is associated with mutations in the human *GLI3* gene.[48] Patients with these mutations also exhibit malformations involving the central nervous system (hypothalamic hamartoblastoma, pituitary aplasia or dysplasia), craniofacial features, limbs (postaxial polydactyly), kidneys (renal dysplasia), adrenal glands (adrenal hypoplasia), and the heart.[49] Esophageal atresia, tracheoesophageal fistula, esophageal and tracheal stenosis (cartilaginous sleeves), laryngomalacia, tracheomalacia, bronchomalacia, lobar atresia, and pulmonary aplasia have been observed in patients with *Pfeiffer, Apert,* and *Crouzon syndromes*, all of which are associated with mutations in the human *FGFR2* gene.[49-53] Patients with these mutations also exhibit varying degrees of craniosynostosis, or premature closure of the cranial sutures.[51]

Pseudoglandular Stage (5 to 17 Weeks Post Conception)

The *pseudoglandular stage* of lung development is so named because of the distinct glandular appearance of the lung during this period of morphogenesis; that is, the lung is composed of multiple epithelial tubules surrounded by relatively extensive regions of mesenchyme. At the beginning of this stage, the rate of cell proliferation increases, and sequential branching of the airways and vascular structures continues. Formation of the conducting airways, including the terminal bronchioles, is more or less complete by the end of this stage, with 12 to 17 generations of bronchial tubules in the upper lobes, 18 to 23 in the middle lobes, and 14 to 23 in the lower lobes.[54] Numerous *acinar tubules* and *buds*, which give rise to the adult *pulmonary acinus*, are also formed in the periphery of the lung by the end of this stage, arising as distal branches of the terminal bronchioles.[55,56] The pulmonary acinus includes two to four respiratory bronchioles, each ending in six to seven generations of branched alveolar ducts and sacs.

The bronchial tubules are lined initially by a pseudostratified columnar epithelium. These cells are morphologically undifferentiated and contain large pools of intracellular glycogen, deriving most of their energy needs from anaerobic glycolysis. A prominent basement membrane, rich in laminin and collagen Type IV, underlies the epithelium. Mesenchymal cells adjacent to these tubules differentiate into myofibroblasts by 7 weeks PC and align themselves in a circumferential orientation that is perpendicular to the long axis of the tubules. The ECM is composed

of various types of glycosaminoglycans and proteoglycans, such as chondroitin, dermatan, and heparan sulfate, as well as laminin, fibronectin, tenascin, and Type I and Type III collagen.[7, 12] These macromolecules are important for cell proliferation, migration, adhesion, and differentiation during lung development. As branching progresses, the pseudostratified columnar epithelium is reduced to a tall columnar epithelium in the proximal airways and to a cuboidal epithelium in the distal acinar tubules and buds. Cytodifferentiation of the conducting airway epithelium occurs in a centrifugal direction with ciliated, nonciliated (serous), goblet, neuroepithelial, and basal cells appearing first in the more proximal airways.[57,58] Isolated neuroepithelial cells, the first bronchial epithelial cells to differentiate, can be detected in the proximal airways by 8 to 9 weeks PC.[59] Clusters of neuroepithelial cells, called *neuroendocrine bodies*, are detected by 9 to 10 weeks PC. These are located at branch points along the bronchial tree and are innervated by sympathetic and sensory nerve fibers. Ciliated cells appear in the epithelium of the trachea by 10 weeks, in the mainstem bronchi by 12 weeks, and in the segmental bronchi by 13 weeks. Cartilage appears in the trachea and bronchi by 10 weeks and in the segmental bronchi by 16 weeks.[60] Mucous glands appear in the trachea by 11 to 12 weeks and in the bronchi by 13 weeks, with active mucus production by 14 weeks.[61] By the end of this developmental stage, cartilaginous structures extend as far as the segmental bronchi, and airway smooth muscle extends as far as the alveolar ducts. Spontaneous contractility of fetal airway smooth muscle can be observed in cultured human fetal lung explants at this stage of development.[62] The smooth muscle layer enveloping the conducting airways is invested by an extensive network, or plexus, of neural ganglia and nerve bundles that is detected as early as 7.5 to 8 weeks PC.[63] Elastic fibers are detected in the walls of the trachea and the mainstem bronchi, the pleura, and the pulmonary artery.[7] Epithelial cell differentiation is initiated in the distal acinar structures with the onset of surfactant protein B (SP-B) and C (SP-C) expression. These two hydrophobic, lung-specific proteins are expressed selectively in the distal respiratory epithelium by 12 to 14 weeks PC.[64]

The intrapulmonary arterial system develops along with the bronchial and bronchiolar tubules, branching in parallel with these airways.[8, 9, 65] The pulmonary veins and lymphatics take a different pathway through the lung, coursing in between the airways in the connective tissue septa that divide and surround each pulmonary segment.[66] All the preacinar, or distal, arteries and veins are formed by the end of this period.[67-69] Formation of these structures takes place through the process of *vasculogenesis*, that is, by the coalescence of nascent endothelial cells, or *angioblasts* (derived from the mesenchyme), into endothelial tubes. These tubes gradually become invested with smooth muscle cells, so by the end of this developmental stage, smooth muscle actin and myosin can be detected in all the vasculature.[70-72]

Various congenital defects in branching morphogenesis may arise during the pseudoglandular stage of lung development, including bronchopulmonary sequestration, congenital cystic adenomatoid malformations (CCAMs), cyst formation, acinar dysplasia or aplasia, and pulmonary hypoplasia. The pleuroperitoneal cavity also closes early in the pseudoglandular period. Failure to close the pleural cavity is often accompanied by herniation of the abdominal contents, leading to secondary pulmonary hypoplasia (see later).

Molecular Mechanisms Regulating Branching Morphogenesis

During the pseudoglandular stage of lung development, FGF-10 signaling continues to be critical for branching morphogenesis. FGF-7 (also called KGF) is also expressed in the mesenchyme at this time and binds to FGFR2 receptors in the epithelium. FGF-7 influences branching morphogenesis by promoting epithelial growth and differentiation. Overexpression of FGF-7 in transgenic mice results in the formation of large, fluid-filled, cystlike structures,[73, 74] whereas *Fgf7* null mutants have no abnormalities, a finding suggesting that FGF-7 signaling in the lung overlaps with that of other growth factors.[75] FGF-9 is also expressed at high levels during this stage of lung development, but it is synthesized in the pulmonary epithelium, not in the mesenchyme. FGF-9 signaling is mediated through FGFR1 receptors, which are expressed in the mesenchyme. Targeted disruption of *Fgf9* in null mutant mice results in pulmonary hypoplasia due to a reduction in mesenchymal tissue and decreased branching of the airways, although sacculation of the peripheral air spaces and cytodifferentiation of alveolar epithelial cells are not perturbed.[76]

Additional growth factors that promote branching morphogenesis and growth of the lung include the following: (1) FGF-1 (also known as acidic FGF) and FGF-2 (also known as basic FGF), which up-regulate FGF-7; (2) epidermal growth factor (EGF) and transforming growth factor-α (TGF-α), which stimulate branching morphogenesis, cell proliferation, and cytodifferentiation through their receptor, EGFR; (3) hepatocyte growth factor (HGF), which is a potent mitogen; (4) insulin-like growth factor (IGF), which facilitates signaling of other growth factors; (5) platelet-derived growth factor (PDGF), which is a potent mitogen and chemoattractant for mesenchymal cells; and (6) vascular endothelial growth factor (VEGF), which regulates vascular growth and patterning.[16, 17]

Factors that tend to antagonize or limit FGF signaling, in addition to SHH, include transforming growth factor-β (TGF-β), bone morphogenetic protein 4 (BMP4), and the Sprouty (*Spry2* and *Spry4*) genes, which may also modulate the EGF and TGF-β pathways.[16, 17] TGF-β modulates branching morphogenesis in the lung by limiting epithelial bud formation. TGF-β accumulates in the mesenchyme adjacent to the proximal airways and at sites of cleft formation (between the branching airways), where it inhibits FGF-10 expression and promotes the synthesis and deposition of ECM components. Deposition of ECM components stabilizes the proximal airways and prevents further branching at these sites. Induction of SMAD family members, downstream mediators of TGF-β, also inhibits cell proliferation, as well as FGF-10 expression.[16] Members of the TGF-β family are also important for proximal-distal differentiation and left-right patterning in the lung. Weaver and colleagues[77] showed that disruption of BMP4 signaling in mice alters proximal-distal differentiation patterns in the developing pulmonary epithelium. BMP4 is expressed at high levels in the distal epithelium and counteracts FGF-10–induced bud formation. Overexpression of the BMP antagonist, *Xnoggin*, or blockade of BMP4 signaling in transgenic mice by using a dominant-negative BMP receptor (*dnAlk6*), resulted in a reduction of distal alveolar cell types with a concomitant increase in bronchiolar cell types (ciliated cells and Clara cells).[77] Overexpression of GREMLIN, a secreted protein that binds to BMP4 and prevents it from interacting with its receptor, resulted in a similar phenotype in transgenic mice,[78] whereas reduction of GREMLIN expression in cultured lungs increased branching morphogenesis, epithelial cell proliferation, and cytodifferentiation of Type II cells.[79]

Left-right asymmetry is accomplished by a signaling cascade involving four other members of the TGF-β family: LEFTY-1, LEFTY-2, NODAL, and GDF1.[17] LEFTY-1 restricts the expression of LEFTY-2 and NODAL to the left side. Inactivation of *Lefty-1* in mice leads to bilateral expression of *Lefty-2*, resulting in left pulmonary isomerism. In this condition, the lobation pattern normally seen on the right side (four lobes) is replaced by the left-sided pattern (one lobe), resulting in bilateral single, or "left," lobes.[80] In contrast, targeted deletion of *Nodal* or *Gdf1* results in right isomerism of the lung.[81, 82] Other factors that may be involved in left-right patterning in the lung include retinoic acid signaling and FOXj1 (also known as HFH-4) expression. Targeted disruption of retinoic acid signaling in compound *RARα1–/–;*

RARβ2–/– null mutant mice results in agenesis of the left pulmonary lobe,[41] whereas targeted disruption of the nuclear transcription factor *Foxj1* results in random left-right asymmetry, as well as the complete absence of cilia.[83] This phenotype is similar to that seen in the human congenital disorder *Kartagener syndrome*, in which situs inversus, bronchiectasis, and immotile cilia are found.[49]

Molecular Mechanisms Regulating Vascular Development

Vascular growth and patterning is regulated by VEGF, which is synthesized in the epithelium and is secreted into the mesenchyme, where it binds to its receptors, VEGFR-1 (also known as Flt-1 in the mouse), VEGFR-2 (also known as Flk-1 in the mouse, or KDR in humans), and VEGFR-3, found on primitive endothelial cells.[84] Targeted inactivation of the *Vegf* gene in mice results in impaired angiogenesis and is lethal in the fetal period,[85] whereas targeted mutation of the VEGF receptor, *Flt-1*, is also lethal because of disrupted vascular formation in the embryo.[86] Recently, Ruhrberg and colleagues[87] engineered a transgenic mouse expressing an isoform of VEGF-A (*Vegf120/ 120*), which lacked heparin-binding, or ECM interaction domains. These mice survived beyond the neonatal period and exhibited a specific decrease in capillary branch formation. Expression of this isoform in the lung impaired lung microvascular development and delayed air space maturation.[88]

Vascular development is also dependent on interactions with surrounding ECM components. Fibronectin, which binds to endothelial cells via integrin receptors, is a component of the capillary basement membrane and is important for early capillary tube formation. Fibronectin also promotes cell migration and proliferation and prevents apoptosis, or cell death. Mice that lack the fibronectin gene fail to develop normal vasculature and die *in utero*.[89] Laminin, a large, noncollagenous glycoprotein, is another important basement membrane component that promotes cell attachment, migration, differentiation, cell growth, and vascular tube formation.[90] Type IV collagen, which is the major structural component of mature basement membranes, also binds to endothelial cells through specific integrin receptors and promotes cell attachment and cytodifferentiation. Type IV collagen is expressed later than fibronectin and laminin, and its appearance coincides with a reduction in endothelial cell division, promoting tube formation and stabilizing the structure of newly formed vessels. Adhesion molecules, such as E-selectin, also promote capillary tube formation.

Additional growth factors that modulate vascular development include PDGF-A and PDGF-B, which function as mitogens and chemoattractants for other mesenchymal cells that will be incorporated into the vessel wall. Once these cells contact the endothelium, they differentiate into smooth muscle cells, most likely through the activation and secretion of TGF-β, which, in turn, inhibits further endothelial cell proliferation and stimulates ECM deposition (elastin and collagen) by the smooth muscle cells. A similar phenomenon occurs with the recruitment of smooth muscle cells by the developing bronchial tubules. In addition to PDGF and TGF-β, endothelial cells secrete various other growth factors and inhibitors that are important for cell proliferation and differentiation. These include EGF/TGF-α, FGF-1, FGF-2, IGF-I, and IGF-II, all of which stimulate cell proliferation; and tumor necrosis factor-α and heparan sulfate, which inhibit cell proliferation. The deposition of ECM components (collagen and elastin) appears to be stimulated by both PDGF and TGF-β, as well as by IGF-I and IGF-II.[65]

Canalicular Stage (16 to 26 Weeks Post Conception)

The *canalicular stage* is so named because of the appearance of vascular canals, or capillaries, that multiply in the interstitial compartment to form the *air-blood barrier*, or *alveolar-capillary respiratory membrane*, the future gas-exchange surface of the lung.[1] Development of the alveolar-capillary membrane, along with the synthesis and secretion of pulmonary surfactant, is critical for extrauterine survival of the immature fetus, if delivered prematurely near the end of this stage. Gas exchange cannot occur in the premature infant unless these capillaries are close enough to the adjacent alveolar epithelium. Rapid expansion of the capillary bed, with condensation and thinning of the mesenchyme, is the first critical step in the formation of the gas-exchange regions of the lung. During this stage of lung development, the total surface area of the alveolar-capillary membrane increases exponentially with a concomitant decrease in the mean mesenchymal wall thickness, thereby increasing the potential for gas exchange in the immature lung.[1] Disturbances in this stage of lung development result in severe hypoxemia and are not compatible with life after birth.

At the beginning of the canalicular stage, formation of the bronchial tree is complete, and the terminal bronchioles have divided into two or more respiratory bronchioles that have subdivided further into small clusters of short acinar tubules and buds lined by cuboidal epithelium. These structures undergo further differentiation to become the adult respiratory unit, or *pulmonary acinus,* consisting of alveolarized respiratory bronchioles, alveolar ducts, and alveoli. Clusters of acinar tubules and buds grow by further lengthening, subdividing, and widening at the expense of the surrounding mesenchyme. The proportion of dividing epithelial and endothelial cells increases, and the number of dividing interstitial cells (fibroblasts) falls. Epithelial growth drops in the larger airways, and cell proliferation occurs predominantly in the peripheral acinar tubules and buds. This peripheral growth is accompanied by the growth and development of intra-acinar capillaries (derived from angioblastic cells in the interstitium), which align themselves around the air spaces, establishing contact with the adjacent epithelium to form the primitive alveolar-capillary membrane. Epithelial cell differentiation becomes increasingly complex and is especially apparent in the distal regions of the lung parenchyma, where alveolar Type I and Type II cells can be detected. Bronchiolar cells begin to express differentiated features and to synthesize cell-specific proteins, such as the Clara cell secretory protein (CCSP).[23, 91-93] Cuboidal Type II cells lining the distal tubules express increasing amounts of surfactant proteins and phospholipids.[23, 64, 94-99] Nascent lamellar bodies, the storage form of pulmonary surfactant, are seen in association with rich glycogen stores in cuboidal pre-Type II cells lining the acinar tubules and buds.[100-103] Cells of the proximal acinar tubules become flattened and attenuated, acquiring features of typical, squamous, Type I alveolar epithelial cells. Type I cell differentiation occurs in conjunction with the formation of the alveolar-capillary membrane, that is, wherever endothelial cells of the developing capillary system come into contact with adjacent acinar epithelial cells. Where this occurs, the intercellular junctional complexes, originally localized around the epithelial cell apex, shift to the basolateral aspect of the intercellular cleft. The cells develop thin cytoplasmic attenuations, differentiating into squamous Type I cells and losing features previously associated with pre-Type II cells. By the end of the canalicular stage of lung development, the potential alveolar-capillary membrane (air-blood barrier) is thin enough to support gas exchange.

Abnormalities of lung development associated with the canalicular stage include acinar dysplasia, alveolar capillary dysplasia, and pulmonary hypoplasia. Pulmonary hypoplasia is often caused by diaphragmatic hernia or compression by thoracic or abdominal masses, by prolonged rupture of membranes causing oligohydramnios, or by renal agenesis (Potter syndrome) in which amniotic fluid production is impaired. Whereas postnatal gas exchange can be supported late in the canalicular stage, infants born during this period generally suffer severe complica-

tions related to decreased levels of pulmonary surfactant, which cause respiratory distress syndrome (RDS) and hyaline membrane disease. The administration of exogenous surfactants improves survival in these infants, but bronchopulmonary dysplasia, a complication secondary to ventilatory therapy for RDS, frequently develops later. Surfactant synthesis and mesenchymal thinning can be accelerated by glucocorticoids,[104-106] which are administered to mothers to prevent RDS when a premature birth is anticipated.[107]

Saccular Stage (24 to 38 Weeks Post Conception)

During the *saccular stage* of lung development, the terminal clusters of acinar tubules and buds begin to dilate and expand into thin, smooth-walled, transitory alveolar saccules and ducts; there is a marked reduction, or condensation, of the surrounding mesenchymal (interstitial) tissue. The lung continues to grow peripherally by branching and growth of the transitory alveolar ducts, so by the end of this period, three additional generations of alveolar ducts ending in terminal saccules have formed. These peripheral regions of the lung also increase in size as a result of lengthening and widening of all of the segments distal to the terminal bronchioles. Intersaccular and interductal septa develop that contain delicate collagen fibers and a double capillary network.[1] Overall cell proliferation slows as a result of a sharp drop in division of the epithelial cell population. With the reduction in epithelial cell proliferation comes ultrastructural evidence of cytodifferentiation. Maturation of Type II epithelial cells continues and is associated with increased synthesis of surfactant phospholipids[97, 108, 109] and the surfactant-associated proteins A, B, C, and D.[23, 64, 94, 96, 98, 99, 111] Glycogen content is reduced, and mitochondrial enzyme activity increases, indicating a shift to aerobic oxidative pathways. Lamellar bodies increase in number and size, and increasing amounts of tubular myelin (the secretory form of pulmonary surfactant) are seen in the terminal air spaces.[100, 102] The concentration of pulmonary surfactant is still low, however, and its phospholipid composition differs significantly from that at term.[108]

Squamous Type I cells continue to differentiate and line an increasing proportion of the surface area of the distal lung. Enlargement of the potential gas exchange surface is dependent on the development of Type I cells with their attenuated, flattened, squamous cell shape. Capillaries become associated more closely with the squamous Type I cells, decreasing the diffusion distance between the air spaces and the capillary bed. Basal lamina of the epithelium and endothelium fuse to form the thin-walled, alveolar-capillary membrane. In the newborn and adult lung, the mean thickness of the alveolar-capillary membrane is 0.6 μm, a size that permits passive diffusion of oxygen and carbon dioxide between the alveolar lumen and the capillary bed.[1] Near the end of this stage, the stroma, or interstitial tissue, contains increasing amounts of ECM, and elastin is deposited in areas where future interalveolar septa will form, thus subdividing the terminal alveolar saccules into true alveoli. The immature lung contains relatively few elastin and collagen fibers, has little elastic recoil, and can be easily ruptured at this stage.[7]

By the beginning of the saccular stage of lung development, the conducting airways have developed both mucous cells and ciliated cells. Cartilage and submucosal glands extend as far down the airway as they do in the adult lung. The epithelial cells are capable of producing fetal lung fluid.

Abnormalities associated with the saccular stage of lung development are similar to those associated with the canalicular stage of lung development, including pulmonary hypoplasia, acinar dysplasia or aplasia, alveolar capillary dysplasia, RDS, hyaline membrane disease, and bronchopulmonary dysplasia in the premature infant.

Alveolar Stage (36 Weeks Post Conception to 2 Years Postnatally)

The *alveolar stage* is the last stage of lung development and is marked by the formation of secondary alveolar septa, which partition the terminal ducts and saccules into true alveolar ducts and alveoli, and by maturation of the alveolar-capillary membrane. This process greatly increases the surface area of the lung available for gas exchange. At the beginning of this stage, the alveolar septa are relatively thick and contain a capillary network on each side of a central core of connective tissue, often referred to as a double capillary network.[1] The secondary interalveolar septa consist of short buds or projections of connective tissue that also contain a double capillary network and interstitial cells that are actively synthesizing collagen and elastin. Restructuring of the terminal saccule into a true alveolus consists of lengthening and thinning of the secondary septa, reduction of septal interstitial tissue, and remodeling of the capillary bed by fusion of the two septal capillary networks into one.[1] Pulmonary vascular resistance decreases as remodeling of the pulmonary vasculature and capillary bed occurs. This stage is accompanied by a phase of rapid cellular proliferation in both the epithelial and mesenchymal cell populations. Interstitial fibroblasts actively proliferate early in this stage, but then they slow down as synthesis and deposition of collagen, elastin, and fibronectin begin to increase. Endothelial growth is brisk throughout this stage, and dividing endothelial cells are located primarily in the developing secondary septal crests. Both Type II and Type I cells increase in number during this stage, but only Type II cells are proliferating actively, a feature suggesting that Type I cells are derived from Type II cells. Type I cells are thought to be terminally differentiated and to lack the capacity for mitosis. Although Type II cells account for two-thirds of the total number of alveolar epithelial cells in the adult human lung, the larger squamous Type I cells actually occupy 93% of the total alveolar surface. Type I cells form a tight epithelial barrier that is impervious to extracellular fluid and ions; however, they are easily injured by oxidants, barotrauma, and infection, readily detaching from the alveolar wall when injured. Injury to the lung during this stage of development can result in abnormal remodeling of the lung with a reduction in the number of alveoli and the development of interstitial fibrosis. An additional factor that may cause disturbances in alveolarization is administration of glucocorticoids, which inhibits cellular proliferation, thereby reducing septation and formation of alveoli. Conversely, glucocorticoid administration enhances thinning of the alveolar septa, increases maturation of Type II cells, and enhances the production of surfactant in the premature lung and in fetal lung explants.[104-106]

Disorders associated with disturbances in the alveolar stage of lung development, which present at birth, include persistent fetal circulation and pulmonary hypertension of the newborn, lobar emphysema, meconium aspiration syndrome, pneumonia, and RDS associated with genetic surfactant protein B deficiency.[112,113]

Molecular Mechanisms Regulating Alveolar Development

Although many studies describing the effects of exogenous substances or mechanical ventilation on alveolar development in the premature lung have been published, little is known about the molecular mechanisms that regulate morphogenesis and cytodifferentiation during the canalicular, saccular, and alveolar stages of normal lung development. Factors that modulate elastin formation in the developing lung have been shown to play an important role in the process of alveologenesis. *Alveologenesis* is characterized by the development of secondary septa that subdivide the terminal air sacs into definitive alveoli. This process appears to be driven by the synthesis and deposition of elastin by alveolar myofibroblasts located at the tips of the developing

septa. PDGF, a potent mitogen and chemoattractant for mesenchymal cells, is expressed in the pulmonary epithelium, whereas its receptor, PDGFRα, is found on presumptive alveolar smooth muscle cells, or myofibroblasts. In mice with a targeted deletion of the *Pdfg-A* gene, myofibroblasts fail to multiply and migrate into the primary alveolar septa.[114,115] This results in postnatal development of emphysema, or enlarged alveolar saccules, owing to a complete failure of alveologenesis, as well as reduced deposition of elastin in the lung parenchyma. Mice with a targeted deletion of the elastin gene (*Eln-/-*) also develop emphysema in the postnatal period because of the absence of elastin synthesis and deposition, which also results in the complete failure of alveologenesis.[116] Retinoic acid has been shown to enhance ongoing alveologenesis by up-regulating the transcription of tropoelastin, the soluble precursor of elastin.[117] Mice bearing compound null deletions in the retinoic acid receptors, RAR-γ-/-, RXR-α+/-, demonstrate a decrease in elastin gene expression and elastic tissue with a reduction in alveolar formation in the postnatal lung.[118]

FGF signaling has also been implicated in the process of alveologenesis. The lungs of compound null mutant mice, homozygous for targeted deletion of both the *FgfR-3* and *FgfR-4* genes, are completely blocked in alveologenesis and do not form definitive alveoli.[119] In contrast to the *Pdfg-A* and *Eln* null mutant mice, no abnormalities in the alveolar myofibroblast cell population or in elastin synthesis and deposition during alveologenesis were observed. However, increased elastin deposition was detected later in the postnatal period (day 21), suggesting that elastin synthesis was increased. Although the double mutant mice were 50% smaller than normal mice, were sickly, and died within the first few months of life, no differences in cell proliferation, cell death, or surfactant protein production were found in their lungs.[119]

As described earlier, the nuclear transcription factor GATA-6 has been shown to be important for development of the foregut endoderm. Targeted deletion of the *Gata-6* gene in mice disrupts formation of the foregut endoderm and all its developmental derivatives including the lung.[25] GATA-6 has also been implicated in the regulation of gene expression in the lung. *In vitro* studies have shown that GATA-6 enhances transcription of TTF-1, as well as SP-A and SP-C.[120-122] Lung-specific expression of a GATA-6-Engrailed, dominant-negative, fusion protein in transgenic mice inhibited maturation of the alveolar epithelium during the saccular and alveolar periods of lung development.[123,124] Transgenic mice lacked detectable alveolar Type I cells, with decreased expression of the Type I cell markers aquaporin-5 and T1α. Although the distal airways were dilated, squamous differentiation of the alveolar epithelium was disrupted. Instead, the distal airways were lined with cuboidal alveolar Type II cells. The alveolar septa were thickened, with a relatively undeveloped capillary network. Expression of SP-B, SP-C, CCSP, and FOXj1 was also decreased.

ABNORMAL DEVELOPMENT OF THE LUNG AND CONDUCTING AIRWAYS

As can be seen from Table 76-1, most pulmonary malformations arise during the embryonic and pseudoglandular stages of lung development. These malformations represent a spectrum of closely related abnormalities associated with the early stage of lung bud formation, branching morphogenesis, separation of the trachea from the esophagus, and failure of the pleuroperitoneal cavity to close properly. Abnormalities in other organ systems, such as renal agenesis, dysplastic growth of the kidney, or congenital diaphragmatic hernia, may also affect branching morphogenesis of the lung during these early developmental stages. During the canalicular and saccular stages of lung development, abnormalities related to growth and maturation of the respiratory parenchyma and its vasculature predominate, leading to abnormalities in acinar development, alveolar capillary dysplasia, pulmonary hypoplasia, and respiratory insufficiency. Infants born prematurely, during the saccular and early alveolar stages of development, are subject to clinical complications and syndromes that are related primarily to biochemical immaturity of the lung, or surfactant deficiency. *Surfactant deficiency* causes respiratory distress in the immediate postnatal period and has been associated with hyaline membrane disease. Acute lung injury in the neonatal period may alter subsequent alveolar growth and differentiation, resulting in bronchopulmonary dysplasia or chronic interstitial lung disease. Mutations in the SP-B gene have been associated with respiratory distress and failure in full-term infants,[112,113] whereas mutations in the SP-C gene have been associated with the onset of chronic interstitial lung disease in the first year of life.[125]

Congenital Malformations of the Tracheobronchial Tree

Tracheoesophageal Fistulas

Most congenital malformations of the tracheobronchial tree arise during formation of the respiratory diverticulum and branching morphogenesis of the lung. One of the most critical events in the formation of the respiratory system is the initial separation of the primitive foregut into the respiratory and alimentary tracts. This process begins during the third week of gestation and is complete by the sixth week. Failure of this process to proceed normally results in the formation of a *tracheoesophageal fistula*, one of the most commonly encountered abnormalities of the trachea. Tracheoesophageal fistulas are usually found in combination with various forms of esophageal atresia. The most common combination is esophageal atresia with a lower, or distal, tracheoesophageal fistula: the upper segment of the esophagus ends in a blind pouch, whereas the lower segment originates from the trachea just above the bifurcation. This combination accounts for 80 to 90% of all cases.[126] Tracheoesophageal fistula in low birth weight infants is often associated with various other malformations, and it carries a high risk of a poor outcome. In comparison, survival of term infants with isolated tracheoesophageal fistula is almost 100%. Tracheoesophageal fistula is found in VACTERL syndrome, in association with vertebral anomalies, anal atresia, congenital cardiac disease, renal anomalies, and limb abnormalities.[49,126] From their mutant analysis of the *Gli* genes, which encode transcription factors mediating SHH signal transduction, Kim and colleagues[127,128] observed that defective SHH signaling leads to a spectrum of developmental anomalies in mice strikingly similar to those of VACTERL syndrome. These investigators proposed that VACTERL syndrome could be caused by defective SHH signaling during human embryogenesis.

Tracheal Agenesis, Tracheal Stenosis, and Tracheomalacia

Tracheal agenesis is a rare, but fatal, anomaly thought to be caused by displacement of the tracheoesophageal septum. Classification of anatomic variations in this malformation is based on the length of the agenetic segment and the presence or absence of an esophageal fistula.[129,130] The most common variation is complete absence of the trachea below the larynx, with a fistula connecting fused mainstem bronchi and the esophagus. Other variations include tracheal agenesis with fistulas connecting each mainstem bronchi to the esophagus, agenesis of the proximal trachea with mainstem bronchi fused to form the distal trachea (with or without a fistulous connection to the esophagus), and a short segment of tracheal agenesis between the proximal and distal segments of the trachea, linked by an atretic fibrous band of tissue.

Tracheal stenosis is a rare malformation in which the trachea is narrowed, either because of intrinsic abnormalities in cartilage formation or by external compression from abnormal vessel formation or vascular rings.[129,130] Narrowing of the trachea by compression results in local obstruction to the passage of air, whereas cartilage deformities may cause obstruction of the airway on both inspiration and expiration. The major underlying causes of intrinsic tracheal stenosis are abnormalities in cartilaginous ring formation, either from posterior fusion of the normally C-shaped rings or from formation of a complete cartilaginous sleeve. The latter malformation has been reported in children with craniosynostosis syndromes, including *Crouzon*, *Apert*, and *Pfeiffer syndromes*.[50,51] These syndromes involve abnormal fusion of skeletal or osseous structures and are associated with mutations in *FGFR2*.[40,52] These malformations represent mesenchymal defects in which the cells do not respond normally to FGF signaling. Extrinsic stenosis of the trachea is caused by external compression of the trachea, usually associated with abnormally situated blood vessels, termed vascular rings.

Tracheomalacia occurs when there is an absence or "softening" of the cartilaginous rings that causes the trachea to collapse on expiration, creating an obstruction. In the normal trachea, the cartilage/soft tissue ratio is 4.5:1, a ratio that remains constant throughout childhood.[129] In tracheomalacia, there is a reduction in this ratio, in some instances as low as 2:1.[129] This malformation may be segmental or diffuse. In most cases, tracheomalacia is associated with other congenital malformations, such as tracheoesophageal fistula and vascular rings.

Bronchial Atresia, Bronchial Stenosis, and Bronchomalacia

Bronchial atresia is a rare anomaly. The most commonly affected lobe is the left upper lobe, but atresia of the right upper and lower lobes has also been reported. The segmental bronchus is the most common site of atresia, but subsegmental and lobar bronchi can also be affected.[129,130] The distal lung is hypoplastic, emphysematous, or hyperinflated. Often, there is a deficiency of bronchi and vessels in the affected lobe, as well as an absence of segmentation and interlobular septa. Like tracheal stenosis, *bronchial stenosis* may be intrinsic or caused by extrinsic compression.[129,130] Intrinsic bronchial stenosis is rare and is usually associated with anomalous cartilage segmentation. Extrinsic bronchial stenosis from compression is usually associated with congenital heart disease. Compression occurs when the pulmonary arteries enlarge in response to pulmonary hypertension, thus compressing the left upper lobe bronchus. An enlarged left atrium, a bronchogenic cyst, or a teratoma may also compress the left main bronchus. *Bronchomalacia* is caused by abnormalities in the bronchial cartilage that lead to collapse, or bronchiectasis, of the affected airway during respiration. Bronchomalacia may be associated with other anomalies, various skeletal dysplasias, or widespread congenital cartilage deficiency.[129,130]

Bronchopulmonary Sequestration

Bronchopulmonary sequestration develops as a mass of abnormal pulmonary tissue, which is not connected to the tracheobronchial tree and receives its blood supply from one or more anomalous systemic arteries arising from the aorta.[129–131] There are two forms of bronchopulmonary sequestration. *Intralobar sequestrations* occur within the visceral pleural lining of a pulmonary lobe, and *extralobar sequestrations* are found outside the pleural lining. Both types of sequestration occur more frequently on the left side, sometimes in association with diaphragmatic defects. Rarely, a sequestration may be connected to the esophagus or to the stomach.

Intralobar sequestrations are found most frequently in the posterior basal segment of the left lower lobe. The blood supply is derived from either the thoracic or abdominal aorta, whereas the venous drainage is to the pulmonary vein of the affected lobe. Embryologically, there appears to be a failure of the pulmonary artery to supply a peripheral portion of the lung. Instead, the arterial supply is derived from a persistent ventral branch of the primitive dorsal aorta. Although many cases of intralobar sequestration occur in children, at least half of affected patients are more than 20 years old when the diagnosis is made. Clinically, these patients present with recurrent pulmonary infection, cough, or chest pain. The affected tissue is often cystic, lined with either columnar or cuboidal epithelium, and filled with mucus. Again, there is a continuous accumulation of mucus secretions, which gives rise to acute or chronic infections and inflammation.

Extralobar sequestration develops as a complete, separate segment of pulmonary tissue, or accessory lobe, which is enclosed within its own pleural sac. Although the embryologic origin of this malformation is unknown, it may develop from the primitive gut as an extra, more distally placed, lung bud, which is then sealed off from the gut. Extralobar sequestration usually occurs on the lower left side of the thorax, often between the left lower lobe and the diaphragm. Other extrapulmonary sites of sequestration include paraesophageal, mediastinal, or paracardiac regions. Extralobar sequestration can also occur within the muscle of the diaphragm and below the diaphragm in the retroperitoneum. The arterial supply arises from the abdominal aorta or one of its branches, whereas the venous drainage is into the systemic venous system, thus creating a left-to-right shunt. This malformation is frequently associated with other congenital anomalies, especially congenital diaphragmatic defects, which occur in more than half of the cases. Most extralobar sequestrations are found in children less than 1 year of age, but the lesion occurs in older children and adults as well. Clinically, extralobar sequestration is usually asymptomatic and is often discovered during repair of a diaphragmatic defect. If the sequestration is located in the wall of the esophagus, however, it may cause dysphasia and hematemesis. Mediastinal or hilar locations may also cause symptoms because of bronchial obstruction and overinflation of the lobe, or, conversely, because of compression of normal pulmonary parenchyma. If the sequestered lobe becomes infected, it may appear to be a chronic pulmonary abscess accompanied by fever, chest pain, cough, and bloody, purulent sputum. Histologically, the lesion may be composed of normal lung or of immature or dysplastic pulmonary parenchyma, with absent or reduced number of cartilaginous bronchi and an irregular pattern of bronchiole-like structures resembling a cystic adenomatoid malformation (see later).

Congenital Bronchogenic Cysts

Bronchogenic cysts are caused by abnormal budding and branching of the tracheobronchial tree during its development.[129-131] Most bronchogenic cysts are found in paratracheal, carinal, hilar, or paraesophageal regions (middle mediastinum), but they may also be found in the lungs as pulmonary cysts, which communicate with the tracheobronchial tree. In neonates, communication between a cyst and the tracheobronchial tree may incorporate a check valve mechanism, which results in rapid expansion of the cyst. Sometimes the cyst becomes so large that it compresses the mediastinum, thus compromising the heart and resulting in death. Mediastinal cysts, conversely, rarely communicate with the tracheobronchial tree. They are often lined with ciliated columnar epithelial cells and rarely contain distal lung parenchyma. These cysts are filled with a clear, serous fluid unless they become infected. The walls of these cysts generally contain smooth muscle, cartilage, and mucous glands.

Congenital Lobar Emphysema (Pulmonary Overinflation)

Congenital lobar emphysema, or pulmonary overinflation, can be divided into two types: (1) congenital lobar overinflation; and (2) regional, or segmental, pulmonary overinflation.[129-131] In congenital lobar overinflation, either an upper or a middle lobe of the lung is hyperinflated and compresses the remaining ipsilateral lung or lobes. If there is a marked shift of the mediastinum to the opposite side, a ventilatory crisis ensues with dyspnea, cyanosis, and sometimes circulatory failure. Most cases are caused by partial bronchial obstruction. Extrinsic bronchial obstruction may be caused by dilated pulmonary vessels, and other cardiac defects that cause increased pulmonary blood flow. Intrathoracic masses, such as bronchogenic cysts, extralobar sequestrations, enlarged lymph nodes, and neoplasms, may also cause bronchial compression. Intrinsic bronchial obstruction is most often related to defects in the bronchial cartilage with absent or incomplete rings. These abnormal bronchi collapse during expiration, which causes distal air trapping and overinflation of the affected lobe. In regional, or segmental, pulmonary overinflation, only a small segment of the lung is hyperinflated.

Congenital Malformations of the Distal Lung Parenchyma

Pulmonary Agenesis and Aplasia

Pulmonary agenesis and aplasia represent two different forms of arrested lung development that result in the absence of the distal lung parenchyma.[129-131] *Pulmonary agenesis* is the complete absence of one or both lungs, including bronchi, bronchioles, vasculature, and respiratory parenchyma. In *pulmonary aplasia,* only rudimentary bronchi are present, each of which ends in a blind pouch, with no pulmonary vessels or respiratory parenchyma. The incidence of these anomalies is rare and represents failure of one of the primitive foregut branches to develop during the early, embryonic stage of lung development. Developmental arrest at a later stage may result in lobar agenesis or pulmonary dysplasia; some bronchial elements are present, but there are no alveoli.

Bilateral pulmonary agenesis is very rare and is caused by developmental arrest in the outgrowth of the respiratory primordium during the embryonic stage of lung development. Several cases of bilateral agenesis of the lung have been reported in the literature.[129,130] In one case, a trachea with 10 cartilaginous rings remained connected to the esophagus throughout its length. There were no lung buds or pleural cavities. In another case, the trachea was separated from the esophagus, but it ended blindly with only two cartilaginous rings. In other cases, branching morphogenesis was arrested at the bronchial bud stage.

Unilateral pulmonary agenesis is more common than bilateral pulmonary agenesis, and it may represent an imbalance in the growth of the lung buds. If balanced growth is not established between the left and right lung buds, then one side will develop normally, whereas the other will fail completely (aplasia) or will undergo limited development (dysplasia or hypoplasia). These defects arise early in lung development, when the respiratory primordium bifurcates into the right and left primitive lung buds at the end of the fourth week of gestation. These malformations suggest an absence or imbalance in the number of progenitor cells located in the two primitive lung buds that results in differential growth or arrest of lung development. Unilateral pulmonary agenesis may affect either lung, although the right side is more commonly involved. There are usually no serious clinical consequences, owing to compensatory growth, or hyperplasia, of the contralateral lung. Pulmonary agenesis is frequently associated with other congenital anomalies, such as tracheal stenosis, esophageal atresia, tracheoesophageal fistula, bronchogenic cysts, patent ductus arteriosus, tetralogy of Fallot, and anomalies of the great vessels.[129]

Pulmonary Hypoplasia

Pulmonary hypoplasia develops as a result of other abnormalities in the developing fetus. It occurs in infants with renal agenesis or dysplasia, urinary outlet obstruction, loss or reduction of amniotic fluid from premature rupture of membranes, diaphragmatic hernia, large pleural effusions, congenital anomalies of the neuromuscular system, and chromosomal abnormalities, including trisomy 13, 18, and 21.[129] Many of these abnormalities reduce the volume of the pleural cavity and physically restrict growth or expansion of the peripheral lung. In *congenital diaphragmatic hernia*, the pleuroperitoneal cavity fails to close. This allows the developing abdominal viscera to bulge into the pleural cavity and stunts the growth of the lung. The left side of the diaphragm is involved more often than the right, probably because the left pericardioperitoneal canal is larger and closes later than the right. The severity of the resulting pulmonary hypoplasia varies, depending on the timing of the onset of compression. With early, severe compression of the lung, there is marked hypoplasia. This is accompanied by a decrease in alveolar number and size, decreased gas-exchange surface area, and a proportional decrease in the pulmonary vasculature. Often, there is evidence of severe pulmonary hypertension, most likely because of an increased proportion of muscular arteries in the periphery of the lung, which results in increased pulmonary vascular resistance.

Oligohydramnios, or an insufficient amount of amniotic fluid, is thought to cause pulmonary hypoplasia by mechanical restriction of the fetal chest wall, that is, by allowing the uterine wall to compress the fetal thorax. Beginning at about 16 weeks of gestation, a substantial fraction of amniotic fluid is contributed by the fetal kidney. Therefore, renal agenesis, or any cause of decreased fetal urine output, results in oligohydramnios and, secondarily, in pulmonary hypoplasia. Reduced amniotic fluid for an extended period in the absence of renal anomalies, such as in prolonged rupture of the amniotic membranes, has also been associated with pulmonary hypoplasia.

Congenital Cysts of the Lung

Unlike bronchogenic cysts, *bronchiolar cysts* are in communication with the more proximal branches of the bronchial tree, as well as with distal alveolar ducts and alveoli, although the connections may be small and tortuous.[129,130] Bronchiolar cysts are lined with ciliated pseudostratified epithelium and may have mucous glands, smooth muscle, and cartilage in their walls. These cysts are usually multiple and are restricted to a single lobe. They may be filled with air, fluid, or both. Alveolar cysts are lined with cuboidal or squamous epithelium. No muscle or cartilage appears in the walls, but there may be connective tissue hyperplasia. Both types of cysts affect the right lung more frequently than the left and the lower lobes more frequently than the upper. Because congenital pulmonary cysts may be difficult to distinguish from acquired cysts, the pathogenesis of these structures is still obscure.

Congenital Cystic Adenomatoid Malformations

CCAMs are most often found in the lungs of infants and have features of both immaturity and malformation of the small airways and distal lung parenchyma.[131] There are five types of CCAMs, which are classified on the basis of gross appearance and histologic features. Type 0 lesions are rare and are composed of 0.5-cm, bronchial-like, cystic structures with abundant cartilage in their wall. Type 1 lesions are the most common, accounting for more than 50% of the cases, and are composed of one or more large cysts ranging from 3 to 10 cm in diameter. These lesions contain fibrous septa lined by pseudostratified, ciliated columnar or cuboidal cells, with clusters of mucus-filled cells resembling goblet cells. Cartilaginous foci are also present in 5 to 10% of these lesions. Type 2 lesions are the second most common and are characterized by evenly spaced, uniform cysts that are usually less than 2 cm in diameter. These bronchiolar-like structures are lined by cuboidal or ciliated columnar cells. Striated muscle may be present in the septa or adjacent to the cysts. Type 3 lesions are composed of a solid mass of tissue with multiple microscopic cysts of less than 0.2 cm that are lined by cuboidal or low columnar epithelial cells. Type 4 lesions are found in the peripheral lung and are characterized by large (≥7 cm in diameter), thin-walled cysts that are lined by alveolar epithelial cells. Immunohistochemical analysis of cytodifferentiation markers for specific pulmonary epithelial cells revealed that CCAM Types 1, 2, and 3 contained clusters of gastrin-releasing peptide—positive neuroendocrine cells and CCSP-positive Clara cells, a finding demonstrating a bronchiolar origin for these cysts.[132] The epithelial lining of CCAM Type 4 cysts was immunopositive for a Type I cell–associated surface antigen and the Type II cell, surfactant-associated proteins, SP-A, SP-B, and SP-C.[132] These findings suggest that CCAM Types 1, 2, and 3 arise during the pseudoglandular stage of branching morphogenesis, whereas CCAM Type 1 arises during the canalicular or saccular stage of acinar development.

Alveolar Capillary Dysplasia

Alveolar capillary dysplasia, with misalignment of the pulmonary veins, is characterized by inadequate vascularization of the alveolar parenchyma resulting in a reduced number of capillaries in the alveolar wall. In addition, the pulmonary lobules are malformed, and the pulmonary veins are displaced, or misaligned, in that they course with the pulmonary arteries in the peribronchiolar connective tissue instead of in the interlobular septa. This malformation causes persistent pulmonary hypertension in the neonate and is fatal.[129–131]

Congenital Pulmonary Lymphangiectasis

Congenital pulmonary lymphangiectasis is an extremely rare condition, consisting of markedly distended or dilated pulmonary lymphatics, which are found in the bronchovascular connective tissue, along the interlobular septa, and in the pleura. The dilated lymphatic channels are thin walled, are lined by endothelial cells, and form a network of communicating channels. This condition has been associated with *Noonan, Ulrich-Turner*, and *Down syndromes*. Males are more frequently affected than females (2:1). Pulmonary lymphangiectasis can be divided into three main categories: primary, secondary, and generalized lymphangiectasis.[129,131] Primary lymphangiectasis is a fatal developmental defect in which the pulmonary lymphatics fail to communicate with the systemic lymphatics. Affected infants present with RDS and pleural effusions and die shortly after birth. Secondary pulmonary lymphangiectasis is associated with cardiovascular malformations, including anomalous pulmonary venous return, atrioventricular valve defects, ostium secundum, pulmonary stenosis, ventricular septal defect, mitral atresia, hypoplastic left heart, cor triatriatum, and atresia of the common pulmonary veins.[129] Generalized pulmonary lymphangiectasis is characterized by proliferation of the lymphatic spaces and occurs in the lung as part of a systemic abnormality in which multiple lymphangiomas are also found in the bones, viscera, and soft tissues.

REFERENCES

1. Burri PH: Structural aspects of prenatal and postnatal development and growth of the lung. *In* McDonald JA (ed): Lung Growth and Development. New York, Marcel Dekker, 1997, p 1.
2. Langston C, et al: Human lung growth in late gestation and in the neonate. Am Rev Respir Dis 1984;129:607.
3. Davies G, Reid L: Growth of alveoli and pulmonary arteries in childhood. Thorax 1970;25:669.
4. Hislop AA, et al: Alveolar development in the human fetus and infant. Early Hum Dev 1986;13:1.
5. Zeltner TB, et al: The postnatal development and growth of the human lung. I. Morphometry. Respir Physiol 1987;67:247.
6. Smith EI: The early development of the trachea and esophagus in relation to atresia of the esophagus and tracheoesophageal fistula. Contrib Embryol Carnegie Inst Wash 1957;36:41.

7. Crouch EM, et al: Collagen and elastic fiber proteins in lung development. *In* McDonald JA (ed): Lung Growth and Development. New York, Marcel Dekker, 1997, p 327.

8. Congdon, ED: Transformation of the aortic arch system during development of the human embryo. Carnegie Inst Contrib Embryol 1922;14:47.

9. Hislop A, Reid L: Intrapulmonary arterial development during fetal life: branching pattern and structure. J Anat 1962;113:35.

10. Hislop A, Reid L: Fetal and childhood development of the intrapulmonary veins in man: branching pattern and structure. Thorax 1973;28:313.

11. Hilfer SR: Morphogenesis of the lung: control of embryonic and fetal branching. Annu Rev Physiol 1996;58:93.

12. Shannon JM, Deterding RR: Epithelial-mesenchymal interactions in lung development. *In* McDonald JA (ed): Lung Growth and Development. New York, Marcel Dekker, 1997, p 81.

13. Taderera JV: Control of lung differentiation in vitro. Dev Biol 1967;16:489.

14. Spooner BS, Wessells NK: Mammalian lung development: interactions in primordium formation and bronchial morphogenesis. J Exp Zool 1970;175:445.

15. Masters JRW: Epithelial-mesenchymal interaction during lung development: the effect of mesenchymal mass. Dev Biol 1976;51:98.

16. Perl A-KT, Whitsett JA: Molecular mechanisms controlling lung morphogenesis. Clin Genet 1999;56:14.

17. Kaplan F: Molecular determinants of fetal lung organogenesis. Mol Genet Metabol 2000;71:321.

18. Cardoso WV: Molecular regulation of lung development. Annu Rev Physiol 2001;63:471.

19. Costa RH, et al: Transcription factors in mouse lung development and function. Am J Physiol 2001;280:L823.

20. Ang SL, et al: The formation and maintenance of the definitive endoderm lineage in the mouse: involvement of HNF3/forkhead proteins. Development 1993;119:1301.

21. Lai E, et al: Hepatocyte nuclear factor 3 forkhead or "winged helix" proteins: a family of transcription factors of diverse biologic function. Proc Natl Acad Sci USA 1993;90:10421.

22. Monaghan AP, et al.: Postimplantation expression patterns indicate a role for the mouse forkhead/HNF-3 alpha, beta and gamma genes in determination of the definitive endoderm, chorda-mesoderm and neuroectoderm. Development 1993;119:567.

23. Zhou L, et al: Thyroid transcription factor-1, hepatocyte nuclear factor-3β, surfactant protein B, C, and Clara cell secretory protein in developing mouse lung. J Histochem Cytochem 1996;44:1183.

24. Stahlman MT, et al: Temporal-spatial distribution of hepatocyte nuclear factor-3beta in developing human lung and other foregut derivatives. J Histochem Cytochem 1998;46:955.

25. Morrisey EE, et al: GATA-6 regulates HNF-4 and is required for differentiation of visceral endoderm in the mouse embryo. Genes Dev 1998;199:55.

26. Ang SL, Rossant J: HNF-3β is essential for node and notochord formation in mouse development. Cell 1994;78:561.

27. Weinstein DC, et al: The winged-helix transcription factor HNF-3 beta is required for notochord development in the mouse embryo. Cell 1994;78:575.

28. Lazzaro D, et al: The transcription factor TTF-1 is expressed at the onset of thyroid and lung morphogenesis and in restricted regions of the foetal brain. Development 1991;113:1093.

29. Stahlman MT, et al: Expression of thyroid transcription factor-1 (TTF-1) in fetal and neonatal human lung. J Histochem Cytochem 1996;44:673.

30. Kimura S, et al: The T/ebp null mouse: thyroid specific enhancer-binding protein is essential for organogenesis of the thyroid, lung ventral forebrain, and pituitary. Gene Develop 1996;10:60.

31. Minoo, P, et al: Defects in tracheoesophageal and lung morphogenesis in NKx2.1 (−/−) mouse embryos. Dev Biol 1999;209:60.

32. Villavicencio EH, et al: The sonic hedgehog-patched-Gli pathway in human development and disease. Am J Hum Genet 2000;67:1047.

33. Litingtung Y, et al: Sonic hedgehog is essential for the development of the foregut. Nat Genet 1997;17:259.

34. Motoyama J, et al: Essential function of Gli2 and Gli3 in the formation of lung, trachea, and oesophagus. Nat Genet 1998;20:54.

35. Min H, et al: Fgf-10 is required for both limb and lung developmental and exhibits striking functional similarity to *Drosophila* branchless. Genes Dev 1998;12:3156.

36. Sekine K, et al: Fgf10 is essential for limb and lung formation. Nat Genet 1999;21:138.

37. Arman E, et al: Fgfr2 is required for limb outgrowth and lung branching morphogenesis. Proc Natl Acad Sci USA 1999;86:11895.

38. De Moerlooze L, et al: An important role for the IIIb isoform of fibroblast growth factor receptor 2 (FGFR2) in mesenchymal-epithelial signaling during mouse organogenesis. Development 2000;127:483.

39. Peters K, et al: Targeted expression of a dominant negative FGF receptor blocks branching morphogenesis and epithelial differentiation of the mouse lung. EMBO J 1994;13:3296.

40. Hajihosseini MK, et al: A splicing switch and gain-of-function mutation in FgfR2-IIIc hemizygotes causes Apert/Pfeiffer-syndrome–like phenotypes. Proc Natl Acad Sci USA 2001;98:3855.

41. Mendelsohn C, Lohmes D, Decimo D et al: Function of the retinoic acid receptors (RARs) during development. II. Multiple abnormalities at various stages of organogenesis in RAR double mutants. Development 1994;120:2749.

42. Malpel S, et al: Regulation of retinoic acid signaling during lung morphogenesis. Development 2000;127:3057.

43. Volpe MV, et al: Hoxb-5 control of early airway formation during branching morphogenesis in the developing mouse lung. Biochim Biophys Acta 2000;1475:337.

44. Kappen C: Hox genes in the lung. Am J Respir Cell Mol Biol 1996;15:56.

45. Volpe MV, et al: Association of bronchopulmonary sequestration with expression of the homeobox protein Hoxb-5. J Pediatr Surg 2000;35:1817.

46. Aubin J, et al: Early postnatal lethality in Hoxa-5 mutant mice is attributable to respiratory tract defects. Dev Biol 1997;192:432.

47. Moens CB, et al: A targeted mutation reveals a role for N-myc in branching morphogenesis of the embryonic mouse lung. Genes Dev 6;691.

48. Kang S, et al: GLI3 frameshift mutations cause autosomal dominant Pallister-Hall syndrome. Nat Genet 1997;15:266.

49. Jones KL: Smith's Recognizable Patterns of Human Malformation, 5th ed. Philadelphia, WB Saunders Co, 1997.

50. Cohen MM Jr, Kreiborg S: Visceral anomalies in the Apert syndrome. Am J Med Genet 1993;15:45:758.

51. Noorily MR, et al: Congenital tracheal anomalies in the craniosynostosis syndromes. J Pediatr Surg 1999;34:1036.

52. Kan SH, et al: Genomic screening of fibroblast growth-factor receptor 2 reveals a wide spectrum of mutations in patients with syndromic craniosynostosis. Am J Hum Genet 2002;70:472.

53. Scheid SC, et al: Tracheal cartilaginous sleeve in Crouzon syndrome. Int J Pediatr Otorhinolaryngol 2002;65:147.

54. Wells LJ, Boyden EA: Development of the bronchopulmonary segments in human embryos of Horizons XVII–XIX. Am J Anat 1954;95:163.

55. Ten-Have Opbroek AAW: The development of the lung in mammals: an analysis of concepts and findings. Am J Anat 1981;162:201.

56. Kitaoka H, et al: Development of the human fetal airway tree—analysis of the numerical density of airway endtips. Anat Rec 1996;244:207.

57. Scarpelli EM: Lung cells from embryo to maturity. *In* Scarpelli EM (ed): Pulmonary Physiology: Fetus, Newborn, Child, and Adolescent, 2nd ed. Philadelphia, Lea & Febiger, 1990, pp 42–82.

58. Thurlbeck WM: Pre- and postnatal organ development. *In* Chernick J, Mellins RB (eds): Basic Mechanisms of Pediatric Respiratory Disease: Cellular and Integrative. Philadelphia, BC Decker, 1991, pp 23–35.

59. Sunday ME: Neuropeptides and lung development. *In* McDonald JA (ed): Lung Growth and Development. New York, Marcel Dekker, 1997, p 401.

60. Bucher U, Reid L: Development of the intrasegmental bronchial tree: the patterns of branching and development of cartilage at various stages of intrauterine life. Thorax 1961;16:207.

61. Jeffery PR, Reid LM: Ultrastructure of airway epithelium and submucosal gland development. *In* Hodson WA (ed): Development of the Lung. New York, Marcel Dekker, 1979, p 87.

62. McCray PB Jr: Spontaneous contractility of human fetal airway smooth muscle. Am J Respir Cell Mol Biol 1993;8:573.

63. Sparrow MP, et al: Development of the innervation and airway smooth muscle in human fetal lung. Am J Respir Cell Mol Biol 1999;20:550.

64. Khoor A, et al: Temporal-spatial distribution of SP-B and SP-C proteins and mRNAs in the developing respiratory epithelium of the human lung. J Histochem Cytochem 1994;42:1187.

65. Morrell NW, et al: Development of the pulmonary vasculature. *In* Gaultier C, et al (eds): Lung Development. New York, Oxford University Press, 1999, p 152.

66. Verbeken EK, et al: Membranous bronchioles and connective tissue network of normal and emphysematous lungs. J Appl Physiol 1996;81:2468.

67. deMello DE, Reid LM: Embryonic and early fetal development of human lung vasculature and its functional implications. Pediatr Dev Pathol 2000;3:439.

68. Hall SM, et al: Origin, differentiation, and maturation of human pulmonary veins. Am J Respir Cell Mol Biol 2002;26:333.

69. Hall SM, et al: Prenatal origins of human intrapulmonary arteries: formation and smooth muscle maturation. Am J Respir Cell Mol Biol 2000;23:194.

70. Leslie KO, et al: Alpha smooth muscle actin expression in developing and adult human lung. Differentiation 1990;44:143.

71. Woodcock-Mitchell J, et al: Myosin isoform expression in developing and remodeling rat lung Am J Respir Cell Mol Biol 1993;8:617.

72. Miano JM, et al: Smooth muscle myosin heavy chain exclusively marks the smooth muscle lineage during mouse embryogenesis. Circ Res 1994;75:803.

73. Simonet WS, et al: Pulmonary malformation in transgenic mice expressing human keratinocyte growth factor in the lung. Proc Natl Acad Sci USA 1995;92:1246.

74. Tichelaar JW, et al: HNF-3/forkhead homologue-4 influences lung morphogenesis and respiratory epithelial cell differentiation in vivo. Dev Biol 1999;213:405.

75. Guo L, et al: Keratinocyte growth factor is required for hair development but not for wound healing. Genes Dev 1996;10:165.

76. Colvin JS, et al: Lung hypoplasia and neonatal death in Fgf9-null mice identify this gene as an essential regulator of lung mesenchyme. Development 2001;128:2095.

77. Weaver M, et al: BMP signaling regulates proximal-distal differentiation of endoderm in mouse lung development. Development 1999;126:4005.

78. Lu MM, et al: The bone morphogenic protein antagonist gremlin regulates proximal-distal patterning of the lung. Dev Dyn 2001;222:667.

79. Shi W, et al: Gremlin negatively modulates BMP-4 induction of embryonic mouse lung branching morphogenesis. Am J Physiol 2001;280:L1030.

80. Meno C, et al: Lefty-1 is required for left-right determination as a regulator of lefty-2 and nodal. Cell 1998;94:287.

81. Rankin CT, et al: Regulation of left-right patterning in mice by growth/differentiation factor-1. Nat Genet 2000;24:262.

82. Gaio, U, et al: A role of the cryptic gene in the correct establishment of the left-right axis. Curr Biol 1999;9:1339.

83. Chen J, et al: Mutation of the mouse hepatocyte nuclear factor/forkhead homologue 4 gene results in an absence of cilia and random left-right asymmetry. J Clin Invest 1998;102:1077.

84. Carmeliet P, Collen D: Role of vascular endothelial growth factor and vascular endothelial growth factor receptors in vascular development. Curr Topics Microbiol Immunol 1999;237:133.

85. Gerber HP, et al: VEGF is required for growth and survival in neonatal mice. Development 1999;126:1149.

86. Fong GH, et al: Role of Flt-1 receptor kinase in regulating the assembly of vascular endothelium. Nature 1995;376:66.

87. Ruhrberg C, et al: Spatially restricted patterning cues provided by heparin-binding VEGF-A control blood vessel branching morphogenesis. Genes Dev 2002;16:2684.

88. Galambos C, et al: Defective pulmonary development in the absence of heparin-binding vascular endothelial growth factor isoforms. Am J Respir Cell Mol Biol 2002;27:194.

89. George EL, et al: Defects in mesoderm, neural tube and vascular development in mouse embryos lacking fibronectin. Development 1993;117:1079.

90. Kubato Y, et al: Role of laminin and basement membrane in the morphological differentiation of human endothelial cells in capillary-like structures. J Cell Biol 1988;107:1589.

91. Singh G, et al: Identification, cellular localization, isolation, and characterization of human Clara cell–specific 10 kd protein. J Histochem Cytochem 1988;36:73.

92. Strum JM, et al: Immunochemical localization of Clara cell protein by light and electron microscopy in conducting airways of fetal and neonatal hamster lung. Anat Rec 1990;227:77.

93. Ten Have-Opbroek AAW, DeVries ECP: Clara cell differentiation in the mouse: ultrastructural morphology and cytochemistry for surfactant protein A and Clara cell 10 kD protein. Microsc Res Tech 1993;26:400.

94. Schellhase DE, et al: Ontogeny of surfactant proteins in the rat. Pediatr Res 1989;26:167.

95. Otto-Verberne CJM, et al: Expression of the major surfactant-associated protein, SP-A, in Type II cells of human lung before 20 weeks of gestation. Eur J Cell Biol 1990;53:13.

96. Endo H, Oka T: An immunohistochemical study of bronchial cells producing surfactant protein A in the developing human fetal lung. Early Hum Dev 1991;25:149.

97. Batenburg JJ, Hallman M: Developmental biochemistry of alveoli. In Scarpelli EM (ed): Pulmonary Physiology: Fetus, Newborn, Child, and Adolescent. Philadelphia, Lea & Febiger, 1991, p 106.

98. Weaver TE, Whitsett JA: Function and regulation of expression of pulmonary surfactant-associated proteins. Biochem J 1991;273:249.

99. Khoor A, et al: Developmental expression of SP-A and SP-A mRNA in the proximal and distal respiratory epithelium in the human fetus and newborn. J Histochem Cytochem 1993;41:1311.

100. Williams MC, Mason R: Development of the Type II cell in the fetal rat lung. Am Rev Respir Dis 1977;115:37.

101. Hilfer SR: Development of terminal buds in the fetal mouse lung. Scanning Electr Microsc 1983;111:1378.

102. Chi EY: The ultrastructural study of glycogen and lamellar bodies in the development of fetal monkey lung. Exp Lung Res 1985;8:275.

103. Ten Have-Opbroek AAW, et al: Ultrastructural characteristics of inclusion bodies of Type II cells in late embryonic mouse lung. Anat Embryol 1990;181:317.

104. Whitsett JA, et al: Glucocorticoid enhances surfactant proteolipid Phe and pVal synthesis and RNA in fetal lung. J Biol Chem 1987;262:15618.

105. Ballard PL: Hormonal regulation of pulmonary surfactant. Endocr Rev 1989;10:165.

106. Mendelson CR, Boggaram V: Hormonal control of the surfactant system in fetal lung. Annu Rev Physiol 1991;53:415.

107. Yeomans ER: Prenatal corticosteroid therapy to prevent respiratory distress syndrome. Semin Perinatol 1993;17:253.

108. Rooney SA, et al: Molecular and cellular processing of lung surfactant. FASEB J 1994;8:957.

109. Crouch E, et al: Developmental expression of pulmonary surfactant protein D (SP-D). Am J Respir Cell Mol Biol 1991;5:13.

110. Wohlford-Lenane CL, Snyder JM: Localization of surfactant-associated protein (SP-C) mRNA in fetal rabbit tissue by in situ hybridization. Am J Respir Cell Mol Biol 1992;6:239.

111. Wohlford-Lenane CL, et al: Localization of surfactant-associated proteins SP-A and SP-B mRNA in fetal rabbit tissue by in situ hybridization. Am J Respir Cell Mol Biol 1992;7:335.

112. Nogee LM, et al: A mutation in the surfactant protein B gene responsible for fatal neonatal respiratory disease in multiple kindred. J Clin Invest 1994;93:1860.

113. Nogee LM, et al: Allelic heterogeneity in surfactant protein B (SP-B) deficiency. Am J Respir Crit Care Med 1999;161:973.

114. Bostrom H, et al: PDGF-A signaling is a critical event in lung alveolar myofibroblast development and alveogenesis. Cell 1996;85:863.

115. Lindahl P, et al: Alveogenesis failure in PDGF-A–deficient mice is coupled to lack of distal spreading of alveolar smooth muscle cell progenitors during lung development. Development 1997;124:3943.

116. Wendel DP, et al: Impaired distal airway development in mice lacking elastin. Am J Respir Cell Mol Biol 2000;23:320.

117. McGowan SE, et al: Endogenous retinoids increase perinatal elastin gene expression in rat lung fibroblasts and fetal explants. Am J Physiol 1997;273:L410.

118. McGowan S, et al: Mice bearing deletions of retinoic acid receptors demonstrate reduced lung elastin and alveolar numbers. Am J Respir Cell Mol Biol 2000;23:162.

119. Weinstein M, et al: FGFR-3 and FGFR-4 function cooperatively to direct alveogenesis in the murine lung. Development 1998;125:361.

120. Shaw-White JR, et al: GATA-6 activates transcription of thyroid transcription factor-1. J Biol Chem 1999;274:2658.

121. Bruno MD, et al: GATA-6 activates transcription of surfactant protien A. J Biol Chem 2000;275:1043.

122. Liu C, et al: GATA-6 and thyroid transcription factor-1 directly interact and regulate SP-C gene expression. J Biol Chem 2002;277:4519.

123. Yang H, et al: GATA6 regulates differentiation of distal lung epithelium. Development 2002;129:2233.

124. Liu C, et al: GATA-6 is required for maturation of the lung in late gestation. Am J Physiol 2002;283:L468.

125. Nogee LM, et al: Mutations in the surfactant protein C (SP-C) gene associated with interstitial lung disease. N Engl J Med 2001;344:573.

126. Skandalakis JE, et al: The esophagus. In Skandalakis JE, Gray SW (eds): Embryology for Surgeons, 2nd ed. Baltimore, Williams & Wilkins, 1994, p 65.

127. Kim J, et al: The VACTERL association: lessons from the sonic hedgehog pathway. Clin Genet 2001;59:306.

128. Kim PC, et al: Murine models of VACTERL syndrome: role of sonic hedgehog signaling pathway. J Pediatr Surg 2001;36:381.

129. Gould SJ, Hasleton PS: Congenital abnormalities. In Hasleton PS (ed): Spencer's Pathology of the Lung, 5th ed. New York, McGraw-Hill, 1996, p 57.

130. Skandalis JE, et al: The trachea and the lungs. In: Skandalis JE, Coray SW, eds. Embryology for Surgeons, 2nd ed. Baltimore: Williams and Wilkins, 1994, p 414.

131. Katzenstein A-LA : Katzenstein and Askin's Surgical Pathology of Non-Neoplastic Lung Disease, 3rd ed. Philadelphia, WB Saunders Co, 1997, p 361.

132. Morotti RA, et al: Congenital cystic adenomatoid malformation of the lung (CCAM): evaluation of the cellular components. Hum Pathol 1999;30:618.

77

Jeanne M. Snyder

Regulation of Alveolarization

The alveolus is the primary functional unit of the lung, the site where oxygen and carbon dioxide are exchanged between inspired air and the blood. Alveolar growth is optimized to provide an enormous surface area where the blood in pulmonary capillaries circulates within a few micrometers of the inspired air. The blood in alveolar capillaries and the inspired air are separated by the thin wall of a capillary endothelial cell, a fused basal lamina, and the attenuated cytoplasm of an alveolar Type I epithelial cell.[1] There are about 300×10^6 alveoli in adult human lungs, most of which are formed by about 18 months of age.[2, 3] Further growth and development of the distal lung parenchyma involve the thinning of the alveolar wall, an increase in capillary density, and a modest increase in the diameter of the alveoli.[2,3]

The postnatal formation of alveoli is impaired in bronchopulmonary dysplasia (BPD), a disease of prematurity that is thought to be caused by injury resulting from mechanical ventilation, hyperoxia, and inflammation.[4,5] Husain and co-workers described the "new" BPD as a chronic lung disease, prominent in very low birth weight infants who have been treated with surfactant replacement therapy, that is characterized by impaired alveolarization.[4,5] Experimentally, premature baboons that have been mechanically ventilated with elevated oxygen levels also have lungs with alveoli that are decreased in number and larger than normal.[6] It is hypothesized that mechanical ventilation or exposure of the lung to high levels of oxygen very early in development leads to impaired alveolarization and eventually chronic lung disease.[5] Although surfactant therapy has lessened the impact of some of the characteristics of the lung injury (fibrosis and inflammation), it has not affected the impairment of alveolarization.[5]

When one lung is removed, new alveoli can form in the remaining lung.[7,8] It also appears that the number of alveoli in the lung can change in response to physiologic stimuli, such as starvation, age, oxygen tension, or hormonal status.[9] In addition, it has been reported that treatment with retinoic acid can increase the number of alveoli in neonatal and adult rats.[10,11] However, we do not fully understand the processes that regulate the formation of new alveoli in the developing lung, nor do we know how to affect these processes in humans. The ability to program the human lung to form new alveoli is a major and elusive goal in pulmonary biology.

STRUCTURE OF THE ALVEOLAR WALL

The alveolar wall consists of a connective tissue core in which many capillaries are suspended.[1] The capillary bed in the lung alveoli is probably the largest in the body. The cells present within the alveolar wall (i.e., primarily fibroblasts and myofibroblasts) produce an extracellular matrix that is particularly rich in elastin and also contains collagen, proteoglycans, and glycosaminoglycans.[12]

The surface of the alveolar wall is lined by two epithelial cell types, alveolar Type I and Type II.[13] Type I cells are extremely attenuated squamous cells whose cytoplasm forms part of the air-blood gas exchange barrier. About 90% of the alveolar surface is lined by alveolar Type I cells.[14] Type II cells are cuboidal secretory cells, often located at the corner of an alveolus, that produce pulmonary surfactant, a lipoprotein substance that lowers surface tension in the alveolus and plays an important role in lung host defense mechanisms.[15] Although Type II cells form only a small proportion of the alveolar surface area, there are approximately equal numbers of alveolar Type I and II cells in the alveolus.[14]

FORMATION OF ALVEOLI IN THE DEVELOPING LUNG

In the human, some alveoli form prenatally (~20%); however, most alveoli form after birth.[2,3] Studies suggest that most human alveoli are formed within the first 18 months.[16,17] Much of our understanding of the processes involved in alveolar formation is derived from studies in rodents, primarily in the rat and mouse (Fig. 77-1).[9] In these species, alveolarization occurs during the first 2 weeks of postnatal life.[9]

OVERVIEW OF EARLY LUNG DEVELOPMENT

Pseudoglandular Phase

Very early lung development, before the formation of alveoli, is characterized by branching morphogenesis, which occurs during the pseudoglandular phase.[18] The lung buds and trachea originate as diverticula from the endoderm-lined foregut. The lung buds then undergo repeated dichotomous branching to give rise to the conducting airways of the lungs. It has been estimated that approximately 22 orders of branching airways are formed by about 16 weeks of gestation in the human. The branching ducts in the developing lung are lined by tall columnar epithelial cells that begin to differentiate into ciliated and secretory cells proximally but remain undifferentiated at the distal aspects of the branching tree system.[13] Within the epithelium of the conducting airways, at their most distal aspect, are cellular progenitors that will give rise to the alveolar region of the lung.[19]

Canalicular Phase

From 16 to 24 weeks of gestation in the human, during the canalicular phase of lung development, the distal aspect of the branching tubes in the developing lung undergoes considerable remodeling.[18] The epithelium that lines the ducts changes from tall columnar to low columnar/cuboidal in shape. The number of blood vessels, primarily capillaries, in the connective tissue between the ducts increases strikingly. Starting at weeks 20 to 22, some of the epithelial cells begin to differentiate into alveolar Type II cells that synthesize and secrete pulmonary surfactant.[13] In addition, the distal lung epithelial cells that are close to the underlying capillaries begin to thin and differentiate into alveolar Type I cells.[13]

Saccular Phase

The terminal portion of the branching duct system in the embryonic lung lengthens and will eventually give rise to the alveolar ducts and alveolar sacs, the spaces from which true alveoli will form via septation.[9,18] This phase of lung development, called the saccular phase, extends from about 24 weeks to term in the human.[18] Simultaneously with changes in the structure of the epithelium-lined ducts, profound remodeling occurs in the connective tissue surrounding the primitive lung ducts. The relative amount of ductal lumen (the future air space) in the distal lung tissue increases dramatically while the relative amount of connective tissue (both cells and extracellular matrix components) simultaneously decreases as a component of the distal lung tissue.[18]

FORMATION OF ALVEOLI IN THE DEVELOPING LUNG

The formation of pulmonary alveoli in the human fetus begins prenatally; however, most alveoli are formed after birth (~80%).[16,17] Premature human infants who are born when their lungs are quite immature structurally (i.e., in the range of 24 to 28 weeks) can still respire enough to maintain viability.[5] In guinea pigs, sheep, pigs, and cows, almost all alveolarization occurs *in utero*.[9] In rodents such as mice and rats, alveoli are formed during the first few weeks of postnatal life.[20,21] During development, the formation of alveoli increases the pulmonary gas exchange surface area in proportion to the growth of the whole organism.[9] The mechanisms by which the growth of an organism promotes a corresponding increase in the formation of its lung alveoli are not well understood.[9]

Beginning at the end of gestation in the human, and postnatally in rodents such as mice or rats, the terminal sacs in the developing lung begin to undergo septation to form true alveoli.[9,22] The conducting airway system ends at the level of the respiratory bronchiole, which is a structure characterized by occasional alveoli interrupting the airway wall.[1] The epithelium of a respiratory bronchiole is columnar proximally and gradually transitions to the typical alveolar epithelium that lines the alveolar ducts, alveolar sacs, and alveoli. The entire functional unit (the

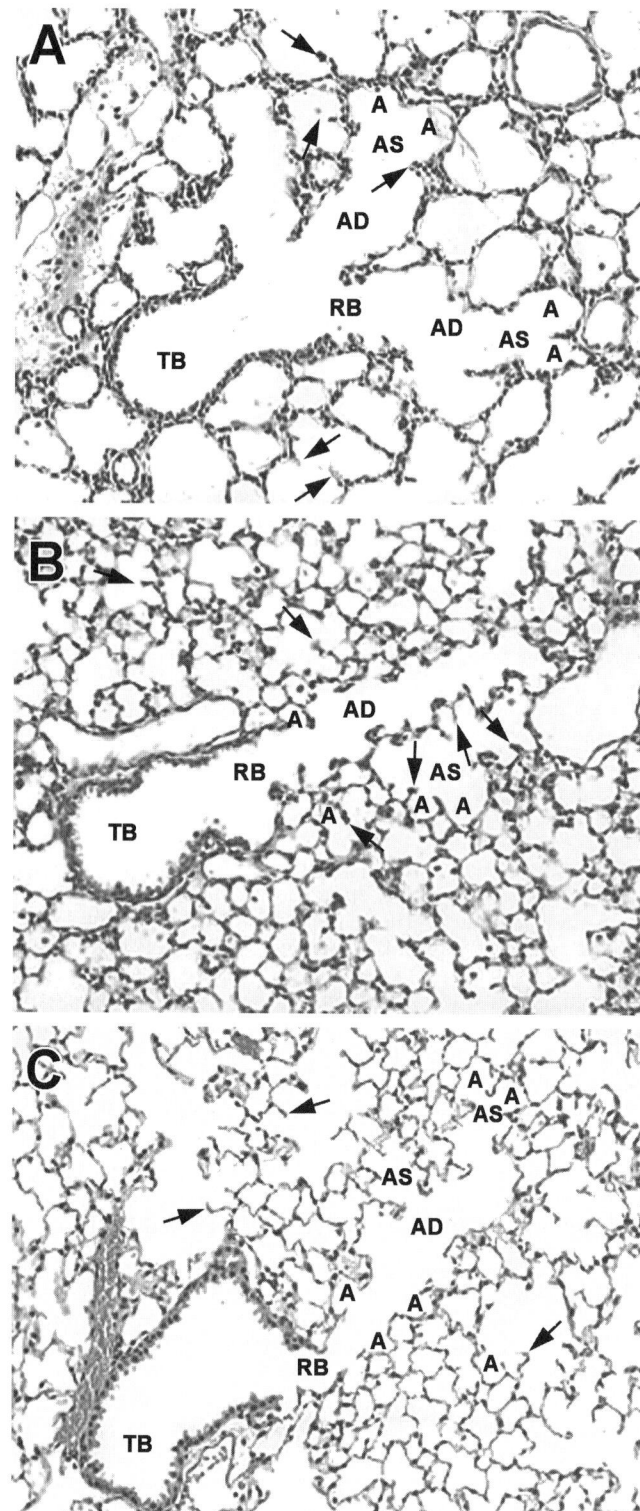

Figure 77–1. Alveolarization in mouse lung tissue. Mouse lung tissue was harvested at postnatal days 0, 12, and 56 (**A, B,** and **C,** respectively), inflation fixed at constant pressure, paraffin embedded, sectioned, and then stained with hematoxylin and eosin. Terminal bronchioles (TB) in the lung open into respiratory bronchioles (RB), which, in turn, open into alveolar ducts (AD) ending in alveolar sacs (AS). Alveoli (A) are found at every level of the respiratory acinus. At day 0 postnatally (**A**), the walls of the alveolar ducts and sacs are the primary septa. Secondary septa (*arrows*) grow into the lumen and begin dividing the primitive alveolar duct and sac air spaces into alveoli. By 12 days postnatally (**B**), the number of secondary septa (*arrows*) has increased dramatically, and many alveoli have been formed, thus increasing the surface area in the lung available for gas exchange. Note the decrease in the wall thickness of the alveoli from day 0 to day 12. At 56 days postnatally (**C**), the alveolar septa (*arrows*) are much thinner and longer than observed at the earlier postnatal stages of development.

ole, alveolar duct, or alveolar sac. It is believed that all these alveoli are equally functional.

In the prenatal human lung and in the postnatal mouse lung, alveoli form by the growth of secondary septa that project from the wall of the terminal saccule.[9] The secondary septa are evenly spaced and extend into the saccule to a similar extent. The growth of secondary septa into the lumen of the terminal saccule is mediated, at least in part, by the proliferation of fibroblasts.[24] A subset of interstitial fibroblasts in the developing lung is characterized by cytoplasmic lipid droplets.[25] The function of these cells is not fully understood, but they probably play an important role in the morphogenesis of the alveolar wall.[25] At the tip of the secondary septa is a myofibroblast, a cell type that produces elastin and other important extracellular matrix components present in the alveolar wall.[26] This particular cell type probably plays a key role in alveolarization, because the absence of myofibroblasts results in a failure to produce alveoli in postnatal life and an emphysematous lung phenotype.[27,28]

The connective tissue core of the secondary alveolar septa is characterized by abundant elastin, probably laid down by the myofibroblast.[29] The elastin fibers are arranged in an orderly and predictable manner within the alveolar septa.[30-32] Elastin gene expression peaks during the period of postnatal alveolarization.[33,34] The cross-linking of elastin monomers is a critical process in alveolarization because inhibition of this process leads to a decreased surface area in the lung.[35] Elastin fiber deposition also involves the coordinated expression of fibrillins, emelin, fibulin, and microfibril–associated glycoproteins.[29] In addition, collagens Type I, III, and IX are produced by connective tissue cells and are deposited in the alveolar wall during the formation of the secondary septa, where they convey mechanical strength.[36] Glycosaminoglycans, such as hyaluronic acid, chondroitin sulfate, and heparin sulfate, are also present in the alveolar wall and make important contributions to its mechanical properties.[37] Finally, proteoglycans, adhesive glycoproteins such as fibronectin, and components of the basal lamina, including laminins and Type IV collagen, also are produced and are laid down during alveolarization in a regulated and integrated manner.[38]

REGULATION OF ALVEOLARIZATION

Vascular Endothelial Growth Factor

The process of alveolarization includes the morphogenesis of an elaborate pulmonary capillary bed in the distal lung, which must form in concert with the differentiation of the alveolar epithelium and the eruption of secondary septa. The growth and

respiratory acinus) consists, in order, of a respiratory bronchiole (several orders of respiratory bronchioles are possible), alveolar ducts (again, several orders or branches of alveolar ducts can be present), and alveolar sacs.[1] Alveolar ducts can constitute a major portion of the gas exchange tissue in the lung, as much as approximately 30% in some species.[23] Alveoli branch from the alveolar ducts, either singly or in clusters from an alveolar sac, which is the terminus of the alveolar duct. Alveoli are present at every level of the respiratory acinus, in the respiratory bronchi-

differentiation of pulmonary vasculature begin in the fetal lung coincident with the canalicular and saccular stages of lung development.[39] Initially, the capillaries in the wall of the septa are a double capillary system; that is, one capillary is associated with each surface of the forming alveolar septa.[40] As alveolarization proceeds, however, the alveolar wall thins, and a single capillary system forms in the alveolar wall with the capillaries coming to lie very close to one of the surfaces of the alveolar wall.[40]

Vascular endothelial growth factor (VEGF) is a growth factor that acts as a mitogen for endothelial cells.[41] VEGF stimulates angiogenesis and vasculogenesis and also regulates endothelial permeability.[41] VEGF binds to at least two receptors: Flk-1 (VEGF receptor 2) and Flt-1 (VEGF receptor 1).[41] VEGF and its receptors are expressed in the developing lung in a coordinated fashion that peaks at the end of gestation and during early neonatal life.[42, 43] There are several VEGF isoforms of different molecular weights; however, VEGF 188 predominates in the fetal lung.[43] Transgenic mice that overexpress VEGF in alveolar epithelial cells have disrupted lung development, that is, disrupted branching morphogenesis, hypertrophy of blood vessels, decreased number of terminal saccules, and decreased connective tissue.[44]

VEGF increases cell division in human fetal lung Type II cells.[45] It was shown that anti-VEGF receptor 2 antibodies, administered *in utero*, delay fetal mouse lung development.[46] Conversely, lung development in mice, as assessed by the production of surfactant, structural changes, and survival, was accelerated by the prenatal or postnatal administration of VEGF.[46] In a study conducted in adult rats, treatment with a VEGF receptor blocker, SU5416, led to an enlargement of alveoli and a decrease in alveolar surface area, a pattern similar to that observed in emphysema.[47] When the same VEGF inhibitor was administered to newborn rats, alveolar formation was significantly impaired.[48] The inhibitory effects of treatment with SU5416 for 24 hours on the second day after birth persisted until 3 to 4 months of age.[49] Other inhibitors of angiogenesis, for example, thalidomide and fumagillin, administered to neonatal rats during the peak period of alveolarization, also inhibit the formation of alveoli.[49] Together, these results suggest that VEGF probably plays a key role in the process of alveolarization.

The growth of pulmonary capillaries and the formation of alveoli during the period of alveolarization are closely linked in the postnatal lung. The functional relationship between these processes is unknown, but defects in the formation of blood vessels and alveolarization are characteristic of BPD.[4, 50] In a primate model of BPD, the premature baboon, decreased numbers of endothelial cells and a disrupted microvasculature were observed in the distal lung.[6] Maniscalco and co-workers observed both decreased numbers and an abnormal distribution of capillaries in the alveolar septa of patients with BPD.[51] The lung tissue of infants with known BPD was also characterized by decreased VEGF and VEGF-2 receptor gene expression.[51] Other animal models in which alveolarization has been impaired are also characterized by decreased numbers of alveolar capillaries (e.g., in neonatal rats exposed to high oxygen and in premature ventilated lambs).[23, 52] The role of vascular growth factors in hyperoxia-induced injury in the developing lung has been reviewed.[53]

Other Regulators of Angiogenesis

In addition to VEGF and its receptors, there are many other mediators of angiogenesis and vasculogenesis whose roles in lung development are still relatively unexplored. For example, angiopoietins, ephrins, and semaphorins, all of which have been shown to play a role in angiogenesis in other systems, are present in the developing lung and may play an important role in alveolarization.[54-56] Angiopoietins 1 to 4 bind to Tie 2 receptors in endothelial cells and act together with VEGF and its receptors to influence angiogenesis.[54] Angiopoietin 1 is expressed in the developing lung but apparently does not change in concentration during development.[57, 58] Ephrins are growth factors that bind to tyrosine kinase–linked receptors and are involved in vasculogenesis and angiogenesis.[55] The role of these growth factors and their receptors in lung development is unknown. Semaphorins are a more recently described class of growth factors, initially noted in the central nervous system, that bind to receptors called neuropilins.[56] Neuropilins may act as co-receptors with VEGF receptor 2 and play a role in angiogenesis.[56] Both semaphorins and neuropilins have been detected in the developing lung.[59] Blockade of neuropilins in the newborn rat results in defects in alveolarization.[60]

Platelet-Derived Growth Factors

Platelet-derived growth factors (PDGFs) are dimers of A and/or B polypeptide chains that bind to two receptor tyrosine kinases, PDGF-Rα and PDGF-Rβ.[61] PDGF is a potent mitogenic factor for connective tissue cells.[61] PDGF-A is expressed by epithelial cells in the developing lung.[62] PDGF-A homozygous gene-deleted mice die postnatally because of failure of postnatal alveolarization.[27, 28] The PDGF-A knock-out mice lack alveolar myofibroblasts that express PDGF-Rα in their primary septa.[27, 28] In addition, these mice do not have normal elastin deposition pattern in their lungs and do not form secondary septa.[27, 28] These data are suggestive that the PDGF-Rα–positive myofibroblasts in the developing postnatal lung play a major role in alveolar septation and that PDGF-A is an important regulator of alveolarization.[63]

Glucocorticoids

Glucocorticoids are steroid hormones produced by the adrenal gland in response to adrenocorticotropic hormone, a peptide produced by the pituitary.[64] Release of adrenocorticotropic hormone from the pituitary is, in turn, regulated by another peptide, corticotropin-releasing hormone (CRH), which is produced in the hypothalamus.[64] Glucocorticoids bind to glucocorticoid receptors (GR), which are members of the steroid hormone receptor family of transcription factors.[64] Antenatal glucocorticoids, administered to the mother at risk of delivering prematurely, can accelerate lung development and reduce the risk of neonatal respiratory distress syndrome.[65,66] Respiratory distress syndrome is caused by surfactant deficiency; thus, glucocorticoids presumably act by increasing the production of surfactant in differentiated alveolar Type II cells.[64] However, glucocorticoids have many other effects on the developing lung.[64]

Antenatal glucocorticoids accelerate structural maturation of the lung, in particular thinning of the alveolar wall.[67, 68] In rats, which undergo alveolarization postnatally, glucocorticoids inhibit alveolarization.[67] The formation of secondary alveolar septa is impaired in the lungs of glucocorticoid-treated neonatal rats, with the result of fewer and larger alveoli in the mature lung.[67] Similar findings were obtained when glucocorticoids were administered to the rats antenatally.[69] The glucocorticoid effects on lung structure appear to be permanent, at least in the rat.[69] The effects of glucocorticoids on primate lung development are consistent with observations made in the rat model; that is, glucocorticoids impair alveolarization in the developing lung.[70]

The concept that glucocorticoids play a key role in lung development is supported by the observation that mice that are CRH gene deleted die of respiratory failure resulting from inadequate lung development.[71] The effect of the CRH gene deletion on lung development is probably structural because surfactant components are not as strongly affected by the CRH gene deletion.[71] A similar observation was made in GR-deficient mice; that is, the effects of the GR gene deletion include immature structural development of the lung, whereas surfactant components such as the surfactant proteins are not as strongly affected.[72]

BPD is caused by multiple factors; however, mechanical ventilation, oxygen toxicity, and inflammation have key roles in the pathophysiology of this disease.[73] Glucocorticoids are effective in treating BPD, perhaps because of their antiinflammatory effects.[64] The long-term effects of glucocorticoid treatment of premature infants with BPD are still not fully understood and are of great concern. It is known, however, that the lungs of infants with BPD have fewer and larger alveoli, an observation that makes the use of glucocorticoids, which impair alveolarization, to treat these infants problematic.[4,74]

Retinoic Acid

Retinoic acid plays a key role in the differentiation and maintenance of differentiation of all respiratory epithelia, from the trachea to the alveolus.[75,76] All-*trans* retinoic acid, which is the best characterized, most abundant, biologically active retinoid, binds to retinoic acid receptors (RARs) and to retinoid-X receptors (RXRs).[77] RARs and RXRs are members of the steroid hormone receptor family of transcription factors.[77] There are three RAR genes (RARα, β, and γ) and three RXR genes (α, β and γ), each of which produces several isoforms.[77] The RARs form heterodimers with RXRs and bind to *cis*-acting elements in retinoic acid responsive genes.[77]

Massaro and Massaro and co-workers showed that all-*trans* retinoic acid plays a key role in regulating alveolarization in rats and mice.[10,11,78] In their initial report concerning the effects of retinoic acid, postnatal rats were treated with all-*trans* retinoic acid or dexamethasone.[10] Dexamethasone administration to postnatal rats inhibits alveolarization.[79] Treatment with retinoic acid alone caused an increase in the number of alveoli, but it had no effect on lung gas exchange surface area when compared with controls.[10] In addition, retinoic acid abolished many of the inhibitory effects of glucocorticoids on alveolarization.[10] Specifically, treatment with retinoic acid plus glucocorticoid resulted in greater numbers of alveoli and greater surface area (corrected for body weight) in the lung than in the glucocorticoid-alone condition.[10] In another study by the same investigators, adult rats were treated with intratracheal elastase to create a model of emphysema.[11] When the rats were treated with all-*trans* retinoic acid, the effects of the elastase on the number of alveoli and amount of gas exchange surface area were reversed.[11] It has been reported that treatment of newborn rats with retinoic acid during exposure to hyperoxia protected their lungs from the deleterious effects of hyperoxia on alveolar formation.[80]

Morphometric studies in transgenic mice revealed that the lungs of RARβ gene-deleted mice have more, but smaller, alveoli.[78] However, gas exchange surface area is the same in the RARβ gene-deleted and wild-type mice.[78] In the same article, it was shown that treatment of postnatal rats with an RARβ agonist impairs the formation of alveoli.[78] Together, these observations suggest that RARβ may be an endogenous inhibitor of alveolarization.[78] In another transgenic mouse model, McGowan and co-workers showed that RARγ probably mediates some of the effects of retinoic acid on alveolarization.[81] RARγ gene-deleted mice had lungs with fewer and larger alveoli than age-matched wild-type mice.[81] The effects of RARγ gene deletion were magnified in mice that were heterozygous for the deletion of RXRα.[81] Together, these data support a role for RARγ/RXRα heterodimers in the regulation of alveolarization.[81]

Elastin is an important component of the alveolar wall that is involved in alveolarization and is regulated by all-*trans* retinoic acid.[29,82] Retinyl esters increase in the lung during development and decrease thereafter.[83] The retinyl esters are concentrated in lipid-laden fibroblasts, a prominent cell type in the connective tissue component of the primary septa in the developing lung.[84]

McGowan and co-workers showed that endogenous retinoids in the developing lung increase lung elastin gene expression.[82] Retinoids also increase elastin gene expression *in vitro* in isolated, cultured lipid-laden fibroblasts.[82] In RARγ gene-deleted mice, a decrease in elastin mRNA was observed in lipid-laden fibroblasts isolated from postnatal lung when compared with the elastin mRNA levels in fibroblasts isolated from wild-type, control mice.[81] In addition, there was a marked decrease in elastin fibers in the alveolar walls of mice from RARγ gene-deleted mice when compared with control lungs.[81] Together, these data suggest that retinoic acid regulates elastin gene expression and elastin fiber deposition, two important events in alveolarization in the postnatal lung.

The plasma concentration of vitamin A (retinol, the metabolic precursor to all-*trans* retinoic acid) is significantly lower in very low birth weight, premature infants.[85] Some of the histologic characteristics of lung tissue in vitamin A–deficient models and in BPD are similar.[75,76] Kennedy and co-workers described a meta-analysis of four small clinical trials in which vitamin A supplementation in very low birth weight infants decreased mortality and the incidence of BPD.[86] The results of a more recent, large clinical trial suggest that vitamin A supplementation in extremely low birth weight infants decreases their risk of subsequent chronic lung disease.[87] These clinical data illustrate the potential usefulness of retinoids in accelerating lung development and in decreasing the incidence of BPD in newborn infants. One of the beneficial effects of the clinical use of retinoids may be in promoting alveolarization; however, this point has yet to be established.

The loss of sufficient numbers of alveoli in the adult lung leads to inadequate gas exchange surface area and the ensuing pathophysiology of emphysema.[88] No clinical treatment that promotes the regeneration of alveoli in the adult lung is available as yet. In light of observations in rats indicating that retinoic acid treatment leads to *de novo* alveolarization, clinical trials in which all-*trans* retinoic acid is administered to patients with emphysema are currently under way.[89] In preliminary findings, retinoid treatment was well tolerated and was associated with relatively few side effects.[89] Unfortunately, no effects of the retinoid treatment on pulmonary function or lung structure (as assessed using computed tomography) were observed in this pilot study.[89]

Estrogen and Testosterone

Lung development is influenced by the sex of the fetus. It has been shown that lung maturation is delayed in male fetuses when compared with females.[90] The incidence of respiratory distress syndrome and infant mortality is greater in males than in females.[91] It has been hypothesized that androgens, present primarily in the male, delay lung development in the male fetus.[90] However, the lungs of androgen-receptor negative male mice were shown to have the same body weight–adjusted surface area as wild-type male mice.[92]

There may also be a sex difference in the formation of alveoli in the neonatal lung.[93] Massaro and co-workers reported that female rats and mice (60 days old) have smaller and more numerous lung alveoli and that their body weight–adjusted lung surface area is significantly greater than in male rats.[93] In another study, these same investigators showed that estrogen mediates the sex-linked effects on lung structure in rats.[92] Treatment of female newborn rats with androgens did not alter their lung structure.[92] Together, these data suggest that estrogen regulates alveolarization in the postnatal lung.

During pregnancy, the fetus (male or female) is exposed to very high levels of estrogens, which drop dramatically after birth.[94] Some clinicians have suggested that preterm infants may benefit from estrogen replacement therapy. In fact, some benefit of estrogen therapy in terms of the incidence of chronic lung disease has been reported.[95] It is not known whether these effects reflect differences in alveolar formation.

Nutrition

Caloric restriction reduces the metabolic rate and physiologic requirement for oxygen.[96] Studies performed primarily in rats showed that caloric restriction of adults increases the size of their alveoli and reduces the lung gas exchange surface area available for respiration.[97] Refeeding apparently reverses these changes.[97] These observations were confirmed in a morphometric study in adult mice.[98] Observations of the inhabitants of the Warsaw ghetto during World War II are consistent with a similar process occurring in humans; that is, an emphysema-like morphology was observed in the lungs of severely malnourished adults.[99]

Massaro and co-workers hypothesized that during periods of low oxygen requirements (e.g., caloric restriction), alveoli are destroyed, whereas during refeeding, which would increase oxygen needs, alveolar regeneration is activated.[9]

Oxygen

The lung alveolar surface area functions as a gas exchange unit, and oxygen has a potent influence on the formation of alveoli in the developing lung.[9] Dimensions of the surface area available for gas exchange are directly related to the oxygen needs of the organism.[100] In general, in newborn rats undergoing alveolarization, hyperoxia tends to decrease the alveolar surface area.[9] Burri and Weibel showed that neonatal rats reared in 40% oxygen had decreased alveolar surface area when compared with air-breathing controls.[101] Similar observations were made by Randell and co-workers in a study in which neonatal rats were reared in 95% oxygen for the first 7 days after birth.[102] Exposure to high oxygen for 7 days followed by rearing in room air until 40 days of age also resulted in impaired alveolarization, that is, a decreased alveolar surface area in the oxygen-exposed animals when compared with controls reared in room air.[23] The signaling pathway in the developing lung that senses oxygen levels and regulates alveolar surface area is unclear at present. However, it has been shown that hyperoxia inhibits the expression of VEGF in neonatal rabbit lung.[103] Hyperoxia also increases apoptosis in the distal lung of neonatal mice.[104] Hypoxia is also a potent regulator of alveolar formation.[9,105] Blanco and Massaro and their co-workers showed that rearing newborn rats in 13% oxygen results in fewer alveoli and decreased gas exchange surface area.[106,107]

Inflammation

Alveolarization in premature human newborns is thought to be inhibited by many factors, including mechanical ventilation, oxygen, inadequate nutrition, glucocorticoids, and, possibly, infection. All these stimuli can result in inflammation. Thus, many investigators have hypothesized that inflammatory mediators impair alveolarization.[108-110] Intrauterine infection is a common cause of preterm birth, and it is now apparent that such infections may also influence postnatal lung development.[111] A final common pathway in many inflammatory states is the activation of matrix metalloproteinases, a process that results in the destruction of extracellular matrix components and consequent changes in lung structure and function.[112] An important function of the pulmonary surfactant proteins A and D (SP-A and SP-D) may be to regulate inflammation in the lung alveolus.[113] In this regard, SP-D gene–deleted mice and SP-A/SP-D double gene–deleted mice develop emphysema postnatally.[114,115] In addition, inflammation is now closely linked to the destruction of alveoli in adult lung that is frequently observed in chronic obstructive pulmonary disease.[116-118]

Other Mediators of Alveolarization

Treatment of newborn rats with thyroid hormone accelerates the formation of lung alveoli and results in smaller alveoli and an increase in gas exchange surface area.[119] Conversely, a drug that inhibits thyroxine, propylthiouracil, impairs the formation of alveoli and decreases respiratory surface area.[119] Thus, thyroid hormone should be added to the list of mediators that influence the formation of lung alveoli in the developing lung.

Fibroblast growth factors (FGF) comprise a family of peptides that play an important role in many aspects of lung development.[120] These factors bind to one of several tyrosine kinase receptors (FGFR).[120] Mice that are deficient in FGFR-3 and FGFR-4 fail to form normal alveoli during postnatal life.[121]

Many other growth factors, growth factor receptors, and transcription factors are known to regulate aspects of lung development.[19,122,123] Many of these mediators affect lung development at multiple sites and at several stages of development. Therefore, it is difficult to ascribe a specific role for some of these factors in the formation of alveoli. However, it is likely that many of these regulatory factors do influence the formation of alveoli in the developing lung.

CONCLUSIONS

Our understanding of the formation of pulmonary alveoli has advanced greatly, but it is still in its infancy. We now have careful morphologic and morphometric descriptions of the alveolarization process in many species; however, human data remain incomplete. We now know that the formation and destruction of alveoli are responsive to several physiologic stimuli including nutritional status, oxygenation, and removal of one or part of a lung (Table 77-1). There is also strong evidence that many regulatory factors including retinoic acid, glucocorticoids, estrogen, and growth factors such as VEGF and PDGF can influence the formation of alveoli in the developing lung. However, there are still no clinically proven therapies that can be used to increase the formation of alveoli in humans, either in the neonate or in the adult lung. The transgenic mouse has been an extremely fruitful model for studying lung development, including the formation of alveoli. However, the study of the formation of alveoli in the lung would greatly benefit from the availability of an *in vitro* model of alveolarization as well as from the establishment of biochemical end-points that could be used to assess the degree of alveolarization in *in vitro* and *in vivo* model systems. A better understanding of the regulatory link between pulmonary vasculogenesis and alveolarization is also greatly needed. Finally, we need to elucidate the hierarchy of genes that influence alveolarization, starting with

TABLE 77-1

Mediators of Alveolarization

Regulators	References
Positive	
Vascular endothelial growth factor	47
Neuropilins	61
Platelet-derived growth factor A	28
Retinoic acid	11, 12
Estrogen	92
Thyroid hormone	119
Fibroblast growth factor	121
Nutrition	97
Negative	
Glucocorticoids	68
Oxygen	102
Inflammation	109

the transcription factors that may act as master regulators. Powerful new tools such as microchip gene array analysis and availability of mouse genome sequences will facilitate the search for key regulators of alveolarization.[124,125]

REFERENCES

1. Weibel ER, Taylor CR. (1998) Functional design of the human lung for gas exchange. In: Fishman GP (ed.) *Fishman's Pulmonary Diseases and Disorders.* McGraw-Hill, New York, pp. 21-61.
2. Langston C, Kida K, Reed M, Thurlbeck WM. (1984) Human lung growth in late gestation and in the neonate. *Am Rev Respir Dis 129:* 607-613.
3. Hislop AA, Wigglesworth JS, Desai R. (1986) Alveolar development in the human fetus and infant. *Early Hum Dev 13:* 1-11.
4. Husain AN, Siddiqui NH, Stocker JT. (1998) Pathology of arrested acinar development in postsurfactant bronchopulmonary dysplasia. *Hum Pathol 29:* 710-717.
5. Jobe AH, Ikegami M. (2001) Prevention of bronchopulmonary dysplasia. *Curr Opin Pediatr 13:* 124-129.
6. Coalson JJ, Winter V, deLemos RA. (1995) Decreased alveolarization in baboon survivors with bronchopulmonary dysplasia. *Am J Respir Crit Care Med 152:* 640-646.
7. Gilbert KA, Petrovic-Dovat L, Rannels DE. (1997) Hormonal control of compensatory lung growth. In: MacDonald JA (ed.) *Lung Growth and Development, Lung Biology in Health and Disease.* Marcel Dekker, New York, pp. 627-666.
8. Takeda S, Hsia CC, Wagner E, Ramanathan M, Estrera AS, Weibel ER. (1999) Compensatory alveolar growth normalizes gas-exchange function in immature dogs after pneumonectomy. *J Appl Physiol 86:* 1301-1310.
9. Massaro D, Massaro GD. (2002) Invited Review: pulmonary alveoli: formation, the "call for oxygen," and other regulators. *Am J Physiol 282:* L345-358.
10. Massaro GD, Massaro D. (1996) Postnatal treatment with retinoic acid increases the number of pulmonary alveoli in rats. *Am J Physiol 270:* L305-310.
11. Massaro GD, Massaro D. (1997) Retinoic acid treatment abrogates elastase-induced pulmonary emphysema in rats. *Nat Med 3:* 675-677.
12. Weibel ER, Crystal RG. (1997) Structural organization of the pulmonary interstitium. In: R.G. Crystal, et al. (ed.) *The Lung: Scientific Foundations.* Lippincott-Raven, Philadelphia, pp. 685-695.
13. Mallampalli RK, Acarregui MJ, Snyder JM. (1997) Differentiation of the alveolar epithelium in the fetal lung. In: MacDonald JE (ed.) *Lung Growth and Development.* Marcel Dekker, New York, pp. 119-162.
14. Crapo JD, Young SL, Fram EK, Pinkerton KE, Barry BE, Crapo RO. (1983) Morphometric characteristics of cells in the alveolar region of mammalian lungs. *Am Rev Respir Dis 128:* S42-46.
15. Frerking I, Gunther A, Seeger W, Pison U. (2001) Pulmonary surfactant: functions, abnormalities and therapeutic options. *Intensive Care Med 27:* 1699-1717.
16. Zeltner TB, Burri PH. (1987) The postnatal development and growth of the human lung. II. Morphology. *Respir Physiol 67:* 269-282.
17. Margraf LR, Tomashefski JF Jr, Bruce MC, Dahms BB. (1991) Morphometric analysis of the lung in bronchopulmonary dysplasia. *Am Rev Respir Dis 143:* 391-400.
18. Snyder JM, Mendelson CR, Johnston JM. (1985) The morphology of human fetal lung development. In: Nelson GH (ed.) *Pulmonary Development in Transition from Intrauterine to Extrauterine Life.* Marcel Dekker, New York, pp. 19-46.
19. Perl AK, Wert SE, Nagy A, Lobe CG, Whitsett JA. (2002) Early restriction of peripheral and proximal cell lineages during formation of the lung. *Proc Natl Acad Sci USA 99:* 10482-10487.
20. Burri PH, Dbaly J, Weibel ER. (1974) The postnatal growth of the rat lung. I. Morphometry. *Anat Rec 178:* 711-730.
21. Amy RW, Bowes D, Burri PH, Haines J, Thurlbeck WM. (1977) Postnatal growth of the mouse lung. *J Anat 124:* 131-151.
22. Massaro GD, Massaro D. (1996) Formation of pulmonary alveoli and gas-exchange surface area: quantitation and regulation. *Annu Rev Physiol 58:* 73-92.
23. Randell SH, Mercer RR, Young SL. (1990) Neonatal hyperoxia alters the pulmonary alveolar and capillary structure of 40-day-old rats. *Am J Pathol 136:* 1259-1266.
24. Kauffman SL. (1980) Cell proliferation in the mammalian lung. *Int Rev Exp Pathol 22:* 131-191.
25. McGowan SE, Torday JS. (1997) The pulmonary lipofibroblast (lipid interstitial cell) and its contributions to alveolar development. *Annu Rev Physiol 59:* 43-62.
26. Kapachi Y GG. (1997) Contractile cells in pulmonary alveolar tissue. In: R.G. Crystal, et al. (ed.) *Scientific Foundations.* Lippincott-Raven, Philadelphia, pp. 697-707.
27. Bostrom H, Willetts K, Pekny M, et al. (1996) PDGF-A signaling is a critical event in lung alveolar myofibroblast development and alveogenesis. *Cell 85:* 863-873.
28. Lindahl P, Karlsson L, Hellstrom M, et al. (1997) Alveogenesis failure in PDGF-A-deficient mice is coupled to lack of distal spreading of alveolar smooth muscle cell progenitors during lung development. *Development 124:* 3943-3953.
29. Mariani TJ, Pierce RA. (1999) Development of lung elastic matrix. In: Gaultier C, Bourbon JR, Post M (eds.) *Lung Development.* Oxford University Press, New York, pp. 28-45.
30. Mercer RR, Crapo JD. (1990) Spatial distribution of collagen and elastin fibers in the lungs. *J Appl Physiol 69:* 756-765.
31. Bairos V, Goncalves C, Figueiredo M. (1995) Study of the elastic fibres' framework of the rat lung. *Ital J Anat Embryol 100 Suppl 1:* 431-439.
32. Honda T, Ishida K, Hayama M, Kubo K, Katsuyama T. (2000) Type II pneumocytes are preferentially located along thick elastic fibers forming the framework of human alveoli. *Anat Rec 258:* 34-38.
33. Noguchi A, Firsching K, Kursar JD, Reddy R. (1990) Developmental changes of tropoelastin synthesis by rat pulmonary fibroblasts and effects of dexamethasone. *Pediatr Res 28:* 379-382.
34. Bruce MC. (1991) Developmental changes in tropoelastin mRNA levels in rat lung: evaluation by in situ hybridization. *Am J Respir Cell Mol Biol 5:* 344-350.
35. Kida K, Thurlbeck WM. (1980) Lack of recovery of lung structure and function after the administration of beta-amino-propionitrile in the postnatal period. *Am Rev Respir Dis 122:* 467-475.
36. Crouch E, Mecham R, Davila R, Noguchi A. (1997) Collagens and elastic fibers in lung development. In: MacDonald J (ed.) *Lung Growth and Development, Lung Biology in Health and Disease.* Marcel Dekker, New York, pp. 327-364.
37. Tanaka R, Al-Jamal R, Ludwig MS. (2001) Maturational changes in extracellular matrix and lung tissue mechanics. *J Appl Physiol 91:* 2314-2321.
38. Sannes PL, Wang J. (1997) Basement membranes and pulmonary development. *Exp Lung Res 23:* 101-108.
39. deMello DE, Sawyer D, Galvin N, Reid LM. (1997) Early fetal development of lung vasculature. *Am J Respir Cell Mol Biol 16:* 568-581.
40. Burri PH, Tarek MR. (1990) A novel mechanism of capillary growth in the rat pulmonary microcirculation. *Anat Rec 228:* 35-45.
41. Ferrara N. (2000) Vascular endothelial growth factor and the regulation of angiogenesis. *Recent Prog Horm Res 55:* 15-35; discussion 35-16.
42. Lassus P, Turanlahti M, Heikkila P, et al. (2001) Pulmonary vascular endothelial growth factor and Flt-1 in fetuses, in acute and chronic lung disease, and in persistent pulmonary hypertension of the newborn. *Am J Respir Crit Care Med 164:* 1981-1987.
43. Ng YS, Rohan R, Sunday ME, Demello DE, D'Amore PA. (2001) Differential expression of VEGF isoforms in mouse during development and in the adult. *Dev Dyn 220:* 112-121.
44. Zeng X, Wert SE, Federici R, Peters KG, Whitsett JA. (1998) VEGF enhances pulmonary vasculogenesis and disrupts lung morphogenesis in vivo. *Dev Dyn 211:* 215-227.
45. Brown KR, England KM, Goss KL, Snyder JM, Acarregui MJ. (2001) VEGF induces airway epithelial cell proliferation in human fetal lung in vitro. *Am J Physiol 281:* L1001-1010.
46. Compernolle V, Brusselmans K, Acker T, et al. (2002) Loss of HIF-2alpha and inhibition of VEGF impair fetal lung maturation, whereas treatment with VEGF prevents fatal respiratory distress in premature mice. *Nat Med 8:* 702-710.
47. Kasahara Y, Tuder RM, Taraseviciene-Stewart L, et al. (2000) Inhibition of VEGF receptors causes lung cell apoptosis and emphysema. *J Clin Invest 106:* 1311-1319.
48. Le Cras TD, Markham NE, Tuder RM, Voelkel NF, Abman SH. (2002) Treatment of newborn rats with a VEGF receptor inhibitor causes pulmonary hypertension and abnormal lung structure. *Am J Physiol 283:* L555-562.
49. Jakkula M, Le Cras TD, Gebb S, et al. (2000) Inhibition of angiogenesis decreases alveolarization in the developing rat lung. *Am J Physiol 279:* L600-607.
50. Jobe AH, Bancalari E. (2001) Bronchopulmonary dysplasia. *Am J Respir Crit Care Med 163:* 1723-1729.
51. Bhatt AJ, Pryhuber GS, Huyck H, Watkins RH, Metlay LA, Maniscalco WM. (2001) Disrupted pulmonary vasculature and decreased vascular endothelial growth factor, Flt-1, and TIE-2 in human infants dying with bronchopulmonary dysplasia. *Am J Respir Crit Care Med 164:* 1971-1980.
52. Albertine KH, Jones GP, Starcher BC, et al. (1999) Chronic lung injury in preterm lambs: disordered respiratory tract development. *Am J Respir Crit Care Med 159:* 945-958.
53. D'Angio CT, Maniscalco WM. (2002) The role of vascular growth factors in hyperoxia-induced injury to the developing lung. *Front Biosci 7:* d1609-1623.
54. Loughna S, Sato TN. (2001) Angiopoietin and Tie signaling pathways in vascular development. *Matrix Biol 20:* 319-325.
55. Kullander K, Klein R. (2002) Mechanisms and functions of Eph and ephrin signalling. *Nat Rev Mol Cell Biol 3:* 475-486.
56. Neufeld G, Cohen T, Shraga N, Lange T, Kessler O, Herzog Y. (2002) The neuropilins: multifunctional semaphorin and VEGF receptors that modulate axon guidance and angiogenesis. *Trends Cardiovasc Med 12:* 13-19.
57. Maniscalco WM, Watkins RH, Pryhuber GS, Bhatt A, Shea C, Huyck H. (2002) Angiogenic factors and alveolar vasculature: development and alterations by injury in very premature baboons. *Am J Physiol 282:* L811-823.
58. Chinoy MR, Graybill MM, Miller SA, Lang CM, Kauffman GL. (2002) Angiopoietin-1 and VEGF in vascular development and angiogenesis in hypoplastic lungs. *L60-66.*
59. Kagoshima M, Ito T. (2001) Diverse gene expression and function of semaphorins in developing lung: positive and negative regulatory roles of semaphorins in lung branching morphogenesis. *Genes Cells 6:* 559-571.

60. Ito T, Kagoshima M, Sasaki Y, et al. (2000) Repulsive axon guidance molecule Sema3A inhibits branching morphogenesis of fetal mouse lung. *Mech Dev 97:* 35-45.

61. Betsholtz C, Karlsson L, Lindahl P. (2001) Developmental roles of platelet-derived growth factors. *Bioessays 23:* 494-507.

62. Han RN, Mawdsley C, Souza P, Tanswell AK, Post M. (1992) Platelet-derived growth factors and growth-related genes in rat lung. III. Immunolocalization during fetal development. *Pediatr Res 31:* 323-329.

63. Bostrom H, Gritli-Linde A, Betsholty C. (2002) PDGF-A/PDGF alpha-receptor signaling is required for lung growth and the formation of alveoli but not for early lung branching morphogenesis. *Dev Dyn 223:* 155-162.

64. Bolt RJ, van Weissenbruch MM, Lafeber HN, Delemarre-van de Waal HA. (2001) Glucocorticoids and lung development in the fetus and preterm infant. *Pediatr Pulmonol 32:* 76-91.

65. Liggins GC. (1969) Premature delivery of foetal lambs infused with glucocorticoids. *J Endocrinol 45:* 515-523.

66. Liggins GC, Howie RN. (1972) A controlled trial of antepartum glucocorticoid treatment for prevention of the respiratory distress syndrome in premature infants. *Pediatrics 50:* 515-525.

67. Massaro D, Massaro GD. (1986) Dexamethasone accelerates postnatal alveolar wall thinning and alters wall composition. *Am J Physiol 251:* R218-224.

68. Willet KE, McMenamin P, Pinkerton KE, et al. (1999) Lung morphometry and collagen and elastin content: changes during normal development and after prenatal hormone exposure in sheep. *Pediatr Res 45:* 615-625.

69. Massaro D, Teich N, Maxwell S, Massaro GD, Whitney P. (1985) Postnatal development of alveoli: regulation and evidence for a critical period in rats. *J Clin Invest 76:* 1297-1305.

70. Bunton TE, Plopper CG. (1984) Triamcinolone-induced structural alterations in the development of the lung of the fetal rhesus macaque. *Am J Obstet Gynecol 148:* 203-215.

71. Muglia LJ, Bae DS, Brown TT, et al. (1999) Proliferation and differentiation defects during lung development in corticotropin-releasing hormone-deficient mice. *Am J Respir Cell Mol Biol 20:* 181-188.

72. Cole TJ, Blendy JA, Monaghan AP, et al. (1995) Targeted disruption of the glucocorticoid receptor gene blocks adrenergic chromaffin cell development and severely retards lung maturation. *Genes Dev 9:* 1608-1621.

73. Jobe AH. (1993) Pulmonary surfactant therapy. *N Engl J Med 328:* 861-868.

74. Jobe AH. (2001) Glucocorticoids, inflammation and the perinatal lung. *Semin Neonatol 6:* 331-342.

75. Chytil F. (1992) The lungs and vitamin A. *Am J Physiol 262:* L517-527.

76. Chytil F. (1996) Retinoids in lung development. *FASEB J 10:* 986-992.

77. Chambon P. (1995) The molecular and genetic dissection of the retinoid signaling pathway. *Recent Prog Horm Res 50:* 317-332.

78. Massaro GD, Massaro D, Chan WY, et al. (2000) Retinoic acid receptor-beta: an endogenous inhibitor of the perinatal formation of pulmonary alveoli. *Physiol Genomics 4:* 51-57.

79. Massaro GD, Massaro D. (1992) Formation of alveoli in rats: postnatal effect of prenatal dexamethasone. *Am J Physiol 263:* L37-41.

80. Veness-Meehan KA, Pierce RA, Moats-Staats BM, Stiles AD. (2002) Retinoic acid attenuates O_2-induced inhibition of lung septation. *Am J Physiol 283:* L971-980.

81. McGowan S, Jackson SK, Jenkins-Moore M, Dai HH, Chambon P, Snyder JM. (2000) Mice bearing deletions of retinoic acid receptors demonstrate reduced lung elastin and alveolar numbers. *Am J Respir Cell Mol Biol 23:* 162-167.

82. McGowan SE, Doro MM, Jackson SK. (1997) Endogenous retinoids increase perinatal elastin gene expression in rat lung fibroblasts and fetal explants. *Am J Physiol 273:* L410-416.

83. Shenai JP, Chytil F. (1990) Vitamin A storage in lungs during perinatal development in the rat. *Biol Neonate 57:* 126-132.

84. McGowan SE, Harvey CS, Jackson SK. (1995) Retinoids, retinoic acid receptors, and cytoplasmic retinoid binding proteins in perinatal rat lung fibroblasts. *Am J Physiol 269:* L463-472.

85. Shenai JP, Kennedy KA, Chytil F, Stahlman MT. (1987) Clinical trial of vitamin A supplementation in infants susceptible to bronchopulmonary dysplasia. *J Pediatr 111:* 269-277.

86. Kennedy KA, Stoll BJ, Ehrenkranz RA, et al. (1997) Vitamin A to prevent bronchopulmonary dysplasia in very-low-birth-weight infants: has the dose been too low? The NICHD Neonatal Research Network. *Early Hum Dev 49:* 19-31.

87. Tyson JE, Wright LL, Oh W, et al. (1999) Vitamin A supplementation for extremely-low-birth-weight infants: National Institute of Child Health and Human Development Neonatal Research Network. *N Engl J Med 340:* 1962-1968.

88. Walter R, Gottlieb DJ, O'Connor GT. (2000) Environmental and genetic risk factors and gene-environment interactions in the pathogenesis of chronic obstructive lung disease. *Environ Health Perspect 108 Suppl 4:* 733-742.

89. Mao JT, Goldin JG, Dermand J, et al. (2002) A pilot study of all-trans-retinoic acid for the treatment of human emphysema. *Am J Respir Crit Care Med 165:* 718-723.

90. Nielsen HC, Torday JS. (2000) Sex difference in fetal lung development. In: Mendelson CR (ed.) *Endocrinology of the Lung.* Human Press, Totowa, NJ, pp. 141-159.

91. Torday JS, Nielsen HC, Fencl M de M, Avery ME. (1981) Sex differences in fetal lung maturation. *Am Rev Respir Dis 123:* 205-208.

92. Massaro GD, Mortola JP, Massaro D. (1996) Estrogen modulates the dimensions of the lung's gas-exchange surface area and alveoli in female rats. *Am J Physiol 270:* L110-114.

93. Massaro GD, Mortola JP, Massaro D. (1995) Sexual dimorphism in the architecture of the lung's gas-exchange region. *Proc Natl Acad Sci USA 92:* 1105-1107.

94. Challis JRG, Matthews SG, Gibb W, Lye SJ. (2000) Endocrine and paracrine regulation of birth at term and preterm. *Endocr Rev 21:* 514-550.

95. Trotter A, Maier L, Pohlandt F. (2001) Management of the extremely preterm infant: is the replacement of estradiol and progesterone beneficial? *Paediatr Drugs 3:* 629-637.

96. Gonzales-Pacheco DM, Buss WC, Koehler KM, Woodside WF, Alpert SS. (1993) Energy restriction reduces metabolic rate in adult male Fisher-344 rats. *J Nutr 123:* 90-97.

97. Sahebjami H, Wirman JA. (1981) Emphysema-like changes in the lungs of starved rats. *Am Rev Respir Dis 124:* 619-624.

98. Massaro G, Radaeva S, Clerch LB, Massaro D. (2002) Lung alveoli: endogenous programmed destruction and regeneration. *Am J Physiol 283:* L305-309.

99. Massaro D MG. (2001) Pulmonary alveolus formation: critical period, retinoid regulation and plasticity. *Novartis Found Symp:* 229-241.

100. Tenney SM, Remmers JE. (1963) Comparative quantitative morphology of the mammalian lung diffusing area. *Nature 197:* 54-56.

101. Burri PH, Weibel ER. (1971) Morphometric estimation of pulmonary diffusion capacity. II. Effect of Po$_2$ on the growing lung, adaption of the growing rat lung to hypoxia and hyperoxia. *Respir Physiol 11:* 247-264.

102. Randell SH, Mercer RR, Young SL. (1989) Postnatal growth of pulmonary acini and alveoli in normal and oxygen-exposed rats studied by serial section reconstructions. *Am J Anat 186:* 55-68.

103. Maniscalco WM, Watkins RH, D'Angio CT, Ryan RM. (1997) Hyperoxic injury decreases alveolar epithelial cell expression of vascular endothelial growth factor (VEGF) in neonatal rabbit lung. *Am J Respir Cell Mol Biol 16:* 557-567.

104. McGrath-Morrow SA, Stahl J. (2001) Apoptosis in neonatal murine lung exposed to hyperoxia. *Am J Respir Cell Mol Biol 25:* 150-155.

105. Moore LG. (2001) Human genetic adaptation to high altitude. *High Alt Med Biol 2:* 257-279.

106. Blanco LN, Massaro D, Massaro GD. (1991) Alveolar size, number, and surface area: developmentally dependent response to 13% O_2. *Am J Physiol 261:* L370-377.

107. Massaro GD, Olivier J, Dzikowski C, Massaro D. (1990) Postnatal development of lung alveoli: suppression by 13% O_2 and a critical period. *Am J Physiol 258:* L321-327.

108. Speer CP. (1999) Inflammatory mechanisms in neonatal chronic lung disease. *Eur J Pediatr 158 Suppl 1:* S18-22.

109. Jobe AH, Ikegami M. (2001) Antenatal infection/inflammation and postnatal lung maturation and injury. *Respir Res 2:* 27-32.

110. Clark RH, Gerstmann DR, Jobe AH, Moffitt ST, Slutsky AS, Yoder BA. (2001) Lung injury in neonates: causes, strategies for prevention, and long-term consequences. *J Pediatr 139:* 478-486.

111. Lyon A. (2000) Chronic lung disease of prematurity: the role of intra-uterine infection. *Eur J Pediatr 159:* 798-802.

112. Parks WC, Shapiro SD. (2001) Matrix metalloproteinases in lung biology. *Respir Res 2:* 10-19.

113. Crouch E, Wright JR. (2001) Surfactant proteins A and D and pulmonary host defense. *Annu Rev Physiol 63:* 521-554.

114. Wert SE, Yoshida M, LeVine AM, et al. (2000) Increased metalloproteinase activity, oxidant production, and emphysema in surfactant protein D gene-inactivated mice. *Proc Natl Acad Sci USA 97:* 5972-5977.

115. Hawgood S, Ochs M, Jung A, et al. (2002) Sequential targeted deficiency of SP-A and -D leads to progressive alveolar lipoproteinosis and emphysema. *Am J Physiol 283:* L1002-1010.

116. Jeffery PK. (2001) Lymphocytes, chronic bronchitis and chronic obstructive pulmonary disease. *Novartis Found Symp 234:* 149-161; discussion 161-148.

117. Chung KF. (2001) Cytokines in chronic obstructive pulmonary disease. *Eur Respir J Suppl 34:* 50s-59s.

118. Barnes PJ. (2001) Cytokine modulators as novel therapies for airway disease. *Eur Respir J Suppl 34:* 67s-77s.

119. Massaro D, Teich N, Massaro GD. (1986) Postnatal development of pulmonary alveoli: modulation in rats by thyroid hormones. *Am J Physiol 250:* R51-55.

120. Ware LB, Matthay MA. (2002) Keratinocyte and hepatocyte growth factors in the lung: roles in lung development, inflammation, and repair. *Am J Physiol 282:* L924-940.

121. Weinstein M, Xu X, Ohyama K, Deng CX. (1998) FGFR-3 and FGFR-4 function cooperatively to direct alveogenesis in the murine lung. *Development 125:* 3615-3623.

122. Warburton D, Schwarz M, Tefft D, Flores-Delgado G, Anderson KD, Cardoso WV. (2000) The molecular basis of lung morphogenesis. *Mech Dev 92:* 55-81.

123. Costa RH, Kalinichenko VV, Lim L. (2001) Transcription factors in mouse lung development and function. *Am J Physiol 280:* L823-838.

124. Mariani TJ, Reed JJ, Shapiro SD. (2002) Expression profiling of the developing mouse lung: insights into the establishment of the extracellular matrix. *Am J Respir Cell Mol Biol 26:* 541-548.

125. Waterston RH, et al. (2002) Initial sequencing and comparative analysis of the mouse genome. *Nature 420:* 520-562.

Richard Harding and Stuart B. Hooper

78

Physiologic Mechanisms of Normal and Altered Lung Growth

Survival at birth depends on the ability of the lung to exchange respiratory gases at a level that adequately provides for the metabolic demands of the neonate. The ability of the neonatal lung to perform this role is dependent on the fetal lung's having grown sufficiently and having developed unique structural, physiologic, and biochemical features by the time of birth. The lung must have developed an intricate system of airways to allow low-resistance airflow to and from the respiratory zone; the internal surface area must be large and separated from a dense vascular network by a thin sheet of tissue. The mechanical properties of the lung must have matured to allow expansion of the lung during inspiration with little effort but must retain sufficient recoil to drive expiration, while preventing collapse of the lung at end expiration. In healthy term infants, these features are usually present by the time of birth, even though the lungs play no functional role in gas exchange *in utero*. However, if fetal lung development has been compromised, the neonate may experience respiratory insufficiency, the most common cause of morbidity and mortality in the neonatal period. Respiratory insufficiency can arise either from an insufficient period of development *in utero*, owing to preterm birth, or from environmental or genetic factors that disrupt lung development. In this chapter, we consider the physiologic processes that determine the normal growth and structural maturation of the fetal lung and discuss how these processes can become perturbed *in utero*, thus giving rise to compromised lung development and lung function after birth.

During fetal life, the future air spaces of the lungs are filled with a unique liquid that is produced by the lung epithelium. This liquid, a product of net chloride flux across the pulmonary epithelial cells[1] (see Chapter 83), plays a critical role in fetal lung development by maintaining the future air spaces in a distended state; it also limits the entry into the lungs of amniotic fluid, which can potentially have damaging effects. The volume of liquid within the future air spaces and its flux to and from the lower airways are influenced by fetal muscular activity as well as by postural changes and other factors that influence transpulmonary pressure.[2] By maintaining the lungs in a distended state, fetal lung liquid serves as an internal "splint" around which the distal air spaces of the lungs develop.[2-4] It is also apparent that, without this underlying degree of expansion, the fetal lung is unable to grow and structurally mature.[2] As a result, much attention has focused on understanding how the basal degree of lung expansion is controlled and the mechanisms by which it influences growth and remodeling of fetal lung tissue. Investigators have recognized that the fetal metabolic and endocrine environments, including the availability of micronutrients such as retinoic acid, also play an important role in fetal lung development. However, these factors appear mainly to influence and modulate the processes that regulate normal lung growth and development, particularly physical factors such as lung expansion. Because it is clear that physical factors underlie many common disorders of fetal lung development, they will be the major focus of this chapter.

PHYSIOLOGIC CONTROL OF FETAL LUNG EXPANSION

Data on fetal lung liquid dynamics and lung expansion are almost entirely derived from studies of chronically catheterized fetal sheep using indicator dilution techniques to assess lung liquid volumes,[2, 4, 5] as well as purpose-built flow meters to measure liquid flow within the trachea.[6,7] During the latter half of ovine gestation, the volume of liquid retained within the fetal lungs markedly increases and, during the last weeks of gestation, is greater than the functional residual volume of the air-filled lung after birth (Fig. 78-1).[2, 4] Basal lung luminal volumes are 35 to 45 mL/kg in late-gestation fetal sheep,[2, 8-10] whereas the functional residual volume in newborn lambs is 25 to 30 mL/kg.[11] The high level of fetal lung expansion is maintained by fetal activity, particularly fetal breathing movements (FBMs)[12, 13] and adductor activity of the glottis,[2] features indicating that the fetus actively participates in maintaining its lung volume (Fig. 78-2). It is also influenced by the transpulmonary pressure gradient, which, in turn, is influenced by the amount of available intrathoracic and intrauterine space (see later). Thus, values that have been reported from dead, anesthetized, exteriorized, or paralyzed fetuses will necessarily underestimate lung luminal volumes because lung liquid is lost under these conditions (see Fig. 78-2).[2, 12] Similarly, measurements of lung liquid volumes in chronically catheterized fetuses are questionable unless the measurements were made in the absence of fetal hypoxemia or labor and in the presence of normal amniotic fluid volumes.[8, 14] Both labor and reduced amniotic fluid volumes reduce lung luminal volumes by compressive forces on the fetus that increase transpulmonary pressure.[8, 14, 15]

In the absence of labor, the volume of lung liquid in healthy fetuses is mainly determined by fetal muscular activity and the transpulmonary pressure gradient; alterations in the secretion rate of fetal lung liquid have no significant effect on luminal volume because they simply cause corresponding changes in the efflux of liquid.[16, 17] The rate of liquid efflux from the fetal lung via the trachea is dependent on the pressure gradient between the lung lumen and the amniotic sac (transpulmonary pressure) as well as the resistance to liquid efflux through the upper airway, particularly by the glottis.[18, 19] In the absence of FBMs (i.e., fetal apnea), the pulmonary intraluminal pressure is 1 to 2 mm Hg higher than amniotic sac pressure,[20] owing to the inherent recoil of lung tissue and the resistance of the glottis.[19] During apnea, the efflux of liquid via the trachea is, on average, lower than its rate of production, and liquid accumulates within the lungs (Fig. 78-3).[6] During episodes of FBM, the resistance to liquid efflux is reduced because of phasic abduction of the glottis,[19] which permits an increased rate of liquid flow from the lungs.[6] Thus, despite rhythmic contractions of the diaphragm, there is a net loss of liquid from the lungs during FBMs that is two- to threefold greater than the loss during intervening apneic periods.[18, 21] Although liquid sometimes enters the fetal lungs during accentuated FBMs and changes in upper airway function, the net flow is out of the lungs.[18] This essentially unidirectional flux maintains a constant chemical environment within the developing air spaces,[22] thus restricting the entry of potentially harmful substances in amniotic fluid (e.g., meconium).

The transpulmonary pressure gradient and therefore the efflux of lung liquid are also influenced by factors external to the lungs such as abdominal pressure.[14] Changes in fetal posture (e.g., trunk flexion), which increase abdominal pressure, increase the transpulmonary pressure gradient and lead to a reduction in

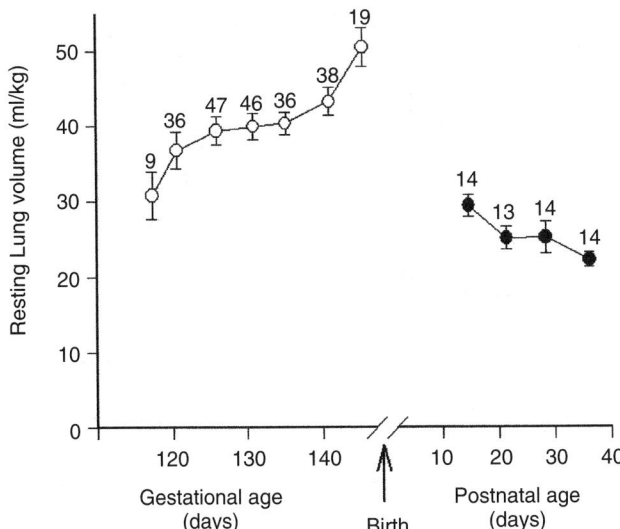

Figure 78–1. Basal lung volumes in the ovine fetus and neonate. The lung volume measurements made in the fetus (*open symbols*; numbers of measurements above symbols) are a measure of the volume of lung liquid retained within the future airways and were made using an impermeant indicator dilution technique. The postnatal lung volume measurements (*closed symbols*) are a measure of the volume of air remaining within the lungs at end expiration (functional residual capacity; FRC) and were made using the helium dilution technique.

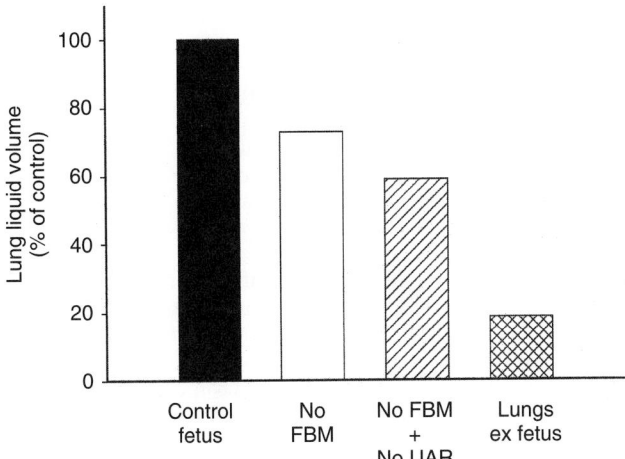

Figure 78–2. The influence of fetal muscular activity on the volume of liquid retained within the future airways. Compared with control fetuses, the inhibition of fetal breathing movements (FBM) by either fetal spinal cord transection[13] or selective blockade of the phrenic nerves[12] causes an approximately 25% decrease in fetal lung liquid volume, which demonstrates the importance of the fetal diaphragm in maintaining the volume of fetal lung liquid. When the fetal upper airway is bypassed, eliminating upper airway resistance (UAR) in addition to the abolition of FBM, the volume of lung liquid is reduced further, and this demonstrates the independent effect of the fetal upper airway in maintaining fetal lung liquid volumes. The further reduction in lung luminal volume after the removal of the lungs from the fetus demonstrates the contribution that the fetal chest wall makes to maintaining fetal lung liquid volumes. (From Harding R, Hooper SB: J Appl Physiol 81:209, 1996.)

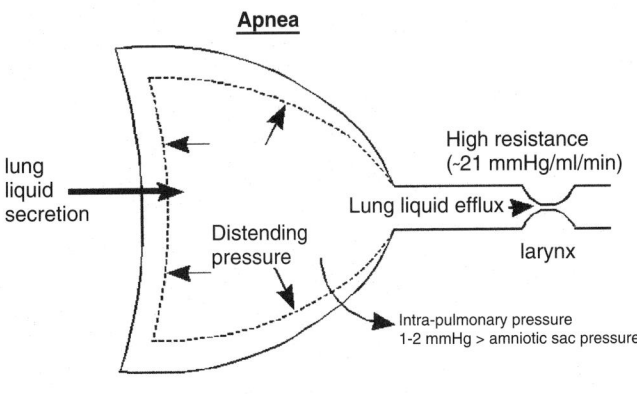

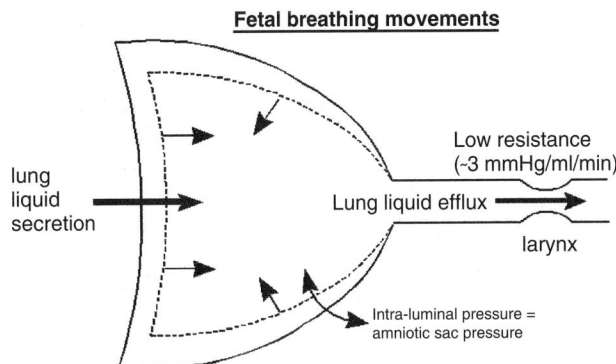

Figure 78–3. Diagram showing the function of the fetal upper airway in regulating the efflux of lung liquid during periods of apnea (*upper panel*) and fetal breathing movements (FBM; *lower panel*). During periods of apnea, the resistance to lung liquid efflux through the upper airway is high (owing to lack of laryngeal abductor activity and tonic adductor activity) and, as a result, liquid tends to accumulate within the future airways and causes the lungs to expand; this liquid accumulation is responsible for generating a transpulmonary pressure gradient of 1 to 2 mm Hg (intraairway > amniotic sac pressure). During periods of FBM, the resistance to lung liquid efflux through the upper airway decreases (owing to phasic dilator activity of glottic abductor muscles and lack of sustained activity in adductor muscles), and therefore liquid leaves the lungs at an increased rate. As a result, the transpulmonary pressure gradient usually decreases to 0 mm Hg during episodes of FBM.

lung volume.[14] Such changes in fetal posture can arise from fetal movement or can be imposed on the fetus by uterine contractions or when intrauterine space is limited by oligohydramnios.[14] Oligohydramnios forces the fetus into a posture that increases its spinal curvature (Fig. 78-4);[14, 23] this flexion increases fetal abdominal pressure and transpulmonary pressure, leading to increased lung liquid efflux and a reduced lung volume.[14, 15] This is the likely cause of lung hypoplasia associated with oligohydramnios.[14]

Most evidence indicating that the degree of fetal lung expansion regulates the growth and development of the fetal lungs has been derived from experiments in which (1) the fetal lung was chronically drained of liquid to cause lung "deflation" or (2) the fetal trachea was obstructed to cause liquid accumulation within the future airways.

EFFECTS OF REDUCED LUNG EXPANSION ON FETAL LUNG GROWTH

Sustained reductions in fetal lung expansion can cause severe lung hypoplasia, retard structural development of the lung, and

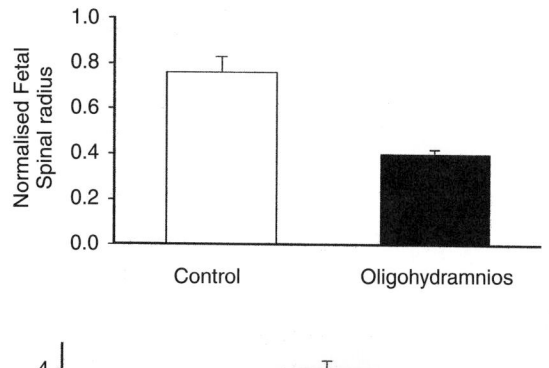

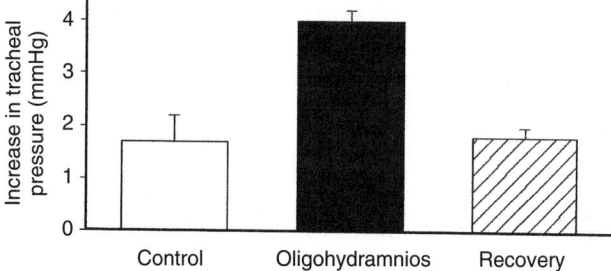

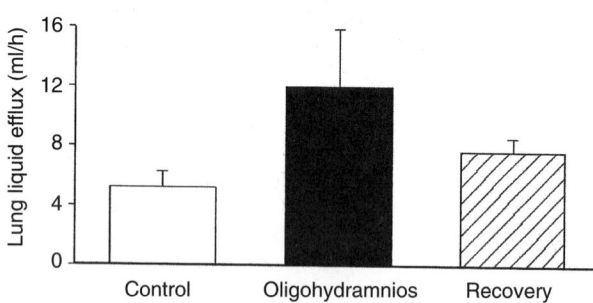

Figure 78–4. Effect of oligohydramnios, induced by the drainage of amniotic fluid, on the degree of spinal cord flexion (measured as a normalized spinal radius) in fetal sheep (*top panel*); a smaller normalized spinal radius is indicative of a greater curvature of the spine. Shown are the effect of oligohydramnios on fetal tracheal pressure (*middle panel*) and lung liquid efflux (*bottom panel*) associated with non-labor uterine contractions during a control period, 48 hours of oligohydramnios, and a recovery period. These data demonstrate that when intrauterine volume is reduced, non-labor-related uterine contractions increase abdominal pressure (data not shown) and tracheal pressure, resulting in an increase in liquid efflux from the fetal lungs. (Data from Harding R, et al: A mechanism leading to reduced lung expansion and lung hypoplasia in fetal sheep during oligohydramnios. Am J Obstet Gynecol 1990;163:1904.)

cause major changes in the proportions of alveolar epithelial cell (AEC) phenotypes. These effects appear to depend on the degree to which lung expansion is decreased. A prolonged 25% reduction in lung expansion causes an approximately 25% reduction in lung growth,[13] whereas total lung deflation causes lung tissue growth effectively to cease.[3, 24, 25] The mechanisms for the reduction in lung growth are currently unknown, although a reduction in the expression of insulin-like growth factor II (IGF-II) has been observed in two separate models of reduced lung expansion.[13, 26] The normal remodeling of lung parenchyma, which characterizes structural development of the lung, is also severely retarded by prolonged reductions in fetal lung expansion.[3] In particular, interalveolar tissue volumes and distances are greatly increased,[3] leading to increased blood gas diffusion barriers and therefore

reduced diffusing capacities for respiratory gases. Furthermore, the process of alveolarization is greatly attenuated, resulting in markedly reduced alveolar numbers[3,27] and, importantly, altered elastin deposition in the saccule walls (normally, elastin is deposited at the tips of secondary septal crests and is a key feature in the process of alveolarization).[28] Fetal lung hypoplasia is also characterized by reduced development of the pulmonary vascular bed, indicating that prolonged reductions in fetal lung expansion also influence pulmonary vascular growth.[29]

The alveolar epithelium of the fetal lung is also affected by prolonged reductions in fetal lung expansion.[3, 30] Evidence indicates that reduced lung expansion promotes differentiation of Type I into Type II cells,[30] and this supports *in vitro* evidence suggesting that Type I cells are not terminally differentiated and can transdifferentiate into Type II cells.[31, 32]

EFFECTS OF INCREASED LUNG EXPANSION

Prolonged overexpansion of the fetal lungs is a potent stimulus for fetal lung growth and tissue remodeling, and it is usually induced experimentally by obstructing the fetal trachea.[3, 33] The increase in lung cell proliferation is time dependent[34] and is restricted to the expanded lung tissue.[24] The fetal lung growth response after tracheal obstruction differs according to the stage of fetal lung development. During the alveolar stage in fetal sheep, lung DNA content increases within 2 days of tracheal obstruction,[35] and the stimulated increase in growth is completed within 7 days, resulting in an almost doubling (~70% increase) in DNA content[26, 34]; the eventual cessation of accelerated growth is likely the result of restraint by the chest wall, thus preventing further lung expansion. In contrast, during the late pseudoglandular/early canalicular stage of ovine lung development (80 to 110 days; 0.5 to 0.7 of term), the increase in lung DNA content is undetectable at 2 days of tracheal obstruction,[35] but eventually it results in a greater increase in lung DNA content (~200%) than later in fetal life[36]; similar results have been obtained in fetal rabbits.[37,38] The lower rate of accelerated lung growth after tracheal obstruction in younger fetuses is thought to be the result of a lower lung compliance and hence a lower rate of lung expansion.[35, 36] However, the eventual greater increase in lung DNA content at the younger age is likely caused by a more compliant chest wall, allowing the lungs eventually to expand to a greater degree than in older fetuses.[36]

The characteristics of the lung growth response to an increase in lung expansion also differ according to the stage of lung development. During the alveolar stage, increased lung expansion causes the proliferation of most major cell types,[33] but during the late pseudoglandular/early canalicular stage, it primarily causes mesenchymal cell proliferation,[36] leading to a large increase in the distance between air spaces.[36] In contrast, during the later stages of fetal lung development, prolonged increases in fetal lung expansion accelerate structural maturation of the lung; the proportion of tissue space is reduced, owing to a reduction in interalveolar tissue, whereas alveolar number and surface area are increased.[3, 33, 37-39] The mechanisms by which an increase in fetal lung expansion stimulates septation and alveolarization are unknown but are probably linked to the increase in tropoelastin expression induced by this stimulus.[28] Thus, the effects of increased fetal lung expansion will depend on the stage of development at which the stimulus is applied.

Sustained increases in fetal lung expansion also have a major impact on AEC differentiation.[3] Type II AECs are induced to differentiate, via an intermediate cell type, into Type I AECs such that within 10 days of pulmonary overexpansion in fetal sheep, fewer than 2% of AECs are of the Type II phenotype, whereas more than 90% are of the Type I phenotype.[40] Thus, at least in the fetus, the phenotypes of AECs appear to be plastic and profoundly influenced by the degree of lung expansion.

ROLE OF FETAL BREATHING MOVEMENTS IN FETAL LUNG DEVELOPMENT

FBMs begin early in fetal life and, in the healthy fetus, occur in discrete episodes that become associated with a fetal behavioral state resembling rapid eye movement sleep.[41, 42] The principal inspiratory muscles used in FBMs include the diaphragm and abductor muscles of the glottis;[19] as in postnatal rapid eye movement sleep, the intercostal muscles are largely quiescent. During the latter half of gestation, the overall incidence of FBMs is 40 to 50%,[43] separated by periods of apnea, when the glottis is closed by sustained adductor muscle activity.[19] Typically, individual FBMs lower intrathoracic pressure by up to 5 mm Hg and cause small oscillations of fluid (see later) within the fetal trachea[44,45] and nasal passages.[46, 47] Much interest has focused on FBMs because they are an important determinant of fetal lung development, although their precise role *in vivo* has been difficult to determine.[2,4]

In exploring the functional role of FBMs, numerous techniques have been used to eliminate or blunt their effects, including fetal paralysis,[48] sectioning[49,50] and reversible blockade of the phrenic nerves,[12] sectioning of the fetal spinal cord above the outflow of the phrenic motoneurons,[13, 51, 52] and replacing sections of the thoracic wall with a compliant membrane.[53] These studies must be interpreted with caution, however, because the procedures also have effects that are additional to the abolition of FBMs; for example, phrenic nerve section causes the diaphragm muscle to atrophy and to lengthen, whereas thoracoplasty may allow lung compression; fetal paralysis abolishes glottic adductor activity and may alter fetal posture, thereby causing lung compression. To understand the role of FBMs themselves in lung development, it is necessary to alter only FBMs and to measure fetal lung luminal volume. When this is done, it is apparent that the reduction in lung growth induced by the abolition of FBMs can be explained by the associated decrease in the basal level of fetal lung expansion;[12,13] indeed, the percentage of decrease in lung expansion is similar to the percentage of decrease in lung growth.[13] The decrease in lung expansion after abolition of the thoracic component of FBMs can be explained by persistence of glottic dilator activity.[13] As a result, the loss of lung liquid is increased during centrally generated "FBMs," when compared with intact fetuses.[12,13] Thus, in intact fetuses, activation of the diaphragm apparently plays a key role during FBMs by restricting the loss of lung liquid when the resistance to lung liquid efflux is lowered by dilatation of the glottis.[4] Collectively, these data demonstrate that fetal muscular activities, whether active glottic adduction during apnea or activation of the diaphragm during FBMs, help to defend fetal lung liquid volumes and therefore the degree of lung expansion (see Fig. 78-2). At present, there is no *in vivo* evidence to suggest that phasic stretch, as such, of the lung during FBMs is an important determinant of fetal lung growth.

Numerous *in vitro* studies have shown that phasic stretch of fetal lung cells in culture, in a manner purported to simulate FBMs *in vivo*, stimulates lung cell proliferation.[54] These experiments have provided important information on the transduction pathways by which phasic mechanical stimuli initiate lung cell proliferation. However, the stimulus used (~5% stretch) does not simulate FBMs *in vivo*. *In vivo*, individual breathing movements are essentially isovolumetric, and therefore the percentage of length change experienced by a cell with each FBM will be negligible. This is because the fetal chest wall is very compliant, fetal lung liquid is very viscous compared with air, and, because of its bulk, fetal lung liquid has a large inertia. Thus, although activation of the diaphragm causes a reduction in intrathoracic pressure, very little liquid is inhaled with each inspiratory effort because other sections of the chest wall are simultaneously drawn in,[55] and liquid has to be present within the pharynx before any liquid can be inhaled.[19] As a result, the tidal volume in the fetus

is very small; in late-gestation fetal sheep, the tidal volume is usually less than 0.5 mL[44, 45] at FBM rates of up to three per second. In human fetuses during the last trimester, the mean FBM frequency is approximately one per second,[46] although respiratory cycle times of up to 1.5 to 2.0 seconds have been reported. Color Doppler ultrasound has been used to measure fluid flow velocity waveforms in the trachea and nasopharynx of human fetuses, although the contribution of this fluid movement to lung volume changes is currently unclear.[47] Thus, at least in the sheep, fetal tidal volume is less than 1% of resting lung volume, but it markedly increases immediately after birth to approximately 20% of resting lung volume.

MECHANOTRANSDUCTION MECHANISMS

All cells, tissues, and even whole organs are subjected to physical forces *in vivo*, including shear stress, strain, stretch, and compression; such forces can result from gravity, osmotic pressures, fluid flow, intracellular tensile forces, body movements, and changes in the internal volume of an organ (e.g., intestine, stomach, uterus, heart, bladder, and lung). It has been proposed that cells exist in a state of isometric tension that is generated by the intracellular contractile filaments of the cell.[56] Thus, externally applied forces are thought to be imposed on a preexisting equilibrium of forces, causing changes in cell shape and intracellular structural fiber alignment until the force equilibrium is reestablished.[56,57]

It has been recognized for many years that physical forces play an important role in cellular growth and differentiation and are also critical regulators of three-dimensional tissue structure,[57] particularly in the lung.[4,58] Thus, physical forces are an important means by which cells interact with their environment,[56,57,59] and the transduction pathways by which these forces are translated into chemical stimuli, leading to changes in cell function, are beginning to be understood. The discovery of cell-surface receptors that bind to various extracellular matrix proteins has greatly advanced the understanding of mechanotransduction mechanisms. For example, the integrin family of transmembrane proteins clusters at focal adhesion sites and binds to a specific sequence, arg-gly-asp (RGD), that is common in many extracellular matrix proteins.[60] The intracellular domains of these receptors are mechanically linked to fibrillar-actin bundles via various cytoskeletal-associated proteins (e.g., talin, vinculin, paxillin) and are associated with certain protein kinases.[60] Because actin bundles are a major component of the intracellular structural scaffolding, it is clear that the intracellular and extracellular structural components are mechanically coupled, via extracellular matrix receptors, to form a structural continuum (Fig. 78-5). It is via these physical couplings that mechanical forces can be detected and translated into intracellular chemical signals.[57,60,61] Although the intracellular signaling pathways are less well defined, they likely include stretch-activated ion channels, activation of intracellular second-messenger systems, and the direct activation of RNA polymerases and DNA synthetic enzymes via changes in nuclear shape.

It is possible that increased expansion of the fetal lung stimulates the synthesis and release of specific growth factors that act locally, in a paracrine manner, to stimulate cellular proliferation in the expanded tissue. The fetal lung produces numerous growth factors, including platelet-derived growth factor, vascular endothelial growth factor, IGF-II, keratinocyte growth factor, and transforming growth factor-β_1. Although IGF-II expression is increased after 7 days of increased lung expansion,[26] it is important to know whether the expression of IGF-II (as well as the other growth factors) parallels the increase in DNA synthesis rates; DNA synthesis is maximal at 2 days of tracheal obstruction[34] and then declines to control values by 10 days (Fig. 78-6). Similarly, it is important to understand how the expression of specific growth factor receptors changes in response to an

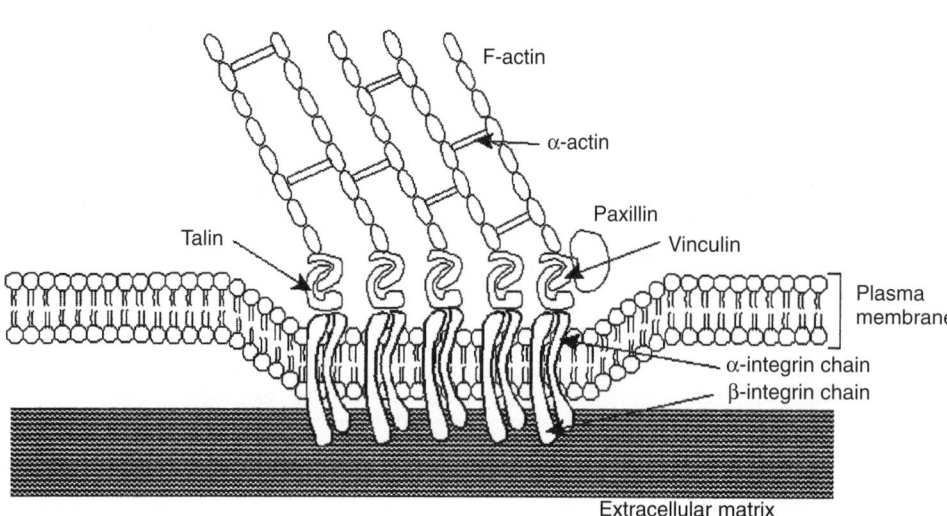

Figure 78–5. A schematic diagram demonstrating how the extracellular matrix receptors (integrins) mechanically couple the intracellular microfilaments with the extracellular matrix to form a structural continuum. Proteins associated with the intracellular domain are associated with numerous intracellular signaling pathways that may mediate the response to alterations in fetal lung expansion. (Data from Ingber D, et al: *In* Fransas JA (ed): Physical Forces and the Mammalian Cell. San Diego, Academic Press, 1993, p 61; and Rubin K, et al: *In* Comper WD (ed): Extracellular Matrix. Amsterdam, Harwood Academic Publishers, 1997, p 262.)

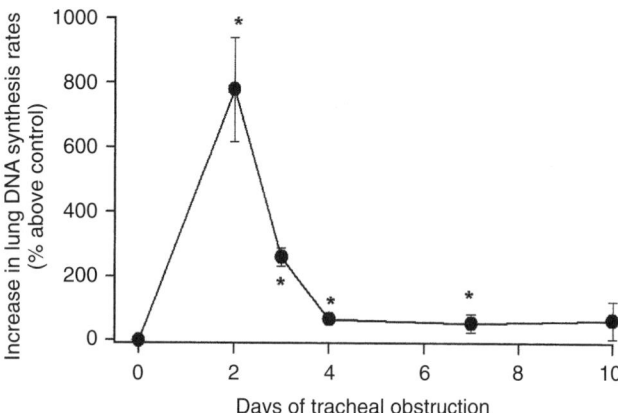

Figure 78–6. Time course for the increase in DNA synthesis rates in the fetal lung during sustained obstruction of the fetal trachea. Peak DNA synthesis rates occur at approximately 2 days of tracheal obstruction, a finding indicating that the mechanisms responsible for the increase in cellular proliferation are most active at this time.

increase in fetal lung expansion or whether the release of extracellularly bound growth factors is involved. Indeed, the fetal lung undergoes marked structural remodeling in response to a sustained increase in lung expansion, which may lead to the liberation of growth factors bound to the extracellular matrix. This is supported by the finding that the replacement of lung liquid with saline reduces the lung growth response to tracheal obstruction, indicating that growth promoting factors may be released into lung liquid,[62] although this has not specifically been examined.

PHYSICAL CAUSES OF FETAL LUNG HYPOPLASIA

By definition, *lung hypoplasia* refers to a significant reduction in lung weight or cellular content that affects lung function. Various seemingly diverse disorders of pregnancy result in pulmonary hypoplasia during fetal development. These include the following: oligohydramnios, a significant reduction in the volume of amniotic fluid; congenital diaphragmatic hernia (CDH); thoracic space-occupying lesions such as pulmonary cysts, tumors, and pleural effusions; and numerous fetal musculoskeletal deformities. It is now apparent that these disorders share a common mechanism by which they induce fetal lung hypoplasia,[23] namely, a prolonged reduction in the degree of fetal lung expansion.

Oligohydramnios

Oligohydramnios occurs in approximately 10% of all pregnancies and is usually caused by premature rupture of the fetal membranes. Another cause is inadequate production of fetal urine resulting from fetal urinary tract disorders including bilateral renal agenesis, renal dysplasia, and agenesis or stenosis of the ureters, urethra, or urethral valve.[23] The severity of the lung growth deficit depends on numerous factors, particularly the gestational age at onset and the duration of oligohydramnios.[63] In its most severe form, pulmonary hypoplasia is lethal within hours of birth, but it can be subclinical and undetected during the neonatal period in less severe forms. The likely physiologic mechanism by which oligohydramnios causes pulmonary hypoplasia is a reduction in fetal lung expansion.[14, 15] In the absence of amniotic fluid, the intrauterine space available to the fetus is reduced; the uterus compresses the fetus and causes increased flexion of the fetal spine between the thoracic and lumbar segments (see Fig. 78-4).[14,23] This leads to an increase in abdominal pressure, elevation of the diaphragm, compression of the lungs, and the loss of lung liquid (see Fig. 78-4);[14] the rate of lung liquid loss is increased during non–labor-related uterine contractions, which further increase the degree of fetal spinal flexion. The degree of compression imposed by the uterus can be so severe that it causes marked facial and limb disorders.[64]

Congenital Diaphragmatic Hernias

CDH is less common than oligohydramnios and is often associated with other anomalies, but it usually results in severe, often fatal, pulmonary hypoplasia. The mortality rates associated with this disorder vary widely among studies, arguably because of the inclusion or exclusion of subjects, but these rates are usually reported as greater than 50%.[65,66] CDH is a result of failure of the embryonic diaphragm to close (at ~12 weeks of gestation), thus allowing abdominal contents to migrate into the thorax; in the most severe form of CDH, the liver can also herniate into the chest.[67] The hernias can either be unilateral (both left-sided and right-sided) or bilateral, causing the lung chronically to collapse on the affected side. Owing to the perforated thoracic compartment (which allows unimpeded lung recoil), the lung on the side of the hernia is unable to expand, thus causing lung growth to fail. In addition, the abdominal contents may also compress the contralateral lung, as well as the ipsilateral lung, owing to a shift in the mediastinal ligament. Because the defect occurs early in fetal life, it usually results in severe pulmonary hypoplasia and causes major alterations in airway structure and function.

Musculoskeletal Disorders

Various musculoskeletal disorders in the fetus also result in severe pulmonary hypoplasia,[23] and although the precise mechanisms depend on the type of disorder, they likely involve a prolonged reduction in lung expansion. Any disorder that chronically reduces the ability of the fetus to defend its lung volume (see earlier) will likely result in pulmonary hypoplasia. Because the the diaphragm and glottic adductor muscles play crucial roles in maintaining fetal lung expansion,[14] interference with their activities would be expected to affect fetal lung growth.

EFFECTS OF CORTICOSTEROIDS ON FETAL LUNG GROWTH AND DEVELOPMENT

During development, the fetal lung is naturally exposed to corticosteroids of maternal and fetal origin, particularly during late gestation and under conditions of fetal distress. Much attention has focused on the role of corticosteroids in fetal lung development, owing to their therapeutic value in enhancing lung maturity, although their precise effects on lung development *in vivo* are still unclear. In the fetal lung, it is well established that elevated circulating corticosteroid levels have important effects on (1) structural development of the lung, (2) the surfactant system, and (3) the reabsorption of lung liquid. Other suggested effects of corticosteroids include a reduction in lung tissue growth and a stimulation of Type II AEC differentiation, although these latter effects are the subject of debate. Here, we focus on the role of cortisol in lung growth and structural maturation.

It is often assumed that corticosteroids induce lung maturation at the expense of lung growth, but the *in vivo* data are contradictory and are likely a reflection of species differences as well as differences in dose, number of doses used, and route of administration. Most studies have used synthetic glucocorticoids (betamethasone or dexamethasone), which have a 30- to 40-fold greater bioactivity than cortisol. When administered to the mother, betamethasone[68,69] causes a decrease in both fetal body and lung growth[70,71]; this effect increases with increasing number of doses. However, when it is administered directly to the fetus, a greater dose of betamethasone does not affect fetal body or lung growth.[72] Similarly, physiologic doses of cortisol, infused directly into the fetus to simulate the preparturient increase in fetal plasma cortisol levels, induce structural maturation of the lung without affecting either fetal lung or body growth.[73,74] These data suggest that the effect of maternally administered betamethasone on fetal body and lung growth is dose dependent or mediated via an effect on the placenta.

The removal or abolition of the endogenous source of corticosteroids in the fetus has also led to conflicting results on fetal lung growth. Adrenalectomy[75] and hypophysectomy[76] in fetal sheep significantly reduce lung weight, resulting from a reduction in protein content, rather than a reduction in DNA

content.[75] This finding indicates that endogenous cortisol may contribute to lung growth, particularly protein accumulation, late in gestation. In contrast, knock-out of the corticotropin-releasing hormone (CRH) gene in mice increases fetal lung DNA content and rates of cellular proliferation, particularly in epithelial cells,[77] a finding suggesting that endogenous corticosteroids may suppress pulmonary cell proliferation in late gestation. However, adrenalectomy and hypophysectomy only abolish the endogenous surge of cortisol near term because the transplacental flux of cortisol from the maternal compartment sustains low circulating levels in these fetuses.[75] Similarly, only -/- CRH knock-out mice fetuses from -/- mothers are glucocorticoid deficient and, as a result, die at birth as a result of respiratory insufficiency. In contrast, -/- CRH knock-out fetuses from heterozygote +/- mothers survive birth, probably because of the transplacental transfer of corticosteroids from the +/- mothers.[78] Thus, it appears that the survival of newborn mice at birth is not dependent on exposure to the preparturient increase in circulating corticosteroids, as it is in humans and sheep, although some circulating corticosteroids are required. These data reveal the conflicting nature of the reported roles for endogenous corticosteroids in regulating fetal lung development. Data on lung growth from glucocorticoid receptor (GR) knock-out fetal mice may help to resolve some of these issues.

One of the principal effects of corticosteroids on lung development is altered architecture, resulting in improved lung mechanics after birth.[79] In particular, both natural and synthetic corticosteroids markedly reduce interalveolar wall thickness and lead to a reduction in percentage of tissue space, a reduction in cellularity (cell density per tissue volume), and a marked increase in potential air space volume; these changes would be expected to increase lung compliance. In contrast, adrenalectomy in fetal sheep, hypophysectomy in fetal pigs,[80] and knock-outs of both the GR and CRH increase interairway distances, decrease air space volumes, and increase cellularity, resulting in respiratory failure at birth, presumably owing to a reduction in lung compliance. Although this is arguably the major beneficial effect of corticosteroids on the developing lung, the mechanisms remain unknown in spite of intensive investigation.[79]

Corticosteroids can also affect alveolarization, although this effect may be dose or species dependent because betamethasone administered to rats has been shown to arrest alveolarization,[81,82] whereas physiologic doses of cortisol administered to fetal sheep increase alveolar number (R. Boland and S. Hooper, unpublished observations). In addition, the increase in lung compliance induced by corticosteroids interacts with the relationship between lung expansion and lung growth and causes an enhanced increase in lung growth after an increase in lung expansion.[74]

EFFECTS OF METABOLIC FACTORS ON FETAL LUNG GROWTH AND MATURATION

Impaired nutrient and oxygen delivery during fetal life can affect the developing lung. Studies of respiratory function in infants,[83,84] children,[85,86] and adults[87,88] suggest that lung development may be affected by intrauterine conditions that induce fetal growth restriction (FGR), and many animal studies have explored the relationship between reduced nutrient or oxygen availability and lung development.[89-91] A problem in interpreting such studies is that nutritional restriction or hypoxia can induce a range of endocrine changes that could in themselves affect lung development; such changes include elevated circulating levels of corticosteroids, catecholamines, and prostaglandins.[92,93] When examined separately, the effects of fetal hypoxemia differ from those of nutrient restriction. Prolonged hypoxemia in the absence of hypoglycemia leads to reduced DNA synthesis rates in ovine fetal lungs.[94] In rats, fetal hypoxia from early in gestation caused the lungs to be small relative to body weight;[95] however, hypoxia later in gestation did not appear to affect fetal lung growth.[95,96]

Impaired nutrition during early life can influence alveolar formation; for example, in rats, in which alveolar formation occurs largely after birth,[97] intermittent starvation soon after birth caused enlarged alveoli, thicker septa, and a reduction in elastin deposition.[98] In sheep, hypoxemia and nutritional restriction during late gestation (coinciding with pulmonary saccular and alveolar formation)[99,100] led to a reduced number of alveoli per respiratory unit and thicker alveolar septa after birth.[101] Thus, it appears that adequate nutrition is necessary for normal alveolar formation; similar findings have been made in undernourished postnatal rats[98] and in guinea pigs undernourished during late gestation and in early neonatal life.[102] The potential causes of impaired alveolar formation in the presence of FGR include hypoxemia, hypoglycemia, and increased circulating glucocorticoid concentrations.[92] Furthermore, glucose transport to the lungs of growth-restricted fetal rats is reduced,[103] and this could decrease metabolic activity within lung cells.

The alveolar blood-air barrier can also be affected by undernutrition during fetal life. FGR in late gestation increases the blood-air barrier thickness in fetal sheep, relative to controls, and this effect persisted for at least 2 years after birth.[104] In guinea pig offspring subjected to maternal undernutrition during pregnancy, the alveolar surface area was reduced, leading to a reduced diffusing capacity. Although this effect was related to the smaller body size,[102] a smaller surface area was still apparent at 126 days after birth in spite of catch-up growth in body weight and lung volume.

Structural elements of the lung, such as elastic fibers, collagens, proteoglycans, and basement membrane proteins are laid down during early lung development and may be affected by nutritional status. Elastin is necessary for airway and alveolar development and affects lung compliance.[105] Tropoelastin is expressed principally by fibroblasts, particularly during alveolar formation.[106-108] Owing to the long half-life of elastin,[109] alterations in elastin deposition may exert persistent effects on the mechanical properties of the lung. It is now apparent that nutritional factors can affect elastin deposition; for example, in growing rats, protein restriction sufficient to restrict growth caused a loss of lung desmosine and an increase in alveolar dimensions.[92,110] In humans, elastin accumulates in the lungs between 25 weeks of gestation and 15 weeks after birth, and it is apparent that this accumulation is not significantly affected by FGR.[111] Similarly, pulmonary tropoelastin expression and elastin content were not altered in fetal sheep subjected to late-gestational FGR.[112] During fetal and postnatal life, both hypoxia and fetal undernutrition may be associated with increased levels of corticosteroids[113]; these may affect elastin synthesis because it has been shown that exogenous corticosteroids can both increase[108] and decrease[114] elastin formation in the fetal lungs. Elastin deposition in the lung may also be affected by hypoxia because hypoxia down-regulates tropoelastin gene expression[115] in pulmonary fibroblasts and tropoelastin synthesis in pulmonary artery smooth muscle cells.[116] Paradoxically, hypoxia (12 to 13% oxygen) also increases pulmonary lysyl oxidase activity, the extracellular enzyme responsible for cross-linking elastin and collagen.[117,118] However, an inhibitory effect of hypoxia on elastin synthesis was not observed in growing rats.[119]

Collagens, which are produced within the lung by fibroblasts and other cell types, provide the lung with mechanical strength.[120] In contrast to elastin, lung collagen is synthesized and degraded throughout life,[120] and it is well established that collagen metabolism is affected by nutritional status.[121] Lung collagen content was significantly reduced in postnatal rats fed a low-protein diet.[110,122] Collagen IV is a major component of base-ment membranes, and therefore it affects the strength and function of the blood-air barrier.[123] It is of interest that procollagen gene expression in lung fibroblasts is increased by hypoxia,[124] which is a feature of FGR.

Proteoglycans are a major component of lung extracellular matrix, yet no data apparently exist on the influence of impaired nutrition or oxygenation on proteoglycan synthesis in the developing lung. In vascular tissue, hypoxia has been shown to decrease proteoglycan production by bovine pulmonary artery endothelial cells[125] and by human aortic smooth muscle cells.[126]

Development of pulmonary surfactant is also affected by nutritional factors. Undernutrition of pregnant rats results in impaired surface tension–lowering properties of fetal lung extracts[127]; the maturation of Type II AECs in these offspring is also delayed because their glycogen content increases and the volume density of lamellar bodies decreases.[128] Prolonged periods of fetal hypoxia, induced by placental restriction, also increase surfactant protein-A and surfactant protein-B (SP-A and SP-B) expression at 0.88 of gestation[129] but not near term.[130] This finding suggests that FGR or nutrient restriction may have beneficial effects on lung maturity in preterm infants, but not in those born at term. The effects of undernutrition and hypoxia on Type II cells are likely to differ according to gestational timing and alterations in cortisol levels.

Certain micronutrients are now know to be essential for normal lung development. Vitamin A (retinol) and retinoic acid play important roles early in lung development, during embryogenesis and organogenesis. Retinoic acid appears to be the most active of the retinoids[131] and affects many aspects of lung development including early airway branching, alveolar formation, and the synthesis of surfactant and surfactant proteins.[132] For example, vitamin A deficiency during gestation reduces the expression of surfactant proteins A, B, and C in fetal rat lungs.[133] Considerable interest has been directed toward understanding the effects of retinoic acid on alveolar formation and surfactant synthesis. This effect must include elastogenesis because inhibitors of retinoid metabolism decrease tropoelastin expression in fetal rat lung explants,[134] and vitamin A deficiency during pregnancy reduces elastin staining in fetal rat lungs.[135] There is some evidence that a reduction in alveolar formation during early development may be reversible, because treatment with retinoic acid is able to increase alveolar numbers, at least in rats and mice.[136,137]

Vitamin D can affect the developing lung, possibly via binding sites on Type II AECs[138]; it can advance maturation of Type II cells as indicated by a reduction in glycogen content and increased surfactant synthesis.[139] Selenium is also important because it is necessary for the activity of glutathione peroxidase, an important antioxidant defense enzyme. Selenium deficiency in rats led to altered lung development, particularly alveolar septation.[140]

POTENTIAL TREATMENTS FOR LUNG GROWTH DISORDERS

Fetal Treatments

It is clear that fetal lung development is a consequence of a complex interaction of various mechanical, endocrine, and metabolic factors. The challenge is to translate this knowledge into therapeutic treatments that will improve the outcome for both preterm infants and newborn infants who have hypoplastic lungs. The finding that increased fetal lung expansion is a potent stimulus for fetal lung growth and structural maturation has prompted the suggestion that it may be used as an *in utero* therapeutic treatment for fetuses with severely hypoplastic lungs. Indeed, experimental studies have shown that increases in fetal lung expansion induced by tracheal obstruction can rapidly reverse fetal lung growth deficits *in utero*[25,141-143] and can restore respiratory function postnatally in conditions that would otherwise be fatal.[144] However, clinical trials in human fetuses with severe pulmonary hypoplasia resulting from CDH have had mixed success, although some marginal improvements in outcomes have been reported.[145] The major problems relate to preterm labor, failure to stimulate fetal lung growth in some cases, and postnatal respiratory insufficiency in other cases, despite induced lung growth.[145] Thus, a significant discrepancy exists between the results obtained from clinical trials and those obtained from animal experiments. Although the reasons for these discrepancies are unknown, they may relate to the stage of lung development at which the treatment was applied, the duration of the tracheal obstruction, and the severity of the fetal lung hypoplasia. For example, most tracheal obstruction procedures in humans have been carried out at less than 28 weeks of gestation, when the lungs are at the early to mid-canalicular stage of development.[145-148] However, when tracheal obstruction is performed at this stage of lung development in fetal sheep, the induced lung growth is abnormal, causing marked mesenchymal cell proliferation and increased interairway distances.[36] Similarly, sustained increases in fetal lung expansion can severely reduce the numbers of Type II AECs[40] and surfactant protein gene expression.[149-152] Although this reduction in Type II AECs[30] and surfactant protein gene expression is reversible, it is dependent on being able to release the obstruction before birth,[149,153] so the fetus will spend sufficient time *in utero* for the AECs to transdifferentiate and reestablish near-normal proportions. Thus, inappropriate growth and reduced Type II cell numbers may help to explain why infants subjected to prolonged tracheal obstruction *in utero* can suffer respiratory insufficiency after birth, despite having a normal or larger lung.

The failure to stimulate lung growth by tracheal obstruction in human fetuses with CDH may also be explained by the inability of fetal lung liquid secretion to expand the fetal lungs. Because the severely hypoplastic fetal lung is highly noncompliant, compared with a normally grown lung, it is more difficult to expand. Thus, if the internal distending pressure required to expand it is greater than the osmotic pressure driving lung liquid secretion, which is only approximately 4 to 5 mm Hg,[34] the lung will not expand, despite the trachea's being occluded. Because ongoing lung liquid secretion and increased lung expansion are requirements for accelerated fetal lung growth,[34,74] without continued lung liquid secretion, the mechanical mechanism that induces the growth response will not be activated.[154]

Another complication associated with tracheal obstruction for the correction of CDH in fetal humans is the development of fetal hydrops.[146,154] This phenomenon has also been observed in fetal sheep,[36] but only when the tracheal obstruction is performed during the pseudoglandular/canalicular stages of lung development; it does not occur during the alveolar stage. The hydrops is thought to result from the greater increase in lung expansion and lung growth that occurs in the immature fetus; this is thought to result from an immature chest wall that allows the lungs eventually to expand to a much greater degree.[36] The resultant hydrops that occurs in immature fetuses is likely caused by restricted venous return or by the expanded lungs constraining the heart. Taken together, these data indicate that if tracheal obstruction is to be used successfully to stimulate lung growth in fetal humans, (1) the obstruction is better performed later in gestation, (2) the obstruction needs to be reversible, and (3) it may be beneficial to improve lung compliance, by the use of corticosteroids, before the onset of obstruction.

Potential Postnatal Treatments

The mechanisms controlling lung growth in the early neonatal period, particularly in infants with pulmonary hypoplasia, is not well known or understood. It is possible that lung expansion is an important determinant, as it is before birth, although the mechanical forces exerted on the air-filled lung are considerably more complex, particularly in the ventilated neonate. Nevertheless, continuous positive airway pressure, which would be expected to increase the basal degree lung expansion by increasing end-expiratory lung volumes, has been shown to enhance lung growth in growing ferrets.[155] Similarly, the compensatory lung growth induced by partial resection of the air-filled lung after birth is thought to be expansion dependent.[156] Combined, these findings indicate that lung growth after birth is, at least partially, regulated by the basal degree of lung expansion. Consequently, because positive end-expiratory pressures are commonly used in neonatal intensive care units to enhance oxygenation and to prevent lung collapse and injury in preterm infants and infants with pulmonary hypoplasia, it is likely that this approach will have the added beneficial effect of enhancing postnatal lung growth. However, a potential complication of increasing end expiratory lung volumes in ventilated infants is an alteration in the proportion of AECs leading to a reduction in the number of Type II AECs, although this effect has not been verified in experimental animals.

SUMMARY

Growth and structural maturation of the fetal lung result from a complex interaction of physical, endocrine, and metabolic factors. The physical expansion of the fetal lung appears to be crucial for normal lung development; during the later stages of gestation, the basal level of lung expansion becomes significantly greater than the resting or end-expiratory lung volumes in the air-breathing newborn. This high degree of fetal lung expansion is actively maintained, and it depends on fetal diaphragmatic and glottic activity, and therefore factors that reduce or inhibit these muscular activities result in a reduction in fetal lung expansion. A reduction in lung expansion is now recognized as underlying various disorders resulting in pulmonary hypoplasia in human infants. Although the mechanisms by which alterations in fetal lung expansion accelerate or retard the growth and development of the lung are largely unknown, they are vital areas of research that may have substantial clinical benefits.

REFERENCES

1. Strang LB: Fetal lung liquid: secretion and reabsorption. Physiol Rev 1991;71:991.
2. Harding R, Hooper SB: Regulation of lung expansion and lung growth before birth. J Appl Physiol 1996;81:209.
3. Alcorn D, et al: Morphological effects of chronic tracheal ligation and drainage in the fetal lamb lung. J Anat 1977;123:649.
4. Hooper SB, Harding R: Fetal lung liquid: a major determinant of the growth and functional development of the fetal lung. Clin Exp Pharmacol Physiol 1995;22:235.
5. Olver RE, Strang LB: Ion fluxes across the pulmonary epithelium and the secretion of lung liquid in the foetal lamb. J Physiol (Lond) 1974;241:327.
6. Harding R, et al: The regulation of flow of pulmonary fluid in fetal sheep. Respir Physiol 1984;57:47.
7. Wickham PJD, Harding R: Flowmeter for slow-flowing physiological liquids. Med Biol Eng Comput 1984;22:406.
8. Lines A, et al: Lung liquid production rates and volumes do not decrease before labor in healthy fetal sheep. J Appl Physiol 1997;82:927.
9. Cassin S, Perks AM: Estimation of lung liquid production in fetal sheep with blue dye dextran and radioiodinated serum albumin. J Appl Physiol 2002;92:1531.
10. Pfister RE, et al: Volume and secretion rate of lung liquid in the final days of gestation and labour in the fetal sheep. J Physiol (Lond) 2001;535:889.
11. Davey MG, et al: Postnatal development of respiratory function in lambs studied serially between birth and 8 weeks. Respir Physiol 1998;113:83.
12. Miller AA, et al: Role of fetal breathing movements in control of fetal lung distension. J Appl Physiol 1993;75:2711.
13. Harding R, et al: Abolition of fetal breathing movements by spinal cord transection leads to reductions in fetal lung liquid volume, lung growth and IGF-II gene expression. Pediatr Res 1993;34:148.

14. Harding R, et al: A mechanism leading to reduced lung expansion and lung hypoplasia in fetal sheep during oligohydramnios. Am J Obstet Gynecol 1990;163:1904.

15. Dickson KA, Harding R: Decline in lung liquid volume and secretion rate during oligohydramnios in fetal sheep. J Appl Physiol 1989;67:2401.

16. Hooper SB, et al: Lung liquid secretion, flow and volume in response to moderate asphyxia in fetal sheep . J Dev Physiol 1988;10:473.

17. Dickson KA, Harding R: Restoration of lung liquid volume following its acute alteration in fetal sheep. J Physiol (Lond) 1987;385:531.

18. Harding R, et al: Influence of upper respiratory tract on liquid flow to and from fetal lungs. J Appl Physiol 1986;61:68.

19. Harding R, et al: Upper airway resistances in fetal sheep: the influence of breathing activity. J Appl Physiol 1986;60:160.

20. Vilos GA, Liggins GC: Intrathoracic pressures in fetal sheep. J Dev Physiol 1982;4:247.

21. Dickson KA, et al: State-related changes in lung liquid secretion and tracheal flow rate in fetal lambs. J Appl Physiol 1987;62:34.

22. Adamson TM, et al: Composition of alveolar liquid in the foetal lamb. J Physiol (Lond) 1969;204:159.

23. Harding R, Albuquerque CA: Pulmonary hypoplasia: role of mechanical factors in prenatal lung growth. In Gaultier C, et al (eds): Lung Development. Oxford, Oxford University Press, 1999, p 364.

24. Moessinger AC, et al: Role of lung fluid volume in growth and maturation of the fetal sheep lung. J Clin Invest 1990;86:1270.

25. Nardo L, et al: Lung hypoplasia can be reversed by short-term obstruction of the trachea in fetal sheep. Pediatr Res 1995;38:690.

26. Hooper SB, et al: Changes in lung expansion alter pulmonary DNA synthesis and IGF-II gene expression in fetal sheep. Am J Physiol 1993;265:L403.

27. Davey MG, et al: Stimulation of lung growth in fetuses with lung hypoplasia leads to altered postnatal lung structure in sheep. Pediatr Pulmonol 2001;32:267.

28. Joyce BJ, et al: Sustained changes in lung expansion alter tropoelastin mRNA levels and elastin content in fetal sheep lungs. Am J Physiol 2003;284:L643.

29. DiFiore JW, et al: Experimental fetal tracheal ligation and congenital diaphragmatic hernia: a pulmonary vascular morphometric analysis. J Pediatr Surg 1995;30:917.

30. Flecknoe SJ, et al: Determination of alveolar epithelial cell phenotypes in fetal sheep: evidence for the involvement of basal lung expansion. J Physiol (Lond) 2002;542:245.

31. Danto SI, et al: Reversible transdifferentiation of alveolar epithelial cells. Am J Respir Cell Mol Biol 1995;12:497.

32. Shannon JM, et al: Modulation of alveolar type II cell differentiated function in vitro. Am J Physiol 1992;262:L427.

33. Nardo L, et al: Changes in lung structure and cellular division induced by tracheal obstruction in fetal sheep. Exp Lung Res 2000;26:105.

34. Nardo L, et al: Stimulation of lung growth by tracheal obstruction in fetal sheep: relation to luminal pressure and lung liquid volume. Pediatr Res 1998;43:184.

35. Keramidaris E, et al: Effect of gestational age on the increase in fetal lung growth following tracheal obstruction. Exp Lung Res 1996;22:283.

36. Probyn ME, et al: Effect of increased lung expansion on lung growth and development near midgestation in fetal sheep. Pediatr Res 2000;47:806.

37. De Paepe ME, et al: Temporal pattern of accelerated lung growth after tracheal occlusion in the fetal rabbit. Am J Pathol 1998;152:179.

38. De Paepe ME, et al: Lung growth response after tracheal occlusion in fetal rabbits is gestational age-dependent. Am J Respir Cell Mol Biol 1999;21:65.

39. Kitano Y, et al: Tracheal occlusion in the fetal rat: a new experimental model for the study of accelerated lung growth. J Pediatr Surg 1998;33:1741.

40. Flecknoe S, et al: Increased lung expansion alters the proportions of type I and type II alveolar epithelial cells in fetal sheep. Am J Physiol 2000;278:L1180.

41. Dawes GS, et al: Breathing in fetal lambs: the effect of brain stem section. J Physiol (Lond) 1983;335:535.

42. Dawes GS: Fetal breathing movements and sleep in sheep. Ann Rech Vet 1977;8:413.

43. Harding R: Fetal breathing movements. In Crystal RG, et al. (eds): The Lung: Scientific Foundations, 2nd ed. Philadelphia, Lippincott–Raven, 1997, p 1655.

44. Dawes GS, et al: Respiratory movements and rapid eye movement sleep in the foetal lamb. J Physiol (Lond) 1972;220:119.

45. Maloney JE, et al: Diaphragmatic activity and lung liquid flow in the unanesthetized fetal sheep. J Appl Physiol 1975;39:423.

46. Badalian SS, et al: Fetal breathing-related nasal fluid flow velocity in uncomplicated pregnancies. Am J Obstet Gynecol 1993;169:563.

47. Kalache KD, et al: Differentiation between human fetal breathing patterns by investigation of breathing-related tracheal fluid flow velocity using Doppler sonography. Prenat Diagn 2000;20:45.

48. Moessinger AC: Fetal akinesia deformation sequence: an animal model. Pediatrics 1983;7:857.

49. Fewell JE, et al: Effects of phrenic nerve section on the respiratory system of fetal lambs. J Appl Physiol 1981;51:293.

50. Alcorn D, et al: Morphological effects of chronic bilateral phrenectomy or vagotomy / the fetal lamb lung. J Anat 1980;130:683.

51. Liggins GC, et al: The effect of spinal cord transection on lung development in fetal sheep. J Dev Physiol 1981;3:267.

52. Wigglesworth JS, Desai R: Effects on lung growth of cervical cord section in the rabbit fetus. Early Hum Dev 1979;3:51.

53. Liggins GC, et al: The effect of bilateral thoracoplasty on lung development in fetal sheep. J Dev Physiol 1981;3:275.

54. Liu M, et al: Mechanical strain-enhanced fetal lung cell proliferation is mediated by phospholipase C and D and protein kinase C. Am J Physiol 1995;268:L729.

55. Harding R, Liggins GC: Changes in thoracic dimensions induced by breathing movements in fetal sheep. Reprod Fertil Dev 1996;8:117.

56. Chicurel ME, et al: Cellular control lies in the balance of forces. Curr Opin Cell Biol 1998;10:232.

57. Ingber D, et al: Mechanochemical transduction across extracellular matrix and through the cytoskeleton. In Fransas JA (ed): Physical Forces and the Mammalian Cell. San Diego, Academic Press, 1993, p 61.

58. Wirtz HR, Dobbs LG: The effects of mechanical forces on lung functions. Respir Physiol 2000;119:1.

59. Sims JR, et al: Altering the cellular mechanical force balance results in integrated changes in cell, cytoskeletal and nuclear shape. J Cell Sci 1992;103:1215.

60. Rubin K, et al: Molecular recognition of the extracellular matrix by cell surface receptors. In Comper WD (ed): Extracellular Matrix. Amsterdam, Harwood Academic Publishers, 1997, p 262.

61. Ingber DE: The riddle of morphogenesis: a question of solution chemistry or molecular cell engineering. Cell 1993;75:1249.

62. Papadakis K, et al: Fetal lung growth after tracheal ligation is not solely a pressure phenomenon. J Pediatr Surg 1997;32:347.

63. Moessinger AC, et al: Oligohydramnios-induced lung hypoplasia: the influence of timing and duration in gestation. Pediatr Res 1986;20:951.

64. Thomas IT, Smith DW: Oligohydramnios, cause of the nonrenal features of Potter's syndrome, including pulmonary hypoplasia. J Pediatr 1974;84:811.

65. Adzick NS, et al: Diaphragmatic hernia in the fetus: prenatal diagnosis and outcome in 94 cases. J Pediatr Surg 1985;20:357.

66. Adzick NS, et al: Fetal diaphragmatic hernia: ultrasound diagnosis and clinical outcome in 38 cases. J Pediatr Surg 1989;24:654.

67. Harrison MR, et al: Correction of congenital diaphragmatic hernia in utero. V. Initial clinical experience. J Pediatr Surg 1990;25:47.

68. French NP, et al: Repeated antenatal corticosteroids: size at birth and subsequent development. Am J Obstet Gynecol 1999;180:114.

69. Ikegami M, et al: Repetitive prenatal glucocorticoids improve lung function and decrease growth in preterm lambs. Am J Respir Crit Care Med 1997;156:178.

70. Schellenberg J-C, et al: Growth, elastin concentration, and collagen concentration of perinatal rat lung: effects of dexamethasone. Pediatr Res 1987;21:603.

71. Adamson IY, King GM: Postnatal development of rat lung following retarded fetal lung growth. Pediatr Pulmonol 1988;4:230.

72. Jobe AH, et al: Fetal versus maternal and gestational age effects of repetitive antenatal glucocorticoids. Pediatrics 1998;102:1116.

73. Wallace MJ, et al: Effects of elevated fetal cortisol concentrations on the volume, secretion and reabsorption of lung liquid. Am J Physiol 1995; 269:R881.

74. Boland RE, et al: Cortisol pretreatment enhances the lung growth response to tracheal obstruction in fetal sheep. Am J Physiol 1997;273:L1126–L1131.

75. Wallace MJ, et al: Role of the adrenal glands in the maturation of lung liquid secretory mechanisms in fetal sheep. Am J Physiol 1996;270 : R1.

76. Deayton JM, et al: Early hypophysectomy of sheep fetuses: effects on growth, placental steroidogenesis and prostaglandin production. J Reprod Fertil 1993;97:513.

77. Muglia LJ, et al: Proliferation and differentiation defects during lung development in corticotropin-releasing hormone-deficient mice. Am J Respir Cell Mol Biol 1999;20:181.

78. Muglia L, et al: Corticotropin-releasing hormone deficiency reveals major fetal but not adult glucocortoid need. Nature 1995;373:427.

79. Jobe AH, Ikegami M: Lung development and function in preterm infants in the surfactant treatment era. Annu Rev Physiol 2000;62:825.

80. Pinkerton KE, et al: Hypophysectomy and porcine fetal lung development. Am J Respir Cell Mol Biol 1989;1:319.

81. Johnson JW, et al: Long-term effects of betamethasone on fetal development. Am J Obstet Gynecol 1981;141:1053.

82. Massaro GD, Massaro D: Retinoic acid treatment partially rescues failed septation in rats and in mice. Am J Physiol 2000;278:L955.

83. Lum S, et al: The association between birthweight, sex, and airway function in infants of nonsmoking mothers. Am J Respir Crit Care Med 2001; 164:2078.

84. Tyson JE, et al: The small for gestational age infant: accelerated or delayed pulmonary maturation? Increased or decreased survival? Pediatrics 1995;95:534.

85. Nikolajev K, et al: Effects of intrauterine growth retardation and prematurity on spirometric flow values and lung volumes at school age in twin pairs. Pediatr Pulmonol 1998;25:367.

86. Rona RJ, et al: Effects of prematurity and intrauterine growth on respiratory health and lung function in childhood. BMJ 1993;306:817.

87. Barker DJP, et al: Relation of birth weight and childhood respiratory infection to adult lung function and death from chronic obstructive airways disease. BMJ 1991;303:671.

88. Stein CE, et al: Relation of fetal growth to adult lung function in south India. Thorax 1997;52:895.

89. Edelman NH, et al: Nutrition and the respiratory system: Chronic obstructive pulmonary disease (COPD). Am Rev Respir Dis 1986;134:347.

90. Gaultier C: Malnutrition and lung growth. Pediatr Pulmonol 1991;10:278.

91. Sahebjami H: Nutrition and lung structure and function. Exp Lung Res 1993;19:105.

92. Gagnon R, et al: Fetal endocrine responses to chronic placental embolization in the late-gestation ovine fetus. Am J Obstet Gynecol 1994;170:929.

93. Gagnon R, et al: Fetal sheep endocrine responses to sustained hypoxemic stress after chronic fetal placental embolization. Am J Physiol 1997;272:E817.

94. Hooper SB, et al: DNA synthesis is reduced in selected fetal tissues during prolonged hypoxemia. Am J Physiol 2002;261:508.

95. Faridy EE, et al: Fetal lung growth: influence of maternal hypoxia and hyperoxia in rats. Respir Physiol 1988;73:225.

96. Larson JE, Thurlbeck WM: The effect of experimental maternal hypoxia on fetal lung growth. Pediatr Res 1988;24:156.

97. Massaro D, et al: Postnatal development of alveoli: regulation and evidence for a critical period in rats. Anat Rec 1974;180:77.

98. Das RM: The effects of intermittent starvation on lung development in suckling rats. Am J Pathol 1984;117:326.

99. Joyce BJ, et al: Compromised respiratory function in postnatal lambs following placental insufficiency and intrauterine growth restriction. Pediatr Res 2001;50:641.

100. Wignarajah D, et al: Influence of intra-uterine growth restriction on airway development in fetal and postnatal sheep. Pediatr Res 2002;51:681.

101. Maritz GS, et al: Effects of fetal growth restriction on lung development before and after birth: a morphometric analysis. Pediatr Pulmonol 2001;32:201.

102. Lechner AJ: Perinatal age determines the severity of retarded lung development induced by starvation. Am Rev Respir Dis 1985;131:638.

103. Simmons RA, et al: Intrauterine growth retardation: fetal glucose transport is diminished in lung but spared in brain. Pediatr Res 1992;31:59.

104. Maritz GS, et al: Altered lung structure persists until maturity following fetal growth restriction. Am J Respir Crit Care Med (in press).

105. Nardell EA, Brody JS: Determinants of mechanical properties of rat lung during postnatal development. J Appl Physiol 1982;53:140.

106. Shibahara S, et al: Modulation of tropoelastin production and elastin messenger ribonucleic acid activity in developing sheep lung. Biochemistry 1981;20:6577.

107. Pierce RA, et al: Elastin in lung development and disease. Ciba Found Symp 1995;192:199.

108. Pierce RA, et al: Glucocorticoids upregulate tropoelastin expression during late stages of fetal lung development. Am J Physiol 1995;268:L491.

109. Mecham RP: Elastic fibers. In Crystal RG, et al. (eds): The Lung: Scientific Foundations, 2nd ed. Philadelphia, Lippincott-Raven, 1997, p 729.

110. Matsui R, et al: Connective tissue, mechanical, and morphometric changes in the lungs of weanling rats fed a low protein diet. Pediatr Pulmonol 1989;7:L159.

111. Desai R, et al: Assessment of elastin maturation by radioimmunoassay of desmosine in the developing human lung. Early Hum Dev 1988;16:61.

112. Joyce BJ, et al: Tropoelastin expression and elastin content in fetal and postnatal lung following intra-uterine growth restriction. Am J Respir Crit Care Med 2002;164:A642.

113. Dwyer CM, Stickland NC: The effects of maternal undernutrition on maternal and fetal serum insulin-like growth factors, thyroid hormones and cortisol in the guinea pig. J Dev Physiol 1992;18:303.

114. Willet KE, et al: Lung morphometry and collagen and elastin content: changes during normal development and after prenatal hormone exposure in sheep. Pediatr Res 1999;45:615.

115. Berk JL, et al: Hypoxia downregulates tropoelastin gene expression in rat lung fibroblasts by pretranslational mechanisms. Am J Physiol 1999;277:L566.

116. Stenmark KR, et al: Cellular adaptation during chronic neonatal hypoxic pulmonary hypertension. Am J Physiol 1991;261:97.

117. Brody JS, et al: Lung lysyl oxidase activity: relation to lung growth. Am Rev Respir Dis 1979;120:L1289.

118. Brody JS, Vaccaro C: Postnatal formation of alveoli: interstitial events and physiologic consequences. Fed Proc 1979;38:215.

119. Sekhon HS, Thurlbeck WM: Lung growth in hypobaric normoxia, normo-baric hypoxia, and hypobaric hypoxia in growing rats. J Appl Physiol 1995;78:L124.

120. Chambers RC, Laurent GJ: The lung. In Comper WD (ed): Extracellular Matrix. Amsterdam, Harwood Academic Publishers, 1996, p 378.

121. Berg RA, Kerr JS: Nutritional aspects of collagen metabolism. Annu Rev Nutr 1992;12:369.

122. Myers BA, et al: Protein deficiency: effects on lung mechanics and the accumulation of collagen and elastin in rat lung. J Nutr 1983;113:2308.

123. West JB, Mathieu-Costello O: Structure, strength, failure, and remodeling of the pulmonary blood-gas barrier. Annu Rev Physiol 1999;61:543.

124. Zhao L, et al: Effect of hypoxia on proliferation and alpha 1(I) procollagen gene expression by human fetal lung fibroblasts. Chung Kuo I Hsueh Ko Yuan Hsueh Pao 1998;20:109.

125. Humphries DE, et al: Effects of hypoxia and hyperoxia on proteoglycan by bovine pulmonary artery endothelial cells. J Cell Physiol 1986;126:249.

126. Figueroa JE, et al: Effect of hypoxia and hypoxia/reoxygenation on proteoglycan metabolism by vascular smooth muscle cells. Atherosclerosis 1999;143:135.

127. Faridy EE: Effect of maternal malnutrition on surface activity of fetal lungs in rats. J Appl Physiol 1975;39:535.

128. Curle DC, Adamson IY: Retarded development of neonatal rat lung by maternal malnutrition. J Histochem Cytochem 1978;26:401.

129. Gagnon R, et al: Changes in surfactant-associated protein mRNA profile in growth-restricted fetal sheep. Am J Physiol 1999;276:L459.

130. Cock ML, et al: Effects of intrauterine growth restriction on lung liquid dynamics and lung development in fetal sheep. Am J Obstet Gynecol 2001;184:209.

131. Chytil F: Retinoids in lung development. FASEB J 1996;10:986.

132. Zachman RD: Role of vitamin A in lung development. J Nutr 1995;125:1634S.

133. Chailley-Heu B, et al: Mild vitamin A deficiency delays fetal lung maturation in the rat. Am J Respir Cell Mol Biol 1999;21:89.

134. McGowan SE, et al: Endogenous retinoids increase perinatal elastin gene expression in rat lung fibroblasts and fetal explants. Am J Physiol 1997;273:L410.

135. Antipatis C, et al: Effects of maternal vitamin A status on fetal heart and lung: changes in expression of key developmental genes. Am J Physiol 1998;275:L1184.

136. Massaro GD, Massaro D: Postnatal treatment with retinoic acid increases the number of pulmonary alveoli in rats. Am J Physiol 1996;270:L305.

137. Massaro GD, Massaro D: Retinoic acid treatment partially rescues failed septation in rats and mice. Am J Physiol 2000;278:L955.

138. Marin L, et al: 1,25(OH)2D3 stimulates phospholipid biosynthesis and surfactant release in fetal rat lung explants. Biol Neonate 1990;57:257.

139. Marin L, et al: Maturational changes induced by 1 alpha,25-dihydroxyvitamin D3 in type II cells from fetal rat lung explants. Am J Physiol 1993;265:L45.

140. Kim HY, et al: The role of selenium nutrition in the development of neonatal rat lung. Pediatr Res 1991;29:440.

141. Bealer JF, et al: The "PLUG" odyssey: adventures in experimental fetal tracheal occlusion. J Pediatr Surg 1995;30:361.

142. Hedrick MH, et al: Plug the lung until it grows (PLUG): a new method to treat congenital diaphragmatic hernia in utero. J Pediatr Surg 1994;29:612.

143. Kitano Y, et al: Fetal tracheal occlusion in the rat model of nitrofen-induced congenital diaphragmatic hernia. J Appl Physiol 1999;87:769.

144. Davey MG, et al: Respiratory function in lambs after in utero treatment of lung hypoplasia by tracheal obstruction. J Appl Physiol 1999;87:2296.

145. Flake AW, et al: Treatment of severe congenital diaphragmatic hernia by fetal tracheal occlusion: clinical experience with fifteen cases. Am J Obstet Gynecol 2000;183:1059.

146. Graf JL, et al: Fetal hydrops after in utero tracheal occlusion. J Pediatr Surg 1997;32:214.

147. Harrison MR, et al: Fetoscopic temporary tracheal occlusion by means of detachable balloon for congenital diaphragmatic hernia. Am J Obstet Gynecol 2001;185:730.

148. Vanderwall KJ, et al: Fetando-Clip: a fetal endoscopic tracheal clip procedure in a human fetus. J Pediatr Surg 1997;32:970.

149. Bin SW, et al: The effects of tracheal occlusion and release on type II pneumocytes in fetal lambs. J Pediatr Surg 1997;32:834.

150. Piedboeuf B, et al: Deleterious effect of tracheal obstruction on type 2 pneumocytes in fetal sheep. Pediatr Res 1997;41:473.

151. Lines A, et al: Alterations in lung expansion affect surfactant protein A, B, and C mRNA levels in fetal sheep. Am J Physiol 1999;276:L239.

152. Saddiq WB, et al: The effects of tracheal occlusion and release on type-II pneumocytes in fetal lambs. J Pediatr Surg 1997;32:834.

153. Lines A, et al: Re-expression of pulmonary surfactant proteins following tracheal obstruction in fetal sheep. Exp Physiol 2001;86:55.

154. Flake AW, et al: Treatment of severe congenital diaphragmatic hernia by fetal tracheal occlusion: clinical experience with fifteen cases. Am J Obstet Gynecol 2000;183:1059.

155. Zhang S, et al: Strain-induced growth of the immature lung. J Appl Physiol 1996;81:1471.

156. Rannels DE: Role of physical forces in compensatory growth of the lung. Am J Physiol 1989;257:L179.

Minke van Tuyl and Martin Post

79

Molecular Mechanisms of Lung Development and Lung Branching Morphogenesis

Lung development can be subdivided into five distinct stages (Table 79-1).[1] The early stages of lung development comprise the embryonic and pseudoglandular periods of lung development, after which the prospective conductive airways have been formed, and the acinar limits can be recognized. During the pseudoglandular period, the primitive airway epithelium starts to differentiate, and neuroendocrine, ciliated, and goblet cells appear, whereas mesenchymal cells have begun to form cartilage and smooth muscle cells. In the subsequent canalicular period, the airway branching pattern is completed, and the prospective gas exchange region starts to develop. During this period, respiratory bronchioli appear, interstitial tissue decreases, vascularization of peripheral mesenchyme increases, and distal cuboidal epithelium differentiates into Type I and Type II cells. In the saccular (terminal sac) period, growth of the pulmonary parenchyma, thinning of the connective tissue between the air spaces, and maturation of the surfactant system are the most important steps toward *ex utero* life. Although already functional, the lung is structurally still in an immature condition at birth. The air spaces present are smooth-walled transitory ducts and saccules with primitive septa that are thick and contain a double capillary network. During the alveolar period, alveoli are formed through a septation process that greatly increases the gas exchange surface area, and the capillaries fuse to form a single layer. A hallmark throughout lung development is the signaling between the epithelial and mesenchymal tissue layers. The combination and concentration of signals, depending on position and time in gestation, determine lung morphogenesis (branching, growth, and differentiation). Since the 1980s, molecular studies of lung development have started to shed light on the complex series of events that control proper formation of the lung. In this chapter, we summarize the current thoughts on the molecular mechanisms that determine lung pattern formation.

EARLY LUNG DEVELOPMENT

Lung development starts as an endodermal outgrowth of the ventral foregut around the fourth week of human development. This foregut mass rapidly elongates into a single tube dividing into a ventral esophagus and a dorsal trachea that, in turn, bifurcates into a right and a left primary lung bud. This process is modified in the mouse, in which the respiratory system develops from paired endodermal buds in the ventral half of the primitive foregut, just anterior to the developing stomach at 9.5 days of gestation. The two buds elongate in a posterior-ventral direction. At the same time, starting at the primary branch point, the single gut tube begins to pinch into two tubes, the dorsal esophagus and the ventral trachea. In humans, the left lung bud gives rise to two mainstem bronchi, whereas the right lung bud gives rise to three mainstem bronchi. In the mouse, the right lung characteristically has four stem bronchi, whereas the left lung consists of one stem bronchus. The main bronchi branch and rebranch in a dichotomous manner, a process called *branching morphogenesis,* and they eventually form the airway tree. Endoderm-derived epithelial cells line the airways, whereas the surrounding mesenchyme provides the elastic tissue, smooth muscle, cartilage, vascular system, and other connective tissues. The formation of

the bronchial tree is finished at 16 days of gestation in the mouse and at 16 weeks of gestation in humans. At this stage of development, the tracheobronchial tree from the trachea to the terminal bronchioles resembles a system of branching tubules that terminate in exocrine gland–like structures.

MOLECULAR BASIS OF LUNG BUD AND LOBE FORMATION

The outgrowth of the ventral foregut, the formation of the trachea, and the outgrowth of the main pulmonary bronchi take place during the embryonic period of lung development. The crucial event at this stage is the initiation of lung formation at the right place along the anterior-posterior axis of the foregut. What determines the position of the lung, anterior to the abdominal organs but posterior to the thyroid (all of which are derived from the foregut)? Genetic studies have implicated several transcription factors and morphogens, including peptide growth factors and their cognate receptors, in specifying the morphogenetic progenitor field of the lung along the foregut axis (Fig. 79-1). One important transcription factor in this process is hepatocyte nuclear factor-3β (HNF-3β).[2] HNF-3β belongs to the winged helix/forkhead family, which has been renamed the Forkhead Box (Fox) family.[3] *Hnf3β (foxa2)* is expressed in ventral foregut endoderm before and immediately at the start of lung bud formation.[4-6] Targeted ablation of *foxa2* in mice leads to embryonic death between E6.5 and E9.5, which is before lung formation.[7, 8] However, chimeras rescued for the embryonic-extraembryonic constriction showed that *foxa2* was essential for foregut and lung formation.[9]

Fibroblast growth factor-10 (FGF-10) is a member of the large family of FGFs that are involved in multiple processes during embryonic development.[10-12] In the murine lung, *fgf10* mRNA is dynamically expressed in the distal mesenchyme adjacent to the primitive lung buds.[13] The importance of FGF-10 for lung development was shown in *fgf10*-deficient mice that die at birth as a result of severe respiratory failure.[14, 15] The *fgf10*-deficient mice exhibit complete lung agenesis (i.e., lung development had stopped after the formation of the trachea).[14,15] FGFs bind to and signal via FGF tyrosine kinase receptors (FGFr).[10, 11, 16] The FGF-10 receptor (*Fgfr2-IIIb*), a *fgfr2* splice variant, is expressed in lung bud epithelium.[17] The appositional expression of *fgf10* and *fgfr2-IIIb* is in line with the dependence of lung patterning on mesenchymal-epithelial interactions.[17] FGFr-2b is capable of binding FGF-1 and FGF-7, which have also been implicated in lung development.[10, 13, 18] Because a targeted mutation of *fgfr2* results in an early lethal phenotype owing to placental insufficiency,[19,20] *fgfr2*-/- chimeras were created to overcome this early lethality and to allow lung development to be analyzed.[17] As in *fgf10*-deficient mice, only a trachea was formed without any further pulmonary branching.[17] Similarly, transgenic mice that overexpress a dominant negative *fgfr2-IIIb* splice variant in distal lung epithelium showed a severe pulmonary defect with only the formation of the trachea and two main bronchi, but without any lateral branches.[21] Moreover, cre-mediated excision to generate mice lacking the *IIIb* form of *fgfr2* while retaining expression of the *IIIc* splice form resulted in mice that had no

TABLE 79-1

Stages of Lung Development

Stage	Gestational Age Human (wk)	Gestational Age Mouse (d)	Main Events	Epithelial Differentiation State
Embryonic	3.5-7	9.5-14.2	Formation of lung bud, trachea, left and right primary bronchus, and major airways	Undifferentiated columnar epithelium
Pseudoglandular	5-17	14.2-16.6	Establishment of the bronchial tree; all preacinar bronchi are formed	Proximal: columnar epithelium, ciliated, nonciliated, basal, neuroendocrine cells Distal: cuboidal epithelium; precursor Type II cells
Canalicular	16-26	16.6-17.4	Formation of the prospective pulmonary acinus, increase of capillary bed	Proximal: columnar epithelium, ciliated, nonciliated, basal, neuroendocrine cells Distal: differentiation of cuboid Type II to squamous Type I cells
Saccular	24-38	17.4-5 postnatal	Formation of saccules, alveolar ducts, and alveolar air sacs	Proximal: ciliated, nonciliated Clara, basal, neuroendocrine cells Distal: Type I cells flatten and Type II cells mature
Alveolar	36-2 y postnatal	5-30 postnatal	Formation of alveoli by septation of alveolar air sacs, thinning of interaveolar septa, and fusion of the capillary bed to a single layered network	Proximal: columnar epithelium; ciliated, nonciliated, basal, neuroendocrine cells Distal: mature Type I and II cells

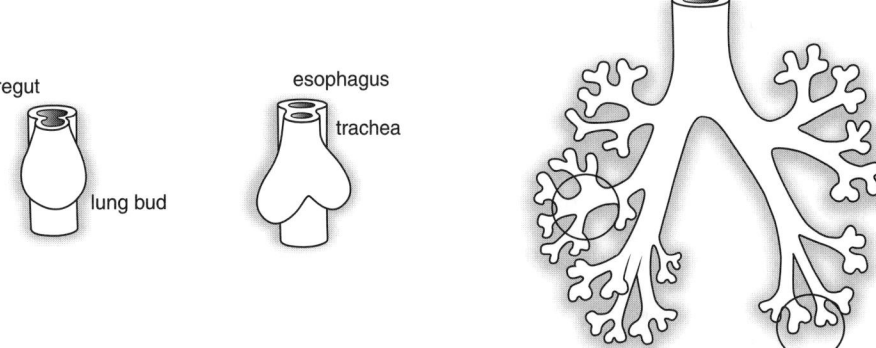

Outgrowth of foregut	Formation of primary bronchi	Branching morphogenesis	Alveolarization
Foxa2	Fgf10	Shh	PdgfA
Gli2/Gli3	Fgfr-IIIb	Gli2	Pdgfrα
		RA	RA
		RAR	RAR/RXR
		Hox	Fgfr3/4
		TTF-1	TTF-1
		Gata-6	
		N-myc	
		Fgf (1,7,9,10)	
		Tgfβ (1,3)	

Figure 79-1. Transcription and growth factors regulating lung development (drawings represent human lungs, which in the normal situation consist of two lobes on the left and three lobes on the right side). See text for details.

lungs and died at birth.[22] Taken together, these data indicate that FGF-10 signaling via FGFr-2-IIIb plays a crucial role in the initiation of lung bud formation (see Fig. 79-1). The "no lung" phenotype as a result of inhibited FGF-10 signaling shows a striking similarity to a phenotype resulting from the loss of function of either *Branchless* (*bnl*) or *Breathless* (*btl*) in *Drosophila*. *Bnl* encodes an FGF homologue that functions as a ligand for *btl*, which encodes a *Drosophila* homologue of FGFr. Loss of function of either *bnl* or *btl* prevented tracheal branching in the fly.[23,24]

Sonic hedgehog (Shh) is a secreted signaling molecule and is a mammalian homologue of *Drosophila* Hh involved in many fundamental processes during embryonic development.[25] *Shh* is expressed in early pulmonary epithelium, with highest gene expression at the tips of developing lung branches.[26] Shh signals via the mesenchymal-located patched (ptc) receptor, a finding suggesting a signaling loop between pulmonary epithelium and mesenchyme during lung development.[26] The importance of Shh for lung development was shown when the *shh* gene was genetically ablated. The *shh* null mutant has a lung bud consisting of only one lobe on each side of the trachea.[27,28] Thus, in contrast to the *fgf10* null mutant, the initiation of lung formation does occur in *shh* null mutants, but they have an incorrect number of lung lobes and a subsequent failure of branching morphogenesis.[27,28] The mesenchyme was the primary target of Shh deficiency, showing decreased cell proliferation and increased cell death in the absence of Shh.[27] The effect of Shh on pulmonary mesenchyme was also demonstrated when Shh was overexpressed in distal lung epithelium using the surfactant protein (SP)-C promoter.[26] Overexpression of Shh resulted in smaller lungs at birth that lacked alveoli but had an increased proportion of mesenchymal mass. Further analysis revealed an increased number of proliferating cells in the mesenchyme of the transgenic lungs.[26] All together, these results support a role for Shh in epithelial-mesenchymal signaling during early lung formation.

Cubitus interruptus has been identified as a downstream target in Hh signaling in *Drosophila*.[25] Mammalian *gli* genes are the putative homologues of *Drosophila* and have also been implicated in mammalian Shh signaling.[25] Three *gli* genes have been described in mice: *gli1*, *gli2*, and *gli3*, all of which are expressed in early pulmonary mesenchyme.[29] In comparison with the *shh* null mutant, an even more dramatic phenotype was observed in mice lacking both *gli2* and *gli3*. These *gli2-/-,gli3-/-* mutant mice have no lung, trachea, or esophagus and die early in gestation.[30] Other foregut derivatives such as thymus, stomach, and pancreas do develop in *gli2-/-,gli3-/-* mutant mice, although these structures are hypoplastic.[30] These data suggest that combined Gli2 and Gli3 signaling is crucial for the initiation of lung bud formation (see Fig. 79-1). The complete absence of trachea and lung formation was already ameliorated by the presence of one *gli3* gene. *Gli2-/-,gli3-/+* mutants had a lung consisting of one hypoplastic lobe.[30] The finding that ablation of both *gli2* and *gli3* resulted in a far worse lung phenotype than the deficiency of *shh* alone may indicate that SHH is not the only regulator of *gli* genes during lung development. The complete absence of a lung in *gli2-/-*, *gli3-/-* mutant mice is similar to the "no lung" phenotype seen in *fgf10*-deficient mice. However, the trachea and esophagus are present in *fgf10*-deficient mice but are absent in *gli2,gli3* deficient mice, a finding implicating different signaling pathways. Other single or compound mutants for the three *gli* genes show a variable degree of lung hypoplasia with an aberrant number of lung lobes and decreased branching morphogenesis.[30-32]

Retinoic acid (RA) plays a crucial role during development and is involved in the developmental process of almost every organ.[33,34] Both a deficiency and an excess of RA cause congenital defects during human development in a variety of organs.[33,34] RA exerts its effects via the RAR and RXR tyrosine kinase receptors, which function as transcriptional regulators of target genes. The RAR family is composed of three genes, which produce several isoforms: RARα$_{1,2}$, RARβ$_{1∠4}$, and RARγ$_{1,2}$, all activated by both all-*trans*-RA and 9-*cis*-RA, whereas the three isoforms from the RXR family (RXRα, RXRβ, and RXRγ) are activated only by 9-*cis*-RA.[34] Mice deficient for only one of the isoforms showed a less severe phenotype than expected on the basis of their expression patterns, a finding indicating a high degree of redundancy among the RA receptors.[34] In contrast, compound mutant mice had similar congenital defects as seen with fetal vitamin A deficiency.[33,34] *RARα-/-;β2-/-* double-mutant mice die soon after birth with agenesis of the left lung and hypoplasia of the right lung.[35] Lung hypoplasia was also reported in *RARα1-/-,β-/-* and *RXRα-/-;RARα-/-* double-mutant mice.[36,37] In addition, RA has profound influences on lung development during branching morphogenesis and alveolarization (see later). Furthermore, RA may regulate *hox* genes.[38-41] *Hox* genes form a large family of homeobox-containing transcription factors that are implicated in the specification of cells that form morphologic structures along an anterior-posterior axis. *Hox* genes are arranged in four chromosomal clusters, and their 3′ to 5′ position of each gene

within a cluster corresponds with their expression along the anterior-posterior axis of the developing body.[42] Specifically, genes of the 3′ regions of the *Hox* clusters *a* and *b* have been shown to be expressed in the developing lung. The *Hoxb* cluster is predominantly expressed in the early pulmonary mesenchyme.[38-41,43-48] Within the mesenchyme, *hoxb* genes express a proximal-distal expression gradient, suggesting a role for *hoxb* genes in specifying proximal from distal pulmonary mesenchyme.[47] Several mutant mice models confirm the role of *hox* genes during lung development. Single-mutant mice for *hox* genes are generally normal, most likely because of redundancy. However, compound *hoxa1-/-,hoxb1-/-* mutants have severe lung hypoplasia ranging from five hypoplastic lung lobes to only two lung lobes.[49] *Hoxa5-/-* mice die perinatally and have laryngotracheal malformations, a reduced tracheal lumen, and lung hypoplasia.[50]

Another homeodomain transcription factor expressed at the onset of lung morphogenesis is thyroid transcription factor-1 (TTF-1), also known as Nkx2.1.[51-53] Expression of *ttf-1* mRNA is localized to epithelial cells of the developing pulmonary tubules and decreases in more proximal conducting airways with advancing gestation.[6,54,55] The *ttf-1* gene continues to be expressed in adult bronchiolar and alveolar epithelial Type II cells, in which it plays an important role in the regulation of Clara cell secreted protein (CCSP) and surfactant protein synthesis (see later). Targeted disruption of *ttf-1* resulted in severe hypoplasia of the thyroid and lung, with a developmental arrest at the pseudoglandular stage of lung development.[56] In contrast to the different null mutants in the Shh-Gli pathway, *ttf-1* null mutants lack distal epithelial cell differentiation.[53,56]

SEPARATING ESOPHAGUS AND TRACHEA

The formation of a tracheoesophageal septum divides the ventral trachea from the dorsal esophagus. A failure to form a septum will result in a tracheoesophageal fistula, a not uncommon congenital defect in humans.[57] Deficiency of all aforementioned growth and transcription factors that are implicated in the etiology of lung agenesis or hypoplasia also results in a tracheoesophageal fistula with different gradations of severity (Table 79-2). *Gli2-/-,gli3-/-* mutant mice have no trachea, nor do they form an esophagus,[30] whereas *gli2-/-,gli3+/-* mutants have a single tracheoesophageal tube connected to the stomach.[30] In *shh-/-* mutant mice, the trachea and esophagus failed to separate, resulting in a tracheoesophageal fistula.[27,28] Mice haploinsufficient for the transcription factor *foxf1* (Hfh8) exhibit foregut abnormalities including narrowing, sometimes, atresia of the esophagus as well as frequent fusion of trachea and esophagus.[58] *Foxf1* expression was absent in foregut derivates (trachea, esophagus, oral cavity, lungs) of *shh-/-* mutants, a finding indicating that SHH signaling is required for activation of *foxf1* in these tissues.[58] Surprisingly, the separation of the trachea and esophagus occurs normally in *fgf10*-deficient mice,[14,15] whereas *ttf-1*–deficient mice have a complete tracheoesophageal defect.[53] *RARα-/-;β2-/-*, *RARα1-/-;β-/-*, and *RXRα-/-;RARα-/-* mutant mice all exhibit a tracheoesophageal septum defect and other tracheal malformations such as disorganized cartilage rings and shortening of the trachea.[35-37]

LEFT-RIGHT ASYMMETRY

At around 5 weeks' gestation, five separate lobes can be identified in the human lung: two on the left and three on the right. In the mouse, the right lung characteristically has four major lobes, whereas the left lung consists of only one small lobe. Such left-right asymmetries during development are an integral part of the establishment of a body plan, and until recently, the molecular basis of left-right asymmetry was not well known. Several distinct yet highly conserved mechanisms have

TABLE 79-2

Separating Trachea and Esophagus*

	Trachea	Esophagus	Remarks
Fgf10$^{-/-}$	+	+	T-E separation, trachea ends blind
Shh$^{-/-}$	+	+	T-E septum defect
Gli2$^{-/-}$	+	+	T-E separation with stenosis
Gli2$^{-/-}$;Gli3$^{-/+}$	+	−	Single (tracheal) tube connecting to the stomach, esophageal atresia
Gli2$^{-/-}$;Gli3$^{-/-}$	−	−	No esophagus, trachea, or lung
RARα$^{-/-}$;β2$^{-/-}$	+	+	T-E septum defect, tracheal cartilage malformations
RARα1$^{-/-}$;β$^{-/-}$			
TTF-1$^{-/-}$	+	+	T-E septum defect

* Transcription and growth factors involved in the separation of esophagus and trachea around gestational week 4 in humans and day 12 in mice. A failure of separation results in a complete or incomplete T-E septum defect, a not uncommon congenital anomaly in humans.
T-E = tracheoesophageal.

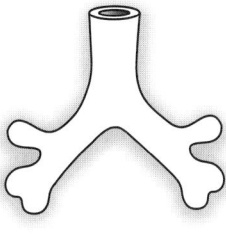

Pulmonary left isomerism

Shh

Gli2

Lefty-1

Pulmonary right isomerism

Pitx2

Gdf-1

ActRIIb

Nodal

Figure 79-2. Transcription and growth factors involved in left-right determination of the developing mouse lung (drawings represent human lungs, which in the normal situation consist of two lobes on the left and three lobes on the right side). See text for details.

since been proposed to initiate the vertebrate left-right axis including the Shh signaling pathway.[59] Molecules such as Shh,[60, 61] FGF-8,[60,62] N-cadherin,[63] activin β, the activin receptor IIB,[64] and foxj1 (HFH4)[65] also influence left-right asymmetry during development (Fig. 79-2). However, it appears that all these pathways converge to influence the expression patterns of genes in the transforming growth factor-β (TGF-β) family of cell-cell signaling factors, called nodal and lefty-1 and 2.[66-69] *Shh* and *lefty-1* mutants have left pulmonary isomerism with only one lobe on each side of the lung.[27,28,61,67] Both Shh and foxa2 are thought to act upstream of lefty-1 and were normal in *lefty-1$^{-/-}$* mice.[67] Although no data are available on the expression of *lefty* in the *shh$^{-/-}$* mutant lung, *lefty-1* is absent in *shh$^{-/-}$* mutant lateral plate mesoderm (LPM).[61] *Lefty-1$^{-/-}$* mice show bilateral expression of *nodal* and *lefty-2* in LPM, which results in ectopic expression of the homeobox transcription regulator pitx2 in the right side of the foregut region.[67] Pixt2 is clearly a powerful determinant of left-right asymmetry because ectopic expression of *pitx2* in the right LPM alters looping of the heart and gut and reverses body rotation in *Xenopus* embryos,[70] whereas the phenotype of *pitx2$^{-/-}$* mice demonstrates right pulmonary isomerism and altered cardiac position.[71-73] Growth/differentiation factor-1 (GDF-1) encodes another member of the TGF-β superfamily, and it is proposed to act upstream of nodal, lefty-1 and lefty-2, and pitx2.[74] Mice deficient for this factor as well as hypomorphic mutants for *nodal* exhibit right pulmonary isomerism.[69,74] It has

not been possible to investigate the role of foxa2 in left-right asymmetry formation of the lung, because null mutant mice die before the onset of lung formation. However, in rescued *foxa2* mutant mice, *shh* was not detected in the foregut region.[9]

BRANCHING MORPHOGENESIS

The early branching of the primary bronchi tends to be monopodal. Starting at the level of the secondary bronchus, each bronchus subsequently undergoes dichotomous branching (i.e., each branch bifurcates repeatedly into two branches). The enlarging bronchial tree branches into the surrounding mesenchyme, which will eventually furrow into the characteristic lobes of the lung: two on the left and three on the right in humans and one left and four right in mice.

Branching of the lung buds is controlled by epithelial-mesenchymal tissue interactions.[75, 76] The mesenchymal component, most likely a soluble factor, dictates the branching pattern of the epithelium.[77] The strong inductive capacity of pulmonary mesenchyme was shown when pulmonary mesenchyme induced a lung epithelial phenotype in epithelial ureter buds.[78] Branching appears also to be regulated by positional information along the anterior-posterior axis of the lung because proximal mesenchyme (trachea and main bronchi) and distal mesenchyme (lung bud) differ in their ability to support epithelial branching morphogenesis.[79-81] Some progress has been made in elucidating the complex mixture of transcription factors and morphogens, which guide proper lung branching (see Fig. 79–1). Although alterations in cell adhesion and matrix remodeling at the epithelial-mesenchymal interface also contribute to lung branching morphogenesis, they are not discussed, and the reader is referred to a published review.[82]

It is evident from the previous discussion that transcription factors belonging to the Hox, Fox, and Nkx families are likely involved in this process. Other transcription factors implicated in lung branching morphogenesis are gata-6 and N-*myc*. Gata-6 belongs to the Gata family of zinc finger–containing transcription factors and is expressed in epithelial and mesenchymal cells of the developing lung bud.[83,84] Gata-6 is essential for endoderm formation because targeted deletion of *gata-6* resulted in embryonic death before lung formation owing to failure of visceral endoderm formation.[85,86] In the lung, gata-6 appears to be important for branching morphogenesis, because inhibition of *gata-6* expression causes decreased branching morphogenesis.[84, 85] More recently, expressing a *gata-6* engrailed dominant negative fusion protein in distal lung epithelium resulted in a lack of alveolar Type I and a perturbation in alveolar Type II cells together with a reduction in the number of proximal airway tubules.[87] Conversely, overexpression of g*ata-6*, using the SP-C promoter, also disrupted branching morphogenesis and caused a lack of distal epithelial cell differentiation.[88] Altogether, these results indicate that balanced gata-6 expression level is important for branching morphogenesis during the pseudoglandular period of lung development but also during later stages of lung development when alveolar Type I and II cells differentiate and the gas exchange area matures. N-*myc* is a member of the *myc* family of proto-oncogenes, which includes N-*myc*, c-*myc*, and L-*myc*. Myc proteins belong to the basic helix-loop-helix (bHLH) class of transcription factors. In the lung, N-*myc* is expressed in pulmonary epithelium.[89, 90] Mice homozygous for the N-*myc* null mutation die at mid-gestation.[89,91] Leaky null mutants for N-*myc* survive to the point when lung development starts; however, pulmonary branching morphogenesis is dramatically reduced, resulting in severe lung hypoplasia.[90,92]

Several growth factors, including FGFs and TGF-βs have been shown to regulate lung branching morphogenesis.[82,93] FGFs are generally produced by the pulmonary mesenchyme, whereas FGFr-1 and FGFr-2 have been localized to embryonic and fetal lung epithelium.[94, 95] Transcripts for FGF-7 are detected in lung mesenchyme at sites of active branching morphogenesis.[96, 97] Exogenous FGF-7 inhibits rat lung branching morphogenesis *in vitro*[98] but stimulates proliferation of Type II pneumocytes *in vitro*[99] and *in vivo*.[100, 101] Surprisingly, mice bearing a null mutation of the *fgf7* gene had no obvious lung abnormalities,[102] a finding suggesting that FGF-7 can be replaced by other factors, such as FGF-1 and FGF-10. FGF-1, which binds to both FGFr-2 splice variants, FGFr-2-IIIb and FGFr-2-IIIc, is crucial for branching of embryonic mouse epithelium in mesenchyme-free culture.[103] FGF-2, which binds to FGFr-2-IIIc, but not to FGF-2-IIIb, did not affect epithelial branching in these cultures, a finding suggesting that the effect of FGF-1 on epithelial branching is mediated via FGFr-2-IIIb receptor, which also binds FGF-7.[104] As mentioned earlier, FGF-10 also binds to FGFr-2-IIIb, and both null mutants for FGFr-2-IIIb and FGF-10 show complete lung agenesis.[14,15,22] *In vitro*, FGF-10 elicits endodermal expansion and bud formation, whereas FGF-7 induces expansion of the endoderm but never progresses to bud formation.[105] This finding suggests that FGF-7 and FGF-10 signals are transduced in different physiologic responses and may explain why FGF-7 cannot compensate for loss of FGF-10. Another member of the FGF family, FGF-9, is expressed in pulmonary mesothelium and epithelium in early development and later only in the mesothelium.[17,106] This expression pattern is different from that of FGF-1, FGF-7, and FGF-10,

which are expressed only in the lung mesenchyme. Targeted deletion of *fgf9* resulted in severe lung hypoplasia and immediate postnatal death.[106] Analysis of the lungs revealed decreased branching morphogenesis and a lack of alveoli; however, the numbers of lung lobes and primary bronchi were normal.[106]

TGF-β belongs to a superfamily that includes activin, bone morphogenic growth factor (BMP), and TGF-β1, 2, and 3. These peptides can exert a variety of biologic effects including regulation of cell growth and differentiation and expression of various proteins. TGF-β1 plays an inhibitory role during lung development. In the lung, TGF-β1 mRNA and protein were found in the mesenchyme and epithelium, respectively.[107-109] Both addition of exogenous TGF-β1 to cultured embryonic mouse lung explants and *in vivo* overexpression of TGF-β1 in distal lung epithelial cells resulted in decreased branching morphogenesis, inhibited distal epithelial cell differentiation, and inhibited formation of the pulmonary vasculature, findings indicating an inhibitory role for TGF-β1 during branching morphogenesis.[110-114] Most, if not all, biologic activities of TGF-β are transmitted via transmembrane Ser/Thr kinase receptors, known as Type I and Type II receptors.[115] Signal transduction requires the formation of a heteromeric complex of Type I (TGF-βrI) and Type II (TGF-βrII) receptors. Inhibition of TGF-βrII signaling stimulated lung morphogenesis in whole lung explants in culture, a finding underlining the negative effects of TGF-β signaling on branching morphogenesis.[116] *In vivo* studies showed that *tgfβ1* null mutants themselves have no gross developmental abnormalities; however, 50% of the null mutants die before E11.5 because of defects in yolk sac vascularization.[117,118] *Tgfβ3* null mutants die postnatally with cleft palate and delayed pulmonary development,[119] whereas *tgfβ2*-deficient mice die postnatally and display a lung phenotype characterized by postnatal collapse of alveoli and terminal airways.[120] Smad proteins are downstream effector proteins in TGF-β signaling.[121] Smad1 to smad3 proteins are expressed in distal lung epithelium, whereas smad4 is expressed in both distal lung epithelium and mesenchyme.[122, 123] Downregulation of *smad2/3* and s*mad4* expression resulted in increased branching morphogenesis in cultured lung explants. Exogenous TGF-β1 did not reverse this inhibitory effect, a finding consistent with TGF-βs being upstream of smad proteins.[123]

EPITHELIAL DIFFERENTIATION

As branching proceeds, numerous different cell phenotypes are formed along the anterior-posterior axis of the developing epithelial tubules and associated mesenchymal components, each with different morphologies and patterns of gene expression. This patterning of differentiated lung cells may also be controlled by epithelial-mesenchymal interactions.[77, 80] Since the early 1990s, some regulatory molecules involved in epithelial morphogenic patterning in the lung have been identified (Fig. 79–3).

Pulmonary neuroendocrine cells (PNECs) are the first cells to differentiate in humans and animals.[124, 125] Mash-1 is a bHLH transcription factor implicated in neural differentiation.[126] In the lung, *mash-1* is expressed in clusters or single progenitor PNECs.[127] Mice deficient for *mash-1* did not develop PNECs, a finding indicating an essential role for this transcription factor in the differentiation of PNECs.[127] Hes-1 encodes a bHLH protein that is up-regulated in response to Notch activation and represses downstream targets such as mash-1, thereby preventing neural differentiation.[128] Indeed, *hes-1*–deficient embryos had increased *mash-1* mRNA expression and PNECs in their lungs.[129] Whether the Notch signaling pathway plays a further role in distal epithelial specification remains to be elucidated. Pod1 is another bHLH protein that acts as a transcriptional regulatory protein that governs cell fate determination and differen-

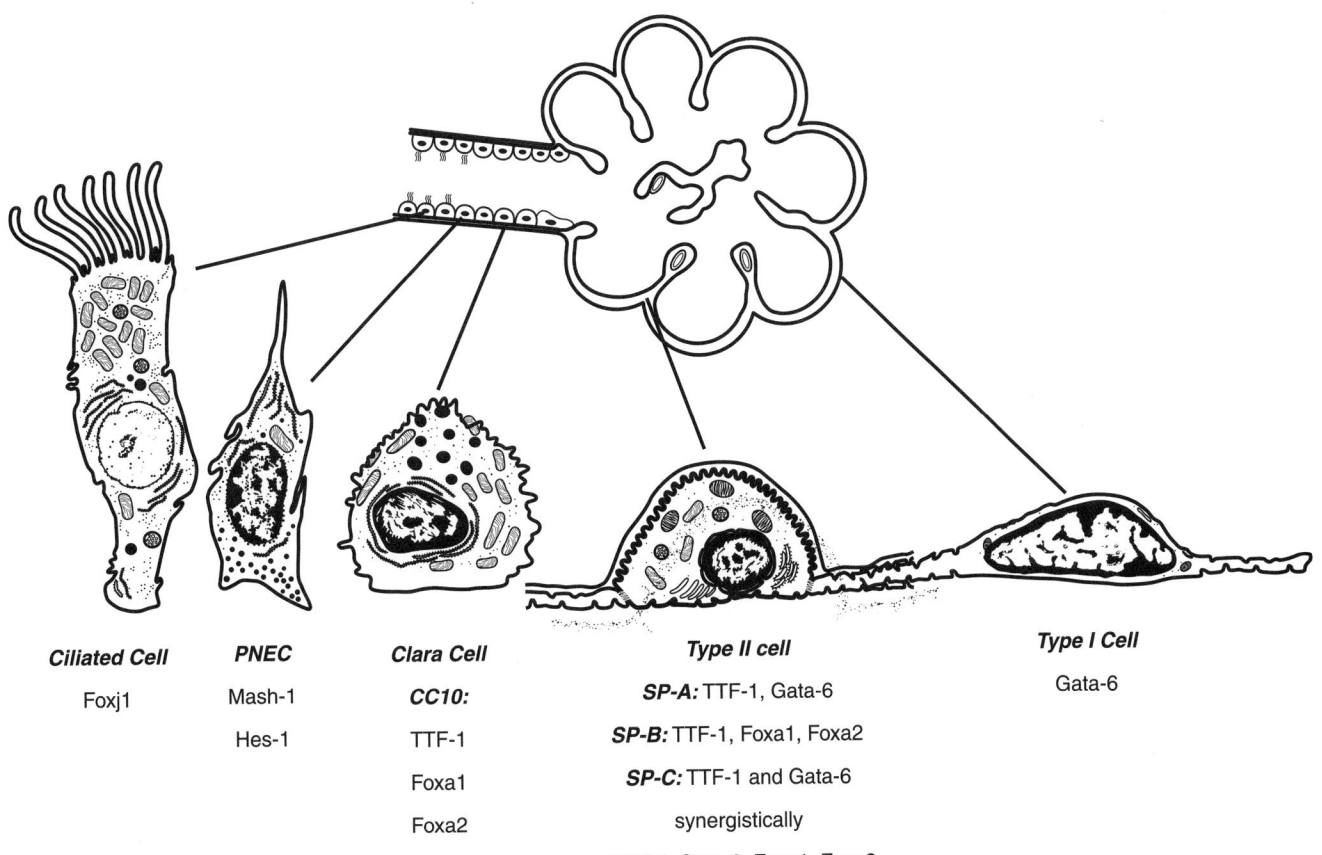

Ciliated Cell

Foxj1

PNEC

Mash-1

Hes-1

Clara Cell

CC10:

TTF-1

Foxa1

Foxa2

Type II cell

SP-A: TTF-1, Gata-6

SP-B: TTF-1, Foxa1, Foxa2

SP-C: TTF-1 and Gata-6

synergistically

TTF-1: Gata-6, Foxa1, Foxa2

Type I Cell

Gata-6

Figure 79–3. Molecular control of epithelial cell differentiation during human lung development. See text for details.

tiation in a variety of tissues. The *pod1* null mutant dies at birth with severely hypoplastic lungs that have a reduced number of tertiary branches and a lack of acinar tubules, terminal air sacs, and alveoli.[130] Marker analysis revealed a disturbance in proximal-distal patterning of the lung epithelium with increased CCSP and decreased SP-C expression.[130]

Epithelial transcription factors such as foxa2, gata-6, and TTF-1 (Nkx2.1) have also been shown to influence lung epithelial specification. In both fetal mouse and human lung, the temporal-spatial distribution of TTF-1 follows the pattern of expression of surfactant proteins.[6, 55] It has been shown that TTF-1 regulates the transcription of SP-A, B, and C[131-135] and CCSP.[131, 136] Consequently, *ttf-1* null mutants lack distal epithelial cell differentiation, whereas the proximal epithelial cell marker foxj1 (HFH4) is unaffected.[137] Taken together, these data underline the importance of TTF-1 for the establishment of the distal epithelial cell phenotype. Moreover, gata-6 transactivates SP-A and TTF-1,[138,139] and it has been shown that gata-6 acts synergistically with TTF-1 to influence the activity of the SP-C promoter.[140] A role for gata-6 in bronchial epithelial specification has been suggested by the observation that *gata-6−/−* ES cells fail to contribute to bronchial epithelial cells.[85] In some respiratory epithelial cells, TTF-1 is co-expressed with members of the fox family of transcription factors. Transcripts for *foxa1* and *foxa2* are detected in foregut cells forming the embryonic lung bud and later in the distal epithelium of the developing and mature lung.[6, 141] Like TTF-1, foxa1 and foxa2 appear to modulate the expression of SP-B and CCSP.[131,141,142] Foxa1 and Foxa2 were proposed to be upstream regulators of TTF-1,[143] and it is possible

that both members of the Fox family confer lung-specific gene expression in the primitive foregut through TTF-1 as the intermediate. HNF3/forkhead homologue 4 (HFH4:foxj1) is a transcription factor of the winged helix/forkhead family, expressed in various tissues during development. In the developing and adult lung, *foxj1* expression is restricted to ciliated cells of the bronchial and bronchiolar epithelium.[137,144] The role of foxj1 in ciliated cell differentiation was clearly demonstrated when *foxj1* was overexpressed in distal pulmonary epithelial cells. High levels of *foxj1* expression inhibited branching morphogenesis and enhanced the development of ciliated cells, whereas the development of distal epithelial cells was inhibited.[145] In contrast, *foxj1* null mutant mice completely lack respiratory ciliated cells.[65,146] These data indicate that foxj1 is essential for the development of pulmonary ciliated cells.

Secreted morphogens such as SHH appear not to be involved in regulating proximal-distal epithelial specification because SP-C and CCSP are expressed in *Shh*-deficient mice.[28] In *Drosophila*, Hh may regulate the expression of *Decapentaplegic* (Dpp), the *Drosophila* counterpart of BMP.[25] In the murine lung, BMP4 is implicated in lung epithelial specification. *Bmp4* is expressed in early distal lung tips and at lower levels in the mesenchyme adjacent to the distal lung buds.[147,148] Overexpression of BMP4 in the distal epithelium *in vivo* resulted in hypoplastic lungs with grossly dilated terminal lung buds separated by abundant mesenchyme.[147] Distal epithelial differentiation was abnormal with decreased SP-C expression, whereas proximal differentiation (CCSP expression) was normal.[147] *In vitro*, however, exogenous BMP4 clearly enhanced peripheral lung epithelial branching morhogenesis and SP-C expression.[149] The secreted BMP antagonist Xnoggin is expressed in distal mouse lung mesenchyme at early development.[148] Overexpression of Xnoggin or the dominant negative BMP receptor dnAlk6 in distal pulmonary epithelium resulted in a proximal epithelial phenotype of the fetal lung.[148] Similar results were obtained when Gremlin, another BMP antagonist, was overexpressed in the distal lung epithelium.[150] These studies clearly indicate a role for BMP4 in proximal-distal epithelial differentiation during lung development and as a result probably argue against SHH as a regulator of BMP4 expression.

ALVEOLAR DEVELOPMENT

Alveolarization is the last step of lung development. Alveoli are produced by septation of the pulmonary saccules that form the immature lung. In both humans and mice, alveolarization occurs predominately after birth. One of the key elements in the alveolarization process (see Fig. 79-1) appears to be one of the three isoforms of the platelet-derived growth factors (PDGFs), namely, PDGF-A.[151] PDGF-A is normally expressed in early pulmonary epithelium and becomes undetectable at later gestations.[152] Its receptor, PDGF-rα, is expressed in the mesenchyme adjacent to the epithelium that expresses PDGF-A, a finding suggesting a paracrine signaling loop between epithelium and mesenchyme.[152-154] In mice, absence of PDGF-A results in prenatal and postnatal death. Postnatal deaths were characterized by emphysematous lungs with areas of atelectasis, without any formation of septa or alveoli. Instead, dilated prealveolar saccules were found.[153,154] In normal mice, alveolar septa contain smooth muscle cell α–smooth muscle actin (α-sma)–positive myofibroblasts. The postnatal *pdgfA* null mutant lungs lack alveolar staining for α-sma, a finding indicating a lack of alveolar myofibroblasts. In addition, they were almost completely devoid of parenchymal elastin fibers, and this most likely contributed to the failure of alveolar formation.[153,154] Myofibroblasts surrounding vessels and bronchioles appeared normal and were tropoelastin positive, a finding suggesting a different developmental lineage.[154] Moreover, PDGF-rα–positive cells were specifically missing from lungs of *pdgfA* null mutants, and it has been proposed that these cells are progenitor cells for alveolar myofibroblasts.[153,154] Taken together, PDGF-A is important for the formation of alveolar myofibroblasts that produce elastin, which, in turn, is important for alveolar formation. *Pdgfrα*-deficient mice die *in utero* with severe skeletal malformations and incomplete cephalic closure. *Pdgfrα*-deficient lungs were hypoplastic; however, primary branching and histology were not affected.[155,156] Obviously, postnatal alveolar formation could not be examined in these mice.

Both *fgfr3* and *fgfr4* are expressed in postnatal pulmonary mesenchyme, whereas their ligands are expressed in pulmonary epithelial cells.[157] Although a null mutation of either *fgfr3* or *fgfr4* caused no obvious lung defects, silencing of both receptors resulted in severe overall body growth retardation and a failure of postnatal alveolar formation.[157] Despite the large dilated saccules without any proper alveolar septation, differentiation (including α-sma–positive myofibroblasts) and proliferation proceeded normally.[157] Besides its role in prenatal lung development, TTF-1 also regulates postnatal lung development and homeostasis. Postnatally, TTF-1 expression decreases dramatically. However, TTF-1 expression remains detectable in adult alveolar Type II cells. Overexpression of TTF-1 in distal lung epithelial cells, using the SP-C promoter, did not affect prenatal lung development, but it perturbed postnatal alveolarization and led to emphysema, severe inflammation, and fibrosis.[158] RA has been shown to increase the number of alveoli in postnatal rats and even abrogates decreased alveolarization seen after the experimental use of dexamethasone or elastase, which decreases alveolar formation, thus making RA a potential powerful factor in "neoalveogenesis" in prematurity or after lung injury.[159-162] Similarly, compound mice homozygous for an *RARγ* and heterozygous for an *RXRα* deletion had a reduced number of alveoli and less elastic fiber in their alveolar walls.[163] RARβ, conversely, appears to be an endogenous inhibitor of septation, and, consequently, the *RARβ* null mutant shows early onset septation resulting in twice as much alveoli in the null mutant lungs when compared with wild-type lungs.[164]

VASCULAR DEVELOPMENT

The lung is composed of a complex network of airways and vessels, and although much has been learned regarding the mechanisms controlling lung bud formation and airway branching, the mechanisms involved in vascular formation during lung development remain obscure. Three processes are believed to control pulmonary vascular development: *angiogenesis,* which is defined as sprouting of new vessels from preexisting ones and gives rise to the central vessels; *vasculogenesis,* which is *de novo* synthesis of blood vessels from blood lakes in the periphery of the lung; and the *fusion of proximal and peripheral vessels* to form the pulmonary circulation.[165] Investigators have shown that, even in the early stages of lung development, vascular connections are well established, and pulmonary vascular development occurs at all developmental stages, with completion of a single capillary network during the alveolar period.[166,167]

The molecular mechanisms involved in vascular formation during lung development are relatively unknown. Members of the vascular endothelial growth factor (VEGF) family,[168,169] the Angiopoietin family,[170,171] and members of the Ephrin family[172] have all been implicated in controlling vascularization of the pulmonary system. VEGF, a potent mitogen for endothelial cells, influences angiogenesis and vasculogenesis.[173] It is essential for embryonic development, and even haploinsufficiency of *vegf* causes embryonic lethality.[174,175] In the embryonic and adult lung, *vegf* mRNA is detected in lung epithelium.[176-178] VEGF signals via two high-affinity receptors, Flt-1 and Flk/KDR, which in the embryonic lung are localized in the mesenchyme.[177,178] The complementary expression patterns of VEGF in lung epithelium and the two VEGF receptors in the mesenchyme suggest a paracrine signaling loop and possible influence on lung development and branching morphogenesis.[179] Overexpression of the VEGF 164 isoform in distal airway epithelium resulted in perinatal death.[180] The lungs appeared abnormal, with dilated respiratory tubules and saccules and a decreased number of terminal buds.[180] Flk-1 expression in the mesenchyme was increased, indicative of a regulatory role of VEGF between pulmonary epithelium and mesenchyme. Mice that lacked the VEGF isoforms 164 and 188 and expressed only isoform 120 had a decrease in peripheral vascular development with fewer air-blood barriers and a general delay in lung development.[181]

Another factor implicated in pulmonary vascular development is foxf1 (also known as HFH8 or fraec1). *Foxf1* null mutant mice die *in utero* because of defects in mesodermal differentiation and cell adhesion.[182] In the lung, *foxf1* is expressed in smooth muscle cells surrounding bronchioles and alveolar endothelial cells.[183,184] Heterozygous mutant mice carrying a disruption of *foxf1* gene, in which foxf1 levels are reduced by 80%, displayed a 55% postnatal mortality with lung hemorrhaging. Analysis of the lungs revealed abnormalities in alveolar formation and pulmonary vasculature.[184] From these studies, it can be concluded that a disruption in pulmonary vascular development goes hand in hand with impaired branching morphogenesis and lung hypoplasia. The question remains whether the airway-branching phenotype is the indirect result of disrupted vessel formation or whether the factors involved in vascular development directly affect pulmonary branching morphogenesis as well.

SYNOPSIS

Molecular studies of lung development have started to unravel the complex series of events that control proper formation of the lung. Observations such as no lung formation are interesting for understanding organogenesis of the lung itself, but the clinical relevance is minimal, because having no lung is incompatible with life. However, the finding that factors implicated in foregut specification are also regulating lung branching morphogenesis is tremendously intriguing for clinical practice (see Fig. 79-1). One of the major complications of preterm birth is immaturity of the lung. Despite modern management, many infants exhibit lung dysfunction characterized by arrested lung development and interrupted alveolarization. A better understanding of the molecular basis of pulmonary development may guide clinicians in the design of strategies to mimic normal lung maturation in a premature infant.

REFERENCES

1. Ten Have-Opbroek AA: Lung development in the mouse embryo. Exp Lung Res 1991;17(2):111.
2. Ang SL, et al: The formation and maintenance of the definitive endoderm lineage in the mouse: involvement of HNF3/forkhead proteins. Development 1993;119(4):1301.
3. Kaestner KH, et al: Unified nomenclature for the winged helix/forkhead transcription factors. Genes Dev 2000;14(2):142.
4. Monaghan AP, et al: Postimplantation expression patterns indicate a role for the mouse forkhead/HNF-3 alpha, beta and gamma genes in determination of the definitive endoderm, chordamesoderm and neuroectoderm. Development 1993;119(3):567.
5. Stahlman MT, et al: Temporal-spatial distribution of hepatocyte nuclear factor-3beta in developing human lung and other foregut derivatives. J Histochem Cytochem 1998;46(8):955.
6. Zhou L, et al: Thyroid transcription factor-1, hepatocyte nuclear factor-3beta, surfactant protein B, C, and Clara cell secretory protein in developing mouse lung. J Histochem Cytochem 1996;44(10):1183.
7. Weinstein DC, et al: The winged-helix transcription factor HNF-3 beta is required for notochord development in the mouse embryo. Cell 1994; 78(4):575.
8. Ang SL, Rossant J: HNF-3 beta is essential for node and notochord formation in mouse development. Cell 1994;78(4):561.
9. Dufort D, et al: The transcription factor HNF3beta is required in visceral endoderm for normal primitive streak morphogenesis. Development 1998;125(16):3015.
10. Goldfarb M: Functions of fibroblast growth factors in vertebrate development. Cytokine Growth Factor Rev 1996;7(4):311.
11. Kato S, Sekine K: FGF-FGFR signaling in vertebrate organogenesis. Cell Mol Biol (Noisy-le-grand) 1999;45(5):631.
12. Ornitz DM, Itoh N: Fibroblast growth factors. Genome Biol 2001;2(3):5.
13. Bellusci S, et al: Fibroblast growth factor 10 (FGF10) and branching morphogenesis in the embryonic mouse lung. Development 1997; 124(23):4867.
14. Sekine K, et al: Fgf10 is essential for limb and lung formation. Nat Genet 1999;21(1):138.
15. Min H, et al: Fgf-10 is required for both limb and lung development and exhibits striking functional similarity to *Drosophila* branchless. Genes Dev 1998;12(20):3156.
16. Ornitz DM, et al: Receptor specificity of the fibroblast growth factor family. J Biol Chem 1996;271(25):15292.
17. Arman E, et al: Fgfr2 is required for limb outgrowth and lung-branching morphogenesis. Proc Natl Acad Sci USA 1999;96(21):11895.
18. Igarashi M, et al: Characterization of recombinant human fibroblast growth factor (FGF)-10 reveals functional similarities with keratinocyte growth factor (FGF-7). J Biol Chem 1998;273(21):13230.
19. Arman E, et al: Targeted disruption of fibroblast growth factor (FGF) receptor 2 suggests a role for FGF signaling in pregastrulation mammalian development. Proc Natl Acad Sci USA 1998;95(9):5082.
20. Xu X, et al: Fibroblast growth factor receptor 2 (FGFR2)-mediated reciprocal regulation loop between FGF8 and FGF10 is essential for limb induction. Development 1998;125(4):753.
21. Peters K, et al: Targeted expression of a dominant negative FGF receptor blocks branching morphogenesis and epithelial differentiation of the mouse lung. EMBO J 1994;13(14):3296.
22. De Moerlooze L, et al: An important role for the IIIb isoform of fibroblast growth factor receptor 2 (FGFR2) in mesenchymal-epithelial signalling during mouse organogenesis. Development 2000;127(3):483.
23. Sutherland D, et al: branchless encodes a *Drosophila* FGF homolog that controls tracheal cell migration and the pattern of branching. Cell 1996;87(6):1091.
24. Klambt C, et al: breathless, a *Drosophila* FGF receptor homolog, is essential for migration of tracheal and specific midline glial cells. Genes Dev 1992;6(9):1668.
25. Ingham PW, McMahon AP: Hedgehog signaling in animal development: paradigms and principles. Genes Dev 2001;15(23):3059.
26. Bellusci S, et al: Involvement of sonic hedgehog (Shh) in mouse embryonic lung growth and morphogenesis. Development 1997;124(1):53.
27. Litingtung Y, et al: Sonic hedgehog is essential to foregut development. Nat Genet 1998;20(1):58.
28. Pepicelli CV, et al: Sonic hedgehog regulates branching morphogenesis in the mammalian lung. Curr Biol 1998;8(19):1083.
29. Grindley JC, et al: Evidence for the involvement of the Gli gene family in embryonic mouse lung development. Dev Biol 1997;188(2):337.
30. Motoyama J, et al: Essential function of Gli2 and Gli3 in the formation of lung, trachea and oesophagus. Nat Genet 1998;20(1):54.
31. Bai CB, Joyner AL: Gli1 can rescue the in vivo function of Gli2. Development 2001;128(24):5161.
32. Park HL, et al: Mouse Gli1 mutants are viable but have defects in SHH signaling in combination with a Gli2 mutation. Development 2000; 127(8):1593.
33. Zile MH: Function of vitamin A in vertebrate embryonic development. J Nutr 2001;131(3):705.
34. Ross SA, et al: Retinoids in embryonal development. Physiol Rev 2000; 80(3):1021.
35. Mendelsohn C, et al: Function of the retinoic acid receptors (RARs) during development. II. Multiple abnormalities at various stages of organogenesis in RAR double mutants. Development 1994;120(10):2749.
36. Luo J, et al: Compound mutants for retinoic acid receptor (RAR) beta and RAR alpha 1 reveal developmental functions for multiple RAR beta isoforms. Mech Dev 1996;55(1):33.
37. Kastner P, et al: Vitamin A deficiency and mutations of RXRalpha, RXRbeta and RARalpha lead to early differentiation of embryonic ventricular cardiomyocytes. Development 1997;124(23):4749.
38. Packer AI, et al: Regulation of the Hoxa4 and Hoxa5 genes in the embryonic mouse lung by retinoic acid and TGFbeta1: implications for lung development and patterning. Dev Dyn 2000;217(1):62.
39. Cardoso WV, et al: Retinoic acid alters the expression of pattern-related genes in the developing rat lung. Dev Dyn 1996;207(1):47.
40. Cardoso WV: Transcription factors and pattern formation in the developing lung. Am J Physiol 1995;269(4):L429.
41. Volpe MV, et al: Hoxb-5 control of early airway formation during branching morphogenesis in the developing mouse lung. Biochim Biophys Acta 2000;1475(3):337.
42. Krumlauf R: Hox genes in vertebrate development. Cell 1994;78(2):191.
43. Kappen C: Hox genes in the lung. Am J Respir Cell Mol Biol 1996;15(2):156.
44. Krumlauf R, et al: Developmental and spatial patterns of expression of the mouse homeobox gene, Hox 2.1. Development 1987;99(4):603.
45. Wall NA, et al: Expression and modification of Hox 2.1 protein in mouse embryos. Mech Dev 1992;37(3):111.
46. Bogue CW, et al: Identification of Hox genes in newborn lung and effects of gestational age and retinoic acid on their expression. Am J Physiol 1994;266(4):L448.
47. Bogue CW, et al: Expression of Hoxb genes in the developing mouse foregut and lung. Am J Respir Cell Mol Biol 1996;15(2):163.
48. Volpe MV, et al: Hoxb-5 expression in the developing mouse lung suggests a role in branching morphogenesis and epithelial cell fate. Histochem Cell Biol 1997;108(6):495.
49. Rossel M, Capecchi MR: Mice mutant for both Hoxa1 and Hoxb1 show extensive remodeling of the hindbrain and defects in craniofacial development. Development 1999;126(22):5027.
50. Aubin J, et al: Early postnatal lethality in Hoxa-5 mutant mice is attributable to respiratory tract defects. Dev Biol 1997;192(2):432.
51. Kimura S, et al: The T/ebp null mouse: thyroid-specific enhancer-binding protein is essential for the organogenesis of the thyroid, lung, ventral forebrain, and pituitary. Genes Dev 1996;10(1):60.
52. Lazzaro D, et al: The transcription factor TTF-1 is expressed at the onset of thyroid and lung morphogenesis and in restricted regions of the foetal brain. Development 1991;113(4):1093.
53. Minoo P, et al: Defects in tracheoesophageal and lung morphogenesis in Nkx2.1(-/-) mouse embryos. Dev Biol 1999;209(1):60.
54. Zhou H, et al: Expression of thyroid transcription factor-1, surfactant proteins, type I cell-associated antigen, and Clara cell secretory protein in pulmonary hypoplasia. Pediatr Dev Pathol 2001;4(4):364.
55. Stahlman MT, et al: Expression of thyroid transcription factor-1(TTF-1) in fetal and neonatal human lung. J Histochem Cytochem 1996;44(7):673.
56. Yuan B, et al: Inhibition of distal lung morphogenesis in Nkx2.1(-/-) embryos. Dev Dyn 2000;217(2):180.
57. Albers GM, Wood RE: The lower respiratory organs: tracheoesophageal fistula. *In* Stevenson RE, et al (eds): Oxford Monographs on Medical Genetics No. 27:

Human Malformations and Related Anomalies, Vol 2. Oxford, Oxford University Press, 1993, p 350.

58. Mahlapuu M, et al: Haploinsufficiency of the forkhead gene Foxf1, a target for sonic hedgehog signaling, causes lung and foregut malformations. Development 2001;128(12):2397.

59. Hamada H, et al: Establishment of vertebrate left-right asymmetry. Nat Rev Genet 2002;3(2):103.

60. Meyers EN, Martin GR: Differences in left-right axis pathways in mouse and chick: functions of FGF8 and SHH. Science 1999;285(5426):403.

61. Tsukui T, et al: Multiple left-right asymmetry defects in Shh(-/-) mutant mice unveil a convergence of the shh and retinoic acid pathways in the control of Lefty-1. Proc Natl Acad Sci USA 1999;96(20):11376.

62. Boettger T, et al: FGF8 functions in the specification of the right body side of the chick. Curr Biol 1999;9(5):277.

63. Garcia-Castro MI, et al: N-Cadherin, a cell adhesion molecule involved in establishment of embryonic left-right asymmetry. Science 2000;288(5468):1047.

64. Oh SP, Li E: The signaling pathway mediated by the type IIB activin receptor controls axial patterning and lateral asymmetry in the mouse. Genes Dev 1997;11(14):1812.

65. Chen J, et al: Mutation of the mouse hepatocyte nuclear factor/forkhead homologue 4 gene results in an absence of cilia and random left-right asymmetry. J Clin Invest 1998;102(6):1077.

66. Meno C, et al: Left-right asymmetric expression of the TGF beta-family member lefty in mouse embryos. Nature 1996;381(6578):151.

67. Meno C, et al: lefty-1 is required for left-right determination as a regulator of lefty-2 and nodal. Cell 1998;94(3):287.

68. Meno C, et al: Diffusion of nodal signaling activity in the absence of the feedback inhibitor Lefty2. Dev Cell 2001;1(1):127.

69. Lowe LA, et al: Genetic dissection of nodal function in patterning the mouse embryo. Development 2001;128(10):1831.

70. Campione M, et al: The homeobox gene Pitx2: mediator of asymmetric left-right signaling in vertebrate heart and gut looping. Development 1999;126(6):1225.

71. Lin CR, et al: Pitx2 regulates lung asymmetry, cardiac positioning and pituitary and tooth morphogenesis. Nature 1999;401(6750):279.

72. Lu MF, et al: Function of Rieger syndrome gene in left-right asymmetry and craniofacial development. Nature 1999;401(6750):276.

73. Gage PJ, et al: Dosage requirement of Pitx2 for development of multiple organs. Development 1999;126(20):4643.

74. Rankin CT, et al: Regulation of left-right patterning in mice by growth/differentiation factor-1. Nat Genet 2000;24(3):262.

75. Alescio TC: Induction in vitro of tracheal buds by pulmonary mesenchyme grafted on tracheal epithelium. J Exp Zool 1962;150:83.

76. Spooner BS, Wessells NK: Mammalian lung development: interactions in primordium formation and bronchial morphogenesis. J Exp Zool 1970;175(4):445.

77. Masters JR: Epithelial-mesenchymal interaction during lung development: the effect of mesenchymal mass. Dev Biol 1976;51(1):98.

78. Lin Y, et al: Induced repatterning of type XVIII collagen expression in ureter bud from kidney to lung type: association with sonic hedgehog and ectopic surfactant protein C. Development 2001;128(9):1573.

79. Wessells NK: Mammalian lung development: interactions in formation and morphogenesis of tracheal buds. J Exp Zool 1970;175(4):455.

80. Shannon JM: Induction of alveolar type II cell differentiation in fetal tracheal epithelium by grafted distal lung mesenchyme. Dev Biol 1994;166(2):600.

81. Shannon JM, et al: Mesenchyme specifies epithelial differentiation in reciprocal recombinants of embryonic lung and trachea. Dev Dyn 1998;212(4):482.

82. Keijzer R, Post M: Lung branching morphogenesis: role of growth factors and extracellular matrix. In Gaultier C, et al (eds): Lung Development. New York, Oxford University Press., 1999, p 1.

83. Morrisey EE, et al: GATA-6: a zinc finger transcription factor that is expressed in multiple cell lineages derived from lateral mesoderm. Dev Biol 1996;177(1):309.

84. Keijzer R, et al: The transcription factor GATA6 is essential for branching morphogenesis and epithelial differentiation during fetal pulmonary development. Development 2001;128(4):503.

85. Morrisey EE, et al: GATA6 regulates HNF4 and is required for differentiation of visceral endoderm in the mouse embryo. Genes Dev 1998;12(22):3579.

86. Koutsourakis M, et al: The transcription factor GATA6 is essential for early extraembryonic development. Development 1999;126(9):723.

87. Yang H, et al: GATA6 regulates differentiation of distal lung epithelium. Development 2002;129(9):2233.

88. Koutsourakis M, et al: Branching and differentiation defects in pulmonary epithelium with elevated Gata6 expression. Mech Dev 2001;105(1-2):105.

89. Stanton BR, et al: Loss of N-myc function results in embryonic lethality and failure of the epithelial component of the embryo to develop. Genes Dev 1992;6(12A):2235.

90. Moens CB, et al: A targeted mutation reveals a role for N-myc in branching morphogenesis in the embryonic mouse lung. Genes Dev 1992;6(5):691.

91. Charron J, et al: Embryonic lethality in mice homozygous for a targeted disruption of the N-myc gene. Genes Dev 1992;6(12A):2248.

92. Moens CB, et al: Defects in heart and lung development in compound heterozygotes for two different targeted mutations at the N-myc locus. Development 1993;119(2):485.

93. Desai TJ, Cardoso WV: Growth factors in lung development and disease: friends or foe? Respir Res 2002;3(1):2.

94. Gonzalez AM, et al: Distribution of fibroblast growth factor (FGF)-2 and FGF receptor-1 messenger RNA expression and protein presence in the midtrimester human fetus. Pediatr Res 1996;39(3):375.

95. Han RN, et al: Expression of basic fibroblast growth factor and receptor: immunolocalization studies in developing rat fetal lung. Pediatr Res 1992;31(5):435.

96. Post M, et al: Keratinocyte growth factor and its receptor are involved in regulating early lung branching. Development 1996;122(10):3107.

97. Mason IJ, et al: FGF-7 (keratinocyte growth factor) expression during mouse development suggests roles in myogenesis, forebrain regionalisation and epithelial-mesenchymal interactions. Mech Dev 1994;45(1):15.

98. Shiratori M, et al: Keratinocyte growth factor and embryonic rat lung morphogenesis. Am J Respir Cell Mol Biol 1996;15(3):328.

99. Panos RJ, et al: Keratinocyte growth factor and hepatocyte growth factor/scatter factor are heparin-binding growth factors for alveolar type II cells in fibroblast-conditioned medium. J Clin Invest 1993;92(2):969.

100. Panos RJ, et al: Intratracheal instillation of keratinocyte growth factor decreases hyperoxia-induced mortality in rats. J Clin Invest 1995;96(4):2026.

101. Ulich TR, et al: Keratinocyte growth factor is a growth factor for type II pneumocytes in vivo. J Clin Invest 1994;93(3):1298.

102. Guo L, et al: Keratinocyte growth factor is required for hair development but not for wound healing. Genes Dev 1996;10(2):165.

103. Nogawa H, Ito T: Branching morphogenesis of embryonic mouse lung epithelium in mesenchyme-free culture. Development 1995;121(4):1015.

104. Orr-Urtreger A, et al: Developmental localization of the splicing alternatives of fibroblast growth factor receptor-2 (FGFR2). Dev Biol 1993;158(2):475.

105. Shannon JM, et al: Induction of alveolar type II cell differentiation in embryonic tracheal epithelium in mesenchyme-free culture. Development 1999;126(8):1675.

106. Colvin JS, et al: Lung hypoplasia and neonatal death in Fgf9-null mice identify this gene as an essential regulator of lung mesenchyme. Development 2001;128(11):2095.

107. Pelton RW, et al: Expression of transforming growth factor-beta 1, -beta 2, and -beta 3 mRNA and protein in the murine lung. Am J Respir Cell Mol Biol 1991;5(6):522.

108. Pelton RW, et al: Immunohistochemical localization of TGF beta 1, TGF beta 2, and TGF beta 3 in the mouse embryo: expression patterns suggest multiple roles during embryonic development. J Cell Biol 1991;115(4):1091.

109. Heine UI, et al: Colocalization of TGF-beta 1 and collagen I and III, fibronectin and glycosaminoglycans during lung branching morphogenesis. Development 1990;109(1):29.

110. Zhou L, et al: Arrested lung morphogenesis in transgenic mice bearing an SP-C-TGF-beta 1 chimeric gene. Dev Biol 1996;175(2):227.

111. Bragg AD, et al: Signaling to the epithelium is not sufficient to mediate all of the effects of transforming growth factor beta and bone morphogenetic protein 4 on murine embryonic lung development. Mech Dev 2001;109(1):13.

112. Serra R, Moses HL: pRb is necessary for inhibition of N-myc expression by TGF-beta 1 in embryonic lung organ cultures. Development 1995;121(9):3057.

113. Serra R, et al: TGF beta 1 inhibits branching morphogenesis and N-myc expression in lung bud organ cultures. Development 1994;120(8):2153.

114. Zeng X, et al: TGF-beta1 perturbs vascular development and inhibits epithelial differentiation in fetal lung in vivo. Dev Dyn 2001;221(3):289.

115. Wrana JL, et al: Mechanism of activation of the TGF-beta receptor. Nature 1994;370(6488):341.

116. Zhao J, et al: Abrogation of transforming growth factor-beta type II receptor stimulates embryonic mouse lung branching morphogenesis in culture. Dev Biol 1996;180(1):242.

117. Dickson MC, et al: Defective haematopoiesis and vasculogenesis in transforming growth factor-beta 1 knock out mice. Development 1995;121(6):1845.

118. Shull MM, et al: Targeted disruption of the mouse transforming growth factor-beta 1 gene results in multifocal inflammatory disease. Nature 1992;359(6397):693.

119. Kaartinen V, et al: Abnormal lung development and cleft palate in mice lacking TGF-beta 3 indicates defects of epithelial-mesenchymal interaction. Nat Genet 1995;11(4):415.

120. Sanford LP, et al: TGFbeta2 knockout mice have multiple developmental defects that are non-overlapping with other TGFbeta knockout phenotypes. Development 1997;124(13):2659.

121. Attisano L, et al: The Smads. Genome Biol 2001;2:8.

122. Dick A, et al: Expression of Smad1 and Smad2 during embryogenesis suggests a role in organ development. Dev Dyn 1998;211(4):293.

123. Zhao J, et al: Abrogation of Smad3 and Smad2 or of Smad4 gene expression positively regulates murine embryonic lung branching morphogenesis in culture. Dev Biol 1998;194(2):182.

124. Sunday ME: Pulmonary neuroendocrine cells and lung development. Endocr Pathol 1996;7(3):173.

125. Cutz E: Neuroendocrine cells of the lung: an overview of morphologic characteristics and development. Exp Lung Res 1982;3(3-4):185.

126. Casarosa S, et al: Mash1 regulates neurogenesis in the ventral telencephalon. Development 1999;126(3):525.

127. Borges M, et al: An achaete-scute homologue essential for neuroendocrine differentiation in the lung. Nature 1997;386(6627):852.

128. Ishibashi M, et al: Targeted disruption of mammalian hairy and Enhancer of split homolog-1 (HES-1) leads to up-regulation of neural helix-loop-helix factors, premature neurogenesis, and severe neural tube defects. Genes Dev 1995;9(24):3136.

129. Ito T, et al: Basic helix-loop-helix transcription factors regulate the neuroendocrine differentiation of fetal mouse pulmonary epithelium. Development 2000;127(18):3913.

130. Quaggin SE, et al: The basic-helix-loop-helix protein pod1 is critically important for kidney and lung organogenesis. Development 1999;126(24):5771.

131. Bohinski RJ, et al: The lung-specific surfactant protein B gene promoter is a target for thyroid transcription factor 1 and hepatocyte nuclear factor 3, indicating common factors for organ-specific gene expression along the foregut axis. Mol Cell Biol 1994;14(9):5671.

132. Bruno MD, et al: Lung cell-specific expression of the murine surfactant protein A (SP-A) gene is mediated by interactions between the SP-A promoter and thyroid transcription factor-1. J Biol Chem 1995;270(12):6531.

133. Margana RK, Boggaram V: Functional analysis of surfactant protein B (SP-B) promoter. Sp1, Sp3, TTF-1, and HNF-3alpha transcription factors are necessary for lung cell-specific activation of SP-B gene transcription. J Biol Chem 1997;272(5):3083.

134. Kelly SE, et al: Transcription of the lung-specific surfactant protein C gene is mediated by thyroid transcription factor 1. J Biol Chem 1996; 271(12):6881.

135. Glasser SW, et al: Human SP-C gene sequences that confer lung epithelium-specific expression in transgenic mice. Am J Physiol 2000;278(5):L933.

136. Toonen RF, et al: The lung enriched transcription factor TTF-1 and the ubiquitously expressed proteins Sp1 and Sp3 interact with elements located in the minimal promoter of the rat Clara cell secretory protein gene. Biochem J 1996;316(2):467.

137. Tichelaar JW, et al: HNF-3/forkhead homologue-4 (HFH-4) is expressed in ciliated epithelial cells in the developing mouse lung. J Histochem Cytochem 1999;47(6):823.

138. Bruno MD, et al: GATA-6 activates transcription of surfactant protein A. J Biol Chem 2000;275(2):1043.

139. Shaw-White JR, et al: GATA-6 activates transcription of thyroid transcription factor-1. J Biol Chem 1999;274(5):2658.

140. Liu C, et al: GATA-6 and thyroid transcription factor-1 directly interact and regulate surfactant protein-C gene expression. J Biol Chem 2002; 277(6):4519.

141. Bingle CD, et al: Role of hepatocyte nuclear factor-3 alpha and hepatocyte nuclear factor-3 beta in Clara cell secretory protein gene expression in the bronchiolar epithelium. Biochem J 1995;308(1):197.

142. Bingle CD, Gitlin JD: Identification of hepatocyte nuclear factor-3 binding sites in the Clara cell secretory protein gene. Biochem J 1993;295(1):227.

143. Ikeda K, et al: Hepatocyte nuclear factor 3 activates transcription of thyroid transcription factor 1 in respiratory epithelial cells. Mol Cell Biol 1996;16(7):3626.

144. Blatt EN, et al: Forkhead transcription factor HFH-4 expression is temporally related to ciliogenesis. Am J Respir Cell Mol Biol 1999;21(2):168.

145. Tichelaar JW, et al: HNF-3/forkhead homologue-4 influences lung morphogenesis and respiratory epithelial cell differentiation in vivo. Dev Biol 1999;213(2):405.

146. Brody SL, et al: Ciliogenesis and left-right axis defects in forkhead factor HFH-4-null mice. Am J Respir Cell Mol Biol 2000;23(1):45.

147. Bellusci S, et al: Evidence from normal expression and targeted misexpression that bone morphogenetic protein (Bmp-4) plays a role in mouse embryonic lung morphogenesis. Development 1996;122(6):1693.

148. Weaver M, et al: Bmp signaling regulates proximal-distal differentiation of endoderm in mouse lung development. Development 1999; 126(18):4005.

149. Shi W, et al: Gremlin negatively modulates BMP-4 induction of embryonic mouse lung branching morphogenesis. Am J Physiol 2001;280(5):L1030.

150. Lu MM, et al: The bone morphogenic protein antagonist gremlin regulates proximal-distal patterning of the lung. Dev Dyn 2001;222(4):667.

151. Betsholtz C, et al: Developmental roles of platelet-derived growth factors. Bioessays 2001;23(6):494.

152. Orr-Urtreger A, Lonai P: Platelet-derived growth factor-A and its receptor are expressed in separate, but adjacent cell layers of the mouse embryo. Development 1992;115(4):1045.

153. Bostrom H, et al: PDGF-A signaling is a critical event in lung alveolar myofibroblast development and alveogenesis. Cell 1996;85(6):863.

154. Lindahl P, et al: Alveogenesis failure in PDGF-A-deficient mice is coupled to lack of distal spreading of alveolar smooth muscle cell progenitors during lung development. Development 1997;124(20):3943.

155. Bostrom H, et al: PDGF-A/PDGF alpha-receptor signaling is required for lung growth and the formation of alveoli but not for early lung branching morphogenesis. Dev Dyn 2002;223(1):155.

156. Sun T, et al: A human YAC transgene rescues craniofacial and neural tube development in PDGFRalpha knockout mice and uncovers a role for PDGFRalpha in prenatal lung growth. Development 2000;127(21):4519.

157. Weinstein M, et al: FGFR-3 and FGFR-4 function cooperatively to direct alveogenesis in the murine lung. Development 1998;125(18):3615.

158. Wert SE, et al: Increased expression of thyroid transcription factor-1 (TTF-1) in respiratory epithelial cells inhibits alveolarization and causes pulmonary inflammation. Dev Biol 2002;242(2):75.

159. Massaro D, et al: Postnatal development of pulmonary alveoli: modulation in rats by thyroid hormones. Am J Physiol 1986;250(1):R51.

160. Massaro GD, Massaro D: Postnatal treatment with retinoic acid increases the number of pulmonary alveoli in rats. Am J Physiol 1996;270(2):L305.

161. Massaro GD, Massaro D: Retinoic acid treatment abrogates elastase-induced pulmonary emphysema in rats. Nat Med 1997;3(6):675.

162. Massaro GD, Massaro D: Retinoic acid treatment partially rescues failed septation in rats and in mice. Am J Physiol 2000;278(5):L955.

163. McGowan S, et al: Mice bearing deletions of retinoic acid receptors demonstrate reduced lung elastin and alveolar numbers. Am J Respir Cell Mol Biol 2000;23(2):162.

164. Massaro GD, et al: Retinoic acid receptor-beta: an endogenous inhibitor of the perinatal formation of pulmonary alveoli. Physiol Genomics 2000;4(1):51.

165. deMello DE, et al: Early fetal development of lung vasculature. Am J Respir Cell Mol Biol 1997;16(5):568.

166. Schachtner SK, et al: Qualitative and quantitative analysis of embryonic pulmonary vessel formation. Am J Respir Cell Mol Biol 2000;22(2):157.

167. Burri PH: Lung development and pulmonary angiogenesis. In Gaultier C, et al (eds): Lung Development. New York, Oxford University Press, 1999, p 122.

168. Bhatt AJ, et al: Expression of vascular endothelial growth factor and Flk-1 in developing and glucocorticoid-treated mouse lung. Pediatr Res 2000;47(5):606.

169. Healy AM, et al: VEGF is deposited in the subepithelial matrix at the leading edge of branching airways and stimulates neovascularization in the murine embryonic lung. Dev Dyn 2000;219(3):341.

170. Maisonpierre PC, et al: Angiopoietin-2, a natural antagonist for Tie2 that disrupts in vivo angiogenesis. Science 1997;277(5322):55.

171. Colen KL, et al: Vascular development in the mouse embryonic pancreas and lung. J Pediatr Surg 1999;34(5):781.

172. Hall SM, et al: Origin, differentiation, and maturation of human pulmonary veins. Am J Respir Cell Mol Biol 2002;26(3):333.

173. Dvorak HF, et al: Vascular permeability factor/vascular endothelial growth factor, microvascular hyperpermeability, and angiogenesis. Am J Pathol 1995;146(5):1029.

174. Carmeliet P, et al: Abnormal blood vessel development and lethality in embryos lacking a single VEGF allele. Nature 1996;380(6573):435.

175. Ferrara N, et al: Heterozygous embryonic lethality induced by targeted inactivation of the VEGF gene. Nature 1996;380(6573):439.

176. Monacci WT, et al: Expression of vascular permeability factor/vascular endothelial growth factor in normal rat tissues. Am J Physiol 1993;264(4):C995.

177. Breier G, et al: Expression of vascular endothelial growth factor during embryonic angiogenesis and endothelial cell differentiation. Development 1992;114(2):521.

178. Millauer B, et al: High affinity VEGF binding and developmental expression suggest Flk-1 as a major regulator of vasculogenesis and angiogenesis. Cell 1993;72(6):835.

179. Gebb SA, Shannon JM: Tissue interactions mediate early events in pulmonary vasculogenesis. Dev Dyn 2000;217(2):159.

180. Zeng X, et al: VEGF enhances pulmonary vasculogenesis and disrupts lung morphogenesis in vivo. Dev Dyn 1998;211(3):215.

181. Galambos C, et al: Defective pulmonary development in the absence of heparin-binding vascular endothelial growth factor isoforms. Am J Respir Cell Mol Biol 2002;27(2):194.

182. Mahlapuu M, et al: The forkhead transcription factor Foxf1 is required for differentiation of extra-embryonic and lateral plate mesoderm. Development 2001;128(2):155.

183. Peterson RS, et al: The winged helix transcriptional activator HFH-8 is expressed in the mesoderm of the primitive streak stage of mouse embryos and its cellular derivatives. Mech Dev 1997;69(1-2):53.

184. Kalinichenko VV, et al: Defects in pulmonary vasculature and perinatal lung hemorrhage in mice heterozygous null for the Forkhead Box f1 transcription factor. Dev Biol 2001;235(2):489.

Pierre M. Barker and Kevin W. Southern

80

Regulation of Liquid Secretion and Absorption by the Fetal and Neonatal Lung

The fetal lung is filled with liquid secreted by the developing lung epithelia. The rate and volume of liquid secreted into the fetal lung are calibrated to maintain lung volume at about functional residual capacity, and they are major determinants of normal lung growth. At birth, effective transition from placental to pulmonary gas exchange requires removal of liquid from the lung. The process of emptying the lung begins before birth, is augmented by labor, and is mostly complete after 2 hours of independent breathing. Liquid is removed from the lung lumen by a combination of mechanical drainage and liquid absorption across the lung epithelium (Fig. 80-1). The liquid absorption mechanism is switched on by the perinatal epinephrine surge associated with labor and delivery. This epinephrine responsiveness is absent in the immature fetal lung and is induced in the last half of gestation by the rise in active thyroid and steroid hormones in the fetal circulation. The increase in oxygen tension (Po_2) associated with the onset of air breathing at birth consolidates the switch to liquid absorption. Because the absorptive mechanism of the fetal lung develops in the latter part of gestation, infants who are born prematurely may have a restricted ability to clear fluid from their lungs.

DYNAMICS OF LUNG LIQUID FLOW BEFORE AND AFTER BIRTH

Lung Liquid Formation and Flow During Fetal Life

Because it is intuitive that the fetal lung lumen must be filled with liquid rather than air, early debate about the fetal lung revolved around the origins of this liquid. The preferred early hypothesis was that liquid was aspirated by fetal breathing movements into the lung from the amniotic cavity.[1] However, the proposed amniotic origin of lung liquid was disproved in the 1940s by Jost and Pollicard, who observed progressive lung distention in fetal rabbits whose tracheas had been ligated.[2] Further evidence of local production of fetal lung liquid came from the observation, in fetal sheep, that the ionic composition of fetal lung liquid differed from that of amniotic fluid (sodium [Na^+] and chloride [Cl^-] concentrations are lower in amniotic fluid, and potassium [K^+] is higher).[3,4] In addition, the observation that the Cl^- concentration of fetal lung liquid was higher that that of plasma or interstitial fluid[4] was the strongest early evidence that lung liquid may be actively secreted by the pulmonary epithelium.

Liquid Secretion

The source of lung liquid was subsequently shown to derive from an active secretory process by the epithelium lining the developing lung.[5] The rate of liquid secretion was measured in fetal guinea pig, goat, and sheep by collection of diverted tracheal fluid,[6,7] by tracheal flowmeter,[8] and by the indicator dilution method.[5,8-10] There is an apparent increase in the secretion rate in fetal sheep from approximately 1.5 mL/kg/hour at midgestation[11] to approximately 5 mL/kg/hour in late gestation.[12] The secreted liquid is then passively expelled into the trachea and into the oropharynx, where it is either swallowed or expelled into the amniotic cavity. The volume of liquid in the fetal lung lumen is regulated by the distending pressure of

approximately 2 mm Hg (relative to amniotic fluid),[13] generated by liquid secretion and resistance to liquid efflux through the fetal larynx.[14,15] The volume of liquid in the fetal lung increases with growth of the fetus and with the increasing alveolarization of the lung during gestation. In the latter part of gestation, the developing fetal sheep lung is distended to a volume (~30 mL/kg) that approximates functional residual capacity of a full-term newborn infant.[16] The volume to which the fetal lung is distended is apparently crucial for normal lung development. Experimental continuous intrauterine drainage of liquid from fetal sheep lungs resulted in lung hypoplasia, whereas overdistention of the fetal lung by tracheal ligation resulted in hyperplasia.[17-19]

Fetal Breathing Movements

Fetal breathing movements initiated by diaphragmatic contractions result in small oscillations of liquid flow (~0.5 mL) in the conducting airways.[20-22] Disruption of fetal breathing by phrenic nerve section or cervical cord lesions results in lung hypoplasia[23,24] through mechanisms that most likely are related to decreased fetal lung volume.[25] Although it is likely that these breathing movements are important for normal lung growth, they do not influence the rate of liquid secretion or the net movement of lung liquid out of the lung.

Airway Wall Contractions

Peristaltic contractions of the developing airways cause changes in local lung liquid flow and pressure that may also be important in lung development. Striking contractions of embryonic airways were first observed in chick embryos in the 1920s.[26] Studies on various animal models demonstrate that these contractions cause peristalsis of the airway similar to that seen in the gut. These peristaltic waves propagate distal movement of intraluminal liquid and cause expansion of the end-buds.[27] Smooth muscle contractions were inhibited by the calcium (Ca^{2+}) channel blocker nifedipine.[28] However, it is not clear whether the observed lung hypoplasia after nifedipine administration was the result of inhibition of peristalsis or whether liquid secretion was influenced by this intervention.

Surgical Intervention

Given that ligation of fetal airways promotes lung growth distal to that point, surgical obstruction of the fetal airway has evolved as a technique for prevention or correction of potential lung hypoplasia, particularly with lung anomalies associated with congenital diaphragmatic hernia. However, early enthusiasm for fetal surgery has been tempered by poor results.[29] The traditional hypothesis that lung hypoplasia results from compression by herniating abdominal viscera has been challenged[30] because pulmonary anomalies have been observed before herniation of abdominal contents into the chest.[31] The role of ion transport in the pathogenesis lung hypoplasia is not known.

Perinatal Changes in Lung Liquid Flow

At the time of birth, the newborn infant switches from placental to pulmonary gas exchange. This requires an abrupt replacement

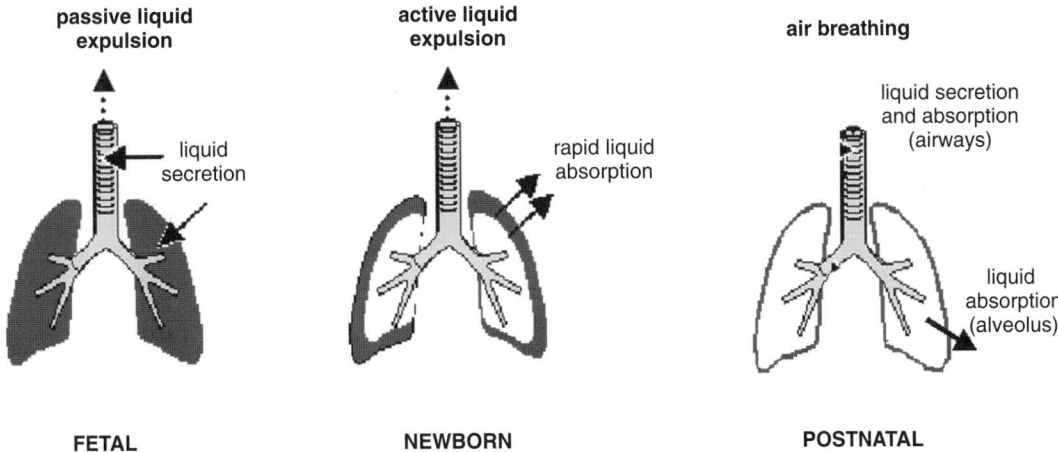

Figure 80–1. Fetal, neonatal, and postnatal phases of liquid flow across lung epithelia.

of the liquid in the lung lumen with air. Within a few hours, approximately 100 mL of fetal lung liquid contained in the human lung lumen must be cleared. This is achieved by the initiation of complex series of mechanical and ion transport events.

Decrease in Lung Liquid Volume Before Labor

Some investigators, working mainly with fetal rabbits and sheep, observed a decrease in both lung liquid volume and secretion rates toward the end of gestation.[6, 8, 12, 32] It is likely that mechanical forces (e.g., active fetal exhalation) may participate in some of the expulsion of liquid in the hours leading up to the onset of labor.[33]

Role of Labor

The finding that delivery by cesarean section (CS) slowed lung liquid clearance,[34] particularly when the procedure was undertaken before the onset of labor,[35] indicated that labor was in some way important to the removal of lung liquid. Rabbits that were born at term, either vaginally or by CS after the onset of labor, had less water in their lungs than did rabbits that were delivered operatively without prior labor (Fig. 80–2). This observation argued against the previously held notion that any significant amount of lung liquid is "squeezed" out of the lungs by thoracic compression during vaginal delivery. These data provided evidence that labor induces other (nonmechanical) mechanisms that must be responsible for lung liquid clearance before birth.

Fate of Lung Liquid During Labor and Delivery

Once labor is initiated, there is rapid removal of liquid from the lung caused by a reversal of the direction of liquid flow across the pulmonary epithelium.[12] The secretory process that dominates fetal life is abruptly switched, to allow absorption of liquid from the lung lumen into the fetal circulation.[12] It is now clear that active transcellular Na+ absorption drives liquid out of the lumen into the interstitial space (see later).[36] Most interstitial liquid moves into the fetal/newborn pulmonary circulation, and some drains via the lung lymphatics.[37] Starling forces that may assist liquid absorption (e.g., osmotic pressure and hydrostatic gradients between the lung interstitium and the lung lumen) do not change during labor, and they are not thought to play a role in removal of fetal lung liquid before birth.

Liquid Movement After Birth

After birth, there is an acceleration of active liquid absorption,[12] and most of the liquid is cleared from the full-term newborn lung

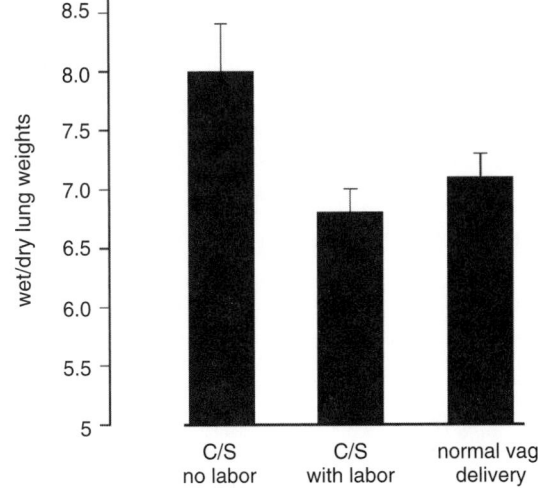

Figure 80–2. Effect of labor on lung water content (wet/dry weight) of newborn rabbit pups born after normal vaginal (vag.) delivery or by cesarean section (C/S). (Data from Bland RD, et al: Am J Obstet Gynecol *135*:364–37, 1979.)

within 2 hours of independent breathing.[38] Egan and co-workers noted a transient increase in solute permeability of the alveolar epithelium at the onset of breathing and speculated that this "window" of decreased paracellular resistance may assist with passive liquid absorption at birth.[39]

BASIC MECHANISMS OF TRANSEPITHELIAL ION TRANSPORT

The ion transport mechanisms located in the pulmonary epithelium drive the secretion and absorption of liquid into and out of the lumen of the fetal and newborn lung. Advances in understanding of perinatal lung liquid flow have derived from better characterization of the function, regulation, and molecular identity of these channels and transporters.

Boston, Humphreys, Olver, and Strang and their associates launched a series of studies in the 1960s and 1970s that described the flow of liquid from the pulmonary circulation to the lung lumen,[40, 41] characterized the barrier properties of the

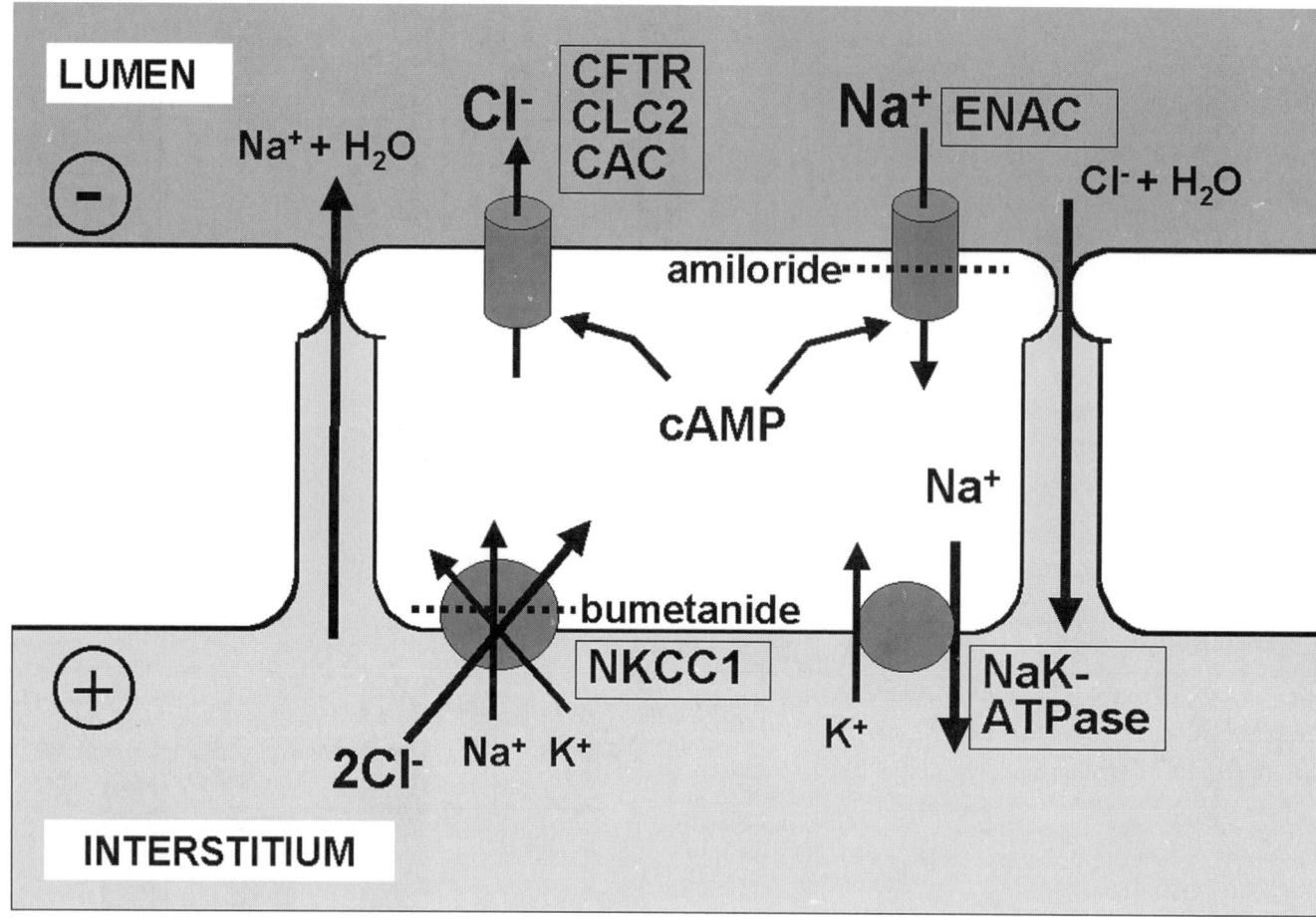

Figure 80–3. Arrangement of ion transporters and pumps in the lung epithelia of fetal lung. Amiloride is a specific inhibitor of the epithelial sodium (Na+) channel (ENAC), and bumetanide blocks Na+, potassium (K+), chloride (Cl-) co-transporter 1 (NKCC1). The *plus* and *minus* signs indicate polarity of the lumen with respect to the interstitium. CAC = calcium-activated channel; cAMP = cyclic adenosine monophosphate; CFTR = cystic fibrosis transmembrane conductance regulator; CLC2 = voltage-gated Cl- channel 2.

epithelium and endothelium,[11,42] and provided the first evidence of secondary active Cl- transport as the mechanism for lung liquid secretion by the fetal lung.[5] These studies showed that the alveolar epithelium was highly restrictive to macromolecules compared with the endothelium. This barrier property accounts for the virtual absence of protein in the fetal lung lumen, in contrast to the interstitium and circulation. Despite this oncotic gradient across the alveolar epithelium, lung liquid is secreted actively by transcellular Cl- transport. Workers from the same laboratory were the first to show that clearance of lung liquid at birth was also driven by an active ion transport process, namely, Na+ absorption.[36]

The basic configuration of ion transporters and channels follows a pattern that is similar to that found in other mammalian ion transporting epithelia. The electrochemical gradient for entry and exit of ions to and from the lung epithelial cells is established by Na+,K+-adenosine triphosphatase (ATPase) at the basolateral membrane. Activity of this transporter results in the low intracellular [Na+] that creates a gradient for Na+ to enter the cell through either the basolateral membrane (entraining Cl- as part of the secretory process) or through apical membrane (first step in the absorptive process). The main identified transporters and channels that result in liquid secretion and absorption are shown in Figure 80-3.

The molecular identities of the main transporters and pumps located on the interstitial facing membrane (Na+ pump, Na+,K+-ATPase, and Na+,K+,2Cl- co-transporter [NKCC1]) are known (see Fig. 80-3). Likewise, the principal Na+ channel on the luminal membrane (epithelial Na+ channel [ENaC]) has been cloned.[43] However, the identity of the principal mechanism responsible for fetal Cl- secretion across the lumen membrane is not known. Candidates for Cl- channels include the cystic fibrosis transmembrane conductance regulator (CFTR, cloned in 1989)[44] and the voltage-gated Cl- channels 2 and 3 (CLC2, CLC3, cloned in 1995),[45] all of which are expressed in the fetal lung.[46,47] There is strong functional evidence for a purinoceptor-Ca2+–activated Cl- channel in fetal lung epithelia,[48,49] but this channel has yet to be cloned.

Chloride Secretion

The "uphill" movement of Cl- from the interstitium to the lung lumen was shown by Olver and Strang[5] to be the driving force for fetal lung liquid secretion. Since then, the identity of the entry and exit steps for Cl- transit across the lung epithelium have been sought. From studies of other Cl--secreting mammalian epithelia, NaK2Cl (NKCC) co-transporter family members were likely candidates for the Cl- entry mechanism through the basolateral membrane. On the apical membrane, it is assumed that Cl^- channels, exchangers, or co-transporters must be responsible for exit of Cl^- into the lumen.

Sodium, Potassium, Chloride Co-transporter

In fetal sheep and guinea pig lung, addition of the loop diuretic bumetanide or furosemide (specific NKCC inhibitors) to fetal lung liquid caused slowing of lung liquid secretion or liquid absorption.[50,51] Loop diuretics also inhibited liquid secretion in vitro by distal lung explants from fetal rat lung,[52,53] and they decreased basal short circuit current by excised fetal canine or rabbit trachea.[54,55] Of the two NKCC isoforms that have been described, mRNA of NKCC1 but not NKCC2 is abundantly expressed in epithelia from all regions of the late-gestation fetal mouse lung.[56] Postnatally, there is a significant decrease in NKCC1 expression by mouse tracheal epithelia.[57] The likely existence of non-NKCC Cl^- entry mechanisms is suggested by the minimal inhibition by bumetanide of basal and cyclic adenosine monophosphate (cAMP)-induced Cl^- secretion across fetal human and mouse distal lung epithelium[48,58] and apparently normal survival and lung health in NKCC1 "knock-out" (NKCC–/–) mice.[56,57,59] Studies of fetal NKCC1–/– did show that maximal (cAMP-mediated) but not basal Cl^- secretion was compromised by NKCC1 deletion. Studies of postnatal NKCC1–/– mice showed that NKCC1-mediated Cl^- secretion by airway epithelium wanes after birth, matching the apparent decrease in NKCC mRNA expression in postnatal airways.[57] The molecular expression of other potential Cl^- entry mechanisms (e.g., Cl^-/bicarbonate exchanger) in fetal lung epithelia have not been reported.

Cystic Fibrosis Transmembrane Conductance Regulator

Studies of postnatal cystic fibrosis (CF) epithelia indicate that CFTR provides a critical apical membrane conduit for Cl^- secretion[60] and is an important regulator of Na^+ transport in lung epithelia after birth.[61] However, non-CFTR mechanisms must exist for liquid secretion by fetal lung epithelia, because the lungs of fetuses with CF are normally developed,[62] and explants of CF-affected human fetal lung are inflated with secreted liquid.[63]

A role for CFTR in fetal lung liquid secretion is suggested by intense expression of CFTR mRNA in all regions of first trimester human fetal lung, with less intense expression in the alveolar and large airway epithelia during the second and third trimesters.[64] In the postnatal lung, CFTR mRNA signal is localized to small airways and submucosal gland epithelium and is not detected in the alveolar epithelium.[65]

Lungs from CFTR–/– mouse fetuses are normally inflated with liquid, and airway explants from these fetuses have basal and cAMP-stimulated anion secretion that is indistinguishable from wild-type littermate controls.[66] There is also evidence of liquid secretion by lung epithelia of human fetuses with CF. However, exposure to cAMP causes no change in liquid volume in CF fetal lung explants, whereas additional liquid secretion was induced by cAMP in normal fetal lung tissue.[63] These studies suggest that CFTR has some role in, but is not required for, basal fetal lung liquid secretion.

Other Fetal Chloride Channels

The identity of non-CFTR anion secretory paths in fetal lung epithelia remains elusive. Purinoceptor-activated Cl^- secretion has been observed in CFTR–/– fetal mouse lung[66] and in wild-type fetal rat and fetal human lung epithelia.[48,49] The molecular identity of the purinoceptor-activated Cl^- channel is not known. The developmental expression pattern of CLC2 and CLC3 indicates a possible role for these channels in fetal lung liquid secretion.[47] However, the absence of functional studies in fetal lung tissues or a knock-out model deficient in CLC2 or CLC3 makes the significance of these channels difficult to determine at present.

Role of Sodium Absorption in Perinatal Lung Liquid Clearance

The observation that spontaneous or epinephrine-induced absorption of fetal lung liquid was associated with a large increase in net Na^+ transport out of the lumen and could be blocked by amiloride, a specific Na^+ channel blocker (Fig. 80–4), provided the first conclusive evidence that perinatal liquid absorption is mediated through Na^+ transport.[36] Some Na^+ and cation channels have been identified by electrophysiologic means (patch clamp or Ussing chamber studies) on the apical membrane of fetal distal lung epithelial (FDLE) cells isolated from rodents.[67] However, the observation that all activated and spontaneous liquid absorption could be inhibited by mixing the Na^+ channel blocker amiloride into fetal lung liquid demonstrated a critical role for amiloride-sensitive Na^+ transport in perinatal lung liquid clearance. This finding was strengthened by the observation that amiloride instilled into the trachea of the newborn guinea pig impaired lung water clearance in a dose-dependent manner,[68] and it was later confirmed by ENaC knock-out murine studies (see later).[69] The roles of the high-energy Na^+,K^+-ATPase pump on the basolateral membrane and ENaC on the apical membrane have been extensively studied since the molecular identity of these genes became known.[43,70]

Na+,K+-Adenosine Triphosphatase

Evidence that labor was also crucial for the activation of the lung epithelial Na^+,K^+-ATPase pump came from measurements of the ouabain-sensitive uptake of rubidium-86 ($^{86}Rb^+$, a surrogate for K^+ uptake) in alveolar Type II cells freshly isolated from newborn rabbit pups. These studies demonstrated that labor was associated with a three- to fourfold increase in pump activity in fetal alveolar Type II cells.[71,72] In rat and mouse whole lung, expression of $\alpha 1$ and $\beta 1$ subunits increases from low levels in early fetal life to a peak around the time of birth.[73,74] Fetal $\alpha 1$ subunit mRNA is expressed in both epithelium and endothelium, whereas $\beta 1$ subunit expression is localized to epithelium only. By the end of the first week of life, epithelial expression of $\alpha 1$ and $\beta 1$ subunit mRNA is localized to small airways and the basolateral surface of alveolar Type II but not Type 1 cells.[74,75]

Epithelial Sodium Channel

ENaC subunit mRNA expression has been studied extensively in developing human and rodent lung epithelia. In both rat and mouse whole lung, an abrupt increase in αENaC mRNA expression in late gestation reaches levels seen in the adult lung shortly after birth.[76,77] In mouse lung, there is a similar increase in expression of γENaC and a more gradual increase in βENaC that peaks in adult lung (Fig. 80–5). Expression of γENaC parallels that of αENaC, with intense expression of subunit mRNA in all regions of the fetal lung, whereas βENaC expression in fetal and early postnatal lung is restricted to the airway epithelium.[76] Studies in guinea pig showed that both αENaC mRNA expression and the sensitivity of lung liquid clearance to amiloride and to β-adrenoceptor blockade were highest shortly after birth, and they declined in parallel with endogenous plasma epinephrine concentration,[78] findings providing further support for the key role of β-adrenoceptor activation of Na^+ channels at birth. Immunocytochemical studies of human fetal lung surprisingly showed significant αENaC protein expression in early mid-trimester fetal lung, at a time when the fetal lung is not thought to be capable of significant Na^+ transport.[79] Whereas the function or location of this protein within the cell is not known, it is possible that there is a discrepancy between developmental ENaC expression in human and rodent lung.

Other Sodium Channels

Other putative amiloride-sensitive Na^+-permeable channels in fetal lung have been described that may contribute to the driving

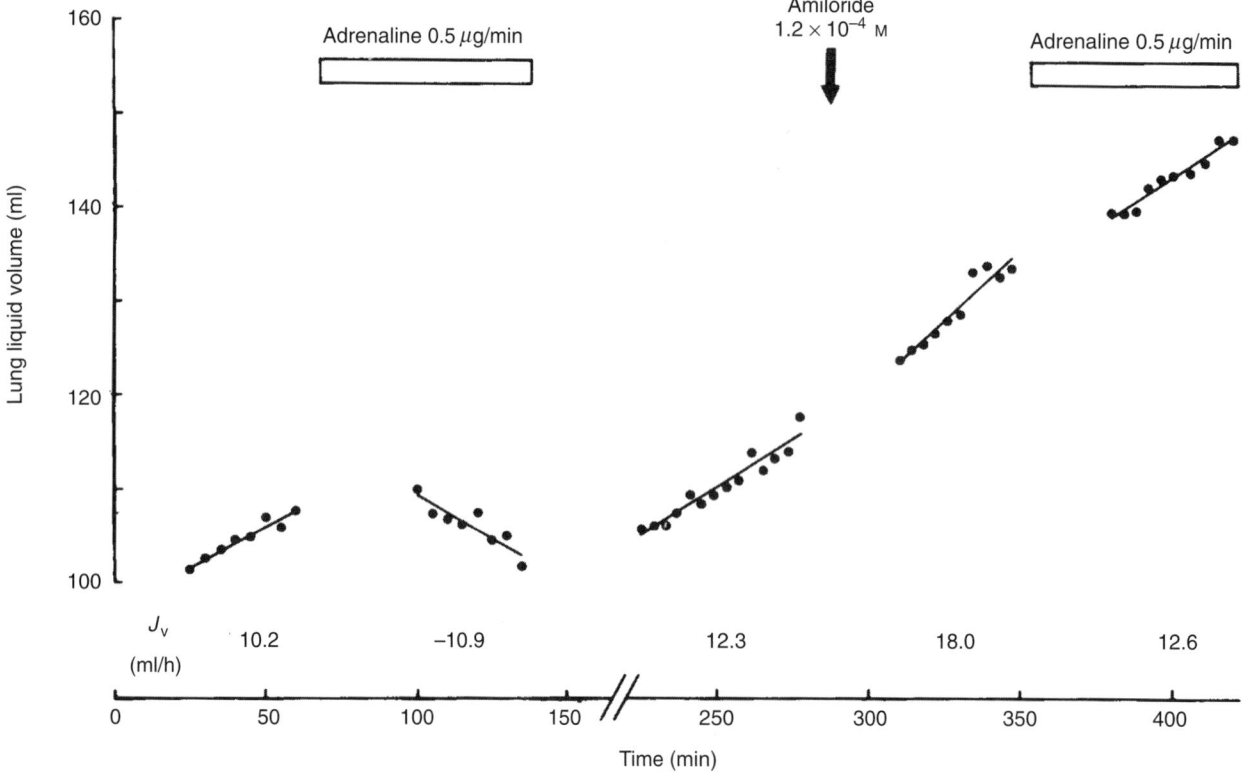

Figure 80–4. Effect of epinephrine (adrenaline) infusion and topical amiloride on cumulative lung volume across the lung epithelium of a near-term fetal sheep. At the start of the study, volume increases because of liquid secretion (J_v 10.2 mL/hour) Epinephrine infusion abruptly causes a decrease in lung volume, reversing the direction of flow (J_v −10.9 mL/hour) from secretion to absorption. Secretion is restored when the epinephrine infusion is discontinued. Addition of the sodium channel blocker amiloride to lung liquid prevents liquid absorption when the epinephrine infusion is restarted. (From Olver RE, et al: J Physiol [Lond] *376*:321–340, 1986.)

force for lung liquid clearance. These include certain amiloride-sensitive poorly/nonselective cation channels: G-protein-regulated,[80] β-adrenoceptor agonist/Ca^{2+}–activated,[81] and cyclic nucleotide-gated channels.[82] According to at least one school of thought,[83] the β-adrenoceptor responsive, nonselective channel may be a multimer of αENaC subunits, and the role of β and γ subunits may be to confer selectivity on the channel. An additional pathway for Na^+ absorption is Na^+,glucose co-transport, which has been reported in fetal sheep lung epithelia.[84]

Knock-out Models of Sodium Transport

Certain knock-out and other transgenic mouse models were used to explore the role of ion transport in the perinatal regulation of lung liquid flow. Knock-out mice for all three ENaC subunits were reported,[69, 85, 86] and additional ENaC mutants were studied.[87,88] The most striking finding was that mutant newborns lacking the aENaC gene were unable to clear lung liquid from the alveolar spaces after birth (Fig. 80-6). These mice were readily identifiable compared with their unaffected littermates by increased work of breathing, failure to feed, and failure to move around. Mice with γENaC or βENaC null mutations had delayed liquid clearance, but they had near normal lung water content 12 hours after birth. All subunit mutations resulted in severe hyperkalemia, which was the most likely cause of death in the early neonatal period. αENaC null mice that were "rescued" with an αENaC transgene were able to clear lung liquid in the newborn period at near-normal rates with approximately 50% Na^+ channel activity.[88] These studies indicate that ENaC function is a critical requirement for clearance of neonatal lung liquid in the new-

born period and suggest that the αENaC subunit is the core, rate-limiting part of the Na^+ channel in lung epithelia. Evidently, neonatal and postnatal lung liquid clearance can be sustained in the murine model with approximately 50% normal Na^+ channel activity.

HORMONAL REGULATION OF ION AND LIQUID TRANSPORT

Cyclic Adenosine Monophosphate–Mediated Liquid Transport

Although cAMP stimulates liquid and Cl⁻ secretion by both proximal and distal regions of the cultured immature human fetal lung,[48, 63] its net effect in late gestation is the opposite, namely, the induction of liquid absorption. Birth is known to be associated with a surge in fetal catecholamine secretion.[89] The link between β-adrenergic stimulation and lung liquid clearance was made in 1978 by Walters and Olver,[90] who discovered that epinephrine and isoproterenol, but not norepinephrine, caused the rapid absorption of lung liquid by late-gestation fetal sheep lungs, and the absorptive response could be inhibited by prior treatment with propranolol. In addition to effects on liquid secretion and lung water, β-adrenoceptor agonists caused release of surfactant,[91, 92] and the two physiologic processes combined to improve early neonatal lung aeration and gas exchange.[93, 94]

These observations were subsequently extended[12] to demonstrate that, at any particular stage of gestation, a log-linear relationship exists between fetal plasma epinephrine concentration

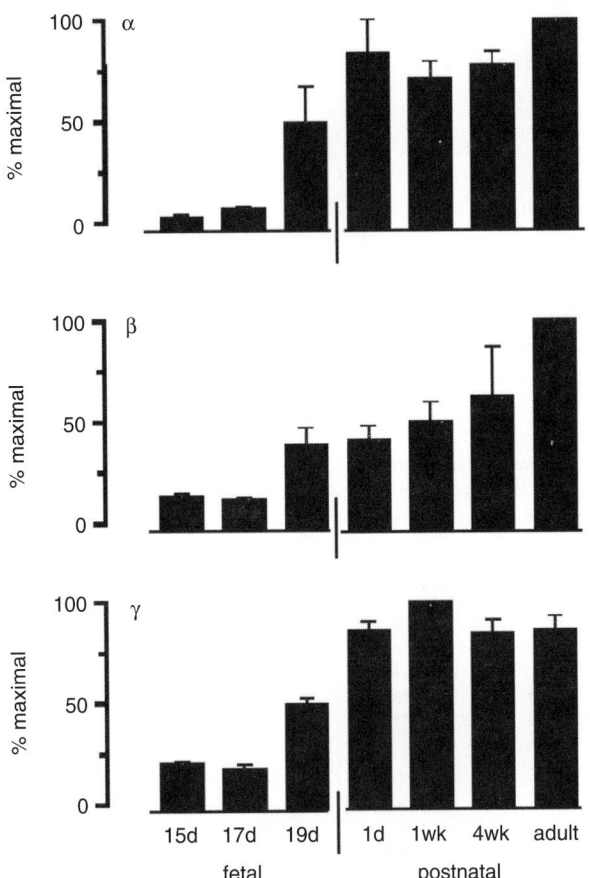

Figure 80–5. α, β, and γ epithelial sodium channel subunit mRNA expression in fetal (term = 19 days) and postnatal whole mouse lung. (From Talbot CL, et al: Am J Respir Cell Mol Biol 1999;20:398–406.)

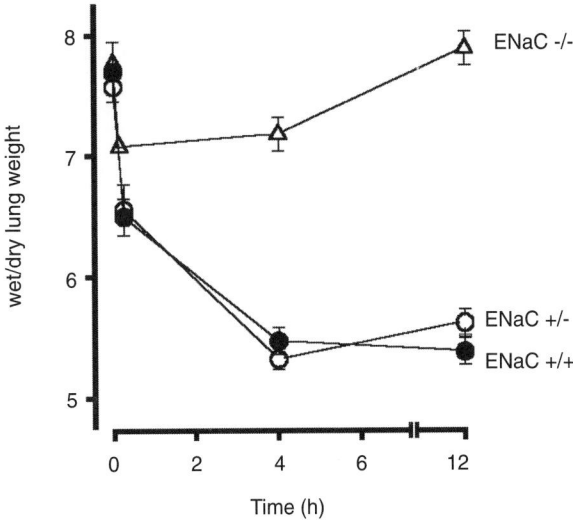

Figure 80–6. Lung water content (wet/dry lung weight) before (0 hour) and after birth (15 minutes, 4 hours, 12 hours) in α–epithelial sodium channel (αENaC) knock-out mice (αENaC -/-) and littermate controls (αENaC +/- and +/+). (From Hummler E, et al: Nat Genet 1996;12:325–328.)

Thyroid and Steroid Hormones

The role of thyroid and glucocorticoid hormones in the maturation of the absorptive response to epinephrine is evident from a series of experiments by Barker and co-workers, whose initial studies showed a profound blunting of the response to epinephrine (and db-cAMP) in thyroidectomized fetal lambs,[100] that was reversed by infusion of triiodothyronine (T_3) alone.[101] Neither T_3 nor hydrocortisone was capable of advancing maturation of the epinephrine response in normal fetuses with intact thyroid glands when they were given separately, but a powerful synergistic effect was observed when they were given concurrently (Fig. 80–8).[102] In thyroidectomized fetal lambs, the response to epinephrine was detectable within 2 hours of the start of infusion of the hormone combination. This induction of epinephrine-sensitive liquid absorption was lost within 24 hours of cessation of hormone administration.[103] These data, together with the observation[104] that T_3 and betamethasone have an additive effect in up-regulating fetal rat lung surfactant synthesis *in vivo*, emphasize the high degree of coordination of development of the lung liquid clearance and surfactant systems for efficient lung adaptation at birth.

The observation[105] that the rise in αENaC expression parallels plasma cortisol (but not T_3) in the late-gestation and newborn guinea pig, and can be blocked by metyrapone after delivery by CS, underscores the pivotal role of this hormone in the regulation of ENaC near term. Tchepichev and colleagues[77] demonstrated that prenatal steroids, but not thyroid hormones, could advance timing of the increase in αENaC mRNA in fetal rat lung, but neither hormone had any effect on expression of βENaC or γENaC subunit mRNA expression. Champigny and associates also reported no effect of thyroid hormones on ENaC mRNA expression, but they did report a potentiation by thyroid hormones of the steroid effect on Na^+ currents in rat alveolar epithelial cells.[106] Otulakowski and colleagues subsequently identified putative binding sites for thyroid and glucocorticoid receptors in the promoter region of αEnaC,[107] and although T_3 alone had no effect on reporter gene activity, it potentiated gene stimulation by steroid hormones.

A similar pattern of regulation has been reported for the subunits of Na^+,K^+-ATPase. Studies of 18-day rat fetal distal lung

and the degree of inhibition of secretion or absorption of liquid. The threshold for absorption falls in late gestation to reach an epinephrine level of 0.12 nmol/mL at term. During spontaneous labor, the relationship between endogenous fetal plasma epinephrine and the rate of liquid absorption is similar to that obtained by epinephrine infusion. Classically, β-adrenoreceptor agonists act via the cAMP/PKA (prekallikrein activator) signaling pathway, and, as predicted, the addition of a lipid-soluble analogue of cAMP, dibutyryl cAMP (db-cAMP), can mimic the effect of epinephrine in the mature fetal lamb.[95] The finding that the response to db-cAMP had a similar gestation dependence indicates that the rate-limiting step involved post-cAMP regulation of Na^+ transport, rather than changes at the β-receptor.

Because cAMP mediates both liquid secretion and liquid absorption in the fetal lung, the potential exists for an epinephrine surge to cause inappropriate lung liquid secretion in neonates born very prematurely. In explants of human fetal lung, cAMP caused a striking increase in liquid volume (Fig. 80-7A). This effect was attenuated by pretreatment of explants with thyroid and steroid hormones (see Fig. 80-7B). The maturational effect of these hormones on liquid secretion and absorption is discussed later.

Another hormone that increases cellular cAMP, arginine vasopressin, rises during labor. Although it can be shown to inhibit lung liquid secretion,[96,97] probably acting via the V_1 receptor and protein kinase C,[98] its effect is weaker than that of epinephrine, and its role is uncertain. It has been suggested that arginine vasopressin may provide back-up for the β-adrenoceptor–dependent pathway and may explain why β-adrenoceptor blockade fails to prevent lung liquid absorption during labor.[99]

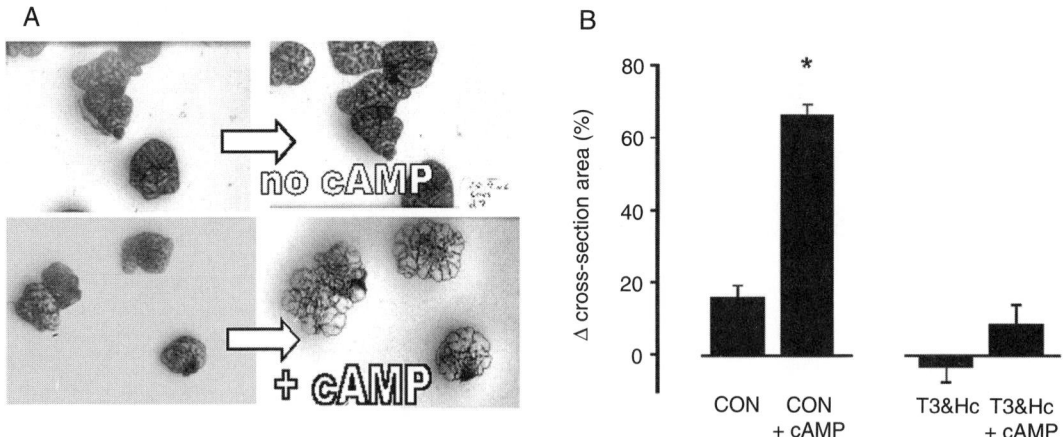

Figure 80–7. These 20-week human fetal lung explants expanded with liquid when they were exposed for 24 hours to 10^{-4} mol chlorophenylthio-cyclic adenosine monophosphate (cAMP) (**A**). This increase in diameter was attenuated in explants preincubated for 48 hours with 10^{-9} mol triiodothyronine (T_3) and 10^{-6} mol hydrocortisone (Hc) (**B**). CON = control.

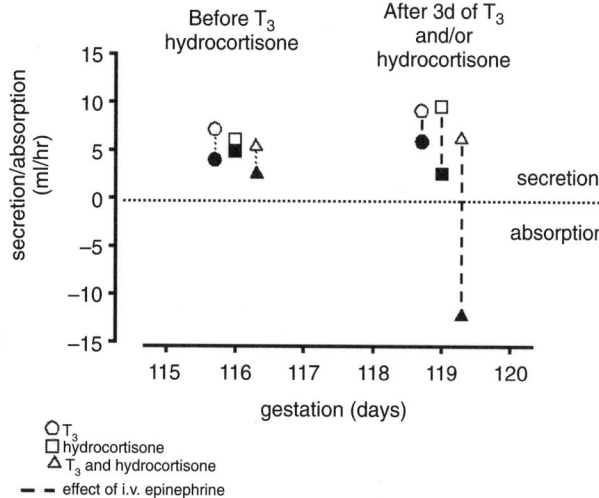

Figure 80–8. Effect of thyroid and steroid hormone on basal secretion (*open symbols*) and the ability of immature fetal sheep (term = 145 days) to respond to epinephrine infusion (*closed symbols*). Thyroid (triiodothyronine [T_3]) and steroid hormone exposure did not affect basal secretion rates. Only fetuses that had been treated with thyroid *and* steroid hormone for 3 days were able to absorb lung liquid during epinephrine infusion. (From Barker PM, et al: Pediatr Res 1990;27:588–591.)

epithelial (FDLE) cells treated with dexamethasone showed a threefold increase in $\alpha1$ and $\beta1$ mRNA expression.[108] Studies of postnatal alveolar cells showed similar effects of steroid hormones on Na^+,K^+-ATPase activity. In addition, there is a large body of evidence in postnatal alveolar cell studies that activity of Na^+,K^+-ATPase can be up-regulated by intracellular cAMP.[109, 110] The similarity of hormonal regulation of ENaC and Na^+,K^+-ATPase implies a coordinated increase in activity of the two principal mechanisms that underlie the perinatal absorptive response.

REGULATION OF ION TRANSPORT BY OXYGEN

O_2 appears to be a particularly important factor in maintaining the liquid absorptive response after birth. The onset of breathing results in a sharp increase in alveolar Po_2 from the fetal level of 23 to 25 mm Hg to about 100 mm Hg postnatally. The potential

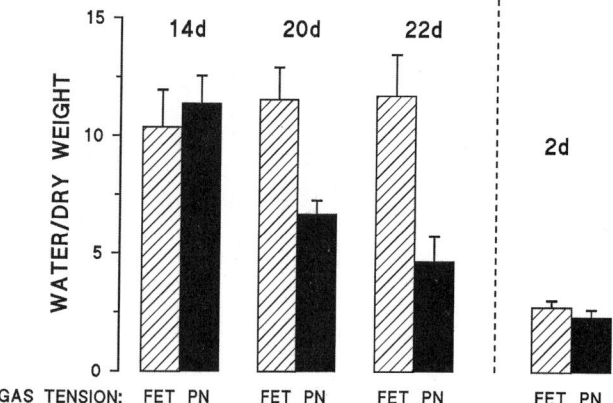

Figure 80–9. Effect of fetal (FET, ambient O_2 of 3%) or postnatal (PN, ambient O_2 of 21%) conditions on liquid volume of distal lung explants derived from fetal mouse lung. (Data from Barker PM, Gatzy JT: Am J Physiol 265:L512–L517, 1993.)

for this change in ambient O_2 to switch the fetal lung from a secretory to an absorptive state was first shown by Barker and Gatzy[111] in studies of fetal rat distal lung explants. A shift from fetal Po_2 (~25 mm Hg) to room air (~150 mm Hg) inhibited liquid secretion (reduction in lung water/dry weight ratios and in the number and size of liquid-filled cysts) by fetal lung explants in late-gestation lung explants, whereas there was no inhibition of liquid secretion by high Po_2 at very early gestations (Fig. 80–9). By contrast, no liquid secretion was induced in postnatal explants with exposure to fetal gas concentrations, a finding suggesting that the switch to liquid absorption may be irreversible 2 days after birth. The effect of O_2 on liquid secretion could be induced in immature explants by co-culture in thyroid and steroid hormones. These studies further demonstrated a crucial role of thyroid and steroid hormones in priming the distal lung epithelium to respond to triggers (epinephrine and O_2) that switch transepithelial liquid flow from secretion to absorption at birth.

Subsequently, studies with rat FDLE monolayers showed that the increase in Na^+ transport induced by raising Po_2 from 30 to 150 mm Hg was accompanied by an increase in ENaC mRNA expression.[112] This shift in Po_2 was accompanied by a temporary fall in epithelial resistance lasting several hours, consistent with the increase in solute permeability noted by Egan and co-workers[39] at the onset of breathing *in vivo* and that may assist passive liquid absorption. Vivona and co-workers[113] showed, in adult rats, that hypoxia decreased alveolar liquid clearance, an effect that was independent of *ENaC* and Na$^+$,K$^+$-ATPase subunit expression. These studies indicate that the mechanisms of postnatal O$_2$-induced neonatal alveolar Na$^+$ and liquid transport include posttranscriptional regulation of ENaC and may be reversible.

Further experiments were undertaken in mature rat FDLE cells to determine how the effects of shifting Po$_2$ from fetal to neonatal levels and the action of hormones are integrated to control lung liquid transport.[114] In these studies, glucocorticoid and thyroid hormones up-regulated Na$^+$ transport and up-regulated β-agonist–induced apical Na$^+$ conductance (G$_{Na}$) independently of ambient Po$_2$. In contrast, a shift to neonatal Po$_2$ was a prerequisite for hormonal up-regulation of Na$^+$,K$^+$-ATPase. These findings contrasted with the reported effects of thyroid hormones and steroids on immature fetal sheep lung, which were restricted to induction of β-agonist–responsive liquid absorption, with no effect on basal secretion rates.[102] Postnatally, steroids and Po$_2$ also have an additive effect in up-regulating expression of ENaC-like Na$^+$ channels in Type II alveolar cells.[115]

The promoter region of α-rENaC contains a consensus nuclear factor-κB (NF-κB) binding element. Further experiments in rat FDLE cells[116] showed that a rise in Po$_2$ to 150 mm Hg induced this redox-sensitive transcription factor, and blocking NF-κB activation reduced the O$_2$-evoked rise in G$_{Na}$.[117] These findings could be interpreted as indicating that Po$_2$ activation of NF-κB up-regulated the expression of ENaC, thus increasing Na$^+$ transport at the onset of breathing. However, subsequent experiments using FDLE monolayers[118,119] demonstrated that a shift from fetal (23 mm Hg) to postnatal (100 mm Hg) alveolar Po$_2$, which induces a maximal Na$^+$ response, resulted in an immediate increase in NF-κB expression and a detectable increase in Na$^+$ pump capacity within 6 hours, whereas activation of the αENaC promoter was not seen until after 24 hours, reaching a maximum (together with G$_{Na}$) at 48 hours.

It therefore appears that the early increase in fluid absorptive capacity in response to the rise in alveolar Po$_2$ at birth is primarily the result of an increase in Na$^+$,K$^+$-ATPase pump capacity, and the increase in G$_{Na}$ may be secondary to this increase in Na$^+$ transport, not its cause. Both components of the response are enhanced by glucocorticoid and thyroid hormones, which are also required for β-adrenoceptor–mediated control of G$_{Na}$. This discrepancy between the effects of these hormones in rat versus sheep studies raises the possibility that thyroid and steroid hormones may inhibit basal secretion rates or increase G$_{Na}$ in late, but not early, gestation. The discrepancy in the time course of activation NF-κB and the rise in αENaC expression indicates that activation of the αENaC promoter requires additional transcription factors.

LUNG LIQUID AND ION TRANSPORT IN NEONATAL RESPIRATORY DISEASE

This section reviews the evidence that inefficient lung water clearance can result in neonatal lung disease and discusses the contribution of abnormal airway ion transport.

Lung Liquid

Animal studies show a clear correlation between intraluminal liquid volume and respiratory function at birth. Berger and colleagues[120] examined the effect of residual lung liquid volume at birth on gas exchange in lambs delivered by CS near term. Animals that had approximately 45% lung liquid volume removed just before delivery had significantly better respiratory function compared with those delivered without liquid removal. The first clinical evidence that lung liquid may play a role in

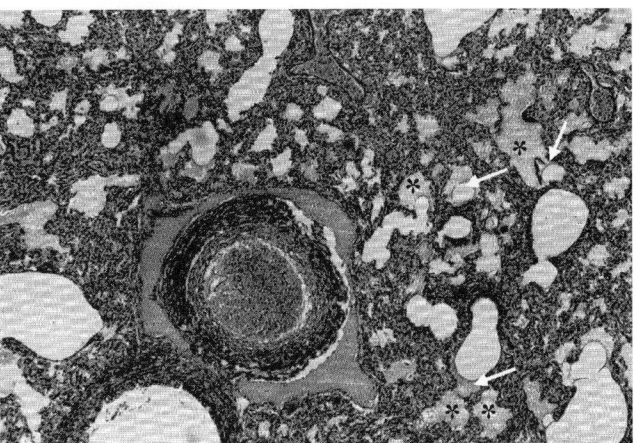

Figure 80–10. Photomicrograph of a lung from a 1300-g infant who died of respiratory distress syndrome at 8 hours without mechanical ventilation. The *arrows* show meniscus of liquid (*asterisk*) contained inside the alveoli. (From DeSa DJ: J Pathol 97:469–478, 1969.)

neonatal respiratory disease came from an analysis by DeSa of postmortem lung findings after perinatal death.[121] Infants who died of idiopathic respiratory distress syndrome (RDS) had significantly higher lung liquid content (determined as the percentage of wet weight of the lung) compared with infants who died of other, nonrespiratory causes.[122] These findings were supported by other evidence of lung liquid excess on histologic examination after RDS (Fig. 80–10).[121]

In an early review, Bland identified certain factors that may predispose the newborn preterm infant to pulmonary edema,[123] as follows:

1. Persistent pulmonary hypertension is more common in this group of infants, particularly if they experience hypoxia or patent ductus arteriosus.
2. A large transpulmonary pressure that drives fluid into the alveolar compartment may develop in areas of the lung with surfactant deficiency. The advent of artificial surfactant therapy has significantly decreased the incidence of RDS, and some of its effect may result from decreased surface tension and improved gas exchange in areas of the preterm lung that are incompletely emptied of alveolar liquid at birth.[124]
3. Mechanical ventilation likely disrupts the epithelial barrier and allows entry to the alveolar space of proteins that, in turn, may increase intra-alveolar fluid.
4. High inspired O$_2$ releases toxic metabolites that may interfere with essential cellular functions, including ion transport.

Against this background of susceptibility to pulmonary edema, a major defense against alveolar flooding, ion transport, is almost certainly incompletely developed in infants born very prematurely.[125]

The correlation between preterm delivery and respiratory distress is clear; however, some clinical studies, both prospective and retrospective, also demonstrated a link between mode of delivery and respiratory condition in the neonate.[126-128] Elective CS without labor is associated with a small but significant increased risk of RDS. This risk is exacerbated by delivery even a couple of weeks before term.[129]

The condition of transient tachypnea of the newborn (TTN) is probably the best-described consequence of inadequate neonatal lung liquid clearance. This self-limiting disease, characterized by an increase in respiratory rate, occurs more frequently in infants delivered by elective CS and is thought to result from delayed activation of liquid clearance in infants not subjected to the stress of labor.[130, 131] These clinical data are consistent with animal studies demonstrating the importance of gestation and labor in perinatal lung water clearance and successful adaptation to air breathing.

Airway Ion Transport Studies

Some investigators have used nasal electrical potential difference (PD) to measure ion transport directly across the upper airway *in vivo*. Nasal PD measures the electrical potential generated by active transport of charged ions (Cl⁻ and Na⁺) across the nasal membrane. The use of nasal PD to infer patterns of ion transport in the lower airways and alveoli has been validated by measurement of similar ion transport patterns in nasal and lower bronchial epithelia for both normal subjects and and those with CF.[132, 133] Furthermore, nasal PD can predict who will be susceptible to high-altitude pulmonary edema.[134] Gowen and colleagues reported that nasal PD could distinguish newborn infants with CF from healthy neonates and those with non-CF respiratory disease.[135] This test also detected ion transport differences that reflected the mode of delivery. Nasal PD was significantly higher in infants born by elective CS compared with those born normally or by CS after labor. Infants with TTN had the highest nasal PD, but they also had decreased amiloride-sensitive Na⁺ transport compared with babies who did not have TTN.[136] These preliminary studies support the notion that TTN may result in persistence of a fetal ion transport phenotype after birth.

In a more recent study, these investigators examined the relationship between airway ion transport at birth and development of RDS in infants at or less than 30 weeks' gestational age.[137] The RDS group had significantly lower maximal PDs and less inhibition after amiloride perfusion (Fig. 80–11), a finding suggesting reduced ENaC-mediated Na⁺ absorption. However, this group demonstrated a close correlation between maximal PD and birth weight, and the lower birth weight of the RDS group could represent a significant confounding variable. Although more studies are needed in this area, the available evidence supports an etiologic role for immature ion transport processes in the evolution of acute and possibly chronic lung disease (CLD) in preterm infants.

Therapeutic Considerations

Our understanding of the role of labor in clearing fetal liquid from the perinatal lung is supported by clinical studies that show a protective effect of labor on subsequent respiratory outcome. Drugs that augment the switch from liquid secretion to liquid absorption at birth are candidates for novel therapies to treat lung disease associated with premature birth. Possible strategies include inhibition of Cl⁻ secretion and augmenting of Na⁺ transport across respiratory epithelia.

Effect of Labor

Respiratory morbidity of both term and preterm infants is related to mode of delivery. In term infants born to mothers undergoing repeat CS, there was a higher incidence of TTN after birth without a trial of labor (6%) compared with those born with a trial of labor (3%). The TTN rate in infants who had a trial of labor was similar to that after routine vaginal births.[138] In both preterm and term infants, the rates of all respiratory problems were significantly higher in infants born by CS without labor compared with those born by either route with labor.[139]

β-Adrenergic Stimulation

In term infants undergoing CS without labor, there was a significant improvement in dynamic lung compliance and a decrease in respiratory rate in infants whose mothers had

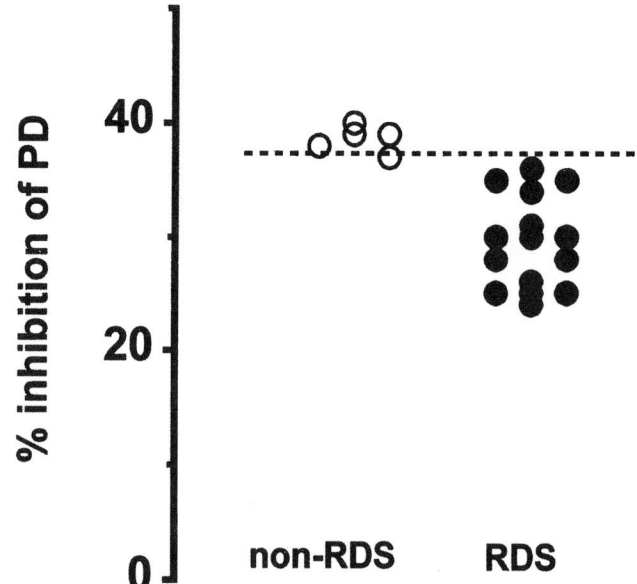

Figure 80–11. The percentage of inhibition of nasal potential difference (PD) by the sodium channel blocker amiloride discriminates between infants who subsequently developed respiratory distress syndrome (RDS) (*closed circles*) and those who did not develop RDS (*open circles*). (Data from Barker PM, et al: Pediatr Res *27*:588–591, 1990.)

received a β-adrenergic agonist in the last 2 hours of labor, compared with infants who had not been exposed to these drugs.[140] These studies confirm the important role of labor in clearing lung liquid in preparation for air breathing, and the finding supports the hypothesis that β-adrenergic stimulation induced by labor plays a key role in triggering the absorptive process. This beneficial effect of prenatal β-adrenergic stimulation on respiratory morbidity was also observed in preterm infants.[141]

Sodium Transport

Steroid and thyroid hormones exert a major maturational effect on Na⁺ transport in the developing fetal lung. Both hormones have been used for prevention and treatment of neonatal lung disease. Meta-analyses of multiple randomized trials suggest that prenatal steroids reduce the risk of RDS by about 50%,[142,143] but, even combined with surfactant therapy, antenatal steroid therapy has not decreased CLD in preterm infants. Some clinical trials examining the addition of thyrotropin-releasing hormone to antenatal steroids have been reported. Early trials suggested some reduction in respiratory morbidity in infants of mothers given the hormone;[144, 145] however, subsequent larger studies have not confirmed these findings and have suggested potentially negative outcomes, both short term and long term, after treatment with thyrotropin-releasing hormone.[146, 147, 148] Postnatal steroid administration has been used extensively to treat ventilator-dependent lung disease in preterm infants,[149] and studies showed that short courses of dexamethasone given early (in the first 2 weeks of life) may prevent bronchopulmonary dysplasia.[150, 151, 152] However, enthusiasm for steroid therapy has been tempered by reports of negative effects of both prenatal and postnatal glucocorticoids on lung development and pathologic findings in multiple organs.[153] These concerns have generated interest in the possibility that lower doses of steroids may be effective and may generate fewer side effects. Pilot studies in very preterm infants suggest that adrenal insufficiency can be reversed and CLD can be prevented with low doses of glucocorticoids.[154, 155, 156] The mechanism of low-dose steroid

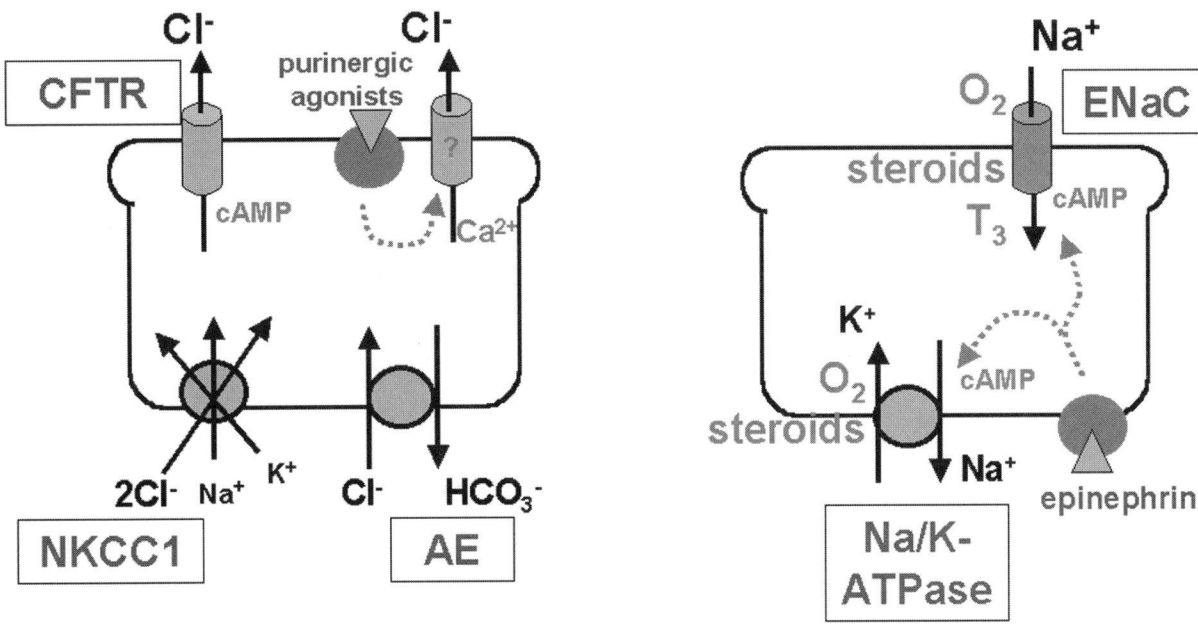

Secretion   **Absorption**

Figure 80–12. Summary of ion transport components and regulations. AE = anion exchanger; cAMP = cyclic adenosine monophosphate; CFTR = cystic fibrosis transmembrane conductance regulator; ENaC = epithelial sodium channel; HCO_3^- = bicarbonate; NKCC1 = sodium-potassium-chloride co-transporter 1; T_3 = triiodothyronine

benefit for CLD is not known. We speculate that this treatment may enhance maturity of the ion transport system and may result in more effective lung water clearance in these preterm infants.

Chloride Secretion

Furosemide, a drug that inhibits Cl⁻ secretion by blocking the basolateral NKCC, has been investigated for the treatment of CLD after preterm delivery. Two systematic reviews for the Cochrane Database examined use of furosemide for CLD after preterm studies. Studies of aerosolized furosemide suggested a short-term benefit in lung mechanics after a single administration; however no data were available on clinical outcome and repeated administration.[157] Similar conclusions were drawn for administration by oral or intravenous routes, although long-term administration by these routes was associated with consistent improvement in lung compliance and oxygenation.[158] Strategies to reduce fetal Cl⁻ secretion will be assisted by better molecular characterization of fetal Cl⁻ pathways.

SUMMARY

Ion transport has a key role in the switch from liquid-filled to air-filled lungs at birth. Although this physiologic process occurs over hours, the adaptive processes that prepare the fetal lung for birth are initiated at a much earlier stage of pregnancy. There is clear evidence that active Cl⁻ secretion underpins fetal lung liquid secretion and that this process is critical for normal lung growth *in utero*. Although there has been progress on elucidating mechanisms for Cl⁻ entry into the airway cells, the molecular identity of the channel or channels involved in transporting Cl⁻ into the lung lumen remains elusive. The functional and molecular basis of liquid absorption has been well characterized, with detailed animal studies and molecular identification of the key components (ENaC and Na⁺,K⁺-ATPase) of this process (Fig. 80–12). Both Cl⁻ secretion and Na⁺ absorption are activated

by a rise in cellular cAMP, and an alternative path for Cl⁻ secretion is activated by a rise in intracellular Ca^{2+}. The sequence of events that switch liquid secretion to liquid absorption is known. In late gestation, a rise in fetal glucocorticoids and active thyroid hormones readies, but does not activate, the Na⁺ absorptive mechanism. In the last few days of gestation, there is some decrease in lung liquid production and intraluminal liquid volume. Labor has an important role in initiating lung liquid clearance in preparation for air breathing. During labor, some liquid is actively exhaled, but the main mechanism for clearing liquid is activation of Na⁺ transport by coordinated induction of ENaC and Na⁺,K⁺-ATPase. A rise in fetal epinephrine levels in response to the stress of contractions and birth appears to trigger the switch from liquid secretion to liquid absorption. After birth, a rise in ambient O_2 augments Na⁺ absorption, which completes the transition to the postnatal state. After birth, the lung retains some liquid secretory capability, and a balance of liquid secretion and liquid absorption sustains a thin film of liquid on the airway surface of the air-filled lung. There is strong circumstantial evidence that incomplete maturation of ion transport contributes to respiratory disease in very preterm infants, but future studies will need to confirm this cause-and-effect relationship. Better understanding of the regulation of ion transport across the fetal and newborn lung will open the possibility of novel therapeutic approaches to acute lung disease and CLD associated with preterm birth.

REFERENCES

1. Preyer W: Specielle Physiologie des Embryo. Leipzig: Greeben Verlag (L. Fernau), 1885, p 149.
2. Jost A, Policard A: Contribution experimentale a l'etude du developpment prenatal du poumon chez le lapin. Arch Anat Micr 1948;37:323-332.
3. Adamson TM, et al: Composition of alveolar liquid in the foetal lamb. J Physiol (Lond) 1969;204:159-168.
4. Adams FH: The tracheal fluid in the fetal lamb. Biol Neonate 1963;5:151-158.

5. Olver RE, Strang LB: Ion fluxes across the pulmonary epithelium and the secretion of lung liquid in the foetal lamb. J Physiol (Lond) 1974;241:327–357.

6. Kitterman JA, et al: Tracheal fluid in fetal lambs: spontaneous decrease prior to birth. J Appl Physiol 1979;47:985–989.

7. Mescher EJ, et al: Ontogeny of tracheal fluid, pulmonary surfactant, and plasma corticoids in the fetal lamb. J Appl Physiol 1975;39:1017–1021.

8. Dickson KA, et al: Decline in lung liquid volume before labor in fetal lambs. J Appl Physiol 1986;61:2266–2272.

9. Perks AM, Cassin S: The rate of production of lung liquid in fetal goats, and the effect of expansion of the lungs. J Dev Physiol 1985;7:149–160.

10. Perks AM, et al: Fluid production by in vitro lungs from fetal guinea pigs. Can J Physiol Pharmacol 1990;68:505–513.

11. Olver RE, et al: Epithelial solute permeability, ion transport and tight junction morphology in the developing lung of the fetal lamb. J Physiol (Lond) 1981;315:395–412.

12. Brown MJ, et al: Effects of adrenaline and of spontaneous labour on the secretion and absorption of lung liquid in the fetal lamb. J Physiol (Lond) 1983;344:137–152.

13. Vilos GA, Liggins GC: Intrathoracic pressures in fetal sheep. J Dev Physiol 1982;4:247–256.

14. Adams F, et al: Physiology of the fetal larynx and lung. Ann Otol Rhinol Laryngol 1967;76:735–743.

15. Harding R, et al: Influence of upper respiratory tract on liquid flow to and from fetal lungs. J Appl Physiol 1986;61:68–74.

16. Klaus M, et al: Lung volume in the newborn infant. Pediatrics 1962;30:111–116.

17. Carmel JA, et al: Tracheal ligation and lung development. Am J Dis Child 1965;109:452–456.

18. Alcorn D, et al: Morphological effects of chronic tracheal ligation and drainage in the fetal lamb lung. J Anat 1977;123:649–60.

19. Moessinger AC, et al: Oligohydramnios-induced lung hypoplasia: the influence of timing and duration in gestation. Pediatr Res 1986;20:951–954.

20. Maloney JE, et al: Diaphragmatic activity and lung liquid flow in the unanesthetized fetal sheep. J Appl Physiol 1975;39:423–428.

21. Harding R, et al: Ingestion in fetal sheep and its relation to sleep states and breathing movements. Q J Exp Physiol 1984;69:477–486.

22. Dickson KA, et al: State-related changes in lung liquid secretion and tracheal flow rate in fetal lambs. J Appl Physiol 1987;62:34–38.

23. Goldstein JD, Reid LM: Pulmonary hypoplasia resulting from phrenic nerve agenesis and diaphragmatic amyoplasia. J Pediatr 1980;97:282–287.

24. Wigglesworth JS, Desai R: Effect on lung growth of cervical cord section in the rabbit fetus. Early Hum Dev 1979;3:51–65.

25. Hooper SB, Harding R: Fetal lung liquid: a major determinant of the growth and functional development of the fetal lung. Clin Exp Pharmacol Physiol 1995;22:235–247.

26. Lewis M: Spontaneous rhythmical contraction of the muscles of the bronchial tubes and air sacs of the chick embryo. Am J Physiol 1924;68:385–388.

27. Schittny JC, et al: Spontaneous peristaltic airway contractions propel lung liquid through the bronchial tree of intact and fetal lung explants. Am J Respir Cell Mol Biol 2000;23:11–18.

28. McCray PB Jr: Spontaneous contractility of human fetal airway smooth muscle. Am J Respir Cell Mol Biol 1993;8:573–580.

29. Porter HJ: Pulmonary hypoplasia. Arch Dis Child 1999;81:F81—F83.

30. Jesudason EC, et al: Pulmonary hypoplasia: alternative pathogenesis and antenatal therapy in diaphragmatic hernia. Arch Dis Child 2000;82:F172.

31. Kluth D, et al: The natural history of congenital diaphragmatic hernia and pulmonary hypoplasia in the embryo. J Pediatr Surg 1993;28:452–462.

32. Bland RD: Edema formation in the lungs and its relationship to neonatal respiratory distress. Acta Paediatr Scand Suppl 1983;305:92–99.

33. Pfister RE, et al: Volume and secretion rate of lung liquid in the final days of gestation and labour in the fetal sheep. J Physiol 2001;535:889–899.

34. Adams FH, et al: The disappearance of fetal lung fluid following birth. J Pediatr 1971;78:837–843.

35. Bland RD, et al: Labor decreases the lung water content of newborn rabbits. Am J Obstet Gynecol 1979;135:364–37.

36. Olver RE, et al: The role of amiloride-blockable sodium transport in adrenaline-induced lung liquid reabsorption in the fetal lamb. J Physiol (Lond) 1986;376:321–340.

37. Bland RD, et al: Studies of lung fluid balance in newborn lambs. Ann NY Acad Sci 1982;384:126–145.

38. Aherne W, Dawkins MJR: The removal of fluid from the pulmonary airways after birth in the rabbit, and the effect on this of prematurity and pre-natal hypoxia. Biol Neonate 1964;7:214.

39. Egan EA, et al: Changes in non-electrolyte permeability of alveoli and the absorption of lung liquid at the start of breathing in the lamb. J Physiol (Lond) 1975;244:161–179.

40. Boston RW, et al: Formation of liquid in the lungs of the foetal lamb. Biol Neonat 1965;12:306–315.

41. Humphreys PW, Strang LB: Effects of gestation and prenatal asphyxia on pulmonary surface properties of the foetal rabbit. J Physiol (Lond) 1967;192:53–62.

42. Normand IC, et al: Passage of macromolecules between alveolar and interstitial spaces in foetal and newly ventilated lungs of the lamb. J Physiol (Lond) 1970;210:151–164.

43. Canessa CM, et al: Amiloride-sensitive epithelial Na+ channel is made of three homologous subunits. Nature 1994;367:463–467.

44. Kerem B, et al: Identification of the cystic fibrosis gene: genetic analysis. Science 1989;245:1073–1080.

45. Lengeling A, et al: Chloride channel 2 gene (Clc2) maps to chromosome 16 of the mouse, extending a region of conserved synteny with human chromosome 3q. Genet Res 1995;66:175–178.

46. McGrath SA, et al: Cystic fibrosis gene and protein expression during fetal lung development. Am J Respir Cell Mol Biol 1993;8:201–208.

47. Murray CB, et al: ClC-2: a developmentally dependent chloride channel expressed in the fetal lung and downregulated after birth. Am J Respir Cell Mol Biol 1995;12:597–604.

48. Barker PM, et al: Bioelectric properties of cultured monolayers from epithelium of distal human fetal lung. Am J Physiol 1995;268:L270—L277.

49. Barker PM, Gatzy JT: Effects of adenosine, ATP, and UTP on chloride secretion by epithelia explanted from fetal rat lung. Pediatr Res 1998;43:652–659.

50. Cassin S, et al: The effects of bumetanide and furosemide on lung liquid secretion in fetal sheep. Proc Soc Exp Biol Med 1986;181:427–431.

51. Carlton DP, et al: Ion transport regulation of lung liquid secretion in foetal lambs. J Dev Physiol 1992;17:99–107.

52. Krochmal EM, et al: Volume and ion transport by fetal rat alveolar and tracheal epithelia in submersion culture. Am J Physiol 1989;256:F397–F407.

53. McCray PB Jr, Welsh MJ: Developing fetal alveolar epithelial cells secrete fluid in primary culture. Am J Physiol 1991;260:L494–L500.

54. Cotton CU, et al: Paths of ion transport across canine fetal tracheal epithelium. J Appl Physiol 1988;65:2376–2382.

55. Zeitlin PL, et al: Ion transport in cultured fetal and adult rabbit tracheal epithelia. Am J Physiol 1988;254:C691—C698.

56. Gillie DJ, et al: Liquid and ion transport by fetal airway and lung epithelia of mice deficient in sodium-potassium-2-chloride transporter. Am J Respir Cell Mol Biol 2001;25:14–20.

57. Grubb BR, et al: Alterations in airway ion transport in NKCC1-deficient mice. Am J Physiol 2001;281:C615–C623.

58. Krochmal-Mokrzan EM, et al: Effects of hormones on potential difference and liquid balance across explants from proximal and distal fetal rat lung. J Physiol (Lond) 1993;463:647–665.

59. Flagella M, et al: Mice lacking the basolateral Na-K-2Cl cotransporter have impaired epithelial chloride secretion and are profoundly deaf. J Biol Chem 1999;274:26946–26955.

60. Welsh MJ, Smith AE: Molecular mechanisms of CFTR chloride channel dysfunction in cystic fibrosis. Cell 1993;73:1251–1254.

61. Stutts MJ, et al: CFTR as a cAMP-dependent regulator of sodium channels. Science 1995;269:847–850.

62. Davis PB, et al: Cystic fibrosis. Am J Respir Crit Care Med 1996; 154:1229–1256.

63. McCray PB Jr, et al: Expression of CFTR and presence of cAMP-mediated fluid secretion in human fetal lung. Am J Physiol 1992;262:L472–L481.

64. Tizzano EF, et al: Regional expression of CFTR in developing human respiratory tissues. Am J Respir Cell Mol Biol 1994;10:355–362.

65. Engelhardt JF, et al: Expression of the cystic fibrosis gene in adult human lung. J Clin Invest 1994;93:737–749.

66. Barker PM, et al: Cl⁻ secretion by trachea of CFTR (+/–) and (–/–) fetal mouse. Am J Respir Cell Mol Biol 1995;13:307–313.

67. Matalon S, et al: Fetal lung epithelial cells contain two populations of amiloride-sensitive Na⁺ channels. Am J Physiol 1993;264:L357–L364.

68. O'Brodovich H, et al: Amiloride impairs lung water clearance in newborn guinea pigs. J Appl Physiol 1990;68:1758–1762.

69. Hummler E, et al: Early death due to defective neonatal lung liquid clearance in alpha-ENaC–deficient mice. Nat Genet 1996;12:325–328.

70. Kawakami K, et al: Primary structure of the alpha-subunit of Torpedo Californica (Na⁺ + K⁺)ATPase deduced from cDNA sequence. Nature 1985;316(6030):733–736.

71. Bland RD, Boyd CA: Cation transport in lung epithelial cells derived from fetal, newborn, and adult rabbits. J Appl Physiol 1986;61:507–515.

72. Chapman DL, et al: Developmental differences in rabbit lung epithelial cell Na(+)-K(+)-ATPase. Am J Physiol 1990;259:L481–L487.

73. O'Brodovich H, et al: Ontogeny of alpha 1- and beta 1-isoforms of Na(+)-K(+)-ATPase in fetal distal rat lung epithelium. Am J Physiol 1993; 264:C1137–C1143.

74. Crump RG, et al: In situ localization of sodium-potassium ATPase mRNA in developing mouse lung epithelium. Am J Physiol 1995;269:L299–L308.

75. Schneeberger EE, McCarthy KM: Cytochemical localization of Na+K+ATPase in rat type II pneumocytes. J Appl Physiol 1986;60:1584–1589.

76. Talbot CL, et al: Quantitation and localization of ENaC subunit expression in fetal, newborn, and adult mouse lung. Am J Respir Cell Mol Biol 1999;20:398–406.

77. Tchepichev S, et al: Lung epithelial Na channel subunits are differentially regulated during development and by steroids. Am J Physiol 1995;269:C805–C812.

78. Finley N, et al: Alveolar epithelial fluid clearance is mediated by endogenous catecholamines at birth in guinea pigs. J Clin Invest 1998;101:972–981.

79. Smith DE, et al: Epithelial Na(+) channel (ENaC) expression in the developing normal and abnormal human perinatal lung. Am J Respir Crit Care Med 2000;161:1322–1331.

80. MacGregor GG, et al: Amiloride-sensitive Na+ channels in fetal type II pneumocytes are regulated by G proteins. Am J Physiol 1994;267:L1–L8.

81. Marunaka Y, et al: Regulation of an amiloride-sensitive Na$^+$-permeable channel by a b$_2$ adrenergic agonist, cytosolic Ca^{2+} and Cl$^-$ in fetal rat alveolar epithelium. J Physiol (Lond) 1999;515:669-683.

82. Junor RWJ, et al: A novel role for cyclic nucleotide-gated cation channels in lung liquid homeostasis in sheep. J Physiol (Lond) 1999;520:255-260.

83. Jain L, et al: Antisense oligonucleotides against the a-subunit of ENaC decrease lung epithelial cation channel activity. Am J Physiol 1999;276:L1046-L1051.

84. Barker PM, et al: Pulmonary glucose transport in the fetal sheep. J Physiol (Lond) 1989;409:15-27.

85. Barker PM, et al: Role of gammaENaC subunit in lung liquid clearance and electrolyte balance in newborn mice: insights into perinatal adaptation and pseudohypoaldosteronism. J Clin Invest 1998;102:1634-1640.

86. McDonald FJ, et al: Disruption of the beta subunit of the epithelial Na$^+$ channel in mice: hyperkalemia and neonatal death associated with a pseudohypoaldosteronism phenotype. Proc Natl Acad Sci USA 1999;96:1727-1731.

87. Pradervand S, et al: Salt restriction induces pseudohypoaldosteronism type 1 in mice expressing low levels of the beta-subunit of the amiloride-sensitive epithelial sodium channel. Proc Natl Acad Sci USA 1999;96:1732-1737.

88. Hummler E, et al: A mouse model for the renal salt-wasting syndrome pseudohypoaldosteronism. Proc Natl Acad Sci USA 1997;94:11710-11715.

89. Lagercrantz H, Bistoletti P: Catecholamine release in the newborn infant at birth. Pediatr Res 1977;11:889-893.

90. Walters DV, Olver RE: The role of catecholamines in lung liquid absorption at birth. Pediatr Res 1978;12:239-242.

91. Enhorning G, et al: Isoxsuprine-induced release of pulmonary surfactant in the rabbit fetus. Am J Obstet Gynecol 1977;129:197-202.

92. Lawson EE, et al: The effect of epinephrine on tracheal fluid flow and surfactant efflux in fetal sheep. Am Rev Respir Dis 1978;118:1023-1026.

93. Bergman B, et al: Effect of terbutaline on lung mechanics and morphology in the preterm rabbit neonate. Clin Physiol 1983;3:111-121.

94. Faxelius G, et al: Catecholamine surge and lung function after delivery. Arch Dis Child 1983;58:262-266.

95. Walters DV, et al: Dibutyryl cAMP induces a gestation-dependent absorption of fetal lung liquid. J Appl Physiol 1990;68:2054-2059.

96. Perks AM, Cassin S: The effects of arginine vasopressin and epinephrine on lung liquid production in fetal goats. Can J Physiol Pharmacol 1989;67:491-498.

97. Perks AM, et al: Lung liquid production by in vitro lungs from fetal guinea pigs: effects of arginine vasopressin and arginine vasotocin. J Dev Physiol 1993;19:203-212.

98. Albuquerque CA, et al: Mechanism of arginine vasopressin suppression of ovine fetal lung fluid secretion: lack of V2-receptor effect. J Matern Fetal Med 1998;7:177-182.

99. Chapman DL, et al: Changes in lung lipid during spontaneous labor in fetal sheep. J Appl Physiol 1994;76:523-530.

100. Barker PM, et al: The effect of thyroidectomy in the fetal sheep on lung liquid reabsorption induced by adrenaline or cyclic AMP. J Physiol (Lond) 1988;407:373-383.

101. Barker PM, et al: The role of thyroid hormones in maturation of the adrenaline-sensitive lung liquid reabsorptive mechanism in fetal sheep. J Physiol (Lond) 1990;424:473-485.

102. Barker PM, et al: Synergistic action of triiodothyronine and hydrocortisone on epinephrine-induced reabsorption of fetal lung liquid. Pediatr Res 1990;27:588-591.

103. Barker PM, et al: Development of the lung liquid reabsorptive mechanism in fetal sheep: synergism of triiodothyronine and hydrocortisone. J Physiol (Lond) 1991;433:435-449.

104. Gross I, et al: Glucocorticoid-thyroid hormone interactions in fetal rat lung. Pediatr Res 1984;18:191-196.

105. Baines DL, et al: The influence of mode of delivery, hormonal status and postnatal O$_2$ environment on epithelial sodium channel (ENaC) expression in guinea pig lung. J Physiol 2000;522:147-157.

106. Champigny G, et al: Regulation of expression of the lung amiloride-sensitive Na$^+$ channel by steroid hormones. EMBO J 1994;13:2177-2181.

107. Otulakowski G, et al: Structure and hormone responsiveness of the gene encoding the alpha-subunit of the rat amiloride-sensitive epithelial sodium channel. Am J Respir Cell Mol Biol 1999;20:1028-1040.

108. Chalaka S, et al: Na(+)-K(+)-ATPase gene regulation by glucocorticoids in a fetal lung epithelial cell line. Am J Physiol 1999;277:L197-L203.

109. Berthiaume Y: Effect of exogenous cAMP and aminophylline on alveolar and lung liquid clearance in anesthetized sheep. J Appl Physiol 1991;70:2490-2497.

110. Bertorello AM, et al: Isoproterenol increases Na+-K+-ATPase activity by membrane insertion of alpha-subunits in lung alveolar cells. Am J Physiol 1999;276:L20-L27.

111. Barker PM, Gatzy JT: Effect of gas composition on liquid secretion by explants of distal lung of fetal rat in submersion culture. Am J Physiol 1993;265:L512-L517.

112. Pitkanen O, et al: Increased Po2 alters the bioelectric properties of fetal distal lung epithelium. Am J Physiol 1996;270:L1060-L1066.

113. Vivona ML, et al: Hypoxia reduces alveolar epithelial sodium and fluid transport in rats: reversal by beta-adrenergic agonist treatment. Am J Respir Cell Mol Biol 2001;25:554-561.

114. Olver RE, et al: The molecular basis of fluid transport in developing lung. J Physiol (Lond) 2002.

115. Jain L, et al: Expression of highly selective sodium channels in alveolar type II cells is determined by culture conditions. Am J Physiol 2001;280:L646-L658.

116. Rafii B, et al: O$_2$-induced ENaC expression is associated with NF-kappaB activation and blocked by superoxide scavenger. Am J Physiol 1998;275:L764-L770.

117. Haddad JJE, et al: NF-kB Blockade reduces the O$_2$-evoked rise in Na$^+$ conductance in fetal alveolar cells. Biochem Biophys Res Commun 2001;281:987-992.

118. Ramminger SJ, et al: The effects of Po2 upon transepithelial ion transport in fetal rat distal lung epithelial cells. J Physiol (Lond) 2000;524:539-547.

119. Baines DL, et al: Oxygen-evoked Na+ transport in rat fetal distal lung epithelial cells. J Physiol (Lond) 2001;532:105-113.

120. Berger PJ, et al: Effect of lung liquid volume on respiratory performance after caesarean delivery in the lamb. J Physiol (Lond) 1996;492:905-912.

121. DeSa DJ: Microscopy of the pulmonary alveolar lining layer in rabbits and perinatal infants. J Pathol 1969;99:57-66.

122. DeSa DJ: Pulmonary fluid content in infants with respiratory distress. J Pathol 1969;97:469-478.

123. Bland RD: Pathogenesis of pulmonary edema after premature birth. Adv Pediatr 1987;34:175-221.

124. O'Brodovich H: The role of active Na$^+$ transport by lung epithelium in the clearance of airspace fluid. New Horiz 1995;3:240-247.

125. O'Brodovich H: Respiratory distress syndrome: the importance of effective transport (editorial). J Pediatr 1997;130:342-344.

126. Hales KA, et al: Influence of labor and route of delivery on the frequency of respiratory morbidity in term neonates. Int J Gynaecol Obstet 1993;43:35-40.

127. Morrison JJ, et al: Neonatal respiratory morbidity and mode of delivery at term: influence of timing of elective caesarean section. Br J Obstet Gynaecol 1995;102:101-106.

128. Dani C, et al: Risk factors for the development of respiratory distress syndrome and transient tachypnoea in newborn infants: Italian Group of Neonatal Pneumology. Eur Respir J 1999;14:155-159.

129. Wax JR: Contribution of elective delivery to severe respiratory distress at term. Am J Perinatol 2002;19:81-86.

130. O'Brodovich H: Immature epithelial Na$^+$ channel expression is one of the pathogenetic mechanisms leading to human neonatal respiratory distress syndrome. Proc Assoc Am Physicians 1996;108:345-355.

131. Olver RE: Of labour and the lungs. Arch Dis Child 1981;56:656-662.

132. Knowles MR, et al: Measurements of transepithelial electric potential differences in the trachea and bronchi of human subjects in vivo. Am Rev Respir Dis 1982;126:108-112.

133. Smith SN, et al: The in vivo effects of milrinone on the airways of cystic fibrosis mice and human subjects. Am J Respir Cell Mol Biol 1999;20:129-134.

134. Scherrer U, et al: High-altitude pulmonary edema: from exaggerated pulmonary hypertension to a defect in transepithelial sodium transport. Adv Exp Med Biol 1999;474:93-107.

135. Gowen CW, et al: Increased nasal potential difference and amiloride sensitivity in neonates with cystic fibrosis. J Pediatr 1986;108:517-521.

136. Gowen CW Jr, et al: Electrical potential difference and ion transport across nasal epithelium of term neonates: correlation with mode of delivery, transient tachypnea of the newborn, and respiratory rate. J Pediatr 1988;113:121-127.

137. Barker PM, et al: Decreased sodium ion absorption across nasal epithelium of very premature infants with respiratory distress syndrome. J Pediatr 1997;130:373-377.

138. Hook B, et al: Neonatal morbidity after elective repeat cesarean section and trial of labor. Pediatrics 1997;100:348-353.

139. Curet LB, et al: Effect of mode of delivery on incidence of respiratory distress syndrome. Int J Gynaecol Obstet 1988;27:165-170.

140. Eisler G, et al: Randomised controlled trial of effect of terbutaline before elective caesarean section on postnatal respiration and glucose homeostasis. Arch Dis Child 1999;80:F88-F92.

141. Kerem E, et al: Prenatal ritodrine administration and the incidence of respiratory distress syndrome in premature infants. J Perinatol 1997;17:101-106.

142. Crowley P, et al: The effects of corticosteroid administration before preterm delivery: an overview of the evidence from controlled trials. Br J Obstet Gynaecol 1990;97:11-25.

143. National Institutes of Health: Effect of corticosteroids for fetal maturation on perinatal outcomes. NIH Consens Statement 1994;12:1-24.

144. Ballard RA, et al: Respiratory disease in very-low-birthweight infants after prenatal thyrotropin-releasing hormone and glucocorticoid: TRH Study Group. Lancet 1992;339:510-515.

145. Knight DB, et al: A randomized, controlled trial of antepartum thyrotropin-releasing hormone and betamethasone in the prevention of respiratory disease in preterm infants. Am J Obstet Gynecol 1994;171:11-16.

146. Collaborative Santiago Surfactant Group: Collaborative trial of prenatal thyrotropin-releasing hormone and corticosteroids for prevention of respiratory distress syndrome. Am J Obstet Gynecol 1998;178:33-39.

147. Ballard RA, et al: Antenatal thyrotropin-releasing hormone to prevent lung disease in preterm infants: North American Thyrotropin-Releasing Hormone Study Group. N Engl J Med 1998;338:493-498.

148. Crowther CA, et al: Australian Collaborative Trial of Antenatal Thyrotropin-Releasing Hormone: adverse effects at 12-month follow-up. ACTOBAT Study Group. Pediatrics 1997;99:311-317.

149. Bancalari E: Corticosteroids and neonatal chronic lung disease. Eur J Pediatr 1998;157(Suppl 1):S31–S37.
150. Rastogi A, et al: A controlled trial of dexamethasone to prevent bronchopulmonary dysplasia in surfactant-treated infants. Pediatrics 1996;98:204–210.
151. Tsukahara H, et al: Early (4–7 days of age) dexamethasone therapy for prevention of chronic lung disease in preterm infants. Biol Neonate 1999;76:283–290.
152. Garland JS, et al: A three-day course of dexamethasone therapy to prevent chronic lung disease in ventilated neonates: a randomized trial. Pediatrics 1999;104:91–99.
153. Merrill JD, Ballard RA: Antenatal hormone therapy for fetal lung maturation. Clin Perinatol 1998;25:983–997.
154. Hanna C, et al: Hydrocortisone replacement in extremely premature infants with cortisol insufficiency. Clin Res 1989;37:180A.
155. Helbock HJ, et al: Glucocorticoid-responsive hypotension in extremely low birth weight newborns. Pediatrics 1993;92:715–717.
156. Watterberg KL, et al: Prophylaxis against early adrenal insufficiency to prevent chronic lung disease in premature infants. Pediatrics 1999;104:1258–1263.
157. Brion LP, et al: Aerosolized diuretics for preterm infants with (or developing) chronic lung disease. Cochrane Database Syst Rev 2000;2.
158. Brion LP, Primhak RA: Intravenous or enteral loop diuretics for preterm infants with (or developing) chronic lung disease. Cochrane Database Syst Rev 2002;1.

Thomas H. Shaffer and Marla R. Wolfson

81

Upper Airway Structure: Function, Regulation, and Development

Although the conducting airways are formed well before fetal viability is complete, they undergo significant maturational changes during late gestation. Conducting airways are susceptible to damage until they acquire the characteristics of more mature airways. Controversy exists concerning the pathogenesis of bronchopulmonary dysplasia (BPD) in the neonate[1-3]; however, prolonged mechanical ventilation and oxygen toxicity appear to be major contributors to BPD. Serial evaluations of pulmonary function in premature infants surviving BPD have concluded that the duration and pressure magnitude of mechanical ventilation, rather than increased inspired oxygen tension, damage the airways and interfere with their growth.[4,5] Within this context, greater mechanical ventilation requirements of the very premature infant relative to those of the older infant precipitate an age-related predisposition for airway damage. This chapter summarizes the function-structure characteristics and regulation of the developing trachea and bronchi, analyzes the impact of mechanical ventilation on airway function, and reviews the clinical assessment of airway function.

STRUCTURE-FUNCTION CHARACTERISTICS

Airway Embryology

Airway development in humans begins during the fourth week of gestation when the respiratory diverticulum, or lung bud, branches from the embryonic foregut.[6] The esophagotracheal septum forms and separates the foregut into the esophagus dorsally and the trachea ventrally. Thus, the developing airway is of foregut endodermal origin. Elongation of the respiratory diverticulum forms the trachea, whereas the mainstem bronchi are formed by branching. Growth and elongation continue in the caudal direction under the influence of airway secretions and physical forces. By the end of the 16th week of gestation, the branching of the conducting airways is complete.

Maturation of the airway occurs first in the trachea and proceeds distally. Tracheal cartilage formation begins during the seventh week of gestation. Full maturation of the distal airway cartilage is not completed until after birth. Epithelial differentiation begins in the trachea during the 10th week of gestation. Lung fluid secreted from the epithelial cells promotes the growth and development of the respiratory system together with the phasic contractions of the fetal airway smooth muscle (ASM); such contractions are present following the 23rd gesta-

tional week.[7] Fetal lung fluid is a stable, isotonic solution with a low protein content and a high concentration of chloride ions. In addition to maintaining the lung in an expanded state, which is an important role in respiratory development, the fetal lung fluid keeps the lungs free of amniotic fluid and clears the airway lumen of mucus and cellular debris.

Airway Structure

The airway tree is a branched conducting system the major functions of which include the delivery, distribution, and conditioning of gas to the gas exchange units of the lung. The lower airway is composed of three primary components: epithelium, cartilage, and smooth muscle. The epithelium lines the entire length of the airway. From the trachea to the large bronchioles, the airway epithelium is composed of a pseudostratified ciliated columnar epithelium referred to as *respiratory epithelium*. The pseudostratified nomenclature applies because the respiratory epithelium is one cell layer thick and all cells attach to the basement membrane. However, not all cells extend completely to the airway lumen, giving the histologic appearance of multiple cell layers. Beyond the large bronchioles, there is a gradual transition to a simple ciliated columnar epithelium, and finally a cuboidal epithelium. The epithelium is composed of approximately eight different cell types. The primary cell type in the epithelium is the columnar epithelial cell, which contains a layer of cilia on its apical surface. Other cell types present include mucus-secreting cells, brush cells, small granule cells, and basal cells. The brush cells are columnar cells with extensions of the plasma membrane termed *microvilli*. The basal surfaces of these cells have synaptic contact (epitheliodendritic synapse) and are considered receptor cells. Small granule cells are a class of enteroendocrine cells seen in the gut and gut derivatives. Some of these cells are associated with nerves and they function in reflex arcs. Basal cells are cuboidal cells the nuclei of which are located adjacent to the basement membrane. They are the reserve population of cells the function of which is to replace old or displaced cells, enabling the epithelium to regenerate.

Cartilage is present from the trachea to the bronchioles. In the trachea, cartilage exists as C-shaped rings that are open posteriorly. In the bronchi, the cartilage forms plates that encompass the entire airway circumference. At more distal airway generations, the cartilage plates become smaller and more discontinuous, gradually disappearing before the bronchioles. Like the airway cartilage, ASM also varies along progressive airway generations. In the trachea, ASM is confined to the trachealis muscle. The trachealis, along with fibroelastic tissue, bridges the gap between the tips of the C-shaped cartilage rings and forms the posterior wall of the trachea. In contrast, bronchial ASM forms a complete circumferential layer that gradually diminishes and becomes discontinuous at lower generations.

A mucosal layer covers the inner surface of the trachea. The mucosa consists of an epithelial layer supported by a basement membrane. This basement membrane is part of a loose connective tissue layer referred to as the *lamina propria*. The lamina propria is highly cellular, containing lymphocytes and lymphatic tissue, plasma and mast cells, eosinophils, and fibroblasts. Glands that send ducts to the epithelial surface are also included within the mucosal layer.

The submucosa, as its name indicates, lies below the mucosa and is a connective tissue layer containing the distributing blood vessels, lymphatics, and mucus-secreting glands. The submucosa ends when it blends into the perichondrium of the cartilage rings. The outer layer of the trachea consists of adventitia, which binds the trachea to adjacent structures such as the esophagus, neck musculature, and mediastinal structures. The adventitia contains the large blood vessels and nerves supplying the components of the tracheal wall.

The primary innervation of the trachea is cholinergic from the vagus nerve.[8] Vagal stimulation results in contraction of ASM. Additionally, there is nonadrenergic noncholinergic innervation (NANCi) of the trachea, which mediates both bronchoconstrictive and bronchodilatory actions through mediators such as nitric oxide, vasoactive intestinal peptide, neurokinins, and substance P. There is little, if any, direct sympathetic innervation of the airway. Sympathetic control is provided primarily through circulating catecholamines.

Mechanics and Regulation of the Developing Airway

It is well accepted that infant airways are more compliant than adult airways. Early studies in necropsied human tracheobronchial segments indicated that airway pressure-volume relationships are correlated with maturity.[9, 10] Thus, a reduction in airway compliance with maturity results in decreased collapsibility and increased resistance to deformation during positive pressure ventilation. Therefore, the immature airway is more likely to sustain deformational changes resulting from barotrauma as compared with the less compliant airway of the older infant or adult.

Animal tracheas have been used extensively as models to study mechanisms that determine maturational changes in airway function. Using *in vitro* rabbit tracheal segments[11] as shown in Figure 81–1, there is an age-related decrease in compliance in the developing rabbit airway that parallels that seen in neonates.[9] An *in vivo* study of the innervated and perfused trachea of the lamb demonstrated similar developmental changes in airway compliance and a decrease in the tracheal relaxation time constant.[12] In comparison with results of *in vitro* studies, the absolute values of specific tracheal compliance *in vivo* were lower. Contribution of forces of surrounding connective tissue, or neural-humoral influences on ASM tone, may affect the elastic properties of the developing airway and account for these observed differences. In addition, the decrease in relaxation time constant with maturation is also suggestive of age-related differences in smooth muscle tone *in vivo*. Alterations of smooth muscle tone modulate mechanical properties and pressure-flow relationships of the trachea in preterm and newborn lambs.[13-15] In general, tracheas stimulated with acetylcholine become stiffer and are less compressible organs as reflected by decreased resistance to airflow when subjected to compressive

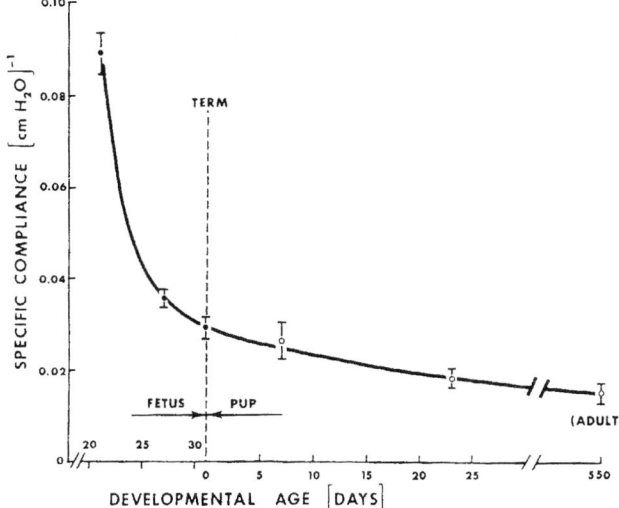

Figure 81–1. Developmental change in specific tracheal compliance in the rabbit. Term = 31 days. (Bhutani VK, et al: Respir Physiol *43*:221, 1981).

forces.[15-17] Specifically, however, the effect of pharmacologic stimulation on airway mechanics is age-dependent and the ability of ASM to decrease airway compliance and increase flow may be limited in the preterm trachea.

The inability of ASM to generate as much force as its adult counterpart probably contributes to this limitation. The effect of postnatal aging on ASM maximal force production and sensitivity to various agonists remains controversial.[18] Some studies show that contractility and sensitivity increase with age,[8,19-20] whereas others suggest that contractility and sensitivity reach their peak early in postnatal life, declining thereafter.[21, 22] When the extremes of the developmental spectrum are compared, however, a clear pattern emerges (Fig. 81–2). Several investigators have shown that maximal contractility of ASM increases between two- and fourfold from preterm or newborn to adult.[8, 15, 16, 19] Furthermore, maximum active stress has been shown to increase significantly during late gestation in both the lamb[19] and pig.[23] This change is not the result of an increase in smooth muscle mass, because normalization for cross-sectional area eliminates that variable.

Developmental changes in force-generation of ASM and non-ASM in various species have been related to an increase in contractile proteins (actin and myosin) per unit area and age-related differences in amounts and types of myosin isoforms.[21,24,25] Age-related increases in contractile responses of vessels have also been related to alterations in the orientation of vascular smooth muscle cells that change from a circular to oblique orientation relative to the long axis of the vessel wall.[26] Furthermore, age-related shifts in the synthetic activity of vascular smooth muscle cells have been identified in neonatal rats. Initially, synthetic activity is primarily secretory, producing extracellular proteins, collagen, and elastin; after 4 weeks of age, synthetic activity is primarily contractile, producing the intracellular protein actomyosin.[27] Driska[28] identified age-related differences in morphometry and similar shortening responses in ASM cells isolated from preterm and adult sheep. Adult cells were similar in size and appearance to adult arterial smooth muscle cells, but velocity of shortening (0.54/sec) was approximately three times faster. Isolated preterm ASM cells were about half as long and thick as adult cells but shortening velocities were similar.

Airway epithelium plays an important role in the modulation of smooth muscle function. Studies of adult airways have shown that airway epithelium generates relaxant and contractile factors

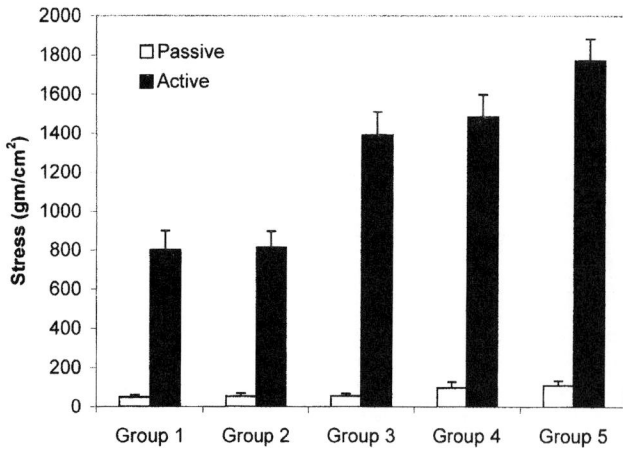

Figure 81–2. Active and passive stress of isolated trachealis muscle strips from preterm, newborn, and adult sheep. Stress normalized for cross-sectional area and for percentage of muscle fibers within the strip. Group 1 = 110 days' gestation ($n = 8$), Group 2 = 111-124 days' gestation ($n = 25$), Group 3 = 125-140 days' gestation ($n = 5$), Group 4 = newborns ($n = 10$), Group 5 = adults ($n = 16$). There was a significant increase in both active and passive stress as a function of age ($p < .001$). *Post hoc* analysis disclosed significant differences in active stress between Group 1 and Groups 3, 4, and 5, and between Group 2 and Groups 4 and 5. Similarly, passive stress increased between Groups 1 to 3 and Group 5. Values are mean ± standard error of the mean. Term is 147 ± 3 days' gestation. (Panitch HB, et al: Pediatr Res *31*:151, 1992.

that modulate the tone of the underlying smooth muscle.[29-33] Furthermore, epithelial damage has been associated with bronchial hyperreactivity.[34] In a similar study of de-epithelialized preterm lamb trachea, force-generation in response to acetylcholine stimulation was increased compared with the intact tracheal smooth muscle strip.[35] These data demonstrate that preterm airway epithelium is able to modulate the responsiveness of smooth muscle. Additionally, the magnitude of the effect was unchanged with maturation (preterms to adults). Thus, even during late gestation, epithelial integrity may be an important determinant of smooth muscle function, bronchial hyperreactivity, and bronchodilator responsiveness. It is not completely understood whether regional differences in airway epithelium exert differential contractile/relaxant influences on ASM in the developing airway.

The observation that the structural arrangement of muscle and cartilage in the adult trachea differs from that in the bronchi suggests that the functional effects of muscle contraction may also be different in these tissues in the adult, and presumably during development as well.[33] Studies of the adult trachea suggest that the elasticity of the passive trachealis muscle and connective tissue is greater than that of the bronchial wall.[36] Tracheal smooth muscle is capable of generating larger circumferential tensions than bronchial muscle, presumably related to the circumferential alignment and relatively greater proportion of the smooth muscle cells in the trachealis muscle compared with helical orientation and fewer smooth muscle cells in the bronchial wall. Regional differences in force-generation have been noted in the premature airway of sheep as well.[35] Passive, active, and total stress development decreased significantly as a function of airway generation, from trachea (0 generation) to the subsegmental bronchi (4th generation). The receptor-mediated response to acetylcholine was significantly lower in generations 0, 1, and 2 than in generations 3 and 4. In addition, the internal radius-to-wall thickness ratio (r/t) decreased from trachea to fourth generation airway. The law of Laplace predicts that

because of this decline in r/t, the trachea would be exposed to the greatest degree of wall stress during positive pressure ventilation (PPV).[35] Taken together, these data help to explain the structural changes as well as physiologic changes in airway reactivity seen in the premature infant after mechanical ventilation.

Although the intact trachea provides a suitable preparation for studying the mechanical function of the muscle and cartilage, it is important to consider the individual differences in ASM function and contribution of cartilage. Along these lines, several authors have suggested that airway cartilage plays an important role in determining airway compressibility and inflatibility.[37-39] Moreno and colleagues[38] softened rabbit tracheas with papain and demonstrated alterations in unstressed tracheal volume and compliance. In a related study using papain-treated rabbits, McCormack and colleagues[40] observed changes in pulmonary function indicative of increased airway collapsibility. The maturational effects of cartilage contribution to airway function was demonstrated by Penn and colleagues, who showed that tracheal cartilage of preterm lambs is extremely compliant relative to that of the adult sheep.[39] It was suggested that these age-related changes in cartilage paralleled developmental differences in tracheal smooth muscle and tracheal mechanics.[14, 19, 41] Therefore, age-related differences in airway mechanical function may reflect an increase in stiffness that occurs in both airway muscle and cartilage.

Effects of Mechanical Ventilation on Airway Function

Although mechanical ventilation undoubtedly increases the survival of patients in respiratory compromise, it is also associated with increased morbidity.[42] The volumes, pressures, and oxygen concentrations that are incumbent in mechanical ventilation provide a mechanism of injury to a respiratory system that is not suited to such exposure.[43] This dilemma is most obvious in the premature and neonatal patient population.[44, 45]

Mechanical ventilation has little effect on adult airways but has been shown to affect the dimensions[46-48] and mechanical properties of the airways in preterms and newborns.[49, 50] The extent of ventilation-induced deformation appears to be directly related to the compliance of the airway and inversely related to age. Following mechanical ventilation, we have observed an increase in tracheal diameter, thinning of cartilage and muscle, disruption of the muscle-cartilage junction, and focal abrasions of the epithelium.[46] As shown in Figure 81-3, in comparison with unventilated trachea, decreased inflation and increased collapsing compliance of the trachea following ventilation produce a structure analogous to that of a fire hose in that it is difficult to expand but easier to collapse.[50] In addition, ventilated tracheae showed greater resistance to airflow. The clinical implications of these studies include increased dead space, flow limitation, elevated airway resistance, increased work of breathing, and gas trapping.[51]

The mechanisms that precipitate the alterations in mechanical properties of the ventilated trachea are unclear. Preliminary studies of ASM force generation are inconclusive and require further study. It is possible that loss of an epithelial relaxant factor due to epithelial disruption might explain the intensive bronchoconstrictor response to inhaled agonists seen in infants with pulmonary dysfunction.[52, 53] Focal abrasion and denudation of the airway epithelium following mechanical ventilation have been reported[51] and are illustrated in Figure 81-4. The airway epithelium plays an important role in the modulation of ASM, through the release of both contractile and relaxant paracrine mediators.[54, 55]

Disruption of the muscle-cartilage junction may reduce the ability of the airway to resist compressive forces, such as excessive supra-atmospheric pressures produced by infants with airflow obstruction. Pressure-induced alterations in the orientation of ASM fibers may affect the ability of smooth muscle con-

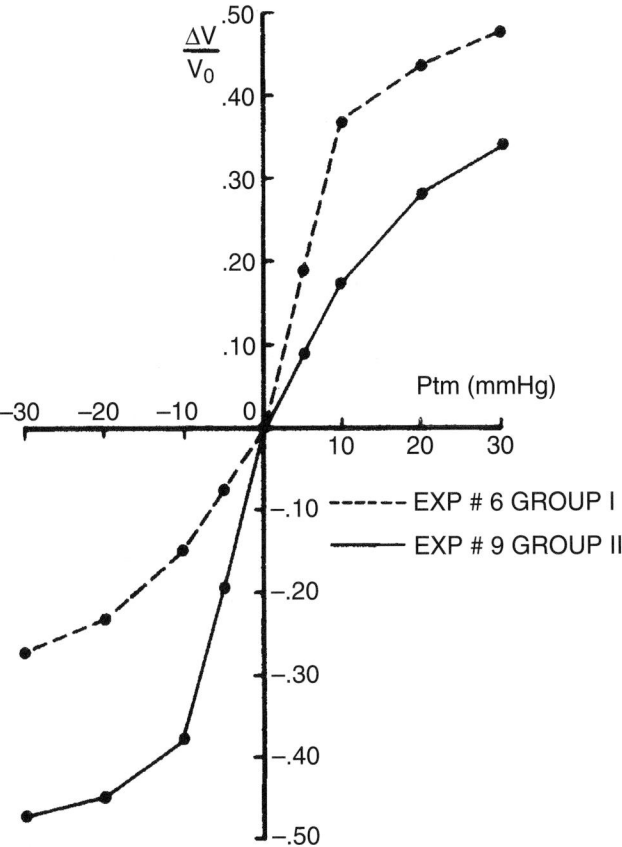

Figure 81–3. Pressure (Ptm) as a function of normalized volume change ($\Delta V/V0$) in a typical unventilated (Group I) and ventilated (Group II) trachea segment. (Penn RB, et al: Pediatr Res *23*:519, 1988.

traction to stiffen the airway, resist deformation, or generate increased force. It is also possible that pressure-induced alterations in the alignment of cartilage components (i.e., proteoglycan-collagen configuration) may attenuate the contribution of cartilage as a structural support for the trachea. In addition to pressure-induced tracheomegaly, histologic studies of ventilated neonatal human and animal lungs describe widening of the peripheral airways.[56, 57] Apart from the qualitative assessment of dimensions, the effects of ventilation on the peripheral airways is not known. Presumably age, regional differences in the amount of cartilage, orientation, force-generating capabilities, and receptor sensitivity of ASM may exacerbate the effect of ventilation on the relatively more compliant distal (compared with proximal) airways. This effect would be further potentiated by ventilatory strategies in which an inspiratory hold is produced by long inspiratory times. Long inspiratory times favor equilibration of pressures throughout the tracheobronchial tree, thereby increasing the length of time that the highly compliant distal airways are subjected to barotrauma. It should be noted, however, that high-frequency jet ventilation (HFJV), evaluated in preterm rabbit airways, demonstrated significant dimensional and mechanical deformation of tracheal segments as well as an increased propensity toward collapsibility following HFJV.[58] Therefore, ventilation techniques that attempt to minimize pulmonary barotrauma might still have some deleterious effect on immature proximal airways.

CLINICAL ASSESSMENT OF AIRWAY FUNCTION

Several modalities exist to evaluate airway function in the pediatric population. These include measurements of lung function during tidal breathing or forced exhalation, radiography, fluoroscopy, and airway endoscopy. Taken together, these tests can be used to identify and quantitate functional abnormalities found in preterm airways exposed to PPV, including elevated airway resistance, decreased forced expiratory flows, airway hyperreactivity, and excessive central airway collapsibility. In addition, these diagnostic procedures have also provided important insight into the effects of early injury on future airway growth and function and can be used to test the effectiveness of newer therapies. Evaluation of airway function is especially useful and should be considered in infants whose course is not one of gradual improvement or is marked by frequent severe pulmonary exacerbations, and in infants who demonstrate stridor, chronic wheezing, or focal areas of chronic atelectasis or hyperinflation.

Pulmonary Function Profile

With the simultaneous measurement of respiratory pressures, volumes, and air flow, pulmonary mechanics can be monitored relatively noninvasively.[59] Pulmonary function profiles can be determined to assess initial disease etiology, the response to therapy, and disease sequelae during follow-up.[60] For example,

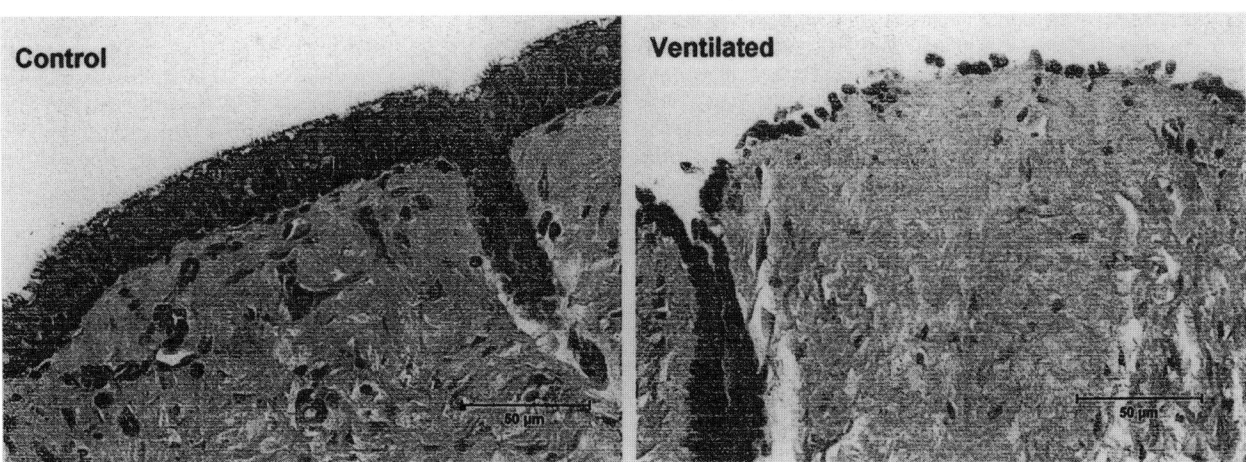

Figure 81–4. Effect of mechanical ventilation on epithelial lining of neonatal lamb trachea. *Left panel*: Nonventilated control. *Right panel*: Mechanical ventilation (mean airway pressure = 15 cm H_2O, duration = 2.8 hours). Scale bar = 50 μm. (Cullen AB, et al: Pediatr Res *47*:355A, 2000 .)

the pressure-volume relationship of a premature infant can identify the degree of respiratory function and monitor the response following surfactant administration. In addition, the evaluation of tidal breath pressure–volume relationships serves as a tool to optimize the parameters of mechanical ventilation. Over time, sequential pulmonary mechanics can be used to monitor the progression and improvement in both lung and airway abnormalities.

Measurements of Airway Function During Tidal Breathing

Dynamic pulmonary compliance as measured by the esophageal balloon and pneumotachometry technique is significantly lower in infants who go on to develop chronic lung disease compared with those of normal infants or of infants who recover uneventfully from neonatal respiratory distress.[60-62] Although these measurements reflect the elastic properties of the lung to some degree, they are also influenced by maldistribution of ventilation associated with regions having differing time constants (frequency dependence of compliance).[61] Thus, dynamic compliance measurements in infants with chronic lung disease probably also reflect some degree of airway obstruction. Quasistatic methods of measuring respiratory system compliance in infants with BPD have verified that alterations in the elastic properties of the lung contribute significantly to the observed decrease in compliance.[63] Studies comparing static and dynamic compliance measurements in this group of infants, however, have not been performed. Thus, it is not clear whether the improvement in dynamic compliance seen in infants with moderate-to-severe BPD studied longitudinally[60,62] represents a change in the characteristics of the lung parenchyma, or whether it reflects a coexistent decrease in respiratory rate or improvement in airway obstruction. Interestingly, both static and dynamic measurements of compliance have been shown to have predictive value regarding the development of BPD in mechanically ventilated preterm infants.[64,65]

Resistance measurements, including airway resistance as determined by plethysmography, pulmonary resistance measured by the esophageal balloon and pneumotachometry technique, or respiratory system resistance determined by the airway occlusion technique, are significantly elevated in infants with BPD.[60,62,66-68] When measurements of resistance or its reciprocal, conductance, have been made serially, values have approached normal over the first 2 to 3 years of life.[60,62] Longitudinal changes in resistance can reflect either resolution of airway obstruction or merely an increase in airway diameter related to growth. To eliminate the influence of growth or changes in lung volume on these measurements, investigators have also reported size-corrected values of resistance or conductance (i.e., specific conductance, defined as the conductance divided by lung volume at FRC). Data reported in this way confirm the presence of airway obstruction in infants with BPD.[60,69] In the latter study, although pulmonary resistance decreased to only one-fourth of the original measurement over the first 3 years of life, specific conductance rose only minimally and remained below normal at the end of the study period.[60] Arad and co-workers[69] found that specific conductance rose from $57 \pm 7\%$ of predicted in infancy to $90 \pm 8\%$ of predicted by 5 to 7 years of age, although the children who required mechanical ventilation in infancy demonstrated air trapping and small airway obstruction in childhood.

Forced Expiratory Flow Measurements

Measurements of tidal mechanics include significant contributions of the nasopharynx, pharynx, and central airways. Earlier investigators have applied either the rapid thoracic compression technique[66,70,71] or the rapid deflation technique[72,73] to infants with BPD to obtain information more reflective of small airways, and to compare data obtained in infancy with spirometric measurements routinely performed later in childhood. Such studies also demonstrate significant airway obstruction in infancy, with

evidence of incomplete recovery with growth. When maximum expiratory flow-volume (MEFV) curves were generated by the rapid deflation technique in a group of preterm infants during the acute phase of BPD, severe small airway obstruction as determined by a marked reduction in V_{max25} was noted, and the shape of the MEFV curve was concave to the volume axis.[72] When patients with moderate BPD who were weaned from mechanical ventilation before 5 months of age were studied longitudinally with the same technique, there was a gradual increase in V_{max25} to approximately 40% of predicted by 3 years of age.[73] In contrast, those patients who required extended periods of mechanical ventilation (> 10 months) showed no increase in V_{max25} over the same time period.

Similar evidence of airway obstruction has been demonstrated using the rapid compression technique.[66, 70] Partial expiratory flow-volume (PEFV) curves were generated over the tidal range of breathing and quantitated by measuring maximal flow at FRC $\dot{V}_{max}FRC$) in young infants with BPD. Furthermore, the separation between tidal and forced flow curves was interpreted as a measure of expiratory flow reserve.[70] As seen, the shape of the PEFV curve was typically concave to the volume axis and there was a smaller expiratory flow reserve compared with findings in infants with normal lungs. Size-corrected forced expiratory flows were only half those of normal controls and did not increase by 14.5 to 22 months of age.[70] Furthermore, the slope of the regression equation for $\dot{V}_{max}FRC$ versus age was lower in the BPD group compared with unaffected infants. These data suggest that early exposure to PPV and high concentrations of oxygen not only caused early airway damage, but also interfered with subsequent normal airway growth.

Values of $\dot{V}_{max}FRC$ are usually considered as representative of small airway function. However, other studies have shown that central airway collapsibility (i.e., tracheomalacia or bronchomalacia) can cause a marked reduction in values of $\dot{V}_{max}FRC$ and appear graphically similar to small airway obstruction.[71, 74] Panitch and coworkers studied five infants with BPD who had bronchoscopic evidence of tracheobronchomalacia with the rapid compression technique.[71] As shown in Figure 81–5, when CPAP was applied to the airway opening, there was an incremental increase in $\dot{V}_{max}FRC$. Additionally, in several patients, there was a change in the shape of the PEFV curve from concave to convex, suggesting that CPAP acted as an intra-airway stent to prevent collapse. Furthermore, the ratio of forced-to-tidal flows at mid-expiration, a reflection of expiratory flow reserve, increased with application of CPAP. Thus, it is possible that reductions in $\dot{V}_{max}FRC$ previously ascribed to small airway damage in infants with BPD may also represent a component of central airway injury.

Assessment of Airway Reactivity

Airway reactivity, as determined by bronchodilator responsiveness, has been well documented in infants with BPD using assessments of both tidal mechanics and forced expiratory flows. Acute decreases in pulmonary, respiratory system, and airway resistance ranging from 23 to 48% have been reported in response to a variety of β-agonist and anticholinergic drugs.[67,68,75-79] The magnitude of this response was even more dramatic when forced flows were tested: Kao and associates[67] reported an increase of 86% over baseline values of $\dot{V}_{max}FRC$ in 15 infants with BPD at a mean age of 15.8 weeks after treatment with metaproterenol, and of 45% over baseline after treatment with atropine. Similarly, Motoyama and partners[72] found an increase of 214% over baseline values of V_{max25} after isoetharine inhalation in 32 intubated and mechanically ventilated infants. Bronchodilator responsiveness could be demonstrated in infants as young as 26 weeks' postconceptional age, and as early as at 12 days' postnatal age.

Other investigators have also demonstrated early evidence of bronchodilator responsiveness. Gomez-Del Rio and colleagues[77]

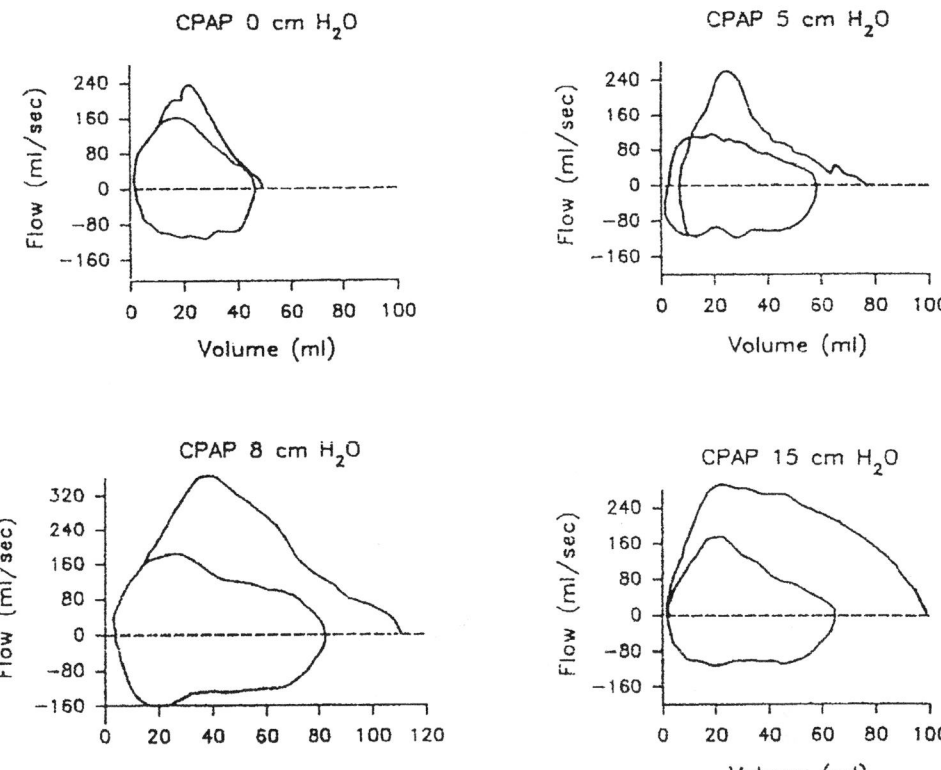

Figure 81–5. Series of partial expiratory flow volume (PEFV) curves from an infant with bronchopulmonary dysplasia and bronchoscopically documented tracheobronchomalacia, showing the effect of increasing levels of continuous positive airway pressure (CPAP). Off CPAP, the curve shape becomes straight, and at higher levels of CPAP it becomes convex. At each level of CPAP, expiratory flow reserve also increases. Values of maximal flow of functional lung reserve capacity ($\dot{V}_{max}FRC$) at each level of CPAP are (mL/sec) 26 (0 cm H_2O), 53 (5 cm H_2O), 120 (8 cm H_2O), and 204 (15 cm H_2O). (Panitch HB, et al: Am J Respir Crit Care Med *150*:1341, 1994.

found significant improvement in pulmonary resistance in 30 mechanically ventilated preterm infants younger than 20 days of age after isoetharine inhalation. The youngest was only 3 days of age, and gestational ages ranged from 27 to 34 weeks. Denjean and co-workers[75] measured significant decreases in respiratory system resistance after salbutamol inhalation in ventilator-dependent preterm infants at 13.3 ± 4.9 days' postnatal age. These observations of early bronchodilator responsiveness suggest that loss of epithelial modulation, as well as ASM hypertrophy, probably contribute to airway hyperreactivity seen in chronically ventilated infants.

Radiographic Evaluation of Airway Injury

Acquired tracheomalacia has been evaluated fluoroscopically and by computed tomography (CT). Sotomayor and colleagues[80] used fluoroscopy in anteroposterior, oblique, or lateral views to document central airway collapse in infants with BPD who required mechanical ventilation for periods of 3 weeks to 4 months. These investigators also employed fluoroscopy to determine the amount of distending pressure required to maintain airway patency in those infants. McCubbin and coworkers[81] studied central airway collapse in 10 infants (3.3–20.5 months of age) with BPD, using cine-CT. A group of 7 children of similar age with glottic or supraglottic obstruction but no evidence of lower airway disease was used as a control group. The median percentage decrease in airway cross-sectional area during exhalation in the BPD group was 63.5% (range, 23–100%), whereas that of the control group was only 9% (range, 5–13%). This significant difference in collapsibility was present in a short segment of airway in six children and was diffuse in the other four patients. Because narrowing was not always diffuse, those authors speculated that the underlying cause of collapse must include local sites of injury as well as transmural pressure changes.

Bhutani and co-workers[48] described roentgenographic evidence of acquired tracheomegaly in very preterm neonates (under 1000 g in birth weight) who had received mechanical

ventilatory support. Increases in tracheal width at the level of the thoracic inlet and carina were present compared with individually weight-matched nonventilated controls. Those authors speculated that the persistent airway dimensional deformation seen in those infants resulted in increased anatomic dead space and contributed to carbon dioxide retention following extubation.

The ability to evaluate small airway pathology with conventional bronchographic agents has been limited by poor resolution of the bronchioles at the secondary lobule level.[82] Because of the density, low surface tension, and radiopacity of the perfluorochemical liquid, perflubron, it has been used as an bronchographic contrast agent for high-resolution CT direct visualization of the airways through the centrilobar bronchioles and their first order branches with definition within 1 mm of the lung surface.[83,84]

Radiographic studies of the perflubron-filled lungs of animals and humans with congenital diaphragmatic hernia have proven informative to delineate qualitatively the degree of pulmonary hypoplasia, distribution, and elimination pattern of the PFC liquid.[85,86] Regional differences in PFC clearing, detected on radiography, were related to localized bronchial obstruction.[85]

The acoustic attenuation in PFC liquids is substantially lower than that of tissue, making these liquids an excellent medium for highlighting lung structure in ultrasound technology. PFCs have the lowest sound speeds of any liquid, and this factor in combination with their acoustic attenuation affords a depth penetration capability ideal for ultrasound imaging.[84]

Endoscopic Evaluation of Airway Injury

Airway endoscopy provides for both diagnosis and treatment of anatomic lesions of supraglottic, glottic, and subglottic regions, as well as of the trachea and bronchi to the segmental level.[87-93] Two prospective studies of infants who required intubation in the newborn period found that the incidence of moderate-to-severe subglottic stenosis was 9.8% and 12.8%[88,89] but the incidence of other fixed anatomic lesions is unknown. Endoscopy of the airway was selected when infants presented with acquired lobar emphysema, persistent lobar atelectasis, or unexplained medical failure.[91, 92, 94-97] Typically, when lobar emphysema occurred, the right lower lobe and right middle lobes were more commonly affected.[91,92,94-96,98]

Direct visualization of the airways during spontaneous breathing is the most direct method of identifying central airway collapse. Although both rigid and flexible fiberoptic bronchoscopy is available for the study of pediatric airways, rigid bronchoscopy must be performed while the patient undergoes general anesthesia. Often, the child receives assisted ventilation during the procedure. Consequently, the patient's effort of breathing decreases and exhalation may be completely passive. Thus, many cases of central airway collapse can be underdiagnosed using this method.

In contrast, flexible bronchoscopy is usually performed using conscious sedation. The patient breathes spontaneously but must breathe around the bronchoscope as well. Variations in expiratory effort can influence the degree of intrathoracic airway collapse. Because of these technical considerations and lack of universally agreed-on criteria, the frequency of diagnosis of central airway collapse will vary from center to center. To circumvent these inconsistencies, some authors have based the diagnosis on percentage of airway narrowing during exhalation.[71, 93, 99] Mair and Parsons[99] have recommended a grading system based on the percentage of airway narrowing present at end-expiration during spontaneous respiration together with an increase in the membrane-to-cartilage ratio. Others have defined tracheobronchomalacia as collapse resulting in more than 50%[71, 100] or more than 75%[80] obstruction during spontaneous breathing with no mention of changes in the proportion of membrane to cartilage. Acquired extrathoracic tracheomalacia has also been described in patients with BPD.[89]

To date, quantitative studies of the inherent characteristics of the developing airway wall have required excision of an airway segment or surgical creation of an isolated segment. One laboratory study demonstrated that airway wall characteristics at various collapsing pressures and attendant changes in stiffness following smooth muscle stimulation could be quantitated bronchoscopically from airway pressure-area relationships.[101] Neonatal lamb tracheal segments were suspended over hollow mounts in a buffer-filled chamber, and subjected to a range (0 to −4.0 kPa) of pressures to determine wall stiffness under collapsing forces before and after stimulation of the trachealis with methacholine (MCh). Luminal images were recorded through a 3.6-mm flexible bronchoscope under the same conditions and the cross-sectional area was quantitated. Both pressure-volume and pressure-area relationships detected significant changes in airway wall stiffness after MCh administration ($p < .002$), and the magnitude of change was similar between methods. More recently, this same method was reported to quantitate airway stiffness in vivo.[102] The speculation is that this technique may be clinically useful to quantitate airway collapsibility, and can differentiate whether deformation is secondary to effort or intrinsic abnormalities of the airway wall.

SUMMARY

Considerable progress has been made in characterizing developmental (preterm, newborn, and adult) differences in airway physiology with respect to pressure-volume and pressure-flow relationships, the effects of mechanical ventilation, and pharmacologic stimulation. In this regard, studies have been conducted using in vivo, in vitro, and muscle bath preparations, and they offer valuable insight into how the very premature infant may differ from the later-term and full-term neonate with respect to airway function. Nevertheless, little is known about how positive airway pressure ventilation alters the cellular, biochemical, and molecular constituents of the components of the immature airway, and why some mechanically ventilated premature infants develop severe airway dysfunction whereas others do not. Ultrastructure studies that assess structural damage with greater sensitivity, and biochemical and molecular analysis that can detect alterations in collagen muscle and connective tissue composition would improve our understanding of the pathogenesis of pressure/stretch-related injury. These laboratory findings coupled with clinical pulmonary function results and anatomic airway studies should provide further understanding of basic biologic development of the airway that can facilitate continual advancement of neonatal and pediatric clinical respiratory management.

REFERENCES

1. Northway WA, Jr, et al: Pulmonary disease following respiratory therapy of hyaline membrane disease. Bronchopulmonary dysplasia. N Engl J Med 276:357, 1967.
2. O'Brodovich HM, Mellins RB: Bronchopulmonary dysplasia: unresolved neonatal acute lung injury. Am Rev Resp Dis 132:684, 1985.
3. Watts JL, et al: Chronic pulmonary disease in neonates after artificial ventilation: distribution of ventilation and pulmonary interstitial emphysema. Pediatrics 60:273-281, 1977.
4. Stocks J, Godfrey S: The role of artificial ventilation, oxygen, and CPAP in the pathogenesis of lung damage in neonates: Assessment by serial measurements of lung function. Pediatrics 57:352, 1976.
5. Stocks J, et al: Airway resistance in infants after various treatments for hyaline membrane disease: Special emphasis on prolonged high levels of inspired oxygen. Pediatrics 61:178, 1978.
6. Harding R, Hooper SB. Regulation of lung expansion and lung growth before birth. J Appl Physiol 81:209, 1996.
7. Schittny JC, et al: Spontaneous peristaltic airway contractions propel lung liquid through the bronchial tree of intact and fetal lung explants. Am J Respir Cell Mol Biol 23:11, 2000.
8. Haxhiu-Poskurica B, et al: Development of cholinergic innervation and muscarinic receptor subtypes in piglet trachea. Am J Physiol 264:L606, 1993.
9. Burnard ED, et al: Pulmonary insufficiency in prematurity. Aust Pediatr J 1:12, 1965.
10. Croteau JR, Cook CD: Volume-pressure and length-tension measurements in human tracheal and bronchial segments. J Appl Physiol 16:170, 1961.
11. Bhutani VK, et al: Pressure-volume relationships of tracheae in fetal newborn and adult rabbits. Respir Physiol 43:221, 1981.
12. Shaffer TH, et al: In vivo mechanical properties of the developing airway. Pediatr Res 25:143, 1989.
13. Bhutani VK: The effect of tracheal smooth muscle tone on neonatal airway collapsibility. Pediatr Res 20:492, 1986.
14. Koslo RJ, et al: The role of tracheal smooth muscle contraction on neonatal tracheal mechanics. Pediatr Res 20:1216, 1986.
15. Penn RB, et al: Effect of tracheal smooth muscle tone on collapsibility of immature airways. J Appl Physiol 65:863, 1988.
16. Coburn RF, et al: Effect of trachealis muscle contraction on tracheal resistance to airflow. J Appl Physiol 16:170, 1972.
17. Knudson RJ, Knudson DE: Effect of muscle constriction on flow-limiting collapse of isolated canine trachea. J Appl Physiol 38:125, 1975.
18. Fisher JT: Airway smooth muscle contraction at birth: In vivo versus in vitro comparisons to the adult. Can J Physiol Pharmacol 70:590, 1992.
19. Panitch HB, et al: Maturational changes in airway smooth muscle structure-function relationships. Pediatr Res 31:151, 1992.
20. Rodriguez RJ, et al: Maturation of the cholinergic response of tracheal smooth muscle in the piglet. Pediatr Pulmonol 18:28, 1994.
21. Sparrow MP, Mitchell HW: Contraction of smooth muscle of pig airway tissues from before birth to maturity. J Appl Physiol 68:468, 1990.
22. Murphy TM, et al: Expression of airway contractile properties and acetylcholinesterase activity in swine. J Appl Physiol 67:174, 1989.
23. Booth RJ, et al: Early maturation of force production in pig tracheal smooth muscle during fetal development. Am J Respir Cell Mol Biol 7:590, 1992.
24. Kawamoto S, Adelstein RS: Characterization of myosin heavy chains in cultured aorta smooth muscle. J Biol Chem 262:7282, 1987.
25. Masaki T, et al: Changes in the smooth muscle myosin isoforms during development of chicken gizzard. In Emerson C, Fischman D, Nadal-Ginard B, Siddiqui M, eds: Molecular Biology of Muscle Development. Vol. 29. New York, Alan R. Liss, 1986, 323-336.
26. Cliff WJ: The aortic tunica media in growing rats studied with the electron microscope. Lab Invest 1967; 17:599-615.
27. Wolinsky H: Long term effects of hypertension on the rat aorta wall and their relation to concurrent aging changes. Circ Res 30:301, 1972.
28. Driska SP, et al: A method for isolating adult and neonatal airway smooth muscle cells and measuring shortening velocity. J Appl Physiol 86:427, 1999.
29. Cuss FM, Barnes PJ: Epithelial mediators. Am Rev Resp Dis 136:S32, 1987.
30. Aizawa H, et al: A possible role of airway epithelium in modulating hyperresponsiveness. Br J Pharmacol 93:139, 1988.

31. Barnes PJ, et al: The effect of airway epithelium on smooth muscle contractility in bovine trachea. Br J Pharmacol *86*:685, 1985.
32. Flavahan NA, et al: Respiratory epithelium inhibits bronchial smooth muscle tone. J Appl Physiol *58*:834, 1985.
33. Stuart-Smith K, VanHoutte PM: Airway epithelium modulates the responsiveness of porcine bronchial smooth muscle. J Appl Physiol *65*:721, 1988.
34. Laitinen LA, et al: Damage of the airway epithelium and bronchial reactivity in patients with asthma. Am Rev Respir Dis *131*:599, 1985.
35. Gauthier SP, et al: Structure-function of airway generations 0 to 4 in the preterm lamb. Pediatr Res *31*:157, 1992.
36. Olsen CR, et al: Rigidity of tracheae and bronchi during muscular constriction. J Appl Physiol *23*:27, 1967.
37. Gunst SJ, Lai-Fook SJ: Effect of inflation on trachealis muscle tone in canine tracheal segments in vitro. J Appl Physiol *54*:906, 1983.
38. Moreno RH, et al: Effect of intravenous papain on tracheal pressure-volume curves in rabbits. J Appl Physiol *60*:247, 1986.
39. Penn RB, et al: Developmental differences in tracheal cartilage mechanics. Pediatr Res *26*:429, 1989.
40. McCormack GS, et al: Lung mechanics in papain-treated rabbits. J Appl Physiol *60*:242, 1986.
41. Panitch HB, et al: A comparison of preterm and adult airway smooth muscle mechanics. J Appl Physiol *66*:1760, 1989.
42. Acute Respiratory Distress Syndrome Network: Ventilation with lower tidal volumes as compared with traditional tidal volumes for acute lung injury and the acute respiratory distress syndrome. N Engl J Med *342*:1301, 2000.
43. Greenspan JS, et al: Assisted Ventilation: Physiologic Implications and Complications. *In* Polin RA, Fox WW (eds): Fetal and Neonatal Physiology. Philadelphia, WB Saunders Co., 1998, 1193–1212.
44. Coalson JJ, et al: Pathophysiologic, morphometric, and biochemical studies of the premature baboon with bronchopulmonary dysplasia. Am Rev Resp Dis 145:872, 1992.
45. Hislop AA, Haworth SG: Airway size and structure in the normal fetal and infant lung and the effect of premature delivery and artificial ventilation. Am Rev Resp Dis *140*:1717, 1989.
46. Deoras KS, et al: Structural changes in the tracheae of preterm lambs induced by ventilation. Pediatr Res *26*:434, 1989.
47. Bhutani VK, et al: Pressure-induced deformation in immature airways. Pediatr Res *15*:829, 1981.
48. Bhutani VK, et al: Acquired tracheomegaly in very preterm neonates. Am J Dis Child *140*:449, 1986.
49. Bhutani VK, Shaffer TH: Time-dependent tracheal deformation in fetal, neonatal, and adult rabbits. Pediatr Res *16*:830, 1982.
50. Penn RB, et al: Effect of ventilation on mechanical properties and pressure-flow relationships of immature airways. Pediatr Res *23*:519, 1988.
51. Cullen AB, et al: Functional characteristics of newborn airway: Effect of Ventilation. Pediatr Res *47*:355A, 2000.
52. Panitch HB, et al:. Epithelial modulation of preterm airway smooth muscle contraction. J Appl Physiol *74*:1437, 1993.
53. Mirmanesh SJ, et al: Alpha-adrenergic bronchoprovocation in neonates with bronchopulmonary dysplasia. J Pediatr *121*:622, 1992.
54. Savla U, et al: Cyclic stretch of airway epithelium inhibits prostanoid synthesis. Am J Physiol *273*:L1013, 1997.
55. Takizawa H: Airway epithelial cells as regulators of airway inflammation. Int J Mol Med *1*:367, 1998.
56. Reynolds EOR, et al: Hyaline membrane disease, respiratory distress, and surfactant deficiency. Pediatrics *42*:758, 1968.
57. Ackerman NB Jr, et al: Pulmonary interstitial emphysema in the premature baboon with hyaline membrane disease. Crit Care Med *12*:512, 1984.
58. Bhutani VK, et al: Effect of high-frequency jet ventilation on preterm and rabbit tracheal mechanics. Pediatr Pulmonol *2*:327, 1986.
59. Shaffer TH, et al: Pulmonary function testing in the critically ill neonate. *In* Lafeber HN, ed: Fetal and Neonatal Physiological Measurements. Amsterdam, Excerpta Medica, 1991.
60. Gerhardt T, et al: Serial determination of pulmonary function in infants with chronic lung disease. J Pediatr *110*: 448, 1987.
61. Bryan MH, et al: Pulmonary function studies during the first year of life in infants recovering from the respiratory distress syndrome. Pediatrics *52*:169, 1973.
62. Morray JP, et al: Improvement in lung mechanics as a function of age in the infant with severe bronchopulmonary dysplasia. Pediatr Res *16*:290, 1982.
63. Tepper RS, et al: Noninvasive determination of total respiratory system compliance in infants by the weighted-spirometer method. Am Rev Respir Dis *130*:461, 1984.
64. Dreizzen E, et al: Passive compliance of total respiratory system in preterm newborn infants with respiratory distress syndrome. J Pediatr *112*:778, 1988.
65. Bhutani VK, Abbasi S. Relative likelihood of bronchopulmonary dysplasia based on pulmonary mechanics measured in preterm neonates during the first week of life. J Pediatr *120*:605, 1992.
66. Kao LC, et al: Oral theophylline and diuretics improve pulmonary mechanics in infants with bronchopulmonary dysplasia. J Pediatr *111*:439, 1987.
67. Kao LC: Effects of inhaled metaproterenol and atropine on the pulmonary mechanics of infants with bronchopulmonary dysplasia. Pediatr Pulmonol *6*:74, 1989.

68. Wilkie RA, Bryan MH. Effect of bronchodilators on airway resistance in ventilator-dependent neonates with chronic lung disease. J Pediatr *111*:278, 1987.
69. Arad I, et al: Lung function in infancy and childhood following neonatal intensive care. Pediatr Pulmonol *3*:29, 1987.
70. Tepper RS, et al: Expiratory flow limitation in infants with bronchopulmonary dysplasia. J Pediatr *109*:1040, 1986.
71. Panitch HB, et al: Effects of CPAP on lung mechanics in infants with acquired tracheobronchomalacia. Am J Resp Crit Care Med *150*:1341, 1994.
72. Motoyama EK, et al: Early onset of airway reactivity in premature infants with bronchopulmonary dysplasia. Am Rev Resp Dis *136*:50, 1987.
73. Mallory GB Jr, et al: Longitudinal changes in lung function during the first three years of premature infants with moderate to severe bronchopulmonary dysplasia. Pediatr Pulmonol *11*:8, 1991.
74. Panitch HB, et al: Effect of altering smooth muscle tone on maximal expiratory flows in patients with tracheomalacia. Pediatr Pulmonol *9*:170, 1990.
75. Denjean A, et al: Dose-related bronchodilator response to aerosolized salbutamol (albuterol) in ventilator-dependent premature infants. J Pediatr *120*:974, 1992.
76. Cabal LA, et al: Effects of metaproterenol on pulmonary mechanics, oxygenation, and ventilation in infants with chronic lung disease. J Pediatr *110*:116, 1987.
77. Gomez-Del Rio M, et al: Effect of a beta-agonist nebulization on lung function in neonates with increased pulmonary resistance. Pediatr Pulmonol *2*:287, 1986.
78. Kao LC, et al: Effect of isoproterenol inhalation on airway resistance in chronic bronchopulmonary dysplasia. Pediatrics *73*:509, 1984.
79. Sosulski R, et al: Physiologic effects of terbutaline on pulmonary function of infants with bronchopulmonary dysplasia. Pediatr Pulmonol *2*:269, 1986.
80. Sotomayor JL, et al: Large-airway collapse due to acquired tracheobronchomalacia in infancy. Am J Dis Child *140*:367, 1986.
81. McCubbin M, et al: Large airway collapse in bronchopulmonary dysplasia. J Pediatr *114*:304, 1989.
82. Murata K, et al: Centrilobar lesions of the lung: demonstration by high-resolution CT and pathologic correlation. Radiology *161*:641, 1986.
83. Stern RG, et al: High-resolution computed tomographic bronchiolography using perfluoroctylbromide (PFOB): An experimental model. J Thorac Imaging *8*:300, 1993.
84. Wolfson MR, et al: Utility of a perfluorochemical liquid for pulmonary diagnostic imaging. *In* Chang TMS, Riess JG, Winslow RM, eds: Biomaterial, Artificial Cells, and Immobilization Technology. New York, Marcel Dekker, 1994.
85. Gross GW, et al: Use of liquid ventilation with Perflubron during extracorporeal membrane oxygenation: Chest radiographic appearances. Radiology *194*:717, 1995.
86. Miller TF, et al: Combined ECMO and partial liquid ventilation (PLV) in human neonates: LiquiVent perfluorochemical (PFC) elimination. Pediatr Res *39*:231A, 1996.
87. Fan LL, et al: Predictive value of stridor in detecting laryngeal injury in extubated neonates. Crit Care Med *10*:453, 1982.
88. Sherman JM, et al: Factors influencing acquired subglottic stenosis in infants. J Pediatr *109*:322, 1986.
89. Downing GJ, Kilbride HW: Evaluation of airway complications in high-risk preterm infants: Application of flexible fiberoptic airway endoscopy. Pediatrics *95*:567, 1995.
90. Sherman JM, Nelson H: Decreased incidence of subglottic stenosis using an "appropriate-sized" endotracheal tube in neonates. Pediatr Pulmonol *6*:183, 1989.
91. Miller RW, et al: Tracheobronchial abnormalities in infants with bronchopulmonary dysplasia. J Pediatr *111*:779, 1987.
92. Greenholz SK, et al: Surgical implications of bronchopulmonary dysplasia. J Pediatr Surg *22*:1132, 1987.
93. Duncan S, Eid N: Tracheomalacia and bronchopulmonary dysplasia. Ann Otol Rhinol Laryngol *100*:856, 1991.
94. Nagaraj HS, et al: Recurrent lobar atelectasis due to acquired bronchial stenosis in neonates. J Pediatr Surg *15*:411, 1980.
95. Grylack LJ, Anderson KD: Diagnosis and treatment of traumatic granuloma in tracheobronchial tree of newborn with history of chronic intubation. J Pediatr Surg *19*:200, 1984.
96. Miller KE, et al: Acquired lobar emphysema in premature infants with bronchopulmonary dysplasia: An iatrogenic disease? Radiology *138*:589, 1981.
97. Hauft SM, et al: Tracheal stenosis in the sick premature infant. Am J Dis Child *142*:206, 1988.
98. Moylan FMB, Shannon DC: Preferential distribution of lobar emphysema and atelectasis in bronchopulmonary dysplasia. Pediatrics *63*:130, 1979.
99. Mair EA, Parsons DS: Pediatric tracheobronchomalacia and major airway collapse. Ann Otol Rhinol Laryngol *101*:300, 1992.
100. Couvreur J, et al: La dyskinesia tracheale (tracheomalacie) chez l'enfant. Reflexions a propos de 127 cas reconnus par endoscopie. Ann Pediatr (Paris) *27*:561, 1980.
101. Panitch HB, et al: Quantitative bronchoscopic assessment of airway collapsibility. Pediatr Res *43*:832, 1998.
102. Panitch, HB, et al: *In vivo* quantitation of airway stiffness. Am J Resp Crit Care Med *157*:A470, 1998.

Regulation of Lower Airway Function

The potential impact of the lower airway on prenatal and postnatal lung function is considerable. However, when compared with healthy and diseased adult airways, little attention has been paid to the diverse neural mechanisms that regulate airway caliber in the perinatal period. This subject has gained considerable interest because of the injurious effects of increased inspired oxygen and positive pressure ventilation on neonatal airway function. It is, therefore, important to gain greater understanding of the normal maturational changes exhibited by airway smooth muscle contractile and relaxant mechanisms superimposed on the immature structural elements that compose airway structures (Fig. 82–1).

OVERVIEW OF AIRWAY INNERVATION

Most studies of central neural output to the airways have focused on the regulation of airway muscles, even though many of the same principles apply to control of secretory glands, mucus production, and blood flow in the airways.[1, 2] In addition to neural mechanisms, physical changes in the thorax may influence the caliber of intrathoracic airways. For example, during lung inflation, lowered intrathoracic pressure and traction from inflating alveoli may result in airway dilatation, and the effects will vary between more proximal and distal contractile elements in the developing lung.

Airway Afferents

Myelinated afferents from the lung (Fig. 82–2) are mediated through two types of receptors: slowly adapting receptors (SARs) and rapidly adapting receptors (RARs); both types of receptors have been described in the newborn canine and feline lung.[3] SARs are situated largely in the smooth muscle of conducting airways and stimulated by lung inflation or stretch. SAR stimulation causes a reflex decrease in vagal efferent outflow to airway smooth muscle (as well as a decrease in respiratory frequency mediated through the Hering-Breuer reflex). RARs, sometimes called irritant receptors, reside primarily in the epithelium and are activated by rapid inflation and deflation maneuvers and airway irritants to cause reflex bronchoconstriction. Vagal afferent pathways from these receptors project to and terminate in the nucleus tractus solitarius of the brain stem. This is also the site of termination for peripheral chemoreceptors, and consistent with the common features shared by efferent output to airway and ventilatory muscles, as discussed later in this chapter. Although both types of afferents have been characterized using neurophysiologic recordings in the newborn, limited information is available on developmental changes in their reflex actions on airway smooth muscle.[4] Presumably, the presence of high end-expiratory and peak pressures associated with mechanical ventilation and resultant inflammation could exert a reflex effect on the magnitude and control of bronchomotor tone in the neonate.

The receptors of unmyelinated afferents are thought to play an important role in reflex responses associated with pulmonary defense and inflammation and have been implicated in the pathophysiology of lung diseases such as asthma and bronchopulmonary dysplasia (BPD).[5] C-fiber afferents contain the neuropeptides substance P, neurokinin A, and calcitonin gene–related peptide that can be released into the airway to induce smooth muscle contraction, mucus secretion, and vascular leak. However, these responses tend to be species specific and their relevance to human, let alone neonatal, disease remains unclear. In addition to the local effects of neuropeptides released from sensory nerve endings, c-fiber excitation may also induce reflex vagally mediated bronchoconstriction and airway secretory responses. A major tool for elucidating the role of c-fibers is the application of capsaicin, the pungent extract of hot peppers, which is a specific stimulant of these receptors. It is not entirely clear whether c-fiber afferents behave similarly in the newborn as in the adult. In 2-week old piglets, the tracheal constrictor response to capsaicin (and laryngeal irritant receptor stimulation) was diminished when compared with more mature animals.[4] Similarly, reflex increase in submucosal gland secretion was significantly lower than in mature piglets.[6] Interestingly, the anticipated phrenic responses of apnea (to both stimuli) was readily elicited in the younger animals, suggesting a differential maturation of airway and ventilatory responses. Subsequent studies did demonstrate a bronchoconstrictor response in newborn canine and porcine lung in vivo, suggesting that proximal and distal airways may not exhibit comparable maturational patterns.[4, 7]

Cholinergic Innervation

Cholinergic innervation controls airway smooth muscle constriction and submucosal gland secretion. These efferent fibers to the airways arise mainly from the nucleus ambiguus and partly from the dorsal motor nucleus of the vagus, both situated in the medulla oblongata.[8-10] They relay in parasympathetic ganglia located within the airways and from which short postganglionic fibers innervate the muscles and glands of the airways as well as vessels (Fig. 82–3). Released acetylcholine (ACh) from the nerve endings may also reach smooth muscle and other targets by diffusion.[11] Stimulation of vagal fibers to airway smooth muscle may also elicit release of inhibitory neurotransmitters, and this so-called nonadrenergic, noncholinergic system is described later in this chapter.

Released ACh activates muscarinic receptors. Muscarinic receptor subtypes, coupled to the family of G proteins, mediate airway contractile responses and their modulation, although there are considerable interspecies differences in the roles of the muscarinic receptor subtypes.[12] M_1 receptors are largely present on neuronal tissue and ganglia, and the selective M_1 receptor antagonist pirenzepine reduces the contractile response to vagal stimulation in newborn animals.[13, 14]

M_2 receptors are located on prejunctional postganglionic cholinergic fibers in airway smooth muscle in some species, and exhibit an autoinhibitory action, whereby the quantal release of ACh in response to nerve stimulation is reduced due to feedback inhibition.[15] Sinus node M_2 receptors also mediate the bradycardia seen with vagal stimulation. Selective blockade, or downregulation, of M_2 receptors may enhance vagally mediated bronchoconstrictor responses and a reduction in the bradycardia response. In newborn animals, M_2 receptors have not been detected in tracheal smooth muscle,[13] although the presumed low density of the receptors may make them difficult to detect. Functional studies of the actions of a selective M_2 antagonist suggest that M_2 autoinhibitory actions may be reduced or absent in the newborn, because blockade of M_2 receptors does not

Figure 82–1. Schematic representation of factors that contribute to maintenance of airway caliber during early postnatal life. Available experimental data suggest that compliant, immature airways are structurally weak but exhibit a well-developed smooth layer characterized by diminished contractile and enhanced relaxant neural pathways.

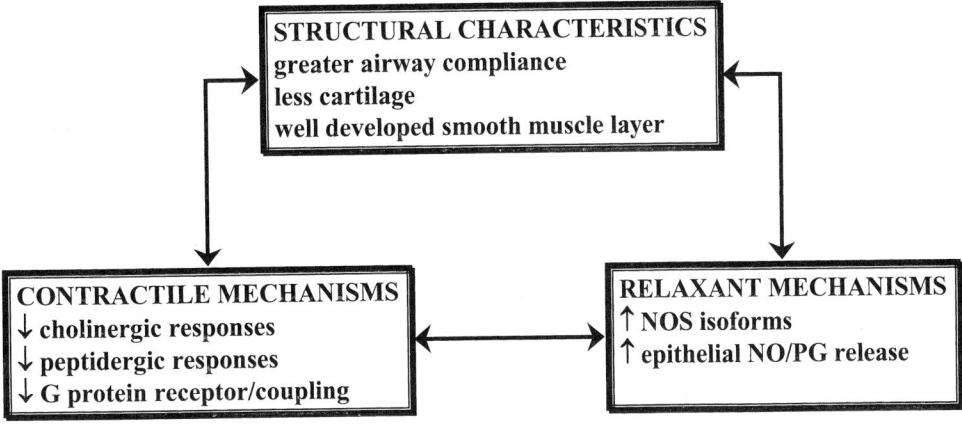

STRUCTURAL CHARACTERISTICS
greater airway compliance
less cartilage
well developed smooth muscle layer

CONTRACTILE MECHANISMS
↓ cholinergic responses
↓ peptidergic responses
↓ G protein receptor/coupling

RELAXANT MECHANISMS
↑ NOS isoforms
↑ epithelial NO/PG release

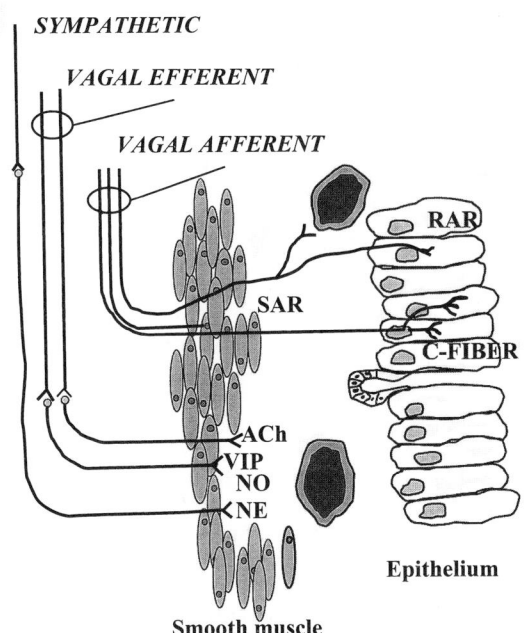

SYMPATHETIC

VAGAL EFFERENT

VAGAL AFFERENT

RAR

SAR

C-FIBER

ACh
VIP
NO
NE

Epithelium

Smooth muscle

Figure 82–2. General airway innervation includes vagal and sympathetic efferents, vagal afferents, and their associated neurotransmitters. Afferent receptors consist of myelinated axons of slowly adapting receptors and rapidly adapting receptors (SARs and RARs, respectively) and unmyelinated axons of c-fibers. SARs increase their activity during lung inflation or stretch, and increased SAR activity reflexively decreases efferent outflow to smooth muscle. RARs are stimulated by lung deflation, inhalation of irritants such as dust, and rapid lung inflation. RARs cause reflex bronchoconstriction. C-fiber receptor stimulation causes reflex bronchoconstriction, mucus secretion, and increased submucosal blood flow.

studies support a developmental change in signal transduction mechanisms; generation of inositol 1,4,5-triphosphate (IP_3) by adolescent animals is increased compared with findings in the adult and is accompanied by an apparent increase in maximal force generation.[18] *In vivo* studies show that M_3 receptor antagonism decreases bronchoconstrictor responses to vagal stimulation in the newborn that, at low dosages, does not affect the bradycardic response.[14] Among the many unanswered questions in the newborn are the extent of receptor subtype differentiation in human neonates, investigation of G-protein signal transduction, the role of M_2 autoinhibitory receptors in modulating airway tone, and the possible impact of inflammatory lung disease on muscarinic receptor regulation and its pharmacologic manipulation.

Transneuronal viral labeling studies have demonstrated that cells innervating airway-related preganglionic parasympathetic neurons extend from the diencephalon to the most caudal brainstem nuclei.[9] Within the ventral medulla oblongata, there is an extensive rostral caudal network of neurons. Included within this network are neurons innervating airway-related vagal preganglionic neurons within the raphe pallidus, the parapyramidal nucleus, the retrotrapezoid nucleus, and the gigantocellular and lateral paragigantocellular reticular nuclei. The observation that the neurons projecting to the airway-related preganglionic cell bodies arise predominantly from the same regions of the ventrolateral medulla known to be involved in cardiovascular and respiratory regulatory functions strongly suggests that these neurons integrate multiple visceral functions and serve as a central coordinator of cholinergic outflow to the lung and respiratory output.[19, 20] This linkage of cholinergic outflow to airways and phrenic output to ventilatory muscles is consistent with the observation in newborn dogs and piglets that hypercapnia increases both ventilatory responses and airway constriction.[4, 21] This is also consistent with observations made in infants with bronchopulmonary dysplasia that hypoxia may elicit airway constriction.[22, 23] However, activation of subsets of neurons within raphe nuclei has qualitatively different effects on cholinergic outflow to the airways, activity of hypoglossal motoneurons, or phrenic nuclei.[24] Namely, released serotonin following chemical stimulation of raphe nuclei inhibits airway smooth muscle tone but increases genioglossus and diaphragm discharge. Differences in response are due to differences in expression of serotoninergic receptor subtypes.

Sympathetic Responses

Sympathetic innervation of airway smooth muscle is highly species specific, and in airway smooth muscle in humans, direct sympathetic innervation appears to be lacking (see Fig. 82–3). Nevertheless, circulating catecholamines activate airway adrenoceptors to exert specific actions that affect smooth muscle contractile function.[5, 25]

enhance bronchoconstrictor responses to vagal stimulation.[14] Further studies are needed that employ autoradiographic, molecular biologic, and *in vitro* techniques to elucidate their functional role in the newborn. The potential role of lung injury and infection in modulating physiologic responses coupled to M_2 receptors in the newborn remains to be explored.

M_3 receptors are present on smooth muscle and mucus glands and airway epithelial cells, where they initiate the events leading to smooth muscle contraction, airway narrowing, and mucus secretion.[16, 17] In the newborn, the density of M_3 receptors has been reported to be similar to that in the adult; however, they do not appear to be tightly coupled to G-protein signal transduction mechanisms that lead to smooth muscle contraction.[13] Other

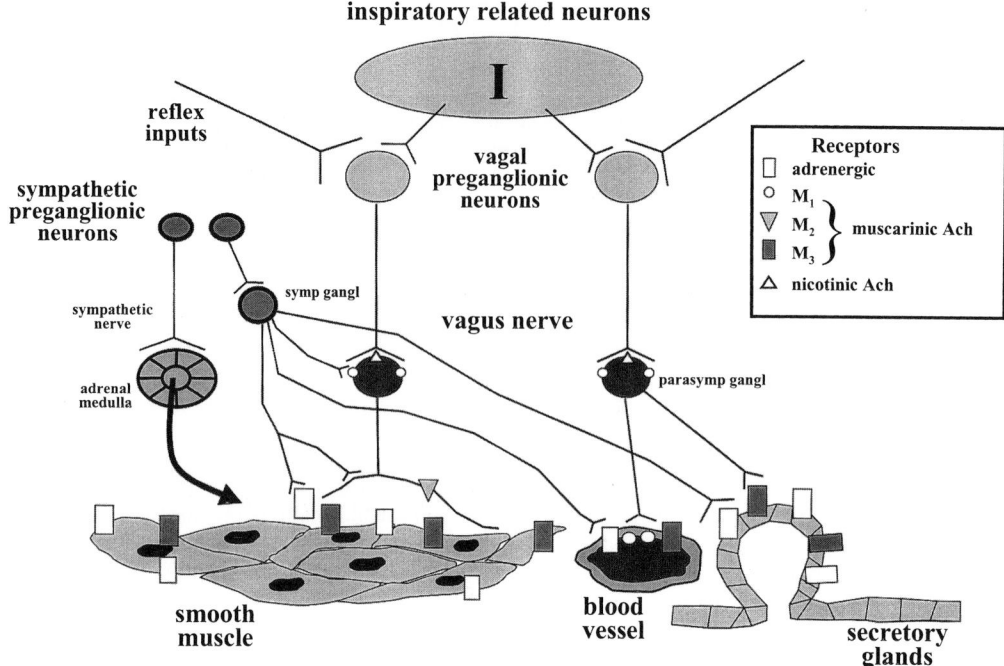

Figure 82–3. Schematic representation of the major parasympathetic, or cholinergic (contractile) and sympathetic or adrenal adrenergic (relaxant) pathways that innervate (or regulate) airway smooth muscle. Efferent output from vagal preganglionic neurons to airways is influenced by various afferent reflex inputs (illustrated in Fig. 82-2), and inspiratory-related neurons (I) in the brain stem. Excitation of parasympathetic efferents also increases the output of submucosal secretory glands and results in relaxation of adjacent vascular structures. See text for the functional roles of the various muscarinic (cholinergic) receptor subtypes.

β-Adrenergic responses in airway smooth muscle are composed of two inhibitory actions: first, relaxation of airway smooth muscle mediated by airway β_2-receptors, which are coupled to the stimulatory G-protein (G_s), and adenylate cyclase, and second, inhibition of ACh release from postganglionic vagal axons through prejunctional α_2-adrenergic and β_1-receptors in some species.[26] Activation of β-adrenergic receptors is the pharmacologic basis for neonatal bronchodilator therapy. Maturational studies have demonstrated that β-adrenergic receptors in lung tissue increase with advancing gestation and subsequent postnatal development, but this may be more important for their role in surfactant synthesis and release.[27,28] The airway relaxant response to β-adrenoreceptor stimulation actually appears to decrease with advancing maturation, and several mechanisms including greater muscarinic antagonism of β-receptor responses have been proposed.[29,30]

The second category of adrenergic responses is attributed to α-adrenoceptors, of which both α_1- and α_2-subtypes play a role. Available data indicate that in adult humans α-adrenergic contractile responses of airway smooth muscle are weak or absent, although this may not hold true for the newborn. A potential role for α-adrenergic receptors in the control of airway smooth muscle in newborn infants with bronchopulmonary dysplasia is supported by observations in preterm infants with chronic lung disease in whom ophthalmic application of the α_1-adrenergic agonist phenylephrine resulted in an increase in total pulmonary resistance and a decrease in compliance.[31] The deterioration in lung mechanics was attributed to α_1-receptor-mediated contraction of airway smooth muscle. Furthermore, adrenergic agonists having mixed α- and β-receptor actions cause airway smooth muscle contraction in newborn puppies,[32,33] and both α_1- and α_2-adrenoreceptors appear to be involved in mediating the response. Neonatal porcine tracheal smooth muscle does not display a contractile response to norepinephrine,[34] a finding similar to that of the adult.[35] Nevertheless, infusion of norepinephrine in newborn pigs increases lung resistance, reminiscent

of the adult response. In the piglet the contractile effects of norepinephrine are evident in *parenchymal* tissue, suggesting that circulating catecholamines may exert an action on gas exchange, at least in this species.[34] The implications of the above-mentioned studies for human infants remain to be seen; however, they may be part of a previously unappreciated component of the pulmonary response to the surge of systemically released catecholamine at parturition.[36] α_2-Adrenergic receptors are present in preganglionic and postganglionic nerve terminals as well as nonmyelinated c-fibers. Their activation inhibits release of ACh and peptidergic mechanisms may be implicated.[37]

Nonadrenergic Noncholinergic (NANC) Innervation

Rather than representing a separate pathway for modulation of airway caliber, the NANC system comprises both inhibitory and excitatory mechanisms modulated by several neurotransmitters located in traditional (e.g., vagal) fibers (Fig. 82-4). Reference to noncholinergic (i.e., NANC) innervation reflects the neurotransmitters known *not* to mediate its effects. The system is highly species specific but has been identified in human airways. The NANC inhibitory component of vagal innervation is demonstrated *in vivo* by measuring the response to vagal stimulation after muscarinic and β-adrenergic effects on airway smooth muscle are blocked by atropine and propranolol, and then airway tone is elevated by an infusion of contractile agonist (e.g., serotonin or histamine).[5] Under these conditions, stimulation of vagal preganglionic axons causes bronchodilation. Vasoactive intestinal peptide was initially proposed as the primary neurotransmitter of the NANC system, but subsequently nitric oxide (NO) was also shown to act as a NANC neurotransmitter, with considerable interspecies variation (Fig. 82-5).

Limited information is available about the ontogeny of this system in the airways.[38] Activation of vagal preganglionic axons results in a NANC-mediated bronchodilation in newborn feline airways, a response that is eliminated by ganglionic blockade

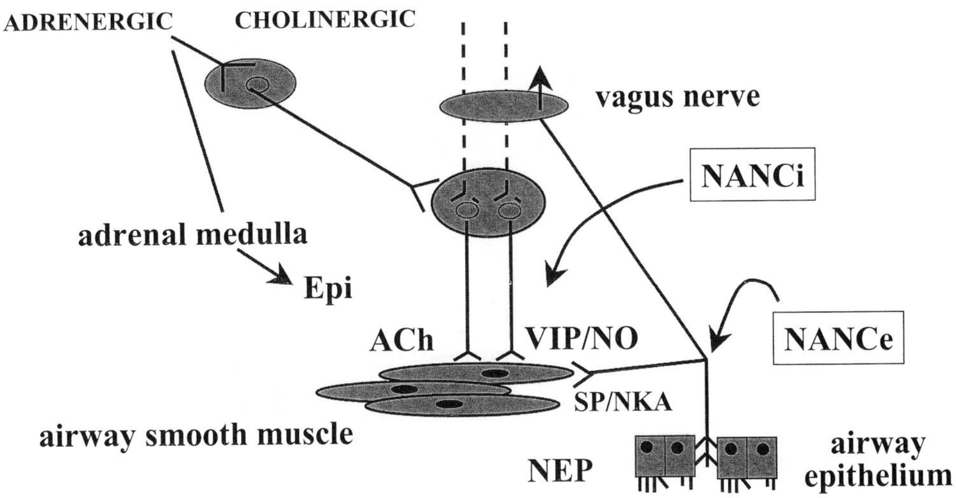

Figure 82–4. Representation of the non-adrenergic non-cholinergic (NANC) innervation of airway smooth muscle and related afferent fibers from airway epithelium that complement traditional cholinergic and adrenergic pathways. The inhibitory component of this system (NANCi) appears to be mediated primarily by release of nitric oxide (NO) and vasoactive intestinal peptide (VIP). NANC excitatory mechanisms (NANCe) are initiated by release of neuropeptides such as substance P (SP) and neurokinin A (NKA) from c-fiber afferent nerve endings, and this is modulated by the neuropeptide degrading enzyme, neutral endopeptidase (NEP), in epithelial cells.

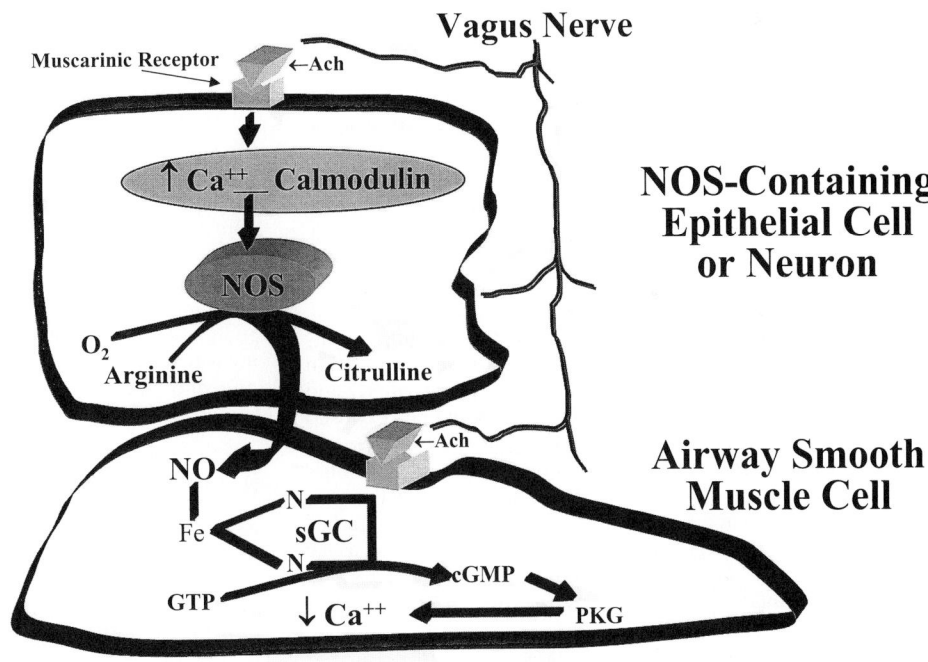

Figure 82–5. Diagrammatic representation of the nitric oxide cyclic guanosine monophosphate (NO-cGMP) pathway that mediates airway smooth muscle relaxation. NO synthase (NOS)-containing epithelial cells or neurons (as well as airway smooth muscle cells) are innervated by cholinergic fibers and express muscarinic receptors. Activation of these NOS-containing cells results in production of NO (from its L-arginine substrate), which diffuses into the smooth muscle layer and interacts with the heme moiety of soluble guanylyl cyclase (sGC), leading to intracellular accumulation of cGMP. This causes activation of protein kinase G (PKG) which, in turn, causes a decrease in inositol 1,4,5-triphosphate ($InsP_3$)-stimulated elevation of intracellular Ca^{2+} and consequent smooth muscle relaxation.

with hexamethonium, confirming the efferent nature of the response.[39] Comparison with the mature response is confounded by the necessity of infusing an agonist to measure a response, and the possibility that neonatal and adult airways may possess different sensitivities to the contractile agonist. NANC inhibitory innervation also appears to be functional in young guinea pigs.[40] In some species, NANC inhibitory responses undergo significant developmental changes, for example, NANC relaxatory responses are not present in rabbits until 2 weeks of age.[41] Interestingly, allergen sensitization significantly reduced the NANC response at 2, 4, and 12 weeks of age,[41] suggesting that host or environmental factors may alter the maturation of the inhibitory NANC system, and predispose to airway reactivity, as discussed later in this chapter. The NANC inhibitory system has not been explored in human neonatal airways; data on other

airway neurotransmitters suggest that it might be expected to be present.[42]

Nitric oxide has received considerable attention for its ability to reverse persistent pulmonary hypertension of the newborn and this has largely overshadowed investigation of its role in control of airway smooth muscle. Nevertheless, some evidence indicates that expression of neuronal NO synthase is developmentally regulated, declining during late gestation but subsequently increasing postnatally in the rat.[43] In developing sheep lungs, all three isoforms of NO synthase are expressed in airway epithelium and so might be expected to modulate underlying contractile responses.[44] It has been shown that release of endogenous NO from airway epithelium opposes cholinergically mediated contraction of piglet tracheal smooth muscle.[17] This phenomenon decreases with advancing postnatal age, requires an intact epithelium, and correlates with a relative up-regulation of M_3 muscarinic receptors in airway epithelium of the youngest animals. In the newborn piglet, nitric oxide inhalation causes a modest decrease in total lung resistance, with decreases in both airway and tissue (lung parenchymal) resistance.[45] In the same animal model, inhibition of NO synthase increases tissue more than airway resistance, suggesting a role for endogenous NO in relaxing primarily distal (parenchymal) areas of lung tissue. Thus, the NANC inhibitory system and NO may play a significant role in modulating airway and lung function in the neonate, and this may be disturbed in response to inflammatory airway disease, as discussed later.

NANC excitatory mechanisms also play a role in modulating airway smooth muscle. Within this system the tachykinin peptides, such as substance P and neurokinin A, have undergone some study during early postnatal development. As already indicated, these tachykinins are synthesized in sensory neurons and transported to sensory nerve endings from which they are released and have the ability to elicit airway contractile responses by several interrelated mechanisms. Tachykinin release from c-fiber nerve endings may directly or reflexly elicit smooth muscle contraction, modulate cholinergic responses through muscarinic receptors, and induce histamine release from mast cells. In young rabbits, substance P-induced modulation of ACh release increases with advancing postnatal age.[46] In newborn piglets, exogenously administered substance P elicits weak contractile responses of tracheal smooth muscle when compared with older animals.[47] This weak smooth muscle contractile response elicited by the neurokinin $(NK)_1$-receptor agonist substance P in newborn pigs is associated with an adult complement of NK_1 receptors in trachea and lung, but with immature G protein coupling,[48] as observed for muscarinic receptors in the piglet airway.[13]

There is some debate about whether increased expression of substance P or other neuropeptides contributes to lung or airway pathophysiology. In mature animal models, chronic exposure to irritant gas increases substance P content; however, it is controversial whether this serves to aggravate airway hyperreactivity or serves a protective role for airway and lung structures.[49, 50] Furthermore, in addition to eliciting airway smooth muscle constriction, substance P may induce relaxation of *preconstricted* neonatal tracheal tissue by release of NO and relaxant prostaglandins.[51] Newborn and 3-week-old rats exposed to hyperoxia exhibit increased tachykinin precursor expression, increased substance P content in the lung, and increased cholinergic responsiveness, although the relationship of the latter to the increased substance P content is not clear.[52] Ongoing studies are focusing on the signaling pathways that modulate airway smooth muscle relaxant responses through NO- and prostaglandin-mediated mechanisms in health and disease (see Fig. 82-5).

MATURATIONAL CHANGES IN AIRWAY PHYSIOLOGIC RESPONSES

Elegant immunohistochemical studies of developing human and porcine fetal airways have been performed from as early as the first trimester.[53] These have revealed the development of an airway smooth layer by the end of the human embryonic period extending from trachea to terminal lung sacs, as well as an extensive nerve plexus comprising nerve trunks and ganglia investing the airways and innervating smooth muscle. This layer of airway smooth muscle is functional in the first trimester as evidenced by phasic spontaneous narrowing and relaxation of airways with back and forth movement of lung fluid.[53, 54] Tonic activity in airway smooth muscle might stimulate lung growth by providing positive intraluminal pressure. These data are consistent with human autopsy findings that airway smooth muscle is present at 23 weeks' gestation at all levels of the conducting airways and

increased in amount during the earliest signs of developing chronic lung disease, as early as 10 days of birth.[55]

Despite clear evidence of an intact airway smooth muscle layer early in gestation, the effect of postnatal maturation on airway contractile responses is somewhat controversial. Studies employing methacholine (cholinergic) challenge have demonstrated greater airway narrowing during bronchoconstriction in immature animals largely attributable to greater airway compliance or distensibility in the walls of distal airways.[56] This was associated with less cartilage and proportionately more muscle in the airway wall of immature versus mature rabbits.[57]

In contrast, physiologic studies employing isolated tracheal smooth muscle strips from several species have demonstrated decreased cholinergic responsiveness in early postnatal life.[13,58,59] These *in vitro* studies are complicated by the need to carefully normalize the airway contractile response for smooth muscle mass and myosin content.[60] Nonetheless, the weight of evidence appears to point to an anatomically intact, but functionally diminished, airway smooth muscle layer superimposed on highly compliant airway structures in early postnatal life.

AIRWAY FUNCTION IN NEONATAL LUNG INJURY

Positive Pressure Ventilation and Mechanical Strain

Both structural and functional changes occur in airway smooth muscle over a wide range of developmental ages. It is known that vagally mediated bronchoconstrictor tone is minimal under baseline conditions in the newborn period.[61] Furthermore, the high deformability or compliance of the trachea in the preterm period appears to be a consequence of decreased airway smooth muscle contractility[62] and diminished cartilaginous support.[57, 63] The obvious result is that tracheas, and possibly lower airways, are vulnerable to deformation during positive pressure ventilation.

Abnormal mechanical stress and its effect on smooth muscle contractility may serve as a useful model for characterizing one aspect of neonatal lung and airway injury.[64] Cultured airway smooth muscle cells exposed to such stress eliminate the confounding effects of deformational strain on surrounding tissues. Such studies have demonstrated strain induced increases in cell myosin light chain kinase (MLCK) accompanied by increased phosphorylation of the myosin light chain, all key steps in the smooth muscle contractile response.[65]

Hyperoxic Exposure

Exposure of the immature airway to increased supplemental oxygen is a common occurrence in neonatal practice and may predispose preterm infants to the development of bronchopulmonary dysplasia, especially in the presence of assisted ventilation. In newborn animal models, most notably the guinea pig and rat pup, hyperoxic exposure has been associated with development of airway hyperreactivity.[66, 67] Although hyperoxic exposure may increase smooth muscle area, this effect is variable and does not, of itself, explain the development of hyperoxia-induced airway hyperresponsiveness.[68,69]

Epithelial injury with loss of airway relaxant factors may contribute to the hyperoxia-induced increase in airway contractile responses. This is supported by data from tracheal strips in preterm sheep, in which epithelium removal was associated with greater cholinergic responsiveness.[70] A similar phenomenon is observed in rat pups in whom the response of lung resistance induced by vagal stimulation was increased after nonspecific blockade of NO synthase in normoxic animals. However, after hyperoxic exposure NOS blockade no longer affected the contractile response induced by vagal stimulation (Fig. 82-6).[71] These findings indicate that NO, released by stimulation of vagal preganglionic fibers, modulates bronchopulmonary contractile

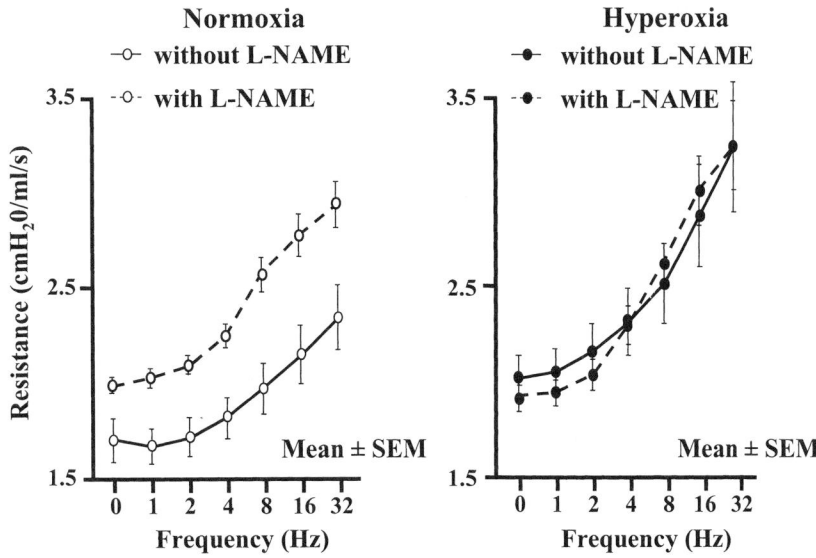

Figure 82–6. Responses of total lung resistance to vagal stimulation in normoxia (*left panel*) and hyperoxia exposed (*right panel*) rat pups. Blockade of nitric oxide synthase NOS with L-NAME potentiated the response of lung resistance in the normoxic group. In the hyperoxic group the resistance response to vagal stimulation was increased when compared to the normoxic animals, but there was no further effect of L-NAME.

responses to endogenously released ACh in rat pups. This effect appears to be lost after prolonged hyperoxic exposure and may contribute to airway hyperreactivity under these conditions. These findings are somewhat analogous to observations made in young ferrets infected with human respiratory syncytial virus in whom nonadrenergic noncholinergic inhibitory responses of tracheal smooth muscle were significantly decreased for a prolonged period.[72]

From these observations, largely in maturing animal models, the balance of airway contractile and relaxant responses plays an important role in optimizing airway patency. This delicate balance may be altered when immature airway structures are exposed to a variety of potentially injurious influences. Future studies need to focus on the signaling pathways underlying such events and the longer term consequences of such exposure in early postnatal life.

ACKNOWLEDGMENT

This chapter was prepared through the financial support of grant HL 56470 from the National Institutes of Health.

REFERENCES

1. Jordan D: Central nervous pathways and control of the airways. Respir Physiol *125*:67, 2001.
2. Coleridge HM, Coleridge JC: Neural regulation of bronchial blood flow. Respir Physiol *98*:1, 1994.
3. Fisher JT, et al: Morphological and neurophysiological aspects of airway and pulmonary receptors. *In* Haddad GG, Farber JP (eds): Developmental Neurobiology of Breathing. New York, Marcel Dekker, 1991, p 219.
4. Haxhiu-Poskurica B, et al.: Maturation of respiratory reflex responses in the piglet. J Appl Physiol *70*:608, 1991.
5. Barnes PJ: Modulation of neurotransmission in airways. Physiol Rev *72*:699, 1992.
6. Haxhiu MA, et al.: Reflex and chemical responses of tracheal submucosal glands in piglets. Respir Physiol *82*:267, 1990.
7. Anderson JW, Fisher JT: Capsaicin-induced reflex bronchoconstriction in the newborn. Respir Physiol *93*:13, 1993.
8. Kalia M, Mesulam MM: Brain stem projections of sensory and motor components of the vagus complex in the cat: II. Laryngeal, tracheobronchial, pulmonary, cardiac, and gastrointestinal branches. J Comp Neurol *193*:467, 1980.
9. Haxhiu MA, et al.: CNS innervation of airway-related parasympathetic preganglionic neurons: a transneuronal labeling study using pseudorabies virus. Brain Res *618*:115, 1993.
10. Haxhiu MA, Loewy AD: Central connections of the motor and sensory vagal systems innervating the trachea. J Auton Nerv Syst *57*:49, 1996.
11. Burnstock G: Studies of autonomic nerves in the gut-past, present and future. Scand J Gastroenterol *71*(Suppl):135, 1982.
12. Zaagsma J, et al: Muscarinic control of airway function. Life Sci *60*:1061, 1997.
13. Haxhiu-Poskurica B, et al.: Development of cholinergic innervation and muscarinic receptor subtypes in piglet trachea. Am J Physiol *264*:L606, 1993.
14. Fisher JT, et al: Muscarinic contractile competence of airway smooth muscle in the newborn dog. Can J Physiol Pharmacol *74*:603, 1996.
15. Barnes PJ: Muscarinic receptor subtypes in airways. Life Sci *52*:521, 1993.
16. Mak JCW, et al: Localization of muscarinic receptor subtype mRNAs in human lung. Am J Respir Cell Mol Biol *7*:344, 1992.
17. Jakupaj M, et al.: Role of endogenous NO modulating airway contraction mediated by muscarinic receptors during development. Am J Physiol *273* (Lung Cell Mol Physiol 17): L531, 1997.
18. Rosenberg SM, et al.: Maturational regulation of inositol 1,4,5-trisphosphate metabolism in rabbit airway smooth muscle. J Clin Invest *88*:2032, 1991.
19. Haxhiu MA, et al: Medullary effects of nicotine and GABA on tracheal smooth muscle tone. Respir Physiol *64*:351, 1986.
20. Martin RJ, et al: Neurochemical control of tissue resistance in piglets. J Appl Physiol *79*:812, 1995.
21. Waldron MA, Fisher JT: Differential effects of CO_2 and hypoxia on bronchomotor tone in the newborn dog. Respir Physiol *72*:271, 1988.
22. Tay-Uyboco JS, et al.: Hypoxic airway constriction in infants of very low birth weight recovering from moderate to severe bronchopulmonary dysplasia. J Pediatr *115*:456, 1989.
23. Teague WG, Pet al.: An acute reduction in the fraction of inspired oxygen increases airway constriction in infants with chronic lung disease. Am Rev Respir Dis *137*:861, 1988.
24. Haxhiu MA, et al.: Behavioral state control and airway instability. Adv Exp Med Biol *499*:445, 2001.
25. Barnes PJ: Beta-adrenergic receptors and their regulation. Am J Respir Crit Care Med *152*:838, 1995.
26. Nijkamp FP: β-Adrenergic receptors in the lung: an introduction. Life Sci *52*:2073, 1993.
27. Whitsett JA, et al: β-Adrenergic receptors in the developing rabbit lung. Am J Physiol *240* (Endocrinol Metab 3):E351, 1981.
28. Lyon ME, et al: Characterisation of the β adrenergic response cascade in fetal guinea pig lung. Thorax 1994; *49*:664.
29. Schramm CM, et al: Role of muscarinic M2 receptors in regulating _-adrenergic responsiveness in maturing rabbit airway smooth muscle. Am J Physiol *269*(Lung Cell Mol Physiol 13):L783, 1995.
30. Varlotta L, Schramm CM: Maturation of catecholamine response and extraneuronal uptake in rabbit trachea. Am J Physiol *266* (Lung Cell Mol Physiol 10):L217, 1994.
31. Mirmanesh SJ, et al: Alpha-adrenergic broncho provocation in neonates with broncho pulmonary displace. J Pediatr *121*:622, 1992.
32. Pandya KH: Postnatal developmental changes in adrenergic receptor responses of the dog tracheal muscle. Arch Int Pharmacodyn Ther *230*:53, 1977.
33. Watanabe H, et al: Alpha adrenergic receptor contractile responses in the newborn dog. Can J Physiol Pharmacol *72*:483, 1994.

34. Dreshaj JA, et al: Norepinephrine increases lung resistance by constricting lung parenchyma without changing airway caliber in piglets (abstract). Pediatr Res 35:331A, 1994.

35. Leff AR, et al: Autonomic response characteristics of porcine airway smooth muscle in vivo. J Appl Physiol 58:1176, 1985.

36. Faxelius G, et al: Catecholamine surge and lung function after delivery. Arch Dis Child 58:262, 1983.

37. Biyah K, Advenier C: Effects of three alpha 2-adrenoceptor agonists, rilmenidine, UK 14304 and clonidine on bradykinin- and substance P-induced airway microvascular leakage in guinea-pigs. Neuropeptides 29:197, 1995.

38. Waldron MA, Fisher JT: Neural control of airway smooth muscle in the newborn. In Haddad G, Farber JP (eds): Developmental Neurobiology of Breathing. New York, Marcel Dekker, 1991, p 483.

39. Waldron MA, et al: Nonadrenergic inhibitory innervation to the airways of the newborn cat. J Appl Physiol 66:1995, 1989.

40. Clerici C, et al: Nonadrenergic bronchodilation in newborn guinea pigs. J Appl Physiol 67:1764, 1989.

41. Colasurdo GN, et al: Maturation of nonadrenergic noncholinergic inhibitory system in normal and allergen-sensitized rabbits. Am J Physiol (Lung Cell Mol Physiol) 267:L739, 1994.

42. Fayon M, et al: Human airway smooth muscle responsiveness in neonatal lung specimens. Am J Physiol 267 (Lung Cell Mol Physiol 11):L180, 1994.

43. North AJ, et al: Nitric oxide synthase type I and type III gene expression are developmentally regulated in rat lung. Am J Physiol 266:L635, 1995.

44. Sherman TS, et al.: Nitric oxide synthase isoform expression in the developing lung epithelium. Am J Physiol 276 (Lung Cell Mol Physiol 20):L383, 1999.

45. Potter CF, et al.: Effect of exogenous and endogenous nitric oxide (NO) on the airway and tissue components of lung resistance in the newborn piglet. Pediatr Res 41:886, 1997.

46. Tanaka DT, Grunstein MM: Maturation of neuromodulatory effect of substance P in rabbit airways. J Clin Invest 83:345, 1990.

47. Haxhiu-Poskurica B, et al: Tracheal smooth muscle responses to substance P and neurokinin A in the piglet. J Appl Physiol 72:1090, 1992.

48. Yohannan MD, et al: Ontogeny of neurokinin-1 receptors in the porcine respiratory system. Peptides 220:1454, 1999.

49. Kwong K, et al.: Chronic smoking enhances tachykinin synthesis and airway responsiveness in guinea pigs. Am J Respir Cell Mol Biol 25:299, 2001.

50. Killingsworth CR, et al: Substance P content and preprotachykinin gene-I mRNA expression in a rat model of chronic bronchitis. Am J Respir Cell Mol Biol 14:334, 1996.

51. Mhanna MJ, et al.: Mechanism for substance P-induced relaxation of precontracted airway smooth muscle during development. Am J Physiol 276 (Lung Cell Mol Physiol 20):L51, 1999.

52. Agani FH, et al: Effect of hyperoxia on substance P expression and airway reactivity in the developing lung. Am J Physiol: Lung Cell Mol Physiol 40–45, 1997.

53. Sparrow MP, et al: Development of the innervation and airway smooth muscle in human fetal lung. Am J Respir Cell Mol Biol 20:550, 1999.

54. Schittny JC, et al: Spontaneous peristaltic airway contractions propel lung liquid through the bronchial tree of intact and fetal lung explants. Am J Respir Cell Mol Biol 23:11, 2000.

55. Sward-Comunelli SL, et al.: Airway muscle in preterm infants: changes during development. J Pediatr 130:570, 1997.

56. Shen X, et al.: Effect of transpulmonary pressure on airway diameter and responsiveness of immature and mature rabbits. J Appl Physiol 89:1584, 2000.

57. Ramchandani R, et al.: Differences in airway structure in immature and mature rabbits. J Appl Physiol 89:1310, 2000.

58. Panitch HB, et al: A comparison of preterm and adult airway smooth muscle mechanics. J Appl Physiol 1989; 66:1760.

59. Rodriguez RJ, Dreshaj IA, Kumar G, et al.: Maturation of the cholinergic response of tracheal smooth muscle in the piglet. Pediatr Pulmonol 1994; 18:28.

60. Murphy TM, Mitchell RW, Halayko A, et al.: Effect of maturational changes in myosin content and morphometry on airway smooth muscle contraction. Am J Physiol 260 (Lung Cell Mol Physiol 4):L471, 1991.

61. Clement MG, et al.: Effects of vagotomy on respiratory mechanics in newborn and adult pigs. J Appl Physiol 60:1992, 1986.

62. Panitch HB, et al: Maturational changes in airway smooth muscle structure-function relationships. Pediatr Res 31:151, 1992.

63. Penn RB, et al: Developmental differences in tracheal cartilage mechanics. Pediatr Res 26:429, 1989.

64. Smith PG, et al.: Mechanical strain increases force production and calcium sensitivity in cultured airway smooth muscle cells. J Appl Physiol 89:2002, 2000.

65. Smith PG, et al: Mechanical strain increases contractile enzyme activity in cultured airway smooth muscle cells. Am J Physiol 268(Lung Cell Mol Physiol 12):L999, 268.

66. Agani FH, et al.: Effect of hyperoxia on substance P expression and airway reactivity in the developing lung. Am J Physiol 273(Lung Cell Mol Physiol 17):L40, 1997.

67. Uyehara CFT, et al.: Hyperoxic exposure enhances airway reactivity of newborn guinea pigs. J Appl Physiol 74:2649, 1993.

68. Szarek JL, et al.: Time course of airway hyperresponsiveness and remodeling induced by hyperoxia in rats. Am J Physiol 269 (Lung Cell Mol Physiol 13):L227, 1995.

69. Hershenson MB, et al.: Exposure of immature rats to hyperoxia increases tracheal smooth muscle stress generation in vitro. J Appl Physiol 76:743, 1994.

70. Panitch HB, et al.: Epithelial modulation of preterm airway smooth muscle contraction. J Appl Physiol 74:1437, 1993.

71. Iben SC, et al.: Role of endogenous nitric oxide in hyperoxia-induced airway hyperreactivity in maturing rats. J Appl Physiol 89:1205, 2000.

72. Colasurdo GN, et al.: Human respiratory syncytial virus produces prolonged alterations of neural control in airways of developing ferrets. Am J Respir Crit Care Med 157:1506, 1998.

83

Gary C. Sieck, Carlos B. Mantilla, and Mohamed A. Fahim

Functional Development of Respiratory Muscles

In this chapter, we focus on the fetal and neonatal development of the diaphragm muscle (DIAm), the major inspiratory muscle in mammals. The DIAm is a complex structure separating the thoracic and abdominal cavities, hence the Greek derivation of its name meaning "to span a partition." The DIAm appears rather late in evolution; it is present only in mammals, whereas other vertebrates use different means of ventilation. The DIAm has multiple sites of origin and insertion reflecting its complex embryologic derivation. The mechanical actions of the DIAm are as complex as its multiple sites of origin and insertion. Its major function is in inspiration, although the DIAm is also involved in several nonventilatory motor behaviors including coughing, defecation, emesis, micturition, parturition, sneezing, vocalization, and weight lifting.

As in other skeletal muscles, neural control of the DIAm is based on recruitment and frequency coding of motor units, each comprising a motoneuron and the muscle fibers it innervates. Motor units in the adult DIAm vary considerably in their mechanical, histochemical, and biochemical properties,[1-4] and this heterogeneity provides the range of control of muscle force generation that occurs during different motor behaviors. The cumulative contractile and fatigue properties of the motor unit pool determine the constraints under which the DIAm responds to the various mechanical demands placed on it during different ventilatory and nonventilatory behaviors. Clearly, these motor demands can change during development, and the DIAm must adapt or remodel to accommodate these changing demands.

The DIAm becomes rhythmically active during late fetal development (fetal respiratory movements), and at birth, it must be ready to sustain ventilation. Postnatally, the DIAm is one of the most active skeletal muscles, with a duty cycle (time active versus relaxed) of approximately 40%, compared with limb muscles (duty cycles ranging from 2 to 15%). It is not surprising, therefore, that fetal and neonatal disorders of the DIAm often lead to ventilatory failure and premature death. Despite the vital importance of the DIAm, previous studies have provided mostly descriptive information about its development and growth. However, accumulating information about myogenesis and

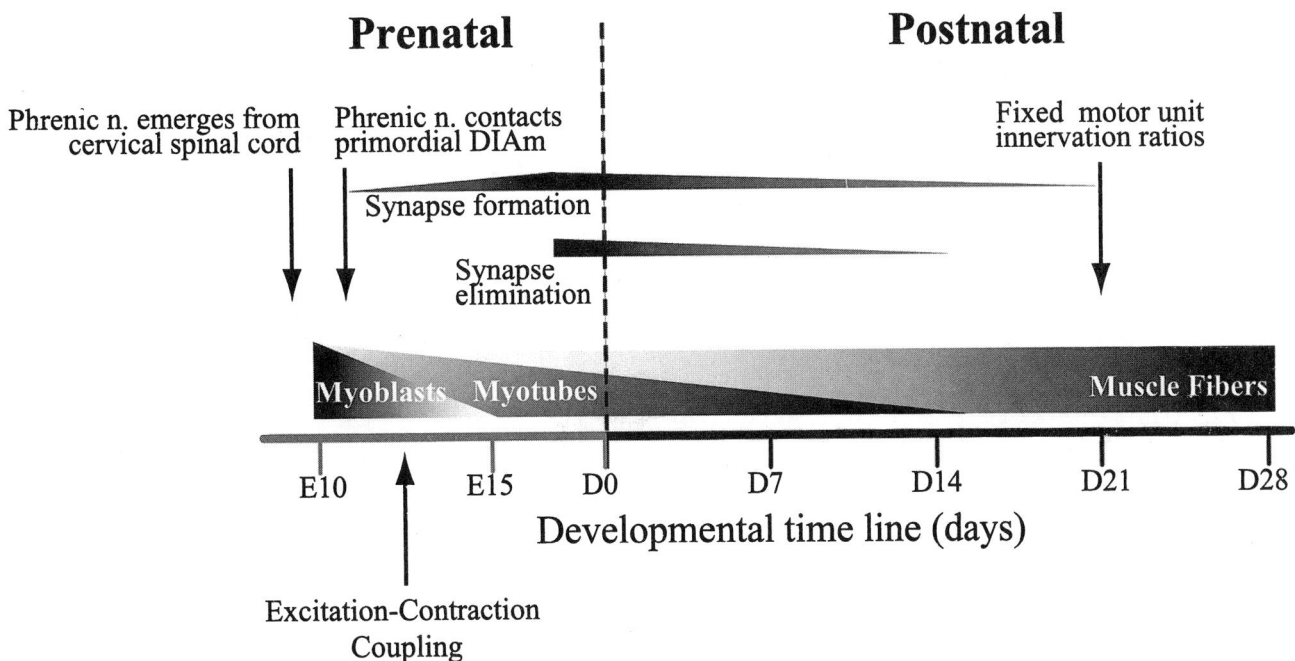

Figure 83–1. Schematic illustration showing the timeline for major events in the development of the mouse diaphragm muscle (DIAm). Similar seminal events occur in the embryonic and early postnatal development of the DIAm in other mammals including humans, although temporal characteristics and inter-relationships may vary.

neural development that derives from *in vitro* model systems may be applicable to the mechanisms regulating DIAm development *in vivo*. Yet the applicability of these *in vitro* results regarding the basis of myogenesis and neural development remains to be established, especially in the context of maturation of other systems, such as the central nervous system, the lung, and the thoracic and abdominal walls. Unfortunately, such integrative information is lacking.

Increasingly, rodent models are used to explore the genetic basis for developmental plasticity in neuromotor control. Accordingly, in this chapter, we focus on results obtained in rats and mice. Benchmarks for the development of the mouse DIAm are summarized in Figure 83-1. The fetal and neonatal developmental benchmarks in rats are generally comparable to those in mice, and at present there is much more information specific to the DIAm in rats. In mice, developmental benchmarks for the DIAm begin at approximately embryonic day 11 or 12 (E11, E12), when the phrenic nerve makes initial contact with the primordial DIAm. These developmental benchmarks in the rat, although offset by a few days, are generally comparable. In both species, the final pattern of adult motor units and muscle fiber types is not achieved until postnatal day 28 (D28). During this 5- to 6-week span, dramatic changes in DIAm innervation, contractile protein expression, and function occur. Obviously, the timeline for such developmental benchmarks in humans is far more protracted, but it is likely that a similar convergence of neural and myogenic events also occurs. Therefore, much can be learned by studying the integrated aspects of myogenesis and neural development of the DIAm in rodent models.

EMBRYOLOGIC DERIVATION AND INNERVATION OF THE DIAPHRAGM MUSCLE

Myogenesis

Skeletal muscle fibers, including those in the DIAm, are formed in two stages: (1) commitment (also known as determination), in which mesodermal progenitor cells are transformed to myoblasts; and (2) terminal differentiation, in which myoblasts fuse to form myotubes and myofibers (Fig. 83-2). Myogenesis may proceed via an intrinsic genetic program, or it may require either the presence of positive extrinsic signals or the removal of inhibitory signals.[5] None of these potential mechanisms can be excluded at present. However, there is converging evidence that myogenesis is induced in various nonmuscle cells by the expression of proteins belonging to the basic helix-loop-helix (bHLH) superfamily.[6,7] Collectively, these are known as muscle regulatory factors (MRFs) and include MyoD,[8] myogenin,[9] Myf-5,[10] and MRF4.[11] In human muscle, MRF4 is also known as Myf-6.[12] In addition to providing a molecular mechanism for the regulation of myogenesis in fetal and neonatal muscle, MRFs are also involved in determining the expression of myosin heavy chain (MHC) isoforms in adult muscle.[13]

Genetic determinants of myoblast commitment have been most extensively studied in *Drosophila*, but this information is likely to be directly applicable to myoblast commitment in the mammalian DIAm as well. In *Drosophila*, it has been shown that neural-derived proteins (e.g., sonic hedgehog and Wnt 1, 3, and 4) promote commitment to myoblasts within a myotome.[5, 14] Expression of sonic hedgehog and other signals commit mesodermal cells to form myoblasts, possibly by releasing suppression of the expression of specific MRFs.[15] The process of myoblast commitment is marked by the expression of the paired-box protein Pax-3, which appears to regulate MRF expression positively. For example, it has been shown that ectopic expression of Pax-3 induces both MyoD and Myf-5 in embryonic tissue.[16] The consequent increase in MRFs then initiates a cascade of signals that continues through differentiation and thus sustains myogenesis. The MRFs function as molecular switches, initiating myogenesis by inducing expression of muscle-specific genes through binding of the bHLH motif to *cis*-acting DNA control elements of muscle-specific genes, known as E-boxes.[17] The E-box is a CANNTG sequence-containing motif present in the promoter regions of many skeletal muscle–specific genes.[18] Transcriptional regulation mediated by MRFs may also involve interactions of MRFs with the family of MADS-box proteins termed myocyte

Commitment

Terminal Differentiation

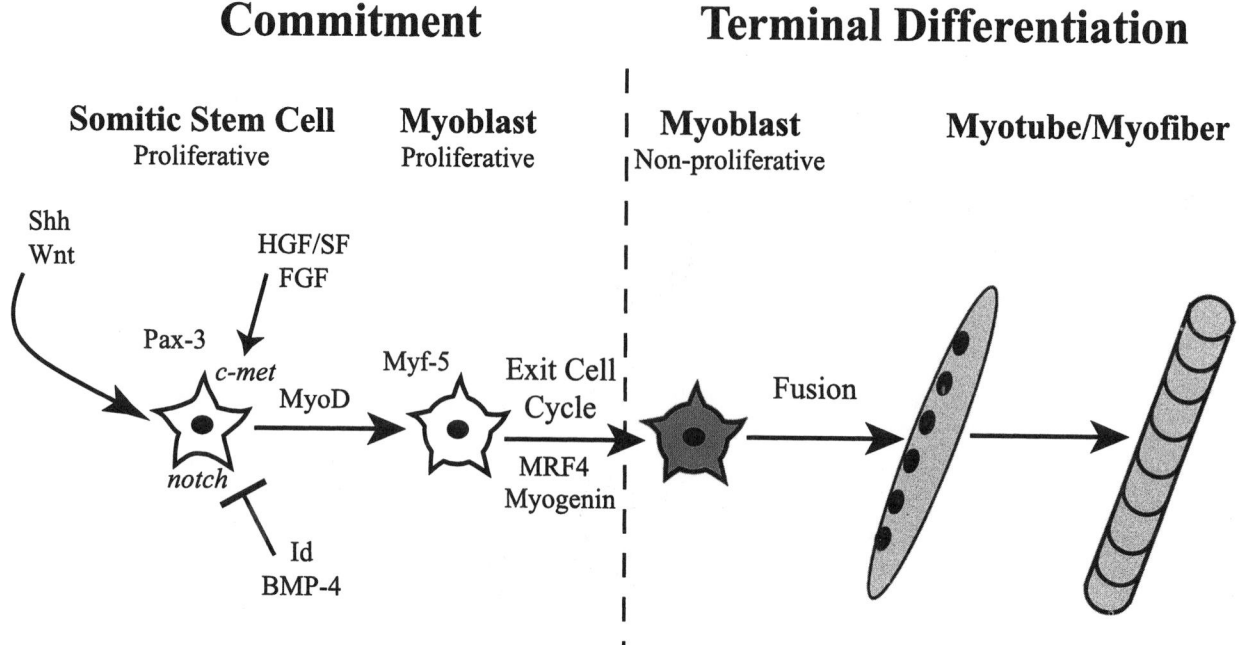

Figure 83–2. Schematic illustration demonstrating the two major stages of myogenesis: commitment and terminal differentiation. During commitment, somitic stem cells proliferate and are committed to myoblasts, a process marked by MyoD and Myf-5 expression. This process ends when proliferating myoblasts exit the cell cycle, influenced by expression of muscle regulatory factor 4 (MRF4) and myogenin. The exit of myoblasts from the cell cycle marks the beginning of the differentiation stage. Thereafter, nonproliferative myoblasts fuse to form myotubes and, with the formation of distinct sarcomeres, myofibers. The differentiation process continues until adult fiber types are established. BMP-4 = bone morphogenic protein 4; FGF = fibroblast growth factor; HGF/SF = hepatocyte growth factor/scatter factor.

enhancer factor 2 (MEF2A-D). MEF2 may determine muscle-specificity for genes lacking MRF binding domains. Binding sites for MEF2 are located in the promoter regions of many muscle-specific genes including myogenin. However, MEF2 binding alone is not sufficient to induce myogenesis.

It is also possible that myoblast commitment is prevented by the presence of inhibitory signals that suppress MRF expression or activity. For example, a class of HLH proteins, termed Id factors (Id1-Id4), inhibits MRF activity by forming heterodimers with E2 products (ubiquitously expressed HLH-containing proteins encoded for by E2 genes). These products prevent dimerization with MRFs and subsequent activation of skeletal muscle–specific genes.[19] The Id proteins lack the basic DNA binding domain; therefore, heterodimerization of bHLH proteins with Id proteins prevents the strong binding to DNA by either E-proteins or MRFs.[20] Another example is the twist protein, which, in mice, inhibits MRFs by sequestering E-proteins and thus prevents the formation of MRF-E protein heterodimers.[21] Yet another inhibitory factor is Mist1, which binds with MyoD to form an inactive heterodimer.[22] It is possible that such inhibitory influences on the myogenic program exist to prevent myogenesis in nonmyotomal somite cells and thus ectopic formation of skeletal muscle.

In hypaxial muscles (e.g., limb muscles, chest and abdominal wall muscles, and DIAm), MyoD is the first MRF to be expressed. MyoD expression then initiates a cascade resulting in subsequent expression of Myf-5, MRF4, and myogenin.[23] The sequence of MRF expression appears to be critical for the development of normal muscle. MyoD and Myf-5 are highly expressed in proliferating myoblasts, a finding suggesting a primary role for these MRFs during this stage of myogenesis.[8] In mutant mice lacking MyoD[24] or MRF4,[25] there is no apparent effect on normal skeletal muscle development, but Myf-5 and myogenin are upregulated, respectively. Therefore, it is possible that redundant

MRF expression may rescue normal skeletal muscle phenotype in these animals. Similarly, Myf-5–deficient mice appear to have normal skeletal muscle, but they succumb to asphyxiation soon after birth because of rib cage abnormalities.[26] In contrast, myogenin-deficient mice have only myoblasts without the development of myotubes/myofibers,[27, 28] a finding suggesting that myogenin is indispensable for differentiation of myotubes/myofibers. In mice lacking both Myf-5 and MyoD, no myoblasts are present, a finding suggesting that expression of both these MRFs is required for myoblast commitment.[29] Mice lacking Myf-5 and MRF4 resemble Myf-5 knock-outs, a finding suggesting that MRF4 regulates later aspects of myogenesis.

With terminal differentiation, committed mononucleated myoblasts are nonreversibly transformed into multinucleated myotubes/myofibers with expression of contractile proteins (see Fig. 83–2). Thus, terminal differentiation represents the irreversible exit of proliferating myoblasts from the cell cycle. Yet not all myoblasts lose their ability to proliferate, because a pool of myoblasts (satellite cells) persists into adulthood, and their proliferative capacity is important in processes of injury and repair as well as in other conditions of muscle remodeling. Throughout life, proliferating myoblasts are susceptible to apoptosis (i.e., programmed cell death) until they are terminally differentiated and exit the cell cycle. The balance between proliferation and apoptosis may play an important role in controlling the total number of muscle fibers of a given type.[30] Terminal differentiation of myoblasts in hypaxial muscles does not occur *in vivo* until myoblasts have migrated from the myotome to their final location (e.g., thoracic or abdominal walls or the limbs). As myoblasts migrate from the lateral dermomyotome, they express Myf-5 and c-met (a tyrosine kinase receptor for hepatocyte growth factor/scatter factor), which thus can be used as markers for this process of differentiation. In hypaxial muscles, including the DIAm, expression of Myf-5 and c-met begins at approximately E10 and continues through E12.[31] Expression of MyoD is also important in the process of terminal differentiation, and it can be inhibited *in vitro* by bone morphogenic protein 4 or fibroblast growth factor 5,[15] both of which have been implicated in maintenance of the myoblast proliferative capacity and inhibition of differentiation.

Terminal differentiation of mononucleated myoblasts leads to their fusion and formation of multinucleated myotubes/myofibers. Although the formation of myotubes/myofibers is coincident with the initial appearance of innervation in hypaxial muscles, converging evidence from *in vitro* and *in vivo* models indicates that terminal differentiation can be initiated in the absence of neural influence. Myotubes/myofibers can form *in vitro* in the absence of innervation, but at a much slower pace compared with that observed *in vivo*. This finding suggests that neural influence may facilitate the normal process of terminal differentiation and formation of myotubes/myofibers. This potential facilitating influence of innervation needs to be explored further. There is evidence, based on *in vitro* model systems, that terminal differentiation into myotube/myofiber formation depends on the expression of several other nonneural proteins, including those present in the extracellular matrix (e.g., fibronectins and laminins), basal lamina (e.g., muscle cell adhesion molecule, neural cell adhesion molecule, and M-cadherin), cell membrane (e.g., β_1-integrin), and cytoskeleton (e.g., actin and desmin).[32] Obviously, terminal differentiation and myotube/myofiber formation involve very complex interactions between differentiating cells and their surrounding environment. Current research is only starting to unravel these complex interactions. Even though the process of myoblast fusion into myotubes/myofibers is called terminal differentiation, there is subsequent differentiation of these nascent muscle fibers into adult muscle fiber types (see later).

In addition to the hormonal and biochemical milieu, other factors may also influence myogenesis. For example, *in vitro* passive mechanical strain results in both myotube hyperplasia and hypertrophy.[33,34] Thus, both proliferation and differentiation of myoblasts are affected by passive strain. Passive stretching can also prevent the atrophy of myotubes, which normally occurs in culture media containing no growth factors. The transduction of passive strain into a proliferative or trophic influence is unclear, but it may involve mediators such as prostaglandin $F_{2\alpha}$, insulinlike growth factor I, or other cytokines.[34] Although these *in vitro* studies employed passive strain, these results suggest that early mechanical activation of the fetal DIAm (e.g., fetal respiratory movements) may be important in promoting further myogenesis.

Myosin Heavy Chain

Myosin is a hexameric protein (MW 480 kDa) comprising two heavy chains and four light chains. At the rod-shaped COOH-terminus end of the myosin molecule, the two heavy chains (MW 200 kDa) dimerize into a 200-nm α-helical tail. At the NH_3-terminus, the heavy chains separate and form two distinct heads (S-1), which contain both actin and nucleotide binding domains of the myosin molecule. The S-1 converts chemical energy into mechanical work through a process that involves stereospecific docking of S-1 with actin, thereby reversing the intramolecular conformational changes induced by adenosine triphosphate (ATP) hydrolysis.[35,36] Numerous MHC isoforms exist, all of which are encoded by a highly conserved multigene family located on chromosome 17 (human) or 11 (mouse).[37] The rate of ATP hydrolysis at the S-1 varies among the different MHC isoforms, and this provides the molecular basis for fiber type differences in mechanical properties.[38-41] The essential (MLC_{20}) and regulatory myosin light chains (MLC_{17}) provide structural support and possibly modulate mechanical performance of the MHC.[42] For example, different MLC isoforms exist, and it has been suggested

that these different isoforms modulate the kinetic properties of MHC.[43] There is also evidence that either calcium (Ca^{2+}) binding to or phosphorylation of MLC_{17} results in modulation of S-1 ATPase activity.[44-46]

Adult skeletal muscle fibers are classified histochemically as Type I, IIa, and IIb, based on the pH lability of myofibrillar ATPase staining.[47] Muscle fiber type classification in the adult corresponds with the expression of different MHC isoforms; fibers classified as Type I express MHC_{Slow}, IIa fibers express MHC_{2A}, and IIb fibers express MHC_{2B} or MHC_{2X}.[37,48-50] Such histochemical classification of muscle fiber types is not possible during fetal and neonatal development. During this period, there are dramatic transitions in MHC isoform expression, with a high incidence of coexpression of MHC isoforms that precludes ready distinction of different muscle fiber types.[51-54] In the fetal mouse and rat DIAm, an embryonic MHC isoform (MHC_{Emb}) is predominantly expressed together with MHC_{Slow} and MHC_{2A}. At or close to birth, the predominant isoform expression switches to a neonatal MHC isoform (MHC_{Neo}), again together with MHC_{Slow} and MHC_{2A}. Thereafter, MHC_{Neo} expression gradually disappears and is totally absent in the mouse and rat DIAm by D28. Expression of MHC_{2X} and MHC_{2B} isoforms emerges only after D14 in the mouse and rat DIAm, and the proportion of fibers expressing these isoforms increases until about D28, when the adult pattern of MHC isoform expression is fully established. This dramatic postnatal transition in MHC isoform expression in the DIAm represents an important stage of muscle fiber differentiation, especially with respect to the development of mature contractile properties (see later). Beyond D28, the relative contribution of each MHC isoform changes because of the disproportionate growth of DIAm fibers (e.g., the growth of fibers expressing MHC_{2X} and MHC_{2B} is approximately two- to threefold greater than that of fibers expressing MHC_{Slow} and MHC_{2A} isoforms).[1,55,56] Based on the temporal associations between innervation and the major developmental events in myogenesis (see later), it would seem reasonable that the nervous system can either directly (e.g., activity, nerve traffic) or indirectly (e.g., secretion of neurotrophins) influence DIAm development.[57] However, the precise mechanisms by which activation history and neurotrophins influence DIAm development remain largely unknown. The time course for developmental transitions in MHC isoform expression in the DIAm is also influenced by the hormonal milieu (e.g., thyroid hormones, growth hormone, insulin-like growth hormone) surrounding the fibers. For example, MHC expression is sensitive to thyroid hormone levels.[58,59] Nutritional status can also affect myogenesis and MHC isoform expression.[55]

Embryologic Origins

The DIAm derives from three embryonic structures: the septum transversum, the pleuroperitoneal membranes, and the esophageal mesenchyme.[60,61] The septum transversum forms a transverse partition separating the thoracic (superior), containing the developing heart and pericardial cavity, from the abdominal (inferior), containing the future peritoneal cavity, portions of the coelomic cavity. However, the peritoneum and pericardial cavities communicate through two large dorsolateral openings, the pericardioperitoneal canals. The left pleuropericardial canal is larger than the right and closes at a later stage in development; this accounts for the greater incidence of congenital DIAm hernias on the left side. Growth of the embryonic axis causes a progressive caudal displacement of the septum transversum. The anterior edge of the septum transversum eventually becomes attached at the midthoracic level, whereas the dorsal edge becomes attached at the lowest thoracic level. Committed myoblasts migrate within the septum transversum and eventually differentiate to form DIAm myotubes/myofibers. Coincident with myoblast migration, the phrenic nerves exit the cervical spinal cord following the septum transversum and migrating myoblasts.[61, 62] It is possible that instead of the migrating myoblasts, the initial targets of phrenic nerve terminals are the pleuroperitoneal membranes,[63, 64] which are transverse membranes that grow ventrally to fuse with the posterior margin of the septum transversum. As it descends, the phrenic nerve moves toward the central tendon within the pleuropericardial folds to a medial location between the pericardial and pleural cavities. The mechanism by which the phrenic nerve is guided toward the primordial DIAm remains unclear.

Innervation

Although the crural portions of the DIAm have a different derivation (the esophageal mesenchyme) and site of origin (upper lumbar vertebral column) compared with the costal and sternal regions, all regions of the DIAm are innervated by cervical spinal cord segments.[65-68] Innervation of the DIAm displays a somatotopic pattern, with the sternal and more ventral aspects of both costal and crural regions being innervated by phrenic motoneurons located in more rostral segments of the cervical spinal cord. It remains unclear whether the somatotopic pattern of DIAm innervation develops before or after initial synapse formation (i.e., it could reflect either the pattern of phrenic nerve outgrowth or the location of myotubes/myofibers).

In the mouse, the phrenic nerve arrives at the developing DIAm by E11 (see Fig. 83-1; Fig. 83-3), whereas in the rat, the phrenic nerve is only just emerging from the cervical spinal cord at E11 and contacts the primordial DIAm by about E13.[64] Thus, there is about a 2-day difference between mice and rats with respect to the time course of these important developmental benchmarks. After arrival at the primordial DIAm, phrenic motor axons branch, apparently guided by Schwann cells, which make initial contact with myotubes/myofibers (see Fig. 83-3; Fig. 83-4). Both Schwann cells and nerve terminals at this early stage display coated vesicles, a finding suggesting vesicular release (Fig. 83-5). Certain regulatory processes may be involved in guiding Schwann cell and phrenic axon terminal outgrowth, both with respect to the initial targeting to the pleuroperitoneal fold and the subsequent contact with myotubes/myofibers. These regulatory processes may involve components of the extracellular matrix or the release of neurotrophins or chemotactic substances. Schwann cell migration and branching may be essential to the outgrowth and branching of phrenic nerve terminals. Unfortunately, most of the available literature in this important area is limited because it is based on measurements of axonal outgrowth and branching using *in vitro* preparations. Clearly, this is a complex integrated system in which *in vitro* measurements may not accurately reflect *in vivo* conditions.

In both rats and mice, it has been shown that phrenic motoneurons and DIAm express various neurotrophins that could influence neural and DIAm development including neurotrophin-3, neurotrophin-4/5, and brain-derived neurotrophic factor (BDNF).[69, 70] Neurotrophin receptors (i.e., TrkC-neurotrophin-3; TrkB-neurotrophin-4/5, and BDNF) are present in DIAm[69] and phrenic nerve terminals. It remains to be established

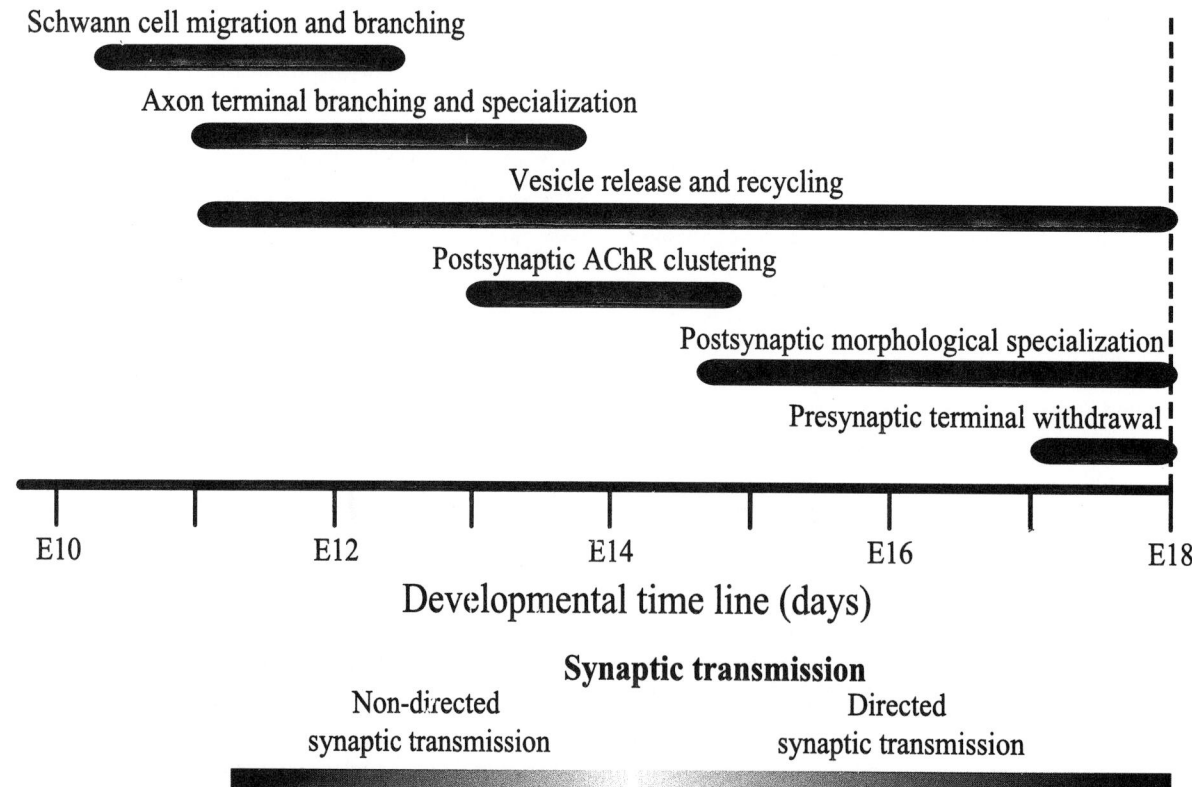

Figure 83–3. Schematic illustration demonstrating the timeline for major events in synapse formation in the mouse diaphragm muscle including differentiation of presynaptic and postsynaptic elements of neuromuscular junctions. Experimental evidence suggests that synaptic transmission is initially "nondirected" toward specific postsynaptic targets (i.e., cholinergic receptor [AChR] clusters that define motor end plates). With cholinergic receptor clustering and differentiation of postsynaptic specializations, synaptic transmission becomes "directed" toward these targets.

how expression of neurotrophins and their receptors changes during embryonic and early postnatal development of the DIAm. However, the presence of these neurotrophins and evidence of vesicular trafficking at early stages of embryonic development suggest that secretion of neurotrophins may at least partially influence nerve terminal outgrowth, synapse formation, or DIAm myogenesis. In this respect, homozygous null mutant mice for neurotrophin-3, BDNF, and TrkB do not survive after birth.[71, 72] Clearly, other abnormalities in the central nervous systems of these mutant animals may affect survivability. Unfortunately, there is no specific information available concerning development of the phrenic nerve, nor have structural abnormalities in the DIAm been explored.

Concurrent with the outgrowth of phrenic nerve terminals, there is also a progression of events on the postsynaptic side,

with the expression and aggregation of cholinergic receptors. In the mouse DIAm, aggregation and clustering of cholinergic receptors are apparent at about E13 (see Fig. 83–3; Fig. 83–6). The process of aggregation of cholinergic receptors has received considerable attention, and it is known that this process involves agrin secretion by the nerve terminal and incorporation into the basal lamina, with subsequent activation of muscle-specific kinase (MuSK) receptors at the postsynaptic membrane and finally rapsyn-mediated cholinergic receptor clustering.[73] However, it has been shown that cholinergic receptor clustering can occur in the absence of neural influence. Yet these early cholinergic receptor clusters are not maintained.[74, 75] After the aggregation of cholinergic receptors, there is further specialization of the postsynaptic membrane, with the formation of synaptic folds and differentiation of the complex neuromuscular

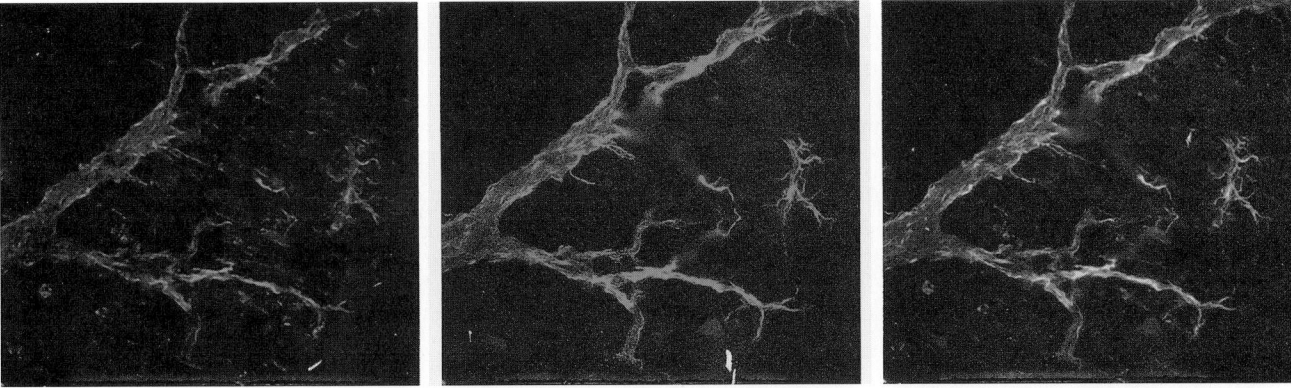

Figure 83–4. Confocal photomicrographs displaying immunoreactivity for neurofilamin (to mark branching nerve fibers in *green*) and S-100 (to mark Schwann cells in *red*) in the mouse diaphragm muscle at E12.5. Note the extensive branching and overlap of both nerve fibers and Schwann cells at this early age. See also color plate section.

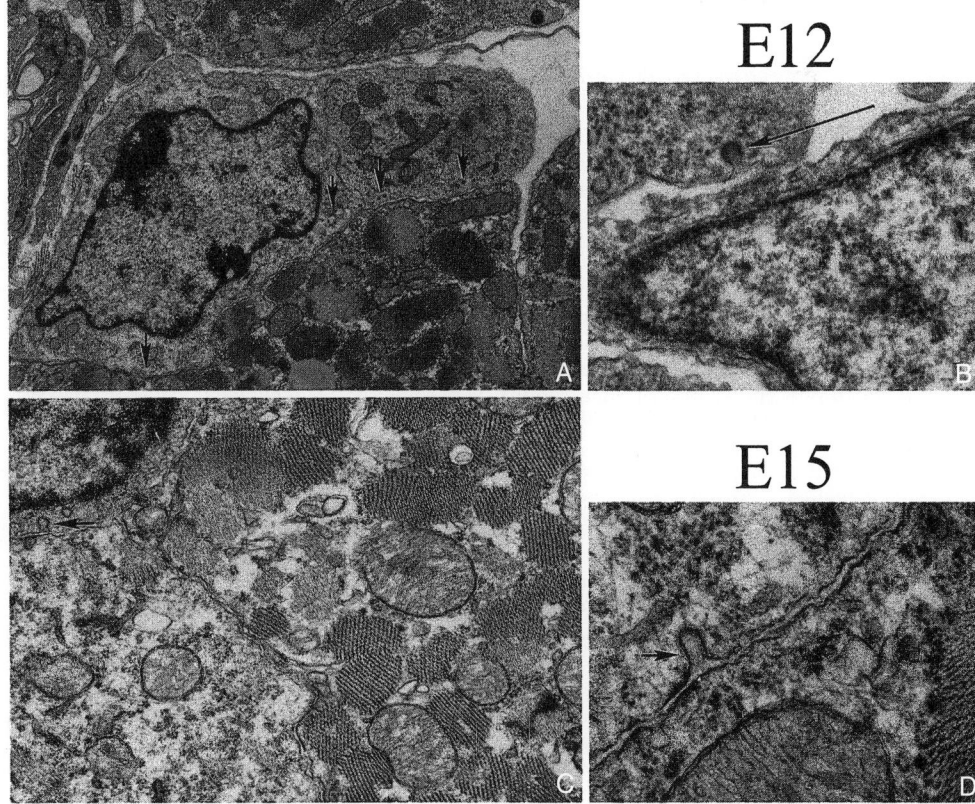

Figure 83–5. Electron photomicrographs showing (**A**) the presence of coated vesicles (*arrows*) in both a nerve terminal and a Schwann cell (noted by the presence of a distinct nucleus) and (**B**) an exocytotic vesicle (*arrow*) at a nerve terminal in a mouse diaphragm muscle at E12. Evidence of nondirected vesicular release (*arrow*) from both nerve terminals (**C**) and Schwann cells (**D**) continues through E15.

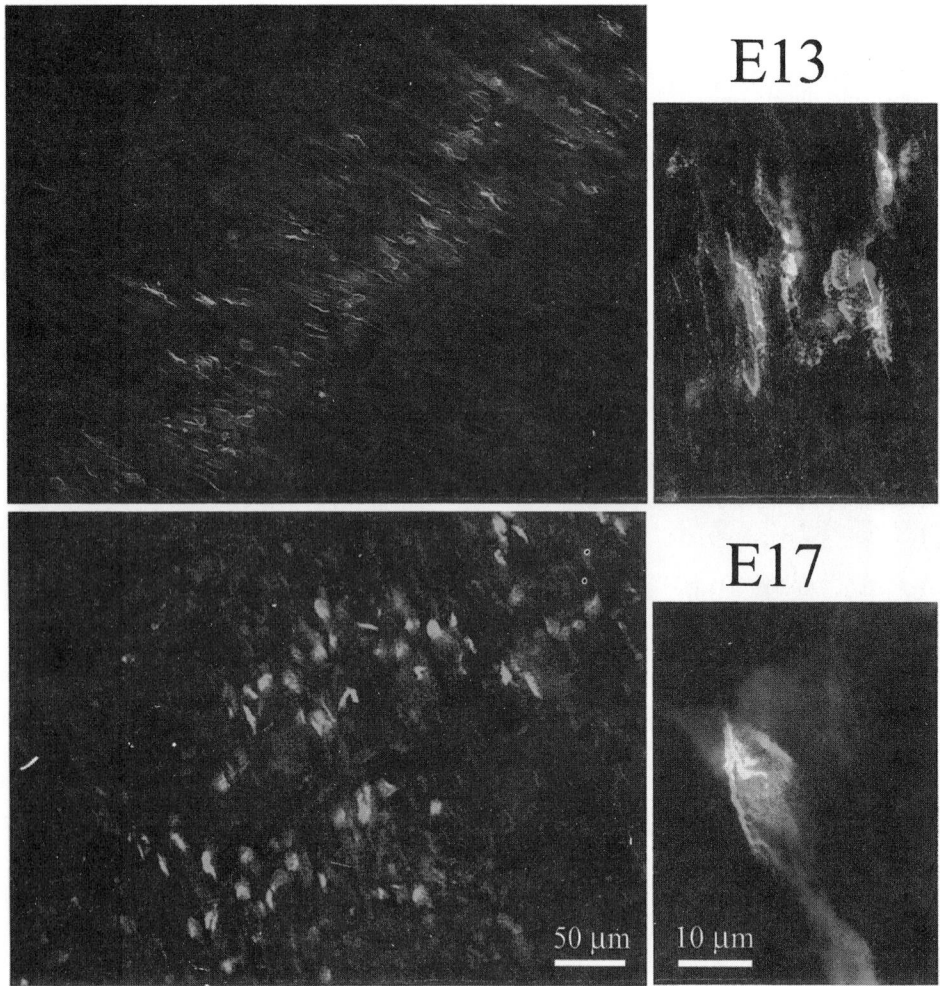

E13

E17

50 μm   10 μm

Figure 83–6. Confocal photomicrographs displaying α-bungarotoxin (BTX) labeling (in *green*) of cholinergic receptors and neurofilamin (NF) labeling (in *red*) of phrenic nerve axons and nerve terminals in the mouse diaphragm muscle at E13 and E17. Note the more diffuse pattern of BTX staining at E13 compared with E17, a finding indicating a progression toward clustering of cholinergic receptors. Also note the greater overlap between nerve terminals (NF staining) and cholinergic receptors (BTX staining) at E17. See also color plate section.

junction structure characteristic of the adult DIAm (see Fig. 83-3; Fig. 83-7). Previously, we demonstrated that in the adult rat DIAm, neuromuscular junction morphology varies across different fiber types (Fig. 83-8), and it is far more complex in fibers expressing MHC_{2X} and MHC_{2B} isoforms as compared with fibers expressing MHC_{Slow} and MHC_{2A} isoforms.[76] The morphology of neuromuscular junctions is much smaller and is far less complex in the fetal and neonatal DIAm (Fig. 83-9), but there is currently very little information regarding the mechanisms responsible for the development of fiber type-specific differences in neuromuscular junction structure.

Initially, a single myotube/myofiber can be contacted by multiple motoneurons (polyneuronal innervation). Subsequently, polyneuronal innervation disappears through the process of synapse elimination, which, in the mouse and rat DIAm, is complete by about D14 (see Fig. 83-1; Fig. 83-10).[74,77-81] The process of synapse elimination is not fully understood. It has been suggested that there may be a competition among motoneurons for target cell innervation that depends on activity (Hebbian competition).[80-82] Accordingly, terminal synapses of more active motoneurons will persist at the expense of less active motoneurons. This theory is confounded by the finding that, in adult muscle, motor units with the largest innervation ratio (i.e., number of muscle fibers innervated by a single motoneuron) are those that are least active (e.g., fast-fatigable motor units).[83-85] Accordingly, either the activity patterns of these motoneurons must change dramatically during development (transitioning from most to least active) or these motoneurons must initially

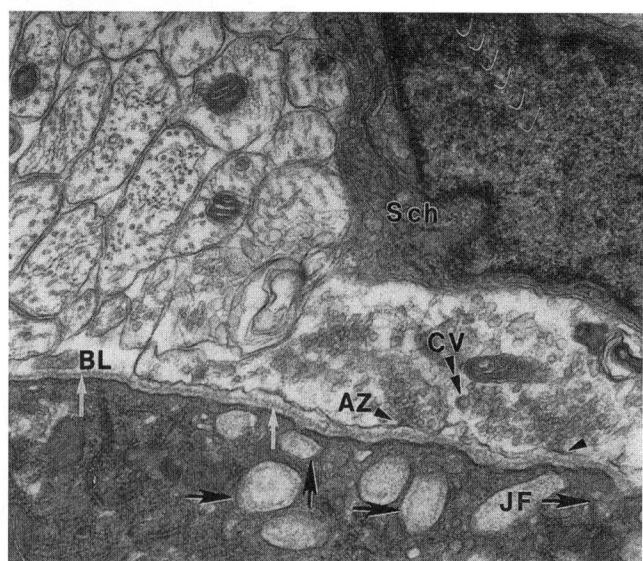

Figure 83–7. Electron photomicrograph illustrating the presence of postsynaptic specializations (e.g., basal lamina [BL], *white arrows*, and junctional folds [JF], *black arrows*) at a neuromuscular junction in the mouse diaphragm muscle at E16. The electron micrograph also displays nerve terminals containing coated synaptic vesicles (CV) aggregating around active zones (AZ) and a Schwann cell (Sch).

Slow
(Type I)

Fast Fatigable
(Type IIb or IIx)

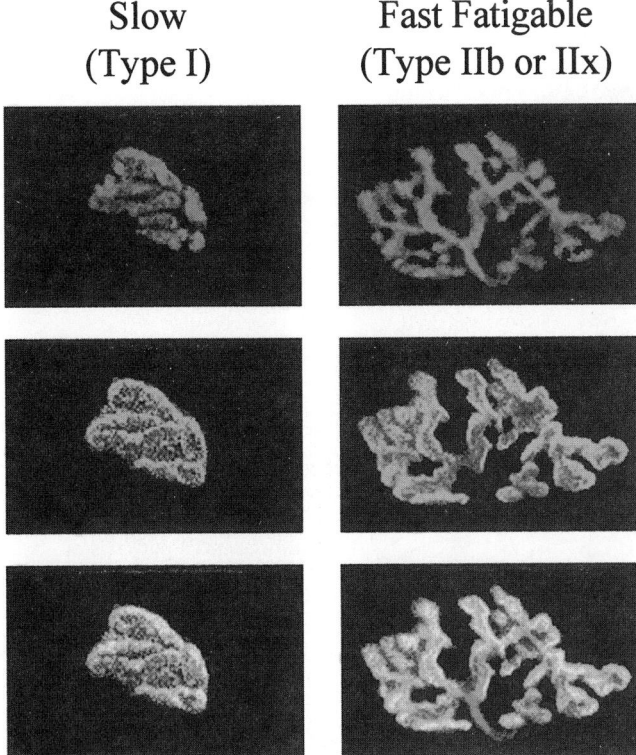

Figure 83–8. Confocal photomicrographs of presynaptic (*red*) and postsynaptic (*green*) elements of neuromuscular junctions in the adult rat diaphragm muscle. Note the differences in complexity and size of neuromuscular junctions that depend on motor unit (muscle fiber) type. See also color plate section.

innervate a greater number of muscle fibers to account for the subsequent greater loss of synaptic contacts (see Fig. 83-10). It is also possible that, instead of total activity, the pattern of activity is more important. More recently, it has been suggested that secretion of synaptotrophins (including neurotrophins) or synaptotoxins at nerve terminals results in maintenance or elimination of synapses, respectively.[74] Another possibility is that muscle fibers use intracellular signals called synaptomedins to maintain contact with selected nerve terminals—this may or may not be dependent on differential activity.[86] None of these possibilities can be excluded at present, and it is likely that a combination of mechanisms is responsible for the final pattern of motor unit innervation. However, because differences in innervation ratio exist across motor unit types, it is likely that these mechanisms underlying synapse elimination are linked to muscle

fiber lineage or MHC isoform expression. In addition to synapse elimination, motor unit composition is also affected by the fact that myogenesis and the formation of myotubes/myofibers continue postnatally (e.g., until the third postnatal week in the rat and mouse DIAm).[55] Thus, the final innervation ratio of motor units is not established in the mouse and rat DIAm until about D28.

Fetal respiratory movements indicating intact inspiratory drive and functional synapses have been observed in numerous species including humans. In the rat, fetal respiratory movements begin at about E17, but the presence and timing of such movements in mice have not been determined. The onset of fetal respiratory movements does not particularly denote the beginning of functional synapses and excitation-contraction coupling in DIAm fibers. We found that intracellular Ca^{2+} and contractile responses could be elicited in the mouse DIAm by indirect nerve stimulation as early as E12.5 (Fig. 83-11). These intracellular Ca^{2+} and contractile responses were blocked by D-tubocurarine and α-bungarotoxin, findings indicating dependence on acetylcholine release and activation of cholinergic receptors. Yet, at this early age, synapses are only primordial at best, with no postsynaptic specialization and limited clustering of cholinergic receptors. These observations are consistent with the presence of coated vesicles and other indications of vesicular release (see Fig. 83-5). Myotubes/myofibers that are forming in the DIAm at this time also display the onset of sarcomeric organization necessary for a mechanical response (Figs. 83-12 and 83-13). Thus, it appears that the nervous system can induce mechanical responses even before well-defined synapses are present. Such mechanical responses may be important in the subsequent development of myofibers in the DIAm (e.g., further sarcomeric organization and alignment of sarcomeres).

Clearly, neuromuscular transmission in the fetal and neonatal DIAm is quite different from that of the adult muscle. In previous studies, it was demonstrated that the neonatal rat DIAm is far more susceptible to neuromuscular transmission failure during repetitive activation than the adult.[87-90] Certainly, the increased susceptibility of the fetal and neonatal DIAm to neuromuscular transmission failure can be attributed, at least in part, to the more extensive branching of phrenic axons (resulting from polyneuronal innervation) and thus the greater likelihood of failure of action potential propagation at axonal branch points.[88,90-92] It is also likely that differences in the number of synaptic vesicles and presynaptic neurotransmitter release or consequent activation of cholinergic receptors could account for neuromuscular transmission failure. In this regard, differences in spontaneous miniature end plate potential frequency and amplitude as well as evoked end plate potential amplitude suggest either reduced neurotransmitter release or disproportionately smaller end plate regions (i.e., fewer cholinergic receptors) in the early postnatal DIAm.[87-89]

Figure 83–9. Confocal photomicrograph showing the morphology of neuromuscular junctions in the mouse diaphragm muscle at E17. In comparison with neuromuscular junctions in the adult diaphragm muscle (see Fig. 83-8), neuromuscular junctions at this age are substantially smaller and far less complex. See also color plate section.

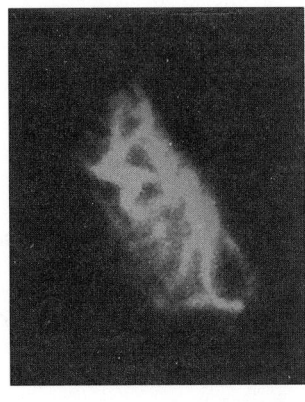
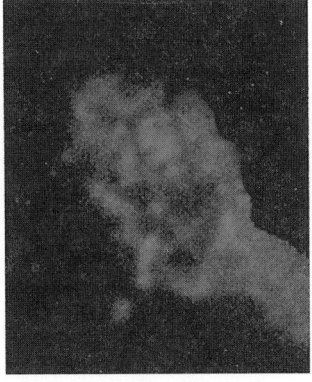
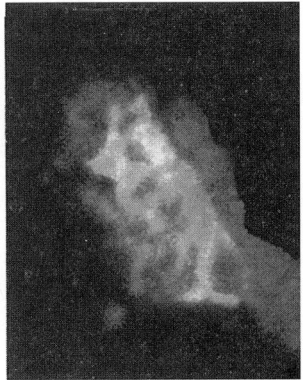

Synapse Elimination

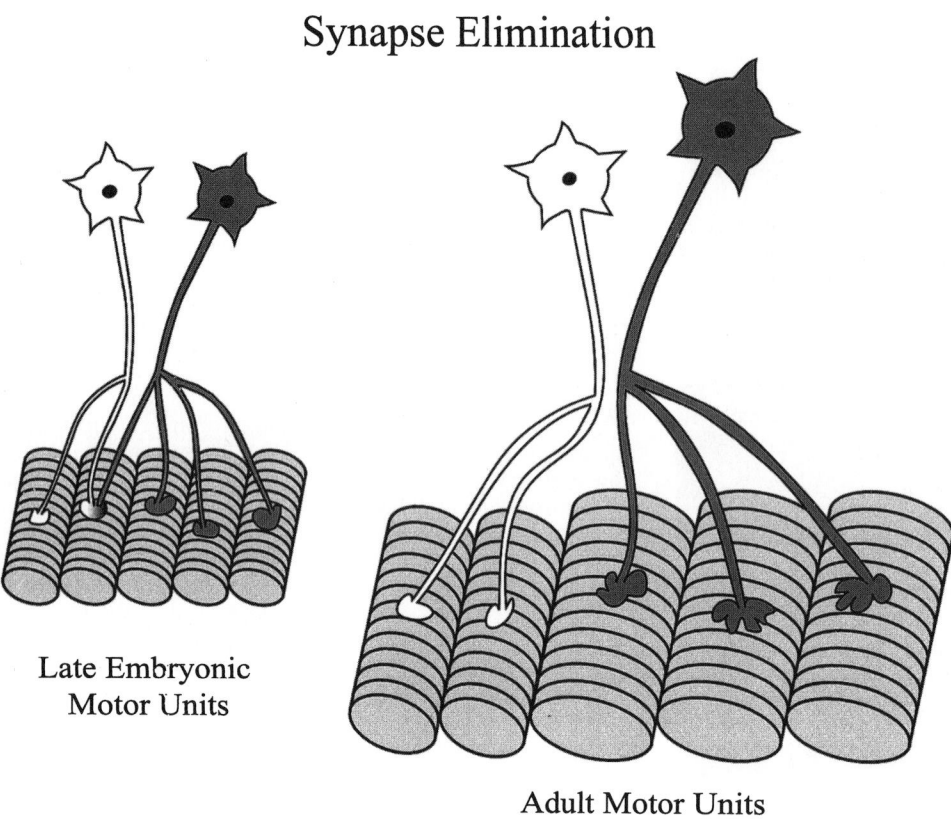

Late Embryonic
Motor Units

Adult Motor Units

Figure 83–10. Schematic illustration of the process of synapse elimination. It is thought that differential patterns of motoneuron activity lead to selective withdrawal of motor axon terminals, which may be regulated by the secretion of synaptotrophins or synaptotoxins by the nerve terminal or production of synaptomedins within myofibers.

E12.5

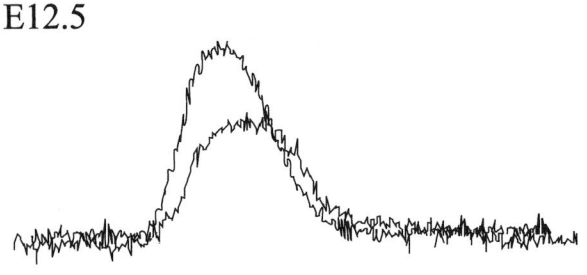

E18

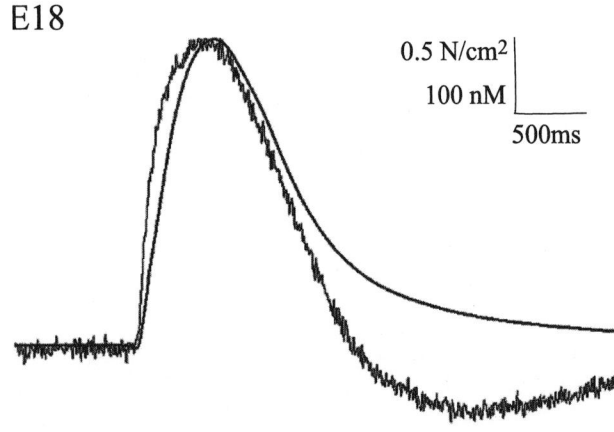

0.5 N/cm^2
100 nM
500ms

Figure 83–11. Simultaneous measurement of force and intracellular calcium responses to phrenic nerve stimulation in the mouse diaphragm muscle at E12.5 and E18. Myofibers mounted between force and length transducers in a flow-through chamber were loaded with Fluo-3AM. Phrenic nerve terminals were stimulated using low-current, short-duration (0.1 ms), square-wave pulses. Responses were blocked using D-tubocurarine (10 μM).

MUSCLE FIBER CONTRACTILE PROPERTIES

Excitation-Contraction Coupling

As mentioned earlier, fetal respiratory movements are present in the rat at about E17; but this does not necessarily reflect the onset of excitation-contraction coupling. In fact, intracellular Ca^{2+} and contractile responses are elicited in the mouse DIAm by indirect nerve stimulation as early as E12.5 (see Fig. 83-11), a finding indicating excitation-contraction coupling. These early mechanical responses are coincident with the earliest formation of myotubes/myofibers, expression of contractile proteins, and the presence of rudimentary sarcomeres (see Figs. 83-12 and 83-13). However, the coordination of these events with the emergence of other structures important in excitation-contraction coupling (e.g., functional synapses, T-tubules, triads, and sarcoplasmic reticulum) is largely unknown. Some studies have focused on the embryologic development of the sarcoplasmic reticulum, T-tubules, and triads and their association with myofibrillar organization.[93-103] In ultrastructural studies, we observed the presence of T-tubules, triads, and sarcoplasmic reticulum in the mouse DIAm at E14 (Fig. 83-14). Takekura and colleagues also presented ultrastructural and confocal evidence of the presence of T-tubules, triads, and sarcoplasmic reticulum in the embryologic mouse DIAm but only as early as E17.[104] These investigators also reported the consistent presence of ryanodine receptor clustering at E15 in the mouse DIAm, a finding indicating the presence of sarcoplasmic reticulum.

Association of Contractile Properties with Fiber Type or MHC Isoform Expression

It is now well established that mechanical properties of skeletal muscle fibers correlate with fiber type and MHC isoform composition.[37, 40, 105-112] In the rat and mouse DIAm, fibers that express MHC_{2X} and/or MHC_{2B} display faster maximum unloaded shortening velocities (V_o) (Fig. 83-15) and greater specific forces (i.e., force generated per muscle cross-sectional area) (Fig. 83-16) than fibers expressing MHC_{Slow} and MHC_{2A}. In the adult rat DIAm, the greater maximum specific force of fibers expressing MHC_{2X} or MHC_{2B} is at least partially explained by differences in MHC protein content per half-sarcomere (i.e., greater number of cross-bridges in parallel) as well as the force per cross-bridge (see Fig. 83-16).[110, 111, 113, 114] Similarly, the faster V_o of adult rat DIAm fibers expressing MHC_{2X} or MHC_{2B} is at least partially explained by faster cross-bridge cycling kinetics and a correspondingly higher rate of ATP consumption.[40, 108]

During fetal and early postnatal development, DIAm fiber contractile properties change dramatically, corresponding with transitions in MHC isoform composition. For example, from E15 to about D28, specific force generated by the rat DIAm increases almost 20-fold (Fig. 83-17),[1, 54-57, 59, 115-117] a finding corresponding with an increase in relative expression of fast MHC isoforms[54, 56, 115] and MHC content per half-sarcomere.[111] The lower specific force of fetal and neonatal DIAm results from both a lower MHC content per half-sarcomere and a reduced force per cross-bridge.[111] During the same developmental period, V_o of the

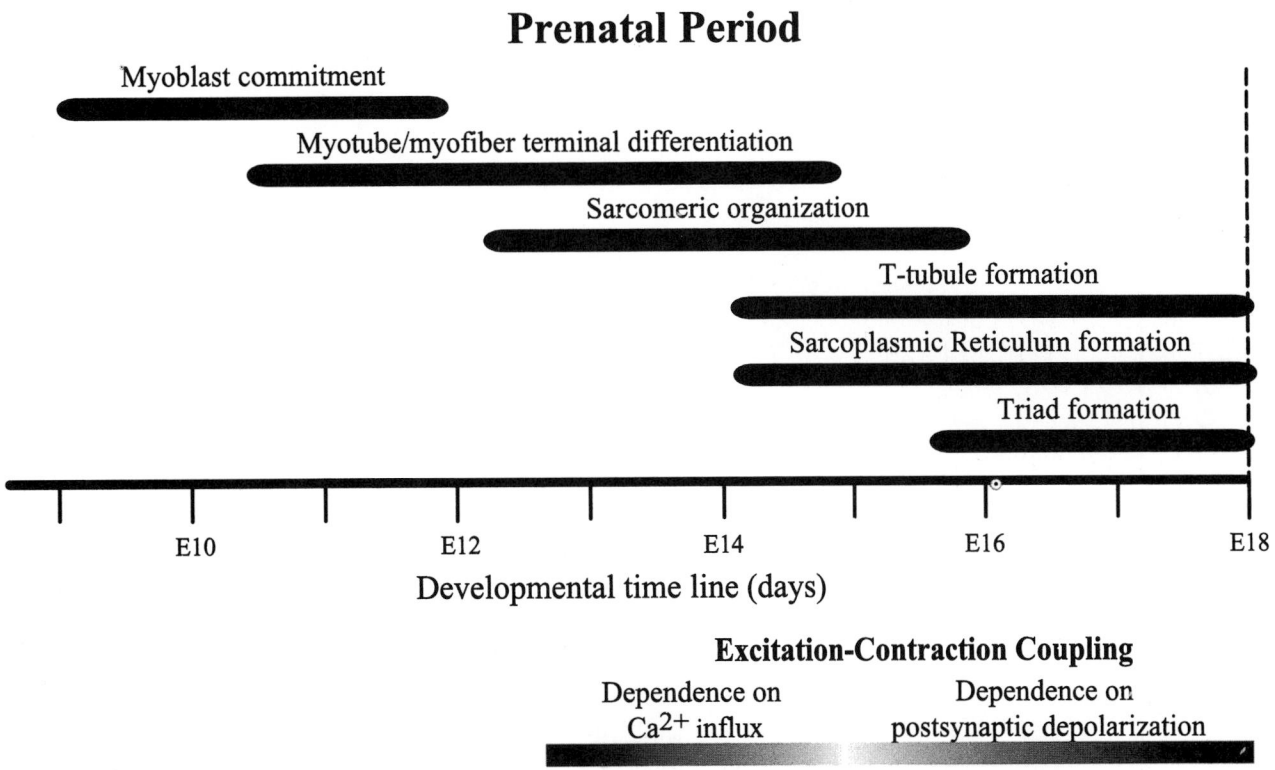

Figure 83-12. Schematic illustration demonstrating the timeline for major embryologic events in the formation of myotubes/myofibers in the mouse diaphragm muscle. It is likely that before the differentiation of distinct T-tubules, triads, and sarcoplasmic reticulum, excitation-contraction coupling is mediated primarily via calcium (Ca^{2+}) influx, whereas in later embryonic stages, mechanisms underlying excitation-contraction coupling resemble those in the adult.

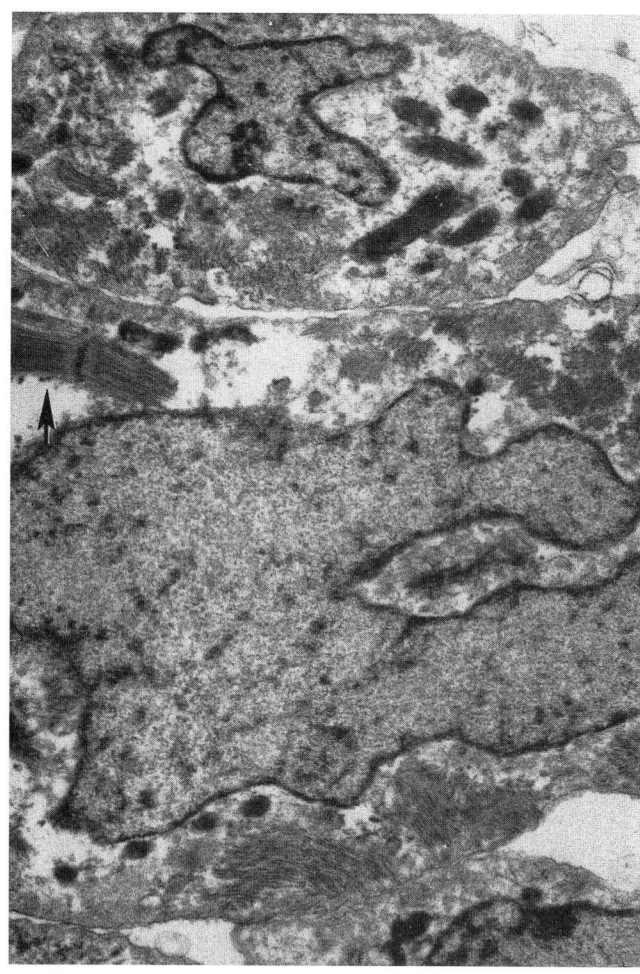

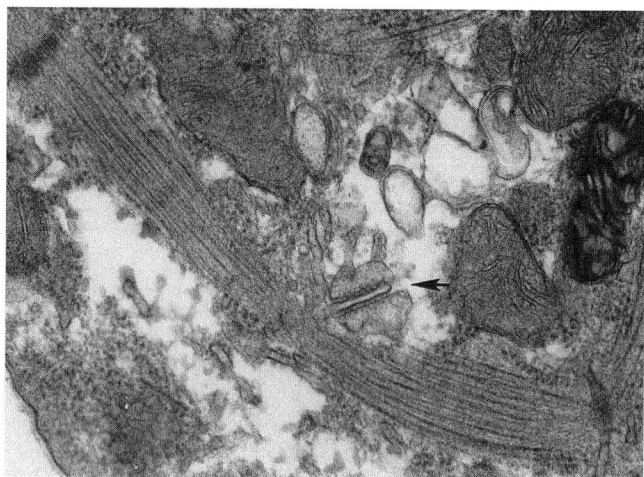

Figure 83–14. Electron photomicrograph showing the presence of a triad (*arrow*) in the mouse diaphragm muscle at E14.

Figure 83–13. Electron photomicrograph displaying rudimentary sarcomeric organization (*arrow*) in the mouse diaphragm muscle at E12.5.

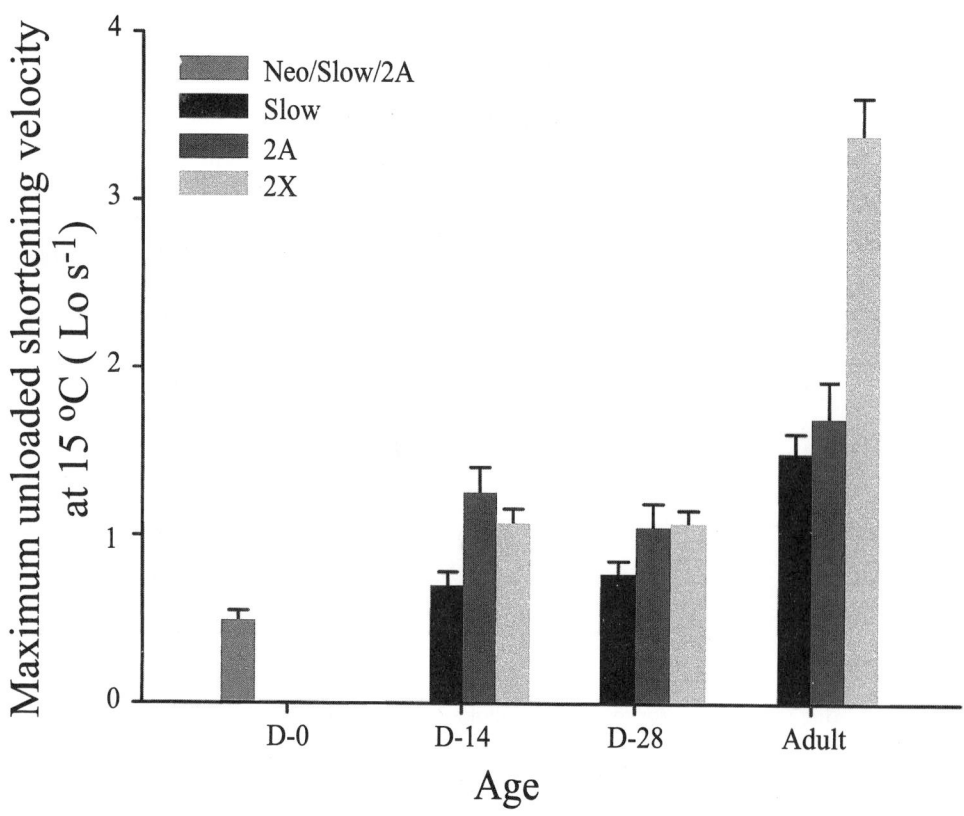

Figure 83–15. Maximum unloaded shortening velocity (expressed as Lo/s) of single triton-X permeabilized rat diaphragm muscle fibers expressing different myosin heavy chain (MHC) isoforms. Maximum unloaded shortening velocity was not solely dependent on MHC isoform expression, but it increased with age for fibers expressing the same MHC isoform.

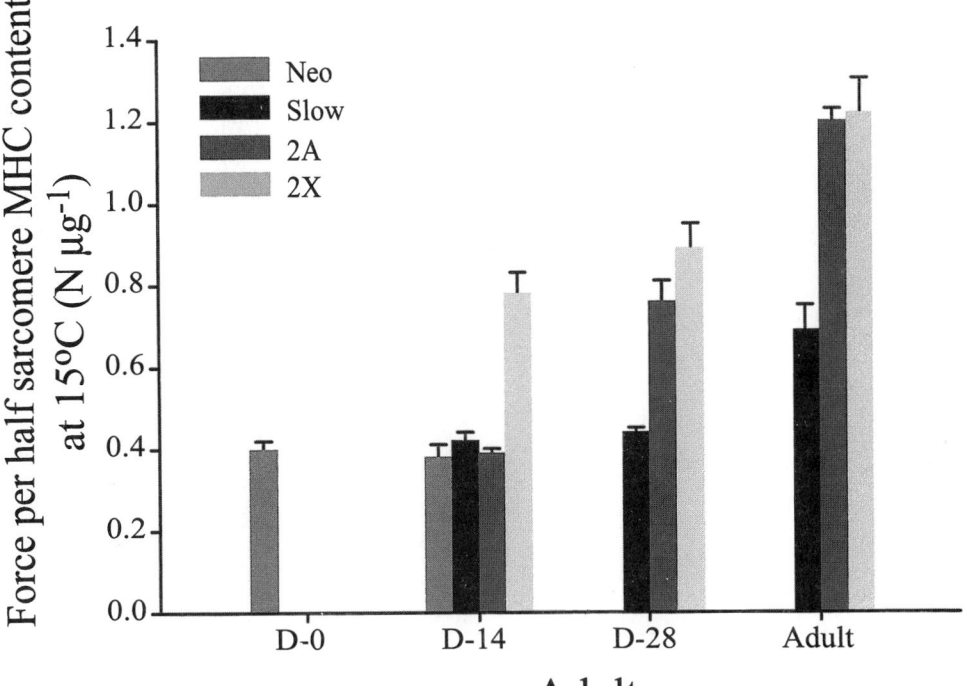

Figure 83–16. Maximum force of single triton-X permeabilized rat diaphragm muscle fibers expressing different myosin heavy chain (MHC) isoforms was normalized for MHC content per half-sarcomere. Maximum force per half-sarcomere MHC content (equivalent to force per cross-bridge) varied with MHC isoform as well as across age groups for a given isoform.

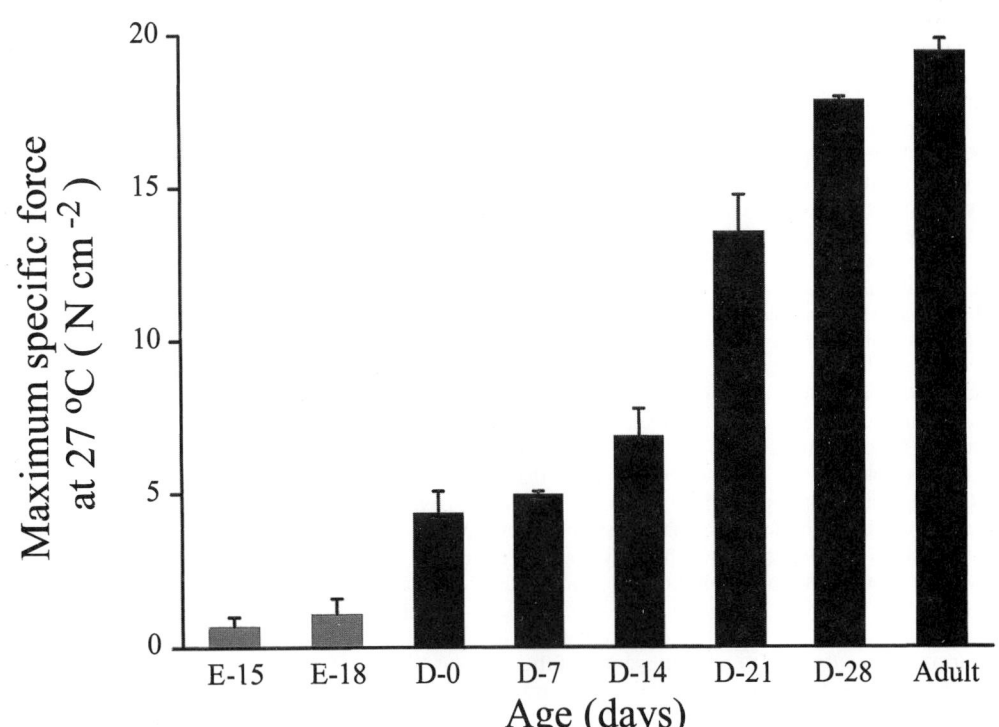

Figure 83–17. Developmental changes in maximum specific force (force per cross-sectional area) of rat diaphragm muscle. Maximum specific force increases almost 20-fold from E15 to adulthood.

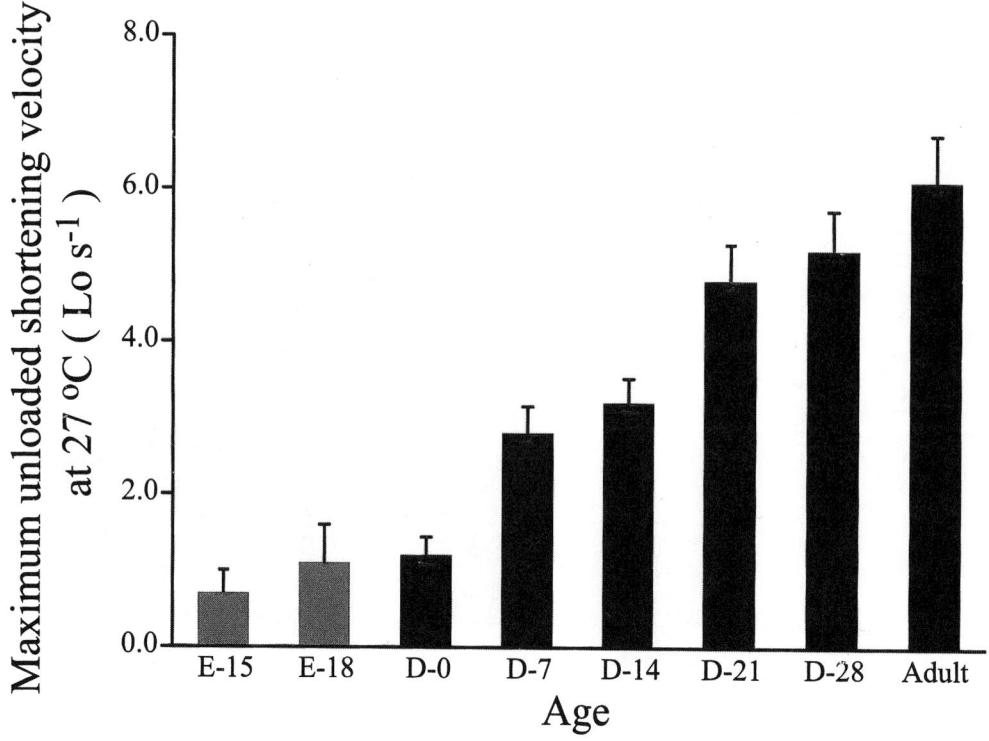

Figure 83–18. Developmental changes in maximum unloaded shortening velocity (expressed as Lo s⁻¹) of the rat diaphragm muscle. Maximum unloaded shortening velocity increases more than sixfold from E15 to adulthood.

DIAm increases by more than sixfold (Fig. 83–18),[56,57,59,117] again corresponding with the increase in relative expression of fast MHC isoforms.[56] The slower V_o of fetal and neonatal DIAm reflects the slower rate of ATP consumption of these fibers, which predominantly express MHC_{Emb} and MHC_{Neo} isoforms (Fig. 83–19).[54] With an increase in both force and velocity, there is an accompanying increase in maximum power output and work performance of the rat DIAm from birth to D28.[117] However, as power output and work performance of the DIAm increase postnatally, fatigue resistance to repeated activation declines.[1,116,117]

Although it is clear that the contractile properties of DIAm undergo profound shifts during early development that correspond to the transitions in MHC isoform expression, the signals driving these changes are not yet known. Changes in contractile properties induced by pathophysiologic conditions may not always be reflected by changes in MHC isoform composition alone. For example, with perinatal hypothyroidism there is a dramatic reduction in maximum specific force and a slowing of V_o in the rat DIAm that cannot be fully attributed to the moderate changes in MHC isoform composition. Similarly, following unilateral denervation of the DIAm at D7, there is a marked reduction in maximum specific force and a slowing of V_o that are not predicted from the slight changes in MHC isoform composition. As mentioned above, the changes in specific force may reflect the total MHC content per half-sarcomere (i.e., number of cross-bridges in parallel) of DIAm fibers,[110] rather than MHC isoform expression as such. The slowing of V_o is more difficult to explain. Clearly, these results indicate that cross-bridge cycling kinetics can be slowed, independent of the MHC isoform expressed. It is possible that these pathophysiologic conditions affect actomyosin ATPase activity of the myosin S-1 fragment or that there is an increased internal resistance to shortening. In support, we observed that, after unilateral denervation of the adult rat DIAm, maximum isometric ATP consumption rate was reduced independent of MHC isoform expression.[118]

MHC Isoform Expression and Cross-Bridge Cycling Kinetics in Single Muscle Fibers

In the original model of muscle contraction proposed by Huxley, cross-bridges cycle between two functional states: a force-generating state, in which cross-bridges are strongly attached to actin; and a non–force-generating state, in which cross-bridges are detached from actin.[119, 120] The transitions between the two primary functional states of cross-bridges are described by two apparent rate constants, one for cross-bridge attachment (f_{app}) and the second for cross-bridge detachment (g_{app}). An increase in isometric force with increasing myoplasmic Ca^{2+} is explained by the recruitment of cross-bridges into the force-generating state (described by f_{app}).[119,120] The transition of cross-bridges from force-generating to non–force-generating states (described by g_{app}) requires the hydrolysis of ATP (actomyosin ATPase). Thus, in the Huxley model, the transduction of chemical to mechanical energy is implicit. Brenner[121-123] proposed an analytical framework based on Huxley's two-state model of cross-bridge cycling in which this transduction of chemical to mechanical energy was more explicitly described. In the Brenner analytical framework, the steady-state fraction of strongly bound cross-bridges in the force generating state (α_{fs}) is given by

$$\alpha_{fs} = f_{app}/(f_{app} + g_{app})$$

Isometric force generated by a muscle fiber is then described by the following relationship:

$$\text{Isometric force} = n \cdot F \cdot \alpha_{fs}$$

where n is the number of cross-bridges in parallel per half-sarcomere, and F is the mean force per cross-bridge in the force-generating state. Assuming the hydrolysis of one ATP molecule during each cross-bridge cycle, isometric ATP consumption rate

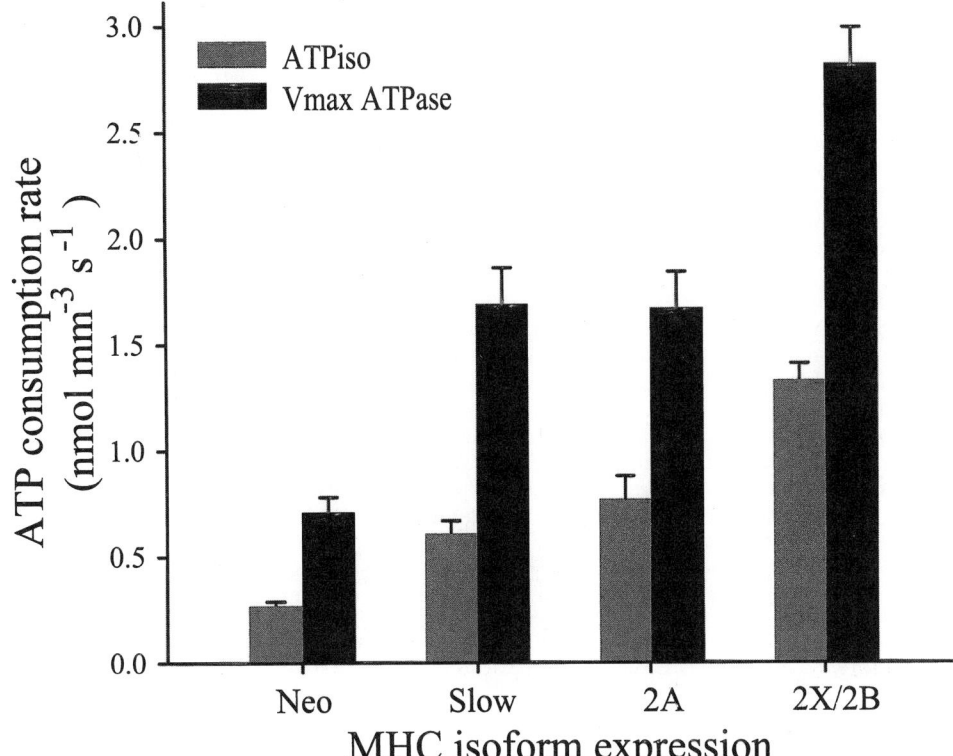

Figure 83–19. Maximum velocity of the actomyosin adenosine triphosphatase (ATPase) reaction (Vmax ATPase) and maximum isometric ATP consumption rate (ATPiso) of the rat diaphragm muscle fibers expressing different MHC isoforms. For each fiber type, Vmax ATPase was greater than ATPiso, a finding indicating substantial reserve capacity for ATP consumption. Although Vmax ATPase and ATPiso varied across MHC isoforms and with age, the reserve capacity for ATP consumption remained relatively constant.

(actomyosin ATPase activity) is described by the following relationship:

$$ATPase = n \cdot b \cdot g_{app} \cdot \alpha_{fs}$$

where b is the number of half-sarcomeres within the fiber. At maximal Ca^{2+} activation, at which α_{fs} remains constant, actomyosin ATPase activity is directly proportional to g_{app}.

Previously, we employed a quantitative histochemical procedure to determine the maximum velocity of the actomyosin ATPase reaction (V_{max} ATPase) in DIAm fibers expressing different MHC isoforms.[40, 108, 124] Fibers expressing MHC_{2X} and MHC_{2B} have higher V_{max} ATPase compared with fibers expressing MHC_{Slow} and MHC_{2A}. To determine the ATP consumption rate of single permeabilized rat DIAm fibers during maximum isometric activation (ATP_{iso}), we used a reduced nicotinamide adenine dinucleotide–linked fluorometric procedure.[40, 108] ATP_{iso} was 30 to 45% lower than V_{max} ATPase, but the dependence on MHC isoform expression was still present, being highest in fibers expressing MHC_{2X} and MHC_{2B} and lowest in fibers expressing MHC_{2A}. This finding reflects a reserve capacity for ATP consumption in DIAm fibers, which is consistent with the well-known fact that ATP consumption rate increases in proportion to work.[125, 126] Difference in reserve capacity for ATP consumption may account, at least in part, for differences in fatigability among DIAm fibers.[40, 108] In another study, we found that the postnatal transition from MHC_{Neo} to adult fast MHC isoform expression in rat DIAm fibers is accompanied by an increase in V_{max} ATPase and ATP_{iso} (see Fig. 83-19).

MHC Isoform Expression and Calcium Sensitivity of Muscle Fibers

In skeletal muscle fibers, force generation depends on myoplasmic $[Ca^{2+}]$. The dependency of force generation of myoplasmic $[Ca^{2+}]$ is usually expressed as the force/pCa ($-\log [Ca^{2+}]$) relationship. We found that the force/pCa relationship of rat DIAm fibers expressing MHC_{Slow} is shifted leftward compared with fibers expressing adult fast MHC isoforms.[109] The greater Ca^{2+} sensitivity of DIAm fibers expressing MHC_{Slow} is consistent with previous observations by other investigators.[127-130]

It is widely recognized that in skeletal muscle, Ca^{2+} binding to the regulatory protein troponin C (TnC) underlies the dependency of force on myoplasmic $[Ca^{2+}]$. Ca^{2+} binding to TnC may simply act to increase the availability of myosin binding sites on actin and may thus increase the probability of cross-bridge formation. Different isoforms of TnC from fast (TnC-f) and slow (TnC-s) muscle fibers have different numbers of regulatory binding sites for Ca^{2+} (two for TnC-f versus one for TnC-s) and different binding affinities for $Ca.^{2+}$ These differences in TnC isoforms may underlie the fiber type differences in force/pCa relationships. In support of this possibility, investigators have shown that there are changes in the force/pCa relationship of rabbit psoas fibers when the TnC-f present in these fibers is substituted with TnC-s.[131,132]

Functional Implications of Developmental Changes in Mechanical Performance of the Diaphragm Muscle

The DIAm plays a vital role in sustaining ventilation from the time of birth onward, concurrent with the maturation of other structures that affect its mechanical performance. For example, with maturation of limb muscles and locomotor function, the ventilatory demands placed on the DIAm increase dramatically, and the DIAm must be capable of meeting the increased range of functional demands that coincide with postnatal development. In addition, compliance of the lung and chest wall changes markedly during early development. The neonatal lung is stiffer as a result of greater alveolar recoil, which is offset by expression of surfactant, whereas the chest and abdominal walls are more compliant. As a result, the DIAm must generate greater relative intrathoracic pressures to produce a given level of inspiratory airflow and tidal volume. Yet the neonatal DIAm generates much lower maximum tetanic force (see Fig. 83-17) and has a much slower maximum unloaded V_o (see Fig. 83-18) compared with the adult. Thus, the functional reserve capacity of the neonatal DIAm is greatly reduced, and a far greater fraction of maximum power output must be recruited to accomplish ventilation. Polyneuronal innervation of DIAm fibers may be particularly important as a neural strategy to accomplish greater fractional recruitment of DIAm motor units. As synapse elimination proceeds, more selective recruitment of DIAm motor units becomes possible, coinciding with the increased range of functions required of the DIAm. In addition, early postnatal expression of MHC_{2X} and MHC_{2B} isoforms in DIAm fibers increases overall functional range, but at the expense of lower energy efficiency and greater susceptibility to fatigue.[2, 4] It is likely that DIAm fibers expressing MHC_{2X} and MHC_{2B} isoforms are recruited only during motor behaviors that require high force output and are of short duration, such as expulsive behaviors.[2, 4] Such motor behaviors of the DIAm may be less necessary in the neonate. Yet the absence of such functional reserve may cause the neonate to be more susceptible to aspiration and asphyxiation. Clearly, greater attention should be focused on the integrative aspects of DIAm development, and it will be important to place the genetic regulation of myogenesis and changing innervation patterns of the DIAm in this more global context.

REFERENCES

1. Sieck GC, Fournier M: Developmental aspects of diaphragm muscle cells: structural and functional organization. *In* Haddad GG, Farber JP (eds): Developmental Neurobiology of Breathing. New York, Marcel Dekker, 1991, pp 375–428.
2. Sieck GC: Neural control of the inspiratory pump. News Physiol Sci 6:260, 1991.
3. Sieck GC: Physiological effects of diaphragm muscle denervation and disuse. Clin Chest Med 15:641, 1994.
4. Sieck GC, Prakash YS: The diaphragm muscle. *In* Miller AD, et al (eds): Neural Control of the Respiratory Muscles. Boca Raton, FL, CRC Press, 1996, pp 7–20.
5. Arnold HH, Braun T: Genetics of muscle determination and development. Curr Top Dev Biol 48:129, 2000.
6. Weintraub H, et al: The myoD gene family: nodal point during specification of the muscle cell lineage. Science 251:761, 1991.
7. Weintraub H, et al: Muscle-specific transcriptional activation by MyoD. Genes Dev 5:1377, 1991.
8. Davis RL, et al: Expression of a single transfected cDNA converts fibroblasts to myoblasts. Cell 51:987, 1987.
9. Braun T, et al: Differential expression of myogenic determination genes in muscle cells: possible autoactivation by the Myf gene products. EMBO J 8:3617, 1989.
10. Braun T, et al: A novel human muscle factor related to but distinct from MyoD1 induces myogenic conversion in 10T1/2 fibroblasts. EMBO J 8:701, 1989.
11. Rhodes SJ, Konieczny SF: Identification of MRF4: a new member of the muscle regulatory factor gene family. Genes Dev 3:2050, 1989.
12. Braun T, et al: Myf-6, a new member of the human gene family of myogenic determination factors: evidence for a gene cluster on chromosome 12. EMBO J 9:821, 1990.
13. Hughes SM, et al: MyoD protein is differentially accumulated in fast and slow skeletal muscle fibres and required for normal fibre type balance in rodents. Mech Dev 61:151, 1997.
14. Borycki AG, et al: Sonic hedgehog controls epaxial muscle determination through Myf5 activation. Development 126:4053, 1999.
15. Cossu G, et al: How is myogenesis initiated in the embryo? Trends Genet 12:218, 1996.
16. Maroto M, et al: Ectopic Pax-3 activates MyoD and Myf-5 expression in embryonic mesoderm and neural tissue. Cell 89:139, 1997.
17. Olson EN: Signal transduction pathways that regulate skeletal muscle gene expression. Mol Endocrinol 7:1369, 1993.
18. Buckingham M: Which myogenic factors make muscle? Curr Biol 4:61, 1994.
19. Benezra R, et al: Id: a negative regulator of helix-loop-helix DNA binding proteins. Control of terminal myogenic differentiation. Ann NY Acad Sci 599:1, 1990.
20. Jen Y, et al: Overexpression of Id protein inhibits the muscle differentiation program: in vivo association of Id with E2A proteins. Genes Dev 6:1466, 1992.
21. Spicer DB, et al: Inhibition of myogenic bHLH and MEF2 transcription factors by the bHLH protein Twist. Science 272:1476, 1996.
22. Lemercier C, et al: The basic helix-loop-helix transcription factor Mist1 functions as a transcriptional repressor of myoD. EMBO J 17:1412, 1998.
23. Sabourin LA, Rudnicki MA: The molecular regulation of myogenesis. Clin Genet 57:16, 2000.
24. Rudnicki MA, et al: Inactivation of MyoD in mice leads to up-regulation of the myogenic HLH gene Myf-5 and results in apparently normal muscle development. Cell 71:383, 1992.
25. Zhang W, et al: Inactivation of the myogenic bHLH gene MRF4 results in up-regulation of myogenin and rib anomalies. Genes Dev 9:1388, 1995.
26. Braun T, et al: Targeted inactivation of the muscle regulatory genes Myf-5 results in abnormal rib development and perinatal death. Cell 71:269, 1992.
27. Hasty P, et al: Muscle deficiency and neonatal death in mice with a targeted mutation in the myogenin gene. Nature 364:501, 1993.
28. Nabeshima Y, et al: Myogenin gene disruption results in perinatal lethality because of severe muscle defect. Nature 364:532, 1993.
29. Rudnicki MA, et al: MyoD or Myf-5 is required for the formation of skeletal muscle. Cell 75:1351, 1993.
30. Walsh K, Perlman H: Cell cycle exit upon myogenic differentiation. Curr Opin Genet Dev 7:597, 1997.
31. Buckingham ME, et al: Myogenesis in the mouse. CIBA Found Symp 165:111, 1992.
32. Knudsen KA: Cell adhesion molecules in myogenesis. Curr Opin Cell Biol 2:902, 1990.
33. Vandenburgh H, et al: Skeletal muscle growth is stimulated by intermittent stretch-relaxation in tissue culture. Am J Physiol 256:C674, 1989.
34. Vandenburgh HH: Mechanical forces and their second messengers in stimulating cell growth in vitro. Am J Physiol 262:R350, 1992.
35. Rayment I, et al: Three-dimensional structure of myosin subfragment-1: a molecular motor. Science 261:50, 1995.
36. Cooke R: The actomyosin engine. FASEB J 9:636, 1995.
37. Schiaffino S, Reggiani Cg: Molecular diversity of myofibrillar proteins: gene regulation and functional significance. Physiol Rev 76:371, 1996.
38. Barany M: ATPase activity of myosin correlated with speed of muscle shortening. J Gen Physiol 50:197, 1967.
39. Stienen GJ, et al: Myofibrillar ATPase activity in skinned human skeletal muscle fibres: fibre type and temperature dependence. J Physiol (Lond) 493:299, 1996.
40. Sieck GC, et al: Cross-bridge cycling kinetics, actomyosin ATPase activity and myosin heavy chain isoforms in skeletal and smooth respiratory muscles. Comp Biochem Physiol 119:435, 1998.
41. Sieck GC, Prakash YS: The diaphragm muscle. *In* Miller AD, et al (eds): Neural Control of the Respiratory Muscles. Boca Raton, FL, CRC Press, 1997, pp 7–20.
42. Rayment I, et al: Structure of the actin-myosin complex and its implications for muscle contraction. Science 261:58, 1993.
43. Reiser PJ, et al: Shortening velocity in single fibers from adult rabbit soleus muscles is correlated with myosin heavy chain composition. J Biol Chem 260:9077, 1985.
44. Perrie WT, et al: A phosphorylated light-chain component of myosin from skeletal muscle. Biochem J 35:151, 1973.
45. Diffee GM, et al: Effects of a non-divalent cation binding mutant of myosin regulatory light chain on tension generation in skinned skeletal muscle fibers. Biophys J 68:1443, 1995.
46. Patel JR, et al: Myosin regulatory light chain modulates the Ca2+ dependence of the kinetics of tension development in skeletal muscle fibers. Biophys J 70:2333, 1996.
47. Brooke MH, Kaiser KK: Muscle fiber types: how many and what kind? Arch Neurol 23:369, 1970.
48. Bar A, Pette D: Three fast myosin heavy chains in adult rat skeletal muscle. FEBS Lett 235:153, 1988.
49. Schiaffino S, et al: Muscle fiber types expressing different myosin heavy chain isoforms: their functional properties and adaptive capacity. *In* Pette D (ed): The Dynamic State of Muscle Fibers. Berlin, De Gruyter, 1990, pp 329–341.
50. Sieck GC: Organization and recruitment of diaphragm motor units. *In* Roussos C (ed): The Thorax, 2nd ed. New York, Marcel Dekker, 1995, pp 783–820.
51. LaFramboise WA, et al: Myosin isoforms in neonatal rat extensor digitorum longus, diaphragm, and soleus muscles. Am J Physiol 259:L116, 1990.
52. LaFramboise WA, et al: Emergence of the mature myosin phenotype in the rat diaphragm muscle. Dev Biol 144:1, 1991.
53. Watchko JF, et al: Postnatal expression of myosin isoforms in an expiratory muscle: external abdominal oblique. J Appl Physiol 73:1860, 1992.
54. Watchko JF, et al: Myosin heavy chain transitions during development: functional implications for the respiratory musculature. Comp Biochem Physiol 119:459, 1998.
55. Prakash YS, et al: Effects of prenatal undernutrition on developing rat diaphragm. J Appl Physiol 75:1044, 1993.
56. Johnson BD, et al: Contractile properties of the developing diaphragm correlate with myosin heavy chain phenotype. J Appl Physiol 77:481, 1994.
57. Sieck GC, Zhan WZ: Denervation alters myosin heavy chain expression and contractility of developing rat diaphragm muscle. J Appl Physiol 89:1106, 2000.
58. Izumo S, et al: All members of the MHC multigene family respond to thyroid hormone in a highly tissue-specific manner. Science 231:597, 1986.
59. Sieck GC, et al: Hypothyroidism alters diaphragm muscle development. J Appl Physiol 81:1965, 1996.
60. Wells LJ: Development of the human diaphragm and pleural sacs. Contrib Embryol 35:107, 1954.
61. Larsen WJ: Human Embryology, 2nd ed. New York, Churchill Livingstone, 1997.
62. Last RJ: Last's Anatomy: Regional and Applied, 9th ed. Edinburgh, Churchill Livingstone, 1994.
63. Allan DW, Greer JJ: Embryogenesis of the phrenic nerve and diaphragm in the fetal rat. J Comp Neurol 382:459, 1997.

64. Greer JJ, et al: An overview of phrenic nerve and diaphragm muscle development in the perinatal rat. J Appl Physiol 86:779, 1999.
65. Gordon DC, Richmond FJ: Topography in the phrenic motoneuron nucleus demonstrated by retrograde multiple-labelling techniques. J Comp Neurol 292:424, 1990.
66. Hammond CG, et al: Motor unit territories supplied by primary branches of the phrenic nerve. J Appl Physiol 66:61, 1989.
67. Fournier M, Sieck GC: Topographical projections of phrenic motoneurons and motor unit territories in the cat diaphragm. In Sieck GC, et al (eds): Respiratory Muscles and Their Neuromotor Control. New York, Alan R. Liss, 1987, pp 215–226.
68. Laskowski MB, Sanes JR: Topographic mapping of motor pools onto skeletal muscles. J Neurosci 7:252, 1987.
69. Mantilla CB, et al: Alterations in neurotrophin receptor expression in rat diaphragm neuromuscular junction following spinal cord hemisection. Soc Neurosci Abstr 25:511, 1999.
70. Johnson RA, et al: Cervical dorsal rhizotomy increases brain-derived neurotrophic factor and neurotrophin-3 expression in the ventral spinal cord. J Neurosci 20: RC 77, 2000.
71. Conover JC, Yancopoulos GD: Neurotrophin regulation of the developing nervous system: analyses of knockout mice. Rev Neurosci 8:13, 1997.
72. Liu X, Jaenisch R: Severe peripheral sensory neuron loss and modest motor neuron reduction in mice with combined deficiency of brain-derived neurotrophic factor, neurotrophin 3 and neurotrophin-4. Dev Dyn 218:94, 2000.
73. Gautam M, et al: Distinct phenotypes of mutant mice lacking agrin, MuSK, or rapsyn. Brain Res Dev Brain Res 114:171, 1999.
74. Sanes JR, Lichtman JW: Development of the vertebrate neuromuscular junction. Ann Rev Neurosci 22:389, 1999.
75. Sanes JR, Lichtman JW: Induction, assembly, maturation and maintenance of a postsynaptic apparatus. Nat Rev Neurosci 2:791, 2001.
76. Prakash YS, et al: Morphology of diaphragm neuromuscular junctions on different fibre types. J Neurocytol 25:88, 1996.
77. Bennett MR, Pettigrew AG: The formation of synapses in striated muscle during development. J Physiol (Lond) 241:515, 1974.
78. Bennett MR, Lavidis NA: Segmental motor projections to rat muscles during the loss of polyneuronal innervation. Dev Brain Res 13:1, 1984.
79. Brown MC, et al: Polyneuronal innervation of skeletal muscle in new-born rats and its elimination during maturation. J Physiol (Lond) 261:387, 1976.
80. Redfern P: Neuromuscular transmission in new-born rats. J Physiol (Lond) 209:701, 1970.
81. Personius KE, Balice-Gordon RJ: Activity-dependent editing of neuromuscular synaptic connections. Brain Res Bull 53:513, 2000.
82. Jansen JKS, Fladby T: The perinatal organization of the innervation of skeletal muscle in mammals. Prog Neurobiol 34:39, 1990.
83. Sieck GC: Diaphragm motor units and their response to altered use. Semin Respir Med 12:258, 1991.
84. Fournier M, Sieck GC: Mechanical properties of muscle units in the cat diaphragm. J Neurophysiol 59:1055, 1988.
85. Bodine SC, et al: Maximal force as a function of anatomical features of motor units in the cat tibialis anterior. J Neurophysiol 57:1730, 1987.
86. Balice-Gordon RJ, Lichtman JW: In vivo observations of pre- and postsynaptic changes during the transition from multiple to single innervation at developing neuromuscular junctions. J Neurosci 13:834, 1993.
87. Feldman JD, et al: Developmental changes in neuromuscular transmission in the rat diaphragm. J Appl Physiol 71:280, 1991.
88. Fournier M, et al: Neuromuscular transmission failure during postnatal development. Neurosci Lett 125:34, 1991.
89. Bazzy AR, Donnelly DF: Failure to generate action potentials in newborn diaphragms following nerve stimulation. Brain Res 600:349, 1993.
90. Sieck GC, Prakash YS: Fatigue at the neuromuscular junction: branch point vs. presynaptic vs. postsynaptic mechanisms. Adv Exp Med Biol 384:83, 1995.
91. Krnjevic K, Miledi R: Failure of neuromuscular propagation in rats. J Physiol (Lond) 140:440, 1958.
92. Krnjevic K, Miledi R: Presynaptic failure of neuromuscular propagation in rats. J Physiol (Lond) 149:1, 1959.
93. Flucher BE, et al: Biogenesis of transverse tubules in skeletal muscle in vitro. Dev Biol 145:77, 1991.
94. Flucher BE, et al: Coordinated development of myofibrils, sarcoplasmic reticulum and transverse tubules in normal and dysgenic mouse skeletal muscle, in vivo and in vitro. Dev Biol 150:266, 1992.
95. Flucher BE: Structural analysis of muscle development: transverse tubules, sarcoplasmic reticulum, and the triad. Dev Biol 154:245, 1992.
96. Flucher BE, et al: Development of the excitation-contraction coupling apparatus in skeletal muscle: association of sarcoplasmic reticulum and transverse tubules with myofibrils. Dev Biol 160:135, 1993.
97. Flucher BE, et al: Molecular organization of transverse tubule/sarcoplasmic reticulum junctions during development of excitation-contraction coupling in skeletal muscle. Mol Biol Cell 5:1105, 1994.
98. Flucher BE, Franzini-Armstrong C: Formation of junctions involved in excitation-contraction coupling in skeletal and cardiac muscle. Proc Natl Acad Sci USA 93:8101, 1996.
99. Franzini-Armstrong C: Simultaneous maturation of transverse tubules and sarcoplasmic reticulum during muscle differentiation in the mouse. Dev Biol 146:353, 1991.
100. Franzini-Armstrong C, Jorgensen AO: Structure and development of E-C coupling units in skeletal muscle. Annu Rev Physiol 56:509, 1994.
101. Franzini-Armstrong C, Protasi F: Ryanodine receptors of striated muscles: a complex channel capable of multiple interactions. Physiol Rev 77:699, 1997.
102. Felder E, et al: Morphology and molecular composition of sarcoplasmic reticulum surface junctions in the absence of DHPR and RyR in Mouse Skeletal Muscle. Biophys J 82:3144, 2002.
103. Takekura H, et al: Development of the excitation-contraction coupling apparatus in skeletal muscle: peripheral and internal calcium release units are formed sequentially. J Muscle Res Cell Motil 15:102, 1994.
104. Takekura H, et al: Sequential docking, molecular differentiation, and positioning of T-tubule/SR junctions in developing mouse skeletal muscle. Dev Biol 239:204, 2001.
105. Schiaffino S, et al: Myosin heavy chain isoforms and velocity of shortening of type 2 skeletal muscle fibres. Acta Physiol Scand 134:575, 1988.
106. Sweeney HL, et al: Velocity of shortening and myosin isozymes in two types of rabbit fast-twitch muscle fibers. Am J Physiol 251:C431, 1986.
107. Bottinelli R, et al: Force-velocity relations and myosin heavy chain isoform compositions of skinned fibres from rat skeletal muscle. J Physiol (Lond) 437:655, 1991.
108. Sieck GC, Prakash YS: Cross bridge kinetics in respiratory muscles. Eur Respir J 10:2147, 1997.
109. Geiger PC, et al: Force-calcium relationship depends on myosin heavy chain and troponin isoforms in rat diaphragm muscle fibers. J Appl Physiol 87:1894, 1999.
110. Geiger PC, et al: Maximum specific force depends on myosin heavy chain content in rat diaphragm muscle fibers. J Appl Physiol 89:695, 2000.
111. Geiger PC, et al: Mechanisms underlying increased force generation by rat diaphragm muscle fibers during development. J Appl Physiol 90:380, 2001.
112. Pette D: Historical Perspectives: plasticity of mammalian skeletal muscle. J Appl Physiol 90:1119, 2001.
113. Geiger PC, et al: Effect of unilateral denervation on maximum specific force in rat diaphragm muscle fibers. J Appl Physiol 90:1196, 2001.
114. Geiger PC, et al: Effects of hypothyroidism on maximum specific force in rat diaphragm muscle fibers. J Appl Physiol 92, 2002.
115. Watchko JF, et al: Contractile properties of the rat external abdominal oblique and diaphragm muscles during development. J Appl Physiol 72:1432, 1992.
116. Watchko JF, Sieck GC: Respiratory muscle fatigue resistance relates to myosin phenotype and SDH activity during development. J Appl Physiol 75:1341, 1993.
117. Zhan W-Z, et al: Isotonic contractile and fatigue properties of developing rat diaphragm muscle. J Appl Physiol 84:1260, 1998.
118. Han YS, et al: Effects of denervation on mechanical and energetic properties of single fibers in rat diaphragm muscle. Biophys J 76:A34, 1999.
119. Huxley AF, Simmons RM: Proposed mechanism of force generation in striated muscle. Nature 233:533, 1971.
120. Huxley AF: Muscle structure and theories of contraction. Prog Biophys Chem 7:255, 1957.
121. Brenner B: Kinetics of the crossbridge cycle derived from measurements of force, rate of force development and isometric ATPase. J Muscle Res Cell Motil 7:75, 1986.
122. Brenner B: The necessity of using two parameters to describe isotonic shortening velocity of muscle tissue: the effect of various interventions upon initial shortening velocity (vi) and curvature (b). Basic Res Cardiol 81:54, 1986.
123. Brenner B, Eisenberg E: Rate of force generation in muscle: Correlation with actomyosin ATPase activity in solution. Proc Nat Acad Sci USA 83:3542, 1986.
124. Blanco CE, Sieck GC: Quantitative determination of calcium-activated myosin adenosine triphosphatase activity in rat skeletal muscle fibres. Histochem J 24:431, 1992.
125. Fenn WO: A quantitative comparison between the energy liberated and the work performed by the isolated sartorius muscle of the frog. J Physiol (Lond) 58:175, 1923.
126. Fenn WO: The relation between the work performed and the energy liberated in muscular contraction. J Physiol (Lond) 58:373, 1924.
127. Danieli-Betto D, et al: Calcium sensitivity and myofibrillar protein isoforms of rat skinned skeletal muscle fibres. Pflugers Arch 417:303, 1990.
128. Greaser ML, et al: Variations in contractile properties of rabbit single muscle fibres in relation to troponin T isoforms and myosin light chains. J Physiol (Lond) 406:85, 1988.
129. Laszewski-Williams B, et al: Influence of fiber type and muscle source on Ca^{2+} sensitivity of rat fibers. Am J Physiol 256:C420, 1989.
130. Metzger JM, Moss RL: Calcium-sensitive cross-bridge transitions in mammalian fast and slow skeletal muscle fibers. Science 247:1088, 1990.
131. Moss RL, et al: Altered Ca^{2+} dependence of tension development in skinned skeletal muscle fibers following modification of troponin by partial substitution with cardiac troponin C. J Biol Chem 261:6096, 1986.
132. Brandt PW, et al: Co-operative interactions between troponin-tropomyosin units extend the length of the thin filament in skeletal muscle. J Mol Biol 195:885, 1987.

Jacopo P. Mortola

Mechanics of Breathing

In the linked events that contribute to the translation of the output of the respiratory rhythm generator into ventilation, mechanical properties of the respiratory system obviously represent a critical step. Following activation of the respiratory muscles, the magnitude of force generated depends on the physical properties of the inspiratory muscles (i.e., the force-length and force-velocity characteristics). The physical translation of force into inspiratory muscle pressure depends on the configuration of the muscle and the mechanical characteristics of the structure to which the force is applied. Finally, of the total muscle pressure generated, part is required to overcome the elastic properties of the respiratory system to change lung volume (V), and part is dissipated to overcome the resistive characteristics of the respiratory system to move air, that is, to generate flow ($\dot{V}$). An additional pressure component required to accelerate the gas and dependent on the inertia of the respiratory system is usually so small that it can be neglected. Hence, the total pressure P generated is equal to the sum of elastic (Pel) and resistive (Pres) components, the former proportional to V and 1/C, the latter proportional to $\dot{V}$ and R,

$$P = Pel + Pres = (V \times 1/C) + (\dot{V} \times R) \qquad [1]$$

where C and R are proportionality factors determined by, respectively, the elastic and resistive characteristics of the system.

During *spontaneous breathing*, the total P for inflation is generated by the respiratory muscles, hence P = Pmus, and inflow can occur whenever (Pmus–Pel) is greater than 0. Normally, during resting breathing, because tidal volume is entirely above the resting volume of the respiratory system (Vr), Pmus is generated by the inspiratory muscles, and expiration is passive. However, in some conditions, like some cases of hyperventilation or artificially elevated lung volumes, the expiratory muscles may become active, and breathing occurs across Vr. In these cases, inspiration is the combined result of the recoil of the respiratory system after expiratory muscle relaxation plus the active contraction of the inspiratory muscles.

During *artificial ventilation*, Pmus = 0, and the driving pressure is generated by the ventilator, which opposes Pel and Pres. Whenever Pmus = 0, we say that the system is in a *passive* mode; this is not only the case during artificial ventilation but also during the latter part of the expiratory phase of the resting spontaneous breathing cycle. At this time, the elastic pressure stored during inspiration (Pel) becomes the driving pressure generating expiratory flow, that is, Pel = Pres = $\dot{V} \times$ Rrs. Whenever Pmus differs from 0, we say that the system is in an *active* mode; this is of course the case during spontaneous inspiration, but it can also occur when $\dot{V}$ = 0, such as during breath holding (in which case Pmus = Pel).

Whenever $\dot{V}$ = 0, Equation 1 simplifies to

$$P = Pel = V \times 1/C \qquad [2]$$

Such a condition is defined as *static*, irrespective of whether Pel is offset by muscle activity (e.g., during breath holding) or by external means with Pmus = 0 (e.g., relaxation against an artificial occlusion of the airways). On the contrary, whenever $\dot{V}$ differs from 0, the system is in a *dynamic* condition, again, irrespective of whether the respiratory muscles are active (inflation during spontaneous inspiration) or not (inflation by a ventilator) (Table 84-1).

A dynamic condition with no changes in V, such that V × 1/C becomes negligible and

$$P = Pres = \dot{V} \times R \qquad [3]$$

can be approached when $\dot{V}$ is very high and V is very small, such as during panting or during high frequency ventilation. During an inspiratory effort against closed airways, because the change in lung volume equals 0 (and therefore $\dot{V}$ = 0), no external work is performed, and the total pressure (P = Pmus) is entirely dissipated as heat.

PASSIVE MECHANICAL PROPERTIES OF THE RESPIRATORY SYSTEM

As already stated, the respiratory system is in a passive mode when Pmus = 0. Obviously, this is the case during artificial ventilation of a paralyzed subject, but it can also occur without paralysis after a period of hyperventilation, that is, when the partial pressure of carbon dioxide is lowered below the threshold for muscle activation. During spontaneous breathing, the passive mode can be achieved by artificial occlusion of the airways at any lung volume above the resting volume of the respiratory system. This maneuver determines relaxation of the inspiratory muscles by the stimulation of the slowly adapting stretch receptors in the airways and the vagally mediated Hering-Breuer inflation reflex. This brief period of artificially provoked muscle relaxation is sufficient to evaluate the passive mechanical properties of the respiratory system in a spontaneously breathing infant.

Passive Respiratory Mechanics During Artificial Ventilation

Measurements of passive respiratory mechanics during artificial ventilation are, in some respects, easier to perform than during spontaneous breathing. In fact, by definition, the conditions of Pmus = 0 required for passive measurements can be more easily tested and fulfilled than during spontaneous breathing. In addition, artificial ventilation through an endotracheal tube bypasses the upper airways, which are often characterized by nonlinear mechanical properties. Therefore, the respiratory system is more likely to behave as a first-order mechanical system, and this substantially simplifies the conceptual approach and analysis of the measurements. Air leaks around the endotracheal tube and accurate estimation of the tube resistance are common but solvable methodologic problems.

In an intubated and artificially ventilated infant, $\dot{V}$ can be easily measured by a pneumotachograph placed in series between the endotracheal tube and the ventilator. The signal, properly amplified, is then electronically integrated to obtain the changes in lung volume (V). Ptotal during artificial ventilation can be conveniently measured at the mouth (Pao). From these measurements, the values of Crs and Rrs are either separately computed or derived from the equation of motion. In fact, because three ($\dot{V}$, V, Pao) of the five variables of Equation 1 are measured, it is possible to mathematically derive the two unknown constants.

Compliance

At end-inflation Crs = ΔV/ΔPao, where ΔV and ΔPao represent the difference in V and Pao between the onset of inflow and the zero-

TABLE 84–1

Glossary of Terms, Units, and Common Terminology

BTPS	Body temperature, ambient pressure, saturated with water vapor
C (CL, Crs, Cw)	Compliance, mL/cm H_2O (e.g., of the lungs, respiratory system, and chest wall)
FRC	Functional residual capacity (end-expiratory volume), mL
P	Pressure, cm H_2O
Pao	Pressure at the airway opening, cm H_2O
Pel	Elastic pressure (proportional to lung volume), cm H_2O
Pmus	Pressure generated by respiratory muscles, cm H_2O
Pres	Resistive pressure (proportional to airflow), cm H_2O
R (RL, Rrs, Rw)	Resistance, cm $H_2O \times mL^{-1} \times s$ (of the lungs, respiratory system, and chest wall)
τrs	Passive time constant of respiratory system, s
τrs(exp)	Expiratory time constant of respiratory system, s
V	Volume, mL (BTPS)
V̇	Flow, mL (BTPS)/s
Vr	Static relaxation volume of respiratory system, mL
Active Mode	Pmus >0, contraction of inspiratory or expiatory muscles
Passive Mode	Pmus = 0, muscle relaxation
Static Condition	V̇ = 0. (a) *Active:* breath holding by muscle contraction above or below Vr;
	(b) *Passive:* relaxation against closed airways above Vr (Pao >0), below Vr (Pao <0), or at Vr (Pao = 0)
Dynamic Condition	V̇ >0. (a) *Active:* spontaneous breathing; (b) *Passive:* artificial ventilation or part of expiration during spontaneous breathing

flow point at end-inflation. If Crs were simply computed as the ratio of V and Pao at end-inflation, it would yield a spuriously low value whenever the infant is ventilated with some positive end-expiratory pressure, which, in fact, is the most frequent condition.

Lung compliance (CL) is similarly computed as the ratio between the change in V and the change in transpulmonary pressure, which is the difference between Pao and pleural pressure; finally, chest wall compliance can also be determined as Cw = 1/(1/Crs–1/CL). Pleural pressure is usually measured in the esophagus, with an esophageal balloon or an esophageal liquid-filled catheter, but whether esophageal pressure can be taken with confidence as representative of the mean change in pleural pressure in infants (especially premature infants) is continuing to be debated.[1-5] Problems are related not only to technical aspects of the measurements (including the frequency response of the esophageal catheter) but also to the degree of chest wall distortion. A common test, in a spontaneously breathing infant, is that of comparing the changes in esophageal pressure with those of Pao during an inspiratory effort against occluded airways.[2,6] Because lung volume and transpulmonary pressure should not change during the inspiratory effort, the Pao-esophageal pressure difference during the effort should remain nil if esophageal pressure is a reliable index of pulmonary pressure. However, in infants, particularly those who are premature, the distortion of the chest is often large and not necessarily the same between an unoccluded inspiration and an occluded inspiratory effort. Therefore, the possibility exists that what appears as a reliable measure during the effort[7] is not equally valid during normal spontaneous breathing.

Compliance measured as thus described is often labeled *dynamic* compliance, a term that may be confusing because it seems to contradict the compulsory requirement of static condition for these measurements. In effect, the word *dynamic* is used to stress the fact that the measurement has been collected by taking advantage of a very brief and transient condition of V̇ = 0 at end-inflation, during the dynamic state of continuous ventilation. In healthy adults, the values of *dynamic* compliances are very close to the *static* measurements, which are obtained by monitoring P for one or a few seconds at constant V. In infants, however, *dynamic* compliances are consistently lower than the *static* values[8-10] mainly because of lung stress relaxation. This latter is a phenomenon characteristic of viscoelastic tissues and is substantially more marked in newborns than in adults.[11, 12] Asynchronous behavior of peripheral lung units also contributes to the *dynamic-static* difference in the values of the newborn's compliances,[13] and probably more so in conditions of marked chest distortion.[14]

Resistance

Inflation. The total resistance of the respiratory system (Rrs) at any given time during the inflation phase can be calculated according to the following formula: Rrs = Prs/V̇ = [Pao – Pel]/V̇, where Prs and Pel are, respectively, the resistive and elastic pressure components of P (Equation 2).[15] The measurement is more accurate at the time of peak flow, which is usually in the middle third of inflation. Alternate analytical approaches are based on the computation by planimetry of Pres, and on various solutions of the Equation of Motion (Equation 1).[16] Chest wall resistance (Rw) can then be calculated as Rrs – RL.

Deflation. To the extent that the respiratory system behaves as a first-order mechanical system, if deflation is unimpeded, the decrease in volume and flow should follow an exponential curve. The semilog representation of either signal during deflation should therefore yield a linear relation, of which the reciprocal of the slope represents the time constant (τrs).[17] From this, Rrs is computed as τrs/Crs.

Passive Respiratory Mechanics in the Spontaneously Breathing Infant

For these measurements, the infant is breathing through a face mask connected to a pneumotachograph. Newborn babies tolerate the mask extremely well, although, were measurements of breathing pattern also desirable, the possible effects introduced by the stimulation of the trigeminal area[18] and by the added dead space should be taken into account. With some practice, the same investigator holding the mask on the infant's face (covering both mouth and nostrils) can manually perform brief occlusions of the pneumotachograph outlet, a maneuver that represents the basis for the measurements of Crs and Rrs to be described. Of course, more sophisticated techniques for airway occlusion can be devised, and the use of a solenoid valve may be desirable for the accurate timing of the occlusion.

Compliance

After occlusion of the airways at end-inspiration or during expiration (Fig. 84–1), Pao rises to the value corresponding to the recoil pressure of the respiratory system at that volume. The time course of the increase in Pao depends on the time of progressive relaxation of the inspiratory muscles. Because inspiratory muscle relaxation is triggered by the activation of the airway slowly adapting stretch receptors (which respond to transpulmonary pressure) the larger the lung volume at which the occlusion is performed,

SPONTANEOUS BREATHING

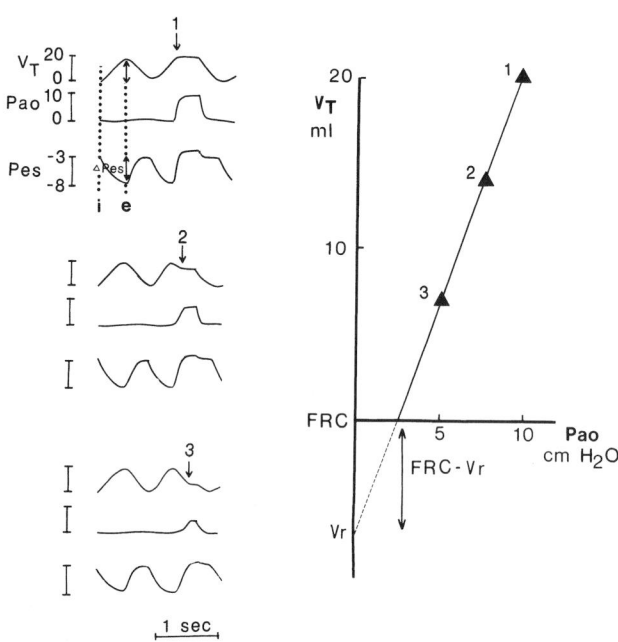

Figure 84–1. Schematic representation of the changes in lung volume (V_T), pressure measured at the mouth (Pao), and esophageal pressure (Pes) in a spontaneously breathing infant. Three conditions are indicated at left, from top to bottom, beginning with a breathing cycle followed by a cycle with occlusion of the airways performed by the investigator. At 1, occlusion is at end inspiration; at 2, in the first third of expiration; at 3, in the second half of expiration. The corresponding Pao-V points are plotted in the diagram at right, and the slope of the linear regression represents the compliance of the respiratory system, and the intercept on the y-axis represents the difference between end-expiratory level (FRC) and resting volume (Vr). Although only three data points are represented, a larger number of points through the whole V_T is desirable to improve the accuracy of the linear regression. If the Pes record is also available (*left panels*), dynamic lung compliance can be computed as V_T/ΔPes, between the two zero-flow points at beginning and end inspiration (*i, e*).

the greater the probability of complete muscle relaxation. The occlusion must be brief because the same vagal reflex inhibiting the inspiratory muscles eventually yields activation of the expiratory muscles by the Hering-Breuer expiratory promoting reflex. An accurate computation of Crs requires measurements of ΔV and ΔPao over as wide a range of V as possible for a more confident estimation of the V-Pao slope.[8, 19–21] In fact, because during spontaneous breathing the lung volume at end expiration (functional residual capacity, FRC) is usually greater than the static relaxation volume (Vr), if Crs was simply measured as dV/dPao (instead of being measured as the slope of the V-Pao curve), it would result in an incorrect low value. The FRC-Vr difference can be calculated by extrapolation of the expiratory $\dot{V}$-V loop (see later); hence, on theoretical grounds, with only one occlusion it should be possible to compute τrs, FRC-Vr, Crs, and Rrs.[22] In practice, the averaging of more than a single breathing cycle is often required for a confident measurement of τrs and FRC-Vr.

An alternate occlusion method has been proposed.[23] A first brief occlusion of the airways is performed to establish a reference V and the corresponding static Pao; a second occlusion is then done at a different V, within the same expiration, or in the following breath. Then, Crs is computed from the V difference

between the two occlusions (ΔV) and the corresponding difference in Pao (ΔPao), as Crs = ΔV/ΔPao. This method circumvents the potential problems introduced by breath-by-breath oscillations in FRC. If the esophageal pressure were also monitored, as schematically indicated in Figure 84-1, Crs could be partitioned into its lung and chest wall components.

Other approaches have been proposed in an attempt to quantify the elastic properties of the respiratory system over a range in volume larger than tidal volume.[24]

Time Constant and Resistance

Because respiratory system compliance and resistance are approximately constant within the tidal volume range, both $\dot{V}$ and V during expiration decrease following an exponential curve. Therefore, a semilog representation of $\dot{V}$, or V, during the expiration following a brief occlusion of the airways at end-inspiration (as in the maneuver described for measurements of Crs) yields a linear relationship, the reciprocal of the slope being the passive time constant of the respiratory system (τrs).[25] Because the ratio of two exponential decays ($\dot{V}$ and V in time) is a constant,[17] τrs can also be calculated from the slope of the V (y-axis) – $\dot{V}$ (x-axis) relationship (Fig. 84–2).[19, 22, 26] From τrs, Rrs is calculated as τrs/Crs. Such a simple and very practical approach is not readily applicable when the expiratory decays of $\dot{V}$ and V do not follow exponential curves. This could be due to respiratory muscle activation or, more likely, to nonlinear mechanical behavior of the upper airways. In these cases, τrs and Rrs vary during expiration, and the $\dot{V}$ at which they are measured needs to be defined.

The extrapolation of the linear segment of the $\dot{V}$-V curve to zero flow represents the dynamic elevation of the end-expiratory level (or FRC-Vr difference) in the spontaneously breathing infant.[19, 20] In fact, if the expiratory time was sufficiently long, expiration would proceed until Vr, and FRC would equal Vr. In infants, however, expiration is too short with respect to τrs, and inspiration begins at a lung volume higher than Vr.[16] The FRC-Vr difference, which can also be computed by extrapolation of the Pao-V curve (see Fig. 84–1), averages 7 to 15 mL in infants a few days old,[19, 20, 27–29] or about 20 to 30% of tidal volume.

As in adults, also in infants pulmonary resistance measurements are sensitive to the absolute lung volume at which they are performed.[30]

ACTIVE MECHANICAL BEHAVIOR OF THE RESPIRATORY SYSTEM

An important question is whether during spontaneous breathing the mechanical properties of the respiratory system are the same as during passive conditions. The answer is that during inspiration and expiration the system does not behave exactly as expected on the basis of passive measurements. During inspiration, the main reason for the difference has to do with the uneven distribution of forces on the chest wall during muscle contraction, leading to distortion. This has several functional implications, including its effect on the energetics of breathing (see next section). The lowering of compliance in dynamic conditions, mentioned earlier, is an additional factor contributing to the difference between active and passive mechanics.

During expiration, neural mechanisms that control the expiratory flow and mean lung volume by regulating the postinspiratory and laryngeal muscle activity effectively increase the expiratory resistance, prolonging the time constant above the passive value.[16]

Mechanics of Chest Wall Distortion

During passive inflation of the respiratory system (e.g., during artificial ventilation) both abdominal and pleural pressures increase. In fact, in the absence of diaphragmatic tension, the

Figure 84–2. Human infant, spontaneously breathing. Flow and volume are continuously recorded and schematically plotted on the x- and y-axes for one breathing cycle *(continuous line)*. Inspiration is at left (negative flows) and expiration is at right (positive flows). At end-inspiration of the second breathing cycle, the airways are briefly occluded *(end-insp. occl.);* following release of the occlusion, the slope of the deflation flow-volume curve *(dashed line)* represents the passive time constant of the respiratory system (τrs). Often, the tidal expiratory flow-volume curve is at left of the passive curve, indicating that the respiratory time constant of expiration during resting breathing, $\tau rs(exp)$, exceeds τrs. When the expiratory flow-volume relationship presents a linear segment, as indicated in the diagram, it is possible to extrapolate the $\tau rs(exp)$ line to zero flow; the intercept on the y-axis represents the volume difference between end expiration (functional residual capacity, FRC) and resting volume (Vr).

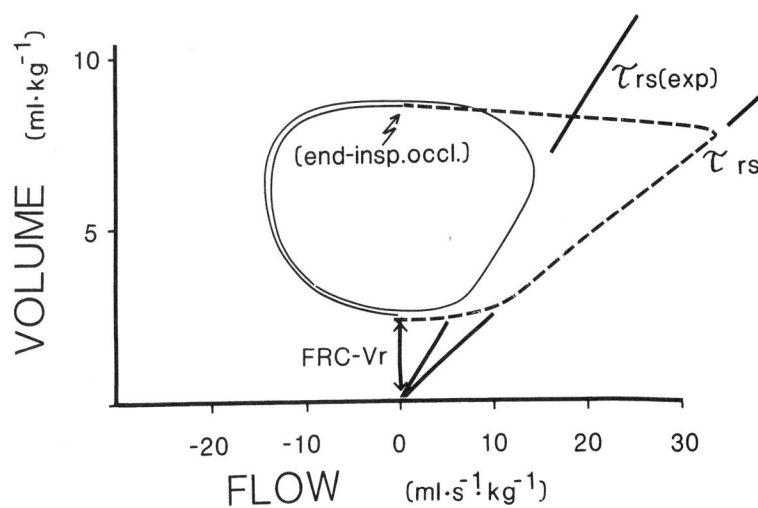

changes in pleural and abdominal pressures are the same, and any region of the chest wall (specifically, its two main compartments, rib cage and abdomen) will be driven by the same uniformly applied pressure.

In active conditions (Pmus >0), when the diaphragm is contracting, abdominal pressure similarly increases, expanding the abdomen. However, the motion of the rib cage depends on the interplay of several factors.[16] First, pleural pressure during spontaneous inspiration is subatmospheric, tending to collapse both the upper and lower regions of the rib cage. This effect on the lower portion of the rib cage could be partly offset by the expanding action of the abdominal pressure, and the direct outward-pulling of the diaphragmatic fibers. Hence, during diaphragmatic contraction, a given increase in abdominal pressure will not necessarily be accompanied by a rib cage expansion similar to the passive inflation. In fact, diaphragmatic contraction alone yields a collapse of the upper rib cage, as in quadriplegic patients who have lost the use of the intercostal muscles[31]; in normal infants, this is likely to occur because their characteristically high Cw implies that the mechanical coupling between upper and lower rib cage regions is not as strong as in adults. It follows that during spontaneous inspiration an expansion of the rib cage to a degree comparable with that observed during passive inflation requires the intervention of the extra-diaphragmatic muscles, namely, the intercostal muscles. In other words, motion of the whole chest wall during active breathing as in passive conditions should not be interpreted as *absence* of distortion, but, rather, as *compensation* for distortion.[32] The two concepts are different when examined in light of the energetics of breathing.

A functional evaluation of the net effect of chest distortion on lung volume can be done by comparing lung volumes between active and passive conditions at the same abdominal pressure (or abdominal motion, because, in absence of abdominal muscle activity, changes in abdominal pressure and abdominal displacement are closely related).[32] A schematic example is presented in Figure 84–3, which refers to a newborn infant breathing spontaneously during sleep; V̇, V, and Pao, in addition to the motion of the abdominal wall, are recorded. At end-inspiration, the airways are artificially occluded; during the short time of the occlusion the respiratory muscles relax, as suggested by the plateau in Pao. Hence, at end-inspiration, the abdomen-V data point reflects the active condition, whereas during the occlusion it reflects the passive situation. The complete abdomen-V passive relationship is constructed by multiple occlusions at different lung volumes during expiration, similar to what was described earlier for the

measurement of Crs during spontaneous breathing. The active points (at end-inspiration) can be compared with the passive relationship, and the difference on the y-axis represents the V difference between active and passive conditions. Normally, in infants during resting breathing, at any given abdominal pressure, tidal volume is less than the passive V, by as much as approximately 50%; this means that breathing in infants involves a substantial *volume loss*.[32] The volume loss is probably even larger in rapid-eye-movement sleep, when the intercostal muscles are less active and the inward movement of the rib cage in inspiration is maximal. In addition, the volume loss is likely to be larger in the supine posture than in the prone position,[33] because abdominal compliance is higher in the former than in the latter case. A very large volume loss could indicate a high Cw:CL ratio, as in premature infants or in bronchopulmonary dysplasia, or in conditions of increased airways resistance. Conversely, a very small volume loss, or a tidal volume exceeding the passive V, indicate increased activity of the extradiaphragmatic muscles, such as it might be seen in hypoxia or in association with other conditions of elevated respiratory drive.

Expiratory Time Constant

One may expect the passive time constant of the respiratory system (τrs, see Fig. 84–2) to be equal to the time constant of tidal expiration, $\tau rs(exp)$, because in resting condition expiration is a passive process. However, this is often not the case,[19, 20, 28] and $\tau rs(exp)$ exceeds τrs mainly for two reasons. First, the inspiratory activity does not cease instantaneously at end-inspiration but proceeds during part of the expiratory phase, effectively reducing the elastic recoil pressure of the respiratory system. Second, the adduction of the vocal folds during expiration increases airway resistance, prolonging τrs. Graphically, the effects of the activity of the inspiratory and laryngeal muscles in expiration can be appreciated by comparing the tidal expiratory flow-volume loop with that obtained after release of an end-inspiratory airway occlusion (see Fig. 84–2).[19, 20] Because the expiratory curve is at the left of the passive curve, $\tau rs(exp)$ is longer than τrs at any volume during expiration.

The prolonged $\tau rs(exp)$ implies that mean lung volume is higher than it would be if expiration was occurring with a time constant equal to τrs. In addition, the next inspiration begins at a volume (FRC) higher than Vr. Indeed, almost 30 years ago, Olinsky and co-workers[34] showed that in infants during short periods of apnea FRC decreased, and suggested that during tidal resting breathing FRC was maintained above Vr. Only a few years

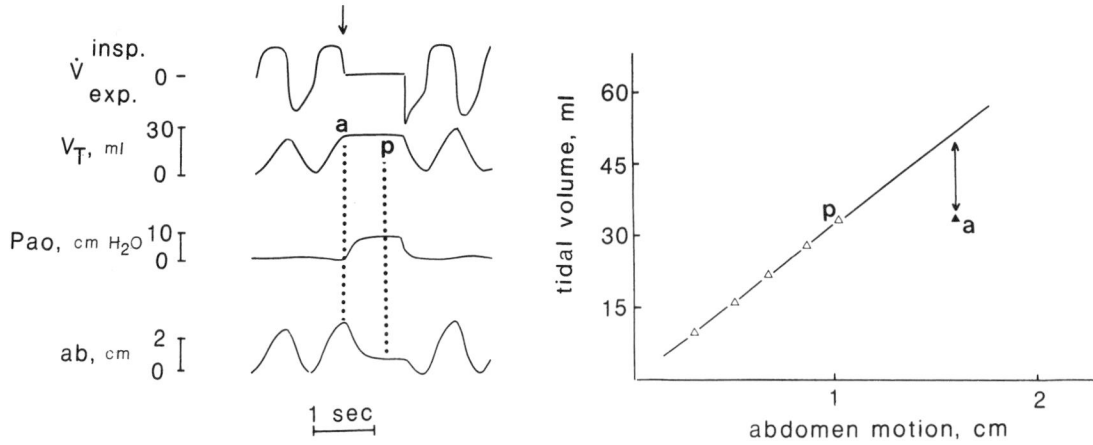

Figure 84–3. Schematic representation of the changes in airflow (V̇), volume (V_T), pressure at the airway opening (Pao), and motion of the abdomen (ab) in a spontaneously breathing infant. At *arrow*, the airways are occluded by the investigator, and muscle relaxation is achieved at plateau of Pao. The active (a, *solid triangle*) and passive (p) V-ab points are plotted at right. The passive relationship (*open triangles*) is obtained by multiple occlusions at different lung volumes during expiration. The vertical distance between a and the passive V (*double arrow*) indicates the volume loss because of distortion.

later it was possible to compute the FRC-Vr difference from analysis of the static pressure-volume curve (see Fig. 84-1) and the expiratory flow-volume curve (see Fig. 84-2).[19, 20, 27-29, 35] The FRC-Vr difference can be explained by the combined effect of the breathing rate (which in infants is high compared to the adults) and of the expiratory action of inspiratory and laryngeal muscles.[36] The elevation of FRC above Vr is particularly important because in infants the high Cw:CL ratio predisposes to a low Vr.[13] These control mechanisms for FRC are lost in infants artificially ventilated through an endotracheal tube. In these cases, an end-expiratory P of a few cm H_2O[37, 38] is added to the expiratory line of the ventilator to prevent deflation of the lungs to Vr.

ASPECTS OF THE ENERGETICS OF BREATHING

From the equation of motion of the respiratory system (Equation 1), it is apparent that once Crs and Rrs are known, it is possible to compute the total pressure required to inflate the lung to a given volume in a given time. From this pressure, the total work can also be calculated, assuming a sinusoidal flow pattern or a squared flow pattern, on the basis of the formula originally proposed by Otis and co-workers.[39] These and other computations have indicated that in newborns, as in adults, breathing frequency occurs within the optimal range of minimal external work.[19] The respiratory work calculated in this way represents the *passive* work of breathing, because it is based on values of Crs and Rrs obtained in passive conditions. When the muscles themselves are producing the pressure that inflates the respiratory system, the *active* work of breathing is likely to exceed the passive value. The main reason for this difference is that the respiratory muscles cannot generate a force as uniformly applied to the system as it is in passive conditions. The inflationary action of the main inspiratory muscle, the diaphragm, can be pictured more like that of a piston expanding the abdomen and simultaneously collapsing the upper rib cage than that of a uniform chest wall expander. The result of this uneven distribution of muscle force is that some force is lost in the distortion of the chest wall, instead of being translated into pressure driving the respiratory system. Furthermore, during contraction, muscles lose some force depending on their length and the velocity of shortening. Therefore, from the point of view of the dynamics and energetics of breathing, one could state that during active

breathing the respiratory system behaves as if its impedance were higher than in passive conditions because of a lower Crs, higher Rrs, or both.

Estimates of the active pressure required to expand the respiratory system have been obtained by measuring the Pao generated during an inspiratory effort against closed airways. In fact, in this condition, the change in lung volume is negligible, and, supposedly, the inspiratory muscles are contracting isometrically. The main assumption underlying this approach is that the Pao generated by the muscles is the same pressure required to generate V and V̇ during normal breathing. Measurements of Pao are made at known time intervals from the onset of the occluded effort and those of flow and volume at the corresponding times from the onset of the preceding open airway breath (Fig. 84-4, *left*).[40]

The slope and intercept of the plot of Pao/V (y-axis) against V̇/V (x-axis) represent, respectively, the *active* Rrs and 1/Crs (see Fig. 84-4, *right*). From several studies that applied this approach or slightly modified ones, it can be concluded that the newborn infant's Crs during spontaneous breathing is about 65% of the passive value, whereas Rrs is approximately the same as in passive conditions. This would mean that the elastic work (and cost) of breathing during spontaneous breathing in an infant is approximately 50% (1/0.65) higher than expected from values of respiratory mechanics obtained in passive conditions.

Notwithstanding the difficulties in quantifying the active mechanical properties of the respiratory system, the estimate of the active work is useful because it represents a more realistic evaluation of the work imposed on the respiratory muscles than passive measurements would provide. In addition, the knowledge of the active values of Crs and Rrs yields more accurate predictions of the ability to maintain ventilation in face of external elastic or resistive loads.[41]

Several techniques, other than those described, are available to provide additional information on the mechanical status of the respiratory pump in infants. These include methods oriented to measure thoracic gas volume, the mechanical properties of the airways, and their interaction with those of the lung. The former are usually done by techniques employing body plethysmography, the latter by forced expiratory maneuvers. Although these measurements can provide useful data, they do present some problems related to the practical application in infants.[42-44] Forced expiratory maneuvers, for example, require sucking from

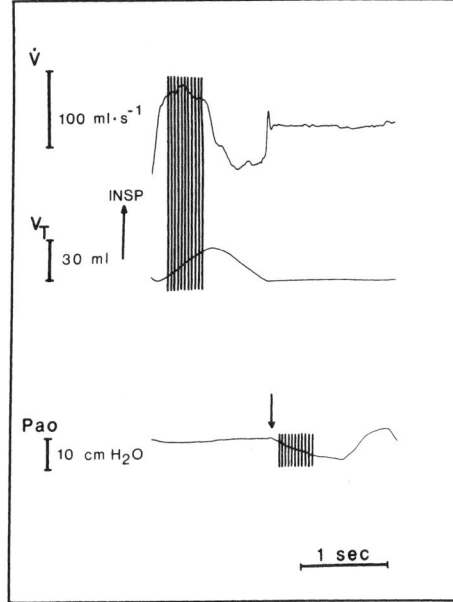
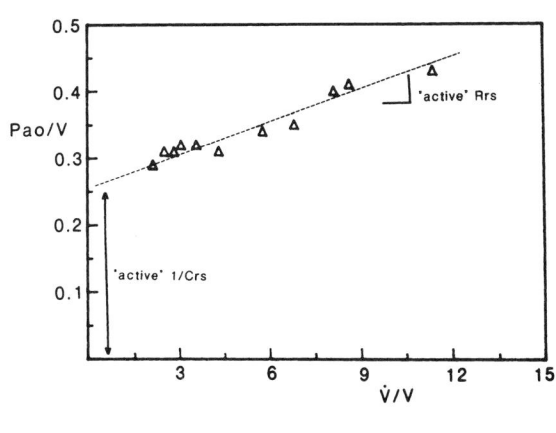

Figure 84–4. *Left,* newborn infant, spontaneously breathing. From top to bottom, records of airflow ($\dot{V}$), tidal volume (V_T), and mouth pressure (Pao). At the time point indicated by the *arrow,* the airways are occluded by the investigator; hence, the infant makes an inspiratory effort, lowering Pao. The vertical lines indicate iso-time measurements of Pao, $\dot{V}$, and V from the onset of the effort (Pao) and from the onset of the preceding breath ($\dot{V}$ and V). *Right,* The individual Pao/$\dot{V}$ – $\dot{V}$/V points are plotted; the slope and the reciprocal of the intercept of the linear regression represent, respectively, the active resistance and active compliance of the respiratory system. (Modified from Mortola JP, Saetta M: Pediatr Pulmonol *3*:123, 1987.)

the airways,[45] or forced squeezing on the thorax[46-47]; either approach yields results that depend greatly on how the pressure is applied and how the maneuver is performed.[48, 49] Thus, these methodologies are usually confined to the research setting. On the contrary, measurements of Crs and Rrs are simple, relatively standard techniques readily applicable to a wide range of healthy and sick infants. Because in infants Cw is very high in comparison to CL, Crs can more easily reflect pathologic changes in CL than it would be possible in adults; hence, its measurement has been found useful in predicting the course and outcome of respiratory problems as well as in classifying the severity of some respiratory diseases.

REFERENCES

1. LeSouef PN, et al: Influence of chest wall distortion on esophageal pressure. J Appl Physiol *55*:353, 1983.
2. Asher MI, et al: Measurement of pleural pressure in neonates. J Appl Physiol *52*:491, 1982.
3. Dinwiddie R, Russell G: Relationship of intraesophageal pressure to intrapleural pressure in the newborn. J Appl Physiol *33*:415, 1972.
4. Milner AD, et al: Relationship of intra-oesophageal pressure to mouth pressure during the measurement of thoracic gas volume in the newborn. Biol Neonate *33*:314, 1978.
5. Heaf DP, et al: The accuracy of esophageal pressure measurements in convalescent and sick intubated infants. Pediatr Pulmonol *2*:5, 1986.
6. Baydur A, et al: A simple method for assessing the validity of the esophageal balloon technique. Am Rev Respir Dis *126*:788, 1982.
7. Coates AL, et al: Liquid filled esophageal catheter for measuring pleural pressure in preterm neonates. J Appl Physiol *67*:889, 1989.
8. Olinsky A, et al: A simple method of measuring total respiratory system compliance in newborn infants. S Afr Med J *50*:128, 1976.
9. Sullivan KJ, Mortola JP: Dynamic lung compliance in newborn and adult cats. J Appl Physiol *60*:743, 1986.
10. Kano S, et al: Fast versus slow ventilation for neonates. Am Rev Respir Dis *148*:578, 1993.
11. Sullivan KJ, Mortola JP: Age related changes in the rate of stress relaxation within the rat respiratory system. Respir Physiol *67*:295, 1987.
12. Pérez Fontán JJ, et al: Stress relaxation of the respiratory system in developing piglets. J Appl Physiol *73*:1297, 1992.
13. Mortola JP: Dynamics of breathing in newborn mammals. Physiol Rev *67*:187, 1987.
14. Sullivan KJ, Mortola JP: Effect of distortion on the mechanical properties of newborn piglet lung. J Appl Physiol *59*:434, 1985.
15. Mead J, Whittenberger JL: Physical properties of human lung measured during spontaneous respiration. J Appl Physiol *5*:779, 1953.
16. Mortola, J. P. Respiratory Physiology of Newborn Mammals. A Comparative Perspective. The Johns Hopkins University Press, Baltimore, 2001, pp 344.
17. McIlroy MB, et al: A new method for measurement of compliance and resistance of lungs and thorax. J Appl Physiol *18*:424, 1963.
18. Dolfin T, et al: Effects of a face mask and pneumotachograph on breathing in sleeping infants. Am Rev Respir Dis *128*:977, 1983.
19. Mortola JP, et al: Dynamics of breathing in infants. J Appl Physiol *52*:1209, 1982.
20. Mortola JP, et al: Muscle pressure and flow during expiration in infants. Am Rev Respir Dis *129*:49, 1984.
21. Fletcher ME, et al: Respiratory compliance in infants—a preliminary evaluation of the multiple interrupter technique. Pediatr Pulmonol *14*:118, 1992.
22. LeSouef PN, et al: Passive respiratory mechanics in newborns and children. Am Rev Respir Dis *129*:552, 1984.
23. Mortola JP, et al: Referencing lung volume for measurements of respiratory system compliance in infants. Pediatr Pulmonol *16*:248, 1993.
24. Grunstein MM, et al: Expiratory volume clamping: a new method to assess respiratory mechanics in sedated infants. J Appl Physiol *62*:2107, 1987.
25. Brody AW: Mechanical compliance and resistance of the lung-thorax calculated from the flow recorded during passive expiration. Am J Physiol *178*:189, 1954.
26. Zin WA, et al: Single-breath method for measurements of respiratory mechanics in anesthetized animals. J Appl Physiol *52*:1266, 1982.
27. Thach BT, et al: Intercostal muscle reflexes and sleep breathing patterns in the human infant. J Appl Physiol *48*:139, 1980.
28. Kosch PC, Stark AR: Dynamic maintenance of end-expiratory lung volume in full-term infants. J Appl Physiol *57*:1126, 1984.
29. Mortola JP, et al: Expiratory pattern of newborn mammals. J Appl Physiol *58*:528, 1985.
30. Miller MJ, et al: Effects of nasal CPAP on supraglottic and total pulmonary resistance in preterm infants. J Appl Physiol *68*:141, 1990.
31. Mortola JP, Sant' Ambrogio G: Motion of the rib cage and the abdomen in tetraplegic patients. Clin Sci Mol Med *54*:25, 1978.
32. Mortola JP, et al: Mechanical aspects of chest wall distortion. J Appl Physiol *59*:295, 1985.
33. Wolfson MR, et al: Effect of position on the mechanical interaction between rib cage and abdomen in preterm infants. J Appl Physiol *72*:1032, 1992.
34. Olinsky A, et al: Influence of lung inflation on respiratory control in neonates. J Appl Physiol *36*:426, 1974.
35. Stark AR, et al: Regulation of end-expiratory lung volume during sleep in premature infants. J Appl Physiol *62*:1117, 1987.
36. Griffiths GB, et al: End-expiratory level and breathing pattern in the newborn. J Appl Physiol *55*:243, 1983.

37. Berman LS, et al: Optimum levels of CPAP for tracheal extubation of newborn infants. J Pediatr 89:109, 1976.
38. Gregory GA, et al: Treatment of the idiopathic respiratory-distress syndrome with continuous positive airway pressure. N Engl J Med 284:1333, 1971.
39. Otis AB, et al: Mechanics of breathing in man. J Appl Physiol 2:592, 1950.
40. Mortola JP, Saetta M: Measurements of respiratory mechanics in the newborn: a simple approach. Pediatr Pulmonol 3:123, 1987.
41. Milic-Emili J, Zin WA: Breathing responses to imposed mechanical loads. In Fishman AP (ed): Handbook of Physiology, Section 3. The Respiratory System, Vol. II, Part 2. Bethesda, American Physiological Society, 1986, pp 751–769.
42. Beardsmore CS, et al: Problems in measurement of thoracic gas volume in infancy. J Appl Physiol 52:995, 1982.

43. Helms P: Problems with plethysmographic estimation of lung volume in infants and young children. J Appl Physiol 53:698, 1982.
44. Stocks J, et al: Pressure-flow curves in infancy. Pediatr Pulmonol 1:33, 1985.
45. Motoyama EK, et al: Early onset of airway reactivity in premature infants with bronchopulmonary dysplasia. Am Rev Respir Dis 136:50, 1987.
46. Adler SM, Wohl MEB: Flow-volume relationship at low lung volumes in healthy term newborn infants. Pediatrics 61:636, 1978.
47. Taussig LM, et al: Determinants of forced expiratory flows in newborn infants. J Appl Physiol 53:1220, 1982.
48. Silverman M, et al: Partial expiratory flow-volume curves in infancy: technical aspects. Bull Eur Physiopathol Respir 22:257, 1986.
49. LeSouef PN, et al: Effect of compression pressure on forced expiratory flow in infants. J Appl Physiol 61:1639, 1986.

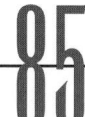

William Edward Truog

85 Pulmonary Gas Exchange in the Developing Lung

Integral to the system of pulmonary gas exchange are mechanisms to maintain matching of pulmonary perfusion and alveolar ventilation, such that atmospheric oxygen and pulmonary capillary blood have intimate contact. Requisite features of the gas exchange apparatus include sustained effective respiratory efforts to replenish the oxygen stores in alveolar gas and free diffusion of both oxygen and carbon dioxide across the alveolar-capillary barrier.

Mechanisms for maintaining the matching of alveolar ventilation ($\dot{V}_A$) and pulmonary perfusion ($\dot{Q}_p$) and the factors that influence changes in intrapulmonary distribution of $\dot{V}_A$ and $\dot{Q}_p$ in neonates are the topics of this chapter. The potential impact of insufficient oxygen-carrying capacity and diminished cardiac output on tissue delivery of oxygen is discussed elsewhere in this text.

A particular feature of postnatal gas exchange to which the lung must accommodate is the different frequency at which $\dot{V}_A$ and $\dot{Q}_p$ occur. The pulmonary circulation maintains forward flow, although at varying velocity, through the pulmonary microvasculature. By contrast, the inhalation of gases is periodic, occurring normally at a rate in neonates that is 20 to 50% of the cardiac rate. Therefore, different sinusoidal patterns of ventilation and perfusion occur within the lung, a factor that must be accommodated in achieving or maintaining optimal gas exchange efficiency.

To help sustain sufficient oxygen and carbon dioxide flux between gas and blood, an adequate alveolar gas volume or functional residual capacity (FRC) must be established shortly after birth and sustained thereafter. Development of the FRC occurs in the process of transition from fetal to neonatal life, as the fluid-filled lung empties itself of liquid and repletes itself with resident gas (Fig. 85–1).[1] The established resident gas volume serves as an intrapulmonary reservoir for oxygen.

The newborn infant is particularly vulnerable to the development of arterial hypoxemia for several reasons. First, because the partial pressure of oxygen in arterial blood (Pa_{O_2}) of normal newborns is low compared with that of adults,[2, 3] there is less intravascular oxygen reserve during periods of no oxygen movement into the lungs (i.e., during apnea). Second, the neonatal lung has an FRC that is close to airway closing volume. *Atelectasis*, or airway closure, may develop easily, especially considering the relative paucity of channels of collateral ventilation in the newborn. Finally, the metabolic demand for oxygen in newborn infants is greater on a per kilogram basis than in adults. Therefore, the infant more quickly depletes oxygen stores in the

blood and in resident alveolar gas in attempting to maintain aerobic metabolism. All these "physiologic" differences are potential contributors to arterial hypoxemia. Their contributions are accentuated in premature babies, who manifest additional problems of susceptibility to apnea because of immaturity of the respiratory centers and to lung segment collapse at end expiration because of extremely compliant chest walls.

ASSESSMENT OF VENTILATION-PERFUSION RELATIONSHIPS

Alveolar and Arterial Oxygen Tension

The measurement of Pa_{O_2} provides an excellent approximation of the efficiency of the lung as a gas-exchanging organ. The idealized alveolar to arterial oxygen gradient can be calculated by solving the alveolar air equation:

$$PA_{O_2} = PI_{O_2} - PA_{CO_2}/R + PA_{CO_2} \times (1 - R)/R$$

where R = respiratory exchange ratio. The alveolar partial pressure of carbon dioxide (PA_{CO_2}) is assumed to be approximately equal to Pa_{CO_2}; the partial pressure of inspired oxygen (PI_{O_2}) is calculated from measured barometric pressure and body temperature and assumes that inspired gas is 100% saturated with water vapor on reaching the acinar space. The calculated alveolar/arterial oxygen partial pressure calculated difference (AaD_{O_2}) in normal adults breathing ambient air at sea level is between 10 and 20 mm Hg. This value is increased with increasing fraction of inspired oxygen (FI_{O_2}). Neonates have large AaD_{O_2} values during ambient air breathing (as high as 40 to 50 mm Hg shortly after birth), even allowing for R values close to 1.0, presumably based on relatively high utilization of carbohydrate. The AaD_{O_2} may remain in the range of 20 to 40 mm Hg for days after birth in term infants who are not distressed.[4, 5]

The AaD_{O_2} quantifies the degree of venous admixture plus alveolar capillary membrane diffusion disequilibrium. However, neither the AaD_{O_2} nor the calculated ratio of arterial to alveolar oxygen tension (Pa_{O_2}/PA_{O_2}) discriminates between these components. Venous admixture includes both intrapulmonary shunt (perfusion of pulmonary capillary blood past nonventilated lung regions before joining the stream of pulmonary venous blood) and perfusion of low $\dot{V}_A/\dot{Q}$ areas in which alveolar ventilation is insufficient to restore PA_{O_2} to the value predicted from the "idealized" PA_{O_2} calculated earlier. Although pulmonary end-capillary

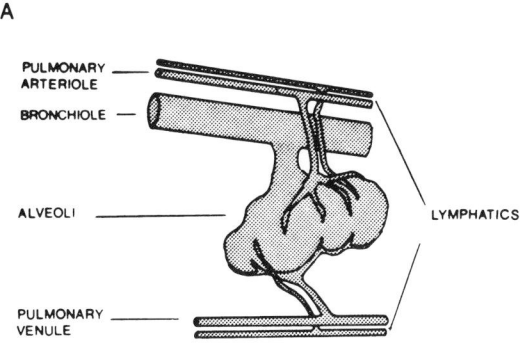

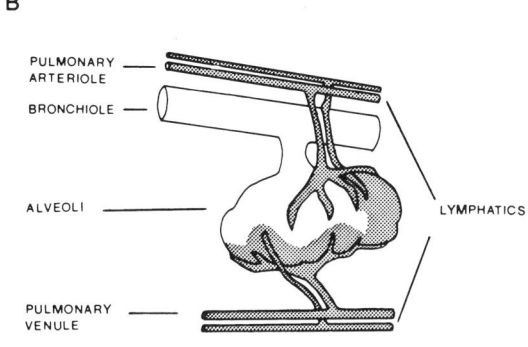

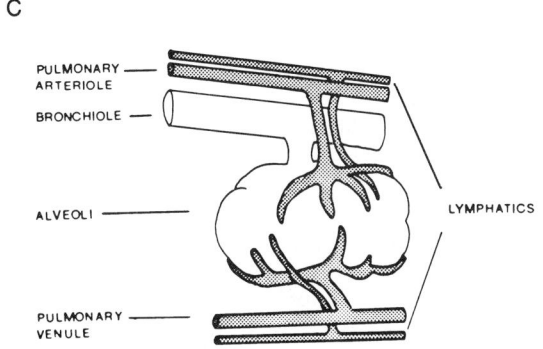

Figure 85–1. Airway fluid is removed from the lungs in several steps during birth. **A,** Fluid secretion from the lung stops during labor, although the air sacs and airways remain fluid filled. **B** and **C,** Fluid remaining in the airways is squeezed out the mouth and nose and is rapidly reabsorbed into the now expanded pulmonary capillary bed as well as into the lymphatic drainage system of the lung. (From Carlo WA, Chatburn BL [eds]: Neonatal Respiratory Care, 2nd ed. Chicago, Year Book Medical Publishers, 1988.)

to alveolar space equilibrium can be predicted to occur for oxygen and carbon dioxide in low $\dot{V}A/\dot{Q}$ areas, because PA_{O_2} is low, only a small rise in Pa_{O_2} occurs as blood traverses the pulmonary microcirculation (Fig. 85–2).[6] Depressed pulmonary end-capillary P_{O_2} is associated with disproportionately depressed oxygen content because of the shape of the oxyhemoglobin curve, leading to an undue depression of the mixed Pa_{O_2} as measured in the left atrium or systemic arteries (assuming no extrapulmonary right-to-left shunts). Therefore, overall pulmonary gas exchange is the flow-weighted and alveolar ventilation–weighted sum of gas exchange occurring in lung regions or groups of

acinar units with a common $\dot{V}A/\dot{Q}$. Lung units with both low $\dot{V}A/\dot{Q}$ and normal $\dot{V}A/\dot{Q}$ relationships are depicted in Figure 85–3). Also shown in Figure Fig. 88–3 is a pulmonary arterial to pulmonary venous connection bypassing any air-filled area, which, in the neonate, could represent shunt through the ductus arteriosus, through the foramen ovale, through connections between pulmonary and bronchial arteries, or through the thebesian circulation. The AaD_{O_2} measured in ambient air summarizes gas exchange, but it tells little about pulmonary reserves or about the cause of an increased difference between PA_{O_2} and Pa_{O_2}.

The presence of a moderate to severe degree of $\dot{V}A/\dot{Q}$ mismatching has an especially depressing effect on Pa_{O_2} when the FI_{O_2} is between 0.3 and 0.7 (Fig. 85–4).[7] The effect of low $\dot{V}A/\dot{Q}$ areas on the calculation of AaD_{O_2} can be eliminated by breathing 100% oxygen to remove nitrogen from any open but underventilated lung regions. However, absorption atelectasis may then develop, thus increasing the size of the shunt, which was the subject of the measurement. There is evidence that increased shunt with oxygen breathing occurs in premature infants[8] and in neonatal lambs but not in adult dogs.[9] These differences have been attributed to different degrees of development of pathways of collateral ventilation. Hence, the Pa_{O_2} determination or the ratio of Pa_{O_2} to PA_{O_2} does not provide detailed knowledge of the state of ventilation-perfusion relationships in the lung.

Nitrogen Gradient

When PA_{O_2} is low because of diminished alveolar ventilation (i.e., insufficient replacement of alveolar oxygen from inspiratory gas relative to the rate of removal by pulmonary capillary blood), the alveolar partial pressure of nitrogen (PA_{N_2}) rises because during "no flow" states (end expiration and end inspiration), the sum of gas partial pressures in the alveolar spaces must equal atmospheric pressure. The pressure of water (PH_2O) and PA_{CO_2} are relatively constant; therefore, when PA_{O_2} is diminished, the PA_{N_2} must be increased. If the elevated PA_{N_2} is sustained, there will be increased absorption of nitrogen into pulmonary capillary blood and development of an arterial to alveolar nitrogen gradient (aAD_{N_2}), which has been used to estimate the presence of low $\dot{V}A/\dot{Q}$ lung regions. Perfusion of nonventilated lung units produces no increase in PA_{N_2}, because the end-capillary and mixed venous partial pressures are the same for oxygen, carbon dioxide, and nitrogen, as well as any other inert gas solution. An aAD_{N_2} can develop because of the presence of either a small area of very low $\dot{V}A/\dot{Q}$ or a larger region of less imbalanced $\dot{V}A/\dot{Q}$, as long as $\dot{V}A/\dot{Q}$ is less than 1.0. Using the aAD_{N_2} to estimate shunt indirectly ($\dot{V}A/\dot{Q} = 0$) may result in an overestimation of shunt because of the sigmoidal shape of the oxyhemoglobin dissociation curve (i.e., small reductions in PA_{O_2} can disproportionately depress the arterial oxygen content when on the steep part of the curve).

Based on measurements of AaD_{O_2} and aAD_{N_2} in healthy newborn infants, Krauss and associates[10, 11] inferred that there was a relatively small low $\dot{V}A/\dot{Q}$ region after 1 to 2 days of postnatal life. Furthermore, the calculated aAD_{N_2} in infants with respiratory distress syndrome showed little contribution from low $\dot{V}A/\dot{Q}$ areas.[12] This observation suggests that the large venous admixture occurring with respiratory distress syndrome results from intrapulmonary or extrapulmonary shunt.

Carbon Dioxide Gradient

Arterial to alveolar differences for carbon dioxide (aAD_{CO_2}) reflect areas of the lungs that are poorly perfused but have a large dead space because they receive a substantial fraction of minute ventilation ($\dot{V}E$). Mismatching of $\dot{V}A/\dot{Q}$ as a cause of carbon dioxide retention has been emphasized to explain the development of respiratory acidosis when $\dot{V}E$ is elevated higher

$\dot{V}_A/\dot{Q}$ Relationships

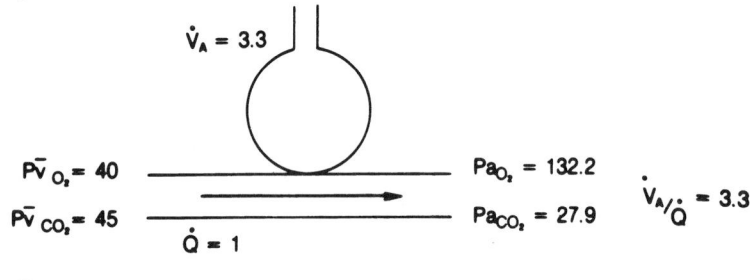

Figure 85–2. Effects of $\dot{V}_A/\dot{Q}$ ratios on blood gas tensions, expressed as mm Hg. **A,** Intrapulmonary shunt leaves mixed venous blood gas tensions unaltered. **B,** Alveolus with low $\dot{V}_A/\dot{Q}$ ratio: only partial oxygenation occurs. **C,** Relatively normal $\dot{V}_A/\dot{Q}$ ratio with satisfactory oxygenation of pulmonary capillary blood. **D,** Underperfused alveolus with high $\dot{V}_A/\dot{Q}$ ratio. (From Thibeault DW, Gregory GA [eds]: Neonatal Pulmonary Care, 2nd ed. Norwalk, CT, Appleton & Lange, 1986.)

than normal.[13] A small aAD_{CO_2} exists in some newborn infants,[5] but once a normal FRC has been established, the magnitude of the gradient is not consistent with a substantial number of high $\dot{V}_A/\dot{Q}$ areas, except in premature infants.[5] Deficiencies in carbon dioxide exchange during illness probably result from excess dead space ventilation with normal or increased total $\dot{V}_E$.[14]

Pulse Doppler Oximetry

The substitution of pulse Doppler oximetry saturation (Sp_{O_2}) for Pa_{O_2} is seductive but often misleading. The Sp_{O_2} is accurate, reproducible, and harmless and painless to obtain. However, change in Sp_{O_2} may not reflect concomitant change in Pa_{O_2}, but rather, shifting position of the oxyhemoglobin dissociation curve. Acute increases in pH and decrease in P_{CO_2} can produce left shift of the curve, raising Sp_{O_2} without changing Pa_{O_2}. Significant transfusions of adult hemoglobin into term and especially preterm infants will alter the oxygen half-saturation of hemoglobin, producing a right shift and a lower Sp_{O_2} with no change in Pa_{O_2}. Lack of awareness of this potential discrepancy may result in clinical harm from inappropriate undertreatment or overtreatment.

Use of Inert Gases to Assess $\dot{V}_A/\dot{Q}$ Matching

A technique employing trace quantities of inert gases to map the continuous distribution of ventilation-perfusion ratios from shunt to dead space ($\dot{V}_A/\dot{Q}$ of 0 to distribute multiple $\dot{V}_A/\dot{Q}$ of infinity) became practical with the application of computer tech-

nology and an understanding of the steady-state behavior of inert gases dissolved in blood.[15] Wagner and associates[16, 17] described a technique that employs six inert gases (which encompass a range of solubility in blood) and in which retention of each gas in blood perfusing the lung can be expressed by the simple relationship:

$$Pa/Pv = Palv/Pv = \lambda/(\lambda + \dot{V}_A/\dot{Q})$$

where λ is the Ostwald blood gas solubility coefficient (unique for each gas) and Pa, Pv, and Palv are the partial pressures of the gas measured in arterial blood, mixed venous blood, and alveolar gas (in reality measured in mixed expired gas and corrected for dead space ventilation). The equation assumes that each gas demonstrates a linear dissociation between blood or plasma and air, that is, behavior unlike that demonstrated by the respiratory gases oxygen and carbon dioxide.

Under conditions of presumed steady-state gas exchange, which is always an approximation of *in vivo* situations, the multiple inert gas elimination technique (MIGET) allows quantification of shunt, dead space, and low and high $\dot{V}_A/\dot{Q}$ lung regions during both normal and experimental conditions. A major advantage of the technique is the quantification of shunt, separate from low $\dot{V}_A/\dot{Q}$ areas, without the need to resort to 100% oxygen breathing. The experimental data consist of the measured ratios of the mixed arterial to mixed venous and mixed expired to mixed venous partial pressure for each of the

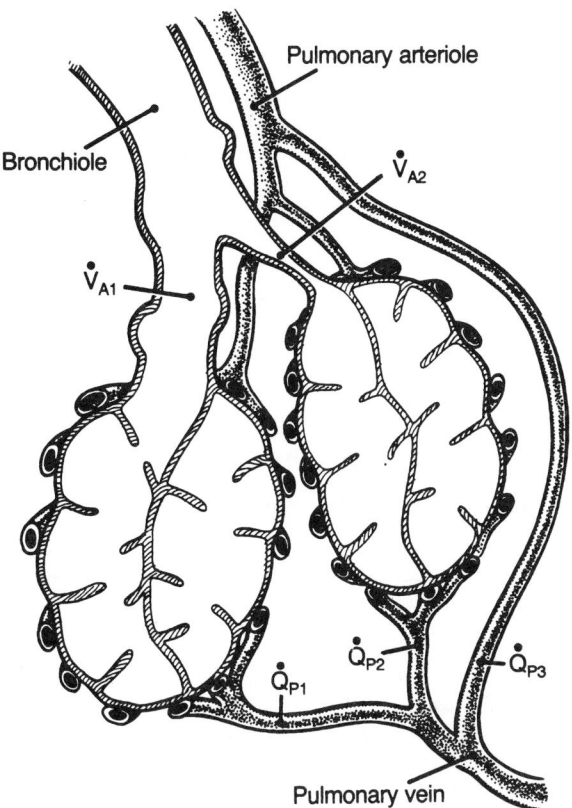

Figure 85–3. Schematic illustration of airway and vascular relationships. The acinar unit, containing many alveolar sacs, is shown with multiple pulmonary capillaries enveloping the saccules, providing maximal gas-exchanging surface area. $\dot{V}_{A_1}/\dot{Q}p_1$ corresponds to an acinar region (containing multiple alveoli) with normal $\dot{V}_A/\dot{Q}$; $\dot{V}_{A_2}/\dot{Q}p_2$ represents an acinar region with a low $\dot{V}_A/\dot{Q}$ and poor gas exchange. The pulmonary arteriole to pulmonary venous connection, $\dot{Q}p_3$, which bypasses any air-containing spaces, could represent intrapulmonary as well as extrapulmonary shunts.

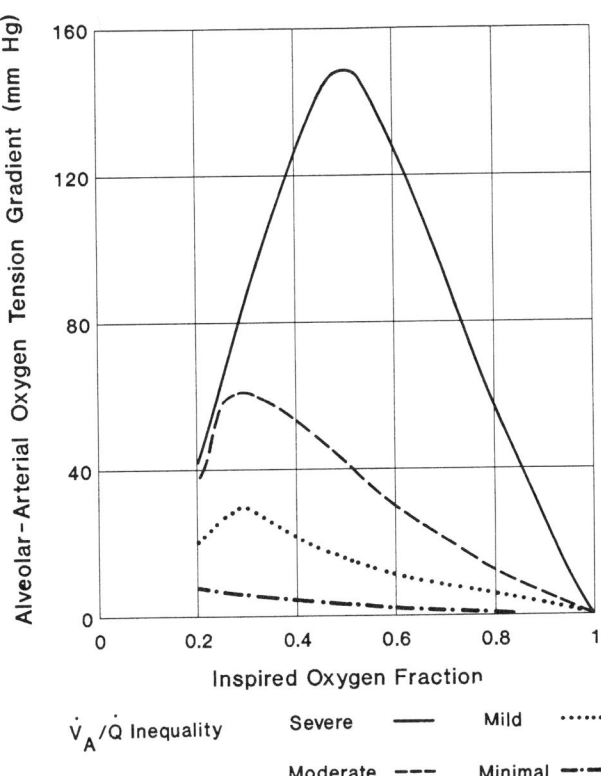

Figure 85–4. The effects of changes in inspired oxygen fraction, shown on the abscissa, on the calculated alveolar-arterial oxygen gradient are plotted for varying degrees of $\dot{V}_A/\dot{Q}$ inequality without any coexisting shunt. (From Dantzker DR: Hosp Pract Jan *15*:135, 1986.)

gases employed (usually sulfur hexafluoride, ethane, cyclopropane, halothane, diethyl ether, and acetone) and the measured solubility of each gas. Translation of these discrete experimental measurements into continuous distributions of ventilation and perfusion provides one method of assessing $\dot{V}$ relationships (Fig. 85–5).[13] Additional methods of interpretation have been devised to respond to concerns about the inherent nonuniqueness of the mathematical solutions describing the 50-compartment lung.[18] Techniques of data analysis now include computation of the area under the curve defined by calculating the aA inert gas partial pressure difference for each gas. The calculated area reflects overall $\dot{V}$ heterogeneity (Fig. 85–6).[19, 20] Calculation of the standard deviation of pulmonary blood flow (SD $\dot{Q}p$) provides a quantitative index of dispersion of $\dot{Q}p$ about the mean $\dot{V}_A/\dot{Q}$ value, separate from shunt and dead space.[18] Under experimental conditions, each of these assessments appears to be consistent with the others in providing semiquantitative estimates of the $\dot{V}_A/\dot{Q}$ heterogeneity of the lung. Current limitations of the MIGET include the lack of on-line analysis capacity for assessment of $\dot{V}_A/\dot{Q}$ relations and the necessity of the assumption of steady-state gas exchange.[18]

Any assessment of ventilation and perfusion must consider the following assumptions:

1. There is uniformity of the inspired gas composition. Inspired gas that is altered in composition by rebreathing of expired gas from more slowly emptying adjacent lung areas in the nonhomogeneously ventilated lung will produce series inequality of ventilation, which is difficult to differentiate from the more familiar parallel inequality.

2. Although the composition of pulmonary arterial blood is relatively uniform, there can be effects on gas exchange from intraregional differences in hematocrit.[21] Gas exchange is retarded when lung units with low $\dot{V}_A/\dot{Q}$ are perfused by blood with high hematocrit. If high neonatal hematocrits predispose to greater pulmonary interregional variability, then this effect could contribute to depressed oxygen exchange. The timing of pulmonary capillary development may be important in promoting the occurrence of this phenomenon.

3. Alveolar end-pulmonary capillary partial pressure disequilibrium, as may occur during a shortened transit time across the pulmonary capillary bed, may limit transport of oxygen (see later). There is less possibility of alveolar end-capillary disequilibrium for inert gases, with their rapid equilibrium time, to transfer respiratory gases.[22]

All the techniques used for gas exchange analysis demonstrate limitations because of invasiveness, inaccuracy, and problems of reproducibility. They all depend on assumptions about steady-state conditions, which in periods of rapid transient change in $\dot{Q}p$ or $\dot{V}_A$, or in the presence of pulmonary disease, may not be true. During rapidly evolving disease states, the techniques may not reflect rapidly changing contributions to overall gas exchange inefficiency. Nonetheless, the application of a technique such as MIGET has allowed new insights about pulmonary gas exchange by illustrating effects on $\dot{V}_A/\dot{Q}$ matching resulting from a variety of pulmonary diseases.[23]

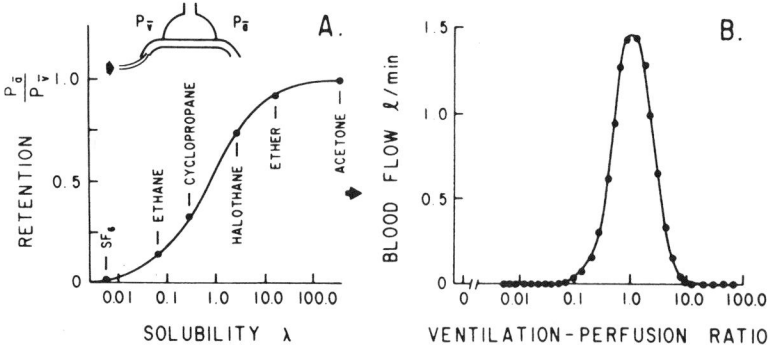

Figure 85–5. A, Retention solubility curve created by the experimental techniques referred to in the text. Each of the six gases is plotted against its measured solubility. Pa = partial pressure of each inert gas in arterial blood; Pv = partial pressure in mixed venous blood. **B,** The retention solubility curve can be used to derive a distribution of fractional perfusion to each of 50 theoretical lung compartments. (From West JB: Am Rev Respir Dis *116*:919, 1977.)

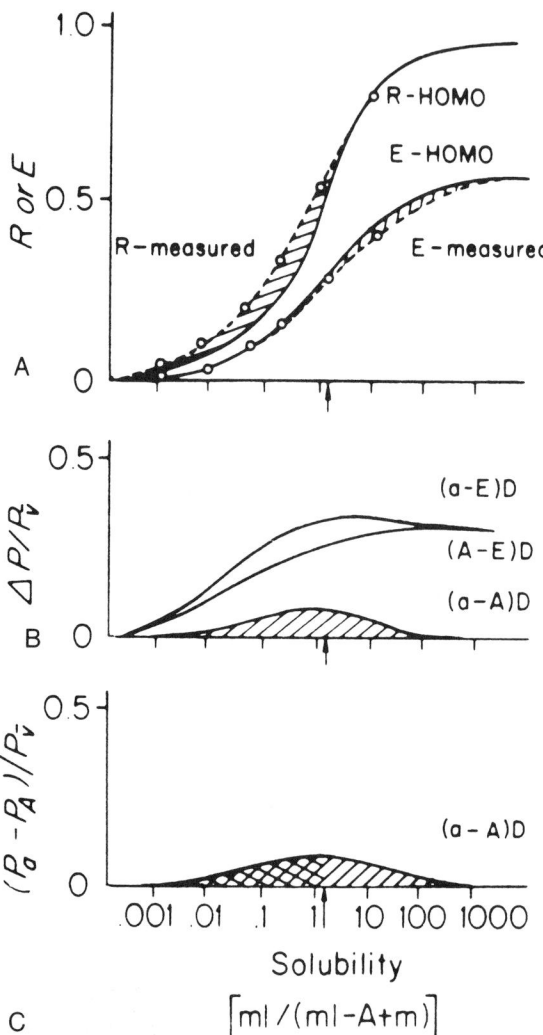

Figure 85–6. A, Measured and homogeneous retention (R) and excretion (E) curves are plotted against solubility, with R and E values shown as *open circles*. The homogeneous curves would occur if there were no $\dot{V}_A/\dot{Q}$ heterogeneity in the lung (i.e., an idealized lung). The *hatched areas* between the measured and homogeneous R and E curves occur because of $\dot{V}_A/\dot{Q}$ heterogeneity. **B,** The sum of the areas under the aAD curve is shown. The area under the (a-A) D curve is calculated by subtracting the (A-E) (D) curve from the (a-E) D curve. The *arrow* on the abscissa indicates solubility that is numerically equal to mean $\dot{V}_A/\dot{Q}$ in the lung. **C,** The area under the curve to the left of the mean $\dot{V}_A/\dot{Q}$, represented by the *double-crosshatch area,* is an index of low $\dot{V}_A/\dot{Q}$ lung areas. (From Truog WE, et al: J Appl Physiol *47*:1112, 1979.)

FACTORS REGULATING VENTILATION-PERFUSION MATCHING IN THE DEVELOPING LUNG

Effects of Increased Pulmonary Arterial Pressure

Pulmonary arterial pressure (Ppa), which equals or exceeds systemic arterial pressure (Psa) during fetal life, declines normally in the hours surrounding birth to a level approximately 50% of Psa. The further decline to adult levels occurs more slowly. It is unknown, however, to what extent increased Ppa or persistent elevation of Ppa undermines or contributes to the stability of ventilation-perfusion matching in the neonatal lung during the normal transition to extrauterine life or during pulmonary diseases. Neonatal pulmonary diseases are commonly characterized by elevated Ppa and pulmonary vascular resistance (PVR). The diseased neonatal lung may also demonstrate collapsed segments or lobes, which can interfere with $\dot{V}_A/\dot{Q}$ matching.

An elevation in Ppa may change the intrapulmonary distribution of Qp. Elevations in Ppa can occur either because of constriction of smooth muscle (or possibly nonmuscularized endothelial cells) lining the vessels that compose the pulmonary microvasculature or because of a passive increase in left atrial pressure. Different vasoactive substances may mediate vasoconstriction at different sites within the microvasculature.[24] If a particular stimulus induces vasoconstriction only in previously dilated small muscular arteries and arterioles (which are conveying blood to well-ventilated areas), and not in already constricted vessels, the ratio in regional resistance of constricted vessels in nonventilated lung areas to resistance in previously dilated vessels in well-ventilated areas would be decreased. One result of this change in the ratio of local vascular resistance could be increased intrapulmonary right-to-left shunt (perfusion of nonventilated intrapulmonary regions) because of a redistribution of Qp favoring flow to nonventilated regions.

Changes in Ppa are relevant to gas exchange in both adults and newborns. However, in establishing and maintaining $\dot{V}_A/\dot{Q}$ matching, neonates appear to respond differently from adults to certain stimuli affecting Ppa, PVR, and, at least theoretically, bronchial and bronchiolar smooth muscle constriction. For instance, lambs have a more vigorous hypoxic pulmonary vasoconstrictive response than do adult sheep, and the onset of the response can be detected at a higher PaO_2.[25] If this phenomenon is also true in humans, it has implications in neonates regarding the effects of even brief apneic episodes on $\dot{V}_A/\dot{Q}$ matching. Inferences about effects of the changes in Ppa in neonates with both regional and generalized lung injury cannot be easily extrapolated from results in adults.

The decline of Ppa and PVR after birth occurs in conjunction with elimination of some of the intraparenchymal pulmonary fluid. Factors modulating the decline in Ppa include the endogenously produced arachidonate metabolite and vasodilator, prostacyclin,[26] and endogenously produced or nitric oxide.[27] Mean Ppa does not approach adult values until days after birth. Wagner[28] suggested that moderate elevation in Ppa may help to maintain

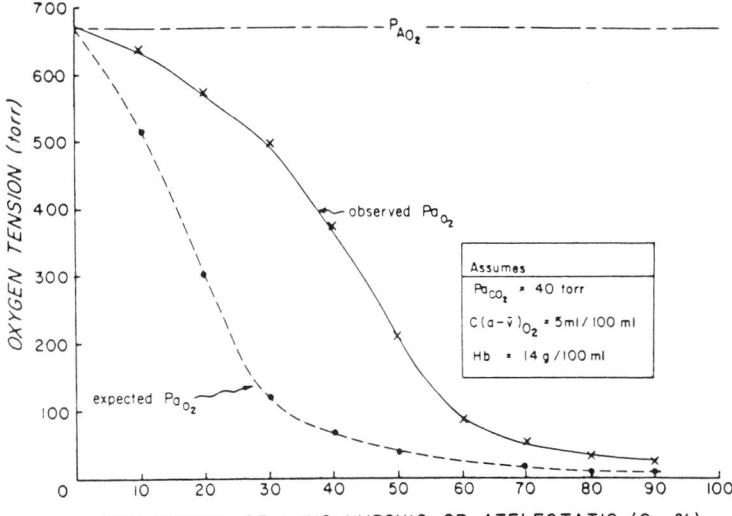

Figure 85-7. The effect of progressively increasing size of atelectatic lung region on arterial oxygen tension is demonstrated by the *dashed line,* which would occur if no redistribution of blood flow away from the atelectatic area occurred. The *solid line* indicates the effects of presumed hypoxic pulmonary vasoconstriction. Note the conversion of the two lines when more than 40% of the lung develops atelectasis. The assumptions regarding O_2 content (Ca_{O_2}) are shown in the *inset.* (From Marshall BE: Adv Shock Res 8:1, 1982.)

$\dot{V}A/\dot{Q}$ matching, given the relatively unstable lung volume of the neonate. However, elevations in PVR also favor passage of vascular fluid into the extravascular alveolar lung spaces, especially if the anatomic site of increased pressure is venular. Such fluid extravasation can have secondary effects on $\dot{V}A/\dot{Q}$ matching by altering bronchiolar dimensions (see Fig. 85-3).

The muscular development of pulmonary arteries during the third trimester creates the possibility of an inappropriately vigorous pulmonary vascular response to vasoconstrictive stimuli applied postnatally. Persistent pulmonary hypertension of the newborn may, in some instances, be a clinical consequence of this phenomenon. In support of this hypothesis, persistent pulmonary hypertension of the newborn has been associated with the accumulation of leukotrienes in tracheal lavage fluid; leukotrienes are potent vasoconstrictor substances.[29]

Because of the changes in resting pulmonary vascular pressure and PVR in the neonatal period, it is important to understand the mechanisms controlling these changes and the consequent effects on gas exchange.

Hypoxic Pulmonary Vasoconstriction and $\dot{V}A/\dot{Q}$ Matching

Hypoxic pulmonary vasoconstriction prevents localized mismatching of ventilation and perfusion by diminishing blood flow locally to those areas of the lungs that are underventilated or not ventilated at all. As regional alveolar and acinar P_{O_2} values decline, because of reduced localized ventilation, blood flow through the local pulmonary microvasculature is inhibited by an increase in resistance in muscular small arteries. Blood flow and, presumably, alveolar ventilation are then redirected into well-ventilated lung regions. The mechanisms by which a decrease in local P_{O_2} induces constriction of vascular smooth muscle remain incompletely understood. Many modulators, including vasoconstrictive leukotrienes, have been described.[30] However, mediation of this response, as opposed to modulation, may depend on changes in calcium and potassium selective membrane channels in the pulmonary vascular smooth muscle cell membrane.[31]

When regional alveolar hypoxia is created by lobar or segmental atelectasis induced by endobronchial balloon obstruction, an inverse correlation can be detected between the increase in resistance and the increase in overall intrapulmonary shunt (Fig. 85-7). Marshall[32] showed that with progressively larger areas of pulmonary parenchymal collapse, up to unilateral atelectasis, the diversion of $\dot{Q}p$ away from atelectatic lung areas and the capacity to maintain satisfactory $\dot{V}A/\dot{Q}$ matching becomes less effective (see Fig. 88-7). These studies are particu-

larly relevant to the neonatal condition, in which both lobar and multiregional atelectasis can develop.

In addition to the size of the collapsed nonventilated segment as a modifier of hypoxic pulmonary vasoconstriction and $\dot{V}A/\dot{Q}$ matching, the presence of local inflammation cells and their products in the affected region has been addressed. Secretions containing bacteria and inflammatory cell products can become trapped in the atelectatic region, possibly inhibiting local hypoxic pulmonary vasoconstriction and resulting in persistent regional blood flow and hypoxemia.

Global or total lung exposure to alveolar hypoxia produces a different challenge for control of pulmonary gas exchange. Under these circumstances, there is the potential for an increase in regional $\dot{Q}p$ to preexisting shunt or low $\dot{V}A/\dot{Q}$ regions. Superimposition of global alveolar hypoxia produces increased resistance to $\dot{Q}p$ in the regions in which resistance beds will become more balanced, with redirection of $\dot{Q}p$ back into low $\dot{V}A/\dot{Q}$ areas. However, in lambs exposed to acute alveolar hypoxia ($F_{I_{O_2}}$ = .12), there was no evidence of an alteration in $\dot{V}A/\dot{Q}$ matching in spite of a doubling (beyond room air baseline values) of Ppa and PVR (Fig. 85-8).[33] Hansen and others[34] demonstrated redistribution of $\dot{Q}p$ in neonatal lambs during acute alveolar hypoxia and provided indirect evidence of heterogeneity of local vascular resistance during elevated PVR.

One effect resulting from an increasing Ppa is recruitment of pulmonary capillaries, particularly in upper lobes. This process increases gas exchange surface area and represents a "reserve" mechanism to help sustain pulmonary gas exchange during adverse conditions. However, there is evidence that neonatal lambs have an already fully recruited microvasculature, at least as assessed by direct vital microscopy during hypoxia (Fig. 85-9).[35] Indirect evidence of full capillary recruitment present under baseline conditions has also been inferred from work in piglets.[36] If these findings can be generalized to newborn humans, they will represent another instance of the decreased reserves available to sustain gas exchange and point to a relative lack of vascular compliance in the neonatal lung.

The role of acute hypoxic vasoconstriction in the maintenance of ventilation-perfusion matching has been tested in neonatal animals subjected to 3 days of breathing more than 90% inspired oxygen.[37] This was done to determine whether hyperoxia-induced blunting of the vascular response to acute alveolar hypoxia ($F_{I_{O_2}}$ = .12) would be associated with worsened $\dot{V}$ matching. Preexposure of animals to hyperoxia did result in diminished hemodynamic response and in deterioration in $\dot{V}A/\dot{Q}$ matching during exposure to acute vasoconstrictive stimuli, such as alveolar hypoxia.

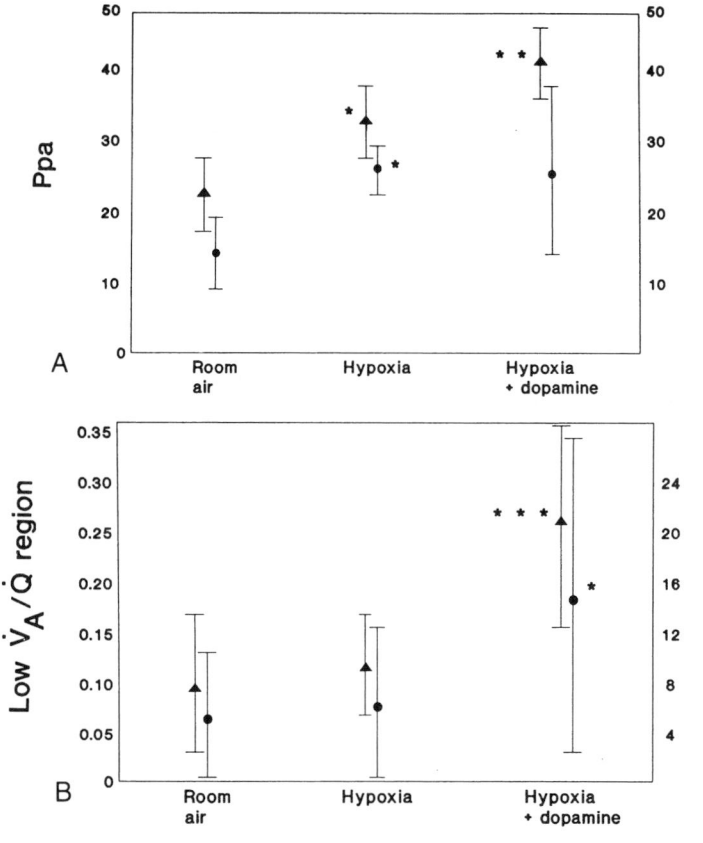

Figure 85–8. A, Pulmonary vascular resistance (PVR; •, expressed as torr/L/min) and mean pulmonary arterial pressure (Ppa; ▲, expressed as mm Hg) are plotted for the experimental conditions of room air, alveolar hypoxia and alveolar hypoxia plus dopamine infusion. Ppa increased with hypoxia ($p < .05$ and increased further [** = $p < .02$] with hypoxia and dopamine) compared with hypoxia alone. PVR increased with hypoxia compared with room air conditions (* = $p < .05$). **B,** Intrapulmonary shunt, which is represented as a dot (•), and the index of low $\dot{V}_A/\dot{Q}$ area (▲) are plotted for the same experimental conditions. The size of the low $\dot{V}_A/\dot{Q}$ region increased (*** = $p < .01$) during hypoxia plus dopamine compared with that found during hypoxia alone. Increased shunt between the same two experimental conditions also developed. (From Truog WE: Biol Neonate *46*:220, 1984, by permission of S Karger AG, Basel.)

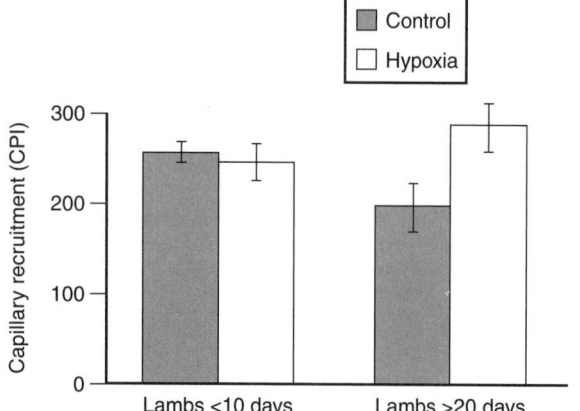

Figure 85–9. The assessment of capillary recruitment during alveolar hypoxia is depicted. Recruitment is measured by a capillary recruitment index (sum of perfused capillaries normalized to alveolar wall area) in lambs less than 10 days and more than 20 days old. Inspired O_2 was .35 during control and was .12 during hypoxia. Pulmonary arterial pressure increased significantly in both older and younger groups. Only the older animals demonstrated evidence of recruitment.[35]

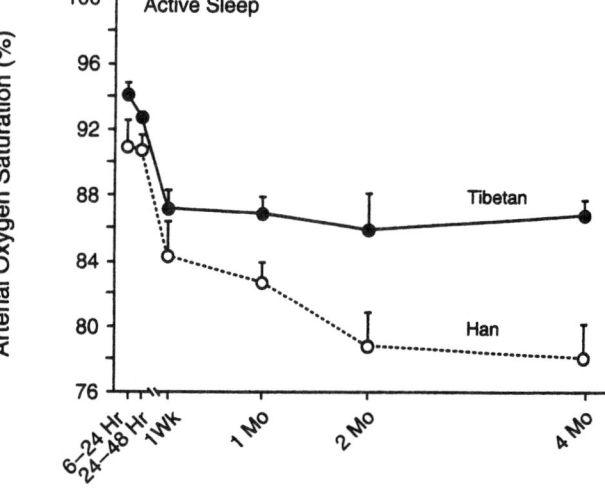

Figure 85–10. Oximetry recorded in multigenerational dwellers' infants at high altitude (Tibetan) versus single-generation dwellers' infants (Han). Data were obtained during active sleep in apparently healthy term infants. (From Niermeyer et al: N Engl J Med 33:1248, 1995.)

Possible genetic contributions to postnatal regulation of gas exchange in a relatively hypoxic environment have been examined.[38] Comparisons of Spo_2 were obtained in healthy term infants born at 3300 m (approximately 11,800 ft) and normalized for activity state. The infants of multigenerational dwellers at altitude demonstrated consistently higher Spo_2 than infants of recent dwellers during all relevant activity states (Fig. 85-10).

Demonstrated in Figure 88-10 is the comparison of Spo_2 during active sleep, the behavioral state associated with irregular breathing effort, and reduced FRC because of changes in intercostal muscle tone. There are multiple contributing factors to Spo_2, and the factors relevant to these findings could not be evaluated. Susceptibility to pulmonary hypertension may be genetically determined, even in very young infants.

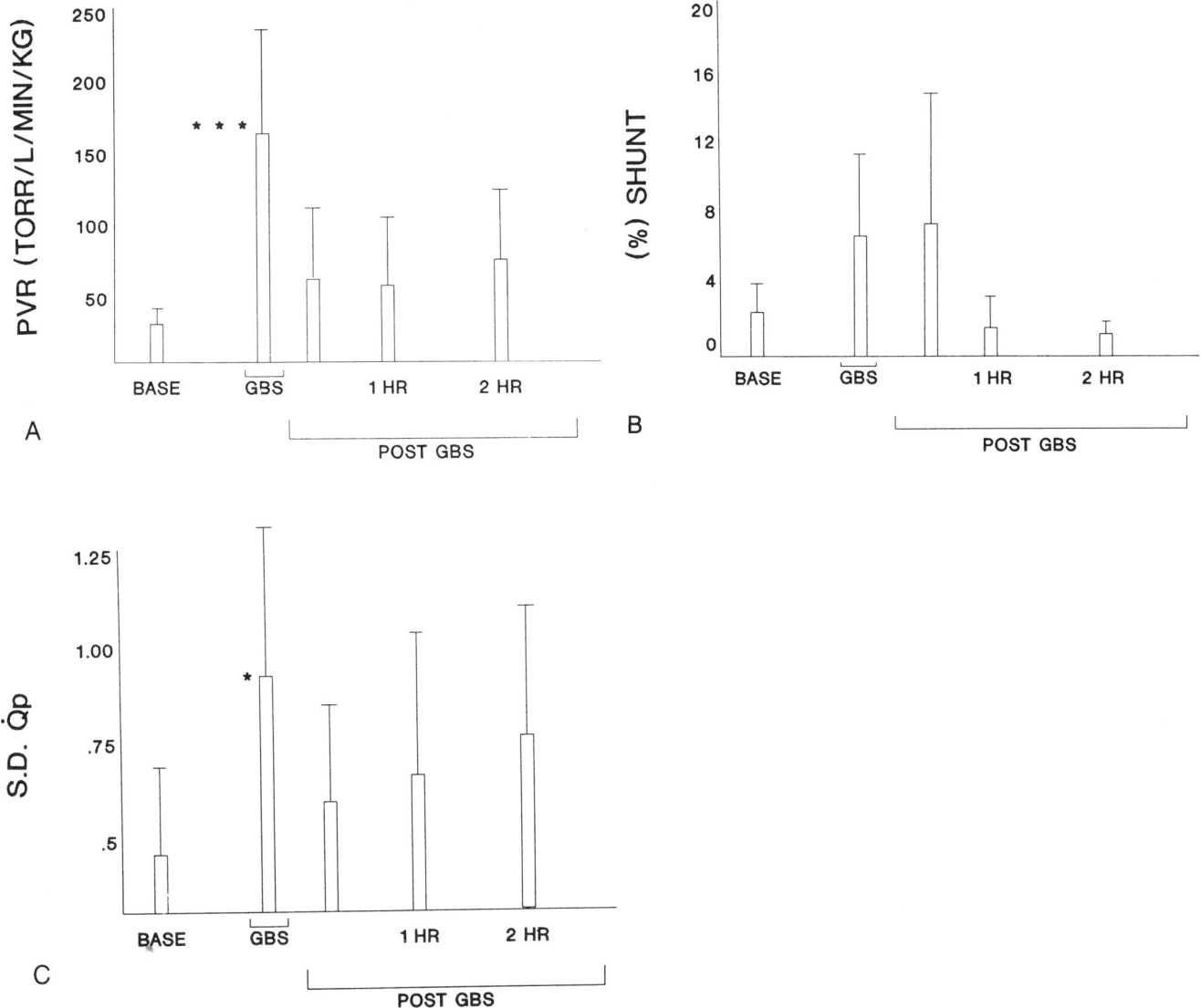

Figure 85–11. A, Calculated pulmonary vascular resistance (PVR) is plotted against experimental conditions before, during, and at 1 and 2 hours after the end of a 20-minute intravenous infusion of group B streptococcus (GBS) into neonatal piglets. Twenty minutes into the intravenous infusion of GBS, the PVR tripled compared with baseline ($p < .001$). **B,** Intrapulmonary shunt and, **C,** the standard deviation of pulmonary blood flow (SD $\dot{Q}p$) are plotted against the same experimental conditions. There is no change in percentage of shunt, but there is an increase in SD $\dot{Q}p$ during the GBS infusion. The increased SD $\dot{Q}p$ is associated with a decline in Pao$_2$ from 90 to 55 mm Hg mean during the GBS infusion. (From Sorensen GK, et al: Pediatr Res *19*:922, 1985.)

Vasoactive Mediators Influencing Peripheral Vascular Resistance and V̇a/Q̇ Matching

Stimuli that produce an acute elevation in Ppa may result in a failure of maintenance of normal V̇a/Q̇ matching in neonates. Vasoactive peptide and phospholipid substances are two classes of such agents. These substances are synthesized and released into the circulation in response to bacterial infusion or endotoxin infusion. Their effect on PVR and gas exchange varies with species and with postnatal age. Intravenous infusion of *Escherichia coli* endotoxin into adult goats produced a 200 to 250% rise in Ppa and PVR, yet it was associated with a small decrease (of 8 to 9 mm Hg) in Pao$_2$.[39] Infant or neonatal animals demonstrate a different response. In piglets, a similar rise in Ppa, associated with infusion of either group B streptococcus or other bacteria, resulted in a 30 to 40 mm Hg decline in Po$_2$.[40, 41] This decline was associated with a generalized mismatching of V̇a/Q̇, with the development of low V̇a/Q̇ areas, but not with an increase in intrapulmonary shunt (Fig. 85-11).[42] The elevation in Ppa induced by bacterial products correlated with increased plasma levels of the vasoconstrictor arachidonic acid metabolite, thromboxane A$_2$, a finding implying that arachidonic acid products can alter distribution of perfusion and ventilation.

The young piglet has served as a useful model for examining the effects on pulmonary gas exchange of potential anti-inflammatory or antiinfective therapies, including antivasoactive agents. When pretreated with an inhibitor of the enzyme thromboxane synthase, piglets demonstrated no immediate increase in Ppa, no decrease in Pao$_2$, and no development of V̇a/Q̇ mismatching[43] during an infusion of group B streptococcus. When administered after 2 hours of bacterial infusion, a thromboxane synthase inhibitor induced a decrease in Ppa and PVR, but without improvement in inert or respiratory gas exchange.[44] These findings imply that regulation of hemodynamics and the regulation of V̇a/Q̇ matching become increasingly independent phenomena under conditions of ongoing bacterial product

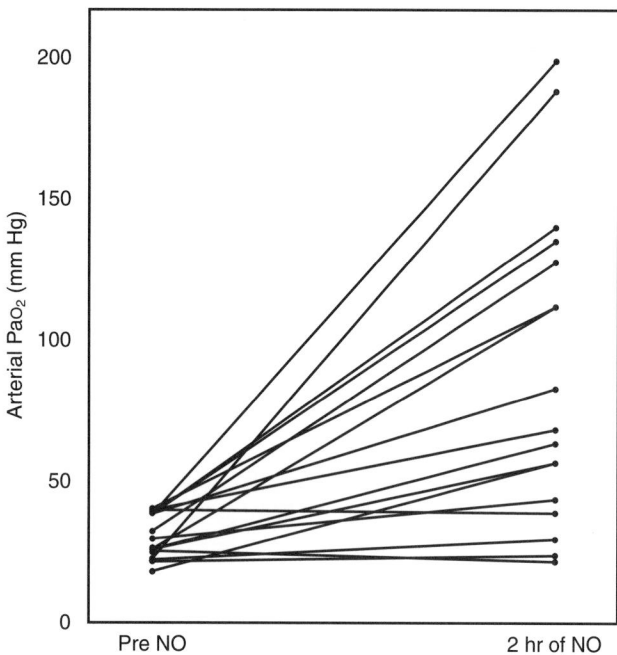

Figure 85–12. The effect of administering inhaled nitric oxide (NO) to 17 full-term or near-term infants with pulmonary parenchymal disease and pulmonary arterial hypertension. The infants received 20 parts per million (ppm) of NO during assisted ventilation with an FI_{O_2} of 1.0. The response, measured by umbilical Pao_2 after 2 hours, was highly variable, suggesting that lowering pulmonary arterial pressure may have a variable effect on venous admixture.

stimulation. Studies in experimental animals by Gibson and co-workers[45] demonstrated, during controlled bacteremia, that multiple vasoactive agents participate in the persistence of elevated PVR.

Catecholamines form another class of substances that can alter $\dot{V}A/\dot{Q}$ matching in the neonate by increasing Ppa. Truog and Standaert[33] demonstrated that when dopamine (25 μg/kg/minute) is administered to neonatal lambs in which Ppa and PVR are already increased because of breathing (FI_{O_2} = .12), there is a further rise in Ppa, coupled with a deterioration in gas exchange associated with an increase in both intrapulmonary shunt and $\dot{V}$ mismatching, separate from shunt (see Fig. 85-8).

Information strongly suggests that products of the endothelium, endothelin and nitric oxide, participate in regulation of $\dot{Q}p$ by changing local vasoconstriction and hence local vascular resistance.[46] The vasoconstricting effects of endothelin-1 are augmented and the vasodilating effects are attenuated with increasing age in sheep.[47] Vasodilating effects are mediated in part by nitric oxide. Administration of inhaled nitric oxide can result in a simultaneous reduction in PVR and an improvement in Pao_2.[48, 49] Other investigators have failed to show significant change in respiratory or inert gas exchange during treatment with inhaled nitric oxide in animals with pulmonary hypertension caused by bacterial infusion.[50] Because nitric oxide may induce both bronchodilatation and pulmonary vasodilation (through its alteration in vascular smooth muscle cGMP concentrations), its impact on gas exchange can be profound, but not easily predictable. This is shown in Figure 85–12. Data were obtained from 17 newborn infants with severe pulmonary hypertension associated with multiple underlying medical disorders except congenital diaphragmatic hernia. A wide range of response is apparent.

The effect of elevated Ppa on gas exchange can be difficult to predict in the clinical setting of a neonate with one of many possible causes of respiratory distress. In addition to the disorders discussed earlier, elevation of Ppa may result from a diminished cross-sectional microvascular area secondary to either a primary developmental failure or delayed growth (or early regression of) the microvasculature. The diminished cross-sectional area increases vascular resistance and results in an extrapulmonary shunt. Further, there is presumably a spectrum of local resistances across the pulmonary microvasculature shortly after the time of birth, as long as lung fluid is being removed from potential gas exchange areas. Sudden vasoactive stimulation may result in a redistribution of $\dot{Q}p$, $\dot{V}A/\dot{Q}$ mismatching, and arterial hypoxemia, producing a vicious cycle with diminished pulmonary venous oxygen pressure (Pv_{O_2}) and a further decline in Pao_2. Low mixed venous Po_2 is a secondary stimulus inducing pulmonary arterial hypertension.[51] In situations characterized by low cardiac output and $\dot{V}A/\dot{Q}$ mismatching, the low Pv_{O_2} increases Ppa and PVR. Intrapulmonary or extrapulmonary shunt through the foramen ovale or ductus arteriosus may result. Measurement of simultaneously obtained pulmonary venous and preductal and postductal Pao_2 would be necessary to differentiate among the anatomic sites for the shunt.

Distribution of Ventilation and $\dot{V}A/\dot{Q}$ Matching

Although many studies have examined postnatal changes in lung mechanics, there is less information available describing the distribution of ventilation.[52] Analysis of $\dot{V}A$ distribution by nitrogen or xenon washout during 100% oxygen breathing is difficult to perform in sick (or well) neonates because of the need for multiple breath analysis and exposure to radioactivity. Analysis of $\dot{V}A$ distribution does demonstrate at least two types of acinar spaces, which empty at different rates.[52] The pulmonary function measurement, called *pulmonary clearance delay*, quantitates the presence of these two acinar compartments. It is difficult to draw conclusions about $\dot{V}A/\dot{Q}$ matching from this index because it relates only to ventilation, irrespective of relative distribution of $\dot{Q}p$. Engel[53] reviewed the theoretical and experimental evidence of incomplete alveolar gas mixing with inspiration that develops because of the interaction between diffusion and convection at airway branch points subtending branches of unequal length. It is unknown whether this problem is diminished or magnified in the much smaller neonatal lung or to what extent the resulting inhomogeneous alveolar gas mixtures contribute to overall $\dot{V}A/\dot{Q}$ heterogeneity in the neonate. Much would depend on the matching of intra-acinar Q distribution and intra-acinar V distribution.

The immature lung, with potential variability in acinar development, has not been well studied with regard to the contribution of "micro" $\dot{V}A/\dot{Q}$ inequality to overall gas exchange abnormalities. Similarly, $\dot{V}A/\dot{Q}$ scans that rely on insoluble radioactive tracers injected intravenously may inaccurately portray $\dot{V}A$ or $\dot{Q}p$ distribution because of both shunt and spatial restrictions imposed by the small chest of the neonate or young infant. Factors that influence bronchial and bronchiolar constriction can alter the distribution of each inhaled breath. Some factors possibly relevant in the newborn are listed in Table 85-1.

Cardiac Function and Pulmonary Vascular Resistance

An additional factor influencing PVR is the diminished cardiac reserve of neonates, especially premature neonates, who depend largely on chronotropy for raising cardiac output. Older children or adults, by contrast, have more effective inotropic mechanisms for increasing cardiac output. The newborn has difficulty doubling the resting cardiac output either by pharmacologic stimulation or by increased sympathetic nervous system activity. Thus, efforts to increase Pao_2 (assuming constant tissue oxygen extraction and an unchanging degree of $\dot{V}A/\dot{Q}$ mismatching) by increasing cardiac output (and Pv_{O_2}) are not usually successful in the newborn.

TABLE 85-1

**Some Factors Capable of Producing Bronchoconstriction
or Bronchiolar Narrowing in the Newborn**

Airway inflammation
Mucosal edema
Excess mucus secretion
Sloughing of damaged epithelial cells
Hyperreactive bronchial smooth musculature
Inspiration of cold, dry gas
Increase in parasympathetic nervous system stimulation
Congenital airway stenosis or deficient cartilage development
Bronchiolar narrowing secondary to vascular engorgement
Presence of any foreign body, including partially occluded
    endotracheal tubes
Trauma from suction catheters
Aspiration of stomach contents into upper airway
Hypoosmolar or hyperosmolar solution in the airway

DIFFUSION AND PULMONARY GAS EXCHANGE

Respiratory gas exchange depends on prompt diffusion of respiratory gases between the tissue and plasma, the erythrocyte and plasma, the plasma and resident alveolar gas, and the alveolar gas and gas in the conducting airways. Of these, *alveolar-capillary membrane diffusion* has been considered the most likely barrier to gas exchange, but it has not been well documented to be abnormal in any neonatal condition, including extreme prematurity, when it is corrected for the size of the gas exchange surface area available.

Gas movement between the alveolar space and pulmonary capillary blood is a passive process, summarized by *Fick's law*, which asserts that the amount of gas transferred is governed by the partial pressure of that gas in the two compartments, the inverse of the square root of the molecular weight of the gas, and the specific characteristics of the diffusion barrier (thickness and surface area). Thus, the transport of gas is expressed by the following:

$$\dot{V} \propto pt\, D_m(P_A - P_b)$$

where D_m = alveolar-capillary membrane diffusion conductance and $(P_A - P_b)$ represents the partial pressure difference across the membrane. To simplify the analysis, it is useful to study a single gas that binds firmly to hemoglobin. Because carbon monoxide combines avidly with hemoglobin, the P_{CO} in pulmonary capillary plasma is virtually zero when small quantities of carbon monoxide are inspired, thus simplifying the analysis of diffusing capacity. In clinical practice, the diffusing capacity of the lung is expressed by the following:

$$D_{mco} = \dot{V}co/P_{A_{CO}}$$

The diffusing capacity of the lung for carbon monoxide is expressed as the volume of carbon monoxide transferred in milliliters of carbon monoxide per minute per millimeter of mercury of alveolar partial pressure of carbon monoxide. The diffusing capacity is usually abbreviated DL_{CO}. Both a single-breath technique (which is difficult to perform in a neonate) and a steady-state technique can be used for assessing $P_{A_{CO}}$.

Use of carbon monoxide as the marker gas does not eliminate other variables in interpretation. Ventilation-perfusion heterogeneity, reduced pulmonary capillary transit time, lung volume, and pulmonary capillary blood volume all can affect interpretation of diffusing capacity, as well as intrinsic properties of the alveolar capillary membrane itself, the actual subject of the measurement. Detailed analysis of the effects of these factors on diffusion measurement is available elsewhere.[54] Comparing serial measurements of DL_{CO} assumes that effective $\dot{Q}p$ ($\dot{Q}p_{total} - \dot{Q}p_{shunt}$) is unchanged. This may represent an insupportable assumption in many neonatal pulmonary diseases. Rapid postnatal lung growth and alveolarization, with change in lung volumes, complicate interpretation of serial measurement of diffusion capacity in the neonatal lung. However, Escourrou and co-workers[55] inferred from cross-sectional studies using MIGET in neonatal and infant piglets that diffusion limitation may contribute to early postnatal hypoxemia in animals breathing room air. Either a reduction in surface area or an increase in thickness of the alveolar capillary membrane can reduce DL_{CO}. Although these conditions may occur in neonatal pulmonary diseases, they probably have little practical significance for transport of oxygen because virtually every pulmonary disease is treated with increased $P_{A_{O2}}$. Hence, the driving pressure (partial pressure gradient) across the membrane becomes very large for oxygen. Even in these circumstances, there may be lung regions in which diffusion disequilibrium may occur because neonatal pulmonary conditions rarely affect the lung uniformly.

DL_{CO} has been measured acutely in premature infants with and without respiratory distress syndrome, and no significant differences have been found.[56] However, in this study, DL_{CO} was notably lower than DL_{CO} values measured in earlier studies conducted in full-term healthy infants.[57] The different results may relate to the smaller quantity of both intrapulmonary gas and blood found in the premature newborn. The differences highlight the problems in interpretation of cross-sectional studies of DL_{CO} in the newborn.

Perhaps the most important diffusing capacity measurements are made after recovery and growth. Hakulinen and co-workers[58] made the observation that children born very prematurely and studied at age 7 to 11 years demonstrated modest but significant reduction in DL_{CO} (single-breath test). This was true for premature infants with or without the diagnosis of bronchopulmonary dysplasia. Some "normal" values for DL_{CO} may have overestimated DL_{CO} in some of these children because airflow obstruction, which was common in the preterm infants, may have produced an overestimation of the true DL_{CO}.

REFERENCES

1. Truog WE: Delivery room management and resuscitation of the newborn. *In* Carlo WA, Chatburn BL (eds): Neonatal Respiratory Care, 2nd ed. Chicago, Year Book Medical Publishers, 1988.
2. Nelson NM, et al: Pulmonary function in the newborn infant: the alveolar-arterial oxygen gradient. J Appl Physiol *18*:534, 1963.
3. Oliver TK Jr, et al: Serial blood gas tensions and acid-base balance during the first hour of life in human infants. Acta Paediatr Scand *50*:346, 1961.
4. Koch G: Alveolar ventilation, diffusing capacity, and the A-a PO_2 difference in the newborn infant. Respir Physiol *4*:168, 1968.
5. Thibeault DW, et al: Alveolar-arterial oxygen O_2 and CO_2 differences and their relation to lung volume in the newborn. Pediatrics *41*:574, 1968.
6. Krauss AN: Ventilation-perfusion relationships in neonates. *In* Thibeault DW, Gregory GA (eds): Neonatal Pulmonary Care, 2nd ed. Norwalk, CT, Appleton & Lange, 1986.
7. Dantzker DR: Physiology and pathophysiology of pulmonary gas exchange. Hosp Pract Jan *15*:135, 1986.
8. Parks CR, et al: Gas exchange in the immature lung. II. Method of estimation and maturity. J Appl Physiol *36*:108, 1974.
9. Parks CR, et al: Gas exchange in the immature lung. I. Anatomical shunt in the premature infant. J Appl Physiol *36*:103, 1974.
10. Krauss AN, Auld PAM: Ventilation-perfusion abnormalities in the premature infant: triple gradient. Pediatr Res *3*:255, 1969.
11. Krauss AN, et al: Adjustment of ventilation and perfusion in the full-term normal and distressed neonate as determined by urinary alveolar nitrogen gradients. Pediatrics *47*:865, 1971.
12. Corbet AJS, et al: Ventilation-perfusion relationships as assessed by $aADN_2$ in hyaline membrane disease. J Appl Physiol *36*:74, 1974.
13. West JB: Ventilation-perfusion relationships. Am Rev Respir Dis *116*:919, 1977.
14. West JB: Causes of carbon dioxide retention in lung disease. N Engl J Med *284*:1232, 1971.
15. Farhi LE: Elimination of inert gas by the lung. Respir Physiol *3*:1, 1967.
16. Wagner PD, et al: Simultaneous measurement of eight foreign gases in blood by gas chromatography. J Appl Physiol *36*:600, 1974.

17. Wagner PD, et al: Measurement of continuous distributions of ventilation-perfusion ratios: theory. J Appl Physiol *36*:588, 1974.
18. Hlastala MP: Multiple inert gas elimination technique. J Appl Physiol *56*:1, 1984.
19. Hlastala MP, Robertson HT: Inert gas elimination characteristics of the normal and abnormal lung. J Appl Physiol *44*:258, 1978.
20. Truog WE, et al: Oxygen-induced alteration of ventilation-perfusion relationships in rats. J Appl Physiol *47*:1112, 1979.
21. Young IH, Wagner PD: Effect of intrapulmonary hematocrit maldistribution on O_2, CO_2, and inert gas exchange. J Appl Physiol *46*:240, 1979.
22. Farhi LE: Ventilation-perfusion relationships. *In* Farhi LE (ed): Handbook of Physiology, Sect 3: The Respiratory System. Baltimore, Williams & Wilkins, 1987, pp 199–215.
23. West JB, et al: Pulmonary gas exchange. Am J Respir Crit Care Med *157*:S82, 1998.
24. Dawson CA: Role of pulmonary vasomotion in physiology of the lung. Physiol Rev *64*:544, 1984.
25. Custer JC, Hales C: Influence of alveolar oxygen on pulmonary vasoconstriction in newborn lambs vs. sheep. Am Rev Respir Dis *132*:326, 1985.
26. Leffler CW, et al: Onset of breathing stimulates pulmonary vascular prostacyclin synthesis. Pediatr Res *18*:932, 1984.
27. Fineman J, et al: *N*-nitro-L-arginine attenuates endothelium dependent pulmonary vasodilation in lambs. Am J Physiol *260*:H1299, 1991.
28. Wagner WW Jr: Pulmonary circulatory control through hypoxic vasoconstriction. Semin Respir Med *7*:124, 1985.
29. Stenmark KR, et al: Leukotriene C_4 and D_4 in neonates with hypoxemia and pulmonary hypertension. N Engl J Med *309*:77, 1983.
30. Goldberg R, et al: Influence of an antagonist of slow reacting substance of anaphylaxis on the cardiovascular manifestations of hypoxia in piglets. Pediatr Res *19*:121, 1985.
31. Weir EK, Archer SL: Mechanism of acute hypoxic pulmonary hypertension. FASEB J *9*:183, 1995.
32. Marshall BE: Importance of hypoxic pulmonary vasoconstriction with atelectasis. Adv Shock Res *8*:1, 1982.
33. Truog WE, Standaert TA: Effect of dopamine infusion on pulmonary gas exchange in lambs. Biol Neonate *46*:220, 1984.
34. Hansen TN, et al: Hypoxia and angiotensin II infusion redistribute lung blood flow in lambs. J Appl Physiol *58*:812, 1985.
35. Means LJ, et al: Pulmonary capillary recruitment in neonatal lambs. Pediatr Res *34*:596, 1993.
36. Gibson RL, et al: Hypoxic pulmonary vasoconstriction during and after infusion of group B streptococcus in neonatal piglets. Am Rev Respir Dis *137*:774, 1988.
37. Truog WE, et al: Effects of hyperoxia on vasoconstriction and VA/Q matching in the neonatal lung. J Appl Physiol *63*:2536, 1987.
38. Niermeyer S, et al: Arterial oxygen saturation and Tibetan and Han infants born in Lhasa, Tibet. N Engl J Med *333*:1248, 1995.
39. Rojas J, et al: Studies on group B beta-hemolytic streptococcus. II. Effects on pulmonary hemodynamics and vascular permeability in unanesthetized sheep. Pediatr Res *15*:899, 1981.
40. Rojas J, et al: Pulmonary hemodynamics and ultrastructural changes associated with group B streptococcal toxemia in adult sheep and newborn lambs. Pediatr Res *17*:1002, 1983.
41. Runkle B, et al: Cardiovascular changes in group B streptococcal sepsis in the piglet: response to indomethacin and relationship to prostacyclin and thromboxane A_2. Pediatr Res *18*:874, 1984.
42. Sorenson GK, et al: Mechanisms of pulmonary gas exchange abnormalities during experimental group B streptococcal infusion. Pediatr Res *19*:922, 1985.
43. Truog WE, et al: Effects of the thromboxane synthetase inhibitor, Dazmegrel (UK 38,485) on pulmonary gas exchange and hemodynamics in neonatal sepsis. Pediatr Res *20*:481, 1986.
44. Truog WE, et al: Neonatal group B streptococcal sepsis: effects of late treatment with Dazmegrel. Pediatr Res *23*:352, 1988.
45. Gibson RL, et al: Group B streptococcal sepsis: effect of combined pentoxifylline indomethacin pretreatment. Pediatr Res *31*:222, 1992.
46. Truog WE: Standaert TA: Effects of dopamine infusion on pulmonary gas exchange in lambs. Biol Neonate *46*:220, 1984.
47. Wong J, et al: Developmental effects of endothelin-1 on the pulmonary circulation in sheep. Pediatr Res *36*:394, 1994.
48. Abman S, et al: Acute effects of inhaled nitric oxide in children with severe hypoxemic respiratory failure. J Pediatr *124*:881, 1994.
49. Putensen J, et al: Improvement in VA/Q distributions during inhalation of nitric oxide in piglets with methacholine-induced bronchoconstriction. Am J Respir Crit Care Med *151*:116, 1995.
50. Berger JI, et al: Effects of inhaled nitric oxide during group B streptococcal sepsis in piglets. Am Rev Respir Dis *147*:1080, 1993.
51. Benumof J, et al: Interaction of PVO_2 with PaO_2 on hypoxic pulmonary vasoconstriction. J Appl Physiol *51*:871, 1981.
52. McCann EM, et al: Pulmonary function in the sick newborn infant. Pediatr Res *21*:313, 1987.
53. Engel LA: Gas mixing within the acinus of the lung. J Appl Physiol *54*:609, 1983.
54. Hlastala MP: Diffusing-capacity heterogeneity. *In* Farhi LE (ed): Handbook on Physiology, Sect 3: The Respiratory System. Baltimore, Williams & Wilkins, 1987.
55. Escourrou PJL, et al: Mechanism of improvement in pulmonary gas exchange during growth in awake piglets. J Appl Physiol *65*:1055, 1988.
56. Krauss AN, et al: Carbon monoxide diffusing capacity in newborn infants. Pediatr Res *10*:771, 1976.
57. Stahlman MT: Pulmonary ventilation and diffusion in the human newborn infant. J Clin Invest *36*:1018, 1957.
58. Hakulinen AL, et al: Diffusing capacity of the lung in school-aged children born very preterm, with and without bronchopulmonary dysplasia. Pediatr Pulmonol *21*:353, 1996.

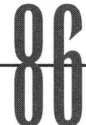

Maria Delivoria-Papadopoulos and Jane E. McGowan

Oxygen Transport and Delivery

OXYGEN TRANSPORT SYSTEM

The oxygen transport system in humans depends on many interrelated factors, including the fraction of oxygen in inspired air, partial pressure of oxygen in inspired air, alveolar ventilation, relation of ventilation to perfusion of the lungs, arterial pH and temperature, cardiac output, blood volume, hemoglobin concentration, and affinity of hemoglobin for oxygen. In normal subjects, this complex system, which adjusts to tissue requirements to maintain an adequate end-capillary oxygen tension, has a reasonable reserve capacity and the ability to respond rapidly to changes in oxygen need. Gestation and the immediate postnatal period tax the oxygen transport system more than any other time period in the human life cycle. In addition to the factors just listed fetal oxygenation also varies with transplacental oxygen transport, which in turn depends on placental perfusion and PVO_2 in the uterine vein, thus indirectly reflecting the state of the maternal cardiorespiratory system. Oxygenation of the newborn infant requires a successful transition from fetal to newborn circulatory patterns and establishment of adequate alveolar respiration.

Aerobic metabolism is critically dependent on a constant and adequate supply of oxygen. Although molecular oxygen participates in numerous types of oxidative reactions necessary for cellular metabolism (e.g., production of prostaglandins via cyclooxygenase), its primary role is as the final electron acceptor in the mitochondrial respiratory chain, the process by which energy produced by glycolysis and the citric acid cycle is stored in high-energy phosphate bonds in the form of adenosine triphosphate (ATP). Although ATP is produced during anaerobic glycolysis, the delivery of oxygen to allow aerobic metabolism results in a more than 15-fold increase in the quantity of ATP produced from glucose metabolism. The diffusion of oxygen from midcapillary to the cell is the last step in oxygen transport and depends on several factors, including the oxygen pressure gradient between capillary and cell, the distance between the closest perfusing capillary and the cell, and the impedance to diffusion of the tissue, called the *diffusion coefficient*. Mitochondrial oxygen supply *in vivo* ultimately depends on a number of factors, including the distance between the closest perfusing capillary and the cell, the tissue impedance to oxygen diffusion, and the oxygen pressure gradient between capillary and mitochondrion. The pressure gradient, which directly affects mitochondrial oxygen uptake, varies with regional oxygen delivery, tissue oxygen consumption, and hemoglobin-oxygen affinity. *In vitro*, mitochondrial function remains at maximal levels at oxygen pressure (Po_2) as low as 0.5 mm Hg; however, there is probably a "critical" Po_2 *in vivo* below which mitochondrial respiration is compromised.[1]

Under basal conditions, the lungs load about 4 mL of oxygen per minute per kilogram of body mass onto hemoglobin but can increase this rate 15-fold through the respiratory response to input from the carotid and aortic bodies (which sense arterial oxygen content) and brain stem chemoreceptors. Arterial blood transports oxygen from the pulmonary capillaries to the tissues. The oxygen content of the arterial blood is usually high enough to meet cellular oxygen demand. When the oxygen content is decreased, however, local perfusion or hemoglobin-oxygen affinity may change to compensate for the lower oxygen content.

The cardiovascular system regulates oxygen supply through variation in cardiac output and distribution of blood flow. Alterations in the metabolic rate of peripheral tissues activate local regulatory mechanisms that modulate arterial blood flow and venous return and, thereby, cardiac output. The distribution of blood flow to specific tissues and organs is also set by local metabolic activity. Consequently, different controls exist for different tissues.[2] Coronary blood flow, for example, reflects the metabolic activity of heart muscle; because the oxygen extraction of cardiac muscle is normally high, changes in cardiac work must be matched closely by concomitant changes in coronary blood flow. When oxygen supply is limited, flow is reduced to tissues with low oxygen extraction (such as kidney and gut) in favor of tissues with high extraction (such as heart and brain). The high-flow–low-extraction areas of the circulation constitute an oxygen reserve system that may be deployed in times of oxygen deprivation.

In contrast, cardiac output does not appear to be directly responsive to moderate changes in either Pao_2 or blood oxygen content[3] (presumably because other mechanisms provide an adequate adjustment) and is virtually unaffected by an increase in $Paco_2$ to 50 mmHg. Blood viscosity and volume are additional determinants of cardiac output. If volume is kept constant and viscosity is altered (e.g., by a change in hematocrit), a reciprocal change in cardiac output occurs. Conversely, cardiac output varies directly with blood volume, presumably through the effect of volume on venous return. The induced alterations in cardiac output that follow changes in viscosity and blood volume are corrected toward normal by subsequent compensatory changes in peripheral vascular resistance. A number of neurohumoral factors also affect cardiac output by direct action on the heart, as reflected in the strength and especially the rate of cardiac contraction.

Hemoglobin concentration is regulated by a renal sensing mechanism that operates to maintain a balance between oxygen supply and oxygen requirement of renal tissues. A decrease in concentration or arterial oxygen saturation of hemoglobin or any increase in hemoglobin affinity for oxygen causes increased erythropoietin production via increased expression of hypoxia-inducible factor.[4,5] The effect of erythropoietin on bone marrow is usually limited by available iron, so that red blood cell production is stimulated to about twice its basal value of 1% of the total red blood cell mass per day. Consequently, red blood cell mass increases slowly in response to hypoxia.[6] Because it increases blood viscosity, a higher hemoglobin concentration at the same total blood volume reduces blood flow and thus oxygen delivery. Normal cardiac output is re-established by increasing plasma volume proportionately (i.e., by increasing total blood volume).[7]

The affinity of hemoglobin for oxygen, in association with flow distribution, translates oxygen flow into oxygen availability.

This characteristic of hemoglobin is classically depicted in the oxygen dissociation curve (oxygen equilibrium curve). Because of its remarkable ability to combine reversibly with large quantities of oxygen, hemoglobin increases the oxygen transport capacity of blood about 70-fold over that of oxygen transported dissolved in plasma. For example, if the entire oxygen requirement of the maternal organism had to be met by physically dissolved oxygen, the required cardiac output would be 100 L/min.

STRUCTURE OF THE HEMOGLOBIN MOLECULE

The hemoglobin molecule contains four heme groups bound to the protein globin. The heme groups, located in crevices near the exterior of the molecule, consist of an organic moiety, protoporphyrin, and an iron atom. The iron in heme binds to the four nitrogens in the center of the protoporphyrin ring (Fig. 86–1). The four oxygen-binding sites of hemoglobin are relatively far apart, with the distance between the two closest sites being 25 Å.

The primary structure of the hemoglobin molecule is genetically determined by the amino acid sequence of the globin chains. The three basic chain structures most important in humans are the α- (141 amino acids), β- (146 amino acids), and γ- (146 amino acids) chains, which form hemoglobin A ($\alpha_2\beta_2$; Hb A) and hemoglobin F ($\alpha_2\gamma_2$; Hb F). The β- and γ-chains differ from each other by only a few amino acid residues. There are nine amino acid positions in the sequence that are the same in all or nearly all species studied thus far. These conserved positions are involved either in the oxygen-binding site directly or in forming hydrogen bonds between helices. The positions of the nonpolar residues in the interior of hemoglobin vary considerably, but substitutions always involve one nonpolar residue for

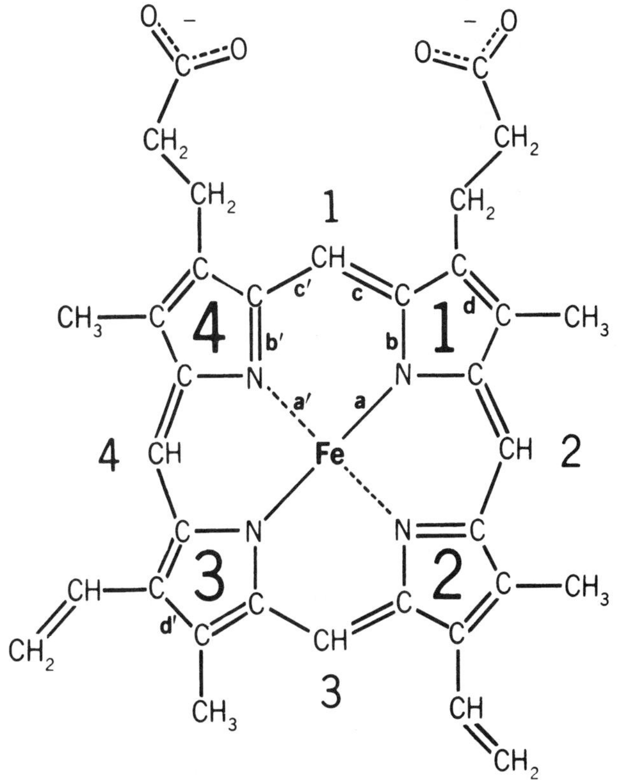

Figure 86–1. The heme group is an essential component in hemoglobins, cytochromes, and enzymes such as catalase and peroxidase. The central porphyrin ring has various side chains: methyl, —CH3; vinyl, —CH—CH2; and propionic acid, —CH—CH2—COOH.

another, thereby conserving the striking nonpolar character of the molecule's interior. Eight α-helices, by convention designated A-H, constitute the secondary structure of the hemoglobin molecule. Helices E and F form a hydrophobic cleft at the insertion of the heme moiety. The position in space of the α-helices with respect to one another provides tertiary structure, whereas the spatial relationship of the subunit globin chains provides the quaternary structure of the hemoglobin molecule.

The quaternary structure of deoxyhemoglobin is termed the *T* or *tense form*, whereas that of oxyhemoglobin is the *R* or *relaxed form*. X-ray crystallographic studies have confirmed that oxygenated and deoxygenated hemoglobin differ in their conformation, with the oxygenated form being more compact.[8] In addition, these conformational changes were found to be crucial for the interactions of hemoglobin with organic phosphates[9] (see later discussion).

In the T form (deoxyhemoglobin), the iron atom is pushed out about 0.6 Å from the heme plane because of steric repulsion between the proximal histidine and nitrogen atoms of the porphyrin. On oxygenation, the iron atom moves into the plane of the protoporphyrin ring, forming a strong bond with oxygen. Oxygenation of the first heme group then favors a switch in the quaternary structure from T to R through the proximal histidine group. The heme group and proximal histidine residue make intimate contact with 15 side chains; oxygenation causes structural changes of the F helix, the EF corner, and the FG corner. These changes are then transmitted to the subunit interfaces (Figs. 86-2 and 86-3). The expulsion of a tyrosine residue from the pocket between the F and H helices leads to the rupture of interchain salt links. Consequently, on oxygenation of the first heme group, the equilibrium is shifted in favor of the R form. Each subsequent molecule of oxygen is bound more strongly because fewer salt links remain to be broken. Because each hemoglobin molecule (tetramer) contains four iron atoms, it can combine with four oxygen molecules. Each mole of hemoglobin thus can combine with four moles of oxygen for a normal blood oxygen capacity of 7.76 mM/L (i.e., 1.94 mM hemoglobin/L × 4 = 7.76). Expressed alternatively, 1 g of hemoglobin can combine with 1.368 mL of oxygen for an oxygen-carrying capacity of about 20 mL/dL when the hemoglobin concentration is 15 g/dL[10] (see following section).

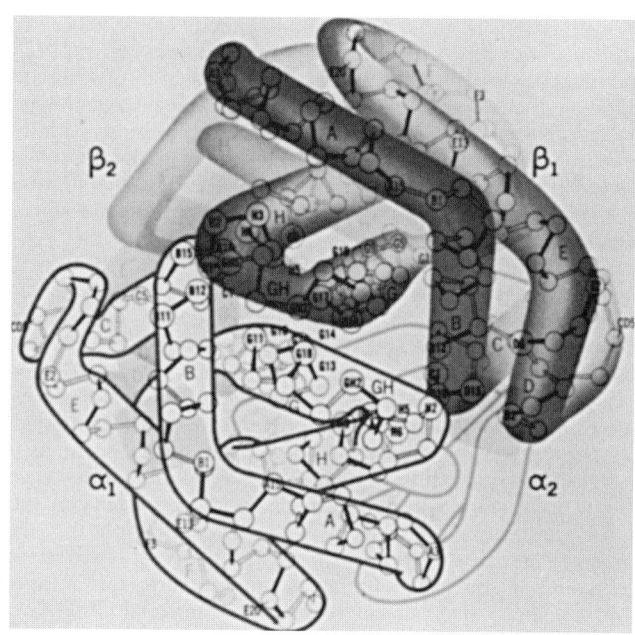

Figure 86–2. Hemoglobin tetramer, $\alpha_1\beta_1$ contacts ($\alpha_2\beta_2$ are identical). The eight α-helices, which constitute the secondary structure, are labeled A to H. The packing of chains in the hemoglobin molecule is such that close interlocking contact of side chains exists between unlike subunits, but there is little contact between α and α or β and β. The $\alpha_1\beta_1$ or $\alpha_2\beta_2$ contacts involving BGH helices and the GH corner are called packing contacts because they represent subunit packing that is unchanged when the hemoglobin molecule goes from its deoxy to its oxy configuration.

HEMOGLOBIN/OXYGEN INTERACTIONS

Hemoglobin-oxygen affinity is the continuous relationship between hemoglobin-oxygen saturation and oxygen tension. It is customarily plotted as the sigmoid-shaped oxygen equilibrium curve, and it can be summarily expressed as the P_{50}, i.e., the

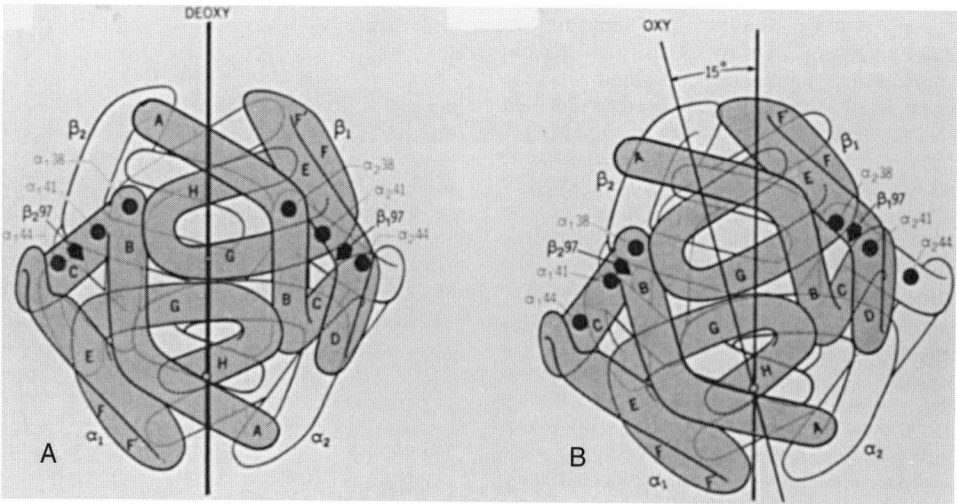

Figure 86–3. Subunit motion in hemoglobin: combination into deoxyhemoglobin and oxyhemoglobin. Two dimers are superimposed in *A* and *B*. *A*, The complete tetramer is shown in its deoxyhemoglobin conformation. Note the position of β97 relative to α41 and α44. B, In oxyhemoglobin, the $\alpha_1\beta_1$ is rotated 15 degrees relative to $\alpha_2\beta_2$. Note the new positions of β97 between α41 and α38.

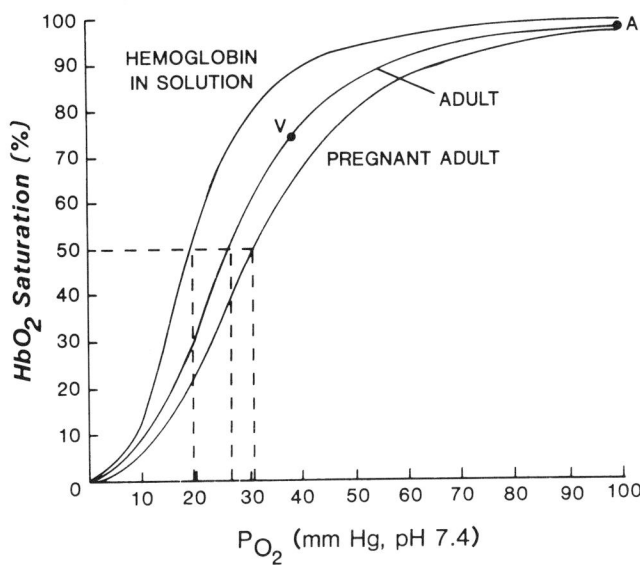

Figure 86–4. Oxyhemoglobin saturation curve under standard conditions for normal blood of pregnant and nonpregnant adults. Also shown is the dissociation curve for hemoglobin in solution.

oxygen tension at which 50% of hemoglobin is saturated with oxygen at standard temperature and pH (Fig. 86-4). The sigmoidal shape of the oxygen-hemoglobin equilibrium curve can be explained only if two assumptions are made: (1) that the heme groups react with oxygen in a fixed sequence, and (2) that the oxygenation and deoxygenation of one heme group profoundly affect the oxygenation and deoxygenation of the others. This phenomenon has been termed *heme-heme interaction*. As each heme group accepts oxygen, it becomes progressively easier for the next heme group of the molecule to pick up oxygen. This concept is implicit in the Hill equation for percent saturation:[11]

$$y/100 = k \times P_{O_2}^n / 1 + (k \times P_{O_2}^n)$$

where y = percent saturation with oxygen, k = equilibrium constant, P_{O_2} = oxygen partial pressure, and the exponent n = the average number of iron atoms per hemoglobin molecule. The value of n for normal hemoglobin is approximately 2.9.

As blood circulates through the normal lung, P_{O_2} increases from about 40 mmHg to about 110 mmHg, a pressure sufficient to ensure at least 95% saturation of hemoglobin with oxygen. The oxygen-hemoglobin equilibrium relationship is such that any further increase of oxygen tension in the lung results in only a small increase in saturation. In the normal adult, when oxygen tension has fallen to approximately 27 mmHg, at a pH of 7.40 and a temperature of 37°C, 50% of hemoglobin is saturated with oxygen (i.e., the P_{50} for whole blood is 27 mmHg).

The steep and flat parts of the curve reflect definitive processes in oxygen unloading. As oxygen diffuses from capillary to tissue, there is at first a rapid fall in P_{O_2} (represented by the flat part of the curve) until the steep part is reached, where capillary P_{O_2} decreases little even though large amounts of oxygen are released. Because oxygen tension at the mitochondrial surface, the point of oxygen utilization, is always about 0.5 to 1.0 mmHg,[1,12] the driving pressure for, and consequently the rate of, oxygen delivery is determined solely by the mean P_{O_2} in capillary blood. This, in turn, is set by the position of the dissociation curve on the P_{O_2} axis and by its steepness, such that relatively little change in driving pressure occurs as the red blood cell

moves through the capillary. As the partial pressure of oxygen decreases, tissue oxygenation may become impaired. The term *critical P_{O_2}* was introduced to indicate the oxygen tension of blood below which diffusion is impaired and organ function is disturbed.[13] A critical P_{O_2} cannot be a well-defined value that applies to all tissues under all conditions. The oxygen requirements of tissues vary, and, in some tissues, such as striated muscles, oxygen requirements are determined by the level of activity. For the brain, an organ in which an adequate oxygen supply is essential for maintaining energy metabolism, the critical P_{O_2} appears to be about 20 mmHg.

When hemoglobin-oxygen affinity is increased (lower P_{50}), the curve is shifted to the left, and oxygen (which is bound more tightly to hemoglobin) is released only at lower partial pressures. For example, whereas a P_{O_2} of 40 mmHg results in an oxygen saturation of 75% at 37°C and pH 7.40, a leftward shift of the curve results in a higher saturation at the same P_{O_2}. The resulting change in oxygen unloading ultimately could result in impaired diffusion. When affinity is decreased (higher P_{50}), the curve is shifted to the right. Consequently, oxygen is bound less tightly to hemoglobin and is released at higher partial pressures, thereby enhancing oxygen unloading at the tissue level. Therefore, the release of oxygen from the blood at the tissue level depends on the position of the oxygen equilibrium curve, which, in turn, is modified by intraerythrocytic pH, P_{CO_2}, temperature, and other factors, including electrolyte concentration, organic phosphate levels, and hemoglobin type.

FACTORS ALTERING BLOOD OXYGEN-HEMOGLOBIN AFFINITY

The effect of temperature on the oxygen equilibrium curve was first noted by Barcroft and King in 1909.[14] Increased temperature shifts the curve toward the right, thereby facilitating the release of oxygen. In addition, changes in temperature alter both the Bohr factor and the 2,3-diphosphoglycerate (DPG) effect[15] (see later).

The Bohr effect is the shift to the right of the oxygen equilibrium curve of both adult and fetal blood in response to an increase in P_{CO_2} or a decrease in pH, or both. Oxygen unloading is determined by the P_{O_2} gradient between blood and tissues. The shift of the oxyhemoglobin dissociation curve to the right as carbon dioxide enters the blood from the tissues tends to raise the oxygen tension, increasing the gradient for any given oxyhemoglobin saturation and facilitating transfer of oxygen to the tissues. The change in log P_{50} per unit change in pH (i.e., $-\Delta\log P_{50}/-\Delta pH$) is known as the Bohr factor. Its value for adult human blood is -0.48, and for the newborn infant it is -0.44. The effective pH is the intracellular pH of the red blood cell, which is usually 0.2 unit less than plasma pH at physiologic levels, although the pH gradient across the red blood cell may vary in disease states. Thus an acute change in pH of 0.1 unit changes P_{50} by approximately 3 mmHg. The effect of pH changes lasting longer than 2 to 3 hours depends largely on the compensatory change in organic phosphate synthesis (see later discussion). The Bohr effect is more pronounced, at least experimentally, as oxygen saturation decreases and is diminished in 2,3-DPG–depleted blood.[16]

The Bohr effect produced by varying P_{CO_2} at constant fixed acid is larger (-0.48) than that induced by alterations in metabolic acids at constant P_{CO_2} (-0.40).[16] The molecular basis of the carbon dioxide effect is twofold. It follows both carbon dioxide–induced changes in pH and the action of carbon dioxide as a ligand, binding reversibly to uncharged amino groups in the hemoglobin molecule to form carbamates.[17-19] Bound carbamates form salt bridges stabilizing the T (deoxy-) conformation of hemoglobin and decreasing hemoglobin-oxygen affinity. In addition, the affinity of other sites on the hemoglobin molecule for H^+ ion is enhanced by transition from oxyhemoglobin to deoxyhemoglobin, allowing deoxyhemoglobin to take up much of the H^+ ion generated from spontaneous decomposition of carbonic acid.

By modifying hemoglobin-oxygen affinity, carbon dioxide also facilitates respiratory gas exchange in the lungs. At the lungs, carbon dioxide is given up by red blood cells into the alveoli. Carbon dioxide concentration falls, thereby shifting the oxygen equilibrium curve to the left; the increase in hemoglobin-oxygen affinity enhances uptake of oxygen from the alveoli.[20] The combined effects of pH, P_{CO_2}, and temperature on the oxygen equilibrium curve can be viewed, in theory, as advantageous for species survival. An increase in tissue metabolism causes increases in local temperature, H^+ ion concentration, and P_{CO_2}, all of which raise P_{50}. The result is a higher gradient of oxygen tension between capillary and mitochondrion at the site (tissue) where oxygen consumption is highest. For example, the *in vivo* oxygen equilibrium curve has been shown to shift markedly rightward during acute exercise as a result of combined Bohr and temperature effects.[21]

EFFECT OF ERYTHROCYTE 2,3-DIPHOSPHOGLYCERATE (2,3-DPG) ON BLOOD OXYGEN-HEMOGLOBIN AFFINITY

It has long been recognized that the oxygen affinity of Hb A in free solution is considerably greater than that of the intact fresh erythrocyte. This difference suggested to many investigators that the red blood cell contained a substance or substances capable of interacting with hemoglobin and reducing its affinity for oxygen. In 1967, it was demonstrated that interaction with a number of organic phosphates decreased the affinity of a hemoglobin solution for oxygen, with 2,3-DPG being the most effective.[22,23] Of the organic phosphates normally found in the human erythrocyte, 2,3-DPG is present in the largest concentrations and thus is both qualitatively and quantitatively the most important phosphate with respect to modulation of hemoglobin-oxygen affinity. The content of 2,3-DPG in the human red blood cell averages 4.5 μmol/mL red blood cells (range 3.4 to 5.2 μmol/mL red blood cells), whereas ATP concentration averages 1.0 μmol/mL red blood cells (range 0.8 to 1.4 μmol/mL red blood cells). The remainder of the organic phosphates generally totals less than 0.4 μmol/mL red blood cells. Hemoglobin-oxygen affinity as indicated by P_{50} is linear with respect to 2,3-DPG concentration over a wide range; a change of 0.43 mmol of 2,3-DPG/mL red blood cells results in a 1-mmHg change in P_{50}.[24]

The highly negatively charged anion 2,3-DPG binds preferentially to deoxyhemoglobin in a 1:1 molar ratio under physiologic conditions of solute concentration and pH. On a molecular basis, 2,3-DPG decreases oxygen affinity by stabilizing the quaternary structure of deoxyhemoglobin through cross-linking of β-chains. 2,3-DPG is stereochemically complementary to a constellation of six positively charged groups located on the β-chains and facing the central cavity of the hemoglobin molecule.[25] A single molecule of 2,3-DPG is anchored by six salt bridges to cations at the entrance of the central cavity. On oxygenation, 2,3-DPG is extruded because the central cavity becomes too small. A second mechanism by which 2,3-DPG reduces oxygen affinity is by altering the intraerythrocytic pH relative to plasma pH. The reduction in pH consequently decreases oxygen affinity by the Bohr effect. It has been shown that both mechanisms apply in the intact erythrocyte and that, at concentrations of 2,3-DPG above normal, the latter mechanism predominates.[26] The concentration of 2,3-DPG in human red blood cells varies with gestational and postnatal age and can be influenced by hemoglobin level, pH, oxygenation, and activity of red blood cell enzymes such as hexokinase and pyruvate kinase.[27]

FETAL OXYGEN TRANSPORT

Fetal blood has a higher affinity for oxygen and lower P_{50} than that of adult blood, an observation first made in 1930.[28] Figure 86-5 shows this relationship for the human fetus near term, in whom P_{50} is about 20 mmHg under standard conditions. Barcroft and Hall and associates[29-31] reported a gradual decrease in the blood oxygen affinity (increase in P_{50}) during the course of gestation, such that the fetal curve progressively approximates the maternal curve. In the placenta, because of the low P_{O_2} at which transfer of oxygen is achieved, the high affinity of fetal hemoglobin favors oxygen uptake in the fetus. The highest P_{O_2} in the fetus is in umbilical venous blood and usually does not go much above 30 mmHg. At that oxygen tension, the saturation of human fetal blood is 6% to 8% higher than the saturation of maternal blood.[32]

These findings raised questions as to the mechanism or mechanisms responsible for the increased oxygen affinity of fetal blood. Hall[31] suggested that this might result from a specific difference in hemoglobin. Korber,[33] in 1866, had first noted that blood from human newborn umbilical vessels denatured less readily in alkaline or acid solutions than did blood from adults, the difference being most pronounced in alkali. In 1930, Haurowitz[34] demonstrated that the difference in alkaline denaturation resides in the globin chains of hemoglobin and proposed the presence of two hemoglobins in newborn blood, an alkali-susceptible adult fraction and a more resistant fetal fraction. In 1963, the human fetal α-chain was shown to have the same amino acid sequence as the α-chain of human adult hemoglobin.[35] In addition to the two α-chains, fetal hemoglobin was found to contain two non–α-chains (labeled γ-chains), which resemble the β-chain and contain the same number of amino acids (146) but differ in sequence by a total of 39 amino acids. Each γ-chain contains four isoleucine residues not found in either the α- or the β-chain. In addition, three proline residues present in the β-chain have been substituted by other amino acids.

A linear correlation between the proportional composition of fetal hemoglobin and the P_{50} at the time of delivery has been noted in humans. At term, Hb A composes about 25% of the total

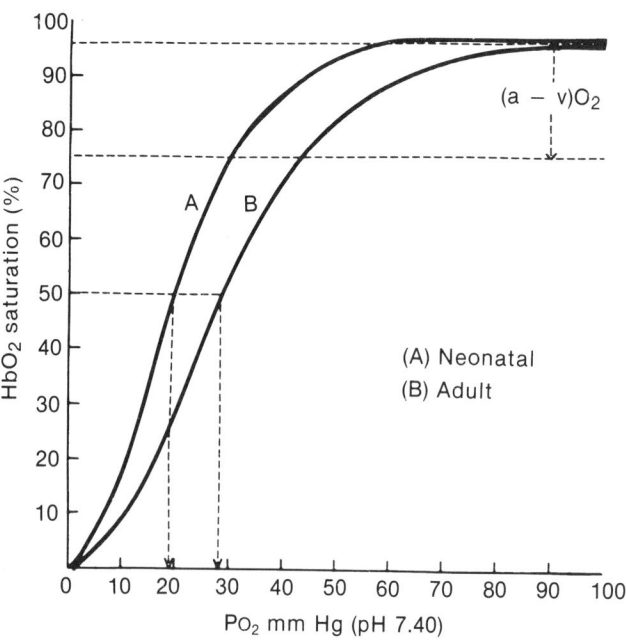

Figure 86–5. Oxyhemoglobin equilibrium curves of blood from term infants at birth and from adults.

hemoglobin, and the fetal P_{50} is about 19 mmHg.[26, 36] Birth, intrauterine hypoxia,[37] and hemolytic disease of the newborn infant do not cause a change in the proportions of Hb A and Hb F at any given gestational age. During the period of accelerated erythropoiesis near term, however, Hb A synthesis predominates. The subcellular events (transcription and translation) responsible for the gradual, orderly change in synthesis from γ- to β-chains are not completely understood.[38, 39] However, recent studies suggest that the interaction of multiple transcription factors with the locus control region (LCR) of the globin gene sequence on chromosome 11 regulates the forms of the globin gene (ε, γ, δ, or β) expressed at each stage of development.[40] The erythroid Kruppel-like factor (EKLF) and the stage selector protein (SSP) seem to be particularly important. Although the specific developmental signals that regulate developmental changes in transcription factor expression have not been identified, changes in expression of hypoxia-inducible factor 1 in response to changes in fetal blood oxygen tension may play a role in this process.[41]

Fetal Blood Oxygen Delivery

Despite an oxygen tension in fetal blood that is only one fifth to one fourth that of the adult, fetal arterial blood oxygen content and oxyhemoglobin saturation at term are not much lower than those of the adult (Fig. 86-6). This, of course, results from a combination of the high oxygen-carrying capacity and increased oxygen affinity of fetal blood. The greater oxygen affinity of fetal blood is generally considered an advantage in that it allows incorporation of oxygen to nearly saturate fetal hemoglobin at relatively low oxygen tensions. The possible disadvantage in oxygen delivery to fetal tissues is offset by the fact that the fetal oxyhemoglobin saturation curve is rather steep, so that a small decrease in oxygen tension results in a major decrement in oxyhemoglobin saturation and unloading of oxygen to the tissues.

The actual oxyhemoglobin saturation curve in vivo as blood flows through the placental exchange capillaries is an additional important consideration. Compared with standard conditions, maternal arterial blood is slightly hypocarbic (P_{CO_2} = 32 mm Hg) and alkalotic (pH 7.42), whereas fetal blood is slightly hypercarbic (P_{CO_2} = 45 mm Hg) and acidotic (pH 7.34). As fetal blood courses through the exchange vessels, it gives up hydrogen ions and carbon dioxide, leading to a rise in pH and fall in P_{CO_2}. The opposite changes occur in the maternal exchange vessels. Thus, in vivo the maternal and fetal oxyhemoglobin saturation curves

may be almost superimposed (see Fig. 86-6). Although the double Bohr effect in the placenta has been credited with significantly augmenting oxygen exchange, theoretical studies suggest that this accounts for only 2% of the total oxygen transferred.[42] As noted earlier, the Bohr effect is expressed by the factor $-\Delta\log P_{50}/-\Delta pH$, which has a value of about -0.48 for both fetal and maternal blood at pH values between 7.2 and 7.8. Below a pH of 7.2, however, the Bohr effect is greater for fetal than for maternal blood. An additional factor tending to shift the in vivo fetal dissociation curve to the right is the temperature of the fetus, which exceeds that of the mother by 0.5 to 1.0°C. In human neonates, the dissociation curve also shifts toward that of the mother as the concentration of Hb F decreases.[32, 43]

Effect of 2,3-DPG on Fetal Hemoglobin-Oxygen Affinity

In 1971, the deoxygenation kinetics of isolated fetal and adult hemoglobin were studied, and significant functional differences were found.[44] Although 2,3-DPG bound to fetal hemoglobin, the binding constant was lower than for adult hemoglobin.[36] Other experiments performed on whole blood demonstrated a significant fall in P_{50} when erythrocytes were depleted of 2,3-DPG, even in samples of blood having a high percentage of fetal hemoglobin.[45] With the use of pure solutions of fetal and adult hemoglobin, it subsequently has been shown that the effect of 2,3-DPG on the P_{50} of fetal hemoglobin is approximately 40% of 2,3-DPG's effect on the P_{50} of adult hemoglobin.[46]

On the basis of these findings, one would expect the P_{50} of whole blood to be related to both the 2,3-DPG level and the relative concentration of adult and fetal hemoglobin. Because the concentrations of adult hemoglobin and 2,3-DPG, and therefore the functioning fraction of DPG (total red blood cell DPG content in nanomoles/milliliter red blood cells times the percentage of adult hemoglobin), increase during gestation, it is not surprising that the P_{50} of whole blood correlates with gestational age (Fig. 86-7). (The term *functioning fraction* is not intended to imply that a compartmentalized portion of the red blood cell's 2,3-DPG is in combination with the hemoglobin but instead is used to underscore the fact that both 2,3-DPG and adult hemoglobin act in concert to determine the oxygen affinity of intracellular hemoglobin.) The correlation of P_{50} with gestational age is even closer than with the functioning fraction of DPG, suggesting that other factors contribute to the rise of P_{50} during gestation.

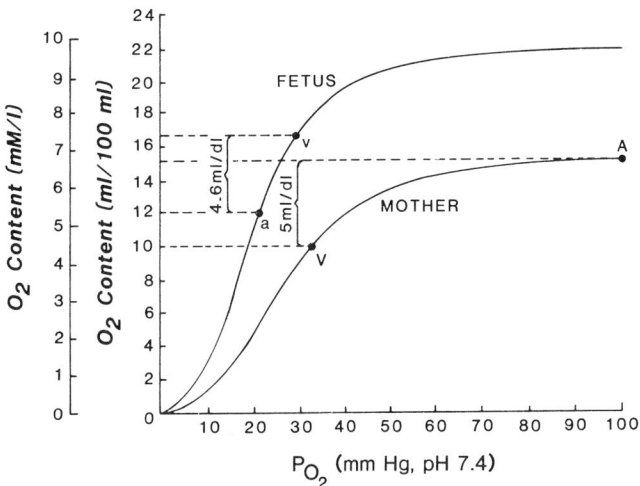

Figure 86–6. Blood oxygen content as a function of oxygen tension for human maternal and near-term fetal blood.

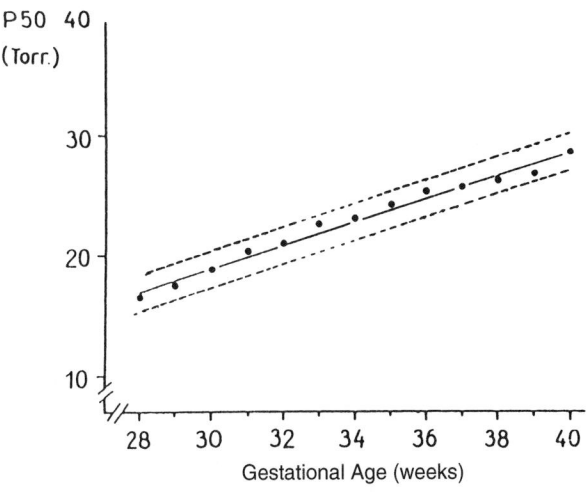

Figure 86–7. Relationship between gestational age and hemoglobin P_{50}. Each point represents mean value for age; dashed lines indicate ± 2 SD.

TABLE 86-1

Oxygen Transport in Term Infants

Number of Infants	Age	Total Hb (g/dl blood)	Hct (%)	MCHC (%)	O2 Capacity (ml/dl blood)	P50 @ pH 7.40 (mmHg)	2,3-DPG (nmol/ ml RBC)	Fetal Hb (% of total)	FFDPG* (nmol/ ml RBC)	Reticulocyte Count (%)
19	1 day	17.8	52.7	34.2	24.7	19.4	5433	77.0	1246	4.70
		±2.0	±7.1	±1.9	±2.8	±1.8	±1041	±7.3	±570	±1.74
18	5 days	16.2	46.9	34.1	22.6	20.6	6580	76.8	1516	2.15
		±1.2	±6.0	±0.8	±2.2	±1.7	±996	±5.8	±495	±1.64
14	3 wk	12.0	33.5	35.9	16.7	22.7	5378	70.0	1614	0.88
		±1.3	±4.3	±1.2	±1.9	±1.0	±732	±7.33	±252	±0.71
10	6-9 wk	10.5	30.2	34.9	14.7	24.4	5560	52.1	2670	1.63
		±1.2	±3.9	±0.6	±1.6	±1.4	±747	±11.0	±550	±0.65
14	3-4 mo	10.2	30.3	33.8	14.3	26.5	5819	23.2	4470	1.36
		±0.8	±2.4	±1.7	±1.2	±2.0	±1240	±16.0	±1380	±0.45
8	6 mo	11.3	34.0	33.4	14.7	27.8	5086	4.7	4840	1.42
		±0.9	±3.6	±0.7	±0.6	±1.0	±1570	±2.2	±1500	±1.15
8	8-11 mo	11.4	34.8	32.8	15.9	30.3	7381	1.6	7260	0.82
		±0.6	±1.9	±0.9	±0.8	±0.7	±485	±1.0	±544	±0.27

* Functioning fraction of 2,3-diphosphoglycerate.
All values are given as mean ± 1 SD.

There is no satisfactory explanation for the rise in 2,3-DPG levels during gestation. It has been speculated, however, that the increase is the result of increased synthesis of adult hemoglobin, because it has been shown in vitro that the reduced hemoglobin of adults is more effective than the reduced hemoglobin of fetuses in stimulating 2,3-DPG synthesis.[47] This hypothesis is also supported by the significant correlation between the percentage of adult hemoglobin and 2,3-DPG content in the neonatal period (Table 86-1).

Postnatal Changes in Oxygen Transport

The high oxygen affinity of fetal blood, which is well adapted to oxygen uptake in the placenta, has disadvantages in postnatal life. Assuming there is adequate postnatal lung function, the pulmonary circulation is exposed to an oxygen tension of 80 mmHg or more, so that high affinity at low oxygen tensions has no advantage for oxygen uptake during the newborn period. At the tissue level, the low P_{50} decreases the driving potential for oxygen diffusion, limiting the rate at which oxygen can be unloaded. The newborn infant needs more oxygen than the fetus, for even in a neutral thermal environment and at minimal activity, the oxygen consumption of most species increases by 100% to 150% in the first few days of life.[48] Colder environments and muscle activity further increase the metabolic demand for oxygen. Hence, a P_{50} adequate for tissue supply in the fetus does not provide a sufficient rate of net oxygen diffusion in the neonate.

To meet the increased oxygen demands after birth, oxygen-carrying parameters of blood change drastically. In most species, postnatal changes take place in both oxygen affinity and oxygen-carrying capacity, but at different rates and by different amounts. Following birth, the infant's blood oxygen affinity decreases rapidly.[26] On the first day of life, the P_{50} in normal infants is 19.4 ± 1.8 mmHg, in contrast to a value of 27.0 ± 1.1 mmHg for the normal adult (all values are mean ± SD). In the term infant, P_{50} increases gradually and reaches normal adult values by 4 to 6 months of life (Fig. 86-8), corresponding to the time course of the replacement of fetal hemoglobin by adult hemoglobin. The red blood cell 2,3-DPG concentration on day 1 averages 5.43 ± 1.04 μmol/mL red blood cells and thus does not differ significantly from the adult value of 5.11 ± 0.42 μmol/mL red blood cells. By the fifth day, 2,3-DPG increases to 6.58 ± 1.00 μmol/mL red blood cells.[35] Although this increment has

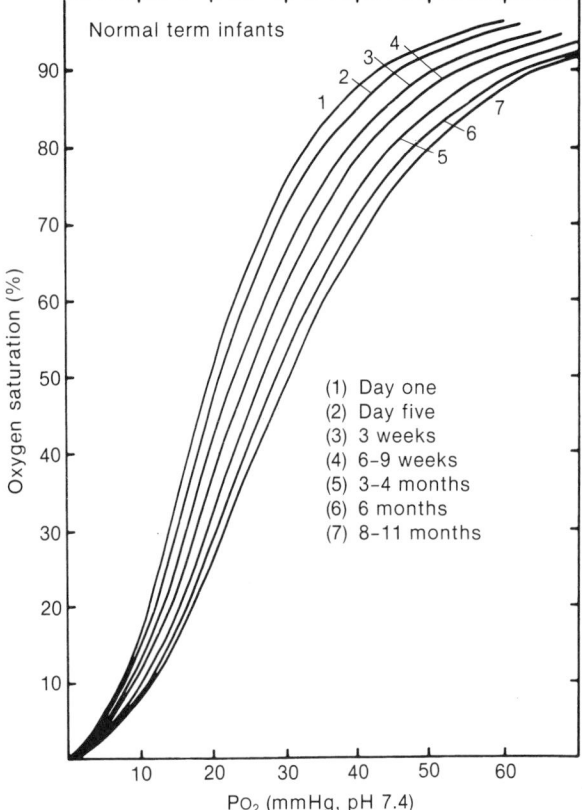

Figure 86-8. Oxygen equilibrium curve of blood from term infants at different postnatal ages.

only a modest direct effect on fetal hemoglobin oxygen affinity, it lowers intracellular pH, thereby decreasing blood oxygen affinity.

For most of the first year of life, Hb F decreases from about 75% to about 2% of the total, whereas 2,3-DPG concentrations in general remain fairly constant at 5 to 6 μmol/mL red blood cells. At 8 to 11 months of age, the concentration of 2,3-DPG rises to about 7 μmol/mL. The P_{50} at this age averages 30.3 mm Hg, which exceeds the value for the normal adult, whereas the fetal

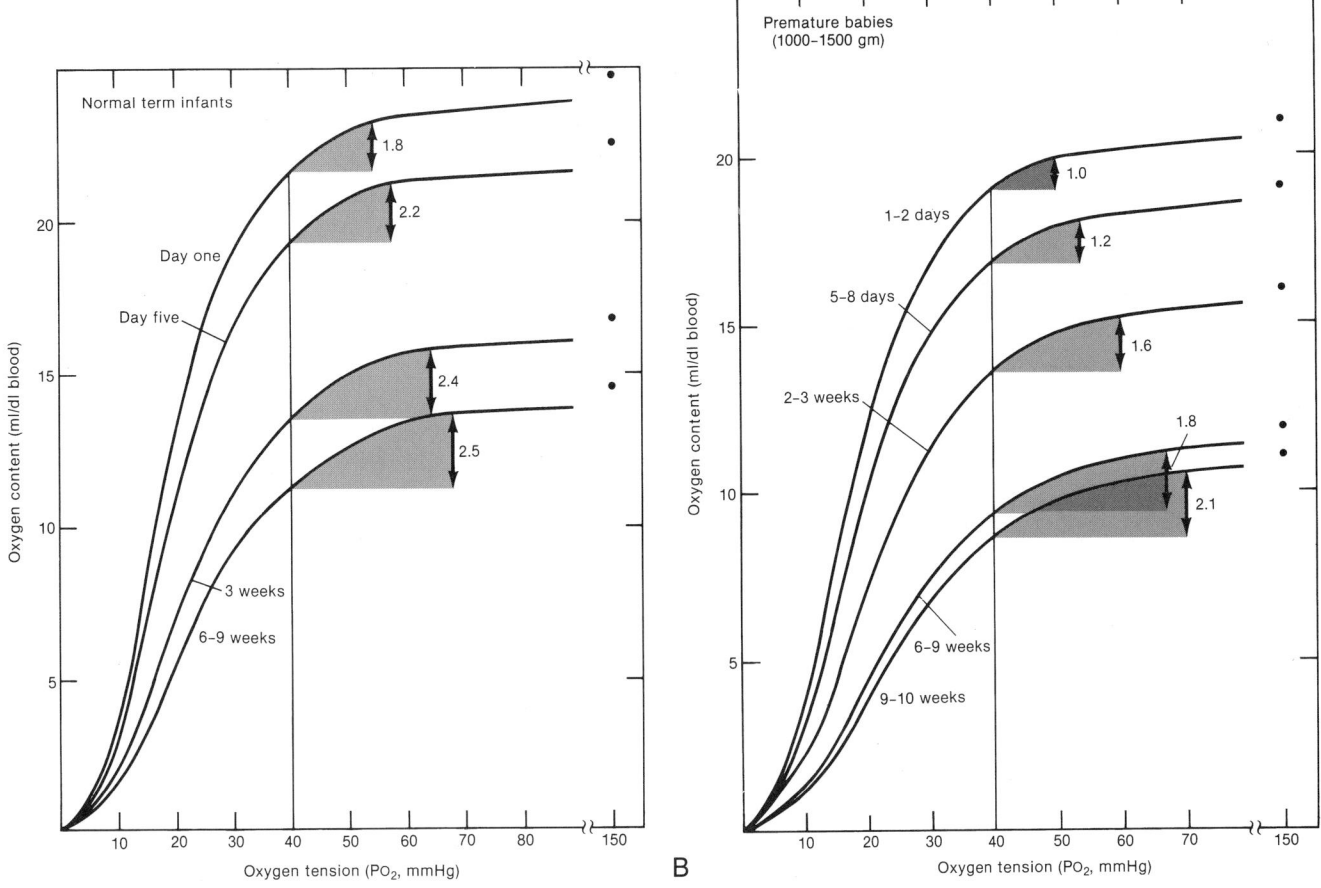

Figure 86–9. Oxygen equilibrium curves of blood from term infants (**A**), and preterm infants, birthweight 1000 to 1500 g (**B**), at different postnatal ages. *Double arrows* represent the oxygen-unloading capacity between a given "arterial" and "venous" Po₂. Points corresponding to 150 mm Hg on the abscissa are the O₂ capacities; each curve represents the mean value of the infants studied in each age group.

hemoglobin concentration is decreased to normal adult levels. Average values for the percentage of fetal hemoglobin, P_{50}, and 2,3-DPG levels for term infants of various postnatal ages are shown in Table 86–1. Thus, the postnatal change in P_{50} correlates neither with the change in red blood cell DPG content alone nor with the decline in fetal hemoglobin alone. Instead, the progressive decrease in oxygen affinity during the first 6 months of life correlates significantly with the functioning DPG fraction. The changes in oxygen affinity during postnatal life should be taken into account when the oxygen saturation or content of arterial blood in the neonate is derived from measurements of Pao₂ and pH. In the absence of other measurements, gestational age can be used for a reasonably accurate estimation of the oxygen affinity.

In general, preterm, low birth weight infants have a lower erythrocyte 2,3-DPG content, lower P_{50}, and higher fetal hemoglobin concentration than their larger term counterparts. During the first several weeks of life, these small infants have functioning fractions of DPG that are significantly lower than those of term infants. Premature infants have a smaller oxygen unloading capacity initially than do term infants and do not catch up during the first 3 months of life[3] (Fig. 86-9).

Effect of Altered Physiologic States on Oxygen Delivery to Tissues

Various alterations in physiology may have a significant effect on oxygen delivery to the tissues. Under such conditions, variations in oxygen-carrying capacity, blood flow, or hemoglobin-

oxygen affinity have the potential to improve or impair tissue oxygenation.

Hypoxemia

The response to hypoxemia changes significantly during maturation. Oxidation of the cytochromes of the electron transport chain during hypoxemia is lower in the newborn infant compared with the adult at any given degree of hemoglobin saturation, presumably because of the presence of fetal hemoglobin in the circulation.[49] The lower level of oxidation preserves mitochondrial metabolism and helps maintain high-energy phosphate production during hypoxemia. The left-shifted hemoglobin-oxygen curve associated with fetal hemoglobin might be expected to be a disadvantage during hypoxemia because release of oxygen to tissues is decreased. On the contrary, tissue oxygen extraction in the fetus and neonate appears to be increased during acute hypoxemia, thus maintaining normal levels of oxygen consumption.[50] In contrast, animal studies suggest that fetal oxygen extraction is not increased during chronic fetal hypoxemia; instead, fetal oxygen consumption is decreased, presumably reflecting a decrease in metabolic rate in response to reduced oxygen delivery.[51] The fetal response to hypoxemia also appears to be organ-specific. For example, studies in animal models have shown that cerebral blood flow increases proportionately more during acute hypoxemia when there is a high fetal hemoglobin concentration, thereby preserving or even increasing oxygen delivery to brain, although this response is blunted during chronic hypoxemia.[51, 52] Similar data are not available for other organs.

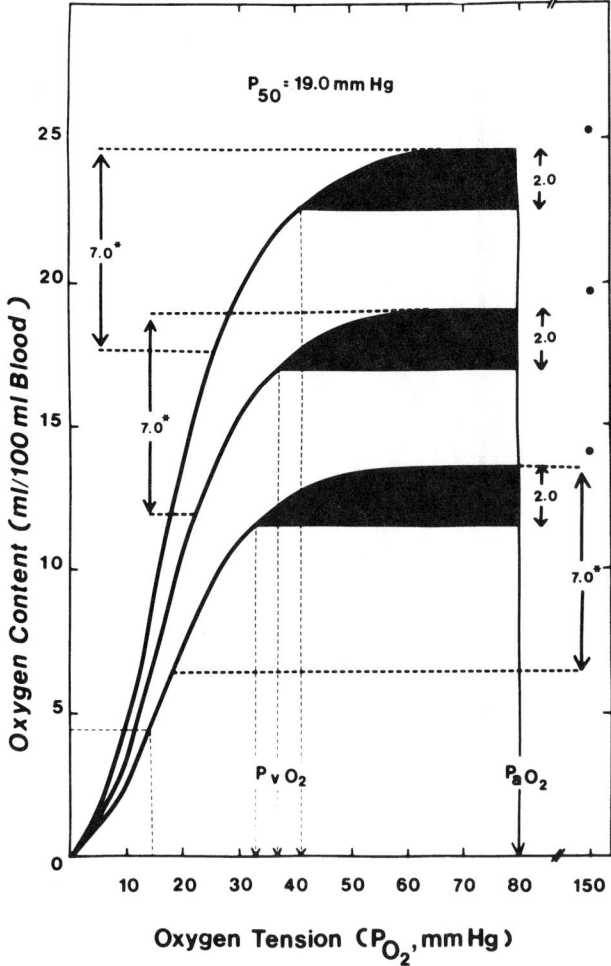

Figure 86–10. The effect of altered hematocrit at a constant P_{50} of 19.0 mm Hg on the tissue oxygen unloading of newborn infants. The asterisk represents the calculated myocardial extraction of oxygen. In this study, the P_{50} equals 19.0 mmHg at a pH of 7.40 and temperature of 37°C.

Sepsis

Bacterial sepsis may also affect tissue oxygen transport. Sepsis caused by group B streptococci, for example, is associated with a higher critical venous oxygen saturation (the levels below which tissue acidosis develops) than is hypoxemia.[53] This seems to be a specific effect of sepsis, rather than a result of the alterations in circulatory status (e.g., increased catecholamine levels) that occur in response to infection. Oxygen consumption is increased during sepsis at the same time that oxygen delivery may be decreased as a result of impairment of myocardial function by endotoxin.[54] There is also evidence suggesting that sepsis may decrease oxygen extraction at the tissue level, further reducing tissue oxygen delivery.

Anemia

Anemia is a common clinical problem in the premature infant. Assuming that an infant is healthy and has no evidence of cardiac disease, pulmonary disease, or increased metabolic needs, a decrease in the oxygen-carrying capacity is a source of concern only if oxygen delivery to the tissues approaches the limit of oxygen stores. As seen in Figure 86–10, infants at birth with significant differences in total oxygen-carrying capacity but similar oxygen affinities exhibit the same arteriovenous oxygen

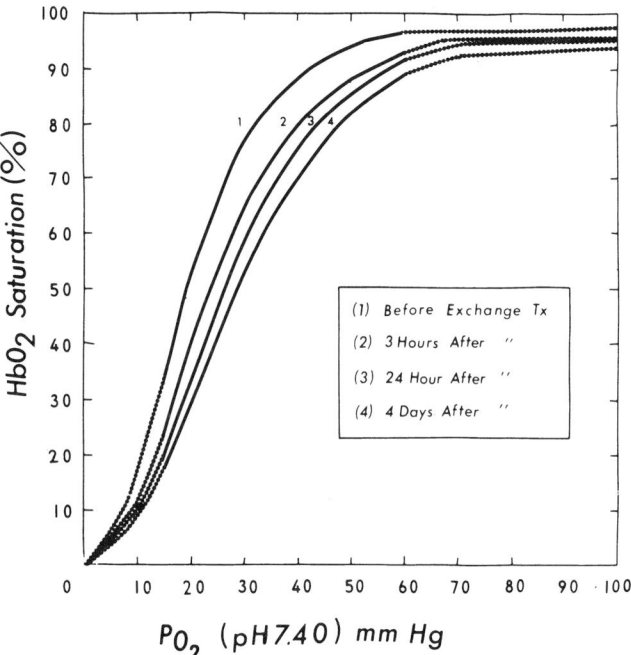

Figure 86–11. The effect of exchange transfusion with fresh adult blood of low oxygen affinity on the oxyhemoglobin dissociation curve of the newborn infant. An acute shift of the curve to the right is seen after such a transfusion.

content differences. It is worth noting that when oxygen-carrying capacity decreases significantly as a result of anemia, sufficient oxygen unloading occurs without lowering the venous oxygen tension below 30 mmHg.

A reduction in oxygen-carrying capacity may be more critical under conditions of impaired oxygen uptake, such as in the presence of lung disease. In the presence of reduced oxygen uptake, tissue oxygen delivery can be improved by optimizing preload, afterload, SaO_2, and oxygen-carrying capacity (i.e., hemoglobin concentration). The effect of a decrease in SaO_2 on oxygen delivery is significantly less than the effect of anemia.[55,56] For example, SaO_2 would have to decrease from 95% to approximately 80% to have an effect on oxygen content comparable to a 2-g decrease in hemoglobin concentration. Thus, in situations of marginal oxygen delivery, maintenance of hemoglobin concentrations high enough to optimize oxygen-carrying capacity is essential.

Exchange Transfusions

An acute rightward shift of the oxyhemoglobin curve of the newborn infant can be produced by exchange transfusion with adult blood, with its lower oxygen affinity[57,58] (Fig. 86–11). The consequences of exchange transfusions with fresh versus stored blood were first demonstrated in 1954, and further delineated in later studies. Infants who underwent exchange transfusion with blood that had been stored for 7 days or longer had a decreased P_{50} compared with infants receiving fresh blood (< 24 hours old).[59] The increase in oxygen affinity occurring with blood storage correlated with a simultaneous fall in 2,3-DPG levels.[60] The calculated oxygen-unloading capacity was decreased in infants receiving 5-day-old blood transfusions, but in those receiving fresh blood it was increased.[36] These studies demonstrated that during the immediate post-transfusion period, the infant's blood reflects the storage characteristics of the blood received.

Further investigations revealed that these findings resulted from use of blood stored in acid-citrate-dextrose; use of this storage medium results in a prompt fall in 2,3-DPG levels and concomitant rapid increase in oxygen affinity. In contrast, the use of citrate-phosphate-dextrose preserves the oxygen affinity and 2,3-DPG content of the stored blood essentially unchanged throughout normal storage periods.[36] These findings have significant physiologic consequences. If blood with a lower P_{50} than normal adult hemoglobin is used for exchange transfusion, the amount of oxygen unloaded is decreased. To compensate for this, the infant must either increase cardiac output or the arteriovenous oxygen difference.[61] The latter situation results in decreased venous oxygen tension, which could thereby impair oxygen diffusion from the capillaries to the tissues. Thus, knowledge of the storage conditions of the blood products to be used for exchange transfusion may be of critical importance in determining the physiologic impact of the procedure, particularly in the infant with compromised cardiorespiratory function.

REFERENCES

1. Chance B: Reaction of oxygen with the respiratory chain in cells and tissue. J Gen Physiol 49:163, 1965.
2. Weisse AB, et al: Late circulatory adjustments to acute normovolemic polycythemia. Am J Physiol 211:1413, 1966.
3. Guyton AC: Regulation of cardiac output. Anesthesiology 29:235, 1971.
4. Krantz SB, Jacobson LO: Erythropoietin and the Regulation of Erythropoiesis. Chicago, University of Chicago Press, 1970.
5. Jelkmann W, Hellwig-Burgel T: Biology of erythropoietin. Adv Exp Med Biol 502:169, 2001.
6. Thorling EB, Ersley AJ: The "tissue" tension of oxygen and its relation to hematocrit and erythropoiesis. Blood 31:332, 1968.
7. Schruefer JJP, et al: Interdependence of whole blood and hemoglobin oxygen dissociation curves from hemoglobin type. Nature (Lond) 196:550, 1962.
8. Perutz MF: The hemoglobin molecule. Sci Am 211:64, 1964.
9. Perutz MF: Stereochemistry of cooperative effects of hemoglobin. Nature 228:726, 1970.
10. Scherrer M, Bachofen H: The oxygen combining capacity of hemoglobin. Anesthesiology 36:190, 1972.
11. Hill AV: J Appl Physiol (Lond) 40 IV, 1910.
12. Chance B, et al: The intracellular oxidation-reduction state. In Dickens F, Neil E (eds): Oxygen in the Animal Organism. London, Pergamon Press, 1964, pp 367–392.
13. Opiz E, Schneider M: Über die Sauerstoffversorgung des Gehirns und der Mechanismus von Mangeliverkungen. Ergebn Physiol 46:126, 1950.
14. Barcroft J, King WOR: The effect of temperature on the dissociation curve of blood. J Physiol 39:374, 1909.
15. Hlastala MP, et al: Influence of temperature on hemoglobin-ligand interaction in whole blood. J Appl Physiol 43:545, 1977.
16. Hlastala MP, Woodson RD: Saturation dependency of the Bohr effect: interactions among H^+, CO_2, and DPG. J Appl Physiol 38:1126, 1975.
17. Margaria R, Green AA: The first dissociation constant, pK_1, of carbonic acid in hemoglobin solutions and its relation to the existence of a combination of hemoglobin with carbon dioxide. J Biol Chem 102:611, 1933.
18. Naeraa N, et al: pH and molecular CO_2 components of the Bohr effect in human blood. Scand J Clin Lab Invest 18:96, 1966.
19. Roughton FJW: Some recent work on the interactions of oxygen, carbon dioxide and haemoglobin. Biochem J 117:801, 1970.
20. Christiansen J, et al: The absorption and dissociation of carbon dioxide by human blood. J Physiol 48:244, 1914.
21. Shappell SD, et al: Adaptation to exercise: role of hemoglobin affinity for oxygen and 2,3-diphosphoglycerate. J Appl Physiol 30:827, 1971.
22. Benesch R, Benesch RE: The effect of organic phosphates from the human erythrocyte on the allosteric properties of hemoglobin. Biochem Biophys Res Commun 26:162, 1967.
23. Chanutin A, Curnish RR: Effect of organic phosphates on the oxygen equilibrium of human erythrocytes. Arch Biochem Biophys 121:96, 1967.
24. Oski FA, et al: The effects of deoxygenation of adult and fetal hemoglobin on the synthesis of red cell 2,3-diphosphoglycerate and its in-vivo consequences. J Clin Invest 49:400, 1970.
25. Arnone A: X-ray diffraction study of binding of 2,3-diphosphoglycerate to human deoxyhaemoglobin. Nature 237:146, 1972.
26. Delivoria-Papadopoulos M, et al: Postnatal changes in oxygen transport of term, premature, and sick infants: the role of red cell 2,3-diphosphoglycerate and adult hemoglobin. Pediatr Res 5:235, 1971.
27. Delivoria-Papadopoulos M, et al: Oxygen-hemoglobin dissociation curves: effect of inherited enzyme defects of the red blood cell. Science 165:601, 1969.
28. Anselmino KY, Joffman F: Die Ursachen des Icterus Neonatorum. Arch Gynalkol 143:477, 1930.
29. Barcroft J, Elsden SR: The oxygen consumption of the sheep foetus. J Physiol (Lond) 105:25P, 1946.
30. Barcroft J, et al: The rate of blood flow and gaseous metabolism of the uterus during pregnancy. J Physiol (Lond) 77:194, 1933.
31. Hall FG: Haemoglobin function in the developing chick. J Physiol (Lond) 83:222, 1935.
32. Beer R, et al: Sauglingen während der ersten Lebensmonate. Arch Ges Physiol 265:526, 1958.
33. Korber E: Über Differenzen des Blutfarbstoffes. Inaugural Dissertation, Dorpat, 1866.
34. Haurowitz F: Zur Chemie des Blutfarbstoffes. Über das Hämoglobin des Menschen. Atschr Physiol Chem 186:141, 1930.
35. Schroeder WA, et al: The amino acid sequence of the α-chain of human fetal hemoglobin. Biochemistry 2:1353, 1963.
36. Delivoria-Papadopoulos M, et al: Exchange transfusion in the newborn infant with fresh and "old" blood. The role of storage of 2,3-diphosphoglycerate, hemoglobin-oxygen affinity, and oxygen release. J Pediatr 6:898, 1971.
37. Cook CD, et al: Measurement of fetal hemoglobin in newborn infants: correlation with gestational age and intrauterine hypoxia. Pediatrics 20:272, 1957.
38. Wood WG, Weatherall DJ: Haemoglobin synthesis during human foetal development. Nature 244:162, 1973.
39. Wood WG, et al: Switch from foetal to adult haemoglobin synthesis in normal and hypophysectomised sheep. Nature 264:799, 1976.
40. Jane SM, Cunningham JM: Br J Haematol 102:415, 1998.
41. Semenza GL: Hypoxia-inducible factor 1: control of oxygen homeostasis in health and disease. Pediatr Res 49:614, 2001.
42. Hill EP, et al: Kinetics of O_2 and CO_2 exchange. In West JB (ed): Bioengineering Aspects of Lung Biology. New York, Marcel Dekker, 1975.
43. Beer R, et al: Die Sauerstoff-Dissoziationskurve des fetalen Blutes und der Gasaustausch in der menschlichen Plazenta. Pflugers Arch Ges Physiol 260:306, 1955.
44. Salhany JM, et al: The deoxygenation of kinetic properties of human fetal hemoglobin: effect of 2,3-diphosphoglycerate. Biochem Biophys Res Commun 45:1350, 1971.
45. Brewer GJ, Eaton JW: Erythrocyte metabolism: interaction with oxygen transport. Science 171:1205, 1971.
46. Riegel KP: Respiratory gas transport characteristics of blood and hemoglobin. In Stave U (ed): Physiology of the Neonatal Period. New York, Appleton-Century-Crofts, 1970.
47. Bauer CH, et al: Different effects of 2,3-diphosphoglycerate and adenosine triphosphate on the oxygen affinity of adult and fetal human haemoglobin. Life Sci 7:1339, 1968.
48. Avery ME: The Lung and Its Disorders, 3rd ed. Philadelphia, WB Saunders, 1974.
49. Sylvia AL, et al: Effect of transient hypoxia on oxygenation of the developing rat brain: relationships among haemoglobin saturation, autoregulation of blood flow and mitochondrial redox state. J Dev Physiol 12:287, 1989.
50. Stein JC, Ellsworth ML: Capillary oxygen transport during severe hypoxia: role of hemoglobin oxygen affinity. J Appl Physiol 75:1601, 1993.
51. Richardson BS, Bocking AD: Metabolic and circulatory adaptations to chronic hypoxia in the fetus. Comp Biochem Physiol A Mol Integr Physiol 119:717, 1998.
52. Ramaekers VT, et al: Brain oxygen transport related to levels of fetal haemoglobin in stable preterm infants. J Dev Physiol 17:209, 1992.
53. Hammerman C: Influence of disease state on oxygen transport in newborn piglets. Biol Neonate 66:128, 1994.
54. Meadow WL, et al: Oxygen delivery, oxygen consumption, and metabolic acidosis during group B streptococcal sepsis in piglets. Pediatr Res 22:509, 1987.
55. Delima LGR, Wynands JE: Oxygen transport. Can J Anaesth 40:R81, 1993.
56. van der Hoeven MA, et al: Relationship between mixed venous oxygen saturation and markers of tissue oxygenation in progressive hypoxic hypoxia and in isovolemic anemic hypoxia in 8- to 12-day-old piglets. Crit Care Med 27:1885, 1999.
57. Delivoria-Papadopoulos M, et al: The role of exchange transfusion in the management of low birth weight infants with and without severe respiratory distress syndrome: I. initial observations. J Pediatr 89:273, 1976.
58. Delivoria-Papadopoulos M, et al: Variations of blood oxygen affinity and content on cardiac output (CO) and oxygen transport to the tissues in newborn lambs (Abstract). Pediatr Res 12:393, 1978.
59. Delivoria-Papadopoulos M, et al: Postnatal changes in oxygen hemoglobin affinity and erythrocyte 2,3-diphosphoglycerate in piglets. Pediatr Res 8:64, 1974.
60. Bunn HF, et al: Hemoglobin function in stored blood. J Clin Invest 48:311, 1969.
61. Delivoria-Papadopoulos M, et al: The pathophysiology of exchange transfusion of the newborn infant with regard to oxygen transport. In Preservation of Red Blood Cells. Washington, DC, National Academy of Sciences, 1973, pp 137–147.

Henrique Rigatto

87

Control of Breathing in Fetal Life and Onset and Control of Breathing in the Neonate

There are at least three important considerations regarding the study of the control of breathing during the fetal and neonatal period. First, the fetus sleeps all the time and the neonate most of the time.[1-4] This means that their control of breathing must be studied during sleep and compared with the control of breathing in adult subjects during sleep and not during wakefulness.[5-8] This was not the norm in the past and accounts for some important misconceptions. Second, the fetus and the neonate are non-cooperative subjects. This means that we must study their respiratory control without their being aware and must try to compare the measurements with those of the adult under similar conditions. This is difficult to do. Third, measurements in the neonate are usually made, by necessity, with the infant in the decubitus position, whereas those in the adult subject are usually made while the adult is in the sitting or standing position.[6,9] The implications of different positions on the control of breathing were also not dealt with in the past. Unless there is some consistency in the methodology, it is difficult to define what is actually distinct or unique about the control of breathing in the neonate. In this chapter, I review some of the concepts and the progress made in the area of control of breathing in the fetus and newborn. I also highlight major developments and critically analyze the scientific foundations of our knowledge in this area.

CONCEPTUAL AND HISTORICAL PERSPECTIVES

Although the major advances in our understanding of the control of breathing generally apply to the fetus and newborn, there are two major aspects that make breathing during this period unique. One is the presence and purpose of fetal breathing, and the other is the physiologic mechanism responsible for the first breath at birth.

In 1970, Dawes and co-workers[10] presented evidence that the fetal sheep makes regular breathing movements during rapid eye movement (REM) sleep. In their work, tracheal pressure changes were measured as an index of fetal breathing. Simultaneously, Merlet and co-workers,[11] using changes in intraesophageal pressure as an index of fetal breathing, demonstrated respiratory activity in fetal sheep. Subsequent work confirmed and expanded these findings by recording the electrical activity of the diaphragm and by clearly showing the central origin of the respiratory output *in utero*.[2,12-16] It is now universally accepted that the fetus makes breathing exercises *in utero* beginning with early pregnancy.[14,15,17-23] Because there is no gas exchange associated with this activity, its purpose is unknown. Dawes[24] suggested, in a teleologic vein, that the breathing *in utero* is important to exercise the respiratory muscles for a vital function after birth.

The discovery of fetal breathing brought a new dimension to the events occurring at birth. What had traditionally been called "the initiation of breathing at birth" must now be called "the establishment of continuous breathing at birth." Breathing begins long before birth. The question now is not what determines the appearance of breathing at birth but what makes it continuous. Or, from another perspective, we may ask what makes fetal breathing episodic, present only during low-voltage electrocortical activity (LVECoG). The answers to these questions remain essentially unknown.

THE FETUS

Breathing Pattern at Rest

Fetal breathing occurs primarily during periods of LVECoG, which accounts for 40% of fetal life during the last trimester of gestation in sheep.[2,10,24-26] In the human fetus, this percentage is similar.[17,21,22] During high-voltage ECoG (HVECoG), there is no established breathing present, but occasional breaths may surface after episodic, generalized, tonic muscular discharges associated with body movements (Fig. 87-1).[2] During LVECoG, breathing is irregular, and the diaphragmatic electromyogram (EMG) is characterized by abrupt onset and ending. Less frequently, there is a progressive increase in envelope amplitude, comparable to the inspiratory slope observed in the anesthetized newborn lamb (Fig. 87-2). A gradual decrease in diaphragmatic EMG at the end of a breath, reflecting postinspiratory activity (as observed in the newborn infant), is rarely seen in the fetus.[2,19,23,27,28] This irregular diaphragmatic activity generates a negative tracheal pressure of about 2 to 5 mm Hg. The corresponding changes in tracheal flow are less than seen postnatally, likely owing to the higher viscosity of lung fluid in the system. The irregular breathing activity observed during this period probably reflects the influence of the reticular formation on breathing so characteristic of REM sleep. The average breath has an inspiratory time of 0.45 second, an expiratory time of 0.74 second, and a total duration of 1.12 seconds.[27,29] The physiologic mechanism responsible for the occurrence of fetal breathing only during LVECoG is unknown.

Fetal State

The occurrence of fetal breathing during LVECoG has led some investigators to believe that the fetus may be awake during part of this period.[30-32] In fact, using electrophysiologic criteria, it was postulated that during the last part of gestation in sheep, the fetus was awake about 5% of the time.[12,13,32,33]

It was further postulated that certain chemical and pharmacologic agents could alter fetal breathing by "arousing" the fetus.[12,32,33] In the late 1970s, I became interested in determining whether the fetus was at times awake *in utero* and whether arousal could be induced by chemical or pharmacologic agents. My colleagues and I found the polysynaptic reflexes obtained from the hindlimbs in the chronic fetal sheep preparation to be unusually intense during transition from LVECoG to HVECoG.[16] We speculated that this could represent fetal wakefulness. We subsequently implanted a window on the left flank of the ewe to observe the fetus *in utero* directly (Fig. 87-3).[2,34] The technique proved to be powerful and has generated substantial new information. *Wakefulness,* defined by open eyes and purposeful movement of the head, was not observed in the fetus under resting conditions. Analysis of videotapes, amounting to more than 5000 hours of observation over 8 years, clearly showed that the fetus alternates between two basic behavioral states, REM (mostly LVECoG) and quiet (mostly HVECoG) sleep.[2,3] Activities such as movement, swallowing, licking, and breathing occur during REM sleep (Fig. 87-4). During quiet sleep, the fetus is still and occasionally shows generalized movements associated with

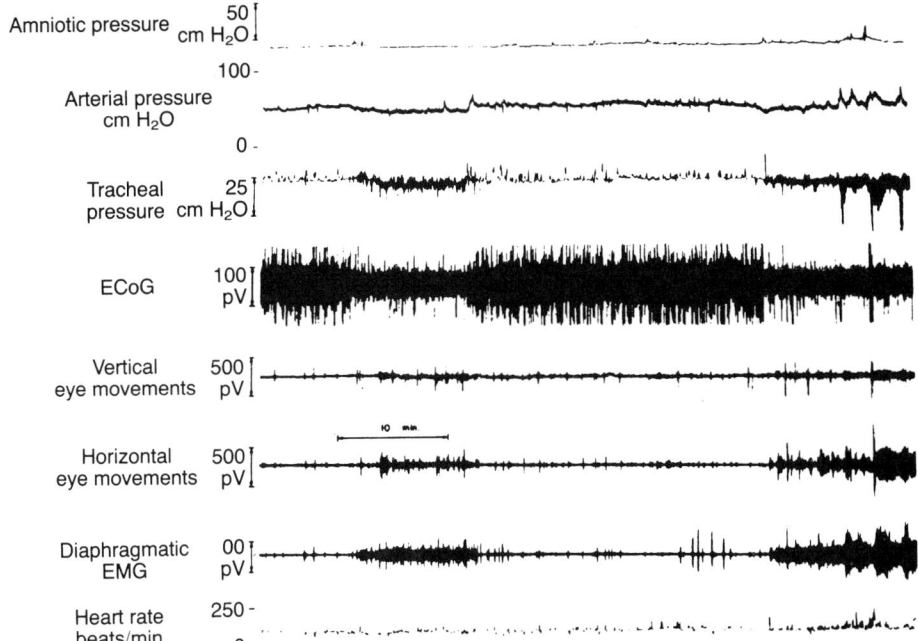

Figure 87–1. Fetal breathing in a fetal lamb at 134 days' gestation. The deflections in tracheal pressure and diaphragmatic activity occur during periods of rapid eye movement (REM) sleep in low-voltage electrocortical activity (ECoG) only. In high-voltage electrocortical activity (quiet sleep), breathing is absent.

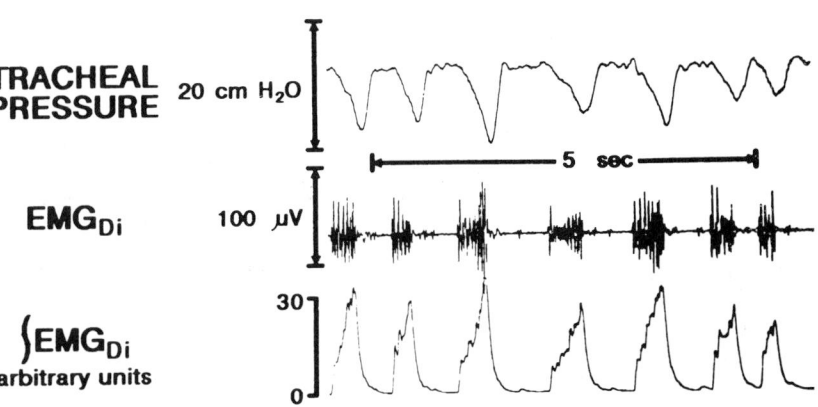

Figure 87–2. Tracheal pressure and diaphragmatic activity (EMG$_{Di}$) in a fetal lamb at 129 days' gestation. Note the abrupt beginning and ending of diaphragmatic activity in some of the breaths and the progressive increase in activity in others. A gradual decrease in diaphragmatic activity, reflecting postinspiratory activity, as seen in the newborn infant, is rarely seen in the fetus.

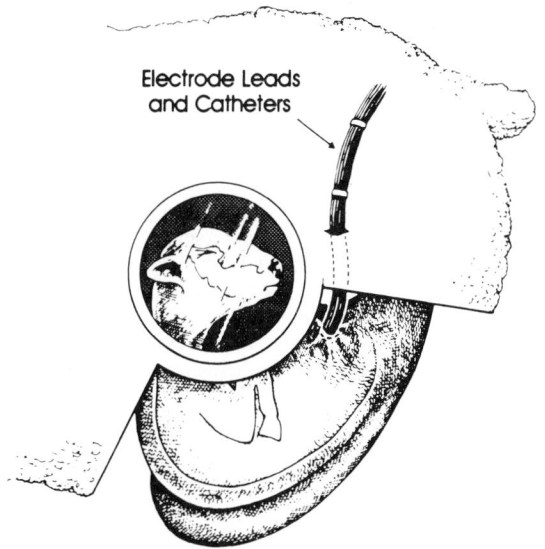

Figure 87–3. View of the head of the fetus as it appears after surgery is completed. The bundle with catheters and electrical leads crosses the abdominal and uterine walls at some distance from the window.

tonic discharges. The enhancement of the polysynaptic reflexes we observed previously was associated with generalized tonic discharges and rotation of the body and head during the transition from LVECoG to HVECoG. It was not associated with wakefulness.[2, 34] This generalized discharge is typical of the transition from LVECoG to HVECoG. We speculate that understanding the neurophysiologic basis for this intense discharge may give us the explanation of how the change from low to high voltage occurs.

Besides the normal irregularity of the respiratory pattern seen in REM sleep, licking and swallowing clearly disturb breathing activity;[2, 19, 28] breathing becomes slower and irregular, and diaphragmatic activity becomes interspersed with clusters of esophageal EMG activity. This digestive tract activity occurs primarily during REM sleep and is translated behaviorally and electrophysiologically as a general increase in EMG activity, blood pressure, and heart rate.

Modulation of Fetal Breathing by Carbon Dioxide, Oxygen, Pulmonary Reflexes, and Pharmacologic Agents

Initially, fetal breathing was thought by some investigators to depend on behavioral influences, because it was observed only during REM sleep and seemed somewhat refractory to chemical stimuli.[35] Subsequent studies, however, clearly showed that the

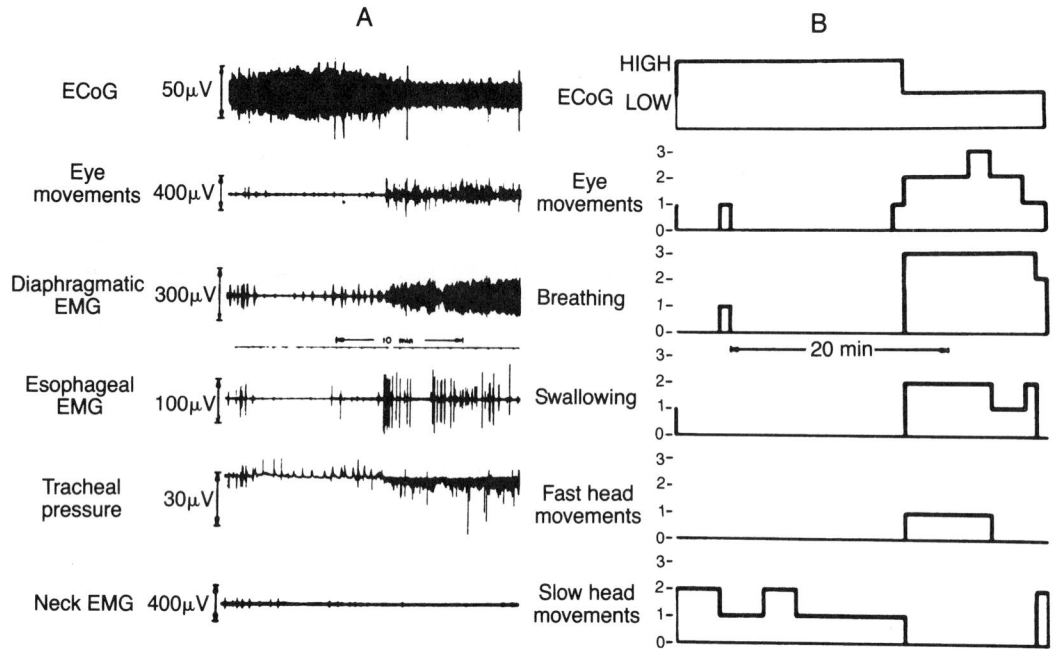

Figure 87–4. A comparative representation of observations made on a polygraph (**A**) and through a double-wall Plexiglas window (**B**). Fetal breathing, eye movements, and swallowing are predominantly present in low-voltage electrocortical activity (ECoG): 0 = absent; 1 = low activity; 2 = medium; 3 = high. EMG = electromyography.

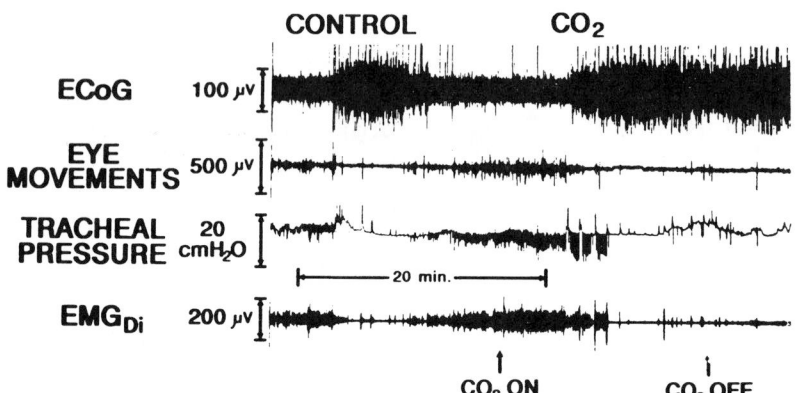

Figure 87–5. Fetal breathing during control and during CO_2 rebreathing. Note the increase in tracheal pressure and diaphragmatic activity during CO_2 rebreathing. Fetal breathing was prolonged into the transitional low-voltage to high-voltage electrocortical activity (ECoG), but it stopped in established high-voltage ECoG. EMG_{Di} = electromyographic diaphragmatic activity.

fetal breathing apparatus is capable of responding well to chemical stimuli and to other agents known to modify breathing postnatally. Thus, it became clear that the fetus responds to an increase in partial pressure of arterial carbon dioxide ($Paco_2$) with an increase in breathing.[17,18,27,29,33,34,36] This increase is associated with increases in tracheal pressure, integrated diaphragmatic activity, and frequency (Fig. 87-5). Both inspiratory and expiratory times decrease, as would be expected from postnatal studies.[29] The increased breathing activity is prolonged into the transitional HVECoG, but it does not continue into the established HVECoG.[29]

We specifically investigated whether we could increase $Paco_2$ during rebreathing or during direct administration of carbon dioxide to the fetus through an endotracheal tube.[29] Breathing activity was always abolished in established HVECoG, and only when $Paco_2$ was unphysiologically high (>100 mm Hg) and pH was low (<7.0) could breathing be initiated in HVECoG. At this level of acidosis, low pH could have been the primary stimulus to initiate breathing, because acidosis has been shown to induce continuous breathing.[37] This increased breathing activity was not associated with wakefulness.[29] Conversely, reducing $Paco_2$ to less

than the *apneic threshold level* abolishes breathing activity,[38] as has been shown in postnatal life.[39,40-43]

Administration of low oxygen to the fetus by having the ewe breathe hypoxic mixtures abolished fetal breathing. This was associated with a decrease of body movements and a decrease in the amplitude of the ECoG.[18,44] Conversely, an increase in arterial partial pressure of oxygen (Pao_2) to levels greater than 200 mm Hg through the administration of 100% oxygen by an endotracheal tube induced continuous fetal breathing in some experiments in sheep.[45] These findings suggest that the low Pao_2 in the fetus at rest may be a normal mechanism contributing to inhibition of breathing *in utero.*

Of the pulmonary reflexes, the inflation reflex of Hering-Breuer is present in fetal life. Lung distention with saline infusion produced decreased frequency of breathing.[14,15] Section of the vagus nerve, however, did not alter breathing pattern, and the relevance of the pulmonary reflexes to fetal breathing is still not clear.[24,31]

Pharmacologic agents, such as indomethacin, pilocarpine, 5-hydroxytryptophan, and morphine, induce continuous breathing in the fetus for a variable duration.[26,29,34,46-49] This continu-

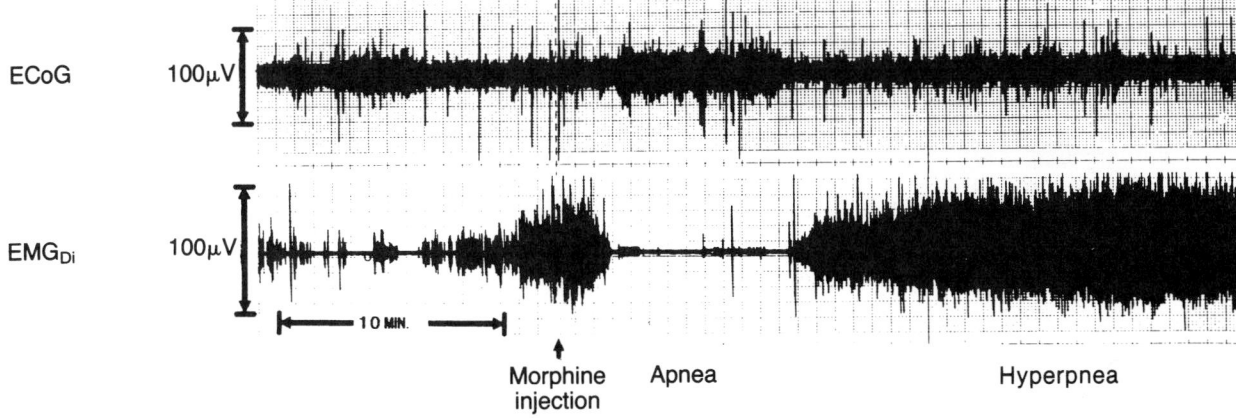

Figure 87–6. The fetal response to intravenous injection of morphine. Administration of morphine-induced apnea was followed by prolonged and intense continuous breathing. Apnea coincided with a change in electrocortical activity (ECoG) from low to high voltage, and, conversely, hyperpnea was associated with a change in ECoG from high to low voltage. During hyperpnea, at times, the fetus showed signs of arousal, such as open eyes, squirming, and licking. EMG_{Di} = electromyographic diaphragmatic activity.

ous breathing classically crosses the ECoG barrier; that is, it occurs with LVECoG and HVECoG (Fig. 87-6). As the response starts to fade, the HVECoG breaks in, and breathing is inhibited. Intense breathing is restricted to periods of LVECoG. Once the pharmacologic effects subside and breathing becomes normal again, the intensity of breathing activity decreases. There are two interesting facts about this prolonged breathing response to pharmacologic agents. First, fetuses in general do not tend to wake except when the stimulus is morphine; and second, prolonged breathing tends to cross the HVECoG barrier. In response to morphine given during a breathing interval, the fetus becomes apneic and simultaneously switches from LVECoG to HVECoG; this state is followed by a prolonged run of continuous breathing, lasting an average of about 2 hours, during which the fetus switches back to LVECoG.[2, 47] During the period of maximal breathing, fetuses may open their eyes, increase body movements, and have some swallowing activity, a behavior suggesting arousal.[47] This effect is transient and accounts for only part of the breathing response to morphine. During administration of pilocarpine, I noticed the fetus opening its eyes on one occasion, but behaviorally the fetus seemed to be in REM sleep.[34] All these pharmacologic agents produce an increase in tracheal pressure and integrated diaphragmatic EMG activity, but only indomethacin, pilocarpine, and morphine increase respiratory frequency. With 5-hydroxytryptophan, breathing was deep and slow.[34] Because endogenous opiates have been hypothesized to inhibit fetal breathing, some investigators have reported that naloxone given to the fetus results in continuous breathing, a lowered threshold for carbon dioxide stimulation of breathing, and increased wakefulness.[33] I could not corroborate these findings in experiments using the window technique.[34] Indeed, in dosages of naloxone equivalent to those used in other experiments,[33] I produced seizures in the fetus that were associated with intense and prolonged body convulsions, followed by limited periods of continuous breathing. I believe that this action is agonist and depends on the central stimulant effects of naloxone, not on its inhibitory action on endogenous opiates.

There is much evidence suggesting that the actions of carbon dioxide and those of the pharmacologic agents are central. The effect of hypoxia is poorly understood, but it also seems to act centrally. The peripheral chemoreceptors were originally thought to be inactive *in utero*; however, the idea that they are completely silent was probably derived from incorrect experimental evidence.[50] Blanco and co-workers[51] clearly documented activity of the peripheral chemoreceptors in the fetal lamb and showed that these chemoreceptors are reset at the time of delivery. Johnston

and Gluckman[52] found that the response to hypoxia in the fetal lamb with a pontine lesion (an area that appears responsible for the response to hypoxia) is mediated through peripheral chemoreceptors. Resection of the carotid bodies does not alter fetal breathing or the fetal state substantially and apparently does not alter the establishment of breathing at birth.[53,54] The exact relevance of peripheral chemoreceptors to intrauterine breathing remains undetermined.

ESTABLISHMENT OF CONTINUOUS BREATHING AT BIRTH

Breathing is intermittent in the fetus and becomes continuous after birth. The mechanism responsible for this transition from intermittent to continuous breathing is unknown. The traditional view about the onset of continuous breathing at birth is that labor and delivery produce transient fetal asphyxia that stimulates the peripheral chemoreceptors to induce the first extrauterine breath. Breathing is then maintained through the input of other stimuli such as cold, touch, and other sensory stimuli.[10, 55-58] This overall view was generated through experiments done decades ago in the acute exteriorized fetal preparation at a time when the general consensus was that the fetus did not breathe *in utero*.

Some observations have made this general view open to question. First, denervation of the carotid and aortic chemoreceptors does not alter fetal breathing or the initiation of continuous breathing at birth (Figs. 87-7 and 87-8).[53,54] Second, continuous breathing can be initiated *in utero*, with manifestations of arousal, by raising Pa_{O_2} with administration of 100% oxygen to the fetus through an endotracheal tube (Fig. 87-9).[45] Continuous breathing does not occur if the Pa_{O_2} does not rise. In fetuses in which Pa_{O_2} does not rise, however, continuous breathing will subsequently initiate on umbilical cord occlusion.[45] This continuous breathing in response to high Pa_{O_2} or cord occlusion is independent of an increase in Pa_{CO_2}, because it remains when P_{CO_2} is kept constant by ventilating the fetus with high-frequency oscillation. These observations during administration of 100% oxygen and cord occlusion suggest that the fetus can resemble a newborn *in utero*. Breathing can occur in the fetus in the absence of transient hypoxemia to stimulate the peripheral chemoreceptors and without any of the sensory stimuli (e.g., cold) thought to be important for the establishment of continuous breathing at birth. Together, these observations suggest that continuous breathing at birth may depend more on a hormone or chemical mediator than on low oxygen or sensory stimuli. It

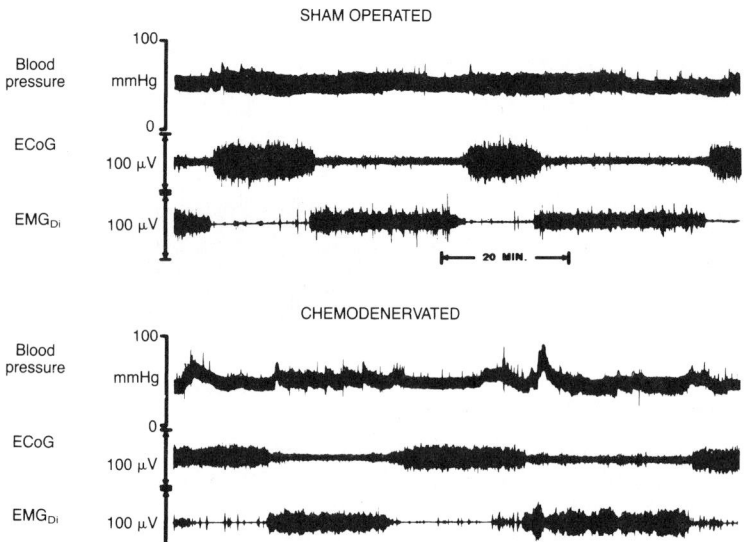

Figure 87–7. Breathing activity in a sham-operated fetal sheep (132 days' gestation) and in a chemodenervated fetal sheep (130 days' gestation). Breathing activity remains intact in the chemodenervated fetus. Blood gases were comparable in the two fetuses. ECoG = electrocortical activity; EMG$_{Di}$ = electromyographic diaphragmatic activity.

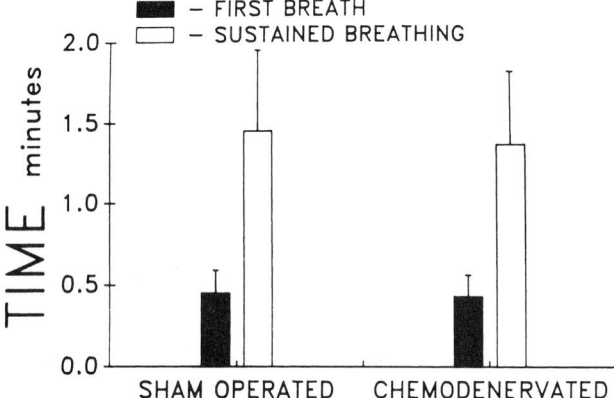

Figure 87–8. Delay in minutes from opening of the window to the appearance of the first breath and to sustained breathing. There were no significant differences between the two groups.

is indeed tempting to speculate that occlusion of the umbilical cord in the presence of appropriate oxygenation is needed to maintain continuous breathing. In the mid-1990s, my colleagues and I investigated the role of placental products on the control of fetal breathing.[59, 60] Initial results suggested that a small peptide was involved in the inhibition of breathing. However, it has since become clear that the inhibitory role of the placental extract relates to the presence of prostaglandin and not of a small peptide (Fig. 87-10). The exact prostaglandin that has a predominant role in this inhibition remains unknown.

THE NEONATE

Breathing Pattern at Rest

The neonate, particularly the premature infant, breathes irregularly. There is great breath-to-breath variability and long stretches of periodic breathing in which breathing and apnea alternate.[9, 61-65] Douglas and Haldane's statement that "the sur-

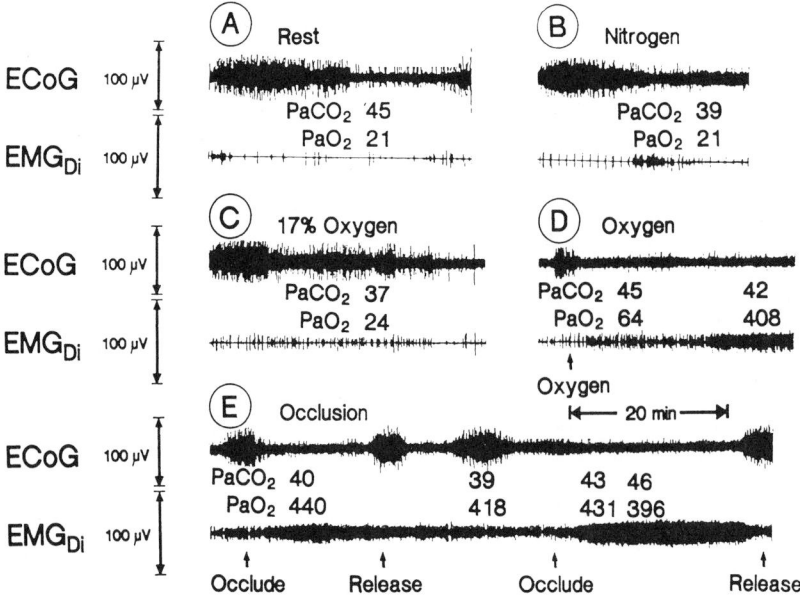

Figure 87–9. Representative tracing showing the effect of various concentrations of O$_2$ on fetal breathing and electrocortical activity (ECoG). **A,** Control cycle showing little breathing in a fetus in early labor at 143 days' gestation. **B,** Lung distention (mean airway pressure 30 cm H$_2$O) and inspired N$_2$ do not affect baseline tracing. **C,** Breathing is not altered by 17% O$_2$. **D,** Administration of 100% O$_2$ induces continuous breathing. **E,** Occlusion on two occasions induces more forceful breathing than that observed with O$_2$ alone. Continuous breathing was elicited despite preventing the rise of Paco$_2$ by ventilating the fetus with high-frequency ventilation (15 Hz, stroke = 7 cm H$_2$O). EMG$_{Di}$ = electromyographic diaphragmatic activity.

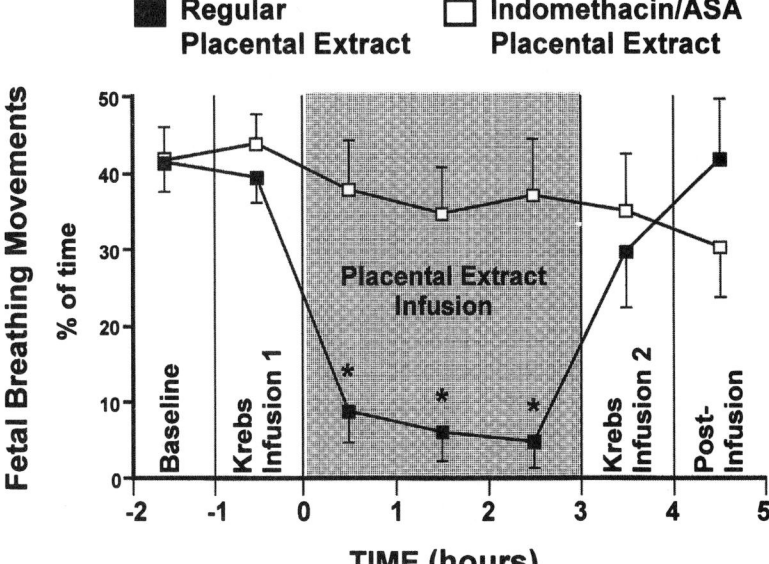

Figure 87–10. Illustration of the effect of eliminating the prostaglandins from the placental extract on fetal breathing. Fetal breathing remained essentially unchanged with the infusion of a regular placental extract (not treated with indomethacin/acetylsalicylic acid [ASA]), whereas it decreased significantly with the infusion of an indomethacin/ASA-treated extract.

prising fact is not that we breathe regularly, but that we do not breathe periodically most of the time" applies more at this age than at any other.[66] The resting breathing pattern of the neonate is not sleep-state dependent, although sleep greatly modulates it.[3,67] Neonates spend 90% of their time in REM sleep at 30 weeks of gestation and 50% at term as compared with 20% in adult subjects.[3-5] Quiet sleep is difficult to define before 32 weeks' gestation, and wakefulness occurs rarely in the newborn. We have shown that periodic breathing, a common breathing pattern in premature infants in which they alternate between breathing intervals and apneas lasting 5 to 10 seconds, occurs in the three states—wakefulness, REM, and quiet sleep—but its prevalence is increased in REM sleep.[3] It is frequently stated in textbooks that in quiet sleep, in analogy with criteria used for adult subjects, breathing is regular. However, our laboratory and others have shown that periodic breathing is common in quiet sleep.[9,68,69] The difference is that periodic breathing in quiet sleep is regular—that is, the breathing and apneic intervals are of similar duration, and it is very irregular in REM sleep. The best-defined periodic breathing observable in small babies is in quiet sleep during tracé alternant electroencephalogram (EEG) (Fig. 87-11). Therefore, there are two major differences between neonates and adults regarding staging of sleep state. One difference relates to the patterns of breathing observed in quiet and REM sleep states and the other to the presence of the tracé alternant EEG during quiet sleep in the neonate. Because this EEG pattern subsides after 44 weeks' postconceptional age, it is not used in adults to characterize quiet sleep. Finally, the overall minute ventilation is increased in REM sleep as compared with quiet sleep, and this is the result of a primary increase in respiratory frequency with little change in tidal volume.[3,6,9]

Periodic Breathing and Apnea

Periodic breathing, defined as pauses in respiratory movements that last for up to 20 seconds alternating with breathing, is common in preterm infants. When the respiratory pause is longer than 20 seconds, it is called *apnea.*[70] Although the duration used to distinguish periodic breathing and apnea is arbitrary, it has proved useful and has been widely adopted. Periodic breathing is not as harmful as apnea because the respiratory pause is short and the decrease in heart rate is minor. In contrast, apnea is a more serious condition; the respiratory pause is longer and is frequently associated with decreases in heart rate to less

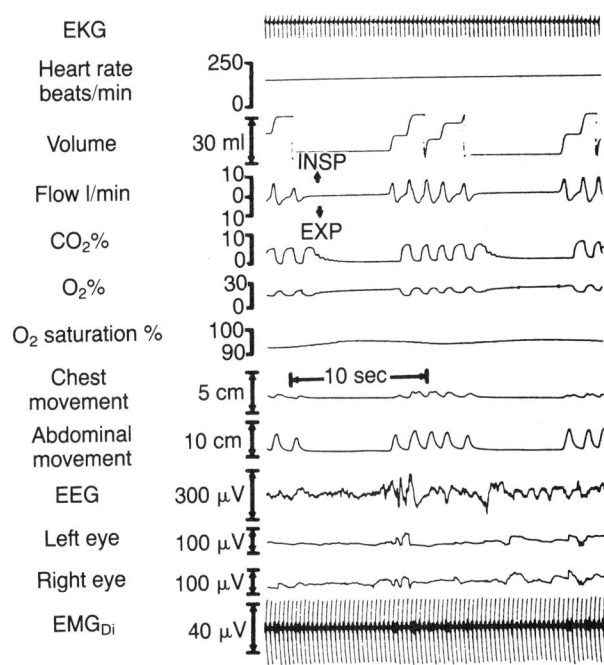

Figure 87–11. Periodic breathing during quiet sleep in an 8-day-old preterm infant born at 32 weeks. Note the regular periodicity of breathing, with both apneic and breathing intervals keeping a constant length. Note also the classic tracé alternant pattern on the electroencephalogram (EEG). ECG = electrocardiogram ; EMG_{Di} = electromyographic diaphragmatic activity.

than 80 beats/minute.[62,70] In very small preterm infants, significant bradycardia can occur with very short apneic pauses. In this instance, therefore, the length of the respiratory pause is not a very useful indicator of severity of the disruption in breathing. For this reason, many centers, including ours, have decided to rely on heart rate as the primary indicator of severity.

Apneic episodes in the neonate are classified according to the absence or presence of breathing efforts during the period of no airflow.[71] Central apneas are those with no flow and no observable breathing efforts. Obstructive apneas are those with no flow

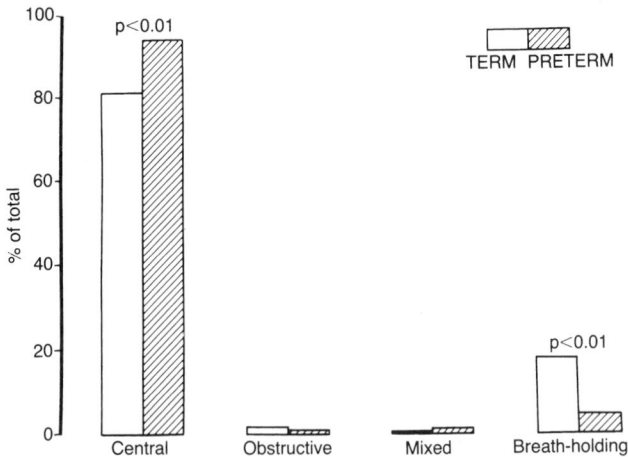

Figure 87–12. Frequency distribution of the various types of apnea in healthy preterm and term infants. Central apneas are predominant. The frequency of breath-holding apneas is greater in term than in preterm infants. Obstructive and mixed types of apnea are rare.

despite breathing efforts. Mixed apneas begin as central and end as obstructive apnea. Breath-holding apneas are those in which flow stops at midexpiration, and the remaining expiration occurs just before breathing starts again. A newer method of classifying apneas, based on a magnified cardiac-induced pulse observed on the respiratory flow tracing, has been described. This method is able to detect the presence and timing of airway obstructions with great precision. Using this method, it is obvious that some apneas, previously classified as central because of absence of respiratory efforts, are indeed obstructive.[72] My colleagues and I have been using this method extensively in our experimental studies, but its use in routine clinical care is not yet established.

In preterm infants with underlying disease who are followed-up longitudinally, central apneas predominate, and purely obstructive apneas are rare (Fig. 87–12).[71] Obstructive apneas are more commonly noted as part of a mixed apneic event. In preterm infants recovering from respiratory support, with some degree of residual lung disease (bronchopulmonary dysplasia), the prevalence of obstructive apneas appears to be increased, comprising up to 48% of the apneas in some studies.[73] There is no clear explanation for the obstruction, but it seems to be at the level of the larynx.[73] Our initial observations suggest that borderline hypoxemia of these infants may be a predisposing factor. One report described obstruction in 80% of the pauses in preterm infants with periodic breathing.[74] In unpublished observations, my colleagues and I have not corroborated this high prevalence, but small preterm infants can exhibit short mixed apneas associated with a significant decrease in heart rate.

Periodic breathing and apnea are clearly consequences of a disturbance of the respiratory control system, but the precise mechanisms are unclear. Investigators in this area tend to believe that the negative feedback loop controlling respiration is affected by multiple factors related primarily to anatomic and physiologic immaturity. For example, arborization of dendrites at 30 weeks' gestation is meager, and neuroconduction and synaptic relay are impaired.[75] Delays in traffic of neuromessages may then make the system oscillate. Unfortunately, we do not know how much immaturity is needed for a given impairment in neurophysiologic traffic. Oscillation in arterial gas tensions, changes in circulation time, incoordination of the respiratory pump owing to a compliant chest wall, and changes in sleep state may all contribute to this instability of the respiratory control system.[70]

Periodic breathing and apnea probably have common physiopathogenic roots; apnea is probably just a more severe manifestation of the disturbance that induces periodic breathing. This was demonstrated more conclusively in studies in which my colleagues and I observed that long apneas (≥ 20 seconds' duration) are not random events. They are almost invariably preceded by apneas of progressively increased duration.[76] In infants who breathe periodically and who develop apnea, the ventilatory system is depressed, as reflected by a high $Paco_2$ and a low minute ventilation. Additionally, the carbon dioxide response curve is shifted to the right, and the slope is slightly decreased in infants with apnea.[63] This physiologic configuration predisposes the system to oscillation. Compared with those in infants who breathe continuously, the peripheral chemoreceptors of infants with periodic breathing and apnea seem hyperactive, as reflected by the longer apneic period and more pronounced immediate decrease in ventilation that periodic breathers manifest on inhalation of high-oxygen mixtures.[62,63] Hypoxia may be a contributing factor, because inhalation of a low-oxygen mixture easily induces periodic breathing and apnea in these infants. In response to a hypoxic inspired mixture, small infants manifest a transient increase in ventilation followed by a decrease (Fig. 87–13);[77,78] apnea usually appears during the late response. In adults, the response is also biphasic, but the decrease in ventilation is less pronounced.[79,80] The initial increase in ventilation reflects peripheral chemoreceptor activity; the mechanism responsible for the late response is controversial.[64] In kittens, the late decrease in ventilation is probably the result of mechanical failure, possibly the result of an increase in pulmonary impedance caused by hypoxia-related bronchoconstriction.[81] The same mechanism may also explain why the ventilatory response to carbon dioxide in neonates is less under hypoxic conditions in comparison with hyperoxic conditions.[82]

The sleep state appears to be a contributing factor, because periodic breathing and apnea are more frequent in REM sleep than in quiet sleep. The neonate sleeps almost uninterruptedly, continuously alternating between REM sleep and quiet sleep. This pattern increases instability in the respiratory control system. Indeed, minor alterations during sleep, such as a startle or a sigh, produce apnea in these infants. The almost continuous change in baseline ventilation during sleep is what Douglas and Haldane called "the hunting of the respiratory centre."[66]

Although sleep modulates breathing, it does not cause apnea; apnea also occurs during wakefulness. The high prevalence of apnea during REM sleep may be related to muscle activity in this stage. During REM sleep, the tone of the intercostal muscles is abolished in conjunction with a decrease in diaphragmatic activity and in the tone of the adductor muscles of the upper airway, a combination of factors likely to induce chest distortion, impairment of the braking mechanism during expiration, pulmonary collapse, and apnea (Fig. 87–14).[70] When chest distortion occurs, diaphragmatic work increases by about 40%, adding to the mechanical impairment. This observation is compatible with the finding that the application of continuous negative pressure around the chest tends to abolish apnea.[83]

Chemical Regulation

Inhalation of carbon dioxide increases ventilation during REM and quiet sleep in newborn infants. The response to steady-state inhalation of carbon dioxide is the same in these two sleep states, but the response during rebreathing of carbon dioxide is less in REM than in quiet sleep (Fig. 87–15).[3,6,8,68] My colleagues and I postulated that the differences in response with these two techniques is related to the finding that when breathing is used, it is possible to measure the response in "phasic" REM only, whereas when the steady-state technique is used, the response always covers both "phasic" and "tonic" REM sleep.[68] Because the carbon dioxide response in "tonic" REM is the same as that during quiet sleep, the results using the steady-state method tend to resemble those in quiet sleep.[7,84]

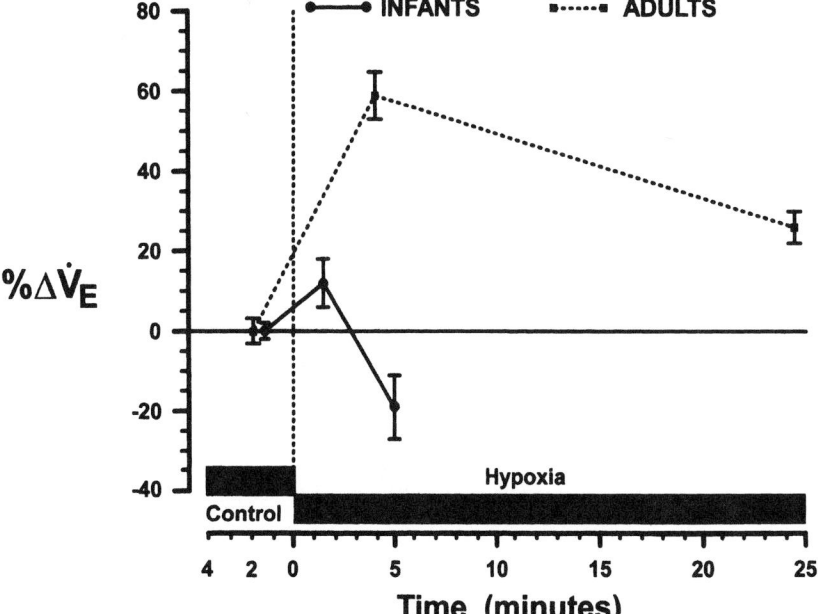

Figure 87–13. Ventilatory response ($\%\Delta\dot{V}_E$) to low inhaled oxygen in preterm infant and adult subjects. Preterm infants were studied during quiet sleep in the prone position; adults were studied during wakefulness in the sitting position. Both responses are biphasic, and the late depression in ventilation is more pronounced in preterm infants. (Adapted from Sankaran K, et al: Immediate and late ventilatory response to high and low O_2 in preterm infants and adult subjects. Pediatr Res *13*:875, 1979; and Easton PA, et al: Ventilatory response to sustained hypoxia in normal adults. J Appl Physiol *61*:906, 1986.)

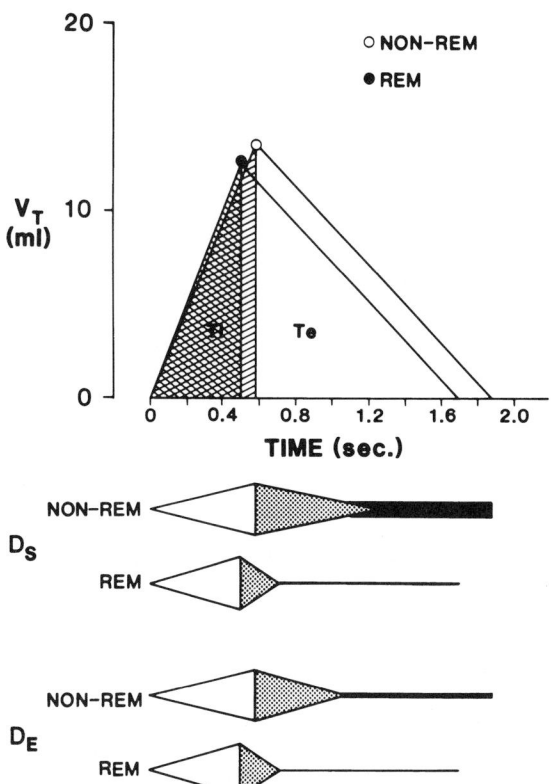

Figure 87–14. Diagrammatic changes in tidal volume, timing, and diaphragmatic EMG in non-rapid eye movement (non-REM) (quiet) and REM (active) sleep. Total phasic activity diminishes from non-REM to REM sleep. Also, in both sleep states, it is shorter in esophageal (De) than in surface (Ds) EMG. Expiratory phase activity as a proportion of total phasic activity decreases significantly from non-REM to REM sleep. V_T = tidal volume.

The pattern of breathing observed with inhalation of carbon dioxide varies with the percentage of carbon dioxide inhaled. If the percentage of inhaled carbon dioxide is low (<2%) during steady-state inhalation, the response will consist primarily of an increase in tidal volume.[9] If the percentage of inhaled carbon dioxide is high (>2%), the response in both sleep states will consist of an increase in respiratory frequency and in tidal volume.[63,68] Periodic breathing is abolished with a small increase in inhaled carbon dioxide of about 1 to 2%.[9,63] This response has been attributed to the increased central drive and to increased stores of carbon dioxide, with better buffering capacity for the oscillations in Pa_{CO_2}.

Inhalation of low oxygen produces an immediate increase in ventilation (1 minute), followed by a later decrease (5 minutes).[61,64,85,86] The response is similar in wakefulness, in REM sleep, and in quiet sleep, although hyperventilation seems slightly more sustained during "late hypoxia" in quiet sleep.[3] The sustained hyperventilation in these infants during quiet sleep reflects the more autonomic control during this sleep state, in which the system is more responsive to chemical stimuli.[7,84] The immediate increase in ventilation reflects peripheral chemoreceptor stimulation and is associated with an increase in frequency and in tidal volume. The late response is primarily manifested by a decrease in frequency.[62,64] The mechanism responsible for this response is still unclear, and it may vary according to species. In humans, it is likely related to central release of inhibitory neuromodulators.[78,79,80] However, experiments in kittens and in newborn monkeys suggest that the late decrease in ventilation may be a mechanical effect rather than a depression of the central respiratory neurons.[81,87,88] In these experiments, diaphragmatic activity and frequency remained elevated during hypoxia, but tidal volume decreased to less than control values during late hypoxia. These experiments were carried out while the subjects were in quiet sleep. The peculiar response of the neonate to low inhaled oxygen is of great clinical significance. Infants who are borderline hypoxic tend to breathe periodically or to develop apneic spells. Hypoxia can

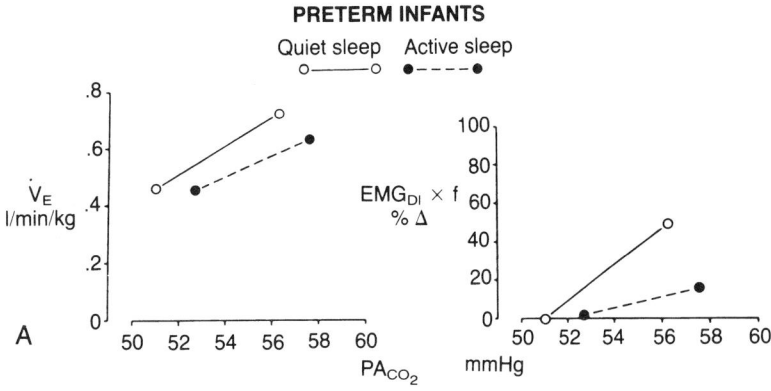

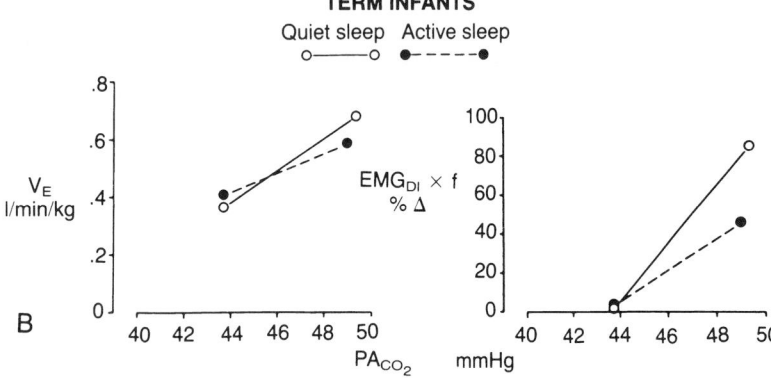

Figure 87–15. The ventilatory response to CO_2 rebreathing in neonates. Preterm (**A**) and term (**B**) infants showed a decreased response to CO_2 in phasic rapid eye movement sleep as compared with quiet sleep. EMG_{Di} = electromyographic diaphragmatic activity; V_E = minute ventilation.

induce periodic breathing in these infants, as shown previously.[58] Relief from these apneic spells, which are frequently associated with bradycardias, can be obtained by increasing the inspired oxygen concentration.[62,63]

Administration of high concentrations of oxygen, conversely, produces an immediate decrease in ventilation followed by hyperventilation, a response that is similar during wakefulness, REM, and quiet sleep. These findings suggest a lack of major differences in the activity of the peripheral chemoreceptors during these sleep states.[70, 89] The immediate decrease in ventilation after the administration of 100% oxygen is related to a decrease in frequency (apnea is common in preterm infants) and a decrease in tidal volume. The late increase in ventilation with oxygen is likely related to cerebral vasoconstriction with an increased hydrogen ion concentration at the chemoreceptor site.[90]

Pulmonary Reflexes

The *inflation reflex of Hering-Breuer* is much more active in the newborn period than in adult life.[91, 92] Small increases in lung volume cause apnea. This response is so powerful in the newborn that many investigators have used this inflation to produce apnea and then to study the mechanical properties of the respiratory system during the passive expiratory phase after apnea. The action of the stretch receptors is influenced by sleep state; it is abolished during REM sleep. The irritant receptors are also poorly developed in preterm infants, and the mediated reflexes are also abolished during REM sleep.[93] Therefore, airway mechanisms responsible for clearing, such as cough, are impaired during REM sleep. The paradoxical *reflex of Head* is commonly observed in the neonate in the form of a sigh.[94] Many investigators attribute the high prevalence of sighs to the greater need for lung recruitment at this age.[95] Sighs are more frequent

in REM than quiet sleep and are also more frequent during periodic than regular breathing. During periodic breathing, a sigh usually appears during the first or second breath after apnea. When it occurs during regular breathing, it tends to be followed by short apneas.[96] Efforts to discover the mechanisms triggering sighs have been fruitless. Thach and Tauesch[95] showed that asphyxia does not seem to be a stimulus. Alvarez and co-workers,[97] however, observed that airway occlusion in the presence of hypoxia predisposes to sighs.

Respiratory Muscles

The activity of the respiratory muscles is much altered by sleep state. Tonic activity of most respiratory muscles is abolished during REM sleep.[19, 28, 98, 99] The disappearance of tone in the intercostal muscles has been suggested as a major factor responsible for the increased chest distortion seen during REM sleep in infants with this condition. Lack of tone leads to chest wall collapse during inspiration, and caudal displacement of the diaphragm has to be twice as great to produce the same lung volume displacement.[98, 100] Because of chest wall collapse, functional residual capacity is decreased in these infants during REM sleep.[98] My colleagues and I have found that distorted and nondistorted breaths produce the same instantaneous ventilation as long as they are of the same duration, although the work of the diaphragm is 40% greater when distortion is present.[100] Postinspiratory activity of the diaphragm is also affected by sleep. This activity controls, in part, the duration of expiratory time.[101, 102] In neonates, this activity is more pronounced in the lateral than in the crural part of the diaphragm, it is longer in quiet than in REM sleep, and it is more prolonged in preterm than in term infants.[103, 104] The length and variability of this activity in preterm infants suggest that because of their highly compliant chest wall, these infants use the postinspiratory diaphragmatic activity as a braking mechanism. The role of the postinspiratory diaphragmatic activity in maintaining lung volume and in controlling expiratory time is much more important in the newborn than in older children and adults. Similarly, sleep state profoundly affects the muscular control of upper airway resistance. Studies in fetal and neonatal lambs suggest that the abductor muscles of the larynx—the posterior cricoarytenoid and cricothyroid—have inspiratory activities parallel to those of the diaphragm during both quiet and REM sleep. Conversely, the adductor muscles of the larynx—the thyroarytenoid, lateral cricoarytenoid, and intra-arytenoid—have a phasic expiratory activity during quiet sleep. This activity is lost during REM sleep in the fetus and in the newborn lamb.[19,28] A reduction in adductor activity of the larynx, in conjunction with decreased intercostal and decreased postinspiratory diaphragmatic activity during REM sleep, may cause the decrease in lung volume observed during this sleep state.

CONCLUSIONS

In summary, although the basic mechanisms involved in the control of breathing during fetal and neonatal life are similar to those investigated more extensively in adults, there are some aspects that make this control unique at this early age. First, sleep seems to have a very profound effect during this period of life, particularly in the fetus, in which breathing is allowed to surface only during REM sleep. Second, breathing activity is present *in utero* beginning early in gestation. Fetal breathing occurs without apparent reason, because it is not responsible for gas exchange. To explain why this episodic breathing *in utero* becomes continuous after birth is the major challenge of the moment. Trying to understand this change at birth may result in the discovery of key mediators that are at the heart of the mechanism controlling breathing in general.

REFERENCES

1. Parmelee AH, et al: Sleep states in premature infants. Dev Med Child Neurol 9:70, 1967.
2. Rigatto H, et al: Fetal breathing and behavior measured through a double-wall Plexiglas window in sheep. J Appl Physiol 61:160, 1986.
3. Rigatto H, et al: Ventilatory response to 100% and 15% O₂ during wakefulness and sleep in preterm infants. Early Hum Dev 7:1, 1982.
4. Stern E, et al: Sleep cycle characteristics in infants. Pediatrics 43:65, 1969.
5. Bülow K: Respiration and wakefulness in man. Acta Physiol Scand Suppl 59:1, 1963.
6. Davi M, et al: Effect of sleep state on chest distortion and on the ventilatory response to CO₂ in neonates. Pediatr Res 13:982, 1979.
7. Phillipson EA: Control of breathing during sleep. Am Rev Respir Dis 118:909, 1978.
8. Reed DJ, Kellogg RH: Changes in respiratory response to CO₂ during natural sleep at sea level and at altitude. J Appl Physiol 13:325, 1958.
9. Kalapesi Z, et al: Effect of periodic or regular respiratory pattern on the ventilatory response to low inhaled CO₂ in preterm infants during sleep. Am Rev Respir Dis 123:8, 1981.
10. Dawes GS, et al: Respiratory movements and paradoxical sleep in the fetal lamb. J Physiol (Lond) 210:47P, 1970.
11. Merlet C, et al: Mise en evidence de mouvements respiratoires chez le foetus d'agneau. C R Acad Sci Ser D 270:2462, 1970.
12. Ioffe S, et al: Respiratory response to somatic stimulation in fetal lambs during sleep and wakefulness. Pflugers Arch 388:143, 1980.
13. Ioffe S, et al: Sleep, wakefulness and the monosynaptic reflex in fetal and newborn lambs. Pflugers Arch 388:149, 1980.
14. Maloney JE, et al: Modification of respiratory center output in the unanesthetized fetal sheep *in utero*. J Appl Physiol 39:552, 1975.
15. Maloney JE, et al: "Fetal breathing" and the development of patterns of respiration before birth. Sleep 3:299, 1980.
16. Rigatto H, et al: The response to stimulation of hindlimb nerves in fetal sheep, *in utero*, during the different phases of electrocortical activity. J Dev Physiol 4:175, 1982.
17. Boddy K, Dawes GS: Fetal breathing. Br Med Bull 31:3, 1975.
18. Boddy K, et al: Foetal respiratory movements, electrocortical and cardiovascular responses to hypoxaemia and hypercapnia in sheep. J Physiol (Lond) 243:599, 1974.
19. Harding R, et al: Laryngeal function during breathing and swallowing in foetal and newborn lambs. J Physiol (Lond) 272:14P, 1977.
20. Maloney JE, et al: Diaphragmatic activity and lung liquid flow in the unanesthetized fetal sheep. J Appl Physiol 39:423, 1975.
21. Patrick J, et al: A definition of human fetal apnea and the distribution of apneic intervals during the last ten weeks of pregnancy. Am J Obstet Gynecol 136:471, 1980.
22. Patrick J, et al: Patterns of human fetal breathing during the last 10 weeks of pregnancy. Obstet Gynecol 56:24, 1980.
23. Hagan RAC, et al: The effect of sleep state on intercostal muscle activity and rib cage motion. Physiologist 19:214, 1976.
24. Dawes GS: Breathing before birth in animals and man: an essay in developmental medicine. N Engl J Med 290:557, 1974.
25. Dawes GS, et al: Respiratory movements and rapid eye movement sleep in the fetal lamb. J Physiol (Lond) 220:119, 1972.
26. Kitterman JA, et al: Stimulation of breathing movements in fetal sheep by inhibitors of prostaglandin synthesis. J Dev Physiol 1:453, 1979.
27. Dawes GS, et al: Effects of hypercapnia on tracheal pressure, diaphragm and intercostal electromyograms in unanesthetized fetal lambs. J Physiol (Lond) 326:461, 1982.
28. Harding R, et al: Respiratory function of the larynx in developing sheep and the influence of sleep state. Respir Physiol 40:165, 1980.
29. Rigatto H, et al: Effect of increased arterial CO₂ on fetal breathing and behavior in sheep. J Appl Physiol 64:982, 1988.
30. Condorelli S, Scarpelli EM: Somatic-respiratory reflex and onset of regular breathing movements in the lamb fetus in utero. Pediatr Res 9:879, 1975.
31. Condorelli S, Scarpelli EM: Fetal breathing: induction in utero and effects of vagotomy and barbiturates. J Pediatr 88:94, 1976.
32. Ruckebusch Y: Development of sleep and wakefulness in the foetal lamb. Electroencephalogr Clin Neurophysiol 32:119, 1972.
33. Moss IR, Scarpelli EM: Generation and regulation of breathing *in utero*: fetal CO₂ response test. J Appl Physiol 47:527, 1979.
34. Rigatto H: A new window on the chronic fetal sheep model. *In* Nathanielsz PW (ed): Animal Models in Fetal Medicine III. Ithaca, NY, Perinatology Press, 1984, pp 57–67.
35. Chernick V: Fetal breathing movements and the onset of breathing at birth. Clin Perinatol 5:257, 1978.
36. Jansen AH, et al: Influence of sleep state on the response to hypercapnia in fetal lambs. Respir Physiol 48:125, 1982.
37. Molteni RA, et al: Induction of fetal breathing by metabolic acidemia and its effect on blood flow to the respiratory muscles. Am J Obstet Gynecol 136:609, 1980.
38. Kuipers IM, et al: Effect of mild hypocapnia on fetal breathing and behavior in unanesthetized normoxic fetal lambs. J Appl Physiol 76:1476, 1994.
39. Phillipson E, et al: Critical dependence of respiratory rhythmicity on metabolic CO₂ load. J Appl Physiol 50:45, 1981.
40. Phillipson EA, Bowes G: Control of breathing during sleep. *In* Fishman AP, et al (eds): Handbook of Physiology, vol II, part 2. Bethesda, MD, American Physiological Society, 1986, pp 649–689.
41. Kolobow T, et al: Control of breathing using an extracorporeal membrane lung. Anesthesiology 46:138, 1977.
42. Canet E, et al: Apnea threshold and breathing rhythmicity in newborn lambs. J Appl Physiol 74:3013, 1993.
43. Khan A, et al: The vulnerability of the "CO₂ apneic threshold" in neonates. Pediatr Res 49:380A, 2001.
44. Clewlow F, et al: Changes in breathing, electrocortical and muscle activity in unanaesthetized fetal lambs with age. J Physiol (Lond) 341:463, 1983.
45. Baier RJ, et al: The effects of continuous distending airway pressure under various background concentrations of oxygen, high frequency oscillatory ventilation, and umbilical cord occlusion on fetal breathing and behavior in sheep. *In* Proceedings of the Society for the Study of Fetal Physiology. Cairns, Australia, Society for the Study of Fetal Physiology, 1988, p 26.
46. Brown ER, et al: Regular fetal breathing induced by pilocarpine infusion in the near-term fetal sheep. J Appl Physiol 50:1348, 1981.
47. Hasan SU, et al: Effect of morphine on breathing and behavior in fetal sheep. J Appl Physiol 64:2058, 1988.
48. Olsen GD, Dawes GS: Morphine effects on fetal lambs. Fed Proc 42:1251, 1983.
49. Quilligan EJ, et al: Effect of 5-hydroxytryptophan on electrocortical activity and breathing movements of fetal sheep. Am J Obstet Gynecol 141:271, 1981.
50. Biscoe TJ, et al: Types of nervous activity which may be recorded from the carotid sinus nerve in the sheep foetus. J Physiol (Lond) 202:1, 1969.
51. Blanco CE, et al: The response to hypoxia of arterial chemoreceptors in fetal sheep and new-born lambs. J Physiol (Lond) 351:25, 1984.
52. Johnston BM, Gluckman PD: Peripheral chemoreceptors respond to hypoxia in pontine-lesioned fetal lambs in utero. J Appl Physiol 75:1027, 1993.
53. Jansen AH, et al: Effect of carotid chemoreceptor denervation on breathing *in utero* and after birth. J Appl Physiol 51:630, 1981.
54. Rigatto H, et al: The effect of total peripheral chemodenervation on fetal breathing and on the establishment of breathing at birth. Presented at the International Symposium on Fetal and Neonatal Development, Oxford, 1987.
55. Barcroft J: The onset of respiratory movement. *In* Researches on Pre-Natal Life. Oxford, Blackwell Scientific Publications, 1977, pp 260–272.
56. Dawes GS: The establishment of pulmonary respiration. *In* Foetal and Neonatal Physiology. Chicago, Year Book Medical Publishers, 1968, pp 125–140.
57. Gluckman PD, et al: The effect of cooling on breathing and shivering in unanesthetized foetal lambs *in utero*. J Physiol (Lond) 343:495, 1983.

58. Harned HS Jr, Ferreiro J: Initiation of breathing by cold stimulation: effects of change in ambient temperature on respiratory activity of the full-term fetal lamb. J Pediatr 83:663, 1973.

59. Alvaro RE, et al: Preliminary characterization of a placental factor inhibiting breathing in the fetal sheep. Pediatr Res 37:324A,1995.

60. Alvaro RE, et al: A placental factor inhibits breathing induced by umbilical cord occlusion in fetal sheep. J Dev Physiol 19:23,1993.

61. Cross KW, Oppé TE: The effect of inhalation of high and low concentrations of oxygen on the respiration of the premature infant. J Physiol (Lond) 117:38, 1952.

62. Rigatto H: Disorders of the control of breathing. In Pediatric respiratory diseases. Publication no. 86-2107. Bethesda, MD, National Institutes of Health, 1986, pp 20–25.

63. Rigatto H, Brady JP: Periodic breathing and apnea in preterm infants. I. Evidence for hypoventilation possibly due to central respiratory depression. Pediatrics 50:202, 1972.

64. Rigatto H, Brady JP: Periodic breathing and apnea in preterm infants. II. Hypoxia as a primary event. Pediatrics 50:219, 1972.

65. Waggener TB, et al: Apnea duration is related to ventilatory oscillation characteristics in newborn infants. J Appl Physiol 57:536, 1984.

66. Douglas CG, Haldane JS: The causes of periodic or Cheyne-Stokes breathing. J Physiol (Lond) 38:401, 1908–1909.

67. Gabriel M, et al: Apneic spells and sleep states in preterm infants. Pediatrics 57:142, 1976.

68. Moriette G, et al: The effect of rebreathing CO_2 on ventilation and diaphragmatic electromyography in newborn infants. Respir Physiol 62:387, 1985.

69. Prechtl HRF: The behavioural states of the newborn infant. Brain Res 76:185, 1974.

70. Rigatto H: Control of breathing in the neonate and the sudden infant death syndrome. In Fishman AP (ed): Pulmonary Diseases and Disorders, 2nd ed. New York, McGraw-Hill, 1988, pp 1363–1372.

71. Lee DSC, et al: A developmental study on types and frequency distribution of short apneas (3 to 15 seconds) in term and preterm infants. Pediatr Res 22:344, 1987.

72. Lemke RP, et al: The use of a magnified cardiac artifact in the respiratory flow tracing to evaluate airway closure may be a superior method of diagnosing types of apnea in neonates. Pediatr Res 37:340A, 1995.

73. Mathew OP, et al: Pharyngeal airway obstruction in preterm infants during mixed and obstructive apnea. J Pediatr 100:964, 1982.

74. Miller MJ, et al: Airway obstruction during periodic breathing in premature infants. J Appl Physiol 64:2496, 1988.

75. Purpura DP: Dendritic differentiation in human cerebral cortex: normal and aberrant development patterns. Adv Neurol 12:91, 1975.

76. Al-Saedi SA, et al: Prolonged apnea and respiratory instability in preterm infants: a discriminative study. Pediatr Res 37:324A, 1995.

77. Sankaran K, et al: Immediate and late ventilatory response to high and low O_2 in preterm infants and adult subjects. Pediatr Res 13:875, 1979.

78. Rehan V, et al: The biphasic ventilatory response to hypoxia in preterm infants is not due to a decrease in metabolism. Pediatr Pulmonol 22:287, 1996.

79. Easton PA, et al: Ventilatory response to sustained hypoxia in normal adults. J Appl Physiol 61:906, 1986.

80. Easton PA, et al: Recovery of the ventilatory response to hypoxia in normal adults. J Appl Physiol 64:521, 1988.

81. Rigatto H, et al: The ventilatory response to hypoxia in the unanesthetized newborn kittens. J Appl Physiol 64:2544, 1988.

82. Rigatto H, et al: The effects of O_2 on the ventilatory response to CO_2 in preterm infants. J Appl Physiol 39:896, 1975.

83. Thibeault DW, et al: Thoracic gas volume changes in premature infants. Pediatrics 40:403, 1967.

84. Phillipson EA, et al: Ventilatory and waking responses to CO_2 in sleeping dogs. Am Rev Respir Dis 115:251, 1977.

85. Brady JP, Ceruti E: Chemoreceptor reflexes in the new-born infant: effects of varying degrees of hypoxia on heart rate and ventilation in a warm environment. J Physiol (Lond) 184:631, 1966.

86. Brady JP, et al: Chemoreflexes in the newborn infant: Effects of 100% oxygen on heart rate and ventilation. J Physiol (Lond) 17:332, 1964.

87. LaFramboise WA, et al: Pulmonary mechanics during the ventilatory response to hypoxemia in the newborn monkey. J Appl Physiol 55:1008, 1983.

88. LaFramboise WA, Woodrum DE: Elevated diaphragm electromyogram during neonatal hypoxic ventilatory depression. J Appl Physiol 59:1040, 1985.

89. Aizad T, et al: Effect of a single breath of 100% oxygen on respiration in neonates during sleep. J Appl Physiol 57:1531, 1984.

90. Davi M, et al: Effect of inhaling 100% O_2 on ventilation and acid-base balance in cerebrospinal fluid in neonates. Biol Neonate 38:85, 1980.

91. Cross KW, et al: The response of the new-born baby to inflation of the lungs. J Physiol (Lond) 151:551, 1960.

92. Olinsky A, et al: Influence of lung inflation on respiratory control in neonates. J Appl Physiol 36:426, 1974.

93. Fleming PJ, et al: Functional immaturity of pulmonary irritant receptors and apnea in newborn preterm infants. Pediatrics 61:515, 1978.

94. Bodani J, et al: The effect of periodic breathing and sleep state on the incidence and "structure" of augmented breaths in neonates. Pediatr Res 18:402A, 1984.

95. Thach BT, Tauesch HW: Sighing in human newborn infants: role of inflation-augmenting reflex. J Appl Physiol 41:502, 1976.

96. Ardila R, et al: Relationship between infantile sleep apnea and preceding hyperventilation event? Clin Invest Med 9:A151, 1986.

97. Alvarez JE, et al: Sighs and their relationship to apnea in the newborn infant. Biol Neonate 63:139, 1993.

98. Henderson-Smart DJ, Read DJC: Reduced lung volume during behavioral active sleep in the newborn. J Appl Physiol 46:1081, 1979.

99. Lopes J, et al: Importance of inspiratory muscle tone in maintenance of FRC in the newborn. J Appl Physiol 51:830, 1981.

100. Luz J, et al: Effect of chest and abdomen uncoupling on ventilation and work of breathing in the newborn infant during sleep. Pediatr Res 16:297A, 1982.

101. Remmers JE, Bartlett D Jr: Reflex control of expiratory airflow and duration. J Appl Physiol 42:80, 1977.

102. Remmers JE, et al: Pathogenesis of upper airway occlusion during sleep. J Appl Physiol 44:931, 1978.

103. Reis FJC, et al: Diaphragmatic activity and ventilation in preterm infants. I. The effects of sleep state. Biol Neonate 65:16, 1994.

104. Reis FJC, et al: Diaphragmatic activity and ventilation in preterm infants. II. The effects of inhalation of 3% CO_2 and abdominal loading. Biol Neonate 65:69, 1994.

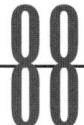

Dan Zhou and Gabriel G. Haddad

Basic Mechanisms of Oxygen-Sensing and Response to Hypoxia

A large body of experimental work has been performed on oxygen-sensing mechanisms and on the cellular events that result from oxygen deprivation. This work has been performed in a variety of cell types, tissues, and organs, and these comparative studies have contributed to our understanding of O_2 sensing. As a result of these investigations, a number of new concepts regarding O_2 sensing have emerged. Neurons, renal and respiratory epithelial cells, hepatocytes, myocardial cells, vascular smooth muscle, endothelial cells—virtually every cell type studied has been shown to sense O_2 one way or another. This type of investigation has also been done at various ages, and age has been very important in determining both sensing and responsiveness to lack of O_2. Since we have generally focused in the past on the study of nerve and glial cells during O_2 deprivation, this chapter focuses on excitable tissues. However, an extensive body of new knowledge has demonstrated recently that much of what is known about the heart's sensing mechanisms can be applied to the central nervous system (CNS), for example, and much of what we know about the renal epithelium can be applied to respiratory cells. It should be recognized, however, that although there are similarities between tissues, there are often major differences. These differences reflect either differing environments or the function of that particular cell type of tissue. In certain instances, when the duration and severity of the stimulus are not too overwhelming, nerve cells may adapt and possibly survive hypoxia. Often, however, when the stress is severe, the response of the cells, from sensing to death, is considerably shortened, and it is often difficult to tease apart the processes that control the various stages of response.

The aim of this chapter is to highlight observations that will demonstrate that there are a number of potential O_2 sensors in nerve cells. We detail results and data regarding ionic flux and controlling ionic flux mechanisms. We also detail some newer observations regarding gene activation during O_2 deprivation that occurs over much longer periods of time.

OXYGEN-SENSING VIA MEMBRANE PROTEINS: IONIC ALTERATIONS

Potassium Ionic Flux and Its Regulation; Short versus Long Exposures

Potassium ion (K^+) channel modulation has been shown to be an integral and important cellular response to O_2 deprivation in nerve and cardiac cells. It is not clear, however, what signals precede the modulation of K^+ channels. This modulation can be direct or indirect.[1,2] Part of this modulation occurs as a result of changes in the concentrations of cytosolic factors (e.g., ATP and Ca^{2+}) that are altered during O_2 deprivation. For example, a number of cytosolic factors change during hypoxia: Ca^+, pH, Na^+, ATP/ADP/AMP ratios, and redox.[3-8] These, in turn, modulate a number of ion channels, including K^+ channels.

If K^+ channels can be modulated by cytosolic changes during hypoxia, one should question whether there are mechanisms originating from changes other than in the cytosol. For example, does the partial pressure of O_2 itself affect plasma membrane channels? To test the hypothesis that membrane-delimited mechanisms participate in the O_2-sensing process and are involved in the modulation of K^+ channel activity in central neurons, experiments were performed using patch-clamp techniques and dissociated cells from the rat neocortex and substantia nigra.[1,2] Oxygen deprivation produced a biphasic response in current amplitude; there was an initial transient increase followed by a pronounced decrease in outward K^+ currents. The reduction in outward currents was a reversible process since perfusion with a normoxic medium with a P_{O_2} greater than 100 mm Hg (1 mm Hg = 133 Pa) resulted in complete recovery. In cell-free excised membrane patches, we have demonstrated that a specific K^+ current (large conductance, inhibited by micromolar concentrations of ATP and activated by Ca^{2+}) was reversibly inhibited by lack of O_2. This was characterized by a marked decrease in channel open-state probability and a slight reduction in unitary conductance. The magnitude of channel inhibition by O_2 deprivation was closely dependent on O_2 tension. These studies demonstrated the selective nature of the hypoxia-induced inhibition of some K^+ channels[1,2,8] (Figs. 88–1 and 88–2) and also provided the first evidence for the regulation of K^+ channel activity by O_2 deprivation in cell-free excised patches of central neurons.[1,2]

It is not well understood how this inhibition occurs. With the use of specific agents that chelate metal, including heme, nonheme iron, and copper, our laboratory has demonstrated that iron-center blockers inhibited the channel in excised patches in a fashion similar to that of low P_{O_2}. These results suggested that K^+ channel activity is modulated during hypoxia by iron-containing proteins, thus providing evidence for an O_2-sensing mechanism in neuronal membranes.

Although most ionic fluxes that have been studied during hypoxia are plasma membrane related, there have been a number of reports on ion channels in mitochondrial membranes.[9,10] However, it is unclear how these are involved in O_2 sensing or in hypoxic injury. We have recently obtained evidence that the maxi-K channels can be found in mitochondrial membranes and that they play a role in apoptotic cell death induced by serum deprivation.[11] Furthermore, data demonstrate that mitochondrial channels (ATP-dependent K^+ channels) are present in myocardial cells and may be important for hypoxic injury.[12]

The observation that the relative "insensitivity" or lack of response of immature cells or tissues to low O_2 tensions compared with the more mature response of differentiated cells is of particular interest. Based on a large number of studies investigating ion fluxes and activities, release of neurotransmitters, or changes in membrane electrophysiologic properties, it is clear that the newborn infant exhibits a blunted response to hypoxia.[3,13-17] Although there is a paucity of cellular and molecular work on this subject in the fetus, it is clear from whole-body studies in the fetus exposed to hypoxia that its response is very blunted, if not totally eliminated. In other types of studies, however, investigating the response of the neonatal lung to hypoxia (compared with that of the adult), the response in terms of septation and alveolar formation was more severe in the neonate than in the adult.[18] For example, hypoxia in the first couple of weeks of life will inhibit septation, whereas the adult there is very little effect on alveolar size.[18] Therefore, depending on the measured variable, the newborn infant may or may not be as responsive as the adult. Since most systems exhibit plasticity at an early stage in life, strong stimuli may affect function and structure much more in the neonate, especially when these stimuli occur over prolonged periods of time. Acute short stresses, however, especially those in the CNS, may not be as significant for the newborn infant.

Sodium Ionic Flux and Its Regulation; Short versus Long Exposures

The concentrations of Na^+ and Cl^- change markedly during hypoxia. Anoxia induces a drop in extracellular Na^+ in brain slices, and removal of extracellular Na^+ prevents the anoxia-induced morphologic changes in dissociated hippocampal neurons.[5,6,19] To understand the mechanisms that sense O_2 and lead to acute neuronal swelling during anoxia, the ionic movements of Cl^- and Na^+ during O_2 deprivation in the hypoglossal (XII) neurons of rat brain slices have been studied. Baseline extracellular Cl^- and Na^+ activities ($[Cl^-]_o$), and $[Na^+]_o$ were measured in adult and neonatal brain slices.[5,6,19] During a period of anoxia (4 min), $[Na^+]_o$ decreased markedly in adult slices whereas $[Na^+]_o$ did not show any significant change in the neonatal slice. Anoxia induced a significant decrease of $[Cl^-]_o$ in both the adult and neonate; however, $[C^-]_o$ dropped seven times more in the adult than in the neonate. Intracellular Cl^- activity ($[Cl^-]_i$) has been studied in adult hypoglossal cells. It is not surprising that there was an increase in $[Cl^-]_i$ with O_2 deprivation. In order to study intracellular Na^+ (Na^+_i) in isolated neurons, we used the fluorophore "sodium green" in freshly dissociated rat neurons, and SBFI, a fluorescent indicator for sodium, in cultured cortical neurons. Ten minutes of anoxia caused an increase in Na^+_i with a latency of about 2 minutes. In these neurons, fluorescence increased by an average of about 20%. We conclude that, during anoxia, (1) intracellular $[Cl^-]$ and $[Na^+]$ increase in the adult, most likely because of entry of extracellular ions into the cytosol, and (2) there is a major maturational difference in mechanisms regulating Cl^- and Na^+ homeostasis between neonate and adult brain tissue.

Although it is well known that Na^+_i increases during hypoxia, the sensors for this ionic alteration are not well documented. It is possible that exchangers/transporters and channels are somehow located within the cascade of events that lead to this

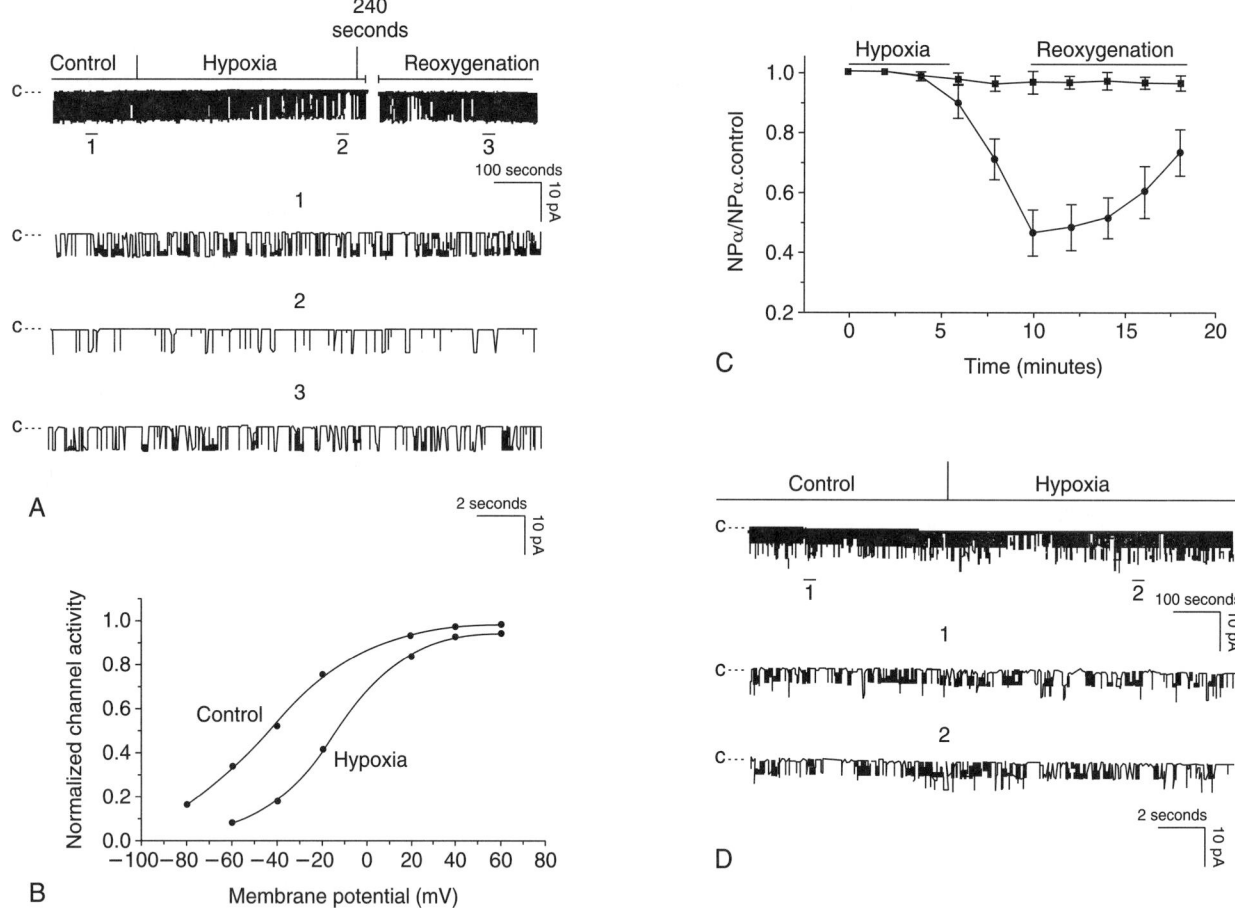

Figure 88–1. Effect of hypoxia on single-channel BK_{Ca} current. **A,** Effect of hypoxia on single BK_{Ca} channel in a cell-attached patch from a neocortical neuron. Current was recorded with high-KCl (140 mM) solution in the pipette and physiologic solution in the bath at a V_m of -30 mV. The channel closed level is indicated by "C". Three parts of the compressed trace are shown, as indicated by numbers 1–3 (fast time resolution). **B,** Effect of hypoxia on the voltage activation of BK_{Ca} channel under the ionic condition just described. The line is fitted to a Boltzmann distribution. $V_{0.5}$ shifted from -42.4 ± 4.8 mV to -18.6 ± 3.5 mV after exposure of hypoxia for 10 minutes. **C,** Time course of the hypoxia-induced effect on NP_o. In cell-attached recordings (*filled squares*), channel inhibition started about 5 minutes after the onset of hypoxia, and a maximum inhibition was reached in about 10 minutes. After that time, NP_o was markedly reduced to about 43% of control level. Reoxygenation led to partial recovery. In inside-out recordings (*filled circles*), NP_o was not significantly affected during hypoxia. **D,** Continuous recording of a single BK_{Ca} channel current from an inside-out patch of a neocortical neuron during hypoxia, using a symmetrical 140-mM KCl on both sides of the membrane, with a V_m of -30 mV. The channel closed level is indicated by "C". Two parts of the compressed trace (indicated by the numbers *1* and *2*) are shown at fast-time resolution. (From Liu H, et al: J Clin Invest *104*:577, 1999.)

increase. The regulation of the voltage-sensitive Na⁺ channels during hypoxia has been investigated using isolated hippocampal neurons.[5, 20] Given the prior data demonstrating an increase in intracellular Na⁺, it is somewhat surprising that hippocampal neurons respond to acute oxygen deprivation with an inhibition of whole-cell Na⁺ currents (I_{Na}).[21, 22] Since kinases can modulate I_{Na} and are activated during hypoxia, we hypothesized that kinase activation may play a role in the hypoxia-induced inhibition of I_{Na}. I_{Na} was recorded at baseline, during exposure to kinase activators (with and without kinase inhibitors), and during acute hypoxia (with and without kinase inhibitors). Hypoxia reduced I_{Na} to about 40% of initial values and shifted the steady-state inactivation in the negative direction.[23] Hypoxia had no effect on activation or fast inactivation. Protein kinase A (PKA) activation with adenosine 3′,5′-cyclic adenosine monophosphate, N^6,O_2-dibutyryl, sodium salt (db-cAMP) resulted in a reduction of I_{Na} to 63%, without an effect on activation or steady-state inactivation. I_{Na} was also reduced by activation of

protein kinase C (PKC) with phorbol 12-myristate 13-acetate (PMA) to 40% or with 1-oleoyl-2-acetyl-*sn*-glycerol (OAG) to 46%. In addition, steady-state inactivation was shifted in the negative direction by PKC activation.

Neither the activation curve nor the kinetics of fast inactivation was altered by PKC activation. The response to PKA activation was blocked by the PKA inhibitor (H-89) and by PKA inhibitory peptide PKA_{5-24} (PKA_i). PKC activation was blocked by the kinase inhibitor (H-7), by the PKC inhibitor calphostin C, and by the inhibitory peptide PKC_{19-31} (PKC_i). The hypoxia-induced inhibition of I_{Na} and shift in steady-state inactivation were greatly attenuated by H-7, calphostin C, or PKC_i, but not with H-89 or PKA_i.[12] We conclude that hypoxia activates PKC in rat CA1 neurons, and that PKC activation leads to the hypoxia-induced inhibition of I_{Na}. These data indicate that kinases can inhibit whole cell Na⁺ currents very much like that observed during hypoxia. However, it is unclear how kinases are activated during hypoxia, and what events occur up-stream.

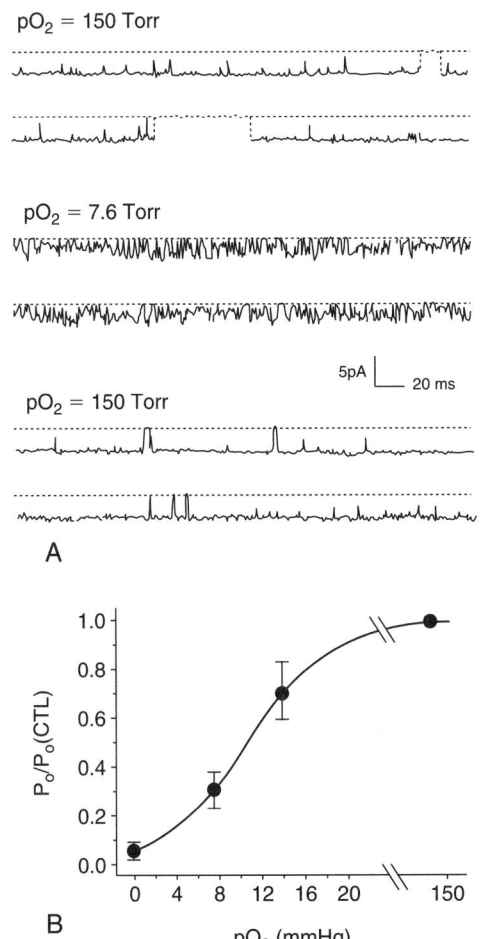

Figure 88–2. A large conductance K$^+$ current is inhibited during O$_2$ deprivation. **A,** Continuous recordings of a single K$^+$ current from an inside-out patch with the same solution (150 mM K$^+$) in both internal and external sides, when the membrane potential was held at 20 mV. During baseline (*top two traces*), this channel had a P_{open} of 0.92 and a unitary conductance of 188 pS. Straight lines indicate the channel closed level. Hypoxia (Po$_2$ ≈ 8 torr) induced a decrease in P_{open} to 0.24 (*middle two traces*). Recovery of P_{open} (0.96) is seen after reperfusion (*lower two traces*). **B,** Dose-dependent inhibition of P_{open} by graded hypoxia. Note the P_{open} was normalized to its control level. Data presented as means ± SEM (n = 3) are fitted with an equation of y = 1/{1 + exp[(K$_d$ − x)/h]}, where y = P_{open}/P_{open} (control), x = Po$_2$, K$_d$ = 11, a Po$_2$ level for 50% inhibition of y, and h = 4. (From Jiangnay C, Haddad GG: Proc Natl Acad Sci U S A *91*:7198, 1994.)

From this analysis, we should highlight a few issues pertaining to O$_2$ sensing. (1) In these studies, sensing is very rapid; whatever the sensor, the reactions that lead to the electrophysiologic responses observed using our techniques and approaches must be very quick, on the order of seconds. (2) Most of the alterations are not genetically mediated, and no gene expression is presumably altered in this short period of time.

Chronic hypoxia has also been studied in our laboratory as well as in others.[24-26] From the point of view of Na$^+$ flux, it seems that Na$^+$ influx increases when neurons are subjected to hypoxia for days.[24, 27] It is important to note that, Na$^+$ influx through voltage-sensitive Na$^+$ channels can lead to cell death, and this form of cell death is most likely due to the activation of cell death genes.[26]

O$_2$ SENSING VIA GENE REGULATION: LONGER PERIODS

Neurons vary widely in their capacity to adapt to a limited oxygen supply, reflecting the diversity of neuronal function and their adaptive mechanisms to oxygen deprivation. The hypoxia-tolerant neurons can be found in every order of vertebrates, such as Crucian carp,[28] tadpoles,[29] turtle,[30] and the naked Kenyan mole rat. Neurons from oxygen-sensitive species such as *Rattus norvegivus* are hypoxia-tolerant during the embryonic and neonatal periods.[31,32] The discovery of the hypoxia-tolerant property of an invertebrate species, *Drosophila melanogaster*, provided researchers with a new model system to study the mechanism of hypoxia-tolerance in neuronal systems.[33] Those studies have prompted a number of questions. How do neurons "sense" the lack of microenvironmental O$_2$? How do they respond? How does sensing O$_2$ deprivation affect the cascade that follows the initial steps?

Multiple O$_2$-sensing systems most likely exist, and, although much remains to be learned about how cells sense and adapt to conditions of oxygen scarcity, it is clear that O$_2$ sensing (and the cascade of events that follow O$_2$ deprivation) largely depend on the regulation of gene transcription. Such mechanisms are fairly quick, and targets can be multiple. Several transcription factors, such as activator protein 1 (AP-1), early growth response protein-1 (EGR-1),[34] nuclear factor κB (NFκB),[35] CAAT enhancer binding protein beta (C/EBPβ/NF-IL-6),[36] and the hypoxia-inducible factor (HIF) were found to be involved in the modulation of gene expression by oxygen. Among these O$_2$-sensitive transcriptional systems, perhaps the best-described O$_2$-sensing pathway is the oxygen-sensitive transcription factor HIF, which activates the gene transcription machinery in an oxygen deprivation–dependent manner.[37]

Hypoxia-inducible factors (HIFs) are heterodimeric transcription factors containing an α and a β-subunit that belong to the basic-helix-loop-helix (bHLH)-PAS protein superfamily. HIF-1α was first cloned from the human Hep3B cell line[38] and is a member of the PAS superfamily 1 (MOP1). The mouse and rat isoforms also have been cloned.[39, 40] Additionally, two other α-subunits have been cloned, from humans, rats, and mice (HIF-2α and HIF-3α). HIF-2α is known as endothelial PAS domain protein 1 (EPAS1), HIF-1α-like factor (HLF), or HIF-related factor (HRF) and is a member of the PAS superfamily 2 (MOP2).[41] HIF-3α is also referred to as MOP7.[41] The β subunits of HIF, HIF-1β, HIF-2β, and HIF-3β, are members of the arylhydrocarbon receptor nuclear translocator, ARNT family, also named as ARNT$_1$, ARNT$_2$, or ARNT$_3$.[42] HIF-1α and β homologues also exist in *Drosophila* tissues, and studies in this species have provided new data on the cellular adaptive responses to chronic hypoxic stress.[13,43] HIF-1 has been most extensively studied (Fig. 88–3).

Previous investigations have shown that HIF-1 mRNA is expressed in the mouse, rat, and human brain.[44] Since the brain is extremely sensitive to hypoxia and ischemia, the regulation of HIF-1 expression is highly relevant. Two of its target gene products in the brain are erythropoietin (EPO) and vascular endothelial growth factor (VEGF).[45,46] In the adult rat brain, HIF-1 mRNA was found in neuronal cells.[47] In hypoxia-treated rats or mice, an increase of HIF-1 mRNA is found in the brain, kidney, and lung. The HIF-1 regulated gene VEGF increased accordingly with an expression pattern similar to that of HIF-1. This provides evidence for a neuroprotective role of HIF-1 in the CNS. HIF-1 has indeed been shown to mediate adaptive responses to reduced O$_2$ availability, including angiogenesis, glycolysis, and ischemia tolerance in the brain.

Control of angiogenesis through HIF-1 and HIF-2 is regulated by growth factors, including VEGF.[48] Numerous studies have demonstrated that chronic hypoxia induces angiogenesis in the adult brain, in association with an increase in VEGF. A time course study, however, has shown that following exposure to 10% O$_2$,

Normoxia   Hypoxia

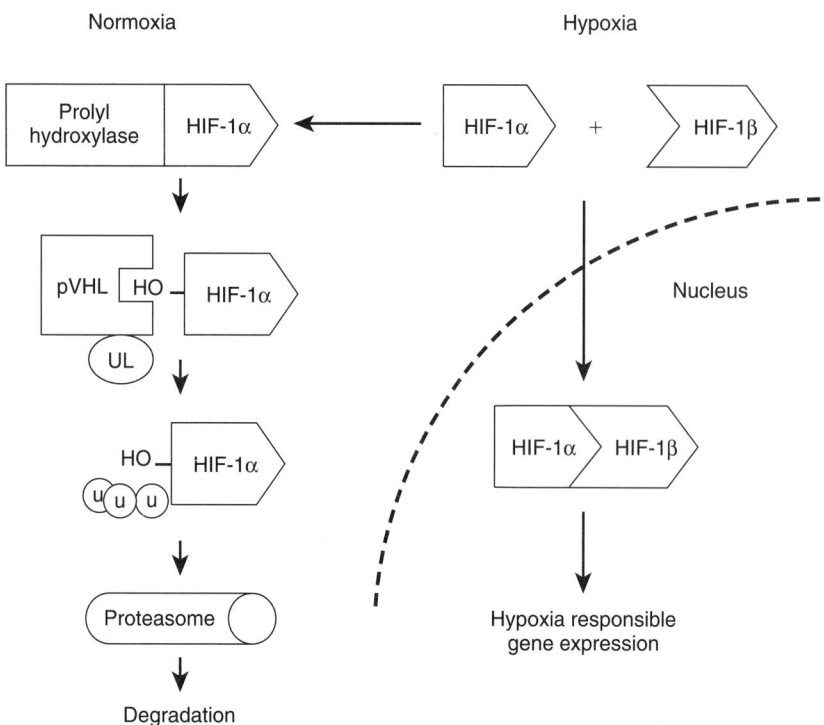

Figure 88–3. A brief schematic summarization of the function and regulation of hypoxia-inducible factor-1 (HIF-1). When the intracellular oxygen tension reaches a critical level, HIF-1α subunits are oxidatively modified by a prolyl hydroxylase. This iron-dependent process results in a hydroxylation of a specific proline residue within HIF-1α's internal oxygen-dependent degradation domain. The hydroxylation of HIF-1α is necessary and sufficient for binding of HIF-1α to pVHL E3 ubiquitin ligase complex. The ubiquitination (u) of HIF-1α leads to degradation of this transcription factor by proteasome. In hypoxic condition, the hydroxylation of proline residue will not occur, and HIF-1α escapes the degradation process, thus HIF-1α forms a stable heterodimer with HIF-1β (ARNT). This HIF-1αβ heterodimer translocates to the nucleus, where it binds to hypoxia-response element and switches on the transcription of hypoxia-responsive genes. pVHL = the protein of the von Hippel–Lindau tumor suppressor gene; UL = E3 ubiquitin ligase.

HIF-1 rapidly accumulated, remained at high levels for only 14 days, and then decreased by 21 days, despite continuous use of a low arterial oxygen tension. This would indicate that either HIF has a long-lasting effect on target genes, or that long-lasting hypoxia or other HIF targets can maintain the induction of genes such as VEGF, since angiogenesis does not regress at a time when HIF has gone back to normal levels.[49] When 21-day-old adapted rats were exposed to a more severe hypoxic challenge (8% oxygen), HIF-1 increased again, indicating that the HIF gene can still be up-regulated with more severe stresses.[49] Thus, HIF-1 and its regulated genes appear to have a role in vascular remodeling and metabolic changes that contribute to adaptation to chronic hypoxia.

It has been found that a noninjurious hypoxic exposure can protect cells from an otherwise lethal hypoxic-ischemic attack several hours or days later. This noninjurious hypoxic stimulation has been termed *preconditioning*. Several studies have suggested that HIF-1 could be an important mediator of hypoxia-induced tolerance to ischemia by preconditioning.[50-52] Indeed, hypoxic preconditioning induced the expression of HIF-1, and its target genes have been found in the neonatal and adult brain. Using DNA microarray methods combined with real-time RT-PCR technologies, a set of HIF-1 but not HIF-2–mediated gene expression has been identified in the neonatal rat brain.[53] In this study, 12 genes were reported to be induced; they include, *VEGF, EPO, GLUT-1, adrenomedullin, propyl 4-hydroxylase, MT-1, MKP-1, CELF, 12-lipoxygenase, t-PA, CAR-1*, and an expressed sequence tag. Some of these genes, such as *GLUT-1, MT-1, CELF, MKP-1*, and *t-PA*, did not show a hypoxic regulation in either neurons or astrocytes, suggesting that other cells are responsible for the up-regulation of these genes in the hypoxic brain. These results also demonstrate that, besides the HIF-1 pathway, a number of other endogenous molecular mechanisms also might be involved in the hypoxic preconditioning-induced tolerance.

Although a great deal of work has been done to understand the biologic role of hypoxia-induced gene expression in the brain, many important questions remain largely unanswered. Which genes are expressed and which are inactivated during hypoxia in different brain regions and cell types is still unknown.

Further research is needed to describe the diversity of oxygen sensors and the mechanisms by which these sensors regulate the gene transcription machinery.

REFERENCES

1. Jiang C, Haddad GG: A direct mechanism for sensing low oxygen levels by central neurons. Proc Natl Acad Sci U S A 91:7198, 1994.
2. Jiang C, et al: O₂ deprivation activates an ATP-inhibitable K⁺ channel in substantia nigra neurons. J Neurosci 14:5590, 1994.
3. Xia Y, Haddad GG: Major difference in the expression of μ- and δ-opioid receptors between turtle and rat brain. J Comp Neurol 436:202, 2001.
4. Ma E, et al: Mutation in pre-mRNA adenosine deaminase markedly attenuates neuronal tolerance to O₂ deprivation in *Drosophila melanogaster*. J Clin Invest 107:685, 2001.
5. Friedman JE, Haddad GG: Removal of extracellular sodium prevents anoxia-induced injury in rat CA1 hippocampal neurons. Brain Res 641:57, 1994.
6. Chidekel AS, et al: Anoxia-induced neuronal injury: role of Na⁺ entry and Na⁺-dependent transport. Exp Neurol 146:403, 1997.
7. Yao H, et al: Intracellular pH regulation of CA1 neurons in Na⁺/H⁺ isoform 1 mutant mice. J Clin Invest 104:637, 1999.
8. Liu H, et al: O₂ deprivation inhibits Ca2⁺-activated K⁺ channels via cytosolic factors in mice neocortical neurons. J Clin Invest 104:577, 1999.
9. Siemen D, et al: Ca²⁺-activated K channel of the BK-type in the inner mitochondrial membrane of a human glioma cell line. Biochem Biophys Res Commun 257:549, 1999.
10. Douglas RM, et al: Voltage-sensitive Na⁺ channels are present in mitochondria of rat brain cells. Soc Neurosc 32:835.8, 2002.
11. Xia S, et al: BSLO is present in mitochondria and may have a role in neuronal apoptosis. Soc Neurosci 32:217.10, 2002.
12. Xu W, et al: Cytoprotective role of Ca2⁺-activated K⁺ channels in the cardiac inner mitochondrial membrane. Science 298:1029, 2002.
13. Ma E, Haddad GG: A *Drosophila* Cdk5α-like molecule and its possible role in response to O₂ deprivation. Biochem Biophys Res Comm 261:459, 1999.
14. Xia Y, Haddad GG: Effect of prolonged O₂ deprivation on Na⁺ channels: differential regulation in adult versus fetal rat brain. Neuroscience 94:1231, 1999.
15. Schmitt BM, et al: Na/HCO₃ cotransporters in rat brain: expression in glia, neurons and choroid plexus. J Neurosci 20:6839, 2000.
16. Gu XQ, et al: Effect of extracellular HCO₃⁻ on Na⁺ channel characteristics in hippocampal CA1 neurons. J Neurophysiol 84:2477, 2000.
17. Jiang C, Haddad GG: Short periods of hypoxia activate a K⁺ current in central neurons. Brain Res 64:352, 1993.
18. Vicencio AG, et al: Regulation of TGF-beta ligand and receptor expression in neonatal rat lungs exposed to chronic hypoxia. J Appl Physiol 93:1123, 2002.
19. Xia Y, Haddad GG: Voltage-sensitive Na⁺ channels increase in number in newborn rat brain after *in utero* hypoxia. Brain Res 635:339, 1994.

20. Friedman JF, Haddad GG: Anoxia induces an increase in intracellular sodium in rat central neurons. Brain Res *663*:329, 1994.
21. Cummins TR, et al: Effect of metabolic inhibition on the excitability of isolated hippocampal CA1 neurons: developmental aspects. J Neurophysiol *66*:1471, 1991.
22. Cummins TR, et al: Human neocortical excitability is decreased during anoxia via sodium channel modulation. J Clin Invest *91*:608, 1993.
23. O'Reilly J, et al: Oxygen deprivation inhibits Na+ current in rat hippocampal neurons via protein kinase C. J Physiol (Lond) *503*:479, 1997.
24. O'Reilly JP, Haddad GG: Chronic hypoxia *in vivo* renders neocortical neurons more vulnerable to subsequent acute hypoxic stress. Brain Res *711*:203, 1996.
25. Banasiak KJ, et al: Mechanism underlying hypoxia-induced neuronal apoptosis. Prog Neurobiol *62*:215, 2000.
26. Banasiak KJ, et al: Activation of voltage-sensitive sodium channels induces caspase-3-mediated neuronal apoptosis. Soc Neurosci *27*:501, 2001.
27. Cummins TR, et al: Comparison of the functional properties of human and rat neocortical sodium currents. Soc Neurosci *18*:1136, 1992.
28. Nillson GE: Surviving anoxia with the brain turned on. News Physiol Sci *16*:217, 2001.
29. West NH, Burggren WW: Gill and lung ventilation responses to steady-state aquatic hypoxia and hyperoxia in the bullfrog tadpole. Respir Physiol *47*:165, 1982.
30. Belkin DA: Anaerobic brain function: effects of stagnant and anoxic anoxia on persistence of breathing in reptiles. Science *162*:1017, 1968.
31. Haddad GG, Donnelly DF: O₂ deprivation induces a major depolarization in brain stem neurons in the adult but not in the neonatal rat. J Physiol *429*:411, 1990.
32. Haddad GG, Jiang C: O₂ deprivation in the central nervous system: on mechanisms of neuronal response, differential sensitivity and injury. Prog Neurobiol *40*:277, 1993.
33. Haddad GG, Ma E: Neuronal tolerance to O₂ deprivation in *Drosophila*: novel approaches using genetic models. Neuroscientist 7:538, 2001.
34. Yan SF, et al: Hypoxia-associated induction of early growth response-1 gene expression. J Biol Chem *274*:15030, 1999.
35. Koong AC, et al: Hypoxia causes the activation of nuclear factor kappa B through the phosphorylation of I kappa B alpha on tyrosine residues. Cancer Res *54*:1425, 1994.
36. Yan SF, et al: Nuclear factor interleukin 6 motifs mediate tissue-specific gene transcription in hypoxia. J Biol Chem *272*:4287, 1997.
37. Wang GL, Semenza GL: Purification and characterization of hypoxia-inducible factor 1. J Biol Chem *270*:1230, 1995.
38. Wang GL, et al: Hypoxia-inducible factor 1 is a basic-helix-loop-helix-PAS heterodimer regulated by cellular O₂ tension. Proc Natl Acad Sci U S A *92*:5510, 1995.
39. Wenger RH, et al: Nucleotide sequence, chromosomal assignment and mRNA expression of mouse hypoxia-inducible factor-1 alpha. Biochem Biophys Res Commun *223*:54, 1996.
40. Kietzmann T, et al: Perivenous expression of the mRNA of the three hypoxia-inducible factor alpha-subunits, HIF1 alpha, HIF2alpha and HIF3alpha, in rat liver. Biochem J *354(Pt 3)*:531, 2001.
41. Hogenesch JB, et al: Characterization of a subset of the basic-helix-loop-helix-PAS superfamily that interacts with components of the dioxin signaling pathway. J Biol Chem *272*:8581, 1997.
42. Semenza GL: Regulation of mammalian O₂ homeostasis by hypoxia-inducible factor 1. Annu Rev Cell Dev Biol *15*:551, 1999.
43. Lavista-Llanos S, et al: Control of the hypoxic response in *Drosophila melanogaster* by the basic helix-loop-helix PAS protein similar. Mol Cell Biol *22*:6842, 2002.
44. Weiner CM, et al: *In vivo* expression of mRNAs encoding hypoxia-inducible factor 1. Biochem Biophys Res Commun *225*:485, 1996.
45. Sakanaga M, et al: *In vivo* evidence that erythropoietin protects neurons from ischemic damage. Proc Natl Acad Sci U S A *95*:4635, 1998.
46. Jin KL, et al: Vascular endothelial growth factor: direct neuroprotective effect in *in vitro* ischemia. Proc Natl Acad Sci U S A *97*:10242, 2000.
47. Bergeron M, et al: Induction of hypoxia-inducible factor-1 (HIF-1) and its target genes following focal ischemia in rat brain. Eur J Neurosci *11*:4159, 1999.
48. Carmeliet P: Mechanisms of angiogenesis and arteriogenesis. Nat Med *6*:389, 2000.
49. Chavez JC, et al: Expression of hypoxia-inducible factor-1alpha in the brain of rats during chronic hypoxia. J Appl Physiol *89*:1937, 2000.
50. Bergeron M, et al: Role of hypoxia-inducible factor-1 in hypoxia-induced ischemic tolerance in neonatal rat brain. Ann Neurol *48*:285, 2000.
51. Jones NM, Bergeron M: Hypoxic preconditioning induces changes in HIF-1 target genes in neonatal rat brain. J Cereb Blood Flow Metab *21*:1105, 2001.
52. Bernaudin M, et al: Normobaric hypoxia induces tolerance to focal permanent cerebral ischemia in association with an increased expression of hypoxia-inducible factor-1 and its target genes, erythropoietin and VEGF, in the adult mouse brain. J Cereb Blood Flow Metab *22*:393, 2002.
53. Bernaudin M, et al: Brain genomic response following hypoxia and re-oxgenation in the neonatal rat. J Biol Chem *277*:3972, 2002.

Martha J. Miller and Richard J. Martin

89

Pathophysiology of Apnea of Prematurity

EPIDEMIOLOGY AND DEFINITION OF APNEA

Definition

Apnea is a perplexing disorder of respiratory control that is very common in small premature infants. Infants of all ages may experience respiratory pauses of varying duration, in conjunction with startles, movement, defecation, or swallowing during feeding. Short respiratory pauses are typically self-limiting and are not associated with bradycardia (<100 beats/minute). More prolonged respiratory pauses lasting 20 seconds or longer and short pauses associated with bradycardia, cyanosis, or pallor were historically defined as clinically significant apnea by the American Academy of Pediatrics Task Force on prolonged apnea.[1]

Apnea should be distinguished from *periodic breathing,* in which the infant exhibits regular cycles of respiration of approximately 10 to 18 seconds in length, interrupted by pauses at least 3 seconds in duration; this pattern recurs for at least 2 minutes.[2] Periodic breathing has been considered a benign respiratory pattern in the premature or young term infant. The respiratory pause of apnea, unlike that of periodic breathing, may not be self-limiting and may produce significant physiologic changes, which we consider in detail in the following discussion.

Classification

Apneic events are distinguished not only by their duration but also by the presence or absence of airway obstruction during the episode of apnea. Thach and Stark[3] initially described an increase in the frequency of apnea when the premature infant's neck was flexed. Subsequently, upper airway obstruction was found to accompany apnea in preterm babies, even though neck flexion was not present.[4] The location within the upper airway at which obstruction occurs is usually within the pharynx, but it may vary. Mathew and co-workers[5] noted that obstruction occurred within the pharynx in 93% of cases of apnea, at the level of the larynx in 1%, and in 6% at both the larynx and pharynx. The presence or absence of upper airway obstruction forms the basis of the classification of apnea into three types (Fig. 89–1). *Mixed apnea* is the most commonly observed clinically significant event in small premature infants and consists of obstructed inspiratory efforts as well as a central pause greater than or equal to

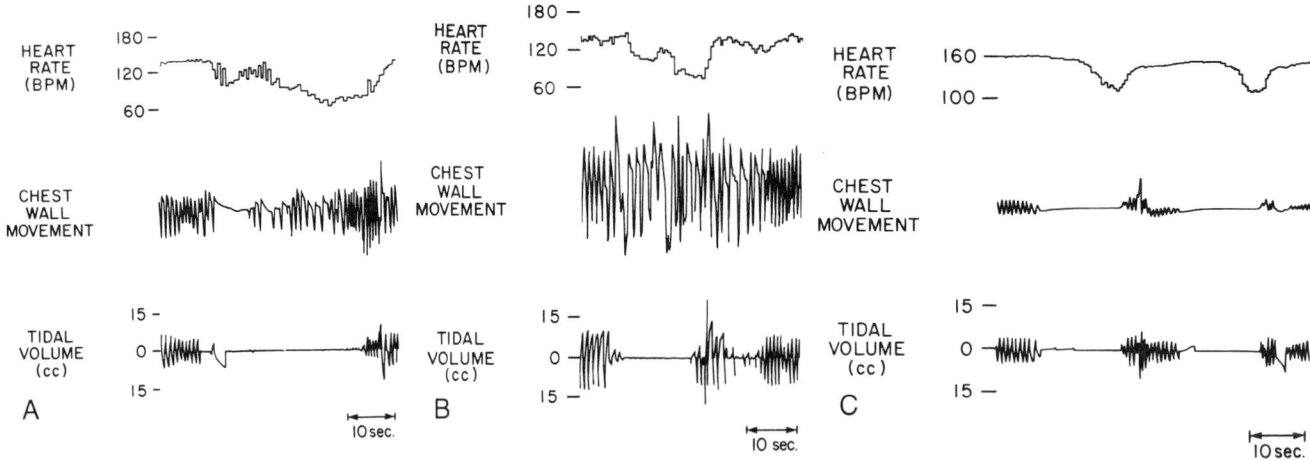

Figure 89–1. **A,** Mixed apnea. Obstructed breaths precede and follow a central respiratory pause. **B,** Obstructive apnea. Breathing efforts continue, although no nasal airflow occurs. **C,** Central apnea. Both nasal airflow and breathing efforts cease simultaneously. (From Miller MJ: *In* Edelman N, Santiago T [eds]: Breathing Disorders of Sleep. New York, Churchill Livingstone, 1986.)

2 seconds in duration (see Fig. 89-1*A*). In *obstructive apnea,* obstructed breaths characterized by chest wall motion without nasal airflow continue throughout the entire apnea (see Fig. 89-1*B*). In *central apnea,* inspiratory efforts cease entirely, and obstructed breaths are not observed (see Fig. 89-1*C*). Mixed apnea accounts for approximately 50 to 75% of all apnea in premature infants; obstructive apnea, 10 to 20%; and central apnea, 10 to 25%.[6] The mechanism by which these three types of apnea are produced is incompletely understood, as discussed later, and their distribution may change with advancing postconceptional age. Furthermore, the proportion of mixed apnea progressively increases (and that of purely central apnea decreases) the longer the apnea endures.

Apnea duration and classification may also correlate with the neurologic status of the infant. Butcher-Puech and co-workers[7] found that infants who exhibited obstructive apnea of more than 20 seconds' duration had a higher incidence of intraventricular hemorrhage, hydrocephalus, prolonged mechanical ventilation, and abnormal neurologic development after the first year of life. It is possible that apnea in some infants is a symptom of a diffuse neurologic insult in prenatal or postnatal life that leads to disordered control of breathing in the premature infant. In most infants, underlying neuropathology is unlikely, because apnea frequency decreases over time as the infant matures. Hypothetically, apnea may resolve when central and peripheral chemoreceptors develop to the point at which appropriate responses occur to change in blood gas status. A further important developmental phenomenon may be the increasing ability of medullary respiratory control centers over time to activate upper airway dilating musculature in synchrony with increasing ventilatory drive.

Hypoxemic events resembling apnea have also been detected in intubated, mechanically ventilated preterm infants. Bolivar and co-workers[8] described episodes of hypoxemia preceded by an increase in total pulmonary resistance and a decrease in compliance, analogous to changes described by Miller and associates before apnea in unintubated infants.[9] Furthermore, Dimaguila and others[10] reported that such episodes may be preceded by subtle spontaneous movement and are characterized by both central respiratory depression and obstruction to airflow (the latter features analogous to mixed apnea). These hypoxemic episodes in intubated infants are a consequence of hypoventilation, frequently associated with arousal,[11] and they further illustrate the vulnerability of premature infants to imbalance of central respiratory control and altered pulmonary function.

Physiologic Effects

Cessation of respiration during apnea has significant ventilatory and reflex cardiovascular consequences for the preterm infant. Both hypoxia and hypercarbia accompany prolonged apnea. The decrease in oxygenation in term infants with apnea has been observed to be directly related to the duration of the apnea and to be significantly greater in obstructive than in central apnea (Fig. 89-2).[12] In most premature infants, apnea, if appropriately treated, is not thought to produce significant long-term complications. However, in a retrospective analysis, Kitchen and associates[13] did note a significant correlation between apnea of infancy requiring treatment with theophylline and later development of cerebral palsy. This correlation could reflect early (apnea) and late (cerebral palsy) manifestations of diffuse cerebral hypoxic-ischemic injury in a small subset of premature infants, as discussed later.

The reflex effects of apnea include characteristic changes in heart rate, blood pressure, and pulse pressure. Bradycardia may begin as early as 1.5 to 2 seconds after the onset of apnea[14] (Fig. 89-3). The bradyarrhythmia is most often sinus in character, with an occasional infant showing a nodal escape.[15] Henderson-Smart and co-workers[16] noted a significant correlation between the decrease in oxygen saturation and heart rate and postulated that bradycardia during apnea could result from hypoxic stimulation of the carotid body chemoreceptors. Daly and Scott[17] determined the effect of hypoxic perfusion of the isolated carotid body on heart rate in the dog. When ventilation was allowed to increase in response to hypoxia, tachycardia occurred. However, when this reflex increase in ventilation was prevented, bradycardia resulted. In the spontaneously breathing subject, the decrease in heart rate owing to hypoxic stimulation of the carotid body may be masked by a cardiac accelerator response that may derive from stretch receptors in the lung as well as cycling of the respiratory control center in the medulla.[18] At the onset of apnea, at which time cessation of ventilation and onset of hypoxia occur almost simultaneously, hypoxia would be expected to produce bradycardia.

Other reflex input may accentuate the bradycardia during hypoxemia. For example, the reflex effects of apnea in infants have also been compared with the diving response of the seal.[19] During reflex apnea in these animals, upper airway afferent input from superior laryngeal and trigeminal nerve stimulation may produce greatly enhanced bradycardia. The contribution of upper airway reflexes to the bradycardia that occurs during

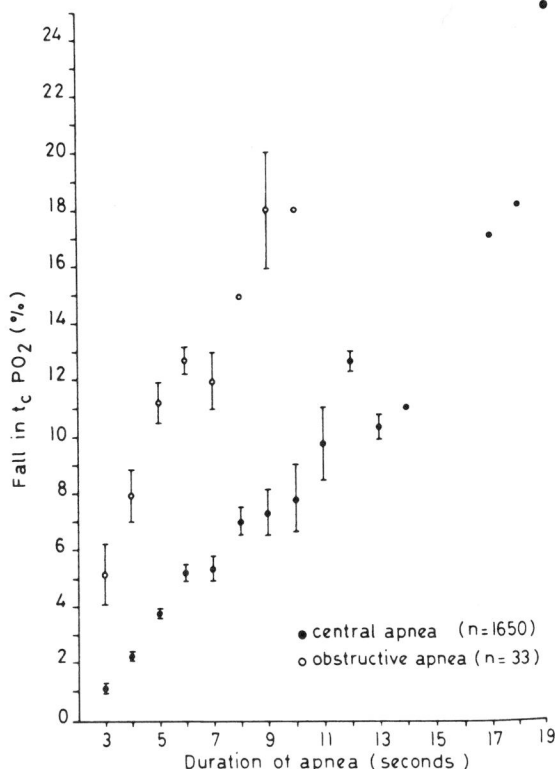

Figure 89–2. Relationship between duration of apnea and decrease in transcutaneous partial pressure of oxygen (tcPo$_2$). The fall in tcPo$_2$ over time is greater during obstructive than central apnea. (From Kahn A, et al: Pediatrics 70:852, 1982. Reproduced by permission of Pediatrics.)

apnea has not been studied in human infants. In summary, the rapid onset of bradycardia during apnea may be a complex reflex deriving from multiple sources, including trigeminal receptors and carotid chemoreceptors.

A change in blood pressure also accompanies apnea in newborn infants. Girling[20] noted that the decrease in heart rate during apnea was accompanied by a concomitant rise in pulse pressure, usually owing to an increase in systolic pressure, occasionally accompanied by a fall in diastolic pressure. During bradycardia, filling volume of the heart may increase, leading to a rise in stroke volume and pulse pressure in accordance with Starling's law. With more severe apnea and bradycardia (<80 beats/minute), a decrease in systemic blood pressure may occur, accompanied by a fall in cerebral diastolic and systolic blood flow velocity (Fig. 89-4).[21] In infants without cerebrovascular autoregulation, cerebral blood flow may mirror systemic blood flow, and cerebral perfusion may decrease to very low levels during prolonged apnea. Resolution of apnea may be accompanied by cerebral hyperperfusion.[22] Thus, very prolonged apnea could be analogous to a hypoperfusion-hyperperfusion type of brain insult and could lead to hypoxic-ischemic brain injury in susceptible premature infants.

Epidemiology

In defining the epidemiology and developmental correlates of apnea, part of the difficulty lies in the numerous definitions of apnea that have been used by various investigators. However, some trends do emerge. Apnea is more frequent in more immature infants. Twenty-five percent of infants who weigh less than 2500 g at birth and 84% of infants who weight less than 1000 g

may experience apnea during the neonatal period.[23] Carlo and associates[24] showed that the onset of apnea may occur on day 1 of life in infants without respiratory distress syndrome (Fig. 89-5). In contrast, spontaneously breathing infants with respiratory distress syndrome may show a delay in the peak frequency of apnea until day 7 of life. Thereafter, both the frequency and duration of apnea decrease between 1 and 20 weeks of postnatal age,[25] as discussed later (Fig. 89-6). These observations serve to emphasize the developmental immaturity of respiratory control that underlies infantile apnea, as well as the resolution of this disorder over time.

Idiopathic apnea is usually related to prematurity at delivery. In rare infants, underlying specific familial neuropathology may be identified. Adickes and co-workers[26] described a family in which three of six siblings presented between 18 and 26 months of age with sleep apnea and subsequently died of this disorder. Neuropathologic evaluation revealed that the affected persons suffered from Leigh disease (subacute necrotizing encephalomyelopathy). In this disease, spongiform degeneration may be present in the areas of the brain stem that regulate ventilation, including the nucleus reticularis and nucleus gigantocellularis. Other disorders affecting the brain stem that may present with apnea include olivopontocerebellar atrophy, myotonic dystrophy, and syringobulbia, as well as brain stem infarction resulting from asphyxia.[27] In the ongoing search for the underlying cause of idiopathic apnea, examination of familial cases of apnea with discrete brain stem lesions may offer valuable clues to the areas of the brain stem that could be dysfunctional in premature infants.

Apnea can recur in premature infants after the neonatal period in response to specific clinical situations in which the respiratory drive is altered. Respiratory syncytial viral infection is well known to elicit apnea, which may be of the typical mixed or obstructive type or may have a pattern more reminiscent of periodic breathing.[28] These spells may be severe, and may require endotracheal intubation. The cause of respiratory depression in respiratory syncytial viral infection is unknown. However, the apnea resolves with recovery from this infection.

Former premature infants may also experience apnea during recovery from general anesthesia.[29] This most commonly occurs in the first few months of life, particularly when either ketamine sedation or general anesthesia is used during surgery. For this reason, during the acute postoperative period, cardiorespiratory monitoring of former preterm infants is an important part of their care.

PHYSIOLOGIC FACTORS

Alteration in Central Drive

Immaturity or depression of central inspiratory drive to the muscles of respiration has traditionally been accepted as a key factor in the pathogenesis of apnea of prematurity. Vulnerability of the bulbopontine respiratory centers in the brain stem to inhibitory mechanisms could explain why apneic episodes are precipitated in preterm infants by such a wide diversity of specific clinicopathologic events, as outlined in Figure 89-7.[30] In other words, apnea may reflect the final common response of incompletely organized and interconnected respiratory neurons to a multitude of afferent stimuli. It has been proposed that immature circuits within neuronal networks may be highly susceptible to inhibitory neurotransmitters and neuroregulators such as adenosine and γ-aminobutyric acid (GABA). Unfortunately, the maturation of central respiratory integrative mechanisms and of their biochemical neurotransmitters is inaccessible to study in human infants, and no ideal animal model that exhibits spontaneous apnea has been identified for study in the nonanesthetized state.

Using noninvasive techniques, Henderson-Smart and co-workers[31] documented that brain stem conduction times of

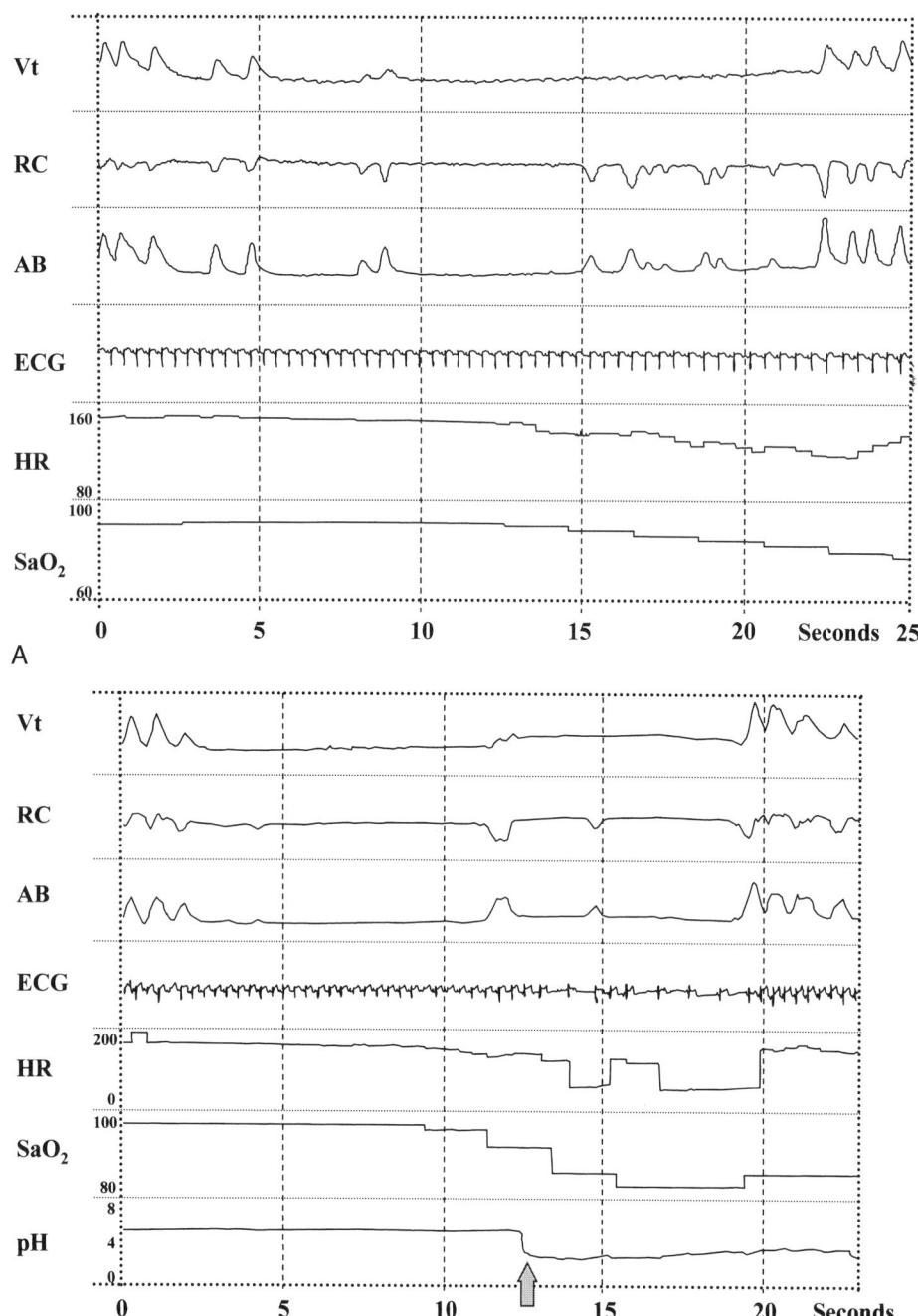

Figure 89–3. A, Relationship between apnea and bradycardia. During this mixed apnea, the heart rate (HR) begins to decrease approximately 5 seconds after the apnea begins. **B,** Relationship between apnea and gastroesophageal reflux. Reflux occurs after the onset of apnea, as indicated by the decrease in lower esophageal pH (*arrow*). AB = abdomen motion; ECG = electrocardiogram; RC = rib cage motion; Sao$_2$ = arterial oxygen saturation; Vt, tidal volume (estimated).

auditory-evoked responses are longer in infants with apnea than in matched premature infants without apnea. These observations provide some indirect evidence that infants with apnea exhibit greater than expected immaturity of brain stem function on the basis of postconceptional age and support the concept that stability of central respiratory drive improves as dendritic and other synaptic interconnections multiply in the maturing brain.

The absence of respiratory muscle activity during central apnea unequivocally points to the depression of respiratory center output. In support of this concept, Gauda[32] documented a decrease in diaphragm electromyographic (EMG) activity during spontaneously obstructed inspiratory efforts that characterize mixed apnea, as discussed later. Thus, both central and mixed apneic episodes share an element of decreased respiratory center output to the respiratory muscles. The role played by

the balance of neurotransmitter substances in modulating this inhibition is not yet known. GABA is considered a ubiquitous major inhibitory neurotransmitter within the brain. Physiologic studies in neonatal animal models have implicated GABA in declines in respiratory frequency and decreased ventilatory responses during hypercapnia, hypoxia, and superior laryngeal nerve stimulation.[33-35] Therefore, GABA has the potential to play a key role in the vulnerability of preterm infants to apnea. Dopaminergic receptors have been implicated as playing an inhibitory role in both peripheral chemoreceptor responses and central neural mechanisms elicited by hypoxia.[36] There is evidence from neonatal animal studies that endogenous endorphins may depress central respiratory drive; however, this depression occurs only during the first few postnatal days, and these agents become much less important with advancing age.[37] Endogenous

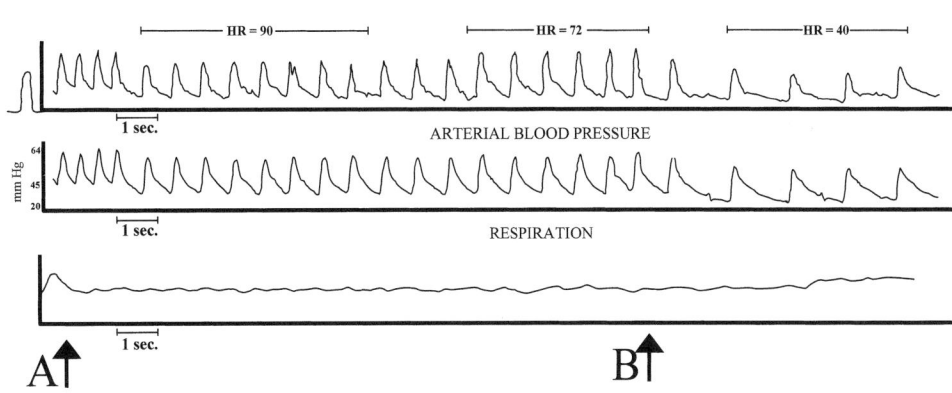

Figure 89–4. Relationship of apnea, cerebral blood flow velocity, and blood pressure. The apnea begins at *A*. At *B*, approximately 16 seconds into the apnea, systemic blood pressure falls, and cerebral blood flow velocity decreases. HR = heart rate. (From Perlman JM et al: Pediatrics 76:333, 1985.)

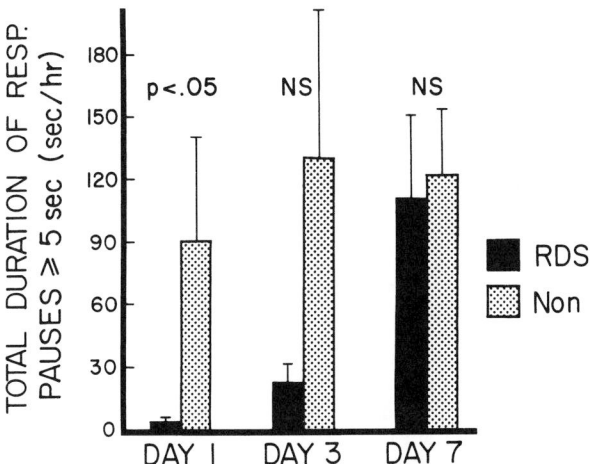

Figure 89–5. A comparison of the total duration of respiratory pauses lasting 5 seconds or longer between infants with and without respiratory distress syndrome (RDS). (From Carlo WA, et al: Am Rev Respir Dis *126*:103, 1982.)

opiates may modulate the ventilatory response to hypoxia in newborn primate animals[38]; however, a competitive opiate receptor antagonist, naloxone, has no benefit in resuscitation of the asphyxiated human neonate,[39] nor does naloxone appear to play a therapeutic role in apnea of prematurity. Thus, the final output of the respiratory control nuclei in the medulla may be a complex function of many inhibitory and stimulatory inputs, both humoral and neural. The exact manner in which these are altered during apnea of prematurity remains to be elucidated.

Role of Sleep State

It became apparent in the mid-1970s that respiratory control is influenced by sleep state in infants. It was observed that apnea occurs more commonly during active (or rapid eye movement) and indeterminate (or transitional) sleep, when respiratory patterns are irregular in both timing and amplitude.[40] It is less common for apnea to be observed during quiet sleep, when respiration is characteristically regular with little breath-by-breath change in tidal volume or respiratory frequency, although periodic breathing may actually occur predominantly in quiet sleep. In term neonates, respiratory variability alone can be employed

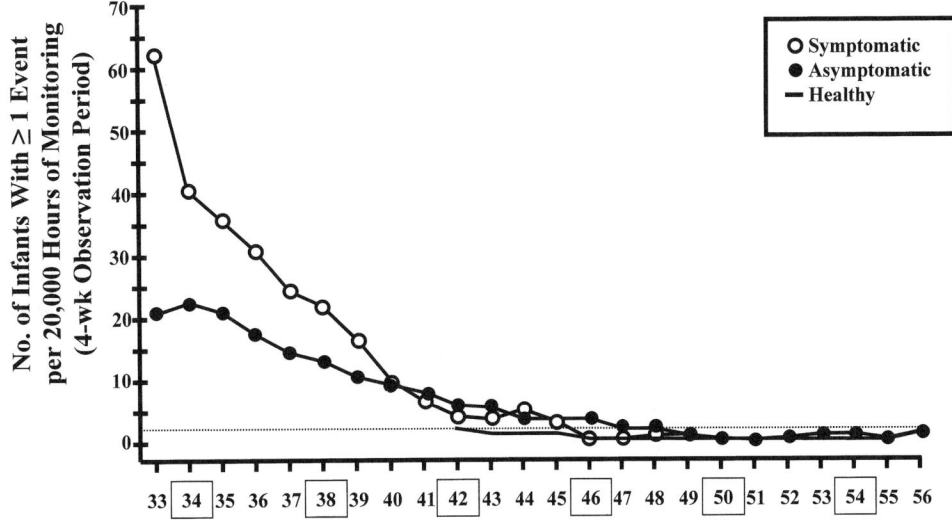

Figure 89–6. The number of infants who experienced at least one apneic episode lasting 30 seconds accompanied by bradycardia decreased with advancing postconceptional age (PCA). Data are presented for symptomatic and asymptomatic preterm infants, depending on the persistence of cardiorespiratory events before discharge, and a healthy term group. (From Ramanathan et al, 2001.)

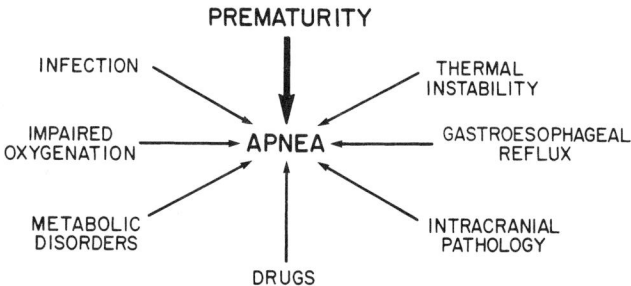

Figure 89–7. Some diverse factors known to precipitate development of apneic episodes in predisposed preterm infants. (From Martin RJ, et al: J Pediatr 109:733, 1986).

to stage sleep with a high degree of accuracy.[41] However, sleep state is not easily definable by any criteria before 32 weeks of gestation, when apnea occurs most frequently.

The higher incidence of apnea during active sleep is probably the result of the variability of respiratory rhythmicity that characterizes that state. Other factors may enhance the infants' vulnerability to apnea during active sleep. Chest wall movements are predominantly asynchronous (or paradoxical) during active sleep, in contrast to quiet sleep.[42] Specifically, abdominal expansion during inspiration is almost always accompanied by inward movement of the rib cage during active sleep, whereas during quiet sleep, rib cage and abdomen expand together. These paradoxical chest wall movements during active sleep appear to be the result of decreased intercostal muscle activity, secondary to spinal motoneuron inhibition.[43] In very preterm infants, however, the paucity of quiet sleep, together with an extremely compliant rib cage, makes paradoxical chest wall movements almost a constant feature. Asynchronous chest wall movements may predispose to apnea by decreasing functional residual capacity and impairing oxygenation.[44] The compensatory increase in diaphragm activity that results may increase diaphragmatic work and predispose to diaphragmatic fatigue[45] and collapse of the pharyngeal airway.[46] Thus, the enhanced vulnerability to apnea during active sleep may simultaneously operate at several levels of respiratory function.

Influence of Chemoreceptor and Mechanoreceptor Responses

The ventilatory and respiratory muscle responses to increases in inspired carbon dioxide reflect predominantly central chemoreceptor activity and are less well developed in the immature infant who is less than 33 weeks of postconceptional age.[47]

It is unclear whether this reduced ventilatory response to carbon dioxide in small preterm infants is primarily the result of decreased central chemosensitivity or mechanical factors preventing an appropriate increase in ventilation. Unlike adults, preterm infants do not increase frequency of ventilation during hypercapnia, and this is accompanied by prolongation of expiratory duration.[48] It has been shown that the carbon dioxide response curve has a decreased slope (indicating a less steep ventilatory response to increasing carbon dioxide concentrations) in preterm infants who exhibit apnea (Fig. 89–8),[49] but a cause-and-effect relationship between decreased carbon dioxide responsiveness and apnea of prematurity has not been clearly established. Both may simply reflect decreased respiratory drive. Administration of carbon dioxide would be expected to relieve apnea, as it does periodic breathing, but this is probably not therapeutically feasible in human infants.

As in adult animal models, the newborn piglet has been employed to identify the physiologic consequences of decreased central (carbon dioxide) chemosensitivity. This has been done by

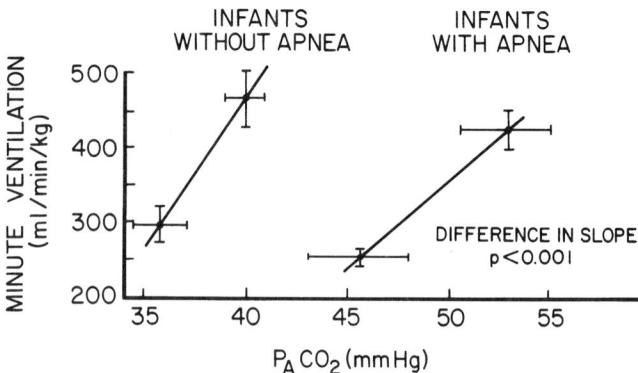

Figure 89–8. Comparison of carbon dioxide sensitivity obtained from ventilatory responses to changing alveolar partial pressure of carbon dioxide ($P_{A_{CO_2}}$) in preterm infants with and without apnea. Note the less steep ventilatory response in the apneic group. (From Gerhardt T, Bancalari E: Pediatrics 74:58, 1984. Reproduced by permission of Pediatrics.)

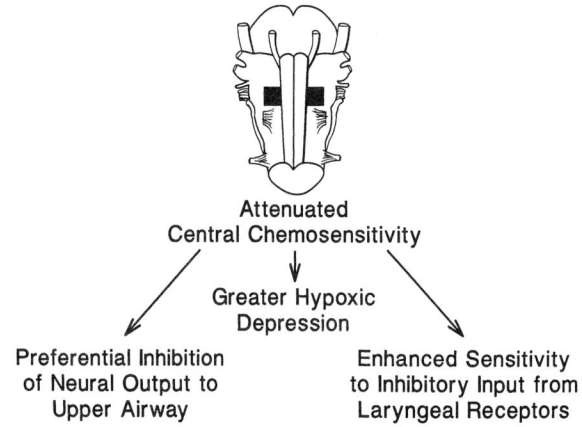

Figure 89–9. Hypothetical framework for mechanisms whereby attenuated central (carbon dioxide) chemosensitivity enhances vulnerability to neonatal apnea. The *black squares* indicate the intermediate area of the ventral medullary surface of the brain stem.

cooling a discrete area (the intermediate area) of the ventral medullary surface.[50, 51] Cooling at this site (or microinjection of inhibitory neurotransmitters) inhibits central chemosensitivity, possibly by directly affecting chemosensitive cells at this site but also by inhibiting neural transmission between central chemosensitive cells and respiratory rhythm generators situated in the brain stem. There are obvious limitations in extrapolating data from anesthetized newborn piglets to apneic human infants. Nonetheless, as seen in Figure 89–9, attenuated central chemosensitivity may underlie some of the physiologic characteristics of neonatal respiratory control. These include preferential inhibition of neural output to the upper airway muscles as compared with the diaphragm, enhanced sensitivity to inhibitory afferents from upper airway (e.g., laryngeal) receptors, and greater hypoxic depression of breathing (as discussed later).

It has been known for many years that preterm infants respond to a fall in inspired oxygen concentration with a transient increase in ventilation over approximately 1 minute, followed by a return to baseline or even depression of ventilation.[52] The characteristic response to low oxygen in infants appears to result from initial peripheral chemoreceptor stimulation, followed by overriding depression of the respiratory center as a result of hypoxemia. Consistent with these findings is the observation that a progressive decrease in inspired oxygen concentration causes a significant flattening of carbon dioxide responsiveness in preterm infants.[53] This unstable response to low inspired oxygen may play an important role in the origin of neonatal apnea. It offers a physiologic rationale for the decrease in incidence of apnea observed when a slightly increased concentration of inspired oxygen is administered to apneic infants. The biphasic ventilatory response to low inspired oxygen, however, does not appear unique to apneic infants and probably serves to increase their vulnerability to apnea, rather than causing the problem. Consistent with the prolonged vulnerability of respiratory control in preterm infants is the observation that the characteristic biphasic ventilatory response to hypoxia persists into the second month of postnatal life.[54]

Afferent neural input from pulmonary stretch receptors is capable of substantially modulating respiratory timing in human neonates. This vagally mediated response is called the *Hering-Breuer reflex.* It acts to inhibit inspiration, prolong expiration, or both, with increasing lung volume.[55] Active shortening of expiratory duration with decrease in lung volume may provide a neonatal breathing strategy to preserve functional residual capacity in the presence of a highly compliant chest wall. Another manifestation of this reflex response to lung inflation is that inspiratory duration is typically prolonged after end-expiratory airway obstruction when lung inflation is prevented. This ability of neonates to increase the duration of an obstructed inspiratory effort appears to be an appropriate compensatory mechanism during airway occlusion. More important, upper airway obstruction contributes substantially to apneic episodes in preterm infants, and upper airway muscles show preferential reflex activation in response to airway obstruction in infants.[56] Gerhardt and Bancalari[57] compared the ability of preterm infants with and without apnea to respond to end-expiratory airway occlusion. Prolongation of the occluded inspiratory effort was significantly longer in the nonapneic group, a finding suggesting a more mature respiratory reflex response resulting in a greater ability to respond to airway obstruction.

Apnea in premature infants is accompanied by complex changes in pulmonary mechanics and ventilatory timing.[9] Before apnea occurs, an increase in total pulmonary resistance has been observed in association with a decrease in tidal volume and a prolongation in expiratory time. Such changes may be noted before mixed, obstructive, and central apnea. These observations suggest that a diminution in respiratory drive precedes apnea, reminiscent of the cyclic alterations in drive observed by Waggener and co-workers.[58] After the apnea resolves and respiration is resumed, the respiratory drive in premature infants is initially increased (reflected in a higher ratio of tidal volume to inspiratory time), which may result from cumulative hypoxia and hypercapnia. Total pulmonary resistance is increased and supraglottic resistance is also elevated, possibly in response to a fall in lung volume and collapse of the upper airway when respiratory drive declines during the apnea. Remarkably, within two to three breaths after apnea, the premature infant is noted to restore pulmonary resistance and respiratory drive to normal preapnea values. Thus, the neural systems that restore respiratory homeostasis appear capable of adequate response, even in premature infants with apnea.

Relation of Apnea to Periodic Breathing

Periodic breathing, defined earlier as recurrent sequences of pauses in respiration, is so common as to be considered normal in preterm infants.[59] It can be abolished by increasing environmental oxygen,[59] but because periodic breathing is considered harmless, this is not recommended. Apnea and periodic breathing share many characteristics, but some specific differences have been noted. Both forms of respiratory instability decline in

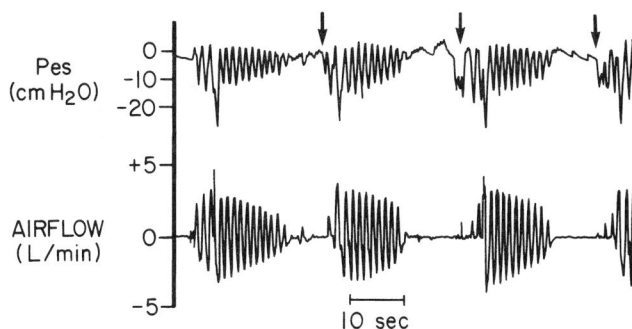

Figure 89–10. During this epoch of periodic breathing, obstructed breaths occur at the onset of each ventilatory cycle, as indicated by esophageal pressure (Pes) swings in the absence of nasal airflow. (From Miller MJ, et al: J Appl Physiol *64*:2496, 1988.)

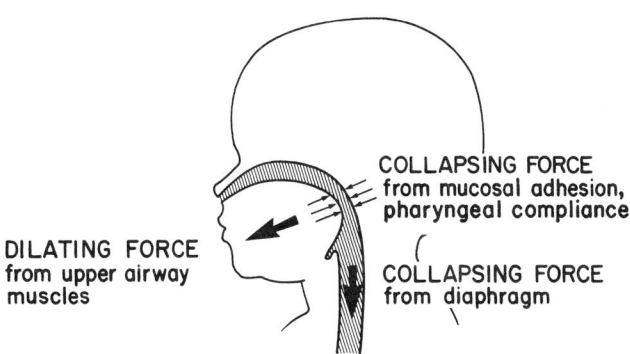

Figure 89–11. Sagittal section of the upper airway, demonstrating various forces operating either to collapse the pharynx or to maintain its patency during normal respiration. (Modified from Thach BT: *In* Tilden JT, et al [eds]: Sudden Infant Death Syndrome. New York, Academic Press, 1983.)

frequency after birth, over a 5- to 10-week period. The respiratory pause in both apnea and periodic breathing is preceded by a decline in tidal volume and by a prolongation of respiratory time reminiscent of the cyclic changes in ventilation described by Waggener and co-workers[58]; both may be accompanied by obstructed breaths before the onset of respiratory cycles (Fig. 89–10).[9,60] Apnea and periodic breathing do differ in the following respects: the respiratory pauses of apnea are not limited in duration, and they are accompanied by frequent swallows, which are not observed during periodic breathing. Thus, the physiologic correlates of these forms of respiratory instability differ in several ways. The specific central neuronal pathways that lead to each have yet to be determined.

Differential Responses of Upper Airway and Chest Wall Muscles

Because premature infants exhibit pharyngeal or laryngeal obstruction during spontaneous apnea, much interest has focused on the interactions among the various respiratory muscle groups in maintaining airway patency. A model was proposed for the pathogenesis of neonatal apnea by Thach,[46] a modification of which is shown in Figure 89–11. This model proposes that negative luminal pressures generated during inspiration in the upper airway predispose a compliant pharynx to collapse. Patency can be maintained by activation of upper airway muscles that may increase tone within the extrathoracic airway through tonic or phasic contraction in synchrony with

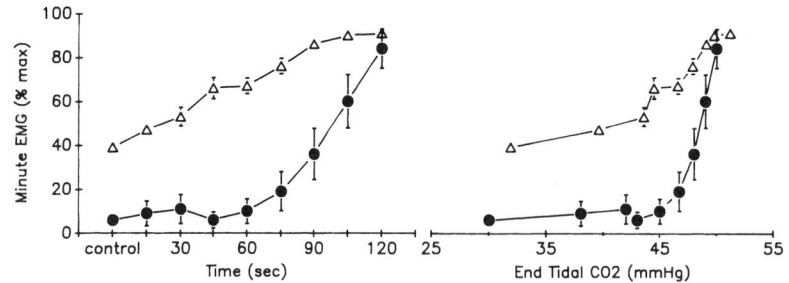

Figure 89–12. *Left,* Time course of average minute electromyogram (EMG) in response to hyperoxic carbon dioxide (CO_2) rebreathing expressed as the percentage of maximum activity (mean ± SE) for the diaphragm (*triangles*) and genioglossus (*circles*) in preterm infants. (Because maximum activity occasionally occurred before the last epoch of CO_2 rebreathing, mean values just before the off response do not always reach 100% of maximal activity.) The linear response of the diaphragm EMG contrasts with the delayed genioglossus response. *Right,* Average minute EMG in relation to end-tidal CO_2 during hyperoxic rebreathing. An increase in genioglossus EMG occurred only after a CO_2 threshold of approximately 45 mm Hg had been reached. (From Carlo WA, et al: J Appl Physiol 65:2434, 1988.)

the chest wall muscles. The relative role played by active upper airway muscle contraction and passive rigidity of the anatomic framework of the upper airway in maintaining pharyngeal patency in preterm infants is unclear.

Whereas many upper airway muscles, including the alae nasi and laryngeal abductor and adductor muscles, modulate patency of the extrathoracic airway, failure of genioglossus activation has been most widely implicated in mixed and obstructive apnea in both adults and infants. Carlo and co-workers[61] compared activity of the genioglossus muscle with that of the diaphragm in response to hypercapnic stimulation. Consistent with data obtained in animal models,[62] genioglossus activation in preterm infants was delayed for about 1 minute after initiation of carbon dioxide rebreathing and occurred only after a carbon dioxide threshold of approximately 45 mm Hg had been reached (Fig. 89-12).[61] In contrast, diaphragm EMG activity increased linearly with progressive hypercapnia. Thus, it is possible that an absent, small, or delayed upper airway muscle response to hypercapnia may result in upper airway instability when accompanied by a linear increase in chest wall activity. This may predispose to obstructed inspiratory efforts after a period of central apnea. Consistent with this hypothesis is the observation that short apneic episodes are more likely to be central, and longer (>15 seconds) episodes are more likely to be examples of mixed apnea. Furthermore, airway obstruction often occurs toward the end of the longer episodes of mixed apnea, when diaphragmatic activity may be enhanced before that of the upper airway muscles.

Neonates typically exhibit a modest prolongation of inspiratory time when lung inflation is prevented by end-expiratory airway occlusion; as indicated earlier, this is a manifestation of the Hering-Breuer reflex. Studies in animals demonstrated that this vagally mediated inhibition of normal lung inflation has a greater influence on the upper airway muscles than on the diaphragm.[63] This vagal inhibition is released when the airway is occluded. Consequently, airway occlusion results in a greater increase of upper airway muscle activity, as compared with the diaphragm, when an obstructed inspiratory effort is compared with the corresponding preocclusion breath. A similar preferential increase in amplitude of the submental (genioglossus) versus diaphragm EMG has been noted in healthy preterm infants during end-expiratory airway occlusion.[56] It is theoretically possible that exaggerated vagal inhibition of the dilator muscles of the upper airway may contribute to the origin of obstructive apnea.

Gauda and co-workers[64] employed sublingual surface electrodes (placed over the insertion of the genioglossus within the mandible) to compare the genioglossus responses with end-expiratory airway occlusion between preterm infants with mixed and

obstructive apnea and nonapneic control infants. In both groups of infants, genioglossus EMG activity was typically absent during unobstructed breathing. As seen in Figure 89-13, occlusion resulted in immediate release of this inhibition, with resultant augmentation of the genioglossus in the nonapneic infants. Infants with apnea, however, had significantly delayed activation of their genioglossus in response to occlusion. The cause of the delay in activation of the genioglossus after airway obstruction observed in apneic infants is not currently understood. This observation suggests that vagal inhibition of the dilator muscles of the upper airway does not contribute to the initiation of apnea. Subsequently, Gauda and co-workers[32] evaluated the activity of the genioglossus and diaphragm during spontaneously occurring mixed and obstructive apneic episodes. During mixed apnea, the amplitude of the diaphragm EMG activity decreased on the initial obstructed inspiratory effort and did not exceed that of the breath preceding apnea until flow was reestablished (Fig. 89-14). Genioglossus activity accompanied approximately only 20% of breaths immediately preceding spontaneous apnea, and this frequency did not increase significantly until resolution of the apnea, with genioglossus activity present during 40% of breaths associated with reestablishment of airflow. Thus, decreased diaphragmatic activity is a major component of spontaneous apnea associated with airway obstruction, and neither diaphragm nor genioglossus activity is increased until resolution of apnea. These findings suggest that central, mixed, and obstructive apnea are caused by a common mechanism, a reduction in central drive affecting the diaphragm and dilating muscles of the upper airway. However, the finding that only 40% of spontaneous apneic episodes were terminated with genioglossus activation indicates that this is not the sole mechanism by which upper airway obstruction is relieved in premature infants.

Upper Airway Reflexes

Reflexes originating from the upper airway may directly alter the pattern of respiration in infants and may play a crucial role in both the initiation and termination of apnea. The walls of the nasal cavity, nasopharynx and oropharynx, and larynx contain many sensory nerve endings that may respond to a variety of chemical and mechanical stimuli. Sensory input from these upper airway receptors travels to the central nervous system through cranial nerves V, VI, IX, X, XI, and XII and may have powerful effects on respiratory rate and rhythm, heart rate, and vascular resistance.[65] In human infants, interest has focused on two aspects of control of respiration by sensory input from the upper airway, that is, the response elicited from the nasopharynx to changes in luminal pressure and apnea produced by liquid

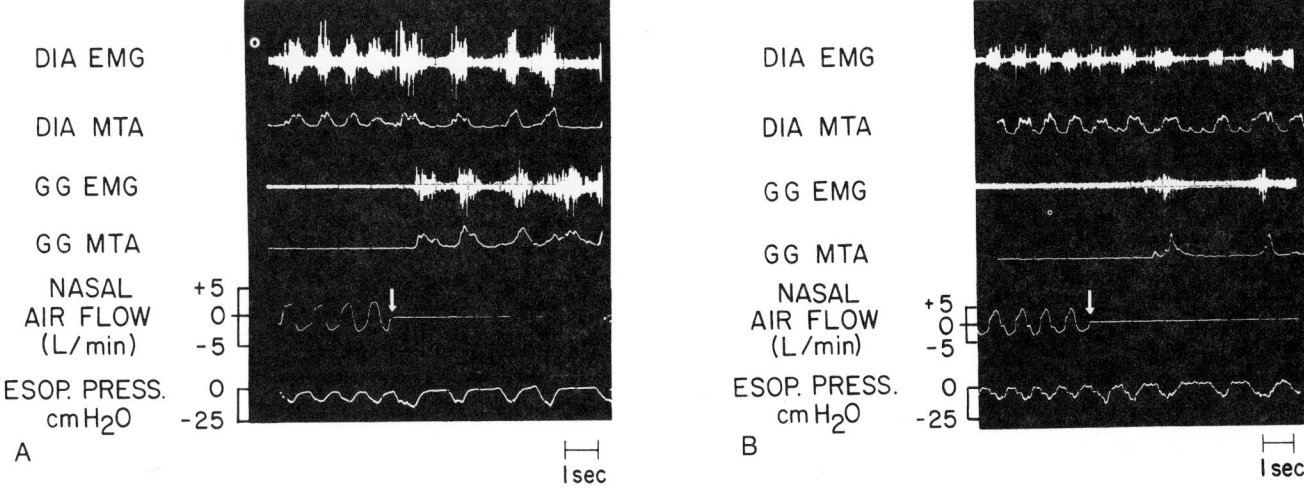

Figure 89–13. **A,** Typical response of the genioglossus (GG) electromyogram (EMG) in a nonapneic infant before and during occlusion. The *arrow* depicts the start of an end-expiratory airway occlusion. Both raw and moving time averaged (MTA) signals are presented for the GG EMG and the diaphragm (DIA) EMG. Each occluded inspiratory effort is associated with a GG EMG. **B,** Typical response of the GG EMG in an apneic infant before and during occlusion. The GG EMG does not appear until the third occluded inspiratory effort and reappears with the fifth occluded inspiratory effort. ESOP. PRESS. = esophageal pressure. (From Gauda EB, et al: Pediatr Res *22*:683, 1987.)

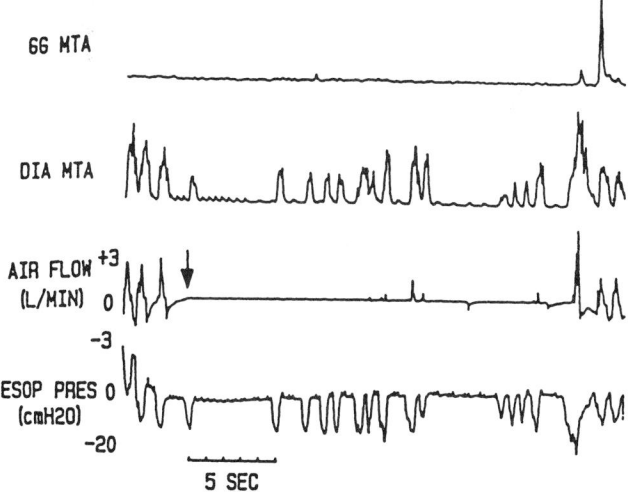

Figure 89–14. A representative tracing of the genioglossus (GG) and diaphragm (DIA) response during spontaneous apnea. The *arrow* denotes the onset of mixed apnea. The DIA amplitude of the initial obstructed inspiratory effort is less than the DIA amplitude of the breath preceding apnea, whereas the DIA amplitude of the breath at resolution of the apnea exceeds that of the preapneic breath. The GG electromyogram appears only at resolution of the apnea. The moving time averaged (MTA) signals for both the GG and DIA are depicted. ESOP PRES = esophageal pressure. (From Gauda EB, et al: Pediatr Res *26*:583, 1989.)

stimulation of chemoreceptors in and around the larynx and hypopharynx. Abu-Osba and co-workers[66] observed that sensory deprivation of the entire upper airway, including the larynx in rabbits, resulted in pharyngeal collapse. Similarly, topical anesthesia of the upper airway mucous membranes eliminated airway reflex response to pressure and was associated with pharyngeal obstruction, as well as death of the animal. These observations suggest that afferent sensory input from the upper airway is necessary for airway patency. In contrast, in kittens and puppies, steady airflow through the entire upper airway actually has been found to depress respiration.[67] Thus, depending on the species and experimental conditions, inhibitory or excitatory stimuli may originate from the upper airway.

In human infants who have undergone tracheostomy, Thach and others[68] showed that negative pressure within the isolated upper airway depressed ventilation. In adult rabbits, Mathew and Farber[69] examined the effect of upper airway negative pressure on respiratory timing. Application of negative pressure to the isolated upper airway resulted in prolonged diaphragmatic inhibition; however, phasic upper airway muscle activity continued. The ability of the upper airway muscles to respond to increasing negative pressure may be augmented by chemoreceptor drive and inhibited by input from pulmonary stretch receptors.[70] The net balance of these reflex inputs may ultimately determine the patency of the upper airway at a specific time. These observations may be relevant to the processes that initiate and resolve obstructive apnea. For example, during apnea, upper airway occlusion would result in increased negative airway pressure below the site of the obstruction. Reflex inhibition of diaphragmatic contraction resulting from increasing negative pressure in the airway lumen could produce the central pause characteristic of mixed apnea (see Fig. 89-1) and also could result in a decrease in luminal pressure, which would allow the airway to reopen.

A second important area of sensory reception in the upper airway lies in and around the larynx. Menon and co-workers[71] described apnea associated with overt regurgitation of gastric contents into the upper airway of human infants. Presumably, acidic stomach contents that enter the larynx excite chemoreceptors that cause both apnea and swallowing. These receptors have been studied in the lamb. Chemoreceptors in the region of the larynx send afferent neural output to the medulla: when these receptors are stimulated by water or ammonium chloride, apnea can be elicited.[72] Menon and co-workers[73] and, more recently, Miller and DiFiore[74] made an observation that may link idiopathic apnea of prematurity with inhibitory reflexes arising within the upper airway. Swallows were found to be much more common during apnea than during comparable periods of uninterrupted sleep (Fig. 89-15). Furthermore, swallowing during the respiratory pause is unique to apnea and does not occur during periodic breathing.[74] The origin of these swallows is unclear.

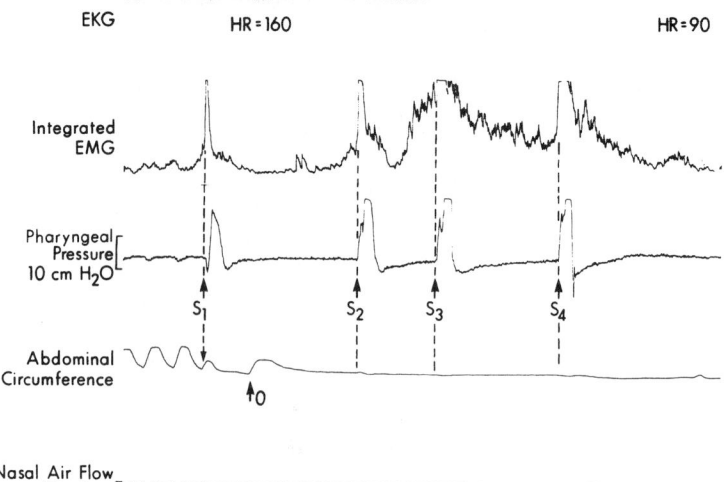

Figure 89–15. A typical prolonged apneic spell with swallowing (S1) occurring at the onset of the apnea as well as during the apnea (S2, S3, S4). An obstructed breath (0) is also noted at the beginning of the apnea. EKG = electrocardiogram; EMG = electromyogram; HR = heart rate. (From Menon AP, et al: Am Rev Respir Dis 130:969, 1984.)

Apneic episodes of varying duration have been elicited, resembling central or obstructive apnea, by introducing saline boluses into the oropharynx during sleep.[75] Accumulation of saliva in the pharynx could prolong apnea via a chemoreflex mechanism and also elicit swallowing movements.

Gastrointestinal Reflux

Although *gastroesophageal reflux* is often incriminated in causing neonatal apnea, caution should be exercised when attributing apnea to reflux. Despite the frequent coexistence of apnea and gastroesophageal reflux in preterm infants, investigations into the timing of reflux in relation to apneic events indicate that they are not commonly temporally related. Monitoring studies demonstrate that when a relationship between reflux and apnea is observed, apnea may precede rather than follow reflux (see Fig. 89-2).[76, 77] This suggests that loss of respiratory neural output during apnea may be accompanied by a decrease in lower esophageal tone and gastroesophageal reflux. Such a phenomenon is supported by data in a newborn piglet model, in which apnea was accompanied by a fall in lower esophageal sphincter pressure.[78] Although physiologic experiments in animals reveal that reflux of gastric contents to the larynx induces reflex apnea, there is no clear evidence that treatment of reflux will affect frequency of apnea in most preterm infants.[79] Therefore, pharmacologic management for reflux with agents that decrease gastric acidity or enhance gastrointestinal motility should be generally reserved for the preterm infants who exhibit signs of emesis or regurgitation of feedings, regardless of whether apnea is present.

PHYSIOLOGIC RATIONALE FOR THERAPEUTIC INTERVENTIONS

Continuous Positive Airway Pressure

Continuous positive airway pressure (CPAP) delivered by nasal prongs, nasal mask, or face mask at 2 to 5 cm H_2O pressure has proved effective in the treatment of apnea in preterm infants. Initial studies suggested that the beneficial effects of CPAP were mediated by means of an alteration of the Hering-Breuer reflex, stabilization of the chest wall with consequent reduction of the intercostal-phrenic inhibitory reflex, or increase in oxygenation.[80] Although such mechanisms may play a role, nasal CPAP reduces only mixed and obstructive apnea, with little or no effect on central apnea in infants (Fig. 89-16).[6] Therefore, it

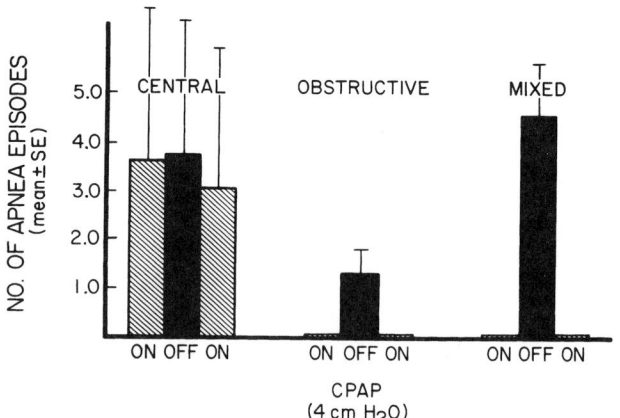

Figure 89–16. Effect of continuous positive airway pressure (CPAP) on the number of apneic episodes lasting 10 seconds or longer in 10 infants. Mixed and obstructive apnea decreased significantly during both periods of CPAP; however, no effect on central apnea was noted. (From Miller MJ, et al: J Pediatr 106:91, 1985.)

appears that CPAP exerts its beneficial effect in infants by splinting the upper airway with positive pressure throughout the respiratory cycle, and nasal cannula flow at 1 to 2.5 L/minute may serve the same purpose.[81] Animal studies have demonstrated that genioglossus activity decreases with CPAP administration[82]; therefore, reflex activation of upper airway dilating muscles is unlikely to be involved in the relief of apnea by CPAP.

Pharmacologic Agents

The methylxanthines (theophylline, caffeine) have proven effective in treatment of apnea in the newborn infant.[83] Several mechanisms have been proposed whereby methylxanthines decrease the incidence of apnea (Table 89-1). Available evidence points to central respiratory stimulation rather than bronchodilatation as the major site of action. In infants, caffeine has been shown to increase minute ventilation by increasing mean inspiratory flow (a measure of inspiratory drive) without altering respiratory timing.[84] This is consistent with the data obtained in premature infants receiving therapeutic doses of aminophylline. Gerhardt and associates[85] observed an increase in respiratory center output in premature infants receiving aminophylline, as meas-

TABLE 89-1

Effects of Xanthines

Physiologic
  Increased minute ventilation
  Shift of CO_2 response curve to left ± increased slope
  Greater efficiency of diaphragmatic contraction
  Improved pulmonary mechanics
  Decreased hypoxic ventilatory depression
Biochemical
  Adenosine receptor antagonism
  Inhibition of phosphodiesterase
  Enhancement of calcium flux across sarcolemma (?)

ured by an increase in esophageal pressure change per breath, and a lowering of the threshold of the respiratory center to carbon dioxide. At the dose of aminophylline employed in this study, no increase in carbon dioxide sensitivity or improvement in pulmonary mechanics was observed. A concurrent increase (approximately 20%) in metabolic rate was noted, however, and was recently confirmed with caffeine.[86] This could be considered an adverse effect in preterm infants, who are frequently nutritionally compromised. These findings are in agreement with the central stimulatory effect of theophylline, which has been reported in animals and human adults. Animal data suggest that systemically administered theophylline acts directly on brain stem neurons, because respiratory stimulation occurs in the absence of peripheral (carotid body or vagus) reflex mechanisms, medullary chemoreceptor responses, or suprapontine brain structures.[87] Additional stimulatory effects of aminophylline on peripheral chemoreceptor activity were demonstrated by Cattarossi and others[88] in the newborn human. Thus, in the infant, aminophylline may exert its effects at both the peripheral and central chemoreceptors.

The xanthines inhibit phosphodiesterase, which normally breaks down cyclic adenosine monophosphate (cAMP), although the relationship of cAMP accumulation with relief of apnea in infants is unclear. Adenosine and its analogues cause respiratory depression, and adenosine antagonism has also been proposed as the major mechanism to explain the therapeutic effect of theophylline.[34] In support of this concept, Darnall[89] documented that aminophylline partially reduces the ventilatory depression induced by hypoxia in newborn piglets. Xanthines may, however, have additional effects on the respiratory system. In adult patients with emphysema, theophylline appears to enhance diaphragmatic strength, as measured by transdiaphragmatic pressure generated against an occluded airway, while reducing EMG evidence of diaphragmatic fatigue.[90] Enhancement of calcium transport across the sarcolemma is a proposed mechanism by which theophylline increases diaphragm contractility, although the relevance of this action to human infants with apnea is not known.[91]

Doxapram, known to be a potent respiratory stimulant with predominantly peripheral chemoreceptor effects, has been used in neonates with idiopathic apnea of prematurity.[92] This drug may have a limited therapeutic role in infants with apnea refractory to xanthine derivatives, although potential side effects appear to limit its usefulness.[93] Despite the widespread use of methylxanthines for treatment of apnea, many questions remain to be answered concerning selection for therapy, duration of therapy, and potential long-term effects on growth and development.[94]

Relation of Apnea to Sudden Infant Death Syndrome

One of the controversial aspects of apnea has been its proposed relation to the *sudden infant death syndrome* (SIDS). Many observations on the epidemiology and physiology of SIDS point to an abnormality of control of ventilation as one underlying cause of this multifactorial disorder. Early reports of the neuropathology of SIDS suggested the presence of tissue changes consistent with chronic hypoxia within the areas of the brain stem that regulate breathing and within the carotid body.[95, 96] Prolonged apnea has been reported in infants with *near-miss SIDS* (now referred to as *apparent life-threatening event*), a proportion of whom subsequently died of SIDS.[97] Short apneic episodes, periodic breathing, and mixed and obstructive apnea have all been identified in near-miss SIDS infants.[98] In addition, a decreased ventilatory response to hypercarbia and hypoxia has been observed in infants at risk of SIDS.[99] All these observations suggested that an abnormality of ventilatory control could contribute to death from SIDS. Such considerations prompted the development of polygraphic monitoring in which variables such as heart rate, nasal airflow, chest and abdominal movement, and transcutaneous oxygen tension or oxygen saturation were measured in an attempt to predict the risk of SIDS in vulnerable infants. However, studies evaluating large cohorts of infants have failed to demonstrate that monitoring of cardiorespiratory variables could prospectively identify SIDS victims.[100] Although evidence implicates an abnormality of ventilatory control in SIDS, the nature of this abnormality is unknown. Indeed, more than one underlying cause of cardiorespiratory instability may eventually be implicated in this disorder. For example, it has been proposed that approximately 2% of infants who die of SIDS may have a sodium channel mutation with resultant predisposition to the long QT syndrome and potentially fatal arrhythmia.[101, 102]

Body Position

A reduction in postneonatal mortality and in the rate of sudden infant death has been associated with sleeping in the supine position. This finding has been substantiated in many countries and has generated public education campaigns designed to promote supine and avoid prone sleeping.[103] The physiologic mechanisms that underlie this relationship between SIDS and prone positioning are currently under active investigation. These include softness and porosity of bedding, which may encourage carbon dioxide rebreathing,[104] and thermal stress, which may destabilize respiratory control by as yet undetermined mechanisms.[105]

Several studies have documented physiologic benefits for prone versus supine positioning in preterm infants, especially in the presence of residual lung disease. These include modest improvement in transcutaneously measured partial pressure of oxygen,[106] more time in quiet sleep,[107] decreased energy expenditure,[108] less apnea,[109] and greater ventilatory responses to inspired carbon dioxide[110] in the prone as compared with the supine position. These findings suggest that respiratory control may be vulnerable in preterm infants who are placed supine, even when there is no longer overt respiratory distress. Nonetheless, supine positioning should also be recommended for such infants in the home, and it should be initiated before hospital discharge. Prenatal and postnatal exposure to smoking also predisposes to SIDS, although extensive physiologic studies have failed to reveal an underlying mechanism consistently.[111]

Apnea as a Continuum from the Infant to the Child and Adult and Neurodevelopmental Outcome

Apnea of prematurity generally resolves by about 36 to 40 weeks of postconceptional age. However, in the most premature infants (24 to 28 weeks' gestation), apnea frequently persists beyond 36 weeks of postconceptional age, and in occasional infants it may persist beyond 40 weeks of postconceptional age. Cardiorespiratory events in such infants return to the baseline "normal" level at about 43 to 44 weeks of postconceptional age.

In other words, beyond 43 to 44 weeks of postconceptional age, the incidence of cardiorespiratory events in preterm infants does not significantly exceed that in term babies (see Fig. 89-5).[25]

Many preterm infants have resolved their apnea and bradycardia by the time they are ready for hospital discharge as determined by maturation of temperature control and feeding pattern. An apnea-free observation period, usually ranging from 3 to 7 days, is used as a criterion for determining discharge date. For a subset of infants, however, the persistence of cardiorespiratory events may delay discharge from the hospital. In these infants, apnea lasting longer than 20 seconds is rare; rather, they exhibit frequent episodes of desaturation to less than 80% or bradycardia to less than 70 or 80 beats/minute with short respiratory pauses. The reason that some infants exhibit marked desaturation and bradycardia with short pauses is unclear.[112-114] For such infants, home cardiorespiratory monitoring until 43 to 44 of weeks postconceptional age may offer an alternative to a prolonged hospital stay.

Because idiopathic apnea is most often seen in high-risk preterm infants, separating the consequences of premature birth from the effects of apnea of prematurity has proven difficult. Infants born prematurely often have multiple problems, and many of these conditions, particularly periventricular leukomalacia and intraventricular hemorrhage, may contribute to poor neurodevelopmental outcome. In one study of preterm infants followed-up to early school age, factors that predicted poor neurodevelopmental outcomes included apnea of prematurity.[115] In another series of very low birth weight infants followed-up to 24 months of age, predischarge apnea and desaturation during apnea correlated with mental and motor neurodevelopmental scores. It is possible that recurrent hypoxia is the detrimental feature of the breathing abnormalities exhibited by preterm infants.[116] Ongoing studies are addressing the question whether pharmacologic treatment of apnea affects longer-term neurodevelopmental outcome.

A respiratory disorder similar to apnea of infancy, termed *sleep apnea syndrome,* also occurs in adults. Both obese and non-obese adults may present with mixed, obstructive, or central sleep apnea.[117, 118] Just as in infantile apnea, adults with sleep apnea syndrome experience upper airway obstruction within the pharynx. Sleep apnea syndrome may be accompanied by daytime somnolence, hypoxemia, cardiac arrhythmias, polycythemia, hypertension, morning headaches, and intellectual deterioration. CPAP has been used effectively to relieve mixed, obstructive, and central apnea in adults.[119] Thus, it would seem that the pathophysiology of sleep apnea in adults and infants may share some common elements, including failure of maintenance of patency of the upper airway. Adults and infants do differ in two respects. In adults, obstructive apnea fails to respond to theophylline therapy.[120] This lack of response may reflect an underlying dissimilarity in the balance of inhibitory and excitatory neurotransmitters that regulate respiration in humans at different ages. Alternatively, the degree of narrowing of the upper airway may be more critical for development of obstructive apnea in adults than in infants. In addition, apnea in adults is not accompanied by an increase in spontaneous swallows. In childhood, sleep-disordered breathing is receiving greater attention, and its potential relation to apnea of prematurity is under study.

The long-term outcome of infants with persistent sleep apnea is not well understood. Guilleminault and co-workers[121] described children 6 months to 17 years old who had obstructive sleep apnea syndrome. The presenting complaints included sleepiness, fatigue, personality changes, and poor school performance. All children had continuous heavy snoring during sleep. Twenty-two children with secondary sleep apnea had an obvious cause of their apnea such as micrognathia, neuromuscular disorders such as Arnold-Chiari malformation, or syringobul-

bia. Twenty-six children with primary sleep apnea exhibited no clear cause of their disorder, although mildly enlarged adenoids were reported. Thus, apnea as a manifestation of instability of respiratory control of the diaphragm and upper airway during sleep has been described in infants, young children, and adults. The underlying complex of factors that produce apnea, including cyclic fluctuation in respiratory center output, imbalance of drive to the upper airway musculature, and anatomic narrowing of the upper airway, may differ in each age group, but the final outcome, apnea, is remarkably similar. Sleep apnea thus emerges as a not so silent disorder that accompanies humanity from the cradle to the grave.

FUTURE DIRECTIONS

Initiation of Apnea

Two questions may be fundamental both to the cause of apnea and to the nature of the respiratory dysfunction in SIDS:

1. How is apnea initiated?
2. By what mechanisms is apnea terminated?

Cyclic instability of ventilation has been observed in both infants and adults with sleep apnea. Cherniack and Longobardo[122] proposed that apnea may derive from instability in the automatic feedback control of breathing. In this model, cyclic variation in ventilation, such as observed in periodic breathing, could derive from increased circulation time, increased chemoreceptor sensitivity, or the inherently low stores of oxygen in the circulation. For example, apnea could occur when the respiratory control center in the medulla overcompensates in response to a brief increase in ventilation, resulting in a *central* respiratory pause, or apnea. Obstructive apnea could be produced when, in addition, an imbalance of central drive exists to the upper airway dilating muscles and diaphragm, as described earlier in this chapter.

Initiation of apnea could also involve a global alteration in the central regulation of ventilation and muscular function. During all stages of sleep (particularly active sleep), a generalized decrease in skeletal muscle tone occurs. A more profound depression of muscle tone may occur during apnea. Schulte and others[123] reported that monosynaptic reflex excitability decreases during prolonged apnea and speculated that these changes may result from a decrease in output from the reticular activating system to the brain stem as well as higher brain structures. Thus, unstable feedback control of ventilation, an imbalance in activity of upper airway muscles and the diaphragm, and a decrease in output from the reticular activating system have all been proposed as mechanisms that may initiate apnea, but which factor is most crucial has yet to be demonstrated.

Termination of Apnea

Increasing hypoxia and hypercarbia during apnea would be expected to lead to increased ventilatory drive to the diaphragm and upper airway, resulting in eventual resolution of apnea. Why, then, do some infants apparently fail to respond appropriately to these stimuli? As previously discussed, auditory brain stem conduction times are prolonged in infants with apnea, possibly reflecting decreased synaptic efficiency and myelination.[31] The delayed response of the apneic infant to hypercapnia and hypoxia may simply be the result of immaturity in processing afferent chemosensory information at the brain stem level. The decreased carbon dioxide response observed in apneic infants is consistent with this hypothesis.

Arousal from sleep may also play a role in the ability of the infant to terminate apnea quickly. The nature of the infant's sleep state may determine whether arousal occurs in response to apnea; this issue was investigated by Baker and Fewell[124] in the lamb. In active sleep, arousal was dependent on the rate of change in arterial oxygen concentration. A synergy appeared to exist between arterial carbon dioxide and oxygen levels, the most rapid arousal occurring when both were changing.[125] Repeated exposure to hypoxemia during sleep resulted in evidence of adaptation, that is, increased time to arousal and decreased saturation at arousal. Such habituation to repeated hypoxic exposure has not been studied in human infants. However, depression of reflex response to hypoxia could provide a mechanism by which multiple sequential apneas could occur. Thus, several important variables, including peripheral and central chemoreceptor responses, sleep state, and previous exposure to hypoxia, could affect the infant's ability to terminate apnea. Exactly which of these influences is most crucial in resolution of apnea in the human infant remains an important question for future research.

ACKNOWLEDGMENT

This work is supported by National Institutes of Health grant HL62527.

REFERENCES

1. Task Force on Prolonged Apnea: Prolonged apnea. Pediatrics *61*:651, 1978.
2. Rigatto H, Brady JP: Periodic breathing and apnea in preterm infants, evidence for hypoventilation possibly due to central respiratory depression. Pediatrics *50*:202, 1972.
3. Thach BT, Stark AR: Spontaneous neck flexion and airway obstruction during apneic spells in preterm infants. J Pediatr *94*:275, 1979.
4. Milner AD, et al: Upper airway obstruction and apnea in preterm babies. Arch Dis Child *55*:22, 1980.
5. Mathew OP, et al: Pharyngeal airway obstruction in preterm infants during mixed and obstructive apnea. J Pediatr *100*:964, 1982.
6. Miller MJ, et al: Continuous positive airway pressure selectively reduces obstructive apnea in preterm infants. J Pediatr *106*:91, 1985.
7. Butcher-Puech MC, et al: Relation between apnoea duration and type and neurological status of preterm infants. Arch Dis Child *60*:953, 1985.
8. Bolivar J, et al: Mechanisms for episodes of hypoxemia in mechanically ventilated preterm infants. Pediatr Res *35*:A1287, 1994.
9. Miller MJ, et al: Changes in resistance and ventilatory timing that accompany apnea in premature infants. J Appl Physiol *75*:720, 1993.
10. Dimaguila MAVT, et al: Characteristics of hypoxemic episodes in intubated very low birthweight infants. J Pediatr *130*:577, 1997.
11. Lehtonen L et al: Relationship of sleep state to hypoxemic episodes in ventilated ELBW infants. J Pediatr *141*:363–9, 2002.
12. Kahn A, et al: Effects of obstructive sleep apneas on transcutaneous oxygen pressure in control infants, siblings of sudden infant death syndrome victims and near miss infants: comparison with the effects of central sleep apneas. Pediatrics *70*:852, 1982.
13. Kitchen WH, et al: Collaborative study of very-low-birth-weight infants. Am J Dis Child *137*:555, 1983.
14. Haddad GG, et al: Heart rate pattern during respiratory pauses in normal infants during sleep. J Dev Physiol *6*:329, 1984.
15. Valimaki I, Tarlo PA: Heart rate patterns and apnea in newborn infants. Am J Obstet Gynecol *110*:343, 1971.
16. Henderson-Smart DJ, et al: Incidence and mechanism of bradycardia during apnoea in preterm infants. Arch Dis Child *61*:227, 1986.
17. Daly M de B, Scott MJ: The effect of stimulation of the carotid body chemoreceptors on heart rate in the dog. J Physiol (Lond) *144*:148, 1958.
18. Davidson NS, et al: Respiratory modulation of baroreceptor and chemoreceptor reflexes affecting heart rate and cardiac vagal efferent nerve activity. J Physiol (Lond) *259*:523, 1976.
19. Angell-James JE, et al: Lung inflation: effects on heart rate, respiration, and vagal afferent activity in seals. Am J Physiol *240*:H190, 1981.
20. Girling DJ: Changes in heart rate, blood pressure, and pulse pressure during apnoeic attacks in newborn babies. Arch Dis Child *7*:405, 1972.
21. Perlman JM, Volpe JJ: Episodes of apnea and bradycardia in the preterm newborn: impact on cerebral circulation. Pediatrics *76*:333, 1985.
22. Ramalkers VT, et al: Cerebral hyperperfusion following episodes of bradycardia in the preterm infant. Early Hum Dev *34*:199, 1993.
23. Alden ER, et al: Morbidity and mortality of infants weighing less than 1000 grams in an intensive care nursery. Pediatrics *50*:40, 1972.
24. Carlo WA, et al: The effect of respiratory distress syndrome on chest wall movements and respiratory pauses in preterm infants. Am Rev Respir Dis *126*:103, 1982.
25. Ramanathan R, et al: Cardiorespiratory events recorded on home monitors: Comparison of healthy infants with those at increased risk for SIDS. JAMA *285*:2199, 2001.
26. Adickes ED, et al: Familial lethal sleep apnea. Hum Genet *73*:39, 1986.
27. Brazy JE, et al: Central nervous system structure lesions causing apnea at birth. J Pediatr *111*:163, 1987.
28. Pickens DL, et al: Characterization of prolonged apneic episodes associated with respiratory syncytial virus infection. Pediatr Pulmonol *6*:195, 1989.
29. Welborn LG, et al: Postoperative apnea in former premature infants: prospective comparison of spinal and general anaesthesia. Anaesthesiology *72*:838, 1990.
30. Martin RJ, et al: Pathogenesis of apnea in preterm infants. J Pediatr *109*:733, 1986.
31. Henderson-Smart DJ, et al: Clinical apnea and brainstem neural function in preterm infants. N Engl J Med *308*:353, 1983.
32. Gauda EB, et al: Genioglossus and diaphragm activity during obstructive apnea and airway occlusion in infants. Pediatr Res *26*:583, 1989.
33. Abu-Shaweesh JM, et al: Changes in respiratory timing induces by hypercapnia in maturing rats. J Appl Physiol *87*:484, 1999.
34. Abu-Shaweesh JM, et al: Central GABAergic mechanisms are involved in apnea induced by SLN stimulation in piglets. J Appl Physiol *90*:1570, 2001.
35. Miller MJ, et al: Recurrent hypoxic exposure and reflex responses during development in the piglet. Respir Physiol *123*:51, 2000.
36. Suguihara C, et al: Effect of dopamine on hypoxic ventilatory response of sedated piglets with intact and denervated carotid bodies. J Appl Physiol *77*:285, 1994.
37. Long WA, Lawson EE: Developmental aspects of the effect of naloxone on control of breathing in piglets. Respir Physiol *51*:119, 1983.
38. Mayock DE, et al: Role of endogenous opiates in hypoxic ventilatory response in the newborn primate. J Appl Physiol *60*:2015, 1986.
39. Chernick V, et al: Clinical trial of naloxone in birth asphyxia. J Pediatr *113*:519, 1988.
40. Hoppenbrouwers T, et al: Polygraphic studies of normal infants during the first six months of life. III. Incidence of apnea and periodic breathing. Pediatrics *60*:418, 1977.
41. Haddad GG, et al: Determination of sleep state in infants using respiratory variability. Pediatr Res *21*:556, 1987.
42. Curzi-Dascalova L: Thoracico-abdominal respiratory correlations in infants: constancy and variability in different sleep states. Early Hum Dev *2*:25, 1978.
43. Bryan AC, Bryan MH: Control of respiration in the newborn. Clin Perinatol *5*:269, 1978.
44. Martin RJ, et al: Arterial oxygen tension during active and quiet sleep in the normal neonate. J Pediatr *94*:271, 1979.
45. Muller N, et al: Diaphragmatic muscle fatigue in the newborn. J Appl Physiol *46*:688, 1979.
46. Thach BT: The role of pharyngeal airway obstruction in prolonging infantile apneic spells. *In* Tilden JT, et al (eds): Sudden Infant Death Syndrome. New York, Academic Press, 1983, p 279.
47. Rigatto H, et al: Chemoreceptor reflexes in preterm infants. II. The effect of gestational and postnatal age on the ventilatory response to inhaled carbon dioxide. Pediatrics *55*:614, 1975.
48. Noble LM, et al: Transient changes in expiratory time during hypercapnia in premature infants. J Appl Physiol *62*:1010, 1987.
49. Gerhardt T, Bancalari E: Apnea of prematurity. I. Lung function and regulation of breathing. Pediatrics *74*:58, 1984.
50. Martin RJ, et al: Hypoglossal and phrenic responses to central respiratory inhibition in piglets. Respir Physiol *97*:93, 1994.
51. Martin RJ, et al: Role of the ventral medullary surface in modulating respiratory responses to reflex stimulation in piglets. *In* Trouth OL, et al (eds): Ventral Brainstem Mechanisms and Control of Respiration and Blood Pressure. New York, Marcel Dekker, 1995, p 625.
52. Cross KW, Oppe TE: The effect of inhalation of high and low concentrations of oxygen on the respiration of the premature infant. J Physiol *117*:38, 1952.
53. Rigatto H, et al: Effects of O_2 on the ventilatory response to CO_2 in preterm infants. J Appl Physiol *39*:896, 1975.
54. Martin RJ, et al: Persistence of the biphasic ventilatory response to hypoxia in preterm infants. J Pediatr *132*:960, 1998.
55. Martin RJ, et al: Effect of lung volume on expiratory time in the newborn infant. J Appl Physiol *45*:18, 1978.
56. Carlo WA, et al: Differential response of respiratory muscles to airway occlusion in infants. J Appl Physiol *59*:847, 1985.
57. Gerhardt T, Bancalari E: Apnea of prematurity. II: respiratory reflexes. Pediatrics *74*:63, 1984.
58. Waggener TB, et al: Oscillatory breathing patterns leading to apneic spells in infants. J Appl Physiol *52*:1288, 1982.
59. Fenner A, et al: Periodic breathing in premature and neonatal babies: incidence, breathing pattern, respiratory gas tensions, response to changes in the composition of ambient air. Pediatr Res *7*:174, 1973.
60. Miller MJ, et al: Airway obstruction during periodic breathing in premature infants. J Appl Physiol *64*:2496, 1988.
61. Carlo WA, et al: Differences in CO_2 threshold of respiratory muscles in preterm infants. J Appl Physiol *65*:2434, 1988.
62. Haxhiu MA, et al: Responses to chemical stimulation of upper airway muscles and diaphragm in awake cats. J Appl Physiol *56*:397, 1984.

63. van Lunteren E, et al: Phasic volume-related feedback on upper airway muscle activity. J Appl Physiol 56:730, 1984.

64. Gauda EB, et al: Genioglossus response to airway obstruction in apneic versus nonapneic infants. Pediatr Res 22:683, 1987.

65. Long WA, Lawson EE: Maturation of the superior laryngeal nerve inhibiting effect. Am Rev Respir Dis 123:A166, 1981.

66. Abu-Osba YK, et al: An animal model for airway sensory deprivation producing obstructive apnea with postmortem findings of sudden infant death syndrome. Pediatrics 68:796, 1981.

67. Al-Shway S, Mortola JP: Respiratory effects of airflow through the upper airways in newborn kittens and puppies. J Appl Physiol 53:805, 1982.

68. Thach BT, et al: Negative upper airway pressure decreases inspiratory airflow and tidal volume in tracheostomized sleeping human infants. Am Rev Respir Dis 131:A295, 1985.

69. Mathew OP, Farber JP: Effect of upper airway negative pressure on respiratory timing. Respir Physiol 54:259, 1983.

70. Gauda EG, et al: Mechano- and chemoreceptor modulation of respiratory muscles in response to upper airway negative pressure. J Appl Physiol 76:2656, 1994.

71. Menon AP, et al: Apnea associated with regurgitation in infants. J Pediatr 106:625, 1985.

72. Storey T, Johnson P: Laryngeal water receptors initiating apnea in the lamb. Exp Neurol 47:42, 1975.

73. Menon AP, et al: Frequency and significance of swallowing during prolonged apnea in infants. Am Rev Respir Dis 130:969, 1984.

74. Miller MJ, DiFiore JM: A comparison of swallowing during apnea and periodic breathing in premature infants. Pediatr Res 37:796, 1995.

75. Pickens DL, et al: Prolonged apnea associated with upper airway protective reflexes in apnea of prematurity. Am Rev Respir Dis 137:113, 1988.

76. Arad-Cohen N, et al: The relationship between gastroesophageal reflux and apnea in infants. J Pediatr 137:321, 2000.

77. Peter CS, et al: Gastroesophageal reflux and apnea of prematurity: no temporal relationship. Pediatrics 109:8, 2002.

78. Kiatchoosakun P, et al: Effects of hypoxia on respiratory neural output and lower esophageal sphincter pressure in piglets. Pediatr Res 52:50–55, 2002.

79. Kimball AL, Carlton DP: Gastroesophageal reflux medications in the treatment of apnea in premature infants. J Pediatr 138:355, 2001.

80. Martin RJ, et al: The effect of a low continuous positive airway pressure on the reflex control of respiration in the preterm infants. J Pediatr 90:976, 1977.

81. Sreenan C, et al: High-flow nasal cannulae in the management of apnea of prematurity: a comparison with conventional nasal continuous positive airway pressure. Pediatrics 107:108, 2001.

82. Mathew OP, et al: Influence of upper airway pressure changes on genioglossus muscle respiratory activity. J Appl Physiol 52:438, 1982.

83. Henderson-Smart DJ, Steer P: Methylxanthine treatment for apnea in preterm infants. Cochrane Database Syst Review 3:CD00140, 2001.

84. Aranda JV, et al: Effect of caffeine on control of breathing in infantile apnea. J Pediatr 103:975, 1983.

85. Gerhardt T, et al: Effect of aminophylline on respiratory center activity and metabolic rate in premature infants with idiopathic apnea. Pediatrics 63:537, 1979.

86. Bauer J, et al: Effect of caffeine on oxygen consumption and metabolic rate in very low birth weight infants with idiopathic apnea. Pediatrics 107:660, 2001.

87. Eldridge FL, et al: Mechanism of respiratory effects of methylxanthines. Respir Physiol 53:239, 1983.

88. Cattarossi L, et al: Aminophylline and increased activity of peripheral chemoreceptors in newborn infants. Arch Dis Child 69:52, 1993.

89. Darnall RA Jr: Aminophylline reduces hypoxic ventilatory depression: possible role of adenosine. Pediatr Res 19:706, 1985.

90. Murciano D, et al: Effects of theophylline on diaphragmatic strength and fatigue in patients with chronic obstructive pulmonary disease. N Engl J Med 311:349, 1984.

91. Aubier M, et al: Diaphragmatic contractility enhanced by aminophylline: role of extracellular calcium. J Appl Physiol 54:460, 1983.

92. Yamazaki T, et al: Low dose doxapram therapy for apnea of prematurity. Pediatr Int 43:124, 2001.

93. Barrington KJ, et al: Physiologic effects of doxapram in idiopathic apnea of prematurity. J Pediatr 108:124, 1986.

94. Schmidt B: Methylxanthine therapy in premature infants: Sound practice, disaster, or fruitless byway. J Pediatr 135:526, 1998.

95. Naeye RL: Brainstem and adrenal abnormalities in the sudden infant death syndrome. Am J Clin Pathol 66:526, 1976.

96. Naeye RL, et al: Carotid body in the sudden infant death syndrome. Science 191:567, 1976.

97. Cornwell AC, et al: Ambulatory and in-hospital continuous recording of sleep state and cardiorespiratory parameters in near-miss for the sudden infant death syndrome and control infants. Biotelemetry 5:113, 1978.

98. Guilleminault C, et al: Apneas during sleep in infants: possible relationship with sudden infant death syndrome. Science 190:677, 1975.

99. Shannon DC, et al: Abnormal regulation of ventilation in infants at risk for sudden infant death syndrome. N Engl J Med 297:747, 1977.

100. United States Department of Health and Human Services: Infantile apnea and home monitoring: report of a consensus development conference. NIH publication no. 87-2905. Bethesda, MD, National Institutes of Health, 1987.

101. Schwartz PJ, et al: Molecular diagnosis in a child with sudden infant death syndrome. Lancet 358:1342, 2001.

102. Ackerman MJ, et al: Postmortem molecular analysis of SCN5A defects in sudden infant death syndrome. JAMA 286:2264, 2001.

103. Willinger M, et al: Infant sleep position and risk for sudden infant death syndrome: report of meeting held January 13 and 14, 1994, National Institutes of Health, Bethesda, MD. Pediatrics 93:814, 1994.

104. Kemp JS, Thach BT: Quantifying the potential of infant bedding to limit CO_2 dispersal and factors affecting rebreathing in bedding. J Appl Physiol 78:740, 1995.

105. Fleming PJ, et al: Interactions between thermoregulation and the control of respiration in infants: possible relationship to sudden infant death. Acta Paediatr Suppl 389:57, 1993.

106. Martin RJ, et al: Arterial oxygen tension during active and quiet sleep in the normal neonate. J Pediatr 94:271, 1979.

107. Brackbill Y, et al: Psychophysiologic effects in the neonate of prone versus supine placement. J Pediatr 82:82, 1973.

108. Masterson J, et al: Prone and supine positioning effects on energy expenditure and behavior of low birth weight neonates. Pediatrics 80:689, 1987.

109. Heimler R, et al: Effect of positioning on the breathing pattern of preterm infants. Arch Dis Child 67:312, 1992.

110. Martin RJ, et al: Vulnerability of respiratory control in healthy preterm infants placed supine. J Pediatr 127:609, 1995.

111. Sundell H: Why does maternal smoke exposure increase the risk of sudden infant death syndrome? Acta Pediatr 90:718, 2001.

112. Upton CJ, et al: Apnoea, bradycardia, and oxygen saturation in preterm infants. Arch Dis Child 66:381, 1991.

113. Poets CF, et al: Prolonged episodes of hypoxemia in preterm infants undetectable by cardiorespiratory monitors. Pediatrics 95:860, 1995.

114. DiFiore JM, et al: Cardiorespiratory events in preterm infants referred for apnea monitoring studies. Pediatrics 108:1304, 2001.

115. Taylor HG, et al: Predictors of early school age outcomes in very low birth weight children. J Dev Behav Pediatr 19:235, 1998.

116. Cheung P-Y, et al: Early childhood neurodevelopment in very low birth weight infants with predischarge apnea. Pediatr Pulmonol 27:14, 1999.

117. Guilleminault C, Dement WC: Sleep apnea syndrome and related sleep disorders. In Williams RL, Koracan I (eds): Sleep Disorders: Diagnosis and Treatment. New York, John Wiley, 1978, p 9.

118. Bradley TD, et al: Clinical and physiologic heterogeneity of the central sleep apnea syndrome. Am Rev Respir Dis 134:217, 1986.

119. Remmers JE, et al: Nasal airway positive pressure in patients with occlusive sleep apnea. Am Rev Respir Dis 130:1152, 1984.

120. Guilleminault C, Hayes B: Naloxone, theophylline, bromocriptine, and obstructive sleep apnea: negative results. Bull Eur Physiopathol Respir 19:632, 1983.

121. Guilleminault C, et al: A review of 50 children with obstructive sleep apnea syndrome. Lung 159:275, 1981.

122. Cherniack NS, Longobardo GS: Cheyne-Stokes breathing: an instability in physiologic control. N Engl J Med 288:952, 1973.

123. Schulte FJ, et al: Rapid eye movement sleep, motoneurone inhibition, and apneic spells in preterm infants. Pediatr Res 11:709, 1977.

124. Baker SB, Fewell JE: Effects of hyperoxia on the arousal response to upper airway obstruction in lambs. Pediatr Res 21:116, 1987.

125. Fewell JE, Konduri G: Repeated exposure to rapidly developing hypoxemia influences the interaction between oxygen and carbon dioxide in initiating arousal from sleep in lambs. Pediatr Res 24:28, 1988.

90

Evaluation of Pulmonary Function in the Neonate

The ability to measure lung function is essential for understanding basic physiology, confirming the diagnosis of pathologic conditions, and evaluating the effect of therapeutic interventions. Pulmonary function testing in adults and children has been effectively used as a research and clinical tool since the 1950s.[1] Although infant pulmonary function testing was introduced about the same time,[2] its practical use has lagged behind due to technical limitations, lack of cooperation from patients, long-term duration of testing and time-consuming analysis methods.[3-7] The availability of computerized pulmonary function systems and on-line volume-pressure data has moved infant pulmonary function testing from the research laboratories to the patient bedside, while efforts to weed out the physiologic and technical factors that can distort accurate measurements continue.

PHYSIOLOGIC BACKGROUND

Each respiratory cycle is governed by the volume of air, driving pressure, and time (Fig. 90-1). The volume of air that enters or leaves the respiratory tract over a period of time determines airflow.

The driving force required for initiation of inspiratory airflow is generated by contraction of the respiratory muscles and outward movement of the thorax. This results in a transient decrease in alveolar pressure from atmospheric pressure at end expiration to subatmospheric level and peak flow at midinspiration. Inspiratory flow continues until alveolar pressure returns to atmospheric pressure at the end of the inspiratory phase. The expiratory driving force is generated by relaxation of the respiratory muscles and inward recoil of the lung, resulting in an increase in alveolar pressure and causing expiratory airflow. Flow reaches a peak at midexpiration and returns to zero at the end of the expiratory cycle when alveolar pressure returns to zero again, at which point another respiratory cycle commences.

Therefore, change in alveolar pressure is determined by airway resistance and airflow, and alveolar pressure cycles from a negative to a positive value relative to atmospheric pressure. Pleural pressure, however, remains subatmospheric throughout the respiratory cycle due to a balance of the opposing forces of lung elastic recoil and chest wall outward recoil. Pleural pressure decreases during spontaneous inspiration. The magnitude of the change in pleural pressure is determined by airflow, tissue resistances, and elastic forces. Because there is no airflow at the end-inspiratory and end-expiratory points of the breathing cycle, there are no flow-resistive losses; at these time points, pleural pressure depends only on elastic forces (in healthy lungs during normal tidal breathing). At mid breathing cycle, however, airflow and resistance are maximal. Basic evaluation of pulmonary functions is therefore, based on measurements of the interaction of driving pressure (P), flow ($\dot{V}$), and volume (V). The equation of motion[8] that has been used to describe the mechanics of air flow and driving pressure is:

$$P = EV + R\dot{V}V + I\ddot{V}$$

where
E = Elastance of the respiratory tract (equivalent to the reciprocal of compliance [C] or E = 1/C).
R = Frictional resistance of respiratory tract.
I = Inertance of the respiratory tract, due to airflow acceleration ($\ddot{V}$).

This linearized relationship of driving pressure to volume and flow has been considered an ideal elemental equation[8] and has been a basic principle of respiratory physiology. However, it is well appreciated that the respiratory system is not a linear system. Resistance and compliance are not constants, and both depend on volume, volume history, and flow. In addition, the respiratory system is a complex system consisting of multiple components with differing mechanical properties. This is particularly pertinent in the preterm neonate.[9-11] Despite its inexactitude, and because of the complexities of dealing with nonlinear modeling, a simple linear model makes the fewest assumptions and provides a useful framework for examining the dynamic behavior of the normal respiratory system.

INSTRUMENTATION

Instrumentation to measure the airflow and driving pressure signals is required to meet basic physical capabilities for accuracy, precision, and response. The standard specifications for resolution and the ranges for airflow, pressure and volume observed in neonatal pulmonary function testing are shown in Table 90-1. Techniques to evaluate the equipment characteristics (e.g., linearity, hysteresis, frequency response, damping characteristics) (Fig. 90-2), and proper calibration to improve accuracy have been studied extensively.[12]

MEASUREMENTS

The techniques for neonatal pulmonary evaluation that are available for clinical use are described next.

Static Lung Volumes

Definition

The components of static lung volumes are illustrated in Figure 90-3. The classical definitions that are relevant for neonates are listed next:

Residual Volume. Volume of air remaining in the respiratory system at the end of maximum possible expiration.

Functional Residual Capacity. Volume of air in the respiratory system at the resting level or at the end of tidal volume expiration, which is in continuity with the airways. *Functional residual capacity* (FRC) is that volume maintained by the opposing forces of lung elastic recoil and chest wall elastic recoils.

Expiratory Reserve Volume. Volume of air that comprises the difference between FRC and residual volume.

Thoracic Gas Volume. The total amount of gas in the lung at end expiration; irrespective of whether the gas is in communication with the airways. In healthy infant without air trapping, FRC is equivalent to thoracic gas volume.

Total Lung Capacity. Gas volume in the respiratory system at the end of maximum inspiration.

Techniques of Measurement

Whole body plethysmography is the standard criterion for measurement of lung volumes, but it is not a practical technique for newborn infants. FRC is the only volume that can be measured accurately in infants by tracer gas techniques. Both a closed-circuit helium dilution system[13-19] and an open-circuit nitrogen

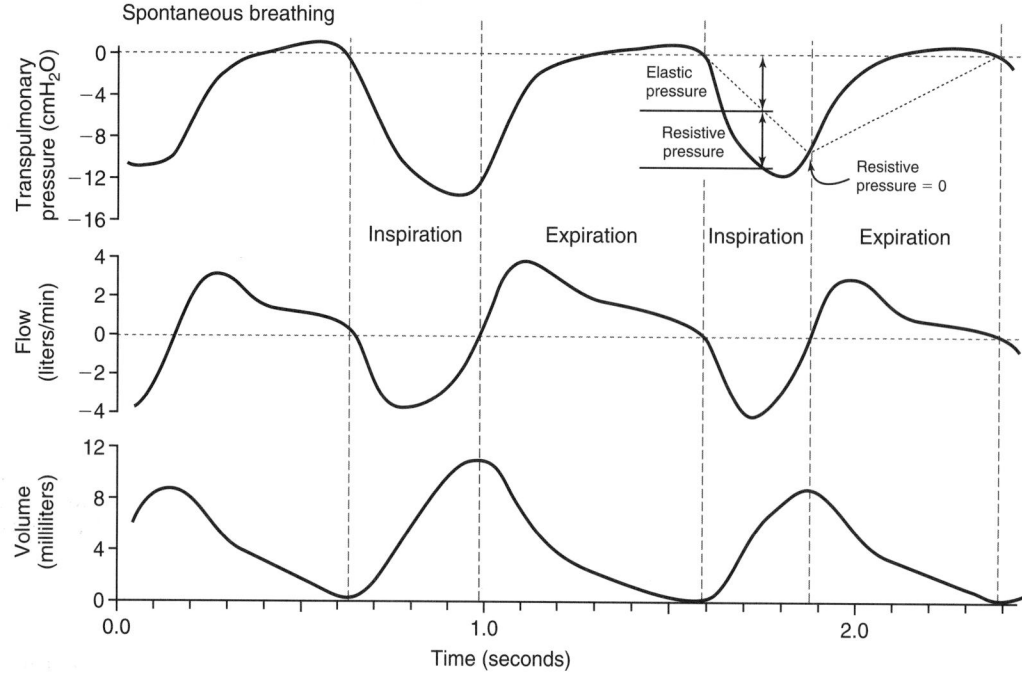

Figure 90–1. Pressure, flow, and volume signals of a respiratory cycle.

TABLE 90-1

Standard Specifications of Equipment for Neonatal Pulmonary Function Testing

	Nonlinearity (%)	Range	Resolution
Flow	± 2.5	± 0.17 L/sec*	3 mL/sec
Volume	± 2.5	0-75 mL	0.02 mL
Pressure	± 0.6	± 75 cm H_2O	0.1 cm H_2O

* ± 1 L/sec for forced expiratory maneuvers

washout system[20-22] have been used. However there is about 15% underestimation of FRC value compared with measurements with whole body plethysmography. The difference may represent airway closure during tidal breathing, given that neither tracer gas technique measures gas in areas of the lung that are trapped in a cyst or behind obstructed airways, or in lung compartments with a very long time constant.

Helium Dilution Technique. The infant's airway is connected to a closed circuit of a known helium concentration at the end of a normal, restful expiration. The infant breathes from the circuit for 30 to 60 seconds during which time the helium concentration is diluted to a lower value (Fig. 90–4). This decrease in helium concentration is proportional to the lung volume. If no helium has been lost from the closed system, the amount of helium present before connection is equivalent to the amount after connection, thus the mass balance equation:

$$V_i C_i = (V_f + FRC) C_f$$

where

V_i = Initial volume of the closed breathing circuit before patient connection.
C_i = Initial helium concentration in V_i.
V_f = Final volume of the closed breathing circuit after equilibration with the patient's FRC.
C_f = Final helium concentration after equilibration with the patient's FRC.
Thus, FRC = $V_i C_i / C_f$ - V_f.

The volume V_f in the last equation includes volume changes due to the patient's carbon dioxide production, oxygen consumption, and dead space in the system. Carbon dioxide can be continuously removed from the system by passing the gas stream through a carbon dioxide absorbent. To compensate for the patient's oxygen consumption, oxygen is added to the breathing circuit to maintain a constant volume. Alternately, volume lost during oxygen consumption can be computed by measuring the volume of the breathing circuit after disconnecting the patient at end expiration.[14]

Technical Limitations. Sick infants with airway disease and poor distribution of ventilation have prolonged equilibration time (i.e., long respiratory time constants),[14] which may lead to hypoxia and CO_2 retention. Leaks around the endotracheal tube or face mask and high inspired oxygen concentration are also a frequent source of error, and methods have been developed that attempt to correct for this error.[24] Measurement accuracy may be improved by reducing the total volume of the breathing circuit resulting in larger changes in helium concentration, and using same gas mixture used during the test for calibration.

Nitrogen Washout Technique. FRC can be calculated by measurement of the total expired nitrogen by a mass spectrometer[22, 25] or a nitrogen analyzer, while the infant breathes either 100% oxygen[21] or an oxygen-helium mixture[26,27] to wash out the nitrogen present in the lung at end expiration. The basic principle is described by the mass balance equation:

$$FRC = V_{N2} / (C_{iN2} - C_{fN2})$$

where

V_{N2} = Volume of nitrogen washed out.
C_{iN2} = Initial alveolar nitrogen fractional concentration (assumed to be 0.79).
C_{fN2} = Final alveolar nitrogen fractional concentration (assumed to be 0.0).

V_{N2} can be obtained by collecting all of the expired volume and measuring its mixed nitrogen concentration. Alternately, V_{N2} can be computed from the integration of the product of instantaneous flow (V(t)) and the instantaneous nitrogen concentration (C_{N2}(t)) signals over time:

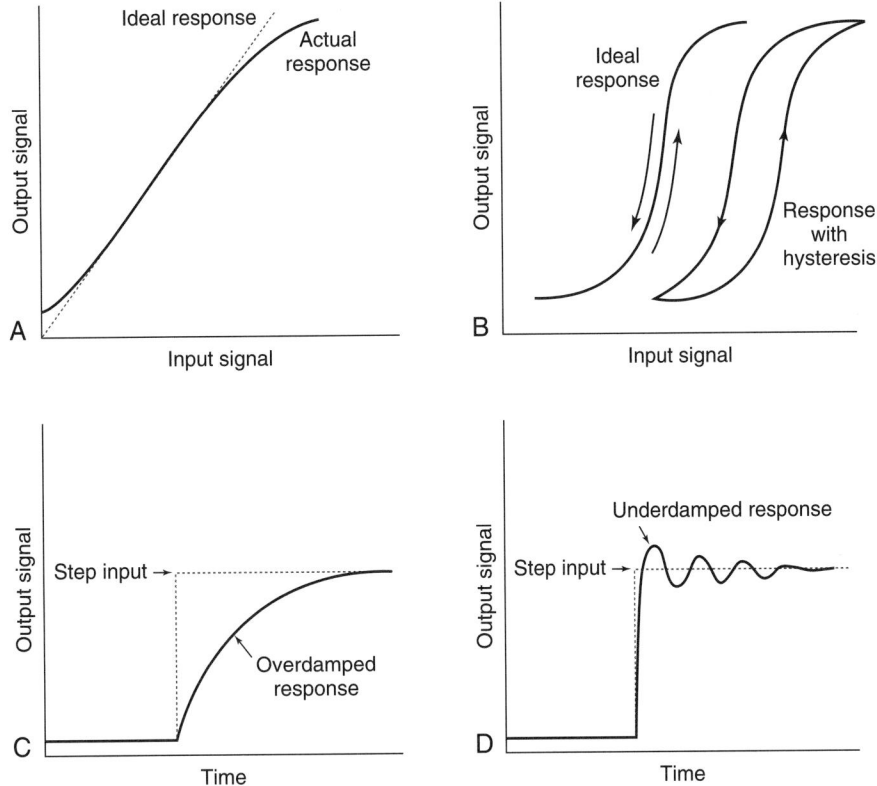

Figure 90–2. Technical considerations for instrumentation: **A**, nonlinearity. **B**, hysteresis. **C**, overdamping. **D**, underdamping.

$$V_{N_2} = \int \dot{V}(t) \cdot C_{N_2}(t)\,dt$$

Although instantaneous flow can be measured using a pneumotachometer, V_{N_2} can also be determined using a simplified method that assumes that the average of the inspiratory and expiratory flow remains constant over the washout period,[21] thus:

$$V_{N_2} = \dot{V} \int C_{N_2}(t)\,dt$$

In this method the expired gas is passed through a mixing chamber to produce a multiple breath averaged nitrogen washout curve.

The nitrogen washout technique has been compared with the helium dilution technique[26] and found to produce comparable measurements of FRC in infants and very young children.

Technical Limitations. Breathing high oxygen concentrations may result in hyperoxia or absorption atelectasis in areas of lung with low ventilation. A heliox mixture may be used in place of 100% oxygen, although this option has not been evaluated thoroughly.

The open circuit nitrogen washout technique as just described cannot be easily implemented in ventilated infants. Although an adaptation been developed,[28] it cannot be used in infants who are receiving inhaled oxygen greater than 70%. As with the helium dilution method, this technique is also prone to gas leakage errors.

Other Techniques to Measure FRC. Inductive plethysmography and occlusion techniques (multiple or single) have been reported for FRC determination.[29] An alternative tracer gas technique that uses sulfur hexaflouride (SF_6) washout has also been developed that can be used on ventilated infants on high oxygen concentrations.[30, 31]

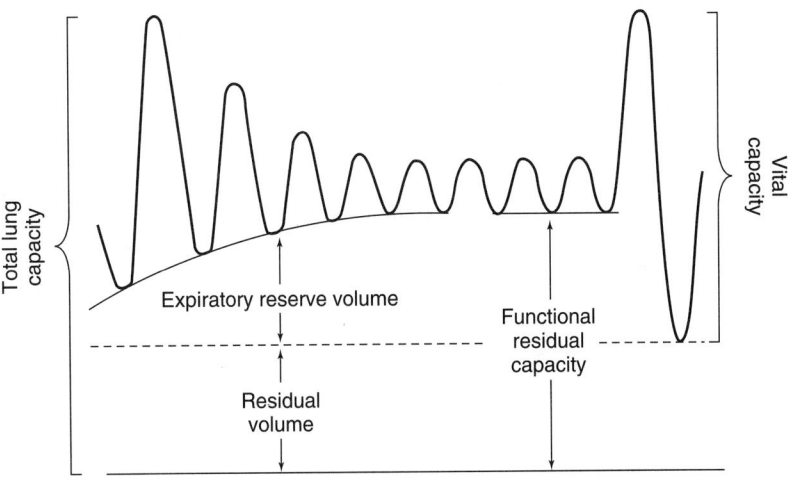

Figure 90–3. Static lung volumes.

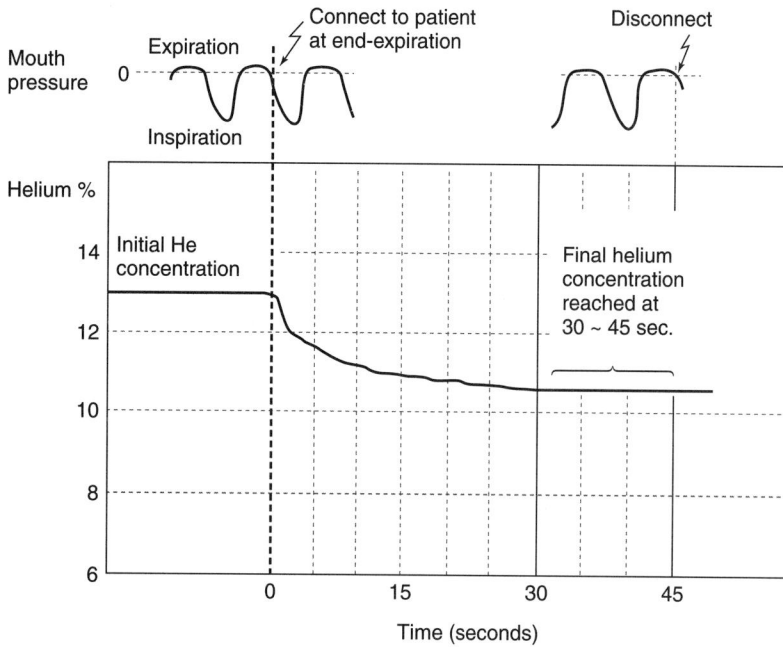

Figure 90–4. Typical time course of helium concentration during FRC measurement by helium dilution. The mouth pressure signal is used to automatically switch a solenoid valve at end expiration.

Dynamic Lung Volumes

Definitions

Tidal Volume and Minute Ventilation. *Tidal volume* is defined as the volume of gas entering and leaving the respiratory tract with each breath. The volume varies with the activity of the baby. *Minute ventilation* is defined as the total volume of gas expired over a period of 1 minute. Accurate measurement of tidal volume (no leak around endotracheal tube or face mask) and respiratory frequency allows measurement of minute ventilation. When *minute ventilation* is combined with the measurement of expired CO_2 concentration, dead space ventilation can be calculated and differentiated from alveolar ventilation.

Measurement

Plethysmography (body box),[32-36] inductive plethysmography,[37-39] impedance pneumography,[40-41] and pneumotachography are different techniques used for measurement of tidal volume.

Pneumotachography. Pneumotachography is the most commonly used technique to measure tidal volume in neonates.[42-44] The pneumotachograph is an instrument used to measure respiratory flow instantly by acting as a linear resistor to gas flow. Thus, gas flow through a pneumotachograph is directly proportional to the pressure drop across the resistive element. A differential pressure transducer converts this pressure drop to an electronic flow signal. Respiratory volume changes can be obtained by electronic integration of the flow signal over time.

Technical Limitations. Accurate determination of gas flow requires a linear output signal, which may only be feasible by selecting a pneumotachograph according to the infant's size and with a flow range slightly higher than the maximum expected to keep dead space to a minimum.[45-47] The pneumotachograph should be calibrated using the same connectors, adapters, and gas composition used for actual measurements, and heated to 37 to 38°C to prevent condensation and errors due to temperature and humidity differences between inspired and expired gas.[48-51]

The differential pressure transducer used in conjunction with the pneumotachograph must also be linear over the range of pressure being measured[52-54] and must have sufficient frequency response characteristics.

Pulmonary Compliance

Definition

Lungs, airways, and thorax are elastic; these tissues stretch due to changes in pressure during inspiration; when the pressure change ceases, the tissues return or recoil to their resting positions. The systematic change in both pressure and volume during inflation and deflation allows a static pressure-volume curve of the lungs to be plotted. The curves that the lungs follow during inflation and deflation are different and are also influenced by surface tension. This physical property of the lungs is known as hysteresis. The compliance of a tissue is defined as the change in volume resulting from a given change in the pressure.[55]

Static Compliance

Static compliance is an accurate determinant of lung elastic properties. It measures the change in volume for a given pressure at static (i.e., nonflow) conditions. A sufficient equilibration period is required to ensure that the actual pressure change is recorded.

Dynamic Compliance

Dynamic compliance is the determination of the change in volume and pressure during the respiratory cycle and is predominantly influenced by breathing frequency. During rapid breathing, there may not be sufficient equilibration time to determine the actual change in volume and pressure accurately.

Pulmonary Resistance

Pulmonary resistance results predominantly from the frictional resistance to airflow. Airflow requires a driving pressure generated by the changes in alveolar pressure. When alveolar pressure is lower or higher than atmospheric pressure, air flows into or out of the lungs accordingly. Resistance to airflow is defined as the pressure gradient between alveolar and atmospheric pressure divided by the resulting airflow value.

The airway resistance, which may be responsible for as much as 80% of the total pulmonary resistance in a normal lung, is influenced by the velocity and pattern of airflow, geometry of the airways, and the density and viscosity of the gas itself.[55] The tissue frictional resistance normally accounts for about 20% of the pulmonary resistance and is influenced by the configuration

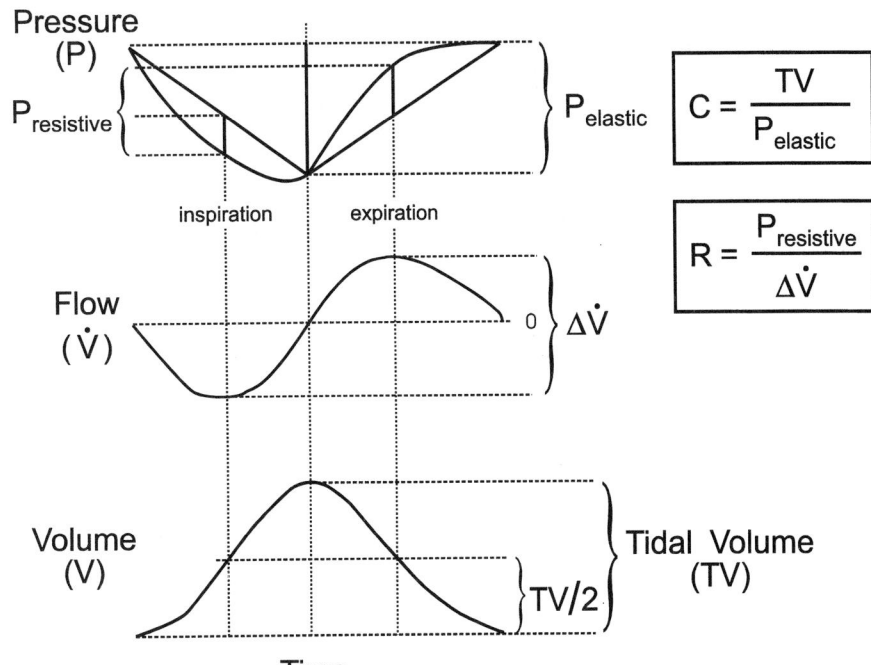

Figure 90–5. Determination of pulmonary mechanics on the basis of pressure, air flow, and volume signals when a linear respiratory model is assumed. C = compliance; R = resistance.

of the chest wall and the lung as well as by the fluid content of the pulmonary tissue. Inertial resistance that is less than 1% of pulmonary resistance is usually more dependent on the breathing frequency and the density of the gas.[55]

Pulmonary Energetics

The cumulative product of pressure and volume at any instant during a respiratory cycle is the work of breathing. The latter is also defined by the hysteresis of the dynamic pressure-volume loop.

Measurement of Pulmonary Mechanics

Pulmonary mechanics are calculated by measurement of transpulmonary pressure (pressure at airway opening minus pleural pressure) and flow and volume changes throughout respiratory cycle.

Airflow and volume are measured by pneumotachography. Pleural pressure can be estimated by esophageal pressure[56-60] measured by a pressure transducer connected to an air-filled balloon[61,62] or a fluid-filled catheter,[63,64] or by a microtransducer-tipped catheter. The accuracy of the esophageal pressure measurement can be evaluated by an occlusion test.[59,61,65-67]

The calculation of compliance and resistance are based on the assumption of a linear model.[10] Thus, the driving pressure is always the sum of the elastic and resistive pressure. The calculations may be performed by the traditional "chord" analysis as shown in Figure 90–5.[10,56-58] or by any of several computerized techniques, such as the least mean squares analysis method.[11]

Technical Limitations

Reliable esophageal pressure measurement by esophageal balloon catheter depends on proper size, positioning, and inflation of the balloon. Water-filled catheters need to be free of gas bubbles and accumulation of secretions at the tip. Placement of catheters may generate peristalsis, resulting in an initial pressure drift. Because measured esophageal pressure reflects pleural pressure at that specific location, its accuracy depends on assuming that the pressure change at the site represents mean pleural pressure changes. Altered patterns of inspiratory muscle contraction or esophageal muscle tone and distortion of the chest wall could result in uneven pleural pressure distribution.[63,65-67]

Accuracy of measurements is also dependent on body position. Measurements should be done in supine, neutral head posi-

tion, and only during quiet sleep.[68] Flexion or extension of the neck in small infants can effect the airflow resistance.[69] Feeding volume may also effect the measurements and should be standardized in repeated studies.[70, 71] In mechanically ventilated infants, the ventilatory support should be kept the same during sequential studies to prevent shifting of the tidal volume to a different portion on the pressure-volume curve.

Commercially available equipment may have variable frequency response; phase shift errors between signals and drifting calibration values should be tested with a calibrated lung simulator to ensure accuracy at the expected infant tidal volumes and frequencies prior to its clinical use.

Airflow Mechanics

The tone of tracheobronchial smooth muscle provides a mechanism to stabilize the airways and prevent airway collapse.[72-74] Plugging of the airways, edema, and weakening of the airway walls, and resulting tracheobronchomalacia alter airflow.[75-77] In addition, the increased driving pressure secondary to the high elastic and resistive loads during tidal breathing in infants with bronchopulmonary dysplasia often leads to self-induced expiratory flow limitation.

Measurement

Resistance to airflow is measured by calculation of pulmonary mechanics, the tidal flow-volume relationship, and forced expiratory flow generated by rapid thoracic compression.

Tidal Flow: Volume Relationship

The on-line graphic display of a tidal flow–volume loop is useful for evaluating changes in inspiratory and expiratory airflow-volume response during tidal breathing. In addition to the determination of the peak flow values, the patterns of airflow and tidal volumes indicative of turbulence and/or flow limitation may also be evaluated (Fig. 90–6).[78]

Forced Expiratory Flow

Forced expiration is commonly used to detect obstructive lung disease by determining the lung volume at which small airways begin to close. During expiration, flow is limited by airway

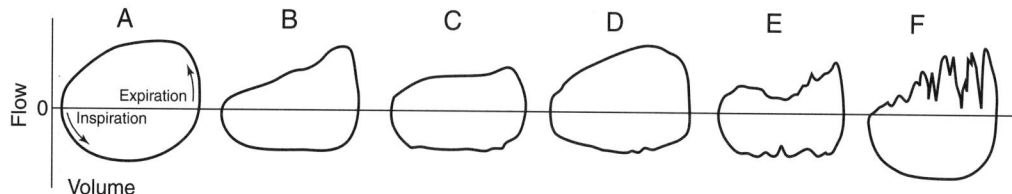

Figure 90–6. Tidal flow volume relationships; **A,** Normal infant. **B,** Extrathoracic upper airway obstruction. **C,** Fixed upper airway obstruction. **D,** Inspiratory limitations of small airway disease. **E,** Broncheomalacia. **F,** Secretion in the airway.

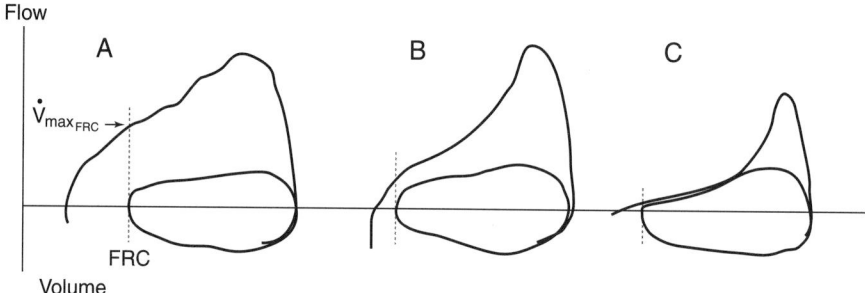

Figure 90–7. Schematics of partial forced expiratory flow relationship: Normal infants (**A**) and infants with moderate (**B**) and severe chronic lung disease (**C**).

TABLE 90-2

Mean Normal Values of Neonatal Pulmonary Function Parameters During the First Month

Ref. No.	GA (wk)	AGE (d)	VT (ml/kg)	FRC (ml/kg)	DCL (ml/cmH₂O)	CRS (ml/cmH₂O)	Resistance (cm H₂O/l/sec)	WOB (g-cm/kg)	$\dot{V}_{max}$ (ml/sec)	$\dot{V}_{max}$FRC
83	28–30	2–3	5.9	—	2.0	—	Exp 50.1	—	—	—
84	28–34	2–3	6.3	—	2.4	—	Total 54.0	12.0	—	—
85	28–30	5–7	6.6	—	2.3	—	Exp 70.0	—	—	—
64	31–36	3–30	—	16.7	2.2	—	Exp 86.8	—	—	—
19	34	4–28	—	29.5	—	—	—	—	—	—
86	34	1–28	—	—	—	2.4	—	—	—	—
87	Preterm	1–16	—	38.7	—	—	—	—	—	—
Coll.	Term	1–30	5.3–7.2	17.1–52.6	3.2–5.7	3.2–3.8	total 26–57.8	13.0–20.5	185–186	1.82–1.90

GA = gestational age, VT = tidal volume, FRC = functional residual capacity, DCL = dynamic lung compliance, CRS = total respiratory system compliance, resistance = pulmonary resistance, WOB = work of breathing, $\dot{V}_{max}$ = maximal flow, $\dot{V}_{max}$FRC = maximal flow at functional residual capacity, exp = expiratory, Coll. = refs. 13, 20, 29, 32, 64, 78, 79, 83, and 86–93.

compression, which is determined by the elastic recoil of the lung, the resistance of the airway, and airway wall mechanics. In infants, forced expiratory flow is generated by rapid thoracic compression, or negative pressure forced deflation. Rapid thoracic compression is preferred for being a noninvasive technique that does not require intubation, paralysis, or deep sedation to generate partial expiratory flow-volume loops (PEFV). Parameters that are used to characterize PEFV include peak expiratory flow, forced expiratory flow at functional residual capacity ($\dot{V}_{max}$FRC), and the shape of the expiratory flow curve (Fig. 90–7).[79-82]

Technical Limitations. This technique generates only a partial rather than a complete flow-volume loop, which limits the evaluation of true flow limitation in response to the appropriate compression pressure for each infant. The major limitation is the variability of FRC in young infants because inspiration may start before the completion of a full expiration.

NORMAL VALUES

Normal values for pulmonary function parameters are essential for meaningful clinical interpretation. In adults, these values have been predicted on the basis of age, gender, relationship to height and weight, as well as considerations of race and ethnic background. Similar data in neonates have not yet been established.

Values for normal term babies have been obtained by different techniques and are presented in Table 90-2. Preterm neonates who are considered normal and who have not received mechanical ventilatory support[83-85] are infrequent; data from such infants are also tabulated in Table 90-2.

In comparing values, one needs to take into account the study population and the conditions that affects measurements such as body and neck posture, the effect of feeding, and sleep state.

CLINICAL APPLICATIONS

The clinical usefulness of neonatal pulmonary functions is that it defines the magnitude and pattern of respiratory compromise. Individual disease processes are not differentiated by pulmonary function data. Infants with hyaline membrane disease, pulmonary edema, or pneumonia have low lung compliance, whereas infants with increased airway resistance have an obstructive disease process such as meconium aspiration syndrome or bronchopulmonary dysplasia. However pulmonary function data can be used to determine the severity of the pathology, its resolution, and the effect of the treatment. Airway abnormalities such as malacia and intrathoracic and extrathoracic obstructive lesions may be determined by the alterations in the shape of the flow-volume loops during tidal breathing (see Fig. 90–6).[94-96]

The recent addition of the pneumotachometers and waveform graphics to infant ventilators provides clinicians with pulmonary function data at the bedside. This information can be used to assist in management of ventilatory support such as adjustment of tidal volume to prevent overdistention,[97, 98] determination of optimal inspiratory time,[99] estimation of optimal end distending pressure,[98] the appropriateness of manual ventilation,[100] airways reactivity,[101, 102] and the effect of therapeutic interventions.[103-110] Respiratory energetics such as resistive work of breathing can also be determined measured from the hysteresis of the pressure-volume loop during spontaneous breathing to estimate respiratory loss of calories.[111]

The serial evaluation of pulmonary outcome in the immediate postnatal period[112, 113] and during infancy[114-117] provides the information necessary for detection of late onset complications, resolution of the acute lung injury and response to treatment.

REFERENCES

1. Hutchinson J: On the capacity of the lungs, and on the respiratory functions, with a view of establishing a precise and easy method of detecting disease by the spirometer. Med Chir Soc (Lond) Trans 29:137, 1846.
2. Karlberg P, et al: Studies of respiratory physiology in the newborn infant: Acta Paediat Scan 43:397, 1954.
3. Clutario BC: Clinical pulmonary function. In Scarpelli EM (ed): Pulmonary Physiology of the Fetus, Newborn and Child. Philadelphia, Lea & Febiger, 1975, pp 299-325.
4. Bryan AC, Wohl MB: Respiratory mechanics in children. In Geiger SR (ed): Handbook of Physiology, Section 3: The Respiratory System. Macklem PT, Mead J (vol. eds), Volume III, Mechanics of Breathing, Part I, Fishman AP (section ed). Bethesda, MD, American Physiological Society, 1986, pp 179-191.
5. Bancalari E: Pulmonary function testing and other diagnostic laboratory procedures in neonatal pulmonary care. In Thibeault DW, Gary GA (eds): Neonatal Pulmonary Care, 2nd ed. East Norwalk, CT, Appleton-Century Crofts, 1986, pp 195-234.
6. Gerhardt T, et al: Panel Discussions: Physiological and technical considerations. In Bhutani VK, et al (eds): Neonatal Pulmonary Function Testing: Physiological, Technical and Clinical Considerations. Ithaca, NY, Perinatology Press, 1988, pp 127-158.
7. McCann EM, et al: Pulmonary function in the sick newborn infant. Pediatr Res 21:313, 1987.
8. Rodarte JR, Rehder K: Dynamics of respiration. In Geiger SR (ed): Handbook of Physiology, Section 3: The Respiratory System, Macklem PT, Mead J (vol. eds), Volume III, Mechanics of Breathing, Part I, Fishman AP (section ed). Bethesda, MD, American Physiological Society, 1986, pp 131-144.
9. Neergard K, Wirz K: Uber eine Methode zur Messung der Lungenelastizitat am lebenden Menschen, ins besondere beim Emphysem. Z Klin Med 105:51, 1927.
10. Mead J, Whittenberger JL: Physical properties of human lungs measured during spontaneous respiration. J Appl Physiol 5:779, 1953.
11. Bhutani VK, et al: Evaluation of neonatal pulmonary mechanics and energetics: A two factor least mean square analysis. Pediatr Pulmonol 4:150, 1988.
12. Butler JP, et al: Principles of measurement: Applications to pressure, volume, and flow. In Geiger SR (ed): Handbook of Physiology, Section 3: The Respiratory System, Macklem PT, Mead J (vol. eds), Volume III, Mechanics in Breathing, Part I, Fishman AP (section ed). Bethesda, MD, American Physiological Society, 1986, pp 15-33.
13. Berglund G, Karlberg P: Determination of the functional residual capacity in newborn infants. Acta Paediat Scand 45:541, 1956.
14. Krauss AN, Auld PAM: Measurement of functional residual capacity in distressed neonates by helium rebreathing. J Pediatr 77:228, 1970.
15. Fox WW: Measurement of functional residual capacity in infants using the helium dilution method. In Bhutani VK, et al (eds): Neonatal Pulmonary Function Testing: Physiological, Technical and Clinical Considerations. Ithaca, NY, Perinatology Press, 1988, pp 81-90.
16. Schwartz JG, Fox WW, Shaffer TH. A method for measuring functional residual capacity in neonates with endotracheal tubes. IEEE Trans Biomed Eng 25:304, 1978.
17. Da Silva WJ, et al: Role of positive end-expiratory pressure changes on functional residual capacity in surfactant treated preterm infants. Pediatr Pulmonol 18:89, 1994.
18. Beardsmore CS, et al: Measurement of lung volumes during active and quiet sleep in infants. Pediatr Pulmonol 7:71, 1989.
19. Ronchetti R, et al: An analysis of a rebreathing method for measuring lung volume in the premature infant. Pediatr Res 9:797, 1975.
20. Sivieri EM, et al: Functional residual capacity in preterm neonates. Eur Respir J 8: 363s, 1995.
21. Gerhardt T, et al: A simple method for measuring functional residual capacity by N_2 washout in small animals and newborn infants. Pediatr Res 19:1165, 1985.
22. Sivan Y, et al: Functional residual capacity in ventilated infants and children. Pediatr Res 28:451, 1990.
23. Koen PA, Moskowitz GD, Shaffer TH. Instrumentation for measuring functional residual capacity in small animals. J Appl Physiol 43: 755, 1977.
24. Fox WW, et al: Effects of endotracheal tube leaks on functional residual capacity determination in intubated neonates. Pediatr Res 13:60, 1979.
25. Strang LB, McGrath MW: Alveolar ventilation in normal newborn infants studied by air wash-in after oxygen breathing. Clin Sci 23:129, 1962.
26. Tepper RS, Asdell S: Comparison of helium dilution and nitrogen washout measurements of functional residual capacity in infants and very young children. Pediatr Pulmonol 13:250, 1992.
27. Richardson P, Anderson M: Automated nitrogen-washout methods for infants: Evaluated using cats and a mechanical lung. J Appl Physiol 52:1378, 1982.
28. Sivan Y, et al: An automated bedside method for measuring functional residual capacity by N_2 washout in mechanically ventilated children. Pediatr Res 28:446, 1990.
29. Mortola JP, et al: Dynamics of breathing in infants. J Appl Physiol 52:1209, 1982.
30. Jonmarker C, et al: Measurement of functional residual capacity by sulfur hexafluoride washout. Anesthesiology 63:89, 1985.
31. Schulze A, et al: Measurement of functional residual capacity by sulfur hexafluoride in small-volume lungs during spontaneous breathing and mechanical ventilation. Pediatr Res 35:494, 1994.
32. Polgar G: Airway resistance in the newborn infant. J Pediatr 59:915, 1961.
33. Nelson NM, et al: Pulmonary function in the newborn infant. I. Methods: Ventilation and gaseous metabolism. Pediatrics 30:963, 1962.
34. Polgar G: Opposing forces to breathing in newborn infants. Biol Neonat 11:1, 1967.
35. Polgar G, Lacourt G: A method for measuring respiratory mechanics in small newborn (premature) infants. J Appl Physiol 32:555, 1972.
36. Karlberg P, et al: Respiratory studies in newborn infants. Acta Paediat 49:345, 1960.
37. Duffty P, et al: Respiratory induction plethysmography (Respitrace): An evaluation of its use in the infant. Am Rev Respir Dis 123:542, 1981.
38. Dolfin T, et al: Calibration of respiratory induction plethysmography (Respitrace) in infants. Am Rev Respir Dis 126:577, 1982.
39. Tabachnik E, et al: Measurement of ventilation in children using the respiratory inductive plethysmograph. J Pediatr 99:895, 1981.
40. Newton PE, et al: Measurement of ventilation using digitally filtered transthoracic impedance. J Appl Physiol 54:1161, 1983.
41. Goldensohn ES, Zablow L: An electrical impedance spirometer. J Appl Physiol 14:463, 1959.
42. Fleisch A: Pneumotachograph: Apparatus for recording respiratory flow. Arch Ges Physiol 209:713, 1925.
43. Silverman L, Whittenberger JL: Clinical pneumotachograph. In Comroe JH (eds): Methods in Medical Research. Vol 2. Chicago, Year Book Medical Publishers, 1950, pp 104-112.
44. Lilly JC: Flow meter for recording respiratory flow of human subjects. In Comroe JH (ed): Methods in Medical Research. Vol 2. Chicago, Year Book Medical Publishers, 1950, pp 113-121.
45. Finucane KE, et al: Linearity and frequency response of pneumotachographs. J Appl Physiol 32:121, 1972.
46. Grenvik A, et al: Problems in pneumotachography. Acta Anaesthesiol Scand 10:147, 1966.
47. Rigatto H, Brady JP: A new nosepiece for measuring ventilation in preterm infants. J Appl Physiol 32:423, 1972.
48. Wall MA: Infant endotracheal tube resistance: Effects of changing length, diameter, and gas density. Crit Care Med 8:38, 1980.
49. Turner MJ, et al: The effects of temperature and composition on the viscosity of respiratory gases. J Appl Physiol 67:472, 1989.
50. Turney SZ, Blumenfeld W: Heated Fleisch pneumotachometer: a calibration procedure. J Appl Physiol 34:117, 1973.
51. Muller NL, Zamel N: Pneumotachograph calibration for inspiratory and expiratory flows during HeO_2 breathing. J Appl Physiol Respirat Environ Exercise Physiol 51:1038, 1981.
52. Kafer ER: Errors in pneumotachography as a result of transducer design and function. Anesthesiology 38:275, 1973.
53. Churches AE, et al: Measurement errors in pneumotachography due to pressure transducer design. Anaesth Intensive Care 5:19, 1977.
54. Abrahams N, et al: Errors in pneumotachography with intermittent positive pressure ventilation. Anaesth Intensive Care 3:284, 1975.
55. Comroe JH: Mechanical factors in breathing. In Physiology of Respiration. 2nd ed. Chicago, Year Book Medical Publishers, 1974, pp 94-141.
56. American Thoracic Society and the European Respiratory Society: Respiratory mechanics in infants: physiologic evaluation in health and disease. Am Rev Respir Dis 147:474, 1993.
57. American Thoracic Society and the European Respiratory Society: Respiratory function measurements in infants: symbols, abbreviations, and units. Am J Respir Crit Care Med 151:2041, 1995.
58. Dinwiddie R, Russell G: Relationship of intraesophageal pressure to intrapleural pressure in the newborn. J Appl Physiol 33:415, 1972.
59. Asher MI, et al: Measurement of esophageal pressure in neonates. J Appl Physiol 52:491, 1982.
60. Senterre J, Geubelle F: Measurement of endoesophageal pressure in the newborns. Biol Neonat 16:47, 1970.
61. Beardsmore CS, et al: Improved esophageal balloon technique for use in infants. J Appl Physiol 49:735, 1980.
62. Heldt GP: Development of stability of the respiratory system in preterm infants. J Appl Physiol 65:441, 1988.

63. LeSouef PN, et al: Influence of chest wall distortion on esophageal pressure. J Appl Physiol 55:353, 1983.
64. Gerhardt T, et al: Pulmonary mechanics in normal infants and young children during first 5 years of life. Pediatr Pulmonol 3:309, 1987.
65. Bryan MH, et al: Chest wall instability and its influence on respiration in the newborn infant. In Stern L, et al (eds): Intensive Care of the Newborn. New York, Masson, 1976, pp 249–258.
66. Heaf DP, et al: The accuracy of esophageal pressure measurements in convalescent and sick intubated infants. Pediatr Pulmonol 2:5, 1986.
67. Baydur A, et al: A simple method for assessing the validity of the esophageal balloon technique. Am Rev Respir Dis 126:788, 1982.
68. Stocks JC, et al: Infant lung function; measurement conditions and equipement. Eur Respir J 1989; 2:123–129.
69. Reiterer F, et al: Influence of head-neck posture on airflow and pulmonary mechanics in preterm neonates. Pediatr Pulmonol 17:149–54, 1994.
70. Blondheim O, et al: Effect of enteral gavage feeding rate on pulmonary functions of very low birthweight infants. J Pediatr 122:751, 1993.
71. Heldt GP, The effect of gavage feeding on the mechanics of lung, chestwall and diaphragm of preterm infants. Pediatr Res 24:55, 1988.
72. Bhutani VK, et al: The influence of smooth muscle tone on neonatal lamb tracheal mechanics. Pediatr Res 20:492, 1986.
73. Koslo RJ, et al: Effect of trachealis muscle contraction on neonatal lamb tracheal mechanics. Pediatr Res 20:1216, 1986.
74. Duara S, et al: Extrathoracic airway stability during resistive loading in preterm infants. J Appl Physiol 63:1539, 1987.
75. Deoras KS, et al: Structural changes in the tracheae of preterm lambs induced by ventilation. Pediatr Res 26:434, 1989.
76. Bhutani VK, et al: Determination of alterations in tracheobronchial airflow mechanics in preterm infants following mechanical ventilation. Fetal Neonatal Physiological Measurements 3:419, 1989.
77. Jones JG, et al: Effect of changing airway mechanics on maximum expiratory flow. J Appl Physiol 38:1012, 1975.
78. Adler SM, Wohl MEB: Flow-volume relationship at low lung volumes in healthy term newborn infants. Pediatrics 61:636, 1978.
79. Taussig LM, et al: Determinants of forced expiratory flows in newborn infants. J Appl Physiol 53:1220, 1982.
80. Tepper RS: Tidal expiratory flow-volume curves: A simple noninvasive test of pulmonary function in sick and healthy infants. Am Rev Respir Dis 127:217, 1983.
81. Taussig LM, et al: Lung function in infants and young children. Am Rev Respir Dis 116:233, 1977.
82. LeSouef PN, et al: Effect of compression pressure on forced expiratory flow in infants. J Appl Physiol 61:1639, 1986.
83. Abbasi S, Bhutani VK. Pulmonary mechanics and energetics of normal, non-ventilated low birthweight infants. Pediatr Pulmonol 8:89, 11990.
84. Abbasi S, Bhutani VK. Lung function in preterm infants without any lung disease or ventilatory intervention. Pediatr Res 33:313A, 1993.
85. Anday EK, et al: Sequential pulmonary function measurements in very low-birth weight infants during the first week of life. Pediatr Pulmonol 3:392, 1987.
86. Migdal M, et al: Compliance of the total respiratory system in treating preterm and full-term newborns. Pediatr Pulmonol 3:214, 1987.
87. Nelson NM, et al: Pulmonary function in the newborn infant: Trapped gas in the normal infant lung. J Clin Invest 42:1850, 1963.
88. Cook CD, et al: Studies of respiratory physiology in the newborn infant. III Measurements of mechanics of respiration. J Clin Invest 36:440, 1957.
89. Strang LB, McGrath MW: Alveolar ventilation in normal newborn infants studied by air wash-in after oxygen breathing. Clin Sci 23:129, 1962.
90. Feather E, Russell G: Respiratory mechanics in infants of low birth weight and the effects of feeding. Biol Neonate 24:117, 1974.
91. Taeusch MW, et al: Respiratory regulation after elastic loading and CO_2 rebreathing in normal term infants. J Pediatr 88:102, 1976.
92. Mortola JP, et al: Muscle pressure and flow during expiration in infants. Am Rev Respir Dis 129:49, 1984.
93. Gerhardt T, et al: Functional residual capacity in normal neonates and children up to 5 years of age determined by an N_2 washout method. Pediatr Res 20:668, 1986.
94. Sotomayor JL, et al: Large airway collapse due to acquired tracheobronchomalacia in infancy. Am J Dis Child 140:367, 1986.
95. McCubbin M, et al: Large airway collapse in bronchopulmonary dysplasia. J Pediatr 114:304,1989.
96. Tepper RS, et al: Expiratory flow-limitation in infants with bronchopulmonary dysplasia. J Pediatr 109:1040, 1986.
97. Fisher JB, et al: Quantitative identification of lung overdistention from pressure-volume curves. Pediatr Pulmonol 8:203, 1988.
98. Mammel MC, et al: Determining optimum inspiratory time during intermittent positive pressure ventilation in surfactant-depleted cats. Pediatr Pulmonol 7:223, 1989.
99. Carlo WA, et al: Efficacy of computer-assisted management of respiratory failure in neonates. Pediatrics 78:139, 1986.
100. Sivieri E, et al: On-line pulmonary graphics for assistance in the manual ventilation of neonates. Fetal and Neonatal Physiological Measurement 3:425, 1989.
101. Mirmanesh J, et al: Effect of a-adrenergic stimulation in infants with bronchopulmonary dysplasia. J Pediatr 121:622, 1992.
102. Tepper RS: Airway reactivity in infants: A positive response to methacholine and metaproterenol. J Appl Physiol 62:1155, 1987.
103. Kao LC, et al: Oral theophylline and diuretics improve pulmonary mechanics in infants with bronchopulmonary dysplasia. J Pediatr 111:439, 1987.
104. Davis JM, et al: Changes in pulmonary mechanics following caffeine administration in infants with bronchopulmonary dysplasia. Pediatr Pulmonol 6:49, 1989.
105. Rotschild A, et al: Increased compliance in response to salbutamol in premature infants with developing bronchopulmonary dysplasia. J Pediatr 115:894, 1989.
106. Pappagallo M, et al: Effect of inhaled dexamethasone in ventilator dependent preterm infants. Pediatr Res 27:219A, 1990.
107. Sosulski R, et al: Physiologic effects of terbutaline on pulmonary function of infants with bronchopulmonary dysplasia. Pediatr Pulmonol 2:271, 1986.
108. Wilkie RA, Bryan MH: Effect of bronchodilators on airway resistance in ventilator-dependent neonates with chronic lung disease. J Pediatr 111:278, 1987.
109. Greenough A, et al: Response to bronchodilators assessed by lung mechanics. Arch Dis Child 61:1020, 1986.
110. Davis JM, et al: Changes in pulmonary mechanics after the administration of surfactant to infants with respiratory distress syndrome. N Engl J Med 319:476, 1988.
111. Wolfson MR, et al: The mechanics and energetics of breathing helium in infants with bronchopulmonary dysplasia. J Pediatr 104:752, 1984.
112. Goldman SL, et al: Early prediction of chronic lung disease by pulmonary function testing. J Pediatr 102:613, 1983.
113. Graff MA, et al: Compliance measurement in respiratory distress syndrome: The prediction of outcome. Pediatr Pulmonol 2:332, 1986.
114. Morray JP, et al: Improvement in lung mechanics as a function of age in the infants with severe bronchopulmonary dysplasia. Pediatr Res 16:290, 1982.
115. Master IB, et al: Longitudinal study of lung mechanics in normal infants. Pediatr Pulmonol 3:3, 1987.
116. Bryan MH, et al: Pulmonary function studies during the first year of life in infants recovering from the respiratory distress syndrome. Pediatrics 52:169, 1973.
117. Gerhardt T, et al: Long-term study of pulmonary function in infants surviving with chronic lung disease (CLD). Pediatr Res 18:392A, 1984.

Robert B. Cotton

91 Pathophysiology of Hyaline Membrane Disease (Excluding Surfactant)

Hyaline membrane disease is a disorder of newborn premature infants that is characterized by respiratory failure beginning at birth. Unless modified by surfactant treatment, the disease progresses to maximal severity by 24 to 48 hours after birth. Almost all the 5 to 10% mortality associated with hyaline membrane disease occurs during the acute phase of progressive respiratory failure and is limited, for the most part, to extremely immature infants weighing less than 1000 g at birth. Of those who survive the initial course of acute respiratory failure, most improve rapidly over a period of 3 to 5 days. Fifteen percent to 30% of survivors experience a prolonged course of ventilatory failure known as *bronchopulmonary dysplasia,* which may last

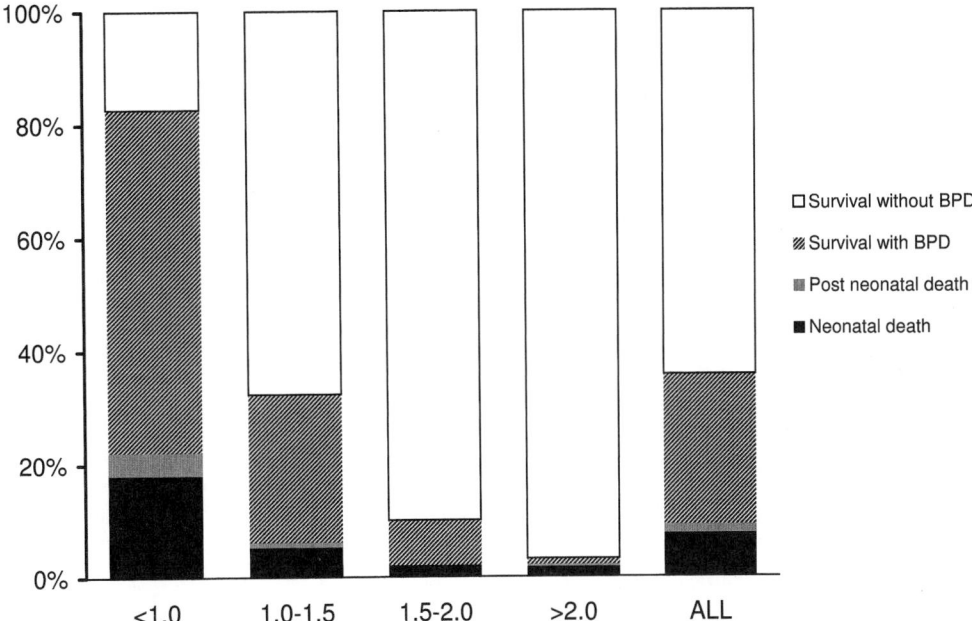

Figure 91–1. Outcome of 807 infants with hyaline membrane disease who were admitted to the Vanderbilt Newborn Intensive Care Unit in Nashville, Tennessee, during the 5-year period 1997 to 2001. BPD = bronchopulmonary dysplasia.

months, or longer, and occasionally ends in death. Figure 91-1 illustrates the strong influence of birth weight on the outcome of hyaline membrane disease.

Hyaline membrane disease, respiratory distress syndrome, and idiopathic respiratory distress syndrome are interchangeable labels for the same disease. By calling attention to an important histopathologic feature of the disorder, the term *hyaline membrane disease* is a useful reminder that its pathogenesis includes destruction of terminal airway epithelium. This finding is not seen in the various syndromes of transient respiratory distress, which largely have run their course by 24 to 48 hours after birth. *Respiratory distress syndrome* is the most commonly encountered label for this disease. The modifier "idiopathic" has been dropped now that the importance of surfactant deficiency in the pathophysiology of the disease has become widely accepted.

The stage was set for our current understanding of the pathophysiology of hyaline membrane disease by investigations in the 1950s and 1960s that described the disease based on classic models of pulmonary function. It was also during this era that the role of persistent fetal circulatory pathways in hyaline membrane disease was discovered. Further understanding of the mechanisms underlying impaired gas exchange during hyaline membrane disease came in the 1970s, as investigators sought to explain the spectacular success of constant distending airway pressure on oxygenation and survival. In the 1980s, conclusive demonstrations of the efficacy of surfactant replacement validated the idea put forth by Avery and Meade[1] in 1959 that "lack of a normal lining material in the lungs of infants would contribute to the atelectasis seen in hyaline membrane disease...."

This chapter describes the mechanisms involved that underlie the clinical manifestations of hyaline membrane disease. In regard to surfactant, this chapter limits the discussion to the major pathophysiologic consequences of deficiency of this material. The biochemistry of surfactant, mechanisms governing its production, release, and action, and issues surrounding its use in prevention and treatment of hyaline membrane disease are discussed elsewhere in this volume.

PATHOLOGY

Total lung volume is not decreased in hyaline membrane disease. Postmortem examination of human infants dying during the acute phase of this disorder reveals lungs that are described as full[2] or even voluminous.[3] They are often compared with liver to emphasize their appearance as a solid, airless organ that is congested and dark purplish red. On microscopic examination, there is marked capillary and venous congestion. Interstitial edema is widespread and is especially prominent in the adventitia surrounding small arterioles, which are markedly constricted early in the disease. Dilated lymphatic spaces are frequently seen adjacent to respiratory bronchioles and arterioles. Hyaline membrane formation, which represents a coagulum of sloughed cell debris in a protein matrix, occurs characteristically at the junction of respiratory bronchioles and alveolar ducts. Hyaline membranes are visible evidence that this disease involves a massive exudation of plasma proteins occurring in association with a destructive injury of the epithelial lining of the terminal conducting airways. The fully formed membrane often has the appearance of an eschar plastered against the denuded epithelial basement membrane. The respiratory bronchioles and alveolar ducts are frequently dilated and may be filled with protein-rich edema fluid in association with membrane formation early in the course of the disease.

The pathologic "lesion" of hyaline membrane disease is highly localized to the extent that visible epithelial disruption and destruction are limited to the terminal conducting airway at the junction of the respiratory bronchioles and alveolar ducts. Distal to this lesion, the structure of the terminal air sacs, which are the site of gas exchange, appears intact, except for a generalized reduction in volume. Based on these histopathologic features, the limitation to gas exchange by the lung in hyaline membrane disease appears to be determined more by events at the gateway to the gas exchange unit than within the unit itself.

The pathologic appearance of the lung of infants dying early in the course of hyaline membrane disease presents a picture of lung injury characterized by vascular engorgement and interstitial edema in association with terminal airways filled with protein-containing fluid. These features are consistent with physiologic findings that include delayed clearance of fetal lung liquid,[4-6] increased permeability of both epithelial[4, 7, 8] and endothelial barriers,[6] delayed lung lymph protein clearance,[5, 6] and a grossly increased pulmonary blood volume.[9] These physiologic observations confirm that the pathologic appearance of the lung in hyaline membrane disease results from disruption of the normal segregation of gas and liquid compartments.

LUNG INJURY AND PERMEABILITY PROBLEMS

In the presence of hyaline membrane disease, total lung water, which includes water in the airways and vascular spaces as well as interstitial and intracellular water, is increased almost 50% in premature lambs.[9] When compared with control animals, lambs with hyaline membrane disease have more than twice as much extravascular water and 50% more intravascular blood volume (Fig. 91-2).[9] The increased extravascular water represents both delayed clearance of fetal lung liquid and an accumulation of water resulting from increased transvascular filtration of fluid across the pulmonary capillary bed. The marked increase in lung lymph protein clearance, the appearance of proteinaceous edema fluid within the terminal conducting airways, and the subsequent widespread development of hyaline membranes all signify the escape of protein as well as water from the microvascular circulation in a process involving increased vascular permeability.[6]

Permeability of the epithelial lining of terminal airways is also increased in hyaline membrane disease.[4,7,8] A large bidirectional protein flux can be demonstrated between the airways and circulation of prematurely delivered lambs,[8] a finding totally consistent with the microscopic findings of widespread destruction of terminal airway epithelium at the respiratory bronchioles and alveolar ducts that leaves only the basement membrane as a barrier between air space and interstitium. Surfactant deficiency and ischemia are two mechanisms that contribute to this injury.

Surfactant Deficiency

Evidence indicates that *surfactant deficiency* per se is responsible for the epithelial lesion of hyaline membrane disease. Endotracheal surfactant treatment of premature newborn rabbits before positive pressure ventilation prevents the widespread necrosis and desquamation of bronchiolar epithelium seen in untreated littermates.[10] In the presence of inadequate surfactant at gas-liquid interfaces, the high pressure required to overcome surface tension forces in terminal conducting airways leads to epithelial injury and necrosis. The respiratory bronchioles and alveolar ducts are poorly supported structures in the immature lung and, under these conditions, are particularly susceptible to disruption as a result of overdistention, a characteristic histopathologic finding in hyaline membrane disease. Based on comparisons between surfactant-deficient rabbits ventilated with conventional mechanical ventilation and those receiving high-frequency ventilation, the degree of epithelial damage appears to be related to the magnitude of pressure swings, rather than mean pressure within the airways.[11] In addition, surfactant deficiency and accompanying high surface tensions at gas-liquid interfaces in terminal conducting airways may cause hydrostatic pressure gradients that interfere with the expedient disposal of fetal lung liquid or promote interstitial accumulation of edema fluid filtered from the microvascular circulation.

Ischemic Damage

Under some circumstances, the pathologic lesion of hyaline membrane disease may represent *ischemic necrosis* of the epithelial lining of terminal airways at the junctions of respiratory bronchioles and alveolar ducts. Both experimental and epidemiologic findings link acute asphyxia to the incidence and severity of this disease. Occasionally, hyaline membrane disease occurs in the near-term infant with a mature amniotic fluid lecithin/sphingomyelin ratio. Similarly, premature infants with immature lecithin/sphingomyelin ratios do not always have hyaline membrane disease. Infants with a prolapsed umbilical cord, bleeding placenta previa, or placental abruption have an increased incidence of hyaline membrane disease. There is also an increased incidence and severity of the disease in the second-born twin. These factors all point to the possible role of acute perinatal stress in the pathogenesis of hyaline membrane disease. Moreover, the tightly constricted arteriole characteristically adjacent to a respiratory bronchiole that is undergoing epithelial slough provides histopathologic evidence that ischemia may be involved in a process in which surfactant deficiency may be a secondary consequence of injury and necrosis of the epithelial lining.[12]

PATENT DUCTUS ARTERIOSUS

During the 1950s, many investigators considered hyaline membrane disease to be the result of left ventricular failure and pulmonary congestion caused by left-to-right shunting through the ductus arteriosus.[13-15] The presence of this shunt during the course of hyaline membrane disease, suspected on the basis of physical and radiographic findings, was confirmed by indicator dilution studies.[16, 17] In 1960, Dr. Clement Smith[18] stated, "Although the primary cause [of hyaline membrane disease] may be elsewhere, we continue to think that circulatory factors lie somewhere near the center of this puzzling and important problem."

During the acute phase of hyaline membrane disease, traditional clinical signs of a patent ductus arteriosus such as prominent murmur and precordial hyperactivity are usually absent. Nevertheless, left-to-right ductus shunting can be demonstrated in this setting by indicator dilution studies[17] or by Doppler ultrasound examinations[19,20] in most, if not all, newborn infants with hyaline membrane disease. A quantitative description of flows at different sites in the central circulation during hyaline membrane disease is shown in Figure 91-3.[21] In this composite example, which is based on studies of newborn premature lambs with the disease, 39% of left ventricular output is diverted back across the ductus and is recirculated through the pulmonary vascular bed. Figure 91-3 also illustrates the possibility of simultaneous right-to-left shunting across the foramen ovale. Indeed, bidirectional shunting (right-to-left at the foramen ovale and left-to-right at the ductus arteriosus) is probably not uncommon.

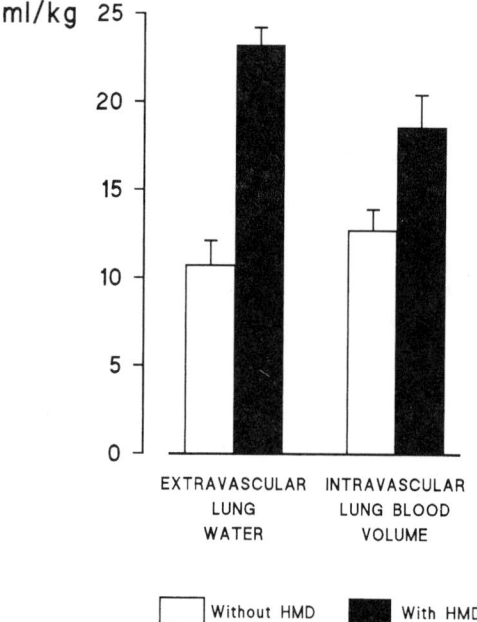

Figure 91-2. Extravascular lung water and intravascular lung blood volume measured in premature lambs with hyaline membrane disease (HMD) using a multiple indicator dilution method. (Data from ref. 9.)

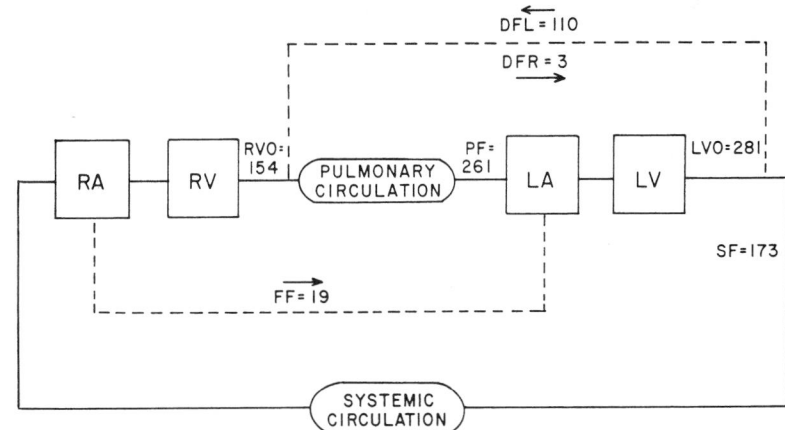

Figure 91–3. Mean values for components of cardiac output in 10 premature lambs with hyaline membrane disease. Flows are expressed as mL/kg/min. DFL and DFR = left-to-right and right-to-left flow through the ductus arteriosus; FF = right-to-left flow across the foramen ovale; LA = left atrium; LV = left ventricle; RA = right atrium; RV = right ventricle; SF = systemic flow. (From Cotton RB, et al: J Appl Physiol *43*:355, 1977.)

The lungs of infants with hyaline membrane disease are characteristically fluid laden for reasons described earlier in this section. As discussed later, hypoxemia occurs in large part because of venous admixture resulting from right-to-left shunts through terminal airway units that are fluid filled or collapsed. The problem of fluid and protein accumulation by the lungs is further exacerbated by left-to-right ductus shunting.[8] Indeed, some investigators have considered that the clinical expression of hyaline membrane disease in extremely immature infants is dominated by the consequences of left-to-right ductus shunting, rather than by surfactant deficiency.[22]

MECHANISMS OF HYPOXEMIA IN HYALINE MEMBRANE DISEASE

The principal mechanism of *hypoxemia* in hyaline membrane disease is venous admixture resulting from both intrapulmonary shunting and right-to-left shunting across the foramen ovale. Venous admixture is quantified by assuming that the oxygen content of arterial blood is the result of adding venous blood to blood equilibrated with alveolar gas. Venous admixture, an expression of the percentage of this mixture made up of venous blood, can be derived from the standard shunt equation:

$$VA\ (\%) = (Cc'_{O_2} - Ca_{O_2})/(Cc'_{O_2} - Cv_{O_2}) \times 100$$

where VA = venous admixture, Cc'_{O_2} = the end-pulmonary capillary blood oxygen content, Ca_{O_2} = the arterial blood oxygen content, and Cv_{O_2} = the mixed venous blood oxygen content.[23] Figure 91–4 shows how arterial partial pressure of oxygen (Pa_{O_2}) responds to changes in the fraction of inspired oxygen (Fi_{O_2}) at selected amounts of venous admixture.[24] When venous admixture is less than 40%, increasing the Fi_{O_2} will usually result in an adequate Pa_{O_2}. When venous admixture is 50% or more, increasing Fi_{O_2} from room air to 1.0 increases Pa_{O_2} by only a few millimeters of mercury, and adequate oxygenation is not achieved.

Intrapulmonary Shunting

In hyaline membrane disease, intrapulmonary venous admixture occurs largely as a result of the perfusion of terminal airways that are partially collapsed, collapsed, or fluid filled. For the most part, these terminal airways are either extremely underventilated or not ventilated at all as a result of epithelial slough, exudation, and hyaline membrane formation at the junction of the respiratory bronchioles and alveolar ducts. The effect of this pathologic process on terminal airway collapse is compounded by the associated surfactant deficiency, whether primary or secondary in origin. Based on studies of alveolar-arterial gradients of nitrogen

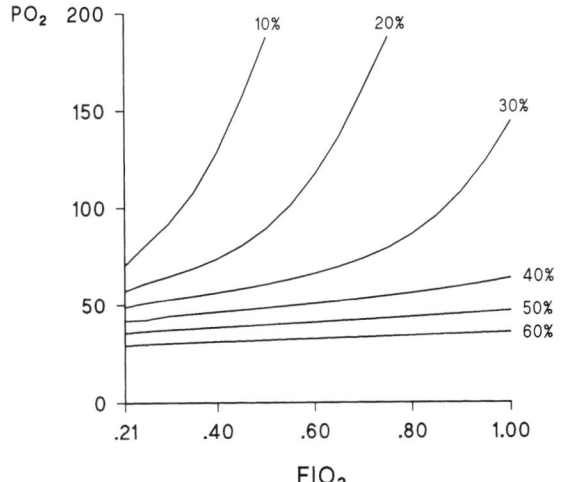

Figure 91–4. Arterial oxygen pressure (Po_2) response to changes in inspired oxygen fraction (Fi_{O_2}) at selected amounts of venous admixture between 10 and 60%. (Data obtained using computer software provided by Daniel P. Lindstrom and Torsten Olsson.)

and carbon dioxide, the lung in hyaline membrane disease can be modeled as comprising three compartments.[25, 26] One compartment is made up of terminal gas exchange units that are intact and are adequately ventilated and perfused. The second compartment is characterized by terminal airways that are open but markedly underventilated. These units may be perfused, but only if local alveolar hypoxia can be relieved by breathing 100% oxygen. The third compartment is totally unventilated but perfused. It includes those units with terminal conducting airways that are severely affected by epithelial damage, exudate, and slough. In addition, this compartment also represents any anatomic right-to-left shunt that is present.[27]

Extrapulmonary Shunting

There is a complex but predictable pattern of shunting through persistent fetal circulatory pathways that evolves during the natural course of hyaline membrane disease.[17] During the first 12 hours after birth, the predominant shunt is from right to left, from the inferior vena cava across the foramen ovale into the left atrium. Even though the ductus is widely patent, there is little flow through it in either direction until after 12 to 24 hours of age, when a left-to-right shunt of increasing magnitude occurs as a result of falling pulmonary vascular resistance. Significant right-to-left shunting at the ductus does not occur unless pulmonary vascular resistance is markedly elevated in the presence of severe hypoxemia, hypercarbia, or acidosis or when systemic vascular pressure is extremely low.

PULMONARY FUNCTION IN HYALINE MEMBRANE DISEASE

Functional Residual Capacity

Functional residual capacity (FRC) is decreased in hyaline membrane disease.[28-32] In newborn infants without lung disease, FRC is approximately 30 mL/kg,[29, 32] a volume coinciding with the volume of fetal lung liquid present in the airways before birth.[33] Loss of FRC occurs in hyaline membrane disease as a result of surfactant deficiency and displacement of gas volume by pulmonary vascular congestion, interstitial edema, and airway flooding with proteinaceous fluid.

During the course of hyaline membrane disease, FRC is influenced by numerous factors, including the patient's spontaneous ventilatory effort, the stability of the chest wall, and the patient's ability to muster an effective grunt. Defense of FRC against encroachment by a rising tide of lung water is the principal strategy of management for this disorder. When the patient's own defenses are overcome, FRC can be recovered and protected by the addition of distending airway pressure in the form of continuous positive pressure or intermittent mandatory ventilation.

Changes in FRC mirror the improvement in oxygenation that occurs with the addition of distending airway pressure or with spontaneous recovery beginning on the second or third day after birth.[30, 34-36] During recovery, there is a striking correlation between improving arterial oxygenation and increasing FRC and diuresis as excess lung water recedes into the circulation and is cleared by the kidneys.[34, 37]

Mechanical Properties of the Lung

The abnormal mechanical properties of the lung in hyaline membrane disease are the consequence of interacting pathophysiologic events.[38] The marked decrease in *lung compliance,* one of the hallmarks of hyaline membrane disease, is the consequence of two factors: (1) a decrease in the number of ventilated terminal air spaces (i.e., *derecruitment*); and (2) an increase in the recoil pressure of ventilated terminal air spaces. In addition, dynamic, but not static, compliance is further reduced in hyaline membrane disease owing to changes in the viscoelastic properties of lung tissue and the presence of inhomogeneity of ventilation.[39]

Derecruitment and the consequent loss of FRC occur as a result of the collapse of unstable terminal air spaces or as a result of alveolar flooding and tissue injury. The effects of air space instability on compliance and lung volume are discussed further later. The elastic recoil pressure of ventilated air spaces in hyaline membrane disease may be increased for a variety of reasons. Surface elastic forces are increased in hyaline membrane disease as a result of surfactant deficiency, inhibited surfactant function, or both (see Section XIII of this text). Alveolar flooding[40, 41] may also increase surface elastic forces. Tissue elastic forces may be increased with engorgement of the pulmonary vascular bed,[42] but it is unclear that this is the mechanism of decreased compliance observed in patients with hyaline membrane disease complicated by symptomatic patent ductus arteriosus.[43] Increased elastic recoil resulting from both surface forces and tissue elastic forces occurs when the infant with hyaline membrane disease is ventilated high on the volume axis of the lung's pressure-volume curve, either inadvertently or out of necessity. In the presence of extensive derecruitment, the small compartment of ventilated air

spaces that remains must provide more than its normal share of ventilation to achieve adequate gas transport. The smaller the ventilated compartment is, the more distended will its terminal air spaces become at end inspiration for a given tidal volume. At high volume, surface forces are minimally reduced by surfactant, and tissue elastance increases as the elastin network, which dominates at low- and middle-volume ranges, gives way to the structural influence of poorly compliant collagen.[44]

Like FRC, compliance also mirrors the course of pulmonary insufficiency in hyaline membrane disease.[34] Intercostal and sternal retractions in the infant capable of a spontaneous ventilatory effort provide a visual assessment of compliance at the bedside. As compliance improves, with manipulations of mechanical ventilation, surfactant replacement therapy, or evolution of the natural course of disease, chest wall retractions diminish, a finding indicating that less transpulmonary pressure is required to expand the lung.

Lung resistance, which is the sum of airway resistance and lung tissue resistance, is three to six times greater in infants with hyaline membrane disease than in newborn infants with normal lungs.[38] Although some of the increase in resistance may result from damage to conducting airways or from peribronchial edema,[45] the major cause of increased resistance is a decrease in the cross-sectional area of patent conducting airways leading to ventilated lung.[38]

Effect of Alveolar Instability on Lung Volume and Compliance

Alveolar instability refers to the tendency for an alveolus to switch abruptly between the inflated state and the collapsed state.[46] When pressure across the alveolus exceeds the critical opening pressure, an unstable alveolus inflates suddenly. During deflation, an unstable alveolus collapses abruptly when transalveolar pressure falls to less than the critical closing pressure. Figure 91-5 illustrates the stabilizing effect of surfactant treatment on an unstable alveolus with a critical opening pressure of slightly more than 11 cm H_2O and a critical closing pressure of just less than 7 cm H_2O.

Because the dimensions of the terminal air spaces are not uniform throughout the lung, all alveoli do not behave uniformly in surfactant deficiency. Under these conditions, there is a range of critical opening and closing pressures. As a result, there are several populations or compartments of terminal air spaces. One compartment remains collapsed throughout inspiration and expiration, another is ventilated during inspiration but collapses during each expiration, and a third is ventilated and stable to the extent that gas volume is retained at end expiration. The distribution of these compartments is affected by a variety of factors, especially treatment with surfactant replacement or with distending airway pressure. How changes in the relative size of these compartments affect lung volumes and compliance during fixed conditions of pressure-limited mechanical ventilation is illustrated in Figure 91-6. In this model, stabilization alone results in increased FRC and decreased compliance. Tidal volume and compliance do not improve until there is recruitment of new terminal air spaces from the previously unventilated compartment.

Ventilation

Infants with hyaline membrane disease who can be managed without intermittent positive pressure ventilation have spontaneous tidal volumes of 4 to 6 mL/kg, the same or only slightly less than the tidal volume of newborn infants with normal lung function. In contrast to infants with normal lungs, dead space makes up a much larger portion of tidal volume, 60 to 80% versus 30 to 40%.[47-49] After subtracting dead space from tidal volume, infants

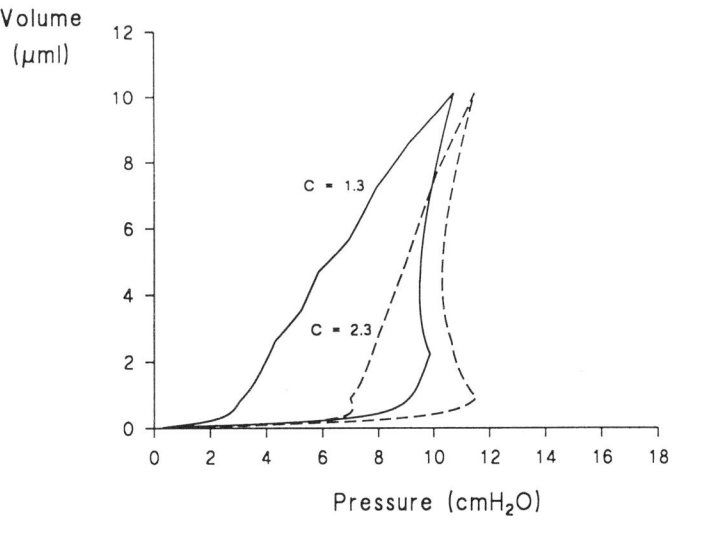

Figure 91–5. Pressure volume characteristics of a model alveolus when lined by extract from a premature infant's lung *(broken line)* or when lined by extract from an adult human lung *(solid line).* The data and model used to construct these pressure volume curves were taken from Clements and colleagues (J Appl Physiol *16*:444, 1961). (From Cotton R: Semin Perinatol *18*:19, 1994.)

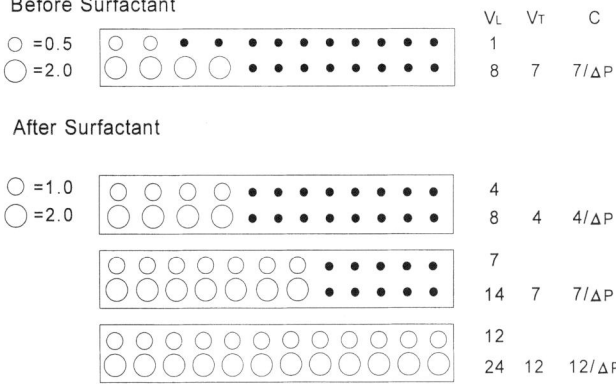

Figure 91–6. Alveolar stabilization and recruitment. Model of a 12-alveolus lung in which the *top row of each panel* represents the volume of each alveolus at end expiration and the *bottom row* represents the volume of each alveolus at end inspiration. The *solid circles* indicate alveolar collapse. The *open circles* indicate alveoli that are not collapsed. The end-expiratory volume and end-inspiratory volume of an individual alveolus are shown to the *left* of *panels 1 and 2.* Before surfactant treatment, there are two ventilated alveoli that are stable, two ventilated alveoli that are unstable, and eight collapsed alveoli that constitute an unventilated compartment. In *panel 2,* after surfactant, the two ventilated alveoli that were unstable before surfactant have become stabilized. The unventilated compartment of eight collapsed alveoli remains the same as before surfactant. In *panel 3,* three alveoli from the unventilated compartment have been recruited and stabilized. In *panel 4,* the unventilated compartment has been fully recruited, and all alveoli are ventilated and stable. The stepwise effect of this process of stabilization and recruitment on lung volume (V_L), tidal volume (V_T), and compliance (C) is shown to the *right* of the panels. (From Cotton R: Semin Perinatol *18*:19, 1994.)

with hyaline membrane disease are left with a decreased alveolar portion of tidal volume for which they compensate by breathing faster. As a result of increasing respiratory rate, a nearly normal alveolar ventilation and arterial carbon dioxide tension can be attained. A decreased alveolar portion of tidal volume is the expected pathophysiologic consequence of encroachment on terminal air spaces by lung water and is consistent with the well-documented loss of FRC in this disease.

Physiologic dead space is derived from systemic arterial carbon dioxide tension; *anatomic dead space* is derived from an estimate of alveolar carbon dioxide tension obtained from end-tidal gas analysis. The difference between the two dead spaces is referred to as *alveolar dead space.* (Physiologic dead space = anatomic dead space + alveolar dead space.[49]) In newborn infants with normal lungs, there is no detectable difference between physiologic and anatomic dead space because their arterial-alveolar carbon dioxide gradient is close to zero. Infants with hyaline membrane disease have a significant gradient of 12 to 16 mm Hg in carbon dioxide tension between arterial blood and alveolar gas, which results in an increase in measured physiologic dead space. This gradient has been explained as the result of a relative underperfusion of ventilated alveoli.[25,49] When terminal airway units are totally obstructed by epithelial slough and exudate, dilated respiratory bronchioles proximal to the obstruction behave as unperfused but ventilated "alveoli."

TREATMENT: PATHOPHYSIOLOGIC CONSIDERATIONS

Surfactant replacement therapy has become a standard part of the treatment of hyaline membrane disease and has proven to be enormously successful in bringing about highly significant reductions in mortality and pulmonary complications, especially air-leak syndromes. Chapters 104 and 106 are devoted to the subject of surfactant replacement therapy. The following discussion of treatment of hyaline membrane disease is limited to the role of oxygen therapy and the mechanical effects of distending airway pressure on the pathophysiology of this disorder.

The primary challenge in managing the pulmonary insufficiency of hyaline membrane disease is achieving an adequate Pa_{O_2}. If oxygenation can be achieved, carbon dioxide removal is only a matter of increasing minute ventilation sufficiently to make up for an inadequate alveolar portion of tidal volume. Management of the hypoxemia of hyaline membrane disease should be approached by recognizing the impact of venous admixture on Pa_{O_2} as a function of $F_{I_{O_2}}$ (see Fig. 91–4). Oxygenation can be achieved under conditions of modest venous admixture up to 30 or 40% by increasing $F_{I_{O_2}}$. With severe disease characterized by venous admixture above 40%, something must be done to reduce right-to-left shunt before adjustments in $F_{I_{O_2}}$ will have any significant effect on Pa_{O_2}.

Effects of Fraction of Inspired Oxygen

Some reduction in venous admixture can be realized by increasing the $F_{I_{O_2}}$ to 100%.[25,26] In part, this reduction in venous admixture reflects events in a lung compartment made up of gas exchange units that are extremely poorly ventilated. When the patient breathes 100% oxygen, local alveolar hypoxia is relieved, and perfusion is restored to those units that are open. In addition to reducing right-to-left intrapulmonary shunting, it is also possible to manipulate the magnitude of right-to-left shunt across fetal pathways by changing $F_{I_{O_2}}$.[17]

Even though simple oxygen administration without adding positive airway pressure can lead to a reduction in venous admixture, oxygen therapy by itself is often of limited efficacy. Before use of mechanical ventilation, survival from hyaline membrane disease was predicated more on effective grunting and increased respiratory effort than on oxygen therapy. Unless a patient could sustain adequate spontaneous ventilation and an effective grunt, the hypoxemia of hyaline membrane disease could not be overcome, even by hyperbaric oxygen therapy (Fig. 91–7).[50]

Effects of Distending Airway Pressure

Application of distending airway pressure to the airway of patients with hyaline membrane disease brings about a prompt reduction in venous admixture. The reduction in venous admixture results from a decrease in intrapulmonary right-to-left shunting as well as a decrease in right-to-left shunting across the foramen ovale.

Distending airway pressure may be applied in a variety of ways. In the original report[51] of its successful use in hyaline membrane disease, constant distending pressure was applied to an indwelling endotracheal tube by means of a continuous flow through an anesthesia bag that had an adjustable leak in its tail. In addition to this "Gregory continuous positive airway pressure apparatus," positive distending pressure can also be applied by face mask, nasal prongs, or head chamber. Distending airway pressure has also been delivered by surrounding the thorax with subatmospheric pressure, either with a chamber surrounding the entire body below the neck or with a cuirass around the thorax. All these methods deliver a continuous distending pressure during which ventilation depends on spontaneous breathing by the patient.

In patients whose ventilation is supplemented or taken over mechanically, distending airway pressure includes both the positive pressure provided for inspiration and positive end-expiratory pressure (PEEP). During positive pressure ventilation with PEEP, mean airway pressure measured at the endotracheal tube adapter is considered to represent effective distending airway pressure.

With increasing distending airway pressure, FRC increases[30] and venous admixture decreases as a result of stabilization and recruitment of effective ventilatory units. There is a significant

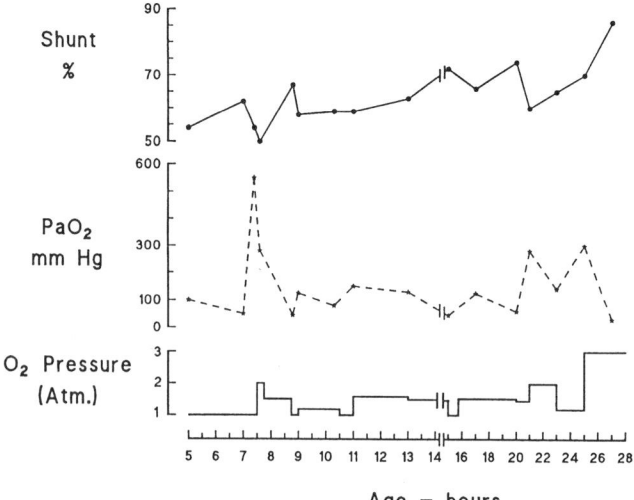

Figure 91–7. Serial arterial oxygen tensions in an infant with hyaline membrane disease treated with hyperbaric oxygen. The increase in arterial partial pressure of oxygen (Pa_{O_2}) after each increment in inspired oxygen pressure is transient. The overall course is one of progressive venous admixture (shunt %) despite the administration of 100% oxygen at pressures up to 3 atmospheres. (From Cochran WD, et al: N Engl J Med *272*:349, 1965. Reprinted by permission of the New England Journal of Medicine.)

decrease in the gradients of carbon dioxide[25] and nitrogen[52] between alveolar gas and arterial blood, indicating an improved perfusion of ventilated units and an improved ventilation of perfused units, respectively. In patients able to sustain spontaneous ventilation, application of distending airway pressure is followed by a reduction in minute ventilation. For the most part, this reduction can be accounted for by a decrease in tidal volume;[35,51] to a lesser extent, a decrease in the rate of breathing plays a role.[35] When distending airway pressure is applied, there is little or no change in arterial partial pressure of carbon dioxide,[35,51] signifying that alveolar ventilation is maintained in spite of the reduction in minute ventilation. This suggests that the dead space/tidal volume ratio is also decreased by distending airway pressure. The decrease in dead space/tidal volume ratio results from an increase in the alveolar portion of tidal volume caused by stabilization and recruitment of terminal air spaces.

Although application of distending airway pressure causes a prompt increase in arterial oxygen tension as a result of decreasing right-to-left shunt, there is no corresponding increase in dynamic lung compliance.[51] In fact, dynamic compliance may decrease after the application of distending airway pressure.[35] This response in dynamic compliance, which is similar to that reported after surfactant replacement therapy,[53–55] can be explained by the stabilizing effect of distending airway pressure on terminal air spaces. Figure 91–6 illustrates the effects of stabilization and recruitment on lung volumes and compliance. The results are similar, regardless of whether those effects are mediated by surfactant replacement or by increased end-expiratory pressure.

It has been recommended that the optimal level of distending airway pressure should be that level at which compliance increases.[56,57] Above this optimal level of distending airway pressure, compliance decreases, signifying that the dominant effect has become an overdistention of open gas exchange units rather than recruitment of new units. At an optimal level of distending airway pressure, the pattern of breathing becomes more regular, and the chest wall becomes more stable, with a decrease in inter-

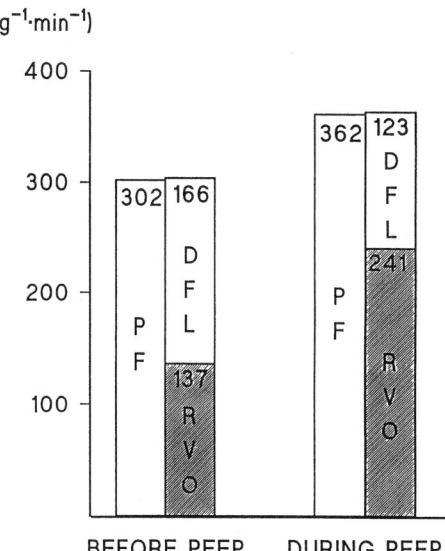

Figure 91–8. Effect of positive end-expiratory pressure (PEEP) on the components of pulmonary blood flow (PF) in premature lambs with hyaline membrane disease. DFL = left-to-right blood flow across the ductus arteriosus; RVO = right ventricular output. (From Cotton RB: *In* Stern L [ed]: Hyaline Membrane Disease: Pathogenesis and Pathophysiology. Orlando, FL, Grune & Stratton, 1984, p 184.)

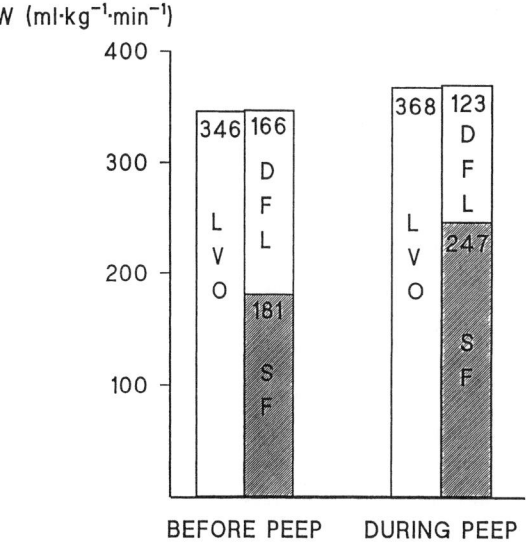

Figure 91–9. Effect or positive end-expiratory pressure (PEEP) on the components of left ventricular output (LVO) in premature lambs with hyaline membrane disease. DFL = left-to-right blood flow across the ductus arterious; SF = systemic blood flow. (From Cotton RB: *In* Stern L [ed]: Hyaline Membrane Disease: Pathogenesis and Pathophysiology. Orlando, FL, Grune & Stratton, 1984, p 184.)

costal and sternal retractions. These clinical observations imply an improvement in compliance and provide a handy bedside assessment of optimal levels of distending pressure.

Outside the lung, distending airway pressure has a beneficial effect on the distribution of cardiac output and on right-to-left shunting through the foramen ovale. In hyaline membrane disease, left ventricular output exceeds right ventricular output as a result of the bidirectional shunting discussed earlier. One increment in the extra volume load of the left ventricle can be accounted for by the portion of left ventricular output that is diverted back through the pulmonary circulation through the ductus arteriosus. A second increment results from the portion of systemic venous return that is shunted from the inferior vena cava across the foramen ovale into the left atrium. When additional distending airway pressure in the form of PEEP is added to the positive pressure ventilation of newborn premature lambs with hyaline membrane disease, a series of effects on the circulatory pattern can be demonstrated (Figs. 91–8 and 91–9).[58] The triggering event is thought to be a reduction in right-to-left shunting across the foramen ovale. The rerouted right-to-left foramen shunt appears as additional right ventricular output, which displaces a major part of the left-to-right ductus shunt from the pulmonary circulation forward into the systemic circulation. Pulmonary vascular resistance, pulmonary blood flow, and left ventricular output do not change appreciably. Right ventricular output and systemic blood flow increase. The net result of these changes is an increase in systemic Pao_2 caused by reduced venous admixture at the foramen ovale, as well as decreased lung congestion and protein leak subsequent to the reduction in left-to-right ductus shunting.

REFERENCES

1. Avery ME, Mead J: Surface properties in relation to atelectasis and hyaline membrane disease. Am J Dis Child 95:517, 1959.
2. Stahlman MT: Respiratory disorders in the newborn. *In* Kendig EL, Chernick V (eds): Disorders of the Respiratory Tract in Children. Philadelphia, WB Saunders Co, 1977, pp 271–290.
3. Avery ME, Taeusch HW: Hyaline membrane disease. *In* Schaffer's Diseases of the Newborn. Philadelphia, WB Saunders Co, 1984, pp 133–147.
4. Egan EA, et al: Fetal lung liquid absorption and alveolar epithelial solute permeability in surfactant deficient, breathing fetal lambs. Pediatr Res 14:314, 1980.
5. Normand ICS, et al: Flow and protein concentration of lymph from lungs of lambs developing hyaline membrane disease. Arch Dis Child 43:334, 1968.
6. Sundell HW, et al: Lung lymph studies in newborn lambs with hyaline membrane disease. *In* Jones CT, Nathanielsz PW (eds): Physiology of the Developing Fetus and Newborn. London, Academic Press, 1985, pp 331–335.
7. Egan EA, et al: Lung solute permeability and lung liquid absorption in premature ventilated fetal goats. Pediatr Res 14:314, 1980.
8. Jobe A, et al: Permeability of premature lamb lungs to protein and the effect of surfactant on that permeability. J Appl Physiol 55:169, 1983.
9. Sundell HW, et al: Lung water and vascular permeability: surface area in premature newborn lambs with hyaline membrane disease. Circ Res 60:923, 1987.
10. Nilsson R, et al: Lung surfactant and the pathogenesis of neonatal bronchiolar lesions induced by artificial ventilation. Pediatr Res 12:249, 1978.
11. Hamilton PP, et al: Comparison of conventional and high-frequency ventilation: oxygenation and lung pathology. J Appl Physiol 55:131, 1983.
12. Stahlman MT, et al: Pathophysiology of respiratory distress in newborn lambs. Am J Dis Child 108:375, 1964.
13. Burnard ED: Changes in heart size in the dyspnoeic newborn baby. BMJ 1:1495, 1959.
14. Lendrum FC: The "pulmonary hyaline membrane" as a manifestation of heart failure in the newborn infant. J Pediatr 47:149, 1955.
15. Stahlman MT: Digitalis in hyaline membrane syndrome. *In* Oliver TK (ed): Adaptation to Extrauterine Life. Report of the 31st Ross Conference on Pediatric Research. Columbus, OH, Ross Laboratories, 1959, pp 92–92.
16. Rudolph AM, et al: Studies on the circulation in the neonatal period: the circulation in the respiratory distress syndrome. Pediatrics 27:551, 1961.
17. Stahlman MT, et al: Circulatory studies in clinical hyaline membrane disease. Biol Neonate 1972; 20:300–320.
18. Smith CA: Circulatory factors in relation to idiopathic respiratory distress (hyaline membrane disease) in the newborn. J Pediatr 56:605, 1960.
19. Reller MD, et al: Review of studies evaluating ductal patency in the premature infant. J Pediatr 122:S59, 1993.
20. Seppanen MP, et al: Doppler-derived systolic pulmonary artery pressure in acute neonatal respiratory distress syndrome. Pediatrics 93:769, 1994.
21. Cotton RB, et al: Quantitation of cardiac output components in the presence of bidirectional shunts. J Appl Physiol 43:352, 1977.
22. Jacob J, et al: The contribution of PDA in the neonate with severe RDS. J Pediatr 96:79, 1980.
23. Comroe JH. The Lung. Chicago, Year Book Medical Publishers, 1977.
24. Rojas J, et al: A quantitative model for hyaline membrane disease. Pediatr Res 16:35, 1982.

25. Hansen TN, et al: Effects of oxygen and constant positive pressure breathing on aADCO$_2$ in hyaline membrane disease. Pediatr Res *13*:1167, 1979.

26. Corbet AJ, et al: Ventilation-perfusion relationships as assessed by a ADN$_2$ in hyaline membrane disease. J Appl Physiol *36*:74, 1974.

27. Parks CR, et al: Gas exchange in the immature lung. I. Anatomical shunt in the premature infant. J Appl Physiol *36*:10, 1974.

28. Krauss AN, Auld PAM: Measurement of functional residual capacity in distressed neonates by helium rebreathing. J Pediatr *77*:228, 1970.

29. Berglund G, Karlberg P: Determination of the functional residual capacity in newborn infants. Acta Paediatr Scand *45*:541, 1956.

30. Bose CL, et al: Measurement of cardiopulmonary function in ventilated neonates with respiratory distress syndrome. Pediatr Res *20*:316, 1986.

31. Jackson JC, et al: Changes in lung volume and deflation stability in hyaline membrane disease. J Appl Physiol *59*:1783, 1985.

32. McCann EM, et al: Pulmonary function in the sick newborn infant. Pediatr Res *21*:313, 1987.

33. Normand ICS, et al: Permeability of lung capillaries and alveoli to non-electrolytes in the foetal lamb. J Physiol (Lond) *219*:303, 1971.

34. Heaf DP, et al: Changes in pulmonary function during the diuretic phase of respiratory distress syndrome. J Pediatr *101*:103, 1982.

35. Bancalari E, et al: Effects of continuous negative pressure on lung mechanics in idiopathic respiratory distress syndrome. Pediatrics *51*:485, 1973.

36. Richardson CP, Jung AL: Effects of continuous positive airway pressure on pulmonary function and blood gases of infants with respiratory distress syndrome. Pediatr Res *12*:771, 1978.

37. Engle WD, et al: Diuresis and respiratory distress syndrome: Physiologic mechanisms and therapeutic implications. J Pediatr *102*:912, 1983.

38. Cotton RB, Olsson T: Lung mechanics in respiratory distress syndrome. *In* Robertson B, Taeusch HW (eds): Surfactant Therapy for Lung Disease. New York, Marcel Dekker, 1995, pp 121–149.

39. Sullivan KJ, Mortola JP: Dynamic lung compliance in newborn and adult cats. J Appl Physiol *60*:743, 1986.

40. Cook CD, et al: Pulmonary mechanics during induced pulmonary edema in anesthetized dogs. J Appl Physiol *14*:177, 1959.

41. O'Brodovich H, Hannam V: Exogenous surfactant rapidly increases PaO$_2$ in mature rabbits with lungs that contain large amounts of saline. Am Rev Respir Dis *147*:1087, 1993.

42. Hauge A, et al: Interrelations between pulmonary liquid volumes and lung compliance. J Appl Physiol *38*:608, 1975.

43. Clyman RI, et al: Cardiovascular effects of patent ductus arteriosus in preterm lambs with respiratory distress. J Pediatr *111*:579, 1987.

44. Hoppin FGJ, et al: Lung recoil: elastic and rheological properties. *In* Macklem PT, et al (eds): Handbook of Physiology, Sect 3: The Respiratory System, Vol 3. Bethesda, MD, American Physiological Society, 1986, pp 195–215.

45. Goldman SL, et al: Early prediction of chronic lung disease by pulmonary function testing. J Pediatr *102*:613, 1983.

46. Greaves IA, et al: Micromechanics of the lung. In: Macklem PT, et al (eds): Handbook of Physiology, Sect 3: The Respiratory System, Vol 3. Bethesda, MD, American Physiological Society, 1986, pp 217–231.

47. Chu J, et al: Neonatal pulmonary ischemia. I. Clinical and physiological studies. Pediatrics *40*:709, 1967.

48. Cook CD, et al: Studies of respiratory physiology in the newborn infant. II. Observations during and after respiratory distress. Acta Paediatr Scand Suppl *43*:397, 1954.

49. Nelson NM, et al: Pulmonary function in the newborn infant. II. Perfusion estimation by analysis of the arterial-alveolar carbon dioxide difference. Pediatrics *30*:975, 1962.

50. Cochran WD, et al: A clinical trial of high oxygen pressure for the respiratory distress syndrome. N Engl J Med *272*:347, 1965.

51. Gregory GA, et al: Treatment of the idiopathic respiratory-distress syndrome with continuous positive airway pressure. N Engl J Med *284*:1333, 1971.

52. Corbet AJS, et al: Effect of positive-pressure breathing on aADN$_2$ in hyaline membrane disease. J Appl Physiol *38*:33, 1975.

53. Edberg KE, et al: Immediate effects on lung function of instilled human surfactant in mechanically ventilated newborn infants with IRDS. Acta Paediatr Scand *79*:750, 1990.

54. Goldsmith LS, et al: Immediate improvement in lung volume after exogenous surfactant: alveolar recruitment versus increased distention. J Pediatr *113*:424, 1991.

55. Cotton RB, et al: The physiologic effects of surfactant treatment on gas exchange in newborn premature infants with hyaline membrane disease. Pediatr Res *34*:495, 1993.

56. Bonta BW, et al: Determination of optimal continuous positive airway pressure for the treatment of IRDS by measurement of esophageal pressure. J Pediatr *91*:449, 1977.

57. Suter PM, et al: Optimum end-expiratory airway pressure in patients with acute pulmonary failure. N Engl J Med *292*:284, 1975.

58. Cotton RB, et al: Effect of positive end-expiratory pressure on right ventricular output in lambs with hyaline membrane disease. Acta Paediatr Scand *69*:603, 1980.

92

Richard L. Auten, Jr.

Mechanisms of Neonatal Lung Injury

OVERVIEW

This chapter concentrates on the mechanisms that initiate lung injury, on their probable interactions, and on therapeutic strategies in use and under investigation that are aimed at preventing and treating lung injury, with a particular emphasis on premature infants, because that population represents the great majority of those who suffer long-term sequelae. The subject is covered in great detail in the book by Bland and Coalson,[1] so this chapter focuses on broad physiologic principles.

Mounting evidence points to the etiologic role of antenatal inflammation and oxidative stress in some cases of lung injury in premature newborns (see Chap. 94). Mechanical injury is sustained after positive pressure ventilation—even during initial resuscitation—compounding and accelerating these mechanisms. Mechanical ventilation designed to mimic neonatal intensive care practices in very premature baboons and sheep (without preterm labor or antenatal inflammation) causes acute lung inflammation and edema and is succeeded by persistence of underdeveloped and enlarged alveoli.[2,3]

The inflammatory processes that accompany mechanical lung injury in newborn lungs share some, but not all, of the patterns observed in older patients, and the relevant distinctions are discussed later.

VULNERABILITIES OF THE PREMATURE LUNG

Babies at highest risk to develop bronchopulmonary dysplasia (BPD) are born at approximately 70% gestation, at a time when the fetal lung is completing the canalicular stage and beginning the saccular or alveolar stage of development. Alveoli are relatively thick walled, and pulmonary capillaries are incompletely branched and do not extend to the ends of the alveolar septa. Surfactant synthesis and secretion are incomplete. Enzymatic antioxidants, superoxide dismutase, catalase, and glutathione peroxidase are relatively low and less inducible. Nutritional antioxidants such as vitamin E and β-carotene are also relatively low. With these liabilities, the extremely premature newborn lung is subjected to positive pressure ventilation, supplemental oxygen, and endotracheal intubation, all of which can injure developing lung and lead to impaired alveolar development and BPD.

SEQUELAE OF LUNG INJURY: INTERPRETING CLINICAL BRONCHOPULMONARY DYSPLASIA STUDIES: APPLES AND ORANGES?

Many of these premature newborns and most full-term newborns do not develop BPD after initial respiratory failure. It should be possible to discover the differences between patients who develop BPD and those who avoid it and to use this knowledge to devise treatments to prevent and treat lung injury, thus reducing the risk of BPD. Because of the long-standing practice of defining clinical BPD in the literature according to its treatment, namely, supplemental oxygen, it is difficult to interpret and compare outcomes. Ellsbury and colleagues[4] pointed out in a survey that the target oxygen saturation limits used to initiate or discontinue supplemental oxygen vary widely. For example, according to the oxygen use/requirement definition, which was used historically, a patient receiving supplemental oxygen at 36 to 40 weeks of postconceptual age would be classified as suffering from BPD, even if the oxygen therapy were only 0.1 L/minute by nasal cannula, whereas a patient receiving multiple diuretics and bronchodilators—but not receiving oxygen—would not necessarily be so classified in a clinical study. Efforts are under way to describe a physiologic definition of BPD that may allow more rational comparisons of outcomes in the future.

MECHANICAL MECHANISMS OF INJURY

Mechanical Lung Injury at Birth

Animal studies have shown that structural damage and inflammatory response can be generated after only a few overdistending breaths.[5] Significant lung injury can take place after brief periods of mechanical ventilation of the incompletely recruited lung. Forced recruitment may be harmful. Bjorklund and colleagues[6-8] showed, in a series of studies conducted in preterm, surfactant-treated lambs, that initial recruitment maneuvers with tidal volumes varying from 8 to 30 mL/kg had no benefit and caused dose-dependent histologic damage with increasing volumes. Lung volumes less than optimal functional residual capacity require higher than optimal peak pressures in later breaths to rerecruit alveoli fully. Gradual recruitment has been advocated as a strategy aimed to avoid this pitfall.[9] Early use of continuous positive airway pressure (CPAP), within a minute or two of delivery (in the spontaneously breathing infant), may avert lung injury by allowing gradual recruitment and avoiding the need for synchronized intermittent mandatory ventilation, and it has been advocated by investigators since its introduction by Wung and colleagues, who reported low rates of surfactant and endotracheal intubation use.[9-11]

Surfactant to Prevent Injury

Early use (<1 hour of age) of selective, empiric surfactant therapy of very premature newborns, typically less than 26 weeks of estimated gestational age, has been shown in several studies to reduce the risk of pneumothorax and BPD.[12-14] Uniform distribution of surfactant may be enhanced by administration at a time when alveolar fluid is incompletely resorbed. Preventilatory surfactant is beneficial in animal studies of premature delivery,[15] but it is not superior to early surfactant treatment (<1 hour of age), possibly because concurrent infection or inflammation may partly inactivate surfactant function. The clinical response to surfactant therapy is therefore variable. Uneven or asymmetric surfactant distribution may contribute to the heterogeneous clinical response, and it may further contribute to lung injury by directing positive airway pressure preferentially to the compliant parts of the lung. This often injures the compliant lung and spares (for a while) the noncompliant, non–surfactant-treated lung. Prompt use of exogenous surfactant, within the first hour of birth, clearly improves survival and avoids air leak—pneumothorax and pulmonary interstitial emphysema—in the smallest premature newborns.[14]

Continuous Positive Airway Pressure Versus Surfactant

Studies that have directly tested effects of very early or immediate surfactant treatment for newborns judged to be at high risk to develop respiratory distress syndrome (RDS) or BPD have shown short-term benefits. Failure to demonstrate robust prevention of BPD supports the selective use of surfactant treatment. Larger preterm infants who can be stabilized with CPAP in the delivery room may be candidates for expectant management. Reported survival advantages of very early or immediate surfactant treatment in the least mature newborns (estimated gestation age <26 weeks) would argue strongly for its uniform use in that group. A "bedside" or immediately available functional test of surfactant, such as a microbubble test of surface tension, can predict the development of RDS and can be performed reliably on tracheal aspirates and gastric aspirates.[16-18] The latter would potentially allow expectant management in the CPAP-treated very preterm newborn until the likelihood of substantial benefit of surfactant treatment was established.

Derecruitment

Maintaining lung recruitment to avoid injury is important. The mechanisms of mechanical lung injury attributable to derecruitment are summarized in Figure 92-1. Trauma to delicate airways can easily result if the lung is derecruited to volumes lower than functional residual capacity, resulting in alveolar collapse, and excessive pressure delivered to terminal airways to rerecruit alveoli in subsequent assisted breaths, and this subject has been reviewed in detail.[19] The details of appropriate mechanical ventilation strategies designed to avert this are discussed in Chapter 96, and they have been reviewed by Bhutani and others.[20, 21] However, there is significant controversy about the precise means that should be used. The accurate monitoring of delivered tidal volumes and airway pressures using in-line flow sensors and pneumotachographs can be hampered by the typically large, variable endotracheal tube leaks, particularly in the smallest newborns.

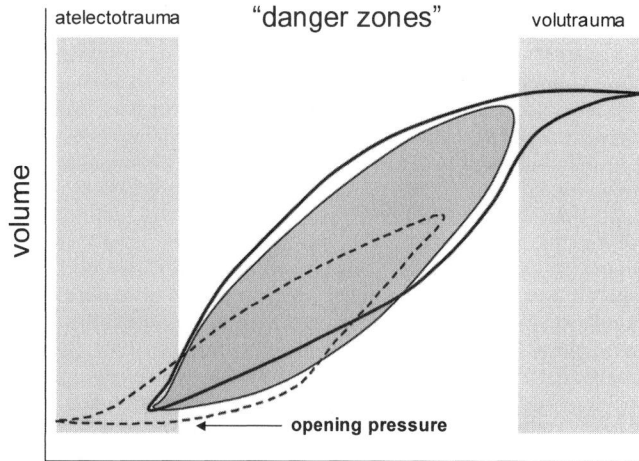

Figure 92–1. Static pressure-volume loop after recruitment (*solid line, gray fill*) of lung volume higher than functional residual capacity. After derecruitment, the pressure-volume loop demonstrates decreased hysteresis (*dashed line*), decreased slope, and loss of lung volume at end deflation, predisposing to "atelectotrauma." Overinflation (*dark solid line*) of the lung leads to increased luminal pressure without increased accumulation of lung volume, increasing shear stress to airways, and predisposing to "volutrauma."

Overexpansion

As the mechanical breath volume increases to approach the total lung capacity, increased airway pressure and mechanical shear force are applied to the airways and alveoli without a proportional increase in lung volume (see Fig. 92-1, at the upper inflection point). Unfortunately, there is scant objective evidence from clinical trials that can guide the specific choice of mechanical ventilation strategy. Only randomized clinical trials that are designed with a protocol-governed approach to mechanical ventilation can be readily interpreted. To date, there are no such trials using conventional intermittent mandatory ventilation, synchronized or not, that have been designed to test the ability of an open lung strategy to prevent lung injury and to avoid chronic lung disease in newborns. The role of nonconventional ventilation, such as high-frequency ventilation, is considered later.

Patient-Triggered Ventilation to Avoid Atelectasis

Avoiding patient-ventilator dyssynchrony is demonstrably important to avoiding derecruitment and hyperpnea. Intermittent hypoxemic episodes in mechanically ventilated premature newborns are often attributable to patient-ventilator dyssynchrony.[22] Patient-triggered ventilation has shown some short-term physiologic advantages,[23] but no well-designed clinical trials have shown clear long-term benefit. The specific method of patient triggering may need to be tailored to the dominant pathophysiologic features, as reviewed by Greenough.[24] A meta-analysis of studies designed to evaluate patient-triggered ventilation showed decreased length of ventilation requirement and reduced incidence of pneumothorax, but it was unable to define the mechanisms responsible for these benefits, because few patients received the respiratory mechanical monitoring necessary to delineate them.[25]

High-Frequency Ventilation to Stabilize Recruitment and Avoid Injury

The use of high-frequency ventilation theoretically avoids repetitive derecruitment and rerecruitment that lead to airway injury. The mechanics and principles are discussed in detail in Chapter 97. By leaving the lungs filled with gas at all times, the lung volume does not fall to less than functional residual capacity. Likewise, the phasic variations in airway pressure that are present at the wye of the ventilator circuit are dampened in the distal airways and alveoli. This principle has led some clinicians to advocate empiric use of high-frequency ventilation to maintain optimal lung volume stably and therefore ventilation-perfusion matching. In the prematurely delivered baboon, high-frequency oscillation preserved lung inflation and prevented lung inflammation in the short-term, but it did not confer long-term benefits to alveolar development as determined by lung morphometry.[26]

Clinical studies that employed a strategy of optimizing lung volume using high-frequency ventilation demonstrated modest benefits when compared with conventional tidal ventilation,[27-29] and some have shown no benefit.[30,31] There were no differences in inflammatory responses in newborns randomized to high-frequency ventilation versus conventional ventilation, possibly because of the likely role of inflammation in spontaneous preterm birth.[32] At present, there are not enough long-term studies of lung development and lung physiology in convalescent newborns and infants to determine whether empiric high-frequency ventilation treatment prevents abnormalities of pulmonary function and later chronic respiratory problems. Indeed, meta-analyses of clinical trials of high-frequency ventilation used as primary therapy in premature newborns with respiratory failure have concluded that short-term pulmonary benefits are modest (reduced need for oxygen at 36 weeks of postconceptual age), and risks, which are primarily neurodevelopmental, owing to uncontrolled hypocarbia adversely affecting cerebral blood flow, are significant.[33,34]

The presumed mechanical advantages of avoiding atelectotrauma may be of greatest benefit to those patients who are most likely to require the longest course of mechanical ventilation, namely, the most immature. Conversely, those patients are most likely to have the least control of cerebrovascular regulation. Proper assessment of the risks and benefits will require prospective stratification of mechanical ventilatory strategies among risk groups.

To Ventilate or Not to Ventilate

Mechanical ventilation can certainly initiate and exacerbate lung injury, particularly with inhomogeneous lung disease that results in wide variability of time constants throughout the lung. The magnitude of its contribution to BPD is unclear and likely varies depending on how it is employed. Selective use of mechanical ventilation, even in extremely low birth weight premature newborns, may avoid this risk.[35] However, even though relatively brief periods of mechanical ventilation can initiate injury and inflammation, there are no published clinical studies that evaluate the duration or severity of this response. The role of mechanical ventilation in the propagation of BPD remains to be proved. Indeed, neonatal intensive care centers that routinely intubate and mechanically ventilate the smallest, highest-risk newborns demonstrate rates of BPD that are similar to those centers that routinely avoid intubation (E. Bancalari, personal communication). Fortunately, there are ongoing prospective, randomized, controlled trials designed to answer this important question definitively.

Lung Water and Patent Ductus Arteriosus Contribute to Mechanical Lung Injury

Inhomogeneity of time constants and regional variability of lung compliance invite volutrauma. The patent ductus arteriosus (PDA) contributes to this mechanism. PDA has uniformly been identified in virtually all clinical studies as a powerful contributor to chronic lung disease of prematurity, and it is considered in detail elsewhere. Early, definitive closure of the PDA reduces BPD. Fluid and electrolyte management would be expected to affect uniformity of lung compliance and therefore reduce the susceptibility of the lung to mechanical overdistension. Meta-analysis of four randomized, controlled trials limiting fluid administration and insensible water losses demonstrated lower rates of death, development of PDA, and necrotizing enterocolitis and a trend toward reduced incidence of BPD.[36]

Persistence or recurrence of PDA is highly correlated with the development of BPD, probably because of the same principle of uneven effects on lung compliance. Alternatively, recurrence of PDA is often associated with sepsis, which itself may contribute to inflammatory lung injury.[37] Chorioamnionitis and fetal inflammation may also contribute to the production of prostaglandins that promote ductal patency by the same mechanisms. Early, aggressive treatment of PDA is therefore likely to reduce the risk of lung injury by improving lung mechanics, thus allowing decreased exposure to oxygen and mechanical ventilation.

HUMORAL LUNG INJURY: CONGENITAL, PERINATAL, AND POSTNATAL INFECTION

Infection is recognized as a very common initiator of inflammatory lung injury.[38] Neonatal pneumonias, particularly group B streptococcal infections, can be fatal, and they are a frequent cause of severe respiratory failure necessitating extracorporeal membrane oxygenation as lifesaving treatment. Although the respiratory failure is often severe, it is typically the hemodynamic instability that is fatal. Herpes simplex, adenovirus, and enteroviruses are less common etiologic agents that accompany or cause severe respiratory failure in the newborn. In all these cases, the systemic inflammatory response is accompanied by significant pulmonary neutrophil influx, alveolar-capillary leak, and, in some cases, necrotizing tracheobronchitis. Despite severe respiratory failure caused by these agents, term newborns typically recover completely and uncommonly exhibit long-term sequelae. Premature newborns are more likely to develop BPD as a consequence, likely owing to death or dysregulation of progenitor cells ordinarily destined to complete repair and development.

Ureaplasma infection has been suspected to play a role in the development of BPD by this mechanism, and it was first implicated in reports from the late 1980s.[39-41] The evidence implicating *Ureaplasma* species is suggestive. Horowitz and colleagues[42] reported up to 25% colonization rates in premature infants at high risk to develop BPD and found higher colonization in newborns who developed BPD. *Ureaplasma* induces secretion of inflammatory cytokines in type II pneumocytes,[43] and it impairs expression of antiinflammatory cytokines in monocytes *in vitro*.[44] Maternal colonization with *U. urealyticum* is associated with elevated concentrations of interleukin-8 (IL-8) in amniotic fluid,[45] with an indication of IL-8 in cultured newborn lung fibroblasts,[46] and with elevated IL-8 and monocyte chemoattractant protein-1 (MCP-1, a macrophage-attracting chemokine) in the tracheal aspirates of newborns who later developed BPD.[47] However, clinical trials of antibiotic therapy have not yet shown conclusive benefit.[48, 49] Study of associations of *Ureaplasma* colonization with chronic lung disease has yielded contradictory results.[50, 51] Conversely, the clinical trials conducted so far may not have been sufficiently powered to test the hypothesis.

An autopsy study of premature newborns with pneumonia linked the presence of *U. urealyticum* in the lung to profibrotic histologic changes often found in advanced BPD, as demonstrated in Figure 92-2.[52] The role of *U. urealyticum* in apparent exacerbations of respiratory failure in very low birth weight premature infants may be underestimated, and more sensitive techniques employing polymerase chain reaction identification of *Ureaplasma* DNA identified infected patients who were culture negative.[53, 54] Likewise, experimental infection in newborn animals can cause lung injury and abnormal develop-

ment (R. Viscardi, personal communication). Whether it does so in humans remains to be determined.

Sick newborns, particularly mechanically ventilated premature newborns, are at high risk to develop these and other nosocomial infections. Late-onset sepsis in premature newborns has been strongly predictive of later development of BPD in several studies.[37, 55, 56] Infection may represent another instance of the "second hit" that exacerbates inflammation and contributes to dysregulated lung development and repair discussed in Chapter 93.

ASPIRATION INJURY

Meconium Aspiration

Biochemical contents of meconium are toxic to the lung. Fatty acids, oleic acid in particular, can be directly toxic to epithelial membranes. *In vitro*, neutrophils exposed to meconium release IL-8, which may serve to amplify the inflammatory response by recruiting more neutrophils and by stimulating the respiratory burst.[57-59] Oleic acid, hemoglobin, and other components may inactivate lung surfactant, thereby leading to alveolar instability.[60] Experimental and clinical treatment with exogenous surfactant restores minimum surface tension, improves oxygenation, and reduces the need for extracorporeal membrane oxygenation.[61-63]

Amniotic Fluid Aspiration

At first glance, it may seem paradoxical that amniotic fluid, which is produced in part by the fetal lung, would be toxic to pulmonary epithelium. However, the aspiration of cellular debris and the components of dead cells are likely to provoke an inflammatory response by the same mechanisms attributed to meconium aspiration: direct cellular toxicity, release of humoral mediators, and surfactant inactivation. Although the net flux of pulmonary fluid in fetal life is away from the lung, there is mixing during labor, particularly if the fetus gasps in response to hypoxia. Infected amniotic contents have been reported frequently in postmortem examinations. The exposure of the fetal lung to proinflammatory cytokines derived from inflamed fetal membranes is discussed in more detail in Chapter 94.[64]

LEUKOCYTE-MEDIATED INJURY

How does inflammation—regardless of its initiating cause—exacerbate newborn lung injury? Several features of inflammation are unique to the lung. The proximity of the lung to the environment and its exposure to toxins and pathogens discussed earlier necessitate host defense mechanisms that are poised to respond quickly to microbial invasion and then to down-regulate the inflammatory response to avoid cytotoxicity from a rampant immune response. Lewis Thomas,[65] in *Lives of a Cell,* observed: "It is our response to...[bacterial] presence that makes the disease. Our arsenals for fighting off bacteria are so powerful, and involve so many different defense mechanisms, that we are in more danger from them than from the invaders. We live in the midst of explosive devices; we are mined."

Resident alveolar macrophages and the innate immune system, typified by complement and surfactant proteins A and D, do not require the generation of specific antibodies, because they all possess molecular recognition domains that bind chemical motifs found on some pathogens and permit clearance from air spaces.[66] The role of the macrophage in the initial response to injury is not firmly established. Different injuries or exposures can alter the timing and sequence of inflammatory cell influx. In neonatal surfactant deficiency and in experimental oxygen toxicity in newborn rats, resident alveolar macrophages both precede and succeed the influx of neutrophils that are isolated from bronchoalveolar lavage fluid.[67, 68] Cellular inflammatory

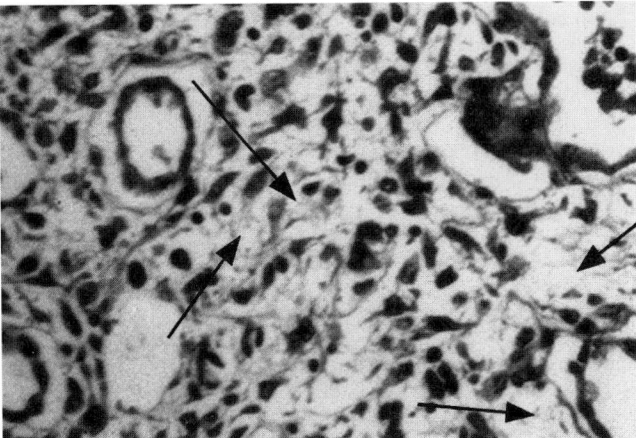

Figure 92–2. Fibrosis is identified with pentachrome staining (*arrows*) in histologic lung sections obtained at autopsy from a ventilator-dependent newborn in whom *Ureaplasma urealyticum* was identified post mortem by polymerase chain reaction assay. Magnification 400×. (Courtesy of R.M. Viscardi.)

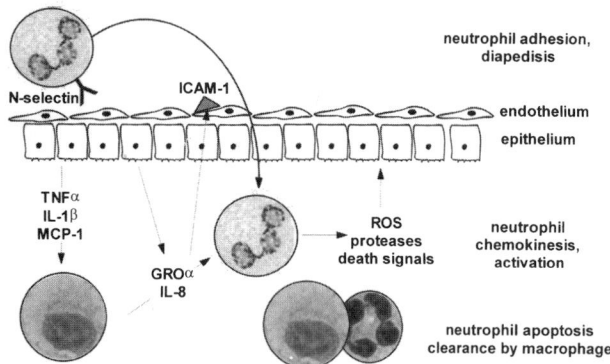

Figure 92–3. Damaged cells release proinflammatory cytokines that up-regulate adhesion molecules on circulating leukocytes and endothelium. Both epithelium and macrophages produce neutrophil chemokines, such as growth-related oncogene-α (GROα) and interleukin-8 (IL-8), that further up-regulate adhesion of neutrophils and regulate chemotaxis, chemokinesis, and the reactive oxygen producing respiratory burst. On activation, the neutrophil requires continuous chemokine signal transduction without which the neutrophil undergoes apoptosis and is cleared by alveolar macrophages. Activated neutrophils release reactive oxygen species (ROS), proteases, and other toxic materials that can damage adjacent cells. ICAM-1 = intercellular adhesion molecule-1; MCP-1 = monocyte chemoattractant protein-1; TNFα = tumor necrosis factor-α.

responses to mechanical or oxidative injury in the lung are prompted by release of prostanoids or by the binding of pathogens to signal molecules that activate proinflammatory cytokines, such as IL-1β or tumor necrosis factor-α (TNF-α). These, in turn, stimulate expression of monocyte chemokines, such as MCP-1,[69] known to be expressed in alveolar epithelium,[70] which recruits macrophages into the lung. The recruitment of leukocytes in general and neutrophils in particular into the lung hinges on the complex interplay of cytokines, chemokines, and cellular adhesion molecules that is summarized in Figure 92–3.

Large animal models designed to mimic clinical BPD by the use of appropriate oxygen therapy, moderate ventilation, and surfactant treatment after premature delivery showed a similar sequence of the development of injury and inflammation, even though they lack antecedent labor. Premature newborns who later develop BPD are likely to have elevations of proinflammatory cytokines and chemokines in tracheal aspirate samples.[71-73] These elevations may be present on the day of birth, a finding suggesting that the inflammatory response began antenatally or shortly after delivery, perhaps during the initial resuscitation.

NEONATAL VULNERABILITIES TO INFLAMMATION

Duration of Inflammation Determines the Injury

Antenatal exposure to inflammation may be the first "hit" of the two-hit injury sequence postulated by Barker and colleagues[74] that conditions the lung for later abnormal development. The newborn has particular developmental distinctions that characterize initiation and resolution of inflammation. The duration of inflammation—whether present at birth or after later mechanical injury—may determine the impact of this hit. Activation of the IL-8 receptor (CXCR2) by IL-8 dooms the neutrophil to apoptosis or necrosis. Activated neutrophils have shorter life spans, and blockade of the neutrophil IL-8 receptor CXCR2 accelerates neutrophil apoptosis.[75] Whether neutrophils in newborns are as susceptible to apoptosis on activation is unknown. Antiinflamma-

tory cytokines that take part in the termination of inflammation, such as IL-10, are relatively sparse in the tracheal aspirates of premature newborns who are at high risk to develop BPD.[76] Premature newborns are slow to initiate inflammation, but they are also slow to resolve it. This may explain part of the difference in the pulmonary outcomes between immature and mature newborns after lung injury.

Inflammatory Processes Interrupt Lung Development

Damage to the developing lung may be sustained during a critical period, leading to death of particular progenitor cells necessary to orderly transition from the canalicular to the alveolar stage of lung development. Indirect effects of reactive oxygen species produced by leukocytes may damage lung cell DNA in certain proliferating cell types, thereby necessitating DNA repair and delaying orderly mitosis and tissue development.[77] This may occur by disrupting the normal order of cell proliferation or by accelerating pathologic lung cell apoptosis, possibly through elaboration of cell death signaling molecules, such as Fas-Fas ligand.[78,79]

INTERRUPTING INFLAMMATION TO PREVENT LUNG INJURY AND ITS SEQUELAE

Selective interruption of inflammation may protect lung development. Animal and clinical studies demonstrated short-term benefits of glucocorticoid treatment to prevent or treat lung injury or to prevent or treat BPD. The mechanisms by which they confer these short-term benefits are manifold, but only the antiinflammatory role is considered here. Glucocorticoids down-regulate the mRNA transcription of IL-1, TNF-α, IL-6, and IL-8, among others. They prevent neutrophil degranulation and activation.[80] However, clinical trials did not demonstrate that glucocorticoid treatment can *safely* prevent BPD: growth restriction, neurodevelopmental impairment, and increased susceptibility to infection[81-83] led the American Academy of Pediatrics and the Canadian Pediatric Society in 2002 to recommend against the use of glucocorticoids to prevent or treat BPD outside of randomized, controlled clinical investigations.[84]

Selective Immunomodulation

Can more selective modification of inflammation avoid the undesired effects of steroids on growth and development? Nonsteroidal antiinflammatory treatment with cromolyn reduced inflammatory mediators in high-risk newborns but did not prevent BPD as defined.[85] Leukotriene inhibitors have been used in experimental models but not in clinical trials to prevent BPD.[86,87] Most clinical studies of newborn lung injury have implicated the proinflammatory cytokines and the C-X-C chemokine pathway.[71-73, 88] Experimental studies that blocked the C-X-C neutrophil chemokine pathway in newborn rat lung preserved alveolar development,[89,90] possibly by reducing neutrophil-borne oxidative stress,[91] or by accelerating neutrophil apoptosis.[75] Because the inflammatory response is mediated by cytokines and chemokines, they and their receptors would appear to be logical therapeutic targets.

Numerous lung injury models of sepsis-associated injury, ventilator-induced lung injury, and acute RDS have shown benefit by blocking one or more proinflammatory cytokines or chemokines, and many of these are reviewed thoroughly elsewhere.[92] However, only a few have attempted to interrupt or prevent BPD or its components in newborn models, and there are no published clinical trials. Newborn animals increase pulmonary neutrophil chemokine expression in response to hyperoxia exposure and to normoxic mechanical ventilation.[2, 3, 70, 89] Treatment with neutralizing antibodies directed against the chemokines after the initiation of the injury by hyperoxia, but before significant elevations of the chemokines occurred, preserved alveolar development in newborn rats,[90] possibly by avoiding oxidative impairment of lung cell proliferation.[91]

Monocytes recruited to the lung secrete neutrophil chemokines,[93] as well as cytokines that later contribute to fibrosis and repair. The role of resident alveolar macrophages in this inflammatory process in preterm newborns is not completely understood. Blocking monocyte influx may serve as an indirect tactic to prevent neutrophil influx, and it was reported to attenuate hyperoxia-induced protein damage in newborn rats.

Blocking neutrophil influx or neutrophil function is not safe during acute bacterial or fungal infections, and blocking macrophage function during the resolution of acute inflammation delays neutrophil clearance from the airways, thus increasing the likelihood that neutrophil-derived reactive oxygen species or proteolytic enzymes will contribute further to lung injury. Topical treatment with immune modulators may avoid systemic impairment of immunity.

Modulation of Inflammatory Effects: Protease-Mediated Injury

Destruction of biomolecules is the purpose of neutrophil-mediated proteases such as elastase, cathepsin G, and others.[29] Newborns, and premature infants in particular, are relatively deficient in antiproteases such as α_1-antiprotease and secreted leukocyte protease inhibitor.[94-96] Clinical substitution of antitrypsin has not had a robust benefit, but this may be because aerosol delivery of the antiprotease fails to reach the vulnerable target, namely, the lung matrix, which may be an important target of interstitial release of leukocyte-borne proteases. Catalytic cleavage of matrix molecules may further amplify the inflammatory cascade and lung injury.[97,98] Failure to protect matrix from proteolytic attack may not interrupt the release of leukocyte chemoattractants and may thereby perpetuate the vicious cycle.

OXIDATIVE STRESS, ACUTE NEWBORN LUNG INJURY, AND BRONCHOPULMONARY DYSPLASIA

Deficiency of Antioxidant Defenses in Prematurity

Antioxidant defenses in premature newborns are likely inadequate to meet the challenges of high oxidative stress. The transition from the fetal milieu, wherein the oxygen delivery at relatively low arterial partial pressure of oxygen is adequate to the metabolic demands, to the extrauterine existence with its significantly higher metabolic demands, is typically accompanied by supplemental oxygen treatment. Studies in premature animals showed that the enzymatic activity and gene expression of superoxide dismutases, catalase, and glutathione peroxidase are decreased.[99,100] Naturally, this invokes the notion of antioxidant deficiency in the presence of relatively increased oxidant stress, leading to impaired cellular metabolism, direct biomolecular damage, and structural cellular damage. However, the nature of the contribution of oxidant stress depends on the relevant biologic compartments and relationships among potential molecular substrates. This was reviewed in detail by Smith and Welty.[101] Serum glutathione stores are diminished (relative to adults) in premature newborns at risk to develop BPD. Oxidation of proteins isolated from tracheal aspirates of newborns destined to develop BPD provides some indirect evidence of inadequate antioxidant defense.[102]

Metals and Oxidant-Mediated Lung Injury

Likely oxidant-stress mechanisms involved in the initiation and propagation of lung injury include oxidation and nitrosylation of proteins, lipids, and nucleic acids. In addition, free metals such as iron or complexed iron can take part in many different reactions that are likely to produce reactive oxygen species or to damage critical catalytic components of enzymes or cofactors, for example[103]:

I. $Fe^{3+} + O_2^{-\bullet} \rightarrow Fe^{2+} + O_2$
Formation of ferrous iron

II. $Fe^{2+} + H_2O_2^{-\bullet} \rightarrow Fe^{3+} + OH^- + HO^\bullet$
Formation of hydroxyl radical

III. $Fe^{2+} + LOOH \rightarrow Fe^{3+} + LO^\bullet + OH^-$
Catalysis of lipid peroxidation "chain reaction"

Normally, iron is handled very carefully by cells, owing to its powerful redox capacity for catalyzing these potentially damaging reactions. Direct and indirect evidence points to this pathway as a contributor to lung injury. Free iron contributes to lipid peroxidation in ischemia-reperfusion injury.[104] Newborns who developed chronic lung disease were found to have higher serum ceruloplasmin and ferritin levels, and they had twice as many blood transfusions as age-matched control patients who did not have chronic lung disease.[105] Low plasma antioxidant activity and frequent red blood cell transfusions have been associated with an increased risk of BPD.[106] Erythropoietin treatment in hyperoxia-exposed rabbits increased the resistance of blood and tracheal aspirates to lipid peroxidation.[107] This finding, coupled with the relatively decreased inducibility of heme oxygenase-1 in newborns, a principal chelator of free iron, suggests that iron may contribute to oxidant-mediated lung damage in newborns.

In vitro, superoxide, hydrogen peroxide, peroxyl radical, singlet oxygen, and hydroxyl radical *can* develop in particular compartments within the lung and inside lung cells. These compounds can damage lipid, protein, carbohydrate, and nucleic acid cell components. What is unknown at present is whether they *do* occur in sufficient measure to cause lung cell injury leading to BPD.[108] The strength of the evidence implicating each reactive species in the pathology of newborn lung injury is variable.

Reactive Oxygen Species: Physiologic Role

Jankov and colleagues[109] pointed out that the evidence implicating oxidative stress in the cause of BPD in humans is not definitive. Preventing lung injury by antioxidant treatment may be ineffective if such therapy impairs appropriate cell division and repair. The redox state of the cell is tightly regulated, and its disturbance may alter the ability of the cell to divide or differentiate. Antioxidant treatment has actually impaired lung growth in hyperoxia-exposed newborn rats.[110] Hydrogen peroxide in particular has been shown to regulate certain receptor signal-transduction pathways, acting as a second messenger. Because it is freely diffusible, its production by superoxide dismutases, for example, could potentially have wide-ranging effects on numerous cell physiologic pathways.[111-113] Large changes in intracellular flux of reactive oxygen species may have unpredictable effects on lung injury and development.

SUMMARY

The mechanisms of lung injury in newborns are interdependent, as shown in Figure 92–4. Because the mechanisms of lung injury that lead to abnormal lung development are manifold, we should expect that preventive treatments will have to be individualized, depending on the dominant pathophysiologic features. Nevertheless, cellular injury followed by inflammation and further oxidative injury is the sequence common to all the mechanisms discussed. Future investigations will likely focus on avoidance of

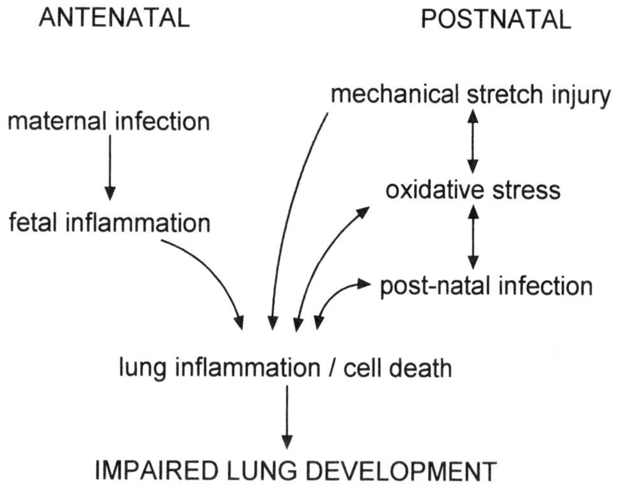

ANTENATAL   POSTNATAL

Figure 92–4. Combined antenatal and postnatal cellular injuries at critical phases of development contribute to BPD.

mechanical injury, selective inflammatory blockade, and individualized supplementation of antioxidants.

REFERENCES

1. Bland RD, Coalson JJ (eds): Chronic Lung Disease in Early Infancy, Vol 137. *In* L'Enfant C (series ed): Lung Biology in Health and Disease. New York, Marcel Dekker, 2000.
2. Coalson JJ, et al: Neonatal chronic lung disease in extremely immature baboons. Am J Respir Crit Care Med *160*:1333, 1999.
3. Albertine KH, et al: Chronic lung injury in preterm lambs: disordered respiratory tract development. Am J Respir Crit Care Med *159*:945, 1999.
4. Ellsbury DL, et al: Variability in the use of supplemental oxygen for bronchopulmonary dysplasia. J Pediatr *140*:247, 2002.
5. Jackson JC, et al: Effect of high-frequency ventilation on the development of alveolar edema in premature monkeys at risk for hyaline membrane disease. Am Rev Respir Dis *143*:865, 1991.
6. Bjorklund LJ, et al: Lung recruitment at birth does not improve lung function in immature lambs receiving surfactant. Acta Anaesthesiol Scand *45*:986, 2001.
7. Ingimarsson J, et al: The pressure at the lower inflexion point has no relation to airway collapse in surfactant-treated premature lambs. Acta Anaesthesiol Scand *45*:690, 2001.
8. Bjorklund LJ, Werner O: Should we do lung recruitment maneuvers when giving surfactant? Pediatr Res *50*:6, 2001.
9. Lundstrom KE: Initial treatment of preterm infants: continuous positive airway pressure or ventilation? Eur J Pediatr *155*(Suppl 2):S25, 1996.
10. Wung JT, et al: A new device for CPAP by nasal route. Crit Care Med *3*:76, 1975.
11. Sahni R, Wung JT: Continuous positive airway pressure (CPAP). Indian J Pediatr *65*:265, 1998.
12. Kendig JW, et al: A comparison of surfactant as immediate prophylaxis and as rescue therapy in newborns of less than 30 weeks' gestation. N Engl J Med *324*:865, 1991.
13. Hudak ML, et al: A multicenter randomized masked comparison trial of synthetic surfactant versus calf lung surfactant extract in the prevention of neonatal respiratory distress syndrome. Pediatrics *100*:39, 1997.
14. Soll RF, Morley CJ: Prophylactic versus selective use of surfactant in preventing morbidity and mortality in preterm infants. Cochrane Database Syst Rev CD000510, 2001.
15. Cummings JJ, et al: Pre- versus post-ventilatory surfactant treatment in surfactant-deficient preterm lambs. Reprod Fertil Dev 7:1333, 1995.
16. Boo NY, et al: Usefulness of stable microbubble test of tracheal aspirate for the diagnosis of neonatal respiratory distress syndrome. J Paediatr Child Health *33*:329, 1997.
17. Friedrich W, et al: The stable microbubble test on tracheal aspirate samples from newborn babies for diagnosis of surfactant deficiency and/or surfactant malfunction. Biol Neonate *73*:10, 1998.
18. Teeratakulpisarn J, et al: Prediction of idiopathic respiratory distress syndrome by the stable microbubble test on gastric aspirate. Pediatr Pulmonol *25*:383, 1998.
19. Auten RL, et al: Volutrauma: what is it, and how do we avoid it? Clin Perinatol *28*:505, 2001.
20. Bhutani VK, Sivieri EM: Clinical use of pulmonary mechanics and waveform graphics. Clin Perinatol *28*:487, 2001.
21. Wiswell TE, Donn SM: Update on mechanical ventilation and exogenous surfactant. Clin Perinatol *28*(3):487, 2001.
22. Bolivar JM, et al: Mechanisms for episodes of hypoxemia in preterm infants undergoing mechanical ventilation. J Pediatr *127*:767, 1995.
23. Donn SM, et al: Patient triggered assisted ventilation of newborns. J Perinatol *12*:312, 1992.
24. Greenough A: Update on patient-triggered ventilation. Clin Perinatol *28*:533, 2001.
25. Greenough A, et al: Synchronized mechanical ventilation for respiratory support in newborn infants. Cochrane Database Syst Rev CD000456, 2001.
26. Yoder BA, et al: High-frequency oscillatory ventilation: effects on lung function, mechanics, and airway cytokines in the immature baboon model for neonatal chronic lung disease. Am J Respir Crit Care Med *162*:1867, 2000.
27. Gerstmann DR, et al: The Provo multicenter early high-frequency oscillatory ventilation trial: improved pulmonary and clinical outcome in respiratory distress syndrome. Pediatrics *98*:1044, 1996.
28. Keszler M, et al: Multicenter controlled clinical trial of high-frequency jet ventilation in preterm infants with uncomplicated respiratory distress syndrome. Pediatrics *100*:593, 1997.
29. Plavka R, et al: A prospective randomized comparison of conventional mechanical ventilation and very early high frequency oscillatory ventilation in extremely premature newborns with respiratory distress syndrome. Intensive Care Med *25*:68, 1999.
30. Rettwitz-Volk W, et al: A prospective, randomized, multicenter trial of high-frequency oscillatory ventilation compared with conventional ventilation in preterm infants with respiratory distress syndrome receiving surfactant. J Pediatr *132*:249, 1998.
31. Thome U, et al: Randomized comparison of high-frequency ventilation with high-rate intermittent positive pressure ventilation in preterm infants with respiratory failure. J Pediatr *135*:39, 1999.
32. Thome U, et al: Comparison of pulmonary inflammatory mediators in preterm infants treated with intermittent positive pressure ventilation or high frequency oscillatory ventilation. Pediatr Res *44*:330, 1998.
33. Thome UH, Carlo WA: High-frequency ventilation in neonates. Am J Perinatol *17*:1, 2000.
34. Henderson-Smart DJ, et al: Elective high frequency oscillatory ventilation versus conventional ventilation for acute pulmonary dysfunction in preterm infants. Cochrane Database Syst Rev CD000104, 2001.
35. Lindner W, et al: Delivery room management of extremely low birth weight infants: spontaneous breathing or intubation? Pediatrics *103*:961, 1999.
36. Bell EF, Acarregui MJ: Restricted versus liberal water intake for preventing morbidity and mortality in preterm infants. Cochrane Database Syst Rev CD000503, 2001.
37. Stoll BJ, et al: Late-onset sepsis in very low birth weight neonates: a report from the National Institute of Child Health and Human Development Neonatal Research Network. J Pediatr *129*:63, 1996.
38. Fanaroff AA, et al: Incidence, presenting features, risk factors and significance of late onset septicemia in very low birth weight infants: the National Institute of Child Health and Human Development Neonatal Research Network. Pediatr Infect Dis J *17*:593, 1998.
39. Wang EE, et al: Role of *Ureaplasma urealyticum* and other pathogens in the development of chronic lung disease of prematurity. Pediatr Infect Dis J 7:547, 1988.
40. Cassell GH, et al: Does *Ureaplasma urealyticum* cause respiratory disease in newborns? Pediatr Infect Dis J 7:535, 1988.
41. Sanchez PJ, Regan JA: *Ureaplasma urealyticum* colonization and chronic lung disease in low birth weight infants. Pediatr Infect Dis J 7:542, 1988.
42. Horowitz S, et al: Respiratory tract colonization with *Ureaplasma urealyticum* and bronchopulmonary dysplasia in neonates in southern Israel. Pediatr Infect Dis J *11*:847, 1992.
43. Kruger T, Baier J: Induction of neutrophil chemoattractant cytokines by *Mycoplasma hominis* in alveolar type II cells. Infect Immun *65*:5131, 1997.
44. Manimtim WM, et al: *Ureaplasma urealyticum* modulates endotoxin-induced cytokine release by human monocytes derived from preterm and term newborns and adults. Infect Immun *69*:3906, 2001.
45. Ghezzi F, et al: Elevated interleukin-8 concentrations in amniotic fluid of mothers whose neonates subsequently develop bronchopulmonary dysplasia. Eur J Obstet Gynecol Reprod Biol *78*:5, 1998.
46. Stancombe BB, et al: Induction of human neonatal pulmonary fibroblast cytokines by hyperoxia and *Ureaplasma urealyticum*. Clin Infect Dis *17*:S154, 1993.
47. Baier RJ, et al: Monocyte chemoattractant protein-1 and interleukin-8 are increased in bronchopulmonary dysplasia: relation to isolation of *Ureaplasma urealyticum*. J Invest Med *49*:362, 2001.
48. Lyon AJ, et al: Randomised trial of erythromycin on the development of chronic lung disease in preterm infants. Arch Dis Child *78*:F10, 1998.
49. Buhrer C, et al: Role of erythromycin for treatment of incipient chronic lung disease in preterm infants colonised with *Ureaplasma urealyticum*. Drugs *61*:1893, 2001.
50. Agarwal P, et al: *Ureaplasma urealyticum* and its association with chronic lung disease in Asian neonates. J Paediatr Child Health *36*:487, 2000.
51. Heggie AD, et al: Identification and quantification of ureaplasmas colonizing the respiratory tract and assessment of their role in the development of chronic lung disease in preterm infants. Pediatr Infect Dis J *20*:854, 2001.

52. Viscardi RM, et al: Lung pathology in premature infants with *Ureaplasma urealyticum* infection. Pediatr Dev Pathol 5:141, 2002.
53. Da Silva O, et al: Role of *Ureaplasma urealyticum* and *Chlamydia trachomatis* in development of bronchopulmonary dysplasia in very low birth weight infants. Pediatr Infect Dis J 16:364, 1997.
54. Nelson S, et al: Detection of *Ureaplasma urealyticum* in endotracheal tube aspirates from neonates by PCR. J Clin Microbiol 36:1236, 1998.
55. Rojas MA, et al: Changing trends in the epidemiology and pathogenesis of neonatal chronic lung disease. J Pediatr 126:605, 1995.
56. Gonzalez A, et al: Influence of infection on patent ductus arteriosus and chronic lung disease in premature infants weighing 1000 grams or less. J Pediatr 128:470, 1996.
57. de Beaufort AJ, et al: Effect of interleukin 8 in meconium on in-vitro neutrophil chemotaxis. Lancet 352:102, 1998.
58. Yamada T, et al: Meconium-stained amniotic fluid exhibits chemotactic activity for polymorphonuclear leukocytes in vitro. J Reprod Immunol 46:21, 2000.
59. Yamada T, et al: Chemotactic activity for polymorphonuclear leukocytes: meconium versus meconium-stained amniotic fluid. Am J Reprod Immunol 44:275, 2000.
60. Moses D, et al: Inhibition of pulmonary surfactant function by meconium. Am J Obstet Gynecol 164:477, 1991.
61. Auten RL, et al: Surfactant treatment of full-term newborns with respiratory failure. Pediatrics 87:101, 1991.
62. Findlay RD, et al: Surfactant replacement therapy for meconium aspiration syndrome. Pediatrics 97:48, 1996.
63. Lotze A, et al: Multicenter study of surfactant (Beractant) use in the treatment of term infants with severe respiratory failure: Survanta in Term Infants Study Group. J Pediatr 132:40, 1998.
64. Newnham JP, et al: The fetal maturational and inflammatory responses to different routes of endotoxin infusion in sheep. Am J Obstet Gynecol 186:1062, 2002.
65. Thomas L: The Lives of a Cell: Notes of a Biology Watcher. New York, Viking Press, 1974.
66. Watford WT, et al: Complement-mediated host defense in the lung. Am J Physiol 279:L790, 2000.
67. Jackson JC, et al: Sequence of inflammatory cell migration into lung during recovery from hyaline membrane disease in premature newborn monkeys. Am Rev Respir Dis 135:937, 1987.
68. Sherman M, Truog WE: Macrophages. *In* Bland RD, Coalson JJ (eds): Chronic Lung Disease in Early Infancy, Vol 137. New York, Marcel Dekker, 2000, p 1062.
69. Standiford TJ, et al: Alveolar macrophage-derived cytokines induce monocyte chemoattractant protein-1 expression from human pulmonary type II–like epithelial cells. J Biol Chem 266:9912, 1991.
70. D'Angio CT, et al: Chemokine mRNA alterations in newborn and adult mouse lung during acute hyperoxia. Exp Lung Res 24:685, 1998.
71. Kotecha S, et al: Increase in interleukin-8 and soluble intercellular adhesion molecule-1 in bronchoalveolar lavage fluid from premature infants who develop chronic lung disease. Arch Dis Child 72:F90, 1995.
72. Kotecha S, et al: Increase in interleukin (IL)-1 beta and IL-6 in bronchoalveolar lavage fluid obtained from infants with chronic lung disease of prematurity. Pediatr Res 40:250, 1996.
73. Kotecha S, et al: Increase in the concentration of transforming growth factor beta-1 in bronchoalveolar lavage fluid before development of chronic lung disease of prematurity. J Pediatr 128:464, 1996.
74. Barker DJ, et al: Weight in infancy and death from ischaemic heart disease. Lancet 2:577, 1989.
75. Auten RL, et al: Nonpeptide CXCR2 antagonist prevents neutrophil accumulation in hyperoxia-exposed newborn rats. J Pharmacol Exp Ther 299:90, 2001.
76. Jones CA, et al: Undetectable interleukin (IL)-10 and persistent IL-8 expression early in hyaline membrane disease: a possible developmental basis for the predisposition to chronic lung inflammation in preterm newborns. Pediatr Res 39:966, 1996.
77. O'Reilly MA: DNA damage and cell cycle checkpoints in hyperoxic lung injury: braking to facilitate repair. Am J Physiol 281:L291, 2001.
78. Serrao KL, et al: Neutrophils induce apoptosis of lung epithelial cells via release of soluble Fas ligand. Am J Physiol 280:L298, 2001.
79. Matute-Bello G, et al: Recombinant human Fas ligand induces alveolar epithelial cell apoptosis and lung injury in rabbits. Am J Physiol 281:L328, 2001.
80. Schleimer RP, et al: An assessment of the effects of glucocorticoids on degranulation, chemotaxis, binding to vascular endothelium and formation of leukotriene B4 by purified human neutrophils. J Pharmacol Exp Ther 250:598, 1989.
81. Barrington KJ: The adverse neuro-developmental effects of postnatal steroids in the preterm infant: a systematic review of RCTs. BMC Pediatr 1:1, 2001.
82. Murphy BP, et al: Impaired cerebral cortical gray matter growth after treatment with dexamethasone for neonatal chronic lung disease. Pediatrics 107:217, 2001.
83. Barrington KJ: Postnatal steroids and neurodevelopmental outcomes: a problem in the making. Pediatrics 107:1425, 2001.
84. Committee on Fetus and Newborn: Postnatal corticosteroids to treat or prevent chronic lung disease in preterm infants. Pediatrics 109:330, 2002.
85. Viscardi RM, et al: Cromolyn sodium prophylaxis inhibits pulmonary proinflammatory cytokines in infants at high risk for bronchopulmonary dysplasia. Am J Respir Crit Care Med 156:1523, 1997.
86. Manji JS, et al: Timing of hyperoxic exposure during alveolarization influences damage mediated by leukotrienes. Am J Physiol 281:L799, 2001.
87. Boros V, et al: Leukotrienes are indicated as mediators of hyperoxia-inhibited alveolarization in newborn rats. Am J Physiol 272:L433, 1997.
88. Kotecha S: Cytokines in chronic lung disease of prematurity. Eur J Pediatr 155(Suppl 2):S14, 1996.
89. Deng H, et al: Lung inflammation in hyperoxia can be prevented by antichemokine treatment in newborn rats. Am J Respir Crit Care Med 162:2316, 2000.
90. Auten RL Jr, et al: Anti-neutrophil chemokine preserves alveolar development in hyperoxia-exposed newborn rats. Am J Physiol 281:L336, 2001.
91. Auten RL, et al: Blocking neutrophil influx reduces DNA damage in hyperoxia-exposed newborn rat lung. Am J Respir Cell Mol Biol 26:391, 2002.
92. Strieter RM, et al: Chemokines in lung injury: Thomas A. Neff Lecture. Chest 116:103S, 1999.
93. Vozzelli M, et al: Monocyte chemoattractant protein-1 mediates hyperoxia induced macrophage accumulation in newborn rat lung. Pediatr Res 47:379A, 2000.
94. Watterberg KL, et al: Secretory leukocyte protease inhibitor and lung inflammation in developing bronchopulmonary dysplasia. J Pediatr 125:264, 1994.
95. Sluis KB, et al: Proteinase-antiproteinase balance in tracheal aspirates from neonates. Eur Respir J 7:251, 1994.
96. Ohlsson K, et al: Protease inhibitors in bronchoalveolar lavage fluid from neonates with special reference to secretory leukocyte protease inhibitor. Acta Paediatr 81:757, 1992.
97. Wallaert B, et al: Activated alveolar macrophages in subclinical pulmonary inflammation in collagen vascular diseases. Thorax 43:24, 1988.
98. Shock A, Laurent GJ: Adhesive interactions between fibroblasts and polymorphonuclear neutrophils in vitro. Eur J Cell Biol 54:211, 1991.
99. Frank L, Sosenko IR: Failure of premature rabbits to increase antioxidant enzymes during hyperoxic exposure: increased susceptibility to pulmonary oxygen toxicity compared with term rabbits. Pediatr Res 29:292, 1991.
100. Chen Y, Frank L: Differential gene expression of antioxidant enzymes in the perinatal rat lung. Pediatr Res 34:27, 1993.
101. Smith CV, Welty SB: Mechanisms of oxygen-induced lung injury. *In* Bland RD, Coalson JJ (eds): Chronic Lung Disease in Early Infancy, Vol 137. New York, Marcel Dekker, 2000, pp 749–777.
102. Varsila E, et al: Early protein oxidation in the neonatal lung is related to development of chronic lung disease. Acta Paediatr 84:1296, 1995.
103. McCord JM: Iron, free radicals, and oxidative injury. Semin Hematol 35:5, 1998.
104. Zhao G, et al: Role of iron in ischemia-reperfusion oxidative injury of rat lungs. Am J Respir Cell Mol Biol 16:293, 1997.
105. Cooke RW, et al: Blood transfusion and chronic lung disease in preterm infants. Eur J Pediatr 156:47, 1997.
106. Silvers KM, et al: Antioxidant activity, packed cell transfusions, and outcome in premature infants. Arch Dis Child 78:F214, 1998.
107. Bany-Mohammed FM, et al: Recombinant human erythropoietin: possible role as an antioxidant in premature rabbits. Pediatr Res 40:381, 1996.
108. Frank L, Sosenko IR: Oxidants and antioxidants: what role do they play in chronic lung disease? *In* Bland RD, Coalson J (eds): Chronic Lung Disease in Early Infancy, Vol 137. New York, Marcel Dekker, 2000, pp 257–284.
109. Jankov RP, et al: Antioxidants as therapy in the newborn: some words of caution. Pediatr Res 50:681, 2001.
110. Luo X, et al: Effect of the 21-aminosteroid U74389G on oxygen-induced free radical production, lipid peroxidation, and inhibition of lung growth in neonatal rats. Pediatr Res 46:215, 1999.
111. Sundaresan M, et al: Requirement for generation of H_2O_2 for platelet-derived growth factor signal transduction. Science 270:296, 1995.
112. Chiba Y, et al: Activation of rho is involved in the mechanism of hydrogen-peroxide–induced lung edema in isolated perfused rabbit lung. Microvasc Res 62:164, 2001.
113. Roberts ML, Cowsert LM: Interleukin-1 beta and reactive oxygen species mediate activation of c-Jun NH2-terminal kinases, in human epithelial cells, by two independent pathways. Biochem Biophys Res Commun 251:166, 1998.

Kurt H. Albertine and Theodore J. Pysher

93 Impaired Lung Growth After Injury in Premature Lung

Premature birth is any delivery, regardless of birth weight, that occurs before 37 completed weeks from the first day of the last menstrual cycle (term is 40 weeks in humans).[1] Gestational age is dated from the first day of the last menstrual cycle. Gestational age is about 2 weeks more than developmental age, which is dated from conception. Pregnancies that end prior to 20 to 22 completed weeks of gestation are termed *abortions*. A reasonable definition of premature birth, therefore, is any delivery that occurs between 20 and 37 weeks of gestation. In the United States and Canada, the overall rate of prematurity is approximately 10%,[2, 3] despite the extensive use of tocolytic agents to arrest premature labor.[4-6]

Premature infants who are born as early as 22 weeks gestational age may survive if supported by intensive medical care, important components of which are antenatal steroids and postnatal surfactant replacement, mechanical ventilation, and supplemental oxygen. These therapies and others are required because the gas-exchange regions of the lungs of the prematurely born infant are not structurally or functionally developed to support extrauterine life. The goal of this chapter is to describe the impact of premature birth on lung growth, with emphasis on alveolar formation.

LUNG STRUCTURE OF THE DISTAL LUNG IN THE CONTEXT OF THE LUNG'S PRINCIPAL FUNCTION

Exchange of oxygen and carbon dioxide in the mature lung occurs in relatively large units that are referred to as terminal respiratory units. These units consist of alveolar ducts, together with their accompanying alveoli, that stem from a respiratory bronchiole.[7] In the adult human lung, such units contain approximately 100 alveolar ducts and 2000 anatomic alveoli and are approximately 5 mm in diameter, with a volume of about 0.02 mL at functional residual capacity. Together, the two lungs of the adult human contain about 150,000 terminal respiratory units.[8] Their function is such that diffusion of oxygen and carbon dioxide in

the gas phase is so rapid that the partial pressures of each gas are uniform throughout the unit. From each inspired breath, oxygen that reaches the alveolar duct gas diffuses into all the associated alveoli because the incoming air has a higher oxygen concentration than that of the alveolar gas. Oxygen subsequently diffuses through the air-blood barrier into red blood cells, where it combines with hemoglobin as the red blood cells flow along the capillaries. Carbon dioxide diffuses in the opposite direction.

In the normal adult human lung, the air-blood barrier is exceedingly thin, about 1.5 μm, which facilitates gas diffusion through the barrier.[8, 9] For oxygen, the air-blood barrier's structural components are, in order, alveolar epithelium and its subjacent basal lamina, alveolar wall interstitium, basal lamina of the capillary endothelium, capillary endothelium, plasma, membrane of red blood cells, and, finally, hemoglobin molecules. For carbon dioxide, the obstacles to diffusion are encountered in the opposite sequence.

STRUCTURE OF THE PREMATURE LUNG

The terminal respiratory units of the prematurely born infant are incompletely developed, and the air-blood barrier is too thick to allow efficient exchange of oxygen and carbon dioxide. This structural problem is greater with more immature premature infants because the development of the terminal respiratory units occurs during the second half of gestation and the thickness of the air-blood barrier is inversely related to gestational age. A brief review of the stages of lung development for humans illustrates these points (Fig. 93-1).[10]

Branching of the bronchial tree and major pulmonary vessels is complete by 16 weeks' gestation in humans. Prior to 17 weeks of gestation, the future bronchi and bronchioles extend into a core of relatively undifferentiated mesenchyme that contains few blood vessels (see Fig. 93-1*a*). This period of lung development is called the pseudoglandular stage. From week 17 to week 28 of gestation, the human fetal lung is at the canalicular stage.

Figure 93–1. Comparison of normal lung histology during development in humans with lung histopathology associated with acute lung injury or chronic lung disease of prematurity. See also color plate section. **Panels a through d**: Ontogeny (H & E stain). All the lungs were fixed at low lung volume at autopsy. *Panel a*: Infant stillborn at 12 to 14 weeks' gestation. Considerable autolysis (postmortem degeneration) is evident; airways (*AW*) are lined by columnar epithelium that is largely desquamated. There is no development in the intervening mesenchyme (*M*), which is devoid of blood vessels. *Panel b*: Infant stillborn at 20 weeks' gestation. Smooth-walled respiratory bronchioles and alveolar ducts lined by low cuboidal epithelium (*arrow*) are visible beyond the larger AW. Numerous capillaries (*arrowhead*) are visible deep within the developing mesenchyme. *Panel c*: Infant stillborn at 29 weeks' gestation. The distal air spaces are subdivided by many capillaries (*arrowhead*), which are present in the thick primary septum (*arrow*). An AW is visible. *Panel d*: Infant stillborn at 40 weeks' gestation (term). Alveolar development has progressed to thinner primary septa and secondary septa (crests; *arrow*) protrude into the developing alveoli. The alveolar walls have numerous capillaries. **Panels e and f**: Hyaline membrane disease (HMD) (H & E stain). *Panel e*: Birth at 25 weeks' gestation, followed by 6 hours of mechanical ventilation. In the first few hours of life, the premature, mechanically ventilated lung shows uneven expansion of the distal air spaces, vascular congestion, and interstitial edema. Hyaline membranes (*arrowhead*) are uniformly present. Some patchy hemorrhage also may be present. *Panel f*: HMD, birth at 29 weeks' gestation, followed by 2 days of mechanical ventilation. The distribution of ventilation is uneven, with centriacinar expansion and peripheral collapse. **Panels g and h**: Chronic lung disease (CLD). *Panel g*: Birth at 22 weeks' gestation, followed by 44 days of mechanical ventilation (28 to 29 weeks postconceptual age) (Masson's trichrome stain). In this specimen, the distal air spaces appear filled with cellular debris (∗). Thick, cellular M separates the adjacent air spaces. *Panel h*: Birth at 24 weeks' gestation, followed by 151 days of mechanical ventilation (45 weeks' postconceptual age) (H & E stain). Simplification and overdistention of the distal air spaces is clearly evident. Primary septa are thick and cellular. Secondary septa (crests; *arrow*) are infrequently visible; visible ones are short, thick, and devoid of capillaries near their tip. *Panels a through g* are the same magnification: scale bar, 100 μm. *Panel h* scale bar is 50 μm in length). AW = airways; M = mesenchyme; PA = pulmonary artery.

Ontogeny   ## Lung Injury

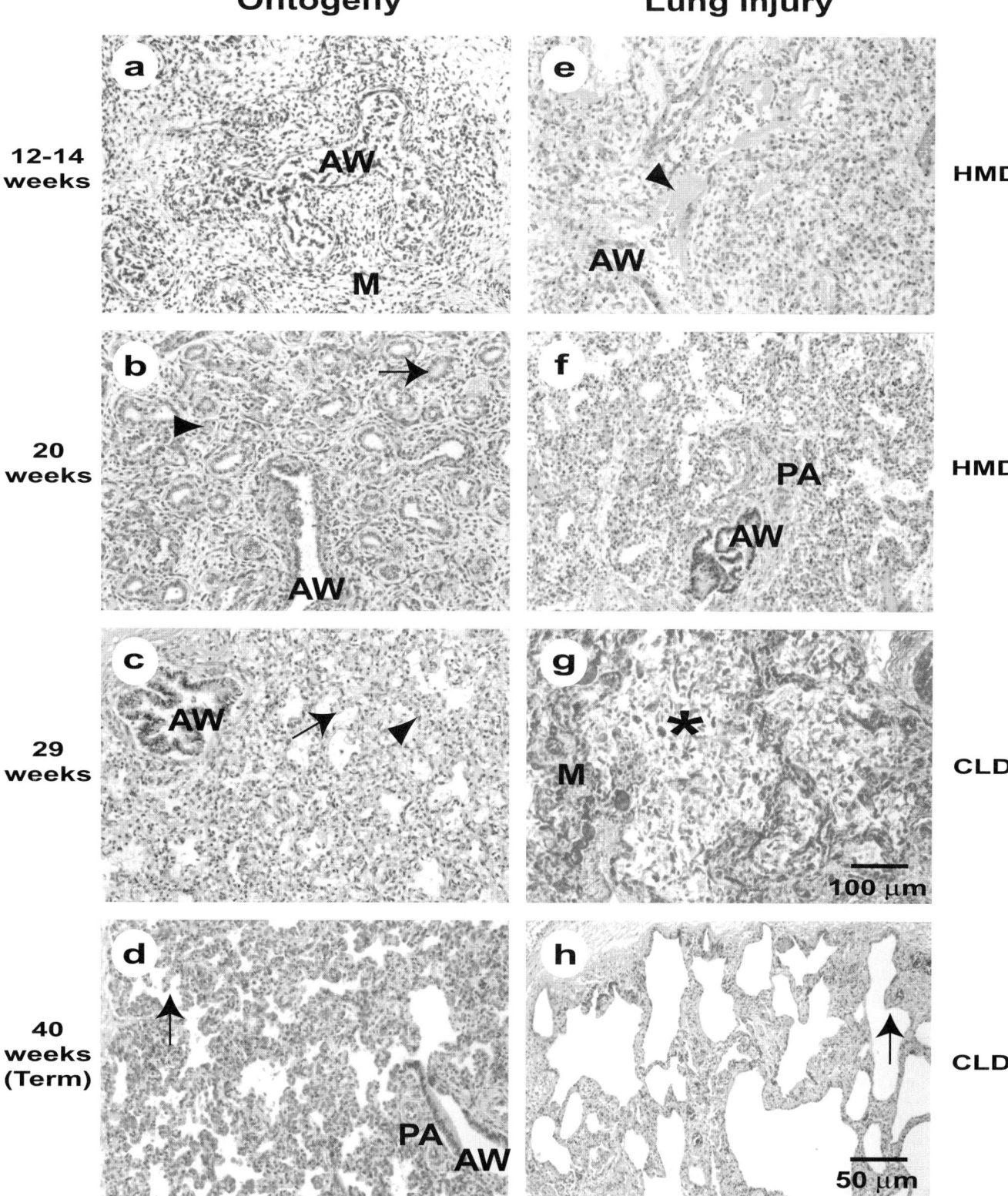

12-14
weeks

20
weeks

29
weeks

40
weeks
(Term)

HMD

HMD

CLD

CLD

Lung architecture at this stage is characterized by more elongated profiles of the distalmost airways and proliferation of capillaries. Although capillary proliferation is robust, the developing capillaries are distant from the distal airways (see Fig. 93-1b). During this period, the cells lining the distalmost airways become cuboidal and show ultrastructural evidence of differentiation toward alveolar Type II epithelial cells in the form of osmiophilic lamellar bodies.[11] Arising from cuboidal epithelial cells are alveolar Type I (squamous) epithelial cells. These terminally differentiated cells, although fewer in number than their cuboidal counterpart, cover about 90% to 95% of the alveolar surface area of the peripheral lung in the adult.[12] Both structural attributes of alveolar Type I epithelial cells provide a large, thin cellular barrier specialized for gas exchange.

From about weeks 24 to 36 of gestation, lung development is at the saccular stage. During this stage, the initially cylindrical distalmost airways become divided by primary septa into which capillaries extend, resulting in more numerous and thinner air-blood interfaces. Continual growth results in further thinning of the mesenchyme. The result of these structural changes is a marked increase in the potential gas-exchange surface of the lung. From about 32 weeks of gestation and continuing through the first 18 to 24 months of postnatal life, alveoli are formed by progressive expansion and subdivision of the terminal air sacs (see Fig. 93-1c). Subdivision occurs during the process of secondary septation (also called secondary crest formation). During the alveolar stage, the air-blood barrier attains its adult thinness by further reduction of the connective tissue compartment in the developing alveolar walls and juxtaposition of the alveolar walls and alveolar capillaries.

Alveolar Type II epithelial cells, and the surfactant phospholipids and apoproteins that they synthesize, secrete, and recycle, are essential for normal lung function. In the human lung, Type II cells that contain lamellar bodies are histologically recognizable at the transition from the canalicular to the saccular stages of lung development (weeks 20 to 24 of gestation). Surfactant synthesis normally begins later, during the saccular stage (about 30 weeks of gestation)[13] but can be induced earlier, as discussed later. From the saccular stage to the end of term gestation, the concentrations of dipalmitoyl phosphatidylcholine and other surfactant phospholipids increase in lung tissue, lung lavage liquid, and amniotic liquid. Surfactant apoproteins (SP) A, B, and C, expressed only in lung tissue, also are developmentally regulated but not concordantly. Human SP-A mRNA and protein in lung tissue are not detectable until the saccular stage of lung development (about 30 weeks' gestation).[13-16] Human SP-B and SP-C mRNAs are detectable in lung tissue at very low levels earlier than are SP-A, during the canalicular stage (about 24 weeks' gestation).[17] Detection of SP-B and SP-C proteins, however, occurs later in development, during the saccular stage (about 30 weeks' gestation).[15] To our knowledge, human SP-D protein has been detected only in amniotic liquid during the saccular stage of lung development (about 24 weeks' gestation).[18,19] Thus, the cellular and biochemical machinery to reduce surface tension at air-liquid interfaces in the future air spaces develops during the third trimester in humans. Many premature infants are born before the third trimester and therefore are at risk for respiratory failure because their lungs are deficient in surfactant. To assess lung development prior to birth, one measures these secretory products in amniotic liquid.[20]

Another impediment to gas diffusion in the lungs of premature infants is the presence of liquid in the interstitium and potential air spaces. Fluid is an impediment, because diffusion is much faster in the gas phase than in water. For example, the solubility of oxygen in water is low (0.03 mL/L × mm Hg P_aO_2) compared with carbon dioxide, the solubility of which is about 20 times more than oxygen (0.7 mL/L × mm Hg P_aCO_2). The advantage for carbon dioxide persists even though the driving pressure for carbon dioxide diffusion is only one tenth that for oxygen entering the blood. Therefore, oxygen diffusion is much slower in the relatively overhydrated environment of the premature lung.

Normal intrauterine lung growth requires appropriate distention by lung luminal liquid.[21] The fetal lungs are filled with liquid that flows from the pulmonary vascular compartment, through the interstitium, to the potential air spaces. Liquid flows from the interstitium into the fetal potential air spaces because chloride is secreted across the fetal respiratory epithelium into the potential air spaces,[22] causing an osmotic concentration gradient that promotes the flow of water. Lung luminal liquid is propelled centrally along the conducting airways to the oropharynx, where the liquid is either swallowed or expelled into the amniotic sac. Balance between adequate production of lung luminal liquid and its drainage is required for normal intrauterine lung growth.[21] When drainage exceeds production, the fetal lung is not exposed to continuous liquid distending pressure, so lung growth is inhibited. This occurs, for example, in fetuses with oligohydramnios due to prolonged rupture of amniotic membranes.[23] Other conditions that disturb lung growth include diaphragmatic hernia[24] or such conditions that result in a mass effect compressing the developing lung, or pulmonary artery occlusion.[25] Near term birth, the secretory activity of the respiratory epithelium switches from a predominantly chloride-secreting membrane to a predominantly sodium-absorbing membrane.[26-28] This molecular switch reverses water movement, thereby drying the potential air spaces for gaseous diffusion.

Structural and functional characteristics of the airways also may be affected by premature birth. During the canalicular and saccular stages of lung development, the airways have little smooth muscle in their wall, the epithelium is immature, and cell-cell adhesion is weak. Physiologic studies of human tracheobronchial segments ex vivo indicate that pressure-volume relations are affected by maturity,[29,30] so that airway compliance is inversely related to maturity. The reduced compliance of the airways of premature infants may explain the need for higher airway pressures, while increased volume is needed to inflate the collapsed gas exchange regions compared with the airways of term infants.[31] The dearth of smooth muscle and weak adhesion between cells of the immature airway increases the susceptibility to injury by the increased pressures and volumes that are required to effect ventilation. Injury is manifested by reactive and metaplastic airway epithelial cells in tracheal aspirates and lung lavage liquid, as well as development of air leaks (interstitial emphysema and pneumothorax).

ACUTE LUNG INJURY OF PREMATURITY (RESPIRATORY DISTRESS SYNDROME)

When an infant is born prematurely, the structurally immature lungs are deficient in surfactant. Therefore, surface tension forces are high, and the alveoli are unstable,[32] which results in alveolar collapse (atelectasis), causing ventilation-perfusion mismatch. Such mismatch results, in turn, in intrapulmonary shunting and thus contributes to poor oxygenation.[33] Opening the collapsed air spaces requires high ventilatory pressures that are transmitted to the immature distal airways and gas exchange regions of the lung. In effect, the extreme effort required to expand the lungs with the first breath must be repeated with each breath because surfactant is not present to prevent collapse of the distal air spaces. Prematurely born infants who have these characteristics tire quickly and develop respiratory distress syndrome (RDS).

RDS affects about 30,000 infants annually in the United States. The incidence is about 50% to 60% of infants who are born before 30 weeks' gestation[34] and increases with decreasing gestational age.[35-37] RDS is more prevalent and severe in male compared with female premature infants, for unclear reasons.

Because RDS is a predictable consequence of lung immaturity, strategies have been developed to accelerate lung development before premature delivery. Administration of hormones, such as glucocorticoids,[38-41] is one. The seminal studies of Liggins and colleagues demonstrated that glucocorticoids accelerated lung maturation of fetal sheep and decreased the incidence of RDS in human infants after antenatal corticosteroid therapy.[42, 43] The maturational effect of corticosteroid treatment on lung structure was first described by Kikkawa and colleagues.[44] Corticosteroids (betamethasone or dexamethasone) accelerate maturation of alveolar Type II epithelial cells, which are the source of pulmonary surfactant. For these reasons, mothers in premature labor who are at risk of giving birth to a premature infant between 24 and 35 weeks' gestation are treated antenatally with glucocorticoids.[45]

A treatment strategy to reduce lung stiffness (increase lung compliance) after premature birth is to instill surfactant into the airways.[46] Surfactant replacement therapy is beneficial because once it becomes widely and thinly distributed in the lung, the exogenous surfactant reduces surface tension at air-liquid interfaces, thereby stabilizing alveoli when they are deflated. After surfactant replacement, oxygenation improves swiftly, followed for several hours by progressive improvement in gas exchange and lung mechanics.[47-49] Other improvements, at least in premature lambs, are reduced vascular injury and edema.[50] Thus, surfactant replacement therapy reduces the incidence and severity of RDS following premature birth. Instilled surfactant is not recycled as efficiently as native surfactant, but by reducing the lung injury associated with RDS, this therapy improves the opportunity for the premature lung to repair and grow.

The pathologic findings in RDS are similar to those of adults with acute respiratory distress syndrome (ARDS),[51] superimposed on the immature lung.[52] Lesions in the lungs reflect both the disease and its treatment with mechanical ventilation and supplemental oxygen. Within the first 3 to 4 hours, the lungs may show only uneven ventilation of distal air spaces resulting from surfactant deficiency, interstitial edema resulting from incomplete removal of fetal lung liquid, or acute injury to microvascular endothelial cells, and congestion of capillaries (see Fig. 93-1d). By 12 to 24 hours, necrosis of alveolar and bronchiolar epithelial cells develops and the denuded walls become coated by characteristic hyaline membranes, which are brightly eosinophilic transudates of plasma proteins admixed with necrotic epithelial cells and fibrin (see Fig. 93-1e).[53] Hyaline membranes accumulate especially at branch points. These pathologic features are similar to the exudative phase of ARDS in adults, but the alveolar Type II epithelial cell hyperplasia that constitutes the proliferative phase of ARDS in adults, as seen in autopsy slides, is not as prominent in hyaline membrane disease seen in autopsy slides in premature infants.

Mechanical ventilation of premature infants can result in ventilator-induced lung injury,[54] even following repeated doses of exogenous surfactant. The injurious effects of mechanical ventilation depend on a number of factors, among which are the magnitude of airway pressure (barotrauma) and lung volume (volutrauma)[55, 56] and the concentration of inspired oxygen (oxygen toxicity). Several experimental animal studies have compared indices of ventilator-induced lung injury between conditions that raised airway pressure and increased lung volume.[57-59] These studies suggest that large lung volumes, rather than high peak airway pressures, are the cause of ventilator-induced lung injury. For this reason, volutrauma is used to describe the injury that is associated with mechanical ventilation.

How does volutrauma induce lung injury, especially following premature birth? Evidence suggests that some of the circumstances just described are exacerbated. For example, regional overinflation increases microvascular permeability, either directly or indirectly (through release of inflammatory mediators from

sequestered leukocytes in the lung), which leads to alveolar flooding. Alveolar flooding, in turn, is associated with inactivation of surfactant, which in turn leads to atelectasis and less compliant lungs. If these cycles are not broken, lung injury recurs, necessitating higher airway pressure, larger tidal volume, and more supplemental oxygen. As the extent and duration of mechanical ventilation with supplemental oxygen increases, and lung volutrauma persists or increases, acute lung injury may progress to chronic lung disease.

CHRONIC LUNG DISEASE OF PREMATURITY

Survival of prematurely born infants with RDS has significantly increased since the introduction of antenatal steroid and postnatal surfactant replacement therapies and gentler ventilation strategies.[36, 60-62] As described earlier, 84% of premature infants weighing 500 to 1500 g at birth now survive. Unfortunately, about 8000 to 10,000 premature infants who develop RDS in the United States annually, and who receive antenatal glucocorticoids and postnatal surfactant replacement, go on to develop chronic lung disease (CLD) of prematurity (also called bronchopulmonary dysplasia or BPD). The reported incidence of CLD ranges between 15% and 60% of premature infants.[63-65] As expected, smaller infants are at greater risk than larger premature infants. After adjusting for a number of risk factors, development of CLD is associated most with need for high inspired oxygen 96 hours after birth, high peak inspiratory pressure, and high fluid intake.

The original description of BPD was made by Northway and colleagues.[66] The principal clinical criteria were the requirement for supplemental oxygen for at least 28 days after birth (a duration selected because it was a month; Northway, personal communication). The major radiologic criteria were cyst formation and hyperexpansion mixed with atelectasis. The characteristic pathologic findings at autopsy depended upon the duration of disease prior to death. Classic hyaline membrane disease was seen in the first 2 to 3 days. A regenerative phase was seen over the next week that consisted of necrosis and regeneration of bronchiolar and alveolar epithelium, in addition to hyaline membranes. Over the next 10 days, hyperplasia of bronchiolar and arteriolar smooth muscle, fibrosis, and dilated or collapsed distal air sacs ensued. In the final stage, these alternating areas of overdistention and atelectasis became fixed. The term *bronchopulmonary* was chosen because it identified airway and blood vessel involvement; *dysplasia* was chosen because it described the failure of the distal air sacs to develop into normal anatomic alveoli (Northway; personal communication). Today, CLD is usually defined clinically as either oxygen dependency at 28 days of life with appropriate radiologic findings or oxygen dependency at 36 weeks postconceptional age.[67,68]

BPD originally described by Northway and colleagues was diagnosed in premature infants who did not recover from RDS. However, treatment of respiratory failure from other causes, including meconium aspiration pneumonia,[69] neonatal pneumonia,[70] congestive heart failure,[71] or congenital diaphragmatic hernia,[72] may be associated with CLD.

Prematurely born infants who develop CLD today are much younger (23 to 26 weeks of gestation) and smaller (< 1000 g) than those who developed BPD over 30 years ago (31 to 34 weeks of gestation and ~2000 g at birth), and the radiologic and pathologic features of their lung disease are less severe. Today, the radiologic findings include lung hyperinflation, emphysema, and interstitial densities, and the principal autopsy pathologic findings are dilated and simplified distal air sacs[73,74] (see Fig. 93-1f and g). Usually missing are the pathologic changes in the central airways. Recognition of these distinctions between contemporary CLD and BPD that was described over 30 years ago has prompted clinicians and investigators to call today's CLD "new" BPD. Debate continues whether the disease that is seen today is "new" or a less severe variant of BPD.

IMPAIRED ALVEOLAR FORMATION AFTER INJURY IN PREMATURE LUNG

Simplification of distal air sacs is characteristic of the histopathology in premature lungs. Simplification is related to failure of alveolar secondary septa (crests) to sprout into the distal air sacs. The mechanisms that participate in normal or abnormal secondary septation of alveoli are not known and are a topic of intense investigation today.[67]

Alveolar formation is initiated near the end of the fetal period and continues postnatally after term gestation.[10,75-79] At term gestation, alveolar formation is less complete in humans, baboons, and mice[10,75-79] compared with sheep and other ruminants.[80-82]

Alveolar formation is structurally manifest by evagination of partitions along the smoothly curved saccular walls during late gestation and/or early postnatal life.[10] Regardless of the speed with which alveolar formation occurs among species, low ridges elongate into secondary septa. Capillary loops accompany these septal evaginations, resulting in a thin air-blood interface on either side of the septa and attenuation of the mesenchymal core through apoptosis.[83] These processes create an increased surface area of thin air-blood barriers that minimally impede the diffusion of oxygen and carbon dioxide.[84]

The late initiation of and prolonged period for alveolar formation have limited the success of knockout or transgenic mice as models to identify regulatory molecules during alveolar formation. Such approaches often affect the earliest stages profoundly and sometimes result in embryonic or fetal death before alveolar formation is initiated. An important exception is the platelet-derived growth factor (PDGF)-A-null mouse.[85] Some of the PDGF-A -/- mice survive through the postnatal period, but these mice lack both alveolar myofibroblasts and alveolar elastin. Their lungs have simplified distal air spaces. Another exception is the elastin null mouse.[86] These mice survive through the first several days of postnatal life, but the postnatal mice are cyanotic. Their lungs have reduced airway and vascular generations, and their distal air spaces are developmentally arrested at the saccular stage.

Because CLD occurs almost exclusively after premature birth and weeks of mechanical ventilation with supplemental oxygen, reproducing the human disease in animal models requires intensive, large-animal protocols. Coalson and coworkers developed a primate model that has the pathologic features of CLD, including alveolar simplification.[87-90] These investigators showed that early application of high-frequency ventilation may reduce the severity of the histopathologic changes[91-93] and speculated that hyperoxia and tidal ventilation of the premature lung leads to lung overstretch and release of inflammatory mediators that cause loss of alveoli and alveolar capillary surface area.[89,94] Bland and colleagues also developed a model of CLD, using preterm lambs.[95-98] Mechanical ventilation of preterm lambs for 3 to 4 weeks, using large tidal volume (15 mL/kg body wt), resulted in inhibition of alveolar formation and alveolar capillary growth, disruption of gas exchange, diminished numbers of microvessels, persistent muscularization of resistance arterioles, increased pulmonary vascular resistance, and decreased expression of endothelial nitric oxide synthase protein.[96-98] Management of premature lambs with high-frequency jet ventilation, on the other hand, was associated with improved structural formation of alveoli and alveolar capillary growth.[99]

A consequence of failed septation is reduced surface area for gas exchange, including the capillary surface area.[94,97] However, the latter observation in experimental animals with evolving CLD has not been confirmed in autopsy tissue from infants who died with established CLD.[100] One explanation for this discor-

dance is the time frame of the CLD. Experimental animal studies are relatively short (up to 4 weeks; evolving CLD), whereas premature infants with CLD may be managed with mechanical ventilation and supplemental oxygen for much longer periods (months; established CLD), suggesting that capillary proliferation may be an adaptive response to impaired septation in CLD.

Studies using premature lambs with evolving CLD also indicated that the tropoelastin gene is excessively and continuously up-regulated.[95] Up-regulation of tropoelastin gene expression occurred on the third day of continuous mechanical ventilation[101] and remained elevated for the 3- to 4-week studies. Although the results from the premature lambs with evolving CLD and elastin knockout mice[86] (described earlier) seem contradictory, they may suggest that tropoelastin gene expression must be tightly regulated for normal septation, and that too much or too little tropoelastin gene expression may impair normal septation.

Appropriate stretch of the developing lung appears to be of key importance for formation of normal alveoli. Overstretch leads to distortion of cells and extracellular matrix in the developing lung. The distortion may lead to the local synthesis and release of regulatory molecules that affect cellular division, phenotype, and metabolic activity. High lung inflation (overstretch), for example, increases mRNA levels for transforming growth factor (TGF)-β_1 fourfold and basic fibroblast growth factor (bFGF; or FGF2) by 60%, compared with low lung inflation in adult rabbits.[102] PDGF is involved in stretch-mediated signaling, and elastin is also a stretch-responsive gene. These data emphasize the importance of mechanical stretch in alveolar formation.

Among the mediators proposed to link overstretch and arrested alveolar formation are growth factors, cytokines, and matrix-degrading proteinases released by epithelial and mesenchymal cells, as well as resident and infiltrating inflammatory cells. For example, the developing lung has the ability to synthesize and release vascular endothelial growth factor (VEGF),[103] FGFs,[104] PDGFs,[105,106] TGFs,[107,108] insulin-like growth factors,[109,110] and epidermal growth factor (EGF),[111,112] as well as their receptors. Of these growth factors, VEGF[113-117] and related vascular growth signaling molecules,[118,119] FGF signaling,[120,121] and PDGF-A[85,106] are implicated in alveolar formation.

VEGF is a potent multifunctional cytokine and angiogenic factor. Its actions include stimulating angiogenesis by promoting proliferation of endothelial cells and pericytes, increasing endothelial cell permeability, inducing transient accumulation of endothelial cell cytoplasmic calcium, shape change, division and migration, and altering gene expression. In the lung, VEGF is prominently expressed by alveolar Type II cells and airway epithelial cells. The role of specific VEGF isoforms in pulmonary vascular growth appears to be spatially regulated because mice that express only VEGF 120 (and therefore do not express the heparan sulfate-binding VEGF164 and 188 isoforms) have normal pre-acinar pulmonary vessels and arrested formation of acinar microvessels.[122] Those mice also have delayed air space maturation and reduced numbers of air-blood barriers. Other signaling molecules also may participate in pulmonary vascular morphogenesis, such as Notch signaling.[119,123] However, information is limited.

In various cells, VEGF expression is regulated by other growth factors, such as TGF-β,[124] PDGF,[125] and dexamethasone.[103] The biologic function of VEGF in disease states may rely on altered amounts of VEGF protein, as well as altered VEGF receptor (VEGF-R) number and affinity. For example, hypoxia induces pulmonary production of VEGF and its receptor, VEGF-R2[103,126]; the converse is true for hyperoxia,[127] which is a risk factor for failed alveolar formation.[128,129] In this regard, disruption of pulmonary blood vessel formation in rats, by blocking binding of VEGF to its receptor, results in lung histopathologic changes that look like CLD.[113,114] Recovery of neonatal and adult rabbits from hyperoxia is associated with increased VEGF mRNA expression by alveolar epithelial cells.[127,130] These findings suggest a role for VEGF in regulating alveolar capillary proliferation normally and after oxidant injury; the latter plays a central role in the pathogenesis of CLD.

Deficiency of retinol or retinol-binding protein after premature birth may contribute to the development of CLD in neonates.[131-134] Clinical trials of retinol treatment of neonates at risk for CLD, however, have yielded conflicting results. In a randomized, double-blind controlled trial,[135] infants who received vitamin A had a significantly lower incidence of CLD and reduced need for supplemental O_2, mechanical ventilation, and intensive care. In a subsequent study, retinol supplementation had no effect on the incidence of CLD in preterm infants.[136] Recently, however, large multicenter studies of retinol versus placebo treatment of tiny preterm infants showed a small but significant reduction in the incidence of CLD among the retinol-treated infants.[137,138] Experimental animal studies have provided promising results in this regard. One study showed that retinoid signaling is required for alveolar formation.[139] Another study used pregnant rats repeatedly treated with dexamethasone to inhibit lung development *in utero*.[140] The newborn pups, treated with all-*trans*-retinoic acid postnatally, had greater alveolar formation than did untreated control rat pups. A third study showed that retinoids reversed steroid-induced suppression of lung growth and epithelial cell proliferation in cultured fetal rat lung.[141] A fourth study showed that retinoic acid treatment of adult rats with elastase-induced pulmonary emphysema was associated with reversal of emphysematous lesions.[142] Our initial studies using premature lambs with evolving CLD of prematurity have shown that daily treatment with vitamin A is associated with greater formation of alveoli and alveolar capillaries and increased expression of VEGF and VEGF-R2.[117] The molecular mechanism(s) by which vitamin A up-regulates expression of VEGF and VEGF-R2 are being investigated by our group.

SUMMARY

The structural and functional immaturity of the premature infant's lung necessitates use of antenatal steroids, perinatal surfactant replacement therapy, postnatal mechanical ventilation and oxygen supplementation, and other supportive measures. Acute lung injury often occurs as a result of lung immaturity and the therapy that it necessitates. If recovery does not ensue, the affected premature infants progress to CLD. Although CLD continues to be one of the most serious of pediatric public health issues, important progress has been made. For example, CLD of prematurity occurs infrequently today in the larger (≥ 2 kg) and more mature (≥ 32 weeks) premature infants, the population that Northway and colleagues described in the original paper on BPD.[66] Moreover, the severity of CLD is less today than it was 30 years ago. These encouraging changes reflect better understanding of lung developmental biology and improvements in clinical management of prematurely born infants. Nonetheless, challenges remain because the incidence of premature birth is increasing, the size of the premature infants that can be supported is much smaller, and the incidence of CLD among the smallest premature infants remains very high.

REFERENCES

1. American Academy of Pediatrics and the American College of Obstetricians and Gynecologists: Guidelines for Perinatal Care. Elk Grove Village, IL, 1997.
2. Advance Report on Final Natality Studies: Monthly Vital Statistics Report *40*:8, 1991.
3. Copper RL, et al: A multicenter study of preterm birth weight and gestational age-specific neonatal mortality. Am J Obstet Gynecol *168*:78, 1993.
4. Leveno KJ, et al: The national impact of ritodrine hydrochloride for inhibition of preterm labor. Obstet Gynecol *76*:12, 1990.
5. The Canadian Preterm Labor Investigators Group: Treatment of preterm labor with the beta-adrenergic agonist ritodrine. N Engl J Med *327*:308, 1992.
6. Goldenberg RL, et al: Prevention of premature birth. N Engl J Med *339*:313, 1998.
7. Hayek H: The Human Lung. New York, Hafner, 1960.
8. Weibel ER: Morphometry of the Lung. New York, Academic Press, 1963.
9. Crapo JD: Morphometric characteristics of cells in the alveolar region of mammalian lungs. Am Rev Respir Dis *128*:S42, 1983.
10. Burri PH: Structural aspects of prenatal and postnatal development and growth of the lung. In McDonald JA (ed): Lung Growth and Development. New York, Marcel Dekker, 1997, pp 1-35.
11. Albertine KH, et al: Anatomy of the lungs. In Murray JF, et al (eds): Textbook of Respiratory Medicine. Philadelphia, WB Saunders, 2000, pp 3-33.
12. Crapo JD, et al: Cell number and cell characteristics of the normal human lung. Am Rev Respir Dis *125*:332, 1982.
13. King RJ, et al: Appearance of apoproteins of pulmonary surfactant in human amniotic fluid. J Appl Physiol *39*:735, 1975.
14. Ballard PL, et al: Regulation of pulmonary surfactant apoprotein SP 28-36 gene in fetal human lung. Proc Natl Acad Sci U S A *83*:9527, 1986.
15. Pryhuber GS, et al: Ontogeny of surfactant proteins A and B in human amniotic fluid as indices of fetal lung maturity. Pediatr Res *30*:597, 1991.
16. Liley HG, et al: Surfactant protein of molecular weight 28,000-36,000 in cultured human fetal lung: cellular localization and effect of dexamethasone. Mol Endocrinol *1*:205, 1987.
17. Liley HG, et al: Regulation of messenger RNAs for the hydrophobic surfactant proteins in human lung. J Clin Invest *83*:1191, 1989.
18. Miyamura K, et al: Surfactant proteins A (SP-A) and D (SP-D): levels in human amniotic fluid and localization in the fetal membranes. Biochim Biophys Acta *1210*:303, 1994.
19. Inoue T, et al: Enzyme-linked immunosorbent assay for human pulmonary surfactant protein D. J Immunol Methods *173*:157, 1994.
20. Clements JA, et al: Assessment of the risk of the respiratory-distress syndrome by a rapid test for surfactant in amniotic fluid. N Engl J Med *286*:1077, 1972.
21. Harding R, et al: Regulation of lung expansion and lung growth before birth. J Appl Physiol *81*:209, 1996.
22. Olver RE, et al: Ion fluxes across the pulmonary epithelium and the secretion of lung liquid in the foetal lamb. J Physiol *241*:327, 1974.
23. Adzick NS: Experimental pulmonary hypoplasia and oligohydramnios: relative contributions of lung fluid and fetal breathing movements. J Pediatr Surg *19*:658, 1984.
24. Harrison MR, et al: Correction of congenital diaphragmatic hernia *in utero*. II. Simulated correction permits fetal lung growth with survival at birth. Surgery *88*:260, 1980.
25. Wallen LD, et al: Morphometric study of the role of pulmonary arterial flow in fetal lung growth in sheep. Pediatr Res *27*:122, 1990.
26. Chapman DL, et al: Changes in lung liquid during spontaneous labor in fetal sheep. J Appl Physiol *76*:523, 1994.
27. O'Brodovich H, et al: Amiloride impairs lung liquid clearance in newborn guinea pigs. J Appl Physiol *68*:1758, 1990.
28. Olver RE, et al: The role of amiloride-blockable sodium transport in adrenaline-induced lung liquid reabsorption in the fetal lamb. J Physiol *376*:321, 1986.
29. Croteau JR, et al: Volume-pressure and length-tension measurements in human tracheal and bronchial segments. J Appl Physiol *16*:170, 1961.
30. Burnard ED, et al: Pulmonary insufficiency in prematurity. Aust Paediatr J *1*:12, 1965.
31. Frank L: Pathophysiology of lung injury and repair: special features of the immature lung. *In* Polin RA, et al (eds): Fetal and Neonatal Physiology. Philadelphia, WB Saunders, 1992, pp 914-926.
32. Reynolds EO, et al: Hyaline membrane disease, respiratory distress, and surfactant deficiency. Pediatrics *42*:758, 1968.
33. Avery ME, et al: Surface properties in relation to atelectasis and hyaline membrane disease. Am J Dis Child *97*:517, 1959.
34. Kendig JW, et al: A comparison of surfactant as immediate prophylaxis and as rescue therapy in newborns of less than 30 weeks' gestation. N Engl J Med *324*:865, 1991.
35. Angus DC, et al: Epidemiology of neonatal respiratory failure in the United States: projections from California and New York. Am J Respir Crit Care Med *164*:1154, 2001.
36. Lemons JA, et al: Very low birth weight outcomes of the National Institute of Child Health and Human Development Neonatal Research Network, January 1995 through December 1996. NICHD Neonatal Research Network. Pediatrics *107*:E1, 2001.
37. Stoll BJ, et al: Late-onset sepsis in very low birth weight neonates: the experience of the NICHD neonatal research network. Pediatrics *110*:285, 2002.
38. Doyle LW, et al: Effects of antenatal steroid therapy on mortality and morbidity in very low birth weight infants. J Pediatr *108*:287, 1986.
39. Van Marter LJ, et al: Maternal glucocorticoid therapy and reduced risk of bronchopulmonary dysplasia. Pediatrics *86*:331, 1990.
40. Pierce RA, et al: Glucocorticoids upregulate tropoelastin expression during late stages of fetal lung development. Am J Physiol *268*:L491, 1995.
41. Ballard PL, et al: Glucocorticoid regulation of surfactant components in immature lambs. Am J Physiol *273*:L1048, 1997.
42. Liggins GC: Premature delivery of foetal lambs infused with glucocorticoids. J Endocr *45*:515, 1969.

43. Liggins GC, et al: A controlled trial of antepartum glucocorticoid treatment for prevention of the respiratory distress syndrome in premature infants. Pediatrics 50:515, 1972.

44. Kikkawa Y, et al: Morphologic development of fetal rabbit lung and its acceleration with cortisol. Am J Pathol 64:423, 1971.

45. National Institutes of Health (NIH) Consensus Conference: Effects of corticosteroids for fetal maturation. JAMA 273:412, 1995.

46. Jobe AH: Pulmonary surfactant therapy. N Engl J Med 328:861, 1993.

47. Kwong MS, et al: Double-blind clinical trial of calf lung surfactant extract for the prevention of hyaline membrane disease in extremely premature infants. Pediatrics 76:585, 1985.

48. Enhorning G, et al: Prevention of neonatal respiratory distress syndrome by tracheal instillation of surfactant: a randomized clinical trial. Pediatrics 76:145, 1985.

49. Husain AN, et al: Pathology of arrested acinar development in postsurfactant bronchopulmonary dysplasia. Hum Pathol 29:710, 1988.

50. Carlton DP, et al: Surfactant and lung fluid balance. In Robertson B, et al (eds): Surfactant Therapy for Lung Disease. New York, Marcel Dekker, 1995, pp 33–46.

51. Albertine KH: Histopathology of pulmonary edema and the acute respiratory distress syndrome. In Matthay MA, et al (eds): Lung Biology in Health and Disease. New York, Marcel-Dekker, 1998, pp 37–84.

52. Wigglesworth JS: Pathology of neonatal respiratory distress. Proc R Soc Med 70:861, 1977.

53. Stocker JT: The respiratory tract. In Dehner LP, et al (eds) Pediatric Pathology, 2nd ed. Philadelphia; Lippiincott-Williams, 2001, pp 445–517.

54. Dreyfuss D, et al: Ventilator-induced lung injury: lessons from experimental studies. Am J Respir Crit Care Med 157:294, 1998.

55. deLemos RA, et al: Ventilatory management of infant baboons with hyaline membrane disease: the use of high frequency ventilation. Pediatr Res 21:594, 1987.

56. Davis JM, et al: Differential effects of oxygen and barotrauma on lung injury in the neonatal piglet. Pediatr Pulmonol 10:157, 1991.

57. Dreyfuss D, et al: High inflation pressure pulmonary edema. Respective effects of high airway pressure, high tidal volume, and positive end-expiratory pressure. Am Rev Respir Dis 137:1159, 1988.

58. Carlton DP, et al: Lung overexpansion increases pulmonary microvascular protein permeability in young lambs. J Appl Physiol 69:577, 1990.

59. Adkins WK, et al: Age affects susceptibility to pulmonary barotrauma in rabbits. Crit Care Med 19:390, 1991.

60. Merritt TA, et al: Randomized, placebo-controlled trial of human surfactant given at birth versus rescue administration in very low birth weight infants with lung immaturity. J Pediatr 118:581, 1991.

61. Hodson WA: Ventilation strategies and bronchopulmonary dysplasia. In Bland RD, et al (eds): Chronic Lung Disease in Early Infancy. New York, Marcel Dekker, 2000, pp 173–208.

62. LeFlore JL, et al: Association of antenatal and postnatal dexamethasone exposure with outcomes in extremely low birth weight neonates. Pediatrics 110:275, 2002.

63. Avery ME, et al: Is chronic lung disease in low birth weight infants preventable? A survey of eight centers. Pediatrics 79:26, 1987.

64. Palta M, et al: Multivariate assessment of traditional risk factors for chronic lung disease in very low birth weight neonates. The Newborn Lung Project. J Pediatr 119:285, 1991.

65. Van Marter LJ, et al: Rate of bronchopulmonary dysplasia as a function of neonatal intensive care practices. J Pediatr 120:938, 1992.

66. Northway WH Jr, et al: Pulmonary disease following respiratory therapy of hyaline membrane disease: bronchopulmonary dysplasia. N Engl J Med 276:357, 1967.

67. Jobe AH, et al: Bronchopulmonary dysplasia. Am J Respir Crit Care Med 163:1723, 2001.

68. Northway WH Jr: Bronchopulmonary dysplasia: thirty-three years later. Pediatr Pulmonol 23:5, 2001.

69. Rhodes PG, et al: Chronic pulmonary disease in neonates with assisted ventilation. Pediatrics 55:788, 1975.

70. Campognose P, et al: Neonatal sepsis due to nontypable Haemophilus influenzae. Am J Dis Child 40:117, 1986.

71. Mayes L, et al: Severe bronchopulmonary dysplasia: a retrospective review. Acta Paediatr Scand 72:225, 1983.

72. Bos AP, et al: Radiographic evidence of bronchopulmonary dysplasia in high-risk congenital diaphragmatic hernia survivors. Pediatr Pulmonol 15:231, 1993.

73. Hislop AA, et al: Pulmonary vascular damage and the development of cor pulmonale following hyaline membrane disease. Pediatr Pulmonol 9:152, 1990.

74. Margraf LR, et al: Morphometric analysis of the lung in bronchopulmonary dysplasia. Am Rev Respir Dis 143:391, 1991.

75. Boyden EA: The mode of origin of pulmonary acini and respiratory bronchioles in the fetal lung. Am J Anat 141:317, 1974.

76. Davies G, et al: Growth of the alveoli and pulmonary arteries in childhood. Thorax 25:669, 1970.

77. Langston C, et al: Human lung growth in late gestation and in the neonate. Am Rev Respir Dis 129:607, 1984.

78. Emery JL, et al: The postnatal development of the lung. Acta Anat 65:10, 1966.

79. Dunnill MS: Postnatal growth of the lung. Thorax 17:329, 1962.

80. Alcom DG, et al: A morphologic and morphometric analysis of fetal lung development in the sheep. Anat Rec 201:655, 1981.

81. Davies P, et al: Postnatal growth of the sheep lung: a morphometric study. Anat Rec 220:281, 1988.

82. Docimo SG, et al: Pulmonary development in the fetal lamb: quantitative histologic study of the alveolar phase. Anat Rec 229:495, 1991.

83. Bruce MC, et al: Lung fibroblasts undergo apoptopsis following alveolarization. Am J Respir Cell Mol Biol 20:228, 1999.

84. Albertine KH: Structural organization and quantitative morphology of the lung. In Cutillo AM (ed): Application of Magnetic Resonance to the Study of Lung. Mount Kisko, NY, Futura Publishing Company, 1996, pp 73–114.

85. Lindahl P, et al: Alveogenesis failure in PDGF-A-deficient mice is coupled to lack of distal spreading of alveolar smooth muscle cell progenitors during lung development. Development 124:3943, 1997.

86. Wendel DP, et al: Impaired distal airway development in mice lacking elastin. Am J Respir Cell Mol Biol 23:320, 2000.

87. Escobedo MB, et al: A baboon model of bronchopulmonary dysplasia. I. Clinical features. Exp Mol Pathol 37:323, 1982.

88. Coalson JJ, et al: A baboon model of bronchopulmonary dysplasia. II. Pathologic features. Exp Mol Pathol 37:335, 1982.

89. Coalson JJ, et al: Diffuse alveolar damage in the evolution of bronchopulmonary dysplasia in the baboon. Pediatr Res 24:357, 1988.

90. Coalson JJ, et al: Pathophysiologic, morphometric, and biochemical studies of the preterm baboon with bronchopulmonary dysplasia. Am Rev Respir Dis 145:872, 1992.

91. Bell RE, et al: High-frequency ventilation compared to conventional positive-pressure ventilation in the treatment of hyaline membrane disease in primates. Crit Care Med 12:764, 1984.

92. Meredith KS, et al: Role of lung injury in the pathogenesis of hyaline membrane disease in premature baboons. J Appl Physiol 66:2150, 1989.

93. Yoder BA, et al: High-frequency oscillatory ventilation: effects on lung function, mechanics, and airway cytokines in the immature baboon model for neonatal chronic lung disease. Am J Respir Crit Care Med 162:1867, 2000.

94. deLemos RA, et al: The contribution of experimental models to our understanding of of the pathogenesis and treatment of bronchopulmonary dysplasia. Clin Perinatol 19:521, 1992.

95. Pierce RA, et al: Chronic lung injury in preterm lambs: disordered pulmonary elastin deposition. Am J Physiol 272:L452, 1997.

96. Albertine KH, et al: Chronic lung injury in preterm lambs: disordered respiratory tract development. Am J Respir Crit Care Med 159:945, 1999.

97. Bland RD, et al: Chronic lung injury in preterm lambs: abnormalities of the pulmonary circulation and lung fluid balance. Pediatr Res 48:64, 2000.

98. MacRitchie AN, et al: Reduced endothelial nitric oxide synthase protein in pulmonary arteries and airways of chronically ventilated preterm lambs. Am J Physiol 281:L1011, 2001.

99. Payne J, et al: High frequency, low volume mechanical ventilation enhances alveolar formation in chronically ventilated preterm lambs. J Invest Med 48:25A, 2000.

100. Olsen SL, et al: Platelet endothelial cell adhesion molecule-1 and capillary loading in premature infants with and without chronic lung disease. Pediatr Pulmonol 33:255, 2002.

101. Pierce R, et al: Lung tropoelastin expression increases in lambs after premature birth and 3 days of mechanical ventilation. FASEB J 11:A557, 1997.

102. Berg JT, et al: High lung inflation increases mRNA levels of ECM components and growth factors in lung parenchyma. J Appl Physiol 83:120, 1997.

103. Klekamp JG, et al: Vascular endothelial growth factor is expressed in ovine pulmonary vascular smooth muscle cells in vitro and regulated by hypoxia and dexamethasone. Pediatr Res 42:744, 1997.

104. Han RNN, et al: Expression of basic fibroblast growth factor and receptor: immunolocalization studies in developing rat fetal lung. Pediatr Res 31:435, 1992.

105. Han RNN, et al: Platelet-derived growth factors and growth-related genes in rat lung. III. Immunolocalization during fetal development. Pediatr Res 31:323, 1992.

106. Bostrom H, et al: PDGF-A signaling is a critical event in lung alveolar myofibroblast development and alveogenesis. Cell 85:863, 1996.

107. Border WA, et al: Transforming growth factor β in tissue fibrosis. N Engl J Med 331:1286, 1994.

108. Ruocco S, et al: Expression and localization of epidermal growth factor, transforming growth factor-α, and localization of their common receptor in fetal human lung development. Pediatr Res 39:448, 1996.

109. Moats-Staats BM, et al: Regulation of the insulin-like growth factor system during normal rat lung development. Am J Respir Cell Mol Biol 12:56, 1995.

110. Wallen LD, et al: Cellular distribution of insulin-like growth factors I and II during development of rat lung. Am J Physiol 267:L531, 1994.

111. Strandjord TP, et al: Expression of TGFα, EGF, and EGF receptor in fetal rat lung. Am J Physiol 267:L384, 1994.

112. Warburton D, et al: Epigenetic role of epidermal growth factor expression and signaling in embryonic mouse lung morphogenesis. Dev Biol 149:123, 1992.

113. Le Cras TD, et al: Treatment of newborn rats with a VEGF receptor inhibitor causes pulmonary hypertension and abnormal lung structure. Am J Physiol 283:L555, 2002.

114. Jakkula M, et al: Inhibition of angiogenesis decreases alveolarization in the developing rat lung. Am J Physiol Lung Cell Mol Physiol 279:L600, 2000.

115. Maniscalco WM, et al: Angiogenic factors and alveolar vasculature: development and alterations by injury in very premature baboons. Am J Physiol *282*:L811, 2002.

116. Albertine KH, et al: Retinol treatment of fetal lambs with continuous drainage of lung luminal and amniotic liquids is associated with enhanced development of distal lung parenchyma. Pediatr Res *51*:60A, 2002.

117. Albertine KH, et al: Retinol treatment from birth increases expression of vascular endothelial growth factor (VEGF) and its receptor, fetal liver kinase-1 (FLK-1), and is associated with greater lung capillary surface density in chronically ventilated preterm lambs. Pediatr Res *51*:60A, 2002.

118. Schachtner SK, et al: Qualitative and quantitative analysis of embryonic pulmonary vessel formation. Am J Respir Cell Mol Biol *22*:157, 2000.

119. Taichman DB, et al: Notch1 and Jagged1 expression by the developing pulmonary vasculature. Dev Dyn *225*:166, 2002.

120. Wicher C, et al: Alveolar formation in the developing lung is reduced in hypomorphic *fgf*8 mice. J Invest Med, in press.

121. Peters K, et al: Targeted expression of a dominant negative FGF receptor blocks branching morphogenesis and epithelial differentiation of the mouse lung. EMBO J *13*:3296, 1994.

122. Galambos C, et al: Defective pulmonary development in the absence of heparin-binding vascular endothelial growth factor isoforms. Am J Respir Cell Mol Biol *27*:194, 2002.

123. Xue Y, et al: Embronic lethality and vascular defects in mice lacking the Notch ligand Jagged1. Hum Mol Genet *8*:723, 1999.

124. Pertovaara L, et al: Vascular endothelial growth factor is induced in response to transforming growth factor-beta in fibroblastic and epithelial cells. J Biol Chem *269*:6271, 1994.

125. Finkenzeller G, et al: Platelet-derived growth factor–induced transcription of the vascular endothelial growth factor gene is mediated by protein kinase C. Cancer Res *52*:4821, 1992.

126. Tuder RM, et al: Increased gene expression for VEGF and the VEGF receptors KDR/Flk and Flt in lungs exposed to acute or to chronic hypoxia. Modulation of gene expression by nitric oxide. Clin Invest *95*:1798, 1995.

127. Maniscalco WM, et al: Vascular endothelial growth factor mRNA increases in alveolar epithelial cells during recovery from oxygen injury. Am J Respir Cell Mol Biol *13*:377, 1995.

128. Maniscalco WM, et al: Hyperoxic injury decreases alveolar epithelial cell expression of vascular endothelial growth factor (VEGF) in neonatal rabbit lung. Am J Respir Cell Mol Biol *16*:557, 1997.

129. Klekamp JG, et al: Exposure to hyperoxia decreases the expression of vascular endothelial growth factor and its receptors in adult rat lungs. Am J Pathol *154*:823, 1999.

130. Maniscalco WM, et al: Vascular endothelial growth factor mRNA increases in alveolar epithelial cells during recovery from oxygen injury. Am J Respir Cell Mol Biol *13*:377, 1995.

131. Brandt RB, et al: Serum vitamin A in premature and term neonates. J Pediatr *92*:101, 1978.

132. Hustead VA, et al: Relationship of vitamin A (retinol) status to lung disease in the preterm infant. J Pediatr *105*:610, 1984.

133. Shenai JP, et al: Vitamin A status of neonates with bronchopulmonary dysplasia. Pediatr Res *19*:185, 1985.

134. Shenai JP, et al: Plasma retinol-binding protein response to vitamin A administration in infants susceptible to bronchopulmonary dysplasia. J Pediatr *116*:607, 1990.

135. Shenai JP, et al: Clinical trial of vitamin A supplementation in infants susceptible to bronchopulmonary dysplasia. J Pediatr *111*:269, 1987.

136. Pearson E, et al: Trial of vitamin A supplementation in very low birth weight infants at risk for bronchopulmonary dysplasia. J Pediatr *121*:420, 1992.

137. Tyson JE, et al: Vitamin (Vit.) A supplementation to increase survival without chronic lung disease (CLD) in extremely low birth weight (ELBW) infants: a 14-center randomized trial. Pediatr Res *43*:199A, 1998.

138. Tyson JE, et al: Vitamin A supplementation for extremely-low-birth-weight infant. N Engl J Med *340*:1962, 1999.

139. McGowan S, et al: Mice bearing deletions of retinoic acid receptors demonstrate reduced lung elastin and alveolar numbers. Am J Respir Cell Mol Biol *23*:162, 2000.

140. Massaro GD, et al: Postnatal treatment with retinoic acid increases the number of pulmonary alveoli in rats. Am J Physiol *270*:L305, 1996.

141. Oshika E, et al: Antagonistic effects of dexamethasone and retinoic acid on rat lung morphogenesis. Pediatr Res *43*:315, 1998.

142. Massaro GD, et al: Retinoic acid treatment abrogates elastase-induced pulmonary emphysema in rats. Nature Med *3*:675, 1997.

Alan H. Jobe and Suhas Kallapur

94 Antenatal Factors That Influence Postnatal Lung Development and Injury

SPECTRUM OF LUNG DISEASE IN PRETERM INFANTS

The normal fetal lung at 26 weeks of gestation is in an early saccular stage of development and severely surfactant deficient. Surfactant treatment and the use of gentler approaches of assisted ventilation have resulted in populations of very preterm infants with a wide range of lung diseases not easily classifiable into the traditional categories of respiratory distress syndrome (RDS), lung immaturity, or normal. Data from the National Institute of Child Health and Human Development Neonatal Network indicated that mortality for infants weighing 501 to 1500 g at birth was only 14%, but *bronchopulmonary dysplasia* (BPD), defined as the need for oxygen at 36 weeks, occurred in 23% of these infants.[1] In the population of very preterm infants in the 750- to 1000-g birth weight range (average gestational age of 26 weeks), 37% of the infants did not have RDS, but 42% ultimately developed BPD. Many infants develop BPD without having RDS. In one series of 177 surviving infants with birth weights less than 1250 g, 115 infants had RDS, and 61 of these infants developed BPD.[2] However, 27 infants either resolved the RDS or had no initial lung disease and subsequently developed BPD. Therefore, 30% of the infants with BPD had clinical courses that were not characteristic of the normal progression from RDS to BPD in ventilated infants. There is a complex interplay of antenatal and postnatal factors affecting postnatal lung development (Fig. 94-1). The goal of this chapter is to explore some of the antenatal factors that may modulate lung development and thus alter the postnatal clinical course of lung disease in preterm infants.

CHORIOAMNIONITIS

The fetal lungs are protected from the traditional mechanisms of lung injury, but infection or inflammation can reach the fetal lung. Genital infections can ascend through the cervix and spread between the chorioamnion and the uterine wall and are common associations with early preterm labor.[3] Inflammation of the chorioamnion, termed *chorioamnionitis,* is a histologic diagnosis. Clinical chorioamnionitis is diagnosed using a combination of indicators such as elevated maternal temperature, uterine tenderness, malodorous vaginal discharge, maternal leukocytosis, and fetal tachycardia.[4] Spread of the inflammation to the amniotic fluid can be evaluated by amniocentesis to sample fluid for culture on cell counts, or by the measurement of proinflammatory mediators. Further spread of the infection or inflammation to the fetus can be by two routes.[5] The fetus can swallow and aspirate the inflammatory products in the amniotic fluid and can develop pneumonia or sepsis syndromes, or the fetus may receive inflammatory signals from the inflamed fetal placenta

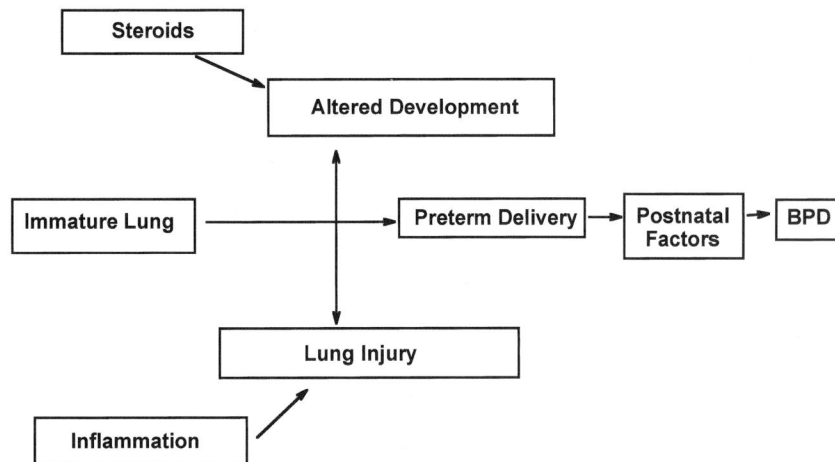

Figure 94–1. The interactions of steroids and inflammation on lung development and lung injury. The interplay of these factors and exposures modulates the development of bronchopulmonary dysplasia (BPD) in preterm infants.

and chorioamnion. The fetal inflammatory response to chorioamnionitis has been defined as an elevation of interleukin-6 (IL-6) in fetal cord blood obtained by cordocentesis or in cord blood after delivery.[6] *Funisitis,* or inflammation of the umbilical cord, correlates with elevated cord IL-6 levels and signs of generalized fetal inflammation.

The rapidly progressive chorioamnionitis or infection caused by organisms such as *Escherichia coli, Listeria monocytogenes,* or group B streptococci is relatively infrequent in the preterm population. In contrast, clinically asymptomatic histologic chorioamnionitis caused by low-virulence or commensal organisms increases in frequency as gestational age at delivery decreases. In one series, about 70% of infants (<30 weeks of gestation) delivered by cesarean section with intact membranes had histologic chorioamnionitis.[3] This clinically inapparent chorioamnionitis is associated with recurrent preterm deliveries, and indicators of inflammation may be present before mid-gestation. Amniotic fluid sampled before 20 weeks of gestation for genetic diagnostic indications can contain elevated proinflammatory mediators and may be culture positive for low-virulence pathogenic organisms.[7] Often, these infants have no overt signs of infection at delivery.

The diagnosis of chorioamnionitis and the evaluation of its impact on the newborn are problematic because of the frequency of chorioamnionitis and the spectrum of the disease. Neonatal morbidity associated with elevated plasma IL-6 occurred with the diagnosis of clinical chorioamnionitis in 19% of cases and in 71% of cases with histologic chorioamnionitis.[6] However, no morbidity occurred with clinical or histologic chorioamnionitis 29% of the time. Nevertheless, the most common cause of fetal death or death soon after birth for very low birth weight infants was sepsis or pneumonia in an autopsy series.[8] The effects of chorioamnionitis on the preterm fetus range from severe infection or death to normal fetal development with histologic chorioamnionitis as an incidental finding.

Fetal Lung Injury

The traditional concept is that fetal infection or inflammation associated with chorioamnionitis can result in an aspiration pneumonia syndrome and sepsis. Gomez and colleagues[6] proposed that the fetal inflammatory response was equivalent to acute RDS in adults with systemic inflammatory mediators targeting the lungs. However, other fetuses are exposed to inflammation in the amniotic fluid and do not have elevated plasma IL-6 levels. Elevated IL-1β, IL-6, and IL-8 in amniotic fluid measured within 5 days of preterm delivery predicted the subsequent development of BPD.[9] Histologic chorioamnionitis was not useful retrospectively in this series because it was present in

92% of infants who developed BPD and in 62% of infants without BPD. RDS was also a poor predictor of BPD. In another report, severe histologic chorioamnionitis and elevated tumor necrosis factor-α (TNF-α) in amniotic fluid was associated with an increased incidence of RDS and subsequently BPD.[10] In a comparison of the predictive values for the development of BPD, elevated cord plasma IL-6 was a better predictor than was elevated IL-6 in the amniotic fluid.[11] Fetal exposure to inflammation is associated with a lung injury process that results in an increased incidence of BPD. There is a graded increasing risk of BPD from histologic chorioamnionitis to elevated inflammatory mediators in amniotic fluid and to a fetal inflammatory response with elevated IL-6 in fetal blood.

Clinical Lung Maturation

Although chorioamnionitis is generally considered as having adverse effects on the fetus, some reports indicate beneficial effects for the fetus. Watterberg and colleagues[12] reported that histologic chorioamnionitis and high IL-1β in airway samples on the first day after delivery predicted a decreased incidence of RDS but an increased incidence of BPD. Infants who were culture positive for *Ureaplasma urealyticum* also had less RDS but more BPD than infants who were culture negative.[13] Higher cord plasma levels of IL-6 predicted less RDS in another report.[14] Although these small clinical series may reflect a reporting bias, the presence of chorioamnionitis was associated with improved survival for 881 infants born at less than 26 weeks of gestation in the United Kingdom and Ireland in 1995.[15] The associations of chorioamnionitis with outcomes such as RDS and BPD are likely to be quite complex. In a large epidemiologic report, histologic chorioamnionitis predicted a decreased incidence of BPD unless the infant received mechanical ventilation or developed postnatal sepsis, which, in combination with histologic chorioamnionitis, increased the risk of BPD. This study implies that fetal exposure to inflammation can mature the lung, but a subsequent injury (ventilation or sepsis) promotes an enhanced injury response resulting in BPD.

Animal Models

Bry and colleagues[16] reported that intra-amniotic injections of recombinant IL-1α induced the mRNA for surfactant protein A (SP-A) and SP-B and improved the pressure-volume curves in preterm rabbits. IL-1α also increased the mRNA for SP-A, B, and C in early gestation explants of rabbit lungs.[17] To explore the relationships between inflammation and maturation further, *E. coli* endotoxin was given by intra-amniotic injection in sheep.[18] The

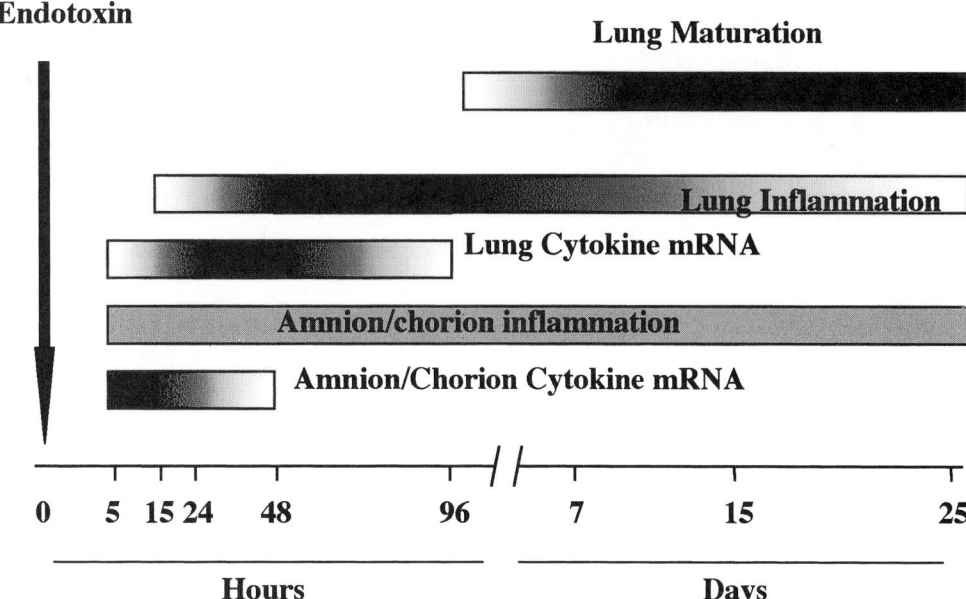

Figure 94–2. The time course of lung inflammation and maturation after intra-amniotic endotoxin in preterm lambs. The *shading* within each box is roughly proportional to the intensity and magnitude of the response. (Based on data from refs. 21 and 23.)

fetal sheep lung responded to intra-amniotic endotoxin with a large increase in compliance and lung gas volume within 5 to 7 days. These improvements in lung function after preterm birth were accompanied by persistent increases in the mRNA for SP-A, SP-B, SP-C, and SP-D and hundredfold increases in the SPs in the air spaces.[19] The processing of SP-B was induced, the amount of surfactant lipid increased, and the antioxidant enzymes increased.[20]

In the preterm lamb model, "clinical maturation" was a late response of the lung to inflammation (Fig. 94–2). Within hours of the intra-amniotic injection of endotoxin, white blood cells producing the mRNA for the proinflammatory cytokines IL-1β, IL-6, and IL-8 infiltrated the chorioamnion and, subsequently, the amniotic fluid.[21] The cells in amniotic fluid expressed the mRNA for IL-1α and IL-8 for at least 1 week after the endotoxin exposure. Within 5 hours of intra-amniotic endotoxin, the fetal lung contained activated granulocytes, and the airways expressed heat shock protein 70.[22] The amount of hydrogen peroxide in cells lavaged from the lungs was maximal at 24 hours, and both the lung tissue and lavage cells expressed proinflammatory cytokines.[23] Apoptosis increased at 24 hours, and cell replication increased by 72 hours. This response of the fetal lung was characteristic of an acute but modest generalized inflammatory response that resolved by clinical maturation in that lung function was strikingly improved after preterm delivery and ventilation.

The lung maturational response in the preterm lamb model did not occur in the absence of chorioamnionitis and lung inflammation. A low dose of endotoxin that induced very mild inflammation did not result in lung maturation.[21] The inflammation in the chorioamnion and lung did not result in increased plasma cortisol or a significant systemic inflammatory response.[18] Therefore, the inflammation-mediated mechanisms for inducing lung maturation were independent of the adrenal axis. The fetal sheep responded to recombinant ovine IL-1α or IL-1β with chorioamnionitis and lung maturation.[24] Intra-amniotic endotoxin–induced chorioamnionitis had no effect on the fetal lung when the fetal lung was surgically isolated from the amniotic fluid.[25] In contrast, endotoxin infused over 24 hours into the fetal lung fluid resulted in striking lung maturation. Therefore, endotoxin or the products of inflammation induced by endotoxin or IL-1 induced the lung

maturation without the requirement for a systemic fetal inflammatory response.

CYTOKINES AND ALTERED LUNG DEVELOPMENT

Preterm infants who have increased proinflammatory cytokines in bronchoalveolar lavage have an increased risk of developing BPD.[26] Animal experiments showed that exposure of the developing lung to cytokines alters both the lung architecture and the components of the surfactant system. Transgenic mice over-expressing TNF-α,[27] transforming growth factor-α,[28] IL-6,[29] and interferon-γ[30] have fewer and larger alveoli. Although each over-expression resulted in different associated lung abnormalities, the common theme was interference with alveolar development. Cytokines also regulate surfactant homeostasis. Mice that lack granulocyte-macrophage colony-stimulating factor (GM-CSF) or the GM-CSF receptor have alveolar proteinosis resulting from decreased catabolism of saturated phosphatidylcholine and SP-A.[31] Similarly, mice that over-express IL-4 in Clara cells have alveolar proteinosis.[32]

Preterm fetal rabbits or lambs exposed to intra-amniotic IL-1α or endotoxin have increased surfactant pool sizes and improved lung compliance.[16] IL-1 and endotoxin injected in amniotic fluid induce comparable maturational changes in fetal lamb lung.[24] Although the mechanism of lung maturation in this model is not known, both IL-1 receptor and the toll receptor involved in endotoxin signal transduction share common components.[33] Although the endotoxin-induced lung maturation is striking in the preterm lamb, these changes are also accompanied by structural changes of fewer and larger alveoli, a pathologic hallmark of BPD.[25,34]

The fetal lung response to a proinflammatory stimulus also is dependent on the gestation and the developmental milieu of the fetus. Exposure of explants of preterm fetal rabbit lung to IL-1 caused increased SP mRNA, whereas IL-1 inhibited SP mRNA in explants from term lungs.[17] Similarly, postnatal exposure to endotoxin decreased SP-B mRNA synthesis in mouse lung, whereas intrauterine exposure to endotoxin increased SP-B synthesis in lamb lungs.[19] Thus, the preterm infant probably responds to proinflammatory stimuli in a complex fashion with changes in the developmental program of the saccular lung.

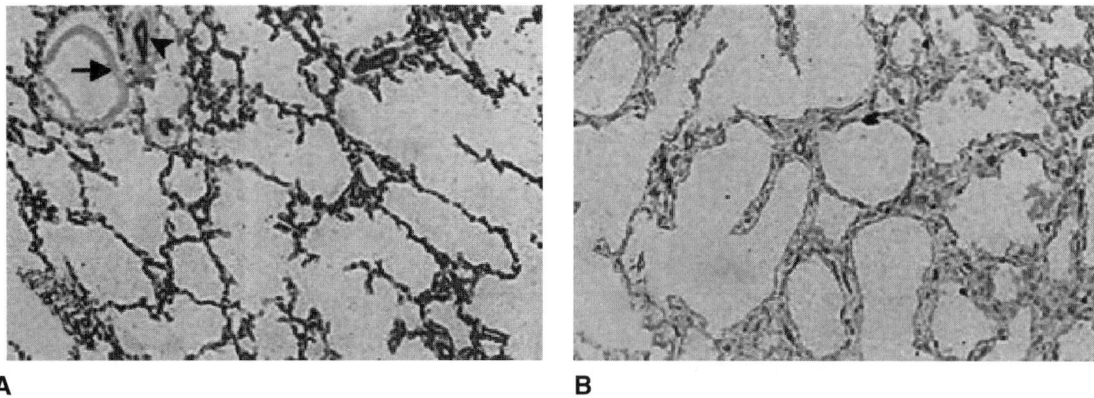

Figure 94–3. Lung sections from infants dying of nonlung causes (**A**) and of bronchopulmonary dysplasia (BPD) (**B**) were immunostained for PECAM-1 (CD31) antigen, which is specific for vascular endothelium. Staining for PECAM was decreased and aberrant in infants with BPD, a finding indicating impaired vascular growth. The *arrow* shows PECAM staining in the alveolar wall. (From Bhatt AJ, et al: Am J Respir Crit Care Med *164*:1971, 2001.)

Some of these changes are beneficial to *ex utero* survival of the preterm, whereas other changes may predispose the fetus to development of BPD.

ANTENATAL INFECTION AND VASCULAR INJURY

Infants with BPD have decreased and disorganized lung microvasculature with decreased angiogenic growth factors such as vascular endothelial growth factor (VEGF) and its receptors (Fig. 94–3).[35, 36] This decreased microvascular development was also seen in the preterm lamb and baboon models of BPD induced by mechanical ventilation.[37, 38] In recombination experiments with rat embryo tissue, epithelial cells were required to maintain Flk-1 (a marker of endothelial cells) expression in the distal lung mesenchymal cells.[39] In transgenic mice that overexpressed VEGF or in mice lacking the higher-molecular-weight heparin-binding VEGF isoforms, alveolar development was disrupted.[40, 41] Abnormalities of pulmonary circulation were associated with lung hypoplasia in animal models.[42, 43] Neonatal rat pups, in which VEGF signaling was disrupted with pharmacologic inhibitors of the Flk-1/KDR receptor, had impaired alveolarization.[44] These experiments suggest that there is cross-talk between the mediators of vascular and alveolar development in the lung. Intra-amniotic endotoxin caused impaired alveolarization in lambs (Fig. 94–4).[34, 45] The chemokines IP-10 (interferon-inducible protein) and MIG (monokine induced by gamma interferon), known to inhibit vascular development in other animal models, are robustly induced in the lungs of preterm lambs exposed to intra-amniotic endotoxin.[46] These experiments suggest the possibility that antenatal infections could induce vascular injury in the developing lung, which could predispose the preterm infant to BPD.

EVENTS AFTER FETAL LUNG INFLAMMATION

The preterm fetal lung normally does not mount inflammatory responses, and the multiple components that make up a mature response to injury are deficient. The preterm fetal lung contains almost no macrophages or granulocytes, and normal host defense proteins such as SP-A and SP-D are present in very low amounts. When challenged with intrauterine endotoxin or IL-1, fetal lambs recruited activated granulocytes rapidly.[21] The fetal lung was also capable of suppressing fulminant inflammation because repeated doses or continuous intra-amniotic infusions of endotoxin did not result in severe or progressive lung inflammation.[18, 45] Nevertheless, granulocytes and increased numbers of monocytes/macrophages and lymphocytes persisted in the fetal airways for several weeks after the intra-amniotic

endotoxin exposure, a finding indicating that resolution of the inflammation was delayed.[21]

The lungs of fetal sheep exposed to endotoxin 30 days before preterm delivery had an amplified inflammatory response to mechanical ventilation relative to normal preterm lambs.[47] This result was consistent with the clinical observation that the risk of BPD was increased when a preterm infant exposed to chorioamnionitis was ventilated after birth.[48] Another variable that may contribute to lung injury is the fate of inflammatory mediators that are in the lungs of the infant at delivery. The uninjured fetal lung is quite impermeable to proteins and large-molecular-weight substances such as endotoxin. However, gentle mechanical ventilation of the preterm lung with endotoxin or IL-1 in the air spaces resulted in the transfer of the proinflammatory mediators to the systemic circulation and a systemic inflammatory response.[49]

Glucocorticoid Effects on the Fetal Lung

Although antenatal glucocorticoids decrease the incidence of RDS, they do not decrease the incidence of BPD in survivors.[50] This lack of clear benefit for BPD has been attributed to the increased survival of very preterm infants most at risk of BPD. However, an alternative possibility is the decreased alveolar septation that occurs after antenatal glucocorticoid treatment. Exposure of fetal monkeys or sheep to glucocorticoids decreased the lung mesenchyme, thinned the alveolar capillary barrier, and increased potential lung gas volume, but decreased alveolar septation (see Fig. 94–4).[34, 51] Monkeys exposed to a relatively high dose of antenatal glucocorticoids had a more functionally mature lung that held more gas after preterm birth, but that lung was smaller with fewer and larger alveoli at term.[52] Alveolar septation also was decreased in the fetal sheep lung by maternal betamethasone.[53] The magnitude of the arrest in alveolar septation was similar for either antenatal intra-amniotic endotoxin or maternal betamethasone in sheep.[34] Although the mechanisms resulting in altered alveolar septation are not known, it is provocative that both proinflammatory and antiinflammatory stimuli that induce clinical lung maturation have as adverse effects inhibition of alveolar septation. As with endotoxin, antenatal glucocorticoids may alter the fetal lung responses to injury and may initiate the anatomic changes characteristic of BPD.

Interactions of Antenatal Glucocorticoids and Inflammation

In clinical practice, most women at risk of very preterm delivery with chronic histologic chorioamnionitis and low-grade

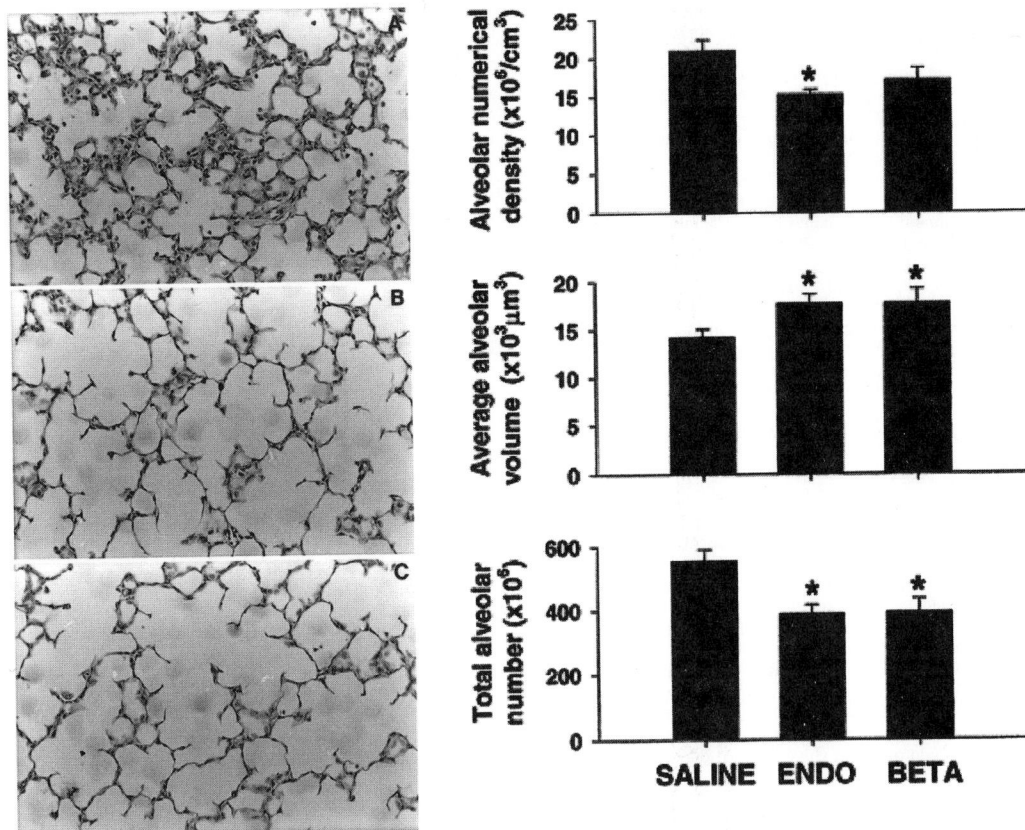

Figure 94–4. Preterm lamb lungs at 125 days gestation and 7 days after control saline (A), intra-amniotic endotoxin (Endo) (B), or maternal betamethasone (Beta) (C) administration. The *bar graph* shows indices of alveolar development in treated versus control groups of preterm lambs. Both endotoxin and maternal betamethasone impaired alveolar development. *$p < .05$ versus controls. (From Willet KE, et al: Pediatr Res *48*:782, 2000.)

infection are asymptomatic. Based on current recommendations, these women receive antenatal glucocorticoids without an amniocentesis to evaluate for infection or inflammation. This clinical practice is based on good clinical data indicating that antenatal glucocorticoids improved neonatal outcomes despite histologic chorioamnionitis or preterm rupture of membranes.[14,54] Antenatal glucocorticoids decreased plasma IL-6 and IL-8 in newborns born to mothers with chorioamnionitis, a finding suggesting that the fetal inflammatory response could be decreased.

Interactions between experimental chorioamnionitis and antenatal glucocorticoids have been minimally explored. Fetal sheep responded to antenatal betamethasone with improved lung function and decreased body weights and thymic weights.[55] In contrast, the more striking lung maturation induced by intra-amniotic endotoxin occurred without decreased body or thymic weights. Exposure of the fetus to antenatal glucocorticoids and intra-amniotic endotoxin resulted in a large lung maturation response without adverse growth effects on body and thymic weights. Maternal betamethasone initially suppressed the endotoxin-induced inflammation in the fetal lungs, but there was a subsequent rebound inflammation.[56] There is no experimental information about how these combined mediator systems could influence postnatal lung development. The benefit of less RDS may result in more or more severe BPD if there are persistent effects on alveolar septation.

REFERENCES

1. Lemons JA, et al: Very low birth weight outcomes of the National Institute of Child Health and Human Development Neonatal Research Network, January 1995 through December 1996. Pediatrics *107*:E1, 2001.
2. Charafeddine L, et al: Atypical chronic lung disease patterns in neonates. Pediatrics *103*:759, 1999.
3. Goldenberg RL, et al: Intrauterine infection and preterm delivery. N Engl J Med *342*:1500, 2000.
4. Chaiworapongsa T, et al: Evidence for fetal involvement in the pathologic process of clinical chorioamnionitis. Am J Obstet Gynecol *186*:1178, 2002.
5. Romero R, et al: Infection in the pathogenesis of preterm labor. Semin Perinatol *12*:262, 1988.
6. Gomez R, et al: The fetal inflammatory response syndrome. Am J Obstet Gynecol *179*:194, 1998.
7. Wenstrom KD, et al: Elevated second-trimester amniotic fluid interleukin-6 levels predict preterm delivery. Am J Obstet Gynecol *178*:546, 1998.
8. Barton L, et al: Causes of death in the extremely low birth weight infant. Pediatrics *103*:446, 1999.
9. Yoon BH, et al: Amniotic fluid cytokines (interleukin-6, tumor necrosis factor-alpha, interleukin-1 beta, and interleukin-8) and the risk for the development of bronchopulmonary dysplasia. Am J Obstet Gynecol *177*:825, 1997.
10. Hitti J, et al: Amniotic fluid tumor necrosis factor-alpha and the risk of respiratory distress syndrome among preterm infants. Am J Obstet Gynecol *177*:50, 1997.
11. Yoon BH, et al: A systemic fetal inflammatory response and the development of bronchopulmonary dysplasia. Am J Obstet Gynecol *181*:773, 1999.
12. Watterberg KL, et al: Chorioamnionitis and early lung inflammation in infants in whom bronchopulmonary dysplasia develops. Pediatrics *97*:210, 1996.
13. Hannaford K, et al: Role of *Ureaplasma urealyticum* in lung disease of prematurity. Arch Dis Child *81*:F162, 1999.
14. Shimoya K, et al: Chorioamnionitis decreased incidence of respiratory distress syndrome by elevating fetal interleukin-6 serum concentration. Hum Reprod *15*:2234, 2000.
15. Costeloe K, et al: The EPICure study: outcomes to discharge from hospital for infants born at the threshold of viability. Pediatrics *106*:659, 2000.
16. Bry K, et al: Intraamniotic interleukin-1 accelerates surfactant protein synthesis in fetal rabbits and improves lung stability after premature birth. J Clin Invest *99*:2992, 1997.
17. Glumoff V, et al: Degree of lung maturity determines the direction of the interleukin-1-induced effect on the expression of surfactant proteins. Am J Respir Cell Mol Biol *22*:280, 2000.
18. Jobe AH, et al: Endotoxin induced lung maturation in preterm lambs is not mediated by cortisol. Am J Respir Crit Care Med *162*:1656, 2000.

19. Bachurski CJ, et al: Intra-amniotic endotoxin increases pulmonary surfactant components and induces SP-B processing in fetal sheep. Am J Physiol 280:L279, 2001.

20. Sosenko IR, Jobe A: Intra-amniotic endotoxin: promotion of lung antioxidant enzyme activity in preterm lambs precedes maturation of lung function and surfactant. Pediatr Res 49:383A, 2001.

21. Kramer BW, et al: Dose and time response after intra-amniotic endotoxin in preterm lambs. Am J Respir Crit Care Med 164:982, 2001.

22. Kramer BW, et al: Injury, inflammation and remodeling in fetal sheep lung after intra-amniotic endotoxin. Am J Physiol 283:L452, 2002.

23. Kallapur SG, et al: Intra-amniotic endotoxin: Chorioamnionitis precedes lung maturation in preterm lambs. Am J Physiol 280:L527, 2001.

24. Willet K, et al: Intra-amniotic injection of IL-1 induces inflammation and maturation in fetal sheep lung. Am J Physiol 282:L411, 2001.

25. Moss TM, et al: Intra-amniotic endotoxin induces lung maturation by direct effects on the developing respiratory tract in preterm sheep. Am J Obstet Gynecol 187:1059, 2002.

26. Speer CP, Groneck P: Oxygen radicals, cytokines, adhesion molecules and lung injury in neonates. Semin Neonatol 3:219, 1998.

27. Miyazaki Y, et al: Expression of a tumor necrosis factor-alpha transgene in murine lung causes lymphocytic and fibrosing alveolitis. J Clin Invest 96:250, 1995.

28. Hardie WD, et al: Postnatal lung function and morphology in transgenic mice expressing transforming growth factor-β. Am J Pathol 151:1075, 1997.

29. DiCosmo BF, et al: Airway epithelial cell expression of interleukin-6 in transgenic mice: uncoupling of airway inflammation and bronchial hyperreactivity. J Clin Invest 94:2028, 1994.

30. Wang Z, et al: Interferon gamma induction of pulmonary emphysema in the adult murine lung. J Exp Med 192:1587, 2000.

31. Ikegami M, et al: Surfactant metabolism in transgenic mice after granulocyte macrophage-colony stimulating factor ablation. Am J Physiol 270:L650, 1996.

32. Ikegami M, et al: Interleukin-4 increases surfactant and regulates metabolism in vivo. Am J Physiol 278:L75, 2000.

33. O'Neill LA, Dinarello CA: The IL-1 receptor/toll-like receptor superfamily: crucial receptors for inflammation and host defense. Immunol Today 21:206, 2000.

34. Willet KE, et al: Antenatal endotoxin and glucocorticoid effects on lung morphometry in preterm lambs. Pediatr Res 48:782, 2000.

35. Bhatt AJ, et al: Disrupted pulmonary vasculature and decreased vascular endothelial growth factor, Flt-1 and Tie-2 in human infants dying with bronchopulmonary dysplasia. Am J Respir Crit Care Med 164:1971, 2001.

36. Lassus P, et al: Pulmonary vascular endothelial growth factor and Flt-1 in fetuses, in acute and chronic lung disease, and in persistent pulmonary hypertension of the newborn. Am J Respir Crit Care Med 164:1981, 2001.

37. Albertine KH, et al: Chronic lung injury in preterm lambs. Am J Respir Crit Care Med 159:945, 1999.

38. Coalson JJ, et al: Neonatal chronic lung disease in extremely immature baboons. Am J Respir Crit Care Med 160:1333, 1999.

39. Gebb SA, Shannon JM: Tissue interactions mediate early events in pulmonary vasculogenesis. Dev Dyn 217:159, 2000.

40. Zeng X, et al: VEGF enhances pulmonary vasculogenesis and disrupts lung morphogenesis in vivo. Dev Dyn 211:215, 1998.

41. Ng YS, et al: Differential expression of VEGF isoforms in mouse during development and in the adult. Dev Dyn 220:112, 2001.

42. Le Cras TD, et al: Abnormal lung growth and the development of pulmonary hypertension in the fawn-hooded rat. Am J Physiol 277:L709, 1999.

43. Le Cras TD, et al: Neonatal dexamethasone treatment increases the risk for pulmonary hypertension in adult rats. Am J Physiol 278:L822, 2000.

44. Jakkula M, et al: Inhibition of angiogenesis decreases alveolarization in the developing rat lung. Am J Physiol 279:L600, 2000.

45. Moss TM, et al: Early gestational Intra-amniotic endotoxin: Lung function, surfactant and morphometry. Am J Respir Crit Care Med 165:805, 2002.

46. Kallapur SG, et al: Increased IP-10 and MIG expression after intra-amniotic endotoxin in Preterm lamb lung. Am J Respir Crit Care Med 167:779, 2003.

47. Ikegami M: Postnatal lung inflammation increased by ventilation of preterm lambs exposed antenatally to E. coli endotoxin. Pediatr Res 52:356, 2002.

48. Van Marter LJ, et al: Chorioamnionitis, mechanical ventilation, and postnatal sepsis as modulators of chronic lung disease in preterm infants. J Pediatr 140:171, 2002.

49. Kramer BW, et al: Intratracheal endotoxin causes systemic inflammation in ventilated preterm lambs. Am J Respir Crit Care Med 165:463, 2002.

50. Crowley P: Antenatal corticosteroid therapy: a meta-analysis of the randomized trials: 1972–1994. Am J Obstet Gynecol 173:322, 1995.

51. Bunton TE, Plopper CG: Triamcinolone-induced structural alterations in the development of the lung of the fetal rhesus macaque. Am J Obstet Gynecol 148:203, 1984.

52. Johnson JWC, et al: Glucocorticoids and the rhesus fetal lung. Am J Obstet Gynecol 130:905, 1978.

53. Willet KE, et al: Lung morphometry after repetitive antenatal glucocorticoid treatment in preterm sheep. Am J Respir Crit Care Med 163:1437, 2001.

54. Shimoya K, et al: Interleukin-8 in cord sera: a sensitive and specific marker for the detection of preterm chorioamnionitis. J Infect Dis 165:957, 1992.

55. Newnham JP, et al: The interactive effects of endotoxin with prenatal glucocorticoids on short-term lung function in sheep. Am J Obstet Gynecol 185:190, 2001.

56. Kallapur SG, et al: Maternal glucocorticoids increase endotoxin-induced lung inflammation in preterm lambs.

95

Eduardo Bancalari

Pathophysiology of Bronchopulmonary Dysplasia

Bronchopulmonary dysplasia (BPD) is one of the most frequent sequelae in infants who survive after prolonged mechanical ventilation. It is characterized by chronic respiratory failure, and in more severe cases it may be associated with pulmonary hypertension and cor pulmonale. The infants with BPD described originally required prolonged mechanical ventilation because of severe respiratory failure resulting from hyaline membrane disease.[1] Today, most infants who have BPD are small premature babies who require prolonged mechanical ventilation because of poor respiratory effort and apnea.[2] The most important pathogenic factors that contribute to chronic lung damage include prematurity with incomplete lung development, mechanical trauma, oxygen toxicity, perinatal and nosocomial infections, patent ductus arteriosus (PDA) and pulmonary edema, and airway injury and obstruction. The interaction of these multiple factors leads to the final morphologic and functional alterations of the lungs observed in these infants.

Although mechanical trauma and oxygen toxicity are still considered important pathogenic factors in the development of the more severe form of BPD, currently, with the increased use of prenatal steroids and the administration of exogenous surfactant, the initial respiratory course is usually milder, and therefore, infants are exposed to much lower airway pressures and oxygen concentrations. Still, many of them gradually develop increasing oxygen requirements and show persistent radiographic changes compatible with BPD. Although it is possible that these low levels of airway pressure and oxygen exposure may be sufficient to damage the immature lung, it is likely that other factors play a more important role in the development of the milder lung damage observed in these infants.

Increasing evidence suggests that inflammation plays a major role in the pathogenesis of BPD.[3] This inflammatory response can be triggered by numerous factors including ventilation with excessive tidal volumes,[4] free oxygen radicals,[5-7] increased pulmonary blood flow from PDA,[8] and various antenatal and postnatal infections.[9-15] The possible role of antenatal infections has been suggested by publications showing an increased risk of BPD in infants born to mothers with evidence of chorioamnionitis.[16-18] Several inflammatory cytokines were found in higher concentrations in the amniotic fluid of mothers who delivered infants who developed BPD.[19,20] In addition, data suggest a higher risk of BPD in infants whose airways are colonized with *Ureaplasma urealyticum* or other bacteria.[21-23] A significant increase in inflammatory cells, eicosanoids, and various cytokines has been demonstrated in the airways of infants who subsequently develop BPD.[24-31] The increase in cytokine concentrations has been documented from the first days after birth, a finding supporting the contention that the inflammatory process can start before birth and is secondary to an infection of the amniotic cavity and the fetal lung. Among the markers of inflammation that have been found in high concentrations in tracheobronchial secretions of infants who develop BPD are neutrophils,[24, 25] macrophages,[26] leukotrienes,[28] platelet-activating factor,[27] interleukin-6,[29, 31] interleukin-8,[30] and tumor necrosis factor.[31] Evidence of pulmonary alveolar macrophage activation has also been reported in infants who subsequently developed BPD.[32] These activated pulmonary alveolar macrophages have been suggested as a source of neutrophil chemoattractants, especially when exposed to hyperoxia.[33] Neonates who develop BPD also have elevated concentrations of fibronectin in lung lavage fluid.[34, 35] This high molecular weight protein is released from pulmonary alveolar macrophages, epithelial and endothelial cells, and fibroblasts and is associated with the development of pulmonary fibrosis. An increase in elastase and an imbalance between elastase and a protease inhibitor in the lung have also been postulated as an important mechanism for the development of neonatal lung injury.[36-39] Urine excretion of elastic degradation products is greater in neonates who develop BPD than in controls.[40] This is of particular concern in light of evidence of a marked reduction in alveolar septation in lungs of infants who died of severe BPD.[41, 42]

In extremely low birth weight infants, systemic nosocomial infections and episodes of symptomatic PDA are strong predictors for the development of BPD.[2, 43] Furthermore, when both complications (infection and PDA) occur at the same time, there is a synergistic interaction that further increases the risk of developing BPD (Fig. 95-1).[44] As a consequence of the left-to-right shunting through the PDA, pulmonary blood flow and lung fluid increase, negatively affecting lung function and gas exchange, and this also increases the risk of BPD.[45] The presence of a PDA has been associated with elevated concentrations of myeloperoxidase in the tracheobronchial fluid, a finding suggesting that the increased pulmonary blood flow may result in damage of the pulmonary endothelium with adhesion and migration of polymorphonuclear leukocytes into the lung tissue.[8]

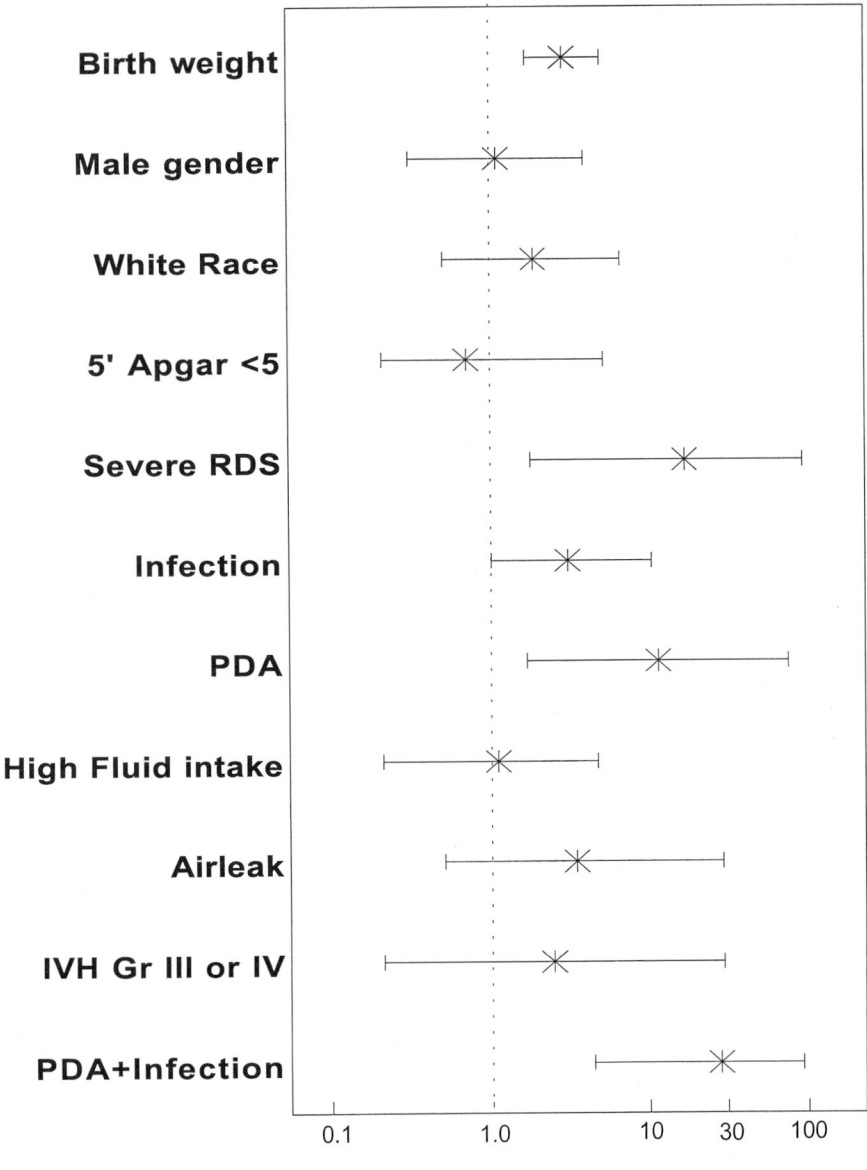

ODDS RATIO FOR CLD

Figure 95–1. Odds ratios and their 95% confidence intervals for bronchopulmonary dysplasia, from logistic regression analysis of infants who survived 28 or more days after birth (*n* = 105). CLD = chronic lung disease; IVH = intraventricular hemorrhage; PDA = patent ductus arteriosus; RDS = respiratory distress syndrome. (From Gonzalez A, et al: *J Pediatr* *128*:470, 1996.)

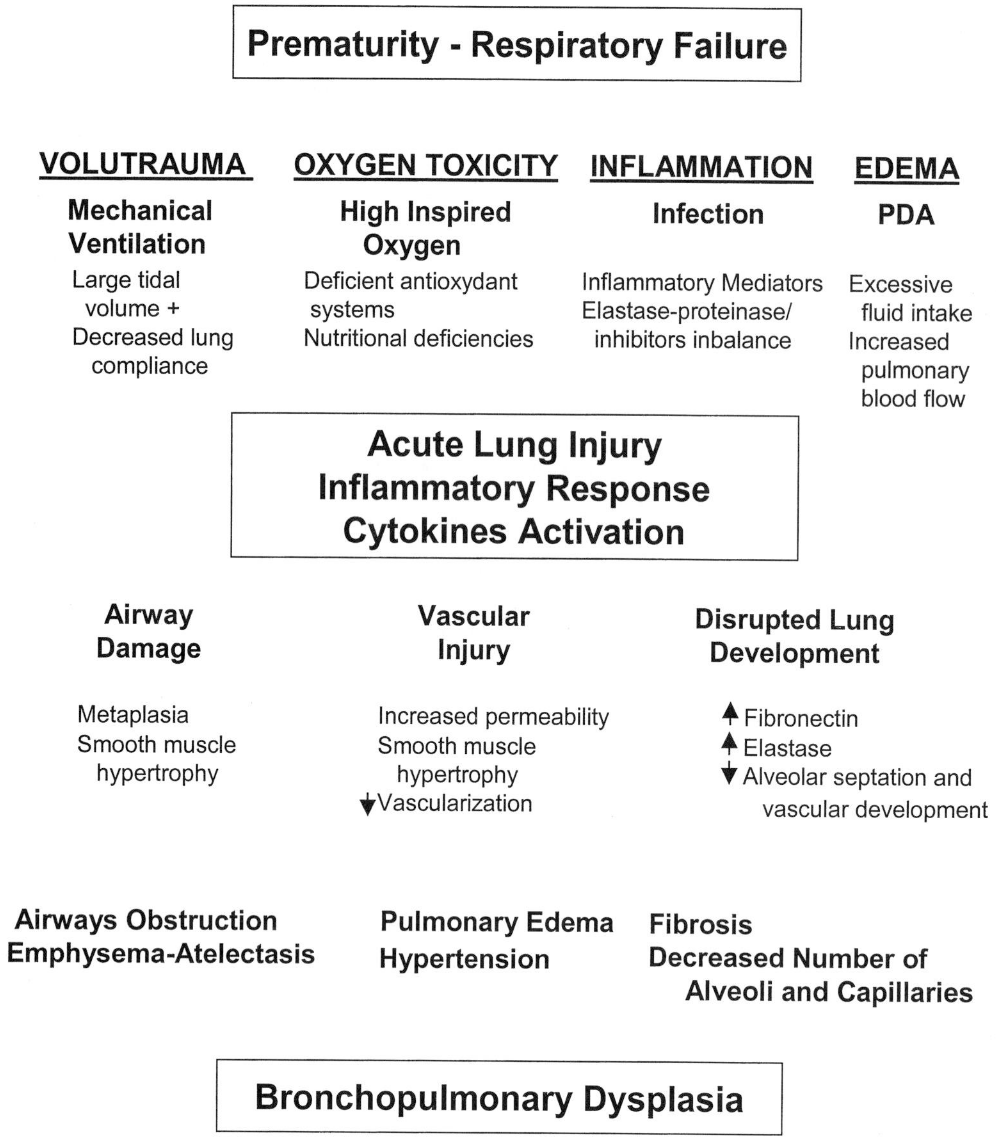

Prematurity - Respiratory Failure

VOLUTRAUMA

Mechanical Ventilation

Large tidal volume + Decreased lung compliance

OXYGEN TOXICITY

High Inspired Oxygen

Deficient antioxydant systems
Nutritional deficiencies

INFLAMMATION

Infection

Inflammatory Mediators
Elastase-proteinase/ inhibitors inbalance

EDEMA

PDA

Excessive fluid intake
Increased pulmonary blood flow

Acute Lung Injury Inflammatory Response Cytokines Activation

Airway Damage

Metaplasia
Smooth muscle hypertrophy

Vascular Injury

Increased permeability
Smooth muscle hypertrophy
▼Vascularization

Disrupted Lung Development

▲ Fibronectin
▲ Elastase
▼ Alveolar septation and vascular development

Airways Obstruction Emphysema-Atelectasis

Pulmonary Edema Hypertension

Fibrosis Decreased Number of Alveoli and Capillaries

Bronchopulmonary Dysplasia

Figure 95–2. Pathophysiology of bronchopulmonary dysplasia. PDA = patent ductus arteriosus.

Other factors have been proposed as having a pathogenic role in BPD. Vitamin A deficiency has been proposed to play a role, because of evidence that infants who develop BPD have lower vitamin A levels than those who recover without chronic lung damage.[46] This possible association is supported by the similarities between some of the airway epithelial changes observed in both BPD and in vitamin A deficiency and by clinical evidence that vitamin A administration in the first weeks of life affords some degree of protection against BPD.[47, 48] Another factor suggested to play a role in the development of BPD in extremely premature infants is early adrenal insufficiency. Infants with lower cortisol levels in the first week of life have an increased incidence of lung inflammation and BPD, and early treatment with low-dose hydrocortisone increases survival without BPD.[49-51]

The major problem in the prevention of BPD is that as the initial lung damage develops, it produces a progressive deterioration in lung function and gas exchange that makes necessary the use of higher peak airway pressures and inspired oxygen concentrations. This initiates a cycle in which the required treatment—mechanical ventilation and oxygen therapy—induces more lung damage and exacerbates the respiratory failure. Figure 95-2 summarizes some of the most important pathogenic factors in BPD.

PULMONARY FUNCTION IN INFANTS WITH BRONCHOPULMONARY DYSPLASIA

The alterations in pulmonary function in infants with BPD are nonspecific and reflect the severe disruption of lung architecture that occurs in these infants. The degree of abnormality in lung function may range from mild to severe, paralleling the clinical and radiographic presentation. There are few studies that describe the early changes in lung function in infants who subsequently develop BPD or that have followed longitudinally the course of these infants' lung function.

Lung Function in Early Bronchopulmonary Dysplasia

Infants who develop BPD appear to have different lung function early in the evolution of their respiratory failure than do infants who recover without lung sequelae. Higher airway resistance was found during the first weeks of life in infants who subsequently developed BPD than in infants who recovered without lung damage.[52, 53] This finding suggests that early airway obstruction may be a marker or a predisposing factor for the development of more severe pulmonary damage. Measurements of lung

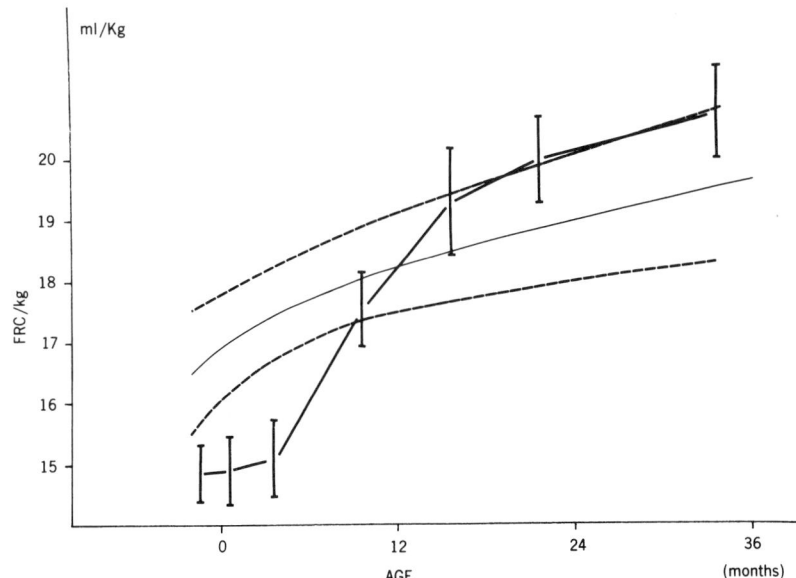

Figure 95–3. Sequential measurements of functional residual capacity (FRC) per kilogram in infants with chronic lung disease (mean ± SE, *heavy line*). Measurements were shifted to the left to correct for preterm birth. For comparison, curve for physiologically normal infants *(thin line)* and its 95% confidence limits *(dashed lines)* are shown. (From Gerhardt T, et al: J Pediatr *110:*448, 1987.)

compliance during the first week of life have also shown lower values in infants who later developed BPD.[54-56]

Lung mechanics measurements during the first week of life have been used to improve the accuracy of BPD prediction models.[57, 58] Although the added predictive value of pulmonary resistance has been inconsistent, models that include gestational age and pulmonary compliance have displayed the highest predictive accuracy. The low initial pulmonary compliance in infants who ultimately develop BPD is most likely a reflection of the severity of the acute respiratory illness in these infants.

Lung Function in Established Bronchopulmonary Dysplasia

Ventilation

Tidal volume is normal or reduced, and respiratory rate is increased in most of these infants, and the result is normal or increased minute ventilation.[59] This can lead to increased dead space ventilation that contributes to the hypercapnia observed in infants with severe BPD.

Distribution of Ventilation. The morphologic alterations in the lungs of infants with BPD result in a severe disruption of the relationship between ventilation and perfusion. The damage to the small airways produces different time constants in different areas of the lungs that alter the distribution of the inspired gas.[60] The disturbed ventilation/perfusion relationships lead to an increased arterial-alveolar gradient for carbon dioxide in areas that are ventilated but poorly perfused (high ventilation/perfusion ratio) and an increased alveolar-arterial oxygen gradient caused by poorly or nonventilated areas that receive blood flow (low ventilation/perfusion ratio). Studies evaluating regional excretion of xenon have demonstrated very limited ventilation of the overdistended areas, whereas perfusion is relatively preserved.[61] Nitrogen clearance delay studies have confirmed the presence of slowly ventilated compartments in infants with severe BPD.[60]

Lung Volume

Lung volume measurements in infants with BPD have given variable results, depending on the age of the infants. Functional residual capacity values lower than normal were reported during the first month of life, but they increased to above normal by 6 to 16 months of age (Fig. 95-3).[62,63] The later increase in lung volume in infants with BPD may reflect gas trapping secondary to small airways obstruction.

Lung Compliance

Dynamic lung compliance is consistently decreased in infants with BPD (Fig. 95-4).[62,63] This may reflect changes in the elastic properties of the lung secondary to fibrosis and interstitial fluid accumulation. Compliance may also be reduced by alterations in surfactant metabolism, which have been described in infants with BPD.[64] The decrease in dynamic compliance also reflects the increase in small airway resistance that produces frequency dependence of compliance. Overdistention of portions of the lung resulting from gas trapping can further contribute to the decrease in compliance.

Therapeutic intervention with diuretics, bronchodilators, and systemic steroids results in a reduction in airway resistance and improves lung compliance in these infants.[65-69] Similar results have been reported after the administration of inhaled nebulized furosemide[70] or beclomethasone.[71]

Airway Resistance

One of the most striking and consistent changes in lung function in infants with severe BPD is increased airway resistance (see Fig. 95-4). This can lead to severe maldistribution of the inspired gas,[60] lung overdistention from gas trapping, and hypoventilation secondary to increased work of breathing.

The mechanisms for increased airway resistance include several factors that contribute to airway damage and obstruction. During the initial stages of BPD, there is cell damage, with hyperplasia and squamous metaplasia of the airway epithelial lining. Infection and inflammatory reaction in the airways increase mucus secretion. In addition, there may be a decreased clearance of mucus resulting from depression of ciliary activity. Infants with severe BPD have hypertrophy of the smooth muscle surrounding the airways,[1,72] and this plays an important role in the increased airway resistance and airway hyperactivity observed in these infants. Increased production of inflammatory mediators, such as leukotrienes and platelet-activating factor, may also contribute to airway smooth muscle constriction and increased pulmonary resistance.[28, 73, 74] A more frequent family history of asthma in infants with BPD raises the possibility that genetically determined airway hyperactivity may also contribute to the development of BPD in some cases.[75, 76] The increase in airway resistance is not specific to infants with BPD, but it is

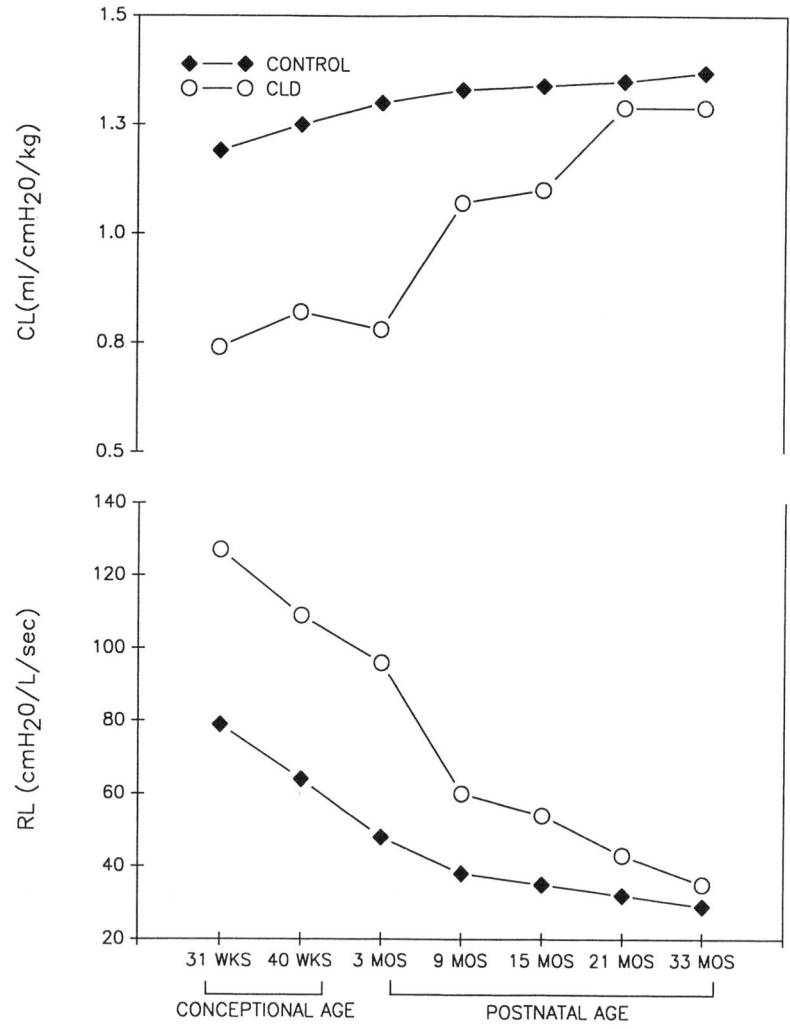

Figure 95–4. Sequential measurements of lung compliance (CL) and resistance (RL) in infants with chronic lung disease and in normal controls. (Modified from Gerhardt R, et al: J Pediatr *110*:448, 1987.)

observed in most infants who receive mechanical ventilation, regardless of whether they develop BPD.[77] The increase in airway resistance combined with lower compliance is responsible for a marked increase in the work of breathing and alveolar hypoventilation and carbon dioxide retention that are characteristic of these infants. The degree of airway damage is not uniform throughout the lung; this variability determines the abnormal distribution of ventilation and the development of areas of overdistention alternating with areas of collapse observed in cases of severe BPD.

The exact location of the obstruction has not been defined, but forced expiratory flows at functional residual capacity are decreased.[78] This finding suggests that the damage is at the level of the small airways. In infants with severe BPD, large airways are also compromised and may demonstrate increased collapsibility that develops during active expiration as a result of tracheomalacia or bronchomalacia.[79,80] This alteration is responsible for the severe deterioration in gas exchange observed in some of these infants during periods of agitation, when they generate positive intrathoracic pressure. These episodes can be ameliorated by using sedation or by maintaining a relatively high positive endexpiratory airway pressure.[81,82]

Of interest are observations that demonstrate increased airway resistance and functional residual capacity in infants with BPD in response to a reduction in their inspired oxygen concentration.[83,84] This could also explain the episodic airway obstruction often observed in infants with BPD. Cold air or methacholine challenge also produces a marked increase in pulmonary resistance in these patients.[85-87]

The increased airway resistance in infants with BPD is partially reversible with bronchodilators[88-94] or diuretic therapy.[67,95-99] This finding suggests that the increased airway resistance results from a combination of airway hyperreactivity and interstitial pulmonary edema, both of which play a role in the obstruction of the small airways. The administration of systemic or inhaled steroids has also been demonstrated to reduce the airway obstruction in infants with BPD.[66,69,71]

Gas Exchange

Most infants with severe BPD exhibit marked hypoxemia and hypercapnia and require supplemental oxygen to maintain a normal partial pressure of oxygen. This hypoxemia is mainly the result of an abnormal ventilation/perfusion relationship and alveolar hypoventilation. The oxygen requirement decreases gradually as the disease process subsides, but it may increase during sleep, feedings, physical activity, or episodes of pulmonary infection or edema.

The increased partial pressure of carbon dioxide is secondary to alveolar hypoventilation and to an increased arterial-alveolar carbon dioxide gradient produced by a mismatch of ventilation and perfusion and increased alveolar dead space. The chronic hypercapnia is often accompanied by an increased serum bicarbonate concentration that tends to compensate for the respiratory acidosis. This increase in plasma base can be exaggerated by diuretics, which are frequently used in infants with BPD.

Metabolic Rate

Infants with BPD have an increased metabolic rate, close to 25% higher than that of matched controls.[100] This increase in oxygen consumption is at least in part the result of the increased work of breathing and is one of the factors that may interfere with normal growth in these infants.[101] The increased metabolic rate can also impose an extra load on the respiratory system and can contribute to respiratory failure in infants with severe BPD. This may become evident when carbon dioxide production is suddenly increased, such as during a glucose load, which can aggravate hypercapnia in these infants.[102]

Long-Term Lung Function in Infants With Bronchopulmonary Dysplasia

Few studies have evaluated long-term lung function in infants with BPD. Because the initial damage occurs at a time when the lung is in one of the most active phases of growth and development, it is very likely that some of the alterations in lung structure and function will persist through adulthood.

Gerhardt and colleagues[63] performed serial pulmonary function evaluations in a group of infants up to 3 years of age with relatively mild BPD. Lung function showed gradual improvement over time, and at the end of the follow-up period, the values for compliance and resistance were close to the normal range (see Fig. 95–4). In infants with severe BPD, persistent alterations in lung function have been reported beyond 3 years of age,[103] whereas in some patients abnormalities persist at the end of the first and second decades,[85, 86] a finding suggesting that the lung damage, when severe, persists into adulthood.

Morphometric studies performed in lungs from children who died of severe BPD between the ages 2 and 28 months revealed a striking reduction in the number of alveoli compared with the lungs of control subjects.[42] This abnormality results in a significant reduction in the lung surface area available for gas exchange. In contrast, pulmonary function studies done in children with BPD who have reached school age suggest continued lung growth, as indicated by an increase in total lung capacity and improved airway function.[104]

CARDIOVASCULAR FUNCTION IN INFANTS WITH BRONCHOPULMONARY DYSPLASIA

Pulmonary Hypertension: Cor Pulmonale

Pulmonary hypertension and right ventricular hypertrophy are commonly observed in infants with severe BPD, and in many instances, pulmonary hypertension is responsible for a deterioration in the clinical condition or the demise of these infants.[72, 105] Pulmonary hypertension has been documented by direct pressure measurements during cardiac catheterization and indirectly by echocardiography.[105-107] The specific mechanisms that result in increased pulmonary vascular resistance in these infants are many and include alveolar hypoxia, increased alveolar pressure and overdistention, and release of mediators of inflammation such as platelet-activating factor and leukotriene B_4.[27] Postmortem examination of the lungs of infants with BPD frequently reveals hypertrophy of the smooth muscle in the pulmonary vessels and muscle extension into intra-acinar arteries.[72] In some cases, there is also evidence of thromboembolism in the lumina of pulmonary vessels.[108] A slowing in the growth and development of the pulmonary vessels may also occur in these infants and may contribute to the increased pulmonary vascular resistance. The bronchial arteries in infants with BPD are abnormally prominent,

and communications exist between those arteries and the pulmonary circulation through precapillary collateral vessels.[109] These anastomoses may develop in preexisting channels that dilate, or they may occur in granulation tissue seen in the lungs of patients with BPD. More importantly, they may aggravate the existing pulmonary hypertension. The pulmonary hypertension in infants with BPD is usually responsive to an increase in the inspired oxygen concentration, demonstrating a reactive pulmonary vascular bed.[106,107,110] Nevertheless, the values frequently remain substantially higher than normal, a finding reflecting the loss in cross-sectional area resulting from inadequate development or structural remodeling of the pulmonary vascular bed.

Systemic hypertension has also been described in infants with BPD.[111] The mechanism for this hypertension is not clear, but it may contribute to the left ventricular dysfunction and hypertrophy observed in many of these patients.[112] This hypertrophy can also be secondary to an increased afterload of the left ventricle. Left ventricular overload results from the higher negative intrathoracic pressure generated by these infants to overcome the increased mechanical impedance of their respiratory system. Right ventricular hypertrophy can also interfere with left ventricular function and can contribute to the hypertrophy of this ventricle. Decreased pulmonary vascular clearance of catecholamines has been reported in infants with severe BPD, and it may contribute to the systemic hypertension observed in some of these patients.[113] The use of vasodilators such as the calcium channel blocker nifedipine can be effective in improving cardiovascular function in infants with severe BPD.[114,115] Inhaled nitric oxide has also been used in infants with BPD to decrease pulmonary vascular resistance and to improve ventilation perfusion matching. Nitric oxide may also modulate the inflammatory process in the lung. Although results have not been consistent, some studies have shown an improvement in oxygenation during nitric oxide administration.[116-118]

REFERENCES

1. Northway WH Jr, et al: Pulmonary disease following respirator therapy of hyaline membrane disease: bronchopulmonary dysplasia. N Engl J Med 276:357, 1967.
2. Rojas M, et al: Changing trends in the epidemiology and pathogenesis of neonatal chronic lung disease. J Pediatr 126:605, 1995.
3. Pierce MR, et al: The role of inflammation in the pathogenesis of bronchopulmonary dysplasia. Pediatr Pulmonol 19:371, 1995.
4. Dreyfuss D, Saumon G: Ventilator-induced lung injury: lessons from experimental studies. Am J Respir Crit Care Med 157:294, 1998.
5. Saugstad OD: Bronchopulmonary dysplasia and oxidative stress: are we closer to an understanding of the pathogenesis of BPD? Acta Paediatr 86:1277, 1997.
6. Banks BA, et al: Plasma 3-Nitrotyrosine is elevated in premature infants who develop bronchopulmonary dysplasia. Pediatrics 101:870, 1998.
7. Ogihara T, et al: New evidence for the involvement of oxygen radicals in triggering neonatal chronic lung disease. Pediatr Res 39:117, 1996.
8. Varsila E, et al: Closure of patent ductus arteriosus decreases pulmonary myeloperoxidase in premature infants with respiratory distress syndrome. Biol Neonate 67:167, 1995.
9. Coalson JJ, et al: Bacterial colonization and infection studies in the premature baboon with bronchopulmonary dysplasia. Am Rev Respir Dis 144:1140, 1991.
10. Cassell GH, et al: Perinatal mycoplasmal infectious. Clin Perinatal 18:241, 1991.
11. Piedra PA, et al: Description of an adenovirus type 8 outbreak in hospitalized neonates born prematurely. Pediatr Infect Dis J 11:460, 1992.
12. Numazaki K, et al: Chronic respiratory disease in premature infants caused by Chlamydia trachomatis. J Clin Pathol 39:84, 1986.
13. Ballard RA, et al: Acquired cytomegalovirus in preterm infants. Am J Dis Child 133:482, 1979.
14. Watts DH, et al: The association of occult amniotic fluid infection with gestational age and neonatal outcome among women in preterm labor. Obstet Gynecol 79:351, 1992.
15. Couroucli XI, et al: Detection of microorganisms in tracheal aspirates of preterm infants by polymerase chain reaction: association of adenovirus infection with bronchopulmonary dysplasia. Pediatr Res 47:225, 2000.
16. Watterberg KL, et al: Chorioamnionitis and early lung inflammation in infants in whom bronchopulmonary dysplasia develops. Pediatrics 97:210, 1996.

17. Matsuda T, et al: Necrotizing funisitis: clinical significance and association with chronic lung disease in premature infants. Am J Obstet Gynecol 177:1402, 1997.

18. Van Marter LJ, et al: For the developmental epidemiology: chorioamnionitis, mechanical ventilation, and postnatal sepsis as modulators of chronic lung disease in preterm infants. J Pediatr 140:171, 2002.

19. Yoon BH, et al: Amniotic fluid cytokines (interleukin-6 tumor necrosis factor-α, interleukin-1ß, and interleukin-8) and the risk for the development of bronchopulmonary dysplasia. Am J Obstet Gynecol 177:825, 1997.

20. Yoon BH, et al: A systemic fetal inflammatory response and the development of bronchopulmonary dysplasia. Am J Obstet Gynecol 181:773, 1999.

21. Cassell GH, et al: Association of Ureaplasma urealyticum infection of the lower respiratory tract with chronic lung disease and death in very low birth weight infants. Lancet 2:240, 1998.

22. Wang EEL, et al: Association of Ureaplasma urealyticum colonization with chronic lung disease of prematurity: results of a metaanalysis. J Pediatr 127:640, 1995.

23. Groneck P, et al: Bronchoalveolar inflammation following airway infection in preterm infants with chronic lung disease. Pediatr Pulmonol 31:331, 2001.

24. Merritt TA, et al: Cytologic evaluation of pulmonary effluent in neonates with respiratory distress syndrome and bronchopulmonary dysplasia. Acta Cytol 25:631, 1981.

25. Todd DA, et al: Cytological changes in endotracheal aspirates associated with chronic lung disease. Early Hum Dev 51:13, 1998.

26. Clement A, et al: Alveolar macrophage status in bronchopulmonary dysplasia. Pediatr Res 23:470, 1988.

27. Stenmark KR, et al: Potential role of eicosanoids and PAF in the pathophysiology of bronchopulmonary dysplasia. Am Rev Respir Dis 136:770, 1987.

28. Mirro R, et al: Increased airway leukotriene levels in infants with severe bronchopulmonary dysplasia. Am J Dis Child 144:160, 1990.

29. Grigg JM, et al: Increased levels of bronchoalveolar lavage fluid interleukin-6 in preterm ventilated infants after prolonged rupture of membranes. Am Rev Respir Dis 145:782, 1992.

30. Groneck P, et al: Association of pulmonary inflammation and increased microvascular permeability during the development of bronchopulmonary dysplasia: a sequential analysis of inflammatory mediators in respiratory fluids of high- risk preterm neonates. Pediatrics 93:712, 1994.

31. Jónsson B, et al: Early increase of TNFα and IL-6 in tracheobronchial aspirate fluid indicator of subsequent chronic lung disease in preterm infants. Arch Dis Child 77:F198, 1997.

32. Irving LB, et al: Alveolar macrophage activation in bronchopulmonary dysplasia. Am Rev Respir Dis 133(Suppl A):207, 1986.

33. Harada RN, et al: Macrophage effect or function in pulmonary oxygen toxicity: hyperoxia damages and stimulates alveolar macrophages to make and release chemotaxis for polymorphonuclear leukocytes. J Leukoc Biol 35:373, 1984.

34. Watts CL, Bruce MC: Effect of dexamethasone on fibronectin and albumin levels in lung secretion of infants with BPD. J Pediatr 121:597, 1992.

35. Gerdes JS, et al: Tracheal lavage and plasma fibronectin: relationship to respiratory distress syndrome and development of bronchopulmonary dysplasia. J Pediatr 108:601, 1986.

36. Watterberg KL, et al: Secretory leukocyte protease inhibitor and lung inflammation in developing bronchopulmonary dysplasia. J Pediatr 125:264, 1994.

37. Ogden BE, et al: Neonatal lung neutrophil and elastase/proteinase inhibitor imbalance. Am Rev Respir Dis 130:817, 1984.

38. Walti H, et al: Persistent elastase/proteinase inhibitor imbalance during prolonged ventilation of infants with BPD: evidence for the role of nosocomial infections. Pediatr Res 26:351, 1989.

39. Bruce MC, et al: Risk factors for the degradation of lung elastic fibers in the ventilated neonate. Am Rev Respir Dis 146:204, 1992.

40. Bruce MC, et al: Altered urinary excretion of elastin cross-links in premature infants who develop bronchopulmonary dysplasia. Am Rev Respir Dis 131:568, 1985.

41. Husain AN, et al: Pathology of arrested acinar development in postsurfactant bronchopulmonary dysplasia. Hum Pathol 29:710, 1998.

42. Margraf LR, et al: Morphometric analysis of the lung in BPD. Am Rev Respir Dis 143:391, 1991.

43. Marshall DD, et al: Risk factors for chronic lung disease in the surfactant era: a North Carolina population-based study of very low birth weight infants. Pediatrics 104:1345, 1999.

44. Gonzalez A, et al: Influence of infection on patent ductus arteriosus and chronic lung disease in premature infants weighting 1000 grams or less. J Pediatr 128:470, 1996.

45. Gerhardt T, Bancalari E: Lung compliance in newborns with patent ductus arteriosus before and after surgical ligation. Biol Neonate 38:96, 1980.

46. Shenai JP, et al: Vitamin A status of neonates with bronchopulmonary dysplasia. Pediatr Res. 19:185, 1985.

47. Shenai JP: Vitamin A supplementation in very low birth weight neonates: rational and evidence. Pediatrics 104:1369, 1999.

48. Tyson JE, et al: Vitamin A Supplementation for extremely-low-birth-weight infants. N Engl J Med 340:1962, 1999.

49. Watterberg KL, Scott SM: Evidence of early adrenal insufficiency in babies who develop bronchopulmonary dysplasia. Pediatrics 95: 120, 1995.

50. Watterberg KL, et al: Prophylaxis against early adrenal insufficiency to prevent chronic lung disease in premature infants. Pediatrics 104:1258, 1999.

51. Watterberg KL, et al: Links between early adrenal function and respiratory outcome in preterm infants: airway inflammation and patent ductus arteriosus. Pediatrics 150:320, 2000.

52. Goldman SL, et al: Early prediction of chronic lung disease by pulmonary function testing. J Pediatr 102:613, 1983.

53. Motoyama EK, et al: Early onset of airway reactivity in premature infants with bronchopulmonary dysplasia. Am Rev Respir Dis 136:50, 1987.

54. Graff MA, et al: Compliance measurement in respiratory distress syndrome: the prediction of outcome. Pediatr Pulmonol 2:332, 1986.

55. Greenspan JS, et al: Sequential changes in pulmonary mechanics in the very low birth weight (≤1000 grams) infant. J Pediatr 113:732, 1988.

56. Van Lierde S, et al: Pulmonary mechanics during respiratory distress syndrome in the prediction of outcome and differentiation of mild and severe bronchopulmonary dysplasia. Pediatr Pulmonol 17:218, 1994.

57. Bhutani VK, Abbasi S: Relative likelihood of bronchopulmonary dysplasia based on pulmonary mechanics measured in preterm neonates during the first week of life. J Pediatr 120:605, 1992.

58. Freezer NJ, Sly PD: Predictive value of measurements of respiratory mechanics in preterm infants with HMD. Pediatr Pulmonol 16:116, 1993.

59. Morray JP, et al: Improvement in lung mechanics as a function of age in the infant with severe bronchopulmonary dysplasia. Pediatr Res 16:290, 1982.

60. Watts JL, et al: Chronic pulmonary disease in neonates after artificial ventilation: distribution of ventilation and pulmonary interstitial emphysema. Pediatrics 60:273, 1977.

61. Moylan FMB, Shannon DC: Preferential distribution of lobar emphysema and atelectasis in bronchopulmonary dysplasia. Pediatrics 63:130, 1979.

62. Bryan MH, et al: Pulmonary function studies during the first year of life in infants recovering from respiratory distress syndrome. Pediatrics 52:169, 1973.

63. Gerhardt T, et al: Serial determination of pulmonary function in infants with chronic lung disease. J Pediatr 110:448, 1987.

64. Clement A, et al: Decreased phosphatidylcholine content in bronchoalveolar lavage fluids of children with bronchopulmonary dysplasia: a preliminary investigation. Pediatr Pulmonol 3:67, 1987.

65. Brundage KL, et al: Dexamethasone therapy for bronchopulmonary dysplasia: improved respiratory mechanics without adrenal suppression. Pediatr Pulmonol 12:162, 1992.

66. Gladstone IM, et al: Pulmonary function tests and fluid balance in neonates with chronic lung disease during dexamethasone treatment. Pediatrics 84:1072, 1989.

67. Kao LC, et al: Randomized trial of long-term diuretic therapy for infants with oxygen-dependent bronchopulmonary dysplasia. J Pediatr 124:772, 1994.

68. Rotschild A, et al: Increased compliance in response to salbutamol in premature infants with developing bronchopulmonary dysplasia. J Pediatr 115:984, 1989.

69. Yoder MC Jr, et al: Effect of dexamethasone on pulmonary inflammation and pulmonary function of ventilator-dependent infants with bronchopulmonary dysplasia. Am Rev Respir Dis 143:1044, 1991.

70. Rastogi A, et al: Nebulized furosemide in infants with bronchopulmonary dysplasia. J Pediatr 125:976, 1994.

71. LaForce WR, Brudno S: Controlled trial of beclomethasone dipropionate by nebulization in oxygen- and ventilator-dependent infants. J Pediatr 122:285, 1993.

72. Taghizadeh A, Reynolds EOR: Pathogenesis of bronchopulmonary dysplasia following hyaline membrane disease. Am J Pathol 82:241, 1976.

73. Motoyama E, et al: Early appearance of neutrophil chemotaxis leuktorine B₄(LTB₄) and airway reactivity in infants with bronchopulmonary dysplasia. Am Rev Respir Dis 133:A207, 1986.

74. Stenmark KR, et al: Recovery of platelet activating factor and leukotrienes from infants with severe bronchopulmonary dysplasia: clinical improvement with cromolyn treatment. Am Rev Respir Dis 131:A236, 1985.

75. Bertrand JM, et al: The long term pulmonary sequelae of prematurity: the role of familial airway hyperreactivity and the respiratory distress syndrome. N Engl J Med 312:742, 1985.

76. Nickerson BG, Taussig LM: Family history of asthma in infants with bronchopulmonary dysplasia. Pediatrics 65:1140, 1980.

77. Stocks J, Godfrey S: The role of artificial ventilation, oxygen, and CPAP in the pathogenesis of lung damage in neonates: assessment by serial measurements of lung function. Pediatrics 57:352, 1976.

78. Tepper RS, et al: Expiratory flow limitation in infants with bronchopulmonary dysplasia. J Pediatr 109:1040, 1986.

79. Miller RW, et al: Tracheobronchial abnormalities in infants with bronchopulmonary dysplasia. J Pediatr 111:779, 1987.

80. Sotomayor JL, et al: Large-airway collapse due to acquired tracheobronchomalacia in infancy. Am J Dis Child 140:367, 1986.

81. McCoy KS, et al: Spirometric and endoscopic evaluation of airway collapse in infants with bronchopulmonary dysplasia. Pediatr Pulmonol 14:23, 1992.

82. Panitch HB, et al: Effects of CPAP on lung mechanics in infants with acquired tracheobronchomalacia. Am J Respir Crit Care Med 150:1341, 1994.

83. Teague WP, et al: An acute reduction in the fraction of inspired oxygen increases airway constriction in infants with chronic lung disease. Am Rev Respir Dis 137:861, 1988.

84. Tay-Uyboco JS, et al: Hypoxic airway constriction in infants of very low birth weight recovering from moderate to severe bronchopulmonary dysplasia. J Pediatr *115:*456, 1989.

85. Smyth JA, et al: Pulmonary function and bronchial hyper-reactivity in long-term survivors of bronchopulmonary dysplasia. Pediatrics *68:*336, 1981.

86. Northway WH, et al: Late pulmonary sequelae of bronchopulmonary dysplasia. N Engl J Med *323:*1793, 1990.

87. Greenspan JS, et al: Airway reactivity as determined by a cold air challenge in infants with bronchopulmonary dysplasia. J Pediatr *114:*452, 1989.

88. Brundage KL, et al: Bronchodilator response to ipratropium bromide in infants with bronchopulmonary dysplasia. Am Rev Respir Dis *142:*1137, 1990.

89. Cabal LA, et al: Effects of metaproterenol on pulmonary mechanics, oxygenation, and ventilation in infants with chronic lung disease. J Pediatr *110:*116, 1987.

90. Gomez-Del Rio M, et al: Effect of a beta-agonist nebulization on lung function in neonates with increased pulmonary resistance. Pediatr Pulmonol *2:*287, 1986.

91. Kao LC, et al: Effect of isoproterenol inhalation on airway resistance in chronic bronchopulmonary dysplasia. Pediatrics *73:*509, 1984.

92. Stefano JL, et al: A randomized placebo-controlled study to evaluate the effects of oral albuterol on pulmonary mechanics in ventilator-dependent infants at risk of developing BPD. Pediatr Pulmonol *10:*183, 1991.

93. Wilkie RA, Bryan MH: Effect of bronchodilators on airway resistance in ventilator-dependent neonates with chronic lung disease. J Pediatr *111:*278, 1987.

94. Kao LC, et al: Effects of inhaled metaproterenol and atropine on the pulmonary mechanics of infants with bronchopulmonary dysplasia. Pediatr Pulmonol *6:*74, 1989.

95. Engelhardt B, et al: Short- and long-term effects of furosemide on lung function in infants with bronchopulmonary dysplasia. J Pediatr *109:*1034, 1986.

96. Kao LC, et al: Effect of oral diuretics on pulmonary mechanics in infants with chronic bronchopulmonary dysplasia: results of a double-blind crossover sequential trial. Pediatrics *74:*37, 1984.

97. Kao LC, et al: Oral theophylline and diuretics improve pulmonary mechanics in infants with bronchopulmonary dysplasia. J Pediatr *111:*439, 1987.

98. McCann EM, et al: Controlled trial of furosemide therapy in infants with chronic lung disease. J Pediatr *106:*957, 1985.

99. Rush MG, et al: Double-blind, placebo-controlled trial of alternate-day furosemide therapy in infants with chronic bronchopulmonary dysplasia. J Pediatr *117:*112, 1990.

100. Weinstein MR, Oh W: Oxygen consumption in infants with bronchopulmonary dysplasia. J Pediatr *99:*958, 1981.

101. Kurzner SI, et al: Growth failure in bronchopulmonary dysplasia: elevated metabolic rates and pulmonary mechanics. J Pediatr *112:*73, 1988.

102. Yunis KA, Oh W: Effects of intravenous glucose loading on oxygen consumption, carbon dioxide production, and resting energy expenditure in infants with bronchopulmonary dysplasia. J Pediatr *115:*127, 1989.

103. Mallory GB, et al: Longitudinal changes in lung function during the first three years of premature infants with moderate to severe bronchopulmonary dysplasia. Pediatr Pulmonol *11:*8, 1991.

104. Blayney M, et al: Bronchopulmonary dysplasia: improvement in lung function between 7 and 10 years of age. J Pediatr *118:*201, 1991.

105. Harrod JR, et al: Long-term follow-up of severe respiratory distress syndrome treated with IPPB. J Pediatr *84:*277, 1974.

106. Abman SH, et al: Pulmonary vascular response to oxygen in infants with severe bronchopulmonary dysplasia. Pediatrics *75:*80, 1985.

107. Berman W, Jr, et al: Evaluation of infants with bronchopulmonary dysplasia using cardiac catheterization. Pediatrics *70:*708, 1982.

108. Tomashefski JF, et al: BPD: a morphometric study with emphasis on the pulmonary vasculature. Pediatr Pathol *2:*469, 1984.

109. Goodman G, et al: Pulmonary hypertension in infants with bronchopulmonary dysplasia. J Pediatr *112:*67, 1988.

110. Halliday HL, et al: Effects of inspired oxygen on echocardiographic assessment of pulmonary vascular resistance and myocardial contractility in bronchopulmonary dysplasia. Pediatrics *65:*536, 1980.

111. Abman SH, et al: Systemic hypertension in infants with bronchopulmonary dysplasia. J Pediatr *104:*928, 1984.

112. Melnick G, et al: Normal pulmonary vascular resistance and left ventricular hypertrophy in young infants with bronchopulmonary dysplasia: an echocardiographic and pathologic study. Pediatrics *66:*589, 1980.

113. Abman SH, et al: Pulmonary vascular extraction of circulating norepinephrine in infants with bronchopulmonary dysplasia. Pediatr Pulmonol *3:*386, 1987.

114. Brownlee JR, et al: Acute hemodynamic effects of nifedipine in infants with bronchopulmonary dysplasia and pulmonary hypertension. Pediatr Res *24:*186, 1988.

115. Johnson CE, et al: Pharmacokinetics and pharmacodynamics of nifedipine in children with bronchopulmonary dysplasia and pulmonary hypertension. Pediatr Res *29:*500, 1991.

116. Banks BA, et al: Changes in oxygenation with inhaled nitric oxide in severe bronchopulmonary dysplasia. Pediatrics *103:*610, 1999.

117. Lonnqvist PA, et al: Inhaled nitric oxide in infants with developing or established chronic lung disease. Acta Paediatr *84:*118, 1995.

118. Clark PL, et al: Safety and efficacy of nitric oxide in chronic lung disease. Arch Dis Child *86:*F41, 2002.

Jay S. Greenspan, Thomas H. Shaffer, William W. Fox, and Alan R. Spitzer

96

Assisted Ventilation: Physiologic Implications and Complications

Mechanical ventilation is used in the treatment of neonatal pulmonary insufficiency. Since its introduction in the 1980s, it has been steadily refined, resulting in the successful treatment of many previously fatal diseases and dramatically improving the survival rate of many high-risk neonates. As with many other advances in medicine, however, this therapy has been accompanied by complications, particularly chronic lung injury or bronchopulmonary dysplasia (BPD).[1] This disease, unknown before the use of mechanical ventilation, has produced a population of patients who are ventilator or oxygen dependent, with serious accompanying morbidity and mortality.[2,3] A clear understanding of the physiology of mechanical ventilation is essential for the neonatologist to maximize the benefits and reduce the problems associated with its use.

This chapter provides a review of the physiologic and pathophysiologic processes in conventional mechanical ventilation of the neonate. Because acute and chronic neonatal lung disease is multifactorial in origin, virtually all aspects of neonatal care can be considered part of the ventilation strategy. The prevention of lung injury includes attention to issues such as infection, fluid management, patent ductus arteriosus, nutrition, anemia, and many other aspects of patient management. For the purposes of this chapter, however, the indications and implications of initiating mechanical ventilation are discussed, and some of the newer techniques of ventilation and lung protection are addressed.

PULMONARY PHYSIOLOGY AND PATHOPHYSIOLOGY: CONSIDERATIONS WITH ASSISTED VENTILATION

Although the design of the lung serves multiple functions, the primary structure and its placement within the thorax establish its main purpose as gas exchange. The respiratory system consists of a series of branching tubes that bring fresh gas from the atmosphere to the terminal air spaces, while allowing the elimination of respiratory byproducts of metabolism to flow from the alveoli back into the environment (Fig. 96-1). The diaphragm, the primary muscular force during quiet ventilation, contracts during inspiration, lowering intrapleural pressure. This

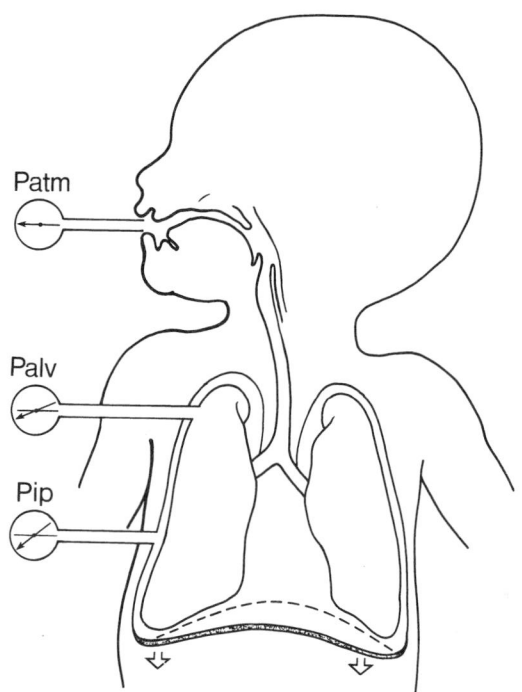

Figure 96–1. Negative pressure gradient produced on inspiration by descent of the diaphragm in spontaneously breathing infant. Pressures measured in interpleural space (Pip) and alveoli (Palv), and at opening of mouth or atmosphere (Patm). Pip < Palv < Patm. (From Harris TN: *In* Goldsmith JP, Karotkin EH [eds]: Assisted Ventilation of the Neonate, 2nd ed. Philadelphia, WB Saunders Co, 1988, p 24.)

contraction, occurring against the anchoring ribcage, results in a pressure gradient that decreases from the mouth to the alveoli and leads to an inward flow of gas. Simultaneously, the increase in intra-abdominal pressure and the physical structure of the thorax limit inspiratory movement until rising intrathoracic pressure terminates flow. During inspiration, a series of elastic elements—the chest wall muscles, diaphragm, airway connective tissue, pleurae, and blood vessels—stretch within the thorax. At the end of inspiration, the energy stored in these stretched elastic elements provides a recoil force that pumps gas out of the lung during expiration. Under normal circumstances, expiration is a passive process. When the respiratory workload is increased, the accessory muscles of the intercostal spaces and the abdominal musculature are recruited, so both inspiration and expiration may become active and require additional energy expenditure. The gas volume in the lungs at the point at which inspiratory effect again begins to oppose the expiratory recoil forces is known as the *functional residual capacity* (FRC).

Neurochemical control of breathing in the newborn and its influence on the process are only partially understood (Table 96–1). Compared with an adult, the brain stem centers of respiratory control in the neonate are immature and are more susceptible to failure, as seen in apnea of infancy.[4] Chemoreceptor responsiveness also appears to be diminished, particularly with respect to hypoxemia.[5-7] In addition, numerous reflex responses present in very young infants disappear rapidly during the first months and years of life.[8] Finally, sleep state, which influences respiratory control, is different in the newborn infant, with predominance of rapid eye movement (REM) sleep.[6,7]

Numerous studies have attempted to establish values for ventilatory volumes in neonates (Table 96–2).[9] Although values for tidal volume and minute ventilation change with growth, physiologic dead space remains relatively constant at about 0.3 throughout life in the healthy person. Pulmonary function

testing, aided by the use of computerized analysis (Fig. 96–2), has produced extensive data on compliance and resistance measurements during states of both health and disease.[9] *Compliance* refers to the lung relationship that correlates a given change in volume to a change in pressure required to produce that volume change. In general, the smaller the lung is, the lower the compliance. If one compares compliance in the healthy newborn with FRC (*specific compliance*), values are comparable to those seen in older children and adults. Little contribution to total lung compliance is made by the newborn chest wall, especially in preterm infants, because thoracic compliances are extraordinarily high.

The airways of young infants are small in caliber, highly distensible, and susceptible to injury during mechanical ventilation.[10-14] *Resistance* (related to the fourth power of the radius of the airway by Poiseuille's law) is rapidly elevated by any reduction in airway caliber. Increased secretions, airway edema, increased collapsibility of the airway, and other related phenomena may result from the use of mechanical ventilation in the small infant.[15] Furthermore, assessment of flow-volume and pressure-volume loops provides important information about airway patency and chest wall distortion.[16] Measurement of FRC, although somewhat more difficult, can also be performed with either a helium dilution method[17] or the nitrogen washout technique.[18] Finally, the lack of infant cooperation during forced expiratory volumes[19] has been resolved by the use of external compression of the thorax (Fig. 96–3). These techniques enable the neonatologist to understand both normal infant ventilation and the alterations produced during mechanical ventilation.

Certain features of the developing lung predispose it to injury during therapy with mechanical ventilation. Surface tension is relatively higher in the alveoli for all infants during the first hours of life, and some degree of atelectasis is common until a monomolecular layer of phospholipids (and their accompanying proteins), collectively known as *surfactant*, is deposited at the air-liquid interface (Table 96–3). Surfactant, primarily composed of phosphatidylcholine, phosphatidylglycerol, phosphatidylinositol, and several other lipid-soluble moieties, decreases the surface tension in the lung at end-expiration.[20-25] The surfactant proteins (SP-A, SP-B, SP-C) play important roles in the stability and recycling of the lipid moieties. Surfactant reduces the tendency of the lung to collapse from increased surface active forces in the alveoli. Surface tension and structural immaturity appear to be the major factors in the premature lung that lead to respiratory insufficiency and result in hyaline membrane disease or respiratory distress syndrome (RDS) (Fig. 96–4). Although primarily a disease of prematurity, RDS does occasionally occur in full-term births. When surfactant deficiency and structural immaturity are present, lung compliance in the newborn is reduced, and ventilator support is frequently necessary.

In addition to lung immaturity, numerous studies have suggested that the ventilatory muscles of newborns are more susceptible to fatigue than those of adults, a factor that may additionally contribute to the respiratory problems of preterm neonates.[26] Studies of histochemical and physiologic properties of respiratory muscle fibers reported age-related differences in human and baboon diaphragm. In comparison with fibers in the full-term baby or adult, the diaphragm in the premature baboon has fewer contractile proteins per fiber area and poorly developed sarcoplasmic reticulum; thus, the premature diaphragm contracts from progressively shorter lengths and develops less tension. When mechanical ventilation is used in infants with respiratory muscle weakness, the work of breathing is reduced, oxygen consumption is decreased, and respiratory muscle fatigue may be prevented. Other factors, such as the fragility of lung tissue, marginal energy reserves, limited ability to increase cardiac output, and lability of pulmonary perfusion from pulmonary hypertension, also may result in both a greater need for mechanical ventilation and additional problems during mechanical ventilation.

TABLE 96-1

Factors Affecting Control of Ventilation in the Spontaneously Breathing Neonate

Neurologic Factors

Maturity of the CNS

   Degree of myelination, which largely determines speed of impulse transmission and response time to stimuli affecting ventilation

   Degree of arborization or dendritic interconnections (synapses) between neurons, allowing summation of excitatory potentials coming in from other parts of the CNS and largely setting the neuronal depolarization threshold and response level of the respiratory center

Sleep state (i.e., REM sleep vs. quiet or non-REM sleep)

   REM sleep is generally associated with irregular respirations (both in depth and in frequency), distortion, and paradoxical motion of the rib cage during inspiration, inhibition of Hering-Breuer and glottic closure reflexes, and blunted response to CO_2 changes

   Quiet sleep is generally associated with regular respirations, a more stable rib cage, and a directly proportional relationship between Pco_2 and degree of ventilation

Reflex responses

   Hering-Breuer reflex, whereby inspiratory duration is limited in response to lung inflation sensed by stretch receptors located in major airways. Not present in adult humans, this reflex is active during quiet sleep of newborns but absent or weak during REM sleep

   Head's reflex, whereby inspiratory effort is further increased in response to rapid lung inflation. Thought to produce the frequently observed biphasic signs of newborns that may be crucial for promoting and maintaining lung inflation (and therefore breathing regularity) after birth

   Intercostal-phrenic reflex, whereby inspiration is inhibited by proprioception (position-sensing) receptors in intercostal muscles responding to distortion of the lower rib cage during REM sleep

   Trigeminal-cutaneous reflex, whereby tidal volume increases and respiratory rate decreases in response to facial stimulation

   Glottic closure reflex, whereby the glottis is narrowed through reflex contraction of the laryngeal adductor muscles during respiration, thereby breaking exhalation and increasing subglottic pressure (as with expiratory grunting)

Chemical Drive Factors (Chemoreflexes)

Response to hypoxemia (falling Pao_2) or to decrease in O_2 concentration breathed (mediated by peripheral chemoreceptors in carotid and aortic bodies)

   Initially, there is increase in depth of breathing (tidal volume), but subsequently if hypoxia persists or worsens, there is depression of respiratory drive, reduction in depth and rate of respiration, and eventual failure of arousal

   For the first week of life at least, these responses are dependent on environmental temperature, i.e., keeping the baby warm

   Hypoxia is associated with an increase in periodic breathing and apnea

Response to hyperoxia (increase in FI_{O_2} concentration breathed): enriched O_2 breathing causes a transient respiratory depression, stronger in term than in preterm infants

Response to hypercapnia (rising $Paco_2$ or $[H^+]$) or to increase in CO_2 concentration breathed (mediated by central chemoreceptors in the medulla)

   Increase in ventilation is directly proportional to inspired CO_2 concentration (or, more accurately stated, to alveolar CO_2 tension), as is the case in adults

   Response to CO_2 is in large part dependent on sleep state: In quiet sleep, a rising $Paco_2$ causes increase in depth and rate of breathing, whereas during REM sleep, the response is irregular and reduced in depth and rate. The degree of reduction closely parallels the amount of rib cage deformity occurring during REM sleep

   Ventilatory response to CO_2 in newborns is markedly depressed during behavioral activity such as feeding and easily depressed by sedatives and anesthesia

CNS = central nervous system; REM = rapid eye movement.
Adapted from Harris TN: *In* Goldsmith JP, Karolkin EH (eds): Assisted Ventilation of the Neonate. Philadelphia, WB Saunders Co, 1988, p 28.

TABLE 96-2

Ventilatory Values in Normal Newborns

Authors	Method	Weight (kg)	Respiratory Rate	V_T (mL)	V_E (mL/min)	V_A (mL/min)	V_D/V_T
Cook, et al	Plethysmography	3.8	38	16.0	—	—	0.32*
Swyer, et al	Pneumotachography	3.0	37	20.6	—	—	—
Strang	Plethysmography	3.3	41	18.1	750	378	0.50†
Nelson, et al	Nonrebreathing valve	2.2	38	12.8	480	309	0.25†
Koch	Nonrebreathing valve	3.6	44 (24 h)	16.5	703	442	0.25*
			39 (7 d)	16.6	632	425	0.24*
Bancalari, et al	Plethysmography	3.3	48	18.1	868	—	—

* Physiologic.
† Anatomic.
V_T = tidal volume; V_E = respiratory minute volume; V_A = alveolar ventilation; V_D/V_T = physiologic dead space.
Adapted from Bancalari E: *In* Thibeault DW, Gregory GA (eds): Neonatal Pulmonary Care. Norwalk, CT, Appleton-Century-Crofts, 1986, p 208.

ETIOLOGY OF LUNG INJURY WITH MECHANICAL VENTILATION

Mechanical ventilation enables the infant to maintain adequate gas exchange until the lung can heal. Although effective, this therapy can induce lung injury, thereby exacerbating the disease process as well as creating new iatrogenic disorders. The lung of the premature infant is more susceptible to injury than the more mature lung. Although the source of iatrogenic injury for the ventilated preterm infant may be similar to that of the older infant, child, or adult, these mechanisms are exacerbated. Current concepts identify lung tissue injury from barotrauma (effect of pressure), volutrauma (effect of tidal volumes), atelectrauma (repetitive opening and closing of lung units from low lung volumes), and toxic reactive oxygen species as causative of this injury.[27-29] Studies of preterm lambs demonstrated alterations in lung function after brief exposure to high ventilation pressure at birth.[30] Furthermore, the histopathology of controlled studies of

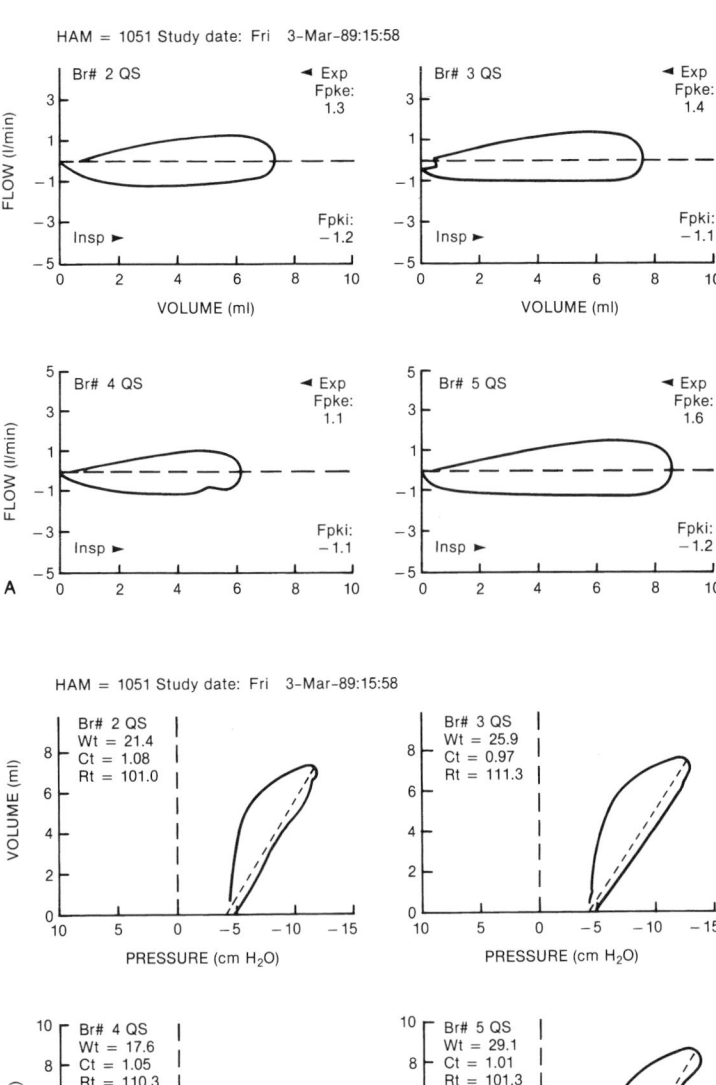

Figure 96–2. Computerized pulmonary function tests demonstrating flow-volume (**A**) and volume-pressure (**B**) loops for four consecutive breaths in an individual infant. The *dotted line* in each volume-pressure loop indicates the slope of the line for the calculated compliance. Ct = total lung compliance; Exp = expiration; Fpke = peak expiratory flow; Fpki = peak inspiratory flow; Insp = inspiration; Rt = total lung resistance; Wt = total work.

preterm animals and infants with chronic lung disease suggests that lung development is arrested by prolonged mechanical ventilation.[31-33] Adult animal studies demonstrate an increase in proinflammatory cytokines and induction of c-*fos* mRNA with mechanical ventilation, with the greatest increases occurring with high inflation pressures and tidal volumes with zero end-expiratory pressure.[34] In addition, studies have demonstrated that this lung injury could alter gene expression in the lung. Thus, noxious stimuli lead to another mechanism of lung injury called *biotrauma.* Nonsurvivors of adult/acute RDS (ARDS) have elevation of bronchoalveolar lavage fluid (BALF) cytokines, suggesting a pulmonary origin for the plasma cytokines.[35] Elevated levels of interleukin-8 in BALF are predictive of severe ARDS, and cytokines are released into the systemic circulation when the alveolar-endothelial barrier is disrupted.[36, 37] This may be the mechanism by which ventilator-induced lung injury leads to multiorgan failure.[38] Because the lung is in contact with the entire cardiac output, the release of active substances can act as a significant attenuator of or contributor to systemic compromise.

Although the circulating neutrophil pool and alveolar macrophage population increase with age,[39, 40] both have been implicated in mechanisms of lung injury of preterm infants. The circulating neutrophil pool size decreases and lung neutrophils increase after the mechanical ventilation of preterm animals.[41-46] The increase in neutrophils in the pulmonary air space is directly related to the decrease in circulating neutrophils, clearance of protein and liquid from the lung, and extravascular lung water. Pulmonary neutrophils therefore play a role in the pathogenesis of lung injury and the creation of lung edema.

Mechanotransduction, the conversion of a mechanical stimulus into structure and functional alterations of tissues, has been shown to affect the lung.[47, 48] Prolonged mechanical gas ventilation of the preterm lamb results in increased elastin expression (mRNA tropoelastin) and abnormal lung development.[49] Some of these alterations can be attenuated with ventilation strategies designed to reduce injury.[50-54]

Once injury is initiated, many factors can contribute to ongoing damage. Pulmonary injury initiates and is accompanied by a series of responses that ultimately lead to varying degrees of residual damage, depending on the duration and level of ventilator support. Desquamation of the epithelial and ciliary apparatus, increased goblet cells and smooth muscle, bronchial necrosis

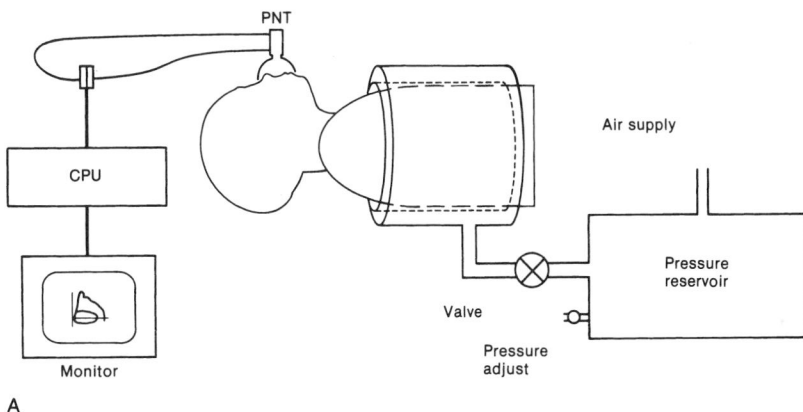

A

Figure 96–3. A, Infant partial expiratory flow volume (PEFV) by rapid thoracic compression set-up showing the compression bag wrapped around the infant's thorax and abdomen and connected to the pressure reservoir. Flow is measured by a pneumotachograph (PNT), processed by computer (CPU), and displayed at a flow-volume loop. **B,** PEFV curves from infants with obstructive lung disease compared with a normal curve demonstrating flow limitation and concavity toward the volume axis. (From Bhutani VK, et al: Neonatal Pulmonary Function Testing. Ithaca, NY, Perinatology Press, 1988.)

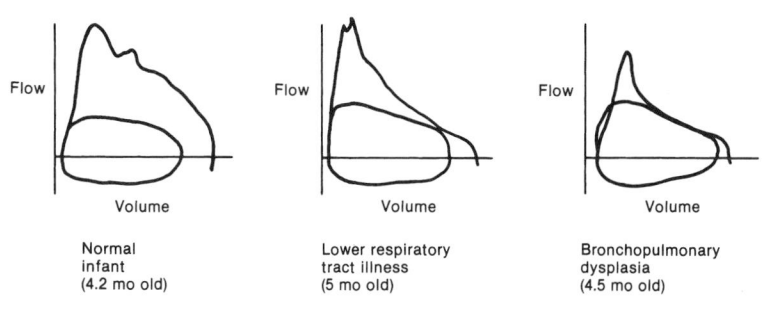

B

TABLE 96-3

Roles of Surfactant in Pulmonary Physiology

Reduce alveolar surface tension
Increase compliance
Decrease work of breathing
Increase alveolar stability
Improve alveolar recruitment
Reduce lung forces that result in pulmonary edema

---

that heals with fibrosis, increased interstitial lung fluid, rupture of alveolar septa, and diffuse inflammatory disease throughout the lung are some of the changes that are apparent with mechanical ventilation.[55-60] These sequelae of lung injury are most often seen in BPD, as evidenced by airway distention, shifting atelectasis on chest roentgenography, hyperinflation of other areas of the lung, ventilation/perfusion (V/Q) inequalities, and impaired cardiac function.[11, 61-64] The use of mechanical ventilation is therefore a two-edged sword: often, there is no other way to save an infant's life, yet the therapy itself almost always produces some degree of lung and airway damage.

INITIATION OF NEONATAL LUNG DISEASE AND THE DECISION TO INITIATE NEONATAL MECHANICAL VENTILATION

Given the risk of injury associated with mechanical ventilation, the decision to place an infant on respiratory support, with the selection of appropriate ventilator settings, is one of the most critical decisions made in medicine. The clinician must understand the reasons behind this decision and the strategy that will be employed. This decision has been made more difficult over the past several years, because a large body of work has begun to redesign the ventilation targets for neonates and to elucidate the ramifications of the decision to ventilate the patient me-

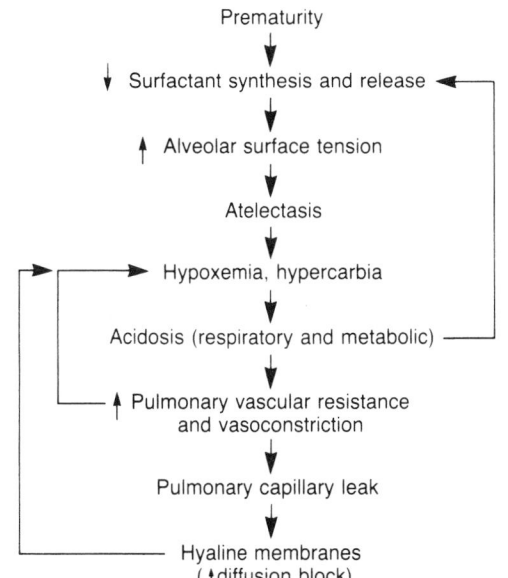

Figure 96–4. The pathogenesis of respiratory distress syndrome. (From Polin RA, Burg MD [eds]: Workbook in Practical Neonatology. Philadelphia, WB Saunders Co, 1983, p. 106.)

chanically. The process that determines the need for mechanical ventilation begins *in utero*, with the initiation of maternal steroid or tocolytic therapy, and proceeds in the delivery room.

The development of adequate pulmonary blood flow, FRC, and V/Q matching, with uniform distribution of lung surfactant, can be affected by the management of these issues in the first few minutes of life. Animal studies demonstrate that airway and lung parenchymal injury can occur with only a few large breaths at the time of birth.[65-68] In addition, tidal breathing in the delivery room can cause alterations in surfactant function. These changes may result from parenchymal disruption with protein leak and surfactant inactivation.[69, 70] Hence, tidal breaths in the delivery room can reduce the efficacy of exogenous surfactant administration while simultaneously disrupting the integrity of the airway structure and the pulmonary parenchyma. As a result, from even shortly after birth, the physician attempting to reduce pulmonary trauma in the neonate may be fighting a losing battle.

Once in the intensive care nursery, the infant who is managed on mechanical ventilator support must be monitored closely. The relatively recent addition of on-line, ventilator-generated lung mechanics measurements allows for rapid assessment, alteration, and sculpting of ventilator breaths. The goal of any strategy is to provide the necessary gas exchange while minimizing lung injury. Defining adequate gas exchange in the newborn infant is no longer clear. Providing for arterial carbon dioxide pressure ($Paco_2$) and pH values that are normal for adult humans may constitute relative overventilation for the newborn. Decreasing $Paco_2$ may result in unnecessary lung injury, and low levels of $Paco_2$ may be detrimental. Permitting higher levels of $Paco_2$, or allowing time for these levels to diminish over time in the newborn, may alleviate the need to initiate mechanical ventilation. Increasingly, programs are evaluating the use of early continuous positive airway pressure (CPAP) and are permitting Pco_2 levels to be relatively elevated to avoid the lung injury associated with mechanical ventilation. Similarly, a high requirement for supplemental oxygen to maintain a level of arterial oxygen pressure (Pao_2) that would be considered normal in a human adult may also not be necessary.[71] The newborn infant's oxygen requirement is in transition from the hypoxemic levels of the fetus to that of the adultlike human. If the expense of achieving higher levels of oxygen is lung injury, perhaps lower levels can be tolerated. Recent work has suggested that tolerating lower blood hemoglobin saturation levels may be beneficial. Hence, understanding the gas-exchange targets not only will affect ventilator management but may eliminate the need to initiate or maintain mechanical ventilator support.

CONVENTIONAL ASSISTED VENTILATION IN THE NEWBORN INFANT

Several different modes of ventilator assistance exist for the treatment of neonatal lung disease (Table 96–4). All types of ventilator support basically serve the same function: to assist in gas exchange to reduce pulmonary insufficiency, an inability of the lung to exchange gas adequately to meet the demands of aerobic

TABLE 96-4

Modes of Ventilatory Assistance in the Newborn

Oxygen therapy
CPAP
   Nasal CPAP
   Endotracheal CPAP
   Face-mask CPAP
Negative end distending pressure
Negative-pressure ventilation
Positive-pressure ventilation
   Pressure limited
   Time-cycle limited
   Volume limited
High-frequency positive pressure ventilation
   Oscillatory
   Flow interrupter
   Jet
High-frequency negative pressure ventilation
Extracorporeal membrane oxygenation
Liquid ventilation

CPAP = continuous positive airway pressure.

metabolism. Common causes of pulmonary insufficiency and respiratory distress in the newborn period are listed in Table 96-5.

Virtually all assisted ventilation currently used in the United States is some variant of positive-pressure ventilation. Negative-pressure ventilators disappeared from most nurseries as very low birth weight infants (<1500 g) increased in number in the nursery population. Although some recent efforts with negative-pressure ventilation in pulmonary hypertension appear to be interesting, this therapy is still uncommon.[72, 73]

In contrast to spontaneous ventilation, positive-pressure mechanical ventilation generates gas flow in a different manner. With positive-pressure breathing, a gradient down the airway is again established by raising pressure in the proximal airway (usually through an endotracheal [ET] tube, occasionally a tracheostomy), compared with the decrease in intrapleural pressure that occurs with spontaneous breathing. Gas still flows in the direction of decreasing pressure, although the mechanism for producing this flow differs significantly. As shown in Figure 96-5, although there is a transpulmonary pressure gradient of a similar direction in both spontaneous and assisted ventilation, the pressure throughout the lung, from the atmosphere

TABLE 96-5

Differential Diagnosis of Respiratory Distress in the Newborn Period*

Respiratory			Extrapulmonary			
Common	*Less Common*	*Rare*	*Heart*	*Metabolic*	*Brain*	*Blood*
Respiratory distress syndrome (hyaline membrane disease)	Pulmonary hemorrhage	Airway obstruction (upper), e.g., choanal atresia	Congenital heart disease	Metabolic acidosis	Hemorrhage	Acute blood loss
Transient tachypnea	Pneumothorax	Space-occupying lesion	Patent ductus	Hypoglycemia	Edema	Hypovolemia
Meconium aspiration	Immature lung syndrome	e.g., diaphragmatic	arteriosus	Hypothermia	Drugs	Twin-twin
Primary pulmonary hypertension (persistent fetal circulation)		hernia, lung cysts	(acquired)	Septicemia	Trauma	transfusion
Pneumonia, especially caused by group B streptococci		Hypoplasia of the lung			Hyperviscosity	

* Presentation with or without cyanosis, grunting, retractions, tachypnea, apnea, shock, lethargy.
Data from Martin RJ, et al: *In* Klaus MH, Fanaroff AV (eds): Care of the High Risk Neonate. 3rd ed. Philadelphia, WB Saunders Co, 1986.

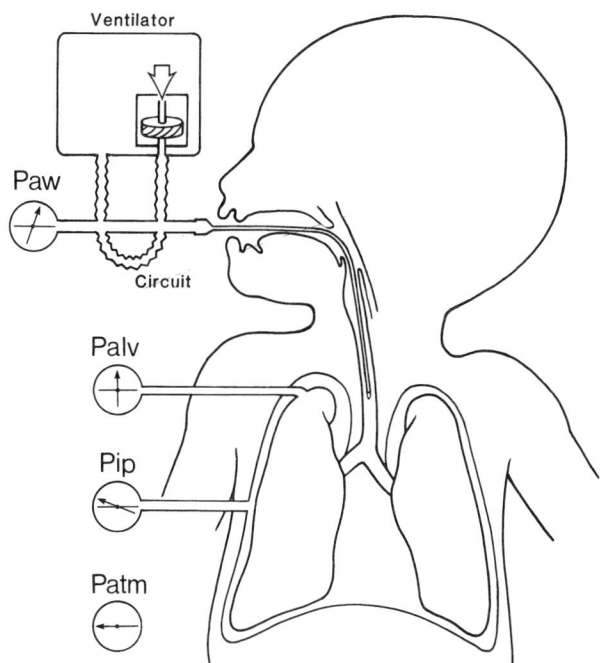

Figure 96–5. Positive pressure gradient produced by ventilator. Pressures measured in airway (Paw) and as in Figure 96-1. Paw > Palv > Pip > Patm. (From Goldsmith JP, Karothin EH [eds]: Assisted Ventilation of the Neonate. Philadelphia, WB Saunders Co, 1988, p 25.)

to the pleural cavity, is higher with mechanical ventilation. As a result, the airways and lungs receive higher pressures than normal. In the young infant with decreased connective tissue and cartilage, the airway becomes distended,[11, 15] and gas flow, which depends partly on rigidity of the airway, may become more turbulent. With increasing turbulence, gas distribution throughout the lung is altered, gas exchange is reduced, and one often has to compensate by further increasing ventilator pressure support.[74,75] This process, occurring over several days, may lead to progressive airway and lung injury. Although positive pressure applied to the fragile preterm pulmonary airway and parenchyma produces lung injury, the specific ventilator variable that induces the greatest injury has remained controversial. Attempts to eliminate lung injury completely in the neonate have been less than successful, and it has become increasingly clear that the process of tidal breathing itself is sufficient to induce injury in the preterm infant. Animal studies suggest that even short-term and limited tidal breathing (volutrauma), as well as ventilation of the atelectatic lung (atelectrauma), causes injury.[71, 76-80] The size of the breath may therefore be more important than the inflating pressure in determining the risk of chronic lung disease. In the atelectatic lung, adequate minute ventilation is achieved by overinflating already expanded lung regions, thereby causing damage to those ventilated regions. Hence, using an adequate amount of end-expiratory pressure, or mean airway pressure (MAP), to optimize alveolar volume recruitment may diminish lung injury.

The goal of therapy therefore is to maximize the benefits of ventilation while minimizing its negative effects. Understanding the controls available with mechanical ventilation can assist in this end.

VARIABLES IN ASSISTED VENTILATION

Several different controls for mechanical ventilation can be manipulated in the care of individual infants (Table 96-6). Each

TABLE 96-6

Control Variables in Assisted Ventilation

Oxygen therapy
Continuous positive airway pressure
Peak inflating pressure
Frequency
Inspiratory/expiratory ratio
　Inspiratory time
　Expiratory time
Mean airway pressure

variable has both physiologic advantages and disadvantages that must be considered.

Oxygen Therapy

Maintenance of adequate tissue oxygenation is one of the primary goals of therapy during mechanical ventilation. The simplest way to achieve adequate oxygenation is to increase the fraction of oxygen in inspired gas. Oxygen must be considered a drug, however, with potential harmful side effects such as retinopathy of prematurity (ROP)[81-83] and BPD.[64] Retinopathy is believed to occur, at least in part, from varying oxygen concentrations in the blood that result in vasoconstriction and subsequent proliferation and abnormal vascular growth in the retina of the immature infant's eye. Other factors, such as prematurity itself, carbon dioxide levels, apnea, blood pressure, and vitamin E levels, as well as some additional (possibly unknown) factors, also appear to be important in the development of this condition.[82] Genetic tendency may also play a role.

BPD appears to be a result of prolonged exposure to high inspired oxygen concentrations and positive-pressure ventilation. It is thought that this condition may have an underlying inherited tendency in some families[84] and is also multifactorial in origin. Generation of superoxide anions from oxygen may be one of the inflammatory processes that initiates the lung response that later results in BPD (Fig. 96-6). Superoxide dismutase (SOD), catalase, glutathione peroxidase, and other enzymes important in the catalytic reduction of these anions are reduced in the premature infant. As a result, the premature lung may be at increased risk from the effects of this oxygen byproduct. Studies with SOD have suggested a therapeutic role for this agent in preventing BPD.

Mammalian cells contain two types of SOD molecules, namely CuZnSOD and MnSOD. Human CuZnSOD, which resides in the cytoplasm of the cell, is a dimeric metalloprotein composed of identical noncovalently lined 16-kDa subunits, each containing one atom of copper and one atom of zinc. An extracellular glycosylated tetrameric form of CuZnSOD also exists. Human MnSOD is localized in the mitochondria and is a homotetramer composed of 22-kDa subunits, each possessing one manganese atom.

Developmental up-regulation of antioxidant enzyme expression occurs in various mammalian species during the last 10 to 15% of gestation and parallels the increase in surfactant levels.[85] *In vitro* and *in vivo* hyperoxic exposure of the lungs of normal immature animals results in a rapid increase in pulmonary SOD activity.[86] In humans, SOD activity in the lung also increases with age; it is lowest in fetal life, increases in term infants, and is highest in adults.[87] Most premature infants without RDS show the expected hyperoxic increase in SOD activity, whereas most infants with RDS do not.[88] This finding suggests that antioxidant deficiency may play a role in neonatal lung disease.

In a prior study, recombinant human (r-h) CuZnSOD was well tolerated, with an adverse experience profile generally comparable to that of placebo. In addition, no between-group differences

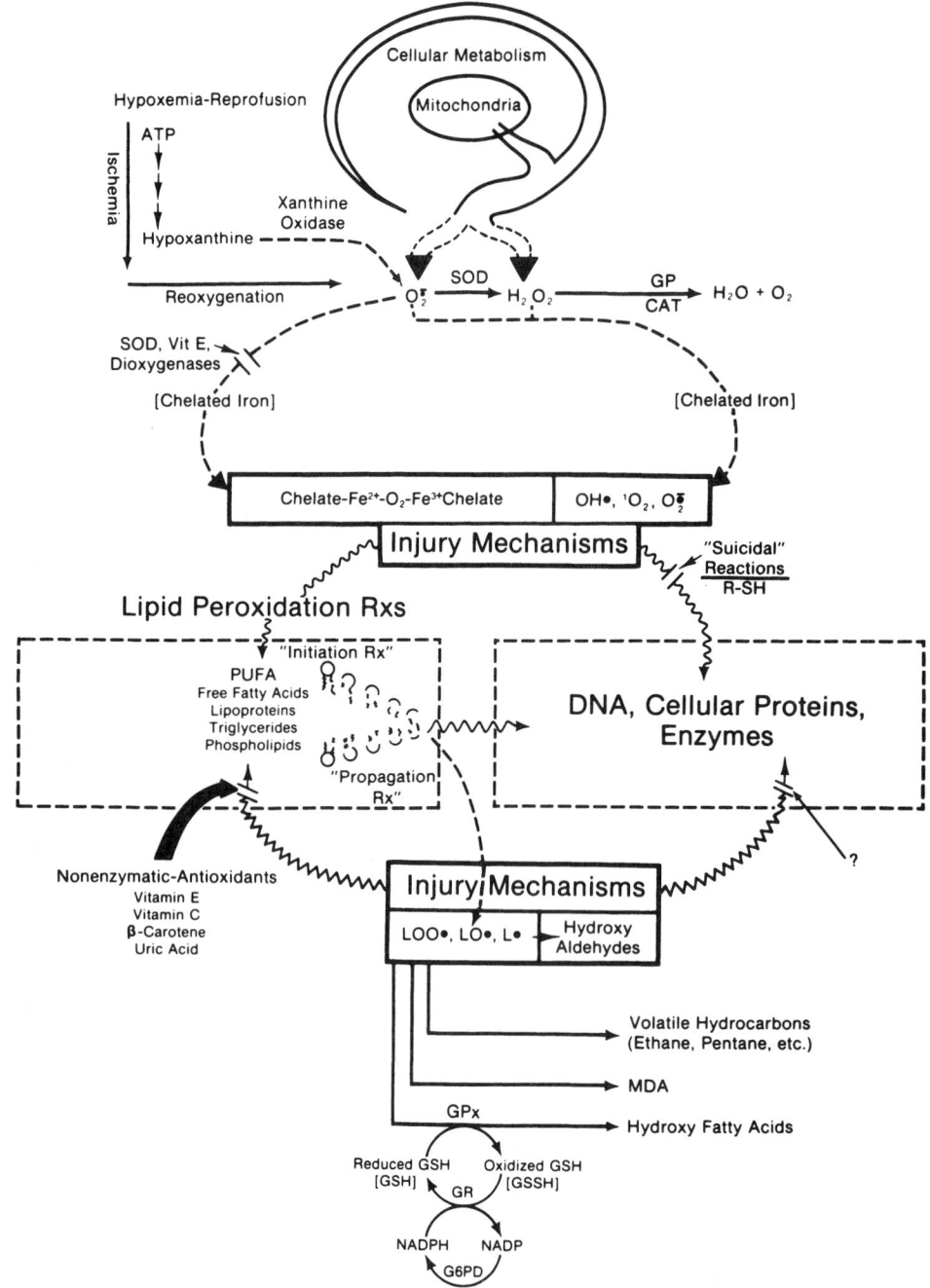

Figure 96–6. Schematic representation of the source and generation of free radicals and reactive intermediates and the enzymatic and nonenzymatic protective systems available to the cell. Additional details are provided in the text. (Adapted from Roberts RJ: Nucleic Acid Res 12[Suppl]:167, 1984.)

in growth parameters or physical or neurologic examination findings were seen at 1 year of corrected age. There were no significant differences between treatment groups in the short-term end-points of BPD, death, or the combined end-point of BPD or death. However, fewer patients who were previously treated with r-h CuZnSOD compared with those patients who were previously treated with placebo used respiratory medications between 6 and 12 months of corrected age. Further, fewer infants in the r-h CuZnSOD group required home nebulizer use. Thus, results from these studies support further prospective evaluation of the long-term effects of r-h CuZnSOD in preterm infants with RDS.[89]

Because of the substantial morbidity from these conditions, oxygen therapy must be cautiously administered and monitored during the neonatal period. Frequent assessment of inspired oxygen concentration, as well as blood oxygen saturation and tension, is recommended.

If hyperoxia leads to major morbidity in the newborn, hypoxia can produce even greater problems. Hypoxemia, if prolonged, results in a change from aerobic to anaerobic metabolism, increased lactic acid production, and, ultimately, cellular and organ demise. Death usually follows soon afterward. These effects are unquestionably time related. A shorter duration of hypoxemia, however, may result in organ injury that can be permanent.[90] The effects of hypoxemia on central nervous system function and development are a constant concern for the neonatologist. The effects of hypoxemia on the developing brain are discussed in more detail elsewhere in this book.

Since the mid-1990s, there has been a gradual change in the approach to oxygen use and acceptable hemoglobin oxygen saturations in the newborn. In the process of resuscitation of the newborn, it is no longer believed that even brief exposures to 100% oxygen are harmless.[91] The risks of high oxygen levels may occur at relatively "normal" oxygen saturations. The fear of low oxygen tensions includes increase in pulmonary vascular and airway resistance and decreased growth and enzymatic activity. Several studies suggest that normal levels of oxygen saturation (96 to 99%) in preterm infants with chronic disease may increase the risk of pneumonia or exacerbation of chronic lung disease or ROP and may prolong the oxygen requirement.[92-94] The optimal arterial oxygen saturation varies with the disease state, but it will probably be lowered over the next several years.[91,95]

Continuous Positive Airway Pressure

Since its introduction by Gregory and colleagues in 1971,[96] the use of CPAP has become a standard part of ventilator care. CPAP is also referred to as *positive end-expiratory pressure* (PEEP) when used in conjunction with a mechanical ventilator (that is supplying a ventilator rate for the infant) or continuous distending pressure. The full effects of this form of therapy are not fully understood, and part of the difficulty may be that CPAP may have variable results in different clinical situations. CPAP is believed to result in progressive alveolar recruitment, inflating collapsed alveoli[96] and reducing intrapulmonary shunt.[97-100]

From Laplace's law:

$$\text{Pressure} = \frac{2 \times \text{tension}}{\text{radius}} \qquad [1]$$

However, one could expect that collapsed alveoli would remain collapsed, and inflated or partially inflated alveoli would become increasingly inflated or overdistended. These findings have never been clearly documented. Some of the effects of CPAP, however, have been measured. CPAP increases gas volume in the lung, including FRC.[97] Initially, as FRC increases, gas exchange improves; arterial Po_2 (Pao_2) increases and arterial Pco_2 ($Paco_2$) decreases. With additional CPAP, however, the volume of the lung increases excessively, and the lung becomes overdistended. In such cases, Pao_2 remains high, but $Paco_2$ also begins to increase as tidal volume diminishes and physiologic dead space is increased. Continued excessive CPAP may ultimately lead to very serious consequences, such as air leak syndromes: pneumomediastinum, pneumothorax, or pneumopericardium.[101] Excessive CPAP may also increase dead space ventilation, leading to a rise in $Paco_2$. Furthermore, although low levels of CPAP may be useful in decreasing pulmonary edema or left-to-right cardiac shunting, high levels of CPAP can lead to a reduction in cardiac output, reduced pulmonary perfusion, and enhanced V/Q mismatching, resulting in a lower Pao_2.[102-104] Depending on levels of CPAP applied and lung compliance, pulmonary vascular resistance may be increased with CPAP, although its use early in the course of RDS may lead to decreased pulmonary vascular resistance.[105]

CPAP has some nonspecific effects on neonatal ventilation as well. Application of CPAP appears to produce a more regular breathing pattern in preterm neonates[106] and has been thought to be mediated through chest wall stabilization and reduction of thoracic distortion. Obstructive apnea is also reduced with CPAP,[107] even when it is applied by nasopharyngeal route. Furthermore, it has been shown that both inspiratory and expiratory times are increased with CPAP. Finally, it is thought that surfactant release may be enhanced by CPAP in RDS. Intracranial

pressure is increased by CPAP and is directly related to the amount of CPAP applied as well as compliance of the lungs.[108] With increased lung compliance, more pressure is transmitted to the cardiovascular system, resulting in a rise in central venous pressure and intracranial pressure. Cerebral perfusion pressure, however, can decrease with application of end-distending pressure, because venous pressure rises and arterial pressure decreases initially. Some compensation is likely to occur over time; however, these changes in intracranial pressure may lead to an increased risk of intracranial hemorrhage, especially in the preterm baby.[90]

Some effects of CPAP on renal function have been documented.[109] These include a decrease in glomerular filtration rate, reduction of urinary sodium excretion, and diminished urinary output.[110, 111] These findings also appear to be mediated through transmission of pressure to the cardiovascular system with reduction in renal blood flow. As renal blood flow decreases, there may be some redistribution of intrarenal blood flow to the inner renal cortex and outer medulla.[112] Aldosterone appears to increase with application of CPAP,[113] and antidiuretic hormone secretion may increase as well,[114] although there have also been reports of decreased antidiuretic hormone with CPAP. These contradictory findings may again be a reflection of the finding that CPAP may improve or worsen lung compliance, resulting in either increase or decrease in intracranial perfusion (Table 96-7).[115] One trend in respiratory support of the premature newborn is the use of noninvasive ventilation strategy. At the forefront of this approach is permissive hypercapnia and the early use of CPAP in lieu of mechanical ventilation. Reports in the 1980s showed that units that accepted higher values for arterial Pco_2 and used CPAP aggressively had a lower rate of chronic lung disease.[116] The concept of "gentle ventilation" with permissive hypercapnia and the aggressive use of CPAP illustrates one of the most confusing aspects of managing respiratory distress in the newborn, namely, when, and to what degree, to intervene. The introduction of mechanical ventilation is potentially detrimental, and deciding to place an infant on mechanical ventilator support remains a difficult decision. In addition, determining what measurements (e.g., blood gases, graphics monitoring) should guide ventilator changes remains unclear. Permissive hypercapnia in preterm infants seems safe and may reduce the duration of assisted ventilation. This strategy has particular appeal in that hypocarbia may be related to brain injury. However, severe hypercarbia may also cause brain injury, a finding strongly suggesting that nature has excellent physiologic reasons to establish eucapnic ventilation as the normal range. When using a strategy or permissive hypercapnia, it is important to minimize atelectasis, because the recruitment and de-recruitment of lung regions is not optimal. In addition, although data look promising when this strategy is implemented, long-term follow-up of infants managed with high carbon dioxide levels has not been explored.

Peak Inflating Pressure

Peak inflating pressure (PIP) is the primary ventilator variable that determines tidal volume on most time-cycled or pressure-limited ventilators. Since the introduction of neonatal mechanical ventilation, controversy has raged over the optimal approach to the administration of PIP. Many of the effects of PIP are similar to those described previously in the section on CPAP. The introduction of a peak pressure, unlike the constant pressure application of CPAP, may have additional physiologic effects on the neonatal airways and lungs.

Once one begins cycling a ventilator and providing a PIP, physiologic changes occur. Tidal volume and minute ventilation increase. Depending on the type of waveform generated by the ventilator and the duration of inspiratory to expiratory time (I/E ratio) selected, mean airway pressure (MAP) may be altered (Fig. 96-7). Airways expand, and, as noted with CPAP, alveolar distention is

TABLE 96-7

Continuous Positive Airway Pressure

Low (2–3 cm H₂O)		Medium (4–7 cm H₂O)	
Use	*Side Effects*	*Use*	*Side Effects*
Maintenance of lung volume in very low birth weight infants During weaning During hyperventilation for PPHN	May be too low to maintain adequate lung volume or adequate oxygenation CO₂ retention	Increasing lung volume in surfactant deficiency, such as RDS Stabilizing areas of atelectasis Stabilizing obstructed airways	If lungs have normal C$_L$: May overdistend May impede venous return Air leak

High (8–10 cm H₂O)		Ultrahigh (11–15 cm H₂O)	
Use	*Side Effects*	*Use*	*Side Effects*
Preventing alveolar collapse with poor C$_L$ and poor lung volume Improving distribution of ventilation	Pulmonary air leak Decreased C$_L$ if overdistended May impede venous return (metabolic acidosis) May increase PVR CO₂ retention	Tracheal or bronchial collapse Markedly decreased C$_L$ or severe obstruction Preventing white-out or reestablishing lung volume during ECMO	Same as "High" levels, depending on C$_L$

C$_L$ = lung compliance; ECMO = extracorporeal membrane oxygenation; PPHN = persistent pulmonary hypertension of the newborn; PVR = pulmonary vascular resistance; RDS = respiratory distress syndrome.

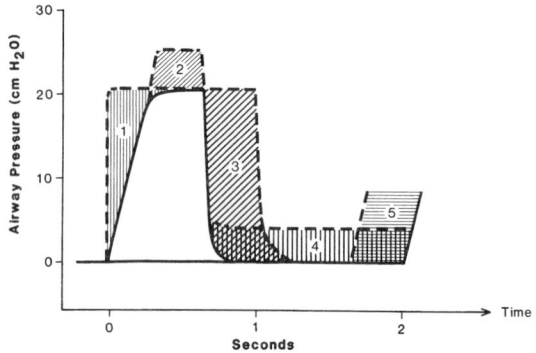

Figure 96–7. Five different ways to increase mean airway pressure: (*1*) increase inspiratory flow rate, producing more of a square-wave inspiratory pattern; (*2*) increase peak inspiratory pressure; (*3*) reverse the inspiratory/expiratory (I/E) ratio or prolong inspiratory time without changing the rate; (*4*) increase positive end-expiratory pressure; and (*5*) increase ventilator rate by reducing expiratory time without changing inspiratory time. (Modified from Reynolds EOR: *In* Goldsmith JP, Karotkin EH [eds]: Assisted Ventilation of the Neonate. Philadelphia, WB Saunders Co, 1988, p 61.)

increased. One of the primary goals of all mechanical ventilation is to achieve the optimal gas exchange at the lowest positive pressure. The neonatologist must constantly examine the benefits derived by the patient versus the risk of pulmonary injury (Table 96-8) with different ventilator approaches. These approaches have become even more complicated with the newer modes of ventilation, all innovated to decrease pulmonary iatrogenic injury.

The causes of injury with mechanical ventilation were previously outlined. No clear data suggest a specific level of PIP that will invariably damage an individual infant. Some infants demonstrate barotrauma at low levels of PIP, whereas other infants may not have any injury even at higher levels of PIP. Size and gestational age clearly influence the response of mechanical ventilation, although babies of equal gestational age, weight, and severity of disease may have different responses to mechanical ventilation. A study of the incidence of chronic lung disease in

perinatal centers in academic institutions confirmed this highly variable incidence of BPD in infants treated with mechanical ventilation.[116] It cannot be overemphasized that one should not attempt to limit PIP to some predetermined pressure value in an attempt to reduce barotrauma while ignoring the importance of adequate gas exchange. In many instances, high peak pressures are necessary to achieve adequate ventilation and oxygenation. Inadequate gas exchange is invariably either fatal or injurious to the central nervous system and must never be ignored while one tries to limit pressure below some arbitrary level.

Additional factors become more important in mechanical ventilation when one adjusts ventilator peak pressure. The length and caliber of an ET tube significantly influence airway resistance. Longer, narrower ET tubes have higher airway resistance. Because of the added resistance, gas trapping can occur because the recoil of the lung does not have sufficient time to evacuate gas from the air spaces. As a result, the lung expands to a higher FRC. Although this increase in lung volume may be of value early in the course of neonatal lung diseases complicated by atelectasis (i.e., RDS), in most cases, air trapping adds to the likelihood of air leaks and pulmonary injury. It has been demonstrated, in studies by Wall,[117] that if one shortens a 2.5-mm inner-diameter (ID) ET tube from 14.8 to 4.8 cm (tracheostomy length), the measured *in vitro* resistance is reduced to that of a full-length 3.0-mm ID ET tube. Therefore, one must select the appropriate size tube for an individual infant to maximize flow and decrease resistance to a minimum. ET tubes are usually supplied in excessive lengths and should be cut to remove any unnecessary dead space after ideal placement has been secured. The effect of the diameter of the ET tube is somewhat surprising in the neonate, given that airways rapidly decrease in caliber to a size far smaller than the ET tube within one or two bronchial divisions. One would consequently expect that the smaller airways of the tracheobronchial tree would contribute far more to resistance than the ET tube. Resistance within the lung is primarily dependent on the total cross-sectional area of all airway branches. Because the total cross-sectional area of the airways of the lung increases rapidly with bronchial subdivisions, these smaller airways contribute far less to resistance than expected. As a result, the larger airways and the ET tube in the newborn infant become the major contributors to resistance, a finding that is especially important in the baby with chronic lung disease who often demonstrates bronchospasm or tracheobronchomalacia.

TABLE 96-8

Waveforms in Neonatal Mechanical Ventilation

Sine Wave		Square Wave	
Advantages	*Side Effects*	*Advantages*	*Side Effects*
Smoother increase of pressure More like normal breathing pattern	Lower mean airway pressure	Higher mean airway pressure for equivalent PIP Longer time at peak pressure may open up atelectasis or improve distribution of ventilation	With high flow, the ventilator may be applying higher pressure to normal alveoli, resulting in barotrauma Could impede venous return if inverse I/E ratio is used

I/E = inspiratory/expiratory; PIP = peak inspiratory pressure.
Adapted from Fox WW, et al: *In* Goldsmith J Karotkin E (eds): Assisted Ventilation of the Neonate. Philadelphia, WB Saunders Co, 1988.

TABLE 96-9

Peak Inspiratory Pressure

Low (<30 cm H$_2$O)		High (≥30 cm H$_2$O)	
Advantages	*Side Effects*	*Advantages*	*Side Effects*
Fewer side effects, especially BPD, PAL Normal lung development may occur more rapidly	Insufficient ventilation; may not control PaCO_2 May have low PaO_2, if too low Generalized atelectasis may occur (may be desirable in some cases of air leaks)	May reexpand atelectasis Increase PaO_2 Decrease PaCO_2 Decrease pulmonary vascular resistance	Associated with PAL, BPD May impede venous return May decrease cardiac output

BPD = bronchopulmonary dysplasia; PAL = pulmonary air leaks.

Furthermore, because work of breathing, or the force needed to expand the lung (pressure times volume displacement), is so closely related to resistance, small changes in airway caliber markedly increase resistance and, in turn, work of breathing. Such problems are important in the consideration of optimal approaches to mechanical ventilation. In many cases of BPD, for example, initial respiratory failure may be related to the finding that the contribution of resistance factors to work of breathing is excessive for the infant over a certain period, although it may not be immediately apparent when one performs pulmonary function testing. Energy expenditure ultimately exceeds limited energy stores, and ventilator failure ensues. Subsequent ventilator management may be complicated by the problems created during ventilator cycling (Table 96-9).

Rate Effects

Respiratory rate is one of the primary determinants of minute ventilation. *Minute ventilation* equals the product of tidal volume and respiratory rate (or frequency). Several schools of thought exist concerning the optimal ventilator frequency for neonatal mechanical ventilation, although these can be divided into two primary modes of therapy: rapid-rate ventilation (>60 breaths/minute)[118] and slower-rate ventilation (<40 breaths/minute).[119] In both instances, the goal has been to try to reduce the complications associated with high inflating pressures. Advantages and disadvantages exist with all forms of treatment (Table 96-10). In attempting to understand the physiologic consequences of rate on ventilation, the concept of time constant must be addressed. The *time constant* of the lung is a measure of how rapidly equilibration between proximal and alveolar pressures occurs, and it

expresses how quickly an infant can move air into or out of the lung. The time constant is expressed by the following equation: time constant = compliance × resistance. Time constants can be determined for both inspiration and expiration, although the neonatologist is particularly interested in the expiratory time constant with mechanical ventilation, because it is very important to have some idea of how rapidly the lung empties after a mechanical breath. Bancalari[120] determined that, in the normal newborn, with a compliance of 0.005 L/cm H$_2$O and a resistance of 30 cm H$_2$O/L/second, one time constant equals about 0.15 second. A single time constant is defined as the time required by the lung to discharge 63% of the tidal volume that was delivered to the terminal air spaces. Three time constants equal the time required for the alveolus to discharge 95% of gas delivered and would therefore be approximately 0.45 second in the normal, spontaneously breathing infant. In diseased lung states, the effects of changes in compliance and resistance must be considered in applying mechanical ventilation. For an infant with RDS who has markedly reduced compliance in the early stages of the disease, the time constant of the lung may be exceedingly short. During that disease stage, one can readily use high rates to ventilate an infant, because the exit time of gas from the lung is so rapid, or one can use a slower rate with a prolonged inspiratory phase, again relying on the short time constant of a very stiff lung to allow gas exit during the short expiratory phase. Difficulty arises, however, with both these therapeutic modalities when the lung begins to heal.

During the recovery period, compliance begins to increase as surfactant release is enhanced and structural maturity occurs, whereas the effects of ventilator therapy, as noted previously, tend to narrow the airway lumen and increase resistance. In these circumstances, the time constant of the lung tends to

TABLE 96–10

Positive End-Expiratory Pressure

Low (2–3 cm H₂O)		Medium (4–7 cm H₂O)		High (≥8 cm H₂O)	
Advantages	*Side Effects*	*Advantages*	*Side Effects*	*Advantages*	*Side Effects*
Used during weaning	May be too low to maintain adequate lung volume	Stabilizes lung volume	May overdistend lungs with normal compliance	Prevents alveolar collapse in surfactant deficiency states with severely decreased C_L	PAL
Maintenance of lung volume in premature infants with low FRC	CO_2 retention	Recruit lung volume with surfactant deficiency states (e.g., RDS)		Improves distribution of ventilation	Decreases compliance if lung overdistends
		Improve ventilation/ perfusion matching			May impede venous return to the heart
					May increase PVR CO_2 retention

C_L = lung compliance; FRC = functional residual capacity; PAL = pulmonary air leaks; PVR = pulmonary vascular resistance; RDS = respiratory distress syndrome.

become increasingly prolonged, and if the rate of ventilation is not changed from the initial approach, gas trapping occurs, leading to a situation referred to as *inadvertent PEEP*.[129] Although some inadvertent PEEP may be of value in maintaining lung volume during periods of atelectasis, progressive air trapping may lead to air dissection and air-leak syndromes and may also be one of the important initiating factors in the development of BPD. Furthermore, as demonstrated by Boros and colleagues,[121] the use of very high ventilator rates with conventional mechanical ventilation at fixed flow rates is limited by the finding that *in vitro* minute ventilation decreases beyond a certain maximum rate for individual ventilators (Fig. 96–8). High-frequency ventilators, which generate inspiratory flow in a different manner from conventional ventilators, are not affected by these rate limitations to the same extent. The high-frequency ventilator, however, can also produce air trapping or inadvertent PEEP when it is used at rates beyond its optimal frequency. In neonatal ventilation, the introduction of continuous-flow circuitry,[122] rather than intermittent flow of gas, permits the use of slow ventilator rates. Before the introduction of this modification, an infant breathing between respirator cycles would simply rebreathe exhaled gas in the breathing circuit, thus increasing work of breathing and raising the $Paco_2$. With the addition of constant flow, periodic ventilator breaths could be combined with spontaneous ventilation in a mode of therapy referred to as *intermittent mandatory ventilation* (IMV).[123] This therapy enables the physician to supply a ventilator rate in the midrange (40 to 60 breaths/minute), thus providing sufficient ventilatory support for the infant while avoiding some of the complications of either high or low rate ventilation. At these midrange rates, the likelihood of air trapping and injury appears to be reduced for most infants. *Again, the management of neonatal ventilator assistance cannot be carried out by following simple rules.* Although the guidelines indicated are helpful in initiating treatment, each child must have care individualized to some degree. Newer ventilators have permitted the use of modalities such as assist/control (A/C) ventilation and pressure-support ventilation that allow the infant to set rate parameters. These techniques generally result in faster respiratory rates and greater synchrony. A comparative evaluation of the benefits of these modalities has not been completed. Experience is therefore an essential ingredient in successful ventilator treatment of neonates.

Mean Airway Pressure

Studies have demonstrated the significance of MAP in the physiology of neonatal mechanical ventilation. MAP is defined as the

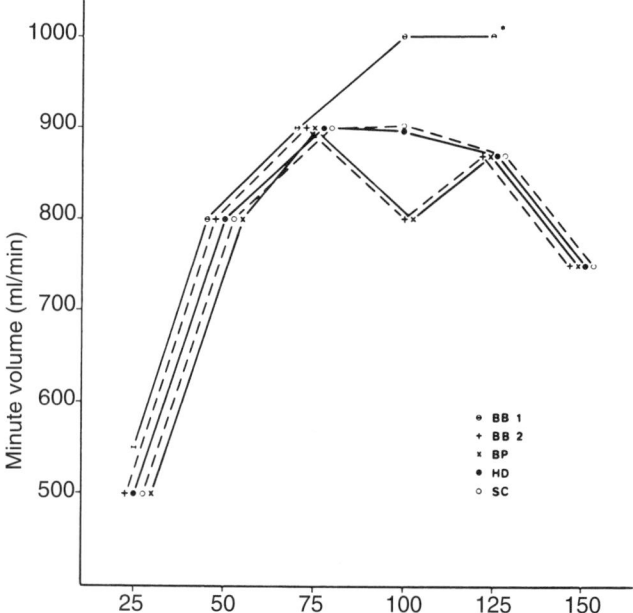

Figure 96–8. Minute volume effects of increasing ventilator rates from 25 to 150 breaths/minute (bpm—*horizontal axis*). Ventilators examined: BB 1, Babybird 1; BB 2, Babybird 2; BP, Bourns BP200; HD, Healthdyne; SC, Sechrist. Ventilator settings: peak inspiratory pressure = 25 cm H₂O; positive end-expiratory pressure = 5 cm H₂O; inspiration to expiration ratio (I/E) = 1:2 (after 75 bpm, ventilator BB 1 minute volumes were measured at 1:1 I/E ratio); flow = 10 Vain. (From Boros SJ, et al: Pediatrics 74:487, 1984.)

mean of instantaneous readings of proximal airway pressure during a single respiratory cycle. In waveform terminology, MAP is equal to the integration of the area under the pressure curve during a respiratory cycle. When one compares the two types of waveforms generated by ventilators, sine waves and square waves, it is obvious that MAP is higher in square wave ventilation compared with sine wave ventilation if inspiratory time (T_i) and PIP are equal (Fig. 96–9). Increasing MAP has been shown to increase oxygenation in neonates with RDS.[124] However, this relationship may not hold true for all methods of increasing MAP (see Fig. 96–7). For example, if MAP is increased by raising the PIP, but with a very short T_i, that increase may be dissipated rapidly in the upper airways and ET tube, thus negating its effect.

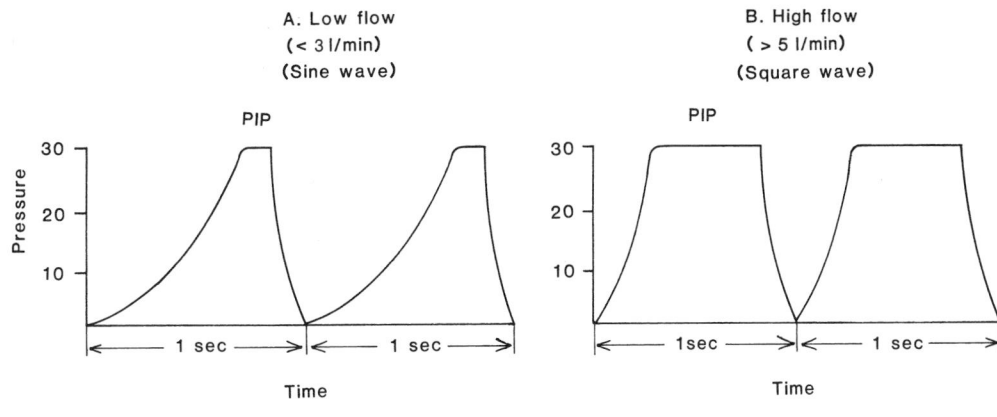

Figure 96–9. Comparison of ventilator waveforms. **A,** Sine wave (relative). **B,** Square wave (relative). (From Goldsmith JP, Karotkin EH [eds]: Assisted Ventilation of the Neonate. Philadelphia, WB Saunders Co, 1988, p 148.)

The primary factors that control MAP are PEEP, I/E ratio, PIP, and waveform. Reynolds[119] demonstrated that prolonging inspiration (increased T_i) during slow-rate ventilation with a square wave increased oxygenation. Additional work by Boros and associates[124] confirmed the value of increasing MAP to improve oxygenation in RDS. As MAP increases, right-to-left shunt and the alveolar-arterial oxygen gradient are progressively reduced. Although high MAP may improve oxygenation during acute phases of neonatal lung disease (which is usually accompanied by decreased compliance), as infants recover and compliance improves, high MAP may cause venous obstruction similar to that seen with high CPAP. In addition, airways may become overdistended, leading to the complication of pulmonary injury described previously. Because MAP is a function of numerous variables and is not specifically set on any conventional ventilator (this control is available on some high-frequency oscillators), one must again be cautious in selecting the optimal ventilatory pattern for this disease state to maximize the effect of MAP on oxygenation while attempting to reduce the negative effects of excessive levels.

In general, the greatest effect on oxygenation can be achieved by increasing PEEP, because MAP will increase in direct proportion to the increase in PEEP (depending on the I/E ratio). If one does not simultaneously change PIP, however, in such circumstances, Paco$_2$ may rise because tidal volume will decrease (secondary to the decrease in the difference between PIP and PEEP). Furthermore, one must consider that oxygenation may paradoxically decrease as one attempts to raise MAP, if one begins to impede venous return to the heart, thereby impairing venous return and cardiac output, while also compressing the pulmonary vasculature. In such cases, the clinician has usually exceeded the optimal level of PEEP for the clinical situation.

Inspiratory/Expiratory Ratio

Many of the effects of I/E ratio have been discussed in sections related to CPAP, PIP, ventilator rate, and MAP. Some of the effects of varying I/E ratio are noted in Table 96–11. Again, it is not possible simply to set an I/E ratio at the onset of ventilator treatment that will maximize oxygenation and ventilation throughout the clinical course of the disease. One must reevaluate the clinical course frequently in this regard. In fact, it may be better to select a T_i as a variable rather than selecting an I/E ratio, because, with an I/E ratio selection, the T_i may become excessively long as the

ventilator rate is slowed during recovery. For example, an I/E ratio equal to 1.0 at a rate of 60 breaths/minute produces a T_i of 0.5 second, but the T_i becomes prolonged to 1.0 second when the rate is slowed to 30 beats/minute. Prolonged T_i may predispose patients to air leaks and BPD if the time constant of the lung is exceeded.

APPROACHES TO RESPIRATORY SUPPORT

As noted previously, the effects of injury associated with neonatal mechanical ventilation can result in substantial morbidity and mortality. Because of the continuing high incidence of BPD, ranging from approximately 10 to 40% at major university medical centers,[116] several alternative approaches to ventilator support have been investigated (see Tables 96–4 and 96–6 through 96–9). We are concentrating on conventional ventilation, although modalities such as high-frequency ventilation, inhalational nitric oxide, and extracorporeal life support remain important tools in the intensive care nursery. These modalities are discussed elsewhere in this book.

Advances in Conventional Ventilation

Many improvements in conventional ventilators have been introduced into the intensive care nursery. The addition of flow sensors permitted on-line respiratory function measurements and more complex monitoring systems. Miniaturization of technologies, available for adult ventilation including pressure-support, A/C, and volume ventilation, are now available for even the smallest neonates.

For the infant receiving intermittent mandatory ventilation (IMV), spontaneous respiratory effort that is not in synchrony with the mechanical breath can be detrimental. The active expiration of the asynchronous breath may diminish tidal volume and may result in barotrauma.[125] Attempts at achieving synchrony have included pharmacologic paralysis, sedation, and the use of a rapid respiratory rate and a short T_i. Variable results have been demonstrated in multiple studies, but, in general, synchronous ventilation diminishes barotrauma and alterations in cerebral blood flow and increases tidal volume and minute ventilation.[126, 127]

Synchrony on IMV can be achieved with rapid rates.[128] Maintaining synchrony in these infants, in the healthier infant, or during weaning is difficult. Patient-triggered ventilation addresses some of these limitations and has now become a standard

TABLE 96–11

Neonatal Mechanical Ventilatory Rates

Slow (< 40 breaths/min)		Medium (40–60 breaths/min)		Rapid (>60 breaths/min)	
Advantages	*Side Effects*	*Advantages*	*Side Effects*	*Advantages*	*Side Effects*
Increased Pao₂ with increased MAP	Must increase PIP to maintain ventilation	Mimics normal ventilatory rate	May not provide adequate ventilation in some cases	Higher Pao₂ (may be the result of air trapping)	May exceed time constant and produce air trapping
Useful in weaning	Increased PIP may cause barotrauma	Effectively treats most neonatal lung diseases		May allow decreased PIP and Vt	May cause inadvertent PEEP
Used with square wave ventilation	Patient may require paralysis	Usually does not exceed time constant of lung, so air trapping is unlikely		Hyperventilation may be useful in PPHN	May result in change in compliance (frequency dependence of compliance)
Used when I/E ratio is inverted				May reduce atelectasis (? air trapping)	Inadequate Vt and minute ventilation if only dead space is ventilated

I/E = inspiratory/expiratory; MAP = mean airway pressure; PEEP = positive end-expiratory pressure; PIP = peak inspiratory pressure; PPHN = persistent pulmonary hypertension of the neonate; Vt = tidal volume.

part of the neonatologist's repertoire. In general, patient-triggered ventilation consists of two forms of mechanical ventilation: *synchronized IMV (SIMV)* and *A/C ventilation.* With SIMV, the ventilator is synchronized to the infant's breathing pattern. If the patient-triggering threshold is met within a specific time (depending on the preset ventilator rate), a ventilator breath is not delivered, and the infant breathes spontaneously. A ventilator breath *is* delivered if the infant fails to breathe. Examination of the baby's breathing pattern with SIMV will reveal both spontaneous breaths and ventilator breaths. The value of this form of support is that pressures within the airway are not stacked, so injury to the airway and the lung is theoretically reduced, and gas is not inadvertently "dumped" from the ventilator because airway pressures are reached prematurely. Although many neonatologists use SIMV as their primary mode of ventilator support for neonates, this technique appears to have greater benefit as a weaning tool or if overdistention is present with A/C ventilation, particularly in the extremely low birth weight infant with either RDS or pulmonary insufficiency of prematurity.

A/C ventilation is also a form of patient-triggered support. With A/C ventilation, each infant breath that reaches the trigger threshold initiates a full ventilator breath. If the infant is apneic, or if the effort is inadequate to trigger a ventilator breath, the ventilator will deliver a preset back-up rate to the baby. All breaths in this form of ventilation appear similar and are entirely ventilator derived, and no spontaneous infant breaths ever occur on A/C support (unless the generated pressure is so low that it fails to trigger the ventilator). With A/C ventilation, the infant is fully synchronized to the ventilator. With the use of termination sensitivity as an adjunct, T$_i$ will be limited to a percentage of maximum flow, and air trapping can usually be reduced or eliminated.

A/C ventilation is a very effective form of initial treatment for many babies with various neonatal lung diseases in the early stages of their illness. The use of A/C ventilation limits pressure exposure for the infants, and they often spontaneously select a rate that is optimal for gas exchange, with a lower pressure than would usually be set on SIMV. Minute ventilation is higher on A/C than on SIMV.[129] It is more difficult, however, to wean babies on A/C ventilation; occasionally, some overdistention will occur if there is excessive neural drive to breathe, and prolonged use of A/C ventilation may lead to some diaphragmatic muscle atrophy and further weaning difficulty. Consequently, we often move

infants from A/C to SIMV when they begin to show signs of recovery from their lung disease. With A/C ventilation, one must also be cautious of autocycling of the ventilator. This problem can occur when there is erroneous triggering of the ventilator from leaks in the system, build-up of humidity in the circuit, or sensing of the cardiac pulsations as breaths. Frequent breaths are delivered unnecessarily to the baby. We have also seen an occasional infant on A/C support who does well while awake, with good gas exchange, but who has inadequate blood gases while sleeping or if sedated. In such cases, it would be helpful to have the capability of using two separate ventilator settings, one for waking periods and one during apneic support when slightly more pressure may be necessary for gas exchange. To date, however, no neonatal ventilator allows for the selection of multiple ventilator settings simultaneously that could automatically trigger under certain conditions.

An adjunct therapy during patient-triggered ventilation is *pressure-support ventilation,* in which spontaneous infant breaths are partially or fully augmented by an inspiratory pressure assist higher than baseline end-distending pressure. This approach eases the work of breathing by allowing additional pressure delivery to overcome the elastic and resistive loads. This form of therapy may be used alone or in association with SIMV ventilation. Because it is synchronized with the infant's ventilation, it can be used in babies who are becoming fatigued from work of breathing, in sedated infants, and in infants in a weaning phase of ventilation who are first beginning to reuse their respiratory musculature. When this technique is used in conjunction with SIMV, it is important that the SIMV rate is not set too high, or the baby will have no impetus to breathe, and one of the primary purposes of pressure support will be nullified.

Tidal volume–guided ventilation or volume-guarantee ventilation is a newer approach to therapy in which the clinician sets a mean tidal volume to be delivered by the ventilator while still allowing management of ventilator pressures. It is a variation of pressure-support ventilation in which volume, not pressure, guides the delivery of an augmented breath. The goal is to minimize variation in delivery of tidal volume, thought to be the cause of pulmonary injury in infants. Volume guarantee is used in conjunction with patient-triggered modalities. When the operator sets the inspiratory pressure limit during patient-triggered support, the ventilator attempts to deliver the set guaranteed tidal volume using the lowest airway pressure possible. When the expired tidal volume exceeds the upper pressure limit, the ventilator will use a lower PIP on the next breath. If the set tidal volume cannot be delivered within the set pressure limit, an alarm alerts the operator to reset the pressure limit to a higher level or to adjust the guaranteed tidal volume to a lower level. Although available data on this technique are limited, it does appear that volume guarantee can achieve similar levels of gas exchange with slightly lower mean levels of inspiratory pressure.[130] Additional modifications may occur in the future, such as guaranteed minute ventilation, in which a desired minute ventilation is designated, with the ventilator providing a mix of guaranteed tidal volume and frequency to provide the desired minute ventilation.

Proportional assist ventilation (PAV) and *respiratory muscle unloading* (RMU) require even more sophisticated computer assistance to achieve their effects. These innovative approaches work to control ventilator pressure throughout inspiration (in the case of PAV) or throughout the entire cycle (during RMU). With both forms of ventilator support, the infant's respiratory effort is continuously monitored. During inspiration, as with pressure support ventilation, pressure rises to more than baseline to produce the desired inspiratory resistive unloading, thereby easing work of breathing. During exhalation, the circuit pressure falls to less than the baseline end-distending pressure, facilitating elastic and resistive unloading throughout that phase of the respiratory cycle. With this form of support, the resulting airway pressure is a variable that changes with the needs of the infant at any point during the respiratory cycle and is a weighted summation of a combination of airflow and tidal volume above baseline pressure. Although infant studies with PAV and RMU are limited at present, the initial work appears very encouraging.[131,132] In a trial that examined the relative effects of low birth weight infants treated with IMV, A/C, and PAV, PAV appeared to maintain equivalent arterial oxygenation at lower airway and transpulmonary pressures than the other two modalities. During PAV, the oxygenation index was also reduced by 28%, with no evidence of more frequent apnea or other complications. There was also a decrease in both systolic and diastolic beat-to-beat variability with PAV, suggesting that there is additional overall cardiovascular stability offered to infants treated with this form of support. Another study indicated that there was less thoracoabdominal synchrony during PAV in preterm infants.[133] Currently, few centers use this form of ventilator support, because it is still in early trials, yet the concepts appear very promising. Additional larger scale trials will unquestionably be seen in the near future.

The additional space required by the ventilator adapter and by the ET tube adds a significant amount of anatomic dead space during mechanical ventilation, particularly to the airway of an extremely low birth weight (<1000 g) infant. Through a mechanism of tracheal gas insufflation, fresh gas is delivered to the more distal part of the ET tube and aids in washing out carbon dioxide from the airway. Peak inspiratory pressure can usually be decreased as well as tidal volume.[134] These factors may reduce barotrauma and volutrauma in these infants, and early trials appear promising.

Adjuncts to Mechanical Ventilation

The care of infants with respiratory failure during the newborn period has been helped immeasurably by additional approaches including the measurement of pulmonary functions and lung volumes by computer, the administration of synthetic or natural surfactant, and early trials of antioxidants such as SOD for the prevention of BPD.

Pulmonary function testing, which enables the determination of such factors as tidal volume, dynamic or static lung compli-

ance, resistance, work of breathing, FRC, and others, has eliminated much of the guesswork that once was standard in neonatal intensive care units. Furthermore, pulmonary function tests have altered our understanding of the management of some diseases.[135] Increased use of pulmonary function testing can better define therapy and should be a standard part of newborn intensive care.

Few therapeutic adjuncts have had the impact of surfactant in the intensive care nursery. Since its widespread introduction, surfactant has significantly decreased the severity and incidence of RDS during the neonatal period while reducing the likelihood of BPD.

The respiratory system influences cardiovascular function through its effects on venous return and pulmonary vascular resistance. Return of venous blood to the heart depends primarily on the gradient between extrathoracic and intrathoracic pressures or transpulmonary pressure. Normally, because intrapleural pressure is subatmospheric (because of the effects of lung recoil and thoracic retraction), there is a favorable pressure gradient for the flow of blood back to the right side of the heart. With the application of positive-pressure ventilation, there is an increase in intrathoracic pressures, thereby reducing venous return and cardiac output. Ventricular performance of the heart may also become compromised owing to compression. The increase in intrapleural pressure that occurs with the introduction of mechanical ventilation depends on the degree of pressure transmitted from the airway to the intrapleural space. Pressure transmission is primarily a factor of lung compliance in infants. Thoracic compliance, important in adults, is relatively insignificant during the neonatal period because it is so high compared with lung compliance. In the patient with RDS, reduction in lung compliance allows significantly less pressure transmission to the intrapleural space. Extrathoracic to intrathoracic pressures are not dramatically altered, so venous return and cardiac output are maintained. Patients with reduced compliance can tolerate significant levels of PIP and PEEP with a minimal decrease in cardiac output. Sudden increase in intrathoracic pressure, however, as seen in a tension pneumothorax, may reduce venous return, even with a poorly compliant lung. This situation, encountered in the very premature infant with surfactant deficiency, may result in an increase in venous pressure in the central nervous system and intraventricular hemorrhage. Furthermore, increasing compliance during RDS recovery may lead to a rapid increase in intrapleural pressure transmission over several hours, as seen during the diuretic phase of RDS. These findings suggest that maintenance of high ventilator pressures may lead to an increased risk of intraventricular hemorrhage and air leaks.

In addition to its effects on venous return and cardiac output, airway pressure during mechanical ventilation is also transmitted to intraparenchymal vessels. This effect is complex and depends on several factors in the newborn infant. Lung compliance again plays an important role, and in neonates there is less transmission of positive pressure with reduced compliance. In RDS, the disease process itself produces a decrease in FRC. This decrease results in an increase in pulmonary vascular resistance, offsetting the beneficial effect of reduced pressure transmission from the airway. In contrast, lung overdistention, as seen in ventilation with large tidal volumes or modes of treatment that lead to gas trapping (i.e., high rate positive-pressure breathing) may pose problems. In these instances, overdistention of the air spaces compresses arterioles and capillaries, leading to increased pulmonary vascular resistance. Maintenance of FRC at near normal levels appears to be optimal for maintaining pulmonary perfusion. In addition to gas volumes, it is evident that another significant part of the equation for pulmonary perfusion must include blood volume. When blood volume is reduced (e.g., in hemorrhage, postasphyxia capillary leak, or sepsis), the influence of mechanical ventilator pressures on pulmonary perfusion is magnified.

Other complications associated with the effects of mechanical ventilation on cardiovascular performance during the neonatal period need further investigation. Investigators have shown that mechanical ventilation may alter relative tone in the autonomic nervous system; levels of various neurohumoral substances, referred to collectively as eicosanoids, may have wide-ranging effects in certain disease states, such as persistent pulmonary hypertension of the newborn (PPHN).[136] In PPHN, there is a persistent elevation of pulmonary vascular resistance (PVR) of unknown etiology. Some evidence suggests that the increase in PVR may be partly mediated through either elevated or decreased amounts of these substances, which have very potent vasodilating and vasoconstricting capabilities. Other none-icosanoids, such as bradykinin, histamine, various hormones, and acetylcholine, as well as numerous other (perhaps some undiscovered) factors, also may have significant influence on pulmonary vascular tone and therefore perfusion. Furthermore, hypoxemia produces some degree of pulmonary arteriolar vasoconstriction, acting either through these vasoactive substances or through some alternative mechanism. Ultimately, a delicate balance emerges in which the infant's blood volume, thoracic gas volume, autonomic control, and humoral factors produce a condition in which effective pulmonary blood flow is controlled. One of the most complicated diseases in which pulmonary hypoperfusion plays an important role is PPHN, or persistent fetal circulation. This syndrome, first characterized during the 1970s by Gersony and other investigators,[137,138] is a disease primarily of full-term infants. The pathophysiology is notable in that the infant fails to demonstrate the normal decrease in PVR that typically occurs after birth. Pulmonary artery pressure is often higher than systemic blood pressure, which results in right-to-left shunting of blood across the foramen ovale and/or the ductus arteriosus. Infants with this syndrome often demonstrate significant differential cyanosis, with high preductal oxygen saturation, whereas postductal saturation may be very low, depending on the degree of shunting. The syndrome is most commonly associated with postdate infants, sepsis, meconium aspiration, small for gestational age infants, pulmonary hypoplasia, and diaphragmatic hernias. In many cases, no specific etiology is discernible. Evidence suggests that some infants may have pulmonary vascular hypoplasia. Additionally, several new syndromes have been described that previously were thought to be PPHN. These syndromes include partial or complete surfactant protein B deficiency in which the synthesis of surfactant-associated proteins is abnormal, resulting in a picture of alveolar proteinosis and chronic respiratory failure, and alveolar-capillary dysplasia, a syndrome diagnosed post mortem by findings. At present, lung transplantation offers the only potential cure for these entities.

Since 1978, when Fox introduced the hyperventilation technique for the treatment of PPHN,[139] mechanical ventilator therapy has been an important part of the care given to these babies. Hyperventilation has been demonstrated to decrease PVR in this syndrome.[136,139,140] It is not entirely clear whether the response is a nonspecific pulmonary vasodilatation caused by a reduction of $Paco_2$, an increase in pH, a mechanical effect of ventilation, or some combination of factors. Subsequent work has demonstrated that hyperventilation does not provide better outcomes than other ventilation schemes in this population. Most likely, the lung injury associated with hyperventilation outweighs the benefit of transient decreases in PVR with hypocarbia. In addition, drugs such as inhaled nitric oxide have replaced hyperventilation as a means of increasing pulmonary blood flow. The disease also has a series of stages through which the baby progresses to a more physiologic circulatory pattern, at which time the ventilatory approach must be altered to avoid ventilator-induced lung injury.[141-144] In milder cases and in some clinical situations, hyperventilation may not be necessary.[142] In many cases, injury occurs early, leading to a need for an alternative therapeutic approach such as high-frequency ventilation or extracorporeal membrane oxygenation (ECMO). Of additional concern are findings that indicate that continued hyperventilation to avoid ECMO may be a primary cause of neurologic injury, cerebral palsy, and developmental delay.[145]

In contrast to pulmonary hypoperfusion, pulmonary hyperperfusion may also have a significant physiologic impact on optimal positive-pressure ventilation. In infants with a ventricular septal defect or in preterm infants with RDS and a patent ductus arteriosus, lung compliance may be adversely affected during ventilation by the excess pulmonary blood volume. With left-to-right shunting at a high rate, the pulmonary lymphatics may not maintain normal rates of fluid reabsorption. Interstitial fluid increases, and alveolar-capillary diffusion of gases may be reduced. These factors invariably lead to a need to increase ventilator support during mechanical ventilation. Failure to intervene by either pharmacologic means or surgery may lead to greater lung injury and may increase the probability of chronic lung disease.[146]

An additional concern in infants receiving mechanical ventilation is that of V/Q mismatching. During the application of CPAP or positive-pressure ventilation, areas of the lung that are atelectatic tend to remain so, whereas inflated or partly inflated regions of the lung tend to become further distended. The circulation generally responds to this situation with improved perfusion to lung segments that are inflated, whereas areas of the lung that are collapsed receive less perfusion. These effects are thought to be locally mediated. When atelectasis is present, the arteriolar bed in that region becomes partially constricted. Although this vasoconstriction is somewhat beneficial, there is still some lung tissue that is not receiving any significant ventilation. V/Q mismatching is then present and is a common phenomenon in neonatal lung disease.

With pulmonary interstitial emphysema, air dissects along distal bronchioles, interfering with circulation and gas exchange in affected segments of the lung that, however, may still be ventilated, resulting in a redistribution of pulmonary blood flow. As the situation progresses, gas exchange worsens, and ventilator support is commonly increased in an attempt to improve gas exchange. Too often, this response produces further overdistention of the already ventilated regions of the lung and increased pulmonary interstitial emphysema and ultimately results in the redistribution of pulmonary perfusion to less distended regions of the lung, owing to local vascular resistance changes in these regions. V/Q mismatching in such situations is often progressive, leading in some instances to tension pneumothorax. In such cases, one has maximum V/Q mismatching. Ventilation is now escaping into the pleural cavity, where no gas exchange can occur, while the perfusion remains confined within the lung, which is being progressively compressed from without by the pneumothorax. Subsequently, the heart may also be constricted as intrathoracic pressure increases. V/Q mismatching under any of the foregoing conditions therefore results in an increase in physiologic dead space and wasted ventilation. To compensate, the clinician must provide additional ventilatory support as well as alternate therapy (e.g., chest tube) in an attempt to reestablish more normal V/Q relationships.

REFERENCES

1. Northway WH Jr, et al: Pulmonary disease following respirator therapy of hyaline membrane disease: bronchopulmonary dysplasia. N Engl J Med 276:368, 1967.
2. Philip AG: Oxygen plus pressure plus time: the etiology of bronchopulmonary dysplasia. Pediatrics 55:44, 1975.
3. Taghezadech A, Reynolds EO: Pathogenesis of bronchopulmonary dysplasia following hyaline membrane disease. Am J Pathol 82:241, 1976.

4. Gibson E: Apnea. *In* Spitzer A (ed): Intensive Care of the Fetus and Neonate. St. Louis, Mosby–Year Book, 1996, pp. 470–481.
5. Rigatto H: A critical analysis of the development of peripheral and central respiratory chemosensitivity during the neonatal period. *In* von Euler C, Lagercrantz H (eds): Central Nervous Control Mechanisms in Breathing. New York, Pergamon Press, 1979.
6. Rigatto H, et al: Ventilatory response to 100% and 15% oxygen during wakefulness and sleep in preterm infants. Early Hum Dev 7:1, 1982.
7. Rigatto H: Control of breathing in the fetus and newborn. *In* Spitzer A (ed): Intensive Care of the Fetus and Neonate. St. Louis, Mosby–Year Book, 1996, pp 458–469.
8. Harris TN: Physiological principles. *In* Goldsmith JP, Karothers EH (eds): Assisted Ventilation of the Neonate. Philadelphia, WB Saunders Co, 1988, p 28.
9. Antunes MJ, Greenspan JS: Pulmonary function testing. *In* Spitzer A (ed): Intensive Care of the Fetus and Neonate. St. Louis, Mosby–Year Book, 1996, pp. 517–530.
10. Bhutani VK, et al: Pressure-induced deformation in immature airways. Pediatr Res 15:829, 1981.
11. Bhutani VK, et al: Acquired tracheomegaly in very preterm neonates. Am J Dis Child 140:449, 1986.
12. Penn RB, et al: Effect of tracheal smooth muscle tone on the collapsibility of extremely immature airways. J Appl Physiol 65:863, 1988.
13. Panitch HB, et al: A comparison of preterm and adult airway smooth muscle mechanics. J Appl Physiol 66:1760, 1989.
14. Antunes MJ, et al: Decreased functional residual capacity predates requirement for ECMO and lung opacification during ECMO. Pediatr Res 31:192A, 1992.
15. Deoras KS, et al: Structural changes in the tracheae of preterm lambs induced by ventilation. Pediatr Res 26:434, 1989.
16. Allen JL, et al: Thoracoabdominal asynchrony in infants with airflow obstruction. Am Rev Respir Dis 141:337, 1990.
17. Fox WW, et al: Effects of endotracheal tube leaks on functional residual capacity determination in intubated neonates. Pediatr Res 13:60, 1979.
18. Gerhardt T, et al: A simple method for measuring functional residual capacity by N_2 washout in small animals and newborn infants. Pediatr Res 19:1165, 1985.
19. Morgan WJ, et al: Partial expiratory flow-volume curves in infants and young children. Pediatr Pulmonol 5:232, 1988.
20. Notter RH, Morrow PE: Pulmonary surfactant: a surface chemistry viewpoint. Am Biomed Eng 3:119, 1975.
21. Notter RN, Shapiro DL: Lung surfactant in an era of replacement therapy. Pediatrics 68:781, 1981.
22. Notter RN, Finkelstein JN: Pulmonary surfactant: an interdisciplinary approach. J Appl Physiol 57:1613, 1984.
23. Raju TK, et al: Double-blind controlled trial of single-dose treatment with bovine surfactant in severe hyaline membrane disease. Lancet 1:651, 1987.
24. Jobe A, et al: Duration and characteristics of treatment of premature levels with natural surfactant. J Clin Invest 67:370, 1981.
25. Vermont-Oxford Neonatal Network: A multicenter, randomized trial comparing synthetic surfactant with modified bovine surfactant extract in the treatment of neonatal respiratory distress syndrome. Pediatrics 97:1, 1996.
26. Wolfson MR, et al: Respiratory muscle function. *In* Tecklin J (ed): Cardiopulmonary Physical Therapy. St. Louis, CV Mosby, 1989.
27. Northway WH: An introduction to bronchopulmonary dysplasia. Clin Perinatol 19:489, 1999.
28. Troug WE, Jackson JC: Alternative Modes of Ventilation in the Prevention and Treatment of Bronchopulmonary Dysplasia. Philadelphia, WB Saunders Co, 1992, pp 621.
29. Slutsky AS: Lung injury caused by mechanical ventilation. Chest 116:9S, 1999.
30. Bjorklund LJ, et al: Manual ventilation with a few large breaths at first compromises the therapeutic effect of subsequent surfactant replacement in immature lambs. Pediatr Res 42:348, 1998.
31. Jobe AJ: The new BPD: an arrest of lung development. Pediatr Res 4:641, 2000.
32. Coalson JJ, et al: Decreased alveolarization in baboon survivors with bronchopulmonary dysplasia. Am J Respir Crit Care Med 152:640, 2000.
33. Albertine KH, et al: Chronic lung injury in preterm lambs. Disordered respiratory tract development. Am J Respir Crit Care Med 159:945, 1999.
34. Tremblay L, et al: Injurious ventilatory strategies increase cytokines and c-fos m-RNA expression in an isolated rat lung model. J Clin Invest 99:944, 1997.
35. Meduri GU, et al: Inflammatory cytokines in the BAL of patients with ARDS: persistent elevation over time predicts poor outcome. Chest 108:1303, 1995.
36. Tutor JD, et al: Loss of compartmentalization of alveolar tumor necrosis factor after lung injury. Am J Respir Crit Care Med 149:1107, 1994.
37. Donnelly SC, et al: Interleukin-8 and development of adult respiratory distress syndrome in at-risk patient groups. Lancet 341:643, 1993.
38. Slutsky AS, Tremblay LN: Multiple system organ failure: is mechanical ventilation a contributing factor? Am J Respir Crit Care Med 157:1721, 1998.
39. Jacobs RF, et al: Factors related to the appearance of alveolar macrophages in the developing lung. Am Rev Respir Dis 131:548, 1985.
40. Christensen RD, et al: Blood and marrow neutrophils during experimental group streptococcal infection: quantification of the stem cell, proliferative, storage and circulating pools. Pediatr Res 16:549, 1982.
41. Carlton DP, et al: Role of neutrophils in lung vascular injury and edema after premature birth in lambs. J Appl Physiol 83:1307, 1997.
42. Merritt TA, et al: Elastase and alpha 1-proteinase inhibitor activity in tracheal aspirates during respiratory distress syndrome: role of inflammation in the pathogenesis of bronchopulmonary dysplasia. J Clin Invest 72:656, 1983.
43. Ogden BE, et al: Neonatal lung neutrophils and elastase/proteinase inhibitor imbalance. Am Rev Respir Dis 130:817, 1984.
44. Ogden BE, et al: Lung lavage of newborns with respiratory distress syndrome: prolonged neutrophil influx is associated with bronchopulmonary dysplasia. Chest 83:31S, 1983.
45. Arnon S, et al: Pulmonary inflammatory cells in ventilated preterm infants: effect of surfactant treatment. Arch Dis Child 69:44, 1993.
46. Groneck P, et al: Association of pulmonary inflammation and increased microvascular permeability during the development of bronchopulmonary dysplasia: a sequential analysis of inflammatory mediators in respiratory fluids of high-risk preterm neonates. Pediatrics 93:712, 1994.
47. Rannels DE: Role of physical forces in compensatory growth of the lung. Am J Physiol 257:L179, 1989.
48. Wirtz HR, Dobbs LG: Calcium mobilization and exocytosis after one mechanical stretch of lung epithelial cells. Science 250:1266, 1990.
49. Pierce RA, et al: Chronic lung injury in preterm lambs: disordered pulmonary elastin deposition. Am J Physiol 272:L452, 1997.
50. Jackson JC: Effect of high-frequency ventilation on the development of alveolar edema in premature monkeys at risk for hyaline membrane disease. Am Rev Respir Dis 143:865, 1991.
51. Kinsella JP, et al: Independent and combined effects of inhaled nitric oxide, liquid perfluorochemical and high-frequency oscillatory ventilation in premature lambs with respiratory distress syndrome. Am J Respir Crit Care Med 159:1220, 1999.
52. Jackson JC: Reduction in lung injury after combined surfactant and high-frequency ventilation. Am J Respir Crit Care Med 150:534, 1994.
53. Ikegami M, et al: Lung injury and surfactant metabolism after hyperventilation of premature lambs. Pediatr Res 47:398, 2000.
54. Naik A, et al: Effects of different styles of ventilation on cytokine expression in the preterm lamb lung. Pediatr Res 4:372A, 2000.
55. Thurlbeck WM: Morphologic aspects of bronchopulmonary dysplasia. J Pediatr 95:842, 1979.
56. Anderson WR, Strickland MB: Pulmonary complications of oxygen therapy in the neonate. Arch Pathol 91:506, 1971.
57. Roberts R, et al: Oxygen-induced alterations in lung vascular development in the newborn rat. Pediatr Res 17:368, 1983.
58. Sobonya RE, et al: Morphometric analysis of the lung in prolonged bronchopulmonary dysplasia. Pediatr Res 16:969, 1982.
59. Rasche RFH, Kuhns LR: Histopathologic changes in airway mucosa of infants after endotracheal intubation. Pediatrics 50:632, 1972.
60. Lee RM, et al: Ciliary defects associated with the development of bronchopulmonary dysplasia, ciliary motility and ultrastructure. Am Rev Respir Dis 129:190, 1984.
61. Anderson WR, Engal RR: Cardiopulmonary sequelae of reparative stages of bronchopulmonary dysplasia. Arch Pathol Lab Med 107:603, 1983.
62. Melnick G, et al: Normal and pulmonary vascular resistance and left ventricular hypertrophy in young infants with bronchopulmonary dysplasia: an echocardiographic and pathologic study. Pediatrics 66:589, 1980.
63. Berman W Jr, et al: Evaluation of infants with bronchopulmonary dysplasia using cardiac catheterization. Pediatrics 70:708, 1982.
64. Walsh WF, Hazinski TA: *In* Spitzer A (ed): Intensive Care of the Fetus and Neonate. St. Louis, Mosby–Year Book, 1996, pp 641–656.
65. Panitch HB, et al: Maturational changes in airway smooth muscle structure-function relationships. Pediatr Res 31:151, 1992.
66. Bhutani VK, et al: Pressure-induced deformation in immature airways. Pediatr Res 15:829, 1981.
67. Shaffer TH, et al: In-vivo mechanical properties of the developing airway. Pediatr Res 25:143, 1989.
68. Bjorklund LJ, et al: Manual ventilation with a few large breaths at birth compromises the therapeutic effect of subsequent surfactant replacement in immature lambs. Pediatr Res 42:348, 1997.
69. Berry D, et al: Leakage of macromolecules in ventilated and unventilated segments of preterm lamb lungs. J Appl Physiol 70:423, 1991.
70. Nilsson R, et al: Lung surfactant and the pathogenesis of neonatal bronchiolar lesions induced by artificial ventilation. Pediatr Res 12:249, 1978.
71. Jobe A, et al: Mechanisms initiating lung injury in the preterm. Early Hum Dev 53:81, 1998.
72. Sills JH, et al: Continuous negative pressure in the treatment of infants with pulmonary hypertension and respiratory failure. J Perinatol 9:43, 1989.
73. Cvetnic WG, et al: Reintroduction of continuous negative pressure ventilation in neonates: two-year experience. Pediatr Pulmonol 8:245, 1990.
74. Watts JL: Chronic pulmonary disease in neonates after artificial ventilation: distribution of ventilation and pulmonary interstitial emphysema. Pediatrics 60:273, 1977.
75. Boros SJ, Orgill AA: Mortality and morbidity associated with pressure and volume-limited infant ventilators. Am J Dis Child 132:865, 1978.
76. Dreyfuss D, Saumon G: Role of tidal volume, FRC, and end-inspiratory volume in the development of pulmonary edema following mechanical ventilation. Am Rev Respir Dis 148:1194, 1993.

77. Slutsky AS. Lung injury caused by mechanical ventilation. Chest 116(1 Suppl):9S, 1999.

78. Muscedere JG, et al: Tidal ventilation at low airway pressures can augment lung injury. Am J Respir Crit Care Med. 149:1327, 1994.

79. Heicher DA, et al: Prospective clinical comparison of two methods for mechanical ventilation of neonates: rapid rate and short inspiratory time versus slow rate and long inspiratory time. J Pediatr 98:957, 1981.

80. Clark RH, et al: Commentary: Lung protective strategies of ventilation in the neonate: what are they? Pediatrics 105:112, 2000.

81. McPherson AR, et al (eds): Retinopathy of Prematurity. Toronto, BC Decker, 1986.

82. Lucey JF, Dangman B: A reexamination of the role of oxygen in retrolental fibroplasia. Pediatrics 73:82, 1984.

83. Cryotherapy for Retinopathy of Prematurity Cooperative Group: Multicenter trial of cryotherapy for retinopathy of prematurity: preliminary results. Arch Ophthalmol 106:471, 1988.

84. Johnson LH, et al: Vitamin E and ROP: the continuing challenge. In Klaus MH, Fanaroff AA (eds): Yearbook of Neonatal-Perinatal Medicine. St. Louis, Mosby-Year Book, 1993, pp xv–xxiv.

85. Frank L, Sosenko IR: Prenatal development of lung antioxidant enzymes in four species. J Pediatr 110:106, 1987.

86. Sosenko IR, et al: Failure of premature rabbits to increase lung antioxidant enzyme activities after hyperoxic exposure: antioxidant enzyme gene expression and pharmacologic intervention with endotoxin and dexamethasone. Pediatr Res 137:469, 1995.

87. Autor AP, et al: Developmental characteristics of pulmonary superoxide dismutase: relationship to idiopathic respiratory distress syndrome. Pediatr Res 10:154, 1976.

88. Frank L, et al: Oxygen therapy and hyaline membrane disease: the effect of hyperoxia on pulmonary superoxide dismutase activity and the mediating role of plasma or serum. J Pediatr 90:105, 1997.

89. Davis JM, et al: Safety and pharmacokinetics of multiple doses of recombinant human CuZn superoxide dismutase administered intratracheally to premature neonates with respiratory distress syndrome. Pediatrics 100:24, 1997.

90. Graziani LJ, et al: Mechanical ventilation in preterm infants: neurosonographic and developmental studies. Pediatrics 90:515, 1992.

91. Saugstad OD: Is oxygen more toxic than currently believed? Pediatrics 108:1203, 2001.

92. STOP-ROP Multicenter Study Group: Supplemental therapeutic oxygen for prethreshold retinopathy of prematurity (STOP-ROP): a randomized, controlled trial. I. Primary outcomes. Pediatrics 105:295, 2000.

93. Van Marter LJ, et al: Do clinical markers of barotrauma and oxygen toxicity explain interhospital variation in rates of chronic lung disease? Pediatrics 105:1194, 2000.

94. Tin W, et al: Pulse oximetry, severe retinopathy, and outcome at one year in babies of less than 28 weeks gestation. Arch Dis Child Fetal Neonatal Ed 84:F106, 2001.

95. Poets CF: When do infants need additional inspired oxygen? A review of the current literature. Pediatr Pulmonol 26:424, 1998.

96. Gregory GA, et al: Treatment of the idiopathic respiratory distress syndrome with continuous positive airway pressure. N Engl J Med 284:1333, 1971.

97. Saunders RA, et al: The effect of continuous positive airway pressure on lung mechanics and lung volumes in the neonate. Biol Neonate 29:178, 1976.

98. Chernick V: Hyaline membrane disease: therapy with constant lung-distending pressure. N Engl J Med 289:302, 1973.

99. DeLemos RA, et al: Continuous positive airway pressure as an adjunct to mechanical ventilation in the newborn with respiratory distress syndrome. Anesth Analg 52:328, 1973.

100. Herman S, Reynolds EO: Methods for improving oxygenation in infants mechanically ventilated for severe hyaline membrane disease. Arch Dis Child 48:612, 1973.

101. Goldberg RN, Abdenour GE: Air leak syndromes. In Spitzer A (ed): Intensive Care of the Fetus and Neonate. St. Louis, Mosby-Year Book, 1996, pp 629–640.

102. Shaffer TH, Delivoria-Papadopoulos M: Alterations in pulmonary function of premature lambs due to positive end-expiratory pressure. Respiration 36:183, 1978.

103. Shaffer TH, et al: Positive end-expiratory pressure: Effects of lung mechanics of premature lambs. Biol Neonate 34:1, 1978.

104. Hobelmann CF Jr, et al: Mechanics of ventilation with positive end-expiratory pressure. Ann Thorac Surg 24:68, 1977.

105. Sturgeon CL Jr, et al: PEEP and CPAP: Cardiopulmonary effects during spontaneous ventilation. Anesth Analg 52:633, 1977.

106. Martin RJ, et al: The effect of a low continuous positive airway pressure on the reflex control of respiration in preterm infants. J Pediatr 90:976, 1977.

107. Miller MJ, et al: Continuous positive airway pressure selectively reduces obstructive apnea in preterm infants. J Pediatr 106:91, 1985.

108. Frost EA: Effects of positive end-expiratory pressure on intracranial pressure and compliance in brain-injured patients. J Neurosurg 47:195, 1977.

109. Jamsberg PD, et al: Effects of PEEP on renal function. Acta Anaesthesiol Scand 22:508, 1978.

110. Murdaugh HV Jr, et al: Effect of altered intrathoracic pressure on renal hemodynamics, electrolyte excretion and water clearance. J Clin Invest 38:834, 1959.

111. Hemmer M, et al: Urinary antidiuretic hormone excretion during mechanical ventilation and weaning in man. Anesthesiology 52:395, 1980.

112. Hall SV, et al: Renal hemodynamics and function with continuous positive pressure ventilation in dogs. Anesthesiology 41:452, 1974.

113. Annat G, et al: Effect of PEEP ventilation on renal function, plasma renin, aldosterone, neurophysins and urinary ADP, and prostaglandins. Anesthesiology 58:136, 1983.

114. Bark H, et al: Elevation in plasma ADH levels during PEEP ventilation in the dog: mechanisms involved. Am J Physiol 239:E474, 1980.

115. Fox WW, et al: Positive pressure ventilation of the neonate. In Goldsmith JP, Karotkin EH (eds): Assisted Ventilation of the Neonate. Philadelphia, WB Saunders Co, 1988, p 146.

116. Avery ME, et al: Is chronic lung disease in low birth weight infants preventable? A survey of eight centers. Pediatrics 79:26, 1987.

117. Wall NM: Infant endotracheal tube resistance: effects of changing length, diameter, and gas density. Crit Care Med 8:38, 1980.

118. Bland RD, et al: High frequency mechanical ventilation in severe hyaline membrane disease: an alternative treatment? Crit Care Med 8:275, 1980.

119. Reynolds EO: Pressure waveform and ventilator settings for mechanical ventilation in severe hyaline membrane disease. Int Anesthesiol Clin 12:259, 1974.

120. Bancalari E: Inadvertent positive end-expiratory pressure during mechanical ventilation. J Pediatr 108:567, 1986.

121. Boros SJ, et al: Using conventional infant ventilators at unconventional rates. Pediatrics 74:487, 1984.

122. Kirby R, et al: Continuous flow ventilation as an alternative to assisted or controlled ventilation in infants. Anesth Analg 51:871, 1971.

123. Downs JB, et al: Intermittent mandatory ventilation: a new approach to weaning patients from mechanical ventilations. Chest 64:331, 1973.

124. Boros SJ: Variations in inspiratory-expiratory ratio and air pressure waveform during mechanical ventilation: the significance of mean airway pressure. J Pediatr 94:114, 1979.

125. Greenough A, et al: Pancuronium prevents pneumothoraces in ventilated premature babies who actively expire against positive pressure inflation. Lancet 1:1, 1984.

126. Perlman JM, et al: Reduction in intraventricular hemorrhage by elimination of fluctuating cerebral blood-flow velocity in preterm infants with respiratory distress syndrome. N Engl J Med 312:1353, 1985.

127. Cooke RW, Rennie JM: Pancuronium and pneumothorax. Lancet 1:286, 1984.

128. Amitay M, et al: Synchronous mechanical ventilation of the neonate with respiratory disease. Crit Care Med 21:118, 1993.

129. Mrozek JD, et al: Randomized controlled trial of volume-targeted synchronized ventilation and conventional intermittent mandatory ventilation following initial exogenous surfactant therapy. Pediatr Pulmonol 29:11, 2000.

130. Cheema IU, Ahluwahia JS: Feasibility of tidal volume-guided ventilation in newborn infants: a randomized, crossover trial using the volume guarantee modality. Pediatrics 107:1323, 2001.

131. Schulze A, et al: Proportional assist ventilation in low birth weight infants with acute respiratory disease: a comparison to assist/control and conventional mechanical ventilation. J Pediatr 135:339, 1999.

132. Schulze A: Enhancement of mechanical ventilation of neonates by computer technology. Semin Perinatol 24:429, 2000.

133. Musante G, et al: Proportional assist ventilation decreases thoracoabdominal asynchrony and chest wall distortion in preterm infants. Pediatr Res 49:175, 2001.

134. Visveshwara N, et al: Patient-triggered synchronized assisted ventilation of newborns: report of a preliminary study and three years' experience. J Perinatol 11:347, 1991.

135. Antunes MJ, et al: Prognosis with preoperative pulmonary function and lung volume assessment in infants with congenital diaphragmatic hernia. Pediatrics 96:1117, 1995.

136. Morin FC III, Davis JM: Persistent pulmonary hypertension. In Spitzer A (ed): Intensive Care of the Fetus and Neonate. St. Louis, Mosby-Year Book, 1996, pp 506–516.

137. Gersony WM, et al: "PFC" syndrome. Circulation 3:40, 1969.

138. Fox WW, et al: Pulmonary hypertension in the perinatal aspiration syndromes. Pediatrics 59:205, 1977.

139. Fox WW: Mechanical ventilation in the management of persistent pulmonary hypertension of the neonate (PPHN). In Proceedings of Ross Symposium on Cardiovascular Sequelae of Asphyxia in the Newborn. Washington, DC, 1981, p 102.

140. Wiswell T, et al: High-frequency jet ventilation in the early management of respiratory distress syndrome is associated with a greater risk for adverse outcomes. Pediatrics 98:1035, 1996.

141. Wung J, et al: Management of infants with severe respiratory failure and persistence of the fetal circulation, without hyperventilation. Pediatrics 76:488, 1985.

142. Drummond WH, et al: The independent effects of hyperventilation, tolazoline, and dopamine on infants with persistent pulmonary hypertension. J Pediatr 98:603, 1981.

143. Fox WW, Duara S: Persistent pulmonary hypertension in the neonate: diagnosis and management. J Pediatr 103:505, 1983.

144. Sosulski R, Fox WW: The transitional phase during mechanical ventilation of infants with persistent pulmonary hypertension. Crit Care Med 13:715, 1985.

145. Graziani LJ, et al: Clinical antecedents of neurologic and audiologic abnormalities in survivors of neonatal ECMO: a group comparison study. J Child Neurol 12:415, 1997.

146. Brown ER, et al: Bronchopulmonary dysplasia: possible relationship to pulmonary edema. J Pediatr 92:982, 1978.

David J. Durand and Jeanette M. Asselin

97

High-Frequency Ventilation

OVERVIEW

During the last two decades, high-frequency ventilation (HFV) has gained increasing acceptance as a tool for managing neonatal respiratory failure.[1] HFV is the use of subnormal tidal volumes at supra-physiologic rates to provide oxygenation and ventilation. Although the Food and Drug Administration defines conventional ventilation as rates less than 150 breaths per minute, and high frequency ventilation as rates above 150 breaths per minute, this oversimplifies a spectrum of respiratory physiology and ventilatory techniques. In most spontaneously breathing infants, respiratory rates range from 20 to 60 breaths per minute, although they can reach as high as 120 breaths per minute. We generally consider mechanical ventilation that relies on the delivery of normal tidal volumes at rates of less than 60 breaths per minute (1 Hz) as "conventional."

As ventilator rates are increased to rates approaching 100 to 150 breaths per minute, ventilation takes on some of the characteristics of HFV discussed next, and is better considered high-frequency positive-pressure ventilation (HFPPV).[2,3] With the increasing acceptance of "true" HFV devices, HFPPV is not as widely used as it was in the 1970s and early 1980s and may be particularly harmful to the lung. Rapid-rate ventilation with a conventional mechanical ventilator has a much different physiology than does HFV.

Although HFV devices can deliver respiratory frequencies from approximately 2.5 to 30 Hz, most HFV in neonates is accomplished with frequencies of between 5 and 15 Hz (300 to 900 breaths per minute).

TYPES OF HIGH-FREQUENCY VENTILATION

The two main types of HFV are high-frequency oscillatory ventilation (HFOV) and high-frequency jet ventilation (HFJV). Currently, the SensorMedics 3100 A HFOV and the Bunnell Life Pulse HFJV are the two main neonatal HFV devices available in the US, although a number of other HFOV devices are available in other countries.

High-Frequency Oscillatory Ventilation

As shown in Figure 97-1, the SensorMedics 3100A HFOV uses an electromagnetically driven diaphragm to generate a sinusoidal pressure pattern within the ventilator circuit, which is attached to the endotracheal tube. There is a continuous flow of fresh gas ("bias flow") into the circuit and of mixed gas out of the circuit. The oscillating movement of the diaphragm causes active inspiratory and expiratory phases that drive the mixing of gas between the circuit and the alveoli. The amplitude of the pressure wave is measured at the hub of the endotracheal tube as delta pressure and is proportional to the volume of the breath. The mean airway pressure, or the average pressure delivered to the endotracheal tube, is governed by the rate of gas flow into the circuit and the resistance to gas flow out of the circuit. As shown in Figure 97-2, the amplitude of the pressure generated by the diaphragm and the mean airway pressure can be adjusted independently.

High-Frequency Jet Ventilation

The Bunnell Life Pulse HFJV delivers high-velocity, low-volume pulses of gas, which are generated by a pinch valve connected to a high-pressure source (Fig. 97-3). These pulses are delivered to the upper airway and are superimposed on a background gas flow from a conventional ventilator that provides positive end-expiratory pressure (PEEP). In addition, conventional breaths may be administered in conjunction with the jet breaths. Earlier versions of the Bunnell HFJV required a triple lumen endotracheal tube, but this is no longer the case. With the current version of the Bunnell HFJV, a triple lumen is attached to a standard endotracheal tube, providing a jet lumen and a pressure-monitoring lumen, as well as the main lumen for the background gas flow.

With HFJV, ventilation is controlled primarily by the amplitude of the high-frequency breaths, which is measured as the delta pressure between the peak inspiratory pressure generated by the HFJV pulses (HFJV positive inspiratory pressure [PIP]) and the PEEP generated by the conventional ventilator. Mean airway pressure in the Bunnell HFJV is determined by multiple factors, including HFJV PIP, HFJV frequency, PEEP, the frequency of conventional breaths, conventional PIP, and conventional inspiratory time.

Major Differences Between High-Frequency Ventilation Devices

Although it is tempting to group all HFV devices, particularly all oscillators, together into a single homogeneous group, this would be an oversimplification. Relatively subtle design differences can cause significant differences in gas exchange properties.[4,5] We suspect that at least some of the divergent results of the various large clinical trials of HFV (discussed later) are due to these design differences.

One important difference in the design of the various HFV devices is the inspiratory:expiratory ratios they generate. The piston-driven HFOV devices have a mandatory 1:1 ratio. The SensorMedics HFOV, although capable of a range of ratios, is usually used with a 1:2 ratio. The Bunnel HFJV is usually used with a 1:6 ratio. The extremely short inspiratory time (approximately 20 msec) of the Bunnell HFJV is at least part of the reason it is so effective in managing patients with interstitial emphysema or a bronchopleural fistula.[6] This short inspiratory time decreases the time during which ruptured airways are maximally distended and decreases the leak of air out of these airways. On the other hand, the short inspiratory time of the Bunnell HFJV is one of the factors that limits the amount of gas it can deliver and makes it a less effective device for managing large infants with severely noncompliant lungs.

OXYGENATION AND VENTILATION WITH HIGH-FREQUENCY VENTILATION

A number of publications have described the relationship between the factors that govern gas exchange during HFV.[7-11] Fortunately, understanding the details of these relationships is not essential to understanding most of what is seen clinically with HFV. It is easiest to think of HFV as a technique that is extremely efficient at mixing gas in the upper airway with gas in the alveoli.

Oxygenation

Diseases such as respiratory distress syndrome (RDS), meconium aspiration, and pneumonia are all associated with a tendency for

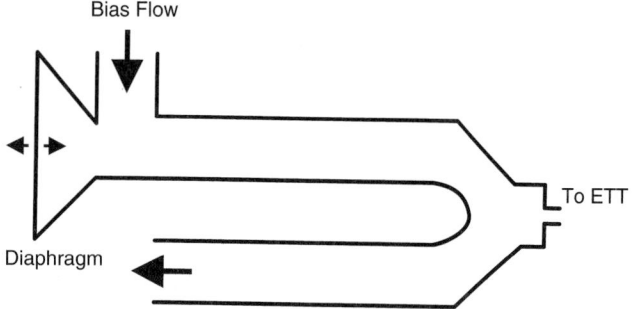

Figure 97–1. Simplified diagram of SensorMedics high frequency oscillating ventilator. The diaphragm applies sinusoidal pressure to the fresh gas, which is added to the circuit as bias flow. This pressure is then transmitted to the endotracheal tube (ETT).

the patient to develop atelectasis. With both conventional ventilation and HFV, increasing mean airway pressure leads to decreased atelectasis, and thus to improved ventilation/perfusion matching and oxygenation. With HFV, a significant increase in mean airway pressure usually also leads to an increase in lung volume, as seen on chest radiographs.

Ventilation

Ventilation, or the removal of CO_2 from the pulmonary blood, primarily depends upon the rate at which fresh gas comes into contact with the pulmonary capillary bed. In the normal lung with spontaneous breathing or conventional ventilation, the rate at which fresh gas comes into contact with pulmonary blood at the alveolar surface is the product of alveolar volume and respiratory frequency. The fundamental difference between CO_2 elimination with conventional ventilation and with HFV is that conventional ventilation delivers fresh gas to the alveoli only by *bulk flow*, while HFV causes both *bulk flow* and *mixing* to occur. In contrast to conventional ventilation in which CO_2 elimination is proportional to the product of respiratory rate (F), and tidal volume (V_T), with HFV CO_2 elimination is proportional to the product of respiratory rate and the *square* of volume delivered to the upper airway ($F \times V_T^2$).[11] With HFV, small changes in V_T have a more profound effect on CO_2 elimination than do small changes in F.

MECHANISMS OF GAS EXCHANGE WITH HIGH-FREQUENCY VENTILATION

The mechanisms by which HFV causes the enhanced gas mixing between the upper airway and the alveoli can be divided into several broad categories, described later. A more detailed description of these mechanisms is presented in the classic paper by Chang.[12]

Bulk Flow

It is commonly thought that HFV is accomplished with tidal volumes that are approximately equal to dead space volume. However, one must remember that dead space is a mathematical approximation that averages the entire respiratory system. In fact, some alveoli are closer to the upper airway than are others. Therefore ventilation with tidal volumes near the theoretical dead space volume will actually deliver fresh gas to some nearly alveoli by bulk flow.

Pendelluft

Pendelluft, a major mechanism of gas exchange in HFV, is the movement of gas between adjacent lung units, caused by driving

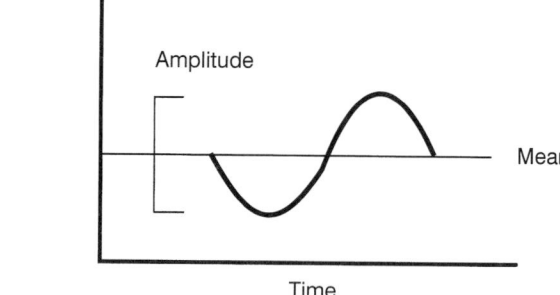

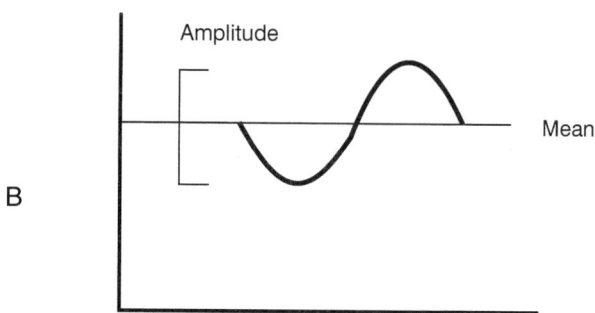

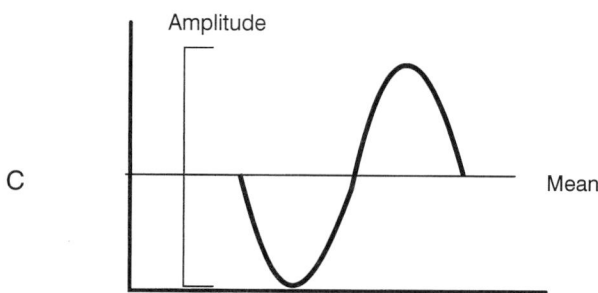

Figure 97–2. Diagram of pressure wave generated by HFOV. A, the mean airway pressure can be increased without affecting the amplitude (**B**), or the amplitude can be increased without affecting the mean airway pressure (**C**).

lung units with different time constants at high rates. The respiratory time constant (τ) is a measure of the amount of time it takes pressure to equalize between the upper airway and the alveoli at end-inspiration or end-expiration. In conventional tidal ventilation, the inspiratory and expiratory times are relatively long compared with τ. Thus, at end-inspiration and end-exhalation, pressure is essentially the same at the upper airway as in each alveolus. As frequency increases, the pressure in the alveolus has less time to reach equilibrium with the pressure in the upper airway.

There are small differences in both the compliance and the airway resistance of different alveolar units, even in uniform diseases such as RDS (Fig. 97–4). Since the respiratory time constant is equal to the product of resistance and compliance ($\tau = R \times C$), there are small differences in the time constants of different alveoli. As respiratory frequencies increase so that T_{insp} and T_{exp} are short relative to τ, there is no longer adequate time for the alveolar pressures to equilibrate with the upper airway pressures. If frequency is further increased so that inspiratory and expiratory time are short relative to the *difference* between the τ of adjacent alveoli, then there will be times in the respiratory cycle when there is a significant pressure gradient between adjacent alveoli. At those times, gas will flow from one alveolus to the

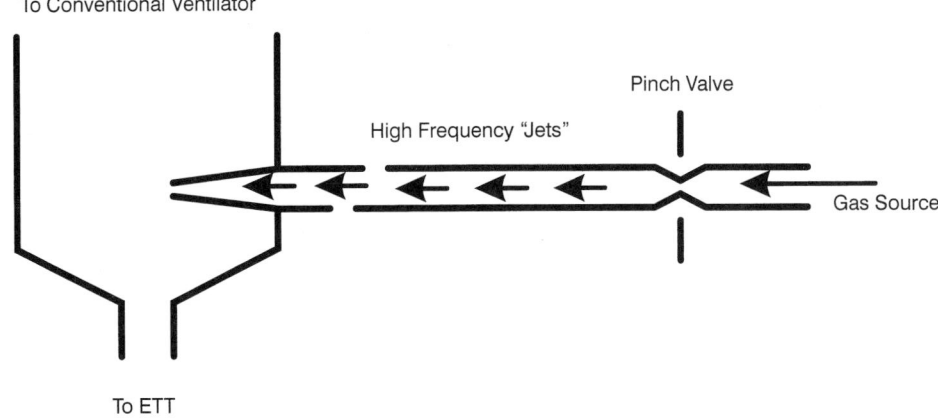

Figure 97–3. Simplified diagram of the Bunnell high frequency jet ventilator, showing pinch valve and endotracheal tube adapter. The pinch valve controls the duration and frequency of the high velocity gas "jets,", which are delivered to the endotracheal tube adapter. The main lumen of the adapter is connected to a conventional tidal ventilator. The pressure monitoring port is not shown in this diagram.

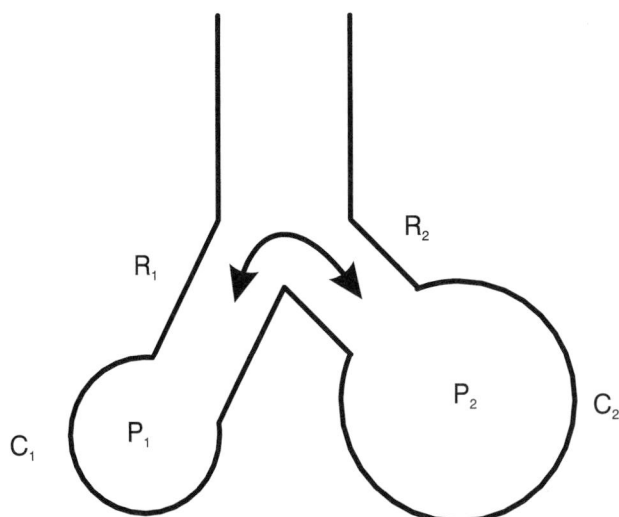

Figure 97–4. Pendelluft. The resistance (R) and compliance (C) of adjacent airways and alveoli are slightly different, resulting in different time constants. At high ventilator rates, this results in a difference in the pressure (P) of the two alveoli, causing gas to move between adjacent alveoli (*arrow*).

other, rather than from the alveolus to the upper airway. When this happens, delivery of relatively small volumes to the upper airway drives mixing between adjacent alveoli. This is the mechanism of the "swinging air" that moves between adjacent alveoli and enhances mixing throughout the lung.

Asymmetric Velocity Profiles

As shown in Figure 97-5, when pressure is suddenly applied to gas in a tube, that gas does not uniformly accelerate. Instead, the gas in the center of the tube accelerates to a velocity greater than the velocity of the gas at the periphery of the tube. The difference between the gas velocity vector at the center (V_c) of the tube and the gas velocity vector at the periphery (V_p), or the asymmetry of the velocity profiles, depends on multiple factors, including the diameter of the tube and the pressure that is applied. When high pressure is suddenly applied to gas at the upper airway, gas in the center of the airway travels at higher velocity, and therefore farther, than gas at the periphery. Thus, some fresh gas will travel much farther into the lung

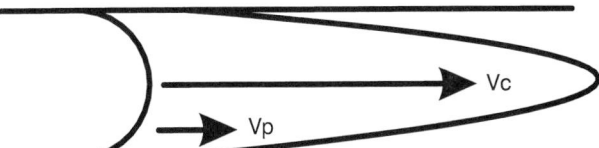

Figure 97–5. Asymmetrical velocity profiles. When pressure is suddenly applied to the gas, the gas in the center of the tube will have a greater velocity (V) than the gas at the periphery (V). Thus, gas in the center will travel farther than the gas at the periphery.

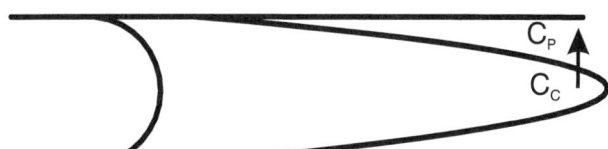

Figure 97–6. Taylor-type dispersion. The asymmetrical velocity profile creates an area of "fresh" gas in the center of the tube, which has a higher concentration of O_2 (C_c) than the "old" gas along the periphery of the tube (C). Therefore, oxygen will diffuse radially from the center to the periphery. The concentration gradient for CO_2 is the opposite, so CO_2 will diffuse from the periphery toward the center.

than if pressure were applied slowly (as in conventional tidal ventilation).

During exhalation, gas is accelerated out of the alveolus, and the process is reversed. However, the diameter of the airways is less during exhalation than during inspiration, so the degree of asymmetry of the velocity profiles is less during exhalation than during inspiration. Thus, the forward (inspiratory) and reverse (expiratory) velocity vectors of a complete HFV cycle do not simply cancel out, returning all gas to its original position.

Taylor-type Dispersion

One of the consequences of markedly asymmetric velocity profiles is that fresh gas in the center of the airway is surrounded by gas from a previous respiratory cycle, at the periphery of the airway. As shown in Figure 97-6, there is a center-periphery concentration gradient for both O_2 and CO_2 (i.e., the concentration in the center of the airway, C_{cent} is different from the concentration at the periphery, C$_{periph}$). This leads to radial diffusion from the periphery of the airway to the center, and from the center to the periphery. This diffusion, caused by the combination of axial asymmetrical velocity vectors and radial concentration gradients, is termed Taylor-type dispersion.

Molecular Diffusion

As with conventional ventilation, molecular diffusion is responsible for the mixing that occurs immediately adjacent to the alveolar surface.

Entrainment

In HFJV, unlike HFOV, small jets of high-velocity gas are injected into an airway. Because of the Venturi principle, these small jets entrain surrounding gas as they travel down the upper airway. This entrainment of gas is part of what allows the very small but very high-velocity jets of gas to cause a significant amount of gas exchange.

DISTRIBUTION OF PRESSURES

The endotracheal tube and airways act as *low-pass filters*. Low-pass filters transmit (pass) low-frequency signals without attenuation, while attenuating high-frequency signals. The degree of attenuation increases as frequency increases. As shown in Figure 97–7, the attenuation of a signal refers to the fact that amplitude is decreased without affecting the mean pressure. Thus, as respiratory frequency increases, less of the pressure delivered to the endotracheal tube is delivered to the alveoli. For example, in an infant with RDS, at a respiratory rate of 0.5 Hz (30 breaths per minute), there is minimal attenuation of the pressure wave from the upper airway to the alveolus. In this case, PIP and PEEP as measured at the upper airway are the same as the PIP and PEEP that would be measured at the alveolus. Somewhere between 1 and 2 Hz (60 to 120 breaths per minute), the endotracheal tube and airways begin to attenuate the amplitude of the pressure wave so that it is smaller when it reaches

the alveoli. When this happens, alveolar PEEP is greater than the PEEP measured at the upper airway, and alveolar PIP is less than the PIP measured at the upper airway.

As frequencies increase, this attenuation of the delta pressure goes from being a clinical annoyance to a fundamental aspect of HFOV. In an experiment involving direct measurement of proximal, tracheal, and alveolar pressure of rabbits receiving HFOV, the endotracheal tube attenuated up to 97% of the amplitude of the oscillation, while the airways imposed an additional 75% decrease in amplitude between the trachea and the alveoli.[13] Increasing oscillatory frequency while maintaining a fixed mean airway pressure and amplitude at the upper airway will increase the amount of attenuation imposed by the endotracheal tube and airways. Thus, an *increase* in frequency will result in a *decrease* in tidal volume delivered to the alveolus. Since V$_E$CO$_2$ is proportional to F × V^2_T, this will result in a *decrease* in CO$_2$ exchange.

The endotracheal tube and airways not only attenuate amplitude or delta pressure but also appear to have an effect on the regional distribution of mean pressure within the lung. Direct measurements of pressures in rabbits ventilated with HFOV showed lower mean airway pressure in the upper lobe than in the lower lobe or the trachea.[13] The magnitude of this difference partially depends on the inspiratory:expiratory ratio.[14]

ADVANTAGES OF HIGH-FREQUENCY VENTILATION

In addition to the theoretical advantages of HFV, there is abundant evidence from animal and clinical studies that HFV is superior to conventional ventilation for at least some neonatal diseases.

Theoretical Advantages of HFV

The left panel of Figure 97–8 shows an oversimplified picture of how the lung, when ventilated with conventional tidal volumes, alternates between end-expiratory volume and end-inspiratory volume. Because of surface forces, a lung that is noncompliant (e.g. as a result of surfactant deficiency or surfactant inactivation) tends to develop alveolar collapse at end-expiration. When this atelectatic lung is then inflated with a normal tidal volume

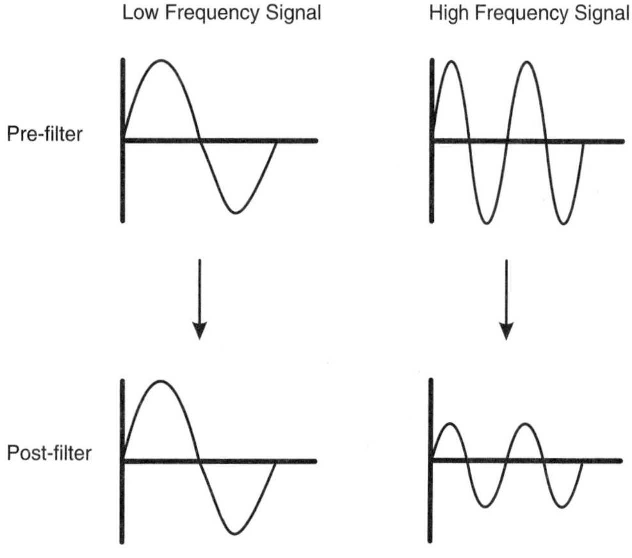

Figure 97–7. Action of a low-pass filter. The low frequency signal on the left is passed without being attenuated, whereas the amplitude of the high frequency signal on the right is dampened or attenuated.

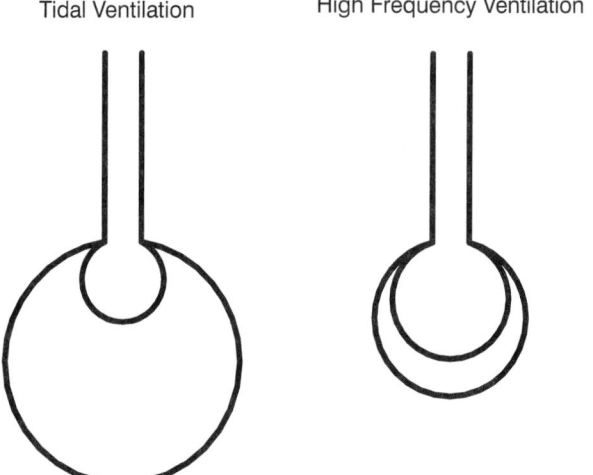

Figure 97–8. The figure on the left depicts the range of volumes through which the lung cycles during tidal ventilation, while the figure on the right depicts the smaller range of volumes that are delivered with HFV.

breath, the result may be overdistention of both the airways and nonatelectatic alveoli. Airway and/or alveolar overdistention can then cause a number of complications, including pulmonary interstitial emphysema, pneumothorax, damage to the alveolar-capillary interface, and release of proinflammatory molecules.

The right panel of Figure 97–8 shows the ideal of HFV, in which lung volumes are maintained between the two extremes seen with tidal ventilation. In this way, both atelectasis and overdistention should be decreased. For patients with a significant component of atelectasis, changing from conventional ventilation to HFV should make it possible to increase the average lung volume, thus decreasing atelectasis, without causing overdistention. Conversely, in patients with overdistention or air leak, it should be possible to decrease the average lung volume, thus decreasing overdistention, without causing end-expiratory collapse.

The early reports of HFV emphasized the advantages of using a low mean airway pressure to treat patients with pulmonary interstitial emphysema and bronchopleural fistula. As the incidence of interstitial emphysema and pneumothorax has decreased, most of the interest in HFV has shifted to its use as a technique to prevent or reverse atelectasis without causing overdistention. This strategy, often referred to as open lung or optimal lung volume, was initially associated with HFOV more than with HFJV. However, it is now clear that strategies aimed at decreasing atelectasis can be applied to both HFOV and HFJV.

Animal Studies of High-Frequency Ventilation

A number of animal studies show that HFV not only provides adequate oxygenation and ventilation in animals with lung disease but also does so in a way that is less traumatic than conventional ventilation. Much of this data comes from an elegant series of studies comparing HFOV to conventional ventilation in premature baboons with RDS.[15-20] These studies, as well as studies using other animal models of lung disease,[21] suggest that HFV causes less damage to the lung than does conventional ventilation. One of the most intriguing studies showed that when premature baboons were treated with HFOV immediately after birth, they were much less likely to develop clinical or histologic evidence of RDS than if they were ventilated with conventional tidal ventilation.[19] Although the early classic studies of HFV were done before the introduction of surfactant replacement therapy, data suggest that, even with surfactant replacement, HFV is superior to conventional ventilation.[22-24]

In addition to the studies on the role of HFV in animal models of RDS, there are data to support its use in other diseases. The many studies that used a surfactant lavage model of RDS in term animals probably can be extrapolated to diseases other than RDS. One study comparing HFV and conventional ventilation in an animal model of meconium aspiration showed that HFV-treated animals had better blood gases, better lung mechanics, and fewer histologic abnormalities.[25]

Clinical Studies of High-Frequency Ventilation

At least 14 controlled trials of HFV have been reported. These trials have used a variety of devices, with a wide range of strategies, to treat a variety of diseases and have (not surprisingly) arrived at different conclusions. The debate over how to interpret these studies is complex, but several broad conclusions are clear. The most important is that the advantages of HFV, while real, are relatively subtle. To see the advantages of HFV, it is essential to match the device and the strategy to the disease process.

A number of case reports and retrospective studies, particularly from the presurfactant era, suggested that HFV offers significant advantages in treating infants with severe air leak,

either pulmonary interstitial emphysema or bronchopleural fistula. One large trial showed that HFJV is superior to tidal ventilation for the treatment of RDS complicated by pulmonary interstitial emphysema.[26] Another large trial showed that HFOV is superior to tidal ventilation for preventing pulmonary interstitial emphysema and pneumothorax in patients with severe RDS.[27]

Recent studies of HFV have focused on its role in preventing chronic lung disease. The most successful studies have used either the Bunnell HFJV[28] or the SensorMedics HFOV,[29-32] both devices with inspiratory:expiratory ratios of less than 1:1. They have also used strategies that emphasized lung recruitment and continuing HFV throughout the ventilatory course. The most encouraging of these studies[32] randomized infants weighing between 601 and 1200 to HFOV or conventional ventilation at less than 4 hours of age, then managed both groups with tightly controlled protocols that emphasized optimizing lung volume, aggressive weaning, and continuing HFV until extubation. In this study, infants treated with HFV were extubated significantly sooner and were significantly less likely to have chronic lung disease at 36 weeks' corrected age. Follow-up studies of infants treated with HFV suggest that HFV treatment led to lung function that was as good as, or better than, lung function in infants treated with conventional ventilation.[33-35]

Although HFV is widely used in diseases other than RDS, there are few data from controlled trials on its role in these populations. The best trial on the role of HFV in term infants with severe pulmonary disease suggested that HFOV offers advantages over conventional ventilation, but it was too small to be conclusive.[36] Both anecdotal experience and data from the Extracorporeal Life Support Organization (ELSO) international extracorporeal membrane oxygenation (ECMO) registry suggest that HFV has become a mainstay of treatment in term and near-term infants with severe lung disease.

In support of its use in populations other than premature infants with RDS, there are now good controlled trials that demonstrated advantages of HFOV in the management of pediatric[37] and adult[38] patients with respiratory failure.

DISADVANTAGES OF HIGH-FREQUENCY VENTILATION

As with all therapies, HFV is not without some disadvantages.

Monitoring

One of the areas in which HFV is clearly inferior to the more sophisticated conventional ventilators is real-time monitoring. The type of simple, accurate graphic monitoring available with conventional ventilation is not an option for HFV. Plethysmography can give an accurate assessment of rapidly changing lung volumes on HFV[39] but is too cumbersome for routine use.

Inadvertent Hyperventilation

Because HFV is so effective at CO_2 removal, it is easy to hyperventilate a patient on HFV. Given the adverse effects of hyperventilation, and of rapid changes in P_{CO_2} on the lungs and the brain, it is essential that patients on HFV be closely monitored. Frequent blood gas determinations or transcutaneous monitoring or both are particularly important when initiating HFV, following surfactant administration, in the operating room, or during any period when the lung mechanics are changing.

Lung Expansion

Because the lung is not constantly cycling through tidal breaths, the visual clues to under-expansion or overdistention are not present. Of particular concern is the fact that over-distention is a significant risk in patients who have had a recent improvement in their lung compliance. Because of the profound effect of τ on the efficacy of HFV, patients with markedly nonhomogeneous lung disease are also at a significant risk of developing regional hyperinflation with HFV. As a general rule, we obtain chest radiographs shortly after starting a patient on HFV, following any large changes in HFV settings, or any time the F_1O_2 has changed by 0.2 or more.

Cardiovascular Effects

The relationship between excessive PEEP and/or mean airway pressure and impairment of cardiac output is well known for conventional ventilation. The same relationship exists with HFV, in which increasing mean airway pressure can decrease cardiac output. Although the use of a lung recruitment strategy theoretically places an infant at risk of decreased cardiac output, in our experience this is not a problem if lung recruitment is done judiciously and with appropriate monitoring of blood gases and chest radiographs.[40] The adverse effects of high mean airway pressure are most often seen in patients with borderline cardiovascular status. In patients with severe pneumonia and septic shock, HFV with a high mean airway pressure may result in improved oxygenation and ventilation, but also in a decrease in cardiac output. Careful titration of mean airway pressure and lung volume, as well as close monitoring of cardiovascular status and judicious use of blood volume expanders is essential in these patients.

Central Nervous System Effects

Several studies have suggested that HFV use was associated with an increased incidence of severe intracranial hemorrhage, periventricular leukomalacia, or both, but most of the clinical trials of HFV, particularly the recent ones, have failed to show any adverse CNS effects. The two most recent trials of HFV included a total of almost 1300 patients and showed no differences in the rate of intracranial hemorrhage or periventricular leukomalacia.[32,41] The most recent study of the neurodevelopmental follow-up of infants treated with HFV showed no detrimental effects of HFV.[30]

REFERENCES

1. Keszler M, Durand DJ: Neonatal high-frequency ventilation: past, present, and future. Clin Perinatol 28:579, 2001.
2. Boros SJ, et al: Using conventional ventilators at unconventional rates. Pediatrics 74:487, 1984.
3. Roithmaier A, et al: Airway pressure measurements during high-frequency positive pressure ventilation in extremely low birth weight neonates. Crit Care Med 22:S71, 1994.
4. Hatcher D, et al: Mechanical performance of clinically available, neonatal, high-frequency, oscillatory-type ventilators. Crit Care Med 26:1081, 1998.
5. Pillow JJ, et al: In vitro performance characteristics of high-frequency oscillatory ventilators. Am J Resp Crit Care Med 164:1019, 2001.
6. Gonzalez F, et al: Decreased gas flow through pneumothoraces in neonates receiving high-frequency jet versus conventional ventilation. J Pediatr 110:464, 1987.
7. Permut S, et al: Model of gas transport during high-frequency ventilation. J Appl Physiol 58:1956, 1985.
8. Venegas JG, et al: Relationship for gas transport during high-frequency ventilation in dogs. J Appl Physiol 59:1539, 1985.
9. Venegas JG, et al: A general dimensionless equation of gas transport by high-frequency ventilation. J Appl Physiol 60:1025, 1986.
10. Venegas JG, et al: Effects of respiratory variables on regional gas transport during high-frequency ventilation. J Appl Physiol 64:2108, 1988.
11. Boynton BR, et al: Gas exchange in healthy rabbits during high-frequency oscillatory ventilation. J Appl Physiol 66:1343, 1989.
12. Chang H: Mechanisms of gas transport during ventilation by high-frequency oscillation. J Appl Physiol 56:553, 1984.
13. Gerstmann DR, et al: Proximal, tracheal, and alveolar pressures during high-frequency oscillatory ventilation in a normal rabbit model. Pediatr Res 28:367, 1990.
14. Pillow JJ, et al: Effect of I/E ratio on mean alveolar pressure during high-frequency oscillatory ventilation. J Appl Physiol 87:407, 1999.
15. Bell RE, et al: High-frequency ventilation compared to conventional positive-pressure ventilation in the treatment of hyaline membrane disease in primates. Crit Care Med 12:764, 1984.
16. deLemos RA, et al: Ventilatory management of infant baboons with hyaline membrane disease: the use of high frequency ventilation. Pediatr Res 21:594, 1987.
17. Gerstmann DR, et al: Influence of ventilatory technique on pulmonary barotrauma in baboons with hyaline membrane disease. Pediatr Pulmonol 5:82, 1988.
18. deLemos RA, et al: Rescue ventilation with high frequency oscillation in premature baboons with hyaline membrane disease. Pediatr Pulmonol 12:29, 1992.
19. Meredith KS, et al: Role of lung injury in the pathogenesis of hyaline membrane disease in premature baboons. J Appl Physiol 66:2150, 1989.
20. Kinsella JP, et al: High-frequency oscillatory ventilation versus intermittent mandatory ventilation: early hemodynamic effects in the premature baboon with hyaline membrane disease. Pediatr Res 29:160, 1991.
21. McCulloch PR, et al: Lung volume maintenance prevents lung injury during high frequency oscillatory ventilation in surfactant-deficient rabbits. Am Rev Respir Dis 137:1185, 1988.
22. Niblett DJ, et al: Comparison of the effects of high frequency oscillation and controlled mechanical ventilation on the development of alveolar edema in premature monkeys at risk for hyaline membrane disease. Am Rev Respir Dis 143:865, 1991.
23. Jackson JC, et al: Reduction in lung injury after combined surfactant and high frequency ventilation. Am J Respir Crit Care Med 150:534, 1994.
24. Froese AB, et al: Optimizing alveolar expansion prolongs the effectiveness of exogenous surfactant therapy in the adult rabbit. Am Rev Respir Dis 148:569, 1993.
25. Wiswell TE, et al: Management of a piglet model of the meconium aspiration syndrome with high-frequency or conventional ventilation. Am J Dis Child 146:1287, 1992.
26. Keszler M, et al: Multicenter controlled trial comparing high-frequency jet ventilation and conventional mechanical ventilation in newborn infants with pulmonary interstitial emphysema. J Pediatr 119:85, 1991.
27. HiFO Study Group: Randomized study of high-frequency oscillatory ventilation in infants with severe respiratory distress syndrome. J Pediatr 122:609, 1993.
28. Keszler M, et al: Multi-center controlled clinical trial of high-frequency jet ventilation in preterm infants with uncomplicated respiratory distress syndrome. Pediatrics 100:593, 1997.
29. Clark RH, et al: Prospective randomized comparison of high-frequency oscillatory and conventional ventilation in respiratory distress syndrome. Pediatrics 89:5, 1992.
30. Gerstmann DR, et al: The Provo multicenter early high frequency oscillatory ventilation trial: improved pulmonary and clinical outcome in respiratory distress syndrome. Pediatrics 98:1044, 1996.
31. Plavka R, et al: A prospective randomized comparison of conventional mechanical ventilation and very early high-frequency oscillatory ventilation in extremely premature newborns with respiratory distress syndrome. Intensive Care Med 25:68, 1999.
32. Courtney SE, et al: Early high frequency oscillatory ventilation vs synchronized intermittent mandatory ventilation for very low birth weight infants. N Engl J Med 347:643, 2002.
33. HiFi Study Group: High-frequency oscillatory ventilation compared with conventional mechanical ventilation in the treatment of respiratory failure in preterm infants: assessment of pulmonary function at 9 months of corrected age. J Pediatr 116:933, 1990.
34. Gerstmann DR, et al: Childhood outcome after early high-frequency oscillatory ventilation for neonatal respiratory distress syndrome. Pediatrics 108:617, 2001.
35. Hofhuis W, et al: Worsening of VmaxFRC in infants with chronic lung disease in the first year of life: a more favorable outcome after high-frequency oscillation ventilation. Am J Respir Crit Care Med 166:1539, 2002.
36. Clark RH, et al: Prospective, randomized comparison of high-frequency oscillation and conventional ventilation in candidates for extracorporeal membrane oxygenation. J Pediatr 124:447, 1994.
37. Arnold JH, et al: Prospective, randomized comparison of high-frequency oscillatory ventilation and conventional mechanical ventilation in pediatric respiratory failure. Crit Care Med 22:1530, 1994.
38. Derdak S, et al: High-frequency oscillatory ventilation for acute respiratory distress syndrome in adults: a randomized, controlled trial. Am J Respir Crit Care Med 166:801, 2002.
39. Weber K, et al: Detecting lung overdistension in newborns treated with high-frequency oscillatory ventilation. J Appl Physiol 89:364, 2000.
40. Durand DJ, et al: Early HFOV vs SIMV in VLBW infants: a pilot study of two ventilation protocols. J Perinatology 21:221, 2001.
41. Johnson AH, et al: High-frequency oscillatory ventilation for the prevention of chronic lung disease of prematurity. N Engl J Med 347:633, 2002.

Thomas H. Shaffer and Marla R. Wolfson

98 Liquid Ventilation

Respiratory insufficiency during early development, whether resulting from immaturity of pulmonary structure and biochemical processes or from aspiration syndromes, calls for the use of assisted ventilation techniques. Exogenous surfactant replacement therapies have demonstrated improvement in gas exchange, decreased ventilatory requirements, and reduction in mortality. Pulmonary function–guided alterations in conventional ventilatory techniques and high-frequency ventilation can facilitate gas exchange at reduced inflation pressures; aggressive measures such as extracorporeal life support eliminate the requirement for pulmonary inflation pressures. In spite of improved survival of the infant with respiratory insufficiency, significant morbidity persists, resulting from barotrauma leading to chronic pulmonary sequelae.[1] Alternative means to support pulmonary gas exchange while preserving lung structure and biochemical development are still required.

Fluid breathing (liquid-assisted ventilation) uses a liquid to replace nitrogen gas as the carrier for oxygen (O_2) and carbon dioxide (CO_2). The air-liquid interface at the alveolar-capillary surface is eliminated, reducing pressure requirements to inflate the lung. To date, perfluorochemicals (PFCs) are the most promising breathing media liquids because of their specific physiochemical properties of low surface tension and high solubility for respiratory gases as well as their chemically and biologically inert nature. After more than 30 years of neonatal and adult animal studies of liquid ventilation,[2-5] the clinical investigations have yielded promising results.

With the evolution of gas breathing in land-dwelling vertebrates, the lung replaced the gill as the gas exchange organ. Mammals make the transition from fluid-filled lungs during fetal life, when gas exchange is performed by the placenta, to gas breathing at birth, when the lungs assume responsibility for breathing. If premature delivery, antenatal or perinatal incident, or postnatal pulmonary insult precludes adequate maturation or impedes function of the pulmonary system, gas exchange insufficiency ensues. Because the lungs developed within a fluid environment, it appears logical that restoration of the fluid-filled environment would provide a natural transitional adjunctive therapy, and the fluid-filled lung might provide an experimental tool to understand lung function. This chapter traces the development of fluid breathing and extended applications from its origin to current areas of investigation.

FLUID AS A VENTILATORY MEDIUM

Saline

Saline was the first liquid employed as a respiratory medium,[6] and it effectively eliminates the gas-liquid interface within the lung. It has been fundamental in elucidating factors that influence alveolar structure, distensibility, stability, ventilation, and pulmonary blood flow.[7-13] Although the detergent-like action of saline has proved useful in removing pulmonary debris, it also removes pulmonary surfactant, which is necessary for lung stability. Furthermore, low respiratory gas solubility and excessive diffusion gradients at atmospheric conditions have limited the applicability of saline to support pulmonary gas exchange.[14-18] Because the O_2 content of saline saturated at 1 atmosphere is only about 3 vol%, it cannot support oxygenation under atmospheric conditions. In 1950, it was suggested that saline saturated with O_2

dissolved under pressure could potentially sustain submersed mammals.[19] Practical application of this concept was first demonstrated in 1962. Additional studies demonstrated that mammals submerged in hyperbaric-oxygenated saline could breathe liquid and resume gas breathing.[15,20-22] Although these studies demonstrated adequate oxygenation, CO_2 retention and profound acidosis occurred, thus rendering saline ventilation physiologically unsound during either normobaric or hyperbaric conditions.

Perfluorochemical Liquids

As an alternative to saline, the utility of other liquids as respiratory media was investigated. Experiments with silicone, vegetable oils, and animal oils demonstrated toxic effects.[23,24] PFCs were first produced during World War II as part of the Manhattan Project and, based on the high solubility of this medium for respiratory gases, were first used to support normobaric respiration in 1966 (Fig. 98-1).[25] This marked the beginning of the use of PFC as an alternative respiratory medium.

A true PFC is formulated from common organic compounds such as benzene, by replacing all the carbon-bound hydrogen atoms with fluorine atoms through techniques such as vapor-phase fluorination, cobalt trifluoride agitation, or electrochemical fluorination.[24] PFC liquids have a strong carbon-fluorine bond that provides them with extreme thermal, chemical, and physical stability. They can be stored at room temperature indefinitely, they can be subjected to antiseptic conditioning without alteration (i.e., autoclave, small pore filtering), and they are clear, odorless, nonbiotransformable, and generally insoluble in aqueous media and nonlipid biologic fluids.

The physicochemical profile and structure of various PFC liquids with potential application for PFC ventilation are shown in Tables 98-1 and 98-2 and Figure 98-2. As a class of liquids, they are unique in two ways: (1) they have the lowest sound speeds of any liquid and (2) gases are exceptionally soluble in the PFC liquids. PFC fluids are characterized by a cyclic or aliphatic structure consisting of 6 to 14 carbon atoms; the physicochemical profile of each compound is influenced by the particular arrangement of the carbon-fluorine bonds.[24,26-28] Gas solubility differs across PFC liquids and type of gas. It is dependent on the sizes of and steric relationships between the PFC and gas molecules.[29-31] Specific to respiratory gas exchange, O_2 and CO_2 are carried only as dissolved gases with solubilities as much as 16 and 3 times greater, respectively, in PFC than water. O_2 solubility ranges from 35 to 70 mL gas/dL at 25°C.[32] Although the carrying capacity for CO_2 is known for fewer compounds, reported values of CO_2 solubility are approximately four times greater than those for O_2, ranging from 122 to 225 mL/dL (i.e., perfluorodecalin [APF-140] = 122 mL/dL, perfluoroalkylpentane [FC-75] = 192 mL/dL, perfluoro-octylbromide [PFOB] = 225 mL/dL). Fewer data are available regarding the diffusivity of specific gases within the PFC liquids.[31,32] It is known that gases diffuse more slowly in liquids than in a gaseous medium and that the gas solubility is not related to the diffusivity within the PFC liquid. Although some properties of these liquids vary, their dielectric strength and resistivity are high, they are denser than both water and soft tissue, and they have relatively low surface tension and viscosity.

Differences in several of the physicochemical properties of the PFC fluids have relevance to their performance as respiratory

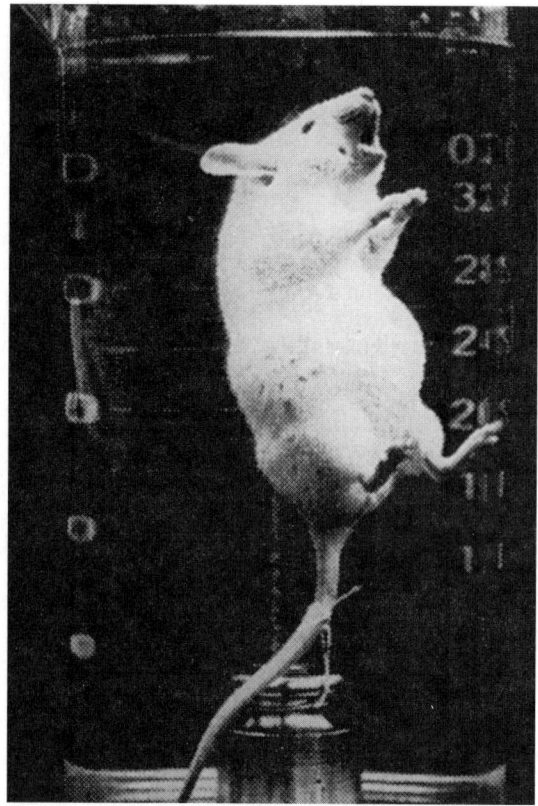

Figure 98–1. The liquid-breathing mouse. This historic mouse is submersed in and breathing a perfluorochemical liquid (FC-75; 3M Corp, St. Paul, MN) saturated with 100% oxygen. (Courtesy of Dr. L. C. Clark, Jr.)

fluids of lower spreading coefficients (i.e., FC-75 > PFOB > APF-140).[33, 34] Fluids of higher viscosity or kinematic viscosity (e.g., viscosity/density) may resist redistribution in the lung and may offer greater flow resistance. Both the carrying capacity (i.e., solubility) and the transfer capacity (i.e., diffusivity of gases within the PFC liquid as determined by the diffusion coefficients) of the liquid are important functional criteria in liquid ventilation. Smaller partial pressure gradients and less time are required for gases to saturate or leave liquids with higher gas diffusion coefficients. The higher the gas solubility, the less fluid volume required to remove or deliver gases. Fluids of higher CO_2 solubility may provide a greater carrying capacity for CO_2 but may require additional ventilation to deplete CO_2 from the reservoir.[35] Each of the physicochemical properties should be considered in the selection of a PFC liquid for specific ventilatory techniques.

Although these fluids are innately nontoxic and weak solvents, material compatibility with ventilator circuitry and endotracheal tubes has been investigated to rule out potential complications associated with leaching of plastics into the PFC and the effect of PFC on the structural integrity of plastic components. PFC liquids have been shown to cause plastic embrittlement of polyvinyl chloride plastics, minimal swelling of polytef (Teflon)-based products, compatibility with medical-grade polyurethane, and solubilization of silicone oil–based materials.[33]

PFC liquids have formed the basis for biologic applications including synthetic bloods, imaging agents, and replacement fluid for the eye.[36-42] Pure medical-grade PFC liquids currently exist for the purpose of liquid ventilation.

BIOPHYSICAL PROFILE AND PHYSIOLOGIC RESPONSES OF THE FLUID-FILLED LUNG

Figure 98–3 provides a summary of the biophysical profile and physiologic responses of the fluid-filled lung.

Pulmonary Structure and Function

The differential effects of tissue forces from surface-active forces on alveolar distensibility have been identified. One study found that more volume was displaced for the same change in pressure in the saline-filled lung than in the gas-filled lung.[13] This effect

media. Fluids of higher vapor pressure (e.g., lower boiling points) tend to volatilize from the lung faster than fluids of lower vapor pressure (e.g., higher boiling points). Fluids of higher spreading coefficients (a parameter related to the surface tension of the liquid and gas-liquid or liquid-liquid interfacial surface tension) may be distributed more readily in the lung than

---

TABLE 98–1

Physicochemical Profile of Various Perfluorocarbons

Perfluorocarbon	Formula	Orientation	O₂ Solution mL/100 mL (25°C)	Vapor Pressure mm Hg (37°C)	Boiling Point °C	Viscosity cS (25°C)	Mol. Wt. g/mol	Density g/mL (25°C)
PP2	C_7F_{14}	Cyclic	57.2	180	76	0.88	350	1.788
PFOB	$C_8F_{17}Br$	Aliphatic	52.7	11	140.5	1	499	1.89
PCI	$C_7F_{15}Cl$	Aliphatic	52.7	48.5	108	0.82	404.5	1.77
P12F	$C_9F_{20}O$	Aliphatic	52.5	39	121	0.95	504.1	1.721
FC-75F	$C_8F_{16}O$	Cyclic	52.2	51	102	0.85	416.1	1.783
FC-75P	$C_8F_{16}O$	Cyclic	52.2	51	102	0.85	416.1	1.783
PFDMA	$C_{12}F_{18}$	Cyclic	39.4	2.6	177.5	4.35	524.1	2
FC47	$C_{12}F_{27}N$	Aliphatic	38.4	2.5	174	2.52	671.1	1.9
PP9	$C_{11}F_{20}$	Cyclic	38.4	5.2	160	3.32	512.1	1.972
APF-57	C_6F_{14}	Cyclic	70	356.4	57.3	—	338	1.58
APF-100	C_8F_{16}	Cyclic	42.1	64.6	98.6	1.11	400	1.84
APF-125	C_9F_{18}	Cyclic	47.7	30	116.6	1.17	450	1.86
APF-140	$C_{10}F_{18}$	Cyclic	49	13.6	142	2.9	462	1.93
APF-145	$C_{10}F_{20}$	Cyclic	45.3	8.9	142.8	1.44	500	1.9
APF-175	$C_{12}F_{22}$	Cyclic	35	1.4	180	3.5	562	1.98
APF-200	$C_{13}F_{24}$	Cyclic	41	1.26	200	5.3	612	1.99
APF-215	$C_{14}F_{26}$	Cyclic	37	0.2	215	8	662	2.02

Data from references 17, 182–184.

Ideal Properties of a Fluid as a Respiratory Medium

High respiratory gas diffusion coefficient
High respiratory gas solubility
Low density and viscosity
Low surface tension
Low lipid solubility
Low vapor pressure
Inertness

was exaggerated when the gas-filled lung with elevated surface tension was filled with saline (Fig. 98–4). On the basis that saline eliminated the gas-liquid interface, and thus interfacial tension, it was concluded that the greater pressure requirements in the air-filled normal and abnormal lung resulted from surface forces.

In the gas-filled lung, alveolar pressures are uniform and vascular pressures are subject to a hydrostatic gradient, but in the saline-filled lung, alveolar and vascular pressures are relatively balanced throughout.[43, 44] This finding suggests that pulmonary blood vessels would be uniformly distended, resulting in more uniform distribution of blood flow and improved matching of ventilation to perfusion in the saline-filled as opposed to the gas-filled lung. In that regard, ultrastructural studies have shown that the capillaries bulge into the alveolar space in the saline-filled lung, whereas the alveolar surface is relatively smooth in the gas-filled lung (Fig. 98–5).[45] This study indicates that because saline eliminates surface tension at the alveolar surface, surface forces are responsible for maintaining the smooth appearance of the alveolar surface, and removal of surface tension supports tissue unfolding. The irregular alveolar surface area is larger in the fluid-filled than in the gas-filled lung of the same volume.

Pulmonary Mechanics

The factors that play a predominant role in maintaining lung volume stability may be divided into components attributable to the tissue properties and surface forces acting at the alveolar-capillary interface. Elastin and collagen confer structural integrity, whereas surface forces dictate stability of gas exchange regions over a wide range of lung volume.

Surface tension at the alveolar-capillary interface created by the interface between two phases (i.e., gas and the lung surface) is the force that resists expansion, and determines the amount of work required to create additional surface for gas exchange. Because the cohesive forces of molecules within a liquid are stronger than those between liquid (i.e., lung surface) and gas (i.e., within alveolus), more work is required to move molecules from within the liquid to a gas-liquid interface than to a liquid-liquid interface. Addition of a surface-active agent, or *surfactant,* to liquid decreases surface tension and reduces the work needed to increase surface area. Replacement of gas with liquid at the lung surface eliminates surface tension. Applying Laplace's law and the bubble model to the lung, $P = 2T/R$, the radius (R) of the alveolus is determined by the pressure gradient (P) across the alveolar wall and surface tension (T) acting on the alveolus; the pressure required to maintain alveolar size is decreased by lowering surface tension. According to this theory, if alveoli at different sizes are subject to the same transmural pressure, surface tension must vary with size to prevent collapse of smaller into larger alveoli. On this basis, an effective pulmonary surfactant must demonstrate a surface tension that varies with surface area.[46]

Alternatively, evidence from morphometric studies has disputed the bubble model theory. If interior alveoli of different sizes share a common wall, the two alveoli have the same internal pressure; thus, there is no driving force to collapse the

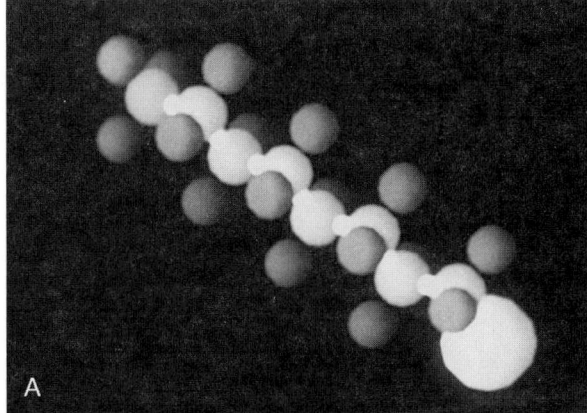
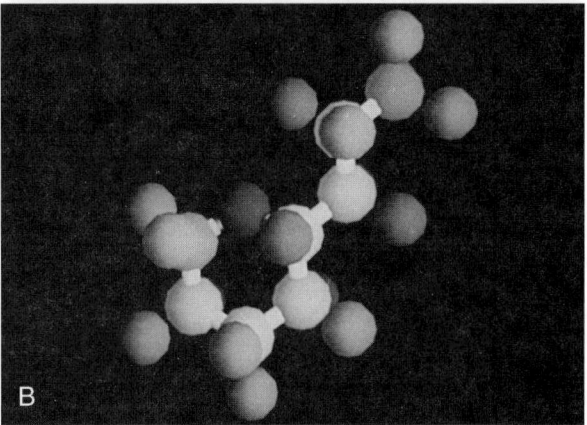
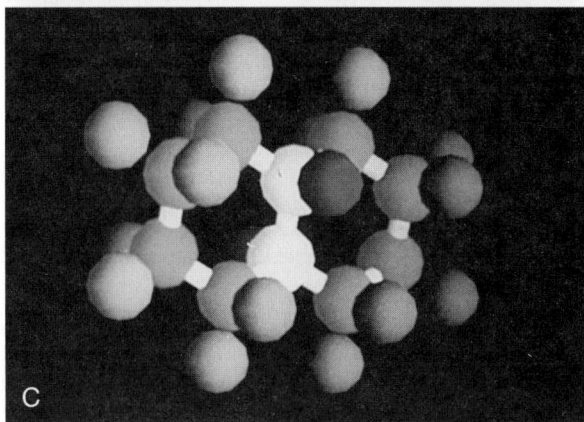

Figure 98–2. Molecular models of perfluorochemicals suitable for liquid ventilation. **A,** *Perfluoro-octylbromide* (i.e., LiquiVent, Alliance Pharmaceutical Corp, San Diego, CA) consists of an 8-carbon skeleton with surround fluorine atoms. Carbon 8 is also bound to a terminal bromide atom. **B,** *Perfluoroalkylpentane* (i.e., a component of RIMAR 101, Miteni Corp, Milan, Italy; FC-75P, 3M Corp, St. Paul, MN) consists of a cyclic portion of five fluorinated carbon atoms and one oxygen atom and a chain of three fluorinated carbon atoms. **C,** *Perfluorodecalin* (APF-140, Air Products and Fine Chemicals Corp, Allentown, PA) consists of a bicyclic molecule of 10 fluorinated carbon atoms.

smaller alveolus. Thus, changes in alveolar size over the respiratory cycle are achieved by unfolding of alveolar membranes.[45] In this situation, any agent capable of lowering surface tension would serve to decrease membrane adhesion and allow membrane unfolding; variable surface tension with area would not be required.[45, 47-49] These principles identify requirements of a modality that would facilitate alveolar stability.

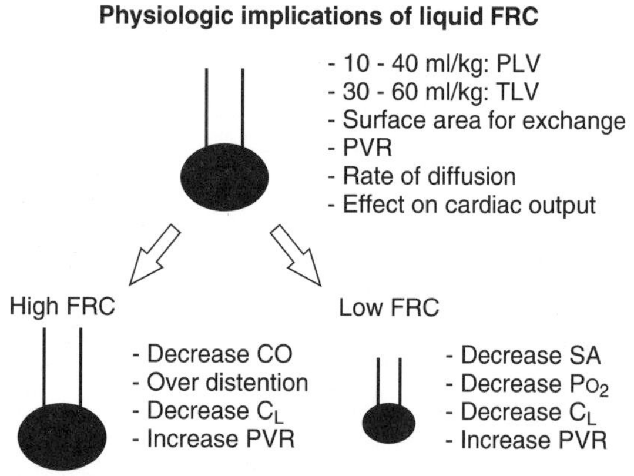

Physiologic implications of liquid FRC

- 10 - 40 ml/kg: PLV
- 30 - 60 ml/kg: TLV
- Surface area for exchange
- PVR
- Rate of diffusion
- Effect on cardiac output

High FRC

- Decrease CO
- Over distention
- Decrease C_L
- Increase PVR

Low FRC

- Decrease SA
- Decrease Po_2
- Decrease C_L
- Increase PVR

Figure 98–3 Biophysical profile and physiologic responses of the fluid-filled lung. C_L = lung compliance; FRC = functional residual capacity; PLV = partial liquid ventilation; PVR = pulmonary vascular resistance; SA = surface area; TLV = tidal liquid ventilation.

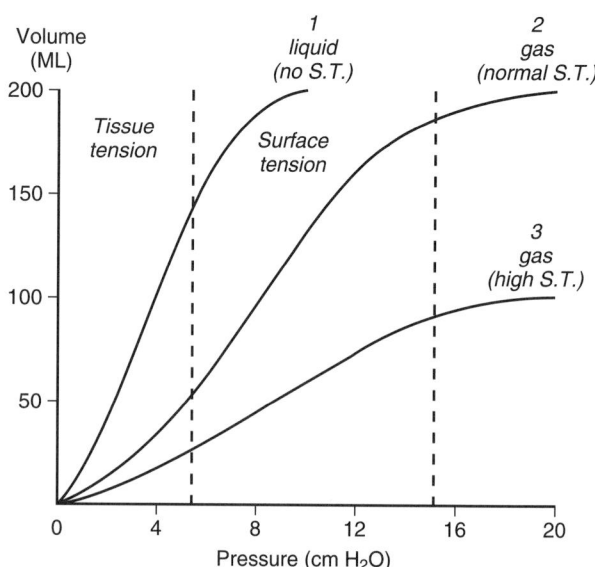

Figure 98–4. Pressure-volume relationship of the gas-filled or liquid-filled lung. S.T. = surface tension. (Redrawn from Comroe JH: Physiology of Respiration. Chicago, Year Book Medical Publishers, 1977.)

The stabilizing role of pulmonary surfactant originated in 1929. It was shown that less pressure (i.e., work) was required to inflate the saline-filled than the air-filled animal lung. This difference resulted from surface forces at the air-liquid interface of the air-filled lung.[13] It was suggested later that phospholipids in the alveolar surface forces reduced surface forces at the air-liquid interface.[50] Subsequently, it was demonstrated that surface tension changed in relation to surface area,[51] and alveolar material obtained from infants dying of respiratory distress syndrome had decreased surfactant activity.[7] These findings suggested that the lack of pulmonary surfactant predisposed infants to atelectasis. Taken together, these studies established the fundamental basis of subsequent work toward exogenous surfactant replacement therapy to reduce inflation pressures for the treatment of respiratory distress syndrome.

Because of the biophysical similarity between the alveolar lining fluid and saline, interfacial tension and surface forces are essentially eliminated in the saline-filled lung. Similar to a completely saline-filled lung, complete insufflation of the lung with a PFC liquid in which gas is carried in the dissolved state elimi-

nates the gas-liquid interface in the lung and reduces, but does not abolish, surface forces. Unlike in the saline-filled lung, and because of physicochemical differences between the alveolar lining fluid and PFC, interfacial tensions remain between alveolar lining fluid and PFC. Therefore, alveolar inflation pressures with PFC are lower than those with gas; however, more pressure is required to inflate the PFC-filled lung than the saline-filled lung. Impairment of lung mechanics after PFC ventilation of healthy, surfactant-sufficient adult animals may be attributable to the additional interfacial tension at the PFC-lung surface and the air-PFC surface.[15, 52-55]

In vivo pulmonary compliance determinations performed in gas-ventilated or PFC-ventilated preterm lambs ranging in age from 106 to 136 days' gestation (term ~150 days) demonstrated significant age-related differences.[5] Although pulmonary compli-

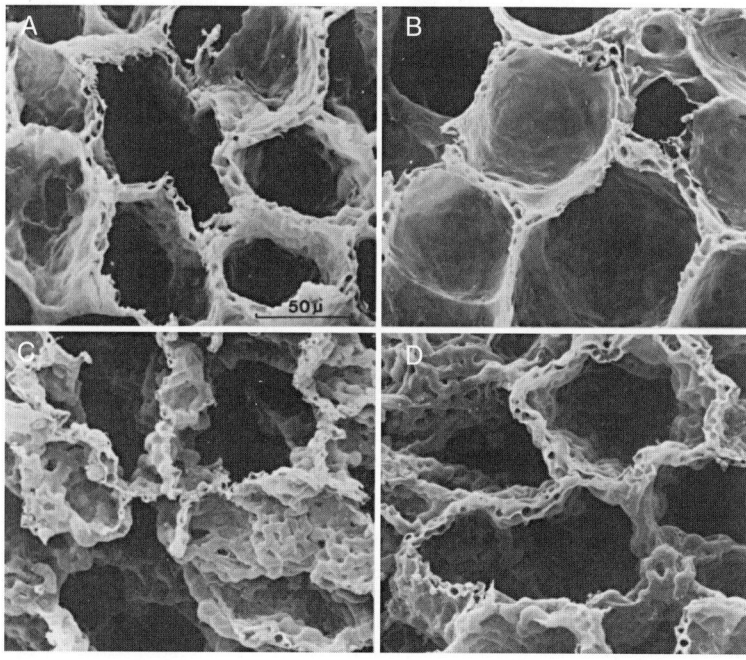

Figure 98–5. Scanning electron micrographs of air-filled (**A** and **B**) and saline-filled (**C** and **D**) lungs at 40% (**A** and **C**) and 80% (**B** and **D**) total lung capacity. (From Gil J, et al: J Appl Physiol *47*:990, 1979.)

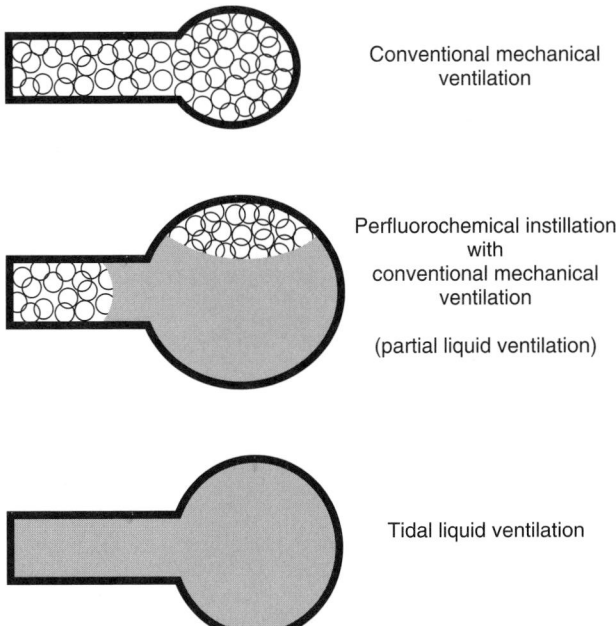

Figure 98–6. Schematic of potential sources of interfacial tensions in the perfluorochemical (PFC)-treated lung during ventilation with tidal volumes of gas (partial liquid ventilation) or PFC liquid (tidal liquid ventilation).

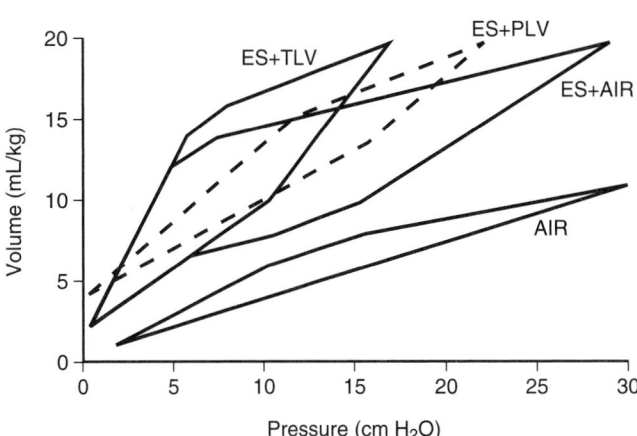

Figure 98–7. Average quasistatic pressure-volume curves of excised preterm lamb lungs exposed to gas ventilation without (AIR) or with (ES + AIR) exogenous surfactant or with perfluorochemical partial liquid ventilation (ES + PLV) or tidal liquid ventilation (ES + TLV). (Redrawn from Tarczy-Hornach P, et al: Pediatr Res 37:353A, 1995.)

ance of the PFC-ventilated lamb was consistently higher than that of the gas-ventilated lamb, this difference was not significant until after approximately 120 days' gestation. This finding suggests that morphologic and tissue properties predominate over surface properties in determining lung distensibility at the earlier stages of development. In addition, it suggests that the structural development (i.e., elastic, collagen, parenchymal interdependence) of the lung limits the effect of a reduction in interfacial surface tension on increasing lung distensibility.

Numerous *in vivo* studies of animals and humans with surfactant deficiency or dysfunction, with or without surfactant pretreatment, have demonstrated improvement in respiratory compliance during tidal liquid ventilation (TLV),[5, 56-76] on recovery to gas ventilation,[67, 71, 78-81] or during gas ventilation after instillation of PFC liquid (partial liquid ventilation [PLV]).[9, 61, 71, 82-101] The greatest reduction in ventilatory pressure requirements and improvement in specific respiratory compliance were noted after (1) the lung was insufflated with PFC liquid to functional residual capacity (FRC), (2) free gas was vented, and (3) ventilation was achieved by moving tidal volumes of PFC.[73] Figure 98–6 illustrates schematically the various interfacial tensions that may exist in the PFC-treated lung during ventilation with tidal volumes of gas or PFC liquid.

Using surfactant-deficient excised lungs of preterm lambs, studies have shown that net interfacial tension is lower in the lung filled with an FRC of PFC liquid than in the gas-filled lung; surfactant pretreatment further reduces net interfacial tension in the PFC-filled lung (Fig. 98–7).[102, 103] When free gas is introduced into the PFC-treated lung, additional interfacial tensions are created at the free gas-PFC and gas-lung surfaces. Although net interfacial tension is increased in the PFC-treated and gas-ventilated lung relative to the liquid-ventilated lung, tension remains lower than in the gas-filled lung and is reduced by surfactant pretreatment.

Gas Exchange

As reviewed earlier, the need for hyperbaric conditions to oxygenate saline adequately, the detergent action of saline (remov-

ing endogenous surfactant), and the inability to remove CO_2 limit the utility of saline as a ventilatory medium. Inadequate CO_2 elimination during saline ventilation has been linked to the slower diffusion rate (greater diffusion coefficients) of CO_2 and the lower maximal expiratory flow associated with elevated density and viscosity in liquids compared with those in gases. These mechanisms were elucidated by theoretical models and experimental data obtained in the saline-filled lung.[14-16,104,105]

One theoretical model viewed the lung as multiple and identical spheric exchange units.[14,15] With each respiratory cycle, the tensions of O_2 and CO_2 change as a function of radial distance from the center of each sphere, diffusion coefficient for the respective gas, and time for diffusion. The partial pressure gradient for each gas decreases over time, resulting in regional differences within each sphere and diffusional dead space (i.e., the center of the sphere has lower CO_2 tensions and higher O_2 tension). Relative to liquid versus gas flow rates, it has been shown that maximal expiratory flow in excised saline-filled animal lungs was one-hundredth of that obtainable in the gas-filled lung.[10, 11] The reduction in maximal expiratory flow was linked to the increase in density and viscosity of saline compared with those of gas and elevated resistive pressures when moving saline and gas at comparable rates. Therefore, to overcome such limitations, the respiratory cycle would ostensibly have to be increased in length and depth for adequate alveolar ventilation to eliminate CO_2. Although the potential for adequate ventilation was identified, strategies for ventilating with saline were not explored further because of the dependence on achieving hyperbaric oxygenation and the detergent-like action of saline in removing native pulmonary surfactant.

There are numerous similarities and differences in the characteristics of PFC liquid and saline relative to gas exchange. Although high respiratory gas solubility of the PFC liquids distinguishes these fluids from saline to support pulmonary gas exchange, theoretical analysis and *in vivo* experimentation demonstrated that low diffusion coefficient for respiratory gases (e.g., gases diffuse into liquids several orders of magnitude slower than into gas) and elevated density and viscosity of liquid (e.g., 10^3 and 10^2 times greater than air) impose rate limitations on alveolar diffusion and expiratory flow.[31,32] Low gas diffusion coefficients and solubilities in PFC have little impact on O_2 exchange because the partial pressure of inspired O_2 can be increased to approximately 700 mm Hg (thereby establishing a sufficient alveolar-arterial O_2 gradient and O_2 content in PFC to meet most metabolic demands). In contrast, the amount of CO_2

removed from the lungs depends primarily on the partial pressure of CO_2 in the blood (usually, 40 mm Hg), thereby limiting the alveolar-arterial CO_2 gradient and CO_2 content. This limitation presents a significant imbalance between the rate of production and elimination of CO_2 from the respiratory system.

Factors contributing to improved matching of ventilation and perfusion in the completely fluid-filled lung also contribute to effective gas exchange during tidal PFC ventilation (see the earlier discussion of pulmonary structure and function). During tidal PFC ventilation, PFC is evenly distributed throughout the lung, and pulmonary blood is redistributed in the completely PFC-filled lung, creating a more homogeneous pattern than during gas breathing.[81,106] The adequacy of gas exchange during gas ventilation of a PFC-filled lung (e.g., PFC-associated gas exchange or PLV) has been related to the "evenness" of bubble oxygenation of PFC and matching of any maldistribution of this pattern to concomitant maldistribution of pulmonary perfusion.[107] Radiographic studies indicate that PFC liquid during gas ventilation is not evenly distributed; stratification occurs, with a primary pattern of gas rising to the nondependent regions and PFC settling to the dependent regions of the lung despite frequent changes in position. Under these conditions, it is currently unknown how much gas exchange occurs in the combined PFC-filled regions of the lung. It is also not known whether improvement in gas exchange in the immature or injured lung occurs in lung regions with only small volumes of PFC liquid (however, these units still may have improved mechanics). Although the high CO_2 solubility in PFC liquids provides an efficient reservoir for CO_2, effective CO_2 elimination during gas ventilation of a PFC-filled lung depends on the distribution of the gas. Nonventilated or poorly ventilated regions and uneven emptying of the lung because of airway obstruction or changing lung mechanics present challenges to this ventilatory approach. Studies of gas ventilation of the PFC-filled normal, immature, or injured lung have demonstrated that inspiratory resistance to gas flow may be normal or increased,[80,98,108] and expiratory resistance to gas flow may be elevated.[92] The expiratory flow profile suggests that the lung empties as multiple compartments.[80,107]

Cardiovascular and Metabolic Responses

Less information is available regarding cardiovascular and metabolic responses during liquid ventilation. Early studies performed in normal adult animals reported decreases in cardiac output, O_2 consumption, CO_2 production, and pH and increases in pulmonary vascular resistance (assessed in the isolated-perfused lung), as well as redistribution of cardiac output and pulmonary blood flow.[109-115] These studies suggested that although liquid ventilation techniques could support effective gas exchange, cardiovascular compromise may be an issue when liquid lung volumes and alveolar pressures are increased to more than normal levels. Similar complications have been noted with excessive use of positive end-distending pressure in the gas-filled lung.[116] It was speculated that most of these findings in the PFC-filled lung were related to the effect of the weight of the PFC to compress the heart, great vessels, or pulmonary vasculature in the dependent region of the lung. More recent studies, performed in adult, neonatal, and premature animals with normal or abnormal lungs, have reported less compromise of cardiopulmonary interaction in the PFC-filled lung.[5,8,81,117-119]

Differences between the earlier and more recent studies reflect improvements in ventilator designs and lung volume management during ventilation. In the earlier studies, measurements were performed shortly after PFC instillation, raising the issue of whether the cardiovascular compromise was related to elevated alveolar or intrathoracic pressures associated with liquid compression of resident gas volumes. Preexisting metabolic acidosis complicated interpretation of several of these studies.[109,110,112,114] In a study of normal neonatal piglets, initial elevations in pul-

monary artery pressure and pulmonary vascular resistance (which resolved within 40 minutes) were related to early respiratory acidosis rather than to vascular compression.[117] This study demonstrated a small decrease in cardiac output in several animals with no difference in cardiac output between gas and tidal liquid breathing in the remaining animals. It was suggested that application of liquid ventilation of the normal animal may require only modest volume expansion (i.e., a single 10 mL/kg bolus) to support normal cardiac output. Furthermore, the earlier studies were conducted in the normal lung, which transmitted ventilatory pressures more readily to the vasculature than a stiff lung. In this regard, studies of adult animals with induced acute respiratory distress syndrome have reported no changes in cardiac index during gas ventilation after PFC instillation.[80,118]

Ventilation/perfusion matching is improved during TLV of the poorly compliant lung of preterm animals.[69,70,74,76,81] Increased oxygenation and reduction in preductal to postductal O_2 tension differences indicate improvement in pulmonary blood flow and reduction of right-to-left ductal shunting. Developmental changes in cardiovascular and metabolic function of the TLV-treated lamb (102 days' gestation to term) parallel developmental changes reported for fetal or gas-ventilated animals.[5] Left ventricular output, absolute pulmonary blood flow, ductal flow, systemic arterial pressure, heart rate, left ventricular ejection and shortening fraction, and velocity of circumferential fiber shortening remain unchanged, whereas meridional wall stress is reduced during gas ventilation of the PFC-filled lung (10 mL/kg).[8,111] Therefore, it is unlikely that the weight of the PFC liquid presents a risk of cardiovascular compromise in the preterm lamb with respiratory distress. As the anteroposterior dimension of the lungs increases, however, hydrostatic pressure gradients may be an issue. Thus, in larger lungs, stratification of gas and PFC liquid during PLV and regional differences in hydrostatic pressure during TLV could play a role in cardiovascular performance.

EXPERIMENTAL AND CLINICAL TECHNIQUES FOR LIQUID-ASSISTED VENTILATION

Table 98–3 lists the techniques for liquid-assisted ventilation. Early investigations of fluid breathing used either total body immersion or gravity-assisted ventilation, which delivered PFC liquid from a reservoir to an intubated animal. These methods were inadequate for extended ventilation of experimental animals because of problems attributed to the differences between gas and liquid physical properties, such as density, viscosity, and gas diffusion rates.[2,15,25,104] Despite more uniform distribution of blood flow in the liquid-filled lung,[44,115] it was demonstrated that expiratory liquid flow and diffusion limitations can preclude sufficient removal of CO_2 when earlier mechanical ventilation schemes are applied.[104,120]

The concept of demand-regulated liquid ventilation was introduced in the early 1970s.[52,121-124] This technique employed the respiratory centers of the experimental animal to control the cycling of the respirator, which circulated oxygenated liquid to and from the lungs. This approach reduced the work of breathing. Early

---

TABLE 98–3

Techniques for Liquid-Assisted Ventilation

Combined gas and liquid ventilation
Tidal liquid ventilation
Lung lavage
Combined gas and liquid ventilation
Perfluorochemical-associated gas exchange
Partial liquid ventilation
Low-dose perfluorochemical instillation (vapor)

experiments with this type of ventilation reported effective oxygenation and better CO_2 removal than immersion or gravity-assisted techniques. Modifications of liquid ventilation systems have evolved, incorporating various designs such as manually controlled flow-assist pneumatic systems[52,121,123,124]; roller pumps with pneumatic, fluidic, and electronic controls[5, 74, 76]; gravity-driven systems[66,125,126]; and modified extracorporeal membrane oxygenation circuits.[127] Control strategies incorporating constant pressure or constant flow, time cycling, and pressure (system, airway, or alveolar) or volume (lung volume, tidal volume) limitation have been explored, with the current approach emphasizing microprocessor-based feedback control (Fig. 98–8).[56,128]

In general, TLV is achieved by cycling fluid from a reservoir to and from the lung. Warmed and oxygenated PFC liquid is pumped from a fluid reservoir into the lung. During expiration, fluid is pumped from the lung with passive assist of the lung recoil; it is filtered and returned to a gas exchanger for oxygenation and CO_2 scrubbing. O_2 concentration is titrated from the inspired O_2 tension,[35] and fluid is returned to the fluid reservoir. PFC vapor in the expired gas is condensed with high efficiency (at 70 to 80%), and noncondensed PFC loss owing to evaporation is measured and returned to the system.[129, 130] During TLV, gas is transported to the alveolar-capillary membrane in dissolved form; O_2 and CO_2 diffuse through the liquid, and the fluid is regenerated extracorporeally. Because the lung is entirely fluid filled, heart sounds are more clearly discerned during TLV. Periodic rotation and suctioning of the patient may be used to facilitate removal of debris. Ventilation/perfusion matching is improved in the lung of a preterm infant with this form of ventilation independent of rotation; however, periodic rotation may further support homogeneous distribution of ventilation and perfusion. This may be more necessary in larger lungs, in which the effect of hydrostatic pressure has a greater influence on the distribution of pulmonary blood flow.

Repeated trials by different investigators confirmed that when mechanical ventilation is performed properly, oxygenation and ventilation can be maintained effectively in the liquid-filled lung.

There is no known physiologic limitation that precludes the duration of TLV. Full-term lambs have been ventilated successfully with physiologic gas exchange for up to 24 hours. Gas exchange data from studies of normal or lung-injured preterm, term, and adult animals have reflected improved liquids and ventilation methods. Along these lines, several researchers have reported alternating conventional ventilator therapy with PFC ventilation in various animal preparations and in human patients with respiratory distress ranging in age from extremely premature infants to adults.[5, 77-81, 88, 89, 107, 131] This form of combined therapy was well tolerated and in many cases demonstrated improvement in lung mechanics.

This combined ventilation scheme (liquid ventilation and gas ventilation) has since been described as PLV,[91, 92] or PFC-associated gas exchange,[111] and is characterized by filling and maintaining the lung with an FRC of PFC liquid while conventional gas ventilation is performed. It has been proposed that the residual PFC liquid within the lung is oxygenated, and CO_2 is exchanged in the lung by means of gas movement provided by the conventional gas ventilator. PLV resembles the situation after the TLV-treated lung is returned to gas ventilation.

BIOCHEMICAL, HISTOLOGIC, AND MORPHOLOGIC FINDINGS IN THE LIQUID-VENTILATED LUNG

Since the 1970s, the aftereffects of liquid breathing have been given a substantial amount of attention. In this regard, it has been demonstrated that adult, newborn, and preterm mammals ventilated with PFC liquids for extended periods were able to return safely to breathing gas without long-term negative effects.

Biochemical Findings

Small but significant levels of PFC have been detected in blood samples from animals either ventilated with PFC liquid or after intratracheal instillation of PFC liquids. Across studies, PFC concentration in the blood ranged from 0.25 to 10 µg PFC/mL of

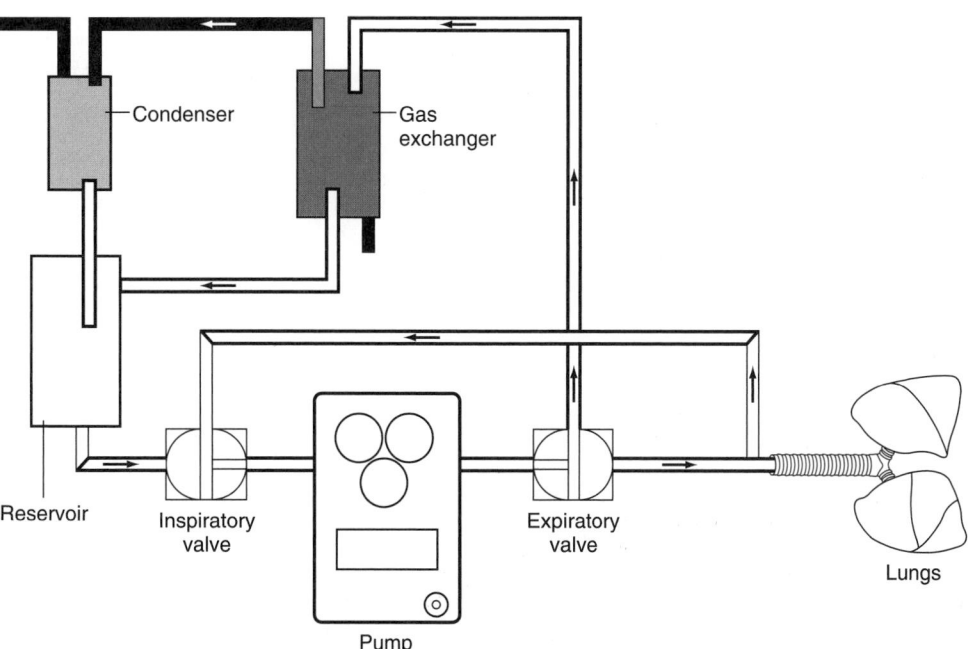

Single pump ventilator

Figure 98–8. Single-pump tidal liquid ventilator. Heater omitted for clarity. *Solid line* = gas flow; *open line* = perfluorochemical liquid flow.

TABLE 98-4

Perfluorochemical Uptake Levels in Arterial Blood After Pulmonary Administration

PFC Compound*	Ventilation Strategy	Exposure Time (h)	Species	PFC Level	Reference Number
LiquiVent	TLV	24	Normal lambs	2.0–3.5 nL/mL	185
LiquiVent	TLV	4	Normal lambs	8.29 ± 0.68 µg/mL	186
LiquiVent	TLV	4	Injured lambs	7.35 ± 0.36 µg/mL	186
LiquiVent	PLV	4	Injured lambs	2.78 ± 0.24 µg/mL	186
LiquiVent	TLV	2	Preterm lambs	1.92–5.97 µg/mL	187
LiquiVent	PLV	2	Preterm lambs	2.88–9.55 µg/mL	187
RIMAR 101	TLV/GV	<1	Preterm humans	0.20–0.69 µg/mL	137
APF-140	TLV	1–3	Adult rats	0.14–2.70 nL/mL	188
APF-140	TLV	1	Preterm lambs	1.38–1.86 nL/mL	101

* LiquiVent, Alliance Pharmaceutical Corp.; RIMAR 101, MitEni; APF-140, Air Products and Fine Chemicals.
GV = gas ventilation; PFC = perfluorochemical; PLV = partial liquid ventilation; TLV = tidal liquid ventilation.

blood and reached a plateau by 15 to 120 minutes of liquid ventilation, depending on the physical properties of the PFC liquid, the technique of PFC administration, and the species or animal preparation studied (Table 98–4). Although there are differences in experimental conditions across studies, results were similar in that they all noted low concentrations of different PFC compounds in the blood after pulmonary exposure to PFC.[101,134-137]

As reported, the concentration of PFC in the tissues with liquid ventilation is organ-dependent, with the highest PFC level typically found in the lungs. In contrast to amounts found in the lungs, there were smaller amounts of PFC reported in other organs. The lowest levels were typically found in organs with low lipid content, and the highest were found in organs with high lipid content.[138] As noted by several investigators,[101,135,136] after return to gas ventilation, there was an overall reduction in PFC levels in organs as a function of gas ventilation duration. This reduction in PFC concentration in tissue was paralleled by a decrease in PFC vapor in expired gas as a function of time after return to gas ventilation.[101,136]

PFC uptake, biodistribution, and elimination were assessed in several infants after liquid ventilation.[137] Similar to results from animal studies, the data demonstrated that PFC uptake and elimination were organ-dependent, PFC concentration in the expired gas samples decayed exponentially to within control range by 8 hours after liquid ventilation, and PFC concentration in the blood was relatively saturated by 15 minutes of liquid ventilation. Tissue values revealed highest residual PFC levels in the lung, with variable but small levels in other organs. In infants surviving for an extended period, levels in the lung markedly diminish, and levels in other organs approach control values.

The overall process of PFC uptake, biodistribution, and elimination has been supported by human studies, experimental animal models, and mathematical models of liquid ventilation.[38,39,101,117,135-137,139,140] Based on the understanding to date, a conceptual interpretation of this process is diagrammed in Figure 98–9, and factors influencing this process are outlined in Table 98–5. Because PFC liquid in general is practically insoluble in water, essentially all the PFC in the blood and tissues is dissolved in lipid.[135,136] Therefore, small quantities of PFC diffuse into the blood passing through the lungs, where PFC dissolves in blood lipid. The uptake process in the blood is dependent on PFC vapor pressure, permeability coefficients in the lung, PFC solubility in blood lipid, and ventilation/perfusion matching. Similar to the distribution of drugs in the body, biodistribution of PFC to the various organs depends on tissue-blood partition coefficients, tissue blood flow, and tissue compartment volume.[137] Therefore, as shown in previous animal and human studies,[101,137,141] vessel-rich organs with high blood flow are saturated more rapidly, and fat-rich organs have a higher capacity for PFC storage. Finally, PFC liquids may be scavenged by

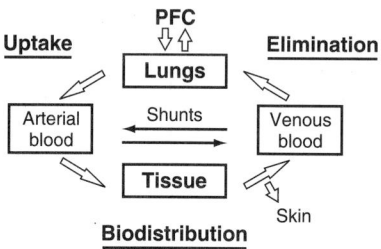

Figure 98–9. Schematic illustration of circulatory processes involved with uptake, biodistribution, and elimination of perfluorochemical (PFC) liquid after intratracheal instillation.

TABLE 98-5

Factors Influencing Perfluorochemical Uptake, Systemic Biodistribution, and Elimination

Perfluorochemical Physicochemical Factors	Physiologic Factors
Uptake	
Vapor pressure	Blood lipid content
Lipid solubility	Lung surface area
Density?	Lung mechanics
Viscosity?	Lung permeability
	Pulmonary blood flow
	Hematocrit
Biodistribution	
Vapor pressure	Blood-organ partition coefficient
Lipid solubility	Organ lipid content
	Cardiac output
	Organ blood flow
Elimination	
Vapor pressure	Alveolar ventilation
Density?	Lung mechanics/pathophysiology
Viscosity?	Positioning
Surface tension?	Dosing requirements
	Duration/type of gas ventilation

macrophages, and because of the unique chemical structure of PFC liquids, they are not metabolized. The essential route of elimination is through the lungs by volatilization in the expiratory gases with the potential for transpiration through the skin.

The elimination of PFC liquid from the respiratory system is based on numerous factors and is still under extensive investigation. Employing a PFC vapor analyzer, studies showed that PFC liquid volume loss and evaporation rate from the lungs corre-

Example 1: Immediately post fill

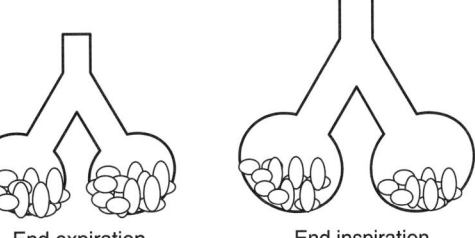

End expiration
FRC_{liquid} = 30 ml/kg
FRC_{gas} = 10 ml/kg

End inspiration
FRC + V_t

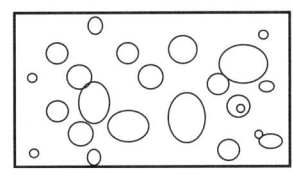

Expired gas
95% saturated

Example 2: Hours post fill

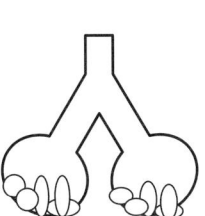

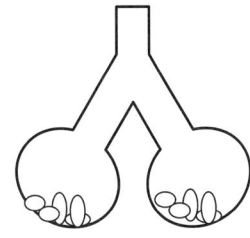

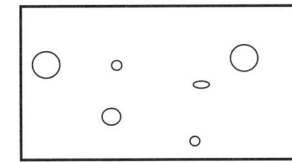

End expiration
FRC_{liquid} = 10 ml/kg
FRC_{gas} = 30 ml/kg

End inspiration
FRC + V_t

Expired gas
30% saturated

Figure 98–10. Influence of perfluorochemical (PFC) liquid or gas lung volume on PFC elimination. FRC = functional residual capacity. (Prepared with the assistance of T. F. Miller, Ph.D.)

lated with time after instillation (Fig. 98-10) and were modulated by changes in PFC physical properties, ventilation strategy, lung pathophysiology, distribution of fluid in the lung (Fig. 98-11), repositioning of the subject, and administration of supplemental PFC doses to the lungs.[129]

Histologic and Morphologic Findings

Morphologic studies of newborn rabbits and immature lambs suggest that liquid ventilation actually seems to minimize damage typically incurred as a result of gas ventilation.[5, 74, 142] Fine structure studies of newborn rabbit lungs ventilated with PFC liquid revealed no indication of damage (Fig. 98-12); the integrity of the epithelial cell membranes and bilaminar plasmalemma suggested maintenance of lung ultrastructure.[143] In addition, it is particularly noteworthy that after liquid ventilation, there was thinning of the epithelial septa, and the epithelial cells appeared flattened and more symmetric. As shown in an electron photomicrograph of lung tissue, these findings were reconfirmed in preterm lambs ventilated with PFC (Fig. 98-13). The exchange spaces are clear, the air-blood interface is thin-walled, the capillaries are intact and thin-walled, and the cytoplasm of epithelial cells is relatively smooth. There is abundant surfactant in lamellar bodies. The salutary effect of PFC ventilation has also been demonstrated in animal preparations of meconium aspiration or hydrochloric acid–induced or oleic acid–induced acute respiratory distress syndrome.[56, 59, 61, 64, 65] Histologic differences between the gas-ventilated lung and the TLV-treated lung were profound, reflecting a substantial reduction in pulmonary consolidation, atelectasis, hemorrhage, disruption of the alveolar-capillary membrane, and absence of inflammatory infiltration in the TLV-treated lung. The histology and morphology of lungs from healthy full-term animals after either prolonged TLV or PLV reflected preserved architecture.[73, 144, 145] Alterations associated with short-term exposure to intrapulmonary PFC liquid could not be detected by histologic or morphologic analysis in human

lungs or other tissues.[146] Marked regional differences in pulmonary histology and morphology were noted in the lungs of preterm lambs with respiratory distress syndrome and in neonatal piglets with induced adult respiratory distress syndrome after PLV.[73,144,145] These changes were associated with stratification of the PFC and gas to the dependent and independent regions of the lung. Prolonged (96 hours) PLV of premature baboons resulted in gas exchange and lung mechanics improvements. There was, however, a trend noted in this study toward delayed pulmonary recovery (based on airway pressures and Type II cell immaturity) in animals ventilated with PLV as compared with historical control animals.[147]

Cellular Findings

In addition to improvement in lung distensibility and gas exchange, studies indicated that, whereas PFC liquids are chemically inert substances, their presence appears to modify certain biologic activity that may reduce pulmonary inflammation and injury associated with respiratory distress syndrome. Pulmonary neutrophil infiltration in rat lungs injured with cobra venom factor or secondary to hemorrhagic shock was significantly reduced during PLV when compared with conventional gas ventilation support.[148, 149] Exposure of alveolar macrophages from rabbit and piglet lungs demonstrated that perflubron liquid *in vitro* decreased the responsiveness of macrophages to potent stimuli.[150] The effects of PFC on neutrophil-epithelial cell interactions have also been evaluated.[151] Neutrophils that were exposed to PFC, washed, and then stimulated retained their ability to generate oxidants, to release proteolytic enzymes, and to adhere to epithelial cells. However, when neutrophils and epithelial cells were simultaneously exposed to PFC, adhesion and target cell injury after stimulation were reduced. The oxidant-generating capacity of cells obtained from PFC-treated humans with acute respiratory distress syndrome was similar to that of peripheral blood neutrophils. Collectively, these findings

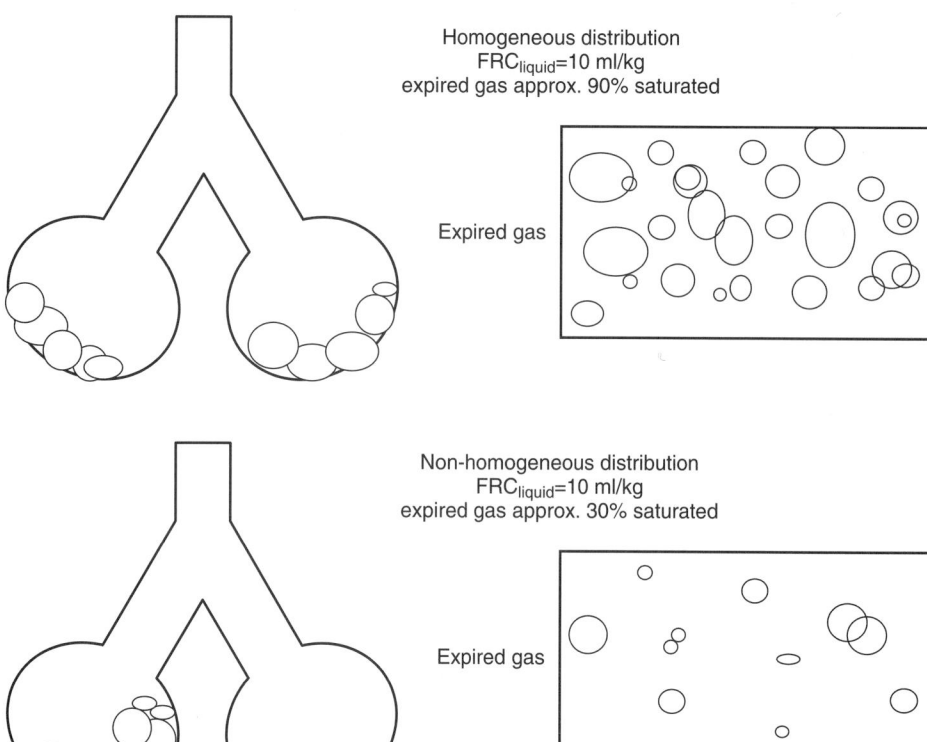

Homogeneous distribution
FRC$_{liquid}$=10 ml/kg
expired gas approx. 90% saturated

Expired gas

Non-homogeneous distribution
FRC$_{liquid}$=10 ml/kg
expired gas approx. 30% saturated

Expired gas

Figure 98–11. Influence of the distribution pattern of perfluorochemical (PFC) liquid on subsequent PFC elimination. FRC = functional residual capacity. (Prepared with the assistance of T. F. Miller, Ph.D.)

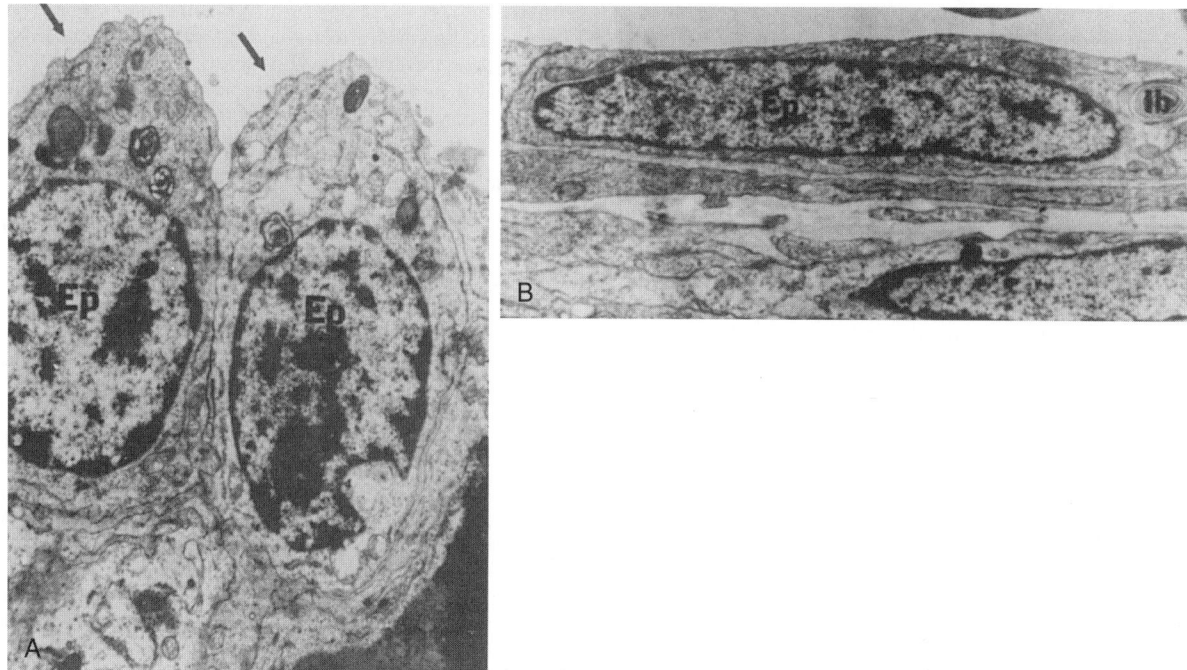

Figure 98–12. Electron micrographs of the lung of a preterm rabbit (27 days' gestation). **A,** Unventilated lung: Note rounded contour of lung epithelium borders (Ep) (×7752). **B,** Liquid ventilated lung. Note the evenness of the luminal border, the flattened and elongated cells with early differentiation, and the lamellar body (lb) (×11,172).

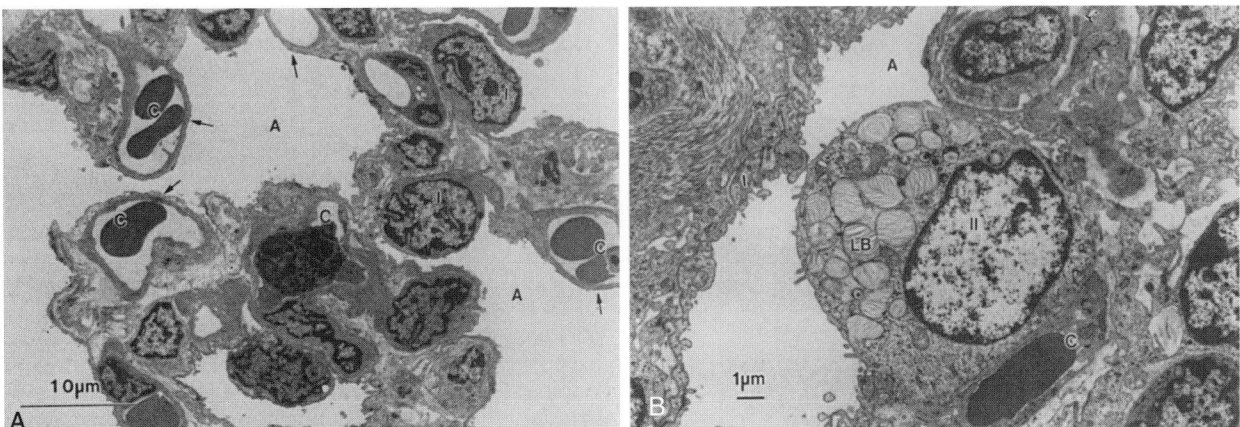

Figure 98–13. Electron micrographs of lung from preterm lamb that was liquid ventilated with perflubron for 1 hour. **A,** Note the clear exchanged spaces (A), thin-walled air-blood interface (red blood cell [C]), and smooth cytoplasm of the epithelial cell. **B,** Abundant surfactant in lamellar bodies (LB) of an alveolar Type II cell. (Courtesy of Drs. Emil Chi and J. Craig Jackson, University of Washington, Seattle.)

suggest that the presence of PFC may provide a mechanical barrier to reduce neutrophil-mediated lung inflammation and injury.

More recent studies compared the cellular effects of PFCs of different properties on human blood cellular elements.[152, 153] At the lowest PFC concentrations, which are comparable to the concentrations found in blood during liquid ventilation, PFC liquids seem to be inert and do not induce leukocyte markers associated with inflammation. In the presence of high perflubron concentrations, simulating the condition within the airways and lungs, monocytes may be induced to produce reactive O_2 species.

The permeability of the alveolocapillary membrane was studied in healthy adult rabbits ventilated with gas alone (control) or by PLV with perflubron.[154] Pulmonary clearance of inhaled technetium-labeled diethylenetriamine penta-acetic acid occurred significantly faster in animals treated with PLV than in animals treated with conventional ventilation alone. The investigators concluded that the faster clearance reflected greater alveolocapillary permeability associated with reversible changes in the surfactant system of healthy animals treated with PLV.

The effect of PFC liquid on surfactant function and metabolism has been examined in healthy and injured animal models. *In vitro* studies have shown that PFC-exposed exogenous surfactant maintains normal surface tension properties.[155, 156] *In vivo* studies of healthy puppies have shown that most of the endogenous surfactant is retained in the lung after a 5-minute PFC lavage.[155] In one study, surfactant synthesis and secretion in surfactant-sufficient lungs were shown to increase after 5 hours of PLV when compared with gas-ventilated controls,[157] whereas the surfactant pool size was unchanged in another study of PLV-treated healthy or injured animals.[158] Preliminary results indicate increased endogenous surfactant phospholipids in broncho-alveolar lavage fluid after 5 hours of PLV in surfactant-deficient lambs.[159]

The effect of PFC ventilation techniques on markers of cell injury, as compared with scheduled physiologically regulated cell death (apoptosis), has been studied in very premature lambs supported with either TLV or conventional mechanical ventilation techniques.[160-162] Animals supported with TLV demonstrated a different pattern of apoptosis than those treated with conventional mechanical ventilation.[160] After conventional mechanical ventilation, apoptotic cells were observed to occlude the lumen of immature air spaces; in contrast, during TLV, apoptosis was limited to small numbers of epithelial cells lining the

air spaces, with only a few cells observed within the lumen. No differences in antioxidant enzyme activity were observed.[161] Histologic evidence of barotrauma was less frequent and urinary desmosine levels, an index of elastin turnover, were significantly lower in animals supported with TLV as compared with conventional mechanical ventilation.[162, 163] Collectively, these studies suggest that the reduction of barotrauma in premature animals supported with TLV as compared with conventional ventilation could be related to cell-specific apoptosis and appears to be independent of antioxidant enzyme activity.

BIOMEDICAL APPLICATIONS

Treatment of Respiratory Insufficiency

Animal Studies

Respiratory Distress. The hypothesis that PFC liquid would minimize surface forces, recruit and promote alveolar stability, and improve gas exchange at lower inflation pressures than with gas ventilation of the surfactant-deficient lung was first tested in 1976 (Fig. 98-14).[69] The first studies were performed with preterm lambs of 132 to 138 days' gestation[69,81] with respiratory distress syndrome. The lambs were delivered by cesarean section, initially supported with gas ventilation, and then briefly ventilated with PFC liquid (≤3 hours) and returned to conventional gas ventilation. Inflation pressures and alveolar-arterial O_2 gradients were reduced, and Pao_2 and pulmonary compliance improved during and after rescue liquid ventilation. $Paco_2$ remained lower on return to gas ventilation, and the youngest animals with the lowest initial pulmonary compliance and Pao_2 showed the most remarkable improvement in Pao_2 and alveolar-arterial O_2 gradient with TLV. In contrast to the gas-filled lung, the low surface tension and spreading capabilities of PFC allow recruitment of lung tissue, which in itself increases lung compliance. Furthermore, because PFC liquid is incompressible and is not absorbed across the lung surface as is gas, alveolar stability is enhanced, thereby providing a liquid positive end-expiratory pressure. These results indicated that TLV could result in a sustained decrease in intrapulmonary shunting and atelectasis.

The ability to support pulmonary gas exchange while protecting the delicate alveolar epithelium of the immature lung with PFC liquid after delivery was demonstrated in several studies using preterm lambs of 102 to 137 days' gestation.[70,74,76] TLV was initiated immediately after birth and was maintained for at least 3 hours. Effective gas exchange and physiologic acid-base status

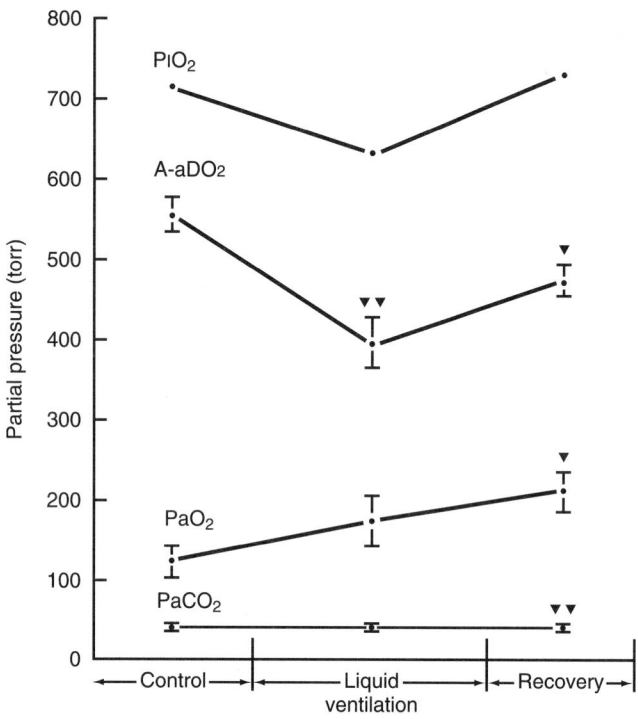

Figure 98–14. Inspired oxygen tension (PI_{O2}), alveolar-arterial oxygen gradient (AaD_{O2}), arterial oxygen tension (Pa_{O2}), and arterial carbon dioxide tension (Pa_{CO2}) during control gas ventilation, tidal liquid ventilation, and recovery to gas ventilation. (Redrawn from Shaffer TH, et al: Pediatr Res *17*:303, 1983.)

were demonstrated, with little age-related variation observed.[76] These studies showed that the alveolar-arterial O_2 gradient during TLV was lower than that reported for gas-ventilated lambs of comparable gestational age, and pulmonary compliance approximated that of older gas-ventilated lambs.

Distinct differences in the clinical, physiologic, and histologic profile between conventional gas-ventilated and liquid-ventilated preterm lambs have been demonstrated (Fig. 98–15).[74] Prophylactic TLV techniques supported gas exchange, acid-base balance, and cardiovascular stability throughout the duration of the experiment and improved survival; gas-ventilated animals

demonstrated progressive deterioration, high morbidity, and poor survival. Differences in profiles were related to the mechanical characteristics of the respiratory system; respiratory compliance was greater, requiring lower inflation pressures in the liquid-ventilated than in the gas-ventilated animals. Thus, maintenance of a liquid-liquid alveolar interface promoted effective cardiopulmonary function and maintenance of the integrity of the pulmonary architecture.

These studies suggest that prophylactic TLV (implemented at birth) may decrease intrapulmonary and extrapulmonary shunting and may attenuate the complications associated with perinatal cardiopulmonary instability of the preterm infant. Evidence obtained in preterm lambs (112 to 128 days' gestation), ventilated prophylactically with PFC liquid at birth and subsequently ventilated with gas, further supports this notion.[79] These animals demonstrated effective pulmonary gas exchange, acid-base status, and cardiovascular stability during TLV. Furthermore, during the period of gas ventilation, pulmonary compliance was noted to be significantly higher than that reported for animals of comparable or older age that had been gas ventilated since birth. Pulmonary compliance was also greater than that of equivalent-age animals rescue-treated with natural surfactant,[164, 165] PFC,[71] or artificial fluorinated surfactant.[166,167]

In addition to the efficacy of tidal PFC ventilation, that of intratracheal instillation of PFC combined with conventional mechanical ventilation has been explored in animals with respiratory distress. Similar to total liquid ventilation, or the recovery phase of liquid ventilation (i.e., return to gas ventilation), PLV uses the alveolar recruitment capabilities of a fluid of low surface tension to establish an adequate FRC as well as the ability of residual PFC to stabilize FRC in a surfactant-deficient or impaired lung. This experimental approach has been studied in acute lung injury models (Fig. 98–16)[80,82,88,89,96–100,118] and in neonatal respiratory distress syndrome models (Fig. 98–17).[61, 73, 83, 90, 92, 119, 147, 168, 169] Although the magnitude of responses varied within the different studies (possibly as a result of differences in techniques and degree of lung injury), it was generally shown that maintenance of an FRC using PFC combined with conventional gas ventilation provided adequate or improved gas exchange at relatively lower airway pressures than conventional gas ventilation alone. In many cases, the histologic pictures of the lungs were greatly improved compared with other forms of respiratory support or untreated control groups.[99]

Aspiration Syndromes. Efficacy of PFC ventilation for the management of aspiration syndromes has also been demonstrated in

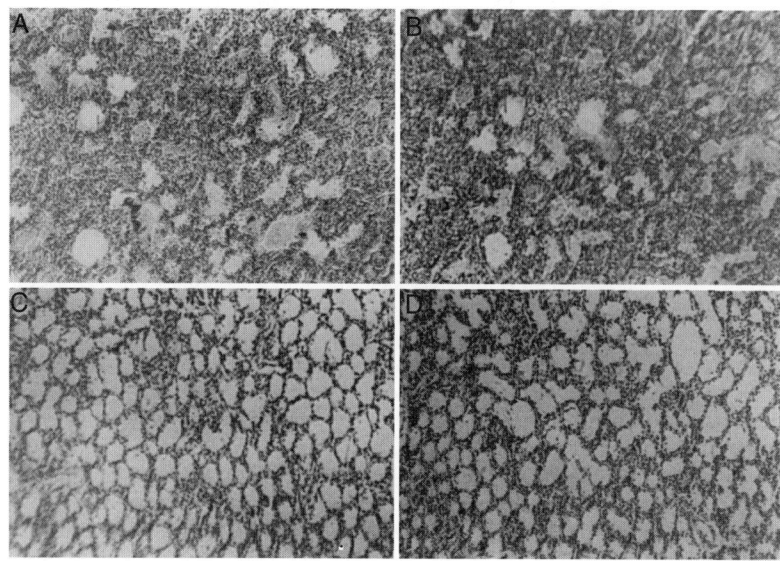

Figure 98–15. Light microscopy of lung sections (**A** and **C**, upper lobes; **B** and **D**, lower lobes) from preterm lambs (110 days' gestation) after 3 hours of gas (**A** and **B**) or tidal liquid ventilation (**C** and **D**). (From Wolfson MR, et al: J Appl Physiol *72*:1024, 1992.)

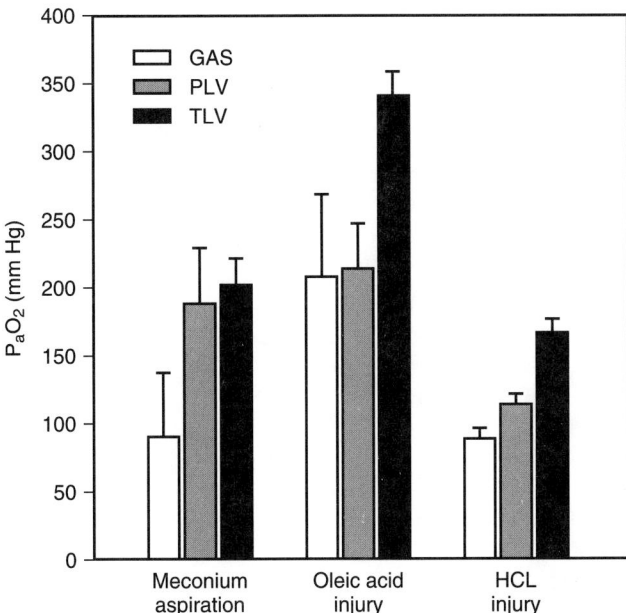

Figure 98–16. Arterial oxygen tension (Pao$_2$) during gas (GAS), partial liquid (PLV), and tidal liquid (TLV) ventilation in animal models of aspiration syndromes and acid-induced adult respiratory distress syndrome. (Data from refs. 54, 56, 57, 70, 75, and 129.)

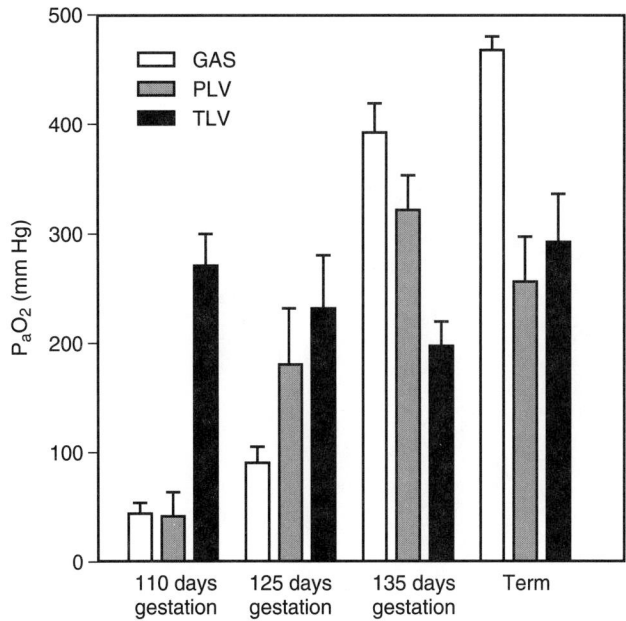

Figure 98–17. Representative "best" arterial oxygen tension (Pao$_2$) during gas (GAS), partial liquid (PLV), and tidal liquid (TLV) ventilation as a function of age in the developing sheep. (Data from refs. 62, 64, 69, 71, 75, 79, 98, 105, 185, and 189.)

neonatal and adult animals.[59, 81, 82, 170] The foundation for this approach is related to removal of caustic substances (i.e., meconium) from the airways and alveolar surface, lung volume recruitment, reduction of surface forces, and improvement in ventilation/perfusion matching. Poor gas exchange, acidosis, and low pulmonary compliance present at birth and during gas ventilation of preterm lambs or induced term animals significantly improved during tidal PFC ventilation[81] or gas ventilation after instillation of PFC liquid (e.g., PLV- or PFC-associated gas exchange).[59, 170] Meconium was observed in the expired liquid during tidal PFC ventilation and floated to the top of the endotracheal tube during PLV. Improvements were noted during tidal PFC ventilation in Pao$_2$, alveolar-arterial O$_2$ gradient, and pulmonary compliance. Pulmonary blood flow was more uniform, and Paco$_2$ was lower during liquid ventilation. Based on these findings, it was concluded that tidal PFC ventilation improved pulmonary perfusion and therefore ventilation/perfusion matching. Similar improvements in pulmonary gas exchange and function have been reported in PLV of term animals with gastric acid–induced or hydrochloric acid–induced acute respiratory distress syndrome with inflammatory processes.[62, 82] Similarly, it appears that PFC ventilation has a role in the management of aspiration syndromes. Early intervention may be useful in breaking the cycle of surfactant inactivation and inhibition and inflammatory processes.

Pulmonary Hypoplasia. Several studies have shown the potential of liquid ventilation for supporting gas exchange and lung mechanics in the presence of pulmonary hypoplasia. The basis of this application is related to low-pressure alveolar recruitment and improved ventilation/perfusion matching. Investigation of a lamb preparation of congenital diaphragmatic hernia supported with PLV, either prophylactically at birth or rescued after a period of gas ventilation, showed improved gas exchange and compliance compared with that of conventional gas ventilation support.[93, 171] The congenital diaphragmatic hernia lamb preparation treated prophylactically with PFC at delivery demonstrated improved function and histology compared with rescue treatment.[9, 171]

Use of Perfluorochemicals in Infants with Respiratory Distress Syndrome

The first human studies of PFC liquid ventilation for the treatment of respiratory distress were performed in near-death infants with severe respiratory failure in 1989.[131, 132] TLV was performed in two 3- to 5-minute cycles separated by 15 minutes of gas ventilation. Although all six infants in these studies ultimately died of their underlying respiratory disease, it was shown that liquid ventilation was able to support gas exchange and residual improvement in pulmonary function after return to gas ventilation in these critically ill patients.[172] Further clinical trials were limited by the need for a medically approved liquid ventilator and medical-grade breathing fluid.

The results of this first human trial and continued success of neonatal and adult animal trials with liquid-assisted gas ventilation promoted initiation of a corporate-sponsored multicenter trial. This trial was designed to examine the safety and efficacy of PLV with LiquiVent (Alliance Pharmaceutical Corporation, San Diego, CA) in the treatment of premature infants with severe respiratory failure in whom conventional therapy had failed.[91] Seven preterm infants 5 days of age or younger (27.8±1.3 weeks' gestation; 1000±166 g) who had received two or more doses of surfactant and were at high risk of mortality were enrolled. During the PLV treatment (Fig. 98–18), all patients demonstrated some improvement in oxygenation, and five of seven patients demonstrated improved CO$_2$ removal and lung compliance; patients experiencing hypercarbia were transferred to high-frequency ventilation. No serious adverse events were related to PLV, and two of the seven patients survived. The remaining infants died of intracranial hemorrhage ($n = 2$) and bronchopulmonary dysplasia ($n = 1$). It was concluded that PLV could be achieved for up to several days in critically ill infants without serious adverse events.

Since this report, six additional patients have been enrolled. From the series of 13 infants studied to date, 10 infants received 24 to 76 hours of PLV, and 3 infants were withdrawn after a short course to receive high-frequency ventilation with residual

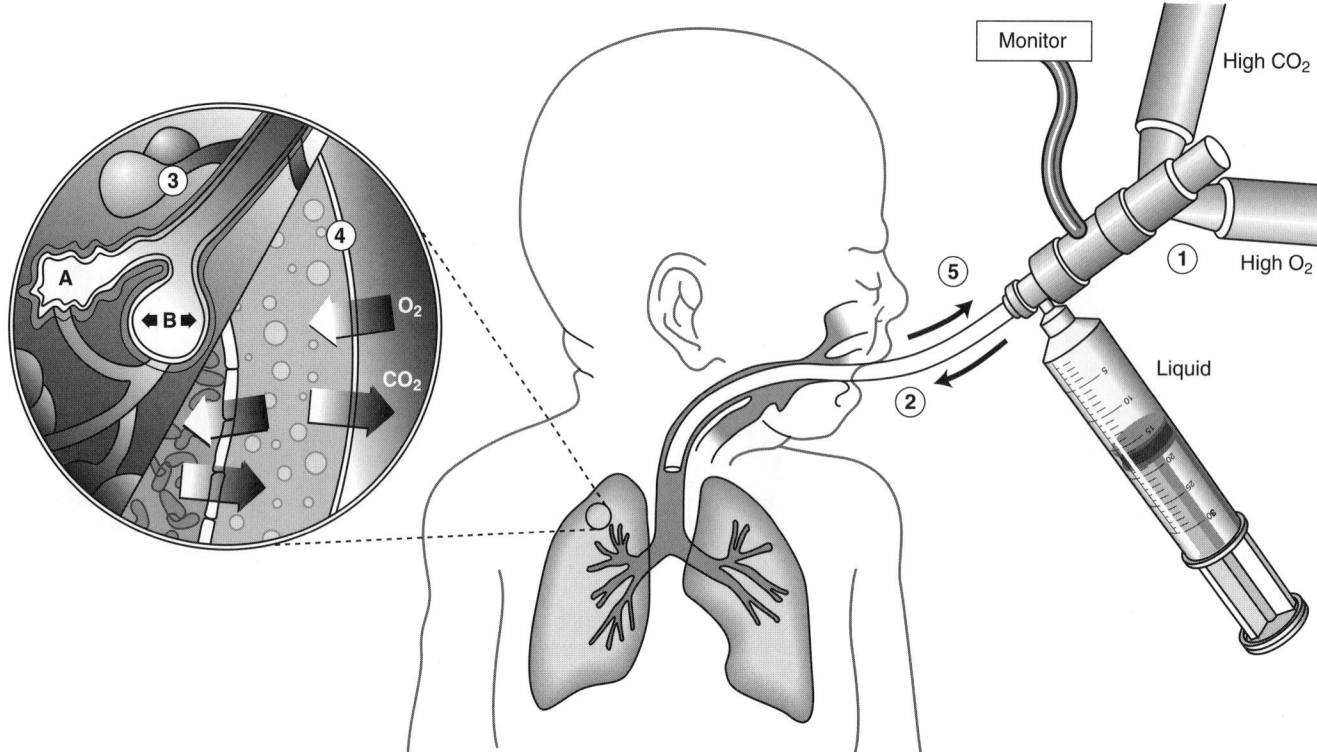

Figure 98–18. Schematic of perfluorochemical dosing and conceptualized gas exchange processes during gas ventilation (i.e., partial liquid ventilation) (Courtesy of Dr. Jay S. Greenspan, Thomas Jefferson University Hospital, Philadelphia.)

PFC in the lung (personal communication, Alliance Pharmaceutical Corporation, San Diego, CA). Eight infants were survivors at 28 days, and seven were discharged. It appears that clinical improvements were clearly demonstrated, with survival in some patients not expected to survive.

Liquid Ventilation as Adjunctive Therapy

The utility of liquid ventilation in the treatment of pulmonary dysfunction extends beyond the lowering of surface tension. In addition to recruiting atelectatic regions of the lung, filling the lungs with PFC has a potential role in delivering both active and inactive agents for treating or diagnosing pulmonary disorders, in preventing further collapse of the lung, and in cleansing the lung, thereby providing a means for improved pulmonary gas transport and mechanics. For these reasons, several investigators have explored the use of liquid ventilation in combination with other forms of respiratory support.

Drug and Tracer Delivery

Several studies have demonstrated the feasibility of using PFC liquid ventilation techniques to deliver aqueous-based pharmacologic agents (i.e., vasopressors, antibiotics) to the lung. Significant physiologic responses and homogeneous distribution of these agents were demonstrated when they were delivered during tidal PFC ventilation in preterm lambs with respiratory distress syndrome and normal or lung-injured full-term lambs[62, 106, 173-179]; limited responses were noted when these agents were delivered during PLV.[174] Despite the lack of miscibility of the aqueous agents in the PFC, the physiologic responses demonstrate that tidal PFC ventilation provided a vehicle to deliver vasoactive agents to the pulmonary and systemic circulation. The delivery of these agents within the PFC tidal volume is consistent with the convective-exchange mechanism[180]; this mechanism is ostensibly absent during PLV.

The physiologic responses to inspired nitric oxide (NO) during PLV were investigated. NO administration in combination with PLV in surfactant-depleted adult pigs produced a significant improvement in gas exchange and decrease in pulmonary artery pressure without deleterious effects on systemic hemodynamic conditions.[181] A study of a congenital diaphragmatic hernia lamb preparation treated prophylactically with PLV demonstrated that NO improved oxygenation and reduced pulmonary hypertension.[171] The ability to deliver NO during PLV is probably related to distribution of NO in the gas-ventilated regions of the lung, the solubility and diffusion of this gas in the PFC, and recruitment of lung volume. These findings on the effective delivery of NO in PFC liquid are consistent with those of earlier studies demonstrating the use of PFC liquid as a vehicle for the delivery of other biologic agents. Based on the transport principles previously described, it appears that the absolute amount of NO delivered to the pulmonary structures is dependent not only on the NO in parts per million in the inspired gas, but also on the amount dissolved in the PFC liquid (PFC liquids have high solubility for most gases; solubility data of NO in PFC have not been reported), the stratification pattern of gas and PFC liquid, the amount and distribution of pulmonary blood flow, and ventilation/perfusion matching. Therefore, for equivalent inspired NO (ppm), the amount of NO delivered to the pulmonary structures of the PFC-filled lung may be different from the amount delivered by gas ventilation. In addition, the clearance of NO from the PFC-filled lung and potential formation of NO_2 during liquid ventilation may also be different as compared with the gas-filled lung.

These studies suggest that PFC-assisted ventilation may be a useful adjunct in delivering therapeutic levels of other agents (i.e., bronchodilators, exogenous surfactant, antibiotics, steroids, chemotherapeutics, mucolytics, antioxidants, and gene therapy products) directly to the lung while protecting nontargeted organs from pharmacologic effects. Alternate combinations of PFC with biologic or nonbiologic agents such as suspensions, micelles, or liposomes may enhance the therapeutic and diagnostic potential of PFC pulmonary delivery techniques. Overall, it appears that this approach has a promising therapeutic role in the management of various neonatal problems, such as surfactant deficiency, consolidation, exudative processes, persistent or acquired pulmonary hypertension, pneumonia, and airway reactivity.

REFERENCES

1. Hack M, et al: Very low birth weight outcomes of the National Institute of Child Health and Human Development Neonatal Network. Pediatrics 87:587, 1991.
2. Shaffer TH: A brief review: liquid ventilation. Undersea Biomed Res 14:169, 1987.
3. Shaffer TH, Wolfson MR: Principles and Applications of Liquid Breathing: Water Babies Revisited. St. Louis, Mosby–Year Book, 1992.
4. Shaffer TH, et al: Liquid ventilation. Pediatr Pulmonol 14:102, 1992.
5. Wolfson MR, Shaffer TH: Liquid ventilation during early development: theory, physiologic processes and application. J Dev Physiol 13:1, 1990.
6. Winternitz MC, Smith GH: Preliminary Studies in Intratracheal Therapy. New Haven, Yale University Press, 1920, pp 144–160.
7. Avery ME, Mead J: Surface properties in relation to atelectasis and hyaline membrane disease. Am J Dis Child 97:517, 1959.
8. Davidson A, et al: Partial liquid ventilation reduces left ventricular wall stress in rescue of surfactant-treated preterm lambs. Chest 3:108, 1995.
9. Fournier L, et al: Morphometric and physiological differences between gas and liquid ventilated lung. Can J Anaesth 42:A29B, 1995.
10. Hamosh P, Luschsinger PC: Maximal expiratory flow in isolated liquid-filled lungs. J Appl Physiol 15:485, 1968.
11. Leith DE, Mead J: Maximum expiratory flow in liquid-filled lungs. Fed Proc 25:506, 1966.
12. Mead J, et al: Surface tension as a factor in pulmonary volume-pressure hysteresis. J Appl Physiol 10:191, 1957.
13. Neergard DV: Neue Auffassungen über einen Grundbegriff der Atemmechanic. Die Retraktionkraft der Lunge, abhangig von der Oberflachenspannung in den Alveolen. Z Gesamte Exp Med 66:373, 1929.
14. Kylstra J: Advantages and limitations of liquid breathing. In Lambertsen CJ (ed): Proceedings of the Third Symposium on Underwater Physiology. Baltimore, Williams & Wilkins, 1967, pp 341–350.
15. Kylstra JA, et al: Pulmonary gas exchange in dogs ventilated with hyperbarically oxygenated liquid. J Appl Physiol 21:177, 1966.
16. Kylstra JA, et al: Gas exchange in saline-filled lungs of man. J Appl Physiol 35:136, 1973.
17. Lynch PR, et al: Decompression incidence in air- and liquid-breathing hamsters. Undersea Biomed Res 10:1, 1983.
18. Wessler EP, et al: The solubility of oxygen in highly fluorinated liquids. J Fluorine Chem 9:137, 1977.
19. Stein SN, Sonnenschein RR: Electrical activity and oxygen tensions of brain during hyperoxic convulsions. J Aviat Med 21:401, 1950.
20. Goodlin R: Fetal incubator. Lancet 1:1356, 1962.
21. Kylstra JA, et al: Of mice as fish. Trans Am Soc Artif Intern Organs 8:378, 1962.
22. Pegg JH, et al: Breathing of pressure-oxygenated liquids. In Second Symposium on Underwater Physiology. Washington, DC, National Academy of Sciences-National Research Council, 1963, pp 166–170.
23. Clark LC Jr: Introduction. Fed Proc 29:1698, 1970.
24. Sargent JW, Seffl RJ: Properties of perfluorinated liquid. Fed Proc 29:1699, 1970.
25. Clark LC Jr, Gollan F: Survival of mammals breathing organic liquids equilibrated with oxygen at atmospheric pressure. Science 152:1755, 1966.
26. Clark LC Jr: Introduction to fluorocarbons. Int Anesthesiol Clin 23:1, 1985.
27. Moore RE, Clark LC Jr: Chemistry of fluorocarbons in biomedical use. Int Anesthesiol Clin 23:11, 1985.
28. Riess JC: Reassessment of criteria for the selection of PFC for second-generation blood substitutes: analysis of structure/property relationships. Artif Organs 8:44, 1984.
29. Reed TM III: Hildebrand theory for gas solubilities in liquids. Fed Proc 29:1708, 1970.
30. Riess JG, LeBlanc M: Solubility and transport phenomena in PFC relevant to blood substitution and other biomedical applications. Pure Appl Chem 54:2383, 1982.
31. Tham MK, et al: Physical properties and gas solubilities in selected fluorinated ethers. J Chem Eng Data 18:385, 1973.
32. Riess JG: Overview of progress in the fluorocarbon approach to in vivo oxygen delivery. Artif Cells Blood Substit Immobil Biotechnol 20:183, 1992.
33. Sekins KM: Lung cancer hyperthermia via ultrasound and PFC liquids: final report. National Institutes of Health Grant R43 CA48611-03. Bethesda, MD, National Institutes of Health, 1995.
34. Weers J, Johnson C: Equilibrium spreading coefficients of perfluorocarbons. San Diego, CA, Alliance Pharmaceutical Corporation Research and Development Report, 1991.
35. Peck GA, et al: Theoretical and experimental assessment of gas exchangers for perfluorochemical (PFC) liquid ventilation. Pediatr Res 37:A396, 1995.
36. Biro GP, Blais P: Perfluorocarbon blood substitutes. CRC Crit Rev Oncol Hematol 6:311, 1987.
37. Haidt SJ, et al: Liquid perfluorocarbon replacement of eye tissue. Invest Ophthalmol 22:233, 1982.
38. Liu MS, Long DM: Biological disposition of perfluorooctylbromide: tracheal administration on alveolography and bronchography. Invest Radiol 11:479, 1976.
39. Long DM, et al: Efficacy and toxicity studies with radiopaque perfluorocarbon. Radiology 105:323, 1972.
40. Mattrey RF: Perfluorooctylbromide: a new contrast agent for CT, sonography and MR imaging. Am J Radiol 152:247, 1989.
41. Mitsuno T, et al: Clinical studies of a PFC whole blood substitute (Fluosol-DA): a summary of 186 cases. Ann Surg 195:60, 1982.
42. Mitsuno T, et al: Development of a PFC emulsion as a blood gas carrier. Artif Organs 8:25, 1984.
43. West JB, et al: Effect of stratified inequality of blood flow on gas exchange in liquid-filled lungs. J Appl Physiol 32:357, 1972.
44. West JB, et al: Distribution of blood flow and ventilation in saline-filled lung. J Appl Physiol 20:1107, 1965.
45. Gil J, et al: Alveolar volume-surface area relation in air and liquid filled lungs fixed by vascular perfusion. J Appl Physiol 47:990, 1979.
46. King RJ, Clements JA: Surface active materials from dog lung. II. Composition and physiologic correlations. J Appl Physiol 223:715, 1972.
47. Adamson AW: Physical Chemistry of Surfaces. New York, John Wiley & Sons, 1982.
48. Sanderson RJ, et al: Morphological and physical basis for lung surfactant action. Respir Physiol 27:379, 1976.
49. Wilson TA, Bachofen H: A model for mechanical structure of the alveolar duct. J Appl Physiol 52:1064, 1982.
50. Pattle RE: Properties, function and origin of the alveolar lining layer. Nature 175:1125, 1955.
51. Clements JA: Surface tension of lung extracts. Proc Soc Exp Biol Med 10:170, 1957.
52. Shaffer TH, Moskowitz GD: Demand-controlled liquid ventilation of the lungs. J Appl Physiol 36:208, 1974.
53. Gollan F, et al: Compliance and diffusion during respiration with fluorocarbon fluid. Fed Proc 29:1725, 1970.
54. Saga S, et al: Pulmonary function after ventilation with fluorocarbon liquid P-12F (caroxin-F). J Appl Physiol 34:160, 1973.
55. Tuazon JG, et al: Pulmonary function after ventilation with fluorocarbon liquid (Caroxin-D). Anesthesiology 38:34, 1973.
56. Shaffer TH: Liquid ventilation. In Ziuschenberger JB, Bartlett RH (eds): Extracorporeal Cardiopulmonary Support in Critical Care. Ann Arbor, MI, Extracorporeal Life Support Organization, 1995.
57. Wolfson MR, et al: Liquid assisted ventilation: an alternative respiratory modality. State of art review. Pediatr Pulmonol 26:42, 1998.
58. Shaffer TH, et al: Liquid ventilation: current status. Pediatr Rev 20:C134, 1999.
59. Greenspan JS, et al: Liquid ventilation. Semin Perinatol 24:396, 2000.
60. Wolfson MR, Shaffer TH: Liquid-assisted ventilation: an update. Eur J Pediatr 158:S27, 1999.
61. Foust R, et al: Liquid assisted ventilation: an alternative ventilation strategy for acute meconium aspiration injury. Pediatr Pulmonol 21:316, 1996.
62. Fox, WW, et al: Liquid ventilation (LV) for pulmonary administration of gentamicin (G) in acute lung injury. Pediatr Res 35:296A, 1994.
63. Hirschl RB, et al: Liquid ventilation provides uniform distribution of perfluorocarbon in the setting of respiratory failure. Surgery 116:159, 1994.
64. Hirschl RB, et al: Liquid ventilation improves pulmonary function, gas exchange, and lung injury in a model of respiratory failure. Ann Surg 221:79, 1995.
65. Hirschl RB, et al: Lung management with perfluorocarbon liquid ventilation improves pulmonary function and gas exchange during extracorporeal membrane oxygenation (ECMO). Artif Cells Blood Substit Immobil Biotechnol 22:1389, 1994.
66. Jackson JC, et al: Full-tidal liquid ventilation with perfluorocarbon for prevention of lung injury in newborn non-human primates. Artif Cells Blood Substit Immobil Biotechnol 22:1121, 1994.
67. Shaffer TH, et al: The effects of liquid ventilation on cardiopulmonary function in preterm lambs. Pediatr Res 17:303, 1983.
68. Shaffer TH, et al: Liquid ventilation. In Boynton BR, et al (eds): New Therapies for Neonatal Respiratory Failure: A Physiological Approach. New York, Cambridge University Press, 1994, pp 279–301.
69. Shaffer TH, et al: Gaseous exchange and acid-base balance in premature lambs during liquid ventilation since birth. Pediatr Res 10:227, 1976.
70. Shaffer TH, et al: Cardiopulmonary function in very preterm lambs during liquid ventilation. Pediatr Res 17:680, 1983.
71. Valls i Soler A, et al: Ventilacion liquida parcial conperfluorocarbonado: comparacion con la adminstracion de surfactante en corderos immadura. I. Correlaciones fisiologicas. An Esp Pediatr 41:190, 1994.
72. Valls i Soler A, et al: Comparison of natural surfactant and brief liquid ventilation rescue treatment in very immature lambs: clinical and physiological correlates. Biol Neonate 69:275, 1996.
73. Wolfson MR, et al: Perfluorochemical rescue of natural surfactant-treated preterm lambs: effect of perflubron dose and ventilatory frequency during gas ventilation. J Appl Physiol 84:624, 1998.
74. Wolfson MR, et al: Physiologic basis of improved lung stability after PFC (PFC) liquid rescue of surfactant treated lambs. Pediatr Res 35:A357, 1994.

75. Wolfson MR, et al: Combined technologies: liquid ventilation (LV) and extracorporeal life support (ECLS) for treatment of meconium aspiration injury. Paper presented at the Eleventh Annual CNMC ECMO Symposium, Keystone, CO, 1995.

76. Wolfson MR, et al: A new experimental approach for the study of cardiopulmonary physiology during early development. J Appl Physiol 65:1436, 1988.

77. Greenspan JS, et al: Liquid ventilation of preterm baby (letter). Lancet 2:1095, 1989.

78. Greenspan JS, et al: Liquid ventilation of human preterm neonates. J Pediatr 117:106, 1990.

79. Bhutani VK, et al: Liquid ventilation: postnatal cardiopulmonary conditioning of very preterm lambs. In Jones CT (ed): Fetal and Neonatal Development. Ithaca, NY, Perinatology Press, 1988, pp 304–308.

80. Richman PS, et al: Lung lavage with oxygenated PFC liquid in acute lung injury. Crit Care Med 21:768, 1993.

81. Shaffer TH, et al: Liquid ventilation: effects on pulmonary function in distressed meconium-stained lambs. Pediatr Res 18:47, 1984.

82. Nesti FD, et al: Perfluorocarbon-associated gas exchange in gastric aspiration. Crit Care Med 22:1445, 1994.

83. Bing DR, et al: Time course of blood gas and lung compliance changes during partial liquid ventilation in an animal model. Pediatr Res 37:A327, 1995.

84. Major D, et al: Improved pulmonary function after surgical reduction of congenital diaphragmatic hernia in lambs. J Pediatr Surg 34:426, 1999.

85. Major D, et al: Morphometrics of normal and hypoplastic lungs in preterm lambs with gas and partial liquid ventilation. Pediatr Surg Int 12:121, 1997.

86. Hernan LJ, et al: Oxygenation during perfluorocarbon associated gas exchange in normal and abnormal lungs. Artif Cells Blood Substit Immobil Biotechnol 22:1377, 1994.

87. Hirschl RB, et al: Liquid ventilation in adults, children and full-term neonates. Lancet 346:1201, 1995.

88. Lachmann B, et al: Perflubron (perfluorooctylbromide) instillation combined with mechanical ventilation: an alternative treatment of acute respiratory failure in adult animals. Adv Exp Med Biol 317:409, 1992.

89. Lachmann B, et al: Intratracheal perfluorooctylbromide (PFOB) in combination with mechanical ventilation. In Proceedings of the International Society for Oxygen Transport to Tissues. Curacao, Willemstand, 1991.

90. Leach CL, et al: Perfluorocarbon-associated gas exchange (partial liquid ventilation) in respiratory distress syndrome: a prospective, randomized, controlled study. Crit Care Med 21:1270, 1993.

91. Leach CL, et al: Partial liquid ventilation with perflubron: a pilot safety and efficacy study in premature newborns with severe RDS who have failed conventional therapy and exogenous surfactant. N Eng J Med 335:761, 1996.

92. Leach CL, et al: Partial liquid ventilation in premature lambs with respiratory distress syndrome: efficacy and compatibility with exogenous surfactant. J Pediatr 126:412, 1995.

93. Major D, et al: Combined ventilation and PFC (PFC) tracheal instillation as an alternative treatment for near-death congenital diaphragmatic hernia. J Pediatr Surg 30:1178, 1995.

94. Papo MC, et al: A medical grade perfluorocarbon used during PAGE improves oxygenation and ventilation in a model of ARDS. Pediatr Res 33:A39, 1993.

95. Pranikoff T, et al: Partial liquid ventilation in newborn patients with congenital diaphragmatic hernia. J Pediatr Surg 31:613, 1996.

96. Tutuncu AS, et al: Intratracheal perfluorocarbon administration as an aid in the ventilatory management of respiratory distress syndrome. Anesthesiology 79:1083, 1993.

97. Tutuncu AS, et al: Gas exchange and lung mechanics during long-term mechanical ventilation with intratracheal perfluorocarbon administration in respiratory distress syndrome. Adv Exp Med Biol 317:401, 1992.

98. Tutuncu AS, et al: Intratracheal perfluorocarbon administration combined with mechanical ventilation in experimental respiratory distress syndrome: dose-dependent improvement of gas exchange. Crit Care Med 21:962, 1993.

99. Tutuncu AS, et al: Comparison of ventilatory support with intratracheal perfluorocarbon administration and conventional mechanical ventilation in animals with acute respiratory failure. Am Rev Respir Dis 148:785, 1993.

100. Tutuncu AS, et al: Dose-dependent improvement of gas exchange by intratracheal perflubron (perfluorooctylbromide) instillation in adult animals with acute respiratory failure. Adv Exp Med Biol 317:397, 1992.

101. Shaffer TH, et al: Liquid ventilation in preterm lambs: uptake, biodistribution and elimination of perfluorodecalin liquid. Reprod Fertil Dev 8:408, 1996.

102. Tarczy-Hornoch P, et al: In-situ interfacial tension during liquid ventilation. Pediatr Res 35:355A, 1994.

103. Tarczy-Hornoch P, et al: Lung compliance during total and partial liquid ventilation vs. exogenous surfactant. Pediatr Res 37:353A, 1995.

104. Schoenfish WH, Kylstra JA: Maximum expiratory flow and estimated CO$_2$ elimination in liquid-ventilated dog's lungs. J Appl Physiol 35:117, 1973.

105. Mead JJ, et al: Significance of the relationship between lung recoil and maximum expiratory flow. J Appl Physiol 22:95, 1967.

106. Wolfson MR, et al: Pulmonary administration of vasoactive substances by perfluorochemical liquid ventilation in neonatal lambs. Pediatrics 97:449, 1996.

107. Fuhrman BP, et al: Perfluorocarbon-associated gas exchange. Crit Care Med 19:712, 1991.

108. Shaffer TH, et al: Pulmonary lavage in preterm lambs. Pediatr Res 12:695, 1978.

109. Harris DJ, et al: Liquid ventilation in dogs: an apparatus for normobaric and hyperbaric studies. J Appl Physiol 54:1141, 1983.

110. Lowe C, et al: Liquid ventilation: cardiovascular adjustments with secondary hyperlactatemia and acidosis. J Appl Physiol 47:1051, 1979.

111. Lowe CA, Shaffer TH: Increased pulmonary vascular resistance during liquid ventilation. Undersea Biomed Res 8:1981.

112. Matthews WH, et al: Steady-state gas exchange in normothermic, anesthetized, liquid-ventilated dogs. Undersea Biomed Res 5:341, 1978.

113. Modell JH, et al: Oxygenation by ventilation with fluorocarbon liquid (FX-80). Anesthesiology 34:312, 1971.

114. Sivieri EM, et al: Instrumentation for measuring cardiac output by direct Fick method during liquid ventilation. Undersea Biomed Res 8:75, 1981.

115. Lowe CA, Shaffer TH: Pulmonary vascular resistance in the fluorocarbon-filled lung. J Appl Physiol 60:154, 1986.

116. Sykes MK, et al: The effects of variations in end-expiratory inflation pressure on cardiopulmonary function in normal hypo- and hypervolemic dogs. Br J Anaesth 42:669, 1970.

117. Curtis SE, et al: Cardiac output during liquid (perfluorocarbon) breathing in newborn piglets. Crit Care Med 19:225, 1991.

118. Curtis SE, et al: Partial liquid breathing with perflubron improves arterial oxygenation in acute canine lung injury. J Appl Physiol 75:2696, 1993.

119. Wolfson MR, et al: Effect of intra-tracheal PFC liquid on pulmonary blood flow in surfactant-treated preterm lambs. Physiol Zool 68:71, 1995.

120. Koen PA, et al: Fluorocarbon ventilation: maximal expiratory flows and CO$_2$ elimination. Pediatr Res 24:291, 1988.

121. Moskowitz GD: A mechanical respirator for control of liquid breathing. Fed Proc 29:1751, 1970.

122. Moskowitz GD, et al: Technical report: demand regulated control of a liquid breathing system. J Assoc Adv Med Instrum 5:273, 1971.

123. Moskowitz GD, et al: Liquid breathing trials and animal studies with a demand-regulated liquid breathing system. Med Instr Art 9:28, 1975.

124. Shaffer TH, Moskowitz GD: An electromechanical demand regulated liquid breathing system. IEEE Trans Biomed Eng 22:412, 1975.

125. Stavis RL, et al: Liquid ventilation (LV): comparison of pressure vs. flow regulated ventilation strategies. Pediatr Res 35:A377, 1994.

126. Troug WE, Jackson JC: Alternative Modes of Ventilation in the Prevention and Treatment of Bronchopulmonary Dysplasia. Philadelphia, WB Saunders Co, 1992.

127. Hirschl RB, et al: Development and application of a simplified liquid ventilator. Crit Care Med 23:157, 1995.

128. Wolfson MR, et al: Multifactorial analysis of exchanger and liquid conservation during perfluorochemical liquid assisted ventilation. Biomed Instrum Technol 33:260, 1999.

129. Shaffer TH, et al: Perfluorochemical (PFC) elimination from the respiratory system. FASEB J 9:A17, 1995.

130. Shaffer TH, et al: Analysis of perfluorochemical elimination from the respiratory system. J Appl Physiol 83:1033, 1997.

131. Puchetti V, et al: Liquid ventilation in man: first clinical experiences on pulmonary unilateral washing using fluorocarbon liquid. Fourth World Congress for Bronchology, 1984, p 115.

132. Winternitz MC, Smith GH: Preliminary Studies in Intratracheal Therapy. New Haven, Yale University Press, 1920, pp 144–160.

133. Stein SN, Sonnenschein RR: Electrical activity and oxygen tensions of brain during hyperoxic convulsions. J Aviat Med 21:401, 1950.

134. Calderwood HW, et al: Residual levels and biochemical changes after ventilation with perfluorinated liquid. J Appl Physiol 39:603, 1975.

135. Modell JH: Liquid ventilation of primates. Chest 69:79, 1976.

136. Modell JH, et al: Distribution and retention of fluorocarbon in mice and dogs after injection or liquid ventilation. Toxicol Appl Pharmacol 26:86, 1973.

137. Wolfson MR, et al: Liquid ventilation of neonates: uptake, distribution, and elimination of the liquid. Pediatr Res 27:A37, 1990.

138. Holaday DA, et al: Uptake, distribution, and excretion of fluorocarbon FX-80 (perfluorobutyl perfluorotetrahydrofuran) during liquid breathing in the dog. Anesthesiology 37:387, 1972.

139. Tuazon AS: Mathematical modeling of tissue uptake and biodistribution of perfluorocarbon chemical (PFC) during liquid ventilation in lambs. Masters thesis, Drexel University, Philadelphia, 1994.

140. Tuazon AS, et al: Tissue uptake of PFC (PFC) during liquid ventilation (LV): a peripheral exchange. FASEB J 8:413A, 1994.

141. Stavis RL, et al: Physiological, biochemical and histological correlates associated with tidal liquid ventilation. Pediatr Res 43:132, 1998.

142. Schwieler GH, Robertson B: Liquid ventilation in immature newborn rabbits. Biol Neonate 29:343, 1976.

143. Forman DL, et al: A fine structure study of the liquid-ventilated rabbit. Fed Proc 43:647, 1984.

144. Smith KM, et al: Partial liquid ventilation: high frequency vs conventional ventilation in an animal model. Pediatr Res 37:A351, 1995.

145. Smith KM, et al: Partial liquid ventilation: histologic differences between high frequency ventilation and conventional ventilation. Pediatr Res 37:A350, 1995.

146. Deoras KS, et al: Liquid ventilation of neonates: tissue histology and morphometry. Pediatr Res 27:A29, 1990.

147. DeLemos R, et al: Prolonged partial liquid ventilation in the treatment of hyaline membrane disease (HMD) in the premature baboon. Pediatr Res 35:A330, 1994.

148. Colton, DM, et al: Neutrophil infiltration is reduced during partial liquid ventilation in the setting of lung injury. Surg Forum *45*:668, 1994.
149. Younger JG, et al: Partial liquid ventilation protects lung during resuscitation from shock. J Appl Physiol *93*:16666, 1997.
150. Smith TM, et al: Liquid perfluorochemical decreases the in vitro production of reactive oxygen species by alveolar macrophages. Crit Care Med *23*:1533, 1996.
151. Varani J, et al: Perfluorocarbon protects lung epithelial cells from neutrophil-mediated injury in an introductory model of liquid ventilation therapy. Shock *6*:339, 1996.
152. Nakstad B, et al: Perfluorochemical (PFC) liquid modulates inflammatory responses in human blood leukocytes. Crit Care Med *29*:1731, 2001.
153. Nakstad B, et al: Perfluorochemical (PFC) liquids do not stimulate endothelin-1 or nitric oxide production in human blood leukocytes. Biol Neonate *80*:267, 2001.
154. Tutuncu AS, et al: Evaluation of lung function after intratracheal perfluorocarbon administration in healthy animals. Crit Care Med *24*:274, 1996.
155. Modell JH, et al: Effect of fluorocarbon liquid on surface tension properties of pulmonary surfactant. Chest *57*:263, 1970.
156. Leach CL, et al: Partial liquid ventilation in premature lambs with respiratory distress syndrome: efficacy and compatibility with exogenous surfactant. J Pediatr *126*:412, 1995.
157. Steinhorn DM, et al: Partial liquid ventilation enhances surfactant phospholipid production. Crit Care Med *24*:1252, 1996.
158. Cleary GM, et al: The effect of partial liquid ventilation on surfactant metabolism in a rat model of meconium aspiration. Pediatr Res *37*:A200, 1995.
159. Leach CL, et al: Partial liquid ventilation with LiquiVent increases endogenous surfactant production in premature lambs with respiratory distress syndrome (RDS). Pediatr Res *35*:220A, 1995.
160. Mantell LL, et al: Distinct patterns of apoptosis in the lung during liquid ventilation compared to gas ventilation. Am J Respir Cell Mol Biol *24*:436, 2001.
161. Foust R, et al: Pulmonary antioxidant enzyme activity during early development: effect of ventilation. Pediatr Crit Care Med *2*:63, 2001.
162. Wolfson MR, et al: Biochemical and histologic indices of reduced pulmonary trauma during perfluorochemical (PFC) liquid ventilation. Pediatr Res *39*;356A, 1996.
163. Wolfson MR, et al: Comparison of gas and liquid ventilation: clinical, physiological and histological correlates. J Appl Physiol *72*:1024, 1992.
164. Ikegami M, et al: Comparison of four surfactants: in vitro surface properties and response of preterm lambs to treatment at birth. Pediatrics *79*:38, 1987.
165. Jobe A, Ikegami M: The prematurely delivered lamb as a model for studies of neonatal adaptation. *In* Nathanielsz PW (ed): Animals in Fetal Medicine, Vol 3. Amsterdam, Elsevier, 1984, pp 4–30.
166. Mercurio MR, et al: Surface tension and pulmonary compliance in premature rabbits. J Appl Physiol *66*:2039, 1989.
167. Gladstone IM, et al: Effect of artificial surfactant on pulmonary function in preterm and fullterm lambs. J Appl Physiol *69*:465, 1990.
168. Lund GC, et al: Effect of inspiratory time (Ti) and ventilatory rate (rate) during partial liquid ventilation (PLV). Pediatr Res *37*:341A, 1995.
169. Smith KM, et al: Partial liquid ventilation using conventional and high frequency techniques. Pediatr Res *37*:351A, 1995.
170. Thompson AE, et al: Perfluorocarbon associated gas exchange (PAGE) in experimental meconium aspiration (MAS). Pediatr Res *33*:A239, 1993.
171. Wilcox DT, et al: Perfluorocarbon associated gas exchange (PAGE) and nitric oxide in the lamb with congenital diaphragmatic hernia model. Pediatr Res *35*:A260, 1994.
172. Shaffer TH, et al: Perfluorochemical liquid as a respiratory medium. Artif Cells Blood Substit Immobil Biotechnol *22*:315, 1994.
173. Zelinka MA, et al: A comparison of intratracheal and intravenous administration of gentamicin during liquid ventilation. Eur J Pediatr *156*:401, 1997.
174. Weis C, et al: Histamine (H) as a selective pulmonary vasodilator during liquid ventilation (LV). Pediatr Res *37*:A356, 1995.
175. Wolfson MR, et al.: Pulmonary administration of vasoactive substances by perfluorocarbon liquid ventilation in neonatal lambs. Pediatr Res *97*:449, 1996.
176. Lisby DA, et al: Enhanced distribution of adenovirus-mediated gene transfer to lung parenchyma by perfluorochemical liquid. Hum Gene Ther *8*:919, 1997.
177. Kimless-Garber DB, et al: Halothane anesthesia during perfluorochemical ventilation. Respir Med *91*:255, 1997.
178. Chappell SE, et al: A comparison of surfactant delivery with conventional mechanical ventilation (CMV) and partial liquid ventilation (PLV) in meconium aspiration injury. Respir Med. *95*:612, 2001.
179. Wolfson MR, Shaffer TH: Pulmonary administration of drugs (PAD): a new approach for drug delivery using liquid ventilation. Fed Proc *4*:A1105, 1990.
180. Scherer PW, Haselton FR: Convective exchange in oscillatory flow through bronchial-tree models. J Appl Physiol *53*:1023, 1982.
181. Houmes RJM, et al: Effects of nitric oxide administration on gas exchange and hemodynamics during perflubron partial liquid ventilation during induced respiratory insufficiency. Am J Respir Crit Care Med *151*:A446, 1995.

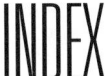

INDEX

Note: Page numbers followed by f refer to figures; those followed by t indicate tables.

A

Abdominal wall, thermoreceptors in, 552
Abortion
  induced, for multifetal reduction, 170f,
    170-171, 171f
  spontaneous
    alcohol consumption and, 235
    early, in multiple pregnancy, 171
Abruptio placentae
  alcohol consumption and, 235
  in multiple pregnancy, 168
Acardia, in multiple pregnancy, 174, 174f
Acclimation, thermal, 560
Acetaminophen
  during lactation, 255
  half-life of, 186t
Acetylcholine
  airway innervation and, 842
  as neurotransmitter, 1709, 1709f, 1875t
  cardiac conduction and, 682, 683f, 684
  umbilicoplacental circulation mediation by,
    752t
Achondroplasia, 1836t, 1837, 1857t
Acid-base balance
  potassium homeostasis and, 1281
  regulation of, 1361-1364
    extracellular buffer system and, 1361,
      1363
    in fetus, 1362
    in neonates, 1363-1364
    intracellular buffer system and, 1361, 1363
    renal compensatory mechanisms and,
      1362
    research compensatory mechanism and,
      1362
  renal tubular function and, prenatal, 1236
  status of, calcium transport and, 1288
Acidemia, cardiac function and, 654
Acidification of urine. See Urinary
  acidification.
Acidosis
  cerebral, in hypoxia-ischemia, 1722-1723,
    1723f
  lactic, 1212t
    in hypoxemia, fetal, 773
  metabolic
    cardiac function and, 654
    fetal, 1362
    neonatal, 1363-1364
    potassium homeostasis and, 1281, 1285
    with hypothermia, 587
  respiratory
    fetal, 1362
    metabolic compensation for, 1329-1330
    neonatal, 1364

Aciduria, arginosuccinic, 595
Acinar buds, 786
Acinar tubules, 786
Acinus(i)
  organization of, 1177
  pancreatic, 1142-1143
ACTH. See Adrenocorticotropic hormone.
Actin filaments, 635
Action potential, cardiac. See Cardiac action
  potential.
Activated partial thromboplastin time
  in adults, 1436t
  in children, 1441t
  in fetuses, 1436t
  in full-term infants, 1436t, 1438t
  in neonates, 1449
  in premature infants, 1437t
  systems for, 1435, 1442t
Activating mutations, 21
Activation potential, 671
Active transport, placental
  of amino acids, 512
  of calcium, 314t, 314-316, 315f
  of drugs, 179, 207
Activin, brain development and, 1786
Activiteá moyenne, 1733
Acute phase reaction, 1563
Acute renal failure, 1335-1339
  causes of, 1338, 1339t
  intrinsic, 1335
  pathophysiologic mechanisms of,
    1335-1338, 1336f
    glomerular transcapillary hydraulic
      pressure difference and, 1337-1338,
      1338f
    golmerular capillary ultrafiltration
      coefficient and, 1338
    plasma colloid osmotic pressure and,
      1338
    plasma flow rate and, 1336-1337
  postrenal, 1335
  prerenal, 1335
  prognosis of, 1339
Acute tubular necrosis, 1335
Acyclovir, during lactation, 256
Adaptive hypometabolism, 541, 542f
ADCC. See Antibody-dependent cellular
  cytotoxicity.
Adenosine
  calcium transport and, 1289
  chemoreceptor-mediated cardiovascular
    responses and, 722
  renal blood flow and, 1244
  thermogenesis and, neonatal, 547t
  umbilicoplacental circulation mediation by,
    752t

Adenosine monophosphate, cyclic
  as second messenger, 1598-1599
  pulmonary liquid transport regulation by,
    826-827, 828f
Adenosine triphosphate
  availability of, apoptosis versus necrosis
    and, 75
  calcium transport and, 1289
ADH. See Vasopressin.
Adhalen, 1854
Adhesion molecules. See Cell adhesion
  molecules; Immunoglobulin gene
  superfamily; Integrins; Selectin(s).
Adipose tissue
  brown, 404-412
    5'-deiodinase and thyroid and, 410f,
      410-411, 411f
    depots of, 405
    development of, prolactin and, 1893
    diseases affecting, 412
    in newborns, 404-405
    recruitment of, 411
    thermogenesis and, 405
      clinical implications of, 411-412
      substrates for, 408-410
      thermogenesis in. See Thermogenesis,
        nonshivering.
    UCP1 and, 405f, 405-408, 406f
      acute regulation of, 406-407, 407f
      adaptive regulation of, 407-408, 408f
      semiacute regulation of, 407
      UCP gene and, 406
  lipids in, 601t
  lipolysis in, 419-420, 420f, 421f
    hypoglycemia and, 495
  white, 405
Admixture lesions, in congenital heart
  disease, 711-712
  single-ventricle physiology with, 711-712
  systemic arterial oxygen saturation
    determinants with, 711
  systemic arterial oxygen saturation versus
    systemic oxygen transport in, 711, 712f
Adrenal cortex, 1915-1923, 1916f. See also
  Corticosteroids; Glucocorticoids;
  Mineralocorticoids; specific
  corticosteroids, e.g. Cortisol.
  adaptation of, to extrauterine life,
    1920-1922, 1922t
  embryogenesis of, 1915
  functional maturation of, fetal, 1915-1919
    fetoplacental steroid metabolism and,
      1918f, 1918-1919, 1919f
    molecular biology of adrenocortical cell
      and, 1915-1917, 1916f
    steroidogenesis and, 1917f, 1917-1918

Aortic stenosis, afterload increase with, 714
Apert syndrome, 48, 786, 790, 1857t
Apgar scoring, resuscitation and, 766, 766t
Apical ectodermal ridge, 1829-1830, 1830f
  in limb development, 1845-1846
Apical membrane, of mammary alveolar cell,
  transport across, 286
Apnea
  central, 906
  continuum from infant to child and adult
    and, 915-916
  idiopathic, 907, 916
  in neonates, 895-896, 896f, 897f
  mixed, 905-906, 906f
  obstructive, 906
  of prematurity, 905-917
    classification of, 905-906, 906f
    definition of, 905
    epidemiology of, 907, 909f
    initiation of, 916
    neurodevelopmental outcome of,
      915-916
    physiologic effects of, 906-907,
      907f-909f
    physiologic factors in, 907-914
      alteration in central drive as, 907-909,
        910f
      chemoreceptor and mechanoreceptor
        responses as, 910f, 910-911
      gastrointestinal reflux as, 914
      periodic breathing as, 911, 911f
      sleep state as, 909-910
      upper airway and chest wall muscle
        responses as, 911-912, 911f-913f
      upper airway reflexes as, 912-914,
        914f
    sudden infant death syndrome and, 915
    termination of, 916-917
    therapeutic interventions for, 914-916
      body position and, 915
      continuous positive airway pressure
        as, 914, 914f
      pharmacologic, 914-915, 915t
Apneic threshold level, 892
Apolipoprotein E, in high density lipoprotein,
  of fetus and newborn, 360
Apoptosis, 72-74
  activation through death receptors, after
    tissue injury, 74
  choice between necrosis and, factors
    determining, 74-75
  following brain injury, molecular evidence
    of, 73-74
  following hypoxia-ischemia, 73
  in cerebral injury, relation between necrosis
    and, 73
  in folliculogenesis, 1945
  in morphologic development of embryo
    and fetus, 72
  in neuronal damage, 73
  mitochondria in, 75-77
    Bcl-2 family members and, 76-77
    mitochondrial permeability transition
      and, 75-76, 76f, 77
  modes of cell death in tissue injury and, 73
  of malignant cells, α-lactalbumin and, 280
  of stem cells, 1369
  preeclampsia and fetal growth impairment
    and, 153
  prevention or suppression of, by
    hypothermia, 586
  T cell, in host defense against viruses,
    neonatal, 1504-1505
  testicular, 1954
  trophoblastic invasion and, 93-94

Apoptosomes, 72
Apoptotic cells, clearance of, complement
  and, 1552
Apparent life-threatening events, 915
Apparent volume of distribution, 192-193
aPTT. See Activated partial thromboplastin
  time.
Aquaporins
  in fetus, urinary concentration and, 1311
  urinary concentration and, 1307t,
    1307-1309
  in neonates, 1314-1316, 1315f
Aqueous pores hypothesis, 198
Arachidonic acid. See also Fatty acids, long
  chain.
  accumulation of, maternal influences on,
    430
  in neonatal pulmonary host defense, 1642
  renal blood flow and, 1246
Arcuate nucleus, hypothalamic, 1872t
ARF. See Acute renal failure.
Arginine
  fetal accretion of, 531t
  in parenteral amino acid mixtures, 533t,
    534t
  normal plasma and urine levels of, 1296t
  requirements for, of low birth weight
    infants, 530t-532t
Arginine vasporessin. See Vasopressin.
Arginosuccinic aciduria, 595
Arm fat area assessment, in neonatal
  nutritional assessment, 295
Arm muscle measurement, in neonatal
  nutritional assessment, 295
Arousal, essential fatty acid deficiency and,
  433
Arterial baroreflex
  humoral interactions on, 720-721
  neonatal, function of, 721
  resetting of, 719-720
  sensitivity of, mechanisms regulating, 718,
    719f
Arterial blood flow, cerebral. See Cerebral
  arterial blood flow velocity.
Arterial oxygen content, cerebral blood flow
  and, 1746
Arteries, trophoblastic invasion of, 94
Artificial ventilation. See Mechanical
  ventilation.
Arylamine N-acetyltransferase 2
  polymorphism, 214-215
Asparagine, requirements for, of low birth
  weight infants, 530t
Aspartate
  fetal accretion of, 531t
  in parenteral amino acid mixtures, 533t,
    534t
  requirements for, of low birth weight
    infants, 530t-532t
Aspartic acid, normal plasma and urine levels
  of, 1296t
Asphyxia
  birth, hyperinsulinism in, 495-496
  glomerular filtration rate and, 1265
  intraventricular hemorrhage and, 1763
Aspirin
  during lactation, 255
  for preterm labor, 109t
Assist/control ventilation, 974
Assisted ventilation. See High-frequency
  ventilation; Liquid ventilation; Mechanical
  ventilation.
Asymmetric cellular division, 57
Atelectasis, prevention of, patient-triggered
  ventilation for, 936

Atenolol, during lactation, 256
Atopic disease, breast-feeding and, 281
Atosiban
  for preterm labor, 109t
  placental transfer of, 207
ATP. See Adenosine triphosphate.
Atria, septation of, 616
Atrial natriuretic peptide
  as neurotransmitter, 1875t
  chorionic, 127
  glomerular filtration rate and, 1258
  renal blood flow and, 1245
  renal hemodynamics and, 1233
  renal sodium transport regulation by, 1276,
    1276f
  renal tubular function and, 1238
  umbilicoplacental circulation mediation by,
    752t
Atrial septal defects, 715
Atrioventricular canal, septation of, 616
Atrioventricular conduction
  atrioventricular conduction system
    formation and, 678-680, 680f, 680t
  before atrioventricular conduction system
    formation, 678, 679f
  physiology of, 680-682, 681f, 682f
Auditory brain stem response, 1809, 1810,
  1812
Auditory system, 1803f, 1803-1816
  behavioral development and, 1813-1815
    sensitivity and, 1814
    sound localization and, 1814-1815
    speech perception and, 1815
  central auditory nervous system and,
    1810-1813, 1812f, 1813f
  ear and, 1803-1810, 1804f
    cochlea of, 1807-1810, 1808f-1811f
    conductive apparatus of, 1804-1807,
      1806f, 1807f
Augmentation gene therapy, 15
Autonomic nervous system
  cardiac conduction and, 682
  hypothalamic control of, 1873
Autoregulation
  hypoxia and, 654
  of cerebral blood flow, 1746
  of glomerular filtration rate, 1258
  of organ blood flow, 776
  of renal blood flow, 1258
    postnatal, 1242-1243
  pressure-flow, 703
AVP. See Vasopressin.
Axons, outgrowth of, 1689-1690
  disorders of, 1689-1690, 1690f
  normal, 1689
Azurophilic granules, 1543, 1543f
  in neonatal pulmonary host defense, 1644

B

B cells
  development of, 1518-1521
    anatomic sites of, 1518
    class switch recombination and, 1521
    commitment to B-cell lineage and,
      1518-1519
    diversification after V(D)J recombination
      and, 1521
    germinal centers and, 1519-1520
    immaturity and, 1521
    ontogeny of V-gene expression and, 1520
    physiological functions of CD5+ B cells,
      1520-1521
    plasma cell differentiation and, 1520

B cells (Continued)
postcommitment, 1519, 1519f
receptor diversity and, 1520
tolerance and, 1521
in host defense, 1478, 1482-1483
against viruses, 1500
neonatal, 1505-1506
in human milk, 1613
in neonatal pulmonary host defense, 1640
proliferation of, T-cell signal for, 1517
Bacteria
colonization by
of gut, necrotizing enterocolitis and,
1170
of skin, skin cleansing and, at birth,
602-603, 603t
normal flora and, in host defense, 1476
Bacterial infection(s)
changing nature of, 1475-1476
host defense against, 1476-1483
B and T lymphocytes in, 1478
components of, 1480-1483
B lymphocytes as, 1482-1483
colony-stimulating factors as, 1482
interferons as, 1482
interleukins as, 1481-1482
natural killer cells as, 1482
T lymphocytes as, 1480-1481
tumor necrosis factor as, 1481
epithelial cells, mucosal barriers, and
normal bacterial flora in, 1476
mast cells in, 1477-1478
monocytes, macrophages, and dendritic
cells in, 1477
natural antimicrobial agents in,
1479-1480
natural opsonins in, 1478-1479
neonatal, complement in, 1554
neutrophils in, 1476-1477
pathogen-associated receptors in, 1479
Bacterial lipopolysaccharide, in host defense,
1479
Bacterial permeability-increasing factor, 1479
Bacterial sepsis, cytokine levels during,
1566-1567
Bactericidal actions
complement-mediated, 1552
of mononuclear phagocytes, 1532
of neutrophils, 1544-1546
nonoxidative, 1546
oxidative, 1545-1546
Bag and mask ventilation, for resuscitation,
limitations of, 769, 770f
Balanced translocation carriers, 7
BALT. See Bronchus-associated lymphoid
tissue.
Barbiturates, maternal use of, 245
Bardet-Biedl syndrome, 20
Baroreflex, arterial
humoral interactions on, 720-721
neonatal, function of, 721
resetting of, 719-720
sensitivity of, mechanisms regulating, 718,
719f
Basal cell layer, of skin, 589
Basal lamina, alveolar, gestational changes in,
1037
Basal metabolic rate, 549
Basal plate, 92
Base deficit, resuscitation and, 768, 769f
Base pairing, 1
Basement membrane, of brain capillaries, 1701
Basic helix-loop-helix protein, 1850
Basolateral membrane, calcium transport
across, 1287

Bayley Scales of Infant Development,
docosahexaenoic acid and, 436
B-cell activating factor, 1519
Bcl-2 protein, apoptotic inhibition by, 76-77
Beckwith-Wiedemann syndrome, 1888
Beds, heated, heat exchange between infant
and environment in, 572
Behavior, essential fatty acid deficiency and,
431-433
Behavioral fever, 567
Behavioral markers, for pain, 1794
Behavioral regulation, of heat loss, 559
Behavioral states
concept of, 1726
electroencephalography and, 1726-1729,
1727t, 1728f, 1728t
Benzodiazepines, maternal use of, 244-245
Beta-adrenergic agents, for preterm labor, 108,
109t
Beta-adrenergic agonists, lung liquid and, 830
Beta-adrenergic blockers, during lactation, 256
Beta-adrenergic receptor polymorphisms, 205
Beta-endorphins, 1875t
fetal regulation of, 1910
pattern during pregnancy, 1909-1910
source of, 1909
Beta-lipotropin
pattern during pregnancy, 1909-1910
source of, 1909
Betamethasone, protein binding of, 205t
Bicarbonate
potassium homeostasis and, 1281
renal bicarbonate threshold and, 1328
tubular reabsorption of
developmental aspects of, 1329
in mature kidney, 1327-1328
Bile
composition of, 1188-1189, 1189f
flow of
cholestasis and. See Cholestasis.
inadequate, consequences of, 1220
ontogeny of, 1218-1219
transporters and, 1190-1192
basolateral, 1190-1191
canalicular, 1191-1192
developmental expression of, 1192
regulation of, 1190-1192, 1191f
formation of, 1187-1188, 1189
neonatal, 1192-1193
Bile acids, 1158, 1179-1184
chemical structure and properties of,
1179-1180
conjugated, placental transfer of, 208
enterohepatic circulation of, 1181-1182,
1182f, 1189-1190, 1190f
alteration in, 1183-1184
during development, 1183, 1184f
in bile, 1188
metabolism of, 1182-1183
altered, 1183-1184, 1184t
placental role in, 1183
physiologic function of, 1179, 1180f, 1180t
synthesis of, 1180f, 1180-1181, 1181f
alteration in, 1184
disorders of, 1193-1194
during development, 1182t, 1182-1183,
1183f
regulation of, 1181, 1181f
Bile ducts
development of, 1176-1177
intrahepatic, formation of, 1188
Bile salt export pump, 1191-1192
Bile salt-stimulated lipase, 1157
Biliary tree, development of, 1188, 1188t,
1189f

Bilirubin, 1199-1204
conjugation of, 1199-1200
genetic variations in, 1200
elevation of, in neonatal
hyperbilirubinemia, 1199, 1200-1201
excretion of, 1200
light absorption by, 1206-1207, 1207f
photochemistry of, 1207-1209
configurational isomerization and,
1207-1208, 1208f
photo-oxidation and, 1208-1209
structural isomerization and, 1208, 1209f
photoproduct formation by, 1209, 1209f
phototherapy and. See Phototherapy, for
jaundice.
production of, 1199
structure of, 1205-1206, 1206f
transport and uptake of, 1199
unconjugated, toxicity of, 1201-1202
affinity for nerve cells and, 1202-1203
bilirubin entry into brain and,
1201-1202, 1202f
cellular, 1203-1204
clinical aspects of, 1204
Bilirubin encephalopathy, 1201, 1204
Biliverdin reductase, 1199
Bioavailability, of drugs, 180-181
Biochemical markers
in neonatal nutritional assessment, 296-298
of glomerular filtration rate, 1258-1259,
1259f, 1260f, 1260t
of inflammation, 1587-1588
of nonshivering thermogenesis, 544-545,
546t
of preterm labor, 107
Bioelectrical impedance analysis, total body,
for body water measurement, 1352-1353
Biomechanical force, angiogenesis and, 55
Biopsychosocial model, anemia of, 1417
Biotransformation, of drugs, 182-184, 183t
in liver, factors affecting, 184
phase I reactions in, 182-183, 183t
phase II reactions in, 183t, 184
Biotrauma, 964
Bipotent stem cells, 1365
Birth. See also Delivery; Labor.
adaptation to extrauterine life and
adrenal, 1920-1922, 1922t
thyroid hormones and, 1930-1932,
1931f
establishment of continuous breathing at,
893-894, 894f, 895f
glomerular filtration rate at, 1262-1263,
1263f
lung injury at, mechanical, 935
lung liquid flow after, 823
myocardial function and, 652-653, 653f
preterm. See Preterm labor.
skin transition at, 600t, 600-604, 601t
acid mantle development and, 601-602,
603f
bacterial colonization and skin cleansing
and, 602-603, 603t
cutaneous immunosurveillance and,
603-604, 604f, 604t
water loss, temperature control, and
blood flow and, 601, 601f-603f
surfactant pool size changes after,
1057-1058, 1058f
sympathetic nervous system activity of,
722-724, 723f, 724f
thermoregulatory system maturity at,
563-565, 564f
thyroid system and, 1930-1932, 1931f
transition to air breathing at, 1037, 1038f

Calcium *(Continued)*
  regulation of, 1287-1289
  transcellular, 1287, 1287f
Calcium-channel blockers, for preterm labor, 108, 109t
Calcium-induced calcium release, 638-639
Calcium-sensing receptor, calcium transport and, 1288
Calcium/sodium exchange system, 317
Calorimetry, in neonates, 298
cAMP. *See* Adenosine monophosphate, cyclic.
Cancer
  apoptosis of malignant cells and, α-lactalbumin and, 280
  childhood, maternal smoking and, 240
  hematopoietic reconstitution in, 1370
  pancreatic, proto-oncogenes and, 1148-1149
  with maldescended testes, 1959
Candidate gene approach, 14
Candidiasis
  invasive, host defense against, 1488-1489
    deficient anticandidal activities of neonatal monocytes and macrophages and, 1488-1489
    phagocytes in, 1488
  mucocutaneous, host defense against, 1487-1488
    deficient T-cell immunity in newborns and, 1488
    virulence factors and surface host defense and, 1487
Cap, in transcription, 3
Capillaries
  integrity of, intraventricular hemorrhage and, 1764
  of brain, 1699. *See also* Blood-brain barrier.
    basement membrane of, 1701
Capillary membrane, volume loading and, 1348
Capsular chorion frondosum, 95
Capsular decidua, 95
Captive bubble tensiometer, 1023
Captopril, during lactation, 256
Carbamazepine
  during lactation, 256
  half-life of, 186t
Carbohydrates. *See also specific carbohydrates, e.g.* Glucose.
  digestion of, 1152-1154
    disaccharides and, 1152-1154
      postnatal, 1153-1154
      prenatal, 1152-1153, 1153f
    pancreatic enzymes in, 1146
    polysaccharides and, 1152
      postnatal, 1152, 1152f
      prenatal, 1152
  metabolism of
    cold exposure and, 543
    disorders of, 1212t
    during pregnancy, 464
    fetal
      energy requirements and, 465-466
      energy substrates and, 469-472, 470t-471f
      metabolic rate and, 467-469, 468t, 469t
      oxygen consumption and, 466t, 466-467, 467f, 468f
    in fetal growth restriction pregnancies, 261-262, 263f, 264f
Carbon balance, 523, 523t
Carbon dioxide
  fetal breathing and, 892, 893
  intraventricular hemorrhage and, 1762-1763
  neonatal breathing and, 896-897

Carbon dioxide gradient, gas exchange and, 871-872
Carbon dioxide tension, cerebral blood flow and, 1746
Carbon monoxide
  in neonatal pulmonary host defense, 1632-1633
  umbilicoplacental circulation mediation by, 752t
γ-Carboxylation system, vitamin K-dependent, 370, 370f
  development of, regulation of, 372, 372f
  maturation of, 371f, 371-372, 372f
Cardiac action potential, 669t, 669-676, 670f, 671t, 672f-674f, 673t
  atrial, 677-678, 678f
  developmental changes in, 673-676
    phase 0 and, 675
    phase 1 and, 675f, 675-676
    phases 2 and 3 and, 676, 676t, 677f
    resting membrane potential and, 673-675
  phase 0 of, 671, 672f
    developmental changes in, 675
Cardiac conduction, 676-687
  atrioventricular
    atrioventricular conduction system formation and, 678-680, 680f, 680t
    before atrioventricular conduction system formation and, 678, 679f
    physiology of, 680-682, 681f, 682f
  autonomic innervation-modulation of, 682
  from sinus node to atrioventricular node, 677-678, 678f
  parasympathetic nervous system and, 682, 683f, 684, 684f
  sympathetic nervous system and, 684-687, 686f
Cardiac function, 635-663. *See also* Myocardial *entries.*
  hypoxic stress and, 653-657
    acidemia and, 654
    circulation and, 654-656
      flow redistribution and, 655-656
      hematologic adjustments and, 654-655
      humoral responses and, 655
      local response and, 654
      metabolism and, 656
      reflex responses and, 655
    failure of adaptation to, 657
    maladaption to, 656
  myocardial contraction and. *See* Myocardial contraction.
  ventricular. *See* Ventricular function.
Cardiac jelly, 615
Cardiac looping, 34
Cardiac malformations, congenital, fetal blood flow patterns with, 657, 658f, 659f
Cardiac muscle. *See also* Myocardial contraction.
  embryology of, 35
Cardiac neural crest, 614-615
Cardiac output
  maternal, in pregnancy, 143, 143t
  neonatal, 776
  oxygen transport and, 881
  resuscitation and, 770
Cardiac tube, formation and looping of, 615
Cardiomegaly, fetal, 659
Cardiomyocyte, 635, 636f, 637f
Cardiopulmonary reflexes, 721-722
Cardiovascular disease
  drug elimination and, 185
  maternal. *See* Maternal cardiovascular disease.

Cardiovascular drugs. *See also* Antihypertensive agents.
  during lactation, 256
Cardiovascular system
  fetal, maternal cocaine use and, 238
  high-frequency ventilation and, 984
  hypothermia and, 586-587
  in bronchopulmonary dysplasia, 959
  in shock. *See* Shock, cardiovascular compromise and.
  intestinal circulation and, 702-703
  maternal. *See* Maternal cardiovascular disease; Maternal cardiovascular system.
  respiratory function and, 975-976
  with liquid ventilation, 990
Carnosine, normal plasma and urine levels of, 1296t
Cartilage
  of growth plate, 1833-1834
  of upper airway, 834-835
k-Casein, in human milk, 280
Caspases, 72
Catabolic activator protein, 41
Catecholamines
  in hypoxemia, fetal, 773-774
  neonatal glucose metabolism and, 479
  regulation of renal sodium transport by, 1275f, 1275-1276
  ventilation-perfusion matching and, 878
Cathelicidins
  in neonatal pulmonary host defense, 1628
  neutrophil, 1544, 1544t
Cathepsins, 528
Cation-Cl cotransporters, 1273
Caudal neuropore, 31
C4b-BP
  in adults, 1436t
  in fetuses, 1436t
  in full-term infants, 1436t
CBF. *See* Cerebral blood flow.
CC chemokines, in neonatal pulmonary host defense, 1650
CCK. *See* Cholecystokinin.
CCSP, in neonatal pulmonary host defense, 1651-1652
CD antigens, on mononuclear phagocytes, 1526, 1527t-1528t, 1528
CD4 T cells
  antigen processing and presentation and, 1533
  cytolytic, in host defense against viruses, 1496-1497
    neonatal, 1503
  IFN-γ production by, in host defense against viruses, neonatal, 1503
  in host defense against viruses, 1490, 1495
    neonatal, 1502-1503
  in human milk, 1613
CD5 B cells, 1520-1521
CD8 T cells
  in host defense against viruses, 1490, 1497f, 1497-1499, 1498f
    neonatal, 1503-1504
  in human milk, 1613
CD11b protein, 1542
CD18 protein, 1542
CD28, in host defense against viruses, 1499
CD40, in host defense against viruses, 1496, 1496f
  neonatal, 1503
CD40-ligand, in host defense against viruses, 1496, 1496f
  neonatal, 1503
CD80-86, in host defense against viruses, 1499

Cholestasis *(Continued)*
  congenital, 1193-1194
  hepatic manifestations of, 1216t
  in metabolic disorders, 1214
  neonatal, 1218-1220
    hepatic injury in, mechanisms of, 1219-1220
    ontogeny of bile flow and, 1218-1219
Cholesterol. *See also* Lipoprotein(s).
  adrenal steroidogenesis and, 1917
  biosynthesis of, 1180, 1181f
    congenital defects and, 381, 382f, 383f
  fetal development and, 380-384
  fetal sources of, 381, 384
  in bile, 1188, 1189f
  metabolism of, 1180-1181
    fetal development and, 441-442, 442f
    postnatal development and, 443
  serum concentrations of
    in fetal development, 440-441
      in experimental animals, 441
      in humans, 440-441, 441f, 441t
    in postnatal development, 442-443
      in experimental animals, 443
      in humans, 442f, 442-443
    perinatal disease and, 443
Cholic acid, 1180, 1180f. *See also* Bile acids.
Cholinergic innervation, of lower airway, 842-843, 844f
Chondrocytes, 1833-1834
  differentiation of, 1831f, 1831-1832, 1832f
  molecular biology of, 1832-1833
Chordal mesoderm, 1675
Chorioamnionitis, 949-951
  animal models of, 950-951, 951f
  brain injury and, 1565-1566
  fetal lung injury due to, 950
  lung maturation and, 950
  preterm birth associated with, 133
  viral, 132
Chorion, definition of, 114t
Chorion frondosum, capsular, 95
Chorionic connective tissue, 95
Chorionic corticotropin-releasing hormone, placental, 126f, 126-127
Chorionic gonadotropin-releasing hormone, placental, 126
Chorionic plate, 94
Chorionic somatostatin, placental, 126
Chorionic thyrotropin-releasing hormone, placental, 126
Chorionicity, 166
  determination of, 166f, 166-167, 167f
Chromatin, 1-2
Chromium-51 ethylenediaminetetra-acetic acid, as glomerular filtration rate marker, 1259
Chromosomal anomalies, in multiple pregnancy, 171
Chromosomal deletions, terminal, 7, 7f
Chromosomal disorders, 9-10
Chromosomal mutations, 7, 7f
Chromosomes, 1-2
  nonmendelian disease and, 22, 23f, 24f
Chymotrypsin
  postnatal, 1155
  prenatal, 1155
Chymotrypsinogen, prenatal, 1155
Cigarette smoking, maternal, 239-240
Ciliary function, in neonatal pulmonary host defense, 1622f, 1622-1623
Cimetidine, during lactation, 257
Ciprofloxacin, during lactation, 256
Circadian rhythms, hypothalamic control of, 1873

Circulation. *See also* Blood flow; Blood pressure; Hemodynamics; Hypertension.
  cerebral, pressure-passive, intraventricular hemorrhage and, 1761-1762
  fetal
    fetal plasma concentration of drugs and, 225
    velocimetry in fetal growth restriction and, 260
  gastrointestinal. *See* Intestinal circulation.
  hypoxic effects on, 654-675
    flow redistribution and, 655-656
    hematologic adjustments and, 654-655
    humoral responses and, 655
    local response and, 654
    metabolic, 656
    reflex responses and, 655
  intestinal. *See* Intestinal circulation.
  maternal, drug transfer into breast milk from, 250-251, 251f
  neonatal, physiology of, 776
  placental. *See* Placental circulation.
  prenatal nutrition and, 727-731
    environmental stimuli and, 728
      transduction of, 730-731
    epidemiologic observations on, 727
    fetal adaptations and, 728-729
    genetics versus environment and, 727-728
    maternal adaptations and, 730
    nutrients and, 728, 728f, 729f
    postnatal adaptations and, 729-730
    timing and, 728
  umbilicoplacental, 749
    anatomy of, 749f, 749-750
    closure of, at birth, 754
  uterine, definition of, 114t
  uteroplacental, maternal adaptations to pregnancy and, 143t, 144
Citrulline, normal plasma and urine levels of, 1296t
Clara cell secretory protein, in neonatal pulmonary host defense, 1651-1652
Cleavage, 29
Clinical description of shock, 777
Cloaca, persistent, 1109
Cloacal membrane, 1109
Clonal deletion, 1521
Clonal ignorance, 1521
Cloning, 12, 12f, 16
Clubfoot
  idiopathic, congenital, 1839, 1841f
  rigid, 1840
Coagulation. *See also* Hemostasis.
  animal models of, 1444
  inhibitors of, consumption of, in disseminated intravascular coagulation, 1462
  intraventricular hemorrhage and, 1764
  vitamin K and, 369
Coagulation factors. *See also* Factor *entries*.
  deficiencies of, inherited, 1450-1452
    combined, 1452
    hemophilia as, 1450-1451, 1452t
    of factor XIII, 1452
    of factors II, V, and X, 1451-1452
Coagulation system
  activation of, during inflammatory response, 1563
  maternal, in multiple pregnancy, 168
Coagulopathy, consumptive, in disseminated intravascular coagulation, 1463
Coarctation of the aorta, afterload increase with, 714
Cocaine
  amino acid transport and, 517

Cocaine *(Continued)*
  detection in fetus, 238-239
  maternal use of, 237-239
    contraindication to, for nursing mothers, 255
  pharmacology of, 237
Cochlea, 1807-1810, 1808f-1811f
Codons, 3
Cognitive development
  maternal alcohol consumption and, 236
  maternal smoking and, 240
Cognitive function
  breast-feeding and, 282
  essential fatty acid deficiency and, 432
  in offspring, preeclampsia and, 154
Cold exposure
  carbohydrate metabolism and, 543
  thermogenesis and, 543
Colinearity, 45
Collagen(s)
  development of, nutrition and, 808
  hematopoiesis and, 1389-1390
Collagenase, in neonatal pulmonary host defense, 1644
Collectins
  in host defense, 1479
  in neonatal pulmonary host defense, 1629-1631, 1630f
  in pulmonary surfactant, 1008-1012, 1009f, 1009t, 1011f
Collodion babies, 591
Colloid oncotic pressure, plasma, in acute renal failure, 1338
Colonic aganglionosis, 1109, 1114-1115, 1679
Colonic motility, 1134f, 1134-1135, 1141
Colony-forming unit(s), 1388
Colony-forming unit-erythrocyte, 1397
Colony-forming unit-erythroid, 1397, 1400f
Colony-forming unit-granulocyte, 1397
Colony-forming unit-macrophage, 1397
Colony-forming unit-megakaryocyte, 1397, 1421
Colony-forming units-erythroid, 1388
Colony-stimulating factors
  in host defense, 1482
  in neonatal pulmonary host defense, 1652, 1652f
Compartments, drug distribution to, 186, 186f
  multicompartment, 187, 187f
  single-compartment, 186
Complement proteins
  biosynthesis of, 1529
  components of, in human milk, 1612
  in host defense, 1478
    against viruses, 1500
      neonatal, 1505-1506
    neonatal, pulmonary, 1626-1627, 1642-1643, 1643f
Complement receptors, 1542, 1551
Complement system, 1549-1554
  activation of, 1551-1552
    anaphylatoxic activity and, 1551
    antibody formation and, 1552
    apoptotic body clearance and, 1552
    bactericidal activity and, 1552
    chemotactic activity and, 1551
    immune complex processing and, 1552
    opsonic activity and, 1551-1552
  alternative pathway of, 1550-1551
    in neonates, 1552, 1553t
  biochemistry of, 1549-1551, 1550f, 1550t
  C3 and terminal component activation and, 1551
  classic pathway of, 1549-1550
    in neonates, 1552, 1553t

Complement system *(Continued)*
    complement receptors and, 1551
    fetal synthesis of components of, 1552
    lectin pathway of, 1551
    neonatal
        component levels and, 1552-1553, 1553f,
            1553t
        functions mediated by, 1553-1554
        host defense and, 1554
Compression isotherm, 1019
Compression reservoirs, 1027
Computed tomography, in intraventricular
    hemorrhage, 1758
Concentration, in isotope studies, 450
Conceptional age, 1726
Congenital anomalies
    cholesterol biosynthesis and, 381, 382f, 383f
    in multiple pregnancy, 171
    requiring surgical repair, anemia with, 1417
Congenital constriction band syndrome, 1838,
    1839f
Congenital cystic adenomatoid
    malformations, 792
Congenital heart disease, 705-716
    admixture lesions and, 711-712
        single-ventricle physiology with, 711-712
        systemic arterial oxygen saturation
            determinants with, 711
        systemic arterial oxygen saturation
            versus systemic oxygen transport in,
            711, 712f
    anemia with, 1417
    bidirectional shunting and, 710-711
    left-to-right shunting and
        at atrial level, 708
        at ventricular or great artery level,
            707-708, 709f
        effects of, on cardiac physiology, 714-715
        lesions with, 715
    phenotypic effects of
        duration of, 707
        no appreciable effect and, 706
        reduction of oxygen transport as,
            706-707
    physiological effects of, 713-714
        afterload and, 714
        left-to-right shunting and, 714-715
        restriction of ventricular filling and,
            715-716
        right-to-left shunting and, 715
        valve regurgitation and, 714
        with adequate pumping capacity,
            713-714
    pulmonary vascular resistance and, 707
    right-to-left shunting and, 708, 710-711
        isolated, 710
        lesions with, 715
        systemic arterial oxygen saturation
            determinants with, 708, 710f-711f
        systemic oxygen delivery with, 708, 710
    transposition physiology in, 712-713, 713f
Conjoined twins, 172, 172f
Connective tissue disorders, 593, 593t
Connexins, 590
Constitutive nitric oxide synthase, 1532
Constriction band syndrome, congenital,
    1838, 1839f
Contiguous gene syndromes, 9-10
Continuous positive airway pressure, 969,
    970t
    for apnea, 914, 914f
    inadvertent PEEP and, 972
    to prevent lung injury, 935
Contractile myofilaments, 1855-1857, 1858f
Contractile proteins, 615

Copper, accumulation of, in cholestasis, 1220
Cor pulmonale, in bronchopulmonary
    dysplasia, 959
Cord blood, platelets in, 1443-1444
Cornified cell envelope, 589
Corona radiata, 27
Coronary heart disease, adult, fetal origins of,
    160-164
    adult living standards related to, 163-164,
        164t
    biologic mechanisms of, 162-163
    congenital heart disease epidemics and, 164
    developmental plasticity and, 161
    growth and, 161f, 161t, 161-162, 162f, 162t
    hypertension and type 2 diabetes and, 162,
        163t
    maternal nutrition and, 164
Corpus callosum, agenesis of, 1689-1690,
    1690f
Corticosteroids. *See also* Glucocorticoids;
    Mineralocorticoids; *specific
    corticosteroids, e.g.* Cortisol.
    brain development and, 1789
    fetal lung development and, 807
    prenatal, surfactant therapy with, 1083f,
        1083-1084
Corticosterone, plasma concentration of, fetal
    and neonatal, 1922t
Corticotropin. *See* Adrenocorticotropic
    hormone.
Corticotropin-releasing hormone
    actions of, 1907
    binding protein for, 1908
    hypothalamic secretion of, 1877, 1877t
    levels during pregnancy, 1908-1909
    sources of, 1907
    umbilicoplacental circulation mediation by,
        752t
Cortisol
    adrenal adaptation to extrauterine life and,
        1921-1922, 1922t
    arterial baroreflex and, 720
    fetoplacental steroid metabolism and, 1918,
        1918f
    functions of, 1923
    plasma concentration of, fetal and neonatal,
        1922t
    renal tubular function and, 1238
    umbilicoplacental circulation mediation by,
        752t
Cortisone, plasma concentration of, fetal and
    neonatal, 1922t
Co-stimulation, 1516
    in host defense against viruses, 1499
    neonatal, 1504
Co-stimulatory molecules, 1516
Cotyledons
    definition of, 114t
    placental, 90, 92f
Cough, host defense and, 1625-1626
CPAP. *See* Continuous positive airway
    pressure.
Cranial neuropore, 31
Craniofacial morphogenesis, 44-48
    growth factors and their cognate receptors
        and, 46-47, 47f
    hindbrain and branchial arch code and, 45
    retinoids and, 47-48
    transcriptional factors and, 45-46, 47f
Craniorachischisis totalis, 1677-1678, 1777f,
    1777-1778
Creatinine
    as glomerular filtration rate marker,
        1258-1259, 1259f, 1260f, 1260t
    clearance of, 1260-1261

CRH. *See* Corticotropin-releasing hormone.
Crigler-Najjar syndrome, types I and II, 1200
Cross-bridges, cycling kinetics of,
    diaphragmatic contractile properties and,
    860-861
Crouzon syndrome, 48, 786, 790, 1837
Cryptorchidism, diagnosis and incidence of,
    1958-1959
CT. *See* Computed tomography.
Cutaneous receptors, 606-607, 607f, 607t
    thermal, neonatal, 550-551, 551f
Cutis laxa, 593
CXC chemokines, in neonatal pulmonary host
    defense, 1650
Cyclic adenosine monophosphate
    as second messenger, 1598-1599
    pulmonary liquid transport regulation by,
        826-827, 828f
Cyclins, 6
Cyclooxygenase
    renal blood flow and, 1246
    umbilicoplacental circulation and, 754t
Cystathionine, normal plasma and urine levels
    of, 1296t
Cystatin C, abnormal glomerular filtration rate
    detection by, 1262, 1262f
Cystic fibrosis, hepatic manifestations of, 1214
Cystic fibrosis transmembrane conductance
    regulator
    bile formation and, 1187-1188
    pulmonary ion transport and, 825
Cyst(e)ine
    fetal accretion of, 531t
    in parenteral amino acid mixtures, 533t, 534t
    normal plasma and urine levels of, 1296t
    requirements for, of low birth weight
        infants, 530t-532t
Cytidylyltransferase, surfactant phospholipid
    and, 1041, 1042, 1044-1047
Cytochrome aa$_3$, brain levels of, in hypoxia,
    1767
Cytochrome P450
    adrenocortical development and, 1916f,
        1916-1917
    CYP2C9 polymorphism and, 214
    CYP2C19 polymorphism and, 214
    CYP2D6 polymorphism and, 213-214, 214t
    drug biotransformation and, 183, 183t
Cytogenetics, 21-22
Cytokine(s), 1555-1568. *See also specific
    cytokines, e.g.* Tumor necrosis factor.
    acute phase reaction and, 1563
    antiinflammatory, 1560-1561
        interleukin-4 as, 1560, 1561f
        interleukin-10 as, 1560
        interleukin-11 as, 1560-1561
        interleukin-13 as, 1560, 1561f
    chorionic, 127
    description of, 1555-1556
    excess, in postnatal wounds, 1608-1609
    fever and, 1563
    in host defense against viruses, 1491-1492
        neonatal, 1501
    in megakaryocytopoiesis, 1422-1424, 1423f
    in neonates, 1564-1568
        inflammatory response and, 1565-1568
        physiology of, 1564
        production of, 1564-1565
    in wound healing, 1607
    inhibiting hematopoiesis, 1377
    intraalveolar networking of
        in neonatal pulmonary host defense,
            1655-1656
        resolution of inflammation and,
            1655-1656

Gastroesophageal reflux (Continued)
  spontaneous free gastroesophageal reflux
    as, 1165–1166
    neonatal, 1166
  sphincteric mechanisms of, 1129, 1130f
Gastrointestinal circulation. See Intestinal
    circulation.
Gastrointestinal contractions, 1111–1116
  intestinal motility and, 1115–1116
  intestinal motor activity and, 1115, 1115f
    development of, 1115–1116
  myogenic control of, 1111, 1111f
  neural control of, 1111–1114
    central nervous system and, 1111–1112,
      1112f
    enteric nervous system and, 1112, 1113f
    neurotransmitters and, 1112–1114
Gastrointestinal drugs, during lactation, 257
Gastrointestinal function, maternal, in
    multiple pregnancy, 168–169
Gastrointestinal hormones, gastrointestinal
    tract growth and, 1098
Gastrointestinal motility, 1125–1135
  anorectal, 1135
    in neonates, 1135
  colonic, 1134f, 1134–1135, 1141
  development of, 1135, 1136f
  esophageal, 1127, 1128f, 1129, 1139
    esophageal body and, 1127
    gastrointestinal reflux and, sphincteric
      mechanisms of, 1129, 1130f
    lower esophageal sphincter and, 1127,
      1129
    upper esophageal sphincter and, 1127
  gastric, 1129, 1131, 1139–1140
    control of gastric emptying and, 1129
    in neonates, 1131
    liquid emptying and, 1129, 1131
    solid emptying and, 1131
  necrotizing enterocolitis and, 1170
  small intestinal, 1131–1134, 1132f,
    1140–1141
    coordination of, 1132, 1132f
    ontogeny of, 1132–1134, 1133f
  suck and swallowing and, 1125–1127, 1126f
    coordination of swallowing with
      breathing and, 1126–1127
    oral phase of swallowing and,
      1125–1126, 1126f, 1127f
    pharyngeal swallowing and, 1126
Gastrointestinal reflux, apnea and, 914
Gastrointestinal tract. See also specific organs.
  calcium transport in, 328–332, 329f, 330f
  development of, 1095–1099
    environmental influences on, 1095–1096,
      1097f
    nature of growth and, 1095, 1096f
    trophic factors in, 1096–1098
      gastrointestinal hormones as, 1098
      glucocorticoids as, 1099
      nutrients and, 1096–1098
      thyroid hormones as, 1099
      tissue growth factors as, 1098–1099
  embryonic development of, homeobox
    genes and, 69–70
  lipolytic activities of
    postnatal, 1157–1158
    prenatal, 1157
  magnesium transport in, 334–338,
    335f–337f
  phosphorus transport in, 332–334, 333f
  potassium homeostasis and, 1285
Gastroschisis, 1106, 1107f
Gastrulation, 30, 30f
  skin development and, 590

GATA-6, lung development and, 789
G-CSF. See Granulocyte colony-stimulating
  factor.
Gelatinase, in neonatal pulmonary host
  defense, 1644
Gene(s). See also specific genes.
  development and, 4–5, 5f
  developmental, disease and, 19–20
  expression of
    apoptosis and, 74
    regulation of, 4
  function of, 2–5
  in hypothalamic development, 1873, 1874t
  regulation and development of
    oxygen-sensing via, 903–904, 904t
  pharmacogenetics and, 215–216
  structure of, 2, 3f
  transcription of, 2–3
  translation of, 3–4
Gene mapping, 13–14, 18–19
Gene mutations, disease-associated, 19–21
  atypical inheritance and, 20
  complex inheritance and, 20–21
  developmental genes and, 19–20
  identification of, 19
Gene therapy, 14–15, 15f, 63–64
Gene transfer, for stem cell therapy, 1370
Genetic code, 3
Genetic disorders, 7–11. See also specific
    disorders.
  chromosomal, 9–10
  heterogeneity in, 10–11
  Mendelian, 7–9
    autosomal dominant, 8, 8f
    autosomal recessive, 7–8, 8f
    X-linked, 8f, 9
  mitochondrial, 10
  multifactorial, 10
  of skin
    of appendages, 595–596
    of dermal-epidermal junction, 594, 594t
    of dermis and subcutis, 593t, 593–594
    of nonkeratinocytes, 591–592, 592t
    prenatal diagnosis of, 596
Genetic engineering, 11
Genetic heterogeneity, 20
Genetics, 1–15. See also Gene(s); specific
    genes.
  cell division and recombination and, 5–6
  genomic organization and, 1–2
  molecular. See Molecular genetics.
  mutation and, 6–7, 7f
  nucleic acid structure and, 1, 2f, 3f
Genitalia. See also specific organs, i.e. Testes.
  male, external, development of, 1936–1937
Genitofemoral nerve, testicular descent and,
  1957
Genome, organization of, 1–2
Genome project, 13
Genomic libraries, 12
GER. See Gastroesophageal reflux.
Germ cell(s)
  development of, 1951–1954, 1952f, 1952t,
    1953f
  embryonic, 1365
Germ cell cysts, 1944
Germinal centers, B-cell development in,
  1519–1520
Germinal matrix
  hemorrhage of, 1745
    intraventricular, 1759, 1765
    subependymal, as site of origin of
      intraventricular hemorrhage, 1759,
      1760f
Germline mosaicism, 8

Gestation. See Pregnancy.
Gestational age, respiratory water and
  evaporative heat loss related to, 577, 581t
Gestational hypertension, 146, 147t
  in multiple pregnancy, 169
Gestational thrombocytopenia, 1429
GFR. See Glomerular filtration rate.
GH. See Growth hormone.
Ghrelin, 1879, 1892
Gilbert syndrome, 1200
Glanzmann's thrombasthenia, 1584–1585
Gli3 gene, in hypothalamic development,
  1874t
Glia, proliferation of, normal, 1683
Glial precursor cells, destruction of,
  intraventricular hemorrhage, 1765
Gliding tendons, 1866
Globin chain synthesis, 1403–1404, 1404f
Globin genes, 1402–1403, 1403f
Glomerular capillary hydraulic pressure, in
  acute renal failure, 1337–1338, 1338f
Glomerular capillary ultrafiltration coefficient,
  in acute renal failure, 1338
Glomerular filtration, of drugs, 184
Glomerular filtration rate
  abnormal, cystatin C detection of, 1262,
    1262f
  at birth, 1262–1263, 1263f
  autoregulation of, 1258
  clearance and, 1258
  glomerular markers and, 1258–1259, 1259f,
    1260f, 1260t
  in acute renal failure, 1335, 1336, 1336f
  in neonates
    clinical assessment of, 1259–1262
      estimation without urine collection
        for, 1261–1262
      standard clearances for, 1259–1261
    development of, 1256–1265
    factors impairing, 1264–1265, 1265f
    increase in, determinants of, 1263–1264,
      1264t
    maturation during first month of life,
      1263, 1263f, 1264f
  physiology of, 1257f, 1257–1258
  prenatal development of, 1234, 1234f, 1235f
  vasoactive agents and, 1257–1258
Glomerular plasma flow rate, in acute renal
  failure, 1336–1337
Glomerulotubular balance, 1254
Glucagon
  calcium transport and, 1288
  neonatal glucose metabolism and, 479
Glucagon peptide 2, gastrointestinal tract
  growth and, 1098
Glucoamylase, 1152
Glucocorticoids. See also Corticosteroids;
  specific glucocorticoids, e.g. Cortisol.
  alveolarization and, 797–798
  antenatal, lung development and, 952–953
  arterial baroreflex and, 720–721
  brain development and, 1789
  gastrointestinal tract growth and, 1099
  neonatal glucose metabolism and, 479
  neonatal growth and, 272
  pancreatic secretion and, 1147
  preeclampsia and fetal growth impairment
    and, 151–152, 152f
  pulmonary liquid and ion transport
    regulation by, 827–828
  surfactant phospholipid biosynthesis and,
    1044–1045
  therapeutic, during pregnancy, 1923
Gluconeogenesis
  acetone as precursor for, 424, 425f

Intestinal blood flow, regulation of,
      necrotizing enterocolitis and, 1170
Intestinal circulation, development of,
      701-704
   blood flow control and, 702-704
      cardiovascular function and, 702-703
      humoral, 703-704, 704t
      local, 704
      neural, 703, 703t
   clinical considerations in, 704
   microcirculation and, 702, 703f
   venous drainage and, 702
Intestinal duplications, 1106, 1108, 1108f
Intestinal motility, development of,
      1115-1116
Intestinal motor activity, 1115, 1115f
Intestinal rotation, incomplete, 1103
Intestinal stenosis, congenital, 1106
Intestines, absorption in, of vitamin E, 356
Intracellular buffer system
      fetal, 1361
      neonatal, 1363
Intracellular water, 1351
      measurement of, 1353
Intracranial hemorrhage, 1454-1455
Intracranial hypertension, 1766
Intralobar sequestrations, 790-791
Intrauterine compression syndromes, 1838t,
      1838-1843
   etiology of, 1838-1842, 1839f-1841f
      theoretical basis for, 1840, 1842
   natural history and treatment of, 1842t,
      1842-1843, 1843f
Intrauterine fetal demise, of one twin,
      174-175
Intrauterine growth restriction, 259-265,
      266-267, 268f
   amino acid transport changes in, 516
   blood flow measurements and, 260-261
      fetal hepatic and ductus venosus, 261,
         262f
      umbilical, 260-261, 261f
      uterine, 260
   fetal velocimetry changes and, 260
   growth factors in, 1887, 1887t
   metabolic changes associated with,
         261-265
      amino acids and, 262-265, 264f
      carbohydrates and, 261-262, 263f, 264f
   mineral transfer in, 320
   placental development and, 259-260
   umbilical blood flow in, 755
Intrauterine infection, 132-138
   ascending
      pathways of, 132
      stages of, 132
   chronic, 133-135
      amniocentesis detection of, 133-134
      preterm labor associated with, 134-135
      sequence-based techniques for detecting,
         135
   etiology of, 138
   fetal inflammatory response syndrome
      with, 137-138, 138f
   maternal host response to, 138
   microbiology of, 132
   preterm labor associated with, 132-133
      molecular mechanisms for, 135-137
         inflammatory cytokines in, 136f,
            136-137
         matrix-degrading enzymes in, 137
         prostaglandins and, 1
      with chronic infection, 134-135
Intrauterine tissues, placental integration
      with, 128-129

Intravascular volume, maternal, in multiple
      pregnancy, 167-168
Intraventricular hemorrhage, 1454, 1455,
      1757f, 1757-1768
   cerebral arterial blood flow and, 1749-1750
   cerebral blood flow measurement in
      with positron-emission tomography,
         1753, 1753f
      with xenon clearance tehcniques,
         1754-1755
   clinical features of, 1757
   complications of, 1766-1768
      hydrocephalus as, 1766-1768, 1767f,
         1767t, 1768f
   diagnosis of, 1757-1759
      computed tomography in, 1758
      magnetic resonance imaging in,
         1758-1759, 1759f
      ultrasound in, 1758, 1758f, 1758t
   mechanisms of brain injury in, 1765-1766
      germinal matrix destruction and glial
         precursors as, 1765
      intracranial hypertension and impaired
         cerebral perfusion as, 1766
      major factors in, 1765, 1765t
      periventricular white matter injury as,
         1765-1766
      preceding hypoxic-ischemic injury as,
         1765
   neuropathology of, 1759-1761
      germinal matrix destruction and, 1759
      hydrocephalus and, 1760
      periventricular hemorrhagic infarction
         and, 1759-1760, 1760f, 1761f
      periventricular leukomalacia and,
         1760-1761, 1761t
      pontine neuronal necrosis and, 1761
      site of origin and, 1759, 1760f
      spread of hemorrhage and, 1759
   pathogenesis of, 1761-1765
      extravascular factors in, 1764-1765
      intravascular factors in, 1761-1764,
         1762f, 1762t
      vascular factors in, 1764
   pathophysiology of, cerebral blood flow
      and, 1745-1746
   prognosis of, 1768, 1768t
Intrinsic factor, parietal cell secretion of, 1120
Intubation, respiratory water and evaporative
      heat exchange and, 577
Inulin
   as glomerular filtration rate marker, 1258
   clearance of, 1259-1260
      method for, without urine collection,
         1261-1262
      constant infusion of, without urine
         collection, for glomerular filtration rate
         estimation, 1261
Inversions, chromosomal, 7, 7f
Inward rectifier, 672
Iodide(s)
   concentration of, thyroid hormone
      synthesis and, 1926-1927
   intrathyroidal, recycling of, 1928
   organification of, 1927
Iodide leak, 1928
Iodine, in human milk, 276t, 277
Iodine-containing compounds,
      contraindication to, for nursing mothers,
      253t, 254
Iodotyrosines
   coupling of, 1927
   deiodination of, 1928
Iohexol, as glomerular filtration rate marker,
      1259

Ion(s)
   alterations in, oxygen-sensing via, 901-903
   transport of, in lung liquid. See Lung liquid,
      ion transport and.
Ion channels, 669
   voltage-gated, 671, 673t
Ionization, of drugs, placental transfer and,
      201-203, 202t, 203t
Iothalamate sodium, as glomerular filtration
      rate marker, 1259
Iron
   lung injury in, 939
   placental transfer of, 207
Iron storage disease, neonatal, 1214-1215
Iron-binding proteins, in neonatal pulmonary
      host defense, 1627
Ischemia
   cerebral acidosis in, 1722-1723, 1723f
   cerebral energy metabolism in, 1721-1723,
      1722f
   hydrocephalus and, 1766
   perinatal, intraventricular hemorrhage and,
      1763
   postnatal, intraventricular hemorrhage and,
      1763-1764
   preceding, intraventricular hemorrhage
      and, 1765
   vulnerability to, intraventricular
      hemorrhage and, 1764
Ischemic necrosis, in hyaline membrane
      disease, 928
Islets, pancreatic, 1143
Isohydric principle, 1361
Isolated growth hormone deficiency, 269
Isoleucine
   fetal accretion of, 531t
   in parenteral amino acid mixtures, 533t,
      534t
   normal plasma and urine levels of, 1296t
   requirements for, of low birth weight
      infants, 530t-532t
Isoniazid, during lactation, 256
Isotope studies. See Stable isotope tracer
      studies.
Isotype switching, 1521
Isoxsuprine hydrochloride, for preterm labor,
      109t
Ito cells, development of, 1177
IUGR. See Intrauterine growth restriction.
IVH. See Intraventricular hemorrhage.

J

Jackson-Weiss syndrome, 1837
JAK protein tyrosine kinases, signal
      transduction by, 1380-1381
Jansen metaphyseal chondrodysplasia, 1836t,
      1837
Jaundice
   neonatal, 1199, 1200-1201
   phototherapy for. See Phototherapy, for
      jaundice.
Jet, placentomes and, 91
Junctional adhesion molecules, 1574t, 1579
Junctional zone, 92

K

Kallikrein-kinin system
   renal hemodynamics and, 1233
   renal tubular function and, 1238
Kallmann syndrome, 1957
Keratinization, 591

Liver disease
coagulopathy in, 1452t, 1454
drug elimination and, 185
Lobar emphysema, congenital, 791
Lobar holoprosencephaly, 1680
Local anesthetics, uteroplacental blood flow
and, 763
Local control, of intestinal circulation, 704
LOD score, 19
Loricin, 589
Low birth weight infants
amino acid requirements for, 529-532,
530t-532t
energy intake of, protein utilization and,
536, 536t
protein intake of, quality of protein and,
535
Low molecular weight heparin, for
thrombosis, neonatal, 1470t
Lower esophageal sphincter, 1127, 1129
gastroesophageal reflux and, 1129, 1130f,
1163, 1164f
Lower genital tract infections, preterm labor
and, 107
Low-pass filters, 982, 982f
Lumbar puncture, in intraventricular
hemorrhage, 1757-1758
Lung(s). *See also* Pulmonary *entries;*
Respiratory *entries.*
canalicular phase of, 1034
derecruitment of
in hyaline membrane disease, 930
to prevent lung injury, 935, 935f
development of, 783-792, 784t
abnormal, 789-792
distal parenchymal malformations and,
791-792
tracheobronchial tree malformations
and, 790-791
adrenal steroids in, 1922
alveolar development in, 818
alveolar stage of, 784t, 789, 813t
molecular mechanisms regulating, 789
antenatal factors influencing
chorioamnionitis as, 949-951
cytokines as, 951-952
infection as, 952, 952f, 953f
branching morphogenesis in, 812,
815-816
canalicular stage of, 784t, 787-788, 795,
813t
corticosteroids and, 807
cytokines and, 951-952
disorders of, treatments for, 808-809
early, 812
embryonic stage of, 783-786, 788t, 813t
homeobox genes and, 67-68
malformations and, 786
molecular mechanisms regulating,
784-786
epithelial differentiation in, 816-818,
817f
esophageal-tracheal separation in,
814-815t
fetal breathing movements and, 805
fetal lung expansion and, 802-805
increased, effects of, 804
mechanotransduction mechanisms
and, 805-806, 806f
physiologic control of, 802-803, 803f,
804f
reduced, effects of, 803-804
fetal lung hypoplasia and, physical causes
of, 806-807
glandular phase of, 1034

Lung(s) *(Continued)*
interruption by inflammatory processes,
938
left-right asymmetry and, 814-815, 815f
lung bud and lobe formation in,
molecular basis of, 812-814, 813f
metabolic factors in, 807-808
nitric oxide in, 733-741
as selective pulmonary vasodilator,
735-737, 736f-738f
in persistent pulmonary hypertension
of the newborn, 737-740, 739f,
740f
in premature neonates, 740-741, 741f
nitric oxide synthases and, 733-735,
735f
vasoregulation by, 733, 734f
prolactin in, 1893
pseudoglandular stage of, 784t, 786-787,
795, 813t
molecular mechanisms regulating,
786-787
saccular stage of, 784t, 788, 795, 813t, 1034
vascular, 818-819
expansion of, 802-805
increased, effects of, 804
mechanotransduction mechanisms and,
805-806, 806f
overexpansion and, 936
physiologic control of, 802-803, 803f, 804f
reduced, effects of, 803-804
with high-frequency ventilation, 983-984
fluid-filled, liquid ventilation and. *See* Liquid
ventilation, fluid-filled lung and.
gas exchange in. *See* Gas exchange;
Ventilation-perfusion relationships.
glucose transporters in, 491
growth of, abnormal, 695-696, 697f
host defense and. *See* Host defense,
pulmonary.
hyaline membrane disease and. *See* Hyaline
membrane disease.
maturity of, in multiple pregnancy, 171
neonatal, ketone bodies in, 426
overexpansion of, 936
premature, 942-947
adult lung structure and function and,
942
injury of, 945-947
acute, 945-946
alveolar function impairment after,
946-947
chronic, 945-946
structure of, 942, 943f, 944
vulnerabilities of, 934-935
structure of, of distal lung, 942
surfactant and. *See* Surfactant, pulmonary;
Surfactant proteins; Surfactant therapy.
Lung compliance, 963
during artificial ventilation, 864-865
during spontaneous breathing, 865-866,
866f
in bronchopulmonary dysplasia,
established, 957, 958f
in hyaline membrane disease, 930
Lung disease
antenatal factors influencing, 949-953
in preterm infants, spectrum of, 949, 950f
Lung hypoplasia, fetal, physical causes of,
806-807
Lung injury
fetal, 950
mechanical ventilation causing, in
respiratory distress syndrome,
1060-1061, 1061f-1064f, 1063

Lung injury *(Continued)*
neonatal, 934-940, 940f
aspiration, 937
humoral, 936-937, 937f
inflammation and, 937-939, 938f
duration of inflammation and, 938
interrupting to prevent, 938-939
interruption of lung development and,
938-939
leukocyte-mediated, 937-938, 938f
lower airway function in, 846-847
mechanical mechanisms of, 935-936
sequelae of, 934-935
vulnerabilities of premature lung and, 934
of premature lung
acute. *See* Respiratory distress syndrome.
chronic. *See* Bronchopulmonary
dysplasia.
with mechanical ventilation, etiology of,
963-965
Lung liquid, 822-831, 823f, 1344
flow of
during fetal life, 822
perinatal changes in, 822-823
formation of, during fetal life, 822
in neonatal respiratory disease, 829f,
829-830
ion transport and, 831, 831f
airway ion transport studies and, 830, 830f
hormonal regulation of, 826-828, 828f
in neonatal respiratory disease, 830f,
830-831
mechanisms of, 823-826, 824f
chloride and, 824-825
sodium and, 825-826, 826f, 827f
oxygen regulation of, 828f, 828-829
lung injury associated with, 936
secretion of, during fetal life, 822
volume of, decrease before labor, 823
Lung resistance, in hyaline membrane disease,
930
Lung transplantation, for surfactant protein
deficiency, 1091
Lung volumes
dynamic, in neonates, 922
in bronchopulmonary dysplasia,
established, 957, 957f
static, in neonates, 919-921, 921f, 922f
Lung water. *See* Lung liquid.
Luteinizing hormone
deficiency of, 1903
functions of, 1898
Leydig cells and, 1951, 1951f
patterns of, in fetus and neonate
general, 1902
mechanisms responsible for, 1903
regulation of, 1898-1901
in adults, 1898f, 1898-1899
in fetus and neonate, 1899-1901
sexual dimorphism and, 1902
Lymph
drainage of, outflow pressure and, 1359
flow of, 1344, 1344f
edema modulation by, 1359
volume of, 1343-1344
Lymphangiectasis, pulmonary, congenital, 792
Lymphangiogenesis, in skin, 594
Lymphatics
fluid volume and, 1348-1349
of skin, 593
Lymphocytes. *See also* B cells; T cells.
homing and response of, in neonatal
pulmonary host defense, 1656-1658,
1657f
maternal, trophoblastic invasion and, 94

Morphogenesis, 29–31, 30f
Mosaicism
  germline, 8
  skin in, 593
Motivation, essential fatty acid deficiency and, 433
MR spectroscopy, cerebral high-energy metabolites and, 1714–1715, 1715f
MRI. *See* Magnetic resonance imaging.
mRNA, 2–3
MRP2 gene, bile flow and, 1192
MRP3 gene, bile flow and, 1190–1191
Mucins
  in human milk, 1612–1613
  in neonatal pulmonary host defense, 1624
Mucociliary function, in neonatal pulmonary host defense, 1624–1625
Mucosa
  barrier function of, in host defense, 1476
  of upper airway, 835
Mucus, in neonatal pulmonary host defense, 1624
Müllerian-inhibiting substance, testicular descent and, 1957–1958
Multicompartment drug distribution, 187, 187f
Multifactorial genetic disorders, 10
Multifetal gestations. *See* Multiple pregnancy.
Multifetal reduction, 170f, 170–171, 171f
Multiple epiphyseal dysplasia, 1836t, 1837
Multiple inert gas elimination technique, 872
Multiple organ failure, in disseminated intravascular coagulation, 1463
Multiple pregnancy, 165–176
  chorionicity and, 166
    determination of, 166f, 166–167, 167f
  dizygotic, 166
  fetal physiology and, 169f, 169–175
    fetal lung maturity and, 171
    fetal pathophysiology and, 171–175, 172f–174f
    growth and, 169–170, 170f
    multifetal reduction and, 170f, 170–171, 171f
  incidence of, 165
  intra-amniotic infection with, 133
  maternal physiology and, 167–169
    cardiovascular, 167
    endocrine, 168
    gastrointestinal, 168–169
    hematologic, 168
    hypertension and, 169
    intravascular volume and, 167–168
    nutrition and, 169
    pulmonary, 168
    renal, 168
    uterine, 167
  monozygotic, 166
  zygosity and, 165–166
Multiple-frequency bioelectrical impedance analysis, for body water measurement, 1353
Multipotent adult stem cells, 1371–1372
Muscle(s)
  cardiac. *See also* Myocardial *entries.*
    embryology of, 35
  chest wall, in apnea, 911–912, 911f–913f
  contraction of. *See also* Gastrointestinal contractions; Myocardial contraction.
    force development and, 635–636, 637f
  glucose transporters in, 492
  myogenesis of, 849–851, 850f
  respiratory. *See* Diaphragm; Respiratory muscle(s).

Muscle(s) *(Continued)*
  striated, 1849–1868
    cellular cytodifferentiation and, 1851–1852, 1851f–1854f, 1854
    contractile myofilaments of, 1855–1857, 1858f
    embryonic origin of, 1849–1850
    fascicular organization of, 1862–1864, 1863f–1865f
    glycogen in, 1855
    historical background of, 1849
    intermediate filaments of, 1857–1859, 1858f, 1859f
    membrane excitability and innervation of, fetal, 1866–1867
    microtubules of, 1859
    muscle spindles and tendon organs and, 1864–1866, 1865f, 1866f
    myofiber differentiation in, metabolic, 1861–1862, 1862f, 1863f
    myofiber growth in, 1860–1861
    myogenic regulatory genes and, 1850–1851
    myotubule degeneration in, 1860
    ribosomes of, 1859
    sarcolemmal nuclei of, 1855, 1855f–1857f
    sarcoplasmic organelles of, 1855
    sarcotubular system of, 1859–1860, 1860f
    suprasegmental neural influences on, 1867–1868
    tendon development and, 1866
  thermoreceptors in, 552
  upper airway, in apnea, 911–912, 911f–913f
Muscle fibers, type of, diaphragmatic contractile properties and, 857, 858f–861f, 860
Muscle spindles, in developing muscle, 1864–1866, 1865f, 1866f
Muscular torticollis, congenital, 1839, 1840f
Musculoskeletal disorders
  intrauterine compression and, 1838t, 1838–1843
    etiology of, 1838–1842, 1839f–1841f
      theoretical basis for, 1840, 1842
    natural history and treatment of, 1842t, 1842–1843, 1843f
  lung hypoplasia and, 807
Musculoskeletal system, embryology of, 35, 36f
Mutations, 6–7
  activating, 21
  chromosomal, 7, 7f
  dominant negative, 21
  dynamic, 7
  frameshift, 6–7, 7f
  missense, 6, 7f
  nonsense, 7, 7f
  point, 6
  single-gene, 6–7, 7f
Myelin, tubular, 1016, 1017f, 1038f, 1038–1039, 1063
Myelination
  in central nervous system, 1693–1694
    disorders of, 1693–1694
    normal, 1693, 1693f
  of brain, fetal, 389
Myelocystocele, 1679
Myeloid dendritic cells, in host defense against viruses, 1493
Myelomeningocele, 1678, 1779–1782
  burden of, 1780–1781
  treatment of, 1781–1782
Myeloperoxidase, 1480
  neutrophil, 1543
Myeloschisis, 1678, 1778

Myoblast(s)
  cytodifferentiation of, 1851–1852, 1851f–1854f, 1854
  in limb development, 1845
  in myogenesis, 849–851, 850f
Myoblast-differentiating factor, 1850
Myocardial contraction, 635–639
  maternal, in pregnancy, 143, 143t
  maturation and, 639–647, 640f
    membrane systems and, 644–645, 645f
    myocardial sympathetic nervous system and, 646–647
    passive mechanical properties and, 644
    sarcolemmal function and, 645–646
    structure and, 639–644
      contractile proteins and, 641–643, 643f
      cytoskeleton and extracellular matrix and, 643–644
      hyperplasia and physiologic hypertrophy and, 639–640, 641f
      myofibrillar, 641
  myofilament and cell structure and, 635, 636f, 637f
    afterload effects and, 638
    excitation-contraction coupling and, 638–639
    force development and, 635–636, 637f
    length and preload effects and, 636–638, 637f
    sarcomere proteins and active force development and, 635
Myocardial function
  birth effects on, 652–653, 653f
  disorders of, shock and, neonatal, 777
  resuscitation and, 769–770
Myocardial ischemia, with tricuspid regurgitation and hypoxemia, in neonates, 662f, 662–663, 663f
Myocytes, 1855–1860
  contractile myofilaments of, 1855–1857, 1858f
  developmental changes in, 639, 640f
  ribosomes of, 1859
  sarcotubular system of, 1859–1860, 1860f
  structure of, developmental changes in, 641
Myofibers
  growth of, 1860–1861
  metabolic differentiation of, 1861–1862, 1862f, 1863f
Myofibrils, structure of, developmental changes in, 641
Myofilaments, 635, 636f
  contractile, 1855–1857, 1858f
  sensitivity of, to calcium, 637
Myogenesis, 849–851, 850f
Myogenic regulatory factors, 1850–1851
Myogenic response, to hypoxic stress, 654
Myogenin, 1850–1851, 1854
Myosin, 635
  developmental changes in, 641–642
  heavy chain, 851
    isoforms of, 851
      diaphragmatic contractile properties and, 857, 858f–861f, 860–861
Myostatin, 1851
Myotubes, 1855–1860
  glycogen in, 1855
  innervation of, 1867
  intermediate filaments of, 1857–1859, 1858f, 1859f
  microtubules of, 1859
  sarcoplasmic organelles of, 1855
  sarcotubular system of, 1859–1860, 1860f

Parenteral nutrition
  amino acid requirements for, 532–534, 533t, 534t
  cholestasis associated with, 1194
  for postnatal infants, lipid emulsions for, 399–400
  lipid emulsions for, for neonates, 417f, 417–418, 418t
  vitamin A and, 350
Parietal cells
  diminished function of, in neonates, 1120
  secretion by, 1119–1120
    of intrinsic factor, 1120
Partial expiratory flow-volume curves, 838
Parturition, adrenal role in initiating, 1923
Parvocellular system, 1877, 1877t
Passive diffusion, of drugs, 179, 220–221, 221f, 222f, 223
Patent ductus arteriosus. See Ductus arteriosus, patent.
Pax genes, 19
PC. See Phosphatidylcholine.
PCR. See Polymerase chain reaction.
PDGF. See Platelet-derived growth factor.
Peak concentration, measured, 195
Peak inflating pressure, 969–971, 970f, 971t
PEEP. See Continuous positive airway pressure.
Peg3 gene, in hypothalamic development, 1874t
Pendelluft, with high-frequency ventilation, 980–981, 981f
Penetrance, incomplete, 8
Pentose phosphate pathway, of erythrocytes, 1406–1407, 1408f
Peptidase, activity of, in small intestine, 1155–1156
Peptide(s). See also specific peptides, e.g. Atrial natriuretic peptide.
  antimicrobial, in neonatal pulmonary host defense, 1628–1629
Peptide YY, gastrointestinal tract growth and, 1098
Perfluorochemicals, for liquid ventilation, 985–986, 986f, 986t, 987f, 987t, 988–989
  in respiratory distress syndrome, 997–998, 998f
  uptake of, 991–993, 992f–994f, 992t
Perfusion. See also Reperfusion; Ventilation-perfusion relationships.
  matching of, to optimize maternal/fetal exchange, 753
  placental, reduced, preeclampsia and fetal growth impairment and, 151
  regional, hypoxia and, 654–655
  systemic, low, in neonates, 661f, 661–662, 662f
Perichondral ring of LaCroix, 1834
Perichondrium, 1831
Periciliary fluid, in neonatal pulmonary host defense, 1614f, 1623–1624
Periodic breathing, 905
  apnea related to, 911, 911f
  in neonates, 895–896, 896f, 897f
Peripheral tolerance, 1521
Peripheral vascular resistance, vasoactive mediators influencing, ventilation-perfusion matching and, 877f, 877–878, 878f
Periventricular hemorrhagic infarction, with intraventricular hemorrhage, 1759–1760, 1760f, 1761f
Periventricular leukomalacia, with intraventricular hemorrhage, 1760–1761, 1761t

Permeability, of placental tissue, 220–221
Peroxisomal disease, hepatic pathology due to, 1215
Peroxisomes, synthesis of, disorders of, 1213t
Persistent truncus arteriosus, 618
PET. See Positron emission tomography.
Pethidine, uteroplacental blood flow and, 763
PFA-100, in neonates, 1449
Pfeiffer syndrome, 48, 786, 790, 1837, 1857t
P-glycoprotein, 1702
Phagocyte(s), in host defense, against invasive candidiasis, 1488
Phagocyte oxidase, 1545
Phagocytic cells, stimulus-response coupling in, 1591–1600
  downstream signaling mechanisms and, 1595–1597
    low molecular weight guanosine triphosphate-binding proteins and, 1595–1596, 1596f
    MAP kinases and Ras-initiated pathways and, 1596–1597
  lipid remodeling and signaling and, 1597–1598
    phosphatidylinositol-3-kinase and, 1597
    phosphoinositide, 1597, 1597f
    phospholipase A_2 and, 1597–1598
    phospholipase D and, 1597
    sphingomyelin and, 1598
  receptor types and, 1592f, 1592–1595, 1593f
    trimeric G-proteins and, 1593f, 1593–1594, 1594t
    tyrosine kinase-initiated signal transduction and, 1594f, 1594–1595, 1595f
  second-messenger-regulated, 1598–1600
    protein kinase C and, 1599–1600, 1601f
    second-messenger generation and, 1598–1599
    second-messenger-regulated kinases and, 1598, 1599
  signal transduction and, 1591–1592
Phagocytosis
  by mononuclear phagocytes, 1530, 1531
  in neonatal pulmonary host defense, 1633–1634, 1634f
  by neutrophils, 1542–1543
  in placental transfer, 118
Pharmacodynamics, 188–189, 189f
  dose-response relationship and, 188–189, 189f
  of adrenergic agents, 229–232, 230f, 231f
    in neonates, 231–232, 232f
  pharmacogenetics and, 213t, 215
  receptor classification and, 188
  receptor regulation and, 188
Pharmacogenetics, 211–216, 212t, 213t
  gene regulation and development and, 215–216
    interaction with ontogeny, 216
    pediatric, clinical, 216
    pharmacodynamics related to, 213t, 215
    pharmacokinetics related to, 212t, 212–213
    phase I drug oxidation polymorphisms and, 213–214
      CYP2C9, 214
      CYP2C19, 214
      CYP2D6, 213–214, 214t
    phase II drug oxidation polymorphisms and, 214–215
      NAT2, 214–215
      TMPT, 215
Pharmacogenomics, 211

Pharmacokinetics, 190–197
  apparent volume of distribution and, 192–193
  bioavailability and, 180–181
  dose adjustments and
    bedside, examples of, 196–197
    mathematical, examples of, 195–196
  drug absorption and, 179–180
    factors affecting, 180
    kinetics of, 180
    membrane transporters and, 180
    transport mechanisms and, 179–180
  drug clearance and, 187, 193, 193f
    first-pass, 193
  drug distribution and, 181–182, 186, 186f
    factors affecting, 181–182, 182t
    multicompartment, 187, 187f
    single-compartment, 186
  drug elimination and, 182–186
    biotransformation and, 182–184, 183t
    disease effects on, 185–186
    first-order, 191f, 191t, 191–192
      multicompartment, 191–192, 192f
    renal, 184–185
    zero-order, 192
  half-lives and, 186, 186t, 187f
  models in, 190–191
  multiple-dose administration and, 194–195
  of adrenergic agents, 228f, 228–229, 229f
    in neonates, 229
  of maternofetal drug exchange, 199, 199f, 199t, 200t
  pharmacogenetics and, 212t, 212–213
  single-dose administration and, by short-duration infusion, 194, 194f
  steady-state conditions and, 193, 194t
  zero-order kinetics of, 187–188
Pharmacologic agents. See Drug(s); Radiopharmaceuticals; specific drugs and drug types.
Phencyclidine, contraindication to, for nursing mothers, 255
Phenobarbital
  contraindication to, for nursing mothers, 253t, 254
  during lactation, 256
  for opioid withdrawal, 243
  half-life of, 186t
  protein binding of, 205t
Phenylalanine
  fetal accretion of, 531t
  in parenteral amino acid mixtures, 533t, 534t
  normal plasma and urine levels of, 1296t
  requirements for, of low birth weight infants, 530t–532t
Phenylbutazone, half-life of, 186t
Phenytoin
  during lactation, 256
  half-life of, 186t
  protein binding of, 205t
Phosphate
  calcium transport and, 1288
  dietary, phosphate transport and, 1292
  renal tubular function and, prenatal, 1236–1237
Phosphatidylcholine
  biosynthesis of, rate of, 1055
  in pulmonary surfactant, 1006–1008, 1007f, 1007t, 1008t
  surfactant, biosynthesis of, 1041, 1042f
    developmental changes in, 1042–1044, 1043f, 1043t
    hormone-induced changes in, 1044–1046
    regulation of, mechanism of, 1046–1048

Placental transfer/transport (Continued)
of glycerol, 379–380, 380f
of heat, 542, 542f
of hematopoietic growth factors,
1383–1384
of ketone bodies, 380
of lipids, 391–392
of magnesium, 319t, 319–320
control of, 320
hormonal regulation of, 320
mechanisms of, 320
of phosphorus, 318t, 318–319
hormonal regulation of, 319
mechanisms of, 319, 319f
of substrates, preeclampsia and fetal growth
impairment and, 151
of water, 118–119
or magnesium
in diabetic pregnancy, 320
in intrauterine growth restriction, 320
transporter protein-mediated, 115–117
amino acids and, 116–117
glucose transfer and, 116
Placental transfusion, during delivery, neonatal
fluid volumes and, 1345
Placentomes, 91
Plasma, volume of, 1341–1343, 1342t, 1343t
during labor and delivery, 1345
measurement of, 1346–1347
regulation of, 1345–1348
Plasma clearance rate, in neonates, 231–232
Plasma colloid oncotic pressure, in acute
renal failure, 1338
Plasma transport, of vitamin A, 347–348, 348f
Plasma water volume measurement, 1353
Plasmids, 16
Plasminogen
in children, 1442t
in full-term infants, 1440t
in premature infants, 1440t
Plasminogen activator inhibitor-1
in children, 1442t
in full-term infants, 1440t
in premature infants, 1440t
Plasticity
developmental, 161
of stem cells, 1366, 1372
Platelet(s), 1443–1444
activation of, during birth process, 1444
disorders of. See also Thrombocytopenia.
qualitative, 1455
in cord blood, 1443–1444
leukocyte mobilization to inflammatory
sites and, 1580–1582, 1582f
megakaryocyte precursors of, 1443
morphology of, in neonates, 1448
neonatal platelet function and, 1444
production of, by megakaryocytes, site of,
1426–1427
Platelet activating factor
in neonatal pulmonary host defense, 1642
intestinal circulation and, 704
necrotizing enterocolitis and, 1171
shock and, neonatal, 775
Platelet aggregation testing, in neonates, 1449
Platelet count, in neonates, 1448
Platelet endothelial adhesion molecule-1,
1574t, 1579
Platelet flow cytometry, in neonates, 1449
Platelet-capillary function, intraventricular
hemorrhage and, 1764
Platelet-derived growth factor
alveolarization and, 797
brain development and, 1786
fetal growth and, 1883

Platelet-derived growth factor (Continued)
growth plate control by, 1835
lung development and, 787, 789
Pleiotropy, 8
of cytokine function, 1382, 1383f
Pluripotent stem cells, 58, 1365
growth factors affecting, 1377
Pneumotachography, for tidal volume
measurement, 922
Pneumothorax, intraventricular hemorrhage
and, 1763
Poikilothermic organisms, 548
Point mutations, 6
Polydactyly, postaxial, type A, 1848t
Polymerase chain reaction, 12–13, 13f, 16
amniotic fluid microorganism detection by,
135
Polymicrogyria, 1688, 1688f
Polymorphonuclear neutrophils, in neonatal
pulmonary host defense, 1634–1635
Polypeptides, placental transfer of, 207
Polyploidization, 1421
Polysaccharides, digestion of, 1152
postnatal, 1152, 1152f
prenatal, 1152
Ponderal index, in neonatal nutritional
assessment, 295–296
Pontine neuronal necrosis, periventricular, 1761
Portal circulation, development of, 1898
Portal vein, preduodenal, 1103
Positive end-expiratory pressure. See
Continuous positive airway pressure.
Positron emission tomography, 1715–1716
cerebral glucose utilization on, 1718f,
1718t, 1718–1719, 1719f
cerebral blood flow and, 1719
for cerebral blood flow measurement,
1751–1753, 1752f, 1753f
Posterior nucleus, hypothalamic, 1872t
Postmitotic compartments, 1390–1392, 1391t,
1392f
Postprandial hyperemia, 703
Potassium
blood-brain barrier transporter for,
1701–1702
homeostasis of, 1279–1285, 1280f
external, regulation of, 1282–1285
gastrointestinal tract and, 1285
renal contribution to, 1282f,
1282–1285, 1283f
internal, regulation of, 1279, 1281t,
1281–1282
acid-base balance and, 1281
hormones and, 1281
plasma potassium concentration and,
1281
with hypothermia, 587
ionic flux of, oxygen-sensing via, 901, 902f,
903f
renal tubular function and, prenatal, 1236
Potassium channel hyperinsulinism, neonatal,
496–497
Potassium currents, voltage-gated, 676, 676t
Power spectral analysis, of baroreflex
function, 721
Prader-Willi syndrome, 10
Prealbumin, serum, in neonatal nutritional
assessment, 297
Prebiotics, in human milk, 281
Precartilage blastema, 1831
Prechordal mesoderm, 1675
Preconditioning, 904
Preeclampsia/eclampsia, 147t, 147–149
fetal growth and development and,
149–154

Preeclampsia/eclampsia (Continued)
growth excess and, 151
growth restriction and, 150f, 150–151
mechanisms of impairment of, 151–154
future risks for offspring and, 154–155
in multiple pregnancy, 169
maternal pathophysiology of, 149, 150t
placental origin of, 147–149
risk factors for, 147, 147t
treatment of, 154
Pregnancy. See also Maternal entries.
carbohydrate metabolism during, 464
complicated, glucocorticoids and, 1071
corticotropin-releasing hormone levels
during, 1908
insulin-like growth factor levels during, 1886
ketonemia in, 419
length of, maternal marijuana use and, 241
loss of
alcohol consumption and, 235
early, in multiple pregnancy, 171
maternal adaptation to, in multiple
pregnancy, 167–169
maternal cardiovascular system during. See
Maternal cardiovascular disease;
Maternal cardiovascular system.
maternal drug abuse during. See Maternal
drug abuse; specific drugs.
multiple. See Multiple pregnancy.
outcome of, maternal marijuana use and,
240–241
twin. See Multiple pregnancy.
vitamin E requirements during, 361, 361f,
362t
Pregnenolone, plasma concentration of, fetal
and neonatal, 1922t
Pregnenolone sulfate, plasma concentration
of, fetal and neonatal, 1922t
Pre-kallikrein
in adults, 1436t
in children, 1441t
in fetuses, 1436t
in full-term infants, 1436t, 1438t
in premature infants, 1437t
Preload
fetal, 649–650, 650f, 651f
myocardial contractility and, 636–638, 637f
Premature infants. See Preterm infants.
Premature labor. See Preterm labor.
Premature rupture of membranes
intra-amniotic infection with, 133
respiratory distress syndrome with,
glucocorticoids and, 1071
Prematurity, ripples of, on
electroencephalography, 1736t, 1737,
1737f
Preoptic area, hypothalamic, 1872t
Preprotachynin A gene, in neonatal
pulmonary host defense, 1643
Prespermatogenesis, 1953
Prespermatogonia, 1952
Pressure gradients, intra-abdominal,
gastroesophageal reflux and, 1165, 1167f
Pressure-flow autoregulation, 703
Pressure-support ventilation, 974
Pressure-volume curve, surfactant therapy
effects on, 1075–1076, 1075f–1077f
Preterm infants. See also Low birth weight
infants; Preterm labor.
anemia in
erythropoietin for
clinical trials in, 1414, 1415t
pharmacokinetics and, 1414, 1416
side effects of, 1416
nutritional supplementation in, 1416

Thyroid hormones *(Continued)*
iodide organification and, 1927
iodotyrosine coupling and, 1927
iodotyrosine deiodination and, 1928
thyroglobulin proteolysis and, 1927
thyroglobulin synthesis and, 1927
Thyroid transcription factor-1, in lung
development, 814, 817
Thyroid-stimulating hormone, placental
production of, 1928
Thyrotropin-releasing hormone
G-cell secretion of, 1120–1121
hypothalamic secretion of, 1877, 1877t
prenatal glucocorticoid combined with, for
respiratory distress syndrome
prevention, 1073
surfactant phospholipid biosynthesis and,
1045
Thyroxine. *See also* Thyroid hormones.
pancreatic secretion and, 1148
Tidal flow:volume relationship, measurement
of, 923, 924f
Tidal liquid ventilation, 989, 991
Tidal volume, 922
Tidal volume-guided ventilation, 974–975
Tie1 and Tie2, vascular development and,
624f, 624–625, 625f
Tight junctions, in lactation, 286–287
Tissue factor pathway inhibitor
in adults, 1436t
in fetuses, 1436t
in full-term infants, 1436t
Tissue growth factors, gastrointestinal tract
growth and, 1098–1099
Tissue injury
apoptotic activation after, through death
receptors, 74
cell death in, modes of, 73
Tissue-type plasminogen activator
for thrombosis, neonatal, 1470t
in children, 1442t
in full-term infants, 1440t
in premature infants, 1440t
Titin, 635
TNF. *See* Tumor necrosis factor.
Tobacco use, maternal, 239–240
Tocolytic therapy
for preterm labor, 108, 109t
uteroplacental blood flow and, 763
α-Tocopherol. *See also* Vitamin E.
protection during antioxidant stress, 355
γ-tocopherol versus, 356–357
γ-Tocopherol
in human nutrition, 357–358
α-tocopherol versus, 356–357
Tolbutamide, during lactation, 257
Tolerance, B cells and, 1521
Torsional deformities, in intrauterine
compression syndromes, 1838
Torticollis, muscular, congenital, 1839, 1840f
Total anomalous pulmonary venous
connection, 716
Total body bioelectrical impedance analysis,
for body water measurement, 1352–1353
Total body chloride content, for body water
measurement, 1353
Total body electrical conductivity, for body
water measurement, 1353
Total lung capacity, 919
Total parenteral nutrition. *See* Parenteral
nutrition.
Totipotent stem cells, 1365
Toxic oxygen species, in neonatal pulmonary
host defense, 1644f, 1644–1645
tPA. *See* Tissue-type plasminogen activator.

TPN. *See* Parenteral nutrition.
Trabeculae, placental, 85, 86f
Trace minerals, in human milk, 276t, 277
Tracers. *See also* Stable isotope tracer
studies.
nonrecycling, 451
reversible (recycling), 451
Trachea
embryology of, 834
structure of, 834–835
Tracheal diverticulum, 1101
Tracheal genesis, 790
Tracheal stenosis, 790
Tracheal suctioning, intraventricular
hemorrhage and, 1763
Tracheobronchial tree, 783
congenital malformations of, 790–791
Tracheoesophageal fistulas, 790, 1101, 1102f
Tracheoesophageal septum, formation of, 824,
825t
Tracheomalacia, 790
Traction tendons, 1866
Transcription, 2–3
Transcription factors, 45–46, 47f
lung development and, 784–786
mutations in, clinical implications of, 48
Transcytosis, lactation and, 286
Transdifferentiation, 63
Transferrin
in neonatal pulmonary host defense, 1627
serum, in neonatal nutritional assessment,
297
Transforming growth factor ß
embryogenesis and, 42
fetal growth and, 1883
gastrointestinal tract growth and, 1099
growth plate control by, 1835
in lung development, 816
in neonatal pulmonary host defense, 1651
in postnatal wounds, 1608
in wound healing, 1607–1609
lung development and, 787
T-cell development and, 1513t
Translation, genetic, 3–4
Translational developmental biology, 57
Translocations, chromosomal, 7, 7f
Transporter(s)
blood-brain, 1701–1702
cation-Cl cotransporters as, 1273
glucose. *See* Glucose transporters.
membrane, 180
monocarboxylic acid, 1720, 1721
Na-Cl cotransporter as, 1274
Na-K-Cl cotransporters as, 1274
organic ion, 1299
sodium bicarbonate co-transporter as,
1272–1273
sodium, potassium, chloride co-transporter
as, 825
sodium/hydrogen transporter, 1271
Transporter genes, bile flow and, 1190–1192,
1191f
Transporter proteins
light chain
anionic, placental transport of amino
acids and, 515
cationic, placental transport of amino
acids and, 515
neutral, placental transport of amino
acids and, 514–515
placental transfer mediated by, 115–117
placental transport of amino acids and,
514t, 514–515
Transposition of the great arteries, physiology
of, 712–713, 713f

Transthyretin, serum, in neonatal nutritional
assessment, 297
Trefoil factors, gastrointestinal tract growth
and, 1099
Treitz, ligament of, 1105
TRH. *See* Thyrotropin-releasing hormone.
Triallelic inheritance, 20
Trichothiodystrophy, 595
Tricuspid regurgitation, myocardial ischemia
with hypoxemia and, in neonates, 662f,
662–663, 663f
Triglycerides. *See also* Lipoprotein(s).
as thermogenesis substrates, 408–409
long chain, postnatal absorption of,
396–397
medium chain
in infant formula, for steatorrhea, 1220
postnatal absorption of, 396–397
metabolism of
fetal development and, 441–442, 442f
postnatal development and, 443
serum concentrations of
in fetal development, 440–441
in experimental animals, 441
in humans, 440–441, 441f, 441t
in postnatal development, 442–443
in experimental animals, 443
in humans, 442f, 442–443
perinatal disease and, 443
Triiodothyronine. *See also* Thyroid hormones.
deiodinase and, 410
thermogenesis and, neonatal, 547t
Triiodothyronine (T_3), *para*-aminohippurate
transport and, 1300, 1300f
Trimeric G-proteins, signaling and, 1593f,
1593–1594, 1594t
tRNA, 3
Trophic feeding, 1096
Trophoblast, 85, 86f, 87–89, 89f
definition of, 114t
Trophoblast invasion, 91–94
arterial, 94
failed, preeclampsia due to, 148, 148f
interstitial, 92–94, 93f
Trophoblastic cell column, 92
Trophoblastic shell, 85
Tropomyosin, developmental changes in, 642
Troponins, 635
developmental changes in, 642–643, 643f
Trough concentration, measured, 195
Truncus arteriosus, persistent, 618
Trypsin, postnatal, 1155
Trypsinogen, prenatal, 1155
Tryptophan
fetal accretion of, 531t
in parenteral amino acid mixtures, 533t,
534t
normal plasma and urine levels of, 1296t
requirements for, of low birth weight
infants, 530t–532t
TSH. *See* Thyroid-stimulating hormone.
T-system
cardiac, 645
in striated muscle, 1860, 1860f
Tuberal nuclei, hypothalamic, 1872t
Tubular myelin, 1016, 1017f, 1038f,
1038–1039, 1063
Tubuloglomerular feedback, 1253–1254
Tumor necrosis factor
acute phase reaction and, 1563
as hematopoietic growth factor, 1376t
characteristics of, 1556
fetal growth and, 1883
fever and, 1563
in host defense, 1481

P/N 9997628268

9 789997 628268